Fishman's Pulmonary Diseases and Disorders

Volume 1

NOTICE

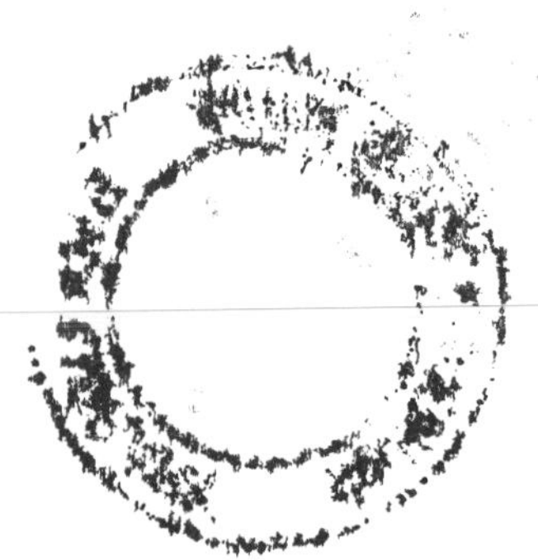

Fishman's Pulmonary Diseases and Disorders

Fifth Edition

Volume 1

EDITOR-IN-CHIEF

Michael A. Grippi, MD

Vice Chairman, Department of Medicine
Pulmonary, Allergy, and Critical Care Division
Perelman School of Medicine at the University of Pennsylvania
Chief Medical Officer, GSPP Specialty Hospital
Philadelphia, Pennsylvania

EDITORS

Jack A. Elias, MD

Dean of Medicine and Biologic Sciences
Frank L. Day Professor of Biology
Professor of Medicine
Professor of Molecular Microbiology and Immunology
Professor of Molecular Biology, Cell Biology, and Biochemistry
Brown University
Warren Alpert School of Medicine
Providence, Rhode Island

Jay A. Fishman, MD

Professor of Medicine
Harvard Medical School
Director, Transplant Infectious Disease and Compromised Host Program
Massachusetts General Hospital
Associate Director, MGH Transplantation Center
Boston, Massachusetts

Robert M. Kotloff, MD

Chairman, Department of Pulmonary Medicine
Respiratory Institute
Cleveland Clinic
Cleveland, Ohio

Allan I. Pack, MBChB, PhD

John Miclot Professor of Medicine
Chief, Division of Sleep Medicine/Department of Medicine
Director, Center for Sleep and Circadian Neurobiology
Perelman School of Medicine at the University of Pennsylvania
Philadelphia, Pennsylvania

Robert M. Senior, MD

Professor of Medicine
Professor of Cell Biology & Physiology
Washington University School of Medicine
St. Louis, Missouri

VIDEO EDITOR

Mark D. Siegel, MD

Professor of Medicine
Department of Internal Medicine
Yale School of Medicine
New Haven, Connecticut

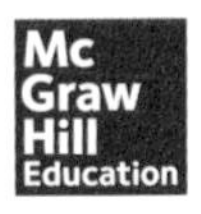

New York Chicago San Francisco Athens London Madrid Mexico City
Milan New Delhi Singapore Sydney Toronto

Fishman's Pulmonary Diseases and Disorders, Fifth Edition

1 2 3 4 5 6 7 8 9 0 DOW/DOW 20 19 18 17 16 15

Set ISBN 978-0-07-180728-9; MHID 0-07-180728-4
Volume 1 ISBN 978-0-07-179672-9; MHID 0-07-179672-X
Volume 2 ISBN 978-0-07-180719-7; MHID 0-07-180719-5

This book was set in Minion by Aptara, Inc.
The editors were Brian Belval and Peter J. Boyle.
The production supervisor was Richard Ruzycka.
Project management was provided by Neera Mehra, Aptara, Inc.
The art manager was Armen Ovsepyan.
The designer was Alan Barnett.
R.R. Donnelley and Sons Co. was printer and binder.

This book was printed on acid-free paper.

Library of Congress Cataloging-in-Publication Data

Fishman's pulmonary diseases and disorders / editor-in-chief, Michael A. Grippi ; co-editors, Jack A. Elias, Jay A. Fishman, Robert M. Kotloff, Allan I. Pack, Robert M. Senior ; video editor, Mark D. Siegel. – Fifth edition.
p. ; cm.
Pulmonary diseases and disorders
Preceded by Fishman's pulmonary diseases and disorders / editor-in-chief, Alfred P. Fishman ; co-editors, Jack A. Elias . . . [et al.]. 4th ed. c2008.
Includes bibliographical references and index.
ISBN 978-0-07-180728-9 (hardcover : set : alk. paper) – ISBN 0-07-180728-4 (hardcover : set : alk. paper) – ISBN 978-0-07-179672-9 (v. 1 : alk. paper) – ISBN 0-07-179672-X (v. 1 : alk. paper) – ISBN 978-0-07-180719-7 (v. 2 : alk. paper) – ISBN 0-07-180719-5 (v. 1 : alk. paper)
I. Grippi, Michael A., editor. II. Title: Pulmonary diseases and disorders.
[DNLM: 1. Lung Diseases. WF 600]
RC756
616.2′4–dc23

2014047567

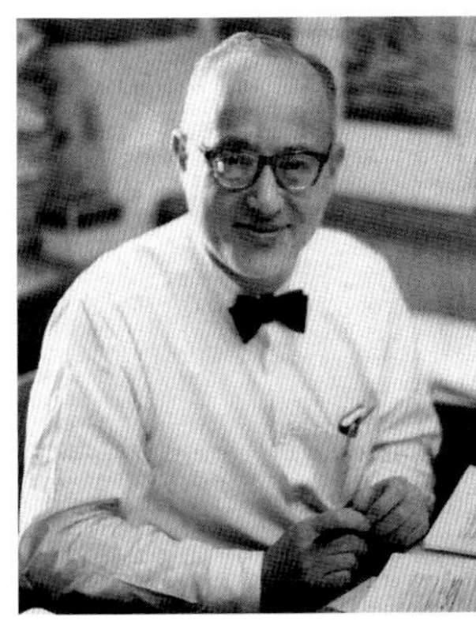 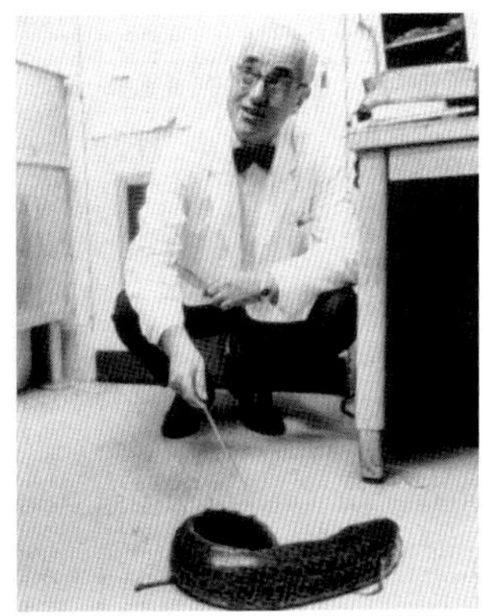

Alfred P. Fishman, MD, 1918–2010

Alfred P. Fishman, MD, was a husband, father, scientist, clinician, author, and consummate editor. The breadth and depth of his intellectual curiosity were great, and his contributions to pulmonary medicine and science of real consequence. He was an exacting task master who set a high bar for all of us, as well as for himself; his commitment to excellence was steadfast. The editors of the fifth edition dedicate this work to Dr. Fishman—the man, the mentor, and the driving force behind the origins of *Pulmonary Diseases and Disorders*.

To Barbara, Kristen, Amy, Emily, Sawyer, Levi, and Kieran
Michael A. Grippi, MD

To Sandy, Lauren, Alma, and Gabby
Jack A. Elias, MD

To Gayle, Aaron, and Brian
Jay A. Fishman, MD

To Debbie, Eric, Brian, and Ethan; and to the memory of Jean and Leon Kotloff
Robert M. Kotloff, MD

To Fran, Alison, Angela, Andrew, and Allan Jr.
Allan I. Pack, MBChB, PhD

To Martha, Jocelyn, Rebecca, Devra, and David
Robert M. Senior, MD

CONTENTS

CONTENTS

PART 7: Other Infiltrative and Airspace Disorders

PART 8: Disorders of the Pulmonary Circulation

VOLUME 2

PART 9: Disorders of the Pleural Space

PART 10: Diseases of the Mediastinum

PART 11: Disorders of the Chest Wall, Diaphragm, and Spine

PART 12: Occupational and Environmental Disorders

SECTION 12 Occupational Disorders

SECTION 13 Environmental Disorders

PART 13: Pulmonary Complications of Nonpulmonary Disorders

PART 14: Sleep and Sleep Disorders

PART 15: Surgical Aspects of Pulmonary Medicine

PART 16: Neoplasms of the Lungs

SECTION 14 Lung Cancer

SECTION 15 Lymphoproliferative Disorders

PART 17: Infectious Diseases of the Lungs

SECTION 16 General Concepts

SECTION 17 Common Syndromes in Pulmonary Infectious Diseases

SECTION 18 Major Pathogens in Pulmonary Infections

PART 18: Acute Respiratory Failure

SECTION 19 Lung Failure

SECTION 20 Respiratory Pump Failure

SECTION 21 Management and Therapeutic Interventions

APPENDIXES

CONTRIBUTORS

Bekele Afessa, MD (Deceased)
Professor of Medicine
Division of Pulmonary and Critical Care Medicine
Mayo Clinic
Rochester, Minnesota
Chapter 95

Abass Alavi, MD (Hon.), PhD (Hon.), DSci (Hon.)
Professor of Radiology and Neurology
Perelman School of Medicine at the University of Pennsylvania
Philadelphia, Pennsylvania
Chapter 32

Micheala A. Aldred, PhD
Genomic Medicine Institute
Cleveland Clinic
Cleveland, Ohio
Chapter 7

Timothy Craig Allen, MD, JD
Professor of Pathology
Director of Anatomic Pathology
The University of Texas Medical Branch
Galveston, Texas
Chapter 67

Murray D. Altose, MD
Professor of Medicine
Case Western Reserve University School of Medicine
Chief of Staff
Cleveland VA Medical Center
Cleveland, Ohio
Chapter 10

Danielle Antin-Ozerkis, MD
Medical Director, Yale Interstitial Lung Disease Program
Associate Professor, Section of Pulmonary and Critical Care Medicine
Yale School of Medicine
New Haven, Connecticut
Chapter 54

Andrea J. Apter, MD, MSc, MA
Professor of Medicine
Chief and Program Director
Section of Allergy and Immunology
Division of Pulmonary, Allergy, and Critical Care Medicine
Perelman School of Medicine
University of Pennsylvania
Philadelphia, Pennsylvania
Chapter 45

Jeffrey J. Atkinson, MD
Division of Pulmonary and Critical Care
Washington University School of Medicine
St. Louis, Missouri
Chapter 40

John R. Bach, MD
Professor of Physical Medicine and Rehabilitation
Professor of Neurosciences
Vice Chairman, Department of Physical Medicine and Rehabilitation,
UMDNJ-New Jersey Medical School
Department of Physical Medicine and Rehabilitation
University Hospital
Newark, New Jersey
Chapter 85

Eduardo J. Mortani Barbosa Jr., MD
Assistant Professor of Radiology
Cardiothoracic Imaging
Perelman School of Medicine at the University of Pennsylvania
Philadelphia, Pennsylvania
Chapter 30

Alan F. Barker, MD
Pulmonary & Critical Care Medicine
Oregon Health & Science University
Portland, Oregon
Chapter 53

Peter J. Barnes, FRS, FMedSci
Margaret Turner-Warwick Professor of Medicine
Head of Respiratory Medicine
Airway Disease Section, National Heart & Lung Institute
Imperial College London
Dovehouse St, London
Chapter 46

Sonja D. Bartolome, MD
Associate Professor, Pulmonary and Critical Care Medicine
UT Southwestern Medical Center
Dallas, Texas
Chapter 98

Cynthia M. Beall, PhD
Distinguished University Professor and S. Idell Pyle Professor of Anthropology
Department of Anthropology
Case Western Reserve University
Cleveland, Ohio
Chapter 92

Matthew C. Bell, MD
Assistant Professor of Medicine & Pediatrics
Department of Pediatrics
Division of Allergy & Immunology
University of Arkansas for Medical Sciences
Arkansas Children's Hospital
Little Rock, Arkansas
Chapter 44

Joshua O. Benditt, MD
Professor of Medicine
Medical Center
University of Washington School of Medicine
Seattle, Washington
Chapter 144

Tithi Biswas, MD
Clinical Associate Professor
Department of Radiation Oncology
Case Western Reserve University School of Medicine
University Hospitals Seidman Cancer Center
Cleveland, Ohio
Chapter 115

Richard C. Boucher, MD
Kenan Professor of Medicine
Director Department of Medicine
Cystic Fibrosis and Pulmonary Research and Treatment Center
University of North Carolina
Chapel Hill, North Carolina
Chapter 6

Ghada Bourjeily, MD
Associate Professor of Medicine, Pulmonary and Critical Care Medicine
The Warren Alpert Medical School of Brown University
The Miriam Hospital
Providence, Rhode Island
Chapter 97

Anthony F. Boyer, MD
Pulmonary Medicine Consultants
Richardson, Texas
Chapter 129

Steven L. Brody, MD
Pulmonary and Critical Care
Department of Medicine
Washington University School of Medicine
St. Louis, Missouri
Chapter 53

Nathan E. Brummel, MD, MSCI
Division of Allergy, Pulmonary, and Critical Care Medicine
Health Services Research
Center for Quality of Aging
Department of Medicine, Vanderbilt University School of Medicine
Nashville, Tennessee
Chapter 150

Ayesha S. Bryant, MSPH, MD
Assistant Professor, Cardiothoracic Surgery
University of Alabama at Birmingham
Birmingham, Alabama
Chapter 105

S. Rodrigo Burguete, MD
Assistant Professor
Division of Pulmonary Diseases & Critical Care Medicine
Department of Medicine
University of Texas Health Science Center San Antonio
San Antonio, Texas
Chapter 78

Bryan M. Burt, MD
Department of Surgery
Division of Thoracic Surgery
Baylor College of Medicine
Houston Texas
Chapter 82

William W. Busse, MD
Professor of Medicine
Department of Medicine
Section of Allergy Pulmonary and Critical Care Medicine
University of Wisconsin School of Medicine and Public Health
Madison, Wisconsin
Chapter 44

Marcus W. Butler, MD, FRCPI
School of Medicine and Medical Sciences
University College Dublin
St Vincent's University Hospital
Dublin, Ireland
Chapter 26

Hilary C. Cain, MD
Associate Professor
Section of Pulmonary and Critical Care Medicine
Department of Internal Medicine
Yale University School of Medicine
VA Connecticut Healthcare System
West Haven, Connecticut
Chapter 66

Jeffrey P. Callen, MD
Professor of Medicine (Dermatology)
Chief, Division of Dermatology
University of Louisville
Louisville, Kentucky
Chapter 29

Edward J. Campbell, MD
HerediLab, Inc.
Salt Lake City, Utah
Chapter 19

Wellington V. Cardoso, MD, PhD
Professor of Medicine and Genetics & Development
Director, Columbia Center for Human Development
Department of Medicine
Columbia University Medical Center
New York, New York
Chapter 4

Laurie L. Carr, MD
Assistant Professor of Medicine
National Jewish Health
Denver, Colorado
Chapter 114

David M. Center, MD
Gordon and Ruth Snider Professor of Pulmonary Medicine
Professor of Medicine and Biochemistry
Associate Provost for Translational Research
Chief, Pulmonary, Allergy, Sleep and Critical Care Medicine
Boston University School of Medicine
Boston Medical Center
Chapter 21

Robert J. Cerfolio, MD, MBA
Professor of Surgery
James H. Estes Endowed Chair Lung Cancer Research
Birmingham, Alabama
Chapter 105

Murali Chakinala, MD, FCCP
Associate Professor of Medicine
Director, Pulmonary Hypertension Center
Co-Director HHT Center
Division of Pulmonary and Critical Care Medicine
Department of Medicine
Washington University School of Medicine
St. Louis, Missouri
Chapter 75

Georgios Chamilos, MD
Department of Internal Medicine
School of Medicine, Stavrakia, Voutes
University of Crete Heraklion
Crete, Greece
Chapter 133

Lydia Chang, MD
Assistant Professor of Medicine
Division of Pulmonary and Critical Care Medicine
University of North Carolina
Chapel Hill, North Carolina
Chapter 112

Lisa Chen, DO
Attending Physician
North Shore University Hospital
Manhasett, New York
Chapter 31

Edward S. Chen, MD
Assistant Professor of Medicine
Johns Hopkins University School of Medicine
Baltimore, Maryland
Chapter 55

Asha N. Chesnutt, MD
Pulmonary and Critical Care Physician
Pulmonary, Critical Care and Sleep Medicine
The Oregon Clinic, PC
Portland, Oregon
Chapter 140

Jason D. Christie, MD
Associate Professor of Medicine and Epidemiology
Division of Pulmonary, Allergy, and Critical Care Medicine
Perelman School of Medicine at the University of Pennsylvania
Philadelphia, Pennsylvania
Chapter 141

Geoffrey L. Chupp, MD
Associate Professor of Medicine, Yale School of Medicine
Director, Yale Center for Asthma and Airway Disease
Director, Pulmonary Function Laboratory, Yale New Haven Hospital
New Haven, Connecticut
Chapters 47 and 48

Andrew Churg, MD
Professor, University of British Columbia
Pathologist, Vancouver General Hospital
University Hospital
Vancouver, BC Canada
Chapter 39

Lauren E. Cohn, MD
Associate Professor of Medicine
Co-Director, Yale Center for Asthma and Airway Diseases
Section of Pulmonary, Critical Care and Sleep Medicine
Yale University School of Medicine
New Haven, Connecticut
Chapter 25

J. Allen D. Cooper Jr., MD
Division of Pulmonary, Allergy and Critical Care Medicine
University of Alabama Medical School
Chief, Pulmonary Section
Birmingham Department of Veterans Affairs Medical Center
Birmingham, Alabama
Chapter 89

Ryan Cooper, MD, MPH
Assistant Professor
Division of Infectious Diseases
University of Alberta
Edmonton, Alberta
Chapter 131

Gregory P. Cosgrove, MD, FCCP
Chief Medical Officer, Pulmonary Fibrosis Foundation
Interstitial Lung Disease Program
Associate Professor
National Jewish Health
University of Colorado-Denver
Denver, Colorado
Chapter 60

Gerard J. Criner, MD
Professor of Medicine
Florence P. Bernheimer Distinguished Service Chair
Chief, Division of Pulmonary and Critical Care
Temple University School of Medicine
Philadelphia, Pennsylvania
Chapter 84

Thomas A. D'Amico, MD
Gary Hock Endowed Professor and Vice-Chair of Surgery
Chief, Section of General Thoracic Surgery
Program Director, Thoracic Surgery
Duke University Medical Center
Durham, North Carolina
Chapter 119

David M. Daughton, MS
Behavioral Researcher, Retired
Pulmonary and Critical Care Medicine
Department of Internal Medicine
Nebraska Medical Center
Omaha, Nebraska
Chapter 41

Daniel T. DeArmond, MD
Assistant Professor
Director of Minimally Invasive Thoracic Surgery
Division of Thoracic Surgery
Department of Cardiothoracic Surgery
University of Texas Health Science Center San Antonio
San Antonio, Texas
Chapter 78

Malcolm M. DeCamp Jr., MD
Fowler McCormick Professor of Surgery
Northwestern University Feinberg School of Medicine
Chief, Division of Thoracic Surgery
Northwestern Memorial Hospital
Chicago, Illinois
Chapter 81

Roy Decker, MD, PhD
Associate Professor of Therapeutic Radiology
Yale University School of Medicine
Attending Physician, Yale-New Haven Hospital
Chapter 59

Marc Decramer, MD, PhD
Professor of Medicine
Chief Executive Officer
University Hospital
University of Leuven
Leuven, Belgium
Chapter 3

Charles S. Dela Cruz, MD, PhD
Assistant Professor
Section of Pulmonary, Critical Care, and Sleep Medicine
Department of Internal Medicine
Yale University School of Medicine
New Haven, Connecticut
Chapters 20 and 109

Horace M. DeLisser, MD
Associate Professor of Medicine
Department of Medicine
Perelman School of Medicine
Translational Research Laboratories
University of Pennsylvania
Philadelphia, Pennsylvania
Chapters 103 and 153

Jerome A. Dempsey, PhD
John Robert Sutton Professor Emeritus of Population Health Sciences
Director, John Rankin Laboratory of Pulmonary Medicine
University of Wisconsin
Madison, Wisconsin
Chapter 18

Jessy Deshane, PhD
Assistant Professor
Department of Medicine
Division of Pulmonary Allergy and Critical Care Medicine
University of Alabama
Alabama, Birmingham
Chapter 27

Clifford S. Deutschman, MS, MD, FCCM
Vice-Chair, Research
Department of Pediatrics
Professor of Pediatrics and Molecular Medicine North Shore-Long Island
Jewish-Hofstra School of Medicine
Steven and Alexandra Cohen Children's Medical Center
New Hyde Park, New York
Investigator
Feinstein Institute for Medical Research
Manhasset, New York
Chapter 142

Burton F. Dickey, MD
Department of Pulmonary Medicine
University of Texas MD Anderson Cancer Center
Houston, Texas
Chapter 6

Karen Doucette, MD, MSc (Epi)
Associate Professor
Division of Infectious Diseases, University of Alberta
Edmonton, Alberta
Chapter 131

Jonathan E. Dowell, MD
Associate Professor
Department of Internal Medicine (Division of Hematology and Oncology)
UT Southwestern Medical Center
Chief, Section of Hematology/Oncology
Dallas Veterans Affairs Medical Center
Dallas, Texas
Chapter 116

M. Bradley Drummond, MD, MHS
Assistant Professor, Pulmonary and Critical Care Medicine
Johns Hopkins University School of Medicine
Baltimore, Maryland
Chapter 42

Ghassan El-Haddad, MD
Assistant Member of Interventional Radiology
H. Lee Moffitt Cancer Center and Research Institute
Assistant Professor of Oncologic Sciences and Radiology
University of South Florida
Tampa, Florida
Chapter 32

Richard I. Enelow, MD
Professor of Medicine, Microbiology, and Immunology
Geisel School of Medicine at Dartmouth
Section of Pulmonary and Critical Care Medicine
Dartmouth-Hitchcock Medical Center
Lebanon, New Hampshire
Chapter 58

Kyle B. Enfield, MD, MS
Assistant Professor of Medicine
Division of Pulmonary and Critical Care Medicine,
Department of Medicine, University of Virginia School of Medicine
Attending Physician and Medical Director, Medical Intensive Care Unit,
University of Virginia Health System
Charlottesville, Virginia
Chapter 127

Perenlei Enkhbaatar, MD, PhD, FAHA
Professor, Department of Anesthesiology
Director of Translational Intensive Care Unit
University of Texas Medical Branch
Galveston, Texas
Chapter 94

Gary R. Epler, MD
Clinical Associate Professor
Harvard Medical School
Pulmonary and Critical Care Medicine
Brigham and Women's Hospital
Boston, Massachusetts
Chapter 51

Loretta Erhunmwunsee, MD
Chief Resident in Thoracic Surgery
Duke University Medical Center
Durham, North Carolina
Chapter 119

Peter F. Fedullo, MD
Director, Medical Intensive Care Unit
Professor of Clinical Medicine
University of California
San Diego, California
Chapter 73

Barry G. Fields, MD
Assistant Professor of Medicine
Division of Pulmonary, Allergy, and Critical Care Medicine
Department of Medicine
Emory University School of Medicine
Atlanta, Georgia
Chapter 99

Thomas M. File Jr., MD, MSc
Chair, Infectious Disease Division
Summa Health System
Akron, OH
Professor, Internal Medicine
Master Teacher, Chair, Infectious Disease Section
Northeast Ohio Medical University
Rootstown, Ohio
Chapter 126

Michael C. Fishbein, MD
Piansky Professor of Pathology and Medicine
Department of Pathology and Laboratory Medicine
UCLA Center for the Health Sciences
Los Angeles, California

Jay A. Fishman, MD
Associate Director, MGH Transplantation Center
Director, Transplant Infectious Disease & Compromised Host Program
Massachusetts General Hospital
Professor of Medicine, Harvard Medical School
Boston, Massachusetts
Chapters 122, 123, 135, and 137

Douglas B. Flieder, MD
Professor of Pathology
Fox Chase Cancer Center
Philadelphia, Pennsylvania
Chapter 120

Barry D. Fuchs, MD
Associate Professor of Medicine
Division of Pulmonary and Critical Care Medicine
Perelman School of Medicine
University of Pennsylvania
Philadelphia, Pennsylvania
Chapters 147 and 152

Ghislaine Gayan-Ramirez, PhD
Department of Pneumology
Katholieke Universiteit Leuven
Leuven, Belgium
Chapter 3

Gregory P. Geba, MD, MPH, DrPH, FACP, FCCP, FAAAAI
Vice President, Clinical Development and Regulatory Affairs
Regeneron Pharmaceuticals, Inc.
Tarrytown, New York
Chapter 47

Warren B. Gefter, MD
Professor of Radiology
Chief, Cardiothoracic Imaging Division
Associate Chair, Department of Radiology
Perelman School of Medicine at University Pennsylvania
Philadelphia, Pennsylvania
Chapter 30

David E. Gerber, MD
Associate Professor
Department of Internal Medicine
(Division of Hematology and Oncology)
Co-Leader, Experimental Therapeutics Program
Harold C. Simmons Cancer Center
UT Southwestern Medical Center
Dallas, Texas
Chapter 116

Alex H. Gifford, MD
Assistant Professor of Medicine
Geisel School of Medicine at Dartmouth
Dartmouth-Hitchcock Medical Center
Chapter 58

Timothy D. Girard, MD, MSCI
Division of Allergy, Pulmonary, and Critical Care Medicine
Center for Health Services Research
Center for Quality of Aging
Department of Medicine, Vanderbilt University School of Medicine
Geriatric Research, Education and Clinical Center (GRECC) Service,
Department of Veterans Affairs Medical Center,
Tennessee Valley Healthcare System
Nashville, Tennessee
Chapter 150

Mark T. Gladwin, MD
Professor of Medicine
Division Chief, Pulmonary, Allergy and Critical Care Medicine
Director, Heart, Lung, Blood and Vascular Medicine
Department of Medicine
Institute of University of Pittsburgh and UPMC Montefiore Hospital
Pittsburgh, Pennsylvania
Chapter 96

Allan R. Glanville, MBBS, MD, FRACP
Director Thoracic Medicine
Medical Director Lung Transplantation
St.Vincent's Hospital
Darlinghurst, Australia
Chapter 107

Alla Godelman, MD
Department of Radiology
Montefiore Medical Center
Assistant Professor of Radiology
Albert Einstein College of Medicine
Chapter 117

Stanley Goldfarb, MD
Associate Dean for Curriculum
Perelman School of Medicine at the University of Pennsylvania
Philadelphia, Pennsylvania
Chapter 17

Mitchell Goldman, MD, FACP
Program Director, Internal Medicine Residency
Professor of Medicine
Division of Infectious Diseases
Indiana University School of Medicine
Indianapolis, Indiana
Chapter 134

Jose L. Gomez, MD, MS
Instructor
Pulmonary, Critical Care and Sleep Section
Yale University School of Medicine
New Haven, Connecticut
Chapter 47

Daniel M. Goodenberger, MD
Professor of Medicine, Washington University School of Medicine
Chief, Medical Service, St. Louis VAMC
Medical Director Emeritus, HHT Centers of Excellence
Washington University and University of Texas Southwestern
St. Louis, Missouri
Chapter 75

Emily K. B. Gordon, MD
Assistant Professor
Department of Anesthesiology and Critical Care
Hospital of the University of Pennsylvania
Philadelphia, Pennsylvania
Chapter 142

Praveen Govender, MD
Assistant Professor of Medicine
Pulmonary, Allergy & Immunology
Associate Director, Sarcoidosis Center at Boston Medical Center
Boston, Massachusetts
Chapter 21

Michael A. Grippi, MD
Vice Chairman, Department of Medicine
Pulmonary, Allergy, and Critical Care Division
Chief Medical Officer, GSPP Specialty Hospital at Rittenhouse
Perelman School of Medicine at the University of Pennsylvania
Philadelphia, Pennsylvania
Chapters 1, 29, 33, 103, 139, and 152

Mridu Gulati, MD, MPH
Departments of Internal Medicine, Section of Pulmonary,
Critical Care and Sleep Medicine
Yale School of Medicine
New Haven, Connecticut
Chapter 57

Indira Gurubhagavatula, MD, MPH
Associate Professor of Medicine
Perelman School of Medicine
University of Pennsylvania
Director, Sleep Disorders Clinic
Philadelphia VA Medical Center
Philadelphia, Pennsylvania
Chapter 101

Andrew R. Haas, MD, PhD
Assistant Professor of Medicine
Chief, Section of Interventional Pulmonology and Thoracic Oncology
Division of Pulmonary, Allergy and Critical Care Medicine
Perelman School of Medicine at the University of Pennsylvania
Philadelphia, Pennsylvania
Chapter 36

Chadi A. Hage, MD
Assistant Professor of Medicine
Indiana University School of Medicine
Pulmonary-Critical Care Medicine
Thoracic Transplant program
Methodist Professional Center-1
Indianapolis, Indiana
Chapter 134

C. William Hanson III, MD
Professor of Anesthesiology and Critical Care
Surgery and Internal Medicine
Perelman School of Medicine at the University of Pennsylvania
Philadelphia, Pennsylvania
Chapter 146

Sergio Harari, MD
Director of Pulmonary Division and Department of Medicine
Unità Operativa di Pneumologia e Terapia Semi-Intensiva Respiratoria
Servizio di Fisiopatologia Respiratoria e Emodinamica polmonare
Ospedale San Giuseppe MultiMedica
Milano, Italy
Chapter 61

John E. Heffner, MD
Professor of Medicine
Garnjobst Chair, Department of Medicine
Oregon Health and Science University
Providence Portland Medical Center
Portland, Oregon
Chapter 76

Erica L. Herzog, MD
Department of Internal Medicine, Section of Pulmonary,
Critical Care and Sleep Medicine
Yale School of Medicine
New Haven, Connecticut
Chapter 57

Søren Hess, MD
Associate Professor, Department of Nuclear Medicine
Odense University Hospital
Denmark
Chapter 32

Robert J. Homer, MD, PhD
Professor of Pathology and Internal Medicine (Pulmonary)
Yale University School of Medicine
New Haven, Connecticut
Pathology and Laboratory Medicine Service
VA CT HealthCare System
West Haven, Connecticut
Chapter 64

Alberto de Hoyos, MD, FCCP, FACS
Director of Alton Ochsner Lung Cancer Center
Director of Thoracic Oncology
Ochsner Medical Center
New Orleans, Louisiana
Chapter 81

Gary B. Huffnagle, PhD
Professor of Medicine
Division of Pulmonary and Critical Care Medicine
University of Michigan Medical Center
Ann Arbor, Michigan
Chapter 121

John T. Huggins, MD
Associate Professor of Medicine
Division of Pulmonary, Critical Care, Allergy and Sleep Medicine
Department of Medicine
Medical University of South Carolina
Charleston, South Carolina
Chapter 77

Louise C. Ivers, MB, BCh, BAO, MPH, DTM&H
Associate Professor of Global Health and Social Medicine
Associate Professor of Medicine
Harvard Medical School
Division of Global Health Equity
Brigham and Women's Hospital
Boston, Massachusetts
Chapter 136

Frank J. Jacono, MD
Associate Professor of Medicine
Division of Pulmonary, Critical Care and Sleep Medicine
Case Western Reserve University
Louis Stokes Cleveland VA Medical Center
Cleveland, Ohio
Chapter 11

Anthony J. Jacques, BS
Department of Population Health Sciences
John Rankin Laboratory of Pulmonary Medicine
University of Wisconsin
Madison, Wisconsin
Chapter 18

James R. Jett, MD
Professor of Medicine
National Jewish Health
Denver, Colorado
Chapter 114

Jian Jing, MD, PhD
Post-Doctoral Fellow
Department of Medicine
University of Colorado School of Medicine
Aurora, Colorado
Chapter 90

David H. Johnson, MD, MACP
Donald W. Seldin Distinguished Chair in Internal Medicine
Professor and Chairman, Department of Internal Medicine
UT Southwestern School of Medicine
Dallas, Texas
Chapter 116

Joshua B. Kayser, MD, MPH
Division of Pulmonary, Allergy and Critical Care
Perelman School of Medicine
University of Pennsylvania
Interim Chief of Medicine
Director, Medical Intensive Care Unit
Philadelphia VA Medical Center
Philadelphia, Pennsylvania
Chapter 153

Michael P. Keane, MD, FRCPI
Professor of Medicine
Chair of Medicine and Therapeutics
University College Dublin
Consultant Respiratory Physician
St Vincent's University Hospital
Dublin, Ireland
Chapter 26

Steven M. Keller, MD
Director Thoracic Surgery, Weiler Hospital
Professor Cardiothoracic Surgery
Albert Einstein College of Medicine
Bronx, New York
Chapter 117

Andrea Kelly, MD
Division of Endocrinology
The Children's Hospital of Philadelphia
Philadelphia, Pennsylvania
Chapter 50

Steven G. Kelsen, MD
Professor of Medicine and Physiology
Division of Pulmonary and Critical Care Medicine
Department of Medicine
Temple University School of Medicine
Philadelphia, Pennsylvania
Chapter 143

Jeffrey A. Kern, MD
Professor of Medicine
Chief, Division of Oncology
Director, Lung Cancer Center
Department of Medicine
National Jewish Health
Denver, Colorado
Professor of Medicine
Pulmonary Sciences and Critical Care Medicine
Department of Medicine
University of Colorado—Denver
Aurora, Colorado
Chapter 108

Talmadge E. King Jr., MD
Julius R. Krevans Distinguished Professor in Internal Medicine
Chair, Department of Medicine
University of California, San Francisco
San Francisco, California
Chapters 61 and 62

Robert A. Klocke, MD
Emeritus Professor and Chair
Department of Medicine
University at Buffalo
Buffalo, New York
Chapters 15 and 16

Michael R. Knowles, MD
Professor of Pulmonary and Critical Care Medicine
Department of Medicine
Marsico Lung Institute/Cystic Fibrosis Center
University of North Carolina
Chapel Hill, North Carolina
Chapter 6

Kenneth S. Knox, MD
Associate Professor of Medicine and Immunobiology
Division Chief, Division of Pulmonary, Allergy,
Critical Care and Sleep Medicine
Department of Medicine, University of Arizona
Tucson, Arizona
Chapter 134

Jonathan L. Koff, MD
Director, Adult Cystic Fibrosis Program
Section of Pulmonary, Critical Care, and Sleep Medicine
Department of Internal Medicine
Yale University School of Medicine
New Haven, Connecticut
Chapter 20

Marin H. Kollef, MD
Director, Critical Care Research
Director, Respiratory Care Services
Barnes-Jewish Hospital
Virginia E. and Sam J. Golman Chair in
Respiratory Intensive Care Medicine
Professor of Medicine Division of Pulmonary and
Critical Care Medicine Washington
University School of Medicine
St. Louis, Missouri
Chapter 129

Dimitrios P. Kontoyiannis, MD, ScD, FACP, FIDSA
Frances King Black Endowed Professor, Infectious Diseases
Deputy Head
Division of Internal Medicine
The University of Texas MD Anderson Cancer Center
Adj Professor Baylor College of Medicine
Adj Professor University of Houston
Houston, Texas
Chapter 133

Robert M. Kotloff, MD
Chair, Department of Pulmonary Medicine
Cleveland Clinic
Cleveland, Ohio
Chapters 95 and 104

Darrell N. Kotton, MD
Professor of Medicine and Pathology
Director, Center for Regenerative Medicine (CReM)
Boston University and Boston Medical Center
Boston, Massachusetts
Chapter 8

Camille Nelson Kotton, MD
Infectious Diseases Division
Massachusetts General Hospital
Boston, Massachusetts
Chapter 138

Mary Elizabeth Kreider, MD, MSCE
Associate Chief for Education and Fellowship Director
Division of Pulmonary and Critical Care Medicine
Clinical Director ILD Program
The Perelman School of the Medicine
University of Pennsylvania
Philadelphia, Pennsylvania
Chapter 87

Michael J. Krowka, MD
Professor, Pulmonary and Critical Care Medicine
Mayo Clinic
Rochester, Minnesota
Chapter 98

Meir H. Kryger, MD, FRCPC
Professor, Pulmonary, Critical Care and Sleep Medicine
Yale School of Medicine
Director, Sleep Medicine Fellowship Program
Physician, VA Connecticut Healthcare System
West Haven, Connecticut
Chapters 49 and 102

Andrew Levinson, MD
Assistant Professor of Medicine (Clinical)
Pulmonary and Critical Care Medicine
The Warren Alpert Medical School of Brown University
The Miriam Hospital and Rhode Island hospital
Providence, Rhode Island
Chapter 97

Howard Li, MD
Assistant Professor
Division of Pulmonary Sciences and Critical Care Medicine
Department of Medicine
Denver VA Medical Center
Denver, Colorado
University of Colorado Anschutz Medical Campus
Aurora, Colorado
Chapter 108

Augusto A. Litonjua, MD, MPH
Associate Professor of Medicine
Channing Division of Network Medicine and
Division of Pulmonary and Critical Care Medicine
Department of Medicine
Brigham and Women's Hospital
Harvard Medical School
Boston, Massachusetts
Chapter 45

Frederic F. Little, MD
Assistant Professor of Medicine
Boston University School of Medicine
Program Director, Allergy/Immunology Fellowship
Medical Director, Pulmonary, Allergy, and Sleep Clinics
Boston Medical Center
Boston, Massachusetts
Chapter 21

Leslie A. Litzky, MD
Professor
Department of Pathology and Laboratory Medicine
Perelman School of Medicine of the University of Pennsylvania
Philadelphia, Pennsylvania
Chapters 79, 111

Christopher Logue, MD
Hyperbaric Medicine Attending Physician
The Institute for Environmental Medicine
The Hospital of the University of Pennsylvania
Emergency Medicine Attending Physician
Penn Presbyterian Medical Center
Philadelphia, Pennsylvania
Chapter 93

Jining Lu, PhD
Assistant Professor of Medicine
Columbia Center for Human Development
Department of Medicine
Columbia University Medical Center
New York, New York
Chapter 4

Nicholas W. Lukacs, PhD
Godfrey Dorr Stobbe Professor of Pathology
Assistant Dean for Faculty Affairs
University of Michigan Medical School
Ann Arbor, Michigan
Chapter 23

Joseph P. Lynch, III, MD
Holt and Jo Hickman Endowed Chair of Advanced Lung Disease
and Lung Transplantation
Professor of Clinical Medicine, Step VIII
Associate Chief, Division of Pulmonary and Critical Care Medicine,
Clinical Immunology, and Allergy
David Geffen School of Medicine at UCLA
Los Angeles, California
Chapter 68

Roberto F. Machado, MD
Associate Professor of Medicine
Section of Pulmonary, Critical Care Medicine, Sleep and Allergy
University of Illinois Chicago
Chicago, Illinois
Chapter 96

Mitchell Machtay, MD
Vincent K. Smith Professor and Chair
Department of Radiation Oncology
Case Western Reserve University School of Medicine
University Hospitals Seidman Cancer Center
Cleveland, Ohio
Chapter 115

Atul Malhotra, MD
Kenneth M. Moser Professor of Medicine
Division of Pulmonary, Critical Care and Sleep Medicine
University of California San Diego
La Jolla, California
Chapter 11

Scott Manaker, MD, PhD
Associate Professor of Medicine
Pulmonary, Allergy, and Critical Care Division
Vice Chair for Regulatory Affairs
Department of Medicine
University of Pennsylvania
Philadelphia, Pennsylvania
Chapter 145

Jess Mandel, MD
Professor of Medicine
Associate Dean for Undergraduate Medical Education
UCSD School of Medicine
La Jolla, California
Chapter 72

Nathaniel Marchetti, DO
Associate Professor of Medicine
Division of Pulmonary and Critical Care Medicine
Temple University School of Medicine
Philadelphia, Pennsylvania
Chapter 84

Paul E. Marik, MD
Chief, Pulmonary and Critical Care Medicine
Department of Internal Medicine
Eastern Virginia Medical School
Norfolk, Virginia
Chapter 69

Thomas J. Marrie, MD, FRCPC, MACP, FRSC
Dean, Faculty of Medicine
Dalhousie University
Halifax, Nova Scotia
Chapter 128

Stanley I. Martin, MD
Associate Professor, Clinical Internal Medicine
Director, Infectious Diseases Fellowship Program
Division of Infectious Diseases
Transplant Infectious Diseases Service
The Ohio State University Wexner Medical Center
Columbus, Ohio
Chapter 135

Fernando J. Martinez, MD, MS
Executive Vice Chairman
Gladys and Roland Harriman Professor of Medicine
Joan and Sanford I. Weill Department of Medicine
Weill Cornell Medical College
NewYork-Presbyterian Hospital/Weill Cornell Medical Center
New York, New York
Chapter 52

Maria Mascarenhas, MD
Division of Gastroenterology, Hepatology and Nutrition
The Children's Hospital of Philadelphia
Philadelphia, Pennsylvania
Chapter 50

Richard A. Matthay, MD
Boehringer Ingelheim Emeritus Professor of Medicine and
Senior Research Scientist in Medicine
Pulmonary and Critical Care Medicine Section
Department of Internal Medicine
Yale University School of Medicine
New Haven, Connecticut
Chapter 109

Michael A. Matthay, MD
Professor, Medicine and Anesthesia
Associate Director, Intensive Care Unit, University of California,
San Francisco
Senior Associate, Cardiovascular Research Institute
San Francisco, California
Chapter 140

Paul H. Mayo, MD
Academic Director Critical Care
Long Island Jewish Medical Center
New Hyde Park, New York
Professor of Medicine
Hofstra North Shore-LIJ School of Medicine
Hempstead, New York
Chapter 31

Jeffrey Mazer, MD
Assistant Professor of Medicine
Pulmonary and Critical Care Medicine
The Warren Alpert Medical School of Brown University
The Miriam Hospital
Providence, Rhode
Chapter 97

John McArdle, MD
Assistant Clinical Professor of Medicine, University of Connecticut
Connecticut Multi-Specialty Group
Hartford, Connecticut
Chapter 65

F. Dennis McCool, MD
Professor of Medicine
Pulmonary Critical Care and Sleep Medicine
Alpert Medical School of Brown University
Memorial Hospital of Rhode Island
Pawtucket, Rhode Island
Chapter 83

Paul McLoughlin, MB, BCh, MRCPI, PhD
Professor of Physiology
University College Dublin
School of Medicine and Medical Sciences
Conway Institute of Biomedical and Biomolecular Research
St. Vincent's University Hospital
Dublin, Ireland
Chapter 26

Eric B. Meltzer, MD
Adjunct Assistant Professor of Medicine
Division of Pulmonary, Allergy and Critical Care Medicine
Department of Medicine
Duke University Medical Center
Durham, North Carolina
Chapter 56

J. Wayne Meredith, MD, FACS
Department of Surgery
Wake Forest Medical Center
Winston-Salem, North Carolina
Chapter 106

Robert E. Merritt, MD
Associate Professor of Surgery
Division of Thoracic Surgery
Ohio State University Medical Center
Columbus, Ohio
Chapter 37

Gaetane Michaud, MS, MD, FRCPC
Associate Professor of Medicine
Yale School of Medicine
New Haven, Connecticut
Chapter 49

Mark E. Mikkelsen, MD, MSCE
Assistant Professor of Medicine
Pulmonary, Allergy and Critical Care Division
Perelman School of Medicine at the University of Pennsylvania
Hospital of the University of Pennsylvania
Philadelphia, Pennsylvania
Chapter 152

David R. Moller, MD
Professor of Medicine
Johns Hopkins University School of Medicine
Baltimore, Maryland
Chapter 55

Edmund K. Moon, MD
Assistant Professor of Medicine
Section of Interventional Pulmonary and Thoracic Oncology
Division of Pulmonary, Allergy, and Critical Care
Department of Medicine
Perelman School of Medicine at the University of Pennsylvania
Philadelphia, Pennsylvania
Chapter 79

Joel Moss, MD, PhD
Deputy Chief, Cardiovascular and Pulmonary Branch
National Heart, Lung, and Blood Institute
National Institutes of Health
Bethesda, Maryland
Chapters 61, 62, and 63

Nathan T. Mowery, MD, FACS
Associate Professor of Surgery
Department of Surgery
Wake Forest Medical Center
Winston-Salem, North Carolina
Chapter 106

Robert Naeije, MD, PhD
Professor and Chairman of the Department of Physiology
and Pathophysiology
Director, Pulmonary Hypertension Clinic, Erasme University Hospital
Department of Physiology
Erasme Campus
Free University of Brussels
Brussels, Belgium
Chapter 13

Patrick J. Neligan, MD, FJFICM
Director of Critical Care Services
Consultant in Anaesthesia and Intensive Care
Galway University Hospitals and National University of Ireland,
Galway, Ireland
Chapter 147

Nikolaus C. Netzer, MD, PhD
University Professor
Hermann Buhl Institute for Hypoxia Research and Sleep Medicine Research
University of Ulm, Department of Internal Medicine, Germany
Faculty of Psychology and Sports Science, University Innsbruck
Innsbruck, Austria
Chapter 92

Kevin P. Newman, MD
Professor of Medicine
Division of Cardiovascular Diseases
University of Tennessee Health Science Center
Memphis, Tennessee
Chapter 34

Michael S. Niederman, MD
Professor of Medicine
SUNY at Stony Brook
Pulmonary and Critical Care
Winthrop-University Hospital
Mineola, New York
Chapter 125

Paul W. Noble, MD
Professor of Medicine
Chair of Medicine
Department of Medicine
Cedars Sinai Medical Center
Los Angeles, California
Chapter 56

Matthias Ochs, MD
Professor and Chair
Institute of Functional and Applied Anatomy
Hannover Medical School
Hannover, Germany
Chapter 2

David Ost, MD, MPH
Professor of Medicine
The University of Texas MD Anderson Cancer Center
Houston, Texas
Chapter 110

Gustavo Pacheco-Rodriguez, PhD
Staff Scientist, Cardiovascular and Pulmonary Branch
National Heart, Lung, and Blood Institute
National Institutes of Health
Bethesda, Maryland
Chapter 63

Allan I. Pack, MBChB, PhD
John Miclot Professor of Medicine
Chief, Division of Sleep Medicine/Department of Medicine
Director, Center for Sleep and Circadian Neurobiology
Perelman School of Medicine at the University of Pennsylvania
Philadelphia, Pennsylvania
Chapter 12

John E. Parker, MD
Professor and Chief, Section of Pulmonary and Critical Care Medicine
Health Sciences Center
West Virginia University Healthcare
Morgantown, West Virginia
Chapter 88

Nicholas J. Pastis, MD
Assistant Professor of Medicine
Division of Pulmonary and Critical Care Medicine
Department of Medicine
Medical University of South Carolina
Charleston, South Carolina
Chapter 118

Jay Peters, MD
Professor and Chief
Division of Pulmonary and Critical Care Medicine
Department of Medicine
University of Texas Health Science Center San Antonio
San Antonio, Texas
Chapter 78

Steve G. Peters, MD
Professor of Medicine
Division of Pulmonary and Critical Care Medicine
Mayo Clinic
Rochester, Minnesota
Chapter 95

Edward L. Petsonk, MD
Professor, Section of Pulmonary and Critical Care Medicine
West Virginia University Healthcare
Health Sciences Center
Morgantown, West Virginia
Chapter 88

Julie V. Philley, MD
Assistant Professor of Medicine
Department of Pulmonary and Critical Care Medicine
University of Texas Health Science Center
Tyler, Texas
Chapter 132

Grace W. Pien, MD, MSCE
Assistant Professor of Medicine
Division of Pulmonary and Critical Care Medicine
Department of Medicine
Johns Hopkins University School of Medicine
Baltimore, Maryland
Chapter 99

Gerald B. Pier, PhD
Professor of Medicine (Microbiology and Immunobiology)
Division of Infectious Diseases
Department of Medicine
Brigham and Women's Hospital
Harvard Medical School
Boston, Massachusetts
Chapter 124

Richard A. Pierce, PhD
Division of Pulmonary and Critical Care
Department of Medicine
Washington University School of Medicine
St. Louis, Missouri
Chapter 40

Jennifer Possick, MD
Assistant Professor of Medicine
Section of Pulmonary, Critical Care and Sleep Medicine
Yale School of Medicine
New Haven, Connecticut
Chapter 65

Bala Prakash, MD
Assistant Professor of Medicine
Pulmonary, Critical Care and Sleep Medicine
Hofstra North Shore- LIJ School of Medicine
Manhasset, New York
Chapter 125

Gregory P. Priebe, MD
Associate Professor
Division of Critical Care Medicine
Department of Anesthesiology, Perioperative and Pain Medicine
Division of Infectious Diseases
Department of Medicine
Boston Children's Hospital
Division of Infectious Diseases
Department of Medicine
Brigham and Women's Hospital
Harvard Medical School
Boston, Massachusetts
Chapter 124

Benjamin A. Raby, MD, MPH
Associate Professor of Medicine
Channing Division of Network Medicine and the Division of Pulmonary and Critical Care Medicine
Director, BWH Pulmonary Genetics Center
Department of Medicine
Brigham and Women's Hospital
Harvard Medical School
Boston, MA
Chapter 9

John P. Reilly, MD, MSCE
Instructor of medicine
University of Pennsylvania
Perelman School of Medicine Division of Pulmonary, Allergy, and Critical Care
Philadelphia, Pennsylvania
Chapter 141

Stephen I. Rennard, MD
Larson Professor of Medicine
Division of Pulmonary, Critical Care, Sleep and Allergy
Nebraska Medical Center
Omaha, Nebraska
Chapter 41

Scott I. Reznik, MD
Associate Professor
Division of Thoracic Surgery
Department of Cardiovascular and Thoracic Surgery
UT Southwestern Medical Center
Temple, Texas
Chapter 113

David Q. Rich, ScD
Associate Professor
Division of Epidemiology, Department of Public Health Sciences
University of Rochester School of Medicine and Dentistry
Rochester, New York
Chapter 91

Andrew L. Ries, MD, MPH
Associate Vice Chancellor for Academic Affairs, Health Sciences
Professor of Medicine and Family and Preventive Medicine
University of California, San Diego
La Jolla, California
Chapter 43

M. Patricia Rivera, MD
Professor of Medicine
Division of Pulmonary and Critical Care Medicine
Medical Director, Bronchoscopy and Pulmonary Function Lab
University of North Carolina
Chapel Hill, North Carolina
Chapter 112

Kenneth B. Roberts, MD
Professor of Therapeutic Radiology
Yale University School of Medicine
Attending Physician, Yale-New Haven Hospital
New Haven, Connecticut
Chapter 59

Carolyn L. Rochester, MD
Associate Professor of Medicine
Section of Pulmonary, Critical Care and Sleep
Yale University School of Medicine
VA Connecticut Healthcare System
New Haven, Connecticut
Chapter 71

Sara Rockwell, PhD
Professor Emeritus of Therapeutic Radiology
Yale University School of Medicine
New Haven, Connecticut
Chapter 59

William N. Rom, MD, MPH
Sol and Judith Bergstein Professor of Medicine
and Environmental Medicine
Director, Division of Pulmonary, Critical Care, and Sleep Medicine
Director, Bellevue Chest Service
New York University School of Medicine
New York, New York
Chapter 86

Ilene M. Rosen, MD, MSCE
Associate Professor of Clinical Medicine
Sleep Medicine Division, Department of Medicine
Perelman School of Medicine, University of Pennsylvania
Philadelphia, Pennsylvania
Chapter 99

Milton D. Rossman, MD
Clinical Professor of Medicine
Division of Pulmonary and Critical Care Medicine
The Perelman School of Medicine
University of Pennsylvania
Philadelphia, Pennsylvania
Chapter 87

Ami N. Rubinowitz, MD
Associate Professor and Co-Chief of Thoracic Imaging
Department of Diagnostic Radiology
Yale University School of Medicine
Yale-New Haven Hospital
New Haven, Connecticut
Chapter 57

Edward T. Ryan, MD, DTM&H
Director, Global Infectious Diseases; Division of Infectious Diseases
Massachusetts General Hospital
Professor of Medicine, Harvard Medical School
Professor of Immunology & Infectious Diseases
Harvard School of Public Health
Boston, Massachusetts
Chapter 136

Steven A. Sahn, MD
Professor of Medicine
Division of Pulmonary, Critical Care, Allergy and Sleep Medicine
Department of Medicine
Medical University of South Carolina
Charleston, South Carolina
Chapter 77

Jonathan M. Samet, MD, MS
Distinguished Professor and Flora L. Thornton Chair
Department of Preventive Medicine
Keck School of Medicine of USC
Director, USC Institute for Global Health
University of Southern California
Los Angeles, California
Chapter 91

Thomas F. Scanlin, MD
Professor and Senior Vice Chair
Department of Pediatrics
Chief, Division of Pulmonary Medicine and Cystic Fibrosis Center
Rutgers Robert Wood Johnson Medical School
New Brunswick, New Jersey
Chapter 50

Edward S. Schulman, MD
Professor of Medicine
Division of Pulmonary, Critical Care and Sleep Medicine
Drexel University College of Medicine
Service Chief, Pulmonary and Critical Care Medicine
Director, Allergy and Asthma Center
Hahnemann University Hospital
Philadelphia, Pennsylvania
Chapter 22

Richard J. Schwab, MD
Professor, Department of Medicine
Division of Sleep Medicine
Pulmonary, Allergy and Critical Care Division
Co-Director, Penn Sleep Center, University of Pennsylvania Medical Center
Philadelphia, Pennsylvania
Chapter 100

David A. Schwartz, MD
Professor of Medicine and Immunology
Robert W. Schrier Chair of Medicine
University of Colorado School of Medicine
Aurora, Colorado
Chapter 90

Marvin I. Schwarz, MD
James Campbell Professor of Pulmonary Medicine
Division of Pulmonary Sciences and Critical Care Medicine
Department of Medicine
University of Colorado
Denver, Colorado
Chapter 60

William D. Schweickert, MD
Assistant Professor of Medicine
Pulmonary, Allergy and Critical Care Medicine
Perelman School of Medicine
University of Pennsylvania
Philadelphia, Pennsylvania
Chapter 151

Mithu Sen, MD, FRCPC, D'ABSM, FCCP, FCCM, FAASM
Associate Professor, Medicine
Divisions of Respirology/Sleep and Critical Care Medicine
Assistant Dean, Schulich School of Medicine and Dentistry
Western University
Ontario, Canada
Chapter 102

Robert M. Senior, MD
Professor of Medicine
Professor of Cell Biology & Physiology
Washington University School of Medicine
St. Louis, Missouri
Chapters 29, 40, Appendices A and B

David S. Seres, MD, ScM, PNS
Associate Professor of Medicine in the Institute of Human Nutrition
Director, Medical Nutrition
Division of Preventive Medicine and Nutrition
Department of Medicine
Columbia University College of Physicians and Surgeons
New York, New York
Chapter 149

Kumar Sharma, MD, FAHA
Professor of Medicine
Director, Institute of Metabolomic Medicine Director
Center for Renal Translational Medicine
University of California, San Diego and VA San Diego HealthCare System
La Jolla, California
Chapter 17

Adrian Shifren, MD
Assistant Professor of Medicine
Department of Internal Medicine
Washington University School of Medicine
Saint Louis, Missouri
Chapters 15 and 16

Joseph B. Shrager, MD
Professor of Cardiothoracic Surgery
Chief, Division of Thoracic Surgery
Stanford University School of Medicine
Stanford Hospitals and Clinics
Stanford, California
Chapter 82

Costi D. Sifri, MD
Associate Professor of Medicine
Division of Infectious Diseases and International Health
Department of Medicine, University of Virginia School of Medicine
Attending Physician and Director, Hospital Epidemiology/Infection
Prevention and Control, University of Virginia Health System
Charlottesville, Virginia
Chapter 127

Gerard A. Silvestri, MD
Professor of Medicine
Division of Pulmonary and Critical Care Medicine
Medical University of South Carolina
Charleston, South Carolina
Chapter 118

Kimberly A. Smith
Department of Pediatrics
Northwestern University
Chicago, Illinois
Chapter 72

CONTRIBUTORS

W. Roy Smythe, MD
Chief Medical Officer, AVIA Health Innovation
Chief Executive Officer, HX360
Chicago, Illinois
Adjunct Professor of Surgery and Molecular Medicine
Texas A&M University Health Science Center College of Medicine
Temple, Texas
Chapter 113

Xavier Soler, MD, PhD
Assistant Professor of Medicine
Associate Director, Pulmonary Rehabilitation
Associate Director, Clinical Trials and Airway Research Center
Division of Pulmonary, Critical Care and Sleep Medicine
University of California, San Diego
La Jolla, California
Chapter 11

Nilam J. Soni, MD
Associate Professor
Division of Hospital Medicine
Department of Medicine
University of Texas Health Science Center San Antonio
San Antonio, Texas
Chapter 78

Akshay Sood, MD, MPH
Associate Professor, Division of Pulmonary and Critical Care Medicine
Department of Medicine
University of New Mexico Health Sciences Center School of Medicine
Albuquerque, New Mexico
Chapter 38

Ulrich Specks, MD
Connor Group Foundation Professor of Medicine
Chair, Division of Pulmonary & Critical Care Medicine
Mayo Clinic
Rochester, Minnesota
Chapter 74

Peter H. S. Sporn, MD
Professor of Medicine and Cell and Molecular Biology
Director, Pulmonary and Critical Care Medicine Fellowship Program
Northwestern University Feinberg School of Medicine
Chicago, Illinois
Chapter 22

Theodore J. Standiford, MD
Professor of Medicine and Chief
Division of Pulmonary and Critical Care Medicine
University of Michigan Medical Center
Ann Arbor, Michigan
Chapter 121

Robert C. Stansbury, MD
Assistant Professor and Medical Director WVUH Sleep Evaluation Center
Section of Pulmonary and Critical Care Medicine
West Virginia University Department of Medicine
Morgantown, West Virginia
Chapter 88

Daniel H. Sterman, MD
Director, Division of Pulmonary, Critical Care, and Sleep Medicine
Professor of Pulmonary Medicine and Cardiothoracic Surgery
New York University School of Medicine
NYU Langone Medical Center
New York, New York
Chapters 35, 36, and 79

Kingman P. Strohl, MD
Center for Sleep Disorders Research
Louis Stokes Cleveland Department of
Veterans Administration Medical Center
Division of Pulmonary, Critical Care, and Sleep Medicine
University Hospitals Case Medical Center and
Case Western Reserve University
Cleveland, Ohio
Chapter 92

Bernie Young Sunwoo, MBBS
Assistant Professor of Clinical Medicine
Department of Medicine
Division of Pulmonary, Allergy and Critical Care
Division of Sleep Medicine
Hospital of the University of Pennsylvania
Philadelphia, Pennsylvania
Chapter 100

Takuji Suzuki, MD, PhD
Assistant Professor
Division of Neonatology and Pulmonary Biology
Cincinnati Children's Hospital Medical Center
Department of Pediatrics
University of Cincinnati College of Medicine
Cincinnati, Ohio
Chapter 70

Darren B. Taichman, MD, PhD
Annals of Internal Medicine
American College of Physicians
Department of Medicine
University of Pennsylvania
Philadelphia, Pennsylvania
Chapter 72

Nichole T. Tanner, MD
Assistant Professor of Medicine
Division of Pulmonary and Critical Care Medicine
Medical University of South Carolina
Health Equity and Rural Outreach Innovation Center
Ralph H. Johnson Veterans Affairs Hospital
Charleston, South Carolina
Chapter 118

Lynn T. Tanoue, MD
Professor of Medicine
Section of Pulmonary, Critical Care and Sleep Medicine
Yale School of Medicine
New Haven, Connecticut
Chapters 65 and 109

Kelan G. Tantisira, MD, MPH
Associate Professor of Medicine
Channing Division of Network Medicine
Brigham and Women's Hospital
Harvard Medical School
Boston, Massachusetts
Chapter 9

Angelo M. Taveira-DaSilva, MD, PhD
Cardiovascular and Pulmonary Branch
National Heart, Lung, and Blood Institute
National Institutes of Health
Bethesda, Maryland
Chapters 62 and 63

Erica R. Thaler, MD
Professor
Department of Otolaryngology—Head and Neck Surgery
Perelman School of Medicine at the University of Pennsylvania
Philadelphia, Pennsylvania
Chapter 146

Victor J. Thannickal, MD
Professor of Medicine
Ben Vaughan Branscomb Chair of Medicine in Respiratory Disease
Division of Pulmonary, Allergy and Critical Care Medicine
Department of Medicine
University of Alabama at Birmingham
Birmingham, Alabama
Chapters 27 and 28

Karen J. Tietze, PharmD
Professor of Clinical Pharmacy
Philadelphia College of Pharmacy
University of the Sciences
Philadelphia, Pennsylvania
Chapter 145

Robert M. Tighe, MD
Assistant Professor of Medicine
Duke University School of Medicine
Department of Medicine
Division of Pulmonary, Allergy and Critical Care
Durham, North Carolina
Chapter 56

Gregory Tino, MD
Chief, Department of Medicine
Penn Presbyterian Medical Center
Associate Professor of Medicine
Pulmonary, Allergy and Critical Care Division
Perelman School of Medicine at the University of Pennsylvania
Philadelphia, Pennsylvania
Chapter 33

Martin J. Tobin, MD
Professor of Medicine
Division of Pulmonary and Critical Care Medicine
Edward Hines Jr. Veterans Affairs Hospital and
Loyola University of Chicago Stritch School of Medicine
Hines, Illinois
Chapter 148

Galen B. Toews, MD (Deceased)
Professor of Medicine
Division of Pulmonary and Critical Care Medicine
University of Michigan Medical Center
Ann Arbor, Michigan
Chapter 121

Olga Torre, MD
Unità Operativa di Pneumologia e Terapia Semi-Intensiva Respiratoria
Servizio di Fisiopatologia Respiratoria e Emodinamica polmonare
Ospedale San Giuseppe MultiMedica
Milano, Italy
Chapter 61

Bruce C. Trapnell, MD
F.R. Luther Professor of Medicine and Pediatrics
University of Cincinnati College of Medicine
Cincinnati Children's Hospital Medical Center
Cincinnati, Ohio
Chapter 70

John Treanor, MD
Professor of Medicine
Infectious Diseases Unit
University of Rochester Medical Center
Rochester, New York
Chapter 130

Homer L. Twigg III, MD
Associate Professor of Medicine
Chief, Division of Pulmonary, Allergy, Critical Care,
and Occupational Medicine
Indiana University Medical Center
Indianapolis, Indiana
Chapter 24

George E. Tzelepis, MD
Professor of Medicine
Department of Pathophysiology
University of Athens Medical School
Athens, Greece
Chapter 83

Omar S. Usmani, MBBS, PhD, FRCP
NIHR Career Development Fellow
Clinical Senior Lecturer & Consultant Physician in Respiratory
& Internal Medicine
National Heart and Lung Institute
Imperial College London & Royal Brompton Hospital
Airways Disease Section (c/o Asthma Lab)
Dovehouse Street, London
Chapter 46

Mark J. Utell, MD
Professor of Medicine
Director of Environmental Medicine
Division of Occupational and Environmental Medicine
University of Rochester School of Medicine and Dentistry
Rochester, New York
Chapter 91

Anil Vachani, MD, MS
Assistant Professor of Medicine
Pulmonary, Allergy, and Critical Care
Perelman School of Medicine at the University of Pennsylvania
Philadelphia, Pennsylvania
Chapter 35

Judith A. Voynow, MD
Edwin L. Kendig Jr. Professor of Pediatric Pulmonary Medicine
Children's Hospital of Richmond at VCU
Richmond, Virginia
Chapter 50

Peter D. Wagner, MD
Department of Medicine
University of California, San Diego
La Jolla, California
Chapter 14

Richard J. Wallace Jr., MD
Professor of Medicine
Chairman, Department of Microbiology
University of Texas Health Science Center
Tyler, Texas
Chapter 132

Tisha Wang, MD
Assistant Clinical Professor
Fellowship Program Director
Associate Chief, Inpatient Services and Training
UCLA Pulmonary and Critical Care Medicine
Los Angeles, California
Chapter 68

Peter A. Ward, MD
Godfrey D. Stobbe Professor
Department of Pathology
University of Michigan Medical School
Ann Arbor, Michigan
Chapter 23

Timothy E. Weaver, MS, PhD
Professor of Pediatrics
Associate Director
Division of Pulmonary Biology
Chair, Institutional Animal Care and Use Committee
Cincinnati Children's Research Foundation and Department of Pediatrics
University of Cincinnati
Cincinnati, Ohio
Chapter 5

Karl T. Weber, MD
Neuton Stern Professor of Cardiovascular Medicine
Division Chief
Division of Cardiovascular Diseases
University of Tennessee Health Science Center
Memphis, Tennessee
Chapter 34

Ewald R. Weibel, MD, DSc (Hon.)
Professor Emeritus
Institut für Anatomie, Universität Bern
Bern, Switzerland
Chapter 2

Arnold N. Weinberg, MD
Infectious Diseases Division
Massachusetts General Hospital
Boston, Massachusetts
Chapter 138

Scott T. Weiss, MD, MS
Professor of Medicine, Harvard Medical School
Associate Director, Channing Laboratory
Department of Medicine, Brigham and Women's Hospital
Director, Partners Center for Personalized Medicine
Boston, Massachusetts
Chapter 45

Matthew Wemple, MD
Clinical Instructor of Medicine
University of Washington School of Medicine
VA Puget Sound Health Care System
Seattle, Washington
Chapter 144

L. Joseph Wheat, MD
MiraVista Diagnostics
Indianapolis, Indiana
Chapter 134

Jeffrey A. Whitsett, MD
Co-Director, Perinatal Institute
Chief, Section of Neonatology, Perinatal and Pulmonary Biology
Interim Director, CCRF, Basic Science
Cincinnati Children's Hospital Medical Center
Cincinnati, Ohio
Chapter 5

Kevin C. Wilson, MD
Associate Professor of Medicine
Division of Pulmonary, Allergy, Sleep, and Critical Care Medicine
Boston University School of Medicine
Boston, Massachusetts
Chapter 21

Robert A. Wise, MD
Professor of Medicine
Pulmonary and Critical Care
Johns Hopkins University School of Medicine
Baltimore, Maryland
Chapter 42

Christine Won, MD, MS
Assistant Professor of Medicine
Section of Pulmonary, Critical Care and Sleep Medicine
Yale University School of Medicine
New Haven, Connecticut
Chapter 49

Daniel Worsley, MD, FRCPSC
Head, Division of Nuclear Medicine
Vancouver General Hospital
Clinical Assistant Professor
Department of Radiology
University of British Columbia
Vancouver, BC Canada
Chapter 32

Joanne L. Wright, MD
Professor, University of British Columbia
Pathologist, St Paul's Hospital
University Hospital
Vancouver, BC Canada
Chapter 39

Cameron D. Wright, MD
Professor of Surgery
Division of Thoracic Surgery
Department of Surgery
MGH Thoracic Surgery
Harvard Medical School
Boston, Massachusetts
Chapter 80

Alissa Jade Wright, MD
Fellow, Transplant Infectious Disease and Compromised Host Program
Division of Infectious Disease
Massachusetts General Hospital (Harvard)
Boston, Massachusetts
Chapter 137

Jason X.-J. Yuan, MD, PhD
Departments of Medicine and Physiology
University of Arizona
Tucson, Arizona
Chapter 72

Gordon L. Yung, MB, BS
Director, Advance Lung Disease Program
Clinical Professor of Medicine
University of California
San Diego, California
Chapter 73

Yong Zhou, PhD
Assistant Professor, Department of Medicine
Division of Pulmonary, Allergy and Critical Care Medicine
University of Alabama
Birmingham, Alabama
Chapter 28

PREFACE

This, the fifth edition of *Fishman's Pulmonary Diseases and Disorders*, represents a substantial departure in content and style from the previous four editions. Notably, this is the first edition in which the founding editor, Alfred P. Fishman (1918–2010), is no longer at the helm. Dr. Fishman, a legend in pulmonary science and medicine, leaves a legacy based on a long and distinguished career. Incredibly, he served as sole editor of the first two editions of the textbook, which initially appeared in print in 1980. Subsequently, he enlisted a number of coeditors, including several from the current group. Those of us who had the opportunity to work with him on the prior two editions remain grateful for his leadership, editorial style, and unrelenting commitment to excellence. His memory inspired us in preparing the current volume. We can only hope that it measures up to his exacting standards.

While many of the elements of the book have changed, one aspect remains firmly entrenched: The book represents a coupling of the body of knowledge of pulmonary and critical care medicine with the underlying basic and applied science upon which the clinical material is based. The book is designed to appeal both to clinicians and investigators who are interested in the science of medicine, including relevant respiratory biology and underlying cellular and molecular mechanisms. We hope that readers will find it authoritative, well referenced, and a suitable platform from which to launch additional inquiry.

The body of knowledge and level of detail in the fifth edition have evolved substantially since the last edition, published in 2008. In virtually all areas of pulmonary medicine, notable advancements have been made, and each is discussed in detail. For example, tremendous progress has occurred in our understanding of the genetics of respiratory disease; indeed, the era of "personalized medicine" is upon us. A full chapter has been devoted to the genetics of pulmonary disease and another to personalized pulmonary medicine—additions from the previous edition. Similarly, growth in immunology and immunosuppressive management, along with technical advances in lung transplantation, has been amply documented in the literature over the last 5 years and is presented in detail. Advances in the science and treatment of pulmonary hypertension have been noteworthy. This area, which was one of great interest to Dr. Fishman, is discussed in a comprehensive chapter on the subject. In addition, the rapid evolution of cardiovascular and pulmonary imaging techniques has been dramatic, and multiple examples of such advanced imaging populate many of the chapters. Utilization of the technology and its attendant costs constitute the basis for considerable debate and ongoing studies regarding applicability in screening patients for underlying pulmonary disease (e.g., lung cancer screening using low-dose CT scanning in at-risk patients). Finally, as another example of noteworthy progress, developments in interventional bronchoscopic techniques continue to evolve and have become increasingly sophisticated over the last 5 years. They are discussed in two related chapters on diagnostic and interventional bronchoscopy.

Within the realm of critical care medicine, significant advances have been reported in the early diagnosis and management of sepsis, multiple organ dysfunction syndrome (MODS), acute respiratory distress syndrome (ARDS), and the newly defined entity of "chronic critical illness." These advances have translated into improved survival of patients with disorders that, at one time, were largely fatal. Patient survival, particularly in the setting of chronic and, sometimes, debilitating, organ dysfunction has generated debate on the appropriateness of application of the technology and affordability of the healthcare thereby engendered. Such considerations inform a discussion of the organization of intensive care units and long-term acute care facilities, topics which have been included in this edition.

Not all of the news has been good. For example, challenges in the medical management of advanced interstitial lung disease, particularly idiopathic pulmonary fibrosis, have remained all too evident. Therapy has been disappointing. Notably, however, several recently completed clinical trials have improved prospects for management.

Those responsible for generating the content of the fifth edition include 278 contributors. They are drawn from among the world's experts in the areas about which they have written. One hundred fifty-nine contributors are new from the last edition, including many from outside the United States, reflecting the vast array of expertise available globally in the areas of pulmonary science and medicine.

Organization and content are not the only metrics that have changed with the fifth edition. Footnoted references are now incorporated extensively. Supplemental content and illustrations are made available by accessing QR codes embedded on the printed pages. Production constraints created by page limitations have been curtailed significantly. Notably, the fifth edition is being made available in an electronic version accessed via the World Wide Web.

An additional technological advance over the prior edition is incorporation of a number of videos designed to complement and, at times, accentuate information contained within the text. Not surprisingly, most of the videos relate to procedures or imaging. They are designed to reflect common or unique findings drawn from "real life" clinical experiences. They, too, are accessible using a QR code reader.

With all of the technological advances in play, at the end of the day, the compilation and synthesis of the information contained within this textbook are a reflection of the commitment, untiring effort, and professionalism of many contributing authors. The editors are enormously grateful for their willingness to "dig deep" and generate authoritative discussions of the complex and expanding fields of pulmonary and critical care medicine.

These same, appreciative editors have, themselves, contributed enormous boluses of time in editing and authoring the chapters that comprise the book. Personally, I found the willingness of my colleagues to step up and orchestrate its preparation extraordinarily gratifying.

Finally, on behalf of all of the editors, I wish to express our thanks for the commitment of key individuals in preparing the fifth edition, including Brian Belval, Executive Editor at McGraw-Hill; Peter Boyle, Sr Project Development Editor; Priscilla Beer, Sr Media Project Manager; and Sarah M. Granlund, Project Manager. Their ability to keep the train on the track was nothing short of exceptional.

Michael A. Grippi, MD

Fishman's Pulmonary Diseases and Disorders

Volume 1

PART 1
Perspectives

CHAPTER 1

Milestones in the History of Pulmonary Medicine*

Michael A. Grippi

The current level of clinical, scientific, and technologic sophistication of medicine has evolved over more than 2000 years. From the inception of medicine, pulmonary medicine has been an integral part of its growth and development. About 300 years ago, progress toward scientific medicine accelerated markedly, and it has continued to gain speed ever since. In the 17th century, research and experimentation began to tilt clinical medicine toward the exact sciences; by the 18th century, pathology had become an integral part of clinical medicine, and clinical–pathologic correlations succeeded empiricism, dogmatism, and metaphysics. The age of the great clinicians dawned in Europe early in the 19th century, when autopsies became legally permissible and socially acceptable, and when physicians who cared for patients actually performed the autopsies.

The road to our current understanding and practice of pulmonary medicine and science has been somewhat convoluted.[1-3] Progress has been punctuated by delays, detours, and reversals. However, it is possible to retrace the scientific trail by examining iconic figures and addressing milestones in drawing the map (Table 1-1). This chapter uses these milestones to trace the course of scientific pulmonary medicine over the last two millennia. By necessity, what follows constitutes a limited overview of *selected* aspects of the history of the field, including alveolar–capillary gas exchange, lung volumes, mechanics of breathing, control of breathing, ventilation–perfusion relationships, and scientific advancements impacting clinical medicine, including chest imaging, lung transplantation, bronchoscopic techniques, and advances in critical care. Indeed, much of the content of the book addresses the many advances in respiratory disorders achieved over the last 50 years.

ALVEOLAR–CAPILLARY GAS EXCHANGE

In reflecting on the history of the science and thinkers largely responsible for our current understanding of the central role of the lungs in gas exchange, the following are considered: the ancient Greeks, William Harvey and the Oxford physiologists, the "phlogiston theory," theories of blood gas diffusion and "secretion" of oxygen, and the physical chemistry of blood gas transport.

■ ANCIENT GREEK MEDICINE

The beginnings of scientific medicine can be traced to ancient Greece in the sixth century BC. At that time, natural philosophers speculated that air, or some essential ingredient in air, was inspired to generate a "vital essence" for distribution throughout the body.

Hippocrates, the "father of medicine," is as much a symbol of the Greek physician of the fifth and fourth centuries BC as the name of a real figure (Fig. 1-1). As an individual, he exemplified the caring physician who kept accurate records, made cautious inferences, and relied more on nature, rest, and diet than on drugs for treatment. His name has been immortalized by affixing it to three major components of Greek medicine, even though none appears to be the work of a single individual.

The first is the *Hippocratic corpus*, a collection of about 70 works that includes case reports, textbooks, lectures, and notebooks. The collection contains a description of Cheyne–Stokes breathing and the use of *Hippocratic succussion* for the diagnosis of fluid and air in the pleural cavity. The second is a collection of aphorisms—a compilation of brief generalizations related to medicine. The third, which is more likely attributable to Pythagoras (c. 530 BC) than Hippocrates (who lived about a century later), is the *Hippocratic oath*, which not only represents the spirit of the physician of ancient Greece, but which has endured to modern times as a reflection of the physician's code of ethics.

Another Greek, Aristotle, not only had an enduring influence on the intellect of humankind in his own time, but also for two millennia, thereafter. Not until the 17th century were Aristotle's doctrine of the four elements (earth, air, fire, and water) and that of Hippocrates (blood, phlegm, yellow bile, and black bile) laid to rest, thereby clearing the way for modern scientific medicine.

Soon after Aristotle, in about 300 BC, an extraordinary medical school was founded at Alexandria in Egypt. One of the first teachers at the school, Erasistratus, postulated that the "pneuma," or spirit essential for life, is generated from interplay between air and blood.

About four centuries after Erasistratus, Galen (Fig. 1-2) drew upon the medical, philosophic, and anatomic knowledge of his day to fashion a remarkable physiologic schema.[3,4] His construct was largely teleologic. Unfortunately, it was so convincing that even though it was ultimately proved to be fanciful, it sufficed to retard scientific progress for a millennium and a half. Galen was a talented individual who was well educated, well read, and well positioned in society to popularize his beliefs. Moreover, his concepts fit well into the tenets of Christianity, which was then in its ascendency; to controvert his authority was tantamount to blasphemy. Among his long-lasting, albeit erroneous, postulates, were the following: invisible pores in the ventricular septum that enabled the bulk of the blood to flow from the right ventricle to the left ventricle, thereby bypassing the lungs; a diminutive pulmonary circulation that served only to nourish the lungs; and two-way traffic in the pulmonary veins that enabled inspired air and "effluent waste vapors" to go their respective ways (Fig. 1-3).

Voices raised in protest to Galen's theories were without lasting effect. In the 13th century, Ibn al-Nafis, writing in his *Canon of Avicenna*, objected that blood does not traverse the ventricular septum from right to left, as Galen had proposed. However, this insight attracted little attention. Three hundred years later, Vesalius voiced similar misgivings. In the 16th century, Michael Servetus, a polymath trained in theology, geography, and anatomy, pictured the pulmonary circulation as the vehicle by which the "inhaled spirit" could be distributed throughout the body. In his theologic treatise, *Christianismi Restitutio*, he pointed out that blood could not traverse the septum between the right and left ventricles, and that the lumen of the pulmonary artery was too large for a nutrient vessel. He became a hunted heretic, wanted for execution by both the Catholic Church and Calvin. He was warned by Calvin to stay out of Geneva. Both Servetus and Calvin then behaved predictably: Servetus showed up at a church where Calvin was preaching and Calvin had him captured and burned at the stake. In 1559, Realdus Columbus of Cremona, a pupil of Vesalius, rediscovered the pulmonary circulation, as did Andreas Caesalpinus in 1571. Despite these challenging observations, Galen's schema was to last for more than another half century—until the physiologic experiments of William Harvey.

■ WILLIAM HARVEY AND THE OXFORD PHYSIOLOGISTS

William Harvey (Fig. 1-4) was led to the discovery of the circulation of the blood[5] by anatomic observations on the valves in systemic

*This chapter constitutes an updated revision of the original chapter written by Alfred P. Fishman.

TABLE 1-1 Landmark Figures in the Evolution of Modern Pulmonary Medicine

Alveolar–Capillary Gas Exchange	Mechanics of Breathing
Ancient Greek Medicine	John Hutchinson (1811–1861)
Hippocrates of CoS (c. 460–359 BC)	Karl Ludwig (1816–1895)
Aristotle (384–322 BC)	Franciscus Cornelius Donders (1818–1889)
Erasistratus of Chios (c. 300–250 BC)	Fritz Rohrer (1888–1926)
Galen of Pergamon (AD 129–99)	Wallace Osgood Fenn (1893–1971)
Ibn al-Nafis (c. 1210–1288)	**Control of Breathing**
Leonardo da Vinci (1452–1519)	*The Central Respiratory Centers*
Miguel Servetus (1511–1553)	Thomas Lumsden (1874–1953)
Andreas Vesalius of Brussels (1514–1564)	Hans Winterstein (1878–1963)
Realdus Columbus of Cremona (1516–1559)	Merkel Henry Jacobs (1884–1970)
Andreas Caesalpinus of Pisa (1519–1603)	*The Peripheral Chemoreceptors*
William Harvey and the Oxford Physiologists	Ewald Hering (1834–1918)
Galileo Galilei (1564–1642)	Joseph Breuer (1842–1925)
William Harvey (1578–1657)	Cornelius Heymans (1892–1968)
Giovanni Alfonso Borelli (1608–1679)	**Scientific Basis of Clinical Medicine**
Marcello Malpighi (1628–1694)	*Pathologic Anatomy*
Robert Boyle (1627–1691)	Gioranni Battista Morgagni (1682–1771)
Richard Lower (1631–1691)	Leopold Auenbrugger (1727–1809)
Robert Hooke (1635–1703)	Jean Nicolas Corvisart (1755–1821)
John Mayow (1640–1679)	René Théophile Hyacinthe Laënnec (1781–1826)
Phlogiston: The Rise and Fall	*Microbiology*
Georg Ernst Stahl (1660–1734)	Robert Koch (1843–1910)
John Black (1728–1799)	*Physiology of the Pulmonary Circulation*
Joseph Priestley (1733–1804)	Claude Bernard (1813–1878)
Carl Wilhelm Scheele (1742–1782)	Auguste Chauveau (1827–1917)
Respiration and Metabolism	Étienne Jules Marey (1830–1904)
Antoine Laurent Lavoisier (1743–1794)	Dickinson W. Richards (1895–1973)
John Dalton (1766–1844)	André Frederic Cournand (1895–1988)
Julius Robert von Mayer (1814–1878)	Werner Forssmann (1904–1979)
Carl von Voit (1831–1908)	*Thoracic Imaging*
Nathan Zuntz (1847–1920)	Wilhelm Conrad Roentgen (1845–1923)
The Blood Gases	Godfrey N. Hounsfield (1919–2004)
Joseph Black (1728–1799)	*Bronchoscopy*
John Dalton (1766–1844)	Gustav Killian (1860–1921)
Heinrich Gustav Magnus (1802–1870)	Chevalier Jackson (1865–1958)
Felix Hoppe-Seyler (1825–1895)	Shigeto Ikeda (1925–2001)
Paul Bert (1833–1886)	*Lung Transplantation*
Christian Bohr (1855–1911)	Vladimir P. Demikhov (1916–1998)
John Scott Haldane (1860–1936)	James D. Hardy (1918–2003)
August Krogh (1874–1949)	Joel D. Cooper
Diffusion or Secretion of Oxygen	
Joseph Barcroft (1872–1947)	
Marie Krogh (1874–1943)	
The Physical–Chemical Synthesis	
Lawrence J. Henderson (1878–1942)	

veins made by his mentor, Fabricus ab Aquapedente. Harvey's small book, *De Motu Cordis*, published in 1628, not only corrected a self-perpetuating error in Galenical teaching, but also marked the birth of modern physiology. The time, however, was not yet ripe to relate the function of the heart to the physiology of breathing. To his dying day, Harvey clung to the idea that the main function of breathing is to cool the heart. Moreover, since he made no use of the microscope, he could not picture how the pulmonary arteries made connections with the pulmonary veins. Galileo invented the compound microscope in 1610. In 1661, using the compound microscope, Marcello Malpighi reported that alveoli were covered by capillaries and that blood and air were kept separate by the continuous alveolar–capillary barrier.

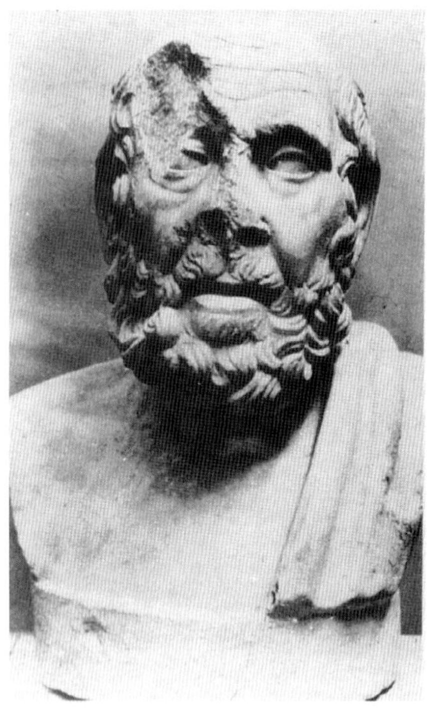
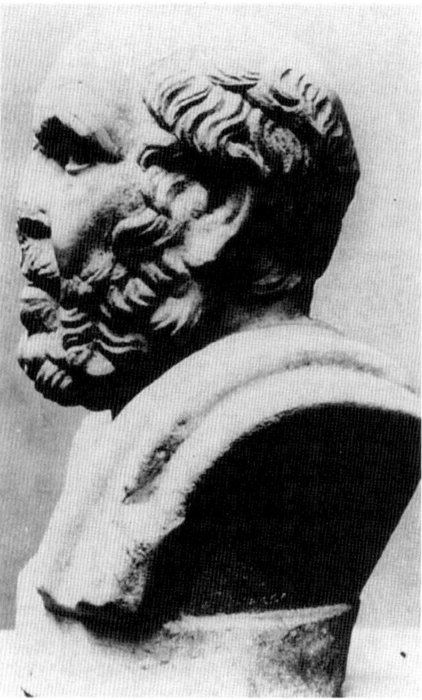

Figure 1-1 The Hippocrates of Ostia. This damaged bust is believed to represent Hippocrates as perceived in antiquity. It was found in a family tomb in excavations near Ostia. *(Used with permission of Dr. Dickinson W. Richards.)*

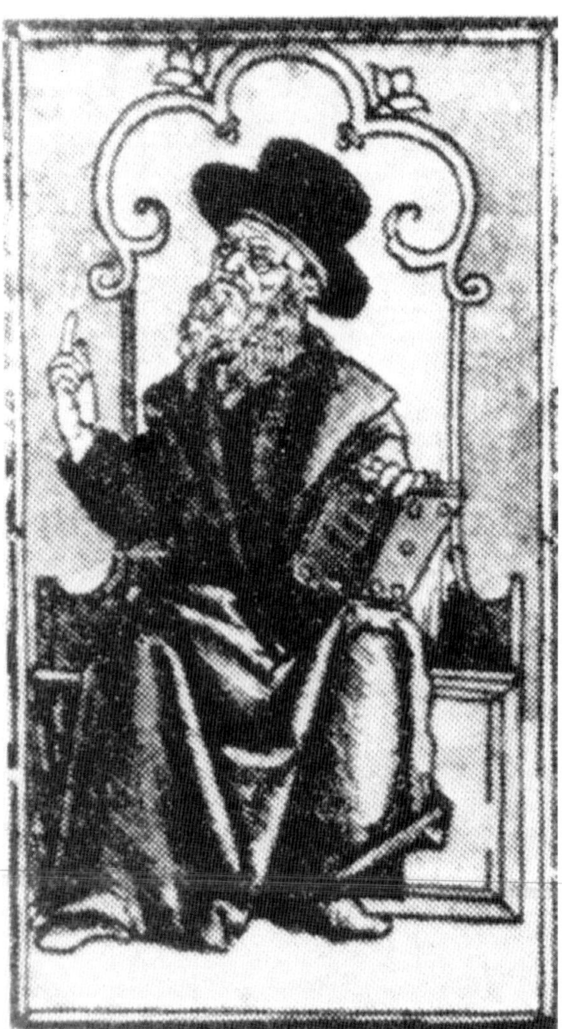

Figure 1-2 Galen of Pergamon as depicted in medieval times. No authentic reproduction exists of Galen in ancient times. *(Used with permission of Galen's Therapeutica, published in Venice in 1500.)*

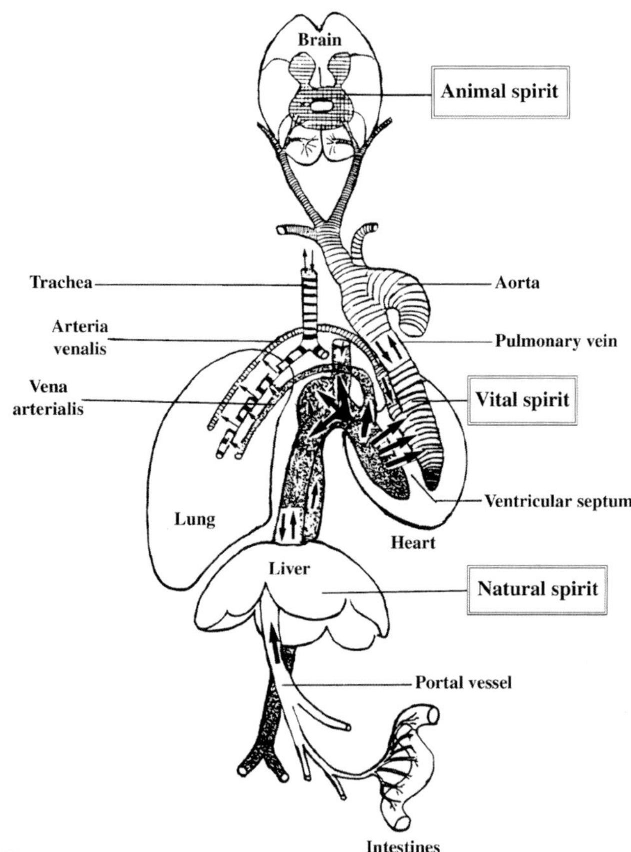

Figure 1-3 Galen's scheme of the circulation. The diagram shows the source and distribution of the three types of spirits. The validity of this scheme depended on invisible pores in the ventricular septum, two-way traffic in the pulmonary vein, and selective permeability of the mitral valve for sooty wastes but not for spirit-containing blood. Vena arterialis, pulmonary vein; arteria venalis, pulmonary artery. *(Modified with permission from Singer C. A Short History of Scientific Ideas to 1900. London: Oxford University Press; 1959.)*

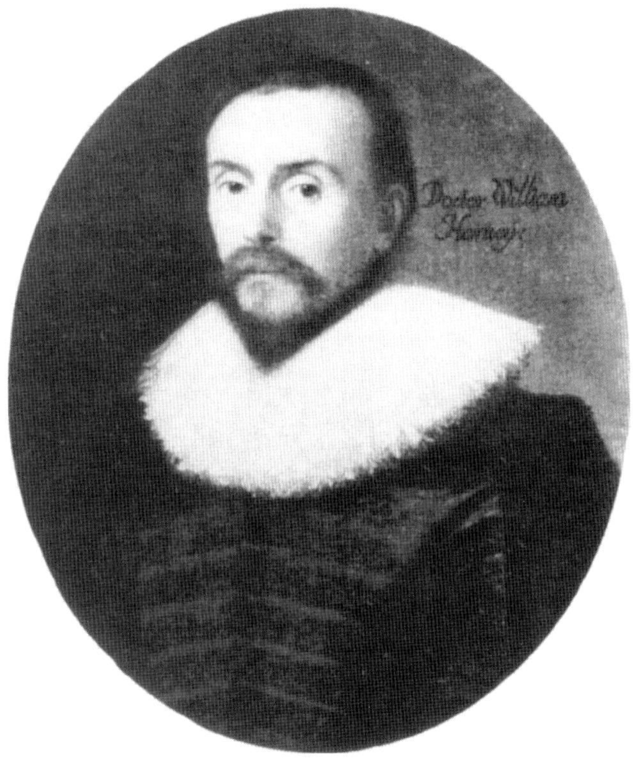

Figure 1-4 William Harvey (1578–1657). This portrait of William Harvey is part of a family group in which William Harvey and his five brothers are gathered around their father, William Harvey.

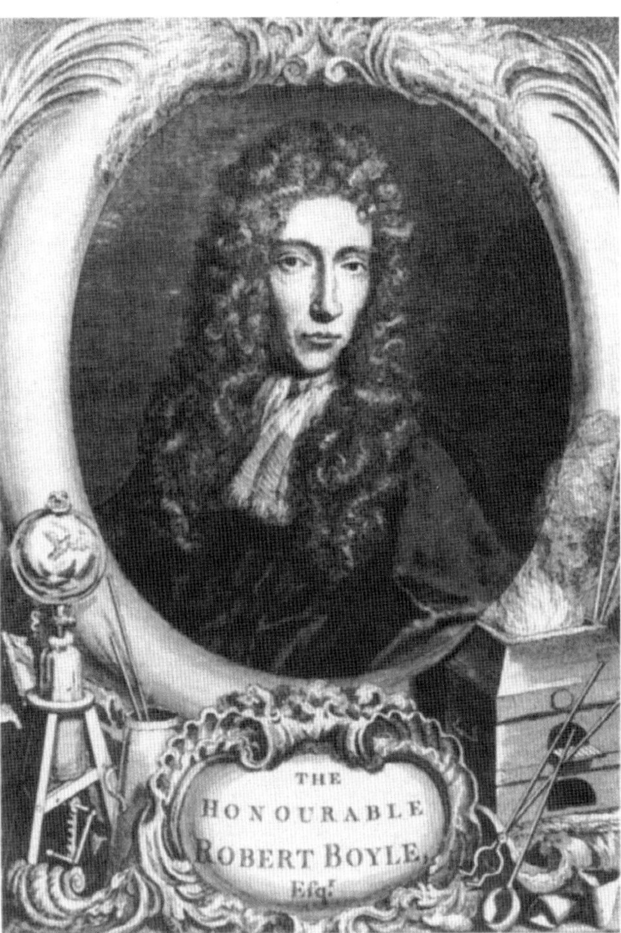

Figure 1-5 Robert Boyle (1627–1691). This engraving, from an original painting by Johann Kerseboom, hangs in the Royal Society, London. Boyle's invention of a pneumatic air pump and his publications concerning "the spring of air and its effect" stimulated considerable research on the physical properties of air and its role in respiration and combustion. He strongly influenced Hooke, Lower, and Mayow at Oxford.

Harvey's description in 1628 of the circulation of the blood had three major consequences for pulmonary medicine: (1) it oriented pulmonary medicine toward the basic sciences and away from philosophy and empiricism; (2) it demolished the Galenic concept of the movement of the blood; and (3) it set the stage for an upcoming generation of physiologists at Oxford University to explore breathing in chemical and physical terms.

The physiologists working at Oxford in the 1660s were greatly impressed by Harvey's disciplined approach to scientific inquiry. Many were medical practitioners who conducted research as a sideline. Four, in particular, began the systematic study of air and its constituents, thereby laying the foundations for contemporary respiratory physiology and medicine: Robert Boyle (Fig. 1-5), Robert Hooke, Richard Lower, and John Mayow.

In 1660, Robert Boyle proved by means of his air pump that air is necessary for life. In 1667, Robert Hooke showed that insufflation of the lungs with air while breathing movements were arrested could keep an open-chest animal alive, that is, that movement of the lungs was not essential for life. Richard Lower, the first to practice blood transfusion, took advantage of Hooke's continuously inflated lung preparation in the dog to observe that dark venous blood becomes bright red as it traverses lungs insufflated with air. In 1674, Mayow interpreted the change in the color of blood from venous to arterial as due to the uptake of "nitroaerial particles" (later to be called "oxygen") from the air.

PHLOGISTON: THE RISE AND FALL

Unfortunately, the discoveries and insights of the Oxford physiologists went largely unnoticed during the century that followed, overshadowed by the "phlogiston theory" of combustion. The theory, advanced by Stahl, postulated that all combustible materials were composed of two ingredients: phlogiston, a principle that transformed into fire when heated, and an ash that was left behind after the fiery phlogiston escaped. The phlogiston theory was sufficiently malleable to accommodate almost every new discovery that could have overthrown it, including the rediscovery of carbon dioxide in 1754 by John Black, and the independent discoveries of oxygen by Priestley and Scheele. Although the respiratory gases had been discovered by the end of the 18th century and many of their properties characterized, the discoveries were misapplied to support, rather than destroy, the phlogiston theory. The phlogiston theory was finally demolished by the experiments of Lavoisier.

RESPIRATION AND METABOLISM

From the time of Hippocrates until early in the 20th century, debate had continued about the site of heat production in the body. In 1777, Lavoisier suggested that air was composed of one respirable gas (which he later named "oxygine") and another (nitrogen) that remained unchanged in the course of respiration. Between 1782 and 1784, Lavoisier and Laplace concluded, on the basis of calorimetric experiments on guinea pigs, that "respiration is therefore a combustion, admittedly very slow, but otherwise exactly similar to that of charcoal" (Fig. 1-6). The similarity between respiration and combustion had previously been recognized by the Oxford physiologists, especially Mayow.[6] By 1783, Lavoisier was accumulating evidence against the phlogiston theory and began to replace it with an entirely new system of chemistry.

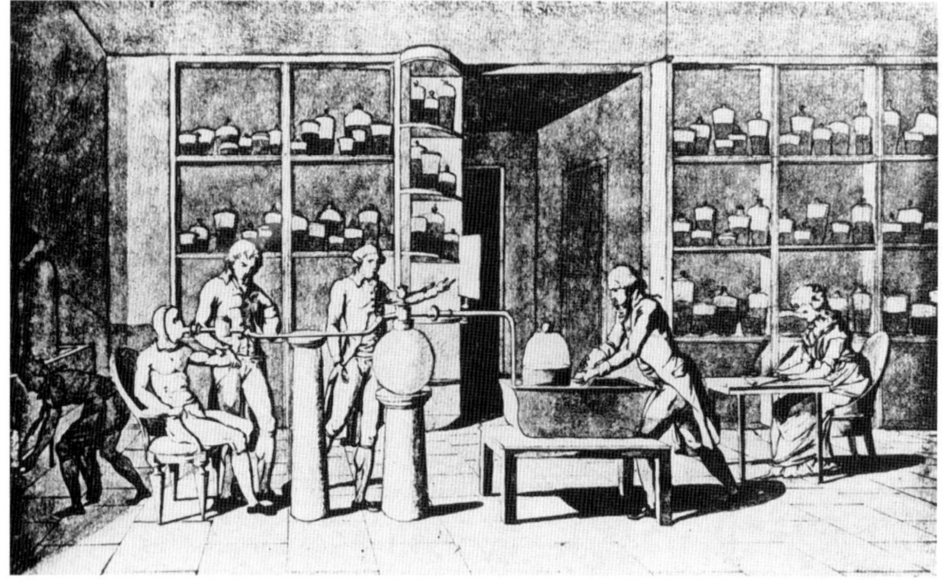

Figure 1-6 Scene from the laboratory of Antoine Laurent Lavoisier (1743–1794). His wife is acting as his assistant, and Sequin is the subject. Studies such as this led to the conclusion that respiration and circulation are similar processes.

As noted previously, the ancients pictured the heart as the heat generator. Lavoisier favored the lungs. Others held that combustion occurred in the blood. Although Spallanzani had shown in the 18th century that isolated tissues take up oxygen and evolve carbon dioxide, the idea that combustion occurred in the tissues was slow to gain acceptance. However, the hypothesis gained strength through the work of Pflüger in 1878. He measured oxygen consumption and carbon dioxide production in dogs and calculated respiratory quotients. His research substantiated a concept that had been enunciated, but not named, by Lavoisier.[7]

Once the idea that oxidation occurred in the tissues had become generally accepted, investigators delved into the processes involved in utilization of foodstuffs by the tissues, energetics, growth, and repair. Carl von Voit and Max von Pettenkofer, using a respiration chamber, drew upon chemical balances and respiratory quotients in humans to distinguish the nature of the foodstuffs being burned and to show that the amounts of fat, protein, and carbohydrate burned varied with the mechanical work done by the subject. Between 1842 and 1845, Julius Robert von Mayer formulated the law of conservation of energy. Subsequently, Max Rubner showed that the law applied to the living body, and Herman von Helmholtz showed that its relevance to metabolism could be demonstrated experimentally. Application of these principles at the bedside was greatly facilitated by the development of a portable metabolic apparatus by Nathan Zuntz. Pioneering bedside studies of metabolic states were conducted by a succession of distinguished investigators, including Magnus-Levy, Graham Lusk, F. G. Benedict, and Eugene F. DuBois.

THE BLOOD GASES

The Oxford physiologists set the stage for the discovery of the blood gases. Using his vacuum pump, Robert Boyle extracted "air" from blood. John Mayow came close to discovering oxygen by showing that only part of air was necessary for life, and that this part, his "nitroaerial spirits," was removed both by respiration and fire (combustion). One of his famous experiments entailed enclosing a mouse and a lighted lamp in an airtight container; the lamp went out first and then the mouse died. However, Mayow did not realize that the "nitroaerial spirits" could be isolated as a gas.[6]

One hundred years after Mayow, Joseph Priestley (Fig. 1-7) exposed a mouse to the gas released from heated mercuric oxide and found that the gas supported life better than air did; he also noticed that a flame burned more vigorously in this gas than in air. Priestley was not alone in his preoccupation with flame. In 1773, about a year before Priestley had obtained oxygen by heating mercuric oxide, Scheele discovered oxygen independently because of his interest in fire, and he designated oxygen as "fire air."

In 1662, Van Helmont, a Capuchin friar and talented chemist, as well as a mystic with a drive to quantify, discovered carbon dioxide, coined the word *gas*, and called carbon dioxide "wild gas" ("gas sylvestre"). In 1755, Joseph Black rediscovered carbon dioxide. He showed that calcium carbonate (limestone) and magnesium carbonate (magnesia alba) lost weight on heating, releasing "fixed air" (CO_2) in the process. This fixed air extinguished both flame and life. Lavoisier knew of the observations of Black and of Priestley and Scheele. He decided in 1778 that the gas obtained from heating

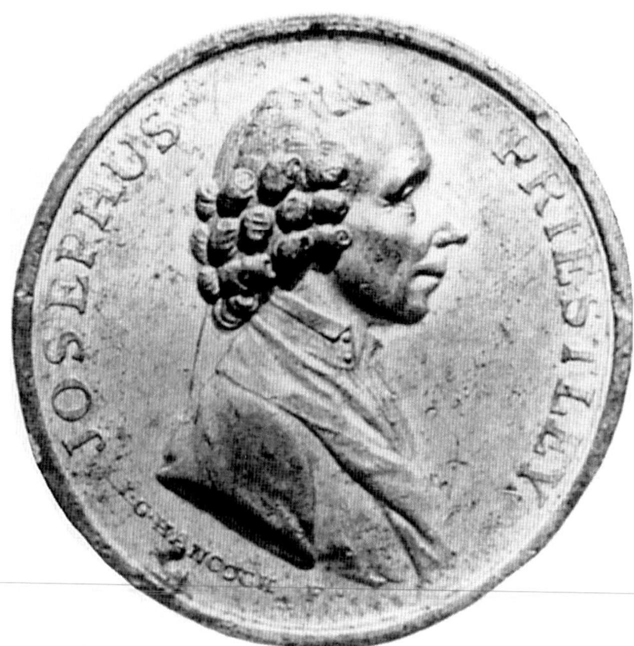

Figure 1-7 Joseph Priestley (1733–1804), the discoverer of oxygen. This figure shows a silver medal struck in his honor in 1783. A Presbyterian minister, he was radical in his religious and political beliefs, inventive in science, and conservative in the interpretation of his findings. *(Reproduced with permission from Fishman AP, Richards DW. Circulation of the Blood: Men and Ideas. New York: Oxford University Press; 1964.)*

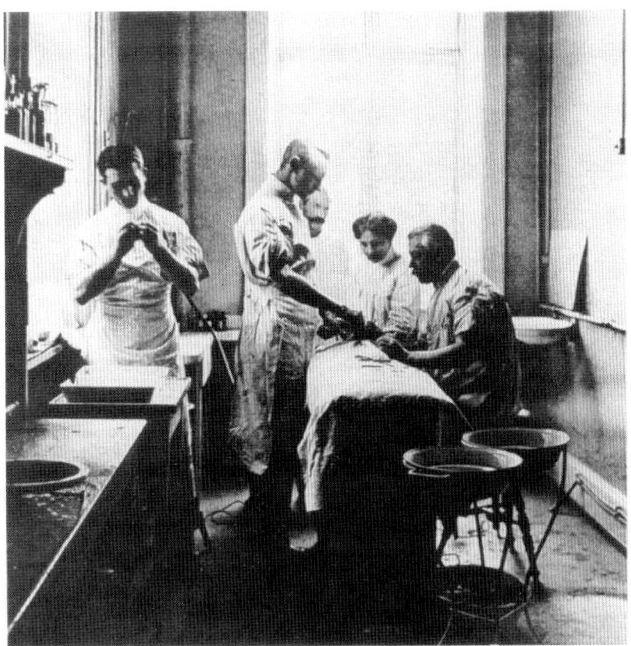

Figure 1-8 Christian Bohr (1855–1911). At work in his laboratory, Bohr *(far right)* and his associates systematically explored the interplay between the respiratory gases and hemoglobin that led to the discovery of the "Bohr effect." *(Reproduced with permission from Fishman AP, Richards DW. Circulation of the Blood: Men and Ideas. New York: Oxford University Press; 1964.)*

mercuric oxide was not "fixed air" or "common air," but "highly respirable air" (oxygen).

The story of hemoglobin, the essential element in the transport of the respiratory gases by the blood, begins with Hoppe-Seyler, who, between 1866 and 1871, crystallized hemoglobin, explored its chemical properties, and assigned it a proper role in the transport of oxygen by the blood. At the turn of the 19th century, Dalton reported his experiments with the respiratory gases, which led to the development of his atomic theory. In 1872, taking advantage of Dalton's law, Paul Bert published the first oxygen dissociation curve, that is, oxygen content at different barometric pressures; he pictured the curve as hyperbolic. Christian Bohr (Fig. 1-8) subsequently identified its s-shaped contour, and in 1904, together with Hasselbach and August Krogh, showed that increasing carbon dioxide tension in blood drives out oxygen, that is, the "Bohr effect." Shortly thereafter, the influence of various factors, for example, temperature and electrolytes, on the affinity of oxygen for hemoglobin (and, consequently, on the position of the oxygen dissociation curve) was explored in detail by Barcroft and associates. In 1914, Christiansen, Douglas, and Haldane reported that an increase in the oxygen tension of the blood drives out carbon dioxide, that is, the "Haldane effect." In 1967, a new dimension was added to the understanding of the position and configuration of the oxygen dissociation curve by the demonstration that diphosphoglycerate, a chemical constituent of red cells, regulates the release of oxygen from oxyhemoglobin.

■ DIFFUSION OR SECRETION OF OXYGEN

Bohr is a central figure as an investigator and mentor in respiratory physiology.[8] In 1904, he raised a troublesome issue that was not easily resolved, primarily because of limitations in methodology at the time. He postulated that even though diffusion could account for oxygen uptake at rest, it could not suffice during strenuous exercise, particularly at altitude. He held that oxygen *secretion* had to be involved.[9] He held to this misconception during his lifetime, a conviction supported by two major lines of evidence. The first was indirect: Oxygen secretion by the swim bladder of fish showed by extrapolation that active transport of oxygen in the lungs was possible. The second was based on observations made during Bohr's expedition to Pike's Peak in 1912, during which it was erroneously demonstrated that with exercise at altitude, arterial oxygen tension exceeded alveolar oxygen tension.

However, even before the report from high altitude, Bohr's former assistant, August Krogh, and his wife, Marie Krogh (Fig. 1-9) had marshaled new evidence to show that "the absorption of oxygen and the elimination of carbon dioxide in the lungs takes place by diffusion and diffusion alone." The final blow to the secretion theory was delivered by Marie Krogh.[10] Based on the single-breath carbon monoxide method for determining diffusing capacity that she and her husband had developed in 1910,[11] she was able to account for oxygen uptake in the lungs by diffusion alone, even during strenuous exercise under conditions of low oxygen tension. Refinements in the carbon monoxide method by Roughton and others extended

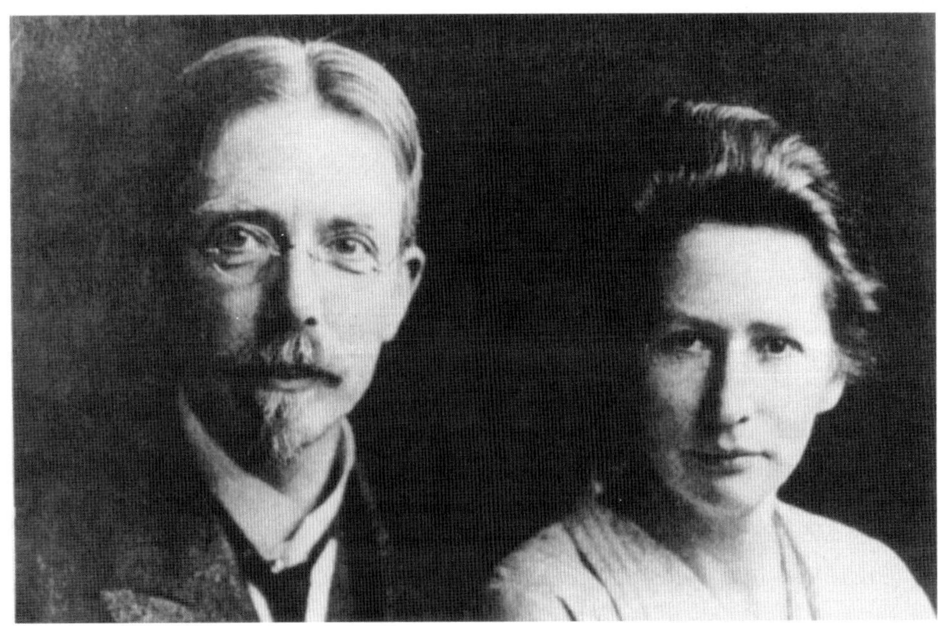

Figure 1-9 August and Marie Krogh in 1922, at the time of their first visit to the United States so that August Krogh could deliver the Silliman Lecture at Yale. They demonstrated that diffusion, without secretion, could account for the transfer of O_2 and CO_2 across the alveolar–capillary membranes of the lungs. *(Used with permission of their daughter, Dr. Bodil Schmidt-Nielsen.)*

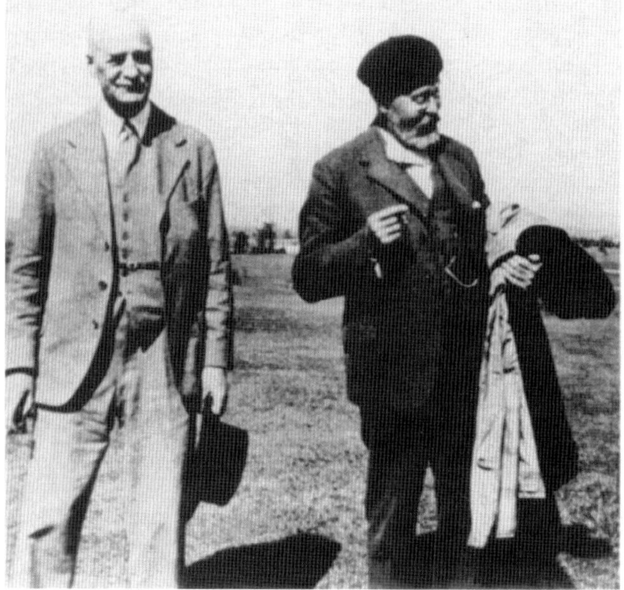

Figure 1-10 Two founders of contemporary respiratory physiology in 1936. Sir Joseph Barcroft (1872–1947) *(left)* proved, in experiments on himself, that diffusion was the mechanism for gas exchange in the lungs and pioneered current understanding of the respiratory functions of the blood. Lawrence J. Henderson (1878–1942) *(right)* provided a mathematical analysis of blood as a physiochemical system and stimulated research on the complex interplay involved in respiratory gas exchange during exercise. *(From Fishman AP, Richards DW. Circulation of the Blood: Men and Ideas. New York, NY: Oxford University Press; 1964, with permission.)*

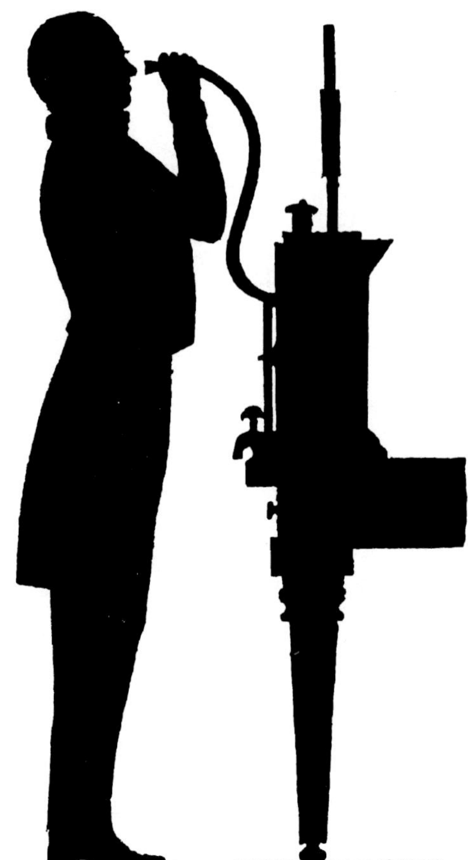

Figure 1-11 John Hutchinson's illustration of a subject about to undergo measurements of lung volumes. *(Reproduced with permission from Hutchinson J: Med Chir Soc (Lond) trans. 1846;29:137.)*

its clinical applicability and provided further evidence against the secretion theory.[12] Despite these observations, Haldane would not let go. Throughout his life, despite mounting evidence to the contrary, he adhered to the idea that oxygen was secreted by the alveolar membrane.

The issue was finally settled by Joseph Barcroft (Fig. 1-10). Using a chamber to reproduce the circumstances of hypoxia and strenuous exercise assessed during the Pike's Peak expedition, he found that under all conditions, the oxygen saturation of arterial blood was less than that of arterial blood exposed to a sample of alveolar gas obtained at the same time. He subsequently confirmed these results by experiments done at high altitude at Cerro de Pasco (1921–1922).

THE PHYSICAL–CHEMICAL SYNTHESIS

Lawrence J. Henderson undertook the herculean task of depicting the reactions of oxygen and carbon dioxide in blood, not as cause and effect, but as interplay among physiochemical variables and functions (Fig. 1-10). His theoretical considerations and practical applications in the Fatigue Laboratory at Harvard University were greatly abetted by close collaboration with Van Slyke, Wu, and McLean at the Rockefeller Institute in New York, who were exploring the exchanges of blood constituents between red cells and plasma. In 1828, Henderson presented his synthesis in the form of a d'Ocagne nomogram that displayed changes in the various elements that entered into the exchange of the respiratory gases between alveolar gas and blood: plasma; the red cell; hemoglobin; and chloride, bicarbonate, and hydrogen ions. He presented nomograms not only for the normal subject at rest and during exercises, but also for individuals with anemia, nephritis, diabetic coma, and other major clinical entities. Henderson dealt with steady-state observations. Roughton and associates enlarged the physiochemical horizons further by discovering carbonic anhydrase in the red cell and addressing transient phenomena related to transport of respiratory gases and carbon monoxide in blood.

LUNG VOLUMES

Although Humphrey Davy had determined his own lung volume using hydrogen as the test gas in 1800,[13] it was not until the 1840s that John Hutchinson laid the groundwork for modern pulmonary function testing. He devised a spirometer and used it to determine the subdivisions of the lung in a large number of healthy subjects, relating the measurements to height and age (Fig. 1-11). The many refinements since then are too numerous for mention in this chapter. A big step forward was the invention of the body plethysmograph many years later, which made possible the determination of the thoracic gas volume and airway resistance.

MECHANICS OF BREATHING

The ancients wondered how air moved into and out of the lungs; as far back as the time of Erasistratus, the diaphragm was recognized as involved in breathing. Galen was aware that the lungs fill the chest cavity and are moved by the actions of the thorax, and that the large airways enlarge and lengthen during inspiration. He marveled at the long course of the nerves to the diaphragm and the innervation of the intercostal muscles. After Galen, interest in the mechanics of breathing waned except for sporadic observations and experiments by anatomists, notably Leonardo da Vinci and Andreas Vesalius. Interest in respiratory mechanics resumed in the 16th century, largely as a result of progress in physics and mathematics, as exemplified in the works of Borelli and Galileo.

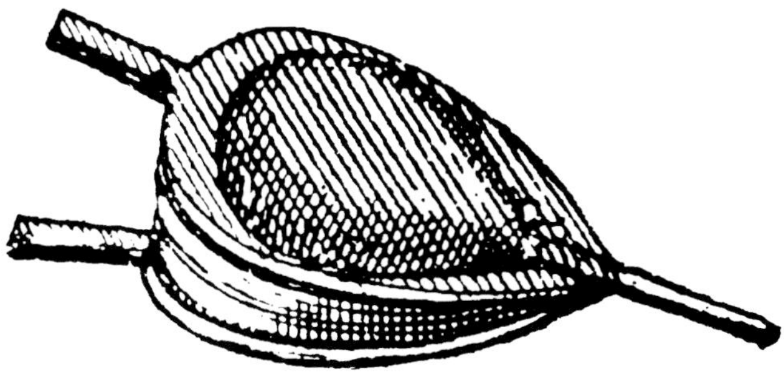

Figure 1-12 Mayow's model of the chest and lungs. The bellows encloses a bladder, the neck of which opens to the outside. A glass window on the upper side makes it possible to observe the bladder during inflation and deflation. *(Reproduced with permission from Mayow J: Medico-Physical Works, Crum A, Brown, Dobbin L (trans). Edinburgh, Alembic Club, Reprints, no 17, 1957. (Translated from Tractatus quinque medico-physics, 1674))*

THE RESPIRATORY MUSCLES

Mayow, one of the Oxford physiologists, drew heavily on the work of colleagues, including Boyle and Hooke, to develop considerable insight into the mechanics of breathing. He also built the first model on record of the chest as a bellows, which contained a bladder within it (Fig. 1-12). He understood that air moved into the lungs as the chest expanded because of the pressure and elasticity of ambient air; he also appreciated that the chest expands because of the action of the intercostal muscles (internal and external), that the diaphragm is the primary muscle of inspiration, and that normal expiration is passive. After Mayow, little research was done on the role of the respiratory muscles in breathing until the mid-19th century, when Donders distinguished between the respective roles played by the inspiratory muscles and elastic forces.

ELASTIC PROPERTIES OF LUNGS AND CHEST

Until the 20th century, observations on the elastic properties of the lungs and chest cage in humans were fragmentary. Access to the pleural space was the major limiting factor. With few exceptions - notably Neergaard and Wirz, who used pleural pressures to determine elastic recoil in normal human subjects, and Christie, who recorded pleural pressures to demonstrate loss of pulmonary elasticity in emphysematous patients - measurements in humans were largely confined either to therapeutic interventions, for example, induction of a pneumothorax or aspiration of pleural fluid, or experiments done at autopsy. The number of observations on the mechanical properties of the lungs increased dramatically when it was shown by Buytendijk, in 1949, and again by Dornhurst and Leathart, in 1952, that esophageal pressures provided an accurate measure of pleural pressures.

The role of alveolar surface tension in determining the elastic forces in the lungs began to be widely appreciated in the late 1950s, although the stage had been set long before. In 1812, Laplace had published the law of surface tension. The implications of this law for the lungs was appreciated initially in 1929 when Neergaard compared pressure–volume curves of lungs filled with air with those filled with fluid. He concluded that unopposed surface tensions would favor alveolar collapse. Then, between 1954 and 1960, a remarkable outpouring of papers from different laboratories showed that a unique surfactant lined the alveoli, and this material was absent in premature infants with hyaline membrane disease (and alveolar collapse); these papers prompted extensive research on the chemical and physical properties of surfactant and on its sites of formation and removal.

AIRWAY RESISTANCE

A giant step forward occurred in 1916 when Rohrer, as part of his doctoral dissertation, presented a conceptual framework for determining flow and resistance in airways. His equations were based on precise anatomic measurements of airway dimensions in a human cadaver, coupled with aerodynamic principles. During the following decade, he and his coworkers, Neergaard and Wirz, applied Poiseuille's law for laminar flow and his equations to the determination of airway resistance. Use of Fleisch's pneumotachygraph, coupled with periodic interruptions of airflow, permitted measurement of alveolar pressure. Clinically useful measurements of alveolar pressure became available in 1956 with the introduction by DuBois and associates of the whole-body plethysmograph, which they coupled with the application of Boyle's law.

SYNTHESIS OF MECHANICS

During the decade between 1915 and 1926, Rohrer and his colleagues provided a remarkably comprehensive synthesis of respiratory mechanics that included a description of the static pressure–volume characteristics of the respiratory system and the work of breathing; they also developed the principle of optimal frequencies of breathing to minimize respiratory work. Together with von Neergaard and Wirz, Rohrer developed and tested, experimentally, concepts involving pressures, flows, and volumes. The full significance of Rohrer's work was not appreciated until the publications by Fenn and his group at the University of Rochester, starting in the 1940s. The contributions of W. O. Fenn, H. Rahn, and A. B. Otis to our present understanding of the mechanics of breathing are significant, and there is little doubt that this group shaped much of the contemporary thinking of respiratory physiologists and pulmonary physicians.[14–17]

CONTROL OF BREATHING

The control of breathing is a complex process that depends on the integrity of the entire respiratory system—lungs, airways, circulation, and control systems.[18] Two dominant control systems exist. One is in the central nervous system; the other is outside the brain. Control mechanisms in the central nervous system are influenced by the state of wakefulness or alertness and are subject to voluntary control. These mechanisms are also influenced reflexively by a variety of peripheral receptors.

LOCALIZATION OF THE CENTRAL RESPIRATORY CENTERS

In 1812, Legallois, apparently intrigued by the gasping movements of the head after decapitation, identified an area in the medulla that was essential for life. In 1923, Lumsden systematically explored the effects of serial sectioning of the brain stem on respiration, marking the beginning of the era of contemporary research on rhythmic breathing. He designated an area in the caudal pons responsible for a sustained inspiratory drive as the "apneustic center," and an area in the rostral and lateral portions of the pons that presumably inhibited the apneustic drive as the "pneumotaxic center"; sectioning of the vagi exaggerated the inhibition of the apneustic drive by the pneumotaxic center. Sixteen years later, Pitts et al.[19], using stereotactic stimulation of the cat medulla, identified inspiratory and expiratory centers and proposed a theory that could account for both rhythmic breathing and apneusis.

CHEMICAL STIMULATION OF THE RESPIRATORY CENTERS

The chemical stimuli to breathing have been known for more than a century. In 1885, Miescher-Ruesch showed in humans that ventilation at rest is primarily regulated by carbon dioxide. Between 1887 and 1901, cross-perfusion experiments by Leon Fredericq underscored the role of carbon dioxide. However, it was not until 1905 to 1909 that Haldane, Priestley, and Douglas paved the way to the modern understanding of the role of carbon dioxide under a variety of experimental conditions.[20] In their experiments on humans, they relied heavily on the Haldane gas analyzer and an alveolar gas sampler of their own invention. However, their experiments did not distinguish clearly between CO_2 and H^+ in the stimulation of the respiratory centers. Winterstein, and later Gesell,[21] advanced the idea that the chemical regulation of respiration is determined by the concentration of hydrogen ions within the respiratory centers.

The Winterstein theories[22] provide a good example of the evolution of ideas prompted by new discoveries and inventions. The original theory in 1911 attributed increments in ventilation caused by hypoxic or hypercapnic inspired mixtures to a single mechanism, that is, acidification of arterial blood by either carbonic acid or lactic acid. In 1921, Jacobs' demonstration of the rapid diffusion of carbon dioxide into starfish eggs implicated acidity within the respiratory centers,[23] as well as arterial blood acidity, as the sites of stimulation. To account for the stimulation of breathing by hypoxia (the peripheral chemoreceptors had not yet been discovered), he invoked the release of asphyxiating substances *(Erstickungsstoffen)* within the respiratory centers themselves. A third theory, postulated in 1949, attempted to incorporate the discovery of the peripheral chemoreceptors, and it finally gave way in 1955 to his fourth theory, which explained the effects of acid or hypoxia on both the central and peripheral chemoreceptors.

A major consequence of Winterstein's research was an impetus to subsequent exploration of the chemical control of breathing. These studies led to the identification of central chemoreceptors, distinct from mechanoreceptors, on the ventral surface of the medulla, and clarification of the role of hydrogen ion activity as the central stimulus to breathing. The studies also prompted a search for a unifying theory for the chemical control of breathing.

THE REFLEX REGULATION OF BREATHING

A considerable and diverse number of peripheral receptors can influence breathing reflexively by supplying information to respiratory centers located in the brain. These include pain receptors, stretch receptors in the muscles and distensible thoracic structures, and organs and chemoreceptors in major systemic arteries.

MECHANORECEPTORS

Until the work of Hering and his student, Breuer, little was known about the role of afferent impulses to the central control mechanisms in the control of breathing, other than the fact that electrical stimulation of the vagus nerves influenced respiration.[24] In 1868, Hering and Breuer reported that inflation of the lungs stopped respiration in expiration and promoted expiration, and that, conversely, a decrease in lung volume ended expiration and promoted inspiration. They inferred that inflation mechanically stimulated nerve endings in the lungs and that the resulting impulses ascending the vagi were inhibitory to inspiration.

PERIPHERAL CHEMORECEPTORS

In 1841, Volkmann suggested the existence of chemoreceptors in the systemic circulation that were sensitive to blood-borne stimulants to respiration. In 1927, J. F. Heymans and C. Heymans first showed that the aortic bodies served this function, and in 1930, C. Heymans and Bouckaert demonstrated the peripheral chemoreceptive function of the carotid bodies. These were physiologic observations that tallied well with the observations of F. De Castro, a student, and later a colleague, of Ramón y Cajal, who was sufficiently impressed by the histologic structure, location, and rich innervation of the carotid body to propose that it might be stimulated by blood-borne substances (Fig. 1-13).[25]

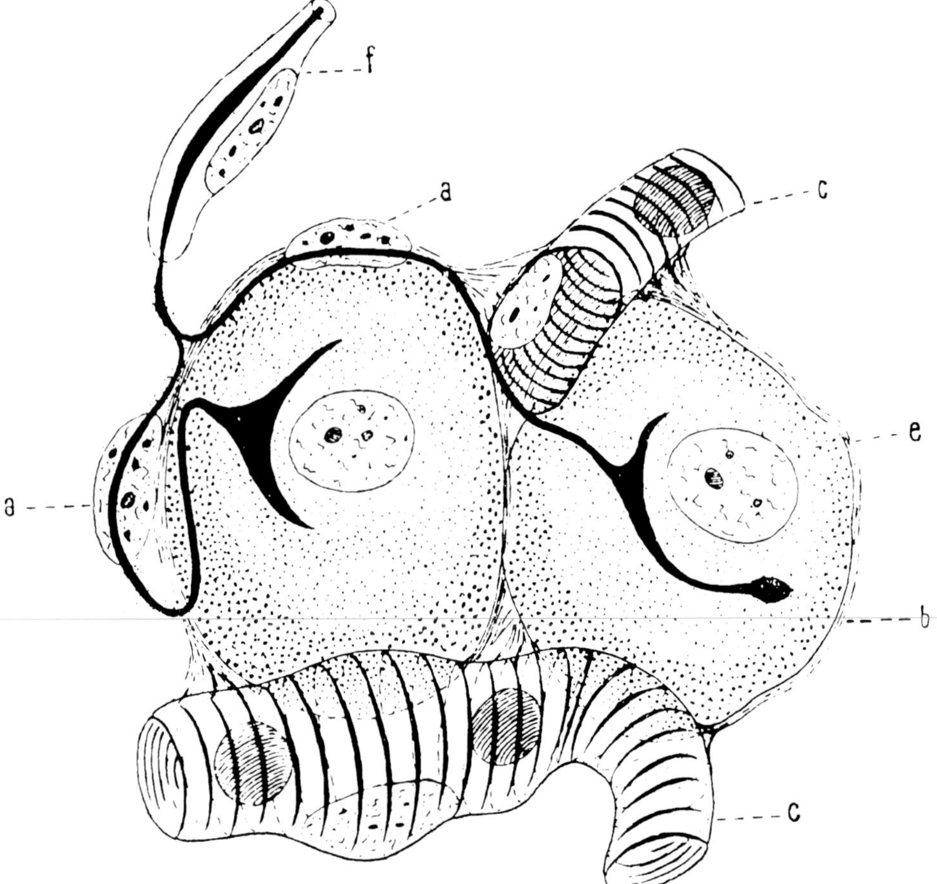

Figure 1-13 Drawing by De Castro showing the structure of the chemoreceptor. The glomus cells (*e*) present an ample cytoplasmic surface for contact with the perfusing blood delivered by the capillary (*c*); sensory nerve fiber (*f*) with sheath of myelin; Schwann cells (*a*) surround the unmyelinated fibers which form the terminal menisci; cell membrane (*b*). *(Reproduced with permission from De Castro F: Sur la structure de la synapse dans les chemoceppteurs: leur mécanisme d'Excitation et R™ le dans la circulation sanguine locale. Acta Physiol Scand. 1951;22(1):14–43.)*

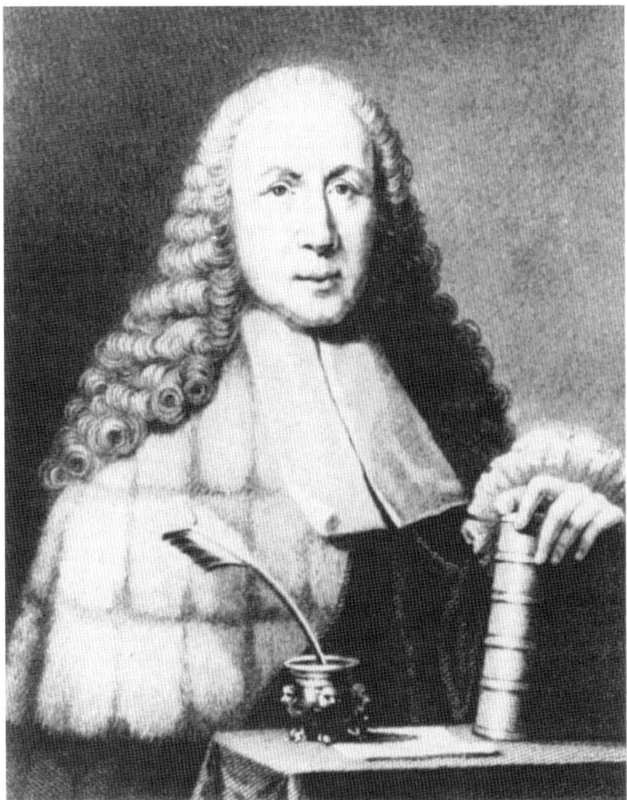

Figure 1-14 Giovanni Battista Morgagni (1682–1771). The five volumes of his *De Sedibus* contain the clinical and pathologic descriptions of approximately 700 cases. *(Courtesy of the Library of the College of Physicians of Philadelphia.)*

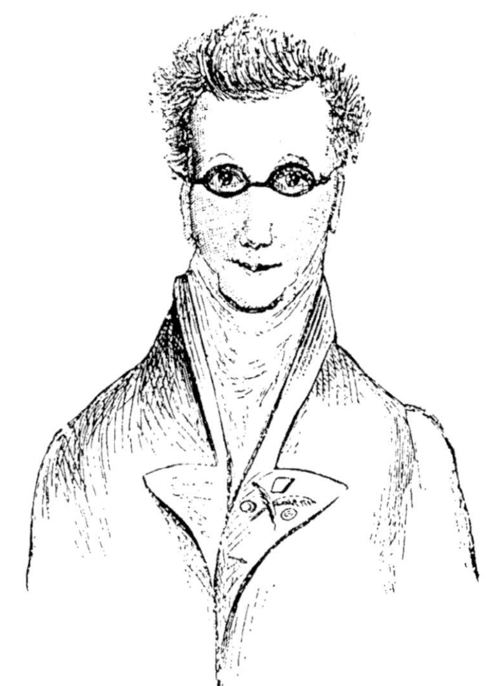

Figure 1-15 Rene T.H. Laënnec (1781–1826). *(Drawn from life in 1825 by Charles James Blasius Williams (1805–1889) and reproduced in his autobiography, Memoirs of Life and Work, London: Smith, Elder & Co; 1884.)*

VENTILATION–PERFUSION RELATIONSHIPS

In 1946, William Dock attributed the apical localization of tuberculosis to hypoperfusion of well-ventilated alveoli in the lung apices in the upright position.[26] Shortly thereafter, ventilation–blood flow relationships were described in quantitative terms in papers by two separate groups: Rahn and Fenn[27] and Riley and Cournand.[28–30]

SCIENTIFIC BASIS OF CLINICAL PULMONARY MEDICINE

Five remarkable figures serve to illustrate different stages in the evolution of the scientific basis of pulmonary medicine: Morgagni, Laënnec, Koch, Cournand, and Richards. They represent key scientists in the areas of pathologic anatomy, microbiology, and physiology.

PATHOLOGIC ANATOMY

Morgagni and Laënnec, almost a century apart, made major contributions to the field of pathologic anatomy. Morgagni (Fig. 1-14), who lived in the 18th century and was a student of Valsalva, veered away from the undisciplined case reports of his predecessors. Instead, he adopted a logical system for relating findings at autopsy to their clinical manifestations. At age 79, he published a compilation of his lifelong experience in his famous work, *De Sedibus et Causis Morborum per Anatomen Indagatis. De Sedibus* includes about 700 cases. The clinical–pathologic correlations in this work benefited greatly from the fact that Morgagni was both a seasoned clinician and a pathologist. One of the compilation's five books is devoted to diseases of the thorax. Among his descriptions were those of a tubercle undergoing liquefaction and the hepatization stage of pneumonia.

René Théophile Laënnec is, perhaps, best known for inventing the stethoscope in 1816 (Fig. 1-15).[31,32] At that time, clinical medicine in Europe, especially in France, was turning from metaphysical concepts and doctrinal systems to pathology as its scientific foundation. Eminent physicians, such as Bichat, Bayle, and Corvisart in France, and William and John Hunter and Baillie in England, were turning to anatomic findings at autopsy to understand the signs and symptoms of their patients. Percussion had been rediscovered by Corvisart. Although Auenbrugger had reported in Latin his "new invention" in 1761, the idea had not caught on until Corvisart – eminent clinician and teacher and personal physician to Napoleon – published a translation in French in 1808. Corvisart's approach to medicine strongly influenced Laënnec. Laënnec applied the stethoscope and Corvisart's "sounding of the chest" to study individual patients with diseases of the lungs and heart throughout their clinical course, along with anatomical examination at autopsy. This was no simple matter. Since there were no pathologists in those days, the physician not only had to provide continuous care during the patient's lifetime, but he also had to arrange for, and perform, the autopsy; he then had to gather all that he had seen and learned and prepare it for publication.

In 1819, two years after the invention of the stethoscope, Laënnec published his famous monograph, *De l'Auscultation médiate*, which drew lessons from carefully documented cases that were studied throughout their clinical course and at autopsy. In this work, Laënnec built upon the monumental tome of Morgagni, who, a generation before, had related the clinical features of the diseases he described to the morbid anatomy, but who had not been able to take the next step of relating the clinical course of individual patients to the anatomic findings after death.

Laënnec's monograph contains descriptions of physical signs, clinical–pathologic correlations for tuberculosis, pneumonia, bronchiectasis, emphysema, and cancer of the lung, and instructions for the treatment of these conditions. The descriptions of tuberculosis were an outstanding contribution to the field and were reported prior to Koch's discovery of the causative agent.

MICROBIOLOGY

Tuberculosis provides a remarkably illuminating example of the impact of a novel basic science on clinical medicine.[33–35] The disease can be traced back to the ancients, who were familiar with the diverse clinical syndromes that we now take for granted as due to tuberculosis; however, they had no way to relate them to a common etiologic agent. A synthesis by Morton in 1685 of all that was then known about tuberculosis focused on cavitary lesions, emaciation ("consumption"), and the tubercle, but it was shrouded in Galenic humors. An understanding of the disease accelerated in the 18th century when clinicians, such as William Cullen, began to sort out the various syndromes relating to phthisis, including hemoptysis, empyema, catarrh, and asthma.

The tempo of discovery increased dramatically in the 19th century after the French Revolution. During the Napoleonic era, distinguished Parisian clinicians, including Bichat, Bayle, Louis, Broussais, and Laënnec, reported clinical-pathologic correlations of tuberculosis (Notably, both Bayle and Laënnec died of tuberculosis.). However, little advance was made in understanding the pathogenesis of tuberculosis until Villemin, who, impressed by the analogy between glanders and syphilis on the one hand, and tuberculosis on the other, and the fact that two of the three diseases had been shown to be infectious in origin, undertook experiments demonstrating that tuberculosis was an infectious disease that could be transmitted from humans to animals, and from animals to animals.

KOCH

In 1876, Koch was a general practitioner in the German township of Wollestein in the province of Posen, where he was responsible for the health care of 4000 inhabitants (Fig. 1-16). Between obstetrical deliveries and satisfying the medical and surgical needs of patients of all ages, he managed to conduct research on the microbial causes of communicable diseases. His laboratory was homemade—based in either the barn or his living room; his major instrument was a microscope used to examine bacteriologic and tissue specimens. In pursuing his research, he kept in mind the dictum of Jacob Henle, one of his teachers in medical school, who counseled that, "before microscopic organisms can be regarded as the cause of contagion in man, they must be found constantly in the contagious material, they must be isolated from it and their strength tested." This lesson was to become the keynote of the future "Koch postulates."

In 1876, Koch, the busy medical practitioner, sent a letter to Professor Ferdinand Cohn, director of the Botanical Institute in Breslau, indicating that he had discovered "the process of development of bacillus anthracis" and requesting permission to present his findings to Professor Cohn, "the foremost authority on bacteria." Koch had discovered the spores of anthrax bacilli. Cohn arranged for him to present his results before a room full of formidable, distinguished scientists, including Julius Cohnheim, Carl Weigert, Moritz Traube, Ludwig Lichtheim, and Leopold Auerbach. Koch's demonstration of the complete life history of the anthrax bacillus, including sporulation, was entirely convincing to these scientists. After the meeting, Cohnheim, upon his return home, announced to his colleagues, "This man has made a splendid discovery which is all the more astonishing because Koch has had no scientific connections and has worked entirely on his own initiative and has produced something absolutely complete. There is nothing more to be done. I consider this the greatest discovery in the field of bacteriology."

During the next 2 years, Koch described novel procedures for the examination, preservation, and photography of bacteria and demonstrated the role of microorganisms in traumatic infections, while continuing his dual existence as a country doctor and an independent investigator. In 1880, Cohn and Cohnheim arranged for him to move to Berlin as a member of the Imperial Sanitary Commission. The move freed more time for research. By 1881, he made another breakthrough—the pour-plate method for isolating pure cultures. The opportunity that this technique afforded to produce transparent solid media, coupled with Koch's invention of new staining methods, paved the way for him to tackle the microbial cause of tuberculosis.

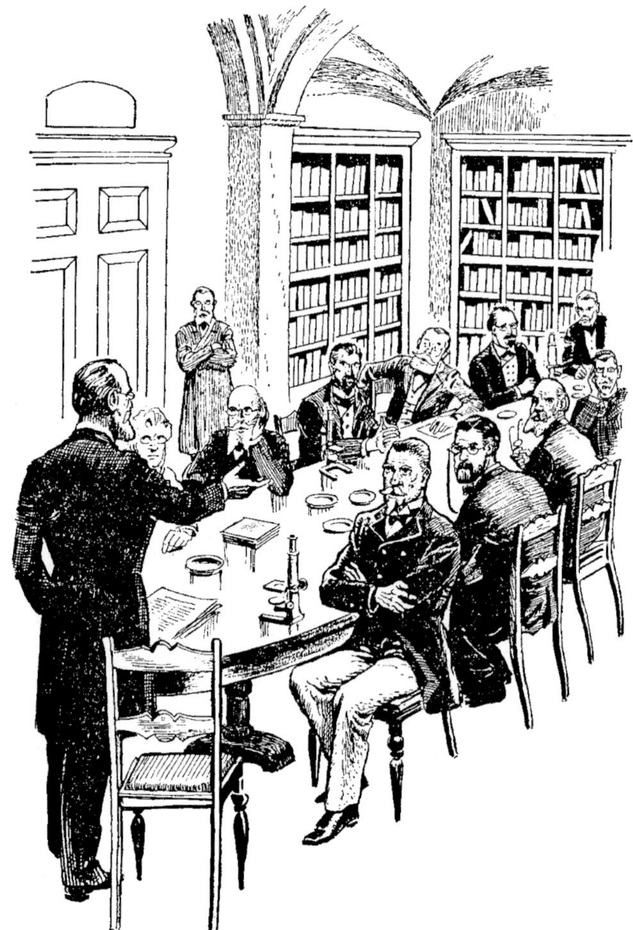

Figure 1-16 Robert Koch (1843–1910), announcing his discovery of the tubercle bacillus as the cause of tuberculosis, Berlin, March 28, 1882. *(Reproduced with permission from Knight D: Robert Koch: Founder of Bacteriology. New York: Franklin Watts, Inc.; 1961:10.)*

Koch's scientific approach, which has been immortalized as "Koch postulates," consisted of four essential steps: (1) To prove that a microbe is the cause of a disease, it must be present in all cases of the disease (Koch showed this for the tubercle bacillus using methylene blue and a counter stain), (2) the microbe must be grown outside of the body in pure culture. (Koch devised blood-serum jelly as a culture medium for the slow-growing tubercle bacillus.), (3) the pure culture must be capable of causing the disease in healthy animals (Koch proved this initially by inoculation and, subsequently, by allowing animals to breathe contaminated air.), (4) the same microbe must then be isolated from the inoculated (infected) animal and grown outside of the body in pure culture.

Koch's discovery of the tubercle bacillus and its modes of transmission revolutionized the treatment of tuberculosis. Before the discovery, tubercular patients were treated in sanitaria, which offered fresh air and altitude. Those who ran the sanitaria did not know that tuberculosis was a contagious disease: Sanitation was unregulated, and neither sterilization nor fumigation was practiced; diagnostic capabilities were limited. Koch's discovery of the tubercle bacillus revolutionized therapy. For the rest of his life, while pursuing the causes of other diseases around the world – rinderpest in South Africa, Texas fever, tropical malaria, blackwater fever, and bubonic plague in Bombay – Koch maintained his interest in tuberculosis.

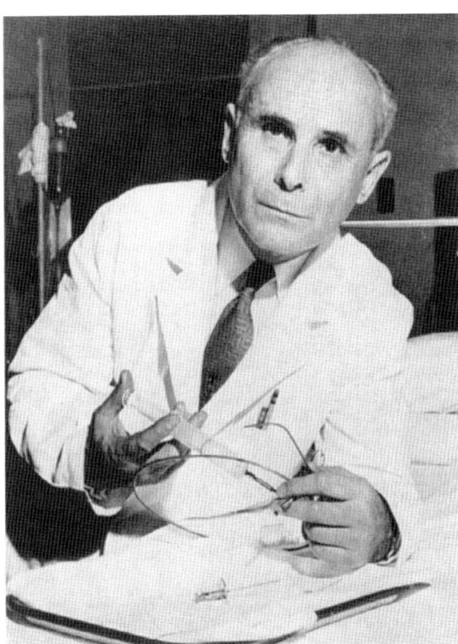

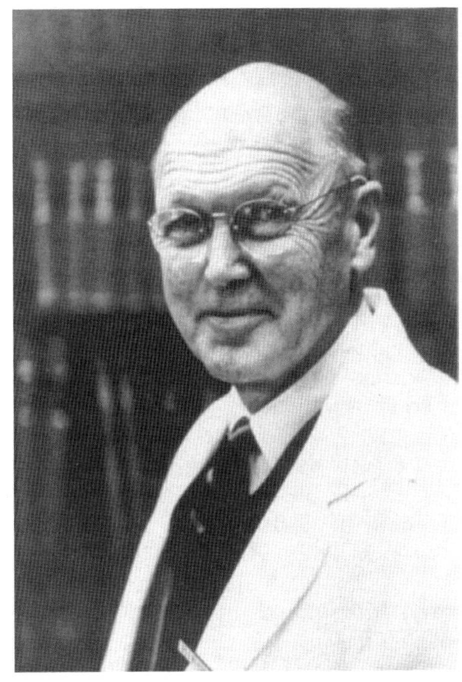

Figure 1-17 André Frederic Cournand (1895–1988) and Dickinson W. Richards (1895–1973). After Forssman's report of the uneventful catheterization of his own right heart, Cournand and Richards pioneered the use of cardiac catheterization for the study of the normal and the abnormal pulmonary circulation and the standardization of pulmonary function tests.

This interest, however, led him into a major mistake—advocacy of tuberculin as a vaccine instead of as a diagnostic test. In 1905, he was awarded the Nobel Prize. On April 7, 1910, the year of his death, he delivered a final address on the epidemiology of tuberculosis before the Berlin Academy of Sciences.

PHYSIOLOGY OF THE PULMONARY CIRCULATION

Starting with William Harvey,[5] studies of the pulmonary circulation have gone hand in hand with advances in pulmonary physiology and medicine. For many years, research on the pulmonary circulation was confined to animal experimentation. A giant step forward was made with the introduction of cardiac catheterization in humans.

Accurate measurement of pulmonary blood flow is a sine qua non for assessing pulmonary and cardiac performance in health and disease. The use of nitrous oxide in humans by Krogh and Lindhard was an important beginning in this direction, but not until mixed venous blood could be sampled for application of the Fick principle could reliable determinations of pulmonary blood flow be made.

Claude Bernard in 1846 and Chauveau and Marey in 1861 had catheterized the right side of the heart in animal experiments. Whether this technique could be used safely in humans was not known until 1929, when Werner Forssmann, a young surgeon in Germany, introduced a ureteral catheter into his own right atrium. In the 1940s, Cournand, Richards, and their colleagues resorted to right heart catheterization to obtain mixed venous blood for the determination of cardiac output by application of the Fick principle (Fig. 1-17). The technique opened the way not only to the accurate determination of cardiac output, but also to exploration of the heart and lungs in a wide variety of clinical disorders.

Until 1946, when von Euler and Liljestrand reported the effects of hypoxia and hypercapnia on the pulmonary circulation in an open-chest preparation of an anesthetized cat, (Fig. 1-18)[36] there was little understanding of the regulation of the pulmonary circulation. However, these studies, coupled with the proposition of local control of the pulmonary circulation by local concentrations of the respiratory gases, paved the way to understanding pulmonary hypertension and the behavior of the pulmonary circulation in normal individuals at rest, after birth, during exercise, and at altitude, and in individuals with heart or lung disease.

The interposition of the pulmonary circulation between the right and left sides of the heart is a prerequisite for gas exchange. However, it also serves a variety of other functions, for example, a

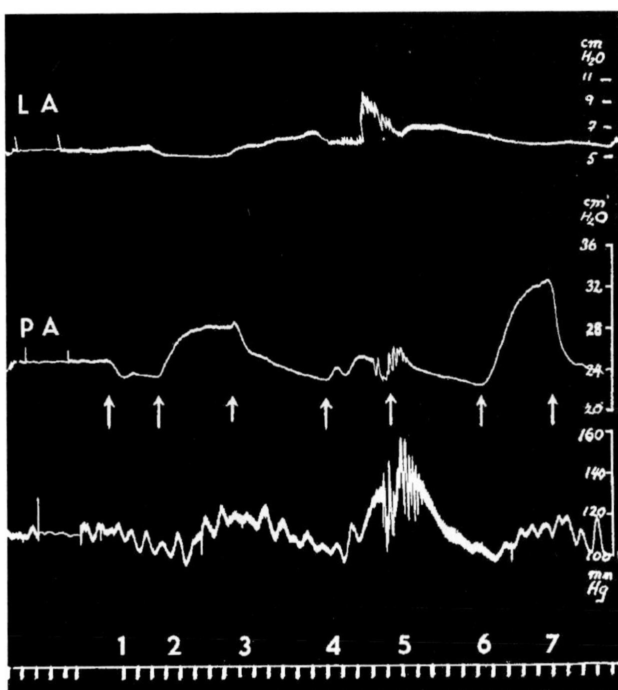

Figure 1-18 Effects of the blood gases on pulmonary arterial pressure in the open-chest cat, artificial respiration. LA, left atrial pressure; PA, pulmonary arterial pressure; lower trace, systemic arterial blood pressure. Numbers along the baseline represent the administration of test gases: 1, O_2 (from air); 2, 6.5% CO_2 in O_2; 3, O_2; 4, 18.7% CO_2 in CO_2; 5, O_2; 6, 10.5% O_2 in N_2; 7, O_2. *(Reproduced with permission from Von Euler, US and Liljestrand, G: Observations on the pulmonary arterial blood pressure in the cat. Acta Physiol Scand. 1946;12(4):301–320.)*

mechanical role, as a filter for particulate matter in blood returning to the heart, and a metabolic role, effecting the synthesis, uptake, and breakdown of biologic compounds. Extensive studies have been conducted in recent decades on the nonrespiratory functions of the lungs. From these studies has emerged considerable understanding of the diverse functions served by the branching pulmonary circulation and its components, including the endothelium and smooth muscle and their interplay.

TECHNOLOGIC ADVANCES THROUGH THE EARLY 20TH CENTURY

The road to contemporary pulmonary medicine could be just as easily traced by using technologic advances as landmarks, instead of people and discoveries. For example, the introduction of the manometer for pressure recording, the use of chambers to simulate high altitude, the development of accurate blood gas analyzers, and the application of sophisticated optical systems for viewing the lumens of the airways and the inside of the chest cavity are all notable milestones. However, probably no better example exists than the discovery of radiographs and the application of this discovery to the diagnosis, prevention, and management of pulmonary tuberculosis.

Wilhelm Conrad Roentgen discovered radiographs in 1895 while experimenting with cathode ray tubes in his physics laboratory at the University of Wurzburg. Although others before him had seen radiographs as early as 1890, Roentgen was apparently the first to grasp the full significance of the discovery, and his publication, quite unpretentious, immediately attracted worldwide attention because of its prospects for the study of anatomic structures and pathologic changes.

Within 2 years after Roentgen's discovery, fluoroscopy of the chest had been introduced into clinical practice, and its value in the early detection of tuberculosis and the diagnosis of pleural effusions was appreciated. In 1901, an atlas of chest radiographs was published, and the use of chest radiography increased greatly with each subsequent improvement in hot cathode radiograph tubes and intensifying screens. The radiographic evaluation of tuberculosis was superior to physical examination for diagnosis and characterization of the disease. By 1910, all patients admitted to sanatoriums had a chest radiographic examination, and by 1917 tuberculosis was classified according to radiographic findings.

MAJOR DEVELOPMENTS SINCE THE MID-20TH CENTURY

Many notable developments have occurred over the last 60 years in pulmonary medicine and the related field of critical care. Measured against the metric of having a broad and deep impact on clinical care, several are particularly noteworthy: advances in thoracic imaging, lung transplantation, bronchoscopy and interventional bronchoscopic techniques, and advances in management of the critically ill.

■ ADVANCES IN THORACIC IMAGING

Following Roentgen's discovery of the x-ray at the turn of the 20th century, another major diagnostic leap forward in pulmonary medicine occurred with development of computerized tomography (CT) in the 1960s.[37–39] In 1967, the first experimental CT scan was generated, with computer reconstruction of an image of a mouse taking 9 days to complete. The first human application was a head CT which demonstrated a brain tumor (Fig. 1-19). In 1973, Dr. Godfrey Hounsfield published a description of CT scanning in the British Journal of Medicine. Along with Dr. Allan Cormack, Hounsfield (Fig. 1-20) was awarded a Nobel Prize in 1979.

Application of CT to lung imaging arose in the mid-1970s; high-resolution techniques were developed in the 1980s. Multislice CT scanning now permits rapid acquisition of high-resolution images from which multiplanar reconstructions can be derived (Fig. 1-21). Elegant characterization and classification of a variety of interstitial and airway diseases is now possible using CT. In addition, when coupled with intravenous contrast injection (CT angiography), rapid, high-resolution scanners provide for the highly accurate diagnosis

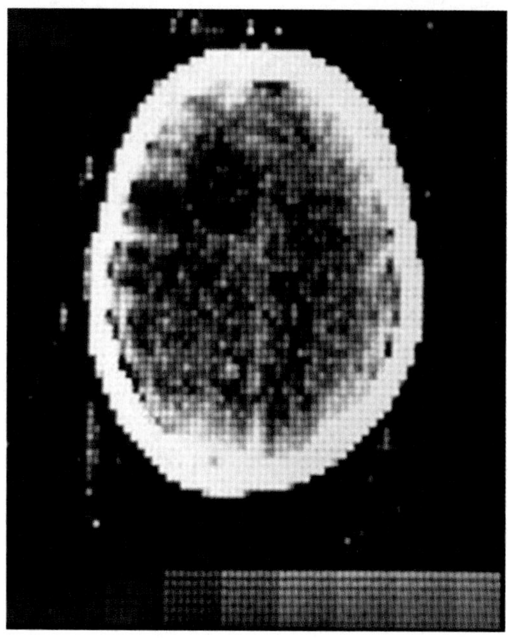

Figure 1-19 The first clinical CT scan, obtained in 1971. The grainy image shows a brain tumor in a frontal lobe (*left side* of image). Advances in image quality over the last four decades have been dramatic. *(Source: impactscan.org.)*

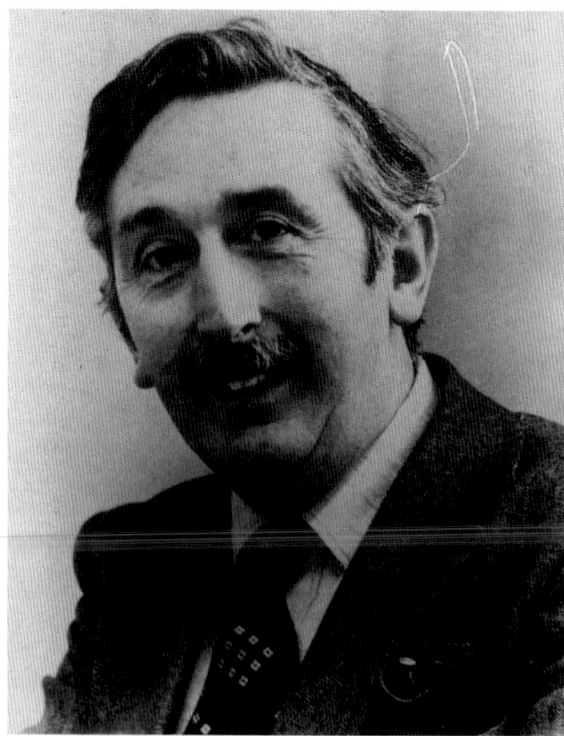

Figure 1-20 Dr. Godfrey Hounsfield, inventor of computerized tomography (CT). Along with Dr. Allan Cormack, Hounsfield was awarded a Nobel Prize in 1979. *(Source: Visible Proofs, National Library of Medicine, National Institutes of Health.)*

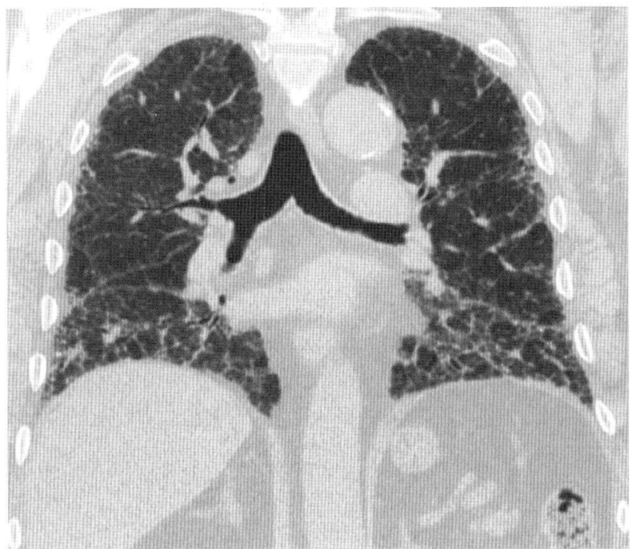

Figure 1-21 A modern day, coronal reconstruction of the chest using CT in a patient with idiopathic pulmonary fibrosis (IPF). Current scanners are capable of rapidly generating high-resolution images from which a variety of computer-generated reconstructions can be derived. *(Used with permission of Dr. Eduardo J. Mortani Barbosa, Jr.)*

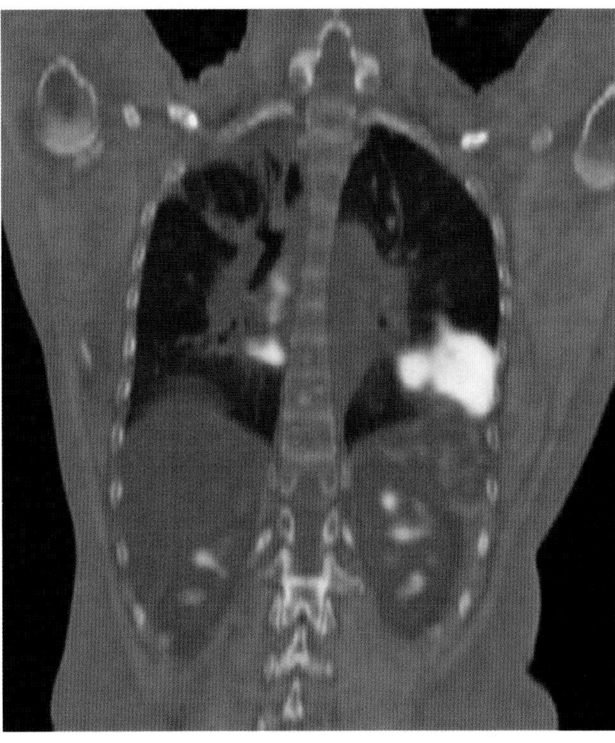

Figure 1-22 A coronal PET/CT image demonstrating metastatic lung cancer, evident as bright areas (in *yellow*) at the left base and the right hilum. The PET and CT images are aligned ("in register") to create precise anatomic localization of the heightened metabolic activity noted in the PET image. *(Used with permission of Dr. Eduardo J. Mortani Barbosa, Jr.)*

of pulmonary embolism[40] and other pulmonary vascular disorders. Advances in multislice techniques (e.g., development of 256-slice or 320-slice scanners) offer the promise of even higher quality imaging.

More recently, aligning the anatomic detail provided by CT with functional images afforded by positron emission tomography (PET) has generated useful information on the staging and clinical assessment of bronchogenic carcinoma, particularly non–small-cell carcinoma.[41–45] Positively charged electrons (positrons), emitted from injected radionuclides are destroyed by electrons and, in the process, produce photons which are detected and imaged by the PET scanner. Malignant cells, by virtue of having increased numbers of cell membrane–based glucose transporters compared with normal cells, accumulate greater levels of the radionuclide,[18] F-fluorodeoxyglucose (F-FDG), which cannot be metabolized further and is trapped within the cells. The tracer-enriched collection of malignant cells stands out against the background of normal tissue. Coupling of the PET-based and CT images provides precise localization of the area of abnormality (Fig. 1-22). PET/CT imaging has been used to evaluate solitary pulmonary nodules, assess local extent of disease (particularly mediastinal and pleural involvement) in lung cancer, and evaluate distant anatomic sites for metastatic disease.

LUNG TRANSPLANTATION

Following on the heels of pioneering animal experimentation conducted by Vladimir Demikhov,[46] the first reported human lung transplantation was conducted by Dr. James Hardy and colleagues in 1963.[47,48] However, it was not until the 1980s that clinically meaningful outcomes were achieved by Dr. Joel Cooper and colleagues with single-lung[49] and bilateral-lung[50] transplantation.

Since the advent of lung transplantation, more than 32,000 procedures have been performed worldwide. Survival of recipients has improved from 4.0 years in the late 1980s and early 1990s to 5.7 years in the last decade. Contemporary, overall survival rates are 79% at 1 year, 63% at 3 years, 52% at 5 years, and 29% at 10 years.[51]

Lung transplantation is associated with improvements in lung function, exercise tolerance, and hemodynamic parameters. Currently, the primary diagnoses for which lung transplantation is most commonly conducted include (in descending order of frequency) idiopathic pulmonary fibrosis (IPF), chronic obstructive pulmonary disease (COPD), cystic fibrosis (CF), and other disorders, including alpha-1-antitrypsin deficiency, sarcoidosis, non-CF bronchiectasis, lymphangioleiomyomatosis (LAM), and primary pulmonary hypertension.[51,52]

Despite tremendous advances in the field, complications of lung transplantation are common and include primary graft dysfunction (noncardiogenic pulmonary edema without other apparent cause occurring in the first 72 hours following transplantation); bronchial stenosis developing at the anastamotic site; a broad array of infectious complications, including CMV infection; acute rejection (occurring in over one-third of recipients); and chronic allograft dysfunction due to bronchiolitis obliterans.[51]

Improved surgical techniques in lung transplantation have been important. However, critical to advances in solid organ transplantation, including lung transplantation, has been development of effective immunosuppressive regimens.The earliest regimens included a limited repertoire of drugs, for example, corticosteroids and azathioprine. Development of calcineurin inhibitors, including cyclosporine in 1977 and tacrolimus in 1983, substantially advanced the field.[53]

While technical and pharmacologic advances in lung transplantation afford many patients with advanced lung disease improved quality of life, a limited supply of suitable donor organs persists. Various approaches have been employed in an attempt to ameliorate the continuous shortage. In addition to obtaining organs from brain-dead donors as the primary source, more recently, many transplant programs have embarked on the somewhat controversial program of donation after cardiac death (DCD) or donation from "non–heart-beating donors," who undergo controlled withdrawal of life support in an operating room. In addition, new technologic developments in organ "reconditioning" offer hope for enlarging the supply of transplantable lungs.[54–56]

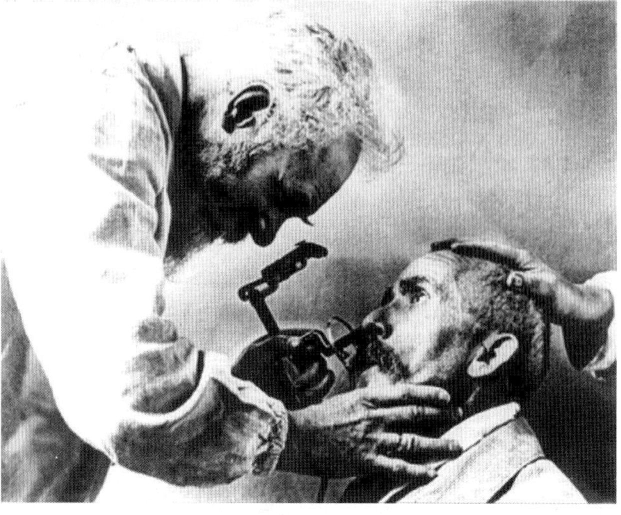

Figure 1-23 Gustav Killian (1860–1921), the father of bronchoscopy. *(Used with permission of Klaus D. Peter, Wiehl, Germany. Released to the public domain, via Wikimedia Commons.)*

BRONCHOSCOPY AND INTERVENTIONAL BRONCHOSCOPIC TECHNIQUES

Application of bronchoscopic techniques, both rigid and flexible, has revolutionized the field of pulmonary medicine, from both diagnostic and interventional perspectives. Credit for invention of the rigid bronchoscope is given to Gustav Killian (Fig. 1-23) in Germany in the late 19th century;[57] in the United States, the field of rigid bronchoscopy was pioneered by Chevalier Jackson in Philadelphia (Fig. 1-24).[58] The next major wave in bronchoscopy arose with development of the flexible fiberoptic technique by Shigeto Ikeda in Japan.[59,60] Since then, significant advances in optics, digital technology, and a variety of interventional techniques, including those based on the fiberoptic method, have been reported.

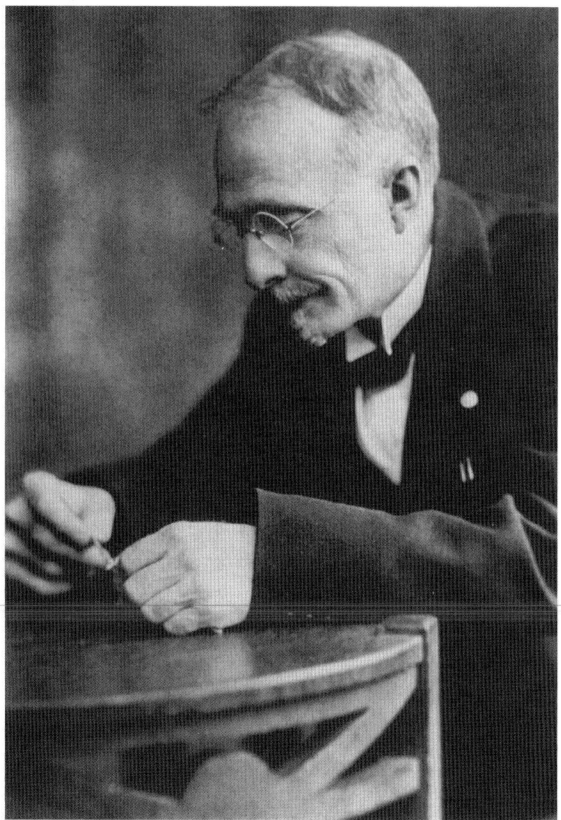

Figure 1-24 Chevalier Jackson (1865–1958), a pioneer in American bronchoesophagology. *(Courtesy of Thomas Jefferson University.)*

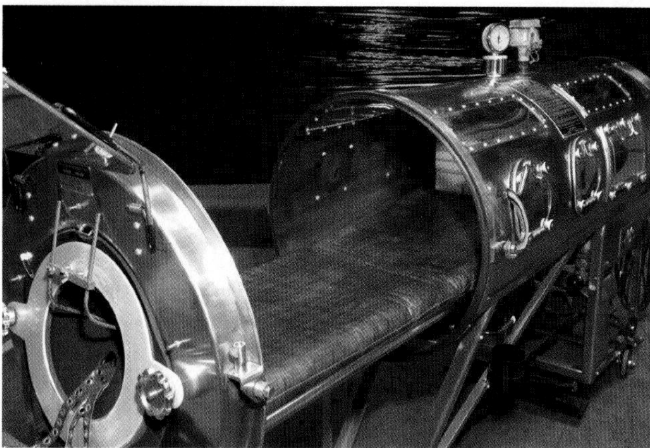

Figure 1-25 An "iron lung." The patient was placed in the hollow cylinder before the device was sealed, with his or her head protruding from one end. *(Used with permission of CDC/GHO/Mary Hilpertshauser. Photo Credit: Jim Gathany.)*

ADVANCES IN CRITICAL CARE

In parallel with the previously noted advances in imaging, transplantation, and bronchoscopy, significant progress in the management of critically ill patients has occurred over the last several decades. One of the most notable is application of mechanical ventilation.[61–63]

The era of the "iron lung," the first widely used negative pressure ventilator, dates back to 1928 (Fig. 1-25).[64–66] Restricted access to the patient was a major limitation to use of the device. The advent of positive pressure ventilators, dramatically evident during the polio epidemic in Copenhagen in 1952, ushered in the "modern" era of mechanical ventilation.[67] Indeed, the clustering of paralyzed patients needing ventilatory support paved the way for development of medical intensive care units. Subsequent invention of the Bennett valve, a result of efforts to establish a means of facilitating high-altitude flight for military purposes, further enhanced clinical use of positive pressure ventilation.[68–71] Many additional refinements in mechanical ventilation, including microprocessor-controlled functions, have evolved over the last quarter century. One noteworthy development in the field deserves special consideration: use of the "low-stretch protocol."

Based on recognition that application of traditionally used tidal volumes of 10 to 15 mL/kg body weight may cause stretch-induced injury in patients with acute lung injury (ALI) and acute respiratory distress syndrome (ARDS), a multicenter prospective trial was undertaken to address whether use of smaller tidal volumes (6 mL/kg), that is, a "low-stretch protocol," would improve outcomes. Indeed, in a landmark study published in 2000, an approximate 25% reduction in mortality using a low-stretch protocol was demonstrated.[72] Additional refinements, including use of higher levels of positive end-expiratory pressure (PEEP)[73] and the so-called "lung recruitment maneuvers"[74] have been added to the contemporary ventilator management scheme for these patients.

In addition to advances in mechanical ventilation, other notable recent refinements in critical care include recognition of the value of venous thromboembolism prophylaxis, prophylaxis against gastrointestinal bleeding, semierect patient positioning to minimize aspiration risk, good (but not excessive) glycemic control, application of spontaneous breathing trials and sedation interruption, and early patient mobilization. However, one particular development warrants special mention: use of early goal-directed therapy (EGDT) in sepsis.

Sepsis is a severe, systemic response to infection and is associated with high mortality. A reflection of the systemic inflammatory response syndrome (SIRS), sepsis may progress to severe sepsis (end-organ dysfunction in the setting of documented or suspected infection) or septic shock (severe sepsis with hypotension unresponsive to intravenous fluid administration). An important study published in 2000 addressed the value of EGDT in the management of septic patients. Such therapy focuses on early and aggressive fluid administration titrated to a goal central venous pressure (CVP), mean arterial blood pressure (MAP), and target central venous oxygen saturation (Scv_{O_2}), and incorporates use of vasoactive agents and transfusion of packed red blood cells as necessary. Application of EGDT has been shown to reduce mortality by as much as one-third[75] and constitutes one of the cornerstones of management of critically ill patients with sepsis, as comprehensively discussed in the "Surviving Sepsis Campaign Guidelines for Management of Severe Sepsis and Septic Shock."[76]

REFERENCES

1. Foster M. *Lectures on the History of Physiology*. London: Cambridge University Press; 1901.
2. Frank RG Jr. *Harvey and the Oxford Physiologists*. Berkeley, CA: University of California Press; 1980.
3. Furley DJ, Wilkie JS. *Galen on Respiration and the Arteries*. Princeton, NJ: Princeton University Press; 1984.
4. Galen C. *Galen: On the Usefulness of the Parts of the Body*. May MT, trans. Ithaca, NY: Cornell University Press; 1968:279–599.
5. Harvey W. *Movement of the Heart and Blood in Animals, an Anatomical Essay*. Franklin KJ, trans. Oxford: Blackwell Scientific Publications; 1957.
6. Mayow J. *Medico-Physical Works*. Crum A, Brown, Dobbin L, trans. Edinburgh: Alembic Club, Reprints, no. 17, 1957. (Translated from Tractatus quinque medico-physics, 1674.)
7. McKie D. *Antoine Lavoissier: Scientist, Economist, Social Reformer*. New York, NY: Schuman; 1952.
8. Bohr C. Ueber die spezifische Tätigkeit der Lungen bei der respiratorischen Gasaufnahme und irh Verhalten zu der durch die Alveolarwand staffindenden Gasdiffusion. *Skand Arch Physiol.* 1904;16:402.
9. Milledge JS. The great oxygen secretion controversy. *Lancet.* 1985;2:1408–1411.
10. Krogh M. The diffusion of gases through the lungs of man. *J Physiol (Lond).* 1915;49:271–300.
11. Krogh A, Krogh M. On the tensions of gases in the arterial blood. *Skand Arch Physiol.* 1910;23:179–192.
12. Roughton FJW. The average time spent by the blood in the human lung capillary and its relation to the rates of CO uptake and elimination in man. *Am J Physiol.* 1945;143:621–633.
13. Davy H. *Researches, Chemical and Philosophical; Chiefly Concerning Nitrous Oxide, or Dephlogisticated Nitrous Air, and its Respiration*. London: J. Johnson; 1800:400–410.
14. Fenn WO. Introduction to the mechanics of breathing. In: Fenn WO, Rahn H, eds. *Handbook of Physiology*. Section 3: Respiration. vol 1. Bethesda, MD: American Physiological Society; 1964:357.
15. Otis AB. History of respiratory mechanics. In: Fishman AP, ed. *Handbook of Physiology*. Section 3: The Respiratory System. vol 3. Mechanics of Breathing; PT Macklem, J Mead (part 1 eds). Bethesda, MD: American Physiological Society; 1986:1.
16. Perkins JF Jr. Historical development of respiratory physiology. In: Fenn WO, Rahn H, eds. *Handbook of Physiology*. Section 3: Respiration. vol 1. Bethesda, MD: American Physiological Society: 1964:1.
17. Rahn H, Otis AB, Chadwick LE, Fenn WO. The pressure-volume diagram of the thorax and lung. *Am J Physiol.* 1946;146: 161–178.
18. Cunningham DJC, Robbins PA, Wolff CB. Integration of respiratory responses to changes in alveolar partial pressures of CO_2 and O_2 and in arterial pH. In: Cherniack NS, Widdicombe JG, eds. *Handbook of Physiology*. Section 3: The Respiratory System. vol 2. Control of Breathing. Bethesda, MD: American Physiological Society; 1986:475.
19. Pitts RF, Magoun HW, Ranson SW. Localization of the medullary respiratory centers in the cat. *Am J Physiol.* 1939;126: 673–688.
20. Haldane JS, Priestley JG. *Respiration*. Oxford: Clarendon Press; 1935.
21. Gesell R. On the chemical regulation of respiration: I. The regulation of respiration with special reference to the metabolism of the respiratory center and the coordination of the dual function of hemoglobin. *Am J Physiol.* 1923;66:40–47.
22. Winterstein H. Die Reactionstheorie der Atmungsregulation. *Arch Ges Physiol.* 1921;187:293–298.
23. Jacobs MH. The production of intracellular acidity by neutral and alkaline solutions containing carbon dioxide. *Am J Physiol.* 1920;53:457–463.
24. Ullmann E. About hering and breuer. In: Porter R, ed. *Breathing: Hering-Breuer Centenary Symposium*. London: J & A Churchill; 1970:3.
25. De Castro F. Sur la structure et l'innervation de la glande intercarotidienne (glomus caroticum) de l'homme et des mammifères et sur un nouveau système d'innervation autonome du nerf glossopharyngien. *Trav Lab Recherches Biol Univ Madrid.* 1926;24:365–432.
26. Dock W. Apical localization of phthisis. *Am Rev Tuber.* 1946;53:297–305.
27. Rahn H. A concept of mean alveolar air and the ventilation-blood flow relationships during pulmonary gas exchange. *Am J Physiol.* 1949;158:21–30.
28. Cournand A. Air and blood. In: Fishman AP, Richards DW, eds. *Circulation of the Blood. Men and Ideas*. Bethesda, MD: American Physiological Society; 1982:3.
29. Cournand A, Ranges HA. Catheterization of the right auricle in man. *Proc Soc Exp Biol Med.* 1941;46(3):462.
30. Riley RL, Cournand A. "Ideal" alveolar air and the analysis of ventilation-perfusion relationships in the lungs. *J Appl Physiol.* 1949;1(12):825–847.
31. Laënnec R. On the diagnosis of diseases of the chest. Forbes J, trans. *A Treatise on the Diseases of the Chest*. London: 1821, Hainer Publishing Co; 1962.
32. Underwood EA. The training of the greatest of chest physicians: Laënnec. *Br J Dis Chest.* 1959:53:109–127.
33. Castiglione A. History of tuberculosis. Recht E, trans. *Medical Life*, 40:148–159, New York, NY: Froben Press; 1933:1–95.
34. Castiglione A. History of tuberculosis. *Med Life.* 1933;40:5–96.
35. Castiglione A. *A History of Medicine*. New York, NY: Alfred A. Knopf; 1947.

36. von Euler US, Liljestrand G. Observations on the pulmonary arterial blood pressure in the cat. *Acta Physiol Scand.* 1946; 12:301–320.

37. Goodman LR. The Beatles, the Nobel prize, and CT scanning of the chest. *Radiol Clin N Am.* 2010;48:1–7.

38. Hounsfield GN. Computerized transverse axial scanning (tomography): part 1. Description of system. *Br J Radiol.* 1973;46:1016–1022.

39. Ambrose J. Computerized transverse axial scanning (tomography): part 2. Clinical application. *Br J Radiol.* 1973;46:1023–1047.

40. Stein PD, Fowler SE, Goodman LR, et al. Multidetector computed tomography for acute pulmonary embolism [PIOPED II]. *N Engl J Med.* 2006;354:2317–2327.

41. Lardinois D, Weder W, Hany TF, et al. Staging of non-small-cell lung cancer with integrated positron-emission tomography and computed tomography. *N Engl J Med.* 2003;348:2500–2507.

42. Kligerman S, Digumarthy S. Staging of non-small cell lung cancer using integrated PET/CT. *AJR Am J Roentgenol.* 2009;193:1203–1211.

43. Padma S, Sundaram PS, George S. Role of positron emission tomography in carcinoma lung evaluation. *J Cancer Res Ther.* 2011;7:128–134.

44. Paul NS, Ley S, Metser U. Optimal imaging protocols for lung cancer staging: CT, PET, MR imaging, and the role of imaging. *Radiol Clin N Am.* 2012;50:935–949.

45. Zhao L, He ZY, Zhong XN, Cui ML. (18)FDG-PET/CT for detection of mediastinal nodal metastases in non-small cell lung cancer: a meta-analysis. *Surg Oncol.* 2012;21:230–236.

46. Langer RM. Vladimir P. Demikhov, a pioneer of organ transplantation. *Transplant Proc.* 2011;43:1221–1222.

47. Hardy JD, Webb WR, Dalton ML Jr, Walker GR Jr. Lung homotransplantation in man. *JAMA.* 1963;186:1065–1074.

48. Dalton ML. The first lung transplantation. *Ann Thorac Surg.* 1995;60:1437–1438.

49. Cooper JD, Pearson FG, Patterson GA, et al. Technique of successful lung transplantation in human. *J Thorac Cardiovasc Surg.* 1987;93:173–181.

50. Cooper JD, Patterson GA, Grossman R, Maurer J. Double-lung transplant for advanced chronic obstructive lung disease. *Am Rev Respir Dis.* 1989;139:303–307.

51. Kotloff RM, Thabut G. Lung transplantation. *Am J Respir Crit Care Med.* 2011;184:159–171.

52. Kreider M, Hadjiliadis D, Kotloff RM. Candidate selection, timing of listing, and choice of procedure for lung transplantation. *Clin Chest Med.* 2011;32:199–211.

53. Linden PK. History of solid organ transplantation and organ donation. *Crit Care Clin.* 2009;25:165–184.

54. Wallinder A, Ricksten S-E, Hansson C, et al. Transplantation of initially rejected donor lungs after ex vivo lung perfusion. *J Thorac Cardiovasc Surg.* 2012;144:1222–1228.

55. Steen S, Ingemansson R, Eriksson L, et al. First human transplantation of a nonacceptable donor lung after reconditioning ex vivo. *Ann Thorac Surg.* 2007;83:2191–2194.

56. Nakajima D, Chen F, Yamada T, et al. Reconditioning of lungs donated after circulatory death with normothermic ex vivo lung perfusion. *J Heart Lung Transplant.* 2012;31:187–193.

57. Killian G. Ueber directe bronchoscopie. *MMW.* 1898;27:844–847.

58. Becker HD. Bronchoscopy: the past, the present, and the future. *Clin Chest Med.* 2010;31:1–18.

59. Tsuboi E, Ikeda S. Transbronchial biopsy smear for diagnosis of peripheral pulmonary carcinomas. *Cancer.* 1967;20:687–698.

60. Ikdea S, Yanai N, Ishikawa S. Flexible bronchofiberscope. *Keio J Med.* 1968;17:1–16.

61. Colice GL. Historical perspective on the development of mechanical ventilation. In: Tobin MJ, ed. *Principles and Practice of Mechanical Ventilation*, 3rd ed. New York, NY: McGraw Hill; 2013:3–41.

62. Snider GL. Historical perspective on mechanical ventilation: from simple life support to ethical dilemma. *Am Rev Respir Dis.* 1989;140:S2–S7.

63. Kacmarek RM. The mechanical ventilator: past, present, future. *Respir Care.* 2011;56:1170–1180.

64. Emerson JH. *The Evolution of Iron Lungs.* Cambridge: JH Emerson; 1978.

65. Drinker P, Shaw LA. An apparatus for the prolonged administration of artificial respiration. *J Clin Invest.* 1929;7:229–247.

66. Drinker P, McKhann CF. The use of a new apparatus for the prolonged administration of artificial respiration. *JAMA.* 1929;92:1658–1660.

67. Lassen HC. A preliminary report on the 1952 epidemic of poliomyelitis in Copenhagen with special reference to the treatment of acute respiratory insufficiency. *Lancet.* 1953;1(6749): 37–40.

68. Motley HL, Cournand A, Eckman M, et al. Physiologic studies on man with the pneumatic balance resuscitator, "Burns model." *J Aviat Med.* 1946;17:431–461.

69. Motley HL, Werko L, Cournand A, et al. Observations on the clinical use of intermittent positive pressure. *J Aviat Med.* 1947;18:417–435.

70. Motley HL, Cournand A, Werko L, et al. Intermittent positive pressure breathing. *JAMA.* 1948;137:370–382.

71. Motley HL, Lang LP, Gordon B. Effect of intermittent positive pressure breathing on gas exchange. *J Aviat Med.* 1950;21:14–27.

72. Ventilation with lower tidal volumes as compared with traditional tidal volumes for acute lung injury and the acute respiratory distress syndrome. The Acute respiratory Distress Syndrome Network. *N Engl J Med.* 2000;342:1301–1308.

73. Brower RG, Lanken PN, MacIntyre N, et al.; The National Heart, Lung, and Blood Institute ARDS Clinical Trials Network. Higher versus lower positive end-expiratory pressures in patients with the acute respiratory distress syndrome. *N Engl J Med.* 2004;351:327–336.

74. Gattinoni L, Caironi P, Cressoni M, et al. Lung recruitment in patients with the acute respiratory distress syndrome. *N Engl J Med.* 2006;354:1775–1786.

75. Rivers R, Nguyen B, Havstad S, et al. Early goal-directed therapy in the treatment of severe sepsis and septic shock. *N Engl J Med.* 2001;345:1368–1377.

76. Dellinger RP, Levy MM, Rhodes A, et al. Surviving sepsis campaign: International guidelines for management of severe sepsis and septic shock, 2012. *Intensive Care Med.* 2013;39: 165–228.

PART 2

Scientific Basis of Lung Function in Health and Disease

SECTION 1 Genetic, Cellular, and Structural Basis of Normal Lung Function

SECTION 2 Physiological Principles of Normal Lung Function

SECTION 3 The Lungs in Different Physiological States

SECTION 4 Lung Immunology

SECTION 5 Lung Injury and Repair

CHAPTER 2

Functional Design of the Human Lung for Gas Exchange

Matthias Ochs
Ewald R. Weibel

At the end of a deep breath, about 80% of the lung volume is air, 10% is blood, and only the remaining 10% is tissue. Because this small mass of tissue is spread over an enormous area – nearly the size of a tennis court – the tissue framework of the lung must be extraordinarily delicate. It is indeed remarkable that the substance of the lung manages to maintain its integrity in the face of the multitude of insults that inevitably accompany a lifetime of exposure to ambient air and the complex necessity of keeping air and blood in intimate contact, but separate, for the sake of gas exchange.

Part of this success is undoubtedly attributable to the unique design of the lung, which ensures mechanical stability as well as nearly optimal conditions for the performance of the lung's primary function: to supply the blood with an adequate amount of oxygen even when the body's demands for oxygen are particularly high, as during heavy work.

THE LUNG AS AN ORGAN

At total lung capacity, the lung fills the entire chest cavity and can reach a volume, in the adult human, of some 5 to 6 L, largely depending on body size. Upon expiration, the lung retracts, most conspicuously from the lower parts of the pleural cavity, the posterior bottom edge of the lung moving upward by some 4 to 6 cm. This preferential lifting of the bottom edge is caused by retraction of the tissue throughout the entire lung, the surfaces of which are freely movable within the thoracic cavity.

The structural background for this mobility of a healthy lung is the formation, during morphogenesis, of a serosal space that is lined on the interior of the chest wall and on the lung surface by a serosa, the parietal and visceral pleurae, respectively (Fig. 2-1). However, this serosal space is minimal, since the visceral pleura is closely apposed to the parietal pleura, with only a thin film of serous fluid intercalated as a lubricant between the two surfaces.[1] Both pleural surfaces are lined by a squamous epithelial layer, often called mesothelium (due to its mesodermal origin), whose surface is richly endowed with long microvilli. The apical microvilli increase the surface area available, suggesting that pleural mesothelial cells are capable of participating in active transserosal transport of solutes. The total volume of pleural fluid is about 15 to 20 mL, with approximately 1700 cells/mm^3 (75% macrophages, 23% lymphocytes, 1% mesothelial cells). The volume and composition of the pleural fluid have to be tightly controlled to ensure an efficient mechanical coupling between chest wall and lung. Pleural fluid originates from pleural capillaries through microvascular filtration. Drainage occurs partly via lymphatic stomata in the parietal pleura. Transcytosis through mesothelial cells in both directions represents another mechanism involved in pleural fluid homeostasis.[2–6]

The connective tissue of the visceral pleura consists of three layers. A superficial layer of predominantly elastic fibers follows the mesothelium, thereby forming an elastic "bag" that enwraps each lobe. A deep sheet of fine fibers follows the outline of alveoli and extends into the depth of the lung. Between these sheets lies a bed of loose connective tissue, containing free cells (histiocytes, plasma cells, and mast cells), that is often close to lymphatics and systemic arterial branches from the bronchial arteries.

The lung is maintained in a stable position within the chest by the hilum, where airways and blood vessels enter from the mediastinum, and by the pulmonary ligament, a long, narrow band of attachment between visceral and mediastinal pleura that extends downward from the hilum. Because of these attachments, a pneumothorax causes the lung to retract and form a lump of tissue that is attached to the mediastinal wall of the thoracic cavity.

The shape of the lung is congruent with that of the fully expanded pleural cavity. This shape is preformed in lung tissue and is hence also evident if an excised lung is inflated, revealing its three faces: the convex thoracic face apposed to the rib cage, the concave diaphragmatic face modeled by the diaphragmatic dome, and the mediastinal face, on which the contours of the heart are impressed beneath the hilum.

As the lung retracts during deflation, the acute edges between the thoracic face and the diaphragmatic and (anterior) mediastinal faces of the lung withdraw; the thoracic and diaphragmatic leaflets of the parietal pleura become apposed, thereby forming a costodiaphragmatic recess on each side (Fig. 2-1). Similarly, as the ventral edge of the lung retracts, the costal and mediastinal pleurae form a

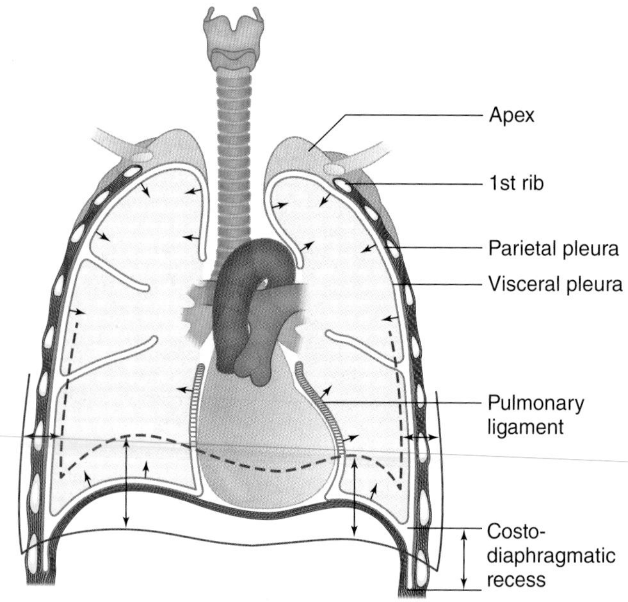

Figure 2-1 Frontal section of chest and lung showing pleural space. *Single arrows* indicate retractive force. *Double arrows* show the excursion of the lung bases and periphery between deep inspiration and expiration.

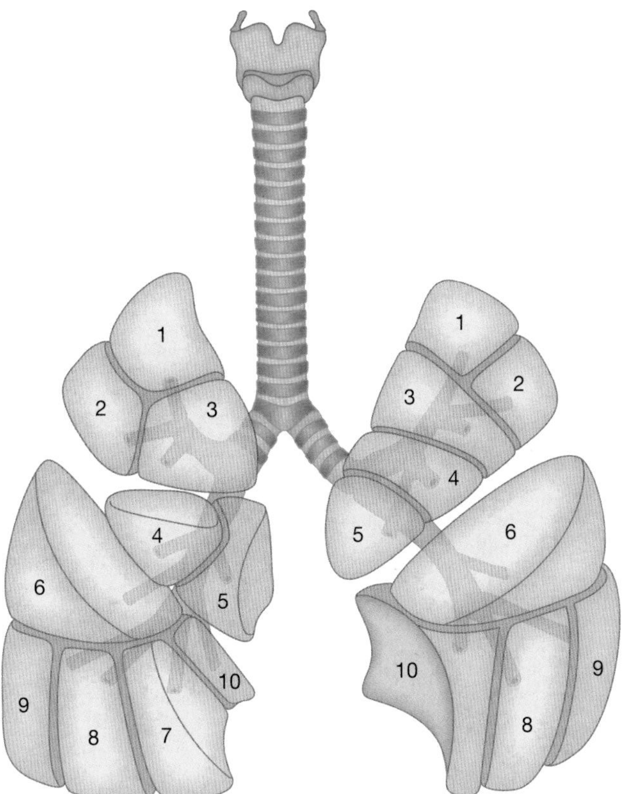

Figure 2-2 Bronchopulmonary segments of human lung. Left and right upper lobes: (1) apical, (2) posterior, (3) anterior, (4) superior lingular, and (5) inferior lingular segments. Right middle lobe: (4) lateral and (5) medial segments. Lower lobes (6): superior (apical), (7) medial–basal, (8) anterior–basal, (9) lateral–basal, and (10) posterior–basal segments. The medial–basal segment (7) is absent in the left lung. (Note: The lungs are represented as turned inward slightly to display part of the lateral face.)

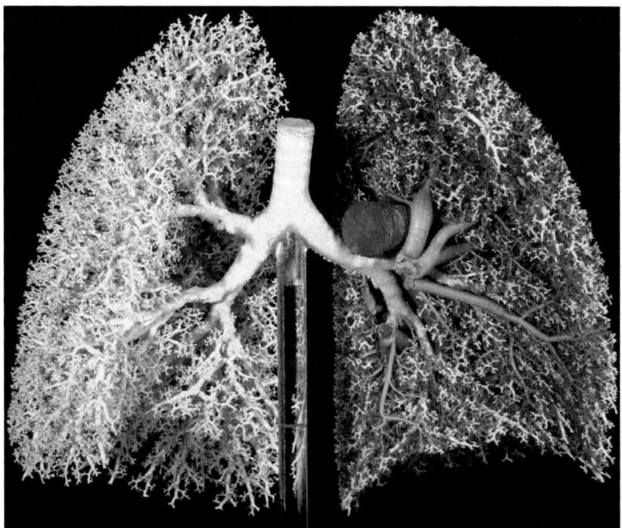

Figure 2-3 A resin cast of the human airway tree shows the dichotomous branching of the bronchi from the trachea and the systematic reduction of airway diameter and length with progressive branching. In the left lung the pulmonary arteries *(red)* and veins *(blue)* are also shown.

recess on each side, corresponding topographically to the borders of the sternum.

The port through which airways and blood vessels enter the lung is the hilum, that is, the attachment of lung tissue to the mediastinum (Fig. 2-1). The airways reach the two hili by the mainstem, or principal, bronchi (Figs. 2-1 and 2-2). The left mainstem bronchus is longer than the right because it must pass under the aortic arch before it reaches the lung. The two principal bronchi course downward and begin to divide sequentially shortly after entering the lung, first releasing the lobar bronchus to the upper lobe (Fig. 2-2). Since a middle lobe is formed only on the right side, there is no middle lobe bronchus on the left; instead, the corresponding parts form the lingula, which receives its airways from the superior bronchus of the upper lobe (Fig. 2-2). The last branch of the stem bronchus goes to the lower lobe.

The branching pattern of the human bronchial tree and of the pulmonary artery and veins are shown in a resin cast in Figure 2-3. The pulmonary artery joins the bronchi while still in the mediastinum (Fig. 2-4A); its trunk lies to the left of the ascending aorta, and the right pulmonary artery turns dorsally to course between ascending aorta and right principal bronchus. In the hilum, the right pulmonary artery lies anterior to the right principal bronchus; the left pulmonary artery, however, "rides" on the principal bronchus and crosses over the superior lobar bronchus to the posterior side. From there on, the pulmonary artery branches in parallel with the bronchi; characteristically, each bronchus is associated with one closely apposed pulmonary artery branch, and this relationship is strictly maintained to the periphery, that is to the respiratory bronchioles.

In contrast, the pulmonary veins (Fig. 2-4B) follow a course independent of the bronchial tree; rather, they lie about midway between two pairs of bronchi and arteries; this position is maintained to the periphery of the airway system. In the hilum, these veins are collected into at least two main veins on either side, which lead into the left atrium located at the back of the heart.

The airways systematically branch over an average of 23 generations of dichotomous branching,[7,8] ending eventually in a blind sac (Fig. 2-5). The last nine generations of these airways are connected to tightly packed alveoli, airway chambers in which gas exchange takes place, whereas the central airways serve the function of conducting the air to the gas-exchange parenchyma. In such a system of sequential branching, the unit of lung parenchyma could be defined according to the portion of parenchyma that is supplied by a particular branch of the bronchial tree, and it is possible to conceive of as many types of units as there are generations unless clear definitions for such units are proposed. However, two units appear to be natural:

1. The lobes, which are demarcated by a more or less complete lining of pleura. There are three lobes on the right (superior, middle, and inferior lobes), and two on the left (superior and inferior lobes).
2. The acinus, which is defined as the parenchymal unit in which all airways have alveoli attached to their wall and thus participate in gas exchange. Along the airway tree, the acinus begins with a transitional bronchiole (Fig. 2-5).[9,10]

Since all other units are somewhat arbitrarily defined, it is not surprising that some ambiguity exists in the literature about their meanings. Nonetheless, a certain convention has been adopted with respect to the following:

1. The lung segments, which are considered as the first subdivisions of lobes. Figure 2-2 shows the location and distribution of the segments to the various lobes. The symmetry is imperfect because on the left the two segments corresponding to the right middle lobe are incorporated into the superior lobe as the lingula (segments 4 and 5) and because the medial–basal segment of the lower lobe is generally missing on the left (segment 7).

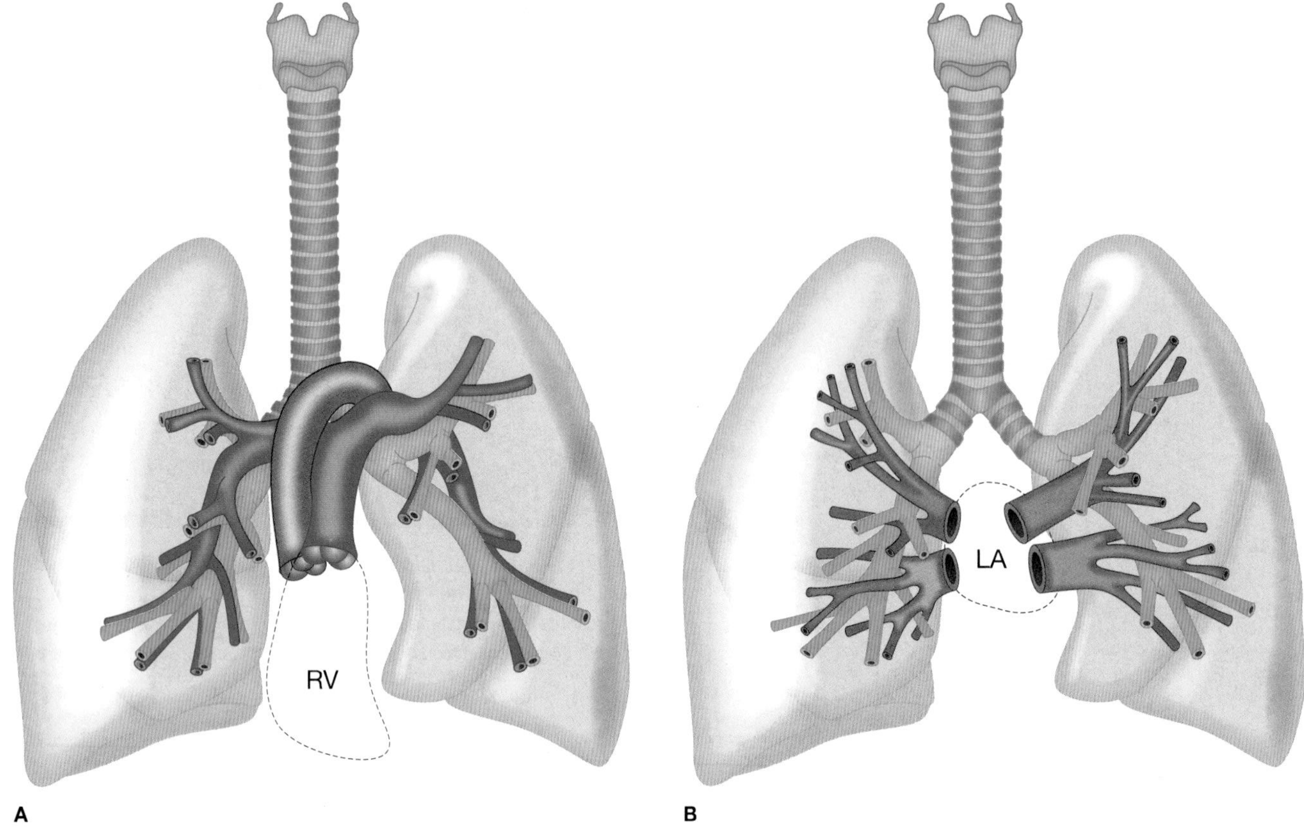

Figure 2-4 Schematic diagrams of the relation of the main branches of pulmonary arteries (**A**) and pulmonary veins (**B**) to the bronchial tree. The arteries follow the airways. Two mainstems of pulmonary vein penetrate independently into the lung on each side. LA, left atrium; RV, right ventricle.

2. The secondary lobule, an old anatomic unit. It was introduced in the 19th century because "lobules" of about 1 cm^3 are visible on the surface of the lung. These lobules are delineated by connective tissue septa that are connected to the pleura. The secondary lobule is difficult to define in terms of the bronchial tree, but it does seem to comprise about a dozen acini. With reference to bronchograms, secondary lobules are supplied by airway branches that are about 1 mm in diameter.

The pulmonary blood vessels show a characteristic relationship to these units (Figs. 2-3 and 2-4). The pulmonary arteries, following the airways, course through the centers of the units and finally fan out into the capillaries located in the delicate alveolar septa of lung parenchyma. In contrast, the veins lie in the boundary between units and collect the blood from at least two or three adjacent units. This arrangement applies to acini and secondary lobules as well as to lung segments.

Therefore, it is evident that the units of lung parenchyma are bronchoarterial units, which share their venous drainage with neighboring units. This architecture has important functional and practical consequences. Except for the lobes, none of the units is separated from each other by complete connective tissue septa.

ORGANIZATION OF LUNG TISSUE

BASIC STRUCTURAL ELEMENTS

While looking at the tissue organization of the lung, we must first consider that the airways and the blood vessels each have their own lining by an uninterrupted cell layer. These layers extend all the way out to the gas-exchange region, but they show different properties in conducting as compared with respiratory structures. Likewise, the connective tissue forms a continuum throughout the lung all the way out to the pleura, but it, too, will be differently organized in the different functional zones; whereas it is reduced to a minimum in the alveolar walls, it contributes a number of different ancillary structures to the wall of conducting airways and blood vessels, such as smooth muscle sheaths or cartilage. This connective tissue space also houses the nutritive vessels and nerves as well as the elaborate defense system related to lymphatic vessels. In the gas-exchange region, however, very few of these accessory structures are found.

The complexity of lung structure is also reflected at the cell biologic level. There is no such thing as a standard "lung cell." Instead, we find some 40 different cell types, highly specialized both structurally and functionally, in the lung.[11–13]

A word of caution is also necessary with respect to the extrapolation of structural findings in experimental animals, especially rodents, to the human lung. Noteworthy species differences include the bronchial circulation, the presence of respiratory bronchioles, the ultrastructural composition and distribution of nonciliated bronchiolar epithelial cells and their protein expression pattern, the frequency of certain cell types like alveolar brush cells and lipid-containing interstitial cells (lipofibroblasts), and the ultrastructural organization of lamellar bodies in type II alveolar epithelial cells. All these structural elements have features characteristic of the human lung that are not found in rodents.[14]

WALL STRUCTURE OF CONDUCTING AIRWAYS

The wall of conducting airways consists of three major components (Figs. 2-6 and 2-7): (1) a mucosa composed of an epithelial and a connective tissue lamina; (2) a smooth muscle sleeve; and (3) an enveloping connective tissue tube partly provided with cartilage.[15]

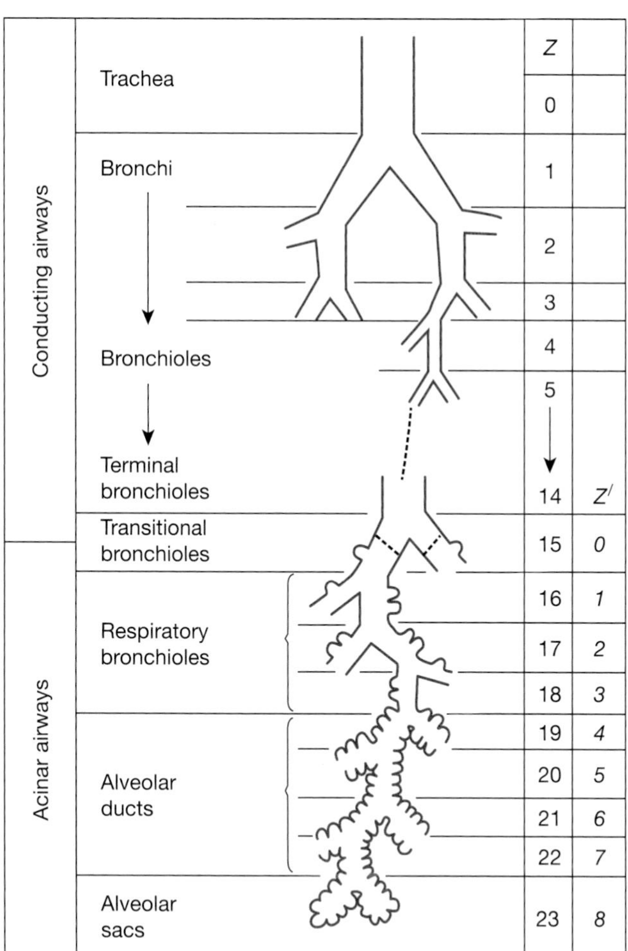

Figure 2-5 Model of airway branching in human lung by regularized dichotomy from trachea (generation z = 0) to alveolar ducts and sacs (generations 19–23). The first 14 generations are purely conducting; transitional airways (generation 15) lead into the acinar airways with alveoli that branch over 8 generations (z′). *(Modified with permission from Weibel ER: Morphometry of the Human Lung. Heidelberg: Springer-Verlag; 1963.)*

EPITHELIUM

Although derived from same anlage,[16,17] the airway epithelium modifies its differentiation characteristics as we proceed from large bronchi over bronchioles to the alveolar region (Fig. 2-6). A simple epithelium exists as a lining of smaller bronchioles: As we move upward toward larger bronchi, the epithelium becomes higher and some basal cells appear, making the epithelium pseudostratified. At the point of transition into the gas-exchange region – that is, at the entrance into the complex of alveoli – the epithelium abruptly becomes extremely thin. Figure 2-6 also shows that the epithelium is not made of a uniform cell population but that it is, at each level, rather a mosaic of at least two cell types, in that secretory cells as well as some rarer special cells are interspersed into the complex of lining cells.[15,18]

If we first have a closer look at the epithelium of larger conducting airways, we see that the lining cells are provided with a tuft of kinocilia at their apical cell face, whereas the secretory cells are goblet cells that produce and discharge to the surface a sticky mucus (Figs. 2-7–2-9). This mucus spreads out as a thin blanket on top of the cilia, which are embedded in a periciliary layer containing a dense network of mucins and mucopolysaccharides tethered to the cilia.[19] The mucus layer is capable of trapping dust particles that are still contained in the air entering the lung. Kinocilia (Fig. 2-10) are motile cell extensions that are known to beat rhythmically in a given direction and at a frequency of about 12 to 20 Hz.[20,21] In the airway epithelium, the cilia are oriented in such a fashion that their beat is directed outward. It is interesting that the cilia of airway epithelia develop at their tip fine claws with which they can grasp the mucus blanket in the phase of their forward beat, whereas on their return to the upright position they glide past the mucus blanket. The result of this is that the mucus blanket, together with trapped foreign material, moves outward or "up the airways" in a steady stream, a feature appropriately called the mucociliary escalator. Since the lining by ciliated cells is uninterrupted from the bronchioles, up the bronchi, to the trachea, this mucociliary escalator ends at the larynx, so that the normal fate of bronchial mucus is to be steadily discharged into the pharynx, whence it is swallowed, usually unnoticed. Only when an excessive amount of mucus accumulates in the trachea or in larger bronchi do we have to assist the system by coughing.

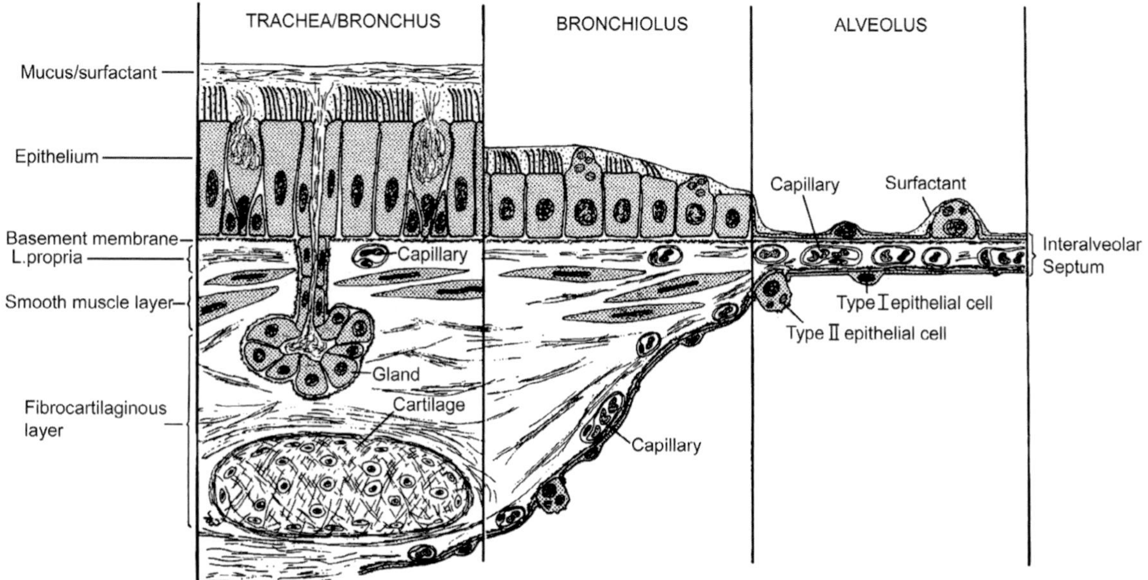

Figure 2-6 Airway wall structure at the three principal levels. The epithelial layer gradually becomes reduced from pseudostratified to cuboidal and then to squamous but retains its organization as a mosaic of lining and secretory cells. The smooth muscle layer disappears in the alveoli. The fibrous layer contains cartilage only in bronchi and gradually becomes thinner as the alveolus is approached.

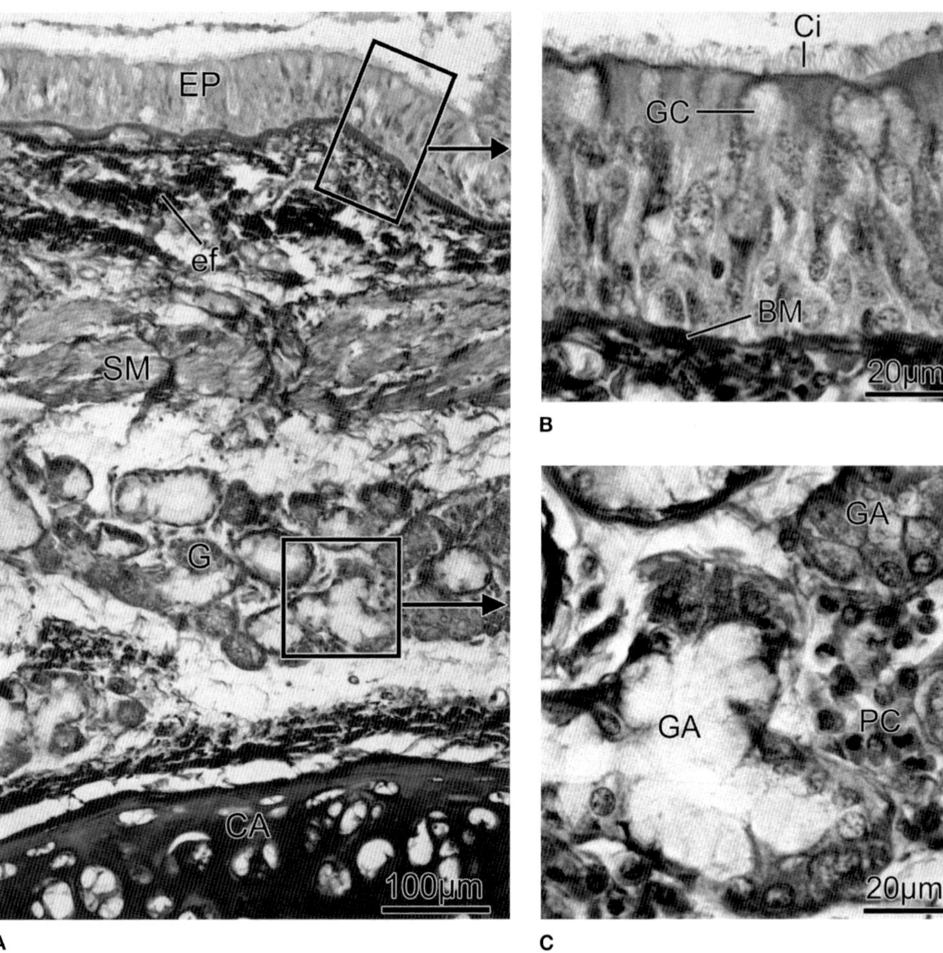

Figure 2-7 Light micrographs of bronchial wall. **A.** The layers from epithelium (EP) to cartilage (CA) with elastic fibers (ef), smooth muscle bundles (SM), and glands (G). **B.** Higher power of pseudostratified epithelium with cilia (Ci). **C.** Details of gland with acini (GA) associated with groups of plasma cells (PC). BM, basement membrane; GC, goblet cell.

The secretory cell population shows a number of specialized features. In the bronchi of all sizes and in larger bronchioles, one finds goblet cells interspersed between the ciliated cells; they form the mucus in their endoplasmic reticulum and Golgi complex, store it as droplets in their apical part, and discharge it in bulk (Figs. 2-8 and 2-9). In larger bronchi, one finds, in addition, small mucus glands located in the connective tissue; they are connected to the bronchial surface by long and narrow ducts (Figs. 2-6 and 2-7). In the normal bronchus, the glandular acini are relatively small and composed of serous and mucus cells; enlargement of the acini and a relative increase of mucus cells are characteristics of chronic bronchitis.

Finally, a special nonciliated secretory cell appears in the smaller bronchioles, the club cell (Clara) (Fig. 2-11).[22,23] This cell population is very heterogeneous, thus displaying both interspecies and intraspecies variations.[24–28] In the human lung, club cells account for about

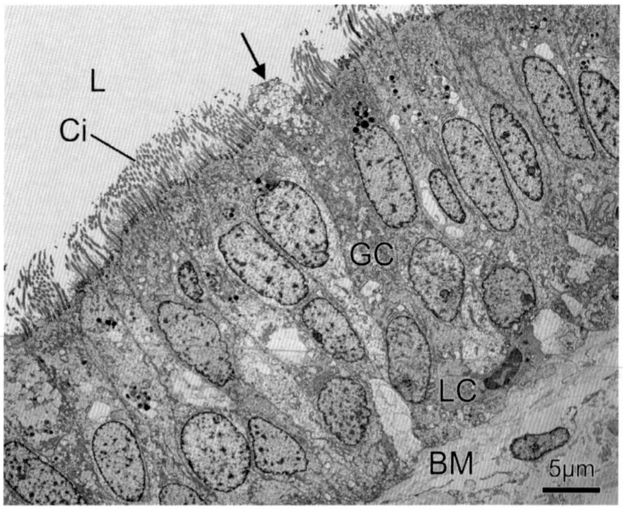

Figure 2-8 Electron micrograph of section across human bronchial epithelium made of high-columnar cells, most of which are ciliated (Ci). A goblet cell (GC) is cut lengthwise; note mucus droplets in process of accumulating at cell apex *(arrow)* and leukocyte (LC) caught in epithelium in process of diapedesis. BM, basement membrane; L, lumen.

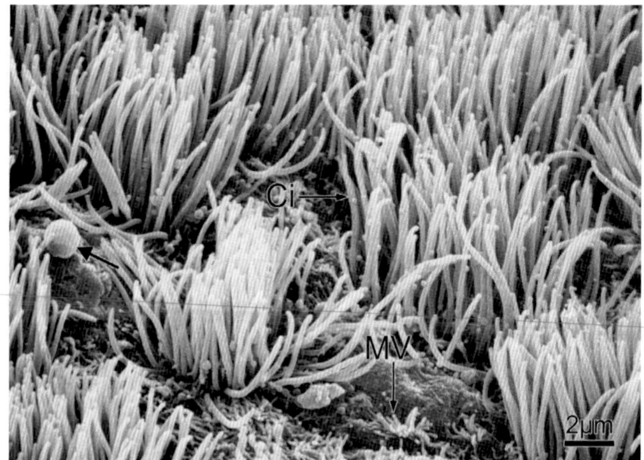

Figure 2-9 Surface view of bronchiolar epithelium shows tufts of cilia (Ci) forming on individual ciliated cells and microvilli (MV) on other cells. Note secretion droplet in process of release from goblet cell *(arrow)*.

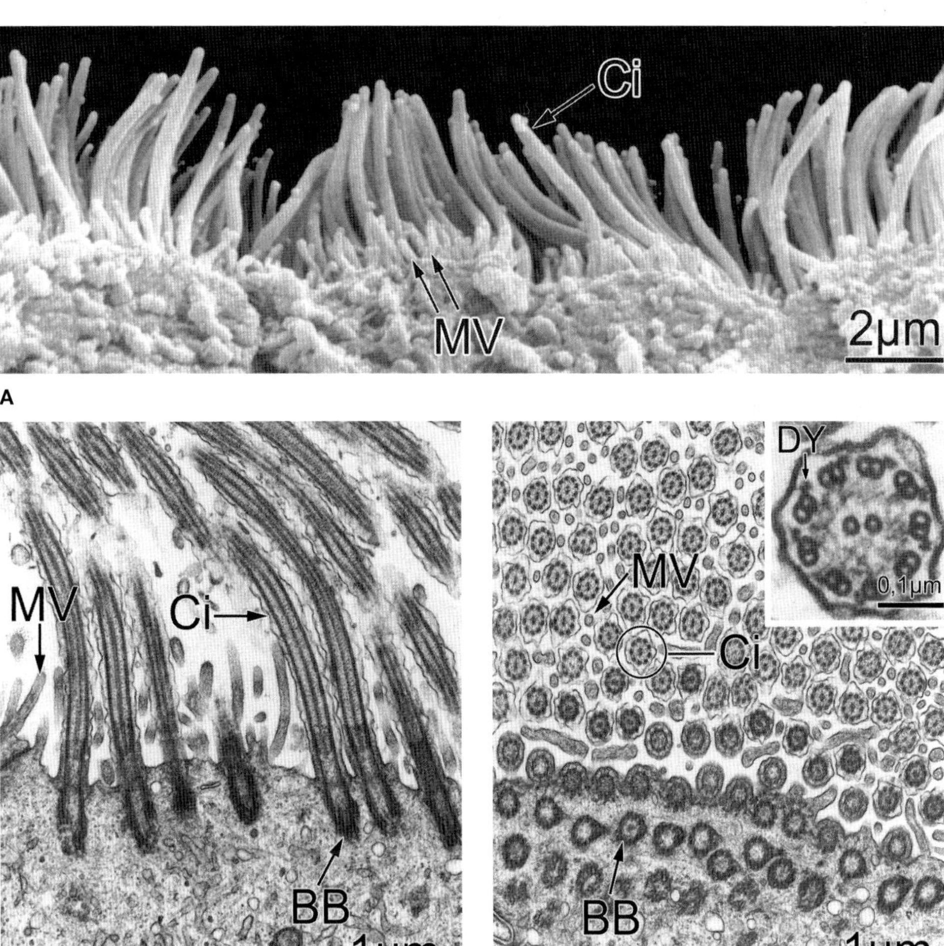

Figure 2-10 Cilia (Ci) from human bronchial epithelium seen on sections of epithelial cells in scanning electron micrograph (**A**), and on thin sections in longitudinal (**B**), and oblique cross section (**C**). They are implanted in the epithelial cell by a basal body (BB). Cross-sectioned cilium at high power (*inset*, **C**) reveals its membrane, which is enveloping a typical set of two axial tubules and nine peripheral duplex tubules with dynein arm (DY) attached. Note abundant short microvilli (MV) interspersed between cilia.

11% and 22% of the total epithelial cell number in terminal and respiratory bronchioles, respectively.[29] Besides the absence of cilia, club cells in conventional preparations are characterized by their dome-shaped apex that protrudes into the airway lumen. In contrast to that in rodents, where this cell is rich in smooth endoplasmic reticulum, club cells in the human lung lack significant amounts of smooth ER. They possess short lateral cytoplasmic extensions while their basal surface that rests on the basement membrane is practically free of infoldings. Membrane-bound electron-dense granules of about 500 to 600 nm diameter are present, which underlines their secretory activity. Our understanding of the functions of club cells is still incomplete. In many aspects, they appear to be functionally related to the secretory cell type of the alveoli, the type II alveolar epithelial cell; ultrastructural features and expression patterns of lung adenocarcinoma cells show characteristics of both club and type II cells. Club cell secretions add to the lining layer of the distal lung. Club cells synthesize and secrete the club cell secretory protein (CCSP),[22] which has been shown to be structurally similar to rabbit uteroglobin. The exact function of CCSP in the human lung still remains to be elucidated. CCSP levels in BAL fluid are decreased in smokers and in patients with COPD or interstitial lung diseases.[30] Animal studies suggest immunomodulatory functions for CCSP.[28] Within the lung, the club cell is the primary site of cytochrome P450 monooxygenase activity. Thus, they are heavily involved in detoxification of xenobiotics. Normal bronchiolar epithelial homeostasis is maintained by proliferation of club cells, whereas a cell population termed "variant Clara cells" or "variant CCSP-expressing cells," which is associated with neuroepithelial bodies or localized at bronchioloalveolar duct junctions, appears to act as progenitor cells for the bronchiolar epithelium under certain pathologic conditions.[28,31]

There are also some additional rarer cells. Neuroendocrine cells are capable of secreting mediators (amines and neuropeptides) into subepithelial capillaries. Prior to secretion, the bioactive substances are stored in dense-cored vesicles (Fig. 2-12). Occasionally, but only rarely in the adult human lung, these cells are organized in extensively innervated groups, and then termed "neuroepithelial bodies." Although it seems clear that neuroepithelial bodies have sensory, most likely oxygen-sensing, properties, their exact physiologic function is still poorly understood.[32–36] Another rare cell type of the airway epithelium is the brush cell. These cells are characterized by the presence of an apical tuft of blunt, broad, and straight microvilli with root-like structures composed of filaments extending into the cytoplasm (Fig. 2-13). Glycogen granules, vesicles, and smooth endoplasmic reticulum are usually present as well. There is species variation in the occurrence of brush cells. While common in rodents (in rats even present in the proximal alveolar epithelium[37]) they are only rarely found in the human lung. Their function is only partly explored. Owing to their ultrastructure and their strategic localization in the airways and at alveolar duct bifurcations, sensory/chemoreceptor as well as sentinel/immune surveillance functions have been proposed.[38,39] Recent evidence suggests that brush cells "taste" the chemical composition of the airway lining fluid.[40,41]

■ INTERSTITIUM

The layer of connective tissue in the bronchial mucosa consists predominantly of elastic fibers that are oriented longitudinally;

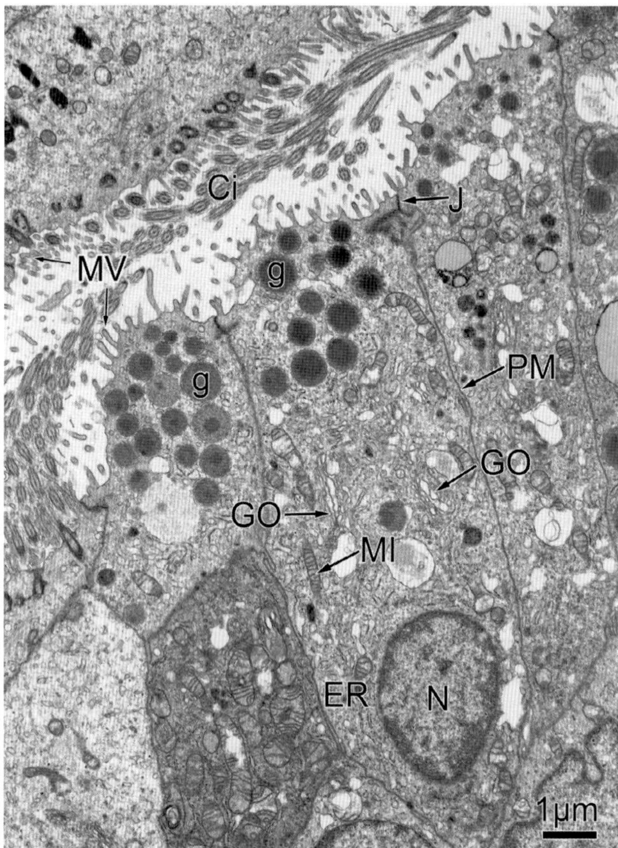

Figure 2-11 Club cells from human bronchiolar epithelium contain dense secretion granules (g) at apex. Note abundant cytoplasmic organelles such as mitochondria (MI), Golgi complex (GO), or endoplasmic reticulum (ER) as well as microvilli (MV) at surface. Cell membranes are closely apposed and form tight junctions (J) at apical edge. Ci, cilia; N, nucleus; PM, plasma membrane.

these fibers serve to maintain a smooth outline of the longitudinal profile of the bronchial lumen no matter how much the bronchi are stretched as the lungs are inflated. In this connective tissue lamina there are foci of lymphoid cells; often they form small lymphoid follicles.[42] However, bronchus-associated lymphoid tissue (BALT) is usually absent in normal adult human lungs and develops only after stimulation when inducible BALT might organize local immune responses.[43–46]

Smooth muscle bundles form a continuous sleeve in the connective tissue underlying the epithelial tube that extends from the major bronchi to the respiratory bronchioles; beyond the respiratory bronchioles, the bundles extend into the wall of alveolar ducts where the muscle fibers lie in the alveolar entrance rings. The bundles have an oblique course and encircle the mucosal tube in a criss-cross pattern; hence, their contraction results primarily in a narrowing of the lumen.

In the small bronchioles there is little else to the airway wall; the smooth muscle layer is ensheathed by a layer of delicate connective tissue that is in direct contact with adjacent alveoli (Fig. 2-6). In the larger bronchioles and even more in the bronchi, the outer connective tissue sheath forms a strong layer of fibers; in the bronchi, rings or plates of cartilage are incorporated into this layer.

The wall structure in the respiratory bronchioles is identical to that of terminal bronchioles except that in some regions the cuboidal epithelium is replaced by an alveolar epithelium of squamous cells (type I cells) closely apposed to capillaries. Very often, these single alveoli constitute outpouchings in these regions; sometimes simple "respiratory patches" form in the bronchiolar wall (see below).

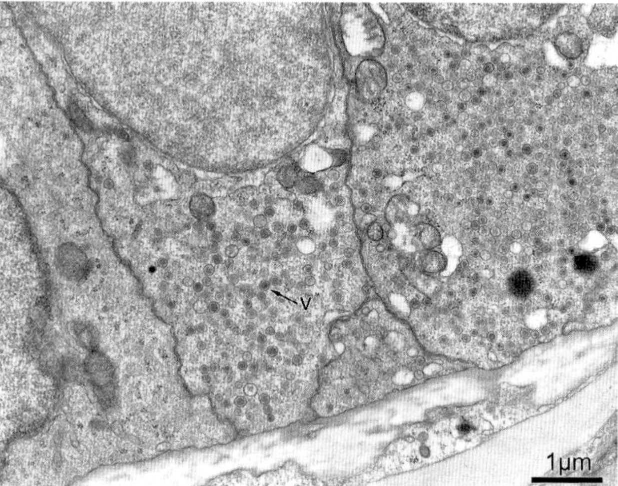

Figure 2-12 Basal part of neuroendocrine cell of human bronchiolar epithelium showing dense-cored vesicles (v). *(Reproduced with permission from Weibel ER. Lung cell biology, in Fishman A, Fisher AB, eds. Handbook of Physiology. Section 3: The Respiratory System. vol 1. Bethesda, MD: American Physiological Society; 1985:47–91.)*

WALL STRUCTURE OF CONDUCTING BLOOD VESSELS

The endothelial lining of pulmonary arteries and veins differs from that of capillaries by some site-specific structural and functional differences.[47–49] The endothelium of conducting blood vessels is thicker, and parts of its cytoplasm are richly endowed with organelles of various kinds (Fig. 2-14). Clearly, these cells are metabolically more active than those of the capillary endothelium. They are particularly rich in membrane-bound rod-shaped granules termed Weibel–Palade bodies,[50,51] which represent the regulated secretory organelles of endothelial cells (Fig. 2-14). The lumen of

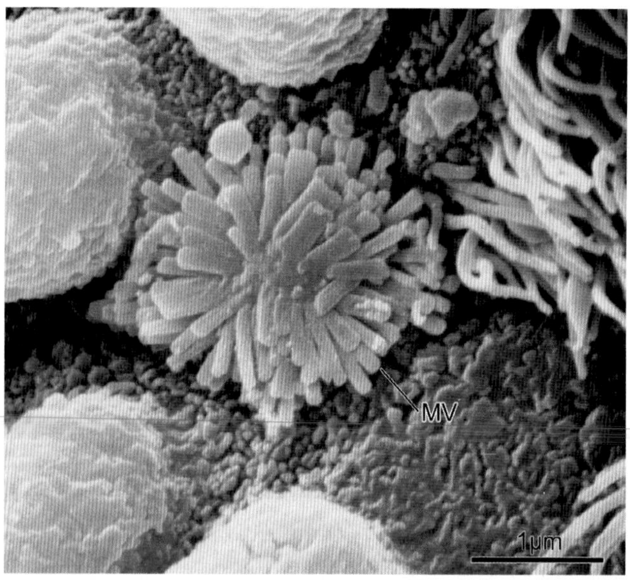

Figure 2-13 Brush cell from small bronchiole of rat lung containing broad microvilli (MV). *(Reproduced with permission from Weibel ER: Lung cell biology, in Fishman A, Fisher AB, eds. Handbook of Physiology. Section 3: The Respiratory System. vol 1. Bethesda, MD: American Physiological Society; 1985:47–91.)*

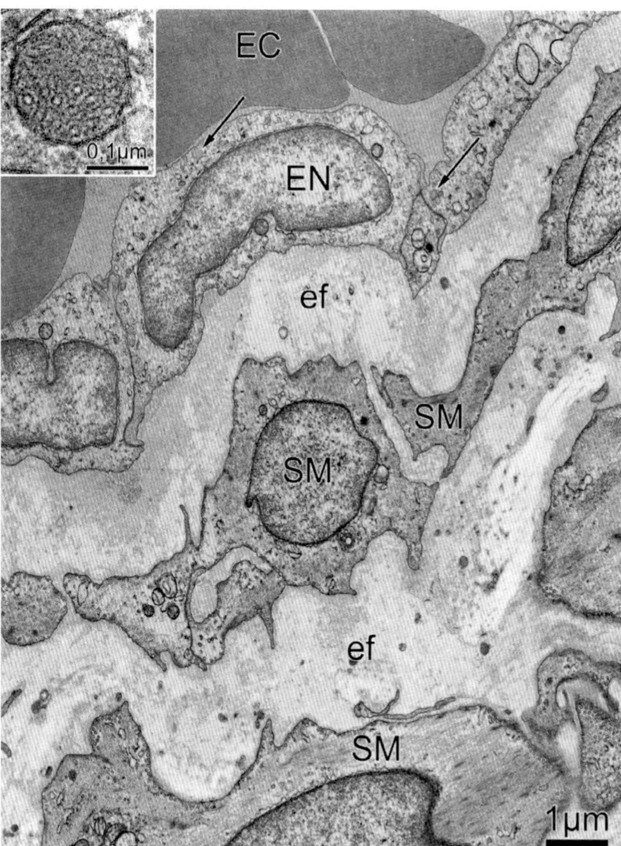

Figure 2-14 Part of wall of pulmonary artery from human lung. Endothelial cells (EN) form thick layer; their cytoplasm is rich in organelles. Specific granules of endothelium *(arrows)*, a cross-section of one of which is shown at high power in the inset, are enveloped by a membrane and contain tubules. The arterial wall is of the elastic type, formed of alternating layers of smooth muscle (SM) and elastic fibers (ef). EC, erythrocyte.

Weibel–Palade bodies is filled with longitudinally arranged tubules. These tubules represent von Willebrand factor,[52] packed in a highly organized spiral that allows rapid secretion into the blood. Other components of Weibel–Palade bodies include tissue-type plasminogen activator, endothelin-1, the leukocyte adhesion receptor P-selectin, interleukin-8, the tetraspanin CD63/LAMP-3, and the small GTPase Rab27a. Thus, Weibel–Palade bodies are actively involved in hemostasis as well as in vasoactive and inflammatory responses.[53–56]

Many of the nonrespiratory metabolic functions of the lung – particularly the transformation of certain bioactive substances, such as angiotensin and prostaglandins – are performed in endothelial cells. Caveolae (or plasmalemmal vesicles) have been implicated in these processes.[57,58] Caveolae are plasma membrane invaginations and associated vesicles with an outer diameter of about 50 to 70 nm. Depending on fixation, the shape of these invaginations appears omega- or cup-like.[59] Their structural framework consists of members of the caveolin family of proteins associated with cholesterol and sphingolipids. Caveolae perform transport and signaling functions and are involved in membrane organization. All endocytic activity mediated by caveolae (thereby bypassing the clathrin-coated vesicle pathway) is pooled under the term potocytosis.[60–63]

Accessory structures develop in the wall in accord with the functional properties of the vessels. Thus, the walls of the major pulmonary arteries that are close to the heart, and therefore exposed to the pressure oscillations of large amplitude prevailing in the outflow tract of the right ventricle, are of the elastic type, that is, layers of elastic lamellae are interconnected with smooth muscle cells as in the aorta; the tone of the smooth muscle regulates the elastic modulus of the vessel wall, thereby controlling the shape of the pulse wave. In the pulmonary arterial tree, this pattern prevails out to branches of about 1 mm diameter.

In contrast, branches less than l mm in diameter are of the muscular type, that is, the smooth muscle fibers encircle the vessel lumen; they can modify the vessel's cross-section and can thus regulate blood flow through this vessel. Compared with systemic arteries, the thickness of the pulmonary arterial wall is reduced about in proportion to systolic pressure, that is, by about a factor of 1:5; in pulmonary hypertension, the wall becomes thicker. Although arterioles are a well-defined entity in the systemic vascular bed, where they constitute the major site of arterial resistance, pulmonary arterioles are more difficult to locate and define. A single muscle layer – the histologic definition of an arteriole – does occur in branches about 100 μm in diameter, but the arterial bed continues out to the precapillaries, which consist of vessels 20 to 40 μm in diameter that are enwrapped by an incomplete smooth muscle sheath. This poverty of smooth muscle contributes importantly to the low resistance to blood flow that is normally afforded by the pulmonary arterial tree.

The structure of pulmonary veins is similar to that of systemic veins in the upper half of the organism. Their walls are rich in connective tissue and contain irregular bundles of smooth muscle. Larger veins contain a large amount of elastic tissue. More extensive in rodents, but to a certain degree also in humans, cardiac muscle tissue from the left atrial myocardium forms sleeves in the adventitia of pulmonary veins where they overlap with the smooth muscle of the venous wall. The arrangement of the myocardial sleeves correlates with the distribution of foci of ectopic beats initiating atrial fibrillation.[64–67]

NUTRITIVE VESSELS AND NERVES

The tissue of lung parenchyma is very well supplied with blood; the fact that it is venous is of no disadvantage, because O_2 is easily obtained from the air. Thus, nutrient supply from pulmonary arteries combined with O_2 supply from air appears to suffice not only for the parenchyma but also for bronchioles and the smaller pulmonary vessels, whose outer surface is almost directly exposed to air. The thicker-walled bronchi, with their glands and cartilage, require a nutrient blood supply from bronchial arteries.[15,68,69] These derive in part directly from anterior branches of the aorta and partly from the upper intercostal arteries. They course alongside the esophagus and penetrate on both sides into the hilum. The bronchial arteries extend to the most peripheral bronchi but not into the walls of bronchioles. On the other hand, some branches supply large pulmonary vessels as vasa vasorum, whereas others course along larger septa to reach the pleura. Some bronchial arteries form anastomoses with peripheral branches of the pulmonary arteries. There have been long discussions about the role that such anastomoses may play. It seems that in the normal lung their importance has been overrated. However, in certain pathologic conditions, such as bronchiectasis and tumors, the bronchial arteries and perhaps the bronchopulmonary anastomoses appear to play an important role. They also enlarge to form a collateral circulation when branches of the pulmonary artery are obliterated. The peribronchovascular space around larger pulmonary artery branches and bronchi with its capillaries from the bronchial circulation has also been proposed as a unique compartment since it is a preferential site of leukocyte infiltration and edema formation under pathologic conditions.[70] Furthermore, the bronchial circulation attenuates ischemia–reperfusion lung injury. Consequently, interruption of the bronchial circulation without revascularization during lung transplantation often leads to bronchial anastomotic complications.

Except for a few bronchial veins in the hilar region, the bronchial system does not have its own venous drainage into the systemic veins. Instead, the bronchial veins, which begin as a peribronchial venous plexus, drain into pulmonary veins; this drainage seems to constitute one source of normal venous admixture to arterial blood.

The lung is innervated by the autonomic nervous system. The parasympathetic fibers are derived from the vagal nerves and the sympathetic fibers from the upper thoracic and cervical ganglia; together they form the pulmonary nervous plexus in the region of the hilum before entering the lung. The fiber bundles follow the major bronchi and blood vessels, finally penetrating into the acini; some nerves also supply the pleura. In addition, motor nerves influence the smooth muscle tone of airways and blood vessels, and sensory nerves are involved in reflex functions (e.g., cough reflex, Hering–Breuer reflex). Moreover, the secretory function of glands as well as of type II alveolar epithelial cells is at least partly under control of this nervous system. Nerve fibers are easily found in the wall of bronchioles and bronchi, where they often follow the course of bronchial arteries. However, fibers in alveolar septa are small and scarce.

THE CELLS OF THE ALVEOLAR REGION

BASIC DESIGN OF THE GAS-EXCHANGE BARRIER

Efficient gas exchange in the lung depends on a very thin barrier of very large surface between air and blood.[16,71] Actually, the barrier is so thin that it cannot be resolved into its constituents by light microscopy. Nevertheless, this barrier must be built of the three minimal tissue layers: an endothelium lining the capillaries, an epithelium lining the airspaces, and an interstitial layer to house the connective tissue fibers. The guiding principle in designing these cells must evidently be to minimize thickness and maximize extent. However, there is definitely a limit to this, set by the need to make the barrier and its constituent cells strong enough to resist the various forces that act on it: capillary blood pressure, tissue tension, and surface tension, in particular. Furthermore, the barrier must remain intact for a lifetime, and this requires continuous repair and turnover of the cells and their components. As a result, about half of the surface of the air–blood barrier is optimized for gas exchange in that the thin epithelial and endothelial cell extensions are only separated by a fused basement membrane. These areas are termed the thin parts of the air–blood barrier. Cell nuclei and connecting tissue fibers are concentrated in the so-called thick parts of the air–blood barrier.

In spite of this delicacy of tissue structure, we find that three-quarters of all the lung cells by volume or weight are contained in the lung parenchyma (Table 2-1). We also note that epithelium and endothelium make up about one-quarter each of the tissue barrier in the alveolar walls, whereas interstitial cells amount to 35%; the interstitial space with the connective tissue fibers makes up no more than 15% of the barrier.[11,72]

TABLE 2-1 Estimated Cell Volumes in the Human Lung

Cell or Tissue	Volume (mL)	Percent Septal Tissue
Tissue (excl. blood)	284	—
Nonparenchyma	99	—
Alveolar septa	185	—
Cells	213	—
Nonparenchyma	50	—
Alveolar septa	163	—
Parenchymal cells	163	—
Alveolar epithelium type I	23	12.6
Alveolar epithelium type II	18	9.7
Capillary endothelium	49	26.4
Interstitial cells	66	35.8
Alveolar macrophages	7	3.9

Source: Reproduced with permission from Weibel ER: The Pathway for Oxygen. Cambridge, MA: Harvard University Press; 1984.

ALVEOLAR EPITHELIUM

The alveolar epithelium is a mosaic of different cell types. The vast majority of the total surface is lined by a single layer of squamous cells; the remaining fraction – only about 3% (Table 2-2) – is occupied by cuboidal secretory cells; one usually calls the squamous lining cells type I and the secretory cells type II alveolar epithelial cells or pneumocytes. Type I and II cells occur with a numerical frequency of about 1:2. A very rare third cell type, the brush cell, can be found in some specific regions near the entrance of the acinus (see above).

The fine structural details of the different types of alveolar epithelial cells can only be fully visualized by electron microscopy, whereas molecular markers selective for either type I or II cells or some of their constituents can be detected and localized by light microscopy (Fig. 2-15; Table 2-3).

Type I Alveolar Epithelial Cells

At first glance, the squamous type I cells show rather simple design features (Fig. 2-16). Their small, compact nucleus is surrounded by a slim rim of cytoplasm, where one finds a modest basic set of organelles, a few small mitochondria, and some cisternae of endoplasmic reticulum, seemingly the picture of a quiescent cell with no great metabolic activity.[11,73]

At the edge of the perinuclear region, a very attenuated cytoplasmic leaflet emerges (Fig. 2-16) and spreads out broadly over the basal lamina. This leaflet is made essentially of the two plasma membranes forming the apical and basal cell face, respectively, with a very small amount of cytoplasmic ground substance interposed (Fig. 2-17). Here one rarely finds any organelles except for the numerous plasmalemmal vesicles implied in the transcellular transport of molecules. In fact, besides capillary endothelial cells, type I alveolar epithelial cells are among the richest in caveolae.

TABLE 2-2 Morphometric Characteristics of Cell Population in Human Pulmonary Parenchyma

Cell Population	Percent of Total Cell Number[a]	Average Cell Volume (μm^3)	Average Apical Cell Surface (μm^2)
Alveolar epithelium			
Type I	8	1764	5098
Type II	16	889	183
Endothelium	30	632	1353
Interstitial cells	36	637	—
Alveolar macrophages	10	2492	—

[a] Total cell number in human lung 230 × 10^9.
Source: Data from Crapo JD, Barry BE, Gehr P, Bachofen M, Weibel ER: Cell number and cell characteristics of the normal human lung. Am Rev Respir Dis. 1982;125:332–337.

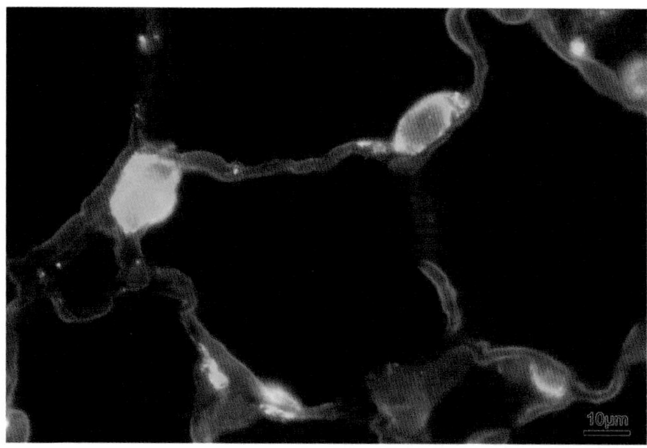

Figure 2-15 Immunofluorescent double labeling of alveolar epithelial cells. Type I cells are stained for Lycopersicon esculentum lectin *(red)*, type II cells are stained for SP-D *(green)*. Compare with Table 2-3. *(Micrograph used with permission of H. Fehrenbach.)*

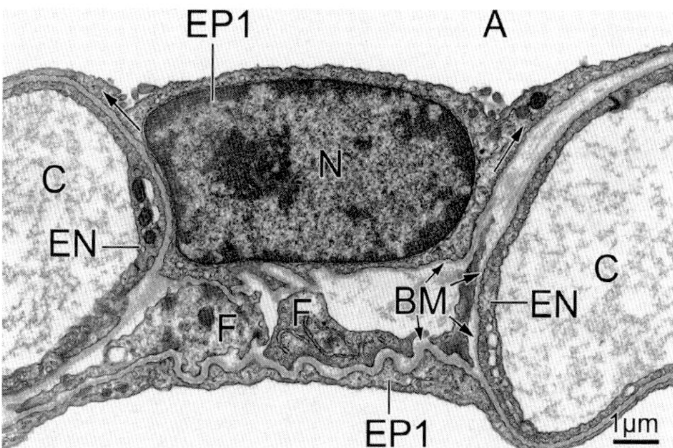

Figure 2-16 A type I alveolar epithelial cell (EP1) from human lung. The nucleus (N) is surrounded by very little cytoplasm, which extends as thin leaflets *(arrows)* to cover the capillaries (C). Note the basement membranes (BM) of the epithelium and endothelium (EN), which become fused in a minimal barrier. Interstitial space contains fibroblast processes (F).

The surface covered by one type I epithelial cell is about 4000 to 5000 μm^2. In some texts one may find the type I cell called the "small alveolar cell" because of its small nucleus; clearly this is a misnomer, as the type I cell is a rather large cell indeed, with respect to both surface and cell volume (Table 2-2). Terminal bars are formed where the cytoplasmic leaflets of epithelial cells meet (Fig. 2-18). If one looks at the surface of the alveolar epithelium in scanning electron micrographs (Fig. 2-19), one notes that the patches covered by single type I cells are variable in size and that even the largest are much smaller than the 4000 to 5000 μm^2 given earlier, a number derived by dividing the total alveolar surface by the total number of type I cell nuclei. Why is this? There seem to be three to four times as many type I cell domains encircled by terminal bars as there are nuclei. Indeed, this observation was already made some 130 years ago by Albert Kölliker; his interpretation was that part of the alveolar surface was lined by "nonnuclear" cytoplasmic plates rather than by complete cells. It turns out that an alternative explanation is possible. One finds that type I cells are not simple squamous cells but rather branched cells with multiple apical faces, as shown diagrammatically in Figure 2-20. Thus, what appears as nonnucleated plates are cytoplasmic domains connected to the perinuclear region by a stalk, spreading out on one side of the alveolar wall or the other; it is evident that several such domains may share a nucleus.[74]

Although type I cells cover about 97% of the alveolar surface area, they have long been neglected as being "silent," providing solely a barrier function. Although their overall function in the human lung remains to be determined, recent animal and in vitro studies strongly suggest that type I cells are actively involved in alveolar ion and fluid homeostasis.[75–77]

TABLE 2-3 Markers for Alveolar Epithelial Cells

Type I Cell	Type II Cell
HTI-56 (human)	Surfactant proteins:
T1α/RTI-40 (rat, mouse)	SP-A
Aquaporin 5	SP-B
Caveolin 1	SP-C
Receptors for advanced glycation end products	SP-D
(RAGE)	ABCA3
Carboxypeptidase M	HTII-280 (human)
Lectins:	RTII-70 (rat)
Lycopersicon esculentum	MMC4 (rat)
Bauhinia purpurea	Alkaline phosphatase
Ricinus communis 1	CD44
	Lectins:
	Maclura pomifera

These markers allow a selective distinction between type I and type II alveolar epithelial cells and can be visualized at a light microscopic level by immunohistochemistry, enzyme histochemistry, or lectin histochemistry. However, other cell types of the distal bronchiolar and alveolar region, e.g., Club cells, capillary endothelial cells, or alveolar macrophages, might also stain positive for some of these markers.
Source: Data from Fehrenbach H. Alveolar epithelial type II cell: defender of the alveolus revisited. Respir Res. 2001;2:33–46; Griffiths MJD, Bonnet D, Janes SM. Stem cells of the alveolar epithelium. Lancet. 2005;366:249–260; Gonzales RF, Allen L, Gonzales L, Ballard PL, Dobbs LG. HTII-280, a biomarker specific to the apical plasma membrane of human lung alveolar type II cells. J Histochem Cytochem. 2010;58:891–901.

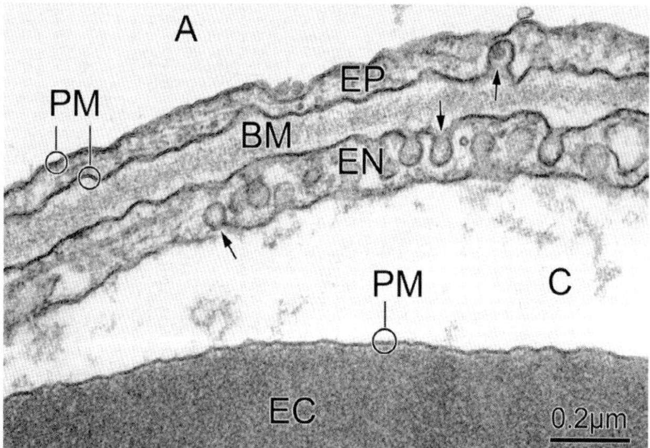

Figure 2-17 Thin, minimal tissue barrier between alveolar air (A) and capillary blood (C) is made of cytoplasmic leaflets of epithelium (EP) and endothelium (EN), joined by fused basement membranes (BM). Note that the epithelial and endothelial leaflets are bounded by plasma membranes (PM), as is the erythrocyte (EC). *Arrows* point to pinocytotic vesicles/caveolae. *(Reproduced with permission from Weibel ER: The Pathway for Oxygen. Cambridge, MA: Harvard University Press; 1984.)*

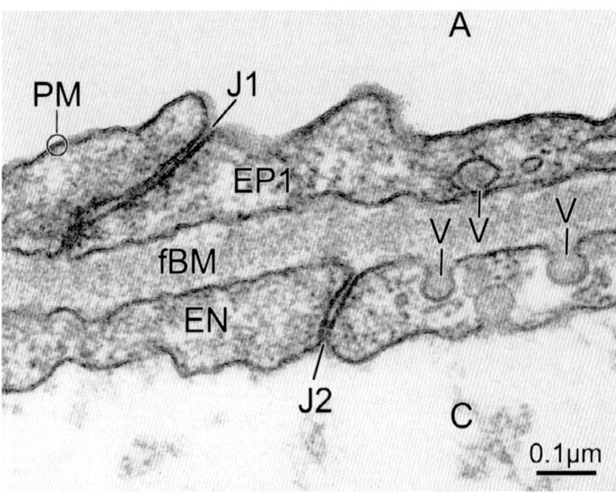

Figure 2-18 Minimal barrier part showing intercellular junctions. Between type I epithelial cells, a "tight" junction (J1) is formed by close apposition of the cell membranes over a comparatively wide band; the junction between endothelial cells (J2) is "leaky" because membranes become apposed over a narrow strip only. Note trilaminar structure of plasma membranes (PM), the occurrence of pinocytotic vesicles/caveolae (V) in both epithelium and endothelium (EN), and the fused basement membranes (fBM). A, alveolus; C, capillary; EP1, type I epithelial cell.

Type I cells are easily damaged, particularly because of their extensive surface area and their complex branching architecture. However, there is an additional problem: one finds that type I cells are not capable of multiplying by mitosis in vivo, neither during lung growth when more cells are needed to coat the expanding alveolar surface nor upon damage in the adult lung when cells need to be replaced. In both instances new type I cells are made by mitotic division and transformation of type II cells, a process that takes about 2 to 5 days.

This seems to work under normal circumstances. There are, however, conditions where this repair mechanism is too slow to cope with excessive damage, so that a syndrome of severe catastrophic

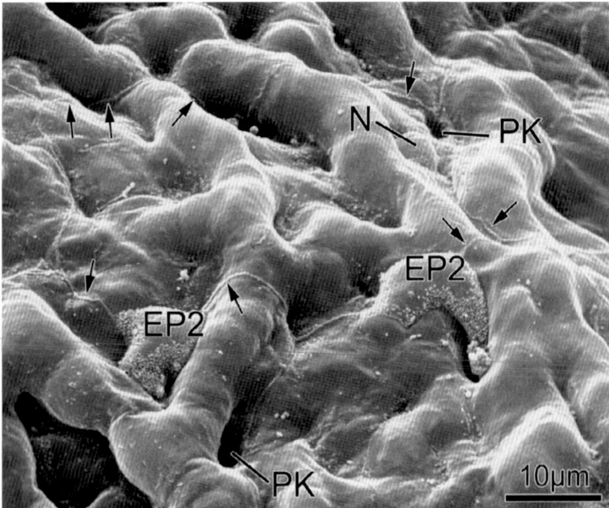

Figure 2-19 Surface of the alveolar wall in the human lung seen by scanning electron microscopy reveals a mosaic of alveolar epithelium made of type I and type II (EP2) cells. *Arrows* indicate boundary of the cytoplasmic leaflet of the type I cell which extends over many capillaries. Note the two interalveolar pores of Kohn (PK). N, nucleus of type I cell.

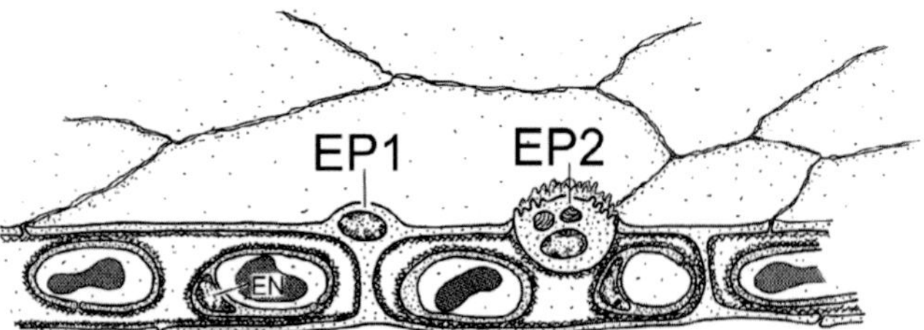

Figure 2-20 Diagram of the alveolar wall showing the complexity of a type I epithelial cell (EP1) and its relation to a type II cell (EP2) and endothelial cell (EN). *(Reproduced with permission from Weibel ER: The Pathway for Oxygen. Cambridge, MA: Harvard University Press; 1984.)*

respiratory failure, acute respiratory distress syndrome (ARDS), develops, which requires intensive care treatment. In such patients one finds large parts of the type I cell lining of the alveolar surface to be destroyed. As a consequence, the barrier has become leaky and the alveoli fill with alveolar edema, so that they can no longer take part in gas exchange.[78,79]

With proper medical care, this alveolar edema can often be resolved within a few days. The alveoli become again filled with air, but in spite of this, gas exchange does not improve. What has happened is that the repair of the severely damaged alveolar epithelium requires a lot of new cells to be made by division of type II cells.[80] These form a rather thick cuboidal lining of the barrier surface, a phenomenon termed cuboidal metaplasia, and this thick barrier offers a high resistance to O_2 flow. It takes several weeks until a thin barrier is restored by transformation of the cuboidal cell lining into delicate type I cells. During this process, the cells go through intermediate stages where they are often positive for both type II and type I cell markers.[81,82]

Type II Alveolar Epithelial Cells

The type II alveolar epithelial cell is a conspicuous but in fact relatively small cell whose mean volume is less than half that of the type I cell (Table 2-2), although it is often called the "large alveolar cell."[11] Its shape is cuboidal, the apical cell surface bulges toward the lumen and is provided, mostly around its periphery, with a tuft of microvilli (Figs. 2-21 and 2-22). Often, type II cells seem to be preferentially located in the corners of alveoli or in

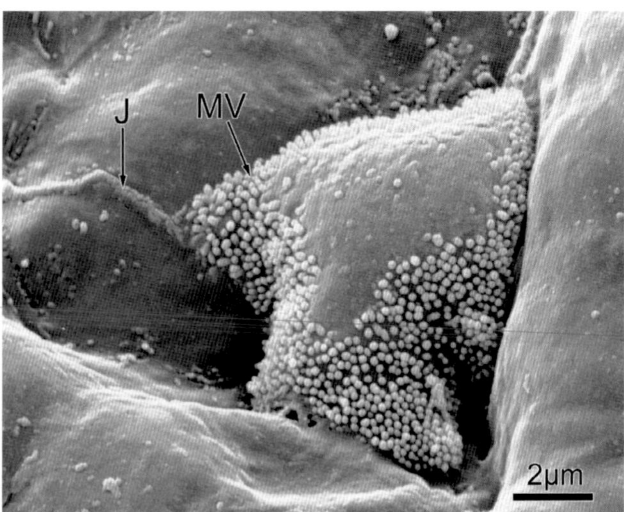

Figure 2-21 Higher magnification of a type II cell reveals a "crown" of short microvilli (MV) and a central "bald patch." Note junction lines of type I cells (J) meeting with the type II cell.

close proximity to interalveolar pores of Kohn. They are usually found as solitary cells; only in cases of alveolar epithelial damage, proliferation of type II cells leads to focal clusters during the repair process. Occasionally, a single type II cell might supply two or even three adjacent alveoli with its apical surface. The basement membrane beneath type II cells is occasionally interrupted. Through these apertures, foot processes of type II cells can extend to the interstitium and come in close proximity to interstitial cells.[83]

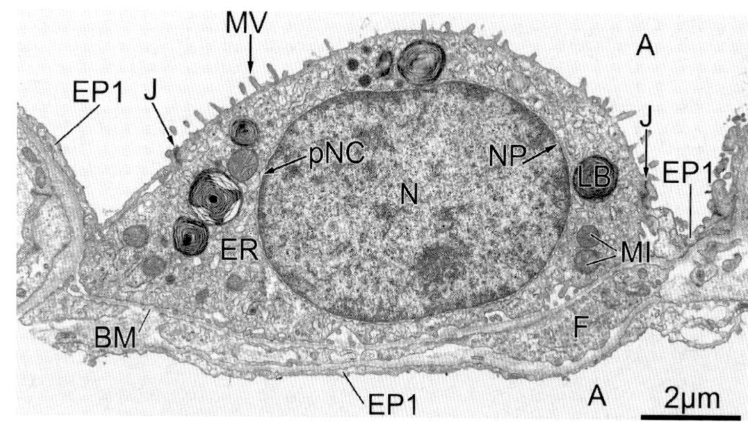

Figure 2-22 A type II epithelial cell from the human lung forms junction (J) with type I epithelial cells (EP1). Its cytoplasm contains osmiophilic lamellar bodies (LB) and a rich complement of organelles: mitochondria (MI), endoplasmic reticulum (ER), and so on. The nucleus (N) is surrounded by a perinuclear cisterna (pNC) which is perforated by nuclear pores (NP). A, alveolus; BM, basement membrane; F, fibroblast; MV, microvilli.

Type II cells contain a wealth of cytoplasmic organelles of all kinds (Fig. 2-22): mitochondria, a lot of endoplasmic reticulum with ribosomes, and a well-developed Golgi complex surrounded by a set of small lysosomal granules among which so-called multivesicular bodies – membrane-bounded organelles containing a group of small vesicles – stand out (Fig. 2-23). In addition, one finds the characteristic lamellar bodies, larger membrane-bounded secretory organelles that contain densely packed phospholipid lamellae. There are notable species differences in the ultrastructural organization of lamellar bodies. In rodents, the lamellae are mostly arranged in parallel stacks whereas in humans, concentrically arranged lamellae are mostly found, which are attached to a projection core consisting of randomly arranged short stacks of densely packed membrane segments (Fig. 2-24).[84] The periodicity of the lamellae is in the range of 4 to 6 nm. One human type II cell contains between 200 and 500 lamellar bodies, making up a total volume of about 2 cm^3 in the entire lung. With a diameter of approximately 1 μm, lamellar bodies are among the largest secretory organelles of all cells in the body. Owing to their equipment with lysosomal enzymes (e.g., acid phosphatase, cathepsins) and proteins (e.g., members of the lysosomal membrane protein (LAMP) family and their acidic pH of about 5.5, lamellar bodies are regarded as secretory lysosome-related organelles.[85]

Type II cells have two main functions: they serve as the cellular source of pulmonary surfactant and they contribute to the regeneration of the alveolar epithelium under physiologic and pathologic conditions. These properties form the basis of the concept of the type II cell as the "defender of the alveolus."[86–88]

Surfactant prevents alveolar atelectasis by a surface area–dependent reduction of the alveolar surface tension (see below).[89–92] Another function of surfactant as a result of the reduction of alveolar surface tension is to prevent the formation of intra-alveolar edema.[93] In addition, certain surfactant components have important immunomodulatory functions in the innate host defense system.[94,95] Taken together, the main functions of surfactant might be summarized as to keep alveoli open, dry, and clean. Surfactant is composed of around 90% lipids, mainly saturated phosphatidylcholine, and around 10% proteins, including the surfactant apoproteins termed SP-A, SP-B, SP-C, and SP-D. Besides its biochemical complexity, surfactant is also morphologically very heterogeneous, consisting of different surfactant subtypes with highly organized structure that represent different stages in metabolism (Figs. 2-24–2-26).[84,96]

The alveolar epithelium (including interalveolar pores of Kohn) is lined by a thin but apparently continuous fluid layer inserted between the apical cell membrane and the surface film, thus forming a duplex lining layer.[97,98] Surfactant functions in and on this layer. It is synthesized, stored, secreted, and to a large extent recycled by type II cells.[84,87,99] Therefore, an intracellular surfactant pool present in type II cells and an intra-alveolar surfactant pool present at the surface of the fluid alveolar lining layer as well as within its hypophase can be distinguished. The intracellular storage form of surfactant is represented by lamellar bodies. Prior to storage, the synthesis of surfactant material involves endoplasmic reticulum, (at least partly) Golgi complex, and multivesicular bodies. In type II cells, multivesicular bodies participate in the posttranslational processing of surfactant proteins as well as in endocytosis and subsequent recycling and/or degradation of surfactant material; thus, most probably representing the junction point between the biosynthetic and endocytotic pathway. In addition, transitional forms between multivesicular bodies and lamellar bodies, termed composite bodies, have been described. Surfactant material present in lamellar bodies is secreted into the alveolar lumen via exocytosis (Figs. 2-25 and 2-26).

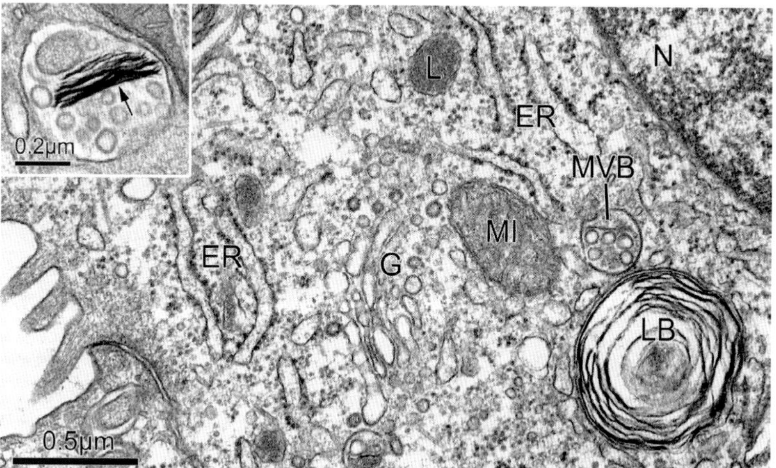

Figure 2-23 Cytoplasmic organelles of the type II cell implicated in the synthesis of surfactant are the endoplasmic reticulum (ER), Golgi complex (G), lysosomes (L), multivesicular bodies (MVB), and finally lamellar bodies (LB). The *inset* shows a large composite body with a stack of phospholipid lamellae *(arrow)*. N, nucleus. *(Reproduced with permission from Weibel ER: The Pathway for Oxygen. Cambridge, MA: Harvard University Press; 1984.)*

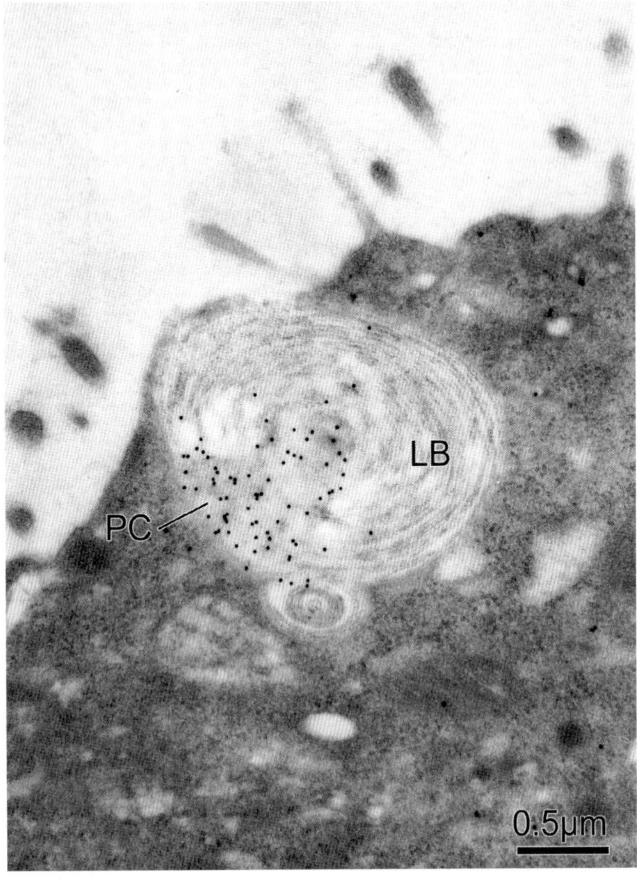

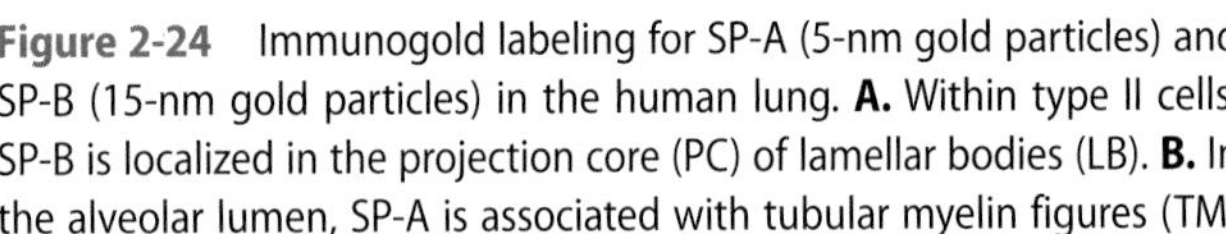

Figure 2-24 Immunogold labeling for SP-A (5-nm gold particles) and SP-B (15-nm gold particles) in the human lung. **A.** Within type II cells, SP-B is localized in the projection core (PC) of lamellar bodies (LB). **B.** In the alveolar lumen, SP-A is associated with tubular myelin figures (TM) whereas SP-B is found in the projection core (PC) of freshly secreted lamellar bodies (LB) and dense core particles *(arrow)* close to tubular myelin. UV, unilamellar vesicle.

Most surfactant components are assembled in lamellar bodies prior to secretion (Figs. 2-24–2-26)—at least the lipid fraction and the hydrophilic surfactant proteins SP-B and SP-C, whereas the hydrophilic surfactant proteins SP-A and SP-D seem to be secreted independently via a constitutive pathway bypassing the regulated exocytosis of lamellar bodies. Lamellar body secretion starts with the fusion of its limiting membrane with the apical plasma membrane, followed by formation of a fusion pore, and finally the slow release of surfactant material through the pore. The diameter of the pore is considerably smaller than that of the lamellar body. Thus, surfactant seems to be squeezed through the pore.[100] The mechanisms that regulate surfactant secretion in vivo are still not fully elucidated. It seems that, among the various stimuli that can act via several different signaling pathways, mechanical stretch during ventilation – either as a direct effect on type II cells or indirectly via type I cells or capillary endothelial cells which may act as "strain sensors" – is the physiologically most relevant.[87,99,101,102]

Intra-alveolar surfactant consists of several subtypes, namely freshly secreted lamellar body-like forms, tubular myelin, the surface film, and small unilamellar vesicles. After secretion, lamellar body-like forms in the hypophase associate with SP-A, which is separately secreted by type II cells,[103] and undergo a major

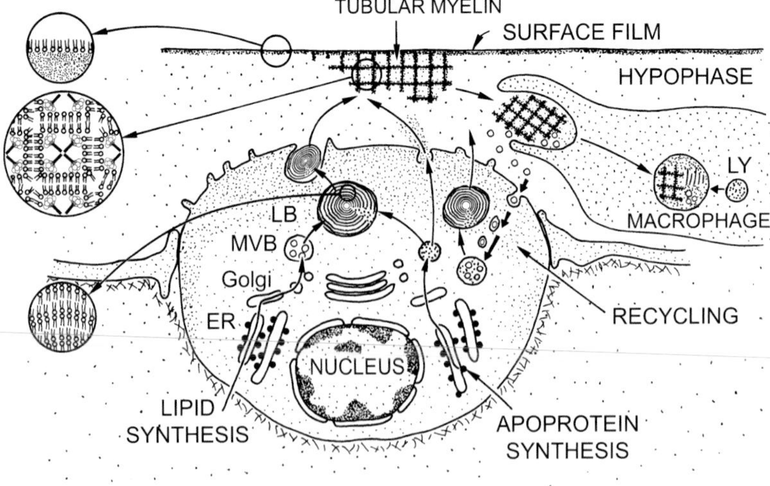

Figure 2-25 Schematic diagram of pathways for synthesis and secretion of surfactant lipids and apoproteins by a type II cell, for their recycling by type II cells, and for their removal by macrophages. Note the arrangement of phospholipids and apoproteins in the lamellar bodies, in tubular myelin, and in the surface film. *(Reproduced with permission from Weibel ER: The Pathway for Oxygen. Cambridge, MA: Harvard University Press; 1985.)*

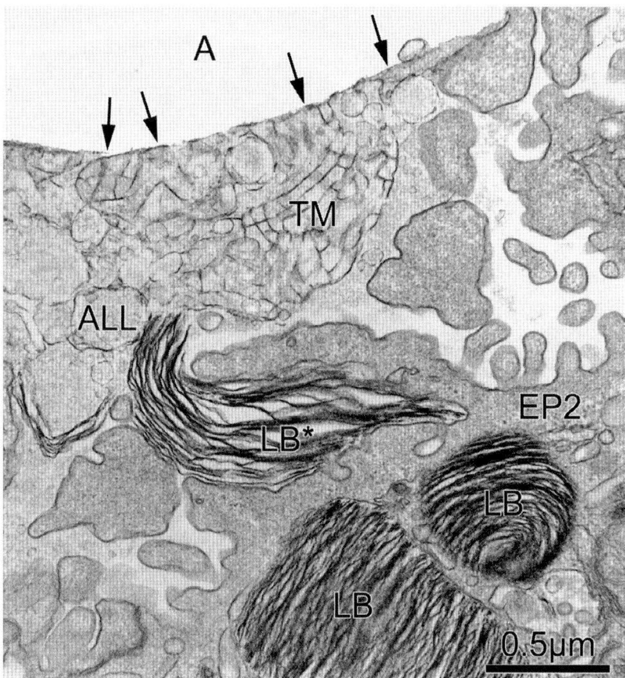

Figure 2-26 Apical part of type II cell (EP2) with lamellar bodies (LB); one of these (LB*) is seen in the process of being secreted into the alveolar surface lining layer (ALL). The free surface of the lining layer is covered by a thin black film of lipids *(arrows)*, which is connected with tubular myelin (TM) in the hypophase. *(Reproduced with permission from Weibel ER, Gil J: Structure-function relationships at the alveolar level, in West JB, ed.: Bioengineering Aspects of the Lung. New York: Springer-Verlag; 1977.)*

structural transformation into tubular myelin figures with a unique lattice-like structure.[104] The precise physiologic function of tubular myelin, however, is still unclear. Tubular myelin is thought to be the immediate precursor of the surface film, although the existence of an additional multilayered surface-associated surfactant reservoir underneath the surface film has been suggested.[96,105] "Spent" surfactant components are found in the hypophase as small unilamellar vesicles. The major route of surfactant clearance is reuptake by type II cells. Within type II cells, surfactant material can either be recycled or degraded. Other routes of surfactant clearance include ingestion and lysosomal degradation by alveolar macrophages and clearance via the airways.

After differential centrifugation of intra-alveolar surfactant material harvested by bronchoalveolar lavage, surface active large aggregates (LA), ultrastructurally largely corresponding to lamellar body-like forms and tubular myelin, and inactive small aggregates (SA), ultrastructurally largely corresponding to unilamellar vesicles, can be distinguished. Thus, the SA/LA ratio can be used to assess the biophysical activity of surfactant.[90,91]

A surfactant film, most likely mainly transported upward from the alveoli, is also present in the airways. Here, surfactant prevents collapse of smaller airways, prevents transepithelial fluid influx, enhances mucociliary transport, and interacts with inhaled pathogens and particles. At least some of the surfactant proteins are also synthesized and secreted by club cells. Club cells express SP-B, but not SP-C, which is exclusively expressed by type II cells. There is some controversy whether club cells express SP-A and SP-D. Although this is obviously the case in rodents, club cells in the normal adult human lung most likely express very low or no SP-A and SP-D.[103,106,107] It seems that club cells are not involved in reuptake or recycling of surfactant components.[108] However, their overall role in surfactant biology is not yet defined.

The surfactant apoproteins as the "smart molecules in the surfactant system"[109] have important functions in surfactant subtype assembly, surfactant biophysics, surfactant homeostasis, and innate immunity.[110–114] The hydrophilic proteins SP-A and SP-D belong to the collectin protein family involved in innate immunity. In addition, SP-A, together with SP-B, is important for tubular myelin formation, thus stabilizing active surfactant forms, whereas the hydrophobic proteins SP-B and SP-C and, in conjunction, SP-A enhance the adsorption of phospholipids into the surface film. SP-A might also inhibit surfactant secretion and stimulate surfactant reuptake by type II cells.

Differences in the ultrastructural organization of intracellular and intra-alveolar surfactant subtypes between humans and rodents are also reflected by a different distribution of surfactant proteins (Fig. 2-24).[84] In the human lung, SP-A within type II cells is mainly found in small vesicles and multivesicular bodies and only rarely at the periphery of lamellar bodies. In the alveolar lumen, SP-A is associated with peripheral membranes of lamellar body-like forms in close proximity to tubular myelin, in the corners of the tubular myelin lattice structure, and partly at the surface film and unilamellar vesicles.[103] SP-B in the human lung is localized in the projection core of lamellar bodies within type II cells and in dense core particles associated with tubular myelin in the alveolar lumen.[115]

The crucial role of the surfactant system for the maintenance of the functional integrity of the lung is clearly demonstrated by surfactant dysfunction disorders, which can be caused either at birth by developmental deficiency (owing to lung immaturity or mutations affecting surfactant synthesis or secretion) or later by acquired dysfunction (owing to damage of type II cells or inhibition/inactivation of intra-alveolar surfactant).[90,91,116] A primary deficiency of surfactant in the immature lungs causes the respiratory distress syndrome of premature neonates (RDS). Surfactant dysfunction mutations causing either acute respiratory failure or chronic lung disease after birth have been identified in the genes encoding for SP-B, SP-C, and the ATP-binding cassette transporter ABCA3, which is present at the limiting membrane of lamellar bodies. Impairment of an originally intact surfactant system is involved in the pathogenesis of a variety of other lung diseases, such as acute lung injury/ARDS as well as obstructive, infectious, and interstitial lung diseases. Mechanisms leading to impaired surfactant activity include apoptotic or necrotic cell death of type II cells, damage of surfactant proteins and lipids by reactive oxygen and nitrogen species, and enzymatic damage by phospholipases or neutrophil elastase. In addition, plasma proteins entering the alveolar space during edema formation are also known to inactivate surfactant.

With a turnover time of about 4 to 10 hours and only a rather small intracellular surfactant reserve available for secretion onto the large alveolar surface, the ability to cope with a lack of active surfactant during lung injury is limited. Hence, there is a rationale to supplement the surfactant material available in cases of surfactant deficiency or damage. One of the major advances in neonatology in our time has been the development of surfactant replacement therapy for the treatment of RDS. The story of the treatment of premature babies with exogenous surfactant is indeed a paradigmatic example in which discoveries from basic research were successfully applied to an important clinical problem.[91,117–119] The indications for surfactant replacement therapy have widened in recent years, with promising results in forms of respiratory failure not caused by a primary deficiency of endogenous surfactant but rather by impairment of an originally intact surfactant system. In these cases, however, the efficacy of exogenous surfactant therapy very much depends on the ability of the surfactant preparation to resist the inhibition/inactivation that caused alterations of the endogenous system.

■ CAPILLARY ENDOTHELIUM

The alveolar septa of the adult lung contain a single capillary network. The capillary endothelium is of the continuous (nonfenestrated) type. Alveolar capillaries are provided with pericytes, but they are rarer and less densely branched than pericytes of the systemic circulation.[120] Pericytes are related to vascular smooth muscle cells in that they both are contractile perivascular cells. Thus, pericytes protect microvessel wall integrity by providing some mechanical support. However, in contrast to vascular smooth muscle cells, pericytes are embedded within the endothelial basement membrane, frequently forming contacts with capillary endothelial cells. They seem to contribute components to the capillary basement membrane and extracellular matrix and secrete vasoactive substances. In addition, pericytes are thought to be involved in the regulation of endothelial cell proliferation and differentiation and to act as progenitor cells for other cell types.[121–124]

Capillary Endothelial Cells

At first glance, capillary endothelial cells resemble type I alveolar epithelial cells, but in contrast to type I cells with their complex branching architecture, capillary endothelial cells form simple sheets (Fig. 2-27).[57] Moreover, compared with the tight occluding junctions between alveolar epithelial cells that constitute a powerful seal of the intercellular cleft, the occluding junctions between capillary endothelial cells are rather leaky, allowing a nearly uninhibited exchange of water, solutes, and even some smaller macromolecules between the blood plasma and the interstitial space (Fig. 2-18). Occluding junctions between capillary endothelial cells are often located at the transition of the thin to the thick part of the air–blood barrier and are often covered by pericytes.

There is another notable and important difference between the two basically similar lining cells on the epithelial and endothelial side of the gas-exchange barrier: their size. Although the capillary surface is some 10% to 20% smaller than the alveolar surface, the capillary endothelial cells are about four times more numerous than type I cells[72]; this means that the surface covered by one type I epithelial cell must be about four times larger, namely 4000 to 5000 μm^2, as compared with about 1000 μm^2 in endothelial cells (Table 2-2).

Numerous caveolae are found in capillary endothelial cells (Figs. 2-17 and 2-18). However, at the bulging part of the capillaries, some parts of the endothelial cell extensions are free of caveolae and are thinned down to a thickness of about 20 to 30 nm, basically consisting of the two plasma membranes with only a minute amount of cytoplasm in between. These areas, rarer in human lungs than in rodents, are termed the avesicular zone of the alveolar capillary endothelium.[11,57] In contrast to the endothelium of conducting vessels, Weibel–Palade bodies are missing in capillary endothelial cells, thereby underscoring the structural and functional differences between alveolar and extra-alveolar endothelial cells.[11,49,125,126]

■ INTERSTITIUM

The interstitium of the alveolar septum is for the most part extremely thin. At the thick parts of the air–blood barrier where epithelial and endothelial basement membranes are separated, one finds elastic fibers and bundles of collagen fibrils in the extracellular matrix as well as interstitial cells, mainly fibroblasts, the cells responsible for production of extracellular matrix components (Figs. 2-28 and 2-29).

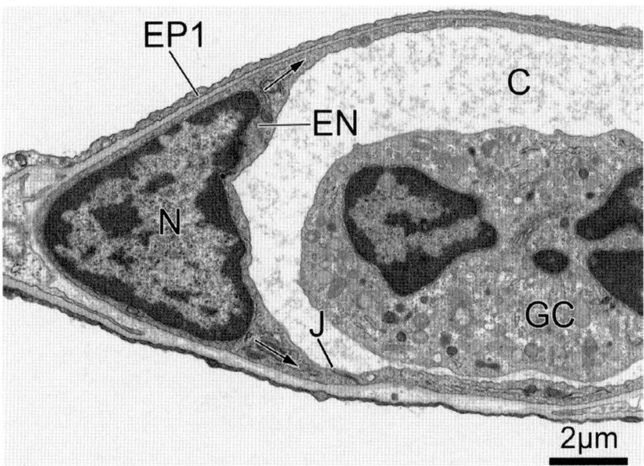

Figure 2-27 An endothelial cell (EN) of capillary (C) is similar in basic structure to a type I epithelial cell (EP1). The nucleus is enwrapped by little cytoplasm but thin leaflets extend as capillary lining *(arrows)*. Note the intercellular junction (J) and a white blood cell/granulocyte (GC), in the capillary. *(Modified with permission from Weibel ER: The Pathway for Oxygen. Cambridge, MA: Harvard University Press; 1984.)*

The precise arrangement of the connective tissue fibers will be discussed later in relation to the mechanical properties of the lung.

Interstitial Cells

The resident interstitial cells of the alveolar septum comprise fibroblasts and contractile cells (myofibroblasts, lipofibroblasts, smooth muscle cells, and pericytes) (Fig. 2-28). Free interstitial cells are part

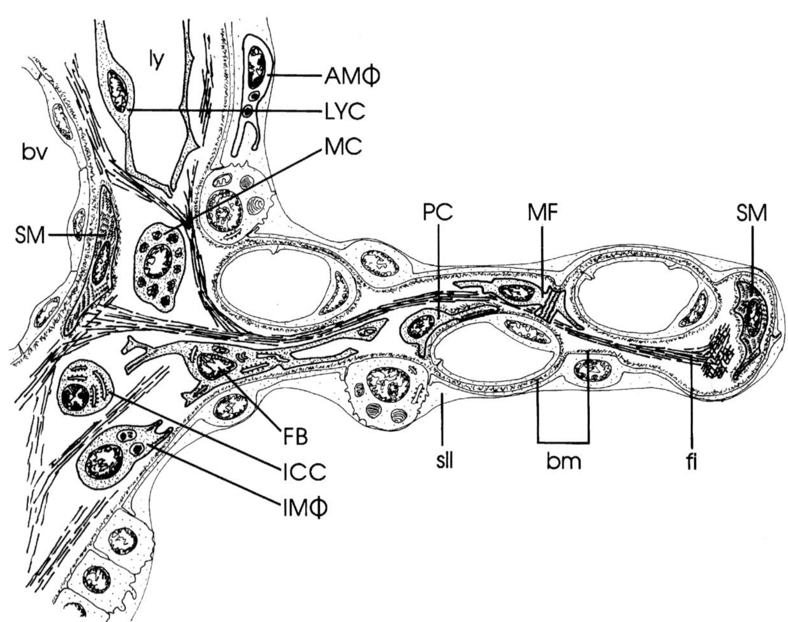

Figure 2-28 Schematic diagram of the structural organization of the alveolar interstitium. The alveolar septum extends between a free edge *(right)* and a perivascular connective tissue sleeve *(left)*, enwrapping a blood vessel (bv). Basement membranes (bm) are associated with epithelium and endothelium, and they bound the interstitial space. Fiber strands (fi) form a continuum. Interstitial cells include: fibroblasts (FB), myofibroblasts (MF), smooth muscle cells (SM), pericytes (PC), various kinds of immune competent cells (ICC), mast cells (MC), lymphatic endothelial cells (LYC), and histiocytes or interstitial macrophages (IMΦ). Alveolar macrophages (AMΦ) are submerged in the alveolar surface lining layer (sll), ly, lymphatic capillary. *(Reproduced with permission from Weibel ER, Crystal RG: Structural organization of the pulmonary interstitium. In: Crystal RG, West JB, Weibel ER, Barmes PJ (eds), The Lung: Scientific Foundations, 2nd ed. New York: Lippincott-Raven; 1997:685–695.)*

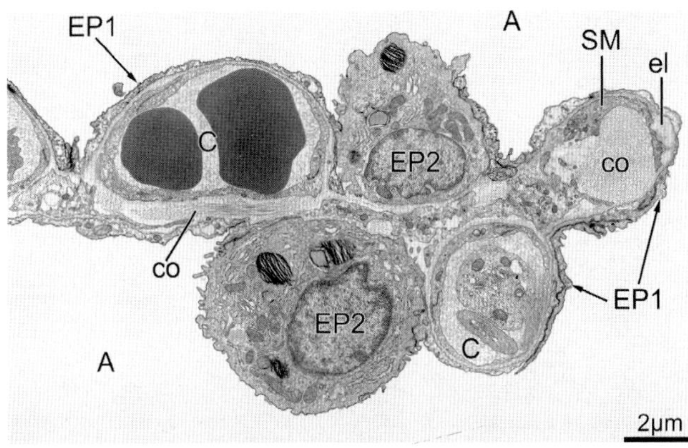

Figure 2-29 Alveolar septum with free edge *(right)* showing reinforced entrance ring with elastic fibers (el), collagen fibrils (co), and smooth muscle cell (SM). The two capillaries (C) are on different sides of the septum, as are the two type II cells (EP2). A, alveolar space; EP1, type I cell. *(Reproduced with permission from Weibel ER, Gil J: Structure-function relationships at the alveolar level, in West JB, ed.: Bioengineering Aspects of the Lung. New York: Springer-Verlag; 1977.)*

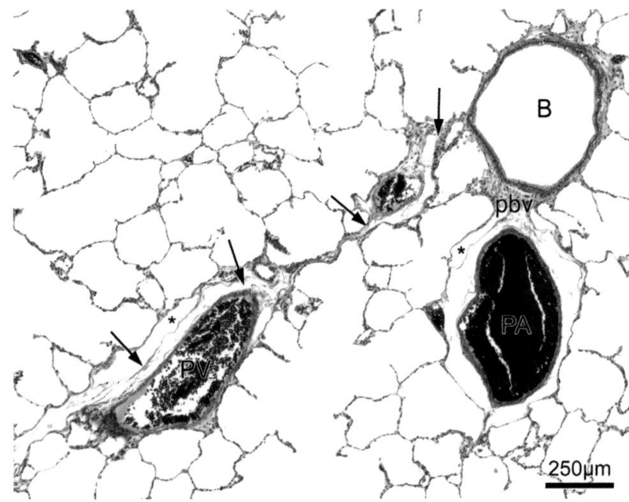

Figure 2-30 Light micrograph of human lung showing connective tissue sleeve *(arrows)* extending from the peribronchovascular space (pbv) around branch of pulmonary artery (PA) and bronchiolus (B) to pulmonary vein branch (PV). Asterisks, lymphatic.

of the defense system usually found in the juxta-alveolar connective tissue sleeves (see below) and include interstitial macrophages (histiocytes), mast cells, and under certain conditions, lymphocytes, plasma cells, and granulocytes.

Fibroblasts are a heterogeneous cell population. Many fibroblasts have notable contractile properties; therefore, they have been termed myofibroblasts. Myofibroblasts contain bundles of microfilaments anchored in patches beneath the plasma membrane. These filament bundles span the entire width of the cell. At the places where the microfilament bundles are connected to the plasma membrane, attachments to the epithelial and/or endothelial basement membrane exist.[11,127,128] Through holes in the basement membranes, myofibroblasts directly link alveolar epithelial and capillary endothelial cells.[83]

Some contractile fibroblasts are equipped with nonmembrane-bound lipid bodies, thus termed lipid interstitial cells or lipofibroblasts.[129,130] These cells are more common in rodent than in human lungs and occur particularly during alveolar development and growth. Lipid bodies consist of an osmiophilic rim of amphipathic phospholipids, glycolipids, sterols and specific proteins, and a hydrophobic core of neutral lipids. In many cell types, lipid bodies represent specialized domains for the synthesis of eicosanoid mediators.[131] Pulmonary lipofibroblasts seem to be related to the lipid-containing perisinusoidal cell (Ito cell) in the liver in that they might serve as a storage depot for retinoids.[130,132] Under certain conditions, lipofibroblasts might provide fatty acid substrates for surfactant synthesis in type II cells.[130]

The occurrence of smooth muscle cells in the alveolar septa is mostly restricted to the free septal edges where they contribute to the network of alveolar entrance rings (Figs. 2-28 and 2-29). Pericytes abut alveolar capillaries (see above).

STRUCTURAL ASPECTS OF THE DEFENSE SYSTEM OF THE LUNG

The large and delicate alveolar surface is constantly challenged by inhaled microorganisms and particulate matter. Thus, normal lung function critically depends on an efficient defense system.[94,113,133-136] At the alveolar level, the primary defense barrier is the alveolar lining layer. Here, alveolar macrophages are the sentinel phagocytic cells of the innate immune system, as we shall discuss later. In addition, protein components of the innate immune system, including the lung collectins SP-A and SP-D as well as a variety of other antimicrobial peptides (e.g., lysozyme, lactoferrin, defensins, cathelicidins), are present in the alveolar lining layer.

Another set of macrophages forms a second defense line just beneath the alveolar epithelium; that is, in the interstitial space of the lung parenchyma. In the normal lung, these interstitial macrophages (histiocytes) are not found in alveolar septa; instead, they occur only in the connective tissue sleeves at the periphery and in the center of acini where the peripheral fiber system connects with the adventitial sheath of bronchioles and pulmonary arteries (Fig. 2-30). Thus, they are found in regions where lymphatics begin their course toward the major airways in the hilar region where lymph nodes are found. In these juxta-alveolar regions of connective tissue, we usually find the common elements of the defense system (Figs. 2-30 and 2-31). These include lymphatic vessels and several mobile cells. Interstitial macrophages are constantly being replenished by blood monocytes migrating into the interstitial space. Sometimes they become permanent residents in the form of storage cells for "indigestible" foreign matter, such as carbon particles and silicates. The relationship

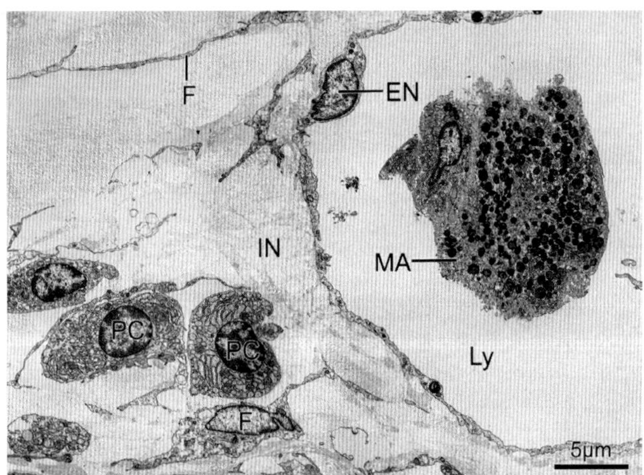

Figure 2-31 Perivascular connective tissue with lymphatic (Ly) containing a macrophage (MA) with heterogeneous population of "lysosomal" granules. Interstitium (IN) contains fibroblasts (F) and plasma cells (PC). EN, lymphatic endothelium.

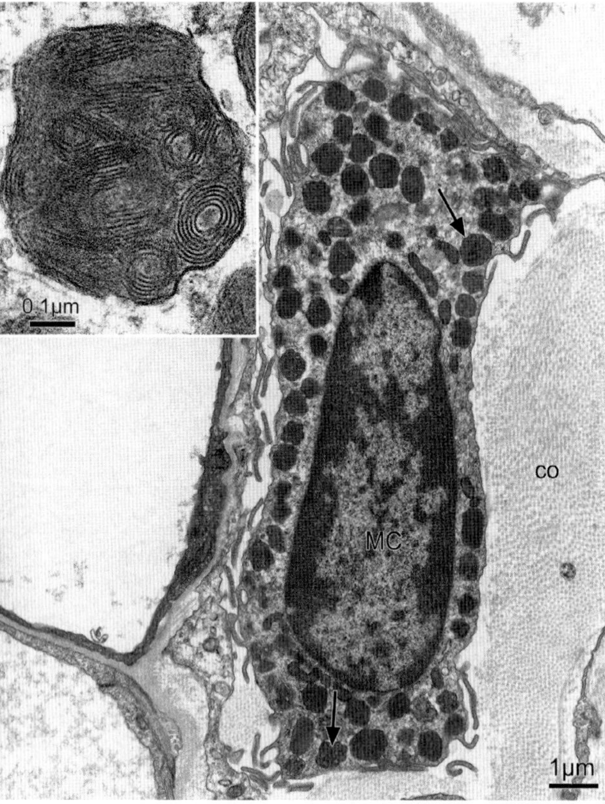

Figure 2-32 Mast cell from human lung containing granules *(arrows)* with scroll-like substructure. *Inset:* Scroll-like substructure of mast cell granule at higher magnification. Co, collagen fibrils. *(Reproduced with permission from Weibel ER: Lung cell biology, in Fishman A, Fisher AB, eds. Handbook of Physiology. Section 3: The Respiratory System. vol 1. Bethesda, MD: American Physiological Society; 1985: 47–91.)*

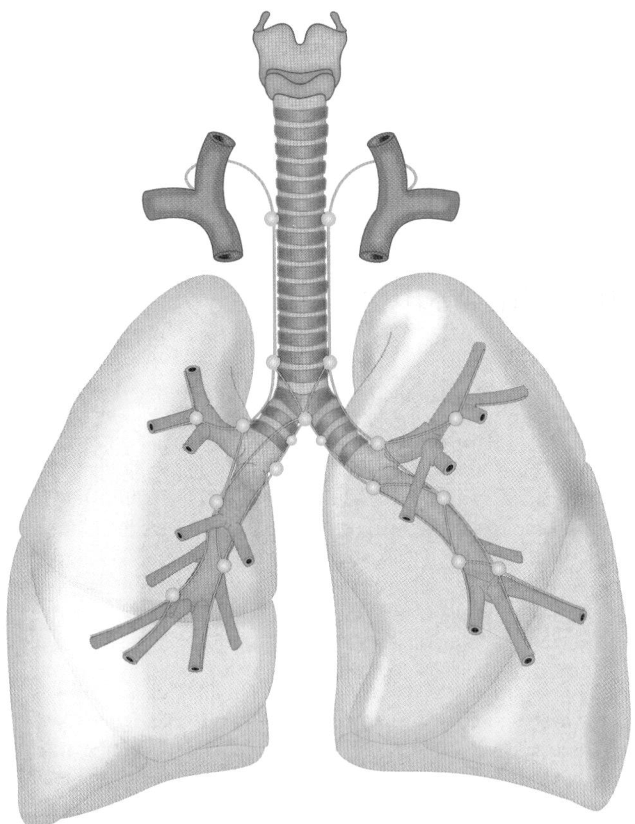
Figure 2-33 Schematic diagram of distribution of lymph nodes and main lymphatic channels along bronchial tree.

between interstitial macrophages and dendritic cells (see below) is under discussion.[137,138] Lymphocytes are less common and are mostly present as T cells whereas B cells and natural killer cells are rare in the normal lung. Granulocytes (neutrophils, eosinophils, and basophils) are present in the human lung, but they are also very rare. Mast cells contain granules storing heparin and histamine as well as peptidases such as tryptases and chymases[139] that, in the human, show a characteristic scroll-like substructure (Fig. 2-32) as well as lipid bodies. According to their anatomic location, they show site-specific characteristics, thus displaying considerable heterogeneity.[140] Antigen-presenting dendritic cells possess long branched dendritic cell processes (hence, their name) and an irregular, folded nucleus. Phagolysosomes are absent. Once activated, dendritic cells migrate to lymph nodes where they induce the proliferation of antigen-specific T cells; thus, providing a link between innate and adaptive immunity. In addition to their presence within the lung parenchyma, dendritic cells are found within the tracheal and bronchial epithelium where they seem to form a network comparable to the Langerhans cells in the epidermis. Like Langerhans cells, airway dendritic cells are characterized by pentalaminar plate-like organelles (Birbeck granules).[141–143] In the ciliated epithelium of bronchi and bronchioles diapedesis is seen; that is, lymphocytes and other leukocytes in the process of penetrating the epithelium to reach the mucus blanket. Plasma cells occur in relatively high numbers around the acini of the seromucous glands of bronchi (Fig. 2-7); hence, it is likely that antibodies are being secreted into the mucus blanket by these glands by a process similar to that occurring in the salivary glands or in the glands of the nasal mucosa.

The third defense line is constituted by the lymph nodes, which are arranged along the major bronchi and extend to subsegmental bronchi about 5 mm in diameter (Fig. 2-33). The most peripheral lymph nodes are tiny, a mere 1 to 2 mm in diameter, but closer to the hilum they become larger, reaching 5 to 10 mm in diameter in the region of the tracheal bifurcation and along the trachea. The lymph nodes from adult human lungs often appear gray or even black because of deposition in the medullary cords of large numbers of macrophages loaded with carbon pigment. This material entered the lung via the airways, primarily as smoke, soot, or coal dust; depending on the size of the particles, they were either deposited on the surface of conducting airways or reached the alveoli. The further down the deposition, the greater the likelihood that this material cannot be eliminated while in the airways, that is, within the mucus blanket. The only exit from the lung parenchyma then is via the lymphatics, but this exit ultimately leads to the blood, a circumstance that is obviously to be avoided. Filtering the lymph in lymph nodes and providing a depository in the medullary cords protects the blood and hence the entire organism from dissemination of indigestible foreign matter and also, in most instances, of infective agents.

Thus, the lymphatic "circulation" in the lung plays an important defense role.[6,42] It is unidirectional. It begins as interstitial fluid that seeps from the capillaries and is efficiently drained along the connective tissue fibers toward those connective tissue sleeves in the center and at the periphery of acini where lymph capillaries begin. From there, lymphatic vessels, endowed with valves and an irregular smooth muscle wall, course in septal structures, in the pleura, and peribronchial and perivascular sheaths toward the hilar region (Fig. 2-33). Lymph nodes are intercalated in the course of the lymphatics, which lead the lymph toward the tracheal bifurcation and then along the trachea into the right and left mediastinal lymph channels. The right channel drains into the right subclavian vein;

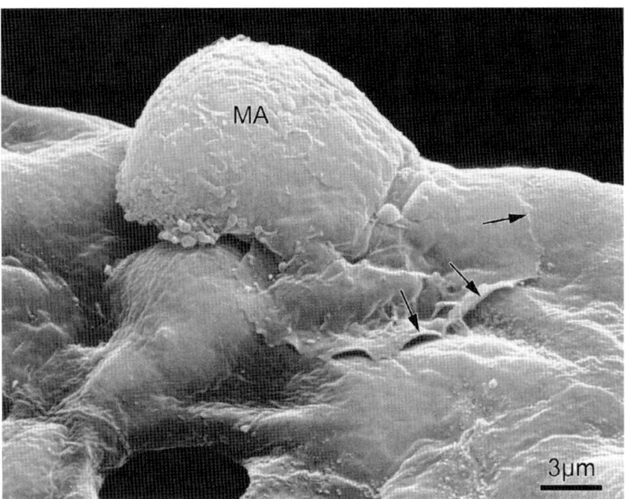

Figure 2-34 Alveolar macrophage (MA) seen sitting on epithelial surface of human lung. Note cytoplasmic lamella *(arrows)* which represents the advancing edge of the cell.

the left, together with the thoracic duct, into the left subclavian vein. Because of the many anastomoses connecting parallel lymphatics, a particular lymph node receives lymph from various lung regions, but the closest regions tend to predominate.

ALVEOLAR MACROPHAGES

Lung macrophages can be differentiated into several populations according to the compartment they are found in: intravascular, interstitial, airway, and alveolar macrophages.[144–146] Of these, the alveolar macrophages, the cell population of the surface lining layer, are of particular importance. They are free cells, endowed with a high phagocytic capacity, which are transiently attached to the surface of the alveolar epithelium by pseudopodia and can crawl over this surface by amoeboid movement (Fig. 2-34). Occasionally, alveolar macrophages can be observed during the passage through an interalveolar pore of Kohn. However, they are submerged beneath the surface film of phospholipids (Fig. 2-35) and, therefore, are part of the surface lining layer of alveoli, more specifically of its hypophase. Alveolar macrophages exert their phagocytic activity within the surface lining layer (Fig. 2-25). Hence, it is not surprising that their vacuoles contain large amounts of ingested surfactant material, in part even tubular myelin. The importance of alveolar macrophages for surfactant removal is underscored by the acquired form of pulmonary alveolar proteinosis, where a defect in surfactant catabolism by alveolar macrophages caused by autoantibodies against granulocyte/macrophage colony-stimulating factor (GM-CSF) leads to an accumulation of surfactant material in the alveoli.[147]

Alveolar macrophages are derived from monocytes – indirectly, therefore, from bone marrow cells – and probably reach the alveoli in two steps: first, by settling in the pulmonary interstitial tissue, and second, by migration from the interstitial tissue into the alveoli where they constitute a partly self-reproducing cell population. Their removal seems to involve two different pathways: (1) some of the macrophages undoubtedly move up the bronchial tree in the mucus blanket and eventually appear in the sputum; and (2) others possibly return into the interstitial space. In the normal lung, however, the second path seems to occur exclusively in those alveoli that abut the connective tissue sleeves around larger vessels and conducting airways or on interacinar septa; that is, where the lymphatic capillaries are located. A preferred location appears to be in the respiratory bronchioles at the entrance into the acinus or in the center of the acinus, where one often finds congregations of dust-laden macrophages; this may be at the origin of centroacinar damage observed in smokers, which lead to progressive emphysema. In these places, macrophages either settle as carbon pigment-loaded histiocytes, or they leave the lung parenchyma via lymphatics (Fig. 2-31) to settle in the lymph nodes. The way in which macrophages and/or their ingested material are transferred from the alveolar surface to the interstitial space is still unknown.

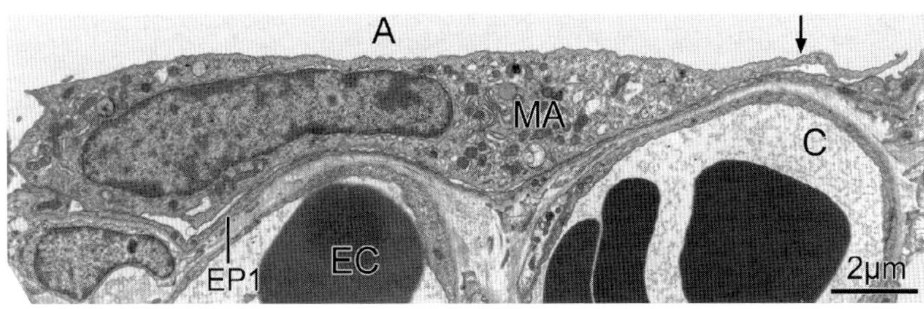

Figure 2-35 Alveolar macrophage (MA) fixed in its natural position of "flat" attachment to the alveolar epithelium. *Arrow* points to advancing cytoplasmic leaflet.

FUNCTIONAL DESIGN OF THE LUNG

From the preceding section it has become apparent that the lung is built of a multitude of cells and tissue elements that all serve specific functions in support of the lung's main function: the exchange of oxygen and carbon dioxide between the air and the blood. But it takes more than cells to make a good lung.[148] The lung's multiple component structures must be integrated to make an efficient and stable gas exchanger, and this demands a blueprint for the integral architecture of the human lung.[7] This must first ensure that the airways and blood vessels are adequately correlated topologically and quantitatively to allow well-matched ventilation and blood flow. It must also realize a complex organization that allows air ventilation, blood perfusion, and gas exchange to function in the most efficient manner. The design principles that govern the architecture of the human lung toward that goal can be characterized as *Complexity, Correlativity, and Connectivity*. Complexity means that the microscopic gas-exchange units are an integral part of the macroscopic airways and vessels; their architectural correlation determines the efficient approximation of air and blood in the gas exchanger; and connecting all the parts into a whole is achieved with a fiber continuum that pervades the entire lung. The implementation of these principles during development is decisive for "making a good lung."

DESIGN OF THE BRANCHING AIRWAY TREE

The entrance to the lung's airways is the trachea (Fig. 2-3), a single tube, the gas-exchange elements where air and blood are brought into close contact are contained in several million units. Between entrance and periphery lies a meticulously designed system of branching airways that serve to conduct the inspired air into those peripheral channels that carry alveoli in their walls and can thus contribute to the exchange of gases between air and blood (Fig. 2-5).[8]

In the mammalian and human lung the airways are built as dichotomous trees.[149] This is the result of lung morphogenesis where the end bud of each airway tube gives rise to two daughter branches. In the human lung this goes on for 23 generations, on average, and, since the number of branches doubles with each generation, there are 2^{23} or about 8 million end branches, generally called alveolar sacs.[8] This is an average value; in reality the number of branching generations needed to reach the alveolar sacs is quite variable, ranging from about 18 to 30. This variability results from the fact that the airways form a space-filling tree (Fig. 2-3) whose endings must be homogeneously distributed in space and reach into every corner and into every gap in the available space, determined by the form of the chest cavity into which the lung develops. Some spaces are filled rapidly and the airways cannot continue to divide, whereas in other places more branches are needed to fill the space.

This branching process is accompanied by growth in length and diameter of the airway segments, the tubes between the branching nodes. The length of the tubes is adjusted to cover the distances needed to fill the space homogeneously with endings, whereas the diameter is, grossly speaking, made proportional to the volume of peripheral lung that is supplied by this branch.

Figure 2-36 shows a portion of a cast of the airway tree from a human lung. It is evident that the airways branch by dichotomy and that the length and the diameter of the tubes become gradually reduced with each generation. At first sight, the airway branching seems quite regular, but there is a certain degree of asymmetry in the sense that the two daughter branches differ in length and diameter; in animal lungs asymmetry is more pronounced than in human lungs.

Despite asymmetric branching some general rules govern the progression of dimensions along the tree. The diameter of daughter branches is smaller than that of the parent in the sense that the diameter reflects the volume of peripheral lung it supplies with air: larger airways serve larger lung units, smaller airways smaller units. The progression of airway diameters follows the law of Hess (1917)[150] and Murray (1926)[151] that, in a dichotomous tree, the diameters of the daughter branches, d_1 and d_2, are related to the parent branch d_0 as:

$$d_0^3 = d_1^3 + d_2^3$$

a law that predicts optimization of the airway diameters for convective air flow, providing lowest resistance for lowest dead space.

For a symmetric tree in which $d_1 = d_2$ this becomes:

$$d_1 = d_0 \cdot 2^{-1/3}$$

which means that the airway diameter becomes reduced by a factor of cube root of 1/2 or about 0.79 with each generation. Considering the progression of airway dimensions along the tree this law should apply to all successive generations so that we predict the average diameter in generation z to be:

$$d(z) = d_0 \cdot 2^{-z/3}$$

Figure 2-37 shows that this is approximately the case for the first 14 generations of conducting airways.

However, a closer look at the airways of the human lung shows that this is only approximately correct.[152] It appears that the smaller bronchioles (beyond generation 10) are provided with some safety factor in that the diameter is reduced by a factor of 0.83 rather than the physically optimal 0.79. This allows regulation of airway cross-section by contraction of the bronchiolar muscle sleeve without unduly increasing flow resistance which is very low in small airways (Fig. 2-38).[153] Design optimization is limited in favor of physiologic robustness.

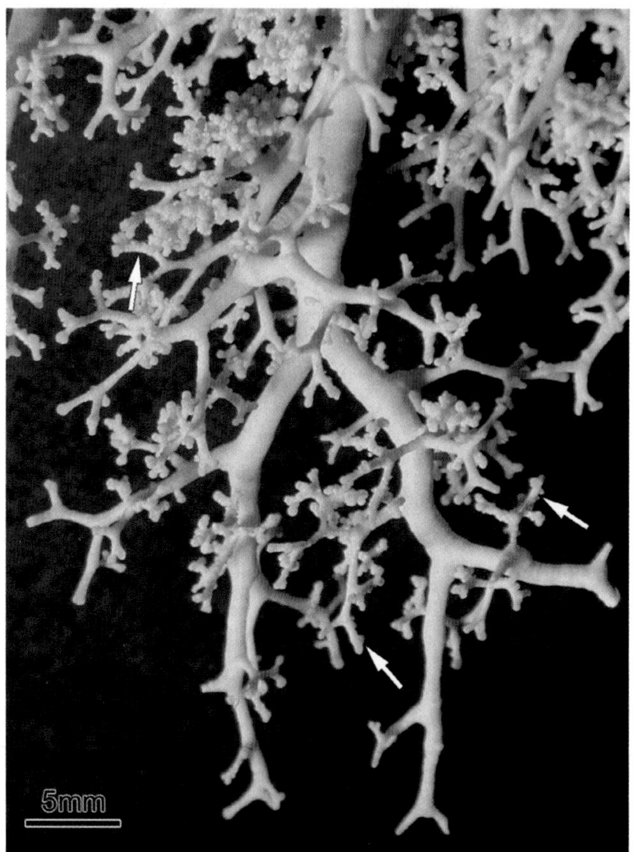

Figure 2-36 Peripheral portion of cast of human airway tree reaching out to the transitional bronchioles and some respiratory bronchioles *(arrows)*.

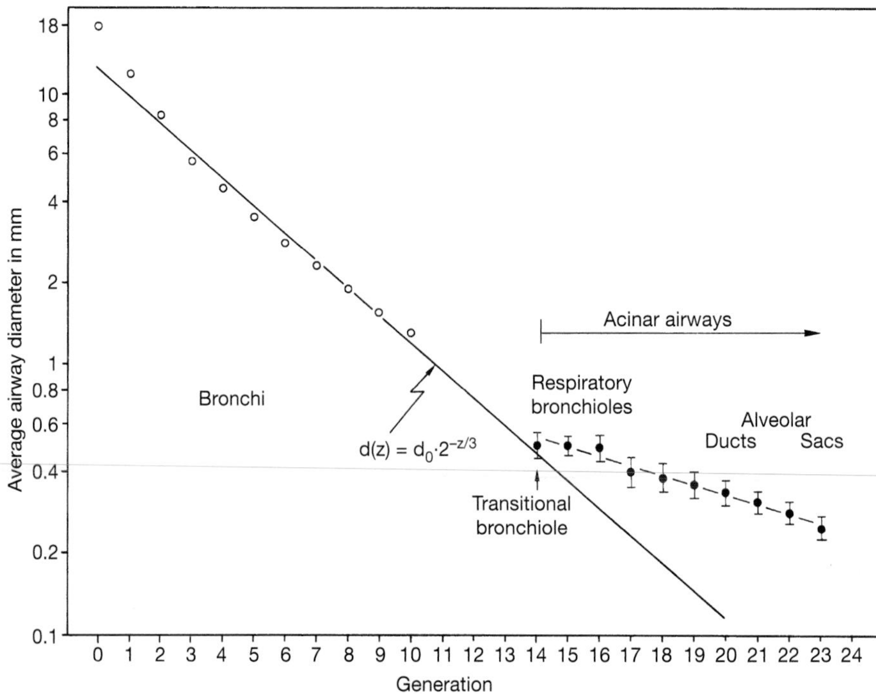

Figure 2-37 Average diameter of airways in human lung plotted by generations of regularized dichotomous branching. *(Reproduced with permission from Haefeli-Bleuer B, Weibel ER: Morphometry of the human pulmonary acinus. Anat Rec. 1988;220(4):401–414.)*

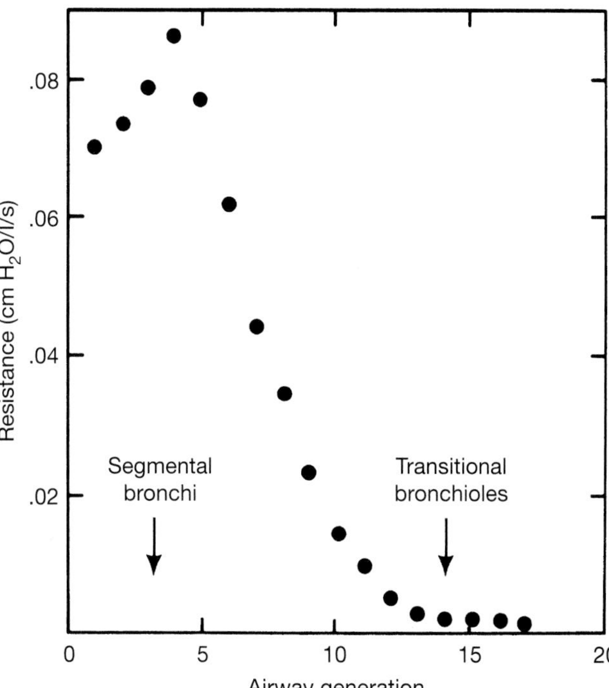

Figure 2-38 Airway resistance to mass air flow is located mostly in the conducting airways and falls rapidly toward the periphery. *(Redrawn with permission from Pedley TJ et al. The prediction of pressure drop and variation of resistance within the human bronchial airways. Respir Physiol. 1970;9(3):387–405.)*

This symmetric airway model reflects the typical pathway along the airway tree. It has been very useful in modeling the basic rules governing the distribution of air flow as well as the deposition of particles entering the lung. However, it disregards the effects of asymmetric branching. It is possible to construct models that take into account irregularities in branching, for example by considering the number of airways of a given diameter, d_u, that exist in each generation, and the length of the bronchial pathway that intervenes between the larynx and particular airways (Fig. 2-39).[8,154]

An alternative approach is to regard the airways as a system of tubes converging from the periphery, the acinus, toward the center, the trachea.[155] By using an ascending ordering system that is employed in analyzing rivers (Strahler system), branches are grouped into orders according to the sequence of convergence, beginning with the smallest most peripheral branches, designated as order 1. This ordering pattern is particularly well adapted to a system of irregular dichotomy because the size of branches in one order varies less than with the generations-down model. This approach does not really account for the asymmetry of branching, however; it rather represents an attempt at extracting average data with less variability in each order. The degree of asymmetric branching is reflected in the branching ratio determined as the ratio of the number of branches in order μ to that in order $\mu + 1$. Remarkably, the progression of diameters through the various orders is again roughly proportional to the cube root of the branching ratio. Hence, from a functional point of view both models yield comparable results.

The general conclusion drawn from this type of analysis is that the diameters of the conducting airways are such as to assure optimal conditions for airflow but relaxing physical optimality conditions in the interest of physiologic robustness; the airways of the lung are thus well designed. The total volume of the conducting airways down to generation 14 (the anatomic dead space) is about 150 mL; it is rapidly flushed by simple gas flow in the course of inhaling 500 mL of fresh air during quiet inspiration. Therefore, for the larger airways, optimization for flow and its distribution to peripheral units are essential for good design.

These are the characteristics of the proximal airways built as smooth-walled tubes to distribute convective air flow into the lung. This design ends more or less abruptly when the airways reach lung parenchyma, the complex of alveoli that are arranged around peripheral airways (Fig. 2-40). The airway tree is thus subdivided into two major functional zones (Fig. 2-5): the first about 14 to 16 generations, on average, are designed as conducting airways where air flow is by convection; this is followed by about 8 generations of acinar airways where an axial channel, called alveolar duct, is enwrapped by a sleeve of alveoli with gas-exchange tissue on their surface.

In the human lung the transition is not abrupt. At some point the smooth bronchiolar wall becomes interrupted by one or two alveoli (Fig. 2-41). This so-called transitional bronchiole (Fig. 2-5) marks the entrance into an acinus.[9] It is followed by some three generations of respiratory bronchioles where an increasing fraction of the wall surface is occupied by alveoli, until the alveolar ducts are reached where the central air duct is completely surrounded by alveoli (Fig. 2-42). These acinar airways continue to branch by dichotomy. Their length and diameter decrease with each generation, but the slope does not follow the law of reduction by the cube root of 1/2; the diameters of respiratory bronchioles and alveolar ducts change very little with each generation.[9] Does this arrangement imply less than an optimal design? On the contrary, the cube-root-of-1/2 law relates to optimizing mass flow of a liquid or air. In the most peripheral airways, mass airflow is only part of the means of transporting O_2 toward the air–blood barrier. Since the airways are blind-ending tubes and since a sizable amount of residual air remains in the lung periphery after expiration, O_2 molecules must move into the residual air by diffusion (Fig. 2-43). However, diffusion of O_2 in the gas phase is best served by establishing as large an interface as possible between residual air and the fresh air that flows in from the trachea.[16] In fact, since the airway diameter remains nearly unchanged, the total airway cross section nearly doubles with each generation beyond generation 14.

The dimensions of the airway tree influence the ventilatory flow of air in a number of ways. First of all, airflow velocity falls along the airway tree because the total cross-sectional area of the airways increases with every generation (Fig. 2-44); whereas the cross-sectional area of the trachea is about 2.5 cm^2, that of the 1024 airways in the 10th generation taken together is 13 cm^2, and as we approach the acinar airways, the total cross section reaches 300 cm^2. However, since the same air volume flows through all generations, the flow velocity falls by more than 100-fold from the trachea to the acini: at rest, the mean flow velocity on inspiration is about 1 m s^{-1} in the trachea and less than 1 cm s^{-1} in the first-order respiratory bronchioles. In exercise, the flow velocities are up to 10 times greater, in proportion to the increased ventilation. This is discussed further when considering the relative importance of convection and diffusion in bringing O_2 to the alveolar surface for gas exchange.

The size of airways also determines the resistance to airflow. However, the overall resistance is rather small; it is given by the reciprocal of the ratio of ventilatory airflow to the pressure difference between the mouth and alveoli, which is normally no greater than about 1 cmH_2O (mbar) or less than 1 mm Hg. It is large enough, however, to potentially affect the distribution of ventilation to the many gas-exchange units. Because, in laminar flow, the resistance is inversely proportional to d^4 the distribution of air flow depends on a delicate balance of the size of parallel airway tracts. Even a slight narrowing of one of the two daughter branches at

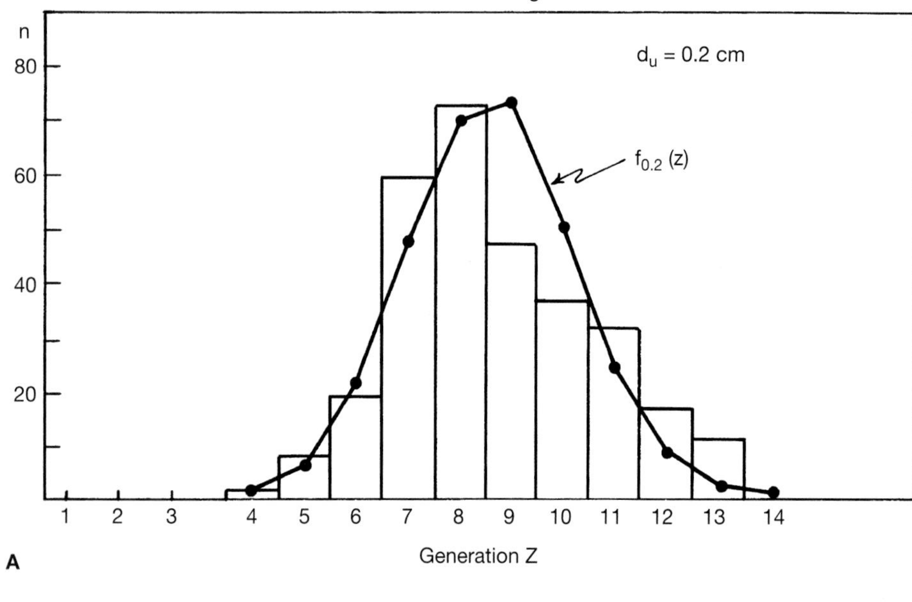

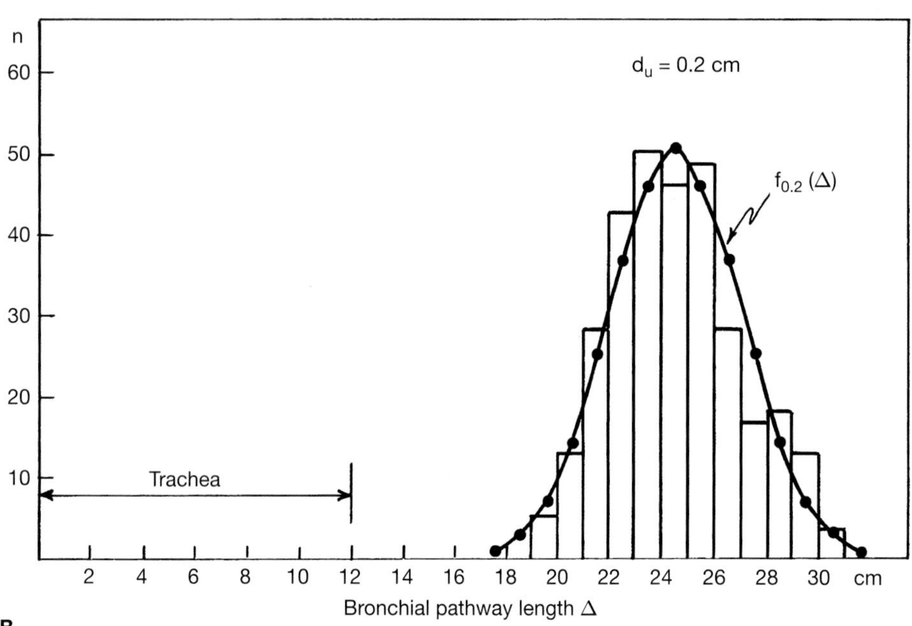

Figure 2-39 Distribution of airways of diameter d_u = 2 mm with respect to (**A**), generations of branching and (**B**), bronchial pathway lengths. *(Reproduced with permission from Weibel ER: Morphometry of the Human Lung. Heidelberg: Springer-Verlag; 1963.)*

a branch point will cause disproportionate air flow to the other branch and thus result in ventilation inhomogeneity.

Since the diameter of airways decreases as they branch (Fig. 2-37), one would suspect that their resistance increases toward the periphery. Apparently this is not the case, as the major pressure drop along the airways occurs in medium-sized bronchi; because the airway diameter decreases with a factor larger than the optimal 0.79 resistance becomes very low in the small bronchioles (Fig. 2-38).[153] This is further accentuated by the fact that the thin-walled bronchioles become widened as the lung expands on inspiration because they are subject to the tissue tensions in the coarse fiber system of the lung. Therefore, airway resistance is seen to fall as lung volume increases. When this effect of tissue tension is disturbed, as in emphysema, some small bronchioles may collapse. This causes ventilation of the peripheral lung units to become highly uneven.

This biophysical way of looking at the significance of the progression of airway dimensions has recently been complemented by the alternative notion that the airway and vascular trees could be determined by the laws of fractal geometry.[156] Fractal trees are formed by repeating the branching pattern from one generation to the next. If the proportion between parent and daughter branches remain the same this is called self-similar branching. In a dichotomous tree the diameter is ideally reduced by a factor of $2^{-1/D_f}$ where D_f is the fractal dimension. Since the airway tree is nearly space-filling $D_f \sim 3$, which means that the Hess–Murray law also follows from fractal geometry as a rule of optimal design, but because the reduction factor is somewhat larger than $2^{-1/3}$ it follows that the actual fractal dimension of the airway tree is a bit larger than 3; this is possible because the tree is "cut off" at the entrance to the acini and the "space" becomes filled with alveoli.[157,158]

■ DESIGN OF THE VASCULAR TREE

In many ways, the course and pattern of dimensional changes in the pulmonary blood vessels resemble those of the airways. Figure 2-3 shows that the pulmonary arteries follow the airways

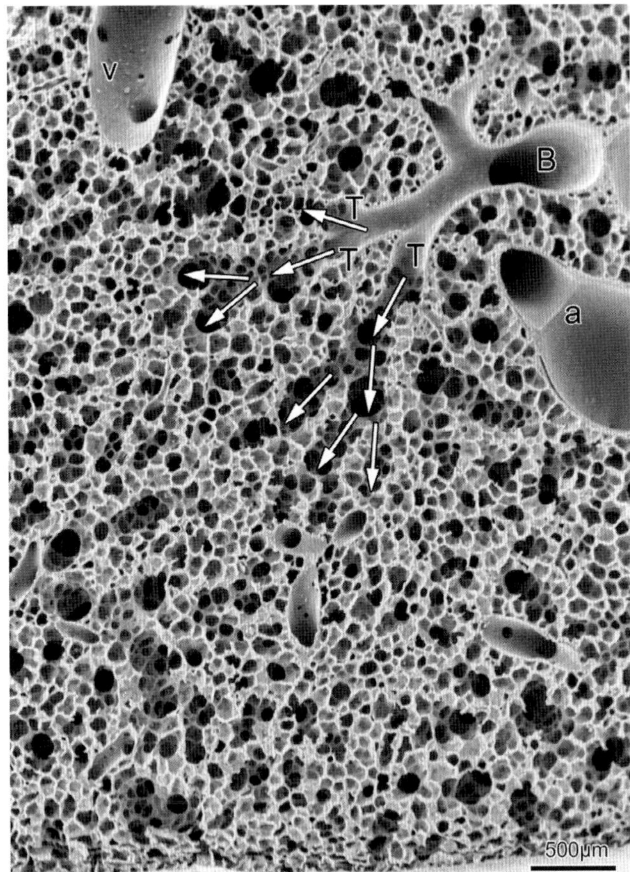

Figure 2-40 Scanning electron micrograph of lung shows branching of small peripheral bronchiole (**B**) into transitional bronchioles (T), from where the airways continue into respiratory bronchioles and alveolar ducts *(arrows)*. Note the location of the pulmonary artery (a) and vein (v) as well as visceral pleura *(bottom)*.

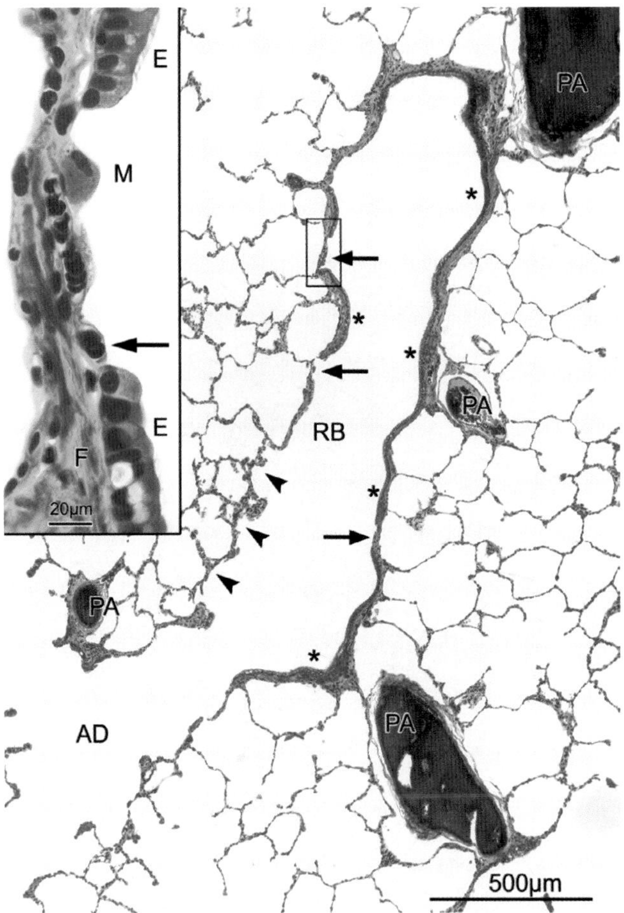

Figure 2-41 Respiratory bronchiole (RB) from human lung cut along its axis toward the transition to alveolar ducts (AD). Note lining by cuboidal airway epithelium *(asterisks)* and the occurrence of respiratory patches *(arrows)* before alveoli proper *(arrowheads)* appear. PA marks branches of pulmonary artery. *Inset:* Higher magnification of one of the respiratory patches in the wall of the respiratory bronchiole with capillaries *(arrow)* and alveolar macrophage (M). The cuboidal epithelium (E) with cilia is replaced by thin squamous epithelium of alveolar type 1 cell. Note thick fibrous layer (F) with smooth muscle cells.

closely, out to the smallest branches; together they form the axis of lung parenchymal units of varying order: acinus, lobule, segment, lobe. As indicated, the veins are differently disposed, lying in the boundary between two or three adjacent units (Figs. 2-30 and 2-45).

The diameter of each pulmonary artery branch also approximates closely that of the accompanying bronchus (Fig. 2-45A). Therefore, it is evident that the diameter law presented earlier for airways must also hold for the first 10 to 16 generations of pulmonary arteries (Fig. 2-37). However, the pulmonary arteries divide more frequently than the airways; very often, small branches leave the artery at right angles and supply blood to the parenchymal units adjacent to the bronchus (Fig. 2-45B). From a count of precapillaries, it seems that the pulmonary arteries divide, on the average, over 28 generations, as compared with 23 for the airways. The diameter of these terminal vessels is about 20 to 50 μm; if this range is plotted onto an extension of the graph of Figure 2-37 to generation 28, it falls on the curve that is obtained by extrapolation from the major branches[8,16]:

$$d(z) = d_0 \cdot 2^{-z/3}$$

This suggests that the pulmonary arteries abide to the cube-root-of-1/2 law from beginning to end. Evidently, the blood is transported to the capillary bed by mass flow only. Therefore, there is no reason to deviate from this fundamental law of design, which minimizes the loss of energy caused by blood flow.

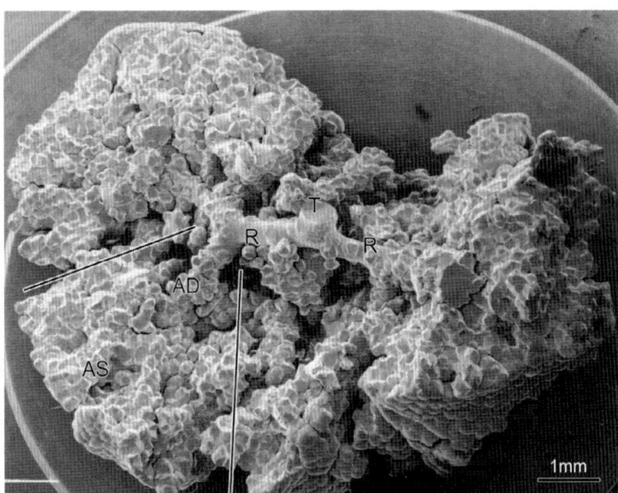

Figure 2-42 Scanning electron micrograph of a complete acinus from a silicon rubber cast of a human lung partly dissected to show transitional (T) and respiratory (R) bronchioles as well as alveolar ducts (AD) and alveolar sacs (AS). Lines mark approximate boundary of 1/8 subacinus. *(Reproduced with permission from Haefeli-Bleuer B, Weibel ER: Morphometry of the human pulmonary acinus. Anat Rec. 1988;220(4):401–414.)*

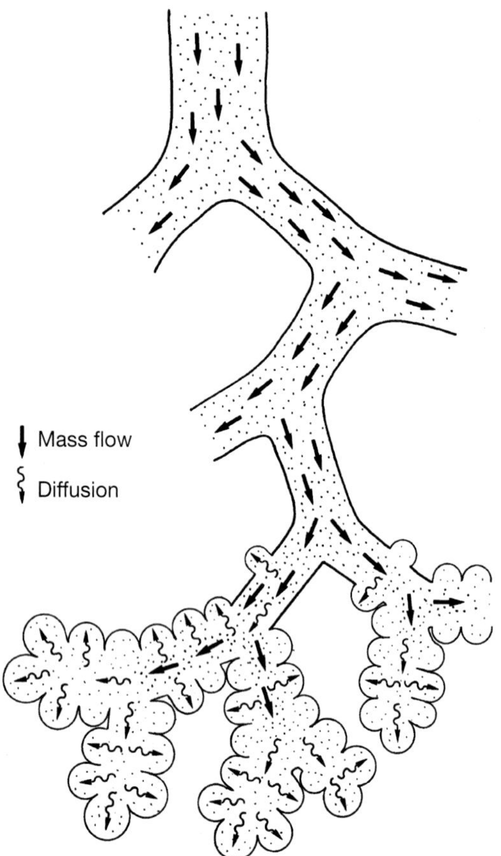

Figure 2-43 Oxygen molecules reach alveoli by combined mass airflow and molecular diffusion, the importance of diffusion increasing toward the periphery.

In a thorough analysis of the pulmonary vascular trees[159] conceived as fractal structures it has been shown that the fractal dimension of both arteries and veins is 2.71, thus somewhat less than 3. The diameter reduction factor is therefore slightly smaller than cube-root-of-1/2, and the diameters follow the regression:

$$d(z) = d_0 \cdot 2^{-z/2.71}$$

Therefore, in contrast to the airways, the resistance to blood flow increases along the pulmonary arteries and is highest in the most peripheral branches or arterioles. The resistance profile of the pulmonary arteries is thus the same as in the systemic circulation.

The alveolar capillary network of the lung is very different from that of the systemic circulation. Whereas in muscle, for example, long capillaries are found to be joined in a loose network, the capillaries of the alveolar walls form dense meshworks made of very short segments (Fig. 2-46).[8,160] The meshes are so dense that some people believe blood flows through the alveolar walls like a sheet rather than through a system of interconnected tubes. In this sheet-flow concept,[161] the sheet is bounded by two flat membranes, the air–blood barrier, connected by numerous "posts." When blood flows through this sheet, it is not channeled in a given direction but has freedom to move in a tortuous way between the posts. Although this concept oversimplifies the actual structural conditions, it does provide a useful description of the pattern of blood flow through the alveolar walls and explains why blood flow is not interrupted when some parts of the capillary bed become squashed flat at high inflation levels (see Fig. 2-58); the capillaries that remain open in the corners are simply some channels of this broad sheet. Furthermore, it is important to note that the capillary network or sheet is continuous through many alveolar walls (Fig. 2-46), probably at least throughout the entire acinus, if not for greater distances.[160] Consequently, it is not possible to isolate microvascular units. One finds, rather, that arterial end branches simply feed into this broad sheet at more or less even distances and that the veins drain these sheets in a similar pattern. However, now we must remember that the arteries reach the acinus along the airways, whereas the veins are in a peripheral location (Fig. 2-45). In principle, therefore, blood flows through the acinar capillary sheet from the center to the periphery of the acinar gas-exchange unit.

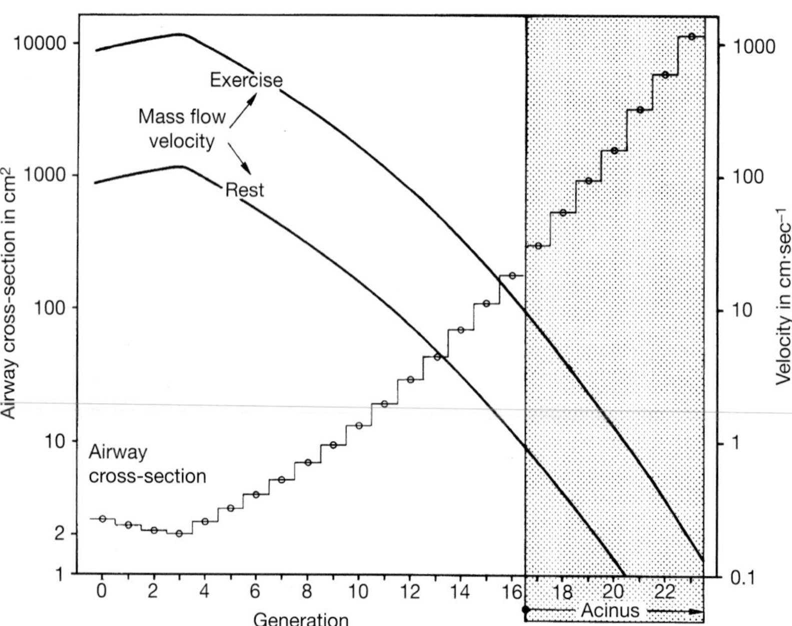

Figure 2-44 As total airway cross-section increases with the generations of airway branching, the mass flow velocity of inspired air decreases rapidly, falling below the molecular velocity of O_2 diffusion in air as we enter the acinus (see Fig. 2-66). *(Reproduced with permission from Weibel ER: The Pathway for Oxygen. Cambridge, MA: Harvard University Press; 1984.)*

DESIGN OF PULMONARY PARENCHYMA

■ ALVEOLI AND CAPILLARIES

The airspaces and blood vessels of lung parenchyma are designed to facilitate gas exchange between air and blood. To this end a very large area of contact between air and blood must be established; for the human lung it is sometimes compared with the area of a tennis court in size. Furthermore, the tissue barrier separating air and blood must be kept as thin as possible—it is found to be about 50 times thinner than a sheet of airmail stationery. This is important, because less than 1 second is available for loading O_2 onto the erythrocytes as they flow through the lung's gas-exchange region.[162]

The first design feature to this end is the formation of alveoli in the walls of all airways within the acinus—that is, in the ventilatory gas-exchange units beginning with a transitional bronchiole (see above) (Fig. 2-40). In the human lung, one estimates that there are about 30,000 acini,[9] and 400 million alveoli[163] so that each of

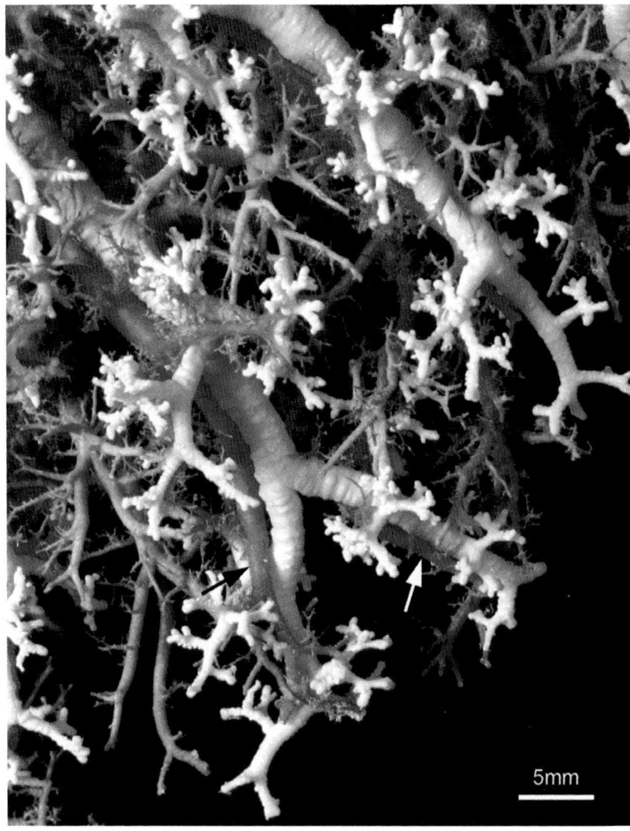

A

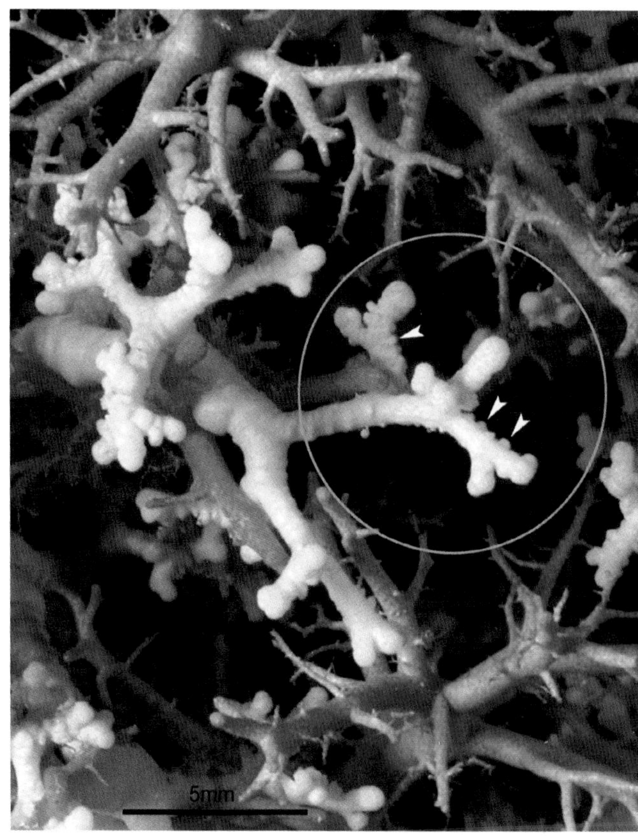

B

Figure 2-45 Casts of airways and blood vessels of human lung. **A.** shows how the pulmonary artery *(red)* closely follows the airways *(yellow)* to the periphery, whereas the pulmonary vein branches *(blue)* lie between the units. Note that the diameter of the pulmonary arteries is similar to that of the accompanying airway, but becomes relatively smaller toward the periphery *(arrow)*; small supernumerary arteries take off at right angles. **B.** Higher power view of group of acini *(circle)*, corresponding about to a secondary lobule, shows how artery penetrates into center of gas-exchange unit with veins collecting the blood around the periphery. *Arrowheads* point to alveolar pouches on transitional and respiratory bronchioles.

the ventilatory gas-exchange units contains some 13,000 alveoli, on average, connected to about seven to nine generations of acinar airways, respiratory bronchioles, and alveolar ducts.[9]

The alveoli are so densely packed that they occupy the entire surface of alveolar ducts; they are separated from each other by delicate alveolar septa that contain the capillary network (Fig. 2-47). About half the space of the septum is taken up by blood, which is thus exposed to the air in two adjacent alveoli (Fig. 2-48A). Although the barrier separating air and blood is extremely thin, we find the capillaries to be provided with a complete endothelial lining, as the alveolar surface of the septum is lined by an epithelium.[11] We have seen earlier that these two cell linings are very much attenuated over the greatest part of the surface.

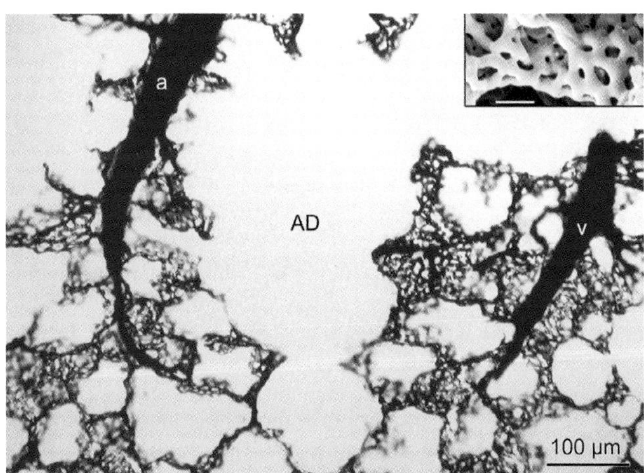

Figure 2-46 Alveolar capillary network demonstrated with gold labeling of blood plasma in a physiologically perfused preparation of a rabbit lung. The dense capillary network spans between end branches of pulmonary artery (a) and vein (v) and extend through many alveolar septa around alveolar duct (AD). *Inset:* Plastic cast shows the dense meshes of the network. Scale bar = 20 μm. *(Inset used with permission of P. Burri.)*

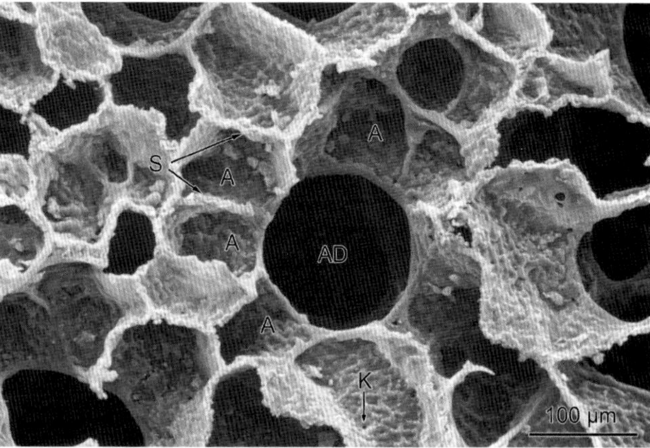

Figure 2-47 Scanning electron micrograph of human lung parenchyma. Alveolar ducts (AD) are surrounded by alveoli (A), which are separated by thin septa (S). K, interalveolar pore of Kohn.

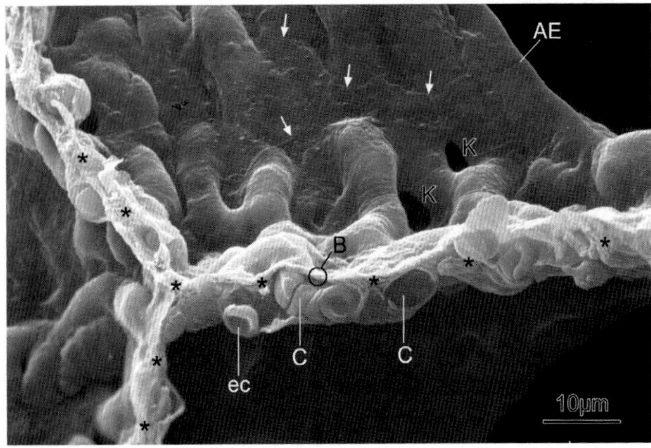

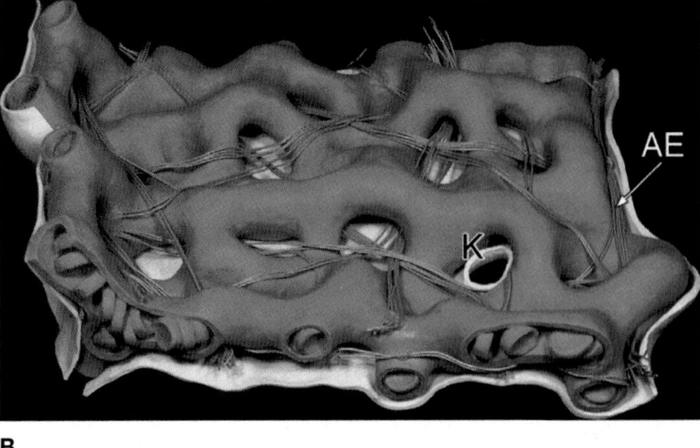

Figure 2-48 In the alveolar wall, shown in (**A**) in a scanning electron micrograph from a human lung, the capillary blood (C) with its erythrocytes (ec) is separated from the air by a very thin tissue barrier (B). *Short arrows* mark intercellular junctions of alveolar epithelium that course toward interalveolar pores of Kohn (K). The model (**B**) shows the capillary network *(red)* to be interwoven with the meshwork of septal fibers *(green)*, the course of which is marked by asterisks in (**A**). The epithelial lining *(yellow)* that crosses the septum at interalveolar pores (K) is removed on the upper surface of the septum to show the capillary. The septal fibers are anchored on the strong fiber bundle marking the free edge of the septum or the alveolar entrance ring (AE). *(Reproduced with permission from Weibel ER: The Pathway for Oxygen. Cambridge, MA: Harvard University Press; 1984.)*

To make the barrier very thin, the interstitial structures must also be reduced to the minimum required (Fig. 2-49). The septal interstitium contains very few cells, mostly slim fibroblast with long extensions; these contain fine bundles of contractile filaments that serve an as yet unknown mechanical function. The septal interstitium usually does not contain cells of the defense system or lymphatics.

INTERNAL SUPPORT OF PARENCHYMAL STRUCTURES: THE PULMONARY FIBER CONTINUUM

This extraordinary reduction of the tissue mass in the alveolar septa inevitably introduces a number of major problems. How is it possible to secure the mechanical integrity of the system if we consider that several forces act on the septal tissue with a tendency to disrupt it? The thin barrier must not only withstand the distending pressure of the capillary blood due to both hemodynamic forces and gravity, particularly in the lower lung zones, but must also keep the capillary bed expanded over a very large surface—a task that is made difficult because surface forces that act on the complex alveolar surface would tend to collapse alveoli and capillaries (see further below). This requires a very subtle, economical design of the fibrous support system.[164,165]

The problem of supporting the capillaries on connective tissue fibers with as little tissue as possible has been solved ingeniously: we find that the fiber network is interlaced with the capillary network.[166] Figure 2-48B shows that when the fibers are taut, the capillaries weave from one side of the septum to the other. This arrangement has a threefold advantage: (1) it allows the capillaries to be supported unit by unit directly on the fiber strands without the need of additional "binders"; (2) it causes the capillaries to become spread out on the alveolar surface when the fibers are stretched; and (3) it optimizes gas-exchange conditions by limiting the presence of fibers, which must interfere with O_2 flow, to half the capillary surface. The thin section of a capillary shown in Figure 2-49 reveals that an interstitial space with fibers and fibroblasts exists on only one side of the capillary, whereas on the other the two lining cells, endothelium and epithelium, become closely joined with only a single common basement membrane interposed. Therefore, over half the surface of the capillary blood is separated from the air merely by a minimal tissue barrier made of epithelial and endothelial cytoplasmic sheets with their basement membranes fused leaving no interstitial space that could enlarge with interstitial pulmonary edema (Fig. 2-17).

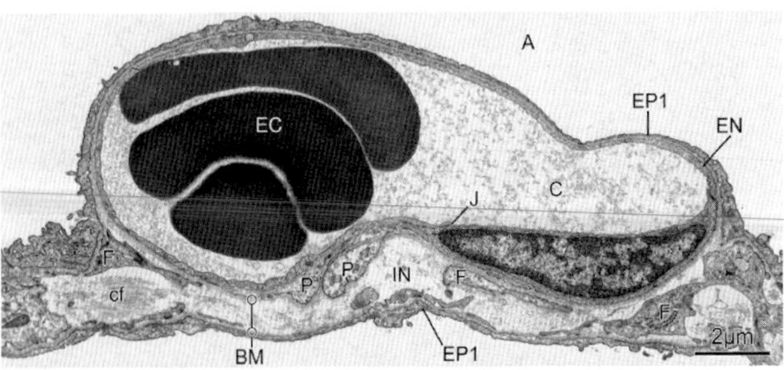

Figure 2-49 Alveolar septum from human lung lined by type I epithelium (EP1) with capillary lined by endothelial cell (EN) that is associated with processes of pericytes (P). Substantial interstitial space (IN) with collagen and elastic fibers (cf) and fibroblasts (F) occurs on one side only, whereas minimal air–blood barrier is formed on other side by fusion of basement membranes (BM) of endothelium and epithelium.

The principal structural "backbone" of the lung is a continuous system of fibers anchored at the hilum and put under tension by the negative intrapleural pressure that tugs on the visceral pleura.[165] The general construction principle follows from the formation of the mesenchymal sheath of the airway units in the developing lung; as the airway tree grows, its branches remain separated by layers of mesenchyme within which blood vessels form. When fiber networks develop within this mesenchyme, they enwrap all airway units and extend from the hilum right to the visceral pleura. The pulmonary fiber system hence forms a three-dimensional fibrous continuum that is structured by the airway system and is closely related to the blood vessels. By virtue of the design of this fibrous continuum, the lung becomes, in fact, subdivided into millions of little bellows that are connected to the airway tree, as represented schematically in Figure 2-50; these structures expand with expansion of the chest because the tension exerted on the visceral pleura by the negative intrapleural pressure becomes transmitted to the bellows' walls through that fiber system.

To try to put some order into this fiber system, we can first single out two major components that can be identified easily (Fig. 2-50).

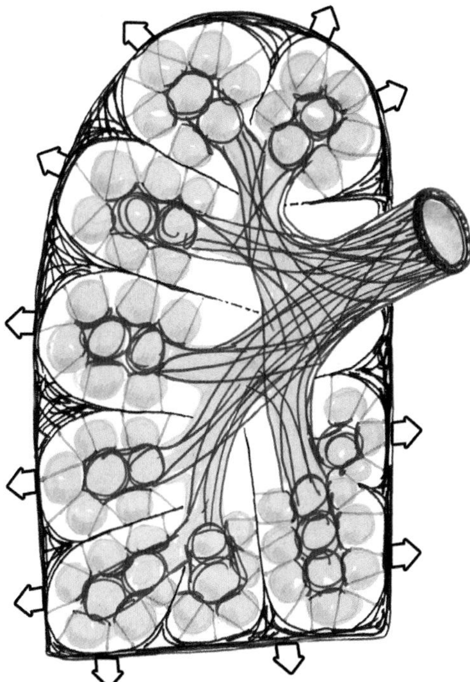

Figure 2-50 The lung's fiber continuum: axial fibers *(red)* extend from airways into the alveolar ducts as a network of entrance rings into alveoli *(yellow)*; peripheral fibers *(black)* extend from the pleura to interlobular septa; the septal fibers *(green)* in the alveolar walls are anchored in peripheral and axial fibers. Arrows indicate the traction on the pleura exerted by thorax and diaphragm. *(Reproduced with permission from Weibel ER: Looking into the lung: What can it tell us? Am J Roentgenol. 1979;133(6):1021–1031.)*

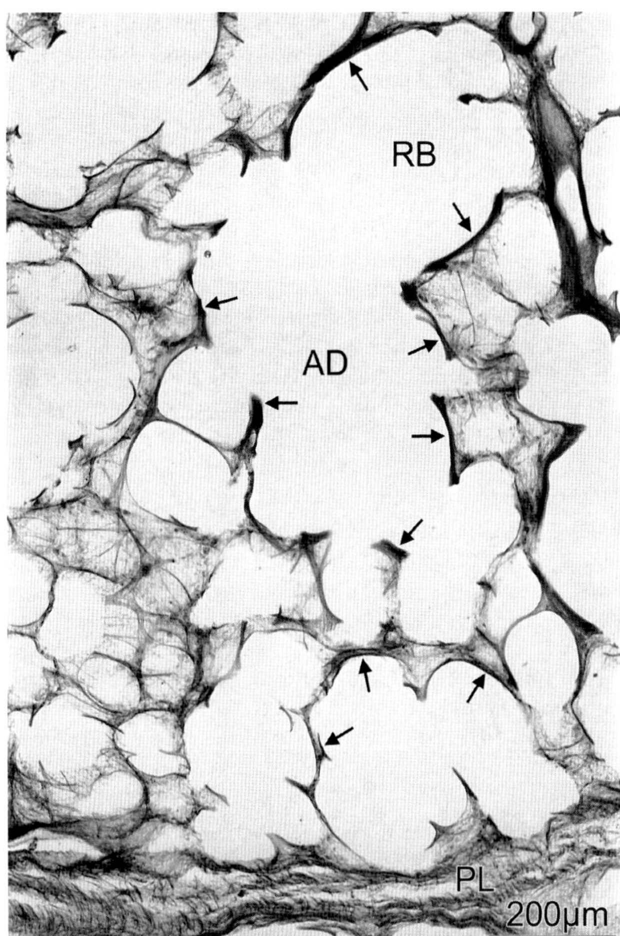

Figure 2-51 Connective tissue stain reveals the strong fiber rings *(arrows)* that demarcate the alveolar ducts (AD) and respiratory bronchioles (RB). Pleura (PL) extends as peripheral fibers into parenchyma. *(Reproduced with permission from Weibel ER: The Pathway for Oxygen. Cambridge, MA: Harvard University Press; 1984.)*

First we find that all airways – from the mainstem bronchus that enters the lung at the hilum out to the terminal bronchioles and beyond – are enwrapped by a strong sheath of fibers. These fibers constitute the axial fiber system; they form the "bark" of the tree whose roots are at the hilum and whose branches penetrate deep into lung parenchyma, following the course of the airways. A second major fiber system is related to the visceral pleura, which is made of strong fiber bags enwrapping all lobes. We then find connective tissue septa penetrating from the visceral pleura into lung parenchyma, separating units of the airway tree. We call these fibers the peripheral fiber system because they mark the boundaries between the units of respiratory lung tissue.

The peripheral fiber system subdivides the lung into a number of units that are not simple to define because they form a continuous hierarchy in accordance with the pattern of airway tree branching. However, as we have seen, two such units appear to be natural: the lobes, which are demarcated by a more or less complete lining by visceral pleura with a serosal cleft interposed (Fig. 2-1); and the acinus, the parenchymal unit in which all airways participate in gas exchange.

The acinus is the functional unit of the pulmonary parenchyma. The airway that leads into the acinus, the transitional bronchiole, continues branching within the acinus for about 6 to 10 additional generations (Figs. 2-5 and 2-40). These intra-acinar airways, called respiratory bronchioles and alveolar ducts, also carry in their wall relatively strong fibers of the axial fiber system, which extend to the end of the duct system. However, since the walls of intra-acinar air ducts are densely settled with alveoli, these fibers are reduced to a kind of delicate network that constitutes the "wall" of the alveolar ducts. The meshes of this network that encircle the alveolar mouths are generally called alveolar entrance rings; it is this fiber network that allows alveoli to be formed as open chambers with free edges of the alveolar septa (Figs. 2-47 and 2-51).[148] These fiber rings are associated with some smooth muscle cells (Fig. 2-29), and they serve as a scaffold for a network of finer fibers that spread within the alveolar septa (Figs. 2-48B and 2-51). However, in a fiber system there may be no loose ends. Accordingly, the septal fiber system must be anchored at both ends—on the network of axial fibers around the alveolar ducts, and on extensions of the peripheral fibers that penetrate into the acinus from interlobular septa. Thus, the fiber system of the lung becomes a continuum that spans the entire space of the lung, from the hilus to the visceral pleura (Fig. 2-50). It is put under varying tension as the pleural bag is expanded by the chest wall and diaphragm. It thus functions as a tensegrity structure where structural integrity is maintained only if the fiber continuum is under tension and undisrupted.[167,168]

The continuous nature of a well-ordered fiber system is an essential design feature of the lung.[148] This becomes evident in emphysema. When some fibers are disrupted, they cannot be kept under tension. They retract and larger airspaces form as the fiber system is rearranged near the damage. Small foci of emphysema form in most lungs in the course of time.

The fiber system serves mainly as a mechanical support for the blood vessels, with which it is intimately associated in an orderly fashion.[148] The pulmonary artery branches in parallel with the airway tree, but it is not related to the axial fiber system. Like the pulmonary veins the pulmonary arteries are associated with those parts of the peripheral fiber system that form an adventitial sheath on the larger vessels of both types and also form a boundary sheath on the outer surface of bronchi where alveolar complexes touch on the bronchial wall. Therefore, it is justified to characterize the connective tissue surrounding bronchi and pulmonary arteries as a peribronchovascular space, which houses the lymphatics as well as the systemic bronchial arteries and their branches. In fact, this space is continuous with the septal connective tissue that enwraps the pulmonary veins (Fig. 2-30) and is continuous with the visceral pleura. However, whereas the arteries penetrate into the acinus, the veins remain at the periphery and are thus located between the airway units (Fig. 2-45). In the alveolar septa, the capillary network spreads out as a broad sheet of vessels whose paths are continuous throughout the system of interconnected alveolar septa (Fig. 2-46). We have seen that these capillaries are intimately related to the septal fiber system (Fig. 2-48B).

PARENCHYMAL MECHANICS AND TISSUE DESIGN

As in all connective tissue, the fibers of the lung are composed of collagen and elastic fibers.[164] The collagen fibers are bundles of fibrils bound together by proteoglycans; they are practically inextensible (less than 2%) and have a very high tensile strength; they rupture at loads of 50 to 70 dyn/cm^{-2}, which means that a collagen fiber of 1-mm diameter can support a weight of over 500 g. In contrast, elastic fibers have a much lower tensile strength but a high extensibility. They can be stretched to about 130% of their relaxed length before rupturing.

In the fiber system of lung parenchyma, collagen and elastic fibers occur in a volume ratio of about 2.5:1, whereas this ratio is 10:1 for the visceral pleura. In a relaxed state, one finds the collagen fibers to be longer than the accompanying elastic fibers, so that they appear wavy. Because of the association between "rubber-like" elastic and "twine-like" collagen fibers, the connective tissue strands behave like an elastic band. They are easy to stretch up to the point where the collagen fibers are taut, but from there on they resist stretching very strongly.

The elastic properties of the lung's fiber system can be studied by filling the airways with fluid so as to eliminate the effects of surface tension. This reveals that the lung's fiber system has a high compliance until high levels of inflation are reached, and that the retractive or recoil force generated by the fiber system amounts to no more than a few millibars at physiologic inflation levels. The actual recoil force in the air-filled lung, reflected by the negative pressure in the pleural space, is appreciably higher, but this is caused by surface tension rather than the retractive force of the fibers.

Surface tension arises at any gas–liquid interface because the cohesive forces between the molecules of the liquid are much stronger than those between the liquid and gas.[169] As a result, the liquid surface tends to become as small as possible. A curved surface, such as that of a bubble, generates a pressure that is proportional to the curvature and the surface tension coefficient γ. The general formula of Gibbs relates this pressure, P_s, to the mean curvature $\overline{K}$:

$$P_s = 2\gamma \cdot \overline{K}$$

In a sphere, the curvature is simply the reciprocal of the radius r (Laplace's law):

$$P_s = \frac{2\gamma}{r}$$

The most critical effect of surface tension is that it endangers stability of the airspace, because a set of connected "bubbles," the alveoli, is inherently unstable: The small ones should contract and the large ones expand. Since the 400 million alveoli are all connected with each other through the airways, the lung is inherently unstable: Why do the alveoli not all collapse and empty into one large bubble? There are two principal reasons.[16,170]

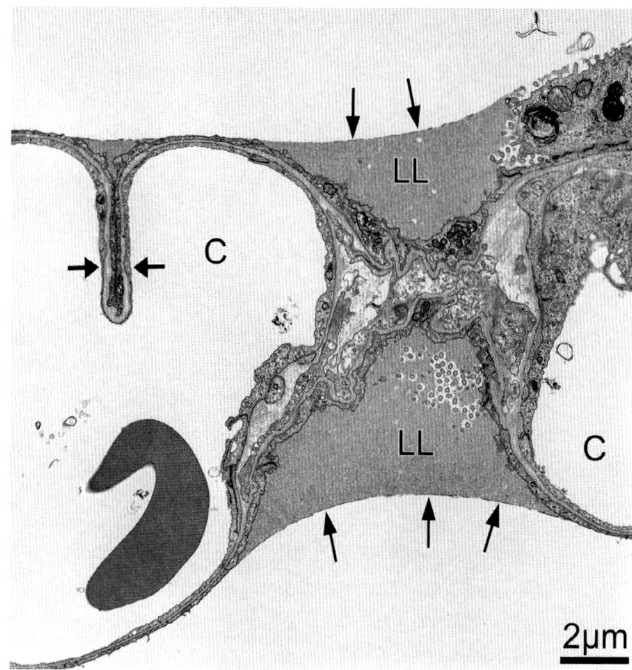

Figure 2-52 Alveolar septum of human lung fixed by perfusion through blood vessels shows alveolar lining layer (LL) in crevices between capillaries (C) topped by surfactant film that appears as a fine black line *(arrows)*. Note the type II cell with lamellar bodies and the fold in thin tissue barrier *(bold arrows)*. *(Used with permission of M. Bachofen and G. Wolff Basel.)*

The first reason is one of tissue structure. The alveoli are not simply soap bubbles in a froth. Rather, their walls contain an intricate fiber system, as we have seen. Thus, when an alveolus tends to shrink, the fibers in the walls of adjoining alveoli are stretched, and this prevents the alveolus from collapsing altogether. It is said that alveoli are mechanically interdependent and this stabilizes them.

The second reason is related to the fact that the alveolar surface is not simply water exposed to air but is lined by surfactant[171] (Figs. 2-25 and 2-52), which has peculiar properties in that its surface tension coefficient γ is variable.[169,172] From a large volume of evidence, it is now established that surface tension falls as the alveolar surface becomes smaller, and that it rises when the surface expands. Because of this feature, which is due to the phospholipoprotein nature of alveolar surfactant (see above), alveoli do not behave like soap bubbles whose surface tension remains constant. When an alveolus begins to shrink, the surface tension of its lining layer falls and the retractive force generated at the surface is reduced or even abolished. Combined with interdependence, this property of surfactant allows the complex of alveoli to remain stable.[170]

Which of the two factors for stabilizing lung structure is now the most important: interdependence or surfactant properties? It turns out that both are essential. If one depletes the lung of its surfactant lining by washing with a detergent, the pressure–volume curve changes dramatically[173] (Fig. 2-53). On deflation, lung volume falls rapidly. If we look at samples from lungs fixed at the same volume (60% total lung capacity) but derived from either normal or detergent-rinsed lungs, we find that surfactant depletion causes the alveoli to collapse. However, this causes the alveolar ducts to enlarge, stretching the strong fiber nets at the mouths of the collapsed alveoli. The ducts do not collapse because of interdependence between adjacent units.

In the normal air-filled lung, surfactant properties and interdependence owing to fiber tension both contribute to stabilizing the

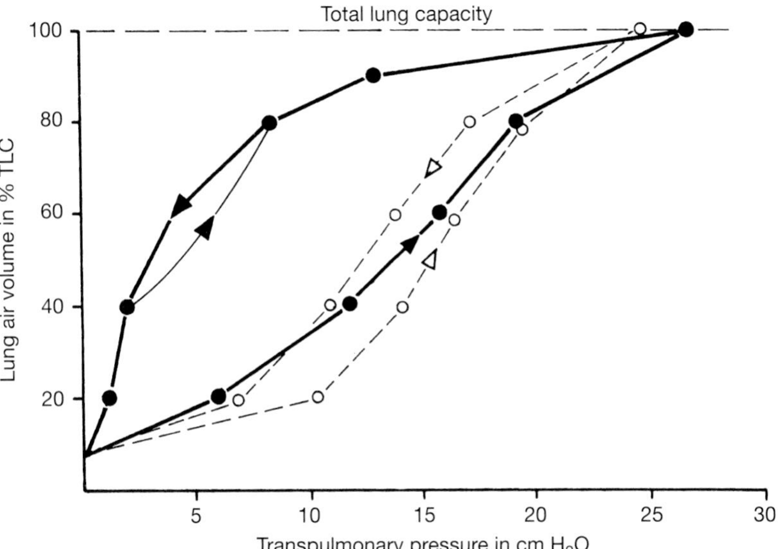

Figure 2-53 Comparison of pressure–volume curve of a normal air-filled rabbit lung *(heavy line)* with that of a surfactant-depleted lung *(broken line)*. The thin line with *paired arrows* represents small hysteresis when breathing between 40% and 80% TLC along the deflation curve.

complex of alveoli and alveolar ducts.[174] To understand this, let us examine Figure 2-54, which shows a highly simplified diagram of a parenchymal unit. Interdependence is established by the continuum of axial, septal, and peripheral fibers. Surface tension exerts an inward pull in the hollow alveoli, where curvature is negative. However, over the free edge of the alveolar septa, along the outline of the duct, the surface tension must push outward because there the curvature is positive.[16] The latter force must be rather strong, because the radius of curvature is very small on the septal edge; but this force is counteracted by the strong fiber strands, usually provided with some smooth muscle cells, that we find in the free edge of the alveolar septum (Figs. 2-29, 2-47, and 2-51). Thus, interdependence is an important factor in preventing the complex hollow of the lung, where negative and positive curvatures coexist, from collapsing. However, its capacity to do so is limited and requires low surface tensions, particularly on deflation when the fibers tend to slack. If surface tension becomes too high, the lung's foam-like structure will partly collapse in spite of fiber interdependence.

This is of considerable physiologic importance. It is sometimes claimed that alveoli pop open when the lung is inflated, collapsing on deflation. That is correct when starting with a deflated lung (Fig. 2-53): collapsed alveoli open up along the inflation curve. But that is not the way we breathe. The normal breathing cycle operates on the deflation slope of the pressure–volume curve (Fig. 2-53) with small hysteresis, a state that is maintained by taking a deep sigh intermittently up to TLC. In this condition the surface tension is kept low because the surfactant lining is spread out[172] and alveoli do not collapse. When we breathe in and out between 80% and 40% of total lung capacity, the range of normal breathing in exercise, alveoli change their size very little. In contrast to the twofold change in air volume the alveolar surface area changes by only about a factor of 1.2.[174] The reason for this is that the main change in air volume does not occur in alveoli, but predominantly in the alveolar ducts as shown in Figure 2-55, and this is very favorable for acinar ventilation. This differential volume change can be explained by the effect of surface forces: at 40% TLC surface tension γ is nearly 0 but it increases to 12 $mN{\cdot}m^{-1}$ at 80% TLC 2. As the lung inflates this causes the positive surface force to become strong on the free edge of alveolar septa (Fig. 2-54), thus causing the duct cross section to widen, while shrinking when the forces decrease on deflation (Fig. 2-55). In this process the alveolar septa become stretched on inflation by only a small degree, a mere 20% in area. The acinus is thus well ventilated whereas the gas-exchange surface is little affected by varying air volume.[148]

MICROMECHANICS OF THE ALVEOLAR SEPTUM

We must finally consider the mechanical factors that shape the alveolar septum in the air-filled lung. As we have seen, the alveolar septum is made of a single capillary network that is interlaced with fibers (Fig. 2-48). When the fibers are stretched, the capillaries bulge alternatingly to one side or the other, and this causes pits and crevices to occur in the meshes of the capillary network.

This irregular surface is to some extent evened out by the presence of an extracellular layer of lining fluid, which is rather thin over the capillaries but forms little pools in the intercapillary pits (Fig. 2-52).[175] This lining consists of an aqueous layer of variable thickness, called the hypophase, and surfactant, which forms a film on the surface of the hypophase. The hypophase seems to contain considerable amounts of reserve surfactant material, which occurs in a characteristic configuration called tubular myelin (Figs. 2-25 and 2-26).

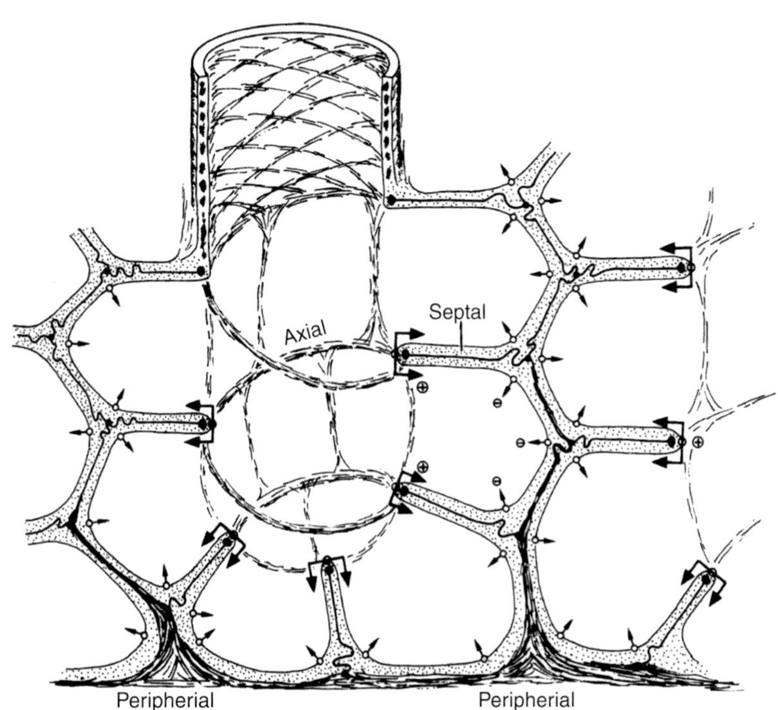

Figure 2-54 Model of the disposition of axial, septal, and peripheral fibers in an acinus showing the effect of surface forces *(arrows)*. *(Reproduced with permission from Weibel ER: The Pathway for Oxygen. Cambridge, MA: Harvard University Press; 1984.)*

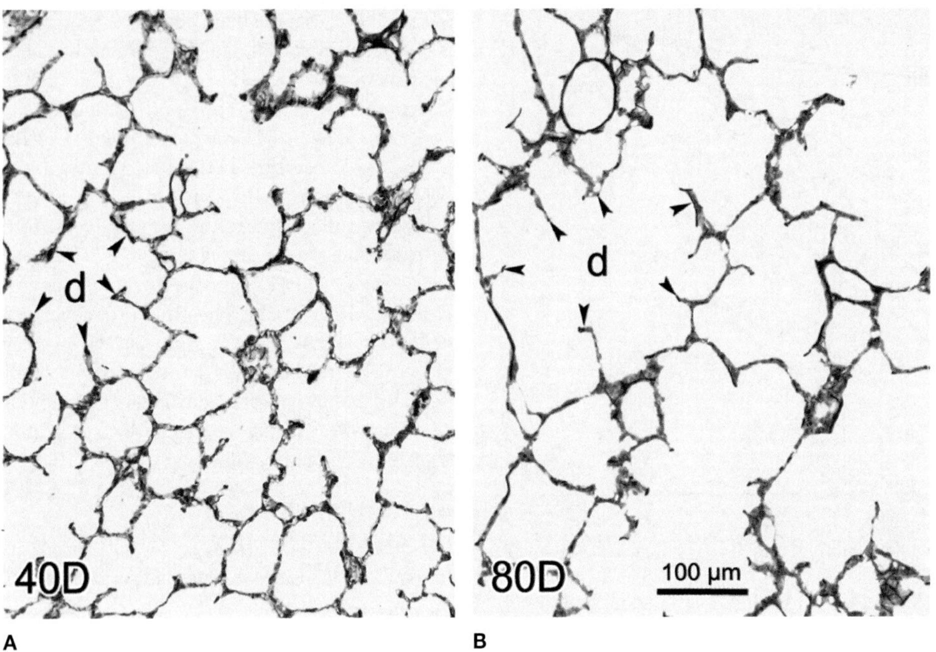

Figure 2-55 Light micrographs of sections of lung parenchyma in rabbit lungs perfusion fixed on deflation to 40% TLC (**A**), and 80% TLC (**B**), respectively (compare Fig. 2-53). Note that the size of the alveolar ducts (d) is markedly enlarged in 80D due to the surface forces acting on the free edges of alveolar septa *(arrow heads). (Preparations used with permission of H. Bachofen, University of Bern.)*

In the alveolar septum, the tissue structures are extremely delicate, as we have seen. Therefore, its configuration is not exclusively determined by structural features but results from the molding effect of various forces that must be kept in balance. Figure 2-56 shows how the three principal mechanical forces – tissue tension, surface tension, and capillary distending pressure – interact in the septum.[16] The fibers of the alveolar septum are under a tension whose magnitude depends on the level of lung inflation. This tends to straighten out the fibers, so that a force (pressure) normal to the fiber axis results, which is responsible for shifting the capillaries to one side of the septum or the other (Figs. 2-48B and 2-56). The walls of the capillaries are exposed to the luminal pressure, which is the result of blood pressure in pulmonary arteries and veins but also depends on gravity, for one finds wider capillaries at the bottom of the lung than at the top. If this distending pressure acts homogeneously over the circumference of the capillary, it will push against the fibers on one side but will cause the thin barrier on the opposite side to bulge outward. This effect is to some extent counteracted by surface tension, which exerts a force normal to the surface (Fig. 2-56). This force depends on two factors. Its direction depends on the orientation of curvature, acting toward the alveolar space over concave regions (negative curvature) and toward the tissue over convexities (positive curvature); and its magnitude depends on the degree of curvature and on the value of the surface tension coefficient γ.

The alveolar septum achieves a stable configuration when all these interacting forces are in balance.[176] Combined forces tend to squash the capillary flat; this happens at high levels of lung inflation when the fibers are under high tension and the surface tension coefficient of surfactant reaches its highest value because of expansion of the surface. On deflation, the fibers are relaxed and surface tension falls drastically. The capillary distending pressure now exceeds both the tissue and the surface forces, with the result that the slack fibers are bent, weaving through the capillary network, whereas the capillaries bulge slightly toward the airspace. Surface tension is apparently so low as to permit a considerable degree of surface "crumpling" to persist (Fig. 2-57).

The importance of the balance between the forces that act on the septum is also shown in Figure 2-58.[177] The specimen of panel B was fixed under zone 3 perfusion conditions, where capillary pressure is larger than alveolar pressure, and all the capillaries are wide, partly bulging toward the airspace, as in Figure 2-57. This is different in panel A, which was fixed under zone 2 conditions where capillary pressure is close to alveolar pressure. In the flat part of the septum, the capillaries are squashed flat, because the surface and tissue forces now exceed the vascular distending pressure. However, it is interesting that the capillaries remain wide in the corners where three septa come together. The distribution of surface forces causes the internal pressure to be lower in the region of these corners, as we can see intuitively from Figure 2-54.

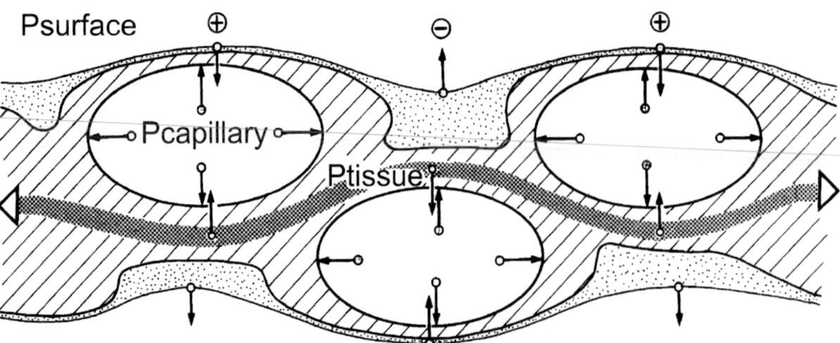

Figure 2-56 Model showing the micromechanical forces of surface tension, tissue tension, and capillary distending pressure that shape the alveolar septum. *(Reproduced with permission from Weibel ER: The Pathway for Oxygen. Cambridge, MA: Harvard University Press; 1984.)*

THE LUNG AS GAS EXCHANGER

The structures discussed so far are designed to ultimately serve the lung's main function, gas exchange between air and blood, in relation to the body's varying O_2 needs.[178] These are set by the energetic demands of the cells and their mitochondria when these produce ATP by oxidative phosphorylation to allow the cells to do work. This process requires a flow of O_2 to be maintained from the lung to the cells, as will be discussed later. It proceeds along the respiratory system through various steps: into the lung by ventilation, to the blood by diffusion, through the circulation by blood flow, from the blood capillaries by diffusion to the cells and

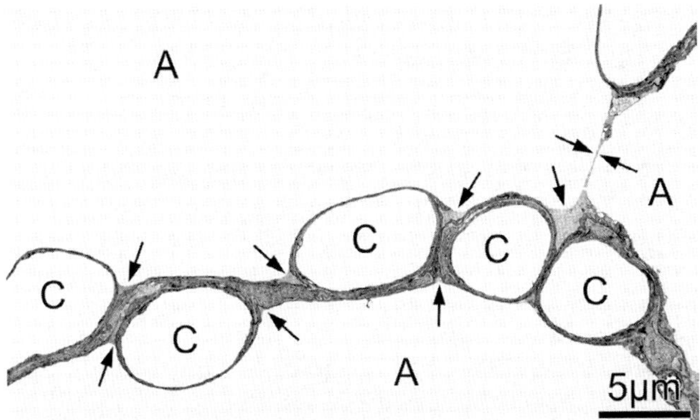

Figure 2-57 Alveolar septum of air-filled rabbit lung perfusion fixed at 60% TLC shows empty capillaries (C), which bulge toward the alveolar airspace (A). Note pools of surface lining layer in the crevices between capillaries *(arrows)* and film spanning across alveolar pore *(double arrows)*. *(Reproduced with permission from Gil J et al. Alveolar volume-surface area relation in air- and saline-filled lungs fixed by vascular perfusion. J Appl Physiol Respir Environ Exerc Physiol. 1979;47(5):990–1001.)*

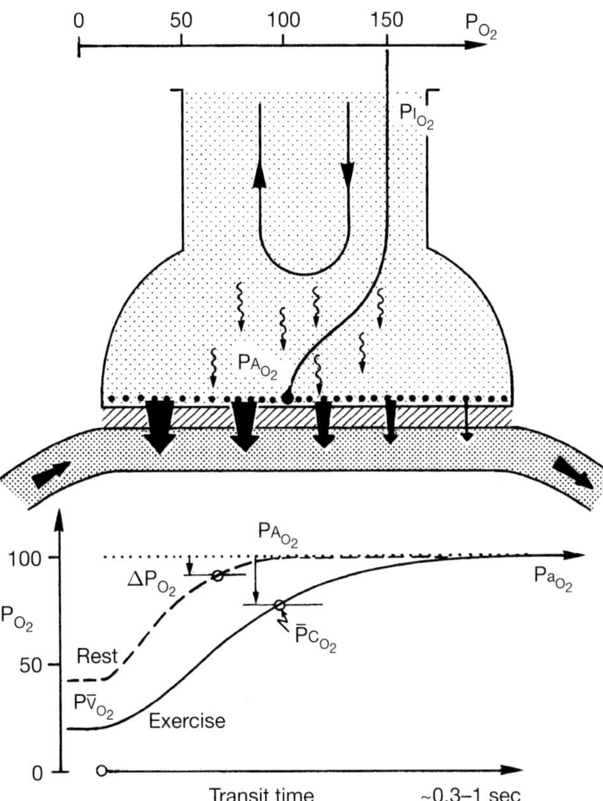

Figure 2-59 Model of gas exchange showing gradual rise of capillary P_{O_2} ($P_{\bar{c}_{O_2}}$) as blood flows through capillary until it approaches alveolar P_{O_2} ($P_{A_{O_2}}$). *(Reproduced with permission from Weibel ER: The Pathway for Oxygen. Cambridge, MA: Harvard University Press; 1984.)*

mitochondria, where it disappears in the process of oxidative phosphorylation.[16] A number of basic features characterize this system[179]: (1) under steady-state conditions the O_2 flow rate, $\dot{V}_{O_2}$ is the same at all levels, that is, O_2 uptake in the lung is equal to O_2 consumption in the tissues; (2) the basic driving force for O_2 flow through the system is a cascade of O_2 partial pressure which falls from inspired P_{O_2} down to near zero in the mitochondria; (3) the O_2 flow rate at each step is the product of a partial pressure difference and a conductance which is related to structural and functional properties of the organs participating in O_2 transfer, as will be discussed below in detail.

With respect to gas exchange in the lung (Fig. 2-59), the O_2 flow rate is determined by the Bohr equation:[180]

$$\dot{V}_{O_2} = (P_{A_{O_2}} - P\bar{c}_{O_2}) \cdot D_{L_{O_2}}$$

Where

$P_{A_{O_2}}$ = P_{O_2} in alveoli,

$P\bar{c}_{O_2}$ = the mean P_{O_2} in pulmonary capillaries, and

$D_{L_{O_2}}$ = the pulmonary diffusing capacity or the lung's O_2 conductance

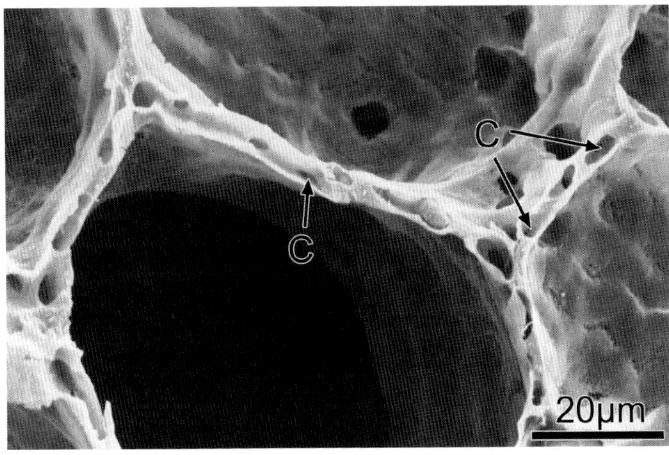

A

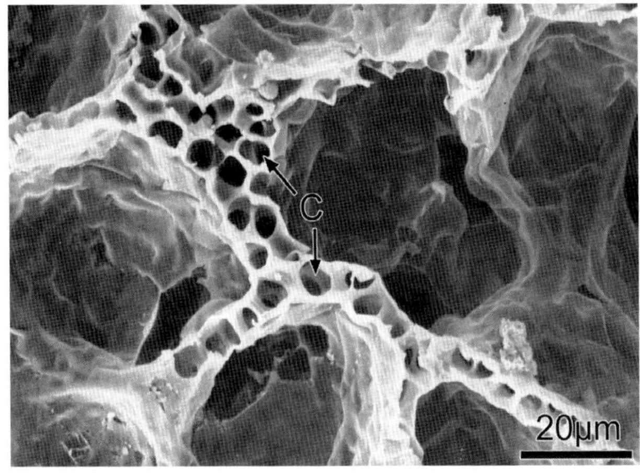

B

Figure 2-58 Scanning electron micrographs of alveolar walls of rabbit lungs fixed under (**A**), zone 2 and (**B**), zone 3 conditions of perfusion. Note that capillaries (C) are wide in zone 3 and slit-like in zone 2, except for "corner capillaries," which are wide in either case. *(Reproduced with permission from Bachofen H et al: Morphometric estimates of diffusing capacity in lungs fixed under zone II and zone III conditions. Respir Physiol. 1983;52(1):41–52.)*

The important point is now that all parameters to the right of this equation may be significantly affected by design features. We will see that DL_{O_2} is largely determined by the surface area and the thickness of the air–blood barrier. The O_2 partial pressure difference is established by ventilation and perfusion of the gas-exchange units, and this may be affected by the design of the airway and vascular trees, particularly in the acinus.[178]

THE PULMONARY DIFFUSING CAPACITY

In the equation mentioned earlier, DL_{O_2} is the total conductance of the gas exchanger for O_2 diffusion from the alveolar air into the capillary erythrocytes until it is bound to hemoglobin. It can be estimated physiologically if we can measure O_2 uptake $\dot{V}_{O_2}$ and estimate the effective P_{O_2} difference between alveolar air and capillary blood, not a trivial undertaking as the change in capillary P_{O_2} as O_2 is being taken up must be integrated (Fig. 2-59). On the other hand the conductance is a physical characteristic. Therefore, it should be possible to calculate a theoretical value of DL_{O_2} from the physical properties of the gas exchanger, its dimensions and material properties.[181,182] To do that we must consider the geometry of the structures involved, alveoli, tissue barrier, and capillary blood, in setting up a physical model of DL_{O_2}. In the first step, we can break the process into two steps (Fig. 2-60):[183] (1) O_2 flow across the barrier or what has been called the membrane conductance DM_{O_2} and (2) O_2 binding to hemoglobin in the red blood cells or the conductance of capillary blood De_{O_2} These two conductances are in series. Accordingly their overall effect on O_2 flow is obtained by adding their resistances or the reciprocal of the conductance:

$$1/DL_{O_2} = 1/DM_{O_2} + 1/De_{O_2}$$

The two conductances DM_{O_2} and De_{O_2} are of very different nature. DM_{O_2} is the conductance of a diffusion barrier that offers "passive" resistance to diffusion and thus depends essentially on the material properties of the barrier, estimated by a diffusion coefficient K, and on the dimensions of the barrier. The larger the surface area S and the thinner the barrier thickness τ the greater DM_{O_2}, according to the formula $DM_{O_2} = K \cdot S/\tau$. In contrast, De_{O_2} is related to a more complex process that involves, besides diffusion, the binding of O_2 to hemoglobin, which is a nonlinear process.

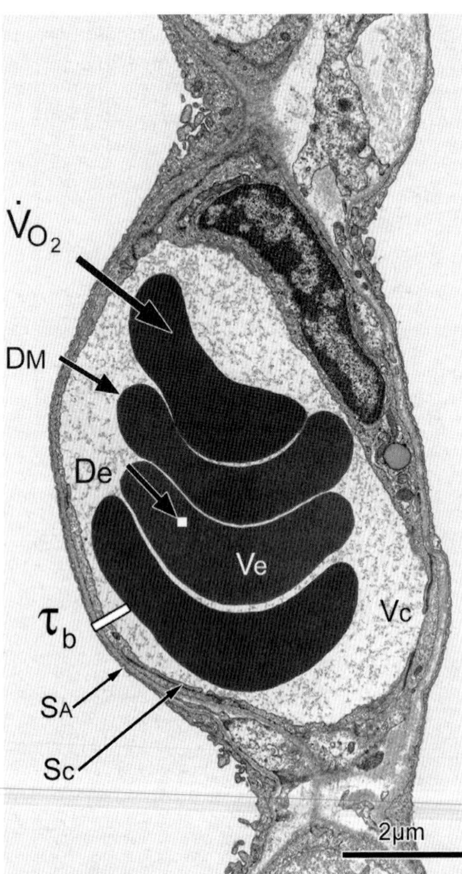

Figure 2-60 Morphometric model for calculating diffusion capacity, DL. Its two components are: (1) the membrane conductance DM, which extends from the alveolar surface (SA) to the nearest erythrocyte membrane traversing the tissue barrier, the capillary surface (Sc), and the plasma layer over the distance τ_b; and (2) the conductance of the erythrocyte interior, De, that depends on the capillary and the erythrocyte volume, Vc and Ve. (See text.)

The Membrane Conductance (DM_{O_2})

The structural characteristics of the membrane conductor are seen in Figure 2-60. It is made of the two layers that separate air in alveoli from the erythrocytes in the capillary: the tissue barrier and the layer of blood plasma. In addition, an alveolar lining layer of varying thickness spreads over the epithelial surface. Even though these layers have distinct characteristics; in effect they act as a single diffusion barrier.[182]

As discussed earlier in this chapter, the tissue barrier is a complex structure. Its two bounding surfaces are formed by independent cell layers, epithelium and endothelium, and they are related to two independent functional spaces, alveoli and capillaries. The two surfaces are not perfectly matched, and the thickness of the barrier varies considerably (Fig. 2-60). Over about half the surface the tissue barrier shows minimal thickness compatible with an intact structure: The thin cytoplasmic leaflets of type I epithelial cells are joined to the thin extensions of endothelial cells by the fused basement membranes leaving no interstitial space. In this region we also find the surface lining layer to be very thin. Over the other half the barrier is thicker because of the occurrence of supporting connective tissue fibers (Fig. 2-49) and the presence of cell bodies of epithelial and endothelial cells as well as fibroblasts, and the lining layer can form deeper pools (Fig. 2-52).

The plasma layer shows even greater variation in its thickness and distribution. Since erythrocytes are of about the same dimension as the capillaries, the plasma layer that separates them from the endothelium can be vanishingly thin where the red cell nearly touches the wall. However, erythrocytes are corpuscular particles and there are "plugs" of plasma of varying size that separate them in the direction of blood flow. Also their distortable disk shape causes the plasma layer between erythrocyte and capillary surface to be quite variable.[184] Furthermore, occasional leukocytes function like plasma plugs in regard to O_2 diffusion to the red cells. Therefore, the diffusion distance from the capillary wall to the red cell membrane can vary from a few nm to several µm.

Strictly speaking, these two layers of the barrier offer O_2 diffusion different resistances so their conductances should be calculated separately. However, this distinction does not appear to be important under normal conditions. Indeed, it is more reasonable to treat them as a single barrier. For one, the flow velocity of the plasma layer is much lower than the diffusion of O_2 so that plasma is quasistatic with respect to diffusion. Furthermore, under normal conditions the surface areas of alveoli, capillaries, and erythrocytes do not differ much, and the diffusion coefficients of tissue and plasma are also quite similar. Therefore, we prefer now to estimate the membrane diffusing capacity by considering O_2 diffusion from the alveolar surface to the erythrocyte membrane as:[182]

$$DM_{O_2} = k_b \cdot S(b)/\tau_{hb} = K_b \cdot (S(A)+S(c))/2 \cdot \tau_{hb}$$

where K_b is Krogh's permeation coefficient estimated at 3.3×10^{-8} $cm^2\ min^{-1}\ mm\ Hg^{-1}$, τ_{hb} is the harmonic mean distance from the alveolar surface to the nearest erythrocyte membrane, and S(b) is the surface area of the barrier that we estimate as the mean of the alveolar and capillary surface areas, S(A) and S(c), respectively, the two most robust measures of the area of air–blood contact. These parameters can be estimated on sections of properly sampled lung tissue by stereologic methods.[185–187]

We should also mention that the presence of a surface lining layer in the living lung may modify the geometry of the barrier as we see it on electron micrographs with the consequence that both the barrier thickness and the alveolar surface are reduced to a similar degree because some thicker parts of the barrier become shifted beneath the surfactant pools (Fig. 2-52).[177] Therefore, the effect on the estimate of DL_{O_2} is negligible.

Erythrocyte Conductance (De_{O_2})

As mentioned, the erythrocyte conductance is of a different nature in that it involves two coupled events,[183] that is, diffusion of molecular oxygen and oxyhemoglobin within the red blood cell as well as the chemical reaction of O_2 with hemoglobin. A way out of this is to obtain an empirical estimate of the rate at which O_2 is bound to whole blood, θ_{O_2}, and to express the erythrocyte conductance De_{O_2} as:

$$De_{O_2} = \theta_{O_2} Vc$$

where Vc is the total capillary blood volume, which can again be estimated on sections by stereologic methods.

The coefficient θ_{O_2} is estimated in vitro on whole blood, but this is difficult because of the effect of variable unstirred layers around the red cells.[188,189] In addition, θ_{O_2} depends on the hematocrit or hemoglobin concentration, and it is not a constant as it falls with increasing O_2–hemoglobin saturation; recent studies have shown that, as blood moves through alveolar capillaries, θ_{O_2} falls gradually from about 4 to 1 mL O_2 mL^{-1}, $torr^{-1}$ so that the correct value can only be found after Bohr integration of capillary P_{O_2}. For normal human lungs and a hemoglobin content of 15 g/100 mL of blood, a value $\theta_{O_2} = 1.8\ mL\,O_2 \cdot mL^{-1}, torr^{-1}$ is a reasonable estimate, but if the actual hemoglobin concentration [Hb] varies a corrected value can be obtained by multiplying this standard value with a factor c = [Hb]/15.

Morphometry of the Human Lung and Diffusing Capacity

With this model in hand, we can now attempt to estimate the diffusing capacity of the human lung on the basis of morphometric data, as listed in Table 2-4. These data, obtained by electron microscopic morphometry on seven young adults,[190] reveal the alveolar surface area to amount to 130 m^2 and the capillary surface to be about 10% smaller. These values are higher than those most commonly quoted in textbooks derived from light microscopic studies, which did not adequately resolve the alveolar surface texture. The harmonic mean thickness of the tissue barrier is 0.6 μm, whereas the total barrier, from alveolar to red cell surface (Fig. 2-60), measures 1.11 μm.[182] The capillary volume is estimated at about 200 mL. With these data we calculate DL_{O_2} for the adult human lung to be about 150 to 200 mL O_2 min^{-1} mm Hg^{-1}, the variation depending on the choice of θ_{O_2}.

These data also allow us to ask the question how the resistance to O_2 diffusion is distributed between the diffusion barrier and the red cells. Table 2-4 shows that the diffusion conductance of the "membrane" and that of the red cells are very similar, which means that the resistance to O_2 uptake is nearly equally divided between membrane and red cells.

These morphometric estimates of the diffusing capacity are based on model assumptions that are considered reasonable. The test of their validity must be to compare them with physiologic estimates. The standard physiologic value of DL_{O_2} of a healthy adult at rest is about 30 mL O_2 min^{-1} mm Hg^{-1}; thus, considerably less than what we find on the basis of morphometric estimates. However, this is not a valid comparison, because, under resting conditions, we take up only one-tenth the amount of O_2 that our lungs are capable

TABLE 2-4 Morphometric Estimate of DL_{O_2} for Young, Healthy Adult Humans of 70-kg Body Weight, Measuring 175 cm in Height

Morphometric data (mean ± 1 SE)			
Total lung volume (60% TLC)	4340	±285	mL
Alveolar surface area	130	±12	m^2
Capillary surface area	115	±12	m^2
Capillary volume	194	±30	mL
Air–blood tissue barrier thickness			
Arithmetic mean	2.2	± 0.2	μm
Harmonic mean	0.62	±0.04	μm
Total barrier harmonic mean thickness	1.11	± 0.1	μm
Diffusing Capacity (mL/min/mm Hg)			
Membrane	DM_{O_2}	350	
Total	DL_{O_2}	158	

Source: Reproduced with permission from Gehr P, Bachofen M, Weibel ER. The normal human lung: Ultrastructure and morphometric estimation of diffusion capacity. Respir Physiol. 1978;32:121–140 and Weibel ER. Symmorphosis: on form and function in shaping life. Cambridge, MA: Harvard University Press; 2000.

of absorbing under conditions of heavy work. There have been a number of estimates of DL_{O_2} in exercising humans,[191] and these have yielded values of the order of 100 mL O_2 min^{-1} mm Hg^{-1}. This estimate should come closer to the "true capacity" of the lung for O_2 transfer to the blood than the value obtained at rest. The fact that this is only about 50% lower than the morphometric estimate is not disturbing, for we do not know whether the "true diffusing capacity" is completely exploited even in heavy exercise. Inhomogeneities in the distribution of ventilation and perfusion would, for example, limit the degree to which "true" DL_{O_2} can be exploited. One aspect of this type of limitation is discussed in the following when we consider the effect of the acinus design on gas exchange.

To test whether the morphometric estimate of DL_{O_2} is reasonable we performed, some years ago, a combined physiologic and morphometric estimation of pulmonary diffusing capacity on four species of canids ranging from 4 to 30 kg in body mass.[192]

Because it is difficult to estimate mean capillary P_{O_2} reliably, most physiologic measurements of the diffusing capacity use carbon monoxide (CO) as a tracer gas; CO binds to hemoglobin so avidly that, for practical purposes, the Pb_{CO} is zero, so that it suffices to measure CO uptake and alveolar CO concentration. It is also possible to revise the morphometric model of diffusing capacity to estimate the conductance for CO instead of O_2 by appropriately changing the permeability coefficients and the rate of CO binding to erythrocytes, θ_{CO}, whereas the morphometric parameters are not changed. In a study on dogs and on other canids, the calculated morphometric value of DL_{O_2} was found to be larger than the physiologic estimate by less than a factor of 1.5, thus confirming the observation made with respect to human lungs.

Therefore, we conclude that the pulmonary gas exchanger is designed with a certain amount of redundancy or excess capacity, but this is by no means unreasonable from an engineering point of view. Indeed, to design the pulmonary gas exchanger with a certain degree of redundancy may make a lot of sense. The lung forms the interface to the environment and its functional performance will thus depend on environmental conditions, such as the prevailing O_2 partial pressure, which falls as we go from sea level to higher altitudes. It has been shown that goats, whose DL_{O_2} is about twice as large as seemingly required, can maintain their maximal level of exercise-induced $\dot{V}_{O_2}$ even under hypoxic conditions whereas the dogs that have very small excess DL_{O_2} cannot. It has also been suggested that human athletes exercising at high altitude may fully exploit their DL_{O_2}. This suggests that the apparent redundancy in DL_{O_2} may be a safety factor to protect the good functioning of the pulmonary gas exchanger even when environmental conditions are not optimal. Recent studies with partial pneumonectomy in dogs have shown that the lung can achieve 85% of its maximal O_2 uptake even when 40% of lung tissue is removed after left pneumonectomy, making use of some of this reserve capacity; but when right pneumonectomy removes 60% of lung tissue, adequate function can be achieved only after compensatory growth of the residual lung tissue to restore diffusing capacity.[193–196]

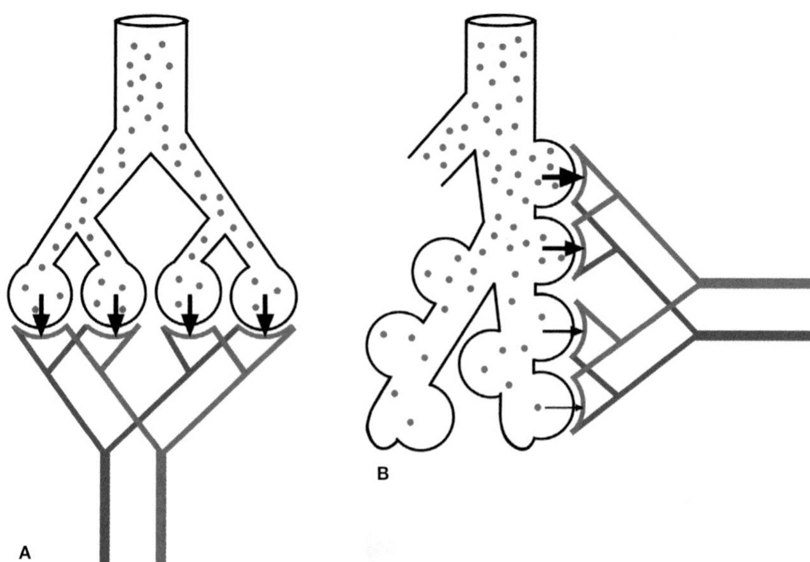

Figure 2-61 Models of ventilation–perfusion relationship in the mammalian pulmonary gas exchanger. **A.** Parallel ventilation/parallel perfusion. **B.** Serial ventilation/parallel perfusion. *(Reproduced with permission from Sapoval B, Filoche M, Weibel ER. Smaller is better, but not too small: A physical scale for the design of the mammalian pulmonary acinus. Proc Natl Acad Sci USA. 2002;99(16):10411–10416. Copyright (2002) National Academy of Sciences, USA.)*

DESIGN OF THE ACINUS AND GAS EXCHANGE

The preceding section considered the overall size of the gas exchanger of the entire lung to compare it with the global performance of this organ. In reality, the surface the size of a tennis court is subdivided into some 400 million gas-exchange units. These are individually perfused with blood because they correspond to the unit capillary network that spans between pulmonary arteriole and venule (Fig. 2-46). The diameter of such a roughly disk-shaped unit is about 500 μm and has a surface area that corresponds approximately to that of an alveolus, even though alveoli and the capillary unit are not congruent as the latter spans over several alveoli and each alveolus is in contact with several capillary units.[162]

These gas-exchange units are arranged along the terminal generations of the airway tree that form the pulmonary acinus (Fig. 2-61B). Note that this arrangement of gas-exchange units to the airway system differs from the common representation of the alveolar–capillary unit as a terminal "bubble" (Fig. 2-61A). This has potential functional consequences because ventilation of alveoli occurs in two steps:[197] (1) upon inspiration oxygen-rich air flows through the airways into the acinus carrying along O_2; (2) in the peripheral airways flow velocity slows down because the airway cross-section increases, and O_2 now moves toward the periphery by diffusion in the air phase, driven by the P_{O_2} gradient that becomes established as O_2 is absorbed at the alveolar surface (Fig. 2-62). Thus, in the peripheral airways diffusion along the airways is combined with diffusive permeation of O_2 into the alveoli and across the tissue barrier to the blood, the actual process of gas exchange. Whereas all capillary network units are individually perfused with venous blood the alveoli are not independent in terms of their O_2 supply, which depends on their location along the airway tree. Therefore, the design of the acinus has significant effects on the gas-exchange conditions.

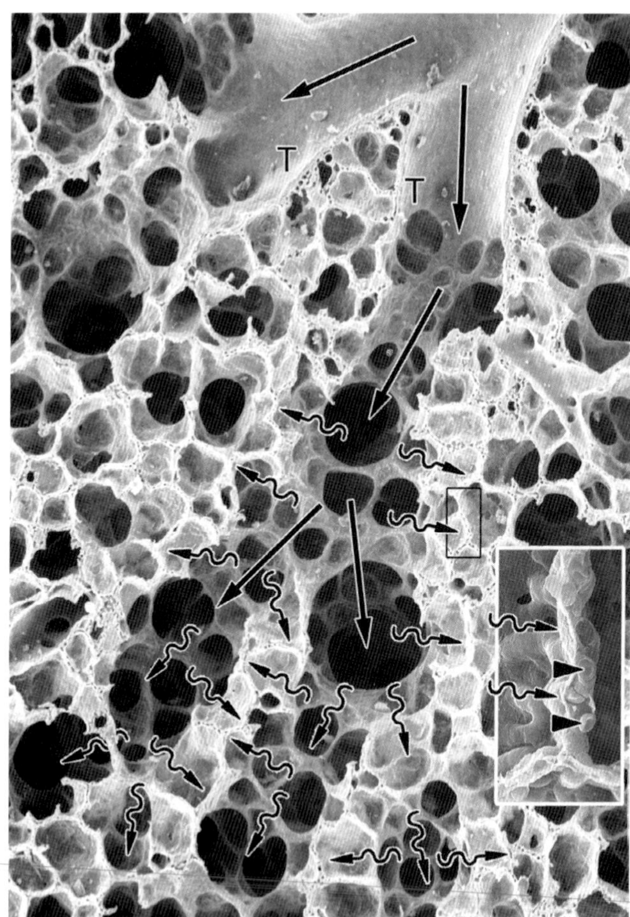

Figure 2-62 Central part of the acinar airways beginning with transitional bronchiole (T) and leading into the branched alveolar ducts. On inspiration air flows in by convection *(straight arrows)*, but as flow velocity falls diffusion of O_2 *(wiggly arrows)* becomes the dominant mechanism for bringing O_2 to the gas-exchange surface. All along acinar airways O_2 is absorbed by the capillary blood in the septa *(inset, arrowheads)*.

THE ACINAR AIRWAY SYSTEM CONNECTED TO THE GAS EXCHANGER

In a systematic study of human lungs[9] the mean volume of acini was found to be 187 mm^3 with a standard deviation of 79 mm^3. The branching pattern for an average size human acinus is shown in Figure 2-63. The segment lengths have been drawn to scale and the terminal clusters of alveoli of the alveolar sacs are marked by a dot. This acinus has been subdivided into eight subacini whose

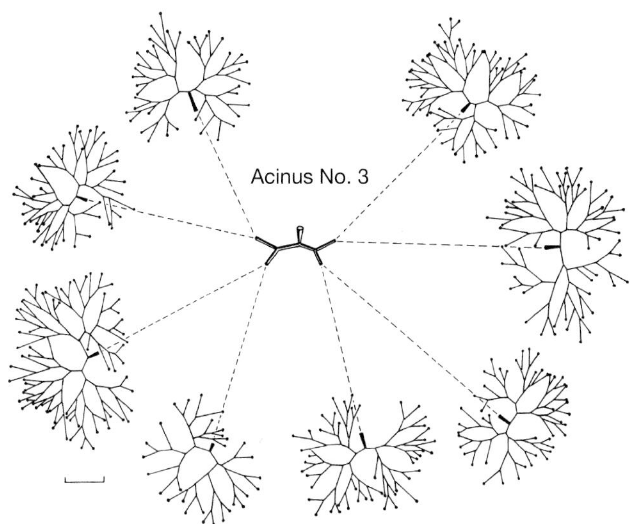

Figure 2-63 Graphic representation of branching pattern of acinar airways in one human acinus of 183 mm^3 volume with the segment lengths drawn to scale. The airways are separated at the third generation thus displaying the branching pattern within each 1/8 subacinus. *(Reproduced with permission from Haefeli-Bleuer B, Weibel ER: Morphometry of the human pulmonary acinus. Anat Rec. 1988;220(4):401–414.)*

substems are located in the third generation of acinar airways. The first three generations of acinar airways following on the transitional bronchiole are respiratory bronchioles, where there are only a few alveoli. In contrast, the alveolar ducts that follow are completely and densely lined with alveoli (Fig. 2-64). The 1/8 subacinus is a unit

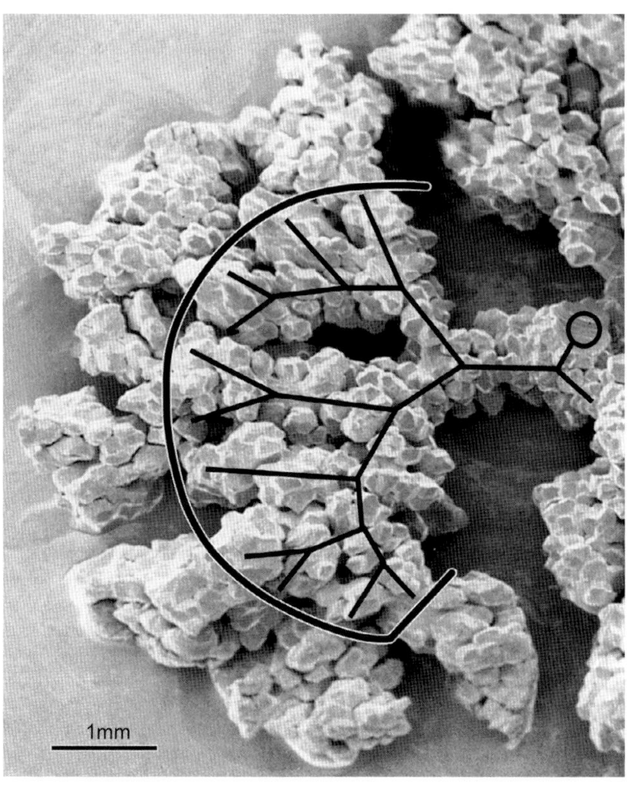

Figure 2-64 Airways of 1/8 subacinus of human lung beginning with generation 18 alveolar duct (circle). The silicon rubber cast has been spread out to show the course of the subsequent branchings. The curved line marks the approximate boundary to the last generation to show that this generation of alveolar sacs (see Fig. 2-5) comprises over half the gas-exchange area of the acinus.

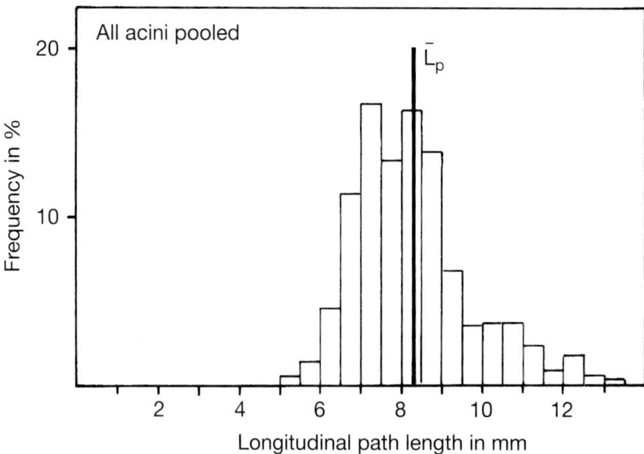

Figure 2-65 Frequency distribution of longitudinal path length from the transitional bronchiole to the alveolar sacs in the human lung. *(Reproduced with permission from Haefeli-Bleuer B, Weibel ER: Morphometry of the human pulmonary acinus. Anat Rec. 1988;220(4):401–414.)*

of functional significance, as we shall see. The intra-acinar airways branch by irregular dichotomy; terminal sacs are located in generations 6 to 11 so that the intra-acinar airways branch over an average of 8 generations (Fig. 2-5).

The morphometry of the intra-acinar airways of the human lung shows a number of characteristic traits. The inner diameter (d_{in}) that characterizes the cross-section of the duct tube decreases from about 490 μm at the transitional bronchiole to 270 μm in the last generations.[9] When this is plotted onto the graph relating airway diameter to generations of branching (Fig. 2-37), we note that this diameter falls less steeply than the cube-root-of-1/2 law we have observed for conducting airways. This is a significant finding in terms of the ventilation of alveoli by O_2 diffusion.

An important morphometric characteristic of acinar airways is the total path length for O_2 diffusion from the entrance at the transitional bronchiole to the terminal cluster of alveoli at the alveolar sac (Fig. 2-5). This path length is determined by two factors: the number of generations and the segment length. The length of alveolar ducts gradually decreases from 1330 to 640 μm in the peripheral generations, the alveolar sacs being a little bit longer. Since the number of branching generations varies somewhat, we can expect the path length to vary even within one acinus. In the human lung, the average longitudinal path length measures 8.3 ± 1.4 mm (Fig. 2-65).[10] Because of the decreasing length of acinar ducts 3.4 mm of this total path length are for the first three generations of respiratory bronchioles, whereas the path length of alveolar ducts and sacs comprised in the 1/8 subacinus (Fig. 2-64) averages 4.7 ± 0.88 mm.

Typical Path Model of Human Acinus

In view of assessing the effect of these structural features on the functional performance of the pulmonary gas exchanger we can attempt to develop what we may call a typical path model for an average human acinus[9,10]; the relevant morphometric data are given in Table 2-5. Such an acinus has a volume of 187 mm^3. Its airways branch over an average of eight generations to reach the terminal alveolar sacs. With each generation the number of branches doubles to end with some 256 terminal alveolar sacs in an average acinus (Fig. 2-63). Locating the transitional bronchiole ($z' = 0$) in generation 14 (Fig. 2-5) the terminal air sacs are in generation 23 of the typical path airway tree. From the estimates of the lengths and inner diameters of the airway segments we can derive overall parameters of functional significance, such as the total airway cross-section per generation, $A_d(z')$, which is a determinant of air flow velocity (Fig. 2-44). Finally,

TABLE 2-5 Typical Path Model of Human Acinus

Generation		Segments			Dimensions per Generation			Path Length
Airways z	Acinus z'	N(z')	l mm	d_{in} mm	$A_d(z')$ mm^2	$V_d(z')$ mm^3	$S_{alv}(z')$ mm^2	$L_p(z')$ mm
15	0	1	1.4	0.50	0.20	0.32	7	1.4
16	1	2	1.33	0.50	0.39	0.52	23	2.73
17	2	4	1.12	0.49	0.75	0.84	67	3.85
18	3	8	0.93	0.40	1.00	0.93	129	4.78
19	4	16	0.83	0.38	1.81	1.50	219	5.61
20	5	32	0.70	0.36	3.26	2.28	349	6.31
21	6	64	0.70	0.34	5.81	4.07	661	7.01
22	7	128	0.70	0.31	9.11	6.38	1204	7.71
23	8	256	0.70	0.29	16.9	13.47	2720	8.41

Source: Modified with permission from Haefeli-Bleuer B, Weibel ER: Morphometry of the human pulmonary acinus. Anat Rec. 1988;220(4):401–414.

we can also estimate the distribution of alveolar surface area to the different generations in proportion to the duct surface $S_d(z')$, but adjusting for the fact that only part of this surface is associated with alveoli in the respiratory bronchioles (generations z' = 1–3). For an estimated alveolar surface of 130 m^2 in the human lung (Table 2-4), there would be about 54 cm^2 of gas-exchange surface per average acinus. It is seen that half this gas-exchange surface is in the last generation (see also Fig. 2-64). A final check of this model is that the path length from the entrance into the transitional bronchiole to the end of the alveolar sacs is 8.4 mm, which agrees well with the mean path length estimated in the human acini (Fig. 2-65).

Implications of Acinar Design for Gas-Exchange Function: The Phenomenon of Diffusion Screening

The gas exchange in the pulmonary acinus involves several physicochemical phenomena that occur within the complex acinar geometry described in the preceding section.[197] As mentioned, in the distal regions of the lung, oxygen is transported toward the alveolar membrane both by convection and molecular diffusion. Oxygen then diffuses through the tissue membrane into the blood, where it is bound by hemoglobin. Several physical parameters govern oxygen uptake at the acinar level, such as air flow velocity, diffusion coefficient of oxygen in air, alveolar membrane permeability, blood hemoglobin content, and its reaction rate with oxygen. Conversely, carbon dioxide is discharged from the blood to the alveolar gas through diffusion across the membrane. It then diffuses backward along the airways to the zone, where convection becomes dominant, and is lastly expelled from the lung. In all these processes, the morphology of the system plays an essential role.

Since oxygen uptake into the blood is driven by the O_2 partial pressure at the alveolar surface we must ask whether this driving force is the same throughout the acinus or whether there could be differences between its central and peripheral parts. Some earlier studies had shown that concentration gradients may exist as a consequence of efficient capture of oxygen by hemoglobin. More recently,[197] we have come to realize that such gradients are strongly influenced by the finite permeability of the membrane that plays a dominant role in the effective properties of the acinus as the ventilatory gas-exchange unit. O_2 molecules entering the unit where diffusion prevails have a larger probability to hit the surface of the alveolar membrane near the entrance than in the more distal regions. If the membrane permeability is large, O_2 molecules are absorbed at the very first hits. As a consequence, O_2 is absorbed into the blood in the first parts of the acinar pathway, a process called *diffusional screening,* so that the gas-exchange units in the deeper part of the acinus would receive less O_2 (Fig. 2-61) or perhaps even not enough for gas exchange to occur. Blood perfusing these regions would not be oxygenated and would thus appear as a shunt. In contrast, if the permeability is small, molecules will be absorbed only after many collisions with the wall. They then have a fair chance to reach the deeper regions and the entire acinar surface can be effective for gas exchange.

To put this into the perspective of structure–function relations this process is related to the balance between two conductances:[197] a diffusion conductance Y_{cross} for O_2 to *cross* the barrier from alveolar air to capillary blood, and a diffusion conductance Y_{reach} for O_2 to *reach* the surface through the airspaces. Both these conductances are determined by the product of: (a) a physical parameter (the permeability coefficient for O_2 in tissue, and the diffusion coefficient for O_2 in air, respectively); and (b) a morphometric parameter (the gas-exchange surface, and the distance along the acinar airways, respectively). The physical coefficients are given quantities, except that the tissue permeability is also affected by the thickness of the tissue barrier, a parameter that varies very little between species. On the other hand, the size and surface of the acinus can be varied during evolution and growth to adjust the two conductances. We can predict that the design of the acinus is optimized if Y_{cross} and Y_{reach} are about equal as this means that both the gas-exchange surface and the acinar air volume, or the diffusion distance, are matched. If Y_{cross} were much smaller than Y_{reach} the low permeability of the gas exchanger would need to be compensated by a larger gas-exchange surface, and this would inevitably entail a larger volume of the acinus to accommodate the surface and by that a longer diffusion distance.

The morphometric study of acini in various mammalian species[9,197,198] revealed that the size of the acini is such that $Y_{cross} \sim Y_{reach}$ so that their morphology seems to be at least partially adapted to minimize the effects of screening. Note that the problem of screening occurs in that part of the acinus where O_2 moves to the surface by diffusion only (Fig. 2-62), in what is called the diffusion cell. The transition between convection and diffusion is determined by the Peclet number (Fig. 2-66), essentially the ratio between air flow and diffusion velocities[197]; diffusion is more effective than convection when the Peclet number is smaller than 1. In the human lung, under resting conditions, this transition occurs in generation 18 and that is the entrance to the 1/8 subacinus (Fig. 2-63); accordingly the diffusion cell corresponds to the 1/8 subacinus. In exercise, where O_2 consumption as well as ventilation is increased, convective transport of O_2 is effective out to generation 21 (Fig. 2-66). So in exercise there are only two to three generations of acinar airways that act as diffusion cell, but that is still highly significant because these generations accommodate 75% of the gas-exchange surface (Fig. 2-64 and Table 2-5).

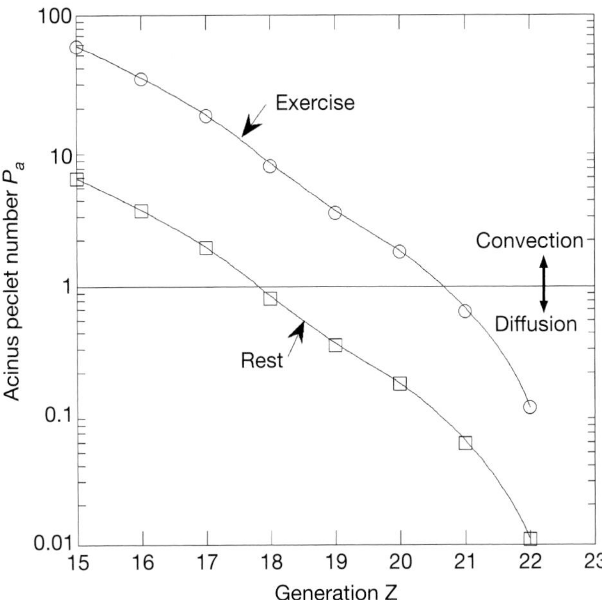

Figure 2-66 In the human acinus the Peclet number, reflecting the relation between convective flow velocity and diffusion velocity of O_2, falls as the airway cross-section increases. Below 1 diffusion becomes the dominant mechanism of alveolar ventilation. This transition point is about in generation 18 at rest and extends out to generation 21 in heavy exercise. *(Reproduced with permission from Sapoval B, Filoche M, Weibel ER. Smaller is better, but not too small: A physical scale for the design of the mammalian pulmonary acinus. Proc Natl Acad Sci USA. 2002;99(16):10411–10416. Copyright (2002) National Academy of Sciences, USA.)*

Note that what has been discussed so far relates essentially to about half the respiratory cycle, namely, inspiration when fresh O_2-rich air is actively brought into the acinus. During expiration things are in a way reversed: CO_2 that has diffused from the blood into the acinar air now dilutes O_2 and the convection–diffusion front is moved toward the bronchi. For this reason, the effective duty cycle of the gas-exchange system is smaller than 1, particularly under the conditions of high O_2 uptake rate in exercise. This must be considered when modeling gas exchange. Recent refined model studies using the same morphometric data together with reasonable assumptions on the physiologic conditions revealed that the size of the human pulmonary acinus is such as to avoid negative effects of diffusional screening.[199]

THE LUNG AS PART OF THE PATHWAY FOR OXYGEN

The lung's main function, gas exchange between air and blood, serves the body's varying O_2 needs as they are set by the energetic demands of the cells and their mitochondria when these produce ATP by oxidative phosphorylation to allow the cells to do work. This process requires a flow of O_2 to be maintained from the lung to the cells[16] which proceeds along the respiratory system through various steps from the lung to the blood, by circulatory blood flow to the cells and mitochondria (Fig. 2-67). A number of basic features characterize this system: (1) under steady-state conditions the O_2 flow rate, $\dot{V}_{O_2}$, is the same at all levels; (2) the basic driving force for O_2 flow through the system is a cascade of O_2 partial pressures, which fall from inspired P_{O_2} down to near zero around the mitochondria; (3) the O_2 flow rate at each step is the product of an O_2 partial pressure difference and a conductance G, which is related to structural and functional properties of the organs participating in O_2 transfer. In the preceding section we have seen that the principal design features of the lung that determine one of the key conductances, the pulmonary diffusing capacity, are sized to just yield a conductance that allows the O_2 uptake required to satisfy the demands of the whole body cell system at work, with a small margin of safety under normal conditions. Therefore, the lung appears designed to serve the body's needs efficiently and economically. The question we may now ask is whether the other parts of the respiratory system, from the heart to the mitochondria are also designed for economic functional performance.[200]

Let us first look at the overall functional performance of the system. We first note that O_2 consumption is highly variable, increasing by about a factor of 10 between resting conditions and heavy exercise when 90% of the O_2 is consumed in the locomotor muscles. Figure 2-68 shows that the oxygen consumption in muscle is proportional to the energy output,[201] measured for example as running speed, and that it reaches a limit $\dot{V}_{O_2max}$ beyond this the running speed can still be increased, but the additional energy required by the higher speed is then supplied through glycolysis or anaerobic ATP production with the result that lactic acid concentration in the blood gradually increases. It is now interesting to note that $\dot{V}_{O_2max}$ is a characteristic of the work capacity of an individual: well-trained athletes reach their $\dot{V}_{O_2max}$ at a higher running speed and a higher level of oxygen consumption, and lactic acid concentration in the blood also begins to increases at the higher performance levels corresponding to $\dot{V}_{O_2max}$ (Fig. 2-68).

One may now raise the question whether this variable limitation of oxidative metabolism is a result of variable functional constraints affecting the regulation of metabolic rate and circulatory transport, or whether it could be set by variations in design constraints characterizing the structural components of the pathway, one possible candidate being the pulmonary diffusing capacity. The answer to this question depends on an integrated study of structure and function of the respiratory system. For this we need a quantitative model of the oxygen pathway that identifies all the functional variables and the design parameters at the four levels of the system[202]: the lung, circulation of blood with the heart, capillaries, and mitochondria (Table 2-6). This model is a further development of the one shown in Figure 2-67 in the sense that, at each level, the equation describing oxygen flow rate sorts out the parameters of functional

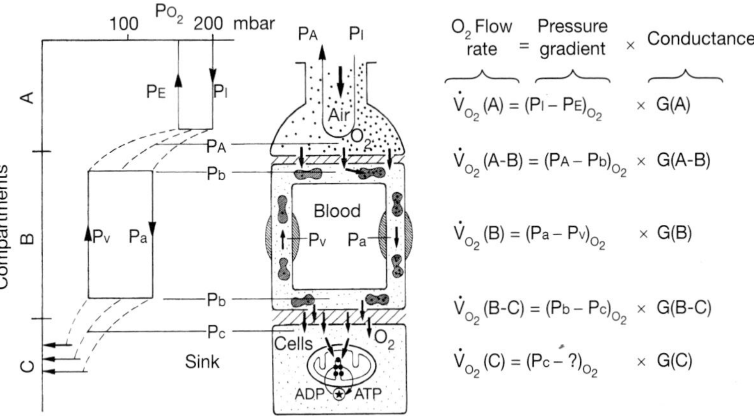

Figure 2-67 Model of the respiratory system from the lung to the cells. Oxygen flow is driven through the system by a cascade of P_{O_2} ranging from inspired PI_{O_2} to near zero at the mitochondria. At each level the flow rate is determined by a partial pressure difference and a conductance. *(Modified with permission from Taylor CR, Weibel ER: Design of the mammalian respiratory system. I. Problem and strategy, Respir Physiol. 1981;44(1):1–10.)*

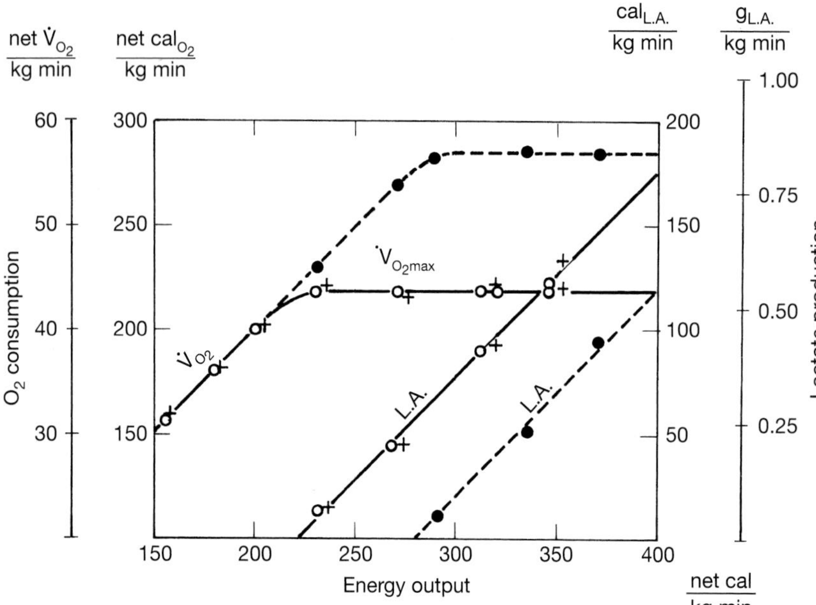

Figure 2-68 Rate of O_2 consumption *(left ordinate)* and lactic acid production *(ordinate at right)* in exercise are plotted as a function of the work intensity and, therefore, of the energy requirement *(abscissa)*. Oxygen consumption increases linearly up to a point corresponding to an energy requirement of 220 cal/kg min^{-1}; if work is pushed beyond that there is no further increase in O_2 consumption ($\dot{V}_{O_2max}$ is reached) but glycolysis now generates the required energy resulting in an increase in lactic acid production. The broken lines refer to athletes (middle- and long-distance runners) whose maximum oxygen consumption is higher; the line of the lactic acid for these subjects is correspondingly shifted to the right. *(Reproduced with permission from Margaria R, Cerretelli P, Diprampero PE, et al. Kinetics and mechanism of oxygen debt contraction in man. J Appl Physiol. 1963;18:371–377.)*

regulation and those of structural design. These are distinguished in the following sense: Functional variables are regulated according to need with short time constants (seconds), whereas structural design parameters are genetically determined static elements that can be adjusted to a certain extent, for example, by training, but with time constants of weeks to months.

Thus, design variables set the capacity of the system because they are determined by structures whose quantitative properties cannot be adjusted at short notice. If the system were designed according

TABLE 2-6 Model of Structure–Function Relations in Pathway for Oxygen Separating Functional and Structural Parameters in the Equations Defining O_2 Flow Rate Through Four Levels

FUNCTION • DESIGN
$\dot{V}_{O_2}\text{(lung)} = (PA_{O_2} - Pb_{O_2})\{t_c, \theta_{O_2}\} \bullet DL_{O_2}\{S(A), S(c), V(c), \tau_{hb}\}$ (1)
$\dot{V}_{O_2}\text{(heart)} = (\sigma_a \cdot Pa_{O_2} - \sigma_{\bar{v}} \cdot P\bar{v}_{O_2}) \cdot f_H \bullet Vs\{V(LV)\} \cdots V_v(ec)$ (2)
$\dot{V}_{O_2}\text{(caps)} = (Pb_{O_2} - Pc_{O_2})\{tc\theta_{O_2}\} \bullet DT_{O_2}\{S(c), V(c), V_v(ec), \delta(c, mi)\}$ (3)
$\dot{V}_{O_2}\text{(mito)} = \dot{V}_{O_2}\{\dot{m}_{ATP}\} \bullet V(mi)\{S_v(im, mi)\}$ (4)

The O_2 flow rate $\dot{V}_{O_2}$ is expressed as the product of functional and design parameters; parameters that affect the factors are shown in italics and placed in braces {.}. The functional parameters include: O_2 partial pressures (P_{O_2}), coefficients of "hematocrit-specific" O_2 capacitance (σ) which depend on O_2-hemoglobin dissociation, O_2 binding rate (θ), heart frequency (f_H), capillary transit time (tc), and mitochondrial O_2 consumption rate as function of ATP flux ($\dot{V}_{O_2}\{\dot{m}_{ATP}\}$). Design parameters include: diffusion conductances (D) of lung and tissue gas exchangers which depend on alveolar and capillary exchange surface areas (S(A), S(c)), capillary volumes (V(c)), hematocrit (V_v(ec)), harmonic mean barrier thickness (τ_{hb}), capillary-mitochondrial diffusion distance (δ(c,mi)), and mitochondrial volume (V(mi)) with inner membrane surface density (S_v(im,mi)).

Source: Data from Weibel ER: Symmorphosis: on form and function in shaping life. Cambridge, MA: Harvard University Press; 2000.

to the principle of symmorphosis we would predict that the design variables are adjusted to $\dot{V}_{O_2max}$ at all levels from the lung to the mitochondria.

The experimental test of this hypothesis requires the integrated measurement of $\dot{V}_{O_2max}$ of the relevant functional parameters, and of all the design parameters, which must then be correlated on the basis of the model of Table 2-6. This cannot be easily done in the human so that is where we can learn from studies in comparative physiology. We know that $\dot{V}_{O_2max}$ is highly variable among mammals. Some species such as dogs, horses, or pronghorn antelopes have a much higher level of $\dot{V}_{O_2max}$ than "normal" species of the same size such as goats or cows; this is called adaptive variation.[203] On the other hand body size matters so that small animals have a higher metabolic rate per unit body mass than large species, which is called allometric variation.[200] These are genetically determined variations, the result of evolution and selection by fitness, in contrast to the changes in overall work capacity and $\dot{V}_{O_2max}$ induced by exercise training in human athletes, which are epigenetic variations.[204,205] In all these cases we can ask how and to what extent the structural design parameters are adjusted to meet the different requirements for O_2 to cover the energetic need at the limit of the aerobic work capacity. If there is a bottleneck, then there will be one and only one parameter whose variation is perfectly matched to the variation in the limit of O_2 flow, $\dot{V}_{O_2max}$, whereas all the parameters that are overdesigned would appear in haphazard relations to the flow limit. On the other hand, if the limiting resistances are distributed all steps would have to be matched to the varying $\dot{V}_{O_2max}$. If we take the bold view that the organisms are economically designed we would predict that the structural parameters at all levels should be sized to the maximal total O_2 flow requirement with no unnecessary excess capacity because that would be a waste. We have called this design principle symmorphosis, meaning that there should be no more structure built into the system than required to serve the functional needs.[179]

Testing the Hypothesis of Symmorphosis

To test such a hypothesis we can first compare mammals that greatly differ in terms of their maximal O_2 consumption. The first type of this variation is found in comparing normal with athletic species, such as dogs with goats or horses with steers.[203] It has been found that such athletic animals can achieve a $\dot{V}_{O_2max}$ that is about

TABLE 2-7 Comparison of Morphometric and Physiologic Parameters of Muscle Mitochondria and Capillaries, and of Heart, Blood and Lung with Variation of $\dot{V}_{O_2max}$ in Three Pairs of Athletic and Sedentary Species. Data per Unit Body Mass

	Mitochondria		Blood	Capillaries		Heart			Lung
Design Function	$\dot{V}_{O_2 max}/M_b$ $mL \cdot min^{-1} \cdot kg^{-1}$	V(mt)/Mb $mL \cdot kg^{-1}$	$V_V(ec)$	V(c)/Mb $mL \cdot kg^{-1}$	V(ec)/Mb $mL \cdot kg^{-1}$	fH min^{-1}	Vs/M_b $mL \cdot kg^{-1}$	$\dot{Q}$(ec)/Mb $mL \cdot min^{-1} \cdot kg^{-1}$	D_{LO_2}/Mb $mL \cdot min^{-1} \cdot mmHg^{-1}$ kg^{-1}
25–30 kg									
Dog	137.4	40.6	0.50	8.2	4.10	274	3.17	434.3	424.8
Goat	57.0	13.8	0.30	4.5	1.35	268	2.07	166.4	288.0
D/G	2.4	2.9	1.68[a]	1.8[a]	3.0	1.02[a]	1.53[a]	2.61	1.48[a]
150 kg									
Pony	88.8	19.5	0.42	5.1	2.14	215	2.50	225.7	284.4
Calf	36.6	9.2	0.31	3.2	0.99	213	1.78	117.5	180.0
P/C	2.4	2.13	1.35[a]	1.6[a]	2.16	1.02[a]	1.40[a]	1.92	1.57[a]
450 kg									
Horse	133.8	30.0	0.55	8.3	4.57	202	3.11	345.5	388.9
Steer	51.0	11.6	0.40	5.3	2.12	216	1.52	131.3	194.4
H/S	2.6	2.6	1.4[a]	0.94[a]	2.16	2.1[a]	2.0[a]	2.63	2.0[a]
Ath/Sed[b]	2.5	2.5	1.5[a]	1.7[a]	2.44	1.0[a]	1.7[a]	2.39	1.7[a]

[a]*These ratios are significantly different from that for* $\dot{V}_{O_2max}$.

[b]*This line presents overall ratios for athletic/sedentary species.*

Source: Data from Taylor, CR, Karas, RH, et al: (1987) Respir. Physiol. 69, 1–127; Jones, JH, Longworth, KE, Lindholm, A et al: (1989) J. Appl. Physiol. 67, 862–870; Constantinopol, M, Jones, JH, Weibel, ER, et al: (1989) J. Appl. Physiol. 67, 871–878; Hoppeler, H, Jones, JH, Lindstedt, SL, et al: (1987) in Equine Exercise Physiology II, eds. Gillespie, JR & Robinson, (Edward Brothers, Ann Arbor, MI), 278–289; Hoppeler, H, Kayar, SR, Claassen, H, et al: (1987) Respir. Physiol. 69, 27–46; Conley JE, Kayar SR, Rosler K, et al: (1987), Respir Physiol 69, 47–64; Karas, RH, Taylor, CR, Rosler, K, et al: (1987) Respir. Physiol. 69, 65–79; Weibel, ER, Marques, LB, Constantinopol, M, et al: (1987) Respir. Physiol. 69, 81–100.

2.5 times higher than that of normal species of the same size. This is much more than what human athletes can achieve. The relevant morphometric data on such species are shown in Table 2-7 for three species pairs.[206] If we go through the respiratory system, beginning at the bottom with the mitochondria, we note that their total volume in the locomotor muscles is also 2.5 times greater in the athletic species with the result that, at $\dot{V}_{O_2max}$ the unit volume of mitochondria consumes the same amount of oxygen in all these six species, namely about 5 mL O_2 per minute and mL mitochondria. In the next level up, the muscle capillaries, we note that the capillary volume is only 1.7 times greater in the athletic species. However we note that in the athletes the hematocrit, that is, the concentration of erythrocytes in the blood, is larger so that as a result the capillary erythrocyte volume, the product of capillary volume with hematocrit, is 2.44 times greater, thus well matched to the mitochondrial O_2 demands. Note that this is what counts because oxygen is delivered exclusively from the capillary red blood cells. When we look at the determinants of total blood flow the heart is the central element. We notice that athletic species have larger hearts resulting in a larger stroke volume Vs, but that the maximal heart frequency is not different between the species pairs so that cardiac output is determined by the stroke volume. This is only 1.7 times greater in the athletic species. However, note that, here again, the hematocrit plays an important role as it determines the amount of O_2 that can be transported to the capillaries. If we calculate the cardiac erythrocyte output $\dot{Q}$ (ec) we find that it is again 2.4 times greater in the athletic species. Thus the design parameters of the internal steps of the O_2 transport cascade are quantitatively adjusted to the needs for O_2 flow under limiting conditions. Thus, it appears that the resistance to O_2 flow is distributed to all levels.

When we then consider the design of the pulmonary gas exchanger we note that the O_2 diffusing capacity of the lung of athletic species is only 1.7 times greater than that of normal species. Considering that we found that the human lung may have some excess capacity by about a factor of 1.5, this may signify that normal sedentary species such as goats or cows have a greater excess capacity than athletic species. Indeed, this can be shown to be the case in two ways:[207] (1) when one calculates the progression of O_2 loading on capillary blood (Bohr integration, Fig. 2-59) one finds that dogs reach saturation just before the blood leaves the capillaries into arterial blood, whereas the goats have some 30% reserve capacity; (2) when goats are run on a treadmill while breathing hypoxic air one finds that they can maintain their $\dot{V}_{O_2max}$ in contrast, dogs cannot run at their established $\dot{V}_{O_2max}$ under such conditions. We concluded from this observation that athletic species have designed a lung to match the requirements for maximal O_2 uptake with no excess capacity while normal sedentary species apparently allow for a certain safety margin which allows them to perform well also under unfavorable hypoxic conditions. If this is now applied to our observations on the human lung this may mean that the excess capacity of the normal lung may just be sufficient to allow athletes to increase their $\dot{V}_{O_2max}$ by training by a factor 1.5, just about what they can achieve (Fig. 2-67).

One has also found that highly trained athletes do not tolerate heavy exercise at very high altitudes as they cannot achieve O_2 saturation of their arterial blood. Thus, it seems that the pulmonary gas exchanger is now the limiting factor for O_2 transfer to the working muscles. The reason for this is that the lung of the adult cannot enlarge its gas-exchange surfaces to match the increased demands of trained muscles. So an athlete must make do with the lung she or he has developed during growth. This contrasts with the changes induced by exercise training in muscle with an increase in mitochondria and capillaries, and in the heart by enlargement of the ventricles, all well matched to the maximal

O_2 demands.[202] Therefore, it is fortunate – and perhaps a sign of good design – that the lung is designed with some excess diffusing capacity to allow the lower, internal, levels of the respiratory system to exploit their capacity to adapt to increased energetic needs.

REFERENCES

1. Agostoni E. Mechanics of the pleural space. *Physiol Rev*. 1972; 52:57–128.
2. Miserocchi G, Negrini D. Pleural space: pressures and fluid dynamics. In: Crystal RG, West JB, Weibel ER, Barnes PJ, eds. *The Lung: Scientific Foundations*, 2nd ed. New York, NY: Lippincott-Raven; 1997:1217–1225.
3. Zocchi L. Physiology and pathophysiology of pleural fluid turnover. *Eur Respir J*. 2002;20:1545–1558.
4. Lai-Fook SJ. Pleural mechanics and fluid exchange. *Physiol Rev*. 2003;84:385–410.
5. Agostoni E, Zocchi L. Pleural liquid and its exchanges. *Respir Physiol Neurobiol*. 2007;159:311–323.
6. Sozio F, Rossi A, Weber E, et al. Morphometric analysis of intralobular, interlobular and pleural lymphatics in normal human lung. *J Anat*. 2012;220:396–404.
7. Weibel ER, Gomez DM. Architecture of the human lung. *Science*. 1962;137:577–585.
8. Weibel ER. *Morphometry of the Human Lung*. Heidelberg: Springer-Verlag; 1963.
9. Haefeli-Bleuer B, Weibel ER. Morphometry of the human pulmonary acinus. *Anat Rec*. 1988;220:401–414.
10. Weibel ER, Sapoval B, Filoche M. Design of peripheral airways for efficient gas exchange. *Respir Physiol Neurobiol*. 2005;148: 3–21.
11. Weibel ER. Lung cell biology. In: Fishman A, Fisher AB, eds. *Handbook of Physiology*. Section 3: The Respiratory System. vol 1. Bethesda, MD: American Physiological Society; 1985:47–91.
12. Massaro D, ed. *Lung Cell Biology*. New York, NY: Marcel Dekker; 1989.
13. Franks TJ, Colby TV, Travis WD, et al. Resident cellular components of the human lung. Current knowledge and goals for research on cell phenotyping and function. *Proc Am Thorac Soc*. 2008;5:763–766.
14. Parent RA, ed. *Comparative Biology of the Normal Lung*. Boca Raton, FL: CRC Press; 1992.
15. Forrest JB, Lee RMKW. The bronchial wall: integrated form and function. In: Crystal RG, West JB, Weibel ER, Barnes PJ, eds. *The Lung: Scientific Foundations*. 2nd ed. New York, NY: Lippincott-Raven; 1997:1081–1091.
16. Weibel ER. *The Pathway for Oxygen*. Cambridge, MA: Harvard University Press; 1984.
17. Morrisey EE, Hogan BLM. Preparing for the first breath: genetic and cellular mechanisms in lung development. *Dev Cell*. 2010; 18:8–23.
18. Breeze RG, Wheeldon EB. The cells of the pulmonary airways. *Am Rev Respir Dis*. 1977;116:705–777.
19. Button B, Cai LH, Ehre C, et al. A periciliary brush promotes the lung health by separating the mucus layer from airway epithelia. *Science*. 2012;337:937–941.
20. Lee RMKW, Forrest JB. Structure and function of cilia. In: Crystal RG, West JB, Weibel ER, Barnes PJ, eds. *The Lung: Scientific Foundations*. 2nd ed. New York, NY: Lippincott-Raven; 1997:459–478.
21. Salathe M. Regulation of mammalian ciliary beating. *Annu Rev Physiol*. 2007;69:401–422.
22. American Thoracic Society. *ATS joins other Societies in Renaming "Clara cell" and "Wegener´s Granulomatosis"*. http://news.thoracic.org/april-2013/ats-joins-other-societies-in-renaming.php New York, NY: 2013.
23. Winkelmann A, Noack T. The Clara cell: a "third reich eponym"? *Eur Respir J*. 2010;36:722–727.
24. Plopper CG, Hyde DM. Epithelial cells of bronchioles. In: Parent RA, ed. *Comparative Biology of the Normal Lung*. Boca Raton, FA: CRC Press; 1992:85–92.
25. Massaro GD, Singh G, Mason RJ, Plopper CG, Malkinson AM, Gail DB. Biology of the Clara cell. *Am J Physiol Lung Cell Mol Physiol*. 1994;266:L101–L106.
26. Plopper CG, Hyde DM, Buckpitt AR. Clara cells. In: Crystal RG, West JB, Weibel ER, Barnes PB, eds. *The Lung: Scientific Foundations*. 2nd ed. New York, NY: Lippincott-Raven; 1997: 517–533.
27. Singh G, Katyal SL. Clara cells and Clara cell 10 kD protein (CC10). *Am J Respir Cell Mol Biol*. 1997;17:141–143.
28. Reynolds SD, Malkinson AM. Clara cell: progenitor for the bronchiolar epithelium. *Int J Biochem Cell Biol*. 2010;42:1–4.
29. Boers JE, Ambergen AW, Thunnissen FB. Number and proliferation of Clara cells in normal human airway epithelium. *Am J Respir Crit Care Med*. 1999;159:1585–1591.
30. Hermans C, Bernard A. Lung epithelium-specific proteins. Characteristics and potential applications as markers. *Am J Respir Crit Care Med*. 1999;159:646–678.
31. Giangreco A, Arwert EN, Rosewell IR, Snyder J, Watt FM, Stripp BR. Stem cells are dispensable for lung homeostasis but restore airways after injury. *Proc Natl Acad Sci USA*. 2009;106:9286–9291.
32. Scheuermann DW. Neuroendocrine cells. In: Crystal RG, West JB, Weibel ER, Barnes PJ, eds. *The Lung: Scientific Foundations*. 2nd ed. New York, NY: Lippincott-Raven; 1997:603–613.
33. Gosney JR. Pulmonary neuroendocrine cell system in pediatric and adult lung disease. *Microsc Res Tech*. 1997;37:107–113.
34. van Lommel A, Bolle T, Fannes W, Lauweryns JM. The pulmonary neuroendocrine system: the past decade. *Arch Histol Cytol*. 1999;62:1–16.
35. Cutz E, Jackson A. Neuroepithelial bodies as airway oxygen sensors. *Respir Physiol*. 1999;115:201–214.
36. Adriaensen D, Brouns I, van Genechten J, Timmermans JP. Functional morphology of pulmonary neuroepithelial bodies: extremely complex airway receptors. *Anat Rec*. 2003;270: 25–40.
37. Chang LY, Mercer RR, Crapo JD. Differential distribution of brush cells in the rat lung. *Anat Rec*. 1986;216:49–54.
38. Reid L, Meyrick B, Antony VB, Chang LY, Crapo JD, Reynolds HY. The mysterious pulmonary brush cell. A cell in search of a function. *Am J Respir Crit Care Med*. 2005;172:136–139.
39. Sbarbati A, Osculati F. A new fate for old cells: Brush cells and related elements. *J Anat*. 2005;206:349–358.
40. Krasteva G, Canning BJ, Hartmann P, et al. Cholinergic chemosensory cells in the trachea regulate breathing. *Proc Natl Acad Sci USA*. 2011;108:9478–9483.
41. Krasteva G, Kummer W. "Tasting" the airway lining fluid. *Histochem Cell Biol*. 2012;138:365–383.

42. Leak LV, Ferrans VJ. Lymphatics and lymphoid tissue. In: Crystal RG, West JB, Weibel ER, Barnes PJ, eds. *The Lung: Scientific Foundations*. 2nd ed. New York, NY: Lippincott-Raven; 1997:1129–1137.
43. Pabst R, Gehrke I. Is the bronchus-associated lymphoid tissue (BALT) an integral structure of the lung in normal mammals, including humans? *Am J Respir Cell Mol Biol*. 1990;3: 131–135.
44. Tschernig T, Pabst R. Bronchus-associated lymphoid tissue (BALT) is not present in the normal adult lung but in different diseases. *Pathobiology*. 2000;68:1–8.
45. Foo SY, Phipps S. Regulation of inducible BALT formation and contribution to immunity and pathology. *Mucosal Immunol*. 2010;3:537–544.
46. Randall TD. Bronchus-associated lymphoid tissue (BALT) structure and function. *Adv Immunol*. 2010;107:187–241.
47. Aird WC. Phenotypic heterogeneity of the endothelium. I. Structure, function, and mechanisms. *Circ Res*. 2007;100:158–173.
48. Aird WC. Phenotypic heterogeneity of the endothelium. II. Representative vascular beds. *Circ Res*. 2007;100:174–190.
49. Stevens T, Phan S, Frid MG, Alvarez D, Herzog E, Stenmark KR. Lung vascular cell heterogeneity. Endothelium, smooth muscle, and fibroblasts. *Proc Am Thorac Soc*. 2008;5:783–791.
50. Weibel ER, Palade GE. New cytoplasmic components in arterial endothelia. *J Cell Biol*. 1964;23:101–112.
51. Weibel ER. Fifty years of Weibel-Palade bodies: the discovery and early history of an enigmatic organelle of endothelial cells. *J Thromb Haemost*. 2012;10:979–984.
52. Wagner DD, Olmsted JB, Marder VJ. Immunolocalization of von Willebrand protein in Weibel-Palade bodies of human endothelial cells. *J Cell Biol*. 1982;95:355–360.
53. van Mourik JA, Romani de Wit T, Voorberg J. Biogenesis and exocytosis of Weibel-Palade bodies. *Histochem Cell Biol*. 2002;117:113–122.
54. Michaux G, Cutler DF. How to roll an endothelial cigar: the biogenesis of Weibel-Palade bodies. *Traffic*. 2004;5:69–78.
55. Metcalf DJ, Nightingale TD, Zenner HL, Lui-Roberts WW, Cutler DF. Formation and function of Weibel-Palade bodies. *J Cell Sci*. 2007;121:19–27.
56. Valentijn KM, Sadler JE, Valentijn JA, Voorberg J, Eikenboom J. Functional architecture of Weibel-Palade bodies. *Blood*. 2011;117:5033–5043.
57. Simionescu M. Lung endothelium: structure and function correlates. In: Crystal RG, West JB, Weibel ER, Barnes PJ, eds. *The Lung: Scientific Foundations*. 2nd ed. New York, NY: Lippincott-Raven; 1997:615–628.
58. Palade GE. Role of plasmalemmal vesicles in microvascular permeability. In: Crystal RG, West JB, Weibel ER, Barnes PJ, eds. *The Lung: Scientific Foundations*. 2nd ed. New York, NY: Lippincott-Raven; 1997:673–683.
59. Schlörmann W, Steiniger F, Richter W, et al. The shape of caveolae is omega-like after glutaraldehyde fixation and cup-like after cryofixation. *Histochem Cell Biol*. 2010;133:223–228.
60. Mineo C, Anderson RG. Potocytosis. *Histochem Cell Biol*. 2001;116:109–118.
61. Cohen AW, Hnasko R, Schubert W, Lisanti MP. Role of caveolae and caveolins in health and disease. *Physiol Rev*. 2004;84:1341–1379.
62. Stan RV. Structure of caveolae. *Biochim Biophys Acta*. 2005;1746: 334–348.
63. Parton RG, del Pozo MA. Caveolae as plasma membrane sensors, protectors and organizers. *Nat Rev Mol Cell Biol*. 2013;14:98–112.
64. Haissaguerre M, Jais P, Shah D, et al. Spontaneous initiation of atrial fibrillation by ectopic beats originating in the pulmonary veins. *N Engl J Med*. 1998;339:659–666.
65. Ho SY, Cabrera JA, Tran VH, Farre J, Anderson RH, Sanchez-Quintana D. Architecture of the pulmonary veins: relevance to radiofrequency ablation. *Heart* 2001;86:265–270.
66. Fynn SP, Kalman JM. Pulmonary veins: anatomy, electrophysiology, tachycardia, and fibrillation. *Pace*. 2004;27:1547–1559.
67. Douglas YL, Jongbloed MR, DeRuiter MC, Gittenberger-de Groot AC. Normal and abnormal development of pulmonary veins: state of the art and correlation with clinical entities. *Int J Cardiol*. 2010;147:13–24.
68. Wagner EM. Bronchial circulation. In: Crystal RG, West JB, Weibel ER, Barnes PJ, eds. *The Lung: Scientific Foundations*. 2nd ed. New York, NY: Lippincott-Raven; 1997; 1093–1105.
69. McCullagh A, Rosenthal M, Wanner A, Hurtado A, Padley S, Bush A. The bronchial circulation - worth a closer look: a review of the relationship between the bronchial vasculature and airway inflammation. *Ped Pulmonol*. 2010;45:1–13.
70. Pabst R. The periarterial space in the lung: its important role in lung edema, transplantation, and microbial or allergic inflammation. *Pathobiology*. 2004;71:287–294.
71. Maina JN, West JB. Thin and strong! The bioengineering dilemma in the structural and functional design of the blood-gas barrier. *Physiol Rev*. 2005;85:811–844.
72. Crapo JD, Barry BE, Gehr P, Bachofen M, Weibel ER. Cell number and cell characteristics of the normal human lung. *Am Rev Respir Dis*. 1982;125:332–337.
73. Schneeberger EE: Alveolar type I cells. In Crystal RG, West JB, Weibel ER, Barnes PJ, eds. *The Lung: Scientific Foundations*. 2nd ed. New York, NY: Lippincott-Raven; 1997; 535–542.
74. Weibel ER. The mystery of "non-nucleated plates" in the alveolar epithelium of the lung explained. *Acta Anat*. 1971;78: 425–443.
75. Williams MC. Alveolar type I cells: molecular phenotype and development. *Annu Rev Physiol*. 2003;65:669–695.
76. Dobbs LG, Johnson MD. Alveolar epithelial transport in the adult lung. *Respir Physiol Neurobiol*. 2007;159:283–300.
77. Dobbs LG, Johnson MD, Vanderbilt J, Allen L, Gonzales R. The great big alveolar TI cell: evolving concepts and paradigms. *Cell Physiol Biochem*. 2010;25:55–62.
78. Bachofen H, Bachofen M, Weibel ER. Ultrastructural aspects of pulmonary edema. *J Thorac Imag*. 1988;3:1–7.
79. Matthay MA, Zemans RL. The acute respiratory distress syndrome: pathogenesis and treatment. *Annu Rev Pathol Mech Dis*. 2011;6:147–163.
80. Bachofen M, Weibel ER. Alterations of the gas exchange apparatus in adult respiratory insufficiency associated with septicemia. *Am Rev Respir Dis*. 1977;116:589–615.
81. McElroy MC, Kasper M. The use of alveolar epithelial type I cell-selective markers to investigate lung injury and repair. *Eur Respir J*. 2004;24:664–673.
82. Clegg GR, Tyrrell C, McKechnie SR, Beers MF, Harrison D, McElroy MC. Coexpression of RTI40 with alveolar epithelial type II cell proteins in lungs following injury: identification

of alveolar intermediate cell types. *Am J Physiol Lung Cell Mol Physiol.* 2005;289:L382–L390.

83. Sirianni FE, Chu FS, Walker DC. Human alveolar wall fibroblasts directly link epithelial type 2 cells to capillary endothelium. *Am J Respir Crit Care Med.* 2003;168:1532–1537.

84. Ochs M. The closer we look the more we see? Quantitative microscopic analysis of the pulmonary surfactant system. *Cell Physiol Biochem.* 2010;25:27–40.

85. Weaver TE, Na CL, Stahlman M. Biogenesis of lamellar bodies, lysosome-related organelles involved in storage and secretion of pulmonary surfactant. *Semin Cell Dev Biol.* 2002;13:263–270.

86. Mason RJ, Williams MC. Type II alveolar cell: defender of the alveolus. *Am Rev Respir Dis.* 1977;115:81–91.

87. Fehrenbach H. Alveolar epithelial type II cell: defender of the alveolus revisited. *Respir Res.* 2001;2:33–46.

88. Mason RJ. Biology of alveolar type II cells. *Respirology.* 2006;11: S12–S15.

89. Hawgood S. Surfactant: composition, structure, metabolism. In: Crystal RG, West JB, Weibel ER, Barnes PJ, eds. *The Lung: Scientific Foundations.* 2nd ed. New York, NY: Lippincott-Raven; 1997;557–572.

90. Griese M. Pulmonary surfactant in health and human lung diseases: state of the art. *Eur Respir J.* 1999;13:1455–1476.

91. Notter RH. *Lung Surfactants. Basic Science and Clinical Applications.* New York, NY: Marcel Dekker; 2000.

92. Perez-Gil J, Weaver TE. Pulmonary surfactant pathophysiology: current models and open questions. *Physiology.* 2010; 25:132–141.

93. Daniels CB, Orgeig S. The comparative biology of pulmonary surfactant: past, present and future. *Comp Biochem Physiol A Mol Integr Physiol.* 2001;129(1):9–36.

94. Wright JR. Immunomodulatory functions of surfactant. *Physiol Rev.* 1997;77:931–962.

95. Wright JR. Immunoregulatory functions of surfactant proteins. *Nat Rev Immunol.* 2005;5:58–68.

96. Perez-Gil J. Structure of pulmonary surfactant membranes and films: the role of proteins and lipid-protein interactions. *Biochim Biophys Acta.* 2008;1778:1676–1695.

97. Weibel ER, Gil J. Electron microscopic demonstration of an extracellular duplex lining layer of alveoli. *Respir Physiol.* 1968;4:42–57.

98. Bastacky J, Lee CY, Goerke J, et al. Alveolar lining layer is thin and continuous: low-temperature scanning electron microscopy of rat lung. *J Appl Physiol.* 1995;79:1615–1628.

99. Mason RJ, Shannon JM. Alveolar type II cells. In Crystal RG, West JB, Weibel ER, Barnes PJ, eds. *The Lung: Scientific Foundations.* 2nd ed. New York, NY: Lippincott-Raven; 1997:543–555.

100. Dietl P, Haller T. Exocytosis of lung surfactant: from the secretory vesicle to the air-liquid interface. *Annu Rev Physiol.* 2005;67:595–621.

101. Rooney SA. Regulation of surfactant secretion. *Comp Biochem Physiol A Mol Integr Physiol.* 2001;129:233–243.

102. Dietl P, Liss B, Felder E, Miklavc P, Wirtz H. Lamellar body exocytosis by cell stretch or purinergic stimulation: possible physiological roles, messengers and mechanisms. *Cell Physiol Biochem.* 2010;25:1–12.

103. Ochs M, Johnen G, Müller KM, et al. Intracellular and intraalveolar localization of surfactant protein A (SP-A) in the parenchymal region of the human lung. *Am J Respir Cell Mol Biol.* 2002;26:91–98.

104. Weibel ER, Kistler GS, Töndury G. A stereologic electron microscope study of "tubular myelin figures" in alveolar lining fluids of rat lungs. *Z Zellforsch Mikrosk Anat.* 1966;69:418–427.

105. Schürch S, Qanbar R, Bachofen H, Possmayer F. The surface-associated surfactant reservoir in the alveolar lining. *Biol Neonate.* 1995;67(suppl 1):61–76.

106. Phelps DS, Floros J. Localization of surfactant protein synthesis in human lung by in situ hybridization. *Am Rev Respir Dis.* 1988;137:939–942.

107. Mason RJ, Greene K, Voelker DR. Surfactant protein A and surfactant protein D in health and disease. *Am J Physiol Lung Cell Mol Physiol.* 1998;275:L1–L13.

108. Savov J, Wright JR, Young SL. Incorporation of biotinylated SP-A into rat lung surfactant layer, type II cells, and Clara cells. *Am J Physiol Lung Cell Mol Physiol.* 2000;279:L118–L126.

109. Hawgood S, Clements JA. Pulmonary surfactant and its apoproteins. *J Clin Invest.* 1990;86:1–6.

110. Hawgood S, Poulain FR. The pulmonary collectins and surfactant metabolism. *Annu Rev Physiol.* 2001;63:495–519.

111. Crouch E, Wright JR. Surfactant proteins A and d and pulmonary host defense. *Annu Rev Physiol.* 2001;63:521–554.

112. Weaver TE, Conkright JJ. Functions of surfactant proteins B and C. *Annu Rev Physiol.* 2001;63:555–578.

113. McCormack FX, Whitsett JA. The pulmonary collectins, SP-A and SP-D, orchestrate innate immunity in the lung. *J Clin Invest.* 2002;109:707–712.

114. Whitsett JA, Weaver TE. Hydrophobic surfactant proteins in lung function and disease. *N Engl J Med.* 2002;347:2141–2148.

115. Brasch F, Johnen G, Winn-Brasch A, et al. Surfactant protein B in type II pneumocytes and intra-alveolar surfactant forms of human lungs. *Am J Respir Cell Mol Biol.* 2004;30: 449–458.

116. Whitsett JA, Wert SE, Weaver TE. Alveolar surfactant homeostasis and the pathogenesis of pulmonary disease. *Annu Rev Med.* 2010;61:105–119.

117. Clements JA. Lung surfactant: a personal perspective. *Annu Rev Physiol.* 1997;59:1–21.

118. Robertson B, Taeusch HW, eds. *Surfactant Therapy for Lung Disease.* New York, NY: Marcel Dekker; 1995.

119. Wrobel S. Bubbles, babies and biology: the story of surfactant. *FASEB J.* 2004;18:1624e. doi: 10.1096/fj.04-2077bkt.

120. Weibel ER. On pericytes, particularly their existence on lung capillaries. *Microvasc Res.* 1974;8:218–235.

121. Shepro D, Morel NM. Pericyte physiology. *FASEB J.* 1993;7:1031–1038.

122. Sims DE. Diversity within pericytes. *Clin Exp Pharmacol Physiol.* 2000;27:842–846.

123. Armulik A, Abramsson A, Betsholtz C. Endothelial/pericyte interactions. *Circ Res.* 2005;97:512–523.

124. Kutcher ME, Herman IM. The pericyte: cellular regulator of microvascular blood flow. *Microvasc Res.* 2009;77:235–246.

125. Stevens T. Molecular and cellular determinants of lung endothelial cell heterogeneity. *Chest.* 2005;128:558S–564S.

126. Effros RM, Parker JC. Pulmonary vascular heterogeneity and the Starling hypothesis. *Microvasc Res.* 2009;78:71–77.

127. Weibel ER, Bachofen H. Structural design of the alveolar septum and fluid exchange. In: Fishman AP, Renkin EM, eds. *Pulmonary Edema.* Bethesda, MD: American Physiological Society; 1979:1–20.

128. Weibel ER, Crystal RG. Structural organization of the pulmonary interstitium. In: Crystal RG, West JB, Weibel ER, Barnes PJ, eds. *The Lung: Scientific Foundations*. 2nd ed. New York, NY: Lippincott-Raven; 1997:685–695.

129. Kaplan NB, Grant MM, Brody JS. The lipid interstitial cell of the pulmonary alveolus. Age and species differences. *Am Rev Respir Dis*. 1985;132:1307–1312.

130. McGowan SE, Torday JS. The pulmonary lipofibroblast (lipid interstitial cell) and its contributions to alveolar development. *Annu Rev Physiol*. 1997;59:43–62.

131. Murphy DJ. The biogenesis and functions of lipid bodies in animals, plants and microorganisms. *Prog Lipid Res*. 2001; 40:325–438.

132. Dirami G, Massaro GD, Clerch LB, Ryan US, Reczek PR, Massaro D. Lung retinol storing cells synthesize and secrete retinoic acid, an inducer of alveolus formation. *Am J Physiol Lung Cell Mol Physiol*. 2004;286:L249–L256.

133. Zhang P, Summer WR, Bagby GJ, Nelson S. Innate immunity and pulmonary host defense. *Immunol Rev*. 2000;173:39–51.

134. Bals R, Hiemstra PS. Innate immunity in the lung: how epithelial cells fight against respiratory pathogens. *Eur Respir J*. 2004;23:327–333.

135. Martin TR, Frevert CW. Innate immunity in the lungs. *Proc Am Thorac Soc*. 2005;2:403–411.

136. Hasenberg M, Stegemann-Koniszewski S, Gunzer M. Cellular immune reactions in the lung. *Immunol Rev*. 2013;251: 189–214.

137. Hume DA. Macrophages as APC and the dendritic cell myth. *J Immunol*. 2008;181:5829–5835.

138. Rees AJ. Monocyte and macrophage biology: an overview. *Semin Nephrol*. 2010;30:216–233.

139. Trivedi NN, Caughey GH. Mast cell peptidases. Chameleons of innate immunity and host defense. *Am J Respir Cell Mol Biol*. 2010;42:257–267.

140. Andersson CK, Mori M, Bjermer L, Löfdahl CG, Erjefält JS. Novel site-specific mast cell subpopulations in the human lung. *Thorax*. 2009;64:297–305.

141. Holt PG. Antigen presentation in the lung. *Am J Respir Crit Care Med*. 2000;162:S151–S156.

142. Masten BJ. Initiation of lung immunity: the afferent limb and the role of dendritic cells. *Semin Respir Crit Care Med*. 2004;25: 11–20.

143. Vermaelen K, Pauwels R. Pulmonary dendritic cells. *Am J Respir Crit Care Med*. 2005;172:530–551.

144. Lohmann-Matthes ML, Steinmüller C, Franke-Ullmann G. Pulmonary macrophages. *Eur Respir J*. 1994;7:1678–1689.

145. Geiser M. Update on macrophage clearance of inhaled micro- and nanoparticles. *J Aerosol Med Pulm Drug Deliv*. 2010;23: 207–217.

146. Schneeberger D, Aharonson-Raz K, Singh B. Pulmonary intravascular macrophages and lung health: what are we missing? *Am J Physiol Lung Cell Mol Physiol*. 2012;302:L498–L503.

147. Trapnell BC, Whitsett JA, Nakata K. Pulmonary alveolar proteinosis. *N Engl J Med*. 2003;349:2527–2539.

148. Weibel ER. It takes more than cells to make a good lung. *Am J Resp Crit Care Med*. 2013;187:342–346.

149. Weibel ER. Design of airways and blood vessels considered as branching trees. In: Crystal RG, West JB, Weibel ER, Barnes PJ, eds. *The Lung: Scientific Foundations*. 2nd ed. New York, NY: Lippincott-Raven; 1997:1061–1071.

150. Hess WR. Das Prinzip des kleinsten Kraftverbrauches im Dienste hämodynamischer Forschung. *Arch. Anat. Physiol.* 1914; 2:1–62.

151. Murray CD. The physiological principle of minimum work. I. The vascular system and the cost of blood. *Proc Nat Acad Sci USA*. 1926;12:207–214.

152. Mauroy B, Filoche M, Weibel ER, Sapoval B. An optimal bronchial tree may be dangerous. *Nature*. 2004;427:633–636.

153. Pedley TJ, Schroter RC, Sudlow MF. The prediction of pressure drop and variation of resistance withion the human bromchial airways. *Respir Physiol*. 1970;9:387–405.

154. Phalen RF, Yeh HC, Schum GM, Raabe OG. Application of an idealized model to morphometry of the mammalian tracheobronchial tree. *Anat Rec*. 1978;190:167–176.

155. Horsfield K. Pulmonary airways and blood vessels considered as confluent trees. In: Crystal RG, West JB, Weibel ER, Barnes PJ, eds. *The Lung: Scientific Foundations*. 2nd ed. New York, NY: Lippincott-Raven; 1997:1073–1079.

156. Mandelbrot B. *The Fractal Geometry of Nature*. New York, NY: Freeman; 1983.

157. Weibel ER. Fractal geometry: a design principle for living organisms. *Am J Physiol Lung Cell Mol Physiol*. 1991;261: L361–L369.

158. West BJ, Barghava V, Goldberger AL. Beyond the principle of similitude: renormalization in the bronchial tree. *J Appl Physiol*. 1986;60:1089–1097.

159. Huang W, Yen RT, McLaurine M, Bledsoe G. Morphometry of the human pulmonary vasculature. *J Appl Physiol*. 1996;81:2123–2133.

160. König MF, Lucocq JM, Weibel ER. Demonstration of pulmonary vascular perfusion by electron and light microscopy. *J Appl Physiol*. 1993;75:1877–1883.

161. Fung YC, Sobin SS. Theory of sheet flow in lung alveoli. *J Appl Physiol*. 1969;26:472–488.

162. Weibel ER. What makes a good lung? The morphometric basis of lung function. *Swiss Med Wkly*. 2009;139:375–386.

163. Ochs M, Nyengaard JR, Jung A, et al. The number of alveoli in the human lung. *Am J Respir Crit Care Med*. 2004;169:120–124.

164. Weibel ER. Functional morphology of lung parenchyma. In: Macklem PT, Mead J, eds. *Handbook of Physiology. Section 3: The Respiratory System*. vol 3/1. Bethesda, MD: American Physiological Society; 1986:89–111.

165. Weibel ER, Bachofen H. The fiber scaffold of lung parenchyma. In: Crystal RG, West JB, Weibel ER, Barnes PJ, eds. *The Lung: Scientific Foundations*. 2nd ed. New York, NY: Lippincott-Raven; 1997:1139–1146.

166. Weibel ER, Gil J. Structure-function relationships at the alveolar level. In: West JB, ed. *Bioengineering Aspects of the Lung*. New York, NY: Marcel Dekker; 1977:1–81.

167. Fuller B. Tensegrity. *Portfolio Artnews Annual*. 1961;4:112–127.

168. Ingber DE. Tensegrity I. Cell structure and hierarchical systems biology. *J Cell Sci*. 2003;116:1157–1173.

169. Clements JA, Hustead RF, Johnson RP, Gribetz I. Pulmonary surface tension and alveolar stability. *J Appl Physiol*. 1961;16: 444–450.

170. Weibel ER, Bachofen H. How to stabilize the pulmonary alveoli: surfactant or fibers? *News Physiol Sci*. 1987;2:72–75.

171. Gil J, Weibel ER. Improvements in demonstration of lining layer of lung alveoli by electron microscopy. *Respir Physiol*. 1969/70;8:13–36.

172. Schürch S, Goerke J, Clements JA. Direct determination of volume and time dependence of alveolar surface tension in excised lungs. *Proc Natl Acad Sci USA*. 1978;75:3417–3421.

173. Bachofen H, Gehr P, Weibel ER. Alterations of mechanical properties and morphology in excised rabbit lungs rinsed with a detergent. *J Appl Physiol*. 1979;47:1002–1010.

174. Bachofen H, Schürch S, Urbinelli M, Weibel ER. Relations among alveolar surface tension, surface area, volume, and recoil pressure. *J Appl Physiol*. 1987;62:1878–1887.

175. Gil J, Bachofen H, Gehr P, Weibel ER. Alveolar volume–surface area relation in air- and saline-filled lungs fixed by vascular perfusion. *J Appl Physiol*. 1979;47:990–1001.

176. Wilson TA, Bachofen H. A model for mechanical structure of the alveolar duct. *J Appl Physiol*. 1982;52:1064–1070.

177. Bachofen H, Weber J, Wangensteen D, Weibel ER. Morphometric estimates of diffusing capacity in lungs fixed under zone II and zone III conditions. *Respir Physiol*. 1983;52:41–52.

178. Weibel ER. Morphological basis of alveolar-capillary gas exchange. *Physiol Rev*. 1973;53:419–495.

179. Taylor CR, Weibel ER. Design of the mammalian respiratory system. I. Problem and strategy. *Respir Physiol*. 1981;44:1–10.

180. Bohr C. Ueber die spezifische Tätigkeit der Lungen bei der respiratorischen Gasaufnahme. *Scand Arch Physiol*. 1909;22:221–280.

181. Weibel ER. Morphometric estimation of pulmonary diffusion capacity. I. Model and method. *Respir Physiol*. 1970/71;11:54–75.

182. Weibel ER, Federspiel WJ, Fryder-Doffey F, et al. Morphometric model for pulmonary diffusing capacity. I. Membrane diffusing capacity. *Respir Physiol*. 1993;93:125–149.

183. Roughton FJ, Forster RE. Relative importance of diffusion and chemical reaction rates in determining rate of exchange of gases in the human lung, with special reference to true diffusing capacity of pulmonary membrane and volume of blood in the lung capillaries. *J Appl Physiol*. 1957;11:290–302.

184. Hsia CC, Chuong CJ, Johnson RL Jr. Critique of the conceptual basis of diffusing capacity estimates: a finite element analysis. *J Appl Physiol*. 1995;79:1039–1047.

185. Weibel ER, Knight BW. A morphometric study on the thickness of the pulmonary air-blood barrier. *J Cell Biol*. 1964;21:367–384.

186. Hsia CC, Hyde DM, Ochs M, Weibel ER. An official research policy statement of the American Thoracic Society / European Respiratory Society: standards for quantitative assessment of lung structure. *Am J Respir Crit Care Med*. 2010;181:394–418.

187. Ochs M. A brief update on lung stereology. *J Microsc*. 2006;222:188–200.

188. Holland RA, Shibata H, Scheid P, Piiper J. Kinetics of O_2 uptake and release by red cells in stopped-flow apparatus: effects of unstirred layer. *Respir Physiol*. 1985;59:71–91.

189. Yamaguchi K, Nguyen-Phu D, Scheid P, Piiper J. Kinetics of O_2 uptake and release by human erythrocytes studied by a stopped-flow technique. *J Appl Physiol*. 1985;58:1215–1224.

190. Gehr P, Bachofen M, Weibel ER. The normal human lung: ultrastructure and morphometric estimation of diffusion capacity. *Respir Physiol*. 1978;32:121–140.

191. Hammond MD, Hempleman SC. Oxygen diffusing capacity estimates derived from measured VA/Q distributions in man. *Respir Physiol*. 1987;69:129–147.

192. Weibel ER, Taylor CR, O'Neil JJ, et al. Maximal oxygen consumption and pulmonary diffusion capacity: a direct comparison of physiologic and morphometric measurements in canids. *Respir Physiol*. 1983;54:173–188.

193. Hsia CC, Fryder-Doffey F, Stalder-Navarro V, Johnson RL Jr, Reynolds RC, Weibel ER. Structural changes underlying compensatory increase of diffusing capacity after left pneumonectomy in adult dogs. *J Clin Invest*. 1993;92:758–764.

194. Takeda S, Hsia CC, Wagner E, Ramanathan M, Estrera AS, Weibel ER. Compensatory alveolar growth normalizes gas exchange function in immature dogs after pneumonectomy. *J Appl Physiol*. 1999;86:1301–1310.

195. Hsia CC, Johnson RL, Weibel ER. Compensatory lung growth:relationship to postnatal growth and adaptation in destructive lung disease. In: Harding R, Pinkerton KE, Plopper CG, eds. *The Lung: Development, Aging and the Environment*. London: Elsevier/Academic Press; 2004:187–199.

196. Hsia CC. Quantitative morphology of compensatory lung growth. *Eur Respir Rev*. 2006;15:148–156.

197. Sapoval B, Filoche M, Weibel ER. Smaller is better – but not too small: a physical scale for the design of the mammalian pulmonary acinus. *Proc Natl Acad Sci USA*. 2001;99:10411–10416.

198. Rodriguez M, Bur S, Favre A, Weibel ER. Pulmonary acinus: geometry and morphometry of the peripheral airway system in rat and rabbit. *Am J Anat*. 1987;180:143–155.

199. Swan AJ, Tawhai MH. Evidence for minimal oxygen heterogeneity in the healthy human pulmonary acinus. *J Appl Physiol*. 2011;110:528–537.

200. Weibel ER, Taylor CR. Design of the mammalian respiratory system: I–IX. *Respir Physiol*. 1981;44:1–164.

201. Margaria R, Cerretelli P, Aghemo P, Saw G. Energy cost of running. *J Appl Physiol*. 1963;18:367–370.

202. Weibel ER. *Symmorphosis. On Form and Function in Shaping Life*. Cambridge, MA: Harvard University Press; 2000.

203. Taylor CR, Karas RH, Weibel ER, Hoppeler H. Adaptive variation in the mammalian respiratory system in relation to energetic demand: I–VIII. *Respir Physiol*. 1987;69:1–127.

204. Hoppeler H, Lüthi P, Claassen H, Weibel ER, Howald H. The ultrastructure of the normal human skeletal muscle. A morphometric analysis on untrained men, women, and well-trained orienteers. *Pfluegers Arch*. 1973;344:217–232.

205. Hoppeler H, Weibel ER. Structural and functional limits for oxygen supply to muscle. *Acta Physiol Scand*. 2000;168:445–456.

206. Weibel ER, Taylor CR, Hoppeler H. The concept of symmorphosis: a testable hypothesis of structure-function relationship. *Proc Natl Acad Sci USA*. 1991;88:10357–10361.

207. Karas RH, Taylor CR, Jones JH, Lindstedt SL, Reeves RB, Weibel ER. Adaptive variation in the mammalian respiratory system in relation to energetic demand. VII. Flow of oxygen across the pulmonary gas exchanger. *Respir Physiol*. 1987;69:101–115.

CHAPTER 3

The Respiratory Muscles

Ghislaine Gayan-Ramirez
Marc Decramer

The respiratory muscles constitute a complex pump system. Several muscles comprise this system, represented schematically in Figure 3-1. Breathing under all circumstances requires a coordinated contraction of different respiratory muscles. The most important inspiratory muscle is the diaphragm. The conditions under which this respiratory muscle system weakens and eventually will fail are addressed in other chapters (see Chapters 83, 85, and 104). This chapter focuses on structural and functional properties of the respiratory muscles, respiratory muscle action, and respiratory muscle interaction.

STRUCTURAL AND FUNCTIONAL PROPERTIES OF RESPIRATORY MUSCLES

The respiratory muscles are skeletal muscles, and, in essence, their structural and functional properties are within the range of other skeletal muscles located in the limbs. Adaptations to their specific function, however, make them distinctly different from other skeletal muscles in a number of respects. First, limb muscles are essentially designed to produce movements, and hence, primarily work against inertial loads. Respiratory muscles mainly have to overcome resistive and elastic loads.

Second, peripheral muscles contract rhythmically during movements, whereas respiratory muscles contract rhythmically and continuously, and they are the only skeletal muscles on which life depends. These vital muscles thus have to be well equipped to sustain continuous rhythmic contraction. These adaptations include high fatigue resistance, high oxidative capacity, greater capillary density, and greater maximal blood flow, and they depend upon structural and functional properties of the muscles.

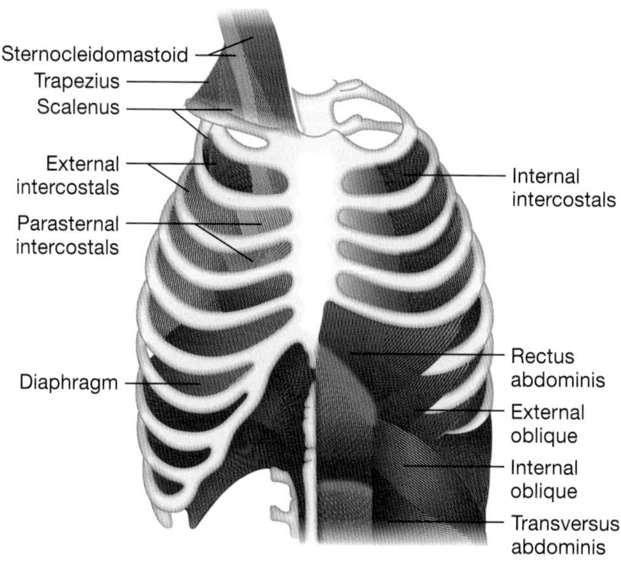

Figure 3-1 Idealized drawing of the respiratory muscles.

STRUCTURAL PROPERTIES

Structural properties of muscles in general, and respiratory muscles in particular, depend upon fiber types present in the muscle, morphological characteristics of the fibers, and motor unit organization.

Fiber Types

Four types of muscle fibers are usually present in skeletal muscles. They are distinguished on the basis of the myofibrillar myosin adenosine triphosphatase (ATPase) activity and its pH dependence and pretreatment with paraformaldehyde.[1,2] Thus, after acid preincubations at pH 4.5, type I fibers are stained dark, type IIa fibers are stained lighter than type IIb and type IIx fibers. In addition, pretreatment with paraformaldehyde after alkaline preincubation at pH 10.4 further allows the distinction between type IIb fibers staining lighter than type IIx fibers. Alternatively, muscle fibers may be distinguished through myosin heavy chain gene expression using electrophoresis and western blotting or via immunostaining.[3] This latter technique has the advantage of revealing the presence of coexpression of different myosin heavy chain isoforms within the same muscle fiber. It has also been revealed that myosin heavy chain 2b is not expressed in human muscle.[4] Type I fibers, or slow oxidative fibers, have a slow contraction profile but are high in endurance and rich in oxidative enzymes.[5] Type II fibers are fast-twitch fibers that develop tension rapidly. They either are fatigue resistant or glycolytic oxidative (IIa), or fatigable or glycolytic (IIb),[5] whereas resistance to fatigue for the type IIx fibers is intermediate between the IIa and IIb fibers. Type II fibers develop greater forces than do type I fibers. Muscles primarily composed of type I fibers have high endurance capacity, whereas those primarily composed of type IIb fibers are designed to develop high forces but have low endurance capacity.[5] Type IIa fibers are intermediate and combine relatively high force development with relatively long endurance.[5] In general, type I fibers have the smallest cross-sectional area, and type IIb fibers tend to have the largest.

The respiratory muscles are mixed muscles containing both fast-twitch and slow-twitch fibers. The human diaphragm contains about 55 ± 5% type I fibers, 21 ± 6% type IIa fibers, and 23 ± 3% type IIx fibers. Other respiratory muscles (i.e., intercostal muscles, abdominal muscles, sternomastoids) contain at least 60% highly oxidative fibers.[6] No data are available on the scalenes. The respiratory muscles thus are generally well equipped to sustain continuous rhythmic contraction.

Morphological Characteristics of the Fibers

The respiratory muscles consist of muscle bundles oriented in a parallel fashion. These bundles consist of hundreds of muscle fibers, each of which in turn consists of hundreds of myofibrils. These myofibrils are made up of hundreds of sarcomeres arranged in series, each sarcomere consisting of a number of myosin (thick filaments) and twice the number of actin (thin) filaments. The capacity of the muscle to produce forces depends upon the number of myofibrils in parallel, since the forces developed by all these myofibrils are additive, whereas the displacement and velocity of shortening depend upon the number of sarcomeres in series. Indeed, the displacements of these sarcomeres arranged in series are additive.

The density of mitochondria in each of the four fiber types tends to be greater than in the same fiber types in limb muscles.[5,7] In addition, in humans, the diaphragm is composed of about 80% oxidative fibers compared with 36% to 46% in the limb muscles of untrained men.[5,7] As a consequence, the volume density of mitochondria in the diaphragm is twofold greater than in the limb muscles.[5,7] Therefore, the oxygen uptake capacity of the diaphragm is considerably greater than that of limb muscles because of the high oxidative fiber content and the greater mitochondrial density.[5,7] Moreover, the maximal blood flow also considerably exceeds that of limb muscles because of the greater capillary density, which is about twice the capillary density in the limb muscle. The diaphragm is thus well equipped to sustain rhythmic contraction at rest through its type I and IIa fibers: The type IIa fibers permit additional recruitment in power and rate during exercise, and the few type IIx fibers permit high power outputs necessary for sneezing and coughing.

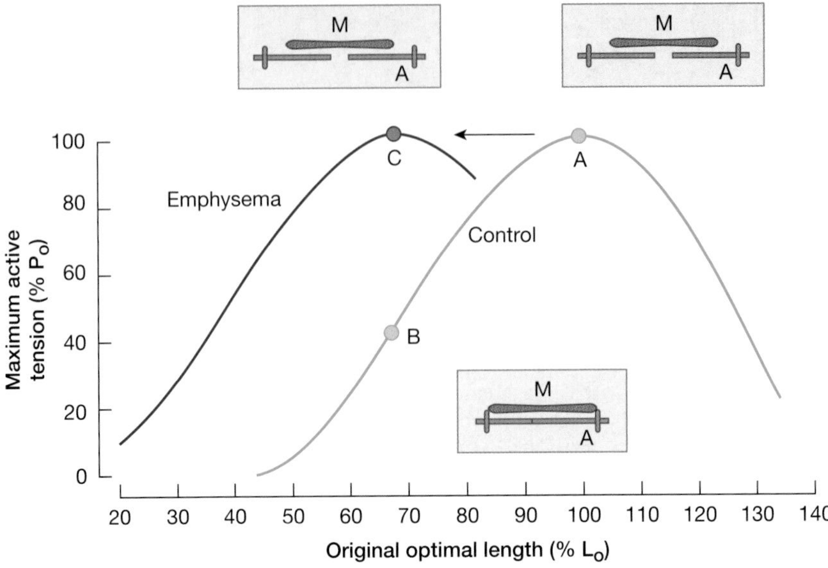

Figure 3-2 Diaphragmatic length–tension curve in normal hamsters and hamsters with elastase-induced emphysema. Tension is expressed as a percentage of maximum tetanic tension, P_O, and length is expressed as a percentage of original optimal length, L_O. The degree of filament overlap among actin (A) and myosin (M) filaments in control (**A**), acute (**B**), and chronic hyperinflation (**C**) is shown. Note that due to sarcomere adaptation in chronic hyperinflation, the degree of filament overlap is the same at a considerably shorter length. *(Reproduced with permission from Farkas G: Functional characteristics of the respiratory muscles. Sem Respir Crit Care Med. 1991;12(4):247–257.)*

Motor Unit Organization

Muscle fibers are organized by their innervations in motor units that vary in their mechanical and fatigue properties. In adults, all muscle fibers within a motor unit are the same fiber type. The muscle fibers within a given motor unit are broadly dispersed throughout a region of the diaphragm. Dispersion occurs both horizontally across the surface of the diaphragm and vertically with fibers at different depths. The innervation ratio (number of fibers supplied by a single motoneuron) is approximately 400 in rat diaphragm[8] compared with an estimated value of 2500 in humans.[9] There are four types of motor units in the respiratory muscles: a motor unit with slower contraction times and resistance to fatigue (type S) and three types of motor units displaying faster contraction times, with various degrees of fatigue resistance. The type S comprises fibers that express the slow isoform of myosin heavy chain. Fast motor units that are fatigue resistant (type FR) comprise muscle fibers expressing the myosin heavy chain 2a; those that are highly fatigable (type FF) comprise muscle fibers expressing myosin heavy chain 2b; and those that are fatigue intermediate (type FInt) comprise muscle fibers that express the myosin heavy chain 2x. Motor units composed of fast fibers are large and develop forces in the range of 110 millinewton (mN). These, however, are considerably smaller than in limb muscles. Motor units composed of slow fibers are smaller and develop forces in the range of 30 to 60 mN. The recruitment pattern of the diaphragm follows the size principle with the smallest motor units being recruited first.

■ FUNCTIONAL PROPERTIES

Functional properties of muscles are generally described in terms of force–length relationships, time-dependent characteristics of the twitch, force–frequency, force–velocity, and power–frequency relationships.

The force–length characteristics of the diaphragm are in essence similar to other muscles. Maximal tension is generated at the optimal length. Three aspects of the force–length curve of the diaphragm are potentially relevant to clinical medicine. First, with hyperinflation, the diaphragm shortens and its capacity to generate force is concomitantly reduced.[10] Second, when hyperinflation occurs chronically, adaptation occurs in the muscle. This adaptation consists of drop out of sarcomeres such that muscle shortening is then accommodated by a reduced number of sarcomeres rather than alterations in filament overlap within the sarcomeres.[11] As a consequence, the force-generating capacity is restored, at least in part, at foreshortened length.[10] This adaptation is summarized in Figure 3-2. The consequences of this adaptation to patients with hyperinflation are discussed in the section "Physiological Conditions Affecting Respiratory Muscle Interaction." Third, although less-than-optimal filament overlap is the primary reason for a reduction in force with muscle shortening, calcium deactivation due to T-tubular failure also plays a role.[12] This is potentially significant for treatment, since inotropic agents restore T-tubular function in foreshortened muscle.[13] Accordingly, inotropic agents exert much greater effects on foreshortened diaphragm than on diaphragm placed at its optimal length.[14] This concept opens up new perspectives for respiratory muscle pharmacotherapy in patients with severe hyperinflation. The length–tension curves of other respiratory muscles and their adaptation to hyperinflation have not been systematically studied.

A particularly interesting question is the relationship between the in situ operational length of the respiratory muscles and the optimal length in vitro. For the diaphragm, the length at functional residual capacity (FRC) comes close to the optimal length.[15,16] The length changes undergone by the diaphragm over the vital capacity range are large, 30% to 40%.[17,18] These length changes are considerably smaller for the parasternal intercostals, the scalenes, and the sternocleidomastoids.[19–21] For the parasternal intercostals, the length at FRC is clearly longer than optimal in supine dogs, so that with hyperinflation, the parasternal intercostals move toward their optimal length.[21,22] Subsequent experiments, however, indicate that the fall in pleural pressure caused by stimulation of the parasternal intercostals in dogs is reduced with increasing lung volume.[23] This discrepancy was shown to result from changes in orientation and motion of ribs with hyperinflation. The scalenes and sternocleidomastoids appear to operate on the ascending limb of their length–tension curves in supine dogs.[20] How hyperinflation in patients affects the force-generating capacity of these muscles remains unclear. According to an analysis, the changes in length during passive inflation are proportional to the mechanical advantage of a particular respiratory muscle.[24] In keeping with this analysis, the mechanical advantage of the diaphragm would be considerably greater than the mechanical advantage of other inspiratory muscles (see in the section "Physiological Conditions Affecting Respiratory Muscle Interaction").

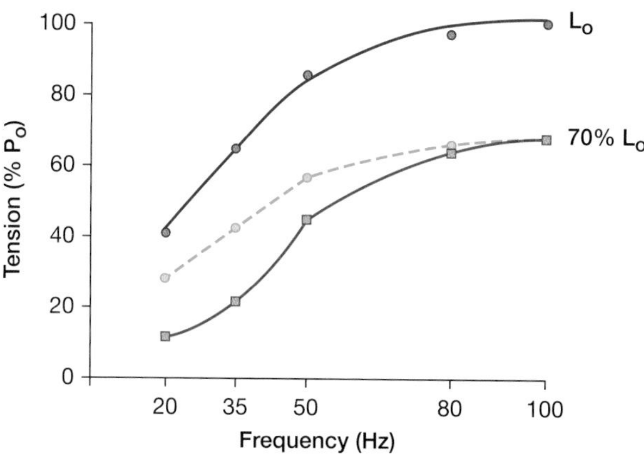

Figure 3-3 Force–frequency curve of human diaphragm at optimal length (L_O) and 70% L_O. Force is expressed as a percentage of maximal tetanic tension, P_O, and frequency is expressed in Hz. *Dashed line* is the predicted line at 70% L_O, whereas the *solid line* is the observed line. The predicted line is based on the assumption that a 30% change in length produces a 35% drop in force at all stimulation frequencies, as is observed for maximal tetanic force. Note that the decrease in force at lower stimulation frequencies is considerably greater than theoretically predicted. *(Reproduced with permission from Farkas G: Functional characteristics of the respiratory muscles. Sem Respir Crit Care Med. 1991;12(4):247–257.)*

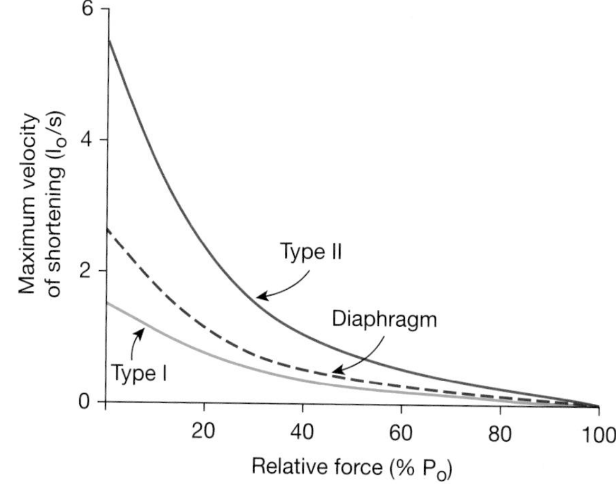

Figure 3-4 Force–velocity curve of human diaphragm *(dashed line)*, which is intermediate between the force–velocity curve of a typical slow muscle (type I) and a typical fast muscle (type II). Maximum velocity is expressed in optimal length (L_O), per second and relative force is expressed as a percentage of maximum tetanic force, P_O.

The force developed by a muscle increases with increasing frequency of stimulation. The increase in force is considerably steeper for a slow muscle in which fusion occurs at lower frequency because of the longer relaxation time than for a fast muscle. The diaphragm is intermediate, so that at in vivo stimulation frequencies (10–30 Hz), a fused tetanic contraction occurs. Particularly interesting is the effect of acute shortening on the force–frequency curve. Since acute shortening is associated with a downward shift of the force–frequency curve, the detrimental effect of acute shortening on the force-generating capacity of the diaphragm appears to be twofold.[10] With muscle shortening there is a clear reduction in maximal tetanic force. However, the decrease in force at submaximal stimulation frequencies is disproportionately greater (Fig. 3-3).

The force–velocity curve of the diaphragm is shown in Figure 3-4. With increasing loads, the velocity of contraction is reduced. The velocity of contraction is a direct function of myosin ATPase activity, and, hence, the force–velocity curve is primarily determined by the muscle fiber composition. The diaphragm is intermediate between the force–velocity curve of a fast and a slow muscle (Fig. 3-4).[6] The production of airflow into the lungs requires power output by the respiratory muscles. Power may be calculated as the product of the values of velocity and force according to the force–velocity relationship (Fig. 3-4). Instantaneous peak power occurs at 30% of maximal force and at 30% of maximal velocity. The frequency–isometric force relationship, frequency–shortening force, and frequency–power relationships show a similar dependency of force and power upon frequency of stimulation.

Fatigue also affects profoundly the force–length, force–frequency, force–velocity, and power–frequency characteristics of the diaphragm. The diaphragm, however, is more resistant to developing fatigue than limb muscles in vivo and in vitro.[25] Of note, the inspiratory muscles recover from fatigue 10 times faster than the elbow flexors performing a similar task.[26] The effects of fatigue on functional properties of the respiratory muscles are discussed in Chapters 84, 85 and 104. The factors determining the development of respiratory muscle fatigue are also discussed in these chapters.

ACTIONS OF RESPIRATORY MUSCLES

THE DIAPHRAGM

The diaphragm is the most important inspiratory muscle. It is innervated by the phrenic nerves supplied by the cervical nerve roots C3 to C5 in humans. It consists of two distinct parts, the costal and crural parts, which have separate actions on the rib cage, separate segmental motor innervations, and a different embryological origin. In respiratory activities, however, the diaphragm frequently operates as a functional unit, and in the following its action is described as such. Diaphragmatic action is schematically represented in Figure 3-5. Diaphragmatic contraction increases chest wall dimensions because of three distinct reasons. First, diaphragmatic descent increases the craniocaudal dimensions of the thorax. Diaphragmatic descent is tightly coupled to outward motion of the free abdominal wall.

Second, diaphragmatic contraction increases the dimensions of the lower rib cage because of the increase in abdominal pressure that it causes. This increase in abdominal pressure acts through the zone of apposition (i.e., the zone in which the diaphragm is immediately apposed to the rib cage) to expand the lower rib cage. This action is the appositional component of diaphragmatic action (Fig. 3-5).[27,28] The magnitude of the appositional component is determined by the magnitude of the zone of apposition, about 25% to 30% of the total internal surface area of the rib cage at FRC in standing humans, and by the magnitude of the increase in abdominal pressure caused by diaphragmatic contraction.[28]

Third, diaphragmatic contraction further increases lower rib cage dimensions because of its insertions into the lower rib cage. The diaphragmatic fibers are oriented axially, and their contraction causes pull on the lower rib cage in an axial direction, leading to cephalad motion and outward rotation of the lower rib and hence, to lower rib cage expansion. This is the *insertional component* of diaphragmatic contraction (Fig. 3-5).[27]

When the diaphragm acts in isolation during diaphragmatic contraction or pacing in high quadriplegics, in whom all inspiratory muscles, except for sternocleidomastoids, are paralyzed,[29,30] it exerts an expiratory effect on the upper rib cage during inspiration.[29,31] These data point out that in normal subjects, quiet inspiration is not accomplished by the diaphragm alone but rather results from the coordinated activity of the diaphragm with the rib cage inspiratory muscles and the abdominal muscles. Indeed, the pattern of chest

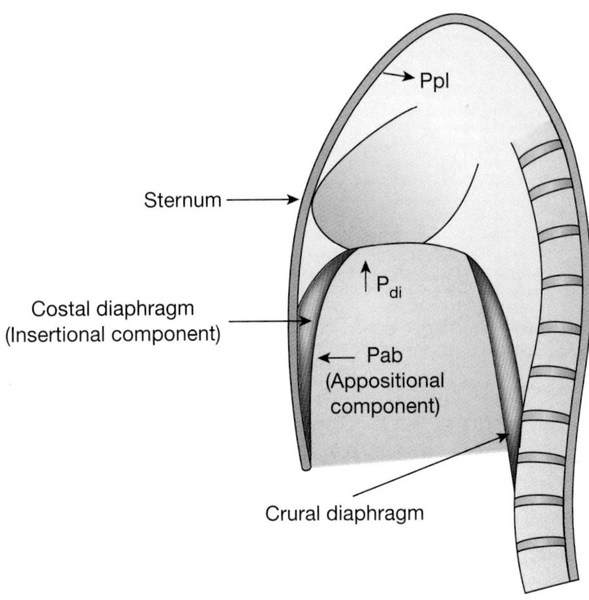

Figure 3-5 Diagram illustrating diaphragmatic action. Lateral view of the thorax. Ppl, pleural pressure; Pab, abdominal pressure; P_{di}, transdiaphragmatic pressure. The costal and the crural diaphragm are shown. See text for further explanation.

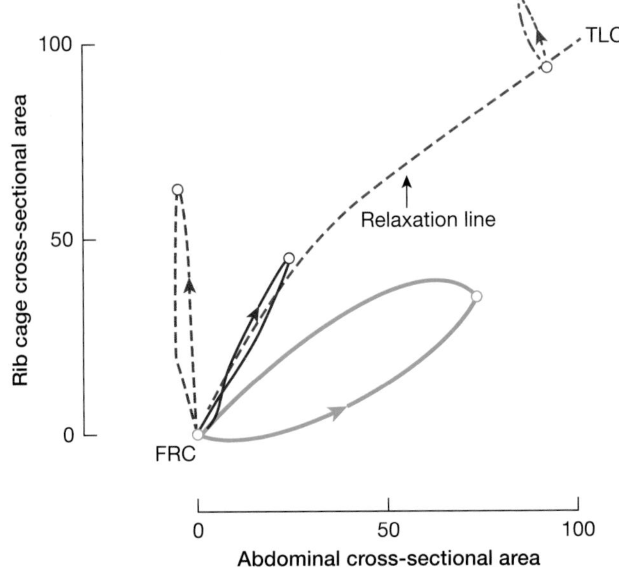

Figure 3-6 Konno–Mead diagram illustrating chest wall motion during quiet breathing *(thin loop)*, diaphragmatic pacing or quiet breathing in tetraplegic patient *(thick loop)*, breathing with diaphragm paralysis *(dash loop)*, and breathing at severely elevated end-expiratory volume *(dash–dot loop)*. Rib cage and abdominal cross-sectional areas are expressed as a percentage of inspiratory capacity. Dashed line is the relaxation line obtained during expiration with muscles relaxed.

wall motion in quadriplegics shown in Figure 3-6 indicates that diaphragmatic contraction alone cannot be responsible for the pattern of chest wall motion observed during quiet breathing (see in the section "Physiological Conditions Affecting Respiratory Muscle Interaction") and hence, that other muscles assist the diaphragm in moving the chest wall during quiet breathing.

THE INTERCOSTAL MUSCLES

The functional anatomy of intercostal muscles is schematically represented in Figure 3-7. Between the chondral portions of the ribs only one layer of intercostal muscles, the parasternal intercostals, is present. Between the osseous portions of the ribs, two layers are present. The outermost layer runs obliquely downward and forward and is called the *external intercostal.* The innermost layer runs obliquely downward and backward and is called the *internal intercostal* (Fig. 3-7, left panel). Note that the internal intercostals and parasternal intercostals have the same fiber orientation. Dorsally only an external intercostal is present. Finally, the fusiform muscle running from the lateral border of the transverse processes of the thoracic vertebra and inserting caudally into the rostral border of the rib below is called the levator costae (Fig. 3-7, right panel).

The parasternal portion of the intercostal musculature, the "parasternals," is consistently active during quiet breathing both in animal and human subjects,[19,32] and is the most important inspiratory portion of the intercostal musculature. The parasternal intercostals have the greatest mechanical advantage, and their contraction produces about 60% of the cephalad motion of the rib during inspiration.[33,34] Within the parasternal intercostals, the medial fibers have a greater mechanical advantage and are activated more consistently and before the middle and lateral fibers.[35]

The action as well as the respiratory role of the interosseus intercostals remain the subject of a longstanding debate. The most commonly accepted view on intercostal muscle action is based on a theory of intercostal muscle fiber orientation and rib geometry. This theory states that the external intercostals are inspiratory in action, and the internal intercostals are expiratory in action.[36] Numerous experiments do not fit with this theory, although a finite element analysis largely confirmed these actions.[36] It is commonly believed that the interosseus intercostals constitute a reserve system that may be recruited with increased ventilatory load. The external intercostals are recruited predominantly during inspiration, primarily in the upper interspaces, whereas the internal intercostals are recruited predominantly during expiration primarily in the lower interspaces.[36] Wilson et al.[34] demonstrated

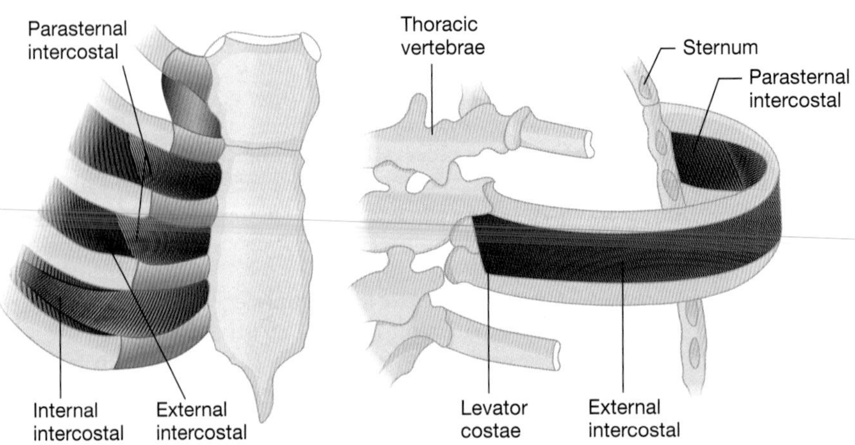

Figure 3-7 Diagram of the functional anatomy of the intercostal muscles, at their anterior *(left)* and posterior *(right)* aspects. Notice the parasternal, internal, and external intercostals, and the levator costae.

by the application of the reciprocity theorem of Maxwell, that the external intercostals in the dorsal portion of the costal interspaces have a large inspiratory mechanical advantage. This advantage decreases in the ventral and caudal directions such that in the ventral portion of the caudal interspaces it is reversed in an expiratory mechanical advantage.[36] Conversely, the internal intercostals in the caudal interspaces have a large expiratory mechanical advantage, but this advantage decreases in the cranial and ventral directions.[36] Because of this pattern of topographic distribution the pattern of neural activation is crucial for the function of these muscles.[36] This pattern was shown to match the pattern of distribution of mechanical advantage, such that the external intercostals have an inspiratory function and the internal intercostals have an expiratory function.[36]

Without question, the levator costae have an inspiratory action on the rib. It is frequently activated even during quiet inspiration in supine dogs.[37] The levator costae's contribution to inspiratory motion of the ribs during quiet breathing, however, appears substantially smaller than that of the parasternal intercostals. This contribution may further increase when the inspiratory motion of the ribs is appreciably increased.

■ THE SCALENES

The scalenes run between the transverse process of the five lower cervical vertebrae and the upper margin of the first (scalenus anterior) and second (scalenus medius and posterior) ribs. The action of these muscles is to raise the first two ribs. The orientation of their axis in the neck causes upward motion of these ribs ("pump handle" motion). Moreover, the scalenes are consistently active during quiet breathing in normal individuals and contribute to chest wall expansion.[38] They may be very important in the case of spinal cord injury. When the injury is below C4 to C8, the scalenes' function is entirely or partially preserved, and they contribute importantly to upper rib cage motion in these patients.[39]

■ THE STERNOCLEIDOMASTOIDS

The sternocleidomastoids run between the mastoid processes of the temporal bone and the manubrium sterni and medial portion of the clavicle. The pressure-generating ability of the sternocleidomastoid muscle in normal humans is about the same as that of the scalene muscles. In humans, these muscles are electrically silent during quiet breathing, but they may be recruited with increased ventilatory load. These muscles are particularly important in high quadriplegics in whom they preserve their function because they are innervated by the 11th cranial nerve and spinal nerves C1 to C2.[29,40] Through training the sternocleidomastoids may develop marked hypertrophy and contribute to several hours of ventilator independence in these patients.[40] They also may be recruited in patients with poliomyelitis and diaphragmatic dysfunction. These muscles are thought to be important in moving the upper rib cage in patients with chronic obstructive pulmonary disease (COPD), even though a clinical experimental study failed to demonstrate consistent activity in these muscles in these patients.[41]

■ THE SHOULDER GIRDLE AND NECK MUSCLES

Several shoulder girdle and neck muscles may contribute to inspiration under particular circumstances. Most of these muscles run from the rib cage to an extrathoracic extension. When the rib cage is fixed in the lean-forward position—a position commonly employed by patients with COPD—these muscles contribute to expansion of the rib cage during inspiration. Muscles that may contribute to inspiration include the trapezius, latissimus dorsi, pectoralis major and minor, erector spinae, teres major, serratus anterior, platysma, mylohyoid, and sternohyoid. Since these muscles commonly contribute to inspiration in patients with severe airflow obstruction, their further use for other activities (e.g., hair combing), may considerably increase dyspnea in these patients.[42]

■ THE CLAVICULAR HEAD OF PECTORALIS MAJOR

The clavicular head of the pectoralis major runs laterally and caudally from the medial half of the clavicle and manubrium sterni to the humerus. If the arms are fixed and braced, contraction causes downward motion of the ribs and sternum, increase in pleural pressure and, hence, expiration. Simultaneously, the lower rib cage and the abdomen move outward. Tetraplegics use this expiratory action when all other expiratory muscles are paralyzed.[43]

■ THE TRIANGULARIS STERNI

The triangularis sterni is the most important expiratory muscle of the rib cage.[44] The muscle runs at the inside of the thorax between the inner aspect of the sternum and the inner aspect of the five lower ribs (Fig. 3-8), and its action is to lower the ribs relative to the sternum and thus to cause expiration. The triangularis sterni is electrically silent in humans breathing quietly,[44] but it is recruited during expiration below FRC.[44] Its neural activation is also coupled with that of the abdominal muscles.[44] Its recruitment threshold is low, lower than the recruitment threshold of most other expiratory muscles.

■ THE ABDOMINAL MUSCLES

The abdominal muscles are composed of four different muscle layers (Fig. 3-1). Ventrally, a muscular sheet running between the lower costal cartilages and the sternum and the pubis, represents the rectus abdominis. This muscle is enclosed in a sheath formed by the aponeuroses of the other three muscles. Laterally, an oblique muscle runs obliquely downward and forward between the lower eight ribs and the iliac crest, inguinal ligament, and linea alba medially, the external oblique. At the inner surface of this muscle lies the internal oblique with a fiber orientation, which is 90 degrees perpendicular to the external oblique. These muscles are homologous to the external and internal intercostals. The innermost layer is the transversus abdominis, a circular muscular sheet surrounding the abdomen, with a fiber orientation that is parallel to the ribs. The transversus abdominis originates from the inner surface of the lower six ribs, where it interdigitates with the costal insertions of the diaphragm. It runs from this origin and the lumbar fascia, iliac crest, and inguinal ligament,

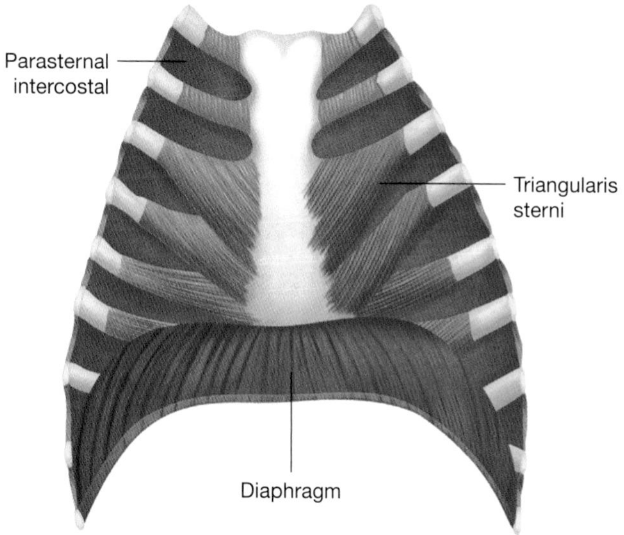

Figure 3-8 Diagram illustrating the functional anatomy of the parasternal intercostal muscles, the triangularis sterni, and the diaphragm.

circumferentially around the abdominal visceral mass to terminate ventrally in the rectus sheet. These muscles all have an expiratory action, by virtue of the inward pull of the abdomen they cause and of the insertions they have in the rib cage. In addition, however, rib cage expansion may occur with contraction of some of these muscles through the increase in abdominal pressure accompanying their contraction.[45]

The abdominal muscles are electrically silent during quiet breathing. Usually, however, tonic activity is present in the abdominal muscles in upright position, particularly in the upper segments.[27] During inspiratory loading, CO_2-induced hyperventilation, exercise, and forced expiration, these muscles are recruited. The transversus abdominis appears to have the lowest recruitment threshold.[46,47]

RESPIRATORY MUSCLE INTERACTION

RESPIRATORY MUSCLE INTERACTION DURING QUIET BREATHING

Respiratory muscle interaction is traditionally studied by means of a Konno–Mead diagram, relating rib cage diameter or cross-sectional area to abdominal diameter or cross-sectional area (Fig. 3-6). First, this relationship is determined in the absence of muscle contraction, during a relaxed expiration, yielding a relaxation line. During quiet breathing in the upright position, the chest wall moves along this relaxation line, which means that proportional expansion of rib cage and abdomen is occurring. In the supine position, abdominal movement is proportionally greater than rib cage movement. Since isolated diaphragmatic contraction in quadriplegics causes abdominal movement without rib cage motion or even inward movement of the upper rib cage (upper rib cage paradox), diaphragmatic contraction alone cannot be responsible for the pattern of motion occurring during quiet breathing (Fig. 3-6). Therefore, this motion requires concomitant contraction of other muscles (i.e., the parasternal intercostals and scalenes). These muscles actively contribute to chest wall motion and cause upper rib cage expansion, whereas diaphragmatic contraction alone would cause upper rib cage paradox. During quiet breathing, the diaphragm probably contributes about 60% to 70% of the tidal volume, and the parasternal intercostals and scalenes contribute the rest.[48]

Posture alters the interaction between the respiratory muscles. For the diaphragm, the resistance of the abdominal contents on diaphragmatic descent is the principal determinant of its action on the rib cage. When changing from a seated to a supine posture in humans, there is a marked increase in abdominal compliance[49] and changes in the diaphragm shape result in less rib expansion. The influence of posture on the lung-expanding action of the diaphragm has been confirmed in patients with upper cervical cord transaction. Indeed, when these patients were supine, the paced diaphragm was able to generate an adequate tidal volume but the latter was progressively and markedly reduced when the patients were gradually tilted head up.[29] The abdominal muscles[50,51] and also the triangularis sterni[44,52,53] are silent in the supine posture in healthy individuals and while the tonic activity of the abdominal muscles in the standing posture is not related to the phases of the respiration, the activity of the triangularis sterni is confined to expiration.[53] Active use of these two sets of expiratory muscles in the standing posture compensates for the adverse effect of this posture on the inspiratory muscles, in particular the diaphragm.

Sleep affects respiratory muscle function negatively but in healthy individuals these physiological changes are not clinically significant. Sleep is associated with a generalized postural muscle hypotonia that is most profound during the phasic events of rapid eye movement (REM) sleep.[54] Therefore, respiratory muscles with a dual respiratory and postural function like the intercostals lose activity during REM sleep whereas the diaphragm, a muscle with only a respiratory function, maintains and even increases its activity to maintain tidal volume during REM sleep.[55] In severe COPD patients where rib cage motion is mainly produced by the inspiratory muscles of the rib cage as the diaphragm is mechanically impaired by hyperinflation, the substantial decrease in the activity of the scalene and sternocleidomastoid muscle during REM sleep is expected to decrease inspiratory pressure development and to lead to hypoventilation.[56]

PHYSIOLOGICAL CONDITIONS AFFECTING RESPIRATORY MUSCLE INTERACTION

Respiratory muscle interaction present during quiet breathing and the chest wall motion resulting from it may be altered in a number of physiological circumstances in which ventilatory load is affected. Indeed, the respiratory muscles participate in tasks that, although not strictly ventilatory in nature, serve important respiratory functions. These tasks of daily life include speech, laughter, swallowing, gagging, vomiting, and coughing. In addition, the interaction of the respiratory muscles is also modified during nonventilatory tasks.

Speech and laughing require the coordination of respiration and structures involved in producing sound features. Spontaneous speech occurs primarily at volume levels below spontaneous end expiration.[57] There is, therefore, a successive recruitment of muscles of expiration to empty the rib cage: first the triangularis sterni muscle[44,57] and the internal intercostal muscles then the external oblique and other muscles of the lateral abdominal wall and finally the rectus abdominis.[46,58,59] At the very end of expiration, the latissimus dorsi is active too.[58,59] Abdominal contraction during speech can optimize the inspiratory function of the diaphragm obliged to contract rapidly between phrases, and will also prevent dissipation of the pressure developed by the rib cage muscles on paradoxical abdominal displacement.[57]

Laughing is a natural maneuver triggered by emotion necessitating the coordination of the laryngeal and respiratory systems to produce a characteristic sound pattern and phasic lung pressure variations superimposed on an active expiratory effort. Laughter generally takes place when lung volume is low, near FRC and is terminated near residual volume.[60] It is characterized by sudden repetitive expiratory efforts leading to a decrease in lung volume due to sudden and sustained increase in gastric and esophageal pressures. The triangularis sterni muscle is recruited during laughing.[44] Higher transdiaphragmatic pressure at the end of the consecutive expiratory efforts indicates that the diaphragm actively prevents part of the increase in abdominal pressure from being transmitted to the chest wall cavity, thereby protecting intrathoracic structures from further mechanical stress and compression.[60] A pilot study suggests that the pattern of diaphragm activation during laughter is different from that induced by coughing or sneezing.[61]

For swallowing, respiration needs to be interrupted. During swallowing, the passive expiration of the diaphragm is interrupted by static activity aimed at preserving respiratory volume for expiration after swallowing.[62] Abdominal activity increases throughout pre- and postswallowing expiration.[62]

Vomiting that is produced by changes in thoracic and abdominal pressures is generated by the coordinated action of the major respiratory muscles. During vomiting, the diaphragm and the external intercostal (inspiratory) muscles cocontract with abdominal (expiratory) muscles in a series of burst of activity that culminates in expulsion while the internal intercostal (expiratory) muscles contract out of phase with these muscles during retching and are inactive during expulsion (see review by Miller[63]). Finally, the portion of the diaphragm surrounding the esophagus relaxes during expulsion, presumably to facilitate rostral movement of the gastric content (see review by Miller[63]).

Coughing, sneezing, and gagging represent complex acts involving both inspiratory and expiratory phases during which most of the respiratory muscles are recruited. Importantly, during those maneuvers, the maximal diaphragm force is reached.[64,65] Voluntary cough in humans is associated with a coordinated activation of the expiratory and accessory muscles. A graded increase in activity and burst duration proportional to cough flow rates is observed. Low cough flow rates are essentially produced by the activation of the expiratory muscles whereas accessory muscles become involved sequentially and increasingly with the production of higher flow rates.[66] The triangularis sterni muscle is actively recruited during coughing[44,67] and also during sneezing.[67]

Finally, understanding the level of muscle recruitment may be particularly relevant when testing respiratory muscle force to evaluate the degree of impairment in some diseases. Indeed, in untrained normal subjects, maximal inspiratory effort against a closed shutter (Müller maneuver or the maximal inspiratory pressure) mainly activates the intercostal muscle and the diaphragm as well as the sternomastoid.[68] The same holds true for the sniff maneuver through the nose.[68] The combined maneuver consisting in a maximal inspiratory maneuver combined with a maximal expiratory effort activates also the expiratory muscles (rectus abdominis) and produces the highest level of diaphragmatic strength as assessed by measuring transdiaphragmatic pressure.[68] The maximal electrical activity of the diaphragm is reached during the sniff maneuver.[68] These data indicate that the pressure generated by these maneuvers reflects a complex interaction between several groups of muscles.

All the above-mentioned effects pertain to ventilatory aspects of the respiratory muscles but, in addition to their respiratory role, the respiratory muscles also contract during postural tasks. The costal and the crural diaphragm are active with a single rapid movement of the contralateral upper limb in humans.[69] Electromyographic activity of the diaphragm increases prior to the onset of the activity of the muscle responsible for movement. This occurs irrespective of the phase of respiration[69] and is associated with an increase in transdiaphragmatic pressure with an initial reduction in length of the costal diaphragm. Similarly, during trunk rotation external and internal intercostal muscles show increased inspiratory activity superimposed on their postural tone[70,71] as do the parasternal intercostals.[72] During repetitive movement, the diaphragm contracts tonically throughout the respiratory cycle and phasic modulation of diaphragm activity at the frequency of limb movement is superimposed on its respiratory and tonic activation.[73] This was also observed in the transversus abdominis muscle.[73] Modulation of the intra-abdominal pressure that occurs through coordinated activity of the diaphragm, abdominal and pelvic floor muscles, may be important for the control of spinal stability when the limbs move.[69,73] When respiratory demand is increased, the activity of the diaphragm and the transversus abdominis associated with movement of an arm is reduced or even abolished, and the associated changes in gastric pressure are reduced.[74] In humans, the postural role of the diaphragm may also be impaired with specific fatigue of the inspiratory muscles.[75] The human triangularis sterni muscle also contracts during postural maneuvers such as head flexion, trunk rotation, and leg lift.[44]

PATHOLOGICAL CONDITIONS AFFECTING RESPIRATORY MUSCLE INTERACTION

Respiratory muscle interaction is profoundly affected by a number of pathological conditions including hyperinflation, reduced or loss of muscle activity.

Hyperinflation is a functional abnormality of lung diseases in which airflow obstruction or loss of elastic recoil are features. Hyperinflation may be particularly severe in patients with COPD, in whom the FRC often exceeds predicted total lung capacity (TLC). An overwhelming amount of evidence shows that hyperinflation reduces the diaphragmatic effectiveness as a pressure generator and reduces diaphragm contribution to chest wall motion. The contribution of the intercostal muscles and scalenes is likely to be increased, such that chest wall motion becomes exclusively or predominantly rib cage motion (Fig. 3-6). The ineffectiveness of the diaphragm may result from diaphragmatic shortening, geometrical alterations, alterations in diaphragm–rib cage interaction, alteration in mechanical arrangements among the costal and crural parts of the diaphragm, reduction in the zone of apposition.[76] Among these, diaphragmatic shortening appears to be the most important. Indeed, with inflation from FRC to TLC, the diaphragm shortens about 30% to 40%,[17,18] whereas the parasternal and upper external intercostal muscles shorten by only 10%,[19,77] the scalene by 2%,[78] and the sternomastoid muscle by 6%.[78] For the diaphragm, this shortening is expected to reduce significantly its pressure-generating capacity. Several studies indicate that diaphragmatic geometry is not affected significantly by hyperinflation, pointing out that the length–force properties of the diaphragm represents the most important factor for the pressure-generating capacity of this muscle.[79,80] The appositional component of diaphragmatic action is reduced substantially due to a reduction in the zone of apposition.[28] The insertional component is affected so that diaphragmatic contraction causes inward retraction of the lower rib cage. This may be noticed clinically in patients with severe hyperinflation.[81,82] The mechanical arrangement between the costal and crural parts of the diaphragm changes from a parallel arrangement at FRC to a series arrangement at TLC.[17] This is likely to further compromise the pressure-generating capacity of the diaphragm independently of its force–length characteristics.

Hyperinflation also impairs the pressure-generating capacity of the inspiratory intercostal muscles (the parasternals and the external intercostals). This effect is mainly related to the orientation and motion of the ribs.[23] The synergistic interaction between the diaphragm and the inspiratory intercostal muscles becomes prominent at high lung volumes.[23] The force-generating capacity of the neck muscles like the scalene and the sternomastoid muscle is maintained with hyperinflation.[78] In dogs, hyperinflation induces lengthening of the abdominal muscles, particularly the transverse abdominis and internal oblique muscle.[83] Consequently, the rise in abdominal pressure obtained by selective stimulation of the abdominal muscles at TLC is greater than that obtained at FRC.[84] This also happens in normal humans during magnetic stimulation of the abdominal muscles.[83]

It should be emphasized, however, that the above pertains to acute hyperinflation. In chronic hyperinflation, the diaphragm adapts to the chronically foreshortened state by dropping out of sarcomeres.[11] As a consequence, the filament overlap within each sarcomere is restored toward optimal overlap. This adaptation is shown in Figure 3-2. This adaptation, however, only partially restores diaphragmatic function. First, because part of the reduction in force with shortening is due to compression of the T-tubular system, blocking exit-electrolyte flow and impeding excitation–contraction coupling.[12] Whether adaptations in T-tubular function also occur with chronic foreshortening remains to be investigated. Second, sarcomere adaptation adapts only to the loss in diaphragmatic function associated with diaphragmatic shortening and not to the loss in function due to geometrical alterations, alterations in diaphragm–rib cage interaction, changes in mechanical arrangement among different parts of the diaphragm, or loss of zone of apposition. Third, although sarcomere adaptation restores the force-generating capacity of a foreshortened diaphragm, it reduces the number of sarcomeres in series. Consequently, sarcomere adaptation compromises the capacity of the diaphragm to undergo changes in length and, hence, its capacity to produce volume changes, presumably its most important function. The fiber length of the parasternal intercostal muscles[85] and of the scalenus muscle[86] are, however, not affected by chronic hyperinflation in animals.

Interventions aimed at reducing hyperinflation such as lung volume reduction surgery (LVRS) and lung transplantation improve diaphragmatic function. The effects of LVRS are primarily due to an increase in the zone of apposition, lengthening of the diaphragm, and improved neuromechanical coupling.[87] To what extent complete sarcomere adaptation is present in patients with COPD and extreme hyperinflation is not clear from the clinical studies with LVRS. After lung transplantation the radius of curvature and the zone of apposition of the diaphragm are also restored. This is primarily due to mediastinal displacement toward the graft.

Expiratory muscle recruitment is frequently observed in COPD patients with severe airflow obstruction.[88] The transversus abdominis is frequently recruited. Expiratory muscle recruitment may contribute to the intrinsic positive end-expiratory pressure ($PEEP_i$) that is frequently observed in these patients. $PEEP_i$ is primarily caused by impaired pulmonary mechanics and consequent dynamic hyperinflation. The functional significance of this expiratory muscle activation is poorly understood. Indeed, in severe airflow obstruction, expiratory flow limitation is frequently present. In the presence of expiratory flow limitation, recruitment of expiratory muscles no longer contributes to expiratory flow.

In patients with pulmonary disease in general and COPD in particular, several factors may contribute to generalized muscle weakness, in which the respiratory muscles partake. These include hypoxemia and hypercapnia, malnutrition, cardiac failure, corticosteroid treatment, infection, electrolyte disturbances, and inactivity with consequent disuse atrophy. A recent study demonstrated that COPD exacerbations contribute to the development of this muscle weakness. Of particular importance appears to be treatment with corticosteroids in repetitive bursts, which is often inadvertently administered to COPD patients. Typically this causes a myopathic pattern characterized by scattered necrotic fibers with an increased number of central and subsarcolemmal nuclei, and generalized muscle fiber atrophy as seen on muscle biopsy[89] instead of selective type IIb fiber atrophy as is seen in animal studies.

The continuous patterns of motor activity associated with respiration make the diaphragm the most active muscle in the body. The daily duty cycle (ratio of active to inactive time) of the diaphragm in most species is about 45% compared to 2% for the extensor digitorum muscle (predominantly composed of type IIb fibers) and 14% for the soleus muscle (mainly a type I muscle).[90] Given the diaphragm is highly active, it is expected to be particularly sensitive to inactivity. It is therefore not surprising that serious diaphragm dysfunction develops rapidly during controlled mechanical ventilation, a situation in which the diaphragm is totally inactive.[91–93] Perturbations in respiratory muscle interaction are also marked in patients with cervical spinal cord injuries. In these patients, the intercostal and abdominal muscle contribution to respiratory function is lost. Diaphragm inspiratory capacity is also often compromised when injury is located at the C3 to C5 levels. During quiet breathing, tetraplegic subjects with injuries at C4 to C7 use their scalene[39,94] that becomes hypertrophied.[94] Patients with high tetraplegia use several neck muscles[40] in addition to the sternocleidomastoids and trapezii to breathe.[29] Quadriplegics are also predisposed to the development of inspiratory muscle fatigue because of reduced muscle strength and endurance.[95] Inspiratory muscle training in these patients increases both strength and endurance and protects against fatigue.[95] Diaphragm contracting alone through phrenic nerve pacing in subjects with upper cervical cord transaction or during spontaneous breathing in subjects with traumatic lower cervical cord transaction exerts both an expiratory action on the upper rib cage and an inspiratory action on the lower rib cage.[29,31,39] Finally because abdominal and expiratory rib cage muscles are paralyzed in subjects with tetraplegia, their ability to raise intrathoracic pressure is markedly reduced. Despite active use of the clavicular portion of the pectoralis major to deflate the rib cage during forced expiration,[43,96,97] cough is ineffective and the clearance of airway secretion is markedly impaired. Strength training of the pectoralis major improves expiratory function,[98] an effect that is expected to increase the effectiveness of coughing that might reduce the prevalence of bronchopulmonary infections in these subjects.

CONCLUSIONS

The act of breathing requires the coordinated action of a number of muscle groups. During quiet breathing, chest wall motion results from the action of the diaphragm but also from the other inspiratory muscles such as the parasternal intercostals and the scalenes in addition to the expiratory muscles. Those respiratory muscles are all well equipped to sustain continuous rhythmic contraction. Respiratory muscle interaction is affected by posture and sleep but also in a number of physiological circumstances in which ventilatory load is altered such as during speech, laughter, swallowing, gagging, vomiting, and coughing. In addition to their respiratory role, the respiratory muscles also contract during postural tasks such as limb muscle movement, leg lift, trunk rotation, and head flexion. Finally, several pathological conditions including hyperinflation, reduced or loss of activity caused by undernutrition, medical treatment (in particular corticosteroids), mechanical ventilation, or spinal cord injury may also affect the function and the interaction of the respiratory muscles. Strategies consisting in reducing hyperinflation (e.g., LVRS, lung transplantation), or improving muscle function through muscle training may help to some extent restoring respiratory muscle function.

ACKNOWLEDGMENTS

The authors thank Mr. Jean Sente for making excellent drawings. They further thank the Fonds voor Wetenschappelijk Onderzoek-Vlaanderen grants #G.0389.03, #G.0386.05, and #G.0197.07, Research Foundation KU Leuven grants #OT/02/44 and #OT/06/52 and Astra Zeneca Pharmaceuticals for their support of the research mentioned in this chapter.

REFERENCES

1. Brooke MH, Kaiser KK. Muscle fiber types: how many and what kind. *Arch Neurol.* 1970;23:369–379.
2. Sieck GC. Organization and recruitment of diaphragm motor units. In: Roussos C, ed. *The Thorax, Part B: Applied Physiology.* 2nd ed. New York, Basel, Hong Kong: Marcel Dekker; 1995:783–820.
3. Gorza L. Identification of a novel type 2 fiber population in mammalian skeletal muscle by combined use of histochemical myosin ATPase and anti-myosin monoclonal antibodies. *J Histochem Cytochem.* 1990;38:257–265.
4. Bottinelli R, Reggiani C. Human skeletal muscle fibres: Molecular and functional diversity. *Prog Biophys Mol Biol.* 2000; 73:195–262.
5. Polla B, D'Antona G, Bottinelli R, Reggiani C. Respiratory muscle fibres: Specialisation and plasticity. *Thorax.* 2004;59:808–817.
6. Edwards RHT, Faulkner JA. Structure and function of the respiratory muscles. In: Roussos C, ed. *The Thorax, Part B: Applied Physiology.* 2nd ed. New York, Basel, Hong Kong: Marcel Dekker; 1995:185–217.
7. McKenzie DK, Bellemare F. Respiratory muscle fatigue. *Adv Exp Med Biol.* 1995;384:401–414.
8. Krnjevic K, Miledi R. Failure of neuromuscular propagation in rats. *J Physiol.* 1958;140:440–461.
9. Rochester DF. The diaphragm: Contractile properties and fatigue. *J Clin Invest.* 1985;75:1397–1402.
10. Farkas GA. Functional characteristics of the respiratory muscles. *Semin Respir Med.* 1991;12:247–257.
11. Farkas GA, Roussos C. Diaphragm in emphysematous hamsters: Sarcomere adaptability. *J Appl Physiol.* 1983;54:1635–1640.

12. Taylor SR, Rüdel R. Striated muscle fibers: Inactivation of contraction induced by shortening. *Science.* 1970;167:882–884.
13. Rüdel R, Taylor SR. Striated muscle fibers: Facilitation of contraction at short lengths by caffeine. *Science.* 1971;172:387–388.
14. Gayan-Ramirez G, Palecek F, Chen Y, Janssens S, Decramer M. Inotropic effects of aminophylline on canine diaphragm are enhanced by hyperinflation. *J Appl Physiol.* 1994;76:39–44.
15. Farkas GA, Rochester DF. Functional characteristics of canine costal and crural diaphragm. *J Appl Physiol.* 1988;65:2253–2260.
16. Road J, Newman S, Derenne JP, Grassino A. In vivo length-force relationship of canine diaphragm. *J Appl Physiol.* 1986;60: 63–70.
17. Decramer M, De Troyer A, Kelly S, Macklem PT. Mechanical arrangement of costal and crural diaphragm. *J Appl Physiol.* 1984;56:1484–1490.
18. Newman S, Road J, Bellemare F, Clozel JP, Lavigne CM, Grassino A. Respiratory muscle length measured by sonomicrometry. *J Appl Physiol.* 1984;56:753–764.
19. Decramer M, De Troyer A. Respiratory changes in parasternal intercostal length. *J Appl Physiol.* 1984;57:1254–1260.
20. Farkas GA, Rochester DF. Contractile characteristics and operating lengths of canine neck inspiratory muscles. *J Appl Physiol.* 1986;61:220–226.
21. Farkas GA, Decramer M, Rochester DF, De Troyer A. Contractile properties of intercostal muscles and their functional significance. *J Appl Physiol.* 1985;59:528–535.
22. Jiang TX, Deschepper K, Demedts M, Decramer M. Effects of acute hyperinflation on the mechanical effectiveness of the parasternal intercostals. *Am Rev Respir Dis.* 1989;139:522–528.
23. De Troyer A, Wilson TA. Effect of acute inflation on the mechanics of the inspiratory muscles. *J Appl Physiol.* 2009;107:315–323.
24. Legrand A, Ninane V, De Troyer A. Mechanical advantage of sternomastoid and scalene muscles in dogs. *J Appl Physiol.* 1997; 82:1517–1522.
25. Gandevia SC, McKenzie DK, Neering IR. Endurance properties of respiratory and limb muscles. *Respir Physiol.* 1983;53:47–61.
26. McKenzie DK, Gandevia SC. Recovery from fatigue of human diaphragm and limb muscles. *Respir Physiol.* 1991;84:49–60.
27. De Troyer A, Estenne M. Functional anatomy of the respiratory muscles. *Clin Chest Med.* 1988;9:175–193.
28. Mead J, Loring S. Analysis of volume displacement and length changes of the diaphragm during breathing. *J Appl Physiol.* 1982; 53:750–755.
29. Danon J, Druz WS, Goldberg NB, Sharp JT. Function of the isolated paced diaphragm and the cervical accessory muscles in C1 quadriplegics. *Am Rev Respir Dis.* 1979;119:909–919.
30. Mead J, Banzett RB, Lehr J, Loring SH, O'Cain CF. Effect of posture on upper and lower rib cage motion and tidal volume during diaphragm pacing. *Am Rev Respir Dis.* 1984;130:320–321.
31. Mortola JP, Sant'Ambrogio G. Motion of the rib cage and the abdomen in tetraplegic patients. *Clin Sci Mol Med.* 1978;54:25–32.
32. De Troyer A, Sampson MG. Activation of the parasternal intercostals during breathing efforts in human subjects. *J Appl Physiol.* 1982;52:524–529.
33. De Troyer A, Farkas GA. Linkage between parasternals and external intercostals during resting breathing. *J Appl Physiol.* 1990; 69:509–516.
34. Wilson TA, De Troyer A. Respiratory effect of the intercostal muscles in the dog. *J Appl Physiol.* 1993;75:2636–2645.
35. De Troyer A, Legrand A. Inhomogeneous activation of the parasternal intercostals during breathing. *J Appl Physiol.* 1995;79: 55–62.
36. De Troyer A, Kirkwood PA, Wilson TA. Respiratory action of the intercostal muscles. *Physiol Rev.* 2005;85:717–756.
37. De Troyer A, Farkas GA. Inspiratory function of the levator costae and external intercostal muscles in the dog. *J Appl Physiol.* 1989;67: 2614–2621.
38. De Troyer A, Estenne M. Coordination between rib cage muscles and diaphragm during quiet breathing in humans. *J Appl Physiol.* 1984;57:899–906.
39. Estenne M, De Troyer A. Relationship between respiratory muscle electromyogram and rib cage motion in tetraplegia. *Am Rev Respir Dis.* 1985;132:53–59.
40. De Troyer A, Estenne M, Vincken W. Rib cage motion and muscle use in high tetraplegics. *Am Rev Respir Dis.* 1986;133:1115–1119.
41. De Troyer A, Peche R, Yernault JC, Estenne M. Neck muscle activity in patients with severe chronic obstructive pulmonary disease. *Am J Respir Crit Care Med.* 1994;150:41–47.
42. Celli BR, Rassulo J, Make BJ. Dyssynchronous breathing during arm but not leg exercise in patients with chronic airflow obstruction. *New Engl J Med.* 1986;314:1485–1490.
43. De Troyer A, Estenne M, Heilporn A. Mechanism of active expiration in tetraplegic subjects. *N Engl J Med.* 1986;314:740–744.
44. De Troyer A, Ninane V, Gilmartin JJ, Lemerre C, Estenne M. Triangularis sterni use in supine humans. *J Appl Physiol.* 1987;62: 919–925.
45. De Troyer A, Sampson M, Sigrist S, Kelly S. How the abdominal muscles act on the rib cage. *J Appl Physiol.* 1983;54:465–469.
46. De Troyer A, Estenne M, Ninane V, Van Gansbeke D, Gorini M. Transversus abdominis muscle function in humans. *J Appl Physiol.* 1990 Mar;68:1010–1016.
47. Abe T, Kusuhara N, Yoshimura N, Tomita T, Easton PA. Differential respiratory activity of four abdominal muscles in humans. *J Appl Physiol.* 1996;80:1379–1389.
48. Rochester DF, Farkas GA. Performance of respiratory muscles in situ. In: Roussos C, ed. *The Thorax, Part B: Applied Physiology.* 2nd ed. New York, Basel, Hong Kong: Marcel Dekker; 1995:1127–1159.
49. Estenne M, Yernault JC, De Troyer A. Rib cage and diaphragm-abdomen compliance in humans: Effects of age and posture. *J Appl Physiol.* 1985;59:1842–1848.
50. Druz WS, Sharp JT. Activity of respiratory muscles in upright and recumbent humans. *J Appl Physiol.* 1981;51:1552–1561.
51. De Troyer A. Mechanical role of the abdominal muscles in relation to posture. *Respir Physiol.* 1983;53:341–353.
52. De Troyer A, Ninane V. Effect of posture on expiratory muscle use during breathing in the dog. *Respir Physiol.* 1987;67:311–322.
53. Estenne M, Ninane V, De Troyer A. Triangularis sterni muscle use during eupnea in humans: effect of posture. *Respir Physiol.* 1988;74:151–162.
54. Remmers JE. Effects of sleep on control of breathing. *Int Rev Physiol.* 1981;23:111–147.
55. Tabachnik E, Muller NL, Bryan AC, Levison H. Changes in ventilation and chest wall mechanics during sleep in normal adolescents. *J Appl Physiol.* 1981;51:557–564.
56. Johnson MW, Remmers JE. Accessory muscle activity during sleep in chronic obstructive pulmonary disease. *J Appl Physiol.* 1984;57: 1011–1017.
57. Estenne M, Zocchi L, Ward M, Macklem PT. Chest wall motion and expiratory muscle use during phonation in normal humans. *J Appl Physiol.* 1990;68:2075–2082.

58. Draper MH, Ladefoged P, Whitteridge D. Expiratory pressures and airflow during speech. *Br Med J.* 1960;1:1837–1843.
59. Draper MH, Ladefoged P, Whitteridge D. Respiratory muscles in speech. *J Speech Hear Res.* 1959;2:16–27.
60. Filippelli M, Pellegrino R, Iandelli I, et al. Respiratory dynamics during laughter. *J Appl Physiol.* 2001;90:1441–1446.
61. Kimata H, Morita A, Furuhata S, Itakura H, Ikenobu K, Kimura Y. Assessment of laughter by diaphragm electromyogram. *Eur J Clin Invest.* 2009;39:78–79.
62. Hårdemark Cedborg AI, Sundman E, Bodén K, et al. Co-ordination of spontaneous swallowing with respiratory airflow and diaphragmatic and abdominal muscle activity in healthy adult humans. *Exp Physiol.* 2009;94:459–468.
63. Miller AD. Respiratory muscle control during vomiting. *Can J Physiol Pharmacol.* 1990;68:237–241.
64. Sieck GC, Fournier M. Diaphragm motor unit recruitment during ventilatory and nonventilatory behaviors. *J Appl Physiol.* 1989;66:2539–2545.
65. Mantilla CB, Seven YB, Zhan WZ, Sieck GC. Diaphragm motor unit recruitment in rats. *Respir Physiol Neurobiol.* 2010;173: 101–106.
66. Lasserson D, Mills K, Arunachalam R, Polkey M, Moxham J, Kalra L. Differences in motor activation of voluntary and reflex cough in humans. *Thorax.* 2006;61:699–705.
67. van Lunteren E, Haxhiu MA, Cherniack NS, Arnold JS. Role of triangularis sterni during coughing and sneezing in dogs. *J Appl Physiol.* 1988;65:2440–2445.
68. Nava S, Ambrosino N, Crotti P, Fracchia C, Rampulla C. Recruitment of some respiratory muscles during three maximal inspiratory manoeuvres. *Thorax.* 1993;48:702–707.
69. Hodges PW, Butler JE, McKenzie DK, Gandevia SC. Contraction of the human diaphragm during rapid postural adjustments. *J Physiol.* 1997;505(Pt 2):539–548.
70. Whitelaw WA, Ford GT, Rimmer KP, De TA. Intercostal muscles are used during rotation of the thorax in humans. *J Appl Physiol.* 1992;72:1940–1944.
71. Rimmer KP, Ford GT, Whitelaw WA. Interaction between postural and respiratory control of human intercostal muscles. *J Appl Physiol.* 1995;79:1556–1561.
72. Hudson AL, Butler JE, Gandevia SC, De TA. Interplay between the inspiratory and postural functions of the human parasternal intercostal muscles. *J Neurophysiol.* 2010;103:1622–1629.
73. Hodges PW, Gandevia SC. Activation of the human diaphragm during a repetitive postural task. *J Physiol.* 2000;522(Pt 1):165–175.
74. Hodges PW, Heijnen I, Gandevia SC. Postural activity of the diaphragm is reduced in humans when respiratory demand increases. *J Physiol.* 2001;537:999–1008.
75. Janssens L, Brumagne S, Polspoel K, Troosters T, McConnell A. The effect of inspiratory muscles fatigue on postural control in people with and without recurrent low back pain. *Spine (Phila Pa 1976).* 2010;35:1088–1094.
76. Decramer M. Hyperinflation and respiratory muscle interaction. *Eur Respir J.* 1997;10:934–941.
77. De Troyer A, Legrand A, Wilson TA. Respiratory mechanical advantage of the canine external and internal intercostal muscles. *J Physiol.* 1999;518(Pt 1):283–289.
78. Farkas GA, Rochester DF. Characteristics and functional significance of canine abdominal muscles. *J Appl Physiol.* 1988;65: 2427–2433.
79. Smith J, Bellemare F. Effect of lung volume on in vivo contraction characteristics of human diaphragm. *J Appl Physiol.* 1987;62:1893–1900.
80. Gauthier AP, Verbanck S, Estenne M, Segebarth C, Macklem PT, Paiva M. Three-dimensional reconstruction of the in vivo human diaphragm shape at different lung volumes. *J Appl Physiol.* 1994;76:495–506.
81. Gilmartin JJ, Gibson GJ. Abnormalities of chest wall motion in patients with chronic airflow obstruction. *Thorax.* 1984;39:264–271.
82. Gilmartin JJ, Gibson GJ. Mechanisms of paradoxical rib cage motion in patients with chronic obstructive pulmonary disease. *Am Rev Respir Dis.* 1986;134:684–687.
83. Estenne M, Pinet C, De Troyer A. Abdominal muscle strength in patients with tetraplegia. *Am J Respir Crit Care Med.* 2000;161: 707–712.
84. D'Angelo E, Prandi E, Bellemare F. Mechanics of the abdominal muscles in rabbits and dogs. *Respir Physiol.* 1994;97:275–291.
85. Kelsen SG, Sexauer WP, Mardini IA, Criner GJ. The comparative effects of elastase-induced emphysema on costal and crural diaphragm and parasternal intercostal muscle contractility. *Am J Respir Crit Care Med.* 1994;149:168–173.
86. Fournier M, Lewis MI. Functional, cellular, and biochemical adaptations to elastase-induced emphysema in hamster medial scalene. *J Appl Physiol.* 2000;88:1327–1337.
87. Gorman RB, McKenzie DK, Butler JE, Tolman JF, Gandevia SC. Diaphragm length and neural drive after lung volume reduction surgery. *Am J Respir Crit Care Med.* 2005;172:1259–1266.
88. Ninane V, Rypens F, Yernault JC, De Troyer A. Abdominal muscle use during breathing in patients with chronic airflow obstruction. *Am Rev Respir Dis.* 1992;146:16–21.
89. Decramer M, De Bock V, Dom R. Functional and histologic picture of steroid-induced myopathy in chronic obstructive pulmonary disease. *Am J Respir Crit Care Med.* 1996;153:1958–1964.
90. Hensbergen E, Kernell D. Daily durations of spontaneous activity in cat's ankle muscles. *Exp Brain Res.* 1997;115:325–332.
91. Gayan-Ramirez G, de Paepe K, Cadot P, Decramer M. Detrimental effects of short-term mechanical ventilation on diaphragm function and IGF-I mRNA in rats. *Intensive Care Med.* 2003;29:825–833.
92. Hermans G, Agten A, Testelmans D, Decramer M, Gayan-Ramirez G. Increased duration of mechanical ventilation is associated with decreased diaphragmatic force: a prospective observational study. *Crit Care.* 2010;14:R127.
93. Jaber S, Petrof BJ, Jung B, et al. Rapidly progressive diaphragmatic weakness and injury during mechanical ventilation in humans. *Am J Respir Crit Care Med.* 2011;183:364–371.
94. Short DJ, Silver JR, Lehr RP. Electromyographic study of sternocleidomastoid and scalene muscles in tetraplegic subjects during respiration. *Int Disabil Stud.* 1991;13:46–49.
95. Gross D, Ladd HW, Riley EJ, Macklem PT, Grassino A. The effect of training on strength and endurance of the diaphragm in quadriplegia. *Am J Med.* 1980;68:27–35.
96. Estenne M, De Troyer A. Cough in tetraplegic subjects: An active process. *Ann Intern Med.* 1990;112:22–28.
97. Estenne M, Gorini M. Action of the diaphragm during cough in tetraplegic subjects. *J Appl Physiol.* 1992;72:1074–1080.
98. Estenne M, Knoop C, Vanvaerenbergh J, Heilporn A, De Troyer A. The effect of pectoralis muscle training in tetraplegic subjects. *Am Rev Respir Dis.* 1989;139:1218–1222.

CHAPTER 4

Molecular Regulation of Lung Development

Wellington V. Cardoso
Jining Lu

INTRODUCTION

This chapter focuses on the mechanisms that control the development of the respiratory tract from the specification of lung endoderm and tracheal progenitors to the formation of the bronchial tree and the alveolar region. Based essentially on histological criteria lung development can be described in four stages: *(a) Pseudoglandular*: Corresponding to the period of formation of the bronchial tree through branching morphogenesis, the lung exhibits a gland-like morphology with epithelial tubules separated by a thick mesenchymal layer; *(b) Canalicular*: Branching is nearly finished and distinct columnar and cuboidal epithelial cells are seen in proximal (large) and distal (small) airways, respectively. Epithelial tubules are separated by a thinner mesenchyme containing blood vessels; *(c) Saccular*: Primitive saccules are seen at the distal end of bronchial tree with widening of the lumens and the appearance of type I (flat-shaped) and type II (cuboidal, surfactant-producing) cells. The intimate approximation of the type I cell to the vascular structures (primitive alveolar–capillary barrier) allows gas exchange during the immediate postnatal period; *(d) Alveolar:* Primitive saccules undergo septation to form numerous smaller mature alveolar structures to increase gas exchange surface.[1,2]

The development of the respiratory system encompasses prenatal and postnatal life, although timing and duration of specific events vary among species. Lung development starts much earlier in humans than in mice and rats; alveolar formation initiates in the human lung by late gestation in contrast to the murine lung, in which alveolization is a postnatal process (see comparison in Fig. 4-1).

HOW RESPIRATORY PROGENITORS ARISE

The lung originates from the anterior portion of the gut tube (foregut), which also gives rise to organs, such as the thyroid, stomach, liver, and pancreas. Respiratory progenitors of the lung and trachea arise from the ventral foregut endoderm in mice at around embryonic day 9 (E9.0, midgestation) and in humans around the 3rd week of gestation. Studies in mice show that these cells can be readily recognized even before a lung primordial bud forms by the expression of Nkx2-1 (Ttf1, thyroid transcription factor 1); this gene, however, is not lung specific and also labels progenitor cells of the thyroid seen in more anterior (cranial) regions of the foregut (Fig. 4-2A).[3] Nkx2–1 is essential for lung cell fate as disruption of this gene in mice results in severe inhibition of branching and no evidence of epithelial cells expressing surfactant protein or other differentiation marker genes typically found in the lung.[3] Questions remain whether in these mutants lung progenitors are never specified or just cannot be maintained in the absence of Nkx2–1. How are these progenitors specified? There is strong evidence that Fgf and Wnt signaling play a key role in this process. Studies in organ culture suggest that Fgf2 at high concentrations is able to induce lung cell fate in the early foregut endoderm.[4] High levels of Fgf1 and 2 are found in the cardiac mesoderm immediately adjacent to the ventral foregut endoderm (Fig. 4-2A). These observations suggest a model in which high levels of Fgfs diffusing from the developing heart induces Nkx2–1-expressing lung progenitor cells.[4] Interestingly, canonical Wnt pathway is also required for lung specification. Both Wnt2 and Wnt2b are present in the foregut mesoderm at the prospective site of lung formation. Loss of canonical Wnt or their ligands prevents the appearance of Nkx2–1-expressing cells.[5,6] Moreover, there is a role for Bmp signaling in the maintenance or expansion of Nkx2–1-expressing lung progenitors.[7]

FORMATION OF THE LUNG AND TRACHEAL PRIMORDIA

Once the Nkx2–1-expressing progenitor cells are specified in the prospective lung region of the foregut, they are subsequently expanded to generate the tracheal and the lung primordia. The primordial lung is identified in human embryos at the beginning of gestation (around the 4th week), much earlier compared to mice (midgestation at E9.5). The two primordial lung buds arise as lateral outgrowths of the ventral foregut endoderm and fuse at the midline, the site where tracheal primordium also starts to form (Fig. 4-2B–D). From then on, the trachea and the digestive tube separate through a mechanism still poorly understood that involves formation of a tracheoesophageal septum.[8,9] Primary lung bud formation is crucially dependent on the local expression of Fgf10 (fibroblast growth factor 10) in the foregut mesoderm.[10,11] Fgf10 diffuses to the nearby endoderm at the prospective lung region and activates Fgfr2b signaling in Nkx2–1-expressing progenitor cells leading to epithelial proliferation and migration toward the Fgf10 source.[12,13] Fgf10-null mice die at birth and have multiple defects. Strikingly, lungs do not form but tracheal development occurs.[10,11] This raises the possibility that tracheal and lung progenitors, although originating from a population of Nkx2–1-expressing endodermal cells, are different at least in their requirement for Fgf10 signaling for expansion or survival.

How is the expression of Fgf10 controlled? How is positioning of the lung primordium along the anteroposterior (AP) axis of the foregut determined? There is accumulated evidence that signaling

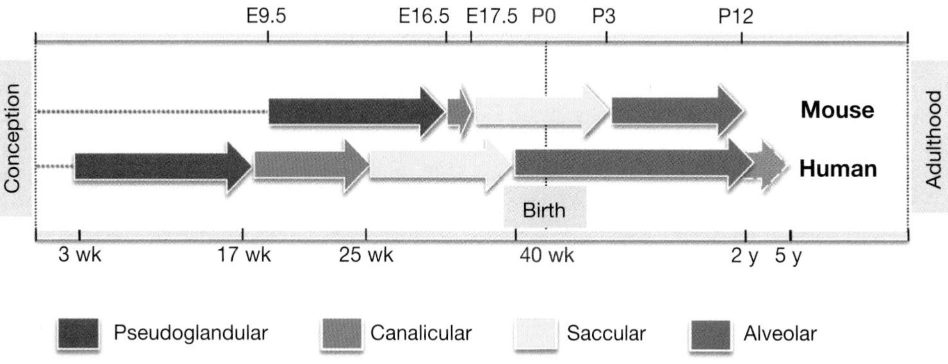

Figure 4-1 Timeline for the developmental stages of mouse and human lungs. Mouse (E, embryonic; P, postnatal days); humans (wk, gestation week; y, year).

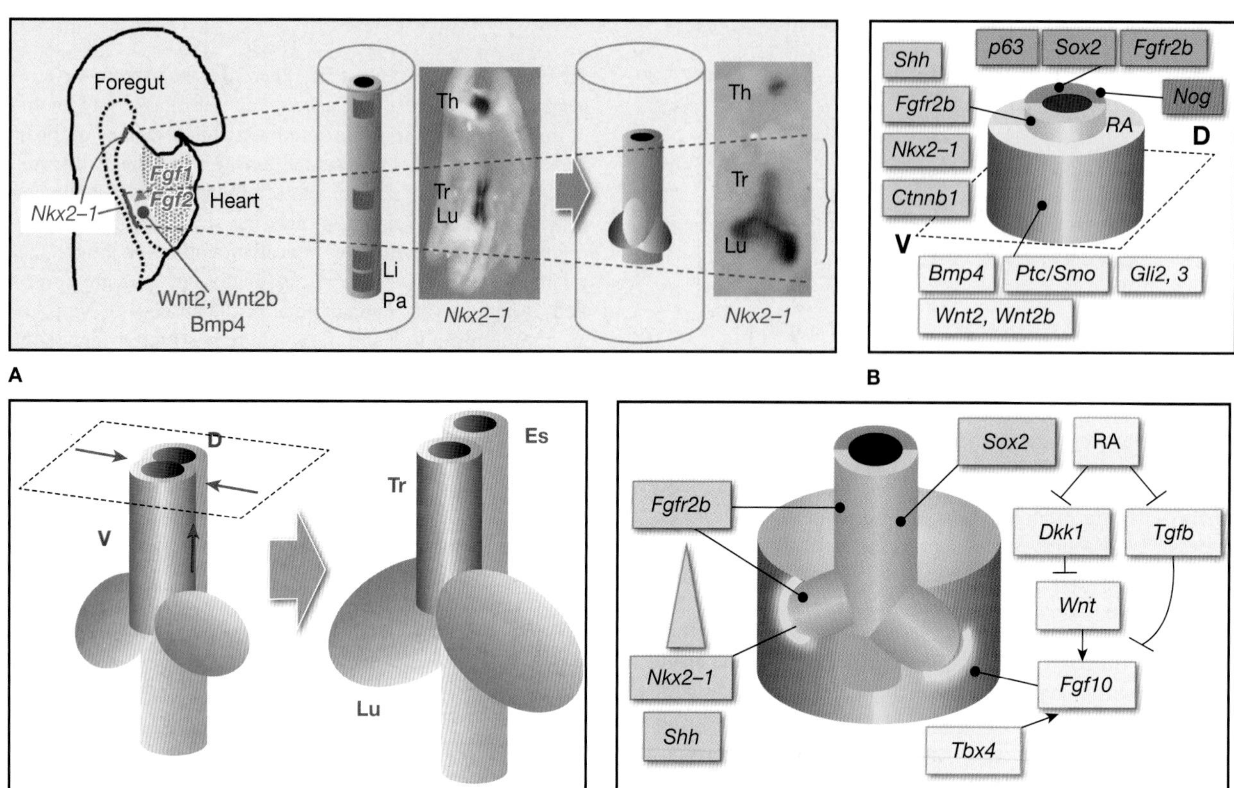

Figure 4-2 Regulation of early lung and tracheal development. **A.** Specification of respiratory progenitors in the foregut by Fgfs *(purple)* from the heart (*red*, Nkx2-1-expressing endoderm) and Wnt2, 2b from foregut mesoderm; expansion of these progenitors initially by Bmp4 signaling. Nkx2–1 ISH labeling respiratory progenitors (Tr, Lu) in the mid foregut endoderm and in the thyroid (Th) primordium of mouse embryos at E9.0 (no signal in the Li, liver and Pa, pancreatic fields). At E9.5, these Nkx2-1-positive cells give rise to the tracheal primordium and primary lung buds. **B.** Ventral–dorsal (V–D) differences in gene expression in the foregut at the onset of lung development. **C.** V–D foregut patterning and tracheoesophageal separation (Es, esophagus). **D.** Regulation of primary lung bud formation in the foregut: Gene network in the mesenchyme *(yellow)* and epithelium (*blue*; highest levels of Nkx2–1 and Shh in the distal bud).

by the vitamin A–derivative retinoic acid (RA) is a major regulator of Fgf10 expression at the onset of lung development.[14] RA synthesis and RA receptor (RAR) activity is prominent in the E8.5–9.5 mouse foregut.[15] Disruption of RA signaling by vitamin A deficiency, or genetic disruption of key components of the RA pathway, or RA antagonists in organ cultures leads to multiple developmental abnormalities, including lung agenesis.[14,16–18] RA integrates multiple pathways in the foregut to regulate primary lung bud morphogenesis. RA signaling in the foregut mesoderm allows activation of the Wnt pathway by suppressing expression of the Wnt inhibitor Dkk1 (Dickkopf-1)[19]; RA also inhibits Tgfβ signaling.[20] The balanced activity of Wnt and Tgfβ leads to proper mesodermal Fgf10 expression required for formation of the lung primordium (Fig. 4-2D). Thus, the disruption of Wnt/Tgfβ/Fgf10 interactions is likely to represent the molecular basis for the failure to form the lung classically reported in vitamin A deficiency. The role of Wnt in the expression of Fgf10 is further supported by the lack of Fgf10 expression in the lung field mesenchyme of foregut in Wnt2a/Wnt2b double null mice.[5]

Other essential regulators of early events associated with the lung primordium are T-box (Tbx) and Gli transcription factors (Fig. 4-2B–D). Multiple T-box genes are expressed in the foregut and particularly Tbx2–Tbx5 have been reported in the developing lung mesenchyme.[21] Studies in chick embryo show that Tbx4 is expressed in the foregut mesoderm at the domain where Fgf10 induces lung bud formation; Tbx4-Fgf10 appear to regulate the posterior boundary of Nkx2–1-expressing lung progenitors.[22] Genetic studies in mice showed a dose-dependent activity of Tbx4 and Tbx5 in regulating primary bud formation, likely through regulation of Fgf10 and Wnt.[23] Gli 1, 2, 3 are known transcriptional effectors of the sonic hedgehog (Shh) signaling detected early in the foregut mesoderm and subsequently in the lung mesenchyme.[24] Disruption of both Gli2 and Gli3 in mice results in dramatic abnormalities that include abrogation of both tracheal and lung primordium.[25] This intriguing phenotype is more severe than that observed in Shh-null mice and thus may represent a disruption of additional Gli-dependent pathways critical for the primary lung buds.[26]

VENTRAL–DORSAL (V–D) PATTERNING AND TRACHEOESOPHAGEAL SEPARATION

Differences in V–D cell fate are already obvious in the prospective lung region of the foregut (Fig. 4-2B) as the ventral endoderm expresses Nkx2–1 (respiratory progenitors) while the dorsal region (prospective esophagus) expresses Sox2 (SRY-box containing gene 2) and the p63.[3,27,28] Epithelial disruption of Sox2 leads to ectopic dorsal expansion of the Nkx2–1 domain and respiratory fate in the esophagus.[27] The Bmp (Bone Morphogenetic Protein) pathway is also important for V–D patterning. Bmp4 is expressed in the ventral foregut mesenchyme prior to and during the emergence of primary buds while its antagonist Noggin is localized to the dorsal endoderm.[7] Conditional deletion of both Bmpr1a and Bmpr1b receptors leads to expansion of a dorsal cell population marked by Sox2 at the cost of the ventral population of Nkx2-1 positive cells. Interestingly this results in tracheal agenesis and formation of lung buds ectopically.[7] Noggin has been proposed to protect the dorsal endoderm from the ventralizing effects of Bmp4.[29]

As the lung and tracheal primordia form, a tracheoesophageal septum extends from the posterior to the anterior region of the foregut and ultimately separates the respiratory from the digestive tracts (Fig. 4-2C). Alternative mechanisms initiating this process have been proposed, including the fusion of endodermal ridges in the midline.[8] Failure to separate these compartments results in tracheoesophageal fistula, a condition of high morbidity relatively frequent in neonatal settings. This defect has been observed as part of the phenotype of several mouse mutants, including the $Shh^{-/-}$, $Nkx2\text{-}1^{-/-}$, Sox2 conditional mutant, $Gli2^{-/-}$; $Gli3^{+/-}$, and the $RAR\alpha^{-/-}$; $RAR\beta^{-/-}$ null-mice.[3,25–27,30]

BRANCHING MORPHOGENESIS: FORMATION OF THE BRONCHIAL TREE AND PATTERNING

The bronchial tree forms through a reiterative process of growth and budding of the epithelial tubules collectively termed as branching morphogenesis. This process initiates right after secondary buds form from the lung primordium, in mice at E10.5. Interestingly, at this time the pattern of lobation of the right and left lungs is also established. The lungs are asymmetric in respect to their right and left axis and their number of lobes varies according to the species. For example, mouse lungs have one left lobe and four right lobes. It is thought that this asymmetry is regulated by left–right (L–R) determinants as part of an early global program of axis specification. Among the signals involved in this process are several Tgfβ-related molecules, such as activin receptor II, Lefty1 and 2, growth differentiation factor 1 (Gdf1), and paired-like homeodomain transcription factor 2 (Pitx2).[31–35] Loss of left–right asymmetry resulting in equal number of lobes in both sides is called pulmonary isomerism and is found in several human conditions.[36,37]

Analysis of the three-dimensional branching pattern of embryonic mouse lungs suggests that the bronchial tree is generated by three geometric branching modes: Domain branching, planar bifurcation, and orthogonal bifurcation, following three sequential orders (Fig. 4-3).[38] All modes are used concurrently during development of the bronchial tree. More than one mode is often used in the individual founder branches to generate the next generation of buds. Domain branching is first used to form founder or parent (secondary) branches. This is followed by permanently switching to an orthogonal bifurcation mode or by a combination of the three modes in a defined sequential order. Results from these analyses

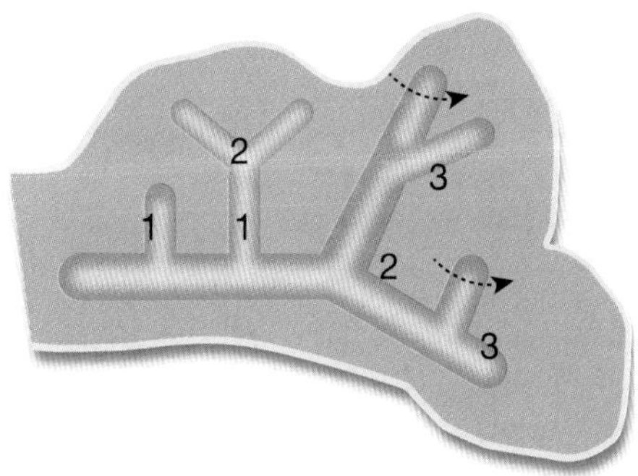

Figure 4-3 Diagram representing the three branching modes: Domain branching (1), planar bifurcation (2), and orthogonal bifurcation (3) (for details see Ref. 38).

strongly suggested that distinct genetically encoded pathways control each branching model. It is likely that these subroutines are also used in the developing human lungs, but this has not been yet demonstrated.

The mechanism generating new buds during branching morphogenesis is similar to that of primary bud morphogenesis and relies on local epithelial activation of Fgfr2b signaling by mesenchymal Fgf10 at the sites of budding.[12,13] Perturbations in levels or distribution of Fgf10 have a major impact in airway morphogenesis and result in smaller than normal hypoplastic lungs. Reduced number of branches among other abnormalities of patterning is found in Fgf10 hypomorphic mice ($Fgf10^{lacZ/-}$).[39] Interestingly, during branching morphogenesis Fgf9 expressed from the pleura and transiently from the distal epithelium serves to expand a population of distal mesenchymal progenitors that expresses Fgf10 (Fig. 4-4A). Mice deficient in Fgf9, have reduced mesenchymal cell population and Fgf10 expression; this leads to disruption of branching morphogenesis and hypoplastic lungs.[40]

How is bud formation controlled during branching morphogenesis? The size and shape of the growing buds is controlled dynamically by exchange of signals between the tip bud epithelium and the immediately adjacent mesenchyme. Shh is a member of the hedgehog family of proteins (sonic, desert, and Indian hedgehog) expressed in the lung predominantly at the tip bud epithelium. Shh signaling is activated in a paracrine fashion in the lung mesenchyme via patched (Ptc)/smoothened (Smo) and its transcriptional effectors Gli (1, 2, 3) proteins where it acts as a critical survival factor for mesenchymal cells.[41–43]

There is accumulated evidence both in vitro and in vivo that Shh has a key role in the developing airways as negative regulator of Fgf10 expression.[41,44] The idea is that during branching, Shh at the tip of growing buds progressively downregulates Fgf10 in distal mesenchymal cells, inhibiting bud outgrowth (Fig. 4-4A). In Shh-null mice there is widespread expression of Fgf10 transcripts and generalized activation of Fgfr2b in lung endoderm that results in severely disrupted branching morphogenesis and cyst-like lungs.[26] A mechanism proposed to maintain the proper balance of Fgf10 levels and prevent excessive Shh signaling is through the Hedgehog interacting protein, Hhip1. Hhip1 is induced by Shh in the mesenchyme adjacent to the distal bud, where it binds to and sequesters Shh ligand preventing it from activating signaling and repressing Fgf10 locally. Indeed Shh activity is aberrantly increased in Hhip-null mice leading to a repression of Fgf10 expression and branching in the developing lung.[45]

The balance of Fgf10 activity in the emerging bud can be regulated by the Sprouty **(Spry)**, a highly conserved family of cysteine-rich proteins (Fig. 4-4A). Spry2 and Spry4 are expressed in the distal lung in the epithelium and mesenchyme, respectively.[46,47] Spry2 negatively regulates the Fgf-mediated activation of receptor tyrosine kinase signaling in the epithelial bud and thus, inhibits bud growth, as demonstrated by functional studies in Drosophila and mice.[48–51] Moreover, Fgf10 protein distribution and receptor binding can be modulated by interactions with heparan sulfate (HS) proteoglycans at sites of budding. Disrupting endogenous gradients of HS or altering HS sulfation in lung culture systems prevents Fgf10 from inducing local responses and can markedly alter lung pattern formation.[52,53]

Another mechanism contributing to airway branching is cleft formation. Here extracellular matrix (ECM) is deposited at branch points, accumulating in the epithelial–mesenchymal interface and preventing local expansion of the epithelium. Clefting has been classically associated with local activity of Tgfβ signaling in the mesenchyme, which suppresses Fgf10 expression and induces synthesis of ECM components (Fig. 4-4B,C). Members of the Tgfβ subfamily Tgfβ1, 2, and 3, their receptors (Tgfβr1 and Tgfβr2)

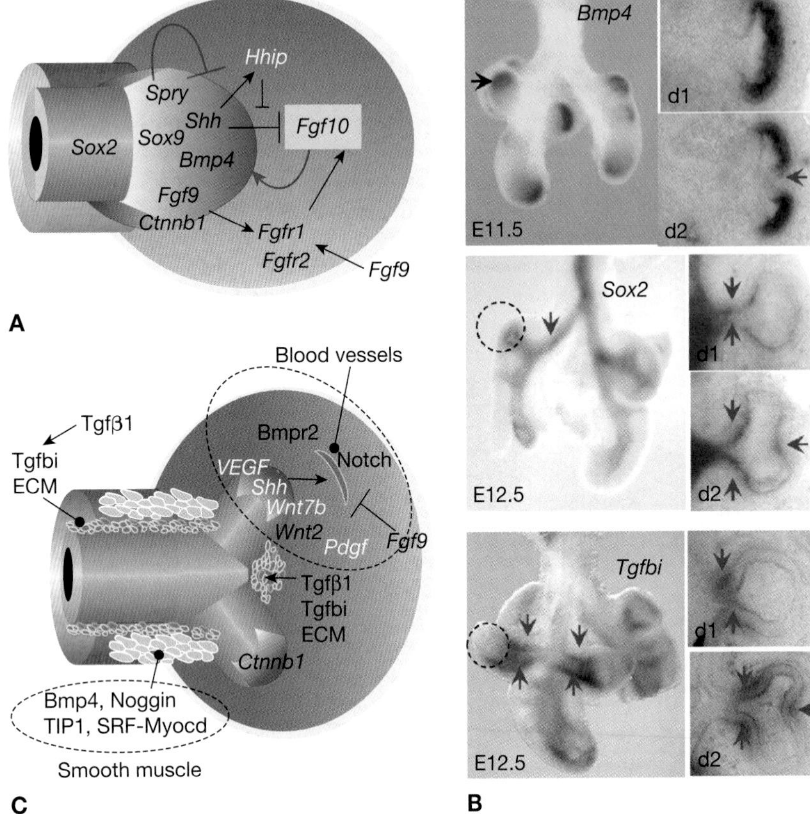

Figure 4-4 Regulation of lung branching morphogenesis, proximal–distal (P–D) patterning and differentiation. **A.** Gene network regulating lung bud elongation. Bud outgrowth is restricted by Fgf10 induction of Bmp4 and Spry2; Spry2 inhibits epithelial Fgf signaling; Bmp4 inhibits epithelial proliferation; Shh inhibits Fgf10 expression through activation of Ptc/Smo signaling. Shh signaling is inhibited by Hhip through a feedback loop. Fgf9 expressed by both mesothelial or distal epithelial cells activate Fgfr1/2 signaling in mesenchyme promoting Fgf10 expression. **B.** ISH of Bmp4, Sox2, and Tgfbi during branching (E11.5–12 in vivo and in E11.5 lungs cultured for 1 and 2 days). Bmp4 labels distal epithelial buds while Sox2 marks the epithelium in stalk and nonbranching proximal regions; Tgfbi labels newly-formed stalks and proximal mesenchyme. **C.** Airway branching and differentiation of mesenchymal components. Localized Tgfβ activity promotes local ECM deposition and cleft formation. Airway and vascular SM requires the input of Shh, Wnt, VEGF, Pdgf notch, and Fgf.

and transducing proteins, Smad 2 and 3 are expressed in different compartments and in a complex pattern during branching morphogenesis. Tgfβ1 transcripts are distributed throughout the lung mesenchyme; however Tgfβ1 protein accumulates in regions between buds and along proximal airways, where ECM components collagen I, III, and fibronectin are abundant.[54] The dynamic activity of Tgfβ during branching is best visualized by expression of its target Tgfbi (Tgfβ-induced or BigH3) in the stalk region of growing buds (Fig. 4-4B,C).[55] Treatment of embryonic lungs in culture with recombinant Tgfβ1 dramatically inhibits branching morphogenesis.[44,56,57] This is likely due to the negative effects on growth and differentiation by epithelial activation Tgfβ signaling, but also from the Tgfβ effects in the mesenchyme. Studies in NIH3T3 fibroblasts, lung and prostate organ cultures demonstrate that Tgfβ1 signaling in mesenchymal cells markedly inhibits Fgf10 expression.[44,58,59] Interestingly Tgfβ1-null mice do not show these defects, presumably due to rescue by maternal transfer of Tgfβ1.[60] Tgfβ2 and Tgfβ3 are expressed in lung epithelium; Tgfβ3 is also found in the developing lung mesenchyme and pleura.[61] Both the Tgfβ2- and Tgfβ3-deficient mice do not have major morphological defects in the lungs at E18.5 but show collapsed lungs postnatally.[62,63]

There is increasing evidence that small noncoding regulatory RNAs are part of the regulatory networks controlling lung development. MicroRNAs (miRNA) are endogenous small noncoding RNAs that regulate target gene expression posttranscriptionally and play important roles in diverse biological processes.[64–67] Individual miRNAs may target multiple message RNAs (mRNAs); conversely, individual mRNAs may contain sequences complementary to multiple miRNA family members.[68] The importance of the miRNA pathway in lung development was demonstrated by the epithelial deletion of Dicer, the key enzyme that processes microRNA precursors into mature miRNAs. Loss of Dicer in the mouse lung epithelium results in drastic arrest of branching morphogenesis and increased epithelial cell death.[69] The increased levels of Fgf10, Bmp4, and Spry-2 in these mutant lungs suggested that the miRNA pathway represses expression of these genes during epithelial–mesenchymal interactions.[69] Interestingly, in humans, DICER mutation has been linked to pleuropulmonary blastoma, a rare pediatric tumor that arises during fetal lung development.[70] It is speculated that loss of DICER in developing lung epithelium alters miRNA-dependent regulation of diffusible growth factors that promote proliferation of both epithelial and mesenchymal cells.

ESTABLISHMENT OF PROXIMAL–DISTAL (P–D) CELL FATE

During lung development, the appearance of distinct fates in epithelial progenitors along the P–D axis is tightly coupled with the branching process. Morphological changes that occur in the epithelial tubules during branching are accompanied by highly dynamic changes in P–D differentiation. For example, the high levels of Bmp4 and Sox9 typically found in the newly formed distal buds are markedly downregulated in the stalks and more proximal regions of the epithelial tubules, which then express Sox2 (Fig. 4-4A,C). Canonical Wnt and Bmp signaling have been implicated as major regulators of P–D cell fate in the lung epithelium.

Wnt ligands, receptors (frizzled), and β-catenin are widely expressed in the developing lung but show distinctive pattern in both epithelium and mesenchyme.[71–73] High activity of Wnt signaling reporter (TOPGAL), nuclear-localized β-catenin, TCF/LEF transcripts, are found in the distal lung buds undergoing branching.[74,75] Targeted disruption of β-catenin, or overexpression of Wnt inhibitor D (Dkk1) in the distal lung epithelium prevents distal bud formation and proximalizes the lung, a phenotype characterized by proximal epithelial phenotypes extending to distal sites. Conversely, activation of canonical Wnt signaling throughout the lung epithelium inhibits Sox2 expression and leads to the appearance of distal fates in proximal airways.[76,77] Thus canonical Wnt plays a key role in the establishment and or maintenance of distal cell fates.

Bmp4 is expressed in lung epithelial progenitors at the tip of growing buds and has been implicated in distal cell fate, potentially through an autocrine activation of Bmpr-Smad signaling.[78] In the lung Bmp4-mediated responses are regulated at multiple levels, for example by Fgf10-Fgfr2b activation in distal buds, which induces Bmp4 expression, or by known Bmp antagonists present in the lung, such as Noggin, Chordin, Gremlin, and the Cerberus-related factor, Cer1.[42,79–82] Bmp4 protein levels in distal epithelium are potentially under the control of the cysteine protease Cathepsin H, which is significantly induced by Fgfr2b signaling.[83] Transgenic mice expressing Bmpr antagonists in lung epithelial progenitors fail to properly form a distal lung and show proximalization.[84] Using a similar genetic approach Bmp4 overexpression results in small lungs containing distal flat cells that are reminiscent of the distal alveolar type I cells.[78] In lung organ cultures Bmp4 antagonizes the proliferative effects of Fgf10 in the distal epithelium; this could presumably foster distal differentiation.[85] Histone deacetylases 1 and 2 (Hdac1/2), enzymes involved in epigenetic modifications, have been recently shown to regulate P–D patterning through controlling expression of Bmp4 and the tumor suppressor Rb1.[86]

miRNAs also play a significant role in lung P–D patterning. For example, the miR-17-92 cluster is expressed during early lung development; gain of function selectively in the developing lung epithelium of transgenic mice results in increased cell proliferation.[87] Conversely, miR-17-92 cluster knockout mice have hypoplastic lungs.[88] In an independent study, miR-17 family members were shown to modulate Fgf10-Fgfr2b downstream signaling by targeting Stat3 and Mapk14.[89] miR-302/367, a direct target of Gata6 transcription factor, coordinates the balance between proliferation and differentiation of lung epithelium and also regulates apical–basal polarity.[90]

FORMATION OF THE VASCULAR AND OTHER MESENCHYMAL COMPONENTS OF THE LUNG

Besides playing a crucial role in epithelial development, the lung mesenchyme gives rise to the vascular, cartilage, and other stromal components of the lung. In turn, expansion and differentiation of mesenchymal progenitors into these different components require diffusible signals from the epithelial and mesothelial (pleural) layers.

The vasculature develops through sprouting angiogenesis from arterial vessels of the aortic arches migrating to the developing lung and formation of a capillary plexus around the distal bud.[91–93] Pulmonary veins arise from the neighbor atrium. Vascular endothelial growth factor (VEGF) signaling plays a major role in vascular development by promoting endothelial cell differentiation (Fig. 4-4B).[94] VEGF-A is found predominantly in the distal lung epithelium but also in the mesenchyme at early stages and signals through VEGFR2 (Flk1) and VEGFR1 (Flt1) in the mesenchyme.[95–97] Among the several VEGF isoforms, VEGF164 is the most active in the lung.[98] Development of lymphatic vessels is still poorly understood. Studies in mice show that VEGF-C and -D acting through their receptor VEGFR-3 promote lymphoangiogenesis.[99,100] VEGFR-3–null mice fail to develop proper lymphatic vessels.[101]

Smooth muscle (SM) is an integral component of vascular and airway epithelium of the lung (Fig. 4-4B). Vascular SM develops by contribution from mesenchymal precursors through signals derived from the epithelium but also from pleural cells migrating to the vascular structures during blood vessel assembly.[102] Significantly reduced mesenchymal cell proliferation and SM differentiation were observed in Shh-null lungs.[43] Interestingly, a signaling cascade involving Shh, miR-206, and Bdnf (brain-derived nerve growth factor) coordinates innervation and formation of the airway SM layer.[103] Wnt7b, acting through Fzd1, Fzd10, and LRP5, is an important epithelial signal required for vascular SM development and the integrity of blood vessels.[104] Wnt7b-null mice show hemorrhagic lungs resulting from rupture of the blood vessels due to SM structural defects.[105] Assembly of the pulmonary arterial wall occurs through controlled migration of SM cells from the inner to the outer layers in a process mediated mostly by PDGFβ.[106] In addition, vascular SM formation depends on Bmp and Notch signaling.[107,108] Bmp4 and Bmpr2 are expressed in SM precursors and disruption of Bmp signaling is associated with increased SM cell proliferation. This phenotype is reminiscent of the excessive SM growth reported in pulmonary hypertension patients with mutations in the Bmpr2 gene.[109–111] Disruption of canonical Notch signaling interferes with specification of arterial SM cells.[107] Notch3 dysregulation is associated with structural changes in the pulmonary artery postnatally and has been implicated in the pathogenesis of adult pulmonary hypertension.[112] The importance of having a precisely matched airway–vascular development is well illustrated by the role of Foxm1, a transcription factor present in the lung mesenchyme. Foxm1-null mice show pulmonary hemorrhage and perinatal death due to misalignment of epithelial and vascular structures.[113] This phenotype closely reminds the abnormalities seen in human congenital alveolar dysplasia.

Airway SM originates from mesenchymal cells of the developing lung when the initial airway start to branch, preceding the appearance of the lung vascular SM. Evidence from a Fgf10-lacZ reporter mouse, which labels Fgf10-derived lineage cells,[114] suggests that a myogenic program of cell fate in developing airways initiates in the distal lung mesenchyme and progresses as these cells are relocated to the bud stalks and more proximal regions.[114,115] This myogenic program is likely to be triggered by high levels of Bmp4 and Shh present at the bud tips (Fig. 4-4C).[41,78] Canonical Wnt signaling is required for the expansion of the SM progenitors in developing airways.[116] Proper differentiation of the airway SM requires input from pathways, including Fgf, TGFβ, as well as physical stretch transduced by tension-induced proteins, such as Tip1.[117–120] Fgf9-Fgfr1/2 signaling suppresses airway SM differentiation through inhibition of myocardin expression.[42,121,122]

During development, SM is responsible for phasic contractility of airways and growth factor production, contributing to maintain normal lung growth. Airway peristalsis influences branching and epithelial differentiation.[123,124] Interfering with process can result in lung hypoplasia.

Cartilage rings present in trachea and proximal airways develop from the precursors in ventral mesenchyme. Proper formation and patterning of cartilage primordia requires signaling by RA (particularly RAR gamma mediated), Foxf1, Shh, Nkx2-1, among others.[125,126]

AIRWAY DIFFERENTIATION

As the epithelial tubules form and branch, they initiate a program of cell fate choice and differentiation that ultimately gives rise to the various airway epithelial cell types. The initial stage is marked by expression of Sox2 throughout the P–D axis of these tubules from trachea to the most distal airways (Fig. 4-4B).[127]

By the middle of the pseudoglandular period, epithelial cells in proximal airways start to express markers of cell commitment to secretory Clara (the secretoglobin Scgb3a2) ciliated (Foxj1) and neuroendocrine (the bltb transcription factor Ascl1) lineages (Fig. 4-5).[128–133] These committed epithelial progenitors then initiate specific programs of differentiation. Foxj1-expressing cells undergo a dramatic organization of their apical compartment and by the end of the canalicular period form multiciliated cells marked by β-tubulin staining.[134] Concomitantly Scgb3a2-expressing cells acquire expression of the Clara cell marker CC10 (Scgb1a1).[135,136] While in humans mucin-secreting goblet cells are seen throughout the respiratory tract epithelium, in mice, they are relatively rare occurring mostly postnatally in trachea and proximal airways. Their presence is largely increased in exposure to environmental agent or infection.[137]

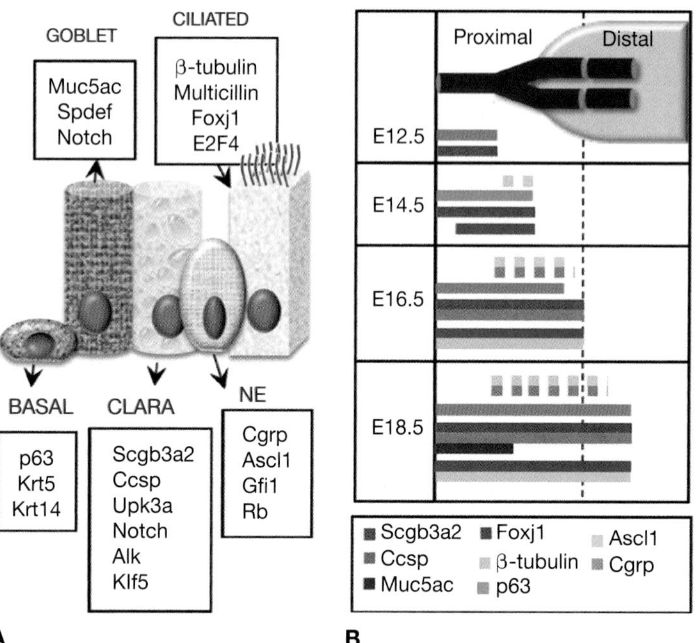

Figure 4-5 Epithelial differentiation in conducting airways. **A.** Cell types and markers associated with or required for the differentiation of specific cells. **B.** Time course of appearance of gene markers associated with different cell lineages in proximal and distal airways of the developing mouse lung.

Ascl1-expressing cells are found in clusters initially in proximal regions and generate neuroendocrine bodies (NEB) and isolated neuroendocrine (NE) cells; they express neural markers such as Cgrp and Pgp9.5. Mice deficient in Ascl1 do not form NE cells or NEB.[130]

Both Clara and basal cells are considered to be progenitor cells of the lung for their ability to self-renew and generate Clara and ciliated cells. Basal cells are recognized by the expression of the transcription factor p63, and also keratins 5 and 14. p63 mutant mice do not form basal cells in the lung or in other regions, such as skin.[138,139] Although p63/Keratin 5-labeled cells can be identified in the embryonic lung, there is no evidence that prenatally they function as lung progenitor cells.

Notch signaling is critical to generate Clara cells and to maintain the balance of the different cell types in the airways.[132] Disruption of Notch signaling in mice results in loss of Clara cells and airways overpopulated by ciliated and NE cells.[107,132,140–141] Conversely, constitutive activation of Notch in the embryonic lung epithelium leads to a decrease in number of ciliated cells and increase in secretory goblet cells.[142] During postnatal life Notch is required to maintain the Clara cell phenotype and prevent them from undergoing goblet cell (mucus) metaplasia.[143] Downregulation of Notch pathway components has been identified in patients with chronic pulmonary obstructive disease (COPD), a condition in which one of the hallmark features is mucus metaplasia.[144] Goblet cell differentiation is also controlled by transcription factors, such as SAM pointed domain-containing ETS transcription factor (Spdef) and Foxa2.[145–147]

Formation of multiciliated cells in the airways depends on expression of the E2F family member E2F4, as well as Foxj1 and multicilin.[148,149] Loss or gain of function of Foxj1 in genetically altered mice leads to absence or ectopic formation of multiciliated cells, respectively.[150,151] miR-449 has been shown to promote the differentiation of ciliated cells by targeting NOTCH1 and the ligand DLL1 in human airway epithelial cells.[152]

FORMATION OF THE GAS EXCHANGE REGION OF THE LUNG

Once branching morphogenesis is completed, distal epithelial buds undergo sacculation. During this morphogenetic process, the lumen of epithelial tubules enlarges at their distal ends to form primitive saccules. Some of the epithelial cells become flattened and very thin, differentiating into type I cells, while the others remain cuboidal and differentiate into surfactant-producing type II cells (Fig. 4-6). Type I cells cover a large area of these saccules and, as the mesenchyme becomes thinner, they come into intimate contact with the capillary network of the primitive saccules to form the primitive alveolar–capillary barrier.[153] Multiple gene knockout mice show defects in sacculation. Among these are T1 alpha,[154] Nfib (nuclear factor I/B),[155] Erk3 (extracellular signal-regulated kinase 3), and Foxm1.[156]

Finally, by late gestation in humans or postnatally in mice the primitive saccules subdivide into smaller units to form the mature alveoli. Alveolization involves formation of secondary septa, which greatly increases the surface area for gas exchange (Fig. 4-6). Alveolar formation is dependent on interstitial myofibroblasts and appear to require tight control of elastin levels. Signaling by Pdgf is necessary to form lung myofibroblasts[157]; Fgfr3 and 4 are required to control proper levels of elastin gene expression.[158] VEGF signaling has also been implicated in maintaining the alveolar structure.[159] Flt1 inhibition leads to immature lungs with decreased alveolar septation. Although there is evidence from some animal models that RA fosters alveolization, some controversies exist and further studies are required to clarify this issue.[160,161] Transcription factors, such as Foxn4 also influence alveolization.[162] Unilateral pneumonectomy (PNX) in mouse stimulates pulmonary capillary endothelial cells (PCECs) to produce angiocrine growth factors that induce

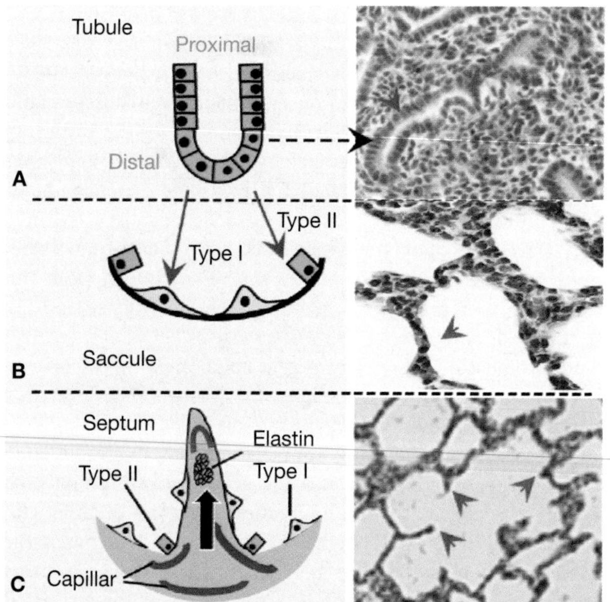

Figure 4-6 Sacculation and alveolar formation, H&E. **A, B.** Distal epithelial tubules expand their lumens and form primitive saccules lined by type I and type II cells. **C.** Septation subdivides saccules into smaller units to form the definitive alveoli.

proliferation of epithelial progenitor cells promoting regenerative alveolization.[163]

FINAL REMARKS

A wealth of information has been generated over the past decades on how growth factors, transcription factors, and matrix components influence lung development. Many of these studies suggest that alterations in developmental pathways reported in animal models are relevant to understand the pathogenesis of human lung conditions. There is also increasing evidence that developmental regulators are recruited in different contexts to mediate normal and aberrant injury–repair responses in the adult lung. Further understanding of these issues will be invaluable in discovery of different therapeutic targets and for the new field of lung regenerative medicine.

REFERENCES

1. ten Have-Opbroek AA, Otto-Verberne CJ, Dubbeldam JA, Dykman JH. The proximal border of the human respiratory unit, as shown by scanning and transmission electron microscopy and light microscopical cytochemistry. *Anat Rec*. 1991; 229(3):339–354.
2. Burri PH. Fetal and postnatal development of the lung. *Annu Rev Physiol*. 1984;46:617–628.
3. Minoo P, Su G, Drum H, Bringas P, Kimura S. Defects in tracheoesophageal and lung morphogenesis in Nkx2.1(–/–) mouse embryos. *Dev Biol*. 1999;209(1):60–71.
4. Serls AE, Doherty S, Parvatiyar P, Wells JM, Deutsch GH. Different thresholds of fibroblast growth factors pattern the ventral foregut into liver and lung. *Development*. 2005;132(1):35–47.
5. Goss AM, Tian Y, Tsukiyama T, et al. Wnt2/2b and beta-catenin signaling are necessary and sufficient to specify lung progenitors in the foregut. *Dev Cell*. 2009;17(2):290–298.
6. Harris-Johnson KS, Domyan ET, Vezina CM, Sun X. beta-Catenin promotes respiratory progenitor identity in mouse foregut. *Proc Natl Acad Sci U S A*. 2009;106(38):16287–16292.
7. Domyan ET, Ferretti E, Throckmorton K, Mishina Y, Nicolis SK, Sun X. Signaling through BMP receptors promotes respiratory identity in the foregut via repression of Sox2. *Development*. 2011;138(5):971–981.
8. van den Brink GR. Hedgehog signaling in development and homeostasis of the gastrointestinal tract. *Physiol Rev*. 2007;87(4): 1343–1375.
9. Jacobs IJ, Ku WY, Que J. Genetic and cellular mechanisms regulating anterior foregut and esophageal development. *Dev Biol*. 2012;369(1):54–64.
10. Min H, Danilenko DM, Scully SA, et al. Fgf-10 is required for both limb and lung development and exhibits striking functional similarity to Drosophila branchless. *Genes Dev*. 1998; 12(20):3156–3161.
11. Sekine K, Ohuchi H, Fujiwara M, et al. Fgf10 is essential for limb and lung formation. *Nat Genet*. 1999;21(1):138–141.
12. Park WY, Miranda B, Lebeche D, Hashimoto G, Cardoso WV. FGF-10 is a chemotactic factor for distal epithelial buds during lung development. *Dev Biol*. 1998;201(2):125–134.
13. Bellusci S, Grindley J, Emoto H, Itoh N, Hogan BL. Fibroblast growth factor 10 (FGF10) and branching morphogenesis in the embryonic mouse lung. *Development*. 1997;124(23):4867–4878.
14. Desai TJ, Malpel S, Flentke GR, Smith SM, Cardoso WV. Retinoic acid selectively regulates Fgf10 expression and maintains cell identity in the prospective lung field of the developing foregut. *Dev Biol*. 2004;273(2):402–415.
15. Malpel S, Mendelsohn C, Cardoso WV. Regulation of retinoic acid signaling during lung morphogenesis. *Development*. 2000;127(14):3057–3067.
16. Wilson JG, Roth CB, Warkany J. An analysis of the syndrome of malformations induced by maternal vitamin A deficiency. Effects of restoration of vitamin A at various times during gestation. *Am J Anat*. 1953;92(2):189–217.
17. Mollard R, Ghyselinck NB, Wendling O, Chambon P, Mark M. Stage-dependent responses of the developing lung to retinoic acid signaling. *Int J Dev Biol*. 2000;44(5):457–462.
18. Kling DE, Schnitzer JJ. Vitamin A deficiency (VAD), teratogenic, and surgical models of congenital diaphragmatic hernia (CDH). *Am J Med Genet C Semin Med Genet*. 2007;145C(2):139–157.
19. Chen F, Cao Y, Qian J, Shao F, Niederreither K, Cardoso WV. A retinoic acid-dependent network in the foregut controls formation of the mouse lung primordium. *J Clin Invest*. 2010; 120(6):2040–2048.
20. Chen F, Desai TJ, Qian J, Niederreither K, Lu J, Cardoso WV. Inhibition of Tgf beta signaling by endogenous retinoic acid is essential for primary lung bud induction. *Development*. 2007;134(16):2969–2979.
21. Chapman DL, Garvey N, Hancock S, et al. Expression of the T-box family genes, Tbx1-Tbx5, during early mouse development. *Dev Dyn*. 1996;206(4):379–390.
22. Sakiyama J, Yamagishi A, Kuroiwa A. Tbx4-Fgf10 system controls lung bud formation during chicken embryonic development. *Development*. 2003;130(7):1225–1234.
23. Arora R, Metzger RJ, Papaioannou VE. Multiple roles and interactions of Tbx4 and Tbx5 in development of the respiratory system. *PLoS Genet*. 2012;8(8):e1002866.
24. Hui CC, Slusarski D, Platt KA, Holmgren R, Joyner AL. Expression of three mouse homologs of the Drosophila segment polarity gene cubitus interruptus, Gli, Gli-2, and Gli-3, in ectoderm- and mesoderm-derived tissues suggests multiple roles during postimplantation development. *Dev Biol*. 1994;162(2):402–413.
25. Motoyama J, Liu J, Mo R, Ding Q, Post M, Hui CC. Essential function of Gli2 and Gli3 in the formation of lung, trachea and oesophagus. *Nat Genet*. 1998;20(1):54–57.
26. Litingtung Y, Lei L, Westphal H, Chiang C. Sonic hedgehog is essential to foregut development. *Nat Genet*. 1998;20(1):58–61.
27. Que J, Luo X, Schwartz RJ, Hogan BL. Multiple roles for Sox2 in the developing and adult mouse trachea. *Development*. 2009;136(11):1899–1907.
28. Daniely Y, Liao G, Dixon D, et al. Critical role of p63 in the development of a normal esophageal and tracheobronchial epithelium. *Am J Physiol Cell Physiol*. 2004;287(1):C171–C181.
29. Que J, Choi M, Ziel JW, Klingensmith J, Hogan BL. Morphogenesis of the trachea and esophagus: current players and new roles for noggin and Bmps. *Differentiation*. 2006;74(7):422–437.
30. Mendelsohn C, Lohnes D, Decimo D, et al. Function of the retinoic acid receptors (RARs) during development (II). Multiple abnormalities at various stages of organogenesis in RAR double mutants. *Development*. 1994;120(10):2749–2771.
31. Kitamura K, Miura H, Miyagawa-Tomita S, et al. Mouse Pitx2 deficiency leads to anomalies of the ventral body wall, heart, extra- and periocular mesoderm and right pulmonary isomerism. *Development*. 1999;126(24):5749–5758.
32. Kosaki R, Gebbia M, Kosaki K, et al. Left-right axis malformations associated with mutations in ACVR2B, the gene for human activin receptor type IIB. *Am J Med Genet*. 1999;82(1):70–76.

33. Meno C, Shimono A, Saijoh Y, et al. lefty-1 is required for left-right determination as a regulator of lefty-2 and nodal. *Cell.* 1998;94(3):287–297.

34. Rankin CT, Bunton T, Lawler AM, Lee SJ. Regulation of left-right patterning in mice by growth/differentiation factor-1. *Nat Genet.* 2000;24(3):262–265.

35. Oh SP, Yeo CY, Lee Y, Schrewe H, Whitman M, Li E. Activin type IIA and IIB receptors mediate Gdf11 signaling in axial vertebral patterning. *Genes Dev.* 2002;16(21):2749–2754.

36. Burn J. Disturbance of morphological laterality in humans. *Ciba Found Symp.* 1991;162:282–296; discussion 296–289.

37. Knowles MR, Leigh MW, Carson JL, et al. Mutations of DNAH11 in patients with primary ciliary dyskinesia with normal ciliary ultrastructure. *Thorax.* 2012;67(5):433–441.

38. Metzger RJ, Klein OD, Martin GR, Krasnow MA. The branching programme of mouse lung development. *Nature.* 2008;453(7196):745–750.

39. Ramasamy SK, Mailleux AA, Gupte VV, et al. Fgf10 dosage is critical for the amplification of epithelial cell progenitors and for the formation of multiple mesenchymal lineages during lung development. *Dev Biol.* 2007;307(2):237–247.

40. Colvin JS, White AC, Pratt SJ, Ornitz DM. Lung hypoplasia and neonatal death in Fgf9-null mice identify this gene as an essential regulator of lung mesenchyme. *Development.* 2001;128(11):2095–2106.

41. Bellusci S, Furuta Y, Rush MG, Henderson R, Winnier G, Hogan BL. Involvement of Sonic hedgehog (Shh) in mouse embryonic lung growth and morphogenesis. *Development.* 1997;124(1):53–63.

42. Weaver M, Batts L, Hogan BL. Tissue interactions pattern the mesenchyme of the embryonic mouse lung. *Dev Biol.* 2003;258(1):169–184.

43. Pepicelli CV, Lewis PM, McMahon AP. Sonic hedgehog regulates branching morphogenesis in the mammalian lung. *Curr Biol.* 1998;8(19):1083–1086.

44. Lebeche D, Malpel S, Cardoso WV. Fibroblast growth factor interactions in the developing lung. *Mech Dev.* 1999;86(1–2):125–136.

45. Chuang PT, Kawcak T, McMahon AP. Feedback control of mammalian Hedgehog signaling by the Hedgehog-binding protein, Hip1, modulates Fgf signaling during branching morphogenesis of the lung. *Genes Dev.* 2003;17(3):342–347.

46. Mailleux AA, Tefft D, Ndiaye D, et al. Evidence that SPROUTY2 functions as an inhibitor of mouse embryonic lung growth and morphogenesis. *Mech Dev.* 2001;102(1–2):81–94.

47. de Maximy AA, Nakatake Y, Moncada S, Itoh N, Thiery JP, Bellusci S. Cloning and expression pattern of a mouse homologue of drosophila sprouty in the mouse embryo. *Mech Dev.* 1999;81(1–2):213–216.

48. Tefft JD, Lee M, Smith S, et al. Conserved function of mSpry-2, a murine homolog of Drosophila sprouty, which negatively modulates respiratory organogenesis. *Curr Biol.* 1999;9(4):219–222.

49. Tefft D, Lee M, Smith S, Crowe DL, Bellusci S, Warburton D. mSprouty2 inhibits FGF10-activated MAP kinase by differentially binding to upstream target proteins. *Am J Physiol Lung Cell Mol Physiol.* 2002;283(4):L700–L706.

50. Perl AK, Hokuto I, Impagnatiello MA, Christofori G, Whitsett JA. Temporal effects of Sprouty on lung morphogenesis. *Dev Biol.* 2003;258(1):154–168.

51. Hacohen N, Kramer S, Sutherland D, Hiromi Y, Krasnow MA. Sprouty encodes a novel antagonist of FGF signaling that patterns apical branching of the Drosophila airways. *Cell.* 1998;92(2):253–263.

52. Izvolsky KI, Zhong L, Wei L, Yu Q, Nugent MA, Cardoso WV. Heparan sulfates expressed in the distal lung are required for Fgf10 binding to the epithelium and for airway branching. *Am J Physiol Lung Cell Mol Physiol.* 2003;285(4):L838–L846.

53. Izvolsky KI, Shoykhet D, Yang Y, Yu Q, Nugent MA, Cardoso WV. Heparan sulfate-FGF10 interactions during lung morphogenesis. *Dev Biol.* 2003;258(1):185–200.

54. Heine UI, Munoz EF, Flanders KC, Roberts AB, Sporn MB. Colocalization of TGF-beta 1 and collagen I and III, fibronectin and glycosaminoglycans during lung branching morphogenesis. *Development.* 1990;109(1):29–36.

55. Lu J, Qian J, Izvolsky KI, Cardoso WV. Global analysis of genes differentially expressed in branching and non-branching regions of the mouse embryonic lung. *Dev Biol.* 2004;273(2):418–435.

56. Serra R, Pelton RW, Moses HL. TGF beta 1 inhibits branching morphogenesis and N-myc expression in lung bud organ cultures. *Development.* 1994;120(8):2153–2161.

57. Zhao J, Bu D, Lee M, Slavkin HC, Hall FL, Warburton D. Abrogation of transforming growth factor-beta type II receptor stimulates embryonic mouse lung branching morphogenesis in culture. *Dev Biol.* 1996;180(1):242–257.

58. Beer HD, Florence C, Dammeier J, McGuire L, Werner S, Duan DR. Mouse fibroblast growth factor 10: cDNA cloning, protein characterization, and regulation of mRNA expression. *Oncogene.* 1997;15(18):2211–2218.

59. Tomlinson DC, Grindley JC, Thomson AA. Regulation of Fgf10 gene expression in the prostate: identification of transforming growth factor-beta1 and promoter elements. *Endocrinology.* 2004;145(4):1988–1995.

60. Letterio JJ, Geiser AG, Kulkarni AB, Roche NS, Sporn MB, Roberts AB. Maternal rescue of transforming growth factor-beta 1 null mice. *Science.* 1994;264(5167):1936–1938.

61. Pelton RW, Johnson MD, Perkett EA, Gold LI, Moses HL. Expression of transforming growth factor-beta 1, -beta 2, and -beta 3 mRNA and protein in the murine lung. *Am J Respir Cell Mol Biol.* 1991;5(6):522–530.

62. Sanford LP, Ormsby I, Gittenberger-de Groot AC, et al. TGFbeta2 knockout mice have multiple developmental defects that are non-overlapping with other TGFbeta knockout phenotypes. *Development.* 1997;124(13):2659–2670.

63. Kaartinen V, Voncken JW, Shuler C, et al. Abnormal lung development and cleft palate in mice lacking TGF-beta 3 indicates defects of epithelial-mesenchymal interaction. *Nat Genet.* 1995;11(4):415–421.

64. He L, Hannon GJ. MicroRNAs: small RNAs with a big role in gene regulation. *Nat Rev Genet.* 2004;5(7):522–531.

65. Stefani G, Slack FJ. Small non-coding RNAs in animal development. *Nat Rev Mol Cell Biol.* 2008;9(3):219–230.

66. Friedman RC, Farh KK, Burge CB, Bartel DP. Most mammalian mRNAs are conserved targets of microRNAs. *Genome Res.* 2009;19(1):92–105.

67. Bartel DP. MicroRNAs: genomics, biogenesis, mechanism, and function. *Cell.* 2004;116(2):281–297.

68. Bartel DP. MicroRNAs: target recognition and regulatory functions. *Cell.* 2009;136(2):215–233.

69. Harris KS, Zhang Z, McManus MT, Harfe BD, Sun X. Dicer function is essential for lung epithelium morphogenesis. *Proc Natl Acad Sci U S A.* 2006;103(7):2208–2213.

70. Hill DA, Ivanovich J, Priest JR, et al. DICER1 mutations in familial pleuropulmonary blastoma. *Science*. 2009;325(5943):965.

71. Lako M, Strachan T, Bullen P, Wilson DI, Robson SC, Lindsay S. Isolation, characterisation and embryonic expression of WNT11, a gene which maps to 11q13.5 and has possible roles in the development of skeleton, kidney and lung. *Gene*. 1998;219(1–2):101–110.

72. Zakin LD, Mazan S, Maury M, Martin N, Guenet JL, Brulet P. Structure and expression of Wnt13, a novel mouse Wnt2 related gene. *Mech Dev*. 1998;73(1):107–116.

73. Tebar M, Destree O, de Vree WJ, Ten Have-Opbroek AA. Expression of Tcf/Lef and sFrp and localization of beta-catenin in the developing mouse lung. *Mech Dev*. 2001;109(2):437–440.

74. Okubo T, Hogan BL. Hyperactive Wnt signaling changes the developmental potential of embryonic lung endoderm. *J Biol*. 2004;3(3):11.

75. De Langhe SP, Sala FG, Del Moral PM, et al. Dickkopf-1 (DKK1) reveals that fibronectin is a major target of Wnt signaling in branching morphogenesis of the mouse embryonic lung. *Dev Biol*. 2005;277(2):316–331.

76. Mucenski ML, Nation JM, Thitoff AR, et al. Beta-catenin regulates differentiation of respiratory epithelial cells in vivo. *Am J Physiol Lung Cell Mol Physiol*. 2005;289(6):L971–L979.

77. Hashimoto S, Chen H, Que J, et al. beta-Catenin-SOX2 signaling regulates the fate of developing airway epithelium. *J Cell Sci*. 2012;125(Pt 4):932–942.

78. Bellusci S, Henderson R, Winnier G, Oikawa T, Hogan BL. Evidence from normal expression and targeted misexpression that bone morphogenetic protein (Bmp-4) plays a role in mouse embryonic lung morphogenesis. *Development*. 1996;122(6):1693–1702.

79. Scott IC, Steiglitz BM, Clark TG, Pappano WN, Greenspan DS. Spatiotemporal expression patterns of mammalian chordin during postgastrulation embryogenesis and in postnatal brain. *Dev Dyn*. 2000;217(4):449–456.

80. Shi W, Zhao J, Anderson KD, Warburton D. Gremlin negatively modulates BMP-4 induction of embryonic mouse lung branching morphogenesis. *Am J Physiol Lung Cell Mol Physiol*. 2001;280(5):L1030–L1039.

81. Lu MM, Yang H, Zhang L, Shu W, Blair DG, Morrisey EE. The bone morphogenic protein antagonist gremlin regulates proximal-distal patterning of the lung. *Dev Dyn*. 2001;222(4):667–680.

82. Michos O, Panman L, Vintersten K, Beier K, Zeller R, Zuniga A. Gremlin-mediated BMP antagonism induces the epithelial-mesenchymal feedback signaling controlling metanephric kidney and limb organogenesis. *Development*. 2004;131(14):3401–3410.

83. Lu J, Qian J, Keppler D, Cardoso WV. Cathespin H is an Fgf10 target involved in Bmp4 degradation during lung branching morphogenesis. *J Biol Chem*. 2007;282(30):22176–22184.

84. Weaver M, Yingling JM, Dunn NR, Bellusci S, Hogan BL. Bmp signaling regulates proximal-distal differentiation of endoderm in mouse lung development. *Development*. 1999;126(18):4005–4015.

85. Weaver M, Dunn NR, Hogan BL. Bmp4 and Fgf10 play opposing roles during lung bud morphogenesis. *Development*. 2000;127(12):2695–2704.

86. Wang Y, Tian Y, Morley MP, et al. Development and regeneration of Sox2+ endoderm progenitors are regulated by a HDAC1/2-Bmp4/Rb1 regulatory pathway. *Dev Cell*. 2013;24(4):345–358.

87. Lu Y, Thomson JM, Wong HY, Hammond SM, Hogan BL. Transgenic overexpression of the microRNA miR-17–92 cluster promotes proliferation and inhibits differentiation of lung epithelial progenitor cells. *Dev Biol*. 2007;310(2):442–453.

88. Ventura A, Young AG, Winslow MM, et al. Targeted deletion reveals essential and overlapping functions of the miR-17 through 92 family of miRNA clusters. *Cell*. 2008;132(5): 875–886.

89. Carraro G, El-Hashash A, Guidolin D, et al. miR-17 family of microRNAs controls FGF10-mediated embryonic lung epithelial branching morphogenesis through MAPK14 and STAT3 regulation of E-Cadherin distribution. *Dev Biol*. 2009; 333(2):238–250.

90. Tian Y, Zhang Y, Hurd L, et al. Regulation of lung endoderm progenitor cell behavior by miR302/367. *Development*. 2011;138(7):1235–1245.

91. deMello DE, Sawyer D, Galvin N, Reid LM. Early fetal development of lung vasculature. *Am J Respir Cell Mol Biol*. 1997;16(5):568–581.

92. Parera MC, van Dooren M, van Kempen M, et al. Distal angiogenesis: a new concept for lung vascular morphogenesis. *Am J Physiol Lung Cell Mol Physiol*. 2005;288(1):L141–L149.

93. Schwarz MA, Caldwell L, Cafasso D, Zheng H. Emerging pulmonary vasculature lacks fate specification. *Am J Physiol Lung Cell Mol Physiol*. 2009;296(1):L71–L81.

94. Pauling MH, Vu TH. Mechanisms and regulation of lung vascular development. *Curr Top Dev Biol*. 2004;64:73–99.

95. Healy AM, Morgenthau L, Zhu X, Farber HW, Cardoso WV. VEGF is deposited in the subepithelial matrix at the leading edge of branching airways and stimulates neovascularization in the murine embryonic lung. *Dev Dyn*. 2000;219(3):341–352.

96. Akeson AL, Greenberg JM, Cameron JE, et al. Temporal and spatial regulation of VEGF-A controls vascular patterning in the embryonic lung. *Dev Biol*. 2003;264(2):443–455.

97. Del Moral PM, Sala FG, Tefft D, et al. VEGF-A signaling through Flk-1 is a critical facilitator of early embryonic lung epithelial to endothelial crosstalk and branching morphogenesis. *Dev Biol*. 2006;290(1):177–188.

98. Ng YS, Rohan R, Sunday ME, Demello DE, D'Amore PA. Differential expression of VEGF isoforms in mouse during development and in the adult. *Dev Dyn*. 2001;220(2):112–121.

99. Kukk E, Lymboussaki A, Taira S, et al. VEGF-C receptor binding and pattern of expression with VEGFR-3 suggests a role in lymphatic vascular development. *Development*. 1996; 122(12):3829–3837.

100. Veikkola T, Jussila L, Makinen T, et al. Signalling via vascular endothelial growth factor receptor-3 is sufficient for lymphangiogenesis in transgenic mice. *EMBO J*. 2001;20(6):1223–1231.

101. Karkkainen MJ, Haiko P, Sainio K, et al. Vascular endothelial growth factor C is required for sprouting of the first lymphatic vessels from embryonic veins. *Nat Immunol*. 2004;5(1):74–80.

102. Que J, Wilm B, Hasegawa H, Wang F, Bader D, Hogan BL. Mesothelium contributes to vascular smooth muscle and mesenchyme during lung development. *Proc Natl Acad Sci U S A*. 2008;105(43):16626–16630.

103. Radzikinas K, Aven L, Jiang Z, et al. A Shh/miR-206/BDNF cascade coordinates innervation and formation of airway smooth muscle. *J Neurosci*. 2011;31(43):15407–15415.

104. Wang Z, Shu W, Lu MM, Morrisey EE. Wnt7b activates canonical signaling in epithelial and vascular smooth muscle cells through interactions with Fzd1, Fzd10, and LRP5. *Mol Cell Biol*. 2005;25(12):5022–5030.

105. Shu W, Jiang YQ, Lu MM, Morrisey EE. Wnt7b regulates mesenchymal proliferation and vascular development in the lung. *Development*. 2002;129(20):4831–4842.

106. Greif DM, Kumar M, Lighthouse JK, et al. Radial construction of an arterial wall. *Dev Cell*. 2012;23(3):482–493.

107. Morimoto M, Nishinakamura R, Saga Y, Kopan R. Different assemblies of Notch receptors coordinate the distribution of the major bronchial Clara, ciliated and neuroendocrine cells. *Development*. 2012;139(23):4365–4373.

108. Jeffery TK, Upton PD, Trembath RC, Morrell NW. BMP4 inhibits proliferation and promotes myocyte differentiation of lung fibroblasts via Smad1 and JNK pathways. *Am J Physiol Lung Cell Mol Physiol*. 2005;288(2):L370–L378.

109. Deng Z, Morse JH, Slager SL, et al. Familial primary pulmonary hypertension (gene PPH1) is caused by mutations in the bone morphogenetic protein receptor-II gene. *Am J Hum Genet*. 2000; 67(3):737–744.

110. Lane KB, Machado RD, Pauciulo MW, et al. Heterozygous germline mutations in BMPR2, encoding a TGF-beta receptor, cause familial primary pulmonary hypertension. *Nat Genet*. 2000; 26(1):81–84.

111. Thomson JR, Machado RD, Pauciulo MW, et al. Sporadic primary pulmonary hypertension is associated with germline mutations of the gene encoding BMPR-II, a receptor member of the TGF-beta family. *J Med Genet*. 2000;37(10):741–745.

112. Li X, Zhang X, Leathers R, et al. Notch3 signaling promotes the development of pulmonary arterial hypertension. *Nat Med*. 2009;15(11):1289–1297.

113. Ustiyan V, Wang IC, Ren X, et al. Forkhead box M1 transcriptional factor is required for smooth muscle cells during embryonic development of blood vessels and esophagus. *Dev Biol*. 2009; 336(2):266–279.

114. Mailleux AA, Kelly R, Veltmaat JM, et al. Fgf10 expression identifies parabronchial smooth muscle cell progenitors and is required for their entry into the smooth muscle cell lineage. *Development*. 2005;132(9):2157–2166.

115. Sparrow MP, Lamb JP. Ontogeny of airway smooth muscle: structure, innervation, myogenesis and function in the fetal lung. *Respir Physiol Neurobiol*. 2003;137(2–3):361–372.

116. Cohen ED, Ihida-Stansbury K, Lu MM, Panettieri RA, Jones PL, Morrisey EE. Wnt signaling regulates smooth muscle precursor development in the mouse lung via a tenascin C/PDGFR pathway. *J Clin Invest*. 2009;119(9):2538–2549.

117. Yang Y, Beqaj S, Kemp P, Ariel I, Schuger L. Stretch-induced alternative splicing of serum response factor promotes bronchial myogenesis and is defective in lung hypoplasia. *J Clin Invest*. 2000;106(11):1321–1330.

118. Jakkaraju S, Zhe X, Pan D, Choudhury R, Schuger L. TIPs are tension-responsive proteins involved in myogenic versus adipogenic differentiation. *Dev Cell*. 2005;9(1):39–49.

119. Cardoso WV, Lu J. Regulation of early lung morphogenesis: questions, facts and controversies. *Development*. 2006;133 (9):1611–1624.

120. Morrisey EE, Hogan BL. Preparing for the first breath: genetic and cellular mechanisms in lung development. *Dev Cell*. 2010; 18(1):8–23.

121. Yi L, Domyan ET, Lewandoski M, Sun X. Fibroblast growth factor 9 signaling inhibits airway smooth muscle differentiation in mouse lung. *Dev Dyn*. 2009;238(1):123–137.

122. White AC, Xu J, Yin Y, Smith C, Schmid G, Ornitz DM. FGF9 and SHH signaling coordinate lung growth and development through regulation of distinct mesenchymal domains. *Development*. 2006;133(8):1507–1517.

123. Jesudason EC, Smith NP, Connell MG, et al. Peristalsis of airway smooth muscle is developmentally regulated and uncoupled from hypoplastic lung growth. *Am J Physiol Lung Cell Mol Physiol*. 2006;291(4):L559–L565.

124. Jesudason EC, Smith NP, Connell MG, et al. Developing rat lung has a sided pacemaker region for morphogenesis-related airway peristalsis. *Am J Respir Cell Mol Biol*. 2005;32(2): 118–127.

125. Mahlapuu M, Enerback S, Carlsson P. Haploinsufficiency of the forkhead gene Foxf1, a target for sonic hedgehog signaling, causes lung and foregut malformations. *Development*. 2001;128(12):2397–2406.

126. Miller LA, Wert SE, Clark JC, Xu Y, Perl AK, Whitsett JA. Role of Sonic hedgehog in patterning of tracheal-bronchial cartilage and the peripheral lung. *Dev Dyn*. 2004;231(1):57–71.

127. Gontan C, de Munck A, Vermeij M, Grosveld F, Tibboel D, Rottier R. Sox2 is important for two crucial processes in lung development: branching morphogenesis and epithelial cell differentiation. *Dev Biol*. 2008;317(1):296–309.

128. Kurotani R, Tomita T, Yang Q, Carlson BA, Chen C, Kimura S. Role of secretoglobin 3A2 in lung development. *Am J Respir Crit Care Med*. 2008;178(4):389–398.

129. Murphy DB, Seemann S, Wiese S, Kirschner R, Grzeschik KH, Thies U. The human hepatocyte nuclear factor 3/fork head gene FKHL13: genomic structure and pattern of expression. *Genomics*. 1997;40(3):462–469.

130. Borges M, Linnoila RI, van de Velde HJ, et al. An achaete-scute homologue essential for neuroendocrine differentiation in the lung. *Nature*. 1997;386(6627):852–855.

131. Blatt EN, Yan XH, Wuerffel MK, Hamilos DL, Brody SL. Forkhead transcription factor HFH-4 expression is temporally related to ciliogenesis. *Am J Respir Cell Mol Biol*. 1999;21(2):168–176.

132. Tsao PN, Vasconcelos M, Izvolsky KI, Qian J, Lu J, Cardoso WV. Notch signaling controls the balance of ciliated and secretory cell fates in developing airways. *Development*. 2009;136(13):2297–2307.

133. Guha A, Vasconcelos M, Cai Y, et al. Neuroepithelial body microenvironment is a niche for a distinct subset of Clara-like precursors in the developing airways. *Proc Natl Acad Sci U S A*. 2012;109(31):12592–12597.

134. Jain R, Pan J, Driscoll JA, et al. Temporal relationship between primary and motile ciliogenesis in airway epithelial cells. *Am J Respir Cell Mol Biol*. 2010;43(6):731–739.

135. Wuenschell CW, Sunday ME, Singh G, Minoo P, Slavkin HC, Warburton D. Embryonic mouse lung epithelial progenitor cells co-express immunohistochemical markers of diverse mature cell lineages. *J J Histochem Cytochem*. 1996;44(2):113–123.

136. Rock JR, Hogan BL. Epithelial progenitor cells in lung development, maintenance, repair, and disease. *Annu Rev Cell Dev Biol*. 2011;27:493–512.

137. Davis CW, Dickey BF. Regulated airway goblet cell mucin secretion. *Ann Rev Physiol*. 2008;70:487–512.

138. Mills AA, Zheng B, Wang XJ, Vogel H, Roop DR, Bradley A. p63 is a p53 homologue required for limb and epidermal morphogenesis. *Nature*. 1999;398(6729):708–713.

139. Yang A, Schweitzer R, Sun D, et al. p63 is essential for regenerative proliferation in limb, craniofacial and epithelial development. *Nature*. 1999;398(6729):714–718.

140. Tsao PN, Chen F, Izvolsky KI, et al. Gamma-secretase activation of notch signaling regulates the balance of proximal and distal fates in progenitor cells of the developing lung. *J Biol Chem*. 2008;283(43):29532–29544.

141. Morimoto M, Liu Z, Cheng HT, Winters N, Bader D, Kopan R. Canonical Notch signaling in the developing lung is required for determination of arterial smooth muscle cells and selection of Clara versus ciliated cell fate. *J Cell Sci*. 2010;123(Pt 2): 213–224.

142. Guseh JS, Bores SA, Stanger BZ, et al. Notch signaling promotes airway mucous metaplasia and inhibits alveolar development. *Development*. 2009;136(10):1751–1759.

143. Tsao PN, Wei SC, Wu MF, et al. Notch signaling prevents mucous metaplasia in mouse conducting airways during postnatal development. *Development*. 2011;138(16):3533–3543.

144. Tilley AE, Harvey BG, Heguy A, et al. Downregulation of the notch pathway in human airway epithelium in association with smoking and chronic obstructive pulmonary disease. *Am J Respir Crit Care Med*. 2009;179(6):457–466.

145. Park KS, Korfhagen TR, Bruno MD, et al. SPDEF regulates goblet cell hyperplasia in the airway epithelium. *J Clin Invest*. 2007; 117(4):978–988.

146. Chen G, Korfhagen TR, Xu Y, et al. SPDEF is required for mouse pulmonary goblet cell differentiation and regulates a network of genes associated with mucus production. *J Clin Invest*. 2009;119(10):2914–2924.

147. Wan H, Kaestner KH, Ang SL, et al. Foxa2 regulates alveolarization and goblet cell hyperplasia. *Development*. 2004;131(4): 953–964.

148. Danielian PS, Bender Kim CF, Caron AM, Vasile E, Bronson RT, Lees JA. E2f4 is required for normal development of the airway epithelium. *Dev Biol*. 2007;305(2):564–576.

149. Stubbs JL, Vladar EK, Axelrod JD, Kintner C. Multicilin promotes centriole assembly and ciliogenesis during multiciliate cell differentiation. *Nat Cell Biol*. 2012;14(2):140–147.

150. Chen J, Knowles HJ, Hebert JL, Hackett BP. Mutation of the mouse hepatocyte nuclear factor/forkhead homologue 4 gene results in an absence of cilia and random left-right asymmetry. *J Clin Invest*. 1998;102(6):1077–1082.

151. Brody SL, Yan XH, Wuerffel MK, Song SK, Shapiro SD. Ciliogenesis and left-right axis defects in forkhead factor HFH-4-null mice. *Am J Respir Cell Mol Biol*. 2000;23(1):45–51.

152. Marcet B, Chevalier B, Luxardi G, et al. Control of vertebrate multiciliogenesis by miR-449 through direct repression of the Delta/Notch pathway. *Nat Cell Biol*. 2011;13(6):693–699.

153. Williams MC. Alveolar type I cells: molecular phenotype and development. *Annu Rev Physiol*. 2003;65:669–695.

154. Ramirez MI, Millien G, Hinds A, Cao Y, Seldin DC, Williams MC. T1alpha, a lung type I cell differentiation gene, is required for normal lung cell proliferation and alveolus formation at birth. *Dev Biol*. 2003;256(1):61–72.

155. Hsu YC, Osinski J, Campbell CE, et al. Mesenchymal nuclear factor I B regulates cell proliferation and epithelial differentiation during lung maturation. *Dev Biol*. 2011;354(2):242–252.

156. Wang IC, Zhang Y, Snyder J, et al. Increased expression of FoxM1 transcription factor in respiratory epithelium inhibits lung sacculation and causes Clara cell hyperplasia. *Dev Biol*. 2010; 347(2): 301–314.

157. Bostrom H, Willetts K, Pekny M, et al. PDGF-A signaling is a critical event in lung alveolar myofibroblast development and alveogenesis. *Cell*. 1996;85(6):863–873.

158. Weinstein M, Xu X, Ohyama K, Deng CX. FGFR-3 and FGFR-4 function cooperatively to direct alveogenesis in the murine lung. *Development*. 1998;125(18):3615–3623.

159. Tang K, Rossiter HB, Wagner PD, Breen EC. Lung-targeted VEGF inactivation leads to an emphysema phenotype in mice. *J Appl Physiol (1985)*. 2004;97(4):1559–1566; discussion 1549.

160. Pierce RA, Michael Shipley J. Retinoid-enhanced alveolization: Identifying relevant downstream targets. *Am J Respir Cell Mol Biol*. 2000;23(2):137–141.

161. Willet KE, Jobe AH, Ikegami M, Newnham J, Sly PD. Antenatal retinoic acid does not alter alveolization or postnatal lung function in preterm sheep. *Eur Respir J*. 2000;16(1):101–107.

162. Li S, Xiang M. Foxn4 influences alveologenesis during lung development. *Dev Dyn*. 2011;240(6):1512–1517.

163. Ding BS, Nolan DJ, Guo P, et al. Endothelial-derived angiocrine signals induce and sustain regenerative lung alveolarization. *Cell*. 2011;147(3):539–553.

CHAPTER 5

Pulmonary Surfactant and Disorders of Surfactant Homeostasis

Jeffrey A. Whitsett

Timothy E. Weaver

INTRODUCTION

Pulmonary surfactant is a complex mixture of phospholipids and proteins that creates a unique interface separating alveolar gas and liquids at the alveolar cell surface, reducing surface tension, and maintaining lung volumes at end expiration. Reduction of the surface tension at the air–liquid interface is a requirement for respiratory function following birth. Deficiency of pulmonary surfactant causes respiratory failure in premature infants, or infantile respiratory distress syndrome (IRDS). The adequacy of pulmonary surfactant is maintained by unique and highly regulated systems mediating the synthesis, secretion, reutilization, and catabolism of surfactant. Loss or inactivation of pulmonary surfactant later in life occurs in the adult respiratory distress syndrome (ARDS), a significant cause of morbidity and mortality following infection, shock, or trauma. Mutations in genes regulating surfactant homeostasis, including SFTPA, SFTPB, SFTPC, ABCA3, TITF1, and CSF2RA cause acute and/or chronic lung disease in newborn infants, children, and adults. Disorders of GM-CSF signaling inhibit surfactant lipid and protein catabolism by alveolar macrophage causing pulmonary alveolar proteinosis (PAP). This chapter reviews the biology of the surfactant system and its implications for the pathogenesis, diagnosis, and treatment of respiratory disease in premature infants and adults. Suggested reviews of these topics are provided in the References section.[1–5]

PHYSICAL FORCES AT THE AIR–LIQUID INTERFACE

In 1929, Van Neergard recognized the critical role of surface tension as a "retractile force" in the lung, observing the marked difference in inflation pressures required to inflate the air- versus water-filled lung. Avery and Mead associated the lack of a lipid-rich material in the lungs of infants dying from idiopathic respiratory distress syndrome with alveolar collapse and respiratory failure.[6] In the absence of pulmonary surfactant, molecular forces at the air–liquid interface create a region of high surface tension because intermolecular forces between water molecules are unopposed at the air–liquid interface, and an area of high retractile force at the surface is created. Forces of 70 dynes/cm^2 are generated at the air–water interface; if unopposed in the alveolus, such forces lead to alveolar collapse and respiratory failure. A surface film composed of multilayered sheets of phospholipids creates a distinct phase separating air and liquid, reducing surface tension to nearly zero and maintaining residual lung volume at end expiration. Complex interactions between surfactant phospholipids and proteins are required to maintain surfactant film throughout life. Pulmonary surfactant lipids and proteins are synthesized and secreted by alveolar type II epithelial cells into the alveoli, where they form multilayered lipid-rich films that reduce surface tension to maintain ventilation (Figs. 5-1 and 5-2).

COMPOSITION OF PULMONARY SURFACTANT

Pulmonary surfactant isolated by lung lavage consists of highly heterogeneous forms of phospholipid–protein aggregates of distinct sizes, structural characteristics, and composition. Tubular myelin is the most abundant form of alveolar phospholipid and consists of large, relatively dense aggregates (termed large aggregate surfactant) composed of phospholipids and surfactant proteins (SPs). Tubular myelin is a highly organized form of surfactant phospholipid, forming square tubular arrays. Tubular myelin represents an extracellular pool of surfactant lipids that rapidly moves to the air–liquid interface and reorganizes to form multilayered sheets that reduce surface tension in the alveolus (Fig. 5-2). Large lamellated structures, with lipid composition similar to that of tubular myelin, are seen within the alveolus and likely represent newly secreted lamellar bodies that unravel to form tubular myelin in the alveoli. The phospholipid composition of lamellar bodies, the intracellular storage form of surfactant, tubular myelin, and lamellated forms present in the alveolus are virtually identical. Smaller, less dense particles (small aggregate surfactant) are also present within the alveolar space, representing remnants or catabolic forms of surfactant that have relatively poor surface activity. Small aggregate surfactant is destined for uptake, reutilization, or catabolism by type II epithelial cells and catabolism by alveolar macrophages.[2,3]

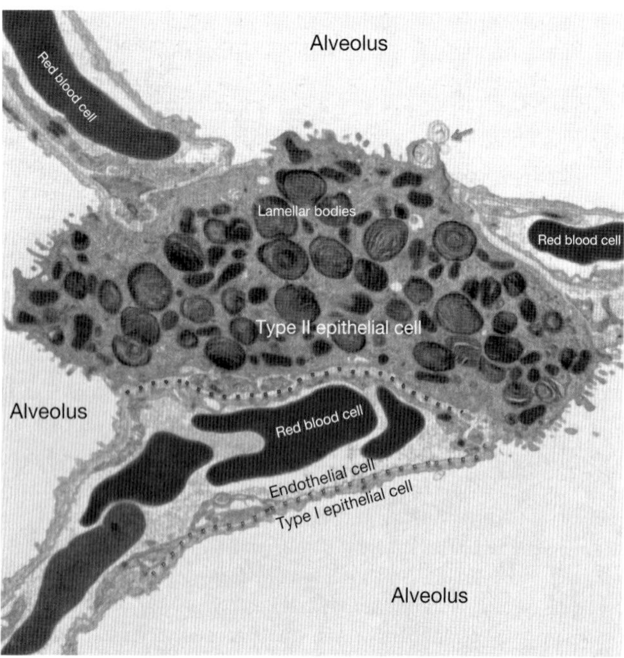

Figure 5-1 Pulmonary alveolar ultrastructure. The air–blood barrier is comprised of the capillary endothelium (above *the dotted orange line*) and the closely apposed type I epithelial cell (below *the dotted orange line*). The dotted blue line delineates the interstitial space between endothelial cells and type II epithelial cells with their specialized secretory lipid organelles (lamellar bodies). Type II cells form tight junctions with type I cells and serve as alveolar progenitor cells. Surfactant lipids and proteins are secreted as lamellar membranes *(arrow)* into the alveolar space forming tubular myelin and lipid membrane multilayers that reduce surface tension, preventing alveolar collapse.

SURFACTANT PHOSPHOLIPIDS AND PROTEINS

The composition of surfactant lipids is similar in all of the structural forms of surfactant isolated from mammalian lungs, with phospholipids generally representing 80% to 90% of the mass of pulmonary surfactant.[3] In the adult lung, phosphatidylcholine (PC) and phosphatidylglycerol (PG) are the most abundant phospholipids, representing approximately 70% to 80% and 5% to 10%, respectively, of the lipid mass. Dipalmitoyl phosphatidylcholine (DPPC) is the most abundant species of PC. Lesser amounts of phosphatidylserine, phosphatidylethanolamine, sphingomyelin, neutral lipids (mostly cholesterol), and glycolipids are also present in surfactant. The lung content of surfactant phospholipids increases markedly with advancing gestation, regulated by a complex signaling and transcriptional network that controls type II alveolar cell differentiation, lipid synthesis, and SP gene expression. Lamellar bodies are secreted into the fetal amniotic fluid. PC, lamellar body counts, DPPC content, and increased lecithin (PC) to sphingomyelin (L/S) ratio, correlate with postnatal respiratory function. These tests are used to predict pulmonary maturity prior to the birth of preterm infants. Lung maturation and synthesis of surfactant components are induced by maternal administration of glucocorticoids, used clinically to prevent respiratory distress prior to premature birth.[7] Proteins represent approximately 5% to 15% of the mass of pulmonary surfactant and include serum proteins and proteins that are synthesized and secreted by type II alveolar epithelial cells. In addition to its specific interaction with SP-B, the anionic phospholipid PG may also play an important role in innate defense. PG constitutes 10 mole% of surfactant lipid, with palmitoyl-oleoyl-PG (PoPG) being the most common species in human surfactant. PoPG specifically suppresses LPS-induced inflammatory responses and prevents infection of epithelial cells by binding RSV or influenza A virus.[8] Thus the unique enrichment of PoPG in the distal airspaces may be an important component of host defense against inhaled pathogens. Four surfactant proteins (SPs), SP-A, SP-B, SP-C, and SP-D, are produced by respiratory epithelial cells, each playing specific roles in surfactant homeostasis and innate host defense.[2,3,9,10]

Surfactant is uniquely enriched in disaturated DPPC. The saturated C16 acyl chains pack densely at an air–liquid interface, reducing tension at the surface. However, dense and stable packing of DPPC occurs at a phase transition of 41°C, far above physiologic temperatures. Thus, at 37°C, pure DPPC maintains a semicrystalline or gel phase that is incapable of moving rapidly with the expansion and compression of the alveoli during the respiratory cycle. The capability of DPPC pulmonary surfactant to move rapidly to the alveolar interface at 37°C and to maintain low surface tension during dynamic compression is conferred by the surfactant-associated

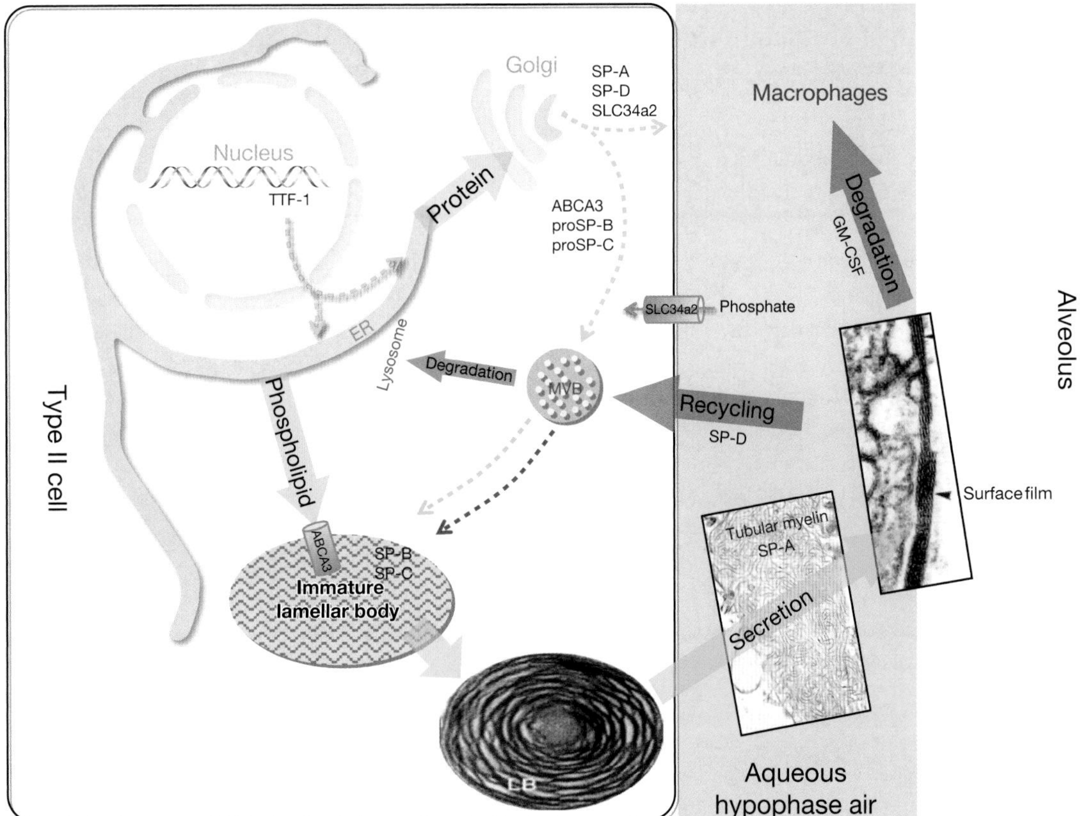

Figure 5-2 Surfactant metabolism. Newly translated surfactant proteins (proSP-B and proSP-C) and lamellar body (ABCA3) proteins traffic from the endoplasmic reticulum (ER) to the Golgi and subsequently to the multivesicular body (MVB). Fusion of the MVB with the lamellar body (LB) is accompanied by proteolytic processing of SP-B and SP-C proproteins to their mature peptides. Surfactant phospholipids (DPPC, PG) are likely transported directly from the ER to the LB by lipid transfer proteins. The contents of the LB are secreted into the alveolar space where they interact with SP-A to form tubular myelin and, ultimately, a phospholipid-rich film (surfactant) at the air–liquid interface. Alveolar surfactant lipids and proteins are cleared through a GM-CSF dependent pathway that regulates alveolar macrophage differentiation and function. Surfactant remnants are also taken up by the type II epithelial cell and recycled to the LB, via the MVB, for resecretion, while a portion is degraded in lysosomes. SP-D plays an important role in regulating alveolar surfactant pool size likely by enhancing its reuptake by type II epithelial cells. The MVB serves to integrate surfactant synthesis, secretion, recycling, and degradation pathways in the type II cell. TTF-1 is a transcription factor critical for differentiation of type II epithelial cells and regulation of expression of Abca3, Slc34a2, and the surfactant proteins. Synthetic pathways are shown in green and catabolic pathways are shown in red.

proteins SP-B and SP-C. PC synthesis in the lung is controlled by genes encoding choline phosphate cytidylyltransferase (PCYTLA) and choline kinase (CHKA), which are required for surfactant lipid synthesis and lung function at birth. DPPC is synthesized in type II alveolar cells via both a de novo pathway and remodeling of lysoPC. The enzyme lysoPC acetyltransferase (LPCAT1) mediates reacylation during surfactant lipid biosynthesis. Surfactant lipids, synthesized in the endoplasmic reticulum (ER) are transferred via a Golgi-independent pathway to lamellar bodies, the major intracellular storage site of surfactant (Fig. 5-2). Transfer of lipids occurs via nonvesicular transport and uptake into lamellar bodies requires the ABCA3 transporter, which selectively transports PC and PG. In contrast, surfactant proteins SP-B and SP-C traffic from the ER to the Golgi and subsequently to multivesicular bodies where proteolytic processing is initiated. Ultimately, multivesicular bodies are incorporated into lamellar bodies with surfactant lipids prior to secretion from type II alveolar cells.[3]

■ STRUCTURE AND FUNCTION OF SURFACTANT PROTEINS

Four distinct surfactant-associated proteins have been isolated from surfactant obtained by lung lavage. Their cDNAs, genes, and structures have been identified and are well characterized (Table 5-1).[9,10] The SPs are expressed in a relatively lung epithelial cell–selective manner and are secreted into the airspaces, where they influence the structure, metabolism, and function of surfactant. Two classes of proteins have been distinguished on the basis of their structures. SP-A and SP-D are relatively abundant, hydrophilic, structurally related proteins and are members of the calcium-dependent lectin family of proteins that have similar amino-terminal collagenous and C-terminal lectin domains.[11] SP-A and SP-D have little "surfactant"-like qualities but are able to bind complex carbohydrates, lipids, and glycolipids, including those on the surface of cells, bacteria, viruses, fungi, and other lung pathogens. SP-A and SP-D influence the structural forms and metabolism of surfactant lipids in the alveolus. They act as opsonins, activate alveolar macrophages, and play important roles in innate host defense in the lung. In contrast, SP-B and SP-C are small, hydrophobic proteins that play critical roles in enhancing the rate of spreading and stability of surfactant phospholipids needed to optimally reduce surface tension.[10] SP-B and SP-C are the sole protein components of the animal-derived surfactant replacement preparations used for the treatment of IRDS at present.[10]

TABLE 5-1 Regulation of Surfactant Homeostasis

Genes/locus	Functions	Inheritance	Presentation	Age at Presentation
ABCA3 16p13.3	Lipid transport Surfactant packaging/function	AR	RDS ILD	Newborns Children
SFTPB 2p12	Surfactant packaging/function	AR	RDS	Newborns
SFTPC 8p21	Surfactant function	AD	ILD > RDS	Infants, children, adults
SFTPA 10q22.2	Tubular myelin, host defense	AD	ILD/lung cancer	Adults
TITF1 14q13	Lung, thyroid, CN morphogenesis, surfactant regulation	AR haploinsufficiency	Thyroid/lung/CNS malformations ILD	Newborns Infants
GM-CSFRα 22.32	Alveolar macrophage function	AR	PAP	Children
GM-CSF 15q31	Alveolar macrophage function	Autoimmune	PAP	Adults

AR, autosomal recessive; RDS, respiratory distress syndrome; ILD, interstitial lung disease; AD, autosomal dominant; PAP, pulmonary alveolar proteinosis.

Surfactant Protein B (SP-B)

SP-B is a hydrophobic, amphipathic 8.8-kDa protein produced from a single gene (SFTPB, OMIM 178640) located on human chromosome 2. The SP-B mRNA is expressed in nonciliated bronchiolar cells and type II alveolar cells and is translated to produce a 40- to 42-kDa precursor that is proteolytically processed in the secretory pathway of type II epithelial cells to form the active 79-amino acid peptide found in alveolar surfactant. In combination with lipids, SP-B can reconstitute most of the surface activity of natural lung surfactant. SP-B contains two regions, (Trp_9-Pro_{23}) and (Ile_{56}-Pro_{67}), predicted to form amphipathic α-helices that interact with the surface of lipid films. Almost 50% of the protein is in an α-helical conformation; the amphipathic domains of SP-B interact with surfactant lipids, and PG in particular, to promote lipid incorporation into and stabilization of the surface film. SP-B contains three intramolecular disulfide bonds that confine the amphipathic helices of SP-B in an antiparallel configuration. Intermolecular disulfide bonds stabilize SP-B dimers. Dimers and higher multimers of SP-B, which are probably stabilized by noncovalent interactions, are readily identified in pulmonary surfactant.

ProSP-B is synthesized in the ER and proteolytically processed in multivesicular and lamellar bodies by cathepsins and other intracellular proteases. The active SP-B peptide is packaged with SP-C and surfactant lipids in lamellar bodies prior to secretion into the alveolus. In the alveoli, the positively charged amino acid residues of SP-B selectively interact with the negatively charged phospholipid DPPG. In a mixed DPPC/DPPG monolayer, SP-B is believed to purify the DPPC monolayer by removal of DPPG. SP-B increases order in the lipid head groups with little effect on order on acyl chains in the lipid membrane interior. The ability to order the lipid head group region is located in the amino- and carboxy-terminal regions of SP-B (1–20) and (53–78), which contain the predicted amphipathic helices. Synthetic peptides that contain these two regions have surface-tension–lowering activity similar to that of native SP-B and peptide mimics have been developed for therapy of respiratory distress in infants. SP-B enhances the insertion (fusion) of phospholipid vesicles into a preformed DPPC/DPPG monolayer, particularly in the presence of divalent cations. SP-B causes lipids in solution to form discoid particles often appearing as stacks or sheets. Together with SP-A, lipids, and Ca^{2+}, SP-B reconstitutes the characteristic ultrastructural features of tubular myelin, producing multilamellar aggregates and square lattice configurations.

SP-B is Required for Survival After Birth Mutations in the gene encoding SP-B (SFTPB, OMIM 265120) cause acute respiratory failure at birth related to surfactant dysfunction.[12,13] Similarly, deletion of Sftpb in the developing lung or its conditional deletion in adult mice causes acute respiratory distress associated with alveolar capillary leak and surfactant deficiency.[14] Pathologic findings of patients with lung disease related to SFTPB mutations are similar to those in mice in which the Sftpb gene is deleted.[14,15] SP-B deficiency is associated with failure to form lamellar bodies, accumulation of abnormal multivesicular bodies within the type II cells, and failure to form tubular myelin or functional surfactant films after secretion into the alveoli.

Hereditary SP-B Deficiency Causes Respiratory Failure at Birth SP-B deficiency is inherited in an autosomal recessive pattern, affected infants developing respiratory failure shortly after birth. While lung morphogenesis proceeds normally in utero, the lack of SP-B results in acute atelectasis and respiratory distress, usually presenting as full-term infants with signs and symptoms of diffuse alveolar collapse after birth. More than 40 distinct SFTPB mutations in patients with SP-B deficiency have been identified.[13,15] The disorder is refractory to surfactant replacement therapy and most patients die from respiratory failure within several months after birth, requiring oxygen and ventilatory support throughout their clinical course. Lung transplantation has been offered to some patients. SP-B deficiency disrupts the formation of lamellar bodies and tubular myelin, and interferes with the processing of proSP-C to the active peptide. Thus, most SP-B–deficient patients lack both SP-B and SP-C peptides in the alveolus. In patients with SFTPB-related disease, proSP-C accumulates in the airspaces, contributing to an alveolar proteinosis–like syndrome. Pathologic diagnoses include desquamative interstitial pneumonitis (DIP), chronic pneumonitis of infancy (CPI) or infantile alveolar proteinosis, histologic changes being influenced by age, and supportive therapies (Fig. 5-3).[16] The definitive diagnosis is made by identification of SFTPB gene mutations, enabling prenatal diagnosis and genetic counseling. While various missense, nonsense, frameshift, and splice variants have been identified, 121ins2 mutation in exon 4 is the most common

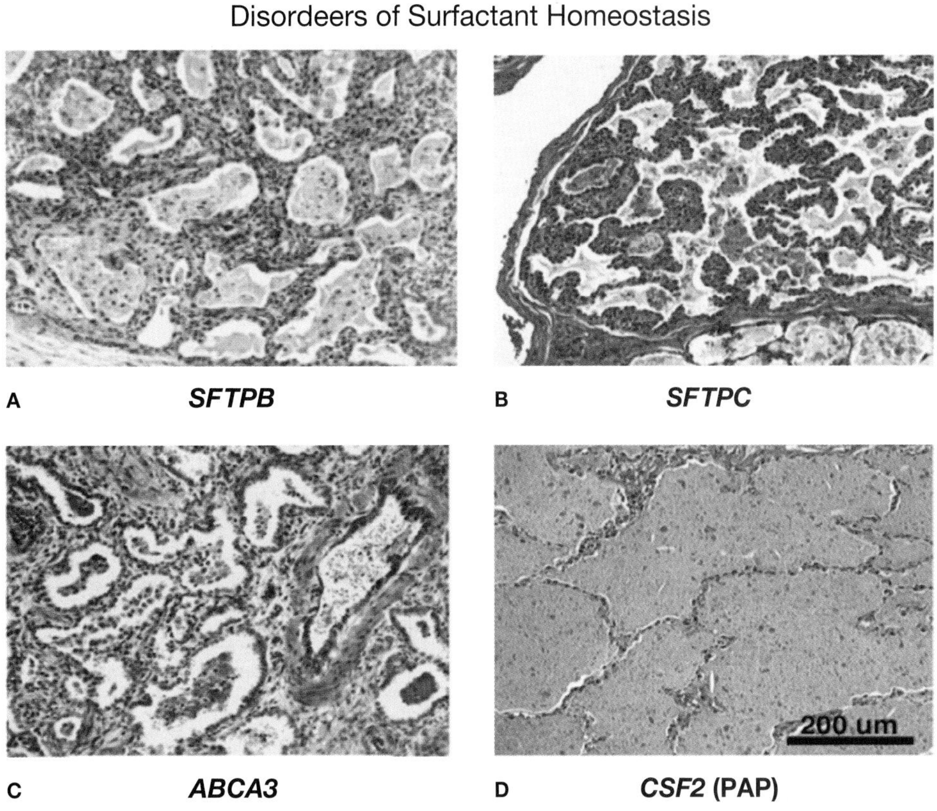

Figure 5-3 Pulmonary histopathology associated with disorders of surfactant homeostasis. Pathologic findings in eonates with mutations in SFTPB (**A**), SFTPC (**B**), and ABCA3 (**C**) are consistent with varying pathologic diagnoses, for example, childhood interstitial pneumonitis (CIP), nonspecific interstitial pneumonitis (NSIP), desquamating interstitial pneumonitis (DIP) or pulmonary alveolar proteinosis (PAP) (**D**). Severe alveolar remodeling, alveolar loss, macrophage infiltration, varying degrees of alveolar proteinosis, and stromal thickening are observed. In contrast, auto-antibodies against GM-CSF or mutations in the GM-CSF receptor (CSFR2A) are associated with pulmonary alveolar proteinosis in which surfactant lipids and proteins accumulate in the alveolus. Alveolar structure is generally well maintained in PAP. *(Reproduced with permission from Whitsett JA, Wert SE, Trapnell BC: Genetic disorders influencing lung formation and function at birth. Hum. Mol. Genet. 2004;13:R207–R215.)*

mutation.[12] In most affected infants, SP-B is lacking in bronchoalveolar lavage fluid and the abnormal proSP-C peptide accumulates in the alveoli, findings that can be verified by immunohistochemistry. Patients with SP-B deficiency do not respond to surfactant replacement and generally succumb from chronic respiratory failure early in infancy in spite of intensive care.

Surfactant Protein C (SP-C) In humans, SP-C is encoded by a single gene (SFTPC, OMIM 178620), located on human chromosome 8.[2,10] SP-C mRNA is expressed exclusively in type II epithelial cells in the lung and is translated to produce a 22-kDa precursor that is palmitoylated and proteolytically processed during intracellular transport to form the active, hydrophobic peptide of 35 amino acids stored in lamellar bodies.[2,3] After secretion, SP-C enhances the surface-active properties of lipid mixtures, lowering surface tension during compression, and enhancing adsorption rate of lipid films at the air–water interface. Both SP-C and SP-B enhance the speed of formation and stability of lipid films. A mixture of surfactant lipids and proteins SP-B and SP-C improves lung inflation and compliance and is useful for treatment of respiratory distress syndrome (RDS) in newborn infants. SP-C is palmitoylated on cysteine residues near the NH_2 terminus. The surface activity of depalmitoylated SP-C is somewhat less than that of palmitoylated SP-C, likely related to reduced stability of the α-helical domain that anchors the peptide within the lipid bilayer. Although the orientation of the palmitoyl groups in a lipid environment is not currently known with certainty, the lipid moiety on SP-C enhances the hydrophobicity of the amino-terminal region enabling its close contact with multilayered lipid films and likely serves to stabilize the α-helical, hydrophobic domain of SP-C. SP-C enhances the uptake of lipids by type II alveolar cells and plays an important role in lipid homeostasis in the alveoli.

In a lipid bilayer, the orientation of the α-helical segment of SP-C is closely parallel with the lipid acyl chains, implying a trans-bilayer orientation. In a surface monolayer, SP-C has a preferential orientation parallel to the interface, as observed by circular dichroism of monolayer films. The positive charges near the NH_2 terminus of SP-C may promote binding of phospholipid vesicles to the monolayer, a step required for insertion of phospholipids into the monolayer. SP-C forms well-defined domains within DPPC/DPPG films below the phase transition temperature of the bulk lipid. SP-C alters the size and shape of lipid vesicles, disrupting vesicular structures, causing the formation of larger vesicles and discoid particles.

Surfactant lipid films fold as a consequence of dynamic compression during the respiratory cycle in a process enhanced by SP-C and SP-B, each interacting with lipids in distinct ways. SP-B serves to stabilize the membrane-to-membrane interactions between the folded lipid layers to create multilayers.[3]

Role of SP-C in the Pathogenesis of Pulmonary Disease Deletion of Sftpc in transgenic mice perturbed surfactant function and caused severe interstitial lung disease (ILD) with advancing age.[17] While $Sftpc^{-/-}$ mice survive after birth, the mice develop emphysema, pulmonary inflammation, and abnormal lipid accumulations in alveolar macrophages, epithelial, vascular, and stromal cells. Surfactant lipid spreading and stability are only modestly perturbed in the absence of SP-C in vivo. The severity of pulmonary disorder related to SP-C deficiency in mice is strongly influenced by genetic strain, age, and other injuries, indicating that both genetic and environmental factors influence lung structure and function in the absence of SP-C. SP-C binds bacterial endotoxin, supporting a role in innate host defense in the lung. SP-C–deficient mice are susceptible to viral and bacterial pathogens and develop severe pulmonary injury in mouse models of pulmonary fibrosis. The finding that $Sftpc^{-/-}$ mice develop an interstitial pulmonary disorder is consistent with findings in humans, wherein SFTPC mutations cause both acute and chronic lung disease.

Mutations in SFTPC Cause Severe Interstitial Lung Disease in Humans Mutations in SFTPC represent a rare cause of acute and chronic lung disease in humans.[18,19] SFTPC mutations are generally inherited as an autosomal dominant gene that has been causally linked to acute respiratory disease in newborn infants and more commonly, to chronic ILD in infants, children, and adults. De novo mutations in the SFTPC gene have been reported. The diagnosis of SFTPC-related lung disease (OMIM 610913) is usually made during infancy, but can present later in life, the severity of disease varying in a single extended family.[19] Most mutations occur in the C-terminal BRICHOS domain of proSP-C that serves as an intramolecular chaperone for the metastable membrane-spanning helical domain.[20] The mutant proSP-C protein is misfolded and/or misrouted resulting in intracellular accumulation. Most mutations result in the lack of synthesis of the active SP-C peptide that may influence the pathogenesis of lung disease. Various forms of ILD have been associated with the disease, including acute RDS in newborns, CPI, nonspecific interstitial pneumonitis (NSIP), and other forms of idiopathic pulmonary fibrosis (IPF) (Fig. 5-3).[16] Lung histopathology associated with SFTPC mutations is likely influenced by age, duration and severity of the disease, treatment, and both genetic and environmental factors. Infants with SFTPC mutations often present with severe respiratory signs and symptoms following viral infections. Definitive diagnosis is made by identification of mutations in the SFTPC gene. The onset and severity of pulmonary disease in humans is highly variable, even in the same kindreds, indicating that genetic and environmental factors strongly influence the disorder. At present, there is no effective therapy for SP-C–related disease. Lung transplantation has been offered for treatment of hereditary SFTPC deficiency in patients with respiratory failure. Mutations in SFTPC are a rare cause of acute and chronic ILD. More than 50 distinct mutations in SFTPC have been associated with clinical lung disease and include missense, frameshift, splice, insertions, and deletions that generally disrupt the structure of the C-terminal BRICHOS domain. The most common mutation, I73T, is found in more than one-third of patients.

ABCA3 Mutations Cause Respiratory Failure at Birth ABCA3 is a large, membrane-spanning transport protein that is present in the limiting membrane of lamellar bodies in type II epithelial cells (Fig. 5-2). More than 140 different mutations associated with severe lung disease in newborn infants have been identified, ABCA3 mutations (OMIM 610921) representing the most common genetic cause of neonatal respiratory failure.[1,4,21,22] While expressed in many tissues, patients with mutations in ABCA3 present with isolated lung disease, and abnormalities in other organ structures or functions have not been observed. Pathologic findings in newborn infants with respiratory failure are similar to those in mice wherein ABCA3 has been genetically deleted. ABCA3-related lung disease is generally inherited as an autosomal recessive disorder (Table 5-1). Affected infants present with severe respiratory failure characteristic of surfactant deficiency within the first days of life. Their lung disease is refractory to conventional therapies, resulting in respiratory failure and death within the first months of life. Pathologic findings are similar to those in SFTPB-related disease, and include alveolar proteinosis, lipoid pneumonia, cuboidal epithelial cell hyperplasia, interstitial thickening, loss of normal alveolar structures, and features of DIP (Fig. 5-3).[16] Older children present with features of NSIP. In newborn infants, respiratory failure is not responsive to surfactant replacement. Lung transplantation has been offered to some patients. ABCA3 is a member of the ATP-dependent, Walker domain–containing proteins that comprise a family of membrane-associated transport proteins that includes the cystic fibrosis transmembrane conductance regulator (CFTR). ABCA3 mediates PC and PG transport into lamellar bodies. The diagnosis of ABCA3-related lung disease is confirmed by nucleotide sequencing of the gene in infants and children with refractory pulmonary disease. While most mutations cause respiratory failure in infancy, the E292V mutation is associated with less severe lung disease, these patients often presenting with ILD later in childhood. Ultrastructural analysis of lung tissue from patients with ABCA3 mutations usually demonstrates the presence of small, atypical lamellar bodies in type II epithelial cells and the absence of tubular myelin in the airways, indicating an abnormality in both intracellular and extracellular lipid homeostasis. The processing of proSP-B is disrupted in some patients with ABCA3-related lung disease.[13]

Role of TITF1 in Surfactant Homeostasis TITF1, encoding the homeodomain-containing nuclear transcription factor, thyroid transcription factor-1 (TTF-1), plays a critical role in lung morphogenesis and the expression of SPs.[23,24] TTF-1 is expressed in the central nervous system, thyroid, and lung and is required for lung formation during embryonic development.[24] TTF-1 regulates the SP genes (SFTPA, B, C, and D), ABCA3, SLC34a2, all expressed in alveolar type II epithelial cells.[23] SLC34a2, is a phosphate transporter associated with the disease pulmonary alveolar microlithiasis.[25] Mutations in TITF1 have been linked to disorders of the central nervous system, thyroid, and lung (OMIM 600635), and more than 150 patients have been reported to date.[26,27] TTF-1–related lung disorders are generally inherited as heterozygous mutations resulting in lung dysfunction of varying severity, ranging from disordered alveolar morphogenesis, surfactant deficiency with respiratory failure in neonates and infants, and ILD in older patients. The majority of patients with TITF1 mutations present with severe lung disease, approximately half of which have a spectrum of brain, thyroid, and lung disease. Histologic findings vary greatly with severe abnormalities in the alveoli, and variable loss of SPs and lipids. Pulmonary disease associated with TITF1 mutations is frequently accompanied by congenital hypothyroidism. The severity of TITF1-related CNS, thyroid, and pulmonary disease varies widely in patients with TITF1 mutations. Diagnosis is made by identification of mutations in the TITF1 gene.

THE PULMONARY COLLECTIONS (SP-A AND SP-D)

■ SURFACTANT PROTEIN A (SP-A)

SP-A is an abundant hydrophilic 26-kDa (monomer) glycoprotein that functions in the host defense, and regulation of extracellular surfactant lipid structure. SP-A mRNA is expressed in nonciliated bronchiolar and alveolar type II epithelial cells in the lung, being translated from two genes (SFTPA1 and 2) located on chromosome 10 in the human.[2,9,11] SP-A in combination with SP-B and SP-C enhances formation of a surface lipid film in the presence of divalent ions, but is not critical for surfactant activity in the alveoli. The amino-terminal third of SP-A is arranged in a collagen-like triple helix, while a carboxy-terminal region has structural similarity to mammalian lectins including SP-D, serum mannose-binding lectin (MBL), and C1q. Protein–protein interactions among SP-A molecules are mediated by the collagen-like domains via intermolecular disulfide bonds that are necessary for SP-A–mediated aggregation of lipids and formation of tubular myelin. Binding and uptake of SP-A by type II alveolar cells and alveolar macrophages are mediated by specific, saturable cell surface receptors; however, the precise nature of the SP-A receptors and their intracellular functions remain unclear.[28] Both collagenous and noncollagenous domains of SP-A bind to isolated type II alveolar cells and immune cells. SP-A increases the association of lipids with type II cells but does not appear to increase internalization of lipid. Deletion of the SP-A gene (Sftpa) in mice does not alter survival or lung function after birth. While tubular myelin is absent, surfactant function, uptake, and secretion are not strongly influenced by deletion of Sftpa in mice.[29] Nevertheless, Sftpa$^{-/-}$ mice are highly susceptible to lung infections by bacterial, viral, and fungal pathogens, indicating that SP-A plays an important role in innate host defense of the lung.[2,9,11]

Usual Interstitial Pulmonary Disease Caused by Mutations in SFTPA2

Missense mutations in the gene encoding SP-A (SFTPA2) have been linked to pulmonary fibrosis pathologically diagnosed as usual interstitial pneumonitis (UIP) (OMIM 178642), generally presenting as ILD in the 4th and 5th decades of life.[30,31] Increased risk of pulmonary adenocarcinoma was observed at more advanced ages. This rare disorder is inherited as an autosomal dominant mutation in which the oligomerization and intracellular trafficking of SP-A(2) is disturbed, resulting in the unfolded protein response and chronic alveolar cell injury.

■ SURFACTANT PROTEIN D (SP-D)

SP-D is a collagenous Ca^{2+}-dependent carbohydrate-binding protein that is structurally related to SP-A and other C-type lectins.[11] SP-D is encoded by a single gene (SFTPD) located near the SFTPA genes on human chromosome 10.[2,9,11] SP-D is synthesized by alveolar type II epithelial cells and nonciliated bronchiolar cells in the lung, but it is also expressed in many other tissues. SP-D forms large oligomers that bind carbohydrates and glycolipids on the surface of bacteria, fungi, and viruses. The interaction of SP-D with microbial pathogens is Ca^{2+}- and carbohydrate-dependent.[11] In contrast to other SPs (SP-A, SP-B, and SP-C), SP-D is not strongly associated with surfactant lipids in the alveolus but plays an important role in determining surfactant structure and homeostasis.

Functions of SP-D In Vivo

Deletion of Sftpd in mice has provided insight into its important role in surfactant and alveolar homeostasis. $Sftpd^{-/-}$ mice survive after birth, but develop severe pulmonary disease associated with macrophage activation, airspace enlargement, and marked accumulation of surfactant lipids in the alveoli.[32,33] SP-D regulates alveolar pools of large and small aggregate surfactant, influencing surfactant particle size and its uptake by type II epithelial cells. Addition of SP-D to surfactant lipid extracts enhances surfactant stability in vitro and protects the preterm lung from endotoxin-induced injury. Infiltration with lipid-laden macrophages, and the induction of synthesis of metalloproteinases 2, 9, and 12 by alveolar macrophages, may contribute to the spontaneous airspace remodeling seen in the $Sftpd^{-/-}$ mice. $Sftpd^{-/-}$ mice are highly susceptible to pulmonary infections and inflammation associated with viral (respiratory syncytial and influenza virus), bacterial, and endotoxin or fungal exposures, indicating that SP-D plays a critical role in innate host defense of the lung.[2,9,11] SP-D binds bacterial, fungal, and viral pathogens, enhancing their opsonization and their killing by alveolar macrophages. Levels of SP-D are low in preterm infants and in infants and older patients with chronic lung disease. SP-D influences immunologic responses to allergens, interacting with alveolar macrophages and lymphocytes in the innate immune system. Thus, SP-D plays an important role in the regulation of surfactant lipid homeostasis, innate host defense of the lung, and prevention of inflammation and alveolar remodeling. Susceptibility to influenza A viral infections has been linked to specific SFTPD alleles, but to date, mutations in SFTPD have not been directly linked to acute or chronic lung disease.

■ RECYCLING AND CATABOLISM OF SURFACTANT LIPIDS AND PROTEINS

Pulmonary surfactant is taken up rapidly in the lung, and much of the lipid is reutilized (Fig. 5-2). After intratracheal administration, labeled lipid appears in type II cells and alveolar macrophages, but is not found in type I cells, indicating that the type II cells actively take up surfactant lipids from the alveolus for recycling or catabolism. Isolated epithelial type II alveolar cells internalize ^{3}H-PC and resecrete the internalized material or degrade it with reincorporation into other lipids. Isolated type II cells endocytose SP-C and SP-B. SP-A also binds to type II epithelial cells and is endocytosed by a receptor-mediated mechanism. While a number of candidate SP-A and SP-D receptors and binding proteins have been identified, whether the proteins are efficiently recycled and mechanisms by which they signal to influence surfactant homeostasis remain unclear.

Pulmonary surfactant as isolated from lavage fluid exists in several forms that can be fractionated based on density. In vivo labeling indicates that phospholipid is initially secreted in the heaviest forms, followed by conversion into distinct heavy and light forms. The most dense or ultraheavy form contains lamellar bodies and tubular myelin. Small aggregate forms are comprised of small unilamellar vesicles. While their lipid composition is similar to that of large aggregates, small aggregates are depleted of SP-A, SP-B, and SP-C, and lack surfactant function. SP-A and SP-D play important roles in the maintenance of the large aggregate surfactant structures. Cycling surfactant by expansion and contraction of a surface film in vitro converts lipids from large to small aggregates that are likely remnants destined for catabolism or recycling. See Perez-Gil and Weaver[3] for review.

REGULATION OF SURFACTANT PRODUCTION

The synthesis of pulmonary surfactant is subject to precise regulatory controls both during development and postnatally.[34] Surfactant phospholipid synthesis increases markedly in late gestation and is enhanced by a variety of hormones, including glucocorticoids in the fetal lung. Lung phospholipid content increases in the latter two-thirds of gestation in preparation for respiratory adaptation at birth. Prenatal glucocorticoids are routinely used to induce lung maturation and surfactant synthesis in infants at risk for preterm delivery.[7] Glucocorticoids reduce the risk of IRDS and enhance the efficacy of surfactant replacement therapy after birth. Like surfactant phospholipids, the SPs are highly regulated, increasing in the latter two-thirds of gestation in the mammalian species studied. Expression of SPs is regulated in complex ways by a variety of hormonal agents. The levels of SP mRNA increase in the perinatal period in association with increased surfactant synthesis and secretion required for postnatal respiratory adaptation. Expression of the SPs is regulated at both transcriptional and posttranscriptional levels, maintaining steady-state protein concentrations within tight constraints in the adult lung. Surfactant production is, in general, enhanced by glucocorticoids, epidermal growth factor (EGF), and cyclic adenosine monophosphate (cAMP) but inhibited by tumor necrosis factor-α (TNF-α), transforming growth factor-β(TGF-β), and insulin, depending on experimental conditions. Transcriptional control of the surfactant genes is modulated by a number of nuclear transcription factors, for example, TTF-1, cyclic AMP-responsive binding protein (CREBPα), members of the forkhead family transcription factors (FOXA2), retinoic acid receptors (RARs), sterol-responsive element-binding protein (SREBP), GATA-binding proteins, Krüppel-like factor 5 (KLF-5), NFATC3, and coactivators associated with these transcription factors.[35] In the lung, surfactant proteins A, B, and D are expressed in nonciliated bronchiolar and type II alveolar cells, while SP-C is expressed exclusively in type II alveolar cells. Transcriptional, epigenetic, and posttranscriptional mechanisms influence the synthesis of SPs and lipids, regulating surfactant concentrations in the airspace during development and repair.

■ SURFACTANT SECRETION

Lamellar bodies containing SPs SP-B and SP-C and lipids are secreted into the alveoli in a process mediated by activation of β-adrenergic receptors and P2×7R purinergic receptors that regulate intracellular cAMP and calcium homeostasis to influence cytoskeletal organization and secretion.[36] Recent studies support a role for the orphan receptor (GPRC116) in the regulation of surfactant secretion, loss of GPRC116 resulting in increased purinoreceptor activity, increased surfactant secretion, and increased alveolar surfactant pool sizes.[37] While secretion of surfactant lipids SP-B and SP-C occurs via lamellar bodies, secretion of surfactant-associated proteins SP-A and SP-D occurs via a distinct, vesicular secretory pathway (Fig. 5-2). Interactions of SP-A and SP-D with lipids occur after their secretion into the alveoli.

GM-CSF Signaling Regulates Surfactant Clearance

Mutations in the genes encoding the GM-CSF receptor (CSFR2A, OMIM 13899) and autoantibodies against CSF2 (GM-CSF) have been associated with early-onset PAP in children and in adults, respectively.[5,38] While less than 10% to 15% of surfactant lipids is cleared by catabolism in alveolar macrophages, this pathway is critical in controlling steady-state surfactant concentrations in vivo. Granulocyte macrophage colony–stimulating factor (GM-CSF or CSF2) and GM-CSF receptors are required for normal surfactant catabolism. See Suzuki et al.[5] and Trapnell et al.[39] for review. SP and lipid clearance are decreased in Csf2 and Csfr2a gene–deleted mice causing PAP in which SPs and phospholipids accumulate in the lung. Findings in the mouse models led to the discovery that GM-CSF signaling abnormalities cause idiopathic PAP.[5,40] Clinical studies demonstrate that idiopathic PAP in adults is usually caused by autoantibodies against GM-CSF.[38] Similar abnormalities in surfactant homeostasis, alveolar macrophage morphology, and function are observed in patients with PAP, whether caused by mutations in GM-CSF receptors or by neutralization of GM-CSF by autoantibodies. Lung lavage and GM-CSF, given systemically or by aerosol, have been successfully used to treat adults with PAP (see Chapter 70).

SURFACTANT HOMEOSTASIS AND REPLACEMENT IN INFANTILE RESPIRATORY DISTRESS SYNDROME

IRDS is associated with prematurity, the risk increasing as gestational age decreases. In addition to the morphologic immaturity of the respiratory tract, lung phospholipid content and surfactant secretion are decreased in preterm infants. While functional surfactant can be isolated from infants with IRDS, surfactant pool sizes are markedly decreased in the preterm compared to the term infant and the surface activity of surfactant from infants with IRDS is decreased. Alveolar–capillary leak of blood or serum proteins inactivate surfactant function. Decreased alveolar surfactant activity associated with pulmonary immaturity causes atelectasis, alveolar collapse, pulmonary hemorrhage, and hypoxemia in preterm infants. A schematic representing factors influencing the pathogenesis of IRDS is provided by Figure 5-4.[41]

Supplemental oxygen and mechanical or assisted ventilation is routinely used to treat IRDS. During the last two decades, widespread use of exogenous surfactant has markedly ameliorated the morbidity and mortality associated with IRDS in preterm infants. Exogenous surfactants – in the form of synthetic mixtures of phospholipids and extracts of lung or surfactant containing bovine or porcine SPs B, C, and phospholipids – have been used extensively for prevention and therapy of RDS in newborn infants.[42] Surfactant replacements with preparations containing SPs B and C act rapidly, increasing lung volumes, and compliance and decreasing the requirements for positive-pressure ventilation and oxygen. Morbidity and mortality from IRDS have been markedly reduced since the application of surfactant replacement for preterm neonates, decreasing barotrauma, pneumothorax, and mortality. Surfactant replacement is given intratracheally resulting in improved lung function and oxygenation. Synthetic surfactants lacking SPs improve lung function in a delayed manner, and treatment with both synthetic and protein-containing surfactants were effective in decreasing morbidity and mortality from IRDS in clinical studies. Animal-based surfactant preparations containing SP-B and SP-C are now standard treatment for IRDS. The effectiveness of surfactant therapy is likely related to the immediate surface tension–reducing properties and to the reuptake and reutilization of the exogenous surfactant lipids by the respiratory epithelium. Following preterm birth, production of endogenous surfactant lipids and proteins by the respiratory epithelium is rapidly induced; therefore, surfactant replacement is primarily utilized in the first few days following birth. Surfactant replacement has been used successfully in the treatment of meconium aspiration and pneumonia in neonates.

SURFACTANT HOMEOSTASIS IN ADULT RESPIRATORY DISTRESS SYNDROME

ARDS occurs in association with trauma, sepsis, long bone fractures, thermal burns, and injury to the lung from aspiration of gastric contents, pneumonia, inhalation of toxic gases, and infection (see Chapter 141). In ARDS, increased permeability of the microvasculature permits leakage of protein and fluid into the lung, inactivating surfactant. Epithelial cell injury may also contribute to surfactant deficiency in ARDS. Various non-SPs and lipids present in elevated concentrations in the lung in ARDS have been implicated in reducing surface activity of pulmonary surfactant; these include immunoglobulins, albumin, fibrinogen, fatty acids, lysophosphatidylcholine, and C-reactive protein. The mechanisms causing the decrease in surfactant activity in ARDS include competition of the proteins for the air–liquid interface, sequestration and dilution of surfactant in non–surface-active particles, and inhibition of SP and lipid synthesis and secretion. Alterations in surfactant composition occur during ARDS and may precede the development of respiratory failure.[43] Phospholipid, SP-A, and SP-B concentrations are decreased, and the minimum surface tension of surfactant tested in vitro is increased

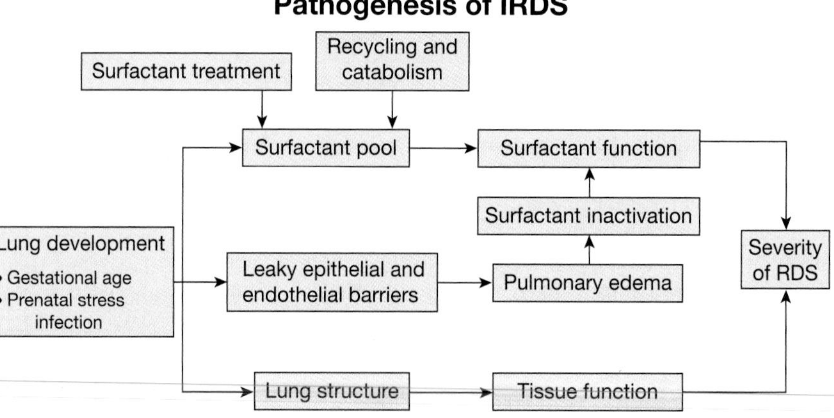

Figure 5-4 Factors influencing the pathogenesis of idiopathic respiratory distress syndrome. The pathogenesis of idiopathic RDS is multifactorial. Immaturity of the alveolar type II cells results in decreased surfactant pools. Lung collapse and injury are caused by surfactant deficiency. Alveolar damage causes leakage of serum proteins and edema that inactivate surfactant, increasing the severity of respiratory distress. Surfactant treatment reduces surface tension, restores phospholipid pool sizes, and improves alveolar–capillary leak to maintain surfactant function. *(Used with permission of Dr. Alan Jobe.)*

in patients at risk for ARDS. In ARDS, total phospholipid, PC, PG, and surfactant proteins SP-A and SP-B are decreased and the ratio of small to large aggregates is significantly increased compared to that in non-ARDS patients. Thus, ARDS leads to both a deficiency in pulmonary surfactant constituents and inhibition of the activity of the remaining surfactant. While surfactant has been effective in ARDS syndromes in laboratory experiments, to date, clinical studies have not supported the routine use of surfactant replacement for RDS in adult patients. In contrast, application of careful ventilatory support has improved outcomes in ARDS.

INHIBITION OF SURFACTANT ACTIVITY DURING LUNG INJURY

Phospholipases A_2 and C and their products, fatty acids, lysoPC, and dipalmitin inhibit surface activity in vitro. These molecules may be released or produced during lung injury. Inhibitory effects of oleic acid may be related to its miscibility with phospholipids, disrupting the interfacial surfactant film, rather than by competition for the interface. The inhibition by PAF, lysoPC, and oleic acid is not reversible, suggesting that their direct interaction with surfactant lipids disrupts lipid organization needed to form stable films. In contrast, palmitic acid improves surfactant function of preparations used for therapy of IRDS. The surface activity of pulmonary surfactant is readily destroyed by phospholipase A_2 or phospholipase C. Oxygen therapy, used routinely for ARDS and IRDS, may influence surfactant homeostasis and function in the alveolus. The rate of synthesis of surfactant lipids and clearance of radiolabeled surfactant extracts decreased in rabbits exposed to 100% O_2 for 64 h. In contrast, exposure of adult rats to 85% O_2 increased expression of surfactant proteins SP-A, SP-B, and SP-C and phospholipids. Oxidants are also released locally in the lung by activated immune cells. Activated alveolar macrophages secrete NO and superoxide, which can then react to form peroxynitrite that can oxidize and inactivate proteins and lipids.[44] Peroxynitrite inhibited the surface activity of surfactant, damaging both lipids and SPs.[42]

■ PLASMA PROTEINS INACTIVATE PULMONARY SURFACTANT

Edema fluid leaks into the airspace in both ARDS and IRDS. Edema fluid obtained from hyperoxia-exposed rabbits contains serum proteins capable of inhibiting surface activity of surfactant extracts, as evaluated in the pulsating bubble apparatus. Thus edema fluid may interfere with surfactant therapy, although the concentration dependence of the inhibition suggests that increased doses of surfactant may aid in overcoming the inhibitory effects of edema fluid. Serum albumin, globulin, and fibrinogen reduce the rate of adsorption, increase the minimum surface tension of the surfactant film, and reduce the hysteresis area between compression and expansion curves in vitro. The mechanism by which plasma proteins inhibit the activity of pulmonary surfactant is likely to be one of competition for the interface, because higher surfactant lipid concentrations overcome albumin inhibition even at high albumin concentrations. Inhibition by C-reactive protein, fibrinogen, and other plasma proteins is reversible. Addition of SP-A and organic surfactant extracts reverses inhibition caused by soluble proteins but not by lysoPC. Both SP-C and SP-B increase the ability of a phospholipid mixture to resist inhibition of surface activity by plasma proteins. SP-B is more effective than SP-C at resisting inhibition by fibrinogen. Optimal resistance to surfactant inhibition by serum protein was observed when both SP-C and SP-B were present.

REDUCTION OF SURFACTANT SYNTHESIS IN ARDS

In addition to the inactivation of pulmonary surfactant by proteins and lipids in edema fluid, a reduction of synthesis of surfactant may contribute to the decreased surfactant activity in ARDS. *Escherichia coli* endotoxin inhibited surfactant synthesis in lung organ cultures. Synthesis of SPs is also influenced by inflammatory responses following lung injury or infection. TNF-α decreased de novo synthesis of SP-A, SP-B, and SP-C mRNA and caused respiratory distress when administered intratracheally to the mouse. TGF-β1, produced during lung injury, decreased the expression of SP-A and SP-C in vitro. Thus, sepsis or lung injury may reduce both the synthesis and functions of surfactant lipids and proteins.

SUMMARY

Pulmonary surfactant is required for airbreathing after birth and for protection of the lung from microbial pathogens and toxicants. Surfactant homeostasis requires the integrated functions of SPs and lipids to reduce surface tension in the alveolus. Decreased production or inactivation of pulmonary surfactant has been associated with both IRDS and ARDS. Mutations in genes mediating surfactant synthesis (ABCA3, SFTPA, SFTPB, SFTPC, TITF1, and CSFR2A receptors) are rare genetic causes of acute or chronic lung diseases.[1–5,15,45] Identification of the genes and proteins mediating alveolar homeostasis provides the knowledge and tools to diagnose and treat rare lung diseases caused by disorders of surfactant homeostasis.

REFERENCES

1. Nogee LM. Genetic basis of children's interstitial lung disease. *Pediatr Allergy Immunol Pulmonol.* 2010;23:15–24.
2. Whitsett JA, Wert SE, Weaver TE. Alveolar surfactant homeostasis and the pathogenesis of pulmonary disease. *Annu Rev Med.* 2010;61:105–119.
3. Perez-Gil J, Weaver TE. Pulmonary surfactant pathophysiology: current models and open questions. *Physiology (Bethesda).* 2010;25:132–141.
4. Gower WA, Nogee LM. Surfactant dysfunction. *Paediatr Respir Rev.* 2011;12:223–239.
5. Suzuki T, Sakagami T, Young LR, et al. Hereditary pulmonary alveolar proteinosis: pathogenesis, presentation, diagnosis, and therapy. *Am J Respir Crit Care Med.* 2011;182:1292–1304.
6. Avery ME, Mead J. Surface properties in relation to atelectasis and hyaline membrane disease. *AMA J Dis Child.* 1959;97: 517–523.
7. Roberts D, Dalziel S. Antenatal corticosteroids for accelerating fetal lung maturation for women at risk of preterm birth. *Cochrane Database Syst Rev.* 2006;(3):CD004454.
8. Numata M, Kandasamy P, Nagashima Y, et al. Phosphatidylglycerol suppresses influenza A virus infection. *Am J Respir Cell Mol Biol.* 2012;46:479–487.
9. Hawgood S. Pulmonary surfactant: a review of protein and genomic structure. *Am J Physiol.* 1989;257(2 Pt 1):L13–L22.
10. Whitsett JA, Weaver TE. Hydrophobic surfactant proteins in lung function and disease. *N Engl J Med.* 2002;347:2141–2148.
11. Crouch EC. Collections and pulmonary host defense. *Am J Respir Cell Mol Biol.* 1989;19:177–201.
12. Nogee LM, Garnier G, Dietz HC, et al. A mutation in the surfactant protein B gene responsible for fatal neonatal respiratory disease in multiple kindreds. *J Clin Invest.* 1994;93:1860–1863.
13. Nogee LM, Wert SE, Proffit SA, et al. Allelic heterogeneity in hereditary surfactant protein B (SP-B) deficiency. *Am J Respir Crit Care Med.* 2000;161:973–981.
14. Clark JC, Wert SE, Bachurski CJ, et al. Targeted disruption of the surfactant protein B gene disrupts surfactant homeostasis, causing respiratory failure in newborn mice. *Proc Natl Acad Sci U S A.* 1995;92:7794–7798.

15. Wert SE, Whitsett JA, Nogee LM. Genetic disorders of surfactant dysfunction. *Pediatr Dev Pathol.* 2009;12:253–274.

16. Deutsch GH, Young LR, Deterding RR, et al. Diffuse lung disease in young children: application of a novel classification scheme. *Am J Respir Crit Care Med.* 2007;176:1120–1128.

17. Glasser SW, Detmer EA, Ikegami M, Na CL, Stahlman MT, Whitsett JA. Pneumonitis and emphysema in sp-C gene targeted mice. *J Biol Chem.* 2003;278:14291–14298.

18. Nogee LM, Dunbar AE, Wert SE, Askin F, Hamvas A, Whitsett JA. A mutation in the surfactant protein C gene associated with familial interstitial lung disease. *N Engl J Med.* 2001;344: 573–579.

19. Thomas AQ, Lane K, Phillips J 3rd, et al. Heterozygosity for a surfactant protein C gene mutation associated with usual interstitial pneumonitis and cellular nonspecific interstitial pneumonitis in one kindred. *Am J Respir Crit Care Med.* 2002;165:1322–1328.

20. Willander H, Askarieh G, Landreh M, et al. High-resolution structure of a BRICHOS domain and its implications for anti-amyloid chaperone activity on lung surfactant protein C. *Proc Natl Acad Sci U S A.* 2012;109:2325–2329.

21. Shulenin S, Nogee LM, Annilo T, Wert SE, Whitsett JA, Dean M. ABCA3 gene mutations in newborns with fatal surfactant deficiency. *N Engl J Med.* 2004;350:1296–1303.

22. Flamein F, Riffault L, Muselet-Charlier C, et al. Molecular and cellular characteristics of ABCA3 mutations associated with diffuse parenchymal lung diseases in children. *Hum Mol Genet.* 2012;21:765–775.

23. Bohinski RJ, Di Lauro R, Whitsett JA. The lung-specific surfactant protein B gene promoter is a target for thyroid transcription factor 1 and hepatocyte nuclear factor 3, indicating common factors for organ-specific gene expression along the foregut axis. *Mol Cell Biol.* 1994;14:5671–5681.

24. Kimura S, Hara Y, Pineau T, et al. The T/ebp null mouse: thyroid-specific enhancer-binding protein is essential for the organogenesis of the thyroid, lung, ventral forebrain, and pituitary. *Genes Dev.* 1996;10:60–69.

25. Ferreira Francisco FA, Pereira e Silva JL, Hochhegger B, Zanetti G, Marchiori E. Pulmonary alveolar microlithiasis. State-of-the-art review. *Respir Med.* 2013;107:1–9.

26. Willemsen MA, Breedveld GJ, Wouda S, et al. Brain-Thyroid-Lung syndrome: a patient with a severe multi-system disorder due to a de novo mutation in the thyroid transcription factor 1 gene. *Eur J Pediatr.* 2005;164:28–30.

27. Galambos C, Levy H, Cannon CL, et al. Pulmonary pathology in thyroid transcription factor-1 deficiency syndrome. *Am J Respir Crit Care Med.* 2010;182:549–554.

28. Kuroki Y, Mason RJ, Voelker DR. Alveolar type II cells express a high affinity receptor for pulmonary surfactant protein A. *Proc Natl Acad Sci U S A.* 1988;85:5566–5570.

29. Korfhagen TR, Bruno MD, Ross GF, et al. Altered surfactant function and structure in SP-A gene targeted mice. *Proc Natl Acad Sci U S A.* 1996;93:9594–9599.

30. Maitra M, Wang Y, Gerard RD, Mendelson CR, Garcia CK. Surfactant protein A2 mutations associated with pulmonary fibrosis lead to protein instability and endoplasmic reticulum stress. *J Biol Chem.* 2010;285:22103–22113.

31. Wang Y, Kuan PJ, Xing C, et al. Genetic defects in surfactant protein A2 are associated with pulmonary fibrosis and lung cancer. *Am J Hum Genet.* 2009;84:52–59.

32. Wert SE, Yoshida M, LeVine AM, et al. Increased metalloproteinase activity, oxidant production, and emphysema in surfactant protein D gene-inactivated mice. *Proc Natl Acad Sci U S A.* 2000;97:5972–5977.

33. Ikegami M, Na C-L, Korfhagen TR, Whitsett JA. Surfactant protein D influences surfactant ultrastructure and uptake by alveolar type II cells. *Am J Physiol Lung Cell Mol Physiol.* 2005; 288:L552–L561.

34. Mendelson CR, Boggaram V. Hormonal control of the surfactant system in fetal lung. *Annu Rev Physiol.* 1991;53:415–440.

35. Maeda Y, Davé V, Whitsett JA. Transcriptional control of lung morphogenesis. *Physiol Rev.* 2007;87:219–244.

36. Andreeva AV, Kutuzov M, Voyno-Yasenetskaya TA. Regulation of surfactant secretion in alveolar type II cells. *Am J Physiol Lung Cell Mol Physiol.* 2007;293:L259–L271.

37. Bridges JP, Ludwig M-G, Mueller M, et al. Orphan G protein-coupled receptor GPR116 regulates pulmonary surfactant pool size. *Am J Respir Cell Mol Biol.* 2013;49(3):348–357. doi: 10.1165/rcmb.2012-0439OC.

38. Kitamura T, Tanaka N, Watanabe J, et al. Idiopathic pulmonary alveolar proteinosis as an autoimmune disease with neutralizing antibody against granulocyte/macrophage colony-stimulating factor. *J Exp Med.* 1999;190:875–880.

39. Trapnell BC, Whitsett JA, Nakata K. Pulmonary alveolar proteinosis. *N Engl J Med.* 2003;349:2527–2539.

40. Dranoff G, Crawford AD, Sadelain M, et al. Involvement of granulocyte-macrophage colony-stimulating factor in pulmonary homeostasis. *Science.* 1994;264:713–716.

41. Jobe AH, Rider EO. Catabolism and recycling of surfactant. In: Robertson B, van Golde LMG, Batenburg JJ, eds. *Pulmonary Surfactant: from Molecular Biology to Clinical Practice.* Amsterdam: Elsevier; 1992:313.

42. Sinclair JC, Haughton DE, Bracken MB, Horbar JD, Soll RF. Cochrane neonatal systematic reviews: a survey of the evidence for neonatal therapies. *Clin Perinatol.* 2003;30:285–304.

43. Gregory TJ, Longmore WJ, Moxley MA, et al. Surfactant chemical composition and biophysical activity in acute respiratory distress syndrome. *J Clin Invest.* 1991;88:1976–1981.

44. Haddad IY, Ischiropoulos H, Holm BA, Beckman JS, Baker JR, Matalon S. Mechanisms of peroxynitrite-induced injury to pulmonary surfactants. *Am J Physiol.* 1993;265:L555–L564.

45. Lawson WE, Loyd JE, Degryse AL. Genetics in pulmonary fibrosis – familial cases provide clues to the pathogenesis of idiopathic pulmonary fibrosis. *Am J Med Sci.* 2011;341:439–443.

CHAPTER 6

Mucociliary Clearance

Burton F. Dickey
Michael R. Knowles
Richard C. Boucher

Mucus forms an essential barrier that protects the lungs from inhaled particles, pathogens, and toxicants. However, excessive mucus accumulation contributes to the pathogenesis of all the common diseases of the airways. Therefore, understanding airway mucus function and dysfunction is important for pulmonary medicine. The airway mucus barrier is mobile, continually propelled in a proximal direction by ciliary beating. Ciliary dysfunction causes disease both because of the failure to clear xenobiotics from the lungs and because it results in mucus accumulation. Mucus and ciliary biology will be considered together in this chapter as they interact to achieve, or fail to achieve, airway clearance.

MUCOCILIARY CLEARANCE IN HEALTH

■ AIRWAY SURFACE LIQUID

Liquid in the airway lumen is distributed between two distinct layers—a mobile mucus layer and a stationary periciliary layer (Fig. 6-1). Secreted polymeric mucins are the principal macromolecular components of the mucus layer, whereas membrane-tethered mucins and nonmucin glycoconjugates are the principal macromolecular components of the periciliary layer.

Mucus Layer

Normal mucus has physical characteristics on the border between a viscous fluid and a soft and elastic solid. Its physical state can vary with the extent of hydration and other conditions as described below in Mucociliary Dysfunction in Disease. Mucus is formed by a network of mucin polymers in water, with water accounting for ~98% of the mass, mucins 0.7%, and salts and nonmucin macromolecules the remainder. Mucins are exceedingly large glycoproteins (monomeric masses up to 3×10^6 Da) that link up to form long chains and branched networks. MUC5AC and MUC5B are the major secreted mucins in the airways.[1–3] They exhibit similar molecular weights and primary structure (Fig. 6-2A), but differ in function (see Secretory Cells) and polymer structure. Whereas MUC5B forms end-to-end polymers (Fig. 6-2B), emerging data suggest that MUC5AC forms branched covalent networks. They have characteristic regions rich in serine and threonine residues linked by their hydroxyl side groups to sugar chains (*O*-glycosylation) that account for 50% to 90% of the mass of mucins.

Mucins are packaged dehydrated in secretory granules. After secretion, they rapidly adsorb several hundred fold their mass of water, so it is critical there be sufficient airway surface liquid.[4] Insufficient liquid results in formation of a gel that is too viscoelastic to be readily cleared by ciliary motion or cough. Once immobile mucus plaques are formed, they swell only very slowly if subsequently exposed to additional liquid because of the high degree of entanglement of the mucin polymers. Besides the need for sufficient surface liquid, adequate bicarbonate must be present in the liquid to allow proper mucus maturation by chelating calcium. In secretory granules, calcium organizes the folding of mucin polymers, and must dissociate to allow mucus expansion.[5–7] Chloride and bicarbonate are both secreted into

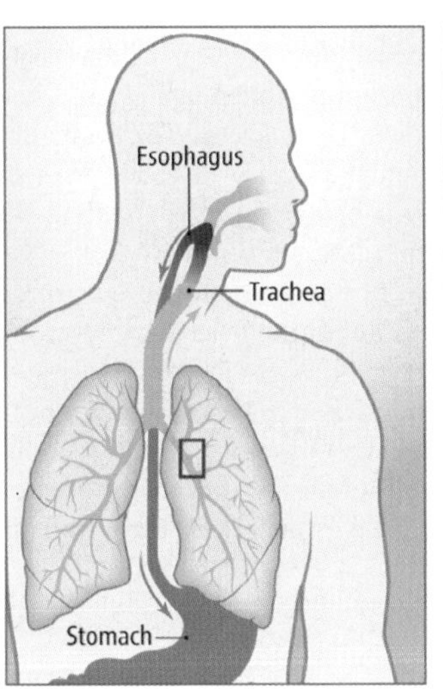

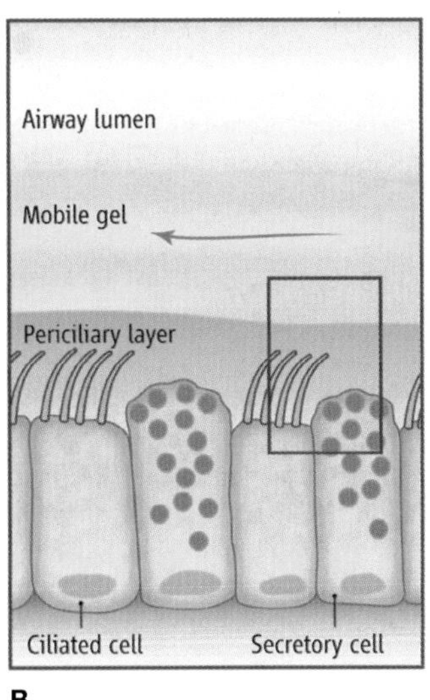

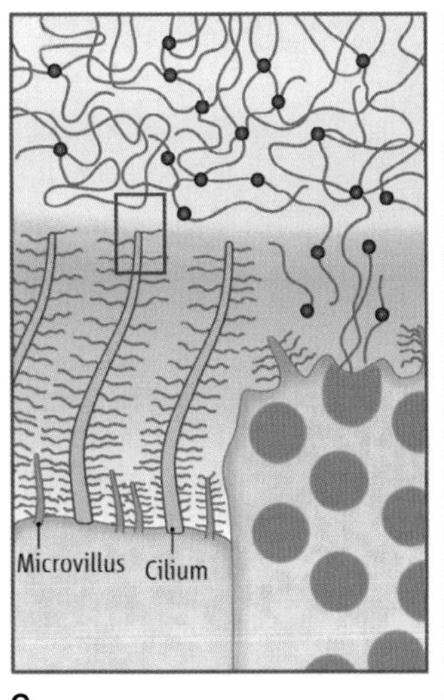

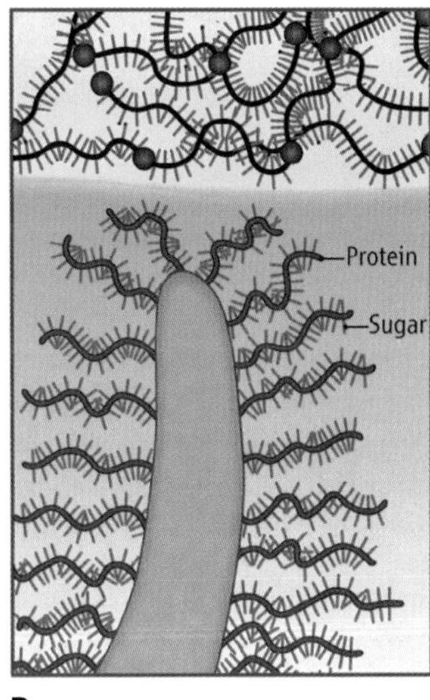

Figure 6-1 Airway surface liquid layers. **A.** Mucus is continuously produced in the conducting airways of the lungs, and swept by ciliary action from distal to proximal airways. After passing through the larynx, mucus is swallowed. **B.** The mobile mucus layer *(light blue)* glides over a periciliary layer of higher osmotic modulus *(dark blue)*. **C.** Airway secretory cells synthesize and secrete mucin polymers that interact with water to form the mobile mucus layer. Ciliated cells are covered by a dense glycocalyx containing glycosaminoglycans, membrane-tethered mucins, and other glycoconjugates that give the periciliary layer its high osmotic modulus. **D.** Mucin polymers are illustrated in the mucus layer with the protein core shown in *black*, sugar side chains in *blue*, and sites of end-to-end polymerization as *black circles*. Membrane-tethered mucins are shown densely coating cilia, while other glycoconjugates are not illustrated. *(Reproduced with permission from Dickey BF: Biochemistry. Walking on solid ground, Science. 2012;337(6097):924–925.)*

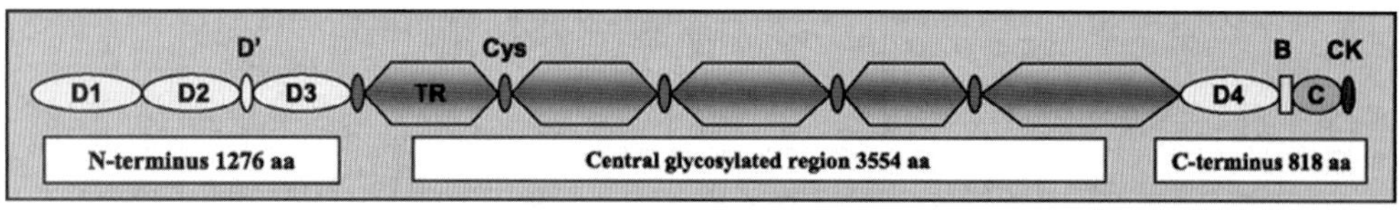

A

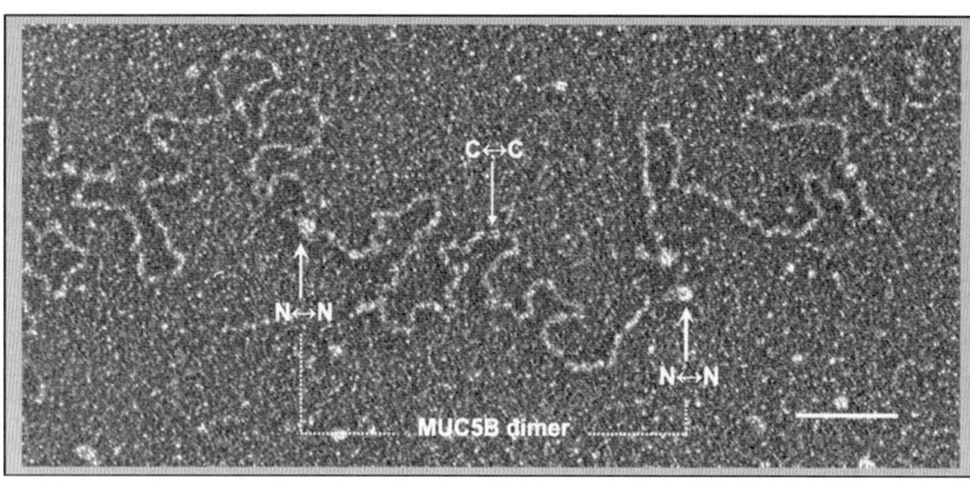

B

Figure 6-2 The structure of MUC5B. **A.** Structural domain representation of the MUC5B monomer. MUC5B has Von Willebrand factor (VWF)-like domains at NH_2- and COOH-terminal regions (D, B, C, and CK domains). The central region contains five heavily glycosylated, tandem repeat (TR), mucin domains and five small cysteine-rich (cys) regions. **B.** Electron microscopy image of a conformationally relaxed, linear MUC5B molecule. The MUC5B intact molecule in mucus is assembled from disulfide bond-mediated interactions between COOH-terminal domains of monomers to form dimers, and subsequent interactions between NH_2-terminal domains to form higher polymer oligomers. The assignment of the structure as a dimer (dotted bar) is made on the basis of the length (850 nm), which is greater than that obtainable by a single MUC5B monomer. The N↔N terminal region and C↔C terminal region can be identified by their size. Scale bar, 100 nm. *(Reproduced with permission from Kesimer M1, Makhov AM, Griffith JD, et al. Unpacking a gel-forming mucin: a view of MUC5B organization after granular release. Am J Physiol Lung Cell Mol Physiol. 2010;298(1):L15-L22.)*

the airway lumen by the cystic fibrosis transmembrane regulator (CFTR). Since the airway epithelium is quite water-permeable, water follows chloride and bicarbonate into the airway lumen.[8] Additional hydration can be provided by other chloride channels as described below in "Mucociliary Dysfunction Disease the sections "Secretory Cells" and "Asthma."

Mucus is produced throughout the conducting airways down to the level of the smallest bronchi and the larger bronchioles, but not in terminal or respiratory bronchioles (Fig. 6-3A). Bronchioles lack submucosal glands, and overall it is estimated that two-thirds of airway mucus is produced by surface epithelial cells and one-third by submucosal glands in primates (Fig. 6-3B).[9] In the most distal airways, the mucus layer is vanishingly thin, but it becomes increasingly thick as it travels proximally, both because additional production adds to its bulk and because the total cross-sectional area of the airways progressively narrows. In the trachea, the mucus gel layer is ~50 μm thick. Besides mucus acting as a simple physical barrier, the mucin sugar side chains act as a combinatorial library to bind particles and pathogens, and a thicker mucus layer has been shown to protect against infection.[10]

Periciliary Layer

It was widely believed until recently that cilia beat in a watery layer of lower density than the overlying mucus layer. However, recent data indicate that the periciliary layer has a higher density than the mucus layer due to a high concentration of membrane-tethered mucins (MUC 1, 4, and 16) and mucopolysaccharides (also called glycosaminoglycans).[11-13] This finding has several important implications for airway function.[14] First, it helps to explain how distinct layers form because dense packing of the grafted glycoconjugates of the periciliary layer tends to exclude the unattached polymeric mucins of the mucus layer (Fig. 6-1C). Second, charged polymers are highly effective lubricants in an aqueous environment, allowing low friction ciliary beating despite the high density of grafted glycoconjugates, and low friction between the periciliary and gel layers. Third, spatial impingement by grafted glycoconjugates may physically couple neighboring cilia to coordinate their beating (Fig. 6-1C). Fourth, glycoconjugates are grafted with increasing density from the top of the periciliary layer to the bottom, which should propel exogenous particles and pathogens out of the periciliary layer for removal by the mobile mucus layer. Fifth, the higher density of water-avid glycoconjugates in the periciliary layer and their grafting to the cell surface results in a nearly constant amount of liquid in this layer except under conditions of severe underhydration. In conditions of overhydration, liquid is transferred to the mucus layer, which is generally well tolerated.

■ AIRWAY EPITHELIAL CELLS

The surface airway epithelium forms a mosaic of two major cell types—secretory and ciliated (Figs. 6-1, 6-4, and 6-5). In addition, basal cells that do not contact the airway lumen serve as progenitors in the proximal airways, and neuroendocrine cells that secrete basolaterally toward sensory neurons are scattered throughout the airways. Secretory and ciliated cells are multilayered and have a tall columnar shape in proximal airways but become single layered and progressively shorter in distal airways until they have a cuboidal shape in bronchioles. Ciliated cells are more abundant than secretory cells in proximal airways, whereas secretory cells are more abundant in distal airways.

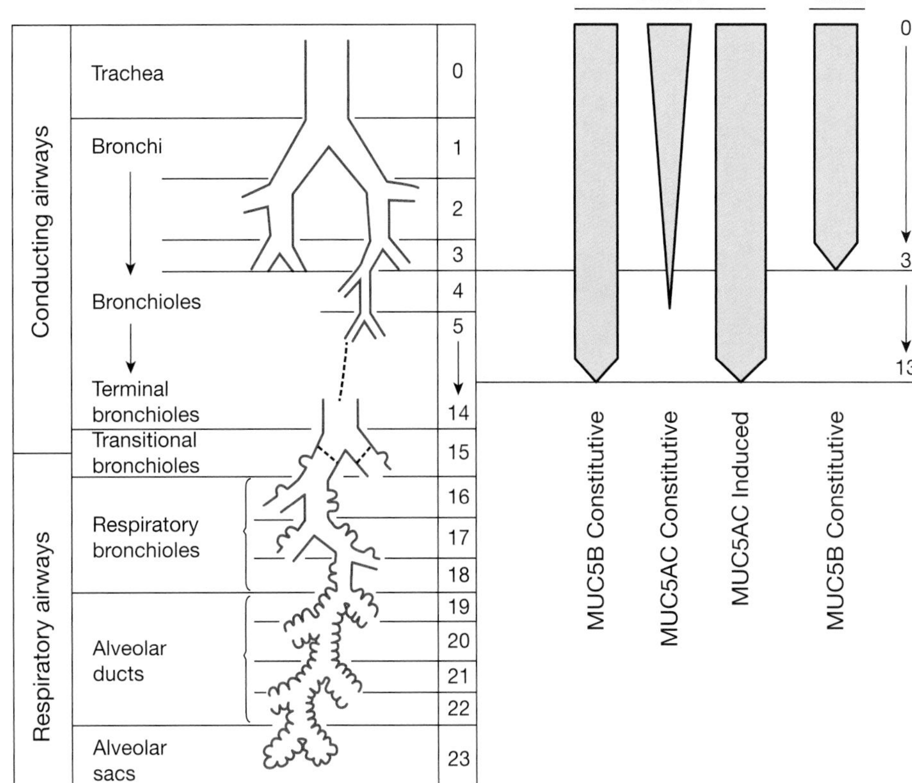

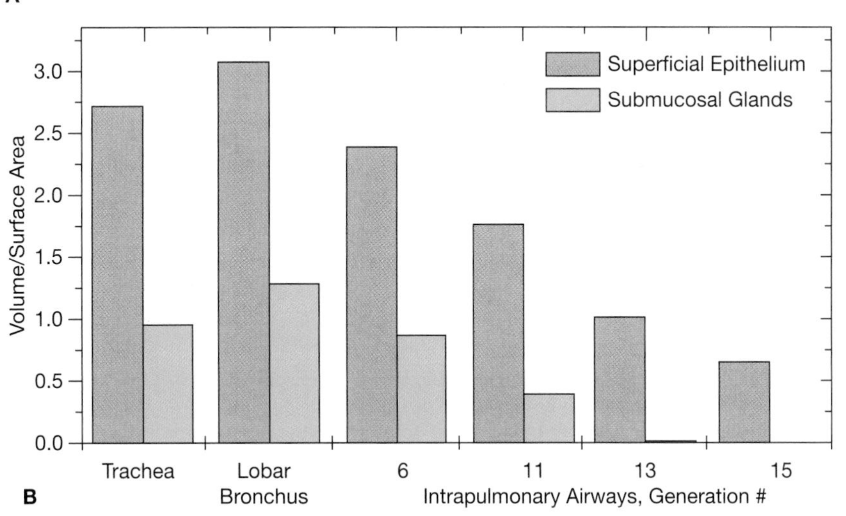

Figure 6-3 Mucin production in conducting airways. **A.** MUC5B is produced constitutively by surface epithelium down to the level of bronchioles proximal to terminal bronchioles, and by submucosal glands present in the trachea and bronchi but not bronchioles. MUC5AC is produced constitutively by surface epithelial cells with a goblet morphology in more proximal airways, and its production can be induced in nongoblet secretory cells that produce MUC5B down to the level of terminal bronchioles. Airway generation is listed numerically in the third column. **B.** The relative amount of mucin produced by surface epithelium and submucosal glands has been estimated by morphometric analysis of the airways of rhesus monkeys stained with Alcian blue/PAS, expressed as the ratio of volume of stained material ($mm^3 \times 10^{-3}$) per unit area of basal lamina (mm^2). *(A: Modified with permission from Weibel ER: Morphometry of the Human Lung. Heidelberg: Springer-Verlag; 1963; B: Reproduced with permission from Plopper CG1, Heidsiek JG, Weir AJ, et al. Tracheobronchial epithelium in the adult rhesus monkey: a quantitative histochemical and ultrastructural study, Am J Anat. 1989;184(1):31–40.)*

Secretory Cells

Subsets of airway secretory cells have been given different names based upon differences in their microscopic appearances, including goblet and club (Clara) cells. However, molecular techniques reveal overlap between these subsets, such as the presence of CCSP (SCGB1A1) in cells with a goblet morphology that express mucin, and the presence of MUC5B in cells with a club morphology.[15–17] Secretory cells are unified by the stable expression of an apical-regulated exocytic machinery,[18,19] whereas the presence of secretory products such as mucins and secretoglobins varies with exposure to extracellular signals that acutely regulate their expression and secretion (Fig. 6-5). Therefore, it is simplest to refer to these cells generically as airway secretory cells, while further specifying their appearance, airway level, and gene expression as appropriate.

Secretory cells in bronchi and proximal bronchioles constitutively express MUC5B (Figs. 6-3 and 6-5), whereas secretory cells in terminal and distal bronchioles do not express MUC5B either constitutively or inducibly.[1,15,20] The same bronchial and proximal bronchiolar secretory cells that express MUC5B can also express MUC5AC, with MUC5AC expressed constitutively in proximal airways but only inducibly in distal airways (Figs. 6-3 and 6-5). Mice with deletion of Muc5b die postnatally from upper and lower respiratory tract inflammation and infection.[21] In contrast, mice with deletion of Muc5ac are healthy at baseline but fail to clear parasitic worms from their guts,[22] and induced expression of Muc5ac in rat lungs prevents worms from transiting the lungs.[23] Thus, Muc5b/MUC5B appears to be the principal mucin functioning in baseline clearance of the airways, while Muc5ac/MUC5AC appears to function principally in parasite defense.

The effector function of Muc5ac in parasite defense dovetails well with the central role of IL-13 in parasite defense and the ability of IL-13 to strongly induce expression of Muc5ac/MUC5AC (>100-fold

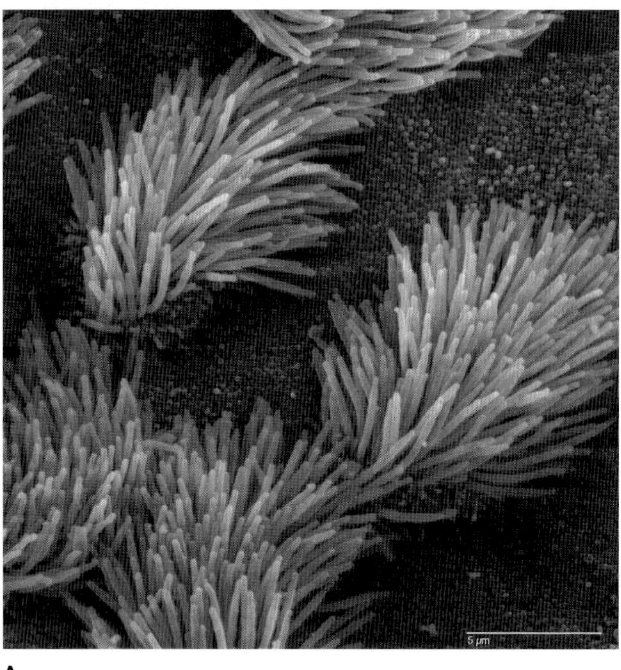

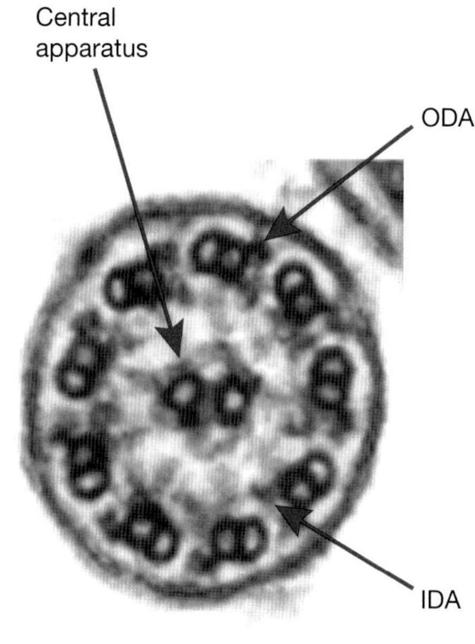

Figure 6-4 Cilia structure. **A.** Scanning electron micrograph of mouse tracheal epithelium showing both ciliated and nonciliated cells. Note the difference in size between the microvilli (on nonciliated cell surfaces) and the cilia. Scale bar, 5 µm. **B.** Transmission electron micrograph of an airway cilium in cross section showing the 9+2 configuration of the microtubules. Arrows point to the central pair of microtubules, and to the outer dynein arms (ODA) and inner dynein arms (IDA) that are critical for ciliary movement and common sites of mutation in PCD. *(A: Photograph used with permission of Charles Daghlian, Dartmouth Electron Microscope Facility. Released to the public domain, via Wikimedia Commons.)*

in cultured human airway cells and 40-fold in mice in vivo).[24–26] Other cytokines that promote mucin gene expression include IL-1β, 4, 6, 9, 23, and 25, but whether they do this directly or by amplifying the intensity of IL-13 signaling is not yet clear.[1] Complement protein C3a, epinephrine, and γ-aminobutyric acid signaling interact with IL-13 signaling to augment Muc5ac expression.[1] ClCa1 is a secreted protein that signals in an autocrine and paracrine fashion in response to IL-13 to increase Muc5ac/MUC5AC expression.[24] A network of transcription factors has been identified that regulates Muc5ac/MUC5AC expression, including STAT6, SPDEF, Foxa2, Foxa3, Notch, β-catenin and XBP-1. While some components of the signaling pathways connecting extracellular ligands with transcriptional regulation are known, such as the key roles of STAT6 downstream of IL-13 and MAPK13 downstream of ClCa1,[24,27] many details remain to be elucidated. The pathways and transcription factors regulating Muc5b/MUC5B expression have been less studied, probably reflecting the fact that expression of this mucin is relatively stable compared to Muc5ac/MUC5AC.[28] However knowledge of the regulation of MUC5B expression during development is likely to give important insight into cell fate specification in the airway, and the recent discovery of aberrant MUC5B expression in interstitial lung diseases highlights its clinical importance (see the section "Interstitial Lung Diseases"). Along with production of the polymeric mucins themselves, specialized enzymes required for glycosylation (e.g., GalNAc-T),[29] folding and polymerization (e.g., AGR2),[30] and other aspects of mucin processing are produced by airway secretory cells.

Mucins are secreted into the airway lumen at a low basal rate and a high stimulated rate. A regulated exocytic mechanism mediates both rates as indicated by abnormal phenotypes in both basal and stimulated secretion when Munc13-2, a sensor of second messengers, is deleted in mice.[16] Additional molecular components of the exocytic mechanism have been identified and their function studied (Fig. 6-6).[18,19,31,32] The rate of mucin secretion is regulated by the second messengers calcium and diacylglycerol, which are generated by a signaling cascade downstream of G-protein–coupled receptors that include the $P2Y_2$ purinergic and A3 adenosine receptors.[18,33,34] ATP is released in autocrine and paracrine fashion and activates $P2Y_2$ receptors and is metabolized to adenosine. It is possible that additional ligands such as histamine and acetylcholine may serve as secretagogues in inflammation, though they may act indirectly by causing smooth muscle contraction and nucleotide release.

As secreted mucins must adsorb large volumes of water to yield mucus of normal viscoelasticity, it is important that adequate airway lumenal water be available. The autocrine/paracrine ligands ATP, adenosine, and ClCa1 regulate the expression and/or activity of CFTR, the calcium-activated chloride channel (CaCC) TMEM16 A, and solute carrier family 26, member 9 (SLC26A9) to control chloride secretion.[24,33,35] As these same ligands regulate mucin production and/or secretion as described earlier, mucin release is thus coordinately regulated with water translocation.

Besides their role in mucin production and secretion, airway secretory cells serve as progenitors of both secretory and ciliated cells.[36] They also express components of the cytochrome P450 system that inactivates toxic inhaled organic compounds by oxidation.[37] They secrete antimicrobial peptides and reactive oxygen species constitutively, and they are capable of sensing pathogens and responding by augmenting their antimicrobial defenses and signaling to leukocytes.[38]

Ciliated Cells

Motile cilia are the defining structural and functional feature of airway ciliated cells (Fig. 6-4) (Video 6-1 Normal). They are evolutionary conserved and share homologous features with flagella of unicellular eukaryotes and mammalian sperm tails. Respiratory cilia have the "9+2" microtubular axonemal structure, which comprises nine peripheral doublets plus a central pair.[39,40] The outer doublets are linked together by proteins that form the dynein regulatory

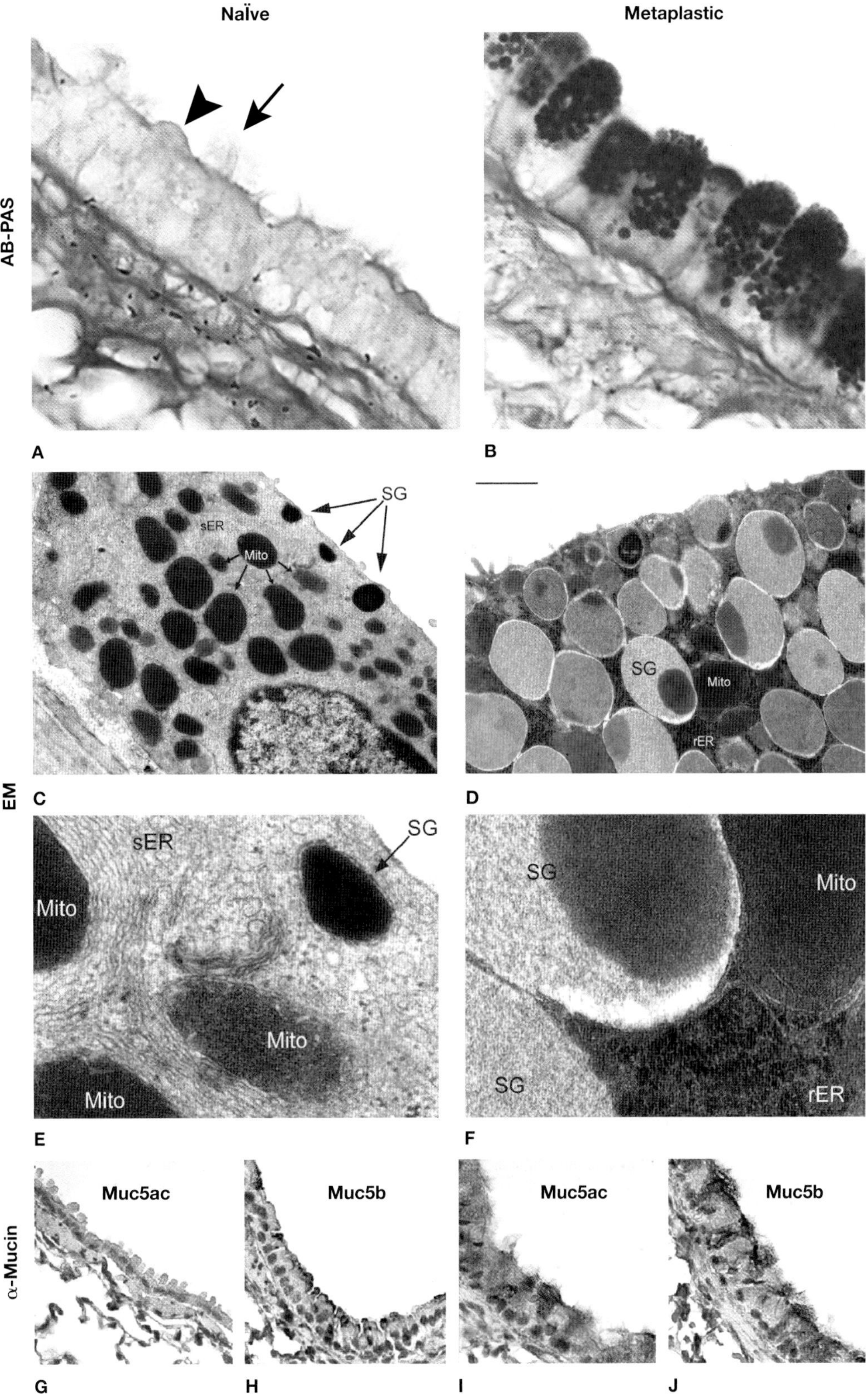

Figure 6-5 Airway epithelial mucus metaplasia. Light micrographs with AB-PAS staining (**A, B**), electron micrographs (EM) (**C–F**; low and high magnification), and immunohistochemical images using mucin-specific antibodies (**G–J**). On the left are images from the airway of a healthy mouse without airway inflammation (naïve), and on the right are images from the airway of a mouse with mucus metaplasia 3 days after the onset of allergic inflammation, as described by Evans et al.[15] Cells in the top row on the left show alternating ciliated *(arrow)* and domed secretory *(arrowhead)* cells, and on the right show prominent mucin granules in secretory cells. Cells in the EM images on the left show small numbers of electron-dense secretory granules (SG) near the apical membrane, numerous mitochondria (Mito), and abundant smooth endoplasmic reticulum (sER). Cells in the EM images on the right show numerous electron-lucent SG containing mucins and an electron-dense core, and abundant rough ER (rER). Images in the bottom row show that Muc5b is present in naïve airways even though it is not apparent by insensitive AB-PAS staining, and that both Muc5ac and Muc5b are present in the thickened metaplastic epithelium. Scale bar in the right middle panel is 10 μm for top row, 1 μm for second row, 150 nm for third row, and 30 μm for bottom row.

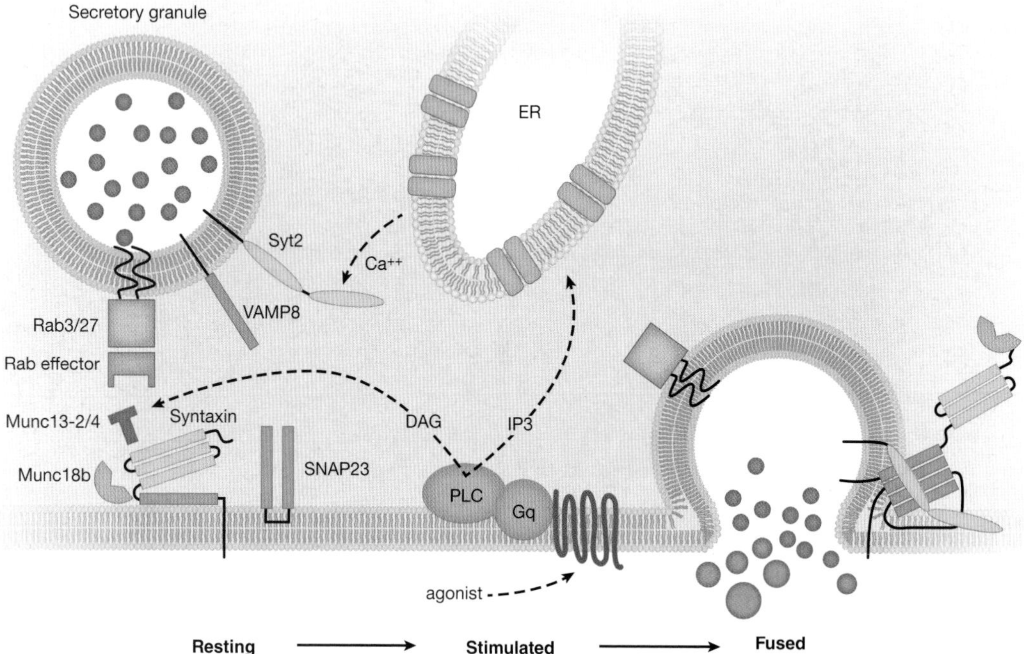

Figure 6-6 Airway mucin secretion. Initially, mucin granules become tethered to the plasma membrane by Rab proteins and their effectors in the vicinity of the exocytic SNARE proteins (VAMP8, SNAP23, and an unknown Syntaxin, shown as black bars) *(Left)*. Activation of heptahelical receptors such as those for ATP ($P2Y_2$) and adenosine (A3R) leads to activation of the trimeric G-protein, Gq, and phospholipase C (PLC), resulting in generation of the second messengers diacylglycerol (DAG) and inositol trisphosphate (IP_3). Diacylglycerol activates the priming protein Munc13-2, and IP_3 induces the release of calcium from apical ER to activate Synaptotagmin-2 (Syt2) *(Center)*. Activation of the regulatory Munc13 and Syt proteins leads to full coiling of the SNARE proteins to induce fusion of the granule and plasma membranes. The interactions of the SNARE proteins take place on a scaffold provided by Munc18b *(Right)*. *(Adapted with permission from Davis CW1, Dickey BF: Regulated airway goblet cell mucin secretion, Annu Rev Physiol. 2008;70:487–512.)*

complex (previously known as "nexin link"), and radial spokes extend from the doublets to the central pair. Taken together, these axonemal components provide the framework for generation of a complex ciliary waveform. The key components for driving ciliary movement are the inner and outer dynein arms, which are present at repetitive multiple units of 96 nm along the length of the peripheral microtubules (doublets) and contain enzymes for ATP hydrolysis to generate force for dynein arm movement. Each cilium contains >300 different proteins and is rooted in the airway epithelial plasma membrane by a basal body, which is a modified centriole. Mutations in genes encoding any part of the axonemal structure or functional components of motile cilia, or components necessary for the biogenesis of cilia, including cytoplasmic proteins, can result in primary ciliary dyskinesia (PCD), as described below in Mucociliary Dysfunction in Disease.

The function of normal motile cilia is to provide mucociliary clearance in the conducting airways, an important innate defense mechanism of the lungs.[41] Cilia provide the coordinated motive force for mechanically clearing mucus containing infectious agents, particles, and toxic substances from the conducting airways. ATP hydrolysis in the dynein arms produces sliding of adjacent axonemal structures and generates the complex ciliary waveform that occurs in human airways.[39,40] Approximately 200 cilia per cell beat in a coordinated fashion on and across cells (Video 6-1). This coordinated vectorial synchrony results from the planar orientation that occurs during ciliogenesis, as well as refinement by cilia-driven fluid flow and the tight packing of cilia due to the negatively charged glycoproteins that coat the ciliary shaft.[11,42] The ciliary forward (power) stroke is more rapid and extends a bit more into the mucus layer than the recovery stroke.[42] Cilia beat at ~6 to 12 Hz, and propel mucus proximally at ~1 mm/min. The regulation of ciliary beat frequency involves a variety of signaling molecules and multiple feedback mechanisms.[39,43] In brief, ciliary beat frequency and mucociliary clearance do not operate at full capacity under basal conditions, but can be stimulated by several intracellular signaling mechanisms including cyclic adenosine monophosphate (cAMP)– and cyclic guanosine monophosphate (cGMP)–dependent phosphorylation of axonemal components, as well as changes in intracellular calcium and pH. In contrast, protein kinase C downregulates ciliary beat frequency.

Video 6-1 Lateral view of normal ciliary activity, using high-speed videomicroscopy. Note the full range of motion (forward and backward) and coordination of ciliary beating within and across ciliated cells. *Access at www.fishmansonline.com*

Besides their role in moving the mucus layer, ciliated cells play additional crucial roles in airway homeostasis. They have a major function in ion transport across the airway luminal surface since both the epithelial Na^+ channel (ENaC) and CFTR are expressed predominantly in ciliated cells. Ciliated cells autoregulate airway surface hydration by sensing both macroscopic (e.g., airflow) and microscopic stresses (e.g., interaction of cilia with the mucus layer) and transmitting these signals into extracellular ATP release. Extracellular ATP regulates the balance between ENaC (inhibits) and CFTR (activates) to constantly adjust airway surface hydration.[44] In addition, ciliated cells are capable of flattening to cover epithelial gaps when secretory cells are injured.[45]

SUBMUCOSAL GLANDS

In bronchial airways, submucosal glands contribute to the secretion of mucins and liquid. Each gland is connected to the airway lumen by a superficial ciliated duct that propels secretions outward and a deeper nonciliated collecting duct.[46] The body of the gland is located between the spiral bands of smooth muscle and the cartilage plates in the airway wall. Mucus cells constitute ~60% of the gland volume, and serous cells, located distal to the mucus cells, make up the remaining ~40%. Glandular mucus cells express MUC5B almost exclusively with very little expression of MUC5AC.[1] The serous cells secrete anions, proteoglycans, and numerous antimicrobial proteins. The rate of submucosal gland secretion can be greatly increased by cholinergic, adrenergic, and peptidergic stimulation. In pathologic states such as COPD and cystic fibrosis (CF), the volume of submucosal glands can increase several fold while maintaining a normal ratio of mucus and serous cells.[47,48]

■ MUCOCILIARY CLEARANCE

Mucus rises up the trachea by ciliary beating, then leaves the lungs by passing through the vocal cords to enter the pharynx to be swallowed (Fig. 6-1A). The vocal cords are covered by squamous epithelium that cannot provide a propulsive surface, but the posterior commissure is covered by mucociliary epithelium and is ideally situated adjacent to the esophagus. Approximately 30 mL of respiratory mucus is propelled out of the lungs daily, carrying inhaled particles and pathogens that are excreted in the gastrointestinal tract.[49]

The rate of mucociliary clearance can be measured in human subjects by a variety of techniques, including direct bronchoscopic observation of the movement of instilled particles and external imaging of the movement of radiolabeled particles. From a practical standpoint, the only commonly used technique is the inhalation of small radiolabeled particles, such as sulfur colloid labeled with technicium-99m, followed by serial imaging with a planar gamma camera.[49,50] The movement of labeled particles from peripheral to central lung regions over the course of several hours is then measured. This technique is used for the evaluation of both disease pathophysiology and the efficacy of therapeutic interventions.[50] Mucus velocity is highest in the trachea and decreases in successive airway generations.[49] Different techniques yield different velocities, but these center around a mucus velocity of 10 mm/min in the trachea of a healthy young adult. Cough clearance provides an important backup mechanism when mucociliary clearance is impaired, and its rate can also be measured using standardized protocols of controlled coughs with imaging of the clearance of inhaled radiolabeled particles.[50]

Mucociliary clearance depends upon a mucus layer of appropriate viscoelasticity, a periciliary layer of appropriate depth, and effective ciliary beating. When these components are interacting optimally, particles and pathogens suspended in the 10,000 L of air that are inspired daily are cleared from the lungs with minimal impact on the underlying epithelium. However failure of any of these components can lead to cascading dysfunction that causes symptoms and contributes to disease pathogenesis.

■ MUCOCILIARY DYSFUNCTION IN DISEASE

The principal symptoms of mucociliary dysfunction are dyspnea and cough. Dyspnea is caused by reduction of the total cross-sectional area of the conducting airways from mucus occlusion. This occurs most commonly from diffuse plugging of small airways, but may also occur when a central airway becomes plugged by mucus due to an underlying anatomical abnormality. Cough is caused by the stimulation of vagal afferents in the intrapulmonary airways or larynx and pharynx. Patients often infer that laryngopharyngeal stimulation, described as "a tickle in the throat," results from postnasal drip because they recognize that mucus descends from the nasopharynx by gravity but are unaware it also ascends from the lungs by ciliary action. Physical signs of impaired mucus clearance include cough, bronchial breath sounds, rhonchi, and wheezes. Radiographically, retained mucus may appear as localized atelectasis or linear and branched opacities. It is important to recognize the role of retained mucus in disease presentation so that symptoms can be relieved and its contribution to disease progression addressed.

Asthma

The central role of diffuse airway obstruction by lumenal mucus in fatal asthma (Fig. 6-7) has been recognized by pathologists for more than 100 years and confirmed in multiple subsequent autopsy case series.[51,52] Mucus occlusion is particularly dangerous

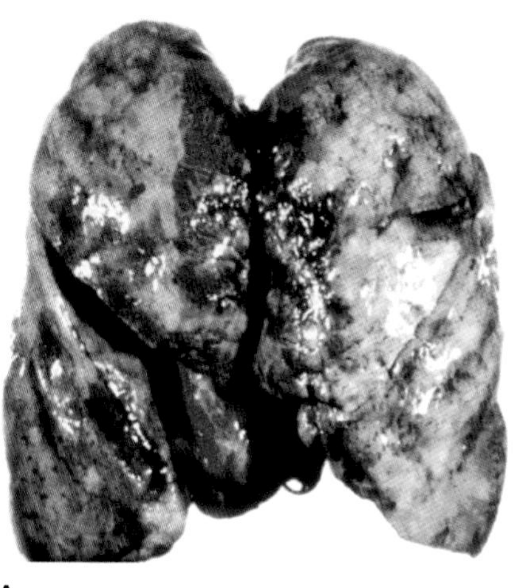
A

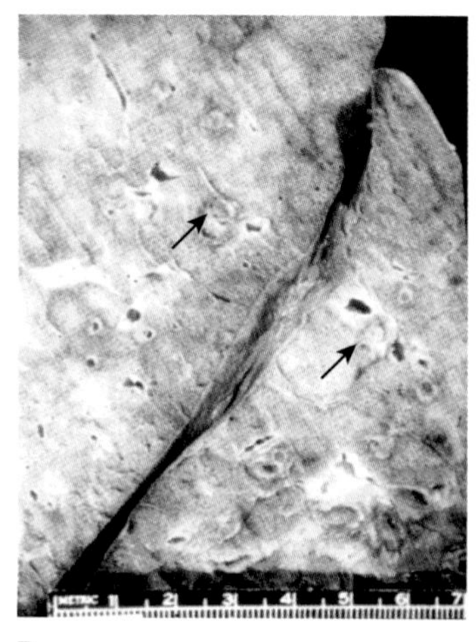
B

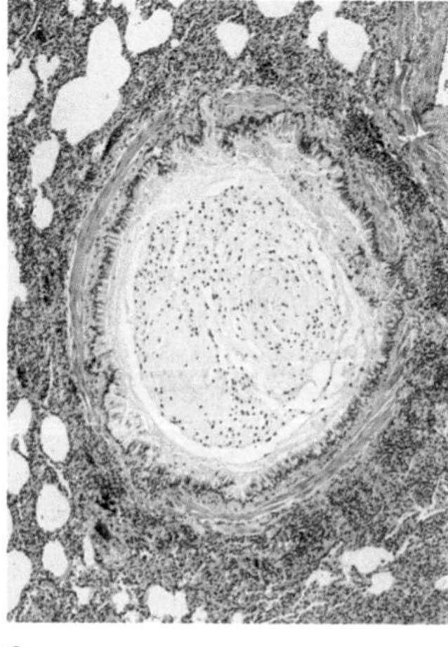
C

Figure 6-7 Airway obstruction by mucus in asthma. **A.** Lungs removed at autopsy from a patient who died from asthma. The lungs did not spontaneously collapse as they normally do because the airways were obstructed by lumenal mucus and bronchoconstriction. **B.** Cut surface of the lungs from the same patient showing mucus plugs *(arrows)* filling the large airways. **C.** Light microscopic image of a small airway from another patient who died from asthma showing infiltration of the airway wall and the lumenal mucus by inflammatory cells. *(**A, B:** Used with permission of James C. Hogg, University of British Columbia; (**C**) Used with permission of Martha L. Warnock, University of California, San Francisco.)*

in asthma because smooth muscle contraction around the lumenal plugs further constricts airflow. The principal underlying cause of mucus dysfunction in asthma is mucin overproduction. This is usually driven by allergic inflammation mediated by IL-13,[53] though IL-17 can also cause mucin overproduction and airway hyperresponsiveness.[54–56] IL-13 can increase the production of MUC5AC in human airway epithelial cells in vitro more than 100-fold,[24,25] and the production of Muc5ac in the lungs of mice in vivo more than 40-fold.[26] In contrast, the production of Muc5b/MUC5B increases minimally or may even decrease at the level of transcripts.[26,57] Mucus plugs in asthma often have a rubbery quality, suggesting that the large quantities of mucins that are produced overwhelm the available airway surface liquid when they are suddenly secreted in response to inflammatory stimuli. This abnormality can occur despite the additional hydration provided by SLC26A9 and ClCa1-dependent CaCC activity that are coordinately upregulated with MUC5AC production by IL-13.[24,35] Additional contributors to abnormal rheologic properties of asthmatic mucus are a high concentration of plasma proteins resulting from increased microvessel density and permeability in the airway wall,[58,59] and the presence of granule and cytoplasmic macromolecules from eosinophils and other leukocytes. The therapeutic focus in addressing mucus dysfunction in asthma should be reducing mucin overproduction and plasma extravasation through the use of anti-inflammatory drugs. Corticosteroids have been the mainstay of treatment, but immunotherapies directed at IgE, IL-13, and IL-5 play increasing roles, and deeper understanding of pathways that control MUC5AC expression may lead to targeted therapies.

Cystic Fibrosis

Complications from the impaired clearance of airway mucus dominate the clinical course of patients with CF. Mutation of the anion channel CFTR causes an imbalance between salt and water absorption mediated by ENaC and secretion mediated by CFTR that results in insufficient airway surface liquid.[60] Defective CFTR function also produces deficient bicarbonate transport that results in impaired mucin unfolding.[5,7] Together these deficiencies lead to the formation of mucus with an abnormally high mucin concentration and viscoelasticity that is poorly cleared by ciliary motion. This problem is compounded when the insufficiency of airway surface liquid becomes so severe that the periciliary layer loses height such that cilia cannot beat and the dehydrated mucus layer adheres to periciliary glycoconjugates.[11,14] Retained lumenal mucus is apparent pathologically in small airways and glandular ducts early in life.[61] Eventually, the failure of mucociliary clearance results in airway colonization with bacteria and fungi, and paradoxically, the mucus gel layer that evolved to protect the lungs from infection instead provides a protected environment for microbial growth. Besides the mechanical problems of mucus clearance in CF, there are likely additional defects in host defenses. For example, the deficiency of bicarbonate secretion results in acidification of airway surface liquid which impairs antimicrobial protein function,[62] and CFTR normally transports thiocyanate that is oxidized by lactoperoxidase to form isothiocyanate, an antimicrobial effector of the innate immune system that is variably reduced in CF.[63] Microbial infection leads to inflammation, and cellular debris such as DNA and actin from necrotic leukocytes further impairs the biophysical properties of mucus. Hydration therapy with aerosolized hypertonic saline solution has become a mainstay of the therapy of CF, together with aerosolized DNase and aerosolized antibiotics. Further discussion of the pathogenesis and therapy of CF is found in Chapter 50.

Video 6-2 Lateral view of defective ciliary function in Primary Ciliary Dyskinesia (PCD) associated with defective outer dynein arms (ODAs). Note the very limited range of motion, which gives the appearance of the cilia being "stiff." *Access at www.fishmansonline.com*

Primary Ciliary Dyskinesia

PCD is a genetically heterogeneous recessive disorder of motile cilia with an estimated incidence of 1 per 10 to 20,000 births.[64] However, due to the inadequacies of diagnostic methods that involve studies of ciliary ultrastructure and/or function, there are only ~1000 patients in the United States with a well-established diagnosis of PCD. Clinical disease reflects defective function of motile cilia in the conducting airways, paranasal sinuses, middle ear (eustachian tube), and the reproductive tract (Video 6-2, ODA defect). Respiratory distress occurs in >80% of full-term neonates with PCD, and infants and children have daily nasal congestion and year-round wet cough occurring soon after birth.[65] Chronic otitis media and recurrent sinus infections are also common. Cough clearance is preserved in PCD compared to CF, which may partially compensate for defective mucociliary clearance; however, recurrent bacterial infections occur in the lower airways, and ~65% of older pediatric patients and all adults have bronchiectasis with predilection for the middle lobe, lingula, and basal segments. Abnormal lung function develops early in life in PCD infants and young children, and spirometry worsens with increasing age.[65] Respiratory microbiology is similar to CF, though chronic *Pseudomonas aeruginosa* infection occurs at an older age in PCD. The prevalence of nontuberculous mycobacterial infection also parallels that seen in CF, with ~15% of adults and a lower percentage of children infected.

The diagnosis of PCD is challenging, because current diagnostic techniques are not standardized or readily available. Identification of PCD requires recognition of key phenotypic features, which include neonatal respiratory distress and situs inversus or ambiguous.[64,65] Identification of ciliary ultrastructural defects by electron microscopy can no longer be the sole "gold standard" for diagnosis because of technical limitations in its routine performance and the fact that at least 30% of PCD patients have normal ultrastructure.[66] The majority of electron microscopic abnormalities involve defective outer dynein arms or combined defects in outer and inner arms. Isolated inner dynein arm defects account for <5% of electron microscopic defects, and false-positive diagnoses commonly occur. Assessment of ciliary motility has been used to confirm a diagnosis of PCD, but technical limitations also preclude this as the sole diagnostic method. Mutations have been described in 21 genes that cover ~65% of PCD patients, and there is strong correlation between mutations in specific genes and defects in ciliary ultrastructure and function. Diagnostic capabilities have recently benefited greatly from measurement of nasal nitric oxide (nNO), which is low in PCD (10%–20% of normal, or <77 nL/min) regardless of the mutated gene.

There are no validated PCD-specific therapies, and treatment for PCD lung disease is extrapolated from other diseases with abnormal mucociliary clearance, particularly CF. Airway clearance therapies, inhaled antibiotics, oral macrolides, and inhaled hypertonic saline solution are useful in CF; thus, these therapies are being used in PCD. Otolaryngologic complications of middle ear disease and sinusitis are managed by standard approaches.

COPD

A role for mucus dysfunction in COPD has long been recognized in the syndrome of chronic bronchitis, defined as a persistent cough that produces sputum for at least 3 months per year in 2 consecutive years. The productive cough probably results from mucus overproduction in proximal airways due to surface epithelial mucus metaplasia and submucosal gland expansion, combined with ciliary dysfunction.[1,67] More recently a second role for mucus dysfunction in COPD has been recognized in the widespread obstruction of small airways identified in pathologic analysis of resected surgical specimens.[68,69] The extent of small airway mucus occlusion correlates with the degree of airflow obstruction, occurs even in patients with an emphysematous phenotype, and predicts longevity. These two mucus phenotypes in COPD – productive cough and airflow obstruction – correlate only weakly.[67] These findings suggest that individuals have differential susceptibility to the effects of cigarette smoke on different aspects of mucociliary clearance, as well as reflecting the independent roles of emphysema and small airway fibrosis in airflow obstruction in COPD.

Mucus overproduction and ciliary dysfunction both result from exposure to toxic products in cigarette smoke and environmental pollutants. Among these products, acrolein is a particularly potent inducer of MUC5AC production.[70] In ciliated cells, cigarette smoke causes both structural and functional changes.[71] Besides these effects, cigarette smoke also decreases airway surface liquid by reducing CFTR function and increasing ENaC function.[72] As is the case in CF, impaired mucociliary clearance results in persistent airway infection, particularly with unencapsulated *Haemophilus influenzae*. Further discussion of the pathogenesis and therapy of COPD is found in Chapters 40 and 42.

Interstitial Lung Diseases

A link between mucus dysfunction and interstitial lung disease was not suspected until a genome-wide association study in 2011 found genetic linkage between a polymorphism in the MUC5B promoter and both familial interstitial pneumonia (FIP) and idiopathic pulmonary fibrosis (IPF). The promoter variant is present in 50% to 60% of individuals with FIP or IPF compared to 19% of unaffected individuals, and increases the risk of disease 7-fold in heterozygotes and 21-fold in homozygotes.[73] Subsequent studies have extended the association to other idiopathic interstitial pneumonitides[74] and subclinical radiographic interstitial abnormalities.[75] The presence of the promoter variant is associated with improved survival in patients with IPF.[76] The promoter variant causes overexpression of MUC5B, but whether disease ensues because of mucus dysfunction in the airway lumen, an epithelial stress response induced the demands of synthesizing such a large and complex molecule, or some other mechanism is not yet known. Further discussion of the pathogenesis and therapy of IPF is found in Chapters 28 and 56.

Other Diseases

Acquired bronchiectasis may be due to a variety of causes including an unrecognized genetic disorder, a respiratory infection early in life, or immunodeficiency. Similar to CF, retained mucus and airway infection dominate the clinical course. Aerosolized 7% hypertonic saline solution treatment has been shown to improve lung function and quality of life.[77]

Viral respiratory infections commonly lead to mucociliary dysfunction, both because of increased mucin production and injury to ciliated cells. In subjects with underlying asthma, viral respiratory infections are a common cause of exacerbation.[78]

Allergic bronchopulmonary aspergillosis (ABPA) can present with symptoms and clinical findings that range from mild to severe. Florid overproduction of MUC5AC resulting from allergic inflammation induced by the persistent fungal infection can lead to atelectasis and mucus impaction of small or large airways. ABPA is addressed in greater detail in Chapter 48

Panbronchiolitis is a syndrome of small airway inflammation and mucus obstruction that occurs predominantly in Asian subjects, and was reported to be associated with a polymorphism in the MUC5B promoter.[79] A molecular mechanism of mucin gene dysfunction has not been identified, nor is it yet known whether there is a relationship between promoter dysfunction in panbronchiolitis and in the interstitial lung diseases.

Localized anatomic abnormalities of the airways, such as the presence of a stricture, a surgical anastomosis, or a therapeutic stent, can result in localized mucus accumulation that can lead to infection or airway closure. It may be possible to remove the localized mucus accumulation by flexible or rigid bronchoscopy, and instillation of sodium bicarbonate solution may partially dissolve the mucus.

Retained mucus is a common problem in intubated patients and those in whom lung mechanics are disrupted as a result of paralysis, immobilization, or surgery; atelectasis and pneumonia are frequent complications in such patients.[1]

Treatment

Therapies for mucus dysfunction can be divided into those that treat mucin production, mucin secretion, mucus clearance, or airway infection.[1] Mucin overproduction has been effectively treated in asthma with the use of corticosteroids and newer drugs that target allergic inflammation, though these agents have not been very effective in neutrophilic airway inflammation as occurs in COPD and CF. Despite evidence of a general role of the EGF receptor in mucin production, an inhibitor did not show benefit in COPD patients.[80] In view of the generally pathologic role of MUC5AC and generally homeostatic role of MUC5B, strategies that selectively target MUC5AC production are attractive. Inhibiting mucin secretion may seem to be an obvious strategy to treat combined overproduction and secretion (mucus hypersecretion), and is being pursued using modified botulinum toxins and MARCKS inhibitors.[1] However it may be difficult to precisely titrate mucin secretion to preserve baseline homeostatic function while inhibiting pathologic secretion, and clinical trials have not so far shown evidence of benefit.

Treatments that promote mucus clearance include physical measures to remove retained secretions and pharmacologic agents to improve mucus rheology.[1] Among physical measures, mechanical insufflation–exsufflation has been shown to effectively clear mucus in patients with weak cough, there is evidence of moderate benefit from multiple measures to increase expectoration in CF, and there is anecdotal evidence of benefit in non-CF bronchiectasis.[81,82] Drugs that effectively improve mucus rheology in specific settings include inhaled dornase alfa, inhaled hypertonic saline solution, and ivacaftor in CF. Inhaled hypertonic saline solution has also shown benefit in non-CF bronchiectasis,[77] and is under investigation in COPD. In contrast, dornase alfa did not show benefit in non-CF bronchiectasis, asthma, or COPD. For the treatment of infected airway mucus, a variety of inhaled, oral and intravenous antibiotic regimens have been shown to have utility in specific situations, particularly in CF and COPD.[1]

REFERENCES

1. Fahy JV, Dickey BF. Airway mucus function and dysfunction. *N Engl J Med.* 2010;363:2233–2247.
2. Rose MC, Voynow JA. Respiratory tract mucin genes and mucin glycoproteins in health and disease. *Physiol Rev.* 2006;86:245–278.

3. Thornton DJ, Rousseau K, McGuckin MA. Structure and function of the polymeric mucins in airway mucus. *Annu Rev Physiol.* 2008;70:459–486.
4. Verdugo P. Supramolecular dynamics of mucus. *Cold Spring Harb Perspect Med.* 2012;2(11):pii: a009597.
5. Quinton PM. Role of epithelial HCO3 transport in mucin secretion: lessons from cystic fibrosis. *Am J Physiol Cell Physiol.* 2010;299:C1222–C1233.
6. Raynal BD, Hardingham TE, Sheehan JK, Thornton DJ. Calcium-dependent protein interactions in MUC5B provide reversible cross-links in salivary mucus. *J Biol Chem.* 2003;278:28703–28710.
7. Ambort D, Johansson ME, Gustafsson JK, Ermund A, Hansson GC. Perspectives on mucus properties and formation–lessons from the biochemical world. *Cold Spring Harb Perspect Med.* 2012;2(11):pii: a014159.
8. Garcia GJ, Boucher RC, Elston TC. Biophysical model of ion transport across human respiratory epithelia allows quantification of ion permeabilities. *Biophys J.* 2013;104:716–726.
9. Plopper CG, Heidsiek JG, Weir AJ, George JA, Hyde DM. Tracheobronchial epithelium in the adult rhesus monkey: a quantitative histochemical and ultrastructural study. *Am J Anat.* 1989;184:31–40.
10. Ehre C, Worthington EN, Liesman RM, et al. Overexpressing mouse model demonstrates the protective role of Muc5ac in the lungs. *Proc Natl Acad Sci U S A.* 2012;109:16528–16533.
11. Button B, Cai LH, Ehre C, et al. A periciliary brush promotes the lung health by separating the mucus layer from airway epithelia. *Science.* 2012;337:937–941.
12. Hattrup CL, Gendler SJ. Structure and function of the cell surface (tethered) mucins. *Annu Rev Physiol.* 2008;70:431–457.
13. Kesimer M, Ehre C, Burns KA, Davis CW, Sheehan JK, Pickles RJ. Molecular organization of the mucins and glycocalyx underlying mucus transport over mucosal surfaces of the airways. *Mucosal Immunol.* 2013;6:379–392.
14. Dickey BF. Walking on solid ground: a gel-on-brush model of airway mucosal surfaces. *Science.* 2012;337:924–925.
15. Evans CM, Williams OW, Tuvim MJ, et al. Mucin is produced by clara cells in the proximal airways of antigen-challenged mice. *Am J Respir Cell Mol Biol.* 2004;31:382–394.
16. Zhu Y, Ehre C, Abdullah LH, et al. Munc13-2−/− baseline secretion defect reveals source of oligomeric mucins in mouse airways. *J Physiol.* 2008;586:1977–1992.
17. Pardo-Saganta A, Law BM, Gonzalez-Celeiro M, Vinarsky V, Rajagopal J. Ciliated cells of pseudostratified airway epithelium do not become mucous cells after ovalbumin challenge. *Am J Respir Cell Mol Biol.* 2013;48:364–373.
18. Davis CW, Dickey BF. Regulated airway goblet cell mucin secretion. *Annu Rev Physiol.* 2008;70:487–512.
19. Kim K, Petrova YM, Scott BL, et al. Munc18b is an essential gene in mice whose expression is limiting for secretion by airway epithelial and mast cells. *Biochem J.* 2012;446:383–394.
20. Wickstrom C, Davies JR, Eriksen GV, Veerman EC, Carlstedt I. MUC5B is a major gel-forming, oligomeric mucin from human salivary gland, respiratory tract and endocervix: identification of glycoforms and C-terminal cleavage. *Biochem J.* 1998;334 (Pt 3):685–693.
21. Roy MG, Livraghi-Butrico A, Fletcher AA, et al. Muc5b is required for airway defence. *Nature.* 2014;505(7483):412–416.
22. Hasnain SZ, Evans CM, Roy M, et al. Muc5ac: a critical component mediating the rejection of enteric nematodes. *J Exp Med.* 2011;208(5):893–900.
23. Tsubokawa D, Goso Y, Nakamura T, et al. Rapid and specific alterations of goblet cell mucin in rat airway and small intestine associated with resistance against Nippostrongylus brasiliensis reinfection. *Exp Parasitol.* 2012;130:209–217.
24. Alevy YG, Patel AC, Romero AG, et al. IL-13-induced airway mucus production is attenuated by MAPK13 inhibition. *J Clin Invest.* 2012;122:4555–4568.
25. Zhen G, Park SW, Nguyenvu LT, et al. IL-13 and epidermal growth factor receptor have critical but distinct roles in epithelial cell mucin production. *Am J Respir Cell Mol Biol.* 2007;36:244–253.
26. Young HW, Williams OW, Chandra D, et al. Central role of Muc5ac expression in mucous metaplasia and its regulation by conserved 5' elements. *Am J Respir Cell Mol Biol.* 2007;37:273–290.
27. Kuperman DA, Huang X, Nguyenvu L, Holscher C, Brombacher F, Erle DJ. IL-4 receptor signaling in Clara cells is required for allergen-induced mucus production. *J Immunol.* 2005;175:3746–3752.
28. Thai P, Loukoianov A, Wachi S, Wu R. Regulation of airway mucin gene expression. *Annu Rev Physiol.* 2008;70:405–429.
29. Bennett EP, Mandel U, Clausen H, Gerken TA, Fritz TA, Tabak LA. Control of mucin-type O-glycosylation: A classification of the polypeptide GalNAc-transferase gene family. *Glycobiology.* 2012;22:736–756.
30. Schroeder BW, Verhaeghe C, Park SW, et al. AGR2 is induced in asthma and promotes allergen-induced mucin overproduction. *Am J Respir Cell Mol Biol.* 2012;47:178–185.
31. Tuvim MJ, Mospan AR, Burns KA, et al. Synaptotagmin 2 couples mucin granule exocytosis to Ca2+ signaling from endoplasmic reticulum. *J Biol Chem.* 2009;284:9781–9787.
32. Singer M, Martin LD, Vargaftig BB, et al. A MARCKS-related peptide blocks mucus hypersecretion in a mouse model of asthma. *Nat Med.* 2004;10:193–196.
33. Lazarowski ER, Boucher RC. Purinergic receptors in airway epithelia. *Curr Opin Pharmacol.* 2009;9:262–267.
34. Young HW, Sun CX, Evans CM, Dickey BF, Blackburn MR. A3 adenosine receptor signaling contributes to airway mucin secretion after allergen challenge. *Am J Respir Cell Mol Biol.* 2006;35:549–558.
35. Anagnostopoulou P, Riederer B, Duerr J, et al. SLC26A9-mediated chloride secretion prevents mucus obstruction in airway inflammation. *J Clin Invest.* 2012;122:3629–3634.
36. Giangreco A, Arwert EN, Rosewell IR, Snyder J, Watt FM, Stripp BR. Stem cells are dispensable for lung homeostasis but restore airways after injury. *Proc Natl Acad Sci U S A.* 2009;106:9286–9291.
37. Lin CY, Wheelock AM, Morin D, et al. Toxicity and metabolism of methylnaphthalenes: comparison with naphthalene and 1-nitronaphthalene. *Toxicology.* 2009;260:16–27.
38. Evans SE, Xu Y, Tuvim MJ, Dickey BF. Inducible innate resistance of lung epithelium to infection. *Annu Rev Physiol.* 2010;72:413–435.
39. Salathe M. Regulation of mammalian ciliary beating. *Annu Rev Physiol.* 2007;69:401–422.
40. Satir P, Christensen ST. Overview of structure and function of mammalian cilia. *Annu Rev Physiol.* 2007;69:377–400.
41. Knowles MR, Boucher RC. Mucus clearance as a primary innate defense mechanism for mammalian airways. *J Clin Invest.* 2002;109:571–577.
42. Sears PR, Thompson K, Knowles MR, Davis CW. Human airway ciliary dynamics. *Am J Physiol Lung Cell Mol Physiol.* 2013;304:L170–L183.

43. Braiman A, Priel Z. Efficient mucociliary transport relies on efficient regulation of ciliary beating. *Respir Physiol Neurobiol.* 2008;163:202–207.

44. Button BM, Button B. Structure and function of the mucus clearance system of the lung. *Cold Spring Harb Perspect Med.* 2013;3(8):pii: a009720.

45. Park KS, Wells JM, Zorn AM, et al. Transdifferentiation of ciliated cells during repair of the respiratory epithelium. *Am J Respir Cell Mol Biol.* 2006;34:151–157.

46. Wine JJ, Joo NS. Submucosal glands and airway defense. *Proc Am Thorac Soc.* 2004;1:47–53.

47. Hays SR, Fahy JV. Characterizing mucous cell remodeling in cystic fibrosis: relationship to neutrophils. *Am J Respir Crit Care Med.* 2006;174:1018–1024.

48. Hogg JC, Macklem PT, Thurlbeck WM. Site and nature of airway obstruction in chronic obstructive lung disease. *N Engl J Med.* 1968;278:1355–1360.

49. Wanner A, Salathe M, O'Riordan TG. Mucociliary clearance in the airways. *Am J Respir Crit Care Med.* 1996;154:1868–1902.

50. Bennett WD, Laube BL, Corcoran T, et al. Multisite comparison of mucociliary and cough clearance measures using standardized methods. *J Aerosol Med Pulm Drug Deliv.* 2013;26:157–164.

51. Hogg JC. The pathology of asthma. *APMIS.* 1997;105:735–745.

52. Kuyper LM, Pare PD, Hogg JC, et al. Characterization of airway plugging in fatal asthma. *Am J Med.* 2003;115:6–11.

53. Elias JA, Lee CG. IL-13 in asthma. The successful integration of lessons from mice and humans. *Am J Respir Crit Care Med.* 2011;183:957–958.

54. Kudo M, Melton AC, Chen C, et al. IL-17 A produced by alpha-beta T cells drives airway hyper-responsiveness in mice and enhances mouse and human airway smooth muscle contraction. *Nat Med.* 2012;18:547–554.

55. Alcorn JF, Crowe CR, Kolls JK. TH17 cells in asthma and COPD. *Annu Rev Physiol.* 2010;72:495–516.

56. Wang YH, Voo KS, Liu B, et al. A novel subset of CD4(+) T(H)2 memory/effector cells that produce inflammatory IL-17 cytokine and promote the exacerbation of chronic allergic asthma. *J Exp Med.* 2010;207:2479–2491.

57. Woodruff PG, Modrek B, Choy DF, et al. T-helper type 2-driven inflammation defines major subphenotypes of asthma. *Am J Respir Crit Care Med.* 2009;180:388–395.

58. Irvin CG, Bates JH. Physiologic dysfunction of the asthmatic lung: what's going on down there, anyway? *Proc Am Thorac Soc.* 2009;6:306–311.

59. Lee CG, Link H, Baluk P, et al. Vascular endothelial growth factor (VEGF) induces remodeling and enhances TH2-mediated sensitization and inflammation in the lung. *Nat Med.* 2004;10:1095–1103.

60. Reddy MM, Stutts MJ. Status of fluid and electrolyte absorption in cystic fibrosis. *Cold Spring Harb Perspect Med.* 2013;3:a009555.

61. Ramsey BW, Banks-Schlegel S, Accurso FJ, et al. Future directions in early cystic fibrosis lung disease research: an NHLBI workshop report. *Am J Respir Crit Care Med.* 2012;185:887–892.

62. Pezzulo AA, Tang XX, Hoegger MJ, et al. Reduced airway surface pH impairs bacterial killing in the porcine cystic fibrosis lung. *Nature.* 2012;487:109–113.

63. Lorentzen D, Durairaj L, Pezzulo AA, et al. Concentration of the antibacterial precursor thiocyanate in cystic fibrosis airway secretions. *Free Radic Biol Med.* 2011;50:1144–1150.

64. Zariwala MA, Knowles MR, Omran H. Genetic defects in ciliary structure and function. *Annu Rev Physiol.* 2007;69:423–450.

65. Sagel SD, Davis SD, Campisi P, Dell SD. Update of respiratory tract disease in children with primary ciliary dyskinesia. *Proc Am Thorac Soc.* 2011;8:438–443.

66. Shoemark A, Hogg C. Electron tomography of respiratory cilia. *Thorax.* 2013;68:190–191.

67. Kim V, Criner GJ. Chronic bronchitis and chronic obstructive pulmonary disease. *Am J Respir Crit Care Med.* 2013;187:228–237.

68. Hogg JC. Pathophysiology of airflow limitation in chronic obstructive pulmonary disease. *Lancet.* 2004;364:709–721.

69. Hogg JC, Chu F, Utokaparch S, et al. The nature of small-airway obstruction in chronic obstructive pulmonary disease. *N Engl J Med.* 2004;350:2645–2653.

70. Bein K, Leikauf GD. Acrolein—a pulmonary hazard. *Mol Nutr Food Res.* 2011;55:1342–1360.

71. Leopold PL, O'Mahony MJ, Lian XJ, Tilley AE, Harvey BG, Crystal RG. Smoking is associated with shortened airway cilia. *PLoS ONE.* 2009;4:e8157.

72. Clunes LA, Davies CM, Coakley RD, et al. Cigarette smoke exposure induces CFTR internalization and insolubility, leading to airway surface liquid dehydration. *FASEB J.* 2012;26:533–545.

73. Seibold MA, Wise AL, Speer MC, et al. A common MUC5B promoter polymorphism and pulmonary fibrosis. *N Engl J Med.* 2011;364:1503–1512.

74. Fingerlin TE, Murphy E, Zhang W, et al. Genome-wide association study identifies multiple susceptibility loci for pulmonary fibrosis. *Nat Genet.* 2013;45:613–620.

75. Hunninghake GM, Hatabu H, Okajima Y, et al. MUC5B promoter polymorphism and interstitial lung abnormalities. *N Engl J Med.* 2013;368(23):2192–2200.

76. Peljto AL, Zhang Y, Fingerlin TE, et al. Association between the MUC5B promoter polymorphism and survival in patients with idiopathic pulmonary fibrosis. *JAMA.* 2013;309(21):2232–2239.

77. Kellett F, Robert NM. Nebulised 7% hypertonic saline improves lung function and quality of life in bronchiectasis. *Respir Med.* 2011;105:1831–1835.

78. Holtzman MJ, Byers DE, Benoit LA, et al. Immune pathways for translating viral infection into chronic airway disease. *Adv Immunol.* 2009;102:245–276.

79. Kamio K, Matsushita I, Hijikata M, et al. Promoter analysis and aberrant expression of the MUC5B gene in diffuse panbronchiolitis. *Am J Respir Crit Care Med.* 2005;171:949–957.

80. Woodruff PG, Wolff M, Hohlfeld JM, et al. Safety and efficacy of an inhaled epidermal growth factor receptor inhibitor (BIBW 2948 BS) in chronic obstructive pulmonary disease. *Am J Respir Crit Care Med.* 2010;181:438–445.

81. Flume PA, Robinson KA, O'Sullivan BP, et al. Cystic fibrosis pulmonary guidelines: airway clearance therapies. *Respir Care.* 2009;54:522–537.

82. McCool FD, Rosen MJ. Nonpharmacologic airway clearance therapies: ACCP evidence-based clinical practice guidelines. *Chest.* 2006;129:250S–259S.

CHAPTER 7

The Genetic Basis of Respiratory Disorders

Micheala A. Aldred

The field of genetics and genomics is advancing at an incredible pace. The completion of the Human Genome Project was just the beginning. Now, thanks to rapid advances in sequencing technology and bioinformatics, we have made significant progress toward sequencing 1000 genomes from around the world, uncovering great genetic diversity and challenging us to understand the biologic relevance. Sequencing the exome (the protein-coding parts of the genome) of a patient with an undiagnosed condition is already a reality. Even beyond human genetics, genomic technologies are making an impact on pulmonary disease, enabling characterization of new respiratory pathogen genomes, such as the SARS virus and pandemic H1N1 influenza, with unprecedented speed. Against this backdrop, a chapter on the genetics of lung diseases could easily be out of date before it is even in print. Thus it does not seek to be encyclopedic, but to give the reader a grounding in the principles of human genetics, an overview of current knowledge in Mendelian lung diseases and a summary of recent progress in understanding genetic factors contributing to common lung conditions. It outlines some of the emerging roles of epigenetic modifications and aims to give a vision of where the field is moving, concluding with current and future prospects for genetically targeted therapies.

PRINCIPLES OF HUMAN GENETICS

GENOME ORGANIZATION

The term "genome" refers to the genetic make-up of an organism (Table 7-1). Mammalian genomes are composed of deoxyribonucleic acid (DNA) and can be subdivided into a nuclear genome - DNA within the nucleus of each cell - and a separate circular genome housed within each mitochondrion. DNA has a double-helix structure, each strand comprises four constituent bases - adenine (A), cytosine (C), guanine (G), and thymine (T) - that pair together, A with T and G with C. DNA needs to be replicated each time a cell divides. This strict base pairing ensures accurate copying of the DNA code.

The human genome is approximately 3.3 billion base pairs in size. This large amount of DNA is wound around proteins known as histones, then packaged into higher-order structures called chromosomes that can be visualized under a light microscope. Most cells of the body contain two copies of each chromosome; one inherited from each parent, and are termed "diploid." Diploid cells contain 23 pairs of chromosomes. During meiosis, these pairs of chromosomes are separated, giving rise to oocytes and sperm that contain a single copy of each chromosome (termed "haploid"). Thus fusion of two haploid gametes gives rise to a new diploid organism, preserving the correct copy number of DNA through the generations. Gender is determined by a pair of sex chromosomes, X and Y; females have two copies of the X-chromosome, whereas males have one each of X and Y. The other 22 pairs of chromosomes are known as the autosomes. Genetic diseases are mainly caused by mutations in autosomal or X-chromosome genes; the Y-chromosome harbors only a few genes and these are mainly involved in determining male characteristics.

GENE STRUCTURE

Only about 1% to 2% of the human genome actually encodes for proteins. The noncoding portion was originally considered to be junk DNA, but it is now increasingly clear that some of it has important regulatory functions. The protein-coding units are called genes. The DNA within a gene is first transcribed into ribonucleic acid (RNA). RNA has a similar base structure to DNA, but is single stranded, has a slightly different sugar backbone and thymine (T) is replaced by uracil (U). Genes are typically divided into coding exons and intervening noncoding introns. The intronic sequences are spliced out of the initial RNA transcript to produce the mature messenger RNA (mRNA) molecule. Some genes have alternative splicing patterns that can give rise to slightly different variants ("isoforms") of the protein. The mRNA is then translated into protein by ribosomes. Ribosomes read the RNA code as a triplet of bases or "codon" and add the corresponding amino acid to the growing protein chain. There is some redundancy in the genetic code and amino acids may be encoded by several different codons. Four codons have a special function: AUG encodes methionine and always marks the initiation site for protein translation, while UGA, UAG, and UAA are stop signals that lead to termination of translation. The DNA flanking the coding region of a gene is not translated but contains important regulatory elements, including the promoter region that regulates transcriptional activity.

CLASSES OF MUTATION

Alterations in the DNA sequence occur when there is an error in DNA replication prior to cell division or DNA damage occurs through environmental exposures such as UV radiation or tobacco smoke. Such mutations may affect a single base (known as a point mutation) or may involve the insertion or deletion of multiple bases. Cells have an extensive DNA repair mechanism that will correct most of these mutations, but any that escape may lead to a permanent change in the sequence that is propagated to daughter cells. Mutations in noncoding regions of the genome often have no detrimental effect and over time, they may become quite common in the population. Variants that are present at a frequency of greater than 1% are known as polymorphisms and have been widely used in genetic mapping studies. Thus the two copies of a gene in any individual are subtly different at the DNA sequence level. These variant forms are known as "alleles." However, mutations that occur in the introns of genes may lead to disease, especially if they disrupt the highly conserved splicing signals immediately flanking an exon. Within the coding region of a gene, the consequence of a point mutation depends on whether it alters the genetic code (Fig. 7-1). Most redundancy lies in the third base of the codon, so for example, a change from GGG to any of GGA, GGC, or GGU still encodes glycine and would not change the sequence of the protein. Such changes are usually silent and may become common polymorphisms. Mutations that lead to an amino acid substitution, for example UGU (cysteine) to UAU (tyrosine), are known as missense mutations. Their effect on protein function depends much on the specific structure and function of that protein. In general, missense mutations in regions that are functionally critical, such as the catalytic domain of an enzyme, will be highly deleterious. These regions are often highly conserved across species, indicating that mutations have not been tolerated during evolution. Missense mutations that affect residues important in secondary structure and protein folding are also likely to have adverse effects, whereas mutations in linker regions may be less critical. Thus interpreting the consequences of genetic changes requires an in-depth knowledge of the protein concerned.

TABLE 7-1 Glossary of Genetic Terms

Term	Definition
Genome	The complete genetic makeup of an organism, including all coding and noncoding DNA
Gene	A discrete protein-coding unit within the genome. Genes are typically subdivided into exons (blocks of protein-coding DNA), introns (intervening noncoding DNA), and flanking regulatory regions
Exome	The entire sequence of all exons within the genome
Somatic	Relating to any cell of the body other than the germ cells. Mutations in somatic cells cannot be passed on to the next generation
Chromosome	A higher order structure into which DNA is packaged. Humans have 23 pairs of chromosomes, 22 autosomes, and a pair of sex chromosome, X and Y, that determine gender
Telomere	The cap at the ends of each chromosome, composed of hundreds of copies of the repeat sequence TTAGGG
Diploid	Containing a full complement of 23 chromosome pairs. All normal somatic cells are diploid
Haploid	Having only a single copy of each chromosome. Mature gametes are haploid, ensuring that a new zygote has the correct chromosome complement
Aneuploid	Cells that have a nondiploid number of chromosomes due to gain or loss of one or more chromosomes during cell division. Aneuploidy commonly occurs in cancer cells, which may become highly abnormal as the tumor progresses
Mutation	Strictly, any change that occurs in the DNA sequence, however in relation to genetic diseases, the term is mainly used to refer to changes that have a deleterious clinical effect
Polymorphism	A genetic variant present at a frequency of at least 1% in a given population, often used synonymously with mutations that have no adverse effect
SNP	Single nucleotide polymorphism: a polymorphism resulting from a single DNA base substitution
Allele	Referring to a specific version of a gene, often used to distinguish between the copies inherited from each parent, or between wild-type and mutant copies
Heterozygote	An individual with one wild-type allele and one variant
Homozygous	An individual with two copies of the same variant allele. In autosomal recessive diseases where an individual inherits two different mutations, one from each parent, the term "compound heterozygote" is used
Genotype	The genetic sequence of the two alleles at a particular gene location
Phenotype	The clinical manifestation of genetic change
Dominant	A mutation that exerts a phenotypic effect in heterozygous form
Recessive	A mutation that is masked by the wild-type allele in a heterozygote and only results in a phenotype when wild-type function is lost
Penetrance	The likelihood that an individual with a mutation will develop clinical disease
Heterogeneity, allelic	The presence of different pathogenic mutations in same gene across different individuals. Most genetic diseases show allelic heterogeneity, unless they are caused by gain of an abnormal function that is only conferred by one specific mutation (e.g., sickle cell disease)
Heterogeneity, genetic	Diseases for which a mutation in one of several different genes can lead to the same clinical phenotype
Heritability	The proportion of trait variance that can be attributed to genetic factors versus the environment
Haplotype/ Haplogroup	A specific combination of SNPs on a contiguous piece of DNA. Haplotype is used when defining the arrangement of SNPs on an individual chromosome; haplogroup refers to groups of ancestrally related variants in mitochondrial genome
Genetic anticipation	A phenomenon in which the age of onset of an autosomal dominant disease becomes earlier with each successive generation. It is most often observed in a group of neuromuscular diseases caused by a unique class of DNA-repeat mutations, but also occurs in familial pulmonary fibrosis associated with telomerase mutations
Imprinting	Epigenetic silencing of an allele based on its parental origin. Relatively few genes are imprinted, but those that are give rise to unusual patterns of inheritance, as the mutation is masked when present on the silenced allele

Mutations that lead to premature truncation of a protein are highly likely to be pathogenic and are a major cause of inherited diseases. Several different types of mutation can lead to premature protein truncation. Nonsense mutations result from a single base change that introduces a stop codon earlier than the natural translation end-point, for example, AGA (arginine) to UGA (stop). Small insertions and deletions can also introduce premature stop codons because if the number of bases added or lost is not a multiple of three, the reading frame for the triplet codon is offset and it is read incorrectly. This is known as a frameshift mutation (Fig. 7-1). Splice-site mutations can lead to retention of an intron, which does not normally code for a protein and, therefore, often contains a stop codon. Alternatively splice-site mutations can lead to exon skipping and again, if the size of the missing exon is not a multiple of three bases, this leads to a downstream frameshift, in addition to losing a whole exon of sequence. The presence of a premature stop codon often triggers a process known as nonsense-mediated mRNA decay (NMD), which leads to degradation of the nonsense-containing mRNA transcript, preventing translation of a truncated protein. This protects the cell from potentially adverse effects of an abnormal protein product. The mechanisms underlying NMD are not fully understood and some transcripts are degraded more efficiently than others. Nonsense mutations in the last exon of a gene do not trigger NMD, due to their proximity

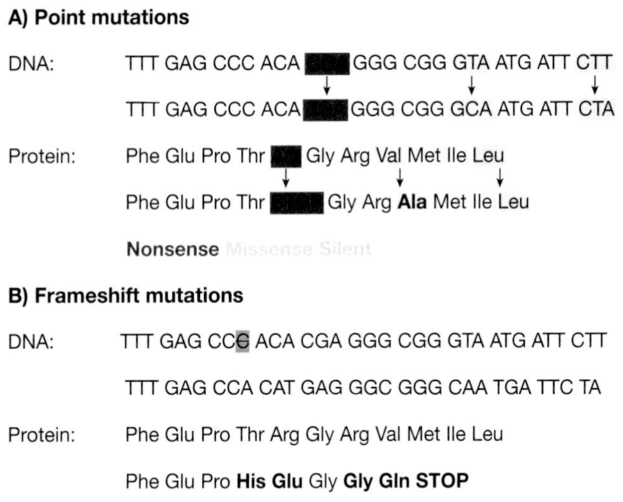

A) Point mutations

DNA: TTT GAG CCC ACA ■■■ GGG CGG GTA ATG ATT CTT

TTT GAG CCC ACA ■■■ GGG CGG GCA ATG ATT CTA

Protein: Phe Glu Pro Thr ■ Gly Arg Val Met Ile Leu

Phe Glu Pro Thr ■■■ Gly Arg **Ala** Met Ile Leu

Nonsense Missense Silent

B) Frameshift mutations

DNA: TTT GAG CCG ACA CGA GGG CGG GTA ATG ATT CTT

TTT GAG CCA CAT GAG GGC GGG CAA TGA TTC TA

Protein: Phe Glu Pro Thr Arg Gly Arg Val Met Ile Leu

Phe Glu Pro **His Glu** Gly **Gly Gln STOP**

Figure 7-1 Classes of genetic mutations. **A.** Single base changes within an exon may lead to premature protein truncation (nonsense mutation, shaded in red), an amino acid substitution (missense mutation, yellow), or there may be no change due to redundancy in the genetic code (silent, blue); **B.** Insertions or deletions lead to frameshift mutations if the number of bases involved is not divisible by three. This almost invariably leads to premature protein truncation downstream of the mutation site.

to the natural stop codon, whereas mutations in first exon, close to the translation initiation codon, may lead to reinitiation at a downstream ATG site.

The last major class of mutation is gene rearrangements, large deletions, or duplications that affect one or more exons. These mutations can be missed by sequence-based methods of DNA analysis and require specialized methods that measure the copy number of DNA across the gene. They typically lead to major disruption of the gene structure and any protein that may be produced is likely to be nonfunctional.

■ MODES OF INHERITANCE

The pattern of inheritance of a genetic disease within a family is determined by the location of the mutation – on an autosome, the X-chromosome, or in the mitochondrial genome – and whether or not a clinical effect (phenotype) is evident when only one copy of the gene is mutated. When mutation of a single allele is sufficient to cause disease, it is known as dominant because the mutation is sufficient to overcome the positive effect of the remaining wild-type allele. Genes that are affected by dominant mutations are typically very sensitive to the 50% reduction in gene dosage that results from inactivating one allele. Alternatively the mutation may cause an abnormal gain of function, or create an abnormal protein that in turn interferes with the function of the wild-type protein, an effect known as dominant negative. In contrast, recessive mutations have no detrimental effect when only one allele is mutated. The remaining wild-type allele is sufficient to maintain normal gene function and a clinical phenotype is only apparent when both alleles are inactivated and the gene function is completely lost. Individuals with a personal or family history of genetic disease should be offered genetic counseling to help them understand their risks and options, and to facilitate appropriate genetic testing.

■ AUTOSOMAL DOMINANT

Autosomal dominant mutations result in a strong pattern of disease in each generation of a family (Fig. 7-2A). An individual with such a mutation has a 50% chance of passing the disease on to each of their children. The hallmarks of autosomal dominant inheritance are approximately equal proportions of males and females affected by the disease and the presence of male-to-male transmission. However, several factors can complicate this model. Some dominant diseases may skip a generation, due to reduced penetrance (Fig. 7-2B). The penetrance of a mutation is defined as the likelihood that someone with the mutation actually develops the disease. If the penetrance is less than 100%, then an individual who inherits the mutation may escape the disease themselves, while still being at 50% risk of passing it on to their children. Independently, the gender ratio may skewed by environmental and/or genetic modifying factors. The most extreme example is inherited diseases affecting sex-specific organs. For example, ovarian cancer can be inherited in an autosomal dominant manner but only females with the mutation actually develop the disease.

■ AUTOSOMAL RECESSIVE

The pattern of inheritance of autosomal recessive diseases is quite different. Individuals with a single copy of the mutation are known as carriers or heterozygotes. Since there is no clinical effect, such individuals are usually unaware of their status. However, when both parents are carriers, each has a 50% chance of passing on the mutation, meaning there is a 25% chance that a child will inherit two copies of the mutation and be affected by the disease. Consequently, autosomal recessive diseases often appear "out of the blue" in a family with no previous history of the condition (Fig. 7-2C). The incidence of recessive diseases largely depends on the heterozygote frequency in the population, but the risk increases in consanguineous families.

■ X-LINKED INHERITANCE

X-linked diseases are caused by mutations in genes on the X-chromosome. Most are recessive, but the different sex-chromosome constitution between females and males, XX versus XY, leads to a unique pattern of inheritance. Males who inherit an X-linked mutation have no wild-type allele on the Y-chromosome to mask its effect, and consequently they develop the disease. Female carriers are generally unaffected, as for autosomal recessive diseases. Thus X-linked diseases are passed through the female line and typically affect only males (Fig. 7-2D). A female carrier has a 50% chance of an affected son. Importantly, males cannot pass the mutation to their sons, so an evidence of male-to-male transmission rules out X-linked inheritance, but all of their daughters will be carriers. In reality, females only have a single X-chromosome active in any given cell, due to a process of X-inactivation in early embryonic development that adjusts the dosage of X-linked genes to be the same as in males. If X-inactivation is random, approximately half of cells in a carrier will express the wild-type allele and half express the mutation, meaning that female carriers usually have no phenotype or are only mildly affected. However, if X-inactivation is highly skewed toward expression of the mutant allele, then female carriers may be as severely affected as males. Rarely, X-linked mutations may be dominant, meaning that all females who inherit the mutation will be affected. Such mutations are often lethal in males. Examples of X-linked recessive conditions that affect the lung include X-linked agammaglobulinemia, an immunodeficiency that can lead to chronic lung disease, and X-linked severe combined immunodeficiency caused by mutations in the *IL2RG* gene that encodes a subunit of the receptor for multiple interleukins.

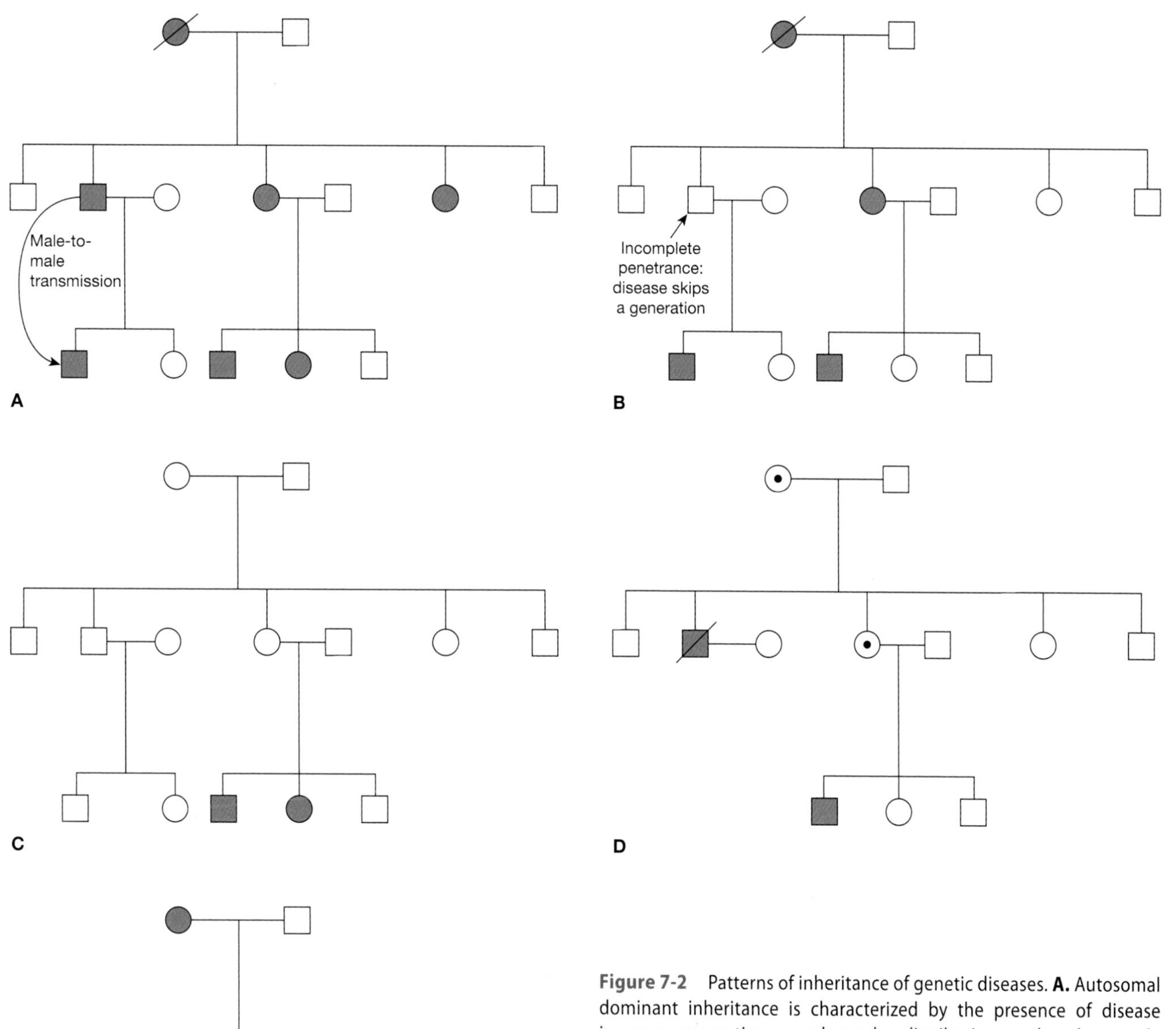

Figure 7-2 Patterns of inheritance of genetic diseases. **A.** Autosomal dominant inheritance is characterized by the presence of disease in every generation, equal gender distribution, and male-to-male transmission; **B.** When an autosomal dominant disease has reduced penetrance, it may skip a generation; **C.** Autosomal recessive disease suddenly appears in the family when both parents are heterozygous mutation carriers; **D.** X-linked recessive diseases are transmitted by carrier females but in general, only males are affected. Male-to-male transmission is impossible; **E.** Mitochondrial diseases are transmitted through the female lineage and can potentially affect all children born to an affected mother. Key: *Squares* denote males; *circles*, females; *solid symbols* denote individuals affected by the disease; *circles with a dot* in the center denote obligate carriers of an X-linked condition.

■ MITOCHONDRIAL MUTATIONS

The mitochondrial genome is a small circular molecule, approximately 16,500 bases long. It encodes some of the proteins required for oxidative phosphorylation and electron transport, together with multiple transfer RNAs and ribosomal RNAs. Mutations in mitochondrial genes adversely affect energy production and thus the clinical consequences are greatest in tissues with high-energy requirements, such as heart, brain, and skeletal muscle. Two characteristics make the inheritance of mitochondrial gene mutations unique. First, mitochondria are almost exclusively transmitted through the maternal lineage; sperm only have mitochondria in the tail for motility and do not enter the oocyte at fertilization. Thus, the pattern of inheritance within a family is similar to X-linked inheritance, with no male-to-male transmission, but differs in that females and males are equally likely to be affected (Fig. 7-2E). In theory, all children born to an affected mother would inherit the mutation and develop the disease. In reality, however, there are many copies of the mitochondrial genome per cell and each cell has a mixture of wild-type and mutant mitochondria (heteroplasmy). The segregation of these mitochondria during cell division is random, so by chance, an oocyte may have a high or low number of mitochondria carrying the mutation. This random drift continues throughout embryonic development and beyond, generating considerable variability in the severity of disease and the tissues that are affected, even among individuals in the same family. Pulmonary involvement is not a major feature of most mitochondrial diseases, but several case reports link pulmonary hypertension with mutation in mitochondrial genes or a nuclear-encoded mitochondrial protein.[1–8] Pulmonary complications of mitochondrial disease are most likely to present as part of a multiorgan syndrome that may also include cardiac and/or skeletal myopathy, neuropathy, retinopathy, renal problems, or metabolic abnormalities.

Another fascinating property of the mitochondrial genome is its high degree of polymorphic variation. Clusters of variants, or "haplogroups," have been used to plot early human migration patterns across the globe. As new variants arose, they were propagated to offspring in the immediate geographic area, but were not present in other populations that had already migrated to different regions. Some of these variants confer subtle functional differences and may have been selectively enriched by helping adaptation to a new environment. They may also modulate risk of disease, particularly for conditions where there is oxidative stress. Data concerning lung diseases are currently limited, but associations with different haplogroups have been reported for atopy and asthma, chronic obstructive pulmonary disease (COPD), high-altitude pulmonary edema, and lung cancer risk.[9–13]

SOMATIC MUTATIONS AND CANCER

Not all of the genetic changes that contribute to disease are inherited. This is particularly true in cancer where, although there may be an inherited predisposition, most genetic changes are somatic and confined to the tumor itself. A later chapter is devoted to the molecular basis of lung cancer, so here we will briefly review the types of somatic changes observed in cancer cells and their relevance to benign lung conditions.

Two major classes of genes may be mutated in cancer: oncogenes and tumor suppressor genes. Oncogenes promote tumorigenesis when they are expressed at an abnormally high level or are inappropriately expressed in tissues where the gene should normally be silent. This may occur due to amplification (extra copies) of the gene, overactivation by upstream transcription factors, a chromosome rearrangement that brings the gene under the control of a strong promoter, or loss of DNA methylation as described in the following section on epigenetics. Alternatively the gene may be mutated in a way that gives the protein a novel gain of function. For example, mutation of a ligand-dependent receptor such that, once activated, it cannot be switched off and continues to signal in the absence of the ligand. These types of oncogenic mutations are usually dominant missense mutations at specific amino acid sites within the protein.

Tumor suppressor genes (TSGs) are like the brakes on the cell; they control cell growth, differentiation, and apoptosis. When their function is lost, the cell proliferates uncontrollably or evades programmed cell death. TSGs are predominantly inactivated by nonsense and frameshift mutations, large gene deletions, or loss of an entire chromosome. They may also be silenced by hypermethylation of their promoter, as described in the next section. In contrast to oncogenes, TSG mutations are often recessive at the cellular level and both copies of the gene must be inactivated before the full cancer-promoting effect is seen. Both mutations may occur as somatic changes in the cell that initiates the cancer, or the first mutation may be inherited, predisposing the individual to the risk of cancer, a model that was first proposed by Alfred Knudson.[14]

As tumors proliferate, their genome may become highly disorganized. Abnormal segregation of the chromosomes during mitosis can lead to aneuploidy, with gains and/or losses of entire chromosomes. There may also be translocations, where segments of different chromosomes are inappropriately joined together, and localized deletions or duplications of large segments of DNA. Such large rearrangements will clearly affect many different genes and can contribute to the activation of oncogenes and/or loss of TSG function.

The study of somatic mutations requires tissue from the affected area, ideally with a comparison to normal tissue from the same patient and also normal tissue from unrelated controls. Due to the difficulty of obtaining such tissues for benign lung diseases, somatic changes have mainly been studied in the context of cancer, but the same approach has recently been applied to pulmonary arterial hypertension (PAH). In addition, somatic epigenetic changes described below are common both in cancer and in several chronic lung diseases, emphasizing the importance of acquiring tissue from the site of disease when this is ethically possible.

EPIGENETICS

DNA AND HISTONE MODIFICATIONS

The term epigenetics refers to factors that influence gene expression without altering the underlying base sequence. Both DNA and histones, the proteins around which DNA is wound, may be epigenetically modified. These changes are usually reversible and play important roles in regulating gene expression and genome stability. The most common DNA modification is methylation of cytosine residues. The promoters of many genes contain a CpG island, a region with a high density of CG dinucleotides. Methylation of CpG sites in these islands leads to a closed chromatin conformation that makes the DNA inaccessible to transcription factors, turning off expression of the gene. Conversely, when most of the cytosines are unmethylated, the DNA is open and actively transcribed. DNA methylation, therefore, plays a critical role in regulating tissue-specific patterns of gene expression. Patterns of DNA methylation are controlled by DNA methyltransferases (DNMTs). DNMT3A and 3B are responsible for de novo methylation of residues that were previously unmethylated. Established patterns of methylation are then maintained by DNMT1. Further fine tuning of gene regulation comes through methylation and acetylation of histones. Acetylation mainly occurs on lysine residues and relaxes the interaction between histone and DNA, leading to increased gene transcription. Deacetylation reverses this and leads to a more tightly closed chromatin conformation. Histone acetylation patterns are controlled by histone acetyltransferases (HATs) and deacetylases (HDACs).

Within noncoding regions of the genome, DNA methylation and chromatin condensation act to suppress repetitive elements that could otherwise recombine and cause structural alterations. In cancer, there is often a global loss of methylation, which can lead to activation of mobile and repetitive elements, predisposing to the genomic instability that is the hallmark of many cancers. Loss of methylation at gene promoters can also activate oncogenes that in turn accelerate the growth of the tumor. At the same time, there may be hypermethylation of specific gene promoters, causing loss of expression of TSGs. It is increasingly clear that more subtle epigenetic changes likely contribute many other diseases, including lung conditions such as idiopathic pulmonary fibrosis (IPF) and COPD.[15,16] Unlike the DNA sequence, epigenetic modifications can change dynamically with age and are influenced by dietary factors such as folate intake. There is also mounting evidence that airborne pollutants such as small diesel particulates and tobacco smoke can directly mediate epigenetic changes.[17,18] Thus the lung may be particularly susceptible to epigenetic changes caused by repeated exposure to these environmental modulators. Importantly, though, some adverse epigenetic changes are reversible with time, for example, smoking-induced changes in DNA methylation gradually revert after quitting.[19] Also, the anti-inflammatory action of corticosteroids is in part epigenetic, recruiting HDAC2 to the site of acetylated (activated) inflammatory genes.[20] Characterizing the role of epigenetics in lung disease is challenging because it requires access to affected and control lung tissues. It may also be difficult to distinguish which changes are causative of disease and not just a reaction to the disease state. However, considerable progress has already been made under the auspices of the NIH Roadmap Epigenomics Consortium and other focused research initiatives.

■ NONCODING RNAs

Noncoding RNAs can directly regulate gene expression at the RNA level without being translated into a protein product. The best characterized family is the microRNAs (miRs), first studied in plants but now also recognized to be important throughout the animal kingdom. Primary miR transcripts are transcribed in the same manner as regular protein-coding genes. In some cases the miR gene may be within an intron of a protein-coding gene and is controlled by the promoter of the "parent" gene. In other cases, miRs may be encoded as separate genes, individually or in a cluster, with their own promoter. The primary miR transcript is then processed into a pre-miR, about 70 to 80 nucleotides in length (Fig. 7-3). The ends of the pre-miR are highly homologous, causing the molecule to loop back on itself in a hairpin-like conformation. This double-stranded RNA structure is then exported from the nucleus into the cytosol, where it is cleaved by the enzyme Dicer into a mature single-stranded miR, approximately 18 to 22 nucleotides long (Fig. 7-3). The mature miR negatively regulates gene expression by binding to the 3′-untranslated region of its target mRNA, which either leads to degradation of the mRNA or inhibits protein synthesis. The seed sequence that initiates binding between the miR and its mRNA target is very short, typically around seven nucleotides, and does not require perfect base pairing. As a consequence, a single miR can potentially target tens or even hundreds of genes.

miRs have been widely studied in cancer and several, such as miR-21, have been dubbed "oncomiRs" because their overexpression promotes tumorigenesis by downregulating tumor suppressor pathways.[21-24] In comparison, relatively little is known about the role of miRs in benign lung diseases. However, it is now an intense area of research and recent data highlight important roles in IPF and PAH, as detailed in the disease-specific sections that follow. The miR pathway is often considered to be an epigenetic mechanism, yet it can be influenced by changes in DNA sequence, either through mutation affecting the miR gene itself, or mutations and polymorphisms that alter the seed sequence in the mRNA target.

Another major class of noncoding RNAs is the long noncoding (lnc) RNAs, greater than 200 bases long. lncRNA transcripts can be thousands of bases in length and, unlike miRs, they may be encoded by large multiexon genes that undergo splicing in the same manner as most protein-coding genes. Well-known examples of lncRNAs are *XIST*, which coats the inactive X-chromosome in female cells, and *TERC*, part of the telomerase complex that maintains the ends of the chromosomes (telomeres). As yet, very little is known about the role of lncRNAs in human disease, the notable exception being *TERC* mutations, one of several causes of IPF described below.

INHERITED LUNG DISEASES

This section provides an overview of the genetic basis of inherited conditions that include lung disease as a major component (Table 7-2). These brief summaries cannot provide exhaustive

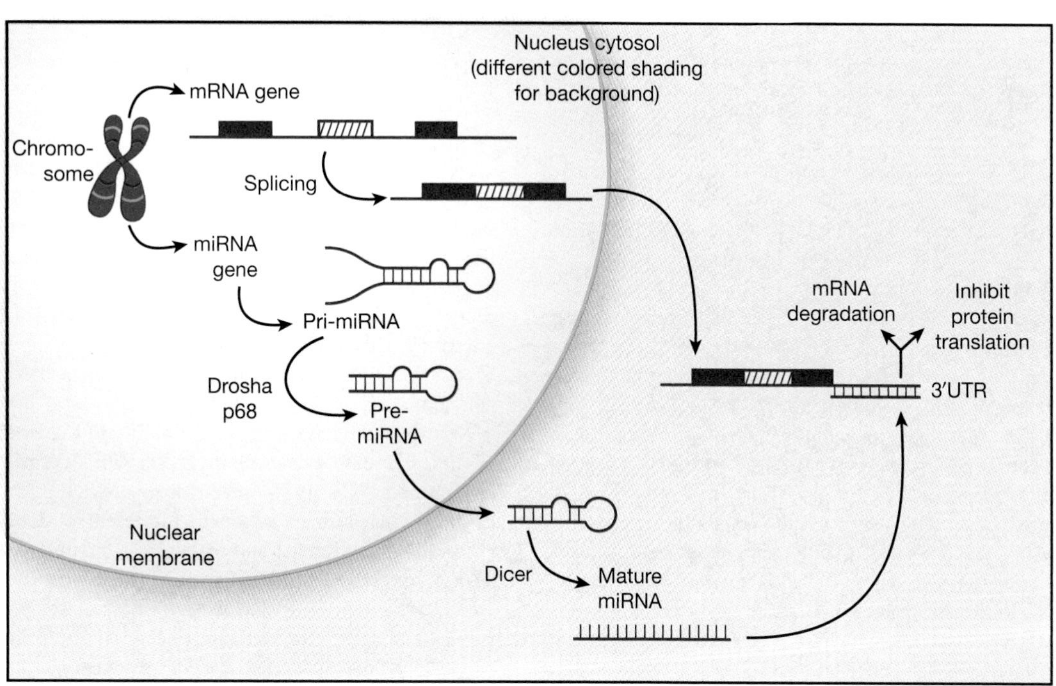

Figure 7-3 microRNA biogenesis. microRNAs that are encoded by independent genes are transcribed by RNA polymerases (mainly RNA pol II) into a primary miRNA transcript with a 5′-cap and 3′-polyadenlyation. The primary miRNA molecule is cleaved by a protein complex, including Drosha and p68, into a double-strand hairpin RNA known as the pre-miRNA. For a subset of microRNAs, recruitment to the p68-Drosha complex is stimulated by activation of the bone morphogenetic protein and transforming growth factor-beta pathways,[67,68] a process that is disrupted by some mutations that cause pulmonary arterial hypertension.[58] Alternatively, some miRNA genes are embedded within the introns of mRNA genes, in which case they are transcribed along with the host gene and the pre-miRNA is generated during mRNA splicing. The pre-miRNA is then exported to the cytosol, where the Dicer complex converts it to the mature single-stranded miRNA molecule. Mature microRNAs negatively regulate expression of their target genes by binding to the 3′-untranslated region of the mRNAs, which either leads to degradation of the mRNA or blocks protein translation.

TABLE 7-2 Mendelian Inherited Lung Diseases

Disease	OMIM	Mode of Inheritance	Gene(s)	Chromosome	Comments
Cystic fibrosis	219700	Autosomal recessive	*CFTR*	7	ΔF508 accounts for ~75% of mutations; many other mutations described at a frequency of 5% or less
Alpha-1 antitrypsin deficiency	613490	Autosomal recessive	*SERPINA1*	14	Z allele (E342K) associated with severe disease, S allele (E264V) is intermediate
Sickle cell disease	603903	Autosomal recessive	*HBB*	11	Predominantly caused by a single mutation, E6V, which leads to an abnormal hemoglobin molecule (HbS)
Pulmonary arterial hypertension	178600	Autosomal dominant, reduced penetrance	*BMPR2* *SMAD9* *ACVRL1* *ENG* *CAV1*	2 13 12 9 7	6–10% of patients have a family history and an additional 15–20% of patients with sporadic idiopathic disease carry a mutation in one of these genes. *BMPR2* mutations account for about 80% of all families and over 200 different mutations have been described
Idiopathic/Familial Pulmonary fibrosis	614742 614743 178500 610913	Autosomal dominant, variable penetrance	*TERT* *TERC* *SFTPA2* *SFTPC*	5 3 10 8	Mutations in *TERT* or *TERC* lead to shortened telomeres. The severity of disease is inversely correlated with telomere length and the age of onset decreases with each succeeding generation (genetic anticipation)
Surfactant metabolism dysfunction	265120 610921 614370 300770	Autosomal recessive X-linked	*SFTPB* *ABCA3* *CSF2RB* *CSF2RA*	2 16 22 X	Disease presentation can range from severe respiratory distress in neonates, through childhood or adult-onset interstitial lung disease. *SFTPC* mutations, listed above under IPF, can also lead to neonatal or childhood surfactant metabolism dysfunction
Alveolar capillary dysplasia	265380	Usually de novo	*FOXF1*	16	Caused by de novo heterozygous mutations or deletions of maternal origin; gene is imprinted; occasionally transmitted as a dominant trait by an unaffected mother
Primary ciliary dyskinesia	Multiple	Autosomal recessive	Multiple	Multiple	Highly heterogeneous disorder with at least 15 different genetic loci
Agammaglobulinemia	300300	X-linked	*BTK*	X	Rare B-cell disorder; recurrent respiratory tract infections
Severe combined immunodeficiency	300400	X-linked	*IL2RG*	X	Rare, affects at least two immune cell types; more severe than agammaglobulinemia; also several autosomal recessive forms

OMIM, Online Mendelian Inheritance in Man; http://omim.org/

reviews of current knowledge, but we refer the reader to entries in Online Mendelian Inheritance in Man (OMIM) and other web resources listed at the end of this chapter, for in-depth information.

■ CYSTIC FIBROSIS

Cystic fibrosis (CF; OMIM 219700) is the most common autosomal recessive disorder in Northern European Caucasians, with a carrier frequency of 1 in 20 to 1 in 25. It is caused by mutations in the cystic fibrosis transmembrane conductance regulator (*CFTR*) gene on chromosome 7, which encodes a transmembrane channel protein important for chloride transport.[25] The most common mutation in Northern Europeans, accounting for about 75% of all CFTR mutations, is a deletion of three base pairs of DNA encoding phenylalanine at codon 508, denoted ΔF508. The frequencies of other mutations are all much lower, each accounting for less than 5% of the total. Thus approximately 56% of individuals with CF will be homozygous for ΔF508 and the majority of others will be compound heterozygotes for two different mutations. In Southern Europeans, ΔF508 is somewhat less common and the mutation spectrum is markedly different in the Ashkenazi Jewish population. Many countries now perform newborn screening for the most common CF mutations, enabling early diagnosis and treatment.

CF mutations can be subdivided into several categories, based on their molecular consequences.[26] Class I mutations, including most nonsense, frameshift, and splice-site mutations and large gene deletions, result in loss of CFTR protein. Class II mutations encode stable proteins that are abnormally processed, leading to retention of the mutant protein in the endoplasmic reticulum. ΔF508 is an example of a Class II mutation. Class III and IV mutations localize correctly to the membrane but they either fail to activate or are inefficient at transporting chloride ions. Class V mutations reduce the rate of CFTR synthesis. Some of these mutations retain a degree of residual function and can mitigate the severity of clinical phenotype.[26,27] Understanding the molecular consequences of these different mutations has been instrumental to developing new therapeutic approaches that seek to correct these defects, as described in the concluding section of this chapter.

Most genetic diseases show variability in the extent and severity of clinical disease, even for individuals with identical mutations. Just as common SNPs may confer risk or protection for common disease, they may also act as genetic modifiers in Mendelian traits. CF is a multisystem disease and with a large enough cohort of patients, it has been possible to identify polymorphisms that modify different aspect of the disease, including pulmonary function (FEV1), bacterial colonization, meconium ileus, and diabetes.[28,29] One particularly interesting polymorphism involves a run of thymine residues in intron 8 of CFTR, commonly present as 9T, 7T, or 5T alleles. These bases are just upstream of exon 9 of the genes and are part of an important signal to regulate mRNA splicing. The shorter alleles splice less efficiently and, in particular, the 5T allele can lead to abnormal splicing that excludes exon 9 from a proportion of the transcripts. Since some full-length CFTR is still made, this is not a severe CF mutation. However, it can lead to a partial phenotype in combination with other mutations and is, therefore, an intragenic modifier. Embryonic development of the vas deferens in males is especially sensitive to the amount of CFTR protein and the 5T allele can contribute to congenital bilateral absence of the vas deferens, even in individuals with little or no lung disease.[30]

ALPHA-1 ANTITRYPSIN DEFICIENCY

Alpha-1 antitrypsin deficiency (AATD; OMIM 613490) is an autosomal recessive disease caused by mutations in the *SERPINA1* gene on chromosome 14, which encodes the protease inhibitor alpha-1 antitrypsin (AAT). AATD was one of the earliest genetic diseases to be understood at the molecular level, since the variant alleles could be identified by protein gel electrophoresis (isoelectric focusing) before the advent of DNA-based genetic testing. Consequently, the alleles are denoted by letters assigned for their relative position on the gel. The wild-type allele is designated M. The most common deficiency allele is Z, a missense mutation that changes glutamic acid to lysine at codon 342 (E342K). Its frequency is highest in Northern European populations. AATD is likely underdiagnosed and the true prevalence may be higher than CF in some countries.[31–33] ZZ homozygotes have low plasma AAT concentrations and are at highest risk for developing lung disease. Accumulation of the mutant protein in the liver can also lead to liver damage. The other most common allele, denoted S (amino acid change E264V), is intermediate in respect to both the level of AAT and disease risk. It is highly prevalent in Southern European populations, with frequencies of 15% to 20% in Spain and Portugal.[33] Clinically, the S allele is of greatest concern in SZ compound heterozygotes, but the severity of lung disease is generally less than for ZZ homozygotes. Individuals with the MZ, MS, or SS genotypes may have slightly impaired lung or liver function. Thus, while overt AATD is considered a recessive condition, the alleles are codominant in their influence on AAT levels and associated risk of disease. There is also a strong gene–environment interaction with tobacco smoking, which can inactivate AAT, further decreasing the level of active protein and greatly increases the risk of lung disease in susceptible genotypes.

Testing for the S and Z alleles may be performed by isoelectric focusing or DNA-based testing. Isoelectric focusing has the advantage that it will pick up other rare alleles that lead to altered protein mobility, whereas the DNA-based tests target only the two known mutations. However, both methods fail to detect rare null mutations that lead to complete loss of protein and, therefore, it is also important to measure the level of AAT in the plasma. This may be followed up with sequencing of the entire *SERPINA1* gene if rare alleles are suspected. Recommendations for genetic testing have been developed by a joint task force of the American Thoracic Society and European Respiratory Society.[34]

PULMONARY ARTERIAL HYPERTENSION

PAH (OMIM 178600) may be idiopathic (IPAH) or associated with an underlying condition such as connective tissue disease, congenital heart defect, or HIV infection (APAH). About 6% of IPAH patients have a family history. PAH is inherited as an autosomal dominant trait with reduced penetrance; on average, only about 27% of mutation carriers will actually develop symptomatic disease. It is more common in females than males and the gender-specific penetrances were recently estimated to be 42% and 14%, respectively.[35] Initial suggestions of genetic anticipation have now been disproved.[35]

Mutations in the bone morphogenetic protein receptor type-II (*BMPR2*) gene account for approximately 80% of familial PAH.[36,37] These are predominantly nonsense, frameshift, or splice-site mutations that lead to premature protein truncation or NMD.[38] Larger gene rearrangements are also frequent.[39,40] Mutations triggering NMD may cause less severe disease than missense mutations resulting in a stable dominant-negative protein, but data from different centers are conflicting.[41,42] *BMPR2* mutations are also found in 11% to 40% of IPAH patients without a family history.[43–45] The revised classification of PAH agreed at the fourth World Symposium created a new category – heritable PAH (HPAH) – that encompasses all patients with a detectable mutation, irrespective of family history.[46,47] *BMPR2* mutations have also been identified in patients with pulmonary veno-occlusive disease[48,39] and in PAH associated with anorexigen exposure,[49,50] congenital heart disease[51] but not in connective tissue disease.

Other genes within the bone morphogenetic protein pathway can also predispose to PAH. Mutations in the type-I receptor ALK1 and its accessory protein endoglin (*ENG*) predominantly cause hereditary hemorrhagic telangiectasia (HHT). However, PAH has been reported in a number of families and may precede the onset of signs or symptoms of HHT.[52–56] Patients with HHT may also develop pulmonary arteriovenous malformations. Several mutations have also recently been identified in the *SMAD9* gene, which encodes Smad8, a downstream mediator of bone morphogenetic protein signaling.[57–59] About 20% of PAH families remain without an identified genetic mutation. Exome sequencing is now being used to determine the cause of PAH in these families and has already led to the identification of two new loci, caveolin-1 (*CAV1*)[60] and a potassium channel gene, *KCNK3*.[61] Whereas *CAV1* mutations were only found in one family and one sporadic case,[60] *KCNK3* mutations were found in three families and 3 of 230 patients with idiopathic PAH.[61] One exciting aspect of this gene discovery is that some mutations could be corrected in vitro by the phospholipase inhibitor ONO-RS-082, raising the possibility of targeted therapeutic intervention for patients carrying a *KCNK3* mutation.[61]

The low penetrance of PAH mutations suggests that additional genetic and/or environmental factors also play a role. The proliferative vascular changes share many features with cancer[62–64] and analysis of affected lung tissues provides molecular support for this hypothesis, with evidence of somatic mutations, microsatellite instability, and aneuploidy.[65,66] miRs likely play an important role in PAH pathogenesis. The bone morphogenetic protein pathway regulates expression of a subset of miRs by promoting processing of the primary miR transcripts.[67,68] This pathway is lost in patients with *BMPR2* or *SMAD9* mutations,[59] whereas several other miRs have also been implicated in PAH, independent of mutation status.[69–74] Overall, despite the progress in understanding HPAH, relatively little is known about the genetic factors that may influence other forms of PAH, particularly APAH, and the heterogeneous nature of the disease remains a challenge.

IDIOPATHIC PULMONARY FIBROSIS

The genetics of IPF (OMIM 178500, 614742, 614743) parallels that of PAH in many respects. A small proportion of cases are familial and the only significant difference in clinical presentation is an earlier age of onset. The pattern of inheritance is autosomal dominant with variable penetrance. Familial pulmonary fibrosis (FPF) is genetically heterogeneous, but unlike PAH, the genes involved do not all fall in a common pathway. Around 3% of families have mutations in either surfactant protein A2 (*SFTPA2*) or surfactant protein C (*SFTPC*) genes, but a much larger proportion of families have mutations affecting telomerase.[75–77] Telomeres are like protective caps on the ends of chromosomes, important in maintaining genome stability. Their DNA sequence comprises many hundreds of copies of the repeat TTAGGG. Due to its position at the end of the chromosome, this sequence cannot be fully replicated and over time the number of repeats gets progressively shorter. Indeed, telomere shortening is believed to be one of the major molecular factors underlying aging. To counteract this, proliferative cells express telomerase, which catalyzes the addition of telomeric DNA. It is especially important in stem cells and germ cells, but is turned off in most differentiated cells. Cancer cells frequently reactivate telomerase. Telomerase is a heteromeric complex composed of a protein with reverse transcriptase activity, encoded by the gene *TERT*, and an lncRNA (*TERC*) that provides the template for synthesizing new telomeric DNA.

The link between IPF and telomerase first came from the identification of genes causing dyskeratosis congenita, a rare multisystem genetic disorder. Patients with dyskeratosis congenita have shortened telomeres and a high incidence of pulmonary fibrosis, prompting analysis of telomere-related genes in FPF.[78] About 18% of families have now been identified with heterozygous mutations in *TERT* and about 1% with *TERC* mutations.[76,77] The average length of the telomeres modifies disease severity and, since the telomeres become progressively shorter with each generation, families with these mutations demonstrate increasingly earlier onset of disease in successive generations, a phenomenon known as "genetic anticipation." Patients with very short telomeres are also at risk for developing aplastic anemia or dyskeratosis congenita.[77] An additional 20% of FPF families have evidence of shortened telomeres but the genetic mutation has not yet been identified. In the remaining 60% of families, the cause of their disease remains unknown.[76]

For patients with IPF (i.e., without a family history), approximately 3% have a *TERT* mutation and less than 1% surfactant protein mutations. However, 25% have a telomere length below the 10th percentile in the general population, suggesting that shortened telomere length is a major risk factor for pulmonary fibrosis, even in the absence of an identifiable mutation.[79] Genomic studies of IPF lung tissue have already yielded considerable insight into the genetic changes contributing to lung fibrosis,[80] including distinct changes in gene expression,[81–83] DNA methylation patterns,[84–86] and miR expression,[87–90] though these have not as yet been translated in new therapeutic approaches.

■ SURFACTANT METABOLISM DYSFUNCTION

Genetic disorders of surfactant metabolism (OMIM 265120, 300770, 610913, 610921, 614370) range from severe neonatal respiratory distress and congenital pulmonary alveolar proteinosis to interstitial lung disease presenting in childhood or adulthood. It is important to note that acquired pulmonary alveolar proteinosis is a distinct autoimmune disorder. Autosomal recessive forms of surfactant metabolism dysfunction are caused by mutations in surfactant protein B gene (*SFTPB*)[91] or the transporter gene *ABCA3*.[92–94] Both lead to severe neonatal respiratory distress. Recessive forms of pulmonary alveolar proteinosis can also be caused by mutations in the granulocyte-macrophage colony-stimulating factor receptor subunits *CSF2RA*, which is X-linked recessive, or *CSF2RB*, autosomal recessive. *SFTPC* mutations are inherited as an autosomal dominant trait with variable penetrance. The phenotype may range from severe neonatal or childhood-onset interstitial lung disease to adult-onset pulmonary fibrosis.[95,96]

■ ALVEOLAR CAPILLARY DYSPLASIA

Alveolar capillary dysplasia (ACD; OMIM 265380) with misalignment of the pulmonary veins is a rare condition caused by heterozygous mutation or deletion of the *FOXF1* gene on chromosome 16.[97] It is usually lethal in infancy and, therefore, mutations are not inherited from an affected parent, rather they occur de novo in the oocyte or sperm, or in the very early embryo. However, one family has been described very recently in which the mother had five affected children and was found to carry a missense mutation in *FOXF1*, despite being unaffected herself.[98] The mutation had arisen de novo on her paternally derived chromosome 16. The authors proposed that *FOXF1* is imprinted on the paternal allele, meaning that it is only expressed from the maternal allele. Thus when the mutation first arose on the paternal allele, its effect was masked because only the normal maternally derived allele was expressed. However, when the mother passed the mutation on to her children, it was now on a maternally derived chromosome and was expressed, leading to ACD and multiple congenital anomalies.

■ PRIMARY CILIARY DYSKINESIA

Primary ciliary dyskinesia (PCD; numerous OMIM numbers) is an autosomal recessive disorder in which abnormalities of the cilia lead to frequent respiratory infections and chronic lung disease. Other manifestations of the condition may include situs inversus and infertility. PCD is genetically very heterogeneous; mutations in at least 15 different genes have so far been identified. Several of these encode components of axonemal dynein, a critical structural component of cilia. Approximately 40% of cases have no identifiable mutation and thus it is expected that many more genes may be identified. This very high level of genetic heterogeneity represents a significant challenge, but the ability to sequence the entire exome of affected individuals holds promise for identifying additional genes.[99–101]

■ SICKLE CELL DISEASE

Sickle cell disease (OMIM 603903) is the most common autosomal recessive disease in Africans and African Americans. Although primarily a blood disorder, it can give rise to significant pulmonary complications, including acute chest syndrome, emboli, and pulmonary hypertension. It is caused by a single A>T mutation in the beta-globin gene that leads to substitution of valine in place of glutamic acid at codon 6. The resulting hemoglobin molecule has reduced solubility compared to the wild-type protein, an example of a mutation that causes gain of an abnormal function. Heterozygous carriers of the mutation have increased resistance to malaria, which is believed to account for the high frequency of the mutation in regions where malaria is or was previously endemic.

GENETIC BASIS OF COMMON LUNG DISEASES

Common lung diseases such as asthma and COPD are not inherited as strong Mendelian traits. However, they may show evidence of familial clustering, suggesting that there is a genetic component to their etiology. The proportion of variation that is estimated to come from genetic factors is termed the "heritability" of the trait, high heritability indicating a strong genetic component. Since common complex diseases do not show clear segregation patterns within families, traditional model-based (parametric) mapping studies cannot be used. Instead, nonparametric methods have been employed across large collections of small family groupings, such as affected sib pairs. Early studies used a candidate gene approach. More recently genome-wide association studies (GWAS) have been used in very large case–control cohorts. Both types of study utilize some of the millions of polymorphic genetic variants throughout the genome and look for a statistically significant association between these genetic markers and the trait of interest. Single nucleotide polymorphisms (SNPs) are now the most commonly used genetic variants, as microarray technology enables simultaneous analysis of more than one million SNPs on a single array. Correlations can also be tested with clinical parameters and biomarkers such as exhaled nitric oxide, serum IgE, and FEV1. Analyzing so many variants across thousands of samples raises the problem of multiple testing, whereby the large number of comparisons between cases and controls greatly increases the likelihood that differences will be identified just by chance. To reduce the number of false-positive results, stringent correction for multiple testing is required. Also, cases and controls must be carefully matched to ensure there is no hidden population stratification that might distort allele frequencies. It is important to note that many of these SNPs are in noncoding regions of the genome and do not directly affect gene regulation or protein function. Rather, they are markers that tag a nearby sequence that may modulate disease risk. In comparison to Mendelian diseases, where mutations confer a high risk of developing the condition, the relative risks for loci identified in GWAS are generally quite small. They have little or no predictive value and so in this respect their clinical utility is limited; the value of these studies is in identifying new pathways and targets for therapeutic intervention.[102] Large amounts of money have been invested in GWAS in a wide range of diseases and the challenge now is to identify the functional variants and fully realize the translational potential of this research. A new and powerful approach is systems biology, which aims to integrate multiple types of "omics" data, such as GWAS, genome-wide expression data, miRs, and epigenomics into networks that identify new pathways and biologic connections.

The literature on GWAS in common lung diseases is large and continues to expand rapidly. In this brief space, it is not possible to discuss these studies in any detail, especially given the complexities of racial and ethnic differences in SNP frequencies and the many subphenotypes that have been studied. We will, therefore, briefly overview some of the major candidate loci and refer the reader to reviews that can be used as a starting point for in-depth reading.

■ ASTHMA

Asthma has a high heritability and has, therefore, been a good candidate for GWAS. Some of the strongest loci identified thus far include HLA-DQ, Orosomucoid-like 3 (*ORMDL3*), and several interleukins and interleukin receptors.[103,104] *ORMDL3* is inducible in the bronchial epithelium and in mice, has been shown to regulate metallloproteinases and several cytokines.[105] SNPs in the same region also modulate expression of a neighboring gene, gasdermin-B (*GSDMB*), part of a family of genes implicated in regulating epithelial cell apoptosis. Through increasingly large studies and meta-analyses, it has been possible to start dissecting the genetic factors associated with specific subgroups, such as childhood asthma, severe asthma, and atopy.[106] Several genes are also associated with response to bronchodilators.[107] Hispanic and African American populations have a higher incidence of severe asthma but are understudied in comparison to Caucasians and represent an important research priority.

Environmental factors such as air pollution and smoking are known to be important modulators of asthma risk. This may be mediated, at least in part, through epigenetic changes affecting DNA methylation, histone acetylation, and miR expression.[16] Changes in DNA methylation directly regulate the arginase–nitric oxide pathway[18,107] and distinct methylation profiles have been identified in asthmatic children compared to controls.[108]

■ CHRONIC OBSTRUCTIVE PULMONARY DISEASE

As described previously, the strongest genetic risk factor for COPD is a mutation in the *SERPINA1* gene that encodes AAT, a risk that is further heightened by tobacco smoke exposure. More common variants with smaller effect size include the nicotine receptors *CHRNA3* and *CHRNA5*, hedgehog-interacting protein (*HHIP*), and *FAM13A*.[109] Smoking is a major risk factor for COPD and as mentioned previously, induces many epigenetic changes in the lung. Altered DNA methylation patterns have been identified in COPD patients in comparison with controls[110] and histone deactylase activity is decreased.[111] Importantly, methylation changes associated with cigarette smoking are reversible with time after quitting[19] and epigenetic changes offer promising targets for drug therapy.[20]

■ SARCOIDOSIS

Relatively little is known about genetic susceptibility to sarcoidosis and despite its prevalence in African Americans, early studies were mainly conducted in cohorts of European ancestry.[112,113] Surprisingly, emerging data suggest common risk loci across multiple different ethnic groups,[114–116] a marked contrast from the heterogeneity in GWAS data for some other diseases. Key loci identified from these studies include the *ANXA11* gene and several HLA subtypes.

TARGETED THERAPIES FOR GENETIC DISEASE

The completion of the human genome project led to high expectations (and in some cases, hype) of a new era of personalized medicine. The first arena in which this has been realized is in the treatment of cancer. Drugs such as imatinib (for chronic myeloid leukemia) and Herceptin (in breast cancer) target specific gene rearrangements or amplifications occurring in these cancers. Several drugs are approved to target epidermal growth factor receptor (EGFR) in non–small-cell lung cancer. Targeted lung cancer therapies are discussed in detail in a later chapter. Progress in other fields has been slower, but some recent advances show great promise, especially for CF.

Initial hopes for gene replacement therapy in CF failed to live up to expectations, but detailed characterization of the types of mutations and their functional consequences are now translating into new therapies. One approach is to promote read-through of nonsense mutations with a small molecule called Ataluren (PTC124).[117] This reduces the recognition of a premature stop codon and allows the ribosome to translate a full-length protein. The same approach has been tried previously with aminoglycoside antibiotics, but Ataluren is more potent and has fewer adverse effects.[118] In theory it should work for any nonsense mutation, but in practice some mutant transcripts are rapidly degraded by nonsense-mediated decay. Logically, therefore, the approach has proven to be most effective for mutations that are relatively stable and not subject to NMD.[119] After positive results in mouse models of CF and Duchenne muscular dystrophy, Ataluren was given orphan drug designation by the FDA and has shown very promising results in phase-II CF clinical trials.[120]

Where a full-length protein is made but it either mislocalizes (class II) or is an inefficient chloride transporter (classes III and IV), drugs are being tested that could improve trafficking to the membrane and improve transporter function. Ivacaftor (VX-770) was found to be effective in rescuing function of the G551D mutation,[121] a class III mutation with a frequency of 3% to 5%. A randomized placebo-controlled trial of Ivacaftor produced exciting results, with highly significant improvements in FEV1, sweat chloride levels, weight, and quality of life scores.[122] Therapies to help the majority of CF patients who are homozygous for ΔF508 are still awaited, but these successes build hope that the vision of personalized medicine, therapies tailored to an individual's personal genetic profile, may become a reality.

Other lung diseases are lagging behind compared with CF, although many do not have the benefit of more than two decades of research on a single gene. However, new therapeutic targets are starting to emerge from some of the research summarized earlier, particularly at the epigenetic level. Several approaches to improving BMPR2 signaling in HPAH are being studied.[123–125] At the epigenetic level, histone deacetylase inhibitors have been proposed as a possible therapy in PAH,[126] whereas corticosteroid-resistant COPD may benefit from increasing HDAC2 activity.[20] As our understanding of the effect of specific genetic mutations and epigenetic modifications increases, the future for targeted therapeutic intervention is bright.

WEB RESOURCES

Online Mendelian Inheritance in Man (OMIM): http://omim.org/
GeneReviews (current expert-authored disease descriptions of inherited diseases): http://www.ncbi.nlm.nih.gov/books/NBK1116/
Genetic Testing Registry: http://www.ncbi.nlm.nih.gov/gtr/
NIH Epigenomics Roadmap Consortium: http://www.roadmapepigenomics.org/
Mitochondrial genome database: http://www.mitomap.org/MITOMAP

REFERENCES

1. Venditti CP, Harris MC, Huff D, et al. Congenital cardiomyopathy and pulmonary hypertension: another fatal variant of cytochrome-c oxidase deficiency. *J Inherit Metab Dis.* 2004;27(6):735–739.
2. Barclay AR, Sholler G, Christodolou J, et al. Pulmonary hypertension–a new manifestation of mitochondrial disease. *J Inherit Metab Dis.* 2005;28(6):1081–1089.
3. Sproule DM, Dyme J, Coku J, et al. Pulmonary artery hypertension in a child with MELAS due to a point mutation of the mitochondrial tRNA ((Leu)) gene (m.3243A > G). *J Inherit Metab Dis.* 2008. [Epub ahead of print.]
4. Van Hove JL, Freehauf C, Miyamoto S, et al. Infantile cardiomyopathy caused by the T14709 C mutation in the mitochondrial tRNA glutamic acid gene. *Eur J Pediatr.* 2008;167(7):771–776.
5. Belostotsky R, Ben-Shalom E, Rinat C, et al. Mutations in the mitochondrial seryl-tRNA synthetase cause hyperuricemia, pulmonary hypertension, renal failure in infancy and alkalosis, HUPRA syndrome. *Am J Hum Genet.* 2011;88(2):193–200.
6. Navarro-Sastre A, Tort F, Stehling O, et al. A fatal mitochondrial disease is associated with defective NFU1 function in the maturation of a subset of mitochondrial Fe-S proteins. *Am J Hum Genet.* 2011;89(5):656–667.
7. Hung PC, Wang HS, Chung HT, Hwang MS, Ro LS. Pulmonary hypertension in a child with mitochondrial A3243G point mutation. *Brain Dev.* 2012;34(10):866–868.
8. Torraco A, Verrigni D, Rizza T, et al. TMEM70: a mutational hot spot in nuclear ATP synthase deficiency with a pivotal role in complex V biogenesis. *Neurogenetics.* 2012;13(4):375–386.
9. Raby BA, Klanderman B, Murphy A, et al. A common mitochondrial haplogroup is associated with elevated total serum IgE levels. *J Allergy Clin Immunol.* 2007;120(2):351–358.
10. Luo YJ, Gao WX, Li SZ, et al. Mitochondrial haplogroup D4 confers resistance and haplogroup B is a genetic risk factor for high-altitude pulmonary edema among Han Chinese. *Genet Mol Res.* 2012;11(4):3658–3667.
11. Zheng S, Qian P, Li F, et al. Association of mitochondrial DNA variations with lung cancer risk in a Han Chinese population from southwestern China. *PLoS One.* 2012;7(2):e31322.
12. Zheng S, Wang C, Qian G, et al. Role of mtDNA haplogroups in COPD susceptibility in a southwestern Han Chinese population. *Free Radic Biol Med.* 2012;53(3):473–481.
13. Zifa E, Daniil Z, Skoumi E, et al. Mitochondrial genetic background plays a role in increasing risk to asthma. *Mol Biol Rep.* 2012;39(4):4697–4708.
14. Knudson AG Jr. Mutation and cancer: statistical study of retinoblastoma. *Proc Natl Acad Sci U S A.* 1971;68(4):820–823.
15. Adcock IM, Tsaprouni L, Bhavsar P, Ito K. Epigenetic regulation of airway inflammation. *Curr Opin Immunol.* 2007;19(6):694–700.
16. Yang IV, Schwartz DA. Epigenetic control of gene expression in the lung. *Am J Respir Crit Care Med.* 2011;183(10):1295–1301.
17. Breton CV, Byun HM, Wenten M, Pan F, Yang A, Gilliland FD. Prenatal tobacco smoke exposure affects global and gene-specific DNA methylation. *Am J Respir Crit Care Med.* 2009;180(5):462–467.
18. Salam MT, Byun HM, Lurmann F, et al. Genetic and epigenetic variations in inducible nitric oxide synthase promoter, particulate pollution, and exhaled nitric oxide levels in children. *J Allergy Clin Immunol.* 2012;129(1):232–239. e231–e237.
19. Wan ES, Qiu W, Baccarelli A, et al. Cigarette smoking behaviors and time since quitting are associated with differential DNA methylation across the human genome. *Hum Mol Genet.* 2012;21(13):3073–3082.
20. Barnes PJ. Targeting the epigenome in the treatment of asthma and chronic obstructive pulmonary disease. *Proc Am Thorac Soc.* 2009;6(8):693–696.
21. Esquela-Kerscher A, Slack FJ. Oncomirs - microRNAs with a role in cancer. *Nat Rev Cancer.* 2006;6(4):259–269.
22. Krichevsky AM, Gabriely G. miR-21: a small multi-faceted RNA. *J Cell Mol Med.* 2009;13(1):39–53.
23. Selcuklu SD, Donoghue MT, Spillane C. miR-21 as a key regulator of oncogenic processes. *Biochem Soc Trans.* 2009;37(Pt 4):918–925.
24. Kumarswamy R, Volkmann I, Thum T. Regulation and function of miRNA-21 in health and disease. *RNA Biol.* 2011;8(5):706–713.
25. Riordan JR, Rommens JM, Kerem B, et al. Identification of the cystic fibrosis gene: cloning and characterization of complementary DNA. *Science.* 1989;245(4922):1066–1073.
26. Welsh MJ, Smith AE. Molecular mechanisms of CFTR chloride channel dysfunction in cystic fibrosis. *Cell.* 1993;73(7):1251–1254.
27. Rowntree RK, Harris A. The phenotypic consequences of CFTR mutations. *Ann Hum Genet.* 2003;67(Pt 5):471–485.
28. Bremer LA, Blackman SM, Vanscoy LL, et al. Interaction between a novel TGFB1 haplotype and CFTR genotype is associated with improved lung function in cystic fibrosis. *Hum Mol Genet.* 2008;17(14):2228–2237.
29. Cutting GR. Modifier genes in Mendelian disorders: the example of cystic fibrosis. *Ann N Y Acad Sci.* 2010;1214:57–69.
30. Chillon M, Casals T, Mercier B, et al. Mutations in the cystic fibrosis gene in patients with congenital absence of the vas deferens. *N Engl J Med.* 1995;332(22):1475–1480.
31. DeCroo S, Kamboh MI, Ferrell RE. Population genetics of alpha-1-antitrypsin polymorphism in US whites, US blacks and African blacks. *Hum Hered.* 1991;41(4):215–221.
32. de Serres FJ. Worldwide racial and ethnic distribution of alpha1-antitrypsin deficiency: summary of an analysis of published genetic epidemiologic surveys. *Chest.* 2002;122(5):1818–1829.
33. de Serres FJ. Alpha-1 antitrypsin deficiency is not a rare disease but a disease that is rarely diagnosed. *Environ Health Perspect.* 2003;111(16):1851–1854.
34. American Thoracic Society, European Respiratory Society statement. American Thoracic Society/European Respiratory Society statement: standards for the diagnosis and management of individuals with alpha-1 antitrypsin deficiency. *Am J Respir Crit Care Med.* 1 2003;168(7):818–900.
35. Larkin EK, Newman JH, Austin ED, et al. Longitudinal analysis casts doubt on the presence of genetic anticipation in heritable pulmonary arterial hypertension. *Am J Respir Crit Care Med.* 2012;186(9):892–896.
36. Deng Z, Morse JH, Slager SL, et al. Familial primary pulmonary hypertension (gene PPH1) is caused by mutations in the bone morphogenetic protein receptor-II gene. *Am J Hum Genet.* 2000;67(3):737–744.
37. The International PPH Consortium, Lane KB, Machado RD, et al. Heterozygous germline mutations in BMPR2, encoding a TGF-beta receptor, cause familial primary pulmonary hypertension. *Nat Genet.* 2000;26:81–84.
38. Machado RD, Aldred MA, James V, et al. Mutations of the TGF-beta type II receptor BMPR2 in pulmonary arterial hypertension. *Hum Mutat.* 2006;27(2):121–132.

39. Aldred MA, Vijayakrishnan J, James V, et al. BMPR2 gene rearrangements account for a significant proportion of mutations in familial and idiopathic pulmonary arterial hypertension. *Hum Mutat.* 2006;27(2):212–213.
40. Cogan JD, Pauciulo MW, Batchman AP, et al. High frequency of BMPR2 exonic deletions/duplications in familial pulmonary arterial hypertension. *Am J Respir Crit Care Med.* 2006;174(5): 590–598.
41. Austin ED, Phillips JA, Cogan JD, et al. Truncating and missense BMPR2 mutations differentially affect the severity of heritable pulmonary arterial hypertension. *Respir Res.* 2009;10:87.
42. Girerd B, Montani D, Eyries M, et al. Absence of influence of gender and BMPR2 mutation type on clinical phenotypes of pulmonary arterial hypertension. *Respir Res.* 2010;11:73.
43. Thomson JR, Machado RD, Pauciulo MW, et al. Sporadic primary pulmonary hypertension is associated with germline mutations of the gene encoding BMPR-II, a receptor member of the TGF-beta family. *J Med Genet.* 2000;37(10):741–745.
44. Koehler R, Grunig E, Pauciulo MW, et al. Low frequency of BMPR2 mutations in a German cohort of patients with sporadic idiopathic pulmonary arterial hypertension. *J Med Genet.* 2004;41(12):e127.
45. Morisaki H, Nakanishi N, Kyotani S, Takashima A, Tomoike H, Morisaki T. BMPR2 mutations found in Japanese patients with familial and sporadic primary pulmonary hypertension. *Hum Mutat.* 2004;23(6):632.
46. Machado RD, Eickelberg O, Elliott CG, et al. Genetics and genomics of pulmonary arterial hypertension. *J Am Coll Cardiol.* 2009;54(1 Suppl):S32–S42.
47. Simonneau G, Robbins IM, Beghetti M, et al. Updated clinical classification of pulmonary hypertension. *J Am Coll Cardiol.* 2009;54(1 Suppl):S43–S54.
48. Runo JR, Vnencak-Jones CL, Prince M, et al. Pulmonary veno-occlusive disease caused by an inherited mutation in bone morphogenetic protein receptor II. *Am J Respir Crit Care Med.* 2003;167(6):889–894.
49. Humbert M, Deng Z, Simonneau G, et al. BMPR2 germline mutations in pulmonary hypertension associated with fenfluramine derivatives. *Eur Respir J.* 2002;20(3):518–523.
50. Abramowicz MJ, Van Haecke P, Demedts M, Delcroix M. Primary pulmonary hypertension after amfepramone (diethylpropion) with BMPR2 mutation. *Eur Respir J.* 2003;22(3):560–562.
51. Roberts KE, McElroy JJ, Wong WP, et al. BMPR2 mutations in pulmonary arterial hypertension with congenital heart disease. *Eur Respir J.* 2004;24(3):371–374.
52. Trembath RC, Thomson JR, Machado RD, et al. Clinical and molecular genetic features of pulmonary hypertension in patients with hereditary hemorrhagic telangiectasia. *N Engl J Med.* 2001;345(5):325–334.
53. Harrison RE, Flanagan JA, Sankelo M, et al. Molecular and functional analysis identifies ALK-1 as the predominant cause of pulmonary hypertension related to hereditary haemorrhagic telangiectasia. *J Med Genet.* 2003;40(12):865–871.
54. Abdalla SA, Gallione CJ, Barst RJ, et al. Primary pulmonary hypertension in families with hereditary haemorrhagic telangiectasia. *Eur Respir J.* 2004;23(3):373–377.
55. Harrison RE, Berger R, Haworth SG, et al. Transforming growth factor-beta receptor mutations and pulmonary arterial hypertension in childhood. *Circulation.* 2005;111(4):435–441.
56. Mache CJ, Gamillscheg A, Popper HH, Haworth SG. Early-life pulmonary arterial hypertension with subsequent development of diffuse pulmonary arteriovenous malformations in hereditary haemorrhagic telangiectasia type 1. *Thorax.* 2008;63(1):85–86.
57. Shintani M, Yagi H, Nakayama T, Saji T, Matsuoka R. A new nonsense mutation of SMAD8 associated with pulmonary arterial hypertension. *J Med Genet.* 2009;46:331–337.
58. Drake KM, Zygmunt D, Mavrakis L, et al. Altered microRNA processing in heritable pulmonary arterial hypertension: an important role for smad-8. *Am J Respir Crit Care Med.* 2011;184:1400–1408.
59. Nasim MT, Ogo T, Ahmed M, et al. Molecular genetic characterization of SMAD signaling molecules in pulmonary arterial hypertension. *Hum Mutat.* 2011;32(12):1385–1389.
60. Austin ED, Ma L, LeDuc C, et al. Whole exome sequencing to identify a novel gene (caveolin-1) associated with human pulmonary arterial hypertension. *Circ Cardiovasc Genet.* 2012;5(3):336–343.
61. Ma L, Roman-Campos D, Austin ED, et al. A novel channelopathy in pulmonary arterial hypertension. *N Engl J Med.* 2013;369(4):351–361.
62. Lee SD, Shroyer KR, Markham NE, Cool CD, Voelkel NF, Tuder RM. Monoclonal endothelial cell proliferation is present in primary but not secondary pulmonary hypertension. *J Clin Invest.* 1998;101(5):927–934.
63. Humbert M, Hoeper MM. Severe pulmonary arterial hypertension: a forme fruste of cancer? *Am J Respir Crit Care Med.* 2008;178(6):551–552.
64. Rai PR, Cool CD, King JA, et al. The cancer paradigm of severe pulmonary arterial hypertension. *Am J Respir Crit Care Med.* 2008;178(6):558–564.
65. Yeager ME, Halley GR, Golpon HA, Voelkel NF, Tuder RM. Microsatellite instability of endothelial cell growth and apoptosis genes within plexiform lesions in primary pulmonary hypertension. *Circ Res.* 2001;88(1):E2–E11.
66. Aldred MA, Comhair SA, Varella-Garcia M, et al. Somatic chromosome abnormalities in the lungs of patients with pulmonary arterial hypertension. *Am J Respir Crit Care Med.* 2010;182(9):1153–1160.
67. Davis BN, Hilyard AC, Lagna G, Hata A. SMAD proteins control DROSHA-mediated microRNA maturation. *Nature.* 2008;454(7200):56–61.
68. Davis BN, Hilyard AC, Nguyen PH, Lagna G, Hata A. Smad proteins bind a conserved RNA sequence to promote microRNA maturation by Drosha. *Mol Cell.* 2010;39(3):373–384.
69. Caruso P, MacLean MR, Khanin R, et al. Dynamic changes in lung microRNA profiles during the development of pulmonary hypertension due to chronic hypoxia and monocrotaline. *Arterioscler Thromb Vasc Biol.* 2010;30(4):716–723.
70. Courboulin A, Paulin R, Giguere NJ, et al. Role for miR-204 in human pulmonary arterial hypertension. *J Exp Med.* 2011;208(3):535–548.
71. Caruso P, Dempsie Y, Stevens HC, et al. A role for miR-145 in pulmonary arterial hypertension: evidence from mouse models and patient samples. *Circ Res.* 2012;111(3):290–300.
72. Parikh VN, Jin RC, Rabello S, et al. MicroRNA-21 integrates pathogenic signaling to control pulmonary hypertension: results of a network bioinformatics approach. *Circulation.* 2012;125(12):1520–1532.
73. Rhodes CJ, Wharton J, Boon RA, et al. Reduced miR-150 is associated with poor survival in pulmonary arterial hypertension. *Am J Respir Crit Care Med.* 2013;187(3):294–302.

74. Kim J, Kang Y, Kojima Y, et al. An endothelial apelin-FGF link mediated by miR-424 and miR-503 is disrupted in pulmonary arterial hypertension. *Nat Med.* 2013;19(1):74–82.

75. Wang Y, Kuan PJ, Xing C, et al. Genetic defects in surfactant protein A2 are associated with pulmonary fibrosis and lung cancer. *Am J Hum Genet.* 2009;84(1):52–59.

76. Garcia CK. Idiopathic pulmonary fibrosis: update on genetic discoveries. *Proc Am Thorac Soc.* 2011;8(2):158–162.

77. Armanios M, Blackburn EH. The telomere syndromes. *Nat Rev Genet.* 2012;13(10):693–704.

78. Armanios MY, Chen JJ, Cogan JD, et al. Telomerase mutations in families with idiopathic pulmonary fibrosis. *N Engl J Med.* 2007;356(13):1317–1326.

79. Cronkhite JT, Xing C, Raghu G, et al. Telomere shortening in familial and sporadic pulmonary fibrosis. *Am J Respir Crit Care Med.* 2008;178(7):729–737.

80. Kass DJ, Kaminski N. Evolving genomic approaches to idiopathic pulmonary fibrosis: moving beyond genes. *Clin Transl Sci.* 2011;4(5):372–379.

81. Kaminski N, Rosas IO. Gene expression profiling as a window into idiopathic pulmonary fibrosis pathogenesis: can we identify the right target genes? *Proc Am Thorac Soc.* 2006;3(4):339–344.

82. Selman M, Pardo A, Barrera L, et al. Gene expression profiles distinguish idiopathic pulmonary fibrosis from hypersensitivity pneumonitis. *Am J Respir Crit Care Med.* 2006;173(2):188–198.

83. Rajkumar R, Konishi K, Richards TJ, et al. Genomewide RNA expression profiling in lung identifies distinct signatures in idiopathic pulmonary arterial hypertension and secondary pulmonary hypertension. *Am J Physiol Heart Circ Physiol.* 2010;298(4):H1235–H1248.

84. Rabinovich EI, Kapetanaki MG, Steinfeld I, et al. Global methylation patterns in idiopathic pulmonary fibrosis. *PLoS One.* 2012;7(4):e33770.

85. Sanders YY, Ambalavanan N, Halloran B, et al. Altered DNA methylation profile in idiopathic pulmonary fibrosis. *Am J Respir Crit Care Med.* 2012;186(6):525–535.

86. Dakhlallah D, Batte K, Wang Y, et al. Epigenetic Regulation of miR-17~92 Contributes to the Pathogenesis of Pulmonary Fibrosis. *Am J Respir Crit Care Med.* 2013;187(4):397–405.

87. Liu G, Friggeri A, Yang Y, et al. miR-21 mediates fibrogenic activation of pulmonary fibroblasts and lung fibrosis. *J Exp Med.* 2010;207(8):1589–1597.

88. Pandit KV, Corcoran D, Yousef H, et al. Inhibition and role of let-7 d in idiopathic pulmonary fibrosis. *Am J Respir Crit Care Med.* 2010;182(2):220–229.

89. Milosevic J, Pandit K, Magister M, et al. Profibrotic role of miR-154 in pulmonary fibrosis. *Am J Respir Cell Mol Biol.* 2012;47(6):879–887.

90. Yang S, Xie N, Cui H, et al. miR-31 is a negative regulator of fibrogenesis and pulmonary fibrosis. *FASEB J.* 2012;26(9):3790–3799.

91. Nogee LM, de Mello DE, Dehner LP, Colten HR. Brief report: deficiency of pulmonary surfactant protein B in congenital alveolar proteinosis. *N Engl J Med.* 1993;328(6):406–410.

92. Shulenin S, Nogee LM, Annilo T, Wert SE, Whitsett JA, Dean M. ABCA3 gene mutations in newborns with fatal surfactant deficiency. *N Engl J Med.* 2004;350(13):1296–1303.

93. Bullard JE, Wert SE, Whitsett JA, Dean M, Nogee LM. ABCA3 mutations associated with pediatric interstitial lung disease. *Am J Respir Crit Care Med.* 2005;172(8):1026–1031.

94. Kunig AM, Parker TA, Nogee LM, Abman SH, Kinsella JP. ABCA3 deficiency presenting as persistent pulmonary hypertension of the newborn. *J Pediatr.* 2007;151(3):322–324.

95. Nogee LM, Dunbar AE 3rd, Wert SE, Askin F, Hamvas A, Whitsett JA. A mutation in the surfactant protein C gene associated with familial interstitial lung disease. *N Engl J Med.* 2001;344(8):573–579.

96. Guillot L, Epaud R, Thouvenin G, et al. New surfactant protein C gene mutations associated with diffuse lung disease. *J Med Genet.* 2009;46(7):490–494.

97. Stankiewicz P, Sen P, Bhatt SS, et al. Genomic and genic deletions of the FOX gene cluster on 16q24.1 and inactivating mutations of FOXF1 cause alveolar capillary dysplasia and other malformations. *Am J Hum Genet.* 2009;84(6):780–791.

98. Sen P, Gerychova R, Janku P, et al. A familial case of alveolar capillary dysplasia with misalignment of pulmonary veins supports paternal imprinting of FOXF1 in human. *Eur J Hum Genet.* 2013;21(4):474–477.

99. Horani A, Druley TE, Zariwala MA, et al. Whole-exome capture and sequencing identifies HEATR2 mutation as a cause of primary ciliary dyskinesia. *Am J Hum Genet.* 2012;91(4):685–693.

100. Olbrich H, Schmidts M, Werner C, et al. Recessive HYDIN mutations cause primary ciliary dyskinesia without randomization of left-right body asymmetry. *Am J Hum Genet.* 2012;91(4):672–684.

101. Knowles MR, Leigh MW, Ostrowski LE, et al. Exome sequencing identifies mutations in CCDC114 as a cause of primary ciliary dyskinesia. *Am J Hum Genet.* 2013;92(1):99–106.

102. Fugger L, McVean G, Bell JI. Genomewide association studies and common disease–realizing clinical utility. *N Engl J Med.* 2012;367(25):2370–2371.

103. Barnes KC. Genetic studies of the etiology of asthma. *Proc Am Thorac Soc.* 2011;8(2):143–148.

104. Cookson WO, Moffatt MF. Genetics of complex airway disease. *Proc Am Thorac Soc.* 2011;8(2):149–153.

105. Miller M, Tam AB, Cho JY, et al. ORMDL3 is an inducible lung epithelial gene regulating metalloproteases, chemokines, OAS, and ATF6. *Proc Natl Acad Sci U S A.* 2012;109(41):16648–16653.

106. Lima JJ, Blake KV, Tantisira KG, Weiss ST. Pharmacogenetics of asthma. *Curr Opin Pulm Med.* 2009;15(1):57–62.

107. Breton CV, Byun HM, Wang X, Salam MT, Siegmund K, Gilliland FD. DNA methylation in the arginase-nitric oxide synthase pathway is associated with exhaled nitric oxide in children with asthma. *Am J Respir Crit Care Med.* 2011;184(2):191–197.

108. Stefanowicz D, Hackett TL, Garmaroudi FS, et al. DNA methylation profiles of airway epithelial cells and PBMCs from healthy, atopic and asthmatic children. *PLoS One.* 2012;7(9):e44213.

109. Cookson WO. State of the art. Genetics and genomics of chronic obstructive pulmonary disease. *Proc Am Thorac Soc.* 2006;3(6):473–475.

110. Qiu W, Baccarelli A, Carey VJ, et al. Variable DNA methylation is associated with chronic obstructive pulmonary disease and lung function. *Am J Respir Crit Care Med.* 2012;185(4):373–381.

111. Ito K, Ito M, Elliott WM, et al. Decreased histone deacetylase activity in chronic obstructive pulmonary disease. *N Engl J Med.* 2005;352(19):1967–1976.

112. Hofmann S, Franke A, Fischer A, et al. Genome-wide association study identifies ANXA11 as a new susceptibility locus for sarcoidosis. *Nat Genet.* 2008;40(9):1103–1106.

113. Fischer A, Schmid B, Ellinghaus D, et al. A novel sarcoidosis risk locus for Europeans on chromosome 11q13.1. *Am J Respir Crit Care Med.* 2012;186(9):877–885.

114. Sato H, Woodhead FA, Ahmad T, et al. Sarcoidosis HLA class II genotyping distinguishes differences of clinical phenotype across ethnic groups. *Hum Mol Genet.* 2010;19(20):4100–4111.

115. Adrianto I, Lin CP, Hale JJ, et al. Genome-wide association study of African and European Americans implicates multiple shared and ethnic specific loci in sarcoidosis susceptibility. *PLoS One.* 2012;7(8):e43907.

116. Levin AM, Iannuzzi MC, Montgomery CG, et al. Association of ANXA11 genetic variation with sarcoidosis in African Americans and European Americans. *Genes Immun.* 2013;14(1):13–18.

117. Welch EM, Barton ER, Zhuo J, et al. PTC124 targets genetic disorders caused by nonsense mutations. *Nature.* 2007; 447(7140):87–91.

118. Hirawat S, Welch EM, Elfring GL, et al. Safety, tolerability, and pharmacokinetics of PTC124, a nonaminoglycoside nonsense mutation suppressor, following single- and multiple-dose administration to healthy male and female adult volunteers. *J Clin Pharmacol.* 2007;47(4):430–444.

119. Linde L, Boelz S, Nissim-Rafinia M, et al. Nonsense-mediated mRNA decay affects nonsense transcript levels and governs response of cystic fibrosis patients to gentamicin. *J Clin. Invest.* 2007;117(3):683–692.

120. Kerem E, Hirawat S, Armoni S, et al. Effectiveness of PTC124 treatment of cystic fibrosis caused by nonsense mutations: a prospective phase II trial. *Lancet.* 2008;372(9640):719–727.

121. Van Goor F, Hadida S, Grootenhuis PD, et al. Rescue of CF airway epithelial cell function in vitro by a CFTR potentiator, VX-770. *Proc Natl Acad Sci U S A.* 2009;106(44):18825–18830.

122. Ramsey BW, Davies J, McElvaney NG, et al. A CFTR potentiator in patients with cystic fibrosis and the G551D mutation. *N Engl J Med.* 2011;365(18):1663–1672.

123. Spiekerkoetter E, Tian X, Cai J, et al. FK506 activates BMPR2, rescues endothelial dysfunction, and reverses pulmonary hypertension. *J Clin Invest.* 2013;123(8):3600–3613.

124. Long L, Yang X, Southwood M, et al. Chloroquine prevents progression of experimental pulmonary hypertension via inhibition of autophagy and lysosomal Bmpr-II degradation. *Circ Res.* 2013;112(8):1159–1170.

125. Drake KM, Dunmore BJ, McNelly LN, et al. Correction of nonsense BMPR2 and SMAD9 mutations by ataluren in pulmonary arterial hypertension. *Am J Respir Cell Mol Biol.* 2013;49(3):403–409.

126. Zhao L, Chen CN, Hajji N, et al. Histone deacetylation inhibition in pulmonary hypertension: therapeutic potential of valproic acid and suberoylanilide hydroxamic acid. *Circulation.* 2012;126(4):455–467.

CHAPTER 8

Stem Cells and Respiratory Disease: Prospects for the Future

Darrell N. Kotton*

INTRODUCTION

Advances in stem cell research offer unprecedented opportunities to develop new treatments, disease models, and drug screens for previously untreatable conditions. These discoveries have captivated the imagination of the lay press and have inspired hope in patients, clinicians, and scientists. Inevitably, in an emerging new field, there are false starts that accompany promising discoveries. If rigorous researchers in the field have difficulty discerning hype from hope, what is a busy clinician to do when confronted with basic questions, such as: "Is stem cell therapy available for my lung disease?" or "Shall I bank my baby's cord blood in case he/she develops cystic fibrosis or emphysema?". This chapter is designed to describe the quickening pace of stem cell and regenerative medicine research related to lung disease and to place the latest discoveries in a historical context, before discussing future prospects.

Stem cells have been found in an increasing number of tissues whose biology is characterized by rapid turnover of differentiated cells. In these tissues, for example, blood, skin, and intestine, a stem cell hierarchy has been described where rare stem cells proliferate occasionally, giving rise to stem cell daughters or to progenitors that can proliferate rapidly, and differentiate into mature cells required for the function of that tissue. These properties of self-renewal and differentiation are the classic hallmarks of stem cells, and their importance in homeostatic maintenance of the blood, skin, and intestine, are well accepted.[1–3] These features also make stem cells attractive vehicles for clinical applications such as the reconstitution of injured or diseased tissues. Several decades of research focused on animals and humans, including the seminal bone marrow transplantation work of Till and McCullough[4] has rigorously proven, for example, that the hematopoietic stem cell, a cell that comprises 1 in 10,000 bone marrow cells, can be delivered to a recipient by simple intravenous infusion, reconstituting all cells of the bone marrow and circulating blood for the life-time of the recipient.[1]

Given the virtually unlimited self-renewing capacity and blood differentiation repertoire of hematopoietic stem cells, most pulmonologists are surprised to learn that cells of similar capacity have not been reproducibly proven to exist in the lung and may not be necessary for the homeostasis of an organ with a quiescent epithelium that contrasts with the rapidly self-renewing epithelia of intestine and skin.

■ LUNG EPITHELIAL RESPONSES TO INJURY

Because the unperturbed adult lung epithelium displays remarkably slow cell turnover, the post-injury or disease responses of human or animal lung have been studied to elucidate both the proliferation potential and differentiation repertoire of various lung cell types. These injury models have been used to search for potential specialized lung cells that might exhibit stem cell properties, such as self-renewal and multipotent differentiation (reviewed by Rawlins and Hogan).[5] Beginning in the 1970s, morphologic studies of human and animal lungs defined subsets of lung epithelia with proliferative capacity, revealing basal, secretory, and club cells (previously called Clara cells) of the proximal airway, and type 2 alveolar cells of the distal lung parenchyma all had the capacity to enter cell

*The author has no financial conflicts of interest to disclose.

cycle in response to lung injury.[6–14] More recently, thymidine-labeling techniques have been replaced by newer methods of identifying proliferating cells or tracking their progeny. These studies have emphasized that most lung epithelial cells, except for airway ciliated cells or type 1 alveolar cells, can proliferate after injury in a remarkably resilient organ where many differentiated epithelial subtypes contribute to tissue repair.[5,15–18]

Beyond assessing the proliferation of cells in the adult lung, the classic developmental biologist's method of "lineage tagging" cells has allowed investigators to follow the origin of lung epithelial cells during development, and to assess where they go upon ageing or after injury.[15,19–21] It is now well established that the many types of epithelial cells in the adult lung arise during development from a few progenitor cells in the embryonic foregut endoderm.[22] The concept has become generally accepted that a limited number of lung epithelial cell types are specified during embryonic development and sustain their committed differentiated state throughout life.[21] In the nascent field of stem cell research, most investigators agree that multipotent, bona fide lung epithelial progenitors exist, if only fleetingly early in embryonic development.[22,23] It remains unclear, however, whether any specialized progenitors or stem cells similar to these embryonic endodermal precursors remain in the lung postnatally or are rederived after injury.

EVOLVING STUDIES IN THE SEARCH FOR LUNG STEM CELLS

With so many proliferation-competent epithelial cells in the adult lung able to participate in post-injury repair, perhaps equally, some investigators have begun to wonder whether some cells are "more equal" than others. The search for specialized reparative lung cells in recent years has been propelled by the emergence of specific and sensitive molecular biology tools and laboratory instruments that can refine our previous understanding of lung biology (Fig. 8-1). New studies suggest that a much greater diversity exists within the previously identified broad classifications of lung airway and alveolar epithelial cells.[24] For example, the response of mouse lung to recover from naphthalene exposure, an injury that depletes the lung of most club cells (identified by the marker club cell secretory protein [CCSP; also known as Scgb1a1 or CC10]), revealed a small subset of airway progenitors, called "variant club cells" (previously variant Clara cells).[25,26] These cells expressed CCSP, but were resistant to naphthalene injury and rapidly reconstituted both secretory and ciliated populations of the injured airway. Most intriguing was the observation that, this rare subset of CCSP+ cells appeared to reside in two specialized microanatomical locations or niches: adjacent to neuroepithelial bodies of the airways and at bronchoalveolar duct junctions. This observation remains one of the most convincing examples to date, suggesting the lung contains progenitor niches, or microanatomical cell compartments with specialized stem or progenitor cells.

One remarkable and controversial study by Kim et al. has proposed that some of these rare CCSP+ progenitors located at the bronchoalveolar duct junction may possess the capacity to reconstitute both airway and alveolar epithelia, suggesting the lung contains rare, multipotent, "bronchoalveolar stem cells" (BASCs).[27] However, the existence of BASCs has been contested in later work by Hogan et al.[19] who employed lineage tagging to trace the progeny of club or variant club cells expressing the CCSP marker which would presumably include the putative BASC population. These investigators found that these cells, either following an injury or during normal fetal lung development, gave rise only to conducting airway but not alveolar epithelia. In later work, Hogan et al. found that under some circumstances, such as following bleomycin-induced lung injury in mice, CCSP+ lineage tagged cells could give rise to alveolar epithelial cells. This confusing literature continues to cause controversy and uncertainty in the field and has dampened enthusiasm for the concept of a lung stem cell

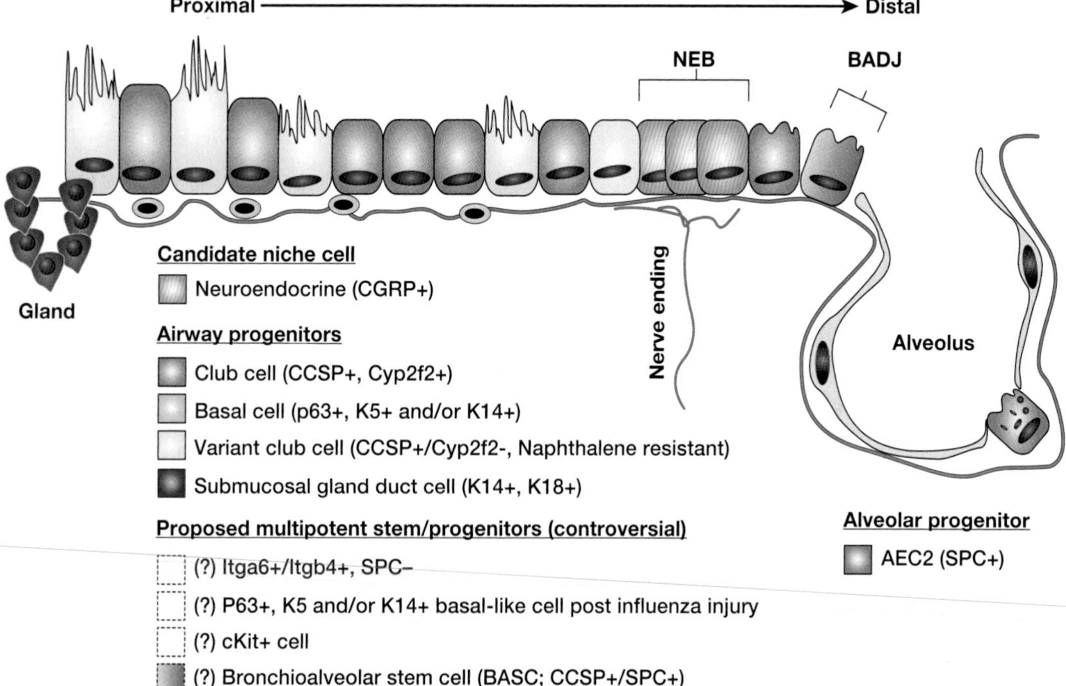

Figure 8-1 Lung epithelial stem and progenitor cell candidates. Schematic of proposed lung epithelial candidate stem or progenitor cells and their niches in the proximal conducting airways and distal alveoli. Cells whose localization or existence is not yet clear or accepted are indicated with dashed boxes and/or question marks. NEB, neuroepithelial body; BADJ, bronchoalveolar duct junction; Gland, submucosal gland duct; AEC2, type 2 alveolar epithelial cell; Marker abbreviations used for each cell subtype include the following: Itg, integrin; K, cytokeratin; CCSP, club cell secretory protein; SPC, surfactant protein-C. *(Modified with permission from Kotton DN: Next-generation regeneration: the hope and hype of lung stem cell research. Am J Respir Crit Care Med. 2012;185(12):1255–1260.)*

hierarchy that might follow the classical paradigm of hematopoietic stem cells of the blood-forming bone marrow.

In the more proximal airways, such as the mouse trachea or human bronchi, investigators have also found remarkable subsets of basal cells that contain extensive proliferative potential and a multipotent differentiation repertoire consisting of the capacity to give rise to basal, secretory, and ciliated lung epithelial cells.[28,29] With the advent of modern flow cytometry, these cells can now be sorted to purity, allowing the cataloging of protein markers (such as p63, NGFR, CK5, or CK14) that identify these cells as well as the delineation of their global transcriptome by microarray analysis.[28,30] The capacity to purify, expand in culture, and differentiate basal cells has resulted in a number of publications in recent years with important implications for those searching for lung cells with stem or progenitor potential.[28,30,31] First, these studies have confirmed that heterogeneity and diversity within the previously limited subsets of lung epithelial cells is indeed much greater than that appreciated a decade ago.[24,32] Second, the studies have revealed the impressive proliferative potential and differentiation repertoire of some subtypes of single lung epithelial cells (such as basal cells), which can expand almost indefinitely in vitro, similar to classically studied stem cells of the skin.[28,31] Taken together, this body of work supports the concept that basal cells can function as tissue-specific stem cells of the proximal conducting airway epithelium.

While there is a quickly growing list of stem/progenitor candidate cells able to reconstitute the conducting airway epithelium, the type 2 alveolar epithelial cell to date remains the best accepted progenitor of the lung alveolus.[33] Basic scientists are on the trail of new candidate alveolar progenitors, however, as evidenced by a notable new study demonstrating the clonal expansion in culture of cells from human or mouse lungs that express basal cell markers yet possess both airway and alveolar differentiation potential in vitro.[31] The authors who described these cells have proposed them as candidate alveolar stem cells, and other labs are working on reproducing these findings before their differentiation repertoire or nomenclature can be established. Most importantly, the p63+ or CK5/14+ lung stem cells described in this exciting study appeared to emerge during recovery from influenza-induced injury in regions of distal lung alveoli, an area of the lung that does not normally harbor cells expressing the basal cell markers p63 or CK5. Other recent studies have utilized flow cytometry to isolate new candidate lung progenitors, identified by coexpression of alpha6 and beta4 integrins.[34] This population appeared to proliferate in response to lung injury, and after purification from mouse lungs displayed remarkable potential for multipotent airway and alveolar differentiation.

While the therapeutic application of these progenitor populations remains years away, it is already clear that the lessons learned from studying the biology of progenitor cells in both mouse models and humans with lung disease can be applied to clinical settings. For example, many publications now demonstrate that communications between some of the best studied lung epithelial progenitors and their neighbors, either in the epithelium or surrounding lung mesenchyme, helps to regulate the fine balance between progenitor self-renewal and differentiation.[17,32,35] Perturbations in these communications, controlled by familiar developmental signaling molecules (such as Wnt, Notch, FGF, retinoic acid, and TGFβ) disturb the balance of lung epithelial homeostasis[36] and contributes to the disordered histopathology and physiology of many lung diseases, including cystic fibrosis, emphysema, idiopathic pulmonary fibrosis, and asthma.[32,37,38] The increased understanding provided by studying the basic biology of lung progenitors and epithelial–mesenchymal interactions has thus allowed a more complete understanding of clinical disease.[37,39] and already is being applied for the development of new pharmaceuticals designed to modulate the above signaling pathways. The long-term goal of achieving sophisticated drug therapies for a variety of lung diseases is likely to ultimately involve activation of endogenous lung progenitors or mature epithelia to accomplish reparative reepithelialization to avoid pathologic lung remodeling.[40]

Common to most of the aforementioned studies evaluating the differentiation repertoire of purified lung progenitor candidates is the suggestion that if an effective technique for grafting these cells into injured lungs were available, these progenitors might be used to regenerate injured epithelia in patients. The prospect of engineering entirely new bioartificial lungs from these cells has also been proposed to meet the needs of growing numbers of patients with end-stage lung diseases who require lung transplantation. Pioneering studies in tissue engineering[41,42] have attempted to develop methods for preparing lung scaffolds or bioartificial lungs that might surmount this highest hurdle in our field: a method for delivering candidate progenitors or lung reparative cells in vivo for engineered lung regeneration. For example, the laboratories of Harald Ott and Laura Niklasson in 2010, both published a technique of engineering bioartificial lungs through the method of detergent-based decellularization of rodent lungs. This method leaves the 3D architecture of the lung matrix intact while stripping away rodent cells. This matrix then served as a scaffold upon which rodent or human cells were adhered to generate "recellularized" lung tissue able to carry out gas exchange in vitro or even in vivo after transplantation.[41,42]

■ CONTROVERSIAL CLAIMS OF PARADIGM SHIFTING STEM CELL RESEARCH DISCOVERIES

This aforementioned studies of lung epithelial injury, proliferation, and regeneration are slowly defining and refining our understanding of candidate lung epithelial progenitors, but there are occasional studies that challenge earlier paradigms of lung development and repair after injury. For example, the laboratory of Anversa et al. in 2011 reported the discovery of a rare cKit+ lung stem cell that they claim can be purified from human lung tissue, can be expanded indefinitely in simple culture media supplemented with serum alone, can be differentiated into multiple lung epithelia by adding dexamethasone, and most importantly, can be injected into injured mouse lungs giving rise to essentially all lung tissues, including mesodermally derived vasculature and endodermally derived airway and alveolar epithelia.[43] This property of naturally occurring pluripotency, defined as the capacity to give rise to multiple cell types across multiple germ layers, is without proven precedent in any adult tissue outside the germline and contradicts many decades of developmental biology research, according to some leaders in this field.[44]

Perhaps it is easiest to understand this new work when placed in the historical context of other prior studies that also initially proposed to shift paradigms in lung biology, including the work of this writer[45] who found that advances in techniques and methods often reveal established paradigms to be correct, and data suggesting paradigm shifts often have simple, alternative explanations that are not obvious at first glance.[46] In the 1990s and early 2000s, for example, a wave of publications claimed that, cells within the bone marrow, such as marrow stromal cells (also known as mesenchymal stem cells [MSCs]) or hematopoietic stem cells, could circulate to the lung and give rise to almost any type of differentiated lung epithelial or vascular endothelial cell. Similar findings were reported when examining injured hearts, brains, livers, and other organs, creating understandable excitement (reviewed by Weiss et al. and Wagers and Weissman[32,47]). Clinical trials were rapidly planned to expose patients to injections of bone marrow–derived cells in the hope of reconstituting degenerative or injured tissues. The opportunity for financial profit inspired companies to promote the banking of cord blood from babies, with glossy pamphlets suggesting to expectant parents that umbilical cord blood containing "stem cells" (now more appropriately called HSCs and MSCs) had the potential to treat diabetes, cystic fibrosis, Parkinson's disease, strokes, or a myriad of other diseases. These diseases might be treated with banked cord blood, if indeed, circulating blood or bone marrow–derived cells could form reconstituting cells for each relevant organ. In hindsight, the launch of some clinical trials and the promotion of cord blood as a panacea was premature as it was based on a first wave of controversially published literature. Advances in laboratory instruments and follow-up laboratory studies begun in 2000, slowly revealed that artifacts, such as autofluorescence, nonspecific antibody labeling, and the fusion of marrow-derived myeloid cells with recipient tissues were actually responsible for the bulk of initial observations and misinterpretations of bone marrow–stem cell engraftment.[46,47]

Clinicians understand that results from an initial, controversial clinical trial require repeating and reproduction of findings before treatment approaches, or established conventions should be radically altered. Likewise, the 2011 published work by Anversa et al. will need to be repeated and reproduced by other scientists before a paradigm shift is warranted. The historical context and false starts of our "lung stem cell field" should make this requirement for reproducibility particularly apparent.

ONE CELL TO RULE THEM ALL: PLURIPOTENT STEM CELLS

Because it remains controversial as to whether an endogenous lung cell possesses broad multipotency or the capacity to produce any type of lung cell, some investigators have chosen to focus their research on the de novo derivation of lung lineages in vitro from pluripotent stem cells, such as embryonic stem (ES) cells, which have well-established potential to generate all cell types in the body,[48] including all lung cells (at least after injection into mouse embryos). The controversy over human ES cell research, unlike other stem cell fields, is not focused on the differentiation potential of the cells, but rather on the ethical debate over whether it is permissible to utilize cells for research that are derived from a pre-implantation human blastocyst embryo (typically those unused from fertility clinics). Despite this ethical controversy, rapid progress is being made in recent years, and ES cells can now be grown indefinitely in culture and then differentiated into lung epithelial lineages upon exposure to defined growth factors.[49–51]

The key advance that has enabled the derivation of lung progenitors from ES cells came with the discovery by Keller et al. that the soluble growth factor, Activin A (hereafter Activin) induced the differentiation of these pluripotent stem cells into the germ layer, definitive endoderm.[52] Since the lung develops from this germ layer, emerging from the anterior foregut endoderm by budding and then branching, the derivation of definitive endoderm from ES cells is a key milestone on the way to generating lung epithelial cells from ES cells.[54] Keller's discovery was based on a careful study of how the embryo develops in vivo. Secreted nodal protein from the node of the embryo is known to differentiate embryonic cells of the epiblast into primitive streak and then into definitive endodermal progenitors within the anterior region of this primitive streak. Since Activin binds similar receptors to nodal protein, Keller et al. found that ES cell cultures exposed to Activin differentiated efficiently into definitive endoderm. Subsequently, investigators in the laboratories of Snoeck,[49] and later Kotton,[50] and Rajagopal[51] found that ES cell–derived endoderm could be patterned into anterior foregut-like precursors that were competent to respond to activated BMP, FGF, and Wnt signaling, differentiating further into primordial lung epithelial progenitors, identified by expression of the transcription factor Nkx2–1 (also known as thyroid transcription factor-1 [TTF1 or Titf1]). Again, these discoveries of how to differentiate stem cells into lung progenitors through activating a sequence of developmental milestones was made possible by mimicking the published inductive signals known to be active during in vivo embryonic endoderm and lung development.[53,54] Once primordial Nkx2–1-expressing primordial lung progenitors have been derived from ES cells (or from induced pluripotent stem [iPS] cells) the cells can be further differentiated into cells expressing a variety of markers of airway and alveolar lineages, including markers of basal cells (p63), ciliated cells (Foxj1 and Cftr), secretory cells (CCSP or mucins), and type 2 or type 1 alveolar epithelia (SPC, SPB, or T1 a), respectively.[50,51] Most intriguing is the finding that ES cell–derived lung epithelia can be used to reconstitute 3D lung tissue scaffolds with cells reminiscent of the morphologic and molecular phenotypes of primary alveolar epithelia.[50]

REPROGRAMMING APPROACHES FOR THE DERIVATION OF LUNG DISEASE-SPECIFIC OR PATIENT-SPECIFIC "INDUCED PLURIPOTENT STEM (iPS) CELLS"

Despite the accepted scientific promise of ES cell research discoveries, there has been a continuing public debate and uncertainty regarding whether it is ethically acceptable to allow public funding of research that uses cells derived through a process that previously involved the destruction of human embryos. The political and ethical concerns that have limited funding or progress in the ES cell research fortunately have found one potential solution in the remarkable discovery of reprogramming technology by Dr. Shinya Yamanaka in 2006. Yamanaka's work revealed that four transcription factors (Oct4, Klf4, Sox2, and cMyc) transferred into cells could reset the epigenetic state of somatic cells, such as skin fibroblasts, into an embryonic like state virtually indistinguishable from ES cells.[55] Reproduction and refinement of this discovery established reprogramming as an accepted technique to engineer iPS cells from dermal fibroblasts or from peripheral blood cells, such as those obtained from simple skin punch biopsies, or banked blood (reviewed by Stadtfeld and Hochedlinger[56]). Like ES cells, the broad differentiation repertoire of iPS cells suggests their potential to form any desired somatic cell type, including lung epithelium.[49] In contrast to ES cells, iPS cells are genetically identical to the individual from whom they are derived, raising the prospect of utilizing iPS cells for autologous cell-based therapies without risk of rejection. Yamanaka, together with his predecessor, Sir Jon Gurdon, who discovered reprogramming approaches in tadpoles 50 years earlier, were awarded the 2012 Nobel Prize in Physiology or Medicine for their paradigm shifting discoveries.[57]

To establish clinically relevant pluripotent stem cell platforms for lung disease research, some investigators have developed new reprogramming technologies able to derive "clinical grade" iPS cells from human skin or blood.[56] and have successfully applied these technologies to generate banks of "lung-disease specific" iPS cell lines from patients with a variety of end-stage lung diseases.[58] In one example of how these cells are being applied to model disease, Rossant et al. generated iPS cells from patients with cystic fibrosis and differentiated these cells in air–liquid interface cultures into cells expressing the Cftr gene responsible for cystic fibrosis, thus modeling Cftr dysfunction using cells of the patients' own genetic background and studying the effects of a pharmaceutical product designed to correct Cftr chloride ion flux.[59] Many other groups are now focused on utilizing patient-specific iPS cell lines (and ES cells) to model lung diseases in vitro, to screen drugs and gene therapy approaches, and to derive de novo replacement lung epithelia and endothelial cells that may one day be transplanted back into the patients from whom they have been derived (Fig. 8-2). The lessons learned from the failed attempts to deliver bone marrow–derived cells to the injured lung epithelium have taught us that delivery of iPS cell–derived lung cells (or any other lung cell) in vivo will not be easy or straightforward. Still, precedent has already been set in rat models of Parkinson's disease and mouse models of sickle cell disease, for example, where iPS-derived replacement neurons and hematopoietic stem cells, respectively, can result in clinical improvementwhen technology for effective differentiation and transplantation of these cells is carefully developed (reviewed in Stadtfeld and Hochedlinger[56]).

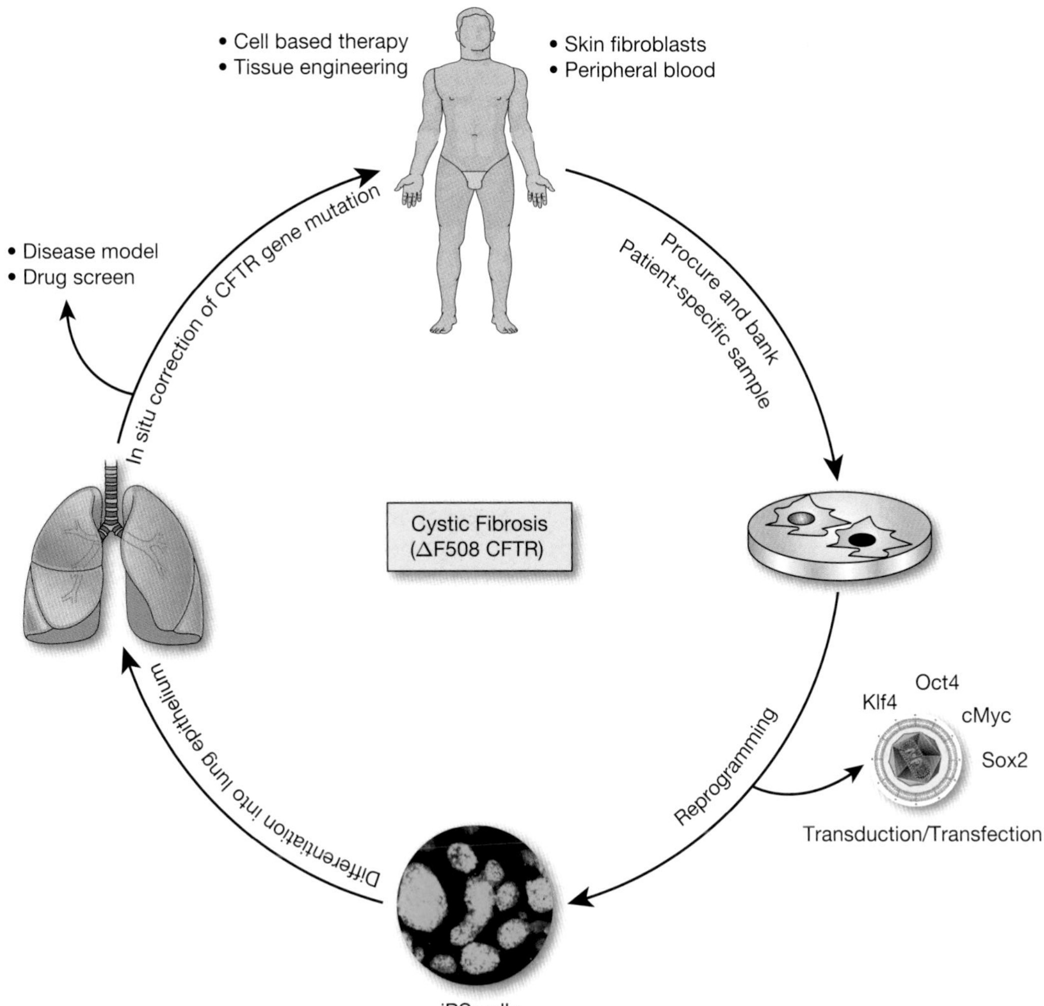

Figure 8-2 Schematic indicating approach for generating patient-specific or disease-specific induced pluripotent stem (iPS) cells from humans with lung disease. Peripheral blood cells or skin fibroblast cells harvested from a patient with lung disease, exemplified by cystic fibrosis, are reprogrammed into iPS cells using defined transcription factors. The resulting iPS cells undergo in vitro "directed differentiation" into lung epithelial or other lung lineages. These lineages can be employed for in vitro studies of disease pathogenesis modeling or high-throughput screening of drugs to predict efficacy. The cells may also undergo correction of any disease-causing gene mutations (such as ΔF508 CFTR) *via* zinc finger nuclease–mediated gene repair. Correction may be performed in the undifferentiated state, or (as shown) following directed differentiation into lung lineages. For future studies, corrected cells may be employed to tissue engineering bioartificial lungs or to develop cell-based therapy by transplantation back into the patient from whom they have been derived. Alternatively, drugs passing in vitro screening can be administered to the patient as personalized medicine.

In almost any field of research where cells reminiscent of the early embryo are employed, such as iPS cells or ES cells, recapitulating the milestones of early development of that tissue lineage has proven to be the most effective and most efficient way to derive desired differentiated lineages in vitro.[48] Unfortunately, little is known about many stages of embryonic lung development, a deficit that limits progress in deriving de novo mature lung epithelia from pluripotent stem cells (be they ES or iPS cells) in vitro and hampers our ability to properly understand and modulate repair after lung injury.

FUTURE PROSPECTS FOCUSED ON THE CLINICAL APPLICATIONS OF STEM CELLS

Given that safe clinical applications of most of the aforementioned exciting stem cell advances remain years away, how is a pulmonologist able to answer questions and respond to the pleas of patients desperate for stem cell therapies? One resource designed to help both physicians and patients access reliable information is the International Society for Stem Cell Research (ISSCR) webpage, which features a downloadable free "Patient Handbook" designed to educate the public about the promise and perils of stem cell research (www.closerlookatstemcells.org). The American Thoracic Society webpage equivalent also helps to objectively caution patients that most stem cell trials charging fees for claimed "treatments" have not been reviewed or substantiated by experts (http://patients.thoracic.org/materials/stem-cells.php).

At the time of publication of this chapter, a number of clinical trials are listed at clinicaltrials.gov for evaluating various cell-based therapies for several lung diseases (reviewed by Weiss et al.[32]). Infusions of MSCs to treat patients suffering from COPD, bronchopulmonary dysplasia, bronchiolitis obliterans, asthma, or acute lung injury, are either planned or underway. Additional trials are listed to test treatments for pulmonary hypertension (employing infusions of endothelial progenitor cells (EPCs) or bone marrow progenitors) and to assess treating pulmonary silicosis utilizing intrabronchial instillations of bone marrow cells.[32] Clinical investigations in Europe, not listed on this website, have also targeted idiopathic pulmonary fibrosis with cell-based therapy.

It is still too early to determine whether any of these trials will prove efficacious, but accumulating data from >100 MSC clinical trials (mostly phase I or II) registered on clinicaltrials.gov for treating diseases affecting other organs suggests that, at least for MSCs, there appears to be little safety risk to participants. That said, there is also little reason to believe that these trials will result in regeneration of lung tissue for participants, as the bulk of basic mechanistic studies in animals suggest the infused cells work mostly via paracrine or immunomodulatory effects on recipient lung tissue.[32] Thus, these trials might be viewed as evaluations of cell-based immunomodulatory drug delivery rather than attempts to regenerate lung tissue.[60] Infused EPCs also appear to have paracrine and perhaps angiogenic effects on recipient tissue,[32] but their capacity to directly form replacement endothelial cells in the lung remains in doubt. When viewed with these results in mind, the term "stem or progenitor cell" – used to refer to the cells being infused in the trials to date – risks misleading clinicians and participants attracted by the promise that these terms imply. The dream of delivering truly regenerative or reconstituting cells to the lung, such as endogenous lung progenitors, ES cells, or iPS cells, will need to be appropriately delayed while these cell populations are fully evaluated in laboratory animals. The impressive differentiation and proliferation potential of the newly described pluripotent stem cell populations also makes them potentially risky and teratogenic in human trials, if deployed before their biology is more fully understood.

All indicators suggest that we are at the onset of realizing the promise of lung regenerative medicine propelled by the quickening pace of stem cell research. Endogenous lung stem or progenitor cell populations, such as basal cells, are just beginning to reveal the mechanisms that control their biology in careful studies at the lab bench.[30,35] New bioartificial lungs generated in the laboratory have already been successfully transplanted into rat recipients,[41,42] and human iPS cells generated from patients with alpha-1 antitrypsin (AAT) deficiency have undergone successful gene correction in vitro followed by hepatic transplantation into rodents.[61] This latter study by Vallier et al. is a conceptual advance for research related to preventing the progression of emphysema caused by AAT deficiency. These researchers demonstrated the full proof of concept of how gene edited iPS cells might be used as a clinical therapy since the research team derived iPS cells from a patient with AAT deficiency, performed gene editing with zinc finger nuclease technology to change the iPS cells from mutant (PiZZ) genotyped cells into gene-corrected (PiMZ or PiMM) cells. The gene-corrected cells were then differentiated into hepatocytes in vitro and then were engrafted in a rodent liver in vivo and secreted human AAT protein. If this approach were applied successfully to humans with AAT deficiency, it would be expected to replace current weekly augmentation therapy treatments and might potentially prevent the progression of emphysema through modulating protease–antiprotease imbalance.

How will the emerging studies focused on lung stem cells impact future clinical care of patients with lung disease? Treatment approaches are likely to involve one or more of several approaches based on the growing literature on endogenous lung progenitors and the newly described lung lineages just now being developed from exogenous pluripotent stem cell sources, such as iPS cells. First, an improved understanding of the pathways that regulate endogenous lung progenitors and control their cell fate decisions to self-renew or differentiate is likely to result in pharmaceutical approaches designed to regulate the behavior of these cell populations during disease pathogenesis. For example, if syndromes such as bronchiolitis obliterans result from an inability to maintain bronchiolar epithelial homeostasis, then an improved understanding of the biology of progenitors of the airways should with time lead to drug approaches for regulating the behavior of these cells toward improved maintenance of homeostasis, epithelial–mesenchymal cross talk, or epithelial barrier integrity. Second, gene therapies aimed at correcting monogenic lung diseases, such as cystic fibrosis or alpha-1 antitrypsin deficiency, likely will involve gene editing[61] or gene correction of lung progenitors or stem cells. A key hurdle limiting progress in lung gene therapy has been the inability to accomplish gene transfer into enough cell numbers. Stem cells provide a potential solution to this problem, since correction of just one stem cell may be sufficient if that cell can self-renew (either in vitro or after engraftment in vivo) extensively enough to reconstitute large numbers of lung epithelial cells via their progeny. Hence, methods for the delivery or engraftment of stem cells into human lung tissue remain a key hurdle still to be solved in order for this hope to come to fruition.

iPS cells are likely to impact lung disease treatments in several ways in the future. First, personalized therapeutic drug regimens can be screened in vitro using lung lineages derived from each patient's iPS cells, potentially predicting effective individualized drug regimens for each individual, rather than the globalized approach currently used to treat disease, where treatments for disease targets are chosen based on trial data from heterogeneous cohorts of patients. If approaches for engrafting or reconstituting lung tissue with exogenously delivered cells are ever successfully developed, iPS-derived cells are one potential source of autologous cell derivatives for potential reconstituting therapies. A particularly attractive, yet far-off goal of some stem cell researchers is the engineering of tissues from stem cells, including the tissue engineering of a whole, functioning, transplantable lung.[41,42] Several groups are working to optimize this approach using iPS cells to derive lung lineages for recellularizing these grafts to optimize tissue engineering of bioartificial lungs for transplantation in future.

While some prospects for employing stem cell–based therapies will take many years to come to fruition, this exciting field of research raises many potential avenues for achieving the long sought-after goal of lung regenerative therapies. Perhaps at this, the most optimistic time in a century of basic science research, we would be most wise to re-emphasize that many of the miraculous advances being made in this field are based on basic science research discoveries realized by investigators who originally had no practical clinical translation in mind. Those who simply wondered what made the Drosophila fly's wing notched, or made the jellyfish glow green, for example, paved the way for today's stem cell discoveries. In 1976, Comroe and Dripps found that the top 10 clinical advances in cardiac and pulmonary medicine derived from 529 key articles, 61.7% of which were classified as "basic science research" and 42% were not clinically oriented at the time the work was done, leading the authors to conclude that "basic science research" pays off in terms of key discoveries.[62] Their report from 38 years ago potentially provides a guide for realizing the full promise of lung-related stem cell research in the years ahead.

SUMMARY

Research discoveries in the fields of stem cell biology and regenerative medicine are beginning to advance and refine an understanding of lung injury and repair. While these emerging studies offer unprecedented opportunities to develop novel therapies for a variety of lung diseases, realization of these therapies will take time and clinical application remains predominantly a future prospect rather than a clinical trial-ready treatment. Given the increasing number of questions from patients about how stem cell research will impact their care, this chapter provides an overview for the clinician or clinician-researcher of the latest advances in lung-related stem cell research and places the new discoveries in a historical context. Established, lineage-restricted, epithelial progenitors of the conducting airways and gas-exchanging alveoli are briefly reviewed, and controversial, newly proposed, tissue-specific candidate lung stem/progenitor cells with broader differentiation repertoire are introduced. Exogenous derivation of lung epithelia from ES cells or iPS cells is also presented as an alternative method for engineering lung tissue de novo in culture.

REFERENCES

1. Morrison SJ, Uchida N, Weissman IL. The biology of hematopoietic stem cells. *Annu Rev Cell Dev Biol.* 1995;11:35–71.
2. Fuchs E, Tumbar T, Guasch G. Socializing with the neighbors: stem cells and their niche. *Cell.* 2004;116(6):769–778.
3. Barker N, van Es JH, Kuipers J, et al. Identification of stem cells in small intestine and colon by marker gene Lgr5. *Nature.* 2007;449(7165):1003–1007.
4. McCulloch EA, Till JE. The radiation sensitivity of normal mouse bone marrow cells, determined by quantitative marrow transplantation into irradiated mice. *Radiat Res.* 1960;13:115–125.
5. Rawlins EL, Hogan BL. Epithelial stem cells of the lung: privileged few or opportunities for many? *Development.* 2006; 133(13):2455–2465.
6. Adamson IY, Bowden DH. The type 2 cell as progenitor of alveolar epithelial regeneration. A cytodynamic study in mice after exposure to oxygen. *Lab Invest.* 1974;30(1):35–42.
7. Adamson IY, Bowden DH. Origin of ciliated alveolar epithelial cells in bleomycin-induced lung injury. *Am J Pathol.* 1977;87(3):569–580.
8. Adamson IY, Bowden DH. Bleomycin-induced injury and metaplasia of alveolar type 2 cells. Relationship of cellular responses to drug presence in the lung. *Am J Pathol.* 1979;96(2):531–544.
9. Bowden DH, Adamson IY, Wyatt JP. Reaction of the lung cells to a high concentration of oxygen. *Arch Pathol.* 1968;86(6):671–675.
10. Cabral-Anderson LJ, Evans MJ, Freeman G. Effects of NO2 on the lungs of rats. I. Morphology. *Exp Mol Pathol.* 1977;27(3):353–365.
11. Evans MJ, Cabral LC, Stephens RJ, Freeman G. Acute kinetic response and renewal of the alveolar epithelium following injury by nitrogen dioxide. *Chest.* 1974;65:Suppl:62S–65S.
12. Evans MJ, Cabral LJ, Stephens RJ, Freeman G. Renewal of alveolar epithelium in the rat following exposure to NO2. *Am J Pathol.* 1973;70(2):175–198.
13. Evans MJ, Cabral LJ, Stephens RJ, Freeman G. Transformation of alveolar type 2 cells to type 1 cells following exposure to NO2. *Exp Mol Pathol.* 1975;22(1):142–150.
14. Evans MJ, Dekker NP, Cabral-Anderson LJ, Freeman G. Quantitation of damage to the alveolar epithelium by means of type 2 cell proliferation. *Am Rev Respir Dis.* 1978;118(4):787–790.
15. Rawlins EL, Ostrowski LE, Randell SH, Hogan BL. Lung development and repair: contribution of the ciliated lineage. *Proc Natl Acad Sci U S A.* 2007;104(2):410–417.
16. Rawlins EL, Hogan BL. Ciliated epithelial cell lifespan in the mouse trachea and lung. *Am J Physiol Lung Cell Mol Physiol.* 2008;295(1):L231–L234.
17. Rawlins EL, Okubo T, Que J, et al. Epithelial stem/progenitor cells in lung postnatal growth, maintenance, and repair. *Cold Spring Harb Symp Quant Biol.* 2008;73:291–295.
18. Borthwick DW, Shahbazian M, Krantz QT, Dorin JR, Randell SH. Evidence for stem-cell niches in the tracheal epithelium. *Am J RespirCell Mol Biol.* 2001;24(6):662–670.
19. Rawlins EL, Okubo T, Xue Y, et al. The role of Scgb1a1+ Clara cells in the long-term maintenance and repair of lung airway, but not alveolar, epithelium. *Cell Stem Cell.* 2009;4(6):525–534.
20. Rock JR, Barkauskas CE, Cronce MJ, et al. Multiple stromal populations contribute to pulmonary fibrosis without evidence for epithelial to mesenchymal transition. *Proc Natl Acad Sci U S A.* 2011;108(52):E1475–E1483.
21. Perl AK, Wert SE, Nagy A, Lobe CG, Whitsett JA. Early restriction of peripheral and proximal cell lineages during formation of the lung. *ProcNatl Acad Sci U S A.* 2002;99(16):10482–10487.
22. Cardoso WV, Lu J. Regulation of early lung morphogenesis: questions, facts and controversies. *Development.* 2006;133(9): 1611–1624.
23. Rawlins EL, Clark CP, Xue Y, Hogan BL. The Id2+ distal tip lung epithelium contains individual multipotent embryonic progenitor cells. *Development.* 2009;136(22):3741–3745.
24. Borok Z, Whitsett JA, Bitterman PB, et al. Cell plasticity in lung injury and repair: report from an NHLBI workshop, April 19–20, 2010. *Proc Am Thorac Soc.* 2011;8(3):215–222.
25. Hong KU, Reynolds SD, Giangreco A, Hurley CM, Stripp BR. Clara cell secretory protein-expressing cells of the airway neuroepithelial body microenvironment include a label-retaining subset and are critical for epithelial renewal after progenitor cell depletion. *Am J Respir Cell Mol Biol.* 2001;24(6):671–681.
26. Giangreco A, Reynolds SD, Stripp BR. Terminal bronchioles harbor a unique airway stem cell population that localizes to the bronchoalveolar duct junction. *Am J Pathol.* 2002;161(1):173–182.
27. Kim CF, Jackson EL, Woolfenden AE, et al. Identification of bronchioalveolar stem cells in normal lung and lung cancer. *Cell.* 2005;121(6):823–835.
28. Rock JR, Onaitis MW, Rawlins EL, et al. Basal cells as stem cells of the mouse trachea and human airway epithelium. *Proc Natl Acad Sci U S A.* 2009;106(31):12771–12775.
29. Hong KU, Reynolds SD, Watkins S, Fuchs E, Stripp BR. *In vivo* differentiation potential of tracheal basal cells: Evidence for multipotent and unipotent subpopulations. *Am J Physiol Lung Cell Mol Physiol.* 2004;286(4):L643–L649.
30. Cole BB, Smith RW, Jenkins KM, Graham BB, Reynolds PR, Reynolds SD. Tracheal Basal cells: a facultative progenitor cell pool. *Am J Pathol.* 2010;177(1):362–376.
31. Kumar PA, Hu Y, Yamamoto Y, et al. Distal airway stem cells yield alveoli in vitro and during lung regeneration following H1N1 influenza infection. *Cell.* 2011;147(3):525–538.
32. Weiss DJ, Bertoncello I, Borok Z, et al. Stem cells and cell therapies in lung biology and lung diseases. *Proc Am Thorac Soc.* 2011; 8(3):223–272.
33. Mason RJ, Williams MC. Type II alveolar cell. Defender of the alveolus. *Am Rev Respir Dis.* 1977;115(6 Pt 2):81–91.
34. Chapman HA, Li X, Alexander JP, et al. Integrin alpha6beta4 identifies an adult distal lung epithelial population with regenerative potential in mice. *J Clin Invest.* 2011;121(7):2855–2862.
35. Rock JR, Gao X, Xue Y, Randell SH, Kong YY, Hogan BL. Notch-dependent differentiation of adult airway basal stem cells. *Cell Stem Cell.* 2011;8(6):639–648.
36. Reynolds SD, Zemke AC, Giangreco A, et al. Conditional stabilization of beta-catenin expands the pool of lung stem cells. *Stem Cells.* 2008;26(5):1337–1346.
37. Guseh JS, Bores SA, Stanger BZ, et al. Notch signaling promotes airway mucous metaplasia and inhibits alveolar development. *Development.* 2009;136(10):1751–1759.
38. Sheppard D. Transforming growth factor beta: a central modulator of pulmonary and airway inflammation and fibrosis. *Proc Am Thorac Soc.* 2006;3(5):413–417.

39. Chen F, Cao Y, Qian J, Shao F, Niederreither K, Cardoso WV. A retinoic acid-dependent network in the foregut controls formation of the mouse lung primordium. *J Clin Invest.* 2010;120(6):2040–2048.

40. Beers MF, Morrisey EE. The three R's of lung health and disease: repair, remodeling, and regeneration. *J Clin Invest.* 2011;121(6):2065–2073.

41. Ott HC, Clippinger B, Conrad C, et al. Regeneration and orthotopic transplantation of a bioartificial lung. *Nat Med.* 2010;16(8):927–933.

42. Petersen TH, Calle EA, Zhao L, et al. Tissue-engineered lungs for *in vivo* implantation. *Science.* 2010;329(5991):538–541.

43. Kajstura J, Rota M, Hall SR, et al. Evidence for human lung stem cells. *N Engl J Med.* 2011;364(19):1795–1806.

44. Hogan BL, Stripp B, Thannickal VJ. Lung stem cells: looking beyond the hype. *Nat Med.* 2011;17(7):788–789.

45. Kotton DN, Ma BY, Cardoso WV, et al. Bone marrow-derived cells as progenitors of lung alveolar epithelium. *Development.* 2001;128(24):5181–5188.

46. Kotton DN, Fabian AJ, Mulligan RC. Failure of bone marrow to reconstitute lung epithelium. *Am J Respir Cell Mol Biol.* 2005;33(4):328–334.

47. Wagers AJ, Weissman IL. Plasticity of adult stem cells. *Cell.* 2004;116(5):639–648.

48. Murry CE, Keller G. Differentiation of embryonic stem cells to clinically relevant populations: lessons from embryonic development. *Cell.* 2008;132(4):661–680.

49. Green MD, Chen A, Nostro MC, et al. Generation of anterior foregut endoderm from human embryonic and induced pluripotent stem cells. *Nat Biotechnol.* 2011;29(3):267–272.

50. Longmire TA, Ikonomou L, Hawkins F, et al. Efficient derivation of purified lung and thyroid progenitors from embryonic stem cells. *Cell Stem Cell.* 2012;10(4):398–411.

51. Mou H, Zhao R, Sherwood R, et al. Generation of multipotent lung and airway progenitors from mouse ESCs and patient-specific cystic fibrosis iPSCs. *Cell Stem Cell.* 2012;10(4):385–397.

52. Kubo A, Shinozaki K, Shannon JM, et al. Development of definitive endoderm from embryonic stem cells in culture. *Development.* 2004;131(7):1651–1662.

53. Morrisey EE, Hogan BL. Preparing for the first breath: genetic and cellular mechanisms in lung development. *Dev Cell.* 2010;18(1):8–23.

54. Kadzik RS, Morrisey EE. Directing lung endoderm differentiation in pluripotent stem cells. *Cell Stem Cell.* 2012;10(4):355–361.

55. Takahashi K, Yamanaka S. Induction of pluripotent stem cells from mouse embryonic and adult fibroblast cultures by defined factors. *Cell.* 2006;126(4):663–676.

56. Stadtfeld M, Hochedlinger K. Induced pluripotency: history, mechanisms, and applications. *Genes Dev.* 2010;24(20):2239–2263.

57. Kotton DN. The 2012 nobel prize in physiology or medicine: democratizing pluripotency for lung researchers. *Am J Respir Crit Care Med.* 2012;186(11):1080–1081.

58. Somers A, Jean JC, Sommer CA, et al. Generation of transgene-free lung disease-specific human ips cells using a single excisable lentiviral stem cell cassette. *Stem Cells.* 2010;28(10):1728–1740.

59. Wong AP, Bear CE, Chin S, et al. Directed differentiation of human pluripotent stem cells into mature airway epithelia expressing functional CFTR protein. *Nat Biotechnol.* 2012;30(9):876–882.

60. Caplan AI. What's in a name? *Tissue Eng Part A.* 2010;16(8):2415–2417.

61. Yusa K, Rashid ST, Strick-Marchand H, et al. Targeted gene correction of alpha(1)-antitrypsin deficiency in induced pluripotent stem cells. *Nature.* 2011;478(7369):391–394.

62. Comroe JH Jr., Dripps RD. Scientific basis for the support of biomedical science. *Science.* 1976;192(4235):105–111.

CHAPTER 9

Personalized Pulmonary Medicine

Benjamin A. Raby

Kelan G. Tantisira

INTRODUCTION

Since the first draft sequences of the human genome were completed in 2001,[1,2] medical research has increasingly focused on the utilization of genetic and genomic profiling in the prediction of disease susceptibility and natural history, as well as drug response and drug development. Personalized medicine can be defined as an approach to medicine in which medical decisions are tailored to the individual patient. In theory, personalized medicine will avoid costly and prolonged trial and error approaches resulting in unwanted therapeutic side effects or diminished treatment efficacy. Diagnostically, personalized medicine uses molecular tracking to signal risk of disease on a genetic level, which may identify disease presence before clinical indications and symptoms appear. Thus, personalized medicine enhances the focus on preventive medicine at the primary, secondary, and tertiary levels. Fully realized, personalized medicine has the potential to facilitate early diagnosis and/or prevention of disease and selection of optimal therapeutic choices with minimal attendant side effects for established disease states. The potential savings, from both a financial and quality-of-life perspective, are enormous.

Much of the efforts to adopt personalized medicine into clinical practice have centered on genetic approaches, as sequence changes in deoxyribonucleic acid (DNA) have been closely associated with a wide range of disease susceptibilities and therapeutic responses. However, the "omics" era includes enhanced focus on cellular and metabolic changes downstream of DNA sequence variation including genomics or transcriptomics (the analysis of gene expression), proteomics (the analysis of protein changes), and metabolomics (the analysis of end products of cellular metabolism). Adding to genomic complexity are the so-called epigenetic changes, the study of changes in gene expression or cellular phenotype caused by mechanisms other than changes in DNA sequence, such as DNA methylation, post-translational modification of gene expression, and microRNA (see further in Chapter 7). Each of these genomic study types has the potential to serve as a biomarker in a personalized medicine context.

In this chapter, the foundations of personalized pulmonary medicine will be reviewed and current approaches designed to facilitate a personalized approach to the diagnosis and treatment of pulmonary disorders will be discussed, including specific examples of personalized approaches currently being implemented in clinical practice. We provide overviews of human genetics, personalized pulmonary diagnostic testing, pharmacogenomics, biomarkers, and future implementation as they relate to personalized respiratory medicine.

DETERMINANTS OF THE CLINICAL UTILITY OF A GENETIC TEST

The predictive power of a genetic test is a function of four interdependent estimable parameters: (1) the *heritability* of the trait; (2) the *penetrance* of the tested genetic variant; (3) *allelic heterogeneity*; and (4) the variant *allele frequency*.

Heritability can be defined as the proportion of disease risk that is explained by genetic determinants. Heritability is highest (~100%) among monogenic diseases like cystic fibrosis (CF), while common diseases such as asthma or obstructive sleep apnea have more modest estimates (30%–60%), with a substantial proportion of disease risk is due to environmental factors. The heritability for many of the commonly measured pulmonary traits is modest (Table 9-1).

Penetrance is defined as the likelihood of the disease among individuals who carry the risk genotype (Fig. 9-1). Penetrance is highest for variants implicated in rare monogenic disorders, approaching 100% for the ΔF508 mutation in CF, and is lowest for more frequent genetic variants associated with common diseases. Wide ranges of intermediate penetrance have also been reported in pulmonary disease, from 90% for FLCN mutations in Birt–Hogg–Dubé syndrome (BHD)[3] to 20% to 50% for *BMPR2* mutations in familial pulmonary hypertension[4] and the *MUC5B* promoter polymorphism in familial pulmonary fibrosis.[5] Penetrance is phenotype-dependent. For example, in BHD, although ~90% of patients with *FLCN* mutations have radiographic evidence of cystic lung disease, dermatologic findings are seen in only ~60%, and spontaneous pneumothorax is observed in only 38% of patients.[3] Similarly, though virtually all PiZ homozygotes have markedly reduced circulating levels of alpha 1-antitrypsin levels, only a subset of these individuals manifests symptomatic emphysema.[6]

TABLE 9-1 Heritability Estimates in Pulmonary Medicine

Trait	Heritability Estimates
Pulmonary diseases	
Cystic fibrosis	1.0
Asthma	0.36–0.72
COPD	0.40–0.77
Sarcoidosis	0.60–0.70
Obstructive sleep apnea	0.33–0.52
Quantitative traits	
FEV_1	0.38–0.77
FVC	0.54–0.91
FEV_1/FVC	0.44–0.46
Airways responsiveness	0.30–0.66
D_{LCO}	0.39–0.46
IgE levels	0.40–0.60

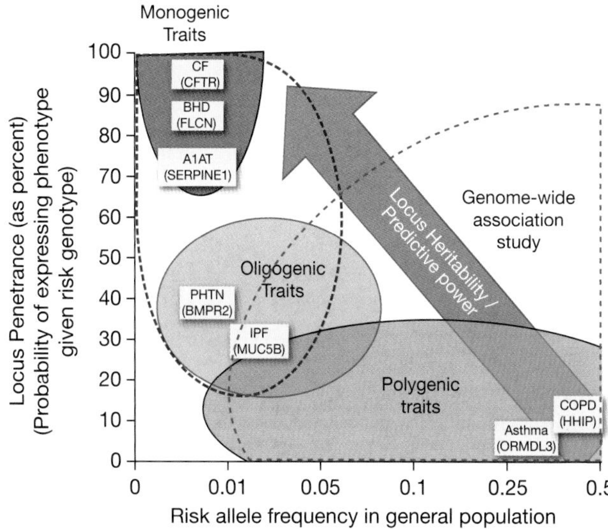

Figure 9-1 The relationship between allele frequency, locus heritability, predictive power, and genetic mapping strategies: Monogenic diseases, such as cystic fibrosis (CF), Birt–Hogg–Dubé syndrome (BHD), and alpha 1-antitrypsin deficiency (A1AT) are caused by highly penetrant, deleterious causal mutations that can be detected by parametric linkage analysis. Polygenic, complex traits, such as asthma and COPD, are caused by numerous genes (dozens to hundreds) harboring variants of much weaker genetic effect. Genome-wide association studies can identify the subset of these variants, but their individual predictive value is low. Oligogenic traits, like familial forms of pulmonary hypertension (PHTN) and idiopathic pulmonary fibrosis (IPF), are caused by variants in a handful of genes with both intermediate frequencies and intermediate penetrance functions.

Allelic heterogeneity refers to the existence of more than one causal allele present in the reference population. Though one variant often predominates as the most prevalent disease allele (e.g., the Z allele in 85% in alpha 1-antitrypsin deficiency), numerous pathogenic variants are typically described, including more than 20 *SERPINE1* mutations in alpha 1-antitrypsin, 50 *FLCN* mutations in BHD, and more than 1800 pathogenic *CFTR* variants in CF. *Locus heterogeneity* is a situation where the same phenotype can manifest through mutations in different genes. For example, familial bronchiectasis resulting from primary ciliary dysfunction has been mapped to no fewer than 18 genes that code for distinct proteins of the ciliary apparatus. There are numerous reports of confirmed primary ciliary dyskinesia where only one of two pathogenic mutations is identified in any one gene,[7,8] suggesting the potential for digenic inheritance, where the combination of two mutations in different genes is sufficient to cause disease.

The influence of variant *allele frequency* on the predictive power of a genetic test is complex, and depends largely on the strength of the genetic effect conferred (the locus heritability) and the disease prevalence. Rare monogenic lung diseases typically result from highly penetrant, low frequency (<1%) variants situated in highly conserved protein-coding sequences. Most common disease susceptibility variants reported are of high frequency (>5% in the general population) but individually are of weak effect. In many instances, the population risk allele frequency exceeds the population disease prevalence (such as the asthma-associated *ORMDL3/GSDMB* risk haplotype, frequency of 62% in asthmatics). In these cases, the specificity of the variant is quite weak. In contrast, rare variants of high penetrance implicated in common disease will have high specificity, yet their low population prevalence diminishes their clinical predictive value, as sensitivity and negative predictive values will be poor.

GENETIC TESTING

All of the major classes of genetic variation – including single nucleotide substitutions, insertions and deletions, copy number variants, and larger, more complex structural variants – have been described in pulmonary disease (Table 9-2), and no single technology has been developed that can reliably survey all these forms simultaneously, though next-generation sequencing (NGS) technologies are emerging as one possible solution. The rapid pace of technological advancement and the vast number of technologies in current use preclude comprehensive survey of all aspects of DNA technologies here. Instead, we emphasize NGS technology as a current and future direction for use in clinical practice.

Whole-genome sequencing. NGS platforms enable DNA sequencing in a highly paralleled fashion, without the need for predefined sequence-dependent hybridization. These methods generate short sequence reads (30–135 bases in length), sampled randomly from the target sample. With these methods, whole-genome sequencing of nearly all genomic regions is now feasible, and is being widely implemented for both research and clinical purposes. The massive parallel nature of these techniques, and their lack of reliance on Sanger chemistries, have resulted in dramatic reductions in cost (now \$1500–\$2000) for whole-genome sequence, favorably raising the prospects for comprehensive genomic testing and personalized medicine.

The major technical challenge, and primary determinant of cost, is achieving sufficient base-calling accuracy. Given the very large numbers of both the bases being called (billions) and polymorphisms per genome (~3–4 million), accuracies of >99.9% are needed to limit the number of spurious findings (both false positive and false negative). Such accuracy can be achieved by ensuring high read depth—the number of times a given base is sequenced. For clinical purposes, minimum average read depths of 30 to 40 times provide reasonable accuracies. For whole genomes, such coverage can only be achieved by performing multiple sequencing runs, increasing costs considerably. More expensive are the downstream costs related to the involved analytical processes of quality assessment, sequence annotation, and variant classification (see below). Additional costs are incurred from the current clinical guidelines that mandate independent technical validation of all actionable (clinically relevant, reportable) variants by Sanger sequencing. Thus, while the technical cost continues to fall, current total charges (often exceeding \$10,000 per clinical genome) preclude widespread adoption of whole genome sequencing at present.

TABLE 9-2 Types of Genetic Variation and their Relative Contribution to Disease Phenotype

Genetic Variation	Definition	Phenotypic Variation %[a]	Example	Pulmonary Manifestation
Chromosomal abnormalities				
Numerical abnormalities	Variations in chromosome number			
Polyploidy	Additional genome copies		69 XXY	Fetal loss
Aneuploidy	Variable number of single chromosome	<1%	Trisomy 21: Down syndrome	Obstructive sleep apnea and pulmonary hypertension
		<1%	Monosomy XO: Turner syndrome	No common pulmonary phenotype
Structural abnormalities	Variations in chromosome structure			
Gross rearrangements	Visible by karyotype/FISH	1%	del(4)(q12): FIP1L1-PDGFRA gene fusion	
Translocations	Aberrant exchange of DNA sequence between two different chromosomes		T(9;22) – Philadelphia chromosome of chronic myelogenous leukemia	Somatic translocations commonly seen in lung cancer tumors
Inversions	Altered sequence orientation		900-kb inversion on 17q21	Glucocorticoid pharmacogenetic response
Copy number variants	Gains or losses of DNA sequence spanning 500 bp or more	9%	GSTM1 null variant	Smoking-related lung function decline
Sequence variants				
Single nucleotide polymorphism	Single base pair substitutions			
Nonsense/Missense	Variant introduces stop codon/ amino acid substitution	55%	FLCN R4496X: Birt-Hogg-Dubé SERPINE1 Glu366Lys (Z) allele	Spontaneous pneumothorax alpha 1-antitrypsin deficiency, emphysema
Splicing	Variant alters normal intron splicing pattern	9.20%	DNAI1 IVS1+3insT: Primary ciliary dyskinesia	Bronchiectasis
Regulatory	Variant alters mRNA transcription or protein translation	2%	17q21 rs12936231 variant alters ORMDL3/GSDMB expression	Asthma
Insertion/Deletion (Indel)	Gain or loss of one or more nucleotides	23%	CFTR ΔF508	Cystic fibrosis
Short tandem repeat	Repetitive element that varies in copy number	0.30%	PHOX2B exon 3 polyalanine repeat expansion	Primary central hypoventilation syndrome

[a] *Percent of total variation listed in Human Gene Mutation Database (http://www.hgmd.cf.ac.uk/ac/index.php, accessed May 30, 2013).*

Targeted sequencing panels. While use of whole-genome sequencing in clinical practice remains modest, there is increasing utility in highly focused, targeted NGS of selected genes or gene regions, which is achieved by "pulling-down" DNA segments of interest using oligonucleotide filters (i.e., probe sets that bind complementary sequence). These filters can be customized to target specific sequences, ranging from a handful of genes to all gene-coding regions (i.e., whole exome filters). This approach markedly reduces the size of targeted sequence length (e.g., an exome sequence is only 3% of the total genome sequence), with numerous advantages for clinical implementation. The marked reduction in target size accommodates clinically reliable read depths in one sequence run, reduces analytic costs (as there is less sequence to annotate), and reduces follow-up validation costs.

Pulmonary-specific sequencing panels. Targeted sequencing of selected genes implicated in pulmonary disease is available commercially through several companies and clinical laboratories. The services provided differ from each other primarily in the gene content of the tests, which are frequently organized in discrete gene panels. Most panels are designed to assess selected gene sets implicated in disorders typified by a particular clinical or radiographic manifestation (i.e., a pulmonary fibrosis panel) or a shared molecular defect (i.e., ciliopathy panel). The largest panels available are those for workup of pulmonary fibrosis and bronchiectasis. Due to technical limitations and the constant pace of novel disease-gene discovery, few panels can be considered fully comprehensive. Yet, most offer coverage of the most commonly implicated genes being considered clinically. Panels of 5 to 20 genes typically cost \$2500 to \$6000, in comparison to the cost of clinical resequencing of individual genes (on average \$1500–\$2000). Thus, when more than one gene is clinically suspected, or for diseases with known locus heterogeneity, diagnostic panels offer greater cost efficiency over single gene resequencing.

More broad sequencing panels may have particular value in the evaluation of patients with more complex presentations (e.g., patients presenting with a combination of bronchiectatic and fibrotic features, or with parenchymal lung disease disproportionate to the degree of concomitant pulmonary hypertension). When a genetic basis is suspected, massively paralleled sequencing across panels of genes may help narrow the differential diagnosis to one or two disorders. Currently, only one laboratory – the Laboratory for Molecular Medicine at the Partners HealthCare Center for Personalized Genetic Medicine – offers combination panel testing, at incremental cost over one panel. Though possibly more cost-effective over current diagnostic strategies, the value of such an approach to the workup of patients with complex presentations remains unclear.

We emphasized that, before ordering more expansive tests, patients must be made aware that surveys of larger panels of genes increase the likelihood of identifying variants of unknown clinical significance (so-called VUS). Patients must be counseled pretest regarding the uncertainty these findings may impart. Genetic test results classify variants according to their likelihood as disease-causing variants. Variants classified as "pathogenic" are those firmly implicated as disease causing due to their demonstrated functional impact, their localization to a highly conserved functional genomic sequence, their presence in affected individuals only, and their strong segregation with disease. So-called "likely pathogenic" variants have many, but not all, of these features. "Benign" variants are those that are common among healthy controls, have no demonstrable function, and do not segregate with disease in families. Counseling of patients regarding these three classes of variants is often unambiguous. In contrast, VUS variants fall into a grey zone, in that they do have features that suggest functional impact but are either observed in unaffected subjects or segregate imperfectly in affected pedigrees (features that suggest incomplete penetrance). Patients must understand the possibility of such findings, and their implications on subsequent workup and management.

Clinical indications for genetic testing. Table 9-3 lists the most common uses of genetic information in clinical practice, both for the patient and at-risk family members. Diagnostic genetic testing is of greatest value when knowledge of the specific gene or mutation will directly impact clinical management. In these cases, genetic testing should be offered to patients in whom the possibility of defining an actionable variant is high, including those with specific disease presentations compatible with the diagnosis of interest, at-risk family members of patients with confirmed molecular diagnoses, and subjects with strong family histories. Some examples are as follows:

- Confirmation of alpha 1-antitrypsin deficiency in patients with emphysema and lung function decline identifies a small subset of COPD patients who may benefit from replacement therapy.
- Identification of Class III CFTR genotypes (particularly the G551R variant) in patients with CF. These patients are candidates for mutation-specific CFTR potentiating therapy with ivacaftor.[9]

TABLE 9-3 Utility of Genetic Information in Clinical Practice

Activity	Paradigmatic Example	Current/*Potential* Utility in Pulmonary Medicine
Preimplantation screening	Tay–Sachs disease	*Primary ciliary dyskinesia*
In utero diagnosis	Trisomy 21	*Congenital diaphragmatic hernia*
Newborn screening	Phenylketonuria	Cystic fibrosis
Diagnostics		LAM vs. Birt–Hogg–Dubé syndrome
Prognostics	Expansion length and age of onset in Huntington's disease	*MUC5B as positive prognostic in IPF*
Presymptomatic interventions	BRCA1 and prophylactic mastectomy/oophorectomy	*BMPR2 and vasodilator therapy*
Surveillance strategies	APC mutations and familial adenomatous polyposis	FLCN mutations and renal cancer screening in Birt–Hogg–Dubé syndrome
Replacement therapies	Gaucher's disease	Alpha 1-antitrypsin deficiency
Mutation-directed therapies	Tyrosine-kinase inhibition in EGFR+ tumors	Ivacaftor in G551R positive cystic fibrosis
Pharmacogenetics	Warfarin dosing	*Polygenic model of inhaled corticosteroid response in asthma*
Gene replacement therapy	X-linked severe combined immunodeficiency	*Surfactant gene replacement in infantile pulmonary fibrosis*

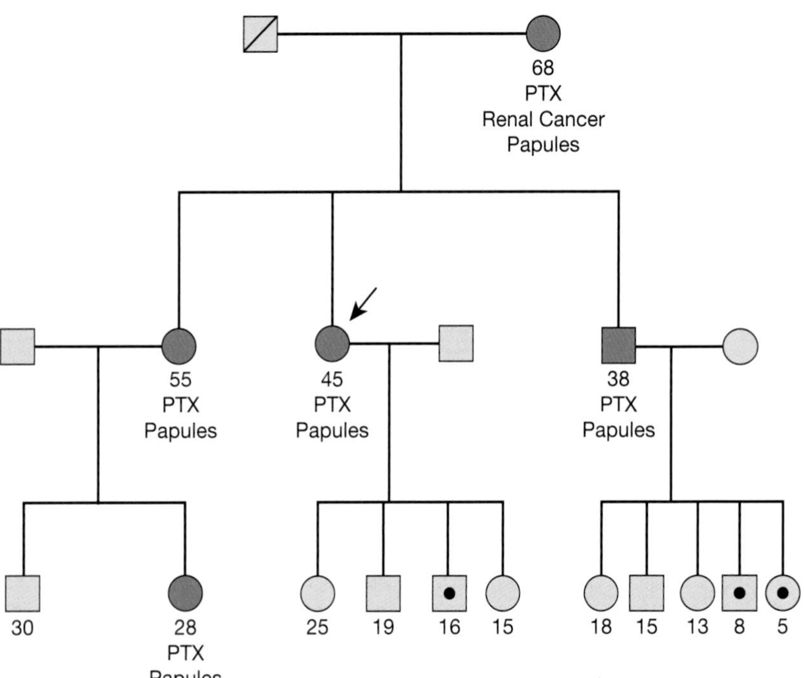

Figure 9-2 Birt–Hogg–Dubé (BHD) syndrome: Index patient *(arrow)* confirmed to harbor a pathogenic FLCN gene mutation. The maternal history of renal cancer places other mutation carriers in this family at risk of both renal and other malignancies. In this pedigree, the large number of reportedly unaffected offspring of two carriers is unusual, given a 50% probability of transmission from carrier to offspring. More likely, the mutation was passed on (hypothetically denoted by *dot*), but these carriers have not yet developed clinical manifestations, possibly due to their younger age. Such individuals would be at risk of eventually developing BHD, including malignancy. Therefore, confirmation of carrier status among at-risk, but seemingly unaffected, family members is warranted.

- Differentiating molecular forms of familial idiopathic pulmonary fibrosis: (1) Patients with *SFTPC* mutations may benefit from hydroxychloroquine treatment[10]; (2) TERC and TERT mutations help identify patients with short telomere syndrome (STS) at risk of marrow and liver failure, including during the post-lung transplant period; (3) Hermansky–Pudlak syndrome (HPS) can often be overlooked clinically due to subtle neurologic (nystagmus) and dermatologic (albinism) features, though these patients are at risk for a potentially severe, but treatable (with DDAVP), bleeding diathesis.

For highly penetrant monogenic diseases, the implications of a positive test result are often profound, even in instances where gene- or mutation-specific therapies are not yet available. Examples include preclinical identification of patients at risk for malignancy (e.g., in BHD or LAM), accelerated lung function decline (in LAM, familial fibrosis), or pulmonary hypertension, who can be more closely followed enabling earlier intervention, and who can be more vigorously counseled regarding the benefits of tobacco smoke avoidance. An illustrative example is provided in Figure 9-2, depicting the value of testing in a family pedigree with BHD. For autosomal dominant diseases of variable penetrance, and for recessive disease, genetic testing offers the ability to identify at-risk carriers prior to the onset of symptoms, providing opportunities for early diagnosis. Negative test results are also of value, providing reassurance to relatives that they are not at risk of developing an illness they may have witnessed afflicting their relatives.

Genetic counseling in pulmonary medicine. The inherently predictive, personal, and irreversible nature of an individual's genetic code distinguishes genetic from other forms of clinical testing. The psychological impact of genetic test results, whether positive or negative, cannot be underestimated. Feelings of inadequacy or imperfection, a sense of inevitable doom and therapeutic nihilism due to a genetic "fate" are not uncommon with a confirmed genetic diagnosis. Conversely, negative results can lead to a false sense of invincibility, leading to unhealthy behaviors (e.g., continuing to smoke). Inherently, the potential impact of genetic testing extends beyond the patient, implicating all blood relatives. Moreover, test results can impact family dynamics and the way in which individual family members react to their test results. For example, though most at-risk family members will be relieved by a negative test result, some experience a deep sense of guilt (so-called "survivors guilt") in relation to their affected family members. Finally, despite legislation at state and federal levels protecting patients from genetic discrimination in the workplace and in access to health care insurance, patients must be informed regarding this risk in other contexts (e.g., the impact on eligibility for life insurance policies).

For all these reasons, it is advised that genetic testing be offered only by, or in consultation with, experienced providers familiar with these issues, including certified genetic counselors, who can adequately address the medical, psychological, and familial implications of test results. We recommend initiating these discussions before testing, so that patients are empowered to provide truly informed consent. Patients should be made aware of the medical implications of both positive and negative results, and should be advised regarding the impact these results may have on them and their family members. Genetic pretest counseling should also address the potential identification of variants of unclear significance.

MUTATION-SPECIFIC THERAPIES IN MONOGENIC LUNG DISEASE

One of the primary goals of genetic classification of disease is the development of mutation-specific therapies. Such activities have traditionally focused on the development of replacement therapies for loss-of-function recessive diseases (i.e., recombinant human alpha 1-proteinase inhibitor replacement therapies). Newer pharmacologic approaches, including small molecule screens and others informed by the functional impact of specific mutations are emerging.

TYROSINE-KINASE INHIBITION FOR HYPEREOSINOPHILIC SYNDROME

Imatinib was identified as a therapy for chronic myelogenous leukemia (CML). However, once the functional mechanisms underlying its therapeutic effects were elucidated, other therapeutic uses were identified. The treatment of hypereosinophilic syndrome (HES) is one such example. Subsets of HES patients harbor a chromosome 4q interstitial deletion that results in the creation of a fusion of the *FIP1L1* and *PDGFRA* genes. The resultant fusion protein has tyrosine-kinase activity similar to that of BCR-ABL, the target site in CML and HES patients positive for the *FIP1L1-PDGFRA* rearrangement respond positively to imatinib therapy.[11,12] *FIP1L1-PDGFRA*-negative HES patients do not. Similar to CML,

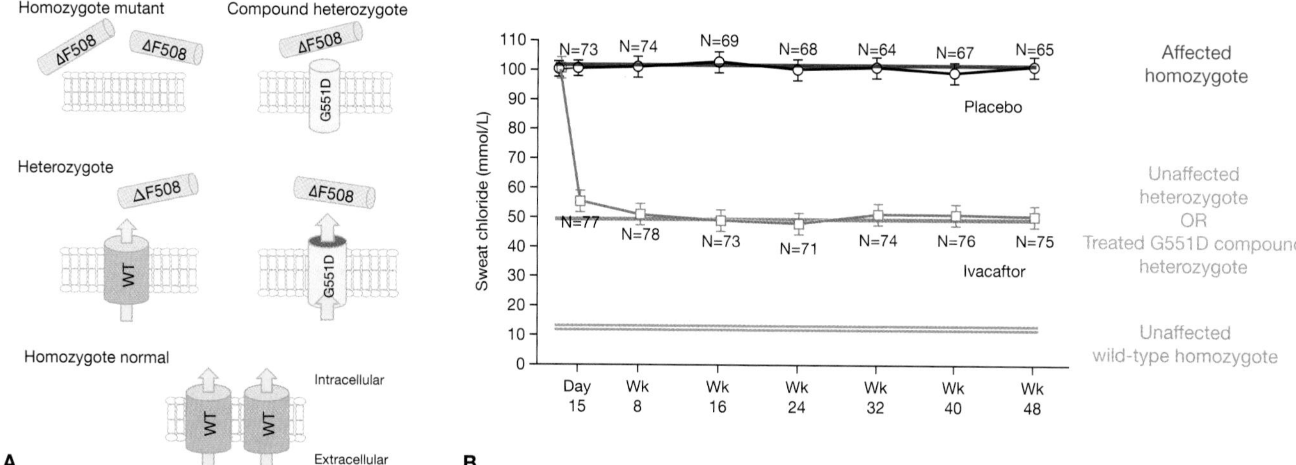

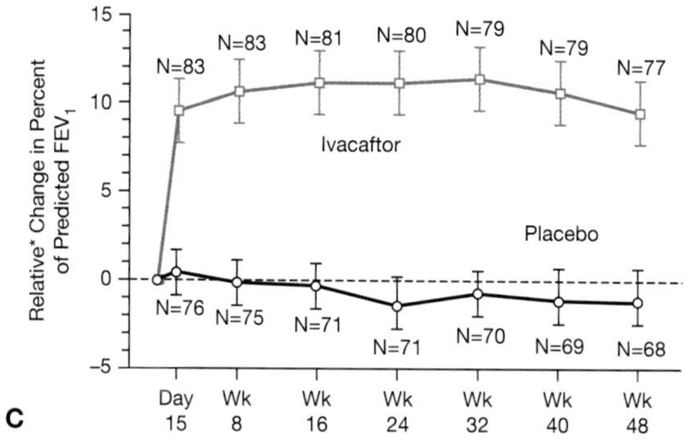

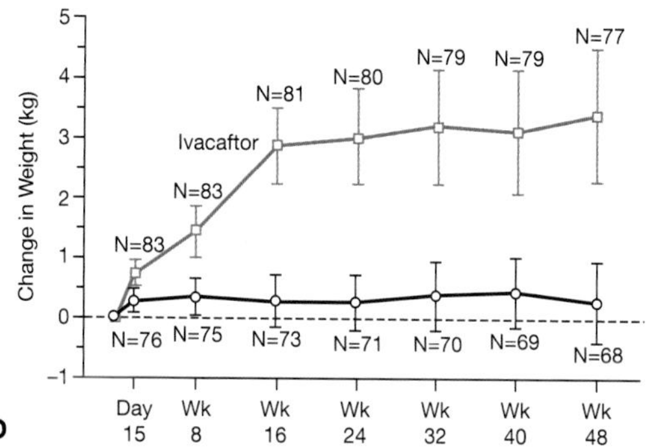

Figure 9-3 Mutation-specific therapeutic action of ivacaftor in cystic fibrosis: **A, B.** The additive effect of CFTR mutations on epithelial chloride efflux and sweat chloride levels, and the effect of ivacaftor. Individuals with two normal alleles have normal chloride efflux *(yellow arrows)*, and a corresponding normal sweat chloride test *(blue double line)*. Individuals with two mutated alleles demonstrate markedly reduced chloride efflux and elevated sweat chloride *(red line)*. Heterozygotes with ~50% normal functional chloride channels on epithelial cell surfaces manifest intermediate reductions in both chloride efflux and sweat chloride responses *(orange line)*. G551D compound heterozygotes treated with ivacaftor *(red disc)* demonstrate sweat chloride levels similar to heterozygote carriers. **C, D.** Therapeutic efficacy of ivacaftor: Patients randomized to ivacaftor demonstrated improvements in relative change in percent of predicted FEV_1 (**C**) and weight (**D**) over 48 weeks, in addition to improvements in symptoms and in quality of life scores (not shown). *Original report erroneously labeled figure as Absolute (not relative) change in percent of predicted FEV_1. *(**B–D.** Reproduced with permission from Ramsey BW, Davies J, McElvaney NG, et al. A CFTR potentiator in patients with cystic fibrosis and the G551D mutation. N Engl J Med. 2011;365(18):1663–1672.)*

mutations of the tyrosine-kinase binding site have been reported upon HES relapse.

MUTATION-SPECIFIC THERAPIES FOR CYSTIC FIBROSIS

In 2011, positive results of a randomized clinical trial of a novel therapy for G551D-positive CF were reported (Fig. 9-3).[9] In a 48-week, randomized, double-blind, placebo-controlled trial, 167 patients received either placebo or ivacaftor—an oral agent that "potentiates" CFTR activity by prolonging channel opening times and augmenting transmembrane chloride transportation. Compared to patients receiving placebo, patients treated with ivacaftor demonstrated significant improvements in FEV_1, fewer respiratory exacerbations, improved quality of life, and a positive weight gain. The ~50% reduction in sweat chloride levels to those approaching those observed in asymptomatic *CFTR* mutation carriers (i.e., heterozygotes) serves as an elegant molecular–clinical correlate, suggesting selective effect on the G551D+ channel, but not ΔF508+ channels. While G551D and other variants likely to benefit via ivacaftor are observed in only ~6% of patients, their identification opens new therapeutic options for this subset of CF patients. The advent of this novel treatment strategy provides motivation for the development of additional agents that target other *CFTR* mutation classes (including the most common *CFTR* mutation—ΔF508), and the application of similar strategies for the treatment of other genetic diseases.

BIOMARKERS IN PULMONARY MEDICINE

Biomarkers have been defined as "biological characteristics that can be objectively measured and evaluated as an indicator of normal biological processes, pathogenic processes, or pharmacological responses to a therapeutic intervention".[13] Ideal biomarker characteristics have been espoused (Table 9-4).[14] There are two major types of biomarkers applicable to clinical medicine: (1) biomarkers of exposure, which are used in risk prediction; and (2) biomarkers of disease, which are used in the screening, diagnosis, and monitoring of disease progression, as well as response to therapy. Thus, biomarkers have the potential to support clinical decisions, from diagnosis to treatment planning; to improve tailored treatment strategies; to avoid over- or undertreatment and adverse side effects; and to enhance prognosis and cost-effectiveness.

While a number of biomarkers have been evaluated in a wide range of pulmonary conditions, including MMP-7, ICAM-1, and IL-8 for interstitial lung disease,[15] procalcitonin for community acquired pneumonia,[16,17] exhaled nitric oxide for asthma and other inflammatory lung disease,[18,19] and RAGE, ICAM-1, and SP-D for ARDS,[20] few are

TABLE 9-4 Ideal Biomarker Characteristics

Easy to measure
Safe to measure
Low cost to measure
Consistent across gender, age, race
Cost of follow-up tests is reasonable
Proven therapy to modify biomarker
Modification of biomarker is proven to protect against disease or outcome

recommended for routine clinical use. This stems largely from their relatively weak predictive power. For instance, at a 5% false-positive rate (specificity 95%), a relative odds of 3.0 between the first and fifth quartiles of a biomarker gives only a 20% detection rate.[21] As such, most current biomarkers cannot substitute other clinical parameters in clinical evaluation, but are used as adjuncts to support clinical judgment.

An example of a biomarker in prominent routine use in pulmonary medicine is the D-dimer and its role in the diagnosis of acute pulmonary embolism (Fig. 9-4). The quantitative rapid enzyme-linked immunosorbent assay (ELISA) has a sensitivity of 95%. In patients with low pretest clinical probability (i.e., 4%–15%), a normal D-dimer rapid ELISA substantially reduces the posttest probability of pulmonary embolism to 0.7% to 2%.[22] Therefore, these patients can safely be excluded from further evaluation.[22–25] Notably, the D-dimer is still used adjunctively to clinical judgment, as both the predictive ability falls in patients with intermediate to high pretest clinical likelihood of pulmonary embolism and the relatively poor specificity (of about 27%)[26] of the D-dimer limit its usefulness outside of low

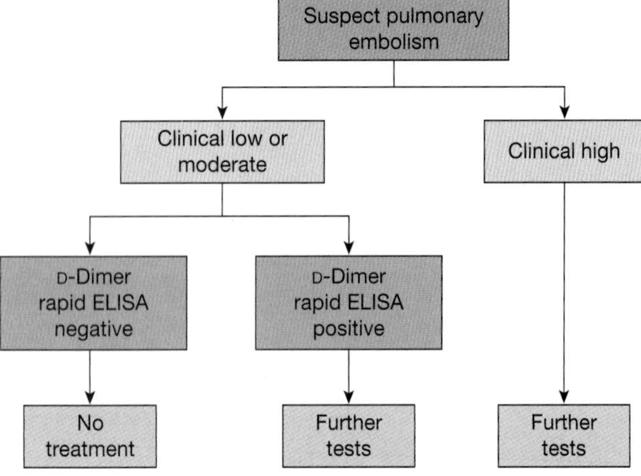

Figure 9-4 Use of D-dimer as a biomarker in the exclusion of pulmonary embolism. The quantitative rapid enzyme-linked immunosorbent assay (ELISA), with a sensitivity of 95%, showed the most clinically useful values among the various D-dimer assays. When used in combination with a low probability objective clinical assessment, which ranges from 4% to 15%, the post-test probability of pulmonary embolism ranges from 0.7% to 2% with a normal D-dimer rapid ELISA. No further testing is required if D-dimer is normal in a patient with a low probability clinical assessment. *(Reproduced with permission from Stein PD, Woodard PK, Weg JG, et al. Diagnostic pathways in acute pulmonary embolism: recommendations of the PIOPED II investigators. Am J Med. 2006;119(12):1048–1055.)*

probability cases. There is, however, evolving evidence that may support the use of the D-dimer in the exclusion of pulmonary embolism, even with intermediate levels of clinical probability.[27–29]

The integration of biomarkers in drug development and their use as a companion diagnostic in clinical practice has been encouraged by regulatory authorities.[30,31] One example of this in clinical practice has been the development of periostin as a biomarker for treatment with lebrikizumab (anti-IL-13). In a study of 42 asthmatic patients and 28 healthy controls, conducted by Woodruff et al.,[32] a three-gene airway epithelial cell expression signature composed of periostin (*POSTN*), chloride-channel regulator 1 (*CLCA1*), and serpin peptidase inhibitor clade B, member 2 (*SERPINB2*), was used as a surrogate marker of T_H2 inflammation. Multivariate cluster analysis defined groups of patients: a T_H2-high cluster (asthmatic patients with high expression of T_H2 cytokine-induced gene expression) and a T_H2-low cluster (asthmatic subjects whose expression analysis was the same as healthy controls). The T_H2-high cluster phenotype was characterized by increased serum IgE levels, allergic inflammation, airways hyperresponsiveness, and increased responsiveness to inhaled corticosteroids.[32]

In a study of lebrikizumab, an IL-13 monoclonal antibody, in 219 adults who had poorly controlled asthma despite inhaled glucocorticoid therapy,[33] high serum periostin levels at baseline predicted a positive treatment response (improvement in FEV_1). Nevertheless, the performance of periostin expression as a clinical predictor has yet to be independently confirmed. Indeed, in a clinical trial of asthmatic subjects not taking inhaled corticosteroids, lebrikizumab did not show any significant improvement in lung function regardless of baseline periostin status.[34]

PHARMACOGENETICS

The response to pharmacologic agents varies tremendously between individuals. For instance, the plasma level of a given medication can vary more than 1000-fold between two individuals having the same weight when treated with the same drug dosage.[35] On average for a given drug, 30% of patients show beneficial effects, 30% fail to improve, 10% only experience side effects, and 30% are noncompliant (which may be related to either lack of efficacy or side effects).[36] Therefore, as many as 70% of all patients are unnecessarily exposed to the potential to develop adverse drug reactions (ADRs).[37–39] In the United States, over 2 million hospitalizations due to serious ADRs and over 100,000 fatal ADRs were noted in 1994, ranking ADRs between the fourth and the sixth leading cause of death.[40] Worldwide, the prevalence of hospitalizations due to ADRs was recently estimated at a median of 5.3% (interquartile range [IQR] 2.7%–9.0%), as based on prospective cohort studies of over 100,000 admissions.[41] Overall, the cost of drug-related morbidity and mortality in the United States exceeded $177.4 billion in 2000,[42] a figure more than double the estimate from 1995.[43] As enormous as these figures are, the burden due to lack of therapeutic response to drug therapy is likely to be much greater.[44]

Pharmacogenetics is the study of variability in drug response due to heredity. Pharmacogenetic variability in drug absorption, drug metabolism, and drug action at the receptor level is well-known. Overall, it is estimated that genetics can account for 20% to 95% of variability in drug disposition and effects.[45] Ideally, pharmacogenetics will allow for "individualized therapy" based upon an individual's genetic makeup that will maximize the potential for therapeutic benefit, while minimizing the risk of adverse effects. The potential for cost savings and for decreasing morbidity and mortality is immense.

PHARMACOGENETIC RESPONSE CATEGORIES

The heritability of many therapeutic agents has been formally established via genetic studies, including the twin studies of Vessel and Page.[46–50] Barring formal genetic studies, the response distribution can also strongly suggest a heritable response. The interindividual response

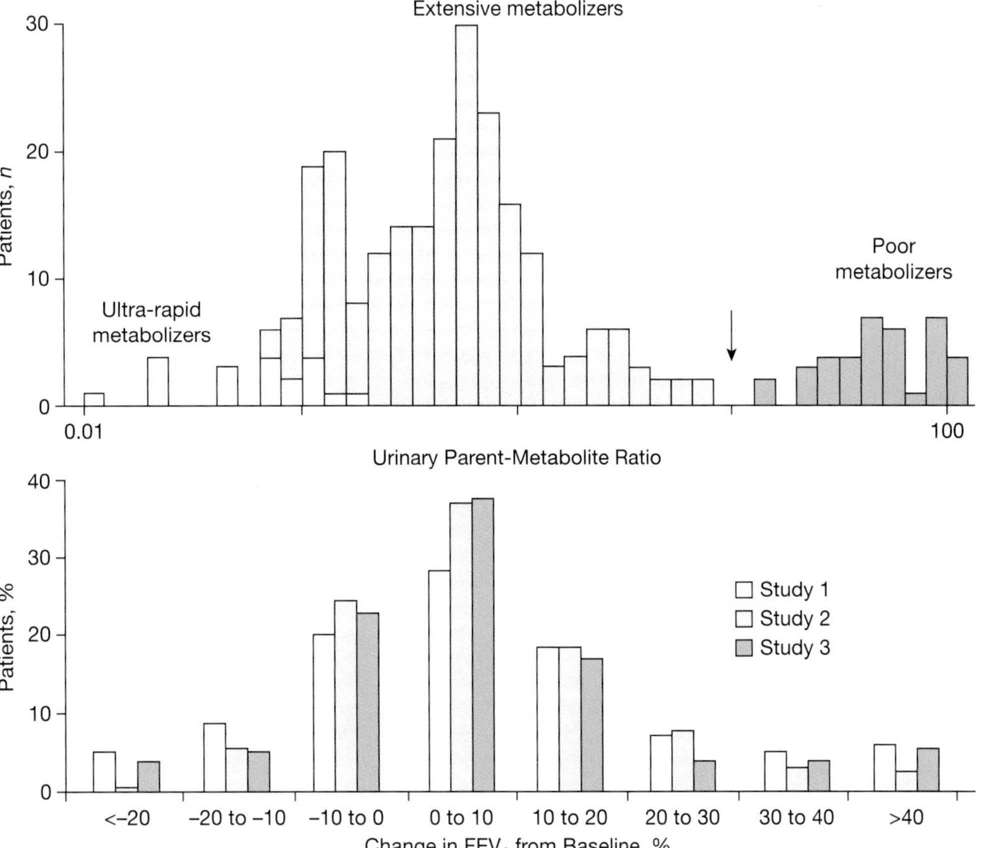

Figure 9-5 Patterns of variation in drug response. *Top.* Multimodal response common to many drug metabolizing enzymes. *Bottom.* Unimodal, yet highly variable, response noted in complex trait drug response. In this case, Studies 1 to 3 refer to three independent clinical trials that measured inhaled corticosteroid response over time. *(Reproduced with permission from Roden DM, Altman RB, Benowitz NL, et al. Pharmacogenomics: challenges and opportunities. Ann Int Med. 2006;145(10):749–757.)*

distribution may be either multimodal or unimodal (Fig. 9-5). A multimodal distribution suggests distinct population subgroups of response, thereby directly supporting a pharmacogenetic basis for response. A unimodal drug response distribution still supports the concept of interindividual variation, with subjects demonstrating both "good" and "poor" responses. The combination of wide interindividual response with high repeatability (the likelihood of a subsequent beneficial/poor response to a drug given a prior response) supports the plausibility of a pharmacogenetic effect.[51]

Pharmacogenetics has traditionally been divided into four categories based upon the effects of genetic variability on the pharmacologic properties of a drug. For instance, one genetic variant can alter the rapidity of drug metabolism (thereby altering bioavailability), whereas another genetic variant can affect binding to a drug receptor (thereby decreasing therapeutic efficacy). The four categories include variation related to pharmacokinetics, pharmacodynamics, idiosyncratic reactions, and disease pathogenesis (Fig. 9-6).[52] Each of these categories will be discussed below, followed by a known example or examples pertinent to pulmonary medicine. Clinical implementation guidelines for several of these examples have been developed.[53–57] Additional examples likely to be encountered by the respiratory practitioner and labeled by the US Food and Drug Administration (FDA) are listed in Table 9-5.

Pharmacokinetics studies the effect of the body upon an administered drug, including the absorption, distribution, tissue localization, biotransformation, and excretion of drugs.[58] Common drug metabolizing enzymes implicated in pharmacogenetics and their estimated effect on drug dosing are shown in Figure 9-7. The cytochrome p450 enzymes (*CYPs*) encode for ~60% to 70% of all phase I (i.e., structural transformation) dependent metabolism and have been the classic examples of drug metabolizing enzymes. The clinically most important *CYPs* are *CYP2C9, CYP2D6,* and *CYP3A4*, with *CYP2C9* discussed in the context of warfarin administration later in this chapter. *CYP* genotypes generally result in three metabolic phenotypes, ultra-rapid metabolizers, extensive (normal) metabolizers, and poor metabolizers (Fig. 9-5).

An example of polymorphic phase II (i.e., drug conjugation) drug metabolizing enzymes is the metabolism of azathioprine by thiopurine-*S*-methyltransferase (*TPMT*).[59] Azathioprine, which is commonly used in the therapy of interstitial lung disease and pulmonary vasculitides, is converted to the active 6-mercaptopurine, which is then metabolized by *TPMT* or converted into 6-thioguanine nucleotides. Decreased *TPMT* activity, as mediated through genetic variation, occurs in about 10% of individuals at intermediate levels, while ~0.3% (1 in 300) have low to absent activity. Clinically, this results in drug-related myelosuppression in 5%, severe leukopenia in 1.2%, and is fatal in 0.3% of subjects taking azathioprine.[60] Both clinical phenotyping (predrug assessment of *TPMT* activity) and genotyping assays are available. Such testing has been noted to be cost-effective

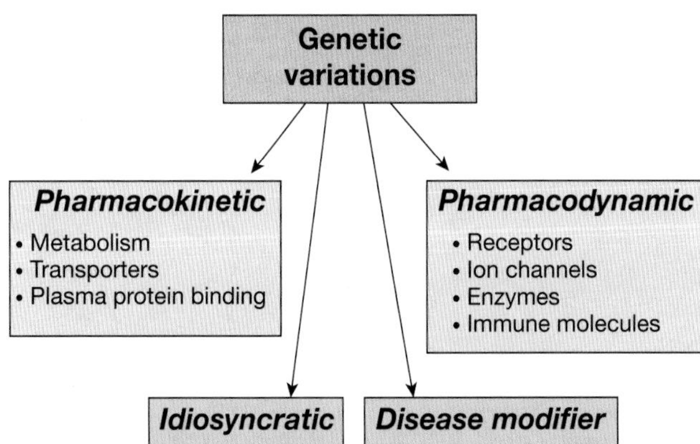

Figure 9-6 Categories of pharmacogenetic response, based upon site of activity of the genetic variant of interest.

TABLE 9-5 Common Pulmonary Medications FDA Labeled for Pharmacogenomic Effects

Drug	Therapeutic Area	Genotype	Variant Genotype Effect
Azathioprine	Interstitial lung disease	*TPMT*	Increased potential for bone marrow suppression
Cisplatin	Oncology	*TPMT*	Children with variants may have an increased risk of ototoxicity
Codeine	Analgesics, cough suppression	*CYP2D6*	Decreased pain relief in poor metabolizers
Dapsone	Anti-infective	*G6PD*	Hemolytic anemia
Erlotinib	Oncology	*EGFR*	EGFR-TK mutation is biomarker of erlotinib efficacy in lung cancer
Gefitinib	Oncology	*EGFR*	EGFR-TK mutation is biomarker of gefitinib efficacy in lung cancer
Imatinib	Pulmonary hypertension	*CYP3A4*	Decreased efficacy in rapid metabolizers, increased toxicity in poor metabolizers
Irinotecan	Oncology	*UGT1A1*	Increased potential for severe diarrhea and fatal neutropenia
Ivacaftor	Pulmonary	*CFTR (G551D)*	G551D genotype is one benefitting from actions of ivacaftor
Lansoprazole	Gastroenterology	*CYP2C19*	Increased efficacy (higher intragastric pH) vs. extensive (normal) metabolizers
Mercaptopurine	Oncology	*TPMT*	Increased potential for bone marrow suppression
Mycophenolic acid	Transplantation	*HGPRT*	Should be avoided in patients with hereditary deficiency of hypoxanthine-guanine phosphoribosyltransferase (HGPRT) such as Lesch–Nyhan or Kelley–Seegmiller syndrome
Omeprazole	Gastroenterology	*CYP2C19*	Increased efficacy (higher intragastric pH) vs. extensive (normal) metabolizers
Isoniazid	Anti-infective	*NAT1; NAT2*	Increased risk of peripheral neuropathy with *NAT1* variation; attenuated with pyridoxine administration; *NAT2* influences drug level
Voriconazole	Antifungals	*CYP2C19*	Possible risk of subtherapeutic voriconazole concentrations, and subsequently of treatment failure
Warfarin	Hematology	*CYP2C9; VKORC1*	Higher warfarin levels and increased potential for adverse effects

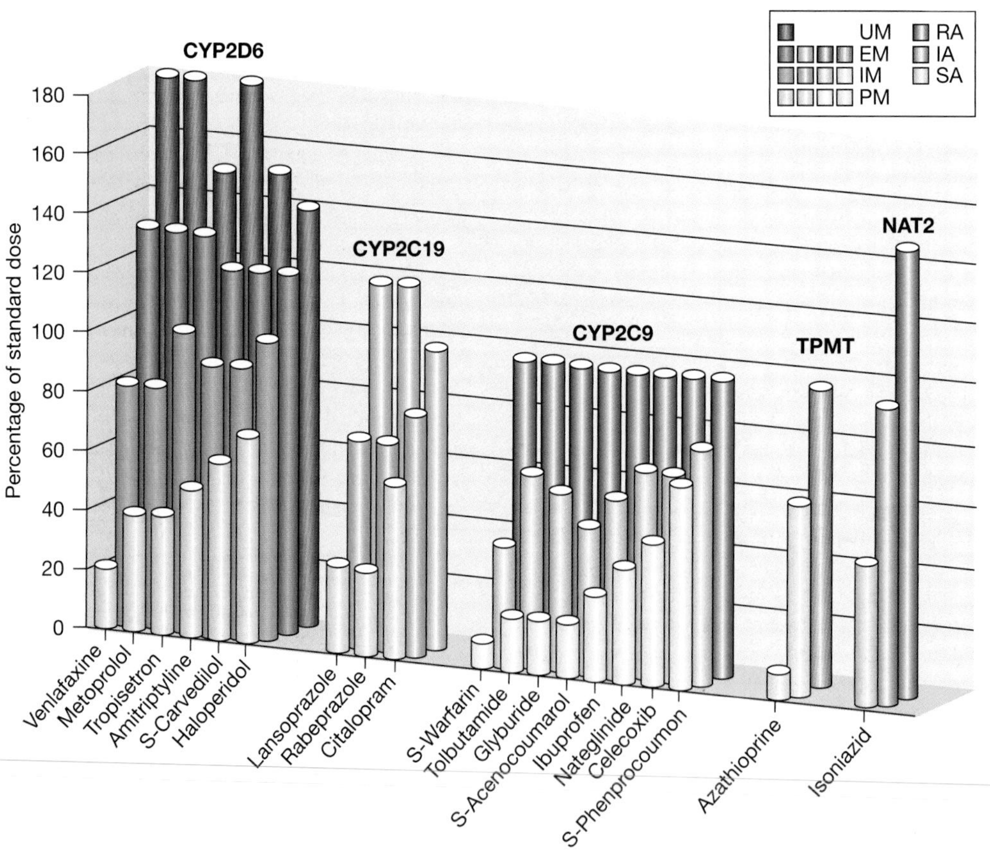

Figure 9-7 Common drug metabolizing enzymes and their standardized effect on drug dosing, according to the difference in pharmacokinetic parameters from clinical studies. Substantial adjustments need to be made to drug dose to achieve the same level of drug exposure in individuals with different genotypes. EM, extensive metabolizer; IA, intermediate acetylator; IM, intermediate metabolizer; PM, poor metabolizer; RA, rapid acetylator; SA, slow acetylator; UM, ultra-rapid metabolizer. *(Reproduced with permission from Kirchheiner J, Fuhr U, Brockmoller J. Pharmacogenetics-based therapeutic recommendations–ready for clinical practice? Nat Rev Drug Discov. 2005;4(8):639–647.)*

in a variety of diseases,[61–63] including recent modeling of azathioprine use in interstitial pulmonary fibrosis.[64] Clinical pharmacogenomic implementation guidelines have been published.[53,56]

Genetics can also influence drug transporters affecting drug absorption, distribution, and excretion. As an example, the solute carrier organic anion transporter family member 2B1 (*SLCO2B1*) mediates the Na(+)-independent transport of organic anions such as leukotriene C4. A nonsynonymous *SLCO2B1* polymorphism (rs12422149) has been associated with significantly reduced plasma concentration of differential response to therapy with montelukast as assessed by change in baseline Asthma Symptom Utility Index scores.[65]

Pharmacodynamics is the study of the biochemical and physiological consequences of the administration of a drug and its mechanism of action,[58] that is, the effect of a drug at its therapeutic target. Genetic variation may lead to response differences despite appropriate concentrations of a drug at its intended target. This category is especially pertinent to pulmonary medicine, since many conditions are treated with inhaled medications which bypass first-pass metabolism by the liver, thereby limiting the effect of pharmacokinetic variants.

Warfarin is the most commonly prescribed anticoagulant medication worldwide and in respiratory medicine is commonly used for the treatment of pulmonary embolism. For warfarin, cytochrome p450 2C9 (*CYP2C9*) is the primary enzyme involved in its metabolism, while vitamin K epoxide reductase complex, subunit 1 (*VKORC1*) is its primary therapeutic target, responsible for the conversion of vitamin K-epoxide to vitamin K. FDA labeling of warfarin includes consideration for testing of variants involved in both pharmacokinetics and pharmacodynamics. "High" and "low" dose risk variants of the *VKORC1* gene, as well as variants of the *CYP2C9* gene have been identified.[66] Overall, *VKORC1* variants account for ~25% of variability in warfarin dosing, with *CYP2C9* adding an additional 6% to 10%.

Multiple early studies supported the ability to predict initial warfarin dosing using a genotype stratified approach.[66–70] Initial guidelines for the clinical implementation of warfarin pharmacogenetics have been detailed.[55,71] However, in two[72,73] of three recently published clinical trials comparing use of a pharmacogenetic algorithm to a clinical dosing strategy, no significant benefit was noted in terms of percentage of time spent within the therapeutic international normalized ratio (INR) range, with the third[74] demonstrating only a modest (67.4%–60.3%) benefit to pharmacogenetics. While disappointing from a pharmacogenetic dosing standpoint, these studies were not powered to address the more important issue of bleeding and thrombotic complications. One study comparing a current genotyped cohort with historical controls demonstrated 31% fewer hospitalizations overall (adjusted hazard ratio [HR]: 0.69, 95% confidence interval [CI]: 0.58–0.82) and 28% fewer hospitalizations for bleeding or thromboembolism (HR: 0.72, 95% CI: 0.53–0.97) based upon pharmacogenetic dosing.[75] Further study in this area is warranted.

Pharmacogenetic tests aimed at combining multiple genetic predictors will likely continue to be a focus going forward. For instance, variants in *CRHR1* and *GLCCI1* have been associated with lung function response to inhaled corticosteroids in multiple asthmatic populations.[76,77] However, these account for just a small proportion of the variability in response to these medications. Nonetheless, combining two variants in the *CRHR1* and *GLCCI1* genes significantly improves the ability to predict response in a replicable fashion.[78]

The **idiosyncratic** category of pharmacogenetic response to drugs includes the individuals that experience an ADR to a therapeutic agent that could not be anticipated based upon the known drug target. Examples of the idiosyncratic category include some compounds that are metabolized by arylamine-*N*-acetyltransferase 2 (*NAT2*). Genetic differences in *NAT2* have been associated with predisposition to the development of peripheral neuropathy in certain individuals taking isoniazid[79] and hypersensitivity reactions to trimethoprim/sulfamethoxazole (including rash, granulocytopenia, and abnormal liver function tests).[79,80] Interestingly, the *NAT2* acetylator phenotype (based upon metabolized level of drugs) may correlate poorly with *NAT2* genotype,[81,82] suggesting that factors other than drug level may explain these idiosyncratic reactions associated with genetic variation.

The final pharmacogenetic category is that of genetic factors influencing **disease pathogenesis**. By modifying the underlying biology/severity of the disease, these genetic factors can also influence which therapies will work or how effective a given medication might be. As a brief example, in CF, the *CFTR* ΔF508 variant has been associated with earlier colonization with *Pseudomonas aeruginosa*,[83] whereas the G551D mutation has a milder clinical phenotype with later *P. aeruginosa* colonization.[84] Therefore, *CFTR* genotype would affect both severity of disease and frequency of antibiotic dosing.

PERSONALIZED PULMONARY MEDICINE: THE CHALLENGE

Despite the availability of personalized diagnostic panels, labeling changes implemented by regulatory agencies (e.g., FDA), and an ever-increasing compilation of genetic, biomarker, and pharmacogenetic studies in the literature, actual translation of personalized pulmonary testing to the bedside has been slower than expected. There are several of reasons for this delay. In the preceding sections, we have outlined how low heritability, variable penetrance, and the need for large effect sizes may affect test performance. Other implementation issues include (1) limitations in the design of published studies, (2) regulatory and ethical concerns, (3) lack of cost-effectiveness analyses, and (4) need to educate both patients and providers.

Study design limitations. Despite the availability of numerous reported genetic and pharmacogenetic associations in the literature, many have not been reproduced in subsequent studies.[85,86] False-positive initial associations may be due to the fact that many pharmacogenetic studies are "spin-offs" from clinical trials or for improperly designed case-control studies and, thus, are underpowered for genetic association. The nature of clinical trials (for pharmacogenetics) and of individualized cohorts (for genetic association) may also result in multiple distinct clinical phenotypes, which vary from study to study. This "phenotypic heterogeneity" combined with "genotypic heterogeneity" (interrogating disparate markers within the same gene) may also contribute to failure to replicate initial findings. These issues were detailed in an evaluation of the pharmacogenetic associations of the β_2-adrenergic receptor (*ADRB2*) gene[87] with β_2-agonist response in asthma. Overall, in 21 studies that focused on the two most common *ADRB2* coding variants (Arg16Gly and Gln27Glu), there were large differences in study design for both genotype definition (e.g., single variant vs. haplotype) and phenotypic outcome. Of a total of 487 interrogated associations, only 2 associations were probed in at least 5 of the studies, for the same endpoint, time of assessment, type of intervention, and genetic group. Not surprisingly, no definitive conclusions have been made regarding the utility of *ADRB2* variants to guide asthma therapy. Clearly, a continued focus on appropriate phenotypes and more precise replication of existing data are needed.

While beyond the scope of this chapter, two additional topics related to study design should be mentioned. The first relates to systems biology and personalized medicine. Given that multiple genetic and environmental factors impact the majority of respiratory disease susceptibility and treatment response, systems approaches seek to integrate data both at the level of data type (e.g., epistasis or gene–gene interactions) and across data types (e.g., integration of biomarker, gene expression, and SNP data) to formulate predictive models.[88–92] While young, this approach is promising with regard to complex trait test development. The second additional point is the ongoing controversy regarding study design and whether prospective, genotype-stratified trials are necessary prior to implementation of pharmacogenetic testing. One perspective is that dosing and administration of drug changes warrant such trials, while the other perspective argues that genotypes are invariant (since people are born with them) and therefore precede even retrospective studies. A potential compromise might be in the use of adaptive clinical trials, with pharmacogenomics included as part of the main trial adaptations.[93]

Regulatory and ethical concerns. As noted earlier the FDA has been proactive in terms of pharmacogenetics, with pharmacogenetic information included on about 10% of labels for drugs approved by the FDA. Nevertheless, questions regarding the regulation of genotyping tests and the extent to which pharmacogenetic analyses should be incorporated into new drug development before or after large clinical trials, remain.[94] While beyond our current scope, one detailed perspective on how pharmacogenetic testing might be included in each phase of clinical drug development has been recently published.[95] Another potential boon to genetic test development is the recent ruling by the US Supreme Court that genes cannot be patented.[96,97]

From an ethics perspective, the longstanding concern has been whether genetic variants could result in stigmatization (e.g., denied insurance).[94] A major step in the protection of individuals' rights came with the passage of H.R. 493, the Genetic Information Nondiscrimination Act of 2008. This law protects Americans against discrimination based on their genetic information in matters related to health insurance and employment and should translate into increased acceptance of personalized testing by the public in the future.

Lack of cost-effectiveness analyses. Despite the multitude of pharmacogenetic association studies in the literature, relatively few cost-effective analyses have been performed. These studies will be crucial prior to the availability of widespread reimbursement for routine personalized pulmonary testing. Circumstances that favor cost-effectiveness of a genetic test include the following: a high prevalence of the genetic variant of interest in the target population, good correlation between phenotype and genotype, satisfactory diagnostic test criteria, disease associated with significant morbidity or mortality if left untreated or undiagnosed, and, for pharmacogenetic variants, significant reduction in ADRs resulting from testing.[98]

Need to educate both patients and providers. Pharmacogenetics and the promise of personalized medicine have been frequently mentioned in the popular lay press. It is therefore incumbent upon both the developers of a given test, as well as healthcare professionals responsible for ordering the test, to be cognizant of the test characteristics and interpretation and to be able to effectively disseminate that information to patients. In turn, in the era of personalized medicine, the need for educating health care providers in both the broad array of potential predictive tools (in addition to genetic variants, genomic, proteomic, and other molecular biomarkers will be increasingly available), as well as the strengths and weakness of each of these approaches, will be needed. The context for these educational efforts is not yet clear. Given available tests, providers will potentially need a diagnostic step to determine which drug is best suited to each patient. Of paramount importance, providers will need to be reassured and cognizant that these tests will not and cannot replace sound clinical judgment.

CONCLUSION

Variation in the susceptibility to disease and response to drugs within pulmonary medicine has a significant heritable component. Although many challenges remain, testing of personalized pulmonary medicine, biomarkers, and pharmacogenetics has begun in earnest. Given the rapidity of new genetic knowledge, we are making progress toward the goal of individualized medicine.

REFERENCES

1. Lander ES, Linton LM, Birren B, et al. Initial sequencing and analysis of the human genome. *Nature.* 2001;409(6822):860–921.
2. Venter JC, Adams MD, Myers EW, et al. The sequence of the human genome. *Science.* 2001;291(5507):1304–1351.
3. Toro JR, Wei M-H, Glenn GM, et al. BHD mutations, clinical and molecular genetic investigations of Birt-Hogg-Dubé Syndrome: a new series of 50 families and a review of published reports. *J Med Genet.* 2008;45(6):321–331.
4. International PPH Consortium, Lane KB, Machado RD, et al. Heterozygous germline mutations in BMPR2, encoding a TGF-beta receptor, cause familial primary pulmonary hypertension. *Nat Genet.* 2000;26(1):81–84.
5. Seibold MA, Wise AL, Speer MC, et al. A common MUC5B promoter polymorphism and pulmonary fibrosis. *New Engl J Med.* 2011;364(16):1503–1512.
6. Silverman EK, Pierce JA, Province MA, Rao DC, Campbell EJ. Variability of pulmonary function in alpha-1-antitrypsin deficiency: clinical correlates. *Ann Intern Med.* 1989;111(12):982–991.
7. Zietkiewicz E, Nitka B, Voelkel K, et al. Population specificity of the DNAI1 gene mutation spectrum in primary ciliary dyskinesia (PCD). *Respir Res.* 2010;11(1):174.
8. Zietkiewicz E, Bukowy-Bieryłło Z, Voelkel K, et al. Mutations in radial spoke head genes and ultrastructural cilia defects in east-european cohort of primary ciliary dyskinesia patients. *PloS One.* 2012;7(3):e33667.
9. Ramsey BW, Davies J, McElvaney NG, et al. A CFTR potentiator in patients with cystic fibrosis and the G551D mutation. *New Engl J Med.* 2011;365(18):1663–1672.
10. Rosen DM, Waltz DA. Hydroxychloroquine and surfactant protein C deficiency. *New Engl J Med.* 2005;352(2):207–208.
11. Cools J, DeAngelo DJ, Gotlib J, et al. A tyrosine kinase created by fusion of the PDGFRA and FIP1L1 genes as a therapeutic target of imatinib in idiopathic hypereosinophilic syndrome. *N Engl J Med.* 2003;348(13):1201–1214.
12. Pardanani A, Brockman SR, Paternoster SF, et al. FIP1L1-PDGFRA fusion: prevalence and clinicopathologic correlates in 89 consecutive patients with moderate to severe eosinophilia. *Blood.* 2004;104(10):3038–3045.
13. Riccardi C, Bruscoli S, Ayroldi E, Agostini M, Migliorati G. GILZ, a glucocorticoid hormone induced gene, modulates T lymphocytes activation and death through interaction with NF-kB. *Adv Exp Med Biol.* 2001;495:31–39.
14. Parikh NI, Vasan RS. Assessing the clinical utility of biomarkers in medicine. *Biomark Med.* 2007;1(3):419–436.
15. Richards TJ, Kaminski N, Baribaud F, et al. Peripheral blood proteins predict mortality in idiopathic pulmonary fibrosis. *Am J Respir Crit Care Med.* 2012;185(1):67–76.
16. Berg P, Lindhardt BO. The role of procalcitonin in adult patients with community-acquired pneumonia–a systematic review. *Dan Med J.* 2012;59(3):A4357.
17. Blasi F, Stolz D, Piffer F. Biomarkers in lower respiratory tract infections. *Pulm Pharmacol Ther.* 2010;23(6):501–507.
18. Petsky HL, Cates CJ, Li A, Kynaston JA, Turner C, Chang AB. Tailored interventions based on exhaled nitric oxide versus clinical symptoms for asthma in children and adults. *Cochrane Database Syst Rev.* 2009;(4):CD006340.
19. Spitale N, Popat N, McIvor A. Update on exhaled nitric oxide in pulmonary disease. *Expert Rev Respir Med.* 2012;6(1):105–115.
20. Bhargava M, Wendt CH. Biomarkers in acute lung injury. *Transl Res.* 2012;159(4):205–217.
21. Pepe MS, Janes H, Longton G, Leisenring W, Newcomb P. Limitations of the odds ratio in gauging the performance of a diagnostic, prognostic, or screening marker. *Am J Epidemiol.* 2004;159(9):882–890.

22. Stein PD, Woodard PK, Weg JG, et al. Diagnostic pathways in acute pulmonary embolism: recommendations of the pioped II investigators. *Am J Med.* 2006;119(12):1048–1055.
23. Carrier M, Righini M, Djurabi RK, et al. VIDAS D-dimer in combination with clinical pre-test probability to rule out pulmonary embolism. A systematic review of management outcome studies. *Thromb Haemost.* 2009;101(5):886–892.
24. Geersing GJ, Erkens PM, Lucassen WA, et al. Safe exclusion of pulmonary embolism using the wells rule and qualitative D-dimer testing in primary care: prospective cohort study. *BMJ.* 2012;345:e6564.
25. van Belle A, Buller HR, Huisman MV, et al. Effectiveness of managing suspected pulmonary embolism using an algorithm combining clinical probability, D-dimer testing, and computed tomography. *JAMA.* 2006;295(2):172–179.
26. Froehling DA, Daniels PR, Swensen SJ, et al. Evaluation of a quantitative D-dimer latex immunoassay for acute pulmonary embolism diagnosed by computed tomographic angiography. *Mayo Clin Proc.* 2007;82(5):556–560.
27. Warren DJ, Matthews S. Pulmonary embolism: investigation of the clinically assessed intermediate risk subgroup. *Br J Radiol.* 2012;85(1009):37–43.
28. Gupta RT, Kakarla RK, Kirshenbaum KJ, Tapson VF. D-dimers and efficacy of clinical risk estimation algorithms: sensitivity in evaluation of acute pulmonary embolism. *AJR Am J Roentgenol.* 2009; 193(2):425–430.
29. Hammond CJ, Hassan TB. Screening for pulmonary embolism with a D-dimer assay: do we still need to assess clinical probability as well? *J R Soc Med.* 2005;98(2):54–58.
30. Amur S, Frueh FW, Lesko LJ, Huang SM. Integration and use of biomarkers in drug development, regulation and clinical practice: a US regulatory perspective. *Biomark Med.* 2008;2(3):305–311.
31. Hong H, Goodsaid F, Shi L, Tong W. Molecular Biomarkers: a US FDA effort. *Biomark Med.* 2010;4(2):215–225.
32. Woodruff PG, Modrek B, Choy DF, et al. T-helper type 2-driven inflammation defines major subphenotypes of asthma. *Am J Respir Crit Care Med.* 2009;180(5):388–395.
33. Corren J, Lemanske RF, Hanania NA, et al. Lebrikizumab treatment in adults with asthma. *N Engl J Med.* 2011;365(12):1088–1098.
34. Noonan M, Korenblat P, Mosesova S, et al. Dose-ranging study of lebrikizumab in asthmatic patients not receiving inhaled steroids. *J Allergy Clin Immunol.* 2013;132(3):567–574.
35. Ingelman-Sundberg M. Pharmacogenetics: an opportunity for a safer and more efficient pharmacotherapy. *J Intern Med.* 2001;250(3):186–200.
36. Maitland-van der Zee AH, de Boer A, Leufkens HG. The interface between pharmacoepidemiology and pharmacogenetics. *Eur J Pharmacol.* 2000;410(2–3):121–130.
37. Vesell ES. Therapeutic lessons from pharmacogenetics. *Ann Intern Med.* 1997;126(8):653–655.
38. Evans WE, Relling MV. Pharmacogenomics: translating functional genomics into rational therapeutics. *Science.* 1999;286 (5439):487–491.
39. Mancinelli L, Cronin M, Sadee W. Pharmacogenomics: the promise of personalized medicine. *AAPS PharmSci.* 2000;2(1):E4.
40. Lazarou J, Pomeranz BH, Corey PN. Incidence of adverse drug reactions in hospitalized patients: a meta-analysis of prospective studies. *JAMA.* 1998;279(15):1200–1205.
41. Kongkaew C, Noyce PR, Ashcroft DM. Hospital admissions associated with adverse drug reactions: a systematic review of prospective observational studies. *Ann Pharmacother.* 2008;42(7):1017–1025.
42. Ernst FR, Grizzle AJ. Drug-related morbidity and mortality: updating the cost-of-illness model. *J Am Pharm Assoc (Wash).* 2001;41(2):192–199.
43. Johnson JA, Bootman JL. Drug-related morbidity and mortality. A cost-of-illness model. *Arch Intern Med.* 1995;155(18):1949–1956.
44. Meisel C, Gerloff T, Kirchheiner J, et al. Implications of pharmacogenetics for individualizing drug treatment and for study design. *J Mol Med (Berl).* 2003;81(3):154–167.
45. Evans WE, McLeod HL. Pharmacogenomics–drug disposition, drug targets, and side effects. *N Engl J Med.* 2003;348(6):538–549.
46. Vesell ES, Page JG. Genetic control of drug levels in man: phenylbutazone. *Science.* 1968;159(3822):1479–1480.
47. Vesell ES, Page JG. Genetic control of drug levels in man: antipyrine. *Science.* 1968;161(3836):72–73.
48. Vesell ES, Page JG. Genetic control of dicumarol levels in man. *J Clin Invest.* 1968;47(12):2657–2663.
49. Vesell ES, Page JG. Genetic control of the phenobarbital-induced shortening of plasma antipyrine half-lives in man. *J Clin Invest.* 1969;48(12):2202–2209.
50. Vesell ES, Passananti GT, Greene FE, Page JG. Genetic control of drug levels and of the induction of drug-metabolizing enzymes in man: individual variability in the extent of allopurinol and nortriptyline inhibition of drug metabolism. *Ann N Y Acad Sci.* 1971;179:752–773.
51. Drazen JM, Silverman EK, Lee TH. Heterogeneity of therapeutic responses in asthma. *Br Med Bull.* 2000;56(4):1054–1070.
52. Silverman ES, Hjoberg J, Palmer LJ, Tantisira KG, Weiss ST, Drazen JM. Application of pharmacogenetics to the therapeutics of asthma. In: Eissa NT, Huston D, eds. *Therapeutic Targets of Airway Inflammation.* Vol 177. New York, NY: Marcel Dekker; 2003:1000.
53. Relling MV, Gardner EE, Sandborn WJ, et al. Clinical pharmacogenetics implementation consortium guidelines for thiopurine methyltransferase genotype and thiopurine dosing: 2013 update. *Clin Pharmacol Ther.* 2013;93(4):324–325.
54. Crews KR, Gaedigk A, Dunnenberger HM, et al. Clinical pharmacogenetics implementation consortium (CPIC) guidelines for codeine therapy in the context of cytochrome P450 2D6 (CYP2D6) genotype. *Clin Pharmacol Ther.* 2012;91(2):321–326.
55. Johnson JA, Gong L, Whirl-Carrillo M, et al. Clinical pharmacogenetics implementation consortium guidelines for CYP2C9 and VKORC1 genotypes and warfarin dosing. *Clin Pharmacol Ther.* 2011;90(4):625–629.
56. Relling MV, Gardner EE, Sandborn WJ, et al. Clinical pharmacogenetics implementation consortium guidelines for thiopurine methyltransferase genotype and thiopurine dosing. *Clin Pharmacol Ther.* 2011;89(3):387–391.
57. Relling MV, Klein TE. CPIC: Clinical pharmacogenetics implementation consortium of the pharmacogenomics research network. *Clin Pharmacol Ther.* 2011;89(3):464–467.
58. Steimer W, Potter JM. Pharmacogenetic screening and therapeutic drugs. *Clin Chim Acta.* 2002;315(1–2):137–155.
59. Yates CR, Krynetski EY, Loennechen T, et al. Molecular diagnosis of hiopurine S-methyltransferase deficiency: genetic basis for azathioprine and mercaptopurine intolerance. *Ann Intern Med.* 1997;126(8):608–614.
60. Gurwitz D, Rodriguez-Antona C, Payne K, et al. Improving pharmacovigilance in Europe: TPMT genotyping and phenotyping in the UK and Spain. *Eur J Hum Genet.* 2009;17(8):991–998.
61. van den Akker-van Marle ME, Gurwitz D, Detmar SB, et al. Cost-effectiveness of pharmacogenomics in clinical practice: A case study of thiopurine methyltransferase genotyping in acute lymphoblastic leukemia in Europe. *Pharmacogenomics.* 2006;7(5):783–792.

62. Winter J, Walker A, Shapiro D, Gaffney D, Spooner RJ, Mills PR. Cost-effectiveness of thiopurine methyltransferase genotype screening in patients about to commence azathioprine therapy for treatment of inflammatory bowel disease. *Aliment Pharmacol Ther.* 2004;20(6):593–599.

63. Marra CA, Esdaile JM, Anis AH. Practical pharmacogenetics: the cost effectiveness of screening for thiopurine S-methyltransferase polymorphisms in patients with rheumatological conditions treated with azathioprine. *J Rheumatol.* 2002;29(12):2507–2512.

64. Hagaman JT, Kinder BW, Eckman MH. Thiopurine S- methyltransferase [corrected] testing in idiopathic pulmonary fibrosis: a pharmacogenetic cost-effectiveness analysis. *Lung.* 2010;188(2):125–132.

65. Mougey EB, Feng H, Castro M, Irvin CG, Lima JJ. Absorption of montelukast is transporter mediated: a common variant of OATP2B1 is associated with reduced plasma concentrations and poor response. *Pharmacogenet Genomics.* 2009;19(2):129–138.

66. Rieder MJ, Reiner AP, Gage BF, et al. Effect of VKORC1 haplotypes on transcriptional regulation and warfarin dose. *N Engl J Med.* 2005;352(22):2285–2293.

67. Gage BF, Eby C, Johnson JA, et al. Use of pharmacogenetic and clinical factors to predict the therapeutic dose of warfarin. *Clin Pharmacol Ther.* 2008;84(3):326–331.

68. Klein TE, Altman RB, Eriksson N, et al. Estimation of the warfarin dose with clinical and pharmacogenetic data. *New Engl J Med.* 2009;360(8):753–764.

69. Scott SA, Edelmann L, Kornreich R, Desnick RJ. Warfarin pharmacogenetics: CYP2C9 and VKORC1 genotypes predict different sensitivity and resistance frequencies in the Ashkenazi and Sephardi Jewish populations. *Am J Hum Genet.* 2008;82(2):495–500.

70. Wadelius M, Chen LY, Lindh JD, et al. The largest prospective warfarin-treated cohort supports genetic forecasting. *Blood.* 2009;113(4):784–792.

71. Avery PJ, Jorgensen A, Hamberg AK, Wadelius M, Pirmohamed M, Kamali F. A proposal for an individualized pharmacogenetics-based warfarin initiation dose regimen for patients commencing anticoagulation therapy. *Clin Pharmacol Ther.* 2011;90(5):701–706.

72. Kimmel SE, French B, Kasner SE, et al. A pharmacogenetic versus a clinical algorithm for warfarin dosing. *New Engl J Med.* 2013;369(24):2283–2293.

73. Verhoef TI, Ragia G, de Boer A, et al. A randomized trial of genotype-guided dosing of acenocoumarol and phenprocoumon. *New Engl J Med.* 2013;369(24):2304–2312.

74. Pirmohamed M, Burnside G, Eriksson N, et al. A randomized trial of genotype-guided dosing of warfarin. *New Engl J Med.* 2013;369(24):2294–2303.

75. Epstein RS, Moyer TP, Aubert RE, et al. Warfarin genotyping reduces hospitalization rates results from the MM-WES (Medco-Mayo Warfarin Effectiveness Study). *J Am Coll Cardiol.* 2010;55(25):2804–2812.

76. Tantisira KG, Lake S, Silverman ES, et al. Corticosteroid pharmacogenetics: association of sequence variants in CRHR1 with improved lung function in asthmatics treated with inhaled corticosteroids. *Hum Mol Genet.* 2004;13(13):1353–1359.

77. Tantisira KG, Lasky-Su J, Harada M, et al. Genomewide association between GLCCI1 and response to glucocorticoid therapy in asthma. *New Engl J Med.* 2011;365(13):1173–1183.

78. McGeachie MJ, Wu AC, Chang HH, Lima JJ, Peters SP, Tantisira KG. Predicting inhaled corticosteroid response in asthma with two associated SNPs. *Pharmacogenomics J.* 2013;13(4):306–311.

79. Spielberg SP. N-acetyltransferases: pharmacogenetics and clinical consequences of polymorphic drug metabolism. *J Pharmacokinet Biopharm.* 1996;24(5):509–519.

80. Zielinska E, Niewiarowski W, Bodalski J. The arylamine N-acetyltransferase (NAT2) polymorphism and the risk of adverse reactions to co-trimoxazole in children. *Eur J Clin Pharmacol.* 1998;54(9–10):779–785.

81. O'Neil WM, Drobitch RK, MacArthur RD, et al. Acetylator phenotype and genotype in patients infected with HIV: discordance between methods for phenotype determination and genotype. *Pharmacogenetics.* 2000;10(2):171–182.

82. Zielinska E, Bodalski J, Niewiarowski W, Bolanowski W, Matusiak I. Comparison of acetylation phenotype with genotype coding for N-acetyltransferase (NAT2) in children. *Pediatr Res.* 1999;45(3):403–408.

83. Levy H, Kalish LA, Cannon CL, et al. Predictors of mucoid pseudomonas colonization in cystic fibrosis patients. *Pediatr Pulmonol.* 2008;43(5):463–471.

84. Comer DM, Ennis M, McDowell C, et al. Clinical phenotype of cystic fibrosis patients with the G551D mutation. *QJM.* 2009;102(11):793–798.

85. Hirschhorn JN, Lohmueller K, Byrne E, Hirschhorn K. A comprehensive review of genetic association studies. *Genet Med.* 2002; 4(2):45–61.

86. Ioannidis JP, Ntzani EE, Trikalinos TA, Contopoulos-Ioannidis DG. Replication validity of genetic association studies. *Nat Genet.* 2001;29(3):306–309.

87. Contopoulos-Ioannidis DG, Alexiou GA, Gouvias TC, Ioannidis JP. An empirical evaluation of multifarious outcomes in pharmacogenetics: beta-2 adrenoceptor gene polymorphisms in asthma treatment. *Pharmacogenet Genomics.* 2006;16(10):705–711.

88. Chen R, Snyder M. Promise of personalized omics to precision medicine. *Wiley Interdiscip Rev Syst Biol Med.* 2013;5(1):73–82.

89. Hood L, Tian Q. Systems approaches to biology and disease enable translational systems medicine. *Genomics Proteomics Bioinformatics.* 2012;10(4):181–185.

90. Wright DW, Wan S, Shublaq N, Zasada SJ, Coveney PV. From base pair to bedside: molecular simulation and the translation of genomics to personalized medicine. *Wiley Interdiscip Rev Syst Biol Med.* 2012;4(6):585–598.

91. Chen R, Snyder M. Systems biology: personalized medicine for the future? *Curr Opin Pharmacol.* 2012;12(5):623–628.

92. Hood L, Flores M. A personal view on systems medicine and the emergence of proactive P4 medicine: predictive, preventive, personalized and participatory. *N Biotechnol.* 2012;29(6):613–624.

93. Antman E, Weiss S, Loscalzo J. Systems pharmacology, pharmacogenetics, and clinical trial design in network medicine. *Wiley Interdiscip Rev Syst Biol Med.* 2012;4(4):367–383.

94. Roden DM, Altman RB, Benowitz NL, et al. Pharmacogenomics: challenges and opportunities. *Ann Intern Med.* 2006;145(10):749–757.

95. Kirchheiner J, Fuhr U, Brockmöller J. Pharmacogenetics-based therapeutic recommendations–ready for clinical practice? *Nat Rev Drug Discov.* 2005;4(8):639–647.

96. Kesselheim AS, Cook-Deegan RM, Winickoff DE, Mello MM. Gene patenting - the supreme court finally speaks. *New Engl J Med.* 2013;369(9)869–875.

97. Ostrer H. Genes: US patent rulings will fuel invention. *Nature.* 2013;499(7456):29.

98. Swen JJ, Huizinga TW, Gelderblom H, et al. Translating pharmacogenomics: challenges on the road to the clinic. *PLoS Med.* 2007;4(8):e209.

CHAPTER 10

Pulmonary Mechanics

Murray D. Altose

For venous blood to be properly arterialized, the distribution of air and blood within the lung is automatically matched to ensure effective gas exchange across alveolar–capillary membranes. Arterialization comprises a series of interrelated processes that begin with the mechanical performance of the ventilatory apparatus—that is, the lungs and the chest wall, including the rib cage, diaphragm, and abdominal wall. The ventilatory apparatus is critical for replenishing fresh air to the lungs for gas exchange. Although the function of each component of the lung and of the chest bellows can be deranged by injury or disease, the design of the ventilatory apparatus provides for considerable reserve. As a result, mechanical derangements are usually quite severe by the time clinical symptoms appear or arterial blood-gas levels become abnormal.

Depending on the nature of the underlying disorder, assessment of the mechanical properties of the ventilatory apparatus provides several different types of information. In some instances, characterization of the mechanical abnormality provides insight into pathogenesis and affords a quantitative measure of severity. In others, once the nature of the mechanical disorder is understood, the mystery surrounding a life-threatening disorder in gas exchange may be dispelled. Finally, certain breathing patterns make sense only if the mechanical performance of the chest bellows is taken into account.

During breathing, the lungs and chest wall operate in unison. The lungs fill the chest cavity so that the visceral pleura are in contact with the parietal pleura of the chest wall. The two pleural surfaces are separated by only a thin liquid film, which provides the bond holding the lungs and chest wall together.

At the end of a normal exhalation when the respiratory muscles are at rest, the ventilatory apparatus is in a state of mechanical equilibrium. The pressure along the entire tracheobronchial tree from the airway opening to the alveoli is equal to atmospheric pressure. The tendency of the lung is to deflate, however, and lung elastic recoil is directed centripetally. This is counterbalanced by the elastic recoil of the chest wall, which is directed centrifugally to favor an increase in volume. These opposing forces generate a subatmospheric pleural pressure of about -5 cmH_2O (Fig. 10-1A). The tendency for the lung to recoil inward and for the chest wall to recoil outward is illustrated by the observation that when the chest is opened at autopsy, the lungs collapse to a nearly airless state and the thorax expands.

Although it is conventional to consider pleural pressure as a single, mean value that reflects mechanical events within the entire ventilatory apparatus, this is clearly an oversimplification on several accounts: (1) pleural pressure is not directly determinable because normally there is only a potential space between the visceral and parietal pleura; (2) on conceptual grounds, distinctions exist between surface and liquid pleural pressures; (3) pleural pressures are not uniform over the surface of the lungs, being strongly affected by gravity; and (4) transmission of pleural pressures at the surface to alveoli located at different depths and loci with the lungs depends on the structural interplay among supporting structures in the alveolar walls (interdependence), which resists any inclination of individual alveoli or even a lobule to collapse.[1] Nonetheless, the concept of mean pleural pressure, as generally used in considerations of respiratory system mechanics, has proved to be of great practical value.[2]

The contraction of the muscles of inspiration produces the forces that permit the flow of gas along the tracheobronchial tree and the expansion of the lungs and chest. The movement of air into the lungs requires a pressure difference between the airway opening and the alveoli sufficient to overcome the resistance to airflow of the tracheobronchial tree. Also, a pressure difference across the alveolar walls (between the alveoli and pleural space) must be generated to overcome elastic recoil and inflate the lungs. During spontaneous breathing, the action of the inspiratory muscles causes an increased outward pull on the chest wall.[3] As a result, the pleural pressure becomes more subatmospheric. This pressure change is transmitted to the interior of the lungs, so alveolar pressure also becomes subatmospheric (Fig. 10-1B). In contrast, during artificial ventilation with a positive-pressure ventilator, a supra-atmospheric pressure applied at the inlet to the airways creates the proper pressure gradient between the airway opening and alveoli for airflow.

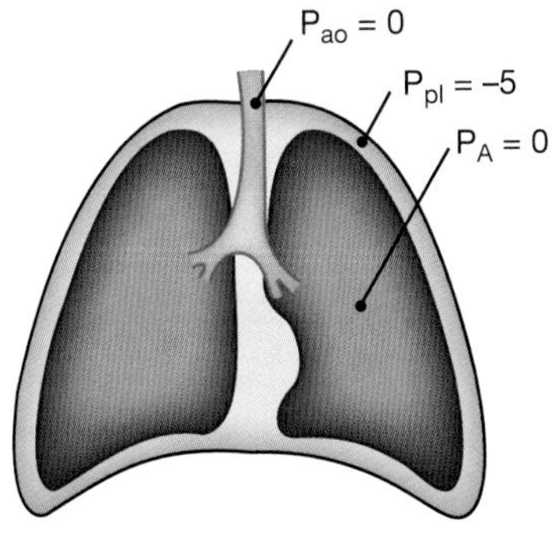

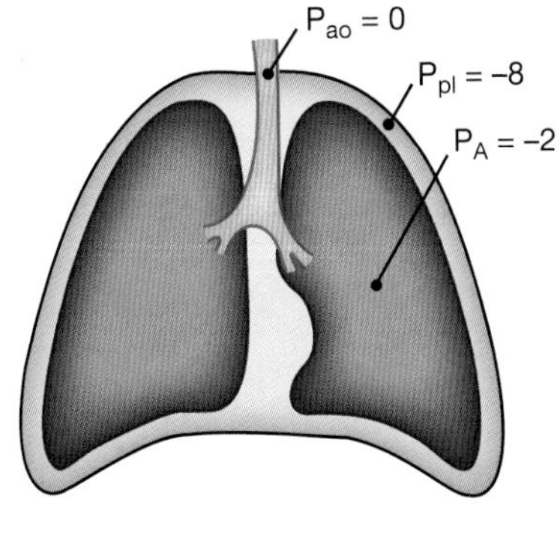

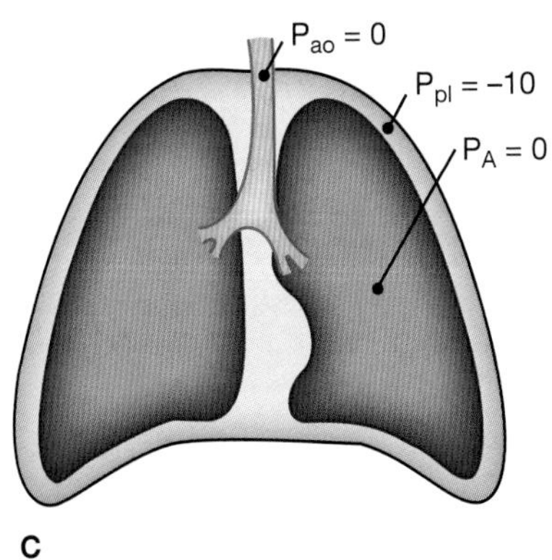

Figure 10-1 Respiratory pressures during a breathing cycle. **A.** End expiration. **B.** During inspiration. **C.** End inspiration. P_{pl}, pleural pressure; P_A, pressure in the alveoli; P_{ao}, pressure at the airway opening.

TABLE 10-1 Lung Volumes and Subdivisions

The *functional residual capacity* (FRC) is the volume of air that remains in the lungs at the end of a normal expiration.
The *tidal volume* (TV) is the volume of air that is drawn into the lungs during inspiration from the end-expiratory position (and also leaves the lungs passively during expiration) in the course of quiet breathing.
The *expiratory reserve volume* (ERV) is the maximum volume of air that can be forcibly exhaled after a quiet expiration has been completed (i.e., from the end-expiratory position).
The *residual volume* (RV) is the volume of air that remains in the lungs after a maximal expiratory effort.
The *inspiratory capacity* (IC) is the maximum volume of air that can be inhaled from the end-expiratory position. It consists of two subdivisions: tidal volume and the *inspiratory reserve volume* (IRV).
The *total lung capacity* (TLC) is the total volume of air contained in the lungs at the end of a maximum inspiration.
The *vital capacity* (VC) is the volume of air that is exhaled by a maximum expiration after a maximum inspiration.

Expansion of alveoli depends on the achievement of an appropriate distending pressure across alveolar walls. This distending pressure or transpulmonary pressure is the difference between alveolar (P_A) and pleural (P_{pl}) pressures. As shown in Figure 10-1A, the transpulmonary pressure at end expiration ($P_A - P_{pl}$) is 5 cmH_2O. At the end of inspiration (Fig. 10-1C), the lungs contain more air and the distending pressure which also represents the recoil pressure is greater.

The energy used during inspiration to overcome the elastic resistance of the lungs is stored. Expiration occurs when these forces are released. When the inspiratory muscles relax, the recoil of the lungs causes the alveolar pressure to exceed the pressure at the mouth, and air flows out of the lungs. Although expiration during quiet breathing is passive, the expiratory muscles are engaged at high levels of ventilation to assist the movement of air out of the lungs.

LUNG VOLUMES

The lung volumes and capacities (Table 10-1) are also considered elsewhere in this book (see Appendix B). The end-expiratory position of the lungs, functional residual capacity (FRC), is the major reference point for the subdivisions of lung volume. This position is set by the opposing recoil forces of the lung and chest wall when the respiratory muscles are at rest.

Total lung capacity (TLC), the total volume of air contained in the lungs after a maximal inhalation, is determined by the balance between the force-generating capacity of the inspiratory muscles and the opposing elastic recoil forces of the lung and chest wall.[4] Weakness of the muscles of inspiration or increased stiffness of the lung reduces TLC. Loss of retractive forces exerted by the lung, as in emphysema, enlarges TLC.

Residual volume (RV), the volume of air remaining in the lungs after a complete exhalation, is set by the balance between the actions of the expiratory muscle and the recoil forces of the lung, which act to decrease lung volume, and the outward recoil forces of the chest wall, which favor lung expansion. In middle-aged and older individuals, closure of airways at low lung volumes, with air trapping in the lung, is an important determinant of RV.[5]

STATIC MECHANICAL PROPERTIES OF THE RESPIRATORY SYSTEM

To assess the elastic properties of the ventilatory apparatus, it is expedient to evaluate the elastic properties of the lungs and chest separately. Elastic properties are conventionally assessed over a fixed range of volumes during periods of arrested airflow.

ELASTIC PROPERTIES OF THE LUNGS (PULMONARY COMPLIANCE)

The change in transpulmonary pressure required to effect a given change in the volume of air in the lungs is a measure of the distensibility, or compliance, of the lungs. Pulmonary compliance is calculated as the ratio of the change in lung volume to the change in transpulmonary pressure—that is,

$$C = \frac{\Delta V_L}{\Delta(P_A - P_{pl})}$$

where

C = lung compliance
$\Delta(P_A - P_{pl})$ = change in transpulmonary pressure
P_A = alveolar pressure and P_{pl} = pleural pressure
ΔV_L = change in lung volume

Compliance denotes distensibility, the ease of stretch or inflation. The inverse of compliance (i.e., elastance) refers to the stiffness or the tendency to resist distortion and to return to the original configuration when the distorting force is removed.

In practice, pulmonary compliance is determined by relating the changes in transpulmonary pressures to the changes in lung volume during interruptions in the course of an expiration after a maximal inspiration (i.e., starting from TLC).

The pressure–volume characteristics of the lung are nonlinear. As lung volume increases, the elastic elements approach their limits of distensibility, and a given change in transpulmonary pressure produces smaller and smaller increases in lung volume.[6,7] Thus, the compliance of the lung is least at high lung volumes and greatest as RV is approached (Fig. 10-2). Elastic recoil forces favoring collapse of the lung can be demonstrated throughout the range of the vital capacity, even at low lung volumes approaching the RV. If the

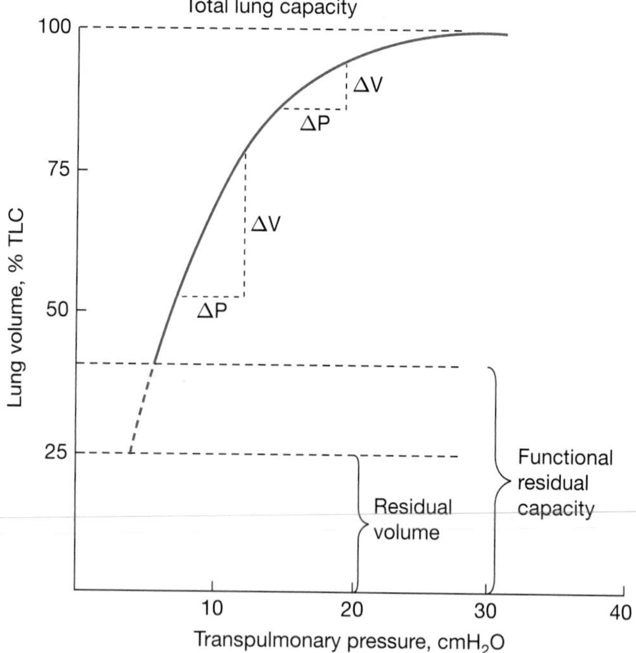

Figure 10-2 Pressure–volume curve of the lung. The static elastic recoil pressure of the lung is approximately 5 cmH_2O at FRC and 30 cmH_2O at TLC. The compliance of the lung ($\Delta V/\Delta P$) is greater at low lung volumes than at high lung volumes.

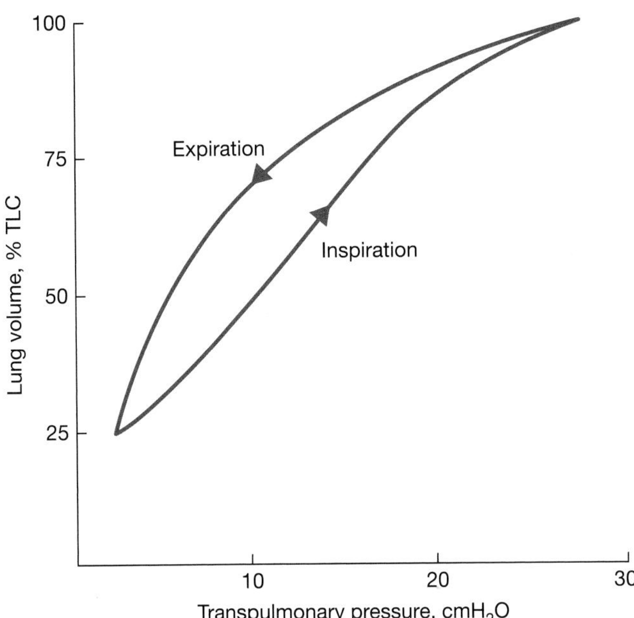

Figure 10-3 Pressure–volume curves of the lung during inspiration and expiration.

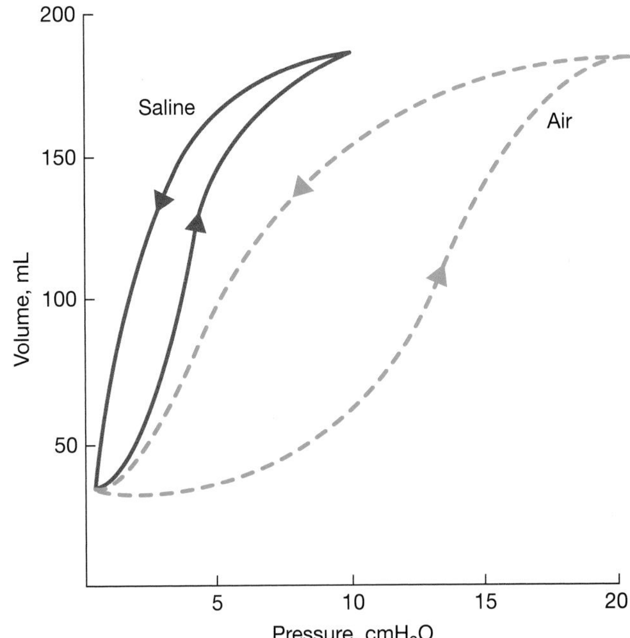

Figure 10-4 Comparison of pressure–volume relationships of air- and saline-filled excised lungs. *Arrows* directed upward indicate inflation; those directed downward indicate deflation. Since saline eliminates surface forces at the liquid–air interface without affecting tissue elasticity, the difference in pressure between the two curves, at any lung volume, is that required to overcome surface forces. To maintain a small lung volume, a large proportion of the pressure is used to overcome surface forces. In contrast, at high lung volumes a greater fraction of the pressure is used to overcome tissue elasticity.

opposing forces of the chest wall on the lungs are eliminated – for instance, by removing the lungs from the thorax or by opening the chest – the lung collapses to a near-airless state. A minimal volume of air does remain in the lungs because of closure of small airways resulting in the trapping of air in more distal airspaces.

If static measurements of transpulmonary pressure are made during lung inflation rather than deflation, the pressure–volume curve has a different configuration (Fig. 10-3). This indicates that the elastic recoil of the lung depends not only on the lung volume at which the determination is made but also on the "volume history" of the lung.[8]

■ HYSTERESIS

Differences in the pathways of the static pressure–volume curve during inspiration (when force is applied) and expiration (when force is withdrawn) are designated as hysteresis, which is a property of all elastic structures. In the lungs, it is due to the surface forces and the properties of the surface material lining the alveolar walls and also to the elastic properties of the tissues. The tissues of the lung are also subject to stress adaptation whereby over time, the pressure required to maintain a given lung volume will decline.[9] An additional factor relates to the closure of small airways at low lung volumes. Once these airways close, the lung units that they serve will not expand during inspiration until a critical opening pressure has been exceeded; only then will the closed units inflate. Recruitment of additional lung units as increasing transpulmonary pressure expands the lungs from low lung volume contributes to the hysteresis of the pressure–volume curve.

The elastic behavior of the lung depends on two factors: the physical properties of the lung tissue, per se, and the surface tension of the film lining of the alveolar walls.

■ SURFACE FORCES

The interior surfaces of the alveoli are lined by a thin liquid layer of osmophilic material. The surface tension at the air–liquid interface of the alveoli, in addition to the elastic properties of the parenchyma, contributes importantly to the elastic recoil of the lungs and acts to decrease lung compliance.[10] The cohesive forces between the molecules of the liquid lining of the alveoli are stronger than those between the film and alveolar gas, thereby causing the film to shrink to its smallest surface area. The behavior of this surface film has been examined in experimental animals by comparison of pressure–volume relationships of air-filled lungs with those of saline-filled lungs; saline eliminates the liquid–air interface without affecting elastic properties of the tissue. A lung distended with saline requires a lower transpulmonary pressure to maintain a given lung volume than a lung that is inflated with air.[11] Also, hysteresis is less in the saline-filled lung. The greater hysteresis in the air-filled lung is explained by the surface tension of the film lining the alveoli, which is higher during inflation as the film expands than it is during deflation as the film is compressed (Fig. 10-4).

By considering the alveolus to be a sphere, Laplace's law can be applied. Laplace's law states that the pressure inside a spherical structure—for example, the alveolus—is directly proportional to the tension in the wall and inversely proportional to the radius of curvature:

$$\text{Alveolar pressure} = \frac{2T}{r}$$

where

T = tension (dyn/cm)
r = radius

Abolition of the liquid–air interface by the instillation of saline into the alveolar spaces eliminates surface forces, thereby reducing the transpulmonary pressure required to maintain a given lung volume.

The surface film lining the alveoli of the lung is termed surfactant.[12] The superficial layer of the film facing the alveolar air is made up of surface-active phospholipids, notably dipalmitoyl lecithin. The deeper layer termed the hypophase consists of surface-active phospholipids linked to protein. Surfactant is generated by type

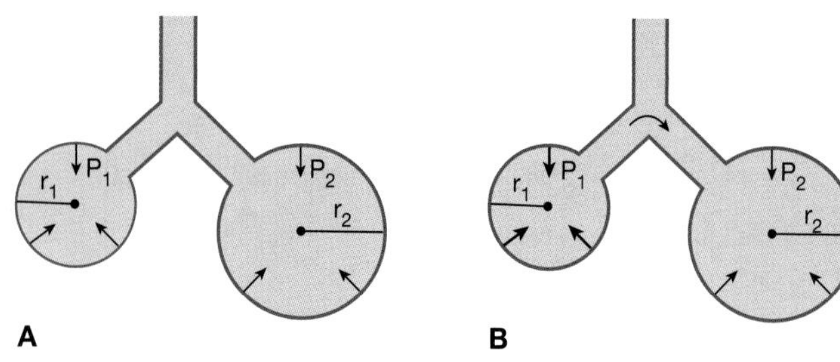

Figure 10-5 The effects of surfactant in maintaining alveolar stability. **A.** Surfactant lowers the tension of the alveolar walls at low lung volumes. Consequently, the transpulmonary pressure (P) of large and small communicating airspaces is the same. $r_1 < r_2, T_1 < T_2, P_1 \leftarrow P_2$. **B.** Without surfactant, the surface tension remains constant as lung volume changes, and the recoil pressure of small airspaces exceeds that of larger ones. As a result, small alveoli tend to empty into larger ones. $r_1 < r_2, T_1 = T_2, P_1 > P_2$.

II alveolar cells and undergoes a continuous cycle of formation, removal, and replenishment.[13]

Surfactant serves several important functions. The surface tension of surfactant is inherently low and decreases even further at low lung volumes when the surface area of the film is reduced. The minimization of surface forces, particularly at low lung volumes, minimizes the adherence of the walls of distal airways that tend to close at low lung volumes and increases the compliance of the lung and decreases the work required to inflate the lungs during the next breath. The automatic adjustment of surface tension as lung volume changes also promotes stability of alveoli at low lung volumes; if the surface tension were to remain constant instead of changing with lung volume, the transpulmonary pressure required to keep an alveolus open would increase as the radius of curvature diminished with decreasing lung volume. Therefore, small alveoli would empty into the larger ones with which they communicate, and atelectasis would be a regular occurrence (Fig. 10-5). Surfactant dysfunction as occurs with acute lung injury results in marked increases in surface tension causing stiffening and instability of alveoli and leads to alveolar collapse.

INTERDEPENDENCE AND COLLATERAL VENTILATION

The low surface tension of surfactant is not the most important determinant of alveolar stability. In reality, the alveoli form a froth rather than individual bubbles.[14] The walls of each alveolus are shared in common with those of adjacent alveoli so that contiguous airspaces attached by their connective tissue framework are tethered to one another and are not free to move independently. The tendency of any one alveolus to collapse is opposed by the traction exerted by the surrounding alveoli. This mechanical interdependence of adjacent airspaces resists the collapse of individual alveoli and serves as a stabilizing influence and ensures uniform inflation.[15] Even when a distal airway is completely obstructed, the alveoli served by the airway can still be ventilated through collateral channels between alveoli (pores of Kohn) and from bronchioles to alveoli (canals of Lambert). This collateral ventilation also prevents alveolar collapse and enhances the uniformity of ventilation, particularly in patients with lung disease.[16]

PHYSICAL PROPERTIES OF LUNG TISSUE

A number of different tissue components contribute to lung elasticity. The pleura, the intralobular septa, peripheral airway smooth muscle tone, and pulmonary vasomotor tone, as well as the tissues of the alveolar walls, play a role in shaping lung elastic recoil.

The major connective-tissue elements of the alveolar walls are the collagen and elastin fibers.[17] Elastin fibers in the alveolar walls and surrounding the bronchioles and pulmonary capillaries have a low tensile strength but can be stretched to over twice their resting length. Elastin fibers are thought to bear most of the stress in the lung at low volumes. Collagen fibers have high tensile strength but are poorly extensible and probably act to limit expansion at high lung volumes.[18] Like a stretched nylon stocking, expansion of the lungs appears to entail an unfolding and geometric rearrangement of the fibers and only slight elongation of individual fibers.

As a result of alterations in the elastin and collagen fibers in the lung, the distensibility of the lungs (measured as compliance) increases with age.[7] This is part of the normal aging process. Pulmonary compliance is also increased by the destruction of alveolar walls and the enlargement of alveolar spaces that characterize pulmonary emphysema. In contrast, the distensibility of the lungs is reduced by pulmonary fibrosis, which stiffens its interstitial tissues.[6]

ELASTIC PROPERTIES OF THE THORAX

The elastic recoil of the chest wall is such that if it were unopposed by the lungs, the chest would enlarge to approximately 70% of TLC. This position represents its equilibrium or resting position.[19] In this position (when the respiratory muscles are completely relaxed), the pressure difference across the chest wall – that is, the difference between pleural pressure and the pressure at the surface of the chest – is zero. If the chest were forced to enlarge beyond its equilibrium position by an increasingly positive pleural pressure or by the application of subatmospheric pressure at the body surface, it would, like the lung, recoil inward, resisting expansion and favoring return to its equilibrium position. Conversely, at volumes less than 70% of TLC, the recoil of the chest is opposite that of the lung and is directed outward (Fig. 10-6).[20] The chest wall can also be

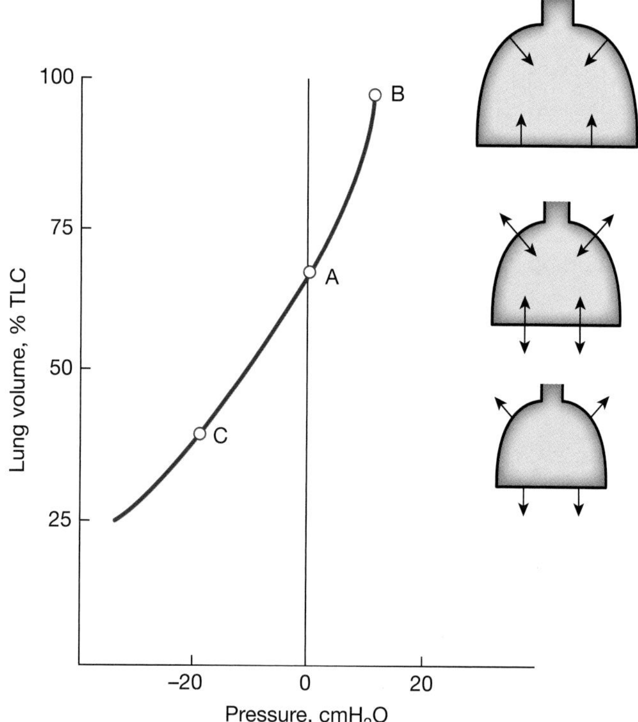

Figure 10-6 Pressure–volume relationships of the isolated chest wall. The direction of the recoil forces across the chest wall is represented by the *arrows*. The equilibrium position of the chest wall at point A, unopposed by the lungs, is approximately 70% of the total lung capacity. In this position, the pressure difference across the chest wall is zero. At larger volumes (B), there is inward recoil of the chest wall; at volumes below the equilibrium position (C), the recoil of the chest wall is directed outward, favoring expansion.

represented as a two-compartment system consisting of the rib cage and the abdomen, and volume changes can be partitioned between the two compartments.[21] Changing from the upright to the supine position at a constant overall lung volume produces a shift in volume from the abdominal to the rib cage compartment. The compliance of the rib cage is similar in the supine and upright positions, but the compliance of the abdominal compartment – particularly at high volumes – is greater in the supine position.[22]

The elastic recoil properties of the chest wall play an important role in determining the subdivisions of lung volume. They may be seriously deranged by disorders affecting the chest wall, such as marked obesity, kyphoscoliosis, and ankylosing spondylitis.

■ ELASTIC PROPERTIES OF THE RESPIRATORY SYSTEM AS A WHOLE

During breathing the lung and the chest wall move together and operate mechanically in series. At any given lung volume the elastic recoil pressure of the total respiratory system (P_{rs}) can be calculated as the algebraic sum of the pressures exerted by the elastic recoil of the lung (transpulmonary pressure) and the elastic recoil of the chest wall.[23]

Since the elastic recoil of the lung is determined (under static conditions of arrested airflow) as the difference between alveolar pressure (P_A) and pleural pressure (P_{pl}) – that is, $P_A - P_{pl}$ – and the elastic recoil of the chest wall is determined (while the respiratory muscles are completely at rest) as the difference between pleural pressure and the pressure at the external surface of the chest (P_{bs})—that is, $P_{pl} - P_{bs}$, the elastic recoil of the entire respiratory system can be expressed as the sum of the two:

$$P_{rs} = (P_A - P_{pl}) + (P_{pl} - P_{bs}) = P_A - P_{bs}$$

Thus, a measure of the elastic recoil of the respiratory system is supplied by the alveolar pressure, provided that the respiratory muscles are completely at rest and the pressure of the body surface is at atmospheric levels. In the absence of airflow into or out of the lung and when the glottis is open, alveolar pressure corresponds to the pressure at the mouth.

Relaxation Pressure–Volume Curve

The elastic properties of the entire respiratory system can be determined from the relaxation pressure–volume curve (Fig. 10-7). FRC represents the equilibrium position of the lung–chest wall system while the respiratory muscles are relaxed. At this point, the opposing recoils of the lung and chest wall are of equal magnitude, and the recoil pressure of the entire respiratory system is zero. With increases in lung volume above FRC, the recoil pressure of the entire system becomes positive, owing to the combination of an increase in centripetal elastic recoil of the lungs and a decrease in the centrifugal recoil of the chest wall. The net effect favors a decrease in lung volume, and lung volume can be maintained with the airway open to the atmosphere only by the action of the inspiratory muscles. As lung volume exceeds 75% of TLC, the recoil of the chest wall also becomes centripetal and the recoil pressure of the chest wall adds to the inward forces acting to diminish lung volume. TLC represents the lung volume at which the inward passive elastic recoil pressure of the respiratory system reaches the maximum force that can be generated by the inspiratory muscles.

At lung volumes below FRC, when the centrifugal recoil of the chest wall exceeds the reduced centripetal recoil of the lungs, the relaxation pressure is negative and this net effect favors an increase in lung volume. Lung volumes below FRC are achieved and maintained by the muscles of expiration.

A switch from the sitting to the supine position decreases FRC because of the effects of gravity. In the upright position, gravity pulls the abdominal contents away from the chest wall. In contrast, in the supine position, the push of the abdominal contents against the diaphragm decreases the centrifugal recoil of the chest wall. The chest wall pressure–volume curve – and, consequently, the pressure–volume curve of the entire respiratory system – is displaced to the right.

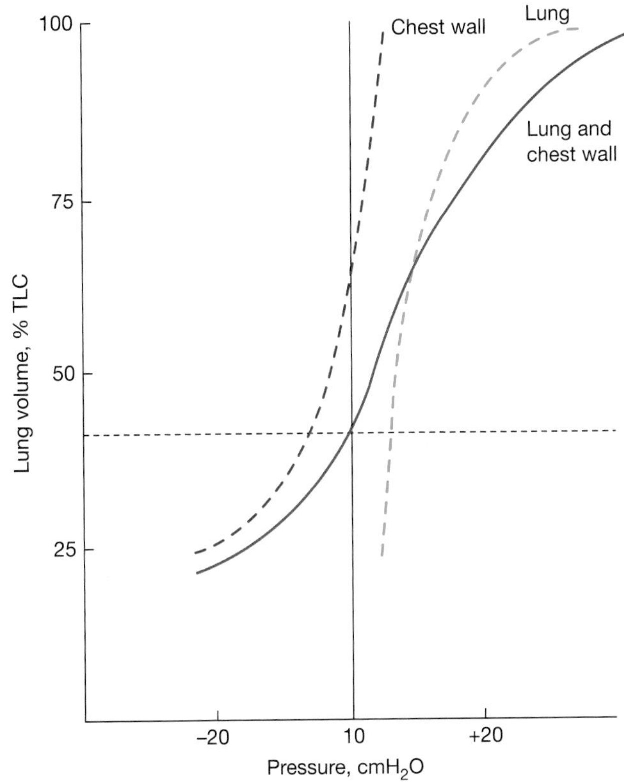

Figure 10-7 Relaxation pressure–volume curves. The lungs and the chest wall function mechanically in series so that the elastic recoil pressures of the total respiratory system, represented by the *solid line*, is the algebraic sum of the separate recoil pressures of the lung and chest wall. At the volume represented by the horizontal *dashed line*, the recoil pressures of the lung and chest wall are equal but in opposite directions. Consequently the net recoil pressure is zero, and the respiratory system is in a position of equilibrium.

DYNAMIC MECHANICAL PROPERTIES OF THE RESPIRATORY SYSTEM

The total nonelastic resistance of the lungs consists of the resistance of the airways to airflow (airway resistance), defined in terms of the driving pressure and the resulting rate of airflow, and the frictional resistance of the lung tissues to displacement during breathing (tissue resistance). Normally, tissue resistance makes up only 10% to 20% of the total pulmonary nonelastic resistance, but in diseases of the pulmonary parenchyma, it may increase considerably.

■ AIRWAY RESISTANCE

A large fraction of the resistance to airflow is in the upper respiratory tract, including the nose, mouth, pharynx, larynx, and trachea. During nasal breathing, the nose constitutes up to 50% of total airway resistance. During quiet mouth breathing, the mouth, pharynx, larynx, and trachea constitute 20% to 30% of the airway resistance; but they account for up to 50% of the total airway resistance when minute ventilation increases—during vigorous exercise, for example. Most of the remainder of airway resistance is in medium-sized lobar, segmental, and subsegmental bronchi up to about the seventh generation of airways.[24,25] Additional branching distally causes a progressive increase in the number of airways in any generation. While the caliber of individual airways in daughter branches compared to the parent branch is reduced, the total cross-sectional area of all of the airways in a given generation increases tremendously with successive generations along the tracheobronchial tree. Consequently, in the normal lung, the small peripheral airways, particularly those less than 2 mm in diameter, constitute only about 10% to 20% of the total airway resistance.[26]

Airway Caliber

The airways, like the pulmonary parenchyma, exhibit elasticity and can be compressed or distended. Therefore, the diameter of an airway varies with the transmural pressure applied to that airway—that is, the difference between the pressure within the airway and the pressure surrounding the airway. The pressure surrounding intrathoracic airways approximates pleural pressure, since these airways are tethered to the parenchymal tissue and are exposed to the expansive forces that are active in overcoming the elastic recoil of the lung.[1]

Airway resistance varies inversely with lung volume. As the lung volume increases, the elastic recoil forces of the lung increase; the traction applied to the walls of the intrathoracic airways also increases, widening the airways and decreasing their resistance to airflow. Conversely, at low lung volumes, the transmural airway pressure is lower and airway resistance increases.[27,28] If the elastic recoil of the lung is reduced – by destruction of alveolar walls in pulmonary emphysema, for instance – the transmural airway pressure at any given lung volume decreases correspondingly; the airways are narrower and airway resistance is greater even though there is no disease of the airways per se.

The effects of a change in transmural pressure on airway caliber depend on the compliance of the airways—which, in turn, is determined by their structural support. The trachea, for example, is almost completely surrounded by cartilaginous rings, which tend to prevent complete collapse even when the transmural pressure is negative. The bronchi are less well supported by incomplete cartilaginous rings and plates, whereas the bronchioles lack cartilaginous support. All airways can be stiffened, albeit to different degrees, by contraction of smooth muscle in their walls.

In patients with airway disease, mucosal edema, hypertrophy and hyperplasia of mucus glands, increased elaboration of mucus, and hypertrophy of smooth muscle further compromise airway caliber and increase airway resistance.

Neural pathways and humoral mechanisms are also important in controlling airway smooth muscle tone and regulating airway caliber. Cholinergic parasympathomimetic stimulation originating from the vagus nerve and mediated through the release of acetylcholine causes airway smooth muscle contraction and airway narrowing. Noncholinergic parasympathetic activity may play a role in airway smooth muscle relaxation through the release of vasoactive intestinal peptide and the subsequent production of nitric oxide.[29] Beta-adrenergic receptors in bronchial smooth muscle activated by various sympathomimetic agents promote airway smooth muscle relaxation and airway dilatation.[30]

Pressure–Flow Relationships: Theoretical Considerations

In the lungs, pressure–flow relationships are extremely complicated because the airways consist of a system of irregular branching tubes that are neither rigid nor perfectly circular. For purposes of simplification, pressure–flow relationships in rigid tubes are generally regarded as a model for those in the airways.

The driving pressure that produces flow of air into and out of the lung must suffice to overcome friction and to accelerate the air. Acceleration in the lungs is of two types: local (i.e., changes in the rate of airflow with time when flow is initiated) and convective (i.e., acceleration of molecules of air over distance while flow is constant). The driving pressure required for convective acceleration

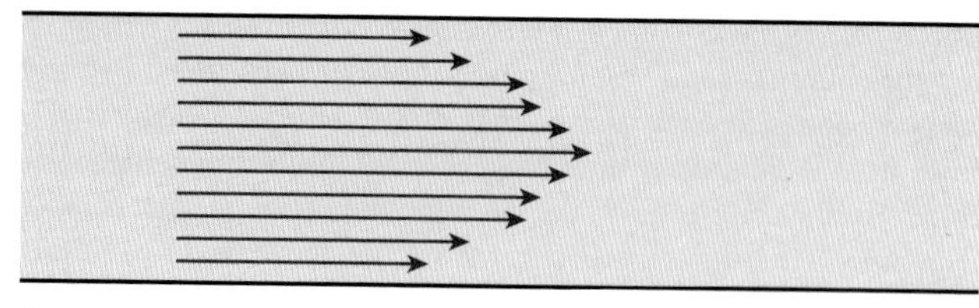
A

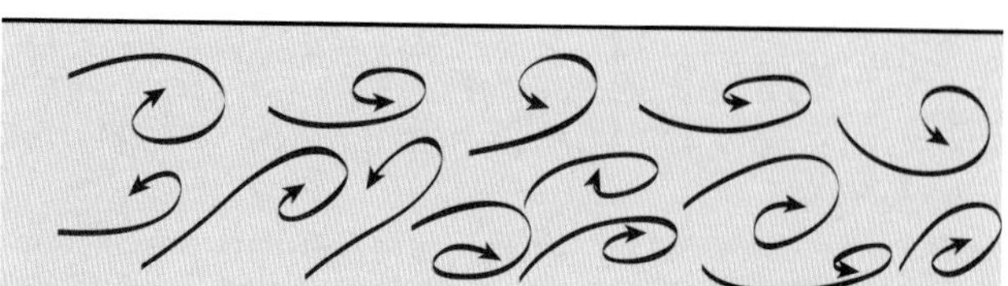
B

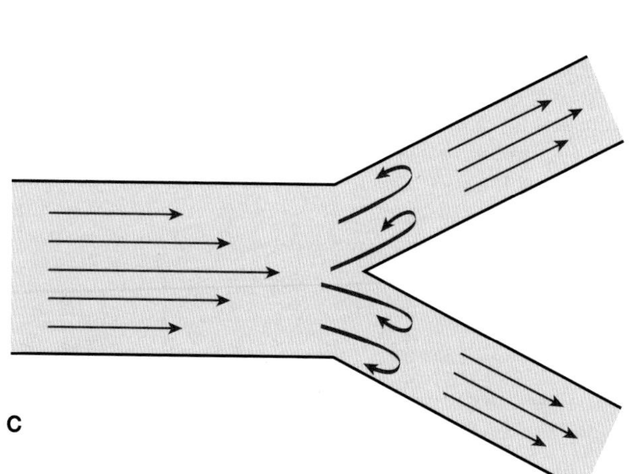
C

Figure 10-8 Patterns of airflow. **A.** Laminar flow. **B.** Turbulent flow. **C.** Transition flow that occurs at bifurcations.

is proportional to the gas density and to the square of the flow rate. It is important during expiration because, as air moves downstream from the alveoli toward the airway opening, the total cross-sectional airway diameter decreases; therefore, molecules of air must accelerate through the converging channels even though the overall flow rate remains unchanged. Also, the driving pressure that produces high expiratory flow rates at large lung volume serves for convective acceleration rather than for overcoming friction.[31,32]

The driving pressure required to overcome friction depends on the rate and the pattern of airflow. Two major patterns of airflow warrant special consideration: laminar and turbulent. Laminar flow is characterized by streamlines that parallel the sides of the tube and are capable of sliding over one another. Also, because the streamlines at the center of the tube move faster than those closest to the walls, the flow profile is parabolic (Fig. 10-8). The pressure–flow characteristics of laminar flow depend on the length (l) and the radius (r) of the tube and the viscosity of the gas (η) according to Poiseuille's equation:

$$\Delta P = \frac{\dot{V} 8 \eta l}{\pi r^4}$$

where

ΔP = the driving pressure (pressure drop between the beginning and the end of the tube)
$\dot{V}$ = the flow rate that the driving pressure produces
r = the radius of the tube

The critical importance of tube radius in determining the driving pressure for a given flow is apparent in the previously mentioned equation. If the radius of the tube is halved, the pressure that is required to maintain a given flow rate must be increased 16-fold. Laminar flow patterns occur only in small peripheral airways, where, because of the enormous overall cross-sectional area, flow through the individual airways is exceedingly slow.

Turbulent flow occurs at high flow rates and is characterized by a complete disorganization of streamlines, so that the molecules of gas move laterally, collide with each other, and change velocities. Under these circumstances, pressure–flow relationships change. In contrast to laminar flow, the rate of turbulent airflow is no longer proportional to the driving pressure. Instead, the driving pressure to produce a given rate of airflow is proportional to the square of flow and is dependent on gas density. Turbulent flow occurs regularly in the trachea.

At lower flow rates during expiration – particularly at branches in the tracheobronchial tree, where flow in two separate tubes comes together into a single channel – the parabolic profile of laminar flow becomes blunted, the streamlines separate from the walls of the tube, and minor eddy formation develops. This is referred to as a mixed, or transitional, flow pattern. In a mixed pattern of airflow, the driving pressure for a given flow depends on both the viscosity and the density of the gas.

Whether airflow is laminar or turbulent is predictable from the Reynolds number (Re), a dimensionless number that depends on the average velocity ($\bar{v}$), the density of the gas (ρ), the viscosity of the gas (η), and the diameter of the tube (D), so that

$$Re = \frac{\bar{v} D \rho}{\eta}$$

In straight, smooth, rigid tubes, turbulence occurs when the Reynolds number exceeds 2000. Therefore, turbulence is most apt to occur when the average velocity is high, gas density is high, gas viscosity is low, and the tube diameter is large. Since most of the resistance to airflow in the normal lung is in large airways, where airflow is largely turbulent and where resistance is density dependent, breathing a mixture of 80% helium and 20% oxygen (a mixture that is 64% less dense than air) reduces the Reynolds number favoring a conversion from turbulent to laminar flow. Consequently airflow increases at a given driving pressure and airway resistance falls.[24]

Calculation of Airflow Resistance

The driving pressure along the tracheobronchial tree – that is, the difference between alveolar pressure and the pressure at the airway opening (mouth) that is required to produce a given rate of airflow into the lungs – provides a measure of the flow resistance of the airways, according to the equation

$$R_{aw} = \frac{P_A - P_{ao}}{\dot{V}}$$

where

$\dot{V}$ = airflow (L/s)
P_A = alveolar pressure (cmH_2O)
P_{ao} = airway-opening pressure (cmH_2O)
R_{aw} = airway resistance ($cmH_2O/L/s$)

Flow–Volume Relationships

Considerable insight into the flow-resistive properties of the airways can be obtained from the relationship between airflow and lung volume during maximal expiratory and inspiratory maneuvers.[33] In practice, a person inhales maximally to TLC; then exhales as forcefully, rapidly, and completely as possible to RV; and then returns to TLC by a rapid, forceful inhalation (Fig. 10-9). During the maximal

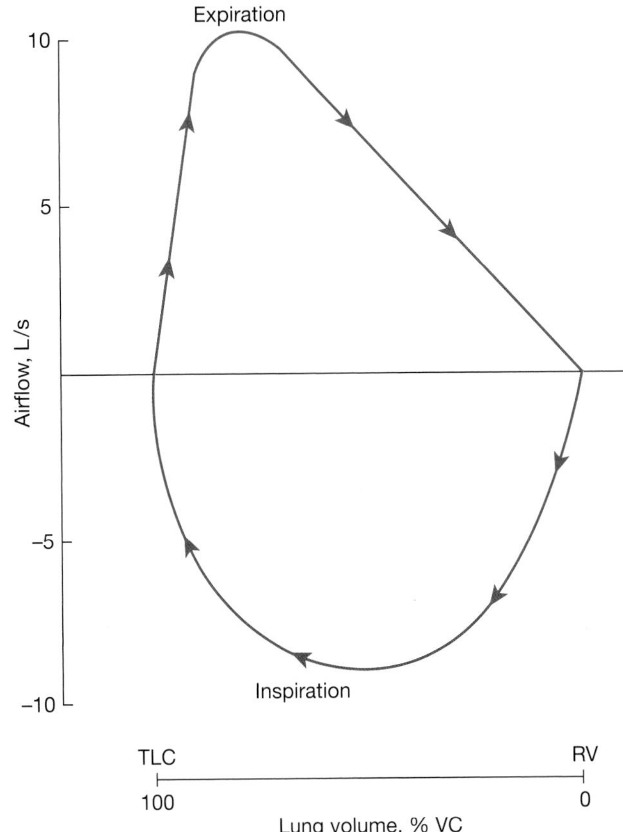

Figure 10-9 Maximal expiratory and inspiratory flow–volume loop.

expiration, the rate of airflow peaks at a lung volume that is close to the TLC; as the lung volume decreases and intrathoracic airways narrow, airway resistance increases, and the rate of airflow decreases progressively.

During maximal inspiration, the pattern of airflow is different. Because of the markedly negative pleural pressure and large transmural airway pressure, the bronchi are wide, and their calibers increase further as lung volume increases. Consequently, inspiratory flow becomes high while the lung volume is still low and remains high over much of the vital capacity, even though the force generated by the inspiratory muscles decreases as they shorten.

A family of flow–volume loops is produced by repeating full expiratory and inspiratory maneuvers over the entire range of the vital capacity using different levels of effort (Fig. 10-10). The greater the effort exerted during inspiration, the greater is the rate of airflow over the entire range—that is, from RV to TLC. Similarly, during expiration, the rate of airflow increases progressively with increasing effort at large lung volumes close to TLC. At intermediate and low lung volumes, the rate of expiratory airflow reaches a maximum while the effort expended is only moderate; thereafter, airflow does not increase further despite increasing expiratory efforts.

ISOVOLUME PRESSURE–FLOW CURVES

Separation of the effects of increasing effort from those of changes in lung volume on the rate of airflow during expiration can be accomplished by using isovolume pressure–flow curves (Fig. 10-11). During repeated expiratory maneuvers performed with varying degrees of effort, simultaneous measurements are made of airflow rate, lung volumes, and pleural pressure. For each lung volume the rate of airflow is plotted against the pleural pressure, as an index of the degree of effort.[34]

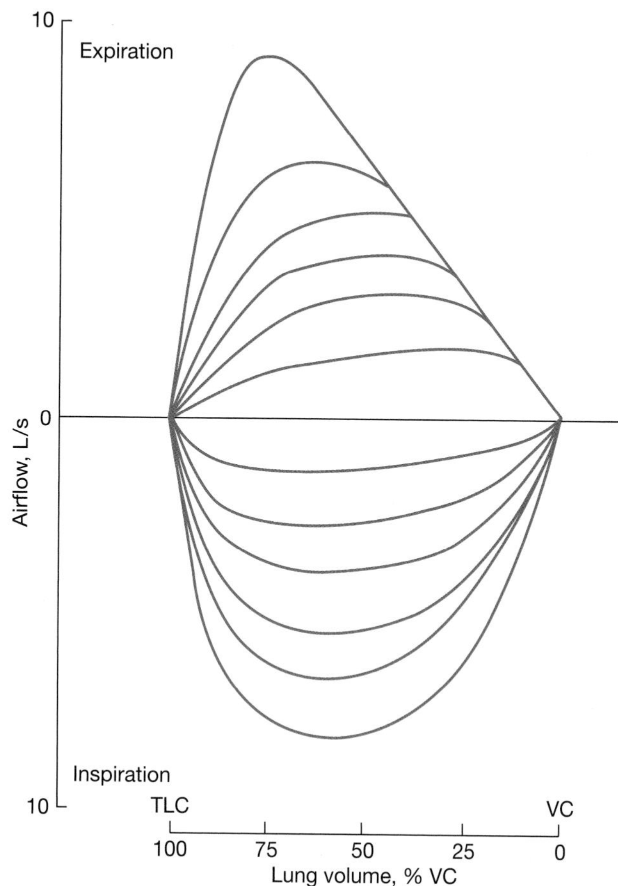

Figure 10-10 Series of flow–volume loops constructed from complete inspiratory and expiratory maneuvers repeated at different levels of effort.

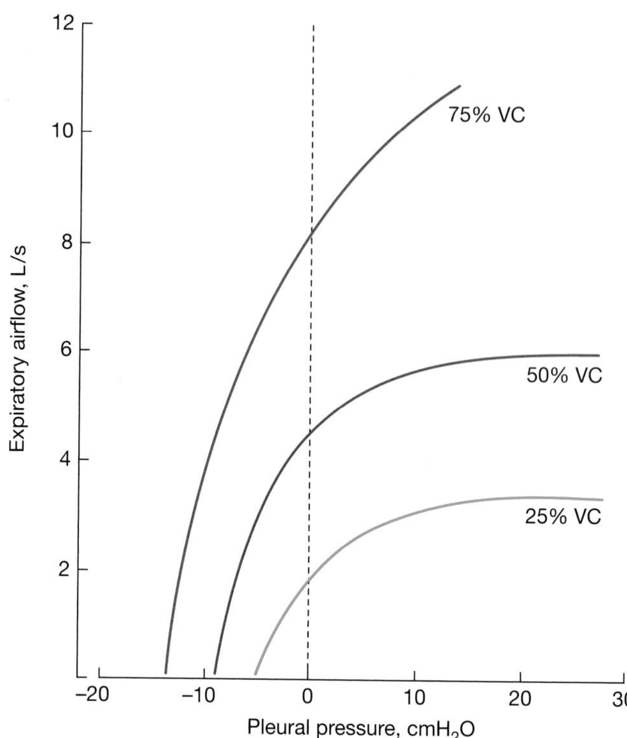

Figure 10-11 Isovolumetric pressure–flow curves. At lung volumes greater than 75% of the vital capacity, airflow is effort dependent; that is, airflow increases progressively with increasing effort. At lower lung volumes, airflow is effort independent; that is, airflow becomes fixed at a maximum level and does not increase despite further increases in effort.

As expiratory effort is increased at any given lung volume, the pleural pressure increases toward, and then exceeds, atmospheric pressure; correspondingly, the rate of airflow increases. At lung volumes above 75% of the vital capacity, airflow increases progressively as pleural pressure increases; it is considered to be effort dependent. In contrast, at lung volumes below 75% of the vital capacity, the rate of airflow levels off as the pleural pressure exceeds atmospheric pressure and becomes fixed at a maximum level. Thereafter, further increases in effort, and in pleural pressure, effect no further increase in the rate of airflow; at these lower lung volumes, airflow is considered to be effort independent. Since the rate of airflow remains constant despite increasing driving pressure, it follows that the resistance to airflow must be increasing in direct proportion to the increase in driving pressure. This increase in resistance is attributed to compression and narrowing of large intrathoracic airways.

EQUAL PRESSURE POINT THEORY: DYNAMIC COMPRESSION OF AIRWAYS

To illustrate the mechanisms that normally limit airflow during a maximal expiratory maneuver, it is useful to consider a model of the lung where the alveoli are represented by an elastic sac and the intrathoracic airways by a compressible tube, both enclosed within a pleural space (Fig. 10-12).[35]

At a given lung volume, when there is no airflow (as during breath holding with the glottis open), pleural pressure is subatmospheric, counterbalancing the elastic recoil pressure of the lung. The alveolar pressure (P_A), which is the sum of the recoil pressure of the lung and pleural pressure (P_{pl}), is zero (Fig. 10-12A). Since airflow has ceased, the pressure along the entire airway is also atmospheric.

At the same lung volume during a quiet expiration, pleural pressure is less subatmospheric. Since lung volume and the elastic recoil pressure of the lung are unchanged, alveolar pressure is now positive with respect to atmospheric pressure; airflow occurs. The alveolar pressure is gradually dissipated along the airway in overcoming resistance so that the pressure at the airway opening (P_{ao}) is zero. All along the airway, however, the airway pressure exceeds pleural pressure and the transmural pressure is positive; the airways remain open, and flow continues (Fig. 10-12B).

A forceful expiration raises pleural pressure above atmospheric pressure and further increases alveolar pressure (Fig. 10-12C). Airway pressure again falls progressively from the alveolus toward the airway opening. But at some point along the airway – the equal pressure point – the drop in airway pressure is equal to the recoil pressure of the lung; intraluminal pressure and the pressure surrounding the airways are equal and the same as pleural pressure. Downstream (i.e., toward the airway opening) the transmural pressure is negative, because the intraluminal airway pressure is less than pleural pressure; the airways are subjected to dynamic compression.

The equal pressure point divides the airways into two components arranged in series: an upstream segment, from the alveoli to the equal pressure point, and a downstream segment, from the equal pressure point to the airway opening. With increasing expiratory effort as the pleural pressure becomes more and more positive with respect to atmospheric pressure, the equal pressure point moves upstream. Once maximum expiratory flow is achieved, the position of the equal pressure point becomes fixed in the region of the lobar or segmental bronchi. Further increase in pleural pressure by increasing expiratory force simply produces more compression of the downstream segment without affecting airflow through the upstream segment.

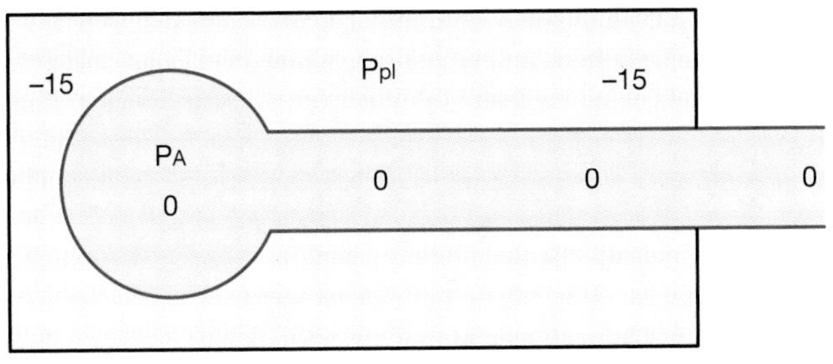

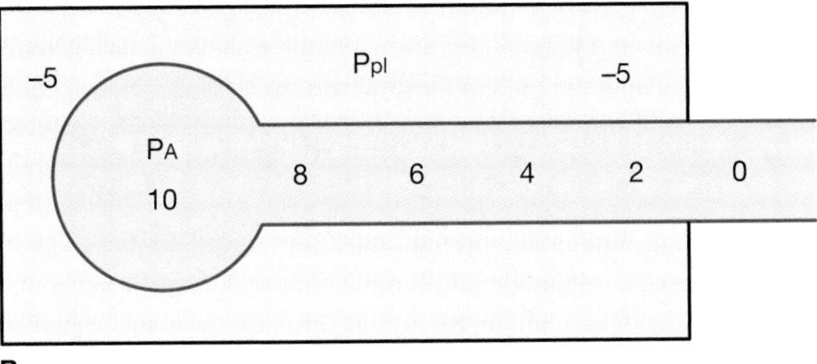

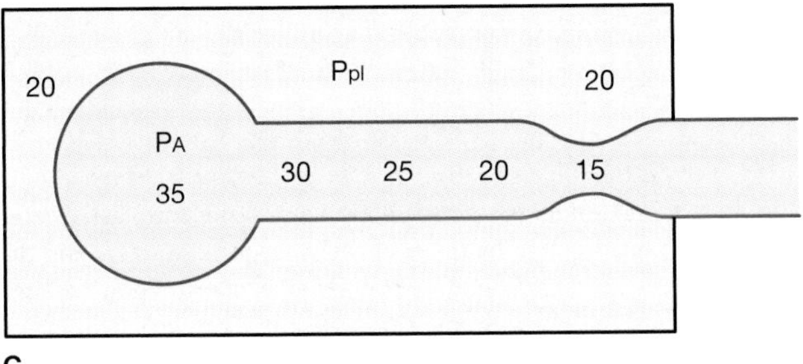

Figure 10-12 Schema of the distribution of pleural, alveolar, and airway pressures at rest and during expiration, illustrating the equal pressure point concept. **A.** End expiration. **B.** Quiet expiration. **C.** Forced expiration.

The driving pressure of the upstream segment – that is, the pressure drop along the airways of that segment – is equal to the elastic recoil of the lung. The maximum rate of airflow during forced expiration ($\dot{V}_{max}$) can be expressed in terms of the elastic recoil pressure of the lung (P_L) and the resistance of the upstream segment (R_{us}), as follows:

$$\dot{V}_{max} = \frac{P_L}{R_{us}}$$

Measurements of the rate of airflow during force expiration form the basis of many tests used to assess the flow-resistive properties of the lung. It is evident, however, that the maximum rate of expiratory airflow depends on many factors: The lung volume at which airflow is determined; the force of expiration (particularly at high lung volumes [i.e., above 75% of vital capacity]); the elastic recoil pressure of the lung; the cross-sectional area of large airways; the collapsibility of large intrathoracic airways; and the resistance of small peripheral airways.

WAVE SPEED LIMITATION THEORY

An alternative explanation for airflow limitation during forced expiration is based on principles of wave speed theory.[36] The wave speed theory proposes that flow is limited by the velocity of propagation of pressure waves along the wall of the tube. The velocity of propagation (v) varies proportionally with the cross-sectional area of the tube (A) and with airway stiffness. At a site where the linear velocity of gas molecules equals the velocity of propagation of pressure waves that is, wave speed, a choke point develops, preventing further increases in flow rate. The flow rate at wave speed is a function of the cross-sectional area of the tube at the choke point (A) and the stiffness of the choke segment (dP/dA), where P is the transmural airway pressure. Where choke points occur in the tracheobronchial tree depends on the lung volume: at large lung volumes, a choke point is situated in the vicinity of the lower trachea; at lower lung volumes, choke points develop more upstream along the bronchial tree. Extension of the neck exerts longitudinal tension and stiffens the trachea, increases wave velocity, and increases maximum expiratory flow rates at large lung volumes.[37]

MECHANICAL DETERMINANTS OF REGIONAL VENTILATION

The lung is not homogeneous, and the mechanical properties of all airways in a given generation and of all alveoli are not the same. This results in important nonuniformities of regional ventilation.

Pleural pressure in the upright person is more subatmospheric at the apex than at the base of the lung, because of the effects of gravity and the weight of the lung.[38] Pleural pressure topography and regional lung expansion are also determined by the shape of the chest wall and by the forces required for the lung to conform to the thoracic cavity shape[9,39] The rate of increase in pleural pressure from top to bottom is approximately 0.25 cmH_2O per centimeter of vertical distance. Consequently, the transpulmonary pressure – that is, alveolar pressure minus pleural pressure – is greater at the top than at the bottom of the lung. Therefore, at most lung volumes, the alveoli at the lung apexes are larger (more expanded) than those at the lung bases (Fig. 10-13).

Because of regional variations in lung compliance, ventilation is not uniform, even in the normal lung. With the use of external scanners after the inhalation of a radioactive gas, such as ^{133}Xenon, it has been demonstrated that within the range of normal tidal volume, lung units are better ventilated, and ventilation per alveolus is greater, at the bottom than at the top of the lung.[40] This is because alveoli near the top of the lung are positioned on the upper, flatter part of the pressure–volume curve and are less compliant than alveoli at the lung bases positioned on the lower, steeper portion of their pressure–volume curves.

At low lung volumes (i.e., near the RV), pleural pressure at the bottom of the lung actually exceeds airway pressure and leads to closure of peripheral airways (Fig. 10-13). During a breath taken from RV, air that enters the lungs first is preferentially distributed to the lung apexes.

The distribution of ventilation within the lungs and the volume at which airways at the lung bases begin to close can be assessed by the single-breath N_2 washout test.[41] This test requires a maximum expiration into an N_2 meter after a maximal inspiration of pure O_2 from RV; the changing concentration of nitrogen is plotted against expired lung volume (Fig. 10-14). Because the inspiration starts at the RV,

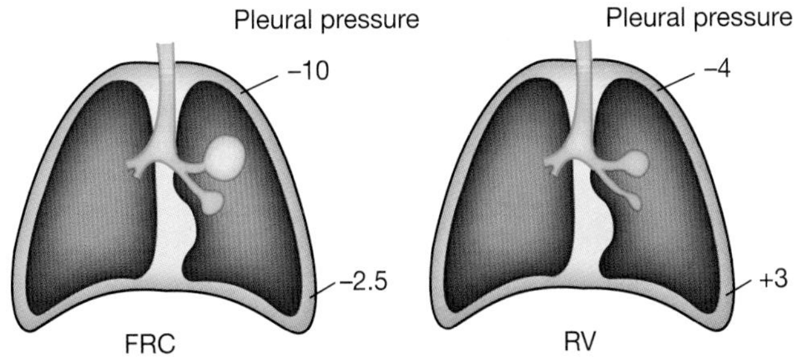

Figure 10-13 Pleural pressure gradients in the upright lung at FRC (left) and at RV (right). The effect of the gradient on alveolar volumes is shown schematically for each case.

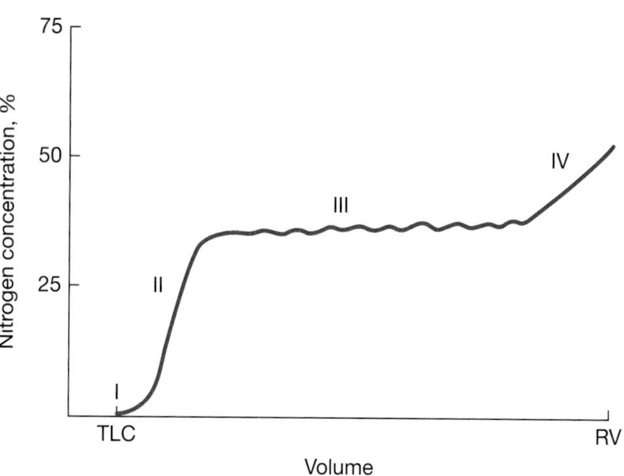

Figure 10-14 Tracing of expired nitrogen concentration during a slow expiration from TLC to RV after a full inspiration of pure O_2. The four phases are indicated. For further details, see text.

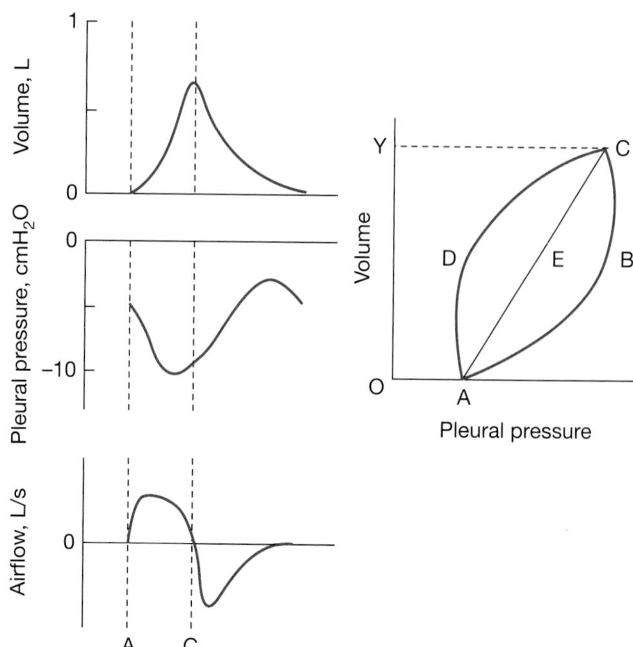

Figure 10-15 Individual tracings of tidal volume, pleural pressure, and airflow, taken simultaneously during a single complete breath, are shown on the left. The relationship between volume and pleural pressure is illustrated by the dynamic pressure–volume loop on the right. Dynamic compliance is determined as the slope of the line AEC. The work of breathing during inspiration to overcome the elastic forces of the lung is represented by the area of the trapezoid OAECY, and the work required to overcome nonelastic forces is represented by the area of the loop ABCEA. The loop AECDE represents the work required to overcome airflow resistance during expiration.

the initial portion of the breath containing dead-space gas, rich in nitrogen, is distributed to alveoli in the upper lung zones. The rest of the breath, which contains only O_2, goes preferentially to lower lung zones. Consequently, the concentration of nitrogen is lower in the alveoli at the lung bases than in the alveoli at the apexes of the lungs.

During expiration, the initial portion of the breath consists of O_2 remaining in the large airways; it contains no N_2 (phase I). As alveolar gas containing N_2 begins to be washed out, the concentration of N_2 in the expired air rises to reach a plateau. The portion of the curve where the concentration of N_2 rises steeply is phase II. The plateau is phase III. Phase III depends on the uniformity of the distribution of ventilation in the lung. If gas enters and leaves alveoli throughout the lung synchronously and equally, phase III is flat. But when the distribution of ventilation is nonuniform, so that gases coming from different alveoli have different N_2 concentration, phase III slopes upward.

At low lung volumes, airways at the lung bases close; only alveoli at the top of the lung continue to empty. Since the concentration of N_2 in the alveoli of upper lung zones is higher than in the alveoli at the lung bases, the slope of the N_2–volume curve increases abruptly, marking the start of phase IV. The volume, above RV, at which phase IV begins is termed the closing volume.[42]

The closing volume increases with advancing age. With diseases of the peripheral airways closing volume may rise to levels above FRC. This results in lung units that are perfused but poorly ventilated leading to reductions in arterial oxygenation.[43,44]

■ DYNAMIC COMPLIANCE OF THE LUNGS

The relationship between changes in volume and changes in pleural pressure during a normal breathing cycle is shown in Figure 10-15. Airflow momentarily ceases at the end of expiration (A) and at the end of inspiration (C); the change in pleural pressure between these two points reflects the increasing elastic recoil of the lung as the volume of air in the lungs increases. The slope of the line connecting the end-expiratory and end-inspiratory points (AEC in the figure) on a pressure–volume loop provides a measure of the dynamic compliance of the lungs.

In normal persons, dynamic compliance closely approximates inspiratory static lung compliance and remains essentially unchanged even when breathing frequency is increased up to 60 breaths per minute. This indicates that lung units that are parallel with each other normally fill and empty uniformly and synchronously, even when airflow is high and the change in lung volume is rapid. The rate of filling and emptying of a lung unit depends on its time constant—that is, the product of its resistance and compliance. Lung units with high resistance and high compliance take longer to fill and empty more slowly compared to units with low resistance and low compliance. In order for the distribution of ventilation in parallel lung units to be independent of the rate of airflow, the resistance and compliance of these units must be matched so that the time constants of individual units throughout the lungs are approximately the same. The time constants of lung units distal to airways 2 mm in diameter are approximately 0.01 second, and fourfold differences in time constants are necessary to cause dynamic compliance to become frequency dependent.[26]

Patchy narrowing of small peripheral airways produces regional differences in time constants. At low breathing frequencies, when the rate of airflow is low, ventilation is fairly evenly distributed. As the breathing frequency increases, however, ventilation tends to be distributed to areas that offer the least resistance to airflow. Therefore, lung units fed by narrowed airways receive proportionally less ventilation than do areas of the lung where the airways remain normal; the change in pleural pressure required to effect the same change in overall lung volume increases. As a result, the dynamic compliance falls.

Measurements of frequency dependence of dynamic compliance are time-consuming and technically difficult, but this test has proved useful in the diagnosis of obstruction in small peripheral airways when results of other conventional tests of lung mechanics are still within normal limits.[45]

WORK OF BREATHING

During breathing, the respiratory muscles work to overcome the elastic, flow-resistive, and inertial forces of the lungs and chest wall.[46] The elastic work of breathing is done to overcome the elastic recoil of the lungs and chest wall; the resistive work is done in overcoming the resistance of airways and tissues. The mechanical work of breathing can be determined by relating the pressure exerted across the respiratory system to the resulting change in volume, since the product of pressure (P) and volume (V) has the dimension of work, according to the equation

$$\text{work} = \int P\, dV$$

Recordings of pleural pressure and lung volume changes during spontaneous breathing can be used to measure the work of breathing; the work of breathing performed on the lungs can be determined from the area of the dynamic pressure–volume loop (Fig. 10-15) and fractionated into its elastic and resistive components. During inspiration, the work done to overcome the elastic forces of the lung is determined from the area of the trapezoid OAECY (Fig. 10-15). The area of the loop ABCEA is the work in overcoming nonelastic forces during inspiration, and the area of the loop OABCY is the total work of breathing during inspiration.

Expiration during quiet breathing is passive, since the elastic recoil of the lung suffices to overcome the expiratory airflow resistance. Some of the stored elastic energy is also used to overcome inspiratory muscle activity that persists into the expiratory phase of breathing. At high levels of ventilation and when airway resistance is increased, additional mechanical work during expiration is required to overcome nonelastic forces. Under these circumstances, the pleural pressure exceeds atmospheric pressure, and the loop AECDA extends beyond the confines of the trapezoid OAECY (Fig. 10-15).

The work of breathing at any given level of ventilation depends on the pattern of breathing. Large tidal volumes increase the elastic work of breathing, whereas rapid breathing frequencies increase the work against flow-resistive forces. During quiet breathing and during exercise, people tend to adjust tidal volume and breathing frequency to values that minimize the force and the work of breathing.[47] Similar adjustments are also seen in patients with pulmonary disorders. Patients with pulmonary fibrosis, which is characterized by an increased elastic work of breathing, tend to breathe shallowly and rapidly; those with airway obstruction and increased nonelastic work of breathing usually breathe more deeply and slowly.

The work done on the chest wall during breathing is calculated by subtracting the work performed on the lung from the total mechanical work of breathing. The total mechanical work of breathing cannot be readily measured during spontaneous breathing because the respiratory muscles that perform the work also make up part of the resistance offered by the chest wall. But the total mechanical work can be determined during artificial ventilation by using either intermittent positive airway pressure or negative pressure applied to the chest, provided that the respiratory muscles are completely at rest. For this determination, the change in lung volume is related to the pressure difference across the respiratory system—that is, differential pressure between the mouth and the body surface. Disturbances of the chest wall, such as kyphoscoliosis and obesity, increase the work of breathing severalfold.

OXYGEN COST OF BREATHING

In order to perform their work, the respiratory muscles require O_2. The O_2 cost of breathing, which reflects the energy requirements of the respiratory muscles, provides an indirect measure of the work of breathing.[48,49] The O_2 cost of breathing is assessed by determining the total O_2 consumption of the body at rest and at an increased level of ventilation produced by voluntary hyperventilation or CO_2 breathing. Provided there are no other factors acting to increase O_2 consumption, the added O_2 uptake is attributed to the increased metabolism of the respiratory muscles.

The O_2 cost of breathing in normal subjects is approximately 1 mL/L of ventilation and constitutes less than 5% of the total O_2 consumption. At high levels of ventilation, however, the O_2 cost of breathing becomes progressively greater. There is a dramatic increase in the O_2 cost of breathing at high levels of ventilation in some diseases of the lung, such as pneumonia, pulmonary fibrosis, and emphysema, and in disorders of the chest wall, such as obesity and kyphoscoliosis. The increase in the energy requirement of the respiratory muscles during increased ventilation, concomitant with a decrease in O_2 supply secondary to arterial hypoxemia, contributes to muscle fatigue, thereby limiting the amount of exertion that these patients can sustain.[3]

REFERENCES

1. Mead J, Takishima T, Leith D. Stress distribution in lungs: a model of pulmonary elasticity. *J Appl Physiol.* 1970;28:596–608.
2. Milic-Emili J, Mead J, Turner JM, Glauser EM. Improved technique for estimating pleural pressure from esophageal balloons. *J Appl Physiol.* 1964;19:207–211.
3. Roussos C, Zakynthinos S. Respiratory muscle energetics. In: Roussos C, ed. *The Thorax.* 2nd ed. Part A. New York, NY: Marcel Dekker Inc.; 1995:681–749.
4. Altose MD, Crapo RO, Wanner A. The determination of static lung volumes. Report of the section on respiratory pathophysiology. *Chest.* 1984;86:471–474.
5. Leith DE, Mead J. Mechanisms determining residual volume of the lungs in normal subjects. *J Appl Physiol.* 1967;23:221–227.
6. Gibson GJ, Pride NB. Lung distensibility: The static pressure-volume curve of the lungs and its use in clinical assessment. *Br J Dis Chest.* 1976;70:143–184.
7. Turner JM, Mead J, Wohl ME. Elasticity of human lungs in relation to age. *J Appl Physiol.* 1968;25:664–671.
8. Hoppin FG Jr, Stothert JC Jr, Greaves IA, Lai YL, Hildebrandt J. Lung recoil: elastic and rheological properties. In: Macklem PT, Mead J, eds. *Handbook of Physiology.* Section 3, The Respiratory System, Vol 3 Part 1, Bethesda, MD: American Physiological Society; 1986:195–216.
9. Marshall R, Widdicombe JG. Stress relaxation of the human lung. *Clin Sci.* 1961;20:19–31.
10. Van Golde LMG, Batenberg JJ, Robertson B. The pulmonary surfactant system: biochemical aspects and functional significance. *Physiol Rev.* 1988;68:374–455.
11. Bachofen H, Hildebrandt J, Bachofen M. Pressure-volume curves of air- and liquid-filled excised lungs surface tension in situ. *J Appl Physiol.* 1970;29:422–431.
12. Clements JA. Surface phenomena in relation to pulmonary function. *Physiologist.* 1962;5:11–28.
13. Whitsett JA, Weaver TE. Hydrophobic surfactant proteins in lung function and disease. *N Engl J Med.* 2002;347:2141–2148.
14. Prange HD. Laplace's law and the alveolus: a misconception of anatomy and a misapplication of physics. *Advan Physiol Educ.* 2003;27:34–40.
15. Zidulka A, Sylvester JT, Nadler S, Anthonisen NR. Lung interdependence and lung–chest wall interaction of sublobar units in pigs. *J Appl Physiol Respir Environ Exerc Physiol.* 1979;46:8–13.
16. Menkes HA, Traystman RJ. Collateral ventilation. *Am Rev Respir Dis.* 1977;116:287–309.
17. Weibel ER. Functional morphology of lung parenchyma. In: Macklem PT, Mead J, eds. *Handbook of Physiology.* Section 3, *The Respiratory System,* Vol 3, Part I. Bethesda, MD: American Physiological Society; 1986:80–112.

18. Stamenovic D. Micromechanical foundations of pulmonary elasticity. *Physiol Rev.* 1990;70:1117–1134.
19. D'Angelo E, Agostoni E. Statics of the chest wall. In: Roussos C, ed. *The Thorax.* 2nd ed. Part A. New York, NY: Marcel Dekker, Inc.; 1995:457–493.
20. Heaf PJD, Prime FJ. The compliance of the thorax in normal human subjects. *Clin Sci (Lond).* 1956;15:319–327.
21. Konno K, Mead J. Measurement of separate volume changes of rib cage and abdomen during breathing. *J Appl Physiol.* 1967;22: 407–422.
22. Sharp JT, Goldberg NB, Druz WS, Danon J. Relative distributions of rib cage and abdomen to breathing in normal subjects. *J Appl Physiol.* 1975;39:608–618.
23. Rahn H, Otis AB, Chadwick LE, Fenn WO. The pressure-volume diagram of the thorax and lung. *Am J Physiol.* 1946;146:161–178.
24. Drazen JM, Loring SH, Ingram RH Jr. Distribution of pulmonary resistance: effect of gas density, viscosity and flow rate. *J Appl Physiol.* 1976;41:388–395.
25. Ferris BG Jr, Mead L, Opie LH. Partitioning of respiratory flow resistance in man. *J Appl Physiol.* 1964;19:653–658.
26. Macklem PT, Mead J. Resistance of central and peripheral airways measured by a retrograde catheter. *J Appl Physiol.* 1967;22:395–401.
27. Hughes JMB, Hoppin FG Jr, Mead J. Effect of lung inflation on bronchial length and diameter in exercise lungs. *J Appl Physiol.* 1972;32:25–35.
28. Stubbs SE, Hyatt RE. Effect of increased lung recoil pressure on maximum expiratory flow in normal subjects. *J Appl Physiol.* 1972;32:325–331.
29. Canning BJ, Fischer A. Neural regulation of airway smooth muscle tone. *Respir Physiol.* 2001;125:113–127.
30. Drazen JM, Gaston B, Shore SA. Chemical regulation of pulmonary airway tone. *Annu Rev Physiol.* 1995;57:151–170.
31. Hyatt RE, Wilson TA, Bar-Yishay E. Prediction of maximal expiratory flow in excised human lungs. *J Appl Physiol Respir Environ Exerc Physiol.* 1980;48:991–998.
32. Schilder DP, Roberts A, Fry DL. Effect of gas density and viscosity on the maximal expiratory flow-volume relationship. *J Clin Invest.* 1963;42:1705–1713.
33. Hyatt RE, Black LF. The flow-volume curve. A current perspective. *Am Rev Respir Dis.* 1973;107:191–199.
34. Fry DL, Hyatt RE. Pulmonary mechanics: a unified analysis of the relationship between pressure, volume and gasflow in the lungs of normal and diseased human subjects. *Am J Med.* 1960;29:672–689.
35. Mead J, Turner JM, Macklem PT, Little JB. Significance of the relationship between lung recoil and maximum expiratory flow. *J Appl Physiol.* 1967;22:95–108.
36. Dawson SV, Elliott EA. Wave-speed limitation on expiratory flow—a unifying concept. *J Appl Physiol Respir Environ Exerc Physiol.* 1977;43:498–515.
37. Mead J. Expiratory flow limitation: a physiologist's point of view. *Fed Proc.* 1980;39:2771–2775.
38. Hoffman EA, Behrenbeck T, Chevalier PA, Wood EH. Estimation of regional pleural surface expansile forces in intact dogs. *J Appl Physiol Respir Environ Exerc Physiol.* 1983;55:935–948.
39. D'Angelo E, Michelini S, Agostoni E. Partition of factors contributing to the vertical gradient of transpulmonary pressure. *Respir Physiol.* 1971;12:90–101.
40. Milic-Emili J, Henderson JAM, Dolovich MB, Trop D, Kaneko K. Regional distribution of inspired gas in the lung. *J Appl Physiol.* 1966;21:749–759.
41. Fowler WS. Intrapulmonary distribution of inspired gas. *Physiol Rev.* 1952;32:1–20.
42. McCarthy DS, Spencer R, Greene R, Milic-Emili J. Measurement of "closing volume" as a simple and sensitive test for early detection of small airway disease. *Am J Med.* 1972;52:747–753.
43. Buist AS. New tests to assess lung function. The single-breath nitrogen test. *N Engl J Med.* 1975;293:438–440.
44. Milic-Emili J, Torchio R, D'Angelo E. Closing volume: a reappraisal (1967–2007). *Eur J Appl Physiol.* 2007;99:567–583.
45. Woolcock AJ, Vincent NJ, Macklem PT. Frequency of dependence of compliance as a test for obstruction on the small airways. *J Clin Invest.* 1969;48:1097–1106.
46. Otis AB. The work of breathing. *Physiol Rev.* 1954;34:449–458.
47. Mead J. Control of respiratory frequency. *J Appl Physiol.* 1960; 15: 325–336.
48. Campbell EJM, Westlake EK, Cherniack RM. Simple methods of estimating oxygen consumption and efficiency of the muscles of breathing. *J Appl Physiol.* 1957;11:303–308.
49. Cournand A, Richards DW Jr, Bader RA, Bader ME, Fishman AP. The oxygen cost of breathing. *Trans Assoc Am Physicians.* 1954;67:162–173.

CHAPTER 11

Control of Ventilation

Frank J. Jacono
Xavier Soler
Atul Malhotra

INTRODUCTION

Breathing is a rhythmic motor act, which is under both conscious and automatic control. This system maintains numerous controlled variables within their homeostatic ranges, but is also responsible for rapidly changing ventilation in response to often unpredictable stimuli. We will discuss the anatomy and physiology of the ventilatory control system, then address integrated responses and illustrative examples of adaptation and dysfunction in the setting of selected disease states.

ANATOMY AND PHYSIOLOGY

The respiratory control system, broadly speaking, comprises a controller, sensors, and a plant (Fig. 11-1). This hierarchical structure, in which there is central processing of afferent input, is important for coordinating respiratory movements with behaviors such as eating, speaking, and moving.[1] The controller is a neuronal network within the central nervous system (CNS), which is responsible for generating and modulating individual breaths and the overall breathing pattern. Often referred to as the respiratory central pattern generator (rCPG), the controller comprises reciprocally connected neuronal populations in the medulla and pons.[2,3] Neural output from the rCPG drives the activity of various motor neuron pools. Motor

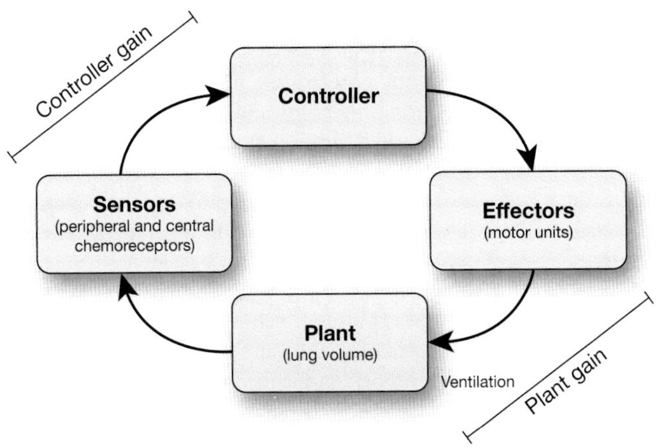

Figure 11-1 Block diagram of the respiratory control system.

neurons in the spinal cord (e.g., phrenic and intercostal) innervate the respiratory pump muscles, while brain stem motor neurons innervate upper airway muscles. The so-called "plant" includes the CO_2 stores, which are made up of lung stores and circulating blood volume including hemoglobin, and is an important component of breathing control. Closed loop feedback to the controller is supplied by chemoreceptors and mechanoreceptors.

The consistent cycling of the ventilatory pattern is generated spontaneously from the spatial and functional architecture of the rCPG. Intrinsic membrane properties of rhythmically active neurons within the rCPG are capable of producing automatic periodicity.[4] In addition, reciprocal (excitatory and inhibitory) synaptic connections between neuronal populations in the medulla and pons are believed to be critical for the automatic generation of the respiratory rhythm.[2,3]

The neural respiratory cycle comprises three phases (Fig. 11-2).[5] Inspiration (T_I) involves ramp-like increases in inspiratory motor neuron firing, which drive phrenic nerve activity throughout this phase. The first phase of expiration (T_{E1}) is often called post-inspiration, because inspiratory motor neurons are still active. Persistent inspiratory motor activity during T_{E1}, which declines throughout this phase, acts to slow the exit of air from the lungs. Finally, during the second phase of expiration (T_{E2}), expiratory muscles are typically electrically silent. During this phase of passive relaxation, gas is expelled as the lungs and chest wall return to their equilibrium state (i.e., functional residual capacity). However, under conditions where respiratory drive is increased, expiratory muscles including the internal intercostal and abdominal muscles become active during T_{E2}. This notion is an example of how the central controller, influenced by sensory feedback, modulates and alters the integrated motor response of the system.

■ BRAIN STEM

Within the medulla and pons, interconnected neuronal populations constitute a network, which is considered necessary for the generation of the respiratory rhythm (Fig. 11-3).[2,3,6] This bilateral pontomedullary respiratory network, which is also responsible for control of the ventilatory pattern, contains the ventral respiratory column (VRC) and the pontine respiratory group (PRG). Afferent signals from lung mechanoreceptors and peripheral chemoreceptors enter the pontomedullary network via the nucleus of the solitary tract (nTS) in the dorsal respiratory group (DRG). The nTS has projections to both pontine and ventral medullary components of the central respiratory network. Taken together, the VRC, DRG, and PRG comprise the brain stem rCPG. The rhythmic output of the rCPG drives the activity of spinal phrenic, intercostal, and lumbar motor neuron pools that innervate the muscles of respiration. Other brain stem motor neurons exhibit respiratory modulation and control muscles of the upper airway. Finally, the rCPG is influenced by higher CNS structures, which allows for conscious control of the ventilatory pattern.

Several regions of rhythmically active neurons in the VRC represent the core circuitry of the rCPG. The pre-Bötzinger complex (pre-BötC) within the VRC is believed to be the main source of rhythmic excitation driving inspiratory premotor neurons and other brain stem circuits. Furthermore, the pre-BötC has been shown to manifest intrinsic rhythmic activity.[4] However, the mechanisms responsible for rhythmic inspiratory pattern generation are complex given the large number of modulatory inputs that converge on the pre-BötC compartment, and are likely to manifest as the result of

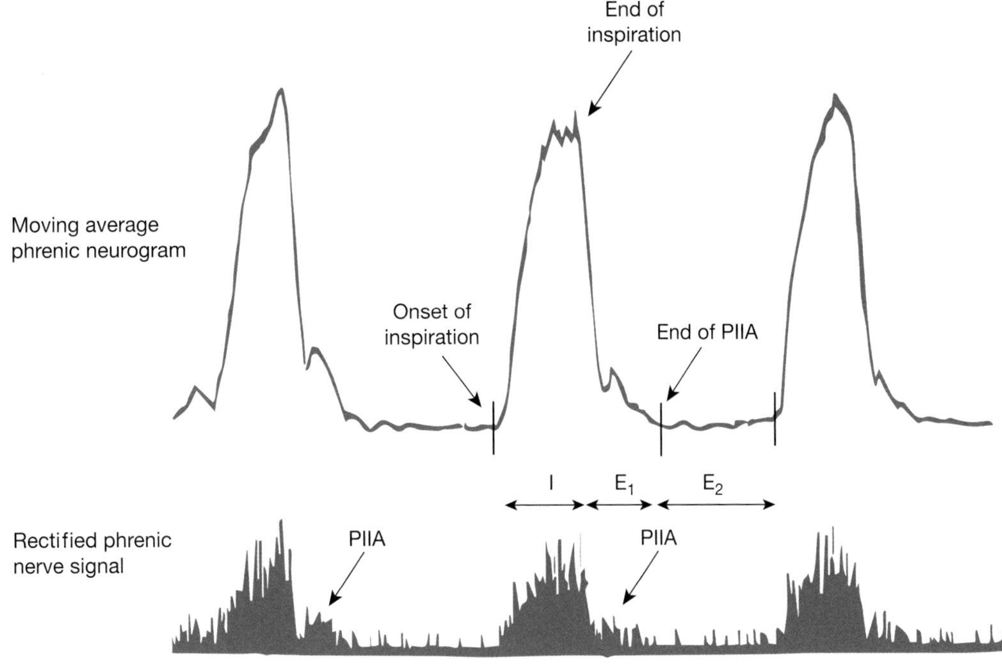

Figure 11-2 Recording of phrenic nerve activity (below) and its moving average (above), which highlights the three phases of the respiratory cycle: (1) Inspiration (I), (2) post-inspiratory activity (expiration, phase 1, E_1), and (3) late expiration (expiration, phase 2, E_2). PIIA, post-inspiratory inspiratory activity.

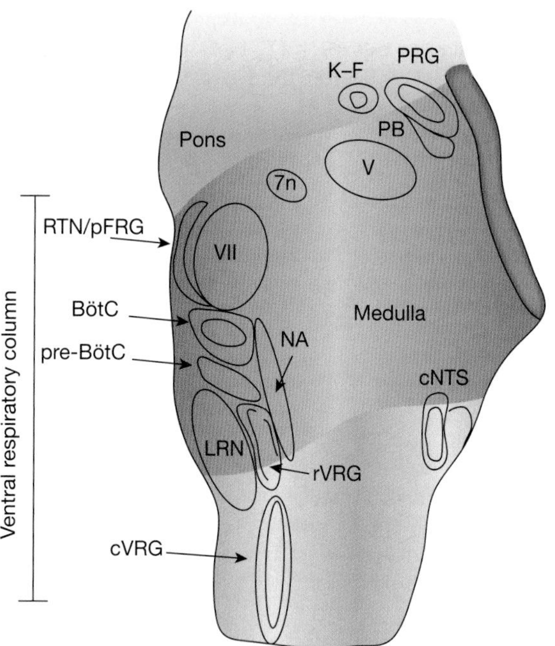

Figure 11-3 Overview of the respiratory central pattern generator (rCPG) within the brainstem. The ventral respiratory column (VRC) is orientated in the rostral-to-caudal direction. The VRC extends from the retrotrapezoid nucleus (RTN) adjacent to the rostral facial nucleus (VII) superiorly, to the caudal ventral respiratory group (cVRG) near the spinomedullary junction inferiorly. The main areas of rhythmically active VRC respiratory neurons are in the Bötzinger complex (BötC), pre-Bötzinger complex (pre-BötC), rostral ventral respiratory group (rVRG), and cVRG. The parafacial respiratory group (pFRG) overlaps anatomically with the RTN, and together these regions include intrinsically bursting neurons which may contribute to rhythm generation. Peripheral chemo- and mechanosensory inputs are transmitted to the nucleus of the solitary tract (nTS) in the dorsal respiratory group (DRG). The pontine respiratory group (PRG) includes the Kölliker–Fuse (K–F) and the parabrachial (PB) nuclei which contain respiratory-modulated neurons. See text for additional details.

network properties. Neuronal populations in the Bötzinger complex (BötC) are the major source of expiratory network activity during normal breathing. Thus, BötC neurons are important for control of the transition between inspiratory and expiratory activities in the rCPG and maintenance of the rhythmicity of normal breathing.

Neurons within the PRG are critical for formation of normal resting breathing patterns. Functional connections between the pons and the rest of the rCPG modulate phase switching (onset and termination of inspiration). For example, the dorsolateral pons (dlPons) is a region within the PRG with respiratory-modulated neurons whose activity varies depending on the presence of vagal afferent feedback. In particular, eupneic breathing patterns are dependent on excitatory drive from pontine neurons to the VRC, emphasizing the importance of the spatial and functional architecture of the brainstem respiratory network. Medullary raphé nuclei likely represent a system of intermediate relays for signaling between the PRG and the VRC. Transmission of an efference copy of ventilatory drive from the VRC is an example of one of these reciprocal connections. These medullary circuits may serve to maintain an overall level of rCPG activity. In addition, certain (particularly rostral) regions within the medullary raphé are chemosensitive, responding to local changes in carbon dioxide or pH, as well as exhibiting altered activity with stimulation of peripheral chemoreceptors.

The rostral ventral respiratory group (rVRG) region within the VRC comprises excitatory neurons that drive spinal phrenic and intercostal inspiratory motor neurons. This group of neurons is inhibited by the BötC during expiration and excited by the pre-BötC during inspiration. These rhythmically alternating influences, along with modulatory inputs from other areas of the pontomedullary network, are responsible for shaping and controlling the pattern of inspiratory rVRG activity. In contrast, the cVRG is thought to be the expiratory counterpart to rVRG activity.

Peripheral chemo- and mechanosensory inputs are transmitted to the nTS, which contains second-order neurons critical for reflex respiratory responses. For example, carotid body chemoreceptor and baroreceptor afferents terminate in the medial and lateral subnuclei of the nTS. Lung mechanoreceptors have projections to "pump cells" in the nTS, resulting in rhythmic activity of these cells which is modulated by lung inflation. The retrotrapezoid nucleus (RTN) is a site of central chemoreception. Chemoresponsive neurons within this region project to other areas of the rCPG and provide excitatory drive to the VRC and PRG. These sensory afferents, and the way in which they modulate breathing, will be discussed in subsequent sections. As part of the respiratory neural network, the nTS modulates breathing via projections to both pontine and ventral medullary components of the central respiratory network. In addition, neurons within the nTS receive inspiratory drive from the VRC and reciprocal pontine projections gate neuronal activity in the nTS.

CHEMORECEPTORS

The carotid and aortic bodies are bilateral sensory organs that detect changes in arterial oxygen. Although very small in size, the reflexes initiated by these tissues (particularly the carotid bodies) are critical for evoking stimulation of breathing during hypoxemia.[7] Stimulation of the carotid body by hypoxia (O_2 sensing) involves stimulus transduction and afferent nerve activation. Carotid bodies are composed of two cell types: type I and type II. Type I cells (also referred to as glomus cells) are of neural crest origin and are considered the putative oxygen-sensing cells. Glomus cells express a variety of neurotransmitters that play critical roles in sensory transmission of hypoxemia. Afferent nerve endings, whose cell bodies lie in the petrosal ganglion, form synaptic contacts with glomus cells and are responsible for afferent signaling to the CNS. The type II cells (also referred to as sustentacular cells) resemble glial cells and they are thought to act primarily as supporting cells.

There are two main pathways by which the carotid body senses hypoxia, although which mechanism is primary remains an area of debate.[8-10] The first main pathway for oxygen sensing involves heme-containing proteins in the glomus cell (metabolic hypothesis). First proposed by Mills and Jobsis, and later supported by studies using exogenous carbon monoxide (CO), there is evidence that mitochondrial cytochrome(s) may act as potential O_2 sensors. Further, several nonmitochondrial heme proteins that are expressed in glomus cells, including NADPH oxidases and heme oxygenase-2 (HO-2), have been proposed as potential oxygen sensors. Finally it has been suggested that hypoxia leads to the formation of iron-containing compounds via chelation as part of the transduction process, although the putative proteins and downstream signaling pathways responsible for afferent nerve activation are not well defined.

The second general mechanism by which hypoxia leads to depolarization of glomus cells is via inhibition of an O_2-sensitive, membrane-bound K^+ channel. This pathway for sensory transduction is based on the neuronal phenotype of the glomus cells and is referred to as the membrane hypothesis. Glomus cells express a variety of O_2-sensitive K^+ channels including outward rectifiers, Ca^{2+}-activated K^+ channels, human-ether-a-go-go (hERG), and twin pore-acid–sensitive K^+ (TASK) channels.[11] There is published evidence supporting and refuting aspects of both the metabolic and membrane hypotheses. Most likely, both pathways complement each other and work in concert to facilitate oxygen sensing by glomus cells. For example, it has been proposed that with increasing severity of hypoxemia, additional pathways are activated, allowing the carotid body to respond to a wide range of arterial oxygen levels.

Regardless of the mechanism(s) involved, hypoxic sensing ultimately leads to a Ca^{2+}-dependent release of neurotransmitters from glomus cells. These signaling molecules activate nerve endings in the carotid sinus nerve leading to an increase in afferent nerve activity (sensory transmission). The carotid body expresses several classes of neurotransmitters, including (1) biogenic amines (acetylcholine [Ach], dopamine, norepinephrine, and 5-hydroxytryptamine), (2) neuropeptides (enkephalins, substance P, and endothelins), (3) adenosine triphosphate (ATP), (4) amino acids (e.g., GABA), and (5) gas transmitters (CO and nitric oxide, NO). Some of the transmitters (e.g., ACh, substance P, ATP) stimulate whereas others (e.g., dopamine, enkephalins) inhibit carotid sinus nerve activity. Identifying which transmitters are primarily responsible for hypoxia-induced afferent nerve activation under physiological conditions remains an area of active research, and it is possible that corelease of multiple molecules, acting in concert, may ultimately be responsible for sensory excitation by hypoxia. While the carotid body is the primary peripheral chemoreceptor responsible for oxygen sensing, carbon dioxide also stimulates the carotid body, but the mechanisms are not fully understood. Finally, the interaction of the central and peripheral chemoreceptors is still debated, but recent evidence supports a hyperadditive model whereby the gain of one group of chemoreceptors can increase the responsiveness of the other (e.g., carotid body stimulation increases the gain of the central chemoreceptors).[12]

MECHANORECEPTORS

The lung, chest wall, and respiratory muscles all contain mechanoreceptors, which provide closed-loop feedback to the rCPG. This afferent input regulates minute ventilation independent from chemical drive. In addition, mechanoreceptor reflexes modulate the respiratory pattern on a breath-by-breath basis by enhancing or terminating inspiration. Afferent axons from lung mechanoreceptors are contained within the vagus nerve, but the importance of these receptors to control of respiration in awake, adult humans is likely small. Additional mechanoreceptors in the respiratory muscles and chest wall have central projections which travel in spinal nerves and the spinal cord. These receptors are important to coordinating the breathing pattern during trunk twisting and during movement between the upright and supine positions.

Several broad categories of mechanoreceptors have been identified which are relevant to ventilatory control:

1. Lung stretch receptors are present in the airway smooth muscle of the distal airways. These slowly adapting receptors are stimulated by lung inflation. Afferent signaling following activation of these receptors tends to terminate inspiration without altering the slope of the inspiratory ramp, as well as to promote expiratory activity. Slowly adapting receptors in the lung are the afferent fibers responsible for the Hering–Breuer reflex, which describes the termination of inspiration (promotion of inspiratory-to-expiratory phase switching) that occurs as a result of lung inflation. In addition, expiratory prolongation and occasional apneas which occur with large and sustained inflation of the lung are a manifestation of this reflex.
2. Rapidly adapting receptors respond to changes in airway mechanical properties that accompany lung inflation and deflation, and become more active as the rate of airflow increases. These receptors are also activated by stimuli that induce bronchospasm, edema, or mucus secretion. For example, they produce cough and laryngeal narrowing in response to stimulation by dust, ammonia, histamine, and other agents, as well as in response to increases in inspiratory airflow. These lung mechanoreceptors are primarily located in the epithelial and submucosal layers of the larger airways, accounting for their sensitivity to inhaled agents. Finally, rapidly adapting receptors lead to increased respiratory frequencies at low lung volumes, due to afferent signaling which increases inspiratory neural activity during lung deflation.
3. Bronchial J receptors are named for their juxtacapillary location. These lung mechanoreceptors project centrally through unmyelinated (in contrast to the first two types) fibers, and respond to pulmonary vascular congestion associated with increases in pulmonary artery and capillary pressure. Stimulation contributes to the increase in respiratory frequency and a decrease in tidal volume in response to pulmonary edema.
4. Bronchial C receptors are named for their sensitivity to capsaicin, and are located in the airway wall. Similar to type J receptors, these lung receptors project centrally through unmyelinated fibers. Activation of C fibers with capsaicin or bradykinin produces cough and a rapid, shallow breathing pattern. Unlike other lung receptors described here, bronchial C receptors are relatively insensitive to mechanical stimulation and changes in lung volume.
5. Muscle spindles transduce muscle length. The diaphragm has few if any muscle spindles, but these mechanoreceptors are plentiful in the intercostal muscles. Muscle spindles tend to augment breathing when activated.
6. Muscle tendon organs are located in series with muscle fibers in the tendon and are activated as muscle fibers generate force. Thus, these mechanoreceptors sense the efficiency of force generation and inhibit breathing when activated. The central tendon of the diaphragm contains tendon organs, as do the tendons of accessory muscles of respiration.
7. The rib cage joints and upper airways (larynx, pharynx, and nasal cavity) also contain receptors that impact control of ventilation. For example, cold air stimulation of the pharynx initiates the cough reflex, and can reduce the ventilatory response to carbon dioxide.

UPPER AIRWAY AND PUMP MUSCLES

The upper airway muscles are described more completely elsewhere but are addressed briefly here for completeness. The pharyngeal dilator muscles can be broadly classified into those with phasic activity (burst with inspiration) and tonic activity (constant activity throughout the respiratory cycle). The genioglossus is a frequently studied muscle as it is a representative phasic muscle which is readily accessible for intramuscular recordings and is controlled by the hypoglossal motor nucleus. The genioglossus is a major dilator muscle, which serves to protrude the tongue and protect pharyngeal patency in the face of collapsing perturbations. The tensor palatini, in contrast, is a representative tonic muscle controlled by trigeminal motor branches. Recent insights from recordings of single motor units have defined the complexity of these various muscles and provided insights into brainstem control in humans.[13] Although robust activity of the pharyngeal dilator muscles have been observed in obstructive sleep apnea patients during wakefulness, the fall in activity of these muscles at sleep onset likely contributes to a propensity to upper airway collapse in susceptible individuals. Some data also support evidence of structural neural remodeling and reinnervation of genioglossus muscle fibers suggesting neural injury may also be present in people with sleep apnea.[14] Given the recent realization that sleep apnea has multiple underlying mechanisms, there is likely a subset of OSA patients who have dysfunction in upper airway muscles as a major pathogenic factor. Various approaches are being considered to augment upper airway dilator muscle activity, including the possibility of pharmacological manipulation of hypoglossal output or electrical stimulation of the hypoglossal nerve. Pharmacological targets are being defined through careful studies of premotor inputs to the hypoglossal motor nucleus, although as yet no human trials have shown clear augmentation of genioglossus activity with pharmacotherapy. While the role of hypoglossal nerve stimulation in treating sleep apnea remains incompletely defined, recent work highlights the clinical promise of this approach.[15]

STABILITY OF VENTILATORY CONTROL: LOOP GAIN

Loop gain is an engineering term that is used to define the stability or instability of a negative feedback control system. Overall loop gain can be thought of as the integration of controller and plant factors and is thus the product of controller gain and plant gain (Fig. 11-1). A system with a high loop gain is prone to instability whereas a system with low loop gain is one which is intrinsically stable. The concept of loop gain can be considered in the context of the thermostat analogy, which is a common example of a negative feedback control system designed to regulate room temperature. Situations that lead to oscillations in room temperature can be considered analogous to situations in humans in which CO_2 levels fluctuate. For example, a highly sensitive thermostat is one that responds to trivial fluctuations in room temperature with major changes in output from the air conditioner or furnace; thus, a very sensitive thermostat will lead to marked fluctuations in room temperature. By analogy, exquisite sensitivity of chemoreceptors will contribute to marked fluctuations in CO_2 levels. Another example is a furnace, which is too powerful such that a minor drop in room temperature leads to major elevations in room temperature as a result of the output of the furnace. By analogy, if a minor increase in Pa_{CO_2} led to major increases in ventilation yielding marked reductions in Pa_{CO_2}, the system would be considered unstable, that is, elevated loop gain. Thus, situations, which lead to fluctuations in room temperature, can be considered to understand the factors underlying CO_2 fluctuations in the human.

In the case of ventilation, the propensity for CO_2 fluctuations is a function of an individual's loop gain. That is, an individual with a high loop gain is prone to developing periodic breathing or Cheyne–Stokes breathing, even with minimal perturbation. On the other hand, an individual with low loop gain will maintain relatively stable breathing patterns even with major perturbations. The mechanism underlying a high loop gain can be highly varied, but can generally be considered due to either an elevation of controller gain or plant gain. Controller gain is also known as chemoresponsiveness, which includes chemosensitivity (i.e., how much chemoreceptors fire with a given CO_2 stimulus) in addition to the actual change in ventilation for a given CO_2 stimulus (e.g.,which includes upper airway patency). In addition, plant gain describes the efficiency of CO_2 excretion, that is, how much the CO_2 actually changes for a given change in ventilation. Individuals with congestive heart failure are at risk of Cheyne–Stokes respiration (CSR) likely due to elevated chemoreflex gain as well as elevated plant gain compared to matched controls.

The delay in the circulation, sometimes defined by a mixing gain, is also an important factor in determining breathing pattern. The ability for the human ventilatory control system to develop instabilities is a result of chemoreceptors being located in the brainstem and carotid bodies rather than in the lung. Circulatory delay can also contribute to an unstable breathing pattern, although most studies suggest that marked prolongation of circulatory delay is not present in CSR patients with congestive heart failure compared to heart failure patients without CSR. In classic Guyton experiments, several minute delays were occasionally required to induce periodic breathing in dogs; such circulatory delays are beyond the range of what occurs in humans even in pathological states (e.g., end-stage congestive heart failure). Thus, circulatory delay is considered necessary but not sufficient to induce periodic breathing or CSR. Some interventional studies suggest improvements in sleep apnea with reduction in circulatory delay, emphasizing the importance of this variable in some individuals.[16]

The measurement of loop gain is cumbersome currently as it requires overnight experimental measurements and considerable expertise. However, the concepts are useful in a qualitative manner even if quantitative data are not available. In addition, efforts are ongoing to simplify the loop gain measurement to determine expeditiously which patients may respond to particular interventions.[17] The importance of loop gain is receiving increasing attention given the recognition of its importance in obstructive sleep apnea,[18] central sleep apnea,[19] periodic breathing at high altitude and other conditions. Indeed, manipulation of loop gain using interventions such as oxygen or acetazolamide can lead to improvements in sleep apnea in small physiological studies.[20,21] Thus, further work on ventilatory loop gain is required to define the optimal diagnostic and therapeutic approaches.

CONTROL OF VENTILATION IN HEALTH AND DISEASE: ILLUSTRATIVE EXAMPLES

The afferent, efferent, and central neural systems described earlier, respond to a variety of challenges that affect both normal individuals and patients with respiratory disease. These pathophysiological changes will affect the level of ventilation, the respiratory rhythm, or both. The impact of ventilatory control on specific disease states is addressed as appropriate in relevant sections elsewhere in this text. Following are illustrative examples which are considered to highlight how the respiratory control system adapts in clinically important conditions.

■ VENTILATORY ACCLIMATIZATION TO OXYGEN DISTURBANCES

There are many pathophysiological mechanisms that cause hypoxemia, and it has been well known for more than a century that hypoxia stimulates the respiratory and cardiovascular systems.[22] Heymans et al., among others, demonstrated the importance of carotid body chemoreceptors for the hypoxic ventilatory response.[23,24] Comroe and Mortimer[6] established the idea that arterial chemoreceptors are the dominant O_2-sensitive chemoreceptors for cardiopulmonary control. Elimination of the carotid and aortic body chemoreceptors elicits hypoventilation and essentially obliterates the acute ventilatory response to hypoxemia.[25] Therefore, it has been assumed that central O_2 sensitivity may not play a major role in this response.[26] In fact, chronic hypoxia reportedly has a depressive effect on the brain, limiting its response to further hypoxia. This hypoxic depression spreads rostral caudally in the brain; and may be the result of slowed removal of inhibitory neurotransmitters like GABA during hypoxia due to the buildup of lactic acid in the brain. However, in some experimental preparations, hypoxia continues to stimulate ventilation and the cardiovascular system in the absence of carotid body chemoreceptors, suggesting that other arterial chemoreceptors or sites in the CNS must be sensitive to hypoxia.[6] Focal hypoxia produced by cyanide in the medulla excites sympathoexcitatory neurons,[27] and experimental evidence supports central O_2 sensitivity in the C1 sympathoexcitatory region of the rostral ventrolateral medulla, the posterior hypothalamus, the pre-BötC, and the nucleus tractus solitarius.[25]

Hypoxic Ventilatory Response: The hypoxic ventilatory response is characterized by discrete, time-dependent mechanisms that depend on the severity, duration, and pattern of hypoxic exposure. A reduction in the partial pressure of oxygen produces an immediate increase in ventilation mediated through the peripheral chemoreceptors.[28] While the ventilatory response to hypoxia is independent of the source of hypoxemia, the brain has multiple time domains of O_2 sensitivity that can elicit different ventilatory responses to acute versus chronic hypoxia. Furthermore, this ventilatory response has several unique forms of respiratory plasticity.[29]

Acute and chronic exposure to high altitude: The hypoxic and hypobaric environment encountered at high altitude results in a reduction

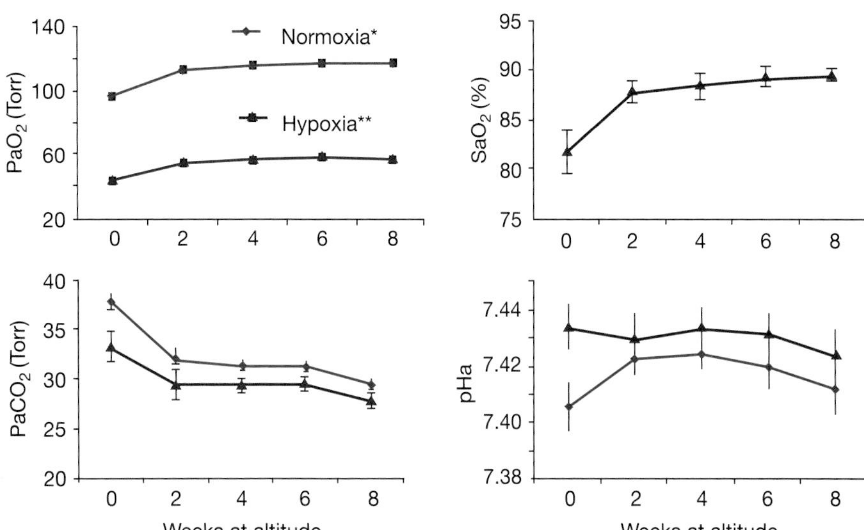

Figure 11-4 Arterial oxygenation increases and arterial CO_2 decreases during time at altitude. These changes persist in normoxia, indicating hyperventilation. pHa is partially compensated during acclimatization. *(Data from Hupperets MD, Hopkins SR, Pronk MG, et al. Increased hypoxic ventilatory response during 8 weeks at 3800 m altitude. Respiratory physiology & neurobiology. 2004;142(2–3):145–152.)* *Normoxia is from data collected breathing at sea level. **Hypoxia is from data collected breathing at 3800-m altitude.

in the available inspired oxygen (inspiratory partial pressure of O_2 [P_{IO_2}]). Acute exposure to altitude results in hypoxemia, which produces an immediate increase in minute ventilation mediated through the peripheral chemoreceptors and characterized by an increase in frequency (respiratory rate) and amplitude (tidal volume). With ongoing exposure, ventilation continues to increase for several days resulting in a sustained gradual decrease in arterial P_{O_2}. Chronic exposure to high altitude, lasting from several hours to months, results in acclimatization. This adaptation to high altitude is characterized by a gradual rise in minute ventilation with a time course depending on the altitude. In humans, at very high altitudes (~8000 m), this process may take at least 30 days. At less extreme altitudes, complete adaptation may be achieved in less than 10 days. However, in one study, ventilation and arterial oxygenation were noted to be greater than during the initial ascent to 3800 m after 8 weeks.[30] In addition, there is an increase in CO_2 sensitivity with exposure to altitude. In people living in high altitude for long periods of time the P_{CO_2} falls to the lower level of normal or even less (Fig. 11-4).[30]

A number of physiological mechanisms of ventilatory acclimatization to hypoxia have been identified. They include (a) plasticity in O_2 sensitivity of the carotid body chemoreceptors, (b) the CNS integration of peripheral O_2-sensitive reflexes (e.g., carotid body chemoreflex), (c) plasticity of CNS mechanisms of acute O_2 sensing, and (d) the CNS integration of other nonchemoreflex ventilatory control pathways such as reflexes from pulmonary vagal chemoreceptors or respiratory rhythm generators.[25,31,32] For example, hypoxia-inducible factor-1 (HIF-1) is a key regulator of O_2-sensitive gene expression in the brain, and increases in HIF-1 have been identified in respiratory nuclei of the CNS as soon as 1 hour after hypoxemia. Hence, O_2 sensing by HIF-1α could be involved in the ventilatory acclimatization to high altitude by increasing the expression of genes with products known to modulate the hypoxic ventilatory response.[33]

OXYGEN-INDUCED HYPERCAPNIA IN CHRONIC OBSTRUCTIVE PULMONARY DISEASE

In severe chronic obstructive pulmonary disease (COPD), transient falls in ventilation and respiratory acidosis have been reported with breathing 100% oxygen for 20 minutes.[34–36] Initially CO_2 retention with oxygen treatment was thought to result from the suppression of the hypoxic drive mediated by carotid chemoreceptors.[37] Subsequently, additional mechanisms have been shown to contribute to oxygen-induced hypercapnia in COPD as follows:

(1) The increase in oxygen tension in lung units with low ventilation/perfusion (V/Q) ratios can blunt hypoxic pulmonary vasoconstriction in these low V/Q lung units, thus diverting perfusion away from high V/Q lung units yielding higher dead space; (2) the Haldane effect, which refers to the reduction in hemoglobin affinity for CO_2 with the binding of oxygen to hemoglobin. With increased blood oxygen levels, the Haldane effect promotes dissociation of carbon dioxide from hemoglobin and leads to a small increase in Pa_{CO_2}; (3) suppression of hypoxic drive as mentioned earlier. Data on P_{CO_2} recruitment threshold in intubated COPD patients support a change in sensitivity of the CNS to CO_2 during hyperoxia; (4) some patients with acute exacerbations of COPD are susceptible to the development of severe hypercapnia due to sleep deprivation that is common in acute illness; patients with associated obstructive sleep apnea might be susceptible since they have high sleep drive and are likely to lose the wakefulness drive to breathe at sleep onset upon initiation of therapy. For example, patients during acute exacerbations of COPD will commonly be sleep deprived and will typically fall asleep once they receive the anxiolytic and antidyspnea effects of oxygen therapy[36,38]; and (5) increases in Fi_{O_2} which occur with noninvasively delivered oxygen as minute ventilation falls. Actual delivered Fi_{O_2} is a function of inspiratory flow demand and room air entrainment; thus, higher oxygen tensions result as ventilatory drive falls for any reason. Occasionally vicious cycles can occur whereby supplemental oxygen leads to a rise in CO_2 level, which contributes to a further increase in oxygen level due to a resultant decrease in inspiratory flow with reductions in room air entrainment.

Understanding these mechanisms has clinical implications, as maintaining the arterial oxygen saturation between 87% and 92% may be a safer approach in patients with a history of respiratory disease, and is unlikely to compromise tissue oxygen delivery.

RESPONSES TO EXTERNAL MECHANICAL LOADS AND BRONCHOCONSTRICTION

In response to external mechanical loads, several compensatory factors act to maintain ventilation[39]: (1) *Responses intrinsic to the respiratory muscles.* The force that the muscle develops for a fixed electrical input depends on the length of the muscle (the force–length relationship). As the muscle shortens, less force is developed. The generated force also decreases as the velocity of shortening increases (force–velocity relationship). With external mechanical impediments (loading), both the magnitude and the velocity of shortening tend to decrease. (2) *Reflex effects.* At the spinal level, less shortening of the inspiratory muscles increases the signal from muscle spindles that, in turn, augments contraction of these muscles. During loading, afferent information from pulmonary mechanoreceptors also changes. Since tidal volume is depressed, inspiratory duration tends to be prolonged (Hering–Breuer inspiratory terminating reflex), but this mechanism is of little importance in humans. (3) *Conscious responses.* Loads increase neuromuscular output even in the face of a constant chemical drive. The magnitude of the increase is related to the severity of the mechanical load. This aspect of load compensation is abolished by anesthesia. Furthermore, the intensity of this load-compensating mechanism is variable, and it is reduced in some chronic lung disease like COPD.

While external loading is used experimentally, major differences exist between the neural responses to bronchoconstriction and external loading. In particular, inspiratory muscle activity increases during bronchoconstriction, even in anesthetized animals. Bronchoconstriction increases breathing frequency via reflex changes in respiratory timing. Expiratory duration (especially the second phase of expiration) shortens more than inspiratory duration. In asthma-induced bronchoconstriction, rapidly adapting receptors are stimulated by mechanical changes in the airways and by substances such as histamine and bradykinin.

RESPONSE TO EXERCISE

The exercise ventilatory response is the most frequently engaged ventilatory response in everyday life.[29] Despite the increase in CO_2 production and O_2 utilization during exercise, ventilatory control mechanisms normally keep arterial P_{CO_2} and $[H^+]$ remarkably constant over a wide range of metabolic rates.[40] This pattern is achieved by graded increases in minute ventilation (V_E) as the rate of CO_2 production increases, and acts to minimize acidosis that would impair cellular function. This response is tightly controlled; respiratory alkalosis does not typically develop during moderate exercise in normal subjects, although it occasionally occurs in pathophysiological states. With increased intensity of exercise, oxygen demand outstrips oxygen supply, anaerobic pathways start to operate and blood lactate levels increase. With exertion above this anaerobic threshold, the exercise-induced metabolic acidosis becomes more marked due to a net increase in lactic acid production. As a result, high-level exercise results in a large increase in ventilation to enhance carbon dioxide excretion and minimize acidemia.

The minute ventilation required to maintain acid–base equilibrium during exercise is defined by (1) the amount of carbon dioxide produced as a result of metabolism (V_{CO_2}); (2) physiological dead space, and (3) the set point at which P_{CO_2} is regulated by the respiratory control system. There is an incomplete understanding of the reflexes responsible for controlling how pulmonary ventilation matches the increases in metabolic demand during exercise without appreciable changes in arterial blood gas composition. The magnitude of oscillations in ventilation is directly related to metabolic CO_2 production. Thus, it has been proposed that a blood-borne signal helps in the coupling of metabolic production of CO_2 and ventilation. Neurally mediated signals from exercising muscles and from higher brain centers are also likely important in the ventilatory response. Finally, this response is responsible for meeting the increased need for oxygen consumption by exercising limb and respiratory muscles.

The initial phase of the exercise response is a rapid increase in ventilation. Proposed sources include signals arising from the cortex (so-called feedforward control), temperature increases, afferent signals arising as a result of muscle contraction (locomotor muscle afferents and respiratory muscle metaboreflex), accumulation of catecholamines, and increases in potassium in the venous blood.[41] There is also evidence that the abrupt initial increase in ventilation at the onset of exercise is a learned response. That is, the primary drive to breathe at the start of exercise will augment respiration in anticipation of impending metabolic needs based on past exercise experiences.[42] Chemoreceptor feedback may act in concert with the feedforward stimulus to minimize disruptions in homeostasis as the intensity of exercise increases. In addition, there is capacity for modulation and plasticity of the mechanisms controlling breathing during exercise. For example, serotonergic modulation of descending drive is a mechanism for long-term modulation of exercise hyperpnea, which may be important in individuals with underlying cardiorespiratory disease.[43]

DISTURBANCES OF RESPIRATORY RHYTHM

Congenital central hypoventilation syndrome (CCHS), occasionally referred to as Ondine's curse, is a rare neurological disorder characterized by inadequate breathing during sleep and, in more severely affected individuals, also during waking periods. Patients congenitally lack or have poor chemosensitivity to both hypercapnia and hypoxia, and suffer from inadequate ventilation. Over 90% of patients with CCHS have an increased polyalanine repeat expansion mutation (PARM) in the paired-like homobox 2B (PHOX2B) gene. Other cases of CCHS are the result of non-PARM mutations of the PHOX2B gene. Most cases are the result of a *de novo* mutation, although patients may have a family history of the disorder. There is a correlation with the number of polyalanine repeat expansion genotype and the need for continuous ventilatory support. The disease typically presents in childhood, but rare adult-onset cases have been reported.[44] A number of conditions are associated with CCHS and reflect the autonomic nervous system dysregulation, including Hirschsprung disease (about 20% of cases) and tumors of neural crest origin (neuroblastomas). While PHOX2B is considered to be the disease-defining gene in CCHS, these patients may have other protein-altering mutations including mutations in the receptor tyrosine kinase, the RET gene, brain derived neurotrophic factor (BDNF), and endothelin1 and 3 genes. Rett syndrome is a neurodevelopmental disorder that occurs almost exclusively in females. After a period of initially normal development, affected patients experience loss of speech and purposeful hand use, stereotypic hand movements, gait abnormalities, and breathing abnormalities among others. Most cases result from mutations in the gene encoding methyl-CpG-binding protein 2 (Mecp2). Loss of Mecp2 function is associated with an irregular breathing pattern. The implicated mechanism has not been established, but may be related to widespread hyperexcitability in respiratory-related regions in the brainstem. Apnea that occurs during wakefulness is typically central, although it may be obstructive. These events may be isolated, or precede or follow hyperventilation. During apneic episodes, the child may stare quietly ahead or smile and appear happy with no evidence of distress, despite severe cyanosis.

Cheyne–Stokes Breathing is one form of periodic breathing characterized by a cyclic rise and fall in ventilation with recurrent periods of apnea or near apnea (Fig. 11-5). It was first observed in patients with cardiac or CNS disease, but it has since been reported in seemingly normal humans. The appearance of Cheyne–Stokes breathing can occur during wakefulness although often masked by behavioral influences, but is more common during nonrapid eye movement (NREM) sleep. The period of the oscillations in ventilation in Cheyne–Stokes breathing often averages 60 to 90 seconds. Cycle length is related to the circulation time measured from the lung to a systemic artery, and increases when circulation time is prolonged. Arousal tends to occur during the hyperpneic phase of the respiratory pattern, a finding which is often associated with paroxysmal nocturnal dyspnea in patients with heart failure.

Cheyne–Stokes breathing has not been consistently produced in animals by lesions in the CNS, but it has been shown to follow manipulations that are likely to produce unstable feedback control of breathing. Cheyne–Stokes breathing is seen in chronic heart failure, as well as in stroke and traumatic brain injury. A similar breathing pattern with a shorter cycle time (~15–30 seconds), often referred to

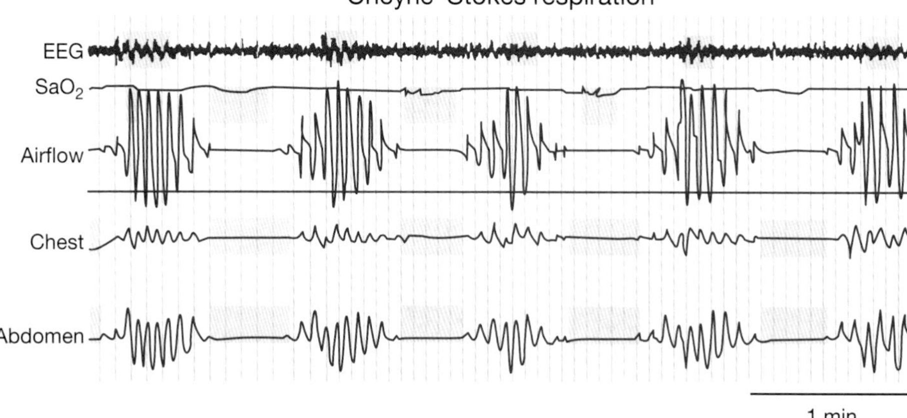

Figure 11-5 An example respiration in a patient with Cheyne–Stokes breathing. Note the characteristic crescendo/decrescendo pattern of breathing, long circulation time (each oxygen desaturation corresponds to the previous apnea), and arousal occurring at the peak of respiratory effort.

as periodic breathing at high altitude, can occur in otherwise healthy individuals at high altitude during the acclimatization period.

Sleep-related abnormalities of ventilatory control: Abnormal ventilatory patterns that can emerge during sleep are increasingly appreciated, including their associations with adverse neurocognitive and cardiovascular consequences. Ventilatory control instability may contribute to both central and obstructive sleep apnea. Indeed, sleep promotes breathing instability because it unmasks a highly sensitive dependence of the respiratory control system on chemoreceptor input. For example, the CO_2 reserve (i.e., the difference between the eupneic Pa_{CO_2} and that required to induce apnea) is labile during sleep and is reduced by hypoventilation, predisposing patients to the development of apneas.[45] Transient cortical arousals promote ventilatory overshoots, upper airway dilator muscle tone is reduced and airway collapsibility is enhanced.[46] In addition, depending on the prevailing pharyngeal mechanics, anatomical factors may cause or contribute to sleep-related disorders. Thus, both basic and clinical investigators have focused on mechanisms that influence upper airway patency during wakefulness and sleep, along with ventilatory control stability during sleep.

There are a number of changes in ventilatory control that occur during sleep; however, most of the same basic mechanisms active during wakefulness are also relevant during sleep. During sleep, there is an elevation of the CO_2 set point (~45 mm Hg as opposed to 40 mm Hg during wakefulness), associated with reduced alveolar ventilation during sleep. In all stages of sleep, there is decreased ability to respond to increments in resistance-load and the work of breathing. Thus, narrowing of the upper airway during sleep is a factor contributing to the rise in Pa_{CO_2}.

Other ventilatory control mechanisms are also affected. Sleep apnea results in recurrent episodes of hypoxemia, which alter the hypoxic ventilatory response resulting in respiratory long-term facilitation (LTF).[47] LTF is a form of neuronal plasticity that is induced by exposure to intermittent hypoxia and causes a persistent increase in ventilation even when normoxia is restored.[29,48] Phrenic (innervating the diaphragm) and hypoglossal (innervating upper airway muscles) nerve activities are both increased. Whereas the impact of LTF on ventilatory stability remains uncertain in the context of sleep apnea at this time, experiments in preclinical animal models suggest that LTF has the potential for both stabilizing and destabilizing influences on breathing that warrant further investigation.[20,49,50]

Apnea is a cessation of airflow for at least 10 seconds, and is probably the most common respiratory rhythm abnormality. Apneas occur often in premature infants and occasionally during sleep in healthy humans. Central apneas arise from complete or partial reductions in central neural outflow to the respiratory muscles during sleep (Fig. 11-6). In contrast to obstructive apneas, in which inspiratory efforts are made against the occluded upper airway, no respiratory effort is generated during central apneas due to cessation of respiratory drive. Thus central apneas are distinguished from obstructive apneas by the absence of respiratory effort, which can be detected by routine monitoring techniques such as respiratory inductive plethysmography combined with assessment of nasal pressure.[19] Mechanisms which can produce central apneas include (1) reduced excitation of chemoreceptors as a consequence of hypocapnia and hyperoxia; (2) functional or actual structural medullary damage which may result in a pattern of grossly irregular ataxic breathing; (3) loss of nonspecific respiratory excitatory stimulation (noise, light, tactile stimuli) in the absence of adequate chemical drive; and (4) active suppression of breathing by respiratory inhibitory reflexes, which is observed in a number of clinical situations including pharmacological therapy with methadone and other opiate medications. Reflex inhibition may arise from the cardiovascular system, from the lung and chest wall, or from somatic and visceral afferents. For example, excitation of receptors located in the upper airway can, via the superior laryngeal nerve, trigger an apnea. Stimulation of J receptors in the lungs by inhaled irritants may produce temporary apnea.

Complex sleep apnea syndrome describes the appearance and persistence of central apneas or hypopneas in patients with obstructive sleep apnea upon successful restoration of airway patency. Patients with complex sleep apnea syndrome present with features of obstructive sleep apnea syndrome. However, when instability of upper airway tone is treated with positive airway pressure therapy, these patients exhibit unstable, chemosensitive ventilatory control leading to repetitive central apneas or periodic breathing during sleep.[51] Adaptive servo-ventilation, which provides both a minimum pressure to hold the airway open as well as a ventilatory assist to minimize persistent cycles of hypo- and hyperventilation, has emerged as an effective treatment. Noninvasive ventilation using bi-level positive airway pressure in the spontaneous-timed mode may also normalize ventilation in some patients.[52]

Central apneas may also occur in critically ill patients as a result of artificial ventilatory support. Application of positive pressure mechanical ventilation may result in a loss of respiratory drive and associated apneas both during and after periods of ventilatory support. This may occur despite normocapnic conditions, and is more frequent during NREM sleep.[52] It is unclear whether these inhibitory effects are dependent on increases in tidal volume (i.e., Hering–Breuer mechanism) or are caused by a resetting of the inherent respiratory rhythm by the externally imposed ventilator frequency.[53,54] In addition, hypocapnia, oversedation, and the presence of CNS disease will also impact the prevalence of apneas during mechanical ventilation.

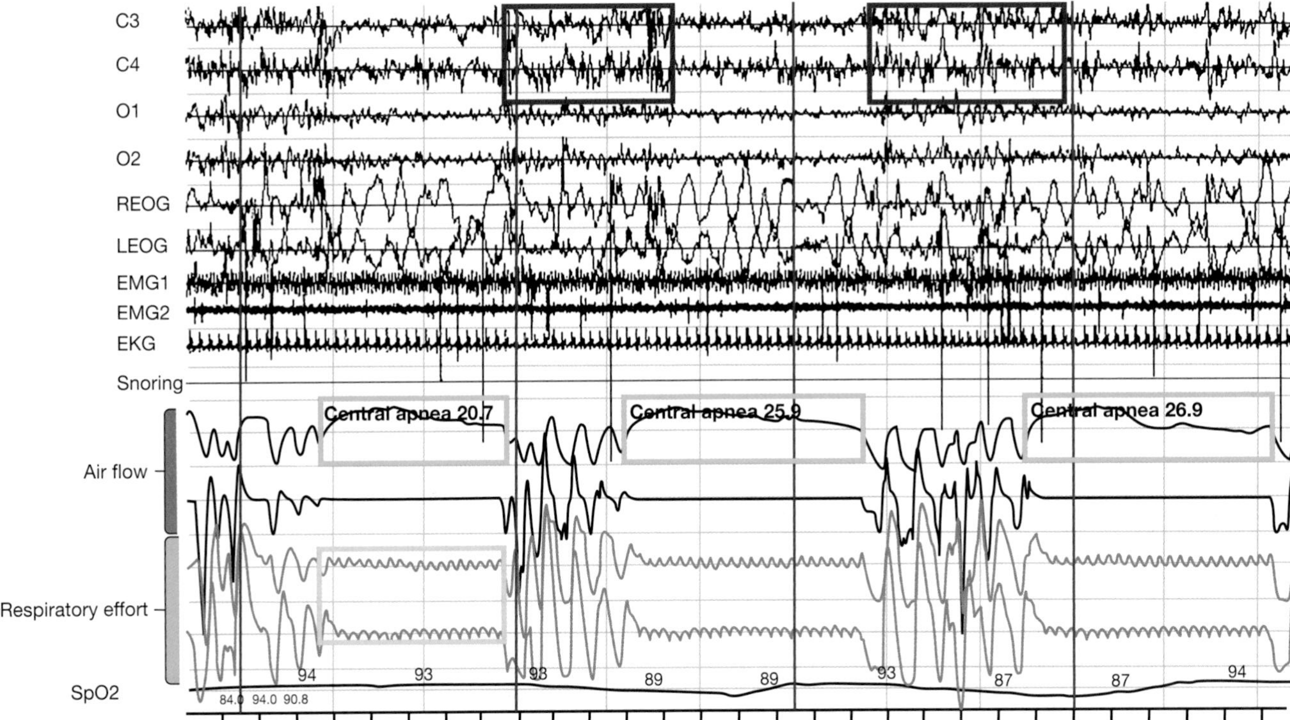

Figure 11-6 An example of respiratory pattern in a patient with central apneas. Note the typical characteristics of central apneas including absence of air flow by both nasal cannula pressure transducer and nasal–oral thermistor (durations in seconds), absence of respiratory effort measured with piezoelectric bands of the thorax and abdomen (orange box), associated oxygen desaturation corresponding to the previous apnea measured by pulse oximeter, and EEG arousal (red box) occurring after an apneic event. EEG channels (C3, C4, O1, O2); electrooculogram channels (REOG, LEOG), chin electromyogram (EMG1), bilateral tibialis anterior EMG2, EKG, snoring microphone.

DYSPNEA AND BREATHLESSNESS

Dyspnea is defined as a subjective sensation of difficulty breathing, frequently termed "shortness of breath." Under normal conditions, breathing is not noticeable. However, with increased demands (e.g., during exercise or with progressive cardiopulmonary disease), respiratory movements and forces become more perceptible. When sufficiently intense, respiratory efforts result in symptoms of dyspnea, and patients with lung disease may complain of dyspnea even at rest. The development of dyspnea is a warning signal, which likely serves to protect the body from harm; but since dyspnea itself can become an incapacitating symptom, considerable attention has been given to its etiology.[55–60] Experiments using breath-holding techniques showed that hypercapnia and hypoxia decrease breath-holding times, supporting the idea that increased levels of chemical drive promote dyspnea. In contrast, increased lung volume (increased oxygen stores) lengthened breath-holding time. Other investigations identified that combined blockade of the phrenic and vagus nerves extends the time apnea can be voluntarily maintained, suggesting that signals from respiratory muscles contribute to the sense of dyspnea. Dyspnea also seems to be related to the effort (as a percentage of maximal capacity) required during breathing. In particular, dyspnea increases as the pressures required for tidal breathing grow greater or the maximal inspiratory pressure decreases (e.g., respiratory muscle paresis or fatigue). Taken together, these data suggest dyspnea may manifest as a sense of air hunger (breath holding) and/or as a sense of excessive effort (breathing against a resistance); and it has been proposed that the two types of dyspnea are produced by different mechanisms with different anatomical pathways. In addition, cognitive and affective factors which determine the relative pleasantness and intensity of sensations may affect the level of dyspnea. A corollary discharge hypothesis has emerged whereby dyspnea is related to a mismatch between the central respiratory output and the actual achieved ventilation. During exercise, dyspnea is not profound since elevations in respiratory drive are associated with increases in the achieved minute ventilation. However, in situations where respiratory mechanics are impaired, for example, airway obstruction, dyspnea can be profound since high drive does not translate into high minute ventilation.

SUMMARY

Considerable progress has occurred in the area of control of breathing both in terms of the basic underlying mechanisms as well as the clinical implications of the applied physiology. Given the ubiquitous nature of the associated diseases and conditions, further efforts into the basic and clinical aspects of this field will likely allow new therapeutic strategies to emerge.

REFERENCES

1. Von Euler C. Brain stem mechanisms for generation and control of breathing pattern. In: Cherniack NS, Widdicombe JG, eds. *Handbook of Physiology; Control of Breathing*. Vol 2. Bethesda, MD: American Physiological Society; 1986:1–67.
2. Lindsey BG, Rybak IA, Smith JC. Computational models and emergent properties of respiratory neural networks. *Compr Physiol.* 2012;2(3):1619–1670.
3. Molkov YI, Bacak BJ, Dick TE, Rybak IA. Control of breathing by interacting pontine and pulmonary feedback loops. *Front Neural Circuits.* 2013;7:16.
4. Feldman JL, Del Negro CA, Gray PA. Understanding the rhythm of breathing: so near, yet so far. *Annu Rev Physiol.* 2013;75:423–452.

5. Richter DW. Generation and maintenance of the respiratory rhythm. *J Exp Biol.* 1982;100:93–107.
6. Comroe JH Jr, Mortimer L. The respiratory and cardiovascular responses of temporally separated aortic and carotid bodies to cyanide, nicotine, phenyldiguanide and serotonin. *J Pharmacol Exp Ther.* 1964;146:33–41.
7. Gonzalez C, Almaraz L, Obeso A, Rigual R. Carotid body chemoreceptors: from natural stimuli to sensory discharges. *Physiol Rev.* 1994;74(4):829–898.
8. Nurse CA, Piskuric NA. Signal processing at mammalian carotid body chemoreceptors. *Semin Cell Dev Biol.* 2013;24(1):22–30.
9. Peers C, Wyatt CN, Evans AM. Mechanisms for acute oxygen sensing in the carotid body. *Respir Physiol Neurobiol.* 2010;174(3):292–298.
10. Prabhakar NR. O2 sensing at the mammalian carotid body: why multiple O2 sensors and multiple transmitters? *Exp Physiol.* 2006;91(1):17–23.
11. López-Barneo J, del Toro R, Levitsky KL, Chiara MD, Ortega-Sáenz P. Regulation of oxygen sensing by ion channels. *J Appl Physiol.* 2004;96(3):1187–1195.
12. Blain GM, Smith CA, Henderson KS, Dempsey JA. Peripheral chemoreceptors determine the respiratory sensitivity of central chemoreceptors to CO(2). *J Physiol.* 2010;588(Pt 13):2455–2471.
13. Trinder J, Woods M, Nicholas CL, Chan JK, Jordan AS, Semmler JG. Motor unit activity in upper airway muscles genioglossus and tensor palatini. *Respir Physiol Neurobiol.* 2013;188(3):362–369.
14. Saboisky JP, Stashuk DW, Hamilton-Wright A, et al. Neurogenic changes in the upper airway of patients with obstructive sleep apnea. *Am J Respir Crit Care Med.* 2012;185(3):322–329.
15. Strollo PJ, Soose RJ, Maurer JT, et al. Upper-airway stimulation for obstructive sleep apnea. *N Engl J Med.* 2014;370(2):139–149.
16. Stanchina ML, Ellison K, Malhotra A, et al. The impact of cardiac resynchronization therapy on obstructive sleep apnea in heart failure patients: a pilot study. *Chest.* 2007;132(2):433–439.
17. Nemati S, Edwards BA, Sands SA, et al. Model-based characterization of ventilatory stability using spontaneous breathing. *J Appl Physiol.* 2011;111(1):55–67.
18. Younes M, Ostrowski M, Thompson W, Leslie C, Shewchuk W. Chemical control stability in patients with obstructive sleep apnea. *Am J Respir Crit Care Med.* 2001;163(5):1181–1190.
19. Eckert DJ, Jordan AS, Merchia P, Malhotra A. Central sleep apnea: pathophysiology and treatment. *Chest.* 2007;131(2):595–607.
20. Edwards BA, Sands SA, Eckert DJ, et al. Acetazolamide improves loop gain but not the other physiological traits causing obstructive sleep apnoea. *J Physiol.* 2012;590(Pt 5):1199–1211.
21. Latshang TD, Nussbaumer-Ochsner Y, Henn RM, et al. Effect of acetazolamide and autoCPAP therapy on breathing disturbances among patients with obstructive sleep apnea syndrome who travel to altitude: a randomized controlled trial. *JAMA.* 2012;308(22):2390–2398.
22. Neubauer JA, Sunderram J. Oxygen-sensing neurons in the central nervous system. *J Appl Physiol.* 2004;96(1):367–374.
23. Heymans C, Delaunois AL, Martini L, Janssen P. The effect of certain autonomic drugs on the chemoreceptors of the carotid body and the baroreceptors of the carotid sinus. *Arch Int Pharmacodyn Ther.* 1953;96(2):209–219.
24. Wang SC, Mazzella H, Heymans C. Hemodynamic studies on the carotid sinus pressoreceptive reflex: effects of occluding efferent branches of carotid bifurcation upon the sinus pressor responses. *Arch Int Pharmacodyn Ther.* 1952;90(1):1–17.
25. Powell FL, Kim BC, Johnson SR, Fu Z. Oxygen sensing in the brain–invited article. *Adv Exp Med Biol.* 2009;648:369–376.
26. Dempsey JA, Forster HV. Mediation of ventilatory adaptations. *Physiol Rev.* 1982;62(1):262–346.
27. Sun MK, Jeske IT, Reis DJ. Cyanide excites medullary sympathoexcitatory neurons in rats. *Am J Physiol.* 1992;262(2 Pt 2):R182–R189.
28. Powell FL, Milsom WK, Mitchell GS. Time domains of the hypoxic ventilatory response. *Respir Physiol.* 1998;112(2):123–134.
29. Mitchell GS, Johnson SM. Neuroplasticity in respiratory motor control. *J Appl Physiol.* 2003;94(1):358–374.
30. Hupperets MD, Hopkins SR, Pronk MG, et al. Increased hypoxic ventilatory response during 8 weeks at 3800 m altitude. *Respir Physiol Neurobiol.* 2004;142(2–3):145–152.
31. Powell FL, Huey KA, Dwinell MR. Central nervous system mechanisms of ventilatory acclimatization to hypoxia. *Respir Physiol.* 2000;121(2–3):223–236.
32. Powell FL. The influence of chronic hypoxia upon chemoreception. *Respir Physiol Neurobiol.* 2007;157(1):154–161.
33. Powell FL, Fu Z. HIF-1 and ventilatory acclimatization to chronic hypoxia. *Respir Physiol Neurobiol.* 2008;164(1–2):282–287.
34. Aubier M, Murciano D, Fournier M, Milic-Emili J, Pariente R, Derenne JP. Central respiratory drive in acute respiratory failure of patients with chronic obstructive pulmonary disease. *Am Rev Respir Dis.* 1980;122(2):191–199.
35. Aubier M, Murciano D, Milic-Emili J, et al. Effects of the administration of O_2 on ventilation and blood gases in patients with chronic obstructive pulmonary disease during acute respiratory failure. *Am Rev Respir Dis.* 1980;122(5):747–754.
36. Calverley PM. Oxygen-induced hypercapnia revisited. *Lancet.* 2000;356(9241):1538–1539.
37. Donald K, Simpson T, McMichael J, Lennox B. Neurological effects of oxygen. *The Lancet.* 1949;254(6588):1056–1057.
38. Malhotra A, Schwartz DR, Ayas N, Stanchina M, White DP. Treatment of oxygen-induced hypercapnia. *Lancet.* 2001; 357(9259):884–885.
39. Cherniack NS. Control of ventilation. In: Fishman AP, ed. *Pulmonary Diseases and Disorders.* 4th ed. Vol 1. New York, NY: McGraw-Hill Companies Inc; 2008:161–172.
40. Wasserman K, Hansen JE, Sue DY, Striger WW, Whipp BJ. *Principles of Exercise Testing and Interpretation.* 4th ed. Philadelphia, PA: Lippincott Williams & Wilkins; 2005.
41. Dempsey JA. New perspectives concerning feedback influences on cardiorespiratory control during rhythmic exercise and on exercise performance. *J Physiol.* 2012;590(Pt 17):4129–4144.
42. Forster HV, Haouzi P, Dempsey JA. Control of breathing during exercise. *Compr Physiol.* 2012;2(1):743–777.
43. Mitchell GS, Babb TG. Layers of exercise hyperpnea: modulation and plasticity. *Respir Physiol Neurobiol.* 2006;151(2–3):251–266.
44. Weese-Mayer DE, Berry-Kravis EM, Ceccherini I, et al. An official ATS clinical policy statement: congenital central hypoventilation syndrome: Genetic basis, diagnosis, and management. *Am J Respir Crit Care Med.* 2010;181(6):626–644.
45. Dempsey JA, Smith CA, Przybylowski T, et al. The ventilatory responsiveness to CO(2) below eupnoea as a determinant of ventilatory stability in sleep. *J Physiol.* 2004;560(Pt 1):1–11.
46. Dempsey JA, Smith CA, Blain GM, Xie A, Gong Y, Teodorescu M. Role of central/peripheral chemoreceptors and their interdependence in the pathophysiology of sleep apnea. *Adv Exp Med Biol.* 2012;758:343–349.
47. Mahamed S, Mitchell GS. Is there a link between intermittent hypoxia-induced respiratory plasticity and obstructive sleep apnoea? *Exp Physiol.* 2007;92(1):27–37.

48. Mateika JH, Sandhu KS. Experimental protocols and preparations to study respiratory long term facilitation. *Respir Physiol Neurobiol.* 2011;176(1–2):1–11.
49. Mahamed S, Mitchell GS. Respiratory long-term facilitation: too much or too little of a good thing? *Adv Exp Med Biol.* 2008; 605:224–227.
50. Owens R, Wellman A, Malhotra A. The chicken-or-egg debate in OSA pathogenesis. *Sleep.* 2009;32(10):1255–1256.
51. Malhotra A, Bertisch S, Wellman A. Complex sleep apnea: it isn't really a disease. *J Clin Sleep Med.* 2008;4(5):406–408.
52. Aurora RN, Chowdhuri S, Ramar K, et al. The treatment of central sleep apnea syndromes in adults: practice parameters with an evidence-based literature review and meta-analyses. *Sleep.* 2012;35(1):17–40.
53. Rice AJ, Nakayama HC, Haverkamp HC, Pegelow DF, Skatrud JB, Dempsey JA. Controlled versus assisted mechanical ventilation effects on respiratory motor output in sleeping humans. *Am J Respir Crit Care Med.* 2003;168(1):92–101.
54. Leevers AM, Simon PM, Dempsey JA. Apnea after normocapnic mechanical ventilation during NREM sleep. *J Appl Physiol.* 1994;77(5):2079–2085.
55. Parshall MB, Schwartzstein RM, Adams L, et al. An official American thoracic society statement: update on the mechanisms, assessment, and management of dyspnea. *Am J Respir Crit Care Med.* 2012;185(4):435–452.
56. Meek PM, Banzett R, Parshall MB, Gracely RH, Schwartzstein RM, Lansing R. Reliability and validity of the multidimensional dyspnea profile. *Chest.* 2012;141(6):1546–1553.
57. Manning HL, Schwartzstein RM. Pathophysiology of dyspnea. *N Engl J Med.* 1995;333(23):1547–1553.
58. O'Donnell DE, Banzett RB, Carrieri-Kohlman V, et al. Pathophysiology of dyspnea in chronic obstructive pulmonary disease: a roundtable. *Proc Am Thorac Soc.* 2007;4(2): 145–168.
59. Wadell K, Webb KA, Preston ME, et al. Impact of pulmonary rehabilitation on the major dimensions of dyspnea in COPD. *COPD.* 2013;10(4):425–435.
60. Laveneziana P, Guenette JA, Webb KA, O'Donnell DE. New physiological insights into dyspnea and exercise intolerance in chronic obstructive pulmonary disease patients. *Expert Rev Respir Med.* 2012;6(6):651–662.

CHAPTER 12

Circadian Rhythms and Sleep Biology

Allan I. Pack

Sleep and circadian rhythm are highly coupled processes. In the original formulation they were considered independent but interacting. Borbely et al.[1–4] posited that the circadian process (Process C) had a 24-hour rhythm that interacted with the sleep drive system (Process S) (Fig. 12-1). Process S is envisaged to be like an old-fashioned egg timer. The drive for sleep is at a very low level following the major sleep bout and increases progressively as wakefulness proceeds, that is, the drive to sleep is related to the duration of prior wakefulness.

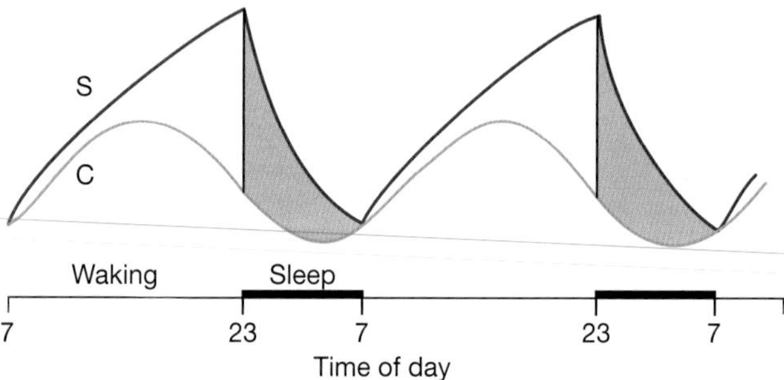

Figure 12-1 Two process model of sleep/wake control. Behavioral state is controlled by the interaction between two processes: (a) Process C, the biological clock and (b) process S, the sleep homeostatic drive. The dark bar below from 23:00 to 07:00 hours is the lights-off period. For further details, see text. *(Reproduced with permission from Kryger MH, Roth T, Dement WC, eds. Principles and Practice of Sleep Medicine, 5th ed. Philadelphia, PA: Elsevier; 2011.)*

Humans are programmed to sustain wakefulness for 16 hours but beyond this develop progressive performance impairments. During the day the drive to sleep is counteracted by an alertness signal from the clock. When this alertness signal declines later in the evening, the sleep drive is unopposed and sleep ensues. During sleep the drive to sleep progressively declines, that is, the egg timer is flipped and the sands recover (Fig. 12-1). The situation is actually more complex than this since sleepiness occurs twice a day, that is, siesta time in early afternoon and late in the evening. While these processes were initially considered independent, they are not at a molecular level.[5,6] Core clock molecules increase their expression in brain when sleep is deprived.[7] Moreover, mutations of a clock-associated gene – DEC2, now called BHLEH41 – result in short sleep in humans (<6 hours) without evidence of daytime performance impairment.[8,9]

In this chapter we describe the basis of the clock and make the point that the lung itself has a clock. We then describe sleep and review recent evidence that sleep alters gene transcription in the lung. The reader will get a background in sleep that will facilitate understanding the cardiopulmonary changes during sleep (see Chapter 101) and sleep-disordered breathing (see Chapter 99).

MOLECULAR MECHANISMS OF THE CLOCK

The fundamental principles of how the clock ticks are conserved across species, although the specific details, that is, genes involved, vary between species (for reviews, see[10,11]).

The original concept that the clock involves a distinct molecular mechanism came from identification of mutant fruit flies (Drosophila) with long circadian periods, short circadian periods, and flies with no circadian rhythm.[12] Subsequently it was determined that these different flies all had different mutations in the same gene which was given the name period (PER), that is, the first clock molecule identified.[13] Later forward genetic studies identified another clock molecule in Drosophila, that is, timeless.[14] The first mammalian clock gene was also identified by forward genetic studies, that is, studying mice that had received a chemical mutagen – ENU – and had an abnormal circadian period.[15] This clock molecule is Clock and is a transcription factor.

In both Drosophila and rodents the major mechanism of oscillation is a negative feedback loop (for mammalian model, Fig. 12-2). There

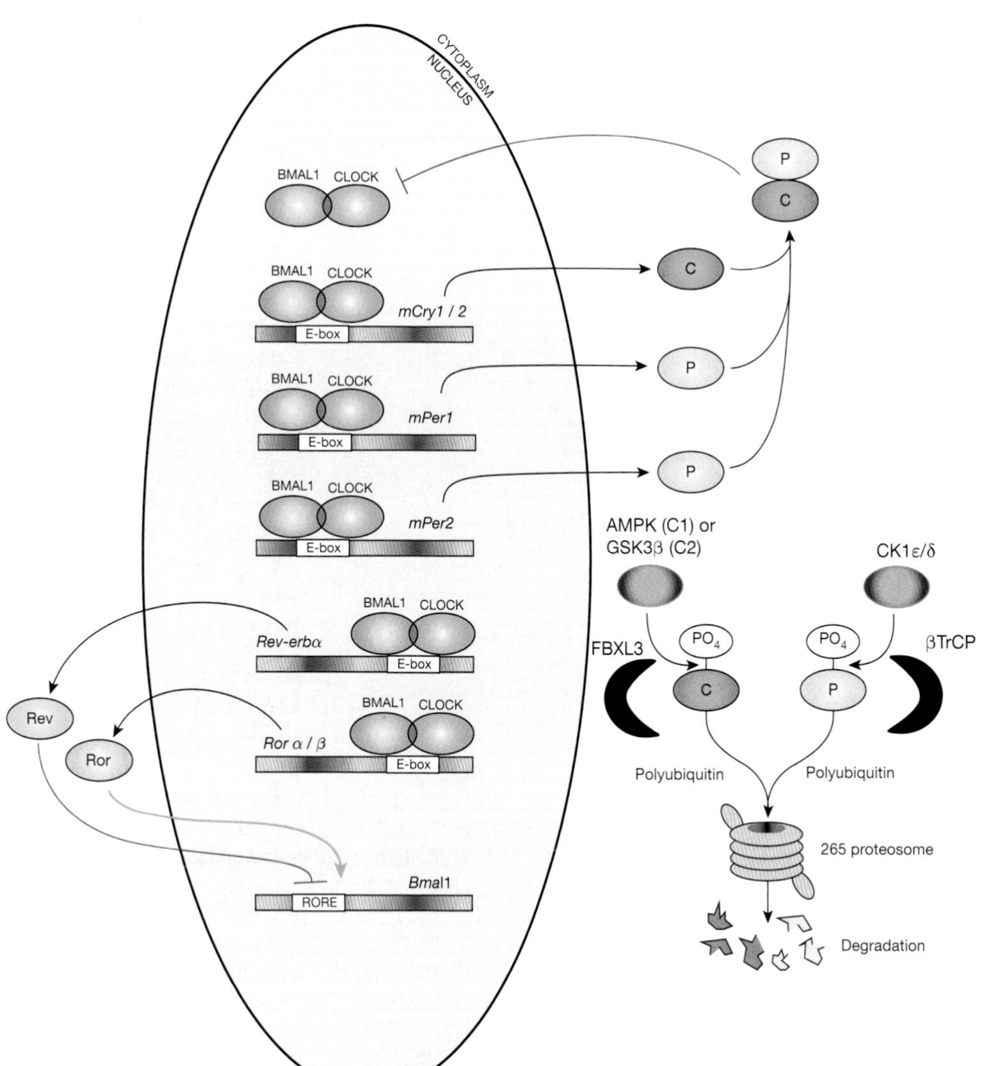

Figure 12-2 The major mechanisms that result in diurnal oscillation of clock genes. For further details, see text. *(Reproduced with permission from Buhr ED, Takahashi JS. Molecular components of the mammalian circadian clock. Handb Exp Pharmacol. 2013;(217):3–27.)*

are also positive feedback loops. In mammals the main clock proteins are the three-period proteins (PER1, PER2, and PER3) and the two cytochrome proteins (CRY1 and CRY2). These proteins form a complex in the cytoplasm that enters the nucleus where they inhibit their own transcription that is controlled by the CLOCK/BMAL1 complex (Fig. 12-2). The degradation of the PER and CRY proteins is important in setting the period of the clock. The PER proteins are phosphorylated by enzymes such as casein kinase 1e and CKII. Once phosphorylated, the PER proteins are targeted for ubiquitination and degradation. In humans mutations in PER2, in the site in which it is phosphorylated[16] and also in CK1 delta,[17] lead to familial phase advance syndrome (for reviews, see[18]). Individuals with this have marked phase advance going to sleep at 7:30 PM and waking up at 4:00 AM.

The other core feedback loop involves the orphan nuclear-receptor genes—REV-ERBα/β and RORα/β. RORs activate BMAL1 while REV-ERBs repress BMAL1 and CLOCK RORs and REV-ERBs are themselves targets of CLOCK-BMAL1 and are negatively regulated by the repressors CRY1 and 2 and PER, particularly PER2.

Thus, the clock is a cell autonomous process and individual cells show circadian oscillation and clock mechanisms can be studied in vitro with cells in culture.

SUPRACHIASMATIC NUCLEUS—THE MASTER CLOCK

The master clock is in the suprachiasmatic nucleus (SCN) of the hypothalamus (for review, see[19]). It contains ~20,000 neurons. Destruction of this nucleus by lesioning results in the animal becoming arrhythmic, that is, with no obvious circadian period.[20,21] The intrinsic period of the clock is not exactly 24 hours and the clock is entrained each day to 24 hours by environmental cues. For the SCN, the main entrainment is by light/dark signals. There is a direct track from the retina to the SCN—the retinohypothalamic tract. Moreover, there is a separate light-sensing mechanism in the eye for entrainment of the clock. This was identified in knockout mice that lacked rods and cones in the retina. While they were blind, there was normal entrainment of the circadian system to light/dark.[22,23] Subsequently, the basis of this light-sensing mechanism was identified (for reviews, see[24,25]). It is the pigment, melanopsin, that is in retinal ganglion cells scattered across the retina.[26–28] This pigment is particularly sensitive to light in the blue color range.[29] This has led to development of blue light boxes, blue light glasses, and glasses that filter out blue light to manipulate the light input to the clock. Following time zone change the output of the master clock is entrained to the new time zone by altered light/dark input. However, this reentrainment is relatively slow with the clock adjusting only about 1 h/d.

PERIPHERAL CLOCKS

Once clock molecules were identified, the surprising result was that they were expressed in all tissues (for review, see[11,30]). It is now realized that there are functioning clocks in all tissues. These peripheral clocks are synchronized with signals from the master clock in the SCN. These peripheral clocks result in rhythmic expression of genes in each tissue and of the order of 3% to 10% of all mRNAs show rhythmic expression in different issues.[31] (The precise number of

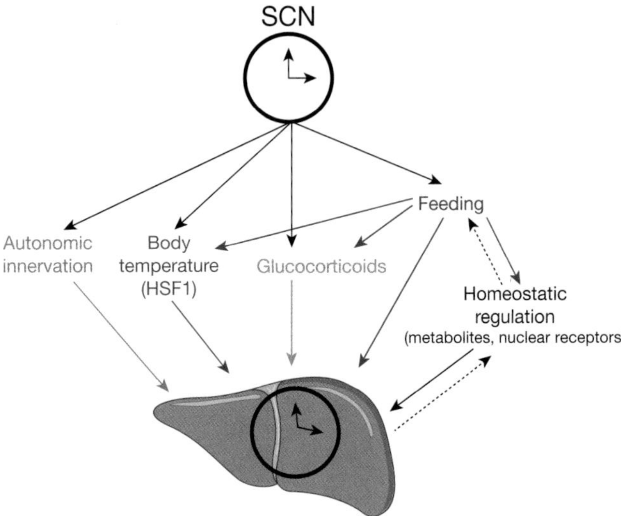

Figure 12-3 There are peripheral clocks in all organs. This diagram is for liver, but there are also clocks in the lung (see text). The "master" clock is in the suprachiasmatic nucleus (SCN) of the hypothalamus. It sends signals to peripheral clocks to synchronize them. There is also local control of clocks by metabolites, etc. *(Reproduced with permission from Mohawk JA, Green CB, Takahashi JS11. Central and peripheral circadian clocks in mammals. Annu. Rev. Neurosci. 2012;35:445–462.)*

genes oscillating depends on the mathematical definition of oscillation such that some estimates of the number of mRNAs oscillating are higher than this.) Thus, there are substantial changes in the molecular functions of different organs at different times of day. The lung is no exception in this regard (see further below).

Peripheral clocks are not only controlled by signals from the master clock but also by signals that occur locally in the particular tissue (Fig. 12-3). Important signals include changes in autonomic nerve activity, body temperature, glucocorticoids, and feeding pattern (Fig. 12-3). Phase shifting of peripheral clocks occurs much more rapidly than for the SCN. Altering the feeding pattern of mice can produce large phase shifts in liver clocks without any effect on the rhythmic expression in genes in the SCN.[32,33]

There is also a molecular clock, not surprisingly, in the lung (for review, see[34]). There is a clock in the Clara cells of the mouse bronchial epithelium.[35] As in other organs, there are a large number of genes that show diurnal changes in expression including genes involved in extracellular matrix, cell cycle, and apoptosis.[36] Genes encoding inflammatory molecules such as chemokine ligands also show diurnal oscillation.[36] The immune response, which is such a critical function of the lung, is under circadian control.[37] Circadian rhythm of other functions of the lung are known to occur, including in FEV_1.[38] Circadian variation also occurs in asthma symptoms[38] as do changes in the cellular content of bronchoalveolar lavage fluids in patients with mild asthma.[39]

Although a new area of inquiry, there are already data that pathological processes may interfere with the normal clock mechanism in the lung. In rats ventilator-induced lung injury results in reduction of REV-ERBα mRNA and protein in lung.[40] The role of REV-ERBα in clock mechanisms at the mRNA and protein level is increased in hyperoxic lung injury.[41] The role of REV-ERBα in clock mechanisms was described briefly earlier. It is likely that in the future the role of clock genes and mechanisms in pathogenesis of lung disease will be further elucidated.

CLOCK GENES AND PHARMACOLOGY

Given that a large part of the genome is regulated by clocks, it is not surprising that clock mechanisms can affect actions of drugs (for reviews, see[42,43]). The absorption of many commonly used drugs show time of day effects as does drug metabolism and drug excretion.[42,43] For example, there is a circadian variation in gene expression of several members of the cytochrome P450 system, the main system for drug oxidation, in liver.[31] Protein levels of cytochrome P450 also oscillate across the day[44] and there is a circadian rhythm of the activity of all cytochrome P450 enzymes.[45]

Thus, efficacy of specific drugs can vary with time of day. The anticoagulant effect of heparin, for example, varies with time of day.[46] When heparin is administered by constant intravenous infusion, the anticoagulant effect varies at different times of day.[46]

The concept of chronopharmacology is most developed for cancer therapy. Levels of plasma 5-fluorouracil vary across the day when the drug is delivered at the same rate.[47–49] There is a circadian variation of the pharmacokinetics of 5-fluorouracil.[50] Clinical trials show that treatment efficacy and toxicity of a chemotherapeutic regimen for metastatic colorectal cancer are enhanced using appropriate chronotherapy compared to constant infusion.[51]

Thus, time of day circadian effects need to be considered in pharmacology. It is likely that there will be a developing interest in this aspect when considering optimal drug regimens.

SLEEP AND ITS STAGES

It is now realized that sleep is universal. While definitions of sleep in mammalian species are based on the electroencephalogram, behavioral criteria[52,53] have led to identification of sleep in many species. In particular, a sleep state has now been identified in Drosophila,[54] zebra fish,[55,56] and most recently in the worm, *Caenorhabditis elegans*.[57] Thus, all model systems are available to study sleep. There are already data that molecular mechanisms regulating sleep are conserved across species.[58]

While there is a suggestion that there are different stages of sleep in Drosophila,[59] rapid eye movement (REM) sleep has only been recognized in mammals and birds. In mammals sleep is divided into two major types—nonrapid eye movement (NREM) sleep and REM sleep (for review, see[60]). REM sleep is a stage with the following: the brain is quite active with flurries of activity resulting in REMs; individuals waking from REM sleep recall their dreams; there is active paralysis of muscles apart from the diaphragm such that normal individuals do not live out their dreams. Individuals with REM behavior disorder do enact their dreams since the atonia of REM sleep is no longer in place. This is a synucleinopathy and a high percentage of individuals with REM behavior disorder go on to develop Parkinson disease (for review, see[61]). Also in REM autonomic instability with variations in heart rate and breathing pattern (for further details, see Chapter 101). NREM sleep is divided into stages based on the electroencephalogram (Fig. 12-4). Originally four stages of NREM sleep were identified but recently stage 3 and stage 4 NREM sleep have been collapsed into one stage—N3. In this stage there is synchronized oscillatory firing of cortical neurons that generate large slow waves which are detected on the electroencephalogram (Fig. 12-4). In all mammalian species there is distinct cycling of the different sleep stages, although the periods of these cycles vary between species. In humans the cycles have approximately a 90-minute duration with episodes of REM sleep occurring every 90 minutes (Fig. 12-5). In the first part of the night individuals cycle down into stage 3 sleep; slow-wave sleep occurs early in the sleep period. Episodes of REM sleep get longer and indeed more phasic, that is, more eye movements etc., as the night progresses. Thus, typically humans are waking up out of REM sleep in the morning. There are major differences in the behavior of the cardiopulmonary system in these different sleep stages. These are discussed in Chapter 101.

MECHANISMS CONTROLLING SLEEP

Sleep is a circuit property, that is, there is no evidence that single neurons sleep, although the intensity of "sleep" may vary across the

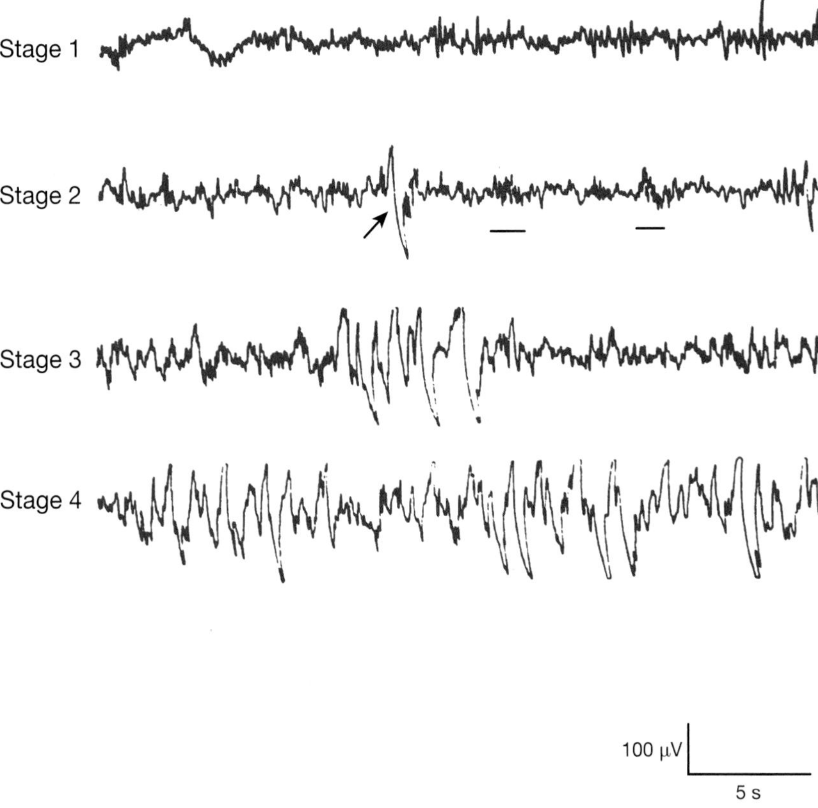

Figure 12-4 Electroencephalographic tracings recorded from a normal young adult demonstrating the four stages of NREM sleep. In the stage 2 recording, the *arrow* points to a characteristic K complex and the underlining to sleep spindles.

brain, that is, local sleep slow waves in NREM sleep are particularly marked over brain regions that have been very active during wakefulness as a result of their involvement in specific tasks.[62,63] Much work over the last two to three decades has identified the neuronal basis for sleep/wake control (for reviews, see[60,64]). Many neuronal groups have increased firing during wakefulness, reduced firing during NREM sleep, and virtually absent firing during REM sleep. These include the following: Cholinergic cells in basal forebrain; orexin (hypocretin) cells in lateral hypothalamus; histamine cells in posterior hypothalamus; dopamine cells in periaqueductal gray; noradrenaline cells in locus coeruleus; and serotonin cells in brain stem raphe nuclei. While these neurons are all more active in waking, they are likely to have different functions during wakefulness. For example, it has been shown that orexin (hypocretin) neurons respond to emotions, for example, positive emotions that result in pleasure increase the level of hypocretin.[65]

While all of these neurons show similar differences in firing between wake and sleep states, there is a different pattern for cholinergic neurons in the pedunculopontine tegmentum (PPT) and lateral–dorsal tegmentum (LDT) in the brain stem. These neurons have reduced firing in NREM sleep compared to wakefulness but higher firing in REM sleep.[60] Thus, REM sleep is thought of as a time with higher cholinergic activity.[60]

While many neurons show increased firing during wakefulness, there are very limited numbers of neurons that increase their activity during sleep. These neurons are in the ventrolateral preoptic (VLPO)[66] and medial preoptic (MPO)[67] area of the hypothalamus. The VLPO has been called the sleep switch.[66] Neurons active during sleep contain the inhibitory neurotransmitter GABA and the neuropeptide galanin.

Since control of wake, sleep and its stage is a circuit property, it has been proposed that behavioral state is controlled by a flip-flop (Fig. 12-6) (for review, see[64]). It is posited that wake-active neurons inhibit sleep-active cells during wakefulness but there are state-dependent changes such that a flip occurs and now sleep cells inhibit wake neurons during sleep. There is a secondary flip-flop that controls oscillation between NREM and REM sleep.[68]

In this proposed mechanism orexin cells play a critical role in stabilizing the flip-flop, that is, preventing too many state transitions. Orexin cells play an important role in narcolepsy. Following the description of this new neuropeptide by two groups – one of which called the neuropeptide, hypocretin[69] while the other called it orexin[70] – it was quickly recognized that it played a key role in narcolepsy. Dogs with a mendelian recessive genetic form of narcolepsy had mutations in the orexin-2 receptor that made it nonfunctional[71] while mice with orexin knockout showed key features of human narcolepsy.[72] Postmortem studies have shown that patients with narcolepsy and cataplexy have loss of orexin (hypocretin) neurons.[73] Thus, narcolepsy is likely an autoimmune disorder in which the main pathogenetic mechanism is destruction of orexin neurons.[74]

Functions of Sleep

Although much effort has been made to understand the neuronal basis of sleep, an equally if not important question is what the

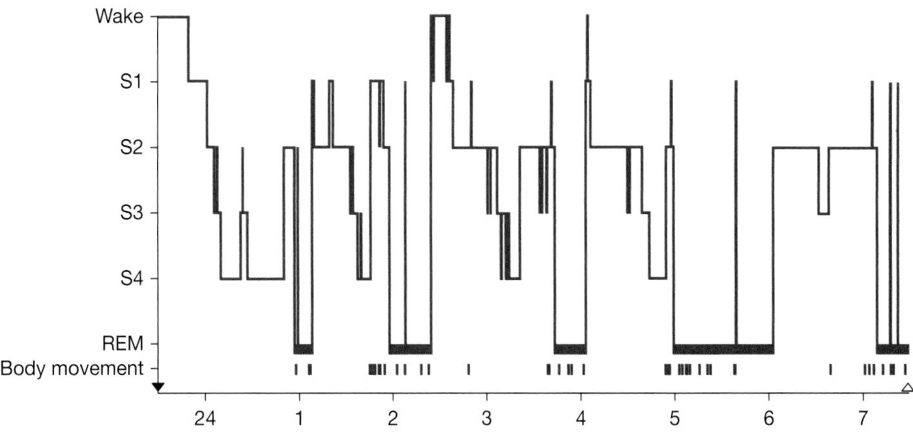

Figure 12-5 The progression of sleep stages across a single night's sleep of a normal young adult. The histogram was drawn on the basis of continuous recordings scored in 30-s epochs.

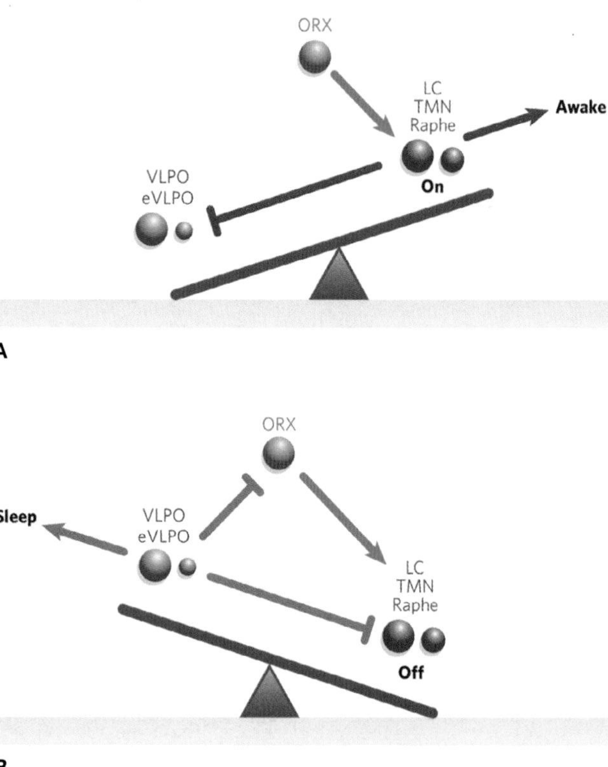

Figure 12-6 A schematic diagram of the flip-flop switch model. During wakefulness (**A**), the monoaminergic nuclei inhibit the ventrolateral preoptic nucleus (VLPO), thereby relieving the inhibition of the monoaminergic cells, and that of the orexin (ORX) neurons, and the cholinergic pedunculopontine (PPT) and laterodorsal tegmental nuclei (LDT). Because the VLPO neurons do not have orexin receptors, the orexin neurons serve primarily to reinforce the monoaminergic tone, rather than directly inhibiting the VLPO on their own. During sleep (**B**), the firing of the VLPO neurons inhibits the monoaminergic cell groups, thereby relieving their own inhibition. This also allows it to inhibit the orexin neurons, further preventing monoaminergic activation that might interrupt sleep. The direct mutual inhibition between the VLPO and the monoaminergic cell groups forms a classic flip-flop switch, which produces sharp transitions in state, but is relatively unstable. The addition of the orexin neurons stabilizes the switch. eVLPO, extended ventrolateral preoptic nucleus.

functions of sleep are. We spend about one-third of our lives sleeping. The question is what benefit do we obtain? Is benefit just for the brain or do other organs, such as the lung, also obtain benefit?

While theories as to the functions of sleep have been proposed for decades, the concepts that have been articulated recently have in large part, although not exclusively, come from microarray studies comparing gene expression between sleeping and wake animals (often enforced with sleep deprivation) sacrificed at the same time of day. The major focus, not surprisingly, has been on the functions of sleep for the brain.

The following functions of sleep for the brain have been proposed.

ENERGY RESTORATION HYPOTHESIS

One of the concepts that has been proposed is the Benington–Heller hypothesis (for review, see[75,76]). It posits that energy stores in brain – primarily glycogen in glia – are depleted during wakefulness and are restored during sleep. There are some data to support this.[77] However, the situation is more complex (for review, see[76]). There is upregulation of key components of the electron transport chain during wakefulness.[78] This is presumably to make ATP to provide increased energy utilization during wakefulness with higher neuronal firing rates.

SYNAPTIC HOMEOSTASIS THEORY

Expression of genes involved in synaptic upscaling such as BDNF and ARC are upregulated during wakefulness and downregulated during sleep.[80] This has led to the concept that there is synaptic upscaling during wakefulness and downscaling during sleep (for review, see[79]). There are data to support this hypothesis. In Drosophila there are increased amounts of synaptic proteins detected during wakefulness and less during sleep.[81]

There is, however, contradictory evidence. In developing animals there is evidence that synaptic plasticity is enhanced during sleep (not wakefulness).[82] It is conceivable, of course, that this phenomenon is specific to the developmental period. Sleep is a critical period for brain development.[83] It is also conceivable that changes in synaptic plasticity with sleep/wake are different in different brain regions (for debate on this, see[84]). Thus, much remains to be determined and it is likely that the situation is more complex than simply strengthening of synapses during wakefulness and downscaling during sleep.

MACROMOLECULAR BIOSYNTHESIS

Microarray studies also suggest that sleep is a stage of macromolecular biosynthesis (for review, see[85]). Among classes of genes whose expression is increased in cerebral cortex and hypothalamus during sleep compared to wakefulness are genes involved in macromolecular biosynthesis.[86] These gene classes are very overrepresented among genes whose expression is increased during sleep.[86] This involves pathways for multiple molecules, for example, all genes in the cholesterol synthesis pathway, six of seven genes in heme synthesis pathway, and genes involved in protein synthesis. Thus, sleep and wake may be part of a metabolic cycle (for concept, see[87]). Energy resources during wakefulness are used for neural activity, that is, ion pumps etc., but during sleep they are used for macromolecular biosynthesis. Thus, sleep is a stage where new molecules are made to restore membranes, vesicles, etc., that is, to prepare for subsequent wakefulness.

RECOVERY FROM ENDOPLASMIC RETICULUM (ER) STRESS

Another concept that arose from microarray studies is that prolonged wakefulness leads to ER stress with protein misfolding.[88,89] This was suggested by the observation that the molecular chaperone, BiP, the master regulator of the unfolded protein response (for review, see[90,91]) is upregulated in multiple brain regions in multiple species with sleep loss.[88,89] The unfolded protein response is a ubiquitous protective mechanism that is activated when ER stress occurs in the ER with misfolding of proteins.[90,91] The UPR results in helping misfolded proteins to fold properly, chaperoning those not folded out for degradation and inhibition of protein translation to reduce protein production (see[90,91]). All components of the unfolded protein response are activated in mouse cerebral cortex following 6 hours of sleep loss.[92] Inhibiting protein translation by administration of the drug salubrinal that is a modulator of the ER stress response, enhances slow-wave sleep and activates sleep promoting neurons in the MPO area.[93]

CLEARANCE OF COMPOUNDS FROM BRAIN

The brain is unique among organs in that it has no lymphatic system (see[94]). Thus, the question is how are compounds cleared from the brain? This has led to the intriguing concept of glia-lymph, that is, glial cells in brain are responsible for clearance of compounds. Recent data show that compounds are much more rapidly cleared during sleep than during wakefulness.[94] Studies with fluorescent-labeled compounds show that there is substantially more convective flux across the brain in sleeping as compared to waking animals.[94] The precise mechanism that allows this increased transport to occur during sleep is unknown, although it seems to be a result of lower levels of the neurotransmitter, noradrenaline during sleep.[94] A compound that is cleared more rapidly during sleep is beta-amyloid that

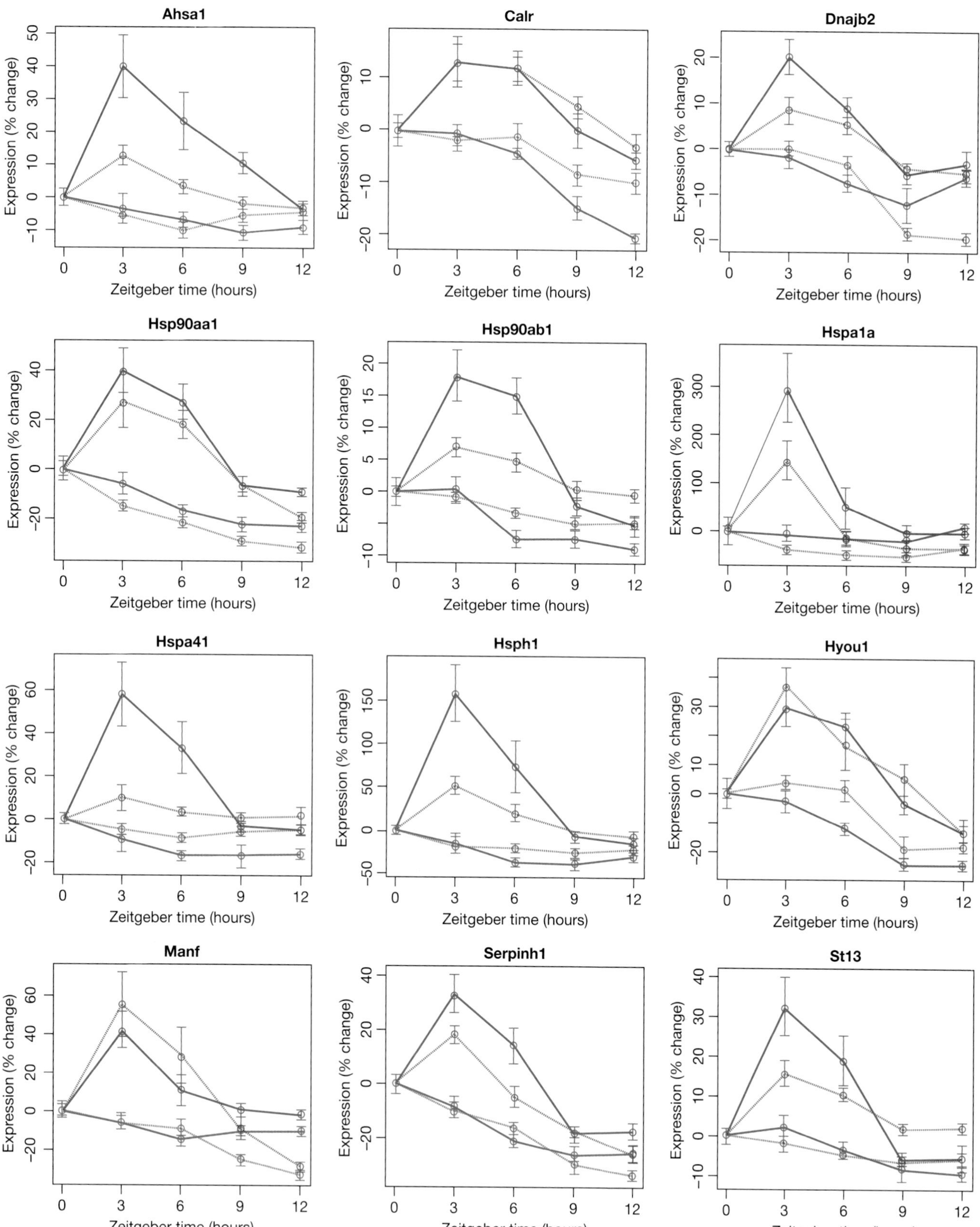

Figure 12-7 Transcript profiles of sleep-repressed genes involved in the unfolded protein response. Temporal profiles of expression for select sleep-responsive genes with annotations relating to protein processing and endoplasmic reticulum (ER) stress. Changes in gene expression from the baseline condition (lights on) are plotted as a percent of baseline expression levels. Maroon curves show data from experimentally sleep-deprived animals and blue curves show data from spontaneously sleeping animals. Data from heart tissue is connected with dashed lines. Data from lung tissue is connected by uninterrupted lines. All genes shown here met statistical criteria for sleep-specific repression in both tissues. Data shown represents mean ± standard error for eight or nine biological replicates. *(Reproduced with permission from Anafi RC, Pellegrino R, Shockley KR, Romer M, Tufik S, Pack AI102. Sleep is not just for the brain: transcriptional responses to sleep in peripheral tissues. BMC Genomics. 2013;362.)*

plays a key role in the pathogenesis of Alzheimer disease. Thus, disturbances of sleep might accelerate Alzheimer's pathology. This has been shown experimentally in mice since sleep loss over many days accelerates plaque development in a mouse model of the disease.[95] Moreover, sleep apnea is now recognized as an independent risk factor for mild cognitive impairment and dementia.[96]

MEMORY CONSOLIDATION

All of the functions described earlier indicate that at a molecular level sleep is an active state with several specific functions (for reviews, see[97,98]). It is not only an active state at a molecular level but also with respect to cognition and memory consolidation. Performance or tasks that require identification of a "hidden rule" are enhanced following sleep, that is, sleep allows the brain to continue to process information and enhances insight.[99] Memory tasks are enhanced after sleep. This is not simply a matter of time since repeating the task several hours later during wakefulness does not result in this enhancement. Enhancement of performance in some tasks is correlated with the amount of slow-wave sleep while for other tasks the correlation is with the amount of REM sleep.[97,98] It has been proposed that REM sleep enhances procedural and emotional memories, while slow-wave sleep enhances declarative memories.[98] Sleep enhancement of memory is reduced with aging.[100]

Thus, sleep seems to have many functions for brain rather than simply one. This is not surprising since it seems logical to ensure maximal benefit from "downtime." The discussion of functions of sleep largely treats sleep as a single entity. We know, however, as described above, that there are specific stages of sleep. Thus, it is conceivable that slow-wave sleep and REM sleep have different functions (see discussion above about memory consolidation). One of the challenges to elucidating function of different stages of sleep is that in mouse models REM sleep episodes are extremely short—of the order of minutes. They are so short that if REM sleep has particular functions they cannot be at the transcriptional level but are likely to be related to posttranslational modifications. It is of interest to consider what the impact of fragmented sleep such as occurs in obstructive sleep apnea (see Chapter 99) will have on the functions described. This has not, however, been studied and is an area of research need and opportunity.

Does the Lung Sleep?

One of the fundamental tenants of sleep biology is that sleep is by the brain and for the brain—a title of a provocative article in *Nature*.[101]

Again, data from microarrays challenge this tenant. Comparing gene expression between sleeping and awake animals sacrificed at the same time of day shows that there are common pathways downregulated in both lung and heart during sleep. As in brain, these pathways are those involved in ER stress, molecular chaperones, and heat shock molecules.[102] There is remarkable similarity in the changes in gene expression in both organs with sleep and sleep deprivation in key genes in these pathways (Fig. 12-7). This suggests that there must be a common signaling mechanism that leads to these dynamic changes in expression of these genes in different tissues in a coordinated way. The nature of this mechanism is unknown. While there are common gene pathways downregulated in sleep in lung and heart, upregulated pathways with sleep are different between organs. In the lung there is upregulation of certain genes for antioxidant enzymes. Thus, is sleep a time for clearing the free radicals produced in the lung during the day? There is a need for more in-depth exploration of the changes in the lung during sleep. These recent data would lead to the conclusion, however, that the lung does indeed sleep.

CONCLUSION

Sleep and circadian biology are dynamic areas of research. New concepts are emerging and some of the fundamental mechanisms are being elucidated. From the point of view of the pulmonologist, there are two major issues. First, both circadian rhythm and sleep have direct effects on molecular mechanisms in the lung. Second, disturbances of sleep like these produced by sleep-disordered breathing will have adverse consequences at a molecular level on the functions of sleep, including potentially in the lung itself.

REFERENCES

1. Borbely AA. A two process model of sleep regulation. *Hum Neurobiol.* 1982;1(3):195–204.
2. Borbely AA. The S-deficiency hypothesis of depression and the two-process model of sleep regulation. *Pharmacopsychiatry.* 1987;20(1):23–29.
3. Borbely AA, Achermann P. Sleep homeostasis and models of sleep regulation. *J Biol Rhythms.* 1999;14(6):557–568.
4. Achermann P. The two-process model of sleep regulation revisited. *Aviat Space Environ Med.* 2004;75(3 Suppl):A37–A43.
5. Franken P. A role for clock genes in sleep homeostasis. *Curr Opin Neurobiol.* 2013;23(5):864–872.
6. Franken P, Dijk DJ. Circadian clock genes and sleep homeostasis. *Eur J Neurosci.* 2009;29(9):1820–1829.
7. Wisor JP, Pasumarthi RK, Gerashchenko D, et al. Sleep deprivation effects on circadian clock gene expression in the cerebral cortex parallel electroencephalographic differences among mouse strains. *J Neurosci.* 2008;28(28):7193–7201.
8. He Y, Jones CR, Fujiki N, et al. The transcriptional repressor DEC2 regulates sleep length in mammals. *Science.* 2009;325(5942):866–870.
9. Pellegrino R, Kavakli IH, Goel N, et al. A novel BHLEH41 variant is associated with short sleep and resistance to sleep deprivation in humans. *Sleep.* 2014;37(8):1327–1336.
10. Zheng X, Sehgal A. Speed control: cogs and gears that drive the circadian clock. *Trends Neurosci.* 2012;35(9):574–585.
11. Mohawk JA, Green CB, Takahashi JS. Central and peripheral circadian clocks in mammals. *Annu Rev Neurosci.* 2012;35: 445–462.
12. Konopka RJ, Benzer S. Clock mutants of Drosophila melanogaster. *Proc Natl Acad Sci U S A.* 1971;68(9):2112–2116.
13. Hall JC, Rosbash M. Oscillating molecules and how they move circadian clocks across evolutionary boundaries. *Proc Natl Acad Sci U S A.* 1993;90(12):5382–5383.
14. Sehgal A, Price JL, Man B, Young MW. Loss of circadian behavioral rhythms and per RNA oscillations in the Drosophila mutant timeless. *Science.* 1994;263(5153):1603–1606.
15. Vitaterna MH, King DP, Chang AM, et al. Mutagenesis and mapping of a mouse gene, Clock, essential for circadian behavior. *Science.* 1994;264(5159):719–725.
16. Toh KL, Jones CR, He Y, et al. An hPer2 phosphorylation site mutation in familial advanced sleep phase syndrome. *Science.* 2001;291(5506):1040–1043.
17. Xu Y, Padiath QS, Shapiro RE, et al. Functional consequences of a CKIdelta mutation causing familial advanced sleep phase syndrome. *Nature.* 2005;434(7033):640–644.
18. Jones CR, Huang AL, Ptacek LJ, Fu YH. Genetic basis of human circadian rhythm disorders. *Exp Neurol.* 2013;243:28–33.
19. Saper CB. The central circadian timing system. *Curr Opin Neurobiol.* 2013;23(5):747–751.
20. Moore RY, Eichler VB. Loss of a circadian adrenal corticosterone rhythm following suprachiasmatic lesions in the rat. *Brain Res.* 1972;42(1):201–206.

21. Stephan FK, Zucker I. Circadian rhythms in drinking behavior and locomotor activity of rats are eliminated by hypothalamic lesions. *Proc Natl Acad Sci U S A.* 1972;69(6):1583–1586.

22. Freedman MS, Lucas RJ, Soni B, et al. Regulation of mammalian circadian behavior by non-rod, non-cone, ocular photoreceptors. *Science.* 1999;284(5413):502–504.

23. Lucas RJ, Freedman MS, Munoz M, Garcia-Fernandez JM, Foster RG. Regulation of the mammalian pineal by non-rod, non-cone, ocular photoreceptors. *Science.* 1999;284(5413):505–507.

24. Foster RG. Neurobiology: bright blue times. *Nature.* 2005; 433(7027):698–699.

25. Peirson S, Foster RG. Melanopsin: another way of signaling light. *Neuron.* 2006;49(3):331–339.

26. Hattar S, Liao HW, Takao M, Berson DM, Yau KW. Melanopsin-containing retinal ganglion cells: architecture, projections, and intrinsic photosensitivity. *Science.* 2002;295(5557):1065–1070.

27. Berson DM, Dunn FA, Takao M. Phototransduction by retinal ganglion cells that set the circadian clock. *Science.* 2002;295(5557):1070–1073.

28. Sekaran S, Foster RG, Lucas RJ, Hankins MW. Calcium imaging reveals a network of intrinsically light-sensitive inner-retinal neurons. *Curr Biol.* 2003;13(15):1290–1298.

29. Dacey DM, Liao HW, Peterson BB, et al. Melanopsin-expressing ganglion cells in primate retina signal colour and irradiance and project to the LGN. *Nature.* 2005;433(7027):749–754.

30. Green CB, Takahashi JS, Bass J. The meter of metabolism. *Cell.* 2008;134(5):728–742.

31. Panda S, Antoch MP, Miller BH, et al. Coordinated transcription of key pathways in the mouse by the circadian clock. *Cell.* 2002;109(3):307–320.

32. Damiola F, Le Minh N, Preitner N, Kornmann B, Fleury-Olela F, Schibler U. Restricted feeding uncouples circadian oscillators in peripheral tissues from the central pacemaker in the suprachiasmatic nucleus. *Genes Dev.* 2000;14(23):2950–2961.

33. Hara R, Wan K, Wakamatsu H, et al. Restricted feeding entrains liver clock without participation of the suprachiasmatic nucleus. *Genes Cells.* 2001;6(3):269–278.

34. Durrington HJ, Farrow SN, Loudon AS, Ray DW. The circadian clock and asthma. *Thorax.* 2014;69(1):90–92.

35. Gibbs JE, Beesley S, Plumb J, et al. Circadian timing in the lung; a specific role for bronchiolar epithelial cells. *Endocrinology.* 2009;150(1):268–276.

36. Sukumaran S, Jusko WJ, Dubois DC, Almon RR. Light-dark oscillations in the lung transcriptome: implications for lung homeostasis, repair, metabolism, disease, and drug action. *J Appl Physiol (1985).* 2011;110(6):1732–1747.

37. Gibbs JE, Blaikley J, Beesley S, et al. The nuclear receptor REV-ERBalpha mediates circadian regulation of innate immunity through selective regulation of inflammatory cytokines. *Proc Natl Acad Sci U S A.* 2012;109(2):582–587.

38. Litinski M, Scheer FA, Shea SA. Influence of the circadian system on disease severity. *Sleep Med Clin.* 2009;4(2): 143–163.

39. Kelly EA, Houtman JJ, Jarjour NN. Inflammatory changes associated with circadian variation in pulmonary function in subjects with mild asthma. *Clin Exp Allergy.* 2004;34(2): 227–233.

40. Li H, Wang C, Hu J, Tan J. A study on circadian rhythm disorder of rat lung tissue caused by mechanical ventilation induced lung injury. *Int Immunopharmacol.* 2014;18(2):249–254.

41. Lagishetty V, Parthasarathy PT, Phillips O, et al. Dysregulation of CLOCK gene expression in hyperoxia-induced lung injury. *Am J Physiol Cell Physiol.* 2014;306(11):C999–C1007.

42. Paschos GK, Baggs JE, Hogenesch JB, FitzGerald GA. The role of clock genes in pharmacology. *Annu Rev Pharmacol Toxicol.* 2010;50:187–214.

43. Musiek ES, Fitzgerald GA. Molecular clocks in pharmacology. *Handb Exp Pharmacol.* 2013;(217):243–260.

44. Lavery DJ, Lopez-Molina L, Margueron R, et al. Circadian expression of the steroid 15 alpha-hydroxylase (Cyp2a4) and coumarin 7-hydroxylase (Cyp2a5) genes in mouse liver is regulated by the PAR leucine zipper transcription factor DBP. *Mol Cell Biol.* 1999;19(10):6488–6499.

45. Gachon F, Olela FF, Schaad O, Descombes P, Schibler U. The circadian PAR-domain basic leucine zipper transcription factors DBP, TEF, and HLF modulate basal and inducible xenobiotic detoxification. *Cell Metab.* 2006;4(1):25–36.

46. Decousus HA, Croze M, Levi FA, et al. Circadian changes in anticoagulant effect of heparin infused at a constant rate. *Br Med J (Clin Res Ed).* 1985;290(6465):341–344.

47. Petit E, Milano G, Levi F, Thyss A, Bailleul F, Schneider M. Circadian rhythm-varying plasma concentration of 5-fluorouracil during a five-day continuous venous infusion at a constant rate in cancer patients. *Cancer Res.* 1988;48(6): 1676–1679.

48. Metzger G, Massari C, Etienne MC, et al. Spontaneous or imposed circadian changes in plasma concentrations of 5-fluorouracil coadministered with folinic acid and oxaliplatin: relationship with mucosal toxicity in patients with cancer. *Clin Pharmacol Ther.* 1994;56(2):190–201.

49. Takimoto CH, Yee LK, Venzon DJ, et al. High inter- and intrapatient variation in 5-fluorouracil plasma concentrations during a prolonged drug infusion. *Clin Cancer Res.* 1999;5(6): 1347–1352.

50. Bressolle F, Joulia JM, Pinguet F, et al. Circadian rhythm of 5-fluorouracil population pharmacokinetics in patients with metastatic colorectal cancer. *Cancer Chemother Pharmacol.* 1999;44(4):295–302.

51. Levi F, Zidani R, Misset JL. Randomised multicentre trial of chronotherapy with oxaliplatin, fluorouracil, and folinic acid in metastatic colorectal cancer. International Organization for Cancer Chronotherapy. *Lancet.* 1997;350(9079):681–686.

52. Tobler I. Effect of forced locomotion on the rest-activity cycle of the cockroach. *Behav Brain Res.* 1983;8(3):351–360.

53. Hendricks JC, Sehgal A, Pack AI. The need for a simple animal model to understand sleep. *Prog Neurobiol.* 2000;61(4): 339–351.

54. Hendricks JC, Finn SM, Panckeri KA, et al. Rest in Drosophila is a sleep-like state. *Neuron.* 2000;25(1):129–138.

55. Shaw PJ, Cirelli C, Greenspan RJ, Tononi G. Correlates of sleep and waking in Drosophila melanogaster. *Science.* 2000;287(5459):1834–1837.

56. Zhdanova IV, Wang SY, Leclair OU, Danilova NP. Melatonin promotes sleep-like state in zebrafish. *Brain Res.* 2001;903(1–2): 263–268.

57. Raizen DM, Zimmerman JE, Maycock MH, et al. Lethargus is a Caenorhabditis elegans sleep-like state. *Nature.* 2008;451(7178): 569–572.

58. Zimmerman JE, Naidoo N, Raizen DM, Pack AI. Conservation of sleep: insights from non-mammalian model systems. *Trends Neurosci.* 2008;31(7):371–376.

59. van Alphen B, Yap MH, Kirszenblat L, Kottler B, van Swinderen B. A dynamic deep sleep stage in Drosophila. *J Neurosci.* 2013;33(16):6917–6927.

60. Jones BE. Basic mechanisms of sleep-wake control. In: Kryger MH, Roth T, Dement WC, eds. *Principles and Practice of Sleep Medicine.* 4th ed. Philadelphia, PA: Elsevier Saunders; 2005:136–153.

61. Mahowald MW, Schenck CH. REM sleep behaviour disorder: a marker of synucleinopathy. *Lancet Neurol.* 2013;12(5):417–419.

62. Krueger JM, Tononi G. Local use-dependent sleep; synthesis of the new paradigm. *Curr Top Med Chem.* 2011;11(19):2490–2492.

63. Rector DM, Schei JL, Van Dongen HP, Belenky G, Krueger JM. Physiological markers of local sleep. *Eur J Neurosci.* 2009; 29(9):1771–1778.

64. Saper CB, Fuller PM, Pedersen NP, Lu J, Scammell TE. Sleep state switching. *Neuron.* 2010;68(6):1023–1042.

65. Blouin AM, Fried I, Wilson CL, et al. Human hypocretin and melanin-concentrating hormone levels are linked to emotion and social interaction. *Nat Commun.* 2013;4:1547.

66. Sherin JE, Shiromani PJ, McCarley RW, Saper CB. Activation of ventrolateral preoptic neurons during sleep. *Science.* 1996;271 (5246):216–219.

67. Alam MA, Kumar S, McGinty D, Alam MN, Szymusiak R. Neuronal activity in the preoptic hypothalamus during sleep deprivation and recovery sleep. *J Neurophysiol.* 2014;111(2):287–299.

68. Lu J, Sherman D, Devor M, Saper CB. A putative flip-flop switch for control of REM sleep. *Nature.* 2006;441(7093):589–594.

69. de Lecea L, Kilduff TS, Peyron C, et al. The hypocretins: hypothalamus-specific peptides with neuroexcitatory activity. *Proc Natl Acad Sci U S A.* 1998;95(1):322–327.

70. Sakurai T, Amemiya A, Ishii M, et al. Orexins and orexin receptors: a family of hypothalamic neuropeptides and G protein-coupled receptors that regulate feeding behavior. *Cell.* 1998;92(4):573–585.

71. Lin L, Faraco J, Li R, et al. The sleep disorder canine narcolepsy is caused by a mutation in the hypocretin (orexin) receptor 2 gene. *Cell.* 1999;98(3):365–376.

72. Chemelli RM, Willie JT, Sinton CM, et al. Narcolepsy in orexin knockout mice: molecular genetics of sleep regulation. *Cell.* 1999;98(4):437–451.

73. Thannickal TC, Moore RY, Nienhuis R, et al. Reduced number of hypocretin neurons in human narcolepsy. *Neuron.* 2000;27(3):469–474.

74. Mahlios J, De la Herran-Arita AK, Mignot E. The autoimmune basis of narcolepsy. *Curr Opin Neurobiol.* 2013;23(5):767–773.

75. Benington JH, Heller HC. Restoration of brain energy metabolism as the function of sleep. *Prog Neurobiol.* 1995;45(4):347–360.

76. Scharf MT, Naidoo N, Zimmerman JE, Pack AI. The energy hypothesis of sleep revisited. *Prog Neurobiol.* 2008;86(3):264–280.

77. Kong J, Shepel PN, Holden CP, Mackiewicz M, Pack AI, Geiger JD. Brain glycogen decreases with increased periods of wakefulness: implications for homeostatic drive to sleep. *J Neurosci.* 2002;22(13):5581–5587.

78. Nikonova EV, Naidoo N, Zhang L, et al. Changes in components of energy regulation in mouse cortex with increases in wakefulness. *Sleep.* 2010;33(7):889–900.

79. Tononi G, Cirelli C. Sleep function and synaptic homeostasis. *Sleep Med Rev.* 2006;10(1):49–62.

80. Cirelli C, Gutierrez CM, Tononi G. Extensive and divergent effects of sleep and wakefulness on brain gene expression. *Neuron.* 2004;41(1):35–43.

81. Gilestro GF, Tononi G, Cirelli C. Widespread changes in synaptic markers as a function of sleep and wakefulness in Drosophila. *Science.* 2009;324(5923):109–112.

82. Frank MG, Issa NP, Stryker MP. Sleep enhances plasticity in the developing visual cortex. *Neuron.* 2001;30(1):275–287.

83. Kayser MS, Yue Z, Sehgal A. A critical period of sleep for development of courtship circuitry and behavior in Drosophila. *Science.* 2014;344(6181):269–274.

84. Frank MG. Why I am not shy: a reply to Tononi and Cirelli. *Neural Plast.* 2013;2013:394946.

85. Mackiewicz M, Zimmerman JE, Shockley KR, Churchill GA, Pack AI. What are microarrays teaching us about sleep? *Trends Mol Med.* 2009;15(2):79–87.

86. Mackiewicz M, Shockley KR, Romer MA, et al. Macromolecule biosynthesis: a key function of sleep. *Physiol Genomics.* 2007; 31(3):441–457.

87. Tu BP, McKnight SL. The yeast metabolic cycle: insights into the life of a eukaryotic cell. *Cold Spring Harb Symp Quant Biol.* 2007;72:339–343.

88. Naidoo N. Cellular stress/the unfolded protein response: relevance to sleep and sleep disorders. *Sleep Med Rev.* 2009;13(3): 195–204.

89. Brown MK, Chan MT, Zimmerman JE, Pack AI, Jackson NE, Naidoo N. Aging induced endoplasmic reticulum stress alters sleep and sleep homeostasis. *Neurobiol Aging.* 2014;35(6): 1431–1441.

90. Zhang K, Kaufman RJ. The unfolded protein response: a stress signaling pathway critical for health and disease. *Neurology.* 2006;66(2 Suppl 1):S102–S109.

91. Schroder M, Kaufman RJ. ER stress and the unfolded protein response. *Mutat Res.* 2005;569(1–2):29–63.

92. Naidoo N, Giang W, Galante RJ, Pack AI. Sleep deprivation induces the unfolded protein response in mouse cerebral cortex. *J Neurochem.* 2005;92(5):1150–1157.

93. Methippara M, Mitrani B, Schrader FX, Szymusiak R, McGinty D. Salubrinal, an endoplasmic reticulum stress blocker, modulates sleep homeostasis and activation of sleep- and wake-regulatory neurons. *Neuroscience.* 2012;209:108–118.

94. Xie L, Kang H, Xu Q, et al. Sleep drives metabolite clearance from the adult brain. *Science.* 2013;342(6156):373–377.

95. Kang JE, Lim MM, Bateman RJ, et al. Amyloid-beta dynamics are regulated by orexin and the sleep-wake cycle. *Science.* 2009;326(5955):1005–1007.

96. Yaffe K, Laffan AM, Harrison SL, et al. Sleep-disordered breathing, hypoxia, and risk of mild cognitive impairment and dementia in older women. *JAMA.* 2011;306(6):613–619.

97. Stickgold R. Parsing the role of sleep in memory processing. *Curr Opin Neurobiol.* 2013;23(5):847–853.

98. Diekelmann S, Born J. The memory function of sleep. *Nat Rev Neurosci.* 2010;11(2):114–126.

99. Wagner U, Gais S, Haider H, Verleger R, Born J. Sleep inspires insight. *Nature.* 2004;427(6972):352–355.

100. Mander BA, Rao V, Lu B, et al. Prefrontal atrophy, disrupted NREM slow waves and impaired hippocampal-dependent memory in aging. *Nat. Neurosci.* 2013;16(3):357–364.

101. Hobson JA. Sleep is of the brain, by the brain and for the brain. *Nature.* 2005;437(7063):1254–1256.

102. Anafi RC, Pellegrino R, Shockley KR, Romer M, Tufik S, Pack AI. Sleep is not just for the brain: transcriptional responses to sleep in peripheral tissues. *BMC Genomics.* 2013;14:362.

CHAPTER 13

Pulmonary Circulation

Robert Naeije

INTRODUCTION: HISTORY AND EVOLUTION

The discovery of the pulmonary circulation was reported in the 13th century by Ibn al-Nafis (1213–1288) in the "Commentary on Anatomy in Avicenna's Canon" and, probably independently, in the 16th century by Michael Servetus (1511–1553) in the "The Restoration of Christianity."[1] However, it has only been recently realized that the pulmonary circulation as a separate high-flow low-pressure system is the end result of an evolutionary process aimed at the optimization of gas exchange of endothermic birds and mammals.[2] Evolution from ancestors of fishes to amphibians, reptiles, and finally birds and mammals has led to progressively greater oxygen consumption requiring thinner pulmonary blood–gas barrier. The alveolocapillary membrane in mammals is a vulnerable structure only 0.3 μm thick. Preservation of the integrity of this barrier has been made possible by the complete separation of the pulmonary circulation from the systemic circulation. This evolution has been accompanied by a progressive unloading and reshaping of the right ventricle (RV) as a thin-walled flow generator.

The extreme potential physiological stresses on the pulmonary circulation are exercise and hypoxia. Exercise increases oxygen uptake and carbon dioxide output up to some 20-fold above resting values, and increases cardiac output up to some sixfold. Strenuous exercise may eventually alter gas exchange because of excessive capillary filtration and stress failure, or expose the RV to excessive loading resulting in a limitation of maximum cardiac output. Hypoxia adds the burden of further increase in pulmonary vascular pressures due to hypoxic pulmonary vasoconstriction.

PULMONARY VASCULAR PRESSURES AND RESISTANCE

■ LIMITS OF NORMAL

The pulmonary circulation is characterized by an inflow pressure or pulmonary artery pressure (Ppa), an outflow pressure or left atrial pressure (Pla), and a pulmonary blood flow (Q) approximately equal to systemic cardiac output. Pulmonary vascular pressures and flows are pulsatile. However, a simple and clinically useful description of the functional state of the pulmonary circulation may be provided by a calculation of pulmonary vascular resistance (PVR) from mean values of Ppa (mPpa), Pla, and Q.

$$PVR = (mPpa - Pla)/Q$$

Measurements of pulmonary vascular pressures and cardiac output are usually performed during a catheterization of the right heart with a fluid-filled balloon-tipped thermodilution catheter (Fig. 13-1). This procedure allows for the estimation of Pla from a balloon-occluded (Ppao) or wedged (Ppw) Ppa and Q by thermodilution.

■ METHODOLOGICAL ASPECTS

The frequency response of fluid-filled catheters is considered to be sufficient for meaningful measurements of systolic and diastolic Ppa (sPpa and dPpa), and derived calculation of mPpa. However, errors may be caused by overdamping or underdamping of signals related to the insufficient or excessive flushing or excessive length of tubing systems.[3] A comparison of pulse pressure (PP, or sPpa − dPpa) measured with fluid-filled catheters compared to gold standard high fidelity micromanometer-tipped catheters in eight dogs with pulmonary hypertension induced either by ensnarement of the pulmonary arteries or injection of microbeads is illustrated in Figure 13-2.[4] Measurements of PP were highly correlated, with an analysis according to Bland and Altman[5] showing almost no bias, indicating excellent accuracy. However, the limits of agreement reached ± 8 mm Hg, which may be insufficiently precise in certain clinical circumstances.

Estimations of Pla by Ppw are generally believed to be accurate based on earlier reports of high levels of correlations.[6] This was recently revisited in a large quality-control study in almost 4000 patients with pulmonary hypertension who underwent measurements of Ppw during a right heart catheterization and Pla estimated by left ventricular (LV) end-diastolic pressure during a left heart catheterization.[7] The results showed a bias of −3 mm Hg, corresponding to an expected pressure gradient from small pulmonary veins to the left ventricle at end diastole, thus indicating excellent accuracy, but limits of agreement ranged from −15 to +9 mm Hg, indicating insufficient precision for cut off number-derived individual diagnosis.

Thermodilution Q compared to gold standard direct Fick measurements has been reported to present with little bias, ±0.1 L/min, and thus excellent accuracy, even in patients with severe pulmonary hypertension and tricuspid regurgitation (TR). The limits of agreement were ±1 L/min, which is relatively large but probably often of minor clinical relevance.[8]

Fluid-filled catheters measure vascular pressures with a zero-leveled external manometer. The best reference is the hydrostatic indifference point, at the level of the tricuspid valve, where pressure is independent of body position.[9] This is midchest or 5 cm below the Louis angle in the supine position, with midaxillary intersection at the two inferior fourths of the rib cage to consider when measurements are in the upright position. Zero leveling at the catheterization table is associated with an overestimation of Ppa and Ppw.

Measurements are generally performed at end expiration, when the lungs are at functional residual capacity (FRC). Lung volumes below or above FRC are associated with increased PVR, because of predominant increased alveolar vessel resistance at high lung volumes, and increased extra-alveolar vessel resistance at lower lung volumes.[10] Thus patients with obstructed airways as a cause of increased FRC may present with an increased PVR. Furthermore, these patients have important intrathoracic pressure swings, which are predominantly positive during expiration.[11] This is illustrated in Figure 13-3. Measurements at end expiration may then overestimate Ppa and Ppw.

Sometimes a measurement of Pla or Ppao cannot be obtained, and a *total* PVR (TPVR) is calculated as:

$$TPVR = mPpa/Q$$

Since Pla is not negligible with respect to Ppa, TPVR is larger than PVR and this difference may be flow dependent. Thus TPVR is not a correct characterization of the flow-resistive properties of the pulmonary circulation when Pla is increased. On the other hand, TPVR may be a more realistic estimate of RV afterload. The RV is exposed to Ppa and not to the difference between Ppa and Pla.

PULMONARY CAPILLARY PRESSURE

While wedged or occluded Ppa measurements (Ppw) are acceptable estimates of Pla, micropuncture studies have shown that pulmonary

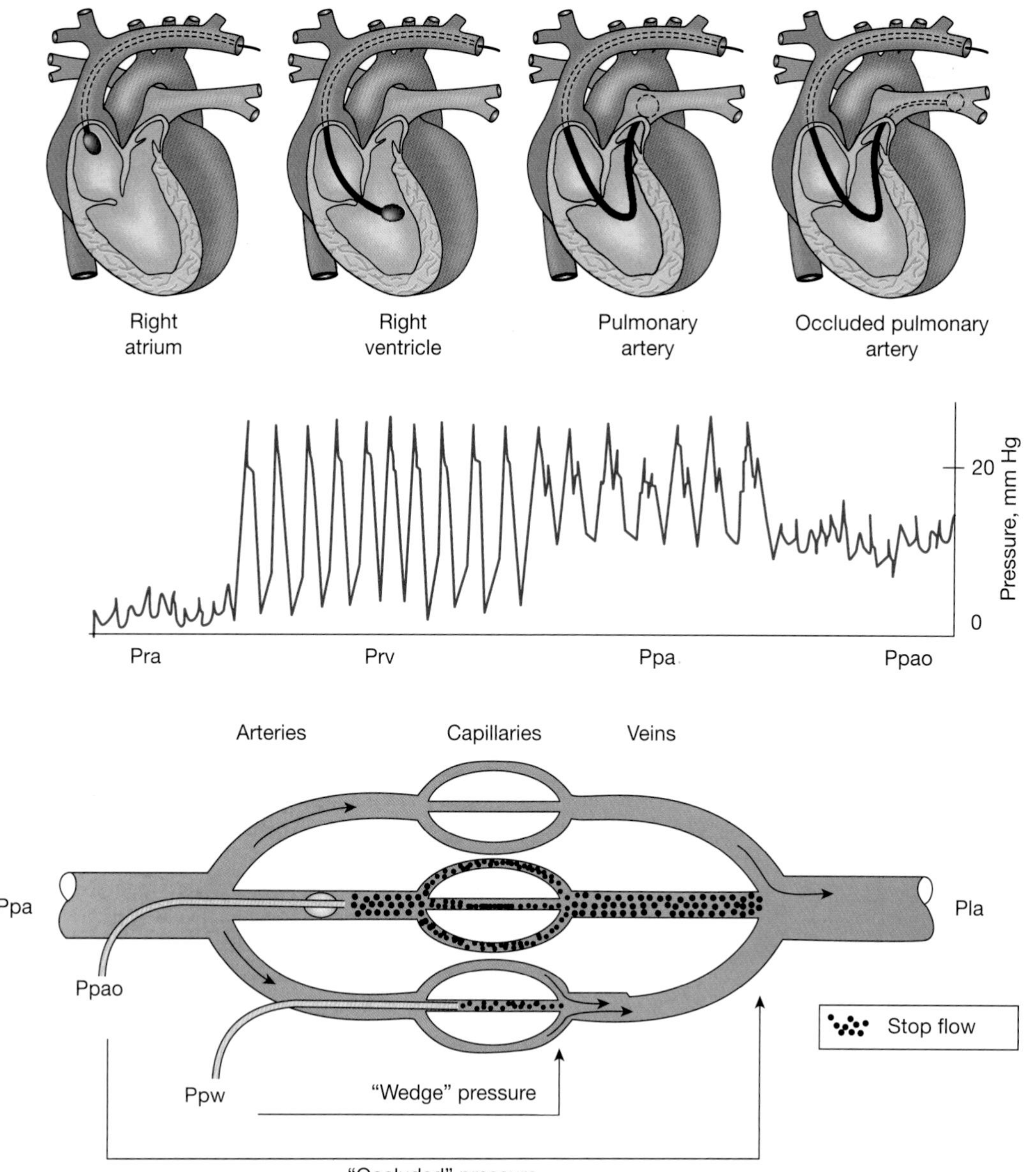

Figure 13-1 Right heart catheterization with flow-directed balloon-tipped catheter with successive measurements of right atrial pressure (Pra), right ventricular pressure (Prv), pulmonary artery pressure (Ppa), and occluded Ppa (Ppao). Because of the fractal structure of the arterial and venous branching of the pulmonary vascular tree, occluded or wedged Ppa prolongs the fluid column of the catheter until same diameter pulmonary vein, which is a satisfactory estimate of left atrial pressure or left ventricular end-diastolic pressure.

capillary pressure (Ppc) is higher than Ppw, about halfway between arterial and venous pressures.[12] Thus wedged or occluded Ppa should not be called "capillary" or "capillary-wedge" pressure. Estimates of Ppc can be obtained from the analysis of Ppa decay curves after arterial occlusion (Fig. 13-4).[13] The limits of normal of Ppc measured in healthy volunteers at rest using single arterial occlusion[14] are shown in Table 13-1. Based on measured distribution of resistances in perfused normal lungs, with 60% arterial resistance and 40% capillary plus venous resistance, Ppc can be estimated from the equation:

$$\text{Ppc} = \text{Pla} + 0.4 \times (\text{mPpa} - \text{Pla})$$ [15]

■ THE CALCULATION OF PVR

A vascular resistance calculation derives from the physical law that governs laminar flows of newtonian fluids through nondistensible, straight cylindric tubes, originally proposed by the French physician Poiseuille and later put in mathematical equation by the German physicist Hagen. Poiseuille showed experimentally that flow was inversely related to the fourth power of the internal radius, and confirmed previous demonstrations that arterial pressure remains high in arteries down to 2 mm in diameter while venous pressure is low in animals. The Hagen–Poiseuille law states that resistance R to flow of a single tube is equal to the product of the length l of the tube and viscosity η and a constant 8 divided by the product of π and the fourth power of the internal radius r. More generally R can be calculated as a pressure drop ΔP to flow Q ratio:

$$R = l\eta 8/\pi r^4 = \Delta P/Q$$

The ratio of pressure drop to flow through an entire vascular bed accounts for the resistances in series and in parallel of the individual vessels. The fact that *r* in the equation is to the fourth power explains why *R* is exquisitely sensitive to small changes in caliber of these

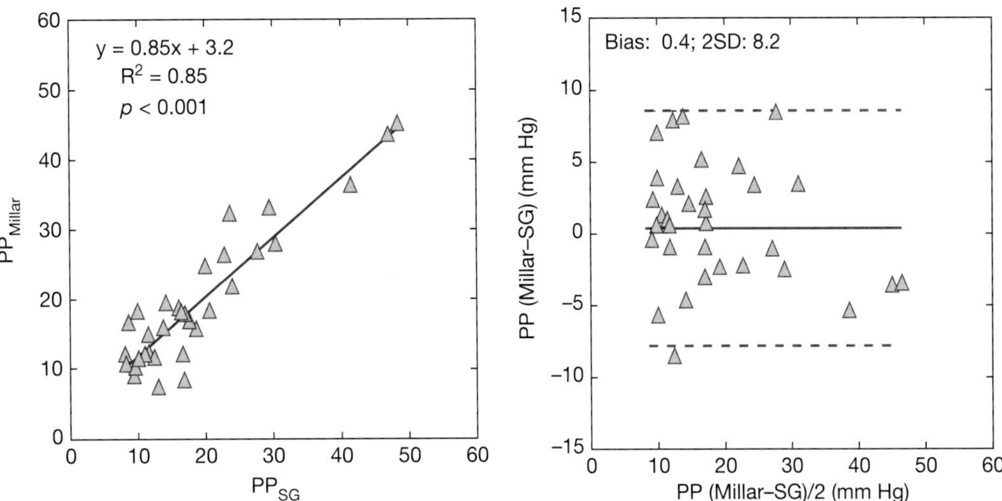

Figure 13-2 Correlation between pulmonary arterial pulse pressure (PP) measured using fluid-filled Swan–Ganz (SG) versus high-fidelity micromanometer-tipped Millar catheters and same measurements presented as Bland and Altman plots. The bias was negligible, indicating accuracy of fluid-filled catheter measurements, but the limits of agreement were of ± 8 mm Hg, indicating limited precision. *(Data from Pagnamenta A, Vanderpool R, Brimioulle S, Naeije R. Proximal pulmonary arterial obstruction decreases the time constant of the pulmonary circulation and increases right ventricular afterload. J Appl Physiol. 2013;114:1586–1592.)*

small vessels (a 10% change in radius results in almost 50% change in resistance). Accordingly, PVR is a good indicator of the state of constriction or dilatation of pulmonary-resistive vessels and is useful for detecting changes in arteriolar vessel caliber due to changes in tone and/or structure.

EFFECTS OF AGE, SEX, AND BODY POSITION

The limits of normal of resting pulmonary vascular pressures and flows as derived from invasive measurements in 60 resting supine young adult healthy volunteers[14,16–18] are shown in Table 13-1. In that study population, cardiac output was lower in women, who are smaller than men, and thus PVR in women was higher. However, there were no sex differences in pulmonary hemodynamics after correction for body dimensions. These data have been confirmed by a recent review of invasive measurements reported in 47 studies on a total of 1187 individuals, of whom 225 were identified as women and 717 as men.[19]

Aging is associated with an increase in PVR. This is due to a slight increase in mPpa and a more important decrease in cardiac output leading to a doubling of PVR over a period of five decades.[20,21]

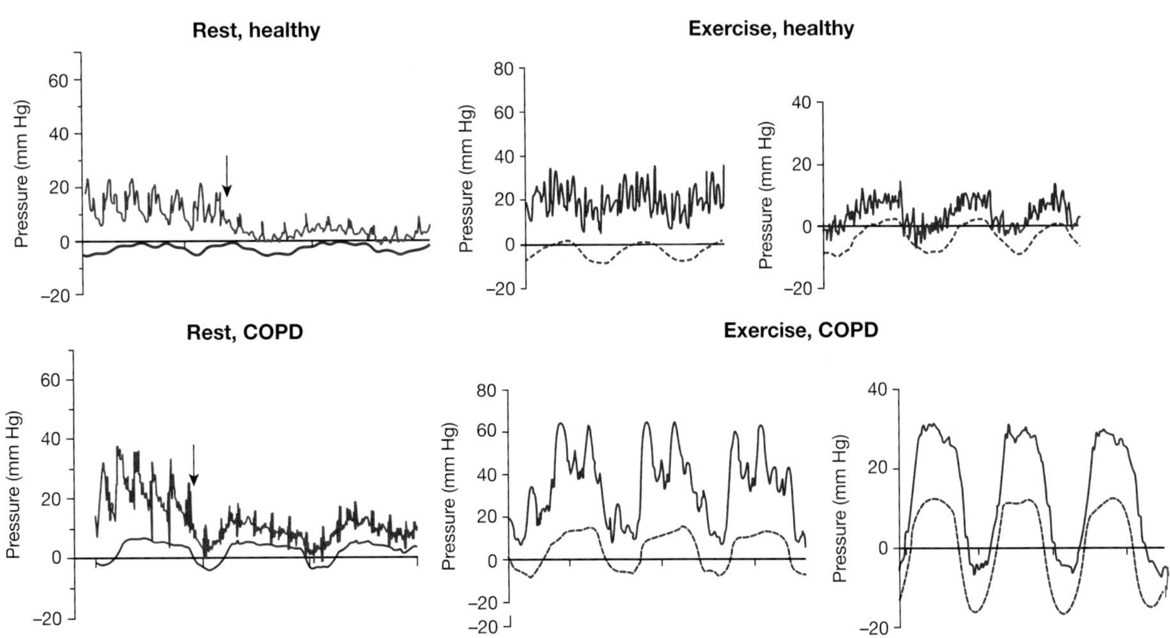

Figure 13-3 Simultaneous pressure recordings of pulmonary artery pressure (Ppa) and wedged Ppa (Ppw) with esophageal pressure (Pes) in a healthy subject and a patient with chronic obstructive pulmonary disease (COPD), at rest and at exercise. The *arrows* represent the moment of balloon inflation. Note the large influence of intrathoracic pressure on the Ppa and Ppw during exercise in COPD. *(Reproduced with permission from Robert Naeije and Bart G. Boerrigter. Pulmonary hypertension at exercise in COPD: does it matter? Eur Respir J. 2013;41:1002–1004.)*

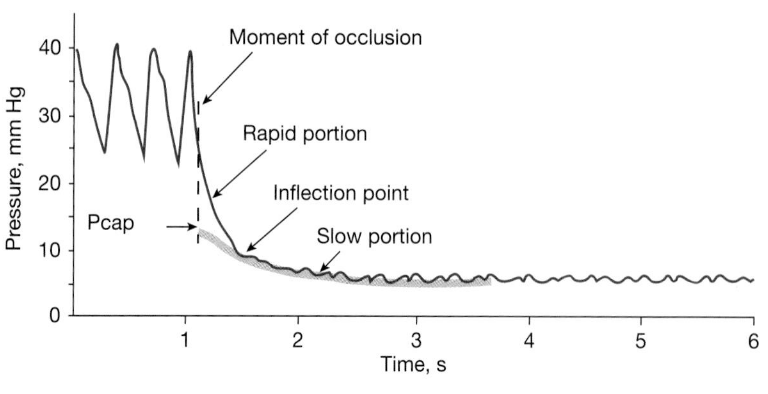

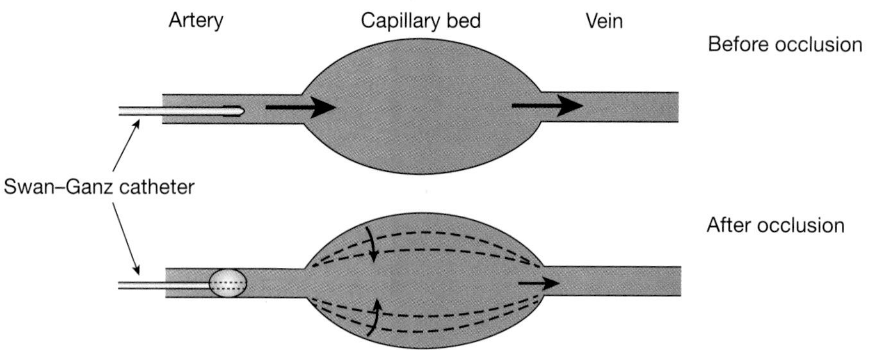

Figure 13-4 Analysis of the pressure transient after pulmonary arterial occlusion for the estimation of pulmonary capillary pressure (Pcap) either by the intersection of the fast and the slow components of the pressure decay curve, or by the extrapolation of the exponential fitting of the slow component of the pressure decay curve to the moment of occlusion.

EFFECTS OF PULMONARY BLOOD FLOW

The inherent assumption in a PVR calculation is that the mPpa–flow relationship is constant and crosses the pressure axis at a value equal to Pla (such that when flow is zero, theoretically, mPpa = Pla). Then, PVR is constant, independent of the absolute pressure or flow.

The relationship between (mPpa–Pla) and Q has been shown to be reasonably well described by a linear approximation over a limited "physiological" range of flows, with a zero extrapolated pressure intercept in well-oxygenated lungs in supine resting intact animals including man, suggesting complete recruitment and minimal distension of the normal well-oxygenated pulmonary circulation. However, hypoxia and a number of cardiac and respiratory diseases increase both the slope and the extrapolated intercepts of multipoint mPpa–Q plots.[23]

While an increase in the slope of mPpa–Q is easily understood as being caused by a decreased cross-sectional area of pulmonary-resistive vessels, the nonzero and typically positive extrapolated pressure intercept has inspired various explanatory models.

However, measurements in healthy elderly individuals are few, so that the exact limits of normal of the pulmonary circulation as a function of age are not exactly known.

Body position affects PVR through associated changes in systemic venous return. In the upright position, Pla, right atrial pressure (Pra), and cardiac output are lower in the supine position. Because of pulmonary vascular derecruitment, mPpa remains essentially the same. Accordingly, PVR is higher upright. This difference in upright versus supine PVR is important to keep in mind when examining PVR changes during exercise performed upright as compared to supine (Fig. 13-5).[22]

TABLE 13-1 Limits of Normal of Pulmonary Vascular Pressures and Pulmonary Blood Flow at Rest

Variables	Mean	Limits of Normal
Q L/min	6.4	4.5–8.5
Heart rate, bpm	67	40–100
Ppa systolic, mm Hg	19	13–26
Ppa diastolic, mm Hg	10	6–16
Ppa, mean, mm Hg	13	8–20
Ppw, mm Hg	9	5–12
Ppc, mm Hg	10	8–12
Pra, mm Hg	5	1–8
PVR, dyne·s·cm^{-5}	55	12–100

Q, pulmonary blood flow; Ppa, pulmonary artery pressure; Ppw, wedged pulmonary artery pressure; Ppc, pulmonary capillary pressure; Pra, right atrial pressure; PVR, pulmonary vascular resistance.

THE STARLING RESISTOR MODEL OF THE PULMONARY CIRCULATION

To explain the nonzero and positive pressure intercept, Permutt et al.[24] conceived a vascular "waterfall" or "Starling resistor" model made of parallel collapsible vessels with a distribution of nonzero and positive closing pressures. The waterfall analogy refers to the fact that the flow rate (Q) over a waterfall is independent of

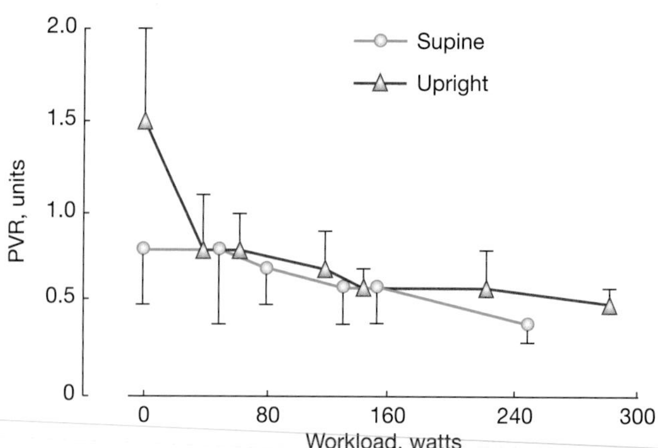

Figure 13-5 Pulmonary vascular resistance (PVR) at rest and during progressively increased workload in healthy volunteers in the upright *(triangles)* versus the supine position *(circles)*. Resting PVR was higher in the upright position. As soon as at moderate workload, upright and supine PVR converge, with mild further decline with increasing levels of exercise. Vertical bars indicate SDs. *(Data from Reeves JT, Dempsey JA and Grover RF. Pulmonary circulation during exercise. In: Pulmonary Vascular Physiology and Physiopathology. Edited by Weir EK and Reeves JT. New York: Marcel Dekker; 1989:107–133.)*

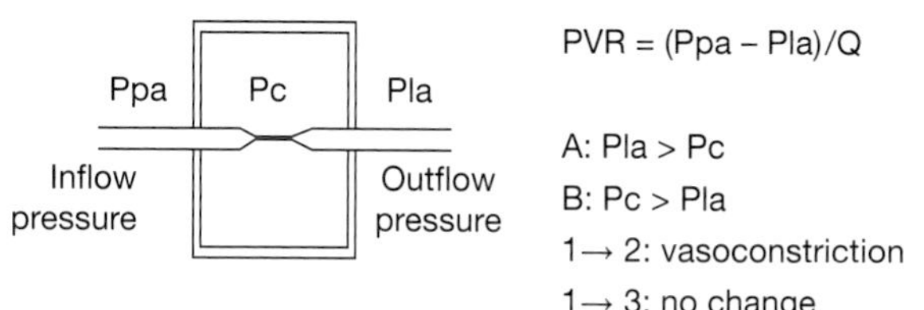

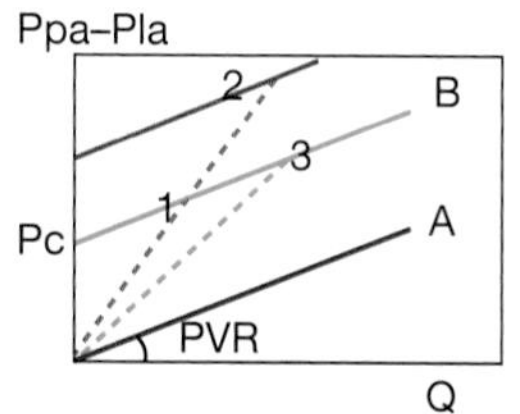

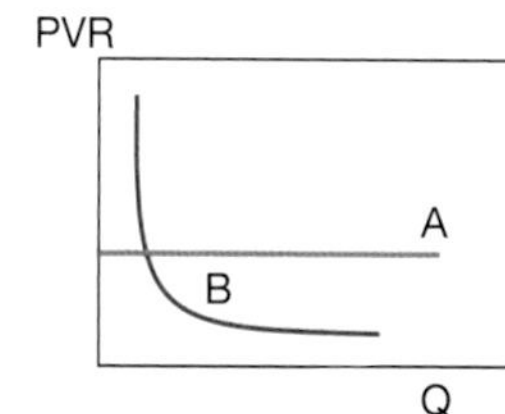

Figure 13-6 Starling resistor model to explain the concept of closing pressure within a circulatory system. Flow (Q) is determined by the gradient between an inflow pressure or mean pulmonary artery pressure (Ppa), and an outflow pressure which is either closing pressure (Pc) or left atrial pressure (Pla). When Pla > Pc, the (Ppa – Pla)/Q relationship crosses the origin (A curve) and PVR is constant. When Pc > Pla, the (Ppa – Pla)/Q relationship has a positive pressure intercept (B curve), and PVR decreases curvilinearly with increasing Q. The B curve is curvilinear a low flow representing recruitment. Also shown are possible misleading PVR calculations: PVR, the slope of (Ppa – Pla)/Q may remain unchanged in the presence of a vasoconstriction (from 1 to 2) or decrease (from 1 to 3) with no change in the functional state of the pulmonary circulation (unchanged pressure/flow line). *(Adapted with permission from Naeije R. Pulmonary vascular resistance: a meaningless variable? Intens Care Med. 2003;29:526–529.)*

its height (the pressure difference between upstream and downstream). Instead, an "external" factor (in the case of a waterfall, fluid momentum) controls the flow rate. The Starling resistor itself was actually a device: A collapsible tube inside of a closed chamber that could be pressurized, thus providing an "external" control over the flow rate through the collapsible tube. Starling used this device in the circuit of his heart–lung preparation to control blood pressure. Permutt postulated that in the pulmonary circulation, as flow decreased, arteries would be progressively derecruited, accounting for a low-flow mPpa-Q curve that is concave to the flow axis, and intercepts the pressure axis at the lowest closing pressure needed to be overcome to generate a flow. At higher flows, complete vessel recruitment and negligible distension account for a linear mPpa-Q curve with an extrapolated pressure intercept representing a weighted mean of closing pressures. In this model, the mean closing pressure is the effective outflow pressure of the pulmonary circulation. At higher flows, Pla is equal to the mean closing pressure. However, at lower flows, Pla is less than the mean closing pressure and becomes irrelevant to flow, analogous to the height of water below a waterfall (Fig. 13-6).

A characteristic typical of a vascular system made up of collapsible vessels is the functional dissociation between inflow pressures, outflow pressures, and flow rate when the closing pressure is higher than the (apparent) outflow pressure (Fig. 13-7). The functional dissociation of inflow and outflow pressures is a feature of derecruited upright upper lung zone 1 described by West et al.[25] It has been reported in pulmonary hypertension associated with acute lung injury[26,27] and in patients who have undergone a cardiac transplantation.[28]

Thu Starling resistor model of the pulmonary circulation appears adequate to explain pressure–flow relationships in derecruited lung regions in healthy states and possibly in certain pathological states associated with an increased surrounding pressure of the small pulmonary-resistive arterioles, such as in lung edema. However, the model has failed to predict correctly mPpa-Q relationships in embolic pulmonary hypertension or after changes in hematocrit.[29] Therefore distensibility models at variable hematocrit have been developed.

DISTENSIBLE MODELS OF THE PULMONARY CIRCULATION

Zhuang modeled the feline pulmonary circulation taking into account not only morphometry but also mechanics (i.e., distensibility) of the pulmonary vascular tree and rheological properties of each of its branched segments.[30] The authors predicted mPpa-Q curves with a slight curvilinearity concave to the flow axis over physiological ranges of flow that was progressively enhanced at decreasing flow. This curvilinearity was generated via arterial, capillary, and venous distensibility based on experimental data with no need to invoke a closing pressure. The distensible or compliant model of Zhuang has been shown to predict parallel shifts of Ppa-Q plots to higher pressures, induced by various interventions such as embolism, changes in lung volume, and hypoxia, and even a functional dissociation between Ppa and Pla at constant Q.[30–32] The model was effective in accurate predictions of mPpa-Q curves at various levels of angiographically determined embolic pulmonary vascular obstruction[33] (Fig. 13-8).

Linehan reasoned that previously reported compliant models were too complex, requiring a large number of parameters not identifiable from pressure and flow measurements alone.[29] Accordingly, he developed a simpler distensibility model and showed its adequacy to describe mPpa-Q relationships at variable hematocrits in

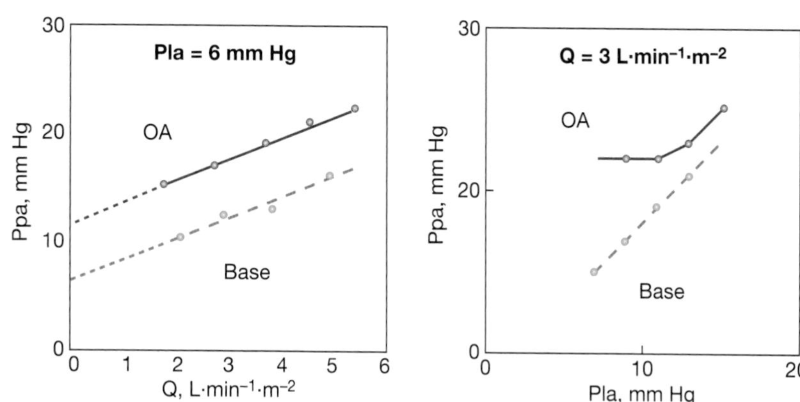

Figure 13-7 Mean pulmonary artery pressure (Ppa) as a function of cardiac output (Q) at constant left atrial pressure (Pla), *left panel*, and Ppa as a function of Pla at constant Q in an anesthetized dog before *(stippled line)* and after *(full line)* injection of oleic acid (OA) to produce an acute lung injury. Lung injury was associated with a shift of linear Ppa–Q relationship to higher pressures, with increased extrapolated pressure intercept *(small stipple line)*. Pla was transmitted to Ppa in a close to 1/1 relationship before oleic acid, but only at a pressure equal to the extrapolated pressure intercept of Ppa–Q after oleic acid, which is compatible with an increased closing pressure becoming the effective downstream pressure of the pulmonary circulation. *(Reproduced with permission from Leeman M, Lejeune P, Closset J, Vachiéry JL, Mélot C and Naeije R. Nature of pulmonary hypertension in canine oleic acid pulmonary edema. J Appl Physiol. 1990;69:293–298.)*

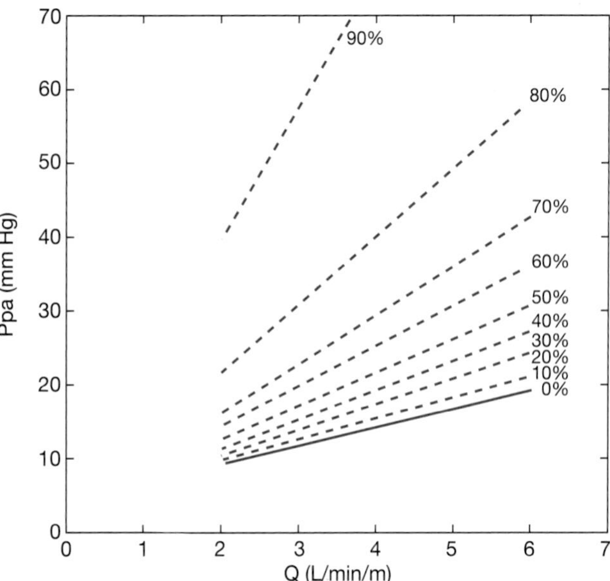

Figure 13-8 Mean pulmonary artery pressure (Ppa)–cardiac output (Q) relationships predicted by the viscoelastic model of Zhuang at increasing levels of angiographically determined embolic obstruction. An increase in mean Ppa above 25 mm Hg corresponding to the definition of pulmonary hypertension occurs after approximately 50% obstruction of the pulmonary vascular bed. A mean Ppa of 50 mm Hg as seen in severe pulmonary hypertension corresponds to 80% obstruction. These estimates are for a Q of 5 L/min, the Ppa–obstruction relationship is flow dependent. *(Data from Mélot C, Delcroix M, Lejeune P, Leeman M and Naeije R. Starling resistor versus viscoelastic models for embolic pulmonary hypertension. Am J Physiol. 1995;267 (Heart Circ Physiol 36):H817–H827.)*

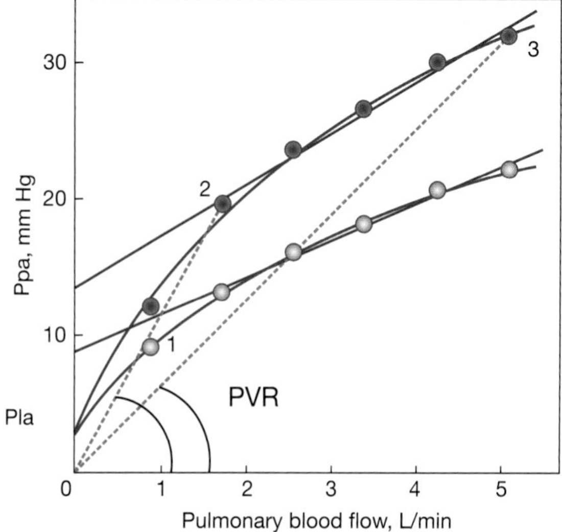

Figure 13-9 Pulmonary artery pressure (Ppa) as a function of blood flow (Q) in normoxia *(empty circles)* and in hypoxia *(full circles)*. Left atrial pressure was 6 mm Hg. Pressure–flow relationships show a slight curvilinearity. Linear adjustment of data points is a cause of positive extrapolated pressure intercepts, and misleading pulmonary vascular resistance (PVR) calculations. Hypoxia-induced increase in Ppa because of hypoxic vasoconstriction is accompanied by unchanged PVR (from 1 to 2) or decreased PVR (from 1 to 3) depending on increased flow. *(Data from Nelin LD, Krenz GS, Rickaby DA, Linehan JH and Dawson CA. A distensible vessel model applied to hypoxic pulmonary vasoconstriction in the neonatal pig. J Appl Physiol. 1992;73:987–994.)*

perfused dog lung lobes. In this model, PVR is calculated with the introduction of a pulmonary-resistive vessel distensibility factor α:

$$\text{PVR} = [(1+\alpha\text{Ppa})^5 - (1+\alpha\text{Pla})^5]/5\alpha Q$$

The distensibility factor α corresponds to the % increase in diameter D_0 per mm Hg increase in pressure:

$$D = D_0 + \alpha P$$

This model allows for prediction of mPpa at given levels of resistance Pla, Q, hematocrit, and distensibility.[34]

Multipoint mPpa-Q plots disclose a slight curvilinearity, which is explained by the natural distensibility of resistive vessels (Fig. 13-9). When generated over a limited physiological range of flows, such curves can still be described by a linear approximation. It is then possible to calculate slope for the estimation of average resistance and an extrapolated pressure intercept to suggest a closing pressure. The slope of multipoint mPpa–Q plots offers a refined definition of the resistive properties of the pulmonary circulation, superior to isolated PVR calculations.[23] Extrapolated pressure intercepts are of unclear significance and would overestimate any possible pulmonary closing pressure in proportion to increased distensibility (Fig. 13-9).

Alternatively, from a given set of values of resistance, Ppa_m, Pla, and Q and at rest and during exercise, the Linehan equation permits recalculation of the distensibility coefficient α. Reeves et al.[35] used reported pulmonary hemodynamic data obtained by right heart catheterization at rest and during exercise in healthy volunteers, and were able to recalculate a value of α equal to 2 ± 0.2%/mm Hg in normoxia. This value was remarkably identical on average to the 2%/mm Hg measured on isolated vessels from a variety of various mammalian species.[36] Reeves also showed that α tends to decrease with aging, and with chronic but not acute hypoxic exposure.[35] Similar values of α were calculated by Argiento et al.[37] from Doppler echocardiographic measurements of pulmonary vascular pressures and flows in normal volunteers. In that study, α was lower in men compared to premenopausal women and decreased with age. The same noninvasive approach revealed a decreased α with chronic hypoxic exposure.[38]

VISCOSITY

Chronic hypoxic exposure is associated with an increased expression of erythropoietin, resulting in increased red blood cell mass, hematocrit, and hemoglobin levels. The upper limits of normal of hemoglobin in healthy subjects chronically exposed to hypobaric hypoxia at high-altitude dwellers has been estimated to be at 21 g/dL in men and 19 g/dL in women.[39] In the Poiseuille-Hagen equation, resistance is directly proportional to viscosity.

The most often used reference equation describing a linear relationship between resistance and hematocrit was reported by Whittaker and Winton based on studies on hind limb vessels[40]:

$$R_0(45\%) = R_0(\text{HCT})\frac{1-\varphi^{1/3}}{0.234}$$

where R_0 is PVR at a hematocrit (HCT) of 45% and φ the measured hematocrit.

Linehan et al.[29] reported an exponential relationship to explain the effect of hematocrit on mPpa–Q relationships in isolated dog lung experiments,

$$R_0(45\%) = R_0(HCT)\frac{1}{\exp(2(\varphi - 0.45))}$$

The effect of altered hematocrit on representative mPpa-Q relationships in healthy sea level and high-altitude dwellers[38] is

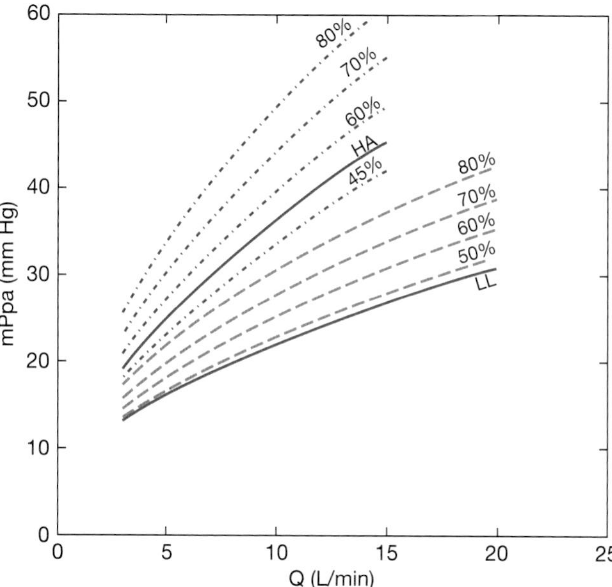

Figure 13-10 Averaged mean pulmonary artery pressure (mPpa)–flow (Q) relationships measured at high altitude in 15 high altitude dwellers (HA) and in 15 lowlander sojourners (LL), *full lines* at the hematocrit of 45% for LL and 52% for HH. The mPpa–Q curves where shifted to higher pressures due to increased hematocrits up to 80%, as modeled from measurements at increasing levels of exercise[37] adjusted with the distensible model of Linehan and associated corrections for hematocrit.[28] Increased hematocrit may be a cause of marked pulmonary hypertension at high altitudes.

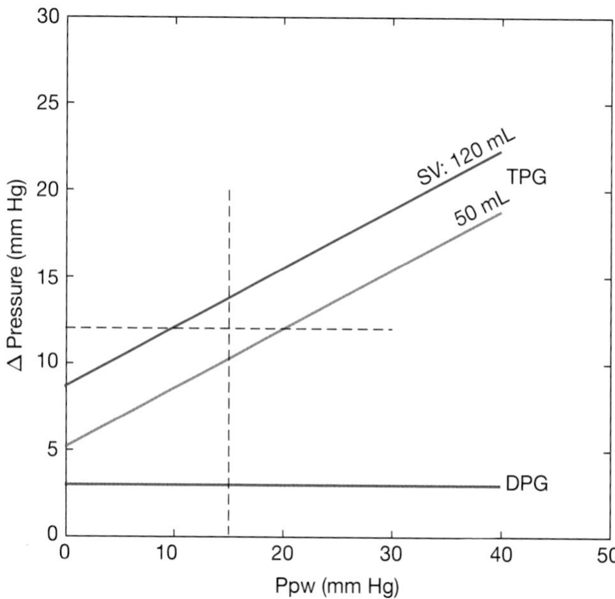

Figure 13-11 Effects of increased pulmonary artery wedge pressure (Ppw) on systolic, diastolic, and mean pulmonary artery pressures (sPpa, dPpa, mPpa) showing progressive increase of the transpulmonary pressure gradient mPpa − Ppw (TPG) with almost unchanged diastolic pressure gradient dPpa − Ppw (DPG). *(Data from Naeije R, Vachiery J, Yerly P, Vanderpool R. The transpulmonary pressure gradient for the diagnosis of pulmonary vascular disease. Eur Respir J. 2013;41:217–223.)*

shown in Figure 13-10. Hematocrit was increased from 45% to 80% in both groups. There was a proportionally more important contribution of increased hematocrit to slope of mPpa–Q in the high-altitude dwellers due to their less distensible pulmonary circulation. Thus the impact of hematocrit on mPpa is enhanced in less distensible pulmonary circulations, for example, typically in old and chronically hypoxic subjects.

LEFT ATRIAL PRESSURE AND THE TRANSPULMONARY PRESSURE GRADIENT

An increase in Pla is transmitted upstream to mPpa. The PVR equation assumes that this is in a 1/1 ratio at any given level of Q. Chronic increase in Pla may induce pulmonary vascular remodeling, and therefore lead to an "out of proportion" increase in mPpa.[41] For this reason, clinicians like to reason in terms of a transpulmonary pressure gradient (TPG) for the differential diagnosis of purely passive increase in mPpa and increased mPpa resulting from pulmonary vascular disease.[42] The TPG is equal to the difference between mPpa and Pla.

$$TPG = mPpa - Pla$$

The upper limit of normal of the TPG is usually assumed to be 12 mm Hg.[42] This corresponds to a PVR of 1.5 Wood units at a cardiac output at the upper limit of normal of 8 L/min. However, it has been recently realized that the TPG is often higher than 12 mm Hg in patients with left heart failure in whom purely passive upstream transmission could be demonstrated by observing an acute return of the TPG to <12 mm Hg after active diuresis or after a cardiac transplantation.[28] In steady-flow conditions, an increase in Pla is transmitted upstream in a less than 1:1 ratio because the pulmonary-resistive vessels are distensible.[43] In pulsatile flow conditions, an increased Pla increases pulse pressure (PP, or sPpa − dPpa) because of a decreased pulmonary arterial compliance.[44] The latter effect is largely predominant.[43] Furthermore, the TPG increases with Q because at any increase in flow mPpa increases more than Pla.[43] These problems are limited or even avoided by using the gradient between dPpa and Pla, or the diastolic pressure gradient (DPG) instead.[43] The upper limit of normal of the DPG is ~5 mm Hg. The effects of increased Ppw on the TPG versus the DPG are modeled in Figure 13-11. Assuming an unchanged dPpa as a function of Ppw, which is reasonable, it can be seen that high Ppw is associated with a passive increase in TPG to more than 12 mm Hg because of a proportionally greater increase in mPpa.[43]

GRAVITY

Pulmonary blood flow increases almost linearly from nondependent to dependent lung regions. This inequality of pulmonary perfusion is best demonstrated in an upright lung.[25] The vertical height of a lung is on average about 30 cm. The difference in pressure between the extremities of a vertical column of blood of the same size amounts to 23 mm Hg, which is large compared to the mean perfusion pressure of the pulmonary circulation. Accordingly, the physiological inequality of the distribution of perfusion of a normal lung can be explained by a gravity-dependent interplay between arterial, venous, and alveolar pressures. At the top of the lung, alveolar pressure (P_A) is higher than mPpa and pulmonary venous pressure (Ppv). In this *zone 1*, flow may be present only during systole, or not at all. Zone 1 is extended in clinical situations of low flow, such as hypovolemic shock, or increased alveolar pressure such as during ventilation with a positive end-expiratory pressure. Further down the lung there is a *zone 2* where $Ppa > P_A > Ppv$. In this zone 2, alveolar pressure is an effective closing pressure, and the driving pressure for flow is the gradient between mean mPpa and P_A. As mentioned before, such a flow condition can be likened to a waterfall since Ppv, the apparent outflow pressure, is irrelevant to

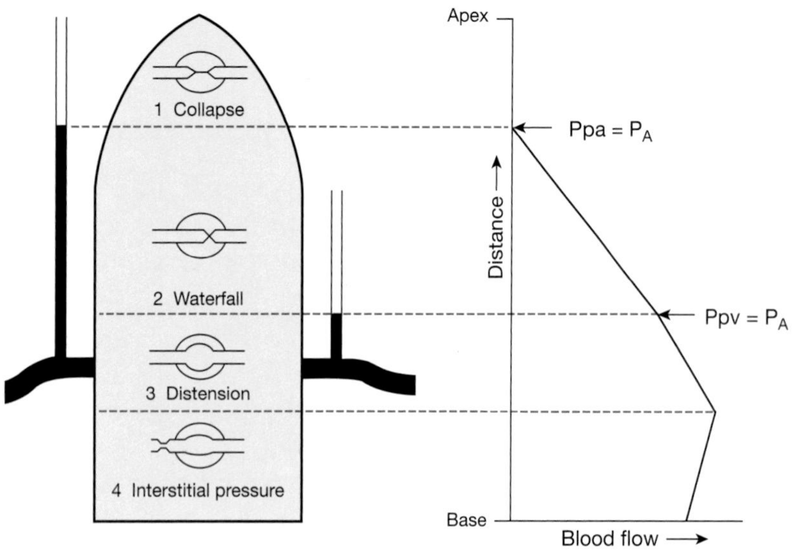

Figure 13-12 Zonal distribution of pulmonary perfusion in an upright lung as determined by the interrelationships between arterial (Part), alveolar (Palv), and venous pressures (Pv), explaining a gravity-determined progressive increase in perfusion from zones 1 and 2 to 3. There is a zone 4 of decreased perfusion at the most dependent part of the lung. *(Adapted with permission from Hughes JM, Glazier JB, Maloney JR, West JB. Effect of lung volume on the distribution of pulmonary blood flow in man. Respir Physiol. 1968;4:58–72.)*

flow as is the height of a waterfall. In *zone 3*, Ppv is higher than P_A, so that the driving pressure for flow is mPpa − Ppv. West's zones are illustrated in Figure 13-12.

At the most dependent regions of upright lung, there is an additional region where flow decreases.[45] This *zone 4* has been attributed to an increase in the resistance of extra-alveolar vessels, because this zone expands when lung volume is reduced or in the presence of lung edema. Active tone may be an additional explanation for zone 4 as it is also reduced by the administration of vasodilators.

The vertical height of lung tissue in a supine human subject is of course reduced compared to the upright position, and accordingly, the lung is then normally almost completely in zone 3. There is however a still measurable increase in flow from nondependent to dependent lung regions (Fig. 13-13).

Three-dimensional reconstructions using single photon emission computed tomography have shown that there is also a decrease in blood flow from the center of the lung to the periphery.[46] High-resolution methods and fractal modeling of the pulmonary circulation have actually led to the notion of a nongravity-dependent distribution of pulmonary blood flow.[47] Subtle differences in arterial branching ratios may indeed influence flow distribution with increased heterogeneity as the scale of the inquiry narrows.[48] However, the overwhelming evidence remains in favor of the thesis that gravity is the single most important determinant of pulmonary blood flow distribution.[48] Vascular geometry-related small unit heterogeneity of pulmonary blood flow distribution has not been shown to be relevant to gas exchange.

HYPOXIA

There is an active intrapulmonary control mechanism able to some extent to correct the passive gravity-dependent distribution of pulmonary blood flow: A decrease in P_{O_2} increases pulmonary vascular tone. Hypoxic pulmonary vasoconstriction was first demonstrated on isolated cat lungs by von Euler and Liljestrand,[49] who proposed a functional interpretation that can still be considered valid. In lung tissue, P_{O_2} is determined by a ratio between O_2 carried to the lung by alveolar ventilation (V_A) and O_2 carried away from the lung by blood flow (Q):

$$P_{O_2} = V_A/Q$$

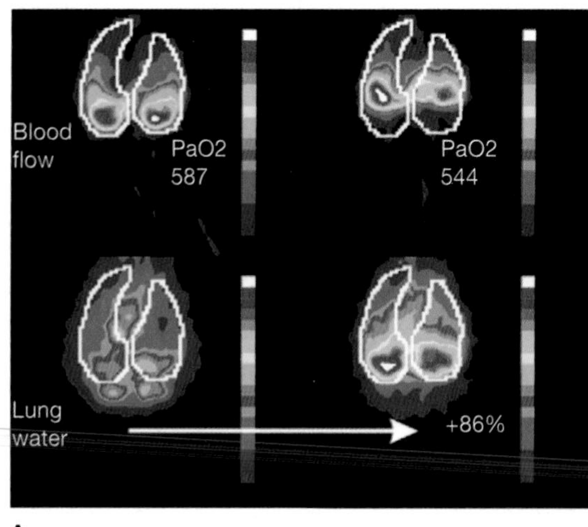

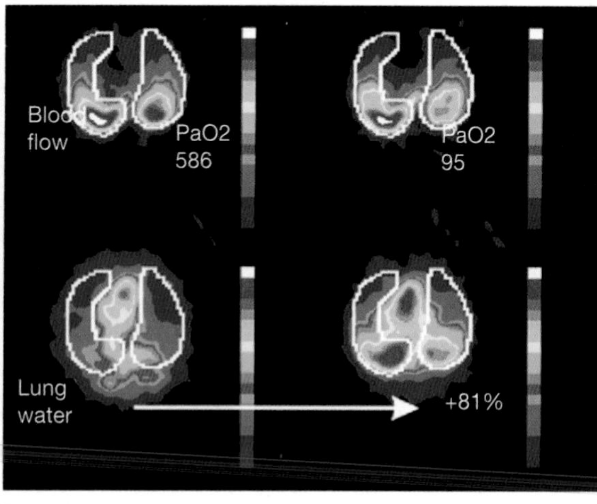

Figure 13-13 PET scan measurements of blood flow and lung water in a supine dog before and after induction of acute lung injury, with preserved hypoxic vasoconstriction (**A**) or without hypoxic vasoconstriction (**B**). In the normal lung, blood flow and water increase to the most dependent lung regions (from *blue* to *red*). Acute lung injury approximately doubles lung water, but arterial P_{O_2} (Pa_{O_2}) is preserved because of a hypoxic vasoconstriction redirecting flow to better aerated lung regions. Prevention of hypoxic vasoconstriction increases flow to the dependent edematous lung regions, and this is associated with a marked decrease in Pa_{O_2}. *(Reproduced with permission from Gust R, Kozlowski J, Stephenson AH, et al. Synergistic hemodynamic effects of low-dose endotoxin and acute lung injury. Am J Respir Crit Care Med. 1998;157(6 Pt 1):1919–1926.)*

In contrast, in systemic tissue, local P_{O_2} is accordingly determined by a ratio of O_2 carried to the tissues by blood flow (Q) and local O_2 consumption (V_{O_2})

$$P_{O_2} = Q/V_{O_2}$$

The attributes of hypoxic pulmonary vasoconstriction have been recently extensively reviewed.[50] The hypoxic pulmonary pressor response is universal in mammals and in birds, but with considerable interspecies and interindividual variability. It is intense in pig, horse, and cow, moderate in rodents and humans, and very low in dog, guinea pig, yak, and llama. Chronic hypoxia induces pulmonary hypertension, in proportion to initial vasoconstriction. Initial hypoxic vasoconstriction is a quasi-immediate response with subsequent modulation depending on the experimental model or preparation. Hypoxic vasoconstriction strengthens during the first few hours of hypoxic exposure in humans. The temporal sequence of hypoxia-induced remodeling is less well known. After 6 hours of hypoxic exposure, reoxygenation immediately decreases PVR, without however a complete return to normal.[51] The reversibility of increased PVR with reoxygenation is largely lost after 24 to 48 hours exposure to hypoxia.[14]

Hypoxic vasoconstriction is observed in lungs devoid of nervous connections, and indeed also in isolated pulmonary arterial smooth muscle cells.[50] The response is enhanced by acidosis, a decrease in mixed venous P_{O_2}, repeated hypoxic exposure (in some experimental models), perinatal hypoxia, decreased lung segment size, cyclooxygenase inhibition, nitric oxide inhibition, and certain drugs or mediators that include almitrine and low-dose serotonin. The response is inhibited by alkalosis, hypercapnia, an increase in pulmonary vascular or alveolar pressures, vasodilating prostaglandins, nitric oxide, complement activation, low-dose endotoxin, calcium channel blockers, β_2-stimulants, nitroprusside, and, paradoxically, by peripheral chemoreceptor stimulation. The hypoxic pressor response is biphasic, with a progressive increase as P_{O_2} is progressively decreased to approximately 35 to 40 mm Hg, followed by a decrease ("hypoxic vasodilatation") with more profound hypoxia.

The hypoxia-induced increase in PVR is mainly caused by a constriction of precapillary small arterioles.[50] Small pulmonary veins also constrict in response to hypoxia, but this should not normally contribute to more than 20% to 30% of the total change in PVR.[52]

While hypoxic pulmonary vasoconstriction has been shown to be an only moderately efficient feedback mechanism,[18,53] it may still produce substantial improvements in arterial oxygenation of patients with inhomogenous lungs such as in chronic obstructive pulmonary disease (hypoxemia mainly explained by low V_A/Q ratios) or in the acute respiratory distress syndrome (hypoxemia mainly explained by V_A/Q ratios equal to zero, or shunt).[54]

Topographical blood flow distribution measured by PET scan and arterial P_{O_2} can be shown to conform to the expected functional effects of hypoxic pulmonary vasoconstriction in experimental acute lung injury models, as an inhibition of the response prevents redistribution of blood flow to nondependent lung regions and markedly aggravates shunt and arterial hypoxemia.[55] This is illustrated in Figure 13-13, in an experiment which also shows the predominant effects of gravity on the distribution of pulmonary blood flow and its relevance to gas exchange.

The biochemical mechanism of hypoxic pulmonary vasoconstriction remains incompletely understood.[50] Current thought is that a decrease in P_{O_2} inhibits smooth muscle cell voltage-gated potassium channels, resulting in membrane depolarization, influx of calcium, and cell shortening. However, the nature of the low P_{O_2}-sensing mechanism remains elusive. Mitochondria and nicotinamide adenine dinucleotide phosphate oxidases are discussed as oxygen sensors. Reactive oxygen species, redox couples, and adenosine monophosphate-activated kinases are candidate mediators. The reversal of hypoxic vasoconstriction by profound hypoxia, in the range of 25 to 30 mm Hg and lower, is due to an activation of ATP-dependent potassium channels.

MAINTENANCE OF VASCULAR TONE

Normal as well as abnormal pulmonary vascular tone is modulated by a series of endothelium-derived and circulating mediators.[50] Endothelium-derived relaxing factors include nitric oxide, prostacyclin, and the endothelium-derived hyperpolarizing factor. The major endothelium-derived contracting factor is endothelin. These observations have been on the basis of efficient treatments of pulmonary arterial hypertension with prostacyclin derivatives, phosphodiesterase-5 inhibitors to enhance nitric oxide signaling, and endothelin receptor blockers.

The pulmonary circulation is richly innerved by the autonomic nervous system, which includes adrenergic, cholinergic, and nonadrenergic noncholinergic signaling systems.[56] However, the role played by the autonomic nervous system in the control of pulmonary vascular tone appears to be minor. Sympathetic innervation of the pulmonary arterial tree is predominantly proximal and plays a role in the modulation of proximal compliance.

EXERCISE

■ PULMONARY ARTERY PRESSURE

Exercise stresses the pulmonary circulation by an increase in cardiac output and in left atrial pressure.[22] In 1989, Reeves et al.[57] reviewed the published data on invasive pulmonary hemodynamic measurements during supine or upright exercise in a total of nearly 100 normal subjects. This analysis established that supine exercise is associated with a slight decrease in PVR, which is explained by pulmonary vascular distension of fully recruited lungs in West's zone 3 conditions. In the upright position, the resting PVR was found to be higher, which is explained by pulmonary vascular derecruitment caused by a lower cardiac output (via decreased venous return). A higher resting PVR accounts for the more marked and hyperbolic decrease of PVR with exercise reported in upright subjects (Fig. 13-5).

Reeves et al. were able to find measurements at rest and at least two levels of exercise in 63 subjects (including 21 women), so that they could calculate linear regressions relating mPpa to Q in each of them. On average, each liter per minute of increase in cardiac output was accompanied by 1 mm Hg increase in mPpa in young adult men and women. Advanced age (60–80 years) was found to be associated with a more than doubling of the slope of mPpa–Q relationships, to an average of 2.5 mm Hg/L/min. However, there was large interindividual variation, with standard deviations on the order of the means, which makes it difficult to estimate the limits of normal.

A more recent review of the literature of invasive pulmonary hemodynamic data in normal subjects confirmed this data.[58] Invasive measurements of PVR were found in only 13 subjects aged more than 50 years. The review otherwise confirmed an only moderate decrease in PVR with exercise, which was, however, less important or absent in older subjects; and slopes of mPAP–Q of ~1 mm Hg/L/min in subjects of less than 50 years.[58]

The pulmonary circulation during exercise has been more recently reevaluated, using Doppler echocardiography in a total of 177 healthy subjects[37,38,59,60] and a right heart catheterization in 24 other healthy volunteers.[61] In these studies at least four mPpa–Q coordinates were measured at increasing levels of workload. There was a perfect agreement between invasive and noninvasive measurements The results confirmed that the linear adjustment of multipoint mPpa–Q relationships should not exceed 3 mm Hg/L/min, which corresponds to an mPpa at a Q <10 L/min, or a maximum exercise TPVR <3 Wood units. Fitting the data using

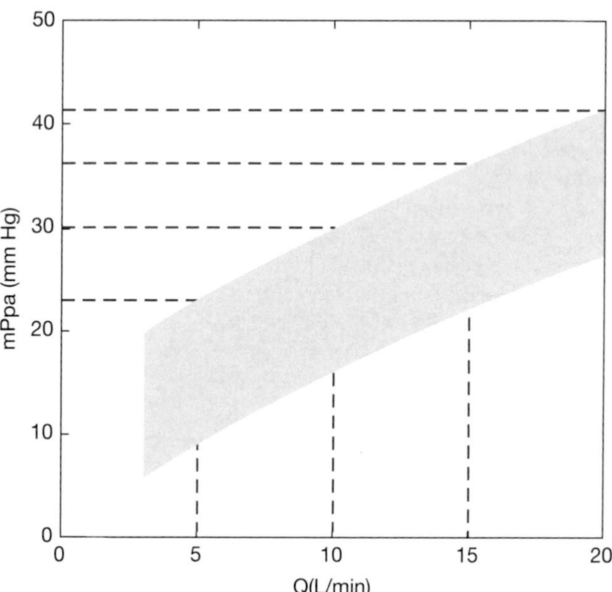

Figure 13-14 Limits of normal of mean pulmonary artery pressure (mPpa) as a function of increasing flow (Q) with exercise in healthy young adults, constructed from noninvasive and invasive data reported.[60] *Stippled lines* indicate upper limits of mPpa increasing from 25 mm Hg at a Q of 5 L/min to 45 mm Hg at Q of 20 L/min. *(Data from Bossone E, D'Andrea A, D'Alto M, et al. Echocardiography in pulmonary arterial hypertension: from diagnosis to prognosis. J Am Soc Echocardiogr. 2013;26(1):1–14.)*

Linehan's distensible model of the pulmonary circulation allowed for the calculation of normal α values <2%/mm Hg, decreasing at increasing levels of exercise.[37,38,59,60] These results have also been recently confirmed by invasive measurements,[61] allowing for a definition of the limits of normal of mPpa as a function of Q at exercise (Fig. 13-14).

After exercise, mPpa and Q rapidly return to resting values. Measurements within 5 minutes after a maximum exercise test in normal subjects are nearly back to resting normal.[59] Rapid return to normal of pulmonary vascular pressures and flows decreases the relevance of postexercise measurements as a reflection of exercise-induced changes. On the other hand, the workload–Q relationship is quite variable.[37] It is therefore preferable to express mPpa at exercise as a function of cardiac output rather than of workload to define the functional state of the pulmonary circulation.[61]

■ LEFT ATRIAL PRESSURE

Left atrial pressure increases with exercise. Strenuous exercise may be associated with very high Pla, up to 20 to 30 mm Hg in athletes.[20,21,62,63] At levels of exercise corresponding to increases in Q to less than 15 L/min, Pla remains more or less within the limits of normal or slightly above.[22] Increased Pla at very high levels of exercise is explained by progressive decrease in LV diastolic compliance in part related to competition for space with the RV within a nonacutely distensible pericardium.[64]

■ SHUNTING OF AGITATED CONTRAST

In 2004, Eldridge and Stickland independently reported on the occurrence of exercise-induced shunting demonstrated by agitated saline contrast echocardiography in subjects with otherwise no evidence of intrapulmonary or intracardiac shunt at rest.[65,66] In these studies, exercise-induced pulmonary shunting of bubbles was shown to be correlated with cardiac output, mPpa, and alveolar-to-arterial P_{O_2} gradient at exercise, suggesting an impact on gas exchange.[66] Agitated saline or gelatine contrast echocardiography is standard practice for the detection of cardiac right-to-left shunts. The contrast bubbles are of 10 to 35 μm in size, and do not normally traverse the pulmonary circulation. In the case of a cardiac right-to-left shunt, the appearance of contrast in the left heart chambers is immediate. In the case of pulmonary shunt, the appearance of contrast in the left heart chambers is delayed by 3 to 5 beats. The most likely explanation for positive pulmonary transit of agitated contrast is pulmonary capillary distension.[60,67]

In addition to variable LV diastolic compliance resulting in variable increase in Pla transmitted upstream to Ppa, much of the variability of the mPpa and PVR responses is related to pulmonary-resistive vessel distensibility. Data are emerging supporting the notion that low PVR at high levels of exercise is associated with an increased pulmonary vascular reserve defined by a combination of high α and lung diffusing capacity and positive pulmonary transit of agitated saline at Doppler echocardiography.[60,67]

PULSATILE FLOW PULMONARY HEMODYNAMICS

The study of the pulmonary circulation as a steady-flow system is a simplification. Pulmonary pulse pressure, or the difference between sPpa and dPpa, is proportionally much higher than systemic pulse pressure. Instantaneous pulmonary blood flow varies from a maximum at midsystole to around zero in diastole.

The morphology of pulmonary pressure and flow waves changes with the development of pulmonary hypertension. In patients with severe pulmonary hypertension, the RV pressure wave is characterized by a sharp initial upstroke, followed by a short plateau, and by a late systolic peaking, and the Ppa pressure wave is characterized by a huge pulse pressure and a late systolic peaking as well,[68] while the pulmonary flow wave presents with a shortened acceleration time and late or midsystolic deceleration.[69] In the most severe forms of pulmonary hypertension the pulmonary artery pressure wave looks "ventricularized."[68] These morphological aspects are entirely explained by the combined effects of decreased compliance[70] and wave reflection.[71]

■ PULMONARY VASCULAR IMPEDANCE

A complete evaluation of pulmonary vascular function relies on the calculation of the relationship between pulsatile pressure and flow or pulmonary vascular impedance (PVZ) instead of the relationship between mean pressure and flow (PVR). PVZ is calculated from a spectral analysis of the pulmonary arterial pressure and flow waves.[72] This analysis is possible because the pulmonary circulation behaves nearly linearly. This means that a purely sinusoidal flow oscillation produces a purely sinusoidal pressure oscillation of the same frequency. The sinusoidal pressure and flow waves can be related by the ratio of their amplitudes (modulus) and the difference in their phases (phase angle). A typical PVZ spectrum in a dog is illustrated in Figure 13-15.

Pulmonary arterial impedance at zero Hz, Z_0, (the ratio of mean pressure to mean flow, mPpa/Q) corresponds to TPVR. This parameter is mainly determined by the small resistance vessels as well as Pla. As frequency increases, the impedance is affected by more proximal elements of the arterial tree. The modulus of the impedance decreases from Z_0 rapidly to a first minimum at 2 to 3 times the heart rate and then oscillates about a constant value. The impedance phase increases from a negative value at low frequencies, indicating that flow leads pressure to zero at higher frequencies. The precipitous fall in modulus and the negative phase of the impedance are a measure of the total arterial compliance. At high frequencies the rather constant modulus and nearly zero phase angle are a measure of the proximal arterial compliance.

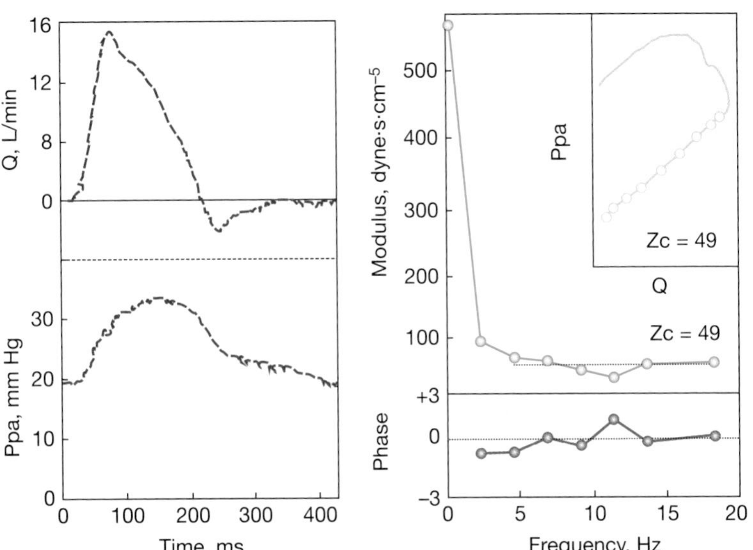

Figure 13-15 Pulmonary artery flow (Q) and pressure (Ppa) waves and pulmonary arterial input impedance spectrum. At 0 Hz the total PVR is obtained (mean pressure over mean flow). Between 0 and 4 Hz the impedance is mainly determined by total arterial compliance. The averaged input impedance for high frequencies, usually taken between 4 and 8 Hz, equals the characteristic impedance (Zc). The oscillation of the impedance about the characteristic impedance results from wave reflection. Zc is also the slope of early-systolic Ppa–Q relationship.

The impedance modulus at high frequencies, when impedance phase is nearly zero and therefore wave reflections can be ignored, is the characteristic impedance Zc. It is typically measured as the average modulus at higher frequencies (usually 10–20 times the heart rate). It can also be measured as the slope of the early systolic pulmonary artery pressure–flow relationship in the time domain (Fig. 13-15).[73]

The oscillations of the impedance modulus about its mean value result from distinct wave reflections. Increased magnitude of these oscillations implies increased reflections. A shift of the first minimum of modulus to higher frequencies indicates an increased wave velocity or a decreased distance to the dominant reflection site.

Characteristic impedance depends on the ratio of inertia to compliance of the proximal pulmonary circulation, and can be approximated by the equation:

$$Zc = [(\rho/\pi r^4)/(\Delta\pi r^2/\Delta P)]$$

where ρ is the density of blood, r the mean internal radius, $\rho/\pi r^4$ the inertance, and $\Delta\pi r^2/\Delta P$ the compliance of the pulmonary arterial tree.

The human PVZ spectrum has the same pattern as reported in canine studies, but with lower Z_0 and Zc values due to greater body size and thus relatively higher pulmonary blood flow.

Distal small vessel obstruction such as caused by microembolism, hypoxia, or pulmonary arterial hypertension increases Z_0 but have limited effects on the PVZ spectrum, with some shift of first minimum and maximum of Ppa/Q to higher frequencies, but unchanged or sometimes even a decrease in Zc.[71,74] Proximal vessel disease such as by experimental proximal ensnarement of the pulmonary arteries or clinical chronic thromboembolic pulmonary hypertension shifts the entire PVZ spectrum to higher ratios of pressure and flow moduli.[71,74] Very high Ppa due to major peripheral small vessel obstruction may also increase Zc because of extreme stiffening of the pulmonary arteries and increased reflected wave speed.[75,76]

Exercise has been reported in an animal study to decrease PVR but to shift the PVZ spectrum to higher pressure and flow moduli at all frequencies with an increase in Zc, a shift of the first minimum of the ratio of pressure and flow moduli to higher frequencies and more negative phase angle.[77] The authors explained the increase in Zc by a decreased area compliance of the proximal pulmonary arterial tree because of increased distending pressure related to increased flow, with possibly a contribution of exercise-associated sympathetic nervous system activation. It had indeed already been shown experimentally that sympathetic nervous system activation may increase Zc without significantly changing PVR.[78] However, the authors could not exclude a spurious increase in Zc caused by too tight fitting of the electromagnetic flow probe placed around the main pulmonary artery.[77]

There has been one small study on the effects of exercise on pulmonary arterial compliance (Ca), Zc, and PVR in eight normal subjects.[79] Exercise was associated with a 50% decrease in PVR and a 30% increase in pulmonary arterial compliance (Ca), while Zc did not change (Fig. 13-16). The apparent discrepancy between changes in Zc and Ca is explained by the sensitivity of Zc to proximal stiffness and dimensions, while Ca integrates the distensibility of the entire pulmonary circulation. Thus unchanged Zc would be explained by the balanced effects of proximal stiffening and increased cross-sectional area.

THE TIME CONSTANT OF THE PULMONARY CIRCULATION

A few decades ago, Reuben[80] had noted an inverse relationship between PVR and Ca in the normal or diseased pulmonary circulation. This was recently revisited in a series of studies that showed that the product of PVR and Ca, or the time constant (RC-time) of the pulmonary circulation remains constant over a wide range of severities, etiologies, and treatments of pulmonary hypertension (Fig. 13-17).[81–83] This remarkable property of the pulmonary circulation has two consequences. The first is that Ca becomes a more important determinant of RV afterload than PVR when mPpa and

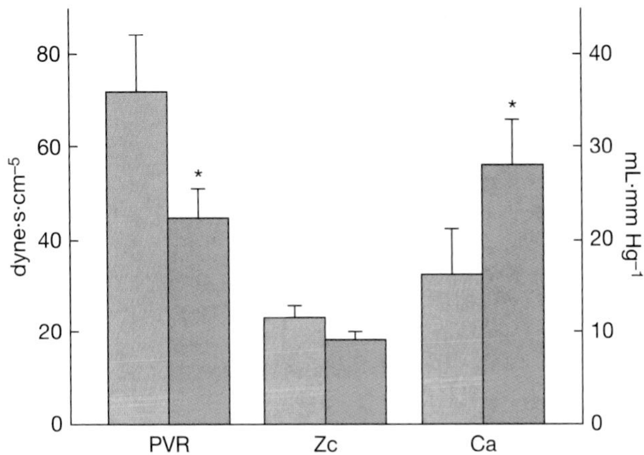

Figure 13-16 Effects of exercise on pulmonary vascular resistance (PVR), characteristic impedance (Zc), and arterial compliance (Ca) in healthy human subjects. Compared to resting state (blue bars), exercise (red bars) decreased PVR and increased Ca, while there was no significant (*) change in Zc. *(Data from Slife DM, Latham RD, Sipkema P and Westerhof N. Pulmonary arterial compliance at res and at exercise in normal humans. Am J Physiol. 1990;258 (Heart Circ Physiol 27): H1823–H1828.)*

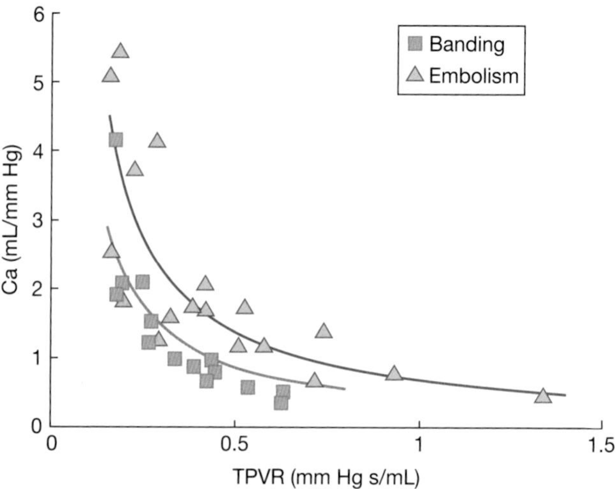

Figure 13-17 Pulmonary arterial compliance (Ca) as a function of total pulmonary vascular resistance (TPVR) in dogs with pulmonary hypertension induced either by an ensnarement of the pulmonary arteries (banding, proximal obstruction) or the injection of microbeads (embolism, distal obstruction). The time constant Ca × TPVR is shorter with proximal obstruction.

PVR are only modestly elevated.[84] The second is that RV oscillatory power (Wosc) remains a constant fraction of total power (Wtot) irrespective of Ppa.[80,85]

The only noticeable exception to the constancy of RC-time is pulmonary hypertension secondary to LV failure.[86] In these patients, RC-time is decreased because of a stiffer pulmonary arterial tree caused by increased pulmonary venous pressure.[43] One would expect proximal obstruction of the pulmonary circulation, like in patients with proximal chronic thromboembolic pulmonary hypertension, to be a cause of shorter RC-time as well (Fig. 13-17). A slight but significant decrease in RC-time has indeed recently been reported in such patients[87] like in experimental pulmonary hypertension on proximal pulmonary arterial banding.[4] It must however be underscored that a constancy or near constancy of RC-time in the pulmonary circulation contrasts with the absence of relationship between resistance and compliance in the systemic circulation.

The stability of the time constant of the pulmonary circulation explains the reported tight correlation between systolic, diastolic, and mean Ppa in normal subjects and in patients with pulmonary hypertension of all possible etiologies.[88] Accordingly, mPpa can be calculated from sPpa using a simple formula:

$$mPpa = 0.6 \times sPpa + 2$$

This notion is of practical relevance as noninvasive evaluations of the pulmonary circulation in clinical practice often rely on the measurement of a maximum velocity of TR to calculate a sPpa using the simplified form of the Bernoulli equation and a measurement or estimate of Pra[89]:

$$sPpa = (TR^2 + 4) + Pra$$

RIGHT VENTRICULAR FUNCTION

The RV is functionally coupled to the pulmonary circulation.[90] Because of the normally low pulmonary vascular pressures taking the entire cardiac output, the RV acts as a thin-walled flow generator. The structural and functional characteristics of the RV allow for the accommodation of large increases in flow, less so small increases in afterload. However, the basic laws of the heart remain applicable, that is rapid beat-to-beat heterometric adaptations (Starling law of the heart) and otherwise progressive structural and inotropic homeometric adaptations (Anrep's law of the heart) to changes in loading conditions.[91] Thus the RV adaptation to pulmonary hypertension is homeometric with increased contractility, eventual hypertrophy, and preserved dimensions. Failure of this mechanism depends on rate of onset and magnitude of increase in Ppa and results in heterometric adaptation, with increased RV dimensions and systemic congestion.[88,89]

RIGHT VENTRICULAR HYDRAULIC LOAD

Increased Ppa requires increased RV hydraulic power to sustain adequate forward flow. Hydraulic power is made of two components: The energy per unit time (power) to produce steady flow, which is the product of mPpa and Q, and the power to produce the pulsatile component of Ppa and Q. The latter can be calculated from the difference between the product of the integrations of instantaneous Ppa and Q waves and the product of mPpa and Q. Since mean flow determines oxygen transport, mean power may be considered useful whereas oscillatory power is "wasted." As a consequence, the ratio of oscillatory to mean power, or oscillatory to total (mean plus oscillatory) power, should preferably be small.[92]

Because of the proportional relationship between systolic, diastolic, and mPpa, one would expect the ratio of oscillatory to total RV power to remain constant. This was indeed recently reported in a study of 49 patients with pulmonary hypertensions of variable severities.[85] Total power increased with severity of pulmonary hypertension, but the ratio of oscillatory to total power remained reasonably constant, at 23%. Accordingly, the authors proposed that the total power of the RV should be equal to 1.3 times mean power in all circumstances. As the proportionality of pulmonary artery pressures appears to be maintained at exercise[93] the calculation of total RV power as 1.3 times mean power is probably transposable, but this will require confirmation by further studies. On the other hand, situations of shortened RC-time like heart failure[87] or purely proximal pulmonary arterial obstruction[4,87] are associated with an increased oscillatory component of total RV power.

RIGHT VENTRICULOARTERIAL COUPLING

The calculation of power includes a measurement of cardiac output, and thus depends not only on the mechanical properties of the pulmonary circulation, but also on ventricular function. It has been suggested that power transfer and ventricular efficiency are near maximal in normal subjects. A simplified approach to test this has been given by Sunagawa et al.[94] These authors proposed a graphical analysis based on the right ventricular pressure–volume diagram[91,95] and a characterization of the arterial system by means of its arterial elastance (Fig. 13-18).

The diagram allows for the determination of maximal ventricular elastance (Emax), which is the best possible load-independent measurement of contractility, and of arterial elastance, Ea, as a measurement of afterload as it is "seen" by the ventricle, and the calculation of an Emax/Ea ratio as a measurement of the coupling of ventricular to arterial function.

Mathematical modeling shows that the optimal matching of systolic ventricular and arterial elastances occurs at an Emax/Ea ratio around 1.5. Isolated increase in Ea, or decrease in Emax, decreases the Emax/Ea ratio, indicating uncoupling of the ventricle from its arterial system. Everything else being the same, a decrease in Emax/Ea is necessarily accompanied by a decrease in stroke volume. On the other hand, an isolated increase in preload is associated with an increase in stroke volume with unaltered ventriculo-arterial coupling.[91]

However, the complex geometry of the RV makes functional evaluations with measurement of instantaneous volume changes

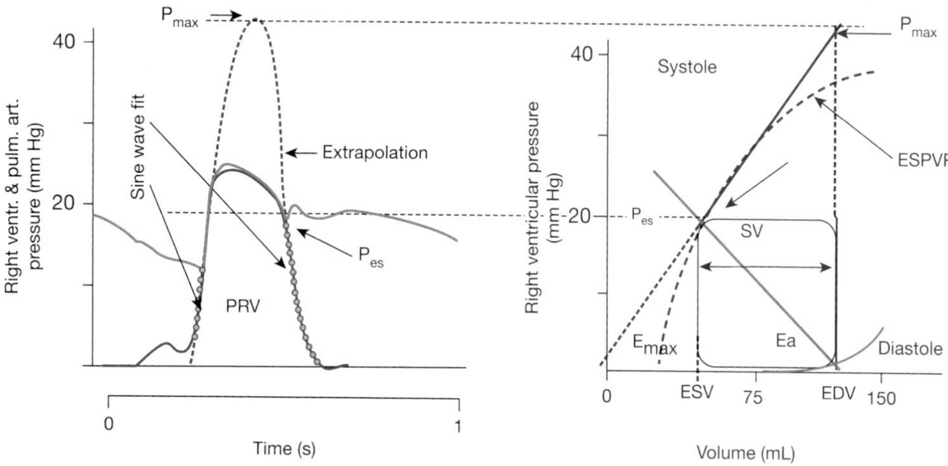

Figure 13-18 Single-beat method to measure right ventriculoarterial coupling. A maximum pressure (*Pmax*) is calculated from nonlinear extrapolation of early and late isovolumic portions of the right ventricular pressure curve. A *straight line* is drawn from *Pmax* and the end-diastolic volume (EDV) to *Pes* and the end-systolic volume (ESV), thus *Emax* = (*Pmax* − *Pes*)/SV, where SV is the stroke volume. The arterial elastance *Ea* is defined by the ratio *Pes*/SV. ESPVR, end-systolic pressure-volume relationship.

technically difficult, and the determination of Emax may be unreliable because of the particular shape of the RV pressure–volume loop and noncoincidence of end-ejection and end-systole. This problem can be overcome by measuring pressure–volume loops at several levels of preload,[96] but bedside manipulations of venous return are too invasive to be ethically acceptable. In addition, when applied to intact beings, changes in venous return are associated with reflex sympathetic nervous system activation, which affects the ventricular function that is measured.

These concerns have been addressed by a single-beat method allowing for a direct quantification of the coupling of the RV to the pulmonary circulation.[97] The approach had been initially proposed for the left ventricle.[98] In its principle, the method avoids absolute volume measurements and related technical complexities, to calculate Emax and Ea from instantaneous RV pressure and flow output measurements. As shown in Figure 13-18, a Pmax is estimated from a nonlinear extrapolation of the early- and late-systolic isovolumic portions of the right ventricular pressure curve. This estimated Pmax has been shown to be tightly correlated with Pmax directly measured during a nonejecting beat.[97] A straight line drawn from Pmax to the RV pressure versus relative change in volume curve allows for the determination of Emax. A straight line drawn from the Emax point to the end-diastolic relative volume point determines Ea.

The Emax/Ea ratio as determined by the single-beat method has been shown to be decreased by propranolol and increased by dobutamine, and maintained in the presence of increased Ea due to hypoxic pulmonary vasoconstriction.[97] In fact, Emax increases adaptively to increased Ea in hypoxia, even in the presence of adrenergic blockade, which is compatible with the notion of homeometric adaptation of right ventricular contractility. The method has been used to show that acutely administered prostacyclin does not have a positive inotropic effect as the explanation for the increased cardiac output associated with its use.[99]

Kuehne et al.[100] used magnetic resonance imaging (MRI) together with RV pressure measurements with Pmax calculations to generate pressure–volume loops and Emax and Ea determinations in patients with pulmonary arterial hypertension. As compared to controls, Emax was almost doubled, but Emax/Ea was decreased, indicating insufficient homeometric adaptation and pending RV failure. The importance of RV systolic function adaptation for the preservation of RV–arterial coupling in patients with severe pulmonary hypertension PAH has been confirmed by a study that used conductance catheter measurements of pressure and volume, and the Valsalva maneuver to decrease venous return and generate a family of pressure–volume loops.[101]

Since Emax/Ea can be simplified to a ratio of volumes, Sanz et al. reported on the estimation of RV–arterial coupling estimated by the ratio of stroke volume to end-systolic volume measured by MRI in 139 patients referred for pulmonary hypertension. The resulting “Emax/Ea” was shown to decrease progressively with increasing severity of pulmonary hypertension.[102]

An alternative approach was developed by Elzinga and Westerhof in 1978.[103] The authors described RV pump function curves by plotting mean RV pressure as a function of stroke volume. As shown in Figure 13-19, the pump function curve is built from measurements of mean RV pressure and stroke volume, a calculated maximum pressure at zero stroke volume, and a parabolic extrapolation to a zero pressure stroke volume. In this representation, an increase in preload shifts the curve to greater stroke volumes with no shape change, while an increased contractility leads to a higher maximum pressure with no change in maximum stroke volume. This analysis has been used to explain the more severe RV failure in pulmonary arterial hypertension associated with systemic sclerosis,[104] in agreement with pressure–volume loop-derived estimations of RV–arterial coupling.[101] A derived simplified measure of the adequacy of RV systolic function adaptation to afterload is contractile reserve, defined by the increase in RV systolic pressure during an exercise stress. RV

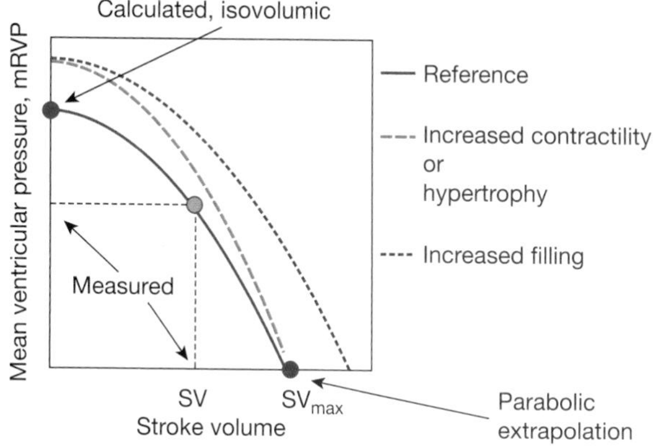

Figure 13-19 Pump function curve defined by mean right ventricular pressure as a function of stroke volume. The zero stroke volume point is calculated from a maximum pressure determination (see Fig. 13-18). The zero pressure point results from a parabolic extrapolation, from measured and zero stroke volume points. *(Data from Elzinga G, Westerhof N. The effect of an increase in inotropic state and end-diastolic volume on the pumping ability of the feline left heart Circ Res. 1978;42:620–628.)*

contractile reserve has been reported to be an important predictor of survival in patients with severe pulmonary hypertension.[105]

ACKNOWLEDGMENTS

Rebecca Vanderpool and Bart Boerrigter helped in the preparation of this chapter.

REFERENCES

1. West JB. Ibn al-Nafis, the pulmonary circulation and the Islamic Golden Age. *J Appl Physiol.* 2008;105:1877–1880.
2. West JB. The role of the fragility of the pulmonary blood-gas barrier in the evolution of the pulmonary circulation. *Am J Physiol Regul Integr Comp Physiol.* 2013;304:R171–R176.
3. Gibbs NC, Gardner RM. Dynamics of invasive pressure monitoring systems: clinical and laboratory evaluation. *Heart Lung.* 1988;17:43–51.
4. Pagnamenta A, Vanderpool R, Brimioulle S, Naeije R. Proximal pulmonary arterial obstruction decreases the time constant of the pulmonary circulation and increases right ventricular afterload. *J Appl Physiol.* 2013;114:1586–1592.
5. Bland JM, Altman DG. Statistical methods for assessing agreement between two different methods of clinical measurement. *Lancet.* 1986;1:307–310.
6. Connolly DC, Kirklin JW, Wood EH. The relationship between pulmonary artery wedge pressure and left atrial pressure in man. *Circ Res.* 1954;2:434–440.
7. Halpern SD, Taichman DB. Misclassification of pulmonary hypertension due to reliance on pulmonary capillary wedge pressure rather than left ventricular end-diastolic pressure. *Chest.* 2009;136:37–43.
8. Hoeper MM, Maier R, Tongers J, et al. Determination of cardiac output by the Fick method, thermodilution, and acetylene rebreathing in pulmonary hypertension. *Am J Respir Crit Care Med.* 1999;160:535–541.
9. Guyton AC, Jones CE, Coleman TG. *Circulatory Physiology: Cardiac Output and its Regulation.* 2nd ed. Philadelphia, PA: WB Saunders; 1973.
10. Howell JB, Permutt S, Proctor DF, Riley RL. Effect of inflation of the lung on different parts of the pulmonary vascular bed. *J Appl Physiol.* 1961;16:71–76.
11. Naeije R, Boerrigter BG. Pulmonary hypertension at exercise in COPD: does it matter? *Eur Respir J.* 2013;41:1002–1004.
12. Battacharya J, Nanjo S, Staub NC. Micropuncture measurement of lung microvascular pressure during 5-HT infusion. *J Appl Physiol.* 1982;52:634–637.
13. Cope DK, Grimbert F, Downey JM, Taylor AE. Pulmonary capillary pressure: A review. *Crit Care Med.* 1992;20:1043–1056.
14. Maggiorini M, Mélot C, Pierre S, et al. High altitude pulmonary edema is initially caused by an increased capillary pressure. *Circulation.* 2001;103:2078–2083.
15. Gaar KA Jr, Taylor AE, Owens LJ, Guyton AC. Pulmonary capillary pressure and filtration coefficient in the isolated perfused lung. *Am J Physiol.* 1967;213:910–914.
16. Naeije R, Mélot C, Mols P, Hallemans R. Effects of vasodilators on hypoxic pulmonary vasoconstriction in normal man. *Chest.* 1982;82:404–410.
17. Naeije R, Mélot C, Niset G, Delcroix M, Wagner PD. Improved arterial oxygenation by a pharmacological increase in chemosensitivity during hypoxic exercise in normal subjects. *J Appl Physiol.* 1993;74:1666–1671.
18. Mélot C, Naeije R, Hallemans R, Lejeune P, Mols P. Hypoxic pulmonary vasoconstriction and pulmonary gas exchange in normal man. *Respir Physiol.* 1987;68:11–27.
19. Kovacs G, Berghold A, Scheid S, Olschewski H. Pulmonary artery pressure during rest and exercise in healthy subjects: a systematic review. *Eur Respir J.* 2009;34:888–894.
20. Granath A, Jonsson B, Strandell T. Circulation in healthy old men, studied by right heart catheterization at rest and during exercise in supine and sitting position. *Acta Med Scand.* 1964;176:425–446.
21. Granath A, Strandell T. Relationships between cardiac output, stroke volume, and intracardiac pressures at rest and during exercise in supine position and some anthropometric data in healthy old men. *Acta Med Scand.* 1964;176:447–466.
22. Naeije R, Chesler NC. Pulmonary circulation at exercise. *Compr Physiol.* 2012;2:711–741.
23. Naeije R. Pulmonary vascular resistance: a meaningless variable? *Intens Care Med.* 2003;29:526–529.
24. Permutt S, Bromberger-Barnea B, Bane HN. Alveolar pressure, pulmonary venous pressure and the vascular waterfall. *Med Thorac.* 1962;19:239–260.
25. West JB, Dollery CT, Naimark A. Distribution of blood flow in isolated lung: relation to vascular and alveolar pressures. *J Appl Physiol.* 1964;19:713–724.
26. Leeman M, Lejeune P, Closset J, Vachiéry JL, Mélot C, Naeije R. Nature of pulmonary hypertension in canine oleic acid pulmonary edema. *J Appl Physiol.* 1990;69:293–298.
27. Zapol WM, Snider MT. Pulmonary hypertension in severe acute respiratory failure. *N Engl J Med.* 1977;296:476–480.
28. Naeije R, Lipski A, Abramowicz M, et al. Nature of pulmonary hypertension in congestive heart failure. Effects of cardiac transplantation. *Am J Respir Crit Care Med.* 1997;147: 881–887.
29. Linehan JH, Haworth ST, Nelin LD, Krenz GS, Dawson CA. A simple distensible model for interpreting pulmonary vascular pressure-flow curves. *J Appl Physiol.* 1992;73:987–994.
30. Zhuang FY, Fung YC, Yen RT. Analysis of blood flow in cat's lung with detailed anatomical and elasticity data. *J Appl Physiol.* 1983;55:1341–1348.
31. Marshall BE, Marshall C. A model for hypoxic constriction of the pulmonary circulation. *J Appl Physiol.* 1988;64:68–77.
32. Bshouty Z, Younes M. Distensibility and pressure-flow relationship of the pulmonary circulation. II. Multibranched model. *J Appl Physiol.* 1990;68:1514–1527.
33. Mélot C, Delcroix M, Lejeune P, Leeman M, Naeije R. Starling resistor versus viscoelastic models for embolic pulmonary hypertension. *Am J Physiol.* 1995;268(*Heart Circ Physiol 36*): H817–H827.
34. Nelin LD, Krenz GS, Rickaby DA, Linehan JH, Dawson CA. A distensible vessel model applied to hypoxic pulmonary vasoconstriction in the neonatal pig. *J Appl Physiol.* 1992;73:987–994.
35. Reeves JT, Linehan JH, Stenmark KR. Distensibility of the normal human lung circulation during exercise. *Am J Physiol Lung Cell Mol Physiol.* 2005;288:L419–L425.
36. Krenz GS, Dawson CA. Flow and pressure distributions in vascular networks consisting of distensible vessels. *Am J Physiol Heart Circ.* 2003;284:H2192–H2203.
37. Argiento P, Vanderpool RR, Mule M, et al. Exercise stress echocardiography of the pulmonary circulation: limits of normal and sex differences. *Chest.* 2012;142:1158–1165.

38. Groepenhoff H, Overbeek MJ, Mulè M, et al. Exercise pathophysiology in patients with chronic mountain sickness. *Chest.* 2012;142:877–884.

39. Penaloza D, Arias-Stella J. The heart and pulmonary circulation at high altitudes: healthy highlanders and chronic mountain sickness. *Circulation.* 2007;115:1132–1146.

40. Whittaker SR, Winton FR. The apparent viscosity of blood flowing in the isolated hindlimb of the dog, and its variation with corpuscular concentration. *J Physiol.* 1933;78: 339–369.

41. Moraes DL, Colucci WS, Givertz MM. Secondary pulmonary hypertension in chronic heart failure. The role of endothelium in pathophysiology and management. *Circulation.* 2000;102: 1718–1723.

42. Hoeper MM, Barberà JA, Channick RN, et al. Diagnosis, assessment, and treatment of non-pulmonary arterial hypertension pulmonary hypertension. *J Am Coll Cardiol.* 2009;54(1 suppl):S85–S96.

43. Naeije R, Vachiery J, Yerly P, Vanderpool R. The transpulmonary pressure gradient for the diagnosis of pulmonary vascular disease. *Eur Respir J.* 2013;41:217–223.

44. Harvey RM, Enson Y, Ferrer MI. A reconsideration of the origins of pulmonary hypertension. *Chest.* 1971;59:82–94.

45. Hughes JM, Glazier JB, Maloney JR, West JB. Effect of lung volume on the distribution of pulmonary blood flow in man. *Respir Physiol.* 1968;4:58–72.

46. Hakim TS, Lisbona R, Michel RP, Dean GW. Role of vasoconstriction in gravity-nondependent central-peripheral gradient in pulmonary blood flow. *J Appl Physiol.* 1993;63: 1114–1121.

47. Glenny R. Counterpoint: Gravity is not the major factor determining the distribution of blood flow in the healthy human lung. *J Appl Physiol.* 2008;104:1533–1535.

48. Hughes M, West JB. Point:Counterpoint: Gravity is/is not the major factor determining the distribution of blood flow in the human lung. *J Appl Physiol.* 2008;104:1531–1533.

49. von Euler US, Liljestrand G. Observations on the pulmonary arterial blood pressure in the cat. *Acta Physiol Scand.* 1946;12:301–320.

50. Sylvester JT, Shimoda LA, Aaronsen PI, Ward JP. Hypoxic pulmonary vasoconstriction. *Physiol Rev.* 2012;92:367–520.

51. Dorrington KL, Clar C, Young JD, Jonas M, Tansley JG, Robbins PA. Time course of the human pulmonary vascular response to 8 hours of isocapnic hypoxia. *Am J Physiol.* 1997;273: H1126–H1134.

52. Hillier SC, Graham JA, Hanger CC, Godbey P, Glenny RW, Wagner WW. Hypoxic vasoconstriction in pulmonary arterioles and venules. *J Appl Physiol.* 1997;82:1084–1090.

53. Grant BJB. Effect of local pulmonary blood flow control on gas exchange: theory. *J Appl Physiol Respir Environ Exerc Physiol.* 1982;53:1100–1109.

54. Brimioulle S, Lejeune P, Naeije R. Effects of hypoxic pulmonary vasoconstriction on gas exchange. *J Appl Physiol.* 1996;81:1535–1543.

55. Naeije R, Brimioulle S. Physiology in medicine: the importance of hypoxic pulmonary vasoconstriction in maintaining arterial oxygenation during acute lung injury. *Crit Care.* 2001; 5:67–71.

56. Downing SE, Lee JC. Nervous control of the pulmonary circulation. *Annu Rev Physiol.* 1980;42:199–210.

57. Reeves JT, Dempsey JA, Grover RF. Chapter 4. Pulmonary circulation during exercise. In: Weir EK, Reeves JT, eds. *Pulmonary Vascular Physiology and Physiopathology.* New York, NY: Marcel Dekker; 1989:107–133.

58. Kovacs G, Olschewski A, Berhold A, Oschewski H. Pulmonary vascular resistance during exercise in normal subjects: a systematic review. *Eur Respir J.* 2012;39:131–318.

59. Argiento P, Chesler N, Mulè M, et al. Exercise stress echocardiography for the study of the pulmonary circulation. *Eur Respir J.* 2010;35:1273–1278.

60. Lalande S, Yerly P, Faoro V, Naeije R. Pulmonary vascular distensibility predicts aerobic capacity in healthy individuals. *J Physiol.* 2012;590:4279–4288.

61. Naeije R, Vanderpool R, Dhakal B, et al. Exercise-induced pulmonary hypertension: physiological basis and methodological concerns. *Am J Respir Crit Care Med.* 2013;187:576–583.

62. Bevegaard S, Holmgren A, Jonsson B. Circulatory studies in well trained athletes at rest and during heavy exercise, with special reference to stroke volume and the influence of body position. *Acta Physiol Scand.* 1963;57:26–50.

63. Holmgren A, Jonsson B, Sjostrand T. Circulatory data in normal subjects at rest and during exercise in the recumbent position, with special reference to the stroke volume at different working intensities. *Acta Physiol Scand.* 1960;49: 343–363.

64. Stickland MK, Welsh RC, Petersen SR, et al. Does fitness level modulate the cardiovascular hemodynamic response to exercise? *J Appl Physiol.* 2006;100:1895–1901.

65. Eldridge MW, Dempsey JA, Haverkamp HC, Lovering AT, Hokanson JS. Exercise-induced intrapulmonary arteriovenous shunting in healthy humans. *J Appl Physiol.* 2004;97: 797–805.

66. Stickland MK, Welsh RC, Haykowsky MJ, et al. Intrapulmonary shunt and pulmonary gas exchange during exercise in humans. *J Physiol.* 2004;561:321–329.

67. La Gerche A, MacIsaac AL, Burns AT, et al. Pulmonary transit of agitated contrast is associated with enhanced pulmonary vascular reserve and right ventricular function at exercise. *J Appl Physiol.* 2010;109:1307–1317.

68. Cournand A, Bloomfield RA, Lawson HD. Double lumen catheter for intravenous and intracardiac blood sampling and pressure recording. *Proc Soc Exp Biol Med.* 1945;60:73–75.

69. Kitabatake A, Inoue M, Asao M, et al. Noninvasive evaluation of pulmonary hypertension by a pulsed Doppler technique. *Circulation.* 1983;68:302–330.

70. Elzinga G, Piene H, de Jong JP. Left and right ventricular pump function and consequences of having two pumps in one heart. *Circ Res.* 1980;46:564–574.

71. Furuno Y, Nagamoto Y, Fujita M, Kaku T, Sakurai S, Kuroiwa A. Reflection as a cause of mid-systolic deceleration of pulmonary flow wave in dogs with acute pulmonary hypertension: comparison of pulmonary artery constriction with pulmonary embolisation. *Cardiovasc Res.* 1991;25:118–124.

72. Bergel DH, Milnor WR. Pulmonary vascular impedance in the dog. *Circ Res.* 1966;16:401–415.

73. Dujardin JP, Stone DN, Forcino CD, Paul LT, Pieper HP. Effects of blood volume changes on characteristic impedance of the pulmonary artery. *Am J Physiol.* 1982;242:H197–H202.

74. Wauthy P, Pagnamenta A, Vassali F, Brimioulle S, Naeije R. Right ventricular adaptation to pulmonary hypertension. An

interspecies comparison. *Am J Physiol Heart Circ Physiol.* 2004;286:H1441–H1447.

75. Laskey WK, Ferrari VA, Palevsky HI, Kussmaul WG. Pulmonary artery hemodynamics in primary pulmonary hypertension. *J Am Coll Cardiol.* 1993;21:406–412.
76. Huez S, Brimioulle S, Naeije R, Vachiéry JL. Feasibility of routine pulmonary arterial impedance measurements in pulmonary hypertension. *Chest.* 2004;125:2121–2128.
77. Elkins RC, Milnor WR. Pulmonary vascular response to exercise in the dog. *Circ Res.* 1971;29:591–599.
78. Pace JB. Sympathetic control of pulmonary vascular impedance in anesthetized dogs. *Circ Res.* 1971;29:555–567.
79. Slife DM, Latham RD, Sipkema P, Westerhof N. Pulmonary arterial compliance at rest and at exercise in normal humans. *Am J Physiol.* 1990;258 (*Heart Circ Physiol* 27):H1823–H1828.
80. Reuben SR. Compliance of the pulmonary arterial system in disease. *Circ Res.* 1971;29:40–50.
81. Lankhaar JW, Westerhof N, Faes TJ, et al. Quantification of right ventricular afterload in patients with and without pulmonary hypertension. *Am J Physiol Heart Circ Physiol.* 2006;291:H1731–H1737.
82. Lankhaar JW, Westerhof N, Faes TJ, et al. Pulmonary vascular resistance and compliance stay inversely related during treatment of pulmonary hypertension. *Eur Heart J.* 2008;29:1688–1695.
83. Saouti N, Westerhof N, Helderman F, et al. RC time constant of single lung equals that of both lungs together: a study in chronic thromboembolic pulmonary hypertension. *Am J Physiol Heart Circ Physiol.* 2009;297:H2154–H2160.
84. Bonderman D, Martischnig AM, Vonbank K, et al. Right ventricular load at exercise is a cause of persistent exercise limitation in patients with normal resting pulmonary vascular resistance after pulmonary endarterectomy. *Chest.* 2011;139:122–127.
85. Saouti N, Westerhof N, Helderman F, et al. Right ventricular oscillatory power is a constant fraction of total power irrespective of pulmonary artery pressure. *Am J Respir Crit Care Med.* 2010;182:1315–1320.
86. Tedford RJ, Hassoun PM, Mathai SC, et al. Pulmonary capillary wedge pressure augments right ventricular pulsatile loading. *Circulation.* 2012;125:289–297.
87. Mackenzie Ross RV, Toshner MR, Soon E, Naeije R, Pepke-Zaba J. Decreased time constant of the pulmonary circulation in chronic thromboembolic pulmonary hypertension. *Am J Physiol Heart Circ Physiol.* 2013;305:H259–H264.
88. Chemla D, Castelain V, Provencher S, Humbert M, Simonneau G, Hervé P. Evaluation of various empirical formulas for estimating mean pulmonary artery pressure by using systolic pulmonary artery pressure in adults. *Chest.* 2009;135:760–768.
89. Yock P, Popp R. Noninvasive estimation of right ventricular systolic pressure by Doppler ultrasound in patients with tricuspid regurgitation. *Circulation.* 1984;70:657–662.
90. Champion HC, Michelakis ED, Hassoun PM. Comprehensive invasive and noninvasive approach to the right ventricle-pulmonary circulation unit: state of the art and clinical and research implications. *Circulation.* 2009;120:992–1007.
91. Sagawa K, Maughan L, Suga H, Sunagawa K. *Cardiac Contraction and the Pressure-Volume Relationship.* New York, NY: Oxford University Press; 1988.
92. Milnor WR, Bergel DH, Bargainer JD. Hydraulic power associated with pulmonary blood flow and its relation to heart rate. *Circ Res.* 1966;19:467–480.
93. Syyed R, Reeves JT, Welsh D, Raeside D, Johnson MK, Peacock AJ. The relationship between the components of pulmonary artery pressure remains constant under all conditions in both health and disease. *Chest.* 2008;133:633–639.
94. Sunagawa K, Maughan WL, Sagawa K. Optimal arterial resistance for the maximal stroke work studied in the isolated canine left ventricle. *Circ Res.* 1985;56:586–595.
95. Suga H, Sagawa K, Shoukas AA. Load independence of the instantaneous pressure-volume ratio of the canine left ventricle and the effect of epinephrine and heart rate on the ratio. *Circ Res.* 1973;32:314–322.
96. Maughan WL, Shoukas AA, Sagawa K, Weisfeldt ML. Instantaneous pressure-volume relationship of the canine right ventricle. *Circ Res.* 1979;44:309–315.
97. Brimioulle S, Wauthy P, Ewalenko P, et al. Single-beat estimation of right ventricular end-systolic pressure-volume relationship. *Am J Physiol Heart Circ Physiol.* 2003;284:H1625–H1630.
98. Sunagawa K, Yamada A, Senda Y, Kikuchi Y, Nakamura M, Shibahara T. Estimation of the hydromotive source pressure from ejecting beats of the left ventricle. *IEEE Trans Biomed Eng.* 1980;57:299–305.
99. Kerbaul F, Brimioulle S, Rondelet B, Dewachter C, Hubloue I, Naeije R. How prostacyclin improves cardiac output in right heart failure in conjunction with pulmonary hypertension. *Am J Respir Crit Care Med.* 2007;175:846–850.
100. Kuehne T, Yilmaz S, Steendijk P, et al. Magnetic resonance imaging analysis of right ventricular pressure-volume loops: in vivo validation and clinical application in patients with pulmonary hypertension. *Circulation.* 2004;110:2010–2016.
101. Tedford RJ, Mudd JO, Girgis RE, et al. Right ventricular dysfunction in systemic sclerosis associated pulmonary arterial hypertension. *Circ Heart Fail.* 2013;6(5):953–963.
102. Sanz J, García-Alvarez A, Fernández-Friera L, et al. Right ventriculo-arterial coupling in pulmonary hypertension: a magnetic resonance study. *Heart.* 2012;98:238–243.
103. Elzinga G, Westerhof N. The effect of an increase in inotropic state and end-diastolic volume on the pumping ability of the feline left heart. *Circ Res.* 1978;42:620–628.
104. Overbeek MJ, Lankhaar JW, Westerhof N, et al. Right ventricular contractility in systemic sclerosis-associated and idiopathic pulmonary arterial hypertension. *Eur Respir J.* 2008;31:1160–1166.
105. Grunig E, Tiede H, Enyiamayew EO, et al. Assessment and prognostic relevance of right ventricular contractile reserve in patients with pulmonary arterial hypertension. *Circulation.* 2013;128(18):2005–2015.

CHAPTER 14

Ventilation, Pulmonary Blood Flow, and Ventilation–Perfusion Relationships

Peter D. Wagner

This chapter and the two succeeding it together share responsibility for presenting the physiological basis of normal pulmonary gas exchange. Gas exchange occurs by an integrated series of gas transport steps between the environmental air we breathe and the Hb molecule of the red cells passing through the pulmonary capillaries. These transport steps are of two types—diffusive and convective, and a number of conceptually separate diffusive as well as convective processes interact to accomplish the gas exchange mission. This is true both for gases that are taken up from the environment into the blood (i.e., O_2 and occasional toxic gases or volatile anesthetics) and for gases that are eliminated from the body (i.e., CO_2 and volatile anesthetic agents).

This chapter deals principally with the convective processes and Chapter 16 with those involving diffusion. However, since the two types of process occur simultaneously they are closely linked.

BASIC OUTLINE OF THE GAS EXCHANGE PATHWAY

This section dwells on O_2, being the gas of principal physiological interest. However, the pathway components are of course identical for all gases and furthermore do not depend on whether the gas is being taken up (O_2) or eliminated (CO_2). On the other hand, distinct quantitative differences in the uptake or elimination patterns of different gases exist, but those are readily explained by differences in their fundamental physical or chemical properties, and not by transport pathway differences.

To understand the gas transport pathway one must first appreciate the anatomy of the lungs, laid out in detail in Chapter 2. The salient functional features are presented in Figure 14-1.

The chest wall (rib cage and diaphragm) contains muscles that on contraction expand the volume of the chest cavity and thus reduce the hydrostatic pressure of the pleural space, expanding the

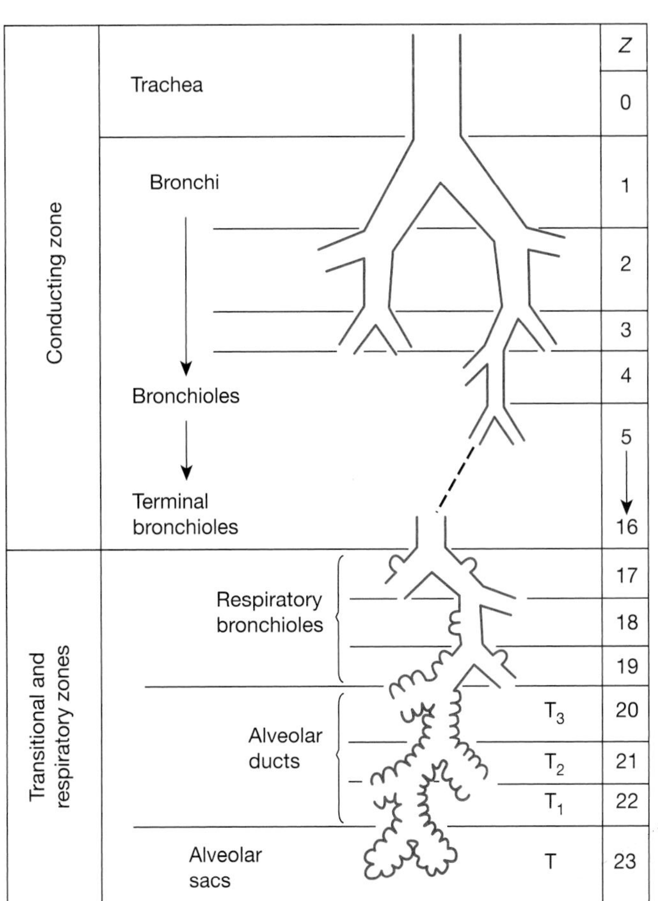

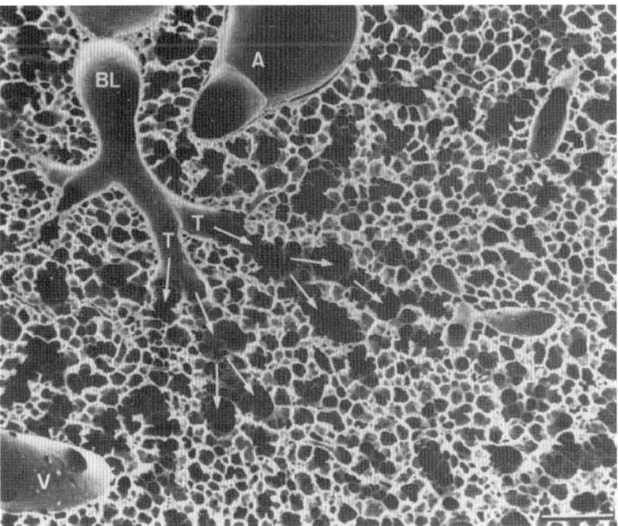

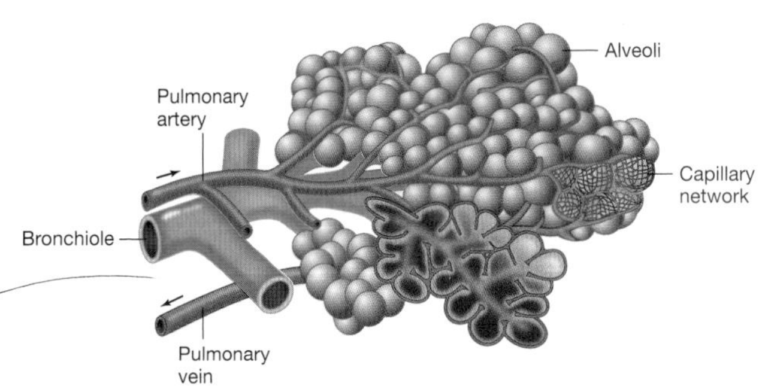

Figure 14-1 Principal anatomical features of the lung related to gas exchange. **A** shows the organization of branching airways, mirrored by a photograph of a lung slice showing terminal and respiratory bronchioles and the alveolar parenchyma (see also **B**) *(**A.** Modified with permission from Weibel ER: Morphometry of the Human Lung. Heidelberg, Springer-Verlag; 1963).* **C** shows how the capillaries are wrapped around alveoli and **D** is a scanning electron micrograph indicating the rich capillary networks in the alveolar walls (PA, pulmonary artery). **E** is a transmission electron micrograph showing the capillaries (C) and the three layers of the blood–gas barrier (EN, endothelium; BM, basement membrane; and EPI, epithelium). *(**B, D,** and **E.** Reproduced with permission from Weibel ER. The Pathway for Oxygen. Cambridge, MA: Harvard University Press; 1984.) (continued)*

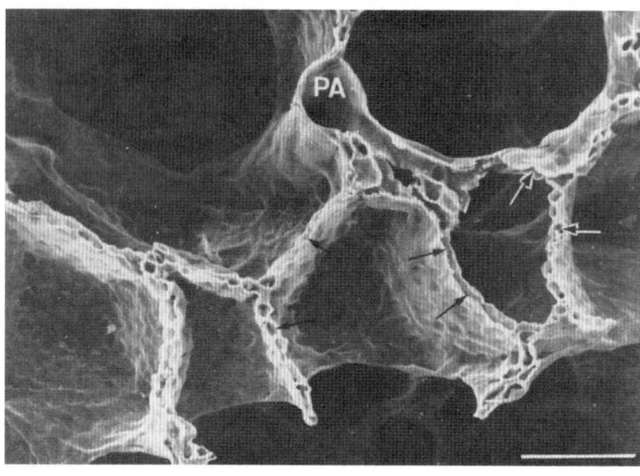

D

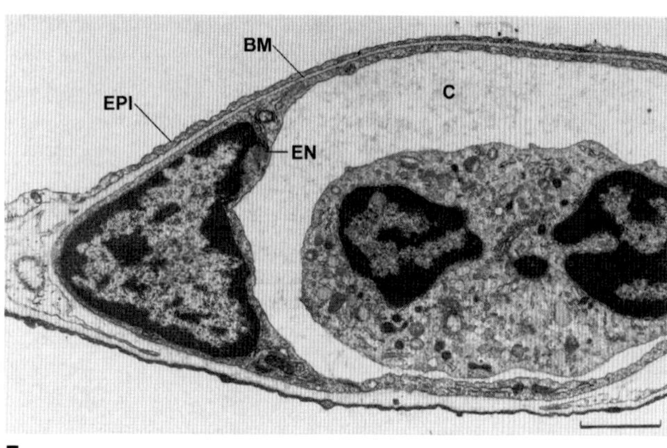

E

Figure 14-1 *(Continued)*

lungs with air drawn in via the mouth and nose. Although there is but a single air passage in the neck (i.e., the trachea), this soon branches into right and left main bronchi. These also divide many times, essentially dichotomously. There are some 16 such orders of branching of these bronchi, resulting in a structure that resembles an inverted deciduous tree without its leaves in winter.[1] With each successive branch the airways become shorter and narrower, but ever greater in number, usually doubling at each branching. Thus, although the cross-sectional area of any one airway becomes smaller with each branching, the greater number of airways more than makes up for loss of individual cross-sectional area such that the sum of cross-sectional areas of all airways of a given generation rises essentially exponentially with each branching (Fig. 14-2). The total volume of gas in these 16 conducting airway generations is called the anatomic or conducting airway dead space, and approximates 1 mL per pound of body weight. After these 16 or so successive branches, the tubular, purely conducting airways begin to show alveolar units in their wall (generations 17–19 or so) and these finally give way to fully alveolated structures (in succession: alveolar ducts, alveolar sacs, and alveoli). There are some 300 million alveoli, each about 300 μm in diameter. They are blind structures so that ventilation has to be accomplished by a tidal, in-and-out process (rather than a flow-through process as for pulmonary blood flow). The alveoli can be seen in Figure 14-1, from a different perspective. For gas exchange to occur, O_2 must be moved from the mouth all the way to the alveoli—it is only within alveoli that gas exchange occurs.

Each alveolus is densely covered in a capillary network, seen from various perspectives in Figure 14-1. This network is closely applied to the alveolar gas space as Figure 14-1 shows, with on average only about 1/2 μm of cellular and interstitial tissue between the blood inside the capillary and the alveolar gas outside.[2] The capillary network is fed by the pulmonary arterial tree which branches alongside the airways in a very similar pattern as the airways. The capillaries then drain into venules that join to form larger and larger vessels, eventually becoming the pulmonary veins that drain oxygenated blood into the left atrium. This coalescence of venous vessels forms a similar branching tree to the pulmonary arteries and airways, but in reverse. The right ventricle is responsible for unidirectional pumping of blood through this vascular system.

The gas exchange pathway from the lips to the left atrium is therefore highly complex structurally, and understanding how gases pass along the pathway requires following the events an O_2 molecule must participate in between the lips and the left atrium.

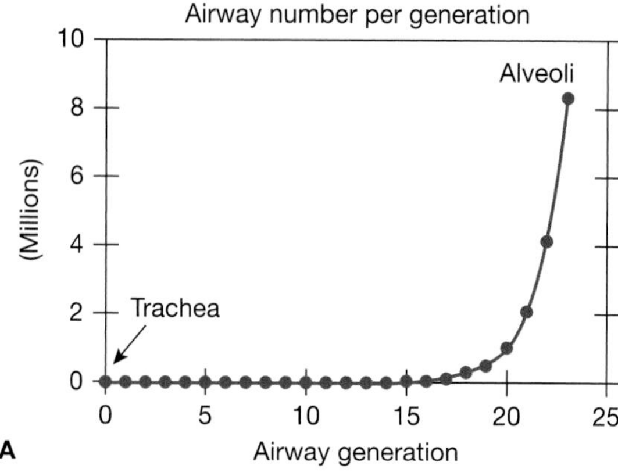

A

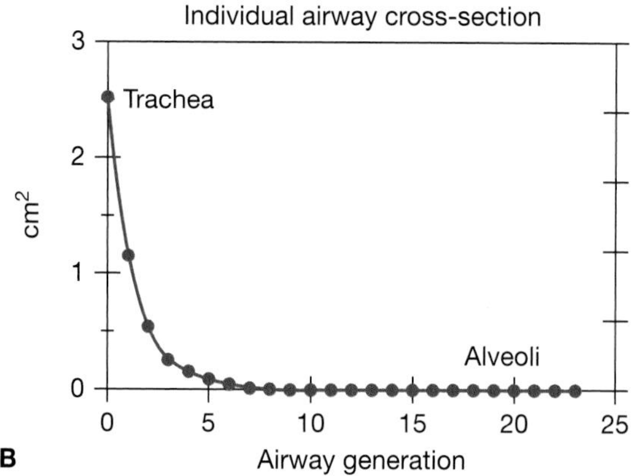

B

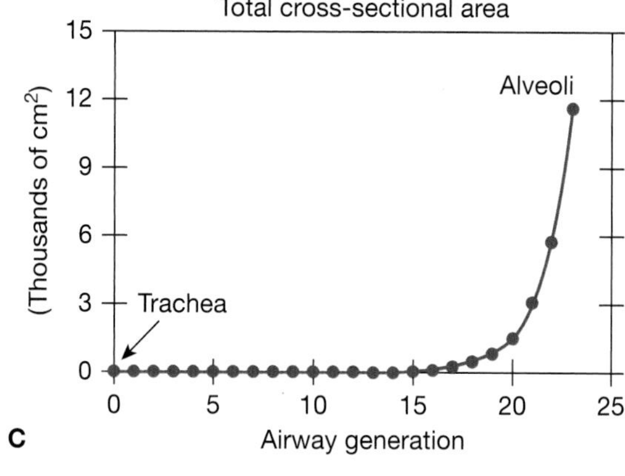

C

Figure 14-2 Relationship between number (**A**) and cross-sectional area (**B**) of the airways at a given generation. Note that total airway cross-sectional area (**C**) increases extremely rapidly beyond airway generation 15 or so, the beginning of the respiratory zone for gas exchange.

1. The first step is inspiration of air into the trachea via mouth and nose. Accomplished by inspiratory chest wall muscle contraction which reduces intrathoracic pressure, this step is convective (like water flowing from a region of high to low pressure along a garden hose). All the respired air must pass the trachea but at the first branch point some air goes to the right lung, the rest to the left. At each successive branch point, similar mass-conserving distribution of air must occur between the daughter branches of each parent pathway. Remembering that there are some 23 total branchings from the mouth to the 300 million alveoli, there is a very real risk of quite uneven distribution of that inspired air amongst those alveoli.[3] The principal determinants of how air is distributed at branch points (i.e., between daughter branches) are the mechanical properties of the respiratory system: the compliance (elastic properties), the resistance, and the inertial properties. These concepts are more fully treated in Chapter 10.
2. During normal resting inspiration, flow is laminar in most of the airways. Thus inspired gas develops a parabolic profile due to higher molecular velocities in the center than periphery of the airway (Fig. 14-3). The parabolic "tongue" of inspired gas in Figure 14-3 moves down an airway, while around the tongue is gas remaining from the previous expiration. The tongue therefore has O_2 at a concentration of 21% and essentially no CO_2. The gas around the tongue, having undergone gas exchange during the preceding breath, has about 14% O_2 and 5% CO_2. Consequently, during forward motion of this tongue toward the alveoli, O_2 will diffuse from the tongue to its surrounding gas while CO_2 will diffuse in the opposite direction. This is called Taylor dispersion,[4] and it reduces the forward transport of O_2 produced by the onward convective movement of the tongue. This effect however is considered quite small and is generally not of significance to overall gas exchange.

   Note that if inspiration occurs at high rates as in exercise, such laminar flow may not occur in the larger airways—it may be turbulent and then Taylor dispersion is essentially noncontributory, as the turbulent mixing evens gas concentrations across the airway lumen.
3. Figure 14-2 shows the exponential increase in airway cross-sectional surface area as one proceeds deeper and deeper into the lungs. The significance of this curve is that since the mass flow rate of inspired gas is the same at every generation (because the airways are simply a conducting system), the forward velocity of O_2 molecules falls (since flow rate is the product of velocity and cross-sectional area). As it happens, by about generations 17 to 19, where the alveoli are just beginning to appear, this forward velocity has become so low that passage of O_2 from here on out to the alveoli is heavily dependent on simple gaseous diffusion, not just on continuing convective flow.
4. If alveoli are not equally ventilated with gas (and equally perfused with blood), their alveolar O_2 concentration will differ, as explained later in this chapter. Because adjacent alveoli are so physically close, there can be considerable diffusion of O_2 between such alveoli when their O_2 levels are different. This passive process tends to reduce concentration differences between these alveoli. However, although it can be detected experimentally, it is of probably minor clinical significance. Step 3 (and to some extent Step 4) are responsible for most of the alveolar gas mixing that must occur for gas exchange to take place—that is, the mixing of each breath of newly inspired gas with alveolar gas still present from prior breaths.
5. The heart acts as a massaging pump to further enhance gas mixing into the alveolar gas spaces. Alternate filling and emptying of the cardiac chambers respectively facilitates exhaling and inhaling of airway gas into those alveoli physically close to the heart,[5] but has little effect on more distant alveoli. Although a well-known and easily demonstrated phenomenon, this so-called cardiogenic mixing is probably also of minimal physiological impact for gas exchange.
6. Once the dominant convective and diffusive gas transport steps have brought O_2 from the lips to the alveolar gas spaces, O_2 physically dissolves in the tissues separating alveolar gas from capillary blood, the blood–gas barrier (Fig. 14-1). O_2 then moves by diffusion through the blood–gas barrier and into the plasma. Over 98% of these O_2 molecules diffuse further, that is, into the red cell interior, and then bind rapidly to hemoglobin. The remaining 2% or so remain physically dissolved in the plasma and red cell water.

   This transport process from alveolar gas to hemoglobin is accomplished passively by simple diffusion: No convective forces or active transport processes are involved. The diffusion process is discussed more fully in Chapter 16. In normal lungs at rest, this process is very rapid and causes no O_2 transport limitation.
7. Finally, the red cells are transported convectively by cardiac pumping action out of the pulmonary capillaries and into the pulmonary veins and then to the left atrium, and left ventricle, finally reaching the various body tissues.

Parabolic (laminar) flow profile

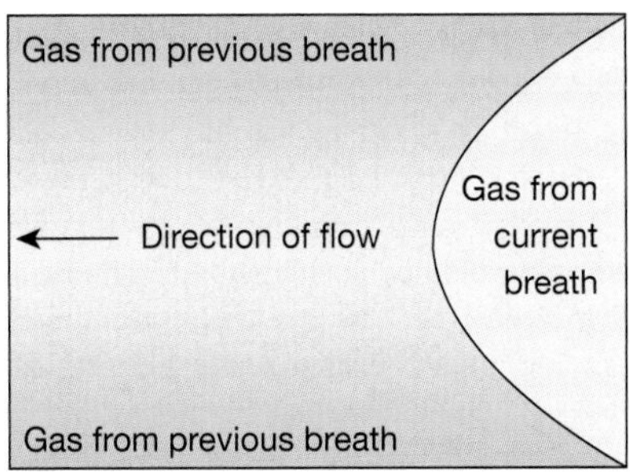

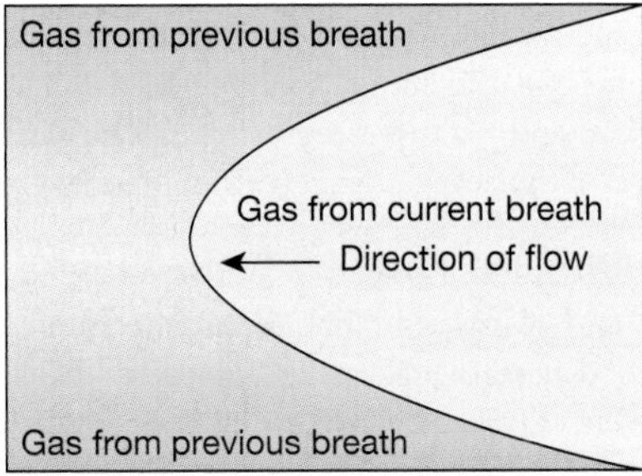

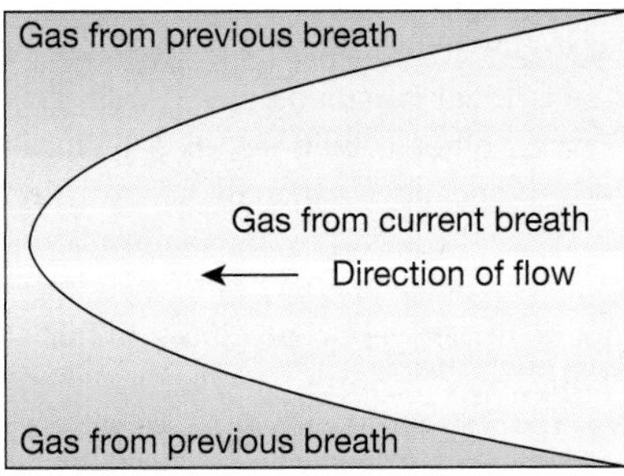

Figure 14-3 The parabolic profile of laminar flow. The three panels indicate sequential points in time during a single inspiration proceeding from right to left. Because the gas remaining from the previous breath has a low oxygen concentration and high CO_2 concentration relative to that of the inspired gas in the current breath, there will be diffusive exchange between the parabolic tongue and the surrounding gas (Taylor dispersion).

POTENTIAL DISRUPTIONS OF THE GAS TRANSPORT PATHWAY

If all the above elements of the transport pathway mentioned previously were functionally perfect, the partial pressure of O_2 (and other gases) would be identical in the gas of all 300 million alveoli and equal to that in systemic arterial blood. The system comes close to perfection in health,[6] but there is never complete equivalence of alveolar and arterial pressures, even in healthy young, normal people. Aging further leads to a progressive impairment of the pathway with arterial P_{O_2} falling from 95 to 100 mm Hg at age 20 to 75 to 80 mm Hg at age 80 or thereabouts.[7] However, alveolar P_{O_2} tends to be invariant with age. Thus, the difference between alveolar and arterial P_{O_2} steadily increases from about 5 to 10 mm Hg to about 20 to 25 mm Hg over this age range. Pulmonary diseases such as asthma, emphysema and bronchitis, fibrosis, pneumonia, and many others can greatly disrupt gas transport to the point of causing death from insufficient tissue O_2 supply.

Consequently, it is essential to have a good understanding of the O_2 transport pathway and what may affect it even in health, in order to appreciate the problems seen in pulmonary diseases.

A traditional view of how to consider abnormalities of the transport pathway has evolved over the years and is very useful as a framework for discussion. It is based upon the end result of gas exchange – the arterial P_{O_2} – and there are different reasons why this variable can fall below normal values.

Four principal potential mechanisms of failure of the O_2 transport pathway can lead to a reduced arterial P_{O_2} (i.e., to arterial hypoxemia):

1. Hypoventilation
2. Diffusion limitation
3. Shunt
4. Ventilation–perfusion ($\dot{V}A/\dot{Q}$) inequality.

These are the so-called "intrapulmonary" factors that directly cause hypoxemia. Modulating "extrapulmonary" factors are also important. These include changes in inspired O_2 concentration, in total cardiac output, in overall metabolic rate, and in Hb concentration.

The four "intrapulmonary" factors are now defined and discussed.

HYPOVENTILATION

Normal levels of ventilation produce a tightly regulated arterial P_{CO_2} at 40 ± 2 mm Hg in normal subjects with several control systems in place to ensure this (for details, see Chapter 11). However, if overall ventilation is reduced for any reason, alveolar P_{CO_2} (PA_{CO_2}), and therefore arterial P_{CO_2}, must rise to maintain constant the elimination of metabolically produced CO_2. Reciprocally, alveolar P_{O_2} (PA_{O_2}), and hence arterial P_{O_2}, will fall (and by relatively similar amounts as P_{CO_2} will rise). The alveolar gas equation[8] quantitatively relates PA_{O_2} and PA_{CO_2}, and is used to calculate how much PA_{O_2} will change for a change in PA_{CO_2}:

$$PA_{O_2} = PI_{O_2} - \frac{Pa_{CO_2}}{R} + PA_{CO_2} \cdot FI_{O_2} \cdot \frac{(1-R)}{R} \qquad (1)$$

PI_{O_2} and FI_{O_2} are inspired O_2 partial pressure and fractional concentration, respectively, and R is the respiratory exchange ratio, normally 0.8.

Hypoventilation represents a failure of step 1 of the gas transport pathway (see above) and can occur for several reasons: (1) the control centers in the nervous system that regulate ventilation could malfunction due to trauma, diseases, drugs, or anesthetics; (2) there could be neuronal or neuromuscular dysfunction of the nerves supplying the chest wall muscles of respiration; (3) the chest wall muscles could be fatigued, damaged, or paralyzed; or (4) the airways or chest wall could be disrupted from trauma or other mechanical derangement such as compression, or in the case of airways, obstruction.

Conceptually this type of problem is usually thought of as a whole-lung issue, usually with obvious causes, and can be reversed by recognizing the cause and taking appropriate reparative and/or ventilatory supportive steps.

DIFFUSION LIMITATION

Whereas diffusive transport plays a recognizable, if small, role within the airways and alveolar gas (see above), the concept of diffusive limitation affecting arterial P_{O_2} is more usually associated with transport step 6 – diffusion of O_2 from alveolar gas into the capillary and red cell.

This topic is specifically the focus of Chapter 16 and is not dealt with here. Indeed, the ensuing discussion of other factors sets aside diffusion limitation of O_2 transport for the sake of simplicity and assumes that the diffusive exchange of O_2 (and CO_2) between alveolar gas and capillary blood proceeds to completion within a single red cell's passage through the pulmonary microcirculation. This is reasonable under most conditions. Diffusion limitation in health is seen at sea level in some but not all athletes[9] but only at or near maximal exercise. It is universally seen in normal subjects exercising at altitude.[10,11]

SHUNT

A shunt is a blood pathway that does not allow any contact between alveolar gas and red cells, so that no gas exchange occurs in the affected region. Consequently, blood passes through a shunt maintaining a mixed venous blood composition. When this blood reaches pulmonary veins, the left atrium and eventually arterial blood, it mixes with other blood that has undergone alveolar gas exchange. The result is a fall in arterial P_{O_2} and potentially an increase in arterial P_{CO_2} (arterial P_{CO_2} may not increase if the patient raises his or her level of ventilation, but hypoxemia will persist).

Classical pathophysiological scenarios giving rise to shunts are: (1) pulmonary edema, which fills alveoli with fluid, thereby abolishing their ventilation and any gas exchange; (2) alveolar filling with cellular and micro-organismal debris as in pneumonia, with the same result as in edema; (3) collapse of a region of lung due to pneumothorax, gas absorption distal to a fully obstructed airway, or to external compression; (4) rarely, the presence of abnormal arteriovenous vascular channels in the lungs, that can occur in, for example, hepatic cirrhosis; and (5) direct right-to-left vascular communications at the level of the heart or great (extrapulmonary) blood vessels.

VENTILATION–PERFUSION ($\dot{V}A/\dot{Q}$) INEQUALITY

The exquisite and complex branching architecture of the airways and of the blood vessels makes the lungs very susceptible to the potential problem of nonuniform distribution of alveolar ventilation and of pulmonary blood flow. Whenever alveoli are ventilated at less than average rates, for example if their feeding airways become partially obstructed for any reason, the ratio of ventilation to blood flow ($\dot{V}A/\dot{Q}$ ratio) will fall (assuming their blood flow does not fall similarly). In certain other conditions, lung regions may suffer a reduction in local blood flow rather than ventilation, so that the $\dot{V}A/\dot{Q}$ ratio rises above the average value in those areas.

Whenever there is a range of $\dot{V}A/\dot{Q}$ ratios in a lung such that the $\dot{V}A/\dot{Q}$ ratio is not identical everywhere, it is said that $\dot{V}A/\dot{Q}$ inequality exists. The pathological cause of $\dot{V}A/\dot{Q}$ inequality does not matter in this definition, nor whether the problem originates in the airways or blood vessels. The principal concept is that, compared to a lung having the same total alveolar ventilation and blood flow, a lung that has $\dot{V}A/\dot{Q}$ inequality will exchange (all) gases in an inefficient manner.[12] The result is hypoxemia and, potentially, hypercapnia (raised arterial P_{CO_2}). A large section of this chapter presents the physiological reasons for this effect of $\dot{V}A/\dot{Q}$ inequality.

Understanding of $\dot{V}A/\dot{Q}$ inequality can be demanding, but no matter what its pathologic origins, the concepts are similar. $\dot{V}A/\dot{Q}$

inequality can occur at many different scales. Not uncommonly, it can be manifest on a large scale as differences between the right and left lungs. Classical examples of this include unilateral atelectasis, pneumothorax, pulmonary embolus, or pneumonia. All these are relatively common phenomena that can lead to severe gas exchange disturbances. At the other end of the scale, there can be $\dot{V}A/\dot{Q}$ ratio differences between essentially adjacent alveoli. However, research has shown that small groups of contiguous alveoli can maintain functional homogeneity of $\dot{V}A/\dot{Q}$ ratios via rapid gas diffusion rates, possibly augmented by collateral ventilation and/or blood flow.[13] It is likely that all alveoli distal to individual respiratory (or perhaps terminal) bronchioles can retain functional homogeneity for gas exchange through these mechanisms.[14]

In between these two extremes of scale, vascular or airway obstruction at all levels will produce $\dot{V}A/\dot{Q}$ inequality that, depending on how widespread it is, causes hypoxemia and potentially hypercapnia.

Even the young normal lung usually contains $\dot{V}A/\dot{Q}$ inequality, which explains the 5 to 10 mm Hg P_{O_2} difference between alveolar gas and arterial blood generally observed in healthy young subjects.[15] There are several mechanisms for the existence of such $\dot{V}A/\dot{Q}$ inequality.

Gravity-Based Inequality

Ventilation, and, even more so, blood flow are unevenly distributed in a manner systematically influenced by gravity.[6,16] This is due respectively to the weight of the lungs and of the blood in the blood vessels. Thus, dependent lung regions receive far more blood flow than nondependent regions, a finding that is in concept independent of body position. It turns out that the gravitational gradient in blood flow considerably exceeds that of ventilation. As a result, the nondependent lung regions are of higher than average $\dot{V}A/\dot{Q}$ ratio, and the dependent regions are of lower than average $\dot{V}A/\dot{Q}$ ratio.[6] Average $\dot{V}A/\dot{Q}$ ratio is about 1.0, because total alveolar ventilation and blood flow are similar. At the apex of the upright human lung, the $\dot{V}A/\dot{Q}$ ratio is about 3; at the base it is about 0.6, 5-fold lower. There is a smooth gradation between the two extremes as depicted in Figure 14-4. This large-scale apex-to-base gradient in $\dot{V}A/\dot{Q}$ ratios does not produce more than about a 4 mm Hg drop in arterial P_{O_2} (compared to expectations in the absence of this phenomenon), and thus a 4 mm Hg alveolar–arterial P_{O_2} difference.[6]

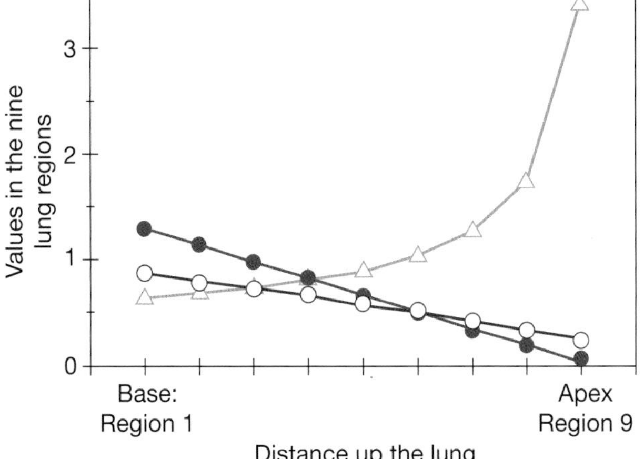

Figure 14-4 Topographical relationships between ventilation and blood flow as a function of distance up and down the upright lung (divided into nine contiguous regions). Although both ventilation and blood flow are higher at the base than at the apex, the ventilation–perfusion ratio ($\dot{V}A/\dot{Q}$) rises exponentially from the bottom to the top of the lung. *(Adapted with permission from West JB. Ventilation/blood flow and gas exchange, 5th ed. Chicago, IL. Blackwell Scientific Publications; 1990.)*

Fractally Based $\dot{V}A/\dot{Q}$ Inequality

The branching airway and blood vessel structure of the lung constitutes a fractal system that is innately susceptible to $\dot{V}A/\dot{Q}$ inequality independent of gravity.[17] A fractal system is one in which the geometric pattern (e.g., of airway branching) is repeated at ever smaller scales. In the case of the airway tree it means in essence that the division of an airway into two "daughter" branches is a repeating feature from the large to the small airways. With some 23 sequential orders of branching, very small random inequalities in gas or blood flow distribution repeated at each branch point of the system can rapidly escalate into very significant degrees of nonuniform ventilation or blood flow. To illustrate, consider a branching system of just 16 dichotomous sequences—at each of the 16 branch points, air is not precisely split 50/50 between each daughter pair. Rather, suppose a 49%/51% split—a nonuniform effect of trivial proportions at any one airway branch. The most poorly ventilated regions (receiving 49% of the split at every one of the 16 branchings) end up with only about half as much ventilation as the best ventilated regions that receive 51% of the split at each branch.

Unless the fractal structure somehow distributes both ventilation and blood flow in a correlated manner to preserve $\dot{V}A/\dot{Q}$ ratios (even as $\dot{V}A$ or $\dot{Q}$ individually vary), significant hypoxemia could result. Understanding the consequences of the fractal nature of the lung is a topic of much current interest. It appears that there must be correlation of $\dot{V}A$ with $\dot{Q}$ since the large potential for fractally based hypoxemia is not generally realized.

Longitudinally Based Inequality

As airways and blood vessels progressively narrow with each branch point, resistance to gas and blood flow increases. Not all alveoli receive gas or blood from airways that have gone through the exact same number of branchings. Hence, some alveoli will be more and some will be less distant from the mouth. Such simple principles suggest the possibility of reduced $\dot{V}A$ and/or $\dot{Q}$ of those alveoli further from the mouth compared to more proximal alveoli, and therefore the chance of a central to peripheral, or longitudinal, gradient in ventilation and blood flow. Although not universally observed, there is a fair amount of evidence that such inequality exists,[18] but its contribution to gas exchange is hard to establish. To the extent that similar physical principles apply to both gas and blood flow in the present context, one can theorize that more distant alveoli have both less ventilation and blood flow, so that again there is a natural tendency to preserve the $\dot{V}A/\dot{Q}$ ratio between central and peripheral regions.

Anatomically Based Inequality

Another potential reason for nonuniform gas or blood flow distribution is intrinsic anatomical differences between lung regions. Perhaps the best example is in the dog and horse where, independent of body position in relation to gravity, the dorsal regions of the lower lobes often can be shown to have an unduly high share of total pulmonary perfusion. This tendency, presumably based on the overall branching architectural differences between lobes or within lobes, becomes important in concept when patients are moved from one body position to another, in order to best understand consequent changes in gas exchange.[19]

Collateral Ventilation and Blood Flow

To this point, a picture has been painted of a branching architecture that has no lateral connections between either adjacent airways or blood vessels at any level of branching. Such lateral connections can exist at several airway levels from large airways down to alveoli.[13,20] This is a species-dependent phenomenon, so that while the pig has little or no such collateral pathway structures, the dog has extensive collateral ventilatory channels. Humans are somewhere between these extremes.

Whatever the evolutionary pressure for collateral channel development, the ability to move gas around obstructions in airways by the use of collateral channels appears to be a useful property of human lungs. This is because total airway obstruction in the absence of collateral channels often leads to rapid alveolar gas absorption into the blood from the alveoli distal to the obstructed airway, and this in turn leads to atelectasis and therefore vascular shunts and hypoxemia. Remarkably, chronic human lung diseases typified by airway obstruction – chronic obstructive pulmonary disease (COPD), asthma – produce $\dot{V}_A/\dot{Q}$ inequality due to presence of poorly ventilated areas, but only uncommonly lead to true shunts.[21,22] The likely explanation for the paucity of shunts in COPD and asthma is the existence of collateral ventilation.

Collateral ventilation in man therefore appears to be a naturally occurring structural phenomenon that can to some extent counteract the gas exchange consequences of diseases.

Collateral perfusion must also occur in the alveolar capillary network. This is deduced simply from the richly interconnecting microvascular network that has the potential to allow blood to flow easily around microvascular obstructions into adjacent vessels. Just how much collateral blood flow potential exists at a larger scale is not clear, being difficult to study. However, well-documented connections occur between the bronchial and pulmonary circulations,[23] creating a different kind of collateral circulatory network. The importance of this connection is evident when the pulmonary artery is either absent or embolized. Then, the bronchial circulation expands considerably and can support function of the affected lung regions long term.

Reactive Vasoconstriction and Bronchoconstriction

The distribution of ventilation or blood flow in the lung can be modified by vasoreactive or bronchoreactive functional changes that appear triggered by changes in alveolar gas composition. The most well-documented phenomenon is that of hypoxic pulmonary vasoconstriction.[24,25] Here, in response to local alveolar hypoxia produced by locally reduced ventilation, local pulmonary arterial constriction reduces blood flow in the hypoxic region. Whether this system developed to counteract disease or to cope with intrauterine life and the abrupt transition to air-breathing is arguable, although most people favor the latter explanation.

Irrespective of the reasons, the effect of hypoxic vasoconstriction is to help return the local ratio of ventilation to blood flow towards normal. This automatic effect (mediated by O_2-sensitive potassium channels in pulmonary arterial smooth muscle cells) is rarely able to fully restore $\dot{V}_A/\dot{Q}$ ratios to normal, but even partial improvements in $\dot{V}_A/\dot{Q}$ ratio facilitate gas exchange significantly. The negative aspect of hypoxic vasoconstriction is a rise in pulmonary vascular resistance. If this is substantial and protracted over time, pulmonary arterial hypertension can develop, eventually leading to right heart failure. However, factors other than hypoxic vasoconstriction are then also generally present – microvascular destruction and alveolar distortion – and these may be more important to heart failure than hypoxia per se. However, hypoxic vasoconstriction has provided a rationale for enriched O_2 therapy in patients with chronic disease to reduce the severity, or to delay the progression, of pulmonary hypertension.

To a much less obvious extent, a counterpart to hypoxic vasoconstriction occurs in the airways: hypocapnic bronchoconstriction.[26] Here, especially when pulmonary embolism occurs, the $\dot{V}_A/\dot{Q}$ ratio in the embolized area rises due to loss of blood flow from vascular obstruction. This increase in $\dot{V}_A/\dot{Q}$ ratio leads to a lower local P_{CO_2} (see below), which causes bronchoconstriction in the local area. This reduces local ventilation and thus tends to normalize the local $\dot{V}_A/\dot{Q}$ ratio. Radioactive tracer ventilation scans may show evidence of this as a modest reduction in the ventilation of embolized regions.

THE $\dot{V}_A/\dot{Q}$ RATIO AND GAS EXCHANGE

To this point, much space has been given to the concepts underlying the distribution of ventilation ($\dot{V}_A$), blood flow ($\dot{Q}$), and hence their ratio, $\dot{V}_A/\dot{Q}$. The reason for this lies in the importance of $\dot{V}_A/\dot{Q}$ ratios to the basic function of the lung—to exchange O_2 and CO_2 between the blood and the air. $\dot{V}_A/\dot{Q}$ inequality, no matter what its physiological basis or pathological cause, interferes with gas exchange and causes hypoxemia and sometimes hypercapnia.

The following section will explain the relationship of $\dot{V}_A/\dot{Q}$ inequality to gas exchange. The subject is complex and must be considered at several "concentric" levels. To start, we will consider how the $\dot{V}_A/\dot{Q}$ ratio in a small local lung region controls local P_{O_2}, P_{CO_2}, and therefore how much O_2 and CO_2 are exchanged in that region. This isolated approach requires at first some key assumptions. Removing the restrictions of these assumptions is the next "concentric" step in understanding $\dot{V}_A/\dot{Q}$ relationships. A final outer shell of modifying factors that can further affect gas exchange forms a third level of the analysis.

THE $\dot{V}_A/\dot{Q}$ RATIO OF A SMALL HOMOGENEOUS UNIT OF LUNG AND GAS EXCHANGE

How the $\dot{V}_A/\dot{Q}$ ratio determines gas exchange is best explained by considering the flux of O_2 from the environment into and out of the alveolus with each breath as well as from the alveolar gas into the capillary blood. Equations that describe these processes and follow the fundamental principle of mass conservation must be used. Original descriptions of these appeared more than 50 years ago.[8,27–30] Figure 14-5 provides a model of the lung and specifies the total ventilation ($\dot{V}_A$) and blood flow ($\dot{Q}$) of this model together with the key locations of the relevant O_2 levels. It can be used to consider a small homogeneous unit of lung.

Convention has long considered ventilation over a period of time as a constant in spite of the tidal nature of breathing. This is in fact a very reasonable approximation that has stood the test of

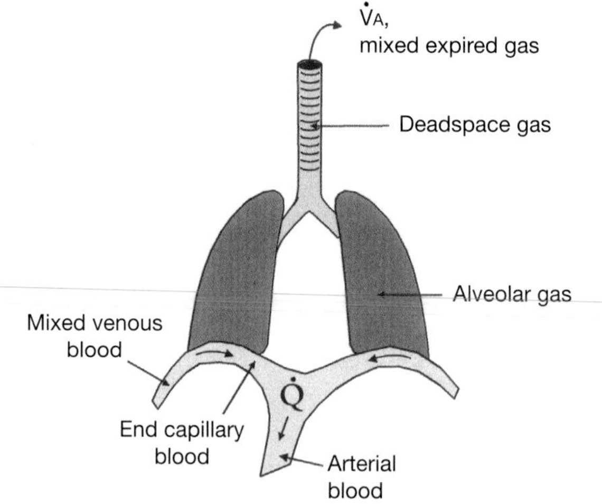

Figure 14-5 Conceptual model of the lungs indicating main sites in which oxygen and carbon dioxide partial pressures are different, together with the principal convective processes accomplishing gas exchange, ventilation ($\dot{V}_A$), and blood flow ($\dot{Q}$).

time. Similarly, blood flow is considered constant, and this too has proved reasonable. If $\dot{V}A$ and $\dot{Q}$ are therefore considered as alveolar minute ventilation and blood flow of a small homogeneous unit respectively, the following simple mass conservation equations can be written for O_2:

$$\dot{V}_{O_2} = \dot{V}I \cdot FI_{O_2} - \dot{V}A \cdot FA_{O_2} \quad (2)$$

and

$$\dot{V}_{O_2} = Q \cdot Cc'_{O_2} - \dot{Q} \cdot C\overline{v}_{O_2} \quad (3)$$

In these equations, $\dot{V}_{O_2}$ is amount of O_2 transferred from the environment into the blood per unit time and, given the assumption of steady state conditions, this, when summed over all such units in the lungs, equals metabolic rate. $\dot{V}I$ and $\dot{V}A$ are, respectively, the inspired and expired volumes of gas respired per minute, less than the amount remaining in the conducting airways. As anticipated, $\dot{V}I$ and $\dot{V}A$ are close to being identical, otherwise the lungs would blow up or collapse in a short period of time. However, $\dot{V}I$ does not generally equal $\dot{V}A$ because slightly more O_2 is consumed per minute than is CO_2 produced (i.e., the respiratory quotient is in general not 1.0). Thus, $\dot{V}A = \dot{V}I - \dot{V}O_2 + \dot{V}_{CO_2}$. Mostly, the inequality of $\dot{V}I$ and $\dot{V}A$ can be ignored because the difference is only about 1%—if $\dot{V}I$ is 6 L/min and $\dot{V}O_2$ is 300 mL/min with $\dot{V}_{CO_2}$ at 240 mL/min, $\dot{V}A =$ 5.94 L/min. Although this small difference is not ignored in research applications, it can be for the present purposes, so that $\dot{V}I$ is replaced by $\dot{V}A$ in Equation (1), simplifying the analysis. In Equation (1), FI_{O_2} and FA_{O_2} are the fractional concentrations (F) of O_2 in inspired (I) and exhaled alveolar (A) gas, respectively, from a small unit in Figure 14-5. In Equation (2), Cc'_{O_2} and $C\overline{v}_{O_2}$ are the O_2 concentrations (C) in the oxygenated end capillary blood leaving (c′) and the deoxygenated blood entering ($\overline{v}$) the vasculature respectively. The abbreviation c′ stands for end capillary blood; $\overline{v}$ for mixed venous (pulmonary arterial) blood.

Since Equations (1) and (2) both describe the same O_2 flux rate ($\dot{V}_{O_2}$) they may be set equal to each other:

$$\dot{V}A\,[FI_{O_2} - FA_{O_2}] = \dot{Q}\,[Cc'_{O_2} - C\overline{v}_{O_2}] \quad (4)$$

and rearranged so that:

$$\dot{V}A/\dot{Q} = [Cc'_{O_2} - C\overline{v}_{O_2}]/[FI_{O_2} - A_{O_2}] \quad (5)$$

It should further be noted that because diffusion equilibration of O_2 transfer across the alveolar–capillary membrane is assumed to be complete, alveolar P_{O_2} and end capillary P_{O_2} are identical. Hence, the relationship between FA_{O_2} and Cc'_{O_2} is uniquely dictated by the O_2-Hb dissociation curve such that knowing FA_{O_2} allows us to determine directly Cc'_{O_2} (or vice versa).

Equation (5) is very revealing and explains directly the role of the $\dot{V}A/\dot{Q}$ ratio in governing alveolar gas exchange. This equation states that for a given set of what may be called boundary conditions (i.e., composition of inspired gas and mixed venous blood, represented here by FI_{O_2} and $C\overline{v}_{O_2}$, respectively) and for a known O_2–Hb dissociation curve, alveolar (and thus end capillary) P_{O_2} is uniquely determined by the ratio of alveolar ventilation ($\dot{V}A$) to blood flow ($\dot{Q}$).

Under the given assumptions, summarized as (1) continuous and constant ventilation and blood flow; (2) steady state conditions; (3) diffusion equilibration of alveolar–capillary exchange; and (4) equality of inspired and expired ventilation, equations identical in construct to Equation (5) can be written for any gas being exchanged by the lung.

For CO_2, this produces Equation (6):

$$\dot{V}A/\dot{Q} = [C\overline{v}_{CO_2} - Cc'_{CO_2}]/[FA_{CO_2} - FI_{CO_2}] \quad (6)$$

The order of bracketed terms on the right is reversed to maintain positive numbers, since CO_2 is being eliminated from the blood. Of course, FI_{CO_2} is essentially zero and thus drops out of the equation.

Unfortunately, neither Equation (5) nor (6) is amenable to simple quantitative solutions, because of the complexity of the O_2 and CO_2 dissociation curves. The equations are however readily explored by appropriate computerized numerical analyses.[31–35] Using such programs, one can explore the relationship between $\dot{V}A/\dot{Q}$ ratio and alveolar P_{O_2} and P_{CO_2}, and this is done in Figure 14-6. These relationships are important because they indicate what degrees of $\dot{V}A/\dot{Q}$ abnormality are required to affect gas exchange for both O_2 and CO_2. The four panels of Figure 14-6 show alveolar P_{O_2} and P_{CO_2} as well as end capillary O_2 and CO_2 concentrations. The latter better reflect total gas exchange as a function of $\dot{V}A/\dot{Q}$ ratio. Specific conditions for Figure 14-6 are that mixed venous blood P_{O_2} is 40 mm Hg and P_{CO_2} 45 mm Hg, normal resting values. Also, inspired gas is room air, and [Hb] is 15 g/dL. In each panel, the three solid circles are positioned at the normal $\dot{V}A/\dot{Q}$ ratio (of about 1.0) and at $\dot{V}A/\dot{Q}$ ratios 10 times greater and less. All four relationships are highly non-linear. Focusing on the two lower panels, it is evident for O_2 that a 10-fold reduction in $\dot{V}A/\dot{Q}$ greatly reduces local O_2 transport, whereas a 10-fold increase barely improves it. Furthermore, as $\dot{V}A/\dot{Q}$ falls even lower than 0.1, there is little further loss in O_2 transport. There is however little protection against a fall in $\dot{V}A/\dot{Q}$ below 1.0, because the curve is very steep below a $\dot{V}A/\dot{Q}$ of 1.0, as the lower left panel shows. For CO_2, the curves are opposite in slope (P_{CO_2} falls as $\dot{V}A/\dot{Q}$ increases).

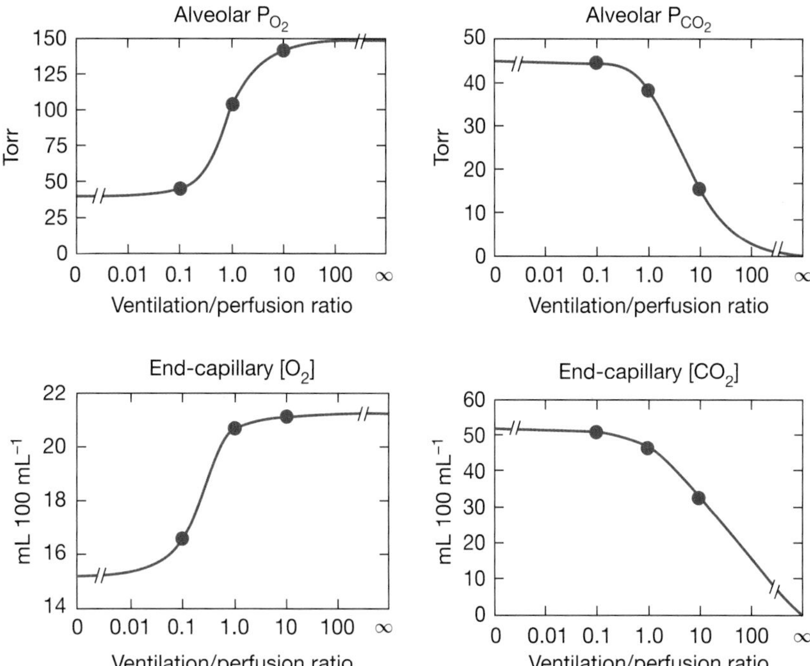

Figure 14-6 Calculated relationships between alveolar P_{O_2} and P_{CO_2} and the ventilation–perfusion ratio *(top panels)* and their corresponding end-capillary blood concentrations *(lower panels)*. The three solid circles in each case represent values for ventilation–perfusion ratios of 0.1, 1.0, and 10. (See text for further details.)

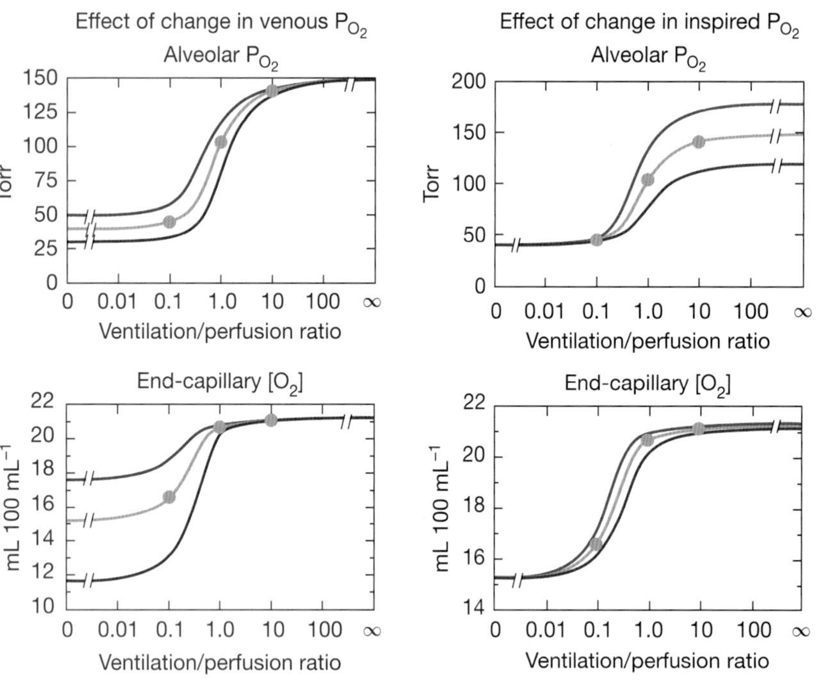

Figure 14-7 Effects of changes in mixed venous P_{O_2} *(left panels)* or inspired P_{O_2} *(right panels)* on alveolar P_{O_2} and associated end-capillary oxygen concentrations. Note that changes in venous P_{O_2} mostly affect values associated with low ventilation–perfusion ratios, whereas changes in inspired P_{O_2} affect units throughout the $\dot{V}_A/\dot{Q}$ range, especially those with medium to high $\dot{V}_A/\dot{Q}$ ratios.

However, unlike the case for O_2, there is little difference between a $\dot{V}_A/\dot{Q}$ of 1.0 and a 10-fold reduction, whereas an increase in $\dot{V}_A/\dot{Q}$ considerably reduces alveolar P_{CO_2} and end capillary CO_2 concentration. The reason for the differences between O_2 and CO_2 lies mainly in the slopes of their dissociation curves: that for CO_2 is about 10-fold greater than that for O_2. It has been shown that the higher the slope of the dissociation curve (or equivalently for an anesthetic gas, its solubility) the more it is sensitive to areas of high $\dot{V}_A/\dot{Q}$. The lower the slope or solubility, the more the gas is affected by areas of low $\dot{V}_A/\dot{Q}$. Consequently, areas of low $\dot{V}_A/\dot{Q}$ predictably cause more reduction in arterial P_{O_2} than increase in arterial P_{CO_2}. Although Figure 14-6 is true strictly only for the stated "boundary" conditions (i.e., mixed venous blood and inspired gas composition), the principles hold even for different such conditions, as shown in Figure 14-7 for O_2. The left panels illustrate how changes in mixed venous P_{O_2} alone will affect alveolar P_{O_2} and end capillary $[O_2]$ via Equation (4). The right panels correspondingly show how change in inspired P_{O_2} affects O_2. Venous P_{O_2} is selected at 30, 40, and 50 mm Hg, and inspired P_{O_2} is chosen to be 120, 150, and 180 mm Hg. Changes in venous P_{O_2} dramatically affect P_{O_2} and $[O_2]$ in unventilated and poorly ventilated regions as well as regions approaching normal, but have no real effect on high $\dot{V}_A/\dot{Q}$ alveoli. Altering inspired P_{O_2} (but not venous) has the converse effect if P_{O_2} is examined (top right panel), but, due to the nonlinear shape of the O_2–Hb dissociation curve, effects on $[O_2]$ are minimal in high $\dot{V}_A/\dot{Q}$ areas, small in very low $\dot{V}_A/\dot{Q}$ areas, and more significant between $\dot{V}_A/\dot{Q}$ ratios of 0.1 and 1.0 (bottom right panel). This figure shows how the inspired and mixed venous "boundary conditions" alter the magnitude (but not basic patterns) of alveolar gas exchange.

If one returns to the normal boundary conditions ($P\bar{v}_{O_2}$ = 40 mm Hg, PI_{O_2} = 150 mm Hg), one can explore the consequences of $\dot{V}_A/\dot{Q}$ inequality on gas exchange. In reality, the complex structure of the lungs defies a simple analysis but conceptually even a two-compartment model is an invaluable aid to understanding this conceptually difficult area.

Figure 14-8 shows such a simple two-compartment model in three configurations: (1) each compartment equally ventilated and perfused such that there is no $\dot{V}_A/\dot{Q}$ inequality; (2) the left compartment hypoventilated due to airway obstruction, causing $\dot{V}_A/\dot{Q}$ inequality; and (3) the left compartment hypoperfused from vascular obstruction. Table 14-1 shows the corresponding O_2 and CO_2 calculations for each compartment. Specific assumptions common to all three models are (1) the mixed venous P_{O_2} remains at 40 mm Hg; inspired P_{O_2} is constant at 150 mm Hg; total alveolar ventilation summed over both compartments is constant as is total blood flow, both taken to be 6 L/min; [Hb] is constant at 15 g/dL. Further, airways obstruction reduces L-hand compartmental ventilation from 3.0 to 0.3 L/min, redistributing the balance to the R-hand compartment. Vascular obstruction is of the same order as the right panel of the figure shows. Note that for both obstructive models, one compartment has developed a $\dot{V}_A/\dot{Q}$ ratio less than average and the other a $\dot{V}_A/\dot{Q}$ ratio greater than average, irrespective of the location of the obstruction.

Using the curves of Figure 14-6, for $P\bar{v}_{O_2}$ = 40 mm Hg and PI_{O_2} = 150 mm Hg, $P\bar{v}_{CO_2}$ = 45 mm Hg and PI_{CO_2} = 0 mm Hg, alveolar P_{O_2} and P_{CO_2} are listed for each compartment of Figure 14-8 in Table 14-1.

In Table 14-1, alveolar diffusion equilibration is assumed to be complete such that alveolar P_{O_2} (PA_{O_2}) equals end capillary P_{O_2} (Pc'_{O_2}); the same holds for P_{CO_2}. In each obstructive model, the low $\dot{V}_A/\dot{Q}$ compartment has a lower-than-average P_{O_2} and higher-than-average P_{CO_2} as Figure 14-6 dictates. The converse is seen for the compartment of high $\dot{V}_A/\dot{Q}$ ratio. Corresponding end capillary O_2 and CO_2 concentrations are also listed in Table 14-1.

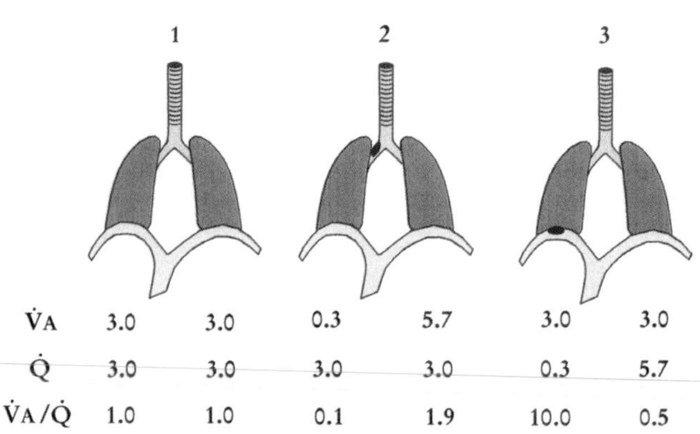

Figure 14-8 Three two-compartment models of ventilation–perfusion relationships. *Model 1* represents an ideal lung without ventilation–perfusion mismatch. *Model 2* represents a lung in which one compartment has a 90% reduction in its alveolar ventilation due to airway obstruction, and *Model 3* is a lung in which one compartment has a 90% reduction in capillary blood flow due to vascular obstruction. Ventilation, blood flow, and ventilation–perfusion ratio of each compartment are indicated. Total ventilation and total blood flow remain the same among the three models. (See text for further details.)

TABLE 14-1 O_2 and CO_2 Calculations for the Models of Figure 14-8

	Normal		Airway Obstruction Model		Vascular Obstruction Model	
	Left	Right	Left	Right	Left	Right
P_{AO_2}, Pc'_{O_2}, mm Hg	103.0	103.0	45.0	120.0	142.0	77.0
P_{ACO_2}, Pc'_{CO_2}, mm Hg	38.8	38.8	44.9	32.5	15.5	42.7
Cc'_{O_2}, mL·dL^{-1}	20.7	20.7	16.7	20.9	21.1	20.1
Cc'_{CO_2}, mL·dL^{-1}	46.9	46.9	50.8	43.9	32.5	48.8
Ca_{O_2}, mL·dL^{-1}	20.7		18.8		20.1	
Ca_{CO_2}, mL·dL^{-1}	46.9		47.5		48.0	
Pa_{O_2}, mm Hg	103.0		55.0		77.0	
Pa_{CO_2}, mm Hg	38.8		39.0		40.9	
$P\bar{A}_{O_2}$, mm Hg	103.0		118.0		110.0	
$P\bar{A}_{CO_2}$, mm Hg	38.8		33.7		29.2	
Total O_2 exchange, mL·min^{-1}	328.0		212 (65%)		294 (90%)	
Total CO_2 exchange, mL·min^{-1}	270.0		234 (87%)		203 (75%)	
$P\bar{A}_{O_2}$−Pa_{O_2}, mm Hg	0.0		63.0		33.0	
Pa_{CO_2}−$P\bar{A}_{CO_2}$, mm Hg	0.0		5.0		11.7	

The question is what will the mixed arterial blood and mixed expired gas O_2 and CO_2 levels change to as a result of obstruction of one compartment, and how will this affect the ability of the total system to exchange O_2 and CO_2? To answer these questions one applies simple mixing questions to the two individual compartments [left (L) and right (R)]:

For O_2:

$$P\bar{A}_{O_2} = (PAO_{2L} \cdot \dot{V}A_L + PAO_{2R} \cdot \dot{V}A_R)/(\dot{V}A_L + VA_R)$$

$$Ca_{O_2} = (Cc'O_{2L} \cdot \dot{Q}_L + Cc'O_{2R} \cdot \dot{Q}_R)/(\dot{Q}_L + \dot{Q}_R) \quad (7)$$

For CO_2, identical equations apply. These mixing equations conserve mass and use the principle that the two gas or blood streams combine in a manner proportional to their relative ventilation and blood flow, respectively. Table 14-1 lists the results of these calculations, giving mixed alveolar partial pressure ($P\bar{A}_{O_2}$, $P\bar{A}_{CO_2}$) and mixed arterial concentrations (Ca_{O_2}, Ca_{CO_2}). From the blood–gas concentration, corresponding arterial partial pressures (Pa_{O_2}, Pa_{CO_2}) are read directly off the O_2 and CO_2 dissociation curves. Finally, whole-lung computations of O_2 and CO_2 exchange rates (mL/min) are determined using either Equations (1) or (2) and the mixed alveolar or arterial data respectively, and the mixed alveolar to arterial partial pressure differences expressed for each gas.

The results are very instructive. Both obstructive models result in hypoxemia and slight hypercapnia, but the effects on arterial P_{O_2} and on the alveolar–arterial P_{O_2} difference greatly exceed those for CO_2 due to both shape and slope differences between the dissociation curves of the two gases. Airways obstruction produces more hypoxemia but *less* hypercapnia than the identical degree of vascular obstruction. This reflects the 10-fold greater dissociation curve slope of CO_2 compared to O_2, rendering O_2 relatively more susceptible to the lower $\dot{V}A/\dot{Q}$ areas seen in the airway obstruction model (0.1 vs. 0.5) (Fig. 14-8) and CO_2 relatively more susceptible to the higher $\dot{V}A/\dot{Q}$ areas of vascular obstruction (10.0 vs. 1.9) (Fig. 14-8) as Figure 14-6 would predict.

Both models have impaired overall O_2 and CO_2 exchange (recall that venous blood, inspired gas, total ventilation, and blood flow were all considered fixed and identical for all three models) as a result of the development of $\dot{V}A/\dot{Q}$ mismatch. In keeping with the differential sensitivity of O_2 and CO_2 to regions of low and high $\dot{V}A/\dot{Q}$ discussed earlier, total O_2 transport is diminished to a greater extent in the airway obstruction model than in the vascular obstruction model (Table 14-1). The converse is true for CO_2, also shown in Table 14-1.

The principal effects of $\dot{V}A/\dot{Q}$ inequality as they apply to O_2 and CO_2 exchange may thus be listed.

$\dot{V}A/\dot{Q}$ inequality:

a. Affects both gases, no matter what the pathological basis of the inequality.
b. Causes arterial hypoxemia and hypercapnia.
c. Causes usually more severe hypoxemia than hypercapnia.
d. Affects O_2 more than CO_2 when very low $\dot{V}A/\dot{Q}$ regions develop.
e. Affects CO_2 more than O_2 when very high $\dot{V}A/\dot{Q}$ regions develop.
f. Impairs total O_2 and CO_2 exchange by the lung.
g. Creates alveolar–arterial differences for both gases.

COMPENSATION FOR THE EFFECTS OF $\dot{V}A/\dot{Q}$ MISMATCH

The preceding analysis shows that if no changes in total ventilation, blood flow, mixed venous blood, or inspired gas composition occur, O_2 and CO_2 transfer across the lung is compromised. This is not viable in the steady state: the lungs must find a way to restore total O_2 and CO_2 transfer to levels equal to metabolic use of O_2 and production of CO_2. This leads to the next concentric level of consideration of $\dot{V}A/\dot{Q}$ inequality referred to at the start of this section.

Here we ask what compensatory mechanisms exist to achieve restoration of O_2 and CO_2 transfer assuming that the initial pathophysiological insults have persisted unchanged. The same models as in Figure 14-8 and Table 14-1 will be used.

CHANGES IN MIXED VENOUS BLOOD

The only possible short-term compensatory changes are in mixed venous blood, total ventilation, and cardiac output. (Hb change in response to tissue hypoxia requires days to weeks to develop and then is by no means always observed; changing inspired P_{O_2} is not usually an option until the patient seeks medical attention.) To reduce complexity, changes in venous blood alone are first addressed.

TABLE 14-2 Gas Exchange Effects of Passive Changes in Mixed Venous Blood—Gas Values Required to Restore $\dot{V}O_2$ and $\dot{V}CO_2$ to Normal in the Models of Figure 14-8

	Airway Obstruction Model		Vascular Obstruction Model	
	Before Change	After Change	Before Change	After Change
$P\bar{v}_{O_2}$, mm Hg	40.0	30.4	40.0	39.5
$P\bar{v}_{CO_2}$, mm Hg	45.0	50.7	45.0	62.4
Pa_{O_2}, mm Hg	55	46	77	67
Pa_{CO_2}, mm Hg	39.0	44.5	40.9	55.6
$\dot{V}_{O_2}$, mL·min^{-1}	212.0	328 (normal)	294.0	328.0 (normal)
$\dot{V}_{CO_2}$, mL·min^{-1}	234.0	270 (normal)	203.0	270.0 (normal)

If it is assumed that there is no limit to how much O_2 can be extracted from the arterial blood by the peripheral tissues, it is evident that $\dot{V}A/\dot{Q}$ inequality will passively lead to a reduced venous P_{O_2} and increased venous P_{CO_2}. This is deduced simply from the hypoxemia and hypercapnia initially produced by the $\dot{V}A/\dot{Q}$ insult, together with the need to extract the same amount of O_2 from (and add CO_2 to) each mL of blood perfusing the tissues as before the $\dot{V}A/\dot{Q}$ insult developed.

If venous P_{O_2} falls (and P_{CO_2} rises), Figure 14-7 indicates that alveolar P_{O_2} will fall in each $\dot{V}A/\dot{Q}$ compartment (as will P_{CO_2} rise). Thus a circle of events is set up such that if a single red cell were followed around the circulation, at each passage through the lungs and then tissues, P_{O_2} would fall progressively with each circuit of the body.

Although not intuitively obvious, this reduction in both arterial and venous P_{O_2} will not "bottom out" at zero (or in the case of CO_2 rise toward infinity) unless the $\dot{V}A/\dot{Q}$ insult was fatally overwhelming in the first place. Both arterial and venous P_{O_2} will restabilize at new lower values (P_{CO_2} values will be higher) than were present immediately after the $\dot{V}A/\dot{Q}$ insult developed. In so doing, $\dot{V}_{O_2}$ and $\dot{V}_{CO_2}$ will have been restored to normal values.

To explore this quantitatively, we will continue on with the models of Figure 14-8 and Table 14-1 to show just what changes in venous and arterial P_{O_2} and P_{CO_2} must occur as a result of this process in order to restore pulmonary O_2 and CO_2 exchange to normal. The values are shown in Table 14-2. For the airways obstruction model, the passive blood gas changes are greater for O_2 than CO_2, consonant with the greater initial decrement in O_2 exchange caused by airways obstruction in the first place. For the vascular obstruction model, the effects are more marked for CO_2, for corresponding reasons. To restore $\dot{V}_{O_2}$ and $\dot{V}_{CO_2}$ in the airways obstruction model, hypoxemia is now more severe, but hypercapnia is mild. However, with vascular obstruction, hypoxemia remains mild while hypercapnia is severe. In both cases, the lung is meeting the original healthy requirement of transferring 328 and 270 mL/min of O_2 and CO_2, respectively.

The speed of passive venous blood composition changes is very rapid, taking place in seconds to minutes as the blood moves continuously around the vascular system between lungs and tissues. The principal effects of the changes can be summarized as follows:

a. Following development of $\dot{V}A/\dot{Q}$ mismatch, and a fall in $\dot{V}_{O_2}$ and $\dot{V}_{CO_2}$ at the lungs, mixed venous P_{O_2} will fall and mixed venous P_{CO_2} will rise to restore pulmonary $\dot{V}_{O_2}$ and $\dot{V}_{CO_2}$ to equal the original metabolic requirements for O_2 and CO_2 transport.

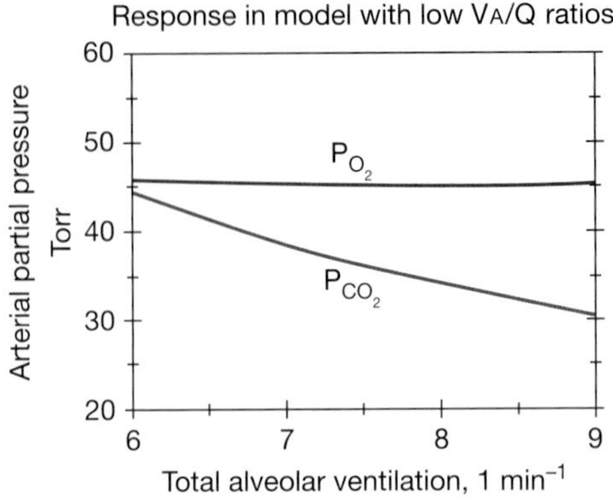

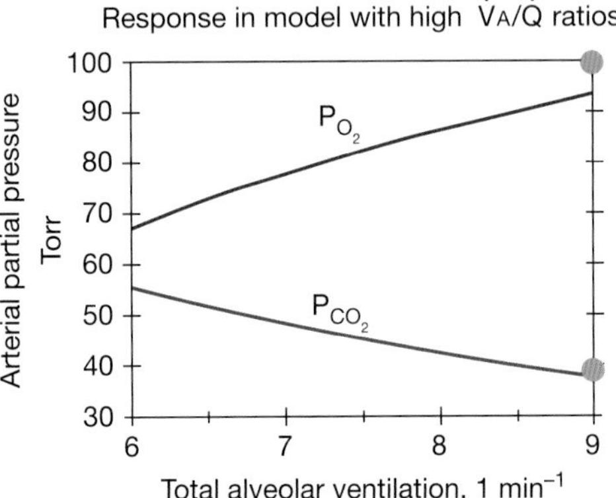

Figure 14-9 Effect of increasing alveolar ventilation on arterial P_{O_2} and P_{CO_2} in the two models with ventilation–perfusion inequalities in Figure 14-8. *Top panel* is that for Model 2 and *bottom panel* is that for Model 3. Increasing ventilation is ineffective in restoring arterial P_{O_2} in the low $\dot{V}A/\dot{Q}$ Model 2, but much more effective in the high $\dot{V}A/\dot{Q}$ Model 3. Both models respond in terms of P_{CO_2}.

b. As a result, there will always be a further fall in arterial P_{O_2} and rise in arterial P_{CO_2}, compared to conditions prior to mixed venous blood changes.

c. When the $\dot{V}A/\dot{Q}$ insult primarily involves development of extremely low $\dot{V}A/\dot{Q}$ areas, those effects are more marked for O_2 than for CO_2.

d. When the $\dot{V}A/\dot{Q}$ insult primarily consists of high $\dot{V}A/\dot{Q}$ areas, CO_2 is affected more than O_2.

CHANGES IN TOTAL VENTILATION

When either low or high $\dot{V}A/\dot{Q}$ areas develop and the mixed venous and arterial adjustments occur as described earlier, there is hypoxemia and hypercapnia. Either or both may well stimulate an immediate increase in total ventilation,[36] which will alleviate to some extent both the hypoxemia and hypercapnia. Figure 14-9 shows for the same two examples used earlier how increases in alveolar ventilation (distributed in the same proportions as in each of the two $\dot{V}A/\dot{Q}$ models of Fig. 14-8) variably improves arterial P_{O_2} and P_{CO_2}. In the low $\dot{V}A/\dot{Q}$ (airways obstruction) model, a 50% increase in total alveolar ventilation from the normal value of 6 to 9 L/min drops arterial P_{CO_2} to almost 30 mm Hg, well below the normal standard value of 40 mm Hg. Arterial P_{O_2}, however, is not affected at all. This is because even a 50% increase in ventilation of the very poorly ventilated unit fails to significantly increase end capillary P_{O_2} of that unit (Fig. 14-6), whereas in the better ventilated unit of that model, Hb in the end capillary blood was already virtually fully saturated before the increase in ventilation.

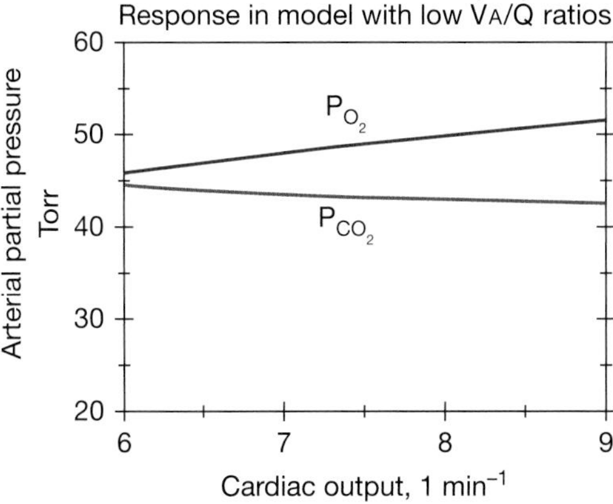

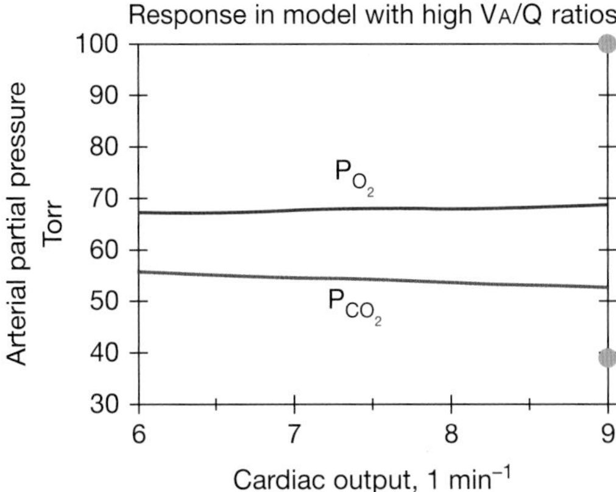

Figure 14-10 Effects of increases in cardiac output on arterial P_{O_2} and P_{CO_2} in Models 2 and 3 of Figure 14-8. Cardiac output produces a significant rise in P_{O_2} in the presence of regions of very low ventilation–perfusion ratio *(top panel)* but has little influence in the presence of higher ventilation–perfusion ratios *(bottom panel)*. P_{CO_2} is affected only minimally in either case.

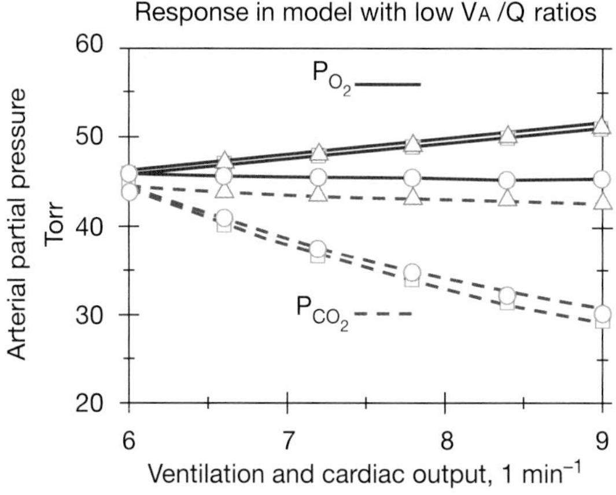

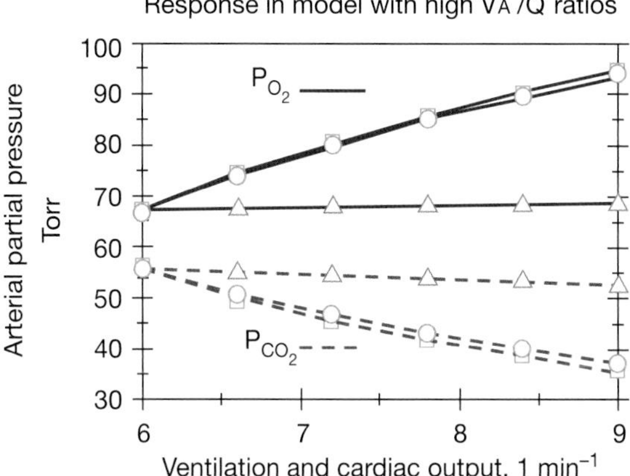

Figure 14-11 Responses to simultaneous increases in ventilation and cardiac output (compared to responses to individual increases as shown in Figs. 14-9 and 14-10). Simultaneous increases do not provide for significantly more improvement than with either alone. o-o, response to increased ventilation only; Δ-Δ, response to increased cardiac output only; □-□, response to simultaneously increased ventilation and cardiac output.

For the model with vascular obstruction, a 50% increase in alveolar ventilation returns both P_{O_2} and P_{CO_2} to near-normal values (Fig. 14-9, lower panel). The difference in the two model responses to ventilation reflects the original $\dot{V}A/\dot{Q}$ ratios of the two compartments—that is, where they lie on the curves of Figure 14-6.

■ CHANGES IN CARDIAC OUTPUT

One final compensatory adjustment is possible—an increase in cardiac output. Adrenergic stimulation by arterial hypoxemia can raise cardiac output by 50% or more, and this will also tend to improve arterial blood gases by raising mixed venous P_{O_2} (and lowering mixed venous P_{CO_2}). Figure 14-10 shows the effects on arterial P_{O_2} and P_{CO_2} of such increases, as was done for ventilation in Figure 14-9, again assuming that the relative distribution of blood flow remains unaltered between the two compartments as total blood flow is increased. For a lung with airways obstruction causing very low $\dot{V}A/\dot{Q}$ regions (upper panel), an increase in cardiac output significantly improves arterial oxygenation—more so than does the same relative increase in ventilation. However, arterial P_{CO_2} is only slightly improved. In stark contrast, increases in cardiac output barely alter arterial P_{O_2} and P_{CO_2} in the high $\dot{V}A/\dot{Q}$ ratio model, especially when it is recalled (Fig. 14-9) how effective an increase in ventilation is in restoring arterial P_{O_2} and P_{CO_2}.

When both ventilation and cardiac output are simultaneously increased, there is no real synergistic effect (Fig. 14-11): P_{O_2} and P_{CO_2} are improved as predicted from the individual changes (i.e., as shown in Figs. 14-9 and 14-10).

In all the calculations depicted in Figures 14-9 to 14-11, the two-compartment models are exchanging the necessary amounts of O_2 and CO_2 to sustain normal metabolism. Depending on (a) the ventilatory and cardiovascular responses to the original insult causing $\dot{V}A/\dot{Q}$ mismatch and (b) the fundamental pattern of $\dot{V}A/\dot{Q}$ mismatch (i.e., the preponderance of low and/or high $\dot{V}A/\dot{Q}$ areas), it is possible to observe hypercapnia, normocapnia, or hypocapnia. However, it is very uncommon for arterial P_{O_2} to be fully normalized by the compensatory mechanisms, and the observed degree of hypoxemia can be extremely variable. As an important clinical corollary, it becomes difficult to establish the severity of the $\dot{V}A/\dot{Q}$ insult per se when the extent of compensating mechanisms cannot be easily established, since these two aspects are so intertwined in their resulting effect on gas exchange.

ASSESSMENT OF VENTILATION–PERFUSION INEQUALITY

Whereas the preceding discussion highlights the complexity of how $\dot{V}A/\dot{Q}$ inequality impairs gas exchange, there is a need for methods to assess the extent of such mismatch in the clinical setting. The multiple inert gas elimination technique was developed expressly for this purpose.[37,38] Although the technique provides the necessary descriptions of the extent and pattern of inequality, it remains a complex technique that is not well suited to routine clinical use. Several traditional quantifying indices of $\dot{V}A/\dot{Q}$ mismatch remain useful on a daily basis. They all make use of O_2 and CO_2 as indicator gases:

1. The first is the alveolar–arterial P_{O_2} difference, $PA_{O_2} - Pa_{O_2}$. This is the difference between alveolar P_{O_2} (PA_{O_2}, calculated from the alveolar gas equation presented subsequently) and the measured arterial P_{O_2} (PA_{O_2}). The $PA_{O_2} - Pa_{O_2}$ is therefore given by

$$PI_{O_2} - Pa_{CO_2}/R + Pa_{CO_2} \cdot FI_{O_2} \cdot (1-R)/R - Pa_{O_2} \quad (8)$$

Use of this equation requires knowledge of inspired P_{O_2} and $[O_2]$, the respiratory exchange ratio R, and the ideal alveolar P_{CO_2}, which is the P_{CO_2} that would be observed in alveolar gas of a homogeneous lung having the R value of the patient's actual lung at the time. Three problems arise with the application of this equation: First, the result is very dependent on PI_{O_2} even when the amount of $\dot{V}A/\dot{Q}$ inequality does not change as PI_{O_2} is varied. Second, the value of R is generally not known and must be assumed. Suppose $P_{CO_2} = 40$ mm Hg and $Pa_{O_2} = 90$ mm Hg for a subject breathing sea level air. If R were 0.7, $PA_{O_2} - Pa_{O_2}$ would be 7 mm Hg (Equation 8). But if R were 1.0, $PA_{O_2} - Pa_{O_2}$ would be 20 mm Hg, a quite different value. Third, in some cases, the usual substitution for the ideal alveolar P_{CO_2}, the measured arterial P_{CO_2}, leads to a systematic error because arterial P_{CO_2} can be significantly higher than the ideal alveolar value. However, $PA_{O_2} - Pa_{O_2}$ remains a very useful index of $\dot{V}A/\dot{Q}$ inequality providing these limitations are kept in mind.
2. The second index is simply the ratio of arterial P_{O_2} to FI_{O_2} which in a perfectly normal lung is virtually insensitive to PI_{O_2}, a major advantage. However, even that is an over-simplification, because this ratio may not be as constant as hoped for depending on the pattern of $\dot{V}A/\dot{Q}$ inequality present.
3. A third index is venous admixture (QsQT) or, equivalently, physiological shunt. This is a parameter that expresses what magnitude shunt would have to be present in a particular case to explain a patient's arterial P_{O_2} if that shunt were the sole cause of hypoxemia. The formula is:

$$\% \text{ QsQT} = 100 \cdot [Cc'_{O_2} - Ca_{O_2}]/[Cc'_{O_2} - C\bar{v}_{O_2}] \quad (9)$$

where Cc'_{O_2} is the calculated end capillary $[O_2]$ of blood perfusing a hypothetical alveolus exchanging gas at the overall respiratory exchange ratio of the patient's actual lungs. Ca_{O_2} is arterial and $C\bar{v}_{O_2}$ mixed venous $[O_2]$, respectively. This parameter, working in the O_2 concentration domain (rather than the partial pressure domain of the $PA_{O_2} - Pa_{O_2}$), better reflects the degree of the gas exchange defect but requires knowledge of the ideal alveolar conditions to calculate Cc'_{O_2}, as well as [Hb]. It also is sensitive to PI_{O_2} in that when $\dot{V}A/\dot{Q}$ inequality is present, its contribution to QsQT diminishes progressively as PI_{O_2} is raised. The most limiting aspect of this parameter however is the need to know the value of $C\bar{v}_{O_2}$, reflecting mixed venous blood. If this must be assumed rather than measured, the value of QsQT will be only as good as the assumption, which may be extremely misleading if changes in $C\bar{v}_{O_2}$ in fact occur but are not accounted for in the QsQT calculation.
4. Finally, as a fourth index, using the arterial and mixed expired partial pressures of CO_2 (Pa_{CO_2}, $P\bar{E}_{CO_2}$, respectively), a very similar calculation to QsQT can be performed to compute the percentage of total ventilation that is wasted on nongas exchanging ("deadspace") areas of the lungs. As for QsQT, the calculation determines the magnitude of the deadspace that would have to be present to dilute the alveolar P_{CO_2} down to the mixed expired level if that deadspace were the only abnormality in ventilation. Expressed as deadspace (VD)/tidal volume (VT) percentage,

$$\% \text{ VD/VT} = 100 \cdot [Pa_{CO_2} - P\bar{E}_{CO_2}]/[Pa_{CO_2}] \quad (10)$$

This parameter is independent of PI_{O_2}, but is weakened by the fact that the normal airway conducting volume is included in the computed result. Thus it may be difficult to separate how much the VD/VT value represents this normal anatomic deadspace as opposed to reflecting $\dot{V}A/\dot{Q}$ inequality amongst the alveoli. This problem is amplified because even normally VD/VT is very dependent on the size of the tidal volume even if the deadspace volume itself is essentially constant. Thus, for a deadspace volume of 150 mL and a tidal volume of 500 mL, VD/VT is 30%, but if tidal volume were to drop to 400 mL, VD/VT now becomes 38%—not because $\dot{V}A/\dot{Q}$ inequality has developed, but simply because smaller breaths are being taken.

In summary, no index of $\dot{V}A/\dot{Q}$ inequality is without potentially significant limitations, both quantitative and qualitative. However, if these limitations are recognized and the data interpreted accordingly, they still remain very useful indices of clinical gas exchange function.

REFERENCES

1. Weibel ER. *Morphometry of the Human Lung*. Berlin: Springer-Verlag; 1963.
2. Weibel ER. *The Pathway for Oxygen*. Cambridge, MA: Harvard University Press; 1984.
3. Engel LA. Chapter 32: Dynamic distribution of gas flow. In: Fishman AP, Macklem PT, Mead J, Geiger SR, eds. Section 3: *The Respiratory System, Handbook of Physiology. Vol. III. Mechanics of Breathing, Part 2*. Bethesda, MD: American Physiological Society; 1986:575–593.
4. Taylor G. Dispersion of soluble matter in solvent flowing slowly through a tube. *Proc R Soc Lond A*. 1953;219(1):186–203.
5. West JB, Hugh-Jones P. Pulsatile gas flow in bronchi caused by the heart beat. *J Appl Physiol*. 1961;16(4):697–702.
6. West JB. *Ventilation/Blood Flow and Gas Exchange*. Oxford and Philadelphia: Blackwell Scientific Publications and Lippincott; 1990.
7. Raine JM, Bishop JM. A-a difference in O_2 tension and physiological dead space in normal man. *J Appl Physiol*. 1963;18(2):284–288.
8. Rahn H, Fenn WO. *A Graphical Analysis of the Respiratory Gas Exchange*. Washington, DC: American Physiological Society; 1955.
9. Powers SK, Lawler J, Dempsey JA, Dodd S, Landry G. Effects of incomplete pulmonary gas exchange on $\dot{V}_{O_2}$ max. *J Appl Physiol*. 1989;66(6):2491–2495.
10. Wagner PD, Gale GE, Moon RE, Torre-Bueno J, Stolp BW, Saltzman HA. Pulmonary gas exchange in humans exercising at sea level and simulated altitude. *J Appl Physiol*. 1986;61(1):260–270.
11. Wagner PD, Sutton JR, Reeves JT, Cymerman A, Groves BM, Malconian MK. Operation Everest II: pulmonary gas exchange during a simulated ascent of Mt. Everest. *J Appl Physiol*. 1987;63(6):2348–2359.
12. West JB. Ventilation-perfusion inequality and overall gas exchange in computer models of the lung. *Respir Physiol*. 1969;7(1):88–110.
13. Menkes HA, Traystman RJ. Collateral ventilation. *Am Rev Respir Dis*. 1977;116(2):287–309.
14. Young I, Mazzone RW, Wagner PD. Identification of functional lung unit in the dog by graded vascular embolization. *J Appl Physiol*. 1980;49(1):132–141.
15. Wagner PD, Laravuso RB, Uhl RR, West JB. Continuous distributions of ventilation-perfusion ratios in normal subjects breathing air and 100% O_2. *J Clin Invest*. 1974;54(1):54–68.

16. Hakim TS, Dean GW, Lisbona R. Effect of body posture on spatial distribution of pulmonary blood flow. *J Appl Physiol.* 1988;64(3):1160–1170.

17. Glenny RW, Lamm WJ, Albert RK, Robertson HT. Gravity is a minor determinant of pulmonary blood flow distribution. *J Appl Physiol.* 1991;71(2):620–629.

18. Wagner P, McRae J, Read J. Stratified distribution of blood flow in the secondary lobule of the lung. *J Appl Physiol.* 1967;22(6):1115–1123.

19. Albert RK, Leasa D, Sanderson M, Robertson HT, Hlastala MP. The prone position improves arterial oxygenation and reduces shunt in oleic-acid-induced acute lung injury. *Am Rev Respir Dis.* 1987;135(3):628–633.

20. Macklem PT. Airway obstruction and collateral ventilation. *Physiol Rev.* 1971;51(2):368–436.

21. Wagner PD, Dantzker DR, Dueck R, Clausen JL, West JB. Ventilation-perfusion inequality in chronic obstructive pulmonary disease. *J Clin Invest.* 1977;59(2):203–216.

22. Wagner PD, Hedenstierna G, Bylin G. Ventilation-perfusion inequality in chronic asthma. *Am Rev Respir Dis.* 1987;136(3): 605–612.

23. Deffebach ME, Widdicombe J. The bronchial circulation. In: Crystal RG, West JB, Barnes PJ, et al., eds. *The Lung: Scientific Foundations.* New York, NY: Raven Press; 1991:741–757.

24. von Euler US, Liejestrand G. Observations on the pulmonary arterial blood pressure in the cat. *Acta Physiol Scand.* 1946;12(4):301–320.

25. Barer GR, Howard P, Shaw JW. Stimulus-response curves for the pulmonary vascular bed to hypoxia and hypercapnia. *J Physiol (Lond).* 1970;211(1):139–155.

26. Newhouse MT, Becklake MR, Macklem PT, MacGregor M. Effect of alterations in end-tidal CO_2 tension on flow resistance. *J Appl Physiol.* 1964;19(4):745–749.

27. Fenn WO, Rahn H, Otis AB. A theoretical study of composition of alveolar air at altitude. *Am J Physiol.* 1946;146:637–653.

28. Riley RL, Cournand A. "Ideal" alveolar air and the analysis of ventilation-perfusion relationships in the lung. *J Appl Physiol.* 1949;1(12):825–847.

29. Riley RL, Cournand A. Analysis of factors affecting partial pressures of oxygen and carbon dioxide in gas and blood of lungs; theory. *J Appl Physiol.* 1951;4(2):77–101.

30. Riley RL, Cournand A, Donald KW. Analysis of factors affecting partial pressures of oxygen and carbon dioxide in gas and blood of lungs; methods. *J Appl Physiol.* 1951;4(2):102–120.

31. Kelman GR. Digital computer subroutine for the conversion of oxygen tension into saturation. *J Appl Physiol.* 1966;21(4):1375–1376.

32. Kelman GR. Digital computer procedure for the conversion of P_{CO_2} into blood CO_2 content. *Respir Physiol.* 1967;3(1): 111–115.

33. Kelman GR. Computer program for the production of O_2-CO_2 diagrams. *Respir Physiol.* 1968;4(2):260–269.

34. Olszowka AJ, Farhi LE. A system of digital computer subroutines for blood gas calculations. *Respir Physiol.* 1968;4(2):270–280.

35. Olszowka AJ, Farhi LE. A digital computer program for constructing ventilation-perfusion lines. *J Appl Physiol.* 1969; 26(1):141–146.

36. Cunningham DJC, Robbins PA, Wolff CB. Chapter 15: Integration of respiratory responses to changes in alveolar partial pressures of CO_2 and O_2 and in arterial pH. In: Fishman AP, Chrniack NS, Widdicombe JG, Greiger SR, eds. *The Respiratory System, Handbook of Physiology.* Vol. II. *Control of Breathing, Part 2.* Bethesda, MD: American Physiological Society; 1986:475–528.

37. Wagner PD, Saltzman HA, West JB. Measurement of continuous distributions of ventilation/perfusion ratios: theory. *J Appl Physiol.* 1974;36(5):588–599.

38. Evans JW, Wagner PD. Limits on $\dot{V}_A/\dot{Q}$ distributions from analysis of experimental inert gas elimination. *J Appl Physiol.* 1977;42(6):889–898.

CHAPTER 15

Blood-Gas Transport

Adrian Shifren
Robert A. Klocke

OXYGEN TRANSPORT

Oxygen is relatively insoluble in aqueous solutions like blood. Dissolved oxygen alone is insufficient to meet the demands of tissue metabolism. Therefore, an alternate means of transporting oxygen is essential. Oxygen binds reversibly to hemoglobin, enhancing the effective solubility of O_2 in blood, and enabling the transport of significant amounts of oxygen—approximately 20 mL/100 mL of blood at a hemoglobin concentration of 150 g/L.

OXYGEN DISSOCIATION CURVE

The oxygen dissociation curve represents the relationship between the oxygen content of blood and the partial pressure of oxygen to which it is exposed (Fig. 15-1).[1] Oxygen content is expressed as the volume of oxygen contained in 100 mL of blood, but may also be expressed as either volumes % or mL/dL. The standard oxygen dissociation curve (Fig. 15-1) demonstrates the effects of oxygen–hemoglobin interaction at standard pH (7.40), temperature (37°C), and atmospheric pressure (760 mm Hg). The blue line at the bottom of the graph in Figure 15-1 shows the amount of oxygen dissolved in blood, and the red line shows the total amount of oxygen in blood at any given oxygen tension. Almost the entire quantity of oxygen transported in blood is bound to hemoglobin. However, the role of dissolved oxygen cannot be ignored. Oxygen diffuses across the alveolar-capillary membrane, enters the plasma, traverses the red cell membrane, and enters the erythrocyte interior—all while dissolved in aqueous solutions. It then combines with hemoglobin enabling the transport of large amounts of oxygen to the metabolizing tissues. Dissolved oxygen, although present in very low concentration in blood, is a critical component of the process of O_2 exchange.

Changes in the quaternary structure of hemoglobin that accompany oxygen binding result in a sigmoid, rather than hyperbolic, oxygen dissociation curve. The S-shaped dissociation curve is the result of changes in oxygen affinity of unbound heme groups following the binding of oxygen to another heme group in the same

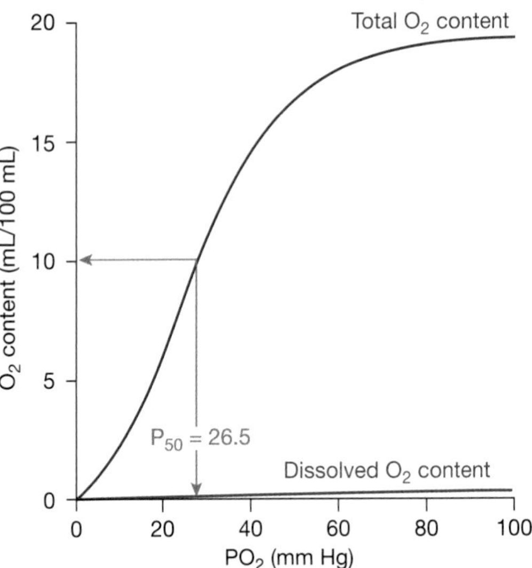

Figure 15-1 Oxygen dissociation curve. Relationship between oxygen content and pressure in normal human blood. The total oxygen content of blood as a function of the partial pressure of oxygen is indicated by the *red line*. The *blue line* indicates the content of dissolved oxygen resulting from changes in P_{O_2}. The partial pressure of oxygen (P_{50}) necessary to saturate one-half of hemoglobin in blood is indicated in *green*.

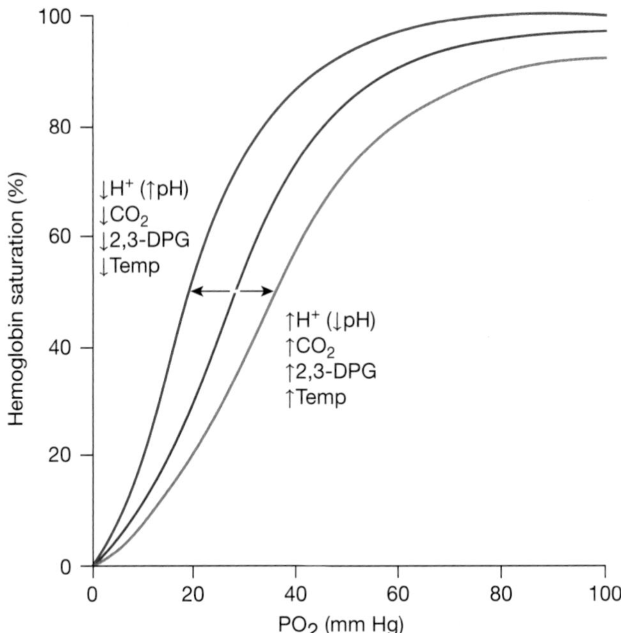

Figure 15-2 Oxygen dissociation curve. The ordinate is % saturation, the percentage of the maximum possible oxygen content. The normal oxygen dissociation curve is shown in *red*. The *blue curve* is shifted to the left of the normal curve (increased oxygen affinity of hemoglobin) as a result of decreased blood hydrogen ion, decreased carbon dioxide, and 2,3-DPG concentrations or decreased temperature. The *green curve* is shifted to the right (decreased oxygen affinity) of the normal curve caused by increases of these factors.

hemoglobin molecule. As illustrated in Figure 15-1, once the partial pressure of oxygen reaches 90 to 100 mm Hg, hemoglobin is almost completely saturated with bound oxygen. There is little additional oxygen binding even at higher oxygen tensions. The flatness of the curve in the arterial oxygen tension range is an advantage because reductions in arterial P_{O_2} (as might be caused by lung disease) will still allow for a relatively normal arterial O_2 content as long as arterial P_{O_2} remains ≥60 mm Hg. The normal partial pressure of oxygen in mixed venous blood at rest is ~40 mm Hg with an oxygen content of ~75% of maximum oxygen capacity. Thus, at rest only one-quarter of the oxygen delivered to body tissues is extracted from blood. However, oxygen extraction varies widely in different tissues. In addition, oxygen utilization changes appreciably during states of increased metabolism. In the tissues, the steep slope of the oxygen dissociation curve between 20 and 60 mm Hg facilitates the release of large amounts of oxygen with relatively moderate decrease in oxygen tension. This permits maintenance of blood oxygen tensions that promote diffusion of oxygen from the capillary blood into metabolizing tissues.

The maximum quantity of oxygen transported in blood is dependent upon hemoglobin concentration, which varies moderately in normal circumstances and substantially in disease states. To facilitate comparison of oxygen dissociation curves with different hemoglobin concentrations, the ordinate of the curve can be normalized by expressing oxygen content at any given pressure as a percentage of the maximum possible oxygen content. This approach substitutes % saturation of hemoglobin for oxygen content, as illustrated in Figure 15-2. Using this format, all normal oxygen dissociation curves are superimposable, regardless of differing hemoglobin concentrations.

ALTERATIONS OF OXYGEN AFFINITY

The relationship between oxygen content and pressure can be affected by several factors. Increases in temperature, carbon dioxide pressure, hydrogen ions (decreased pH), and 2,3-diphosphoglycerate (2,3-DPG) all shift the oxygen dissociation curve to the right.[1] This results in a decrease in the affinity of hemoglobin for oxygen, that is, a greater oxygen tension is required to bind the same amount of oxygen to hemoglobin (Fig. 15-2). Conversely, decreases in temperature, carbon dioxide tension, hydrogen ion (increased pH), and 2,3-DPG shift the curve to the left, that is, increase the affinity of hemoglobin for oxygen.[1] The degree of shift of the oxygen dissociation curve is described by the P_{50}, the partial pressure of oxygen required to achieve 50% oxygen saturation of hemoglobin. The normal P_{50} for human blood is 26.5 mm Hg (Fig. 15-1). The basic sigmoid nature of the relation between oxygen and hemoglobin does not change with alterations in the P_{50}. Rather, the curve is uniformly either stretched or compressed along the P_{O_2} axis.

The human erythrocyte contains large quantities of 2,3-DPG, an organic phosphate that binds to hemoglobin and affects O_2 affinity. The normal concentration of 2,3-DPG in erythrocytes is approximately 5 mM. However, this concentration can change significantly, markedly altering the P_{50}. There is a substantial change in the configuration of the hemoglobin molecule between the oxygenated and deoxygenated states. Oxygen and 2,3-DPG bind at different sites on the hemoglobin molecule, and binding of both molecules changes the overall configuration of hemoglobin, but in different ways. The β-chains are more widely separated in the deoxygenated state than in the oxygenated state, and have positive charges surrounding the central cavity of the hemoglobin tetramer. The widened gap between the β-chains of the deoxygenated molecule enables the highly negatively charged 2,3-DPG molecule to enter the cavity between the β-chains and bind electrostatically to positively charged amino acids of the hemoglobin molecule. This tends to stabilize the hemoglobin molecule in the deoxygenated configuration. Higher pressures of oxygen are thus required to force the change in molecular configuration to the oxygenated form, resulting in a shift of the dissociation curve to the right along the P_{O_2} axis.

The Donnan effect results from the presence of charged macromolecules on one side of a semipermeable membrane failing to distribute evenly across the membrane. This leads to an uneven distribution of charge across the membrane that, in turn, affects the distribution of small, permeable ions across the same membrane. At body pH 2,3-DPG has four negative charges and reduces intraerythrocytic pH by the Donnan effect since 2,3-DPG does not cross the cell membrane. The reduction in intracellular pH resulting from the presence of intracellular 2,3-DPG causes a decrease in oxygen affinity of hemoglobin through the Bohr effect (see below Carbon Dioxide).

Most abnormal hemoglobins have normal oxygen equilibrium curves despite differences in amino acid sequences. Although some hemoglobinopathies are accompanied by changes in oxygen affinity, this usually is due to other factors, such as altered DPG concentration or mean corpuscular hemoglobin concentration. Some relatively rare mutant hemoglobins are exceptions to this rule and exhibit increased O_2 affinity that is accompanied by erythrocytosis. Previously, measurements of P_{50} were advocated to investigate erythrocytosis, but identification of mutant hemoglobins with current molecular techniques is far more likely to identify this rare cause of erythrocytosis.

Large quantities of carbon monoxide (CO) bound to hemoglobin can increase the affinity for oxygen of the remaining unbound sites on hemoglobin. The adverse effects of CO poisoning are twofold: (1) Binding of CO to hemoglobin interferes with oxygen binding and produces a functional anemia; and (2) binding of CO to hemoglobin also increases the affinity of hemoglobin for oxygen, thereby shifting the oxygen equilibrium curve to the left. This increased affinity hinders the release of oxygen in the tissues, but is not as important as the functional anemia caused by CO binding.

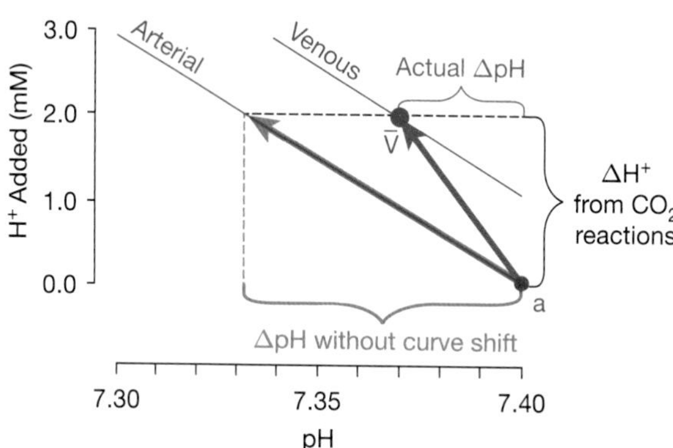

Figure 15-3 Buffer curves (change in pH produced by binding of hydrogen ions) of normal arterial (a) and mixed venous ($\bar{V}$) blood. With release of oxygen bound to hemoglobin in tissues, buffering sites on the hemoglobin molecule increase their affinity for hydrogen ions, thereby shifting the buffer curve upward. The quantity of hydrogen ions (ΔH^+) added to blood by production of CO_2 in normal metabolizing tissues at rest is indicated by the *black bracket*. The figure shows the change in pH *(green bracket)* that would occur if buffering occurred only along the arterial buffer curve *(green arrow)*. The actual, much smaller change in pH *(purple bracket)* that accompanies buffering *(purple arrow)* is due to the upward shift of the arterial buffering curve to the venous relationship that accompanies release of oxygen in the tissues. *(Reproduced with permission from Klocke RA: Encyclopedia of Respiratory Medicine. Philadelphia: Elsevier; 2007.)*

BOHR EFFECT

The shift of the oxygen dissociation curve produced by changes in P_{CO_2} and pH is known as the Bohr effect, after the individual who first described this phenomenon. Similar to 2,3-DPG, both hydrogen ions and carbon dioxide bind at sites on the hemoglobin molecule that differ from the oxygen-binding sites.[2] However, binding of these two moieties at different sites alters the oxygen affinity of hemoglobin through their effects on the configuration of the hemoglobin molecule.[3]

It has been speculated that the increased carbon dioxide tension and hydrogen ion content in blood perfusing metabolizing tissues facilitate the release of oxygen bound to hemoglobin at a higher P_{O_2} by shifting the oxygen dissociation curve to the right.[4] However, quantitative analysis indicates that this mechanism results in minimal augmentation of oxygen release in tissues at rest (2%–3%) because of the minute difference in pH between arterial and venous blood (0.03–0.05 pH units).[5] This effect does become significant during exercise, with the addition of lactic acid, from muscle to venous blood.[6] This is an adaptive response for improving oxygen delivery at high levels of exercise. However, the main benefit of the Bohr effect is the increased buffering capacity of hemoglobin that accompanies deoxygenation of the molecule.[2,4] Figure 15-3 illustrates the buffering curves of normal arterial and venous blood. Both exhibit effective, but parallel, buffering curves. As hemoglobin is deoxygenated, its buffering curve shifts upward and significant amounts of hydrogen ion can be buffered with a smaller change in pH.[2] Approximately half of the hydrogen ions released in aerobic metabolism are buffered in this manner (see section Haldane Effect).

CARBON DIOXIDE TRANSPORT

Carbon dioxide (CO_2) is primarily the by-product of aerobic metabolism. It is also generated through the buffering of hydrogen ions (H^+) from organic acids, such as lactic acid and ketoacids. This buffering occurs through chemical reaction of H^+ ions with intracellular and extracellular bicarbonate ions (HCO_3^-). The CO_2 produced by these reactions diffuses into capillary blood and is carried in both chemical combination and physical solution to the lungs, where it is eliminated through expired ventilation (see Chapter 16, p. 200). Similar to O_2 transport, most CO_2 in blood is not carried as gas, but rather in chemical forms directly or indirectly dependent on hemoglobin.

THE CARBON DIOXIDE DISSOCIATION CURVE

Carbon dioxide is transported in three forms in blood: Dissolved CO_2, bicarbonate ions, and carbamate compounds. The relationship between the blood content and partial pressure of CO_2 differs noticeably from that of O_2. The total quantity of CO_2 contained in arterial blood is more than twice that of O_2 despite the lower partial pressures of CO_2. The CO_2 dissociation curve is very steep (Fig. 15-4). As a result, the difference in partial pressures of CO_2 between arterial and venous blood is small when compared to the large arterial–venous differences in blood P_{O_2}.[7] The total content of blood CO_2, that is, the vertical axis of the CO_2 dissociation curve, is the sum of all three forms of CO_2 (dissolved CO_2, bicarbonate, and carbamate).

DISSOLVED CO_2

Carbon dioxide is 20 times more soluble in aqueous solution than oxygen.[8] However, this increased solubility is insufficient to facilitate transport of all the CO_2 produced by metabolism. Approximately 5% of total CO_2 content in blood exists as dissolved CO_2 in plasma and red cell water. Despite this, dissolved CO_2 has a critical role in gas exchange since only dissolved CO_2 crosses the alveolar–capillary membrane. Therefore, regardless of how CO_2 is transported in blood, each molecule must be converted into the dissolved form for excretion through ventilation. The quantity of dissolved CO_2 is directly proportional to the partial pressure of carbon dioxide in blood, that is, the P_{CO_2}.

BICARBONATE

Carbon dioxide combines with water to form carbonic acid, which dissociates into hydrogen and bicarbonate ions. At normal blood

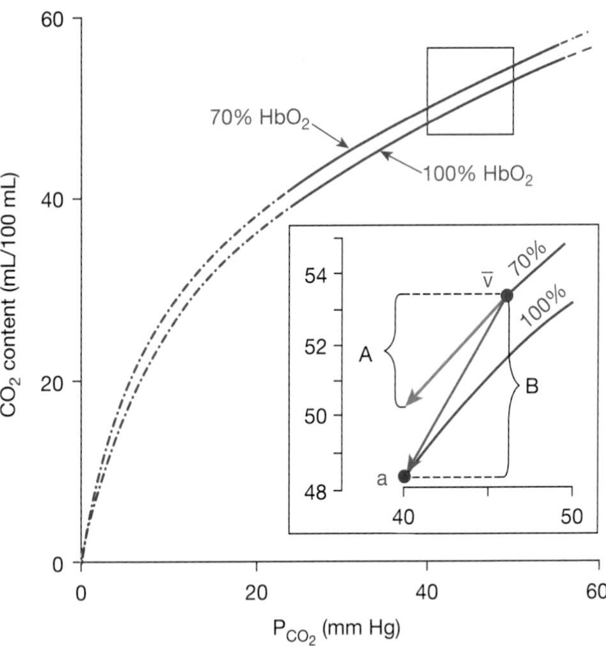

Figure 15-4 The Haldane effect showing the carbon dioxide dissociation curves of blood with 70% *(blue)* and 100% *(red)* oxygen saturations. The portions of the curves most commonly involved in gas exchange are drawn with *solid lines*. The P_{CO_2} and CO_2 contents of mixed venous ($\bar{v}$) and arterial blood (a) normally present at rest are shown in the enlarged inset. If there were no change in the CO_2 dissociation curve with oxygenation in the lung, the decrease in P_{CO_2} would take place along the venous curve *(green arrow)*. This would produce a decrease in blood CO_2 content indicated by the vertical bracket A. The course of CO_2 exchange between arterial and mixed venous points is shown by the *magenta arrow*. The enhanced CO_2 exchange produced by the Haldane effect is indicated by the greater vertical height of bracket B.

pH, carbonic acid dissociates into hydrogen ions and bicarbonate ions.

$$CO_2 + H_2O \xleftrightarrow{CA} H_2CO_3 \leftrightarrow H^+ + HCO_3^- \quad (1)$$

The pKa for reaction (1), including hydration and dissociation, is 6.1.[8] The natural rate of formation of carbonic acid from CO_2 and water is slow and takes seconds to minutes to reach completion in simple aqueous solutions. Under the influence of the carbonic anhydrase (CA) enzyme in the cytosol of erythrocytes, this reaction is increased by a factor of approximately 15,000.[7] CA occurs as two isoenzymes: CA I is present in high concentrations in erythrocytes, but its activity is inhibited by intracellular chloride ions. CA II is present at one-sixth the concentration of CA I within red cells, but is not inhibited by chloride ion and has a sevenfold greater intrinsic activity than CA I. CA II is therefore responsible for almost all the CO_2–bicarbonate catalysis in vivo.[7]

CARBAMATE

Carbon dioxide is also transported as carbamate compounds. Less than 10% of all CO_2 binds to hemoglobin as carbamate, which are salts of carbamic acid formed by the reaction of CO_2 with amino groups on proteins. CO_2 combines with uncharged terminal amino groups on the α and β chains of hemoglobin.

$$\text{R-NH}_3^+ \rightarrow H^+ + \text{R-NH}_2 \quad (2)$$

$$\text{R-NH}_2 + CO_2 \rightarrow \text{R-NHCOOH} \rightarrow \text{R-NHCOO}^- + H^+ \quad (3)$$

where R represents either an α or β chain of hemoglobin.[7] While any NH_2 group on hemoglobin can potentially bind CO_2 as a carbamate compound, only the terminal amino groups of the α and β chains participate in carbamate generation. At the pH present inside red cells, carbamic acid (R-NHCOOH) dissociates completely into a carbamate ion and a hydrogen ion. These H^+ ions, like those liberated by the formation of bicarbonate ions, are buffered principally by hemoglobin (see section Haldane Effect).

Changes in the quaternary structure of hemoglobin accompanying binding and release of oxygen affect the pK's of reactions (2) and (3), altering the equilibrium between the NH_2 and NH_3^+ forms of the terminal amino groups. Because deoxygenated hemoglobin binds more CO_2 than oxygenated hemoglobin, more CO_2 can be carried in venous blood at any given P_{CO_2} than in oxygenated (arterial) blood. The change in CO_2 binding between oxygenated and deoxygenated hemoglobin accounts for approximately one-eighth of the difference between the arterial and venous CO_2 contents during normal gas exchange. The physiological importance of this process would be twice as great but is reduced by interactions between DPG and hemoglobin that limit carbamate formation.[7] Binding of the highly negatively charged DPG molecule to hemoglobin induces change of the amino-NH_2 moieties to the positively charged amino-NH_3^+ forms that do not bind CO_2 as carbamate.

HALDANE EFFECT

Oxygenated blood at any partial pressure of CO_2 contains less total CO_2 content than deoxygenated blood at the same partial pressure (Fig. 15-4). This is known as the *Haldane effect*, after one of the investigators who first described the phenomenon.

Transport of CO_2 in blood as bicarbonate or carbamate is altered by blood oxygenation. These changes are described as "oxylabile" since they are dependent upon the state of hemoglobin oxygenation.[7] Changes in configuration of the hemoglobin molecule accompanying the release of oxygen facilitate binding of CO_2 to hemoglobin as carbamate, that is, *oxylabile carbamate formation*. This increases the total CO_2 content in deoxygenated blood compared with oxygenated blood.[9]

Formation of both bicarbonate ions and carbamate compounds releases large quantities of hydrogen ions. It is essential to buffer these hydrogen ions effectively to promote CO_2 transport. Deoxygenation of hemoglobin also results in a shift of the buffering curve of hemoglobin since deoxygenated hemoglobin is a stronger base than oxyhemoglobin. This shift permits binding of a greater number of hydrogen ions (Fig. 15-3). This *oxylabile buffering*, in turn, facilitates formation of larger quantities of carbamate and bicarbonate.[9]

The synergistic effects of oxygen and carbon dioxide transport result in a change in the carbon dioxide dissociation curve as oxygen is bound and released.[10] Approximately equal changes in bicarbonate and carbamate concentrations are responsible for the Haldane effect. Quantitatively, the Haldane effect has a far greater physiological effect on gas transport than does the Bohr effect. Without the change between the oxygenated and partially reduced CO_2 dissociation curves (the Haldane effect), the difference between arterial and venous CO_2 tensions would be approximately twice the normal value, thereby increasing tissue P_{CO_2}. Model calculations and in vitro data suggest that the Haldane effect accounts for 40% to 50% of total CO_2 exchange in the lung under normal conditions.[7–9]

REFERENCES

1. Baumann R, Bartels H, Bauer C. Blood oxygen transport. In: Farhi LE, Tenney SM, eds. *Handbook of Physiology*. Vol 4. Section 3: *The Respiratory System*. Bethesda, MD: American Physiological Society; 1987:147–172.
2. Klocke RA. Carbon dioxide. In: Lauent GJ, Shapiro SD, eds. *Encyclopedia of Respiratory Medicine*. Oxford: Elsevier; 2007:320–324.

3. Hlastala MP, Woodson RD. Saturation dependency of the Bohr effect interactions among H+, CO_2, and DPG. *J Appl Physiol.* 1975;38:1126–1131.
4. Jensen FB. Red blood cell pH, the Bohr effect, and other oxygenation-linked phenomena in blood O_2 and CO_2 transport. *Acta Physiol Scand.* 2004;182:215–227.
5. Hill EP, Power GG, Longo LD. Mathematical simulation of pulmonary O_2 and CO_2 exchange. *Am J Physiol.* 1973;224:904–917.
6. Stringer W, Wasserman K, Casaburi R, Pórszász J, Maehara K, French W. Lactic acidosis as a facilitator of oxyhemoglobin dissociation during exercise. *J Appl Physiol.* 1994;76:1462–1467.
7. Klocke RA. Carbon dioxide transport. In: Farhi LE, Tenney SM, eds. *Handbook of Physiology*. Vol 4. Section 3: *The Respiratory System*. Bethesda, MD: American Physiological Society; 1987:173–197.
8. Geers C, Gros G. Carbon dioxide transport and carbonic anhydrase in blood and muscle. *Physiol Rev.* 2000;80:681–715.
9. Klocke RA. Mechanism and kinetics of the Haldane effect in human erythrocytes. *J Appl Physiol.* 1973;35:673–681.
10. Grant BJ. Influence of Bohr-Haldane effect on steady-state gas exchange. *J Appl Physiol.* 1982;52:1330–1337.

CHAPTER 16

Diffusion, Chemical Reactions, and Diffusing Capacity

Robert A. Klocke
Adrian Shifren

Uptake of oxygen and excretion of carbon dioxide require rapid, efficient exchange in the lung. The quantities of exchanged gases are staggering. For example, a 1800-calorie diet requires absorption of 375 L of oxygen per day, as well as excretion of a slightly smaller volume of carbon dioxide. Because blood remains in the pulmonary capillary bed for a limited time, the process of exchange must be accomplished in less than 0.75 second at rest and 0.5 second during exercise. This rapid, high-volume exchange occurs efficiently despite numerous interacting processes of diffusion and chemical reaction that occur in the lung. The rates of these processes are not only affected by intrinsic characteristics of blood but also determined by a host of other factors, including inspired oxygen fraction, alveolar gas tensions, cardiac output, and metabolic activity. The ease of exchange of respiratory gases belies the complexity of the overall process.

DIFFUSION

The concentration (C) of a gas dissolved in fluid depends upon its partial pressure (P) and solubility (α)

$$C = \alpha P \tag{1}$$

Gases diffuse from a higher to a lower partial pressure, not necessarily from a higher to a lower concentration. This fact is especially pertinent when a gas diffuses between two phases, as occurs when O_2 and CO_2 are exchanged between alveolar gas and blood. For example, dissolved CO_2 diffuses down a partial pressure gradient from blood (46 mm Hg) into the alveolus (40 mm Hg), even though its actual concentration (millimoles of molecular CO_2 per liter of gas or blood) is greater in alveolar gas (2.5) than it is in venous blood (1.4).

■ INFLUENCE OF PHYSICAL PROPERTIES

The rate of a gas diffusing through an aqueous membrane such as that separating alveolar gas and capillary blood is influenced by five factors. The rate is directly proportional to the surface area of the membrane, but inversely proportional to the thickness of the membrane. The rate increases in direct proportion to the difference in gas pressure between alveolar gas and capillary blood, and the diffusion and solubility coefficients of the gas in the membrane.

The diffusion coefficient of a gas in the alveolar–capillary membrane is largely a function of the size of the gas molecule, which is inversely proportional to the square root of its molecular weight (MW). Oxygen (MW 32) has a slightly greater diffusion coefficient than carbon dioxide (MW 44) in the alveolar membrane. However, the solubility of CO_2 in water, the major component of tissue composing the membrane, is much greater than the solubility of O_2. This difference far outweighs the effect of the slightly smaller size of the oxygen molecule. Thus, the rate of CO_2 transfer across the alveolar membrane is approximately 20 times greater than that of O_2 when both gases diffuse under the same partial pressure gradient. As a result, a much greater P_{O_2} gradient across the membrane is required to maintain O_2 transfer equal to that of CO_2.

On the other hand, the rate of carbon monoxide (CO) transfer is very similar to that of oxygen when both gases diffuse across the alveolar–capillary membrane under the same partial pressure gradient. CO (MW 28) is a slightly smaller molecule than oxygen so its diffusion coefficient is slightly greater. This diffusive advantage is offset by a slightly lower aqueous solubility of CO compared to oxygen. As a result, CO and O_2 transfer across the membrane have approximately equal rates at the same transmembrane partial pressure gradient.

The rate of diffusion is affected by the viscosity of the medium through which the diffusion occurs. Diffusion of a gas in air occurs at a rate that is four orders of magnitude greater than diffusion in water. Diffusion coefficients in tissues are only moderately less than those in water, since most tissues are composed primarily of water. The interior of the erythrocyte is an exception to this general rule. As a consequence of the high concentration of hemoglobin inside the red cell, the viscosity of the cell contents is substantially greater than that of water. This greater viscosity reduces the diffusion coefficient for oxygen to one-third of its aqueous coefficient. The combination of increased viscosity and the large size of the hemoglobin molecule decreases the diffusion coefficient of hemoglobin within the red cell to less than 10% of its diffusion coefficient in a dilute aqueous solution. As a result, significant diffusion gradients are thought to exist within the red cell even though the distance between the cell membrane and the innermost portion of the cell is only a few microns.

■ EFFECT OF DIFFERENT CAPACITANCES

The alveolar–capillary membrane provides a barrier to diffusion of gases between the alveoli and the capillaries. The rate of approach to diffusion equilibrium of a gas in the lung is dependent on the capacitances of the gas in the alveoli and blood relative to its solubility in the alveolar–capillary membrane. Normal ventilation of alveoli results in a large reservoir of oxygen with a pressure of ~100 mm Hg to promote diffusive transfer across the alveolar–capillary membrane. The ability of hemoglobin to bind O_2 increases the oxygen capacity of blood by two orders of magnitude compared with that of the alveolar–capillary membrane. This large capacitance for oxygen in blood requires substantial oxygen transfer across the membrane to reach diffusion equilibrium. Because the solubility of oxygen in the membrane is small relative to the large capacitances in alveolar gas and blood, oxygen exchange across the membrane requires 0.2 to 0.4 second to reach equilibrium.[1] Fortunately, this delay in reaching equilibrium is less than the average of 0.75 second that blood remains in the pulmonary capillary bed. These same conditions are present during carbon monoxide transfer. The large capacitance and the low aqueous solubility of CO lead to similar impediments in gas exchange.

In contrast to oxygen and carbon monoxide, the solubility of carbon dioxide in the membrane is sufficiently great compared to the capacitances of CO_2 in blood and alveoli to permit rapid equilibration of CO_2 across the alveolar–capillary membrane. As discussed (see below Carbon Dioxide) CO_2 exchange requires a finite time for completion, but this delay is the result of the time needed to complete chemical and transport processes in blood, and is not the result of slow diffusive transport across the alveolar–capillary membrane.

Gases transported in blood only in dissolved form are exchanged almost instantaneously across the alveolar–capillary membrane. As long as gas solubilities in the membrane and blood are similar, diffusion equilibrium between alveolar contents and blood is reached within 0.01 second because the normal alveolar–capillary membrane is extremely thin (median thickness of 0.3 μm). Only gases such as oxygen and carbon monoxide that have large alveolar and blood capacitances and reduced solubility in the alveolar–capillary membrane will require a finite time to reach diffusive equilibrium.

CHEMICAL REACTIONS OF GASES

Transport of respiratory gases entails numerous chemical reactions with components of the blood. Like diffusive transport of oxygen, these chemical reactions are not instantaneous and require finite periods of time to reach completion. It is commonly thought that diffusion provides the greatest time-dependent impediment to gas exchange, but in actuality, chemical processes, especially those occurring in combination with diffusion or other chemical reactions, are more likely to slow rates of exchange.

OXYGEN AND CARBON MONOXIDE

From a stoichiometric viewpoint, the successive binding of O_2 to the heme moieties of hemoglobin is described by successive steps, each with separate association and dissociation rate constants. If the heme rings acted independently, these constants would be the same for each heme ring and the resulting dissociation curve would have a hyperbolic shape. However, binding of oxygen to one of the heme rings affects the affinity for O_2 of the remaining heme moieties of the molecule, leading to the familiar sigmoid shape of the oxygen dissociation curve.

Reactions of oxygen and hemoglobin during capillary transit are further complicated by the rate of oxygen diffusion through the viscous interior of the red cell. The chemical reactions of oxygen and hemoglobin occur quite rapidly in dilute hemoglobin solutions but proceed more slowly in red cell suspensions. Because of the large size of the hemoglobin molecule and increased viscosity of the red cell contents, hemoglobin remains relatively immobile. As the red cell enters the pulmonary capillary, oxygen molecules bind to reduced hemoglobin molecules just inside the erythrocyte membrane. As these hemoglobin molecules become saturated, subsequent oxygen molecules entering the red cell must diffuse more deeply into the interior of the cell to reach reduced hemoglobin molecules. This combination of diffusion and chemical reaction causes oxygen uptake to occur as an "advancing front" that proceeds at a rate that is an order of magnitude slower than O_2 uptake in well-mixed, dilute hemoglobin solution. This combined process is complex and not easily described from a theoretical standpoint. As a result, the rate of oxygen uptake by hemoglobin contained in red cells is described by a single overall descriptive parameter, θ_{O_2}, which incorporates all the processes into a single phenomenological value. θ_{O_2} varies with oxygen saturation, pH, and hemoglobin type. The same approach is used to describe carbon monoxide uptake in blood. The rate at which CO replaces bound O_2 in blood with a normal hemoglobin concentration is described by θ_{CO}.

The rates of O_2 and CO uptake by erythrocyte suspensions are determined in vitro and assumed to be representative of the rates of gas exchange in vivo. However, measurements of these rate constants in red cell suspensions in vitro may be affected adversely by methodological artifacts. The actual rates of combination of O_2 and CO with red cells in vivo have not been measured and this lack of data leads to uncertainties in our understanding of exchange of the two gases in the lung.

CARBON DIOXIDE

CO_2 is transported in blood as dissolved molecular CO_2, bicarbonate ion, and carbamate ion.[2] The latter is a salt of a carbamic acid formed by reaction of CO_2 with terminal amino groups of the four chains comprising the hemoglobin molecule. The relation between the partial pressure of CO_2 and the total content of CO_2 in all forms is described by the CO_2 dissociation curve of blood (see Chapter 15, Fig. 15-4). Because CO_2 is more soluble than O_2 in the alveolar–capillary membrane, it often is assumed that CO_2 exchange occurs much more rapidly than O_2 exchange. However, only dissolved CO_2 can cross the alveolar–capillary membrane, and conversion of bicarbonate and carbamate to dissolved CO_2 limits the rate of CO_2 exchange. As indicated in Figure 16-1, *Upper Panel*, when a bolus of dissolved CO_2 is injected into an isolated lung perfused with saline buffer, CO_2 is rapidly exchanged similar to the inert gas acetylene.[3] In contrast, when a bicarbonate bolus is injected into the same preparation (Fig. 16-1, *Lower Panel*), CO_2 exchange lags behind acetylene excretion because a finite period of time is required to convert bicarbonate into dissolved CO_2 that can cross the alveolar–capillary membrane.

As blood enters the pulmonary capillary bed, dissolved CO_2 immediately diffuses into the alveoli and capillary blood P_{CO_2} falls to the level present in the alveolar gas. The majority (>85%) of the CO_2 content in blood entering the capillary bed exists as bicarbonate ion.[2,4] The rapid decrease in capillary P_{CO_2} disturbs the equilibrium between bicarbonate ion and dissolved CO_2 in both the plasma and the red cell. Bicarbonate ion combines with hydrogen ion extremely rapidly to form carbonic acid (H_2CO_3). The natural rate of dehydration of carbonic acid to CO_2 and water is a slow process, requiring 60 to 90 seconds to reach completion. However, the reaction is catalyzed inside the red cell by a factor of ~15,000 by the large concentration of carbonic anhydrase (CA) in red cells.

$$HCO_3^- + H^+ \rightarrow H_2CO_3 \xrightarrow{CA} CO_2 + H_2O \qquad (2)$$

The substantial buffering capacity of hemoglobin inside the erythrocyte, augmented by the simultaneous conversion of reduced to oxygenated hemoglobin, provides the hydrogen ions required for this reaction.[4] The dissolved CO_2 formed by this reaction inside the red cell immediately leaves the blood and enters the alveoli.

There is a minimal amount of CA attached to the interior surface of the pulmonary capillaries, but its activity is <1% of the erythrocytic enzyme. As a result, little or no conversion of bicarbonate to dissolved CO_2 occurs in the plasma during the short

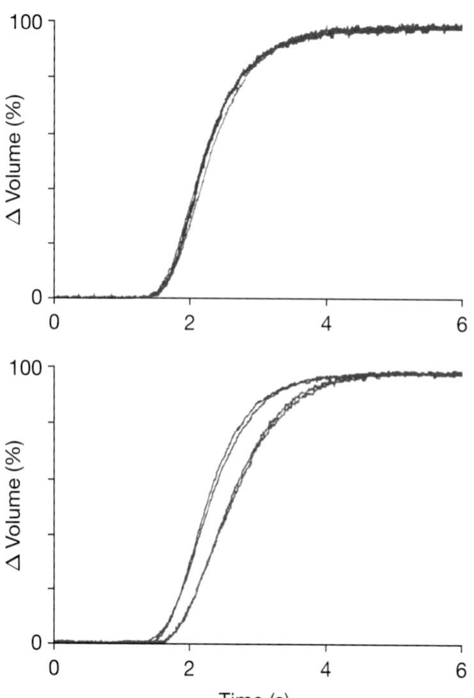

Figure 16-1 Rates of acetylene *(blue curves)* and CO_2 *(red curves)* excretion after two pairs of injections into the pulmonary artery of a single isolated lung preparation perfused with buffer. Volume changes are normalized to facilitate comparison. *Upper Panel*: The excretion of both acetylene and CO_2 proceed at the same rate after injections of buffer containing either dissolved CO_2 or acetylene. Differences in mean transit times for CO_2 and acetylene were −0.027 second for first pair and +0.022 second for second pair of injections. Thus, CO_2 crosses the alveolar–capillary membrane at the same rapid rate as the inert gas acetylene. *Lower Panel*: The excretion of CO_2 generated from injections of bicarbonate *(red curves)* lags behind the excretion of dissolved acetylene (*blue curves*) by +0.301 second in the first set of paired injections of acetylene and bicarbonate and 0.312 second in the second set of paired injections. This slower excretion of CO_2 is caused by the time required to convert bicarbonate to CO_2 with catalysis in this experiment provided by carbonic anhydrase localized to the capillary endothelium. *(Reproduced with permission from Schunemann HJ, Klocke RA: Influence of CO_2 kinetics on pulmonary carbon dioxide exchange. J Appl Physiol. 1993;74:715.)*

pulmonary capillary transit time (0.75 second at rest, 0.5 second during exercise). Inside the red cell, the catalyzed formation of dissolved CO_2 rapidly (~0.1 second) depletes the concentration of intracellular bicarbonate and the production of CO_2 slows substantially[1,5] However, as the intracellular concentration of bicarbonate decreases, plasma bicarbonate enters the cell in exchange for intracellular chloride. Bicarbonate–chloride movement across the erythrocyte membrane occurs in an electrically neutral, one-for-one exchange that is facilitated by an anion exchange protein present in the erythrocyte membrane.[2] Despite the presence of approximately one million anion exchangers with an extremely rapid turnover (50,000 ions per second) in each red cell membrane, bicarbonate–chloride exchange requires 0.3 to 0.4 second to reach completion.[1]

Besides exchange of dissolved CO_2 and bicarbonate, a modest amount of CO_2 excretion (13%) results from release of CO_2 bound to hemoglobin as carbamate.[2] The release of CO_2 bound as carbamate is caused by the alteration of the molecular conformation of hemoglobin that accompanies oxygenation. The carbamate reaction is complete in 0.2 to 0.3 second, but cannot occur until hemoglobin is first oxygenated. The process of oxygenation further delays conversion of carbamate to dissolved CO_2.

Thus, exchange of CO_2 in the lung is thought to require at least ~0.4 to 0.5 second because of the series of processes that are necessary to convert CO_2 carried as bicarbonate and carbamate to dissolved CO_2.[1,5] In fact, computational models of CO_2 exchange suggest that in some circumstances exchange is not quite completed prior to blood leaving the pulmonary capillary.[1,5] Even in the worst case, the degree of disequilibrium is small and a minimal increase in ventilation can easily compensate for a slight impairment of CO_2 exchange.

■ SOURCES OF CO_2 EXCRETED IN THE LUNGS

Bicarbonate accounts for the majority (>85%) of the total CO_2 content transported in arterial and venous blood. Dissolved CO_2 (~5%–6%) and carbamate (<10%) contribute substantially less to the total CO_2 content of blood. The quantity of bicarbonate transported in plasma is much greater than that carried within the red cells for three reasons. First, plasma volume constitutes 55% and erythrocytes only 45% of the total blood volume. Second, bicarbonate is present only in the volume of water in each component; plasma water content (95%) is substantially greater than erythrocyte water content (72%). Third, because of the Donnan distribution of anions across the erythrocyte membrane, bicarbonate concentration inside the red cell is only 63% of the plasma concentration.

The relative contributions of each form of CO_2 content to the quantity of CO_2 excreted during gas exchange in the lung are not exactly proportional to their blood contents. Analysis of the differences between arterial and venous blood CO_2 contents can be used to calculate the amounts of each form of carbon dioxide content excreted in expired ventilation.[2,6,7] This analysis of differences between arterial and venous blood CO_2 contents is shown in Figure 16-2. The vast majority of expired CO_2 enters the lung as bicarbonate and is converted into CO_2 during capillary transit. The contribution of plasma bicarbonate (49%) is greater than the erythrocytic bicarbonate (30%) that is converted into CO_2 and excreted in expired ventilation. Essentially all the CO_2 derived from bicarbonate, whether in plasma or erythrocytes, has to be exposed to CA within the red cells to allow for reaction catalysis during the

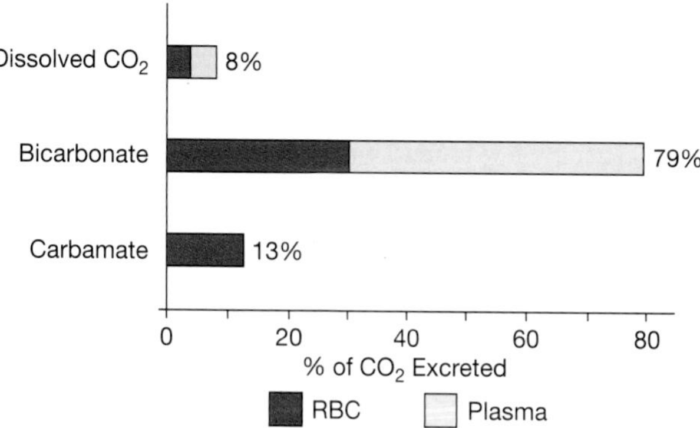

Figure 16-2 Sources of carbon dioxide excreted during passage of blood through the lungs in resting humans. The bars indicate the quantities of the different sources of CO_2 leaving blood from red cells *(red)* and plasma *(yellow)*. Bicarbonate contributes the overwhelming majority of CO_2 to the expired ventilation. As indicated in the figure, the majority of excreted bicarbonate enters the lung in plasma and is exchanged for chloride to reach carbonic anhydrase and hemoglobin buffering capacity within the red cell. *(Data from Klocke RA. Carbon Dioxide Transport, in Handbook of Physiology. Section 3, The Respiratory System, vol 4, edited by LE Farhi, SM Tenney SM. Bethesda: American Physiological Society; 1987.)*

brief capillary transit. This emphasizes the importance of anion exchange across the erythrocyte membrane in the process of carbon dioxide excretion.

The contributions of dissolved CO_2 and carbamate to the quantity of CO_2 in expired ventilation are modest, but are slightly greater than their relative concentrations in blood. Slightly more dissolved CO_2 originates in the plasma than in the red cells because of the greater amount of water in plasma. All excreted CO_2 derived from carbamate entered the lung bound to hemoglobin inside the erythrocytes.

DIFFUSING CAPACITY

The pulmonary diffusing capacity (DL) of a gas provides an estimate of its rate of transfer from the alveoli into capillary blood. Initially investigators thought that only diffusion of gas across the membrane limited exchange. This is the case for inert gases and, as noted earlier, equilibrium of these gases is achieved rapidly even in disease. However, transfer of gases that combine with hemoglobin are limited both by diffusion across the alveolar membrane and by the rate of reactions inside red blood cells.[8] The only gases that have measurable diffusing capacities are those with low solubility in the pulmonary membrane and high capacitance in blood as a result of binding to hemoglobin. These gases include oxygen (O_2), carbon monoxide (CO), and nitric oxide (NO).

DIFFUSING CAPACITY OF OXYGEN (D_{LO_2})

The diffusing capacity is calculated as the volume of gas absorbed by pulmonary blood per unit time ($\dot{V}$) divided by the pressure gradient between alveolar gas (PA) and pulmonary capillary blood (Pcap).

For oxygen,

$$D_{LO_2} = \frac{\dot{V}_{O_2}}{PA_{O_2} - Pcap_{O_2}} \quad (3)$$

Measurement of D_{LO_2} is difficult because, in addition to diffusion, O_2 transfer may be limited by other mechanisms, such as ventilation–perfusion mismatching and shunting. The measurement is further complicated by a changing capillary P_{O_2} during capillary transit that cannot be accurately determined. These difficulties have led investigators to abandon attempts to measure the diffusing capacity of oxygen.

DIFFUSING CAPACITY OF CARBON MONOXIDE (D_{LCO})

Carbon monoxide provides an excellent alternative to measuring diffusing capacity because CO normally is present in minimal amounts in blood and binds to hemoglobin similar to O_2. Because capillary P_{CO} is extremely low in usual circumstances, it can be assumed to be negligible and D_{LCO} is calculated by dividing CO uptake ($\dot{V}_{CO}$) by alveolar P_{CO}. However, like oxygen, CO uptake is limited both by diffusion across the alveolar–capillary membrane and by chemical reaction of CO with intracellular hemoglobin. As described by Roughton and Forster,[8] D_{LCO} comprises two elements:

$$\frac{1}{D_{LCO}} = \frac{1}{Dm_{CO}} + \frac{1}{\theta_{CO} V_c} \quad (4)$$

where

Dm_{CO} = the diffusing capacity of the alveolar–capillary membrane for CO

θ_{CO} = the rate of displacement of O_2 from intracellular hemoglobin by CO

V_c = the volume of blood in the pulmonary capillary bed

Because O_2 and CO compete for binding sites on hemoglobin, CO binding is inhibited by increases in P_{O_2}. Thus, D_{LCO} and θ_{CO} vary inversely with P_{O_2}. Using known in vitro values of θ_{CO} and two measurements of D_{LCO} at normal and elevated inspired O_2 concentrations, Eq. (4) can be solved to provide values of both Dm_{CO} and V_c. Calculation of the diffusing capacity is based on the assumption that the lung is homogeneous, that is, all portions of the lung have the same relative ventilation, perfusion, alveolar volume, and diffusing capacity.

DIFFUSING CAPACITY OF NITRIC OXIDE (D_{LNO})

Nitric oxide binds to hemoglobin at the same sites as O_2 and CO, but the rate of NO binding is much more rapid. Since NO binds to hemoglobin in solution two orders of magnitude faster than the rate of CO binding, it has been postulated that θ_{NO} is much greater than θ_{CO} and approaches a value of infinity. If this is the case, then the term $1/\theta_{NO}V_c$ (analogous to Eq. (4) for CO) approaches zero and the diffusing capacity measured with NO should reflect only the resistance to gas transfer provided by the alveolar–capillary membrane, that is, the Dm_{CO} component of the CO diffusing capacity. If NO binds to intracellular hemoglobin instantaneously, DL (and hence Dm) measured with NO should be 1.97 times Dm measured with CO because NO has a greater aqueous solubility and a minimally larger diffusion coefficient than CO. Phansalkar et al.[9] performed simultaneous measurements of D_{LNO} and the components of D_{LCO} in both normal individuals and patients with sarcoidosis at varying levels of exercise intensity. The ratio of D_{LNO}/Dm_{CO} did not differ in the two groups and averaged 2.42, moderately greater than the theoretical value of 1.97 (Fig. 16-3, *Lower Panel*). The ratio of

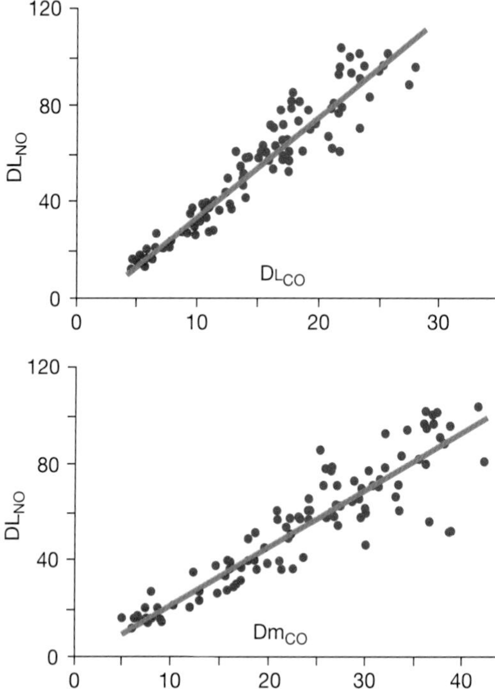

Figure 16-3 Relationships between simultaneous measurements of *(Upper Panel)* D_{LNO} and D_{LCO} and *(Lower Panel)* D_{LNO} and Dm_{CO} in patients with sarcoidosis *(red circles)* and normal subjects *(blue circles)*. The units of all parameters in the figure are mL/min/mm Hg/m^2. D_{LCO} was expressed under standardized conditions of hemoglobin concentration (14.6 mg/dL) and alveolar O_2 tension (P_{ACO_2} 120 mm Hg). Regression lines through the pooled data are *(Upper Panel)* $D_{LNO} = 4.16D_{LCO} - 6.82$, $r^2 = 0.918$ and *(Lower Panel)* $D_{LNO} = 2.42\ Dm_{CO} - 1.87$, $r^2 = 0.865$. *(Reproduced with permission from Phansalkar AR, Hanson CM, Shakir AR, et al. Nitric oxide diffusing capacity and alveolar microvascular recruitment in sarcoidosis. Am J Respir Crit Care Med. 2004;169(9):1034–1040.)*

DL_{NO}/DL_{CO} in both groups did not differ and averaged 4.16 (Fig. 16-3, *Upper Panel*).

More recent work challenges the postulate that θ_{NO} has a value of infinity and DL_{NO} can be used to calculate Dm_{CO}. Borland et al.[10] have shown that DL_{NO} increases progressively as red blood cells are replaced with hemolyzed blood or cell-free heme-based blood substitute, an observation that should not occur if θ_{NO} truly has a value of infinity. As a result, it is premature to speculate on the potential clinical value of measurements of DL_{NO} until the underlying physiology of the measurement of DL_{NO} is clarified. The technique of the measurement itself varies among laboratories. In addition, it requires sophisticated equipment and technical expertise that only are present in research settings.

METHODS FOR MEASURING THE DIFFUSING CAPACITY

Several different techniques are used to measure the carbon monoxide diffusing capacity. In clinical settings the single breath method is utilized almost exclusively. The steady-state and rebreathing methods of determining DL_{CO} are employed primarily in research. The steady-state method usually is performed in subjects who are exercising, thereby limiting its clinical application in patients with restricted ability to exercise. The rebreathing methodology requires rapid-responding gas analyzers and has technical requirements that are not available in most clinical laboratories.

Single Breath Method

With the single breath technique the subject exhales to residual volume, inhales a maximal breath of 0.3% CO, a tracer gas (usually 10% helium), 21% oxygen, and balance nitrogen. The breath is held for approximately 10 seconds followed by a maximal exhalation. After sufficient expiration to clear the dead space, a gas sample is collected to estimate final alveolar CO and helium fractions. After inspiration, the alveolar partial pressure of CO falls exponentially as CO enters the capillary blood. The volume of CO absorbed in the lungs can be calculated from the alveolar volume and the initial and final concentrations of CO in alveolar gas. The rate of CO uptake during the breath-hold is a function of the alveolar PA_{CO}, which falls exponentially during the breath-hold. Capillary CO pressure is assumed to be equal to zero. The single-breath diffusing capacity is calculated by:

$$DL_{CO} = \frac{60VA}{t_{bh}(PB - 47)} \ln \frac{FA_{CO\ initial}}{FA_{CO\ final}} \tag{5}$$

where

60 = the number of seconds per minute
VA = the alveolar volume of gas (mL_{STPD}) present in the lung at the start of the breath-hold
t_{bh} = the duration of the breath-hold (seconds)
P_B = the barometric pressure (mm Hg)
FA_{CO} = the alveolar fraction of carbon monoxide at the initial and final times of the breath-holding period

The insoluble inert gas (usually helium) included in the inspired volume is not absorbed in capillary blood and is diluted in the residual volume present at the start of the maximal inspiration. VA is calculated from the dilution of the helium and the inspired volume (VI):

$$VA = VI \frac{FI_{He}}{FA_{He}} \tag{6}$$

where

FI_{He} and FA_{He} = the inspired and alveolar helium concentrations

The alveolar fraction of He and the final alveolar CO fraction are obtained by measuring CO and He concentrations in the expired alveolar gas sample. The initial alveolar CO fraction is calculated from the dilution of the inspired CO in the volume of gas present in the lung during the breath-hold,

$$FA_{CO} = FI_{CO} \frac{VI}{VA} \tag{7}$$

where

FI_{CO} = the inspired CO fraction

The single breath method requires some degree of patient cooperation to perform the necessary respiratory maneuvers. A patient with an extremely reduced lung volume may not have a vital capacity large enough to clear the dead space and provide a sufficient sample for analysis of alveolar gas concentrations. The ability to hold the breath for 10 seconds also limits applicability to some patients. Finally, this method can be employed only in the resting state since few patients can hold their breath during exercise. Despite these limitations, the single breath DL_{CO} is the most practical and widely used method for measuring DL_{CO}. The technical aspects of the test have been standardized so that the same methodology is utilized in most laboratories.[11]

MEASUREMENT OF Dm AND V_C

Using values of θ_{CO} measured in vitro and values of DL_{CO} determined with different inspired O_2 concentrations, Eq. (4) can be solved for the membrane diffusing capacity (Dm_{CO}) and capillary blood volume (V_c).[8] However, there is considerable uncertainty regarding values of θ, the rate of red cell uptake of gases that bind to hemoglobin. Most in vitro measurements of θ have utilized rapid reaction techniques that may be flawed due to unstirred layers of fluid surrounding the red cells in the experimental apparatus. This artifact is greater the more rapidly that the gas reacts with hemoglobin (NO > O_2 > CO). Furthermore, the rate of gas uptake by erythrocytes may be influenced by the ability of the red cells to be deformed during passage through the pulmonary capillaries, a factor not present during in vitro measurements of θ. Mathematical models suggest that the rate of uptake of gases also depends on erythrocyte orientation and spacing within capillaries. Since the characteristics of erythrocyte transit in the capillary bed have not been defined, extrapolation of in vitro measurements to the in vivo situation introduces elements of uncertainty. Despite these reservations, solution of Eq. (4) using values of θ_{CO} determined in vitro yields values of Dm_{CO} and V_c that agree with independent estimates of these variables using alternate techniques.

Calculation of pulmonary capillary blood volume (V_c) from measurements of DL_{CO} is dependent upon the value of θ_{CO} chosen for the computation. Using in vitro data for θ_{CO} yields values at rest of 75 to 100 mL for men and slightly less for women. V_c measured by the CO method is dependent upon the quantity of hemoglobin present in the capillary bed in addition to the actual capillary volume. Calculation of V_c assumes a normal hemoglobin concentration in capillary blood and variation in this parameter affects the $\theta_{CO}V_c$ component of DL_{CO}.

Dm and V_c have been estimated from morphometric data obtained from excised, fixed canine lungs.[12] Calculations of DL_{CO} using these postmortem morphometric values and in vitro values of θ_{CO} have yielded estimates of DL_{CO} that are much greater than measurements of DL_{CO} under resting conditions in the same intact animal. This discrepancy arises because morphometric measurements are obtained in maximally inflated lungs. The morphometric estimates reflect a fully recruited alveolar surface area and V_C, a circumstance seen during maximal oxygen uptake during exercise. When DL_{CO} calculated from morphometric data is compared to DL_{CO} measured in intact animals under conditions of maximum exercise, there is good agreement between the two estimates.

FACTORS INFLUENCING DIFFUSING CAPACITY

The CO diffusing capacity originally was thought to reflect the resistance of the alveolar–capillary membrane to transfer of CO from the alveoli to capillary blood. The classic work of Roughton and Forster[8] elucidated the influence of chemical reactions on transfer of CO. DL_{CO} may be a measure of decreased gas transfer caused by abnormal diffusion, but also can reflect reduction in hemoglobin concentration, nonuniform distribution of physiological properties throughout the lung, loss of lung tissue, or artifacts in measurement. Because multiple factors in addition to diffusion can affect DL_{CO}, in Europe this test is often termed the CO transfer factor, rather than the CO diffusing capacity.

Hemoglobin Concentration

Capillary blood volume (V_c) is a prime variable in the diffusing capacity; its importance is due to the quantity of hemoglobin available to combine with CO within the capillary bed. The calculated value of V_c can be reduced directly by diseases that decrease capillary volume, but also can vary with the concentration of hemoglobin in blood. For this reason, the predicted DL_{CO} can be corrected for alterations in hemoglobin concentration.[11] For adult males and adolescents:

$$\text{Predicted } DL_{CO} \text{ (Corrected)} = \text{Predicted } DL_{CO}\,(1.7\ \text{Hb}/(10.22 + \text{Hb})) \quad (8)$$

where

Hb = hemoglobin concentration expressed in g/dL

For adult women and children less than age 15, the factor of 10.22 in Eq. (8) is replaced by a factor of 9.38. However, most clinical laboratories do not correct the predicted value of DL_{CO} for abnormal hemoglobin values.

Partial Pressure of Alveolar Oxygen

As indicated previously, θ_{CO} depends on P_{O_2}. Increased alveolar P_{O_2} will reduce measured DL_{CO}. Therefore, DL_{CO} will be lowered if patients receive supplemental oxygen during the measurement. Conversely, reduced alveolar P_{O_2} will lead to an increment in measured DL_{CO}. This has led to the suggestion to apply a correction to DL_{CO} if the measurement was made with an altered inspired oxygen fraction or at altitude. Even when alveolar P_{O_2} is kept at a sea level value during the measurement, lifelong residents of a community located 10,000 ft above sea level have demonstrated moderately greater diffusing capacities than sea-level residents.[13] Short-term residence (6 weeks) at altitude does not cause an increase in DL_{CO}. Beagles raised at altitude, even after reacclimation to sea level, still have moderately greater diffusing capacities than beagles raised at sea level. However, adult dogs taken to altitude for 3 years do not exhibit an increased DL_{CO}, suggesting that residence at altitude during growth is the basis for the increased DL_{CO}.

Body Position

DL_{CO} is 5% to 15% greater in the supine position than in the erect position. Blood volume shifts from the lower trunk and legs to the lungs when in the supine position. Most of the increase in DL_{CO} appears to be due to a 13% to 27% increase in V_c accompanying the fluid shift. However, there is also a minimal increase in Dm_{CO} in the supine position, possibly the result of recruitment of capillaries by the increased intravascular volume. The effect of posture on DL_{CO} decreases with age, but the reasons underlying this observation remain unknown.

Exercise

DL_{CO} can increase as much as twofold during exercise. This increase is attributed to proportionally equal increases in both Dm and V_c. Both alveolar–capillary surface area and capillary volume are recruited by the increase in cardiac output that accompanies exercise. The transit time through the capillary bed decreases, but not to the same degree as would be predicted in a vascular bed with fixed resistance. The potential reduction in transit time is partially offset by recruitment and distention of the pulmonary capillary bed.

Theoretically, DL_{CO} must have a maximum that cannot be exceeded when the entire pulmonary capillary bed and alveolar surface have been recruited. This should lead to a plateau in measured DL_{CO} even though the level of exercise continues to increase. This has never been observed in humans. Using a unique animal model of conscious greyhounds exercising on a treadmill, Carlin et al.[12] could not demonstrate a plateau in DL_{CO} with increasing exercise even though oxygen uptake reached a level of approximately 120 mL/kg/min. This level of O_2 uptake is almost twice that is seen in highly trained humans. Thus, it seems unlikely that the diffusing capacity in humans reaches a plateau during maximal exercise, but this does not rule out the possibility that gas exchange is limited by diffusion in this circumstance. Disequilibrium may occur before maximum recruitment of the diffusing capacity because capillary transit time may be less than the time required for O_2 exchange to be completed. Evidence in humans suggests that blood may leave the capillary bed without attaining complete equilibrium between alveolar P_{O_2} and capillary P_{O_2} at sea level in some patients with lung disease during exercise and in some highly trained athletes during maximal exercise. This also can occur in normal individuals at extremely high altitude with a marked reduction in the inspired P_{O_2}.

Alveolar Volume

DL_{CO} decreases with reduction in alveolar volume due to accompanying decreases in Dm_{CO} and V_c. This occurs with an inadequate inspiration to total lung capacity in persons with normal lungs, or with maximal inspiration in patients whose total lung capacities have been reduced by disease. In an effort to correct for alterations in alveolar volume rather than a true loss of diffusing capacity, some clinicians and investigators normalize DL_{CO} by dividing the observed DL_{CO} by the alveolar volume present during the measurement. This ratio of DL_{CO}/VA will be a useful index only if two assumptions are valid. First, there must be an approximately linear relation between DL_{CO} and VA. This assumption is reasonable at lung volumes greater than 50% of total lung capacity, but not at lower lung volumes. Second, the relation between DL_{CO} and VA must be directly proportional (i.e., a graph of DL_{CO} vs. VA must pass through the origin of the graph). This clearly is not the case. DL_{CO}/VA is not constant in normal persons and varies as alveolar volume changes.[14] Although frequently used, the DL_{CO}/VA ratio alone does not provide a valid index of the effect of changes in alveolar volume.[14,15]

Nonuniform Distribution of Physiological Properties

Calculation of DL_{CO}, regardless of the method used to make the measurement, implicitly assumes that the lung is completely uniform with regard to ventilation, alveolar volume, perfusion, and diffusive properties. This requires that each gas exchange unit possesses the same relationship between all these physiological properties, an assumption that is not completely valid even in normal, healthy persons. The most important factor determining CO uptake is the relationship of local diffusing capacity to local blood flow, the ratio of DL_{CO}/Q. Nonuniform distribution of important physiological variables throughout the lung produces a decrease in diffusing capacity and, by analogy, a reduced ability to transfer oxygen from the inspired air to capillary blood. Transfer is further complicated by the nonlinear nature of the processes involved. For example, the oxygen dissociation curve of hemoglobin has a sigmoid shape and a change in alveolar P_{O_2} may have a large or a minimal effect on the quantity of O_2 exchanged depending on the absolute value of the P_{O_2}. Disruptions of these complex relationships among physiological parameters have variable effects on O_2 transfer. The contributions of individual pathophysiological deviations cannot be assessed by a global measurement such as the diffusing capacity. Thus, DL_{CO} provides a means of assessing overall oxygen exchange but does not indicate specific defects in gas exchange.

TECHNICAL CONSIDERATIONS

Measurements of DL_{CO} have greater variation than spirometric observations such as the forced vital capacity (FVC) or forced expiratory volume in 1 second (FEV_1). Criteria for acceptable measurements of DL_{CO} have been based upon relative or absolute differences between repeated measurements. The American Thoracic Society/European Respiratory Society (ATS/ERS) consensus statement[11] recommends reporting the average of two measurements, both of which agree within 3.0 mL/min/mm Hg or within 10% of the higher measured value. Punjabi et al.[16] reported that an absolute difference of 2.5 mL/min/mm Hg between duplicate measurements could be achieved in 96% of patients. This criterion was deemed more reasonable than a percentage variation because it remained constant over a wide range of measured values in contrast to a changing percentage criterion. The strength of this study is in its size (over 6000 patients) and its performance during routine pulmonary testing in a single clinical setting. A drawback to its universal application is that three or more determinations of DL_{CO} were required in one-half of patients to meet criteria of acceptability. It is important to note that some clinical laboratories will perform only a single diffusing capacity measurement and report this value rather than reporting the mean of at least two acceptable determinations. This obviously increases the variability of reported values and lessens the ability to compare measurements over a period of time.

There is considerable variation in measurements of DL_{CO} among different clinical laboratories. These differences can be overcome by following strict technical protocols. In a carefully controlled multicenter (33 sites) clinical trial, Wise et al.[17] reported that 75% and 95% of the differences between duplicate DL_{CO} determinations with acceptable subject efforts (4797 pairs) were within <1 and <2 mL/min/mm Hg, respectively (Fig. 16-4). Acceptable criteria included inspired volume >90% of the FVC and a breath-hold time between 9 and 11 seconds.

The time of the breath-holding maneuver in the single breath method requires patient cooperation. Because of nonuniform distribution of physiological variables, CO uptake does not occur in a strictly exponential fashion even in healthy persons. As a result, measured DL_{CO} decreases slightly with prolonged breath-hold in normal subjects. This decrement can be substantially greater in patients with lung disease. The empirical breath-holding time of 10 seconds was chosen as a practical compromise to permit measurable CO uptake but still be feasible for patients to perform. Many laboratories set a breath-hold range of 9 to 11 seconds as acceptable, although the ATS/ERS consensus report[11] accepts a range of 8 to 12 seconds. Patients with lung disease often cannot perform rapid respiratory maneuvers mandated by the single breath DL_{CO} measurement. Slower flow rates prolong the time required for inspiration and expiration. As a result, instantaneous, uniform mixing of alveolar contents assumed in the calculation of DL_{CO} is not achieved. This may lead to a decrement in the reported measurement.

Most laboratories request that patients refrain from smoking for variable periods of time prior to measurement of DL_{CO} to avoid accumulation of CO in blood. Significant elevation of carboxyhemoglobin reduces measured DL_{CO} in two ways. First, the presence of carboxyhemoglobin produces a functional anemia, lessening the capacity of hemoglobin to bind O_2 or CO. This reduces the $\theta_{CO}V_c$ component of DL_{CO}. Second, calculation of DL_{CO} assumes that the back pressure of CO in the capillary is zero, and the gradient for CO transfer is equal to PA_{CO}. The presence of carboxyhemoglobin in blood produces an actual alveolar–capillary PCO gradient less than that assumed in the calculation, thereby leading to a lower calculated value of DL_{CO}. Graham et al.[18] measured the effect of experimental elevation of carboxyhemoglobin in normal individuals. Values of DL_{CO} obtained with the usual single breath calculation decreased approximately 1.5% from the true value for each 1.0% elevation of blood carboxyhemoglobin. Although algorithms are available to correct observed DL_{CO} for carboxyhemoglobin effects, it is preferable to make the measurement without a significant elevation of carboxyhemoglobin. At a minimum, 12 hours of abstinence from smoking is advisable in patients who smoke extensively because carboxyhemoglobin levels as great as 6% to 12% are observed immediately following tobacco usage.

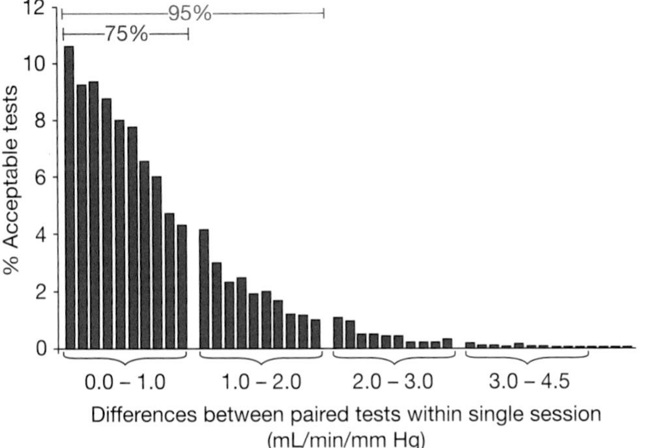

Figure 16-4 Differences between pairs of DL_{CO} measured within a single session in 4732 patients who had acceptable DL_{CO} efforts. The bars in the figure include differences in 75% of paired measurements *(purple)* and the differences in 95% of paired measurements *(red)*. *(Data from Wise RA, Teeter JG, Jensen RL, et al. Standardization of the single breath diffusing capacity in a multicenter clinical trial. Chest. 2007;132:1191.)*

CONTROVERSIES IN INTERPRETATION OF DL_{CO}

As noted previously, DL_{CO} is affected by a number of circumstances. Alveolar P_{O_2} and body position do not present significant problems since a standard inspired P_{O_2} and the sitting position are utilized during measurements in most clinical laboratories. Equations to correct for alterations of alveolar P_{O_2} are available if needed. Empirical equations also can adjust the predicted value of DL_{CO} to compensate for anemia or polycythemia.

Variability in cardiac output and the alveolar volume present during the measurement provides more significant problems. The increases in DL_{CO} observed during exercise are the result of large increases in cardiac output. Increasing cardiac output together with enlargement of the capillary bed increases not only V_c, but also increases Dm because capillary volume and surface area of the alveolar–capillary membrane are related variables. Clinical measurements of DL_{CO} are accomplished under resting conditions, minimizing but not obviating, variability in cardiac output. In addition, disease can alter the distribution of blood flow in the lung in patterns that do not match the distribution of diffusive properties. Unfortunately, measurements of pulmonary blood flow and its distribution are not conveniently measured in clinical laboratories. As a result, the effect of cardiac output on DL_{CO} may not be appreciated in routine determinations. The only practical alternative is to minimize conditions that might alter pulmonary blood flow.

Reduction in alveolar volume by disease is the largest potential source of error in interpreting DL_{CO}. Correction for the effect of altered alveolar volume has been attempted by reporting the ratio of DL_{CO}/VA. However, this attempt to normalize measurements by alveolar volume leads to errors because DL_{CO}/VA does not remain constant as alveolar volume changes. Stam et al.[14] reported values of DL_{CO} and DL_{CO}/VA obtained at several alveolar volumes in normal subjects. They recommend using predicted values of DL_{CO} or DL_{CO}/VA for patients with reduced alveolar volumes equal to values in normal subjects measured at the same reduced alveolar volume. This assumes that disease processes that reduce alveolar volume in patients produce the same changes in DL_{CO} as voluntary reduction in alveolar volume in normal subjects. In a subsequent report,[19] they demonstrated this to be the case in patients with normal lung function tested before, during, and after undergoing treatment with bleomycin for malignancies. In these patients, the linear relationship of DL_{CO}/VA measured at different alveolar volumes shifted downward in parallel fashion as bleomycin produced lung injury. This finding supports the adjustment of predicted values on the basis of reduced alveolar volumes in normal subjects since the slope of the DL_{CO}/VA ratio in relation to VA was the same before and after lung injury. These data were obtained by measuring DL_{CO} at a variety of alveolar volumes prior to and after the pulmonary insult, a situation that is rarely possible in clinical practice. Data obtained in patients with sarcoidosis also support the concept of using predicted values obtained at lower lung volumes in normal subjects.[9] However, other reports in different clinical conditions suggest that some diseases may not affect DL_{CO} in the same manner as voluntary changes in normal subjects. These uncertainties have led to substantial controversy regarding the value of the ratio DL_{CO}/VA.[15,20] Final judgment will require collection of extensive data in a variety of disease states. Regardless of the outcome of this controversy, it is apparent that if DL_{CO}/VA is used in the interpretation of measurements of DL_{CO}, there must be some adjustment of predicted values of DL_{CO}/VA to reflect reductions in alveolar volume. DL_{CO}/VA, whether expressed as a ratio of these two linked measurements or as a rate constant for CO uptake (K_{CO}), is basically the same. The value of using either expression for clinical use is uncertain.

Measurements of Dm_{CO} and V_c can be useful in a carefully controlled, research setting, but there is little or no value of using isolated measurements of these two parameters to aid in diagnosis and clinical management.[21] Calculation of Dm_{CO} and V_c involves both a number of assumptions and extrapolations of data in the literature to a specific clinical setting. Even more cogent is the lack of sufficient data to validate the use of these measurements in clinical practice.

REFERENCES

1. Bidani A. Analysis of abnormalities of capillary CO_2 exchange in vivo. *J Appl Physiol.* 1991;70:1686–1699.
2. Klocke RA. Carbon dioxide transport. In: Farhi LE, Tenney SM, eds. *Handbook of Physiology*. Vol 4. Section 3, *The Respiratory System*. Bethesda, MD: American Physiological Society; 1987:173–197.
3. Schunemann HJ, Klocke RA. Influence of CO_2 kinetics on pulmonary carbon dioxide exchange. *J Appl Physiol.* 1993;74:715–721.
4. Klocke RA. Carbon dioxide. In: Lauent GJ, Shapiro SD, eds. *Encyclopedia of Respiratory Medicine*. Oxford: Elsevier; 2006:320–324.
5. Bidani A, Crandall ED, Forster RE. Analysis of postcapillary pH changes in blood in vivo after gas exchange. *J Appl Physiol.* 1978;44:770–781.
6. Geers C, Gros G. Carbon dioxide transport and carbonic anhydrase in blood and muscle. *Physiol Rev.* 2000;80:681–715.
7. Wieth JO, Andersen OS, Brahm J, Bjerrum PJ, Borders CL Jr. Chloride-bicarbonate exchange in red cells: physiology of transport and chemical modification of binding sites. *Philos Trans R Soc Lond B Biol Sci.* 1982;299:383–399.
8. Roughton FJ, Forster RE. Relative importance of diffusion and chemical reaction rates in determining rate of exchange of gases in the human lung, with special reference to true diffusing capacity of pulmonary membrane and volume of blood in lung capillaries. *J Appl Physiol.* 1957;11:290–302.
9. Phansalkar AR, Hanson CM, Shakir AR, Johnson RL Jr, Hsia CC. Nitric oxide diffusing capacity and alveolar microvascular recruitment in sarcoidosis. *Am J Respir Crit Care Med.* 2004;169:1034–1040.
10. Borland CD, Dunningham H, Bottrill F, et al. Significant blood resistance to nitric oxide transfer in the lung. *J Appl Physiol.* 2010;108:1052–1060.
11. Macintyre N, Crapo RO, Viegi G, et al. Standardization of the single-breath determination of carbon monoxide uptake in the lung. *Eur Respir J.* 2005;26:720–735.
12. Carlin JI, Hsia CC, Cassidy SS, Ramanathan M, Clifford PS, Johnson RL Jr. Recruitment of lung diffusing capacity with exercise before and after pneumonectomy in dogs. *J Appl Physiol.* 1991;70:135–142.
13. Hsia CC. Recruitment of lung diffusing capacity. *Chest.* 2002;122:1774–1783.
14. Stam H, Hrachovina V, Stijnen T, Versprille A. Diffusing capacity dependent on lung volume and age in normal subjects. *J Appl Physiol.* 1994;76:2356–2363.
15. Van den Lee I, Zanen P, van den Bosch JM, Lammers JW. Pattern of diffusion disturbance related to clinical diagnosis: the K_{CO} has no diagnostic value next to the DL_{CO}. *Respir Med.* 2006;100:101–109.
16. Punjabi NM, Shade D, Patel AM, Wise RA. Measurement variability in single-breath diffusing capacity of the lung. *Chest.* 2003;123:1082–1089.
17. Wise RA, Teeter JG, Jensen RL, et al. Standardization of the single-breath diffusing capacity in a multicenter clinical trial. *Chest.* 2007;132:1191–1197.
18. Graham BL, Mink JT, Cotton DJ. Effects of increasing carboxyhemoglobin on the single breath carbon monoxide diffusing capacity. *Am J Respir Crit Care Med.* 2002;165:1504–1510.
19. Stam H, Splinter TA, Versprille A. Evaluation of diffusing capacity in patients with a restrictive lung disease. *Chest.* 2000;117:752–757.
20. Hughes JM, Pride NB. Examination of the carbon monoxide diffusing capacity (DL_{CO}) in relation to its K_{CO} and VA Components. *Am J Respir Crit Care Med.* 2012;186:132–139.
21. Plummer A. The carbon monoxide diffusing capacity: clinical implications, coding and documentation. *Chest.* 2008;134:663–667.

CHAPTER 17

Acid–Base Balance

Stanley Goldfarb
Kumar Sharma

Regulation of $[H^+]$ is of crucial importance for maintenance of normal cellular functions. The normal $[H^+]$ is maintained at about 40 nEq/L. When there is even a small change in the $[H^+]$, intracellular proteins gain or lose H^+ ions resulting in alterations in charge distribution which may affect molecular structure and protein function. The hydrogen ion concentration in bodily fluids is largely regulated by the ratio of the concentrations of carbon dioxide and bicarbonate. This is predicated upon the relationship demonstrated in the Henderson–Hasselbalch equation:

$$pH = pKa + \frac{[HCO_3^-]}{0.03P_{CO_2}} \quad (1)$$

where pH $= -\log[H^+]$ (the H^+ concentration measured in moles per liter) and pKa $= 6.10$. The lungs are responsible for modulating arterial P_{CO_2}, whereas the kidneys are primarily responsible for modulating the concentration of bicarbonate in plasma. In concert, these organs maintain a stable extracellular acid–base milieu that is readily assessed by measuring arterial pH.

The normal internal environment is maintained within narrow limits: The arterial blood pH is kept remarkably close to 7.40, the bicarbonate concentration is maintained around 24.5 mEq/L, and the P_{CO_2} is maintained at about 40 mm Hg. Deviations of the pH with accompanying changes in the P_{CO_2} and $[HCO_3^-]$ result in the four major categories denoted in Table 17-1. Metabolic acidosis is characterized by acidemia (pH < 7.35) that is due to reduced plasma $[HCO_3^-]$. Metabolic alkalosis is characterized by an alkalemia (pH > 7.45) that results from an elevation in the plasma $[HCO_3^-]$. Respiratory acidosis is due to hypoventilation resulting in a net increase in P_{CO_2} (hypercapnia) and a concomitant fall in pH. Respiratory alkalosis is due to primary hyperventilation leading to a fall in P_{CO_2} (hypocapnia) and a rise in pH.

TABLE 17-1 Patterns of P_{CO_2} and HCO_3 Changes in Acid–Base Disorders

Primary Disturbance	Initial Abnormality	Compensatory Response	Expected Compensation
Metabolic acidosis	Decreased pH, decreased $[HCO_3^-]$	Decreased P_{CO_2}	$P_{CO_2} = 1.5 \times [HCO_3^-] + 8 \pm 2$ (Winter's formula)
Metabolic alkalosis	Increased pH, increased $[HCO_3^-]$	Increased P_{CO_2}	P_{CO_2} increases 0.6 mm Hg per mEq/L rise in $[HCO_3^-]$
Respiratory acidosis	Decreased pH, increased P_{CO_2}	Increased $[HCO_3^-]$	Acute: $[HCO_3^-]$ increases 1 mEq/L per 10 mm Hg rise in P_{CO_2} Chronic: $[HCO_3^-]$ increases 3.5 mEq/L per 10 mm Hg rise in P_{CO_2}
Respiratory alkalosis	Increased pH, increased P_{CO_2}	Decreased $[HCO_3^-]$	Acute: $[HCO_3^-]$ falls 2 mEq/L per 10 mm Hg fall in P_{CO_2} Chronic: $[HCO_3^-]$ falls 5 mEq/L per 10 mm Hg fall in P_{CO_2}

In this chapter, we first review the basic physiologic roles that the kidneys and lungs play in maintaining acid–base balance and then discuss their adaptation in primary acid–base disorders. The following section then focuses on clinical application of physiologic concepts in analyzing acid–base problems as encountered by the clinician.

BASIC PHYSIOLOGY OF THE ROLE OF THE KIDNEY IN ACID–BASE BALANCE

Normal metabolism generates large quantities of volatile acid (CO_2) and nonvolatile acid daily. The complete metabolism of carbohydrates and fats generates 15,000 mmol of CO_2 daily. This leads to acid generation as the CO_2 combines with H_2O to form carbonic acid (H_2CO_3). As the volatile fraction is excreted by the lungs during respiration, acid accumulation does not occur. The nonvolatile or "fixed" fraction is produced at a rate of 1 mEq/kg per day. The major source of the nonvolatile acid fraction is the oxidation of sulfur-containing proteins from the diet to sulfuric acid. If this amount of nonvolatile acid is not excreted, life-threatening metabolic acidosis ensues; therefore, for a normal individual to maintain acid–base balance, 50 to 100 mEq of nonvolatile acid must be excreted daily by the kidneys.

The addition of 50 to 100 mEq of acid requires initial buffering before it can be excreted. Whole-body buffering capacity is composed of interacting buffer systems: the bicarbonate and nonbicarbonate buffers (Buf^-), consisting primarily of hemoglobin, proteins, and phosphates. The sum of the buffer anions $[HCO_3^-]$ and $[Buf^-]$ is the total buffer base and defines total-body buffering capacity. Since all body buffer systems are in equilibrium, a change in the serum $[HCO_3^-]$ reflects concurrent changes in the other body buffer systems. The importance of bicarbonate in buffering is due to its relationship with CO_2. As H^+ ions are buffered by HCO_3^-, there is a decrease in the $[HCO_3^-]$ and a concurrent increase in the dissolved $[CO_2]$. As the $[CO_2]$ can be excreted by the lungs to maintain a constant $[CO_2]$, this substantially increases the buffering capacity of bicarbonate. Since the kidney plays a major role in controlling the $[HCO_3^-]$ and $[HCO_3^-]$ is easily measured in serum, the HCO_3^- anion is a useful parameter to evaluate the renal response to an acid load.

The H^+ ions released from the dissociation of sulfuric acid are titrated by blood bicarbonate and nonbicarbonate buffers.

$$H_2SO_4 + 2NaHCO_3 \rightarrow Na_2SO_4 + 2H_2CO_3 \rightarrow 2H_2O + CO_2 \quad (2)$$

Although the added H^+ is excreted via CO_2 elimination by the lungs, this occurs at the cost of depletion of $[HCO_3^-]$. To *replenish* the consumed base, bicarbonate is reabsorbed by the kidneys and returned to the blood. This process does not accomplish the replacement of consumed base, since continuous metabolic production of acid will ultimately decrease the available base present. The process of renal *regeneration* of base requires the urinary excretion of acid or H^+ ions in the absence of any urinary bicarbonate. For every H^+ ion excreted, a bicarbonate is returned to the body. If there is any bicarbonate in the urine, there will be a net gain of H^+. Therefore the kidney has two major functions in this context: (1) reabsorption of all the filtered bicarbonate—this takes place primarily in the proximal tubule and (2) the base consumed by metabolism must be generated in the process of urinary acid excretion. This takes place in the distal portions of the nephron, the distal collecting tubule, and the collecting ducts.

BICARBONATE RECLAMATION

The proximal tubule is responsible for reclaiming 70% to 90% of the filtered bicarbonate. This may occur either by direct bicarbonate absorption at the proximal tubule or via proton secretion into the lumen of the tubule. The latter mechanism appears to be the predominant pathway.[1] Acid excretion across the apical membrane of the proximal tubule occurs by an Na^+/H^+ antiporter (NHE3)[2] and to a lesser extent by a proton pump. The secreted proton enters the tubular fluid and combines with filtered bicarbonate ions leading to carbonic acid formation. Under the influence of carbonic anhydrase, carbonic acid is then split into CO_2 and H_2O. The CO_2 diffuses into the cell where it is rehydrated to carbonic acid and then again split into protons and bicarbonate. The bicarbonate ion exits from the cell through the basolateral membrane into the interstitium via a $3HCO_3/Na$ (NBCe1) symporter, while the proton is secreted into the lumen. The basolateral membrane Na^+/K^+ ATPase antiporter, maintaining a low intracellular sodium concentration, further enhances the NHE3 activity.

In summary, reabsorption of bicarbonate is a cyclic phenomenon and requires carbonic anhydrase and is strictly associated to sodium reabsorption.

Biochemical studies show that total NHE3 and NBCe1 protein abundance are upregulated by chronic respiratory acidosis.[3] However, the main mechanism responsible for the elevation in serum bicarbonate is the increased excretion of titratable acid and ammonium which are stimulated by persistently elevated P_{CO_2} (see Fig. 17-1).[4] It is important to understand that this process reclaims filtered bicarbonate but does not result in a net gain of bicarbonate. At the end of the proximal tubule there is a lowering of the luminal pH from 7.26 to 6.70, and the bicarbonate concentration is lowered from 24 mEq/L to 8 mEq/L.[5] The fluid delivered to the distal tubule is essentially the same with respect to pH and bicarbonate concentration as that which leaves the proximal tubule. The reclamation of the remaining bicarbonate occurs in the thick ascending limb and in the outer medullary collecting tubule. At the collecting tubule, H^+ secretion occurs primarily by an H^+ ATPase pump at the luminal membrane and bicarbonate entry to the blood is via a Cl^-/HCO_3^- exchanger at the basolateral membrane.[6]

The crucial role of carbonic anhydrase is demonstrated by the fact that carbonic anhydrase inhibitors, that is, acetazolamide, result in bicarbonate wasting and the generation and maintenance of metabolic acidosis. The most physiologically important regulators of reclamation of bicarbonate are the pH, the P_{CO_2}, and the extracellular volume status of the patient. In states of acidosis, there is enhanced luminal Na^+/H^+ exchange that may be mediated by an increase in intracellular H^+ ions and by increasing the number of new exchangers and increased activity of the Na^+/HCO_3^- cotransporter at the basolateral membrane. Elevation of the P_{CO_2} will promote higher proximal tubular concentration of CO_2 and lead to intracellular acidosis, giving rise to further secretion of H^+ ions and reclamation of bicarbonate. If there is volume depletion, there will be avid Na^+ reabsorption at the proximal tubule in exchange for H^+ and thus greater reabsorption of bicarbonate. Other factors that are important include the luminal bicarbonate concentration, the tubular flow rate, and the serum potassium.

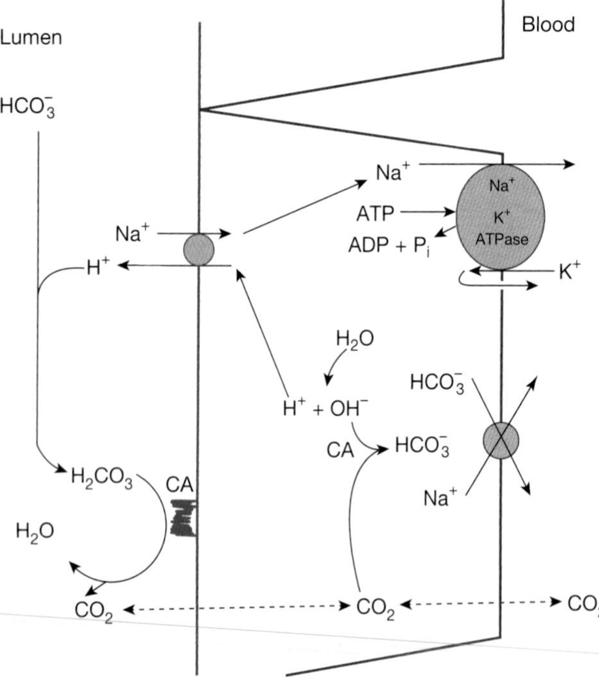

Figure 17-1 Schematic representation of proximal tubular reclamation of filtered bicarbonate. In the lumen, filtered bicarbonate reacts with secreted H^+, generating carbonic acid, which is dehydrated by carbonic anhydrase, CA, located on the brush border. The cell secretes H^+ by a process that exchanges H^+ for filtered Na^+. The source of secreted H^+ is water, which in turn generates OH^- and subsequently bicarbonate because of the presence of intracellular CA. Bicarbonate exits the basolateral side of the cell linked in some fashion with Na^+; sodium is also actively pumped out of the cell.

NET RENAL ACID EXCRETION

Net excretion of acid occurs primarily in the distal nephron and is largely mediated by the active secretory pumps, H^+-K^+ ATPase and H^+ ATPase. The latter appears to be linked in some way to Cl^- reabsorption to preserve electroneutrality. By definition, to produce net H^+ excretion the secreted H^+ will have to be excreted in processes that do not consume bicarbonate.

To achieve net secretion of protons in the luminal fluid of the distal nephron requires association of the protons with urinary buffers other than bicarbonate. Although secreted protons lower the urinary pH to 4.5 resulting in a 3 pH unit differential from arterial pH (a 1000-fold increase in H^+ concentration), the quantity of acid excreted as free H^+ is trivial. For example, daily excretion of 2 L of urine with a pH of 5 would result in excretion of only 0.02 mEq of dissociated H^+ ions in contrast to the 50 to 100 mEq of H^+ generated each day from dietary sources. The nonbicarbonate buffers present in the urine that carry out the role of net acid excretion are the titratable buffers, primarily phosphate, which accounts for 40% of net acid excretion, and ammonia, which accounts for the remainder.

The ability of phosphate to act as proton acceptor in the urine is based on its pKa of 6.8. As the urine pH is lowered below the pKa of 6.8, there is conversion of HPO_4^- to H_2PO_4. This transfer continues until the urine pH reaches 5.5, at which point almost all the phosphate present is in the associated form, H_2PO_4. Other components of this system are uric acid (pKa = 5.75) and creatinine (pKa = 4.97). Although the titratable buffers account for a sizable fraction of net basal acid excretion, they cannot increase in amount to enhance acid excretion in settings of acid loading since phosphate excretion depends on phosphate intake and not on synthesis as is the case for ammonia excretion.

The rate of ammonium (NH_4^+) production and excretion can, however, be varied according to physiologic needs. Ammonia (NH_3) combines with H^+ to form ammonium, which is trapped in the collecting tubule lumen and excreted in the urine. The pKa for this reaction is 9.0. The majority of ammonia is synthesized in the proximal tubular cell by the enzymatic breakdown of glutamine.

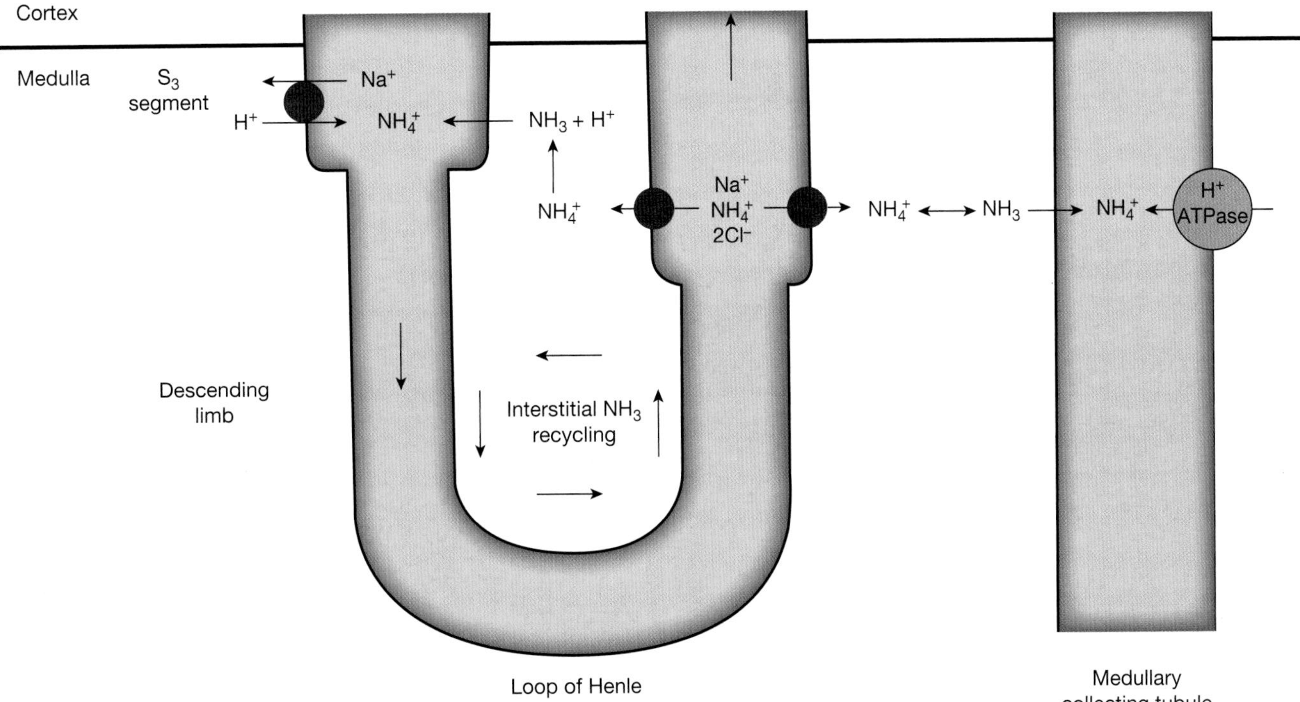

Figure 17-2 Schematic representation of ammonia recycling within the renal medulla. Although NH_4^+ production occurs predominantly in the proximal tubule, most of the NH_4^+ is then reabsorbed in the thick ascending limb, apparently by substitution for K^+ on the Na^+-K^+-$2Cl^-$ carrier in the luminal membrane. Partial dissociation into NH_3 and H^+ then occurs in the less acid tubular cell. The NH_3 diffuses into the medullary interstitium, where it reaches relatively high concentrations; it then diffuses back into those segments that have the lowest pH and therefore have the most favorable gradient: the S_3 segment of the late proximal tubule and, more important, the medullary collecting tubule, where the secreted NH_3 is trapped as NH_4^+ and then excreted. *(Reproduced with permission from Rose B. Clinical Physiology of Acid-Base and Electrolyte Disorders, 4th ed. New York: McGraw-Hill; 1994.)*

Glutamine is actively taken up by the proximal tubule at the apical and basolateral membranes and transported to mitochondria.[1] Deamidation by glutaminase forms ammonium and glutamate. The latter is further metabolized by glutamate dehydrogenase to form ammonium and α-ketoglutarate. Metabolism of α-ketoglutarate to bicarbonate in the liver leads to return of bicarbonate to the systemic circulation (Fig. 17-2).

The ammonium that is formed is transported into the proximal tubular lumen via the Na^+-H^+ antiporter, working in this case as an Na^+–NH_4^+ antiporter. The ammonium is then reabsorbed in the thick ascending limb by substitution of NH_4^+ for K^+ on the Na^+–K^+–$2Cl^-$ carrier. The intracellular ammonium in the thick ascending limb cell is then dissociated into ammonia and H^+. The ammonia accumulates in the medullary interstitium and is finally secreted into the lumen of the medullary collecting tubule. At this site, due to the low lumen pH (4.5–5) the ammonia accepts an H^+ and is trapped in the lumen and excreted in the urine as NH_4Cl.

The importance of the ammonia system is that it can be regulated by the systemic acid–base state. An acid load initially leads to an increase in ammonium excretion within 2 hours due to formation of a more acidic urine which enhances ammonia diffusion into the lumen at the collecting duct. After 5 to 6 days there is maximal NH_4^+ excretion due to increased glutamine uptake and enhanced activity of phosphate-dependent glutaminase and glutamate dehydrogenase to produce more ammonium in the proximal tubule.[6] This is presumably mediated by intracellular acidosis of the proximal tubular cell. The net effect is that NH_4^+ excretion can increase from about 30 mEq per day to as much as 300 mEq/d in severe metabolic acidosis. The plasma potassium is an important regulator of ammonia synthesis as hyperkalemia will result in a transcellular influx of K^+ in exchange for H^+ resulting in lowering of the intracellular H^+ concentration, thus causing an intracellular alkalosis with consequent inhibition of ammonia synthesis. Hypokalemia would have the opposite effect. Urinary acidification is also very important, since an inability to lower urinary pH will result in a reduction in NH_3 trapping in the collecting duct lumen and a subsequent inhibition of the degree of ammonium formation. Inadequate acidification of the urine will also inhibit H_2PO_4 formation.

RESPIRATORY CONTRIBUTION TO ACID–BASE BALANCE

The major roles of the lungs in acid–base balance are to excrete the CO_2 produced daily by aerobic metabolism and to compensate for primary metabolic acid–base disturbances by altering the rate and depth of ventilation. The CO_2 generated by the tissues diffuses into the plasma, at the peripheral capillaries, and is present in the blood in three compartments. Part of the CO_2 remains in the gas phase, but the amount is limited by the solubility coefficient of CO_2 (0.03 mM/mm Hg). CO_2 may also react with amino groups of proteins and form carbamino compounds. The majority of the CO_2 is carried within red blood cells.[7] The red cells contain carbonic anhydrase, which hydrates the CO_2 and thus forms carbonic acid, which dissociates to H^+ and HCO_3^-. The protons are buffered by hemoglobin which has an increased affinity for H^+ at the low oxygen tension present in the peripheral capillaries and venous blood. The bicarbonate produced in the red cell leaves the cell in exchange for chloride. This chloride shift is a characteristic response to elevation of CO_2 in the blood resulting in an acute elevation of bicarbonate in exchange for a drop in serum chloride. When the blood enters the pulmonary circulation, the enhanced oxygenation of hemoglobin promotes release of bound H^+. The H^+ and HCO_3^-, via carbonic anhydrase, combine to reform CO_2, which passively diffuses from the blood into the pulmonary interstitium where the CO_2 tension is very low. Subsequently, CO_2 is lost into the alveolar space.

The rate of minute ventilation is controlled by two sets of chemoreceptors: Those in the respiratory center in the brain stem and those in the carotid and aortic bodies located at the bifurcation of the carotid arteries and in the aortic arch, respectively. The central chemoreceptors are stimulated by an increase in the P_{CO_2} or by metabolic acidosis, both of which appear to be sensed by a fall in the pH of the surrounding cerebral interstitial fluid. The peripheral chemoreceptors are primarily stimulated by hypoxemia, although they may also respond to acidemia. The level of alveolar or effective ventilation varies in accord with the total minute ventilation. Level of total ventilation changes as a function of metabolic demand. Under normal circumstances, P_{CO_2} is well controlled between 38 and 42 mm Hg according to the relationship:

$$P_{CO_2} = \frac{\dot{V}_{CO_2}}{\dot{V}_A} \quad (3)$$

where $\dot{V}_{CO_2}$ is CO_2 production (reflecting metabolic rate) and $\dot{V}_A$ is alveolar ventilation (reflecting CO_2 clearance).

Under basal conditions the volatile acid production or CO_2 that is metabolically generated is completely eliminated by the lungs. The mechanism of the central stimulation of respiration in response to an elevated CO_2 is a topic of intense debate and will not be focused upon in this section (see further details in Chapter 11). However, intracranial adjustments to pH have been consistently observed and have interesting parallels to the effects of acidosis on the proximal tubular cell in the kidney. Increased concentrations of CO_2 in the cerebrospinal fluid (CSF) result in intracellular acidosis, an increase in CSF bicarbonate concentration, and an equimolar reduction in CSF chloride concentration.[7] As brain cells increase their bicarbonate concentration, there is increased buffering, and intracellular brain pH is returned toward normal. The major group of cells within the central nervous system (CNS) responsible for acid–base regulation are the glial cells and the cells of the choroid plexus.[7,8] These cells contain carbonic anhydrase[9] which converts intracellular CO_2H_2O to H^+ and HCO_3^-. The H^+ is exchanged for Na^+ on the blood side, allowing the intracellular pH to increase. The administration of acetazolamide into the cerebral ventricles blocks the expected increase in CSF bicarbonate in response to hypercapnia.[8] In addition to changes in bicarbonate concentration in the CSF in response to hypercapnia, there are also changes in the levels of ammonia.[10] Brain and CSF ammonia increase in hypercapnia; ammonia acts to enhance H^+ buffering thereby preventing a fall in the bicarbonate concentration.

ACUTE AND CHRONIC ADAPTATION TO RESPIRATORY ACIDOSIS

Figure 17-3 depicts the acute steady-state relationships among P_{CO_2}, plasma bicarbonate concentration, and plasma hydrogen concentration during graded degrees of acute hypercapnia.[11,12] These observations were obtained by sequentially exposing unanesthetized normal human volunteers to increasing concentrations of inspired carbon dioxide in a large environmental chamber. Increasing degrees of hypercapnia are associated with a curvilinear rise in plasma bicarbonate concentration, with higher levels of P_{CO_2} resulting in lesser incremental changes in bicarbonate concentration. This acute rise in bicarbonate is largely due to the chloride shift as described earlier. As a result of the modest increment in bicarbonate, the average rise in plasma $[H^+]$ is limited to 0.75 nEq/L per mm Hg rise in P_{CO_2} rather than the 1 nEq/mm Hg rise that would have occurred if the plasma bicarbonate concentration did not change.[13]

The quantitative aspects of the adaptive response to acute hypercapnia are influenced markedly by the baseline acid–base

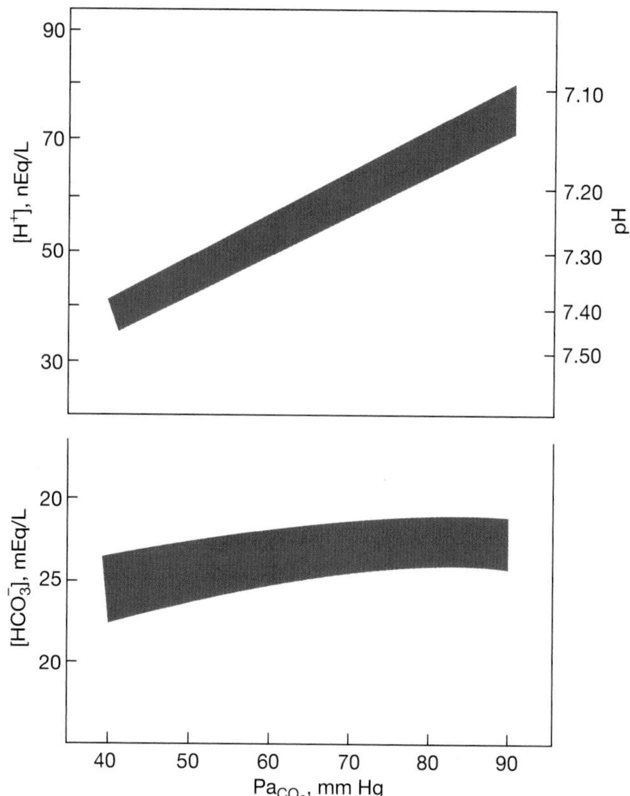

Figure 17-3 Ninety-five percent confidence bands for plasma hydrogen ion and bicarbonate concentrations during acute hypercapnia in normal humans. *(Adapted with permission from Brackett NC Jr, Cohen JJ, Schwartz WB. Carbon dioxide titration curve of normal man: effect of increasing degrees of acute hypercapnia on acid-base equilibrium. New Engl J Med. 1965;272:6–12.)*

status. Acute hypercapnia induces a larger increment in both plasma bicarbonate and H^+ ion concentrations in animals with pre-existing hypobicarbonatemia (whether from metabolic acidosis or from chronic respiratory alkalosis) than in animals with pre-existing hyperbicarbonatemia (whether from metabolic alkalosis or from chronic respiratory acidosis).[14] This points out that the factor controlling the amount of bicarbonate generated from an acute rise in P_{CO_2} is not only the initial pH but also the initial bicarbonate concentration. Although the rise in bicarbonate in response to hypercapnia limits the fall in pH acutely, to excrete the gain of H^+ produced from the rise in P_{CO_2} requires renal compensatory mechanisms.

During the initial period of respiratory acidosis, renal compensation takes about 3 to 5 days, during which time there is enhanced reabsorption of proximal tubular bicarbonate, enhanced secretion of H^+, and increased ammonia production.[15]

These processes will lead to an increase of the serum bicarbonate concentration and a rise in the systemic pH toward normal. However, when a steady state is achieved and a stable P_{CO_2} is present, there is no longer an increase in ammonia production. As filtered bicarbonate is increased, there is enhanced proximal secretion of H^+ and a normalization of intracellular pH removing the stimulus for ammonia synthesis.[15]

RENAL ADAPTATION TO RESPIRATORY ALKALOSIS

The adaptive responses to respiratory alkalosis occur in two distinct steps, in close analogy with respiratory acidosis. Hypocapnia reduces the carbonic acid concentration and causes a prompt fall in H^+.[16] Acutely, this alkalemia is ameliorated by a secondary, adaptive reduction in plasma bicarbonate concentration that stems principally from titration of nonbicarbonate body buffers.[17] During protracted hypocapnia, renal adaptive mechanisms yield a further and larger secondary reduction in plasma bicarbonate that results in still greater amelioration of the alkalemia.[17]

In acute uncomplicated respiratory alkalosis the plasma bicarbonate concentration falls by approximately 0.2 mEq/L for each mm Hg reduction in P_{CO_2}. Thus, a reduction in plasma bicarbonate of 3 to 4 mEq/L occurs within minutes after P_{CO_2} is lowered to 20 to 25 mm Hg. The resulting change in plasma H^+ concentration is approximately 0.75 mEq/L for each mm Hg fall in P_{CO_2}, similar to the relationship between P_{CO_2} and H^+ in acute hypercapnia.

When hypocapnia persists beyond the acute phase, the additional decrement in plasma bicarbonate concentration is a consequence of renal adaptive responses and reflects a dampening of hydrogen ion secretion by the renal tubule.[5] As a result, a transient suppression of net acid excretion occurs, largely manifested by a fall in ammonium excretion and by an increase in net bicarbonate excretion. These changes lead, in turn, to a positive hydrogen ion balance and a reduction in the body's bicarbonate stores. Persistence of the resulting hypobicarbonatemia is explained by the continued inhibition of tubular hydrogen ion secretion and suppression of bicarbonate reabsorption.

The adaptive retention of acid during chronic hypocapnia is normally accompanied by a loss of sodium into the urine; the resultant decrease in the extracellular volume promotes chloride retention and the typical hyperchloremia of chronic respiratory alkalosis.[18] Upon reaching a new steady state, the net excretion of acid returns to control levels, and the altered anionic concentration of the extracellular fluid (ECF), namely hypobicarbonatemia and hyperchloremia, is maintained by a reduced bicarbonate reabsorption and enhanced chloride reabsorption. On average, the combined effect of cell buffers and renal compensation results in a new steady state in which the plasma HCO_3^- concentration falls approximately 4 mEq/L for each 10 mm Hg reduction in the P_{CO_2}.[19] The renal adaptation to persistent hypocapnia appears to be mediated by some direct effect of P_{CO_2} itself, not the systemic pH. In animals in which plasma bicarbonate was reduced by HCl loading prior to adaptation to sustained hypocapnia, the renal response to a primary reduction in P_{CO_2} was the same as in normal individuals, even though the net effect of this adaptation was an overt fall in pH.

RESPIRATORY ADJUSTMENT TO METABOLIC ACIDOSIS

Metabolic acidosis stimulates both central and peripheral chemoreceptors to increase alveolar ventilation and decrease P_{CO_2} to limit the fall in pH. Although peripheral chemoreceptors appear to play a small role, in animal experiments the same degree of respiratory compensation occurs with intact and with ablated peripheral chemoreceptors. The increase in ventilation begins within 1 to 2 hours and reaches its maximal level at 12 to 24 hours. The stereotype is Kussmaul's breathing in acute diabetic ketoacidosis, in which tidal volume is characteristically large with minute ventilation increasing by as much as 35 L. On average, studies in otherwise normal patients with metabolic acidosis reveal that the P_{CO_2} will fall 1.2 mm Hg for every 1.0 mEq/L reduction in plasma HCO_3^- down to a minimum P_{CO_2} of 10 to 15 mm Hg.[20]

On the other hand, failure to mount the expected ventilatory response to metabolic acidosis is an important indicator of respiratory decompensation. Daniel et al.[21] in 140 critically ill trauma patients with metabolic acidosis applied the traditional formula derived from patients with chronic metabolic acidosis. Those whose Pa_{CO_2} exceeded the predicted Pa_{CO_2} by 2 mm Hg or more were 4.2 times more likely to be intubated and compensation status was an independent predictor of intubation as early as 60 minutes after episodes of significant hypotension.

RESPIRATORY ADJUSTMENT TO METABOLIC ALKALOSIS

The development of metabolic alkalosis is sensed by the respiratory chemoreceptors resulting in a decline in alveolar ventilation and an elevation of the P_{CO_2}. On average, the P_{CO_2} rises 0.7 mm Hg for every 1.0 mEq/L increment in the plasma HCO_3^- concentration.[18] Values significantly different from the predicted value represent superimposed respiratory acidosis or alkalosis. However, it is unclear whether this response significantly protects the pH from rising. In experimental animals, the rise in P_{CO_2} in metabolic alkalosis increases net H^+ excretion leading to an increase in the HCO_3^- concentration. The effect after several days is that the arterial pH is the same as it would have been if there had been no respiratory compensation.[6,18]

Ventilation may be strongly affected by influences other than acid–base balance. Among these influences are body temperature, increases in circulating catecholamines, changes in cerebral blood flow, changes in systemic blood pressure, and changes in metabolic activities of different organs (e.g., liver), as well as the physiologic state of the lung itself. Perhaps for teleologic reasons, the defense of chronic metabolic acid–base imbalances by ventilatory compensation is not of major importance.

ALTERNATIVE CONCEPTS OF ACID–BASE BALANCE

The preceding discussion has tacitly assumed that the systemic pH is the final control that affects the renal and respiratory response to an acid–base disorder; however, this issue is certainly not settled. The proximal tubular cell of the kidney can often have effects that are more predictably based on the P_{CO_2} rather than the arterial pH. If P_{CO_2} is elevated, the proximal tubular cells act to secrete protons and reabsorb bicarbonate whether or not there is systemic alkalosis or acidosis. This may be explained if an elevation in P_{CO_2} results in intracellular acidosis and the cell is responding appropriately to its internal milieu.[6,18] Similarly, in the central control of respiration, it is controversial as to whether it is CSF pH, interstitial pH, P_{CO_2}, or the bicarbonate concentration that stimulates compensatory changes in ventilation.[7]

In addition to the previously mentioned observations, it is also known that changes in salt and water balance may affect acid–base status. For example, Schwartz's group[18] found that a low dietary sodium chloride intake in dogs with a stable amount of water intake results in hypoventilation, increased P_{CO_2}, and increased HCO_3^- concentration. Studies in dogs have demonstrated that increasing dietary NaCl with a fixed water intake increases the acidity of body fluids, whereas decreasing the NaCl in diet with a fixed water intake decreases the acidity of body fluids.[22]

An alternative view to understanding acid–base disorders and the regulatory response of the lungs and kidneys is offered by the theories initially proposed by Stewart.[23,24] Based on physicochemistry, Stewart emphasized the important principle that H^+ and HCO_3^- as well as the acidic and anionic forms of weak acids are actually dependent variables in a solution. The three independent variables, P_{CO_2}, the strong ion difference (SID), and the total weak anion concentration, can be manipulated externally and serve to determine the concentration of the dependent variables, H^+ and HCO_3^-. The major components of the weak anions in plasma are the albumin and inorganic phosphate concentrations. The SID is the difference between the sums of all strong cations and all strong anions:

$$[SID] = [Na^+] + [K^+] + [Ca^{2+}] + [MG^{2+}] - [CL^-] - [\text{Other Strong Anions}] \qquad (4)$$

This equation is based on the principles of: (1) electroneutrality, (2) dissociation equilibria of all incompletely dissociated substances, and (3) conservation of mass. This concept appears to better explain the basis for renal and ventilatory response in a variety of states which also affects acid–base balance. Practically, it is observed that the plasma SID is primarily regulated by the kidneys, whereas the P_{CO_2} is regulated by alveolar ventilation. The weak anion concentration is generally not regulated and may often be assumed to be stable.

This concept has primarily been used by investigators in relation to the study of central regulation of ventilation.[7] As albumin and other proteins are not present in the CSF, it is the SID and P_{CO_2} that determine the concentration of weakly dissociating electrolytes, H^+, OH^-, and HCO_3^-. In analyzing various acid–base disturbances, it appears that the change in CSF SID can predict the concentration of CSF bicarbonate.[7]

In evaluating acid–base balance in many species, there is a consistent inverse relationship between the pH and body temperature, whereas the CO_2 content remains stable.[4,25] To explain this relationship Reeves and his coworkers provided evidence that the imidazole ring structure of histidine is responsible for the pH–temperature relationship.[26] This is because imidazole has a pKa in the physiologic range (7.00), is relatively ubiquitous, and has total energy of ionization (7 kcal/mol). To integrate acid–base regulation with receptor function and control of respiration, Reeves and Rahn[4] have proposed the hypothesis that it is not the arterial or intracellular pH that is being regulated per se but rather the constancy of the fractional dissociation of the imidazole moiety of histidine contained in proteins throughout the body.

α-Imidazole is defined as the ratio of the absolute amount of unprotonated imidazole (Im) to total imidazole (HIm + Im):

$$\alpha\text{-Imidazole} = \frac{\text{Im}}{\text{HIm} + \text{Im}} \tag{5}$$

α-Imidazole regulation (alphastat regulation) would have the effect of maintaining cellular protein charge states and enzymatic functions constant. It would also maintain the OH^-/H^+ ratio constant in all compartments. There is also evidence that alphastat regulation directly influences ventilatory status. For example, application of an imidazole blocker to the chemosensitive area of the medulla in cats blocked increases in ventilation caused by local application of acid.[27] Thus, changes in P_{CO_2}, reflecting alveolar ventilation, may be determined by alphastat regulation, which maintains the OH^-/H^+ ratio constant in membranes of the cells in the chemosensitive areas of the medulla.

The difficulty with using these concepts lies in the practical measurement of the relevant molecules. For example, although the imidazole moiety of histidine is considered the most important of the intracellular buffers,[26] its pKa and total energy of ionization may vary widely due to the influence of the local configuration of molecules into which they are incorporated. Thus, even in lower animals such as fish under different temperatures, calculations based on the alphastat model do not accurately predict the acid–base disturbance, since the pKa and enthalpy of ionization vary with temperature and are difficult to measure.

Similarly, measurement of the plasma SID is problematic and is often replaced by the "SID effective," which is roughly equal to the bicarbonate concentration plus albumin and inorganic phosphate.[23] Calculation of the anion gap (AG) – $[Na^+] - [Cl^-] - [HCO_3^-]$ – accounts for the roles of the strong ions Na^+ and Cl^- as well as bicarbonate but does not account for the role of inorganic phosphate or plasma proteins. Although the bicarbonate concentration may not be, strictly speaking, an independent variable, the AG calculation does indicate the quantity of unmeasured anions and hence is an indirect measure of the SID. If one considers the impact of serum proteins and inorganic phosphate in the unmeasured anion pool, the AG gives a very useful parameter in evaluating acid–base disturbances. Many studies have compared the utility of SID versus corrected AG (corrected for the level of serum albumin) and found that it was no more accurate in making a diagnosis. One study of patients in an intensive care unit, reported that Stewart's method diagnosed underlying metabolic acidosis in 22 patients (of the total of 152 patients in the study) with normal plasma bicarbonate level. However, when the AG was corrected for hypoalbuminemia, it was elevated in all of the samples with normal bicarbonate showing the effectiveness of the traditional approach.[28] In another study of 935 ICU patients, the Stewart method detected metabolic acidosis in 14% patients with normal bicarbonate levels, whereas the traditional method made a similar diagnosis in 13% of patients.[29] A recent study in patients with septic shock and liver transplantation found an excellent correlation between SID and corrected AG.[30]

Thus, as will be described in more detail in the following section, the use of the AG is still the most clinically useful tool to determine the contribution of different metabolic etiologies of metabolic acidosis.

APPROACH TO PATIENTS WITH AN ACID–BASE DISTURBANCE

In this section, we examine the diagnostic approach to disorders of acid–base balance with a particular emphasis on the ventilatory response and its role in mitigating or exacerbating acid–base disorders. We will also review the approach to the patient with complex acid–base disorders.

ANALYSIS OF CLINICAL INFORMATION

Table 17-1 summarizes the pattern of abnormality of arterial blood acid–base parameters in the four classic acid–base disorders. It also indicates the physiologic or compensatory response induced in pulmonary or renal function in response to the initial disturbance.

Base Excess and Base Deficit Notations

Base excess and *base deficit* are terms applied to an analytic method for determination of the appropriateness of responses to disorders of acid–base metabolism.[31] The base excess or deficit is determined by measuring blood pH against ambient P_{CO_2} and against a P_{CO_2} of 40 mm Hg. If the calculated HCO_3^- is below 25 when the P_{CO_2} is 40 mm Hg and the original pH is low, a base deficit is indicated. The magnitude of the deficit is expressed as the number of mEq of bicarbonate needed to restore the serum bicarbonate to 25 mEq/L at a P_{CO_2} of 40 mm Hg compared to that at the ambient P_{CO_2}. The use of notations for base excess and deficit has been debated in the medical literature. This notation is favored in the evaluation of acid–base status in the operating room because acute changes in P_{CO_2} and in HCO_3^- can be simply evaluated by this approach. However, this notation can be misleading in chronic respiratory alkalosis or acidosis, since the patient with chronic respiratory alkalosis will be categorized as suffering from a base deficit because of the low serum bicarbonate induced as compensation for the reduced P_{CO_2}. In fact, a "base deficit" is a normal physiologic response to the chronic reduction in P_{CO_2}. Unfortunately, lack of familiarity with the complete analytical paradigm used for this analysis of acid–base disorders has led some to focus on the designations "base deficit" and "base excess" as guides to bicarbonate or acid therapy in chronic respiratory disorders. In addition, discrepancies between the buffering characteristics of plasma, blood, and whole body have also been cited as potential weaknesses in a system for assessing acid–base disorders which relies on in vitro CO_2 titration methods. We, therefore, recommend that the physiologic evaluation of the patient be the mode of analysis of acid–base disorders rather than an emphasis on derived formulae.

Use of Nomograms

As indicated earlier, the body buffers and the kidneys respond in a predictable fashion to a change in P_{CO_2} whereas ventilatory response to changes in $[HCO_3^-]$ is also predictable. Also, the resulting changes in bicarbonate and pH are time dependent so that a larger change occurs in several days than in the first hours. The confidence bands for changes in P_{CO_2} or HCO_3^- in response to primary disturbances are shown in Figure 17-4.[7] Any deviation can be interpreted as a reflection of processes other than a compensatory response. For example, in a patient with chronic obstructive airways disease, other factors affecting the acid–base status are the concentration of potassium in the plasma, the size of ECF volume, chloride depletion, diuretics, renal hypoperfusion, and coexisting renal disease. The special case of posthypercapnic alkalosis is discussed in the next section.

In evaluating an acid–base disorder, the history and physical examination are invaluable in focusing attention on potential pathologic processes.[32] The composition of blood, with respect to serum electrolytes and blood gases, is then examined for consistency with clinical impressions. However, in using the acid–base map (Fig. 17-4), remember that the map is based on data from individuals who had a single disorder. Therefore, the map does not take into account the possibility of multiple disorders. For example, in a patient with chronic obstructive airways disease whose sputum has turned purulent and who develops nausea and vomiting, the possibility arises of coexistent metabolic alkalosis and acute respiratory acidosis. However, ill-advised application of the arterial blood-gas values from this patient (e.g., pH = 7.25 and P_{CO_2} = 75 mm Hg) to the acid–base map would lead to the erroneous conclusion that a chronic respiratory acidosis is present. Thus, the clinician needs to integrate laboratory data with clinical assessments to properly analyze clinical disorders of acid–base balance.

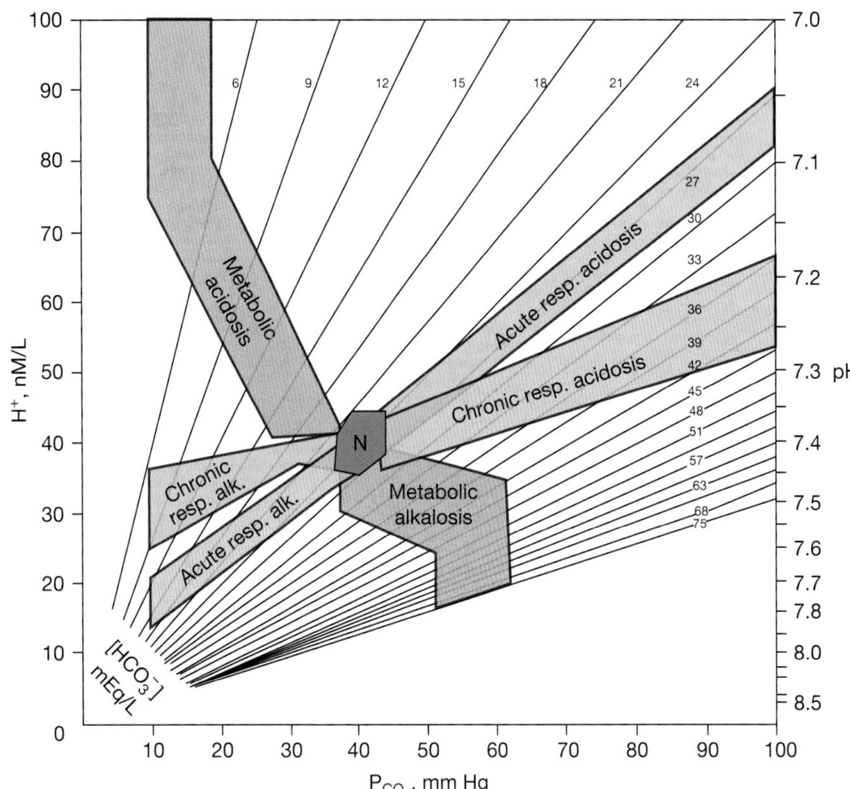

Figure 17-4 Acid–base map showing the normal range (N) and the confidence bands for acute or chronic respiratory and metabolic acid–base disturbances. The ordinates are the partial pressure of CO_2 and the hydrogen-ion activity given in nmol/L and pH units. Isopleths for bicarbonate concentration, in mEq/L, are also shown. *(Reproduced with permission from Goldberg M, Green SB, Moss ML, et al. Computer-based instruction and diagnosis of acid-base disorders. A systematic approach. JAMA. 1973;223(3):269–278.)*

APPROACH TO THE PATIENT WITH METABOLIC ACIDOSIS

An increase in the H^+ concentration of the ECF will result in a series of predictable responses which allow the clinician to ascertain the appropriateness of organized homeostatic responses to the perturbation.[20] The pathophysiologic basis for the initiation of metabolic acidosis and homeostatic responses in the defense of systemic pH have been defined earlier in descriptions of the buffering of newly introduced acid [see Eq. (1)] and in the demonstration of the normal confidence band for the ventilatory response to metabolic acidosis as detailed in the acid–base nomogram (Fig. 17-4).

A key clinical distinction in the pathogenesis of metabolic acidosis is whether the production of the acidosis is rapid or slow. If the etiology of the metabolic acidosis is merely the continued ingestion of a diet which generates a variety of fixed acids such as H_2SO_4 [see Eq. (2)] from the metabolism of methionine residues, then the serum HCO_3^- will fall slowly as only that fraction of the 50 to 100 mEq of H^+ generated from diet that is not excreted would be added to the body fluids each day. However, if the addition occurs because of an acute increase in the acid load such as may occur with lactic acidosis, the kidney capacity can be rapidly overwhelmed, and serum bicarbonate may fall precipitously. See Table 17-2 for the common causes of metabolic acidosis.

Utility of the AG

As seen in Eq. (6), the buffering of mineral acids will result in the production of the salt of the acid, NaA.

$$NaHCO_3 + HA \rightarrow NaA + H_2CO_3^- + H^+ \rightarrow CO_2 + H_2O + NaA \quad (6)$$

TABLE 17-2 Causes of Metabolic Acidosis (Common)

Failure to generate new bicarbonate to replace that consumed in buffering dietary acid load
Diminished NH_4^+ production and excretion
Reduced renal mass
Chronic hyperkalemia
Chronic aldosterone deficiency
Decreased H^+ ion secretion (primary)
Distal renal tubular acidosis
Increased H^+ ion production
Lactic acidosis
Ketoacidosis
Toxic ingestion
Bicarbonate or equivalent losses from body fluids
Renal-proximal RTA, carbonic anhydrase inhibitors
GI-diarrhea, villous adenoma, fistula

If the kidney is able to excrete this salt or, in the case of the production of the salts of organic acids such as lactic acid, if the liver can metabolize the anion to HCO_3^-, then there will be no accumulation of the anion in the ECF. Typically, anions associated with strong organic acids are not measured with routine electrolyte determinations and contribute to the so-called anion gap (AG). Determination of the plasma AG is primarily used in the differential diagnosis of metabolic acidosis. However, the AG also changes in other conditions, a finding that may be of diagnostic importance.

The plasma AG is calculated from the following formula based on routine laboratory determination[33]:

$$AG = (\text{cations}) - (\text{anions})$$

Since Na^+ is the primary measured cation and Cl^- and HCO_3^- are the primary measured anions:

$$AG = [Na^+] - ([Cl^-] + [HCO_3^-]) \tag{7}$$

The normal value is 12 ± 2 mEq/L.

An increase in the AG can be produced by an increase in unmeasured anions or by a reduction in unmeasured cations. Hypokalemia, hypocalcemia, or hypomagnesemia can only raise the AG by a few mEq/L, since these ions can only deviate from normal by a mEq/L or less and maintain a physiologic condition. The predominant extracellular unmeasured anion is actually albumin with many negative charge sites per molecule. Hence, a mild elevation in the AG can occur in conditions in which the albumin concentration or the charge characteristics of albumin are altered, for example, in metabolic alkalosis. In that instance, a number of factors may contribute to the increment, including a rise in the plasma albumin concentration due to extracellular volume depletion and contraction of plasma constituents, an increase in the number of negative charges per albumin molecule induced by the rise in extracellular pH titrating protons off the albumin molecule, and a tendency for systemic alkalemia to induce an increase in lactate production. This latter response serves a homeostatically beneficial function.

In forms of metabolic acidosis in which there is buffering of excess hydrochloric acid by extracellular bicarbonate, then

$$HCl + NaHCO_3 \rightarrow NaCl + H_2CO_3 \rightarrow CO_2 + H_2O \tag{8}$$

Bicarbonate is replaced on an equimolar basis by chloride, and there is no change in the AG; this disorder is also called a *hyperchloremic acidosis* because of the rise in the plasma chloride concentration. Both diarrhea and type 2 (proximal) renal tubular acidosis can lead to the loss of $NaHCO_3$. The kidneys compensate by retaining NaCl in an attempt to preserve volume, with the net effect being a mEq-for-mEq exchange of chloride for bicarbonate.

If the retained acid is not HCl but an organic acid whose anion is not routinely measured such as lactic acid, then the increase in the unmeasured lactate anion will raise the AG. It is important to emphasize that the acidosis is due to the retained proton; the anion is irrelevant to the change in acid–base status or systemic pH but is important as a diagnostic tool. The major causes of a high AG metabolic acidosis include those listed in Table 17-2 under disorders of increased H^+ production. Although renal failure produces an acidosis because of failure of H^+ excretion and bicarbonate production, most patients with severe renal failure retain both hydrogen and anions, such as sulfate, phosphate, and urate, and hence demonstrate a high AG.

The diagnostic utility of a high AG is greatest when the AG is above 20 mEq/L; in this setting, renal failure, lactic acidosis, or evidence of a toxic ingestion will almost always be present. When the AG is less than 20 mEq/L, identifying the anions which contribute to the mild elevation[33] is often impossible.

Urine AG

Estimation of the urinary ammonia content may be a useful clue to the etiology of metabolic acidosis as the value will increase in diseases in which kidney function affecting acid–base balance is completely intact but in which bicarbonate is lost from the body fluids.[13] The calculation of the urinary AG is shown in Eq. (9):

$$\text{Urine AG} = (\text{Urine } [Na^+] + \text{Urine } [K^+]) - \text{Urine } [Cl^-] \tag{9}$$

The usual value will be negative, between −25 and −50 mEq/L, as the ammonium content of the urine is typically in this range, and ammonium accounts for the apparent discrepancy between the level of cations and anions in the urine. In states of metabolic acidosis due to diarrhea or to chronic acid ingestion, the value will be >50 mEq/L as ammonium production is stimulated.

In some conditions, the urine AG will be very low or even positive in the face of metabolic acidosis. In all forms of renal insufficiency, ammonia production by the kidney will be deficient and significantly contribute to a reduced urinary AG and to metabolic acidosis. In type I distal RTA, inability to maintain a steep gradient for protons in the distal tubular lumen and in the collecting duct results in a deficiency in ammonia trapping in the luminal fluid and therefore a decreased excretory rate for ammonia. This in turn leads to metabolic acidosis, a low ammonia excretion, and an abnormally low urinary AG. Finally, type IV RTA, a condition in which hyperkalemia and mild renal insufficiency are found, hyperkalemia suppresses renal ammonia production, and a low urinary AG is found.

In any condition associated with hypokalemia, increased intracellular proton accumulation (which results from the exchange of cellular potassium for extracellular protons) will lead to an exaggerated ammonia production in the kidney. Hence, the use of the AG in the urine will be particularly useful to differentiate classic type I RTA from hypokalemia and acidosis due to diarrhea. The former will show a very low urine AG. Typically, a careful history will elicit the crucial information, and measurement of the urine AG will be confirmatory.

Clinical Assessment of Metabolic Acidosis

In approaching a patient with metabolic acidosis, the clinician should first assess the history and clinical circumstances. For example, patients with renal failure or with uncontrolled diabetes may be presumed to have a metabolic acidosis until disproved by laboratory analysis. The next step is to evaluate the serum electrolytes to determine the level of the serum HCO_3^- and the presence of an AG of greater than 12 ± 2 mEq/L. If both are present, then one must consider the possibility of a metabolic acidosis secondary to increased acid production as listed in Table 17-2. If the HCO_3^- is reduced but the serum AG is normal, then one is dealing with either a respiratory alkalosis or a metabolic acidosis due to reduced renal capacity to generate replacement HCO_3^- to compensate for that lost as a result of decreased acid excretion or increased HCO_3^- loss.

At this point arterial blood gases should be assessed to determine the pH and the ventilatory response. Finding a low pH establishes the diagnosis of metabolic acidosis. Reference to the acid–base nomogram (Fig. 17-4) will verify whether the clinical response is consistent with a simple metabolic acidosis with a normal ventilatory response or whether some other disturbance in ventilation is present.

■ APPROACH TO THE PATIENT WITH METABOLIC ALKALOSIS

Two separate processes are involved in metabolic alkalosis: an excess load of base that is generated either endogenously or exogenously (see Table 17-3) and maintenance of an abnormally high

TABLE 17-3 Causes of Metabolic Alkalosis

Gastrointestinal hydrogen loss
Removal of gastric secretions
Renal hydrogen loss
Primary mineralocorticoid excess
Loop or thiazide diuretics
Posthypercapnic alkalosis
Intracellular shift of hydrogen
Hypokalemia
Alkali administration
Contraction alkalosis

concentration of bicarbonate in the plasma.[5] During hypercapnia, the load of base is the result of renal compensation and *de novo* bicarbonate generation; in posthypercapnic alkalosis, the key abnormality is maintaining the bicarbonate level in plasma at inordinately high levels, as will be discussed below.

Generation of Metabolic Alkalosis

Causes of metabolic alkalosis are predominantly events that remove H^+ ions from the body but also include circumstances in which excess base is added to the body fluids. Hydrogen loss can occur from the gastrointestinal tract or in the urine. Each mEq of hydrogen lost generates 1 mEq of bicarbonate, as the source of hydrogen ions in cells which produce and secrete protons is:

$$H_2O \rightarrow H^+ + OH^- + OH^- + CO_2 \rightarrow HCO_3^- \quad (10)$$

When vomiting or tube drainage prevents stomach acid from reaching the duodenum and combining with HCO_3^- released from pancreatic secretions, the net balance of bicarbonate in body fluids becomes positive, and serum HCO_3^- begins to rise.

Increased renal acid losses may result from enhanced distal hydrogen secretion. Aldosterone acts both by directly stimulating the secretory H^+ ATPase pump and, via the stimulation of sodium reabsorption, by making the lumen more electronegative, thereby favoring hydrogen ion secretion. Increased distal nephron delivery and reabsorption of sodium further stimulates hydrogen ion secretion as the accompanying anion is less avidly reabsorbed than is sodium, and the lumen of the distal nephron becomes more negatively charged. Excess secretion of mineralocorticoids can lead to metabolic alkalosis by this pathway. In patients treated with loop-active or thiazide diuretics, enhanced distal delivery of sodium and increased secretion of aldosterone are usually present, thereby enhancing renal bicarbonate production as a result of enhanced hydrogen ion secretion. This pattern commonly leads to the development of metabolic alkalosis.

Chronic respiratory acidosis leads to a secondary increase in renal hydrogen secretion, as the subsequent rise in the plasma bicarbonate concentration will restore the pH toward normal as a compensatory response. If the patient undergoes a therapeutic maneuver such as rapid lowering of the P_{CO_2} by mechanical ventilation, a posthypercapnic form of metabolic alkalosis will ensue as the patient is left with an elevated plasma bicarbonate concentration.

Hypokalemia is a frequent finding in patients with metabolic alkalosis and may not only be the consequence of some of the disorders which lead to the initiation of metabolic alkalosis but may also actually induce an alkalotic tendency. Gastric drainage, diuretics, and mineralocorticoid excess, all induce potassium as well as hydrogen losses through the GI tract and kidney, respectively. Hypokalemia also induces a transcellular shift in which potassium is exchanged in an electroneutral fashion for hydrogen ions in the ECF. This exchange directly raises the extracellular pH, lowers the intracellular pH, and mitigates the hypokalemia. Intracellular acidosis in renal tubular cells promotes hydrogen secretion and therefore bicarbonate reabsorption (see Section Bicarbonate Reclamation p. 208).

Administering large amounts of alkali does not maintain metabolic alkalosis in normal individuals because of rapid urinary excretion, but it may induce the initiation stage of metabolic alkalosis if factors are active to sustain a high rate of renal HCO_3^- reabsorption. A form of metabolic alkalosis termed *contraction alkalosis* occurs when there is loss of relatively large volumes of bicarbonate-free fluid. Administration of a loop diuretic to induce rapid fluid removal in a markedly edematous patient is the most common cause of a contraction alkalosis. The plasma bicarbonate concentration rises in this setting because there is contraction of the extracellular volume around a relatively constant quantity of extracellular bicarbonate. The degree to which this occurs is in part minimized by intracellular buffering, as the release of hydrogen ions from cell buffers lowers the plasma bicarbonate concentration toward the baseline value. Even this form of alkalosis is probably critically dependent on increases in renal bicarbonate production for its manifestation, since the diuretics promote excess renal hydrogen ion secretion as noted earlier.

Maintenance Phase of Metabolic Alkalosis

Maintenance of metabolic alkalosis requires an increase in the reabsorption of bicarbonate by the renal tubule.[27] Four factors are known to be important in the maintenance phase of metabolic alkalosis: extracellular volume depletion, chloride depletion, hypokalemia, and mineralocorticoid excess.[34]

A reduction in ECF volume and possibly a fall in the glomerular filtration rate (GFR) secondary to extracellular volume depletion are major stimuli for increasing the proximal reabsorption of bicarbonate. The enhanced proximal tubular bicarbonate reabsorption is likely the most important factor. This reabsorption is stimulated by extracellular volume depletion which is a frequent accompaniment of metabolic alkalosis. Enhanced proximal tubular reabsorption of sodium ions is a major factor in the enhanced rate of proton secretion, a key factor in the proximal tubular reabsorptive pathway for bicarbonate. Enhanced activity of the sodium–proton exchanger in the luminal membrane of the proximal tubule is an important component of the transport system.

In addition, an important role is played by the distal nephron in maintaining metabolic alkalosis by way of the secondary phenomena of chloride depletion, extracellular volume depletion, and hypokalemia.[35] Cells of the cortical collecting tubule can either reabsorb or secrete bicarbonate depending on homeostatic requirements. For example, during excess bicarbonate ingestion, the secretory process predominates, and excess bicarbonate is lost into the urine. Chloride depletion enhances the bicarbonate reabsorptive pathway by reducing chloride availability at an anion exchange site on the luminal membrane of the type A intercalated cell. This exchange process normally allows bicarbonate entry into the urine in exchange for chloride absorption. Chloride depletion thus blocks bicarbonate loss.

Hypokalemia acts to stimulate bicarbonate reabsorption through several mechanisms. First, loss of potassium from the ECF leads to a shift of protons into the cell as potassium leaves the cell. Hence, intracellular pH falls, driving enhanced tubular bicarbonate reabsorption. Also, severe potassium depletion produces a defect in tubular fluid chloride reabsorption thus mimicking a chloride depletion state. Finally, excess mineralocorticoid hormone, either as a result of primary overproduction or due to a variety of secondary hyperreninemic states, stimulates H^+ secretion in the cortical collecting tubule and thereby stimulates increased renal tubular bicarbonate production and helps maintain metabolic alkalosis.

Typically, all four components coexist in patients with metabolic alkalosis secondary to vomiting or gastric drainage following gastric intubation. If any of the factors is present in a patient with metabolic alkalosis, therapy will be only partially successful until all the factors have been eliminated.

Depression of ventilation in metabolic alkalosis is a normal physiologic response to the elevation in serum bicarbonate but is difficult to assess clinically and may not be found in many patients as detailed earlier.[36]

Posthypercapnic Metabolic Alkalosis

In response to sustained hypercapnia, the increased excretion of hydrogen ion in the urine and the increased bicarbonate generated by the acid secretory process increase the concentration of bicarbonate in the plasma as described earlier. During this process, the total sodium content of the body remains stable as does the ECF volume (unless there is a separate reason for a volume abnormality, e.g., right ventricular failure and the use of diuretics). If correction of hypercapnia occurs, for example, through the use of mechanical ventilation without simultaneous replacement of sodium chloride, the urinary loss of sodium bicarbonate may lag for several hours or days. This is particularly true if there is concomitant depletion of the ECF volume. This leads to an increase in the reabsorption of solute, including sodium bicarbonate, by the proximal tubule, sustaining the high bicarbonate concentration in blood. This process is similar to the maintenance phase of metabolic alkalosis described earlier; the other processes outlined also could pertain to this posthypercapnic state and produce a persistent metabolic alkalosis following correction of hypercapnia.[37]

APPROACH TO THE PATIENT WITH A MIXED ACID–BASE DISORDER

The approach to patients with mixed acid–base disorders, that is, more than one disturbance in acid–base metabolism, is particularly challenging because no nomogram, calculation of base excess or deficit, or other formula can allow the clinician to parse the pathophysiologic disorders and allow a rational therapeutic plan.[18] Rather, it is the combination of clinical assessment, application of expected compensatory responses, assessment of the AG, and application of principles of physiology that together allow a successful analysis.

To determine the presence of a mixed or complex acid–base disorder, the clinician must follow a rigorous approach that integrates clinical observation with assessment of a variety of laboratory parameters. No single nomogram or other shortcut device will suffice. The initial step is to perform a history and physical examination to seek processes which could contribute to acid–base disorders. For example, any patient who has vomited has the potential for developing a metabolic alkalosis, and any patient with chronic renal failure surely has metabolic acidosis as an ongoing process for which compensation will be necessary. Moreover, many clinical conditions are typically characterized by the presence of more than one concurrent disorder. Patients with severe liver failure will usually experience respiratory alkalosis as a consequence of hepatic encephalopathy so that any other conditions associated with abnormalities of acid–base balance which may develop in these patients will result in mixed acid–base disorders. Septic shock is associated with the mixed disorders of respiratory alkalosis and metabolic acidosis due to lactic acid production. Immediately, following cardiac arrest, patients will have both a respiratory and a metabolic acidosis. Patients with renal failure who undergo gastric drainage will manifest both metabolic alkalosis and metabolic acidosis as a result of the underlying conditions. The clinician must consider these expected abnormalities in acid–base balance when addressing laboratory results.

The second step in the process is to evaluate a venous blood sample for determination of the electrolytes, blood urea nitrogen (BUN), creatinine, and other parameters indicative of liver function. Here, the evaluation of the $[HCO_3^-]$ and analysis of the AG is invaluable. Decrements or elevations of $[HCO_3^-]$ will point toward a disturbance in the body's buffering system. The AG measurement, if elevated, will clarify whether a metabolic acidosis is present, as described earlier. Also, analyzing the AG together with the venous $[HCO_3^-]$ can provide important information. Because the anions which accumulate in most forms of organic acidosis (lactic acidosis, ketoacidosis, many toxic ingestions) can be metabolized in the liver to bicarbonate through the Kreb's cycle, adding the unmeasured anion concentration to the current plasma HCO_3^- concentration indicates the level of $[HCO_3^-]$ prior to the onset of the metabolic acidosis.

ILLUSTRATIVE CASES

The following cases illustrate the clinical approach to the patient with acid–base disturbances.

METABOLIC ACIDOSIS

A 75-year-old patient presented with a 7-day history of intermittent diarrhea and a 5-lb weight loss. The rest of the history was unrevealing. Physical examination only revealed signs of volume depletion. Laboratory values were as follows:

$$[BUN] = 18 \text{ mg/dL}$$
$$[Na^+] = 138 \text{ mEq/L}$$
$$[K^+] = 3.0 \text{ mEq/L}$$
$$[Cl^-] = 110 \text{ mEq/L}$$
$$[HCO_3^-] = 13 \text{ mEq/L}$$

At this point, the lack of an elevated AG (12 mEq/L) and the reduced bicarbonate concentration together suggest the possibility of either respiratory alkalosis or metabolic acidosis of the non–AG variety, that is, in which the chloride concentration has risen as bicarbonate has been utilized in buffering reactions or has been lost from body fluids. The history of diarrhea strongly suggests that a metabolic acidosis is the culprit in the disorder. The relatively low BUN supports the theory that diarrhea, and not renal insufficiency, is the main etiologic factor.

Arterial blood gases are then obtained:

$$pH = 7.24$$
$$P_{CO_2} = 27 \text{ mm Hg}$$
$$P_{O_2} = 100 \text{ mm Hg}$$
$$[HCO_3^-] = 13 \text{ mEq/L}$$

The low serum bicarbonate in association with a low arterial blood pH indicates that the patient has a metabolic acidosis. Finding that the rate of ventilation produces a P_{CO_2} of 27 is consistent with the expected P_{CO_2} of 27.5 ± 2 mm Hg calculated from Winter's formula (see Table 17-1). Reference to the acid–base nomogram (see Fig. 17-4) reveals the graphical equivalent of this calculation as the values for pH, P_{CO_2}, and $[HCO_3^-]$ fall in the confidence band for metabolic acidosis. Other possible etiologies for this form of non–AG metabolic acidosis would include mild renal insufficiency, wherein the decline of GFR has not reached a level where the unmeasured anions such as SO_4^{2-} would begin to accumulate in plasma, and the ingestion of salts such as ammonium chloride which are metabolized in the liver to urea and hydrochloric acid. Urinary electrolyte analysis confirms the diagnosis:

$$[Na^+] = 50 \text{ mEq/L}$$
$$[K^+] = 20 \text{ mEq/L}$$
$$[Cl^-] = 140 \text{ mEq/L}$$
$$\text{Urine volume} = 2 \text{ L}$$
$$\text{Urinary AG} = -70 \text{ mEq/L}$$

The discrepancy between the sum of urine cations and anions in the negative range indicates that an unmeasured cation, in this case ammonium, is being excreted into the urine.[13] It is the excretion of protons in association with ammonia that allows the renal excretion of the accumulated acid load and the attempted regeneration of body HCO_3^- stores. If this value was not greater than −20 to −50 mEq/L, a defect in ammonia production or excretion such as could be found in renal insufficiency or in renal tubular acidosis could be present. In this case, the large urinary cation gap suggests that diarrhea is the culprit.

METABOLIC ALKALOSIS

A 65-year-old patient experienced severe and unremitting vomiting for 4 days. He has had a history of peptic ulcer disease, but he decided to medicate himself with an antacid, which he could not keep from vomiting. There was no other significant past medical history. Physical examination showed a moderate degree of orthostatic hypotension as blood pressure fell from 100/70 mm Hg supine to 90/60 mm Hg when seated. The rest of the examination was not remarkable except for some abdominal tenderness.

Laboratory results revealed the following:

$$[BUN] = 28 \text{ mg/dL}$$
$$[Na^+] = 43 \text{ mEq/L}$$
$$[K^+] = 3.0 \text{ mEq/L}$$
$$[Cl^-] = 85 \text{ mEq/L}$$
$$[HCO_3^-] = 39 \text{ mEq/L}$$

The elevation in HCO_3^- content is consistent with either metabolic alkalosis or with chronic respiratory acidosis with renal compensation. The clinical circumstances strongly imply that metabolic alkalosis will be found, since the patient has been vomiting and has therefore been generating new alkali in the body fluids as gastric hydrochloric acid is lost. Also, the vomiting-induced deficit in ECF volume and in body fluid chloride content will likely act to help sustain the metabolic alkalosis by stimulating a high rate of renal bicarbonate transport by the proximal tubule and inhibiting distal nephron bicarbonate secretion.

Arterial blood gases are then obtained:

$$pH = 7.52$$
$$P_{CO_2} = 46 \text{ mm Hg}$$
$$[HCO_3^-] = 36 \text{ mEq/L}$$

These confirm the diagnosis. Note that the hypoventilatory response is modest, probably because of the degree of hypokalemia which tends to acidify the intracellular fluid and stimulate ventilation. Correction of this abnormality will require both replacement of fluid with sodium and chloride and adequate intake of potassium to fully restore acid–base balance to normal.

MIXED ACID–BASE DISTURBANCE

An insulin-dependent diabetic patient with several days of vomiting developed diabetic ketoacidosis. The following set of electrolytes is obtained:

$$[Na^+] = 140 \text{ mEq/L}$$
$$[K^+] = 5 \text{ mEq/L}$$
$$[Cl^-] = 90 \text{ mEq/L}$$
$$[HCO_3^-] = 15 \text{ mEq/L}$$
$$\text{Anion gap (AG)} = 35 \text{ mEq/L}$$

Since the normal AG is 12 ± 2 mEq/L, this individual has utilized 23 mEq/L of HCO_3^- to buffer the ketoacids. If the production of ketoacids ceases and hepatic metabolism is restored through insulin administration, then 23 mEq/L of HCO_3^- could be added to body fluids. The new set of electrolytes would be:

$$[Na^+] = 140 \text{ mEq/L}$$
$$[K^+] = 5 \text{ mEq/L}$$
$$[Cl^-] = 90 \text{ mEq/L}$$
$$[HCO_3^-] = 38 \text{ mEq/L}$$
$$\text{Anion gap (AG)} = 12 \text{ mEq/L}$$

By assessing the value – (AG increment above 12 mEq/L) + (serum $[HCO_3^-]$) – and finding a value greater than 30, one can infer that some process has previously raised the bicarbonate content above normal even if the ambient total CO_2 level is subnormal at the current moment. Hence either metabolic alkalosis or respiratory acidosis is a component process of the acid–base disorder. Conversely, finding a value less than 20 suggests that the patient had a pre-existent metabolic acidosis or a respiratory alkalosis prior to the onset of the organic acidosis. Finally, the clinician may assess the alveolar–arteriolar O_2 gradient to determine the effectiveness of oxygenation as an initial assessment of respiratory gas exchange efficiency.

At this point the clinician is able to ascertain a tentative diagnosis and perform an arterial blood gas determination to conclude the process. Measurement of the blood gas will show whether the respiratory response to a metabolic disturbance (metabolic alkalosis or metabolic acidosis) or the metabolic (renal) response to a respiratory disturbance is as expected. The acid–base disorder could still be labeled a simple disturbance if the initial assessment of the clinical condition and the AG support that conclusion. Consulting the acid–base map (see Fig. 17-4) will provide the expected compensatory response to each disturbance. In the previously mentioned case of a patient with diabetic ketoacidosis and an initially increased (AG + total CO_2) concentration, the following arterial blood gases were obtained:

$$pH = 7.18$$
$$P_{CO_2} = 38 \text{ mm Hg}$$
$$[HCO_3^-] = 15 \text{ mEq/L}$$

In pure metabolic acidosis the ventilatory response to an $[HCO_3^-]$ lowered to 15 mEq/L would be a P_{CO_2} of 25 mm Hg (see Table 17-1 and Fig. 17-4). In this example, the patient shows a P_{CO_2} that is higher than the expected value of 25 for a patient with pure metabolic acidosis and a depressed HCO_3^- value of 15 mEq/L. Hence this patient demonstrates a so-called triple disturbance, metabolic acidosis (low HCO_3^-, high AG), a metabolic alkalosis ($[HCO_3^-$ + AG increment above 12] >30 mEq/L) and a respiratory acidosis (P_{CO_2} higher than expected value given the lowering of HCO_3^- level as determined from the acid–base nomogram or the formula for expected compensation). Therapy for this patient will require awareness of these various processes, since removal of one of multiple disturbances can induce a more severe expression of the still-present abnormality.

REFERENCES

1. Moe OW, Rector FC, Alpern RJ. Renal regulation of acid-base metabolism. In: Narins RG, ed. *Maxwell & Kleeman's Clinical Disorders of Fluid and Electrolyte Metabolism*, 5th ed. New York, NY: McGraw-Hill; 1994:203–242.
2. Aronson PS, Nee J, Suhm MA. Modifier role of internal H^+ in activating the Na^+-H^+ exchanger in renal microvillus membrane vesicles. *Nature.* 1982;299:161–163.
3. Alpern RJ, Moe OW, Preisig PA. Chronic regulation of the proximal tubular Na/H antiporter: from HCO_3 to SRC. *Kidney Int.* 1995;48:1386–1396.
4. Reeves RB, Rahn H. Patterns in vertebrate acid-base regulation. In: Wood S, Lenfant C, eds. *Evolution of the Respiratory Process: a Comparative Approach.* New York, NY: Dekker; 1979:225–252.
5. Kassirer JP, Schwartz WB. The response of normal man to selective depletion of hydrochloric acid. Factors in the genesis of persistent gastric alkalosis. *Am J Med.* 1966;40:10–18.

6. Rose B. *Clinical Physiology of Acid–Base and Electrolyte Disorders*, 4th ed. New York, NY: McGraw-Hill; 1994.
7. Kazemi H, Hitzig B. Control of ventilation: central chemical drive. In: Narins RG, ed. *Maxwell & Kleeman's Clinical Disorders of Fluid and Electrolyte Metabolism*, 5th ed. New York, NY: McGraw-Hill; 1994:175–186.
8. Wichser J, Kazemi H. CSF bicarbonate regulation in respiratory acidosis and alkalosis. *J Appl Physiol.* 1975;44:504–511.
9. Giacobini E. Cytochemical study of the localization of carbonic anhydrase in the nervous system. *J Neurochem.* 1962;9:169–177.
10. Goldberg M, Green SB, Moss ML, et al. Computer-based instruction and diagnosis of acid–base disorders. A systematic approach. *JAMA.* 1973;223:269–278.
11. Brackett NC Jr, Cohen JJ, Schwartz WB. Carbon dioxide titration curve of normal man: effect of increasing degrees of acute hypercapnia on acid-base equilibrium. *N Engl J Med.* 1965; 272:6–12.
12. Bruno CM, Valenti M. Acid-base disorders in patients with chronic obstructive pulmonary disease: a pathophysiological review. *J Biomed Biotechnol.* 2012;2012:915150.
13. Batlle DC, Hizon M, Cohen E, Gutterman C, Gupta R. The use of the urine anion gap in the diagnosis of hyperchloremic metabolic acidosis. *N Engl J Med.* 1988;318:594–599.
14. Adrogué HJ, Madias NE. Influence of chronic respiratory acid-base disorders on acute CO_2 titration curve. *J Appl Physiol.* 1985;58:1231–1238.
15. Trivedi B, Tannen RL. Effect of respiratory acidosis on intracellular pH of the proximal tubule. *Am J Physiol.* 1986;250:F1039–F1045.
16. Arbus GS, Hebert LA, Levesque PR, Etsten BE, Schwartz WB. Characteristics and clinical application of the "significance band" for acute respiratory alkalosis. *N Engl J Med.* 1969;280:117–123.
17. Gennari FJ, Goldstein MB, Schwartz WB. The nature of the renal adaptation to chronic hypocapnia. *J Clin Invest.* 1972;51:1722–1730.
18. Madias NE, Adrogue HJ, Cohen JJ, Schwartz WB. Effect of natural variations in P_{CO_2} on plasma $[HCO_3^-]$ in dogs: a redefinition of normal. *Am J Physiol.* 1979;236:F30–F35.
19. Gennari FJ, Kassirer JP. Respiratory alkalosis. In: Cohen JJ, Kassirer JP, eds. *Acid-Base.* Boston, MA: Little, Brown and Co.; 1982:349–376.
20. Albert MS, Dell RB, Winters RW. Quantitative displacement of acid-base equilibrium in metabolic acidosis. *Ann Intern Med.* 1967;66:312–322.
21. Daniel SR, Morita SY, Yu M, Dzierba A. Uncompensated metabolic acidosis: an underrecognized risk factor for subsequent intubation requirement. *J Trauma.* 2004;57:993–997.
22. Jennings DB. The physicochemistry of $[H^+]$ and respiratory control: roles of P_{CO_2}, strong ions, and their hormonal regulators. *Can J Physiol Pharmacol.* 1994;72:1499–1512.
23. Fencl V, Leith DE. Stewart's quantitative acid-base chemistry: applications in biology and medicine. *Respir Physiol.* 1993;91: 1–16.
24. Stewart PA. (Ed.) How to understand acid-base balance. In: *A Quantitative Acid-Base Primer for Biology and Medicine.* New York, NY: Elsevier; 1981.
25. Cameron JN. Acid-base status of fish at different temperatures. *Am J Physiol.* 1984;246:R452–R459.
26. Reeves RB. The interaction of body temperature and acid-base balance in ectothermic vertebrates. *Ann Rev Physiol.* 1977; 39:559–586.
27. Nattie EE. Intracisternal diethylpyrocarbonate inhibits central chemosensitivity in conscious rabbits. *Respir Physiol.* 1986; 64:161–176.
28. Fencl V, Jabor A, Kazda A, Figge J. Diagnosis of metabolic acid-base disturbances in critically ill patients. *Am J Respir Crit Care Med.* 2000;162:2246–2251.
29. Dubin A, Menises MM, Masevicius FD, et al. Comparison of three different methods of evaluation of metabolic acid-base disorders. *Crit Care Med.* 2007;35:1264–1270.
30. Ali Y, Abouelnaga S, Khalaf H, Kamel Y. Physical chemical approach versus traditional technique in analyzing blood gases and electrolytes during liver transplant surgery. *Transplant Proc.* 2010;42:861–864.
31. Severinghaus JW. Acid-base balance nomogram: a Boston Copenhagen detente. *Anesthesiology.* 1976;45:539–541.
32. McCurdy DK. Mixed metabolic and respiratory acid-base disturbances: diagnosis and treatment. *Chest.* 1972;62:35S–44S.
33. Gabow PA. Disorders associated with an altered anion gap. *Kidney Int.* 1985;27:472–484.
34. Sabatini S, Kurtzman NA. The maintenance of metabolic alkalosis: factors which decrease bicarbonate excretion. *Kidney Int.* 1984;25:357–361.
35. Galla JH, Bonduris DN, Luke RG. Effects of chloride and extracellular fluid volume on bicarbonate reabsorption along the nephron in metabolic alkalosis in the rat. Reassessment of the classic hypothesis on the pathogenesis of metabolic alkalosis. *J Clin Invest.* 1987;80:41–52.
36. Javaheri S, Kazemi H. Metabolic alkalosis and hypoventilation in humans. *Am Rev Respir Dis.* 1987;136:1011–1016.
37. Schwartz WB, Hays RM, Polak A, Haynie GD. Effects of chronic hypercapnia on electrolyte and acid-base equilibrium: recovery, with special reference to the influence of chloride intake. *J Clin Invest.* 1961;40:1238–1249.

CHAPTER 18

Respiratory System Response to Exercise in Health

Jerome A. Dempsey
Anthony J. Jacques

The increases in muscular oxygen consumption ($\dot{V}_{O_2}$) and carbon dioxide production ($\dot{V}_{CO_2}$) accompanying whole-body exercise present a greater challenge to the maintenance of pulmonary gas exchange than any other physiologic stressor. This chapter discusses the responses of the healthy respiratory system to exercise with an emphasis on the following problems: What neurochemical mechanisms regulate the ventilatory response to exercise and what are the consequences of this hyperpnea to the work and to the fatigue of the respiratory muscles? What mechanisms underlie the widening of the alveolar to arterial partial pressure of oxygen (P_{O_2}) difference during exercise? How do the unique characteristics of the pulmonary circulation determine its response to exercise? How does respiration impact the cardiovascular response to exercise? Under what circumstances might the respiratory system provide a limitation to O_2 transport and/or exercise performance? We consider these problems primarily in the healthy, young, normally fit adult, with reference to special cases of the highly trained athlete and to the effects of healthy aging, high altitude hypoxia, and physical training.

EXERCISE HYPERPNEA

In healthy humans, breathing in all physiological states is remarkably well controlled. Accordingly, the partial pressures of oxygen and carbon dioxide, in systemic arterial blood along with its acidity, are regulated precisely throughout mild to moderate exercise.[1-4]

These relationships are shown in the following alveolar gas equations, where alveolar gas partial pressures are approximately equal to the ratio of the metabolic requirement to alveolar ventilation.

$$P_{A_{CO_2}} = [\dot{V}_{CO_2} \div \dot{V}_A] \cdot K \quad (1)$$

$$P_{A_{O_2}} = P_{I_{O_2}} - [\dot{V}_{O_2} \div \dot{V}_A] \cdot K \quad (2)$$

where:

$P_{A_{CO_2}}$ and $P_{A_{O_2}}$ = alveolar carbon dioxide and oxygen partial pressures (it is assumed $P_{A_{CO_2}} \approx$ arterial P_{CO_2})

$\dot{V}_{CO_2}$ and $\dot{V}_{O_2}$ = volumes of carbon dioxide produced and oxygen consumed

$\dot{V}_A$ = alveolar ventilation

$P_{I_{O_2}}$ = inspired partial pressure of oxygen

K = constant (0.863). This constant allows alveolar gases to be calculated from these equations if $\dot{V}_{O_2}$ and $\dot{V}_{CO_2}$ are expressed in mL/min and $\dot{V}_A$ in L/min.

Table 18-1 illustrates the interrelation of these variables, as one goes from rest to exercise. With exercise, there is an increased metabolic rate, with alveolar ventilation increasing to regulate arterial blood gases near resting levels. In health, dead space (V_D) increases slightly as intrathoracic airways stretch and dilate with increased tidal volume (V_T) – but V_T rises out of proportion; thus, V_D/V_T falls to about one-half its resting value during exercise. In order that $P_{A_{CO_2}}$ be precisely controlled, overall minute ventilation ($\dot{V}_E$) during exercise must be regulated in such a fashion so as to compensate both for the increasing CO_2 production as well as a reduced V_D/V_T. Accordingly, the ratio of $\dot{V}_E$ to $\dot{V}_{CO_2}$ falls from rest to moderate exercise, whereas the $\dot{V}_A$:$\dot{V}_{CO_2}$ ratio and arterial P_{CO_2} are maintained constant until heavy exercise intensities, during which both ratios rise and $P_{A_{CO_2}}$ is reduced. Note the impressive magnitude of ventilatory response required to maintain arterial P_{CO_2} homeostasis during exercise, amounting to a 20-fold increase above resting in the untrained at $\dot{V}_{O_2 max}$ and 30-fold in the highly trained.

REGULATION OF EXERCISE HYPERPNEA

More than a century of highly innovative research on this question has left us with three major stimuli as the primary regulators of exercise hyperpnea. The schematic diagram shown in Figure 18-1 includes these three potential stimuli in a ventilatory control system which features three components, namely a central rhythm generator/integrator in the medulla, mechanical and chemical feedback and feedforward inputs to this integrator, and control of the distribution of efferent output to muscles of both the upper airway and chest and abdominal wall.

CO_2 FLOW

The primary suspects for mediation of the exercise hyperpnea include **humoral stimuli** in the form of CO_2 flow to the lung or the product of blood flow and mixed venous CO_2 content. While still controversial (and mysterious) there is compelling evidence in support of a significant fundamental role for this feedback mechanism. When extracorporeal perfusion is used to increase (or reduce) CO_2 flow to the lung in a resting animal, alveolar ventilation is changed in proportion to $\dot{V}_{CO_2}$ and an isocapnic hyperpnea (or reduced ventilation) is achieved.[5] In human quadriplegic patients, increasing locomotor muscle CO_2 production via electrical stimulation of muscle contraction, increases ventilation. Similarly, increasing $\dot{V}_{CO_2}$ and the respiratory quotient with bicarbonate ingestion in resting humans will increase $\dot{V}_A$ in an isocapnic fashion. Furthermore, when sinusoidal exercise regimens are employed at changing frequencies, the ventilatory response follows the change in $\dot{V}_{CO_2}$ rather than the change in work rate, per se. The case against this purely humoral feedback stimulus in the mediation of exercise hyperpnea is that it has only been tested over a very narrow range of $\dot{V}_{CO_2}$ near resting levels and the exact nature of the stimulus or its site of action has not been identified. Recently, c-fiber receptors in the lung interstitium have been implicated, responding to an increased transport of plasma water into the lung interstitium, secondary to the effects of both increased venous CO_2 content on the osmotic state of blood plasma and increased blood flow on pulmonary capillary pressure.[6] We suspect that $\dot{V}_{CO_2}$ plays an important modulatory role in the control of breathing near resting levels, but it is unlikely to provide sufficient drive to be considered as a primary drive to hyperpnea during exercise.[7]

CENTRAL COMMAND

A purely feedforward input to medullary respiratory controller neurons originates from supramedullary regions of the motor cortex and hypothalamus and operates along synaptic pathways in parallel with

TABLE 18-1 Group Mean Values of Healthy Untrained and Trained Subjects Cardiorespiratory Responses to Steady-State Exercise

	Untrained									
	Relative Exercise Intensity (% Maximal Oxygen Uptake)								Trained A	Trained B
	Rest	15	30	45	60	75	90	100	100	100
$\dot{V}_{O_2}$ (L/min)	0.24	0.45	0.9	1.35	1.8	2.25	2.7	3	5.25	5.25
$\dot{V}_{CO_2}$ (L/min)	0.19	0.4	0.77	1.21	1.71	2.31	3	3.3	6.04	6.04
$\dot{V}_E$ (L/min)	6	14	22	35	51	75	100	115	183	168
$\dot{V}_A$ (L/min)	4	9	18	28	41	60	81	94	150	138
V_T (L)	0.6	0.9	1.2	1.6	2.2	2.5	2.6	2.6	3.1	2.9
fR (breaths·min^{-1})	10	15	18	22	23	30	38	44	59	58
V_D/V_T	0.35	0.28	0.21	0.2	0.19	0.18	0.18	0.18	0.18	0.18
EELV (% TLC)	0.5	0.49	0.46	0.45	0.44	0.43	0.42	0.42	0.48	0.48
Gas exchange										
Pa_{O_2} (mm Hg)	95	95	93	93	92	94	94	94	90	70
$P_{A_{O_2}}$ (mm Hg)	101	101	101	101	107	112	114	117	117	112
Pa_{CO_2} (mm Hg)	41	41	41	41	39	35	33	31	31	38
A-aDO_2 (mm Hg)	6	6	8	8	15	18	20	23	27	42
pH	7.40	7.40	7.38	7.36	7.34	7.30	7.29	7.28	7.25	7.25
Sa_{O_2} (%)	97	97	97	97	96	96	95	95	93	86
$\dot{V}_A/\dot{Q}$	0.8	1.3	2	2.5	2.9	3.5	4.1	4.5	4.7	4.3
Pulmonary circulation										
$\dot{Q}$ (L·min^{-1})	5	7	9	11	14	17	20	21	32	32
PCBV (mL)	83	95	107	119	137	155	173	180	180	180
Transit time (s)	1	0.81	0.71	0.65	0.59	0.55	0.52	0.51	0.33	0.33
PAP (mm Hg)	13	15	17	20	23	27	29	32	30	35
PAWP (mm Hg)	8	9	10	12	13	15	17	21	14	18
PVR (mm Hg·min^{-1}·s^{-1})	60	51.4	46.7	43.7	42.8	42.4	36	31.4	30	33

$\dot{V}_{O_2}$, oxygen uptake; $\dot{V}_{CO_2}$, expired carbon dioxide; $\dot{V}_E$, minute ventilation; $\dot{V}_A$, alveolar ventilation; V_T, tidal volume; fb, breathing frequency; V_D/V_T, dead space to tidal volume ratio; EELV, end-expiratory lung volume as a percentage of total lung capacity; Pa_{O_2}, arterial P_{O_2}; $P_{A_{O_2}}$, alveolar P_{O_2}; Pa_{CO_2}, arterial P_{CO_2}; A-aDO_2, alveolar to arterial oxygen partial pressure difference; Sa_{O_2}, arterial oxyhemoglobin saturation; $\dot{V}_A/\dot{Q}$, global ventilation to perfusion ratio; $\dot{Q}$, cardiac output; PCBV, pulmonary capillary blood volume; transit time, mean pulmonary capillary transit time; PAP, mean pulmonary artery pressure; PAWP, pulmonary artery wedge pressure; PVR, pulmonary vascular resistance. Two columns of values for highly trained subjects are shown, both with equal $\dot{V}_{O_{2max}}$ values. Group A experiences little arterial hypoxemia while Group B experiences substantial hypoxemia in heavy intensity exercise.

the motor control of locomotor muscles. Animal models using electrical or pharmacological stimulation of these supramedullary sites show powerful cardioventilatory responses even in the face of paralyzed locomotor muscles, that is, in the absence of neural feedback.[8] Further, in hypnotized humans even the "suggestion" of exercise – while still at rest – elicits exercise-like cardioventilatory responses with coincident PET imaging studies showing an increased blood flow to motor control regions of the cortex.[9] On the other hand, the "exercise-like" ventilatory response to electrical stimulation of the limbs shows that feedforward central command is not obligatory to the hyperpnea and a normal ventilatory response to exercise is also observed in decorticate animals, that is, in the absence of key hypothalamic regions of purported cardioventilatory central command.

■ MUSCLE AFFERENT FEEDBACK

Lightly and unmyelinated afferents from locomotor muscle sensitive to the metabolic milieu, mechanical deformation, and even vascular distension in the muscle, project via the dorsal horn of the spinal cord and then via the nucleus of the solitary tract to the medullary cardiorespiratory controller neurons. When their effect on ventilation is studied in isolation, using electrical stimulation of muscle, a proportionate increase in $\dot{V}_E$ occurs. However, evidence against a role for muscle afferents in the intact human include the failure of imposed vascular occlusion causing accumulation of muscle metabolites to augment ventilation during recovery from exercise, the failure of spinal cord lesioning to alter the ventilatory response to muscle stimulation, or of epidural anesthesia to reduce the cardioventilatory response to rhythmic exercise. On the other hand, if afferent blockade techniques are employed – such as intrathecal fentanyl which blocks only muscle afferents and leaves efferent motor pathways intact, hypoventilation occurs throughout mild and moderate exercise – uncovering a significant obligatory role for muscle afferents in the steady-state exercise hyperpnea (see Fig. 18-2).[10,11] This inhibitory effect of muscle afferent blockade on exercise hyperpnea has also been shown in patients with COPD and CHF.[12,13] Interestingly, in COPD patients muscle afferent blockade during exercise reduced primarily V_D ventilation, suppressed dyspneic sensations, and substantially improved exercise performance.[12]

In summary, the dilemma of exercise hyperpnea is that findings using isolation of each of these three stimuli support a significant contributory role for each of these mechanisms to the isocapnic hyperpnea of moderate intensity exercise—but there is contradictory evidence against an obligatory major role for any of them. Accordingly, most models emphasize the powerful redundancy of the hyperpnea mechanisms operating under steady-state conditions of exercise or emphasize the importance of compensatory feedback

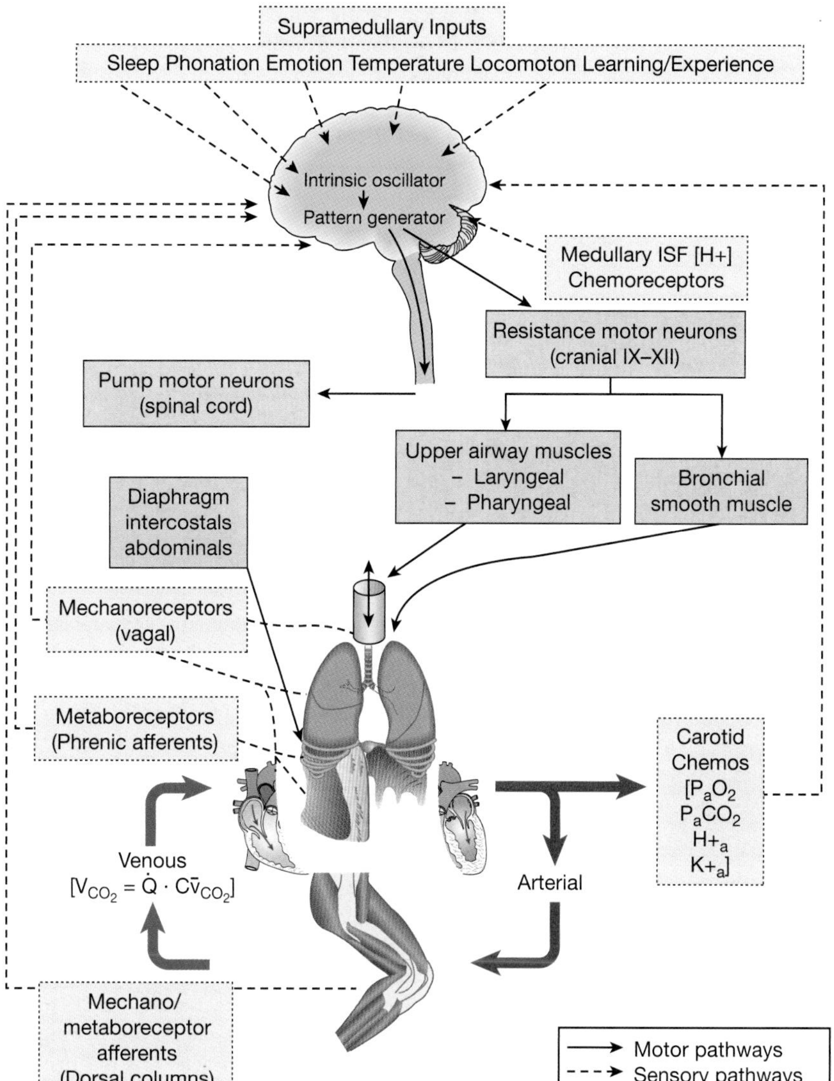

Figure 18-1 Schematic depicting multiple structures contributing to the control of breathing. It is hypothesized that respiratory rhythm originates within a brain stem oscillator which activates brain stem pattern generating neurons that provide for the proper sequential activation of respiratory pump (diaphragm, intercostal, and abdominal) and airway (laryngeal and pharyngeal) muscles. These brain stem neurons receive excitatory and inhibitory input from multiple sources during exercise, including supramedullary central command and mechano/metaboreceptor-initiated spinal afferents from limb and respiratory skeletal muscles. In addition, the brain stem controller neurons receive carotid and intracranial chemoreceptor (RTN, retrotrapezoid nucleus) and vagal mechanoreceptor input critical to meet the appropriate ventilatory and breathing pattern responses to exercise. *(Reproduced with permission from Taylor N. Physiological Bases of Human Performance during work and exercise. New York: Churchill Livinstone; 2008.)*

from carotid and central chemoreceptors if blockade of any of these primary mechanisms was sufficient to cause transient CO_2 retention. There are also suggestions that feedback mechanisms are likely of little consequence; rather, the ventilatory response to exercise depends critically on a "stored memory" of the appropriate ventilatory response by the motor cortex as a result of repetitive trial and error during maturation.[14] We hypothesize – with limited direct evidence – that each of these three mechanisms have an important obligatory role, with CO_2 flow to the lung providing the essential underpinning to ventilatory control in all physiologic states and the interaction of feedforward (central command) and feedback (from muscle afferents) mechanisms providing the primary "exercise" stimulus. The proof for this awaits the appropriate experimental tools – such as was done with the use of opiate receptor agonists (see Fig. 18-2) – to test a specific mechanism without altering the remaining elements of the control system.

Finally, we need to emphasize that this hypothesis applies only to the isocapnic hyperpnea achieved in mild to moderate steady-state levels of exercise. For the hyperventilatory response to heavier intensity exercise we need to add additional mechanisms: an important input from carotid chemoreceptors responding to the changing hydrogen ion, potassium, norepinephrine, temperature, etc. of the arterial blood induced by heavy intensity exercise; the additional powerful inputs from central command responding to the need to recruit more motor units in the presence of fatiguing locomotor muscles; and muscle afferents responding to accumulating ionic changes in the muscle interstitium. Even an obligatory role for carotid chemoreceptors and the hyperventilatory response to heavy exercise has been challenged by the fact that preventing the blood-borne acidity during heavy exercise (via depleting muscle glycogen and preventing acid production) did not prevent the hyperventilatory response.[7] Again multiple, redundant mechanisms are apparently at play. This hyperventilatory response is extremely important in partially compensating for the metabolic acidosis incurred with increasing lactic acid levels in heavy exercise and also for raising alveolar P_{O_2} to maintain arterial P_{O_2} in the face of a widening alveolar to arterial P_{O_2} difference.[15]

■ BREATHING PATTERN DURING EXERCISE

During low to moderate intensity exercise both V_T and breathing frequency (fb) increase roughly in proportion to intensity, while at higher intensities V_T attains a plateau and further increases in $\dot{V}_E$ are accomplished by increases in fb alone (see Fig. 18-3). The increase in fb is accomplished by decreases in both inspiratory time (T_I) and expiratory time (T_E). However the ratio of T_I to total breath cycle duration (T_{TOT}), known as the duty cycle (T_I/T_{TOT}), increases only slightly during exercise (~0.40 at rest to ~0.50 during high-intensity exercise). The fact that the duty cycle remains low is important and beneficial, because prolonged diaphragmatic contractions hinder blood flow to this muscle and may precipitate excessive diaphragmatic fatigue.[16]

The increase in V_T at the onset of exercise is accomplished by both an increase in end-inspiratory lung volume (EILV) and a decrease in end-expiratory lung volume (EELV). However, as exercise intensity increases, EILV does not normally increase beyond 85% to 90% TLC. Beyond this point lung compliance decreases markedly and the respiratory pressure production required for a given change in volume is very large. This inefficiency at high operating lung volumes leads to neuromechanical uncoupling in that a mismatch develops between the required "effort" to inspire and the actual volume of air inhaled. This hyperinflation (secondary to expiratory flow limitation) underlies much of exertional dyspnea, that is, "unsatisfied inspiratory effort" in COPD patients.[17] In health, EELV decreases at the onset of all levels

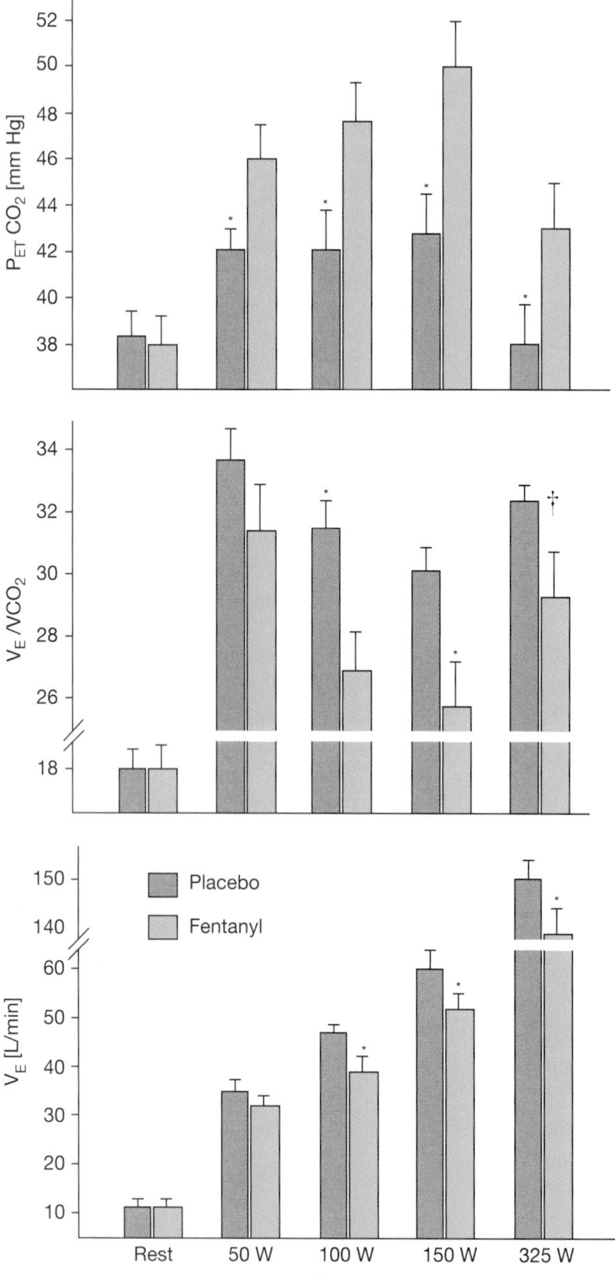

Figure 18-2 Effect of blockage of μ-opioid sensitive type III–IV muscle afferents via intrathecal fentanyl on the steady-state ventilatory response to 3 minutes of cycling exercise at each of four work rates. ($*p < 0.05$, $^{\dagger}p < 0.08$). The fentanyl-induced hypoventilation was due to a reduced breathing frequency. Heart rate, mean arterial blood pressure, and $\dot{V}_E$ were significantly reduced at each work rate. Taking into account the reduced exercise $\dot{V}_E$ with fentanyl plus the ventilatory equivalent of the concomitant rise in P_{ETCO_2}, it is estimated that the partial blockage of muscle afferents accounted for 47%, 45%, and 15% of the total exercise hyperpnea at 100, 150, and 325 W, respectively. *(Modified with permission from Amann M, Blain GM, Proctor LT, Sebranek JJ, Pegelow DF, Dempsey JA. Group III and IV muscle afferents contribute to ventilatory and cardiovascular response to rhythmic exercise in humans. J Appl Physiol. 2010;109(4):966–976.)*

of exercise due to active recruitment of the expiratory muscles, and its decrease is roughly proportional to exercise intensity.[18] The drop in EELV maintains operating lung volumes within the linear portion of the pressure–volume relationship, which minimizes the reduction in respiratory system compliance and associated dyspnea that develops at high lung volumes. The reduced EELV also serves to lengthen the diaphragm and place it in a more optimal range of its length–tension relationship. Thus the maximum dynamic capacity of the inspiratory muscles for force production is improved during tidal breathing and they are required to produce only about one-half of their capacity for force production at maximum exercise in the untrained subject (see Fig. 18-3).[19] A reduced EELV also reduces inspiratory muscle work during the ensuing inspiration due to outward recoil of the rib cage at the onset of inspiration.

Tidal exercise flow–volume loops plotted within the maximal volitional flow–volume envelope provide a simple and useful method to analyze alterations in flow rates, V_T, and operating lung volumes during exercise (Fig. 18-4). In normal, healthy untrained young adult humans the maximal attainable flow rates at any given lung volume are usually much greater than the spontaneous tidal flow rates reached during exercise of all intensities. Thus, as shown in Figure 18-4 (at $\dot{V}_{E\,max}$ in the 100–120 L/min range) there is usually a large reserve for increasing $\dot{V}_E$ even at maximal exercise.

CONTROL OF AIRWAY CALIBER DURING EXERCISE

■ UPPER AIRWAY CALIBER

The upper airway comprises the nose, mouth, pharynx, and larynx, and provides the majority of resistance to airflow at rest and during exercise. In addition, each region of the upper airway has the potential to independently contribute to any alterations in airway resistance during exercise. The work required to produce the large increases in airflow during exercise would become excessive during even low-intensity exercise if several mechanisms were not in place to reduce resistance to airflow in the upper airway during exercise.

First, the route of airflow switches from predominately nasal to oronasal breathing when $\dot{V}_E$ reaches approximately 30 L/min.[20] Second, nasal resistance decreases during exercise in an intensity- and duration-dependent manner secondary to sympathetically mediated vasoconstriction of the nasal mucosal vasculature.[21] Third, the nasal dilator muscles and presumably the skeletal muscles of the pharyngeal and laryngeal regions contract in phase with, but slightly preceding, inspiratory pump muscle recruitment, and this drive to the upper airway muscles is increased at increasing $\dot{V}_E$, resulting in decreased resistance and a larger diameter, stiffer, less collapsible upper airway.[22] Finally, the glottic narrowing that normally occurs during expiration is attenuated during exercise due to laryngeal abductor muscle activation, in addition to a widened mean glottic aperture throughout the respiratory cycle.[23] Thus, the work required to produce the increased airflow that occurs during whole-body exercise is minimized by a variety of adjustments that occur in the upper airway, all of which act to decrease resistance to airflow.

■ BRONCHIAL CALIBER

Bronchial dilation in response to exercise has been well documented in healthy humans.[24] Furthermore, this bronchodilator influence occurs at exercise onset and is very powerful, as evidenced by the prevention of an increase in pulmonary resistance during exercise after histamine inhalation in asthmatic subjects who exhibited large increases in resistance during histamine inhalation at rest.[25] In addition, forced expiratory volume in 1 second (FEV_1) and the maximum volitional flow:volume envelope increase immediately after exercise in both normal[26] and asthmatic subjects.[27] There are several potential mechanisms contributing to the bronchodilator effect of exercise, including neural, mechanical, and locally released mediator mechanisms.

A primary component of the exercise-induced increase in airway caliber is withdrawal of vagal parasympathetic tone to the airways that occurs at the immediate onset of exercise, resulting in bronchial smooth muscle relaxation.[24] The withdrawal of cholinergic tone is thought to be mediated in part by the stimulation of muscle mechano- and chemosensitive afferents (i.e., the same muscle afferents

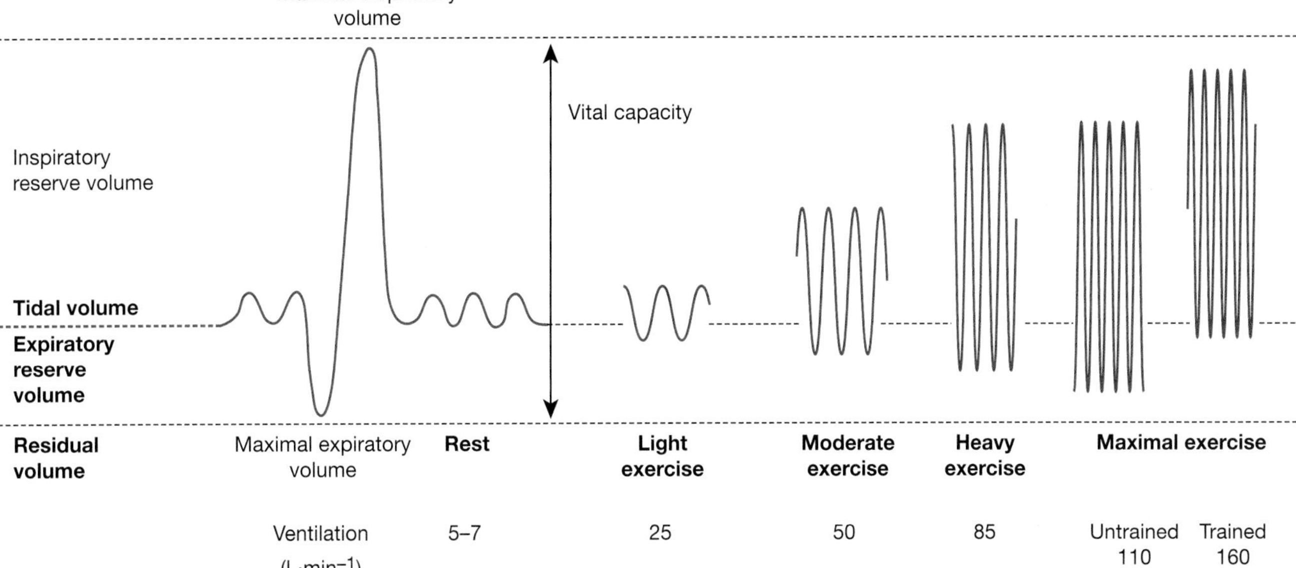

Figure 18-3 Changes in breathing pattern during exercise. The spirograph on the left is from a resting subject showing normal tidal volume, maximum expiration to residual lung volume, then maximal inspiration to total lung capacity. With light to heavy exercise (in both untrained and highly trained subjects) the increase in ventilation is achieved by increasing breathing frequency and tidal volume. Tidal volume increases by encroaching on the expiratory and inspiratory reserve volumes. The reduced end-expiratory lung volume is maintained at maximal exercise in the normally fit subject (maximal oxygen uptake [$\dot{V}_{O_{2max}}$] 45 mL kg^{-1} L min^{-1}). In the trained subject ($\dot{V}_{O_{2max}}$ = 75 mL kg^{-1} L min^{-1}), ventilation, breathing frequency, and tidal volume are all higher and maximal exercise end-expiratory lung volume is increased to near resting values due to expiratory flow limitations. *(Reproduced with permission from Farrell PA, Joyner MJ, Caiozxo VJ. ACSM's Advanced Exercise Physiology, 2nd ed. Philadelphia, PA: Lippincott Williams & Wilkins; 2012.)*

believed to be involved in the pressor and ventilatory responses to exercise) (see Fig. 18-2).[28] Increased lung stretch and activation of slowly adapting pulmonary stretch receptors (that occurs as EILV is increased during exercise) may contribute to this withdrawal of vagal tone.

Mechanical influences may also play a substantial role in increasing airway caliber during exercise. The airways are tethered open by the lung parenchyma, and the increase in EILV and operating lung volumes during exercise will enlarge airway diameter simply as a result of this airway–parenchymal interdependence. Further, the

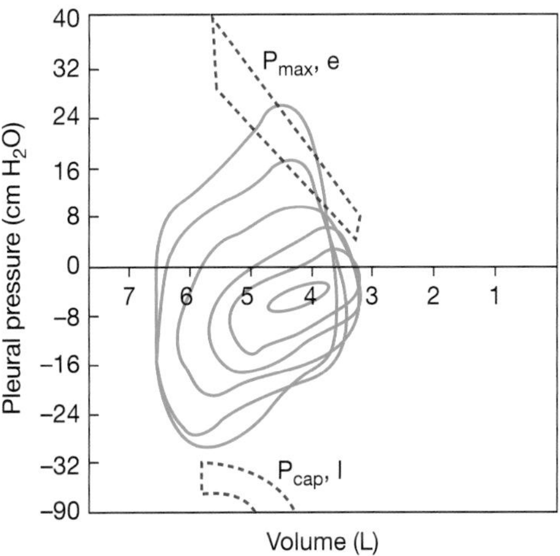

Figure 18-4 Flow–volume and pressure–volume relationships in a young healthy adult, at rest and during exercise. The maximal (outer envelope) flow–volume relationship is obtained via maximal volitional inspiratory and expiratory efforts, before *(solid line)* and immediately following exercise *(broken line)*. For the pressure–volume relationships, only tidal breaths from rest through to maximal exercise are shown. In addition, the maximum inspiratory pleural pressures (P_{cap}, I) are shown at the specific peak volume and flows achieved during tidal breathing in heavy exercise. For minute ventilations up to 115 L min^{-1}, approximating peak exercise in an untrained adult, the inspiratory muscles are activated to only ~40% to 50% of capacity. The more highly trained subject is shown achieving ventilations >150 L min^{-1} at higher metabolic rates. Under these conditions, the tidal flow–volume loop often encroaches on the maximum flow–volume envelope, end-expiratory lung volume rises, and the inspiratory muscles approach 90% of their dynamic capacity for force output and shortening velocity. The broken area on the expiratory side indicates expiratory pressures for any given lung volume (P_{max}, e), beyond which extraexpiratory muscle effort will not produce a higher flow. In almost all instances up to ventilations of ~150 L min^{-1}, this critical expiratory pressure is not exceeded but it is exceeded slightly in the highly trained athlete at maximum exercise. *(Modified with permission from Johnson BD, Saupe KW, Dempsey JA. Mechanical constraints on exercise hyperpnea in endurance athletes. J Appl Physiol. 1992;73(3):874–886.)*

increased outward radial force exerted by the parenchyma on the airways during exercise may induce bronchodilation by a separate mechanism operating at the level of the crossbridges of bronchial smooth muscle.[29] Airway stretch modulates bronchial smooth muscle crossbridge formation, resulting in decreased bronchial smooth muscle force and stiffness and relaxation of airway smooth muscle. Finally, airway mast cells, macrophages, neutrophils, eosinophils, epithelial cells, and smooth muscle cells all have the potential to release a variety of chemical mediators that may alter airway caliber.

WORK, METABOLIC AND CIRCULATORY COST OF BREATHING

During exercise the inspiratory and expiratory muscles perform work on the lung, the abdominal wall, and the rib cage. The work on the lung is composed of elastic work – a function of both the V_T and lung compliance and flow resistive work – a function of airway caliber and flow rate. As the diaphragm descends during inspiration, work is performed on the abdominal wall—a function of abdominal wall compliance. This work maximally contributes about 25% to the total work of breathing during exercise—but in the presence of expiratory flow limitation abdominal muscle tension will persist well into the inspiration which will markedly increase work done by the diaphragm on the abdominal compartment. As shown in Figure 18-5 the total work of breathing rises linearly with the isocapnic hyperpnea of mild and moderate intensity exercise and then rises alinearly with the hyperventilation of heavy intensity exercise.

This severalfold increase in respiratory muscle work requires increases in respiratory muscle $\dot{V}_{O_2}$ and blood flow. Thus, at maximal $\dot{V}_{O_2}$ (~45 mL/kg/min) and cardiac output (~20 L/min) and $\dot{V}_E$ (100–120 L/min), about 8% to 10% of $\dot{V}_{O_2}$ and cardiac output are devoted to breathing in the untrained human and up to 14% to 16% of $\dot{V}_{O_2}$ and cardiac output in the highly trained ($\dot{V}_{O_2max}$ ~65 mL/kg, $\dot{V}_E$ >150 L/min, and CO ~30 L/min—see Table 18-1). Respiratory muscle blood flow, was determined directly by using distribution of infused microspheres in exercising animals[30] and indirectly in humans by the reduction in total cardiac output and increased blood flow to the exercising limb muscles measured when respiratory muscle work was reduced during maximal exercise using a mechanical ventilator (see Fig. 18-6).[31,32]

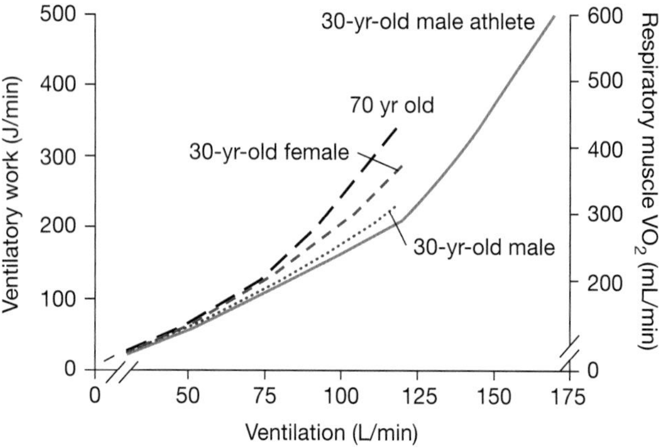

Figure 18-5 Ventilatory work and respiratory muscle $\dot{V}_{O_2}$ during exercise of increasing intensity plotted as a function of $\dot{V}_E$ for sedentary men, active young females, and trained young and older men. In young adult males the O_2 cost of exercise hyperpnea was determined by having subjects mimic the pressure–volume loop, breathing frequency, duty cycle, and ventilation they experienced during submaximal and maximal exercise and measuring the change in $\dot{V}_{O_2}$ from resting eupnea.[108,109] *(Reproduced with permission from Harms CA, Dempsey JA. Cardiovascular consequences of exercise hyperpnea. Exerc Sport Sci Rev. 1999;27:37–62.)*

Several lines of evidence are available in support of the concept that during heavy intensity exercise a metaboreflex is triggered from the diaphragm which travels in phrenic nerve afferent fibers to increase efferent vasoconstrictor outflow from sympathetic neurons in the medulla. For example, studies in healthy humans using muscle microneurography and Doppler blood flow measurements of limb muscle blood flow demonstrated increases in muscle sympathetic nerve activity together with reduced limb vascular conductance and blood flow in the face of inspiratory or expiratory muscle fatigue induced by volitional hyperpnea against increased airway resistive loads.[33] In animals specific acidification of the diaphragm or pharmacologic stimulation of diaphragm afferents caused vasoconstriction in limb muscle and these effects were prevented via ganglionic blockade.[34,35] The finding that vasoconstriction occurs under these conditions of heightened sympathetic outflow in the locomotor muscle vasculature and not in the diaphragm is supported by in situ studies which show feed arteries in the diaphragm to undergo substantially less norepinephrine-induced vasoconstriction than that which occurs in vessels isolated from limb muscle.[36] Apparently these reflex mechanisms and vascular response characteristics combine to protect blood flow to the respiratory muscles during intense exercise.

EXERCISE-INDUCED RESPIRATORY MUSCLE FATIGUE

The structural and functional properties of the respiratory muscles appear to be well suited to the substantial ventilatory requirements of exercise. For example, the human at rest can voluntarily sustain up to 6 to 8 times the resting diaphragmatic pressure production for 10 to 15 minutes without inducing significant fatigue or task failure of the diaphragm.[37] Furthermore, pressures and velocities of shortening sustained by the diaphragm that are 1.5 to 2 times greater than those reached during exhaustive exercise are required to cause diaphragm fatigue when the subject is in the resting state and increases ventilation voluntarily.[37] Nevertheless, significant 15% to 50% reductions in the transdiaphragmatic pressure response to bilateral super maximal phrenic nerve stimulation, across a wide range of stimulation frequencies (1–100 Hz) and lung volumes (residual volume to TLC), have been observed following constant-load, whole-body endurance exercise at >85% $\dot{V}_{O_2max}$ to exhaustion.[38–41] Recent studies using phrenic nerve stimulation at multiple time points during high-intensity exercise shows that significant diaphragm fatigue actually begins to occur fairly early in the time course of the exercise.[42] The magnitude of exercise-induced diaphragm fatigue is determined in part by the amount of diaphragm work contributing to the exercise hyperpnea. Thus, substantially reducing the pressures produced by the diaphragm during endurance exercise using a proportional assist ventilator prevented diaphragm fatigue.[40] Whole-body exercise itself appears to lower the threshold of force output by the diaphragm required for its fatigue, likely because a finite blood flow must be distributed to both locomotor and respiratory muscles.[32] Such a disparity between O_2 supply and demand to the diaphragm appears to occur in subjects of varying fitness levels, but only at workloads exceeding 85% of $\dot{V}_{O_2max}$,[41] or when arterial O_2 saturation is decreased.[43]

CARDIOVASCULAR EFFECTS OF INTRATHORACIC PRESSURE

Respiration has important and complex effects on stroke volume and cardiac output during exercise through changes in intrathoracic and transventricular pressures. This has been demonstrated in human and animal studies by manipulating inspiratory and expiratory pressures during exercise. During inspiration the negative pressure generated in the intrathoracic space widens the pressure gradient across the walls of the right heart thereby augmenting ventricular filling of venous return from the limbs by lowering the pressures within the heart's chambers and augmenting cardiac preload. Conversely, during expiration ventricular filling is impeded by

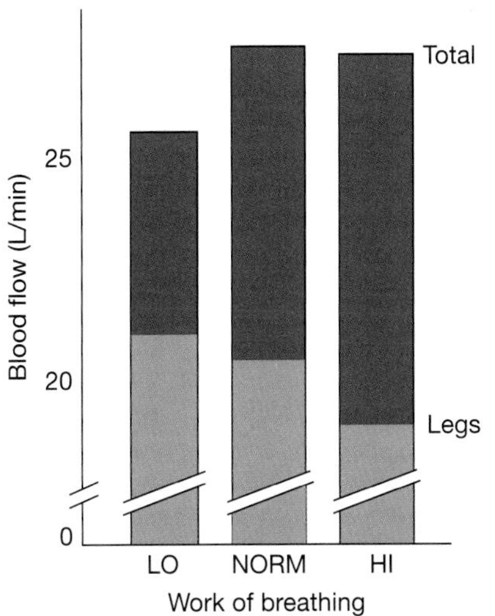

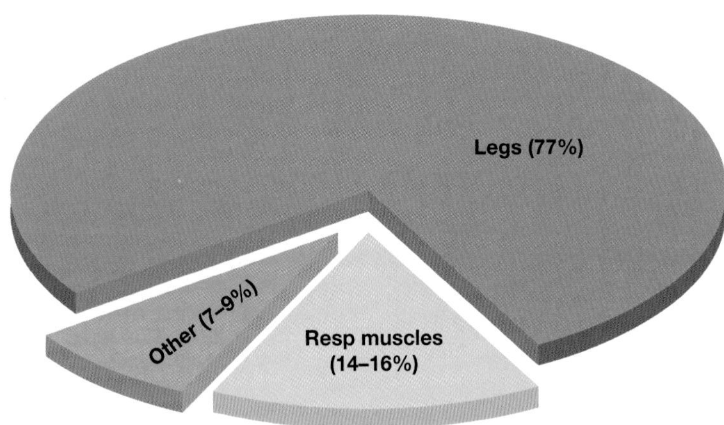

Figure 18-6 Effects of respiratory muscle work during exercise on cardiac output and its distribution in highly fit adult male subjects cycling at $\dot{V}_{O_{2max}}$ ($\dot{V}_{O_2}$ = 65 mL/kg/min, cardiac output = 28 L/min), "LO, NORM, HI" refer to the relative level of the work of breathing present during heavy intensity exercise under normal physiologic conditions, with added resistive loads ("HI") and during unloading of the respiratory muscles via mechanical ventilation ("LO"). The top of each bar indicates the total cardiac output and each bar is divided into blood flow to the limbs and to the rest of the body. The estimated distribution of blood flow to the limb locomotor and to the respiratory muscles is shown in the pie chart. These estimates come from three sources: 1. The oxygen cost of breathing at maximum exercise[108]; 2. Measurements based on microsphere distribution to the respiratory muscles during maximum exercise in the equine[110]; and 3. The change in cardiac output and in limb muscle blood flow determined in response to unloading of the respiratory muscles during maximum exercise.[31,32] These effects of respiratory muscle unloading at maximum exercise on limb blood flow and on total cardiac output are shown in the insert. Note that with reduced respiratory muscle work, that is, unloading, the total cardiac output falls and the limb muscle blood flow (and vascular conductance) rises; whereas with respiratory muscle loading and increased work of breathing at maximum exercise the maximum cardiac output remains unchanged whereas the limb blood flow (and vascular conductance) is reduced. *(Reproduced with permission from Farrell PA, Joyner MJ, Caiozxo VJ. ACSM's Advanced Exercise Physiology, 2nd ed. Philadelphia, PA: Lippincott Williams & Wilkins; 2012.)*

a narrowing of the transmural pressure gradient across the ventricle due to a positive shift in intrathoracic pressure (ITP) which reduces the pressure gradient for venous return. In the steady state these modulatory effects of ITP will be limited by intrinsic "autoregulatory" cardiac mechanisms termed ventricular interdependence, by which the filling of one ventricle shifts the common wall – the IV septum – toward the opposite ventricle which in turn limits its filling. Nevertheless, during exercise – especially in heavy intensity exercise with huge negative shifts in ITP, if positive pressure mechanical ventilation is introduced, stroke volume and cardiac output are reduced – likely due to a less negative inspiratory ITP limiting cardiac preload, that is, reducing ventricular transmural pressure during diastole.[32] Alternatively, with active expiration in heavy exercise – especially in the presence of excessive positive expiratory pressures accompanying expiratory flow limitation – transventricular wall pressures are reduced, diastolic filling is impaired, and stoke volume and cardiac output are compromised.[44,45]

PULMONARY CIRCULATION AND GAS EXCHANGE

The lungs are unique in that they are the only organ that receives all the blood pumped from the heart and thus, the lungs must accommodate the entire increase in cardiac output during exercise. The pulmonary circulation is under limited adrenergic[46] or endothelial[46–51] control during exercise and therefore, because of its unique in-series relationship, the pulmonary circulation is tightly coupled to left (downstream) ventricular function. At the same time, the pulmonary microcirculation has been engineered to maximize gas-exchange efficiency and as a result, vessel walls are very thin, strong, and distensible. Correspondingly, pulmonary vascular resistance and perfusion pressures are about one-fifth of those observed in the systemic circulation at rest.

With upright exercise, there is an increase in venous return to the heart, causing a central shift of blood volume into the thorax.[52] This increases both right and left ventricular filling pressures,[53] helping to maintain, or increase, both end-diastolic volume and stroke volume, despite reductions in filling time secondary to exercise-induced tachycardia. The dominant determinant of pulmonary artery pressure during exercise is left ventricular filling pressure.[54]

The rise in both pulmonary arterial and pulmonary capillary wedge pressures with exercise recruits previously unperfused and distended pulmonary capillaries, increasing capillary blood volume and reducing pulmonary vascular resistance. This increases the surface area for gas diffusion[55] and helps to maintain the red blood cell capillary transit time necessary for complete gas exchange (>0.25 seconds). (Mean pulmonary capillary transit time [seconds] is equal to the ratio of pulmonary capillary blood volume and blood flow [cardiac output].) At peak exercise in untrained subjects, despite the fourfold increase in pulmonary flow (cardiac output) from rest, capillary transit time at maximum exercise is reduced to only about one-half that at rest, due to a doubling of the pulmonary capillary blood volume (see Table 18-1).

It is important for the lung to remain relatively dry for gas exchange. At rest, there is a small outward flow of plasma fluid (~10–20 mL h^{-1}) from the capillaries into the interstitial space of the alveolar wall. The fluid passes into the perivascular and peribronchiolar spaces of the lung, with the lymphatic system transporting this fluid to the hilar lymph nodes. With exercise, thoracic lymph flow increases substantially, due to augmented pulmonary capillary pressures and capillary surface area.[56] In addition, the augmented ventilation with exercise increases lymph flow, acting as a safety mechanism to oppose edema formation in the alveoli or interstitial space.[57] Thus, the lymphatic system is vitally important in preventing exudation of fluid into the alveoli during exercise.

The efficiency of gas exchange for O_2 within the lung is defined and quantified as the difference in P_{O_2} between the alveolar gas and the arterial blood, and is known as the alveolar to arterial P_{O_2} difference (A-aDO_2). If gas exchange within the lung were perfect, the A-aDO_2 would be equal to zero. However, the A-aDO_2 normally amounts to 5 to 10 mm Hg at rest in young, healthy subject.[58] During exercise, the efficiency of gas exchange worsens in an intensity-dependent manner, and the A-aDO_2 increases to values of 15 to 25 mm Hg or more at maximal exercise (see Table 18-1). In contrast, fixed workload endurance exercise does not result in a time-dependent worsening of gas exchange when compared to the first minute of exercise,[59] indicating that the magnitude of the A-aDO_2 is determined primarily by metabolic rate as opposed to exercise duration.

The A-aDO_2 is a complex physiologic variable and as such is determined by a variety of mechanisms during rest and exercise. The worsening of gas-exchange efficiency during exercise is primarily due to an exaggeration of mechanisms present at rest. The principle contributor to the A-aDO_2 during both rest and exercise is the imperfect matching of the distributions of alveolar ventilation ($\dot{V}_A$) and pulmonary blood flow ($\dot{Q}$), otherwise known as the $\dot{V}_A/\dot{Q}$ ratio (see full discussion on $\dot{V}_A/\dot{Q}$ in Chapter 14). The ratio of $\dot{V}_A$ to $\dot{Q}$ can be partitioned into that occurring *among* lung regions (i.e., interregional, primarily dependent on gravity) and to that *within* an isogravitational plane of the lung (i.e., intraregional, or independent of the effects of gravity). The distributions for $\dot{V}_A$ and $\dot{Q}$ were once thought to be dominated by gravity, however, recent studies have resulted in the realization that there is also a great deal of pulmonary blood flow heterogeneity within an isogravitational plane of the lung.[60] Presumably, much intraregional heterogeneity exists for alveolar ventilation as well. These intraregional inhomogeneities are likely due simply to the normal anatomical heterogeneity of vessel and airway diameters, compliances, and resistances within specific lung regions.

During exercise, overall $\dot{V}_A/\dot{Q}$ nonuniformity increases slightly as measured by the multiple inert gas elimination technique (a technique that is not able to partition the $\dot{V}_A/\dot{Q}$ into separate inter- and intraregional distributions).[61,62] Despite this increasing nonuniformity, both $\dot{V}_A$ and $\dot{Q}$ become more uniform from lung apex to base resulting in a more uniform interregional $\dot{V}_A/\dot{Q}$ distribution.[63] Thus, the increased overall $\dot{V}_A/\dot{Q}$ nonuniformity observed during exercise can be attributed almost entirely to a more maldistributed intraregional $\dot{V}_A/\dot{Q}$, which contributes to the decreased efficiency of gas exchange (i.e., widening of A-aDO_2) at increasing exercise intensities. Counteracting the greater nonuniformity of the $\dot{V}_A/\dot{Q}$ distribution during exercise is the fact that overall $\dot{V}_A$ increases out of proportion to $\dot{Q}$ at increasing exercise intensities (see Table 18-1).[62] Thus, even though the distribution of $\dot{V}_A/\dot{Q}$ becomes more nonuniform, the higher overall $\dot{V}_A/\dot{Q}$ assures that little if any of the lung will be markedly underventilated (i.e., $\dot{V}_A/\dot{Q} < 0.8$). Alveolar P_{O_2} is therefore maintained high throughout the lung and this assures maintenance of end-capillary P_{O_2} near resting levels, even in the face of a progressive reduction in mixed venous O_2 content.

A second contributing factor to the A-aDO_2 is the mixing of shunted blood (i.e., venous blood that does not pass a ventilated alveolus) with arterial blood. There are two types of shunt that may contribute to the A-aDO_2 in health. The first type is known as an extrapulmonary shunt, and – in health – primarily consists of Thebesian venous drainage from the coronary circulation, which drains deoxygenated blood directly into the left ventricle.[64] Extrapulmonary shunts as small as 1% to 2% of the cardiac output have been calculated to account for about half of the A-aDO_2 during moderate intensity exercise.[62] Importantly, these shunts would be expected to increase total venous admixture during exercise of increasing intensity due to both a decreased O_2 content of Thebesian effluent (as a result of increased myocardial O_2 extraction)[65] as well as increased total Thebesian flow.

A second type of shunt that may contribute to the A-aDO_2 is commonly referred to as an intrapulmonary shunt, and is the result of direct anatomic connections between pulmonary arterial and venous vessels. These arteriovenous connections have been shown to exist in isolated, perfused whole human lungs.[66,67] and would be expected to have a greater influence on Pa_{O_2} during exercise of increasing intensity as $P\bar{v}_{O_2}$ falls. To date only indirect methods – using a delayed echo-Doppler visualization of intravenous infused microbubbles in the left atrium – support the concept that the intrapulmonary shunt pathway opens during exercise in healthy humans.[68] While the distensibility of this shunt pathway may modify the rise in pulmonary artery pressure during exercise, there is no evidence to indicate that it influences pulmonary O_2 exchange.[69]

SUMMARY: THE OVERBUILT HEALTHY RESPIRATORY SYSTEM

Based on our discussion to date of the respiratory system response to exercise in the untrained healthy adult there appears to be few exceptions to the conclusion that the respiratory system is substantially "overbuilt" and precisely regulated in meeting metabolic requirements of up to 10 to 12 times the resting levels. Key lines of supportive evidence include the following:

- At least three primary and redundant interrelated feedforward and feedback mechanisms combine – along with carotid chemoreceptors involvement with heavy exercise – to ensure near proportional ventilatory responses up to 10- to 12-fold increases in metabolic CO_2 production, that is, a highly precise isocapnic and mechanically efficient "just right" ventilatory response.
- Exercise-induced bronchodilation minimizes the increase in flow resistance respiratory muscle work and precise regulation of increases in V_T and f and reductions in EELV minimize increases in elastic work and V_D ventilation.
- A 20-fold increase in $\dot{V}_E$ is accomplished using less than 50% of the dynamic capacity of inspiratory muscles for force generation and requiring less than 10% of maximum $\dot{V}_{O_2}$ and cardiac output and with tidal flows and volumes which are well within the healthy airways maximal flow:volume envelope.
- Slight increases in overall $\dot{V}_A$:$\dot{Q}$ maldistribution and a small shunt of desaturated mixed venous blood results in a widened alveolar to arterial P_{O_2} difference signifying some degree of inefficiency in pulmonary gas exchange during exercise. However, high overall $\dot{V}_A$:$\dot{Q}$ raises alveolar P_{O_2} sufficiently to avoid severely low $\dot{V}_A$:$\dot{Q}$ regions and prevent arterial hypoxemia.
- The thin-walled and extensive capillary network and "passive" regulation of the pulmonary circulation during exercise, combined with a high capacity thoracic lymphatic "sump pump" in the lung interstitium, means that up to a fourfold increase in cardiac output and pulmonary blood flow do not result in critical reductions in mean red cell transit time or in accumulation of edematous fluid in the alveoli.

The result of these special structural characteristics and neuroregulation in the healthy lung parenchyma, airways, vasculature, and respiratory muscles is that the respiratory system contributes little to the limitation of O_2 transport to working locomotor muscles or to the symptoms of effort perception accompanying exercise and therefore to the limitation of either $\dot{V}_{O_2max}$ or endurance exercise performance.

EXCEPTIONS TO THE RULE—RESPIRATORY SYSTEM LIMITATIONS

There are a growing number of instances being reported in which the healthy respiratory system response to acute exercise appears to be less than "adequate" or inefficient, thereby contributing to exercise limitation and that repeated bouts of high-intensity exercise experienced in the elite endurance-trained athlete may even be maladaptive.

- In a significant number of highly trained endurance athletes exercise-induced arterial hypoxemia (EIAH) occurs (Sa_{O_2} rest to exercise, ~−5 to −10%) secondary primarily to an excessively widened alveolar to arterial O_2 difference and often in combination with a limited hyperventilatory response (see Fig. 18-7 and Table 18-1).[58,70] Preventing this hypoxemia (via increased $F_{I_{O_2}}$) raises $\dot{V}_{O_{2max}}$ (up to 15%) or with longer endurance-type performances reduces the rate of development of limb locomotor muscle fatigue and improves performance time.[71,72] Accumulation of edematous fluid and red cells in the alveoli has also been reported at these high work rates – suggesting a disruption in the alveolar–capillary barrier because of excessive pulmonary capillary hydrostatic pressures.[73] There are a number of continuing mysteries surrounding EIAH including, why the excessive A-aDO_2, that is, diffusion, shunt and/or $\dot{V}_A$:$\dot{Q}$ nonuniformity? …why does the hypoxemia first appear in submaximal exercise? … and why is there such marked heterogeneity in its occurrence among subjects of equal high fitness levels[15,74]?
- Heavy exercise-induced expiratory flow limitation with some degree of hyperinflation occurs at high ventilations in many young trained athletes and even at not so high ventilations in healthy fit elderly and in female athletes (see examples below under "Healthy Aging").This incurs a limitation to expiratory flow and to ventilation, causes high rates of inspiratory and expiratory muscle force generation (see Fig. 18-4, right) and high levels of expiratory ITP which compromises stroke volume and cardiac output. Increasing the maximal flow–volume loop via breathing low-density gases such as He:O_2 prevents this expiratory flow limitation and increases the ventilatory response to heavy exercise.[75]
- When cardiac output exceeds 25 L/min during exercise in endurance athletes mean pulmonary arterial pressures will often exceed 35 to 40 mm Hg because of the limited capability of the pulmonary vasculature (relative to the systemic vasculature) to reduce its vascular resistance.[69,76] Accordingly, a substantial stress is placed on the right ventricle wall which greatly exceeds that on the left ventricle.[77] With prolonged heavy intensity exercise this substantial vascular load results in reduced RV (but preserved LV) function as reported following a marathon or triathlon.[78]
- If the exercise is of very high intensity and sustained, significant fatigue occurs in the diaphragm and expiratory muscles thereby promoting increases in sympathetic vasoconstrictor activity and a reduction in limb vascular conductance and blood flow. Use of positive pressure mechanical ventilation during exercise to prevent respiratory muscle fatigue, also reduces the rate of limb muscle fatigue development and improves endurance performance.[79,80]

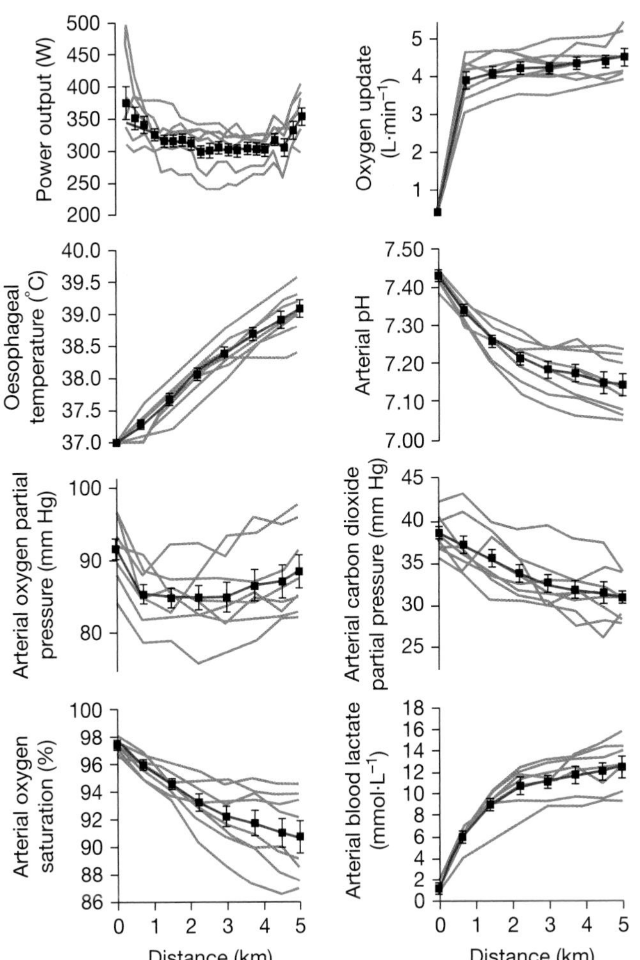

Figure 18-7 Effects of a 5-km time trial (cycle ergometer) in a normoxic environment on the physiological responses of trained cyclists. Thin lines are individual data ($n = 8$), with thick lines showing mean responses. Mean performance time was 483.4 ± 7.5 seconds (range, 437.5–478.4 seconds). Hemoglobin concentration was 14.4 ± 0.5 g L^{-1} and arterial oxygen content was 19.8 ± 0.8 mL O_2 100 mL^{-1} at rest and 16.4 ± 0.7 mL O_2 100 mL^{-1}/20.9 ± 1.0 mL O_2 100 mL^{-1} at 5 km. Note the progressive reduction in arterial hemoglobin O_2 saturation, due to a reduced Pa_{O_2} in the early stage of exercise, and thereafter to a progressive metabolic acidosis and increasing blood temperature. Also note the marked heterogeneity among subjects in their regulation of arterial P_{O_2}, Sa_{O_2}, and P_{CO_2}. *(Modified with permission from Amann M, Eldridge MW, Lovering AT, Stickland MK, Pegelow DF, Dempsey JA. Arterial oxygenation influences central motor output and exercise performance via effects on peripheral locomotor muscle fatigue in humans. J Physiol. 2006;575(Pt 3):937–952.)*

SPECIAL CASES OF RESPIRATORY SYSTEM LIMITATION TO EXERCISE PERFORMANCE

Healthy aging. Beginning in the second decade of life the healthy nonsmoking lung begins to lose elastic recoil (see Fig. 18-8A). This leads, during exercise, to expiratory flow limitation—with sequelae as described earlier such as ventilatory limitation, maldistribution of inspired ventilation, compromised stroke volume, and a significant prevalence of arterial hypoxemia (see Fig. 18-8B).[81] As mentioned earlier, expiratory flow limitation and its sequelae also occur during heavy/maximum exercise in the young highly trained athlete but with aging this occurs at much lower metabolic rates and ventilations than in the young (see Fig. 18-8B and contrast to Fig. 18-4 in younger athletes). Loss of elastic recoil also influences ventilation distribution in the lung resulting in a high V_D/V_T in the elderly. The V_D/V_T undergoes the normal decline during exercise but at a higher absolute V_D/V_T. This means that the healthy elderly must increase their $\dot{V}_E$ not only in proportion to the rising $\dot{V}_{CO_2}$ but also to accommodate the raised V_D. Remarkably this "extra" hyperpnea does indeed occur and $P_{A_{CO_2}}$ is regulated at resting levels, but this homeostatic regulation also means greater ventilatory work and higher flow rates thereby increasing the probability of flow limitation—especially in the highly fit older subject during heavy intensity exercise.

Gender differences. Exercise-induced expiratory flow limitation is more prevalent in young healthy females versus males and occurs at lower levels of metabolic and ventilatory demand.[82] The explanation for this gender difference appears – as based on CT scan evidence – to be one of airway structure limitation, that is, the so-called airway dysanapsis wherein the diameter of intralobar airways is narrowed for any given lung volume in the female.[83] This gender difference blunts the ventilatory response to heavy exercise[82] and may also lead to maldistribution of inspired ventilation which may explain at least

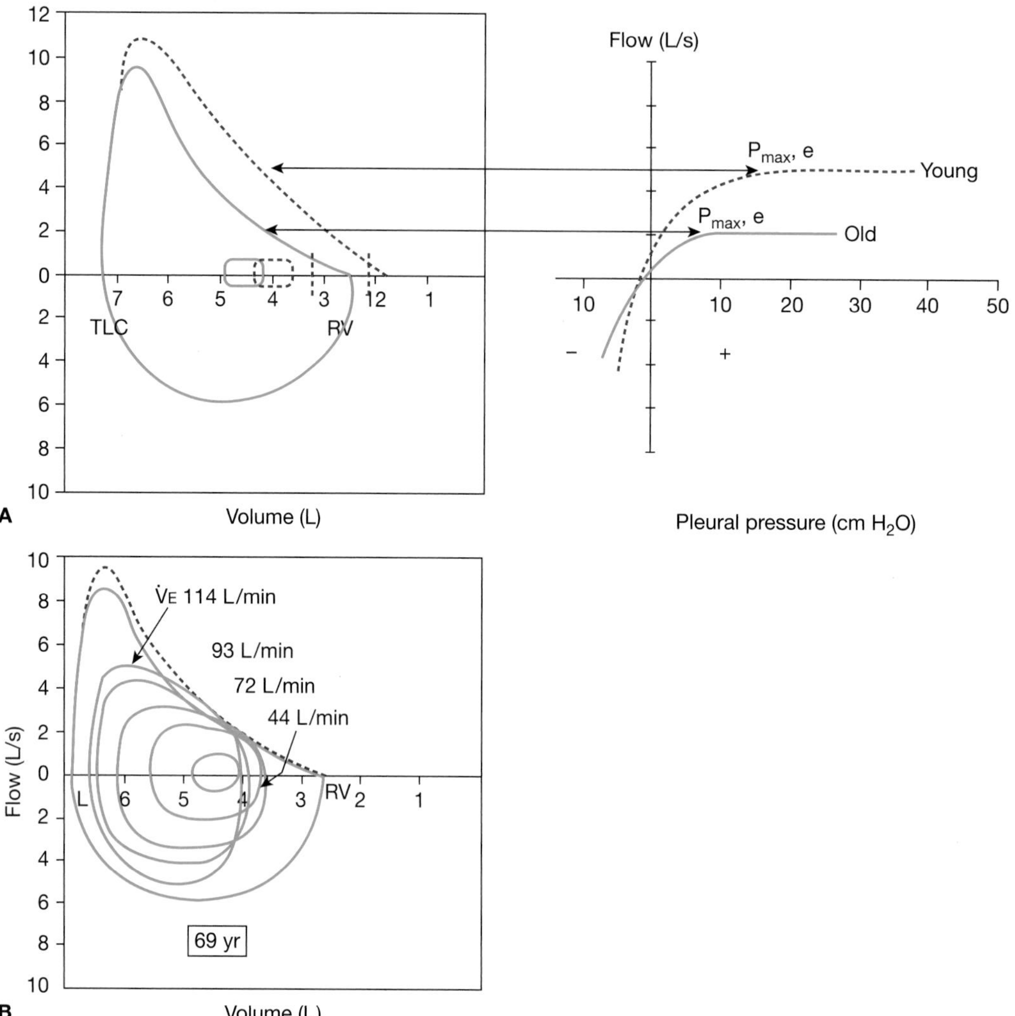

Figure 18-8 **A.** Maximum flow:volume loops and the isovolume pressure:flow relationships in the 30-year-old *(dashed line)* and 70-year-old nonsmoking male *(solid line)*. Note in the older subject the "scooping" in the expiratory limb of the maximum flow:volume loop indicating that airways are narrowing thereby reducing flow rate at any given lung volume during most of a forced expiration. The diagram on the right hand side shows that expiratory flow increases with increasing expiratory effort up to the critical closing pressure (P_{max}, e), at which point, despite additional expiratory effort, airways narrow and close and no increase in flow rate is achieved. Note the much lower P_{max}, e in the older subjects. Also note in the left hand figure that the end-expiratory lung volume is higher in the aged as is the airway closing volume *(solid line)*. These changes in the flow:volume loop and in airway closing volume and in the critical closing airway pressure occur with aging because of reduced lung elastic recoil. **B.** Flow:volume relationships at increasing levels of ventilation during steady-state exercise in the highly fit 69-year-old person. Contrast these with Figure 18-4 in the younger subject. The largest flow:volume envelope shown is that achieved via maximum volitional effort at rest, preexercise *(solid line)* and postexercise *(dashed line)* and the flow:volume loops within this maximal loop are from tidal breaths at rest and during increasing exercise intensities. In older subjects significant expiratory flow limitation begins at exercise ventilations (70 L/min or less) that are much lower than in the younger subject (>100 L/min.) Also note in the older subject that with the onset of the intersection of the tidal with the maximum expiratory flow–volume loop, end-expiratory lung volume increases back to and even in excess of resting levels. *(Reproduced with permission from Johnson BD, Reddan WG, Seow KC, Dempsey JA. Mechanical constraints on exercise hyperpnea in a fit aging population. Am Rev Respir Dis. 1991;143(5 Pt 1):968–977.)*

some of the occurrence of the widened A-aDO_2 and hypoxemia at lower work rates in female- versus male-trained athletes.

Athletic species differences. The thoroughbred horse with a $\dot{V}_{O_2 max}$ >160 mL/kg/min or more than twice that of the highest fit humans are the epitome of respiratory system limitations as shown by substantial arterial hypoxemia and CO_2 retention, pulmonary hypertension, and alveolar–capillary barrier disruption developed by these equine athletes during exercise.[84] Thus the lung appears to be truly "under built" in these amazing athletes in terms of its capability for accepting the very high cardiac outputs and ventilations required by their large cardiovascular and locomotor muscle driven metabolic requirements. This respiratory system limitation to exercise contrasts sharply with other highly aerobic animals such as the prong-horned antelope whose $\dot{V}_{O_2 max}$ is almost double that of the thoroughbred horse but has substantial upregulation of its lung alveolar–capillary surface area that is capable of accommodating their high metabolic requirements.[85]

Extrathoracic, upper airway flow limitation. A growing number of reports demonstrate that some athletes undergo sudden onset, paradoxical narrowing of the glottic aperture (vocal cord dysfunction or VCD) during exercise of severe intensity demanding high rates of airflow. This event immediately precipitates flow limitation, CO_2 retention, hypoxemia, and dyspnea. Evidence is accumulating to suggest that a highly significant portion of these VCD cases are wrongly diagnosed as asthma and therefore improperly treated—often with high doses of inhaled corticosteroids over many years.[86–88] Exercise-induced VCD seems to be especially prevalent in the highly competitive young adult or adolescent endurance athlete of both sexes. In a large group of elite endurance athletes about 5% experienced symptoms of inspiratory stridor during heavy exercise and about one-half of these cases showed both VCD and exercise-induced asthma.[89]

The key to detecting exercise-induced VCD is to understand that this problem involves extrathoracic airway narrowing in both inspiration and expiration and that it most commonly occurs only *during* heavy intensity exercise with sudden onset when flow rates are high. Immediately following cessation of exercise, as air flow rate falls precipitously, the extrathoracic airway diameter is usually no longer compromised. Therefore, an appropriate (noninvasive) test to detect VCD is to examine the characteristics of the breath-by-breath, tidal flow:volume envelope *during* exercise—because the usual means of examining forced maximum expiratory maneuvers, pre- and/or postexercise, will most often miss the event.[88] Accompanying sudden increases in end-tidal P_{CO_2} and reductions in Sa_{O_2} are also helpful markers of VCD. For diagnostic purposes, it is especially important that heavy intensity exercise demanding high flow rates be employed.

Perhaps the starting point here is for the clinician to recognize that not all symptoms of exercise-induced shortness of breath in the competitive athlete are attributable to the intrathoracic airway. Furthermore, the failure of routine spirometry or acute bronchodilator or airway provocation tests to detect significant asthma may not just be due solely to the high intra and inter individual variability in these tests. Please consider the upper airway.

Training effects on the respiratory system – an enigma. The examples of the respiratory system limitations in the equine and human athletes cited earlier raise the question of why the respiratory system has not – apparently – adapted to meet the increased maximum metabolic requirements in the highly trained. After all, there is ample evidence of alveolar and capillary growth in response to chronic hypoxia in the maturing human and canine lung.[90,91] Even caloric restriction with refeeding and partial pneumonectomy elicit substantial compensatory growth in the lung's diffusion surface of rodents.[92] In contrast, there is substantial evidence that chronic physical training does not enhance structure or function of the lungs airways, diffusion surface, or pulmonary vasculature.[93–95] Even the normal age-dependent loss of lung elastic recoil and diffusion capacity and the occurrence of exercise-induced expiratory flow limitation were unaltered by chronic habitual physical training, as demonstrated via longitudinal study of long-distance runners in their sixth and seventh decades of life.[96] To the contrary, evidence is now accumulating to show that reactive, asthmatic airways are highly prevalent in elite endurance-trained athletes. Further, longitudinal training studies – including the use of repeated airway biopsies in elite cross-country skiers – revealed that much of this hypersensitivity may result from hyperpnea-induced epithelial airway injury and subsequent airway repair and remodeling (see Fig. 18-9). Airway dehydration and shear stress along with increased transmural pressure gradients occurring repeatedly with sustained heavy exercise may be the cause of epithelial injury.[97–99] These negative effects on the airway of high-intensity physical training stand in contrast to evidence showing an alleviation of airway hyperresponsiveness in mildly asthmatic children achieved via moderate intensity level training.[100] One potential mechanism accounting for these training-induced reductions in airway responsiveness may be a reduced tone of airway smooth muscle secondary to hyperpnea-induced repeated stretching of the airway. This positive training effect on the airways has also been observed in nonasthmatic sedentary children.[101]

In contrast to the lung, the inspiratory muscles of the chest wall do undergo substantial changes in strength and aerobic capacity with intense training as induced by either whole-body training or specific respiratory muscle training.[102] This training effect on the respiratory muscles might improve exercise performance in health and disease.[103,104] One such mechanism for this improvement

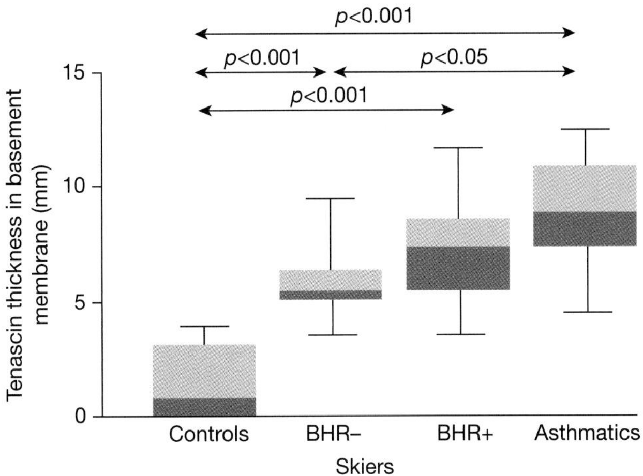

Figure 18-9 Thickness of tenascin immunoreactive band in subepithelial basement membrane zone in controls, in cross-country skiers with (+) and without (–) bronchial hyperresponsiveness (BHR), and in asthmatic subjects. Horizontal bar = median value. The basement membrane thickness is increased in all skiers relative to control subjects, indicating airway remodeling from chronic exercise training. In addition, skiers with asthma-like airway hyperresponsiveness tended to have a greater degree of remodeling. *(Reproduced with permission from Karjalainen EM, Laitinen A, Sue-Chu M, Altraja A, Bjermer L, Laitinen LA. Evidence of airway inflammation and remodeling in ski athletes with and without bronchial hyperresponsiveness to methacholine. Am J Respir Crit Care Med. 2000;161:2086–2091.)*

may involve a delay in diaphragm fatigue during prolonged heavy exercise, which would be expected to reduce metaboreflex effects on sympathetic, vasoconstrictor outflow and prevent reductions in blood flow and oxygen transport to limb locomotor muscles. This hypothesis has not yet been tested during whole-body exercise.

Hypoxic environments. Even mild elevations in altitude, that is, to only 1000 m or so have significant detrimental effects on $\dot{V}_{O_2max}$ and endurance performance. This is especially true in the highly trained athlete who may experience or be very close to significant arterial O_2 desaturation even at sea level and will undergo diffusion limitation and severe O_2 desaturation during exercise at even mild elevations in altitude (see Fig. 18-10).[58] Three major factors come into play as limiting factors to exercise performance at altitude in both acute and long-term hypoxic exposures. First, exercise-induced arterial O_2 desaturation and reduced O_2 transport will exacerbate fatigue of limb locomotor muscles, which in turn feeds back via limb afferents to inhibit cortical motor output, that is, "peripheral" leading to "central" fatigue.[105] Second, the marked hyperventilatory response to exercise in hypoxia is critically important to minimizing arterial O_2 desaturation – but at the same time comes at the cost of increasing respiratory muscle work. This increased respiratory muscle work hastens the onset of diaphragm fatigue, activation of the respiratory muscle metaboreflex triggering sympathetically mediated vasoconstriction of the locomotor muscle vasculature. Thus, a greater share of the cardiac output will be devoted to respiratory locomotor muscle blood flow and limb fatigue is exacerbated.[106] Third, CNS hypoxia, per se, depresses brain neurotransmitter turnover and inhibits motor output to locomotor muscles, that is, the so-called "central fatigue."[107]

Thus, in hypoxic environments both exercise-induced arterial O_2 desaturation and excessive blood flow requirements of the respiratory muscles would contribute significantly to exercise performance limitations by compromising O_2 transport to locomotor muscle ("peripheral" fatigue) and to the brain ("central" fatigue). CNS hypoxia, per se, appears to increase its relative contributions to exercise limitation as the severity of hypoxemia intensifies.

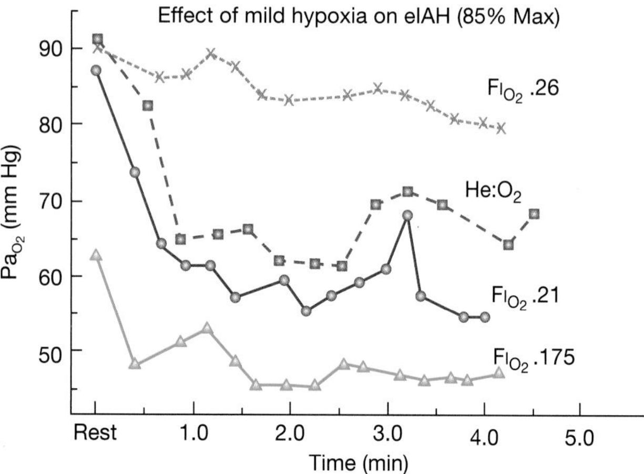

Figure 18-10 Effects of varying FI_{O_2} and of normoxic helium breathing on Pa_{O_2} during constant treadmill running at 15 mph (0% grade) i.e., 4 min. mile pace, in one fit subject ($\dot{V}_{O_2}$ = 4.54 L/min, or 97% $\dot{V}_{O_{2max}}$) ×, 0.26 O_2:N_2; o, 0.209 O_2:N_2; Δ, 0.175 O_2:N_2; □, 0.21 O_2:He; (b) the increase in Pa_{O_2} with He:O_2 breathing (vs. air) reflects the higher ventilation because the low air density gas decreased airway resistance and expanded the maximum flow:volume envelope, thereby reducing expiratory flow limitation during exercise; and (c) the prevention of arterial hypoxemia during exercise with mild inspired hyperoxia (0.26 FI_{O_2}), indicating that the hypoxemia was not secondary to an extrapulmonary shunt. Note the marked arterial hypoxemia during exercise which accompanied the exposure to mild acute hypoxia (0.175 FI_{O_2}). *(Modified with permission from Dempsey JA, Hanson PG, Henderson KS. Exercise-induced arterial hypoxaemia in healthy human subjects at sea level. J Physiol. 1984;355:161–175.)*

SUMMARY

With few exceptions it is safe to generalize that the healthy respiratory system – especially in youth and at sea level – is truly "overbuilt" to efficiently meet the considerable gas transport demands imposed by exercise. The key responses of the respiratory system insuring this homeostatic response include prevention of arterial O_2 desaturation and minimizing the work and therefore metabolic and circulatory costs of breathing. In turn these appropriate respiratory responses are insured by both the very special anatomical structure of the airways, lung parenchyma, pulmonary vasculature, and respiratory musculature as well as the precision with which ventilation is matched to metabolic requirements by the multifaceted autonomic control system. Among highly trained endurance athletes with near-normal respiratory system capacities but supernormal cardiovascular and locomotor capacities, the high demands for systemic O_2 transport do – in rare instances – exceed the lung's gas-exchange capabilities. More often in the highly trained, the high ventilatory requirements demand excessive respiratory muscle work and blood flow. So in these instances, the respiratory system will contribute significantly to exercise limitation. However, even in these cases cardiovascular system limitations remain the major "weak link" in O_2 delivery. Finally, there are instances where inadequacies within the healthy respiratory system impose more significant limitations to locomotor muscle O_2 transport and to exercise performance, including normal aging and gender effects on lung elastic recoil and/or airway resistance and upper airway patency during heavy intensity exercise. Again, the highly trained are more susceptible to these severe respiratory limitations because of their high demand for O_2 transport. Finally, the hypoxic environment through its effects on pulmonary diffusion limitation and ventilatory requirements greatly enhances the contribution of the respiratory system to O_2 transport and exercise performance limitations.

REFERENCES

1. Dempsey JA, Forster HV, Ainsworth DM. The regulation of hyperpnea, hyperventilation and respiratory muscle recruitment during exercise. In: Dempsey JA, Pack AI, eds. *The Regulation of Breathing.* New York, NY: Marcel Dekker; 1995;1065–1134.
2. Kaufman MP, Forster HV. Reflexes controlling circulating ventilatory and airway responses to exercise. In: Rowell LB, Shepherd JT, eds. *Handbook of Physiology.* New York, NY: Oxford University Press; 1996:381–447.
3. Waldrop TG, Eldridge FL, Iwamoto GA, Mitchell JH. Central neural control of respiration and circulation during exercise. In: Rowell LB, Shepard JT, eds. *Exercise: Regulation and Integration of Multiple Systems.* New York, NY: Oxford University Press; 1996:333–380.
4. Ward SA. Peripheral and central chemoreceptor control of ventilation during exercise in humans. *Can J Appl Physiol.* 1994;19: 305–333.
5. Phillipson EA, Duffin J, Cooper JD. Critical dependence of respiratory rhythmicity on metabolic CO_2 load. *J Appl Physiol Respir Environ Exerc Physiol.* 1981;50:45–54.
6. Luijendijk SCM. *Osmotic State of Blood Plasma as a Stimulus for Breathing; A model Study.* Maastricht, The Netherlands: Universitaire Pers Maastricht; 2012.
7. Forster HV, Haouzi P, Dempsey JA. Control of breathing during exercise. *Compr Physiol.* 2012;2:743–777.
8. Eldridge FL, Millhorn DE, Waldrop TG. Exercise hyperpnea and locomotion: parallel activation from the hypothalamus. *Science.* 1981;211:844–846.
9. Thornton JM, Guz A, Murphy K, et al. Identification of higher brain centres that may encode the cardiorespiratory response to exercise in humans. *J Physiol.* 2001;533:823–836.
10. Amann M, Blain GM, Proctor LT, Sebranek JJ, Pegelow DF, Dempsey JA. Group III and IV muscle afferents contribute to ventilatory and cardiovascular response to rhythmic exercise in humans. *J Appl Physiol (1985).* 2010;109:966–976.
11. Amann M, Blain GM, Proctor LT, Sebranek JJ, Pegelow DF, Dempsey JA. Implications of group III and IV muscle afferents for high-intensity endurance exercise performance in humans. *J Physiol.* 2011;589(Pt 21):5299–5309.
12. Gagnon P, Bussieres JS, Ribeiro F, et al. Influences of spinal anesthesia on exercise tolerance in patients with COPD. *Am J Respir Crit Care Med.* 2012;186:606–615.
13. Dempsey JA. New perspectives concerning feedback influences on cardiorespiratory control during rhythmic exercise and on exercise performance. *J Physiol.* 2012;590:4129–4144.
14. Somjen GG. The missing error signal–regulation beyond negative feedback. *News Physiol Sci.* 1992;7:184–185.
15. Dempsey JA, Wagner PD. Exercise-induced arterial hypoxemia. *J Appl Physiol.* 1999;87:1997–2006.
16. Bellemare F, Grassino A. Effect of pressure and timing of contraction on human diaphragm fatigue. *J Appl Physiol Respir Environ Exerc Physiol.* 1982;53:1190–1195.
17. O'Donnell DE, Revill SM, Webb KA. Dynamic hyperinflation and exercise intolerance in chronic obstructive pulmonary disease. *Am J Respir Crit Care Med.* 2001;164:770–777.
18. Henke KG, Sharratt M, Pegelow D, Dempsey JA. Regulation of end-expiratory lung volume during exercise. *J Appl Physiol (1985).* 1988;64:135–146.
19. Johnson BD, Saupe KW, Dempsey JA. Mechanical constraints on exercise hyperpnea in endurance athletes. *J Appl Physiol (1985).* 1992;73:874–886.

20. Dempsey JA, Adams L, Ainsworth D, et al. Airway, lung and respiratory muscle function during exercise. In: Rowell LB, Shepherd JT, eds. *Handbook of Physiology*. New York, NY: Oxford University Press; 1996;448–515.
21. Forsyth RD, Cole P, Shephard RJ. Exercise and nasal patency. *J Appl Physiol Respir Environ Exerc Physiol.* 1983;55:860–865.
22. Connel DC, Fregosi RF. Influence of nasal airflow and resistance on nasal dilator muscle activities during exercise. *J Appl Physiol (1985).* 1993;74:2529–2536.
23. England SJ, Bartlett D Jr. Changes in respiratory movements of the human vocal cords during hyperpnea. *J Appl Physiol Respir Environ Exerc Physiol.* 1982;52:780–785.
24. Warren JB, Jennings SJ, Clark TJ. Effect of adrenergic and vagal blockade on the normal human airway response to exercise. *Clin Sci (Lond).* 1984;66:79–85.
25. Stirling DR, Cotton DJ, Graham BL, Hodgson WC, Cockcroft DW, Dosman JA. Characteristics of airway tone during exercise in patients with asthma. *J Appl Physiol Respir Environ Exerc Physiol.* 1983;54:934–942.
26. Cordain L, Rode EJ, Gotshall RW, Tucker A. Residual lung volume and ventilatory muscle strength changes following maximal and submaximal exercise. *Int J Sports Med.* 1994;15:158–161.
27. Gauvreau GM, Ronnen GM, Watson RM, O'Byrne PM. Exercise-induced bronchoconstriction does not cause eosinophilic airway inflammation or airway hyperresponsiveness in subjects with asthma. *Am J Respir Crit Care Med.* 2000;162:1302–1307.
28. Kaufman MP, Rybicki KJ, Mitchell JH. Hindlimb muscular contraction reflexly decreases total pulmonary resistance in dogs. *J Appl Physiol (1985).* 1985;59:1521–1526.
29. Fredberg JJ, Inouye D, Miller B, et al. Airway smooth muscle, tidal stretches, and dynamically determined contractile states. *Am J Respir Crit Care Med.* 1997;156:1752–1759.
30. Manohar M. Blood flow in respiratory muscles during maximal exertion in ponies with laryngeal hemiplegia. *J Appl Physiol (1985).* 1987;62:229–237.
31. Harms CA, Babcock MA, McClaran SR, et al. Respiratory muscle work compromises leg blood flow during maximal exercise. *J Appl Physiol (1985).* 1997;82:1573–1583.
32. Harms CA, Wetter TJ, McClaran SR, et al. Effects of respiratory muscle work on cardiac output and its distribution during maximal exercise. *J Appl Physiol (1985).* 1998;85:609–618.
33. Sheel AW, Derchak PA, Pegelow DF, Dempsey JA. Threshold effects of respiratory muscle work on limb vascular resistance. *Am J Physiol Heart Circ Physiol.* 2002;282:H1732–H1738.
34. Hussain SN, Chatillon A, Comtois A, Roussos C, Magder S. Chemical activation of thin-fiber phrenic afferents. 2. Cardiovascular responses. *J Appl Physiol (1985).* 1991;70:77–86.
35. Rodman JR, Henderson KS, Smith CA, Dempsey JA. Cardiovascular effects of the respiratory muscle metaboreflexes in dogs: rest and exercise. *J Appl Physiol(1985).* 2003;95:1159–1169.
36. Aaker A, Laughlin MH. Diaphragm arterioles are less responsive to alpha1- adrenergic constriction than gastrocnemius arterioles. *J Appl Physiol (1985).* 2002;92:1808–1816.
37. Babcock MA, Pegelow DF, McClaran SR, Suman OE, Dempsey JA. Contribution of diaphragmatic power output to exercise-induced diaphragm fatigue. *J Appl Physiol.* 1995;78: 1710–1719.
38. Babcock MA, Pegelow DF, Johnson BD, Dempsey JA. Aerobic fitness effects on exercise-induced low-frequency diaphragm fatigue. *J Appl Physiol (1985).* 1996;81:2156–2164.
39. Babcock MA, Pegelow DF, Taha BH, Dempsey JA. High frequency diaphragmatic fatigue detected with paired stimuli in humans. *Med Sci Sports Exerc.* 1998;30:506–511.
40. Babcock MA, Pegelow DF, Harms CA, Dempsey JA. Effects of respiratory muscle unloading on exercise-induced diaphragm fatigue. *J Appl Physiol (1985).* 2002;93:201–206.
41. Johnson BD, Babcock MA, Suman OE, Dempsey JA. Exercise-induced diaphragmatic fatigue in healthy humans. *J Physiol.* 1993;460:385–405.
42. Walker DJ, Walterspacher S, Schlager D, et al. Characteristics of diaphragmatic fatigue during exhaustive exercise until task failure. *Respir Physiol Neurobiol.* 2011;176:14–20.
43. Babcock MA, Johnson BD, Pegelow DF, Suman OE, Griffin D, Dempsey JA. Hypoxic effects on exercise-induced diaphragmatic fatigue in normal healthy humans. *J Appl Physiol (1985).* 1995;78:82–92.
44. Miller JD, Smith CA, Hemauer SJ, Dempsey JA. The effects of inspiratory intrathoracic pressure production on the cardiovascular response to submaximal exercise in health and chronic heart failure. *Am J Physiol Heart Circ Physiol.* 2007;292:H580–H592.
45. Stark-Leyva KN, Beck KC, Johnson BD. Influence of expiratory loading and hyperinflation on cardiac output during exercise. *J Appl Physiol (1985).* 2004;96:1920–1927.
46. Kane DW, Tesauro T, Koizumi T, Gupta R, Newman JH. Exercise-induced pulmonary vasoconstriction during combined blockade of nitric oxide synthase and beta adrenergic receptors. *J Clin Invest.* 1994;93:677–683.
47. Duncker DJ, Stubenitsky R, Tonino PA, Verdouw PD. Nitric oxide contributes to the regulation of vasomotor tone but does not modulate O(2)-consumption in exercising swine. *Cardiovasc Res.* 2000;47:738–748.
48. Lindenfeld J, Reeves JT, Horwitz LD. Low exercise pulmonary resistance is not dependent on vasodilator prostaglandins. *J Appl Physiol Respir Environ Exerc Physiol.* 1983;55:558–561.
49. Manohar M, Goetz TE. L-NAME does not affect exercise-induced pulmonary hypertension in thoroughbred horses. *J Appl Physiol (1985).* 1998;84:1902–1908.
50. Merkus D, Houweling B, Zarbanoui A, Duncker DJ. Interaction between prostanoids and nitric oxide in regulation of systemic, pulmonary, and coronary vascular tone in exercising swine. *Am J Physiol Heart Circ Physiol.* 2004;286:H1114–H1123.
51. Newman JH, Butka BJ, Brigham KL. Thromboxane A2 and prostacyclin do not modulate pulmonary hemodynamics during exercise in sheep. *J Appl Physiol (1985).* 1986;61:1706–1711.
52. Flamm SD, Taki J, Moore R, et al. Redistribution of regional and organ blood volume and effect on cardiac function in relation to upright exercise intensity in healthy human subjects. *Circulation.* 1990;81:1550–1559.
53. Reeves JT, Groves BM, Cymerman A, et al. Operation Everest II: cardiac filling pressures during cycle exercise at sea level. *Respir Physiol.* 1990;80:147–154.
54. Reeves JT, Dempsey JA, Grover RT. Pulmonary circulation during exercise. In: Weir EK, Reeves JT, eds. *Pulmonary Vascular Physiology and Pathophysiology*. New York, NY: Marcel Dekker, Inc.; 1989:107–133.
55. Johnson RLJ, Spicer WS, Bishop JM, Forster RE. Pulmonary capillary blood volume, flow and diffusing capacity during exercise. *J Appl Physiol.* 1960;15:893–902.
56. Coates G, O'Brodovich H, Jefferies AL, Gray GW. Effects of exercise on lung lymph flow in sheep and goats during normoxia and hypoxia. *J Clin Invest.* 1984;74:133–141.

57. Koizumi T, Roselli RJ, Parker RE, Hermo-Weiler CI, Banerjee M, Newman JH. Clearance of filtered fluid from the lung during exercise: role of hyperpnea. *Am J Respir Crit Care Med.* 2001;163:614–618.

58. Dempsey JA, Hanson PG, Henderson KS. Exercise-induced arterial hypoxaemia in healthy human subjects at sea level. *J Physiol.* 1984;355:161–175.

59. Wetter TJ, St Croix CM, Pegelow DF, Sonetti DA, Dempsey JA. Effects of exhaustive endurance exercise on pulmonary gas exchange and airway function in women. *J Appl Physiol (1985).* 2001;91:847–858.

60. Glenny RW, Bernard S, Robertson HT, Hlastala MP. Gravity is an important but secondary determinant of regional pulmonary blood flow in upright primates. *J Appl Physiol (1985).* 1999;86:623–632.

61. Wagner PD, Gale GE, Moon RE, Torre-Bueno JR, Stolp BW, Saltzman HA. Pulmonary gas exchange in humans exercising at sea level and simulated altitude. *J Appl Physiol (1985).* 1986;61:260–270.

62. Gledhill NC, Froese AB, Dempsey JA. Ventilation to perfusion distribution during exercise in health. In: Dempsey JA, Reed CE, eds. *Muscular Exercise and the Lung.* Madison: University of Wisconsin Press; 1977:325–344.

63. Bryan AC, Bentivoglio LG, Beerel F, Macleish H, Zidulka A, Bates DV. Factors affecting regional distribution of ventilation and perfusion in the lung. *J Appl Physiol.* 1964;19:395–402.

64. Ravin MB, Epstein RM, Malm JR. Contribution of thebesian veins to the physiologic shunt in anesthetized man. *J Appl Physiol.* 1965;20:1148–1152.

65. Kitamura K, Jorgensen CR, Gobel FL, Taylor HL, Wang Y. Hemodynamic correlates of myocardial oxygen consumption during upright exercise. *J Appl Physiol.* 1972;32:516–522.

66. Lovering AT, Stickland MK, Kelso AJ, Eldridge MW. Direct demonstration of 25- and 50-micron arteriovenous pathways in healthy human and baboon lungs. *Am J Physiol Heart Circ Physiol.* 2007;292:H1777–H1781.

67. Tobin CE. Arteriovenous shunts in the peripheral pulmonary circulation in the human lung. *Thorax.* 1966;21:197–204.

68. Eldridge MW, Dempsey JA, Haverkamp HC, Lovering AT, Hokanson JS. Exercise-induced intrapulmonary arteriovenous shunting in healthy humans. *J Appl Physiol (1985).* 2004;97:797–805.

69. Lalande S, Yerly P, Faoro V, Naeije R. Pulmonary vascular distensibility predicts aerobic capacity in healthy individuals. *J Physiol.* 2012;590:4279–4288.

70. Harms CA, McClaran SR, Nickele GA, Pegelow DF, Nelson WB, Dempsey JA. Exercise-induced arterial hypoxaemia in healthy young women. *J Physiol.* 1998;507(Pt 2):619–628.

71. Amann M, Eldridge MW, Lovering AT, Stickland MK, Pegelow DF, Dempsey JA. Arterial oxygenation influences central motor output and exercise performance via effects on peripheral locomotor muscle fatigue in humans. *J Physiol.* 2006;575:937–952.

72. Harms CA, McClaran SR, Nickele GA, Pegelow DF, Nelson WB, Dempsey JA. Effect of exercise-induced arterial O_2 desaturation on $\dot{V}_{O_2max}$ in women. *Med Sci Sports Exerc.* 2000;32:1101–1108.

73. Hopkins SR, Johnson EC, Richardson RS, Wagner H, De RM, Wagner PD. Effects of inhaled nitric oxide on gas exchange in lungs with shunt or poorly ventilated areas. *Am J Respir Crit Care Med.* 1997;156:484–491.

74. Dempsey JA, Amann M, Harms CA, Wetter TJ. Respiratory system limitations to performance in the healthy athlete: some answers, more questions! *Dtsch Z Sportmed.* 2012;63:157–162.

75. McClaran SR, Harms CA, Pegelow DF, Dempsey JA. Smaller lungs in women affect exercise hyperpnea. *J Appl Physiol (1985).* 1998;84:1872–1881.

76. La Gerche A, MacIsaac AI, Burns AT et al. Pulmonary transit of agitated contrast is associated with enhanced pulmonary vascular reserve and right ventricular function during exercise. *J Appl Physiol (1985).* 2010;109:1307–1317.

77. La Gerche A, Heidbüchel H, Burns AT et al. Disproportionate exercise load and remodeling of the athlete's right ventricle. *Med Sci Sports Exerc.* 2011;43:974–981.

78. La Gerche A, Burns AT, Mooney DJ et al. Exercise-induced right ventricular dysfunction and structural remodelling in endurance athletes. *Eur Heart J.* 2012;33:998–1006.

79. Harms CA, Wetter TJ, St Croix CM, Pegelow DF, Dempsey JA. Effects of respiratory muscle work on exercise performance. *J Appl Physiol (1985).* 2000;89:131–138.

80. Romer LM, Lovering AT, Haverkamp HC, Pegelow DF, Dempsey JA. Effect of inspiratory muscle work on peripheral fatigue of locomotor muscles in healthy humans. *J Physiol.* 2006;571:425–439.

81. Johnson BD, Reddan WG, Seow KC, Dempsey JA. Mechanical constraints on exercise hyperpnea in a fit aging population. *Am Rev Respir Dis.* 1991;143:968–977.

82. McClaran SR, Wetter TJ, Pegelow DF, Dempsey JA. Role of expiratory flow limitation in determining lung volumes and ventilation during exercise. *J Appl Physiol.* 1999;86:1357–1366.

83. Sheel AW, Guenette JA, Yuan R, et al. Evidence for dysanapsis using computed tomographic imaging of the airways in older ex-smokers. *J Appl Physiol (1985).* 2009;107:1622–1628.

84. Bayly WM, Hodgson DR, Schulz DA, Dempsey JA, Gollnick PD. Exercise-induced hypercapnia in the horse. *J Appl Physiol (1985).* 1989;67:1958–1966.

85. Lindstedt SL, Hokanson JF, Wells DJ, Swain SD, Hoppeler H, Navarro V. Running energetics in the pronghorn antelope. *Nature.* 1991;353:748–750.

86. Fallon KE. Upper airway obstruction masquerading as exercise induced bronchospasm in an elite road cyclist. *Br J Sports Med.* 2004;38:E9.

87. McFadden ER Jr, Zawadski DK. Vocal cord dysfunction masquerading as exercise-induced asthma. A physiologic cause for "choking" during athletic activities. *Am J Respir Crit Care Med.* 1996;153:942–947.

88. Haverkamp H, Miller J, Rodman J, et al. Extrathoracic obstruction and hypoxemia occurring during exercise in a competitive female cyclist. *Chest.* 2003;124:1602–1605.

89. Rundell KW, Spiering BA. Inspiratory stridor in elite athletes. *Chest.* 2003;123:468–474.

90. Cerny FC, Dempsey JA, Reddan WG. Pulmonary gas exchange in nonnative residents of high altitude. *J Clin Invest.* 1973;52:2993–2999.

91. ad hoc Statement Committee, American Thoracic Society. Mechanisms and limits of induced postnatal lung growth. *Am J Respir Crit Care Med.* 2004;170:319–343.

92. Massaro D, Massaro GD. Invited Review: pulmonary alveoli: formation, the "call for oxygen," and other regulators. *Am J Physiol Lung Cell Mol Physiol.* 2002;282:L345–L358.

93. Dempsey JA. J.B. Wolffe memorial lecture. Is the lung built for exercise? *Med Sci Sports Exerc.* 1986;18:143–155.

94. Ross KA, Thurlbeck WM. Lung growth in newborn guinea pigs: effects of endurance exercise. *Respir Physiol.* 1992;89:353–364.

95. Wagner PD. Why doesn't exercise grow the lungs when other factors do? *Exerc Sport Sci Rev.* 2005;33:3–8.

96. McClaran SR, Babcock MA, Pegelow DF, Reddan WG, Dempsey JA. Longitudinal effects of aging on lung function at rest and exercise in healthy active fit elderly adults. *J Appl Physiol (1985).* 1995;78:1957–1968.

97. Kippelen P, Fitch KD, Anderson SD, et al. Respiratory health of elite athletes - preventing airway injury: a critical review. *Br J Sports Med.* 2012;46:471–476.

98. Kippelen P, Anderson SD. Airway injury during high-level exercise. *Br J Sports Med.* 2012;46:385–390.

99. Karjalainen EM, Laitinen A, Sue-Chu M, Altraja A, Bjermer L, Laitinen LA. Evidence of airway inflammation and remodeling in ski athletes with and without bronchial hyperresponsiveness to methacholine. *Am J Respir Crit Care Med.* 2000;161:2086–2091.

100. Scichilone N, Morici G, Zangla D, et al. Effects of exercise training on airway closure in asthmatics. *J Appl Physiol (1985).* 2012;113:714–718.

101. Rosenkranz SK, Rosenkranz RR, Hastmann TJ, Harms CA. High-intensity training improves airway responsiveness in inactive nonasthmatic children: evidence from a randomized controlled trial. *J Appl Physiol.* 2012;112:1174–1183.

102. Powers SK, Lawler J, Criswell D, Lieu FK, Martin D. Aging and respiratory muscle metabolic plasticity: effects of endurance training. *J Appl Physiol (1985).* 1992;72:1068–1073.

103. Patel MS, Hart N, Polkey MI. CrossTalk proposal: training the respiratory muscles does not improve exercise tolerance. *J Physiol.* 2012;590:3393–3395.

104. McConnell AK. CrossTalk opposing view: respiratory muscle training does improve exercise tolerance. *J Physiol.* 2012;590:3397–3398.

105. Amann M, Runnels S, Morgan DE, et al. On the contribution of group III and IV muscle afferents to the circulatory response to rhythmic exercise in humans. *J Physiol.* 2011;589:3855–3866.

106. Amann M, Pegelow DF, Jacques AJ, Dempsey JA. Inspiratory muscle work in acute hypoxia influences locomotor muscle fatigue and exercise performance of healthy humans. *Am J Physiol Regul Integr Comp Physiol.* 2007;293:R2036–R2045.

107. Amann M, Romer LM, Subudhi AW, Pegelow DF, Dempsey JA. Severity of arterial hypoxaemia affects the relative contributions of peripheral muscle fatigue to exercise performance in healthy humans. *J Physiol.* 2007;581:389–403.

108. Aaron EA, Seow KC, Johnson BD, Dempsey JA. Oxygen cost of exercise hyperpnea: implications for performance. *J Appl Physiol (1985).* 1992;72:1818–1825.

109. Harms CA, Dempsey JA. Cardiovascular consequences of exercise hyperpnea. *Exerc Sport Sci Rev.* 1999;27:37–62.

110. Manohar M. Blood flow to the respiratory and limb muscles and to abdominal organs during maximal exertion in ponies. *J Physiol.* 1986;377:25–35.

CHAPTER 19

Aging of the Respiratory System

Edward J. Campbell

The fastest growing segment of the US population consists of individuals of age 65 and older. In the 2010 census, this segment comprised 16% of the population. Since the 1950s, the median age of the US population has increased by 20 years.

The largest decrements in age-adjusted death rates have been occurring in older patients. With the increasing longevity of human population, it is necessary to understand the effects of aging on the respiratory system in healthy people. Perhaps more importantly, because the age-related decrements in respiratory system function can be unmasked by disease, it is critically important to point out that the aged: (1) have an enhanced predisposition to lung disease; (2) have a decreasing reserve of respiratory system function that decreases their ability to cope with the stresses of illness, injury, and surgery; and (3) may have differing responses to therapy when compared with their younger counterparts.

Even in individuals who enjoy apparently good health, there are measurable decrements in function of the respiratory system with age. These changes occur progressively as a healthy individual grows older and are most marked beyond 60 years of age. Cross-sectional studies show clear differences between elderly and young persons with regard to the structure and function of the components of the respiratory system (Table 19-1). As we will see, however, caution must be exercised in ascribing observed changes to age alone. It is also necessary to be aware that longitudinal studies of "healthy" individuals followed to old age are essentially not available. Where appropriate, methodologic problems in the available cross-sectional studies are described.

Although age-associated changes can be measured easily by objective testing, it is important to note that the routine activities of healthy elderly persons are not limited by the decreasing respiratory system function. However, whereas youthful persons have a marked excess of functional capacity over the amount required to meet metabolic needs at rest or with stress (physiologic reserve), the respiratory system draws on this reserve as its function declines with age. Thus, the physiologic reserve, especially for alveolar gas exchange, is reduced with aging. This leaves elderly individuals vulnerable to stresses, diseases, and injuries that are weathered much more easily in the young.

ARE CHANGES IN THE RESPIRATORY SYSTEM CAUSED BY AGING OR RELATED TO AGE IN OTHER WAYS?

For decades, the phenomena explained purely by aging have been required to satisfy specific principles. Roughly according to Hayflick,[1] the changes must be (1) intrinsic (as opposed to environmentally mediated); (2) universal; (3) progressive; and (4) usually detrimental to the organism. Developing an understanding of changes to the lung over time is complicated by the fact that the lung is an open system that is exposed to environment. As such, it is assaulted by respiratory infections and by a constant barrage of particulates and other air pollutants. In addition, the lungs are commonly exposed to tobacco smoke, to occupational dusts and fumes, and to effects of aspiration. At times, environmental influences are inextricably involved in the changes that are observed in the respiratory system over time. However, it is important to draw a distinction between alterations

TABLE 19-1 Respiratory System: Functional Divisions and Changes with Aging

Functional Division	Components	Function	Change(s) with Aging
Conducting airways	All airways not involved in gas exchange (mouth to terminal bronchioles)	Gas movement between environment and alveolar space	Slight changes in size; calcification; glandular hypertrophy
Lung parenchyma	Gas-exchanging airways and vessels; connective tissue framework	Gas exchange between alveolar space and capillary blood	Enlarged terminal airspaces; ventilation/perfusion mismatching
Bellows apparatus	Chest wall and muscles of respiration	Provide mechanical forces for ventilation	Increased rigidity of chest wall; decreased respiratory muscle strength
Ventilatory control	Respiratory control center (pons and medulla); carotid and aortic bodies	Maintaining homeostasis by altering ventilation to match metabolic needs	Markedly decreased responses to hypercapnia and hypoxemia
Cardiovascular system	Heart and systemic vasculature	Blood transport and tissue exchange of respiratory gases	Decreased maximal heart rate and cardiac output; decreased responsiveness to hypoxemia

purely related to aging and those associated with older individuals. Purely age-related changes are biologic phenomena and irreversible. Other alterations associated with increasing age have the potential to be preventable, treatable, and/or reversible.

CHANGES IN THE UPPER AIRWAY

There is a clearly increased risk of aspiration in the elderly that is thought to be a consequence of a number of age-related factors, including comorbid illnesses and debility, medications, and the aging process itself. With regard to purely age-related changes, attention has been focused upon the cough and swallowing reflexes, both of which are protective against aspiration. In the past, these reflexes have been thought to be controlled primarily by the brainstem, but there is now evidence that cortical and subcortical structures play critical roles in their control.[2] By their nature, reflexive cough and swallowing activate both sensory and motor areas in the cortex. The sensory component, including the sensory cortex in reflexive circuits, seems to be more vulnerable to aging than the motor component, including the motor cortex. Therefore, strategies to restore effective cough and swallowing reflexes should be focused upon compensations of sensory components.

Variable amounts of aspiration of both oropharyngeal contents (food particles, saliva, and oropharyngeal organisms), and also gastric contents (food particles and gastric secretions including gastric acid), are increasingly common with aging. Aspiration is particularly common in the very old. Because of the sensory alterations discussed earlier, aspiration in elderly individuals can be associated with few, or no, symptoms.[3]

A potentially important contributor to aspiration is gastroesophageal reflux. In accordance with the earlier discussion of sensory impairments, reflux esophagitis severity increases with age while heartburn severity decreases with age.[4] Consequences of gastroesophageal reflux may be exacerbated by esophageal motor abnormalities associated with aging. Recurrent aspiration of gastric contents in the elderly can lead to airway inflammation, bronchiectasis, and pneumonia.

STRUCTURAL CHANGES IN THE LUNG

Studies of the aging lung have shown changes in shape, with increase in anteroposterior diameter that lead to a "rounding" shape of the lung. These changes are presumably secondary to changes in the shape of the surrounding thoracic cage that are very common after the age of 75. In a study of 100 chest radiographs from individuals ranging in age from 75 to 93 years, 25% had severe kyphosis (>50 degrees) and 43% had moderate kyphosis (35–50 degrees) from vertebral fractures.[5]

CONDUCTING AIRWAYS

The conducting airways consist of the air passages from mouth to the level of respiratory bronchioles. Their volume comprises the anatomic dead space, and their geometry is a primary determinant of airway resistance. The larger cartilaginous airways show a modest increase in size with age, resulting in slight but probably functionally insignificant increase in anatomic dead space. Although calcification of cartilage in the walls of the central airways and hypertrophy of bronchial mucus glands is seen in advanced age, these changes in the extraparenchymal conducting airways appear to have little or no physiologic significance.

Ciliary motility is significantly decreased in subjects over the age of 60, which likely further increases the risk of lower respiratory infection and inflammation.[6]

LUNG PARENCHYMA

After the age of 30 or 40, the respiratory bronchioles and alveolar ducts undergo progressive enlargement (Fig. 19-1). This change has been termed "ductectasia" because of the prominent finding of enlargement of alveolar ducts.[7] The proportion of the lung made up of alveolar ducts increases, and alveolar septa become shortened, leading to a "flattened" appearance of the alveoli. With the change in geometry, the distance between alveolar walls (known to morphologists as the mean linear intercept, or MLI) increases, while the surface-to-volume ratio of the lung decreases.[8] The age-related enlargement of the terminal respiratory units also produces a decrease in the percentage of parenchymal air contained within the alveoli.[9] The net result of these structural changes is that the alveolar surface area decreases by approximately 15% by age 70.

Pulmonary emphysema is also characterized by an increase in the size of terminal airspaces, an increase in MLI, and a decrease in surface area; however, destruction of alveolar septa with fusion of terminal airspaces is a defining characteristic of emphysema. There have been some reports of emphysematous lesions in aged lungs, but it is not certain that smokers were excluded from these studies. Since the fate of individual alveolar septa during the aging process has been somewhat controversial, some have referred to the histologic changes in aged lungs as "senile emphysema." A National Heart, Lung, and Blood Institute Workshop on the definition of emphysema[10] weighed the available evidence, and decided not to include age-related changes in the lung parenchyma under the definition of *emphysema*. To simplify terms and avoid confusion, they recommended use of the term *aging lung* to apply to the uniform airspace enlargement that develops with increasing age. Despite the continued use of "senile emphysema," this term should be avoided.

Computed tomography of the chest in individuals over 75 years of age has shown a surprising prevalence (60%) of a subpleural

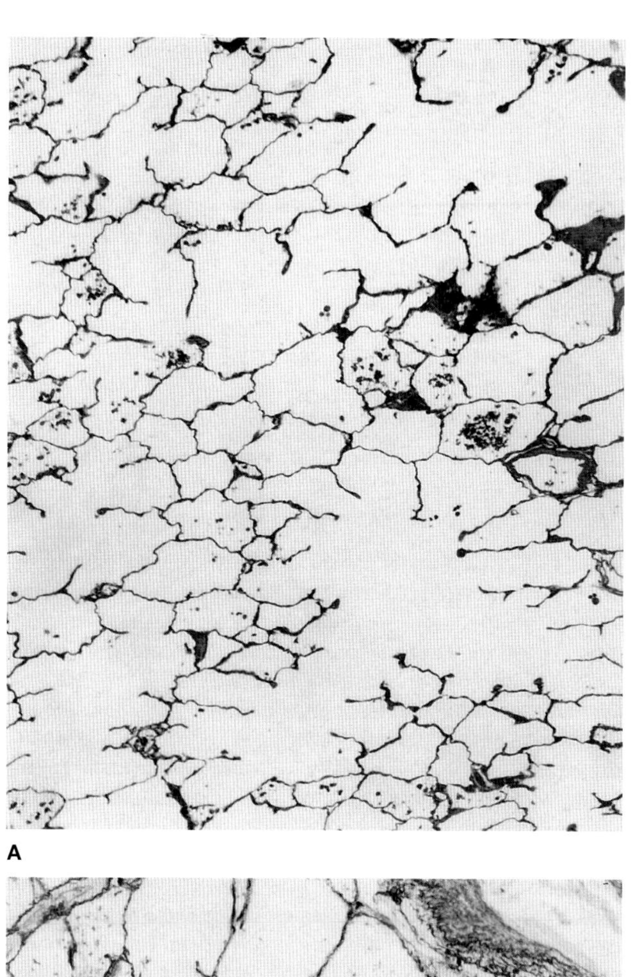

A

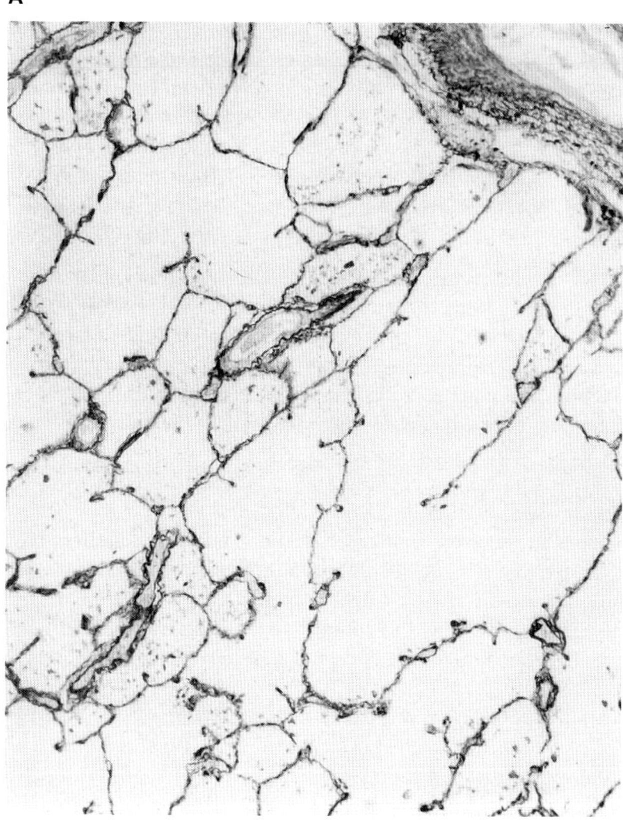

B

Figure 19-1 Histologic changes in the aging lung. **A.** Normal lung of a 36-year-old woman. **B.** Lung of a 93-year-old woman. In (**B**), the alveolar ducts are dilated, and shortening of inter-alveolar septa is observed. *(Used with permission of the Mayo Foundation; photomicrographs used with permission of Charles Kuhn III, MD.)*

basilar reticular pattern that was absent from images from a control population that was less than 55 years old. Lung cysts were seen in 25% of the elderly subjects, but none of the controls.[11] These findings are usually associated with interstitial lung disease, but in the elderly they seem not to reflect a clinically relevant disease process. Caution must be exercised to avoid overreacting to similar image findings in older patients.

CHANGES IN MECHANICAL PROPERTIES OF THE LUNGS

Both the Lungs and chest wall are elastic. The resting volume of excised lungs is smaller than that contained within an intact thoracic cage, because the lungs are held at an increased volume by the outward recoil forces of the chest wall. Thus, in the intact thoracic cage, the lungs exert an inward recoil force. The retractile force of the lungs, or the "elastic recoil," can be measured during life by estimating the pleural pressure with an esophageal balloon at progressively decreasing lung volumes from total lung capacity to functional residual capacity (FRC), when the airways are open and there is no air flow. The negative pleural pressure is generated by the lungs' elastic recoil forces.

The pressure measurements may be displayed on a pressure–volume diagram (Fig. 19-2). Figure 19-2 compares, at the same volume, the elastic recoil pressures of a young man, a normal elderly adult, and a patient with emphysema. The normal elderly individual and the patient with emphysema, both have a greater decrease in elastic recoil pressure than does a young person.[12] This is reflected in the leftward shift of their pressure–volume curves.[13–16] This loss of elastic recoil is the physiologic hallmark of emphysema. However, emphysema is characterized by a much greater loss of elastic recoil than is caused by aging alone.

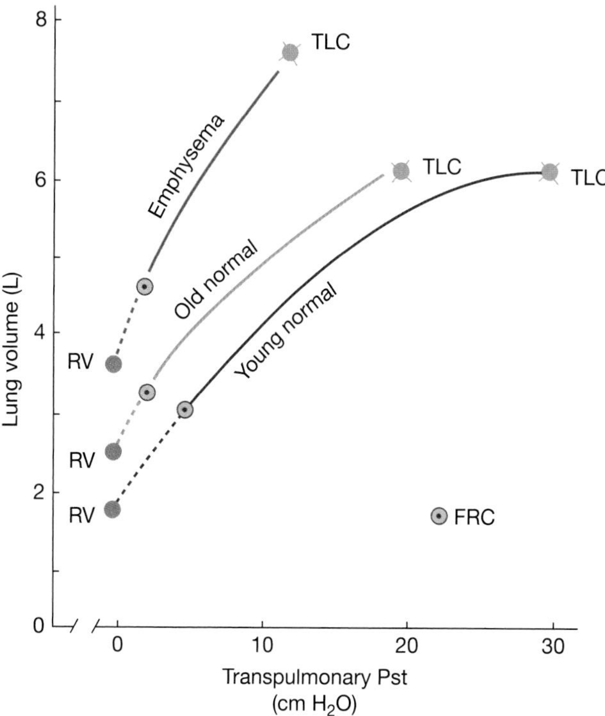

Figure 19-2 Static pressure–volume curves of the lungs. Static recoil pressure, expressed as transpulmonary pressure measured at various lung volumes, is plotted against lung volume on the ordinate. Note that at any lung volume, the recoil pressure is less in the aged individual than in the young, normal control, resulting in a pressure–volume curve that is shifted upward and to the left. For comparison, a curve for a patient with emphysema is shown. In emphysema, recoil pressures are reduced much more, and lung compliance (the slope of the pressure–volume relationship) is clearly abnormal. *(Reproduced with permission from Pride NB. Pulmonary distensibility in age and disease. Bull Physiopathol Respir. 1974;10(1):103–108.)*

There has been some disagreement regarding the effects of aging on lung compliance (Δ volume/Δ pressure; that is , the slope of the pressure–volume relationship Fig. 19-2). The question is whether there is a parallel leftward shift of the pressure–volume curve with aging (no change in compliance), or, instead, a steeper slope in addition to a shift (indicating an increase in compliance), as seen in emphysema. In aged individuals, the static pressure–volume curve is slightly steeper and is more concave in relation to the pressure axis. However, there is a general agreement that changes in lung compliance with aging are not physiologically significant.

Two forces in the lung parenchyma are responsible for producing the elastic recoil of the lungs. The greatest part of the elastic recoil forces is provided by the surface tension at the curved air–fluid interface of the small airways and alveoli. The second retractive force is that produced when the fibrous skeleton of the lung (primarily the elastic fibers) is stretched.

■ CHANGES IN SURFACE FORCES

Most of the loss in lung recoil with age is likely to be related to the decrease in lung surface area with age The loss of surface area that accompanies aging can be expected to reduce the area of gas–liquid interface, resulting in a decrease in the surface tension forces and, ultimately, a decrease in the total elastic recoil of the lung. Whether it is due to loss of air–liquid interface or to changes in lung structural macromolecules the reduced elastic recoil has important consequences for the function of the intraparenchymal airways and, ultimately, on alveolar gas exchange and forced expiratory flow (see "Pulmonary Function Tests").

■ CHANGES IN STRUCTURAL MACROMOLECULES

Weibel has produced elegant studies of the "integral fiber continuum" that extends from the hila to the pleura. This consists of axial fibers extending to the alveolar septae, and septal fibers extending to the pleura.[17] Although most proteins in the lung turn over relatively rapidly, the structural proteins, elastin and collagen, in the lung fibrous network provide a very stable, long-lived skeletal structure for the lung.

Elastic fibers consist in large part of an extremely hydrophobic, highly cross-linked, and very elastic macromolecule (elastin). These fibers are thought to contribute substantially to lung elasticity. Analysis of whole lungs has revealed that the elastin content actually increases (rather than decreases) with age. More recent evidence indicates that the increase in lung elastin with age is accounted for by an increase in pleural elastin; parenchymal elastin does not change.

Careful studies of the elastic fibers in the lung parenchyma have shown that they are remarkably stable following postnatal lung growth. Certain biochemical changes in very long-lived proteins (change of amino acids into their mirror-image structures, or racemization) provide a type of "biological clock" that permits an estimate of the time that has elapsed since the proteins were synthesized. Because of the constraints of the protein synthetic mechanisms, only L-amino acids are incorporated into newly synthesized proteins. With the passage of years at body temperature, however, there is a readily measurable accumulation of D-aspartic acid. When all of the lung proteins are examined together, minimal D-aspartic acid is found. In purified lung elastin, however, there is an age-related accumulation of D-aspartic acid,[18] indicating that lung elastin is turning over very slowly if at all (Fig. 19-3). It has also been possible to estimate lung elastin turnover by measurement of the incorporation into elastic fibers of carbon 14 (^{14}C) from atmospheric nuclear weapons testing. For example, individuals who completed their postnatal lung growth prior to the nuclear age show no excess ^{14}C in their lung elastin, indicating absence of new elastin synthesis. In contrast, an appropriate excess of ^{14}C is found in the lung elastin of individuals whose lungs were growing in the post–weapons testing era. Modeling of the radiocarbon data indicates that the "mean carbon residence time" in elastin is 74 years.[18]

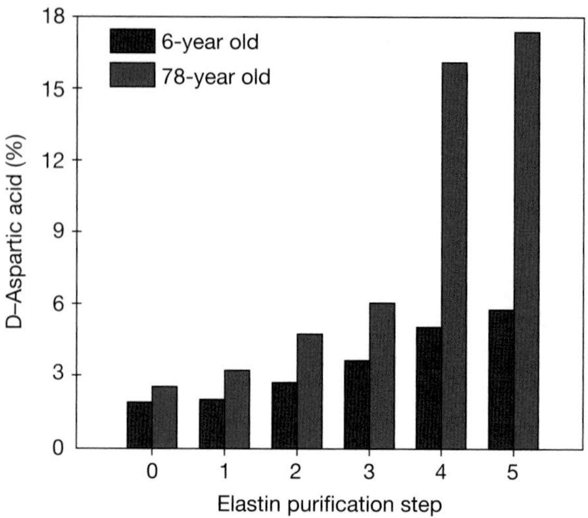

Figure 19-3 Longevity of human lung parenchymal elastin, as evidenced by in vivo racemization of aspartic acid. Each pair of bars shows results from two individuals with greatly differing ages at time of death. Step 0 of elastin purification represents whole lung parenchyma, while step 5 is purified elastin. D-aspartic acid detected in the 6-year-old specimen can be attributed to racemization that occurs during the analytical procedures, whereas, the difference in prevalence of D-aspartic acid between the young and old individual has resulted from racemization in vivo. Note that results from whole-lung hydrolysates (step 0) are similar for both specimens, reflecting their composition of proteins, having predominantly rapid turnover. However, purified elastin from the oldest specimen has racemized extensively in vivo, indicating that it was synthesized many decades before death. These data for elastin agree well with results for other very long–lived proteins. *(Reproduced with permission from Shapiro SD, Endicott SK, Province MA, et al. Marked longevity of human lung parenchymal elastic fibers deduced from prevalence of D-aspartate and nuclear weapons–related radiocarbon. J Clin Invest. 1991;87(5):1828–1834.)*

Taken together, the amino acid racemization and radiocarbon data indicate that lung parenchymal elastin is stable over the human life span, and it appears that the elastin content of the lung parenchyma not only does not change with age, but the individual fibers persist for at least many decades.

Other studies of lung elastic fibers have shown changes in the location and orientation of individual fibers with age as well as changes in the cross-linking of elastin. Thus, some authors have suggested that remodeling of the lung architecture may occur without replacement of elastic fibers. In any case, at the present time, the age-related changes in connective tissue do not provide a sufficient explanation for the decrease in elastic recoil forces observed in the elderly.

Studies of collagen in alveolar walls of humans, as measured by hydroxyproline, have failed to show a consistent change in its quantity during aging.[19] Although human studies have not been done, studies in rodents and birds suggest that lung collagen fibers, like elastic fibers, are very long-lived.[20] Finally, although some qualitative changes in collagen during aging have been described (decreases in solubility and increases in intermolecular cross-links), these appear to have no relationship to changes in lung elastic recoil.

Although convincing evidence for very slow compensatory human lung growth (over many years) has been provided following pneumonectomy,[21] under more ordinary circumstances it appears that the lung adapts to changing dimensions of thorax by realignment of its fibrous skeleton rather than by molecular remodeling.

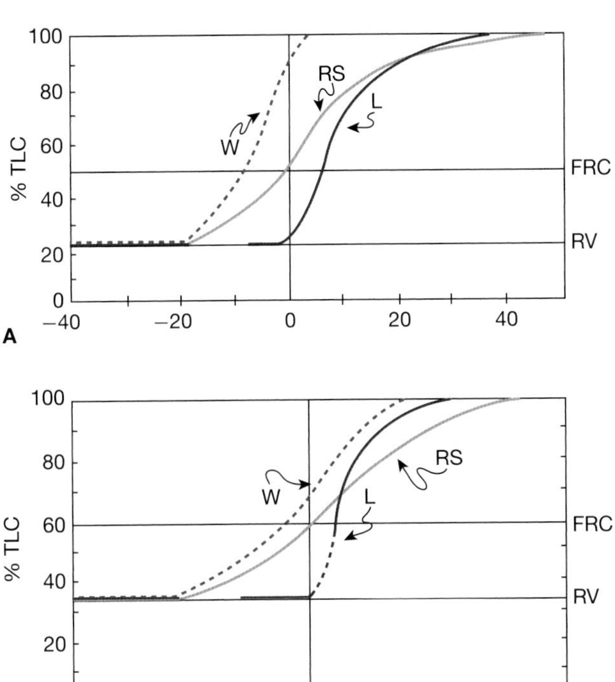

Figure 19-4 Static compliance relationships of the components of the respiratory system. (L, lungs; W, chest wall; RS, total respiratory system.) **A.** A 20-year-old man. **B.** A 60-year-old man. Note that the static compliance of the chest wall is substantially decreased (reduced slope) in the older individual, while functional residual capacity (the resting volume of the respiratory system, or the point at which the pressure gradient across the respiratory system is zero) increases. As in Figure 18-2, it is also apparent that the static recoil pressure of the lungs is reduced in the older subject. *(Data from Mittman C, Edelman NH, Norris AH, et al. Relationship between chest wall and pulmonary compliance and age. J Appl Physiol. 1965;20:1211–1216; and Turner JM, Mead J, Wohl ME. Elasticity of human lungs in relation to age. J Appl Physiol. 1968;25:664–671.)*

■ CHANGES IN CHEST WALL

There is good evidence that the chest wall becomes more rigid with advancing age.[22] As may be seen in Figure 19-4, the static pressure–volume curve of the chest wall is shifted to the right and is less steep with increasing age. The articulations of the ribs with the sternum and the spinal column may become calcified, and the compliance of the rib articulations decreases. The changes in rib articulations may be compounded by the development of kyphosis due to osteoporosis. The decreasing compliance of the chest wall demands greater work from the respiratory muscles. For example, in a 70-year-old person, approximately 70% of the total elastic work of breathing is expended on the chest wall, whereas this value is 40% in a 20-year-old person.

Figure 19-4 also demonstrates that the compliance of the total respiratory system decreases with age because the decrease in lung elastic recoil is outweighed by the changes in the mechanical properties of the chest wall.

CHANGES IN MUSCLES OF RESPIRATION

Age-related changes in nonrespiratory skeletal muscle include decreased work capacity due to alterations in the efficiency of muscle energy, metabolism, atrophy of motor units, and electromyographic abnormalities. Based upon lessons learned with other skeletal muscles, it appeared likely that age-related abnormalities in respiratory muscles also would be found.

An early study by Black and Hyatt appeared to confirm age-related decrements in respiratory muscle function by measuring maximal inspiratory pressure (PI_{max}) and maximal expiratory pressure (PE_{max}) in 120 normal individuals (both smokers and nonsmokers) between the ages of 20 and 70.[23] Maximal respiratory pressures in females were 65% to 70% of those in males. No significant age-related changes were observed in individuals under the age of 55. Trends toward reduced maximal respiratory pressures with age were seen in both genders and with both PI_{max} and PE_{max}. With the number of males studied, the change with age in PI_{max} was not statistically significant for male gender.

More recently, McElvaney and coworkers came to a different conclusion in a similar study of 104 healthy individuals over the age of 55.[24] They found a large variation in maximal respiratory pressures from individual to individual (as by Black and Hyatt), but no significant correlation with age. In contrast, in a third population of 160 healthy individuals who ranged in age from 16 to 75 years, Chen and Kuo found significant gender differences in maximal respiratory pressures as well as trends toward decrements with age for PI_{max} and PE_{max} in both genders. The age-related change in PE_{max} in males was not statistically significant with the sample size studied. When the 40 individuals of both genders in the youngest age group (16–30 years) were compared with the 40 individuals in the oldest group (61–75 years), the decrement in PI_{max} was 32% to 36%, while the decrement in PE_{max} was 13% to 23%.[25] Representative findings for maximal respiratory pressures in women are illustrated in Figure 19-5.

Chen and Kuo also measured inspiratory muscle endurance against a resistive load, and found significant decrements with age. Physically active men had greater inspiratory muscle endurance than sedentary men.

In summary, it appears that when populations of healthy individuals of widely differing ages are studied, moderate age-related decrements in respiratory muscle strength and endurance can be

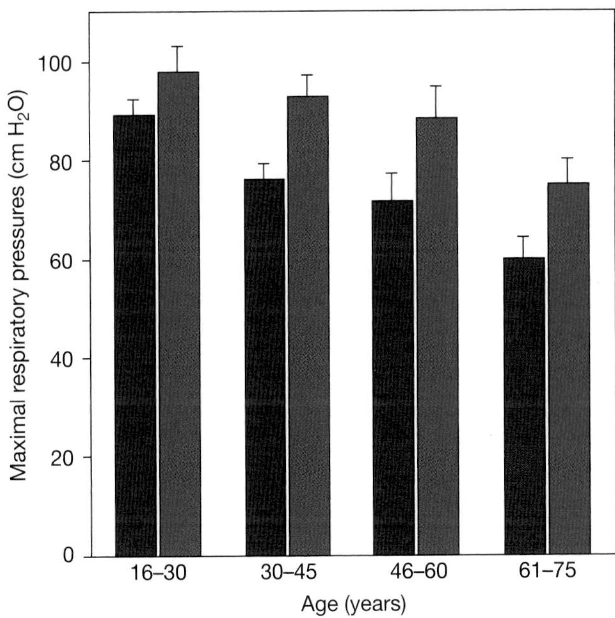

Figure 19-5 Representative variations in maximal respiratory pressures with age among women. Inspiratory and expiratory measurements were made at residual volume and total lung capacity, respectively. Maximal inspiratory pressure *(open bars)* and maximal expiratory pressure *(hatched bars)*. Error bars are standard errors of the mean. Although quantitatively moderate, variations with age were statistically significant for both measurements. *(Data from Chen H-S, Kuo C-S. Relationship between respiratory muscle function and age, sex, and other factors. J Appl Physiol. 1989;66(2):943–948.)*

found. These studies usually define *healthy* only by the absence of disease and do not control for physical activity. They are complicated by marked interindividual variability, and longitudinal studies have not been reported. Continuous respiratory muscle activity may have a training effect that leads to better preservation of respiratory muscle function when compared with other skeletal muscles. Finally, physical activity may have an additional training effect that enhances inspiratory muscle endurance in all age groups.

CONTROL OF BREATHING

In young individuals, minute ventilation is matched with metabolic demands. As a result, arterial blood gas values remain stable throughout a wide range of activities from rest to strenuous exertion, while oxygen consumption and carbon dioxide production are varying widely. Similarly, when the efficiency of gas exchange is diminished by lung disease or congestive heart failure, appropriate increases in minute ventilation minimize the resulting hypercapnia and/or hypoxemia in healthy young individuals. The ventilatory control system is described in detail in Chapter 11.

Ventilatory control mechanisms are typically tested by stressing the respiratory system, by inducing either hypoxemia or hypercapnia while monitoring ventilatory parameters (and often cardiac parameters as well). Such tests have shown striking differences between young and elderly individuals in both ventilatory and cardiac responses.

DIMINISHED VENTILATORY RESPONSE TO HYPERCAPNIA

Kronenberg and Drage compared the ventilatory responses to hypercapnia in eight young (mean age, 25.6 years) and eight elderly (mean age, 69.6 years) individuals.[26] During the tests, the subjects were asked to rebreathe 5% CO_2, while their PA_{O_2} was held above 200 mm Hg by supplemental oxygen to eliminate hypoxic ventilatory drive. Measurements were made while PA_{C_2} was allowed to rise to 65 mm Hg. Although there was considerable individual variation and some overlap between the groups, the elderly individuals had a significantly diminished ventilatory response to hypercapnia, measured as the slope of the relationship between ventilation and PA_{C_2}.

DIMINISHED VENTILATORY RESPONSE TO HYPOXIA

When Kronenberg and Drage measured the ventilatory response to hypoxia at constant CO_2, they found even more striking differences between the young and elderly subjects (Fig. 19-6). For example, the ventilatory response to a PA_{O_2} of 40 mm Hg was uniformly smaller in the older subjects, and there was no overlapping between the groups.[26] The mean minute ventilation at a PA_{O_2} of 40 mm Hg was 40.1 and 10.2 L/min in the young and old groups, respectively.

DIMINISHED OCCLUSION PRESSURE RESPONSES

Peterson et al. confirmed the previously discussed observations and have shown that the differences in responses of elderly subjects to both hypercapnia and hypoxia are due to a lesser increase in tidal volume while the ventilatory rate increases normally. Since this observation could be caused by differences in respiratory muscle strength or increases in chest wall stiffness, the authors also measured airway occlusion pressures, which are valuable indices of respiratory drive that are not affected by respiratory muscle strength or respiratory mechanics.[27] The measurement (P_{100}) is the negative pressure at the mouth, measured 100 ms after the start of inspiration against an occluded airway. The occlusion pressure responses to both hypoxia and hypercapnia (Fig. 19-7) were significantly reduced in the 10 elderly subjects studied by Peterson (mean age, 73.3 years) when compared to nine young control subjects (mean age, 24.4 years). Although the elderly individuals had reduced respiratory muscle strength (mean, 24% lower maximal static inspiratory pressure), the differences in occlusion pressure persisted when normalized for these differences.

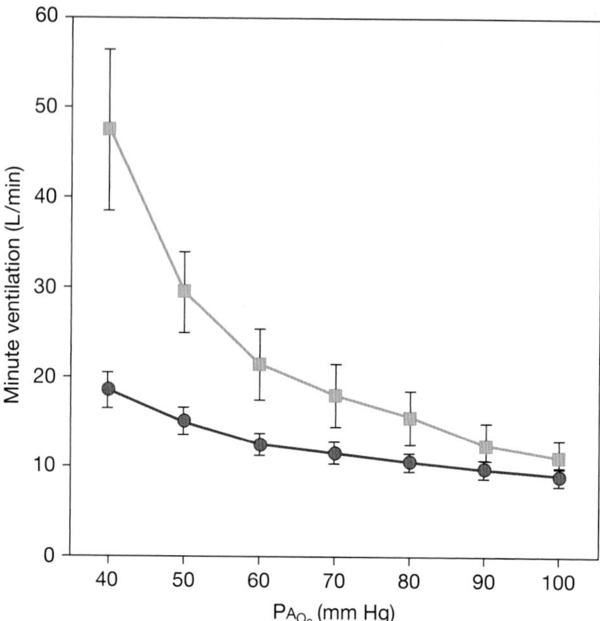

Figure 19-6 Variations with age in ventilatory responses to hypoxia. Eight normal men aged 64 to 73 *(circles)* and eight controls aged 22 to 30 *(squares)* were subjected to isocapnic progressive hypoxia by a rebreathing method. Data values are means, with standard errors of the mean shown by the error bars. Note that the ventilatory responses differ strikingly between the elderly individuals and the controls. *(Reproduced with permission from Kronenberg RS, Drage CW. Attenuation of the ventilatory and heart rate responses to hypoxia and hypercapnia with aging in normal men. J Clin Invest. 1973;52(8):1812–1819.)*

The previously mentioned seminal studies of ventilatory control have been discussed in some detail out of respect for their groundbreaking conceptual importance. Subsequent studies have created some confusion that appears likely to be due to methodologic differences, ages of subjects, and small sample sizes. However, in 14 of 16

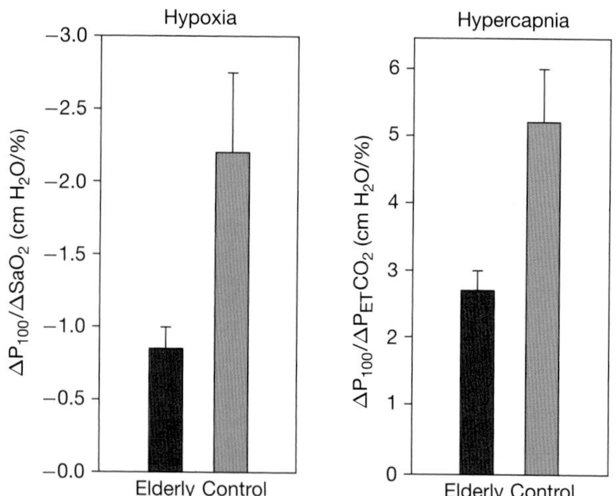

Figure 19-7 Variations with age in occlusion pressure responses to hypoxia and hypercapnia. Data shown are slopes of relationships between occlusion pressure responses and either Sa_{O_2} or end-tidal P_{CO_2}; error bars are standard errors of the mean. Elderly individuals had significantly diminished occlusion pressures in response to both hypoxia and hypercapnia. Both differences were significant, with $p < 0.01$. *(Reproduced with permission from Peterson DD, Pack AI, Silage DA, et al. Effects of aging on the ventilatory and occlusion pressure responses to hypoxia and hypercapnia. Am Rev Respir Dis. 1981;124(4):387–391.)*

studies reviewed by Lalley, ventilatory responses in the elderly were found to be abnormal.[28]

In summary, the reduced responsiveness in tidal volume to either hypoxemia or hypercapnia with age is apparently due to a reduced responsiveness of ventilatory drive or neural output from the respiratory center. It has not been determined whether the diminished ventilatory drive results from altered chemoreceptor function or from altered function of the respiratory center. Kronenberg and Drage favored altered receptor function based on their observation that elderly subjects responded to an alveolar oxygen tension of 40 torr with only an 11% increase in heart rate, whereas the young subjects responded with a 34% increase.

RESPIRATORY LOAD COMPENSATION AND DYSPNEA

Reflex compensation for a change in respiratory mechanical load (as in lung disease, changes in posture, and mouth versus nose breathing) normally serves to maintain ventilation constant during the change. Akiyama et al. measured responses to inspiratory flow-resistive loading in young and elderly individuals and found significant differences.[29] In the young control group, inspiratory loading resulted in an increase in P_{100} at each level of induced hypercapnia, such that inspiratory loading did not change the ventilatory response to hypercapnia when compared with unloaded responses. In marked contrast, the P_{100} in the elderly group did not change when an inspiratory load was applied. In the absence of a compensatory change in ventilatory drive, ventilatory responses to hypercapnia were reduced during inspiratory loading in the elderly group.

At each level of P_{CO_2}, the intensity of perceived dyspnea in response to inspiratory loading was greater in the elderly than in the control group. Thus, the sensation of dyspnea was intact or enhanced in the elderly subjects, while their compensatory responses were reduced. This suggests the possibility that, elderly individuals may complain of a greater dyspnea than younger individuals with similar pathophysiologic deterioration.

SENSITIVITY TO RESPIRATORY DEPRESSION BY OPIOIDS AND SEDATIVES

Older individuals are substantially more sensitive to respiratory depression by opioids and sedatives. This phenomenon demands extra vigilance when these medications are prescribed in nonintubated elderly patients. The enhanced drug effect has been shown to be multifactorial, and the various mechanisms involved are beyond the scope of this chapter.[30–32] However, the dangers associated with higher levels and more prolonged effects of these drugs are real and potentially catastrophic.

PULMONARY CIRCULATION

Invasive physiologic studies of pulmonary artery catheterization have typically been biased by including only subsets of patients whose signs and symptoms led to referral for heart catheterization and who, therefore, may not be representative of a "healthy" cohort. Further, age-related changes in the pulmonary circulation are difficult or impossible to separate from changes due to heart disease or age-related changes in cardiac function.

Ehrsam et al. reported a retrospective analysis of right heart catheterization studies performed in 125 asymptomatic subjects who ranged from 14 to 68 years of age.[33] Small increases in right atrial, pulmonary artery, and pulmonary artery wedge pressures observed in the highest age group disappeared when values were adjusted for sex, weight, and height. No significant age-related changes were found in cardiac output, stroke volume, or oxygen uptake. Age explained 10% or less of the total variation in the hemodynamic and pressure variables when assessed by multiple regressions. During supine exercise with a bicycle ergometer, however, pulmonary artery and wedge pressures increased with age, particularly in subjects over the age of 45. The changes were highly significant with age accounting for 12% to 30% of the total variation when assessed by multiple regressions. Finally, pulmonary artery resistance showed a highly significant increase with age, whether measured at rest or during exercise, with age contributing 12% to 27% to the total variation in pulmonary artery resistance. Although the cohort studied were all asymptomatic and ambulatory, it is possible that silent coronary artery disease was present in some of the subjects, and the prevalence of coronary artery disease can be expected to increase with age. Moreover, younger patients tended to be referred for evaluation of a heart murmur, whereas the older patients were referred for "pulmonary investigation" that included coin lesions, hilar lymphadenopathy, "previous pulmonary infiltrates," and smoke inhalation. Cigarette smoking history was not discussed. Thus, it is not certain that the younger and older patients were strictly comparable.

More recently, Davidson and Fee reported the results of right-heart catheterization at rest in 47 normal subjects who were free of coronary disease and had normal left ventricular systolic function.[34] Smokers were included. The investigators found highly significant but quantitatively modest age-related increases in mean pulmonary artery pressure, pulmonary vascular resistance, and pulmonary/systemic vascular resistance ratio, but they found no age-related differences in pulmonary artery wedge pressure. The authors felt that the most likely explanation for the age-related changes in pulmonary artery pressure and pulmonary vascular resistance was a primary abnormality of the pulmonary vascular bed, but they could not exclude the effects of subtle abnormalities in left ventricular function.

In summary, studies of pulmonary hemodynamics with aging are limited by retrospective design, bias in patient selection, and potential effects of smoking. Minor increases in pulmonary vascular resistance and age-related increases in pulmonary artery wedge pressure during exercise have been reported. These age-related changes may not be physiologically significant.

PULMONARY FUNCTION TESTS

Lung function and exercise capacity decline with age in concert with numerous other physiologic, morphologic, and biochemical changes. Descriptions of "normal" age-related changes are confounded by an increasing prevalence of disease, chronic illness, medication use, and an increasingly sedentary lifestyle. Further, chronologic age only approximates physiologic age; the two often differ significantly. Chronologic age is, therefore, an imperfect measure for indexing changes with senescence. While it would be desirable to isolate the effects of biologic aging (aging in the absence of disease), it is essentially impossible to do so. The best studies to do so are longitudinal, tracing change with time, because they avoid the obvious biases of cross-sectional studies. Longitudinal studies, however, have methodologic problems and biases of their own, the most obvious being that the healthy elderly represent a healthy survival population. If, as a group, they have better than average lung function, they would not represent the general population of elderly people well.

LUNG VOLUMES

Figure 19-8 illustrates typical lung volume changes with aging based on cross-sectional studies. With the exception of vital capacity, the effect of aging on lung volumes is based on cross-sectional rather than longitudinal data because there are almost no longitudinal studies of static lung volumes. Total lung capacity (TLC), the volume of air in the lungs at the end of a maximal inspiration, is marked by the point at which the recoil pressure exerted by the respiratory system is exactly counterbalanced by the maximal inspiratory pressure generated by the respiratory muscles. Since both the compliance of respiratory system (lung and chest wall combined) and maximum inspiratory pressure fall with aging, TLC might also be expected to fall. However, in seven cross-sectional studies of TLC summarized

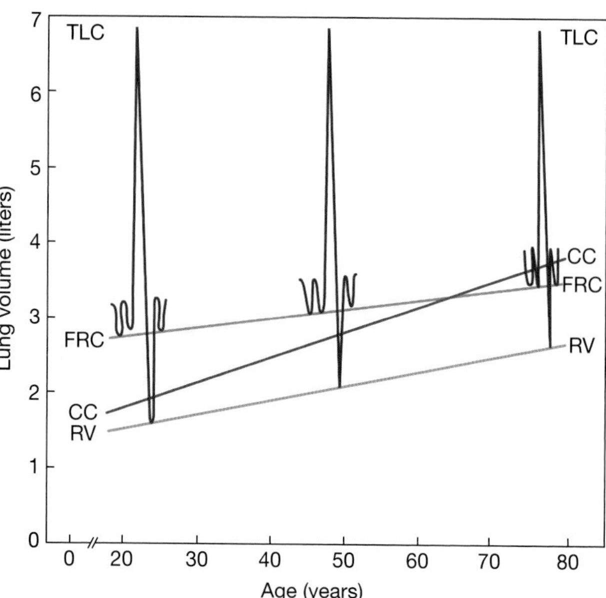

Figure 19-8 Schematic illustration of lung volume changes with age based on cross-sectional studies in seated individuals. (TLC, total lung capacity; FRC, functional residual capacity; RV, residual volume; CC, closing capacity.) Although not labeled, vital capacity (VC) is TLC minus RV. The most consistent changes are an increase in RV and a decrease in VC. *(Reproduced with permission from Peterson DD, Fish-man AP. Aging of the respiratory system, in Fishman AP (ed). Update: Pulmonary Diseases and Disorders. New York, McGraw-Hill, 1992, pp 1–17.)*

by the European Coal and Steel Community, four of the studies in men and three of those in women did not find a significant age coefficient.[35] The remaining studies found only small declines in TLC with age, on the order of −8 to −19 mL/yr. When these study results were combined into average equations, no significant age coefficients were reported for either men or women. McClaran et al. measured lung volumes twice in 18 healthy, fit men.[36] The first measurement was at a mean age of 67 and the second was 6 years later. Although average TLC fell 25 mL/yr, the change was not statistically significant. The study was small and the interval was short.

In summary, current cross-sectional studies suggest that TLC either does not decline with age or declines very slowly. It is interesting to speculate on the possibility that cross-sectional studies of TLC might be confounded because they typically index TLC to both age and height. Height declines with aging, and maximum height during a life span appears to increase with successive generations. The author believes that longitudinal studies of TLC with age are likely to show small but significant declines with age.

Both slow and forced vital capacity (FVC) decline with age, more rapidly in men than women. Average decrements in vital capacity per year vary considerably; in cross-sectional studies, declines range from 21 to 33 mL/yr in men and 18 to 29 mL/yr in women. Theoretically, longitudinal studies should provide better estimates of the effect of aging on lung function. Ware et al., in a study containing both longitudinal and cross-sectional computations, found cross-sectional falls in FVC for men and women to be −34 and −27.8 mL/yr, respectively.[37] The longitudinal estimates were −40 mL and −31.3 mL/yr, respectively. This study contradicts the generally held concept that longitudinal studies show smaller declines in FVC than cross-sectional studies. Currently, it is not certain whether longitudinal studies are all that much different from cross-sectional studies in describing declines in FVC and forced expiratory volume in 1s (FEV_1). Longitudinal studies tend to show an acceleration in the rate of loss in FVC and FEV_1 as age advances.

Cross-sectional studies of residual volume (RV) and the RV/TLC ratio consistently show increases with age. In the young, RV, the volume of air in the lungs at the end of a maximal expiration, is the volume at which the outward static recoil pressure of the respiratory system is counterbalanced by the maximal pressure exerted by the expiratory muscles. In older subjects, expiratory flow never completely reaches zero and the determination of RV is made partly by the length of time an individual can maintain expiratory effort.[38] Other factors leading to an increased RV with aging include loss of lung recoil, decreased chest wall compliance, decreased expiratory muscle force, and increased small airway closure (air trapping) in dependent lung zones. Time of exhalation and increase in air trapping are probably more important than changes in lung and chest wall compliance in explaining the increase in RV with aging.

FRC is also determined by the balance of the elastic recoil forces of the lung and chest wall; but, in this instance, the equilibrium occurs at the end of a quiet (unforced) exhalation. Since lung recoil falls and the chest wall stiffens with age, one would expect FRC to increase. Cross-sectional studies, however, show inconsistent results, with most showing no change in FRC with aging. Studies that find an increase in FRC with aging show a small positive age coefficient on the order of 7 to 16 mL/yr. McClaran's longitudinal study found FRC to increase 40 mL/yr, but again, the change was not significant.[36] Despite the conflicting data, it is generally believed that FRC increases with aging.

Loss of lung recoil also changes the volume at which airway closure occurs. When adults exhale fully, small airways close in the region of the terminal bronchioles in dependent lung zones. The lung volume at which this closure begins is measured as closing volume or, if it is added to RV, closing capacity. Closing volume increases linearly with age from about 5% to 10% of TLC at age 20 to about 30% of TLC at age 70.[39] The loss of lung elastic recoil, a possible decrease in the recoil of the intrapulmonic airways, and decreases in small airway diameter probably explain most of the changes in CV.

Closing volume encroaches on tidal volume by about age 44 when subjects are supine and about age 65 when they are seated (Fig. 19-8). Airway closure during tidal breathing explains most of the decrease in arterial oxygen tension (PA_{O_2}) observed with aging[40,41] and may contribute to an aging-related increased frequency dependency of compliance.

AIRFLOW

While essentially all expiratory flows measured during a maximum expiratory maneuver decrease with age, the declines are most evident at lower lung volumes (Fig. 19-9). Nunn and Gregg, in a study of 225 male and 228 healthy female nonsmokers,[42] reported a modest, nonlinear decrease in peak expiratory flow (PEF) with aging (Fig. 19-10), which reached a high point at age 30 to 35; a decline became evident at about age 45. After age 50, the average decline was about 4 L/min per year in men, about 2.5 L/min per year in women.

Figure 19-11, from Paoletti et al.,[43] illustrates changes in FEV_1 during growth, maturation, and senescence. Changes in FVC are similar. In one model of aging, FVC and FEV_1 increase progressively during the growth phase until about age 12. In the maturation phase (during adolescence), there is an acceleration of these increases. Increases in FVC and FEV_1 are seen up to about 20 years in women and about 25 years in men; increases in lung volumes occur even after somatic growth ceases. There appears to be a plateau phase where there is little or no change in FVC or FEV_1 prior to the onset of a decline. However, Robbins et al. demonstrated that, while the plateau correctly represents average data, lung function is often increasing or decreasing in individuals (Fig. 19-12). Their study confirms the suspicion that the "plateau" phase represents the merging of slower maturation-related increases in FVC and FEV_1 in some subjects, with subtle decreases in others.[44] In the decline phase, there appears to be acceleration in the rate of loss of FVC and FEV_1 as age progresses.

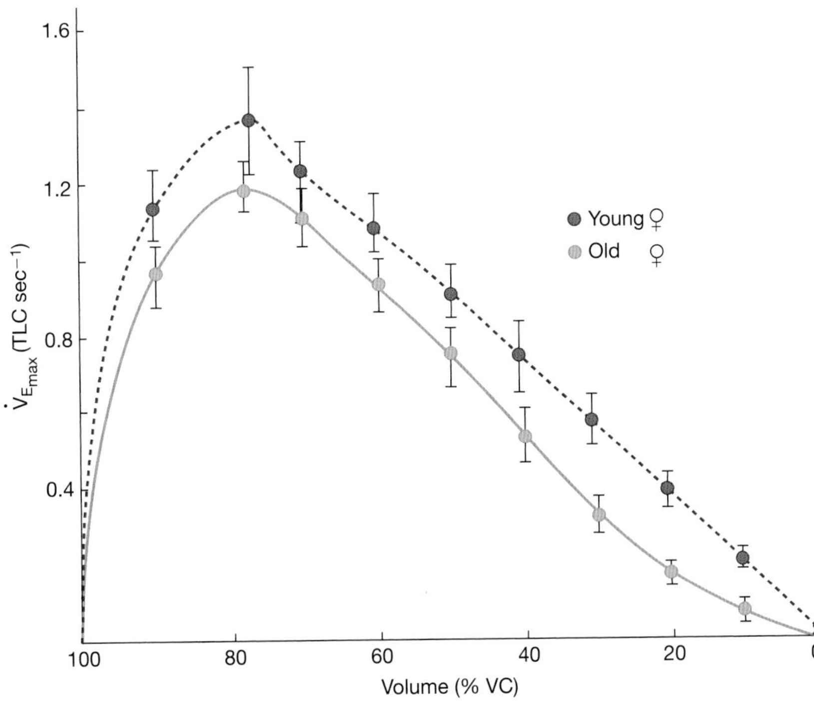

Figure 19-9 Illustrative maximal flow–volume curves for healthy "elderly" women (mean age, 63 years) and healthy young women (mean age, 25 years). Although all flows tend to be reduced with aging, the reduction in flow is most evident at lower lung volumes, where the flow–volume curve is clearly concave to the volume axis. *(Reproduced with permission from Peterson DD, Fish-man AP. Aging of the respiratory system, in Fishman AP (ed). Update: Pulmonary Diseases and Disorders. New York, McGraw-Hill; 1992:1–18.)*

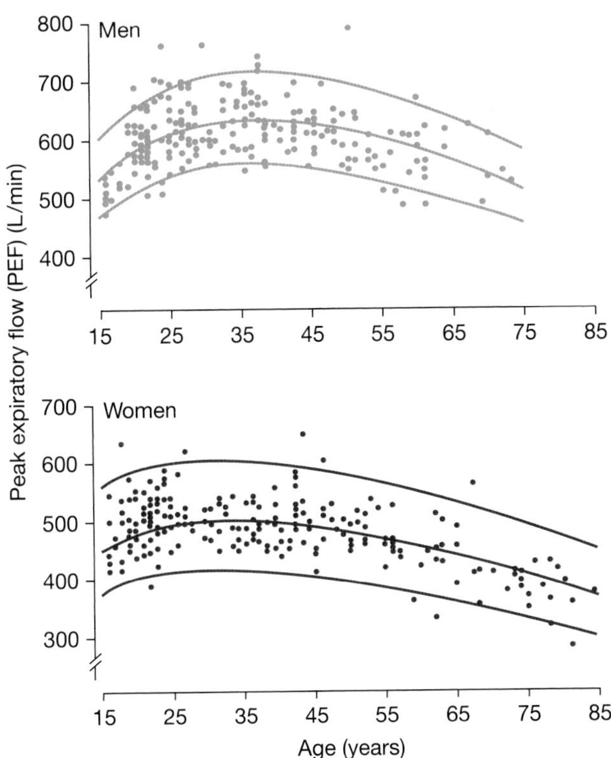

Figure 19-10 Changes in peak expiratory flow in 225 males and 228 females who were healthy nonsmokers. The *center line* is a regression curve representing mean data and the boundaries are 90% confidence intervals. *(Reproduced with permission from Nunn AJ, Gregg I. New regression equations for predicting peak expiratory flow in adults. Br Med J. 1989;298(6680):1068–1070.)*

An accelerated rate loss at older ages is, however, not found in all studies. The rate of decline in FVC and FEV_1 with age tends to be greater: (1) in men; (2) in taller individuals; (3) in individuals with larger baseline values; and (4) in individuals with increased airway reactivity.

AIRWAYS RESISTANCE

Total airway resistance measured at FRC does not change with aging. Since upper airways increase and smaller airways decrease in size with aging, it is likely that peripheral airway resistance increases and central airway resistance decreases. That total airway resistance does not change with aging may be a function of the counterbalancing of these two opposite changes. However, since about 90% of total airway resistance resides in the upper airways, significant changes in peripheral airway resistance might not be readily reflected in total airway resistance. Significant increases in peripheral airway resistance with age also would be consistent with the more dramatic decreases in maximum flow observed at low lung volumes.

GAS EXCHANGE

The carbon monoxide diffusing capacity (DL_{CO}), also known as transfer factor (TL_{CO}), declines with age. Earlier cross-sectional studies report a linear decline in DL_{CO} of about −0.2 mL CO/min per mm Hg per year for men and −0.15 mL CO/min per mm Hg per year for women. These declines are roughly 0.5% per year. In a large representative sample of US adult men, Neas and Schwartz found an almost linear fall in DL_{CO}.[45] In women, however, they found a nonlinear, quadratic decline in DL_{CO} with age. After age 47, the nonlinear component was not significant and the decline in DL_{CO} was identical to that in the earlier studies. The decline in DL_{CO} with age did not vary with race.

The decline in DL_{CO} with age is not explained by increased nonhomogeneity of gas distribution. Measured DL_{CO} falls as alveolar P_{O_2} increases, and venous hemoglobin concentration falls. Neither alveolar P_{O_2} nor hemoglobin concentration varies enough with age to explain the aging decline in DL_{CO}. The magnitude of the decline in DL_{CO} corresponds fairly well to the magnitude of the known aging-related decrease in the internal surface area of the lung.

The components of DL_{CO} are membrane diffusing capacity (Dm) and pulmonary capillary blood volume (Vc). Both Dm and Vc decrease with age. In a cross-sectional reference value study of 54 male and 36 female healthy nonsmokers, the decline in Dm and Vc with age were found to be linear.[46] Membrane diffusing capacity fell at about 0.6% per year in both men and women. Pulmonary capillary blood volume fell at about 0.3% per year.

Although alveolar oxygen pressure (PA_{O_2}) remains constant with age, arterial P_{O_2} (Pa_{O_2}) decreases and the alveolar–arterial oxygen tension gradient ($PA - a_{O_2}$ increases with aging (Fig. 19-13).[47] The decline in Pa_{O_2} with aging is more pronounced when subjects are studied in a recumbent as contrasted with an upright position. The most likely explanation for the decline in Pa_{O_2} with aging is increased mismatching of ventilation to blood flow ($\dot{V}E/\dot{Q}$) as airway closure begins to occur during tidal breathing. Increased ($\dot{V}E/\dot{Q}$) mismatching with aging is also associated with an increase in physiologic dead space.[48,49] Hypoventilation does not contribute to the age-related fall in Pa_{O_2}, since Pa_{CO_2} and pH do not change with age (Fig. 19-13).

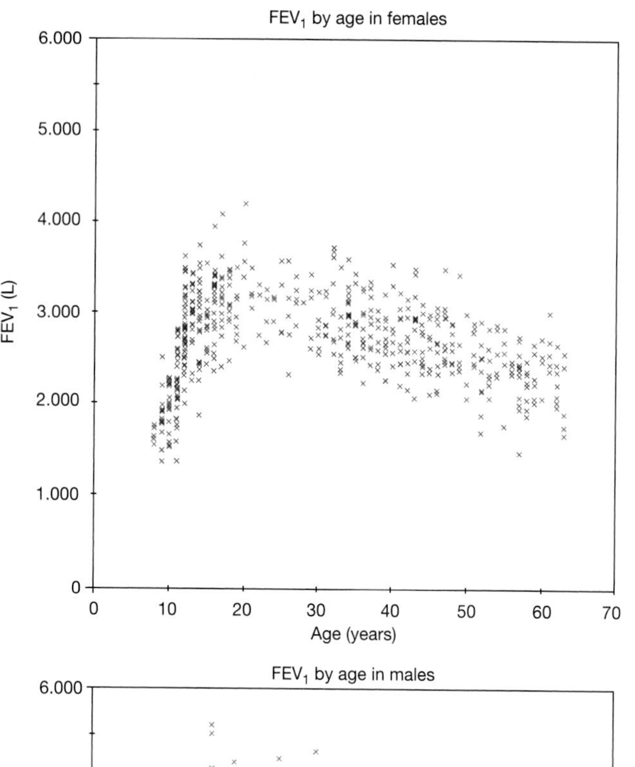

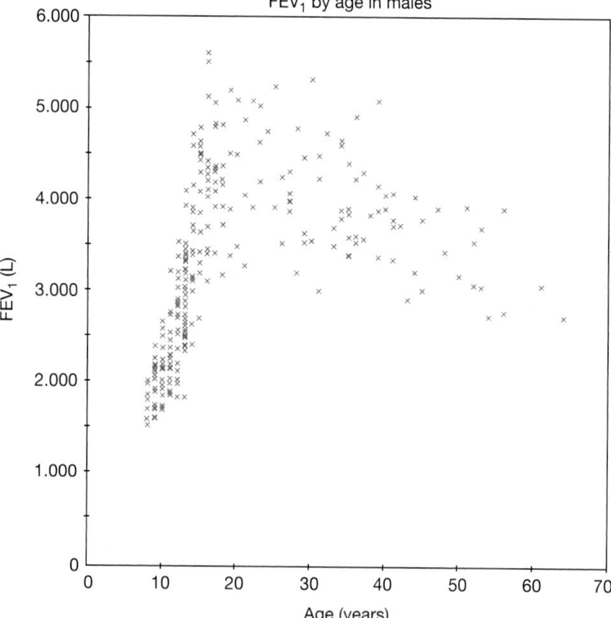

Figure 19-11 Change in FEV_1 with age from a cross-sectional study of 538 females and 263 males selected as "normal" from a larger study of 3289 subjects. Changes in FVC are similar. *(Reproduced with permission from Paoletti P, Pistelli G, Fazzi P, et al. Reference values for vital capacity and flow-volume curves from a general population study. Bull Eur Physiopathol Respir. 1986;22(5):451–459.)*

EXERCISE CAPACITY

Peak $\dot{V}_{O_2}$ ($\dot{V}_{O_2peak}$) and maximum work capacity decrease with aging in both sedentary and active individuals.[50] $\dot{V}_{O_2peak}$ (L/min) increases until about age 20. Declines are evident at about age 25 in both men and women and continue at about 1% per year (Fig. 19-14). If one expresses $\dot{V}_{O_2peak}$ as a function of body weight (L/kg per min), the decline is evident much earlier, perhaps in the first decade of life. The magnitude of the decline in $\dot{V}_{O_2peak}$ tends to be greater in longitudinal than in cross-sectional studies and occurs roughly twice as fast in sedentary than in physically active persons. Most, but not all, studies report linear declines in $\dot{V}_{O_2peak}$ with age, even though a nonlinear decline would be expected based on the number and type of variables that affect exercise capacity.

The decline in exercise capacity with age occurs as a result of normal aging but is accelerated by lifestyle issues. Aging is associated with significant changes in body configuration. Specifically, there is an increase in total body weight, primarily representing an increase in fat mass, since fat-free mass (mostly muscle mass) decreases with aging. The changes are most pronounced in sedentary persons. Muscle mass decreases, with a preferential atrophy of type II muscle fibers, and is associated with a decrease in muscle capillarization and oxidative activity. Muscle strength decreases on the order of 2%/yr from ages 20 to 70. Variables associated with loss of exercise capacity with aging are listed in Table 19-2.

While exercise capacity declines with aging, it is also clear that the ability to respond to exercise conditioning is well maintained even at very advanced ages. Elderly individuals respond to both endurance and resistive training with improvements similar in magnitude to those seen in the young.[50–52] There are equivalent increases in $\dot{V}_{O_2\,peak}$, muscle mass, capillarization of muscle tissue, muscle oxidative activity, and general muscle strength.

LUNG AND AIRWAY INFLAMMATION

In recent years, there has been considerable interest in the presence and control of lung inflammation in elderly individuals, and this has become a confusing subject. A variety of quantitative abnormalities in mediators of inflammation have been described in elderly individuals that have mostly been in the direction of increased lung parenchymal and airway inflammation. However, these differences from younger subjects must be viewed in the context that elderly individuals have impaired cough, increased evidence of gastroesophageal reflux, and decreased effectiveness of the ciliary escalator. All of these abnormalities can be expected to lead to an increased load of particulates and microorganisms in the lower respiratory tract, and/or recurrent episodes of aspiration. As a striking example of studies of airway inflammation, the mean quantity and percentage of neutrophils in broncho-alveolar lavage fluid have been found to be increased in elderly individuals, but many of the studied elderly subjects were indistinguishable from young normals.[53] The increased mean values in the elderly were strongly influenced by outlying high values in a subpopulation, and thus presumably did not result from a direct effect of aging.

SLEEP

Sleep complaints from elderly patients present a difficult problem for the clinician, who must determine whether the complaints are related to the normal aging process, sleep hygiene issues, or the presence of pathology.[54,55] Problems with sleep are widespread among elderly persons, with 25% to 40% complaining about sleep difficulties. There is no evidence to confirm the widely held belief that the need for sleep declines with age. However, sleep quality decreases, and the frequency of various primary sleep disorders increases. The most common age-related change in sleep pattern is a striking increase in the number of nocturnal awakenings, resulting in lower total sleep time and lower sleep efficiency (total sleep time/time in bed). Whether or not sleep latency changes with aging is equivocal. The amount of time spent in stage 1 nonrapid eye movement (NREM or light) sleep tends to increase with age. The decrease in total sleep time at night is associated with an increase in unwanted daytime naps. Disrupted sleep in the elderly is, in large part, explained by medical and psychological issues and the lack of structured physical and social activity during the day. Chronic illnesses, nocturia, medication and alcohol use, periodic leg movements, bereavement, and depression also play a role. Not surprisingly, the elderly are more likely to use sedatives or hypnotics; their use is more frequent in elderly women than in elderly men. While

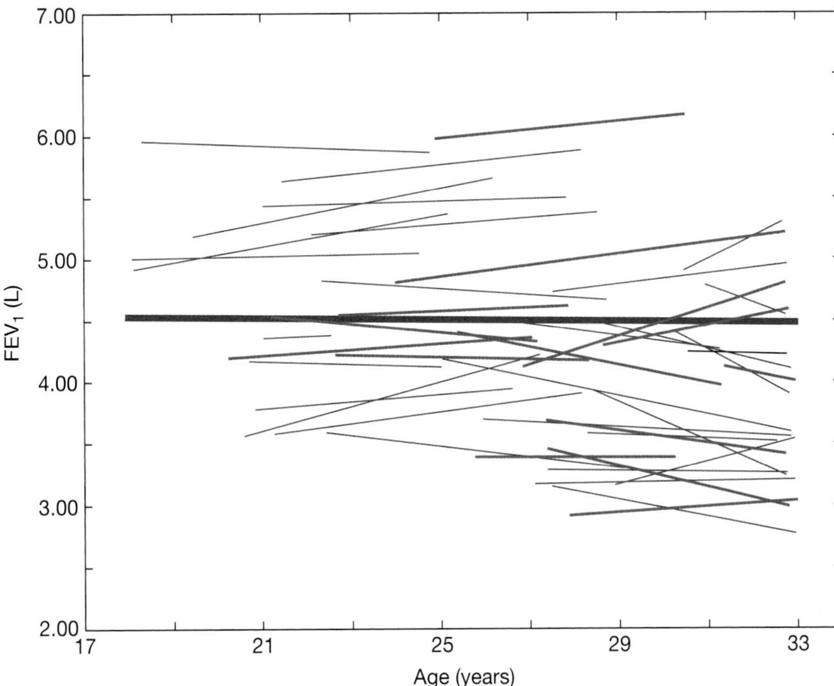

Figure 19-12 Predicted FEV_1 trajectories from 44 men based on linear regressions of longitudinal data. Nonsmokers *(fine lines)* and smokers *(dashed lines)*. The heavy line is based on the entire group's data. While the group's data show no change with age, data for individuals show both increases and declines with age during this time period, when a plateau in lung function was theorized to occur. *(Reproduced with permission from Robbins DR, Enright PL, Sherrill DL. Lung function development in young adults: Is there a plateau phase? Eur Respir J. 1995;8(5):768–772.)*

hypnotics and sedatives are occasionally necessary, their chronic use may contribute to sleep disruption and aggravate certain sleep disturbances, such as sleep apnea. Increased autonomic activity, increased sensitivity to external stimuli (which may increase arousals as a result of environmental factors), decreased exposure to outdoor light, inactivity, and daytime napping also play a role in sleep disruptions in the elderly. Alterations in endogenous circadian rhythms for variables like temperature and cortisol or thyroid-stimulating hormone (TSH) levels may also contribute to sleep disruption in the elderly.

The neural system that regulates sleep is, like most other systems, subject to the aging process, and sleep disruption occurs in the elderly in the absence of any pathologic process. The amount of stages 3 and 4 sleep (slow- or delta-wave sleep) declines with aging, although some argue that the aging decline is mostly a technical issue related to how delta-wave amplitude is defined. Changes in slow-wave sleep appear to be evident early, perhaps by 20 years of age. Arguments have been made both for and against declines in the amount of REM sleep with age. The persistent controversy about REM sleep and aging suggests that if REM sleep does change with aging, the magnitude of decline is so small that it does not overwhelm the confounding factors in studies.

Sleep disorders such as sleep apnea and restless limb syndrome, with periodic limb movements, appear to be more prevalent in older persons, and they are also marked more among nursing home residents than the independent elderly. For example, using an apnea index of five per hour as a threshold, one study found evidence of sleep apnea in 42% of elderly nursing home residents, in contrast to 24% of the independent elderly. A community-based study of individuals aged 71 to 87, showed a 55% prevalence of sleep-disordered breathing that was documented by polysomnography, including 38% obstructive sleep apnea and 17% central sleep apnea.[56] However, longitudinal follow-up of these individuals did not show an independent correlation with either cardiovascular disease or mortality.

INTERPRETING PULMONARY FUNCTION TESTS IN THE ELDERLY

Several issues complicate the interpretation of lung function tests in the elderly, as reviewed by Vaz Fragoso and Gill.[57] The elderly are not well represented in most reference value reports; the number of subjects usually falls off significantly after age 60. The number of

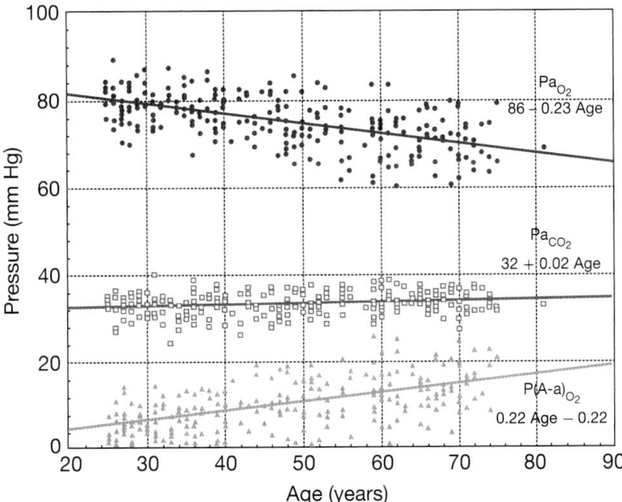

Figure 19-13 Change in Pa_{O_2}, Pa_{CO_2} and A-a gradient $P(A-a)_{O_2}$ with age. Data were obtained from 200 healthy men and women living in Salt Lake City, UT (altitude = 1400 m). Sea-level data would be similar, with a small upward shift in Pa_{O_2} and Pa_{CO_2}.

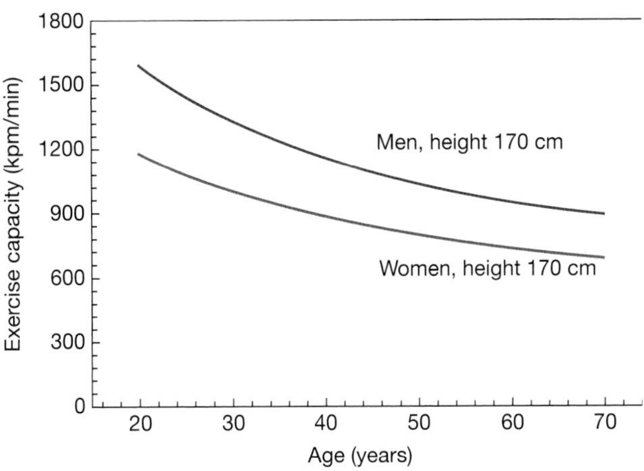

Figure 19-14 Decline in maximum exercise capacity with age. Exercise capacity declines nonlinearly with age. Maximum work capacity correlates strongly with peak oxygen uptake. *(Reproduced with permission from Jones NL, Summers E, Killian KG. Influence of age and stature on exercise capacity during incremental cycle ergometry in men and women. Am Rev Respir Dis. 1989;140(5):1373–1380.)*

TABLE 19-2 Variables Associated with a Decline in Exercise Capacity with Age

Variable	Comment
Decreased muscle mass	These changes especially affect $\dot{V}_{O_2}$ calculated per kg of body weight
Increased fat mass	
Decreased tissue oxygen delivery Decreased maximal heart rate Decreased stroke volume Decreased maximal $C(a - \bar{v})_{O_2}$ difference	As a result of the decreased cardiac output and maximal $C(a - \bar{v})_{O_2}$, delivery and extraction are reduced; decreased cardiac output is a major contributor to the age-related decline in exercise capacity
Maximum voluntary ventilation	
Increased ventilation at each workload	At each workload, older individuals breathe more and work harder for each breath than younger persons; however, the effect is small and contributes little to the decline in exercise capacity with aging
Increased oxygen cost of breathing	
Sedentary lifestyle	Lifestyle issues play a large role in the rate at which exercise capacity is lost with age; the good news is that, like other deconditioned groups, the elderly respond very well to exercise training
Decreased training intensity in active persons	
Decreased willingness to work to maximal level during tests	

subjects over age 80 is usually so small that mean values calculated from regression equations are essentially an extrapolation of the data for younger persons. This means that the average or "predicted" value may not be as representative for the elderly as it is for middle-aged persons. The fall in sample size with aging likely reflects the reduced total number of candidates for participation and the larger number of individuals who fail screening criteria. In reference value studies, individuals are screened so as to be free of symptoms and illnesses that alter lung function. These selection criteria may eliminate more older than younger candidates because of their increased prevalence of illness. Also, test quality is carefully standardized. Cognitive impairment may compromise test quality. As a result, older individuals may have more difficulty meeting test quality criteria, increasing their likelihood of exclusion and potentially increasing the variability of reference data for the elderly. In summary, the selection processes may make the older individuals who participate in reference studies less representative of the individuals who present for clinical lung function testing.

These same issues also affect the limits applied to determine whether a tested individual is within the "normal" range. Limits are often defined assuming that the distribution of data is Gaussian. Although tests of this assumption are sparse, there is reason to suspect that it is more likely to fail in the elderly. Even when the "normal" range is defined using methods that avoid assumptions about data distribution, data from the elderly are often lumped with those of the younger subjects. The result may be an erroneous "normal" range. All these reference value issues suggest that increased caution should be used in interpreting lung function tests in the elderly. This caution is especially important for those over age 80 and in any elderly person whose data lie near the limits of a "normal" range.

REFERENCES

1. Hayflick L. Biological aging is no longer an unsolved problem. *Ann NY Acad Sci.* 2007;1100:1–13.
2. Brooks SM. Perspective on the human cough reflex. *Cough.* 2011;7:10. http://www.coughjournal.com/content/7/1/10.
3. Ebihara S, Ebihara T, Kohzuki M. Effect of aging on cough and swallowing reflexes: implications for preventing aspiration pneumonia. *Lung.* 2012;190:29–33.
4. Becher A, Dent J. Systematic review: ageing and gastro-oesophageal reflux disease symptoms, oesophageal function and reflux oesophagitis. *Aliment Pharmacol Ther.* 2011;33:442–454.
5. Edge J, Millard F, Reid L, Simon G. The radiographic appearance of the chest in persons of advanced age. *Br J Radiol.* 1964;37:769–774.
6. Houtmeyers E, Gosselink R, Gayan-Ramirez G, Gayan-Ramirez G, Decramer M. Regulation of mucociliary clearance in health and disease. *Eur Respir J.* 1999;13:1177–1188.
7. Ryan SF, Vincent TN, Mitchell RS, Ductectasia; An asymptomatic pulmonary change related to age. *Med Thorac.* 1965;22:181–187.
8. Verbeken EK, Cauberghs M, Mertens I, Clement J, Lauweryns JM, Van de Woestijne KP. The Senile Lung. Comparison with normal and emphysematous lungs. 1. Structural aspects. *Chest.* 1992;101:793–799.
9. Thurlbeck WM, Angus GE. Growth and aging of the normal human lung. *Chest.* 1975;67:3S–7S.
10. The definition of emphysema. Report of a National Heart, Lung, and Blood Institute, Division of Lung Diseases workshop. *Am Rev Respir Dis.* 1985;132:182–185.
11. Copley SJ, Wells AU, Hawtin KE, et al. Lung morphology in the elderly: comparative CT study of subjects over 75 years old versus those under 55 years old. *Radiology.* 2009;251:566–573.
12. Pierce JA. The elastic performance of the lungs in health and disease. *Biochem Clin.* 1964;4:9–16.
13. Frank NR, Mead J, Ferris BG. The mechanical behavior of the lungs in healthy elderly persons. *J Clin Invest.* 1957;36:1680–1687.
14. Knudson RJ, Clark DF, Kennedy TC, Knudson DE. Effect of aging alone on mechanical properties of the normal adult human lung. *J. Appl Physiol: Respirat Environ Exercise Physiol.* 1977;43:1054–1062.
15. Gelb AF, Zamel N. Effect of aging on lung mechanics in healthy nonsmokers. *Chest.* 1975;68:538–541.
16. Bode FR, Dosman J, Martin RR, Ghezzo H, Macklem PT. Age and sex differences in lung elasticity, and in closing capacity in nonsmokers. *J. Appl Physiol.* 1976;41:129–135.
17. Weibel ER. It takes more than cells to make a good lung. *Am J Respir Crit Care Med.* 2013;187:342–346.

18. Shapiro SD, Endicott SK, Province MA, Pierce JA, Campbell EJ. Marked longevity of human lung parenchymal elastic fibers deduced from prevalence of D-aspartate and nuclear weapons–related radiocarbon. *J Clin Invest*. 1990;87:1828–1834.
19. Lang MR, Fiaux GW, Gillooly M, Stewart JA, Hulmes DJ, Lamb D. Collagen content of alveolar wall tissue in emphysematous and non-emphysematous lungs. *Thorax*. 1994;49:319–326.
20. Pierce JA, Resnick H, Henry PH. Collagen and elastin metabolism in the lungs, skin, and bones of adult rats. *J Lab Clin Med*. 1967;69:485–492.
21. Butler JP, Loring SH, Patz S, Tsuda A, Yablonskiy DA, Mentzer SJ. Evidence for adult lung growth in humans. *N Engl J Med*. 2012;367:244–247.
22. Mittman C, Edelman NH, Norris AH, et al. Relationship between chest wall and pulmonary compliance and age. *J Appl Physiol*. 1965;20:1211–1216.
23. Black LF, Hyatt RE. Maximal respiratory pressures: normal values and relationship to age and sex. *Am Rev Respir Dis*. 1969;99: 696–702.
24. McElvaney G, Blackie S, Morrison NJ, Wilcox PG, Fairbarn MS, Pardy RL. Maximal static respiratory pressures in the normal elderly. *Am Rev Respir Dis*. 1989;139:277–281.
25. Chen H, Kuo C. Relationship between respiratory muscle function and age, sex, and other factors. *J Appl Physiol*. 1989;l66:943–948.
26. Kronenberg RS, Drage CW. Attenuation of the ventilator and heart rate responses to hypoxia and hypercapnia with aging in normal men. *J Clin Invest*. 1973;52:1812–1819.
27. Peterson DD, Pack AI, Silage DA, Fishman AP. Effects of aging on ventilatory and occlusion pressure responses to hypoxia and hypercapnia. *Am Rev Respir Dis*. 1981;124:387–391.
28. Lalley PM. The aging respiratory system—Pulmonary structure, function, and neural control. *Respir Physiol Neurobiol*. 2013;187: 199–210.
29. Akiyama Y, Nishimura M, Kobayashi S, Yamamoto M, Miyamoto K, Kawakami Y. Effects of aging on respiratory load compensation and dyspnea sensation. *Am Rev Respir Dis*. 1993;148:1586–1591.
30. Mann C, Pouzeratte Y, Eledjam JJ. Postoperative patient-controlled analgesia in the elderly: risks and benefits of epidural versus intravenous administration. *Drugs Aging*. 2003;20:337–345.
31. Freye E, Levy JV. Use of opioids in the elderly—Pharmacokinetic and pharmacodynamic considerations. *Anasthesiol Intensivmed Notfallmed Schmerzther*. 2004;39:527–537.
32. Dowling GJ, Weiss SRB, Condon TP. Drugs of abuse and the aging brain. *Neuropsychopharmacology*. 2008;33:209–218.
33. Ehrsam RE, Perruchoud A, Oberholzer M, Burkart F, Herzog H. Influence of age on pulmonary hemodynamics at rest and during supine exercise. *Clin Sci*. 1983;65:653–660.
34. Davidson WR, Fee E. Influence of aging on pulmonary hemodynamics in a population free of coronary artery disease. *Am J Cardiol*. 1990;65:1454–1458.
35. Quanjer PH, Temmelling GJ, Cotes JE, Pedersen OF, Peslin R, Yernault JC. Lung volumes and forced ventilatory flows: Report working party standardization of lung function tests, European Community for Steel and Coal. Official statement of the European Respiratory Society. *Eur Respir J*. 1993;Suppl 16:5–40.
36. McClaran SR, Babcock MA, Pegelow DF, Reddan WG, Dempsey JA. Longitudinal effects of aging on lung function at rest and exercise in healthy active fit elderly adults. *J Appl Physiol*. 1995;78: 1957–1968.
37. Ware JH, Dockery DW, Louis TA, Xu XP, Ferris BG Jr, Speizer FE. Longitudinal and cross-sectional estimates of pulmonary function decline in neversmoking adults. *Am J Epidemiol*. 1990;132: 685–700.
38. Leith DE, Mead J. Mechanisms determining residual volume of the lungs in normal subjects. *J Appl Physiol*. 1967;23:221–227.
39. Bode FR, Dosman J, Martin RR, Ghezzo H, Macklem PT. Age and sex differences in lung elasticity, and in closing capacity in nonsmokers. *J Appl Physiol*. 1976;41:129–135.
40. Holland J, Milic-Emili J, Macklem PT, Bates DV. Regional distribution of pulmonary ventilation and perfusion in elderly subjects. *J Clin Invest*. 1968;47:81–92.
41. Edelman NH, Mittman C, Norris AH, Shock NW. Effects of respiratory pattern on age differences in ventilation uniformity. *J Appl Physiol*. 1968;24:49–53.
42. Nunn AJ, Gregg I. New regression equations for predicting peak expiratory flow in adults. *BMJ*. 1989;298:1068–1070.
43. Paoletti P, Pistelli G, Fazzi P, et al. Reference values for vital capacity and flow-volume curves from a general population study. *Bull Eur Physiopathol Respir*. 1986;22:451–459.
44. Robbins DR, Enright PL, Sherrill DL. Lung function development in young adults: is there a plateau phase? *Eur Respir J*. 1995;8:768–772.
45. Neas LM, Schwartz J. The determinants of pulmonary diffusing capacity in a national sample of U.S. adults. *Am J Respir Crit Care Med*. 1996;153:656–664.
46. Crapo RO, Morris AH, Gardner RM. Reference values for pulmonary tissue volume, membrane diffusing capacity, and pulmonary capillary blood volume. *Bull Europ Physiopathol Resp*. 1982;18:893–899.
47. Sorbini CA, Grassi V, Solinas E, Muiesan G. Arterial oxygen tension in relation to age in healthy subjects. *Respiration*. 1968;25:3–13.
48. Raine JM, Bishop JM. A-a difference in O_2 tension and physiological dead space in normal man. *J Apppl Physiol*. 1963;18:284–288.
49. Wagner PD, Laravuso RB, Uhl RR, West JB. Continuous distributions of ventilation-perfusion ratios in normal subjects breathing air and 100 per cent O_2. *J Clin Invest*. 1974;54:54–68.
50. Couser JI, Guthmann R, Abdulgany HM, Kane CS. Pulmonary rehabilitation improves exercise capacity in older elderly patients with COPD. *Chest*. 1995;107:730–734.
51. Malbut KE, Dinan S, Young A. Aerobic training in the 'oldest old.' The effect of 24 weeks of training. *Age Ageing*. 2002;31:255–260.
52. Vaitkevicius PV, Ebersold C, Shah MS, et al. Effects of aerobic exercise training in community-based subjects aged 80 and older: a pilot study. *J Am Geriatr Soc*. 2002;30:2009–2013.
53. Meyer KC, Rosenthal NS, Soergel P, Peterson K. Neutrophils and low-grade inflammation in the seemingly normal aging lung. *Mech Ageing Dev*. 1998;104:169–181.
54. Gislason T, Reynisdottir H, Kristbjarnson H, Benediktsdóttir B. Sleep habits and sleep disturbances among the elderly: an epidemiological survey. *J Intern Med*. 1993;234:31–39.
55. Prinz PN, Vitello MV, Raskind MA, Thorpy MJ. Geriatrics: sleep disorders and aging. *N Engl J Med*. 1990;323:520–526.
56. Johansson P, Alehagen U, Svanborg E, Dahlström U, Broström A. Clinical characteristics and mortality risk in relation to obstructive and central sleep apnea in community-dwelling elderly individuals: a 7-year follow-up. *Age Aging*. 2012;41:468–474.
57. Vaz Fragoso CA, Gill TM. Respiratory impairment and the aging lung: a novel paradigm for assessing pulmonary function. *J Gerontol A Biol Sci Med Sci*. 2011;67:264–275.

CHAPTER 20

Innate and Adaptive Immunity in the Lung

Charles S. Dela Cruz
Jonathan L. Koff

The lung is constantly exposed to foreign agents. As a result it is faced with the challenge of distinguishing nonpathogenic moieties in ambient air from potentially pathogenic antigens derived from microorganisms. Here, we use the term "pathogens" to refer to infectious agents, allergens, toxins, and other inhaled antigens unless stated otherwise. The lung protects itself using local tissue structures such as the mucus layer, ciliary ladder, and smooth muscles. It also employs complex immune defenses that are both innate and adaptive.[1,2] The immune responses need to be able to recognize and to react to a wide variety of stimuli. They must be able to recognize and to eliminate unwanted pathogens to keep pulmonary structures free of infection. On the other hand, they must not overreact to inhaled stimuli to avoid potential excessive inflammation and lung injury. This need to control the intensity and duration of such responses is required to preserve normal lung structure, especially the highly vascularized and fragile alveolar epithelial surface that is required for gas exchange. Alterations of these lung protective mechanisms lead to many of the pulmonary diseases physicians face in their patients. Therefore, understanding the innate and adaptive immune responses in the lung is important in our attempts to understand the pathophysiology and to improve the management of many pulmonary diseases. The anatomic and immune defenses will be reviewed in this chapter.

ANATOMIC MECHANISMS

Given the lungs' large surface area, it is exposed to many inhaled environmental challenges, because the air we breathe contains infectious agents, toxic gases, and fine particulate matter (Fig. 20-1). The alveolar and capillary membrane barriers are important for gas exchange, and need to be defended from the injurious effects of incoming toxic and infectious pathogens. If the consequences of these exposures are not controlled, this can lead to excessive inflammation, lung edema, as well as propagation of infectious agents. This can, in turn, lead to alveolar destruction, abnormal fibrotic repair, and compromised gas exchange. Air is inhaled through the nose or the mouth into the extrathoracic portion of the trachea before it enters the thorax. The nose filters and conditions the inhaled air for humidity and body temperature as it flows through the nasal turbinates. Nasal hairs also provide a barrier that traps larger particulates. The nasal secretions lining the airway mucosa contain many substances such as lysozyme, immunoglobulins (such as secretory immunoglobulin A [sIgA]), and antimicrobial peptides that bind to, and inactivate invading microbes. For example, sIgA accounts for 15% of the total protein in upper airway secretions and plays a significant role in neutralizing and preventing epithelial attachment of invading viruses and bacteria.[3] The conducting airway mucosa is also coated with acidic viscous fluid and mucus secreted by Clara cells, goblet cells, and bronchial glands (Fig. 20-1). This fluid makes up an important airway surface lining that coats the bronchial epithelium and forms a barrier between the outside world and the lung parenchyma.

INNATE IMMUNITY IN THE LUNG

The innate immune response is an evolutionarily conserved system of host defense evident in all multicellular organisms. In the constant battle between host and pathogens, the purpose of the innate immune system is to provide a rapid response, in contrast to the adaptive immune system, which provides a more specific response but takes longer to respond (see Section "Adaptive Immune Responses in the Lung"). Because humans breathe approximately 10 L of air per day (12 to 15 breaths/min × 500 mL tidal volume), we are constantly exposed to pathogens (e.g., viruses, bacteria, and fungi), allergens (e.g., house dust mites, dander), and toxins (e.g., cigarette smoke and pollutants). The innate immune system allows humans to respond to these stimuli even if they have not been exposed to them previously.

Because of the constant exposure to the environment, similar to other mucosal surfaces (e.g., gut and skin), the innate immune system must maintain a balanced response. Ideally, this should include (1) pathogen recognition, (2) initiation of an appropriate response, which is typically manifested by inflammation, and (3) resolution of inflammation. An inappropriately regulated innate response contributes to the pathogenesis of lung diseases as diverse as asthma, emphysema, and interstitial lung disease.

The most important property of the innate immune system is its response to pathogens regardless if there has been a prior exposure. Thus, an acquired immunologic memory against the pathogen is not required. The anatomic and antimicrobial structures that prevent infection and injury noted earlier can be thought of as part of the innate response. Therefore, one of the most important roles of the lung innate immune system is its function as a barrier to inhaled pathogens.[4] The epithelial surface of the lung creates a barrier with tight junctions between neighboring cells that prevent pathogen entry (Fig. 20-1). In addition to this barrier function, the epithelium has a coordinated system for the removal of inhaled pathogens. Goblet cells and secretory glands produce mucus that engulfs pathogens. A coordinated system of ciliated cells moves mucus up the mucociliary "ladder" to be expectorated during coughing. A disturbance in this essential function leads to significant pathology. In primary ciliary dyskinesia (PCD), cilia function is impaired and individuals develop bronchiectasis with recurrent bacterial infection.[5] In cystic fibrosis (CF), an abnormality in epithelial chloride channel function causes changes in the airway surface liquid that prevents effective mucus clearance, which also leads to chronic inflammation, bronchiectasis, and recurrent bacterial infections.[6,7] The mucociliary "ladder" is particularly effective for large molecules, but smaller molecules (<5 μM) are able to directly descend to the distal alveolar epithelium. Here, instead of mucociliary clearance, particles encounter secreted surfactant proteins (specifically SP-A and SP-D; also known as pulmonary collectins) that act as opsonins, and assist resident macrophage in phagocytosis.[8] Finally, the epithelium also produces a variety of innate immune antimicrobial molecules that activate alveolar macrophages (AMs) to kill pathogens.[9]

■ PATHOGEN RECOGNITION

The innate immune response allows the host to respond to a wide array of pathogens. However, the mechanism(s) that the host uses to recognize these pathogens was poorly understood until the 1980s. At that time, a seminal advance in our understanding of the immune system occurred when it was proposed that the host detects, and responds to these

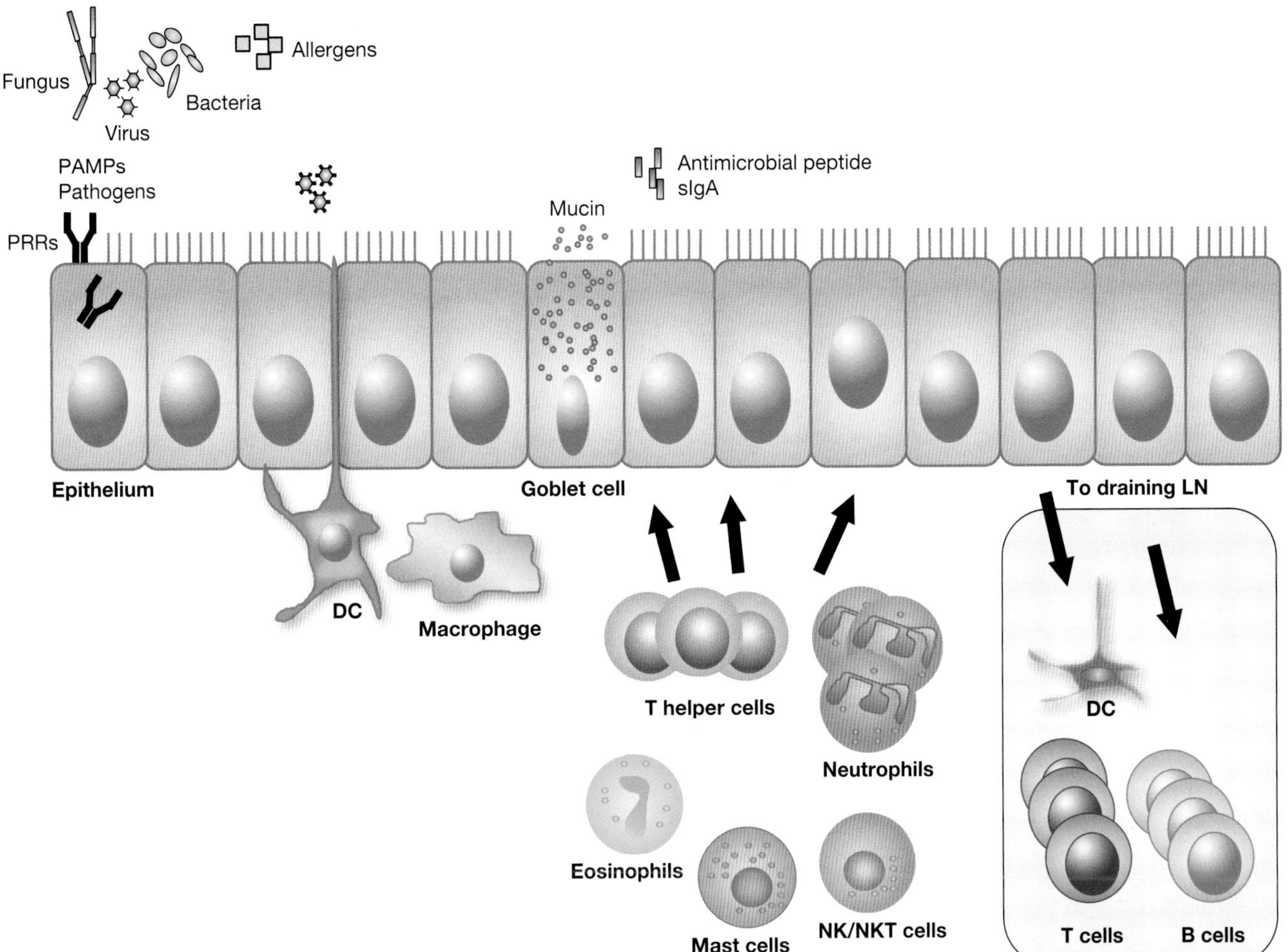

Figure 20-1 Innate recognition of pathogen or PAMPs on airway epithelium. Pathogens such as fungus, virus, or bacteria (or their associated pattern-associated molecular proteins [PAMPs]) and environmental allergens are first detected by membrane bound, cytosolic and/or endosomal innate sensors or pattern recognition receptors (PRRs). The respiratory epithelial cells provide a physical barrier between the airway luminal antigens and the underlying respiratory tissues in their control of immune defense and tolerance. Specialized epithelial cells can have cilia, produce a mucus layer and secrete antimicrobial proteins and secretory IgA (sIgA) that limit pathogen exposure to the epithelial cells. Dendritic cells (DCs) interdigitating between and lying near the epithelium, as well as tissue macrophages, are well positioned to sample and ingest incoming antigen. Recognition of the antigen by the innate immune receptors leads to production of pro-inflammatory cytokines and chemokines which recruits immune cells such as neutrophils, T cells, NK cells, NKT cells, eosinophils, or mast cells. Activated DCs that have taken up the inhaled antigen migrate to nearby draining lymph nodes. In the lymph nodes, the DCs help integrate the signals from the inhaled substance and the innate immune response into signals that direct cells of the adaptive immune system. The DCs encounter appropriate naïve $CD4^+$ T cells where factors such as the phenotype of the antigen-presenting cells (APCs) and cytokine milieu modulate differentiation of $CD4^+$ T cell subsets with their characteristic cytokine and functional profiles. These immune cell functions and cytokine production determine whether an activating or a tolerant response will develop.

pathogens via a cadre of receptors that recognize conserved sequences called pathogen-associated molecular patterns (PAMPs), which exist in pathogens, and are not present in the host (Fig. 20-2).[10,11] Experiments in *Drosophila* (fruit flies) in 1996 identified pattern recognition receptors (PRRs) that recognized PAMPs and supported the concept of innate receptors.[12] Subsequently, PRRs were identified in humans,[13] and more recently, additional PRRs have been shown to recognize endogenous molecules released from damaged cells, which are referred to as damage-associated molecular patterns (DAMPs).[14,15] The major types of PRRs are described in sections "Toll-Like Receptors", "RIG-I-Like Receptors", "Nod-Like Receptors" and "C-Type Lectin Receptors".

Toll-Like Receptors

The mammalian Toll-like receptor (TLR) family received its name from the *Drosophila* Toll gene. Early studies that involved the genetic manipulation of Toll resulted in dramatic defects in innate immune responses (Table 20-1; Fig. 20-2).[12,16] Since this discovery, the TLRs are appreciated to be the prototypical PRR molecules.[13,17] It is now known that some TLRs are present on the cell surface, and others are in endosomes (intracellular vesicles). As a group, they are characterized by N-terminal leucine-rich repeats that recognize pathogens, a transmembrane region, and a cytoplasmic domain that is highly homologous to the interleukin (IL)-1 receptor and the IL-18 receptor.[18] To date, 11 TLRs have been identified in humans, with different TLRs recognizing distinct PAMPs.[19] In general terms, TLR recognition of PAMPs is based upon cellular compartmentalization. Recognition of viral RNA and DNA occurs in endosomes by TLR3, TLR7, and TLR9, while TLR2 and TLR4 have been shown to recognize viral proteins. The remaining TLRs recognize bacteria, parasite, and host

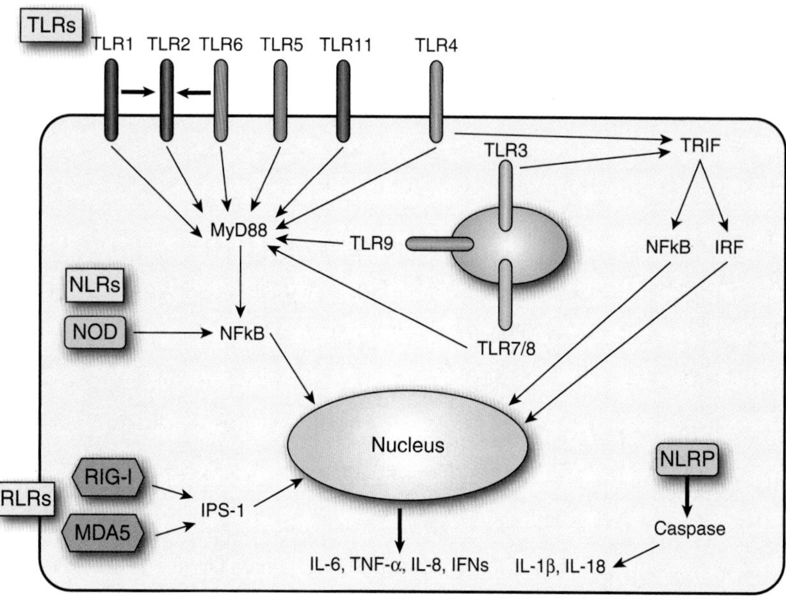

Figure 20-2 Pattern recognition receptors (PRRs). Classes of PRRs include Toll-like receptors (TLRs), retinoic acid–inducible gene-I–like receptors (RLRs) and nucleotide oligomerization domain–like receptors (NLRs). Not shown are C-type lectin receptors (CLRs). TLRs, RLRs (e.g., RIG-I, MDA5, and other sensors), and NLRs (e.g., NOD1, NOD2, NLRP3, etc.) are innate immune sensors that recognize danger signals derived from pathogens (PAMPs), damaged cells (DAMPs), or associated nucleic acids at the cell surface, in endolysosomes or in the cytoplasm. Signaling by these sensors promotes, either the activation and nuclear translocation of transcription factors (IRFs, NFκB and AP-1) that drive expression of cytokines (IFN-α/β, TNF, and pro-IL-1β), or the assembly of the caspase-1 inflammasome and subsequent maturation of IL-1β from pro-IL-1β. IFN, interferon; IL, interleukin; IRFs, interferon regulatory factors; MDA5, melanoma differentiation–associated gene-5; NFκB, nuclear factor κB; NLRP, NLR with a pyrin domain; NOD, nucleotide oligomerization domain; RIG-I, retinoic acid–inducible gene-I; TNF, tumor necrosis factor; TRIF, TIR-domain–containing adapter-inducing interferon-β.

proteins (e.g., DAMPs), while TLR7 and TLR9 recognize DNA from bacteria or protozoa.

TLR Signaling Pathways

TLR recognition of PAMPs stimulates signaling pathways that ultimately lead to activation of gene transcription and protein production. The responses that are elicited can be cell type specific. They also utilize two distinct pathways based on which of two adaptor molecules they employ: (1) myeloid differentiation primary response gene 88 (MyD88) and (2) TIR-domain–containing adapter-inducing interferon-β (TRIF). With the exception of TLR3, and one of the pathways downstream from TLR4, MyD88 is required for the downstream signaling of TLRs. MyD88 interacts with the IL-1R–associated kinase (IRAK)-4, and other IRAK family members, before they dissociate from MyD88 and interact with TNFR-associated factor 6 (TRAF6). IκB kinase (IKK)-β and MAP kinases are activated, leading to another complex of IKK molecules that are degraded and release nuclear factor kappa-light-chain-enhancer of activated B cells (NF-κB). NF-κB is a critical transcription factor for TLR-induced genes in inflammation. In addition, activation of the MAP kinase cascade leads to another transcription factor, AP-1, which is associated with activation of cytokines. TRIF-dependent signaling was found to be responsible for TLR3 signaling and, more recently, TRIF was implicated in TLR4 signaling.[20] TRIF interacts with TRAF3 and TRAF6, and leads to TNF receptor (R)-associated death domain protein (TRADD), ultimately leading to activation of NF-κB. Interestingly, TLR4 was found to activate MyD88 at the surface of the plasma membrane, while TRIF activation occurred when TLR4 was in endosomes.[20] Downstream from TRIF is activation of interferon regulatory factors (IRFs), which lead to interferon production and activation of interferon-dependent genes.

TABLE 20-1 Toll-Like Receptors

TLRs	PAMP	Cellular Location
TLR1	Lipoprotein (bacteria)	Plasma membrane
TLR2	Lipoprotein (e.g., bacteria, viruses, parasites, host damage)	Plasma membrane
TLR3	dsRNA	Endosome
TLR4	LPS (bacteria, virus, host damage)	Plasma membrane
TLR5	Flagellin (bacteria)	Plasma membrane
TLR6	Lipoprotein (bacteria, virus)	Plasma membrane
TLR7 (human TLR8)	ssRNA (virus, bacteria, host damage)	Endosome
TLR9	CpG-DNA (virus, bacteria, protozoa, host damage)	Endosome
TLR10	Unknown	Endosome
TLR11	Profilin-like molecule (protozoa)	Plasma membrane

RIG-I–Like Receptors

The RIG-I–like receptor (RLR) family presently includes three members: retinoic acid–inducible gene-I (RIG-I), melanoma differentiation–associated gene 5 (MDA5), and laboratory of genetics and physiology 2 (LGP2) (Table 20-2).[21] RLRs are expressed at a basal level by all nucleated cells, suggesting a central role in innate immune recognition and response to viral infection. A measure of their importance can be seen in the evolution of viral mechanisms to evade or suppress RLRs.[22] In the 1950s, interferons were discovered to be a critical antiviral innate immune response to viral infection produced by infected cells, and important in the recruitment and activation of natural killer (NK) cells and lymphocytes that recognize and kill virus-infected cells.[23] While the presence of an intracellular TLR receptor for dsRNA was hypothesized in 1969,[24] and subsequently identified, the discovery of RLRs introduced a second family of PRRs that are cytoplasmic sensors of viral nucleic acids that contribute to antiviral host defense by inducing interferon production. RIG-I was initially discovered in 1997 as a gene induced in acute promyelocytic leukemia cells after stimulation

TABLE 20-2 RIG-I-Like Receptors

RLRs	PAMP	Cellular Location
RIG-I	Short dsRNA	Cytoplasm
MDA5	Long dsRNA	Cytoplasm
LGP2	Unknown	Cytoplasm

with retinoic acid.[25,26] Several years later, RIG-I was found to be activated by interferon.[27] Similarly, MDA5 was identified in 1999,[28] and was later found to be induced by interferon.[29] LGP2 was suggested to function as a RIG-I inhibitor, exerting a regulatory role on antiviral innate immune responses,[30] but recent experiments suggest that LGP2 may modify viral RNA to assist RIG-I and MDA5 recognition of dsRNA.[19] Three genes encode RLRs in mice and humans, and all share a conserved helicase domain. Briefly, RIG-I and MDA5 are composed of two N-terminal caspase recruitment domains (CARDs), a central DEAD box helicase/ATPase domain, and a C-terminal regulatory domain.[31] LGP2 retains the helicase domain but lacks the CARD domain.[31] Their cytoplasmic location allows for recognition of dsRNA viruses and dsRNA intermediates generated during ssRNA viral replication. In addition, there is evidence that ssRNA is detected from viruses that do not produce significant amounts of dsRNA.[19] Importantly, eukaryotic cells avoid self-activation of RLRs by RNA in mitochondria, and RNA released into the cytosol is packaged to avoid RLR recognition.[22]

In the human lung, RLRs have been found to respond to a range of respiratory viruses, from rhinovirus (common cold virus) to influenza virus. In response to viruses, activation of intracellular signaling ultimately leads to interferon production and the activation of interferon-dependent genes. RLR signaling is dependent on CARDs, which interact with the interferon-β–promoter stimulator 1 (IPS-1, also known as MAVS, CARDIF, or VISA). IPS-1 is localized on the mitochondrial membrane. IPS-1 activates TRAF3 and TRADD, which are common molecules for IFN-inducible gene expression.[19] In addition, NF-κB signaling has been implicated.[32]

NOD-Like Receptors

Nucleotide oligomerization domain (NOD)-like receptors (NLRs) are another family of cytoplasmic pathogen sensors that were discovered in the 1990s (Table 20-3).[33] Briefly, the molecular structure of NLRs includes a central nucleotide-binding domain and C-terminal leucine-rich repeats. The N-terminal portions of most NLRs contain protein-binding motifs (e.g., CARDs, a pyrin domain, and a baculovirus inhibitor of apoptosis protein repeat [BIR] domain).[19] NLRs activate important signaling pathways mediated by NF-κB and MAP kinases, and activate caspases. The result is activation of diverse signaling pathways that induce innate immune responses.[34]

NOD1 and NOD2 identify bacterial PAMPs by recognition of peptidoglycan from gram-negative bacteria, gram-positive bacteria, and mycobacteria. The importance of NLRs was highlighted by the evidence that NOD polymorphisms are associated with increased severity of atopy, eczema, and asthma,[35] as well as other inflammatory diseases (e.g., Crohn disease,[36] tuberculosis,[37] and lung cancer[38]). This suggests that a defect in bacterial clearance may influence the host microbiome and subsequent pathophysiology of disease. Distinct from NOD1 and NOD2 are a group of NLRs that activate caspases, such as caspase-1. Caspase-1 is the prototypical caspase that has been shown to be required for cleavage and processing of inflammatory cytokines (IL-1β, IL-18) into their active forms. This signaling pathway is now commonly referred to as the "inflammasome," and has been shown to be critical for effective innate immune responses against a wide range of microbial pathogens, cancer, and inflammatory, metabolic, and autoimmune diseases.[39] Specific to the lung, the inflammasome is critical for responses to important pathogens such as influenza A virus,[40,41] *Streptococcus*,[42,43] *Pseudomonas aeruginosa*,[44] and *Mycobacterium tuberculosis*.[45] In addition, activation of the inflammasome has been suggested to contribute to the pathogenesis of asthma,[46] chronic obstructive pulmonary disease (COPD),[47] and pulmonary fibrosis.[48]

TABLE 20-3 NOD-Like Receptors

NLRs	PAMP	Cellular Location
NOD1	Gram-negative > Gram-positive bacteria	Cytoplasm
NOD2	Gram-negative, Gram-positive bacteria, mycobacteria	Cytoplasm
NLRP 1–14	Viruses, bacteria, mycobacteria	Cytoplasm

C-Type Lectin Receptors

The C-type lectin receptors (CLRs) were identified in the early 1900s, and represent a diverse family that includes over one thousand members.[49] The CLRs were initially characterized as Ca^{2+}-dependent (C-type) carbohydrate-binding (lectin) proteins[49] but, subsequently, some CLRs were found to not bind carbohydrate ligands or require Ca^{2+}-dependent signaling.[50] Currently, CLRs have been classified into 17 groups.[50] Structurally, CLRs are characterized by a carbohydrate-recognition domain (CRD) that is highly conserved.[49] Despite this conserved CRD structure, CLRs are involved in cell functions as diverse as adhesion, repair, endocytosis, and phagocytosis, as well as innate immune pathogen recognition. CLRs recognize carbohydrates on a wide variety of pathogens including viruses, bacteria, and fungi. Several of the canonical CLRs include dectins, mannose-binding lectin (MBL) receptors, and surfactant protein (SP). Dectin-1 and Dectin-2 are important PRRs for recognition of fungi.[51] Upon recognition of fungal PAMPs, intracellular signaling pathways involve activation of NF-κB and MAP kinases.[52] MBL receptors function as PRRs by recognition of carbohydrate motifs on pathogens, which leads to complement activation.[18] MBL recognizes diverse pathogens that include gram-positive and gram-negative bacteria, yeast, parasites, mycobacteria, and viruses.[53] SP was first identified as a critical phospholipid for maintaining alveolar compliance to prevent atelectasis.[54] However, in the 1980s after the discovery of MBLs, sequencing of SP revealed significant structural similarities.[55] In accord with these similarities, SP-A and SP-D, secreted by alveolar epithelium, have been shown to function as agglutinins, opsonins, and inflammatory modulators[8] in response to viruses, bacteria, mycobacteria, and fungi.[56]

■ PATHOGEN-INDUCED INNATE IMMUNE RESPONSES

Inhaled pathogens may circumvent the mucociliary "ladder" on airway epithelium, which is typically the first responder to pathogens by virtue of its location and distribution. Antigen-presenting cells (APCs) such as dendritic cells (DCs) provide a critical role for pathogen recognition by extending projections into the airway between epithelial cells to sample the environment. On both airway epithelium and DCs, there is a wide repertoire of PRRs that recognize pathogens.[57] Upon recognition of PAMPs, PRRs activate signaling pathways that lead to subsequent inflammatory responses. An important component of this inflammatory response is the production of chemokines to recruit hematopoietic cells (e.g., neutrophils, eosinophils, macrophages, and lymphocytes including NK, and NKT cells) that are critical effector cells for the initiation and resolution of inflammation. In addition to chemokine production, PRR activation stimulates the production of a variety of cytokines (e.g., tumor necrosis factor (TNF)-α, IL-1β, IL-6, TGF-β, IL-10) that activate effector cells and contribute to the regulation of innate and adaptive responses in the lung.[57] PRR activation influences the balance of oxidation and proteases present in the lung. Importantly, dysregulation of oxidation has been shown to contribute to the pathogenesis of COPD,[58] while defective antiproteases, best exemplified by α1-antitrypsin deficiency, is a significant risk factor for the development of asthma, bronchiectasis, and emphysema.[59] Antimicrobial peptides are also produced by epithelial cells, as well as recruited hematopoietic cells, in response to PRR activation

(Fig. 20-1).[60] In humans, two significant groups of antimicrobial peptides are the cathelicidins[61] and defensins.[60] These small cationic peptides have antimicrobial activity against gram-negative and gram-positive bacteria, fungi, parasites, and viruses.[62] Epithelial and hematopoietic cells (e.g., neutrophils) produce both cathelicidins and defensins, and in addition to their antimicrobial properties, these peptides have been implicated in the induction of inflammation, influencing adaptive immune responses and wound repair.[61,62] Therefore, antimicrobial peptides are an excellent example of an innate immune response, initiated by PRR recognition of pathogens or PAMPs, which results in a protective response, regulates inflammation, and bridges innate and adaptive immunity. Recently a group of innate immune cells, known as innate lymphoid cells (ILCs), have been identified that lack specific antigen receptors but can produce an array of effector cytokines.[63,64] These ILCs have morphologic characteristics of lymphoid cells and can respond to a variety of signals and play an important role in immunity against microorganisms, tissue homeostasis, and repair of damaged tissues. Currently, there are three subsets of ILCs identified: ILC1s include IL-15–dependent NK cells; ILC2s are characterized by their production of T helper (Th) 2 cytokines (IL-5 and IL-13); and ILC3s express the nuclear hormone receptor retinoic acid receptor–related receptor (ROR)γt and produce cytokines IL-17 and IL-22.[63,65] These cells are important in innate immunity and very likely will be discovered to contribute to the development of effective adaptive responses.

CELLULAR RESPONSES IN THE LUNG

When pathogens bypass the initial lung mucosal barriers, the host's immune system responds in an orchestrated defense that involves a number of specialized cells that target the threat, neutralize it, and cleanup remnants to prevent the tissue injury. Macrophages function as phagocytes to engulf pathogens (viable and nonviable microorganisms), as well as apoptotic and necrotic cells that have undergone physiologic and pathologic cell death.[66] Ultimately, the lung must perform these tasks in a selective manner to avoid unnecessary inflammation that can cause continued tissue destruction. The innate immune system, as described earlier, is made up of a humoral arm (lactoferrins, lysozyme, sIgA, SPs, MBLs, and defensins) as well as a cellular arm (AMs, DCs, neutrophils, ILCs, etc.) that express numerous PRRs and or phagocytic receptors important for their diverse functions.

■ MACROPHAGES

Macrophages, initially described in the 1880s, are large mononuclear phagocytic cells. They play an important role in host defense based on their ability to phagocytize inhaled moieties, maintain tissue homeostasis, and function as APCs which are important in adaptive humoral and cell-mediated responses.[67] Macrophage precursors arise from committed hematopoietic stem cells in the bone marrow and are released into the circulation as monocytes before they differentiate into macrophages and DCs as they migrate into the lung. Tissue-resident macrophages form a specialized population based on their local anatomic location. Once called dust cells for their ability to engulf particulates, AMs, named for their presence in the pulmonary alveolus, frequently contain granules of various exogenous materials.[68] One example is particulate matter such as the black carbonaceous granules seen in lungs from smokers and long-term city dwellers. Routine bronchoalveolar lavage will identify these resident airway and AMs. However, pulmonary interstitial macrophages from lung tissue can only be collected by tissue dispersion techniques.[69] Of note, AMs are inferior APCs when compared to DCs.[70]

AMs secrete numerous products (e.g., cytokines, chemokines, and peptides) and directly interact with other cells and molecules through the expression of a variety of surface receptors.[71] AMs have multiple functions that include phagocytosis of cells undergoing apoptosis and necrosis, clearance of ingested pathogens or particulates, routine clearance of surfactant, and suppressing inappropriate inflammation and immune responses to harmless inhaled antigens. Macrophages ingest and phagocytose microbial or environmental particulate matter, which is then enclosed in intracellular vesicular phagosomes that undergo fusion with primary or secondary lysosomes to form phagolysosomes. In these AMs vacuoles, intracellular killing takes place through mechanisms that include antimicrobial proteins, degradative enzymes, oxidation, reactive oxygen intermediate generation, and "respiratory burst" known as nicotinamide adenine dinucleotide phosphate (NADPH) oxidase degradation. Macrophages facilitate many innate recognition functions because they express diverse PRRs (e.g., TLRs, NLRs, and CLRs) to assist host defense in combating invading pathogens. The recognition and clearance of invading pathogens can also occur via opsonin-mediated phagocytosis through the Fcγ receptors. These receptors allow macrophages to be selective in their response to phagocytosed antigen, minimize damaging effects on normal cells, and limit responses to harmless moieties that can be frequently encountered in the airway.

While AMs have greater respiratory burst capacity than other phagocytes,[72] there are certain organisms that have evolved to evade AMs to improve their growth and survival. For example, mycobacteria prevent the fusion of phagosomes and lysosomes, escaping the harmful effects of the lysosomal hydrolases, and thus are resistant to the effects of macrophages. Some inhaled pathogens such as *M. tuberculosis* and environmental particulates such as silica are resistant to AM function and remain in intracellular lysosomal vacuoles for the duration of the macrophage life span. Macrophages also produce inflammatory cytokines and chemokines to recruit other specialized cells to assist in PRR recognition and host defense, in turn, helping to shape the adaptive immune response that follows.

Lung resident AMs are continuously encountering inhaled substances because of their unique position in the alveolar lumen (Fig. 20-1). Because of this location and the potential to cause harm to surrounding delicate and sensitive lung structures (e.g., alveolar epithelium), AMs are normally kept in a quiescent state to limit unnecessary inflammation and injury to nearby structural type I and surfactant producing type II pneumocytes when they encounter harmless antigens. Compared to AMs, DCs are less capable phagocytes with lower levels of expression of phagocytic receptors such as CD11b. In contrast, AMs produce lower levels of pro-inflammatory cytokines and suppress adaptive immune responses through their effects on neighboring DCs and T cells. It has been shown that depletion of AMs can lead to exuberant lung inflammation in response to otherwise innocuous antigens.[73] These AMs, when mixed with DCs in vitro, can suppress T cell function through the release of factors such as nitric oxide, IL-10, TGF-β, and various prostaglandins.[74]

■ DENDRITIC CELLS

If the relatively nonspecific mechanisms of the innate immune system fail, there is a highly developed network of DCs that is responsible for mobilizing the adaptive immune response, especially against invading pathogens and unwanted antigens.[70,75] DCs are also important phagocytic cells and, in general, are better APC than macrophages.[70] DCs are critical at bridging innate and adaptive immunity because of their extensive interdigitating physical extensions that reach between cells to provide a tight surveillance network within intraepithelial and subepithelial structures of the respiratory tract. Via this network, DCs continuously sample what the lung encounters. Because of their distribution, they are ideally positioned to participate in determining whether an inhaled moiety results in pulmonary immunity or tolerance. DCs express MHC and accessory molecules such as CD80, CD86, and CD40 making them excellent professional APCs to incoming naïve T cells.[76,77]

They also express a number of innate immune receptors including TLRs, NLRs, and CLRs for the recognition of various patterned motifs from inhaled antigen and pathogens. Lung DCs also express prostaglandin receptors that affect migratory behavior and cell maturation. They also express inflammatory receptors that detect DAMP proteins such as uric acid, ATP, and high-mobility group box (HMGB)-1. Their ability to sense, take up, process incoming molecules, and migrate to nearby draining lymph nodes for antigen presentation, allows DCs to bridge innate and adaptive immunity in the lung. In the lymph nodes, DCs present MHC peptide antigen complexes to T cell receptors (TCRs) on naïve T cells and in the appropriate context of costimulatory molecules on their cell surface and cytokines in the local microenvironment, naïve T cells are activated and proliferate. In the absence of appropriate costimulation or cytokines, DC and T cell interaction can lead to tolerance to an antigen, a mechanism that likely helps to avoid harmful immunologic response to harmless inhaled antigens.

DCs have been divided into several subsets based on their cell surface protein expression, origin, location, and specialized function.[78] In mice, three major subsets of DCs have been described: resident conventional DCs (cDCs), plasmacytoid DCs (pDCs), and inflammatory DCs. The resident cDCs expresses CD11c markers and have been divided into those that express CD11b, and those that are CD11b negative. At baseline, cDCs expressing MHC and CD11c line the conducting airways and are able to extend their dendrites into the airway lumen between tight junctions. In murine models, these cDCs can also express langerin and the mucosal integrin CD103. cDCs have good antigen presentation function. A migratory cDCs subset migrates to nearby lymph nodes after capturing inhaled antigen in the airway lumen, while lymphoid tissue resident cDCs reside in the lymph nodes and spleen and respond to antigen delivered via the draining lymphatics. pDCs are characterized by the expression of the surface marker Siglec-H (a bone marrow stromal antigen-1) and abundance of endosomal innate receptors TLR7 and TLR9, which make pDCs particularly important antiviral effectors because of their type I interferon production in response to viruses and bacterial DNA. Residing in the alveolar space are alveolar DCs, which classically express MHC class II and CD11c, and can have CD103 subsets. These alveolar DCs have been described to resemble human Langerhans cells.[79]

In response to innate and inflammatory stimuli, DCs are able to increase their numbers with rapid recruitment. These DCs have similar abilities to undergo antigen processing, to migrate to draining lymph nodes, and to modulate naïve T cells for either activation or tolerance. The inflammatory cDCs are normally not present in the lung. However, in the setting of inflammation and/or infection, circulating monocyte-derived $CD11b^+$ DCs upregulate CD11c, retain Ly6C, and can rapidly be recruited to the lung as inflammatory cDCs to respond to the stimulus. Comparable subsets of DCs in human lungs have been described such as myeloid type of DC that express both blood dendritic cell antigen (BDCA)1 or BDCA3 and HLA-DR and pDCs that express BDCA2 and CD123.[80–82]

Overall, DCs rely on neighboring structural cells, such as the airway epithelial cells, to influence the type of antigen-specific immune response. This epithelial–DC interaction in the lung plays an important role in immune homeostasis as well as the initiation and transition of innate immunity toward antigen-specific adaptive immunity. Some have proposed that extracellular matrix surrounding epithelial cells and DCs produces certain chemokines that allow for the activation properties of DCs.[83] Antigen presentation by APCs such as AMs and DCs is a required priming event for T cell activation to occur.

■ NEUTROPHILS

Neutrophils are derived from the bone marrow and require granulocyte colony–stimulating factor (G-CSF) for their proliferation and differentiation into their mature form. In times of stress or infection, neutrophils are mobilized from the bone marrow into the blood stream and eventually to sites of inflammation such as the lungs.[84] During this process, neutrophils become activated, generate free radicals, release granule contents, and participate in phagocytosis and degradation of invading microbes. Neutrophils are one of the first phagocytes recruited to sites of acute lung diseases, but they have a limited life span after their release from the bone marrow and within hours they are cleared with the resolution of the inflammation or disease process. However, in chronic lung diseases, neutrophils can be persistently recruited to the lung. Recruited tissue neutrophils are thought to live substantially longer, up to several days, than circulating neutrophils.[85] These neutrophils, which are modulated by the local microenvironment, are important for antipathogen responses, but they can cause significant lung tissue damage when they accumulate over longer time periods and release granule contents that can be toxic when released in an uncontrolled manner.[86,87] Neutrophils are able to respond to a number of particulate and soluble stimuli. They also have the ability to be primed prior to exposure to stimuli.[88] For example, neutrophils can be primed, or pre-activated, by stimuli such as IL-8, granulocyte macrophage colony–stimulating factor, platelet activating factor, and reactive oxygen species. This process helps prepare neutrophils for subsequent contact with pathogens by extending their life span, upregulating cell surface integrins (such as CD11b), optimizing NADPH oxidase assembly, and prolonging neutrophil functional longevity.[89,90] Neutrophils play an important role in innate immune response to infection, as these phagocytic cells also possess an impressive array of microbicidal weapons against invading pathogens that include toxic oxygen radical species and proteolytic enzymes. Local infiltration and tissue accumulation of neutrophils are mediated by chemokines that are produced by inflamed tissues. At sites of inflammation, mediators such as IL-1 or TNF-α induce or augment the expression of adhesion molecules on endothelial cells and circulating granulocytes. Intravascular circulating neutrophils slow down, roll along, and then anchor on the endothelium allowing entry to the lung interstitium and subsequently the alveolar space. Ultimately, inflammation will cease and, with successful containment of pathogens, resolution of inflammation often follows. This resolution of inflammation requires wound healing and restoration of the lung's normal structure and function. Mechanisms for resolution of tissue inflammation are not as well established, but include substances such as sphingosine-1-phosphate for restoring endothelial barrier and vascular permeability after endotoxin injury or natural mediators derived from essential fatty acids such as ω-3 fatty acids with their anti-inflammatory and pro-resolving properties.[91] Cytokines such as IL-10, TGF-β, and IL-1 receptor antagonist have also been implicated as important mediators of inflammatory resolution. An inability to resolve inflammation can lead to chronic inflammation in the lung as seen in a number of pulmonary diseases.

ADAPTIVE IMMUNE RESPONSES IN THE LUNG

An essential prerequisite for a successful host immune response is the ability to discriminate between self and nonself.[92,93] Adaptive immune responses, which can also be described as acquired, refer to antigen-specific immunity that often takes several days to mature and to develop a targeted response to a specific antigen. Ultimately, the goal of this adaptive response is to react with, and subsequently remove, a specific antigen. This type of immunity is one that develops throughout life and is the premise behind vaccination for pulmonary infections caused by pathogens such as influenza virus and *Streptococcus pneumoniae*.[94,95] From an immunologic standpoint, an antigen is defined to be a substance that reacts to antibody molecules or antigen receptors on lymphocytes. For example, B cells recognize antigen through specific B cell receptor (BCR) (and in this case immunoglobulin [Ig]), while T cells recognize antigen through specific TCR.

This recognition is through specific epitopes on the antigen being recognized. For T cells to recognize antigenic epitopes through TCR, cells recognize peptide epitopes from antigen only when presented by APCs (e.g., DCs and macrophages) in the context of appropriate MHC molecules. Adaptive immune responses are often divided into two major branches: humoral immunity and cell-mediated immune responses. Humoral immune responses rely on the production of antibodies in response to encountered antigens and are mediated by B lymphocytes. Cell-mediated immune responses involve various immune cells such as T lymphocytes, cytotoxic T lymphocytes, activated macrophages, and/or activated NK cells. Activated macrophages and NK cells destroy intracellular pathogens and stimulate nearby structural cells to secrete cytokines that influence other cells of the immune system. Cytotoxic T lymphocytes (often $CD8^+$ cells) are capable of destroying host cells that display foreign antigens on the cell surface, such as cells infected with viruses or intracellular bacteria, or cancer cells that display tumor antigens.

The adaptive arm of the immune response relies on specific recognition of antigens by B and T lymphocytes. These cells are highly equipped to be specific because of their receptors, thus the immune system is capable of recognizing a large number of antigens. The functionality of adaptive immunity is based on specific gene rearrangement that results in the generation of over 10^{11} different species of antigen receptors on the cell surface of T and B cells.[96–98] In addition to adaptive immune responses, this defense system targets pathogens that have evolved mechanisms to evade or to counteract innate immune responses. Therefore, the adaptive immune response builds upon, is shaped by, and itself shapes innate immune responses resulting in a strong interplay between the innate and adaptive arms of our immune system.[99] Adaptive immunity helps protect the lungs not only against a range of pathogens, but environmental inhalants, such as cigarette smoke, dusts, as well as allergens. The adaptive immune response is quite versatile, relies on exquisite specificity, and takes advantage of robust memory. This is especially evident when it comes to countering airborne antigens. It is estimated that our human body has the ability to recognize 10^7 or more different epitopes and can make up to 10^9 different antibodies, each with different specificity. These epitopes are antigenic determinants that are part of the antigen that is recognized by the antibodies generated by B cells, or by receptors on B and T cells. To recognize the immense number of different epitopes, the human body produces 10^7 or more distinct clones of both B and T lymphocytes, each with their unique BCR or TCR, respectively.[85,100] Among the large variety of BCRs and TCRs, there is bound to be at least one that has the epitope-binding site capable to recognize any antigen the immune system eventually encounters. Thus, the body is able to recognize any conceivable antigen it may eventually encounter, allowing for an adaptive immune response. However, only a few B and or T cells can recognize any one epitope, and these cells require an appropriate stimulus to allow for rapid proliferation. This process typically takes several days to occur. During this time, to achieve an effective and mature adaptive immunity, the invading pathogen could cause considerable damage, which is why innate immune responses are important at the early stage of infection, unless the host has already encountered the antigen before and has developed a specific adaptive immune response against the antigen. In this situation, during a repeated encounter with an antigen, adaptive immunity, which already has an established memory response, will take a shorter period of time to mobilize the adaptive effector cells to counter the invading antigen.

A majority of T cells express TCR with $\alpha\beta$ variable chains, which permits them to recognize short peptide epitope of an antigen. Typically, precursor $\alpha\beta$ T cells are recruited out of the bone marrow to the thymus. In the thymus, they undergo the process of positive, then negative selection to assure that the resultant T cells appropriately respond to peptide in the context of self-MHC, but not strong enough to cause potentially damaging autoreactivity. It is also during this thymic maturation that the T cells acquire the expression of either CD4 (allowing it to recognize peptide in the context of class II MHC) or CD8 (allowing it to recognize peptide in the context of class I MHC). Of note, only a small fraction, <5% of all precursor T cells, complete this process of thymic education and maturation. These cells become naïve T cells that circulate throughout the host to encounter their specific antigen for antigenic stimulation. Thymus-independent T cells do exist and have been identified in the gut, but are less well understood in the lung. However, these cells are limited in their diversity and recirculatory capacity and cannot compensate for the lack of thymus-dependent T cells.[101]

T cell development occurs in the thymus where bone marrow–derived premature naïve T cell precursors congregate.[102–104] These T cells start off as double negative cells (CD4 and CD8 negative). Upon acquisition of successful rearrangement of α- and β-TCRs, as well as expression of both CD4 and CD8 (making them double positive cells), these developing T cells undergo positive and negative selection. Since TCRs recognize antigen only in the context of MHC molecules, T cells must be "educated" to first recognize host MHC. During positive selection, double positive T cells that can recognize self-MHCs are selected for proliferation, and those T cells that do not recognize self-MHCs are removed through apoptotic cell death pathways. Positive selection also assures that the appropriate TCR selection will associate with the appropriate CD4 or CD8. For example, TCRs specific for MHC class II need to retain CD4, and lose CD8. If the reverse occurs, they will die via apoptosis. The same is true for T cells that are specific for MHC class I, which need to retain CD8 and lose CD4. Single positive thymocytes (either $CD4^+$ or $CD8^+$) undergo negative selection to remove potential autoreactive cells. Those T cells that have high affinity for binding self-proteins presented on self-MHCs are induced to upregulate genes that drive apoptosis, eliminating them in the thymus. However, if they escape this elimination process, they may subsequently react against self-antigens, which can result in autoimmunity. Positive selection identifies T cells that react with self-MHC and self-antigen.[105] Negative selection eliminates those that react strongly with self-MHC and self-antigen. Therefore, a successful T cell differentiation selects for MHC restricted TCRs with low affinity for self-antigens.

The underlying premise of the adaptive immune response that allows the system to recognize an unlimited scope of antigens that the host ultimately can encounter is the generation of antigen receptor diversity through gene translocation and recombination processes.[106] This process helps shape each receptor (either TCRs on T cells or BCRs, or the Igs on B cells). The TCRs have α- and β-chains, where there are many different V and J genes that can make up the TCR α-chain, and many V, D, and J genes that can recombine to form the variable TCR β-chain. Similarly, BCR undergoes similar gene recombination, including junctional diversity and somatic hypermutation that help generate a wide scope of BCR diversity. In the end, each T or B cell will exhibit a unique receptor capable of recognizing its unique antigen. For B cells, the BCR (Ig) recognizes specific epitopes of the antigen. For T cells, $CD8^+$ or $CD4^+$ T cells will express unique cognate complementary shaped peptide that is bound to either MHC class I or MHC class II molecules, respectively.

GENERATION OF AN IMMUNE RESPONSE

Upon cognate recognition of T cells with antigen/peptide presented on MHC molecules on APCs, the activated lymphocytes rapidly proliferate to produce large clonal populations (Fig. 20-3). Circulating memory T cells have the capacity to persist in the host for a long time and become mobilized and reactivated during a repeat encounter with the same antigen. This subsequent exposure of antigen leads to a more rapid and persistent production of effector cells in a process called clonal expansion. This allows the limited

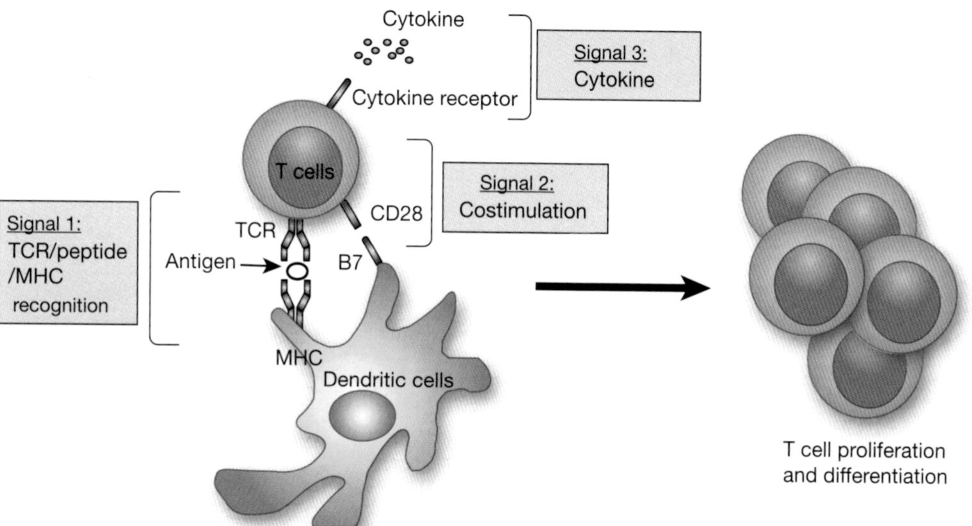

Figure 20-3 Generation of an immune response. Dendritic cells (DCs) and other antigen-presenting cells (such as macrophages) link the innate and adaptive immune response. DCs from the innate immune system present their antigen to naïve T cells at local draining lymph nodes; in the case of the respiratory tract, these are the mediastinal draining lymph nodes. T cell receptor (TCR) ligation to MHC molecules associated with peptides processed from antigen (e.g., pathogen, allergen, toxin) by DCs provide "signal 1." The binding of costimulatory molecule CD28 on lymphocyte to CD80 and CD86 expressed by DCs ("signal 2") leads to T cell activation and cell lineage differentiation. "Signal 3" is provided by the polarizing cytokine signals from nearby innate immune cells and local tissue environment. Depending on the type of antigen that is presented and the nature of cytokines in the microenvironment, innate DC cells direct the development of various T helper lymphocyte lineages that play crucial role in adaptive immune system.

T cell number, with the appropriate antigen recognition and specificity, to expand and proliferate when necessary. During adaptive immunity, pathogens encountered in the mucosal surfaces and, in the lung, the airway mucosa, are transported to draining lymphoid organs where antigen is recognized by naïve B and T lymphocytes, which leads to cell activation. These activated B and T cells proliferate and differentiate into effector cells.

Naïve T cells undergo development and maturation in the thymus and circulate out of the thymus to mucosal surfaces and lymph nodes to encounter antigens.[107,108] APCs, such as macrophages and DCs from the innate immune system, present endocytosed foreign antigen to naïve T cells at local draining lymph nodes. APCs present MHC class II–associated peptides processed from pathogens to CD4$^+$ T cells that express specific TCR against the particular antigen peptide/MHC complex. The TCR–CD3 complex binds to the antigen peptide MHC complex on APC, and this interaction triggers intracellular signaling pathways that provide the first signal, "signal 1," of T cell activation. Upon a subsequent encounter with the same antigen, memory T cells are reactivated using these same TCR pathways.[107] A second signal, "signal 2," is required to ensure that naïve T cells are responding to foreign antigen. This process involves binding of CD28 on lymphocytes to costimulatory molecules CD80 and CD86 that are expressed only by activated APCs. "Signal 2" leads to T cell lineage differentiation. Without "signal 2," during the initial antigen exposure, T cells become anergic and are unable to respond to subsequent antigen encounters, a process that avoids or minimizes production of autoreactive cells, and thus autoimmunity against self-antigens. Once T cells are activated by the two signals, only "signal 1" is required for subsequent future activation; an example of this is seen with memory T cells providing a faster immune response. After two-signal activation, Th cells proliferate and produce multiple cytokines, and this includes IL-2 production for autocrine activation by upregulation of the IL-2 receptor, CD25. "Signal 3" involves polarizing cytokine signaling from innate immune cells that allow for the development of specific types of immune responses.[109] Inflammatory cytokines such as IL-12 can act directly on naïve T cells to provide a third signal, along with antigen and IL-2, to optimally activate differentiation and clonal expansion. CD4$^+$ Th cells play an important role in mediating various types of immune responses through their cytokine release. There are also other CD4-expressing T cells that are not Th cells; these include some cytotoxic T cells, NKT cells, and regulatory T (Treg) cells.

■ ACTIVATION OF NAÏVE HELPER T CELLS

CD4$^+$ T cells play an important role in adaptive immune responses. Proliferating Th cells that develop into effector T cells can differentiate into one of several lineages (Fig. 20-4).[110] Depending on the type of antigen that is presented, the strength of the TCR signal, and the nature of cytokines in the microenvironment, innate APCs (typically DCs) direct the development of various Th lymphocyte lineages. The differentiation of each CD4$^+$ T cell subset is associated with the expression of specific transcription factors that lead to production of an array of cytokines that help orchestrate a specific host response. CD4$^+$ Th cells, based on their cytokine production, help dictate this type of response. The most studied and established Th subset is the dichotomy between type 1 and type 2 responses, often called T helper 1 (Th1) and T helper 2 (Th2) responses.

Th1 cells promote cell-mediated immune responses and are required for host defense against viral and intracellular bacterial pathogens. Th1 responses can be characterized by the secretion of IFN-γ, IL-12, IL-10, and TNF-α/β, and stimulation of classically activating macrophages to tackle intracellular pathogens.[111] These cytokines promote macrophage activation, nitric oxide production, and cytotoxic T lymphocyte proliferation, leading to phagocytosis and destruction of microbial pathogens. Th1 responses in the lung are important because AMs encounter antigens to activate these specific effector responses. IL-27 signaling in naïve CD4$^+$ T cells induces STAT1-dependent expression of the Th1-specific transcription factor, T-bet, which promotes expression of IFN-γ and IL-12 receptors. Subsequent activation stimulates STAT4-dependent

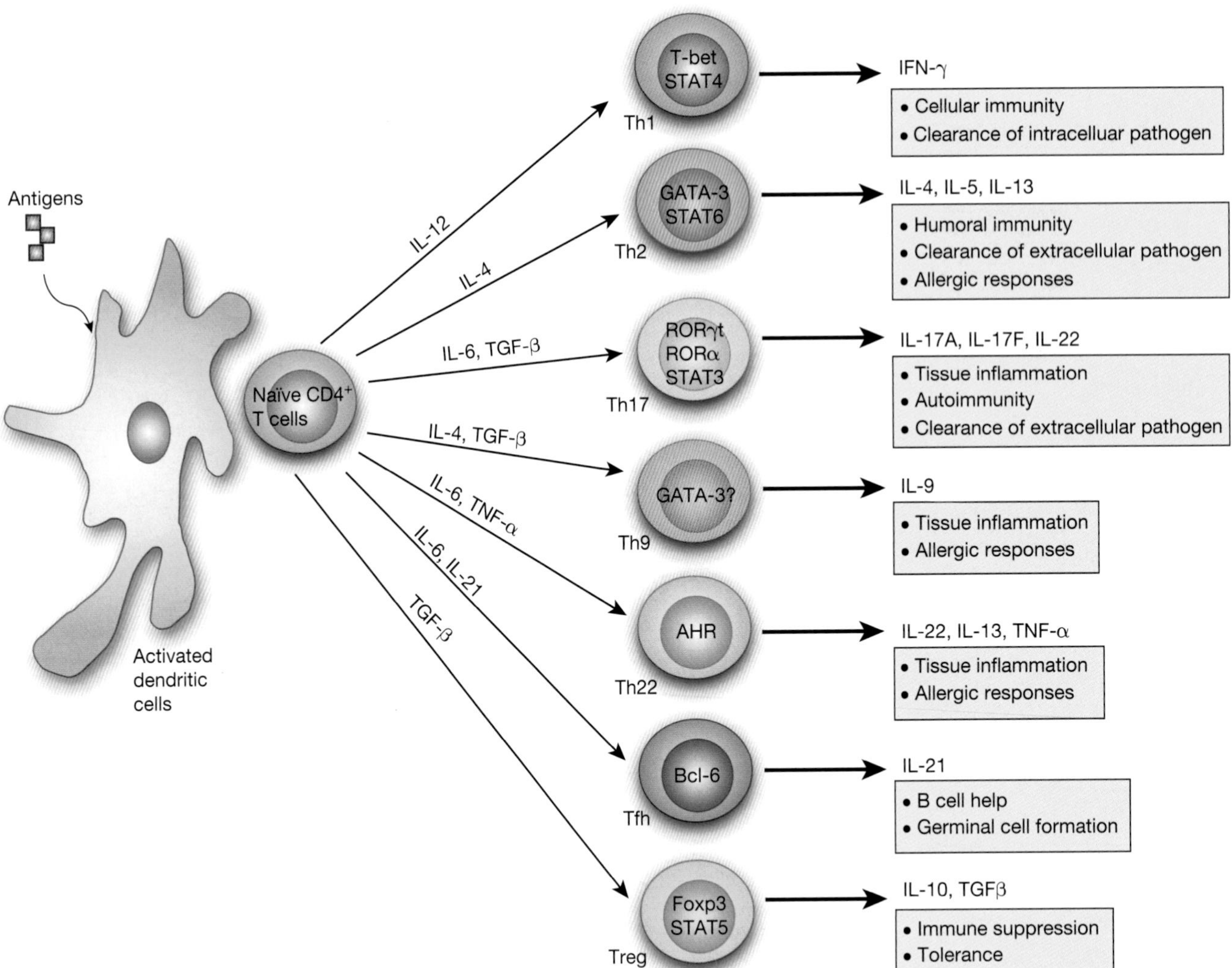

Figure 20-4 T cell differentiation. Naïve CD4$^+$ T cells differentiate into one of several T helper (Th) cell lineage based on signals from innate immune cells induced by antigenic and inflammatory stimuli as presented by activated DCs. The resultant products of differentiated T cells subsequently help tailor the immune response to various encountered antigen scenario. Th cell differentiation is classically regarded as a dichotomy between two main cell types, termed Th1 and Th2. Th1 cells produce IFN-γ as the signature cytokine and are predominantly involved in cell-mediated immunity against intracellular pathogens. In contrast, Th2 cells do not produce IFN-γ and instead produce IL-4, IL-5, and IL-13. Th2 cells are effective activators of B cell proliferation and antibody production, mediating humoral immunity essential for the eradication of extracellular pathogens as well as mediating allergic type of inflammation. Th17 cells have been described as a distinct Th subset characterized by the production of IL-17A, IL-17F, and IL-22, contributing to host defence against extracellular pathogens particularly on mucosal surfaces, as well as in the pathogenesis of autoimmune diseases. Recently, more Th cell subsets have been described such as Th9 and Th22 cells that participate in allergic type of immune responses. Other stimuli cause CD4$^+$ T cells to become regulatory T (Treg) cells that help dampen immune responses. Other stimuli allow CD4$^+$ T cells to reside in lymph nodes, differentiate into follicular helper T (Tfh) cells and provide help to B cells. The various Th subsets require activation of specific master regulator transcription factors such as T-bet, GATA-3, RORγt, Bcl-6, and Foxp3 as well as various STAT molecules for their differentiation as indicated in the diagram. Bcl-6, B cell lymphoma-6; Foxp3, forkhead box p3; ROR, retinoid-related orphan receptor; AHR, aryl hydrocarbon receptor; STAT, signal transducer and activation of transcription.

IFN-γ production and Th1 differentiation. While Th1 cells are critical for the clearance of intracellular pathogens, exaggerated Th1 responses can result in lung pathology (e.g., autoimmune disease, interstitial lung disease, and COPD). Th2 responses are characterized by production of IL-4, IL-5, IL-9, IL-13, and IL-25, and these cytokines favor antibody production and class switching to IgE and IgG. Th2 cells are required for humoral immunity and play an important role in coordinating immune responses to extracellular pathogens.[112] Th2 differentiation occurs in the presence of IL-4 and either IL-2, IL-7, or thymic stromal lymphopoietin (TSLP). IL-4 stimulates naïve CD4$^+$ T cells to induce STAT6-dependent expression of GATA-3, the transcriptional regulator of Th2 cells, which promotes IL-5 and IL-13 expression, and stimulates the expansion of Th2 cells, while suppressing the differentiation of other T cell subtypes. In addition to IL-4–induced activation of GATA-3, IL-2, IL-7, or TSLP is required during Th2 differentiation to activate STAT5, which cooperates with GATA-3 to promote T cell production of IL-4. IL-4 regulates clonal expansion of Th2 cells and, along with IL-13, promotes B cell production of IgE and alternative macrophage activation. Th2 cells also produce IL-5 to stimulate eosinophil activation and survival, or IL-9 to promote mast cell activation. Th2 responses are typically important host immune responses to extracellular pathogens such as parasites or helminths. However, excessive Th2 signaling has been implicated in the development of chronic allergic inflammation and asthma.

T helper 17 (Th17) cells are involved in the immune response against specific fungi and extracellular bacteria.[113] Th17 cells develop from naïve $CD4^+$ T cells in the presence of TGF-β and IL-6, cytokines that induce STAT3-dependent expression of IL-21 and the transcription factor RORγt. IL-21 and IL-23 help establish, regulate, and develop (via clonal expansion) Th17 cells. RORγt-induced gene expression leads to the secretion of IL-17A, IL-17F, and IL-22. Cytokines secreted by Th17 cells stimulate chemokine secretion by resident cells, leading to the recruitment of neutrophils and macrophages to sites of inflammation. These cells produce additional cytokines and proteases that further augment immune responses. For human Th17 differentiation, Th17 polarization requires IL-1β, IL-6, IL-21, and IL-23, and is less dependent upon TGF-β. While Th17 cells play a central role in eliminating harmful microbes, persistent secretion of Th17 cytokines can promote chronic inflammation and has been implicated in lung diseases such as COPD, sarcoidosis, and granulomatous diseases. The role of cytokine polarization in lung diseases has been studied in transgenic animal modeling systems where specific cytokines are over-expressed, or cytokine receptors or transcriptional factors such as GATA-3 and T-bet are modified. These studies have helped to elucidate the effector function of individual cytokines and their pathophysiologic consequences in the lung.[114]

T helper 9 (Th9) cells secrete high levels of IL-9, CCL17, CCL22, and in mouse, IL-10. Th9 cell differentiation requires the presence of TGF-β and IL-4, which induce transcription factors PU.1/Spi-1 and IRF 4 that regulate IL-9.[115] Cytokines such as IL-1β, IL-6, IL-21, and type I interferons all enhance Th9 differentiation, and IL-2 and IL-25 promote IL-9 secretion. Different from Th2 cells, Th9 cells do not express IL-4, IL-5, or IL-13. Th9 cells are important for host defense against parasitic and helminthic infections, but they are also associated with the development of chronic allergic inflammation, airway remodeling, and autoimmune diseases.[115,116] T helper 22 (Th22) cells primarily secrete IL-22, IL-13, and TNF-α. Similar to Th17 cells, Th22 cells express IL-22, but in contrast, they express several fibroblast growth factors (FGFs) and do not express IL-17, IL-4 (Th2 marker), or IFN-γ (Th1 marker).[117] Th22 cells differentiate in the presence of IL-6 and TNF-α, and their differentiation is inhibited by TGF-β.[118] Th22 cells can be regulated by the aryl hydrocarbon receptor (AHR) transcription factor. IL-22 secreted by Th22 cells primarily affects epithelial and stromal cells rather than other hematopoietic cells, which lack a functional IL-22 receptor. Th22 cells contribute to allergic inflammation in the lung, but their role in skin immunity is better established.

Another subset of $CD4^+$ T helper cells are follicular helper T cells (Tfh) which regulate the development of antigen-specific B cell immunity.[119,120] These Tfh cells help B cells generate antibody-producing plasma cells and long-lived memory B cells. Tfh cells are identified by Bcl-6 (a transcriptional repressor) expression and IL-21 secretion. IL-6 and autocrine IL-21 signaling induce Th cells to express Bcl-6, which controls Tfh cell differentiation and suppresses differentiation of Th1, Th2, and Th17 cells. These Tfh cells have been implicated in several autoimmune diseases, including systemic lupus erythematosus and Sjögren syndrome. The actions of Th cells are balanced by Treg cells, a subpopulation of CD4-expressing cells that specializes in suppression of T cell–mediated immune responses.[121,122] Treg cells are identified by their expression of CD25 and the transcription factor Foxp3. Treg cells are capable of regulating and suppressing immune responses. They produce cytokines such as TGF-β and IL-10 that have immune suppressive activities. Of note, failure to activate an appropriate T cell response can lead to chronic infection, while exaggerated T cell responses can cause excessive tissue damage and are associated with inflammatory and autoimmune diseases. During lung infections, Th1 may mediate lung damage in response to infection. Thus, downregulation of such Th1 responses may help preserve lung integrity. Th2 responses are known to be important during the wound healing process, but if this response is prolonged and uncontrolled, it can worsen the injury and contribute to fibrosis.

Considering the diverse and important roles Th cells play in the immune system, it is not surprising that these cells influence the immune response in many pulmonary diseases. Th cells can make occasional mistakes or generate responses that would be considered harmful. In the worst-case scenario, Th cell responses may be disastrous and prove fatal to the host. Fortunately, this is a very rare occurrence. The adaptive immune system must achieve a balance of sensitivity to respond appropriately to foreign antigens, without responding to host antigens and damaging self. When the immune system responds to very low antigen levels that it should not respond to, a hypersensitivity response, such as seen in airway allergies and autoimmune lung diseases, ensues. There are four general types of hypersensitivity reactions that have been described: Type 1 reactions, such as in asthma and allergic lung diseases, involve IgE antibodies and a Th2 response; Type 2 and Type 3 hypersensitivity responses involve the role of autoimmune and low affinity antibodies (and, in some instances, it is felt that Th2 cytokines promote such disorders); and Type 4 reactions, also known as delayed-type hypersensitivity, are the result of chronic inflammation and activation of lymphocytes and macrophages, typically a Th1 cytokine response. Another T cell subtype more recently discovered and less well studied is the γδ T cell subset.[123,124] These T cells have TCR with γδ-chains, rather than the conventional TCR chains. They represent 1% to 5% of circulating lymphocytes and are often found in mucosal surfaces, such as the airways. γδ TCRs have more limited repertoire diversity, and are considered, at times, invariant because they are only able to recognize limited types of antigens. These γδ T cells have been shown to be important in maintaining normal airway responsiveness or tone, as well as in their immunoregulatory role in numerous infectious and noninfectious diseases in the lung.[123,125]

CONCLUSIONS

The lung is a vast organ composed of conducting airways, alveoli, and tissue parenchyma that is highly specialized to sample the diverse antigens that we breathe in. The lung is equipped with a well-orchestrated immune system to clear particulate debris and to eliminate inhaled pathogens and toxins to protect the delicate capillary–alveolar barrier system that is critical for gas exchange. The immune system in the lung has evolved complex and diverse innate and adaptive immune responses to accomplish these critical functions of host defense.

REFERENCES

1. Thompson AB, Robbins RA, Romberger DJ, et al. Immunological functions of the pulmonary epithelium. *Eur Respir J.* 1995;8(1):127–149.
2. Hirota JA, Knight DA. Human airway epithelial cell innate immunity: relevance to asthma. *Curr Opin Immunol.* 2012;24(6):740–746.
3. Corthésy B. Role of secretory immunoglobulin A and secretory component in the protection of mucosal surfaces. *Future Microbiol.* 2010;5(5):817–829.
4. Bartlett JA, Fischer AJ, McCray PB Jr. Innate immune functions of the airway epithelium. *Contrib Microbiol.* 2008;15:147–163.
5. Storm van's Gravesande K, Omran H. Primary ciliary dyskinesia: clinical presentation, diagnosis and genetics. *Ann Med.* 2005;37(6):439–449.

6. Hartl D, Gaggar A, Bruscia E, et al. Innate immunity in cystic fibrosis lung disease. *J Cyst Fibros.* 2012;11(5):363–382.
7. Lobo J, Rojas-Balcazar JM, Noone PG. Recent advances in cystic fibrosis. *Clin Chest Med.* 2012;33(2):307–328.
8. McCormack FX, Whitsett JA. The pulmonary collectins, SP-A and SP-D, orchestrate innate immunity in the lung. *J Clin Invest.* 2002;109(6):707–712.
9. Hickman-Davis JM, Fang FC, Nathan C, Shepherd VL, Voelker DR, Wright JR. Lung surfactant and reactive oxygen-nitrogen species: antimicrobial activity and host-pathogen interactions. *Am J Physiol Lung Cell Mol Physiol.* 2001;281(3):L517–L523.
10. Janeway CA Jr. Approaching the asymptote? Evolution and revolution in immunology. *Cold Spring Harb Symp Quant Biol.* 1989;54 Pt 1:1–13.
11. Medzhitov R. Approaching the asymptote: 20 years later. *Immunity.* 2009;30(6):766–775.
12. Lemaitre B, Nicolas E, Michaut L, Reichhart JM, Hoffmann JA. The dorsoventral regulatory gene cassette spätzle/Toll/cactus controls the potent antifungal response in Drosophila adults. *Cell.* 1996;86(6):973–983.
13. Medzhitov R, Preston-Hurlburt P, Janeway CA Jr. A human homologue of the Drosophila Toll protein signals activation of adaptive immunity. *Nature.* 1997;388(6640):394–397.
14. Casanova JL, Abel L, Quintana-Murci L. Human TLRs and IL-1Rs in host defense: natural insights from evolutionary, epidemiological, and clinical genetics. *Annu Rev Immunol.* 2011; 29:447–491.
15. Kovach MA, Standiford TJ. Toll like receptors in diseases of the lung. *Int Immunopharmacol.* 2011;11(10):1399–1406.
16. Puel A, Yang K, Ku CL, et al. Heritable defects of the human TLR signalling pathways. *J Endotoxin Res.* 2005;11(4):220–224.
17. Poltorak A, He X, Smirnova I, et al. Defective LPS signaling in C3H/HeJ and C57BL/10ScCr mice: mutations in Tlr4 gene. *Science.* 1998;282(5396):2085–2088.
18. Netea MG, van der Meer JW. Immunodeficiency and genetic defects of pattern-recognition receptors. *N Engl J Med.* 2011; 364(1):60–70.
19. Takeuchi O, Akira S. Pattern recognition receptors and inflammation. *Cell.* 2010;140(6):805–820.
20. Kagan JC, Su T, Horng T, Chow A, Akira S, Medzhitov R. TRAM couples endocytosis of Toll-like receptor 4 to the induction of interferon-beta. *Nat Immunol.* 2008;9(4):361–368.
21. Loo YM, Gale M Jr. Immune signaling by RIG-I-like receptors. *Immunity.* 2011;34(5):680–692.
22. Gerlier D, Lyles DS. Interplay between innate immunity and negative-strand RNA viruses: towards a rational model. *Microbiol Mol Biol Rev.* 2011;75(3):468–490, second page of table of contents.
23. Isaacs A, Lindenmann J. Virus interference. I. The interferon. *Proc R Soc Lond B Biol Sci.* 1957;147(927):258–267.
24. Colby C, Chamberlin MJ. The specificity of interferon induction in chick embryo cells by helical RNA. *Proc Natl Acad Sci U S A.* 1969;63(1):160–167.
25. Sun YW. RIG-I, a human homolog gene of RNA helicase, is induced by retinoic acid during the differentiation of acute promyelocytic leukemia cell [Thesis]. Shanghai: Shanghai Second Medical University; 1997.
26. Barral PM, Sarkar D, Su ZZ, et al. Functions of the cytoplasmic RNA sensors RIG-I and MDA-5: key regulators of innate immunity. *Pharmacol Ther.* 2009;124(2):219–234.
27. Yoneyama M, Kikuchi M, Natsukawa T, et al. The RNA helicase RIG-I has an essential function in double-stranded RNA-induced innate antiviral responses. *Nat Immunol.* 2004;5(7):730–737.
28. Huang F, Adelman J, Jiang H, Goldstein NI, Fisher PB. Differentiation induction subtraction hybridization (DISH): a strategy for cloning genes displaying differential expression during growth arrest and terminal differentiation. *Gene.* 1999; 236(1):125–131.
29. Kang DC, Gopalkrishnan RV, Wu Q, Jankowsky E, Pyle AM, Fisher PB. mda-5: an interferon-inducible putative RNA helicase with double-stranded RNA-dependent ATPase activity and melanoma growth-suppressive properties. *Proc Natl Acad Sci U S A.* 2002;99(2):637–642.
30. Komuro A, Horvath CM. RNA- and virus-independent inhibition of antiviral signaling by RNA helicase LGP2. *J Virol.* 2006;80(24):12332–12342.
31. Takeuchi O, Akira S. Innate immunity to virus infection. *Immunol Rev.* 2009;227(1):75–86.
32. Seth RB, Sun L, Ea CK, Chen ZJ. Identification and characterization of MAVS, a mitochondrial antiviral signaling protein that activates NF-kappaB and IRF 3. *Cell.* 2005;122(5):669–682.
33. Inohara N, Nuñez G. The NOD: a signaling module that regulates apoptosis and host defense against pathogens. *Oncogene.* 2001;20(44):6473–6481.
34. Kanneganti TD, Lamkanfi M, Núñez G. Intracellular NOD-like receptors in host defense and disease. *Immunity.* 2007; 27(4):549–559.
35. Hysi P, Kabesch M, Moffatt MF, et al. NOD1 variation, immunoglobulin E and asthma. *Hum Mol Genet.* 2005;14(7):935–941.
36. Hugot JP, Chamaillard M, Zouali H, et al. Association of NOD2 leucine-rich repeat variants with susceptibility to Crohn's disease. *Nature.* 2001;411(6837):599–603.
37. Kleinnijenhuis J, Oosting M, Joosten LA, Netea MG, Van Crevel R. Innate immune recognition of Mycobacterium tuberculosis. *Clin Dev Immunol.* 2011;2011:405310.
38. Kutikhin AG. Association of polymorphisms in TLR genes and in genes of the Toll-like receptor signaling pathway with cancer risk. *Hum Immunol.* 2011;72(11):1095–1116.
39. Davis BK, Wen H, Ting JP. The inflammasome NLRs in immunity, inflammation, and associated diseases. *Annu Rev Immunol.* 2011;29:707–735.
40. Thomas PG, Dash P, Aldridge JR Jr, et al. The intracellular sensor NLRP3 mediates key innate and healing responses to influenza A virus via the regulation of caspase-1. *Immunity.* 2009;30(4):566–575.
41. Ichinohe T, Lee HK, Ogura Y, Flavell R, Iwasaki A. Inflammasome recognition of influenza virus is essential for adaptive immune responses. *J Exp Med.* 2009;206(1):79–87.
42. Harder J, Franchi L, Muñoz-Planillo R, Park JH, Reimer T, Núñez G. Activation of the Nlrp3 inflammasome by Streptococcus pyogenes requires streptolysin O and NF-kappa B activation but proceeds independently of TLR signaling and P2×7 receptor. *J Immunol.* 2009;183(9):5823–5829.
43. Dela Cruz CS, Liu W, He CH, et al. Chitinase 3-like-1 promotes Streptococcus pneumoniae killing and augments host tolerance to lung antibacterial responses. *Cell Host Microbe.* 2012;12(1):34–46.
44. Sutterwala FS, Mijares LA, Li L, Ogura Y, Kazmierczak BI, Flavell RA. Immune recognition of Pseudomonas aeruginosa mediated by the IPAF/NLRC4 inflammasome. *J Exp Med.* 2007; 204(13):3235–3245.

45. Master SS, Rampini SK, Davis AS, et al. Mycobacterium tuberculosis prevents inflammasome activation. *Cell Host Microbe.* 2008;3(4):224–232.

46. Kool M, Willart MA, van Nimwegen M, et al. An unexpected role for uric acid as an inducer of T helper 2 cell immunity to inhaled antigens and inflammatory mediator of allergic asthma. *Immunity.* 2011;34(4):527–540.

47. Doz E, Noulin N, Boichot E, et al. Cigarette smoke-induced pulmonary inflammation is TLR4/MyD88 and IL-1R1/MyD88 signaling dependent. *J Immunol.* 2008;180(2):1169–1178.

48. Gasse P, Mary C, Guenon I, et al. IL-1R1/MyD88 signaling and the inflammasome are essential in pulmonary inflammation and fibrosis in mice. *J Clin Invest.* 2007;117(12):3786–3799.

49. Zelensky AN, Gready JE. The C-type lectin-like domain superfamily. *FEBS J.* 2005;272(24):6179–6217.

50. Kerrigan AM, Brown GD. Syk-coupled C-type lectins in immunity. *Trends Immunol.* 2011;32(4):151–156.

51. Saijo S, Iwakura Y. Dectin-1 and Dectin-2 in innate immunity against fungi. *Int Immunol.* 2011;23(8):467–472.

52. Geijtenbeek TB, Gringhuis SI. Signalling through C-type lectin receptors: shaping immune responses. *Nat Rev Immunol.* 2009;9(7):465–479.

53. Fraser IP, Koziel H, Ezekowitz RA. The serum mannose-binding protein and the macrophage mannose receptor are pattern recognition molecules that link innate and adaptive immunity. *Semin Immunol.* 1998;10(5):363–372.

54. Pattle RE. Properties, function and origin of the alveolar lining layer. *Nature.* 1955;175(4469):1125–1126.

55. Drickamer K, Dordal MS, Reynolds L. Mannose-binding proteins isolated from rat liver contain carbohydrate-recognition domains linked to collagenous tails. Complete primary structures and homology with pulmonary surfactant apoprotein. *J Biol Chem.* 1986;261(15):6878–6887.

56. Kuroki Y, Takahashi M, Nishitani C. Pulmonary collectins in innate immunity of the lung. *Cell Microbiol.* 2007;9(8):1871–1879.

57. Parker D, Prince A. Innate immunity in the respiratory epithelium. *Am J Respir Cell Mol Biol.* 2011;45(2):189–201.

58. Barnes PJ. Chronic obstructive pulmonary disease. *N Engl J Med.* 2000;343(4):269–280.

59. Carrell RW, Lomas DA. Alpha1-antitrypsin deficiency–a model for conformational diseases. *N Engl J Med.* 2002;346(1): 45–53.

60. Ganz T. Defensins: antimicrobial peptides of innate immunity. *Nat Rev Immunol.* 2003;3(9):710–720.

61. Yang D, Biragyn A, Hoover DM, Lubkowski J, Oppenheim JJ. Multiple roles of antimicrobial defensins, cathelicidins, and eosinophil-derived neurotoxin in host defense. *Annu Rev Immunol.* 2004;22:181–215.

62. Tecle T, Tripathi S, Hartshorn KL. Review: defensins and cathelicidins in lung immunity. *Innate Immun.* 2010;16(3): 151–159.

63. Spits H, Cupedo T. Innate lymphoid cells: emerging insights in development, lineage relationships, and function. *Annu Rev Immunol.* 2012;30:647–675.

64. Walker JA, McKenzie A. Innate lymphoid cells in the airways. *Eur J Immunol.* 2012;42(6):1368–1374.

65. Spits H, Artis D, Colonna M, et al. Innate lymphoid cells–a proposal for uniform nomenclature. *Nat Rev Immunol.* 2013; 13(2):145–149.

66. Plüddemann A, Mukhopadhyay S, Gordon S. Innate immunity to intracellular pathogens: macrophage receptors and responses to microbial entry. *Immunol Rev.* 2011;240(1):11–24.

67. Wynn TA, Chawla A, Pollard JW. Macrophage biology in development, homeostasis and disease. *Nature.* 2013;496(7446):445–455.

68. Pedace EA, Bachmann AE, Ruiz-Morena G. Contribution to the study of the reticulo endothelial origin of dust cells or alveolar macrophagi. VI. Some histochemical aspects in the lungs of normal guinea pigs, and others submitted to acetylcholine, histamine, or anaphylactic shock, and so-called experimental asthma. *J Allergy.* 1952;23(3):265–276.

69. Lehnert BE, Valdez YE, Holland LM. Pulmonary macrophages: alveolar and interstitial populations. *Exp Lung Res.* 1985;9(3–4): 177–190.

70. Guilliams M, Lambrecht BN, Hammad H. Division of labor between lung dendritic cells and macrophages in the defense against pulmonary infections. *Mucosal Immunol.* 2013;6(3): 464–473.

71. Lambrecht BN. Alveolar macrophage in the driver's seat. *Immunity.* 2006;24(4):366–368.

72. Stafford JL, Neumann NF, Belosevic M. Macrophage-mediated innate host defense against protozoan parasites. *Crit Rev Microbiol.* 2002;28(3):187–248.

73. Poole JA, Gleason AM, Bauer C, et al. CD11c(+)/CD11b(+) cells are critical for organic dust-elicited murine lung inflammation. *Am J Respir Cell Mol Biol.* 2012;47(5):652–659.

74. Strickland DH, Thepen T, Kees UR, Kraal G, Holt PG. Regulation of T-cell function in lung tissue by pulmonary alveolar macrophages. *Immunology.* 1993;80(2):266–272.

75. Webb TJ, Sumpter TL, Thiele AT, Swanson KA, Wilkes DS. The phenotype and function of lung dendritic cells. *Crit Rev Immunol.* 2005;25(6):465–491.

76. Lambrecht BN, Hammad H. Lung dendritic cells in respiratory viral infection and asthma: from protection to immunopathology. *Annu Rev Immunol.* 2012;30:243–270.

77. Hammad H, Lambrecht BN. Dendritic cells and airway epithelial cells at the interface between innate and adaptive immune responses. *Allergy.* 2011;66(5):579–587.

78. Lambrecht BN, Hammad H. Biology of lung dendritic cells at the origin of asthma. *Immunity.* 2009;31(3):412–424.

79. Pollard AM, Lipscomb MF. Characterization of murine lung dendritic cells: similarities to Langerhans cells and thymic dendritic cells. *J Exp Med.* 1990;172(1):159–167.

80. Demedts IK, Brusselle GG, Vermaelen KY, Pauwels RA. Identification and characterization of human pulmonary dendritic cells. *Am J Respir Cell Mol Biol.* 2005;32(3):177–184.

81. Van Pottelberge GR, Bracke KR, Joos GF, Brusselle GG. The role of dendritic cells in the pathogenesis of COPD: liaison officers in the front line. *COPD.* 2009;6(4):284–290.

82. Iwasaki A. Mucosal dendritic cells. *Annu Rev Immunol.* 2007;25: 381–418.

83. Baratelli FE, Heuzé-Vourc'h N, Krysan K, et al. Prostaglandin E2-dependent enhancement of tissue inhibitors of metalloproteinases-1 production limits dendritic cell migration through extracellular matrix. *J Immunol.* 2004;173(9):5458–5466.

84. Nathan C. Neutrophils and immunity: challenges and opportunities. *Nat Rev Immunol.* 2006;6(3):173–182.

85. Parkin J, Cohen B. An overview of the immune system. *Lancet.* 2001;357(9270):1777–1789.

86. Abraham E. Neutrophils and acute lung injury. *Crit Care Med.* 2003;31(4 Suppl):S195–S199.

87. Ricevuti G. Host tissue damage by phagocytes. *Ann N Y Acad Sci.* 1997;832:426–448.

88. Swain SD, Rohn TT, Quinn MT. Neutrophil priming in host defense: role of oxidants as priming agents. *Antioxid Redox Signal.* 2002;4(1):69–83.

89. DeLeo FR, Renee J, McCormick S, et al. Neutrophils exposed to bacterial lipopolysaccharide upregulate NADPH oxidase assembly. *J Clin Invest.* 1998;101(2):455–463.

90. Lee A, Whyte MK, Haslett C. Inhibition of apoptosis and prolongation of neutrophil functional longevity by inflammatory mediators. *J Leukoc Biol.* 1993;54(4):283–288.

91. Levy BD, Vachier I, Serhan CN. Resolution of inflammation in asthma. *Clin Chest Med.* 2012;33(3):559–570.

92. Sprent J, Cho JH. Self/non-self discrimination and the problem of keeping T cells alive. *Immunol Cell Biol.* 2008;86(1):54–56.

93. Sioud M. Innate sensing of self and non-self RNAs by Toll-like receptors. *Trends Mol Med.* 2006;12(4):167–176.

94. Braciale TJ, Sun J, Kim TS. Regulating the adaptive immune response to respiratory virus infection. *Nat Rev Immunol.* 2012;12(4):295–305.

95. Krishna S, Miller LS. Innate and adaptive immune responses against Staphylococcus aureus skin infections. *Semin Immunopathol.* 2012;34(2):261–280.

96. Strominger JL. Developmental biology of T cell receptors. *Science.* 1989;244(4907):943–950.

97. Kreuwel HT, Sherman LA. The T-cell repertoire available for recognition of self-antigens. *Curr Opin Immunol.* 2001;13(6): 639–643.

98. Herzog S, Jumaa H. Self-recognition and clonal selection: autoreactivity drives the generation of B cells. *Curr Opin Immunol.* 2012;24(2):166–172.

99. Medzhitov R, Janeway CA Jr. Innate immune recognition and control of adaptive immune responses. *Semin Immunol.* 1998;10(5):351–353.

100. Turner SJ, La Gruta NL, Kedzierska K, Thomas PG, Doherty PC. Functional implications of T cell receptor diversity. *Curr Opin Immunol.* 2009;21(3):286–290.

101. Goud SN, Kaplan AM, Subbarao B. Primary antibody responses to thymus-independent antigens in the lungs and hilar lymph nodes of mice. *Infect Immun.* 1990;58(7):2035–2041.

102. Koch U, Radtke F. Mechanisms of T cell development and transformation. *Annu Rev Cell Dev Biol.* 2011;27:539–562.

103. Ciofani M, Zúñiga-Pflücker JC. A survival guide to early T cell development. *Immunol Res.* 2006;34(2):117–132.

104. Ciofani M, Zúñiga-Pflücker JC. Determining $\gamma\delta$ versus $\alpha\beta$ T cell development. *Nat Rev Immunol.* 2010;10(9):657–663.

105. Starr TK, Jameson SC, Hogquist KA. Positive and negative selection of T cells. *Annu Rev Immunol.* 2003;21:139–176.

106. Nishana M, Raghavan SC. Role of recombination activating genes in the generation of antigen receptor diversity and beyond. *Immunology.* 2012;137(4):271–281.

107. Bretscher P. The two-signal model of lymphocyte activation twenty-one years later. *Immunol Today.* 1992;13(2):74–76.

108. Rothenberg EV. Cell lineage regulators in B and T cell development. *Nat Immunol.* 2007;8(5):441–444.

109. Keppler SJ, Rosenits K, Koegl T, Vucikuja S, Aichele P. Signal 3 cytokines as modulators of primary immune responses during infections: the interplay of type I IFN and IL-12 in CD8 T cell responses. *PLoS One.* 2012;7(7):e40865.

110. Zhu J, Paul WE. Heterogeneity and plasticity of T helper cells. *Cell Res.* 2010;20(1):4–12.

111. Damsker JM, Hansen AM, Caspi RR. Th1 and Th17 cells: adversaries and collaborators. *Ann N Y Acad Sci.* 2010;1183: 211–221.

112. Paul WE. What determines Th2 differentiation, in vitro and in vivo? *Immunol Cell Biol.* 2010;88(3):236–239.

113. Kuchroo VK, Awasthi A. Emerging new roles of Th17 cells. *Eur J Immunol.* 2012;42(9):2211–2214.

114. Dela Cruz CS, Kang MJ, Cho WK, Lee CG. Transgenic modelling of cytokine polarization in the lung. *Immunology.* 2011;132(1):9–17.

115. Tan C, Gery I. The unique features of Th9 cells and their products. *Crit Rev Immunol.* 2012;32(1):1–10.

116. Stassen M, Schmitt E, Bopp T. From interleukin-9 to T helper 9 cells. *Ann N Y Acad Sci.* 2012;1247:56–68.

117. Akdis M, Palomares O, van de Veen W, van Splunter M, Akdis CA. TH17 and TH22 cells: a confusion of antimicrobial response with tissue inflammation versus protection. *J Allergy Clin Immunol.* 2012;129(6):1438–1449; quiz1450–1431.

118. Zhang N, Pan HF, Ye DQ. Th22 in inflammatory and autoimmune disease: prospects for therapeutic intervention. *Mol Cell Biochem.* 2011;353(1–2):41–46.

119. Crotty S. Follicular helper CD4 T cells (TFH). *Annu Rev Immunol.* 2011;29:621–663.

120. King C. New insights into the differentiation and function of T follicular helper cells. *Nat Rev Immunol.* 2009;9(11): 757–766.

121. Ohkura N, Kitagawa Y, Sakaguchi S. Development and maintenance of regulatory T cells. *Immunity.* 2013;38(3):414–423.

122. Shevach EM. Biological functions of regulatory T cells. *Adv Immunol.* 2011;112:137–176.

123. Born WK, Lahn M, Takeda K, Kanehiro A, O'Brien RL, Gelfand EW. Role of gammadelta T cells in protecting normal airway function. *Respir Res.* 2000;1(3):151–158.

124. Haas W, Pereira P, Tonegawa S. Gamma/delta cells. *Annu Rev Immunol.* 1993;11:637–685.

125. Carding SR, Egan PJ. Gammadelta T cells: functional plasticity and heterogeneity. *Nat Rev Immunol.* 2002;2(5):336–345.

CHAPTER 21

Lymphocyte- and Macrophage-Mediated Inflammation in the Lung

Praveen Govender
Frederic F. Little
Kevin C. Wilson
David M. Center

INTRODUCTION

The lung receives a continual flow of foreign infectious and non-infectious antigens during respiration. Like the gut, genitourinary tract, and skin the lung is one of the interfaces of the sterile body with the environment. The lung's immune defense system and inflammatory mechanisms are poised to deal with this role. In this chapter we will consider the inflammatory and immune roles of two key cells of hematopoietic origin: the lung lymphocyte and the lung macrophage.

While these two cell types interact extensively and might even be considered co-dependent in many situations, they represent two very different arms of the inflammatory response. The macrophage, as a phagocytic cell, is of ancient phylogenetic lineage. It is a sentinel of the innate immune system. As such, it is not antigen specific but it is triggered by many inflammatory stimuli through both specific and pattern recognition receptors. Lymphocytes are present only in vertebrates and represent a significant refinement in the inflammatory response by the ability to recognize and adapt to specific antigens and discriminate between self and nonself. The functional distinction between these two arms of the immune system is blurring with the recent discovery of innate lymphoid-derived immune cells and the appreciation of multiple functions of macrophages in the inflammatory response.

Macrophages or dendritic cells (DCs) are required for optimal presentation of antigens to lymphocytes, and for optimal lymphocyte activation and cytokine production. Conversely macrophage microbicidal function and release of arachidonate and oxygen metabolites is influenced by cytokines produced by activated T lymphocytes and phagocytosis is markedly enhanced by antibodies produced by B lymphocytes. The cooperation between these two cell types represents a cornerstone of lung defense against noninfectious antigen challenge or microbial infection. Another chapter will deal with acute lung inflammation mediated by neutrophilic leukocytes. In this chapter we will present a brief overview of the macrophage and lymphocytes in the human lung, their function and interactions, and a synthesis of their role in lung inflammation and disease.

We will assume a basic knowledge of immunology. However, an explanation of the terminology used in this chapter is appropriate. Many surface receptors expressed by immunologic cells have had multiple names based on different functions. In the past 30 years these terms have been grouped together in a series of standardized "clusters of differentiation" (CD) for the purpose of standard nomenclature. A list of the CD markers referred to in this chapter, other names used for them, and their putative functions are included in Table 21-1.

TABLE 21-1 Cluster of Differentiation Antigens and Surface Molecules Discussed in this Chapter

Name/CD Designation	Function
CD1	Accessory molecule for antigen presentation on APCs
Sheep RBC receptor/CD2	Accessory molecule for T lymphocyte activation, adhesion receptor (ligand LFA-3)
CD3	Signaling subunit of TCR
αβ TCR	T-cell receptor for antigen
γδ TCR	Alternate form of the T-cell receptor for antigen
CD4	T-cell coreceptor (ligand MHC Class II); marker for helper/inducer cells
CD8	T-cell coreceptor (ligand MHC Class I); marker for cytotoxic cells
CD11a,b,c	α chains of the β2 integrin/CD18; CD11a (LFA-1); CD11b (Mac-1/CR3); CD11c (CR4)
CD14	Macrophage receptor for lipopolysaccharide
CD18	β2 integrin chain
CD25	p55 IL-2 receptor; T-cell activation antigen (TAC)
HLA-DR	Class II MHC; expressed on APCs; activation antigen for T cells
CD28	Stimulatory accessory molecule for T lymphocyte activation (ligands B7–1/CD80, B7–2/CD86)
CTLA-4/CD152	Inhibitory accessory molecule for T lymphocyte activation (ligands B7–1/CD80, B7–2/CD86)
CD29	Common β chain of the β1 integrins
VLA-1–6/CD49a–f	Adhesion molecules; α chains of the β1 integrins (ligands ECM proteins)
VLA-4/α4β1 integrin	Adhesion molecule (ligand VCAM-1 expressed on endothelium, fibronectin)
α4β7 integrin	Adhesion molecule (ligand VCAM-1, fibronectin)
HML-1/αEβ7 integrin	Adhesion molecule (ligand epithelial cell carbohydrate antigen)
ICAM-1/CD54	Cell adhesion molecule for cell–cell interaction (ligand LFA-1/CD11a/CD18)
B7–1/CD80, B7–2/CD86	Accessory molecules for T-cell activation; ligands CD28 (enhances) CTLA-4 (inhibits)
CD95/Fas	Receptor for Fas ligand, induction of apoptosis
VCAM-1/CD106	Adhesion molecule expressed on activated endothelium (ligand α4 integrins)
CCR3	Chemokine receptor (CKR) for CCL11/eotaxin
CCR4	CKR for CCL17/TARC (thymus and activation-regulated chemokine)
CCR5	CKR for CCL4
CCR7	CKR for CCL21/SLC (secondary lymphoid-tissue chemokine)/TCA-4 (T-cell activation-4)

CD, cluster of differentiation; RBC, red blood cell; TCR, T-cell receptor; VLA, very late activation antigen; LFA, lymphocyte function–associated antigen; APC, antigen-presenting cells; MHC, major histocompatibility complex antigen; CR, complement receptor; ECM, extracellular matrix; ICAM, intercellular adhesion molecule; VCAM, vascular cell adhesion molecule; CCR, chemokine CC type receptor; CCL, chemokine CC type ligand.

LYMPHOCYTES IN THE LUNG

Lymphocytes are much more abundant in the lung than previously documented. Recent estimates from CD3+ stained cells in histologic sections of normal human lung approximate the resident T-cell pool to be 10 billion T cells, which is comparable to the number of T cells in human blood.[1] These resident T cells have been examined in detail (see[2]) and are primarily memory T cells with a resident effector phenotype (rTem). In the normal lung these lymphocytes are distributed in one of four compartments (Fig. 21-1). The compartments include lymphocytes at the epithelial surface (LES) including those in the bronchoalveolar space; lymphocytes associated with the epithelium in lymphoid aggregates (also known as bronchus-associated lymphoid tissue [BALT]); interstitial and intraepithelial lymphocytes (IELs); and an intravascular pool. Although the presence of BALT in normal human lung is controversial, it is clear that BALT is present in the setting of infection and possibly with chronic airway inflammation.[3,4] Each compartment has a distinct phenotypic and functional repertoire. It is not yet clear whether there is a sequential influx of lymphocytes from the blood/intravascular pool to interstitium or BALT and finally to the epithelial surface, or whether lymphocytes are destined to reside in one or another of these pools from the time of maturation and/or activation. The absence of afferent lymphatics to the lung dictates that the intravascular pool is the original source of lymphocytes destined to one of the pulmonary compartments. The exact nature of influx and turnover of normal lung lymphocyte populations is not clear. However, the identification of organ- and lung-specific homing chemotactic cytokines (chemokines) with selective distribution of their cognate receptors raises the possibility that the origins of the populations of each compartment are distinct and for intercompartmental trafficking to occur, there must be site-specific signals that alter the chemotactic receptor repertoire in situ.

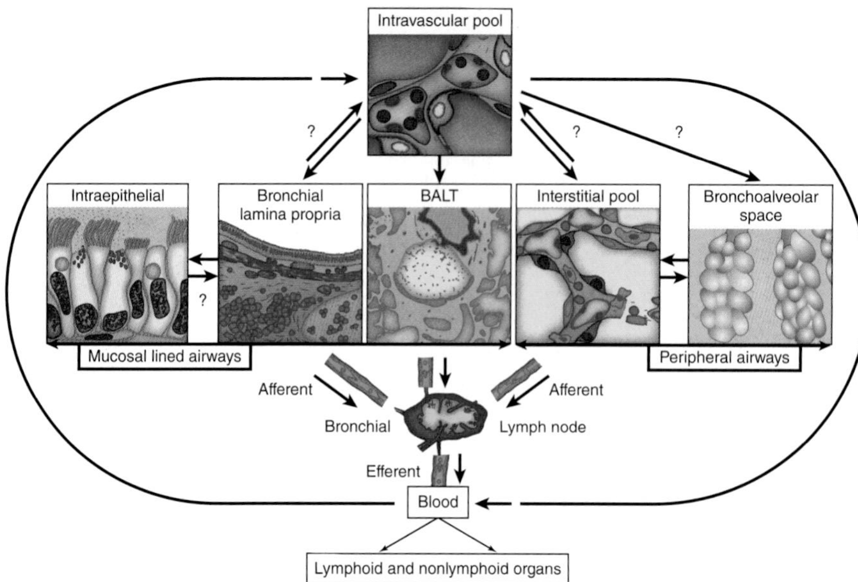

Figure 21-1 Lymphocytes are found in the lung in distinct sites. These include LES (including those at the bronchoalveolar surface); the interstitial and intraepithelial lymphocytes (IELs), bronchus-associated lymphoid tissue (BALT) which are centers of airway antibody production; and an intravascular pool. Lymphocytes travel from lymph nodes to blood and into lung via interaction with lung endothelial cells. Arrows indicate hypothesized trafficking from one pulmonary compartment to another. Some lymphocytes from these various compartments may be able to exit the lung back to lymph nodes, and others become effete and die. For further explanation see text. *(Reproduced with permission from Pabst R. IS BALAT a major component of the human lung immune system? Immunology Today. 1992;13(4):119–122.)*

LYMPHOCYTES AT THE EPITHELIAL SURFACE (LES)

LES and IELs are best studied as lymphocytes from the bronchoalveolar space, are easily recovered from the lung using bronchoalveolar lavage (BAL). Although in normal nonsmoking individuals lymphocytes make up only about 5% to 15% of the 10^5 cells found per milliliter of BAL fluid, lymphocyte numbers may increase dramatically during an inflammatory response.[5–7] LES differ markedly from blood lymphocytes suggesting either a selection bias or organ-specific maturation process that occurs between the blood and lung (Table 21-2). Approximately 70% of LES are T cells; the CD4/CD8 ratio of T cells is approximately the same as in the blood, though with a larger scatter among individuals.[8] Over 70% of BAL T cells are of the previously activated memory type as determined by expression of a low–molecular-weight form of the leukocyte common antigen CD45 (CD45RO),[9,10] and many have been chronically activated as shown by expression of the $\alpha1\beta1$ integrin. The balance of BAL T cells are naive, based on their expression of one of the chemokine receptors CCR7,[11] which primarily identifies T cells that have not come into contact with their cognate antigen. It is unclear what the T-cell representation in BAL is of IEL compared to LES. LES are more likely than blood T cells to express the activation antigen HLA-DR, and CD8+ (cytotoxic/suppressor) and LES are more likely to express markers associated with cytotoxic cell function.[5] An unusual population of memory cytotoxic cells which lack the accessory molecule CD28 has also been described in normal LES.[12] In the neonatal rodent lung the majority of T cells express the gamma-delta T-cell receptor, and account for about 20% of resident (whole lung) pulmonary T cells in adult mice—a percentage that is markedly upregulated with infection.[13] By contrast, the vast majority of human T cells at the epithelial surface are alpha-beta+. The function of the small population of gamma-delta LES T cells in humans remains unknown, but functional similarities to homologous mouse cells suggest that their primary role is to regulate the primary immune response.[14] There are a variable number of natural killer (NK) (including NK-T) cells in this compartment as might be expected in an area of microbial and antigen assault. However, the bulk of NK activity in the lung is found in the interstitial population.[15,16] B cells are also present in the LES population derived by BAL. They have been documented to produce antibodies of all types, with their primary role being to provide mucosal immunity through the secretion of IgA.[5] It is unknown whether there are selected B cell populations among LES.

The source and fate of these T and B cells are unknown. It seems reasonable to hypothesize that epithelial surface T cells (and other lung T cells) emerge from the circulation, perhaps proliferate locally and differentiate further while in the lung, and then die or recirculate.[17] The appearance of labeled blood T cells in LES have been found in the circulation. The predominant memory phenotype of epithelial surface and interstitial T cells strongly suggests that such differentiation occurs before entry into the lung. Once in the epithelial compartment it

TABLE 21-2 Characteristics of Lung Lymphocytes[a]

Location	Number	Cell Type	Comments
Epithelial surface	10^4/mL BAL; approx 10^8 total	CD4/CD8 ratio = blood 70% T cells >90% memory cells 40% express $\alpha_E\beta7$ integrin (70% of CD8+) Memory CTL NK phenotype present, decreased function	Specialized for interaction with epithelial cells. First line of defense?
BALT	? If present in normal (i.e., uninflamed) human lung	B cells in center T cells scattered in center and surrounding follicle	Local antigen sampling and antibody production
Interstitium	10^7/g lung tissue; approx 6×10^9 total	CD4/CD8 ratio < blood >90% memory T cells Bulk of NK activity	With intravascular, equal to total blood lymphocyte pool.
Intravascular	? Characteristics in human	?	Possible mobilizeable cells poised for lung entry

BAL, bronchoalveolar lavage; CD, cluster of differentiation; CTL, cytotoxic T lymphocyte; BALT, bronchus-associated lymphoid tissue.
[a]For a review, see Reference.[15]

appears that bronchial IEL T cells can be long lived potentially surviving within the epithelium for several months, in contrast to the short life span of lymphocytes in the lamina propria.[18,19]

Many LES adhere to and interact with airway epithelial cells through the expression of a unique adhesion molecule (HML-1/$\alpha e\beta 7$ integrin).[20,21] This integrin is expressed on 40% of LES (60% of CD8+ cells are HML-1+ while fewer CD4+ cells express it) and on intestinal lymphocytes, but only rarely on blood or lung interstitial lymphocytes. It is likely that local influences, such as epithelial-derived cytokines like transforming growth factor beta-1 (TGFβ1), result in the expression of this molecule on LES.[22-24] Epithelial cells are directly stimulated by bacteria to release specific chemokines and cytokines (e.g., interleukin (IL)-8, MIP2α (CXCL2), MIP3α (CCL20), IL-7, IL-15) depending on the organism and pathogenicity.[25] These ligands can bind surface chemokine and cytokine receptors on adjacent LES, suggesting that these cells are not necessarily effete or dying cells, which are present in the airway only to be cleared by the mucociliary escalator and expectorated. Rather, they include a specialized lymphocyte population involved in the surveillance of the airway and interaction with epithelial cells. The possibility that LES re-enter the interstitium and lymphoid tissue has been confirmed experimentally in rats.[26] In addition to their interaction with airway epithelial cells, LES directly interact with mucosal DCs, whose phenotype directs further T-cell phenotype evolution (see Lymphocyte Activation in the Lung, below)

LES can be stimulated to proliferate, produce cytokines and antibodies, and to perform cytolytic functions. However, they are in general hyporeactive in proliferative or antibody responses to antigen or mitogens when compared to blood T cells or even when compared to memory T cells in lung interstitium. The reason for this is not known, but may relate to immunosuppressive influences in the airways, including alveolar macrophages (AMs),[27] local production of TGFβ1,[28] the immunosuppressive activity of pulmonary surfactant lipids or proteins,[29] and the possible presence of other immunomodulatory cytokines like IL-10 and IL-16.

■ BRONCHUS-ASSOCIATED LYMPHOID TISSUE (BALT)

BALT is the term applied to localized subepithelial collections of lymphocytes in the airways, and is a secondary lymphoid tissue analogous to other types of mucosa-associated lymphoid tissue (reviewed by Berman et al.,[6] in-depth review by Randall[30]). BALT is present in normal rodent airway and increases in amount with age. Current evidence suggests these structures are uncommon or absent in adult humans but are present in childhood and may appear and proliferate later in life in response to infection or chronic inflammation.[3,30-35] These data suggest that inflammation or infection induces the development of these lymphoid aggregates in humans, and are termed inducible BALT (iBALT) to distinguish them from the classically defined BALT observed in rodents, which is believed to be formed independent of antigen.[36]

Classically defined BALT is similar to gut-associated lymphoid tissue (GALT; e.g., Peyer's patches) in appearance, association with epithelium and a blood vessel, presence of specialized cuboidal or high endothelial venules characteristic of lymphoid tissues, and a specialized thinned overlying epithelium facilitating antigen entry from the bronchial lumen and exit of lymphocytes and lymphocyte products. Immunohistochemistry has revealed a preponderance of B cells staining with IgM, IgG, and IgA, with a scattering (approximately 20%) of T cells, especially CD4+ helper cells within and surrounding the aggregate. BALT lacks organized germinal centers found in other secondary lymphoid tissue. The resemblance of BALT to GALT, as well as the similarity of lymphocyte recirculation patterns from lung- and gut-associated lymphoid tissue has suggested to some authors that these structures represent a common mucosal immune system. In this paradigm, recirculating blood lymphocytes exit into these structures which provide an efficient exposure to antigens sampled from the environment. Activated memory cells are then a source of local antibody production, and they may disperse through the circulation to other mucosal sites to provide dissemination of immunologic memory.

Despite these observations that have been made in rodents, several issues continued to limit what we can infer about BALT function in humans. They include its near absence in normal human airways and limited presence in experimental animals which are primarily observed in pathogen-free colonies. In fact, the infrequent appearance of BALT in humans and mice has led some to doubt whether BALT is an important secondary lymphoid organ.[31] However, there is accumulating evidence that iBALT plays a role in the adaptive immune response to infection.[36] In this new paradigm, infection and inflammation trigger the development of these localized lymphoid tissues through recruitment and priming of naive lymphocytes thereby generating antigen-specific lymphocytes in situ. At the same time, infection and inflammation activate local antigen-presenting cells, which migrate to conventional secondary lymphoid organs (i.e., lymph nodes) for priming and activation of effector cells. Thus, these local lymphoid tissues are capable of not only expanding effector cells that were primed in conventional secondary lymphoid organs but also initiating primary immune responses in situ. In support of this paradigm, splenectomized lymphotoxin-α-null mice that lack the ability to form any secondary lymphoid tissues are still able to develop iBALT[36] in response to infection suggesting distinct mechanisms govern over these lymphoid tissues.

The uniqueness of iBALT in humans and mice is highlighted by the structural difference compared to constitutive BALT in rodents. The iBALT can vary in organization from small clusters of B cells, T cells, and DCs to well-developed follicular aggregates and unlike constitutive BALT, which is found in the upper airway of rodents, iBALT is found in perivascular, peribronchial, and even interstitial areas in the lower airways of the lung.[36] In humans, the specialized overlying epithelium has not been characterized.[37] B-cell follicles, which are seen in iBALT, are centered around CD21-expressing follicular dendritic cells (FDCs)[36] and separated by interfollicular regions containing resident CD11c+ DCs and both CD4+ and CD8+ T cells.[38] The lymphocyte homing chemokines CXCL13 and CCL21 are required for recruitment of naive lymphocytes at HEVs, but unlike conventional lymphoid organs their secretion appears to be independent of LTα.[36] IL-17–producing T cells[33] and CCR7-dependent Tregs[39] have been shown to be important for development of iBALT.

Knowledge of the role of iBALT in the lung is still evolving. BALT development appears to be part of the normal immune response to infectious antigens. The role of BALT expansion in a wide variety of chronic lung diseases such as hypersensitivity pneumonitis, chronic obstructive pulmonary disease, and idiopathic pulmonary fibrosis is less clear.[40]

■ INTERSTITIAL LYMPHOCYTES

Lymphocytes are rarely seen in histologic sections of normal human lung, and there are no established techniques to study these cells as an exclusive, pure population. However, several investigators have prepared lymphocytes from human lungs extensively washed to remove airway surface cells using minced tissue and enzymatic digestion. The resulting population of pulmonary infiltrating lymphocytes in normal humans appears to be distinct from lymphocytes recovered from normal BAL.[41,42] Specifically, approximately 20×10^6 mononuclear cells were found per gram of wet lung tissue; of these 70% were lymphocytes, of which 90% were CD2+ T lymphocytes. There was enrichment for memory T cells similar to that seen in LES, but the CD4/CD8 ratio among IL T cells was lower than that seen in blood or LES. Memory T lymphocytes from the interstitial compartment can be stimulated to produce cytokines, and to proliferate in response to IL-2 despite a decreased proliferative response to mitogens.[43] Most, if not all NK activity in the lung has been localized to the interstitial compartment.[44] The exact origin, fate, and function of interstitial lymphocytes are not known.

■ INTRAVASCULAR LYMPHOCYTES

The presence of this lymphocyte pool has been convincingly shown in animals, especially the pig.[32] Experimental data includes lung perfusion studies showing the continued slow elution of lymphocytes from lung following elimination of red blood cells. The presence of an intravascular lymphocyte pool in humans has not been directly confirmed. However, labeled lymphocytes injected into humans are "held up" in the lung whether injected intravenously or intra-arterially (reviewed by Berman et al.[6]). These data confirm the more recently detected presence of homing receptors on the surface of lymphocytes that match cognate organ-specific chemokine expression.[45] Therefore, this phenomenon likely represents margination of lymphocytes in capillaries due to adhesion molecule interactions. Complete phenotypic characterization of this pool in the human is unknown, as is the size and role of this pool in populating interstitial or epithelial lymphocytes.

■ LYMPHOCYTE RECRUITMENT TO THE LUNG

Lymphocytes are recruited to extravascular sites through a complex process involving adhesion to endothelial cells (ECs), release from adhesion, transendothelial migration, interaction with cellular matrix, and response to locally produced chemoattractants.[6,46,47] This sequential process is characterized by an initial capture step that is mediated by selectins and integrins, followed by arrest/activation mediated by chemokine and cytokine receptors and other integrins.[45,48] The role of chemokines has emerged as central to the regulation of tissue-specific lymphocyte homing and retention. These are low–molecular-weight proteins that share a cysteine repeat motif (e.g., C-C or C-X-C), near the N-terminus. As a class, these proteins have cationic charge, and therefore bind heparin.[49] Chemokine function is mediated through cognate seven transmembrane-spanning receptors. There is significant promiscuity between chemokine receptors and their ligands, such that any specific chemokine may have several ligands and vice versa. Because of their physicochemical properties, the chemokines may bind to heparin-like regions of EC membrane receptors, preventing dilution of locally produced chemoattractant signal by blood flow and facilitating concentration gradients, a phenomenon known as haptotaxis. Chemokines have been shown to enhance both adhesion to ECs and endothelial transmigration of multiple leukocyte types including T-cell subsets and monocytes. Recently, chemokines have also been found to act as accessory growth factors for T-lymphocytes.[50] While CXCL15 (lungkine) appears to be selectively expressed in mouse lung, there does not appear to be a unique human lung–specific lymphocyte directed chemokine profile. However, certain chemokines (see below) are preferentially expressed in TH2 and TH1 type immune responses in the lung.

The interaction of adhesion molecules expressed on blood T cells with complementary adhesion molecules on EC is the critical first step to T-cell emigration from the blood. This step is closely regulated at the level of expression of adhesion molecules by T cells at different stages of development, and by transiently increased adhesion molecule function following T-cell activation. Similarly, expression of adhesion molecules by EC may be increased markedly by organ site and location, or by proinflammatory cytokines, especially tumor necrosis factor (TNF)-α, IL-1, and interferon-γ (IFN).[51–54] Treatment of EC with these cytokines markedly alters the adhesiveness of EC for leukocytes, including certain subsets of T cells. The result of such EC activation by local production of cytokines or other factors is that the exit of T cells from the blood is not random, but rather is restricted to sites such as lymphoid tissues, mucosal sites, or tissue sites of inflammation.

The specific events involved in T-cell transendothelial migration have been dissected at the cellular level, while their characterization in human lung is incomplete. T lymphocytes first appear to "roll" along the endothelium, an interaction which requires loose adhesion via T-cell α4β1 integrin/endothelial VCAM-1 and P-selectin/PSGL-1.[15] A signal is required to produce formal "capture" via other integrin molecules, particularly lymphocyte LFA-1 (αLβ2 integrin) interaction with ICAM-1 or other ligands on endothelium. This latter signal enhances the avidity of integrins for ligand, strengthening adhesion. Other interactions, including decay of integrin affinity, homotypic interaction of T cell and endothelial PECAM (CD31) at EC junctions, and release of matrix degrading enzymes, permit release of firm adhesion and T-cell migration into matrix.[47] Preliminary evidence in TH2-cell migration suggests that this step is mediated by T-cell CCR3/endothelial CCL11 and CCR4/CCL17, respectively.[16,55,56]

T cells are constantly recirculating from blood to tissue and back, with an average half-life in the blood of only about 18 hours.[57] In addition, the sites of migration in vivo appear to be quite different for naive/virgin cells, as opposed to previously activated memory cells. Due to a high level of CCR7 expression, naive cells preferentially traffic to lymphoid tissue where they are likely to encounter antigen,[58] while memory cells traffic to nonlymphoid tissues such as skin or lung.[53,59]

The normal lung vasculature may have unique properties that facilitate the retention of circulating lymphocytes. Whether injected intravenously or intra-arterially, labeled lymphocytes are held up in the lung disproportionately in comparison to other organs. Thus, this is not just a "first-pass" clearance effect from capillary passage.[6] Several investigators have found that antibodies to adhesion molecules, particularly lymphocyte function–associated antigen (LFA)-1, decrease lymphocyte retention in the lung. However, capillary size may determine trapping of activated cells since cytoskeletal changes occurring coincident with activation reduce cellular deformability; this has been shown to be a significant force in the lung trapping of activated neutrophils and monocytes. Lymphocytes also become larger, and lose deformability with activation, but the role of this process in lung retention of lymphocytes is not yet defined.

Lymphocyte chemoattractants represent another step in the regulation of the exit of adherent or trapped T cells from the capillary circulation. As noted earlier, varied T-cell chemoattractants have been described which are relevant to the lung, many of which also alter the growth and activation of T cells (reviewed in References[6,49,50,60]). A partial listing of known chemoattractants may be found in Table 21-3. In lung diseases multiple T-cell chemoattractants have been found in BAL or in tissue specimens, including the chemotactic growth factors IL-2,[29,61] IL-16,[62] IL-33,[63,64] insulin-like growth factor I[13], the C-X-C chemokine IL-8 (CXCL8), and the C-C chemokines macrophage chemotactic protein (MCP)-1 (CCL2), RANTES (CCL5), and macrophage inflammatory protein (MIP)-1α (CCL3).[62,65,66] These chemokines have multiple cellular origins, including macrophages, ECs, and epithelial cells. IL-2 is presumed to be of lymphocyte origin while IGF-1 and IL-16 have multiple potential cellular sources including T cells, eosinophils, and epithelial cells.[67,68] IL-33 is an epithelial-derived alarmin which in addition to being a chemoattractant to TH2 cells via ST2/IL1RAcP receptor also attracts ILC2, eosinophils, and mast cells. Its central role in TH2 immune deviation in asthma in response to epithelial cell necrosis to a variety of injuries is becoming increasingly appreciated.[69–72] It has also been noted that CXCL9, 10, and 11 appear to be important in TH1 responses in the lung, but their expression may relate more to induction by interferon-γ rather than a lung-related phenomena.

Recruitment of lymphocytes to the lung along chemotactic gradients is a complex phenomena involving multiple chemotactic factors, gradients, and responding cell receptors. The final complexion of the lymphocyte population in any compartment is therefore the sum of the responsiveness of each phenotype sequentially responding to and then releasing from chemotactic gradients to respond again. The hierarchy of responses involves regulation of expression of receptors and responsiveness, a phenomena termed chemotactic factor receptor cross desensitization. This can explain retention of T cells (lack of responsive chemotactic receptors) and relocation (sequential responsiveness to induced or constitutive chemotactic gradients). Examples of these modulatory steps are present in human[74–76] and mouse T cells of all phenotypes and likely this is one of the prime factors for accumulation of T cells in organized lymphoid tissues in the thorax and lung (e.g., lymphadenopathy) during infection and inflammation. Moreover, chemotactic gradients and receptor desensitization can be induced by exogenous chemotactic factors of infectious origin, which can in turn regulate responses to endogenous chemotactic factors. For example, HIV-1 gp120 can downregulate the responsiveness of thoracic lymph node lymphocytes to sphingosine-1-phosphate, resulting in lack of normal egress.[74,75,77]

TABLE 21-3 Lymphocyte Chemoattractants[a]

Interleukins	Activation Stimuli
IL-1	Antibody to T-cell receptor (T cells)
IL-2	Antisurface immunoglobulin (B cells)
IL-6	Phorbol esters
IL-10	
IL-15	
IL-16	
IL-33	
Chemokine Chemoattractants	**Growth Factors**
CXCL8/IL-8	Insulin
CCL5/RANTES	IGF-1
CCL3/MIP1-α, CCL4/MIP-1β	TGFβ1
CCL2/MCP-1, CCL8/MCP-2, CCL7/MCP-3	
CXCL10/IP-10	
CL11/eotaxin	
Matrix Proteins	**Miscellaneous Chemoattractants**
Laminin	Lysophosphatidylcholine
Fibronectin	fMLP, mycobacterial lipoarabinomannan
Amyloid protein AA	Casein/denatured protein
Sphingosine 1 phosphate	

[a]Not a complete listing.

IL-, interleukin; RANTES, regulated activated normal T cells expressed, secreted; MIP, macrophage inflammatory protein; MCP, monocyte chemotactic peptide; IGF, insulin-like growth factor; TGF, transforming growth factor. For reviews, see References.[11,52,73]

LYMPHOCYTE FUNCTION IN THE LUNG

Lymphocytes in the lung serve four major functions: (1) antibody production; (2) cytotoxic activity including lysis of virally infected cells, cells that have bound antibody, and tumor cells; (3) cytokine production; (4) immune tolerance. These functions are summarized in Table 21-4 and in a number of references cited.[5,49,78]

Antibody production in the lung by B lymphocytes serves to bind antigen and facilitate inactivation of bioactive material and phagocytosis by macrophages. Mucosal IgA is of particular interest in its active transepithelial transport to the bronchial lumen. Antibody production by lung B cells has been extensively studied in mouse lung. Following challenge, antigen is removed to regional lymph nodes by motile phagocytic cells (macrophages and DCs) where optimal activation of T and B cells occurs. Activated cells relocate into the circulation and migrate into the lung at areas of inflammation, and local antibody production results. Rechallenge with antigen results in a more rapid local response derived from resident memory cells.[5,6,79] While the duration of pulmonary memory lymphocytes is unknown, systemic B lymphocytes can persist for over 100 days in the absence of antigen,[80] as is the case with memory CD4+ and CD8+ T cells.[81]

The lung contains multiple types of cytotoxic cells, including NK cells (not antigen restricted), antigen-restricted cytotoxic cells, and cells exhibiting antibody-dependent cytotoxicity. One unusual aspect of lung cytotoxic cells is the pre-eminence of CD3+ cytotoxic T cells

TABLE 21-4 Function of Lung Lymphocyte Subpopulations[a]

Cell Type	Function	Secreted Products
TH1 cell	Intracellular microbes, (i.e., intracellular bacteria, antiviral and antifungal defense) granuloma formation, graft rejection	IL-2, IFN-γ, IL-3, IL-6, IL-12, IL-16, GM-CSF, TGFβ1
TH2 cell	Allergic inflammation, antiparasite (e.g., helmiths) defense	IL-2, IL-4, IL-5, IL-9, IL-10, IL-3, IL-13 IL-16, GM-CSF, TGFβ1
TH17 cell	Extracellular bacteria and certain fungi. Neutrophilic inflammation	IL-17 A(IL-17), IL-17 F, IL-21, IL-22, TNFα GMCSF, IL-26 (human TH17)
TCTL (CD8 cell)	Antigen-restricted lysis of viral- or mycobacteria-infected macrophages or epithelia; lysis of fungi, tumor cells	TH1 cytokines, perforin, IL-4
T REG cell	Peripheral tolerance (various phenotypes). Maintenance of immature DC	IL-10, TGF-β1, IL-35
NK cell	Nonantigen-restricted lysis of virally infected and tumor cells	Perforin, granzymes, α-defensins, IFNγ, TNFα/β, CCL3, CCL4, CCL5, also IL-17A, IL-22
NKT cell	Restricted $\alpha\beta$TCR interacting With cells presenting glycolipids associated to CD1d	IFN-γ, IL-4, IL-13, IL-2
B cell	Antibody production	IgM, IgG subtypes 1–4, IgE, IgA, IL-10

[a]Not a complete listing. Listed are cytokines or other products produced under in vitro conditions or documented in lung disease.
TH1, T helper type 1; TH2, T helper type 2; CTL, cytotoxic T lymphocyte; NK, natural killer cell; IL-, interleukin-; CMI, cell-mediated immunity; GM-CSF, granulocyte macrophage colony–stimulating factor; TGFb1, transforming growth factor beta 1; DC, dendritic cell.
For reviews, see References.[15,55]

with NK activity (nonantigen-receptor–mediated killing of tumor cell targets). This is in contradistinction to the blood, where the majority of cells expressing NK activity are CD3–.[5] These natural killer T cells (NKT cells) make up less than 0.2% of human peripheral blood T cells and, contrary to an earlier report,[82] are low in number in bronchial tissue and BAL in health and disease. In asthmatics, it is approximated they account for, at most, 1.7% and 0.2% in bronchial tissue and BAL, respectively.[83] They have an invariant TCRα–receptor chain receptor (variable [V] and joining chain [J] Vα14 Jα18 in mice and Vα24 Jα18 in humans) combined with a limited, but not invariant TCRβ-chain repertoire (Vβ8.2, Vβ7, or Vβ2 in mice and Vβ11 in humans), and conventionally are referred to as iNKT or type 1 NKT cells. They recognize foreign and self-glycolipid antigens presented by MHC-class-I-like CD1d antigen-presenting molecule (reviewed by Godfrey, Stankovic, and Baxter[84]). While a role for iNKT cells in host defense to a variety of infectious antigens (e.g., Cryptococcus neoformans)[85] and in modulating the inflammatory response in asthma[86] has been suggested, details of their function have to be elucidated.

NK activity is found in the interstitial compartment of lung T cells and NK cells are present among LES accounting for approximately 10% of tissue lymphocytes. The majority (80%) are phenotypically the cytotoxic subset (CD56dimCD16high) in humans and resting pulmonary NK cells have been found to be functionally impotent.[44,87–89] The impairment of cytotoxic capacity of resting pulmonary NK cells in BAL and lung tissue is believed to be due to the suppressive effects of cytokines such as TGFβ and other mediators such as prostaglandins from AMs, pulmonary surfactant[90] and respiratory epithelial products such as IL-15.[91] The importance of this regulation of NK cells in the lung is exemplified in certain genetic deficiencies which result in either chronic activation of NK cells leading to granulomatous inflammation or recurrent viral and bacterial infections that can involve the upper and lower respiratory tract.[92–94]

Cytokine production by lung T helper cells (TH) has emerged as a major focus of investigation in lung inflammation. In contrast to antibody production by B cells, T cells produce cytokines. Broad ranges of cytokines have been documented to be produced by lung T cells in inflammatory disease (Table 21-4). In general, the complexion of the inflammatory response correlates with the cytokines produced by T cells, suggesting that T cells orchestrate many inflammatory responses.

Activated T-helper (TH) cells produce a distinct spectrum of cytokines.[95–97] The repertoire of a single T cell to produce cytokines appears to be limited and stereotyped, depending on the circumstances of activation. According to data accumulated in mice, naive T cells produce mainly IL-2 in response to activation. After proliferation and switch to memory cell phenotype, T cells differentiate and produce one of four major clusters of effector cytokines, the best characterized being TH1 (interferon-γ, IL-2), TH2 (IL-4, IL-5, IL-10, IL-13), TH17 (IL-17, 23, 25), and Treg (TGFβ, IL-10, PGE). These TH phenotypes share mutually exclusive transcriptional programs, regulated by the transcription factors T-bet (TH1) and GATA-3 (TH2), RORγ/STAT3 (TH17), and FoxP3 (Treg), respectively.[98–100]

Historically, the division between TH1 and TH2 phenotypes was derived by exclusion of the alternate type and led to confusion in the distinction between these phenotypes particularly in humans where the distinction is not as predictable as in the mouse.[95] These two major phenotypes roughly conform to polarized expressions of cell-mediated immune responses: granuloma formation with activation of mononuclear phagocytes and production of opsonizing IgG2 antibody (TH1); or optimal antibody response including IgE formation, often with associated eosinophilia (TH2).

Certain immune responses in the lung are dominated by either a TH1 or TH2 response, while others are mixed. For example, in human asthma T cells producing TH2 cytokines predominate,[101] but IFN-γ producing cells are found in the airways suggesting a mixed response.[102] In contrast, granulomas at sites of tuberculin reactions in skin show evidence for production of IFN-γ and IL-2 but not IL-4.[103] In leprosy or leishmaniasis an ineffective host reaction is associated with a TH2 response, and an effective granulomatous response is associated with a TH1 response. In addition, treatment of ineffective responses to leishmania with IFN-γ have been reported to increase the efficacy of chemotherapy.[96] In sarcoidosis, airway and granuloma cells, particularly activated CD4+ (HLA-DR+) T cells, have been found to produce both IL-2 and IFN-γ, suggesting the predominance of a TH1 response. There is considerable cross-regulation of TH1 and TH2 subsets even after commitment to production of these cytokines, leading to the general concept that the character of an immune response as well as its termination may depend on the sequential predominance of TH1 or TH2 responses. Indeed, the functional distinction between TH1 and TH2 cells is less distinct in humans as it is in the mouse. As a result of these earlier studies, it is now clear that other T-cell phenotypes participate in all these inflammatory events in the lung beyond traditional TH1 and TH2 dichotomy.

First, there is an important role of T cells (and T-regulatory cells in particular) in mediating mucosal tolerance and immune homeostasis.[104,105] This function in the mucosa is directly related to their interaction with mucosal DCs.[78,106,107] While the phenotypic classification of these cells is evolving, the peripheral pool of regulatory T cells (Tregs) is a mixture of natural thymus-derived Tregs (nTregs) and induced Tregs (iTregs), which originate from naive CD4+ T cells under conditions of low antigenic stimulation or by cytokines primarily transforming growth factor beta (TGFβ). While the relative contribution of each type of Treg to immune suppression and homeostasis is not clear, the fact that their TCR repertoire is different suggests a nonredundant complementary role.[108] There appear to be multiple phenotypes within the Treg population with overlapping mechanisms of action. However, the transcriptional factor forkhead box protein 3(Foxp3) appears essential for the suppressive function of this T-cell subset. Deletion of Foxp3 in mice (Scurfy) and humans (IPEX syndrome) results in a lethal condition of autoimmunity and inflammation emphasizing the critical role of Tregs in immune homeostasis and IL-2 in the growth and expansion of Treg. The majority of studies examining the regulatory potential of T cells in inflammatory lung disease, however, have been in *ex vivo* manipulation, depletion, and adoptive transfer experiments in the mouse.[109,110] The evidence for intraparenchymal (i.e., mucosal or interstitial) human Treg cells is not direct, but the requirement for maintenance of peripheral tolerance in the lung and systemic inducibility of tolerance to inhaled antigen[111] provides the basis for their speculated presence in the epithelium. In addition, intratracheal treatment of mice with the immunomodulatory cytokine IL-16[112,113] elicits an expansion of lung CD4+CD25+ T cells.[114]

TGFβ is required for the development of iTregs, but dual stimulation of TGFβ with either IL-4 or IL-6 (IL1β in humans) can alter the cytokine profile of peripheral T cells from suppressive Tregs to proinflammatory TH9 or TH17 cells, respectively. Similar to TH1 and TH2 development, TH9/TH17 and Treg cell development is cross-regulated at the transcription factor level, an important mechanism for maintaining immune homeostasis in the periphery.[115] At the functional level, this requirement of TGF-β for the induction of both Foxp3+ Tregs and TH17 cells provides a system for efficient balance between tolerance and immunity. In the steady state, TGFβ induces Foxp3 and Tregs, inhibits inflammation, and maintains self-tolerance, but once IL-6 is produced by innate immune cells in response to microbial triggers, Treg generation is prevented and the function of nTregs is suppressed while TH17 cells are induced to produce a strong proinflammatory response characterized by neutrophilia.[115]

While a distinct functional role of predominantly IL-9 secreting TH9 cells in the lung is unknown, the TH17 cell cytokine cluster (IL-17A, IL-17 F, IL-22, and IL-21) is understood to help protect the lung against extracellular bacteria and fungi.[116] However, the observed elevations of IL-17A and IL-17F in sputum and blood/BAL in asthma[117,118] indicate that TH17 cells contribute to chronic inflammatory disease as well. TH17 cells, like TH1 and TH2 cells, accomplish some of their role by recruiting cells of the granulocytic–monocytic lineage: TH1 cells recruit monocytes/macrophage, TH2 cells recruit eosinophils, basophils, and mast cells, and importantly TH17 cells recruit neutrophils. Given that up to 50% of asthmatics are nonatopic[116] and IL-17 mediates neutrophilic inflammation, there has been interest in understanding TH17 role in difficult to treat asthma. Interestingly, in vitro experiments have shown that the neutrophilic airway inflammation and bronchial hyperresponsiveness caused by TH17 cells was steroid resistant, consistent with the clinical phenotype.[119] While sarcoidosis is classically thought of as a TH1 disease, IL-17–producing cells are also elevated in peripheral blood and bronchoalveolar lung fluid of these patients.[120] Moreover, both single IL-17A+ and double IL-17/IFNγ+ cells have been reported in sarcoid granulomatous tissue.[121] Thus TH17 cytokine cluster helps understand the heterogeneity in classical TH1 and TH2 disease in the lung.

However, T cells are not the only source of IL-17, innate lymphoid cells (ILCs) such as NKT cells, NK cells and γδ T cells produce IL-17.[115] There is great interest in understanding the contribution of ILCs to immune homeostasis and pathology in the lung. Three features define ILCs: the absence of recombination-activating gene (RAG)-dependent rearranged antigen receptors; a lack of myeloid cell and DC phenotypic markers; and their lymphoid morphology. While the prototypical ILC population is NK cells (see previous section), several other distinct ILC populations have recently been described, all of which appear to originate from a common lymphoid (Id2+) progenitor cell and all, like conventional T cells, produce cytokines.

A particular source of confusion is the number of different names that have been used to characterize these different ILC populations. For example, ILCs that produce TH2-cell–associated cytokines have been variously called natural helper cells,[122] nuocytes,[123] and innate helper 2 (Ih2) cells[124] without clear evidence of uniqueness. A functional nomenclature system based on cytokines produced[125] has recently been proposed: Group 1 ILCs produce IFNγ, Group 2 produce type 2 cytokines (including IL-5 and IL-13), and Group 3 ILCs produce IL-17 and IL-22. ILCs are changing our view of how lymphocytes function in lung inflammation. For example, ILC2 have been shown to contribute IL-13 not IL-4 production in ovalbumin-induced lung inflammation mouse models[126,127] and in IL-13 –/– mice, which are resistant to allergic lung inflammation and virus-induced airway hyperresponsiveness transfer of IL-13 expressing ILC2 s was sufficient to restore airway hyperresponsiveness in both models[126,128] A human equivalent of ILCs have been found in patients with chronic rhinosinusitis.[129]

B-lymphocyte biology has also significantly advanced in recent years and now B cells are known to be comprised of different populations and proven to be pleiotropic in function (Ref.[130] summarizes the current understanding of B-cell lineages in the lung.) Briefly, in mice the majority of B cells are B2 B cells, which originate from the adult bone marrow precursor, traffic through peripheral lymphoid tissue, interact with cognate antigen, and after activation develop into either memory B cells or antibody-secreting plasma cells. In the human lung, the majority of B cells are these mature naive B2 B cells and they reside in BALT (see previous section) or draining lymph nodes. In mice, there is a family of innate-like B cells: marginal zone B cells, B1α and B1β B cells that contribute to rapid immune responses against pathogens and other stimuli. B1 B cells are a small self-renewing subset of B cells that originate from the fetal liver and secrete most, if not all, natural antibodies (IgM and IgA isotype) in the apparent absence of antigenic challenge. Natural antibodies are often polyreactive and bind to foreign antigens as well as to self-components (ex rheumatoid factor) and are important for early pathogen recognition and maintenance of tissue homeostasis.[131] B1 B cells constitute a minor fraction of the spleen and secondary lymphoid tissues but are enriched in the pleural and peritoneal cavities. It is not known whether B1 B cells residing in the pleural cavity migrate into the lung. Human B1 B cells do exist and are found to have marker profile of CD20+CD27+CD43+CD70– and could either be CD5+ or CD5–.[132]

The central role of B cells is the production of immunoglobulins, both within the parenchyma and for export to the mucosal surface of the airway, in the case of polymeric IgA and IgM. In addition, B cells are now known to function as antigen-presenting cells and producers of both inflammatory and regulatory cytokines (i.e., IL-10–producing B-regulatory cells [B-regs]). Very little is known about either of these functions in the lung by B cells. Much of disease immunopathology in the lung is based on T-cell biology, but there is an expanding appreciation of B-cell contribution to diseases such as hypersensitivity pneumonitis, COPD, autoimmune connective tissue diseases, and idiopathic pulmonary fibrosis (see the review by Kato et al.[130] for details). But overall, all these diseases illustrate the potential for the lung to generate an exuberant B-cell response to antigen, either inhaled or self-antigen.

■ LYMPHOCYTE ACTIVATION IN THE LUNG

T lymphocytes are designed to require specific (antigenic) signals for activation, restricting their involvement in inflammation to situations where antigen overwhelms the mucociliary escalator and macrophage and neutrophil defenses. Lymphocytes are activated following engagement of an antigen receptor of remarkably fine specificity. This receptor is unique to a given lymphocyte clone, and is generated by recombination of gene segments in the antibody (for B cells) or T-cell–receptor genes. B-cell receptors consist of single membrane-spanning antibody molecules of the same specificity as the B cell, while T-cell receptors consist of a heterodimeric receptor (dimers of alpha and beta or gamma and delta chains). The T-cell receptor is highly antigen specific and has structural homology to the immunoglobulin molecule. Lymphocytes are activated by cross-linking of membrane antibody by antigen (B cells) or by engagement of the antigen receptor by antigen bound to major histocompatibility complex (MHC) molecules on the surface of so-called antigen presenting cells (APCs), also known as accessory cells. APCs provide many "accessories" for T-cell activation including: (1) a source of MHC molecules to which antigen can bind; (2) internalization and "processing" of antigen including protease digestion into antigenic fragments; (3) multiple cell adhesion molecules which bind to complementary adhesion molecules on T cells and serve to strengthen T-cell–accessory cell interactions and transduce activation signals required for optimal lymphocyte activation; and (4) production of cytokines that amplify activation including IL-1 (reviewed by Cruikshank et al.[112]).

APCs in the lung include pulmonary macrophages of all varieties, however, DCs and Langerhans cells are most efficient in this function (see below). These cells express important "accessory" cell adhesion molecules important to accessory cell function, including ICAM-1, LFA-2, LFA-3, and the CD28 ligands B7–1, B7–2, and CTLA-4.[68,133,134] Other cells, which may be induced to express Class II MHC molecules, may also act as weak accessory cells. Such cells include local B cells, epithelial cells, smooth muscle cells, and fibroblasts. Uncommitted naive T cells require intense accessory cell interaction to be activated by antigen, while previously activated (memory) T cells require less accessory cell input and might be influenced by interaction with such weak accessory cells. Due to naive CCR7+ T cells' inability to cross postcapillary venules, as mentioned earlier most lung T cells are memory cells, which suggests that the relatively weak lung accessory cells may indeed play a role in T-cell activation in the lung inflammatory response (Table 21-5).

As discussed earlier, the lung has proved to contain major immunosuppressive elements, which may serve to prevent inappropriate or excessive T-cell activation in an area of the body, characterized by constant antigen bombardment. These influences include surfactant lipids which have been shown to inhibit T-cell activation, proliferation, and cytokine production[136]; basal production (perhaps by epithelial cells) of the potent immunosuppressive cytokine TGF-β1[28]; and an inhibitory effect of AMs.[27] These inhibitory effects may be moderated, reduced, or increased in various disease states.[137] The role of DC phenotype and degree of maturation in directing activation versus tolerance in T cells is emerging as a key determining step in pulmonary T-cell differentiation. DCs can be broadly described as activating or tolerogenic, and this distinction appears to be related to the maturity of the DC and functionally to the presence of costimulatory molecules on the cell surface (e.g., CD80, CD86, CD40).[106,107] Typically, DCs process inhaled antigen and migrate to draining lymph nodes to present antigen to naive T cells. (The role of BALT in this process is unknown, see earlier discussion.) Thereafter, the nature and concentration of processed antigen determines the fate of cognate T cells: TH1, TH2, TH17, or Treg.[138,139] Presumably, TH cells that have encountered Ag in secondary lymphoid tissue acquire cell surface markers that direct homing and permit postcapillary emigration to lung interstitium and epithelium, either as regulatory or effector cells. There is evidence that the communication between DC and T cells is not exclusively toward T cells; differentiated T cells communicate with local DC via cytokines and cell surface markers to alter DC phenotype. This phenomenon has been described in a mouse diabetes model,[140] and proposed in murine allergic airway inflammation.[141] In light of the emerging central role of DCs in immunologic lung disease and growing knowledge of their plasticity, future directions will likely approach modulating DC phenotype and function as targets for therapy.

■ LYMPHOCYTE CLEARANCE AND DEATH IN THE LUNG

The means by which lymphocytes exit the lung or are cleared during homeostasis or following an inflammatory response is largely unknown. Certainly apoptosis and autophagy play a role in clearing of senescent cells, but signals unique to lung diseases in activating these pathways are less clear. It is not known how long memory T or B cells reside in the lung in any of the compartments, nor is the extent of lymphocyte exit from the lung via lymph to nodes or to the circulation. However, it is clear from studies in the mouse that programmed cell death, or apoptosis, is involved in the termination of antigen-induced inflammatory responses. In lymphocytes, this energy-requiring form of cell death leading to the fragmentation of the nucleus and DNA may result from one of three events: (1) "neglect" or absence of stimulation; (2) stimulation out of context, or without the appropriate second signals (such as CD28 or matrix interactions); or (3) signaling via Fas (CD95) engagement with Fas ligand. Such regulation of cell death appears to be critically important for the termination of an immune response once

TABLE 21-5 Function of Lung Macrophage Populations

Cell Type	Phagocytosis	Microbial Killing	AG Presentation	Cytokine Production
Alveolar macrophage	++++	++++	+/– (suppression)	++++
Interstitial macrophage	++	++	++	++
Dendritic cell	+	+	++++	++
Langerhans cell	++	+	++++	++
Blood monocyte	++	++	+++	+++

Source: Data from Erle DJ, Brown T, Christian D, Aris R. Lung epithelial lining fluid T cell subsets defined by distinct patterns of beta 7 and beta 1 integrin expression. Am J Respir Cell Mol Biol. 1994;10:237–244; Ford WL, Simmonds SJ. The tempo of lymphocyte recirculation from blood to lymph in the rat. Cell Tissue Kinet. 1972;5:175–189; Johnston RB, Jr. Current concepts: immunology. Monocytes and macrophages. N Engl J Med. 1988;318:747–752.

antigen has been cleared, preventing the accumulation of activated lymphocytes.[142]

MACROPHAGES IN THE LUNG

Macrophages reside in many organs. However, they are especially prominent in the lung and perform many functions. Macrophages ingest inhaled particles or antigens and are then removed on the mucociliary escalator. They also serve as "professional" APCs, traveling to regional lymph nodes where they sensitize T and B lymphocytes. Lung macrophages release a variety of cytokines and biologically active arachidonate metabolites, which influence the function of nearby cells including T cells, B cells, ECs, and fibroblasts. Finally, macrophages ingest microorganisms and, when stimulated, kill them using a variety of means including toxic oxygen metabolites and nitric oxide.

Macrophages or macrophage-like cells are found in several lung compartments including the epithelial lining fluid, interstitium, epithelium, and intravascular compartment. These cells have varying functional repertoires and are typically categorized as AMs, interstitial macrophages (IMs), DCs, Langerhans cells, blood monocytes, or blood macrophages, respectively. Each of these cell types, their recruitment, and their activation will be discussed.

■ MACROPHAGE TYPES

Alveolar Macrophages (AMs)

Derivation of AMs from blood monocytes was initially suggested by an experiment in which the quantity of AM declined 20 to 30 days after bone marrow ablation despite in situ proliferation and increased cell stability.[143] Conversely, similar experiments, but with shielding of the chest during bone marrow ablation, have now found that even by 8 months bone marrow monocytes contribute little to the alveolar macrophage compartment during steady-state conditions.[144,145] It is now appreciated in mice at least that lung macrophages have a chimeric origin being derived from the fetal yolk sac and bone marrow–derived blood monocytes and certain subtypes may persist for the mouse lifetime.[146,147] The differentiation of AM derived from blood monocytes is regulated by the tissue microenvironment.[21,135,148,149] However, the molecular details of this differentiation remain largely unknown.[150]

If quantity implies importance, then one would surmise that AMs play an essential role in the lung's defense against foreign invaders. Found in air spaces throughout the lung, it is estimated that macrophages make up 90% of cells found in the alveolar spaces of both smokers and nonsmokers. The absolute quantity of AM, however, is approximately four-fold greater in smokers than nonsmokers.[148] The increased quantity of AMs in smokers is likely due to both recruitment of blood monocytes from the bone marrow and their differentiation into AMs. In one study, AMs were exposed to ambient particles and their supernatant collected. The supernatant promoted transit of monocytes through the bone marrow and their release into the circulation. Analysis of the supernatant revealed large amounts of inflammatory mediators including granulocyte macrophage colony–stimulating factor (GM-CSF), macrophage colony–stimulating factor (M-CSF), macrophage inflammatory protein (MIP)-1beta (CCL4), monocyte chemotactic protein (MCP)-1 (CCL2), IL-6, and ICAM-1.[151] Many of these mediators are known to increase monocyte turnover in the bone marrow and to enhance their recruitment into peripheral tissues.

AMs have a diverse repertoire of functions. Importantly, AMs are the first line of defense against inhaled antigens and pathogens. As such, they have well-developed phagocytic activity that is enhanced when activated by opsonization or inflammatory signals (e.g., IFN-γ).[6,51,152] Activated AMs release more inflammatory mediators and have superior microbial killing than their unstimulated counterparts.[143,150,151] It is impossible to accurately assess the

TABLE 21-6 Cytokines and other Bioactive Substances Released from Lung Macrophages[a]

Arachidonate Metabolites	Cytokines	
Thromboxane A_2	IL-1[b]	IL-10[v]
PGE_2, D_2, $F_{2\alpha}$	IL-1RA	IL-12[b]
LTB_4	IL-6[b]	IL-15
5-HETE	TNF-α[b]	IL-23[b]
IFN-α/β	MIF	
	Ym1,2[v]	TGF-β[v]
Reactive Oxygen Metabolites[b]	**Nitric Oxide[b]**	
Superoxide anion (O_2^-)	Constitutive	
H_2O_2	Inducible?	
hydroxyl radical (OH−)		
Chemokines		
Enzymes[b]	CCL3,4,5[b]	
Metalloproteases	IL-8(CXCL8)[b]	
Elastase	IP-10 (CXCL10)[b]	
Procoagulant activity	CCL17, 18, 22[v]	

[a]*Not a complete listing.*

PG, prostaglandin; LT, leukotriene; IL-, interleukin; HETE, hydroxy tetraenoic acid; TNF, tumor necrosis factor;; IFN, interferon; MIF, macrophage migration inhibitory factor; TGF, transforming growth factor; CCL, chemokine (C-C motif) ligand; CXCL, chemokine (CXC-motif) ligand; IP-10, Interferon gamma-induced protein 10 kd; Ym1, Chitinase 3-like protein 3; Ym2, Chitinase 3-like protein 4.

[b]*Bioactive substances associated with classically activated macrophages v bioactive substances associated with alternatively activated macrophages. See References.*[79,135,136,154]

phagocytic and microbicidal capabilities of AM compared to other lung macrophages because many of the accessible AMs may have been depleted of a portion of their functional capabilities due to previous activation. In general, smaller AMs are more efficient at phagocytosis and microbial killing than larger AMs. The smaller AM may represent younger, recently emigrated phagocytes and the larger AM may represent previously activated AM.[143]

AMs release a variety of inflammatory mediators including arachidonate products, cytokines, and enzymes (see Table 21-6). These mediators impact extracellular matrix, fibrin deposition, and the function of leukocytes and lung cells at sites of inflammation.[21,143,153] Many also play key roles in the pathogenesis of lung diseases. As an example, IFN-γ–inducible protein 10 (IP-10; CXCL10), monokine induced by IFN-γ (MIG; CXCL9), and IFN-inducible T-cell α chemoattractant (I-TAC; CXCL11) are released by AMs and stimulate the release of matrix metalloproteinases-9 and -12 in emphysema.[73]

A wide array of receptors are expressed by AMs, of which most mediate AM activation, migration, or phagocytosis. Perhaps most important are the toll-like receptors (TLRs) which are pattern recognition receptors for microbial cell wall lipids, DNA repeats, and other components of infectious agents. They provide the recognition function of the innate immune system that links to CD14 and subsequent inflammatory cytokine release (e.g., IL-1, IL-6, TNFα) secretion reviewed by Basu and Fenton[155]). These cytokines are essential in controlling infection with intracellular organisms like *Mycobacterium tuberculosis*. For example, AMs express TLR-2 which, when activated, induces killing of intracellular *Mycobacterium tuberculosis*.[156] MARCO is a scavenger receptor

TABLE 21-7 Ligands Recognized by Alveolar Macrophage Receptors[a]

Immunoglobulins (Fc Receptors)	Complement Receptors for:
IgG1, IgG2a (murine)	C3b, iC3b, C4b, C3d, C5a
IgG2b, IgG3 (murine)	
IgG1, IgG3 monomers (human)	
IgE, IgA (murine, human)	
Protein, Cytokine, and Matrix Receptors	**Lipoprotein Receptors for:**
Fibronectin R	Low-density lipoprotein
Fibrin R	Beta–very-low-density lipoprotein
Lactoferrin R, transferrin R	
GM-CSF R	
IFN-γR, IL-2R, IL-4R, IL-1R, IL-1RA	
Insulin	
Chemotactic factor receptors	
Other Receptors and Adhesion Molecules	**Lectin Receptors for:**
Class II MHC (HLA-DR, -DP, -DQ)	α-linked galactose residues
CD4	N-acetyl galactosamine residues
β2 Integrins (CD18; CD11a, b, c)	N-acetyl galactosamine residues
β1 Integrins (CD29; CD49a, b, c, e, f)	α-Linked fucose residues
CD54 (ICAM-1)	N-acetyl neuraminic acid residues
CD14 (Lipopolysaccharide receptor)	Mannose residues (mannose receptor)

[a]Not a complete listing.

Fc, complement binding fragment of immunoglobulin; Ig, immunoglobulin; R, receptor; GM-CSF, granulocyte macrophage colony-stimulating factor; IFN, interferon; IL, interleukin; RA receptor antagonist; MHC, major histocompatibility complex antigen; CD, cluster of differentiation.

Source: Data from Hunninghake GW, Bedell GN, Zavala DC, Monick M, Brady M. Role of interleukin-2 release by lung T-cells in active pulmonary sarcoidosis. Am Rev Respir Dis. 1983;128:634–638; Palecanda A, Paulauskis J, Al-Mutairi E, et al. Role of the scavenger receptor MARCO in alveolar macrophage binding of unopsonized environmental particles. J Exp Med. 1999;189:1497–1506.

expressed by AMs that facilitates phagocytosis of unopsonized particles.[157] In the absence of MARCO, pulmonary infection and inflammation is markedly increased.[158] Other receptors expressed by AMs include chemokine receptors, cytokine receptors, Fc receptors that recognize opsonizing antibodies, complement receptors that facilitate phagocytosis, lectin receptors, bacterial endotoxin (CD14) receptors, and mannose receptors (see Table 21-7).

Under certain circumstances, AMs function as APCs and facilitate memory T lymphocyte activation. This ability is enhanced in disease states such as HIV, transplant graft rejection, and sarcoidosis. In alternative situations, AM may impact the immunologic synapse to suppress T lymphocyte activation. This supposition is corroborated by one animal model in which AM depletion enhanced lymphocyte activation, suggesting that AMs can suppress T lymphocyte activation in normal lung homeostasis.[27]

Interstitial Macrophages (IMs)

IMs are a population of macrophages found in the interstitium of the lung instead of the airway lumen. They may be precursors of AMs in transit from the vasculature to the air spaces.[143] Little is known about human IMs because they are not readily accessible for study. In murine models, IMs have been shown to be functionally different from AMs and suggest IMs have a unique role in immune homeostasis in the lung by protecting against aberrant immune responses to nonpathogenic environmental antigens, even in the presence of proinflammatory stimuli.[159] To this end, IMs have been shown to be more immunoregulatory than microbiocidal in comparison with AMs and one mechanism postulated is by inhibition of maturation and migration of DCs.[159,160] Conversely, IMs can exert a supportive influence on pulmonary DC immune function by preprocessing particulate antigen into smaller peptides that are then loaded on the surface of neighboring DCs.[161]

DCs and Langerhans Cells

DCs are potent APCs that reside within airway epithelium and lung parenchyma. Like AMs, they likely originate in the bone marrow, travel via the blood (0.5% of blood mononuclear cells are DCs), then translocate into tissue. Although chemokines and other factors like IL-16 that are chemotactic for DCs have been identified, the precise stimulus for translocation of lung DCs is unknown.[143] DCs are most numerous in large airway epithelium and decrease in quantity as the airways become smaller.[133] Histologic sections along the long axis of airways have revealed a meshwork of DC processes ideal for antigen sampling and interaction with T cells. A similar meshwork is found in BALT in the mouse.[162] It is unknown whether DCs proliferate in the lung.

DCs are highly mobile and travel from the airway to regional lymph nodes where they interact with lymphocytes.[162] DCs are 10- to 100-fold more potent than monocytes at presenting antigens to naive T lymphocytes. DCs express cell surface proteins that are essential for antigen presentation and lymphocyte activation including MHC, cell–cell adhesion molecules (e.g., ICAM/CD54, LFA-3/CD58, β1 and β2 integrins), CD4, and the CD28 ligands.[134,162] Specialized DCs with distinctive invaginations of the plasma membrane called Langerhans cells also exist in the lung, especially those of smokers. Like DCs, Langerhans cells are potent APCs but are less efficient at phagocytosis, microbial killing, and cytokine secretion compared to macrophages.[133] In mouse lungs, it has been shown that langerin+ DCs are able to sample the content of the airway lumen while keeping the epithelium barrier function intact through expression of tight-junction proteins claudin-1, claudin-7, and zonula-2, which form tight junctions with the airway epithelial cells.[163]

The importance of DCs to the pathogenesis of lung diseases was highlighted by a murine model in which CD11c+ DC depletion during an allergen trial resulted in abrogation of the characteristics of an asthmatic response eosinophilic inflammation, goblet cell hyperplasia, and bronchial reactivity.[164] Their role with T-cell education in the lung is discussed earlier. For the interested reader, one is directed to a state-of-the-art review on DCs in the lung.[161]

Blood Monocytes and Intravascular Macrophages

As discussed earlier, blood monocytes are likely the precursors of both lung macrophages (alveolar and interstitial) and intravascular macrophages with differentiation being directed by the microenvironment. This is supported by the observation that blood monocytes can be induced in vitro to express receptors characteristic of AM over a period of days if cultured in the correct microenvironment. The average monocyte spends 1 to 3 days in the circulation and then exits the circulation to differentiate into a macrophage. During inflammation, translocation from blood to tissue increases.[165]

Intravascular macrophages are found within the vasculature of the lung. They are located in postcapillary venules, strongly adherent, and face the flow of blood. Like IMs, these cells are not readily accessible and, therefore, are difficult to study.[166] They are presumed to act as intravascular inflammatory sentinels, ingesting antigens in the form of microbes, erythrocytes, fibrin, cellular debris and immune cells,[167] and releasing mediators in response to inflammatory stimuli which reach the lung via the blood.[168]

■ RECRUITMENT OF MONOCYTES AND MACROPHAGES

Monocytes are motile cells that adhere to ECs and then migrate with extraordinary efficiency. Monocyte adherence to ECs is promoted by the monocyte "rolling" along vascular walls to increase the likelihood that its β2 integrins (αLβ2, αMβ2, and 4β1) will bind the EC selectins.[43,51,169] Following adhesion, translocation into the lung parenchyma occurs. Once the monocytes have entered the tissue, they differentiate into IMs and continue to migrate via their β1 integrins. Both differentiation and migration are influenced by local tissue-specific factors including chemokines, cytokines, matrix components, complement fragments, antigens, and interactions with other cells.[43,143,149,165]

Monocytes respond to a variety of chemotactic influences including complement fragments (e.g., C5 a), bacterial peptide f-MLP, leukotriene B4, and the chemokines CCL2, CCL3, CCL4, and CXCL8 ((IL-8).[143] The importance of chemokines for monocyte migration is illustrated by a study that investigated the impact of CCR2 (the receptor for CCL2; MCP-1) deletion in a murine model of pulmonary granulomatous inflammation.[170] Following deletion, there was marked decrease in granuloma size and a dramatic decrease in the level of interferon-γ in draining lymph nodes. These findings suggest that CCL2 is vital for monocyte/macrophage migration to sites of inflammation.

Motility of AMs and DCs has also been studied. When labeled DCs and AMs are introduced into the airways, DCs but not AMs are readily found in draining lymph nodes, suggesting that DCs are far more motile than AMs.[133,162] DC migration is likely chemokine mediated. In one set of experiments, IL-13 and IFNγ were administered intranasally, resulting in increased numbers of DCs accumulating in draining lymph nodes, similar to the experiment previously described.[171] Compared to untreated mice, the treated mice had more expression of chemokines including CCL5, CCL2, and CCL7 (MCP-3). In addition, chemokine receptor expression was increased including CCR2, CCR5, and CCR10.

■ ACTIVATION OF LUNG MACROPHAGES

A major feature of tissue macrophages is the ability to be "activated."[21,143,150] Activation of macrophages is a key event in the inflammatory cascade in the lung and defines a functional state characterized by extrusion of pseudopodia and an increase in cell size and membrane ruffling. Examples of stimuli that interact with receptors on the macrophage's surface to induce activation include antigen–antibody complexes (via the macrophage's Fc receptors), complement fragments (via the macrophage's complement receptors), and cytokines (e.g., interferon-γ) and TLR ligands (e.g., LPS lipopolysaccharide) When activated, macrophage phagocytosis, receptor expression, and production of toxic oxygen metabolites are markedly enhanced. The activated macrophage is a secretory cell, releasing cytokines, toxic oxygen metabolites, and enzymes. Finally, antigen presentation is optimized in activated macrophages but increased expression of Class II MHC.[150]

Using several surface markers ([154]), activated macrophages can be further characterized as exhibiting an M1 phenotype (classically activated macrophages, i.e., induced typically by IFNγ) or an M2 phenotype (alternatively activated macrophages, i.e., induced by IL-4/IL-13). M1 macrophages are generally associated with TH1 (and TH17) immune responses, the production of reactive oxygen intermediates, proinflammatory cytokines, and robust antimicrobial activity. M2 macrophages are associated with TH2 immune response, immune response to helminthes, tissue healing, collagen production, and fibrosis (see Table 21-6). However, this binary view of macrophage activation and its functional alignment with TH1 and TH2 lineages is an oversimplification; a third class of macrophages called "regulatory macrophages" has also been described. These macrophages can be activated by TLR agonists in the presence of immunoglobulin G (IgG) immune complexes, apoptotic cells, and prostaglandins, and are defined by production of the immunosuppressive cytokines IL-10 and TGF-β1.[172] These cells are poor antigen-presenting cells and have a propensity to induce TH2 and some believe T regulatory cell responses. Rather than discrete stable subpopulations, many studies have documented flexibility in macrophage programming, with macrophages readily switching from one functional phenotype to another in response to new microenvironmental signals.[172]

These signals result in activated macrophages playing a prominent role in many lung diseases. While it is unclear whether macrophage activation is a cause or result of lung disease, it is probably both. As an example, in emphysema, macrophage activation is initiated by cigarette smoke exposure and results in the release of inflammatory mediators and byproducts that are toxic to lung parenchyma. These inflammatory mediators, in turn, activate additional macrophages, establishing a vicious cycle of macrophage activation and parenchymal lung destruction.

LYMPHOCYTE–MACROPHAGE INTERACTIONS IN THE LUNG

The interactions between lymphocytes and macrophages, and their effects on lung inflammatory cells and on lung inflammation are summarized in Figure 21-2. Lung macrophages and lymphocytes each perform important functions and influence the differentiation and function of a large variety of cells. Lung macrophages and lymphocytes also interact via direct cell–cell contact during T-cell activation and are greatly codependent. The interaction between bronchial DCs, which are highly effective APCs and typically more effective at antigen presentation than macrophages, is not detailed herein as DC's primary action in regulating pulmonary inflammation, as noted earlier, is following migration to regional lymph nodes.

AM and related cells are the initial sentinels of the innate immune response, phagocytizing and eliminating invading antigens and microbes. After interaction with microbial invaders, and especially in conditions of overwhelming invasion, lung macrophage activation via TLRs and CD14 and other receptors (see Table 21-6) results in the release of inflammatory mediators which activate adhesion molecule expression on ECs, and promote the migration and activation of blood leukocytes including polymorphonuclear leukocytes (PMNs), monocytes, lymphocytes, and eosinophils (*left half* of Fig. 21-2). Rapid induction of selectin molecules stored in Weibel–Palade bodies of endothelium results in the rolling adhesion of neutrophils and monocytes. Migration of these leukocytes may be rapidly modulated by rapid release of arachidonate products such as LTB4, bacterial products themselves like the peptide f-MLP, complement fragments, and chemokines. More time is required for optimal expression of adhesion molecules, which enhance lymphocyte entry, especially VCAM and expression of the chemokine chemoattractant cytokines. One exception is the release within hours of IL-16 from epithelium or resident T cells in response to mast cell–derived histamine.[62]

Interaction of resident or infiltrating T cells with APCs (mainly DC, Langerhans cells and monocytes) results in optimal T-cell activation with resultant production of cytokines, which act upon a variety of cytokine-receptor bearing cells (*right half* of Fig. 21-2). This results in the activation of endothelium, optimal B-cell production of antibody, generation of cytotoxic effector T cells, and depending on the nature of the cytokines produced a delayed-type hypersensitivity or granulomatous (type 1 cytokines), allergic (type 2 cytokines), or other T-cell immune response including neutrophilic TH17 inflammation. Fibrosis or repair may also be influenced by the production of neutral proteases by AM,[151,173] or by the elaboration of the fibrogenic cytokine TGFβ1 by T cells or other

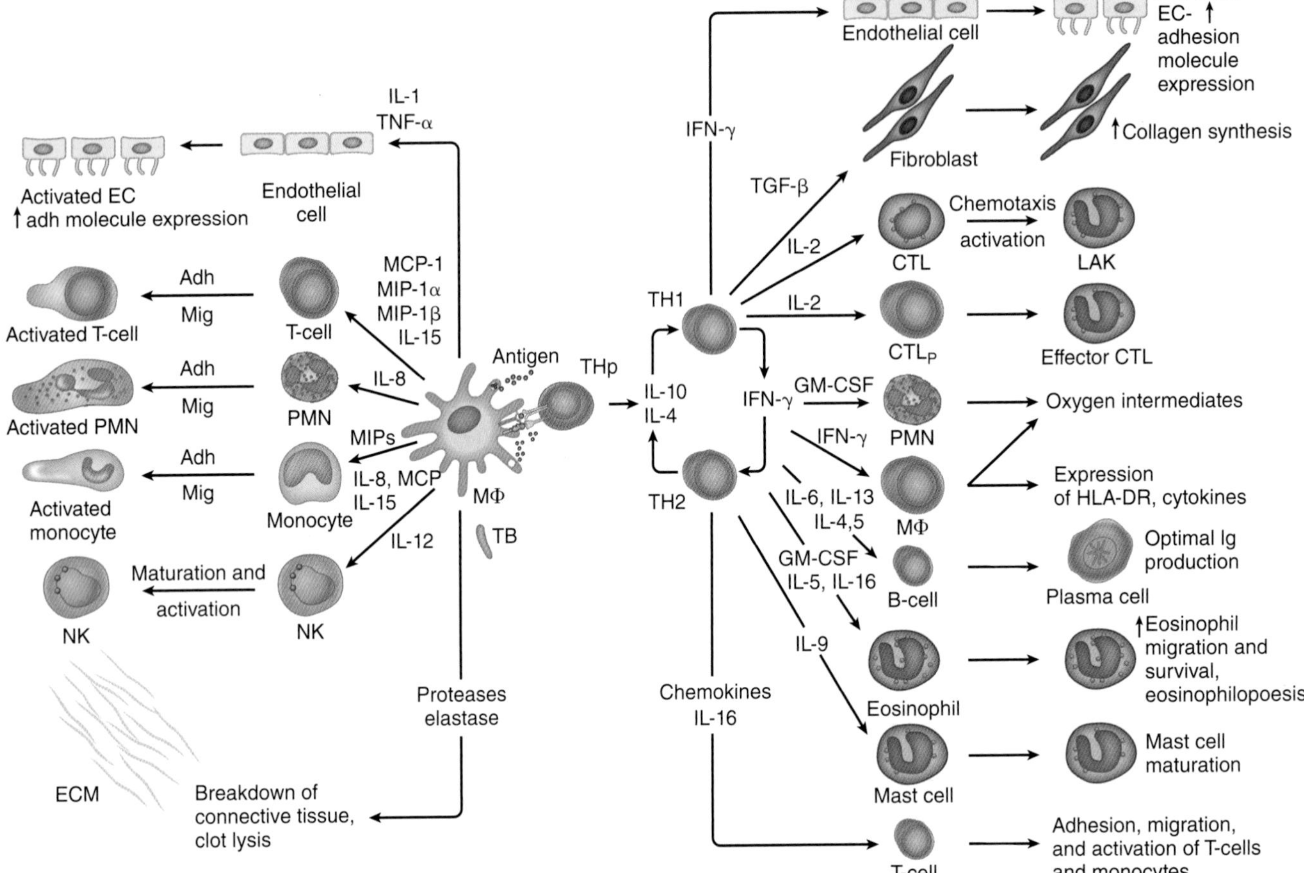

Figure 21-2 Lymphocyte and macrophage interactions in lung inflammation. Lymphocytes and macrophages interact directly and indirectly to influence lung inflammation. These interactions are complex, as illustrated in this diagram, which contains a necessarily incomplete sampling of these processes. Lymphocytes and macrophages interact directly in the process of lymphocyte activation; macrophages also are immunosuppressive in some circumstances. Activated T lymphocytes express a broad range of cytokines, which interact with a variety of effector cells; B lymphocytes produce antibodies. T lymphocytes also may interact with infected epithelial or phagocytic cells or with tumor cells to effect cell lysis. Macrophages similarly produce a large number of cytokines, which alter the functions of a variety of cells. Macrophages also release arachidonate metabolites, reactive oxygen species, nitric oxides, and a large number of proteases, which alter the function of surrounding cells, kill invading microorganisms and degrade matrix proteins. See text for further explanation. *(Adapted with permission from Agostini C, Chilosi M, Zambello R, Trentin L, Semenzato G. Pulmonary immune cells in health and disease: lymphocytes. Eur Respir J. 1993; 6(9):1378–1401.)*

cells depending upon the TH skewing. Of particular interest for the future are the ways the lung macrophage–lymphocyte inflammatory access is "turned off." The networks responsible for control and/or resolution of inflammation to prevent lung damage are likely to be as complex as those that initiate the inflammatory responses in infectious and noninfectious lung diseases.

Overall, the mammalian lung is uniquely poised to protect the environment of the lower respiratory tract and its essential gas exchange units though the presence of a complex network of monocyte/macrophage and lymphocytes selectively sequestered in various anatomical compartments. Together, they coordinate early innate responses to microbial infection and subsequent specific acquired immune responses (e.g., to viruses) that have evolved to protect the organ. Of particular interest in certain noninfectious or autoimmune lung diseases is the similarity of inflammatory responses to those in response to infections where the consequences are deleterious rather than beneficial. Thus, understanding ways to control lung innate and acquired immune responses will be essential in developing appropriate therapies for inflammatory lung diseases. Unfortunately, the converse is also true. Individuals treated with antibodies to TNFα to control the inflammation of rheumatoid arthritis or inflammatory bowel disease are at risk for reactivating latent *Mycobacterium tuberculosis* infections, an infectious disease clearly controlled by early innate and late acquired immunity. More detailed understanding of these processes, how to regulate them quantitatively and how to replace essential elements, is clearly needed to adjust the balance in individuals whose immune systems are compromised or in those whose immune systems are overwhelmed by infection or self-antigens.

REFERENCES

1. Purwar R, Campbell J, Murphy G, Richards WG, Clark RA, Kupper TS. Resident memory T cells (T(RM)) are abundant in human lung: diversity, function, and antigen specificity. *PLoS One*. 2011;6:e16245.
2. Sathaliyawala T, Kubota M, Yudanin N, et al. Distribution and compartmentalization of human circulating and tissue-resident memory T cell subsets. *Immunity*. 2013;38:187–197.
3. Pabst R, Gehrke I. Is the bronchus-associated lymphoid tissue (BALT) an integral structure of the lung in normal mammals, including humans? *Am J Respir Cell Mol Biol*. 1990;3:131–135.
4. Tschernig T, Pabst R. What is the clinical relevance of different lung compartments? *BMC Pulm Med*. 2009;9:39.

5. Agostini C, Chilosi M, Zambello R, Trentin L, Semenzato G. Pulmonary immune cells in health and disease: lymphocytes. *Eur Respir J.* 1993;6:1378–1401.
6. Berman JS, Beer DJ, Theodore AC, Kornfeld H, Bernardo J, Center DM. Lymphocyte recruitment to the lung. *Am Rev Respir Dis.* 1990;142:238–257.
7. Meyer KC, Raghu G, Baughman RP, et al; American Thoracic Society Committee on BALiILD. An official American Thoracic Society clinical practice guideline: the clinical utility of bronchoalveolar lavage cellular analysis in interstitial lung disease. *Am J Respir Crit Care Med.* 2012;185:1004–1014.
8. Harbeck RJ. Immunophenotyping of bronchoalveolar lavage lymphocytes. *Clin Diagn Lab Immunol.* 1998;5:271–277.
9. Dominique S, Bouchonnet F, Smiejan JM, Hance AJ. Expression of surface antigens distinguishing "naive" and previously activated lymphocytes in bronchoalveolar lavage fluid. *Thorax.* 1990;45:391–396.
10. Upham JW, McMenamin C, Schon-Hegrad MA, Robinson BW, Holt PG. Functional analysis of human bronchial mucosal T cells extracted with interleukin-2. *Am J Respir Crit Care Med.* 1994;149:1608–1613.
11. Kallinich T, Schmidt S, Hamelmann E, et al. Chemokine-receptor expression on T cells in lung compartments of challenged asthmatic patients. *Clin.Exp.Allergy.* 2005;35:26–33.
12. Saukkonen JJ, Kornfeld H, Berman JS. Expansion of a CD8+ CD28-cell population in the blood and lung of HIV-positive patients. *J Acquir Immune Defic Syndr.* 1993;6:1194–1204.
13. Sim GK, Rajaserkar R, Dessing M, Augustin A. Homing and in situ differentiation of resident pulmonary lymphocytes. *Int Immunol.* 1994;6:1287–1295.
14. Lahn M. The role of gammadelta T cells in the airways. *J Mol Med.* 2000;78:409–425.
15. Ainslie MP, McNulty CA, Huynh T, Symon FA, Wardlaw AJ. Characterisation of adhesion receptors mediating lymphocyte adhesion to bronchial endothelium provides evidence for a distinct lung homing pathway. *Thorax.* 2002;57:1054–1059.
16. Sallusto F, Mackay CR, Lanzavecchia A. Selective expression of the eotaxin receptor CCR3 by human T helper 2 cells. *Science.* 1997;277:2005–2007.
17. Tschernig T, Hoffmann A, Pabst R. Local proliferation contributes to lymphocyte numbers in normal lungs. *Exp Toxicol Pathol.* 2001;53:187–194.
18. Goto E, Kohrogi H, Hirata N, et al. Human bronchial intraepithelial T lymphocytes as a distinct T-cell subset: their long-term survival in SCID-Hu chimeras. *Am J Respir Cell Mol Biol.* 2000;22:405–411.
19. Schuster M, Tschernig T, Krug N, Pabst R. Lymphocytes migrate from the blood into the bronchoalveolar lavage and lung parenchyma in the asthma model of the brown Norway rat. *Am J Respir Crit Care Med.* 2000;161:558–566.
20. Cepek KL, Shaw SK, Parker CM, et al. Adhesion between epithelial cells and T lymphocytes mediated by E-cadherin and the alpha E beta 7 integrin. *Nature.* 1994;372:190–193.
21. Fels AO, Cohn ZA. The alveolar macrophage. *J Appl Physiol.* 1986;60:353–369.
22. Erle DJ, Brown T, Christian D, Aris R. Lung epithelial lining fluid T cell subsets defined by distinct patterns of beta 7 and beta 1 integrin expression. *Am J Respir Cell Mol Biol.* 1994;10:237–244.
23. Pabst R, Binns RM, Licence ST, Peter M. Evidence of a selective major vascular marginal pool of lymphocytes in the lung. *Am Rev Respir Dis.* 1987;136:1213–1218.
24. Picker LJ, Martin RJ, Trumble A, et al. Differential expression of lymphocyte homing receptors by human memory/effector T cells in pulmonary versus cutaneous immune effector sites. *Eur J Immunol.* 1994;24:1269–1277.
25. Hayday A, Viney JL. The ins and outs of body surface immunology. *Science.* 2000;290:97–100.
26. Pabst R, Binns RM. Lymphocytes migrate from the bronchoalveolar space to regional bronchial lymph nodes. *Am J Respir Crit Care Med.* 1995;151:495–499.
27. Thepen T, Kraal G, Holt PG. The role of alveolar macrophages in regulation of lung inflammation. *Ann NY Acad Sci.* 1994;725:200–206.
28. Yamauchi K, Martinet Y, Basset P, Fells GA, Crystal RG. High levels of transforming growth factor-beta are present in the epithelial lining fluid of the normal human lower respiratory tract. *Am Rev Respir Dis.* 1988;137:1360–1363.
29. Hunninghake GW, Bedell GN, Zavala DC, Monick M, Brady M. Role of interleukin-2 release by lung T-cells in active pulmonary sarcoidosis. *Am Rev Respir Dis.* 1983;128:634–638.
30. Randall TD. Bronchus-associated lymphoid tissue (BALT) structure and function. *Adv Immunol.* 2010;107:187–241.
31. Moyron-Quiroz J, Rangel-Moreno J, Carragher DM, Randall TD. The function of local lymphoid tissues in pulmonary immune responses. *Adv Exp Med Biol.* 2007;590:55–68.
32. Pabst R. IS BALAT a major component of the human lung immune system? *Immunology Today.* 1992;13(4):119–122.
33. Rangel-Moreno J, Carragher DM, de la Luz Garcia-Hernandez M, et al. The development of inducible bronchus-associated lymphoid tissue depends on IL-17. *Nat Immunol.* 2011;12:639–646.
34. Richmond I, Pritchard GE, Ashcroft T, Avery A, Corris PA, Walters EH. Bronchus associated lymphoid tissue (BALT) in human lung: its distribution in smokers and non-smokers. *Thorax.* 1993;48:1130–1134.
35. Tschernig T, Pabst R. Bronchus-associated lymphoid tissue (BALT) is not present in the normal adult lung but in different diseases. *Pathobiology.* 2000;68:1–8.
36. Moyron-Quiroz JE, Rangel-Moreno J, Kusser K, et al. Role of inducible bronchus associated lymphoid tissue (iBALT) in respiratory immunity. *Nat Med.* 2004;10:927–934.
37. Pabst R, Tschernig T. Bronchus-associated lymphoid tissue: an entry site for antigens for successful mucosal vaccinations? *Am J Respir Cell Mol Biol.* 2010;43:137–141.
38. Woodland DL, Randall TD. Anatomical features of anti-viral immunity in the respiratory tract. *Semin Immunol.* 2004;16:163–170.
39. Kocks JR, Davalos-Misslitz AC, Hintzen G, Ohl L, Forster R. Regulatory T cells interfere with the development of bronchus-associated lymphoid tissue. *J Exp Med.* 2007;204:723–734.
40. Carragher DM, Rangel-Moreno J, Randall TD. Ectopic lymphoid tissues and local immunity. *Semin Immunol.* 2008;20:26–42.
41. Holt PG, Robinson BW, Reid M, et al. Extraction of immune and inflammatory cells from human lung parenchyma: evaluation of an enzymatic digestion procedure. *Clin Exp Immunol.* 1986;66:188–200.
42. Marathias KP, Preffer FI, Pinto C, Kradin RL. Most human pulmonary infiltrating lymphocytes display the surface immune phenotype and functional responses of sensitized T cells. *Am J Respir Cell Mol Biol.* 1991;5:470–476.

43. Jonjic N, Jilek P, Bernasconi S, et al. Molecules involved in the adhesion and cytotoxicity of activated monocytes on endothelial cells. *J Immunol.* 1992;148:2080–2083.

44. Weissler JC, Nicod LP, Lipscomb MF, Toews GB. Natural killer cell function in human lung is compartmentalized. *Am Rev Respir Dis.* 1987;135:941–949.

45. Campbell DJ, Debes GF, Johnston B, Wilson E, Butcher EC. Targeting T cell responses by selective chemokine receptor expression. *Semin Immunol.* 2003;15:277–286.

46. Picker LJ. Control of lymphocyte homing. *Curr Opin Immunol.* 1994;6:394–406.

47. Springer TA. Traffic signals for lymphocyte recirculation and leukocyte emigration: the multistep paradigm. *Cell.* 1994;76: 301–314.

48. Wardlaw AJ, Guillen C, Morgan A. Mechanisms of T cell migration to the lung. *Clin Exp Allergy.* 2005;35:4–7.

49. Miller MD, Krangel MS. Biology and biochemistry of the chemokines: a family of chemotactic and inflammatory cytokines. *Crit Rev Immunol.* 1992;12:17–46.

50. Taub DD, Proost P, Murphy WJ, et al. Monocyte chemotactic protein-1 (MCP-1), -2, and -3 are chemotactic for human T lymphocytes. *JClinInvest.* 1995;95:1370–1376.

51. Bevilacqua MP. Endothelial-leukocyte adhesion molecules. *Annu Rev Immunol.* 1993;11:767–804.

52. Pober JS. Warner-Lambert/Parke-Davis award lecture. Cytokine-mediated activation of vascular endothelium. Physiology and pathology. *Am J Pathol.* 1988;133:426–433.

53. Shimizu Y, Newman W, Tanaka Y, Shaw S. Lymphocyte interactions with endothelial cells. *Immunol Today.* 1992;13:106–112.

54. van Dinther-Janssen AC, van Maarsseveen TC, Eckert H, Newman W, Meijer CJ. Identical expression of ELAM-1, VCAM-1, and ICAM-1 in sarcoidosis and usual interstitial pneumonitis. *J Pathol.* 1993;170:157–164.

55. Kim CH, Rott L, Kunkel EJ, et al. Rules of chemokine receptor association with T cell polarization in vivo. *J Clin Invest.* 2001;108:1331–1339.

56. Miotto D, Christodoulopoulos P, Olivenstein R, et al. Expression of IFN-gamma-inducible protein; monocyte chemotactic proteins 1, 3, and 4; and eotaxin in TH1- and TH2-mediated lung diseases. *J Allergy Clin Immunol.* 2001;107:664–670.

57. Ford WL, Simmonds SJ. The tempo of lymphocyte recirculation from blood to lymph in the rat. *Cell Tissue Kinet.* 1972;5: 175–189.

58. von Andrian UH, Mempel TR. Homing and cellular traffic in lymph nodes. *Nat Rev Immunol.* 2003;3:867–878.

59. Ebert LM, Schaerli P, Moser B. Chemokine-mediated control of T cell traffic in lymphoid and peripheral tissues. *Mol Immunol.* 2005;42:799–809.

60. Taub DD, Turcovski-Corrales SM, Key ML, Longo DL, Murphy WJ. Chemokines and T lymphocyte activation: I. Beta chemokines costimulate human T lymphocyte activation in vitro. *J Immunol.* 1996;156:2095–2103.

61. Kornfeld H, Berman JS, Beer DJ, Center DM. Induction of human T lymphocyte motility by interleukin 2. *J Immunol.* 1985;134:3887–3890.

62. Cruikshank WW, Long A, Tarpy RE, et al. Early identification of interleukin-16 (lymphocyte chemoattractant factor) and macrophage inflammatory protein 1 alpha (MIP1 alpha) in bronchoalveolar lavage fluid of antigen-challenged asthmatics. *Am J Respir Cell Mol Biol.* 1995;13:738–747.

63. Prefontaine D, Lajoie-Kadoch S, Foley S, Audusseau S, et al. Increased expression of IL-33 in severe asthma: evidence of expression by airway smooth muscle cells. *J Immunol.* 2009; 183:5094–5103.

64. Prefontaine D, Nadigel J, Chouiali F, et al. Increased IL-33 expression by epithelial cells in bronchial asthma. *J Allergy Clin Immunol.* 2010;125:752–754.

65. Car BD, Meloni F, Luisetti M, Semenzato G, Gialdroni-Grassi G, Walz A. Elevated IL-8 and MCP-1 in the bronchoalveolar lavage fluid of patients with idiopathic pulmonary fibrosis and pulmonary sarcoidosis. *Am J Respir Crit Care Med.* 1994;149:655–659.

66. Standiford TJ, Rolfe MW, Kunkel SL, et al. Macrophage inflammatory protein-1 alpha expression in interstitial lung disease. *J Immunol.* 1993;151:2852–2863.

67. Bellini A, Yoshimura H, Vittori E, Marini M, Mattoli S. Bronchial epithelial cells of patients with asthma release chemoattractant factors for T lymphocytes. *J Allergy Clin Immunol.* 1993;92:412–424.

68. Lim KG, Wan HC, Bozza PT, et al. Human eosinophils elaborate the lymphocyte chemoattractants. IL-16 (lymphocyte chemoattractant factor) and RANTES. *J Immunol.* 1996;156:2566–2570.

69. Borish L, Steinke JW. Interleukin-33 in asthma: how big of a role does it play? *Curr Allergy Asthma Rep.* 2011;11:7–11.

70. Grotenboer NS, Ketelaar ME, Koppelman GH, Nawijn MC. Decoding asthma: translating genetic variation in IL33 and IL1RL1 into disease pathophysiology. *J Allergy Clin Immunol.* 2013; 131:856–865.

71. Le Goffic R, Arshad MI, Rauch M, et al. Infection with influenza virus induces IL-33 in murine lungs. *Am J Respir Cell Mol Biol.* 2011;45:1125–1132.

72. Pitman N, Asquith DL, Murphy G, Liew FY, McInnes IB. Collagen-induced arthritis is not impaired in mast cell-deficient mice. *Ann Rheum Dis.* 2011;70:1170–1171.

73. Barnes PJ, Cosio MG. Characterization of T lymphocytes in chronic obstructive pulmonary disease. *PLoS Med.* 2004;1:e20.

74. Green DS, Center DM, Cruikshank WW. Human immunodeficiency virus type 1 gp120 reprogramming of CD4+ T-cell migration provides a mechanism for lymphadenopathy. *J Virol.* 2009;83:5765–5772.

75. Mashikian MV, Ryan TC, Seman A, Brazer W, Center DM, Cruikshank WW. Reciprocal desensitization of CCR5 and CD4 is mediated by IL-16 and macrophage-inflammatory protein-1 beta, respectively. *J Immunol.* 1999;163:3123–3130.

76. Rahangdale S, Morgan R, Heijens C, et al. Chemokine receptor CXCR3 desensitization by IL-16/CD4 signaling is dependent on CCR5 and intact membrane cholesterol. *J Immunol.* 2006;176:2337–2345.

77. Van Drenth C, Jenkins A, Ledwich L, et al. Desensitization of CXC chemokine receptor 4, mediated by IL-16/CD4, is independent of p56 lck enzymatic activity. *J Immunol.* 2000;165:6356–6363.

78. Stumbles PA, Upham JW, Holt PG. Airway dendritic cells: co-ordinators of immunological homeostasis and immunity in the respiratory tract. *APMIS.* 2003;111:741–755.

79. Curtis JL, Kaltreider HB. Characterization of bronchoalveolar lymphocytes during a specific antibody-forming cell response in the lungs of mice. *Am Rev Respir Dis.* 1989;139:393–400.

80. Maruyama M, Lam KP, Rajewsky K. Memory B-cell persistence is independent of persisting immunizing antigen. *Nature.* 2000;407:636–642.

81. Sprent J, Surh CD. Cytokines and T cell homeostasis. *Immunol Lett.* 2003;85:145–149.

82. Akbari O, Faul JL, Hoyte EG, et al. CD4+ invariant T-cell-receptor+ natural killer T cells in bronchial asthma. *N Engl J Med.* 2006;354:1117–1129.

83. Vijayanand P, Seumois G, Pickard C, et al. Invariant natural killer T cells in asthma and chronic obstructive pulmonary disease. *N Engl J Med.* 2007;356:1410–1422.

84. Godfrey DI, Stankovic S, Baxter AG. Raising the NKT cell family. *Nat Immunol.* 2010;11:197–206.

85. Boyton R. The role of natural killer T cells in lung inflammation. *J Pathol.* 2008;214:276–282.

86. Thomas SY, Chyung YH, Luster AD. Natural killer T cells are not the predominant T cell in asthma and likely modulate, not cause, asthma. *J Allergy Clin Immunol.* 2010;125:980–984.

87. Carrega P, Ferlazzo G. Natural killer cell distribution and trafficking in human tissues. *Front Immunol.* 2012;3:347

88. Robinson BW, Pinkston P, Crystal RG. Natural killer cells are present in the normal human lung but are functionally impotent. *J Clin Invest.* 1984;74:942–950.

89. Wang J, Li F, Zheng M, Sun R, Wei H, Tian Z. Lung natural killer cells in mice: phenotype and response to respiratory infection. *Immunology.* 2012;137:37–47.

90. Wilsher ML, Hughes DA, Haslam PL. Immunomodulatory effects of pulmonary surfactant on natural killer cell and antibody-dependent cytotoxicity. *Clin Exp Immunol.* 1988;74:465–470.

91. Culley FJ. Natural killer cells in infection and inflammation of the lung. *Immunology.* 2009;128:151–163.

92. Hanna J, Mussaffi H, Steuer G, et al. Functional aberrant expression of CCR2 receptor on chronically activated NK cells in patients with TAP-2 deficiency. *Blood.* 2005;106:3465–3473.

93. Moins-Teisserenc HT, Gadola SD, Cella M, et al. Association of a syndrome resembling Wegener's granulomatosis with low surface expression of HLA class-I molecules. *Lancet.* 1999;354:1598–1603.

94. Zimmer J, Donato L, Hanau D, et al. Activity and phenotype of natural killer cells in peptide transporter (TAP)-deficient patients (type I bare lymphocyte syndrome). *J Exp Med.* 1998;187:117–122.

95. Mosmann TR, Sad S. The expanding universe of T-cell subsets: Th1, Th2 and more. *Immunol Today.* 1996;17:138–146.

96. Romagnani S. Lymphokine production by human T cells in disease states. *Annu Rev Immunol.* 1994;12:227–257.

97. Seder RA, Paul WE. Acquisition of lymphokine-producing phenotype by CD4+ T cells. *Annu Rev Immunol.* 1994;12:635–673.

98. Rengarajan J, Szabo SJ, Glimcher LH. Transcriptional regulation of Th1/Th2 polarization. *Immunol Today.* 2000;21:479–483.

99. Szabo SJ, Sullivan BM, Stemmann C, Satoskar AR, Sleckman BP, Glimcher LH. Distinct effects of T-bet in TH1 lineage commitment and IFN-gamma production in CD4 and CD8 T cells. *Science.* 2002;295:338–342.

100. Zheng W, Flavell RA. The transcription factor GATA-3 is necessary and sufficient for Th2 cytokine gene expression in CD4 T cells. *Cell.* 1997;89:587–596.

101. Robinson DS, Hamid Q, Ying S, et al. Predominant TH2-like bronchoalveolar T-lymphocyte population in atopic asthma. *N Engl J Med.* 1992;326:298–304.

102. Krug N, Madden J, Redington AE, et al. T-cell cytokine profile evaluated at the single cell level in BAL and blood in allergic asthma. *Am J Respir Cell Mol Biol.* 1996;14:319–326.

103. Tsicopoulos A, Hamid Q, Varney V, et al. Preferential messenger RNA expression of Th1-type cells (IFN-gamma+, IL-2+) in classical delayed-type (tuberculin) hypersensitivity reactions in human skin. *J Immunol.* 1992;148:2058–2061.

104. Josefowicz SZ, Lu LF, Rudensky AY. Regulatory T cells: mechanisms of differentiation and function. *Annu Rev Immunol.* 2012;30:531–564.

105. Sakaguchi S, Yamaguchi T, Nomura T, Ono M. Regulatory T cells and immune tolerance. *Cell.* 2008;133:775–787.

106. Kuipers H, Lambrecht BN. The interplay of dendritic cells, Th2 cells and regulatory T cells in asthma. *Curr Opin Immunol.* 2004;16:702–708.

107. Rutella S, Lemoli RM. Regulatory T cells and tolerogenic dendritic cells: from basic biology to clinical applications. *Immunol Lett.* 2004;94:11–26.

108. Haribhai D, Williams JB, Jia S, et al. A requisite role for induced regulatory T cells in tolerance based on expanding antigen receptor diversity. *Immunity.* 2011;35:109–122.

109. Suto A, Nakajima H, Kagami SI, Suzuki K, Saito Y, Iwamoto I. Role of CD4(+) CD25(+) regulatory T cells in T helper 2 cell-mediated allergic inflammation in the airways. *Am J Respir Crit Care Med.* 2001;164:680–687.

110. D'Alessio FR, Tsushima K, Aggarwal NR, et al. CD4+ CD25+ Foxp3+ Tregs resolve experimental lung injury in mice and are present in humans with acute lung injury. *J Clin Invest.* 2009;119:2898–2913.

111. Zuleger CL, Gao X, Burger MS, Chu Q, Payne LG, Chen D. Peptide induces CD4(+)CD25+ and IL-10+ T cells and protection in airway allergy models. *Vaccine.* 2005;23:3181–3186.

112. Cruikshank WW, Lim K, Theodore AC, Cook J, Fine G, Weller PF. Center DM. IL-16 inhibition of CD3-dependent lymphocyte activation and proliferation. *J Immunol.* 1996;157:5240–5248.

113. Pinsonneault S, El BS, Mazer B, Cruikshank WW, Laberge S. IL-16 inhibits IL-5 production by antigen-stimulated T cells in atopic subjects. *J Allergy Clin Immunol.* 2001;107:477–482.

114. McFadden C, Morgan R, Rahangdale S, et al. Preferential migration of T regulatory cells induced by IL-16. *J Immunol.* 2007;179:6439–6445

115. Korn T, Bettelli E, Oukka M, Kuchroo VK. IL-17 and Th17 Cells. *Annu Rev Immunol.* 2009;27:485–517.

116. Weaver CT, Elson CO, Fouser LA, Kolls JK. The Th17 pathway and inflammatory diseases of the intestines, lungs, and skin. *Annu Rev Pathol.* 2013;8:477–512.

117. Bullens DM, Truyen E, Coteur L, et al. IL-17 mRNA in sputum of asthmatic patients: linking T cell driven inflammation and granulocytic influx? *Respir Res.* 2006;7:135.

118. Kawaguchi M, Onuchic LF, Li XD, et al. Identification of a novel cytokine, ML-1, and its expression in subjects with asthma. *J Immunol.* 2001;167:4430–4435.

119. McKinley L, Alcorn JF, Peterson A, et al. TH17 cells mediate steroid-resistant airway inflammation and airway hyperresponsiveness in mice. *J Immunol.* 2008;181:4089–4097.

120. Facco M, Cabrelle A, Teramo A, et al. Sarcoidosis is a Th1/Th17 multisystem disorder. *Thorax.* 2011;66:144–150.

121. Ten Berge B, Paats MS, Bergen IM, et al. Increased IL-17 A expression in granulomas and in circulating memory T cells in sarcoidosis. *Rheumatology (Oxford).* 2012;51:37–46.

122. Moro K, Yamada T, Tanabe M, et al. Innate production of T(H)2 cytokines by adipose tissue-associated c-Kit(+)Sca-1(+) lymphoid cells. *Nature.* 2010;463:540–544.

123. Neill DR, Wong SH, Bellosi A, et al. Nuocytes represent a new innate effector leukocyte that mediates type-2 immunity. *Nature.* 2010;464:1367–1370.

124. Price AE, Liang HE, Sullivan BM. Systemically dispersed innate IL-13-expressing cells in type 2 immunity. *Proc Natl Acad Sci U S A.* 2010;107:11489–11494.

125. Spits H, Artis D, Colonna M, et al. Innate lymphoid cells–a proposal for uniform nomenclature. *Nat Rev Immunol.* 2013;13:145–149.

126. Barlow JL, Bellosi A, Hardman CS, et al. Innate IL-13-producing nuocytes arise during allergic lung inflammation and contribute to airways hyperreactivity. *J Allergy Clin Immunol.* 2012;129:191–198. e1–e4.

127. Klein Wolterink RG, Kleinjan A, van Nimwegen M, et al. Pulmonary innate lymphoid cells are major producers of IL-5 and IL-13 in murine models of allergic asthma. *Eur J Immunol.* 2012;42:1106–1116.

128. Chang YJ, Kim HY, Albacker LA, et al. Innate lymphoid cells mediate influenza-induced airway hyper-reactivity independently of adaptive immunity. *Nat Immunol.* 2011;12:631–638.

129. Mjosberg JM, Trifari S, Crellin NK, et al. Human IL-25- and IL-33-responsive type 2 innate lymphoid cells are defined by expression of CRTH2 and CD161. *Nat Immunol.* 2011;12: 1055–1062.

130. Kato A, Hulse KE, Tan BK, Schleimer RP. B-lymphocyte lineage cells and the respiratory system. *J Allergy Clin Immunol.* 2013;131:933–957; quiz 958.

131. Baumgarth N. The double life of a B-1 cell: self-reactivity selects for protective effector functions. *Nat Rev Immunol.* 2011;11:34–46.

132. Griffin DO, Holodick NE, Rothstein TL. Human B1 cells in umbilical cord and adult peripheral blood express the novel phenotype CD20+ CD27+ CD43+ CD70. *J Exp Med.* 2011;208:67–80.

133. Hance AJ. Pulmonary immune cells in health and disease: dendritic cells and Langerhans' cells. *Eur Respir J.* 1993;6:1213–1220.

134. Nicod LP, el Habre F. Adhesion molecules on human lung dendritic cells and their role for T-cell activation. *Am J Respir Cell Mol Biol.* 1992;7:207–213.

135. Johnston RB Jr. Current concepts: immunology. Monocytes and macrophages. *N Engl J Med.* 1988;318:747–752.

136. Kremlev SG, Umstead TM, Phelps DS. Effects of surfactant protein A and surfactant lipids on lymphocyte proliferation in vitro. *Am J Physiol.* 1994;267:L357–L364.

137. Weissler JC, Mendelson C, Moya F, Yarbrough WC Jr. Effect of interstitial lung disease macrophages on T-cell signal transduction. *Am J Respir Crit Care Med.* 1994;149:191–196.

138. Bach JF. Regulatory T cells under scrutiny. *Nat Rev Immunol.* 2003;3:189–198.

139. George TC, Bilsborough J, Viney JL, Norment AM. High antigen dose and activated dendritic cells enable Th cells to escape regulatory T cell-mediated suppression in vitro. *Eur J Immunol.* 2003;33:502–511.

140. Serra P, Amrani A, Yamanouchi J, et al. CD40 ligation releases immature dendritic cells from the control of regulatory CD4+CD25+ T cells. *Immunity.* 2003;19:877–889.

141. Fainaru O, Woolf E, Lotem J, et al. Runx3 regulates mouse TGF-beta-mediated dendritic cell function and its absence results in airway inflammation. *EMBO J.* 2004;23:969–979.

142. Williams GT. Apoptosis in the immune system. *J Pathol.* 1994; 173:1–4.

143. Bitterman PB, Saltzman LE, Adelberg S, Ferrans VJ, Crystal RG. Alveolar macrophage replication. One mechanism for the expansion of the mononuclear phagocyte population in the chronically inflamed lung. *J Clin Invest.* 1984;74:460–469.

144. Janssen WJ, Barthel L, Muldrow A, et al. Fas determines differential fates of resident and recruited macrophages during resolution of acute lung injury. *Am J Respir Crit Care Med.* 2011;184:547–560.

145. Murphy J, Summer R, Wilson AA, Kotton DN, Fine A. The prolonged life-span of alveolar macrophages. *Am J Respir Cell Mol Biol.* 2008;38:380–385.

146. Wynn TA, Chawla A, Pollard JW. Macrophage biology in development, homeostasis and disease. *Nature.* 2013;496:445–455.

147. Yona S, Kim KW, Wolf Y, et al. Fate mapping reveals origins and dynamics of monocytes and tissue macrophages under homeostasis. *Immunity.* 2013;38:79–91.

148. Lohmann-Matthes ML, Steinmuller C, Franke-Ullmann G. Pulmonary macrophages. *Eur Respir J.* 1994;7:1678–1689.

149. Naito M, Umeda S, Yamamoto T, et al. Development, differentiation, and phenotypic heterogeneity of murine tissue macrophages. *J Leukoc Biol.* 1996;59:133–138.

150. Wu HM, Jin M, Marsh CB. Toward functional proteomics of alveolar macrophages. *Am J Physiol Lung Cell Mol Physiol.* 2005;288:L585–L595.

151. Nathan CF. Secretory products of macrophages. *J Clin Invest.* 1987;79:319–326.

152. Adams DO, Hamilton TA. The cell biology of macrophage activation. *Annu Rev Immunol.* 1984;2:283–318.

153. Ishii H, Hayashi S, Hogg JC, et al. Alveolar macrophage-epithelial cell interaction following exposure to atmospheric particles induces the release of mediators involved in monocyte mobilization and recruitment. *Respir Res.* 2005;6:87.

154. Mosser DM, Edwards JP. Exploring the full spectrum of macrophage activation. *Nat Rev Immunol.* 2008;8:958–969.

155. Basu S, Fenton MJ. Toll-like receptors: function and roles in lung disease. *Am J Physiol Lung Cell Mol Physiol.* 2004;286:L887–L892.

156. Thoma-Uszynski S, Stenger S, Takeuchi O, et al. Induction of direct antimicrobial activity through mammalian toll-like receptors. *Science.* 2001;291:1544–1547.

157. Palecanda A, Paulauskis J, Al-Mutairi E, et al. Role of the scavenger receptor MARCO in alveolar macrophage binding of unopsonized environmental particles. *J Exp Med.* 1999;189:1497–1506.

158. Arredouani M, Yang Z, Ning Y, et al. The scavenger receptor MARCO is required for lung defense against pneumococcal pneumonia and inhaled particles. *J Exp Med.* 2004;200:267–272.

159. Bedoret D, Wallemacq H, Marichal T, et al. Lung interstitial macrophages alter dendritic cell functions to prevent airway allergy in mice. *J Clin Invest.* 2009;119:3723–3738.

160. Franke-Ullmann G, Pfortner C, Walter P, et al. Characterization of murine lung interstitial macrophages in comparison with alveolar macrophages in vitro. *J Immunol.* 1996;157:3097–3104.

161. Vermaelen K, Pauwels R. Pulmonary dendritic cells. *Am J Respir Crit Care Med* 2005;172:530–551.

162. Havenith CE, van Miert PP, Breedijk AJ, Beelen RH, Hoefsmit EC. Migration of dendritic cells into the draining lymph nodes of the lung after intratracheal instillation. *Am J Respir Cell Mol Biol.* 1993;9:484–488.

163. GeurtsvanKessel CH, Lambrecht BN. Division of labor between dendritic cell subsets of the lung. *Mucosal Immunol.* 2008;1:442–450.

164. van Rijt LS, Jung S, Kleinjan A, et al. In vivo depletion of lung CD11 c+ dendritic cells during allergen challenge abrogates the characteristic features of asthma. *J ExpMed.* 2005;201:981–991.

165. Ohgami M, Doerschuk CM, Gie RP, English D, Hogg JC. Monocyte kinetics in rabbits. *J Appl Physiol.* 1991;70:152–157.

166. Dehring DJ, Wismar BL. Intravascular macrophages in pulmonary capillaries of humans. *Am Rev Respir Dis.* 1989;139:1027–1029.

167. Schneberger D, Aharonson-Raz K, Singh B. Pulmonary intravascular macrophages and lung health: what are we missing? *Am J Physiol Lung Cell Mol Physiol.* 2012;302:L498–L503.

168. Warner AE, Brain JD. The cell biology and pathogenic role of pulmonary intravascular macrophages. *Am J Physiol.* 1990;258: L1–L12.

169. Springer TA. Traffic signals on endothelium for lymphocyte recirculation and leukocyte emigration. *Annu Rev Physiol.* 1995;57:827–872.

170. Warmington KS, Boring L, Ruth JH, et al. Effect of C-C chemokine receptor 2 (CCR2) knockout on type-2 (schistosomal antigen-elicited) pulmonary granuloma formation: analysis of cellular recruitment and cytokine responses. *Am J Pathol.* 1999;154:1407–1416.

171. Thomas ED, Ramberg RE, Sale GE, Sparkes RS, Golde DW. Direct evidence for a bone marrow origin of the alveolar macrophage in man. *Science.* 1976;192:1016–1018.

172. Galli SJ, Borregaard N, Wynn TA. Phenotypic and functional plasticity of cells of innate immunity: macrophages, mast cells and neutrophils. *Nat Immunol.* 2011;12:1035–1044.

173. Shapiro SD. Elastolytic metalloproteinases produced by human mononuclear phagocytes. Potential roles in destructive lung disease. *Am J Respir Crit Care Med.* 1994;150:S160–S164.

CHAPTER 22

Mast Cells and Eosinophils

Edward S. Schulman
Peter H. S. Sporn

INTRODUCTION

For more than a century physicians have noted a clear connection between mast cell (MC) activation and the subsequent appearance of eosinophils both within the circulation and in tissues. Only recently, however, have basic insights been gained into the mechanisms of this cellular collusion. In keeping with this association, human MCs and eosinophils are considered together in this chapter.

MCs and eosinophils were discovered in the 1870s by the same observer, Paul Ehrlich. He noted that some cells stained in a peculiar fashion when incubated with standard aniline dyes such as toluidine blue and alcian blue. He used the term metachromasie or metachromasia to describe the peculiar color modifications that occurred and the term Mastzellen, meaning "well fed" or "fattened" in German, to describe what we now call MC. Interestingly, this latter term is now known to be a misnomer, since MC cytoplasmic granules are not phagocytosized but rather synthesized during cell growth and again during regranulation. Ehrlich also noted that some cells stained intensely when incubated with the acidic dye eosin. As a result, these cells were called eosinophils. Studies of these two cell types, over the ensuing years, have provided great insight into their roles in biology. They have also highlighted the differences that exist in these cells among different species and their heterogeneity even within a single species and even within single organs.

MAST CELLS

The capacity of strategically localized human MC to rapidly release a panoply of powerful chemical mediators makes this cell a unique member of the body's immune response network. Although most frequently discussed in the context of hypersensitivity immune responses, MCs are also known to participate in normal physiological processes including gastric acid secretion,[1] angiogenesis,[2,3] and lipid clearance.[4–8] Increasing evidence supports a role in the innate immune response, especially serving bacterial defense.[9] MCs also participate in nonallergic pathophysiological processes such as inflammatory bowel disease,[10,11] arthritis,[12] scleroderma,[13,14] tumors, interstitial pulmonary fibrosis,[15–18] envenomation,[3,19–22] and atherosclerosis.[4,5,23,24] Over the years, basophils have been confused with MC in a number of contexts.[25] This confusion is due, in part, to a number of similarities between the cells, including the shared expression of FcRI (high-affinity receptor for Fc fragment of IgE), release of preformed histamine, and metachromatic staining. However, MCs are mononuclear cells and are almost exclusively localized to tissues. In contrast, basophils are circulating polymorphonuclear cells that are found occasionally in tissue reactions, including the late-phase allergic response. In addition, significant differences in the two-cell populations exist in cell lineage, ultrastructure, mediator release biochemistry, mediator profiles, pharmacology, and surface antigenicity.

ANATOMIC LOCALIZATION

MCs are present in all organs but are particularly abundant in the nose, skin, gastrointestinal tract, and lung. They reside primarily near blood vessels, within the adventitia of arteries, and also near lymph vessels and nerves.[26–28] Estimated concentrations of human lung MCs (HLMCs) range from 500 to 4000 mm^{-3}. In nonasthmatics, HLMCs localize to submucosal connective tissues and not epithelium or smooth muscle. Though data in asthmatics are conflicting as to whether numbers are increased versus nonasthmatics, MCs localize to three critical sites: bronchial epithelium,[29] airway mucus glands,[30] and within smooth muscle.[31–34] Mediator release from the small numbers of HLMCs within the epithelium may subserve initial antigen recognition and also be strategically placed to respond to nonantigenic signals, including hyperosmolarity,[35] as well as "endogenous" mediators, including extracellular adenosine and adenosine 5′ monophosphate (ATP).[36–38] In the case of aeroallergens, permeabilization resulting from epithelial MC mediators enhances further antigen penetration to deeper airway smooth muscles and mucus glands, which in turn, promotes bronchoconstriction and mucus secretion, respectively. The finding of HLMC within the smooth muscle layer appears to be a common and critical finding in asthmatics. It is an uncommon finding in nonasthmatics and in patients with eosinophilic bronchitis. Other than MC localization to ASM, the latter condition has virtually identical structural remodeling changes to asthma but is not associated with obstruction or airway hyperresponsiveness (AHR).[31,39] In the lung periphery, abundant MCs reside within small airways and in the alveolar septa, within a few microns of the alveolar lumen.[37] The small numbers of MC in bronchoalveolar lavage (BAL) fluid ($\leq$0.1% of all cells) likely result from epithelial shedding.[27,40]

■ ORIGINS OF MAST CELLS

MCs are believed to be derived from pleuripotent hematopoietic stem cells.[41] Tryptase-negative MC-colony–forming cells leave the marrow and circulate with a surface phenotype that is CD (cluster of differentiation) 34+, c-kit (CD117)+, LY–, CD14–, and CD17–. The progenitors home in a tissue-specific manner where they undergo differentiation, maturation, and synthesis of granule proteases in response to microenvironmental factors, including the matrix and chemokines from fibroblasts, endothelial cells, airway smooth muscle cells, and possibly T cells. The microenvironmental factor most critical in chemotaxis, differentiation, adhesion, proliferation, maturation and survival is stem cell factor (SCF or c-kit ligand), the ligand for the c-kit tyrosine kinase receptor. This receptor is expressed on the MC surface throughout its life span.[42,43]

■ MAST CELL HETEROGENEITY

Striking differences in the morphology, T cell dependence, resident proteoglycans, and responsiveness to secretagogues and drugs have been described in human MC.[44–51] The ontogeny of this heterogeneity, as well as the differing roles these MC play in physiology and disease remain speculative.

The most commonly recognized system for classifying human MC is based on the expression of protease profiles as determined by immunohistochemical staining using monoclonal antibodies. According to this system, the serine proteinase tryptase (T) is expressed in virtually all human MC, and a subset, predominantly in the submucosa of the gut and in the skin and within asthmatic airway smooth muscle also express chymase (C) and multiple other proteases including carboxypeptidase A and cathepsin G. Those that express tryptase alone are classified as the MC_T type, and those with additional proteases, as the MC_{TC} type.[52–54] Because significant numbers of both types can be found in the same organ (e.g., lung), tissue location alone cannot dictate the protease type. In the lung, only 8% to 35% of MCs are MC_{TC}, 1% is MC_C, and the remainder are MC_T. The protease system does follow some rules of distribution and function. MC_T are preferentially localized in bronchi, bronchioles, at mucosal surfaces, alveolar parenchyma, lamnia propia, in areas of T-cell infiltration and are reduced in immunodeficiency syndromes. The MC_{TC} phenotype does not appear immune related and more prevalent in pulmonary vessels and pleura. As detected by immunohistochemical staining, the subtype more selectively expresses interleukin (IL)-4 (85% MC_{TC} vs. 15% MC_{TC}). IL-5 and IL-6 are almost exclusively restricted to the MC_T subtype. Within human lung different compartments appear to show site-specific expression of FcεRIα, IL-9 receptor, histidine decarboxylase (higher in MC_T of bronchi than MC_T of alveoli), 5-lipoxygenase, leukotriene C_4 (LTC_4) synthase, vascular endothelial growth factor (VEGF), basic fibroblast growth factor (FGF)[55] and renin.

HLMC diameters vary between 8 and 18 µm with the majority being 12 to 15 µm. Histamine contents of 2.5 to 10.0 pg/MC vary directly with cell diameter. HLMC densities vary from 1.053 to 1.123 g/mL with the majority (67%) between 1.077 g/mL and 1.088 g/mL. These diameter and density-based subtypes also are distinct with respect to mediator content and function. MC location also subserves function: Airway and parenchymal MC differ in their releasibility. At the ultrastructural level, marked heterogeneity has been described (see Morphology below). Finally, at least two types of proteoglycans are present in HLMC: chondroitin sulfates, predominantly chondroitin sulfate E, and heparin. HLMCs are both positive and negative for the heparin-sensitive dye berberine sulfate, whereas stomach MCs synthesize exclusively chondroitin sulfate E and not heparin.[56,57]

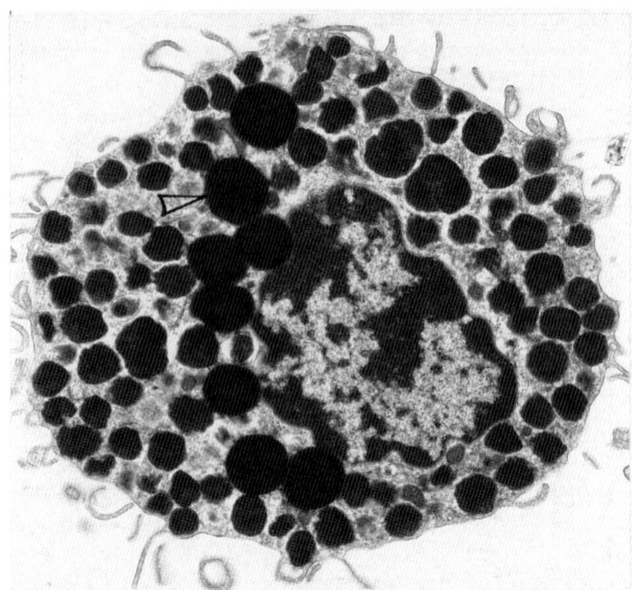

Figure 22-1 Ultrastructure of the human lung mast cell after purification. The mast cell is a mononuclear cell packed with multiple dense cytoplasmic granules that vary in size and shape. Eight electron-dense lipid bodies *(open arrow)* are bunched near the nucleus (×15,000). *(Reproduced with permission from Dvorak AM. Recovery of human lung mast cells from anaphylactic degranulation utilizes a mixture of conservation and synthetic mechanisms, in Galli SJ, Austen KF (eds). Mast Cell and Basophil Differentiation and Function in Health and Disease. New York: Raven; 1989.)*

■ MORPHOLOGY

All MCs are mononuclear cells with heterogeneous cytoplasmic granules (Fig. 22-1). A variety of granule-filling patterns occur within individual cells: scrolls, crystals, particles (the least seen in pure form), and combinations (mixed). The appearance of individual patterns can be influenced by cross section. Granules are outlined by a perigranular membrane. Cell membranes are outlined by short, narrow surface folds.[58–62]

■ MORPHOLOGY OF DEGRANULATION AND REGRANULATION

Following IgE-mediated (anaphylactic) activation of HLMC, granules swell and their perigranular membranes fuse to form canaliculi that open through multiple pores to the cell exterior. Within 20 minutes of activation, granular matrix materials solubilize within these intracytoplasmic channels and empty. In HLMC, only rarely is extrusion of nonsolubilized granules observed. Lipid bodies, which are electron-dense nonmembrane-bound organelles,[63–66] remain adjacent to these channels. They appear to serve as repositories of arachidonic acid and occasionally release lipid into the degranulation channels. In vivo, a process termed "piecemeal degranulation" is more frequently observed than anaphylactic degranulation.[67] This process involves the budding of small vesicles from granule membranes and their movement to the cell surface. Piecemeal degranulation may be more typical of the ongoing MC release observed in chronic asthma.

Depending on the extent to which an individual cell has degranulated, one of two predominant types of regranulation are observed individually or in combination. In partially degranulated cells, the channel (formerly perigranular) membranes are reutilized, and regranulation events resemble degranulation in reverse. In cells with more complete degranulation, the channel membranes are placed in continuity with the plasma membrane and externalized. This results in the appearance of elongated, activated cell surface folds. These excessive folds can be internalized or shed. Shedding results in cells that are initially small (7 μm), but then enter a rapidly expanding recovery cycle to produce a fully mature cell.[62]

ACTIVATION

Immunological activation of MC is the mechanism most studied.[68] It results from antigen cross-linking of antigen-specific cell surface IgE molecules and subsequent aggregation of the high-affinity receptors (FcεRI) to which they are attached.[69,70] Receptor dimerization is the minimum cross-linkage requirement for IgE-mediated activation. In vitro, immunological activation can be achieved using antibodies directed against human IgE or the FcεRI-receptor itself. The mechanism(s) involved in chronic HLMC activation characteristic of asthma are not known but likely may reflect low-level allergen activation. Recent evidence contends that monomeric IgE alone, in the absence of antigen, can also induce prolonged mediator release, a mechanism that may be operative within the asthmatic airway.[71]

Non–IgE-mediated release triggers of MC are also well characterized. In general, the profile of agents that degranulate MC from human intestine and synovium is similar to that of HLMC but different from skin MC.[62,72,73] These non–IgE-mediated secretagogues include ionophores, hyperosmolar stimuli, and "histamine-releasing activities" derived from human alveolar macrophages and other cells.[74–77] The purified anaphylatoxin C5a, an active trigger of human basophils and dermal MC, is generally inactive in HLMC,[78,79] although CD88, the receptor for C5, has been reported in the MC_{TC}.[80] Consistent degranulators of dermal but not HLMC include substance P, morphine, polyamines such as 48/80, and SCF. Even within lung compartments, responsiveness to triggers may vary. Compound 48/80 is reported to degranulate BAL MC, whereas those from lung parenchyma are minimally responsive. To date, neuropeptides have been shown to be inactive in degranulating HLMC. Bee venom phospholipase (PL) A_2 and antigens from dust mites, cockroaches, pollens and fungal spores contain phospholipases and proteases, which can lead to MC release through the protease-activated receptor (PAR) 2.[81,82] Finally, expression in both mouse MC and human progenitor–derived MC of several innate pattern recognition receptors, including the Toll-like receptor-2 (TLR-2) and TLR-4, has been reported.[83,84] The expression of TLR and effects on activation of HLMC are as yet poorly defined. Human peripheral blood–derived cultured MCs are reported to produce type I IFNs following exposure to double-stranded RNA and/or virus, the former implicating TLR-3 expression.[83]

MODULATORS OF ACTIVATION

Although not acting as direct release triggers, a number of endogenous chemicals in the MC microenvironment can influence activation. Extracellular ATP and its breakdown product, adenosine, are potent modulators of HLMC degranulation, although neither directly activates HLMC in vitro.[36–38,85] In asthmatics, aerosolized adenosine induces bronchoconstriction, an effect not observed in other groups of pulmonary patients or normals.[86] The ability of antihistamines to inhibit this response has directly implicated activation of allergically primed airway MC by adenosine.[87,88] Components of the local connective tissue matrix such as fibronectin also modulate MC reactivity.[89]

BIOCHEMICAL ANALYSIS OF HLMC ACTIVATION

Elegant studies defining the biochemical events following IgE-mediated activation have been performed in rodent MCs or cell lines.[90,91] Evaluations of similarities and differences in HLMC activation await future investigations. Two receptors for IgE have been identified. The high-affinity IgE receptor (FcεRI) on MC and basophils is expressed in a tetrameric form ($\alpha\beta\gamma 2$) and on antigen-presenting cells is present in a trimeric form ($\alpha\gamma 2$). The Fc fragment of IgE binds to the α-chain of FcεRI. Expression of the β-chain amplifies signaling. A low-affinity IgE receptor (FcεRII; CD23) is present on B cells but not on MC or basophils.[92] Serum IgE levels correlate with basophil expression of FcεRI, likely indicating a role for IgE in stabilizing the FcεRI on the cell surface. As noted earlier, receptor dimerization is the minimum cross-linkage requirement for antigen-mediated allergen activation through the FcεRI. Following receptor aggregation, multiple signal transduction pathways are activated. Since FcεRI possesses no inherent tyrosine kinase activity, critical to the sequential activation are two tyrosine kinases, lyn which is associated with the β chain and syk. Lyn binds to the β-chain–associated immunoreceptor tyrosine-based activation motifs (ITAMs), which are phosphorylated after FcεRI aggregation. For degranulation to proceed, syk then binds to the γ-chain–linked ITAM, which are also phosphorylated after receptor aggregation. The lynsyk-driven pathway directly or indirectly stimulates tyrosine phosphorylation of several adapter proteins, including the transmembrane adaptor molecule linker for activation of T cells (LAT) among others. These events lead to the generation of inositol triphosphate (IP_3) which induces Ca^{2+} mobilization from intracellular rough endoplasmic reticulum (RER) stores. Also activated are phospholipase C-γ1 and PLC-γ2.[93–101] In this context, at 2 minutes following FcεRI aggregation, extracellular calcium influx occurs through CRACM channels (Ca^{2+} release–activated Ca^{2+} [CRAC] modulator 1),[102,103] which is a prerequisite for degranulation to proceed over the next 5 to 20 minutes. Other "early-phase" granule-associated and lipid mediators (e.g., arachidonate metabolites) are also released over 20 minutes. Over the ensuing 1 to 24 hours, mRNAs for select cytokines are generated followed by their protein synthesis and release.

CHEMICAL MEDIATORS

The clinical expression of MC-mediated responses may reflect the individual mediators or in certain instances, the interplay of the multiple mediators these cells release (Table 22-1). The temporal sequence of their release appears critical to the development of both the early- and late-phase responses after antigen challenge (Fig. 22-2). Certain mediators are virtually unique to MC (e.g., tryptase, chymase, heparin), and others are shared with one or more other cells (e.g., histamine, LTC_4, and IL-5).

Mediators released within minutes after activation are divided into preformed, or secretory, granule-associated mediators (e.g., histamine) and nonpreformed, or newly synthesized mediators (e.g., lipids). It is now known that tumor necrosis factor alpha (TNFα) may be both preformed and newly synthesized. Other cytokine mediators, including IL-5 and IL-13, are only detected over hours and may be critical to the evolution of the "late-phase" response.

PREFORMED MEDIATORS

Mast cells contain a number of preformed mediators. Each is discussed below.

Histamine

Histamine measurements have served as a classic marker of MC-mediated events. The pleiotrophic effects of histamine are mediated through the differential expression, regulation, and distinct intracellular signals evoked by four distinct receptors, H1, H2, H3, and H4. The actual role of histamine in asthma remains less clear, although levels in BAL fluid are many-fold higher in asthmatics, and plasma levels rise three- to fivefold following airway antigen challenge. Most histamine-induced allergic respiratory reactions are mediated via the H1 histamine receptor subclass, producing enhancement of vascular permeability, mucus production, initiation of neurogenic reflexes, and bronchial smooth muscle contraction. The reasons for the marginal value of the H1 receptor-blocking drugs in asthma may be due to high local tissue concentrations of histamine that exceed the inhibitory

TABLE 22-1 Human Mast Cell and Eosinophil Mediators

	Mast Cells	Eosinophils
Granule-associated (preformed) mediators	Histamine Heparin Chondroitin-sulfate E TNFα	MBP ECP EDN EPO CLC protein
Enzymes	Tryptase Chymase Cathepsin G Elastase Carboxypeptidase-A	EPO ECP, EDN Collagenase MMP-9 Indoleamine 2,3-dioxygenase
Acid hydrolases	β-hexosaminidase β-glucuronidase Arylsulfatase	β-glucuronidase Arylsulfatase B
Lipid mediators (nonpreformed)	PGD_2 LTC_4 LTB_4 PAF Thromboxane-A_2	LTC_4 15-HETE 5-oxo-ETE PAF
Cytokines	IL-4, IL-5, IL-13 IL-6, IL-8 TNFα TGFβ bFGF	IL-1α, IL-2, IL-3 IL-4, IL-5, IL-6, IL-8 IL-10, IL-12, IL-13 IL-16, IL-17 GM-CSF TNFα TGFα TGFβ SCF NGF PDGF VEGF
Chemokines		CCL3 CCL5 CCL13 CCL11
Reactive oxygen products	None detected	O_2^-, H_2O_2, OH HOBr, HOCl

capacity of these agents and/or the redundancy of histamine actions with the multiple other mediators that are released.

Proteoglycans

MC proteoglycans serve as the major determinant for the metachromatic tinctorial properties of the cell and form the granule backbone to which other preformed mediators, including histamine and neutral proteases, are bound. HLMCs synthesize heparin and chondroitin sulfate E proteoglycans in roughly a 2:1 ratio.[56] In humans, heparin appears to be unique to MC. In addition to anticoagulant activity, heparin possesses both anti-inflammatory and immunoregulatory properties.[104–106] Heparin may limit allergic responses in the skin, nose and lung and exert protective effects on exercise-induced asthma (EIA). The inhibitory effects may be related to the

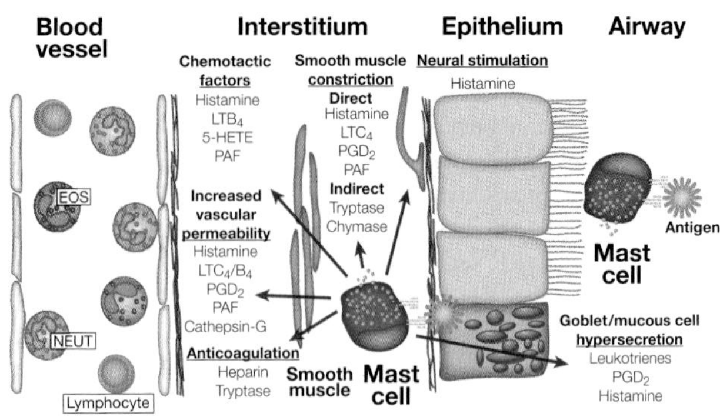

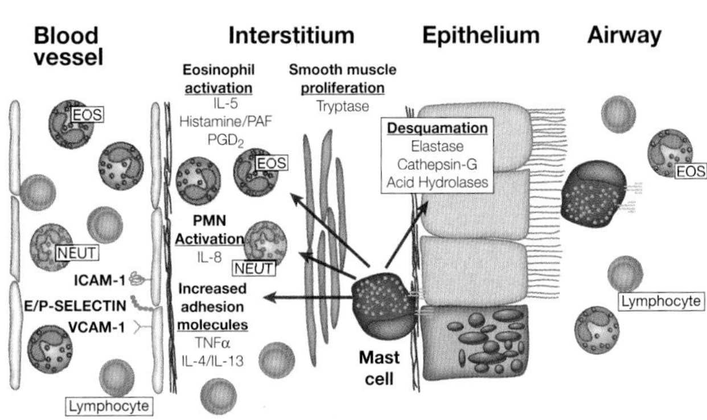

Figure 22-2 Effects of mast cell mediators in the early- and late-phase responses following airway allergen challenge. **A.** Early phase: Mediators are released within minutes following antigen cross-linking of allergen-specific IgE on the cell surface. Mechanisms of the initial airflow obstruction that persists for 30 to 60 minutes include smooth muscle constriction, edema formation due to increased vascular permeability, nerve stimulation, and mucus hypersecretion from both goblet cells and submucosal glands. **B.** Late phase. Within hours, the effects of newly synthesized and released cytokine mediators along with delayed effects of early-phase mediators produce recurrent airway obstruction. Mast cell mediators and cytokines can increase the expression of adhesion molecules on endothelial cells, both recruit and activate leukocytes (particularly eosinophils), contribute to epithelial desquamation, and stimulate smooth muscle proliferation.

extracellular binding and inhibition of multiple mediators, including histamine and cytokines.

Chemotactic Factors

Within hours of MC activation, airway inflammation (the late-phase response) at the tissue level is characterized by the infiltration of leukocytes. This response is principally eosinophilic but also contains neutrophils and, over time, lymphocytes. Chemotactic mediators may be derived directly from MC and/or other cells through secondary stimulation. Early-phase MC-derived eosinophilic chemotactic activities include leukotriene B_4 (LTB_4), platelet-activating factor (PAF), and histamine.[107] HLMCs robustly express IL-8, which along with LTB_4, attracts neutrophils. MCs are responsive to chemokines released from other cells. Airway smooth muscle secretes a number of chemotactic factors including CXCL8, -10, -11, and -12. It appears that the CXCR3/CXCL10 axis predominately mediates the HLMC migration into the airway smooth muscle observed in asthmatic airways.[108,109]

Proteases

Large quantities of neutral proteases are contained within MC and constitute the predominant protein component of the secretory granule. The proteases include tryptase, chymase, cathepsin G, carboxypeptidase A, and elastase.[52–54,110]

Tryptase is the predominant neutral protease of the MC granule. It is a tetramer that is stabilized by its association with proteoglycan. The concentration of tryptase in pulmonary MC is 11 pg/MC. Since the concentrations of tryptase in circulating basophils (α tryptase, see below) are negligible, responses characterized by the presence of histamine but not tryptase at the reaction site or in the circulation implicate mediation by basophils and not MC. Two forms of tryptase (α and β) have been identified. The α tryptase is constitutively secreted in an inactive form and reflects systemic MC burden. The active β form is packaged in the secretory granule and acutely rises in anaphylactic reactions. Postulated roles for tryptase in pathophysiology remain to be established. Described actions include the degradation of the neuropeptide vasoactive intestinal peptide (VIP), mitogenic effects on smooth muscle and epithelial cells, and inactivation of procoagulant proteins.

Chymase is associated with heparin in a manner similar to tryptase. The role of chymase in asthma and other disorders is not clearly defined. Chymase may play a role in tissue remodeling. Substrates include angiotensin I, converting it to the angiotensin II, VIP (inactivates), substance P, bradykinin, and kallidin (inactivates). Other activities include activation of matrix metalloprotease and stimulation of tissue neutrophilia and eosinophilia.

Cathepsin G is a neutral protease with chymotryptic specificities. The concentration of cathepsin G in HLMC is roughly 100 to 700 ng/10^6 cells. An elastase released from HLMC appears to be identical to human neutrophil elastase. A measurement of 40 to 170 ng/10^6 cells assumes all HLMCs contain this enzyme, although it may be localized to an HLMC subset. Among carboxypeptidases, the MC carboxypeptidase A, a metalloexopeptidase, is unique. Granule-associated acid hydrolases include β-hexosaminidase, β-glucuronidase, and arylsulfatase.

NONPREFORMED MEDIATORS

Arachidonic acid metabolites are generated within minutes of MC activation and play a crucial role in the early phases of the asthmatic response. Cyclooxygenase metabolism in MC generates large quantities of prostaglandin (PG) D_2 and a small quantity of thromboxane A_2.[37,111] PGD_2 is the most potent bronchoconstrictor of the cyclooxygenase metabolites. Additional actions of PGD_2 include induction of chemotaxis in eosinophils, basophils, and Th2 cells; increase in capillary permeability and vasodilation. Although all tissue MCs generate PGD_2, not all generate significant quantities of 5-lipoxygenase products (e.g., lung > skin). The major 5-lipoxygenase pathway products of HLMC are LTC_4, and LTB_4, with lesser quantities of 5-HETE. In IgE-mediated human lung challenges, MCs constitute the major source of released LTC_4.[112]

PAF is an early-phase phospholipid bronchoconstrictor that consists of a family of molecules. In contrast to the other lipid mediators, MCs appear to retain PAF intracellularly or demonstrate rapid reuptake of any that may be released.

HLMCs synthesize and release TH2-type cytokines, including IL-5, and -13, which are felt to be central to the evolution of the late-phase response.[113,114] Additional multifunctional cytokines, including IL-3, -6, -8, transforming growth factor beta (TGFβ), basic fibroblast growth factor (bFGF) and TNFα, are also synthesized by HLMC. In general, cytokine protein products are released over a 1- to 24-hour period following allergic activation. IL-4, a cytokine that virtually defines Th2 immunity, is immunolocalized to HLMC, which are rich in surface IL-4 receptors. However, generation of IL-4 mRNA and protein release has been reported by some, but not all, investigators.[113,115] TNFα, stored preformed within MC granules is in a unique position to exert diverse host defense effects in allergy and innate immunity.[116] Recent studies suggest that increased expression of TNFα within HLMC may play a role in asthmatic airway inflammation and correlates with asthma severity.[117,118]

Amphiregulin, a member of the epidermal growth factor family, is secreted following FcεRI-mediated activation. Its effects include increasing mucin gene expression, which may contribute to the epithelial cell metaplasia and mucus hypersecretion of asthma.[119]

PHARMACOLOGIC MODULATION OF MAST CELL FUNCTION

Only a limited number of pharmacologic agents have been tested in vitro on HLMC activation–secretion. In general, these agents have been tested on human parenchymal MC rather than those in bronchi or resident in BAL.[36,37,120] Moreover, inhibitory potency has been evaluated with anaphylactic degranulation rather than piecemeal degranulation, the latter being more characteristic of asthma.[121,122] Several receptors that inhibit MC activation contain immunoreceptor tyrosine-based inhibition motifs (ITIMs). Following inhibitory receptor activation these regions are phosphorylated, and then recruit phosphatases that dephosphorylate key-signaling molecules.[123] The common classes of antiallergic and/or antiasthmatic drugs used in clinical practice have received most evaluation. To date, the β-agonist pharmacologic agents, as typified by fenoterol and salmeterol, are reported to be among the most potent global inhibitors of HLMC mediator release with concentrations that inhibit histamine release by 50% (IC_{50}) of $\leq 10^{-8}$ M. Less effective inhibitors include the theophylline-like phosphodiesterase inhibitor isobutylmethylxanthine ($IC_{50} = 0.5$ mM) and PGE_2 ($IC_{50} = 10^{-5}$ M). Although widely touted as "MC stabilizers," disodium cromoglycate and nedocromil sodium, which recently have been shown as agonists at G-protein–coupled receptor 35 (GPR35)[124] poorly inhibit purified HLMC histamine release.[47,125] Inhibition of BAL MC activation by these agents is reportedly more striking.[126]

The effects of glucocorticosteroids on MC are diverse, including both stimulatory and inhibitory effects on the transcription of select genes. Release of early-phase mediators (e.g., histamine, LTC_4) in vitro and acute airway responses in vivo are unaffected by short pretreatment (up to 24 hours) with these drugs. In contrast, IgE-mediated generation of TH2-type late-phase cytokine mRNA and protein (e.g., IL-5, -13) are suppressed ($IC_{50} = 10^{-8}$–10^{-9} M).[127]

FK-506, a macrolide that binds to a specific binding protein, inhibits HLMC mediator release at low concentrations (0.1–300 nM). Cyclosporin A, which binds to cyclophilin, and auranofin, an orally absorbable gold compound, both inhibit HLMC mediator release.

Specific inhibitors of leukotriene generation include direct 5-lipoxygenase enzyme inhibitors, such as A-60477 (Zileuton), and indirect inhibitors, such as MK-886, which bind to a protein termed 5-lipoxygenase–activating protein (FLAP). Interestingly, PGD_2 release is markedly enhanced by FLAP inhibiton. This phenomenon has been termed a reverse shunt effect. Generally, 5-lipoxygenase pathway inhibitors do not affect HLMC histamine release. Cyclooxygenase-1 inhibition plays a critical role in a certain subset of "aspirin-sensitive" asthmatic patients (see below). Agents such as indomethacin potently inhibit HLMC PGD_2 generation ($IC_{50} = 5.5 \times 10^{-10}$ M) while producing significant enhancement of LTC_4 release.

MAST CELLS IN PULMONARY DISEASE

MCs have been implicated in a variety of pulmonary disorders based, to a great extent, on their presence in increased numbers and/or percentages in diseased tissues and the recovery of increased concentrations of MC-derived mediators, particularly histamine, in BAL fluid. Implicated pulmonary disorders include asthma, idiopathic pulmonary fibrosis, sarcoidosis, extrinsic allergic alveolitis, and chronic bronchitis.[51,128–131]

Asthma

MCs within airway epithelium are in an ideal sentinel position to be exposed to inhaled inciting stimuli. Intraepithelial MCs (IEMCs) express tryptase but seldom chymase except in severe asthma[27,29] and were traditionally thought to represent the classic MC_T phenotype. Recent reports assert that intraepithelial MC_T in "Th2-high" asthma also expresses carboxypepeptidase A3 (CPA3), which had previously been identified only in association with MC_{TC}. At baseline, even very mild asthmatics show evidence of continuous MC degranulation in bronchial mucosa and increased histamine content in BAL. Analysis of BAL in allergen-challenged atopic subjects and asthmatics demonstrates increased release of histamine, tryptase, and PGD_2. Increased numbers of lumenal MC are also noted and correlate with mediator content, airflow obstruction, eosinophil numbers, and bronchial hyperresponsiveness. In general, asthmatic MCs exhibit ultrastructural evidence of degranulation. In nonfatal asthma, there is a significant increase of MC within airway smooth muscle and mucosal gland stroma.[30] Multiple redundant MC mediators likely contribute to increased mucus gland secretion and smooth muscle constriction. Following chronic corticosteroid treatment, allergic reactions are diminished in association with depletion of MC in both the epithelium and submucosa.

Although much attention has been given to IgE-mediated mechanisms of asthmatic airway activation, it is likely that multiple other MC-triggering mechanisms operate under a variety of immunologic, occupational, and environmental conditions. One mechanism proposed for EIA relates to airway cooling and the generation of hyperosmolarity on the dried airway surface leading to MC degranulation.

Up to 10% of asthmatics are intolerant of aspirin and other nonstructurally related nonsteroidal anti-inflammatory drugs (NSAIDs). In vitro pretreatment of human airway tissues with indomethacin results in increased LTC_4 generation following IgE-mediated stimulation. MCs are the principal cells expressing LTC_4 synthase in the airways of aspirin-exacerbated asthmatics[132] and these patients have increased Cox-2 expressing bronchial MC numbers.[133]

Fibrosis

The cellular composition of diffuse fibrotic reactions includes striking increases in MC numbers. MCs synthesize and release important mediators of fibrosis, including TGFβ and hFGF.[15–18,134] The hypothesis that MCs and their mediators are critical to the development of fibrotic reactions is supported by animal models in which MC hyperplasia has been a constant finding in pulmonary fibrosis induced by bleomycin, ionizing radiation, and asbestos. Bronchial remodeling with subepithelial fibrosis is also a prominent feature of the asthmatic airway. It is not clear whether MC proliferation and activation drive and/or are secondary to the fibrotic process. The latter mechanism could be effected through fibroblast generation of SCF, producing MC proliferation, chemotaxis, and inhibition of apoptosis.

EOSINOPHILS

While eosinophils are considered leukocytes, like MC, they in fact reside primarily in the tissues. Indeed, the ratio of tissue to blood eosinophils is estimated to be 100:1 or greater. Under normal circumstances, the major resident population of eosinophils is in the lamina propria of the gastrointestinal tract. Eosinophils are also present in the thymus, as well as the uterus and developing mammary gland in females. In the absence of disease, very few eosinophils are found in the lung. On the other hand, large numbers of eosinophils traffic to the lungs and other tissues in the setting of allergic diseases, helminthic parasite infections and certain other pathological states.

EOSINOPHIL DEVELOPMENT

Eosinophils develop in the bone marrow from hematopoietic stem cell precursors. The immediate eosinophil precursor is a common eosinophil–basophil progenitor. Specific differentiation to the eosinophil lineage involves coordinated expression of the transcription factors, GATA-1, PU.1, and C/EBP. Among these, GATA-1 plays a central role, since mice with deletion of a high-affinity GATA-binding site in the GATA-1 promoter (ΔdblGATA1 mice) completely lack eosinophils, without loss of other hematopoietic lineages.[135] The cytokines, IL-3, granulocyte-macrophage/colony-stimulating factor (GM-CSF) and IL-5 stimulate growth and differentiation of eosinophils in the bone marrow. IL-5, the only one of these that is eosinophil specific, plays an essential role in stimulating bone marrow production of eosinophils and triggering their release into the circulation.[136] IL-5 is produced by lymphocytes and endothelial cells in the bone marrow, as well as by lymphocytes and parenchymal cells in the lung and other tissues. The importance of IL-5 in eosinophil production is demonstrated by the fact that transgenic mice overexpressing IL-5 develop profound blood and tissue eosinophilia.[137] On the other hand, IL-5 knockout mice have markedly reduced numbers of eosinophils at baseline, and fail to develop eosinophilia in response to allergen sensitization and challenge.[138] These and other findings have provided the impetus for development of IL-5 and IL-5 receptor–targeted monoclonal antibodies, which are under study for therapy of asthma and other eosinophilic diseases, as discussed below.

MORPHOLOGY AND STRUCTURE

The mature human eosinophil has a diameter of 12 to 17 μm, slightly larger than the neutrophil. The nucleus is usually bilobed, and the cytoplasm contains characteristic granules that stain yellow-pink with eosin. The distinctive features of eosinophil granules can be seen clearly by electron microscopy (Fig. 22-3). Primary granules, which appear during the promyelocytic stage of development, are round, membrane-limited structures that contain Charcot–Leyden crystal (CLC) protein.[139] Secondary (also termed specific or cytoplasmic crystalloid) granules appear later during eosinophil differentiation.[140] These are more numerous and appear as oval or elongated membrane-bound structures with a dense crystalline core and less dense matrix. The secondary granule core contains major basic protein (MBP), while other granule proteins are in the matrix. Lipid bodies are non-membrane-bound, lipid-rich organelles that localize arachidonic acid-metabolizing enzymes and serve as sites of eicosanoid synthesis.[141]

GRANULE PROTEINS

Eosinophils contain a number of cationic granule proteins that have toxic effects on parasitic helminths and RNA viruses, as well as on host cells. In addition, a variety of other proteins, including enzymes and cytokines, are stored in and released from eosinophil granules. MBP, a highly basic protein that accounts for more than half of eosinophil granule protein mass, is found in the crystalline core of specific granules.[142] MBP is synthesized as a preproprotein, which is cleaved to a 13.8-kD highly cationic molecule during eosinophil maturation. The pro-peptide, which is anionic, is thought to protect the developing eosinophil from the toxic effects of the highly cationic mature MBP. Low levels of MBP are expressed in basophils, consistent with their close lineage relationship to eosinophils. MBP is directly toxic to larvae of Schistosoma mansoni, Trichinella spiralis, and other helminths, supporting a role in host defense against parasites.[143] Several lines of evidence have suggested that MBP could be an important mediator of asthma. MBP inhibits ciliary function and is toxic to respiratory epithelial cells.[144,145] When administered to the airways of monkeys, MBP caused transient bronchoconstriction followed by persistent bronchial hyperresponsiveness.[146] In addition, MBP was shown to bind to and inhibit M2 muscarinic receptors, increasing vagally mediated bronchoconstriction in guinea pigs.[147] On the other hand, mice deficient in MPB showed no attenuation of airway histopathological changes or airway hyperreactivity in an allergen-induced asthma model,[148] suggesting that

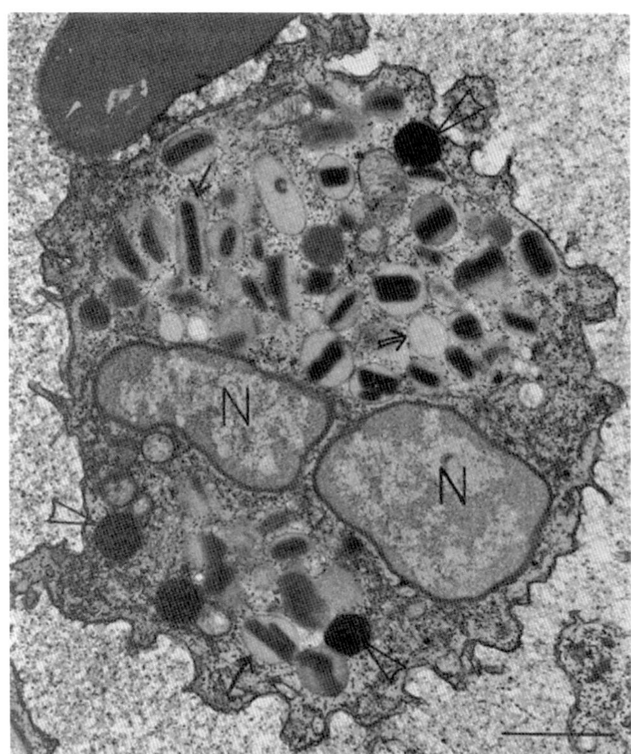

Figure 22-3 Ultrastructure of a mature human blood eosinophil. The bilobed nucleus (N), specific granules *(closed arrows)*, primary granules *(open arrow)*, lipid bodies *(open arrowheads)*, mitochondria, and irregular surface processes are seen. Dark cytoplasmic particles represent glycogen. *(Reproduced with permission from Dvorak AM, Ackerman SJ, Weller PF. Subcellular morphology and biochemistry of eosinophils, in Harris JR (ed). Megakaryocytes, Platelets, Macrophages, and Eosinophils, vol 2. New York: Plenum Press; 1991.)*

MBP does not play an essential role in allergic airway disease, at least in the mouse.

Eosinophil cationic protein (ECP) and eosinophil-derived neurotoxin (EDN) are both highly basic proteins found in the matrix of specific granules. ECP and EDN are homologous proteins (67% amino acid sequence identity), the result of gene duplication, that are also similar to human pancreatic ribonuclease (RNase) A.[143] Indeed, both ECP and EDN are active RNases, with the ability to inactivate RNA viruses, such as respiratory syncytial virus (RSV).[143] EDN was initially described as a neurotoxin that causes severe damage to myelinated neurons, a property possessed by ECP, as well. This activity may account for the neurological abnormalities seen in patients with hypereosinophilic syndrome (HES) and CSF eosinophilia. Like MBP, ECP and EDN are both helminthotoxic.[143] Levels of ECP are elevated in blood, BAL fluid, and sputum in patients with asthma, and have been found to correlate with disease activity.[149] For this reason, ECP levels in blood or sputum are often monitored in asthma clinical trials as a means of assessing response to treatment.

Eosinophil peroxidase (EPO) is another highly basic protein found in the matrix of specific granules. EPO is a unique peroxidase, expressed only in eosinophils. In the presence of H_2O_2, EPO oxidizes halide ions to form highly reactive hypohalous acids. Bromide is the preferred substrate, leading to hypobromous acid (HOBr), an extremely potent oxidant that damages DNA and other critical cellular targets. EPO plus H_2O_2 and halide ions can kill multiple parasites, bacteria, mycobacteria, and also MC and tumor cells.[150] The potential role of EPO in allergic airway disease has been explored in mice with targeted deletion of the EPO gene. In this study, despite a marked reduction in bromo-oxidation of lung proteins, EPO deficiency did not result in any attenuation of allergen-induced airway inflammation or bronchial hyperresponsiveness,[151] indicating that EPO is not essential for development of allergic pulmonary pathology in the mouse.

CLC protein localizes to the primary eosinophil granule, and is also expressed in basophils. The protein readily crystalizes to form bipyramidal CLCs, often seen in affected tissues and considered a hallmark of eosinophil-associated diseases. Previously thought to possess lysophospholipase activity, CLC protein has been shown to belong to the galactose-binding lectin family (galectins) and to avidly bind the sugar mannose.[152] Despite the long-recognized association of CLCs with eosinophil infiltration of tissues, the role of CLC protein in eosinophil-related pathology is unknown.

Eosinophils also contain within their granules various other enzymes, including β-glucuronidase, arylsulfatase B, and matrix metalloproteinase-9 (MMP-9), as well as preformed cytokines and chemokines, which can be released in regulated fashion, as discussed further below.

CHEMICAL MEDIATORS

Eosinophils may produce a number of important chemical mediators, each of which is discussed below.

Lipid Mediators

Upon stimulation, eosinophils produce large quantities of the 5-lipoxygenase–derived eicosanoid, LTC_4. Synthesis of LTC_4 in eosinophils occurs at the nuclear membrane.[153,154] and in cytoplasmic lipid bodies.[155] Following secretion, LTC_4 is converted extracellularly to LTD_4 and LTE_4. These cysteinyl leukotrienes act through $cysLT_1$ and $cysLT_2$ receptors to cause bronchoconstriction, stimulate mucus secretion, promote synthesis of Th2 cytokines, and contribute to airway remodeling.[156] The ability to block these effects underlies the beneficial actions of cysLT receptor antagonists and leukotriene synthesis inhibitors in asthma. Other biologically active lipids produced in substantial quantities by eosinophils include 15-HETE, 5-oxo-ETE, and PAF. However, the roles of these products in asthma and other eosinophil-associated diseases remain unclear.

Cytokines and Chemokines

Classically, eosinophils were considered terminal effector cells of inflammatory responses, acting by secretion of granule proteins and the acute release of other mediators. However, it is now recognized that eosinophils synthesize a wide array of cytokines and chemokines, equipping them to participate in the regulation of immune and inflammatory responses. The major cytokines and chemokines expressed in eosinophils are listed in Table 22-1. Interestingly, a number of these factors have autocrine or paracrine effects on eosinophils themselves. Most notably, IL-3, GM-CSF, and IL-5, which are produced by activated T lymphocytes and other cells, including MCs and eosinophils themselves, enhance eosinophil survival and activate eosinophil function in vitro and in vivo.[154,157–164] In another example, IL-16, a product of eosinophils and other cells, triggers rapid eosinophil release of CCL5 (RANTES), which generates autocrine signals that augment release of LTC_4 and IL-4.[165] A number of cytokines and chemokines synthesized by eosinophils are stored within granules. When cells are stimulated, these preformed cytokines are released by a regulated process involving piecemeal degranulation, which is described further below.

Eosinophil-derived cytokines likely contribute to regulation of inflammatory responses in eosinophil-associated diseases and drive specific pathophysiological responses. For example, elaboration of Th2 cytokines amplifies allergic responses, and is likely important in host defense against parasites and in pulmonary fibrosis. TGFα released by eosinophils is a potent stimulus for synthesis of mucins by airway epithelial cells,[166] which contributes to asthma and other eosinophilic airway diseases. Also, accumulating evidence implicates eosinophil-derived TGFβ as a driver of airway remodeling in asthma,[167] and suggests a link to pulmonary fibrosis, as well.[168] A clearer understanding of the roles of eosinophil cytokines in human diseases will emerge as therapeutic agents designed to target specific cytokines, their receptors and downstream signaling pathways are tested in clinical trials.

Reactive Oxygen Metabolites

Like neutrophils, eosinophils synthesize superoxide anion ($\bullet O_2^-$) and H_2O_2 through the action of NADPH oxidase. Notably, NADPH oxidase components are more highly expressed and more readily activated in eosinophils than neutrophils, endowing stimulated eosinophils with a greater capacity to produce $\bullet O_2^-$ and H_2O_2.[169] As discussed previously, eosinophils produce HOBr through the action of EPO on bromide and H_2O_2.[150] In a reaction involving HOCl and $\bullet O_2^-$, EPO also catalyzes formation of hydroxyl radical ($\bullet$OH), the most reactive of all oxygen metabolites. As noted, EPO-derived oxidants kill parasites and other microorganisms, and thus may be important for host defense. By contrast, EPO appears not to play a key role in allergic airway disease in mice.[148,151] The importance of eosinophil-derived oxidants in human health and disease is at present uncertain, and requires further study.

Eosinophil Recruitment

Current knowledge about the mechanisms of eosinophil recruitment into tissues is based largely on studies of asthma and allergic diseases, but these mechanisms may operate in other eosinophilic disorders as well. The initial step in eosinophil recruitment involves priming, which converts the resting cell to an adhesive, migratory and activation-sensitive phenotype. Priming likely results from exposure to IL-3, IL-5, GM-CSF and chemokines such as CCL11 (eotaxin-1), particularly in allergic individuals, in whom these factors are elevated in the circulation.[170–173] TNFα, leukotrienes, and other inflammatory mediators may prime eosinophils as well. Once primed, eosinophils make contact with the blood vessel wall and undergo rolling, mediated by E- and P-selectins on endothelial cells, which can be upregulated by IL-1 and TNFα, and L-selectin that is constitutively expressed on the eosinophil.[174–177] Rolling activates eosinophil integrins, which mediate tight adhesion through high-affinity binding to endothelial cell adhesion molecules. The eosinophil integrins, VLA-4 (α4β1 or CD49d/CD29) and CD11b/CD18, and their respective endothelial counterligands VCAM-1 and ICAM-1, comprise the most important binding pairs responsible for firm adhesion to the vessel wall. IL-4 and IL-13 increase VCAM-1 expression on endothelial cells.[178,179] Because VLA-4, the binding partner for VCAM-1, is highly expressed on eosinophils, but not neutrophils, this represents a mechanism for selective eosinophil recruitment to sites of allergic inflammation.[175,180] Integrin-mediated firm adhesion is followed by diapedesis, or transmigration across the endothelium. Eosinophils are further activated by endothelial transmigration, which also increases their ability to survive.[181] Based on in vitro studies, eosinophils can probably survive in tissues for 2 weeks or longer.

Upon entering tissue, eosinophils shift from β_1- to β_2-integrin–dominated interactions under the influence of chemokines such as CCL24 (eotaxin-2),[182] and migrate along chemoattractant gradients. Multiple factors are known to be chemotactic for eosinophils, including PAF, LTB_4, complement factors C3a and C5a, GM-CSF, IL-3, IL-5, IL-16, and the chemokines CCL3 (MIP-1α), CCL5, CCL7 (MCP-3), CCL11, CCL24, CCL26 (eotaxin-3), and CXCL8 (IL-8). Among these, IL-5 and the eotaxins (CCL11, CCL24, and CCL26) are the most highly selective for eosinophils, making them attractive as potential therapeutic targets. Indeed, clinical trials of agents directed against IL-5, CCL11, and their receptors in patients with asthma have recently been reported or are underway. The results of some of these studies are discussed at the end of this chapter.

Eosinophil Activation and Degranulation

The priming process required for eosinophil recruitment also represents the initial phase of eosinophil activation. IL-5 is the most important cytokine for priming of eosinophils in vivo.[170,171,183] IL-5 binds to heterodimeric receptors on the eosinophil surface, consisting of a ligand-specific α chain and common β chain that is also used in the receptors for IL-3 and GM-CSF. Binding of IL-5 to its receptor triggers a variety of intracellular signaling cascades, which enhance multiple eosinophil functions, including the response to chemotactic factors, integrin-mediated adhesion, agonist-stimulated LTC_4 and superoxide generation, phagocytosis, and helminthotoxic activity.[154,158,160,171,173,184] IL-3 and GM-CSF are capable of enhancing these functions, as well. As noted earlier, IL-5, IL-3, and GM-CSF also enhance eosinophil survival. The effects of all three cytokines are antagonized by glucocorticoids, which also induce eosinophil apoptosis.[185,186]

Priming of eosinophils in the circulation is enhanced in patients with asthma and hypereosinophilic states, resulting in greater functional responses when blood eosinophils from such individuals are studied in vitro, in comparison to cells from normal controls.[171] In vivo priming has also been demonstrated in eosinophils obtained by BAL following antigen instillation into the lungs of allergic subjects (segmental allergen challenge).[164]

Eosinophils express a panoply of surface receptors that can mediate cell activation. These include receptors for immunoglobulins (IgA, IgG, and IgE), complement components (C3a and C5a), eicosanoids (LTB_4, cysteinyl leukotrienes, and PGD_2) and PAF, and numerous cytokines and chemokines. Priming can upregulate cell surface expression and/or activation of specific receptors,[187] and may induce new expression of receptors not normally present on resting eosinophils, such as the high-affinity IgE receptor FcεRI.[188] Ligand binding to many of these receptors triggers responses that include degranulation, lipid mediator synthesis, and generation of reactive oxygen species. Various ligands activate distinct signaling cascades within the cell, resulting in stimulus-specific differential activation of eosinophil effector functions.

As in MC, the principal mode by which granule-associated proteins are released from human eosinophils is piecemeal degranulation.[140,189–191] This process involves secretion of specific granule contents in discrete packets, without granule-to-granule or granule-to-plasma membrane fusion. An eosinophil undergoing piecemeal degranulation in vitro is illustrated in Figure 22-4. Electron microscopic studies reveal that piecemeal degranulation is associated with the development of complex vesiculotubular networks within emptying granules.[190,191] Interestingly, it has been shown that intracellular cytokine receptors within granules and secretory vesicles play a key role in transporting and guiding selective secretion of their cognate cytokines, allowing for stimulus-specific, selective and sequential release of cationic granule proteins and stored cytokines and chemokines.[192] In addition, receptors for cysteinyl leukotrienes have been demonstrated on eosinophil granule membranes, where they may mediate secretion of granule contents from intact cells in response to endogenously generated LTC_4 or secretion from cell-free granules triggered by extracellular LTD_4.[193]

Besides piecemeal degranulation, the secretion of whole granules, referred to as compound exocytosis, has been described, although this process is not usually observed in vivo. Compound exocytosis involves SNARE family transport docking and vesicle fusion proteins.[194] Finally, cytolytic degranulation is a term used to account for the presence of cell-free eosinophil granules seen in tissue in certain eosinophilic diseases.[140] Whether this is a regulated process or the result of eosinophil necrosis at sites of inflammation is not known.

MAST CELL–EOSINOPHIL INTERACTIONS

Since shortly after their discovery, it has been recognized that MC and eosinophils home to many of the same tissues, particularly in the setting of allergic and other inflammatory conditions. Not surprisingly, therefore, researchers have identified a variety of cooperative interactions between the two cell types. For example, the eosinophil granule proteins MBP and ECP can trigger histamine, PGD_2, and cytokine

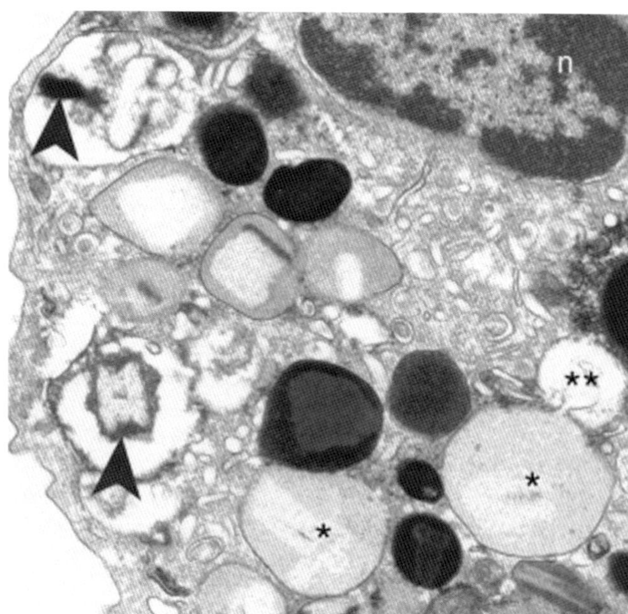

Figure 22-4 Ultrastructure of a human blood eosinophil activated in vitro with CCL11 (eotaxin). Specific granules undergoing piecemeal degranulation exhibit lucent areas in their cores, matrices, or both. Granules with residual cores *(arrowheads)*, reduced internal electron density (*) and membrane empty chambers (**) are shown. *(Reproduced with permission from Melo RCN, Perez SAC, Spencer LA, et al. Intragranular vesiculotubular compartments are involved in piecemeal degranulation by activated human eosinophils. Traffic. 2005;6(10):866–879.)*

release from human MC.[195,196] Eosinophils also produce important MC survival and activation factors, such as SCF and nerve growth factor (NGF).[197] Conversely, MC-derived TNFα induces eosinophil GM-CSF release and autocrine survival enhancement,[198] and MC tryptase induces eosinophil IL-6 and IL-8 secretion.[199] Also, the MC mediators histamine and PGD_2 have been shown to augment synthesis of LTC_4 in human eosinophils.[200] In addition, MC chymase suppresses eosinophil apoptosis and increases adhesion molecule expression, chemokinesis, and cytokine and chemokine release by human eosinophils.[201] Not all MC–eosinophil interactions are proinflammatory, however, as it has been shown that MC tryptase can cleave and inactivate the eosinophil chemokines CCL5 and CCL11.[202] Thus, MCs and eosinophils communicate bidirectionally in complex ways that may amplify or potentially modulate the inflammatory response.

■ EOSINOPHILS AND HOST DEFENSE

Many years ago, histopathological evidence of eosinophils surrounding dying helminths in tissue biopsy specimens led to the hypothesis that eosinophils play a role in the immune response to multicellular parasites. Subsequently, it was demonstrated that, in the presence of antibodies or complement, eosinophils can kill parasites in vitro, as can purified eosinophil granule proteins.[203] Further support of a role for eosinophils in host defense against helminths came from epidemiological studies that correlated high eosinophil counts with resistance to posttreatment reinfection with Schistosoma spp. in humans.[204] Moreover, studies of experimental helminth infections in mice depleted of eosinophils by IL-5 neutralization or gene targeting have indicated that IL-5 and eosinophils are important for protective innate immunity against a variety of parasites,[205–207] although the results are not all consistent.[208] Other studies of mice deficient in CCL11 or treated with a monoclonal antibody targeting CCR3 (the receptor for CCL11 and other eosinophil-active chemokines) have also demonstrated that eosinophils are important for clearance of parasites in vivo.[209,210] A recent study using mice made eosinophil-deficient by expressing the diphtheria toxin A gene under control of the EPO promoter (*PHIL* mice),[211] as well as mice lacking either MBP or EPO, showed that eosinophils kill parasite larvae during primary *Strongyloides stercoralis* infection by a mechanism dependent on MBP.[212] A consistent finding in a number of these studies is that eosinophils play an important role in host defense during primary parasite infection, whereas they appear not to be essential for adaptive responses leading to protective secondary immunity.[207,209,210,212] Interestingly, other recent studies showed that survival of *Trichinella spiralis* was actually reduced in mice genetically ablated of eosinophils, and that parasite growth and survival were restored when the mutant mice were reconstituted with eosinophils by intravenous transfer; in this model, eosinophils enhanced parasite survival by promoting accumulation of Th2 lymphocytes and preventing induction of inducible NO synthase in macrophages and neutrophils at sites of disease.[213,214] Thus, while substantial evidence indicates that eosinophils are protective in the innate immune response to many parasites, the roles they play in helminthic infections are complex and depend on interactions with other immune cells.

As noted earlier, human ECP and EDN are both RNases, and can inactivate RSV in vitro.[143] Mouse eosinophils express a diverse array of eosinophil-associated RNases (EARs) with the ability to inactivate pneumonia virus of mice (PVM),[215] a major pathogen in rodents that is closely related to RSV. More recently, it has been demonstrated that hypereosinophilic IL-5 transgenic mice exhibit enhanced virus clearance when infected with RSV,[216] and that activated eosinophils recruited to the lung in a model of allergen-induced airway disease are profoundly antiviral and promote survival in an otherwise lethal PVM infection.[217] Thus, while they contribute to the pathophysiology of allergic airway disease in the mouse, in the same context activated eosinophils have the capacity to mediate effective antiviral host defense. Further studies are needed to define the role of eosinophils in the immune response to viral infection in humans.

Human MBP and ECP also possess bacteriocidal activity, and various bacteria can induce degranulation of human eosinophils in vitro.[143] In addition, human eosinophils are able to kill *Escherichia coli* in vitro by a mechanism involving NADPH oxidase- and EPO-generated oxidants.[143] Despite these observations, few data exist to implicate a role for eosinophils in host defense against bacterial infections in vivo.

■ IMMUNOREGULATORY CAPACITY OF EOSINOPHILS

Recent investigations have demonstrated that human and mouse eosinophils can process antigen, express major histocompatibility complex II (MHC-II) and co-stimulatory molecules, and function as "professional" antigen-presenting cells.[218,219] In mice, eosinophils within the airway lumen can migrate to regional lymph nodes where they stimulate antigen-specific T-cell proliferation.[220] In addition, eosinophils synthesize, store, and secrete Th2 cytokines and chemokines, endowing them with the capacity to initiate Th2 differentiation of CD4+ T cells as well as recruit Th2 cells to sites of infection or allergen deposition, as demonstrated in several mouse models of allergen-induced airway disease and parasitic infection.[221] Thus, there is now substantial evidence, largely from murine models, that eosinophils play a central role in directing the Th2 immune response. These findings emphasize that, beyond their cytotoxic and destructive potential, eosinophils contribute in complex ways to host defense and the pathophystiology of allergic disease.

■ EOSINOPHIL–DISEASE ASSOCIATIONS

Peripheral blood eosinophilia and eosinophilic lung inflammation are common in a variety of pulmonary conditions, including those listed in Table 22-2. The clinical manifestations and treatment of these disorders are discussed in detail elsewhere in this textbook.

TABLE 22-2 Eosinophilic Lung Diseases

Asthma
Allergic bronchopulmonary aspergillosis/mycosis
Eosinophilic granulomatosis with polyangiitis (Churg–Strauss syndrome)
Simple pulmonary eosinophilia
Chronic eosinophilic pneumonia
Acute eosinophilic pneumonia
Helminthic infections
Drug hypersensitivity reactions
Hypereosinophilic syndrome

Among eosinophilic lung diseases, asthma is by far the most common and most well studied. Over the years, much evidence has accumulated supporting a key role for eosinophils in the pathogenesis of asthma. Among the numerous animal studies addressing this question, most compelling are those involving genetically eosinophil-deficient (ΔdblGATA1 and *PHIL*) mice, which are protected against allergen-induced airway hyperresponsiveness, allergic airway inflammation, mucus hypersecretion, and peribronchiolar collagen deposition.[135,211,222,223] In humans with asthma, eosinophils and their specific products (e.g., ECP) increase in the airway lumen and airway wall during spontaneous exacerbations and following experimental allergen challenge.[149,224,225] Sputum eosinophil numbers and ECP levels also correlate with asthma severity.[149] When asthma improves, either spontaneously or in response to treatment, eosinophils and their products decline.[226,227] Corticosteroids, the most effective therapy for asthma, have potent anti-eosinophil effects.[228] Also, an inhaled corticosteroid treatment strategy directed specifically at reducing sputum eosinophils resulted in significantly better asthma control than treatment based on standard asthma guidelines.[229] Finally, as discussed in the next section, specific eosinophil-targeted therapy with an IL-5–neutralizing monoclonal antibody has been shown to reduce exacerbations and facilitate steroid tapering in patients with severe, oral corticosteroid-dependent asthma with high eosinophils.[230,231]

HES is a rare disorder characterized by persistent marked blood eosinophilia (>1500/μL) or prominent tissue eosinophilia and eosinophil-induced organ damage or dysfunction, in which secondary causes of eosinophilia, such as parasitic or viral infections, allergic diseases, drugs, and hypoadrenalism have been excluded.[232] Pulmonary involvement is seen in 50% of cases. HES is classified as either myeloproliferative or lymphocytic, based on pathophysiology. The myeloproliferative form, exemplified by patients bearing the FIP1L1-PGDFRA fusion gene, which produces a constitutively active tyrosine kinase that drives eosinophil hyperproliferation, represents a type of myeloproliferative neoplasm. The tyrosine kinase inhibitor, imatinib mesylate, is useful in treatment of these patients. In lymphocytic HES, eosinophil proliferation is driven by T-cell overproduction of IL-5 and/or other eosinophil hematopoietins. Corticosteroids are the first line of treatment for these patients. The anti–IL-5 monoclonal antibody, mepolizumab, has also been shown to be effective in steroid-requiring lymphocytic HES.[233]

In addition to the disorders listed in Table 22-2, eosinophils may play a role in the pathogenesis of several pulmonary diseases not normally thought of as eosinophilic in origin. Among these is idiopathic pulmonary fibrosis, in which elevated numbers of eosinophils in BAL fluid have in some studies been associated with a poor prognosis.[234] This is consistent with in vitro and animal data demonstrating the ability of eosinophils to promote tissue fibrosis. Another example is cystic fibrosis, in which increased levels of cationic eosinophil granule proteins correlate with worse pulmonary function, presumably due to toxic effects of these proteins on lung cells.[235]

PHARMACOLOGIC MODULATION OF EOSINOPHILS

Corticosteroids have been the mainstay of pharmacotherapy for eosinophilic disorders for many years. Corticosteroids induce apoptosis of eosinophils, both directly and by inhibiting formation of the prosurvival cytokines, IL-5, IL-3, and GM-CSF.[185,186,228] This leads to rapid reductions of circulating and tissue eosinophils and clinical improvement in the majority of treated patients. Leukotriene receptor antagonists and the anti-IgE monoclonal antibody omalizumab are two other classes of drugs used to treat asthma and allergic diseases that have been shown to reduce circulating eosinophil counts and cause eosinophil apoptosis.[226,236] Of course, these classes of drugs are not specific for eosinophils, so the degree to which their anti-eosinophil activities contribute to their beneficial effects is uncertain.

More recently, highly selective anti-eosinophil therapeutics have been developed and tested in clinical trials. To date, the best studied of these new agents has been the anti–IL-5 monoclonal antibody, mepolizumab, which is highly effective in reducing circulating eosinophil levels in asthma. Although it did not improve clinical endpoints in mild to moderate asthma,[237] mepolizumab has been shown to reduce exacerbation rates, facilitate corticosteroid tapering and improve asthma-related quality of life in patients with severe, oral steroid-dependent asthma and increased sputum eosinophils.[230,231,238] As noted earlier, mepolizumab also led to clinical improvement and facilitated steroid tapering in a randomized trial of patients lymphocytic HES.[233] Similar benefits were seen in an open-label trial of mepolizumab in eosinophilic granulomatosis with polyangiitis (Churg–Strauss syndrome).[239] Other eosinophil-selective therapies in earlier phases of clinical development include monoclonal antibodies, antisense oligonucleotides or small molecule inhibitors targeting the IL-5 receptor, CCL11, CCR3, IL-13, and the IL-4 receptor α chain.[240] An intriguing anti-eosinophil strategy in preclinical development involves targeting Siglec-8, a sialic acid–binding immunoglobulin-like lectin expressed on the surface of human eosinophils and MCs. Engagement of Siglec-8 with cross-linking antibody or glycan ligands triggers selective apoptosis of eosinophils and inhibits inflammatory mediator synthesis and release by MCs (without affecting their survival), suggesting the possibility that activators of Siglec-8 signaling might be particularly effective therapeutic agents by virtue of their ability to target two major cell types that drive allergic respiratory disease.[241]

Ongoing and future investigations involving the novel eosinophil–targeted therapies listed earlier, as well as others yet to be devised, will hopefully lead to safe, new treatments for eosinophilic respiratory disorders. Such studies will also almost certainly yield new and unexpected insights into the complex roles eosinophils play in human health and disease.

REFERENCES

1. Nakamura E, Kataoka T, Furutani K, et al. Lack of histamine alters gastric mucosal morphology: comparison of histidine decarboxylase-deficient and mast cell-deficient mice. *Am J Physiol Gastrointest Liver Physiol.* 2004;287(5):G1053–G1061.
2. Puxeddu I, Ribatti D, Crivellato E, Levi-Schaffer F. Mast cells and eosinophils: a novel link between inflammation and angiogenesis in allergic diseases. *J Allergy Clin Immunol.* 2005;116(3):531–536.
3. Shaik-Dasthagirisaheb YB, Varvara G, Murmura G, et al. Vascular endothelial growth factor (VEGF), mast cells and inflammation. *Int J Immunopathol Pharmacol.* 2013;26(2):327–335.
4. Marone G, de Crescenzo G, Florio G, Granata F, Dente V, Genovese A. Immunological modulation of human cardiac mast cells. *Neurochem Res.* 1999;24(9):1195–1202.

5. Laine P, Kaartinen M, Penttila A, Panula P, Paavonen T, Kovanen PT. Association between myocardial infarction and the mast cells in the adventitia of the infarct-related coronary artery. *Circulation*. 1999;99(3):361–369.
6. Kovanen PT. Mast cells in atherogenesis: actions and reactions. *Curr Atheroscler Rep*. 2009;11(3):214–219.
7. Schulman ES, Quinn TJ, Post TJ, O'Donnell P, Rodriguez A, Gonen B. Low density lipoprotein (LDL) inhibits histamine release from human mast cells. *Biochem Biophys Res Commun*. 1987;148:553–559.
8. Gonen B, O'Donnell P, Post TJ, Quinn TJ, Schulman ES. Very low density lipoproteins (VLDL) trigger the release of histamine from human basophils. *Biochem Biophys Acta*. 1987;917: 418–424.
9. St John AL, Abraham SN. Innate immunity and its regulation by mast cells. *J Immunol*. 2013;190(9):4458–4463.
10. Bischoff SC, Lorentz A, Schwengberg S, Weier G, Raab R, Manns MP. Mast cells are an important cellular source of tumour necrosis factor alpha in human intestinal tissue. *Gut*. 1999;44(5):643–652.
11. Bischoff SC, Wedemeyer J, Herrmann A, et al. Quantitative assessment of intestinal eosinophils and mast cells in inflammatory bowel disease. *Histopathology*. 1996;28(1):1–13.
12. Nigrovic PA, Lee DM. Mast cells in inflammatory arthritis. *Arthritis Res Ther*. 2005;7(1):1–11.
13. Gruber BL. Mast cells in scleroderma. *Clin Dermatol*. 1994;12(3): 397–406.
14. Irani AM, Gruber BL, Kaufman LD, Kahaleh MB, Schwartz LB. Mast cell changes in scleroderma. Presence of MCT cells in the skin and evidence of mast cell activation. *Arthritis Rheum*. 1992;35(8):933–939.
15. Chanez P, Lacoste JY, Guillot B, et al. Mast cells' contribution to the fibrosing alveolitis of the scleroderma lung. *Am Rev Respir Dis*. 1993;147:1497–1502.
16. Wygrecka M, Dahal BK, Kosanovic D, et al. Mast cells and fibroblasts work in concert to aggravate pulmonary fibrosis: role of transmembrane SCF and the PAR-2/PKC-alpha/Raf-1/p44/42 signaling pathway. *Am J Pathol*. 2013;182(6):2094–2108.
17. Cha SI, Chang CS, Kim EK, et al. Lung mast cell density defines a subpopulation of patients with idiopathic pulmonary fibrosis. *Histopathology*. 2012;61(1):98–106.
18. Veerappan A, O'Connor NJ, Brazin J, et al. Mast cells: a pivotal role in pulmonary fibrosis. *DNA Cell Biol*. 2013;32(4):206–218.
19. Metz M, Piliponsky AM, Chen CC, et al. Mast cells can enhance resistance to snake and honeybee venoms. *Science*. 2006; 313(5786):526–530.
20. Akahoshi M, Song CH, Piliponsky AM, et al. Mast cell chymase reduces the toxicity of Gila monster venom, scorpion venom, and vasoactive intestinal polypeptide in mice. *J Clin Invest*. 2011;121(10):4180–4191.
21. Ribatti D, Vacca A, Nico B, Crivellato E, Roncali L, Dammacco F. The role of mast cells in tumour angiogenesis. *Br J Haematol*. 2001;115(3):514–521.
22. Ribatti D, Crivellato E. Mast cells, angiogenesis, and tumour growth. *Biochim Biophys Acta*. 2012;1822(1):2–8.
23. Kovanen PT. Mast cell granule-mediated uptake of low density lipoproteins by macrophages: a novel carrier mechanism leading to the formation of foam cells. *Ann Med*. 1991;23(5):551–559.
24. Kovanen PT. Role of mast cells in atherosclerosis. *Chem Immunol*. 1995;62:132–170.
25. Siracusa MC, Kim BS, Spergel JM, Artis D. Basophils and allergic inflammation. *J Allergy Clin Immunol*. 2013;132(4):789–801.
26. Bradley BL, Azzawi M, Jacobson M, et al. Eosinophils, T-lymphocytes, mast cells, neutrophils, and macrophages in bronchial biopsy specimens from atopic subjects with asthma: comparison with biopsy specimens from atopic subjects without asthma and normal control subjects and relationship to bronchial hyperresponsiveness. *J Allergy Clin Immunol*. 1991; 88(4):661–674.
27. Balzar S, Fajt ML, Comhair SA, et al. Mast cell phenotype, location, and activation in severe asthma. Data from the Severe Asthma Research Program. *Am J Respir Crit Care Med*. 2011;183(3):299–309.
28. Carroll NG, Mutavdzic S, James AL. Distribution and degranulation of airway mast cells in normal and asthmatic subjects. *Eur Respir J*. 2002;19(5):879–885.
29. Dougherty RH, Sidhu SS, Raman K, et al. Accumulation of intraepithelial mast cells with a unique protease phenotype in T(H)2-high asthma. *J Allergy Clin Immunol*. 2010;125(5):1046–1053.
30. Carroll NG, Mutavdzic S, James AL. Increased mast cells and neutrophils in submucosal mucous glands and mucus plugging in patients with asthma. *Thorax*. 2002;57(8):677–682.
31. Brightling CE, Bradding P, Symon FA, Holgate ST, Wardlaw AJ, Pavord ID. Mast-cell infiltration of airway smooth muscle in asthma. *N Engl J Med*. 2002;346(22):1699–1705.
32. El Shazly A, Berger P, Girodet PO, et al. Fraktalkine produced by airway smooth muscle cells contributes to mast cell recruitment in asthma. *J Immunol*. 2006;176(3):1860–1868.
33. Siddiqui S, Mistry V, Doe C, Stinson S, Foster M, Brightling C. Airway wall expression of OX40/OX40 L and interleukin-4 in asthma. *Chest*. 2010;137(4):797–804.
34. Berry M, Morgan A, Shaw DE, et al. Pathological features and inhaled corticosteroid response of eosinophilic and non-eosinophilic asthma. *Thorax*. 2007;62(12):1043–1049.
35. Eggleston PA, Kagey-Sobotka A, Schleimer RP, Lichtenstein LM. Interaction between hyperosmolar and IgE-mediated histamine release from basophils and mast cells. *Am Rev Respir Dis*. 1984;130(1):86–91.
36. Peters SP, Schulman ES, Schleimer RP, MacGlashan DW Jr, Newball HH, Lichtenstein LM. Dispersed human lung mast cells. Pharmacologic aspects and comparison with human lung tissue fragments. *Am Rev Respir Dis*. 1982;126:1034–1039.
37. Schulman ES, MacGlashan DW Jr, Peters SP, Schleimer RP, Newball HH, Lichtenstein LM. Human lung mast cells: purification and characterization. *J Immunol*. 1982;129:2662–2667.
38. Schulman ES, Glaum MC, Post T, et al. ATP modulates anti-IgE-induced release of histamine from human lung mast cells. *Am J Respir Cell Mol Biol*. 1999;20(3):530–537.
39. Siddiqui S, Mistry V, Doe C, et al. Airway hyperresponsiveness is dissociated from airway wall structural remodeling. *J Allergy Clin Immunol*. 2008;122(2):335–341, 341.
40. Forsythe P, McGarvey LP, Heaney LG, MacMahon J, Ennis M. Adenosine induces histamine release from human bronchoalveolar lavage mast cells. *Clin Sci (Colch)*. 1999;96(4):349–355.
41. Gurish MF, Boyce JA. Mast cells: ontogeny, homing, and recruitment of a unique innate effector cell. *J Allergy Clin Immunol*. 2006;117(6):1285–1291.
42. Ashman LK, Cambareri AC, To LB, Levinsky RJ, Juttner CA. Expression of the YB5.B8 antigen (c-kit proto-oncogene product) in normal human bone marrow. *Blood*. 1991;78(1):30–37.

43. Ashman LK. The biology of stem cell factor and its receptor C-kit. *Int J Biochem Cell Biol.* 1999;31(10):1037–1051.

44. Bradding P, Okayama Y, Howarth PH, Church MK, Holgate ST. Heterogeneity of human mast cells based on cytokine content. *J Immunol.* 1995;155:297–307.

45. de Paulis A, Ciccarelli A, Marino I, de Crescenzo G, Marino D, Marone G. Human synovial mast cells. II. Heterogeneity of the pharmacologic effects of antiinflammatory and immunosuppressive drugs. *Arthritis Rheum.* 1997;40:469–478.

46. Schulman ES, Kagey-Sobotka A, MacGlashan DW Jr, et al. Heterogeneity of human mast cells. *J Immunol.* 1983;131: 1936–1941.

47. Schulman ES, Post TJ, Vigderman RJ. Density heterogeneity of human lung mast cells. *J All Clin Immunol.* 1988;82:78–86.

48. Shanahan F, MacNiven I, Dyck N, Denburg JA, Bienenstock J, Befus AD. Human lung mast cells: distribution and abundance of histochemically distinct subpopulations. *Int Arch All Appl Immunol.* 1987;83:329–331.

49. Schulman ES, Pollack RB, Post TJ, Peters SP. Histochemical heterogeneity of dispersed human lung mast cells. *J Immunol.* 1990;144(11):4195–4201.

50. Weidner N, Austen KF. Heterogeneity of mast cells at multiple body sites. Fluorescent determination of avidin binding and immunofluorescent determination of chymase, tryptase, and carboxypeptidase content. *Pathol Res Pract.* 1993;189(2):156–162.

51. Andersson CK, Andersson-Sjoland A, Mori M, et al. Activated MCTC mast cells infiltrate diseased lung areas in cystic fibrosis and idiopathic pulmonary fibrosis. *Respir Res.* 2011;12:139.

52. Irani AA, Schechter NM, Craig SS, DeBlois G, Schwartz LB. Two types of human mast cells that have distinct neutral protease compositions. *Proc Natl Acad Sci U S A.* 1986;83:4464–4468.

53. Irani AM, Goldstein SM, Wintroub BU, Bradford T, Schwartz LB. Human mast cell carboxypeptidase. Selective localization to MCTC cells. *J Immunol.* 1991;147:247–253.

54. Irani AM, Craig SS, DeBlois G, Elson CO, Schechter NM, Schwartz LB. Deficiency of the tryptase-positive, chymase-negative mast cell type in gastrointestinal mucosa of patients with defective T lymphocyte function. *J Immunol.* 1987;138(12):4381–4386.

55. Andersson CK, Mori M, Bjermer L, Lofdahl CG, Erjefalt JS. Novel site-specific mast cell subpopulations in the human lung. *Thorax.* 2009;64(4):297–305.

56. Thompson HL, Schulman ES, Metcalfe DD. Identification of chondroitin sulfate E in human lung mast cells. *J Immunol.* 1988;140:2708–2713.

57. Gilead L, Livni N, Eliakim R, et al. Human gastric mucosal mast cells are chondroitin sulphate E-containing mast cells. *Immunology.* 1987;62(1):23–28.

58. Dvorak AM, Schleimer RP, Schulman ES, Lichtenstein LM. Human mast cells use conservation and condensation mechanisms during recovery from degranulation. In vitro studies with mast cells purified from human lungs. *Lab Invest.* 1986;54:663–678.

59. Dvorak AM, Schulman ES, Peters SP, et al. Immunoglobulin E-mediated degranulation of isolated human lung mast cells. *Lab Invest.* 1985;53:45–56.

60. Dvorak AM, Hammel I, Schulman ES, et al. Differences in the behavior of cytoplasmic granules and lipid bodies during human lung mast cell degranulation. *J Cell Biol.* 1984;99:1678–1687.

61. Dvorak AM, Galli SJ, Schulman ES, Lichtenstein LM, Dvorak HF. Basophil and mast cell degranulation: ultrastructural analysis of mechanisms of mediator release. *Fed Proc.* 1983;42: 2510–2515.

62. Peters SP, Dvorak AM, Schulman ES. Mast Cells in Lung Biology. In: Massaro D, ed. *Lung Biology in Health and Disease.* Vol. 41. New York, NY: Marcel Decker, Inc.; 1989:345–399.

63. Hammel I, Dvorak AM, Peters SP, et al. Differences in the volume distributions of human lung mast cell granules and lipid bodies: evidence that the size of these organelles is regulated by distinct mechanisms. *J Cell Biol.* 1985;100:1488–1492.

64. Dvorak AM, Dvorak HF, Peters SP, et al. Lipid bodies: cytoplasmic organelles important to arachidonate metabolism in macrophages and mast cells. *J Immunol.* 1983;131:2965–2976.

65. Greineisen WE, Shimoda LM, Maaetoft-Udsen K, Turner H. Insulin-containing lipogenic stimuli suppress mast cell degranulation potential and up-regulate lipid body biogenesis and eicosanoid secretion in a PPARgamma-independent manner. *J Leukoc Biol.* 2012;92(3):653–665.

66. Dichlberger A, Schlager S, Lappalainen J, et al. Lipid body formation during maturation of human mast cells. *J Lipid Res.* 2011;52(12):2198–2208.

67. Dvorak AM, Morgan ES, Monahan-Earley RA, et al. Analysis of mast cell activation using diamine oxidase-gold enzyme-affinity ultrastructural cytochemistry. [Review]. *Int Arch All Immunol.* 1995;107:87–89.

68. Rivera J, Fierro NA, Olivera A, Suzuki R. New insights on mast cell activation via the high affinity receptor for IgE. *Adv Immunol.* 2008;98:85–120.

69. Ishizaka T, Conrad DH, Schulman ES, Sterk AR, Ko CG, Ishizaka K. IgE-mediated triggering signals for mediator release from human mast cells and basophils. *Fed Proc.* 1984;43:2840–2845.

70. Ishizaka T, Conrad DH, Schulman ES, Sterk AR, Ishizaka K. Biochemical analysis of initial triggering events of IgE- mediated histamine release from human lung mast cells. *J Immunol.* 1983;130:2357–2362.

71. Cruse G, Kaur D, Yang W, Duffy SM, Brightling CE, Bradding P. Activation of human lung mast cells by monomeric immunoglobulin E. *Eur Respir J.* 2005;25(5):858–863.

72. Fox CC, Kagey-Sobotka A, Schleimer RP, Peters SP, MacGlashan DW Jr, Lichtenstein LM. Mediator release from human basophils and mast cells from lung and intestinal mucosa. *Int Arch Allergy Appl Immunol.* 1985;77(1–2):130–136.

73. Church MK, Clough GF. Human skin mast cells: in vitro and in vivo studies. *Ann Allergy Asthma Immunol.* 1999;83(5):471–475.

74. Schulman ES, Liu MC, Proud D, MacGlashan DW Jr, Lichtenstein LM, Plaut M. Human lung macrophages induce histamine release from basophils and mast cells. *Am Rev Respir Dis.* 1985;131:230–235.

75. Broide DH, Smith CM, Wasserman SI. Mast cells and pulmonary fibrosis. Identification of a histamine releasing factor in bronchoalveolar lavage fluid. *J Immunol.* 1990;145(6):1838–1844.

76. MacDonald SM. Potential role of histamine releasing factor (HRF) as a therapeutic target for treating asthma and allergy. *J Asthma Allergy.* 2012;5:51–59.

77. Kashiwakura JC, Ando T, Matsumoto K, et al. Histamine-releasing factor has a proinflammatory role in mouse models of asthma and allergy. *J Clin Invest.* 2012;122(1):218–228.

78. Schulman ES, Post TJ, Henson PM, Giclas PC. Differential effects of the complement peptides, C5a and C5a des Arg on

human basophil and lung mast cell histamine release. *J Clin Invest*. 1988;81:918–923.

79. Fureder W, Agis H, Willheim M, et al. Differential expression of complement receptors on human basophils and mast cells. Evidence for mast cell heterogeneity and CD88/C5aR expression on skin mast cells. *J Immunol.* 1995;155:3152–3160.
80. Oskeritzian CA, Zhao W, Min HK, et al. Surface CD88 functionally distinguishes the MC_{TC} from the MC_T type of human lung mast cell. *J Allergy Clin Immunol.* 2005;115(6):1162–1168.
81. Dudler T, Machado DC, Kolbe L, et al. A link between catalytic activity, IgE-independent mast cell activation, and allergenicity of bee venom phospholipase A2. *J Immunol.* 1995;155:2605–2613.
82. Machado DC, Horton D, Harrop R, Peachell PT, Helm BA. Potential allergens stimulate the release of mediators of the allergic response from cells of mast cell lineage in the absence of sensitization with antigen-specific IgE. *Eur J Immunol.* 1996;26: 2972–2980.
83. Kulka M, Alexopoulou L, Flavell RA, Metcalfe DD. Activation of mast cells by double-stranded RNA: evidence for activation through Toll-like receptor 3. *J Allergy Clin Immunol.* 2004;114(1): 174–182.
84. Okumura S, Kashiwakura J, Tomita H, et al. Identification of specific gene expression profiles in human mast cells mediated by Toll-like receptor 4 and FcεRI. *Blood.* 2003;102(7): 2547–2554.
85. Peachell PT, Columbo M, Kagey-Sobotka A, Lichtenstein LM, Marone G. Adenosine potentiates mediator release from human lung mast cells. *Am Rev Respir Dis.* 1988;138: 1143–1151.
86. Crimi N, Palermo F, Oliveri R, Polosa R, Settinieri I, Mistretta A. Protective effects of inhaled ipratropium bromide on bronchoconstriction induced by adenosine and methacholine in asthma. *Eur Res J.* 1992;5:560–565.
87. Rafferty P, Beasley R, Holgate ST. The contribution of histamine to immediate bronchoconstriction provoked by inhaled allergen and adenosine 5' monophosphate in atopic asthma. *Am Rev Respir Dis.* 1987;136:369–373.
88. Taylor DA, Jensen MW, Aikman SL, Harris JG, Barnes PJ, O'Connor BJ. Comparison of salmeterol and albuterol-induced bronchoprotection against adenosine monophosphate and histamine in mild asthma. *Am J Respir Crit Care Med.* 1997;156(6):1731–1737.
89. Kruger-Krasagakes S, Grutzkau A, Krasagakis K, Hoffmann S, Henz BM. Adhesion of human mast cells to extracellular matrix provides a co-stimulatory signal for cytokine production. *Immunology.* 1999;98(2):253–257.
90. Rivera J, Olivera A. A current understanding of Fc epsilon RI-dependent mast cell activation. *Curr Allergy Asthma Rep.* 2008;8(1):14–20.
91. Rivera J, Gilfillan AM. Molecular regulation of mast cell activation. *J Allergy Clin Immunol.* 2006;117(6):1214–1225.
92. Acharya M, Borland G, Edkins AL, et al. CD23/ FcεRII: molecular multi-tasking. *Clin Exp Immunol.* 2010;162(1):12–23.
93. Benhamou M, Siraganian RP. Protein-tyrosine phosphorylation: an essential component of Fc epsilon RI signaling. *Immunol Today.* 1992;13(6):195–197.
94. Benhamou M, Ryba NJ, Kihara H, Nishikata H, Siraganian RP. Protein-tyrosine kinase p72syk in high affinity IgE receptor signaling. Identification as a component of pp72 and association with the receptor gamma chain after receptor aggregation. *J Biol Chem.* 1993;268(31):23318–23324.
95. Rivera J. Molecular adapters in Fc(epsilon)RI signaling and the allergic response. *Curr Opin Immunol.* 2002;14(6):688–693.
96. Jouvin MH, Adamczewski M, Numerof R, Letourneur O, Valle A, Kinet JP. Differential control of the tyrosine kinases Lyn and Syk by the two signaling chains of the high affinity immunoglobulin E receptor. *J Biol Chem.* 1994;269:5918–5925.
97. Hundley TR, Gilfillan AM, Tkaczyk C, Andrade MV, Metcalfe DD, Beaven MA. Kit and FcεRI mediate unique and convergent signals for release of inflammatory mediators from human mast cells. *Blood.* 2004;104(8):2410–2417.
98. Tkaczyk C, Okayama Y, Metcalfe DD, Gilfillan AM. FCγ receptors on mast cells: activatory and inhibitory regulation of mediator release. *Int Arch Allergy Immunol.* 2004;133(3):305–315.
99. Tkaczyk C, Horejsi V, Iwaki S, et al. NTAL phosphorylation is a pivotal link between the signaling cascades leading to human mast cell degranulation following Kit activation and Fc epsilon RI aggregation. *Blood.* 2004;104(1):207–214.
100. Siraganian RP. Mast cell signal transduction from the high-affinity IgE receptor. *Curr Opin Immunol.* 2003;15(6):639–646.
101. Kinet JP. A new strategy to counter allergy. *N Engl J Med.* 2005; 353(3):310–312.
102. Vig M, DeHaven WI, Bird GS, et al. Defective mast cell effector functions in mice lacking the CRACM1 pore subunit of store-operated calcium release-activated calcium channels. *Nat Immunol.* 2008;9(1):89–96.
103. Ashmole I, Duffy SM, Leyland ML, Bradding P. The contribution of Orai(CRACM)1 and Orai(CRACM)2 channels in store-operated Ca2+ entry and mediator release in human lung mast cells. *PLoS One.* 2013;8(9):e74895.
104. Baram D, Rashkovsky M, Hershkoviz R, et al. Inhibitory effects of low molecular weight heparin on mediator release by mast cells: preferential inhibition of cytokine production and mast cell-dependent cutaneous inflammation. *Clin Exp Immunol.* 1997;110(3):485–491.
105. Molinari JF, Campo C, Shakir S, Ahmed T. Inhibition of antigen-induced airway hyperresponsiveness by ultralow molecular-weight heparin. *Am J Respir Crit Care Med.* 1998;157(3 Pt 1): 887–893.
106. Vancheri C, Mastruzzo C, Armato F, et al. Intranasal heparin reduces eosinophil recruitment after nasal allergen challenge in patients with allergic rhinitis. *J Allergy Clin Immunol.* 2001; 108(5):703–708.
107. Freeland HS, Schleimer RP, Schulman ES, Lichtenstein LM, Peters SP. Generation of leukotriene B4 by human lung fragments and purified human lung mast cells. *Am Rev Respir Dis.* 1988;138:389–394.
108. Romagnani P, de Paulis A, Beltrame C, et al. Tryptase-chymase double-positive human mast cells express the eotaxin receptor CCR3 and are attracted by CCR3-binding chemokines. *Am J Pathol.* 1999;155(4):1195–1204.
109. Brightling CE, Ammit AJ, Kaur D, et al. The CXCL10/CXCR3 axis mediates human lung mast cell migration to asthmatic airway smooth muscle. *Am J Respir Crit Care Med.* 2005;171(10):1103–1108.
110. Meier HL, Heck LW, Schulman ES, MacGlashan DW Jr. Purified human mast cells and basophils release human elastase and cathepsin G by an IgE-mediated mechanism. *Int Arch All Appl Immunol.* 1985;77:179–183.
111. Peters SP, MacGlashan DW Jr, Schulman ES, Schleimer RP, Hayes EC, Rokach J. Arachidonic acid metabolism in purified human lung mast cells. *J Immunol.* 1984;132:1972–1979.

112. MacGlashan DW Jr, Schleimer RP, Peters SP, et al. Generation of leukotrienes by purified human lung mast cells. *J Clin Invest.* 1982; 70:747–751.

113. Jaffe JS, Glaum MC, Raible DG, et al. Human lung mast cell IL-5 gene and protein expression: temporal analysis of upregulation following IgE-mediated activation. *Am J Respir Cell Mol Biol.* 1995;13:665–675.

114. Jaffe JS, Raible DG, Post TJ, et al. Human lung mast cell activation leads to IL-13 mRNA expression and protein release. *Am J Respir Cell Mol Biol.* 1996;15:473–481.

115. Bradding P, Feather IH, Howarth PH, et al. Interleukin 4 is localized to and released by human mast cells. *J Exp Med.* 1992;176:1381–1386.

116. Bradding P, Roberts JA, Britten KM, et al. Interleukin-4, -5, and -6 and tumor necrosis factor-alpha in normal and asthmatic airways: evidence for the human mast cell as a source of these cytokines. *Am J Respir Cell Mol Biol.* 1994;10(5):471–480.

117. Berry MA, Hargadon B, Shelley M, et al. Evidence of a role of tumor necrosis factor alpha in refractory asthma. *N Engl J Med.* 2006;354(7):697–708.

118. Babu SK, Puddicombe SM, Arshad HH, et al. Tumor necrosis factor alpha (TNF-α) autoregulates its expression and induces adhesion molecule expression in asthma. *Clin Immunol.* 2011; 140(1):18–25.

119. Okumura S, Sagara H, Fukuda T, Saito H, Okayama Y. FcεRI-mediated amphiregulin production by human mast cells increases mucin gene expression in epithelial cells. *J Allergy Clin Immunol.* 2005;115(2):272–279.

120. Schleimer RP, Schulman ES, MacGlashan DW Jr, et al. Effects of dexamethasone on mediator release from human lung fragments and purified human lung mast cells. *J Clin Invest.* 1983; 71:1830–1835.

121. Begueret H, Berger P, Vernejoux JM, Dubuisson L, Marthan R, Tunon-de-Lara JM. Inflammation of bronchial smooth muscle in allergic asthma. *Thorax.* 2007;62(1):8–15.

122. Djukanovic R, Lai CK, Wilson JW, et al. Bronchial mucosal manifestations of atopy: a comparison of markers of inflammation between atopic asthmatics, atopic nonasthmatics and healthy controls. *Eur Respir J.* 1992;5(5):538–544.

123. Karra L, Levi-Schaffer F. Down-regulation of mast cell responses through ITIM containing inhibitory receptors. *Adv Exp Med Biol.* 2011;716:143–159.

124. Yang Y, Lu JY, Wu X, et al. G-protein-coupled receptor 35 is a target of the asthma drugs cromolyn disodium and nedocromil sodium. *Pharmacology.* 2010;86(1):1–5.

125. Fox CC, Wolf EJ, Kagey-Sobotka A, Lichtenstein LM. Comparison of human lung and intestinal mast cells. *J Allergy Clin Immunol.* 1988;81(1):89–94.

126. Pearce FL, Al Laith M, Bosman L, et al. Effects of sodium cromoglycate and nedocromil sodium on histamine secretion from mast cells from various locations. *Drugs.* 1989;37(Suppl 1):37–43.

127. Glaum MC, Jaffe JS, Gillespie DH, et al. IgE-dependent expression of interleukin-5 mRNA and protein in human lung: modulation by dexamethasone. *Clin Immunol Immunopathol.* 1995;75:171–178.

128. Gruber BL. Mast cells in the pathogenesis of fibrosis. *Curr Rheumatol Rep.* 2003;5(2):147–153.

129. Liebler JM, Qu Z, Buckner B, Powers MR, Rosenbaum JT. Fibroproliferation and mast cells in the acute respiratory distress syndrome. *Thorax.* 1998;53(10):823–829.

130. Sepper R, Konttinen YT, Kemppinen P, Sorsa T, Eklund KK. Mast cells in bronchiectasis. *Ann Med.* 1998;30(3):307–315.

131. Ballarin A, Bazzan E, Zenteno RH, et al. Mast cell infiltration discriminates between histopathological phenotypes of chronic obstructive pulmonary disease. *Am J Respir Crit Care Med.* 2012;186(3):233–239.

132. Cai Y, Bjermer L, Halstensen TS. Bronchial mast cells are the dominating LTC_4S-expressing cells in aspirin-tolerant asthma. *Am J Respir Cell Mol Biol.* 2003;29(6):683–693.

133. Sousa A, Pfister R, Christie PE, et al. Enhanced expression of cyclo-oxygenase isoenzyme 2 (COX-2) in asthmatic airways and its cellular distribution in aspirin-sensitive asthma. *Thorax.* 1997;52(11):940–945.

134. Inoue Y, King TE Jr, Tinkle SS, Dockstader K, Newman LS. Human mast cell basic fibroblast growth factor in pulmonary fibrotic disorders. *Am J Pathol.* 1996;149(6):2037–2054.

135. Yu C, Cantor AB, Yang H, et al. Targeted deletion of a high-affinity GATA-binding site in the GATA-1 promoter leads to selective loss of the eosinophil lineage in vivo. *J Exp Med.* 2002;195:1387–1395.

136. Roboz GJ, Rafii S. Interleukin-5 and the regulation of eosinophil production. *Curr Opin Hematol.* 1999;6:164–168.

137. Tominaga A, Takaki S, Koyama N, et al. Transgenic mice expressing a B cell growth and differentiation factor gene (interleukin 5) develop eosinophilia and autoantibody production. *J Exp Med.* 1991;173:429–437.

138. Foster PS, Hogan SP, Ramsay AJ, Matthaei KI, Young IG. Interleukin 5 deficiency abolishes eosinophilia, airways hyperreactivity, and lung damage in a mouse asthma model. *J Exp Med.* 1996;183:195–201.

139. Dvorak A, Letourneau L, Login G, Weller P, Ackerman S. Ultrastructural localization of the Charcot-Leyden crystal protein (lysophospholipase) to a distinct crystalloid-free granule population in mature human eosinophils. *Blood.* 1988;72:150–158.

140. Muniz VS, Weller PF, Neves JS. Eosinophil crystalloid granules: structure, function, and beyond. *J Leukoc Biol.* 2012;92:281–288.

141. Bozza PT, Yu W, Penrose JF, Morgan ES, Dvorak AM, Weller PF. Eosinophil lipid bodies: specific, inducible intracellular sites for enhanced eicosanoid formation. *J Exp Med.* 1997;186:909–920.

142. Peters MS RM, Gleich GJ. Localization of human eosinophil granule major basic protein, eosinophil cationic protein, and eosinophil-derived neurotoxin by immunoelectron microscopy. *Lab Invest.* 1986;54:656–652.

143. Malik A, Batra JK. Antimicrobial activity of human eosinophil granule proteins: involvement in host defence against pathogens. *Crit Rev Microbiol.* 2012;38:168–181.

144. Hastie AT, Loegering DA, Gleich GJ, Kueppers F. The effect of purified human eosinophil major basic protein on mammalian ciliary activity. *Am Rev Respir Dis.* 1987;135:848–853.

145. Hisamatsu K GT, Nakazawa T, Murakami Y, Gleich GJ, Makiyama K, Koyama H. Cytotoxicity of human eosinophil granule major basic protein to human nasal sinus mucosa in vitro. *J Allergy Clin Immunol.* 1990;86:52–63.

146. Gundel RH, Letts LG, Gleich GJ. Human eosinophil major basic protein induces airway constriction and airway hyperresponsiveness in primates. *J Clin Invest.* 1991;87:1470–1473.

147. Evans CM, Fryer AD, Jacoby DB, Gleich GJ, Costello RW. Pretreatment with antibody to eosinophil major basic protein

prevents hyperresponsiveness by protecting neuronal M2 muscarinic receptors in antigen-challenged guinea pigs. *J Clin Invest*. 1997;100:2254–2262.

148. Denzler KL, Farmer SC, Crosby JR, et al. Eosinophil major basic protein-1 does not contribute to allergen-induced airway pathologies in mouse models of asthma. *J Immunol*. 2000;165:5509–5517.

149. Koh GCH, Shek LPC, Goh DYT, Van Bever H, Koh DSQ. Eosinophil cationic protein: is it useful in asthma? A systematic review. *Respir Med*. 2007;101:696–705.

150. Jianguo W, Arne S. Role of eosinophil peroxidase in host defense and disease pathology. *Arch Biochem Biophys*. 2006;445:256–260.

151. Denzler KL, Borchers MT, Crosby JR, et al. Extensive eosinophil degranulation and peroxidase-mediated oxidation of airway proteins do not occur in a mouse ovalbumin-challenge model of pulmonary inflammation. *J Immunol*. 2001;167:1672–1682.

152. Ackerman SJ, Liu L, Kwatia MA, et al. Charcot-Leyden crystal protein (galectin-10) is not a dual function galectin with lysophospholipase activity but binds a lysophospholipase inhibitor in a novel structural fashion. *J Biol Chem*. 2002;277:14859–14868.

153. Brock TG, Anderson JA, Fries FP, Peters-Golden M, Sporn PH. Decreased leukotriene C4 synthesis accompanies adherence-dependent nuclear import of 5-lipoxygenase in human blood eosinophils. *J Immunol*. 1999;162:1669–1676.

154. Cowburn AS, Holgate ST, Sampson AP. IL-5 increases expression of 5-lipoxygenase-activating protein and translocates 5-lipoxygenase to the nucleus in human blood eosinophils. *J Immunol*. 1999;163:456–465.

155. Bandeira-Melo C, Phoofolo M, Weller PF. Extranuclear lipid bodies, elicited by CCR3-mediated signaling pathways, are the sites of chemokine-enhanced leukotriene C4 production in eosinophils and basophils. *J Biol Chem*. 2001;276:22779–22787.

156. Peters-Golden M, Henderson WR. Leukotrienes. *N Engl J Med*. 2007;357:1841–1854.

157. Lopez AF, Williamson DJ, Gamble JR, et al. Recombinant human granulocyte-macrophage colony-stimulating factor stimulates in vitro mature human neutrophil and eosinophil function, surface receptor expression, and survival. *J Clin Invest*. 1986;78:1220–1228.

158. Yamaguchi Y, Hayashi Y, Sugama Y, et al. Highly purified murine interleukin 5 (IL-5) stimulates eosinophil function and prolongs in vitro survival. IL-5 as an eosinophil chemotactic factor. *J Exp Med*. 1988;167:1737–1742.

159. Rothenberg ME, Owen WF Jr, Silberstein DS, et al. Human eosinophils have prolonged survival, enhanced functional properties, and become hypodense when exposed to human interleukin 3. *J Clin Invest*. 1988;81:1986–1992.

160. Kita H, Weiler DA, Abu-Ghazaleh R, Sanderson CJ, Gleich GJ. Release of granule proteins from eosinophils cultured with IL-5. *J Immunol*. 1992;149:629–635.

161. Nakamura Y, Ozaki T, Kamei T, et al. Factors that stimulate the proliferation and survival of eosinophils in eosinophilic pleural effusion: relationship to granulocyte/macrophage colony-stimulating factor, interleukin-5, and interleukin-3. *Am J Respir Cell Mol Biol*. 1993;8:605–611.

162. Ohnishi T, Sur S, Collins DS, Fish JE, Gleich GJ, Peters SP. Eosinophil survival activity identified as interleukin-5 is associated with eosinophil recruitment and degranulation and lung injury twenty-four hours after segmental antigen lung challenge. *J Allergy Clin Immunol*. 1993;92:607–615.

163. Adachi T, Motojima S, Hirata A, Fukuda T, Makino S. Eosinophil viability-enhancing activity in sputum from patients with bronchial asthma, Contributions of interleukin-5 and granulocyte/macrophage colony-stimulating factor. *Am J Respir Crit Care Med*. 1995;151:618–623.

164. Sedgwick JB, Quan SF, Calhoun WJ, Busse WW. Effect of interleukin-5 and granulocyte-macrophage colony stimulating factor on in vitro eosinophil function: comparison with airway eosinophils. *J Allergy Clin Immunol*. 1995;96:375–385.

165. Bandeira-Melo C, Sugiyama K, Woods LJ, et al. IL-16 promotes leukotriene C4 and IL-4 release from human eosinophils via CD4- and autocrine CCR3-chemokine-mediated signaling. *J Immunol*. 2002;168:4756–4763.

166. Burgel PR, Lazarus SC, Tam DC, et al. Human eosinophils induce mucin production in airway epithelial cells via epidermal growth factor receptor activation. *J Immunol*. 2001;167:5948–5954.

167. Kariyawasam HH, Robinson DS. The role of eosinophils in airway tissue remodelling in asthma. *Curr Opin Immunol*. 2007;19:681–686.

168. Huaux F, Liu T, McGarry B, Ullenbruch M, Xing Z, Phan SH. Eosinophils and T lymphocytes possess distinct roles in bleomycin-induced lung injury and fibrosis. *J Immunol*. 2003;171:5470–5481.

169. DeChatelet L, Shirley P, McPhail L, Huntley C, Muss H, Bass D. Oxidative metabolism of the human eosinophil. *Blood*. 1977;50:525–535.

170. Moser R, Fehr J, Olgiati L, Bruijnzeel P. Migration of primed human eosinophils across cytokine-activated endothelial cell monolayers. *Blood*. 1992;79:2937–2945.

171. Sehmi R, Wardlaw A, Cromwell O, Kurihara K, Waltmann P, Kay A. Interleukin-5 selectively enhances the chemotactic response of eosinophils obtained from normal but not eosinophilic subjects. *Blood*. 1992;79:2952–2959.

172. Schweizer R, Welmers B, Raaijmakers J, Zanen P, Lammers J, Koenderman L. RANTES- and interleukin-8-induced responses in normal human eosinophils: effects of priming with interleukin-5. *Blood*. 1994;83:3697–3704.

173. Shahabuddin S, Ponath P, Schleimer RP. Migration of eosinophils across endothelial cell monolayers: interactions among IL-5, endothelial-activating cytokines, and C-C chemokines. *J Immunol*. 2000;164:3847–3854.

174. Dobrina A, Menegazzi R, Carlos TM, et al. Mechanisms of eosinophil adherence to cultured vascular endothelial cells. Eosinophils bind to the cytokine-induced ligand vascular cell adhesion molecule-1 via the very late activation antigen-4 integrin receptor. *J Clin Invest*. 1991;88:20–26.

175. Weller PF, Rand TH, Goelz SE, Chi-Rosso G, Lobb RR. Human eosinophil adherence to vascular endothelium mediated by binding to vascular cell adhesion molecule 1 and endothelial leukocyte adhesion molecule 1. *Proc Natl Acad Sci U S A*. 1991;88:7430–7433.

176. Henriques G, Miotla J, Cordeiro S, Wolitzky B, Woolley S, Hellewell P. Selectins mediate eosinophil recruitment in vivo: a comparison with their role in neutrophil influx. *Blood*. 1996;87:5297–5304.

177. Ulfman LH, Kuijper PH, van der Linden JA, Lammers JW, Zwaginga JJ, Koenderman L. Characterization of eosinophil adhesion to TNF-α-activated endothelium under flow conditions: α4 integrins mediate initial attachment, and E-selectin mediates rolling. *J Immunol*. 1999;163:343–350.

178. Blease K, Seybold J, Adcock IM, Hellewell PG, Burke-Gaffney A. Interleukin-4 and lipopolysaccharide synergize to induce vascular cell adhesion molecule-1 expression in human lung microvascular endothelial cells. *Am J Respir Cell Mol Biol.* 1998;18: 620–630.

179. Terada N, Hamano N, Hohki G, Ikeda T, Sai M, Yamashita T, Konno A. The potential role of interleukin-13 in eosinophilic inflammation in nasal mucosa. *Allergy.* 1998;53:690–697.

180. Bochner BS, Luscinskas FW, Gimbrone MA, et al. Adhesion of human basophils, eosinophils, and neutrophils to interleukin 1-activated human vascular endothelial cells: contributions of endothelial cell adhesion molecules. *J Exp Med.* 1991;173: 1553–1557.

181. Yamamoto H, Sedgwick JB, Vrtis RF, Busse WW. The effect of transendothelial migration on eosinophil function. *Am J Respir Cell Mol Biol.* 2000;23:379–388.

182. Tachimoto H, Burdick MM, Hudson SA, Kikuchi M, Konstantopoulos K, Bochner BS. CCR3-Active chemokines promote rapid detachment of eosinophils from VCAM-1 In vitro. *J Immunol.* 2000;165:2748–2754.

183. Sampson AP. IL-5 priming of eosinophil function in asthma. *Clin Exper Allergy.* 2001;31:513–517.

184. Adachi T, Alam R. The mechanism of IL-5 signal transduction. *Am J Physiol.* 1998;275:C623–C633.

185. Her E, Frazer J, Austen KF, Owen WF Jr. Eosinophil hematopoietins antagonize the programmed cell death of eosinophils. Cytokine and glucocorticoid effects on eosinophils maintained by endothelial cell-conditioned medium. *J Clin Invest.* 1991;88: 1982–1987.

186. Hallsworth MP, Litchfield TM, Lee TH. Glucocorticoids inhibit granulocyte-macrophage colony-stimulating factor-1 and interleukin-5 enhanced in vitro survival of human eosinophils. *Immunology.* 1992;75:382–385.

187. Bracke M, Coffer PJ, Lammers JW, Koenderman L. Analysis of signal transduction pathways regulating cytokine-mediated Fc receptor activation on human eosinophils. *J Immunol.* 1998;161: 6768–6774.

188. Rajakulasingam K, Till S, Ying SU, et al. Increased expression of high affinity IgE (FcεRI) receptor- α chain mRNA and protein-bearing eosinophils in human allergen-induced atopic asthma. *Am J Respir Crit Care Med.* 1998;158:233–240.

189. Melo R, Weller P. Piecemeal degranulation in human eosinophils: a distinct secretion mechanism underlying inflammatory responses. *Histol Histopathol.* 2010;25:1341–1354.

190. Melo RC, Perez SA, Spencer LA, Dvorak AM, Weller PF. Intragranular vesiculotubular compartments are involved in piecemeal degranulation by activated human eosinophils. *Traffic.* 2005;6:866–879.

191. Melo RC, Spencer LA, Perez SA, et al. Vesicle-mediated secretion of human eosinophil granule-derived major basic protein. *Lab Invest.* 2009;89:769–781.

192. Spencer LA, Melo RC, Perez SA, Bafford SP, Dvorak AM, Weller PF. Cytokine receptor-mediated trafficking of preformed IL-4 in eosinophils identifies an innate immune mechanism of cytokine secretion. *Proc Natl Acad Sci U S A.* 2006;103:3333–3338.

193. Neves JS, Radke AL, Weller PF. Cysteinyl leukotrienes acting via granule membrane-expressed receptors elicit secretion from within cell-free human eosinophil granules. *J Allergy Clin Immunol.* 2010;125:477–482.

194. Logan MR, Odemuyiwa SO, Moqbel R. Understanding exocytosis in immune and inflammatory cells: the molecular basis of mediator secretion. *J Allergy Clin Immunol.* 2003;111: 923–932.

195. Patella V, de Crescenzo G, Marinò I, et al. Eosinophil granule proteins activate human heart mast cells. *J Immunol.* 1996;157: 1219–1225.

196. Piliponsky AM, Gleich GJ, Nagler A, Bar I, Levi-Schaffer F. Non-IgE-dependent activation of human lung- and cord blood-derived mast cells is induced by eosinophil major basic protein and modulated by the membrane form of stem cell factor. *Blood.* 2003;101:1898–1904.

197. Hartman M-L, Piliponsky AM, Temkin V, Levi-Schaffer F. Human peripheral blood eosinophils express stem cell factor. *Blood.* 2001;97:1086–1091.

198. Levi-Schaffer F, Temkin V, Malamud V, Feld S, Zilberman Y. Mast cells enhance eosinophil survival in vitro: role of TNF-α and granulocyte-macrophage colony-stimulating factor. *J Immunol.* 1998;160:5554–5562.

199. Temkin V, Kantor B, Weg V, Hartman M-L, Levi-Schaffer F. Tryptase activates the mitogen-activated protein kinase/activator protein-1 pathway in human peripheral blood eosinophils, causing cytokine production and release. *J Immunol.* 2002;169: 2662–2669.

200. Raible DG, Schulman ES, DiMuzio J, Cardillo R, Post TJ. Mast cell mediators prostaglandin-D_2 and histamine activate human eosinophils. *J Immunol.* 1992;148:3536–3542.

201. Wong CK, Ng SS, Lun SW, Cao J, Lam CW. Signalling mechanisms regulating the activation of human eosinophils by mast-cell-derived chymase: implications for mast cell–eosinophil interaction in allergic inflammation. *Immunology.* 2009;126:579–587.

202. Pang L, Nie M, Corbett L, Sutcliffe A, Knox AJ. Mast cell β-tryptase selectively cleaves eotaxin and RANTES and abrogates their eosinophil chemotactic activities. *J Immunol.* 2006;176:3788–3795.

203. Revital S, Jason JX, Lisa AS. Eosinophils in innate immunity: an evolving story. *Cell Tissue Res.* 2010;343:57–83.

204. Hagan P, Blumenthal UJ, Chaudri M, et al. Resistance to reinfection with Schistosoma haematobium in Gambian children: analysis of their immune responses. *Trans R Soc Trop Med Hyg.* 1987;81:938–946.

205. Sasaki O, Sugaya H, Ishida K, Yoshimura K. Ablation of eosinophils with anti-IL-5 antibody enhances the survival of intracranial worms of Angiostrongylus cantonensis in the mouse. *Parasite Immunol.* 1993;15:349–354.

206. Ovington KS, McKie K, Matthaei KI, Young IG, Behm CS. Regulation of primary Strongyloides ratti infections in mice: a role for interleukin-5. *Immunology.* 1998;95:488–493.

207. Herbert DB, Lee JJ, Lee NA, Nolan TJ, Schad GA, Abraham D. Role of IL-5 in innate and adaptive immunity to larval strongyloides stercoralis in mice. *J Immunol.* 2000;165:4544–4551.

208. Herndon FJ, Kayes SG. Depletion of eosinophils by anti-IL-5 monoclonal antibody treatment of mice infected with Trichinella spiralis does not alter parasite burden or immunologic resistance to reinfection. *J Immunol.* 1992;149: 3642–3647.

209. Simons JE, Rothenberg ME, Lawrence RA. Eotaxin-1-regulated eosinophils have a critical role in innate immunity against experimental Brugia malayi infection. *Eur J Immunol.* 2005;35:189–197.

210. Galioto AM, Hess JA, Nolan TJ, Schad GA, Lee JJ, Abraham D. Role of eosinophils and neutrophils in innate and adaptive

protective immunity to larval strongyloides stercoralis in mice. *Infect Immun.* 2006;74:5730–5738.

211. Lee JJ, Dimina D, Macias MP, et al. Defining a link with asthma in mice congenitally deficient in eosinophils. *Science.* 2004;305:1773–1776.

212. O'Connell AE, Hess JA, Santiago GA, et al. Major basic protein from eosinophils and myeloperoxidase from neutrophils are required for protective immunity to strongyloides stercoralis in mice. *Infect Immun.* 2011;79:2770–2778.

213. Fabre V, Beiting DP, Bliss SK, et al. Eosinophil deficiency compromises parasite survival in chronic nematode infection. *J Immunol.* 2009;182:1577–1583.

214. Gebreselassie NG, Moorhead AR, Fabre V, et al. Eosinophils preserve parasitic nematode larvae by regulating local immunity. *J Immunol.* 2012;188:417–425.

215. Rosenberg HF, Domachowske JB. Eosinophils, eosinophil ribonucleases, and their role in host defense against respiratory virus pathogens. *J Leukoc Biol.* 2001;70:691–698.

216. Phipps S, Lam CE, Mahalingam S, et al. Eosinophils contribute to innate antiviral immunity and promote clearance of respiratory syncytial virus. *Blood.* 2007;110:1578–1586.

217. Percopo CM, Dyer KD, Ochkur SI, et al. Activated mouse eosinophils protect against lethal respiratory virus infection. *Blood.* 2013;123(5):743–752.

218. Praveen A, Haibin W, Peter FW. Eosinophils as antigen-presenting cells in allergic upper airway disease. *Curr Opin Allergy Clin Immunol.* 2010;10:14–19.

219. Kita H. Eosinophils: multifaceted biological properties and roles in health and disease. *Immunol Rev.* 2011;242:161–177.

220. Shi H-Z, Humbles A, Gerard C, Jin Z, Weller PF. Lymph node trafficking and antigen presentation by endobronchial eosinophils. *J Clin Invest.* 2000;105:945–953.

221. Spencer LA, Weller PF. Eosinophils and Th2 immunity: contemporary insights. *Immunol Cell Biol.* 2010;88:250–256.

222. Humbles AA, Lloyd CM, McMillan SJ, et al. A critical role for eosinophils in allergic airways remodeling. *Science.* 2004;305:1776–1779.

223. Walsh ER, Sahu N, Kearley J, et al. Strain-specific requirement for eosinophils in the recruitment of T cells to the lung during the development of allergic asthma. *J Exp Med.* 2008;205:1285–1292.

224. Woolley KL, Adelroth E, Woolley MJ, Ellis R, Jordana M, O'Byrne PM. Effects of allergen challenge on eosinophils, eosinophil cationic protein, and granulocyte-macrophage colony-stimulating factor in mild asthma. *Am J Respir Crit Care Med.* 1995;151:1915–1924.

225. Koh YY, Kang H, Kim CK. Ratio of serum eosinophil cationic protein/blood eosinophil counts in children with asthma: comparison between acute exacerbation and clinical remission. *Allergy Asthma Proc.* 2003;24:269–274.

226. Pizzichini E, Leff J, Reiss T, et al. Montelukast reduces airway eosinophilic inflammation in asthma: a randomized, controlled trial. *Eur Respir J.* 1999;14:12–18.

227. Lönnkvist K, Hellman C, Lundahl J, Halldén G, Hedlin G. Eosinophil markers in blood, serum, and urine for monitoring the clinical course in childhood asthma: impact of budesonide treatment and withdrawal. *J Allergy Clin Immunol.* 2001;107:812–817.

228. Walsh G, Sexton D, Blaylock M. Corticosteroids, eosinophils and bronchial epithelial cells: new insights into the resolution of inflammation in asthma. *J Endocrinol.* 2003;178:37–43.

229. Green RH, Brightling CE, McKenna S, et al. Asthma exacerbations and sputum eosinophil counts: a randomised controlled trial. *Lancet.* 2002;360:1715–1721.

230. Haldar P, Brightling CE, Hargadon B, et al. Mepolizumab and exacerbations of refractory eosinophilic asthma. *Engl J Med.* 2009;360:973–984.

231. Pavord ID, Korn S, Howarth P, et al. Mepolizumab for severe eosinophilic asthma (DREAM): a multicentre, double-blind, placebo-controlled trial. *Lancet.* 2012;380:651–659.

232. Simon H-U, Rothenberg ME, Bochner BS, et al. Refining the definition of hypereosinophilic syndrome. *J Allergy Clin Immunol.* 2010;126:45–49.

233. Rothenberg ME, Klion AD, Roufosse FE, et al. Treatment of patients with the hypereosinophilic syndrome with mepolizumab. *Engl J Med.* 2008;358:1215–1228.

234. Meyer KC, Raghu G, Baughman RP, et al. An official American Thoracic Society clinical practice guideline: the clinical utility of bronchoalveolar lavage cellular analysis in interstitial lung disease. *Am J Respir Crit Care Med.* 2012;185:1004–1014.

235. Koller DY, Götz M, Eichler I, Urbanek R. Eosinophilic activation in cystic fibrosis. *Thorax.* 1994;49:496–499.

236. Holgate ST, Djukanović R, Casale T, Bousquet J. Anti-immunoglobulin E treatment with omalizumab in allergic diseases: an update on anti-inflammatory activity and clinical efficacy. *Clin Exp Allergy.* 2005;35:408–416.

237. Flood-Page P, Swenson C, Faiferman I, et al. A study to evaluate safety and efficacy of mepolizumab in patients with moderate persistent asthma. *Am J Respir Crit Care Med.* 2007;176:1062–1071.

238. Nair P, Pizzichini MM, Kjarsgaard M,et al. Mepolizumab for prednisone-dependent asthma with sputum eosinophilia. *N Engl J Med.* 2009;360:985–993.

239. Kim S, Marigowda G, Oren E, Israel E, Wechsler ME. Mepolizumab as a steroid-sparing treatment option in patients with Churg-Strauss syndrome. *J Allergy Clin Immunol.* 2010;125:1336–1343.

240. Fulkerson PC, Rothenberg ME. Targeting eosinophils in allergy, inflammation and beyond. *Nat Rev Drug Discov.* 2013;12:117–129.

241. Kiwamoto T, Kawasaki N, Paulson JC, Bochner BS. Siglec-8 as a drugable target to treat eosinophil and mast cell-associated conditions. *Pharmacol Ther.* 2012;135:327–336.

CHAPTER 23

Leukocyte Accumulation in Pulmonary Disease

Nicholas W. Lukacs
Peter A. Ward

INTRODUCTION

Mediators produced during inflammatory/immune responses dictate the severity and intensity of pulmonary disease. The profile of inflammatory leukocyte populations accumulating in inflamed tissues is initiated by cytokine-induced expression of adhesion molecules on the vascular endothelium. Endothelial adhesion molecules include intracellular adhesion molecule-1 (ICAM-1), vascular cell adhesion molecule-1 (VCAM-1), as well as E- and P-selectins that initiate, and in some cases, mediate the migration of leukocytes into tissues. Subsequently, leukocyte adherence to the endothelium is followed by leukocyte migration into the inflamed tissue, directed by chemotactic molecules at the site of the inflammatory/immune response. Upregulation of these early response mediators is crucial for the initiation of early events that regulate the inciting agent, whether it is infectious or noninfectious in nature. However, the continuous over-production of these mediators can lead to destructive, pathologic consequences due to the continued recruitment and activation of disease-specific leukocyte populations. In human lung, inflammation-induced damage can be observed in numerous inflammatory diseases, including both acute and chronic disease settings. In this chapter, we will examine the mediators that promote inflammatory diseases in lung and outline how specific leukocyte populations can contribute to pulmonary pathology.

LEUKOCYTE ADHESION AND MIGRATION INTO THE LUNG

Important considerations in the biology of leukocyte adhesion and migration into the lung are discussed below.

SELECTIN AND ADHESION MOLECULES IN LUNG INFLAMMATION

The release of early response mediators leads to the upregulation of selectins (E and P) and other adhesion molecules (ICAM-1, VCAM-1, etc.) on surfaces of vascular endothelial cells within the site of inflammation.[1-7] Initially, selectin molecules (P and E) are quickly upregulated on the vascular endothelium and initiate "rolling" of leukocytes on activated endothelium through Ca^{2+}-dependent recognition of cell surface carbohydrates of the *sialyl Lewis X* family and related oligosaccharides. Initial and rapid expression of selectin molecules results in a slowing of leukocyte velocities in the circulatory flow, allowing additional interactions to proceed.[8-11] However, such interactions are required to ultimately allow firm adhesion of leukocytes to endothelial cells. Once the leukocytes have begun the selectin-mediated rolling process, they must next go through a series of activation events to allow them to firmly adhere to other adhesion molecules. Leukocytes ultimately bind firmly to the vascular endothelium via β-integrin receptors on leukocyte surfaces, resulting in a very rapid increase in binding affinity, and engagement of other molecules that are upregulated during inflammatory responses on the vascular endothelium. A number of β-integrin adhesion molecules play a role in the migration process, and they are differentially expressed on subsets of leukocytes.[12-14] The β1α4 integrins (VLA-4), expressed primarily on mononuclear cells and eosinophils, have been shown to bind to vascular cell adhesion molecule-1 (VCAM-1), while β2-integrins (CD11/CD18) are expressed on all leukocytes and bind varyingly to intracellular adhesion molecules-1,2,3 (ICAM-1,2,3), the first of which is highly expressed on endothelial cells. These families of adhesion molecules are able to facilitate leukocyte binding to the activated endothelium and can further dictate the type of leukocytes that bind and extravasate into the inflamed tissue. For example, while neutrophils rely on CD11/CD18 binding to ICAM-1, eosinophils depend upon VLA-4/VCAM-1 interactions to firmly adhere to the endothelial cell surface. Once firmly adherent, leukocytes then enter the tissue following chemotactic gradients through a series of detachment/readherence events typified by the polar expression of integrins specific for the adhesion molecules contained on surfaces of mesenchymal-derived cells.

Cell-to-cell communication during inflammatory events is mediated by cytokines that initiate, maintain, and regulate the inflammatory responses, dictating the intensity of the inflammatory response. The early response cytokines, IL-1 and TNF appear to play a pivotal role in the induction of inflammatory responses through the initiation of cytokine cascades.[15-19] The exuberant production of IL-1 and TNF may lead to multisystem injury and systemic complications, as exemplified in septic shock syndromes. As indicated earlier, IL-1 and TNF initially upregulate selectin (E-selectin) and other adhesion molecules (ICAM-1, VCAM-1) needed for the first step of leukocyte extravasation into tissues. In addition, IL-1 and TNF upregulate other inflammatory cytokines (e.g., IL-6) involved in the chemotactic responses of leukocytes into inflamed tissues. Interestingly, the type of cytokine expressed can dictate the nature of the inflammatory response based upon the adhesion molecule that it induces. For example, while TNF and IL-1 are critical for upregulation of ICAM-1 that facilitates neutrophil and monocyte adhesion, IL-4 produced during allergic responses preferentially upregulates VCAM-1. This adhesion molecule mediates eosinophil adhesion. Thus, the inflammatory/immune cytokine environment in lung can tailor the initiation and adhesion interactions for a particular leukocyte recruitment profile. The production of one of a number of classes of chemotactic factors is required for the movement of leukocytes from the vascular compartment to the extravascular compartment of the lung. We will next describe and characterize the function of chemotactic mediators that are expressed in the lung during specific disease conditions.

CHEMOKINES AND GPCR SIGNALING IN LEUKOCYTE ADHESION

The rapid change in affinity of the β-integrins rely on two events: (1) Initial binding to selectin molecules that activates Syk and MAPK, allowing β-integrin to reach an intermediate affinity state; and (2) activation of leukocyte expressed G-protein coupled receptors (GPCR) on the surface of leukocytes.[20-27] The GPCR ligands, usually chemokines bound to the endothelium via glycosaminoglycans (GAGs), initiate rapid Ca^{2+}-dependent β-integrin activation.[28,29] The β-integrin activation results in a conformational change in its extracellular domain, allowing the active binding site for the putative adhesion molecule to be accessible. If the adhesion molecule is also upregulated and expressed on the activated vascular endothelium, the leukocyte rapidly and firmly adheres and spreads along the endothelial surface due to additional actin polymerization, which is also induced during chemokine-GPCR activation events. Thus, the leukocyte very rapidly transitions from a rolling leukocyte to a cell that is firmly adherent, resulting subsequently in transmigration into the tissue. In addition to the GPCR signal, it also appears that the shear stress experienced by leukocytes also plays a role in development in firm adhesion events. These interactions are described in Figure 23-1.

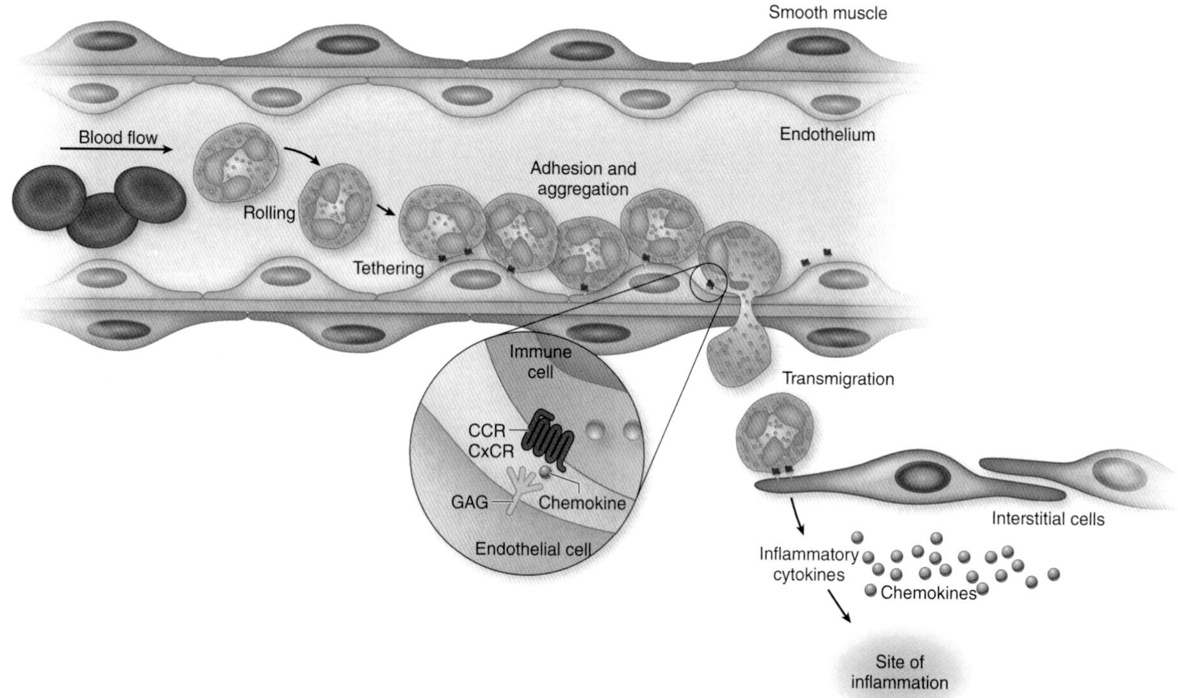

Figure 23-1 Leukocyte migration requires coordinated interactions between adhesion molecules and chemotactic molecules.

A significant amount of research has occurred in recent years, defining critical signaling events that occur during the early stages of leukocyte migration, including selectin-mediated rolling, GPCR-mediated integrin binding, actin polymerization, and leukocyte polarization. One of the most critical events in the transition of leukocytes from rolling to firm adhesion and extravasation is engagement of endothelial bound chemokine ligands with appropriate GPCRs. Chemokine binding activates the Gi-coupled protein-mediated phospholipase C (PLC), which results in inositol-1,4,5 triphosphate (IP_3) formation as well as diacylglycerol (DAG), triggering intracellular Ca^{2+} increases due to translocation from the ER.[30-32] This signaling cascade initiates the activation of Rho GTPases, Rap-1 and Talin1, subsequently mediating integrin affinity increase for their adhesion molecule ligands and allowing clustering following binding. Blockade of events at any stage along this activation pathway can inhibit the β-integrin–mediated adhesion, and interrupting firm adhesion to the activated endothelium.

■ CHEMOATTRACTANTS AND MIGRATION INTO THE LUNG

Below is discussed the role of various chemoattractants in the immune response against pathogens, including complement, arachidonic acid and its derivatives, and chemokines.

Complement

The complement activation cascade plays a significant role in the innate immune response against pathogens, but continual or excessive activation during inflammatory or infectious responses can lead to severe tissue injury. The initiation of the complement cascade can be accomplished via multiple mechanisms, including antibody–antigen complexes, bacterial products, toxins, and lectins (Fig. 23-2). Of the complement activation products, fragments from C3 and C5 have the most profound effects on the inflammatory response. The split products of C3, C3a and C3b, are generated by C3 convertase (other products of C3 cleavage [iC3b, C3d, C3g]) have significant activating roles in the inflammatory pathway. C3a is an anaphylatoxin that induces the activation of mast cells/basophils resulting in mediator release, all of which appear to have direct and indirect effects on vascular permeability.[33-35] C3b acts as a potent opsonizing component, binding to bacteria and allowing accelerated phagocytosis and clearance of pathogens via the C3b receptor on neutrophils and macrophages (Mac-1 [CD11b/CD18]). The split products of C5, C5a and C5b, can subsequently be induced through the sequential participation of C3b and C5 convertase. Similar to C3a, but much more potent, C5a is an anaphylatoxin that interacts with its two receptors (C5aR, C5L2), causing mast cell and basophil degranulation and activation of neutrophils, which collectively induces immediate changes in vascular permeability.[34,36-40] In addition, C5a stimulates vascular smooth muscle contraction and has neutrophil chemotactic and activating characteristics that promote directed migration of these leukocytes toward a concentration gradient.[41,42] C5a can also stimulate neutrophil oxidative metabolism, granule discharge, adhesiveness to vascular endothelium, and assembly on the neutrophil surface of NADPH oxidase (NOX2). C5a can directly stimulate endothelial cells in a G-protein receptor-dependent fashion to cause signal transduction events resulting in increased intracellular Ca^{2+}, induction of superoxide (O_2^-), and expression of P-selectin.[43-45] C3a lacks these activities. Altogether, the functions of C3 and C5 split products indicate that they are potent inflammatory mediators.

Elevated complement component levels in plasma have been described with several pulmonary diseases, including sarcoidosis, idiopathic pulmonary fibrosis (IPF), acute respiratory distress syndrome (ARDS), and chronic obstructive pulmonary disease (COPD).[46,47] Not only can complement initiate GPCR-mediated leukocyte migration but it appears complement activation products can direct the development of immune responses. This can be accomplished via several pathways during initiation of immune responses by regulating IL-12 production.[48] Specifically, C3a appears to drive IL-12 production that then favors type 1 immune responses,[49] while C5a downregulates IL-12 and allows IL-4–mediated type 2 immune responses to be induced.[50] Interestingly, recent studies in $C3^{-/-}$ mice have shown that Th17 responses are also regulated by complement.[51] In contrast, another study suggested that, when C5aR was blocked, there was an exacerbated allergic response that

Leukocyte population	Chemokine receptor
Neutrophil	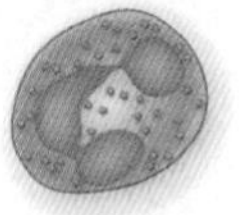 CxCR1 (human only) CxCR2 CCR1
Monocyte	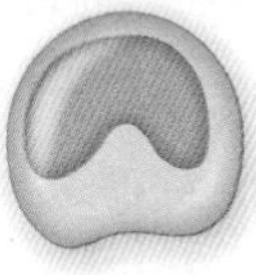 CxCR2 (inflammatory) Cx3CR1 (homeostatic) CCR1 CCR5
Dendritic cell	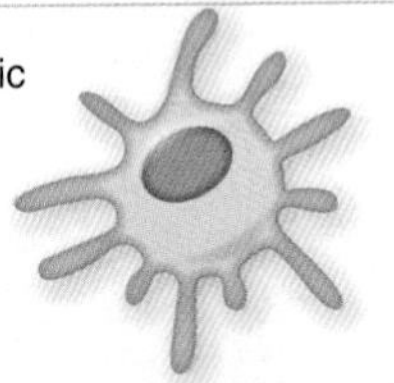 CCR1 CCR2 CCR6 (resting) CCR7 (activated/mature) CxCR4
Basophil	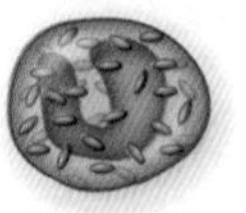 CCR2 CCR3
Eosinophil	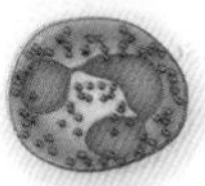 CCR1 CCR3
Th1 cell	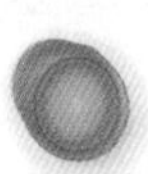 CCR1 CCR5 CxCR3
Th2 cell	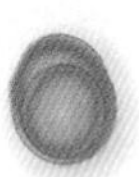 CCR3 CCR4 CCR8
Th17 cell	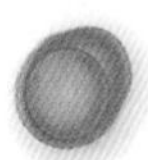 CCR6
Treg cell	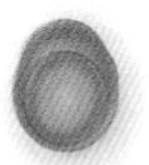 CCR4 CCR8

Figure 23-2 Preferential expression of chemokine receptors on leukocyte subsets can lead to preferential recruitment during pulmonary disease.

also was dependent upon increased IL-17,[52,53] suggesting that the previous study with C3$^{-/-}$ mice was due to inhibition of downstream C5a activation. Thus, while early complement-induced response is critical for containment of infectious organisms, it may be especially important during sensitization to various antigens in determining the phenotype of the pulmonary immune response that will govern the severity of disease outcomes.

The receptors for C3a and C5a have been a source of intense research over the past several years and have led to the resurgence of interest in potentially blocking specific responses during pulmonary disease. The distribution of these receptors depicts their broad role in innate and acquired immune responses. Both C3aR and C5aR are present on alveolar macrophages, DCs, and mast cells, and are also present on sentinel cell populations in the lung that provide important cues for the immediate and prolonged determination of effective immune responses.[54] In particular, activation of these cell populations have been assessed for the differential activation consequences of C3a and C5a. At the same time the expression of C5aR on neutrophils allows an immediate and efficient migration into the lung and activation at the site of inflammation. C5aR is also displayed on cells involved in chronic immune responses, such eosinophils recruited during allergic responses. Thus, activation of the complement system can have potent effects on both acute inflammatory responses as well as chronic inflammation, both of which can lead to long-term pulmonary dysfunction. Interestingly, a second C5a receptor, C5L2, binds C5a and C5a *des arg* extremely efficiently, but C5L2 has no linkage to G proteins.[55] Research examining the possible implications of this second receptor for modulating C5a-mediated responses by competitively binding up C5a during inflammatory responses is the subject of focus from several laboratories. While the function of this second C5a receptor has been controversial, C5L2 appears to mediate several pathologic events, including events in sepsis and perhaps diabetes.[56–60]

Role of Arachidonic Acid and its Products in Lung Responses

The production of arachidonic acid (AA) followed by its enzymatic processing produces a number of lipid mediators that have long been known to be associated with acute and chronic inflammatory responses in the lung.[61–63] Phospholipase A2 degradation of AA leads to its breakdown into platelet activation factor (PAF) that can be immediately processed by 5-LO into 5-HPETE and further processed by 5-LO into leukotriene A4 (Fig. 23-3). 5-HPETE can alternatively be processed into 5-HETE by peroxidases. Leukotriene A4 can be further processed into LTB4 by LTA4 hydrolase or LTC4 by LTC4 hydrolase, followed by continued processing of LTC4 into LTD4, and finally, LTE4. These latter metabolites, C4, D4, and E4 are known as the cysteinyl leukotrienes that are best known to cause airway contractility, causing decreased lung function during large airways disease, such as asthma. Targeting the cysteinyl leukotrienes for blockade has provided significant relief to particular subsets of asthmatic patients.[64]

Of the AA metabolites, PAF and LTB4 have been characterized for their chemotactic activity, promoting migration of leukocytes into sites of inflammation. These mediators were originally identified as potent neutrophil chemoattractants and were associated with acute inflammation-induced airway damage. PAF has a broad range of specificity in its ability to induce leukocyte chemotaxis, since it induces the recruitment of not only neutrophils, but also of monocytes, lymphocytes, and eosinophils.[65,66] During allergic diseases, PAF may have a role in augmentation of eosinophil responses.[67] The actions of PAF on endothelial cells indicate that PAF has a direct role in upregulation of selectin and adhesion molecules and can induce the release of superoxide anion (O_2^-). Instillation of PAF into human, monkey, or guinea pig airways induced an immediate LTC4-independent

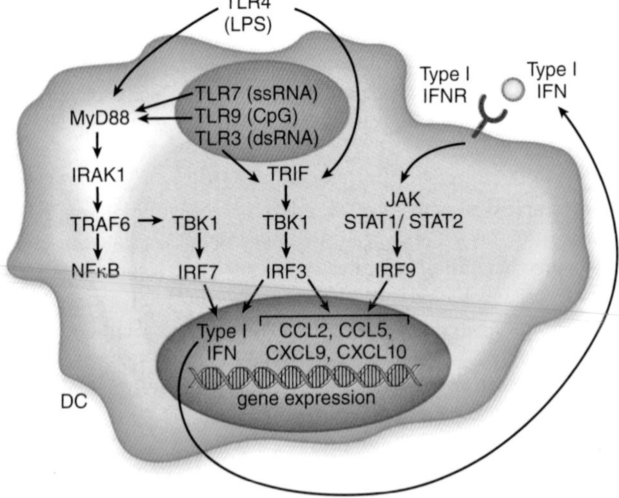

Figure 23-3 Inflammatory gene activation by TLR and type I IFN leads to enhanced leukocyte recruitment.

bronchoconstrictor response, suggesting a possible role in development of pathophysiology in asthmatic responses. Overall, these studies indicate that the signals provided by PAF are not only chemotactic but can also participate in the augmentation of immune/inflammatory pathways in lung. However, over the years several PAF specific inhibitors have been developed, but they have failed to demonstrate effective blocking or attenuating inflammatory responses in human lung.

While leukotrienes in general have broad effects on inflammatory responses, LTB4 is one of the most potent neutrophil chemotactic molecules known and induces O_2^- production. LTB4 can also act to recruit other leukocyte populations, such as monocytes and eosinophils.[68,69] In eosinophil chemotactic assays, LTB4 is more potent than PAF in the activation and degranulation of eosinophils. LTB4 has been found in many disease states, including psoriasis, bacterial peritonitis, inflammatory bowel disease and asthma.[70] LTB4 is rapidly expressed by phagocytic cells (PMNs and macrophages) following stimulation with bacterial LPS or fMLP. More recently, the LTB4 receptor, BLT1, has been implicated in preferential recruitment of Th2 type T lymphocytes during allergic pulmonary responses.[71–73] This receptor has also been implicated in recruitment of T lymphocytes that mediate lung allograft rejection and development of obliterative bronchiolitis in lung allographs in rodents.[74] Thus, LTB4 and BLT1 are now being considered as targets for therapy in chronic immune responses in the lung, in contrast to their traditional roles as potent neutrophil and mononuclear cell chemoattractant in acute lung injury.

Chemokines and Immune Cell Migration

Chemokines (discussed in chapter 26) have been divided into two main families based upon their sequence homology and the position of the first two cysteine residues, C-x-C (alpha) and C-C (beta).[75,76] There are two minor families described each with a single member, the C and Cx3C families. Much of our understanding of chemokines has centered upon their role in mediating leukocyte recruitment to the site of inflammation in lung or specifically directing recirculation of leukocytes during homeostasis. Interestingly, results have indicated that many of these family members also have diverse roles in the activation and differentiation of various immune and nonimmune cell populations. While the chemokine family members' function is diverse, the promiscuous binding relationship between multiple members with a single receptor as well as a specific receptor being able to bind multiple chemokines underscores our relative lack of understanding of the biology of the chemokine family. In particular, it is often difficult to understand how such a vast number of chemotactic molecules, several being produced simultaneously, could coordinate inflammatory responses. Recent studies demonstrate that it may be the overall profile of chemokines being produced that dictates the inflammatory cell response resulting in leukocyte accumulates at a site of injury or infection. This latter aspect can be best displayed during acute inflammatory responses, such as in bacterial infections, when the cellular infiltrate is primarily neutrophilic.[77] Chemokines that bind to CxCR1 and CxCR2 mediates this process. Likewise, when more insidious pathogens are present and acute inflammatory mechanisms cannot effectively control the infectious process, immune cytokines, such as IFN and IL-4, tend to drive the production of chemokines that allow the mononuclear cells, macrophages, and lymphocytes to accumulate at sites of infection, resulting in a more effective immune response for enhanced clearance of the pathogen. Thus, although there are numerous chemokines being produced during any single inflammatory response, the overall profile of the response may be directed to recruitment of cells that are most appropriate to deal with particular stimuli. These "fine tuned" responses mediated by chemokines also depend upon the chemokine receptor profile of the transmigrating leukocyte (Fig. 23-2). For example, while many leukocytes such as PMNs and macrophages tend to have a fairly fixed chemokine receptor expression (CxCR2 for PMNS and CCR2 for inflammatory macrophages),[78–80] T cell subsets (Th1, Th2, Th17, Treg cells) express a differential profile of chemokine receptors that may preferentially allow recruitment to specific types of inflammatory/immune responses.[81–84] Those aspects will be discussed in later sections.

LEUKOCYTE ACCUMULATION AND LUNG PATHOLOGY

A variety of leukocytes may accumulate with the lung. Each is discussed below.

NEUTROPHILS

The accumulation of neutrophils (PMNs) in the lung is the first line of defense against infectious organisms. There are significant numbers of PMNs circulating normally, and they can be quickly mobilized from the bone marrow during inflammatory responses or during acute lung injury. Once activated at the site of inflammation, PMNs preform phagocytic and bacterial/fungal killing functions that promote clearance of bacterial and fungal pathogens. They also can quickly release a number of enzymes, (proteases, etc.), that can have detrimental effects on the local lung tissue and cause physiologic dysfunction and severe damage if not tightly regulated. Individuals with one of many abnormalities in PMN formation, recruitment, or activation defects often develop recurrent, severe infections, both bacterial and fungal.[85,86] As described earlier, PMNs enter the lung via an initial adhesion event that progresses via a selectin-mediated rolling and subsequently through a β_2-integrin (CD11b/CD18)/ICAM-1–induced firm adhesion. While controversial evidence using animals exists, it appears that entry into the lung via the alveolar vasculature may not require the entire adhesion progression since there is low shear stress, allowing leukocytes to migrate into the airspace with less resistance.[87–90] This is because the diameter of the neutrophil and the capillary is nearly the same, which would not allow rolling. Nevertheless, in the alveolar vasculature the adhesion molecules described in section II are still present, functional, and are required for ultimate PMN transmigration. Not surprisingly, numerous chemotactic factors can quickly mobilize and mediate PMN migration into inflamed tissues. These factors include bacterial products such as fMLP, an N-formylated 3 amino acid peptide that is produced by numerous bacteria. fMLP binds to a GPCR (fMLPR). Other chemotactic factors expressed by the host early during pathogen responses include C3a and C5a, as well as the primary lipid mediator, LTB4, all interacting with specific GPCR signaling on the surface of PMNs. Usually, the early migration of PMNs to the lung is likely due to the latter mediators that are quickly cleaved or stored in cells (such as in mast cell granules) and are readily activated or released upon pathogenic or injurious stimuli. Subsequently, the prolonged activation of the pulmonary environment beyond immediate responses (>4 hours) results in cytokine cascades leading to additional and numerous more efficient chemokine protein mediators of migration, including CxCL1 (GROα), CxCL5 (ENA-78), and CxCL8 (IL-8). The CxC family chemokines are produced by both immune and nonimmune cell populations and provide relative specificity for PMN accumulation during lung inflammatory disease via their cognate receptors, CxCR1 and CxCR2, predominantly found on PMNs. Increased numbers of PMNs are often found in severe inflammatory diseases of the lung and likely provide nonspecific damage that may result in lung dysfunction. Several strategies for blocking adhesion as well as chemotactic receptors are currently under development by numerous pharmaceutical companies.

EOSINOPHILS

The role of eosinophils evolutionarily has been linked to chronic parasitic diseases, in which they perform a protective killing response linked to parasite clearance.[91,92] However, as the parasitic burden in humans has been greatly reduced, the immune responses, especially at mucosal surfaces, have led to detrimental chronic responses to inert parasitic antigens. This has led to a number of allergic inflammatory diseases, especially allergic asthma in the lung. Eosinophils are derived in the bone marrow, primarily in the presence of a Th2 type response that provides systemic IL-5 levels that feedback to the bone marrow, directing the maturation and release of eosinophils into circulation. The migration of eosinophils into the lung and other tissues rely on a different subset of adhesion and chemotactic factors for entry into the tissue compartments.[93–99] While the migratory adhesion pathway has not been as thoroughly defined, it appears that it also relies on an initial combination of selectin and β-integrin–mediated adhesion events prior to responding to chemotactic mediators in the lung. While eosinophils are able to utilize CD11b/CD18-ICAM-1–mediated migration pathways, it appears that more efficient and preferential migration is VLA-4 β-integrin–mediated VCAM-1 adhesion. Since VCAM-1 is highly upregulated in the lung during Th2 cytokine–mediated responses, as in asthma, such responses may relate to the inflammatory cytokine environment that stimulates maturation of eosinophils in the bone marrow (IL-5 mediated). Subsequent to adhesion of eosinophils to endothelial cells, eosinophil migration and accumulation in lung can also be regulated by the chemotactic factors that appear to preferentially recruit eosinophils. While C5a and the lipid mediators, LTB4 and PAF, can each provide a stimulus for such migration, it appears that chemokines are the primary stimuli for migration of eosinophils. In particular, CCR3 ligands are the most potent, including CCL5 (RANTES), CCL11 (eotaxin-1), CCL24 (eotaxin-2), and CCL26 (eotaxin-3). CCR3 is the characteristic chemokine receptor expressed on eosinophils and although they also appear to express CCR1, it appears to have only a minor role in the recruitment during chronic disease. Similar to the PMN, eosinophils can induce local damage in lung after their degranulation and release of proteases and enzymes. In addition, eosinophils have been implicated in progression of remodeling diseases, linked to their interaction with fibroblasts.[100,101] Eosinophils have the ability to transform normal fibroblasts into matrix-producing myofibroblasts. Eosinophils have been identified as a significant source of TGFβ, FGF, as well as other pro-fibrotic factors and have been implicated in severe remodeling in chronic allergic and inflammatory diseases.[102,103] Thus, significant effort continues to be made to target eosinophil migration during chronic pulmonary diseases, especially asthma.

MONOCYTES/MACROPHAGES

Resident macrophage populations play an important role in the lung, providing initial protection against pathogenic and noxious damage. The alveolar and interstitial macrophages that reside in and around airways appear to be ideally suited, having optimal ability to phagocytize and kill microorganisms as well as producing regulated levels of inflammatory cytokines. Macrophages also function for uptake of inhaled particles. Phagocytosis requires an intact cytoskeleton and is most efficient when phagocytosis is mediated by Fc receptors. Complement and scavenger receptors such as MARCO are also important mechanisms for mediating clearance of microorganisms.[104–107] During responses to infectious and inflammatory stimuli, the migration of monocytes from the blood can also play an important role in the clearance of the inciting agents. In humans, there appear to be two distinct subsets of circulating monocytes, CD14+ monocytes with high CCR1, CCR2 and CxCR2 expression, and low Cx3CR1 expression as well as a distinct CD16+ population of monocytes with high levels of Cx3CR1 and low levels of CCR2 expression.[108–110] Similar subsets exist in mice and, while not exact, this allows characterization of their different roles in disease once recruited to the site of inflammation allowing extrapolation to human disease. Mice lacking inflammatory, CCR2+ monocytes are highly susceptible to *Listeria monocytogenes* and *Mycobacterium tuberculosis* infections, demonstrating that infiltrating monocytes are important effector cells for the clearance of intracellular bacteria.[111,112] In a similar fashion the inhibition of inflammatory macrophage infiltration into the lung during *Aspergillus fumigatus* and *Cryptococcus* infections can lead to prolonged and detrimental infection by these organisms.[113,114]

The circulating CCR2+ monocyte population also appears to be the progenitor to inflammatory dendritic cells (DC), which express CD11b/CD11c. DC have a different developmental program and upregulate CCR6 on their surfaces for localization to airway epithelium where its ligand, CCL20, is expressed. This distinct subset of DC appears to be crucial for proper T cell activation to infections pathogens mediating Th1 type responses (IFNg producing) for the clearance of *M. tuberculosis*, *Toxoplasmosis gondii*, and *Cryptococcus neoformans* infections in animal models. In contrast, however, inflammatory DC recruitment to the lung (via CCR2) during chronic allergic disease may result in development of Th2 cytokine associated disease. Thus, the role of the inflammatory monocyte accumulation may depend on whether the inciting agent is an intracellular pathogen or a noninfectious stimulus that should optimally be ignored (immunologically tolerated), such as an allergen. Thus, attempts to regulate chronic inflammatory disease by targeting CCR2, its ligands or inflammatory monocytes themselves may cause deviations in lung inflammatory responses that are harmful.

INNATE LYMPHOID CELLS

A new classification of cytokine-producing cells has recently been named for their ability to respond to an inflamed environment in the absence of an antigenic specific stimulus. Innate lymphoid cells (ILC) have been further classified into three types, ILC1 (IFNγ-producing cells), ILC2 (IL-5/IL-13–producing Nuocytes), and ILC3 (IL-17/IL-22–producing cells).[115–117] These subsets are present in relatively low numbers in the lung and respond to innate cytokine signals and information of their accumulation during disease is only now beginning to be explored. ILC1 respond directly to IL-12 and express t-bet, similar to NK and Th1 cells, and have been recently shown to reside at much higher numbers in inflamed intestines of Crohn's disease patients. ILC1 cells appear to be distinct from NK cells, since they do not express granzyme B and other NK cell markers.

ILC2 (a.k.a. Nuocytes) or innate helper cells, respond to epithelial-cell–derived IL-33 and IL-25, express the GATA3 transcription factor, and contain Sca1+, c-kit+, Lin−, and ST2+ (IL-33R) surface markers.[118,119] ILC2 have been clearly implicated in parasite clearance in the intestine, but more recently have been identified in playing a role in models of asthma and influenza-induced disease.[120,121] The ILC2 have been the most extensively characterized and, although there appears to be only a few thousand residing in the mouse lung at baseline, they can produce high levels of Th2 type cytokines, (IL-5 and IL-13), in response to cytokine stimuli, especially IL-33.[122,123] Recent data has suggested that circulatory pools of ILC2 exist in human asthma patients, but further studies need to be explored to determine their relevance in human pulmonary diseases. Early studies suggested that ILC2 (nuocytes) express CCR2 and CCR3, but further study will be required to determine if these receptors mediate accumulation of the cells in the lung.

CD4+ T LYMPHOCYTE SUBSETS

The severity and chronicity of lung disease is dictated by multiple factors including the persistence of stimuli, pathogen or antigenic challenge, as well as the phenotype of the immune response. As discussed earlier and in other chapters, the mediators produced during pulmonary disease may be the most critical in determining the type of inflammation that develops. The discovery of several subsets of CD4+ lymphocytes that are defined by the profile of cytokines produced is critical for selectively responding to various infectious organisms and/or different phase of immune responses.[124,125]

The trafficking of naive lymphocytes from the blood to lymph nodes is pivotal to the maintenance of effective immune surveillance.

However, deciphering the mechanisms involved in lymphocyte recruitment during inflammation may be more pharmaceutically attractive in order to therapeutically regulate chronic debilitating inflammatory diseases. Functional diversity of T cells has been demonstrated by the observation that naive T lymphocytes are activated and differentiate into Th0 type cells that produce different combinations of cytokines. Subsequently, these cells can further differentiate into either Th1 type cells (IL-2 and IFN), Th2 type cells (IL-4, IL-5, and IL-13), Th17 cells (IL-17 and IL-22), or Th9 cells (IL-9) depending upon the cytokine environment that the Th0 cells are exposed. It has become clear that certain diseases are characterized by the Th cytokine phenotype that is produced. For example, allergy and asthma responses have been identified as a largely Th2 type disease, with IL-4, IL-5, and IL-13 promoting the pathogenic phenotype. However, these traditional points of view have begun to break down as we begin to understand that, when we look at an exacerbated disease phenotype, such as a virus or bacterial infection, there appears to be a complex mix of Th cytokine phenotypes.[126–131] In particular, both bacterial- and viral-induced exacerbations appear to enhance the pathology by promoting IL-17 production that, while responding to the pathogenic assault, can also create chronic disease, examples of which are remodeling and mucus hypersecretion responses.[132,133]

Although numerous chemotactic mediators have been implicated in lymphocyte migration, the chemokine mediators appear to preferentially attract specific lymphocyte subsets, both based upon differential receptor display as well as chemokine ligands that are produced in the lung during a particular disease.[125,134,135] For example, IFN and TNF that are produced during Th1 type responses induce CCL3 and CCL5 that bind to CCR1 and CCR5 that are found on Th1 type cells. Other Th1 associated chemokines CxCL9, 10, and 11 all bind specifically to CxCR3 that is also highly expressed on Th1 type cells along with expression on $CD8^+$ cytotoxic T cells. Thus, these profiles of chemokine production are most appropriate for viral and intracellular bacterial infections. Likewise, there are CC chemokines that are preferentially upregulated by Th2 cytokines (IL-4 and IL-13), but not Th1 type cytokines including CCL1, CCL11, CCL17, and CCL22. These chemokine mediators bind to CCRs preferentially found on Th2 cells, including CCR8, CCR3, and CCR4, respectively. Thus, the cytokine environment can reinforce itself by recruiting additional T cells capable of producing chemokines associated with the allergic/asthmatic responses.[136–139] Recent data has also identified other chemokine receptor phenotypes, including CCR6/CCL20 receptor system that appears to be associated with Th17 cell migration.[140,141] Interestingly, CCL20 (LARC) is produced at significant levels by bronchial epithelial cells and attract both inflammatory DC and Th17 type cells that have increased expression of CCR6. Thus, effort continues to be made to identify compounds that might inhibit specific chemokine receptor GPCRs that can be used in specific chronic disease responses.

BACTERIAL INFECTION AND SEPSIS

The early response to infectious organisms is most important when dealing with bacterial infections that can be reversed by preventing colonization and by quickly eliminating the inciting agents. Bacteria, once established, can proliferate at an exponential rate that outpaces the ability to clear bacteria. These events can quickly overwhelm the local sentinel defenses provided by lung macrophage populations. A critical step in early bacterial clearance is the efficient and early recruitment of phagocytic cells (PMNs and monocytes) from the blood. The first response initiated in this case is activation of the complement system quickly resulting in the generation of C3a and C5a.[142] This initiates an early wave of infiltrating leukocytes that may be sufficient for removal of the invading pathogens. In a parallel process of de novo synthesis, continued persistence of the bacteria quickly leads to release of LTB4 from granulocytes, mast cell degranulation, and production of LTB4 from macrophages. LTB4 release effectively maintains the inflammatory influx of PMNs to cope with the presence of bacteria.[143] Subsequently, macrophage populations produce activating cytokines, (IL-1 and TNF), that mediate both adhesion molecule expression on endothelial cells and chemokine production, such as IL-8 and MCP-1, that promote continued influx of phagocytic cells.[144–146] A critical mechanism associated with bacteria-induced inflammatory responses has been shown to be inflammasome activation that induces a caspase-mediated process that cleaves pro-IL-1 to active IL-1 and activates NFkB pathways leading to induction of chemotactic responses that exacerbates inflammation.[147–149] Targeting inflammasome activation and especially IL-1 can significantly attenuate inflammatory diseases.[150–152] Recent evidence suggests that these activation pathways are central to the numerous inflammatory diseases, such as IBD,[153] with recent evidence indicating that pulmonary diseases may also be affected by inflammasome activation.[154–156] Thus, a well-coordinated and multifaceted series of chemoattractants are produced to promote acute inflammatory responses to control the bacterial infection. In addition to bringing about leukocyte migration, these chemoattractants activate PMNs and macrophages to promote enhanced phagocytosis and killing.

One of the harmful consequences of a vigorous and sustained recruitment of PMNs and macrophages, however, is the release of substances that cause tissue damage and necrosis of epithelial cells. Phagocytic cells, in response to the bacterial stimuli and phagocytic action, release proteolytic enzymes, reactive oxygen metabolites, and additional activating cytokines that cause injury to vascular and stromal cells in small and large airways. In particular, elastase release from PMNs may have a devastating effect on tissue.[157] Reports have suggested that the level of PMN-derived elastase in the airway reflects the intensity of PMN accumulation and correlates to the incidence of ARDS development.[158,159] There are numerous causes of PMN activation, including trauma, hemorrhage, burn, etc., all of which can lead to the development of life-threatening ARDS.

ARDS is a common disorder encountered in the ICU and involving septic patients, whether related to bacterial-induced disease or "sterile" inflammatory syndromes. Bacterial infections release danger associated molecules patterns (DAMPs), such as lipopolysaccharide or lipoteichoic acid, which interact with TLRs.[160] Sterile inflammation is a situation in which there is no bacterial inciting agent. This response leads to release of a variety of endogenous products generically referred to as "alarmins." These products interact with NOD receptors the result sometimes being a cytokine storm, multiorgan failure, and death.[160,161] ARDS is an overwhelming inflammatory response ("cytokine storm"), control of which is not possible at this time. These uncontrollable hyperinflammatory responses have been linked to PMN-associated inflammation. Thus, much of the current therapeutic effort has been focused upon attempts to reduce the ongoing influx and activation of PMNs. A number of investigations have examined the potential role of blocking PMN accumulation by blocking CD18 (Mac-1) with antibodies. These studies were largely unsuccessful, emphasizing our inadequate knowledge of lung inflammatory responses.

Given the lack of requirement in some models for adhesion molecule-dependent PMN accumulation, the role of chemotactic molecules has been more widely studied. In animal models of acute lung injury, blockade of C5a and/or its receptor, C5aR, attenuates lung injury, preserving vital lung function.[33,89,162,163] There has been interest in developing new therapies around blocking complement activation cascades as well as development of therapeutic antibodies designed to inhibit the acute inflammatory response. However, since complement and LTB4 mediators are primarily thought to be involved during the initial stages of inflammation and may only constitute a portion of the chemotactic environment, other more stable mediators have been targeted, especially the chemokines. A large body of literature has characterized the significant levels of PMN-associated chemokines, in the CxC family.[164] They have been identified in the airways of ALI and ARDS patients, with the mediators' presence correlating with the severity of the inflammatory response. Numerous animal model studies have demonstrated that, by targeting the CxCR2 or its ligands, or using functionally inert CxCL8 (IL-8) homologs, a reduction in inflammation severity can be achieved. This has led to numerous pharmaceutical attempts for development of efficacious and safe compounds and biologics directed against chemokine ligands and their receptor, CxCR2. The CxCR2 antagonists may not only be useful in ALI or ARDS but in numerous other pulmonary diseases that appear to have PMN infiltration, including COPD, severe asthma, and even cystic fibrosis. Thus, controlling PMN infiltration and activation may be at the core of preserving lung function.

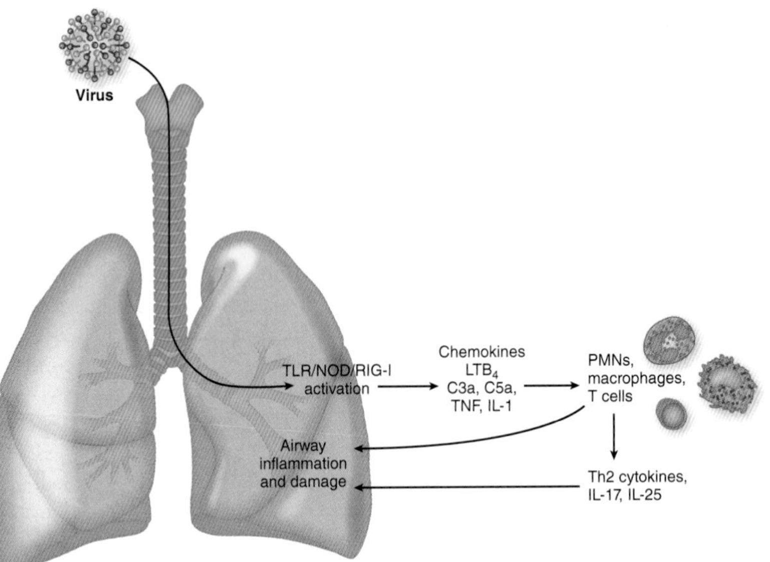

Figure 23-4 Viral exacerbation in pulmonary disease enhances chemotactic and inflammatory cytokine production leading to increased disease severity.

VIRAL EXACERBATION OF LUNG DISEASE

Many causes have been identified to explain exacerbation in patients with underlying lung disease, especially asthma and COPD. Viral infections appear to be the most common cause, such as with influenza, rhinovirus (RV), adenovirus, and respiratory syncytial virus (RSV). While there may be common pathways involved in the exacerbation of pulmonary diseases, activation of chemokines by viral pathogens may be the most prevalent mechanism.[165–168]

Approximately 10% of adults and up to 30% of children are affected by asthmatic disease, making it the most prevalent chronic respiratory disease, whereas COPD is an induced disease most clearly associated with smoking and occurs predominantly in older adults. The mechanism for viral exacerbation of the chronic lung response is unclear, but evidence points to a key role for increased leukocyte recruitment, inflammatory cell activation, and T cell differentiation. The asthmatic condition includes increases in mucus production and epithelial damage along with possible increases in airway remodeling and smooth muscle cell hyperplasia. While many viruses may be causative of asthma and COPD exacerbations, the most common viruses, RV, RSV, and influenza, all appear to function through many common pathways.[169–172] During infections, the upregulation of CxCL8 is significantly increased in sputum samples. CxCL8 is the mediator most frequently associated with exacerbation. Its presence correlates with the number of neutrophils and is productive of the severity of the exacerbation. PMN accumulation and activation lead to the local release of a number of proteases and MPO, with elastase having a significant effect on potentiating mucus production in the airway. In addition, other inflammatory mediators have also been detected during viral-induced exacerbations, including IL-6, LTB4, LTC4/D4, and histamine. Other chemokines that appear include CCL11 (eotaxin) and CCL5 (RANTES). Both have the ability to recruit eosinophils, further intensifying the inflammatory environment in lung.

The commonality of responses between these different RNA viruses likely stems from activation of Toll-like receptors (TLRs).[173,174] Virus-infected epithelial cells and innate immune cells quickly respond to the viral nucleic acid by TLR3 and TLR7/8 activation via dsRNA and ssRNA, respectively.[175,176] The activation of these TLR pathways activate several important mediator pathways including the TRIF adapter pathway leading to IRF3 and MyD88 adapter pathways that lead to NFkB for TLR3 and TLR7 (Fig. 23-3). The NFkB pathway mediates the production of a number of activating and chemotactic proteins, whereas the TRIF pathway primarily upregulates type I IFN and associated chemokine such as RANTES. Interestingly, however, there are differences in the ability of the different viruses to induce different levels of mediators, especially type I IFN. Influenza virus is known to promote high levels of type I IFN, described in animal models, often accompanied by secondary bacterial infection.[177,178] In contrast, RSV promotes comparatively low type I IFN due to specific inhibition of the activation pathways by nonstructural (NS) proteins produced by the virus.[179–182] Since type I IFN can induce additional chemokines together with the lytic nature of influenza, this may explain the intensity of the inflammatory responses that accompany influenza versus RV and RSV infections. Other pathogen recognition pathways, including the helicase (RIG-I) and NOD/inflammasome pathways have also been identified in these responses and contribute significantly to the inflammatory outcome of the responses.[183,184]

In addition to increased chemokines, it appears that other important mediators may also be preferentially expressed during viral exacerbation of asthma and COPD. Both IL-17 A and/or IL-25 (IL-17E) are induced during viral infections. The addition of these two IL-17 family members, both of which share a common receptor chain (IL-17RA), may contribute significantly to the pathogenic environment. Both types of infection induce a steroid-resistant response.[185,186] In the case of IL-17, a neutrophilic inflammation is induced through activation of CxC family chemokines, whereas IL-25 appears to induce an eosinophil accumulation and Th2 cytokine responses that on its own promotes a mucus-rich pathogenic environment. Thus, the addition of these two cytokines may be very important targets during these chronic airway responses where patients often develop steroid resistance in the most severe cases. As depicted in Figure 23-4, the ability of viruses to exacerbate pulmonary disease severity is a consequence of increasing the overall inflammatory response through the activation of several chemotactic mediators via PAMP-mediated pathways, as well as the activation of additional cytokine responses. Similar responses are operative during bacterial-induced disease exacerbation. While this section has outlined several of the critical mediators, other pathways are also important for the overall disease phenotype.

ACKNOWLEDGMENTS

This work was supported by HL114858 (NWL), AI036302 (NWL), GM-29507 (PAW), and GM-61656 (PAW). We would like to thank Robin Kunkel for the outstanding artwork supplied for the figures in this chapter.

REFERENCES

1. Harari OA, McHale JF, Marshall D, et al. Endothelial cell E- and P-selectin up-regulation in murine contact sensitivity is prolonged by distinct mechanisms occurring in sequence. *J Immunol.* 1999;163(12):6860–6866.
2. Bless NM, Tojo SJ, Kawarai H, et al. Differing patterns of P-selectin expression in lung injury. *Am J Pathol.* 1998;153(4): 1113–1122.
3. Borgstrom P, Hughes GK, Hansell P, Wolitsky BA, Sriramarao P. Leukocyte adhesion in angiogenic blood vessels. Role of E-selectin, P-selectin, and beta2 integrin in lymphotoxin-mediated leukocyte recruitment in tumor microvessels. *J Clin Invest.* 1997;99(9):2246–2253.
4. Mizgerd JP, Meek BB, Kutkoski GJ, Bullard DC, Beaudet AL, Doerschuk CM. Selectins and neutrophil traffic: margination and Streptococcus pneumoniae-induced emigration in murine lungs. *J Exp Med.* 1996;184(2):639–645.
5. Mulligan MS, Polley MJ, Bayer RJ, Nunn MF, Paulson JC, Ward PA. Neutrophil-dependent acute lung injury. Requirement for P-selectin (GMP-140). *J Clin Invest.* 1992;90(4):1600–1607.
6. Xu H, Gonzalo JA, St Pierre Y, et al. Leukocytosis and resistance to septic shock in intercellular adhesion molecule 1-deficient mice. *J Exp Med.* 1994;180(1):95–109.
7. Marlin SD, Springer TA. Purified intercellular adhesion molecule-1 (ICAM-1) is a ligand for lymphocyte function-associated antigen 1 (LFA-1). *Cell.* 1987;51(5):813–819.
8. Ley K. Pathways and bottlenecks in the web of inflammatory adhesion molecules and chemoattractants. *Immunol Res.* 2001;24(1): 87–95.
9. Ley K. Molecular mechanisms of leukocyte recruitment in the inflammatory process. *Cardiovasc Res.* 1996;32(4):733–742.
10. Smith CW. Endothelial adhesion molecules and their role in inflammation. *Can J Physiol Pharmacol.* 1993;71(1):76–87.
11. Lukacs NW, Ward PA. Inflammatory mediators, cytokines, and adhesion molecules in pulmonary inflammation and injury. *Adv Immunol.* 1996;62:257–304.
12. Luo BH, Carman CV, Springer TA. Structural basis of integrin regulation and signaling. *Annu Rev Immunol.* 2007;25:619–647.
13. Springer TA. Adhesion receptors of the immune system. *Nature.* 1990;346(6283):425–434.
14. Larson RS, Springer TA. Structure and function of leukocyte integrins. *Immunol Rev.* 1990;114:181–217.
15. Kunkel SL, Remick DG, Strieter RM, Larrick JW. Mechanisms that regulate the production and effects of tumor necrosis factor-alpha. *Crit Rev Immunol.* 1989;9(2):93–117.
16. Larrick JW, Kunkel SL. The role of tumor necrosis factor and interleukin 1 in the immunoinflammatory response. *Pharm Res.* 1988;5(3):129–139.
17. Tracey KJ, Cerami A. Tumor necrosis factor: a pleiotropic cytokine and therapeutic target. *Annu Rev Med.* 1994;45:491–503.
18. Tracey KJ, Lowry SF, Cerami A. Cachectin: a hormone that triggers acute shock and chronic cachexia. *J Infect Dis.* 1988; 157(3):413–420.
19. Cerami A, Beutler B. The role of cachectin/TNF in endotoxic shock and cachexia. *Immunol Today.* 1988;9(1):28–31.
20. Schurpf T, Springer TA. Regulation of integrin affinity on cell surfaces. *EMBO J.* 2011;30(23):4712–4727.
21. Lefort CT, Hyun YM, Schultz JB, et al. Outside-in signal transmission by conformational changes in integrin Mac-1. *J Immunol.* 2009;183(10):6460–6468.
22. Salas A, Shimaoka M, Phan U, Kim M, Springer TA. Transition from rolling to firm adhesion can be mimicked by extension of integrin alphaLbeta2 in an intermediate affinity state. *J Biol Chem.* 2006;281(16):10876–10882.
23. Chigaev A, Buranda T, Dwyer DC, Prossnitz ER, Sklar LA. FRET detection of cellular alpha4-integrin conformational activation. *Biophys J.* 2003;85(6):3951–3962.
24. Chan JR, Hyduk SJ, Cybulsky MI. Detecting rapid and transient upregulation of leukocyte integrin affinity induced by chemokines and chemoattractants. *J Immunol Methods.* 2003; 273(1–2):43–52.
25. Ley K. Integration of inflammatory signals by rolling neutrophils. *Immunol Rev.* 2002;186:8–18.
26. Kuwano Y, Spelten O, Zhang H, Ley K, Zarbock A. Rolling on E- or P-selectin induces the extended but not high-affinity conformation of LFA-1 in neutrophils. *Blood.* 2010;116(4):617–624.
27. Gonzalez-Amaro R, Sanchez-Madrid F. Cell adhesion molecules: selectins and integrins. *Crit Rev Immunol.* 1999;19(5–6): 389–429.
28. Allain F, Vanpouille C, Carpentier M, Slomianny MC, Durieux S, Spik G. Interaction with glycosaminoglycans is required for cyclophilin B to trigger integrin-mediated adhesion of peripheral blood T lymphocytes to extracellular matrix. *Proc Natl Acad Sci U S A.* 2002;99(5):2714–2719.
29. Hirose J, Kawashima H, Yoshie O, Tashiro K, Miyasaka M. Versican interacts with chemokines and modulates cellular responses. *J Biol Chem.* 2001;276(7):5228–5234.
30. Deane JA, Fruman DA. Phosphoinositide 3-kinase: diverse roles in immune cell activation. *Annu Rev Immunol.* 2004; 22: 563–598.
31. Mellado M, Rodriguez-Frade JM, Manes S, Martinez AC. Chemokine signaling and functional responses: the role of receptor dimerization and TK pathway activation. *Annu Rev Immunol.* 2001;19:397–421.
32. Sotsios Y, Ward SG. Phosphoinositide 3-kinase: a key biochemical signal for cell migration in response to chemokines. *Immunol Rev.* 2000;177:217–235.
33. Bosmann M, Ward PA. Role of C3, C5 and anaphylatoxin receptors in acute lung injury and in sepsis. *Adv Exp Med Biol.* 2012;946:147–159.
34. Klos A, Tenner AJ, Johswich KO, Ager RR, Reis ES, Kohl J. The role of the anaphylatoxins in health and disease. *Mol Immunol.* 2009;46(14):2753–2766.
35. Erdei A, Kerekes K, Pecht I. Role of C3a and C5a in the activation of mast cells. *Exp Clin Immunogenet.* 1997;14(1):16–18.
36. Yan C, Gao H. New insights for C5a and C5a receptors in sepsis. *Front Immunol.* 2012;3:368.
37. Ward PA. Role of C5 activation products in sepsis. *ScientificWorldJournal.* 2010;10:2395–2402.
38. Woodruff TM, Ager RR, Tenner AJ, Noakes PG, Taylor SM. The role of the complement system and the activation fragment C5 a in the central nervous system. *Neuromolecular Med.* 2010;12(2):179–192.
39. Ward PA. Functions of C5a receptors. *J Mol Med (Berl).* 2009; 87(4):375–378.
40. Ward PA. Sepsis, apoptosis and complement. *Biochem Pharmacol.* 2008;76(11):1383–1388.
41. Wetsel RA. Expression of the complement C5a anaphylatoxin receptor (C5aR) on non-myeloid cells. *Immunol Lett.* 1995; 44(2–3):183–187.

42. Scheid CR, Webster RO, Henson PM, Findlay SR. Direct effect of complement factor C5a on the contractile state of isolated smooth muscle cells. *J Immunol.* 1983;130(5):1997–1999.

43. Kilgore KS, Ward PA, Warren JS. Neutrophil adhesion to human endothelial cells is induced by the membrane attack complex: the roles of P-selectin and platelet activating factor. *Inflammation.* 1998;22(6):583–598.

44. Foreman KE, Glovsky MM, Warner RL, Horvath SJ, Ward PA. Comparative effect of C3a and C5a on adhesion molecule expression on neutrophils and endothelial cells. *Inflammation.* 1996;20(1):1–9.

45. Foreman KE, Vaporciyan AA, Bonish BK, et al. C5a-induced expression of P-selectin in endothelial cells. *J Clin Invest.* 1994; 94(3):1147–1155.

46. Sarma VJ, Huber-Lang M, Ward PA. Complement in lung disease. *Autoimmunity.* 2006;39(5):387–394.

47. Regal JF. Role of the complement system in pulmonary disorders. *Immunopharmacology.* 1997;38(1–2):17–25.

48. Karp CL, Wills-Karp M. Complement and IL-12: yin and yang. *Microbes Infect.* 2001;3(2):109–119.

49. Kawamoto S, Yalcindag A, Laouini D, et al. The anaphylatoxin C3 a downregulates the Th2 response to epicutaneously introduced antigen. *J Clin Invest.* 2004;114(3):399–407.

50. Wittmann M, Zwirner J, Larsson VA, et al. C5a suppresses the production of IL-12 by IFN-gamma-primed and lipopolysaccharide-challenged human monocytes. *J Immunol.* 1999;162(11): 6763–6769.

51. Ma Q, Li D, Nurieva R, et al. Reduced graft-versus-host disease in C3-deficient mice is associated with decreased donor Th1/ Th17 differentiation. *Biol Blood Marrow Transplant.* 2012;18(8): 1174–1181.

52. Grailer JJ, Bosmann M, Ward PA. Regulatory effects of C5 a on IL-17A, IL-17F, and IL-23. *Front Immunol.* 2012;3:387.

53. Weaver DJ Jr, Reis ES, Pandey MK, et al. C5a receptor-deficient dendritic cells promote induction of Treg and Th17 cells. *Eur J Immunol.* 2010;40(3):710–721.

54. Peng Q, Li K, Sacks SH, Zhou W. The role of anaphylatoxins C3a and C5a in regulating innate and adaptive immune responses. *Inflamm Allergy Drug Targets.* 2009;8(3):236–246.

55. Ohno M, Hirata T, Enomoto M, Araki T, Ishimaru H, Takahashi TA. A putative chemoattractant receptor, C5L2, is expressed in granulocyte and immature dendritic cells, but not in mature dendritic cells. *Mol Immunol.* 2000;37(8):407–412.

56. Rittirsch D, Flierl MA, Nadeau BA, et al. Functional roles for C5 a receptors in sepsis. *Nat Med.* 2008;14(5):551–557.

57. Fisette A, Munkonda MN, Oikonomopoulou K, Paglialunga S, Lambris JD, Cianflone K. C5L2 receptor disruption enhances the development of diet-induced insulin resistance in mice. *Immunobiology.* 2013;218(1):127–133.

58. Zhang X, Schmudde I, Laumonnier Y, et al. A critical role for C5L2 in the pathogenesis of experimental allergic asthma. *J Immunol.* 2010;185(11):6741–6752.

59. Lee H, Whitfeld PL, Mackay CR. Receptors for complement C5a. The importance of C5aR and the enigmatic role of C5L2. *Immunol Cell Biol.* 2008;86(2):153–160.

60. Chen NJ, Mirtsos C, Suh D, et al. C5L2 is critical for the biological activities of the anaphylatoxins C5a and C3a. *Nature.* 2007;446(7132):203–207.

61. McMillan RM. Leukotrienes in respiratory disease. *Paediatr Respir Rev.* 2001;2(3):238–244.

62. Holtzman MJ. Arachidonic acid metabolism. Implications of biological chemistry for lung function and disease. *Am Rev Respir Dis.* 1991;143(1):188–203.

63. Feuerstein G, Hallenbeck JM. Leukotrienes in health and disease. *FASEB J.* 1987;1(3):186–192.

64. Singh RK, Gupta S, Dastidar S, Ray A. Cysteinyl leukotrienes and their receptors: molecular and functional characteristics. *Pharmacology.* 2010;85(6):336–349.

65. Peplow PV. Regulation of platelet-activating factor (PAF) activity in human diseases by phospholipase A2 inhibitors, PAF acetylhydrolases, PAF receptor antagonists and free radical scavengers. *Prostaglandins Leukot Essent Fatty Acids.* 1999;61(2):65–82.

66. Liu L, Mul FP, Kuijpers TW, Lutter R, Roos D, Knol EF. Neutrophil transmigration across monolayers of endothelial cells and airway epithelial cells is regulated by different mechanisms. *Ann N Y Acad Sci.* 1996;796:21–29.

67. Kay AB. Leucocytes in asthma. *Immunol Invest.* 1988;17(8–9): 679–705.

68. Ohnishi H, Miyahara N, Gelfand EW. The role of leukotriene B(4) in allergic diseases. *Allergol Int.* 2008;57(4):291–298.

69. McMillan RM, Foster SJ. Leukotriene B4 and inflammatory disease. *Agents Actions.* 1988;24(1–2):114–119.

70. Osher E, Weisinger G, Limor R, Tordjman K, Stern N. The 5 lipoxygenase system in the vasculature: emerging role in health and disease. *Mol Cell Endocrinol.* 2006;252(1–2):201–206.

71. Peters-Golden M. Expanding roles for leukotrienes in airway inflammation. *Curr Allergy Asthma Rep.* 2008;8(4):367–373.

72. Miyahara N, Miyahara S, Takeda K, Gelfand EW. Role of the LTB4/BLT1 pathway in allergen-induced airway hyperresponsiveness and inflammation. *Allergol Int.* 2006;55(2):91–97.

73. Leff AR. Regulation of leukotrienes in the management of asthma: biology and clinical therapy. *Annu Rev Med.* 2001;52:1–14.

74. Medoff BD, Seung E, Wain JC, et al. BLT1-mediated T cell trafficking is critical for rejection and obliterative bronchiolitis after lung transplantation. *J Exp Med.* 2005;202(1):97–110.

75. Bacon K, Baggiolini M, Broxmeyer H, et al. Chemokine/ chemokine receptor nomenclature. *J Interferon Cytokine Res.* 2002;22(10):1067–1068.

76. Vinader V, Afarinkia K. A beginner's guide to chemokines. *Future Med Chem.* 2012;4(7):845–852.

77. Kobayashi Y. Neutrophil infiltration and chemokines. *Crit Rev Immunol.* 2006;26(4):307–316.

78. Palmqvist C, Wardlaw AJ, Bradding P. Chemokines and their receptors as potential targets for the treatment of asthma. *Br J Pharmacol.* 2007;151(6):725–736.

79. Esche C, Stellato C, Beck LA. Chemokines: key players in innate and adaptive immunity. *J Invest Dermatol.* 2005;125(4):615–628.

80. Sabroe I, Lloyd CM, Whyte MK, Dower SK, Williams TJ, Pease JE. Chemokines, innate and adaptive immunity, and respiratory disease. *Eur Respir J.* 2002;19(2):350–355.

81. Donnelly LE, Barnes PJ. Chemokine receptors as therapeutic targets in chronic obstructive pulmonary disease. *Trends Pharmacol Sci.* 2006;27(10):546–553.

82. Pease JE. Asthma, allergy and chemokines. *Curr Drug Targets.* 2006;7(1):3–12.

83. Proudfoot AE, Power CA, Wells TN. The strategy of blocking the chemokine system to combat disease. *Immunol Rev.* 2000;177:246–256.

84. Cascieri MA, Springer MS. The chemokine/chemokine-receptor family: potential and progress for therapeutic intervention. *Curr Opin Chem Biol.* 2000;4(4):420–427.

85. Schmidt S, Moser M, Sperandio M. The molecular basis of leukocyte recruitment and its deficiencies. *Mol Immunol.* 2013;55(1):49–58.

86. Nauseef WM. How human neutrophils kill and degrade microbes: an integrated view. *Immunol Rev.* 2007;219:88–102.

87. Konrad FM, Reutershan J. CXCR2 in acute lung injury. *Mediators Inflamm.* 2012;2012:740987.

88. Zhou X, Dai Q, Huang X. Neutrophils in acute lung injury. *Front Biosci.* 2012;17:2278–2283.

89. Guo RF, Ward PA. Role of C5a in inflammatory responses. *Annu Rev Immunol.* 2005;23:821–852.

90. Ward PA, Warren JS, Johnson KJ. Oxygen radicals, inflammation, and tissue injury. *Free Radic Biol Med.* 1988;5(5–6):403–408.

91. Jacobsen EA, Taranova AG, Lee NA, Lee JJ. Eosinophils: singularly destructive effector cells or purveyors of immunoregulation? *J Allergy Clin Immunol.* 2007;119(6):1313–1320.

92. Klion AD, Nutman TB. The role of eosinophils in host defense against helminth parasites. *J Allergy Clin Immunol.* 2004;113(1):30–37.

93. Velazquez JR, Teran LM. Chemokines and their receptors in the allergic airway inflammatory process. *Clin Rev Allergy Immunol.* 2011;41(1):76–88.

94. Trivedi SG, Lloyd CM. Eosinophils in the pathogenesis of allergic airways disease. *Cell Mol Life Sci.* 2007;64(10):1269–1289.

95. Leckie MJ. Anti-interleukin-5 monoclonal antibodies: preclinical and clinical evidence in asthma models. *Am J Respir Med.* 2003;2(3):245–259.

96. Pease JE, Williams TJ. Eotaxin and asthma. *Curr Opin Pharmacol.* 2001;1(3):248–253.

97. Busse WW. Leukotrienes and inflammation. *Am J Respir Crit Care Med.* 1998;157(6 Pt 2):S210–S213; discussion S247–S218.

98. Henricks PA, Bloemen PG, Nijkamp FP. Adhesion molecules and the recruitment of eosinophils to the airways. *Res Immunol.* 1997;148(1):18–28.

99. Barthel SR, Johansson MW, McNamee DM, Mosher DF. Roles of integrin activation in eosinophil function and the eosinophilic inflammation of asthma. *J Leukoc Biol.* 2008;83(1):1–12.

100. Xisto DG, Farias LL, Ferreira HC, et al. Lung parenchyma remodeling in a murine model of chronic allergic inflammation. *Am J Respir Crit Care Med.* 2005;171(8):829–837.

101. Ohno I, Nitta Y, Yamauchi K, et al. Transforming growth factor beta 1 (TGF beta 1) gene expression by eosinophils in asthmatic airway inflammation. *Am J Respir Cell Mol Biol.* 1996;15(3):404–409.

102. Tanaka H, Komai M, Nagao K, et al. Role of interleukin-5 and eosinophils in allergen-induced airway remodeling in mice. *Am J Respir Cell Mol Biol.* 2004;31(1):62–68.

103. Zhang K, Flanders KC, Phan SH. Cellular localization of transforming growth factor-beta expression in bleomycin-induced pulmonary fibrosis. *Am J Pathol.* 1995;147(2):352–361.

104. Dahl M, Bauer AK, Arredouani M, et al. Protection against inhaled oxidants through scavenging of oxidized lipids by macrophage receptors MARCO and SR-AI/II. *J Clin Invest.* 2007;117(3):757–764.

105. Arredouani MS, Palecanda A, Koziel H, et al. MARCO is the major binding receptor for unopsonized particles and bacteria on human alveolar macrophages. *J Immunol.* 2005;175(9):6058–6064.

106. Arredouani M, Yang Z, Ning Y, et al. The scavenger receptor MARCO is required for lung defense against pneumococcal pneumonia and inhaled particles. *J Exp Med.* 2004;200(2):267–272.

107. Palecanda A, Paulauskis J, Al-Mutairi E, et al. Role of the scavenger receptor MARCO in alveolar macrophage binding of unopsonized environmental particles. *J Exp Med.* 1999;189(9):1497–1506.

108. Ancuta P, Rao R, Moses A, et al. Fractalkine preferentially mediates arrest and migration of CD16+ monocytes. *J Exp Med.* 2003;197(12):1701–1707.

109. An JL, Ishida Y, Kimura A, Tsokos M, Kondo T. Immunohistochemical detection of CCR2 and CX3CR1 in sepsis-induced lung injury. *Forensic Sci Int.* 2009;192(1–3):e21–e25.

110. Jakubzick C, Tacke F, Ginhoux F, et al. Blood monocyte subsets differentially give rise to CD103+ and CD103- pulmonary dendritic cell populations. *J Immunol.* 2008;180(5):3019–3027.

111. Serbina NV, Pamer EG. Monocyte emigration from bone marrow during bacterial infection requires signals mediated by chemokine receptor CCR2. *Nat Immunol.* 2006;7(3):311–317.

112. Kurihara T, Warr G, Loy J, Bravo R. Defects in macrophage recruitment and host defense in mice lacking the CCR2 chemokine receptor. *J Exp Med.* 1997;186(10):1757–1762.

113. Blease K, Mehrad B, Standiford TJ, et al. Enhanced pulmonary allergic responses to Aspergillus in CCR2-/- mice. *J Immunol.* 2000;165(5):2603–2611.

114. Huffnagle GB, Traynor TR, McDonald RA, et al. Leukocyte recruitment during pulmonary Cryptococcus neoformans infection. *Immunopharmacology.* 2000;48(3):231–236.

115. Scanlon ST, McKenzie AN. Type 2 innate lymphoid cells: new players in asthma and allergy. *Curr Opin Immunol.* 2012;24(6):707–712.

116. Wong SH, Walker JA, Jolin HE, et al. Transcription factor RORα is critical for nuocyte development. *Nat Immunol.* 2012;13(3):229–236.

117. Koyasu S, Moro K. Innate Th2-type immune responses and the natural helper cell, a newly identified lymphocyte population. *Curr Opin Allergy Clin Immunol.* 2011;11(2):109–114.

118. Neill DR, Wong SH, Bellosi A, et al. Nuocytes represent a new innate effector leukocyte that mediates type-2 immunity. *Nature.* 2010;464(7293):1367–1370.

119. Saenz SA, Siracusa MC, Perrigoue JG, et al. IL25 elicits a multipotent progenitor cell population that promotes T(H)2 cytokine responses. *Nature.* 2010;464(7293):1362–1366.

120. Chang YJ, Kim HY, Albacker LA, et al. Innate lymphoid cells mediate influenza-induced airway hyper-reactivity independently of adaptive immunity. *Nat Immunol.* 2011;12(7):631–638.

121. Spits H, Di Santo JP. The expanding family of innate lymphoid cells: regulators and effectors of immunity and tissue remodeling. *Nat Immunol.* 2011;12(1):21–27.

122. Yasuda K, Muto T, Kawagoe T, et al. Contribution of IL-33-activated type II innate lymphoid cells to pulmonary eosinophilia in intestinal nematode-infected mice. *Proc Natl Acad Sci U S A.* 2012;109(9):3451–3456.

123. Price AE, Liang HE, Sullivan BM, et al. Systemically dispersed innate IL-13-expressing cells in type 2 immunity. *Proc Natl Acad Sci U S A.* 2010;107(25):11489–11494.

124. Ebert LM, Schaerli P, Moser B. Chemokine-mediated control of T cell traffic in lymphoid and peripheral tissues. *Mol Immunol.* 2005;42(7):799–809.

125. Schaerli P, Moser B. Chemokines: control of primary and memory T-cell traffic. *Immunol Res.* 2005;31(1):57–74.

126. Kim V, Criner GJ. Chronic bronchitis and chronic obstructive pulmonary disease. *Am J Respir Crit Care Med.* 2013;187(3): 228–237.

127. Jackson DJ, Johnston SL. The role of viruses in acute exacerbations of asthma. *J Allergy Clin Immunol.* 2010;125(6):1178–1187; quiz 1188–1179.

128. Schaller M, Hogaboam CM, Lukacs N, Kunkel SL. Respiratory viral infections drive chemokine expression and exacerbate the asthmatic response. *J Allergy Clin Immunol.* 2006;118(2):295–302; quiz 303–304.

129. Hansbro PM, Beagley KW, Horvat JC, Gibson PG. Role of atypical bacterial infection of the lung in predisposition/protection of asthma. *Pharmacol Ther.* 2004;101(3):193–210.

130. Yamaya M, Sasaki H. Rhinovirus and asthma. *Viral Immunol.* 2003;16(2):99–109.

131. Wedzicha JA. Mechanisms of exacerbations. *Novartis Found Symp.* 2001;234:84–93; discussion 93–103.

132. Zhao Y, Zhang YH, Denney L, et al. High levels of virus-specific CD4+ T cells predict severe pandemic influenza A virus infection. *Am J Respir Crit Care Med.* 2012;186(12): 1292–1297.

133. Mukherjee S, Lindell DM, Berlin AA, et al. IL-17-induced pulmonary pathogenesis during respiratory viral infection and exacerbation of allergic disease. *Am J Pathol.* 2011;179(1): 248–258.

134. Lukacs NW, Miller AL, Hogaboam CM. Chemokine receptors in asthma: searching for the correct immune targets. *J Immunol.* 2003;171(1):11–15.

135. Lukacs NW. Role of chemokines in the pathogenesis of asthma. *Nat Rev Immunol.* 2001;1(2):108–116.

136. Kim CH. Chemokine-chemokine receptor network in immune cell trafficking. *Curr Drug Targets Immune Endocr Metabol Disord.* 2004;4(4):343–361.

137. Kaplan AP. Chemokines, chemokine receptors and allergy. *Int Arch Allergy Immunol.* 2001;124(4):423–431.

138. Campbell JD, HayGlass KT. T cell chemokine receptor expression in human Th1- and Th2-associated diseases. *Arch Immunol Ther Exp (Warsz).* 2000;48(6):451–456.

139. Syrbe U, Siveke J, Hamann A. Th1/Th2 subsets: distinct differences in homing and chemokine receptor expression? *Springer Semin Immunopathol.* 1999;21(3):263–285.

140. Kim CH. Migration and function of Th17 cells. *Inflamm Allergy Drug Targets.* 2009;8(3):221–228.

141. Boniface K, Blom B, Liu YJ, de Waal Malefyt R. From interleukin-23 to T-helper 17 cells: human T-helper cell differentiation revisited. *Immunol Rev.* 2008;226:132–146.

142. Guo RF, Ward PA. Mediators and regulation of neutrophil accumulation in inflammatory responses in lung: insights from the IgG immune complex model. *Free Radic Biol Med.* 2002;33(3): 303–310.

143. Bailie MB, Standiford TJ, Laichalk LL, Coffey MJ, Strieter R, Peters-Golden M. Leukotriene-deficient mice manifest enhanced lethality from Klebsiella pneumonia in association with decreased alveolar macrophage phagocytic and bactericidal activities. *J Immunol.* 1996;157(12):5221–5224.

144. Balamayooran G, Batra S, Fessler MB, Happel KI, Jeyaseelan S. Mechanisms of neutrophil accumulation in the lungs against bacteria. *Am J Respir Cell Mol Biol.* 2010;43(1):5–16.

145. Strieter RM, Belperio JA, Keane MP. Host innate defenses in the lung: the role of cytokines. *Curr Opin Infect Dis.* 2003;16(3): 193–198.

146. Moore TA, Standiford TJ. The role of cytokines in bacterial pneumonia: an inflammatory balancing act. *Proc Assoc Am Physicians.* 1998;110(4):297–305.

147. Rathinam VA, Vanaja SK, Fitzgerald KA. Regulation of inflammasome signaling. *Nat Immunol.* 2012;13(4):333–332.

148. Franchi L, Munoz-Planillo R, Nunez G. Sensing and reacting to microbes through the inflammasomes. *Nat Immunol.* 2012;13(4): 325–332.

149. Franchi L, Eigenbrod T, Munoz-Planillo R, Nunez G. The inflammasome: a caspase-1-activation platform that regulates immune responses and disease pathogenesis. *Nat Immunol.* 2009;10(3): 241–247.

150. Dinarello CA, Simon A, van der Meer JW. Treating inflammation by blocking interleukin-1 in a broad spectrum of diseases. *Nat Rev Drug Discov.* 2012;11(8):633–652.

151. Dinarello CA. Interleukin-1 in the pathogenesis and treatment of inflammatory diseases. *Blood.* 2011;117(14):3720–3732.

152. De Nardo D, Latz E. NLRP3 inflammasomes link inflammation and metabolic disease. *Trends Immunol.* 2011;32(8): 373–379.

153. Zaki MH, Lamkanfi M, Kanneganti TD. The Nlrp3 inflammasome: contributions to intestinal homeostasis. *Trends Immunol.* 2011;32(4):171–179.

154. dos Santos G, Kutuzov MA, Ridge KM. The inflammasome in lung diseases. *Am J Physiol Lung Cell Mol Physiol.* 2012;303(8): L627–L633.

155. Mortaz E, Masjedi MR, Allameh A, Adcock IM. Inflammasome signaling in pathogenesis of lung diseases. *Curr Pharm Des.* 2012; 18(16):2320–2328.

156. Birrell MA, Eltom S. The role of the NLRP3 inflammasome in the pathogenesis of airway disease. *Pharmacol Ther.* 2011; 130(3):364–370.

157. Doring G. The role of neutrophil elastase in chronic inflammation. *Am J Respir Crit Care Med.* 1994;150(6 Pt 2):S114–S117.

158. Moraes TJ, Chow CW, Downey GP. Proteases and lung injury. *Crit Care Med.* 2003;31(4 Suppl):S189–S194.

159. Gadek JE, Pacht ER. The interdependence of lung antioxidants and antiprotease defense in ARDS. *Chest.* 1996;110(6 Suppl):273S–277S.

160. Tolle LB, Standiford TJ. Danger-associated molecular patterns (DAMPs) in acute lung injury. *J Pathol.* 2013;229(2):145–156.

161. Balamayooran T, Balamayooran G, Jeyaseelan S. Review: Toll-like receptors and NOD-like receptors in pulmonary antibacterial immunity. *Innate Immun.* 2010;16(3):201–210.

162. Allegretti M, Moriconi A, Beccari AR, et al. Targeting C5a: recent advances in drug discovery. *Curr Med Chem.* 2005;12(2): 217–236.

163. Ward PA. Role of complement, chemokines, and regulatory cytokines in acute lung injury. *Ann N Y Acad Sci.* 1996;796:104–112.

164. Strieter RM, Keane MP, Burdick MD, Sakkour A, Murray LA, Belperio JA. The role of CXCR2/CXCR2 ligands in acute lung injury. *Curr Drug Targets Inflamm Allergy.* 2005;4(3):299–303.

165. Mackay AJ, Hurst JR. COPD exacerbations: causes, prevention, and treatment. *Med Clin North Am.* 2012;96(4):789–809.

166. Jackson DJ, Sykes A, Mallia P, Johnston SL. Asthma exacerbations: origin, effect, and prevention. *J Allergy Clin Immunol.* 2011; 128(6):1165–1174.

167. Mallia P, Johnston SL. How viral infections cause exacerbation of airway diseases. *Chest.* 2006;130(4):1203–1210.

168. Seemungal TA, Wedzicha JA. Viral infections in obstructive airway diseases. *Curr Opin Pulm Med.* 2003;9(2):111–116.

169. Holtzman MJ, Byers DE, Benoit LA, et al. Immune pathways for translating viral infection into chronic airway disease. *Adv Immunol.* 2009;102:245–276.

170. Celli BR, Barnes PJ. Exacerbations of chronic obstructive pulmonary disease. *Eur Respir J.* 2007;29(6):1224–1238.

171. Traves SL, Proud D. Viral-associated exacerbations of asthma and COPD. *Curr Opin Pharmacol.* 2007;7(3):252–258.

172. Caramori G, Ito K, Contoli M, et al. Molecular mechanisms of respiratory virus-induced asthma and COPD exacerbations and pneumonia. *Curr Med Chem.* 2006;13(19):2267–2290.

173. Raymond T, Schaller M, Hogaboam CM, Lukacs NW, Rochford R, Kunkel SL. Toll-like receptors, Notch ligands, and cytokines drive the chronicity of lung inflammation. *Proc Am Thorac Soc.* 2007;4(8):635–641.

174. Chaudhuri N, Dower SK, Whyte MK, Sabroe I. Toll-like receptors and chronic lung disease. *Clin Sci (Lond).* 2005;109(2): 125–133.

175. Zeytun A, Chaudhary A, Pardington P, Cary R, Gupta G. Induction of cytokines and chemokines by Toll-like receptor signaling: strategies for control of inflammation. *Crit Rev Immunol.* 2010;30(1):53–67.

176. Xagorari A, Chlichlia K. Toll-like receptors and viruses: induction of innate antiviral immune responses. *Open Microbiol J.* 2008;2:49–59.

177. Thitithanyanont A, Engering A, Ekchariyawat P, et al. High susceptibility of human dendritic cells to avian influenza H5N1 virus infection and protection by IFN-alpha and TLR ligands. *J Immunol.* 2007;179(8):5220–5227.

178. Diebold SS, Montoya M, Unger H, et al. Viral infection switches non-plasmacytoid dendritic cells into high interferon producers. *Nature.* 2003;424(6946):324–328.

179. Sluijs KF, Obregon C, Geiser TK, Muhlemann K, Nicod LP. Monocyte differentiation toward regulatory dendritic cells is not affected by respiratory syncytial virus-induced inflammatory mediators. *Am J Respir Cell Mol Biol.* 2011;44(5): 655–664.

180. Oshansky CM, Krunkosky TM, Barber J, Jones LP, Tripp RA. Respiratory syncytial virus proteins modulate suppressors of cytokine signaling 1 and 3 and the type I interferon response to infection by a toll-like receptor pathway. *Viral Immunol.*2009;22(3):147–161.

181. Liu P, Jamaluddin M, Li K, Garofalo RP, Casola A, Brasier AR. Retinoic acid-inducible gene I mediates early antiviral response and Toll-like receptor 3 expression in respiratory syncytial virus-infected airway epithelial cells. *J Virol.* 2007;81(3): 1401–1411.

182. Spann KM, Tran KC, Chi B, Rabin RL, Collins PL. Suppression of the induction of alpha, beta, and lambda interferons by the NS1 and NS2 proteins of human respiratory syncytial virus in human epithelial cells and macrophages [corrected]. *J Virol.* 2004; 78(8):4363–4369.

183. Takeuchi O, Akira S. Innate immunity to virus infection. *Immunol Rev.* 2009;227(1):75–86.

184. Pang IK, Iwasaki A. Inflammasomes as mediators of immunity against influenza virus. *Trends Immunol.* 2011;32(1):34–41.

185. McKinley L, Alcorn JF, Peterson A, et al. TH17 cells mediate steroid-resistant airway inflammation and airway hyperresponsiveness in mice. *J Immunol.* 2008;181(6):4089–4097.

186. Petersen BC, Budelsky AL, Baptist AP, Schaller MA, Lukacs NW. Interleukin-25 induces type 2 cytokine production in a steroid-resistant interleukin-17RB+ myeloid population that exacerbates asthmatic pathology. *Nat Med.* 2012;18(5): 751–758.

CHAPTER 24

Antibody-Mediated Lung Defenses and Humoral Immunodeficiency

Homer L. Twigg III

Antibody-mediated, or humoral, immunity is essential for host defense against respiratory pathogens. Defects in humoral immunity are common and frequently underappreciated. From a respiratory perspective, patients with impaired humoral immunity are susceptible to recurrent bacterial sinopulmonary infections and bronchiectasis. Antibody responses are also the principal mechanism behind the efficacy of vaccination against respiratory pathogens. This chapter focuses on our understanding of the normal B cell environment in the lung, generation of appropriate antibody responses after antigenic challenge, disease states associated with impaired lung humoral immunity, and the pulmonary response to vaccination.

OVERVIEW OF B CELL DEVELOPMENT (ONTOGENY)

The primary cell responsible for generating humoral immunity is the B lymphocyte. There are two phases in the development of antibody responses. The first phase is antigen independent and is called lymphopoiesis. As with the generation of other immune cells, the process begins with a multipotent stem cell in the bone marrow, which undergoes multiple maturation steps leading to mature but antigen naïve B lymphocytes (Fig. 24-1), which express IgM and IgD on the cell surface.[1] This process occurs entirely within the bone marrow (or liver during fetal development). Important cytokines in this process include interleukin (IL)-7,[2] *ckit*-ligand (stem cell factor),[3] and IL-11.[4] Mature B cells express the surface receptors CD19, CD20, CD21, and CD72.[5,6] CD20 is especially relevant as it is the target of the monoclonal antibody rituximab, which is used to deplete B lymphocytes in B cell lymphoproliferative disorders[7] and autoimmune disorders characterized by the production of pathogenic autoantibodies.[8]

At the completion of lymphopoiesis IgM expressing B cells traffic to various lymphoid organs, including lymph nodes in the lung, to await antigenic challenge and enter immunopoiesis.[9,10] Thus, unlike

Lymphopoiesis (antigen independent)

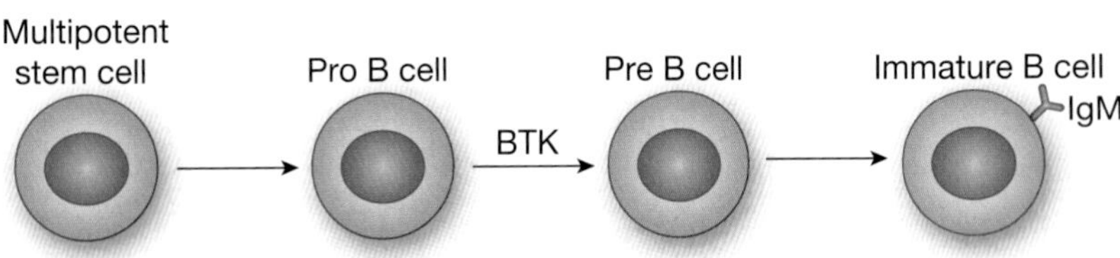

Immunopoiesis (antigen dependent)

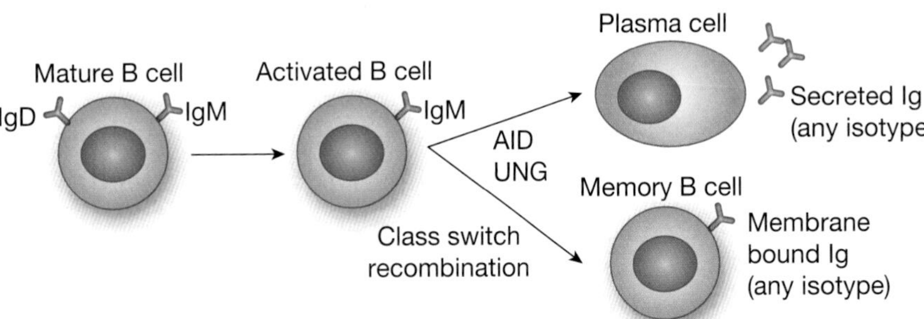

Figure 24-1 Overview of B cell ontogeny. Lymphopoiesis, which occurs in the bone marrow or fetal liver, is an antigen independent process, which begins with a multipotent stem cell and ends with an IgM expressing immature B cell, which will migrate to lymphoid tissues. Immunopoiesis begins with antigen stimulation (hence antigen dependent) and results in antibody secreting plasma cells and antibody expressing memory B cells. Class switch recombination leads to the generation of different immunoglobulin subtypes (IgG, IgA, IgE) from activated IgM expressing B cells. BTK, Bruton's tyrosine kinase, AID, activation-induced cytidine deaminase, UNG, uracil-N-glycosylase.

lymphopoiesis, immunopoiesis is antigen-dependent. The end result of immunopoiesis is the generation of antibody secreting plasma cells[1] and long lived memory B cells, which secrete immunoglobulin only upon re-exposure to antigen.[11] During immunopoiesis class switch recombination and somatic hypermutation occur resulting in the generation of IgA and IgG secreting cells out of IgM precursors and will be discussed in detail below. Immunopoiesis is most efficient in the presence of antigen activated T cells that provide "help" to B cells in the form of cytokines and cell surface activation signals. The most critical latter signal is the interaction between CD40 on B cells and CD40L on activated T cells. In the absence of such signaling (i.e., due to genetic mutations in CD40 or CD40L) class switching fails to occur, resulting in the accumulation of IgM secreting cells and the hyperimmunoglobulin M syndromes, discussed later in this chapter.

IMMUNOGLOBULIN DEVELOPMENT AND STRUCTURE

Below are discussed the basic structure of immunoglobulins and important characteristics of those immunoglobulins found in the lung.

BASIC STRUCTURE

Immunoglobulin (Ig) molecules are made up of two identical protein heavy chains and two identical kappa (κ) or lambda (λ) light chains.[12] Immunoglobulin heavy-chain genes reside on chromosome 14 and immunoglobulin light chains are derived from either the Igκ locus on chromosome 2 or the Igλ locus on chromosome 22. Immunoglobulin heavy chains contain both a variable region that will ultimately contribute to antigen binding and a constant region that binds to cell Fc receptors and complement. Mature immunoglobulin light chains also contain variable and constant regions. Within each variable region, there are hypervariable regions that represent the actual antigen binding site and less variable regions which make up the *framework region.*

The variable domain of the heavy chain is encoded by three sets of genes, the variable (V), diversity (D), and junctional (J) genes, which must be physically rearranged to result in expression of immunoglobulin heavy-chain protein.[13] Similarly, the variable region of the immunoglobulin light-chain protein is encoded by two sets of genes, the V and J genes, which are likewise rearranged to allow transcription of functional protein.[13] The rearrangement of DNA to join V, D, and J heavy-chain genes and V and J light-chain genes also results in elimination of unused V, D, and J sequences and noncoding stretches of DNA or introns. The many possible variable regions resulting from these random rearrangements confer a broad range of potential antigen specificities to the mature immunoglobulin molecules.

CLASS SWITCHING

Once immunopoiesis is initiated B cells alter the isotype of antibody that is produced via *isotype switching.*[13,14] This occurs in *switch regions* on immunoglobulin heavy chains through a process called *class switch recombination.* By translocation of the IgM variable region to *switch regions* adjacent to one of the constant regions coding for IgG, IgA, or IgE, the B cell is able to maintain antigen specificity and at the same time generate different immunoglobulin subtypes with different functional capabilities. Class switch recombination requires an enzyme called activation-induced cytidine deaminase (AID). AID also is critical for *somatic hypermutation*, a process where rapidly proliferating activated B cells have a high rate of point mutations in genes encoding the variable region leading to production of antibodies with different antigen binding affinities.[15] This results in a greatly expanded repertoire of B cells expressing surface IgG of different affinities for the triggering antigen. B cells expressing high affinity antibody on their surface (and thus bind greater amount of antigen) have a survival benefit over B cells coated with weaker affinity to antigen, where less signaling through antigen recognition results in B cell apoptosis. In this way the antibody response moves toward production of higher affinity and more specific immunoglobulin. The importance of AID is reflected in the development of one of the hyperimmunoglobulin M syndromes in patients with defects in this enzyme.[16] The structure of the various immunoglobulin classes is shown in Figure 24-2.

LUNG IMMUNOGLOBULINS

In the lung immunoglobulins comprise the second largest class of proteins present in bronchoalveolar lavage (BAL) fluid after albumin.[17] IgG is the major immunoglobulin in the lower respiratory tract[18] In contrast, IgA is the most abundant immunoglobulin in secretions from the upper respiratory tract, exceeding the concentration of IgG by a ratio of 2.5:1. Smaller amounts of IgE are consistently found in the BAL fluid of normal subjects.[17]

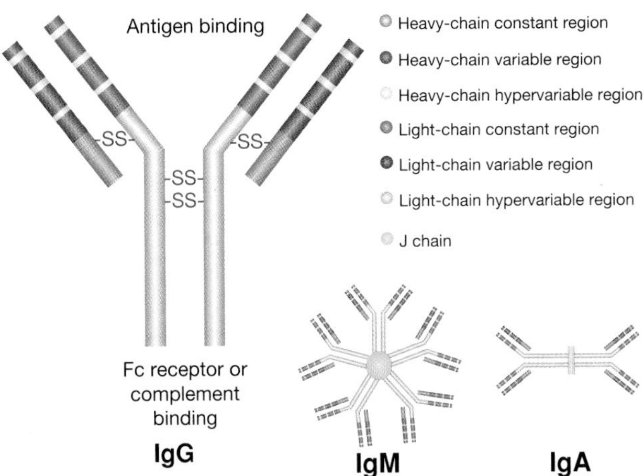

Figure 24-2 Basic immunoglobulin structure. Immunoglobulin molecules consist of two identical protein heavy chains and two identical light chains joined by disulfide bonds. Both heavy and light chains contain a constant and a variable region. Within each variable region there are hypervariable regions that represent actual antigen binding sites. IgM typically exists as a pentamer and IgA as a dimer.

IgG

IgG is the major circulating immunoglobulin found in the vascular compartment. In normal subjects, the amount of IgG measured in BAL (usually expressed as an immunoglobulin/albumin ratio) is in the same proportion as serum, suggesting that under resting conditions most IgG in the lung represents transudation from the vascular compartment.[17,19] This is further supported by the relatively small size of IgG (150,000 D). There are four IgG subclasses found in BAL fluid in approximately the same proportions as found in serum. IgG1 represents approximately 60% to 70% of the IgG present in BAL fluid, IgG2 20% to 25%, and IgG3 and IgG4 are present only in small amounts (<5%).[18] Responses to protein antigens predominantly reside in the IgG1 and IgG3 subclasses while polysaccharide antigens predominantly give rise to IgG2 antibodies.[20,21]

The major function of IgG is to opsonize pathogens and target them for clearance either through uptake by phagocytic cells or by fixing complement. In this regard IgG1 and IgG3 fix complement more avidly than IgG2.[22] Antibody also binds to Fc receptors on phagocytic cells to facilitate uptake. The three primary Fc receptors are FcRI, FcRII, and FcRIII. IgG1 and IgG3 bind FcRIII receptors on phagocytic cells equally well and more potently than IgG2.[23] IgG1 binds to the other Fc receptors more avidly than the other IgG subclasses. Binding of antigen–antibody complexes to Fc receptors is potentially a double-edged sword. On the one hand, not only is uptake of opsonized pathogens through Fc receptors more efficient, so is the intracellular digestion of organisms in phagolysosomes. For example, uptake of opsonized Mycobacterium tuberculosis through the Fc receptor results in intracellular killing of the organism, while uptake through other receptors (i.e., the mannose receptor) allows the organism to escape digestion.[24] On the other hand, uptake of opsonized pathogens through Fc receptors represents an "inflammatory clearance" mechanism that is associated with release of potentially harmful inflammatory mediators into the lung environment.[25]

IgA

In contrast to IgG, IgA is likely locally produced based on an elevated IgA/albumin ratio in BAL compared to serum.[26] IgA can exist as monomeric and polymeric proteins. The latter is usually found as dimeric IgA, characterized by two monomers connected by a J chain.[27] Most IgA in the lung is in dimeric form, with features of secretory IgA (sIgA) characterized by the presence of a J chain and secretory component (SC).[28] The large size of dimeric IgA (385,000 D) also argues against simple transudation of IgA from the vascular compartment into the lung. Finally, the presence of secretory component in BAL is another argument for the local production of IgA in the lung.[29]

IgA has two subclasses: IgA1 and IgA2.[27] IgA1 comprises nearly 80% of serum IgA. In contrast, IgA2 appears to be important in mucosal immunity and nearly half of the IgA present in secretions is IgA2. IgA exerts its protective effect through three mechanisms.[30] First, it serves as an immunologic barrier, inhibiting binding of organisms to mucosal surfaces. Second, the normal movement of IgA from the basilar to apical region of epithelial cells suggests that it may be effective in neutralizing intracellular pathogens. Finally, pathogens bound to IgA may be taken up by airway macrophages through the phagocytic process.

IgM

IgM is present only in very low amounts in respiratory secretions from normal subjects.[17] It exists as a pentamer and the resulting very large size (900,000 D) limit transudation into the lung under normal conditions. Nevertheless, IgM in BAL is greater than would be expected for simple diffusion suggesting some local production.[31] Furthermore, in some disorders characterized by lower respiratory tract inflammation IgM can be detected. However, in this setting it is almost certainly largely derived from serum transudation as part of the inflammatory process.

IgE

Under normal conditions the amount of IgE in BAL is lower than IgG, IgA, or IgM.[31] When present the IgE/albumin ratio suggests local production.[31] IgE–antigen complexes bind the high affinity receptor for IgE (FcRI) on mast cells, basophils, and eosinophils leading to immediate hypersensitivity responses.[32,33] IgE is important for host defense against parasites mediated by eosinophils.[34] However, in developed countries the main role of IgE in pulmonary immunity is in the pathogenesis of allergic and asthmatic disease.[35,36] The severity of disease is correlated with serum IgE in asthma and allergic patients. The importance of this molecule in the pathogenesis of asthma has led to the development of anti-IgE antibodies for patients with resistant IgE-mediated disease.[37] Interestingly, when IgE binds to the low affinity FcRII receptor it inhibits IgE synthesis and reduces inflammation.[38] Thus IgE may also have a role in downregulating the immune response.

CELLULAR INTERACTIONS LEADING TO ANTIBODY SECRETING CELLS

A number of important cellular interactions take place that eventuate in antibody secretion by cells.

B1 AND B2 CELLS

B lymphocytes comprise 1% to 10% of the lung lymphocyte population and can be separated into two main classes. Plasma cells constitutively secrete IgG and other immunoglobulin subclasses.[1,11] In contrast, memory B cells produce immunoglobulin only in response to re-exposure to particular antigens.[11] B cells can be further classified into B1 and B2 cells. B1 cells were first described in the gastrointestinal tract. These cells are IgM+, CD5+ cells that do not require T cell help for development.[39] In the lamina propria B1 cells undergo class switching to an IgA secretory cell. B1 cells home to peritoneal and pleural cavities, respond to common bacterial antigens, and are felt to be very important in the production of IgM and IgA against bacterial pathogens at mucosal sites.[40] As such, they are thought to be important in innate immunity against conserved bacterial antigens. Because of their autonomous ability to secrete antibody, they are also felt to contribute to autoimmune diseases. These cells are difficult to demonstrate in normal lung. As stated earlier, T cells are not necessary for B1 cells to produce antibody, though the presence of T cells appears to augment the immune response.[40–44]

In contrast to B1 cells, B2 cells require T cell help, mainly through secretion of the cytokines interleukin IL-4, IL-5, IL-6, and IL-10, as well as ligation between CD40 on B cells and CD40L on T cells.[45] T cell dependent antibody responses begin with uptake of antigen by accessory cells (AC) and presentation to T cells. AC function can be carried out by mononuclear phagocytes (monocytes, macrophages) or dendritic cells. Submucosal dendritic cells are likely the principal accessory cell in the lung.[46] B cells themselves can also serve as the accessory cell leading to T cell activation.[47] B cells in the lung express surface IgG and IgM. Crosslinking of surface IgG or IgM by antigen results in partial activation of B cells leading to expression of IL-2 receptors and MHC class II molecules,[1] which allows them to serve as accessory cells in T cell activation. With appropriate T cell help activated B cells eventually differentiate into short lived antibody producing plasma cells or memory B cells, the latter characterized by the coexpression of CD20 and CD27.[48] Other surface markers indicating B cell activation and differentiation include CD69, CD80, and CD86.[1] The latter two interact with CD28 and CTLA4 on T cells, respectively, thereby enhancing proliferation of helper T cells. Activation results in production of CD38+ CD138+ plasma cells that secrete IgM (primary response) or other immunoglobulin isotypes (secondary immune responses).[49]

■ COGNATE VERSUS NONCOGNATE RESPONSES

Activated T cells can provide cognate and noncognate B cell help. Cognate B cell help is antigen and MHC restricted and occurs after helper T cells have been activated through T cell receptor (TCR)–MHC class II/antigen complex mechanisms. It was initially thought that B cells were the obligate accessory cells for cognate responses since B cell–T cell contact was occurring through MHC class II/antigen complexes on activated B cells and the TCR on T cells. In contrast, when T cells are stimulated by accessory cells other than B cells or activated in an accessory cell independent manner (i.e., with immobilized anti-CD3), T cells can induce immunoglobulin production in many B cells in a non-MHC or antigen (noncognate) restricted manner. This latter phenomenon results in stimulation of both antigen specific as well as "bystander" B cells leading to a polyclonal antibody response. Subsequent work has shown that this bystander response is only important when the T cells providing B cell help are highly activated and/or differentiated, such as after exposure to IL-4 and IL-6.[49] This latter observation may explain the link between increased IL-6 secretion and nonspecific hypergammaglobulinemia in diseases such as HIV infection.[50] Additional work has shown that this bystander effect is mediated through LFA-1 (CD11a/CD18) on B cells and ICAM-1 (CD54) on activated T cells.[51,52]

■ CYTOKINE SECRETION

Resting T cells provide poor B cell help. T cells that have been stimulated by antigen can be loosely divided into Th1 and Th2 cells based on the cytokine profile they secrete.[53] Th1 cells secrete predominantly interferon-γ (IFN-γ) and interleukin (IL)-2 and are involved primarily in cellular immunity. Th2 cells secrete IL-4, IL-5, and IL-10 and drive humoral immunity. Th2 cells that provide B cell help are called "effector" cells. Signals from T cells to B cells are in two forms: direct cell to cell contact and cytokine secretion. While direct B cell–T cell contact is required for induction of antibody production, both Th1 and Th2 cell membranes can provide this signal.[54] What differentiates these two T cell populations is the cytokine profile they secrete. In particular, IL-4 seems to be an early competence factor that increases the number of B cells responsive to T cell help.[54,55] In contrast, IL-6 is a late factor[55] that promotes continued B cell proliferation and immunoglobulin secretion. IFN-γ downregulates most immunoglobulin secretion.[56] Thus Th2 cells secrete a more favorable cytokine pattern for immunoglobulin production. The one exception is IgG2, which is dependent on IFN-γ secretion.[56]

■ SPECIFIC B CELL AND T CELL RECEPTOR INTERACTIONS AND DOWNREGULATION OF B CELL RESPONSES

Tight regulation of antibody production and secretion is necessary to turn off the response when it is no longer needed and to prevent production of unwanted autoantibodies (Fig. 24-3). This control is mediated through a combination of signaling pathways between T cells and B cells. CD40L is an activation-induced molecule on CD4 T cells that delivers signals to B cells through its counterreceptor CD40, which is constitutively expressed on B cells. Highly activated T cells express increased CD40L. CD40 on B cells in turn downregulates CD40L on activated T cells.[57] These cells are subsequently unable to stimulate resting B cells. Thus this may represent an attempt to downregulate noncognate immunoglobulin production. However, CD40 ligation is still critically important for cognate interactions. Crosslinking of surface immunoglobulin on B cells results in apoptosis of the B cell unless simultaneous binding of CD40 by CD40L occurs.[58] Interestingly, CD40 binding alone induces Fas expression on B cells, an effect that is not inhibited even in the presence of B cell tropic factors such as IL-2, IL-4, and IL-10.[59] Thus ligation of CD40 acts to costimulate B cells that have been activated by binding of specific antigen while simultaneously increasing sensitivity to apoptosis in B cells not crosslinked by antigen. This drives an antigen-specific antibody response.[58]

The role of Fas/FasL interactions in modulating immune responses is well established. Activation of T cells upregulates expression of both Fas and FasL. This is seen as a mechanism to control chronic T cell activation.[60] Fas/FasL interactions are also important in modulating B cell responses.[61] As stated earlier, B cells stimulated through CD40 increase expression of Fas. Thus, these cells are susceptible to apoptosis mediated by FasL expressed by activated T cells. B cell apoptosis induced by FasL is blocked if there is simultaneous crosslinking of surface immunoglobulin by antigen, thereby preserving secretion of protective antibody in the presence of persistent pathogen exposure.

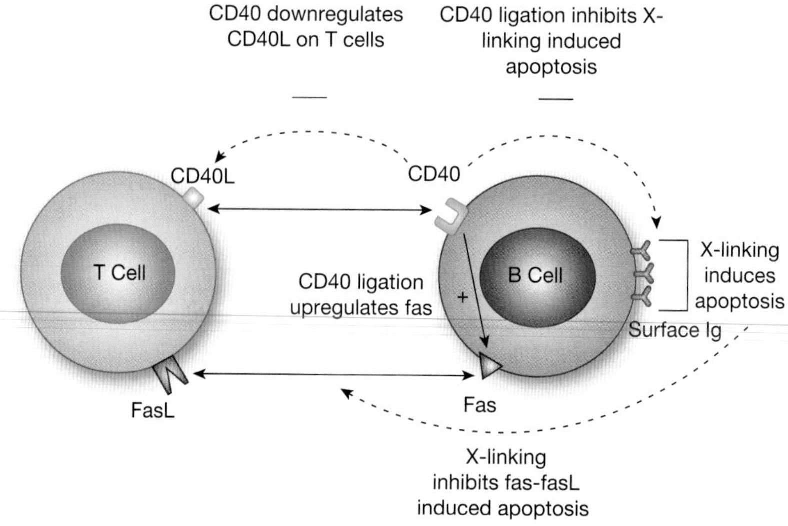

Figure 24-3 Interaction between T cells and B cells during the generation of a humoral response. Multiple signals occur between T cells and B cells. Depending on the presence or absence of crosslinking of surface immunoglobulin on B cells, T cells can either promote B cell growth or induce apoptosis.

PULMONARY ANTIBODY PRODUCTION IN RESPONSE TO ANTIGEN EXPOSURE

Pulmonary immunity to pathogens can be divided into innate and acquired responses. Most pathogens gaining access to the alveolar space are handled by phagocytosis by alveolar macrophages, the principal form of innate immunity. If phagocytosis of pathogens occurs in the absence of opsonizing antibody this usually results in "noninflammatory clearance," with minimal release of inflammatory mediators and preservation of lung structure and function.[62] If phagocytosis is overwhelmed, a specific acquired immune response occurs. This involves the interaction of B and T lymphocytes to produce an antigen-specific cellular and humoral immune response. In the lung, the acquired response has three distinct phases (Fig. 24-4)—afferent antigen processing and transport to regional lymph nodes,[63] presentation to naïve lymphocytes, and efferent migration of activated T lymphocytes and mature B cells back to the site of initial antigen challenge in the lung.[64] This results in the presence of antigen-specific immunoglobulin in the lung lining fluid and consequent increased effectiveness of professional phagocytes such as alveolar macrophages and neutrophils.[65]

This general pathway is similar for IgG and IgA production, though the length of the "circuit" is likely much less for IgA. Rather than having antigen travel to regional lymph nodes, in mucosal immunity IgA can be generated in specialized lymphoid tissue just beneath the mucosal surface, called mucosal-associated lymphoid tissue (MALT), suggesting that IgA secreting plasma cells are produced locally and IgA can readily diffuse back into the airspaces. Such submucosal lymphoid tissue in the upper airway, called nasal-associated lymphoid tissue (NALT), is seen in most animal species, including humans.[66] In contrast, in the lower respiratory tract bronchus-associated lymphoid tissue, or BALT, is readily demonstrable in mice[66] but has been more difficult to find in normal human airways.[67] Prior studies claiming that humans have BALT have generally been in subjects with an inflammatory pulmonary process.[68] Recent investigations may be shedding some light on this controversy, introducing the concept of inducible bronchus-associated lymphoid tissue, or iBALT. In mice lacking secondary lymphoid tissues (spleen, lymph nodes) a robust protective primary pulmonary B and T cell response was demonstrated after influenza infection.[69] This response was associated with induction of B cell follicles centered around follicular dendritic cells in submucosal tissues. Thus collections of antigen presenting cells, B cells, and T cells in the submucosa, which are thought to collectively represent BALT, may only be readily detectable during times of antigenic challenge.

Once antibody producing B cells are formed in secondary lymphoid tissue or MALT, they must traffic back to the original point of entry of the pathogen. This trafficking of lymphocytes back to mucosal sites has been intensely studied, giving rise to a four-step model. The first step is tethering. L-selectin on lymphocytes interacts with addressins on endothelial cells to slow down the movement of lymphocytes through capillaries. In NALT, the responsible endothelial receptor is PNAd[70] while in the lung adhesion is mediated by ICAM-1.[71] Tethering leads to lymphocyte activation mediated by chemokines and their receptors and subsequent firm adhesion to the endothelium. The latter is mediated by LFA-1 binding to ICAM-1 and $\alpha_4\beta_7$ integrin binding to MADCAM-1.[72] Finally, diapedesis through the mucosa occurs, a process that probably involves all the above receptor–counterreceptor interactions.

The end result of this process is the accumulation of antibody secreting plasma cells at the site of initial challenge. Once the invading pathogen has been cleared, plasma cells disappear and are replaced by memory B cells. The great majority of B cells in the normal lung are mature memory B cells. This mirrors the predominance of memory T cells in the lung,[73] suggesting that the lung is primed to respond quickly to antigenic challenges. IgG-, IgM-, and IgA-secreting B cells are present in normal subjects; however, poor correlations exist between the numbers of Ig producing BAL cells and the levels of Ig in BAL fluids.[17,74] In BAL fluid from nonsmokers IgG is present in the same proportion as in serum, leading to speculation that most IgG enters via transudation from the plasma compartments.[17,19] These two observations fit in well with the primary presence of memory B cells in the lung, suggesting that under resting conditions very little local antibody is made. Only after antigenic challenge is local production increased. In support of this is the finding of increased ratios of specific to total antibody in BAL fluid after pneumococcal infection suggesting that local antibody production can be increased after relevant exposures.[75]

DISORDERS OF HUMORAL IMMUNITY AND LUNG DISEASE

Either quantitative or qualitative defects may be associated with disorders of humoral immunity and resultant lung disease. In addition, lung disease has been noted in conjunction with development of autoantibodies. These topics are presented below.

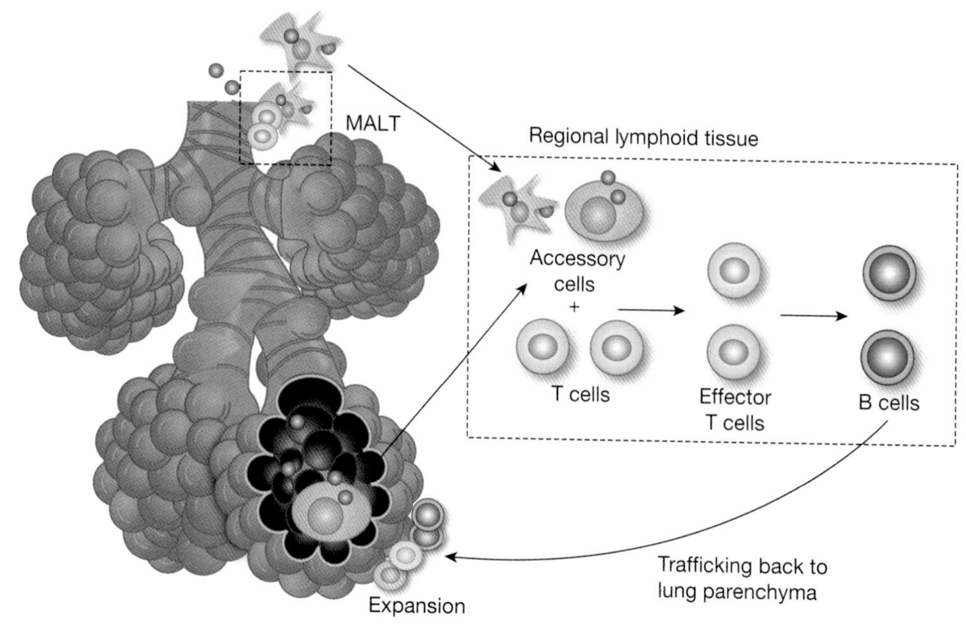

Figure 24-4 Pathway for generation of antigen-specific immune responses in the lung. Foreign antigen is taken up by antigen presenting cells and transported to regional lymph nodes where the primary cellular and humoral immune response is generated. Effector cells then traffic back to the lung to the site of initial antigen challenge. B cells will become antibody secreting plasma cells while others will become memory B cells. This circuit is significantly shorter in the presence of mucosal-associated lymphoid tissue (MALT).

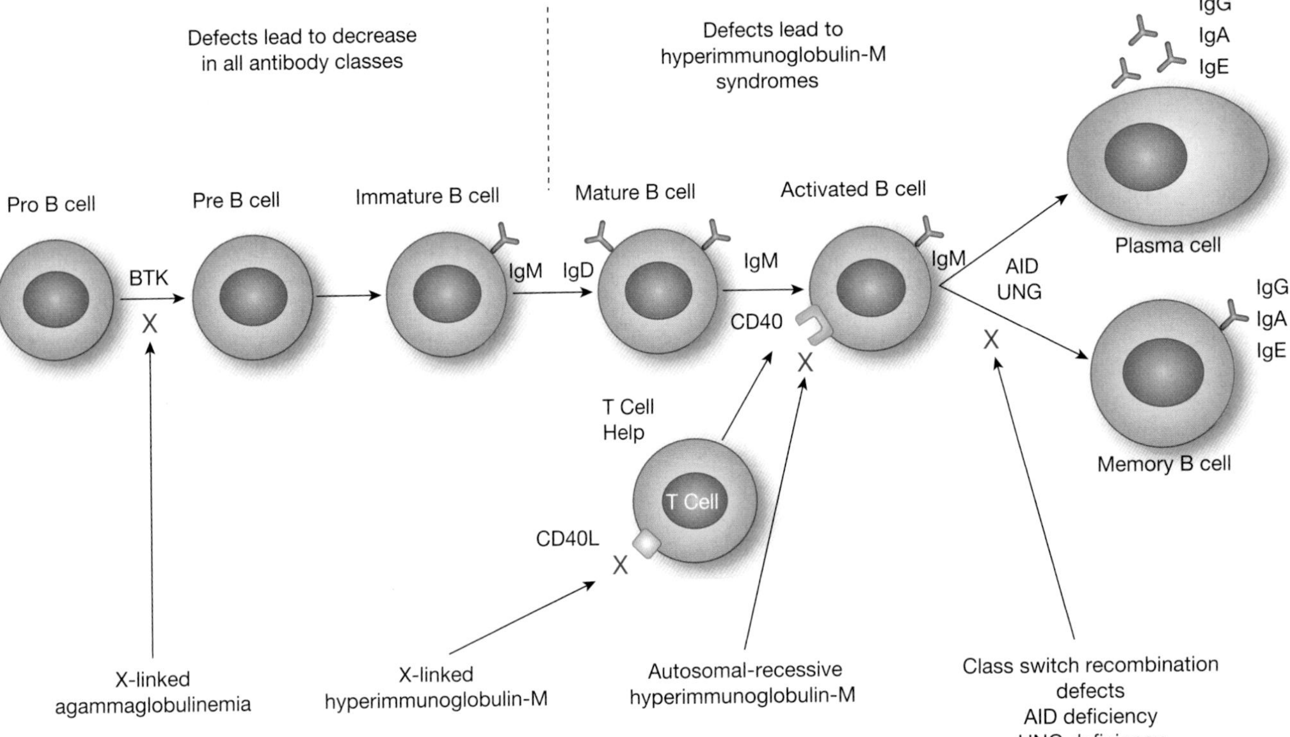

Figure 24-5 Known sites of molecular defects leading to immunoglobulin deficiency. Note defects that occur past the mature B cell stage tend to lead to hyperimmunoglobulin-M syndromes while defects prior to this stage lead to loss of all immunoglobulin classes. BTK, Bruton's tyrosine kinase, AID, activation-induced cytidine deaminase, UNG, uracil-N-glycosylase.

INTRODUCTION

In general, defects in humoral immunity result in an increased susceptibility to bacterial infections, including recurrent sinusitis, bronchitis, pneumonia, otitis media, and even meningitis. In particular, the patients are susceptible to infection with encapsulated organisms such as *Haemophilus influenzae*, *Streptococcus pneumoniae*, *Staphylococcus aureus*, and *Neisseria* species. Chronic diseases such as bronchiectasis and obstructive lung disease can occur as a result of recurrent infection. Antibody defects can be either quantitative (an absolute decrease or loss of antibody) or qualitative (poor antigenic specificity and/or poor opsonic function). In addition, the presence of antibodies against host antigens can lead to autoimmune lung disease. Figure 24-5 shows some of the known molecular defects causing immunoglobulin deficiency. The cause of most of the selective immunoglobulin deficiencies described below is unknown.

QUANTITATIVE DEFECTS

Isolated *IgA deficiency* is the most common primary immunodeficiency in humans, occurring in roughly 1 in 500 individuals.[76] The presence of IgA deficiency is defined by a serum IgA level of less than 5 mg/dL and normal levels of other immunoglobulins. Asthma, IgE-mediated allergic disease, and autoimmune diseases are more common in patients with IgA deficiency.[77] Only about a third of patients with IgA deficiency develop recurrent sinus, pulmonary, and gastrointestinal tract infections, usually with encapsulated bacteria. In the absence of an associated IgG subclass deficiency the development of structural lung disease is rare. These patients almost never require immunoglobulin replacement therapy. However, the coexistence of IgA and IgG subclass deficiency is extremely important to document since the latter may require immunoglobulin infusions. IgA deficient patients are at increased risk for anaphylactic reactions after blood product infusions, including immunoglobulin preparations, because of the presence of IgG anti-IgA antibodies in up to 60% of individuals.[78,79] As such, when the decision is made to give immunoglobulin infusions to an IgG deficient patient with a coexisting low IgA level, immunoglobulin preparations low in IgA must be used.

In contrast to IgA deficiency, patients with *IgG subclass deficiencies* frequently exhibit recurrent sinus and respiratory tract infections with encapsulated organisms regardless of whether it is associated with IgA deficiency.[80] IgG1 deficiency is the most common and it is frequently linked with deficiency of IgG2 and IgG3 as well. Unlike patients with IgA deficiency, the recurrent infections in IgG subclass deficiency can lead to chronic bronchiectasis, and assessment of immunoglobulin deficiency should be part of the standard evaluation of patients with unexplained recurrent infections with destructive lung disease. Patients with IgG2 subclass deficiency have an impaired ability to respond to polysaccharides.[20] As such, their response to the standard polysaccharide pneumococcal vaccine is poor. When IgG subclass deficiency is combined with IgA deficiency the resultant lung disease is more severe than with either deficiency alone.

More severe disease occurs when there are multiple immunoglobulin defects. Perhaps the most common immunodeficiency in this group is *common variable immunodeficiency (CVID)*. Present in 1 in 25,000 individuals, this disease is characterized by hypogammaglobulinemia, decreased antigen-specific antibody responses, and recurrent sinopulmonary infections, frequently leading to chronic lung disease.[81] IgG levels are usually below 300 mg/dL and are accompanied by low IgA and IgM levels as well. Specific antibody responses to common antigens such as tetanus toxoid and pneumococcus are usually very low. Cellular immune defects, primarily lymphopenia with a normal or decreased CD4:CD8 ratio, may also be present. Thus, patients may present with infections typically associated with T cell defects (fungi, mycobacteria) in addition to infections caused by encapsulated bacteria. Proliferation of B cells and T cells in response to strong mitogens is impaired as well. Thus CVID is felt to result from a failure of B cells to terminally differentiate, either due to poor T cell help or an intrinsic B cell defect. The impairment in immunity and immunosurveillance probably contributes to the increased incidence of autoimmune disease, malignancies, and gastrointestinal malabsorption in patients with CVID.[82–84]

Patients with *X-linked agammaglobulinemia (Bruton's agammaglobulinemia)* demonstrate a generalized defect in the ability to make all immunoglobulin classes. This is due to a deficiency of Bruton's tyrosine kinase (BTK), which is essential for early lymphopoiesis.[85] These individuals present in early childhood with recurrent middle ear, sinus, pulmonary, joint, bone, and CNS infections. They almost always develop chronic lung disease, including bronchiectasis, pulmonary fibrosis, and pulmonary hypertension.[86–88] IgG levels are below 200 mg/dL and the other Ig subclasses may be absent. In contrast to patients with CVID, lymphoid tissue is hypoplastic in these patients.

Hyperimmunoglobulin M syndrome refers to several diseases characterized by low concentrations of IgG, IgA, and IgE and a normal or elevated IgM level. As might be expected based on our understanding of normal B cell development, these syndromes result from failure of IgM secreting B cells to undergo class switching. The most common disorder is X-linked hyperimmunoglobulin M syndrome, which arises from a deficiency in the important T cell costimulatory molecule CD40L.[89] Deficiency in the B cell CD40 molecule has also been described, though this is rare.[90] Patients with either of these disorders have severely impaired T cell dependent antibody production. Other hyperimmunoglobulin M disorders are caused by genetic mutations in the enzymes required for class switching, such as AID[91] and uracil nucleoside glycosylase.[92]

Immunoglobulin replacement therapy can prevent recurrent infection and ameliorate some of the long term sequelae of IgG deficiency.[93,94] However, it is important to base treatment decisions on the inability to make specific antibody, not just on an isolated low IgG (or IgG subclass) level. Typically when immunoglobulin deficiency is suspected total IgG, IgA, IgM, and IgG subclass concentrations are checked. A lymphocyte phenotype panel should also be obtained to look for low T and B cell numbers. If low antibody titers are detected, then one should measure common specific antibody titers. Usually tetanus toxoid and pneumococcal antibody titers are assessed because this assesses both the ability to respond to protein (tetanus) and polysaccharide (pneumococcal) antigens. If specific antibody titers are low the patient should be given the tetanus or pneumococcal vaccine and repeat antibody titers obtained 4 weeks later. Failure to increase antibody titers into a "protective" range is indicative of immunoglobulin deficiency and warrants consideration of immunoglobulin replacement therapy. There are several immunoglobulin preparations available. As mentioned earlier, if IgA deficiency is present, a preparation that contains very low IgA should be used to minimize the risk of anaphylaxis.[78] A typical dose of immunoglobulin is 400 mg/kg given once a month, with a goal trough serum immunoglobulin level immediately before the next infusion of 500 mg/dL.

QUALITATIVE DEFECTS

Once antibody is produced in the lung, it must be effective in promoting clearance of the offending pathogen. Just having a vigorous antibody response is insufficient. There are several diseases characterized by poor functioning antibody.

Selective antibody deficiency with normal immunoglobulins (SADNI) was first recognized in the 1980s. The disease is characterized by poor antibody responses to polysaccharide antigens despite normal IgG, IgG subclass, IgM, and IgA concentrations.[95] While many of the primary immunodeficiency diseases described earlier are associated with poor responses to polysaccharide antigens, SADNI should be reserved for patients with only this specific defect. SADNI is one of the most common immunodeficiencies occurring in 5% to 10% of older children and adults presenting with recurrent sinopulmonary infections.[96,97] As with other immunoglobulin deficiencies, these patients also have an increased incidence of atopic disease. Since SADNI is a diagnosis of exclusion, normal IgG, IgG subclass, IgM, and IgA levels must be demonstrated. To demonstrate polysaccharide unresponsiveness, baseline pneumococcal titers are measured and then the 23-valent polysaccharide pneumococcal vaccine is administered.[98] Four weeks later pneumococcal titers are repeated. An appropriate response is indicated by an antibody titer of 1.3 μg/mL or greater in 70% of the serotypes tested.[98] Some patients have an appropriate response to vaccination, but this is followed by a rapid loss of antibody titers over 6 months. These patients fall within the spectrum of patients with SADNI. One of the main reasons for establishing the diagnosis of SADNI versus other immunodeficiencies is the differences in treatment. Patients with SADNI should be administered the 13-valent conjugated pneumococcal vaccine, which is more immunogenic due to the presence of a protein carrier attached to polysaccharide antigens that acts as a hapten.[99] Unlike in more severe humoral immunodeficiencies, immunoglobulin replacement therapy is needed only in a minority of patients with SADNI.

While *HIV infection* is most notably characterized by profound defects in cell-mediated immunity, antibody defects are also present. In fact, the occurrence of two bacterial pneumonias in a year is an AIDS defining illness.[100] HIV infection is characterized by an increased amount of total and pneumococcal-specific antibody in the alveolar space,[75,101] yet invasive pneumococcal disease is prevalent in this population. For example, in HIV-infected Malawians, a population with a high incidence of invasive pneumococcal infection, BAL contains four times the amount of pneumococcal-specific IgG compared to non-HIV-infected subjects. Capsule-specific IgG levels were highest in a group of HIV-infected patients with recent invasive pneumococcal disease, suggesting that despite polyclonal IgG responses in HIV-infected adults, appropriate responses to infection were also present.[75] However, the ability of highly purified BAL IgG from HIV-infected subjects to bind pneumococci is impaired compared to BAL IgG from non-HIV-infected subjects.[102] This parallels the work of other investigators who have demonstrated impaired immunoglobulin opsonic function in HIV-infected subjects, including activity against pneumococcus.[103,104] Thus HIV-infected subjects appear to have dysfunctional pneumococcal antibody in the alveolar space. The reasons for this observation are not known, but could include structural abnormalities in HIV IgG or the lack of a diverse antigenic response (i.e., antibody produced against only a few pneumococcal antigens in HIV-infection compared to a more diverse response in non-HIV-infected subjects).[105] These findings highlight the fact that better correlates are needed for assessing the host response to natural infection or vaccination besides simple measurement of antibody concentrations.[106]

PULMONARY DISEASE ASSOCIATED WITH AUTOANTIBODIES

There are many well-described lung diseases associated with the presence of autoantibodies. Classically these have been described in patients with vasculitic processes such as Goodpasteur's syndrome or granulomatosis with polyangiitis (formerly known as Wegener's granulomatosis), and various connective tissue diseases. A discussion of these disorders is beyond the scope of this chapter. However, a great deal of interest is now turning toward the potential role of autoantibodies in some of the more commonly encountered lung diseases.

Chronic obstructive lung disease (COPD) is increasingly being thought of as an autoimmune disease.[107] Patients with COPD have increased lung titers of autoantibodies against elastin,[108] cytokeratin[109] and against epithelial and endothelial antigens.[110,111] Furthermore, lymphoid follicles consisting of B cells and follicular dendritic cells with adjacent T cells are present in the parenchyma and in bronchial walls of patients with emphysema suggesting that at least some these antibodies may be locally produced.[112] This is further supported by detailed studies demonstrating that the B cells in these aggregates have a limited (oligoclonal) repertoire.[113] That these autoantibodies may be pathogenic is suggested by the presence of immune complex and C3 deposition in the lungs of patients with emphysema.[110] In animal models smoking is able to induce autoantibodies against extracellular matrix proteins in mice,[114] and adoptive transfer of anti-endothelial antibodies can cause emphysema in rats.[115] This discussion would suggest that immunosuppressive medications may be effective in COPD. Indeed, systemic and inhaled corticosteroids result in decreased lymphoid aggregates in the lungs of humans with COPD.[116] Whether reduction in lung B cell immunity is helpful or harmful will depend on whether the B cells are secreting destructive autoantibodies or protective antibodies against microbes that have colonized the airway of these patients.

Another lung disease in which autoantibodies may contribute to pathogenesis is *pulmonary fibrosis*. The current paradigm for the pathogenesis of pulmonary fibrosis starts with lung epithelial and/or microvascular injury leading to an exaggerated inflammatory and fibrotic response. While extensive literature exists on the inflammatory and fibrotic response, much less is known about the inciting event. In pulmonary fibrosis associated with connective tissue disease numerous autoantibodies have been described, including anti-SSA, anti-RNP, and anti-Jo-1.[117–119] Whether similar potential pathogenic roles can be ascribed to autoantibodies in idiopathic pulmonary fibrosis (IPF) is not known. Early on an increase in lung IgG was described in patients with IPF.[120] Up to 30% of patients with IPF have positive antinuclear antibody or rheumatoid factor without other overt signs of autoimmune disease.[121] Anti-phospholipid and anti-endothelial cell antibodies are found in a significant number of patients with IPF.[122] In another study anti-collagen antibodies were found in 81% of patients with IPF.[123] Anti-cytokeratin antibodies are also frequently found in the serum of patients with IPF.[124] Finally, antibodies to heat shock protein 70 identified a group of patients with IPF with a poor prognosis.[125] Thus there is evidence to support a contribution of unchecked humoral immunity in the pathogenesis of fibrotic lung diseases.

Dysregulated humoral immunity also plays a role in lu*ng transplant rejection*. Rejection is associated with upregulation of IgG2 production resulting in an IgG2/IgG1 ratio of greater than 1 in BAL fluid. Since the ratio was normal in serum this strongly argues for local production of IgG2 in the lungs of patients undergoing rejection.[126] In support of this, B cells are a prominent finding in areas of the lung demonstrating obliterative bronchiolitis, the pathologic hallmark of lung rejection,[127] and these cells preferentially produce IgG2.[128] Subsequent work in animal models[129] and humans[130,131] has shown that the major antigens driving this response are collagen V and k-α tubulin. In fact, the presence of circulating anti-collagen V antibody predicts primary graft dysfunction after transplant.[129] That these antibodies may have a pathogenic role in lung transplant rejection is further supported by observations that rituximab or intravenous immunoglobulin therapy reduces the concentration of the autoantibody and reduces the severity of bronchiolitis obliterans syndrome.[130] The current paradigm for lung transplant rejection holds that ischemic injury during the transplant process "uncovers" normally hidden collagen V epitopes that elicit an autoimmune response.[132] This is strongly supported by recent work showing increased collagen V expression in obliterative bronchiolitis lesions and the presence of collagen V antibodies in the lungs of patients who had lung transplant rejection.[133]

PULMONARY ANTIBODY RESPONSES TO VACCINATION

The pulmonary antibody response to vaccination against common pathogens is an important consideration in disease prevention and is discussed below.

■ SYSTEMIC VERSUS MUCOSAL VACCINATION

Vaccination against pulmonary pathogens is a common and effective practice against many diseases. However, the mechanisms behind their effectiveness are not always clear. In theory, both IgA and IgG have a role in protection after vaccination. The presence of pathogen-specific IgA should decrease colonization of the respiratory tract by limiting attachment to respiratory epithelium. Since airway colonization is usually the first step in the development of bacterial pneumonia, decreased colonization should lead to a decreased incidence of pneumonia. When pathogens manage to reach the alveolar space, IgG should take on a greater role as an opsonin in the phagocytosis of organisms. Thus the most effective immunity against bacterial infections should involve both an IgG and IgA response. That being said, the vaccine delivery mechanism impacts the type of immune response generated. In general, systemic administration of a protein antigen results in the generation of circulating IgG, some of which will diffuse into the epithelial lining fluid. In contrast, mucosal antigenic challenge results in a more vigorous IgA response locally at the site of challenge.

Despite the recognition that local antibody may be important in pulmonary host defense, there is little information on humoral responses in the respiratory tract after systemic immunization, the standard approach to vaccine strategies. Much of what we know about mucosal immunity comes from animal models. In a mouse model of mucosal immunity against *Mycoplasma pulmonis*, it has been demonstrated that the site of antigen deposition greatly influences the antibody response and subsequent protective immunity.[134] Intranasal challenge resulted in an increase in IgA antibody forming cells in the nasal submucosa and an increase in mycoplasma-specific IgA in nasal washes. Low numbers of IgA antibody forming cells and IgA concentrations were seen in the lung after isolated nasal challenge, but were increased significantly if animals received both nasal and pulmonary immunization. Both nasal and nasal-pulmonary vaccine exposures resulted in equivalent antigen-specific IgA and IgG in the systemic circulation. Both forms of immunization also significantly reduced the ability of mycoplasma to colonize the nasal passages after experimental exposure to a mycoplasma inoculum. However, animals receiving nasal-pulmonary immunization had significantly fewer organisms in the lungs compared to animals that only received nasal immunization. Since serum mycoplasma-specific IgA and IgG were similar after both types of immunization, this suggests that circulating antibody is less effective in protection against pulmonary pathogens compared to locally produced antibody.

In another animal immunization model against a different pulmonary pathogen, *Moraxella catarrhalis*, the site of specific antibody production and protection after intranasal and subcutaneous challenge was examined.[135] Intranasal administration of *M. catarrhalis* surface proteins resulted in antigen-specific IgA and IgG in both nasal washes and BAL. IgA concentrations far exceeded IgG concentrations in both sites. IgA was significantly higher in BAL and nasal washes than in serum, whereas IgG was higher in serum than both mucosal sites. Immunization was associated with a marked increase in bacterial clearance after intranasal challenge with live *M. catarrhalis* organisms. As might be predicted, subcutaneous administration of the same vaccine resulted in production of far greater antigen-specific IgG compared to IgA, especially in the lung, where moraxella-specific IgG in BAL was nearly 20 times greater than that found in nasal washes. Subcutaneous vaccination induced a marked systemic IgG response, but virtually no antigen-specific IgA in serum, BAL, or nasal washes. Interestingly, despite the brisk systemic and pulmonary IgG response after subcutaneous immunization, intranasal immunization promoted significantly greater bacterial clearance after intranasal challenge with the organisms. These data further support the general premise that while systemic vaccination results in system antigen-specific IgG that may passively diffuse into the epithelial lining fluid in the lung, significant protection will only be afforded if local IgA immune responses are also induced.

The effect of the intranasal and intramuscular polysaccharide pneumococcal vaccine has also been studied in a mouse model.[136] Intranasal vaccination, when accompanied by IL-12 administration (which increases IF-γ production), resulted in increased serum IgG2a anti-pneumococcal antibody, consistent with the known stimulatory effect of IF-γ on IgG2a production.[56] This regimen also resulted in increased pneumococcal-specific IgA in BAL fluid. The serum antibody response was functional in opsonophagocytosis assays. Interestingly, intramuscular vaccination afforded more protection against subsequent intraperitoneal pneumococcal challenge compared to intranasal vaccination. In contrast, intranasal vaccination was more effective in reducing nasopharyngeal colonization after nasal challenge of the organism compared to intramuscular vaccination, despite the higher serum IgG response after the latter. Finally, using IgA knockout mice, these investigators demonstrated that IgA was responsible for reducing pneumococcal colonization after vaccination and intranasal challenge.[136] These results again highlight the general principal that systemic immunization is more effective in providing protection against systemic challenges, while mucosal immunization is more protective against mucosal challenges.

There are significantly fewer studies on the pulmonary response to vaccines in humans. One study compared oral and nasal administration of a cholera toxin B subunit vaccine.[137] Nasal immunization resulted in a fivefold increase in the levels of specific IgA antibodies in BAL fluid. No significant specific IgA responses were seen after oral immunization. Specific IgG antibody concentrations increased eightfold in BAL fluid in the nasally vaccinated subjects, though this was felt to be from transudation from serum rather than local production. Several studies have examined systemic and salivary pneumococcal-specific antibody titers after systemic vaccination in children. Infants given the 7-valent conjugated pneumococcal vaccine at 2, 4, 6, and 15 months had significant plasma IgG responses at 7 months.[138] However, salivary pneumococcal-specific IgG and IgA concentrations were minimal at this time and did not appear till a booster vaccine was given at 15 months. Further studies suggested the salivary IgG was derived from serum while the salivary IgA was locally produced. This same group demonstrated that by age 4 to 5 years, anti-pneumococcal IgA, especially IgA1, was still present in saliva.[139] Interestingly, there was no difference in pneumococcal-specific antibody titers between vaccinated and unvaccinated children at age 4 to 5 years, suggesting that natural environmental exposure also resulted in mucosal immunity. Finally, immunization with the pneumococcal polysaccharide vaccine has been shown to lead to an increase in salivary pneumococcal-specific IgG and IgA in adults as well.[140] In other studies, despite the lack of immunologic correlation, systemic pneumococcal vaccination appears to decrease the incidence of nasopharyngeal carriage of vaccine-specific serotypes.[141]

In total, these studies suggest that in general systemic vaccination induces primarily an IgG response whereas mucosal vaccination induces primarily an IgA response (Fig. 24-6). While it is clear that systemic immunization can result in some local lung IgA production, the strongest mucosal immunity is induced when antigen is introduced directly into the respiratory tract. Intranasal and inhaled vaccines offer advantages in addition to the potential for improved local immunity, including the ability to immunize large populations at less cost.[142] In safety trials of intranasal vaccination against influenza using a virosome formulated inactivated virus the vaccine was associated with high serum concentrations of influenza-specific IgG and the presence of specific IgA in nasal lavage fluid.[143] Similarly, an inhaled measles vaccine has been shown to be immunogenic (as determined by serum measurement of measles-specific IgG) in a large children population.[144]

■ VACCINATION AGAINST PNEUMOCOCCAL DISEASE

There are currently two active vaccines against pneumococcal disease: the 23-valent pneumococcal polysaccharide vaccine (23-PPV) and the 13-valent pneumococcal conjugate vaccine. Because the conjugated vaccine contains protein linked to various polysaccharides, it is theoretically more immunogenic by virtue of its ability to induce T cell help for antibody secretion. The 23-PPV comprises capsular polysaccharide from 23 of the 90 serotypes of *S. pneumoniae*. Cross-reactivity between serogroups and the epidemiology of disease[145,146] suggest that if adequately immunogenic, this vaccine

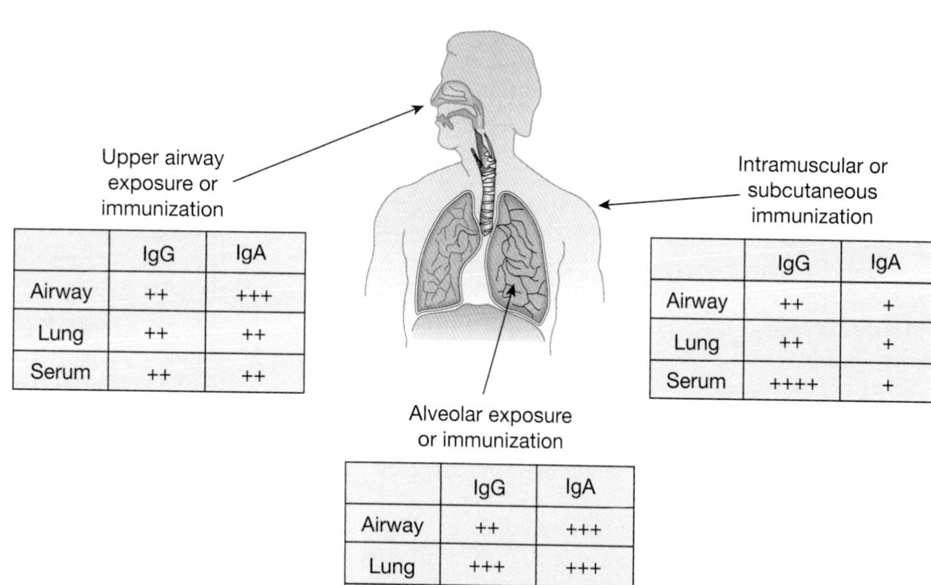

Upper airway exposure or immunization

	IgG	IgA
Airway	++	+++
Lung	++	++
Serum	++	++

Intramuscular or subcutaneous immunization

	IgG	IgA
Airway	++	+
Lung	++	+
Serum	++++	+

Alveolar exposure or immunization

	IgG	IgA
Airway	++	+++
Lung	+++	+++
Serum	+++	++

Figure 24-6 Summary of IgG and IgA concentrations at various sites after upper airway, lower airway, or systemic exposure to bacteria, either as a pathogen or in a vaccine.

should be effective against more than 90% of disease episodes worldwide.[147]

In humans the pneumococcal vaccine is clearly effective in reducing the morbidity and mortality of invasive pneumococcal disease.[148,149] However, studies describing the effect of vaccination on respiratory tract antibody concentrations are lacking. Most studies assessing the immune response to the pneumococcal vaccine focus on serum and salivary antibody titers. Only a few studies have tried to analyse the pulmonary response after vaccination. One study found no difference in the opsonic function of BAL IgG against pneumococcus 1 and 6 months after systemic immunization with the conjugate pneumococcal vaccine.[150] In another study the effect of intramuscular administration of the 23-valent vaccine was compared to inhalation of the same preparation.[151] BAL was performed one month after vaccination. Intramuscular administration resulted in significant increases in serum and BAL pneumococcal-specific IgG titers. Pneumococcal-specific IgA1 titers increased in serum, but not in BAL. This observation supports the concept that mucosal exposure is needed to get a local IgA response. However, no change was seen in any serum or BAL measurement in subjects who inhaled the vaccine. This contrasts with two other studies that found a mild systemic IgG response to inhaled pneumococcal vaccine.[152,153] Lung specific measurements were not assessed in these latter two studies. Thus the conclusion from currently available data suggests effective immunization against pneumococcus still requires systemic (intramuscular) immunization.

VACCINATION AGAINST INFLUENZA

Like the pneumococcal vaccine, vaccination against influenza is highly effective in preventing morbidity and mortality.[154,155] There are two currently available routes for influenza vaccination in humans. The more commonly administered trivalent vaccine consists of neuraminidase and hemagglutinin antigens from three viral strains and is usually given as an intramuscular injection. A second formulation consists of a live attenuated influenza vaccine and is given intranasally. Because it is a live vaccine it is not given to individuals with underdeveloped or impaired immunity. Thus candidates for the nasal vaccine are individuals between the age of 2 and 49 and no existing potentially immunosuppressive condition, including pregnancy.[156]

Because there are systemic and mucosal vaccination options for influenza, more is known about the pulmonary immune response to these vaccines.[157] In one study comparison of inactivated intramuscular and live intranasal influenza vaccines in young children undergoing primary immunization demonstrated that the intranasal preparation induced longer lasting protective antibody concentrations.[158] Nasal secretory IgA developed almost exclusively in nasally vaccinated individuals, whereas nasal IgG was detected in both nasal and intramuscular vaccine recipients. In general, studies show that the trivalent vaccine administered systemically induces a strong IgG response but minimal mucosal influenza-specific IgA. In contrast, the nasal live attenuated vaccine gives a stronger mucosal IgA response. Furthermore, because it results in low level infection, intranasal formulation also induces a specific cellular (cytotoxic T cell) response. Despite these differences, both appear to have similar efficacy in reducing morbidity and mortality from influenza.

Newer vaccine strategies are being developed to enhance population vaccination strategies and improve immunogenicity in individuals with poor antibody responses. In a controlled clinical trial, high dose trivalent influenza vaccination was more immunogenic than standard dose vaccination in subjects over 65, a population known to have a poorer vaccine response.[159] Adjuvants are also being developed to augment the immune response. In humans, using the adjuvant MF59 improves the immune response to the trivalent vaccine.[160] Another innovative approach is to target more conserved influenza antigens, which would obviate the need for yearly vaccination.[161,162] However, many conserved epitopes are poorly immunogenic, indicating that novel delivery methods will be necessary to elicit broad immune responses. In an animal study nucleocapsid and matrix proteins, which are not immunogenic, were able to induce protective antibody responses when administered with nanoparticles coated with papaya mosaic virus as an adjuvant.[163] Very recent animal models are exploring the use of adenovirus vectors to immunize with conserved influenza vaccines.[164] Thus recent advances in vaccine strategies offer hope that newer influenza vaccines will generate broader antigenic coverage, induce both humoral and cellular immunity, and provide longer lasting and better protection against this worldwide pathogen.

CONCLUSION

The humoral immune response is essential for host defense against bacteria. After exposure to potential pathogens, antibody responses in the respiratory tract can occur either quickly through activation of resident memory B cells if there has been prior bacterial exposure, or more slowly through the induction of both systemic and local mucosal immunity if the host is naïve to the organism. The resulting production of antigen-specific IgG and IgA act in concert to help clear the invading pathogen and reduce subsequent colonization of respiratory epithelium. The type and concentration of antibody produced is dependent on the site of exposure. Upper airway exposure results in primarily an IgA response. Organisms that reach the lung after passing through the upper airway induce a more systemic response, including increased production of pathogen-specific IgG. The importance of an effective pulmonary antibody response is highlighted by the significant morbidity associated with diseases characterized by deficient or defective antibody production. Increasing evidence is also pointing toward a key role of autoantibodies in many common lung diseases. Finally, vaccination against respiratory pathogens is dependent on an intact humoral immune system. Systemic vaccination against respiratory pathogens, while effective in generating systemic IgG responses and some mucosal IgA responses, may be less effective than vaccination through mucosal surfaces, which induce a brisk IgA and IgG response both locally and systemically depending on the site of vaccine deposition. Future studies should provide further insight on the pulmonary humoral host response to bacterial challenge and optimal vaccine regimens to minimize the burden of respiratory disease caused by pathogenic bacteria.

REFERENCES

1. Banchereau J, Rousset F. Human B lymphocytes: phenotype, proliferation, and differentiation. *Adv Immunol.* 1992;52:125–262.
2. Muegge K, Vila MP, Durum SK. Interleukin-7: a cofactor for V(D)J rearrangement of the T cell receptor beta gene. *Science.* 1993;261(5117):93–95.
3. Kent D, Copley M, Benz C, Dykstra B, Bowie M, Eaves C. Regulation of hematopoietic stem cells by the steel factor/KIT signaling pathway. *Clin Cancer Res.* 2008;14(7):1926–1930.
4. Paul SR, Bennett F, Calvetti JA, et al. Molecular cloning of a cDNA encoding interleukin 11, a stromal cell-derived lymphopoietic and hematopoietic cytokine. *Proc Natl Acad Sci U S A.* 1990;87(19):7512–7516.
5. Liberg D, Sigvardsson M. Transcriptional regulation in B cell differentiation. *Crit Rev Immunol.* 1999;19(2):127–153.
6. Uckun FM. Regulation of human B-cell ontogeny. *Blood.* 1990; 76(10):1908–1923.
7. Leget GA, Czuczman MS. Use of rituximab, the new FDA-approved antibody. *Curr Opin Oncol.* 1998;10(6):548–551.

8. Gurcan HM, Keskin DB, Stern JN, Nitzberg MA, Shekhani H, Ahmed AR. A review of the current use of rituximab in autoimmune diseases. *Int Immunopharmacol.* 2009;9(1):10–25.

9. LeBien TW, Tedder TF. B lymphocytes: how they develop and function. *Blood.* 2008;112(5):1570–1580.

10. Melchers F. The pre-B-cell receptor: selector of fitting immunoglobulin heavy chains for the B-cell repertoire. *Nat Rev Immunol.* 2005;5(7):578–584.

11. Tsiagbe VK, Linton PJ, Thorbecke GJ. The path of memory B-cell development. *Immunol Rev.* 1992;126:113–141.

12. Alt FW, Blackwell TK, Yancopoulos GD. Development of the primary antibody repertoire. *Science.* 1987;238(4830):1079–1087.

13. Market E, Papavasiliou FN. V(D)J recombination and the evolution of the adaptive immune system. *PLoS Bio.* 2003;1(1):E16.

14. Fried AJ, Bonilla FA. Pathogenesis, diagnosis, and management of primary antibody deficiencies and infections. *Clin Microbiol Rev.* 2009;22(3):396–414.

15. Diaz M, Casali P. Somatic immunoglobulin hypermutation. *Curr Opin Immunol.* 2002;14(2):235–240.

16. Notarangelo LD, Lanzi G, Peron S, Durandy A. Defects of class-switch recombination. *J Allergy Clin Immunol.* 2006;117(4):855–864.

17. The BAL Cooperative Group. Proteins in bronchoalveolar lavage fluid. *Am Rev Respir Dis.* 1990;141:S183–S188.

18. Merrill WW, Naegel GP, Olchowski JJ, Reynolds HY. Immunoglobulin G subclass proteins in serum and lavage fluid of normal subjects. Quantitation and comparison with immunoglobulins A and E. *Am Rev Respir Dis.* 1985;131(4):584–587.

19. Reynolds HY, Merrill WW. Airway changes in young smokers that may antedate chronic obstructive lung disease. *Med Clin North Am.* 1981;65(3):667–689.

20. Siber GR, Schur PH, Aisenberg AC, Weitzman SA, Schiffman G. Correlation between serum IgG-2 concentrations and the antibody response to bacterial polysaccharide antigens. *N Engl J Med.* 1980;303(4):178–182.

21. Stevens R, Dichek D, Keld B, Heiner D. IgG1 is the predominant subclass of in vivo- and in vitro- produced anti-tetanus toxoid antibodies and also serves as the membrane IgG molecule for delivering inhibitory signals to anti-tetanus toxoid antibody-producing B cells. *J Clin Immunol.* 1983;3(1):65–69.

22. Brooks WS, Lee YY, Abell E, Deng JS. Comparison of IgG subclasses and complement binding activity of autoantibodies from patients with bullous pemphigoid and pemphigus. *J Clin Lab Anal.* 1989;3(5):307–311.

23. Bruhns P, Iannascoli B, England P, et al. Specificity and affinity of human Fcgamma receptors and their polymorphic variants for human IgG subclasses. *Blood.* 2009;113(16):3716–3725.

24. Zhang J, Tachado SD, Patel N, et al. Negative regulatory role of mannose receptors on human alveolar macrophage proinflammatory cytokine release in vitro. *J Leukoc Biol.* 2005;78(3):665–674.

25. Canetti C, Hu B, Curtis JL, Peters-Golden M. Syk activation is a leukotriene B4-regulated event involved in macrophage phagocytosis of IgG-coated targets but not apoptotic cells. *Blood.* 2003;102(5):1877–1883.

26. Reynolds HY, Fulmer JD, Kazmierowski JA, Roberts WC, Frank MM, Crystal RG. Analysis of cellular and protein content of bronchoalveolar lavage fluid from patients with idiopathic pulmonary fibrosis and chronic hypersensitivity pneumonitis. *J Clin Invest.* 1977;59(1):165–175.

27. Pilette C, Ouadrhiri Y, Godding V, Vaerman JP, Sibille Y. Lung mucosal immunity: immunoglobulin-A revisited. *Eur Respir J.* 2001;18(3):571–588.

28. Colacicco G, Ray AK, Hendrickson HR, Buckelew AR Jr, Scarpelli EM. Isolation of secretory IgA from a lung surfactant fraction. *Prep Biochem.* 1976;6(6):443–477.

29. Merrill WW, Goodenberger D, Strober W, Matthay RA, Naegel GP, Reynolds HY. Free secretory component and other proteins in human lung lavage. *Am Rev Respir Dis.* 1980;122(1):156–161.

30. Mazanec MB, Nedrud JG, Kaetzel CS, Lamm ME. A three-tiered view of the role of IgA in mucosal defense. *Immunol Today.* 1993;14(9):430–435.

31. Burnett D. Immunoglobulins in the lung. *Thorax.* 1986;41(5):337–344.

32. Sutton BJ, Gould HJ. The human IgE network. *Nature.* 1993;366(6454):421–428.

33. Dombrowicz D, Lin S, Flamand V, Brini AT, Koller BH, Kinet JP. Allergy-associated FcRbeta is a molecular amplifier of IgE- and IgG-mediated in vivo responses. *Immunity.* 1998; 8(4):517–529.

34. Erb KJ. Helminths, allergic disorders and IgE-mediated immune responses: where do we stand? *Eur J Immunol.* 2007;37(5):1170–1173.

35. Sherrill DL, Lebowitz MD, Halonen M, Barbee RA, Burrows B. Longitudinal evaluation of the association between pulmonary function and total serum IgE. *Am J Respir Crit Care Med.* 1995;152(1):98–102.

36. Ericsson CH, Svartengren M, Mossberg B, Camner P. Bronchial reactivity, lung function, and serum immunoglobulin E in smoking-discordant monozygotic twins. *Am Rev Respir Dis.* 1993;147(2):296–300.

37. Busse W, Corren J, Lanier BQ, et al. Omalizumab, anti-IgE recombinant humanized monoclonal antibody, for the treatment of severe allergic asthma. *J Allergy Clin Immunol.* 2001;108(2):184–190.

38. Bettler B, Hofstetter H, Rao M, Yokoyama WM, Kilchherr F, Conrad DH. Molecular structure and expression of the murine lymphocyte low-affinity receptor for IgE (Fc epsilon RII). *Proc Natl Acad Sci U S A.* 1989;86(19):7566–7570.

39. Bao S, Beagley KW, Murray AM, et al. Intestinal IgA plasma cells of the B1 lineage are IL-5 dependent. *Immunology.* 1998;94(2):181–188.

40. Fagarasan S, Honjo T. T-Independent immune response: new aspects of B cell biology. *Science.* 2000;290(5489):89–92.

41. Bluestone JA, Abbas AK. Natural versus adaptive regulatory T cells. *Nat Rev Immunol.* 2003;3(3):253–257.

42. Bondada S, Wu H, Robertson DA, Chelvarajan RL. Accessory cell defect in unresponsiveness of neonates and aged to polysaccharide vaccines. *Vaccine.* 2000;19(4–5):557–565.

43. Buchanan RM, Arulanandam BP, Metzger DW. IL-12 enhances antibody responses to T-independent polysaccharide vaccines in the absence of T and NK cells. *J Immunol.* 1998;161(10):5525–5533.

44. Dullforce P, Sutton DC, Heath AW. Enhancement of T cell-independent immune responses in vivo by CD40 antibodies. *Nat Med.* 1998;4(1):88–91.

45. Defrance T, Vanbervliet B, Briere F, Durand I, Rousset F, Banchereau J. Interleukin 10 and transforming growth factor beta cooperate to induce anti-CD40-activated naive human

B cells to secrete immunoglobulin A. *J Exp Med.* 1992;175(3): 671–682.

46. Constant SL, Brogdon JL, Piggott DA, et al. Resident lung antigen-presenting cells have the capacity to promote Th2 T cell differentiation in situ. *J Clin Invest.* 2002;110(10):1441–1448.
47. Lindell DM, Berlin AA, Schaller MA, Lukacs NW. B cell antigen presentation promotes Th2 responses and immunopathology during chronic allergic lung disease. *PloS One.* 2008;3(9): e3129.
48. Tangye SG, Liu YJ, Aversa G, Phillips JH, de Vries JE. Identification of functional human splenic memory B cells by expression of CD148 and CD27. *J Exp Med.* 1998;188(9): 1691–1703.
49. Croft M, Swain SL. Analysis of CD4+ T cells that provide contact-dependent bystander help to B cells. *J Immunol.* 1992;149(10): 3157–3165.
50. Rautonen J, Rautonen N, Martin NL, Philip R, Wara DW. Serum interleukin-6 concentrations are elevated and associated with elevated tumor necrosis factor-alpha and immunoglobulin G and A concentrations in children with HIV infection. *AIDS.* 1991;5(11):1319–1325.
51. Tohma S, Hirohata S, Lipsky PE. The role of CD11a/CD18-CD54 interactions in human T cell-dependent B cell activation. *J Immunol.* 1991;146(2):492–499.
52. Tohma S, Lipsky PE. Analysis of the mechanisms of T cell-dependent polyclonal activation of human B cells. Induction of human B cell responses by fixed activated T cells. *J Immunol.* 1991;146(8):2544–2552.
53. Street NE, Mosmann TR. Functional diversity of T lymphocytes due to secretion of different cytokine patterns. *Faseb J.* 1991;5(2): 171–177.
54. Noelle RJ, Daum J, Bartlett WC, McCann J, Shepherd DM. Cognate interactions between helper T cells and B cells. V. Reconstitution of T helper cell function using purified plasma membranes from activated Th1 and Th2 T helper cells and lymphokines. *J Immunol.* 1991;146(4):1118–1124.
55. Croft M, Swain SL. B cell response to fresh and effector T helper cells. Role of cognate T-B interaction and the cytokines IL-2, IL-4, and IL-6. *J Immunol.* 1991;146(12):4055–4064.
56. Croft M, Swain SL. B cell response to T helper cell subsets. II. Both the stage of T cell differentiation and the cytokines secreted determine the extent and nature of helper activity. *J Immunol.* 1991;147(11):3679–3689.
57. Yellin MJ, Sippel K, Inghirami G, et al. CD40 molecules induce down-modulation and endocytosis of T cell surface T cell-B cell activating molecule/CD40-L. Potential role in regulating helper effector function. *J Immunol.* 1994;152(2):598–608.
58. Kehry MR. CD40-mediated signaling in B cells. Balancing cell survival, growth, and death. *J Immunol.* 1996;156(7):2345–2348.
59. Garrone P, Neidhardt EM, Garcia E, Galibert L, van Kooten C, Banchereau J. Fas ligation induces apoptosis of CD40-activated human B lymphocytes. *J Exp Med.* 1995;182(5):1265–1273.
60. Kovacs B, Tsokos GC. Cross-linking of the Fas/APO-1 antigen suppresses the CD3-mediated signal transduction events in human T lymphocytes. *J Immunol.* 1995;155(12):5543–5549.
61. Scott DW, Grdina T, Shi Y. T cells commit suicide, but B cells are murdered! *J Immunol.* 1996;156(7):2352–2356.
62. Rubins JB. Alveolar macrophages: wielding the double-edged sword of inflammation. *Am J Respir Crit Care Med.* 2003;167(2): 103–104.
63. Xia W, Pinto CE, Kradin RL. The antigen-presenting activities of Ia+ dendritic cells shift dynamically from lung to lymph node after an airway challenge with soluble antigen. *J Exp Med.* 1995;181(4):1275–1283.
64. Holt PG. Antigen presentation in the lung. *Am J Respir Crit Care Med.* 2000;162(4 Pt 2):S151–S156.
65. Gordon SB, Irving GR, Lawson RA, Lee ME, Read RC. Intracellular trafficking and killing of Streptococcus pneumoniae by human alveolar macrophages are influenced by opsonins. *Infect Immun.* 2000;68(4):2286–2293.
66. McKenzie BS, Brady JL, Lew AM. Mucosal immunity: overcoming the barrier for induction of proximal responses. *Immunol Res.* 2004;30(1):35–71.
67. Pabst R. Is BALT a major component of the human lung immune system? *Immunol Today.* 1992;13(4):119–122.
68. Tschernig T, Pabst R. Bronchus-associated lymphoid tissue (BALT) is not present in the normal adult lung but in different diseases. *Pathobiology.* 2000;68(1):1–8.
69. Moyron-Quiroz JE, Rangel-Moreno J, Kusser K, et al. Role of inducible bronchus associated lymphoid tissue (iBALT) in respiratory immunity. *Nature Medicine.* 2004;10(9):927–934.
70. Csencsits KL, Jutila MA, Pascual DW. Mucosal addressin expression and binding-interactions with naive lymphocytes vary among the cranial, oral, and nasal-associated lymphoid tissues. *Eur J Immunol.* 2002;32(11):3029–3039.
71. Tang ML, Fiscus LC. Important roles for L-selectin and ICAM-1 in the development of allergic airway inflammation in asthma. *Pulm Pharmacol Ther.* 2001;14(3):203–210.
72. Berlin C, Berg EL, Briskin MJ, et al. Alpha 4 beta 7 integrin mediates lymphocyte binding to the mucosal vascular addressin MAdCAM-1. *Cell.* 1993;74(1):185–195.
73. Saltini C, Kirby M, Trapnell BC, Tamura N, Crystal RG. Biased accumulation of T lymphocytes with "memory"-type CD45 leukocyte common antigen gene expression on the epithelial surface of the human lung. *J Exp Med.* 1990;171(4): 1123–1140.
74. Lawrence EC, Blaese RM, Martin RR, Stevens PM. Immunoglobulin secreting cells in normal human bronchial lavage fluids. *J Clin Invest.* 1978;62(4):832–835.
75. Gordon SB, Miller DE, Day RB, et al. Pulmonary immunoglobulin responses to Streptococcus pneumoniae are altered but not reduced in human immunodeficiency virus-infected Malawian adults. *J Infect Dis.* 2003;188(5):666–670.
76. Rosen FS, Cooper MD, Wedgwood RJ. The primary immunodeficiencies (1). *N Engl J Med.* 1984;311(4):235–242.
77. Aytekin C, Tuygun N, Gokce S, Dogu F, Ikinciogullari A. Selective IgA deficiency: clinical and laboratory features of 118 children in Turkey. *J Clin Immunol.* 2012;32(5):961–966.
78. Bjorkander J, Hammarstrom L, Smith CI, Buckley RH, Cunningham-Rundles C, Hanson LA. Immunoglobulin prophylaxis in patients with antibody deficiency syndromes and anti-IgA antibodies. *J Clin Immunol.* 1987;7(1):8–15.
79. Ferreira A, Garcia Rodriguez MC, Lopez-Trascasa M, Pascual Salcedo D, Fontan G. Anti-IgA antibodies in selective IgA deficiency and in primary immunodeficient patients treated with gamma-globulin. *Clin Immunol Immunopathol.* 1988; 47(2): 199–207.
80. Umetsu DT, Ambrosino DM, Quinti I, Siber GR, Geha RS. Recurrent sinopulmonary infection and impaired antibody response to bacterial capsular polysaccharide antigen in

children with selective IgG-subclass deficiency. *N Engl J Med.* 1985;313(20):1247–1251.

81. Watts WJ, Watts MB, Dai W, Cassidy JT, Grum CM, Weg JG. Respiratory dysfunction in patients with common variable hypogammaglobulinemia. *Am Rev Respir Dis.* 1986; 134(4): 699–703.

82. Cunningham-Rundles C, Bodian C. Common variable immunodeficiency: clinical and immunological features of 248 patients. *Clin Immunology.* 1999;92(1):34–48.

83. Quinti I, Soresina A, Spadaro G, et al. Long-term follow-up and outcome of a large cohort of patients with common variable immunodeficiency. *J Clin Immunol.* 2007;27(3):308–316.

84. Mellemkjaer L, Hammarstrom L, Andersen V, et al. Cancer risk among patients with IgA deficiency or common variable immunodeficiency and their relatives: a combined Danish and Swedish study. *Clin Exp Immunol.* 2002;130(3):495–500.

85. Conley ME. Molecular basis of immunodeficiency. *Immunol Rev.* 2005;203:5–9.

86. Lederman HM, Winkelstein JA. X-linked agammaglobulinemia: an analysis of 96 patients. *Medicine (Baltimore).* 1985;64(3):145–156.

87. Bruton OC. Agammaglobulinemia. *Pediatrics.* 1952;9(6):722–728.

88. Chun JK, Lee TJ, Song JW, Linton JA, Kim DS. Analysis of clinical presentations of Bruton disease: a review of 20 years of accumulated data from pediatric patients at Severance Hospital. *Yonsei Med J.* 2008;49(1):28–36.

89. Winkelstein JA, Marino MC, Ochs H, et al. The X-linked hyper-IgM syndrome: clinical and immunologic features of 79 patients. *Medicine (Baltimore).* 2003;82(6):373–384.

90. Lougaris V, Badolato R, Ferrari S, Plebani A. Hyper immunoglobulin M syndrome due to CD40 deficiency: clinical, molecular, and immunological features. *Immunol Rev.* 2005;203:48–66.

91. Quartier P, Bustamante J, Sanal O, et al. Clinical, immunologic and genetic analysis of 29 patients with autosomal recessive hyper-IgM syndrome due to activation-induced cytidine deaminase deficiency. *Clin Immunol.* 2004;110(1):22–29.

92. Imai K, Slupphaug G, Lee WI, et al. Human uracil-DNA glycosylase deficiency associated with profoundly impaired immunoglobulin class-switch recombination. *Nat Immunol.* 2003;4(10):1023–1028.

93. Busse PJ, Razvi S, Cunningham-Rundles C. Efficacy of intravenous immunoglobulin in the prevention of pneumonia in patients with common variable immunodeficiency. *J Allergy Clin Immunol.* 2002;109(6):1001–1004.

94. Stiehm ER. Human intravenous immunoglobulin in primary and secondary antibody deficiencies. *Pediatr Infect Dis J.* 1997;16(7): 696–707.

95. Ambrosino DM, Siber GR, Chilmonczyk BA, Jernberg JB, Finberg RW. An immunodeficiency characterized by impaired antibody responses to polysaccharides. *N Engl J Med.* 1987; 316(13):790–793.

96. Hidalgo H, Moore C, Leiva LE, Sorensen RU. Preimmunization and postimmunization pneumococcal antibody titers in children with recurrent infections. *Ann Allergy Asthma Immunol.* 1996;76(4):341–346.

97. Epstein MM, Gruskay F. Selective deficiency in pneumococcal antibody response in children with recurrent infections. *Ann Allergy Asthma Immunol.* 1995;75(2):125–131.

98. Orange JS, Ballow M, Stiehm ER, et al. Use and interpretation of diagnostic vaccination in primary immunodeficiency: a working group report of the Basic and Clinical Immunology Interest Section of the American Academy of Allergy, Asthma & Immunology. *J Allergy Clin Immunol.* 2012;130(3 Suppl):S1–24.

99. Sorensen RU, Leiva LE, Giangrosso PA, et al. Response to a heptavalent conjugate Streptococcus pneumoniae vaccine in children with recurrent infections who are unresponsive to the polysaccharide vaccine. *Pediatr Infect Dis J.* 1998;17(8):685–691.

100. Schneider E, Whitmore S, Glynn KM, et al. Revised surveillance case definitions for HIV infection among adults, adolescents, and children aged <18 months and for HIV infection and AIDS among children aged 18 months to <13 years–United States, 2008. *MMWR Recomm Rep.* 2008;57(RR-10):1–12.

101. Fahy RJ, Diaz PT, Hart J, Wewers MD. BAL and serum IgG levels in healthy asymptomatic HIV-infected patients. *Chest.* 2001;119(1):196–203.

102. Eagan R, Twigg HL III, Day RB, Zijlstra EE, Molyneux ME, Gordon SB. Purified lung IgG from HIV-infected subjects demonstrates an impaired ability to opsonize pneumococci [abstract]. *Proc Am Thorac Soc.* 2005;2:A453.

103. Janoff EN, O'Brien J, Thompson P, et al. Streptococcus pneumoniae colonization, bacteremia, and immune response among persons with human immunodeficiency virus infection. *J Infect Dis.* 1993;167(1):49–56.

104. Takahashi H, Oishi K, Yoshimine H, et al. Decreased serum opsonic activity against Streptococcus pneumoniae in human immunodeficiency virus-infected Ugandan adults. *Clin Infect Dis.* 2003;37(11):1534–1540.

105. Wisnewski A, Cavacini L, Posner M. Human antibody variable region gene usage in HIV-1 infection. *J Acquir Immune Defic Syndr Hum Retrovirol.* 1996;11(1):31–38.

106. Lee LH, Frasch CE, Falk LA, Klein DL, Deal CD. Correlates of immunity for pneumococcal conjugate vaccines. *Vaccine.* 2003;21(17–18):2190–2196.

107. Agusti A, MacNee W, Donaldson K, Cosio M. Hypothesis: does COPD have an autoimmune component? *Thorax.* 2003;58(10): 832–834.

108. Lee SH, Goswami S, Grudo A, et al. Antielastin autoimmunity in tobacco smoking-induced emphysema. *Nat Med.* 2007;13(5):567–569.

109. Kuo YB, Chang CA, Wu YK, et al. Identification and clinical association of anti-cytokeratin 18 autoantibody in COPD. *Immunol Lett.* 2010;128(2):131–136.

110. Feghali-Bostwick CA, Gadgil AS, Otterbein LE, et al. Autoantibodies in patients with chronic obstructive pulmonary disease. *Am J Respir Crit Care Med.* 2008;177(2):156–163.

111. Karayama M, Inui N, Suda T, Nakamura Y, Nakamura H, Chida K. Antiendothelial cell antibodies in patients with COPD. *Chest.* 2010;138(6):1303–1308.

112. van der Strate BW, Postma DS, Brandsma CA, et al. Cigarette smoke-induced emphysema: A role for the B cell? *Am J Respir Crit Care Med.* 2006;173(7):751–758.

113. Brusselle GG, Demoor T, Bracke KR, Brandsma CA, Timens W. Lymphoid follicles in (very) severe COPD: beneficial or harmful? *Eur Respir J.* 2009;34(1):219–230.

114. Brandsma CA, Timens W, Geerlings M, et al. Induction of autoantibodies against lung matrix proteins and smoke-induced inflammation in mice. *BMC Pulm Med.* 2010;10:64.

115. Taraseviciene-Stewart L, Scerbavicius R, Choe KH, et al. An animal model of autoimmune emphysema. *Am J Respir Crit Care Med.* 2005;171(7):734–742.

116. Hogg JC, Chu FS, Tan WC, et al. Survival after lung volume reduction in chronic obstructive pulmonary disease: insights from small airway pathology. *Am J Respir Crit Care Med.* 2007;176(5):454–459.
117. Hedgpeth MT, Boulware DW. Interstitial pneumonitis in antinuclear antibody-negative systemic lupus erythematosus: a new clinical manifestation and possible association with anti-Ro (SS-A) antibodies. *Arthritis Rheum.* 1988;31(4):545–548.
118. Bernstein RM, Morgan SH, Chapman J, et al. Anti-Jo-1 antibody: a marker for myositis with interstitial lung disease. *Br Med J (Clin Res Ed).* 1984;289(6438):151–152.
119. Wiener-Kronish JP, Solinger AM, Warnock ML, Churg A, Ordonez N, Golden JA. Severe pulmonary involvement in mixed connective tissue disease. *Am Rev Respir Dis.* 1981;124(4):499–503.
120. Weinberger SE, Kelman JA, Elson NA, et al. Bronchoalveolar lavage in interstitial lung disease. *Ann Intern Med.* 1978;89(4):459–466.
121. Raghu G, Brown KK. Interstitial lung disease: clinical evaluation and keys to an accurate diagnosis. *Clin Chest Med.* 2004;25(3):409–419, v.
122. Magro CM, Allen J, Pope-Harman A, et al. The role of microvascular injury in the evolution of idiopathic pulmonary fibrosis. *Am J Clin Pathol.* 2003;119(4):556–567.
123. Nakos G, Adams A, Andriopoulos N. Antibodies to collagen in patients with idiopathic pulmonary fibrosis. *Chest.* 1993;103(4):1051–1058.
124. Dobashi N, Fujita J, Murota M, et al. Elevation of anti-cytokeratin 18 antibody and circulating cytokeratin 18: anti-cytokeratin 18 antibody immune complexes in sera of patients with idiopathic pulmonary fibrosis. *Lung.* 2000;178(3):171–179.
125. Kahloon RA, Xue J, Bhargava A, et al. Patients with idiopathic pulmonary fibrosis with antibodies to heat shock protein 70 have poor prognoses. *Am J Respir Crit Care Med.* 2013;187(7):768–775.
126. Wilkes DS, Heidler KM, Niemeier M, et al. Increased bronchoalveolar IgG2/IgG1 ratio is a marker for human lung allograft rejection. *J Investig Med.* 1994;42(4):652–659.
127. Yousem SA, Martin T, Paradis IL, Keenan R, Griffith BP. Can immunohistological analysis of transbronchial biopsy specimens predict responder status in early acute rejection of lung allografts? *Hum Pathol.* 1994;25(5):525–529.
128. Wilkes DS, Sidner RA, Mathur PN, et al. Preferential production of IgG2 antibodies by parenchymal lung B-lymphocytes during lung allograft rejection. *Transplant Proc.* 1997;29(3):1891–1895.
129. Iwata T, Philipovskiy A, Fisher AJ, et al. Anti-type V collagen humoral immunity in lung transplant primary graft dysfunction. *J Immunol.* 2008;181(8):5738–5747.
130. Hachem RR, Tiriveedhi V, Patterson GA, Aloush A, Trulock EP, Mohanakumar T. Antibodies to K-alpha 1 tubulin and collagen V are associated with chronic rejection after lung transplantation. *Am J Transplant.* 2012;12(8):2164–2171.
131. Bharat A, Saini D, Steward N, et al. Antibodies to self-antigens predispose to primary lung allograft dysfunction and chronic rejection. *Am J Transplant.* 2010;90(4):1094–1101.
132. Sumpter TL, Wilkes DS. Role of autoimmunity in organ allograft rejection: a focus on immunity to type V collagen in the pathogenesis of lung transplant rejection. *Am J Physiol Lung Cell Mol Physiol.* 2004;286(6):L1129–L1139.
133. Vittal R, Fan L, Greenspan DS, et al. IL-17 induces type V collagen overexpression and EMT via TGF-beta-dependent pathways in obliterative bronchiolitis. *Am J Physiol Lung Cell Mol Physiol.* 2013;304(6):L401–L414.
134. Hodge LM, Simecka JW. Role of upper and lower respiratory tract immunity in resistance to Mycoplasma respiratory disease. *J Infect Dis.* 2002;186(2):290–294.
135. Jiao X, Hirano T, Hou Y, Gu XX. Specific immune responses and enhancement of murine pulmonary clearance of Moraxella catarrhalis by intranasal immunization with a detoxified lipooligosaccharide conjugate vaccine. *Infect Immun.* 2002;70(11):5982–5989.
136. Lynch JM, Briles DE, Metzger DW. Increased protection against pneumococcal disease by mucosal administration of conjugate vaccine plus interleukin-12. *Infect Immun.* 2003;71(8):4780–4788.
137. Rudin A, Riise GC, Holmgren J. Antibody responses in the lower respiratory tract and male urogenital tract in humans after nasal and oral vaccination with cholera toxin B subunit. *Infect Immun.* 1999;67(6):2884–2890.
138. Nurkka A, Ahman H, Korkeila M, Jantti V, Kayhty H, Eskola J. Serum and salivary anti-capsular antibodies in infants and children immunized with the heptavalent pneumococcal conjugate vaccine. *Pediatr Infect Dis J.* 2001;20(1):25–33.
139. Nurkka A, Lahdenkari M, Palmu A, Kayhty H. Salivary antibodies induced by the seven-valent PncCRM conjugate vaccine in the Finnish Otitis Media Vaccine Trial. *Vaccine.* 2004;23(3):298–304.
140. Nieminen T, Kayhty H, Virolainen A, Eskola J. Circulating antibody secreting cell response to parenteral pneumococcal vaccines as an indicator of a salivary IgA antibody response. *Vaccine.* 1998;16(2–3):313–319.
141. Klugman KP. Efficacy of pneumococcal conjugate vaccines and their effect on carriage and antimicrobial resistance. *Lancet Infect Dis.* 2001;1(2):85–91.
142. Levine MM. Can needle-free administration of vaccines become the norm in global immunization? *Nat Med.* 2003;9(1):99–103.
143. Glueck R. Pre-clinical and clinical investigation of the safety of a novel adjuvant for intranasal immunization. *Vaccine.* 2001;20(Suppl 1):S42–S44.
144. Dilraj A, Cutts FT, de Castro JF, et al. Response to different measles vaccine strains given by aerosol and subcutaneous routes to schoolchildren: a randomised trial. *Lancet.* 2000;355(9206):798–803.
145. Hausdorff WP, Bryant J, Kloek C, Paradiso PR, Siber GR. The contribution of specific pneumococcal serogroups to different disease manifestations: implications for conjugate vaccine formulation and use, part II. *Clin Infect Dis.* 2000;30(1):122–140.
146. Hausdorff WP, Bryant J, Paradiso PR, Siber GR. Which pneumococcal serogroups cause the most invasive disease: implications for conjugate vaccine formulation and use, part I. *Clin Infect Dis.* 2000;30(1):100–121.
147. Butler JC. Epidemiology of pneumococcal serotypes and conjugate vaccine formulations. *Microb Drug Resist.* 1997;3(2):125–129.
148. Christenson B, Lundbergh P, Hedlund J, Ortqvist A. Effects of a large-scale intervention with influenza and 23-valent pneumococcal vaccines in adults aged 65 years or older: a prospective study. *Lancet.* 2001;357(9261):1008–1011.
149. Cornu C, Yzebe D, Leophonte P, Gaillat J, Boissel JP, Cucherat M. Efficacy of pneumococcal polysaccharide vaccine in immunocompetent adults: a meta-analysis of randomized trials. *Vaccine.* 2001;19(32):4780–4790.

150. Tam JC, Grant NL, Freire-Moran L, Tolmie H, French N, Gordon SB. Opsonic function of bronchoalveolar lavage IgG after pneumococcal vaccination in HIV-infected and uninfected adults. *J Allergy Clin Immunol.* 2009;123(6):1420–1421.

151. Gordon SB, Malamba R, Mthunthama N, et al. Inhaled delivery of 23-valent pneumococcal polysaccharide vaccine does not result in enhanced pulmonary mucosal immunoglobulin responses. *Vaccine.* 2008;26(42):5400–5406.

152. Menzel M, Muellinger B, Weber N, Haeussinger K, Ziegler-Heitbrock L. Inhalative vaccination with pneumococcal polysaccharide in healthy volunteers. *Vaccine.* 2005;23(43):5113–5119.

153. Meyer P, Menzel M, Muellinger B, Weber N, Haeussinger K, Ziegler-Heitbrock L. Inhalative vaccination with pneumococcal polysaccharide in patients with chronic obstructive pulmonary disease. *Vaccine.* 2006;24(31–32):5832–5838.

154. Bridges CB, Thompson WW, Meltzer MI, et al. Effectiveness and cost-benefit of influenza vaccination of healthy working adults: a randomized controlled trial. *JAMA.* 2000;284(13):1655–1663.

155. Nichol KL, Lind A, Margolis KL, et al. The effectiveness of vaccination against influenza in healthy, working adults. *N Engl J Med.* 1995;333(14):889–893.

156. Centers for Disease Control and Prevention(CDC). Prevention and control of influenza with vaccines: recommendations of the Advisory Committee on Immunization Practices (ACIP)–United States, 2012–13 influenza season. *MMWR Morb Mortal Wkly Rep.* 2012;61(32):613–618.

157. Cox RJ, Brokstad KA, Ogra P. Influenza virus: immunity and vaccination strategies. Comparison of the immune response to inactivated and live, attenuated influenza vaccines. *Scand J Immunol.* 2004;59(1):1–15.

158. Johnson PR Jr, Feldman S, Thompson JM, Mahoney JD, Wright PF. Comparison of long-term systemic and secretory antibody responses in children given live, attenuated, or inactivated influenza A vaccine. *J Med Virol.* 1985;17(4):325–335.

159. Falsey AR, Treanor JJ, Tornieporth N, Capellan J, Gorse GJ. Randomized, double-blind controlled phase 3 trial comparing the immunogenicity of high-dose and standard-dose influenza vaccine in adults 65 years of age and older. *J Infect Dis.* 2009;200(2):172–180.

160. Banzhoff A, Nacci P, Podda A. A new MF59-adjuvanted influenza vaccine enhances the immune response in the elderly with chronic diseases: results from an immunogenicity meta-analysis. *Gerontology.* 2003;49(3):177–184.

161. Kaminski DA, Lee FE. Antibodies against conserved antigens provide opportunities for reform in influenza vaccine design. *Front Immunol.* 2011;2:76.

162. Ekiert DC, Bhabha G, Elsliger MA, et al. Antibody recognition of a highly conserved influenza virus epitope. *Science.* 2009;324(5924):246–251.

163. Savard C, Guerin A, Drouin K, et al. Improvement of the trivalent inactivated flu vaccine using PapMV nanoparticles. *PloS One.* 2011;6(6):e21522.

164. Vitelli A, Quirion MR, Lo CY, et al. Vaccination to conserved influenza antigens in mice using a novel simian adenovirus vector, panAd3, derived from the bonobo pan paniscus. *PloS One.* 2013;8(3):e55435.

CHAPTER 25

T Lymphocytes in the Lung

Lauren E. Cohn

The lung is a major site of exposure to the outside world in air-breathing species. Lung immunity has developed to recognize pathogens and activate appropriate responses, to temper inflammation in response to nonpathogenic exposures and turn off immune responses when danger signals have been eliminated. T lymphocytes play a major role in lung immunity predominantly through the induction of CD4 and CD8 T cells in adaptive immunity. A number of smaller subsets of T lymphocytes also play critical roles in early immune responses to pathogens and stimulating adaptive immune responses. Long-lived memory CD4 and CD8 T cells are crucial for host protection from pathogens, but also may drive chronic disease states, such as asthma. In this chapter the basic biology of T lymphocytes and their relevance in the lung in health and disease will be reviewed.

T LYMPHOCYTE SUBSETS

Lymphocytes make up approximately 10% of leukocytes in the blood and nearly 70% of leukocytes in the normal human lung.[1] In both sites, a majority of lymphocytes are T lymphocytes. Lymphocytes include T and B cells and are small, mononuclear cells with a characteristic large nucleus-to-cytoplasm ratio in the resting state. T lymphocytes have their origin in the thymus. T lymphocytes are essential for adaptive immune responses, the type of immunity that develops over a period of days to weeks that fine-tunes an immune response to limit a specific pathogen or insult. The majority of T lymphocytes express alpha-beta (α/β) T cell antigen receptors (TCRs) on the cell surface. The α/β TCR consists of two polypeptide chains with a variable region that binds to antigen, a constant region, and an anchor to the cell membrane. During development in the thymus, T cells undergo TCR gene rearrangement to generate a receptor that has an antigen-binding structure. Each mature T cell bears only this TCR with its unique specificity for antigen binding. Approximately 10^6 different TCRs develop in an individual, thus allowing the individual to respond to an extraordinary range of antigens throughout life. After exposure to a new antigen, TCRs expressed on T lymphocytes develop even finer antigen-binding capabilities through a process called affinity maturation.

The subsets of T lymphocytes that express receptors with less diversity and ability to recognize antigens include natural killer T (NKT) and mucosal-associated invariant T (MAIT) cells that also express an α/β TCR, and gamma-delta (γ/δ) TCR-expressing cells. These subsets of T lymphocytes are more prominent at sites of pathogen exposure, such as the mucosal surfaces. They express preformed receptors that bind to common pathogen components. This preset ability to bind and react to pathogens allows them to respond quickly, leading to early release of cytokines. NKT, MAIT, and γ/δ T cells are part of the innate immune response to pathogens and other insults that provide signals to initiate and direct CD4 and CD8 T cell activation in the adaptive immune response.

In addition to the α/β TCR, T lymphocytes express coreceptors CD4 or CD8. CD4+ T cells are called T helper (Th) cells because of their ability, through production of cytokines, to stimulate other immune cells. Another subset, CD4 regulatory T cells (Treg), downregulate immune responses. CD8 T cells, traditionally called cytotoxic T cells (Tc), release preformed effector molecules that destroy infected cells. They also produce cytokines that aid in local immunity. TCRs on CD4 T cells recognize peptide antigens that bind to domains on MHC Class II molecules that are present on the surface of antigen-presenting cells (APCs). CD8 T cells recognize endogenously derived antigens bound to MHC Class I molecules. MHC Class I molecules are present on the surface of all nucleated cells, whereas MHC Class II molecules are only present on APCs, including dendritic cells (DCs), B cells, and macrophages. Exogenous protein antigens, such as extracellular pathogens and environmental substances, are taken up by APCs and processed into peptides in endocytic vesicles, which are presented on the cell surface bound to MHC II molecules. Endogenous antigens, such as those of intracellular pathogens, including viruses, are processed and presented by Class I MHC molecules.

CD4+ T CELLS

CD4+ T Cell Activation

Mature, naive CD4+ T cells are released from the thymus into the circulation and enter the lymph node through specialized blood vessels, the high endothelial venules (HEVs). Expression of L-selectin (CD62L) on the naive CD4 T cell along with chemokine signals produced by stromal cells within lymphoid tissues permits attachment and transit through the HEVs into the lymph node.[2,3] In the lung, this occurs in the lymph nodes that drain the trachea, bronchi, and lung parenchyma.

Antigens or pathogens that enter the lung are taken up by APCs in the airways and alveoli. DCs are the major APC of the mucosal surfaces. DC in the airway walls and alveoli form a dense network just beneath the epithelium with processes that extend to the airspaces, designed to catch foreign antigens.[4] Macrophages in the airways and lungs also engulf large particles and pathogens through phagocytosis, but they are typically poor stimulators of adaptive immune responses, and likely eliminate antigens or induce regulatory responses, rather than activate immunity. After antigen uptake, APCs break down antigens into peptide fragments in endocytic vesicles, where the peptides are loaded onto Class II MHC proteins and transported to the cell surface. Concurrent with antigen presentation, the APC increases expression of costimulatory molecules and migrates to the lung-draining lymph nodes.

In the T cell area of the lymph node, naive CD4+ T cells move past antigen-expressing APCs, permitting the interaction of TCR and MHC Class II peptide. When the TCR on a CD4+ T cell interacts with its specific antigen on an APC, it ceases to migrate further. T cell activation is initiated upon (1) TCR recognition of MHC class II peptide (signal 1) and (2) costimulatory signaling from the APC (signal 2) (Fig. 25-1). The principal costimulatory molecules expressed on the surface of APCs are CD80 (B7-1) and CD86 (B7-2), which both interact with CD28 on the T cell.[5] If both signal 1 and signal 2 are received, the T cell goes into G1 phase of the cell cycle, begins to produce interleukin-2 (IL-2) and undergoes clonal expansion. This gives rise to a population of effector cells with the identical TCR specificity to the parental cell.

CD4 Helper T Cell Differentiation

Primary Immune Response Antigen-activated CD4+ T cells differentiate into effector cells of different types. CD4 T cell subsets are defined by the cytokines they secrete, and that pattern of cytokines confers its functional properties (Table 25-1). *T helper type 1* (Th1) cells are a subset of CD4+ T cells that secrete the macrophage activating factor, interferon gamma (IFN-γ), and lymphotoxin (LT or TNF-β). *T helper type 2* (Th2) cells produce interleukin-4 (IL-4), IL-5, and IL-13. *T helper type 17* (Th17) cells produce IL-17A, IL-17F, and IL-22. IL-10, an anti-inflammatory cytokine, was originally defined as a Th2 cytokine, but it is now recognized that it can be synthesized by all Th cell subsets upon appropriate activation.[6] Treg produce IL-10 and/or TGF-β1. Since Treg suppress T cell differentiation and APC activation, they are not considered effector cells. Th1 cells stimulate strong cell-mediated immune responses, particularly against intracellular pathogens. Th2 cells, through the production of IL-4 and IL-13, are potent activators of B cell antibody production, particularly immunoglobulin E (IgE). IL-5 secretion by Th2 cells is critical for eosinophil differentiation and maturation. Th2 cells are elicited in immune responses that require a strong humoral component and in antiparasitic responses. Th17 cells stimulate neutrophil mobilization and recruitment, release of antimicrobial peptides, and serve critical host defense functions at mucosal surfaces. An effective immune response to a pathogen commonly results in the induction of a balance of Th1, Th2, and Th17 cells to provide strong cellular and humoral immunity.

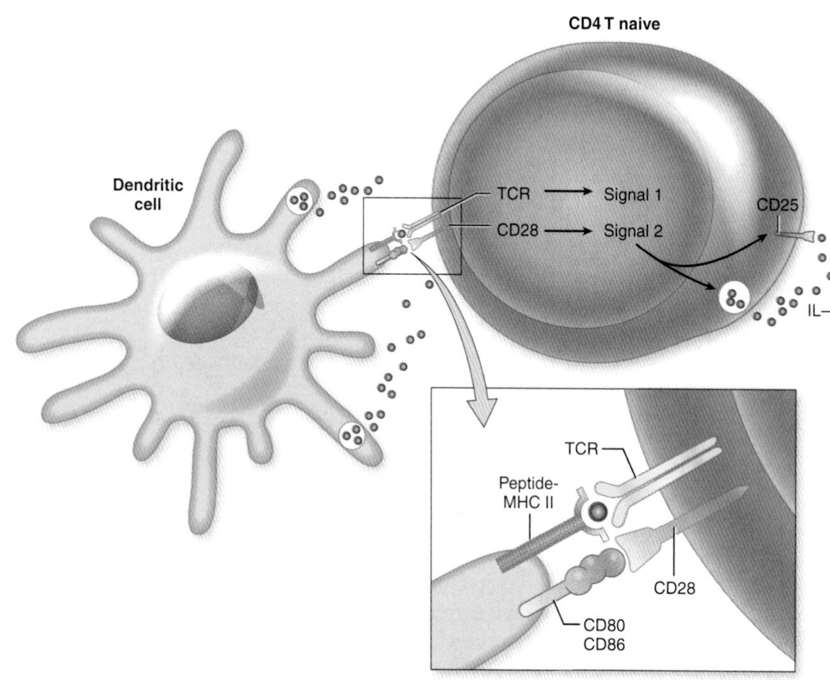

Figure 25-1 Two-signal mechanism of CD4 T cell activation. Antigen-presenting cell (APC) takes up a protein antigen and processes it into peptide fragments that are presented by class II major histocompatibility complex (MHC) molecules. Signal 1 required for CD4 T cell activation is recognized by the T cell antigen receptor (TCR) and engagement of class II MHC-peptide complex. Signal 2 is an interaction of CD28 on the T cell with CD80 or CD86 on the APC, termed costimulation. These signals stimulate interleukin-2 (IL-2) production, IL-2 receptor (IL-2R) expression and induce CD4 T cell proliferation.

CD4+ Treg comprise subsets of cells generated in the thymus (natural Treg) or induced in the secondary lymphoid tissues (inducible (i) Treg) that produce IL-10 and/or TGF-β1 and express the transcription factor Foxp3. They are often identified by their high expression of CD25 and Foxp3.[7] CD4 Treg inhibit the development

TABLE 25-1 T Lymphocyte Subsets and Their Functions

T Lymphocyte		Signals to Activate/Differentiate: Cytokine	Signals to Activate/Differentiate: Transcription Factor	Cytokines and Mediators Produced	Major Functions
CD4 Activated by peptide–MHC Class II	Th1	IFN-γ, IL-12	T-bet	IFN-γ, lymphotoxin	Anti-viral and -mycobacterial effects, activation of macrophages to kill intracellular pathogens
	Th2	IL-4	GATA-3	IL-4, IL-5, IL-13	Antiparasitic responses Stimulation of IgE and other antibody production, increases mucus production, promotes eosinophilia
	Th17	IL-6, TGF-β1, IL-1β (human)	RORγt	IL-17A, IL-17F, IL-22	Antibacterial and anti-fungal effects, recruitment and activation of PMNs
	Treg	TGF-β1, IL-10	Foxp3	TGF-β1, IL-10	Suppression of T cell activation, inhibition of APC function
CD8		Peptide–MHC Class I		IFN-γ, TNF-α Granzyme performin	Cytotoxicity of cells infected with virus or bacteria
NKT		Glycolipids		Extensive range of preformed cytokines that are rapidly released	Shaping adaptive immunity against pathogens
MAIT		Vitamin B metabolites		IFN-γ, TNF-α, IL-17, granzyme	Antimicrobial responses
γ/δ		Mycobacterial lipids, heat-shock proteins		Extensive range of preformed cytokines that are rapidly released	Antimicrobial responses, immune surveillance

of Th1, Th2, and Th17 subsets through actions on both APCs, naive T cells, and effector T cells.[8] Treg exert their suppressive effects by secreting cytokines, including TGF-β1 and/or IL-10, by cell contact leading to cytotoxicity or metabolic disruption or by suppression of APCs.[9]

Molecular Mechanisms of CD4 Th Differentiation Differentiation of naive CD4 T cell into Th1, Th2, Th17, or Treg requires the coordinate action of multiple molecular signals induced by stimulation of the TCR, costimulatory molecules, and cytokine receptors (Fig. 25-2). Major factors in these processes are critical lineage-determining molecules important for stimulation of T cell differentiation, simultaneous inhibition of the opposing phenotypes, T cell proliferation, epigenetic remodeling to modify the chromatin structure and cytosine methylation, and expression of key transcription factors.

T-bet is one of the lineage-determining molecules required for Th1 differentiation. It belongs to the T-box family of transcription factors that regulate multiple developmental processes. T-bet is upregulated in Th1 cells, through effects of IL-12 and activation of STAT4, and IFN-γ and activation of STAT1.[10] Induced expression of T-bet in vitro and in vivo led to IFN-γ production.[11] Thus T-bet drives Th1 development. T-bet also promotes Th1 induction through negative regulation of GATA-3.[12]

The transcription factor GATA-3 is an essential regulator of Th2 differentiation.[13,14] Whereas, GATA-3 is expressed at low levels in naive CD4+ T cells,[13] it is markedly upregulated in cells differentiating along the Th2 lineage and is downregulated in cells differentiating along the Th1 pathway.[13] The differentiation of a naive CD4+ T cell along the Th1 or Th2 pathway is accompanied by extensive reorganization of chromatin structure around the IFN-γ or IL-4/IL-5/IL-13 loci, respectively.[15] GATA-3 appears to be the critical downstream regulator of chromatin remodeling around the IL-4 locus.

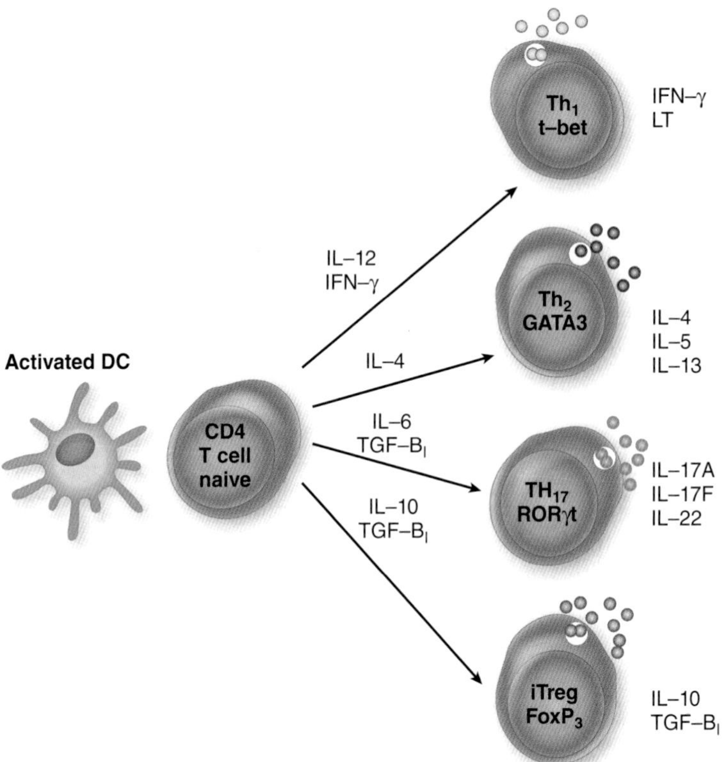

Figure 25-2 Generation of T helper types 1, 2, and 17 (Th1, Th2, Th17) and regulatory T cells (Treg) from a naive CD4+ T cell. A naive CD4+ T cell secretes very low levels of cytokines. Differentiation along the Th1, Th2, Th17, and Treg pathways is triggered when antigen is presented to the T cell receptor in the context of the major histocompatibility complex (MHC) by the appropriate antigen-presenting cell and a second signal imparted by ligation of costimulatory molecules CD80/CD86 and CD28. Dendritic cells (DCs) represent the key APCs for naive T cells. Cytokines produced in innate immune responses activate DC to produce cytokines that direct differentiation of Th subsets leading to induction of critical lineage-determining molecules, T-bet for Th1 cells, GATA-3 for Th2 cells, RORγt for Th17 cells, and Foxp3 for inducible (i)Treg. The cytokines produced by each subset of CD4 T cells are depicted.

The orphan nuclear receptor RORγt induces differentiation of naive CD4+ T cells into Th17 cells.[16] RORγt is required for the expression of IL-17 and the related gene IL-17F in response to IL-6 and TGF-β in mice or IL-1β in humans.

Cytokines, by stimulating production of critical lineage-determining molecules, are the primary factors that affect CD4 Th generation.[17,18] Cytokines produced in innate immune responses modulate how the adaptive immune response will develop. IFN-γ and IL-12 cause induction of Th1 cells. IL-4 and IL-13 drive Th2 cell generation. IL-10 enhances Th2 cell development by inhibiting Th1 cell induction. IL-6, IL-1β, IL-23, and TGF-β1 promote Th17 development.

Other factors that influence CD4 differentiation into Th subsets affect the quality of the signal through the TCR. The dose and structure of the antigen affects the APC–TCR interaction and has been shown to drive Th differentiation along distinct pathways.[19] If peptide–MHC Class II complex on the APC has a high-affinity interaction with the TCR, then a Th1-predominant response results, whereas a weaker-affinity interaction leads to a Th2-like response. Very low doses of soluble protein antigen tend to stimulate Th2-predominant responses, and at higher antigen doses, Th1 responses, suggest that the antigen dose affects the APC–T cell interaction. This may have important implications in atopy, since it has been estimated that exposure to common allergens is so small that it does not exceed 1 μg per year. Another line of investigation suggests that high-affinity interactions lead to preferential generation of Th2 cells.[20] More recent studies show that the fate of Th differentiation is an effect of both antigen dose and TCR–MHC Class II binding.[21] Ultimately, the quality of the signals delivered to the T cell through the TCR influences which Th subsets are activated.

Effector/Memory CD4 T Lymphocytes

It takes 4 to 5 days of proliferation in the lymph node for a naive CD4 T cell to differentiate into an effector cell. Associated with differentiation is a change in expression of cell surface of selectins, integrins, and chemoattractant receptors that permit exit from the lymph node and recruitment to sites of inflammation. With differentiation there is loss of expression of the lymph node homing receptor CD62L and gain of function of tissue homing receptors. Whereas skin and gut effector CD4 T cells each have specific ligands that confer their localization to that tissue through binding to vascular endothelial cells (skin, cutaneous lymphocyte-associated antigen [CLA], small intestine, integrin α4β7), such a lung-specific surface marker has not yet been identified. Human lung effector CD4 T cells are enriched for expression of CCR5, CCR6, chemokine (C-X-C motif) receptor 3 (CXCR3) and the integrins VLA1 (α1β1), CD103 (αEβ7), and VLA4 (α4β1).[22] In addition to expression of receptors that respond to specific signals that direct them to the tissue, subsets of effector CD4 Th cells express different panels of chemokine receptors so they can be called to perform specific duties. The type of injury or invading pathogen leads to release of mediators that recruit appropriate, effective populations of CD4 Th cells to manage the specific problem. Th1 cells typically express CCR5 and CXCR3, Th17 cells express

CCR6, and Th2 cells express CCR4 and CCR8, and the prostaglandin D2 chemoattractant receptor DP_2 (CRTH2) in humans.[22]

Effector cells that were activated in the lymph node arrive at an inflammatory site in the lung where they proliferate and produce cytokines. The major function of CD4 T cells is to produce cytokines to recruit other inflammatory cells and modulate local host-protective responses. Following this robust response, most activated effector CD4+ T cells die, either by a process of apoptosis or necrosis. A small population of CD4+ cells persists as memory cells for the life of the host.

CD4 memory T cells, upon reexposure to specific antigen, respond quickly with a strong response of longer duration. Subsets of CD4 memory T cells have been identified based on tissue localization and circulation patterns, cell surface markers, and functional differences. Effector memory cells (T_{EM}) are found in blood and in nonlymphoid tissues, such as liver and lung. Central memory T cells (T_{CM}) circulate through secondary lymphoid organs, lymphatics and blood, produce higher levels of IL-2 and proliferate more than T_{EM}.[23] The third CD4 memory subset, tissue-resident memory T cells make up large pools of cells in the skin and mucosal tissues, including the lung. T_{RM} remain in the tissue compartment to which they were initially called and do not recirculate. T_{RM} are responsible for barrier protection, exhibit the activation marker CD69 and can be activated locally in the tissue, without trafficking to the lymph node, to provide expedient control of infection.[23]

CD4 Regulatory T Cells

CD4 Treg comprise subsets of cells generated in the thymus (natural Treg) or induced in the secondary lymphoid tissues (inducible (i) Treg) that produce IL-10 and/or TGF-β1 and exhibit high expression of CD25 and the transcription factor Foxp3. They make up 5% to 10% of the peripheral CD4 T cell population. Cytokines produced by CD4 Treg inhibit the development of Th1, Th2, and Th17 subsets through actions on APCs, naive and effector T cells.[8] CD4 Treg are critical for suppressing primary immune responses to self, as indicated by mice and humans deficient in a functional Foxp3 protein that develop autoimmune diseases.[24,25] Treg exhibit additional diverse mechanisms to achieve immune suppression in different inflammatory milieu.[26]

CD8 T CELLS

Pathogens that enter the lung activate tissue-resident DCs and migrate to lymph nodes where they activate naive CD8 T cells. CD8 T cells are activated to differentiate into effector cells through interactions with DCs and the provision of two required activation signals, antigenic peptide presented by MHC Class I molecules and costimulatory signals. Viruses and intracellular bacteria are classical activators of CD8 T cells. Cytokines secreted by DC drive the proliferation and differentiation of CD8 T cells to acquire the ability to become effector CD8 T cells that most commonly secrete IFN-γ and TNF-α and have cytotoxic capabilities through production of granzyme B and perforin.[27] Effector CD8 T cells may also differentiate into subsets of Tc2 cells that secrete IL-4, IL-5, and IL-13 and Tc17 cells that produce IL-17.[28] CD8 memory cells develop from a small subpopulation of cells activated in a primary immune response. Memory CD8, like CD4, T cells include subsets of T_{CM}, T_{EM}, and T_{RM}. While CD8 and CD4 memory T cells may exhibit different homing patterns, memory functions and surface markers appear to mirror observations in CD4 T cells that were described earlier. For example, CD8 T_{RM}, like CD4 T_{RM}, do not recirculate and confer rapid tissue-specific recall responses in the lung.[23,29]

T LYMPHOCYTES WITH RESTRICTED TCR DIVERSITY

T lymphocytes with less diverse arrays of TCRs accumulate in the lung. They respond to different antigens than traditional α/β CD4 and CD8 T cells. Their numbers in tissues are low, but because many respond to the same antigen, they can be activated quickly without further differentiation. Therefore, they participate in innate immunity and some subsets can expand and adapt to exposures. Thus, these T lymphocyte subsets bridge innate and adaptive immunity. There are two small populations of α/β T cells, iNKT cells and MAIT cells that have semi-invariant α chains. Thus, they have undergone somatic mutation in the thymus to generate a TCR, but they have limited diversity due to fewer possible TCR combinations. Both iNKT and MAIT cells are found in high frequencies in mucosal tissues.

Natural Killer T Cells

Type I or invariant (i)NKT cells are a small subpopulation of α/β T cells that express a narrow repertoire of TCRs due to invariant expression of the TCR variable (V)α chain and limited TCR Vβ chains. In humans Vα24-Jα18 pairs almost exclusively with Vβ11, whereas in mice Vα14-Jα18 pair with a limited number of Vβ chains. iNKT cells respond to glycolipid antigens presented on the MHC-like molecule CD-1d, which is a member of a family of nonpolymorphic proteins that bind to lipids, rather than peptide antigens, and is expressed on populations of DCs, B cells, and macrophages.[30]

iNKT cells leave the thymus upon maturation and migrate into tissues. In mice, iNKT cells are enriched in the liver and spleen. In humans iNKT cells are highly enriched in the omentum but have not been well characterized in all tissues.[31] In the bronchoalveolar lavage (BAL) of normal control subjects iNKT cells constituted less than 1% of the lymphocyte population.[32] In mouse, iNKT cells may be 5% to 10% of the lung lymphocytes.[33] Murine studies show that iNKT cells are resident in the lung and, for the most part, do not recirculate to other organs.[34] iNKT cells also reside in the lung microvasculature in the resting state and upon exposure to inhaled lipids, become activated and extravasate into the lung parenchyma where they contribute to lung inflammation.

A hallmark of iNKT cell activation is the rapid elaboration of an extensive array of cytokines and chemokines including IFN-γ, TNF-α, TGF-β, GM-CSF, IL-2, IL-4, IL-5, IL-6, IL-10, IL-13, IL-17, IL-21, RANTES, eotaxin/CCL11, MIP-1α/CCL3, and MIP-1β/CCL4.[30] The early activation of iNKT cells in tissues by specific pathogens is believed to be important in shaping the appropriate adaptive immune response.

MAIT Cells

MAIT cells are another small subpopulation of α/β T lymphocytes that express TCRs with limited diversity. MAIT cells express a semi-invariant α chain, Vα7.2-Jα33, that pairs with a limited number of Vβ chains. MAIT cells are present in humans in the peripheral blood, lamina propria of the intestine, and in the lung.[35] MAIT cell activation requires interaction with the nonpolymorphic MHC I–like molecule MR-1. MR-1 binding of vitamin B metabolites, specifically a precursor of riboflavin synthesis, activates MAIT cells. Since only certain bacteria, fungi, and yeast synthesize this B vitamin, MAIT cells are activated early after exposure to pathogens capable of producing riboflavin.[36,37] Activation of MAIT cells leads to release of cytokines, including IFN-γ, TNF-α, IL-17, granule exocytosis leading to apoptosis, and delivery of antimicrobial peptides.[38,39] MAIT cells help to stimulate effective antipathogen CD4 and CD8 adaptive immune responses. MAIT cells are enriched in the lung in infections, such as tuberculosis, where a fivefold increased frequency, compared to the blood, has been observed.[35]

γ/δ T Cells

Gamma/delta (γ/δ) cells are a subset of T cells that have a TCR composed of γ and δ chains. The γ/δ TCR is generated by VDJ recombination, but unlike the α/β TCR, γ- and δ-chain recombination results in a less diverse repertoire of TCRs. Upon release from the thymus, γ/δ T cells migrate to tissues including lung, skin, intestine, and uterus. γ/δ T cells, like α/β T cells, are found in blood, LN, and spleen. Within specific tissue compartments all γ/δ T cells may express a monoclonal TCR. γ/δ T cells engage a different group of antigens than α/β T cells. γ/δ TCRs respond to a diverse array of antigens including moieties large and small, self and foreign, and peptide and nonpeptide. This includes mycobacterial lipids and heat-shock proteins.[40] γ/δ T cells do not recognize antigens in the context of class I or II MHC; rather, they may recognize their target antigens directly. The full scope of γ/δ TCR-binding antigens remains unknown.[41] γ/δ T cells secrete a range of cytokines and chemokines, many of which are preformed and quickly produced, to recruit inflammatory cells. Their narrow TCR diversity in a tissue compartment, and ability to respond to their stimuli quickly allows for rapid clonal activation without the need for expansion. This suggests that γ/δ T cells play a role in surveillance and protection from infection, and serve as a bridge between innate and adaptive immune responses.

T LYMPHOCYTES IN THE LUNG

T LYMPHOCYTE DISTRIBUTION IN THE LUNG

In the normal human lung, T lymphocytes are found in the airways and alveolar spaces, in the lung parenchyma/interstitium, the pulmonary intravascular spaces, and in lymph nodes, and their numbers differ in each of these compartments. In adult humans, lymphocytes in the lung are not typically organized into lymphoid structures, such as bronchus-associated lymphoid tissue (BALT), whereas BALT is more common in healthy children, in smokers and those with chronic infections and inflammatory diseases, and in normal animals such as rabbits and rats.[42,43] Recent studies show that lymphocytes are not randomly distributed in each lung compartment, but appear to be organized at sites of pathogen entry.[44] T lymphocytes likely have a multidimensional organization in the lung, including close associations with dendritic, epithelial, and mast cells, but these detailed interactions and their structure is not yet well defined. Until recently, analyses of lung lymphocytes have assessed collections of cells from BAL, which includes cells from the airways and alveolar spaces, or in digested lung tissue. Histopathologic assessments afforded, at best, little more than a two-dimensional analysis. Future studies will define the three-dimensional organization of T lymphocytes in the lung, their detailed interactions with both structural cells, including epithelial, endothelial and neuronal, and hematopoietic cells. Kinetic studies will define how lymphocytes transit between compartments in the lung, to secondary lymphoid and other tissues.

Lymphocytes, including T and B cells, make up about 7% of leukocytes isolated from the human lung. It has been estimated that between 2 and 4 × 10^8 lymphocytes reside in the airways and alveolar spaces. Twentyfold more are estimated to make up the pool of lymphocytes in the lung parenchyma in the normal human lung.[45,46] Lymphocytes isolated from the lung parenchyma consist of large populations within the interstitium and the intravascular space.[47]

In the lung parenchyma, T lymphocytes are the predominant lymphocyte population, a majority of which are CD4 T cells (T:B ratio 15:1, CD4:CD8 2:1).[48] Memory CD4 T cells make up a majority of CD4 T cells in the lung and at other mucosal sites. CD8 memory cells make up half of the CD8 T cell population in the lung. With age, the number of lymphocytes and the proportion of lymphocytes with a memory phenotype increase. In the BAL, CD4 T cells comprise about 4% of leukocytes in young adults and 20% in older adults.[49–51] In lung parenchyma, memory CD4 T cells were 65% in young adults and almost 80% in older adults.[48] Thus, the proportion of antigen-experienced CD4 T cells increases in the lung and likely reflects an individual's accumulated respiratory exposure over time.

T LYMPHOCYTES IN LUNG INFECTION

T lymphocytes play critical roles in host defense against bacteria, viruses, and fungi that enter the host through the respiratory tract. This essential function of T lymphocytes is illustrated in HIV infection,[4] in which individuals lack functional T cell subsets leading to susceptibility to pulmonary infection with bacteria, including *Staphylococcus aureus, Streptococcus pneumonia, Haemophilus influenzae*, and mycobacterial species, viruses such as influenza, and fungi such as histoplasmosis and *Cryptococcus neoformans* and pneumocystis jiroveci pneumonia (PJP).[52]

The immunocompetent individual responds to pathogen invasion through activation of NKT, MAIT, and γ/δ T cells along with other first responders, including macrophages, neutrophils, and epithelial cells. These innate immune cells are rapidly activated to secrete cytokines to help contain the pathogen, and to provide signals to activate CD4 and CD8 T cells. The range of cytokines produced by innate immune cells after activation shape the patterns of CD4 and CD8 T cell subsets induced to differentiate to control the invading pathogen. In a primary response to a pathogen, antigen-specific CD4 and CD8 effector T cells begin to arrive from the secondary lymphoid organs in the lung days after the initial infection.

In lung infection, the primary function of CD4 T lymphocytes is to produce cytokines that ultimately lead to elimination of pathogens. CD8 T cells have the additional capacity to kill infected cells. A primary infection results in the development and recruitment of a range of pathogen-specific T cell subsets, including CD4 Th1, Th2, and Th17, and CD8 T cells. Each subset serves a specific purpose in the complex antimicrobial immune response. Yet, in some infections, one subset is essential for antipathogen immunity. Th1 cells are absolutely required for elimination of a number of pathogens, and this reflects Th1 production of IFN-γ. IFN-γ is essential for immunity to respiratory infections because of its myriad antimicrobial functions including macrophage activation, stimulation of microbicidal effectors, and stimulation of antiviral enzymes.[53] Th1 cells are essential for host defense against all mycobacterial species, other intracellular pathogens such as *Chlamydia pneumonia* and *Francisella tularensis*, virus infections including influenza and RSV, gram-negative bacterial infections with *Klebsiella pneumonia*, and fungal infections including coccidiodes, cryptococcosis, and histoplasma.[54] Th2 cells are required for immunity to helminth parasites, and Th17 cells are essential to eliminate the gram-negative bacteria *K. pneumonia* and *Pseudomonas aeruginosa*, chlamydia, *and Mycoplasma pneumonia* and for immunity to various fungal infections including candida.

After a primary infection, pathogen-specific memory CD4 and CD8 T cells develop. Some are retained in the lung as T_{RM} and are presumed to persist there through the life of an individual. Animal studies show that maintenance of the memory CD4 T cell population in the lung in the first year after primary infection required recruitment of new cells from the circulating pool.[44,55] It remains unknown if memory cells continue to be replaced at this rate further out from infection, but it is likely that a dynamic process sustains the population of memory T cells in the lung long after infection.

The population of memory T_{RM} appears to be retained in the lung by surface expression of tissue-specific homing molecules.[56,57] Animal studies show that in different species memory CD4 and CD8 isolated from the lung returned to the lung when reinjected systemically into another animal. One such localization signal is CD103, which is expressed on antigen-specific T cells.[23,58] In both mice and humans, CD69 expression characterized CD4 and CD8 memory T cells that were retained in the lung, rather than those that recirculated.[44] Influenza-specific CD4 and CD8 T_{RM} were compartmentalized in bronchovascular bundles surrounding the airways.[44] Thus, CD4 T_{RM} may be retained adjacent to the tight web of DCs just below the epithelial surface where they can be quickly activated by specific antigen.[59] Virus-specific memory CD8 T cells were observed in or near capillaries in the lung by chemokines secreted by epithelial cells.[55,60] After reexposure to a pathogen in the lung, CD4 and CD8 T_{RM} are activated locally, rather than recirculating to local lymph nodes.[23,44] In humans, T_{RM} produced IFN-γ and

IL-2 upon activation,[48] thus insuring both antimicrobial and proliferation signals at the site of infection. Therefore, T_{RM} in the lung reside in compartments near key sites of exposure that insure rapid recruitment, reactivation, and proliferation upon pathogen reexposure, and they may be skewed toward a memory type 1 phenotype.

T LYMPHOCYTES IN CHRONIC LUNG DISEASES

T lymphocytes serve essential functions in host defense as they respond to specific antigens and are retained in the lung as memory cells, but they may also drive chronic disease when immune responses are generated against nonpathogens such as allergens or self-antigens. The development of immunity against nonpathogenic aeroallergens in allergic asthma is an example of immune dysregulation. While asthma is the most extensively studied T lymphocyte–driven lung disease, many other chronic pulmonary diseases may be caused and/or perpetuated by T lymphocytes, including sarcoidosis, hypersensitivity pneumonitis, autoimmune lung diseases, idiopathic pulmonary fibrosis, pulmonary hypertension and lung cancer, and others.

T Lymphocytes in Allergic Asthma

Long-lived antipathogen responses are protective and reflect useful host immunity. In allergic asthma, the long-lived memory lymphocytes that respond to allergens are deleterious and may remain capable of reactivation throughout the life of the individual. T lymphocytes appear to drive this chronic disease state in the airways. Many T lymphocyte subsets have been implicated in initiating and sustaining asthma.

CD4 T Helper Type 2 Cells in Asthma CD4+ T cells are the predominant lymphocyte population infiltrating the airways and they express markers of activation in asthmatic subjects. CD4+ T cells producing IL-4, IL-5, and IL-13 have been identified in BAL and airway biopsies and are secreted in the airways of patients with mild or asymptomatic asthma.[61] GATA-3 expression was increased in airways of asthmatic patients compared with those in control subjects, indicating the presence of Th2 cells.[62] Antigen challenge in allergic asthmatic patients led to an increase in Th2 lymphocytes in the airways.[63] In asthmatic patients, airway hyperreactivity (AHR) and airway eosinophilia correlated with airway CD4 T cells that produced IL-4 or IL-5 or expressed GATA-3.[62] In conjunction with known effects of IL-4, IL-5, and IL-13, these studies support the hypothesis that Th2 cells drive the characteristic inflammatory response that results in asthma.

Animal studies show that activation of CD4 Th2 cells in the airways leads to pathophysiologic manifestations of asthma. Eosinophilic airway inflammation and AHR have both been shown to be dependent on CD4+ T cells.[64] Studies that employed adoptive transfer of CD4+ T cells from animals with antigen-induced AHR resulted in airway inflammation and hyperresponsiveness in recipient mice, indicating that CD4+ T cells can control many aspects of the disease. CD4+ Th2 cells induced airway eosinophilia, mucus hypersecretion, and AHR, whereas Th1 cells caused a neutrophil-predominant inflammatory response without any of these features of asthma.[64]

Gene association studies also support a role for Th2 cells in asthma. Strong linkages have been identified to flanking markers of the human cytokine gene cluster on chromosomes 5q31 and 16p12, which include genes for IL-4, IL-13, and IL-4Rα.[65] Variants in the IL-4 promoter region are associated with atopy, as are polymorphisms of IL-4Rα, a component of both the IL-4 and IL-13 receptors, and a variant IL-13R.[66] Thus, modifications of IL-4 and/or IL-13 or their signaling, increasing Th2 cell functions, are associated with atopy and asthma.

CD4 T Helper Type 1 Cells in Asthma Th1 cells are also present in the airways of asthmatic patients, but it is still not clear if they serve a protective or pathologic function in asthma. IFN-γ was elevated in the airways of some severe asthmatics, and it was reduced in subsets of other asthmatics[67,68] Some studies show that Th1 cell activation inhibits allergic airway inflammation, whereas other studies suggest that Th1 cells potentiate the inflammatory response in asthma due to the proinflammatory effects of Th1 cytokines.[64]

Human and animal studies suggest that enhancing Th1 cytokines in the lung before or early in the generation of a Th2 response may protect against the development of asthma. IFN-γ–dominated immune responses to viral or mycobacterial infection in childhood are associated with a reduced incidence of asthma.[69] Attendance at day care and exposure to other siblings was protective against wheezing in childhood, which is hypothesized to be from beneficial exposures to respiratory infections. Also, mice immunized in the presence of a Th1-stimulating environment exhibited a reduction in antigen-induced eosinophilic airway inflammation and AHR.[70] Thus, reducing the generation of Th2 cells appears to decrease allergic inflammation. However it is also apparent that a high frequency of virally induced wheezing in early life is a strong predictor for the subsequent development of asthma in children,[71] thus suggesting that timing and nature of infections in early life may be crucial.

Th1 cells can also inhibit the effects of ongoing Th2 cell responses. Th1 cells, through the production of IFN-γ, have been shown to inhibit Th2 cell cytokine production and Th2 cell proliferation in vitro.[72] In mice the Th1 cytokine IFN-γ has inhibitory effects on Th2-induced airway eosinophilia and AHR. When administered before inhaled antigen challenge, IFN-γ reduced the number of CD4+ T cells in the respiratory tract or reduced Th2 cytokine secretion.[73] These effects may result from inhibition of Th2 cell recruitment by IFN-γ. Once Th2 cells are present in the respiratory tract, IFN-γ promotes the resolution of airway eosinophilia and suppresses Th2 cytokine production.[74] Th1 cells, through the production of IFN-γ, can inhibit airway eosinophilia, mucus production, and AHR without an increase in airway inflammation.[75] Although many studies support Th1 cells and IFN-γ as inhibitors of Th2-type responses, other studies show that Th1 cells enhance inflammation and do not ameliorate disease.[76] The proinflammatory effects of Th1 cells are supported by the association of viral respiratory infections, which tend to induce Th1 responses, and exacerbation of symptoms in asthmatic patients. Ultimately, the influence of Th1 cells on allergic airway inflammation may depend on the timing of Th1 relative to Th2 cell activation and the subphenotype of the asthmatic.

CD4 T Helper Type 17 Cells in Asthma Th17 cells, IL-17A and IL-17F are increased in the airways, sputum, and blood of subjects with asthma.[77] Given the heterogeneity of asthmatic airway inflammation and the effects of IL-17A and IL-17F on neutrophil recruitment, it was hypothesized that Th17 cells would be pathogenic in neutrophilic, nonatopic asthma. Yet, there was a positive association of IL-17 and IL-5, and IL-17 with atopic, not with nonatopic asthma.[78] As expected, IL-17A levels were associated with sputum neutrophils and not eosinophils,[79] suggesting that Th17 cells may drive disease in a subset of neutrophilic asthmatics.[80]

Studies to determine the function of Th17 cells have not established a definitive role of Th17 and IL-17A in animal models of asthma. A number of laboratories have shown that Th17 cells, IL-17A and IL-17 receptors are critical for optimal Th2 cell function, AHR, and eosinophilic inflammation. Furthermore, IL-17A was a major determinant in the development of AHR in mice with susceptibility compared to mice with resistance to develop AHR.[81] Yet, other investigators showed neutralization of IL-17 leads to worse disease.[25,82] The complex interplay of Th17 and Th2 cells is highlighted by studies showing that IL-13 inhibits IL-17A production and IL-17A production inhibits IL-25 that drives Th2 function. These studies suggest that disease pathogenesis in asthma may result from a disruption in a critical balance of cytokines that includes IL-17.

Regulatory T Cells in Asthma Foxp3+ Treg likely determine early sensitization to allergen, as suggested by studies of the rare, immune dysregulation, polyendocrinopathy, enteropathy, X-linked syndrome (IPEX), which is caused by mutations in the *Foxp3* gene on the X chromosome. This results in markedly reduced or absent Foxp3+ Treg. Young boys with this condition suffer from both severe autoimmune and allergic symptoms.[24] T cells from these patients show skewing toward a Th2 phenotype. Mice with a mutation in the Foxp3 gene also demonstrate intense multiorgan inflammation, including allergic airway disease, high levels of IgE, eosinophilia, and dysregulated Th1 and Th2 cytokine responses, but they do not exhibit Th2 skewing, as observed in humans with IPEX.[83]

Studies to assess the numbers of CD4+CD25+ T cells in the peripheral blood of healthy, compared to allergic, subjects have not consistently shown differences[8,84] However, some of the methodology used to detect Treg make interpretation of some of these earlier data limited due to the methodologies used to detect Treg. There are data, though, that show impaired CD4+$CD25^{high}$ Foxp3 Treg in allergic disease. In asthmatic children there were reduced numbers of CD4+$CD25^{high}$ T cells in BAL, but not blood, as compared to control children with chronic cough.[85] A lower level of Foxp3 mRNA was reported in asthmatic children. CD4+$CD25^{high}$ T cells in the airways of the asthmatic children correlated with clinical parameters such as lung function, and were restored following corticosteroid treatment. A similar increase in Foxp3 mRNA was reported in the peripheral blood of adult asthma patients following inhaled corticosteroid treatment.[86] Foxp3-expressing Treg are also important negative regulators of asthma and allergic disease in animal models. Treg expressing either IL-10, TGF-β1, or both were required to limit airway inflammation in numerous models of tolerance induction.[87–90] Overall, it appears that impaired Treg responses may contribute to the development of asthma and allergic diseases.

CD8 T Cells in Asthma In atopic asthmatics there were increased CD8 T cells in airway biopsies when compared to biopsies in non-asthmatic, atopic, and normal subjects.[91] Furthermore, the number of CD8 T cells in airway biopsies of atopic asthmatics was associated with a decline in FEV1.[92] During asthma exacerbations and in death from status asthmaticus, there were increased CD8+ T cells in the respiratory tract.[93] These observations suggest that CD8 T cells are detrimental in asthma. Animal studies both support these observations and show that CD8 T cells inhibit allergic airway disease through the production of IFN-γ and induction of IL-12 production. Most likely, CD8 T cells have varying effects in different individuals and under different circumstances.

CD8 T cells recognize endogenous antigens, like viral peptides, rather than allergens. Since asthma exacerbations are most commonly caused by viral respiratory infections, then virus-specific CD8 T cells will be recruited and retained in the lung. Thus, the presence of CD8 T cells in asthmatic lungs may reflect recent infections.

CD8 T cells, like CD4 T cells, can be polarized into subsets. Cytotoxic T cell–type 1 (Tc1) cells are activated in viral infections and generally produce IFN-γ and lymphotoxin. These are classical CD8 T cells. Smaller subsets of CD8 T cells can make other panels of cytokines. For example, when activated in the presence of IL-4, CD8 T cytotoxic–type 2 (Tc2) cells can be induced to produce IL-4, IL-5, and IL-13. Animal studies show that Tc2 cells retain their cytotoxic function, stimulate recruitment of eosinophils, provide B cell help for IgE production, and promote airway hyperresponsiveness.[93] It has been theorized that some respiratory infections may stimulate CD8 Tc2 responses, thus initiating or exacerbating local allergic responses.

REFERENCES

1. Holt PG, Robinson BW, Reid M, et al. Extraction of immune and inflammatory cells from human lung parenchyma: Evaluation of an enzymatic digestion procedure. *Clin Exp Immunol.* 1986;66(1):188–200.
2. Denucci CC, Mitchell JS, Shimizu Y. Integrin function in T-cell homing to lymphoid and nonlymphoid sites: getting there and staying there. *Crit Rev Immunol.* 2009;29(2):87–109.
3. Ebert LM, Schaerli P, Moser B. Chemokine-mediated control of T cell traffic in lymphoid and peripheral tissues. *Mol Immunol.* 2005;42(7):799–809.
4. Schon-Hegrad MA, Oliver J, McMenamin PG, Holt PG. Studies on the density, distribution, and surface phenotype of intraepithelial class II major histocompatibility complex antigen (Ia)-bearing dendritic cells (DC) in the conducting airways. *J Exp Med.* 1991;173(6):1345–1356.
5. Sharpe AH. Mechanisms of costimulation. *Immunol Rev.* 2009;229(1):5–11.
6. Saraiva M, Christensen JR, Veldhoen M, Murphy TL, Murphy KM, O'Garra A. Interleukin-10 production by Th1 cells requires interleukin-12-induced STAT4 transcription factor and ERK MAP kinase activation by high antigen dose. *Immunity.* 2009;31(2):209–219.
7. Chen X, Oppenheim JJ. Resolving the identity myth: key markers of functional CD4+FoxP3 +regulatory T cells. *Int Immunopharmacol.* 2011;11(10):1489–1496.
8. Ray A, Khare A, Krishnamoorthy N, Qi Z, Ray P. Regulatory T cells in many flavors control asthma. *Mucosal Immunol.* 2010;3(3):216–229.
9. Vignali DA, Collison LW, Workman CJ. How regulatory T cells work. *Nat Rev Immunol.* 2008;8(7):523–532.
10. Rao A, Avni O. Molecular aspects of T-cell differentiation. *Br Med Bull.* 2000;56(4):969–984.
11. Szabo SJ, Kim ST, Costa GL, Zhang X, Fathman CG, Glimcher LH. A novel transcription factor, T-bet, directs Th1 lineage commitment. *Cell.* 2000;100(6):655–669.
12. Usui T, Preiss JC, Kanno Y, et al. T-bet regulates Th1 responses through essential effects on GATA-3 function rather than on IFNG gene acetylation and transcription. *J Exp Med.* 2006;203(3):755–766.
13. Zhang DH, Cohn L, Ray P, Bottomly K, Ray A. Transcription factor GATA-3 is differentially expressed in Th1 and Th2 cells and controls Th2-specific expression of the interleukin-5 gene. *J Biol Chem.* 1997;272:21597–21603.
14. Zheng WP, Flavell RA. The transcription factor GATA-3 is necessary and sufficient for Th2 cytokine gene expression in CD4 T cells. *Cell.* 1997;89:587–596.
15. Agarwal S, Rao A. Modulation of chromatin structure regulates cytokine gene expression during T cell differentiation. *Immunity.* 1998;9:765–775.
16. Ivanov II, McKenzie BS, Zhou L, et al. The orphan nuclear receptor RORgammat directs the differentiation program of proinflammatory IL-17+ T helper cells. *Cell.* 2006;126(6):1121–1133.
17. Zhu J, Yamane H, Paul WE. Differentiation of effector CD4 T cell populations (*). *Annu Rev Immunol.* 2010;28:445–489.
18. Lee HJ, O'Garra A, Arai K, Arai N. Characterization of cis-regulatory elements and nuclear factors conferring Th2-specific

expression of the IL-5 gene: a role for a GATA-binding protein. *J Immunol.* 1998;160:2343–2352.

19. Constant SL, Bottomly K. Induction of Th1 and Th2 CD4+ T cell responses: the alternative approaches. *Annu Rev Immunol.* 1997; 15:297–322.
20. Sperling AI, Bluestone JA. The complexities of T-cell co-stimulation: CD28 and beyond. *Immunol Rev.* 1996;153:155–182.
21. Tubo NJ, Pagan AJ, Taylor JJ, et al. Single naive CD4+ T cells from a diverse repertoire produce different effector cell types during infection. *Cell.* 2013;153(4):785–796.
22. Islam SA, Luster AD. T cell homing to epithelial barriers in allergic disease. *Nat Med.* 2012;18(5):705–715.
23. Shin H, Iwasaki A. Tissue-resident memory T cells. *Immunol Rev.* 2013;255(1):165–181.
24. Torgerson TR, Ochs HD. Immune dysregulation, polyendocrinopathy, enteropathy, X-linked: forkhead box protein 3 mutations and lack of regulatory T cells. *J Allergy Clin Immunol.* 2007; 120(4):744–750; quiz 751–752.
25. Sergejeva S, Ivanov S, Lotvall J, Linden A. Interleukin-17 as a recruitment and survival factor for airway macrophages in allergic airway inflammation. *Am J Respir Cell Mol Biol.* 2005;33(3): 248–253.
26. Chaudhry A, Rudensky AY. Control of inflammation by integration of environmental cues by regulatory T cells. *J Clin Invest.* 2013; 123(3):939–944.
27. Russ BE, Denton AE, Hatton L, Croom H, Olson MR, Turner SJ. Defining the molecular blueprint that drives CD8(+) T cell differentiation in response to infection. *Front Immunol.* 2012; 3:371.
28. Cox MA, Harrington LE, Zajac AJ. Cytokines and the inception of CD8 T cell responses. *Trends Immunol.* 2011;32(4):180–186.
29. Kaech SM, Cui W. Transcriptional control of effector and memory CD8+ T cell differentiation. *Nat Rev Immunol.* 2012;12(11): 749–761.
30. Brennan PJ, Brigl M, Brenner MB. Invariant natural killer T cells: an innate activation scheme linked to diverse effector functions. *Nat Rev Immunol.* 2013;13(2):101–117.
31. Lynch L, O'Shea D, Winter DC, Geoghegan J, Doherty DG, O'Farrelly C. Invariant NKT cells and CD1 d(+) cells amass in human omentum and are depleted in patients with cancer and obesity. *Eur J Immunol.* 2009;39(7):1893–1901.
32. Mutalithas K, Croudace J, Guillen C, et al. Bronchoalveolar lavage invariant natural killer T cells are not increased in asthma. *J Allergy Clin Immunol.* 2007;119(5):1274–1276.
33. Thomas SY, Scanlon ST, Griewank KG, et al. PLZF induces an intravascular surveillance program mediated by long-lived LFA-1-ICAM-1 interactions. *J Exp Med.* 2011;208(6):1179–1188.
34. Scanlon ST, Thomas SY, Ferreira CM, et al. Airborne lipid antigens mobilize resident intravascular NKT cells to induce allergic airway inflammation. *J Exp Med.* 2011;208(10):2113–2124.
35. Gold MC, Cerri S, Smyk-Pearson S, et al. Human mucosal associated invariant T cells detect bacterially infected cells. *PLoS Biol.* 2010;8(6):e1000407.
36. Kjer-Nielsen L, Patel O, Corbett AJ, et al. MR1 presents microbial vitamin B metabolites to MAIT cells. *Nature.* 2012;491(7426): 717–723.
37. Gold MC, Eid T, Smyk-Pearson S, et al. Human thymic MR1-restricted MAIT cells are innate pathogen-reactive effectors that adapt following thymic egress. *Mucosal Immunol.* 2013;6(1): 35–44.
38. Dusseaux M, Martin E, Serriari N, et al. Human MAIT cells are xenobiotic-resistant, tissue-targeted, CD161hi IL-17-secreting T cells. *Blood.* 2011;117(4):1250–1259.
39. Le Bourhis L, Martin E, Peguillet I, et al. Antimicrobial activity of mucosal-associated invariant T cells. *Nat Immunol.* 2010;11(8): 701–708.
40. Born WK, Reardon CL, O'Brien RL. The function of gammadelta T cells in innate immunity. *Curr Opin Immunol.* 2006;18(1):31–38.
41. Vantourout P, Hayday A. Six-of-the-best: unique contributions of gammadelta T cells to immunology. *Nat Rev Immunol.* 2013; 13(2):88–100.
42. Randall TD. Bronchus-associated lymphoid tissue (BALT) structure and function. *Adv Immunol.* 2010;107:187–241.
43. Tschernig T, Pabst R. Bronchus-associated lymphoid tissue (BALT) is not present in the normal adult lung but in different diseases. *Pathobiology.* 2000;68(1):1–8.
44. Turner DL, Bickham L, Thome JJT, et al. Lung niches for the generation and maintenance of tissue-resident memory T cells. *Mucosal Immunol.* 2014;7(3):501–510.
45. Hunninghake GW, Gadek JE, Kawanami O, Ferrans VJ, Crystal RG. Inflammatory and immune processes in the human lung in health and disease: evaluation by bronchoalveolar lavage. *Am J Pathol.* 1979;97(1):149–206.
46. Hunninghake GW, Kawanami O, Ferrans VJ, Young RC Jr, Roberts WC, Crystal RG. Characterization of the inflammatory and immune effector cells in the lung parenchyma of patients with interstitial lung disease. *Am Rev Respir Dis.* 1981;123 (4 Pt 1):407–412.
47. Pabst R, Tschernig T. Lymphocytes in the lung: an often neglected cell. Numbers, characterization and compartmentalization. *Anat Embryol (Berl).* 1995;192(4):293–299.
48. Sathaliyawala T, Kubota M, Yudanin N, et al. Distribution and compartmentalization of human circulating and tissue-resident memory T cell subsets. *Immunity.* 2013;38(1):187–197.
49. Meyer KC, Soergel P. Variation of bronchoalveolar lymphocyte phenotypes with age in the physiologically normal human lung. *Thorax.* 1999;54(8):697–700.
50. Burastero SE, Borgonovo B, Gaffi D, et al. The repertoire of T-lymphocytes recovered by bronchoalveolar lavage from healthy nonsmokers. *Eur Respir.* 1996;9(2):319–327.
51. Balbi B, Pignatti P, Corradi M, et al. Bronchoalveolar lavage, sputum and exhaled clinically relevant inflammatory markers: values in healthy adults. *Eur Respir J.* 2007;30(4):769–781.
52. Raju R, Peters BS, Breen RA. Lung infections in the HIV-infected adult. *Curr Opin Pulm Med.* 2012;18(3):253–258.
53. Schroder K, Hertzog PJ, Ravasi T, Hume DA. Interferon-gamma: an overview of signals, mechanisms and functions. *J Leukoc Biol.* 2004;75(2):163–189.
54. Chen K, Kolls JK. T cell-mediated host immune defenses in the lung. *Annu Rev Immunol.* 2013;31:605–633.
55. Anderson KG, Sung H, Skon CN, et al. Cutting edge: intravascular staining redefines lung CD8 T cell responses. *J Immunol.* 2012; 189(6):2702–2706.
56. Binns RM, Licence ST, Pabst R. Homing of blood, splenic, and lung emigrant lymphoblasts: comparison with the behaviour of lymphocytes from these sources. *Int Immunol.* 1992;4(9):1011–1019.
57. Teijaro JR, Turner D, Pham Q, Wherry EJ, Lefrancois L, Farber DL. Cutting edge: tissue-retentive lung memory CD4 T cells mediate optimal protection to respiratory virus infection. *J Immunol.* 2011;187(11):5510–5514.

58. Piet B, de Bree GJ, Smids-Dierdorp BS, et al. CD8(+) T cells with an intraepithelial phenotype upregulate cytotoxic function upon influenza infection in human lung. *J Clin Invest.* 2011;121(6): 2254–2263.

59. Holt PG, Schon-Hegrad MA. Localization of T cells, macrophages and dendritic cells in rat respiratory tract tissue: implications for immune function studies. *Immunology.* 1987;62(3):349–356.

60. Ely KH, Cookenham T, Roberts AD, Woodland DL. Memory T cell populations in the lung airways are maintained by continual recruitment. *J Immunol.* 2006;176(1):537–543.

61. Robinson DS, Hamid Q, Ying S, et al. Predominant TH2-like bronchoalveolar T-lymphocyte population in atopic asthma. *N Engl J Med.* 1992;326(5):298–304.

62. Ray A, Cohn L. Th2 cells and GATA-3 in asthma: new insights into the regulation of airway inflammation. *J Clin Invest.* 1999; 104(8):985–993.

63. Walker C, Kaegi MK, Braun P, Blaser K. Activated T cells and eosinophilia in bronchoalveolar lavages from subjects with asthma correlated with disease severity. *J Allergy Clin Immunol.* 1991;88(6):935–942.

64. Cohn L, Elias JA, Chupp GL. Asthma: mechanisms of disease persistence and progression. *Annu Rev Immunol.* 2004;22:789–815.

65. Ober C, Hoffjan S. Asthma genetics 2006: the long and winding road to gene discovery. *Genes Immun.* 2006;7(2):95–100.

66. Vercelli D. Discovering susceptibility genes for asthma and allergy. *Nat Rev Immunol.* 2008;8(3):169–182.

67. Shannon J, Ernst P, Yamauchi Y, et al. Differences in airway cytokine profile in severe asthma compared to moderate asthma. *Chest.* 2008;133(2):420–426.

68. Woodruff PG, Modrek B, Choy DF, et al. T-helper type 2-driven inflammation defines major subphenotypes of asthma. *Am J Respir Crit Care Med.* 2009;180(5):388–395.

69. Holt PG, van den Biggelaar AH. 99th Dahlem conference on infection, inflammation and chronic inflammatory disorders: the role of infections in allergy: atopic asthma as a paradigm. *Clin Exp Immunol.* 2010;160(1):22–26.

70. Erb KJ, Holloway JW, Sobeck A, Moll H, Le Gros G. Infection of mice with Mycobacterium bovis-Bacillus Calmette-Guerin (BCG) suppresses allergen-induced airway eosinophilia. *J Exp Med.* 1998;187(4):561–569.

71. Martinez FD. Viral infections and the development of asthma. *Am J Respir Crit Care Med.* 1995;151(5):1644–1647; discussion 1647–1648.

72. Fernandez-Botran R, Sanders VM, Mosmann TR, Vitetta ES. Lymphokine-mediated regulation of the proliferative response of clones of T helper 1 and T helper 2 cells. *J Exp Med.* 1988;168: 543–558.

73. Iwamoto I, Nakajima H, Endo H, Yoshida S. Interferon g regulates antigen-induced eosinophil recruitment into the mouse airways by inhibiting the infiltration of CD4+ T cells. *J Exp Med.* 1993;177:573–576.

74. Coyle AJ, Tsuyuki S, Bertrand C, et al. Mice lacking the IFN-g receptor have an impaired ability to resolve a lung eosinophilic inflammatory response associated with a prolonged capacity of T cells to exhibit a Th2 cytokine profile. *J Immunol.* 1996;156: 680–2685.

75. Cohn L, Homer RJ, Niu N, Bottomly K. T helper 1 cells and interferon gamma regulate allergic airway inflammation and mucus production. *J Exp Med.* 1999;190(9):1309–1318.

76. Hansen G, Berry G, DeKruyff RH, Umetsu DT. Allergen-specific Th1 cells fail to counterbalance Th2 cell-induced airway hyperreactivity but cause severe airway inflammation. *J Clin Invest.* 1999;103(2):175–183.

77. Al-Ramli W, Prefontaine D, Chouiali F, et al. T(H)17-associated cytokines (IL-17 A and IL-17 F) in severe asthma. *J Allergy Clin Immunol.* 2009;123(5):1185–1187.

78. Hashimoto T, Akiyama K, Kobayashi N, Mori A. Comparison of IL-17 production by helper T cells among atopic and nonatopic asthmatics and control subjects. *Int Arch Allergy Immunol.* 2005; 137 Suppl 1:51–54.

79. Bullens DM, Truyen E, Coteur L, et al. IL-17 mRNA in sputum of asthmatic patients: linking T cell driven inflammation and granulocytic influx? *Respir Res.* 2006;7:135.

80. Alcorn JF, Crowe CR, Kolls JK. TH17 cells in asthma and COPD. *Annu Rev Physiol.* 2010;72:495–516.

81. Lajoie S, Lewkowich IP, Suzuki Y, et al. Complement-mediated regulation of the IL-17 A axis is a central genetic determinant of the severity of experimental allergic asthma. *Nat Immunol.* 2010;11(10):928–935.

82. Hellings PW, Kasran A, Liu Z, et al. Interleukin-17 orchestrates the granulocyte influx into airways after allergen inhalation in a mouse model of allergic asthma. *Am J Respir Cell Mol Biol.* 2003;28(1):42–50.

83. Lin W, Truong N, Grossman WJ, et al. Allergic dysregulation and hyperimmunoglobulinemia E in Foxp3 mutant mice. *J Allergy Clin Immunol.* 2005;116(5):1106–1115.

84. Lloyd CM, Hawrylowicz CM. Regulatory T cells in asthma. *Immunity.* 2009;31(3):438–449.

85. Hartl D, Koller B, Mehlhorn AT, et al. Quantitative and functional impairment of pulmonary CD4+CD25hi regulatory T cells in pediatric asthma. *J Allergy Clin Immunol.* 2007;119(5): 1258–1266.

86. Karagiannidis C, Akdis M, Holopainen P, et al. Glucocorticoids upregulate FOXP3 expression and regulatory T cells in asthma. *J Allergy Clin Immunol.* 2004;114(6):1425–1433.

87. Rubtsov YP, Rasmussen JP, Chi EY, et al. Regulatory T cell-derived interleukin-10 limits inflammation at environmental interfaces. *Immunity.* 2008;28(4):546–558.

88. Campbell JD, Buckland KF, McMillan SJ, et al. Peptide immunotherapy in allergic asthma generates IL-10-dependent immunological tolerance associated with linked epitope suppression. *J Exp Med.* 2009;206(7):1535–1547.

89. Ostroukhova M, Qi Z, Oriss TB, Dixon-McCarthy B, Ray P, Ray A. Treg-mediated immunosuppression involves activation of the Notch-HES1 axis by membrane-bound TGF-beta. *J Clin Invest.* 2006;116(4):996–1004.

90. Lewkowich IP, Herman NS, Schleifer KW, et al. CD4+CD25+ T cells protect against experimentally induced asthma and alter pulmonary dendritic cell phenotype and function. *J Exp Med.* 2005; 202(11):1549–1561.

91. Azzawi M, Bradley B, Jeffery PK, et al. Identificaiton of activated T lymphocytes and eosinophils in bronchial biopsies in stable atopic asthma. *Am Rev Respir Dis.* 1990;142:1407–1413.

92. van Rensen EL, Sont JK, Evertse CE, et al. Bronchial CD8 cell infiltrate and lung function decline in asthma. *Am J Respir Crit Care Med.* 2005;172(7):837–841.

93. Betts RJ, Kemeny DM. CD8+ T cells in asthma: friend or foe? *Pharmacol Ther.* 2009;121(2):123–131.

CHAPTER 26

Chemokines, Adipokines, and Growth Factors in the Lung

Marcus W. Butler
Paul McLoughlin
Michael P. Keane

Normal development of organ systems, including the lungs, in utero, during subsequent maturation into adulthood, and in health throughout life, requires intricate signals to be exchanged among various tissues, capable of permitting diversity and adaptation in differing cellular and extracellular contexts, while being robust to onslaughts from ever-changing environmental stimuli. Among the mediators involved in such complex cellular signaling, and relevant in the setting of many pulmonary disorders, are chemokines and growth factors. There has been further complexity added with increasing recognition of adipose tissue as a source of systemic bioactive mediators called adipokines, that impact on lung health. While some of these mediators are implicated in the development of disease states, they are more often than not also critical to tissue homeostasis, and are challenging target systems for therapeutic manipulation. Nonetheless, we are now in an era of exciting developments in targeted biologic therapies that offer the potential for substantial progress in the fight against difficult-to-treat pulmonary disorders characterized by pathogenic processes including acute and chronic inflammation, fibrosis, vascular remodeling, and neoplasia.

CHEMOTACTIC CYTOKINES AND THE INFLAMMATORY RESPONSE

The salient feature of inflammation is leukocyte infiltration. These recruited leukocytes contribute to the pathogenesis of chronic inflammation and promote fibrosis via the elaboration of a variety of cytokines. Maintenance of leukocyte recruitment during inflammation requires the expression of cell surface adhesion molecules, and the production of chemotactic molecules, such as chemokines.[1] The chemokines can be divided into four families—CXC, CC, C, and CXXXC—which behave as potent chemotactic factors for neutrophils, eosinophils, basophils, monocytes, mast cells, dendritic cells, NK cells, and T and B lymphocytes (Table 26-1). There is approximately 20% to 40% homology between the members of the four chemokine families.[2] Chemokines are produced by an array of cells, including monocytes, alveolar macrophages, neutrophils, platelets, eosinophils, mast cells, T and B lymphocytes, NK cells, and various structural cells, including keratinocytes, mesangial cells, epithelial cells, hepatocytes, fibroblasts, smooth muscle cells, mesothelial cells, and endothelial cells. Production of chemokines by both immune and nonimmune cells supports the contention that these cytokines may play a pivotal role in orchestrating chronic inflammation.[3]

■ CXC CHEMOKINES

CXC chemokines can be further divided into two groups on the basis of a structure/function domain consisting of the presence or absence of three amino acid residues (Glu-LeuArg; ELR motif) that precede the first cysteine amino acid residue in the primary structure of these cytokines. ELR+CXC chemokines are chemoattractants for neutrophils and act as potent angiogenic factors. In contrast, ELR−CXC chemokines are highly induced by interferons, are chemoattractants for mononuclear cells, and are potent inhibitors of angiogenesis (Table 26-2).[4]

Chemokine activities are mediated through G-protein–coupled receptors. Seven CXC chemokine receptors have been identified (Table 26-3). The ELR+ chemokines bind to CXCR1 and CXCR2 receptors, which are found on neutrophils, T lymphocytes, monocytes/macrophages, eosinophils, basophils, keratinocytes and mast cells, and endothelial cells.[5] CXCR3 is the receptor for CXCL9, CXCL10, and CXCL11, and is expressed on activated T lymphocytes. CXCR3 is also expressed on human umbilical vein endothelial cells (HUMVECs) in a cell cycle–dependent fashion. CXCR4 is the specific receptor for CXCL12 and is the cofactor for lymphotropic HIV-1. In contrast to CXCR3, CXCR4 appears to be expressed on resting T lymphocytes.[5] Two other chemokine receptors have been identified that bind chemokines without a subsequent signal-coupling event. The DARC receptor is similar to other chemokine receptors and it binds both CXC and CC chemokines without apparent signal coupling. This receptor was originally found on human erythrocytes and was thought to represent a "sink" for chemokines.[6] The second nonsignaling chemokine receptor is the D6 receptor, which binds several CC chemokines with high affinity, including CCL2, CCL4, CCL5, and CCL7.[7]

CXC Chemokines in Pulmonary Inflammation

CXC chemokines play a significant role in mediating neutrophil infiltration in the lung parenchyma and pleural space in response to endotoxin and bacterial challenge. CXCL8 is in the bronchoalveolar lavage of patients with community-acquired pneumonia and nosocomial pneumonia and a variety of animal models of pneumonia. In a model of *Aspergillus fumigatus* pneumonia, neutralization of TNF resulted in marked attenuation of the expression of CXCL1 and CXCL2/3 that was paralleled by a reduction in the infiltration of neutrophils and associated with increased mortality.[8] Administration of a TNF agonist peptide to animals that had been intratracheally inoculated with *Klebsiella pneumoniae* led to markedly elevated levels of CXCL2/3 associated with increased neutrophil infiltration.[9] Studies have shown that ventilator-induced lung injury is secondary to stretch-induced chemokine release with a subsequent inflammatory response and neutrophil recruitment.[10] CXCR2 −/− mice are also protected from hyperoxia-induced lung injury. In other studies, the production of CXCL5 in the lung was correlated with the presence of neutrophil-dependent lung injury, and passive immunization with neutralizing CXCL5 antibodies resulted in significant attenuation of lung injury.[11]

Several studies have demonstrated that CXCL8 levels correlate with the development and mortality of ARDS. Early increases in CXCL8 in bronchoalveolar lavage fluid correlated with an increased risk of subsequent development of ARDS, and also demonstrated that alveolar macrophages were an important source of CXCL8 prior to neutrophil influx.[10] Furthermore, there is an imbalance in the expression of ELR+ (CXCL1, CXCL5, CXCL8) as compared with ELR−CXC (CXCL10, CXCL11) chemokines from bronchoalveolar lavage fluid (BALF) of patients with ARDS as compared with controls. This imbalance correlated with angiogenic activity and both procollagen I and procollagen III levels in BALF.[12] These findings suggest that CXC chemokines have an important role in the fibroproliferative phase of ARDS via the regulation of angiogenesis.

TABLE 26-1 The Human C, CC, CXC, and CXXXC Chemokine Families of Chemotactic Cytokines

Systemic Name	Human Ligand Name
C Chemokines	
XCL1	Lymphotactin
XCL2	SCM-1β
CC Chemokines	
CCL1	I-309
CCL2	Monocyte chemotactic protein-1 (MCP-1)
CCL3	Macrophage inflammatory protein-1 alpha (MIP-1α)
CCL4	Macrophage inflammatory protein-1 beta (MIP-1β)
CCL5	Regulated on activation normal T-cell expressed and secreted (RANTES)
CCL7	Monocyte chemotactic protein-3 (MCP-3)
CCL8	Monocyte chemotactic protein-2 (MCP-2)
CCL9	Macrophage inflammatory protein-1 delta (MIP-1δ)
CCL11	Eotaxin
CCL13	Monocyte chemotactic protein-4 (MCP-4)
CCL14	HCC-1
CCL15	HCC-2
CCL16	HCC-4
CCL17	Thymus and activation-regulated chemokine (TARC)
CCL18	DC-CK-1
CCL19	Macrophage inflammatory protein-3 beta (MIP-3β)
CCL20	Macrophage inflammatory protein-3 alpha (MIP-3α)
CCL21	6Ckine
CCL22	MDC
CCL23	MPIF-1
CCL24	MPIF-2
CCL25	TECK
CCL26	Eotaxin-3
CCL27	CTACK
CCL28	MEC
CXC Chemokines	
CXCL1	Growth-related oncogene alpha (GRO-α)
CXCL2	Growth-related oncogene beta (GRO-β)
CXCL3	Growth-related oncogene gamma (GRO-γ)
CXCL4	Platelet factor-4 (PF4)
CXCL5	Epithelial neutrophil–activating protein-78 (ENA-78)
CXCL6	Granulocyte chemotactic protein-2 (GCP-2)
CXCL7	Neutrophil-activating protein-2 (NAP-2)
CXCL8	Interleukin-8 (IL-8)
CXCL9	Monokine induced by interferon-γ (MIG)
CXCL10	Interferon-γ-inducible protein (IP-10)
CXCL11	Interferon-inducible T cell alpha chemoattractant (ITAC)
CXCL12	Stromal cell–derived factor-1 (SDF-1)
CXCL13	B-cell–attracting chemokine-1 (BCA-1)
CXCL14	BRAK/Bolekine
CXCL16	
CXXXC Chemokine	
CXC3CL1	Fractalkine

TABLE 26-2 The CXC Chemokines that Display Disparate Angiogenic Activity

CXC Chemokines that contain the ELR motif	
CXCL1	Growth-related oncogene alpha (GRO-α)
CXCL2	Growth-related oncogene beta (GRO-β)
CXCL3	Growth-related oncogene gamma (GRO-γ)
CXCL5	Epithelial neutrophil–activating protein-78 (ENA-78)
CXCL6	Granulocyte chemotactic protein-2 (GCP-2)
CXCL7	Neutrophil-activating protein-2 (NAP-2)
CXCL8	Interleukin-8 (IL-8)
CXC Chemokines that lack the ELR motif	
CXCL4	Platelet factor-4 (PF4)
CXCL9	Monokine induced by interferon-γ (MIG)
CXCL10	Interferon-γ-inducible protein (IP-10)
CXCL11	Interferon-inducible T-cell alpha chemoattractant (ITAC)
CXCL12	Stromal cell–derived factor-1 (SDF-1)

The Role of CXC Chemokines in Pulmonary Fibrosis

IPF is characterized by the progressive deposition of collagen within the interstitium and subsequent destruction of lung tissue.[13,14] The mechanisms of cellular injury and the role of classic inflammatory cells remain unclear. CXCL8 is significantly elevated in IPF, as compared with either normal or sarcoidosis patients, and correlates with BALF presence of neutrophils. The alveolar macrophage is an important cellular source of CXCL8 in IPF.[15] In addition, BALF levels of CXCL8 in IPF may correlate with a worse prognosis.[16]

Vascular Remodeling in Pulmonary Fibrosis: The Role of CXC Chemokines

The existence of neovascularization in IPF was originally identified in 1963 by Turner-Warwick, who demonstrated that within areas of pulmonary fibrosis there was extensive neovascularization with anastomoses between the systemic and pulmonary microvasculature.[17] Further evidence of neovascularization during the pathogenesis of pulmonary fibrosis has been demonstrated in a rat model of bleomycin-induced pulmonary fibrosis.[18] An imbalance in the levels of angiogenic chemokines (CXCL5, CXCL8), as compared with angiostatic chemokines (CXCL9, CXCL10, CXCL11), favoring net angiogenesis has been demonstrated in both animal models and tissue specimens from patients with IPF (Fig. 26-1).[19] Renzoni[20] has demonstrated vascular remodeling in both IPF and fibrosing alveolitis associated with systemic sclerosis. Cosgrove et al.[21] provided further support for the concept of vascular remodeling in IPF when they demonstrated a relative absence of vessels in the fibroblastic foci of IPF. This appeared to correlate with increased expression of pigment epithelium–derived factor in the fibroblastic foci. Interestingly, they also noted significant vascularity in the areas of fibrosis around the fibroblastic foci, with numerous abnormal vessels in the regions of severe architectural distortion. These findings are similar to those of Renzoni and support the concept of regional heterogeneity of vascularity in IPF. This heterogeneity is not surprising, as usual interstitial pneumonia, which is the pathologic description of IPF, is defined by its regional and temporal heterogeneity.[14]

TABLE 26-3 The CXC Chemokine Receptors

Receptor	Ligand
CXCR1	CXCL6, CXCL7, CXCL8
CXCR2	CXCL1, CXCL2, CXCL3, CXCL5, CXCL6, CXCL7, CXCL8
CXCR3A	CXCL9, CXCL10, CXCL11
CXCR3B	CXCL4, CXCL9, CXCL10, CXCL11
CXCR4	CXCL12
CXCR5	CXCL13
CXCR6	CXCL16
CXCR7	CXCL11, CXCL12

CXC Chemokines in Pulmonary Hypertension

The potential role of the CXCL12/CXCR4/CXCR7 axis in pulmonary hypertension was first suspected when it was reported that CXCR7 expression increased in the lungs of hypoxic hypertensive mice and in the lungs of patients with idiopathic pulmonary arterial hypertension (IPAH).[22] Subsequently, CXCL12 was found to be elevated in the peripheral plasma of patients with pulmonary artery hypertension (PAH), although in a separate study this increase was not observed.[23,24] Increased expression of CXCL12 in remodeled vessels and particularly in the plexiform lesions in explanted IPAH lungs has also been shown.[25]

CXR7 was most prominently expressed in the endothelium of the explanted lungs of hypertensive subjects and, in addition to its well-established role in leukocyte chemotaxis, was shown to play a central role in stimulating endothelial proliferation, whereas CXCR4 was required for endothelial cell chemotaxis.[23] Recruitment of progenitor cells to the remodeled pulmonary vessels is a prominent feature in PAH lungs.[25,26] In vivo blockade of CXCR4 in hypoxic mice reduced the recruitment of progenitor cells to the remodeled vasculature of hypertensive lungs, whereas blockade of CXCR7 did not affect this behavior.[24,26,27]

In rodent models inhibition of CXCL12 action using function-blocking antibodies, or separate selective inhibition of CXCR4 signaling or CXCR7 signaling, attenuates the development of hypoxic pulmonary hypertension.[24,27,28] Taken together these data suggest an important role of CXCL12 signaling, requiring both its cognate receptors, in the pathogenesis of pulmonary hypertension.

CHEMOKINES AND THE TRAFFICKING OF FIBROCYTES TO THE LUNG

Fibrocytes present in the peripheral circulation were first identified in 1994, comprise a minor component of the circulating pool of leukocytes (less than 1%), and express a characteristic pattern of markers, including collagen (Col) I and CD45.[29] Subsequent studies have revealed that circulating fibrocytes express chemokine receptors such as CXCR4 and CCR7 and extracellular matrix (ECM) proteins, such as procollagen I and procollagen III. Fibrocytes migrate in response to CXCL12 and traffic to the lungs in a model of bleomycin-induced pulmonary fibrosis. Treatment of bleomycin-exposed animals with specific neutralizing anti-CXCL12 antibodies inhibits intrapulmonary recruitment of fibrocytes and attenuated lung fibrosis.[30] Levels of circulating CD45+ Col1+ cells are elevated in stable IPF patients versus controls, are transiently higher during an exacerbation and predicted survival.[31] These findings challenge the dogma that fibroblasts and myofibroblasts arise from an intrapulmonary pool of tissue fibroblasts.[32]

THE CC CHEMOKINES

CC chemokines (Table 26-1) are chemoattractants for monocyte, T and B lymphocytes, NK cells, dendritic cells, basophils, mast cells, and eosinophils.[33] The CC chemokines are produced by an array of cells, including monocytes, alveolar macrophages, neutrophils, platelets, eosinophils, mast cells, T cells, B cells, and NK cells, as well as structural cells such as keratinocytes, mesangial cells, epithelial

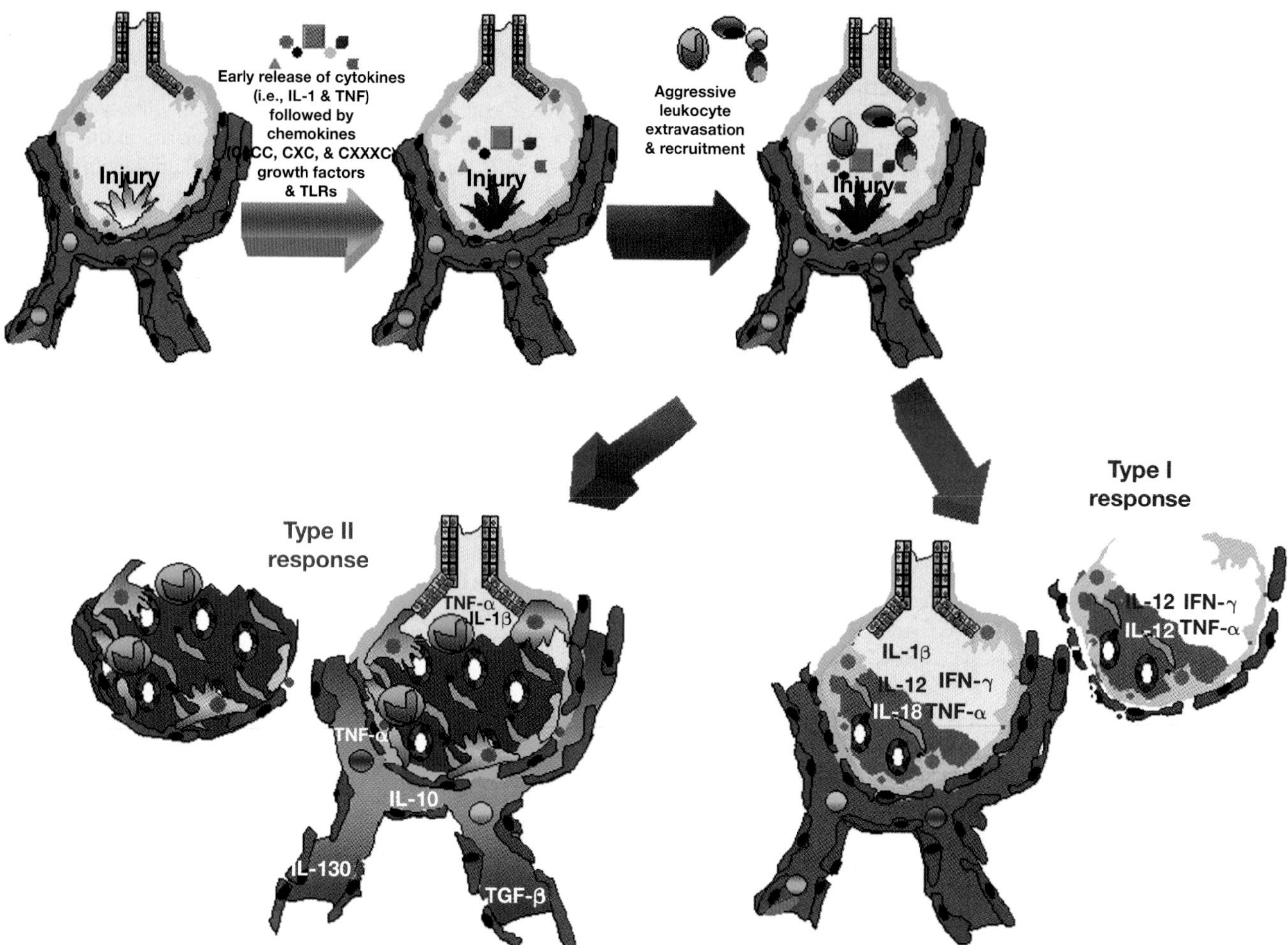

Figure 26-1 The inflammatory response to lung injury. The cytokine profile that is secreted by inflammatory cells during lung injury determines the ultimate outcome following injury. Polarization of the inflammatory response toward a type I response is associated with resolution of lung injury or infection. In contrast chronic infections (e.g., tuberculosis) and chronic inflammatory diseases (e.g., idiopathic pulmonary fibrosis) are associated with a type II profile.

cells, hepatocytes, fibroblasts, smooth muscle cells, mesothelial cells, and endothelial cells.[34]

CC Chemokine Receptors

CC chemokine receptors are structurally homologous and have been identified to have specific ligand-binding profiles (Table 26-4).[34] Naïve T cells express CXCR4 and CCR7 and migrate in response to CXCL12 and CCL19. CXCR3, CXCR6, and CCR5 are expressed at higher levels on type I cells than type II, whereas CCR3, CCR4, and CCR8 are more characteristic of type II cells.[35]

CC Chemokines in Pulmonary Inflammation

The CC chemokines, CCL2, CCL3, CCL4, CCL5 have been implicated in mediating the innate host defense in animal models of pulmonary infection.[36,37] These studies have demonstrated that CC chemokine ligand/receptor biology plays a critical role in innate host defense and development of pulmonary inflammation that is important in eradication of microorganisms.

Mehrad et al. have shown that CCL3 and the recruitment of mononuclear cells play an important role in the eradication of invasive pulmonary aspergillosis. They demonstrated that in both immunocompetent and neutropenic mice CCL3 is induced in the lungs in response to intratracheal inoculation of *A. fumigatus*.[38] These studies indicate that CCL3 and elicitation of mononuclear cells are crucial in mediating host defense against *A. fumigatus* in the setting of neutropenia.[39]

CC Chemokines in Pulmonary Fibrosis

Animal models, such as bleomycin-induced pulmonary fibrosis, have demonstrated the presence and contribution of CC chemokines to the pathogenesis of fibrosis. CCL2 is an important cofactor for the stimulation of fibroblast collagen production and induction of the expression of TGF-β_1. Inhibition of CCL2 or CCL3 resulted in

TABLE 26-4 The CC Chemokine Receptors

Receptor	Ligand
CCR1	CCL2, CCL3, CCL3LI, CCL4, CCL5, CCL7, CCL8, CCL13, CCL14, CCL15, CCL16, CCL23
CCR2	CCL2, CCL7, CCL8, CCL13, CCL16
CCR3	CCL5, CCL7, CCL8, CCL11, CCL13, CCL15, CCL16, CCL24, CCL26, CCL28
CCR4	CCL17, CCL22
CCR5	CCL3, CCL3LI, CCL4, CCL5, CCL7, CCL8, CCL11, CCL13, CCL14, CCL16
CCR6	CCL20
CCR7	CCL19, CCL21
CCR8	CCL1
CCR9	CCL25
CCR10	CCL27, CCL28

a reduction of infiltrating cells into the lungs of bleomycin-treated animals.[40,41]

Furthermore, it has been shown that CCL2 can stimulate interleukin-4 (IL-4) production, indicating that it might be involved in type II polarization.[42] IL-13 promotes bleomycin-induced fibrosis through the elaboration of CCL6.[43] Both CCL17 and CCL22 and their receptor, CCR4, are significantly elevated in the bleomycin model and neutralization of CCL17 attenuates pulmonary fibrosis.[44] Thus, chemokines may have an important role in the switch toward a profibrotic type II phenotype.

Both CCR1 and CCR2 have been shown to play an important role in the pathogenesis in the mouse model of bleomycin-induced pulmonary fibrosis. Treatment with antibodies to CCR1 leads to a reduction in both inflammatory cell infiltrates and the development of fibrosis.[45] Similarly, CCR2 −/− mice are protected from pulmonary fibrosis in response to bleomycin.[46] Furthermore, alveolar epithelial cells from CCR2 −/− mice suppress fibroblast proliferation more than AECs from wild-type mice.[47] CCL2 and CCR2 have an important role in suppression of PGE2, thereby promoting fibroproliferation. Similarly, an important role for CCR2 has been seen in murine model of obliterative bronchiolitis, in which the fibrotic response associated with this disorder was attenuated in CCR2 −/− mice.[48] Similarly, CCL2 and CCL3 are elevated in BALF and lung tissue of ILD patients.[49,50] Accordingly, targeting chemokine receptors may be an efficient way to inhibit pulmonary fibrosis.

Choi et al.[51] described enhanced expression of the chemokines CCL7 and CCL22, in lung tissue of patients with IPF as compared with nonspecific interstitial pneumonia, and nonidiopathic interstitial pneumonia. Furthermore, they describe increased expression of CCL5 in nonspecific interstitial pneumonia as compared with usual interstitial pneumonia. Interestingly, CCL5 protein was identified in nonspecific interstitial pneumonia more prominently than usual interstitial pneumonia. This is all the more interesting as CCL5 is a major stimulus for the production of CCL7 through its interactions with CCR5. These findings raise the possibility that there is a continuum from nonspecific interstitial pneumonia to usual interstitial pneumonia with higher levels of CCL5 in nonspecific interstitial pneumonia leading to subsequent increased CCL7 expression as the disease progresses to usual interstitial pneumonia. There is considerable controversy as to whether nonspecific interstitial pneumonia is an earlier lesion of usual interstitial pneumonia.[52] Several studies have demonstrated the presence of usual interstitial pneumonia and nonspecific interstitial pneumonia patterns in the same patients, which suggests that these are overlapping processes.[52–54] The findings of Choi suggest a transition from a predominance of CCL5 to CCL7 and further support this notion. Of further interest is the previous description that CCL7 can act as a natural antagonist at the CCR5 receptor, which raises the possibility that CCL7 may play a role in regulating its own production.[55]

ADIPOKINES AND PULMONARY INFLAMMATION

With the emergence, in the 20th century, of obesity as a major epidemic linked to systemic metabolic dysfunction, concerted efforts have been made to gain a fuller understanding of the varied functions of adipose tissue, beyond that of being an energy storage organ, and leading to the discovery of various factors that are secreted by adipocytes.[56] These mainly proteinaceous endocrine factors were initially termed adipocytokines, and later, adipokines,[57] and possess pro- and anti-inflammatory activities, potentially of relevance in the context of pulmonary disorders associated with body mass index, including asthma, obstructive sleep apnea syndrome, chronic obstructive pulmonary disease (COPD), PAH, various pulmonary infections, and lung cancer.[58] While the main source of adipocytes in the body is from deposits of subcutaneous and visceral adipose tissue, the development of obesity can give rise to collections of adipose tissue in other locations including the heart, kidneys, bone marrow, the adventitia of major blood vessels, and within the lungs. There is evidence that differential adipokine secretion and functional outcomes can occur at different sites of adiposity within the body, following the stimulus of dietary modification.[59] White adipose tissue, the major form in humans, is predominantly composed of lipid-laden adipocytes, but also adipocyte precursor cells, fibroblasts that generate ECM scaffolding, vascular (smooth muscle and endothelial) cells that provide systemic access for secreted adipokines, and macrophages and T cells that influence the immune phenotype.[60] The cellular composition of adipose tissue can vary in conditions of altered body mass, and macrophages in particular, seem to traffic in larger numbers to adipose tissue under conditions of increased obesity with associated capillary rarefaction and adipose tissue hypoxia.[61]

PROINFLAMMATORY ADIPOKINES

Beyond the "pure" effects of uncomplicated obesity upon respiratory mechanics, pulmonary gas exchange, ventilatory drive, and work of breathing, there is increasing evidence of an association among obesity, adipokines, and pulmonary disease states that are characterized by inflammation.[58] Most of the adipokines identified to date are proinflammatory in their effects (Table 26-5). Some important adipokines that are better known for their other roles, such as TNF-α, IL-6, CCL2, and CXCL5, will not be discussed here.

Leptin

Leptin, coded for by the *ob* gene on chromosome 17, is a 16 KDa protein hormone, mainly secreted by adipocytes,[62] and regulated principally by food intake, whereby fasting reduces leptin levels,

TABLE 26-5 Adipokines Linked to Pulmonary Disease States

Adipokine	Pulmonary Source	Receptor	Lung Disease State
Proinflammatory Adipokines			
Leptin	Alveolar type II pneumocytes, alveolar macrophages, bronchial epithelial cells, lung endothelial cells	Leptin receptor	OSAHS, OHS, COPD, asthma, NSCLC, PAH
Apelin	Lung endothelial cells	Apelin receptor	PAH
Nampt	Lung endothelial cells	Unknown	ALI
Resistin	Unknown	Unknown	Asthma
Anti-inflammatory Adipokines			
Adiponectin	Bronchial epithelial cells	Adiponectin receptors 1 and 2, T-cadherin	COPD, asthma, ALI, PAH

OSAHS, obstructive sleep apnea-hypopnea syndrome; OHS, obesity hypoventilation syndrome; COPD, chronic obstructive pulmonary disease; NSCLC, non–small-cell lung cancer; PAH, pulmonary arterial hypertension; ALI, acute lung injury.

and food consumption transiently increases *ob* gene expression, with leptin being initially regarded as a satiety hormone.[63,64] It is also expressed in human peripheral lung tissue, including alveolar type II pneumocytes, alveolar macrophages, and bronchial epithelial cells,[65,66] and is known to be modulated by gender, sepsis, catecholamines, glucocorticoids, and insulin.[67,68] It is now clear that leptin has pleiotropic effects, which include stimulating TNF and IL-6 production by monocytes, stimulating production of CCL3–5 by macrophages, and stimulating reactive oxygen species production, cell proliferation, and migration. In addition, leptin may have a role in lung development,[56] as it is differentially expressed by fetal rat lung fibroblasts during the time of alveolar differentiation,[69] and capable of stimulating fetal rat surfactant protein synthesis in vitro,[70] although contradictory in vivo findings were observed in fetal sheep and mice lungs.[71]

There have been extensive efforts to relate leptin to respiratory disorders, most notably with obstructive sleep apnea-hypopnea syndrome (OSAHS), COPD, asthma, pneumonia, and other pulmonary infections. Some data suggest leptin has a stimulatory effect on ventilation; for example, the mutant *ob/ob* mouse, which lacks functional leptin and has a phenotype of obesity, hyperphagia, and a low-resting metabolic rate, displays an elevated arterial Pa_{CO_2} independent of obesity onset, which is acutely reversible through exogenous leptin replacement.[72] It has been speculated that OSAHS is a leptin-resistant state, but progress in this field has been hampered by conflicting results of leptin and leptin receptor candidate gene association studies[73,74] and trials of nasal continuous positive airway pressure.[75,76]

In COPD, it has been hypothesized that the known link between the cachexia of COPD and increased mortality, might somehow be related to leptin function. There appears to be an absence of the usual circadian rhythm of circulating leptin in cachectic COPD patients, as opposed to normal weight COPD patients, with associated heart rate variability changes that raise the possibility of a role for leptin in the pathophysiology of COPD cachexia,[77] although further data are needed. The reproducible finding of elevated serum leptin levels during acute exacerbations of COPD, that track markers of the systemic inflammatory response, points to disturbance of the normal leptin feedback loop regulating food intake and energy balance, due to the influence of the acute inflammatory response and systemically administered glucocorticoids, as a possible contributing mechanism to cachexia in COPD.[78] Wild-type mice exposed chronically to cigarette smoke have increased leptin expression in bronchial epithelial cells and pneumocytes versus air-exposed controls. *Ob/ob* mice (lacking functional leptin) that are then exposed acutely or chronically to cigarette smoke exhibit higher neutrophils, CD4+, CD8+, and dendritic cells in BAL and lung tissue than smoke-exposed wild-type mice, compatible with modulation of innate and adaptive immune cell recruitment by leptin in response to smoke.[79] Within human airways, leptin expression is increased in bronchial epithelial cells and alveolar macrophages of ex-smokers with or without severe COPD compared to never smokers, and leptin can induce phosphorylation of the transcription factor STAT3 in lung epithelial cells, supporting the notion of a functioning leptin signaling pathway in these cells.[65]

Obesity is believed to be a risk factor for asthma, but some controversy still surrounds whether or not obesity is a central cause or a confounding comorbidity of asthma.[80,81] Notably, unbiased clustering approaches in severe asthma subjects have identified an obesity-related clinical asthma phenotype typified by obese, female patients with late-onset asthma, and lacking in eosinophilic Th2-mediated inflammation.[82] Ob/ob mice, a model of loss of leptin function, appear to have elevated pulmonary resistance, and increased responses to ozone and methacholine, though this could be mechanical bias from the low lung size of these mutant mice.[68] Interestingly, when a cohort of obese asthmatic women and obese female controls were studied in the setting of bariatric surgery, leptin expression and macrophage inflammation were both increased in visceral adipose tissue of asthmatics independent of BMI, and correlated with airway reactivity, but there was no association with airway inflammation measurements even though the airway epithelial cells expressed receptors for leptin, suggesting that leptin exerts a direct effect on airway epithelium (and not indirectly via enhancing airway inflammation) that is important in the pathogenesis of asthma in obesity.[83] These observations run counter to the hypothesis that leptin is merely a marker for airway inflammation in poorly controlled asthma.[84]

Nampt (PBEF/visfatin)

The gene Nampt codes for a cytokine called pre–B cell colony-enhancing factor (PBEF), also known as visfatin. It is now known to be produced by various cell types including adipocytes, and especially by visceral as opposed to subcutaneous fat, and has gained greater interest by the rediscovery of PBEF as Nampt, the rate-limiting enzyme in the biosynthesis of the essential redox cofactor, NAD. Nampt is inducible in neutrophils and lung microvascular endothelial cells by endotoxin, TNF-α and IL-1β, and in monocytes, it induces production of IL-1β, TNF-α, and IL-6, and the surface expression of costimulatory molecules CD54, CD40, and CD80.[85,86] Against this background of catalyzing the respiratory burst, and its proinflammatory and immunomodulatory capabilities, Nampt has been demonstrated to be found at higher concentrations in serum and BAL fluid from patients with acute lung injury.[87] There have also been a number of independent candidate gene association studies that support a role for Nampt promoter genetic variants in ALI pathogenesis.[87–89]

■ ANTI-INFLAMMATORY ADIPOKINES

Adiponectin

The most intensely studied of the anti-inflammatory adipokines, and with notable evidence of a role in inflammatory lung disorders, is adiponectin, which shares some structural similarity with complement factor C1q, and forms trimers that can go on to form stable hexamers or a high molecular weight form, all of which are detectable in blood.[60] Circulating adiponectin levels are decreased in obesity, particularly in visceral obesity, nonalcoholic fatty liver disease, and type 2 diabetes, being inversely related to insulin resistance. The adipokine is inhibited by proinflammatory factors such as TNF, IL-6, hypoxia, and oxidative stress.[56] There has been considerable interest concerning the involvement of adiponectin in pulmonary disease states. Three described adiponectin receptors (AdipoR1, AdipoR2, and T-cadherin) are expressed in the lungs, with AdipoR1 expressed by lung epithelial cells, and importantly, the baseline phenotype of mice following targeted disruption of the adiponectin gene shows evidence of emphysema-like dilated air spaces and activation of alveolar macrophages.[90,91] These same adiponectin-deficient mice develop pulmonary hypertension with evidence of perivascular inflammation,[92] and an exaggerated form of LPS-inducible acute lung injury that is abrogated by adiponectin.[93]

As further evidence of anti-inflammatory functionality, adiponectin can bind to apoptotic cells and facilitate their phagocytosis by macrophages, analogous to other members of the collectin family, such as C1q and surfactant proteins A and D.[94] In keeping with this intuitive role in airways disease pathobiology, a number of groups have reported increased levels of circulating adiponectin in COPD.[91,95] Adiponectin was found to be elevated in BALF of COPD patients, being highly expressed in their airway epithelium, and the adiponectin receptor AdipoR1 on lung epithelial cells was shown to be functional, releasing IL-8 in the presence of adiponectin.[91] Animal and human data suggest that short-term exposure to cigarette smoke downregulates adiponectin whereas the COPD disease state elevates its expression.[91] In contrast, AdipoR2 is more highly expressed in the airway epithelium of obese asthma patients versus obese control subjects, and the opposite to what is observed for T-cadherin expression.[83] In mice, allergen challenge appears to decrease the pulmonary expression of all three adiponectin receptor types, and T-cadherin may play a role in transporting adiponectin into the lungs.[96] The exact role of adiponectin signaling in asthma will require further study.

■ ADIPOKINES AND PULMONARY HYPERTENSION

The high prevalence of pulmonary hypertension in obese subjects has previously been attributed to hypoxemia resulting from associated obstructive sleep apnea or obesity hypoventilation syndrome.[97–99] However, more recently evidence has been presented that alterations in three specific adipokines (adiponectin, apelin, and leptin) may directly contribute to pulmonary vascular dysfunction.

Adiponectin concentrations are paradoxically reduced in the plasma of obese subjects despite the expansion of adipose tissue.[100] Mice in which adiponectin has been deleted spontaneously develop elevated pulmonary arterial pressure, vascular remodeling, and perivascular inflammation as they grow older.[92] Conversely constitutive overexpression of adiponectin in mice protects against the development of both hypoxia-induced and inflammation-induced (ovalbumin challenge) pulmonary hypertension.[101] These suggest that reduced adiponectin concentrations contribute directly to the development of pulmonary vascular dysfunction in obesity due to a loss of its normal vascular homeostatic action.

Apelin is produced and secreted by adipocytes and acts by binding to the apelin receptor.[102] It is also expressed by a wide variety of other tissues including the pulmonary vasculature.[102] Plasma apelin concentrations are increased in obese individuals.[103] Apelin null mice develop more severe hypoxic pulmonary hypertension than wild-type mice, which is associated with endothelial dysfunction.[104] Leptin concentrations are elevated in patients with both idiopathic PAH and scleroderma-associated PAH and in the pulmonary endothelium from these patients.[105,106] However, the exact role of apelin and leptin in the pulmonary circulation in obese humans remains to be determined.

GROWTH FACTORS

■ TRANSFORMING GROWTH FACTOR-BETA

Mammalian transforming growth factor-beta (TGF-β) belongs to a superfamily of genes and exists as three closely homologous (72%–80%) dimeric isoforms: TGF-β_1, TGF-β_2, and TGF-β_3. Although the three isoforms of TGF-β appear to have overlapping biologic activity, the predominant isoform of TGF-β is TGF-β_1. There are three TGF-β receptors and signal transduction to the nucleus is via the Smad group of proteins. Smad 1, 2, 3, 4, 5, 8, and 9 are activating signals, whereas Smad 6 and 7 are inhibitory signals of TGF-β_1 signaling.[107]

TGF-β is produced by a variety of cells, including platelets, neutrophils, eosinophils, mononuclear leukocytes, fibroblasts, and endothelial cells.[108,109] TGF-β is a pleiotropic cytokine that can modulate inflammatory and immune responses, and orchestrate fibrosis and tissue repair.[110] TGF-β is a potent immunosuppressive agent that inhibits IL-1–dependent lymphocyte proliferation.

TGF-β is chemotactic for fibroblasts and can indirectly induce their proliferation via the expression and autocrine and paracrine activity of PDGF-B. TGF-β is perhaps the most potent and efficacious promoter of ECM production–inducing gene expression and protein production of many of the constituents of ECM. Furthermore, it inhibits the generation of metalloproteinases and augments the expression of tissue inhibitors of metalloproteinases (TIMP).[108,111]

Transient overexpression of active TGF-β_1 results in prolonged and severe interstitial and pleural fibrosis.[112] Transfer of TNF-α or granulocyte macrophage colony–stimulating factor (GM-CSF) to rat lung induces pulmonary fibrosis, due in part to induction of TGF-β_1.[113] Furthermore, transient expression of IL-1β using an adenoviral vector can lead to progressive fibrosis that is associated with a sustained increase in levels of TGF-β_1.[114] Smad 3 −/− mice developed less fibrosis in response to bleomycin compared with wild-type controls.[115] In contrast, IL-7 downregulates TGF-β production and inhibits bleomycin-induced pulmonary fibrosis, and this is mediated via Smad 7 signaling.[116]

In IPF, increased expression of TGF-β has been found in bronchiolar epithelial cells, epithelial cells of honeycomb cysts, and hyperplastic type II pneumocytes. BALF from patients with IPF induces apoptosis in cultured bronchiolar epithelial cells, and this effect is attenuated using anti–TGF-β_1 antibodies.[117] In the bleomycin model, in vivo administration of TGF-β_1 enhanced Fas-mediated epithelial cell apoptosis and lung injury.[117] These studies support the contention that TGF-β is an important mediator of human pulmonary fibrosis.

TGF-beta Superfamily Members and Pulmonary Hypertension

Disturbance of signaling by members of the TGF-β superfamily plays a key role in pulmonary hypertension.[118–121] The bone morphogenetic proteins (BMPs) and their receptors form part of the TGF-β superfamily, whose activities include important proangiogenic and vascular remodeling effects in endothelial and vascular smooth muscle cells.[22,122] The BMPs, like all ligands of the TGF-β superfamily, bind to transmembrane cell surface receptors formed from heterodimerization of a type 1 and type 2 receptor, many of which are expressed in the normal lung and can form a large number of different heteromeric receptor combinations binding with particular BMP ligands. BMP signaling is further modulated by a family of secreted extracellular glycoproteins, accessory proteins that bind directly to BMPs and prevent or enhance their interactions with BMPRs.[123,124]

The requirement for normal BMP function to maintain a healthy pulmonary circulation was first demonstrated by the identification of heterozygote inheritance of mutations in BMPR2 gene as the underlying cause in the rare heritable form of pulmonary arterial hypertension (HPAH) and in a significant proportion (10%–40%) of patients with IPAH without a previous family history.[125–127] These mutations cause attenuation of the normal cellular responses to the BMPs in the lung, where BMP2 and BMP4 signaling through BMP type 1 receptor (BMPR1) and BMPR2 heterodimers play particularly important roles in normal vascular homeostasis, and result in pulmonary hypertension.[121,128–132] Experimentally induced loss of function BMPR2 mutations in mice, or expression of dominant negative BMPR2 constructs, were sufficient to cause the development of pulmonary hypertension alone or increased susceptibility to other well-known causes of PH.[130,132–134] Conversely, overexpression of BMPR2 in the endothelium protected mice against the development of hypoxic pulmonary hypertension.[135] These data show that reduced BMP signaling in the lung either causes pulmonary hypertension or increases susceptibility to other causes of PH.

Later studies reported that reduced BMP signaling was found in many of the common forms of pulmonary hypertension, including hypoxic pulmonary hypertension,[121,131,136] although it was not clear what mechanisms cause reduced BMP signaling in these conditions. More recent work has shown that the glycoprotein BMP antagonist gremlin is markedly and selectively increased in the hypoxic mouse lung and in human lungs with PAH.[22] Genetically manipulated mice with reduced gremlin expression (haplodeficient) are partially protected against the development of hypoxic pulmonary hypertension, suggesting that upregulation of gremlin with a consequent reduction in BMP signaling is an important contributor to the pathogenesis of pulmonary hypertension.[123,137] Furthermore the basal normoxic expression of gremlin is higher in the lung than in any other organ, potentially rendering it more vulnerable to any loss of BMP signaling and may help to explain why the vascular abnormality in hereditary PAH is restricted to the pulmonary circulation even though the expression of mutant BMPR2 is ubiquitous in all vascular beds.[138]

TGF-β are also expressed in the lung as are their type 1 receptors (TGF-βR1) ALK1 and ALK5, and TGF-β receptor type 2 (TGF-βR2) and increased TGF-β signaling has been observed in some forms of pulmonary hypertension.[118–121] Furthermore, PAH develops in a subset of hereditary hemorrhagic telangiectasia patients who have heterozygous mutations in one of the TGF-β type 1 receptors, the ALK1 (activin receptor-like kinase 1).[139,140] Heterozygous mutations in the endoglin (ENG) gene, which codes for a TGF-β coreceptor, are also associated with the spontaneous development of PAH.[139] $ENG^{+/-}$ mice developed pulmonary hypertension associated with loss of peripheral vasculature in adulthood but not in early postnatal life.[141] Taken together these data indicate a requirement for normal TGF-β signaling to prevent the development of pulmonary hypertension.

■ EPIDERMAL GROWTH FACTOR

Epidermal growth factor (EGF) is the prototype member of a family of polypeptide ligands that interact with the ERBB family of four tyrosine kinase receptors (ERBB1–4, also known as human epidermal growth factor receptor, HER1–4).[142,143] All 13 of the EGF extracellular ligands described to date, which include transforming growth factor-α (TGF-α), heparin-binding(HB)-EGF, amphiregulin, epiregulin, and betacellulin among others, contain a conserved EGF domain and are made as a transmembrane protein that is then cleaved by cell surface proteases (ectodomain shedding) to release mature growth factors that bind ERBB, such as the case with EGF which binds to HER1/EGFR.[144] EGF motifs are also found in unrelated proteins including ECM and cell adhesion proteins, blood coagulation factors, and immune response proteins.[145] Control of ERBB family signaling occurs at many levels, including specific cellular patterns of ligand and receptor expression, subcellular segregation of ligands and receptors, and the diversity of intracellular receptor binding proteins that can amplify or attenuate receptor signaling and transcription factor activation, leading to varying cellular outputs of cell proliferation, adhesion, migration, differentiation, or apoptosis.[142] Dysfunctional EGF–ERBB signaling in the lung has consequently been implicated in lung tumorigenesis and lung injury.[146]

EGFR (ERBB1/HER1) is overexpressed in a large number of non–small-cell lung cancers (NSCLCs), and its expression has been correlated with a poor prognosis.[147] NSCLCs will also often express EGFR cognate ligands EGF and TGF-α, leading to receptor hyperactivity in an autocrine fashion.[148] The tyrosine kinase inhibitors gefitinib and erlotinib target the EGF–ERBB complex by acting as competitive inhibitors of ATP binding at the active site of the kinase. It became apparent that drug-responsive cases were enriched for somatic activating mutations in the EGFR kinase domain, with these mutations occurring at a greater frequency in nonsmokers, women, those of Asian genetic ancestry, and in adenocarcinoma.[149]

There is overlap between the signaling events that orchestrate the proliferation, migration, and differentiation of the developing lung epithelia, and those events that are active during lung injury and repair. The importance of EGF motif signaling in lung development is apparent from the HB-EGF(−/−) mouse hypoplastic lung phenotype, characterized by fewer alveoli and less surfactant. Similarly, the EGFR knockout mice display alveolar collapse, reduced alveolarization and loss of surfactant expression, resulting in a phenotype similar to the neonatal respiratory distress syndrome,[150] and exogenous EGF can rescue EGFR(−/−) fetal lambs from such a phenotype.[151] Later in life, there is evidence implicating EGFR signaling in an in vitro model of alveolar epithelial wound repair.[152] and bronchial epithelial repair in asthma.[153] A body of evidence has also implicated EGFR signaling in the pathogenesis of pulmonary fibrosis: For example, TGF-α (−/−) mice are protected from bleomycin-induced fibrosis,[154] as are wild-type mice exposed to bleomycin but administered gefitinib.[155] Given that ERBB tyrosine kinase inhibitors can also cause interstitial lung disease in clinical use,[156] it remains to be seen how best the complex ERBB signaling pathways can be therapeutically manipulated in the lung fibrosis arena.

■ VASCULAR ENDOTHELIAL GROWTH FACTOR

Initially described as a growth factor for endothelial cells, vascular endothelial growth factor (VEGF) is highly expressed in many different lung cell types, and has important roles in lung development and maintenance of lung tissue integrity, through its angiogenic, lymphangiogenic, and hematopoietic roles.[157] VEGF is produced by endothelial cells, fibroblasts, neutrophils, peripheral blood mononuclear cells (PBMCs), and macrophages, and exists as any of five family members, VEGF A, B, C, D, and placenta growth factor (PLGF) and further diversity in biologic activity arises from various alternatively spliced isoforms of family members,[158] including VEGFA121, VEGFA145, VEGFA165, VEGFA189, and VEGFA206, named after the number of coded amino acids. Transcription of VEGF is induced by hypoxia, IL-1β, and by many growth factors including platelet-derived growth factor, TGF-α and -β, insulin growth factor 1, fibrocyte growth factor, and FGF7 (keratinocyte growth factor [KGF]). The VEGF family members have three different VEGF receptors, with VEGFA binding to VEGFR1 and VEGFR2. VEGFR2 −/− mice have lethal defects in vasculogenesis and angiogenesis.[159] The role of VEGF in lung development is complex and can be highlighted by a number of observations. When embryonic murine lungs are cultured, VEGF expression, initially diffuse, is restricted over time and space to subepithelial matrix in the branching tips of the developing airways.[160] Furthermore, aberrant lung morphology has been shown to arise from targeted overexpression or underexpression of VEGF.[161,162] In bronchopulmonary dysplasia, the disease of prematurity and its attending interventions including hyperoxia, there was a demonstrable reduction in lung expression of VEGF, VEGFR1, and Tie-2 associated with disrupted pulmonary vasculature.[163]

There is some evidence to suggest that VEGF may play a protective role in emphysema. Partial and transient inactivation of VEGF gene in murine lungs using an adeno-associated *cre* recombinase virus and conditional VEGF knockout mice, VEGF*loxP*, resulted in apoptosis of alveolar and bronchial cells with ensuing air space enlargement and reduced elastic recoil, reminiscent of emphysema.[164] The low levels of VEGF expressed in human emphysematous lung[165] may be due to upstream factors that cause a reduction in expression of the major controller of VEGF expression, hypoxia-inducible factor (HIF)-1α in COPD lungs.[166]

VEGF and Pulmonary Hypertension

VEGF levels have been variably reported as increased, reduced, or unchanged in pulmonary hypertension with no consistent pattern emerging. However, studies directly examining the effect of inhibiting or stimulating VEGF receptors have produced a coherent picture. Blockade of VEGFR2 using small molecule inhibitors in rats aggravated hypoxic pulmonary hypertension, reduced pulmonary VEGFR2 expression, and increased endothelial cell apoptosis suggesting that VEGFR2 was essential for maintaining and expanding the vascular bed in the hypoxic lung.[167] Moreover, even following return to normoxia and withdrawal of VEGFR2 blockade the pulmonary hypertension was progressive and ultimately fatal. After extended time periods in this model complex plexiform-like lesions similar to those found in human PAH are observed.[168] Mice also show aggravation of hypoxic pulmonary hypertension in the presence of VEGFR2 blockade.[169] Interestingly, pulmonary hypertension has occasionally been reported in patients receiving VEGF inhibitors as part of a cancer chemotherapy treatment program.[170]

Overexpression of VEGFA in the rat lung using adenoviral vectors protected against the development of pulmonary hypertension although no analysis of the capillaries and small intra-acinar vessels (<50 μm) was carried out so it is not possible to know if this protection was accompanied by angiogenesis.[171] Louzier et al.[172] found that overexpression of VEGFB in the hypoxic rat lung using an adenoviral vector strategy protected against the development of hypertension and increased vessel density within the lung. Thus, it is clear that the balanced actions of agonist and inhibitory members of the VEGF family are essential for normal adaptation of the pulmonary circulation to hypoxia although the precise role of the VEGF pathway in human pulmonary hypertension is at present unclear.

■ FIBROBLAST GROWTH FACTOR

The fibroblast growth factor (FGF) family consists of 18 secreted polypeptide ligands that bind to one of four target cell surface FGF receptors (FGFR), that are tyrosine kinase receptors (FGFR1–4), and have many isoforms as a result of exon skipping and alternative splicing, the latter being generally tissue specific.[173] FGF subfamilies are grouped for their shared sequence homology and phylogeny. FGFs regulate diverse biologic processes including angiogenesis and organogenesis including proliferation, cell migration, and paracrine effects on tissue patterning. Two of the FGF ligands have particular relevance to the lung, both within the FGF7 subfamily including FGF7 (KGF) and FGF10.[173,174]

FGF7 is expressed specifically by mesenchymal cells including fibroblasts and vascular smooth muscle cells, and binds exclusively to an epithelial receptor FGFR2-IIIb, suggesting a paracrine loop effect in its epithelial–mesenchymal interactions. Using a dominant-negative mutant to inhibit FGFR2-IIIb results in an absence of branching morphogenesis within the developing murine lung,[175] and FGF7 overexpression results in enlarged bronchial air spaces and papillary cystadenomas.[176] A variety of experimental data have indicated that FGF7 expression increases following acute lung injury and that FGF7 is protective, principally when used as a pretreatment, in the face of injury caused by varied insults including hyperoxia, radiation, graft versus host disease following allogeneic bone marrow transplant, acid, and bleomycin,[174,177–179] but FGF7 may also partially prevent loss of barrier function in airway epithelium when given after an inciting exposure, potentially making FGF7 a more attractive therapeutic intervention were it so.[180,181] Notably, recombinant FGF7 (palifermin) which improves wound healing through cellular proliferation, is FDA approved for the treatment of chemoradiation-induced oral mucositis.[182] In addition to FGF7, FGF10 plays a critical role in lung development, given that FGF10(−/−) mice have defects in branching morphogenesis in lungs and other organs.[183] FGF10 overexpression attenuates bleomycin-induced pulmonary fibrosis in mice.[184] Interestingly, the triple angiokinase inhibitor nintedanib (BIBF 1120), inhibits VEGFR(1-3), platelet-derived growth factor receptors α and β, as well as FGFR1-3, and in a recent phase II clinical trial in patients with idiopathic pulmonary fibrosis, produced clinically meaningful reductions in the decline in forced vital capacity.[185]

■ GRANULOCYTE MACROPHAGE COLONY-STIMULATING FACTOR

GM-CSF is a glycosylated secreted protein produced by a variety of cells including macrophages, endothelial cells, T cells, natural killer cells, mast cells, and fibroblasts. It is defined by its ability to expand in vitro bone marrow precursor cells, via proliferation and differentiation, into colonies of mature myeloid cells, and act as a proinflammatory cytokine.[186–188] Interest from the pulmonary field grew with the initial observation that mice lacking GM-CSF had no major perturbation of hematopoiesis, but had an unexpected finding of compromised maturation of alveolar macrophages resulting in a phenotype of pulmonary alveolar proteinosis (PAP), with defective clearing of surfactant by alveolar macrophages.[189] The major form of human PAP is classified as autoimmune (or primary) PAP, accounting for about 90% of all PAP cases.[190] Autoimmune PAP is characterized by abnormally elevated levels of GM-CSF IgG autoantibodies, that bind GM-CSF with high affinity and neutralize GM-CSF functionality, and results in persistence of dysfunctional alveolar macrophages that are less efficient, with associated neutrophil dysfunction leading to opportunistic infections.[191] While whole lung lavage remains the cornerstone of therapy for PAP, targeted interventions to address the neutralization of GM-CSF are under active study using either (subcutaneous or inhaled) recombinant GM-CSF therapy, rituximab, or plasmapheresis, all with varying success to date.[192]

■ CONNECTIVE TISSUE GROWTH FACTOR

Connective tissue growth factor (CTGF) is a member of the structurally related CCN (ctgf/cyr61/nov) gene family, which contains six genes: ctgf, cyr61, nov, elm1, cop1, and WISP-3.[193] CTGF is produced by vascular smooth muscle cells, fibroblasts, endothelial cells, and epithelial cells, and is activated by a number of factors, particularly TGF-β.[193] CTGF has in vitro activities that include fibroblast proliferation, fibroplasia, and ECM production.[193–195] Furthermore, its presence has been documented in skin lesions of systemic sclerosis, keloids, scar tissue, and eosinophilic fasciitis and in BALF from patients with IPF and sarcoidosis, and it induces ECM in asthmatic airway smooth muscle.[193–196] Transient overexpression of CTGF in a rat model leads to a moderate but reversible pulmonary fibrosis that is associated with increased levels of TIMP-1.[197] Overexpression of TGF-β leads to a concomitant increase in CTGF and TIMP-1, suggesting that CTGF may be a cofactor for the development of fibrosis.[197] CTGF may be responsible for some of the downstream actions of TGF-β and is a potential therapeutic target for the treatment of interstitial lung disease.

CONCLUSIONS

Chemokines, adipokines, and growth factors are now recognized to play fundamental roles in lung development, the lifelong maintenance of lung health, and the development of pulmonary disorders characterized by inflammation and/or fibrosis, some of which are modulated by body mass. The generation of complex, overlapping signaling networks is necessary for both the pathogenesis and resolution of a variety of acute and chronic lung diseases, as these mediators are fundamental to the initiation, maintenance, and final resolution of the inflammatory response. Studies that illuminate the mechanistic role of chemokines, adipokines, and growth factors in mediating lung inflammation are beginning to lead to novel targeted forms of therapies, which will significantly aid in treating enigmatic lung disease.

REFERENCES

1. Thelen M, Stein JV. How chemokines invite leukocytes to dance. *Nat Immunol.* 2008;9(9):953–959.
2. Strieter RM. Interleukin-8: a very important chemokine of the human airway epithelium. *Am J Physiol Lung Cell Mol Physiol.* 2002;283(4):L688–L689.
3. Koelink PJ, Overbeek SA, Braber S, et al. Targeting chemokine receptors in chronic inflammatory diseases: an extensive review. *Pharmacol Ther.* 2012;133(1):1–18.

4. Strieter RM, Polverini PJ, Kunkel SL, et al. The functional role of the ELR motif in CXC chemokine-mediated angiogenesis. *J Biol Chem.* 1995;270(45):27348–27357.
5. Strieter RM, Burdick MD, Mestas J, Gomperts B, Keane MP, Belperio JA. Cancer CXC chemokine networks and tumour angiogenesis. *Eur J Cancer.* 2006;42(6):768–778.
6. Dawson TC, Lentsch AB, Wang Z, et al. Exaggerated response to endotoxin in mice lacking the Duffy antigen/receptor for chemokines (DARC). *Blood.* 2000;96(5):1681–1684.
7. Rot A. In situ binding assay for studying chemokine interactions with endothelial cells. *J Immunol Methods.* 2003;273 (1–2):63–71.
8. Mehrad B, Strieter RM, Standiford TJ. Role of TNF-alpha in pulmonary host defense in murine invasive aspergillosis. *J Immunol.* 1999;162(3):1633–1640.
9. Laichalk LL, Bucknell KA, Huffnagle GB, et al. Intrapulmonary delivery of tumor necrosis factor agonist peptide augments host defense in murine gram-negative bacterial pneumonia. *Infect Immun.* 1998;66(6):2822–2826.
10. Grommes J, Soehnlein O. Contribution of neutrophils to acute lung injury. *Mol Med.* 2011;17(3–4):293–307.
11. Colletti LM, Kunkel SL, Walz A, et al. Chemokine expression during hepatic ischemia/reperfusion-induced lung injury in the rat. The role of epithelial neutrophil activating protein. *J Clin Invest.* 1995;95(1):134–141.
12. Keane MP, Donnelly SC, Belperio JA, et al. Imbalance in the expression of CXC chemokines correlates with bronchoalveolar lavage fluid angiogenic activity and procollagen levels in acute respiratory distress syndrome. *J Immunol.* 2002;169(11):6515–6521.
13. Katzenstein AL, Myers JL. Idiopathic pulmonary fibrosis: clinical relevance of pathologic classification. *Am J Respir Crit Care Med.* 1998;157(4 Pt 1):1301–1315.
14. Raghu G, Collard HR, Egan JJ, et al. An official ATS/ERS/JRS/ALAT statement: idiopathic pulmonary fibrosis: evidence-based guidelines for diagnosis and management. *Am J Respir Crit Care Med.* 2011;183(6):788–824.
15. Mukaida N. Pathophysiological roles of interleukin-8/CXCL8 in pulmonary diseases. *Am J Physiol Lung Cell Mol Physiol.* 2003;284(4):L566–L577.
16. Southcott AM, Jones KP, Li D, et al. Interleukin-8. Differential expression in lone fibrosing alveolitis and systemic sclerosis. *Am J Respir Crit Care Med.* 1995;151(5):1604–1612.
17. Turner-Warwick M. Precapillary systemic-pulmonary anastomoses. *Thorax.* 1963;18:225–237.
18. Keane MP, Belperio JA, Arenberg DA, et al. IFN-gamma-inducible protein-10 attenuates bleomycin-induced pulmonary fibrosis via inhibition of angiogenesis. *J Immunol.* 1999; 163(10):5686–5692.
19. Keane MP, Belperio JA, Burdick MD, Lynch JP, Fishbein MC, Strieter RM. ENA-78 is an important angiogenic factor in idiopathic pulmonary fibrosis. *Am J Respir Crit Care Med.* 2001; 164(12):2239–2242.
20. Renzoni EA. Neovascularization in idiopathic pulmonary fibrosis: too much or too little? *Am J Respir Crit Care Med.* 2004; 169(11):1179–1180.
21. Cosgrove GP, Brown KK, Schiemann WP, et al. Pigment epithelium-derived factor in idiopathic pulmonary fibrosis: a role in aberrant angiogenesis. *Am J Respir Crit Care Med.* 2004;170(3):242–251.
22. Costello CM, Howell K, Cahill E, et al. Lung-selective gene responses to alveolar hypoxia: potential role for the bone morphogenetic antagonist gremlin in pulmonary hypertension. *Am J Physiol Lung Cell Mol Physiol.* 2008;295(2):L272–L284.
23. Costello CM, McCullagh B, Howell K, et al. A role for the CXCL12 receptor, CXCR7, in the pathogenesis of human pulmonary vascular disease. *Eur Respir J.* 2012;39(6):1415–1424.
24. Gambaryan N, Perros F, Montani D, et al. Targeting of c-kit+ haematopoietic progenitor cells prevents hypoxic pulmonary hypertension. *Eur Respir J.* 2011;37(6):1392–1399.
25. Toshner M, Voswinckel R, Southwood M, et al. Evidence of dysfunction of endothelial progenitors in pulmonary arterial hypertension. *Am J Respir Crit Care Med.* 2009;180(8):780–787.
26. Montani D, Perros F, Gambaryan N, et al. C-kit-positive cells accumulate in remodeled vessels of idiopathic pulmonary arterial hypertension. *Am J Respir Crit Care Med.* 2011;184(1):116–123.
27. Young KC, Torres E, Hatzistergos KE, Hehre D, Suguihara C, Hare JM. Inhibition of the SDF-1/CXCR4 axis attenuates neonatal hypoxia-induced pulmonary hypertension. *Circ Res.* 2009;104(11):1293–1301.
28. Sartina E, Suguihara C, Ramchandran S, et al. Antagonism of CXCR7 attenuates chronic hypoxia-induced pulmonary hypertension. *Pediatr Res.* 2012;71(6):682–688.
29. Bucala R, Spiegel LA, Chesney J, Hogan M, Cerami A. Circulating fibrocytes define a new leukocyte subpopulation that mediates tissue repair. *Mol Med.* 1994;1(1):71–81.
30. Phillips RJ, Burdick MD, Hong K, et al. Circulating fibrocytes traffic to the lungs in response to CXCL12 and mediate fibrosis. *J Clin Invest.* 2004;114(3):438–446.
31. Moeller A, Gilpin SE, Ask K, et al. Circulating fibrocytes are an indicator of poor prognosis in idiopathic pulmonary fibrosis. *Am J Respir Crit Care Med.* 2009;179(7):588–594.
32. Mehrad B, Strieter RM. Fibrocytes and the pathogenesis of diffuse parenchymal lung disease. *Fibrogenesis Tissue Repair.* 2012;5(Suppl 1):S22.
33. Luster AD, Alon R, von Andrian UH. Immune cell migration in inflammation: present and future therapeutic targets. *Nat Immunol.* 2005;6(12):1182–1190.
34. Keeley EC, Mehrad B, Strieter RM. Chemokines as mediators of tumor angiogenesis and neovascularization. *Exp Cell Res.* 2011;317(5):685–690.
35. Mantovani A, Sica A, Sozzani S, Allavena P, Vecchi A, Locati M. The chemokine system in diverse forms of macrophage activation and polarization. *Trends Immunol.* 2004;25(12):677–686.
36. Dawson TC, Beck MA, Kuziel WA, Henderson F, Maeda N. Contrasting effects of CCR5 and CCR2 deficiency in the pulmonary inflammatory response to influenza A virus. *Am J Pathol.* 2000;156(6):1951–1959.
37. Strieter RM, Belperio JA, Keane MP. Cytokines in innate host defense in the lung. *J Clin Invest.* 2002;109(6):699–705.
38. Mehrad B, Moore TA, Standiford TJ. Macrophage inflammatory protein-1 alpha is a critical mediator of host defense against invasive pulmonary aspergillosis in neutropenic hosts. *J Immunol.* 2000;165(2):962–968.
39. Phadke AP, Mehrad B. Cytokines in host defense against Aspergillus: recent advances. *Med Mycol.* 2005;43(Suppl 1): S173–S176.
40. Smith RE, Strieter RM, Phan SH, et al. Production and function of murine macrophage inflammatory protein-1 alpha in bleomycin-induced lung injury. *J Immunol.* 1994;153(10):4704–4712.
41. Smith RE, Strieter RM, Phan SH, Kunkel SL. C-C chemokines: novel mediators of the profibrotic inflammatory

response to bleomycin challenge. *Am J Respir Cell Mol Biol.* 1996;15(6):693–702.

42. Hogaboam CM, Lukacs NW, Chensue SW, Strieter RM, Kunkel SL. Monocyte chemoattractant protein-1 synthesis by murine lung fibroblasts modulates CD4+ T cell activation. *J Immunol.* 1998;160(9):4606–4614.
43. Belperio JA, Dy M, Burdick MD, et al. Interaction of IL-13 and C10 in the pathogenesis of bleomycin-induced pulmonary fibrosis. *Am J Respir Cell Mol Biol.* 2002;27(4):419–427.
44. Belperio JA, Dy M, Murray L, et al. The role of the Th2 CC chemokine ligand CCL17 in pulmonary fibrosis. *J Immunol.* 2004;173(7):4692–4698.
45. Tokuda A, Itakura M, Onai N, Kimura H, Kuriyama T, Matsushima K. Pivotal role of CCR1-positive leukocytes in bleomycin-induced lung fibrosis in mice. *J Immunol.* 2000; 164(5):2745–2751.
46. Moore BB, Paine R III, Christensen PJ, et al. Protection from pulmonary fibrosis in the absence of CCR2 signaling. *J Immunol.* 2001;167(8):4368–4377.
47. Moore BB, Peters-Golden M, Christensen PJ, et al. Alveolar epithelial cell inhibition of fibroblast proliferation is regulated by MCP-1/CCR2 and mediated by PGE2. *Am J Physiol Lung Cell Mol Physiol.* 2003;284(2):L342–L349.
48. Belperio JA, Keane MP, Burdick MD, et al. Critical role for the chemokine MCP-1/CCR2 in the pathogenesis of bronchiolitis obliterans syndrome. *J Clin Invest.* 2001;108(4):547–556.
49. Standiford TJ, Rolfe MW, Kunkel SL, et al. Macrophage inflammatory protein-1 alpha expression in interstitial lung disease. *J Immunol.* 1993;151(5):2852–2863.
50. Antoniades HN, Neville-Golden J, Galanopoulos T, Kradin RL, Valente AJ, Graves DT. Expression of monocyte chemoattractant protein 1 mRNA in human idiopathic pulmonary fibrosis. *Proc Natl Acad Sci U S A.* 1992;89(12):5371–5375.
51. Choi ES, Jakubzick C, Carpenter KJ, et al. Enhanced monocyte chemoattractant protein-3/CC chemokine ligand-7 in usual interstitial pneumonia. *Am J Respir Crit Care Med.* 2004;170(5): 508–515.
52. du Bois R, King TE Jr. Challenges in pulmonary fibrosis x 5: the NSIP/UIP debate. *Thorax.* 2007;62(11):1008–1012.
53. Travis WD, Hunninghake G, King TE Jr, et al. Idiopathic nonspecific interstitial pneumonia: report of an American Thoracic Society project. *Am J Respir Crit Care Med.* 2008;177(12): 1338–1347.
54. Katzenstein AL, Zisman DA, Litzky LA, Nguyen BT, Kotloff RM. Usual interstitial pneumonia: histologic study of biopsy and explant specimens. *Am J Surg Pathol.* 2002;26(12):1567–1577.
55. Blanpain C, Migeotte I, Lee B, et al. CCR5 binds multiple CC-chemokines: MCP-3 acts as a natural antagonist. *Blood.* 1999; 94(6):1899–1905.
56. Ouchi N, Parker JL, Lugus JJ, Walsh K. Adipokines in inflammation and metabolic disease. *Nat Rev Immunol.* 2011;11(2): 85–97.
57. Funahashi T, Nakamura T, Shimomura I, et al. Role of adipocytokines on the pathogenesis of atherosclerosis in visceral obesity. *Intern Med.* 1999;38(2):202–206.
58. Sood A. Obesity, adipokines, and lung disease. *J Appl Physiol.* 2010;108(3):744–753.
59. Takaoka M, Nagata D, Kihara S, et al. Periadventitial adipose tissue plays a critical role in vascular remodeling. *Circ Res.* 2009; 105(9):906–911.
60. Tilg H, Moschen AR. Adipocytokines: mediators linking adipose tissue, inflammation and immunity. *Nat Rev Immunol.* 2006;6(10):772–783.
61. Pasarica M, Sereda OR, Redman LM, et al. Reduced adipose tissue oxygenation in human obesity: evidence for rarefaction, macrophage chemotaxis, and inflammation without an angiogenic response. *Diabetes.* 2009;58(3):718–725.
62. Zhang Y, Proenca R, Maffei M, Barone M, Leopold L, Friedman JM. Positional cloning of the mouse obese gene and its human homologue. *Nature.* 1994;372(6505):425–432.
63. Saladin R, De Vos P, Guerre-Millo M, et al. Transient increase in obese gene expression after food intake or insulin administration. *Nature.* 1995;377(6549):527–529.
64. Halaas JL, Gajiwala KS, Maffei M, et al. Weight-reducing effects of the plasma protein encoded by the obese gene. *Science.* 1995;269(5223):543–546.
65. Vernooy JH, Drummen NE, van Suylen RJ, et al. Enhanced pulmonary leptin expression in patients with severe COPD and asymptomatic smokers. *Thorax.* 2009;64(1):26–32.
66. Bruno A, Pace E, Chanez P, et al. Leptin and leptin receptor expression in asthma. *J Allergy Clin Immunol.* 2009;124(2): 230–237, 237.e1–4.
67. Friedman JM, Halaas JL. Leptin and the regulation of body weight in mammals. *Nature.* 1998;395(6704):763–770.
68. Malli F, Papaioannou AI, Gourgoulianis KI, Daniil Z. The role of leptin in the respiratory system: an overview. *Respir Res.* 2010;11:152.
69. Torday JS, Sun H, Wang L, Torres E, Sunday ME, Rubin LP. Leptin mediates the parathyroid hormone-related protein paracrine stimulation of fetal lung maturation. *Am J Physiol Lung Cell Mol Physiol.* 2002;282(3):L405–L410.
70. Kirwin SM, Bhandari V, Dimatteo D, et al. Leptin enhances lung maturity in the fetal rat. *Pediatr Res.* 2006;60(2): 200–204.
71. Sato A, Schehr A, Ikegami M. Leptin does not influence surfactant synthesis in fetal sheep and mice lungs. *Am J Physiol Lung Cell Mol Physiol.* 2011;300(3):L498–L505.
72. O'Donnell CP, Schaub CD, Haines AS, et al. Leptin prevents respiratory depression in obesity. *Am J Respir Crit Care Med.* 1999;159(5 Pt 1):1477–1484.
73. Popko K, Gorska E, Wasik M, et al. Frequency of distribution of leptin receptor gene polymorphism in obstructive sleep apnea patients. *J Physiol Pharmacol.* 2007;58(Suppl 5)(Pt 2): 551–561.
74. Hanaoka M, Yu X, Urushihata K, Ota M, Fujimoto K, Kubo K. Leptin and leptin receptor gene polymorphisms in obstructive sleep apnea syndrome. *Chest.* 2008;133(1):79–85.
75. Hoyos CM, Killick R, Yee BJ, Phillips CL, Grunstein RR, Liu PY. Cardiometabolic changes after continuous positive airway pressure for obstructive sleep apnoea: a randomised sham-controlled study. *Thorax.* 2012;67(12):1081–1089.
76. Chin K, Shimizu K, Nakamura T, et al. Changes in intra-abdominal visceral fat and serum leptin levels in patients with obstructive sleep apnea syndrome following nasal continuous positive airway pressure therapy. *Circulation.* 1999;100(7):706–712.
77. Takabatake N, Nakamura H, Minamihaba O, et al. A novel pathophysiologic phenomenon in cachexic patients with chronic obstructive pulmonary disease: the relationship between the circadian rhythm of circulating leptin and the very low-frequency component of heart rate variability. *Am J Respir Crit Care Med.* 2001;163(6):1314–1319.

78. Creutzberg EC, Wouters EF, Vanderhoven-Augustin IM, Dentener MA, Schols AM. Disturbances in leptin metabolism are related to energy imbalance during acute exacerbations of chronic obstructive pulmonary disease. *Am J Respir Crit Care Med.* 2000;162(4 Pt 1):1239–1245.

79. Vernooy JH, Bracke KR, Drummen NE, et al. Leptin modulates innate and adaptive immune cell recruitment after cigarette smoke exposure in mice. *J Immunol.* 2010;184(12):7169–7177.

80. Wenzel SE. Asthma phenotypes: the evolution from clinical to molecular approaches. *Nat Med.* 2012;18(5):716–725.

81. Figueroa-Munoz JI, Chinn S, Rona RJ. Association between obesity and asthma in 4–11 year old children in the UK. *Thorax.* 2001;56(2):133–137.

82. Moore WC, Meyers DA, Wenzel SE, et al. Identification of asthma phenotypes using cluster analysis in the Severe Asthma Research Program. *Am J Respir Crit Care Med.* 2010;181 (4): 315–323.

83. Sideleva O, Suratt BT, Black KE, et al. Obesity and asthma: an inflammatory disease of adipose tissue not the airway. *Am J Respir Crit Care Med.* 2012;186(7):598–605.

84. Beuther DA. Obesity and asthma. *Clin Chest Med.* 2009;30(3): 479–488, viii.

85. Luk T, Malam Z, Marshall JC. Pre-B cell colony-enhancing factor (PBEF)/visfatin: a novel mediator of innate immunity. *J Leukoc Biol.* 2008;83(4):804–816.

86. Moschen AR, Kaser A, Enrich B, et al. Visfatin, an adipocytokine with proinflammatory and immunomodulating properties. *J Immunol.* 2007;178(3):1748–1758.

87. Ye SQ, Simon BA, Maloney JP, et al. Pre-B-cell colony-enhancing factor as a potential novel biomarker in acute lung injury. *Am J Respir Crit Care Med.* 2005;171(4):361–370.

88. Bajwa EK, Yu CL, Gong MN, Thompson BT, Christiani DC. Pre-B-cell colony-enhancing factor gene polymorphisms and risk of acute respiratory distress syndrome. *Crit Care Med.* 2007;35(5):1290–1295.

89. O'Mahony DS, Glavan BJ, Holden TD, et al. Inflammation and immune-related candidate gene associations with acute lung injury susceptibility and severity: a validation study. *PLoS One.* 2012;7(12):e51104.

90. Summer R, Little FF, Ouchi N, et al. Alveolar macrophage activation and an emphysema-like phenotype in adiponectin-deficient mice. *Am J Physiol Lung Cell Mol Physiol.* 2008;294(6): L1035–L1042.

91. Miller M, Cho JY, Pham A, Ramsdell J, Broide DH. Adiponectin and functional adiponectin receptor 1 are expressed by airway epithelial cells in chronic obstructive pulmonary disease. *J Immunol.* 2009;182(1):684–691.

92. Summer R, Fiack CA, Ikeda Y, et al. Adiponectin deficiency: a model of pulmonary hypertension associated with pulmonary vascular disease. *Am J Physiol Lung Cell Mol Physiol.* 2009;297(3):L432–L438.

93. Konter JM, Parker JL, Baez E, et al. Adiponectin attenuates lipopolysaccharide-induced acute lung injury through suppression of endothelial cell activation. *J Immunol.* 2012;188(2): 854–863.

94. Takemura Y, Ouchi N, Shibata R, et al. Adiponectin modulates inflammatory reactions via calreticulin receptor-dependent clearance of early apoptotic bodies. *J Clin Invest.* 2007;117(2):375–386.

95. Breyer MK, Rutten EP, Locantore NW, Watkins ML, Miller BE, Wouters EF. Dysregulated adipokine metabolism in chronic obstructive pulmonary disease. *Eur J Clin Invest.* 2012; 42(9):983–991.

96. Shore SA, Terry RD, Flynt L, Xu A, Hug C. Adiponectin attenuates allergen-induced airway inflammation and hyperresponsiveness in mice. *J Allergy Clin Immunol.* 2006;118(2):389–395.

97. Golbin JM, Somers VK, Caples SM. Obstructive sleep apnea, cardiovascular disease, and pulmonary hypertension. *Proc Am Thorac Soc.* 2008;5(2):200–206.

98. Mokhlesi B, Tulaimat A. Recent advances in obesity hypoventilation syndrome. *Chest.* 2007;132(4):1322–1336.

99. Haque AK, Gadre S, Taylor J, Haque SA, Freeman D, Duarte A. Pulmonary and cardiovascular complications of obesity: an autopsy study of 76 obese subjects. *Arch Pathol Lab Med.* 2008; 132(9):1397–1404.

100. Arita Y, Kihara S, Ouchi N, et al. Paradoxical decrease of an adipose-specific protein, adiponectin, in obesity. *Biochem Biophys Res Commun.* 1999;257(1):79–83.

101. Weng M, Raher MJ, Leyton P, et al. Adiponectin decreases pulmonary arterial remodeling in murine models of pulmonary hypertension. *Am J Respir Cell Mol Biol.* 2009;45(2):340–347.

102. Castan-Laurell I, Dray C, Attane C, Duparc T, Knauf C, Valet P. Apelin, diabetes, and obesity. *Endocrine.* 2011;40(1):1–9.

103. Boucher J, Masri B, Daviaud D, et al. Apelin, a newly identified adipokine up-regulated by insulin and obesity. *Endocrinology.* 2005;146(4):1764–1771.

104. Chandra SM, Razavi H, Kim J, et al. Disruption of the apelin-APJ system worsens hypoxia-induced pulmonary hypertension. *Arterioscler Thromb Vasc Biol.* 2011;31(4):814–820.

105. Huertas A, Tu L, Gambaryan N, et al. Leptin and regulatory T-lymphocytes in idiopathic pulmonary arterial hypertension. *Eur Respir J.* 2012;40(4):895–904.

106. Tonelli AR, Aytekin M, Feldstein AE, Dweik RA. Leptin levels predict survival in pulmonary arterial hypertension. *Pulm Circ.* 2012;2(2):214–219.

107. Li MO, Wan YY, Sanjabi S, Robertson AK, Flavell RA. Transforming growth factor-beta regulation of immune responses. *Annu Rev Immunol.* 2006;24:99–146.

108. Roberts AB, Sporn MB. The transforming growth factor-betas. In: Sporn MB, Roberts AB, eds. *Peptide Growth Factors and Their Receptors. Handbook of Experimental Pharmacology.* Vol 95. Berlin: Springer-Verlag; 1990:419–472.

109. Rubtsov YP, Rudensky AY. TGFbeta signalling in control of T-cell-mediated self-reactivity. *Nat Rev Immunol.* 2007;7(6): 443–453.

110. Wynn TA. Fibrotic disease and the T(H)1/T(H)2 paradigm. *Nat Rev Immunol.* 2004;4(8):583–594.

111. Bruijn JA, Roos A, de Geus B, de Heer E. Transforming growth factor-beta and the glomerular extracellular matrix in renal pathology. *J Lab Clin Med.* 1994;123(1):34–47.

112. Sime PJ, Xing Z, Graham FL, Csaky KG, Gauldie J. Adenovector-mediated gene transfer of active transforming growth factor-beta1 induces prolonged severe fibrosis in rat lung. *J Clin Invest.* 1997;100(4):768–776.

113. Sime PJ, Marr RA, Gauldie D, et al. Transfer of tumor necrosis factor-alpha to rat lung induces severe pulmonary inflammation and patchy interstitial fibrogenesis with induction of transforming growth factor-beta1 and myofibroblasts. *Am J Pathol.* 1998;153(3):825–832.

114. Kolb M, Margetts PJ, Anthony DC, Pitossi F, Gauldie J. Transient expression of IL-1beta induces acute lung injury

and chronic repair leading to pulmonary fibrosis. *J Clin Invest.* 2001;107(12):1529–1536.

115. Zhao J, Shi W, Wang YL, et al. Smad3 deficiency attenuates bleomycin-induced pulmonary fibrosis in mice. *Am J Physiol Lung Cell Mol Physiol.* 2002;282(3):L585–L593.
116. Huang M, Sharma S, Zhu LX, et al. IL-7 inhibits fibroblast TGF-beta production and signaling in pulmonary fibrosis. *J Clin Invest.* 2002;109(7):931–937.
117. Hagimoto N, Kuwano K, Inoshima I, et al. TGF-beta 1 as an enhancer of Fas-mediated apoptosis of lung epithelial cells. *J Immunol.* 2002;168(12):6470–6478.
118. Eickelberg O, Morty RE. Transforming growth factor beta/bone morphogenic protein signaling in pulmonary arterial hypertension: remodeling revisited. *Trends Cardiovasc Med.* 2007; 17(8):263–269.
119. Morrell NW. Pulmonary hypertension due to BMPR2 mutation: a new paradigm for tissue remodeling? *Proc Am Thorac Soc.* 2006;3(8):680–686.
120. Humbert M, Morrell NW, Archer SL, et al. Cellular and molecular pathobiology of pulmonary arterial hypertension. *J Am Coll Cardiol.* 2004;43(12 Suppl S):13S–24S.
121. Long L, Crosby A, Yang X, et al. Altered bone morphogenetic protein and transforming growth factor-{beta} signaling in rat models of pulmonary hypertension: potential for activin receptor-like kinase-5 inhibition in prevention and progression of disease. *Circulation.* 2009;119(4):566–576.
122. de Jesus Perez VA, Alastalo TP, Wu JC, et al. Bone morphogenetic protein 2 induces pulmonary angiogenesis via Wnt-beta-catenin and Wnt-RhoA-Rac1 pathways. *J Cell Biol.* 2009; 184(1):83–99.
123. Costello CM, Cahill E, Martin F, Gaine S, McLoughlin P. Role of gremlin in the lung: development and disease. *Am J Respir Cell Mol Biol.* 2010;42(5):517–523.
124. Gazzerro E, Canalis E. Bone morphogenetic proteins and their antagonists. *Rev Endocr Metab Disord.* 2006;7(1–2):51–65.
125. Machado RD, Pauciulo MW, Thomson JR, et al. BMPR2 haploinsufficiency as the inherited molecular mechanism for primary pulmonary hypertension. *Am J Hum Genet.* 2001;68(1):92–102.
126. Deng Z, Morse JH, Slager SL, et al. Familial primary pulmonary hypertension (gene PPH1) is caused by mutations in the bone morphogenetic protein receptor-II gene. *Am J Hum Genet.* 2000;67(3):737–744.
127. Lane KB, Machado RD, Pauciulo MW, et al. Heterozygous germline mutations in BMPR2, encoding a TGF-beta receptor, cause familial primary pulmonary hypertension. *Nat Genet.* 2000;26(1):81–84.
128. Anderson L, Lowery JW, Frank DB, et al. Bmp2 and Bmp4 exert opposing effects in hypoxic pulmonary hypertension. *Am J Physiol Regul Integr Comp Physiol.* 2010;298(3):R833–R842.
129. Frank DB, Abtahi A, Yamaguchi DJ, et al. Bone morphogenetic protein 4 promotes pulmonary vascular remodeling in hypoxic pulmonary hypertension. *Circ Res.* 2005;97(5):496–504.
130. Hong KH, Lee YJ, Lee E, et al. Genetic ablation of the BMPR2 gene in pulmonary endothelium is sufficient to predispose to pulmonary arterial hypertension. *Circulation.* 2008;118(7):722–730.
131. Morty RE, Nejman B, Kwapiszewska G, et al. Dysregulated bone morphogenetic protein signaling in monocrotaline-induced pulmonary arterial hypertension. *Arterioscler Thromb Vasc Biol.* 2007;27(5):1072–1078.
132. Song Y, Jones JE, Beppu H, Keaney JF Jr, Loscalzo J, Zhang YY. Increased susceptibility to pulmonary hypertension in heterozygous BMPR2-mutant mice. *Circulation.* 2005;112(4):553–562.
133. Long L, MacLean MR, Jeffery TK, et al. Serotonin increases susceptibility to pulmonary hypertension in BMPR2-deficient mice. *Circ Res.* 2006;98(6):818–827.
134. West J, Harral J, Lane K, et al. Mice expressing BMPR2R899X transgene in smooth muscle develop pulmonary vascular lesions. *Am J Physiol Lung Cell Mol Physiol.* 2008;295(5):L744–L755.
135. Reynolds A, Xia W, Holmes M, et al. Bone morphogenetic protein type 2 receptor gene therapy attenuates hypoxic pulmonary hypertension. *Am J Physiol Lung Cell Mol Physiol.* 2007;292 (5): L1182–L1192.
136. Takahashi K, Kogaki S, Matsushita T, Nasuno S, Kurotobi S, Ozono K. Hypoxia induces alteration of bone morphogenetic protein receptor signaling in pulmonary artery endothelial cell. *Pediatr Res.* 2007;61(4):392–397.
137. Cahill E, Costello CM, Rowan SC, et al. Gremlin plays a key role in the pathogenesis of pulmonary hypertension. *Circulation.* 2012;125(7):920–930.
138. Newman JH, Phillips JA, Loyd JE. Narrative review: the enigma of pulmonary arterial hypertension: new insights from genetic studies. *Ann Intern Med.* 2008;148(4):278–283.
139. Harrison RE, Berger R, Haworth SG, et al. Transforming growth factor-beta receptor mutations and pulmonary arterial hypertension in childhood. *Circulation.* 2005;111(4):435–441.
140. Harrison RE, Flanagan JA, Sankelo M, et al. Molecular and functional analysis identifies ALK-1 as the predominant cause of pulmonary hypertension related to hereditary haemorrhagic telangiectasia. *J Med Genet.* 2003;40(12):865–871.
141. Toporsian M, Jerkic M, Zhou YQ, et al. Spontaneous adult-onset pulmonary arterial hypertension attributable to increased endothelial oxidative stress in a murine model of hereditary hemorrhagic telangiectasia. *Arterioscler Thromb Vasc Biol.* 2010; 30 (3):509–517.
142. Citri A, Yarden Y. EGF-ERBB signalling: towards the systems level. *Nat Rev Mol Cell Biol.* 2006;7(7):505–516.
143. Hayman MJ, Ramsay GM, Savin K, Kitchener G, Graf T, Beug H. Identification and characterization of the avian erythroblastosis virus erbB gene product as a membrane glycoprotein. *Cell.* 1983;32(2):579–588.
144. Harris RC, Chung E, Coffey RJ. EGF receptor ligands. *Exp Cell Res.* 2003;284(1):2–13.
145. Schneider MR, Wolf E. The epidermal growth factor receptor ligands at a glance. *J Cell Physiol.* 2009;218(3):460–466.
146. Finigan JH, Downey GP, Kern JA. Human epidermal growth factor receptor signaling in acute lung injury. *Am J Respir Cell Mol Biol.* 2012;47(4):395–404.
147. Veale D, Ashcroft T, Marsh C, Gibson GJ, Harris AL. Epidermal growth factor receptors in non-small cell lung cancer. *Br J Cancer.* 1987;55(5):513–516.
148. Sharma SV, Bell DW, Settleman J, Haber DA. Epidermal growth factor receptor mutations in lung cancer. *Nat Rev Cancer.* 2007;7(3):169–181.
149. Gettinger S, Lynch T. A decade of advances in treatment for advanced non-small cell lung cancer. *Clin Chest Med.* 2011; 32(4):839–851.
150. Miettinen PJ, Berger JE, Meneses J, et al. Epithelial immaturity and multiorgan failure in mice lacking epidermal growth factor receptor. *Nature.* 1995;376(6538):337–341.
151. Sundell HW, Gray ME, Serenius FS, Escobedo MB, Stahlman MT. Effects of epidermal growth factor on lung maturation in fetal lambs. *Am J Pathol.* 1980;100(3):707–726.

152. Kheradmand F, Folkesson HG, Shum L, Derynk R, Pytela R, Matthay MA. Transforming growth factor-alpha enhances alveolar epithelial cell repair in a new in vitro model. *Am J Physiol*. 1994;267(6 Pt 1):L728–L738.

153. Puddicombe SM, Polosa R, Richter A, et al. Involvement of the epidermal growth factor receptor in epithelial repair in asthma. *Faseb J*. 2000;14(10):1362–1374.

154. Madtes DK, Elston AL, Hackman RC, Dunn AR, Clark JG. Transforming growth factor-alpha deficiency reduces pulmonary fibrosis in transgenic mice. *Am J Respir Cell Mol Biol*. 1999; 20(5):924–934.

155. Ishii Y, Fujimoto S, Fukuda T. Gefitinib prevents bleomycin-induced lung fibrosis in mice. *Am J Respir Crit Care Med*. 2006; 174(5):550–556.

156. Inoue A, Saijo Y, Maemondo M, et al. Severe acute interstitial pneumonia and gefitinib. *Lancet*. 2003;361(9352):137–139.

157. Voelkel NF, Vandivier RW, Tuder RM. Vascular endothelial growth factor in the lung. *Am J Physiol Lung Cell Mol Physiol*. 2006;290(2):L209–L221.

158. Olsson AK, Dimberg A, Kreuger J, Claesson-Welsh L. VEGF receptor signalling - in control of vascular function. *Nat Rev Mol Cell Biol*. 2006;7(5):359–371.

159. Shalaby F, Rossant J, Yamaguchi TP, et al. Failure of blood-island formation and vasculogenesis in Flk-1-deficient mice. *Nature*. 1995;376(6535):62–66.

160. Healy AM, Morgenthau L, Zhu X, Farber HW, Cardoso WV. VEGF is deposited in the subepithelial matrix at the leading edge of branching airways and stimulates neovascularization in the murine embryonic lung. *Dev Dyn*. 2000;219(3):341–352.

161. Akeson AL, Greenberg JM, Cameron JE, et al. Temporal and spatial regulation of VEGF-A controls vascular patterning in the embryonic lung. *Dev Biol*. 2003;264(2):443–455.

162. Gerber HP, Hillan KJ, Ryan AM, et al. VEGF is required for growth and survival in neonatal mice. *Development*. 1999; 126(6):1149–1159.

163. Bhatt AJ, Pryhuber GS, Huyck H, Watkins RH, Metlay LA, Maniscalco WM. Disrupted pulmonary vasculature and decreased vascular endothelial growth factor, Flt-1, and TIE-2 in human infants dying with bronchopulmonary dysplasia. *Am J Respir Crit Care Med*. 2001;164(10 Pt 1):1971–1980.

164. Tang K, Rossiter HB, Wagner PD, Breen EC. Lung-targeted VEGF inactivation leads to an emphysema phenotype in mice. *J Appl Physiol*. 2004;97(4):1559–1566; discussion 1549.

165. Kasahara Y, Tuder RM, Cool CD, Lynch DA, Flores SC, Voelkel NF. Endothelial cell death and decreased expression of vascular endothelial growth factor and vascular endothelial growth factor receptor 2 in emphysema. *Am J Respir Crit Care Med*. 2001;163(3 Pt 1):737–744.

166. Yasuo M, Mizuno S, Kraskauskas D, et al. Hypoxia inducible factor-1 alpha in human emphysema lung tissue. *Eur Respir J*. 2011; 37(4):775–783.

167. Tarasevicience-Stewart L, Kasahara Y, Alger L, et al. Inhibition of the VEGF receptor 2 combined with chronic hypoxia causes cell death-dependent pulmonary endothelial cell proliferation and severe pulmonary hypertension. *FASEB J*. 2001;15(2):427–438.

168. Abe K, Toba M, Alzoubi A, et al. Formation of plexiform lesions in experimental severe pulmonary arterial hypertension. *Circulation*. 2010;121(25):2747–2754.

169. Ciuclan L, Bonneau O, Hussey M, et al. A novel murine model of severe pulmonary arterial hypertension. *Am J Respir Crit Care Med*. 2011;184(10):1171–1182.

170. Garcia AA, Hirte H, Fleming G, et al. Phase II clinical trial of bevacizumab and low-dose metronomic oral cyclophosphamide in recurrent ovarian cancer: a trial of the California, Chicago, and Princess Margaret Hospital phase II consortia. *J Clin Oncol*. 2008;26(1):76–82.

171. Partovian C, Adnot S, Raffestin B, et al. Adenovirus-mediated lung vascular endothelial growth factor overexpression protects against hypoxic pulmonary hypertension in rats. *Am J Respir Cell Mol Biol*. 2000;23(6):762–771.

172. Louzier V, Raffestin B, Leroux A, et al. Role of VEGF-B in the lung during development of chronic hypoxic pulmonary hypertension. *Am J Physiol Lung Cell Mol Physiol*. 2003;284(6): L926–L937.

173. Beenken A, Mohammadi M. The FGF family: biology, pathophysiology and therapy. *Nat Rev Drug Discov*. 2009;8(3):235–253.

174. Ware LB, Matthay MA. Keratinocyte and hepatocyte growth factors in the lung: roles in lung development, inflammation, and repair. *Am J Physiol Lung Cell Mol Physiol*. 2002;282(5): L924–L940.

175. Peters K, Werner S, Liao X, Wert S, Whitsett J, Williams L. Targeted expression of a dominant negative FGF receptor blocks branching morphogenesis and epithelial differentiation of the mouse lung. *EMBO J*. 1994;13(14):3296–3301.

176. Simonet WS, DeRose ML, Bucay N, et al. Pulmonary malformation in transgenic mice expressing human keratinocyte growth factor in the lung. *Proc Natl Acad Sci U S A*. 1995;92(26): 12461–12465.

177. Welsh DA, Summer WR, Dobard EP, Nelson S, Mason CM. Keratinocyte growth factor prevents ventilator-induced lung injury in an ex vivo rat model. *Am J Respir Crit Care Med*. 2000; 162(3 Pt 1):1081–1086.

178. Gomperts BN, Belperio JA, Fishbein MC, Keane MP, Burdick MD, Strieter RM. Keratinocyte growth factor improves repair in the injured tracheal epithelium. *Am J Respir Cell Mol Biol*. 2007;37(1):48–56.

179. Sadovski J, Kuchenbuch T, Ruppert C, et al. Keratinocyte growth factor prevents intra-alveolar oedema in experimental lung isografts. *Eur Respir J*. 2008;31(1):21–28.

180. Crosby LM, Waters CM. Epithelial repair mechanisms in the lung. *Am J Physiol Lung Cell Mol Physiol*. 2010;298(6):L715–L731.

181. Savla U, Waters CM. Barrier function of airway epithelium: effects of radiation and protection by keratinocyte growth actor. *Radiat Res*. 1998;150(2):195–203.

182. Spielberger R, Stiff P, Bensinger W, et al. Palifermin for oral mucositis after intensive therapy for hematologic cancers. *N Engl J Med*. 2004;351(25):2590–2598.

183. Kato S, Sekine K. FGF-FGFR signaling in vertebrate organogenesis. *Cell Mol Biol (Noisy-le-grand)*. 1999;45(5):631–638.

184. Gupte VV, Ramasamy SK, Reddy R, et al. Overexpression of fibroblast growth factor-10 during both inflammatory and fibrotic phases attenuates bleomycin-induced pulmonary fibrosis in mice. *Am J Respir Crit Care Med*. 2009;180(5):424–436.

185. Richeldi L, Costabel U, Selman M, et al. Efficacy of a tyrosine kinase inhibitor in idiopathic pulmonary fibrosis. *N Engl J Med*. 2011; 365(12):1079–1087.

186. Hamilton JA, Stanley ER, Burgess AW, Shadduck RK. Stimulation of macrophage plasminogen activator activity by colony-stimulating factors. *J Cell Physiol*. 1980;103(3):435–445.

187. Burgess AW, Metcalf D. Serum half-life and organ distribution of radiolabeled colony stimulating factor in mice. *Exp Hematol*. 1977;5(6):456–464.

188. Hamilton JA. Colony-stimulating factors in inflammation and autoimmunity. *Nat Rev Immunol.* 2008;8(7):533–544.

189. Dranoff G, Crawford AD, Sadelain M, et al. Involvement of granulocyte-macrophage colony-stimulating factor in pulmonary homeostasis. *Science.* 1994;264(5159):713–716.

190. Inoue Y, Trapnell BC, Tazawa R, et al. Characteristics of a large cohort of patients with autoimmune pulmonary alveolar proteinosis in Japan. *Am J Respir Crit Care Med.* 2008;177(7):752–762.

191. Greenhill SR, Kotton DN. Pulmonary alveolar proteinosis: a bench-to-bedside story of granulocyte-macrophage colony-stimulating factor dysfunction. *Chest.* 2009;136(2):571–577.

192. Borie R, Danel C, Debray MP, et al. Pulmonary alveolar proteinosis. *Eur Respir Rev.* 2011;20(120):98–107.

193. Moussad EE, Brigstock DR. Connective tissue growth factor: what's in a name? *Mol Genet Metab.* 2000;71(1–2):276–292.

194. Allen JT, Spiteri MA. Growth factors in idiopathic pulmonary fibrosis: relative roles. *Respir Res.* 2002;3:13.

195. Brigstock DR. The connective tissue growth factor/cysteine-rich 61/nephroblastoma overexpressed (CCN) family. *Endocr Rev.* 1999;20(2):189–206.

196. Johnson PR, Burgess JK, Ge Q, et al. Connective tissue growth factor induces extracellular matrix in asthmatic airway smooth muscle. *Am J Respir Crit Care Med.* 2006;173(1):32–41.

197. Bonniaud P, Margetts PJ, Kolb M, et al. Adenoviral gene transfer of connective tissue growth factor in the lung induces transient fibrosis. *Am J Respir Crit Care Med.* 2003;168(7):770–778.

CHAPTER 27

Redox Signaling and Oxidative Stress in Lung Diseases

Jessy Deshane
Victor J. Thannickal

INTRODUCTION

Molecular oxygen is a prerequisite to life of all aerobic organisms. The human lung with its large surface area and extensive blood supply is engineered for its primary function in gas exchange. While oxygen is essential for its many roles in human physiology, high concentrations of oxygen or its metabolites, commonly referred to as reactive oxygen species (ROS), have the potential to cause cellular injury and contribute to disease pathogenesis. The most damaging forms of ROS are free radicals. A free radical, by definition, refers to any chemical species containing one or more unpaired electrons in their atomic or molecular orbitals. These unpaired electron(s) give considerable reactivity to free radical species, which can trigger chemical reactions that damage cellular constituents of living organisms. Molecular oxygen (dioxygen) is itself, a radical based on the presence of unpaired electrons in its outermost orbital; however, their parallel spin retrains its reactivity. O_2 can form the superoxide anion radical ($O_2^{\bullet-}$) upon addition of an electron; thus, overcoming this restraint and making $O_2^{\bullet-}$ a highly reactive species.[1,2] The photodynamic activation of oxygen can result in the formation of singlet oxygen, and its reductive activation results in the formation of hydrogen peroxide (H_2O_2) or the highly reactive hydroxyl radical ($^{\bullet}OH$).[3,4] When two free radicals share their unpaired electrons, nonradical species of lower reactivity are generated. Thus, ROS constitute both free radicals and nonradicals.

Nitric oxide ($NO^{\bullet}$) is another small gaseous molecule that serves as an important signaling molecule in diverse physiological processes, including vasorelaxation and immune regulation during chronic inflammation in the lung.[5,6] The regulated production of $NO^{\bullet}$ by lung cells is critical for homeostasis of the lung. However, in some contexts, the reaction of $NO^{\bullet}$ with $O_2^{\bullet-}$ to form reactive nitrogen species (RNS), such as peroxynitrite ($ONOO^-$), may contribute to the pathophysiology of chronic lung diseases.[7–9]

ROS and RNS together play important roles in regulation of cell proliferation, differentiation, and survival.[10–12] ROS/RNS can inactivate enzymes including antiproteases, induce apoptosis, regulate cell proliferation, and modulate the immune-inflammatory system in the lungs and other tissues.[13–16] ROS/RNS have been implicated in initiating inflammatory responses in the lungs through the activation of transcription factors, protein kinase pathways, chromatin remodeling, and gene expression of proinflammatory mediators.[13–16] Under normal physiological conditions, the balance between generation and elimination of ROS/RNS maintains the functional integrity of redox-sensitive signaling cascades regulating cellular phenotypes. In this context, it is important to differentiate the roles of ROS/RNS in "oxidative stress" from "redox signaling." Paradoxically, it appears that nature has co-opted the chemical reactivities of ROS/RNS to function as signaling molecules in homeostasis and normal cellular physiology.

Redox homeostasis of cells/tissues is maintained by the regulated balance of oxidant production and antioxidant systems, both enzymatic and nonenzymatic. However, an increase in oxidant generation in excess of the capacity of cells/tissues to detoxify or scavenge reactive species leads to oxidative stress.[10,17,18] Oxidative stress typically causes damage to cellular components in an indiscriminant manner. Such states are accelerated in the presence of transition metals, such as iron and copper, and/or specific monooxygenases or oxidases.[13,15,16] It is also important to recognize that aberrations in redox signaling or oxidative stress may contribute to the pathogenesis of lung diseases. In this chapter, we review the physiology of ROS and RNS; cellular antioxidant systems; and the role of oxidative stress and redox signaling in the development and progression of selected acute and chronic lung diseases.

METABOLISM OF REACTIVE OXYGEN/NITROGEN SPECIES

■ ENZYMATIC AND NONENZYMATIC SOURCES OF ROS

The primary ROS include superoxide anion ($O_2^{\bullet-}$), hydrogen peroxide (H_2O_2), and hydroxyl radical ($^{\bullet}OH$), which can be generated from both enzymatic and nonenzymatic sources. The human lung is constantly exposed to ambient air, which may contain environmental toxins capable of inducing ROS generation.[13,19] ROS may also be generated by electron transfer reactions in the mitochondria and endoplasmic reticulum (ER), from xenobiotics, and a range of metabolic enzymes that catalyze oxidation reactions.[19] The major endogenous ROS/RNS and the primary mechanisms for their generation are summarized in Table 27-1.

The highly reactive $O_2^{\bullet-}$ formed by the addition of an electron to molecular oxygen is unstable with a half-life of milliseconds. The major site for producing $O_2^{\bullet-}$ is the mitochondria, which is also the primary site for ATP generation in any cell. During mitochondrial

TABLE 27-1 Key Reactive Oxygen and Nitrogen Species

Reactive Species	Formula	Chemical Reaction		
Superoxide	$O_2^{\bullet-}$	NADPH + $2O_2$	$\longleftrightarrow$	NADP+ + $2O_2^{\bullet-}$ + H^+
		$2O_2^{\bullet-}$ + H+	$\longrightarrow$	$O_2 + H_2O_2$
Hydrogen peroxide	H_2O_2	Hypoxanthine + $H_2O + O_2$	$\rightleftarrows$	Xanthine + H_2O_2
		Xanthine + $H_2O + O_2$	$\rightleftarrows$	Uric acid + H_2O_2
Hydroxyl radical	$^{\bullet}OH$	$Fe^2 + H_2O_2$		$Fe^{3+} + OH^- + {}^{\bullet}OH$
Hypochlorous acid	HOCl	$H_2O_2 + Cl^-$	$\longrightarrow$	HOCl + H_2O
Peroxyl radicals	$ROO^{\bullet}$	$R^{\bullet} + O_2$	$\longrightarrow$	$ROO^{\bullet}$
Peroxynitrite	$ONOO^-$	$O_2^{\bullet} + NO$	$\longrightarrow$	$ONOO^-$
		$H_2O_2 + NO_2^-$	$\longrightarrow$	$ONOO^- + H_2O$

electron transport, there is an estimated leak of 1% to 3% of electrons to oxygen resulting in the formation of $O_2^{\bullet-}$.[16] $O_2^{\bullet-}$ generated in the mitochondria, due to its negative charge, does not cross membranes and is released into the mitochondrial matrix where it targets proteins with heme moieties or iron–sulfur clusters to cause loss of protein or enzymatic function.[20] The steady-state levels of intramitochondrial $O_2^{\bullet-}$ concentrations are maintained at very low levels by detoxifying enzymes. ER is another intracellular compartment in which enzymes that detoxify lipid-soluble drugs and other toxic metabolites, reduce molecular O_2 to produce $O_2^{\bullet-}$ and/or H_2O_2, while oxidizing unsaturated fatty acids and xenobiotics.[19,20]

The NADPH oxidase (NOX) gene family encompasses enzymes, the primary function of which is the regulated generation of ROS. NOX enzymes form a membrane-bound multicomponent complex that is present in phagocytes and nonphagocytic cells in the lung.[15,16,18] NOX enzymes play crucial roles in host defense, signal transduction, and hormone synthesis in eukaryotes. There are seven mammalian NOX homologs comprising NOX1 to 5 and the DUOX1 and 2.[21–24] The best characterized NOX isoform is NOX2, which is essential for microbicidal-killing activity of phagocytes. NOX2, upon activation, generates ROS by coordinated assembly and activation of the NOX2 enzymatic complex, which comprises the membrane-associated flavocytochrome b558 (gp91^{phox}), p22^{phox}, and the various cytosolic cofactors (p47^{phox}, p67^{phox}, and p40^{phox}, and the GTPase, Rac1). This complex then mediates the transmembrane electron transfer from the major electron donor, NADPH, to reduce molecular O_2 to $O_2^{\bullet-}$ and H_2O_2.[15,16,18]

Similar to NOX2, activation of NOX1 and NOX3 also requires association with p22^{phox}, and assembly with Rac1 and cytosolic cofactors (p47^{phox} and p67^{phox} or their homologs, NOX organizer 1 (NOXO1) and NOX activator 1 (NOXA1). NOX4 also requires p22^{phox}, but is constitutively active and functions independently of activation of other cofactors.[16,21–24] Expression of NOX1 and NOX4 in nonphagocytic fibroblasts results in increased levels of both $O_2^{\bullet-}$ and H_2O_2, implying that these, unlike the phagocytic NOX2, possess intrinsic basal activity. NOX5 and DUOX1/2 differ from the other NOX homologs and contain additional intracellular Ca^{2+}-binding EF-hand domain regions, and are regulated by Ca^{2+} signaling, independent of p22^{phox} or other cytosolic factors.[16,21–24] The dual oxidases, DUOXs, are composed of the NOX-like region at the C-terminal half, two EF-hands, a membrane-spanning region, and a peroxidase-like domain at the N-terminus. DUOXs do not require cytosolic regulatory components for their activity.[16,21–24] However, transmembrane maturation factors, DUOXA1 and DUOXA2, are essential for ER-to-Golgi transition, maturation, and targeting DUOXs to the plasma membrane as functional complexes. Although initially identified in the thyroid gland, DUOX1 and DUOX2 are the primary sources of H_2O_2 production in the airway epithelium.[25] The NOX/DUOX isoforms are expressed widely in the lung extending from the proximal trachea and large airways to terminal bronchioles and alveoli (Table 27-2).[16,21–25]

In biological systems, dismutation reaction of $O_2^{\bullet-}$ generates H_2O_2, either spontaneously or by enzymatic catalysis by superoxide

TABLE 27-2 Enzymatic Sources for ROS and RNS

Enzyme	Distribution in Lung	Lung Cell Types
DUOX1, DUOX2, NOX2, NOX4	Trachea and upper airways	Airway epithelial cells
NOX1, NOX2, NOX4	Pulmonary vasculature	Pulmonary artery endothelial cells
NOX4	Pulmonary vasculature	Pulmonary artery smooth muscle cells
DUOX1, DUOX2, NOX2, NOX4	Lower airways/ alveolus	Airway epithelial cells
NOX3	Airway alveolus	Endothelial cells
NOX4	Airway alveolus	Myofibroblasts
NOX2, NOX4	Alveolar space/ blood	Monocytes, Macrophages, Neutrophils, Eosinophils
NOS1 (neuronal)	Trachea, bronchus, airways	Airway epithelial cells Neutrophils Neurons
NOS2 (inducible)	Airways, alveolus, alveolar space/ blood	Airway and vascular smooth muscle cells Type II pneumocytes Fibroblasts Macrophages Monocytes Neutrophils Eosinophils Mast cells
NOS3 (endothelial)	Airways, pulmonary vasculature	Airway epithelial cells Type II pneumocytes Pulmonary artery Smooth muscle cells Endothelial cells Macrophages

dismutases (SODs). $O_2^{\bullet-}$ can be generated by molybdenum hydroxylase reactions involving xanthine, sulfite, and aldehyde oxidases, dihydroorotate and flavoprotein dehydrogenases, tryptophan dioxygenases as well as arachidonic acid metabolism.[26,27] Certain oxidases such as monoamine and amino acid oxidases can generate H_2O_2 directly without the intermediate formation of $O_2^{\bullet-}$.[17] During chronic inflammation in the lung, H_2O_2 is produced by both resident and inflammatory cells of the lung.[26,27] The oxidizing potential of H_2O_2 is amplified by inflammatory cell peroxidases such as myeloperoxidase (MPO) and/or eosinophil peroxidase (EPO).[28–32] The hydroxyl radical, $^{\bullet}OH$, is the neutral form of the hydroxide ion that is highly reactive toward cellular constituents, more so than $O_2^{\bullet-}$ or H_2O_2. This radical contributes to most of the reactivity by $O_2^{\bullet-}$ and H_2O_2 in a series of reactions that are catalyzed by transition metal ions. Excess $O_2^{\bullet-}$ targets Fe–S cluster-containing enzymes and catalyzes production of $^{\bullet}OH$ from H_2O_2 by reducing free iron (Fe^{3+} to Fe^{2+}) for Fenton chemistry (see Table 27-1). MPO and EPO enzymes represent an alternate pathway for $^{\bullet}OH$ formation *in vivo*. MPO uses Cl^- as substrate to generate hypochlorous acid, whereas EPO uses Br^- to generate brominating species. The hypohalous acids then generate $^{\bullet}OH$ by reaction with $O_2^{\bullet-}$.[33–38] Both these enzymes can accelerate oxidative modifications of proteins, in particular bromination and chlorination.

ENZYMATIC AND NONENZYMATIC SOURCES OF RNS

An important RNS in the lung is $NO^{\bullet}$, which is endogenously generated by specific nitric oxide synthases (NOSs). These NOS enzymes metabolize L-arginine to $NO^{\bullet}$ and L-citrulline via a five electron oxidation reaction.[6,39–48] This reaction requires a dimeric enzyme, oxygen, NADPH and the cofactors, flavin adenine dinucleotide (FAD), flavin mononucleotide (FMN), tetrahydrobiopterin (BH_4), calmodulin, and iron protoporphyrin. Active NOS enzymes exist in the dimeric form with each monomer consisting of an N-terminal oxygenase domain that binds heme, BH_4, and substrate L-arginine. The cofactors FAD, FMN, and NADPH bind the C-terminal end of the NOS monomer. There are three different NOS forms, all of which are expressed in the lung, the inducible form iNOS or NOS2, neuronal NOS or NOS1, and the endothelial NOS enzyme NOS3 (Table 27-2). The NOS1 and NOS3 enzymes are calcium dependent and produce picomolar levels of NO, while nanomolar levels are generated by the calcium-independent iNOS. $NO^{\bullet}$ synthesis by iNOS is regulated by the availability of the substrate L-arginine and cofactor BH_4. Transfer of electrons occur from the carboxy-reductase domain to the heme iron of the oxygenase domain, which then binds oxygen and oxidizes L-arginine to generate the end products, $NO^{\bullet}$ and citrulline.[6,39–48] Uncoupling of NOS enzymes can contribute to the formation of the $O_2^{\bullet-}$. In a low arginine condition, NADPH is oxidized by the enzyme to generate $O_2^{\bullet-}$. Arginase, an enzyme that competes with the NOSs for L-arginine decreases the arginine availability for NOS. Arginase is a critical enzyme in the urea cycle and converts arginine to ornithine, and then to urea; it can promote uncoupling of NOSs to generate $O_2^{\bullet-}$.[49,50] About 40% of the highly reactive and highly diffusible $NO^{\bullet}$ is consumed in chemical reactions and, when metabolized, give rise to reactive intermediates. $NO^{\bullet}$ reacts with O_2 yielding nitrite (NO_2^-) and recycling of nitrite causes regeneration of bioactive $NO^{\bullet}$. NO_2^- is also a substrate for the heme peroxidases, MPO and EPO, which oxidize nitrite to nitrogen dioxide radical ($NO_2^{\bullet}$). $NO^{\bullet}$ is also oxidized to methemoglobin and NO_3^- by reaction with oxyhemoglobin. $NO^{\bullet}$ reacts with $O_2^{\bullet-}$ to form peroxynitrite ($ONOO^-$), which can mediate tyrosine nitration that may result in either the loss or gain of function of proteins.[7–9,51] In acidic environments, the protonation of $ONOO^-$ results in the formation of ONOOH (peroxynitrous acid), which is then decomposed to both NO_3^- via intermediate $^{\bullet}OH$ and NO_2.[52] ONOOH can also react with thiol residues to form S-nitrosothiols (SNOs) and the reaction is referred to as S-nitrosation or S-nitrosylation. A wide variety of proteins including kinases, channels, and transcription factors are susceptible to S-nitrosylation. SNOs are important molecules in the signaling of $NO^{\bullet}$ bioactivity in the respiratory system.[53–57] SNOs are present in the airway epithelial lining fluid in μmol concentrations, can influence airway tone, and possess substantially greater half-lives than $NO^{\bullet}$ in the lung. It has also been reported that iNOS can specifically bind to cyclooxgenase-2 (COX-2) and S-nitrosylate COX-2, upregulate its catalytic activity and enhance prostaglandin E2 production. Thus, S-nitrosylation represents an important signaling pathway for $NO^{\bullet}$.[53–57] Under physiological conditions, interaction with metal centers of enzymes and S-nitrosylation are the major mechanisms for biological actions of $NO^{\bullet}$. In biological systems, the levels of $O_2^{\bullet-}$ are 10^{-11} to 10^{-10} M while that of NO is 10^{-9} to 10^{-7} M. Under these conditions, $ONOO^-$ is formed at a low rate by the reaction of $NO^{\bullet}$ with $O_2^{\bullet-}$ with a 1:1 stoichiometry.[7–9,51,53–57] However, under pathophysiological conditions, $ONOO^-$ and its derivatives are formed at high levels and may cause irreversible damage to the respiratory chain, inhibit ATP synthesis, and induce cytochrome c release and caspase-dependent apoptosis. RNS may also mediate lipid peroxidation, protein oxidation and nitration, enzyme inactivation, or even cell necrosis.[7–9,51,53–57]

MECHANISMS TO DETOXIFY ROS/RNS

ROS/RNS play a key role in the initiation, amplification, and persistence of inflammation associated with chronic lung diseases.[15–18,58,59] Similar to the formation of ROS/RNS, the removal or detoxification of these species may involve enzymatic and nonenzymatic mechanisms. Nonenzymatic systems constitute the first line of defense against ROS/RNS. The low–molecular-weight nonenzymatic antioxidants in the lung include glutathione, vitamins C and E, β-carotene, uric acid, thiols, and taurine. The larger–molecular-weight antioxidants include lactoferrin, albumin, ceruloplasmin, and transferrin; these molecules mediate their antioxidant function by binding heavy metals, making them unavailable for participation in the Fenton reaction to produce free radicals such as hydroxyl radical.[15,18,26,59,60] Nonenzymatic antioxidant activities range from the hydrophilic quenching of free radicals, protection of critical sulfhydryl groups on proteins to inhibition of lipid peroxidation.

Although nonenzymatic antioxidants are the first line of defense against different ROS, several enzymatic antioxidants work in concert with nonenzymatic antioxidants to form a tightly regulated antioxidant network. The major components of the pulmonary enzymatic antioxidant defense systems are SODs, catalase, and glutathione peroxidases. Peroxiredoxins (PRXs), thioredoxins (TRXs), glutaredoxins, heme oxygenases, and reductases are also involved in cellular adaptation and protection against oxidative stress in the lung. The enzymatic reactions that catalyze the elimination of ROS/RNS are summarized in Figure 27-1.

Superoxide Dismutases: The $O_2^{\bullet-}$ radical is a primary oxidant in chronic lung inflammation.[15,17,61] It participates in the generation of other reactive metabolites, H_2O_2, $^{\bullet}OH$, and $ONOO^-$. SODs represent a key defense against reactive species generated during normal metabolism or inflammatory states. SODs are ubiquitous enzymes that catalyze the dismutation of $O_2^{\bullet-}$ radical to the weaker oxidant, H_2O_2 (see Fig. 27-1). The function of SOD extends beyond its catalysis of $O_2^{\bullet-}$ dismutation to its participation in the regulation of normal cellular homeostasis. H_2O_2 formed from the SOD-catalyzed reaction may function as a signaling molecule at low concentrations. By reducing steady-state concentrations of $O_2^{\bullet-}$, which reacts with $NO^{\bullet}$ to form $ONOO^-$, SOD may serve to promote vasoreactivity and reduce inflammation.[15,61]

There are three mammalian SOD isozymes: the intracellular copper-zinc SOD (CuZn-SOD), the mitochondrial manganese SOD

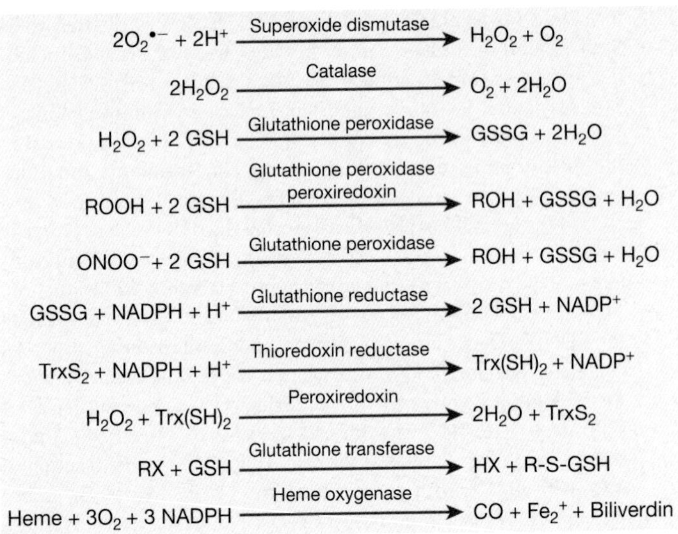

Figure 27-1 Enzymatic mechanisms to detoxify reactive oxygen and nitrogen species.

(Mn-SOD), and extracellular SOD (EC-SOD).[61] The structural and catalytic characteristics of these SOD isozymes are highlighted in Table 27-3.[62–65] Given the complexity of the human lung with its plethora of different cell types, it is conceivable that these isozymes are expressed differentially in specific lung cells with subcellular compartmentalization, as summarized in Table 27-4.[66–79]

Aside from dismutating $O_2^{\bullet-}$ radical by the cyclic oxidation–reduction of its metal ion Cu^{2+}, CuZn-SOD exhibits peroxidase activity.[65] At high levels, H_2O_2 may reduce the Cu^{2+} to either Cu^+-O or Cu^{2+}-OH that may oxidize the histidine residue in the monomer and inactivate or oxidize lung proteins.[80–82] CuZn-SOD also nitrates tyrosine residues in proteins via peroxynitrite,[83–87] and catalyzes the release of NO from nitrosothiols.[88] Although Mn-SOD has similar dismutase activity, it does not elicit peroxidation or nitration, and is inactivated by tyrosine nitration, but not by hydrogen peroxide or cyanide.

EC-SOD is the primary extracellular SOD in the lung[72] containing Cu and Zn ions.[89,90] The EC-SOD has an active site inhibitable by H_2O_2 and cyanide, similar to CuZn-SOD.[74–76] EC-SOD has an arginine- and lysine-rich heparin/matrix-binding domain at its C-terminal region.[91–94] Its extracellular localization is maintained by the interaction of this domain with heparin and heparin sulfate proteoglycans on diverse lung cell types and in the extracellular matrix (ECM) of the lung. This heparin/matrix-binding polybasic region is sensitive to proteolysis, leading to reduced affinity of EC-SOD for ECM and increased release of EC-SOD in plasma.[72,91–97] EC-SOD is abundant in the lung both at the mRNA and protein levels.[91–94] As indicated in Table 27-4, the wide cellular distribution of EC-SOD is consistent with robust EC-SOD activity in the human lung (eightfold > liver, sixfold > brain, two- to threefold > heart, and one- to twofold > kidney)[61]; in comparison, CuZn-SOD and Mn-SOD activities are much lower. The lower activities of CuZn-SOD and Mn-SOD in the lung suggest that cytoplasmic production of $O_2^{\bullet-}$ is lower in lung cells, compared with the metabolically more active cells of the liver and kidney. The dense airway and vascular network in the lung and the higher potential for extracellular inflammatory events resulting from direct exposure of the lung to the external environment may account for high EC-SOD levels in the lung. Even with its high lung localization, EC-SOD is not present at sufficient concentrations to justify its role as the sole scavenger of $O_2^{\bullet-}$ across the entire extracellular space. While CuZn-SOD and Mn-SOD function mainly as bulk scavengers of the $O_2^{\bullet-}$ radicals, the relatively high levels of EC-SOD in the lung and its binding specificity to the ECM components provide protection for the lung matrix.[14,98]

Lack of abnormalities in CuZn-SOD–deficient mice suggest that pathological consequences of mutations are perhaps due to gain of compensatory functions of the enzyme including its peroxidase or nitration reactions and not associated just with the complete loss of SOD activity.[97,99] EC-SOD–overexpressing mice were only partially protected from hyperoxia-induced lung injury, influenza, bleomycin, and hemorrhagic shock,[14,61,98] suggesting that EC-SOD may not be sufficient to attenuate oxidative stress in pathological states in which the EC-SOD system is overwhelmed. Under hyperoxia, mice lacking EC-SOD show shortened survival and extensive lung damage.[14,61,98] Thus, although other antioxidant enzymes may compensate for the loss of EC-SOD under homeostatic conditions, during inflammatory stress, EC-SOD is essential for protecting the lung and limiting injury. Over 90 genetic polymorphisms have been identified in CuZn-SOD, several in association with neurodegenerative diseases.[62] The Arg 213-gly polymorphism in EC-SOD (R213G) is found in 4% to 6% of the human population and influences chronic obstructive pulmonary disease[100,101] and acute lung injury.[102]

Catalase: H_2O_2 is reduced to water by catalase (CAT) and the glutathione peroxidases (see Fig. 27-1). CAT is a metalloprotein oxidoreductase enzyme widely expressed in lung cells (see Table 27-4).[62,103–106] In the presence of excess H_2O_2, CAT undergoes alternate divalent oxidation and reduction at its heme-containing active site. Catalase degrades H_2O_2 to O_2 and water.[62,103–106] Although catalase is the principal scavenger of H_2O_2, it is unable to metabolize large molecular peroxides including lipid peroxides. The gene for catalase is not induced by oxidant stress. However, posttranslational tyrosine phosphorylation of CAT upregulates its activity[107]; whereas, oxidation of tyrosine residues inhibits CAT activity.[8]

Glutathione peroxidases: Glutathione peroxidases (GSH-Pxs) are selenocysteine-containing tetrameric enzymes that utilize reduced glutathione (GSH), a low–molecular-weight tripeptide, as an electron donor and catalyze the biotransformation of various organic and inorganic peroxides, including H_2O_2 and lipid peroxides, to their corresponding alcohols. The detoxification of peroxides by GSH-Pxs occurs via bidirectional second-order kinetics and is a saturation-limited process.[26,108] GSH-Px1, GSH-Px2, GSH-Px3, and GSH-Px4 are the four glutathione peroxidases.[26,108] GSH-Px1 is a ubiquitous intracellular form and is the predominant isoform

TABLE 27-3 Characteristics of Superoxide Dismutases

SOD	Structure	Metal Ions	Type of Enzymatic Activity	Intracellular SOD activity (%)
Mn-SOD	Homotetramer	Mn and Zn	$O_2^{\bullet-}$ Dismutation	10
CuZn-SOD	Homodimer	Cu and Zn	$O_2^{\bullet-}$ Dismutation Peroxidation Nitration	90
EC-SOD	Homotetramer	Cu and Zn	$O_2^{\bullet-}$ Dismutation Peroxidation	0

TABLE 27-4 Enzymatic Mechanisms to Detoxify or Remove ROS/RNS

Antioxidant Enzymes	Acronym	Expression of Antioxidant Enzymes in Lung Cell Types	Cellular Distribution
Superoxide dismutase	SOD		
Mn-SOD		Alveolar type II epithelial cells, septal tip of the alveolar duct, arterioles near the airways, alveolar macrophages	Mitochondria
EC-SOD		Bronchial epithelium, alveolar epithelium, epithelial cells lining intrapulmonary airways, ECM, endothelial cells lining arteries and veins, alveolar macrophages	Plasma membrane
CuZn-SOD		Bronchial epithelium, alveolar epithelium, mesenchymal cells, fibroblasts, arterioles, capillary endothelial cells	Cytosol, nucleus, lysosome, peroxisomes
Catalase	CAT	Airway and alveolar epithelial cells, type II pneumocytes, alveolar macrophages	Peroxisomes, mitochondria
Glutathione peroxidase-1	GSH-Px	Airway epithelial cells, bronchial epithelial cells, alveolar macrophages	Cytosol, mitochondria
Thioredoxin	TRX1 and 2	Bronchial epithelium, alveolar epithelium, macrophages	Cytosol, mitochondria
Thioredoxin peroxidase	TRXPrx	Bronchial epithelial cells, type II pneumocytes, macrophages	Cytosol
Thioredoxin reductase	TRR	Bronchial epithelium, alveolar epithelium, macrophages	Cytosol, mitochondria
Glutaredoxin	Glrx	Bronchial epithelium, alveolar macrophages	Plasma membrane, cytoplasmic vacuoles, nucleus
Glutathione S Transferase	GST	Bronchiolar Clara and alveolar type II cells, bronchial epithelial cells	Plasma membrane, cytosol, microsomes, mitochondria
Peroxiredoxin	PRX	Bronchial epithelium, alveolar epithelium, macrophages	Cytosol, nuclear matrix, peroxisomes, mitochondria
Heme oxygenase	HO	Alveolar type II cells, lung fibroblasts, monocytes, alveolar macrophages	Microsomes, mitochondria, endoplasmic reticulum

that catalyzes the removal of inorganic peroxides, lipid peroxides and hydroperoxides.[26,108–111] GSH-Px2 is localized to the gastrointestinal epithelia with substrate specificities similar to that of GSH-Px1. GSH-Px3 is a secreted form able to reduce lipid hydroperoxides.[110,111] This extracellular isoform accounts for 57% of the GSH-Px activity in the epithelial lining fluid, and GSH-Px1 contributes to 40% activity.[110,111] The fourth isoform, GSH-Px4, is an intracellular peroxidase that preferentially catalyzes the peroxidation of phospholipid hydroperoxides.[109]

Thioredoxins: Thioredoxins (TRXs), which contain an active site cysteine, serve as redox sensors while also reducing H_2O_2.[112,113] H_2O_2 oxidizes the reduced dithiol group (-SH HS-) in TRX to a disulfide bridge (-S-S-). TRXs can reduce protein disulfides (-SH) and protein sulfenic acid intermediates (-SO_3H) by cysteine thiol–disulfide exchanges.[10,11] Two human TRXs are expressed widely in various lung cell types (see Table 27-4). In addition to its direct antioxidant function, TRX, in cooperation with PRXs, augments gene expression of other antioxidant enzymes, including SOD.[114–118] TRXs also participate in refolding of oxidized proteins and activate transcription factors by reducing cysteines present in the DNA-binding site.[119] TRX can be activated by hypoxia, lipopolysaccharide, H_2O_2, microbial infections, and photochemicals. Thus, TRXs are powerful redox modulators, protects cells against oxidative stress, and participates in cell proliferation and survival.[114–118]

Glutaredoxins: Glutaredoxins (GRXs) are thiol–disulfide oxidoreductases with antioxidant capacity in human lung (see Table 27-4).[18,120–123] GRX regulates cellular redox state and redox-dependent signaling pathways via modulation of protein glutathionylation; it regulates the intracellular and extracellular homeostases of glutathionylated proteins and GSH.[18,120–124] These enzymes use glutathione as a cofactor and catalyze the reversible exchange of glutathione with protein thiol groups (see chemical reactions in Fig. 27-1). GRX enzymes are dependent on GSH/GSSG concentrations.[125]

Glutathione-S-Transferases: Glutathione-S-transferases (GSTs) are detoxification enzymes that require intracellular GSH for their catalytic activity. These antioxidant enzymes inactivate secondary metabolites, such as unsaturated aldehydes, epoxides, and hydroperoxides.[126] Three major families of GSTs have been described; the cytosolic GST, mitochondrial GST, and membrane-associated microsomal GST (see Table 27-4).[60] GSTs regulate eicosanoid and glutathione metabolism.[60,127] Under conditions of oxidative stress, cytosolic GST interacts with PRXs.[126] GST family enzymes are expressed in normal lung, mainly in the airways. They protect cells against a number of oxidizing species. GSTs have high genetic variability, and are implicated in the development of smoking-related nonmalignant and malignant diseases.[60,128–131]

Peroxiredoxins: Peroxiredoxins (PRXs) are broad-spectrum peroxidases that detoxify or reduce H_2O_2, peroxynitrite, and organic hydroperoxides (ROOH).[132,133] These are nonseleno-peroxidases whose antioxidant properties are dependent on redox-active cysteines.[133] Six different PRXs have been found in human lung (see Table 27-4).[134,135] These PRXs differ widely in their specificities for H_2O_2, lipid and phospholipid hydroperoxides.[134–138] PRX V and VI function as peroxynitrite reductases, and are protective in ROS/RNS-mediated lung injury.[134–136,139,140] PRXs also regulate peroxide-mediated signaling cascades related to cell proliferation, differentiation, and apoptosis by modulating cytokine-mediated induction of H_2O_2.[18,133,137,138]

Heme oxygenases: Heme oxygenase (HO) catalyzes the breakdown of pro-oxidant heme to generate equimolar amounts of carbon monoxide, ferrous iron, and biliverdin (Fig. 27-1). Biliverdin is then converted by biliverdin reductase to bilirubin, the antioxidant endproduct of the HO reaction.[141–144] CO transported to the lung has vasodilatory and antiapoptotic properties.[145–150] Iron is used for heme synthesis in the cells required for heme-containing proteins or transported to the bone marrow and other tissues.[18,141,144,151,152] There are three isoforms of HO, the inducible HO-1, and the constitutive forms, HO-2 and HO-3. During oxidative stress, transcriptional activation results in rapid induction of HO-1.[141,144,145] This adaptive response of HO-1 confers protection during inflammation and oxidative stress. HO-1 is expressed widely in the lung (see Table 27-4). Consistent with the antioxidant properties of HO-1, mice deficient in HO-1 are more susceptible to oxidative stress.[153,154] Overexpression or induction of HO-1 suppresses inflammation in several models of chronic lung disease.[18,141,144,151,152]

CELLULAR SOURCES AND REGULATION OF ROS/RNS

IMMUNE CELLS

Inflammation is an adaptive response to infectious and noninfectious tissue injury. Recruited inflammatory cells emigrate from the pulmonary microcirculation into the airspaces where they become activated to generate ROS/RNS.

NO• participates in pathogen killing by macrophages.[155] NO• also delays fusion of phagosomes with lysosomes to form a functional phagolysosome, which enhances antigen processing/presentation of macrophages. Macrophages scavenge endogenous dying cells. Phagocytosis of dying cells requires the secretion of alarmins by dying cells to attract and preactivate phagocytes; these signals by dying cells ensures specific recognition and phagocytosis/efferocytosis, all of which involve redox regulation.[156,157]

Beyond the chemical interactions of NO• and ROS that cooperatively eradicate pathogens, these redox-active biomolecules regulate cellular metabolism, inflammation, and tissue-repair functions. Cellular supply of substrates/cofactors for iNOS activity, including arginine, is required for NO• production. However, in the absence of arginine or BH_4, uncoupled NOS becomes an $O_2^{\bullet-}/H_2O_2$ generator. The flavin-binding sites of the reductase domain of iNOS, eNOS, and nNOS are a source of $O_2^{\bullet-}$ generation in the absence of arginine.[155,158–161] Therefore, metabolic pathways that control arginine and BH_4 play a role in determining NO•–$O_2^{\bullet-}$ balance. Cellular arginine levels are dependent on uptake and transport mechanisms and the activation of NOS-arginase enzymatic systems that use arginine. Arginase activation produces ornithine, a starting metabolite for the production of polyamines that are critical molecules supporting DNA stabilization, ion channel transport, and cell proliferation.[155,158–161] Arginase is regulated by NOS and NOX activities; N-hydroxyarginine, a product of NOS, inhibits arginase, while $O_2^{\bullet-}$ increases arginase activity.[155,158–161] High arginase activity is associated with elevated ROS and low NO• fluxes. NO• antagonizes NOX2 assembly through the activation of PPARγ which, in turn, inhibits expression of the p47 subunit required for NOX2 activation.[155,158–161] Thus, $O_2^{\bullet-}$ production is suppressed when NOS activity and NO• levels are high. NO• also inhibits COX2 activity, reducing COX2-dependent ROS production.[162] Thus, as NO• levels decline, ROS generation may increase via multiple mechanisms.

The balance between NO• and ROS may play a key role in the orchestration and resolution of inflammation. RNS and ROS actively control innate and adaptive immune signaling. This aspect of redox function is evident in cells of myeloid lineage, such as monocytes, macrophages, and neutrophils. RNS and ROS produced by these cells participate in induction, maintenance, and/or termination of proinflammatory and anti-inflammatory signaling. Similar to the effect of NO• on pathogen eradication, the temporal and spatial concentration profiles of NO• are key determinants of immune-mediated processes.[155,158–161] A relationship between increasing steady-state levels of NO• has been linked to regulation of expression of tumor suppressor gene p53 and apoptosis in murine and human macrophage cell lines.[163,164] Concentration- and time-dependent changes in the functional profiles of NO• are evident from NO-mediated regulation of cell survival protein signaling cascade[165–169]

Macrophages rely primarily on the NOX2 complex to produce ROS,[5,17,157,168] although the oxidative burst of macrophages is less intense than that of neutrophils. Induction of the proinflammatory phase of an innate immune response is an early response in the immune activation process. This is defined as "classical activation" in macrophages (also called M1 macrophages), and is associated with the production and release of proinflammatory cytokines, proteases including MMP-9, transcription factors such as NF-κB as well as RNS and ROS, including NO• and $O_2^{\bullet-}$. In addition to a role in pathogen eradication, the localized levels of ROS/RNS may dictate integrated signaling and the type of immune activation and determination of cellular phenotypes; ROS/RNS may also regulate crosstalk between proinflammatory and resolution pathways. Classical (proinflammatory) activation of macrophages is followed by an anti-inflammatory healing/tissue-repair phase, which is the ideal outcome of a successful innate immune response. These phases of the innate immune response are initiated by the pathogens or tissue injury, but are rapidly reenforced by the actions of anti-inflammatory cytokines released from macrophages that function in an autocrine manner.[157,158,170–172] These cytokines initiate downregulation of the proinflammatory phase and induction of the repair or tissue remodeling phase.

NO• also affects function of T lymphocytes.[155,173–176] Low NO• concentrations promote differentiation of IFN-γ producing Th1 (T helper 1) in mice and humans, mediated by cGMP activation.[177] During the immune repair/restoration phase, the collective activity of IL-4, IL-13, IL-10, and TGF-β suppress iNOS expression, thereby decreasing NO• and shifting in favor of ROS.[155,173–177] An NO•-independent role for arginase has been identified in the differentiation of alternatively activated macrophages. Although arginase expression in macrophages is prominently associated with Th2 responses, part of its function is to sequester arginine away from effector T cells resulting in a reduced Th2 response; reconstitution with exogenous arginine blocks this reduced Th2 response. In general, low NO• favors Th2 responses, and high NO• augments Th1 responses, suggesting that a NO•/ROS balance may be a critical determinant of immune polarity.[155,178,179] Naïve lymphocytes exposed to high μmol concentrations of NO•, however, regulate the expansion and proliferation of regulatory T cells within lymphoid tissue.[155]

This concentration-dependent regulation by NO• is seen in immunosuppression by heterogeneous immature myeloid cells called myeloid-derived suppressor cells (MDSCs).[180,181] Free radical producing subsets of these MDSCs are critical regulators of allergic airway inflammation.[182,183] NO•-producing cells suppress T cell proliferation and airway hyperresponsiveness (AHR), while $O_2^{\bullet-}$ enhance T cell proliferation and exacerbate AHR.[182,183] Immunosuppression by MDSCs also occurs in the tumor microenvironment in which NO•-mediated increase in cGMP activation, facilitates their binding to cytotoxic lymphocytes to reduce their proliferation.[184,185] Peroxynitrite and H_2O_2 are produced by the combined and cooperative activities of NADPH oxidase, arginase, and iNOS in different MDSC subsets. These drive several molecular blocks in T cells, ranging from the loss of TCRζ-chain expression, interference with IL-2 receptor–mediated signaling and nitration, and subsequent desensitization of the TCR.[184,185] Signal transducer and activator of transcription 3 (STAT3) is a critical regulator of MDSCs. STAT3-mediated upregulation of the NADPH oxidase and ROS levels enhances the suppressive potential of MDSCs.[155,184,185]

Inflammasome activation is an innate immune response to pathogens, but also accompanies the development of autoimmune and chronic inflammatory diseases. Inflammasomes are multicomponent platforms that sense a variety of danger signals, including bacteria, viruses, pathogenic crystals; aggregates through a family of nod-like receptors and consists of caspase-1 to process proinflammatory cytokines for activation.[186–188] Inflammasome activation starts with a priming signal followed by an activation signal. Studies with ROS scavengers suggest a role of ROS in inflammasome activation.[186–190]

EPITHELIAL CELLS

The epithelium of the airways and the alveoli is exposed to high levels of oxygen and to other environmental oxidizing species. Although inflammatory cells are major producers of RNS/ROS, resident lung cells such as epithelial cells, possess enzymatic systems for regulated production of RNS and ROS. DUOX enzymes are the primary contributors of H_2O_2 in the airway epithelium.[25,191] DUOXs are expressed in ciliated surface cells, but not in nonciliated cells or basal cells of the upper airway. The levels of expression of DUOX1 and DUOX2 are selectively regulated by cytokines, with Th1 cytokines regulating DUOX2 and Th2 cytokines regulating DUOX1.[19,21,192,193] The highly inducible DUOX2 mediates host responses to infection and inflammation, while DUOX1 is constitutively expressed in noninflamed airways; DUOX2 plays a role in innate immunity, cell signaling, and mucus production.[19,21,193,194] The airway epithelium participates in innate immune response through the secretion of immune effectors such as mucin, antimicrobial peptides, and ROS to entrap or kill invading microbes. Epithelial cells use microbial pattern recognition receptors for innate immune system recognition to discriminate self from nonself.[19,21,192,193] The release of cytokines/chemokines by the epithelium induces neutrophil recruitment and the activation of transcription factors augmenting the inflammatory response. Lactoperoxidase (LPO) a heme-containing peroxidase in concert with DUOX-generated H_2O_2 generates hypohalous acids that kill pathogens.[25,194] A functional difference between the airway DUOX/LPO system and the phagocytic NOX2/MPO system is that the phagocytic system is active only during the respiratory burst, whereas DUOX generates H_2O_2 continuously.[19,21,192,193]

ENDOTHELIAL CELLS

Endothelial cells (ECs) also participate in innate immunity and crosstalk with immune cells. The importance of ECs in inflammation-induced vascular dysfunction is dependent on their ability to produce and respond to ROS and RNS. Inflammation may alter the balance between $NO^\bullet$ and $O_2^{\bullet -}$ within (and surrounding) ECs, which is necessary for normal vascular function. ROS produced by the endothelium play an important role in vascular pathology.[195,196] ROS can quench $NO^\bullet$ and mediate proinflammatory signaling. Targeting ROS-quenching enzymes catalase and SOD in ECs alleviates toxic effects of excessive ROS and suppresses proinflammatory mechanisms, including endothelial cytokine activation and barrier disruption.[197–199] Pulmonary EC-derived ROS play a pivotal role in EC activation and function. Alterations in EC phenotype contribute to vascular tone, permeability, and inflammatory responses and, thus, have been implicated in lung diseases, including pulmonary hypertension, ischemia-reperfusion (IR) injury, and adult respiratory distress syndrome.[200–202] Contrasting effects of NOS isoforms occur during IR injury, where eNOS appears to be protective and iNOS detrimental. Under homeostatic conditions, the low NO flux generated by eNOS prevents leukocyte recruitment and associated tissue damage through scavenging of ROS. However, when iNOS expression increases, $NO^\bullet$ levels rise and induce tissue injury.[200–202] Thus, the beneficial effects of specific NOS isoforms depend on the type of primary damaging event.

FIBROBLASTS

Fibroblasts and fibroblast-like mesenchymal cells participate in innate immunity and in tissue repair. Such cells are typically resident within the adult human lung[203]; however, studies have reported fibroblasts derived from bone marrow cells[204] or epithelial cells, the latter in a process known as epithelial-to-mesenchymal transition (EMT).[205] EMT is a process regulating cell plasticity, which allows epithelial cells to lose their polarity and specialized junctional structures, to undergo cytoskeletal reorganization, and to acquire morphological and functional features of mesenchymal-like cells. Myofibroblasts are the primary "effector" cells in tissue remodeling and pulmonary fibrosis.[206–208] Activation of the NADPH oxidase isoform, NOX4, mediates generation of H_2O_2, myofibroblast differentiation, contractility, and ECM production in response to TGF-β1.[209] In addition, NOX4 may play a profibrotic role by inducing apoptosis of lung epithelial cells, while myofibroblasts themselves acquire an apoptosis-resistant phenotype. Epithelial cell death may also be mediated indirectly by the paracrine secretion of H_2O_2 by activated myofibroblasts, supporting the concept that NOX4 may be responsible for both myofibroblast activation and epithelial cell disrepair.[210]

OXIDATIVE STRESS IN VARIOUS LUNG DISORDERS

Oxidative stress is implicated in the pathogenesis of both acute and chronic inflammatory and fibrotic lung diseases, some of which are discussed here (Fig. 27-2).

ASTHMA

Asthma is a chronic inflammatory airway disease.[211,212] ROS and RNS have been implicated in the pathogenesis of asthma.[20,213–216] Dysregulation in pathways that lead to oxidative stress or its defense may contribute to the initiation and severity of asthma.[8,20,213–218] Recruitment of inflammatory cells and ROS production have been documented in the airways of asthmatic subjects.[20,112,214,219–222] $O_2^{\bullet -}$ generation was observed highest in airspace cells at the sites of antigen challenge.[213] Leukocyte activation with induction of NADPH oxidase and production of $O_2^{\bullet -}$ and H_2O_2 correlate negatively with FEV_1 in asthmatic subjects.[222] Besides airway macrophages and eosinophils, blood eosinophils and monocytes are also major sources of ROS in asthmatic patients.[213,218,223]

Airway inflammation-associated oxidative stress in asthma may induce oxidative modifications of proteins or lipids.[89,90,224] Increased numbers of eosinophils and neutrophils in association with higher

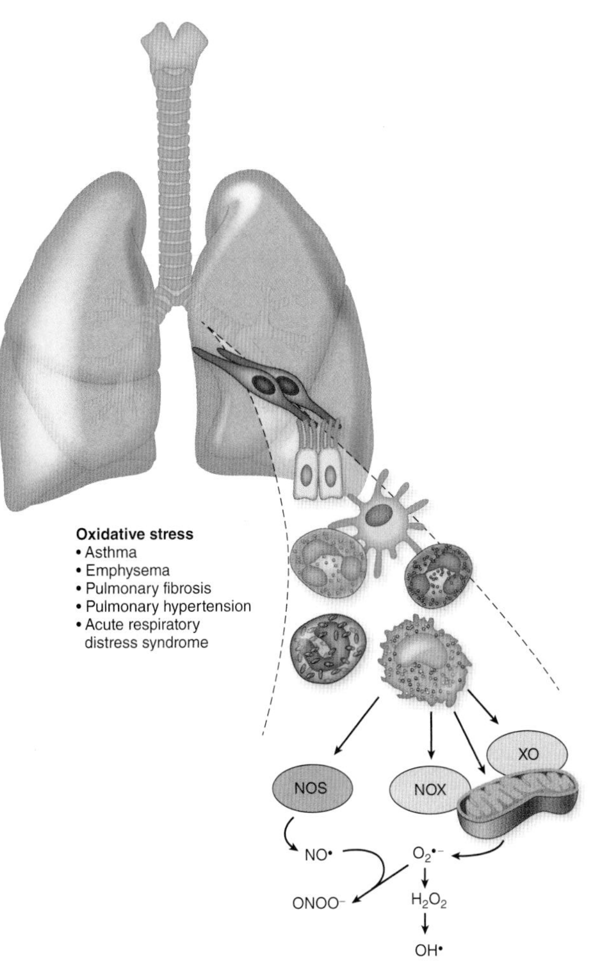

Figure 27-2 Oxidants initiate a number of pathological processes with a multitude of complex mechanisms that contribute to pathogenesis of both acute and chronic inflammatory diseases of the lung. Resident lung cells and recruited inflammatory cells together orchestrate these multilevel processes by regulating enzymatic pathways to balance the generation and metabolism of oxidants.

expression of peroxidases and other markers of eosinophil activation are found in bronchoalveolar lavage fluid (BAL) and bronchial tissues of asthmatics.[225,226] Oxidant products of neutrophil/eosinophil activation, 3-bromotyrosine, and MPO-mediated oxidants, such as chlorotyrosine are increased in asthmatics compared to control subjects; these have been implicated in the pathophysiology of severe asthma.[227,228] Other reactive products including malondialdehyde, thiobarbituric acid-reactive products, and 8-isoprostane, a biomarker of lipid peroxidation are also elevated in exhaled breath condensates of adults and children with asthma.[229–234] The precise mechanisms by which ROS exacerbate asthma is not known, but may involve effects on airway smooth muscle, mucin secretion, and T cell responses.[59,235] ROS can decrease β-adrenergic function in lungs and sensitize airway smooth muscle to acetylcholine-induced contraction.[103,236] H_2O_2 activates mitogen-activated kinases in tracheal myocytes and stimulates contraction of tracheal smooth muscle cells.[235] ROS also stimulates mucin secretion,[103,236] contributes to Th2 cell differentiation,[179] and promotes T cell proliferation via arginase and NADPH oxidase pathways.[182,183] Proinflammatory cytokines are elevated during airway inflammation, which activate oxidases leading to increases in ROS, the targets of which include receptor kinases, phosphatases, phospholipids, or non-receptor tyrosine kinases.[16,237,238]

Another target of ROS is $NO^•$. $NO^•$ metabolism appears to be dysregulated in asthma. Exhaled $NO^•$ is increased in asthmatics and is associated with airway inflammation.[54,55,239] Despite the expression and distribution of all three NOS enzymes in the airway, it is primarily iNOS that contributes to exhaled $NO^•$. Induction of iNOS is observed at both transcriptional and translational levels principally in steroid-naïve patients.[41–43] In mild asthmatics, $NO^•$, nitrate, and SNOs are enhanced in the lower airways.[54] Following antigen challenge, levels of $NO^•$ decrease, while nitrate increases without perturbing levels of nitrite and SNO.[54] Decreasing $NO^•$ levels correlates with increased nitrotyrosine formation from reaction of $NO^•$ with $O_2^{•-}$.[54] Peroxynitrite, thus formed during inflammation, is toxic to microbes; however, it can also cause AHR. Nitrate can be generated from peroxidase-mediated RNS production.[54,240] SNOs are primarily formed during the late asthmatic response.[54,240] Thus, persistent increases in ROS and $NO^•$ lead to RNS formation and subsequent oxidation and nitration of proteins, which contributes to the dysregulation of airway inflammation in asthma.[15] $NO^•$ synthesis can reduce airway resistance mediated by increased production of the bronchodilator S-nitrosoglutathione (GSNO).[241–245] Two mechanisms to co-opt beneficial effects of $NO^•$ signaling are (1) shifting $NO^•$ to a more stable species, such as GSNO; or (2) reducing the local concentrations of ROS, potentially by augmenting the concentration of antioxidant enzymes in the extracellular space. Elevated $NO^•$ has also been attributed to the greater catabolic breakdown of the storage pools of GSNO during changes in the redox state of the lungs.[241–243] GSNOR, a glutathione-dependent formaldehyde dehydrogenase reduces GSNO to hydroxylamine, which is converted to NO by catalase.[245–247] GSNOR-deficient mice are protected from methacholine hyperreactivity following allergen sensitization and challenge, implicating GSNO in controlling airway hyperreactivity.[245–247]

High levels of ROS may overwhelm antioxidant defenses, causing significant loss of antioxidant activity in asthma.[8,67,70,213,217] Global loss of SOD activity, due to SOD deficiency, loss of circulating SOD activity, or inactivation of SOD via oxidative modification reflects the increased oxidative stress in asthmatic patients.[8,67,70,213,217] Oxidative modification-mediated reduction of catalase activity is also observed in asthmatics.[8] Although airway glutathione is increased in asthmatic patients, the ratio of oxidized to reduced glutathione is elevated reflecting an oxidizing microenvironment. Inhalation of exogenous ROS and RNS from exposures to environmental pollutants including ozone, diesel exhaust particles, and oxidant components of tobacco smoke, all contribute to additive oxidative stress, airway hyperreactivity, and inflammation in asthma.

EMPHYSEMA

Emphysema is a dominant phenotype of chronic obstructive pulmonary disease,[248–251] defined pathologically by airspace enlargement and destruction of alveolar septae.[248–251] Important contributing factors to the pathobiology of emphysema include inflammation, alveolar epithelial cell injury/apoptosis, protease–antiprotease and oxidant–antioxidant imbalances.[250–255] Inflammatory cells are recruited to the alveolar environment where they release elastases, cytokines, and oxidants that may then perpetuate the cycle of epithelial injury and inflammation.[250–255] In addition to inflammation, oxidative stress caused by cigarette smoke inhalation contributes to the pathogenesis of emphysema. Cigarette smoke contains $O_2^{•-}$, $^•OH$, and H_2O_2.[256] ROS are also generated by the chronic inflammation, characteristic of emphysema and that persists even after smoking cessation. Activated macrophages and neutrophils present in high numbers in the emphysematous lung are major producers of ROS.[257–262] Oxidative stress originating from constituents of cigarette smoke or products of inflammatory cells can overcome the antioxidative capacity of lung tissues and diminish antiprotease defenses.[263,264] A major consequence of oxidative stress is the activation of the transcription factor nuclear factor-κB (NF-κB), which activates transcription of proinflammatory cytokines.[251,263–265] Cigarette smoke also inhibits histone deacetylase, further promoting the release of proinflammatory cytokines.[266] Therefore, oxidant injury and lung inflammation act in concert to increase alveolar destruction or compromise maintenance and repair of alveolar structure. Antioxidant defenses are determinants of susceptibility to emphysema. A protective role for Nrf2, a transcription factor that regulates multiple critical antioxidant enzymes, has been identified in pulmonary emphysema.[267–270] SOD mimetics abrogate alveolar cell apoptosis and emphysema in mouse models.[271] This blockade of apoptosis prevents oxidative stress and emphysema further supporting the link between oxidative stress and apoptosis.[272,273]

PULMONARY FIBROSIS

Pulmonary fibrosis may result from a number of infectious and noninfectious injuries; by far, the most lethal form is idiopathic pulmonary fibrosis (IPF). IPF is characterized by exuberant ECM deposition, tissue contraction, and apoptosis resistance of (myo) fibroblasts, alongside apoptosis-prone and aberrantly differentiated alveolar type 2 cells.[18,274] This loss of epithelial–mesenchymal homeostasis and communication is central to the pathogenesis of IPF.[206,208] Myofibroblasts are key effector cells in tissue remodeling and fibrosis, typically contained in fibroblastic foci, which are a pathological hallmark of IPF. Chronic inflammation, aberrant wound healing, and degenerative aging processes have all been proposed as contributing to the pathogenesis of IPF.[275] Oxidative stress is common to these processes and is implicated in IPF pathogenesis.[276–278] Lung tissues and bronchoalveolar lavage fluid from IPF patients demonstrate a signature profile of oxidatively damaged proteins.[279–282]

NOX enzymes are a major source of ROS production in pulmonary fibrosis.[207,283–286] Several NOX isoforms, including NOX1,[287–289] NOX2,[290–293] and NOX4[209,285,294] have been implicated in tissue fibrosis. In addition to NOX enzymes, another potential source of ROS implicated in fibrosis is the mitochondria.[295,296] Epithelial cell death is a prominent feature in the IPF lung.[285,297,298] During acute lung injury in mice, NOX1-mediated ROS generation by endothelial and epithelial cells induces cell death.[299,300] NOX4 is expressed in hyperplastic alveolar type II cells in the lungs of IPF patients[294] and may mediate fibrogenic effects by promoting alveolar epithelial cell death.[214] NOX4-deficient mice are protected from bleomycin-induced pulmonary fibrosis through modulation of epithelial cell apoptosis *in vivo*.[214] EMT has been proposed to contribute to the accumulation of myofibroblasts in lung fibrosis.[301,302] ROS has also been shown to promote EMT.[303,304] A role for NOX4 in mediating myofibroblast differentiation and lung fibrosis has been identified.[227] NOX4 mRNA expression is induced by the profibrotic cytokine, transforming growth factor-β1 (TGF-β1), while other NOX/DUOX isoforms were unaffected. NOX4-dependent generation of ROS, specifically H_2O_2, is required for TGF-β1–induced myofibroblast differentiation, ECM generation, and contractility of lung myofibroblasts.[209] Genetic or pharmacological targeting of NOX4 attenuates lung fibrogenesis in murine models of lung injury. Myofibroblasts from IPF patients also produce high levels of H_2O_2 in response to TGF-β1.[210] NOX4 may also contribute to pulmonary vascular remodeling associated with IPF.[305]

ROS generation from alveolar inflammatory cells, primarily neutrophils, and macrophages, may promote alveolar epithelial cell injury in IPF.[276,306] Mice deficient in NOX2 are protected from bleomycin-induced lung injury and fibrosis suggesting a role for inflammatory injury in this model.[307] The protection in $p47^{phox-/-}$ mice was accompanied by enhanced neutrophilic inflammation and MMP-9 activity.[307] Interestingly, airway neutrophils isolated from IPF patients exhibit elevated expression of $p47^{phox}$ and $p67^{phox}$,[308] supporting roles for the NOX2 isoform and neutrophilic inflammation in IPF. MMPs and tissue inhibitors of matrix metalloproteinases play a role in homeostasis and turnover of the ECM. In IPF, oxidation of the cysteine switch of MMPs by ROS activates the latent forms of MMPs.[210,276,309] ROS also regulates MMPs at the transcriptional level.[210,276,309] Thus, oxidative stress, from exogenous sources and multiple endogenous enzymatic sources, contributes to altered cellular homeostasis, including resident cells, recruited inflammatory cells, and their activated products.

PULMONARY HYPERTENSION

Pulmonary arterial hypertension (PAH) is a disorder of the pulmonary circulation characterized by endothelial dysfunction, intimal and smooth muscle proliferation.[310,311] Increased expression of ROS-generating enzymes, uncoupling of NOS enzymes, and mitochondrial dysfunction all contribute to the oxidative stress in PAH.[310,311] Upstream dysregulation of ROS/NO$^\bullet$ redox homeostasis impairs vascular tone, which then triggers the activation of antiapoptotic and mitogenic pathways, leading to cell proliferation and obliteration of the vasculature.[310,311]

ROS derived from the NOX2 and NOX4 isoforms contribute to the long-term responses of the pulmonary vasculature to hypoxia.[312–315] Increased NOX4 expression in pulmonary artery smooth muscle cells (PASMC) has been linked to hypoxia-dependent PAH in mice.[315] Levels of the NOX1 and 2 regulatory proteins, $p47^{phox}$, and Rac1 are increased in both the endothelial and SMC layers of pulmonary arteries[316–318] accompanied by an increase in NOX-derived $O_2^{\bullet-}$.[316–318] NOX-derived ROS is associated with medial thickening, disordered proliferation and migration, impaired angiogenesis, and disturbed fibrinolysis.[316–320] Another source of vascular ROS is xanthine oxidoreductases (XORs), including xanthine dehydrogenase (XD) and xanthine oxidase (XO). In PAH, XO activity dominates over XD activity and is a significant source of ROS production. XO is increased in idiopathic PAH patients compared with healthy controls.[320] In a rat model of chronic hypoxia-induced PAH, lung XO activity was enhanced and inhibition of XO activity with allopurinol reduced the right ventricular hypertrophy and the pulmonary vascular thickening.[316–319,321] Clinical studies have also demonstrated alterations of TGF-β1 expression in adult PAH patients.[322] In hypoxia-dependent PAH in mice, hypoxia increases the expression of TGF-β1 and NOX4 expression.[314,315] TGF-β–induced NOX4 expression and NOX4-mediated ROS production have been implicated in PASMC proliferation.[323,324] TGF-β1 also induces proangiogenic effects by upregulating VEGF.[325] In PASMCs, cyclic stretch induces VEGF expression, both at the mRNA and protein levels[326]; this is preceded by both an increased expression and secretion of TGF-β1 and an increase in ROS generation by the activation of NOX enzymes.[323,324] In models of spontaneously developing PAH, mitochondrial dysfunction and hyperpolarization is associated with reduction in ROS production.[327,328] Decreases in ROS inhibit a $O_2^{\bullet-}$ sensitive K^+ channel leading to pulmonary vascular constriction.[327–329]

Nitrosative stress with increased nitrated eNOS is an early contributor to the development of PAH.[316,330–333] The vasodilatory effects of cGMP are mediated through protein kinase G (PKG).[316,330–333] However, nitration of PKG, attenuates the kinetic activity of PKG, impairs vasodilation, and increases smooth muscle proliferation.[334] This nitration-dependent reduction in PKG activity is observed in lungs of patients with PAH.[334] Nitration of carnitine acetyltransferase, an enzyme that maintains normal mitochondrial function is another indicator of early nitrosative stress in PAH.[335]

Alterations in arginine metabolism have also been noted in models of PAH,[317] where the activity of arginase that catalyzes the hydrolysis of L-arginine to L-ornithine and urea is increased,[158,317,336,337] and the activity of the caveolar enzymes involved in the recycling of L-citrulline and other L-arginine byproducts back to L-arginine are attenuated.[158,317,336,337] Further, increased arginase activity is associated with formation of polyamines and L-proline, which promote smooth muscle cell growth and collagen synthesis. In addition, uncoupling of NOS enzymes occur when L-arginine becomes limited resulting in the production of ROS.[318,338–340] Therefore, high arginase activity may promote aberrant pulmonary vascular remodeling and neointima formation in PAH.[158,336,337]

ACUTE RESPIRATORY DISTRESS SYNDROME

Acute respiratory distress syndrome (ARDS) is a severe form of acute lung injury and a syndrome of acute pulmonary inflammation.[341,342] ARDS is characterized by sudden onset, impaired gas exchange, and an increase in pulmonary capillary permeability.[341–343] Oxidative damage by ROS and RNS has been implicated in the pulmonary vascular endothelial damage that characterizes ARD. Several factors contribute to the intracellular and extracellular oxidant stress in ARDS patients.[341–343] The high inspiratory concentrations of oxygen required to achieve adequate arterial oxygenation, infection, or extrapulmonary inflammation lead to increased ROS production. This, combined with decreased antioxidant capacity of tissues resulting from consumption of the natural antioxidants leads to cellular damage and loss of vasomotor control.[341–343] Measurements of antioxidant concentrations have revealed an oxidant–antioxidant imbalance in ARDS patients. The production of toxic levels of ROS and RNS not only leads to damage of key molecules in cells but can signal changes in cellular responses such as proliferation, apoptosis, and necrosis.[341–343] H_2O_2 has been detected in the exhaled breath, while MPO and oxidized α1-antitrypsin have been detected in BAL of ARDS patients.[341–343] Nitration and oxidation of alveolar space proteins including the surfactants have been identified *ex vivo* in patient samples with ARDS.[341–343] Overabundance of ROS also induces adhesion molecules and cytokines that contribute to endothelial injury.

CONCLUSION

The lungs are exposed to exogenous oxidants from the environment, in addition to endogenous generation of ROS/RNS from resident and recruited inflammatory cells. Several measures of oxidative stress have been used to estimate oxidative stress within the lungs; however, current approaches do not adequately differentiate between different oxidative mechanisms and are used as biomarkers of oxidative damage. Further investigations are needed to discover biomarkers that correlate and differentiate between various types of oxidative injury. While progress has been made to delineate mechanisms through which oxidants initiate and propagate cell and tissue damage, specific signaling pathways and mechanisms of activation are not well understood. Elucidation of these mechanisms may provide strategies for intervention to prevent or protect from disease pathogenesis or progression. A better understanding of factors that influence individual susceptibility will also be useful in risk stratification of patients. Investigations on how early life exposures to oxidants impact airway morphology, immune function, and the airway epigenome may also aid in determining susceptibility, disease expression, and progression.

REFERENCES

1. Miller DM, Buettner GR, Aust SD. Transition metals as catalysts of "autoxidation" reactions. *Free Radic Biol Med.* 1990;8(1):95–108.
2. Halliwell B. Tell me about free radicals, doctor: a review. *J R Soc Med.* 1989;82(12):747–752.
3. Halliwell B. Free radicals, reactive oxygen species and human disease: a critical evaluation with special reference to atherosclerosis. *Br J Exp Pathol.* 1989;70(6):737–757.
4. Halliwell B, Gutteridge JMC. *Free Radicals in Biology and Medicine.* 2nd ed. Oxford: Clarendon Press; 1989.
5. Bergendi L, Benes L, Durackova Z, Ferencik M. Chemistry, physiology and pathology of free radicals. *Life Sci.* 1999;65(18–19): 1865–1874.
6. Stuehr DJ. Structure-function aspects in the nitric oxide synthases. *Annu Rev Pharmacol Toxicol.* 1997;37:339–359.
7. Aulak KS, Miyagi M, Yan L, et al. Proteomic method identifies proteins nitrated in vivo during inflammatory challenge. *Proc Natl Acad Sci U S A.* 2001;98(21):12056–12061.
8. Ghosh S, Janocha AJ, Aronica MA, et al. Nitrotyrosine proteome survey in asthma identifies oxidative mechanism of catalase inactivation. *J Immunol.* 2006;176(9):5587–5597.
9. Masri FA, Comhair SA, Koeck T, et al. Abnormalities in nitric oxide and its derivatives in lung cancer. *Am J Respir Crit Care Med.* 2005;172(5):597–605.
10. Finkel T. Oxygen radicals and signaling. *Curr Opin Cell Biol.* 1998;10(2):248–253.
11. Beckman JS, Koppenol WH. Nitric oxide, superoxide, and peroxynitrite: the good, the bad, and ugly. *Am J Physiol.* 1996; 271(5 Pt 1):C1424–C1437.
12. Gladwin MT, Raat NJ, Shiva S, et al. Nitrite as a vascular endocrine nitric oxide reservoir that contributes to hypoxic signaling, cytoprotection, and vasodilation. *Am J Physiol Heart Circ Physiol.* 2006;291(5):H2026–H2035.
13. Valko M, Leibfritz D, Moncol J, Cronin MT, Mazur M, Telser J. Free radicals and antioxidants in normal physiological functions and human disease. *Int J Biochem Cell Biol.* 2007;39(1):44–84.
14. Crapo JD, Stamler JS. Signaling by nonreceptor surface-mediated redox-active biomolecules. *J Clin Invest.* 1994;93(6):2304.
15. Comhair SA, Erzurum SC. Redox control of asthma: molecular mechanisms and therapeutic opportunities. *Antioxid Redox Signal.* 2010;12(1):93–124.
16. Thannickal VJ, Fanburg BL. Reactive oxygen species in cell signaling. *Am J Physiol Lung Cell Mol Physiol.* 2000;279(6):L1005–L1028.
17. Birben E, Sahiner UM, Sackesen C, Erzurum S, Kalayci O. Oxidative stress and antioxidant defense. *World Allergy Organ J.* 2012;5(1):9–19.
18. Rahman I, Biswas SK, Kode A. Oxidant and antioxidant balance in the airways and airway diseases. *Eur J Pharmacol.* 2006;533(1–3): 222–239.
19. Arnold RS, Lambeth RD. "The NOX Enzymes and the Regulated Generation of Reactive Oxygen Species" In: *Signal Transduction by Reactive Oxygen and Nitrogen Species: Pathways and Chemical Principles,* Kluwer Academic Publishers, The Netherlands, 2003, pp. 102–119.
20. Bast A, Haenen GR, Doelman CJ. Oxidants and antioxidants: state of the art. *Am J Med.* 1991;91(3 C):2S–13S.
21. Leto TL, Morand S, Hurt D, Ueyama T. Targeting and regulation of reactive oxygen species generation by Nox family NADPH oxidases. *Antioxid Redox Signal.* 2009;11(10):2607–2619.
22. Katsuyama M, Matsuno K, Yabe-Nishimura C. Physiological roles of NOX/NADPH oxidase, the superoxide-generating enzyme. *J Clin Biochem Nutr.* 2012;50(1):9–22.
23. Sumimoto H. Structure, regulation and evolution of Nox-family NADPH oxidases that produce reactive oxygen species. *FEBS J.* 2008;275(13):3249–3277.
24. Shono T, Yokoyama N, Uesaka T, et al. Enhanced expression of NADPH oxidase Nox4 in human gliomas and its roles in cell proliferation and survival. *Int J Cancer.* 2008;123(4): 787–792.
25. Geiszt M, Witta J, Baffi J, Lekstrom K, Leto TL. Dual oxidases represent novel hydrogen peroxide sources supporting mucosal surface host defense. *FASEB J.* 2003;17(11):1502–1504.
26. Comhair SA, Erzurum SC. Antioxidant responses to oxidant-mediated lung diseases. *Am J Physiol.* 2002;283(2):L246–L255.
27. Goeptar AR, Scheerens H, Vermeulen NP. Oxygen and xenobiotic reductase activities of cytochrome P450. *Crit Rev Toxicol.* 1995;25(1):25–65.
28. Foote CS, Goyne TE, Lehrer RI. Assessment of chlorination by human neutrophils. *Nature.* 1983;301(5902):715–716.
29. Harrison DG, Chapman MP, Christy JP, Marcus ML. Studies of functional site of origin of native coronary collaterals. *Am J Physiol.* 1986;251(6 Pt 2):H1217–H1224.
30. Klebanoff SJ, Hamon CB. Role of myeloperoxidase-mediated antimicrobial systems in intact leukocytes. *J Reticuloendothel Soc.* 1972;12(2):170–196.
31. Weiss SJ, Test ST, Eckmann CM, Roos D, Regiani S. Brominating oxidants generated by human eosinophils. *Science.* 1986;234(4773):200–203.
32. Weiss SJ. Oxygen, ischemia and inflammation. *Acta Physiol Scand Suppl.* 1986;548:9–37.
33. Holley AE, Cheeseman KH. Measuring free radical reactions in vivo. *Br Med Bull.* 1993;49(3):494–505.
34. Cheeseman KH, Slater TF. An introduction to free radical biochemistry. *British Med Bull.* 1993;49(3):481–493.
35. Candeias LP, Patel KB, Stratford MR, Wardman P. Free hydroxyl radicals are formed on reaction between the neutrophil-derived species superoxide anion and hypochlorous acid. *FEBS Lett.* 1993;333(1–2):151–153.
36. Schmitt D, Shen Z, Zhang R, et al. Leukocytes utilize myeloperoxidase-generated nitrating intermediates as physiological catalysts for the generation of biologically active oxidized lipids and sterols in serum. *Biochemistry.* 1999;38(51):16904–16915.
37. Hazen SL, Hsu FF, Gaut JP, Crowley JR, Heinecke JW. Modification of proteins and lipids by myeloperoxidase. *Methods Enzymol.* 1999;300:88–105.
38. Hazen SL, Zhang R, Shen Z, et al. Formation of nitric oxide-derived oxidants by myeloperoxidase in monocytes: pathways for monocyte-mediated protein nitration and lipid peroxidation in vivo. *Circ Res.* 1999;85(10):950–958.

39. Barnes PJ. Nitric oxide and asthma. *Res Immunol.* 1995;146(9):698–702.

40. Gaston B, Keith JF III. Nitric oxide and bleeding time. *Pediatrics.* 1994;94(1):134–135.

41. Guo FH, Erzurum SC. Characterization of inducible nitric oxide synthase expression in human airway epithelium. *Environ Health Perspect.* 1998;106(suppl 5):1119–1124.

42. Guo FH, De Raeve HR, Rice TW, Stuehr DJ, Thunnissen FB, Erzurum SC. Continuous nitric oxide synthesis by inducible nitric oxide synthase in normal human airway epithelium in vivo. *Proc Nat Acad Sci U S A.* 1995;92(17):7809–7813.

43. Guo FH, Comhair SA, Zheng S, et al. Molecular mechanisms of increased nitric oxide (NO) in asthma: evidence for transcriptional and post-translational regulation of NO synthesis. *J Immunol.* 2000;164(11):5970–5980.

44. Kobzik L, Bredt DS, Lowenstein CJ, et al. Nitric oxide synthase in human and rat lung: immunocytochemical and histochemical localization. *Am J Respir Cell Mol Biol.* 1993;9(4):371–377.

45. Lundberg JO, Lundberg JM, Settergren G, Alving K, Weitzberg E. Nitric oxide, produced in the upper airways, may act in an 'aerocrine' fashion to enhance pulmonary oxygen uptake in humans. *Acta Physiol Scand.* 1995;155(4):467–468.

46. Pou S, Tsai P, Porasuphatana S, et al. Spin trapping of nitric oxide by ferro-chelates: kinetic and in vivo pharmacokinetic studies. *Biochim Biophys Acta.* 1999;1427(2):216–226.

47. Pou S, Keaton L, Surichamorn W, Rosen GM. Mechanism of superoxide generation by neuronal nitric-oxide synthase. *J Biol Chem.* 1999;274(14):9573–9580.

48. Pou S, Pou WS, Bredt DS, Snyder SH, Rosen GM. Generation of superoxide by purified brain nitric oxide synthase. *J Biol Chem.* 1992;267(34):24173–24176.

49. Ignarro LJ, Buga GM, Wei LH, Bauer PM, Wu G, del Soldato P. Role of the arginine-nitric oxide pathway in the regulation of vascular smooth muscle cell proliferation. *Proc Nat Acad Sci U S A.* 2001;98(7):4202–4208.

50. Xu W, Kaneko FT, Zheng S, et al. Increased arginase II and decreased NO synthesis in endothelial cells of patients with pulmonary arterial hypertension. *FASEB J.* 2004;18(14):1746–1748.

51. Andreadis AA, Hazen SL, Comhair SA, Erzurum SC. Oxidative and nitrosative events in asthma. *Free Radic Biol Med.* 2003;35(3):213–225.

52. Hunt JF, Fang K, Malik R, et al. Endogenous airway acidification. Implications for asthma pathophysiology. *Am J Respir Crit Care Med.* 2000;161(3 Pt 1):694–699.

53. Gaston B, Singel D, Doctor A, Stamler JS. S-nitrosothiol signaling in respiratory biology. *Am J Respir Crit Care Med.* 2006;173(11):1186–1193.

54. Dweik RA, Comhair SA, Gaston B, et al. NO chemical events in the human airway during the immediate and late antigen-induced asthmatic response. *Proc Nat Acad Sci U S A.* 2001;98(5):2622–2627.

55. Dweik RA. The promise and reality of nitric oxide in the diagnosis and treatment of lung disease. *Cleve Clin J Med.* 2001; 68(6): 486, 488, 490, 493.

56. Folkerts G, Nijkamp FP. Nitric oxide in asthma therapy. *Curr Pharm Des.* 2006;12(25):3221–3232.

57. Ricciardolo FL, Di Stefano A, Sabatini F, Folkerts G. Reactive nitrogen species in the respiratory tract. *Eur J Pharmacol.* 2006; 533(1–3):240–252.

58. Nadeem A, Masood A, Siddiqui N. Oxidant–antioxidant imbalance in asthma: scientific evidence, epidemiological data and possible therapeutic options. *Ther Adv Respir Dis.* 2008;2(4): 215–235.

59. Bowler RP, Crapo JD. Oxidative stress in allergic respiratory diseases. *J Allergy Clin Immunol.* 2002;110(3):349–356.

60. Rahman I, MacNee W. Oxidative stress and regulation of glutathione in lung inflammation. *Eur Respir J.* 2000;16(3):534–554.

61. Kinnula VL, Crapo JD. Superoxide dismutases in the lung and human lung diseases. *Am J Respir Crit Care Med.* 2003;167(12): 1600–1619.

62. Bartosz G. Superoxide Dismutase and catalase. *The Handbook of Environmental Chemistry.* 2005;2 part O:109–149.

63. Fridovich I. Superoxide dismutases. *Adv Enzymol Relat Areas Mol Biol.* 1986;58:61–97.

64. Fridovich I, Freeman B. Antioxidant defenses in the lung. *Ann Rev Physiol.* 1986;48:693–702.

65. Singh RJ, Goss SP, Joseph J, Kalyanaraman B. Nitration of gamma-tocopherol and oxidation of alpha-tocopherol by copper-zinc superoxide dismutase/H2O2/NO2-: role of nitrogen dioxide free radical. *Proc Nat Acad Sci U S A.* 1998;95(22):12912–12917.

66. Chang LY, Crapo JD. Inhibition of airway inflammation and hyperreactivity by an antioxidant mimetic. *Free Radic Biol Med.* 2002;33(3):379–386.

67. Comhair SA, Ricci KS, Arroliga M, et al. Correlation of systemic superoxide dismutase deficiency to airflow obstruction in asthma. *Am J Respir Crit Care Med.* 2005;172(3):306–313.

68. Crapo JD, Oury T, Rabouille C, Slot JW, Chang LY. Copper, zinc superoxide dismutase is primarily a cytosolic protein in human cells. *Proc Nat Acad Sci U S A.* 1992;89(21):10405–10409.

69. Clyde BL, Chang LY, Auten RL, Ho YS, Crapo JD. Distribution of manganese superoxide dismutase mRNA in normal and hyperoxic rat lung. *Am J Respir Cell Mol Biol.* 1993;8(5):530–537.

70. De Raeve HR, Thunnissen FB, Kaneko FT, et al. Decreased Cu,Zn-SOD activity in asthmatic airway epithelium: correction by inhaled corticosteroid in vivo. *Am J Physiol.* 1997;272 (1 Pt 1):L148–L154.

71. Erzurum SC, Danel C, Gillissen A, Chu CS, Trapnell BC, Crystal RG. In vivo antioxidant gene expression in human airway epithelium of normal individuals exposed to 100% O_2. *J Appl Physiol.* 1993;75(3):1256–1262.

72. Fattman CL, Schaefer LM, Oury TD. Extracellular superoxide dismutase in biology and medicine. *Free Radic Biol Med.* 2003;35(3):236–256.

73. Lakari E, Paakko P, Kinnula VL. Manganese superoxide dismutase, but not CuZn superoxide dismutase, is highly expressed in the granulomas of pulmonary sarcoidosis and extrinsic allergic alveolitis. *Am J Respir Crit Care Med.* 1998;158(2):589–596.

74. Marklund SL. Expression of extracellular superoxide dismutase by human cell lines. *Biochem J.* 1990;266(1):213–219.

75. Marklund SL, Karlsson K. Extracellular-superoxide dismutase, distribution in the body and therapeutic applications. *Adv Exp Med Biol.* 1990;264:1–4.

76. Marklund SL. Analysis of extracellular superoxide dismutase in tissue homogenates and extracellular fluids. *Methods Enzymol.* 1990;186:260–265.

77. Oury TD, Day BJ, Crapo JD. Extracellular superoxide dismutase: a regulator of nitric oxide bioavailability. *Lab Invest.* 1996;75(5):617–636.

78. Oury TD, Crapo JD, Valnickova Z, Enghild JJ. Human extracellular superoxide dismutase is a tetramer composed of two disulphide-linked dimers: a simplified, high-yield purification

of extracellular superoxide dismutase. *Biochem J.* 1996;317(Pt 1): 51–57.

79. Oury TD, Day BJ, Crapo JD. Extracellular superoxide dismutase in vessels and airways of humans and baboons. *Free Radic Biol Med.* 1996;20(7):957–965.

80. Alvarez B, Demicheli V, Duran R, et al. Inactivation of human Cu,Zn superoxide dismutase by peroxynitrite and formation of histidinyl radical. *Free Radic Biol Med.* 2004;37(6):813–822.

81. Singh RJ, Hogg N, Goss SP, Antholine WE, Kalyanaraman B. Mechanism of superoxide dismutase/H(2)O(2)-mediated nitric oxide release from S-nitrosoglutathione–role of glutamate. *Arch Biochem Biophys.* 1999;372(1):8–15.

82. Goss SP, Singh RJ, Kalyanaraman B. Bicarbonate enhances the peroxidase activity of Cu,Zn-superoxide dismutase. Role of carbonate anion radical. *J Biol Chem.* 1999;274(40):28233–28239.

83. Beckman JS, Ischiropoulos H, Zhu L, et al. Kinetics of superoxide dismutase- and iron-catalyzed nitration of phenolics by peroxynitrite. *Arch Biochem Biophys.* 1992;298(2):438–445.

84. Ischiropoulos H, Zhu L, Chen J, et al. Peroxynitrite-mediated tyrosine nitration catalyzed by superoxide dismutase. *Arch Biochem Biophys.* 1992;298(2):431–437.

85. Koppenol WH, Moreno JJ, Pryor WA, Ischiropoulos H, Beckman JS. Peroxynitrite, a cloaked oxidant formed by nitric oxide and superoxide. *Chem Res Toxicol.* 1992;5(6):834–842.

86. Ischiropoulos H, Zhu L, Beckman JS. Peroxynitrite formation from macrophage-derived nitric oxide. *Arch Biochem Biophys.* 1992;298(2):446–451.

87. Crow JP, Ye YZ, Strong M, Kirk M, Barnes S, Beckman JS. Superoxide dismutase catalyzes nitration of tyrosines by peroxynitrite in the rod and head domains of neurofilament-L. *J Neurochem.* 1997;69(5):1945–1953.

88. Jungas T, Motta I, Duffieux F, Fanen P, Stoven V, Ojcius DM. Glutathione levels and BAX activation during apoptosis due to oxidative stress in cells expressing wild-type and mutant cystic fibrosis transmembrane conductance regulator. *J Biol Chem.* 2002;277(31):27912–27918.

89. Karlsson K, Marklund SL. Heparin-, dextran sulfate- and protamine-induced release of extracellular-superoxide dismutase to plasma in pigs. *Biochim Biophys Acta.* 1988;967(1):110–114.

90. Karlsson K, Sandstrom J, Edlund A, Marklund SL. Turnover of extracellular-superoxide dismutase in tissues. *Lab Invest.* 1994; 70(5):705–710.

91. Bowler RM, Gysens S, Hartney C, Ngo L, Rauch SS, Midtling J. Increased medication use in a community environmentally exposed to chemicals. *Ind Health.* 2002;40(4):335–344.

92. Bowler RP, Crapo JD. Oxidative stress in airways: is there a role for extracellular superoxide dismutase? *Am J Respir Crit Care Med.* 2002;166(12 Pt 2):S38–S43.

93. Bowler RP, Nicks M, Warnick K, Crapo JD. Role of extracellular superoxide dismutase in bleomycin-induced pulmonary fibrosis. *Am J Physiol Lung Cell Mol Physiol.* 2002;282(4):L719–L726.

94. Bowler RP, Nicks M, Olsen DA, et al. Furin proteolytically processes the heparin-binding region of extracellular superoxide dismutase. *J Biol Chem.* 2002;277(19):16505–16511.

95. Oury TD, Schaefer LM, Fattman CL, Choi A, Weck KE, Watkins SC. Depletion of pulmonary EC-SOD after exposure to hyperoxia. *Am J Physiol Lung Cell Mol Physiol.* 2002;283(4): L777–L784.

96. Giles BL, Suliman H, Mamo LB, Piantadosi CA, Oury TD, Nozik-Grayck E. Prenatal hypoxia decreases lung extracellular superoxide dismutase expression and activity. *Am J Physiol Lung Cell Mol Physiol.* 2002;283(3):L549–L554.

97. Loenders B, Van Mechelen E, Nicolai S, et al. Localization of extracellular superoxide dismutase in rat lung: neutrophils and macrophages as carriers of the enzyme. *Free Rad Biol Med.* 1998;24(7–8):1097–1106.

98. Folz RJ, Crapo JD. Extracellular superoxide dismutase (SOD3): tissue-specific expression, genomic characterization, and computer-assisted sequence analysis of the human EC SOD gene. *Genomics.* 1994;22(1):162–171.

99. Reaume AG, Elliott JL, Hoffman EK, et al. Motor neurons in Cu/Zn superoxide dismutase-deficient mice develop normally but exhibit enhanced cell death after axonal injury. *Nat Genet.* 1996;13(1):43–47.

100. Juul K, Tybjaerg-Hansen A, Marklund S, Lange P, Nordestgaard BG. Genetically increased antioxidative protection and decreased chronic obstructive pulmonary disease. *Am J Respir Crit Care Med.* 2006;173(8):858–864.

101. Dahl M, Bowler RP, Juul K, Crapo JD, Levy S, Nordestgaard BG. Superoxide dismutase 3 polymorphism associated with reduced lung function in two large populations. *Am J Respir Crit Care Med.* 2008;178(9):906–912.

102. Arcaroli JJ, Hokanson JE, Abraham E, et al. Extracellular superoxide dismutase haplotypes are associated with acute lung injury and mortality. *Am J Respir Crit Care Med.* 2009;179(2):105–112.

103. Rahman I, Adcock IM. Oxidative stress and redox regulation of lung inflammation in COPD. *Eur Respir J.* 2006;28(1):219–242.

104. Deisseroth A, Dounce AL. Catalase: physical and chemical properties, mechanism of catalysis, and physiological role. *Physiol Rev.* 1970;50(3):319–375.

105. Murthy MR, Reid TJ III, Sicignano A, Tanaka N, Rossmann MG. Structure of beef liver catalase. *J Mol Biol.* 1981;152(2):465–499.

106. Reid TJ III, Murthy MR, Sicignano A, Tanaka N, Musick WD, Rossmann MG. Structure and heme environment of beef liver catalase at 2.5 A resolution. *Proc Nat Acad Sci U S A.* 1981;78(8): 4767–4771.

107. Cao C, Leng Y, Kufe D. Catalase activity is regulated by c-Abl and Arg in the oxidative stress response. *J Biol Chem.* 2003; 278(32):29667–29675.

108. Comhair SA, Erzurum SC. The regulation and role of extracellular glutathione peroxidase. *Antioxid Redox Signal.* 2005;7(1–2):72–79.

109. Rhee SG, Yang KS, Kang SW, Woo HA, Chang TS. Controlled elimination of intracellular H(2)O(2): regulation of peroxiredoxin, catalase, and glutathione peroxidase via post-translational modification. *Antioxid Redox Signa.* 2005;7(5–6):619–626.

110. Cantin AM, Fells GA, Hubbard RC, Crystal RG. Antioxidant macromolecules in the epithelial lining fluid of the normal human lower respiratory tract. *J Clin Invest.* 1990;86(3):962–971.

111. Cantin AM, Larivee P, Begin RO. Extracellular glutathione suppresses human lung fibroblast proliferation. *Am J Respir Cell Mol Biol.* 1990;3(1):79–85.

112. Hoshino T, Okamoto M, Takei S, Sakazaki Y, Iwanaga T, Aizawa H. Redox-regulated mechanisms in asthma. *Antioxid Redox Signal.* 2008;10(4):769–783.

113. Xu J, Li T, Wu H, Xu T. Role of thioredoxin in lung disease. *Pulm Pharmacol Ther.* 2012;25(2):154–162.

114. Holmgren A. Thioredoxin and glutaredoxin systems. *J Biol Chem.* 1989;264(24):13963–13966.

115. Ichiki H, Hoshino T, Kinoshita T, et al. Thioredoxin suppresses airway hyperresponsiveness and airway inflammation

in asthma. *Biochem Biophys Res Commun.* 2005;334(4):1141–1148.

116. Burke-Gaffney A, Callister ME, Nakamura H. Thioredoxin: friend or foe in human disease? *Trends Pharmacol Sci.* 2005;26(8): 398–404.

117. Nakamura H. Thioredoxin and its related molecules: update 2005. *Antioxid Redox Signal.* 2005;7(5–6):823–828.

118. Nakamura T, Nakamura H, Hoshino T, Ueda S, Wada H, Yodoi J. Redox regulation of lung inflammation by thioredoxin. *Antioxid Redox Signal.* 2005;7(1–2):60–71.

119. Filomeni G, Rotilio G, Ciriolo MR. Cell signalling and the glutathione redox system. *Biochem Pharmacol.* 2002;64(5–6): 1057–1064.

120. Zhang J, Li YD, Patel JM, Block ER. Thioredoxin overexpression prevents NO-induced reduction of NO synthase activity in lung endothelial cells. *Am J Physiol.* 1998;275(2 Pt 1):L288–L293.

121. Reynaert NL, Wouters EF, Janssen-Heininger YM. Modulation of glutaredoxin-1 expression in a mouse model of allergic airway disease. *Am J Respir Cell Mol Biol.* 2007;36(2):147–151.

122. Mieyal JJ, Gallogly MM, Qanungo S, Sabens EA, Shelton MD. Molecular mechanisms and clinical implications of reversible protein S-glutathionylation. *Antioxid Redox Signal.* 2008;10(11):1941–1988.

123. Shelton MD, Mieyal JJ. Regulation by reversible S-glutathionylation: molecular targets implicated in inflammatory diseases. *Mol Cells.* 2008;25(3):332–346.

124. Lillig CH, Holmgren A. Thioredoxin and related molecules–from biology to health and disease. *Antioxid Redox Signal.* 2007;9(1):25–47.

125. Meyer Y, Buchanan BB, Vignols F, Reichheld JP. Thioredoxins and glutaredoxins: unifying elements in redox biology. *Annu Rev Genet.* 2009;43:335–367.

126. Rushmore TH, Pickett CB. Glutathione S-transferases, structure, regulation, and therapeutic implications. *J Biol Chem.* 1993;268(16):11475–11478.

127. Salinas AE, Wong MG. Glutathione S-transferases–a review. *Curr Med Chem.* 1999;6(4):279–309.

128. Yan F, Chen C, Jing J, Li W, Shen H, Wang X. Association between polymorphism of glutathione S-transferase P1 and chronic obstructive pulmonary disease: a meta-analysis. *Respir Med.* 2010;104(4):473–480.

129. Piacentini S, Polimanti R, Simonelli I, et al. Glutathione S-transferase polymorphisms, asthma susceptibility and confounding variables: a meta-analysis. *Mol Biol Rep.* 2013;40(4): 3299–3313.

130. Polimanti R, Carboni C, Baesso I, et al. Genetic variability of glutathione S-transferase enzymes in human populations: functional inter-ethnic differences in detoxification systems. *Gene.* 2013;512(1):102–107.

131. Shukla RK, Kant S, Mittal B, Bhattacharya S. Polymorphism of cytochrome p450, glutathione-s-transferase and N-acetyltransferases: influence on lung cancer susceptibility. *Niger J Med.* 2010;19(3):257–263.

132. Rhee SG, Kang SW, Chang TS, Jeong W, Kim K. Peroxiredoxin, a novel family of peroxidases. *IUBMB Life.* 2001;52(1–2):35–41.

133. Kinnula VL, Vuorinen K, Ilumets H, Rytila P, Myllarniemi M. Thiol proteins, redox modulation and parenchymal lung disease. 2007;14(2):213–222.

134. Kinnula VL, Lehtonen S, Sormunen R, et al. Overexpression of peroxiredoxins I, II, III, V, and VI in malignant mesothelioma. *J Pathol.* 2002;196(3):316–323.

135. Kinnula VL, Lehtonen S, Kaarteenaho-Wiik R, et al. Cell specific expression of peroxiredoxins in human lung and pulmonary sarcoidosis. *Thorax.* 2002;57(2):157–164.

136. Mutlak H, Zacharowski K. Role of peroxiredoxin 6 in acute lung injury: potential target? *Crit Care Med.* 2011;39(4):899–900.

137. Rhee SG, Chae HZ, Kim K. Peroxiredoxins: a historical overview and speculative preview of novel mechanisms and emerging concepts in cell signaling. *Free Rad Biol Med.* 2005; 38(12):1543–1552.

138. Rhee SG, Kang SW, Jeong W, Chang TS, Yang KS, Woo HA. Intracellular messenger function of hydrogen peroxide and its regulation by peroxiredoxins. *Curr Opin Cell Biol.* 2005;17(2): 183–189.

139. Manta B, Hugo M, Ortiz C, Ferrer-Sueta G, Trujillo M, Denicola A. The peroxidase and peroxynitrite reductase activity of human erythrocyte peroxiredoxin 2. *Arch Biochem Biophys.* 2009;484(2):146–154.

140. Dubuisson M, Vander Stricht D, Clippe A, et al. Human peroxiredoxin 5 is a peroxynitrite reductase. *FEBS Lett.* 2004;571(1–3): 161–165.

141. Deshane J, Wright M, Agarwal A. Heme oxygenase-1 expression in disease states. *Acta Biochim Pol.* 2005;52(2):273–284.

142. Jarmi T, Agarwal A. Heme oxygenase and renal disease. *Curr Hypertens Rep.* 2009;11(1):56–62.

143. Zhou H, Liu H, Porvasnik SL, et al. Heme oxygenase-1 mediates the protective effects of rapamycin in monocrotaline-induced pulmonary hypertension. *Lab Invest.* 2006;86(1):62–71.

144. Hill-Kapturczak N, Chang SH, Agarwal A. Heme oxygenase and the kidney. *DNA Cell Biol.* 2002;21(4):307–321.

145. Raval CM, Lee PJ. Heme oxygenase-1 in lung disease. *Curr Drug Targets.* 2010;11(12):1532–1540.

146. Ryter SW, Otterbein LE, Morse D, Choi AM. Heme oxygenase/carbon monoxide signaling pathways: regulation and functional significance. *Mol Cell Biochem.* 2002;234–235(1–2):249–263.

147. Morse D, Choi AM. Heme oxygenase-1: the "emerging molecule" has arrived. *Am J Respir Cell Mol Biol.* 2002;27(1):8–16.

148. Morse D, Sethi J. Carbon monoxide and human disease. *Antioxid Redox Signal.* 2002;4(2):331–338.

149. Morse D, Sethi J, Choi AM. Carbon monoxide-dependent signaling. *Crit Care Med.* 2002;30(1 suppl):S12–S17.

150. Decaluwe K, Pauwels B, Verpoest S, Van de Voorde J. Divergent mechanisms involved in CO and CORM-2 induced vasorelaxation. *Eur J Pharmacol.* 2012;674(2–3):370–377.

151. Rahman I, Yang SR, Biswas SK. Current concepts of redox signaling in the lungs. *Antioxid Redox Signal.* 2006;8(3–4):681–689.

152. Sikorski EM, Hock T, Hill-Kapturczak N, Agarwal A. The story so far: molecular regulation of the heme oxygenase-1 gene in renal injury. *Am J Physiol Renal Physiol.* 2004;286(3):F425–F441.

153. Poss KD, Tonegawa S. Reduced stress defense in heme oxygenase 1-deficient cells. *Proc Nat Acad Sci U S A.* 1997;94(20):10925–10930.

154. Poss KD, Tonegawa S. Heme oxygenase 1 is required for mammalian iron reutilization. *Proc Nat Acad Sci U S A.* 1997;94 (20):10919–10924.

155. Wink DA, Hines HB, Cheng RY, et al. Nitric oxide and redox mechanisms in the immune response. *J Leukoc Biol.* 2011;89(6):873–891.

156. Kotsias F, Hoffmann E, Amigorena S, Savina A. Reactive oxygen species production in the phagosome: impact on antigen presentation in dendritic cells. *Antioxid Redox Signal.* 2013;18(6):714–729.

157. Brune B, Dehne N, Grossmann N, et al. Redox control of inflammation in macrophages. *Antioxid Redox Signal.* 2013; 19(6):595–637.

158. Maarsingh H, Zaagsma J, Meurs H. Arginine homeostasis in allergic asthma. *Eur J Pharmacol.* 2008;585(2–3):375–384.

159. Maarsingh H, Zaagsma J, Meurs H. Arginase: a key enzyme in the pathophysiology of allergic asthma opening novel therapeutic perspectives. *Br J Pharmacol.* 2009;158(3):652–664.

160. Maarsingh H, Zuidhof AB, Bos IS, et al. Arginase inhibition protects against allergen-induced airway obstruction, hyperresponsiveness, and inflammation. *Am J Respir Crit Care Med.* 2008;178(6):565–573.

161. Maarsingh H, Pera T, Meurs H. Arginase and pulmonary diseases. *Naunyn Schmiedebergs Arch Pharmacol.* 2008;378(2):171–184.

162. Hardy SJ, Ferrante A, Poulos A, Robinson BS, Johnson DW, Murray AW. Effect of exogenous fatty acids with greater than 22 carbon atoms (very long chain fatty acids) on superoxide production by human neutrophils. *J Immunol.* 1994;153(4):1754–1761.

163. Messmer UK, Ankarcrona M, Nicotera P, Brune B. p53 expression in nitric oxide-induced apoptosis. *FEBS Lett.* 1994;355(1):23–26.

164. Messmer UK, Brune B. Modulation of inducible nitric oxide synthase in RINm5 F cells. *Cell Signal.* 1994;6(1):17–24.

165. Sandau KB, Gantner F, Brune B. Nitric oxide-induced F-actin disassembly is mediated via cGMP, cAMP, and protein kinase A activation in rat mesangial cells. *Exp Cell Res.* 2001;271(2):329–336.

166. Sandau KB, Zhou J, Kietzmann T, Brune B. Regulation of the hypoxia-inducible factor 1alpha by the inflammatory mediators nitric oxide and tumor necrosis factor-alpha in contrast to desferroxamine and phenylarsine oxide. *J Biol Chem.* 2001;276(43): 39805–39811.

167. Sandau KB, Fandrey J, Brune B. Accumulation of HIF-1alpha under the influence of nitric oxide. *Blood.* 2001;97(4):1009–1015.

168. Brune B, Zhou J, von Knethen A. Nitric oxide, oxidative stress, and apoptosis. *Kidney Int Suppl.* 2003(84):S22–S24.

169. Brune B, Zhou J. The role of nitric oxide (NO) in stability regulation of hypoxia inducible factor-1alpha (HIF-1alpha). *Curr Medic Chem.* 2003;10(10):845–855.

170. Forman HJ, Torres M. Reactive oxygen species and cell signaling: respiratory burst in macrophage signaling. *Am J Respir Crit Care Med.* 2002;166(12 Pt 2):S4–S8.

171. Forman HJ, Torres M, Fukuto J. Redox signaling. *Mol Cell Biochem.* 2002;234–235(1–2):49–62.

172. Iles KE, Forman HJ. Macrophage signaling and respiratory burst. *Immunol Res.* 2002;26(1–3):95–105.

173. Ridnour LA, Thomas DD, Donzelli S, et al. The biphasic nature of nitric oxide responses in tumor biology. *Antioxid Redox Signal.* 2006;8(7–8):1329–1337.

174. Thomas DD, Ridnour LA, Espey MG, et al. Superoxide fluxes limit nitric oxide-induced signaling. *J Biol Chemi.* 2006;281(36): 25984–25993.

175. Brune B. The intimate relation between nitric oxide and superoxide in apoptosis and cell survival. *Antioxid Redox Signal.* 2005; 7(3–4):497–507.

176. Zhou J, Brune B. NO and transcriptional regulation: from signaling to death. *Toxicology.* 2005;208(2):223–233.

177. Niedbala W, Cai B, Liew FY. Role of nitric oxide in the regulation of T cell functions. *Ann Rheum Dis.* 2006;65(Suppl 3):iii37–iii40.

178. Mills CD, Kincaid K, Alt JM, Heilman MJ, Hill AM. M-1/M-2 macrophages and the Th1/Th2 paradigm. *J Immunol.* 2000;164(12):6166–6173.

179. King MR, Ismail AS, Davis LS, Karp DR. Oxidative stress promotes polarization of human T cell differentiation toward a T helper 2 phenotype. *J Immunol.* 2006;176(5):2765–2772.

180. Nagaraj S, Collazo M, Corzo CA, et al. Regulatory myeloid suppressor cells in health and disease. *Cancer Res.* 2009;69(19): 7503–7506.

181. Gabrilovich DI, Nagaraj S. Myeloid-derived suppressor cells as regulators of the immune system. *Nat Rev Immunol.* 2009;9(3): 162–174.

182. Deshane J, Zmijewski JW, Luther R, et al. Free radical-producing myeloid-derived regulatory cells: potent activators and suppressors of lung inflammation and airway hyperresponsiveness. *Mucosal Immunol.* 2011;4(5):503–518.

183. Arora M, Poe SL, Oriss TB, et al. TLR4/MyD88-induced CD11b+Gr-1 int F4/80+ non-migratory myeloid cells suppress Th2 effector function in the lung. *Mucosal Immunol.* 2010;3(6): 578–593.

184. Lu T, Gabrilovich DI. Molecular pathways: tumor-infiltrating myeloid cells and reactive oxygen species in regulation of tumor microenvironment. *Clin Cancer Res.* 2012;18(18):4877–4882.

185. Gabrilovich DI, Ostrand-Rosenberg S, Bronte V. Coordinated regulation of myeloid cells by tumours. *Nat Rev Immunol.* 2012; 12(4):253–268.

186. Rubartelli A. Redox control of NLRP3 inflammasome activation in health and disease. *J Leukoc Biol.* 2012;92(5):951–958.

187. Martinon F. Signaling by ROS drives inflammasome activation. *Eur J Immunol.* 2010;40(3):616–619.

188. Gross O, Thomas CJ, Guarda G, Tschopp J. The inflammasome: an integrated view. *Immunol Rev.* 2011;243(1):136–151.

189. Aziz M, Jacob A, Yang WL, Matsuda A, Wang P. Current trends in inflammatory and immunomodulatory mediators in sepsis. *J Leukoc Biol.* 2012;93(3):329–342.

190. Matsuda A, Jacob A, Wu R, et al. Novel therapeutic targets for sepsis: regulation of exaggerated inflammatory responses. *J Nippon Med Sch.* 2012;79(1):4–18.

191. Fischer H. Mechanisms and function of DUOX in epithelia of the lung. *Antioxid Redox Signal.* 2009;11(10):2453–2465.

192. Leto TL, Geiszt M. Role of Nox family NADPH oxidases in host defense. *Antioxid Redox Signal.* 2006;8(9–10):1549–1561.

193. Rada B, Leto TL. Oxidative innate immune defenses by Nox/Duox family NADPH oxidases. *Contrib Microbiol.* 2008; 15: 164–187.

194. Morand S, Ueyama T, Tsujibe S, Saito N, Korzeniowska A, Leto TL. Duox maturation factors form cell surface complexes with Duox affecting the specificity of reactive oxygen species generation. *FASEB J.* 2009;23(4):1205–1218.

195. Kalinowski L, Malinski T. Endothelial NADH/NADPH-dependent enzymatic sources of superoxide production: relationship to endothelial dysfunction. *Acta Biochim Pol.* 2004;51(2):459–469.

196. Silva BR, Pernomian L, Bendhack LM. Contribution of oxidative stress to endothelial dysfunction in hypertension. *Front Physiol.* 2012;3:441.

197. Han J, Shuvaev VV, Muzykantov VR. Targeted interception of signaling reactive oxygen species in the vascular endothelium. *Ther Deliv.* 2012;3(2):263–276.

198. Schramm A, Matusik P, Osmenda G, Guzik TJ. Targeting NADPH oxidases in vascular pharmacology. *Vascul Pharmacol.* 2012;56(5–6):216–231.

199. Lee R, Channon KM, Antoniades C. Therapeutic strategies targeting endothelial function in humans: clinical implications. *Curr Vasc Pharmacol.* 2012;10(1):77–93.

200. Van Eeden S, Leipsic J, Paul Man SF, Sin DD. The relationship between lung inflammation and cardiovascular disease. *Am J Respir Crit Care Med.* 2012;186(1):11–16.

201. Lucas R, Verin AD, Black SM, Catravas JD. Regulators of endothelial and epithelial barrier integrity and function in acute lung injury. *Biochem Pharmacol.* 2009;77(12):1763–1772.

202. Sedoris KC, Ovechkin AV, Gozal E, Roberts AM. Differential effects of nitric oxide synthesis on pulmonary vascular function during lung ischemia-reperfusion injury. *Arch Physiol Biochem.* 2009;115(1):34–46.

203. Lama VN, Smith L, Badri L, et al. Evidence for tissue-resident mesenchymal stem cells in human adult lung from studies of transplanted allografts. *J Clin Invest.* 2007;117(4):989–996.

204. Hashimoto N, Jin H, Liu T, Chensue SW, Phan SH. Bone marrow-derived progenitor cells in pulmonary fibrosis. *J Clin Invest.* 2004;113(2):243–252.

205. Willis BC, Liebler JM, Luby-Phelps K, et al. Induction of epithelial-mesenchymal transition in alveolar epithelial cells by transforming growth factor-beta1: potential role in idiopathic pulmonary fibrosis. *Am J Pathol.* 2005;166(5):1321–1332.

206. Hinz B, Phan SH, Thannickal VJ, Galli A, Bochaton-Piallat ML, Gabbiani G. The myofibroblast: one function, multiple origins. *Am J Pathol.* 2007;170(6):1807–1816.

207. Griffith B, Pendyala S, Hecker L, Lee PJ, Natarajan V, Thannickal VJ. NOX enzymes and pulmonary disease. *Antioxid Redox Signal.* 2009;11(10):2505–2516.

208. Tomasek JJ, Gabbiani G, Hinz B, Chaponnier C, Brown RA. Myofibroblasts and mechano-regulation of connective tissue remodelling. *Nat Rev Mol Cell Biol.* 2002;3(5):349–363.

209. Hecker L, Vittal R, Jones T, et al. NADPH oxidase-4 mediates myofibroblast activation and fibrogenic responses to lung injury. *Nat Med.* 2009;15(9):1077–1081.

210. Waghray M, Cui Z, Horowitz JC, et al. Hydrogen peroxide is a diffusible paracrine signal for the induction of epithelial cell death by activated myofibroblasts. *FASEB J.* 2005;19(7):854–856.

211. Horwitz RJ, Busse WW. Inflammation and asthma. *Clin Chest Med.* 1995;16(4):583–602.

212. Busse WW, Kiecolt-Glaser JK, Coe C, Martin RJ, Weiss ST, Parker SR. NHLBI Workshop summary. Stress and asthma. *Am J Respir Crit Care Med.* 1995;151(1):249–252.

213. Calhoun WJ, Reed HE, Moest DR, Stevens CA. Enhanced superoxide production by alveolar macrophages and air-space cells, airway inflammation, and alveolar macrophage density changes after segmental antigen bronchoprovocation in allergic subjects. *Am Rev Respir Dis.* 1992;145(2 Pt 1):317–325.

214. Jarjour NN, Busse WW, Calhoun WJ. Enhanced production of oxygen radicals in nocturnal asthma. *Am Rev Respir Dis.* 1992;146(4):905–911.

215. Comhair SA, Bhathena PR, Farver C, Thunnissen FB, Erzurum SC. Extracellular glutathione peroxidase induction in asthmatic lungs: evidence for redox regulation of expression in human airway epithelial cells. *FASEB J.* 2001;15(1):70–78.

216. Comhair SA, Bhathena PR, Dweik RA, Kavuru M, Erzurum SC. Rapid loss of superoxide dismutase activity during antigen-induced asthmatic response. *Lancet.* 2000;355(9204):624.

217. Comhair SA, Xu W, Ghosh S, et al. Superoxide dismutase inactivation in pathophysiology of asthmatic airway remodeling and reactivity. *Am J Pathol.* 2005;166(3):663–674.

218. Postma DS, Renkema TE, Noordhoek JA, Faber H, Sluiter HJ, Kauffman H. Association between nonspecific bronchial hyperreactivity and superoxide anion production by polymorphonuclear leukocytes in chronic air-flow obstruction. *Am Rev Respir Dis.* 1988;137(1):57–61.

219. Busse WW. Determinants of risk factors for asthma. *Can Respir J.* 1999;6(1):97–101.

220. Gern JE, Lemanske RF Jr, Busse WW. Early life origins of asthma. *J Clin Invest.* 1999;104(7):837–843.

221. Busse W, Elias J, Sheppard D, Banks-Schlegel S. Airway remodeling and repair. *Am J Respir Crit Care Med.* 1999;160(3):1035–1042.

222. Jarjour NN, Calhoun WJ. Enhanced production of oxygen radicals in asthma. *J Lab Clin Med.* 1994;123(1):131–136.

223. Sanders SP. Nitric oxide in asthma. Pathogenic, therapeutic, or diagnostic? *Am J Respir Cell Mol Biol.* 1999;21(2):147–149.

224. Sandstrom J, Nilsson P, Karlsson K, Marklund SL. 10-fold increase in human plasma extracellular superoxide dismutase content caused by a mutation in heparin-binding domain. *J Biol Chem.* 1994;269(29):19163–19166.

225. Olsen RL, Little C. Purification and some properties of myeloperoxidase and eosinophil peroxidase from human blood. *Biochem J.* 1983;209(3):781–787.

226. Wardlaw AJ, Symon FS, Walsh GM. Eosinophil adhesion in allergic inflammation. *J Allergy Clin Immunol.* 1994;94(6 Pt 2): 1163–1171.

227. Wu W, Samoszuk MK, Comhair SA, et al. Eosinophils generate brominating oxidants in allergen-induced asthma. *J Clin Invest.* 2000;105(10):1455–1463.

228. Jatakanon A, Uasuf C, Maziak W, Lim S, Chung KF, Barnes PJ. Neutrophilic inflammation in severe persistent asthma. *Am J Respir Crit Care Med.* 1999;160(5 Pt 1):1532–1539.

229. Montuschi P, Corradi M, Ciabattoni G, Nightingale J, Kharitonov SA, Barnes PJ. Increased 8-isoprostane, a marker of oxidative stress, in exhaled condensate of asthma patients. *Am J Respir Crit Care Med.* 1999;160(1):216–220.

230. Montuschi P, Martello S, Felli M, Mondino C, Chiarotti M. Ion trap liquid chromatography/tandem mass spectrometry analysis of leukotriene B4 in exhaled breath condensate. *Rapid Commun Mass Spectrom.* 2004;18(22):2723–2729.

231. Mondino C, Ciabattoni G, Koch P, et al. Effects of inhaled corticosteroids on exhaled leukotrienes and prostanoids in asthmatic children. *J Allergy Clin Immunol.* 2004;114(4):761–767.

232. Dworski R, Murray JJ, Roberts LJ 2nd, et al. Allergen-induced synthesis of F(2)-isoprostanes in atopic asthmatics. Evidence for oxidant stress. *Am J Respir Crit Care Med.* 1999;160(6): 1947–1951.

233. Pavord ID, Ward R, Woltmann G, Wardlaw AJ, Sheller JR, Dworski R. Induced sputum eicosanoid concentrations in asthma. *Am J Respir Crit Care Med.* 1999;160(6):1905–1909.

234. Morrow JD, Zackert WE, Yang JP, et al. Quantification of the major urinary metabolite of 15-F2t-isoprostane (8-iso-PGF2alpha) by a stable isotope dilution mass spectrometric assay. *Anal Biochem.* 1999;269(2):326–331.

235. Sugiura H, Ichinose M. Oxidative and nitrative stress in bronchial asthma. *Antioxid Redox Signal.* 2008;10(4):785–797.

236. Park HS, Kim SR, Lee YC. Impact of oxidative stress on lung diseases. *Respirol.* 2009;14(1):27–38.

237. Thannickal VJ, Day RM, Klinz SG, Bastien MC, Larios JM, Fanburg BL. Ras-dependent and -independent regulation of reactive oxygen species by mitogenic growth factors and TGF-beta1. *FASEB J.* 2000;14(12):1741–1748.

238. Finlay GA, Thannickal VJ, Fanburg BL, Paulson KE. Transforming growth factor-beta 1-induced activation of the ERK pathway/activator protein-1 in human lung fibroblasts

requires the autocrine induction of basic fibroblast growth factor. *J Biol Chem.* 2000;275(36):27650–27656.

239. Khatri SB, Ozkan M, McCarthy K, et al. Alterations in exhaled gas profile during allergen-induced asthmatic response. *Am J Respir Crit Care Med.* 2001;164(10 Pt 1):1844–1848.
240. Brennan ML, Wu W, Fu X, et al. A tale of two controversies: defining both the role of peroxidases in nitrotyrosine formation in vivo using eosinophil peroxidase and myeloperoxidase-deficient mice, and the nature of peroxidase-generated reactive nitrogen species. *J Biol Chem.* 2002;277(20):17415–17427.
241. Gaston B, Drazen JM, Jansen A, et al. Relaxation of human bronchial smooth muscle by S-nitrosothiols in vitro. *J Pharmacol Exp Ther.* 1994;268(2):978–984.
242. Gaston B, Drazen JM, Loscalzo J, Stamler JS. The biology of nitrogen oxides in the airways. *Am J Respir Crit Care Med.* 1994; 149(2 Pt 1):538–551.
243. Gaston B. Expired nitric oxide in pediatric asthma: emissions testing for children? *J Pediatr.* 1997;131(3):343–344.
244. Fang K, Ragsdale NV, Carey RM, MacDonald T, Gaston B. Reductive assays for S-nitrosothiols: implications for measurements in biological systems. *Biochem Biophys Res Commun.* 1998; 252(3):535–540.
245. Gaston B, Sears S, Woods J, et al. Bronchodilator S-nitrosothiol deficiency in asthmatic respiratory failure. *Lancet.* 1998; 351(9112):1317–1319.
246. Diaz M, Achkor H, Titarenko E, Martinez MC. The gene encoding glutathione-dependent formaldehyde dehydrogenase/GSNO reductase is responsive to wounding, jasmonic acid and salicylic acid. *FEBS Lett.* 2003;543(1–3):136–139.
247. Que LG, Liu L, Yan Y, et al. Protection from experimental asthma by an endogenous bronchodilator. *Science.* 2005;308(5728): 1618–1621.
248. Celli BR. Roger s. Mitchell lecture. Chronic obstructive pulmonary disease phenotypes and their clinical relevance. *Proc Am Thorac Soc.* 2006;3(6):461–465.
249. Halbert RJ, Natoli JL, Gano A, Badamgarav E, Buist AS, Mannino DM. Global burden of COPD: systematic review and meta-analysis. *Eur Respir J.* 2006;28(3):523–532.
250. Tuder RM, Yoshida T, Fijalkowka I, Biswal S, Petrache I. Role of lung maintenance program in the heterogeneity of lung destruction in emphysema. *Proc Am Thorac Soc.* 2006;3(8):673–679.
251. Tuder RM, Yoshida T, Arap W, Pasqualini R, Petrache I. State of the art. Cellular and molecular mechanisms of alveolar destruction in emphysema: an evolutionary perspective. *Proc Am Thorac Soc.* 2006;3(6):503–510.
252. Churg A, Zhou S, Preobrazhenska O, Tai H, Wang R, Wright JL. Expression of profibrotic mediators in small airways versus parenchyma after cigarette smoke exposure. *Am J Respir Cell Mol Biol.* 2009;40(3):268–276.
253. Churg A, Cosio M, Wright JL. Mechanisms of cigarette smoke-induced COPD: insights from animal models. *Am J Physiol Lung Cell Mol Physiol.* 2008;294(4):L612–L631.
254. Taraseviciene-Stewart L, Voelkel NF. Molecular pathogenesis of emphysema. *J Clin Invest.* 2008;118(2):394–402.
255. Yoshida T, Tuder RM. Pathobiology of cigarette smoke-induced chronic obstructive pulmonary disease. *Physiol Rev.* 2007;87(3): 1047–1082.
256. Pryor WA. Cigarette smoke radicals and the role of free radicals in chemical carcinogenicity. *Environ Health Perspect.* 1997;105(Suppl 4):875–882.
257. Dahlgren C, Karlsson A. Respiratory burst in human neutrophils. *J Immunol Methods.* 1999;232(1–2):3–14.
258. Keatings VM, Barnes PJ. Granulocyte activation markers in induced sputum: comparison between chronic obstructive pulmonary disease, asthma, and normal subjects. *Am J Respir Crit Care Med.* 1997;155(2):449–453.
259. Russell RE, Thorley A, Culpitt SV, et al. Alveolar macrophage-mediated elastolysis: roles of matrix metalloproteinases, cysteine, and serine proteases. *Am J Physiol Lung Cell Mol Physiol.* 2002;283(4):L867–L873.
260. Russell RE, Culpitt SV, DeMatos C, et al. Release and activity of matrix metalloproteinase-9 and tissue inhibitor of metalloproteinase-1 by alveolar macrophages from patients with chronic obstructive pulmonary disease. *Am J Respir Cell Mol Biol.* 2002;26(5):602–609.
261. Lacoste JY, Bousquet J, Chanez P, et al. Eosinophilic and neutrophilic inflammation in asthma, chronic bronchitis, and chronic obstructive pulmonary disease. *J Allergy Clin Immun.* 1993;92(4):537–548.
262. Gwinn MR, Vallyathan V. Respiratory burst: role in signal transduction in alveolar macrophages. *J Toxicol Environ Health.* 2006;9(1):27–39.
263. Sharafkhaneh A, Hanania NA, Kim V. Pathogenesis of emphysema: from the bench to the bedside. *Proc Am Thorac Soc.* 2008; 5(4):475–477.
264. Kim V, Rogers TJ, Criner GJ. Frontiers in emphysema research. *Semin Thorac Cardiovasc Surg.* 2007;19(2):135–141.
265. Taraseviciene-Stewart L, Douglas IS, Nana-Sinkam PS, et al. Is alveolar destruction and emphysema in chronic obstructive pulmonary disease an immune disease? *Proc Am Thorac Soc.* 2006;3(8):687–690.
266. Karrasch S, Holz O, Jorres RA. Aging and induced senescence as factors in the pathogenesis of lung emphysema. *Respir Med.* 2008;102(9):1215–1230.
267. Cho HY, Reddy SP, Kleeberger SR. Nrf2 defends the lung from oxidative stress. *Antioxid Redox Signal.* 2006;8(1–2):76–87.
268. Boutten A, Goven D, Boczkowski J, Bonay M. Oxidative stress targets in pulmonary emphysema: focus on the Nrf2 pathway. *Expert Opin Ther Targets.* 2010;14(3):329–346.
269. Boutten A, Goven D, Artaud-Macari E, Boczkowski J, Bonay M. NRF2 targeting: a promising therapeutic strategy in chronic obstructive pulmonary disease. *Trends Mol Med.* 2011; 17(7):363–371.
270. Goven D, Boutten A, Lecon-Malas V, et al. Altered Nrf2/Keap1-Bach1 equilibrium in pulmonary emphysema. *Thorax.* 2008;63(10):916–924.
271. Hillas G, Nikolakopoulou S, Hussain S, Vassilakopoulos T. Antioxidants and mucolytics in COPD management: when (if ever) and in whom? *Curr Drug Targets.* 2012;14(2):225–234.
272. Morissette MC, Parent J, Milot J. Alveolar epithelial and endothelial cell apoptosis in emphysema: what we know and what we need to know. *Int J Chron Obstruct Pulmon Dis.* 2009;4:19–31.
273. Calabrese F, Giacometti C, Beghe B, et al. Marked alveolar apoptosis/proliferation imbalance in end-stage emphysema. *Respir Res.* 2005;6:14.
274. Dikalov S. Cross talk between mitochondria and NADPH oxidases. *Free Rad Biol Med.* 2011;51(7):1289–1301.
275. Ding Q, Luckhardt T, Hecker L, et al. New insights into the pathogenesis and treatment of idiopathic pulmonary fibrosis. *Drugs.* 2011;71(8):981–1001.

276. Cantin AM, North SL, Fells GA, Hubbard RC, Crystal RG. Oxidant-mediated epithelial cell injury in idiopathic pulmonary fibrosis. *J Clin Invest.* 1987;79(6):1665–1673.

277. Kinnula VL, Fattman CL, Tan RJ, Oury TD. Oxidative stress in pulmonary fibrosis: a possible role for redox modulatory therapy. *Am J Respir Crit Care Med.* 2005;172(4):417–422.

278. Crystal RG. Oxidants and respiratory tract epithelial injury: pathogenesis and strategies for therapeutic intervention. *Am J Med.* 1991;91(3 C):39S–44S.

279. Maier K, Leuschel L, Costabel U. Increased levels of oxidized methionine residues in bronchoalveolar lavage fluid proteins from patients with idiopathic pulmonary fibrosis. *Am Rev Respir Dis.* 1991;143(2):271–274.

280. Kuwano K, Nakashima N, Inoshima I, et al. Oxidative stress in lung epithelial cells from patients with idiopathic interstitial pneumonias. *Eur Respir J.* 2003;21(2):232–240.

281. Kuwano K, Hagimoto N, Maeyama T, et al. Mitochondria-mediated apoptosis of lung epithelial cells in idiopathic interstitial pneumonias. *Lab Invest.* 2002;82(12):1695–1706.

282. Lenz AG, Costabel U, Maier KL. Oxidized BAL fluid proteins in patients with interstitial lung diseases. *Eur Respir J.* 1996;9(2):307–312.

283. von Lohneysen K, Noack D, Wood MR, Friedman JS, Knaus UG. Structural insights into Nox4 and Nox2: motifs involved in function and cellular localization. *Mol Cell Biol.* 2010;30(4):961–975.

284. Laleu B, Gaggini F, Orchard M, et al. First in class, potent, and orally bioavailable NADPH oxidase isoform 4 (Nox4) inhibitors for the treatment of idiopathic pulmonary fibrosis. *J Med Chem.* 2010;53(21):7715–7730.

285. Carnesecchi S, Deffert C, Donati Y, et al. A key role for NOX4 in epithelial cell death during development of lung fibrosis. *Antioxid Redox Signal.* 2011;15(3):607–619.

286. Hecker L, Cheng J, Thannickal VJ. Targeting NOX enzymes in pulmonary fibrosis. *Cell Mol Life Sci.* 2012;69(14):2365–2371.

287. Cui W, Matsuno K, Iwata K, et al. NOX1/nicotinamide adenine dinucleotide phosphate, reduced form (NADPH) oxidase promotes proliferation of stellate cells and aggravates liver fibrosis induced by bile duct ligation. *Hepatology.* 2011;54(3):949–958.

288. Paik YH, Iwaisako K, Seki E, et al. The nicotinamide adenine dinucleotide phosphate oxidase (NOX) homologues NOX1 and NOX2/gp91(phox) mediate hepatic fibrosis in mice. *Hepatol.* 2011;53(5):1730–1741.

289. Wang P, Tang F, Li R, et al. Contribution of different Nox homologues to cardiac remodeling in two-kidney two-clip renovascular hypertensive rats: effect of valsartan. *Pharmacol Res.* 2007;55(5):408–417.

290. Looi YH, Grieve DJ, Siva A, et al. Involvement of Nox2 NADPH oxidase in adverse cardiac remodeling after myocardial infarction. *Hypertension.* 2008;51(2):319–325.

291. Masamune A, Watanabe T, Kikuta K, Satoh K, Shimosegawa T. NADPH oxidase plays a crucial role in the activation of pancreatic stellate cells. *Am J Physiol. Gastrointest Liver Physiol.* 2008;294(1):G99–G108.

292. Stas S, Whaley-Connell A, Habibi J, et al. Mineralocorticoid receptor blockade attenuates chronic overexpression of the renin-angiotensin-aldosterone system stimulation of reduced nicotinamide adenine dinucleotide phosphate oxidase and cardiac remodeling. *Endocrinol.* 2007;148(8):3773–3780.

293. Whaley-Connell A, Habibi J, Nistala R, et al. Attenuation of NADPH oxidase activation and glomerular filtration barrier remodeling with statin treatment. *Hypertension.* 2008;51(2):474–480.

294. Amara N, Goven D, Prost F, Muloway R, Crestani B, Boczkowski J. NOX4/NADPH oxidase expression is increased in pulmonary fibroblasts from patients with idiopathic pulmonary fibrosis and mediates TGFbeta1-induced fibroblast differentiation into myofibroblasts. *Thorax.* 2010;65(8):733–738.

295. Mitchell C, Robin MA, Mayeuf A, et al. Protection against hepatocyte mitochondrial dysfunction delays fibrosis progression in mice. *Am J Pathol.* 2009;175(5):1929–1937.

296. Jain M, Rivera S, Monclus EA, et al. Mitochondrial reactive oxygen species regulate transforming growth factor-beta signaling. *J Biol Chem.* 2013;288(2):770–777.

297. Cheresh P, Kim SJ, Tulasiram S, Kamp DW. Oxidative stress and pulmonary fibrosis. *Biochim Biophys Acta.* 2012;1832(7):1028–1040.

298. Liu G, Beri R, Mueller A, Kamp DW. Molecular mechanisms of asbestos-induced lung epithelial cell apoptosis. *Chem Biol Interact.* 2010;188(2):309–318.

299. Thannickal VJ, Horowitz JC. Evolving concepts of apoptosis in idiopathic pulmonary fibrosis. *Proc Am Thorac Soc.* 2006;3(4):350–356.

300. Carnesecchi S, Deffert C, Pagano A, et al. NADPH oxidase-1 plays a crucial role in hyperoxia-induced acute lung injury in mice. *Am J Respir Crit Care Med.* 2009;180(10):972–981.

301. Kim KK, Kugler MC, Wolters PJ, et al. Alveolar epithelial cell mesenchymal transition develops in vivo during pulmonary fibrosis and is regulated by the extracellular matrix. *Proc Nat Acad Sci U S A.* 2006;103(35):13180–13185.

302. Tanjore H, Xu XC, Polosukhin VV, et al. Contribution of epithelial-derived fibroblasts to bleomycin-induced lung fibrosis. *Am J Respir Crit Care Med.* 2009;180(7):657–665.

303. Cannito S, Novo E, di Bonzo LV, Busletta C, Colombatto S, Parola M. Epithelial-mesenchymal transition: from molecular mechanisms, redox regulation to implications in human health and disease. *Antioxid Redox Signal.* 2010;12(12):1383–1430.

304. Radisky DC. Epithelial-mesenchymal transition. *J Cell Sci.* 2005;118(Pt 19):4325–4326.

305. Pache JC, Carnesecchi S, Deffert C, et al. NOX-4 is expressed in thickened pulmonary arteries in idiopathic pulmonary fibrosis. *Nat Med.* 2011;17(1):31–32; author reply 32–33.

306. Strausz J, Muller-Quernheim J, Steppling H, Ferlinz R. Oxygen radical production by alveolar inflammatory cells in idiopathic pulmonary fibrosis. *Am Rev Respir Dis.* 1990;141(1):124–128.

307. Manoury B, Nenan S, Leclerc O, et al. The absence of reactive oxygen species production protects mice against bleomycin-induced pulmonary fibrosis. *Respir Res.* 2005;6:11.

308. Wang CL, Kang J, Li ZH. [Increased expression of NADPH oxidase p47-PHOX and p67-PHOX factor in idiopathic pulmonary fibrosis]. *Zhonghua Jie He He Hu Xi Za Zhi.* 2007;30(4):265–268.

309. Cui Y, Robertson J, Maharaj S, et al. Oxidative stress contributes to the induction and persistence of TGF-beta1 induced pulmonary fibrosis. *Int J Biochem Cell Biol.* 2011;43(8):1122–1133.

310. Tabima DM, Frizzell S, Gladwin MT. Reactive oxygen and nitrogen species in pulmonary hypertension. *Free Radic Biol Med.* 2012;52(9):1970–1986.

311. Wong CM, Bansal G, Pavlickova L, Marcocci L, Suzuki YJ. Reactive oxygen species and antioxidants in pulmonary hypertension. *Antioxid Redox Signal.* 2012;18(14):1789–1796.

312. Liu JQ, Zelko IN, Erbynn EM, Sham JS, Folz RJ. Hypoxic pulmonary hypertension: role of superoxide and NADPH oxidase

(gp91phox). *Am J Physiol Lung Cell Mol Physiol.* 2006;290(1): L2–L10.

313. Fresquet F, Pourageaud F, Leblais V, et al. Role of reactive oxygen species and gp91phox in endothelial dysfunction of pulmonary arteries induced by chronic hypoxia. *Br J Pharmacol.* 2006;148(5):714–723.

314. Fike CD, Slaughter JC, Kaplowitz MR, Zhang Y, Aschner JL. Reactive oxygen species from NADPH oxidase contribute to altered pulmonary vascular responses in piglets with chronic hypoxia-induced pulmonary hypertension. *Am J Physiol Lung Cell Mol Physiol.* 2008;295(5):L881–L888.

315. Mittal M, Roth M, Konig P, et al. Hypoxia-dependent regulation of nonphagocytic NADPH oxidase subunit NOX4 in the pulmonary vasculature. *Circ Res.* 2007;101(3):258–267.

316. Sharma S, Grobe AC, Wiseman DA, et al. Lung antioxidant enzymes are regulated by development and increased pulmonary blood flow. *Am J Physiol Lung Cell Mol Physiol.* 2007;293(4):L960–L971.

317. Sharma S, Kumar S, Sud N, et al. Alterations in lung arginine metabolism in lambs with pulmonary hypertension associated with increased pulmonary blood flow. *Vasc Pharmacol.* 2009;51(5–6):359–364.

318. Sharma S, Smith A, Kumar S, et al. Mechanisms of nitric oxide synthase uncoupling in endotoxin-induced acute lung injury: role of asymmetric dimethylarginine. *Vasc Pharmacol.* 2010;52(5–6):182–190.

319. Hoshikawa Y, Ono S, Suzuki S, et al. Generation of oxidative stress contributes to the development of pulmonary hypertension induced by hypoxia. *J Appl Physiol.* 2001;90(4):1299–1306.

320. Spiekermann S, Schenk K, Hoeper MM. Increased xanthine oxidase activity in idiopathic pulmonary arterial hypertension. *Eur Respir J.* 2009;34(1):276.

321. Jankov RP, Kantores C, Pan J, Belik J. Contribution of xanthine oxidase-derived superoxide to chronic hypoxic pulmonary hypertension in neonatal rats. *Am J Physiol Lung Cell Mol Physiol.* 2008;294(2):L233–L245.

322. Tuder RM, Chacon M, Alger L, et al. Expression of angiogenesis-related molecules in plexiform lesions in severe pulmonary hypertension: evidence for a process of disordered angiogenesis. *J Pathol.* 2001;195(3):367–374.

323. Sturrock A, Cahill B, Norman K, et al. Transforming growth factor-beta1 induces Nox4 NAD(P)H oxidase and reactive oxygen species-dependent proliferation in human pulmonary artery smooth muscle cells. *Am J Physiol Lung Cell Mol Physiol.* 2006;290(4):L661–L673.

324. Ismail S, Sturrock A, Wu P, et al. NOX4 mediates hypoxia-induced proliferation of human pulmonary artery smooth muscle cells: the role of autocrine production of transforming growth factor-{beta}1 and insulin-like growth factor binding protein-3. *Am J Physiol Lung Cell Mol Physiol.* 2009;296(3):L489–L499.

325. Seko Y, Nishimura H, Takahashi N, Ashida T, Nagai R. Serum levels of vascular endothelial growth factor and transforming growth factor-beta1 in patients with atrial fibrillation undergoing defibrillation therapy. *Jpn Heart J.* 2000;41(1):27–32.

326. Zheng W, Seftor EA, Meininger CJ, Hendrix MJ, Tomanek RJ. Mechanisms of coronary angiogenesis in response to stretch: role of VEGF and TGF-beta. *Am J Physiol Heart Circ Physiol.* 2001;280(2):H909–H917.

327. Bonnet S, Michelakis ED, Porter CJ, et al. An abnormal mitochondrial-hypoxia inducible factor-1alpha-Kv channel pathway disrupts oxygen sensing and triggers pulmonary arterial hypertension in fawn hooded rats: similarities to human pulmonary arterial hypertension. *Circulation.* 2006;113(22):2630–2641.

328. Archer SL, Michelakis ED, Thebaud B, et al. A central role for oxygen-sensitive K+ channels and mitochondria in the specialized oxygen-sensing system. *Novartis Found Symp.* 2006;272: 157–171; discussion 171–175, 214–217.

329. Schach C, Xu M, Platoshyn O, Keller SH, Yuan JX. Thiol oxidation causes pulmonary vasodilation by activating K+ channels and inhibiting store-operated Ca2+ channels. *Am J Physiol Lung Cell Mol Physiol.* 2007;292(3):L685–L698.

330. Oishi P, Sharma S, Grobe A, et al. Alterations in cGMP, soluble guanylate cyclase, phosphodiesterase 5, and B-type natriuretic peptide induced by chronic increased pulmonary blood flow in lambs. *Pediatr Pulmonol.* 2007;42(11):1057–1071.

331. Lakshminrusimha S, Wiseman D, Black SM, et al. The role of nitric oxide synthase-derived reactive oxygen species in the altered relaxation of pulmonary arteries from lambs with increased pulmonary blood flow. *Am J Physiol Heart Circ Physiol.* 2007;293(3):H1491–H1497.

332. Oishi PE, Wiseman DA, Sharma S, et al. Progressive dysfunction of nitric oxide synthase in a lamb model of chronically increased pulmonary blood flow: a role for oxidative stress. *Am J Physiol Lung Cell Mol Physiol.* 2008;295(5):L756–L766.

333. Zickus MA, Fonseca FV, Tummala M, Black SM, Ryzhov V. Identification of the tyrosine nitration sites in human endothelial nitric oxide synthase by liquid chromatography-mass spectrometry. *Eur J Mass Spectrom (Chichester, Eng).* 2008;14(4):239–247.

334. Zhao YY, Zhao YD, Mirza MK, et al. Persistent eNOS activation secondary to caveolin-1 deficiency induces pulmonary hypertension in mice and humans through PKG nitration. *J Clin Invest.* 2009;119(7):2009–2018.

335. Sharma S, Sud N, Wiseman DA, et al. Altered carnitine homeostasis is associated with decreased mitochondrial function and altered nitric oxide signaling in lambs with pulmonary hypertension. *Am J Physiol Lung Cell Mol Physiol.* 2008;294(1):L46–L56.

336. Maarsingh H, Bossenga BE, Bos IS, Volders HH, Zaagsma J, Meurs H. L-arginine deficiency causes airway hyperresponsiveness after the late asthmatic reaction. *Eur Respir J.* 2009; 34(1):191–199.

337. Maarsingh H, Leusink J, Zaagsma J, Meurs H. Role of the L-citrulline/L-arginine cycle in iNANC nerve-mediated nitric oxide production and airway smooth muscle relaxation in allergic asthma. *Eur J Pharmacol.* 2006;546(1–3):171–176.

338. Khong SM, Andrews KL, Huynh NN, et al. Arginase II inhibition prevents nitrate tolerance. *Br J Pharmacol.* 2012;166(7): 2015–2023.

339. Wells SM, Holian A. Asymmetric dimethylarginine induces oxidative and nitrosative stress in murine lung epithelial cells. *Am J Respir Cell Mol Biol.* 2007;36(5):520–528.

340. Roe ND, Ren J. Nitric oxide synthase uncoupling: a therapeutic target in cardiovascular diseases. *Vasc Pharmacol.* 2012;57(5–6): 168–172.

341. Bernard GR, Artigas A, Brigham KL, et al. Report of the American-European Consensus conference on acute respiratory distress syndrome: definitions, mechanisms, relevant outcomes, and clinical trial coordination. Consensus Committee. *J Crit Care.* 1994;9(1):72–81.

342. Bernard GR, Artigas A, Brigham KL, et al. The American-European Consensus Conference on ARDS. Definitions, mechanisms, relevant outcomes, and clinical trial coordination. *Am J Respir Crit Care Med.* 1994;149(3 Pt 1):818–824.

343. Ware LB, Matthay MA. The acute respiratory distress syndrome. *N Engl J Med.* 2000;342(18):1334–1349.

CHAPTER 28

Fibroblasts in Lung Homeostasis and Disease

Yong Zhou
Victor J. Thannickal

INTRODUCTION

Fibroblasts are the primary cellular source responsible for synthesis and remodeling of the extracellular matrix (ECM). These cells are in communication with the surrounding microenvironment and play a key role in lung homoeostasis. Following lung injury, fibroblasts are activated and undergo myofibroblast differentiation. Myofibroblasts are key effector cells for lung repair following injury. In addition to fibroblasts, perivascular pericytes and mesenchymal stem cells (MSCs) of bone marrow (BM) origins contribute to myofibroblast population. There is evidence that type II alveolar epithelial cells can differentiate into myofibroblasts in vitro through a process known as epithelial–mesenchymal transition (EMT); however, the role of EMT in fibrogenesis in vivo remains controversial. Myofibroblasts express α-smooth muscle actin (α-SMA), develop robust actin filaments (stress fibers), and acquire contractile activity. The function and behavior of myofibroblasts are regulated by both biochemical and physical cues in the surrounding microenvironment. The fate of myofibroblasts is a key determinant of whether an injury–repair response will resolve or progress into fibrosis. Destruction and aberrant remodeling of the ECM is a common feature of many lung diseases, including pulmonary fibrosis, asthma, chronic obstructive pulmonary disease (COPD), and lung cancer. Targeting myofibroblasts and tissue remodeling may provide a novel and effective strategy for treating a number of chronic lung diseases.

FIBROBLAST BASICS

WHAT ARE FIBROBLASTS?

Fibroblasts were described as early as in the late 19th century, based on their location and their microscopic appearance.[1] These are elongated cells that display a spindle-shaped morphology with extended cell processes.[2] Fibroblasts are ubiquitous in tissues and organs throughout the body and communicate with other cells such as epithelial cells (Fig. 28-1). Despite its discovery over a century, a reliable and specific molecular marker that identifies the fibroblast is currently lacking. Many indicators of fibroblast phenotype have been suggested in the previous studies (e.g., fibroblast-specific protein 1, vimentin, prolyl 4-hydroxylase, procollagen-Iα2, etc.).[3] However, none of them are specific to fibroblasts and/or are present in all fibroblasts. Currently, fibroblasts are identified by their ability to adhere to plastic, and their lack of markers that indicate other cell lineages. Clearly, better cellular markers with absolute specificity for fibroblasts will aid in the study of sources, differentiation, and phenotypic plasticity of fibroblasts.

Tissue-Specific Fibroblasts and Fibroblast Heterogeneity

Fibroblasts isolated from different tissues display a considerable degree of heterogeneity in phenotype and activity.[4] Such diversity is evident by divergent and specific gene expression patterns among fibroblasts isolated from distinct anatomical locations.[5] For example, fetal skin fibroblasts express high levels of collagen types I and V, whereas fetal lung fibroblasts lack collagen I and V expression.[5] Instead, fetal lung fibroblasts exclusively express lung-specific forkhead family transcription factors FOXF1 and FOXP1.[5] Tissue-specific fibroblasts may provide location-specific signaling for a given anatomic origin as well as important positional cues for wound healing and tissue regeneration. Besides the differences in fibroblasts from different anatomical sites, fibroblasts derived from a single tissue are often composed of subsets of different fibroblasts.[6] For example, fibroblast subpopulations isolated from lung differ in expression of surface markers such as Thy-1, cytoskeletal composition, lipid content, and cytokine profile.[7,8] Fibroblasts isolated from lungs with active fibrotic disease such as in the fibroblastic foci of human idiopathic pulmonary fibrosis (IPF) are morphologically and functionally distinct from fibroblasts isolated from normal lungs,[9] suggesting that selective

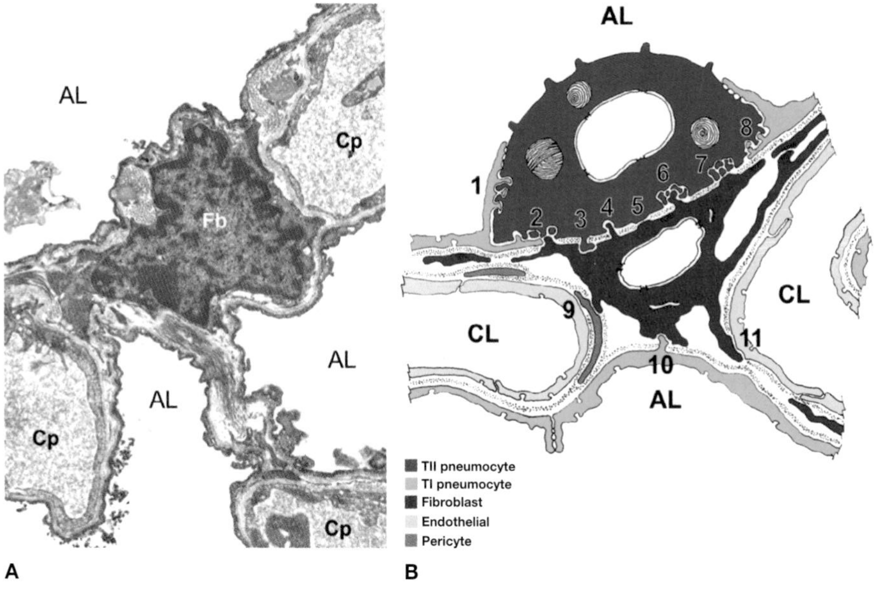

Figure 28-1 An interstitial fibroblast in the alveolar wall. **A.** A transmission electron microscopic image showing the structural organization of the alveolar wall in canine lung. Fb, fibroblast; Cp, capillary; AL, alveolar lumen; (**B**) summary of fibroblast *(red)* relationships with type I *(green)* and type II *(purple)* alveolar epithelial cells, capillary endothelial cells *(yellow)*, and pericytes *(orange)* in human and rabbit alveolar walls. *(Reproduced with permission from Burns AR, Smith CW, Walker DC. Unique structural features that influence neutrophil emigration into the lung. Physiol Rev. 2003;83(2):309–336.)*

expansion of specific fibroblast subsets is associated with the pathogenesis of this disease.

■ FIBROBLAST FUNCTIONS

The important functions of fibroblasts include deposition of ECM, regulation of inflammation, and wound healing.[10] Fibroblasts produce ECM-degrading proteases such as matrix metalloproteinases (MMPs) and their inhibitors, tissue inhibitors of metalloproteinases (TIMPs), supporting their crucial roles in regulating ECM turnover and homeostasis.[11]

ECM Production

One of the major functions of fibroblasts is the production of ECM. The ECM in the lung provides an essential scaffold on which cells can proliferate and differentiate. It also provides the lung with tensile strength and elasticity that are essential for ventilation. Lung ECM is composed of fibrillar proteins, glycoproteins, proteoglycans (PGs), and polysaccharides, each of which has distinct biochemical and biomechanical properties; these include collagens, elastin, fibronectin, PGs, hyaluronan (HA), laminin, vitronectin, and thrombospondin.[12] Type I and type III collagens are the most abundant collagens in the lung interstitium (ratio 3–6:1). Collagen IV is mainly localized to basement membranes. A fibroblast is estimated to synthesize approximately 3.5 million procollagen molecules/cell/day.[13,14] Depending on tissue type and age, 10% to 90% of synthesized procollagens are intracellularly degraded by lysosomal enzymes (e.g., cathepsins B, D, and L). It is postulated that regulation of procollagen-degrading rate may provide an important mechanism for rapid secretion of collagen in response to injury without de novo synthesis of new proteins.

Secretion of Proteolytic Enzymes and Inhibitors

The ECM is a dynamic structure that undergoes constant remodeling. Remodeling of the ECM is regulated by complex mechanisms including stimulatory and inhibitory mediators derived from resident cells in the local environment.[14] Fibroblasts synthesize a variety of proteolytic enzymes and inhibitors that enable them to control the assembly and turnover of the ECM. MMPs are either secreted by fibroblasts as inactive zymogens or anchored to the cell surface. Activation of MMPs occurs by disruption of interactions between the prodomain and the catalytic domain through either the proteolytic cleavage or the conformational change of the proenzymes.[15] MMPs function as proteinases that degrade most ECM proteins. Proteolysis of the ECM macromolecules by MMPs results in the release of cryptic fragments and neoepitopes that promote angiogenesis and cellular migration.[16,17] MMPs also have critical roles in the posttranslational regulation of other proteins including latent growth factors stored within the ECM, membrane receptors, and other proteases.[18] Hence, MMPs impact cell behavior both through modulation of cell–matrix interactions and through regulation of other signaling molecules. MMPs themselves are regulated by their endogenous inhibitors, TIMPs. TIMPs block MMP activity by noncovalently binding to the MMP active site. A tight balance between MMP proteolysis and TIMP expression is required for maintaining lung homeostasis.[19]

Innate Immune Function

Fibroblasts are capable of synthesizing many inflammatory cytokines that are initially thought to be exclusively produced by inflammatory cells.[20] Fibroblast-derived cytokines play an important role in the amplification and perpetuation of the immune response. Fibroblasts generate constitutive and cytokine-induced C-C and C-X-C chemokines that recruit inflammatory and immune cells to the injured cites.[21] Lung fibroblast–derived granulocyte macrophage colony–stimulating factor promotes the survival of eosinophils, which contributes to the fibrotic response in the lung.[22,23] Direct contacts between fibroblasts and T cells promote the production of adhesion molecules and cytokines by the T cells.[24] Interactions between fibroblasts and mast cells facilitate de novo production of eotaxin, a potent eosinophil chemoattractant.[25] The impact of interactions between fibroblasts and inflammatory cells are bidirectional. Th2 cells produce IL-4 that recognizes specific receptors on fibroblasts and modulates fibroblast proliferation and biosynthetic capacity.[26] Eosinophils release mitogens that augment fibroblast proliferation and collagen production.[27,28] Fibroblasts are the main producers of ECM proteins. Since ECM components affect multiple functions and properties of inflammatory and immune cells,[29,30] it suggests a further regulatory role of fibroblasts in innate immune response by the effects on the ECM.

Regulation of Tissue Interstitial Fluid Pressure and Microhemodynamics

Fibroblasts regulate tissue interstitial fluid volume, pressure, and microcirculation hemodynamics by generation of actomyosin-derived forces and transmission of the forces to the ECM via transmembrane integrins.[31] Such mechanical interactions between fibroblasts and matrix are subjected to modulation by soluble factors, such as PDGF that results in increased interstitial fluid pressure, and TNF-α that leads to decreased interstitial fluid pressure.[32,33] Fibroblasts express ecto-5′-nucleotidase (CD73) and soluble guanylyl cyclase (cGC) that affect hemodynamics,[34] suggesting a role of fibroblasts in the regulation of the microcirculation.

MYOFIBROBLASTS: EFFECTOR CELLS IN TISSUE REPAIR

■ HISTORICAL CONTEXT

Myofibroblasts were first identified as fibroblastic cells with a strong muscle cell–like contractile filamentous apparatus in the granulation tissue of healing wounds.[35] These cells are present in organs with increased remodeling, such as in development, inflammation, fibrosis, cancer invasion, and metastasis.[36] Myofibroblasts display prominent cytoplasmic actin microfilaments (stress fibers) (Fig. 28-2). They are connected to one another with adherens and gap junctions as well as to the ECM with focal adhesion (FA) complexes.[37] Myofibroblasts may be further classified into subtypes based on the presence or absence of vimentin, desmin, and/or α-SMA in cytoskeletal filaments. Expression of these proteins varies upon tissue types and is subjected to the regulation by environmental factors.[38] Alternatively, myofibroblasts can be simply classified into two subpopulations, proto-myofibroblasts and mature myofibroblasts.[39]

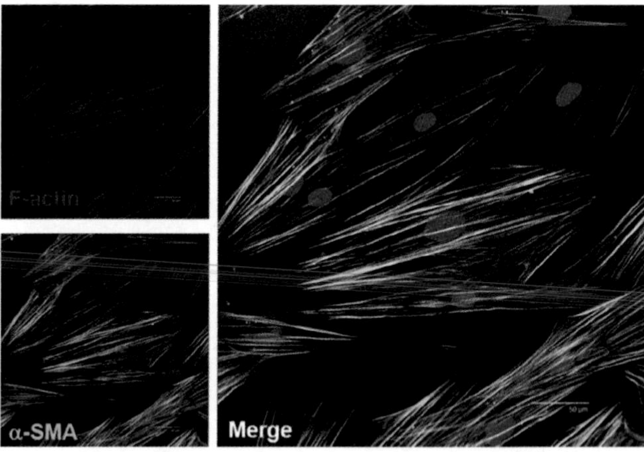

Figure 28-2 Myofibroblasts are characterized by de novo synthesis of α-SMA and incorporation of α-SMA into filamentous actin stress fibers. Scale bar: 50 μm.

TABLE 28-1 Myofibroblast Markers

Marker	Cellular Overlap
Cytoskeletal component	
α-SMA[40]	Smooth muscle cells
Desmin[41]	Hepatic stellate cells, cardiomyocytes
Cofilin[42]	Smooth muscle cells
GB 42-antigen[43]	Smooth muscle cells
Paladin 4Ig[44]	Smooth muscle cells
Tropomyosin-1[45]	Cardiomyocytes
Cell membrane receptor	
Angiotensin II type 1 receptor (AT1R)[46]	Cardiomyocytes, smooth muscle cells
Integrin $a_{11}b_1$[47]	Musculoskeletal cells
Thy-1[48]	Lipofibroblasts
Endosialin[49]	Cardiomyocytes, smooth muscle cells, adipocytes
Cadherin-11[50]	Tenocytes, endothelial cells, mesenchymal cells
Frizzled-2[51]	Smooth muscle cells
Extracellular protein	
Collagen I, III, IV, V, VI[52]	Various cells
Tenascin C[53]	Smooth muscle cells
Fibronectin ED-A[54]	Smooth muscle cells
Osteopontin[55]	Osteoblasts, osteocytes, chondrocytes
Periostin[56]	Preosteoblasts, cardiomyocytes

Proto-myofibroblasts are partly differentiated myofibroblasts that contain α-SMA–negative actin stress fibers, whereas mature myofibroblasts possess extensive network of α-SMA–positive stress fibers and large FAs (termed supermature FAs). α-SMA is the most widely used marker for identification of myofibroblasts (Fig. 28-2). In addition, studies have identified several other markers and modulators of myofibroblasts (Table 28-1). However, a specific and universal myofibroblast marker remains to be identified.

■ ORIGIN OF MYOFIBROBLASTS

The precise origin of myofibroblasts remains unsolved at present. Studies have suggested that local fibroblasts, perivascular pericytes, BM-derived MSCs, tissue MSCs, and epithelial/endothelial cells (through epithelial/endothelial–mesenchymal transition) are among potential cellular sources for myofibroblast population.

Resident Fibroblasts—Mesenchymal Stem Cells

Fibroblasts are the most widely accepted origin for myofibroblasts.[57,58] Fibroblasts influx into injured sites from the surrounding tissue and differentiate into myofibroblasts in response to extracellular stimuli including biochemical and physical cues.[59] These stimuli induce intrinsic changes in gene expression and stress fiber formation that characterizes myofibroblast differentiation.

MSCs that reside in tissues lack hematopoietic and leukocyte markers, but may express α-SMA.[60] Tissue MSCs have been described in the dermal sheath that surrounds the hair follicle facing epithelial stem cells.[61] These MSCs are involved in papilla regeneration and differentiate into myofibroblasts in response to environmental insults. It has been reported that MSCs from subcutaneous fat are responsible for collagen accumulation in scars.[62] Following lung injury, myofibroblasts were found to originate from perivascular and peribronchial sources.[63] It is likely that there are tissue MSCs in the human adult lung,[64] which become activated and undergo myofibroblast differentiation in response to lung injury. In support of this notion, a previous study has provided evidence for isolation of postnatal MSCs from different organs including liver, kidney, and lung.[65]

Pericytes

Pericytes are perivascular cells located on the abluminal side of endothelial cells in microvasculature.[66] These cells share developmental origins with fibroblasts, but differ from fibroblasts by the fact that pericytes anatomically connect with endothelial cells through cell processes within capillary basement membrane, whereas fibroblasts do not directly interact with endothelial cells.[67] The normal function of pericytes includes the regulation of vascular tone and blood flow through expression of contractile microfilaments (actin, myosin) and intermediate filaments (desmin, vimentin).[68] Microvascular pericytes differentiate into myofibroblasts in diffuse cutaneous systemic sclerosis, providing a link between microvascular damage and skin fibrosis.[69] Recent studies using the genetic fate-mapping approach have clearly demonstrated that pericytes are a major cellular source of myofibroblasts in animal models of acute injury to muscle, dermis, and kidney.[70,71] In addition, HSCs, pericyte-like cells in the liver, are the primary myofibroblast progenitors in mouse models of alcoholic and toxic liver fibrosis.[72]

Bone Marrow–Derived Mesenchymal Cells

BM-derived MSCs are self-renewable, multipotent progenitor cells with the capacity to differentiate into lineage-specific cells that form bone, cartilage, fat, tendon, and muscle.[73] Compared with hematopoietic stem cells, MSCs are more radio-resistant and reside mostly in BM stroma. BM-derived MSCs do not express hematopoietic markers and can be isolated as Lin-CD45-CD31-CD34-CD133-Sca-1+Vitamin A-cells.[74] In vitro evidence for a BM origin of myofibroblasts was first presented more than four decades ago. By plating BM cells on culture dishes, colonies consisting of cells exhibiting elongated or polygonal cytoplasm and clear nuclei were formed.[75] Transplantation studies using Y chromosome or green fluorescent protein (GFP) as a marker of donor cells provide in vivo evidence that (myo)fibroblasts in wounded skin, lung fibrosis, and intestinal fibrosis may derive from the BM.[76] There is evidence that monocytes may represent the major BM-derived cell population that contributes to myofibroblasts in fibrotic lesions, at least in some contexts.[77]

Circulating fibrocytes express markers of hematopoietic cells (CD34), leukocytes (CD11b, CD13, and CD45), and fibroblast products (collagens I, III, and fibronectin). These cells are distinguished from monocytes/macrophages, dendritic cells, and B cells by their lack of expression of specific markers for these cell lineages. Circulating fibrocytes migrate into injured tissues and have been identified in a number of fibrotic conditions.[78] Studies have identified the potential for fibrocytes to participate in wound healing and pathological scarring.[78,79] However, the direct contribution of fibrocytes to myofibroblast population during wound healing and fibrosis remains controversial. Evidence for and against fibrocyte-to-myofibroblast differentiation exists.[76,80] It is likely that instead of direct differentiation into myofibroblasts, circulating fibrocytes contribute to fibrosis by production of profibrogenic paracrine mediators that target resident cells.

Epithelial–Mesenchymal Transition

EMT refers to as a process through which fully differentiated epithelial cells lose their epithelial characteristics (e.g., apico-basal polarity, polygonal cell shape, and tight and adherens junctions) and acquire properties of mesenchymal cells (e.g., elongated cell shape, increased motility, and contractility). Epithelial cells undergoing EMT are characterized by downregulation of epithelial markers (e.g., E-cadherin and ZO-1) and concomitant upregulation of mesenchymal markers (e.g., FSP1 and α-SMA) in the injured epithelium.[81] There is overwhelming evidence that primary epithelial cells cultured in vitro undergo EMT in response to a stimulatory input of soluble growth factors (e.g., TGF-β, EGF, and HGF) and/or ECM components (e.g., collagen).[82] However, the concept of in vivo fibrogenic EMT has been challenged by new epithelial lineage tracking studies in a variety of models of kidney, lung, and liver fibrosis in animals.[83]

FACTORS REGULATING FIBROBLAST ACTIVATION AND MYOFIBROBLAST DIFFERENTIATION

Fibroblasts isolated from the site of a healing wound or from fibrotic tissue secrete higher levels of ECM constituents and proliferate more than their normal counterparts isolated from healthy organs.[84] Such an increased activity is referred to as "fibroblast activation." Activated fibroblasts express α-SMA, leading to the term "myofibroblasts." Fibroblast activation and differentiation into myofibroblasts are regulated by various stimuli, including biochemical factors, biophysical cues from the ECM, and epigenetic modifications.

Growth Factor and Cytokine-Mediated Activation

Fibroblasts become activated by stimulation with cytokines such as TGF-β1, PDGF, and FGF2, which are released from injured epithelial cells, infiltrating mononuclear cells such as monocytes and macrophages as well as the ECM.[85–88] TGF-β1 is a pluripotent cytokine that plays a central role in the development of fibrosis. TGF-β1 is sequestered in a latent form (termed latent TGF-β1) in the ECM.[89] Latent TGF-β1 becomes activated in a spatially and temporally regulated fashion in response to injury.[89] Active TGF-β1 binds to its membrane receptors (TGF-βRI and TGF-βRII) and signals through both Smad-dependent canonical pathway and Smad-independent noncanonical pathway that promote fibrotic gene expression.[39] Active TGF-β1 also increases the assembly of stress fibers and FAs that are required for the development of cellular contractility.[39] In addition, prototypic cytokines produced by CD4+ T cells such as IL-13/IL-4 and IL-17 exert profibrotic effects on fibroblasts and play a crucial role in the development of fibrosis.[90,91]

Components of Vascular/Coagulation System

Coagulation proteases such as factor Xa and thrombin activate fibroblasts through receptor-mediated effects elicited by high-affinity thrombin receptor, proteinase-activated receptor (PAR)-1.[92] PAR-1 signaling promotes fibroblast proliferation via the autocrine production of PDGF and CTGF, and drives fibroblast differentiation into myofibroblasts via αvβ5-dependent TGF-β activation.[93,94] Thrombin upregulates expression of the fibrinolysis inhibitor, plasminogen activator inhibitor (PAI)-1, resulting in increased fibrin matrix.[95] Fibrin matrix inhibits surfactant function and contributes to alveolar collapse and traction of remaining airspaces (honeycombing).[92] Lysophosphatidic acid (LPA), a platelet-derived molecule during blood coagulation, promotes fibroblast activation and pulmonary fibrosis by activation of latent TGF-β1 through LPA receptor.[96] Endothelin-1 (ET-1), an activator of extrinsic coagulation cascade, exerts potent mitogenic and profibrotic effects on fibroblasts.[97] Transgenic mice expressing human ET-1 transgene have been shown to develop progressive pulmonary fibrosis.[97]

Reactive Oxygen Species

Accumulating evidence indicates that oxidative stress and reactive oxygen species (ROS) production, mainly in the form of superoxide and hydrogen peroxide, play a significant role in myofibroblast differentiation.[98] The NAD(P)H oxidases of the Nox family have been identified as the enzyme system that is primarily responsible for ROS generation by fibroblasts in response to injury and are recognized as key mediators of myofibroblast differentiation and matrix accumulation in lung fibrosis.[99] Nox4, the most abundant Nox isoform in the lung, has been characterized as a "constitutively active" enzyme, meaning that the enzymatic activity of Nox4 is primarily regulated at the level of gene expression. TGF-β1 increases Nox4 expression and ROS production in lung fibroblasts, which mediates TGF-β1–dependent myofibroblast differentiation.[99] A similar mechanism for myofibroblast differentiation has been demonstrated in cardiac fibroblasts, renal fibroblasts, and mesangial cells.[100,101] Nox4 is also associated with TGF-β1–induced cellular contractility in lung myofibroblasts and cytoskeletal remodeling in vascular smooth muscle cells as well as endothelial cells.[99,102,103] Together, these results indicate that Nox-derived ROS regulate fibroblast morphology, contractility, and differentiation.

Mechanical Stress

Fibroblasts respond to mechanical cues, including externally applied forces, interstitial fluid flow, and matrix rigidity sensed through internally generated forces. Externally applied forces such as stretch provoke diverse fibroblast signaling responses, including activation of mitogen-activated protein (MAP) kinases, [104]Akt,[105] and focal adhesion kinase (FAK). It has been shown that stretch augments TGF-β release and signaling, and promotes the myofibroblast phenotype.[106,107] The continuous interactions between cell-generated forces and the resistance of matrix to cellular forces strengthen cell–matrix contacts and develop α-SMA–positive stress fibers characterizing myofibroblast differentiation.[39,108] Normal lung fibroblasts grown on polyacrylamide gels with a stiffness grade similar to fibrotic lungs undergo myofibroblast differentiation.[109] The effects of matrix stiffening on myofibroblast differentiation may occur through TGF-β–dependent intrinsic and/or TGF-β–independent extrinsic mechanotransduction (see Section "Mechanotransduction in Myofibroblastsinsser").[109,110] Interstitial fluid flow induces fibroblast proliferation, collagen alignment, and fibroblast-to-myofibroblast differentiation in the absence of exogenous mediators.[111,112] $\alpha_1\beta_1$ integrin appears to play an important role in the specific response to interstitial fluid flow.[111] Taken together, these results suggest that fibroblasts are mechanosensitive and are programmed for matrix production, contraction, and differentiation in the presence of mechanical stimuli.

Epigenetic Regulation

The findings that specific signatures of gene profile in myofibroblasts are "memorized" over passages suggest that epigenetic modifications may be involved in the regulation of myofibroblast differentiation.[113] Epigenetic regulation of myofibroblastic phenotype involves DNA methylation, histone modification, and sequence-specific microRNAs (miRNAs). DNA methylation at CpG islands is associated with expression of myofibroblast marker α-SMA in lung cells. Type II alveolar epithelial cells that do not express α-SMA exhibit high levels of methylation at the three CpG islands in the regulatory regions of ACTA2 gene encoding α-SMA protein, whereas lung (myo)fibroblasts exhibit significantly low levels of DNA methylation at these sites.[114] Inhibition of DNA methyltransferase (DNMT) induces α-SMA expression, whereas overexpression of DNMT suppresses α-SMA expression in lung fibroblasts.[114] Inhibition of DNA methylation activates PPARγ and NF-κB, transcription factors known to suppress ACTA2 gene expression,[115] suggesting that modifications of DNA methylation may also indirectly regulate α-SMA expression by inactivation of PPARγ and NF-κB. Histone acetylation has been shown to regulate myofibroblast differentiation. It has been shown that histone deacetylase (HDAC)4 is an essential epigenetic regulator of TGF-β1–induced skin fibroblast-to-myofibroblast differentiation.[116] HDAC8 binds to α-SMA and the binding is likely to regulate actin cytoskeleton–derived cellular contractility.[117]

miRNAs are single-stranded RNA molecules that target multiple mRNAs and induce silencing of multiple transcripts. It has been shown that miR-21 mediates TGF-β1–induced lung myofibroblast differentiation by targeting Smad7, a major inhibitor of TGF-β signaling.[118] In contrast, downregulation of miRNA let-7d expression by TGF-β results in increased mesenchymal gene expression (e.g., ACTA2) in multiple epithelial cell lines, indicative of EMT.[119] miR-132 inhibits MeCP2 and PPARγ expression, resulting in enhanced α-SMA expression in lung fibroblasts.[115]

Other Factors

Wnt ligands induce fibroblast activation and collagen synthesis.[120] β-catenin, a transcription factor and a downstream signal transducer of Wnt signaling, was found to accumulate in the nuclei of cells located in the fibroblastic foci of IPF lungs.[121] Selective inhibition of β-catenin–mediated transcription attenuates lung fibrosis in bleomycin-induced mouse model.[122] These studies suggest a crucial role of the Wnt/β-catenin signal in fibroblast activation and lung fibrosis. Integrins have been implicated in the differentiation of proto-myofibroblasts into mature myofibroblasts.[123] Integrin $\alpha_5\beta_1$ is associated with α-SMA expression in differentiating myofibroblasts.[123] Large clusters of $\alpha_5\beta_1$ are present in the FAs of mature myofibroblasts.[123]In addition, environmental stimuli including hypoxia and hyperglycemia as well as direct contacts between fibroblasts and leukocytes have been reported to be associated with fibroblast activation.[124,125]

MECHANICAL ASPECTS OF MYOFIBROBLASTS

Myofibroblast Contractility

Acquisition of contractility similar to smooth muscle cells is a defining feature of myofibroblasts. Myofibroblasts generate intracellular contractile forces by ATP-powered sliding of actin–myosin filaments.[126] Compared with Ca^{2+}-regulated rapid and reversible contraction in smooth muscle cells, myofibroblast contraction is relatively slow, sustained, and nonreversible.[127] Myofibroblast contractility is primarily regulated by the Rho family of small GTPases (Rho, Rac, and Cdc42) and their downstream targets, primarily myosin light-chain kinase (MLCK) and myosin light-chain phosphatase (MLCP).[39] α-SMA expression and incorporation of α-SMA into stress fibers contribute to myofibroblast contractility.[128] However, the mechanism by which α-SMA regulates myofibroblast contractile force formation is not clear. Myofibroblast contractility facilitates a normal wound healing process by limiting and closing the exposed surface area of the wound. Myofibroblasts disappear from the wound site when a normal repair process is successfully completed. The persistence of myofibroblasts is associated with aberrant wound repair and leads to tissue fibrosis/scarring. Increasing evidence suggests that myofibroblast contractility may provide a feed-forward mechanism (known as mechanotransduction; see Section "Mechanotransduction in Myofibroblasts") that sustains fibrosis. Inhibiting myofibroblast contractility by targeting Rho/Rho kinase (ROCK)/actin cytoskeleton signal pathway selectively activates mitochondria-dependent intrinsic apoptotic pathway in myofibroblasts and ameliorates bleomycin-induced mouse lung fibrosis.[129]

Sensing Matrix Stiffness

The ECM in healthy organs has well-defined mechanical properties that fall within a physiological range.[130] Changes in matrix stiffness that occur in pathological states, such as fibrosis and cancer, have profound effects on cell morphology, proliferation, migration, and gene expression.[130] Characterization of the mechanical properties of normal and fibrotic lung matrix demonstrates increased matrix rigidity in both human IPF and experimental models of lung fibrosis.[131,132] It is believed that protein cross-linking enzymes such as lysyl oxidase (LOXL2) and tissue transglutaminase (TG2) and/or matrix-degrading enzymes such as MMPs regulate the stiffness of ECM, although the precise mechanisms remain to be determined. Fibroblasts sense changes in matrix stiffness by cell–matrix adhesions.[133] Transmembrane integrins at FAs act as direct mechanosensors on the cell membrane by providing a physical link between intracellular actin cytoskeleton and the ECM. The cytoplasmic domain of integrins interacts with signaling molecules at the FA sites (e.g., FAK and c-Src). Thus, integrins also act as indirect mechanosensors to regulate cell function and behavior by modulating FA signals.[134] Matrix stiffness sensing depends largely on cellular contractility and actin cytoskeleton integrity. Fibroblast contractility generates cytoskeletal tension that serves to transmit mechanical information from the ECM. Disruption of actin cytoskeleton–mediated contractility blocks matrix stiffening–induced myofibroblast differentiation.[109]

Mechanotransduction in Myofibroblasts

Mechanotransduction is a process in which cells sense mechanical stimuli and convert mechanical signals into biochemical signals. Recent studies suggest that mechanotransduction in myofibroblasts with prolonged survival/resistance to apoptosis may provide a feed-forward mechanism for progression of fibrosis, as in IPF. It has been reported that lung myofibroblast contraction promotes latent TGF-β activation, the most potent fibrogenic cytokine characterized to date, in the extracellular compartment (Fig. 28-3).[110,135] In this process, the actomyosin apparatus in myofibroblasts generates contractile forces that are transmitted across the cell membrane to the ECM. The force transmission results in a conformational change of the ECM-bound latent TGF-β1 complex, resulting in the release/exposure of active TGF-β1 from the latent complex. The finding suggests an extrinsic mechanotransduction pathway in which mechanical forces derived from intracellular stress fibers are transduced to the ECM and converted into TGF-β1 fibrogenic signal capable of regulating fibrosis.

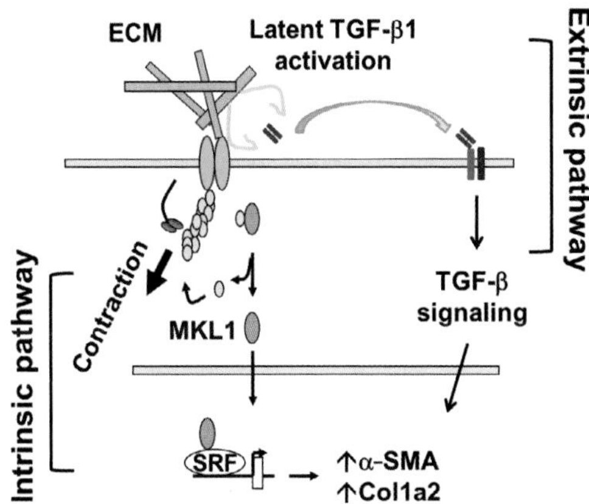

Figure 28-3 Contractile forces promote myofibroblast differentiation via intrinsic and extrinsic mechanotransduction pathways. In the intrinsic mechanotransduction pathway, mechanical stimuli from stiff/fibrotic ECM promote G-actin polymerization into F-actin. This results in the release of MKL1 and its nuclear translocation. MKL1 binds to serum response factor (SRF) in the nucleus to form a transactivation complex and activates fibrotic gene expression that specifies myofibroblast differentiation. In the extrinsic mechanotransduction pathway, actomyosin-generated contractile forces pull against stiff/fibrotic ECM. This results in a conformational change of latent TGF-β1 complex, which releases active TGF-β1 from the latent molecule. Active TGF-β1 then binds to its receptors on the cell membrane and initiates TGF-β signaling that promotes fibrotic gene expression.

In contrast to TGF-β–mediated extrinsic mechanotransduction pathway, an intrinsic mechanotransduction pathway in which the myofibroblast contractile signal is converted into a nuclear signal by transcription factor coactivator megakaryocytic leukemia protein (MKL)1 (also known as MAL/MRTF-A) has also been identified (Fig. 28-3).[109] MKL1 is a serum response factor (SRF) coactivator that constitutively binds to monomeric G-actin in the cytoplasm.[136] In response to matrix stiffening, normal lung fibroblasts undergo extensive actin cytoskeletal remodeling and develop contractile forces. This changes actin cytoskeletal dynamics that favors G-actin polymerization into F-actin. Polymerization of G-actin into F-actin results in the release of MKL1 from G-actin. The liberated MKL1 enters into nucleus, where it binds to SRF and targets to the CArG sequence in the promoter region of ACTA2 gene and col1a2 gene, leading to gene activation.[137] TGF-β neutralizing antibody does not block MKL1-mediated α-SMA expression,[109] suggesting that MKL1-mediated intrinsic mechanotransduction is independent of TGF-β–dependent extrinsic mechanotransduction. In addition to sensing mechanical stimuli, integrins are important mechanotransducers that allow bidirectional transduction and conversion of external forces into intracellular response (outside-in signaling) and internal forces (e.g., stress fiber-derived contractile forces) into extracellular and/or FA signals (inside-out signaling).[39,138] Besides integrins, stretch-activated ion channels, receptor tyrosine kinases (RTKs), CD44, and syndecan-4 are potential mediators of mechanotransduction as well.[139–142] However, mechanical stress may also regulate gene expression in fibroblasts through mechanotransduction-independent mechanisms. It has been shown that cyclic strain increases the mRNA level of tenascin-C within 1 hour in cultured fibroblasts[143] and this induction does not require synthesis of new proteins.[144]

Myofibroblasts in Tissue Homeostasis and Wound Repair

Myofibroblasts play a role in the regulation of differentiation and homeostasis of adjacent epithelia. Such mesenchymal–epithelial interactions are crucial for morphogenesis and organogenesis.[145] Myofibroblasts regulate epithelia by secretion of soluble growth factors and production of basement membrane molecules.[146]

Myofibroblasts play important roles in both normal and aberrant wound repair. As mentioned earlier, myofibroblast contractility facilitates wound closure. During the resolution phase, myofibroblasts produce MMPs and TIMPs that change the local microenvironment from a balance favoring ECM deposition to matrix degradation.[147] Interconnected gap junctions of myofibroblasts allow the electrical signals created by cyclic ion movements to be transmitted through the syncytium and the length of the resident organ.[148] Myofibroblasts sustain their activated state in fibrosis/hypertrophic scarring even when the initial insults have regressed. Myofibroblasts in such a sustained state of activation continue to secrete ECM constituents, growth factors, and cytokines. These result in a self-perpetuating autocrine loop that further stimulates myofibroblast differentiation and prevents normal resolution of tissue injury. In addition to fibrosis/hypertrophic scars, diseases associated with myofibroblastic phenotype include inflammatory pseudotumors, cancer metastasis, and neoplastic transformation of the myofibroblasts themselves.

■ THE FATE OF MYOFIBROBLASTS

The fate of myofibroblasts is a key determinant between normal repair and fibrosis. In normal wound healing, myofibroblasts gradually disappear after wounds are closed. Persistent myofibroblast differentiation is associated with pathological wound healing and fibrosis. Understanding of the physiological clearance of activated fibroblasts is particularly important for developing therapeutic strategies for persistent/progressive fibrosis such as IPF.

Apoptosis

Apoptosis has been suggested as an intriguing possibility for the elimination of myofibroblasts from healing wounds and reversible fibrosis.[149] An earlier study has observed that myofibroblasts undergo apoptosis in granulation tissue on which a vascularized skin flap is grafted.[150] Reduced growth factor and increased MMP expression appear to link to myofibroblast cell death.[151] In addition, disruption of cell–matrix interactions using RGD peptides or soluble fibronectin promotes myofibroblast anoikis, a type of apoptosis that is induced by inadequate or inappropriate cell–matrix interactions.[152] In reversible liver fibrosis, HSC-derived myofibroblasts undergo apoptosis in parallel to the reduction of the total number of HSCs in the recovery phase.[153] Hepatic myofibroblast apoptosis appears to occur by a Fas ligand (APO-1/CD95)–mediated extrinsic pathway.[153] Pharmacological inhibition of ROCK inhibits actin polymerization, downregulates the constitutive expression of antiapoptotic protein, Bcl-2, in IPF lung myofibroblasts; this results in release of cytochrome *c* from mitochondria, triggering mitochondria-dependent intrinsic apoptosis pathway. Furthermore, Fasudil-induced myofibroblast apoptosis ameliorates bleomycin-induced lung fibrosis in mice.[129] This study indicates that targeting mechanosensitive signaling in myofibroblasts may offer an effective approach for treatment of fibrotic disorders (Fig. 28-4).

Dedifferentiation

A recent study showed that HSC-derived myofibroblasts regress to a more quiescent state upon the removal of the fibrogenic stimuli in a carbon tetrachloride–induced mouse model of liver fibrosis.[72] The finding suggests that reversion of myofibroblasts to a more quiescent phenotype may be a second possibility for the clearance of these cells. However, such quiescent HSCs are reactivated more rapidly (in comparison to native HSCs) by subsequent insults, and result in more robust liver fibrosis,[72] suggesting that myofibroblast regression may be an intermediate step toward the resolution of fibrosis. Although regression to an inactive precursor cell may limit the activity of myofibroblasts, this does not appear to completely eliminate the potential for reactivation.

Senescence

Cellular senescence is associated with the loss of the ability of cells to replicate their genome and enter permanent growth arrest in the G1/G0 cell-cycle phase.[154] Although senescent fibroblasts do not respond to mitogens, they remain metabolically active and are resistant to apoptosis. Cellular senescence often occurs by telomere shortening and subsequent activation of p53 and p21 and/or inactivation of pRB and activation of p16.[154] Senescence may also be triggered by other forms of cellular damage, including oxidative stress, DNA damage, and oncogene activation.[154] Myofibroblast senescence has been proposed as an antifibrotic mechanism by limiting the proliferative capacity of fibrogenic fibroblasts and/or by modulating the cellular microenvironment.[155,156] However, this basic assertion is inconsistent with the clinical observation of an increased risk of fibrotic disease with advancing age. This highlights the complexities of cellular senescence in tissue injury repair processes, and supports the concept that the plasticity and fate of senescent cells may be altered with aging which, ultimately, determines the outcome of the tissue repair response.

MYOFIBROBLASTS IN LUNG DEVELOPMENT AND DISEASE

■ ALVEOLOGENESIS

Lung development is a complex process involving reciprocal interactions between mesoderm-derived mesenchyme and endoderm-derived epithelium. Alveolar myofibroblasts are present during alveologenesis, but absent in the adult lung.[157] Myofibroblasts surround

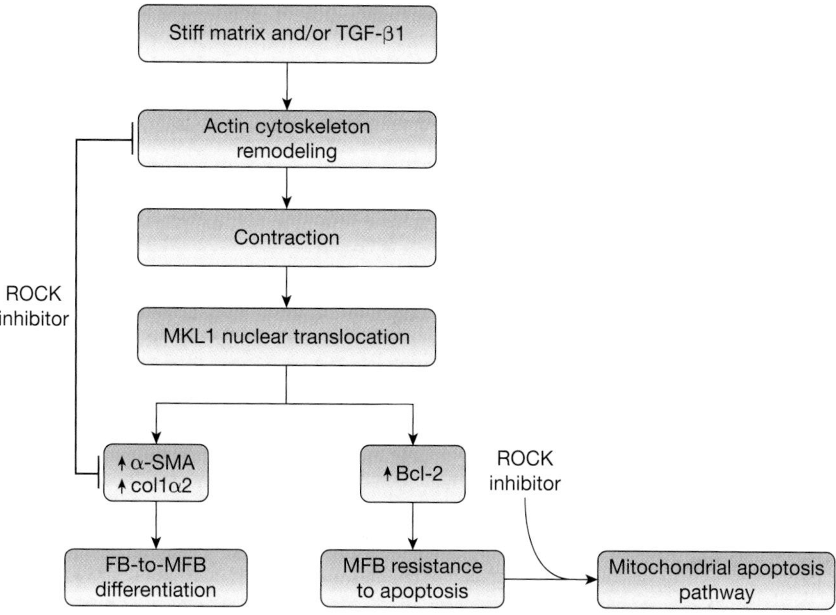

Figure 28-4 Mechanosensitive signaling in myofibroblasts as a target for antifibrotic therapy. In response to extracellular biomechanical and biochemical stimuli, such as matrix stiffness and active TGF-β1, lung fibroblasts undergo actin cytoskeleton remodeling and activation of the actomyosin contractile system, which result in MKL1 translocation from cytoplasm to the nucleus, where it activates fibrogenic genes that specify myofibroblast differentiation. Inhibition of ROCK blocks actin cytoskeletal reorganization, fibroblast acquisition of contractile activity, and MKL1 nuclear translocation, preventing fibroblast-to-myofibroblast differentiation. Inhibition of ROCK activity disrupts the actin cytoskeleton required for myofibroblast contractility. This deactivates constitutively activated MKL1 signaling in myofibroblasts, resulting in downregulation of the antiapoptotic protein, Bcl-2, and activation of the intrinsic apoptotic pathway.

the distal lung epithelial tubules and buds in the pseudoglandular stage of lung development. The absence of alveolar myofibroblasts is associated with deficient secondary septation and the failure of alveolar development.[158] Although alveolar myofibroblasts play an essential role in the morphogenesis of pulmonary alveolar septa, mechanisms involved in the regulation of alveolar myofibroblast survival and clearance in the process of alveologenesis are poorly understood and need further investigation.

PULMONARY FIBROSIS

Pulmonary fibrosis is characterized by excessive synthesis and deposition of ECM proteins in the lung parenchyma, resulting in deficient gas exchange. IPF is the most common and lethal diffuse fibrosing lung disease, with a mortality rate that exceeds that of many cancers. Currently, there is no FDA-approved pharmacological therapy for patients with IPF. The pathogenesis of IPF remains elusive. The current paradigm posits that repeated alveolar epithelial injury and persistent myofibroblast activation are central to the progression of IPF.[159] Regardless of the origins, myofibroblasts isolated from IPF lungs have increased migratory activity, ability to deposit ECM, and prolonged survival/resistance to apoptosis compared to their normal counterparts.[159] Abnormal myofibroblast survival is a key determinant of whether fibrosis will progress or resolve.[160] The survival of IPF myofibroblasts has been found to be regulated by multiple antiapoptotic signals.[48] These include enhanced responsiveness to growth factors and fibrotic cytokines; impaired cyclooxygenase-2 expression and consequential reduction in prostaglandin E2 production; decreased caveolin 1 (CAV1) and PTEN expression; and increased antiapoptotic protein expression as well as signals from the extracellular microenvironment. Myofibroblasts isolated from fibrotic lungs induce cytotoxic effects on epithelial cells. Coculturing of myofibroblasts with lung epithelial cells results in epithelial cell apoptosis by FAS–Fas ligand (FAS–FasL)-dependent and -independent mechanisms.[161,162] Epithelial cell apoptosis can cause further lung injury that augments lung fibrosis. Myofibroblasts produce cytokines and growth factors that signal to the epithelium, resulting in damage to the alveolar basement membrane that prevents reepithelialization.[163] Myofibroblast-produced chemokines promote the recruitment of immune cells and fibrocytes that actively participate in fibrotic progression.[164,165]

ASTHMA

Airway remodeling in patients with asthma encompasses the structural alterations that lead to persistent airflow limitation. Both smooth muscle cells and (myo)fibroblasts have been implicated in the pathogenesis of airway remodeling in asthmatic airways. In asthmatic patients, susceptibility to injury and aberrant repair responses result in fibroblast activation and myofibroblast differentiation, leading to subepithelial fibrosis.[166] Reduced airway remodeling in antileukotriene therapy is due, in part, to diminished myofibroblasts in asthmatic airways.[167] Viral infections are major triggers of acute asthma exacerbations.[168] The susceptibility to viral infections in asthmatic patients is not limited to epithelial cells. Rhinoviruses have been detected in subepithelial cells including fibroblasts, likely due to the disrupted and inflamed epithelium.[169] Fibroblasts from asthmatic patients have enhanced abilities for replication of rhinoviruses and subsequent production of IL-6 and IL-8, resulting in vigorous proinflammatory responses.[170] TGF-β augments rhinovirus replication in fibroblasts isolated from asthmatic patients.[171]

EMPHYSEMA

Emphysema is characterized by the progressive destruction of pulmonary alveoli. A vast majority of cases of pulmonary emphysema is associated with chronic lung injury induced by cigarette smoke. Chronic smoke exposure induces inflammation, protease/antiprotease imbalance, oxidative stress, and death of bronchiolar and alveolar epithelial and endothelial cells.[172] Cigarette smoke reduces lung fibroblast proliferation and migration, and induces fibroblast apoptosis.[173,174] In addition to the cytotoxic effects, cigarette smoke inhibits elastin synthesis and cross-linking in fetal lung fibroblasts.[175,176] Interactions between fibroblasts and alveolar epithelial cells are greatly reduced in the emphysematous lung,[177] suggesting that the repair and regeneration function of fibroblasts are impaired. Emphysema fibroblasts display features of myofibroblast differentiation and senescent phenotype characterized by enlarged morphology and cell-cycle arrest.[178,179]

NON-SMALL-CELL LUNG CANCER

Carcinoma-associated fibroblasts (CAFs) constitute a major portion of reactive tumor stroma. CAFs express α-SMA and high levels of collagens and ED-A FN, indicating that these cells are of myofibroblast characteristics.[180] CAFs are responsible for dense ECM deposition around tumors and thus have been considered as a defense mechanism for tumor growth. In established tumors,

CAFs synthesize cytokines/growth factors (e.g., TGF-β1) and ECM-degrading proteases (e.g., MMPs) that promote angiogenesis, recruitment of inflammatory cells, cancer cell proliferation, invasion, and metastasis.[3] CAF-associated prognostic factors have been identified in non–small-cell lung cancer (NSCLC). In adenocarcinomas, carbonic anhydrase IX expression has been found a better prognostic predictor in CAFs than in cancer cells.[181] Expression of podoplanin, a lymphatic endothelial cell marker, in CAFs is associated with shorter survival in patients with NSCLC.[182] In squamous cell carcinomas, MMP-2 expression in CAFs is found to be a significant unfavorable prognostic factor.[183] While expression of PDGF-B, PDGF-C, and PDGFR-α in cancer cells is associated with a negative prognosis, expression of PDGF-A, PDGF-B, PDGF-D, and PDGFR-α in CAFs is favorable prognostic indicators.[184] In addition, it has been found that stromal expression of PDGF-B, PDGF-D, and PDGFR-α is associated with less nodal metastasis.[185] Clinical prognostic values of TGF-β and FGF in NSCLC have been evaluated in the previous studies.[186–189] Due to the conflicting results, the prognostic roles of TGF-β and FGF2 in NSCLC remain uncertain.

TARGETING MYOFIBROBLASTS AND MATRIX REMODELING FOR LUNG DISEASE THERAPIES

Tissue remodeling in response to injury is a common pathological feature observed in many lung diseases including IPF. Dysregulation of fibroblast function and matrix metabolism are crucial to the aberrant injury repair in IPF lungs. Currently, there are no treatments that specifically target myofibroblast-associated pathologies in IPF.

Pirfenidone inhibits fibroblast proliferation and collagen synthesis and attenuates bleomycin-induced lung fibrosis in mice.[190,191] Two randomized, double-blinded placebo-controlled trials for pirfenidone in patients with IPF (CAPACITY) have been recently completed.[192] In one trial, pirfenidone showed a significant reduction in FVC decline at all study timepoints in patients with IPF compared to the placebo control. In the other trial, an apparent pirfenidone effect on predicted FVC change in IPF patients was observed until week 48. However, the difference between groups was not significant at week 72. These data suggest that pirfenidone has a favorable benefit risk profile and represents a potentially effective treatment for IPF.

PDGF is a potent mitogen and chemoattractant for fibroblasts and induces procollagen production by fibroblasts in vitro. Targeting PDGF receptor with imatinib mesylate, a tyrosine kinase inhibitor, has been shown to prevent bleomycin-induced mouse lung fibrosis.[193] However, a randomized, placebo-controlled trial showed that imatinib does not improve survival or lung function in patients with mild to moderate IPF.[194]

TGF-β1 is the most potent inducer of fibroblast ECM production characterized to date and promotes fibroblast to myofibroblast differentiation. Several types of pharmacotherapy to block TGF-β have been developed including antibodies, soluble receptors, intracellular signaling pathway inhibitors and agents that target the cell surface receptors for TGF-β (TGF-βRI/II).[195,196] A phase I clinical trial with TGF-β–neutralizing antibody (Genzyme) has begun in patients with IPF. Orally active TGF-βRI kinase inhibitors have been shown to attenuate bleomycin-induced mouse lung fibrosis.[197] Since TGF-β has important homeostatic functions in the regulation of immune response and tumor suppression, therapeutic strategies that directly blocks TGF-β may yield undesirable side effects. Alternatively, targeting latent TGF-β activation has become a more favorable approach for the antifibrotic therapy. Integrins are important mediators for in vivo activation of latent TGF-β.[198] $\alpha_v\beta_6$ integrin plays the primary role in regulating epithelial latent TGF-β1 activation.[199] Mouse studies have shown that inhibition of $\alpha_v\beta_6$ integrin blocks bleomycin- and radiation-induced lung fibrosis and this integrin is also abnormally regulated in human fibrotic diseases.[199] Stromedix, a humanized monoclonal antibody to integrin $\alpha_v\beta_6$, is currently in phase II clinical trial in IPF. $\alpha_v\beta_5$ integrin regulates mechanical tension–induced latent TGF-β1 activation in lung (myo)fibroblasts.[110] This integrin is coexpressed with α-SMA–positive myofibroblasts, but absent on hyperplastic epithelial cells in the fibroblastic foci in IPF.[200] The GPI-linked Thy-1 blocks mechanical tension–induced latent TGF-β1 activation, presumably by disruption of the binding of latent TGF-β1 with $\alpha_v\beta_5$ integrin.[135]

Inhibition of excess ECM generation, deposition, and stabilization, and increasing matrix degradation has become important targets for pharmacological therapy. Cytokines including CTGF, PDGF, ET-1, and IGF can induce fibroblast/myofibroblast activation and regulate matrix production. Inhibition of all of these cytokines can inhibit pulmonary fibrosis in a variety of in vivo models of fibrosis.[90,201–203] MMPs including MMP-1, 3, 7 among others have been implicated in the pathogenesis of pulmonary fibrosis,[204] although the exact role of the MMPs in the pathogenesis of pulmonary fibrosis remains not known. Matrix cross-linking enzymes are responsible for the regulation of ECM stabilization. Cross-linking makes matrix potentially more resistant to degradation and may favor fibrosis progression. TG2 induces the cross-linking of collagen and fibronectin, resulting in stabilization of the matrix.[205] TG2 is elevated in many forms of human and murine pulmonary fibrosis.[205] Inhibition of the extracellular cross-linking function of TG2 results in inhibition of ECM generation and cross-linking in the lung.[205] Irreversible inhibitors of TG2 have been developed and are available from several commercial sources. LOXL2, another matrix cross-linking protein, catalyzes the first step in the formation of cross-links in collagens and elastin.[206] LOXL2 cross-links fibrillar collagen, making it more resistant to homeostatic turnover. LOXL2 is induced by TGF-β and is upregulated in IPF.[207,208] Administration of a monoclonal anti-LOXL2 antibody (AB0023) in either a prophylactic manner or a therapeutic manner significantly attenuates bleomycin-induced fibrosis in mice.[208] Phase II clinical studies utilizing the LOXL2 inhibitor GS-6624 are currently carrying out for patients with primary sclerosing cholangitis, nonalcoholic steatohepatitis, and cirrhosis secondary to hepatitis C and/or HIV.

CONCLUSION AND PERSPECTIVES

The understanding of the physiology and pathophysiology of fibroblasts has greatly advanced in the past few decades. It has become increasingly clear that fibroblasts and myofibroblasts play important roles in human health and disease. Despite this, many fundamental questions remain to be answered. The origins of myofibroblasts remain to be clarified. It is not known whether myofibroblasts of various origins exhibit different characteristics and functions in the injury and repair process. Identification of specific markers for fibroblasts will allow their specific isolation and more precise characterization, both in vitro and in vivo. In addition, specific markers could facilitate genetic animal studies allowing the specific targeting of these cells. The independent and interactive roles of cytokines, ECM, and mechanical forces in the regulation of the structure and function of fibroblasts and myofibroblasts need to be characterized.

The identification of myofibroblasts as key cells and potential targets in fibrotic diseases such as IPF has led to the concept that targeting these cells may be a promising approach for disease therapy. Interesting approaches that target myofibroblasts and the ECM include termination of myofibroblast persistence by inducing their apoptosis or their reversion to nonfibrogenic cell phenotypes, interference with collagen cross-linking and ECM stiffening by controlling the activities of protein cross-linking enzymes (e.g., LOXL2 and TG2), and the use of miRNAs as potential therapeutic targets. We believe that these novel approaches will eventually lead to more effective treatments for patients with fibrotic lung diseases.

REFERENCES

1. Hektoen L. The fate of the giant cells in healing tuberculous tissue, as observed in a case of healing tuberculous meningitis. *J Exp Med.* 1898;3:21–52.
2. Tarin D, Croft CB. Ultrastructural features of wound healing in mouse skin. *J Anat.* 1969;105:189–190.
3. Kalluri R, Zeisberg M. Fibroblasts in cancer. *Nat Rev Cancer.* 2006;6:392–401.
4. Irwin CR, Picardo M, Ellis I, et al. Inter- and intra-site heterogeneity in the expression of fetal-like phenotypic characteristics by gingival fibroblasts: potential significance for wound healing. *J Cell Sci.* 1994;107(Pt 5):1333–1346.
5. Chang HY, Chi JT, Dudoit S, et al. Diversity, topographic differentiation, and positional memory in human fibroblasts. *Proc Natl Acad Sci U S A.* 2002;99:12877–12882.
6. Jelaska A, Strehlow D, Korn JH. Fibroblast heterogeneity in physiological conditions and fibrotic disease. *Springer Semin Immunopathol.* 1999;21:385–395.
7. Phan SH. Fibroblast phenotypes in pulmonary fibrosis. *Am J Respir Cell Mol Biol.* 2003;29:S87–S92.
8. Phipps RP, Borrello MA, Blieden TM. Fibroblast heterogeneity in the periodontium and other tissues. *J Periodontal Res.* 1997;32: 159–165.
9. Hagood JS, Prabhakaran P, Kumbla P, et al. Loss of fibroblast Thy-1 expression correlates with lung fibrogenesis. *Am J Pathol.* 2005;167:365–379.
10. Parsonage G, Filer AD, Haworth O, et al. A stromal address code defined by fibroblasts. *Trends Immunol.* 2005;26:150–156.
11. Simian M, Hirai Y, Navre M, Werb Z, Lochter A, Bissell MJ. The interplay of matrix metalloproteinases, morphogens and growth factors is necessary for branching of mammary epithelial cells. *Development.* 2001;128:3117–3131.
12. Ayad S, Boot-Handford R, Humphries M, Kadler K, Shuttleworth A. *The extracellular matrix factsbook.* 2nd ed. San Diego: Academic Press; 1998.
13. McAnulty RJ, Campa JS, Cambrey AD, Laurent GJ. The effect of transforming growth factor beta on rates of procollagen synthesis and degradation in vitro. *Biochim Biophys Acta.* 1991; 1091:231–235.
14. Barnes PJ, Drazen JM, Rennard SI, Thomson NC. *Asthma and COPD: basic mechanisms and clinical management.* Amsterdam, Boston: Academic Press; 2002.
15. Murphy G, Stanton H, Cowell S, et al. Mechanisms for pro matrix metalloproteinase activation. *APMIS.* 1999;107:38–44.
16. Xu J, Rodriguez D, Petitclerc E, et al. Proteolytic exposure of a cryptic site within collagen type IV is required for angiogenesis and tumor growth in vivo. *J Cell Biol.* 2001;154:1069–1079.
17. Schor SL, Ellis IR, Jones SJ, et al. Migration-stimulating factor: a genetically truncated onco-fetal fibronectin isoform expressed by carcinoma and tumor-associated stromal cells. *Cancer Res.* 2003;63:8827–8836.
18. Sternlicht MD, Werb Z. How matrix metalloproteinases regulate cell behavior. *Annu Rev Cell Dev Biol.* 2001;17:463–516.
19. Löffek S, Schilling O, Franzke CW. Series "matrix metalloproteinases in lung health and disease": Biological role of matrix metalloproteinases: a critical balance. *Eur Respir J.* 2011;38: 191–208.
20. Jordana M, Särnstrand B, Sime PJ, Ramis I. Immune-inflammatory functions of fibroblasts. *Eur Respir J.* 1994;7: 2212–2222.
21. Lukacs NW, Kunkel SL, Allen R, et al. Stimulus and cell-specific expression of C-X-C and C-C chemokines by pulmonary stromal cell populations. *Am J Physiol.* 1995;268:L856–L861.
22. Hällgren R, Bjermer L, Lundgren R, Venge P. The eosinophil component of the alveolitis in idiopathic pulmonary fibrosis. Signs of eosinophil activation in the lung are related to impaired lung function. *Am Rev Respir Dis.* 1989;139:373–377.
23. Vancheri C, Gauldie J, Bienenstock J, et al. Human lung fibroblast-derived granulocyte-macrophage colony stimulating factor (GM-CSF) mediates eosinophil survival in vitro. *Am J Respir Cell Mol Biol.* 1989;1:289–295.
24. Bombara MP, Webb DL, Conrad P, et al. Cell contact between T cells and synovial fibroblasts causes induction of adhesion molecules and cytokines. *J Leukoc Biol.* 1993;54:399–406.
25. Jose PJ, Griffiths-Johnson DA, Collins PD, et al. Eotaxin: a potent eosinophil chemoattractant cytokine detected in a guinea pig model of allergic airways inflammation. *J Exp Med.* 1994;179:881–887.
26. Sempowski GD, Beckmann MP, Derdak S, Phipps RP. Subsets of murine lung fibroblasts express membrane-bound and soluble IL-4 receptors. Role of IL-4 in enhancing fibroblast proliferation and collagen synthesis. *J Immunol.* 1994;152:3606–3614.
27. Shock A, Rabe KF, Dent G, et al. Eosinophils adhere to and stimulate replication of lung fibroblasts 'in vitro'. *Clin Exp Immunol.* 1991;86:185–190.
28. Birkland TP, Cheavens MD, Pincus SH. Human eosinophils stimulate DNA synthesis and matrix production in dermal fibroblasts. *Arch Dermatol Res.* 1994;286:312–318.
29. Adair-Kirk TL, Senior RM. Fragments of extracellular matrix as mediators of inflammation. *Int J Biochem Cell Biol.* 2008;40:1101–1110.
30. Bollyky PL, Falk BA, Wu RP, Buckner JH, Wight TN, Nepom GT. Intact extracellular matrix and the maintenance of immune tolerance: high molecular weight hyaluronan promotes persistence of induced CD4+CD25+ regulatory T cells. *J Leukoc Biol.* 2009;86:567–572.
31. Wiig H, Rubin K, Reed RK. New and active role of the interstitium in control of interstitial fluid pressure: potential therapeutic consequences. *Acta Anaesthesiol Scand.* 2003;47: 111–121.
32. Heuchel R, Berg A, Tallquist M, et al. Platelet-derived growth factor beta receptor regulates interstitial fluid homeostasis through phosphatidylinositol-3' kinase signaling. *Proc Natl Acad Sci U S A.* 1999;96:11410–11415.
33. Kristensen CA, Nozue M, Boucher Y, Jain RK. Reduction of interstitial fluid pressure after TNF-alpha treatment of three human melanoma xenografts. *Br J Cancer.* 1996;74:533–536.
34. Kaissling B, Le Hir M. The renal cortical interstitium: morphological and functional aspects. *Histochem Cell Biol.* 2008;130:247–262.
35. Majno G, Gabbiani G, Hirschel BJ, Ryan GB, Statkov PR. Contraction of granulation tissue in vitro: similarity to smooth muscle. *Science.* 1971;173:548–550.
36. Gabbiani G. The biology of the myofibroblast. *Kidney Int.* 1992;41:530–532.
37. Eyden BP. Brief review of the fibronexus and its significance for myofibroblastic differentiation and tumor diagnosis. *Ultrastruct Pathol.* 1993;17:611–622.
38. Powell DW, Mifflin RC, Valentich JD, Crowe SE, Saada JI, West AB. Myofibroblasts. II. Intestinal subepithelial myofibroblasts. *Am J Physiol.* 1999;277:C183–C201.

39. Tomasek JJ, Gabbiani G, Hinz B, Chaponnier C, Brown RA. Myofibroblasts and mechano-regulation of connective tissue remodelling. *Nat Rev Mol Cell Biol.* 2002;3:349–363.

40. Darby I, Skalli O, Gabbiani G. Alpha-smooth muscle actin is transiently expressed by myofibroblasts during experimental wound healing. *Lab Invest.* 1990;63:21–29.

41. Ballardini G, Fallani M, Biagini G, Bianchi FB, Pisi E. Desmin and actin in the identification of Ito cells and in monitoring their evolution to myofibroblasts in experimental liver fibrosis. *Virchows Arch B Cell Pathol Incl Mol Pathol.* 1988;56:45–49.

42. Pho M, Lee W, Watt DR, Laschinger C, Simmons CA, McCulloch CA. Cofilin is a marker of myofibroblast differentiation in cells from porcine aortic cardiac valves. *Am J Physiol Heart Circ Physiol.* 2008;294:H1767–H1778.

43. Kohnen G, Castellucci M, Hsi BL, Yeh CJ, Kaufmann P. The monoclonal antibody GB 42–a useful marker for the differentiation of myofibroblasts. *Cell Tissue Res.* 1995;281:231–242.

44. Rönty MJ, Leivonen SK, Hinz B, et al. Isoform-specific regulation of the actin-organizing protein palladin during TGF-beta1-induced myofibroblast differentiation. *J Invest Dermatol.* 2006;126:2387–2396.

45. Ruhs S, Nass N, Somoza V, et al. Maillard reaction products enriched food extract reduce the expression of myofibroblast phenotype markers. *Mol Nutr Food Res.* 2007;51:488–495.

46. Sun Y, Ramires FJ, Zhou G, Ganjam VK, Weber KT. Fibrous tissue and angiotensin II. *J Mol Cell Cardiol.* 1997;29:2001–2012.

47. Carracedo S, Lu N, Popova SN, Jonsson R, Eckes B, Gullberg D. The fibroblast integrin alpha11beta1 is induced in a mechanosensitive manner involving activin A and regulates myofibroblast differentiation. *J Biol Chem.* 2010;285:10434–10445.

48. Kis K, Liu X, Hagood JS. Myofibroblast differentiation and survival in fibrotic disease. *Expert Rev Mol Med.* 2011;13:e27.

49. Christian S, Winkler R, Helfrich I, et al. Endosialin (Tem1) is a marker of tumor-associated myofibroblasts and tumor vessel-associated mural cells. *Am J Pathol.* 2008;172:486–494.

50. Ehrlich HP, Allison GM, Leggett M. The myofibroblast, cadherin, alpha smooth muscle actin and the collagen effect. *Cell Biochem Funct.* 2006;24:63–70.

51. Cleutjens JP, Blankesteijn WM, Daemen MJ, Smits JF. The infarcted myocardium: simply dead tissue, or a lively target for therapeutic interventions. *Cardiovasc Res.* 1999;44:232–241.

52. Hinz B. Formation and function of the myofibroblast during tissue repair. *J Invest Dermatol.* 2007;127:526–537.

53. Yoshimura H, Michishita M, Ohkusu-Tsukada K, Takahashi K. Appearance and distribution of stromal myofibroblasts and tenascin-C in feline mammary tumors. *Histol Histopathol.* 2011;26:297–305.

54. Serini G, Bochaton-Piallat ML, Ropraz P, et al. The fibronectin domain ED-A is crucial for myofibroblastic phenotype induction by transforming growth factor-beta1. *J Cell Biol.* 1998;142: 873–881.

55. Lenga Y, Koh A, Perera AS, McCulloch CA, Sodek J, Zohar R. Osteopontin expression is required for myofibroblast differentiation. *Circ Res.* 2008;102:319–327.

56. Vi L, Feng L, Zhu RD, et al. Periostin differentially induces proliferation, contraction and apoptosis of primary Dupuytren's disease and adjacent palmar fascia cells. *Exp Cell Res.* 2009;315: 3574–3586.

57. Grinnell F. Fibroblasts, myofibroblasts, and wound contraction. *J Cell Biol.* 1994;124:401–404.

58. Gabbiani G. The myofibroblast in wound healing and fibrocontractive diseases. *J Pathol.* 2003;200:500–503.

59. Hinz B, Phan SH, Thannickal VJ, et al. Recent developments in myofibroblast biology: paradigms for connective tissue remodeling. *Am J Pathol.* 2012;180:1340–1355.

60. Gharzi A, Reynolds AJ, Jahoda CA. Plasticity of hair follicle dermal cells in wound healing and induction. *Exp Dermatol.* 2003;12:126–136.

61. Hoogduijn MJ, Gorjup E, Genever PG. Comparative characterization of hair follicle dermal stem cells and bone marrow mesenchymal stem cells. *Stem Cells Dev.* 2006;15:49–60.

62. van den Bogaerdt AJ, van der Veen VC, van Zuijlen PP, et al. Collagen cross-linking by adipose-derived mesenchymal stromal cells and scar-derived mesenchymal cells: Are mesenchymal stromal cells involved in scar formation? *Wound Repair Regen.* 2009;17:548–558.

63. Zhang K, Rekhter MD, Gordon D, Phan SH. Myofibroblasts and their role in lung collagen gene expression during pulmonary fibrosis. A combined immunohistochemical and in situ hybridization study. *Am J Pathol.* 1994;145:114–125.

64. Lama VN, Smith L, Badri L, et al. Evidence for tissue-resident mesenchymal stem cells in human adult lung from studies of transplanted allografts. *J Clin Invest.* 2007;117:989–996.

65. da Silva Meirelles L, Chagastelles PC, Nardi NB. Mesenchymal stem cells reside in virtually all post-natal organs and tissues. *J Cell Sci.* 2006;119:2204–2213.

66. Allt G, Lawrenson JG. Pericytes: cell biology and pathology. *Cells Tissues Organs.* 2001;169:1–11.

67. Kida Y, Duffield JS. Pivotal role of pericytes in kidney fibrosis. *Clin Exp Pharmacol Physiol.* 2011;38:467–473.

68. Herman IM, D'Amore PA. Microvascular pericytes contain muscle and nonmuscle actins. *J Cell Biol.* 1985;101:43–52.

69. Rajkumar VS, Howell K, Csiszar K, Denton CP, Black CM, Abraham DJ. Shared expression of phenotypic markers in systemic sclerosis indicates a convergence of pericytes and fibroblasts to a myofibroblast lineage in fibrosis. *Arthritis Res Ther.* 2005;7: R1113–R1123.

70. Humphreys BD, Lin SL, Kobayashi A, et al. Fate tracing reveals the pericyte and not epithelial origin of myofibroblasts in kidney fibrosis. *Am J Pathol.* 2010;176:85–97.

71. Dulauroy S, Di Carlo SE, Langa F, Eberl G, Peduto L. Lineage tracing and genetic ablation of ADAM12(+) perivascular cells identify a major source of profibrotic cells during acute tissue injury. *Nat Med.* 2012;18:1262–1270.

72. Kisseleva T, Cong M, Paik Y, et al. Myofibroblasts revert to an inactive phenotype during regression of liver fibrosis. *Proc Natl Acad Sci U S A.* 2012;109:9448–9453.

73. Caplan AI. Mesenchymal stem cells. *J Orthop Res.* 1991;9: 641–650.

74. Simmons PJ, Przepiorka D, Thomas ED, Torok-Storb B. Host origin of marrow stromal cells following allogeneic bone marrow transplantation. *Nature.* 1987;328:429–432.

75. Friedenstein AJ, Chailakhjan RK, Lalykina KS. The development of fibroblast colonies in monolayer cultures of guinea-pig bone marrow and spleen cells. *Cell Tissue Kinet.* 1970;3:393–403.

76. Hashimoto N, Jin H, Liu T, et al. Bone marrow-derived progenitor cells in pulmonary fibrosis. *J Clin Invest.* 2004;113:243–252.

77. Binai N, O'Reilly S, Griffiths B, van Laar JM, Hügle T. Differentiation potential of CD14+ monocytes into myofibroblasts in patients with systemic sclerosis. *PLoS One.* 2012;7:e33508.

78. Bucala R, Spiegel LA, Chesney J, Hogan M, Cerami A. Circulating fibrocytes define a new leukocyte subpopulation that mediates tissue repair. *Mol Med.* 1994;1:71–81.

79. Metz CN. Fibrocytes: a unique cell population implicated in wound healing. *Cell Mol Life Sci.* 2003;60:1342–1350.

80. Roufosse C, Bou-Gharios G, Prodromidi E, et al. Bone marrow-derived cells do not contribute significantly to collagen I synthesis in a murine model of renal fibrosis. *J Am Soc Nephrol.* 2006;17:775–782.

81. Kage H, Borok Z. EMT and interstitial lung disease: a mysterious relationship. *Curr Opin Pulm Med.* 2012;18:517–523.

82. Savagner P. The epithelial-mesenchymal transition (EMT) phenomenon. *Ann Oncol.* 2010;21(Suppl 7):vii89–vii92.

83. Quaggin SE, Kapus A. Scar wars: mapping the fate of epithelial-mesenchymal-myofibroblast transition. *Kidney Int.* 2011;80: 41–50.

84. Castor CW, Wilson SM, Heiss PR, Seidman JC. Activation of lung connective tissue cells in vitro. *Am Rev Respir Dis.* 1979;120: 101–106.

85. Strutz F, Zeisberg M, Hemmerlein B, et al. Basic fibroblast growth factor expression is increased in human renal fibrogenesis and may mediate autocrine fibroblast proliferation. *Kidney Int.* 2000;57:1521–1538.

86. Alvarez RJ, Sun MJ, Haverty TP, Iozzo RV, Myers JC, Neilson EG. Biosynthetic and proliferative characteristics of tubulointerstitial fibroblasts probed with paracrine cytokines. *Kidney Int.* 1992;41:14–23.

87. Alpers CE, Seifert RA, Hudkins KL, Johnson RJ, Bowen-Pope DF. PDGF-receptor localizes to mesangial, parietal epithelial, and interstitial cells in human and primate kidneys. *Kidney Int.* 1993;43:286–294.

88. Zeisberg M, Strutz F, Müller GA. Role of fibroblast activation in inducing interstitial fibrosis. *J Nephrol.* 2000;13(Suppl 3): S111–S120.

89. Giacomini MM, Travis MA, Kudo M, Sheppard D. Epithelial cells utilize cortical actin/myosin to activate latent TGF-β through integrin α(v)β(6)-dependent physical force. *Exp Cell Res.* 2012;318:716–722.

90. Lo Re S, Lecocq M, Uwambayinema F, et al. Platelet-derived growth factor-producing CD4+ Foxp3+ regulatory T lymphocytes promote lung fibrosis. *Am J Respir Crit Care Med.* 2011;184: 1270–1281.

91. Barron L, Wynn TA. Fibrosis is regulated by Th2 and Th17 responses and by dynamic interactions between fibroblasts and macrophages. *Am J Physiol Gastrointest Liver Physiol.* 2011;300: G723–G728.

92. Chambers RC. Procoagulant signalling mechanisms in lung inflammation and fibrosis: novel opportunities for pharmacological intervention? *Br J Pharmacol.* 2008;153(Suppl 1):S367–S378.

93. Blanc-Brude OP, Archer F, Leoni P, et al. Factor Xa stimulates fibroblast procollagen production, proliferation, and calcium signaling via PAR1 activation. *Exp Cell Res.* 2005;304:16–27.

94. Chambers RC, Leoni P, Blanc-Brude OP, Wembridge DE, Laurent GJ. Thrombin is a potent inducer of connective tissue growth factor production via proteolytic activation of protease-activated receptor-1. *J Biol Chem.* 2000;275:35584–35591.

95. Olman MA, Mackman N, Gladson CL, Moser KM, Loskutoff DJ. Changes in procoagulant and fibrinolytic gene expression during bleomycin-induced lung injury in the mouse. *J Clin Invest.* 1995;96:1621–1630.

96. Tager AM, LaCamera P, Shea BS, et al. The lysophosphatidic acid receptor LPA1 links pulmonary fibrosis to lung injury by mediating fibroblast recruitment and vascular leak. *Nat Med.* 2008;14:45–54.

97. Fonseca C, Abraham D, Renzoni EA. Endothelin in pulmonary fibrosis. *Am J Respir Cell Mol Biol.* 2011;44:1–10.

98. Thannickal VJ. Mechanisms of pulmonary fibrosis: role of activated myofibroblasts and NADPH oxidase. *Fibrogenesis Tissue Repair.* 2012;5(Suppl 1):S23.

99. Hecker L, Vittal R, Jones T, et al. NADPH oxidase-4 mediates myofibroblast activation and fibrogenic responses to lung injury. *Nat Med.* 2009;15:1077–1081.

100. Cucoranu I, Clempus R, Dikalova A, et al. NAD(P)H oxidase 4 mediates transforming growth factor-beta1-induced differentiation of cardiac fibroblasts into myofibroblasts. *Circ Res.* 2005;97:900–907.

101. Bondi CD, Manickam N, Lee DY, et al. NAD(P)H oxidase mediates TGF-beta1-induced activation of kidney myofibroblasts. *J Am Soc Nephrol.* 2010;21:93–102.

102. Clempus RE, Sorescu D, Dikalova AE, et al. Nox4 is required for maintenance of the differentiated vascular smooth muscle cell phenotype. *Arterioscler Thromb Vasc Biol.* 2007; 27:42–48.

103. Hu T, Ramachandrarao SP, Siva S, et al. Reactive oxygen species production via NADPH oxidase mediates TGF-beta-induced cytoskeletal alterations in endothelial cells. *Am J Physiol Renal Physiol.* 2005;289:F816–F825.

104. Boudreault F, Tschumperlin DJ. Stretch-induced mitogen-activated protein kinase activation in lung fibroblasts is independent of receptor tyrosine kinases. *Am J Respir Cell Mol Biol.* 2010;43:64–73.

105. Paterno J, Vial IN, Wong VW, et al. Akt-mediated mechanotransduction in murine fibroblasts during hypertrophic scar formation. *Wound Repair Regen.* 2011;19:49–58.

106. Maeda T, Sakabe T, Sunaga A, et al. Conversion of mechanical force into TGF-β-mediated biochemical signals. *Curr Biol.* 2011;21:933–941.

107. Lu F, Ogawa R, Nguyen DT, et al. Microdeformation of three-dimensional cultured fibroblasts induces gene expression and morphological changes. *Ann Plast Surg.* 2011;66:296–300.

108. Hinz B, Gabbiani G. Mechanisms of force generation and transmission by myofibroblasts. *Curr Opin Biotechnol.* 2003;14:538–546.

109. Huang X, Yang N, Fiore VF, et al. Matrix stiffness-induced myofibroblast differentiation is mediated by intrinsic mechanotransduction. *Am J Respir Cell Mol Biol.* 2012;47:340–348.

110. Wipff PJ, Rifkin DB, Meister JJ, Hinz B. Myofibroblast contraction activates latent TGF-beta1 from the extracellular matrix. *J Cell Biol.* 2007;179:1311–1323.

111. Ng CP, Hinz B, Swartz MA. Interstitial fluid flow induces myofibroblast differentiation and collagen alignment in vitro. *J Cell Sci.* 2005;118:4731–4739.

112. Ng CP, Swartz MA. Mechanisms of interstitial flow-induced remodeling of fibroblast-collagen cultures. *Ann Biomed Eng.* 2006;34:446–454.

113. Balestrini JL, Chaudhry S, Sarrazy V, Koehler A, Hinz B. The mechanical memory of lung myofibroblasts. *Integr Biol (Camb).* 2012;4:410–421.

114. Hu B, Gharaee-Kermani M, Wu Z, Phan SH. Epigenetic regulation of myofibroblast differentiation by DNA methylation. *Am J Pathol.* 2010;177:21–28.

115. Mann J, Chu DC, Maxwell A, et al. MeCP2 controls an epigenetic pathway that promotes myofibroblast transdifferentiation and fibrosis. *Gastroenterology*. 2010;138:705–714, 714.e1–714.e4.

116. Glenisson W, Castronovo V, Waltregny D. Histone deacetylase 4 is required for TGFbeta1-induced myofibroblastic differentiation. *Biochim Biophys Acta*. 2007;1773:1572–1582.

117. Waltregny D, Glénisson W, Tran SL, et al. Histone deacetylase HDAC8 associates with smooth muscle alpha-actin and is essential for smooth muscle cell contractility. *FASEB J*. 2005;19:966–968.

118. Liu G, Friggeri A, Yang Y, et al. miR-21 mediates fibrogenic activation of pulmonary fibroblasts and lung fibrosis. *J Exp Med*. 2010;207:1589–1597.

119. Pandit KV, Corcoran D, Yousef H, et al. Inhibition and role of let-7 d in idiopathic pulmonary fibrosis. *Am J Respir Crit Care Med*. 2010;182:220–229.

120. Salazar KD, Lankford SM, Brody AR. Mesenchymal stem cells produce Wnt isoforms and TGF-beta1 that mediate proliferation and procollagen expression by lung fibroblasts. *Am J Physiol Lung Cell Mol Physiol*. 2009;297:L1002–L1011.

121. Königshoff M, Balsara N, Pfaff EM, et al. Functional Wnt signaling is increased in idiopathic pulmonary fibrosis. *PLoS One*. 2008;3:e2142.

122. Henderson WR Jr, Chi EY, Ye X, et al. Inhibition of Wnt/beta-catenin/CREB binding protein (CBP) signaling reverses pulmonary fibrosis. *Proc Natl Acad Sci U S A*. 2010;107:14309–14314.

123. Dugina V, Fontao L, Chaponnier C, Vasiliev J, Gabbiani G. Focal adhesion features during myofibroblastic differentiation are controlled by intracellular and extracellular factors. *J Cell Sci*. 2001;114:3285–3296.

124. Clayton A, Evans RA, Pettit E, Hallett M, Williams JD, Steadman R. Cellular activation through the ligation of intercellular adhesion molecule-1. *J Cell Sci*. 1998;111(Pt 4):443–453.

125. Qi W, Chen X, Poronnik P, Pollock CA. The renal cortical fibroblast in renal tubulointerstitial fibrosis. *Int J Biochem Cell Biol*. 2006;38:1–5.

126. Sanger JW, Sanger JM, Jockusch BM. Differences in the stress fibers between fibroblasts and epithelial cells. *J Cell Biol*. 1983;96:961–969.

127. Desmouliere A, Chaponnier C, Gabbiani G. Tissue repair, contraction, and the myofibroblast. *Wound Repair Regen*. 2005;13:7–12.

128. Hinz B, Celetta G, Tomasek JJ, Gabbiani G, Chaponnier C. Alpha-smooth muscle actin expression upregulates fibroblast contractile activity. *Mol Biol Cell*. 2001;12:2730–2741.

129. Zhou Y, Huang X, Hecker L, et al. Inhibition of mechanosensitive signaling in myofibroblasts ameliorates experimental pulmonary fibrosis. *J Clin Invest*. 2013;123:1096–1108.

130. Chen WL, Simmons CA. Lessons from (patho)physiological tissue stiffness and their implications for drug screening, drug delivery and regenerative medicine. *Adv Drug Deliv Rev*. 2011;63:269–276.

131. Liu F, Mih JD, Shea BS, et al. Feedback amplification of fibrosis through matrix stiffening and COX-2 suppression. *J Cell Biol*. 2010;190:693–706.

132. Booth AJ, Hadley R, Cornett AM, et al. Acellular normal and fibrotic human lung matrices as a culture system for in vitro investigation. *Am J Respir Crit Care Med*. 2012;186:866–876.

133. Chiquet M. Regulation of extracellular matrix gene expression by mechanical stress. *Matrix Biol*. 1999;18:417–426.

134. Ingber D. Integrins as mechanochemical transducers. *Curr Opin Cell Biol*. 1991;3:841–848.

135. Zhou Y, Hagood JS, Lu B, Merryman WD, Murphy-Ullrich JE. Thy-1-integrin alphav beta5 interactions inhibit lung fibroblast contraction-induced latent transforming growth factor-beta1 activation and myofibroblast differentiation. *J Biol Chem*. 2010;285:22382–22393.

136. Miralles F, Posern G, Zaromytidou AI, Treisman R. Actin dynamics control SRF activity by regulation of its coactivator MAL. *Cell*. 2003;113:329–342.

137. Small EM, Thatcher JE, Sutherland LB, et al. Myocardin-related transcription factor-a controls myofibroblast activation and fibrosis in response to myocardial infarction. *Circ Res*. 2010;107:294–304.

138. Burridge K, Chrzanowska-Wodnicka M. Focal adhesions, contractility, and signaling. *Annu Rev Cell Dev Biol*. 1996;12:463–518.

139. Hu H, Sachs F. Stretch-activated ion channels in the heart. *J Mol Cell Cardiol*. 1997;29:1511–1523.

140. Yoneda A, Couchman JR. Regulation of cytoskeletal organization by syndecan transmembrane proteoglycans. *Matrix Biol*. 2003;22:25–33.

141. Gigant-Huselstein C, Hubert P, Dumas D, et al. Expression of adhesion molecules and collagen on rat chondrocyte seeded into alginate and hyaluronate based 3D biosystems. Influence of mechanical stresses. *Biorheology*. 2004;41:423–431.

142. Ruwhof C, van der Laarse A. Mechanical stress-induced cardiac hypertrophy: mechanisms and signal transduction pathways. *Cardiovasc Res*. 2000;47:23–37.

143. Maier S, Lutz R, Gelman L, et al. Tenascin-C induction by cyclic strain requires integrin-linked kinase. *Biochim Biophys Acta*. 2008;1783:1150–1162.

144. Chiquet M, Sarasa-Renedo A, Tunç-Civelek V. Induction of tenascin-C by cyclic tensile strain versus growth factors: distinct contributions by Rho/ROCK and MAPK signaling pathways. *Biochim Biophys Acta*. 2004;1693:193–204.

145. Hogan BL, Yingling JM. Epithelial/mesenchymal interactions and branching morphogenesis of the lung. *Curr Opin Genet Dev*. 1998;8:481–486.

146. Fries KM, Blieden T, Looney RJ, et al. Evidence of fibroblast heterogeneity and the role of fibroblast subpopulations in fibrosis. *Clin Immunol Immunopathol*. 1994;72:283–292.

147. Pilcher BK, Wang M, Qin XJ, Parks WC, Senior RM, Welgus HG. Role of matrix metalloproteinases and their inhibition in cutaneous wound healing and allergic contact hypersensitivity. *Ann N Y Acad Sci*. 1999;878:12–24.

148. Powell DW, Mifflin RC, Valentich JD, Crowe SE, Saada JI, West AB. Myofibroblasts. I. Paracrine cells important in health and disease. *Am J Physiol*. 1999;277:C1–C9.

149. Desmoulière A, Redard M, Darby I, Gabbiani G. Apoptosis mediates the decrease in cellularity during the transition between granulation tissue and scar. *Am J Pathol*. 1995;146:56–66.

150. Rudolph R. Inhibition of myofibroblasts by skin grafts. *Plast Reconstr Surg*. 1979;63:473–480.

151. Darby IA, Bisucci T, Pittet B, Garbin S, Gabbiani G, Desmoulière A. Skin flap-induced regression of granulation tissue correlates with reduced growth factor and increased metalloproteinase expression. *J Pathol*. 2002;197:117–127.

152. Frisch SM, Screaton RA. Anoikis mechanisms. *Curr Opin Cell Biol*. 2001;13:555–562.

153. Saile B, Knittel T, Matthes N, Schott P, Ramadori G. CD95/CD95 L-mediated apoptosis of the hepatic stellate cell. A mechanism terminating uncontrolled hepatic stellate cell proliferation during hepatic tissue repair. *Am J Pathol.* 1997;151:1265–1272.

154. Zhang H. Molecular signaling and genetic pathways of senescence: its role in tumorigenesis and aging. *J Cell Physiol.* 2007;210:567–574.

155. Krizhanovsky V, Yon M, Dickins RA, et al. Senescence of activated stellate cells limits liver fibrosis. *Cell.* 2008;134:657–667.

156. Jun JI, Lau LF. The matricellular protein CCN1 induces fibroblast senescence and restricts fibrosis in cutaneous wound healing. *Nat Cell Biol.* 2010;12:676–685.

157. Yamada M, Kurihara H, Kinoshita K, Sakai T. Temporal expression of alpha-smooth muscle actin and drebrin in septal interstitial cells during alveolar maturation. *J Histochem Cytochem.* 2005;53:735–744.

158. Boström H, Willetts K, Pekny M, et al. PDGF-A signaling is a critical event in lung alveolar myofibroblast development and alveogenesis. *Cell.* 1996;85:863–873.

159. Ding Q, Luckhardt T, Hecker L, et al. New insights into the pathogenesis and treatment of idiopathic pulmonary fibrosis. *Drugs.* 2011;71:981–1001.

160. Thannickal VJ, Horowitz JC. Evolving concepts of apoptosis in idiopathic pulmonary fibrosis. *Proc Am Thorac Soc.* 2006;3:350–356.

161. Golan-Gerstl R, Wallach-Dayan SB, Amir G, Breuer R. Epithelial cell apoptosis by fas ligand-positive myofibroblasts in lung fibrosis. *Am J Respir Cell Mol Biol.* 2007;36:270–275.

162. Aoshiba K, Yasui S, Tamaoki J, Nagai A. The Fas/Fas-ligand system is not required for bleomycin-induced pulmonary fibrosis in mice. *Am J Respir Crit Care Med.* 2000;162:695–700.

163. Yagi Y, Andoh A, Inatomi O, Tsujikawa T, Fujiyama Y. Inflammatory responses induced by interleukin-17 family members in human colonic subepithelial myofibroblasts. *J Gastroenterol.* 2007;42:746–753.

164. Abe R, Donnelly SC, Peng T, Bucala R, Metz CN. Peripheral blood fibrocytes: differentiation pathway and migration to wound sites. *J Immunol.* 2001;166:7556–7562.

165. Huaux F, Liu T, McGarry B, Ullenbruch M, Phan SH. Dual roles of IL-4 in lung injury and fibrosis. *J Immunol.* 2003;170:2083–2092.

166. Holgate ST. The airway epithelium is central to the pathogenesis of asthma. *Allergol Int.* 2008;57:1–10.

167. Kelly MM, Chakir J, Vethanayagam D, et al. Montelukast treatment attenuates the increase in myofibroblasts following low-dose allergen challenge. *Chest.* 2006;130:741–753.

168. Miller EK. New human rhinovirus species and their significance in asthma exacerbation and airway remodeling. *Immunol Allergy Clin North Am.* 2010;30:541–552, vii.

169. Ghildyal R, Dagher H, Donninger H, et al. Rhinovirus infects primary human airway fibroblasts and induces a neutrophil chemokine and a permeability factor. *J Med Virol.* 2005;75:608–615.

170. Bedke N, Haitchi HM, Xatzipsalti M, et al. Contribution of bronchial fibroblasts to the antiviral response in asthma. *J Immunol.* 2009;182:3660–3667.

171. Thomas BJ, Lindsay M, Dagher H, et al. Transforming growth factor-beta enhances rhinovirus infection by diminishing early innate responses. *Am J Respir Cell Mol Biol.* 2009;41:339–347.

172. Tuder RM, Petrache I. Pathogenesis of chronic obstructive pulmonary disease. *J Clin Invest.* 2012;122:2749–2755.

173. Nakamura Y, Romberger DJ, Tate L, et al. Cigarette smoke inhibits lung fibroblast proliferation and chemotaxis. *Am J Respir Crit Care Med.* 1995;151:1497–1503.

174. Ishii T, Matsuse T, Igarashi H, Masuda M, Teramoto S, Ouchi Y. Tobacco smoke reduces viability in human lung fibroblasts: protective effect of glutathione S-transferase P1. *Am J Physiol Lung Cell Mol Physiol.* 2001;280:L1189–L1195.

175. Laurent P, Janoff A, Kagan HM. Cigarette smoke blocks cross-linking of elastin in vitro. *Am Rev Respir Dis.* 1983;127:189–192.

176. Gao S, Chen K, Zhao Y, et al. Transcriptional and posttranscriptional inhibition of lysyl oxidase expression by cigarette smoke condensate in cultured rat fetal lung fibroblasts. *Toxicol Sci.* 2005;87:197–203.

177. Sirianni FE, Milaninezhad A, Chu FS, Walker DC. Alteration of fibroblast architecture and loss of Basal lamina apertures in human emphysematous lung. *Am J Respir Crit Care Med.* 2006;173:632–638.

178. Müller KC, Welker L, Paasch K, et al. Lung fibroblasts from patients with emphysema show markers of senescence in vitro. *Respir Res.* 2006;7:32.

179. Milara J, Serrano A, Peiró T, et al. Aclidinium inhibits cigarette smoke-induced lung fibroblast to myofibroblast transition. *Eur Respir J.* 2013;41:1264–1274.

180. De Wever O, Demetter P, Mareel M, Bracke M. Stromal myofibroblasts are drivers of invasive cancer growth. *Int J Cancer.* 2008;123:2229–2238.

181. Nakao M, Ishii G, Nagai K, et al. Prognostic significance of carbonic anhydrase IX expression by cancer-associated fibroblasts in lung adenocarcinoma. *Cancer.* 2009;115:2732–2743.

182. Kawase A, Ishii G, Nagai K, et al. Podoplanin expression by cancer associated fibroblasts predicts poor prognosis of lung adenocarcinoma. *Int J Cancer.* 2008;123:1053–1059.

183. Ishikawa S, Takenaka K, Yanagihara K, et al. Matrix metalloproteinase-2 status in stromal fibroblasts, not in tumor cells, is a significant prognostic factor in non-small-cell lung cancer. *Clin Cancer Res.* 2004;10:6579–6585.

184. Donnem T, Al-Saad S, Al-Shibli K, Andersen S, Busund LT, Bremnes RM. Prognostic impact of platelet-derived growth factors in non-small cell lung cancer tumor and stromal cells. *J Thorac Oncol.* 2008;3:963–970.

185. Donnem T, Al-Saad S, Al-Shibli K, Busund LT, Bremnes RM. Co-expression of PDGF-B and VEGFR-3 strongly correlates with lymph node metastasis and poor survival in non-small-cell lung cancer. *Ann Oncol.* 2010;21:223–231.

186. Hasegawa Y, Takanashi S, Kanehira Y, Tsushima T, Imai T, Okumura K. Transforming growth factor-beta1 level correlates with angiogenesis, tumor progression, and prognosis in patients with nonsmall cell lung carcinoma. *Cancer.* 2001;91:964–971.

187. Guddo F, Fontanini G, Reina C, Vignola AM, Angeletti A, Bonsignore G. The expression of basic fibroblast growth factor (bFGF) in tumor-associated stromal cells and vessels is inversely correlated with non-small cell lung cancer progression. *Hum Pathol.* 1999;30:788–794.

188. Iwasaki A, Kuwahara M, Yoshinaga Y, Shirakusa T. Basic fibroblast growth factor (bFGF) and vascular endothelial growth factor (VEGF) levels, as prognostic indicators in NSCLC. *Eur J Cardiothorac Surg.* 2004;25:443–448.

189. Boldrini L, Calcinai A, Samaritani E, et al. Tumour necrosis factor-alpha and transforming growth factor-beta are significantly associated with better prognosis in non-small cell lung carcinoma: putative relation with BCL-2-mediated neovascularization. *Br J Cancer*. 2000;83:480–486.

190. Hewitson TD, Kelynack KJ, Tait MG, et al. Pirfenidone reduces in vitro rat renal fibroblast activation and mitogenesis. *J Nephrol*. 2001;14:453–460.

191. Iyer SN, Wild JS, Schiedt MJ, Hyde DM, Margolin SB, Giri SN. Dietary intake of pirfenidone ameliorates bleomycin-induced lung fibrosis in hamsters. *J Lab Clin Med*. 1995;125: 779–785.

192. Noble PW, Albera C, Bradford WZ, et al. Pirfenidone in patients with idiopathic pulmonary fibrosis (CAPACITY): two randomised trials. *Lancet*. 2011;377:1760–1769.

193. Aono Y, Nishioka Y, Inayama M, et al. Imatinib as a novel antifibrotic agent in bleomycin-induced pulmonary fibrosis in mice. *Am J Respir Crit Care Med*. 2005;171:1279–1285.

194. Daniels CE, Lasky JA, Limper AH, et al. Imatinib treatment for idiopathic pulmonary fibrosis: randomized placebo-controlled trial results. *Am J Respir Crit Care Med*. 2010;181: 604–610.

195. Flechsig P, Dadrich M, Bickelhaupt S, et al. LY2109761 attenuates radiation-induced pulmonary murine fibrosis via reversal of TGF-β and BMP-associated proinflammatory and proangiogenic signals. *Clin Cancer Res*. 2012;18:3616–3627.

196. Sime PJ, O'Reilly KM. Fibrosis of the lung and other tissues: new concepts in pathogenesis and treatment. *Clin Immunol*. 2001;99:308–319.

197. Higashiyama H, Yoshimoto D, Kaise T, et al. Inhibition of activin receptor-like kinase 5 attenuates bleomycin-induced pulmonary fibrosis. *Exp Mol Pathol*. 2007;83:39–46.

198. Sheppard D. Integrin-mediated activation of latent transforming growth factor beta. *Cancer Metastasis Rev*. 2005;24:395–402.

199. Munger JS, Huang X, Kawakatsu H, et al. The integrin alpha v beta 6 binds and activates latent TGF beta 1: a mechanism for regulating pulmonary inflammation and fibrosis. *Cell*. 1999;96:319–328.

200. Scotton CJ, Krupiczojc MA, Königshoff M, et al. Increased local expression of coagulation factor X contributes to the fibrotic response in human and murine lung injury. *J Clin Invest*. 2009;119:2550–2563.

201. Bonniaud P, Margetts PJ, Kolb M, et al. Adenoviral gene transfer of connective tissue growth factor in the lung induces transient fibrosis. *Am J Respir Crit Care Med*. 2003;168:770–778.

202. Pilewski JM, Liu L, Henry AC, Knauer AV, Feghali-Bostwick CA. Insulin-like growth factor binding proteins 3 and 5 are overexpressed in idiopathic pulmonary fibrosis and contribute to extracellular matrix deposition. *Am J Pathol*. 2005;166:399–407.

203. Barlo NP, van Moorsel CH, Kazemier KM, van den Bosch JM, Grutters JC. Potential role of endothelin-1 in pulmonary fibrosis: from the bench to the clinic. *Am J Respir Cell Mol Biol*. 2010;42:633.

204. Pardo A, Selman M, Kaminski N. Approaching the degradome in idiopathic pulmonary fibrosis. *Int J Biochem Cell Biol*. 2008;40: 1141–1155.

205. Olsen KC, Sapinoro RE, Kottmann RM, et al. Transglutaminase 2 and its role in pulmonary fibrosis. *Am J Respir Crit Care Med*. 2011;184:699–707.

206. Kagan HM, Li W. Lysyl oxidase: properties, specificity, and biological roles inside and outside of the cell. *J Cell Biochem*. 2003;88: 660–672.

207. Koslowski R, Seidel D, Kuhlisch E, Knoch KP. Evidence for the involvement of TGF-beta and PDGF in the regulation of prolyl 4-hydroxylase and lysyloxidase in cultured rat lung fibroblasts. *Exp Toxicol Pathol*. 2003;55:257–264.

208. Barry-Hamilton V, Spangler R, Marshall D, et al. Allosteric inhibition of lysyl oxidase-like-2 impedes the development of a pathologic microenvironment. *Nat Med*. 2010;16:1009–1017.

PART 3

Symptoms and Signs of Respiratory Disease

SECTION 6 Clinical Approach to the Patient

SECTION 7 Diagnostic Procedures

CHAPTER 29

Approach to the Patient with Respiratory Symptoms

Michael A. Grippi
Robert M. Senior
Jeffrey P. Callen

The most common respiratory complaints prompting medical evaluation are shortness of breath and cough. Less frequent are hemoptysis and thoracic pain. As in any medical assessment, a detailed history and thorough physical examination are of paramount importance. Use of plain chest radiography for routine screening, once popular in the hope of uncovering silent disease amenable to therapy, is not routinely employed, as it has not been proven to decrease mortality or to be cost effective. Chest radiography is now usually reserved for patients who have clinical manifestations of thoracic disease; serial chest radiographs often provide invaluable clues regarding the underlying problem. More sophisticated imaging techniques, including computed tomography (CT),[1,2] along with tests of lung function, help complete the clinical picture.

HISTORY

Although seasoned clinicians may be adept at quickly spotting telltale diagnostic clues, a comprehensive medical history is central to patient evaluation. The history should include a detailed inventory of exposure to air-borne substances that may result in lung injury. One of the most common offenders is cigarette smoke. An attempt should be made to quantify the exposure.

Often, the workplace is the site where toxic air is inhaled. An almost forgotten exposure to a toxic inhalant 20 years ago may explain certain types of pulmonary or pleural diseases. Symptoms that appear to improve during weekends or other periods away from work may be a clue to an occupational exposure that causes a respiratory ailment. A newly installed home humidifier or an air conditioning system that incorporates stagnant pools of water can point the way to resolving a mysterious illness. Brief residence in an area where either cryptococcosis (southwestern United States) or histoplasmosis (southern and midwestern United States) is endemic may help clarify the nature of an illness that mimics tuberculosis. A recent visit to a South or Central American country may bring into focus a more remote possibility (e.g., South American blastomycosis) (Fig. 29-1).

The history should include a thorough evaluation of prior and current medical problems. Rheumatologic disorders, such as systemic sclerosis (scleroderma), may be associated with interstitial lung disease, aspiration pneumonia due to esophageal involvement, or pulmonary vascular disease. Certain malignancies often metastasize to the lung (e.g., breast or colon carcinoma), or predispose to development of venous thromboembolism (e.g., pancreatic carcinoma). Infection with the human immunodeficiency virus (HIV) should not be overlooked, since pulmonary complications are often

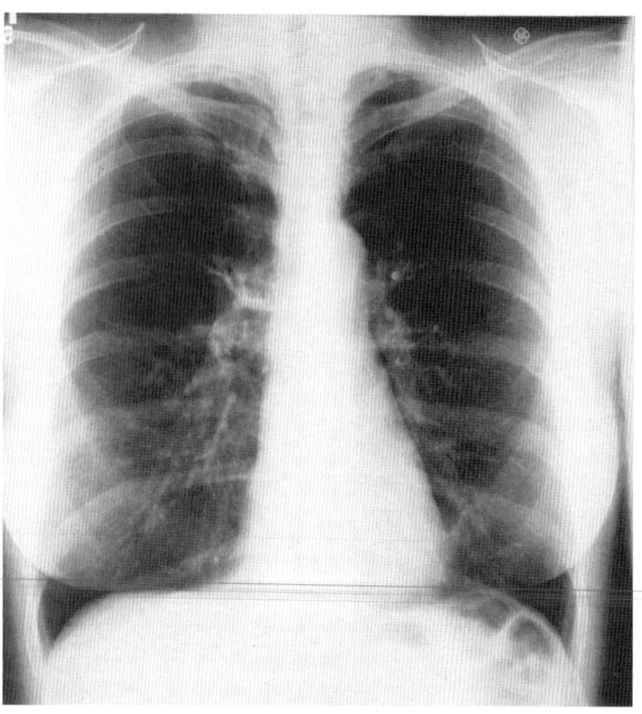

A

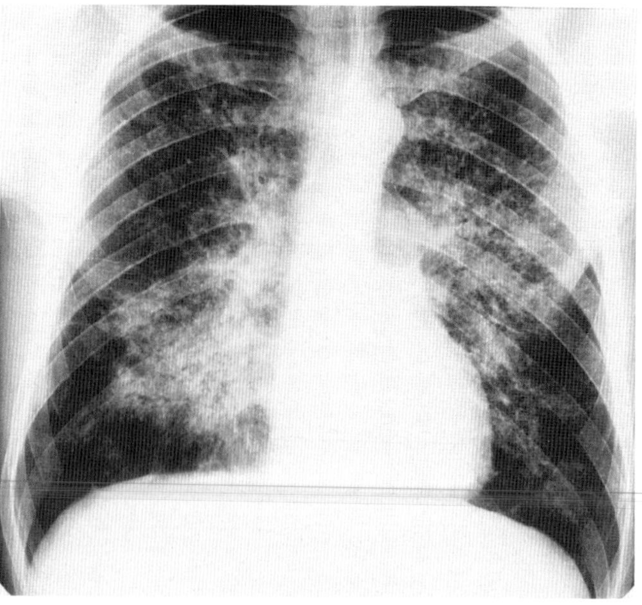

B

Figure 29-1 Exposure in an endemic area. **A.** Clear lung fields. **B.** South American blastomycosis. *(Used with permission of Dr. Nelson Porto.)*

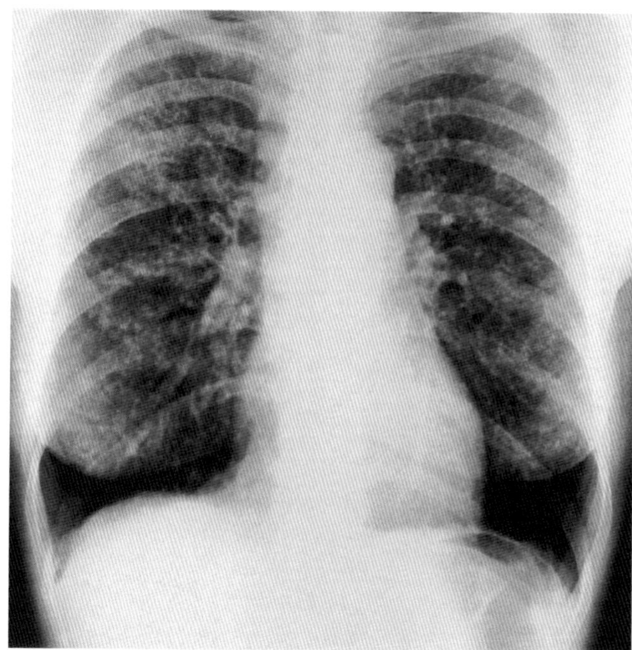

Figure 29-2 Nitrofurantoin hypersensitivity pneumonitis. The ingestion of nitrofurantoin was accompanied by the appearance of patchy interstitial and alveolar changes throughout both lungs.

the initial presentation of acquired immunodeficiency syndrome (AIDS). Other causes of immunodeficiency, such as hematologic malignancy, or prior administration of chemotherapeutic agents, should heighten suspicion of infection as the cause of respiratory symptoms, as well as potential pulmonary drug toxicity.

Indeed, many pharmacologic agents, including chemotherapeutic and nonchemotherapeutic agents, have a propensity for inflicting lung damage (see Chapters 65 and 66). Classic examples include bleomycin, nitrofurantoin, and methotrexate (Fig. 29-2). Beta blockers, administered as part of a cardiac regimen, may evoke bronchoconstriction. Even a common medication, such as aspirin, may, on rare occasion, cause a severe pulmonary disorder (e.g., pulmonary edema).

Finally, the family history is an essential ingredient of the medical inventory. This history can uncover a heritable disease of the lungs (e.g., cystic fibrosis [CF], α_1-antitrypsin deficiency, alveolar microlithiasis, and hereditary telangiectasia).

PHYSICAL EXAMINATION

Before the widespread use of chest radiography, physical examination, along with the history, played a pivotal role in the diagnosis of pulmonary disease. The advent of chest radiography and chest CT imaging has de-emphasized the value of the physical examination. Nonetheless, the physical examination remains a valuable diagnostic measure in the appraisal of chest disease.[3,4]

■ GENERAL ASPECTS

Important clues are often available before examination of the chest. For example, neglected pyorrheal teeth raise the prospect of necrotizing aspiration pneumonia. A lacerated tongue suggests that a convulsive episode may have led to aspiration (Fig. 29-3). Pursing of the lips during expiration ("pursed-lip breathing") may be seen in patients with chronic obstructive pulmonary disease (COPD). Subtle changes in consciousness or coordination may signal that metastasis has occurred to the brain from a primary carcinoma of the lung. In the patient with COPD, a clouded sensorium or a disturbed personality can signify acute elevation in arterial P_{CO_2}.

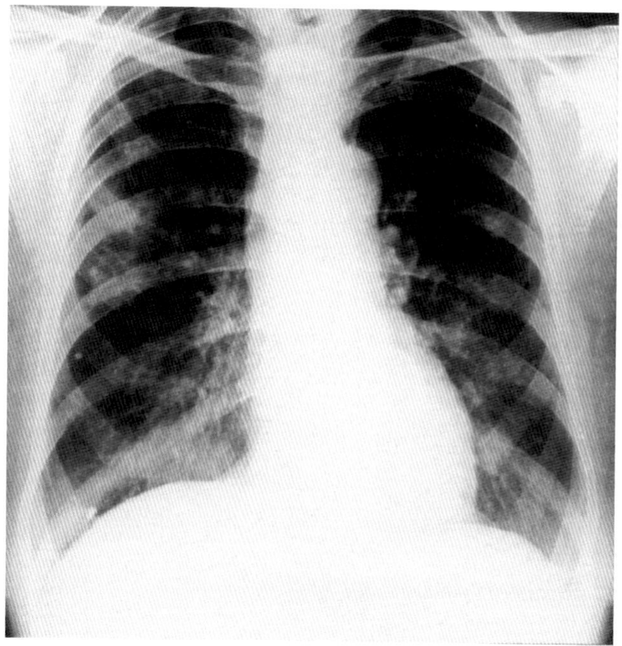

A

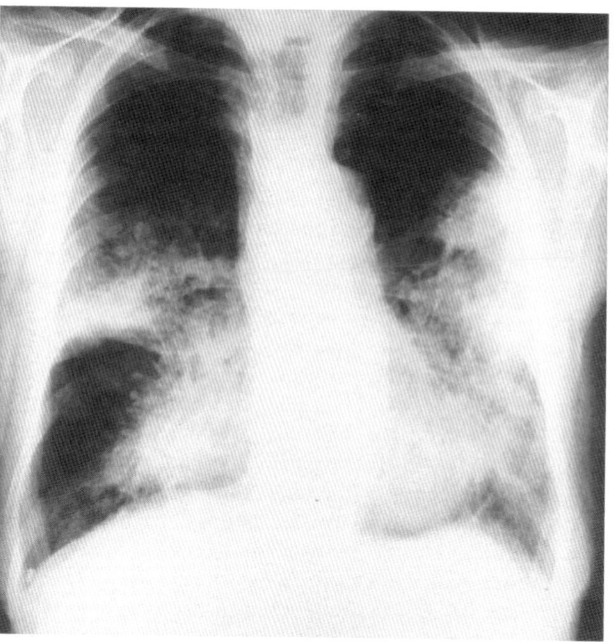

B

Figure 29-3 Chronic aspiration pneumonia. **A.** Chronic aspiration pneumonia in a 72-year-old man hospitalized for repair of hernia. Patchy infiltrates bilaterally. No pulmonary symptoms. Initiating cause was achalasia of esophagus. **B.** Eighteen months later. Persistent cough and breathlessness.

Inspection of the skin often provides clues to diseases of the chest; a more detailed discussion of notable cutaneous manifestations in respiratory disorders is provided later in this chapter. Evidence to support the diagnosis of pulmonary sarcoidosis may be found in the eyes and skin. Petechiae, purpura, necrosis, and/or ulceration of the skin may reflect a systemic vasculitis. The skin lesions of neurofibromatosis type 1 (von Recklinghausen disease) may signify that a solitary pulmonary nodule in the paraspinal region may be a neurofibroma. A minute skin abscess may turn out to be the source of multiple lung abscesses. Distinctive scars over the antecubital veins of a drug addict can help to clarify the etiology of old lesions

TABLE 29-1 Clinical Disorders Commonly Associated with Clubbing of Digits

Pulmonary and thoracic
Primary lung cancer
Bronchiectasis
Cystic fibrosis
Lung abscess
Pulmonary fibrosis
Pulmonary arteriovenous malformations
Empyema
Mesothelioma
Neurogenic diaphragmatic tumors
Cardiac
Congenital
Subacute bacterial endocarditis
Gastrointestinal and hepatic
Hepatic cirrhosis
Chronic ulcerative colitis
Regional enteritis (Crohn's disease)

in the lungs, as well as of a newly discovered lung abscess. Erythema nodosum (EN) is frequently due to sarcoidosis, but may also occur in patients with tuberculosis, histoplasmosis, or coccidioidomycosis. Skin papules in Birt–Hogg–Dube syndrome (see Pulmonary-Cutaneous Syndromes, below) may antedate the pulmonary manifestations of cystic lung lesions and pneumothorax by decades.[5]

A variety of endocrine syndromes may accompany carcinoma of the lung. An altered mental status may be due to hyponatremia caused by the syndrome of inappropriate antidiuretic hormone (SIADH). Clubbing of the digits may accompany various clinical disorders, including idiopathic pulmonary fibrosis, bronchiectasis, and certain carcinomas of the lung (Table 29-1).[6] A puffy face, neck, and eyelids, coupled with dilated veins of the neck, shoulder, thorax, and upper arm (i.e., superior vena cava syndrome) may constitute the first clinical evidence of obstruction of the superior vena cava by a neoplasm of the lung. Although the causes of superior vena cava syndrome are many and diverse, at least 80% are attributable to a primary carcinoma of the lung (Fig. 29-4). In the patient in whom a neoplasm has evoked acute signs and symptoms of increased systemic venous pressure that progresses rapidly (e.g., to laryngeal edema), early diagnosis and prompt treatment of the neoplasm can be lifesaving. The presence of Horner syndrome – unilateral ptosis, miosis, and anhidrosis – in a patient with a carcinoma of the lung suggests a pulmonary sulcus tumor with involvement of the ipsilateral sympathetic pathway within the thorax (Fig. 29-5).

INSPECTION OF THE CHEST

Observation of the chest from the foot of the bed can be informative: a visible lag in expansion of one side of the thorax localizes a pleural effusion, pulmonary infection, or paralyzed diaphragm. The respiratory pattern may be informative: patients with severe airflow obstruction often take slow, deep breaths, whereas rapid and shallow breaths are often seen with restrictive processes, such as interstitial lung disease or kyphoscoliosis. Inspection of the chest and abdomen in the supine position may reveal paradoxical inward movement of the abdomen, indicative of respiratory muscle weakness.[7]

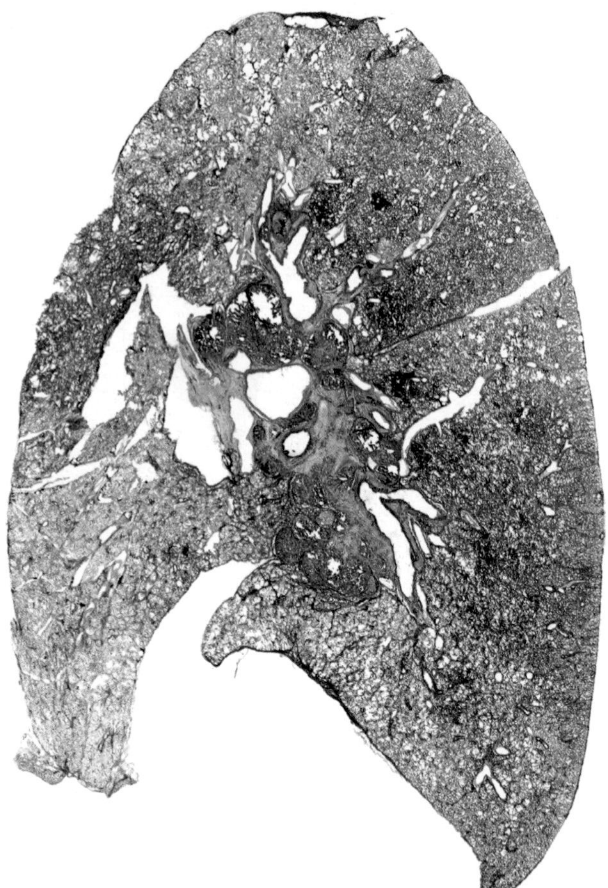

A

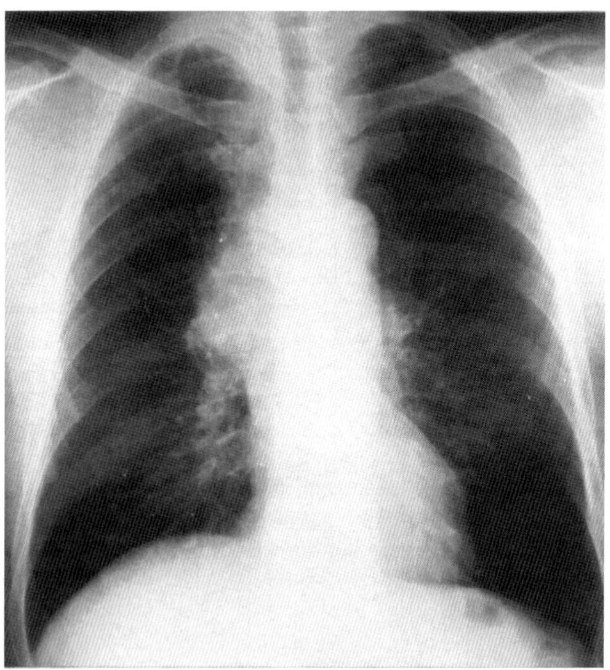

B

Figure 29-4 Local invasiveness of carcinoma of the lung. **A.** Sagittal section of the lung illustrating a carcinoma *(blue)* of the lung in the vicinity of the hilus. **B.** Chest radiograph showing right hilar mass.

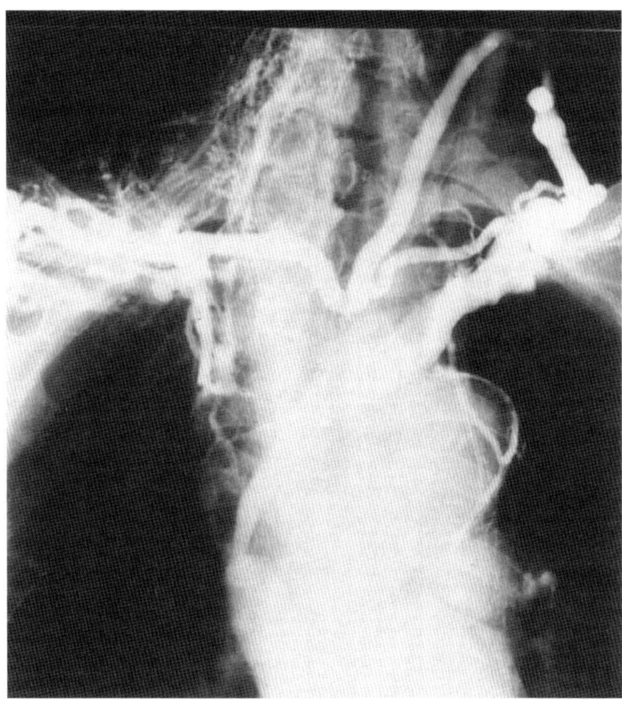

C

Figure 29-4 *(Continued)* **C.** Angiogram showing obstruction and extensive collateral circulation.

■ PALPATION OF THE CHEST

Over the years, the role of palpation in examination of the chest has been considerably devalued. Nonetheless, palpation may provide helpful diagnostic clues as well as confirmatory evidence for other physical signs. For example, the position of the trachea determined by palpation in the suprasternal notch may be helpful in detecting a lateral displacement of the upper mediastinum. Displacement of the apical impulse and of cardiac dullness may be useful indices in detecting shift of the lower mediastinum.

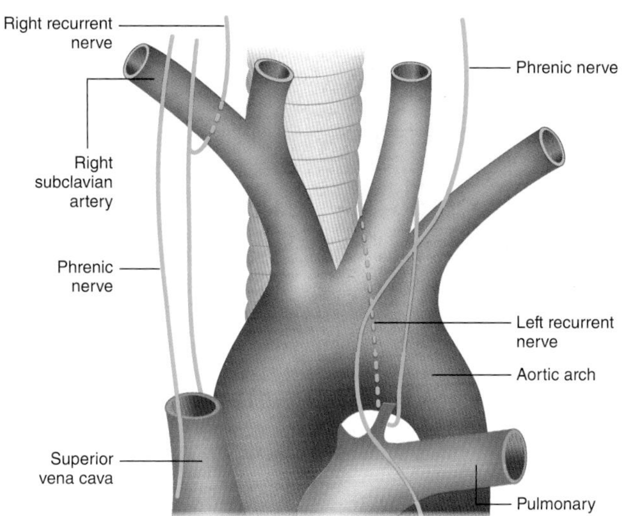

Figure 29-5 Courses of the recurrent laryngeal nerves. Invasion or compression of a nerve by a carcinoma of the lung causes paralysis of the vocal cord.

Tenderness over a rib may reflect a fracture, metastasis, or underlying pleuritis. Enlargement of the right ventricle can be readily detected by palpation in the subxiphoid region. *Hoover sign* may be useful in disclosing a unilateral lag in motion of one side of the chest due to pleuritis or a pleural effusion. The sign is elicited by comparing the displacement from the midline during a patient's deep inspiration of the examiner's hands, each placed lightly over one hemithorax, with thumbs touching beneath the xiphoid at the start of the breath.

An abnormal mass or fullness palpated in the supraclavicular space may be a clue to a neoplasm or an involved lymph node and suggests a convenient location to obtain a biopsy for diagnosis.

Consolidation of the lung, which causes increased transmission of sound, can be detected as fremitus (i.e., as a palpable vibration) over the affected area while the patient repeatedly vocalizes the traditional "one, two, three" as the examiner moves his or her palms systematically over the two hemithoraces. Conversely, impairment of sound transmission, as by a pleural effusion, diminishes vocal fremitus. In some instances, a pleural friction rub is palpable.

■ PERCUSSION OF THE CHEST

Percussion as part of the physical examination follows Auenbrugger sounding of beer barrels to determine their fluid levels. The response to percussion is impaired whenever something other than air-filled lung lies directly beneath the chest wall. Common causes of dullness to percussion are consolidation or atelectasis of the lung, fluid in the pleural space, pleural thickening, and a large mass at the surface of the lung. Widespread hyperresonance may be elicited in emphysema, and circumscribed hyperresonance over a pneumothorax or large bulla.

■ AUSCULTATION OF LUNGS

Ever since the time of Laennec, physicians have applied a stethoscope to the chest in search of sounds of disease.[8] Attention is focused on the intensity and quality of the sounds, as well as on the presence of abnormal (often called "adventitious") lung sounds.[9] Other devices have been used to assess sounds generated by breathing.[10,11] Web sites providing access to audio files demonstrating normal and adventitious breath sounds are available (e.g., www.easyauscultation.com/lung-sounds.aspx).[12]

Changes in the Intensity and Duration of Lung Sounds

The generation of lung sounds requires an ability to move air through patent airways. A global decrease in the intensity of breath sounds over the thorax or a hemithorax may be due to a variety of abnormalities: impaired movement of air due to airways disease (e.g., in emphysema), paralysis of a diaphragm, or complete obstruction of a bronchus. A decrease in audible breath sounds may also occur when the transmission of sounds to the chest wall is impaired (e.g., by a pleural effusion, pleural thickening, or a pneumothorax). A bulla gives rise to a more circumscribed diminution in breath sounds. In a patient with COPD, regional variations in breath sounds correspond to the distribution of ventilation. With adequate pressure of the diaphragm of the stethoscope, it is possible to auscultate the lungs as effectively through thin clothing as over bare skin; of course this approach hinders inspection and percussion.[13]

An abnormal increase in intensity of breath sounds is accompanied by a change in their character (the sounds become either harsh or bronchial). The abnormal sounds are heard over consolidated, atelectatic, or compressed lung as long as the airway to the affected portion of the lung remains patent. Consolidated lung is presumed to act as an acoustic conducting medium that, unlike normal lung, does not attenuate transmission of tracheal sounds to the periphery.

Noting the duration of the inspiratory and expiratory phases of breathing may be useful. Inspiration is normally audible for a longer period, with little, if any, expiratory noise. A prolongation of expiration, often longer than inspiration, is found with obstructed airways.

Changes in the Transmission of Lung Sounds

Changes in voice sounds are often easier to appreciate than changes in breath sounds. Large pleural effusions, pneumothorax, and bronchial occlusion produce distant or inaudible breath sounds. Transmission of voice sounds is enhanced by consolidation, infarction, atelectasis, or compressions of lung tissue. Accompanying the increased transmission is a change in the character of the voice sounds that causes them to be higher pitched and less muffled than normal *(bronchophony)*. When bronchophony is extreme, spoken words assume a nasal or bleating quality *(egophony)* and the sound "ee" is heard through the stethoscope as "ay."[14] Egophony is most common when consolidated lung and pleural fluid coexist; sometimes it is heard over an uncomplicated lobar pneumonia or pulmonary infarction. Transmission of whispered voice sounds with abnormal clarity *(whispered pectoriloquy)* has the same significance as bronchophony.

Changes in the Quality of Lung Sounds

Normal breath sounds have a smooth, soft quality and are described as *vesicular*. Abnormal, or adventitious, lung sounds have traditionally been resistant to meaningful clinical classification. However, a rational, clinically useful set of definitions based on acoustic analysis of tape recordings and the nomenclature introduced by Forgacs is commonly employed (Table 29-2). Using this approach, lung sounds are categorized as continuous (*wheezes, rhonchi,* or *stridor*) or discontinuous *(crackles)*.

Wheezes, rhonchi, and stridor are musical adventitious sounds. Wheezes originate in airways narrowed by spasm, thickening of the mucosa, or luminal obstruction. Although wheezes are more apt to occur during forced expiration (which further narrows airways), they may occur during both inspiration and expiration in asthma. Wheezes presumably originate through a combination of limitation to airflow and vibrations in the walls of the airways. Rhonchi are due to the presence of liquid or mucus in the airways; the quality and location may be readily changed by asking the patient to cough, thus moving the secretions. Stridor is predominantly inspiratory and best heard over the neck. Common causes of stridor are a foreign body in the upper intrathoracic airway or esophagus, an acquired lesion of the airway (e.g., carcinoma in adults), or a congenital lesion in children.

TABLE 29-2 Classification of Common Lung Sounds

Acoustic Characteristics	American Thoracic Society Nomenclature	Common Synonyms
Discontinuous, interrupted explosive sounds; loud, low in pitch	Coarse crackle	Coarse rale
Discontinuous, interrupted explosive sounds; less loud than above and of shorter duration; higher in pitch than coarse crackles or rales	Fine crackle	Fine rale, crepitation
Continuous sounds longer than 250 ms, high-pitched; dominant frequency of 400 Hz or more, hissing sound	Wheeze	Sibilant rhonchus
Continuous sounds longer than 250 ms, low-pitched; dominant frequency about 200 Hz or less, snoring sound	Rhonchus	Sonorous rhonchus

Source: Adapted with permission from Loudon R, Murphy RLH. Lung sounds. Am Rev Respir Dis. 1984;130(4):663–673.

Crackles are generally attributed to a rapid succession of explosive openings of small airways that closed prematurely during the previous expiration.[15] Crackles have been subdivided according to their timing during inspiration (early or late) and by differences in their quality ("wet" or "dry"); at times they have been termed "*rales*." Noting differences in timing has been advocated as a way of distinguishing between possible causes (e.g., "dry" crackles in the fibrosis of interstitial lung disease vs. "wet" crackles in pulmonary edema).[16] Unfortunately, wide variation in the interpretation of these sounds generally renders such attempts at classification of little value and often a cause of confusion. Crackles may accompany alterations in the elastic recoil of airways (emphysema), the presence of secretions (bronchitis or pneumonia), inflammation or fibrosis (interstitial lung disease), or fluid (pulmonary edema). Crackles may also be due to atelectasis, as noted in bedridden patients, and may clear with sequential deep breaths.

Pleural Rub

A pleural friction rub is a coarse, grating, or leathery sound that is usually heard late in inspiration and early in expiration; most often a pleural friction rub is audible low in the axilla or over the lung base posteriorly. The rub sounds close to the ear and usually is not altered by coughing.

DYSPNEA

Dyspnea is the medical term for breathlessness or shortness of breath.[17] The American Thoracic Society has published a comprehensive discussion of the topic.[18] For the patient, dyspnea involves an experience of discomfort in breathing. It is alarming to most and may arouse great concern about a potential dire cause, making it one of the most frequent complaints prompting patients to seek medical evaluation.

In the extensive medical, physiologic, and psychological literature, dyspnea is used variously to designate a variety of sensations, ranging from awareness of breathing on the one hand to respiratory distress on the other. The wide range of meanings is understandable on several counts: (1) dyspnea is a subjective complaint without consistency in objective signs such as tachypnea; (2) few physicians have experienced the respiratory discomfort associated with chest disease, so that most interpretations of the complaint represent extrapolations from normal breathlessness (e.g., after strenuous exercise); (3) most experimental observations relating to dyspnea are based on the study of normal subjects or animals under artificial circumstances; and (4) most physicians apply the term loosely, based on their experience with the predominant patient population that they serve (e.g., patients with COPD or asthma). Despite this variability, in clinical medicine, the complaint of dyspnea almost invariably implies respiratory discomfort.

Because of its subjective nature, the sensation of dyspnea is an amalgam of two components. The first is the sensory input to the cerebral cortex, which consists of information from specialized receptors, predominantly mechanoreceptors, at various sites in the respiratory apparatus (predominantly the upper airways) and face (Fig. 29-6). The different sites of stimulation may contribute to disparities in the sensation. Furthermore, no specific area in the central nervous system (CNS) has been identified as the sensory locus for dyspnea. The input – from airways, lungs (via the vagus nerves), respiratory muscles, chest wall, and chemoreceptors – is processed at consecutive levels of the nervous system (i.e., spinal cord and supraspinal regions en route to the sensorimotor cortex). Additional sensory input, triggered by inadequate oxygen delivery or utilization, is poorly understood. The second component is the perception

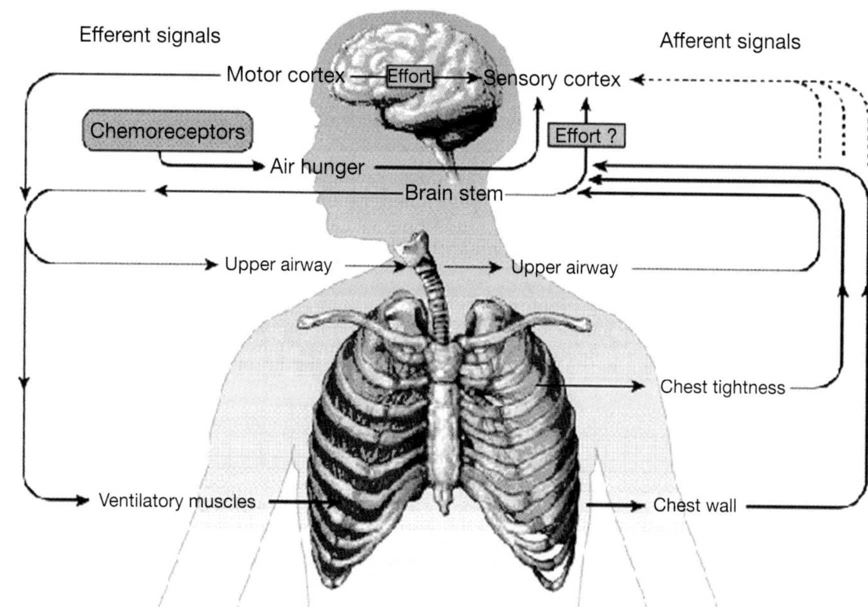

Figure 29-6 Pathways to the sensation of breathlessness. Respiratory effort is believed to originate as a signal transmitted from the motor cortex simultaneously to the sensory cortex and to the motor command to ventilatory muscles. The brain stem may also contribute to the sense of effort. The perception of air hunger is believed to arise, in part, from increased respiratory activity within the brain stem, whereas the sensation of chest tightness probably results from stimulation of vagal irritant receptors. Although afferent information from airway, lung, and chest-wall receptors most likely passes through the brain stem before reaching the sensory cortex, the *dashed lines* indicate uncertainty about whether some afferents bypass the brain stem and project directly to the sensory cortex. *(Reproduced with permission from Manning HL, Schwartzstein RM. Pathophysiology of dyspnea. N Engl J Med. 1995;333(23):1547–1553.)*

of the sensation, which rests heavily on the interpretation of information arriving at the sensorimotor cortex. The interpretation depends greatly on the psychological makeup of the person.

A variety of influences may modify the psychological component of dyspnea. During "Kussmaul breathing" (see below), "air hunger" may seem obvious to the observer, even though the patient does not feel short of breath. In contrast, patients with congestive heart failure or COPD frequently volunteer the complaint of "air hunger." Blunting of the sensorium, as by narcotics or by acute hypercapnia, can eliminate the sensation of breathlessness, even though the abnormal breathing pattern remains. Anxiety may heighten the sense of breathlessness. Indeed, anxiety may be responsible for the clinical syndrome of psychogenic dyspnea, in which the patient experiences "breathing discomfort" that eludes explanation on the basis of a somatic cause. Ill-defined sensations may accompany a full-blown hyperventilation syndrome, consisting of lightheadedness, tingling of the hands and feet, tachycardia, inversion of T waves on the electrocardiogram, and even syncope. Breathing discomfort at rest that decreases with activity is often seen when anxiety or other psychological issues are the cause and is a distinctly unusual pattern for dyspnea due to a cardiopulmonary abnormality.

The quality of dyspnea can vary greatly. In normal persons, as well as in those with chest disease, dyspnea may simply signify the transition from an effortless process that is ordinarily conducted at a subconscious level to the awareness that muscular effort is being expended in breathing.[19] The healthy athlete completing a sprint experiences breathlessness that can be exhilarating, rather than uncomfortable. The asthmatic often interprets breathlessness in terms of "tightness in the chest." The patient with COPD often complains of less severe breathlessness than would be expected from the degree of airway obstruction, possibly reflecting adaptation, either to the chronic obstructive airway disease or to CO_2 retention.

Patients may use different terms to describe breathing discomfort due to various causes.[20–25] In some instances these descriptors may be useful in establishing a differential diagnosis and in assessing the response to therapy.[26] Patients with asthma or myocardial ischemia often refer to "chest tightness."[27] Patients with pulmonary edema may suffer a sensation of "air hunger" or "suffocation."[28] Patients with COPD and hyperinflation of the chest often note an inability to take a deep, satisfying breath. Individuals who are deconditioned may complain of "heavy breathing." Unfortunately, no descriptor has sufficient sensitivity or specificity to be used alone in establishing the cause of a patient's dyspnea. Ethnic and gender differences in the descriptors and perceptions related to dyspnea have been reported.[29,30]

CLINICAL PRESENTATIONS

Dyspnea may be acute, chronic, or paroxysmal (Table 29-3).

TABLE 29-3 Common Causes of Acute and Chronic Dyspnea[a]

Acute
Pulmonary edema
Asthma
Injury to chest wall and intrathoracic structures
Spontaneous pneumothorax
Pulmonary embolism
Pneumonia
Adult respiratory distress syndrome
Pleural effusion
Pulmonary hemorrhage
Foreign body aspiration
Vocal cord dysfunction
Chronic, progressive
Chronic obstructive pulmonary disease
Left ventricular failure
Diffuse interstitial fibrosis
Asthma
Pleural effusions
Pulmonary thromboembolic disease
Pulmonary vascular disease
Psychogenic dyspnea
Anemia, severe
Postintubation tracheal stenosis
Hypersensitivity disorders

[a]*Many chronic processes (e.g., left ventricular failure, asthma, and COPD) may have acute exacerbations.*

Acute Dyspnea

The usual causes of acute dyspnea in children differ from those in adults. In children, upper airway infection (e.g., epiglottis, laryngitis, or acute laryngotracheobronchitis) is a common cause. In adults, the causes of acute dyspnea are much more varied (Table 29-3). Among the most common are acute left ventricular failure, pulmonary thromboembolism, pneumonia, and spontaneous pneumothorax. Less common, but not unusual, is massive collapse of one lung due to inability to clear the airways of thick, tenacious secretions (e.g., in chronic bronchitis or asthma) or the first attack of asthma.

Chronic Dyspnea

Chronic dyspnea is almost invariably progressive. As a rule, this type of dyspnea begins with breathlessness on exertion—which, in time, progresses to dyspnea at rest. Pulmonologists encounter dyspnea in patients who have COPD; cardiologists more often deal with dyspnea in patients who are in chronic congestive heart failure. Especially in older patients, distinction between the heart and lungs in the etiology of dyspnea, or the relative contributions of each, can be difficult to establish.

Asthma is a common cause of recurrent bouts of dyspnea, which are usually accompanied by cough and wheezing. Cardiac dysfunction is another cause of acute bouts of bronchospasm, especially in middle-aged or elderly persons.

PHYSIOLOGIC CORRELATES OF DYSPNEA

Historically, attempts to understand the physiologic bases of dyspnea have evolved along four separate lines: ventilatory performance, the mechanics of breathing, chemoreception, and exercise testing. Exercise testing is presented in Chapter 34.

Ventilatory Performance

Early investigations related the sensation of dyspnea to the level of minute ventilation. Dyspnea was found to correlate with excessive minute ventilation relative to the level of oxygen uptake. Most of the increase in ventilation was accounted for by an increase in respiratory rate, especially in patients with stiff lungs. In patients who continued to ventilate excessively for the level of oxygen uptake (e.g., those with chronic left ventricular failure), the sensation of breathlessness gradually diminished, suggesting adaptation to the continued stimulus.

A second ventilatory measurement that proved to correlate well with dyspnea is the maximum voluntary ventilation (MVV). MVV is decreased by diseases of the lungs, airways, or chest wall. The smaller the MVV, the more likely is dyspnea to occur.

A third time-honored approach to measurement is the "breathing reserve." This value is determined as the difference between the MVV and the actual minute ventilation. In principle, the sensation of breathlessness during the performance of any ventilatory task may be related to the fraction of the maximum breathing capacity (i.e., the MVV) that is used for force generation by the respiratory apparatus. Thus, the closer the minute ventilation is to the maximum breathing capacity, the more likely is the subject to complain of breathlessness. Indeed, when the actual level of ventilation reaches 30% to 40% of the maximum breathing capacity, dyspnea is inevitable. Unfortunately, the breathing reserve correlates better with the dyspnea of normal subjects during exertion than with the dyspnea of chronic bronchitis and COPD or of left ventricular failure. Thus, in COPD the minute ventilation may be a very large fraction of the MVV (>50%) without eliciting dyspnea. In contrast, in acute left ventricular failure, a mild increase in ventilation and a nearly normal MVV may be associated with considerable breathlessness.

Mechanics of Breathing

One teleologic way to regard dyspnea is as a sensation that prompts an unconscious effort to minimize the work, energy cost, or force of breathing. In this light, dyspnea protects the respiratory apparatus from overwork and inefficient operation. This approach has led to exploration of the relationships between dyspnea and the work or oxygen cost of breathing.

Work, Oxygen Cost, and Efficiency of Breathing

It has not been possible to identify a critical level for the work of breathing at which dyspnea will occur. However, a breakdown of the work of breathing into its elastic, resistive, and inertial components has helped to relate physiologic disturbances to particular diseases. For example, in chronic mitral stenosis with pulmonary congestion, the elastic work is greatly increased (Fig. 29-7), whereas in obstructive airway disease, resistive work predominates. Moreover, such observations have reinforced the concept that patterns of breathing are automatically adjusted to minimize the work done by the respiratory muscles in breathing.

The relationship between ventilation and O_2 consumed by the respiratory muscles is curvilinear (Fig. 29-8). This O_2 cost of breathing may increase extraordinarily in patients with COPD or with abnormalities of the chest wall. Indeed, in patients with COPD, the quantity of O_2 delivered to the respiratory muscles during the large ventilatory effort may fail to satisfy their aerobic needs, leading to anaerobic metabolism and lactic acidosis. Although the greater the O_2 cost of breathing the greater the likelihood of dyspnea, the determination of O_2 cost provides no more useful insight into the mechanism of dyspnea than does the work of breathing. Calculation of the efficiency of breathing (i.e., the work of breathing related to energy cost) provides no further clarification.

Length–Tension Inappropriateness

The concept of "length–tension inappropriateness" explains dyspnea as a mismatch between the central motor command to the respiratory muscles (i.e., the motor signal emitted from the brain) and the suboptimal ("inappropriate") shortening of the respiratory muscles elicited by this command (e.g., suboptimal thoracic expansion for any level of central motor command).[31] In essence, this concept pictures a decrease, instead of an increase, in the pressure-generating capacity of the respiratory muscles in the face of the increased need arising from the heightened respiratory drive.

Chemoreception

Chemoreceptors in the medulla respond to changes in pH and Pa_{CO_2} (see Chapter 11). Peripheral receptors in the aortic arch and carotid body also respond to alterations in Pa_{O_2}. Acute hypoxia, hypercapnia, and acidosis are the traditional stimuli for ventilation. For example, upon ascent to altitude, acute hypoxia can stimulate ventilation to the level of awareness that may progress to discomfort during exertion. The effects of these stimuli on breathing decrease if they continue unabated. In addition, side effects, such as blunting of the sensorium during chronic CO_2 retention, diminish the likelihood of dyspnea, even if the level of ventilation is increased. In patients with abnormal pulmonary mechanics, the onset of abnormalities in blood gas composition, as during exercise, may aggravate or contribute to dyspnea. In general, acute hypercapnia is a stronger stimulus for dyspnea than is acute hypoxia.

SCALING

A variety of scaling methods have been devised to quantify dyspnea during exercise and various experimental settings. Some, such as the Borg Category Scale (Table 29-4), use numbers and descriptive terms to depict a change in the intensity of the stimulus ("threshold stimulus detection methods"). Others rely on visual analog scales, which are straight lines, usually 10 cm long, that extend from "not breathless" at one end to "extremely breathless" at the other. The

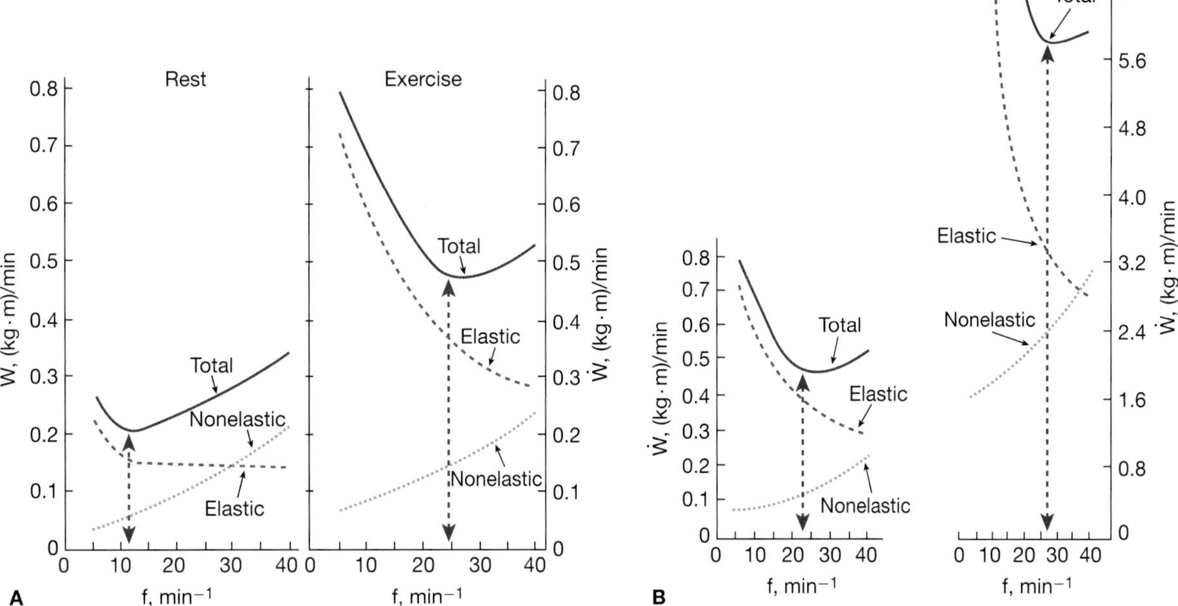

Figure 29-7 Partition of the work of breathing in pulmonary congestion and edema at rest and during exercise. **A.** Normal. The minimal work of breathing at rest was at a respiratory frequency of 12 breaths/min; during exercise, the minimal work was done at a higher frequency (25 breaths/min). **B.** Mitral stenosis. At rest, the frequency for least respiratory work was abnormally high (22 breaths/min); during exercise it increased further (to 28 breaths/min). The *dashed vertical line* (capped by *arrowheads*) in each frame indicates the respiratory frequency at which respiratory work was minimal. f, respiratory frequency. *(Reproduced with permission from Christie RV. Dyspnea in relation to the visco-elastic properties of the lung. Proc R Soc Med. 1953;46(5):381–386.)*

patient marks on the line the intensity of respiratory discomfort elicited by external stimuli, such as resistive loads or exercise testing. The score is measured as the length of the line between "not breathless" and the mark made by the patient. The Shortness of Breath Scale issued by the American Thoracic Society (Table 29-5) has also been used in one form or another, particularly in epidemiologic studies. A recent method of quantifying dyspnea severity that utilizes patient descriptors appears to be applicable and reproducible in a variety of disorders.[32]

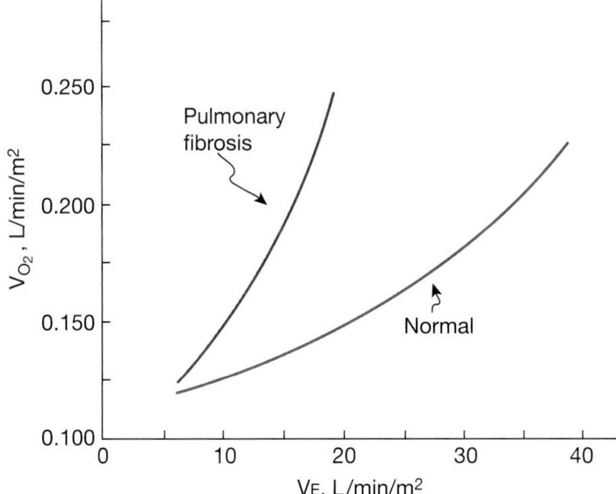

Figure 29-8 Oxygen cost of breathing in restrictive lung disease. Relationship between ventilation and O_2 consumption in pulmonary fibrosis. At each level of ventilation, the patient with pulmonary fibrosis does more work and expends more energy in breathing than does the normal subject.

DYSPNEA IN OBSTRUCTIVE AND RESTRICTIVE PULMONARY DISORDERS

Two common pathophysiologic categories of pulmonary disease in which dyspnea features prominently are chronic obstructive airway disease and restrictive pulmonary disorders.

■ CHRONIC OBSTRUCTIVE AIRWAY DISEASES

Several chronic obstructive airway diseases associated with dyspnea are well recognized, including COPD and asthma.

COPD

COPD refers to a spectrum of airway diseases in which obstruction to airflow is the common denominator (Chapters 39 and 40).

TABLE 29-4 Modified Borg Category Scale

Rating	Intensity of Sensation
0	Nothing at all
0.5	Very, very slight (just noticeable)
1	Very slight
2	Slight
3	Moderate
4	Somewhat severe
5	Severe
6	
7	Very severe
8	
9	Very, very severe (almost maximal)
10	Maximal

TABLE 29-5 American Thoracic Society Shortness of Breath Scale

Descriptions	Grade	Degree
Not troubled by shortness of breath when hurrying on the level or walking up a slight hill	0	None
Troubled by shortness of breath when hurrying on the level or walking up a slight hill	1	Mild
Walks more slowly than people of the same age on the level because of breathlessness or has to stop for breath when walking at own pace on the level	2	Moderate
Stops for breath after walking about 100 yards or after a few minutes on the level	3	Severe
Too breathless to leave the house; breathless on dressing or undressing	4	Very severe

Cigarette smoking is the leading cause of COPD (Chapter 41). The outer limits of the spectrum are marked by chronic bronchitis at one end and emphysema at the other. Most patients with COPD fall into categories between those limits (i.e., they manifest mixtures of chronic bronchitis and emphysema, which vary in degrees) (Fig. 29-9).

Patients with COPD suffer from disturbances in the mechanics of breathing, abnormal lung volumes, and derangements in gas exchange. The minute ventilation, which may be only slightly increased at rest, constitutes an abnormally large fraction of the maximum breathing capacity (i.e., the "breathing reserve" is low).

Abnormalities in the mechanics of breathing dominate the scene: resistance to airflow is high; the thorax assumes a hyperinflated position, placing the inspiratory muscles at mechanical disadvantage; the work of breathing is greatly increased. The O_2 cost of breathing is correspondingly high. Derangements in dead space ventilation and in alveolar–capillary gas exchange add to the afferent stimuli. As a result of the disturbances in mechanics and gas exchange, swings in pleural pressure (a measure of force applied to the lungs) are large, and a considerable muscular effort is expended in breathing; instead of the normal increase of about 1 mL of O_2 uptake per liter of ventilation per minute, the O_2 uptake increases enormously (up to 25 mL/min). Should O_2 delivery to the overworked respiratory muscles be insufficient, fatigue and exhaustion may send nervous and chemical signals of their own to the brain. Finally, if the patient accumulates excess water in the lungs, the juxtacapillary ("J") receptors provide additional sensory input to the central integrating mechanism. As noted above (see "Length–Tension Inappropriateness"), the convergence of these diverse stimuli upon the sensorimotor cortex may generate an inordinate motor command to the respiratory muscles, which cannot mobilize the thorax sufficiently to generate the pleural pressures needed for adequate ventilation.

One enigma is why patients with COPD maintain different levels of ventilation despite equal abnormalities in conventional pulmonary function tests. The "CO_2 retainer," with respiratory acidosis and arterial hypoxemia, often breathes less than does the non–CO_2 retainer in whom blood gas levels are near normal. One teleologic explanation is that the lower ventilation in the CO_2 retainer causes less dyspnea. However, this explanation affords no insight into the physiologic mechanism.

Treatment of the patient with COPD is directed at diminishing airways resistance and restoring arterial blood gases toward normal. Unfortunately, bronchodilators generally have only modest effects, and the basic abnormalities in the mechanics of the lungs and airways remain. Consequently, the load on the respiratory muscles is not readily alleviated by medical management. Management strategies also include consideration of ways in which the performance of the respiratory muscles can be improved. These have generally taken the form of training exercises to facilitate adaptive changes and to increase both muscle strength and endurance. Exercise reconditioning in patients with COPD has been shown to diminish breathlessness, possibly owing to three interactive mechanisms: (1) increased mechanical efficiency of the exercising muscles, which decrease ventilatory requirements; (2) improved function of the respiratory muscles; and (3) increased tolerance of the "dyspneagenic" sensory input to the brain. Attempts to rest the respiratory muscles have no lasting effect on dyspnea.

Asthma

Asthma constitutes a different entity, not only in its clinical expressions but also because it is usually episodic and is often related to allergic manifestations, and generally affects younger individuals (Chapters 45 to 47).

The mechanisms described previously for COPD apply as well to asthma. However, these mechanisms do not account for the sensation of "tightness in the chest" or the inordinate sense of labored breathing that accompanies the breathlessness in asthma.

■ RESTRICTIVE VENTILATORY DEFECTS

Restrictive ventilatory defects are due to a variety of causes, ranging from lung disorders to diseases that affect the pleural space, as well as neuromuscular diseases that affect the function of the thorax (Table 29-6). Diffuse interstitial disease has many different etiologies and may be either acute or chronic (Table 29-7). Characteristically, in widespread interstitial disease the diffusing capacity is low and is accompanied by a considerable decrease in total lung capacity and in vital capacity, as well as lesser decrements in functional residual capacity and residual volume (see Chapter 33). Similar findings occur in severe kyphoscoliosis or encasement of the lung by pleural thickening (Fig. 29-10). In contrast, in pulmonary vascular disease, such as idiopathic pulmonary arterial hypertension, a low diffusing capacity may be accompanied by normal lung volumes. Neuromuscular disease that affects the inspiratory muscles sufficiently to diminish maximum inspiratory pressures may decrease vital capacity and total lung capacity, leaving functional residual capacity and residual volume increased.

Patients with widespread pulmonary fibrosis breathe faster and maintain a higher minute ventilation than do normal subjects, both at rest and during exercise. The work and oxygen cost of ventilating

TABLE 29-6 Common Causes of Restrictive Ventilatory Defects

Cause	Example
Interstitium	
Interstitial fibrosis and/or infiltration	Usual interstitial pneumonitis/idiopathic pulmonary fibrosis
Pulmonary edema	Left ventricular failure
Pleura	
Pleural disease	Fibrothorax
Thoracic cage and abdomen	
Neuromuscular disease	Poliomyelitis
Skeletal abnormalities	Severe kyphoscoliosis
Marked obesity	Grossly overweight

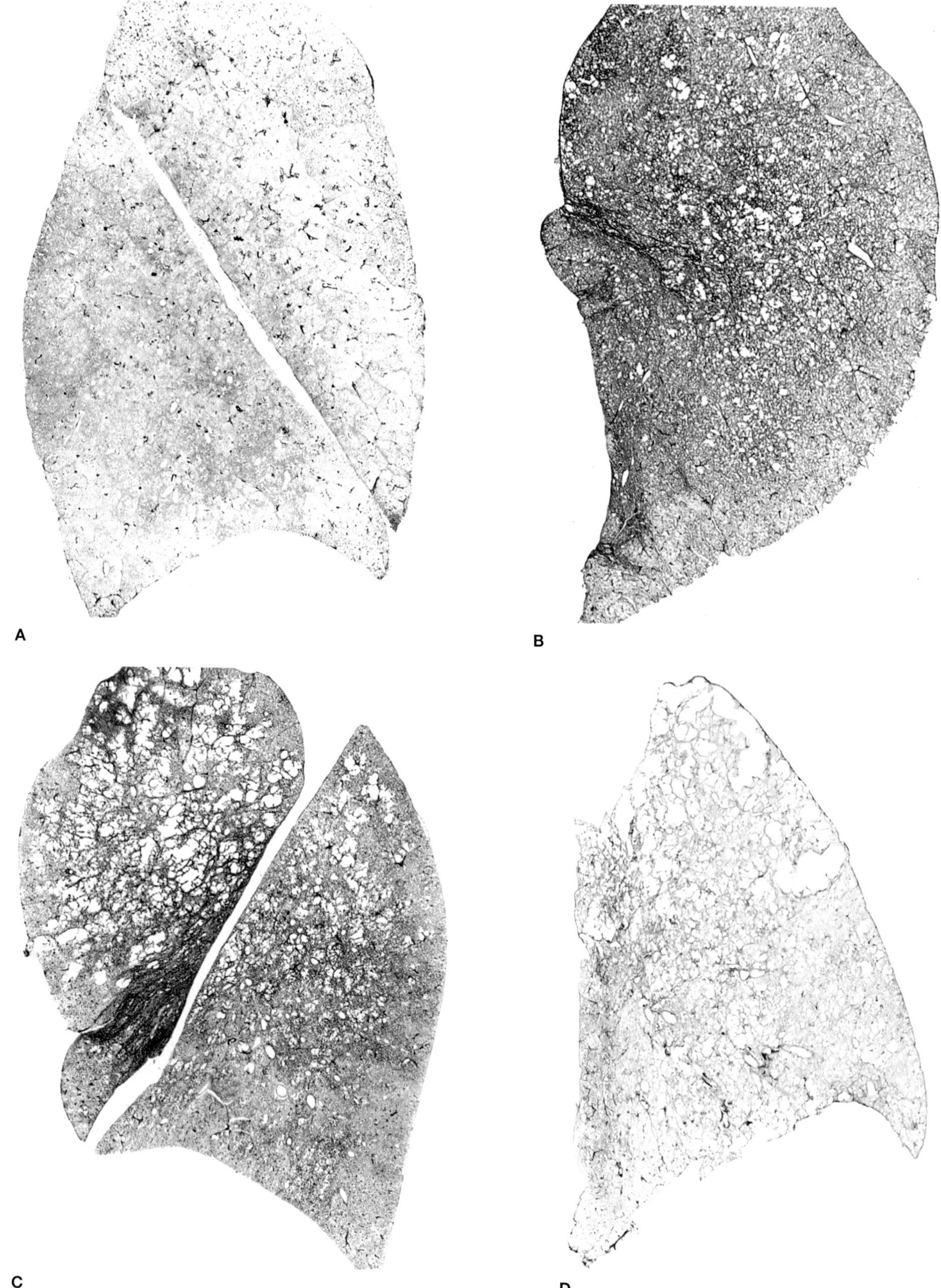

Figure 29-9 Chronic obstructive pulmonary disease (COPD). Sagittal sections showing patterns of emphysema. **A.** Normal lung from a patient who died of unrelated causes. **B.** Predominantly centrilobular emphysema. **C.** Predominantly centrilobular and panlobular emphysema. **D.** Predominantly panlobular emphysema. Centrilobular emphysema is less marked. The three patients with emphysema (**B, C, D**) also had clinical manifestations of chronic bronchitis confirmed by histologic sections.

TABLE 29-7 Some Types of Diffuse Interstitial Diseases

Etiology	Example	Common Features
	Acute	
Infections	Miliary tuberculosis, histoplasmosis	Opportunity for exposure to organism
	Pneumocystis, cytomegalic inclusion virus, fungi	Immunosuppression
Pulmonary edema	Narcotic overdosage, nitrogen dioxide (silo-filler's disease), uremia	Distinctive history
Inhalation	Byssinosis	Monday morning asthma and fever
Aspiration	After loss of consciousness	History of alcoholism or epilepsy
Immunologic	Goodpasture syndrome	Renal and pulmonary involvement
Carcinoma of lung	Adenocarcinoma in situ or minimally invasive adenocarcinoma (previously known as alveolar cell carcinoma)	
	Chronic	
Inhalation	Pneumoconioses	History of exposure to inorganic dust
Radiation therapy	After mastectomy	Gradual evolution after treatment
Lymphangitic spread	Carcinoma of breast, lung, stomach, pancreas	Evidence of primary carcinoma
Medications	Bleomycin, busulfan, cyclophosphamide	History, suggestive chest radiograph
Systemic disorders	Sarcoidosis, connective tissue disorders, eosinophilic granuloma, amyloidosis, tuberous sclerosis	Multiorgan involvement; biopsy
Idiopathic	Idiopathic pulmonary fibrosis	Exclusion of known causes

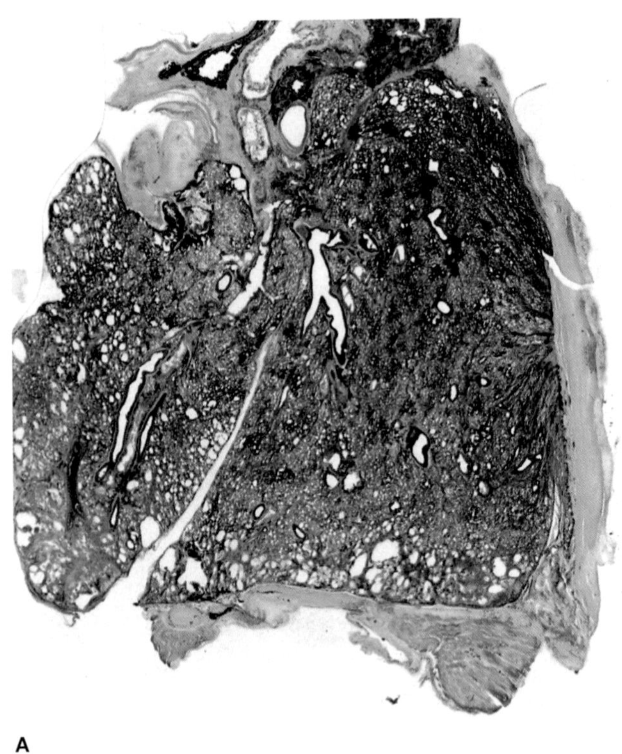

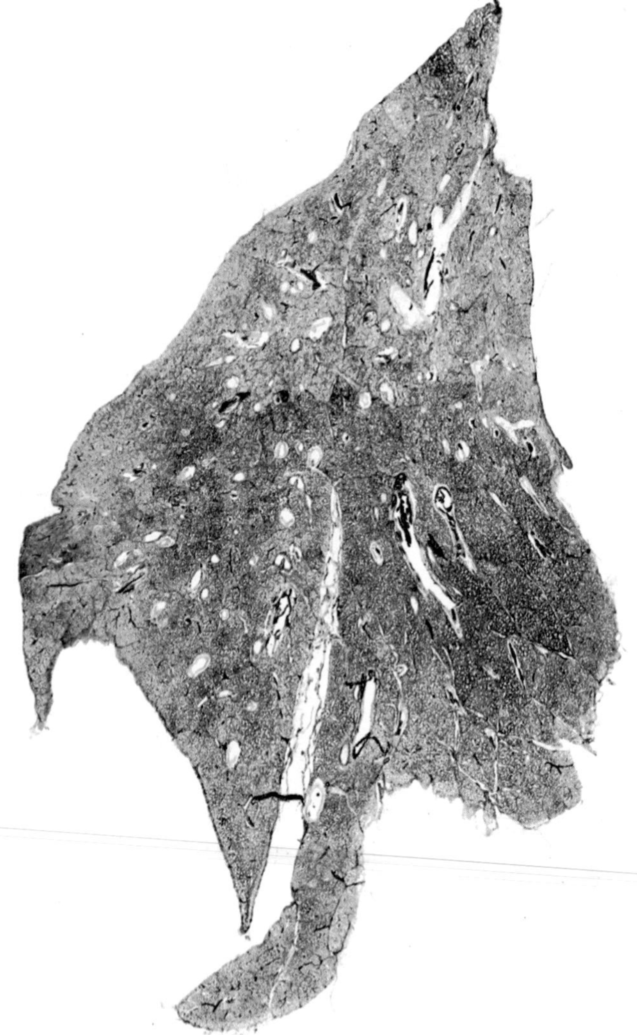

Figure 29-10 Restrictive ventilatory disorders. **A.** Asbestosis with markedly thickened pleura that encases and compresses the lungs. In addition, the lungs were afflicted with diffuse interstitial fibrosis. **B.** Compressed, distorted lung in patient with kyphoscoliosis. The lungs were otherwise normal, so that in this instance restriction was imposed by the chest wall rather than by intrapulmonary or pleural disease.

the stiff lungs are increased. Dyspnea is attributable to the considerable effort by the respiratory muscles in ventilating the stiff lungs and in sustaining the high ventilatory rate. During exercise, dyspnea may become intolerable.

DYSPNEA IN CHRONIC CARDIAC DISEASE

The mechanisms responsible for dyspnea in cardiac disease vary with the extent to which the lungs are stiffened.

Dyspnea occurs in many forms of heart disease that are not associated with congestion of the lungs. Uncomplicated pulmonic stenosis is an excellent example. The symptom is probably related to an inadequate cardiac output during exercise. In Tetralogy of Fallot, dyspnea is sometimes severe and often relieved by assuming a squatting position. In this and other forms of cyanotic heart disease, both dyspnea and fatigue appear during exertion when the arterial oxyhemoglobin saturation decreases appreciably below the resting level.

Cardiac dyspnea is associated with an increase in blood and water content of the lungs. It is a common occurrence in left ventricular failure and mitral stenosis, both of which are accompanied by increases in pulmonary venous and capillary pressures. The engorged pulmonary circulatory bed, coupled with interstitial and alveolar edema, stiffens the lungs (i.e., decreases their compliance) and stimulates the ventilation via "J" receptors. In chronic left ventricular failure, pulmonary fibrosis, consequent to long-standing interstitial edema, contributes to the stiff lungs. Edema of the tracheobronchial mucosa increases airway resistance.

As a result of the stiff lungs and increased airway resistance, swings in pleural pressure during the respiratory cycle are large and the work and energy cost of breathing are increased. Arterial hypoxemia, generally mild, may add to the ventilatory drive. Exercise exaggerates the pulmonary congestion and edema, promotes arterial and mixed venous hypoxemia, and increases the dyspnea.

In patients with pulmonary congestion and edema, tachypnea is a regular feature at rest and increases during exercise. Although tachypnea is consistent, its degree is generally modest and probably not entirely responsible for the dyspnea. Fatigue is a common concomitant of low cardiac output and may stem from diminished O_2 delivery to the respiratory muscles, contributing to respiratory discomfort.

ORTHOPNEA AND OTHER POSITIONAL FORMS OF BREATHLESSNESS

Orthopnea signifies dyspnea in the recumbent, but not in the upright or semiupright, position; it is usually relieved by two or three pillows under the head and back. *Platypnea* signifies dyspnea induced by assuming the upright position and relieved by recumbency.[33]

Platypnea may be seen when, due to gravity, increased blood flow worsens right to left shunting of blood through arteriovenous malformations at the lung bases; it may be accompanied by *orthodeoxia*—desaturation of arterial blood when the patient is upright.

Orthopnea is a hallmark of pulmonary congestion that stiffens the lungs (i.e., decreases their compliance). The decrease in compliance on lying flat is attributable to the fact that more of the lung is located at or below the level of the heart. During recumbency, the swings in pleural pressure, the work of breathing, and the respiratory frequency increase. The increase in respiratory frequency appears to be automatically adjusted to minimize the work of ventilating the more rigid lungs.

Some patients with chronic lung disease or asthma are also intolerant of lying flat. Their discomfort is attributed to the greater difficulty of performing vigorous movements of the chest bellows in the recumbent position.

Finally, patients with asymmetric lung disease may experience *trepopnea*—dyspnea when the affected side of the chest is in the dependent position, thereby promoting ventilation–perfusion mismatch (Chapter 14) and resultant hypoxemia.

PAROXYSMAL NOCTURNAL DYSPNEA

In an episode of paroxysmal nocturnal dyspnea (PND), the patient is aroused from sleep, gasping for air, and must sit up or stand to catch his or her breath; sweating may be profuse. Sometimes the patient opens a room window in an attempt to relieve the oppressive sensation of suffocation. The chest tends to become fixed in the position of forced inspiration. Both inspiratory and expiratory wheezes, often simulating typical asthma, are heard. In some instances, overt pulmonary edema occurs, accompanied by inspiratory crackles. Attacks occasionally recur several times a night, forcing the patient to sleep upright in a chair.

An episode of PND represents precipitous failure of the left ventricle caused by the factors that produce orthopnea (see above), abetted by pulmonary hypervolemia caused by a surge in systemic venous return. Mobilization of peripheral edema from the periphery as the extremities are elevated from the dependent position may contribute to the increase in systemic venous return. The acute increase in pulmonary blood volume increases pulmonary capillary pressures, thereby promoting pulmonary edema, while the surge in venous return imposes an additional burden on the left ventricle.

A variety of factors may trigger an episode of PND: coughing, abdominal distention, the hypercapnic phase of Cheyne–Stokes respiration (see below), a startling noise, or anything that causes a rise in heart rate and further increases the pulmonary capillary and venous pressures. Usually the attack is terminated by assumption of the erect position and a few deep breaths. Cough, an important manifestation of pulmonary congestion, frequently occurs during the attack.

CARDIAC ASTHMA

Asthmatic wheezes, often audible in patients with pulmonary congestion, have given rise to the term *cardiac asthma*. The wheezes are a manifestation of tracheobronchial edema and often are accompanied by overt signs of pulmonary edema. In addition to the reduction in the lumen of the airways and thickening of bronchial walls by edema, the high intrathoracic pressures, which are required to overcome the obstruction during expiration, tend to narrow the airways even further. The resistance to airflow is increased during both inspiration and expiration, and the compliance of the lungs is greatly reduced, reaching values as low as one-tenth of normal. Upon recovery from the acute episode of pulmonary edema, airway resistance and pulmonary compliance return toward normal unless previous episodes have left a residue of pulmonary fibrosis.

DYSPNEA IN ANEMIA

Shortness of breath during exercise or excitement is a common complaint in severe anemia (e.g., hemoglobin concentration under 6–7 g/dL). It is more common in acute than in chronic anemia. Often the dyspnea is associated with dizziness or faintness, and invariably the patient manifests signs of a high cardiac output and low peripheral resistance (i.e., bounding pulse, warm skin, and systolic cardiac murmurs). Although the pathogenesis of the dyspnea is not clear, inadequate oxygen delivery to the respiratory muscles has been proposed.

METABOLIC ABNORMALITIES AND DRUGS

Increases in CO_2 production demand a concomitant rise in ventilation to dispose of the metabolic load and, hence, may result in dyspnea. To prevent acidemia, patients with diabetic ketoacidosis may require an enormous increase in minute ventilation in order to reduce Pa_{CO_2}. Thyrotoxicosis, fever, infection, and pregnancy can also cause an increased minute ventilation, as can drugs, such as aspirin and progesterone.

MISCELLANEOUS DISORDERS

Breathlessness is not uncommon in patients with musculoskeletal disorders. The usual explanation is the heightened motor drive that is needed to activate the weakened respiratory muscles. In the intensive care unit, inadequate ventilator settings for flow and tidal volume may fail to satisfy the intrinsic ventilatory drive of the patient, generating the sensation of breathlessness.

ABNORMAL BREATHING PATTERNS

An important clue to the nature of a clinical problem in pulmonary disease is sometimes provided by bedside observation of a patient's breathing pattern. The pertinent features are the rate, regularity, depth, and apparent effort being expended in breathing. A normal person at rest breathes about 12 to 15 times per minute, with a tidal volume of 400 to 800 mL. As a result, minute ventilation is normally greater than 5 L/min. The pattern is quite regular except for an occasional slow, deep breath, and the respiratory movements appear effortless.

Severe skeletal deformity, as well as massive obesity, can limit chest excursions to cause alveolar hypoventilation (Chapter 83). Neuromuscular weakness, as in myasthenia gravis or Guillain–Barré syndrome, may do the same, not only by diminishing ventilatory excursions as a result of generalized weakness of the respiratory muscles, but also by causing overload of respiratory muscles (e.g., residual effects of poliomyelitis) (Chapters 83 and 84). Unilateral involvement of one pleural space by pneumothorax, effusion, or fibrothorax limits excursions on the affected side. Massive chest trauma may cause flail chest.

In COPD, a slow respiratory rate and large tidal volumes are characteristic. This pattern presumably serves to minimize the work of breathing. Pursed-lip breathing, a self-induced type of positive-pressure breathing, is often part of the picture. In contrast, persons with restrictive ventilator disorders adopt a breathing pattern that is characterized by small tidal volumes and a rapid respiratory rate, often with little apparent effort. This pattern is seen in patients with a decrease in the distensibility of the lung or chest wall or with reduction of the vital capacity from any other cause. During exercise, minute ventilation increases inordinately with respect to the level of O_2 uptake, and respiratory frequency increases more than tidal volume.

Fatigue of the diaphragm and intercostal muscles, sufficient to disturb their coordinated contractions, may give rise to paradoxical breathing, which heralds the onset of respiratory failure.

■ CHEYNE–STOKES RESPIRATION

In the fourth century BC, in a preterminally ill person with fever, sweats, and black urine, Hippocrates described a pattern of breathing in which "the respiration throughout [was] like that of a man correcting himself, and rare and large." Presumably he had observed Cheyne–Stokes breathing, which was described more graphically by William Stokes two millennia later (in 1854) as follows:

"The symptom in question (previously described by Dr. Cheyne) consists in the occurrence of a series of inspirating, increasing to a maximum, and then declining in force and length, until a state of apparent apnea is established. In this condition the patient may remain for such a length of time as to make his attendants believe that he is dead, when a low inspiration, followed by one more decided, marks the commencement of a new ascending and descending series of inspirations."

Cheyne–Stokes breathing is characterized by alternating periods of hypoventilation and hyperventilation (Fig. 29-11). In its typical form, an apneic phase, which lasts for 15 to 60 seconds, is followed by a phase during which tidal volume increases with each successive breath to a peak level and then decreases in a progressive fashion to the apneic phase. At the onset of apnea, CO_2 tension in brachial or femoral arterial blood is at its lowest. As apnea persists, CO_2 tension gradually increases, and respiration is stimulated. CO_2 tension continues to increase until maximum hyperventilation is attained, after which ventilation decreases until apnea again occurs. The arterial oxyhemoglobin saturation varies in an inverse manner, being highest at the onset of apnea and lower during midhyperpnea. During the cycle, CO_2 tension varies by as much as 14 mm Hg and oxyhemoglobin saturation by as much as 18%.

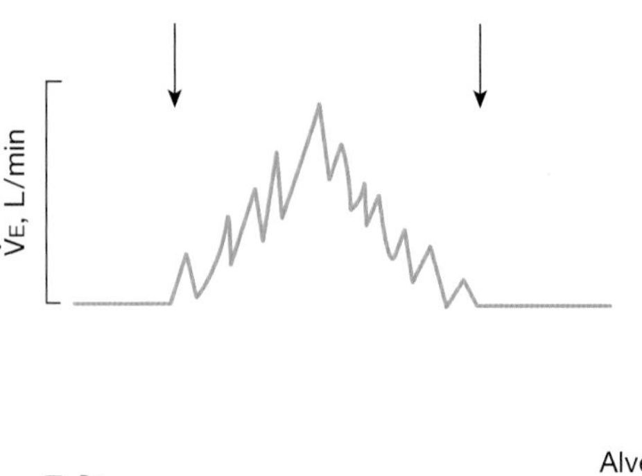

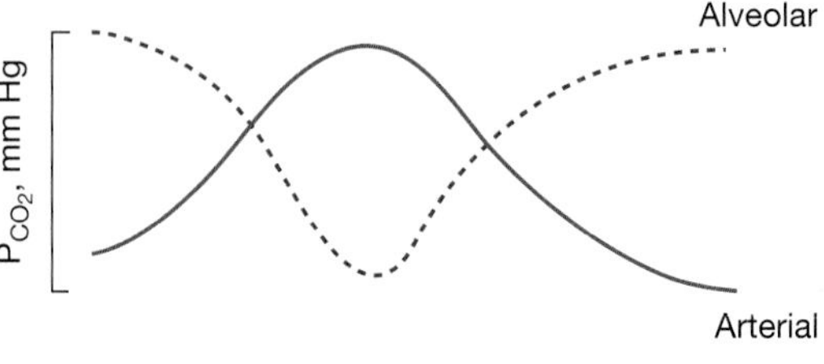

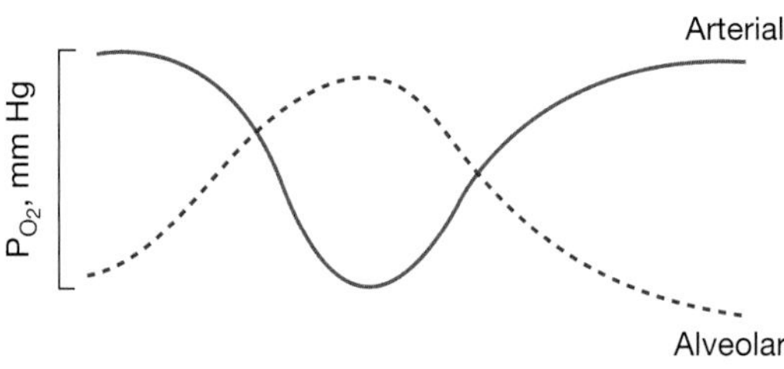

Figure 29-11 Cheyne–Stokes breathing, illustrating the relationship between the ventilation and the blood and alveolar gas tensions during the periods of apnea and hyperpnea. *(Reproduced with permission from Cherniack NS, Fishman AP. Abnormal breathing patterns. Dis Mon. 1975:1–45.)*

In patients with congestive heart failure, the respiratory oscillations are attributable to slowing of the circulation so that the blood gases reaching the respiratory centers in the brain are 180 degrees out of phase with those in pulmonary capillary blood. This mechanism has been verified experimentally by eliciting Cheyne–Stokes breathing in dogs by prolonging the circulation time from heart to brain by way of an extracorporeal circuit.

Fluctuations in mental state and electroencephalographic patterns, and evidence of nervous system dysfunction, may occur during Cheyne–Stokes breathing because of swings in cerebral blood flow. In neurologic disorders, Cheyne–Stokes breathing may be due to supramedullary dysfunction, particularly in patients who have destructive lesions in the tegmentum of the pons.

Less common than in heart failure or neurologic disorders is the occurrence of Cheyne–Stokes respiration in normal infants, in healthy elderly persons, and in normal persons at high altitude. It is also seen occasionally after the administration of respiratory depressants (e.g., morphine), often accompanied by an increase in intracranial pressure, uremia, or coma. At one time, the respiratory center was believed to be depressed in Cheyne–Stokes respiration. This hypothesis has been proved to be in error, since it has been shown that the respiratory response to inhalation of CO_2 is greater than normal in individuals with Cheyne–Stokes respiration. Respiratory alkalosis is common and the arterial P_{CO_2} remains subnormal in both the apneic and hyperpneic phases.

KUSSMAUL BREATHING

In 1874, Kussmaul described three patients with diabetic ketoacidosis who manifested "air hunger": they were breathing with large tidal volumes and so rapidly that there was virtually no pause between breaths. In essence, they were breathing at rest as though they were exercising; breathing was accomplished with little apparent effort. Since then, this pattern of breathing has been observed in other types of severe metabolic acidoses (e.g., alcoholic ketoacidosis). The usual sequence leading to this type of breathing is renal failure with a progressive decrease in plasma bicarbonate and resultant acidosis. The "compensatory" increase in ventilation that Kussmaul described mitigates the fall in systemic pH caused by the fall in plasma bicarbonate (see Chapter 17).

OTHER ABNORMAL PATTERNS

Gasping respirations are characteristic of severe cerebral hypoxia. The pattern consists of irregular, quick inspirations associated with extensions of the neck and followed by a long expiratory pause. It is commonly seen in shock or in other conditions associated with severe reduction in cardiac output.

Hyperventilation is commonly seen in anxious patients without structural disease of the lungs. In some of these patients, striking deep sighs dominate the ventilatory pattern.

DIAGNOSTIC TESTING IN THE EVALUATION OF DYSPNEA

Attention to the history and physical examination findings, as described in the preceding sections, will help to focus the initial approach to diagnosis.[34] In most cases, the initial diagnostic impression can be confirmed or excluded with only a few tests, and appropriate therapy instituted or the hunt for a cause continued (Table 29-8).

A plain chest radiograph is useful in demonstrating changes suggestive of COPD (chest hyperinflation, bullous changes). Vascular engorgement, an enlarged cardiac silhouette, increased interstitial markings, and pleural effusions may indicate left heart failure.

Spirometry is useful in identifying airways obstruction; improvement in values may be noted following administration of a bronchodilator. The measurement of lung volumes or the diffusing capacity may be reserved for when there is suspicion of an interstitial process or other cause of restriction (e.g., muscle weakness). Measurement of arterial oxyhemoglobin saturation both at rest and with exertion is important. While oxyhemoglobin desaturation will not indicate the etiology of the problem, its presence is always an important indicator of the severity of the disease. An echocardiogram can be used to assess ventricular or valvular cardiac function and to estimate pulmonary arterial pressures.

A complete blood count may reveal anemia or suggest an infection. Measurement of serum electrolytes may indicate the presence of an acidosis or renal dysfunction. Measurement of brain natriuretic peptide (BNP) has been useful in helping to exclude heart failure as an acute cause of dyspnea.[35]

Additional testing is usually not required unless the cause of dyspnea remains unclear following basic studies. Further tests often include CT of the chest, which may rarely reveal changes of emphysema or an interstitial process not suggested by plain radiographs or lung function testing. The CT may additionally help to better

TABLE 29-8 Common Tests in the Evaluation of Dyspnea

Test	Some Possible Abnormalities	Some Possible Diagnoses
Plain chest radiograph	Cardiac enlargement	Congestive heart failure
	Vascular enlargement	Pulmonary hypertension
	Abnormal interstitial markings	Pulmonary fibrosis
	Pleural effusions	Malignant pleural effusion
	Hyperinflation	COPD
	Nodules/masses	Neoplastic process
Pulmonary function tests		
Spirometry	Obstructive ventilation defect (decreased FEV_1/FVC, %)	Asthma COPD
	Restrictive ventilatory defect	Interstitial lung disease
Diffusing capacity	Decreased	Interstitial lung disease
		Pulmonary vascular disease
	Increased	Alveolar hemorrhage
Inspiratory and expiratory pressures	Decreased values	Respiratory muscle weakness
Computed tomography	Abnormal interstitial markings	Interstitial lung disease
	Cystic changes	Bullous lung disease
	Lymphadenopathy	Sarcoidosis
	Vascular filling defects	Pulmonary embolism
	Ground-glass opacities	Neoplastic disease
Blood tests	Elevated white blood cell count	Infection
	Anemia	Anemia
	BNP	Heart failure
	Cr	Renal failure
		Respiratory or metabolic acidosis
	ABG	Acidoses or alkaloses (respiratory or metabolic)

COPD, chronic obstructive pulmonary disease; FEV_1/FVC, forced expiratory volume in 1 s/forced vital capacity; BNP, brain natriuretic peptide; Cr, creatine; ABG, arterial blood gas.

characterize an interstitial process identified on plain radiographs. Cardiopulmonary exercise testing (Chapter 34) may be helpful in differentiating between cardiac and respiratory causes of dyspnea, or in excluding a significant abnormality of either system and suggesting deconditioning as the culprit. Arterial blood gas measurements may be necessary to characterize the level of blood oxygenation or to identify hyperventilation or hypercapnia. More invasive testing, including cardiac catheterization or lung biopsy (by either bronchoscopy or surgery), is reserved for situations when the diagnosis remains unsettled and the results will be helpful in guiding therapy or discussions of prognosis.

COUGH

Cough is one of the most frequent causes of visits to the doctor's office.[36,37] Patients are frequently anxious about the possibility of a serious underlying cause. They may also be troubled by the complications of cough, including chest pain from intercostal muscle strain or even a fractured rib. They may be embarrassed by cough-induced urinary or fecal incontinence. Social isolation may also arise from the frequent fear of others that the patient's cough is infectious and communicable.

A cough is an explosive expiration that protects the lungs against aspiration and promotes the movement of secretions and other airway constituents upward toward the mouth. It is a critical element in the self-clearing and protective mechanisms of the lungs—a reflex act that usually, but not invariably, arises from stimulation of the bronchial mucosa somewhere between the larynx and the second-order bronchi. On rare occasions the cause is remote: impacted cerumen in the external auditory canal[38] or an inflammatory process of the pleura (see "Mechanism" below) (Fig. 29-12). The stimuli that may elicit a cough are diverse: inhaled particles, mucus that has been elaborated by the lining of the airways, inflammatory exudate in airways or parenchyma, a new growth or foreign body in an airway, or pressure on the external wall of the bronchus.

A cough may be voluntary, involuntary, or a combination of the two if the subject attempts to control an involuntary cough. Three categories of stimuli are commonly at work in producing an involuntary cough: mechanical, inflammatory, and psychogenic. Mechanical and chemical causes range from inhalation of irritants, such as smoke or dust, to distortions of the airways produced by pulmonary fibrosis or atelectasis. Most often, cough is due to tracheobronchial inflammation. The cigarette smoker is particularly vulnerable to exacerbation of cough by inhaled particles and fumes because of underlying chronic pharyngitis, laryngitis, and tracheobronchitis. As a rule, cough represents organic disease. But on occasion, psychogenic influences are responsible for a dry cough that is related to anxiety. Psychogenic stress can aggravate cough due to organic causes.[39]

The site of origin and significance of a cough may sometimes be ascertained from telltale signs and symptoms (Table 29-9). For example, the cough of acute tracheitis is often associated with retrosternal "burning." Acute laryngitis is usually associated with hoarseness and sore throat, as well as cough. Tuberculosis of the larynx is associated not only with painful swallowing but also with unequivocal evidence of pulmonary tuberculosis. In asthma, cough is part of a constellation of airway obstruction.

Interpretation of the significance of a cough depends on the clinical features with which it is associated. It has to be viewed in context: Is it acute or chronic? Is it productive or nonproductive? How long has it lasted? What is the general condition of the patient, and what comorbidities are present? For example, the acute onset of a hacking, nonproductive cough accompanied by coryza, sore throat, malaise, sweating, and fever generally heralds a viral upper respiratory infection. An episode of asthma may begin with cough and wheezing. In contrast, a persistent cough, even if virtually ignored by the patient, may be a harbinger of serious disease (e.g., carcinoma of the lung). In a cigarette smoker, a change in the nature of the cough from nonproductive to productive may signify the onset of a serious tracheobronchial infection or pneumonia.

A cough that is productive of purulent sputum is generally a reliable indication of infection in the tracheobronchial tree or lungs. When this symptom is associated with an acute illness, the characteristics of the sputum can be of considerable diagnostic help. Rust-colored sputum, which has a distinctive coloration from the even dispersion of blood in yellow, purulent sputum, was previously seen often in pneumococcal pneumonia; it is less commonly seen today due to the widespread use of antibiotics. The classic description of sputum in *Klebsiella* pneumonia is a resemblance to currant jelly; it also contains blood, but it is bright red and more translucent and viscid than the sputum of pneumococcal pneumonia. Purulent sputum with a foul odor usually indicates an anaerobic infection, commonly due to streptococci or *Bacteroides* in a lung abscess. A persistent cough that is productive of purulent sputum occurs in chronic bronchitis, bronchiectasis, and a variety of other suppurative disorders. Sputum that is mucoid may be a consequence of any long-standing bronchial irritant. Copious sputum production *(bronchorrhea)* may be a sign of adenocarcinoma in situ (AIS) or minimally invasive adenocarcinoma (MIA), previously known as bronchoalveolar carcinoma.

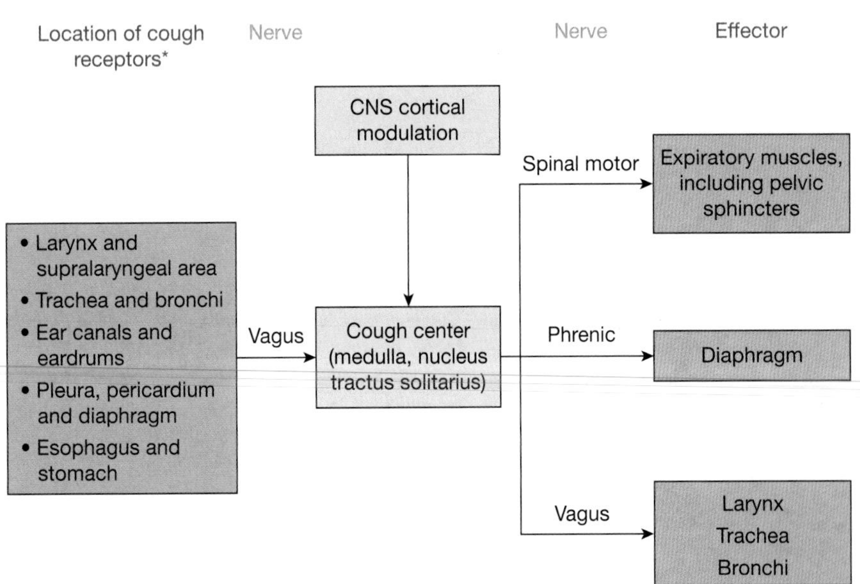

Figure 29-12 Signaling pathways in the development of cough. CN, cranial nerve. *(Reproduced with permission from Silvestri RC, Weinberger SE. Evaluation of subacute and chronic cough in adults. In: UpToDate, Post TW (Ed). UpToDate, Waltham, MA. In: UpToDate, Post TW (Ed). UpToDate, Waltham, MA. (Accessed on November 18, 2014) Copyright © 2014 UpToDate, Inc. For more information visit www.uptodate.com.)*

TABLE 29-9 Some Causes and Characteristics of Cough

Cause	Characteristics
Sinusitis or nasopharyngitis	Cough following an upper respiratory syndrome or sinus symptoms; sensation of a need to clear the throat; postnasal drip
Acute infections of lungs	
Tracheobronchitis	Cough associated with sore throat, running nose, and eyes
Lobar pneumonia	Cough often preceded by symptoms of upper respiratory infection; cough dry, painful at first; later becomes productive
Bronchopneumonia	Cough dry or productive, usually begins as acute bronchitis
Mycoplasma and viral pneumonia	Paroxysmal cough, productive of mucoid or blood-stained sputum associated with flulike syndrome
Exacerbation of chronic bronchitis	Cough productive of mucoid sputum becomes purulent
Chronic infections of lungs	
Bronchitis	Cough productive of sputum on most days for more than 3 consecutive months and for more than 2 y Sputum mucoid until acute exacerbation, when it becomes mucopurulent
Bronchiectasis	Cough copious, foul, purulent, often since childhood; forms layers upon standing
Tuberculosis or fungus	Persistent cough for weeks to months, often with blood-tinged sputum
Parenchymal inflammatory processes	
Interstitial fibrosis and infiltrations	Cough nonproductive, persistent, depends on origin
Smoking and inhalation of irritants	Cough usually associated with injected pharynx; persistent, most marked in morning, usually only slightly productive unless succeeded by chronic bronchitis
Tumors	
Bronchogenic carcinoma	Cough nonproductive to productive for weeks to months; recurrent small hemoptysis common
Adenocarcinoma *in situ* or minimally invasive adenocarcinoma	Cough similar to that with bronchogenic carcinoma except in occasional instances, when large quantities of watery, mucoid sputum are produced
Benign tumors in airways	Cough nonproductive; occasionally hemoptysis
Mediastinal tumors	Cough, often with breathlessness, caused by compression of trachea and bronchi
Aortic aneurysm	Brassy cough
Gastrointestinal	
Gastroesophageal reflux disease (GERD)	Nonproductive cough often following meals or with recumbency; may (or may not) be accompanied by other symptoms of GERD (e.g., heartburn, a bitter oral taste, belching)
Foreign body	
Immediate, while still in upper airway	Cough associated with progressive evidence of asphyxiation
Later, when lodged in lower airway	Nonproductive cough, persistent, associated with localizing wheeze
Cardiovascular	
Left ventricular failure	Cough intensifies while supine, along with aggravation of dyspnea
Pulmonary infarction	Cough associated with hemoptysis, usually with pleural effusion
Medication-induced	
Angiotensin-converting enzyme (ACE) inhibitors	Nonproductive cough, more common in women, may occur at any time (following soon after drug initiation or with years of use)

MECHANISM

A cough begins with a rapid inspiration, followed, in rapid sequence, by closure of the glottis, contraction of the abdominal and thoracic expiratory muscles, abrupt increase in pleural and intrapulmonary pressures, sudden opening of the glottis, and expulsion of a burst of air from the mouth (Fig. 29-13). The high intrathoracic pressures, which often exceed 100 to 200 mm Hg, increase the velocity of airflow through the airways, hastening the propulsion of the offending particles and producing the sound of a cough by setting into vibration airway secretions, the tracheobronchial walls, and the adjacent parenchyma (Fig. 29-14).

Afferent stimuli for a cough originate in irritant receptors and are conveyed centrally by the vagus, glossopharyngeal, trigeminal, and phrenic nerves (Fig. 29-12). In subjects with an idiopathic, persistent, nonproductive cough, increased sensitivity of the afferent nerves of the airways due to neuropeptides stored in them has been proposed.

The vagus nerve carries impulses not only from the larynx, trachea, and bronchi, but also from the pleura and stomach. Receptors in the airways are most concentrated in the larynx, diminish in density in the conducting airways, and are absent from the distal airways, enabling the pooling of secretions in the periphery. The glossopharyngeal nerve carries stimuli from the pharynx; the trigeminal nerve, from the nose and paranasal sinuses; the phrenic nerve, from the pericardium and diaphragm. The motor pathways are even more extensive, comprising not only the cranial and phrenic nerves but also the nerves to the muscles of the rib cage and the accessory muscles. Additional impulses from chemoreceptors are located in the esophagus and carried by the phrenic nerve.

The effectiveness of a cough is strongly influenced by the lung volume at which it occurs. As indicated elsewhere in this volume, cough only removes particles toward the mouth ("downstream"

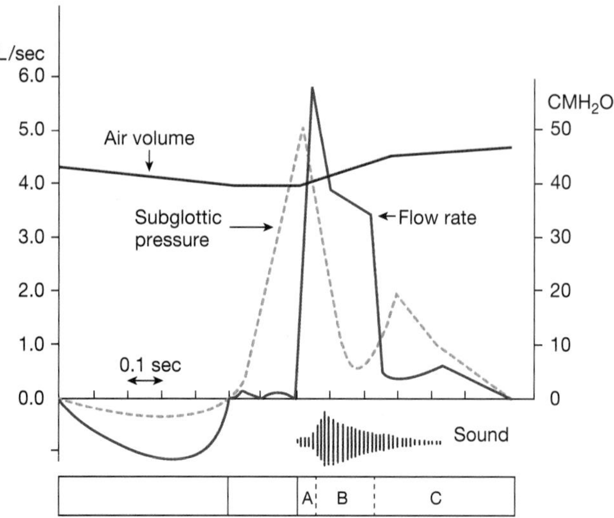

Figure 29-13 Sequence of events during a cough. Simultaneous recordings obtained during a single explosive cough by a normal subject. The three phases of a cough are identified by the boxes at the bottom of the figure. They correspond to (1) a deep initial inspiration, (2) compression of air in the lungs and airways by forceful contraction of the expiratory muscles coupled with tight closure of the glottis and opening of the larynx, and (3) sudden explosive expiration followed by narrowing of the glottis and return of the larynx to its normal inspiratory position. *(Reproduced with permission from Yanagihara N, Von Leden H, Werner-Kukuk E. The physical parameters of cough: the larynx in a normal single cough. Acta Otolaryngol. 1966;61(6):495–510.)*

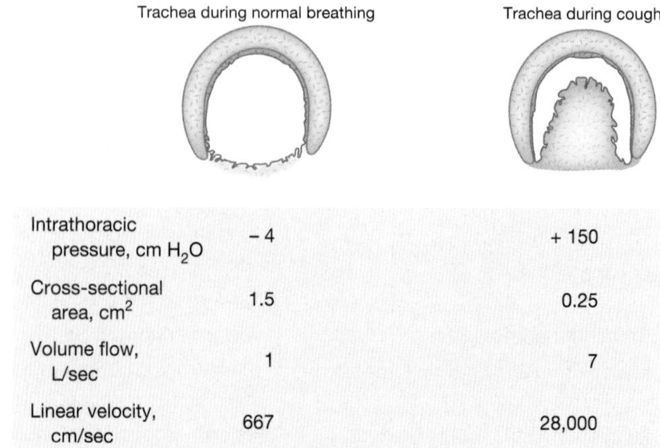

	Trachea during normal breathing	Trachea during cough
Intrathoracic pressure, cm H_2O	− 4	+ 150
Cross-sectional area, cm^2	1.5	0.25
Volume flow, L/sec	1	7
Linear velocity, cm/sec	667	28,000

Figure 29-14 Effects of tracheal narrowing during a cough. The forced expiratory effort during coughing causes invagination of the noncartilaginous part of the intrathoracic trachea by the high intrathoracic pressure. Air rushing with a high linear velocity through the exceedingly narrow trachea dislodges the material to be dispelled and propels it into the throat. *(Reproduced with permission from Comroe. Physiology of Respiration. St. Louis. Mosby-Year Book; 1965.)*

from the "equal pressure points"). In healthy persons at high lung volumes, the equal pressure points are located in the larger airways; they move toward the alveoli ("upstream") as lung volume decreases. A series of coughs without any intervening inspiration moves the equal pressure points even closer to the small airways, helping to clear the depths of the lungs.

The cough reflex may be impaired by interrupting or blunting any step in the sequence. Irritant receptors can be damaged by a local destructive process (e.g., bronchiectasis), or their sensitivity can be diminished by narcotics or anesthetics.

The reflex pathways may be damaged as part of a neurologic disease. Tracheostomy, which eliminates glottic closure, decreases peak intrapulmonary pressures. Contraction of the respiratory muscles may be impaired by weakness due to illness, age, or neuromuscular disease. In general, as long as the patient can achieve maximum expiratory pressures greater than about 60 cm H_2O, the peak flow will suffice to produce effective coughs.

CIRCULATORY CONSEQUENCES

The increase in intrathoracic pressure that is part of the cough mechanism exerts considerable circulatory effects. However, because the increase in intrathoracic pressure is accompanied by an equal rise in vascular (and cerebrospinal fluid) pressures, distending pressures on the vessels of the heart, lungs, and other vital organs are unaltered, so they are normally spared the ill consequences of marked swings in transmural pressures.

The increase in intrathoracic pressure is accompanied by reflex vasodilation of systemic arteries and veins. Both of these effects contribute to a decrease in cardiac output. In patients with cor pulmonale and right heart failure, cough impedes systemic venous return and may result in syncope.

POSTTUSSIVE SYNCOPE

Over 100 years ago, Charcot recognized the syndrome of posttussive syncope in individuals without underlying cardiopulmonary disease. Originally conceived of as a form of epilepsy or a consequence of a laryngeal reflex, it is now attributed to the same circulatory consequences of raised intrathoracic pressures that coughing evokes in a normal person. However, the patient with cough syncope probably coughs more forcefully and longer than does a normal person.

The syncope usually develops within a few seconds after the onset of a paroxysm of coughing and ends quickly once the coughing has stopped. Return to consciousness is without sequelae unless the subject falls and is injured during the faint. Posttussive syncope nearly always occurs in men, probably because they generate a higher intrathoracic pressure and much more profound decrease in cardiac output than do women. It is not clear why this type of fainting occurs in the supine, as well as the upright, position; this occurrence suggests that the reduction in cerebral blood flow during posttussive syncope reflects more than interference with cardiac output. The extent to which intense reflex vasodilation contributes to posttussive syncope is unclear. It is important to distinguish cough syncope from epilepsy and cataplexy.

ETIOLOGY

The most common causes of chronic cough and sputum (defined as lasting longer than 8 weeks) are postnasal drip, gastroesophageal reflux disease (GERD), and asthma. In one series of 71 patients, the cause was determined in 97%, with one cause noted in 38%, two causes in 36%, and three causes in 26%. The spectrum of conditions included postnasal drip in 40%, asthma in 24%, GERD in 15%, and bronchitis in 11%.[40]

In patients treated with angiotensin-converting enzyme (ACE) inhibitors, the drug is very often the cause of a chronic cough (even one developing after years of uncomplicated use). The association of cough and ACE inhibitors may be different among various ethnic groups.[41]

A deliberate evaluation can identify the cause of cough in the vast majority of patients. Usually, the diagnosis is established only by the resolution of the cough following a specific intervention (Fig. 29-15). For example, cough that disappears after antihistamines and inhaled nasal corticosteroid treatment for allergic rhinitis can logically be attributed to postnasal drip. Similarly, cough may disappear after interventions for GERD (e.g., use of H_2-blockers) or asthma (use of inhaled bronchodilators and steroids). A cough that resolves after discontinuation of an ACE inhibitor was presumably caused by the drug. Although the causes of chronic cough are usually benign, a chest radiograph is warranted at the beginning of the evaluation of a chronic cough to assess for serious causes.

HEMOPTYSIS

The coughing up of blood is termed *hemoptysis.*[42] The material and amount produced varies from mere blood streaking of expectorated sputum to massive volumes of pure blood. Massive hemoptysis has been variably defined according to the volume, but its presence

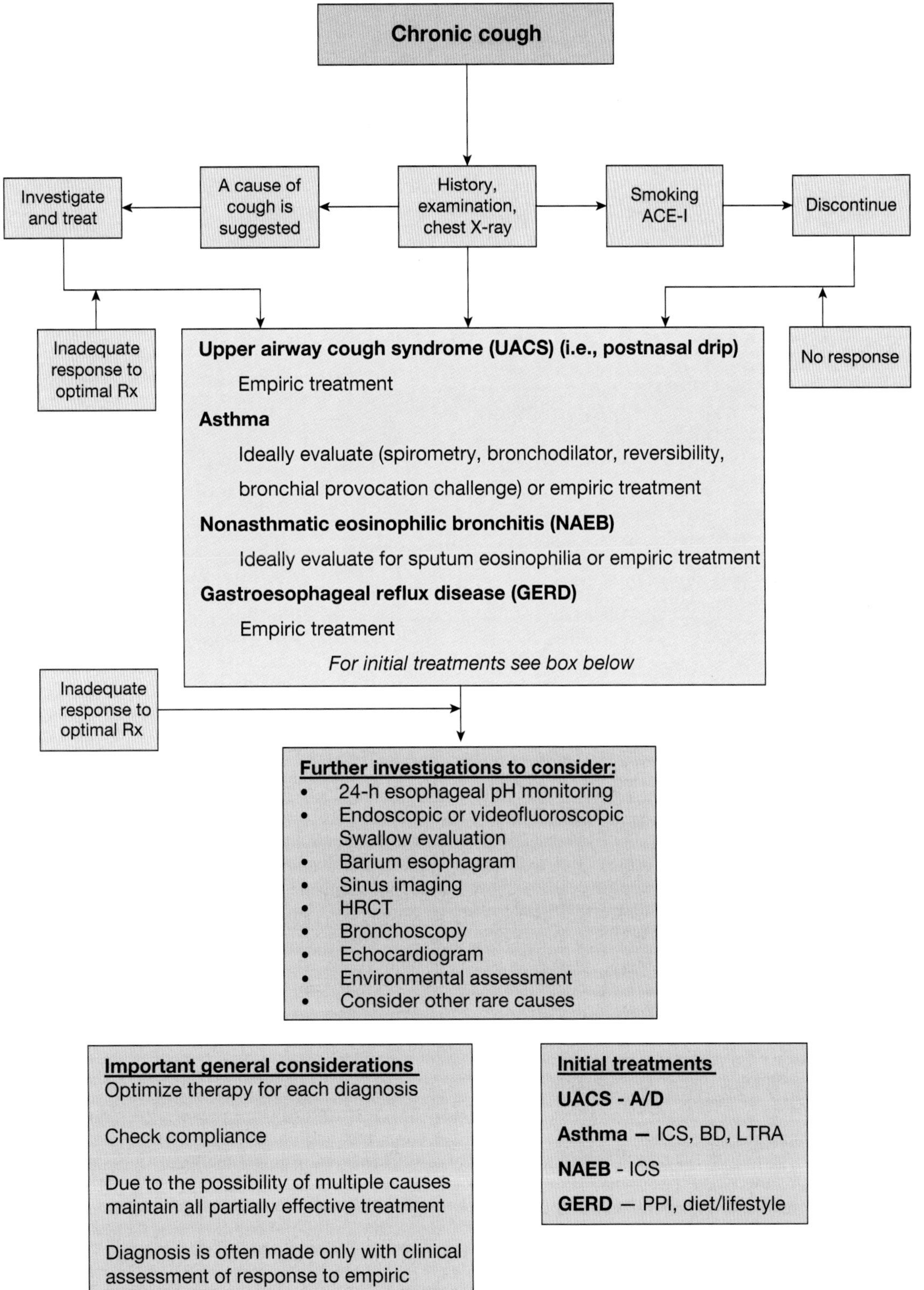

Figure 29-15 Algorithm for the evaluation of chronic cough lasting 8 weeks in adults. ACE-I, ACE inhibitor; BD, bronchodilator; LTRA, leukotrienes receptor antagonist; PPI, proton pump inhibitor; ICS, inhaled corticosteroid; A/D, antihistamine/decongestant; HRCT, high-resolution computed tomography. *(Reproduced with permission from Irwin RS, et al. Diagnosis and management of cough executive summary: ACCP evidence-based clinical practice guidelines. Chest. 2006;129 (1 Suppl):1S–23S.)*

implies a potentially life-threatening process requiring immediate evaluation and treatment.

An initial decision faced by the physician who is told that blood has been coughed up is whether to conclude that the blood is coming from the respiratory tract. Any portion of the respiratory tract can be the source of bleeding including a main bronchus, the lungs, or the nose or throat. On occasion, blood from the nose and throat is inhaled and then expectorated. As long as this possibility is kept in mind, bleeding that originates in the nose, throat, or larynx is not apt to be overlooked.

An additional consideration is distinguishing hemoptysis from hematemesis (vomited blood). Even if the blood is aspirated and then coughed up, the patient can usually tell if the blood originated in the respiratory or alimentary tract. The appearance of the bloody material also helps to distinguish between hemoptysis and hematemesis: blood that originates in the airways is usually bright red, is mixed with frothy sputum, has an alkaline pH, and contains alveolar macrophages that are laden with hemosiderin; in contrast, blood from the stomach usually is dark, has an acid pH, contains food particles, and often occurs in patients with a long history of gastric disease.

Blood arising from the bronchial arteries is more often the source of massive hemoptysis, owing to its higher perfusion pressure, than blood from the pulmonary circulation. The bronchial circulation may be the source of life-threatening bleeding, for example, in patients with bronchiectasis in whom the vessels frequently become distorted and easily ruptured. Dieulafoy's disease of the bronchus, in which there is a submucosal fistula between bronchial and pulmonary arteries, is a rare cause of massive hemoptysis.[43]

The differential diagnosis of hemoptysis includes disorders arising within the airways and the pulmonary parenchyma. Inflammatory processes (e.g., bronchitis and bronchiectasis) and neoplasms are the most common causes of blood arising within the airways. Within the pulmonary parenchyma, common causes are infections, such as tuberculosis, pneumonia, *Aspergillus*, or lung abscess. Inflammatory processes that involve the lung, such as granulomatosis with polyangiitis (formerly known as Wegner's granulomatosis) or Goodpasture syndrome, are also important causes of hemoptysis (Fig. 29-16). Bleeding may be iatrogenic, as for example, after a lung biopsy or when chemotherapy for bone marrow transplantation evokes diffuse alveolar hemorrhage. Vascular disorders, including pulmonary embolism, arteriovenous malfunctions, and mitral stenosis are also to be considered in the differential diagnosis. Unexplained hemoptysis occurs in COPD and usually is not recurrent.[44]

The causes of hemoptysis are numerous and diverse (Table 29-10). The clinical setting is usually helpful in identifying the cause. Hemoptysis before middle age usually brings to mind infections; after 40 to 45 years of age, or if there is a history of smoking, bronchogenic carcinoma heads the list. In patients left with a pulmonary cavity after pulmonary disease that has healed (e.g., tuberculosis), and in regions of the country where pulmonary fungal diseases are prevalent, a bout of hemoptysis is occasionally the first sign of the disease. In patients who have a predisposing cause, such as oral contraceptives or chronic heart failure, pulmonary embolism must be considered.

The evaluation of hemoptysis involves a careful history, physical examination, and a chest radiograph. Initial studies also include a complete blood count. The degree of anemia may influence the rapidity of further testing, and thrombocytopenia may be a contributing factor to hemoptysis. Rapid correction of anemia, thrombocytopenia, or coagulopathy with the transfusion of appropriate blood products may be required promptly depending upon the clinical status and degree of abnormality. Similarly, measurement of coagulation parameters is important. Studies of renal function and a urinalysis may be indicated when a systemic process, which causes a pulmonary-renal syndrome is a possibility. Sputum should be collected and, depending on the circumstance, microbiologic cultures and stains or cytologic examination should be performed. Depending on whether a cause is identified, and the risk factors for a serious cause of bleeding, the evaluation next involves additional studies to search for a source.

TABLE 29-10 Some Causes of Hemoptysis

Infections
Bronchitis
Tuberculosis
Fungal infections
Pneumonia
Lung abscess
Bronchiectasis
Neoplasms
Bronchogenic carcinoma
Bronchial adenoma
Cardiovascular disorders
Pulmonary infarction from thromboembolism
Mitral stenosis
Trauma
Foreign body
Hematologic/immunologic
Disorders of hemostasis
Goodpasture syndrome

Because hunting for the cause and the source of bleeding is generally uncomfortable for the patient and often expensive, the intensity of the search depends on the circumstances. For example, rarely is a search for the bleeding site needed in a patient with acute bronchitis, pneumonia, or bronchopulmonary suppuration. But as a rule, unless the cause is evident, a full-scale investigation is mandatory.

Patients with hemoptysis and a history of tobacco smoking, individuals who are more than 40 years of age, or those who experience hemoptysis that lasts for more than 1 week are at greater risk for a worrisome cause and warrant additional studies. A high-resolution computed tomography (HRCT) of the chest is usually the next step if the patient has no history of tobacco use or if the plain chest radiograph suggests a parenchymal abnormality, such as bronchiectasis or arteriovenous malformation. Patients with a history of tobacco use or other risk factors for a malignancy warrant fiberoptic bronchoscopy (Chapter 35). In practice, HRCT and bronchoscopy are often complementary for visualizing abnormalities that are not apparent on plain chest radiographs. Patients with chronic bronchitis and who are at low risk for malignancy, or in whom the chest radiograph is normal or identifies the cause of hemoptysis (e.g., pneumonia) can usually be treated initially for bronchitis with follow-up appraisals to show prompt resolution of hemoptysis. However, should hemoptysis recur, further evaluation is required.

NEOPLASMS

Nonmassive hemoptysis (<500 cc/24 h) is common in bronchogenic carcinoma; less frequently carcinoma is the cause of massive hemoptysis. The likelihood of a neoplastic cause of hemoptysis is greatly increased in a cigarette smoker. Usually a troublesome cough and vague chest pain precede and accompany the hemoptysis. For hemoptysis to occur, the lesion must communicate with the airways. Most often the bleeding is a consequence of ulceration caused by an expanding tumor; sometimes it is due to a pneumonic process or to an abscess in the lung behind an obstructive lesion. Hemoptysis

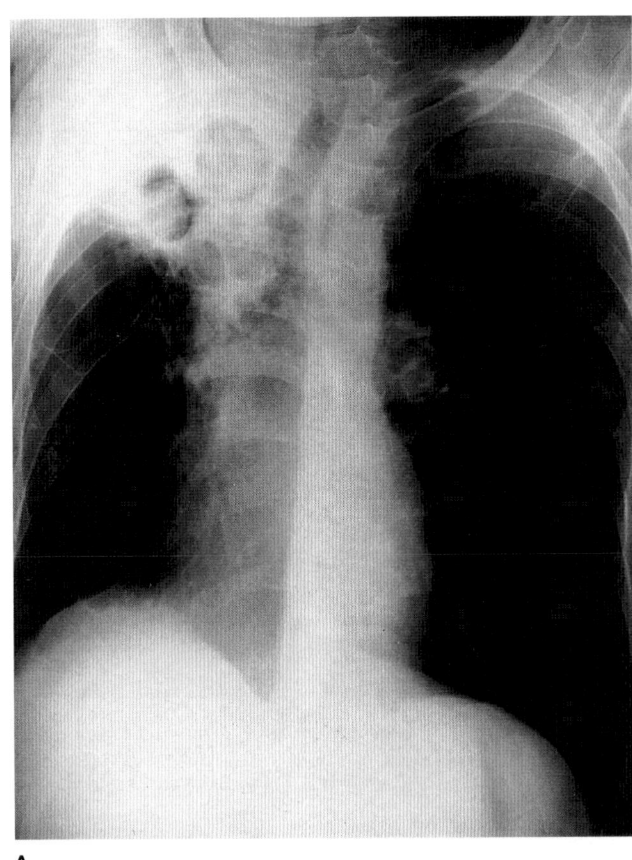

A

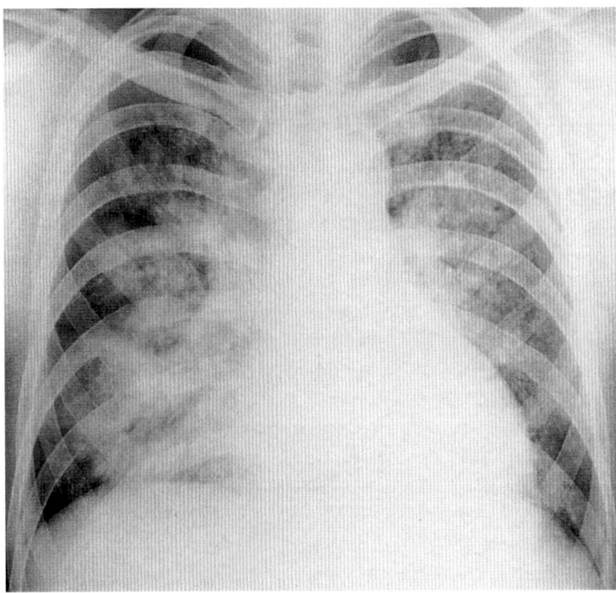

B

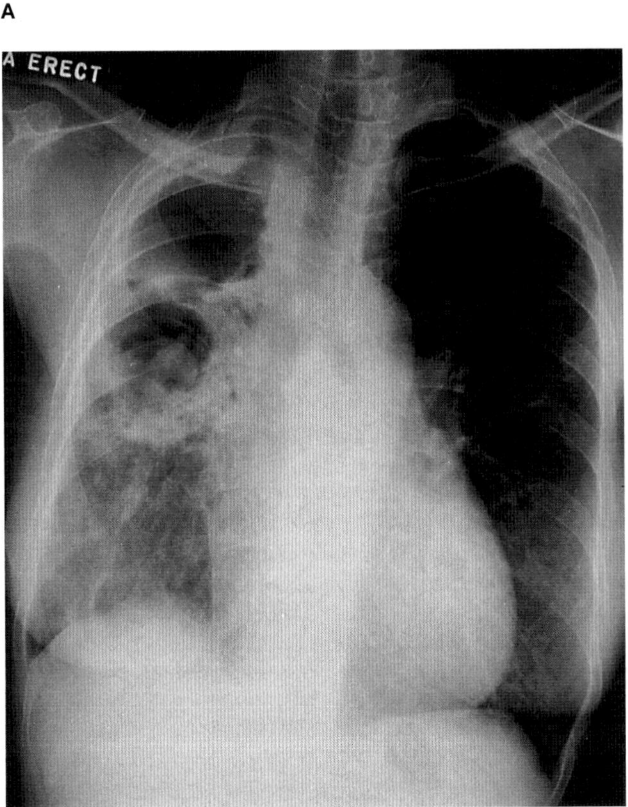

C

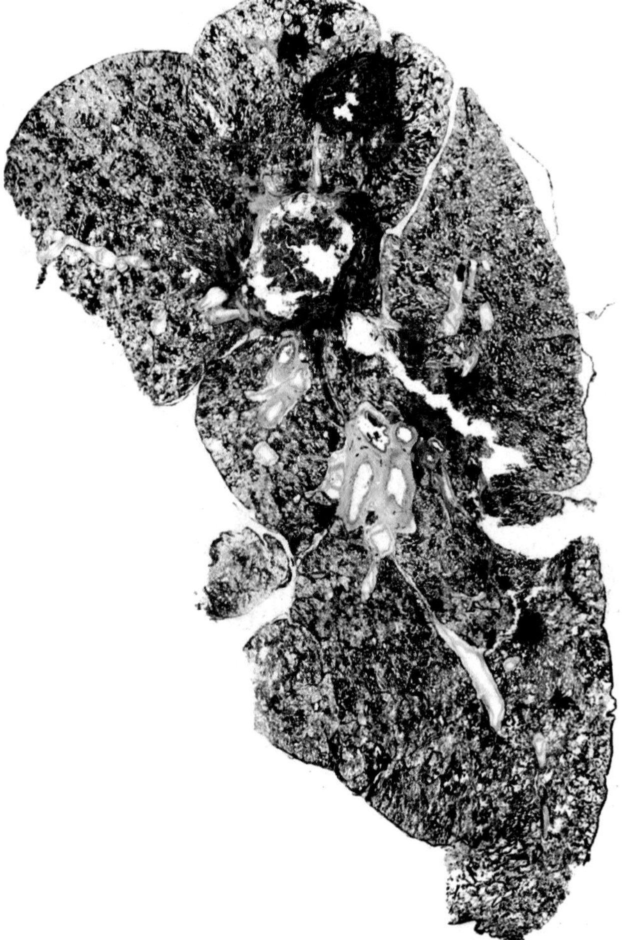

D

Figure 29-16 Causes of hemoptysis. **A.** Old tuberculosis cavities in right apex. They were removed surgically to control hemoptysis. **B.** Goodpasture syndrome. **C.** Fungus ball in coal miner's pneumoconiosis. *(Used with permission of J. Gough.)* **D.** Sagittal section of lung. Fungus ball due to aspergillosis in old tuberculosis cavity. Recurrent hemoptysis was treated with surgical removal of right upper lobe.

rarely complicates metastatic tumors of the lungs (primarily renal and colon carcinomas).

Not only malignant, but also benign, tumors of the lung cause bleeding. The classic example is bronchial carcinoid.

Hemoptysis may accompany a severe infection occurring anywhere from the top to the bottom of the respiratory tract. It is uncommon in the usual viral or bacterial pneumonia. Conversely, it is not uncommon in the pneumonia that complicates bronchogenic carcinoma or in the pneumonia that is caused by staphylococci, influenza virus, or *Klebsiella*.

The infecting organism determines the appearance and composition of the material that is expectorated with the blood. As indicated previously, in pneumococcal lobar pneumonia, the sputum at the onset is characteristically rusty-looking, but sometimes it is faintly or grossly bloody. In staphylococcal pneumonia, the blood is mixed with pus. In *Klebsiella* pneumonia, the bloody sputum may resemble currant jelly. Brisk bleeding is common in lung abscess; the blood is mixed with copious amounts of foul-smelling pus. In lung gangrene, blood is associated with necrotic lung tissue.

Bleeding is common in bronchiectasis. Because it usually originates in a bronchial artery, bleeding is often brisk. While most episodes stop spontaneously, the hemoptysis tends to recur and may be life-threatening.

Fungal infections of the lungs may cause hemoptysis (Fig. 29-16). As in tuberculosis, hemoptysis is generally a consequence of a continuing necrotizing and ulcerating inflammatory process or of bronchiectasis. The most common fungal disorder associated with hemoptysis is a "fungus ball" that resides either in a healed tuberculous or bronchiectatic area or in a cystic residue of sarcoidosis. *Aspergillus* is the usual fungal agent; less often another fungus (e.g., *Mucor*) is the cause.

At one time, the most common source of hemoptysis was an active tuberculosis cavity. Despite the increasing frequency of tuberculosis, hemoptysis is uncommon because of effective antituberculous therapy. If tuberculosis is allowed to progress to the point of extensive fibrosis and cavitation, or becomes complicated by bronchiectasis, hemoptysis can be troublesome and persistent. Hemoptysis may arise from a *Rasmussen aneurysm*, which is an erosion of a small- or medium-sized pulmonary artery into an adjacent tuberculosis cavity.

The "right middle lobe syndrome" is frequently associated with hemoptysis. It is due to a partial or complete obstruction of the right middle lobe bronchus, resulting in atelectasis or pneumonitis in the right middle lobe. The obstruction is more often caused by scarring or inflammation than by physical compression of the lumen by an enlarged lymph node. The cause is usually infectious; the infection may be tuberculosis.

In parts of the world where amebiasis is endemic, hemoptysis follows perforation into the airways of an amebic lung abscess. The sputum resembles anchovy sauce.

■ CARDIOVASCULAR DISORDERS

Pulmonary congestion and alveolar edema sometimes produce blood-tinged sputum. In chronic pulmonary congestion secondary to left ventricular failure or to mitral valve disease, alveolar macrophages in the sputum are often laden with hemosiderin ("heart failure cells"). In severe congestion and edema, the sputum is often pink and frothy. Usually there is no difficulty in recognizing that inadequate performance of the left ventricle is the cause of the bloody sputum.

Pulmonary thromboembolism may produce hemoptysis when associated with infarction (Fig. 29-17). The hemoptysis of pulmonary infarction is usually associated with pleuritic pain and, often, with a small pleural effusion because of the peripheral location of the infarct.

Tight mitral stenosis is sometimes first manifested by a bout of brisk, bright-red hemoptysis that is difficult to control. The source of the bleeding is the submucosal bronchial veins, which proliferate considerably in this disorder. Massive hemoptysis due to mitral stenosis is a medical emergency and is an indication for surgical intervention to relieve the obstruction at the mitral valve.

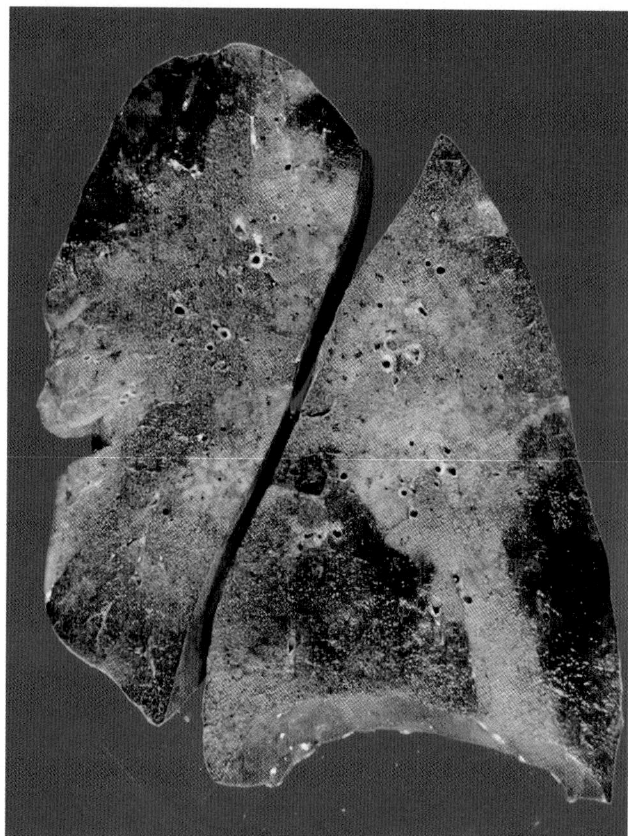

Figure 29-17 Hemorrhagic pulmonary infarcts. Several subpleural areas of infarction are clearly demarcated.

Hemoptysis from other circulatory disorders is much less common. Occasionally, an aortic aneurysm penetrates into the tracheobronchial tree, causing death by exsanguination and asphyxiation. An extraordinary event is the communication of an arteriovenous fistula with a small airway, causing bleeding that is exceedingly difficult to arrest.

■ TRAUMA

Hemoptysis follows a variety of chest injuries: puncture of a lung by a fractured rib, contusions of a lung by severe blunt trauma to the chest, and necrosis of the lining of the tracheobronchial tree by inhaled fumes or smoke. Blunt trauma from the steering wheel during an automobile collision sometimes lacerates or fractures the tracheobronchial tree. Stab or gunshot wounds often tear the lungs or airways. On occasion, mucosal lacerations in the course of severe coughing evoke hemoptysis.

After lobectomy, or now, less commonly, pneumonectomy, a large hemothorax occasionally empties into the airways. This is an alarming and ominous event. Its imminent occurrence is often heralded by the expectoration of blood-stained sputum after a paroxysm of coughing. The hemothorax must be promptly evacuated and the bronchus surgically repaired. Hemoptysis within a few weeks to months after lung resection has different implications: recurrence of tumor, granulation tissue, or bronchial sutures. Prompt bronchoscopy is necessary for accurate appraisal of the situation.

■ MISCELLANEOUS

Other causes of hemoptysis are listed in Table 29-10. They vary greatly in severity, urgency, and prognosis. Sometimes the cause is obscure, as in the occasional instance of hemoptysis that accompanies menstruation (*catamenial hemoptysis*). An aspirated foreign body produces bleeding by damaging the mucosa on impact; if allowed to remain in place, it sometimes causes bronchiectasis, which, in turn, may cause bleeding. Pulmonary calcific foci, either in the pulmonary parenchyma or in lymph nodes, sometimes cause hemoptysis by ulcerating into a bronchus.

Thrombocytopenic purpura and hemophilia and the therapeutic use of anticoagulants are occasional causes of hemoptysis.

Hemoptysis in Goodpasture syndrome (Fig. 29-16) or in idiopathic hemosiderosis is life-threatening.

■ MANAGEMENT OF MASSIVE HEMOPTYSIS

The first priority in the care of a patient with life-threatening hemoptysis is to protect the airway and prevent asphyxiation.[45] Intubation should be contemplated and consideration given to selective intubation of one lung in order to protect it from spillage of blood from the other. When the site of bleeding is known, one simple, initial bedside maneuver is to place the involved side in a dependent position in order to protect the uninvolved lung. Bronchoscopy should be performed promptly in order to identify the source (Chapters 35 and 36). This may also allow bronchoscopic interventions, such as the placement of a balloon catheter to isolate the involved segment, lavage with iced saline, or the application of topical epinephrine (1:20,000). Bronchoscopic localization may help to guide attempts at arresting the bleeding by angiographic embolization. If these modalities fail to stop the bleeding, surgical exploration may be required. Not surprisingly, emergency procedures are accompanied by a high mortality. None of the approaches has been rigorously studied, and the choice is frequently dictated by the urgency, local experience, and availability of bronchoscopy.

CYANOSIS

Cyanosis refers to a bluish discoloration of the skin that is caused by increased amounts of reduced hemoglobin in the subcapillary venous plexus. The discoloration is most apparent in the lobes of the ears, the cutaneous surfaces of the lips, and the nail beds. In patients with dark skin, the mucus membranes and the retina are important sites to examine for cyanosis. Unless flow through the skin is slowed, as in heart failure, cyanosis implies arterial hypoxemia. Cyanosis does not appear in carbon monoxide poisoning or in severe anemia, even though arterial O_2 content is extremely low. This is because there is an insufficient amount of reduced hemoglobin present for the cyanotic discoloration to be visible. The presence of abnormal pigments in blood, such as methemoglobin or bilirubin, complicates the detection of cyanosis.

■ CAPILLARY O_2 CONTENT

An increase in the amount of reduced hemoglobin in the capillaries of the skin, as elsewhere, results from inadequate oxygenation of arterial blood, excessive removal of O_2 from capillary blood (as when the circulation through a region is slowed by vasoconstriction or a very low cardiac output), or from a combination of the two. The concentration of reduced hemoglobin in the skin capillaries must reach about 5 g/dL before cyanosis becomes discernible. Thus, in severe anemia, when hemoglobin concentrations are exceedingly low (on the order of 3–4 g/dL), although virtually all the hemoglobin can be reduced in traversing the skin capillaries, an insufficient amount of reduced hemoglobin remains to produce a visible discoloration. On the other hand, the polycythemic patient develops cyanosis at a higher arterial O_2 saturation than does the normal individual.

■ CAUSES OF CYANOSIS

Several types of cyanosis are usually identified according to the underlying mechanism. They include peripheral cyanosis, cyanosis arising from pulmonary disease, cyanosis from venous admixture, and cyanosis due to abnormal pigments in the blood.

Peripheral Cyanosis

This type of cyanosis is secondary to abnormally large extraction of O_2 from blood flowing through peripheral capillaries. The most common cause is a diminished cardiac output associated with peripheral vasoconstriction. Not only the hands and feet but also the tip of the nose become blue in severe heart failure. Indeed, in patients with intractable heart failure, necrosis occasionally develops at the tip of the nose.

Peripheral vasoconstriction per se, as in Raynaud's disease, also produces cyanosis of the nail beds.

Cyanosis in Pulmonary Disease

Patients with chronic bronchitis and emphysema characteristically manifest derangements in ventilation–perfusion relationships. In some, arterial hypoxemia results. In patients with diffuse interstitial fibrosis, normal arterial oxygenation at rest is succeeded by arterial hypoxemia, and sometimes, by cyanosis, during exercise. Another cause of arterial hypoxemia is the syndrome of alveolar hypoventilation in patients with normal lungs. In any of these situations, cyanosis is intensified if heart failure supervenes and slows blood flow through the skin (i.e., is associated with decreased O_2 delivery).

Cyanosis Due to Venous Admixture

In patients with intracardiac right-to-left shunts, cyanosis arises from a mixture of venous and arterial blood. The effect of venous admixture is particularly striking if the O_2 content of mixed venous blood is inordinately low, as in some types of congenital heart disease and in severe heart failure. Often, secondary polycythemia contributes to the cyanosis. On occasion, regional cyanosis is diagnostic. For example, in patent ductus arteriosus with reversal of blood flow, the lower extremities are deeply cyanotic, whereas the upper extremities are virtually normal in color.

Cyanosis Due to Abnormal Pigments in Blood

Methemoglobinemia is an occasional cause of cyanosis. Methemoglobinemic blood is chocolate brown, and spectrophotometric examination of blood reveals the characteristic pigment. Arterial blood examination discloses a normal P_{O_2}.

The cause of methemoglobinemia may be hereditary (i.e., due to the presence of hemoglobin M or a deficiency in methemoglobin reductase) or, more often, acquired (e.g., by exposure to chemical agents such as aniline dyes, chlorates, nitrates, and nitrites); methemoglobinemia may also result from drugs, such as dapsone, nitroglycerin, phenacetin, or primaquine. Nitrates are a common cause of methemoglobinemia. Nitrates are reduced to nitrites by bacteria in the intestinal tract. Excessive use of nitroglycerin, an organic nitrate, leads to methemoglobinemia.

In methemoglobinemia, the ferrous iron is oxidized to ferric iron, rendering the hemoglobin molecule incapable of binding O_2 or CO_2. Methemoglobin is formed continuously in the normal erythrocyte, but its level within the cell is kept low (<2%) by intracellular reductive mechanisms. High levels of methemoglobin result from hereditary abnormalities (e.g., a deficiency in methemoglobin reductase) or from exposure to drugs or chemicals that increase the rate of oxidation beyond the reductive capacity of the erythrocytes. Clinical manifestations of methemoglobinemia vary with the blood levels. Concentrations of methemoglobin between 10% and 25% usually cause asymptomatic cyanosis. When these levels are exceeded, dizziness, fatigue, and headache appear.

CLUBBING

Clubbing of the digits is a classic finding in medicine that dates back to Hippocrates' awareness of the association between characteristic changes in the fingertips and empyema. Occasionally, it constitutes a valuable clue to clinically inapparent disease of the lungs and pleura. Clubbing of the fingers designates the selective bulbous enlargement of the distal segments of the digits due to an increase in soft tissue (Fig. 29-18). Although most often it is painless, clubbing remains an important finding, as its presence should signal an evaluation for potential serious causes.

When full-blown, clubbing is easy to recognize: (1) the nails, particularly the index finger, become abnormally curved in the longitudinal and coronal planes; (2) the hyponychial angle, viewed

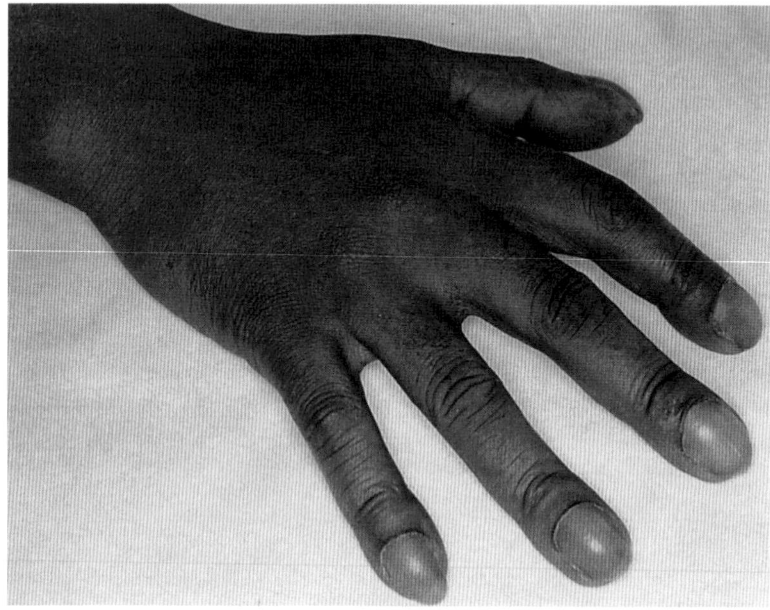

A

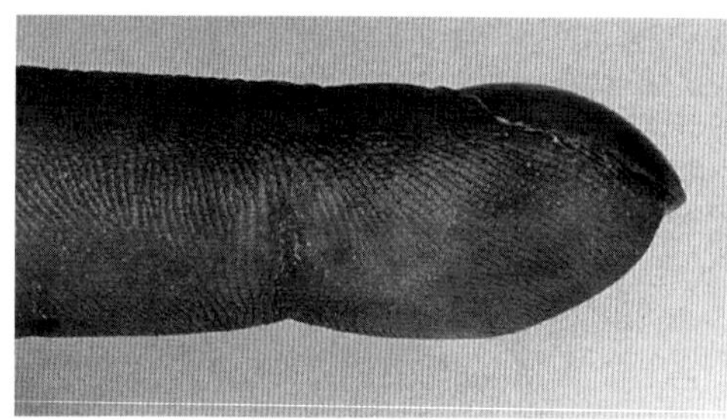

B

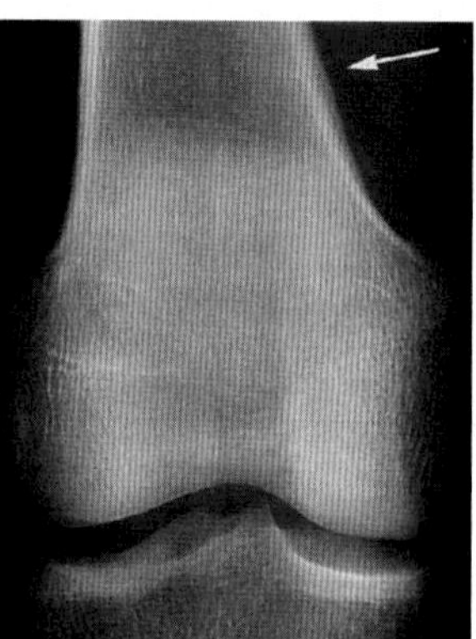

D

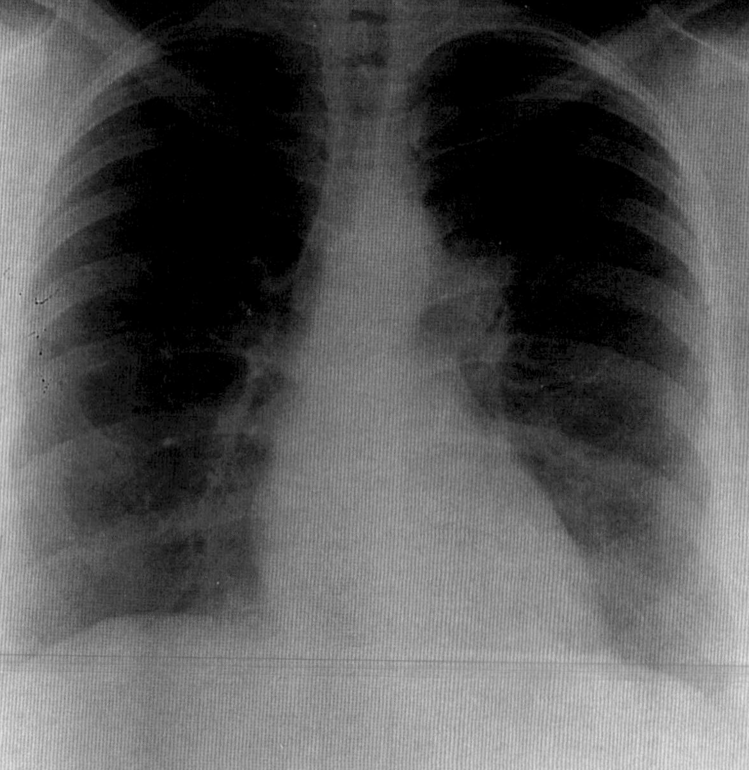

C

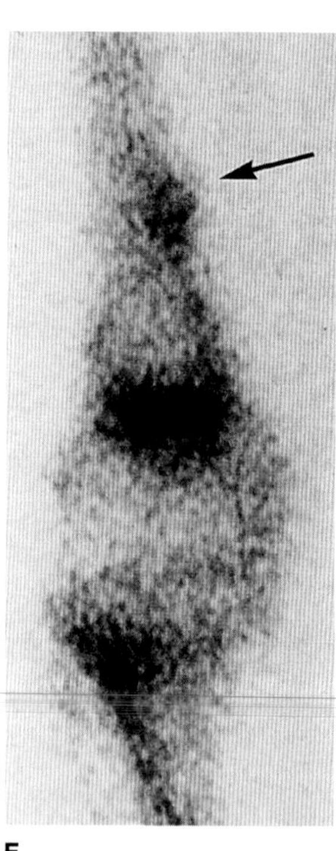

E

Figure 29-18 Clubbing of the digits and hypertrophic osteoarthropathy. A 40-year-old woman developed swelling and tingling of the fingertips in association with painful swelling of both knees. She was a heavy smoker (36 pack-years) and had an 8-month history of a dry cough. **A.** Clubbing of all fingers. **B.** Index finger. **C.** Left hilar mass that proved to be a primary adenocarcinoma of the lung. **D.** Subperiosteal formation of new bone on the medial aspect of the diaphysis of the femur. **E.** Bone scan, using ^{99m}Tc methylene diphosphonate. An abnormal accumulation of isotope is seen in the area of new bone *(arrow)*.

in profile, becomes blunted, often in conjunction with softening and sponginess of the base of the nail; and (3) the undersurface of the terminal digit becomes large and bulbous. Early stages of clubbing are subtle and generally difficult to diagnose. Clubbing often has to be distinguished from simple curvature of the nails and, occasionally, from chronic paronychia and Heberden nodes. A variety of methods have been proposed for quantifying clubbing (e.g., measuring casts of the fingertips), but none has become popular.

Clubbing is generally acquired, but it may be hereditary. Acquired clubbing is seen in a wide variety of disorders, both extrathoracic and thoracic (Table 29-1).

It is important to recognize that clubbing is not caused by all forms of chronic lung disease. COPD, for example, does not cause clubbing. The presence of clubbing in a patient with COPD should alert the clinician to the possibility of a second process, commonly lung cancer. As a rule, clubbing is bilaterally symmetrical, affecting hands and feet; on occasion, local factors, such as injury of a finger or of the median nerve, may cause clubbing that is confined to a single finger. Rarely, clubbing may be confined to the digits of one hand (e.g., in an ipsilateral pulmonary sulcus tumor that has invaded the brachial plexus or following hemiplegia). In certain types of congenital heart disease, a telltale distribution of clubbing is of considerable diagnostic value. For example, in patent ductus arteriosus associated with reversal of shunt through the ductus, clubbing affects only the toes.

■ PATHOGENESIS

The pathogenesis of clubbing is unknown, and no suitable animal model of clubbed fingers has yet been developed, largely because so few species other than primates have fingers. A common denominator in the pathogenesis of clubbing appears to be vasodilation of vessels in the fingertip, including formation of the arteriovenous connections. As a result, hydrostatic pressures increase in the capillaries and venules, promoting the transduction of fluid into the interstitium. The reason for this preferential vasodilation is unclear. A popular notion is that a humoral substance escapes normal deactivation by pulmonary capillaries. This theory could account for clubbing in cyanotic congenital heart disease, in various pulmonary diseases in which proliferation of the bronchial circulation occurs, and in hepatic cirrhosis in which pulmonary arteriovenous anastomoses and right-to-left shunts are common. However, it is difficult to relate this theory to the high incidence of clubbing in subacute bacterial endocarditis.

At present, a single hypothesis that would account for the clubbing that occurs in such diverse disorders as subacute bacterial endocarditis, carcinoma of the lung, hemiplegia, chronic mountain sickness, and purgative abuse is not possible. Indeed, it seems likely that clubbing of the digits is a stereotyped consequence of diverse influences that have in common the capacity to induce marked digital vasodilation and interstitial edema of the soft tissue.

HYPERTROPHIC OSTEOARTHROPATHY

Occasionally, clubbing of the digits is accompanied by hypertrophic osteoarthropathy (HOA), a separate clinical and radiographic entity. Clinically, HOA is manifested by pain and swelling of the soft tissues over the distal ends of the long and tubular bones. Radiographically, the distinctive feature of HOA is the formation of new bone beneath the periosteum of the distal diaphyses of the long bones of the extremities (Fig. 29-18).

The most common disorder associated with HOA is carcinoma of the lung. The incidence is about 5% and is unrelated to the cell type of the cancer, except that small cell carcinoma is rarely implicated; a peripheral carcinoma of the lung is slightly more common than a central one. Joint symptoms precede the local signs of tumor in about one-third of the cases; the interval is sometimes as long as 2 years. Pulmonary metastases rarely cause HOA. Pulmonary tuberculosis is seldom, if ever, associated with HOA. CF and idiopathic pulmonary fibrosis may be accompanied by HOA. Pregnancy may rarely be a cause of HOA, with symptoms resolving promptly with delivery.

As in the case of clubbing of the digits, theories about pathogenesis tend to focus on humoral factors generated elsewhere. However, a neurogenic theory has also been advanced on the basis of two types of observations: (1) in a few patients, vagotomy has relieved the symptoms of inoperable carcinoma of the lung and led to regression of the bony lesions; and (2) in keeping with the observations on the few patients, vagotomy in dogs is usually followed by a decrease in blood flow to the limbs.

In contrast to clubbing of the digits, which is rarely painful, HOA associated with carcinoma of the lung often causes severe rheumatic symptoms. These symptoms vanish after resection of the carcinoma, even though clubbing usually remains. In patients who are treated with radiotherapy for unresectable carcinoma, pain in the vicinity of the joints usually decreases greatly and usually does not recur even if metastases develop in the lungs or elsewhere.

CHEST PAIN

Pain in the chest is a common clinical problem. It may arise from within the thorax (the heart, pericardium, lungs, pleura, chest wall) or be referred from elsewhere (e.g., from below the diaphragm). Characteristic patterns and associations may help to clarify the source of the pain.

First thoughts about chest pain almost invariably turn to the pain of myocardial ischemia. However, cardiac pain is often distinguishable from other types of chest pain because of its viselike nature; its characteristic radiation to the left arm, shoulder, or neck; and its lack of relation to breathing. Extracardiac painful sensations can arise from various sites within the thorax, most often from the pleura, the lungs, or the chest wall. Pain may also be referred to the thorax as a result of GERD.[46–48] In the primary care setting, in stable patients it is usually possible to exclude as the basis for pain cardiac, gastrointestinal, or pulmonary diseases.[49,50]

■ PLEURITIC PAIN

The most characteristic pain associated with the respiratory apparatus is pleural pain. It originates in the parietal pleura and endothoracic fascia; the visceral pleura is insensitive to pain. In contrast to the deep, oppressive substernal pain of myocardial infarction, pleuritic pain is identified by the patient as being close to the thoracic cage. It is predominantly an inspiratory pain, reflecting the stretching of inflamed parietal pleura during movement of the thorax; coughing or laughing is distressing; the patient often clutches the chest to minimize its excursion. The pain is usually local, but sometimes it spreads along the course of the intercostal nerves that supply the affected area. Irritation of the diaphragmatic pleura by an inflammatory process either below or above the diaphragm often causes ipsilateral shoulder pain when the central portion of the diaphragm is involved; sometimes the pain is referred to the abdomen when the outer diaphragmatic pleura is irritated.

As a rule, pleural pain is part of a syndrome of pleural inflammation that includes malaise and fever; an important exception to this generalization is the pleural pain of pulmonary infarction, which is often unassociated with any premonitory signs. In addition to inflammation and malignant etiologies, pleuritic pain occurs with pneumothorax.

■ PULMONARY PAIN

A second distinctive type of respiratory chest pain accompanies a tracheitis or tracheobronchitis. The pain is searing and is most pronounced after cough. Invariably, this central chest pain is associated with evidence of upper respiratory infection. It is aggravated by cough. Cold air may be intolerable.

An uncommon type of chest pain is associated with pulmonary hypertension. It is usually absent at rest and appears during exertion.

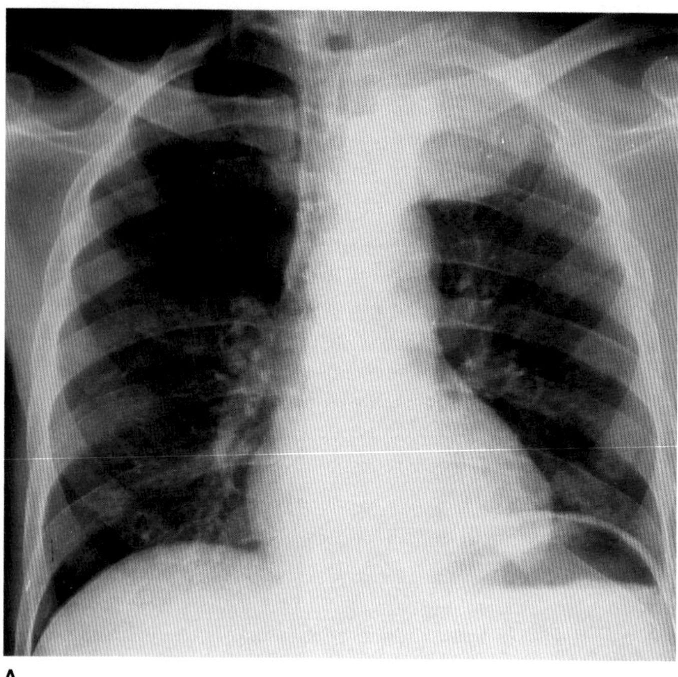

A

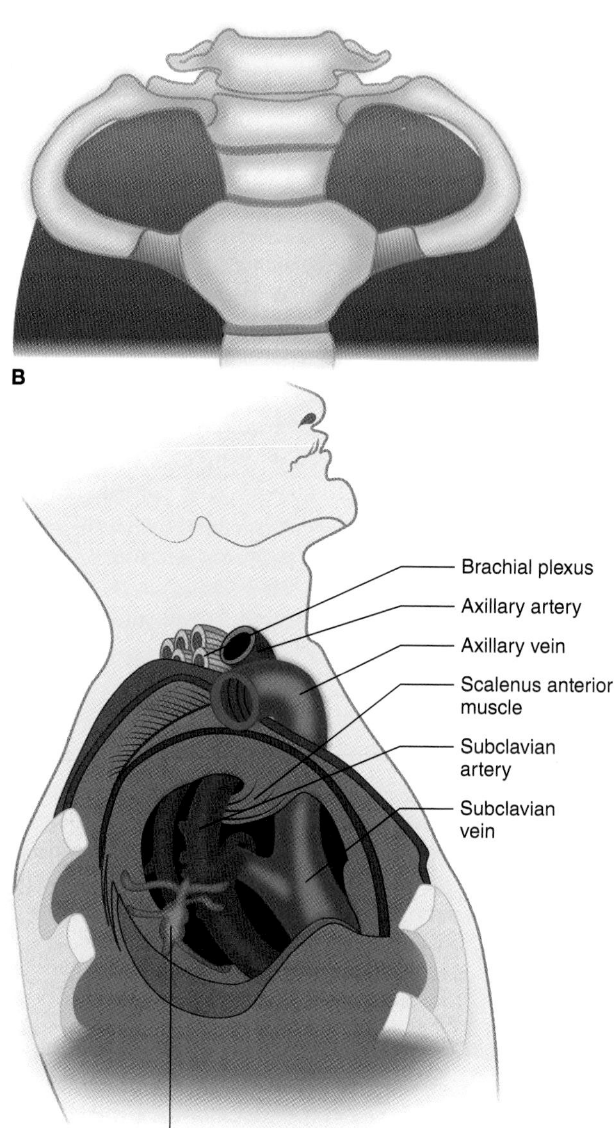

Figure 29-19 Pulmonary sulcus tumor. **A.** Chest radiograph. **B.** Relationships of apex of the lung to adjacent bony structures. **C.** Lateral view of area occupied by apex of lung, showing proximity not only to nerves of brachial plexus but also to sympathetic chain and to blood vessels. A mass that grows posteriorly and laterally can encounter sympathetic chain and bony structures; superiorly, the axillary vessels, brachial plexus, and bony structures; anteriorly, the subclavian vein and its tributaries. *(Reproduced with permission from Pernkopf. Atlas of Topographical and Applied Human Anatomy. Philadelphia, WB Saunders; 1964.)*

The pain is substernal and is associated with dyspnea; it subsides promptly when exercise stops. It is often mistaken for classic angina until the presence of pulmonary hypertension is uncovered. It may be due to right ventricular strain and ischemia.

CHEST-WALL PAIN

Musculoskeletal pain arising in the chest that is also aggravated by breathing may be confused with pleuritic pain. It is rarely severe and incapacitating, is often bilateral, and generally is intensified by changes in body position or flexing the thorax. The affected muscles are often tender to gentle pressure. A fractured rib is often identified as the source of pain by a history of a fall, injury, or trauma. Additional clues are point tenderness and crepitus of the affected area, reproduction of the pain upon manual compression of the chest, or radiographic evidence of a broken rib.

The pain of a pulmonary sulcus tumor, or "Pancoast tumor," (Fig. 29-19) is quite distinctive. This unusual location of a carcinoma of the lung was originally described by Pancoast in 1932. Pain due to the tumor occurs along the distribution of the eighth cervical and first and second thoracic nerves. In addition, Horner syndrome, local destruction of bone by the tumor, and atrophy of hand muscles may be observed. The chest radiograph is distinctive in showing a small, sharply defined shadow at one apex. Destruction of one or more of the upper three ribs posteriorly and of their adjacent transverse processes may also be seen.

CARDIAC PAIN

Attention was called above to the pain of myocardial ischemia. Another type of cardiac pain is that of pericarditis. Pericardial pain is often aggravated by deep breathing and, almost invariably, is accompanied by a telltale rub that is synchronous with the heartbeat. The discomfort may be relieved by leaning forward.

The *postcommissurotomy* or *postpericardiotomy syndrome* is characterized by chest pain that develops within a few days to weeks after cardiac surgery or pericardiotomy. The pain is usually sudden in onset and substernal, with radiation to the left side of the neck; often it is aggravated by deep breathing. Low-grade fever and a high erythrocyte sedimentation rate are regular concomitants.

Chest pain may also be troublesome in patients who have undergone cardiac transplantation. The diagnosis is usually self-evident when account is taken of the antecedent history of cardiac surgery. Indeed, confusion is more apt to arise with the pain of myocardial infarction than with respiratory causes of chest pain.

■ MISCELLANEOUS CAUSES OF PAIN

Other structures in the mediastinum may be the source of chest pain. Noteworthy are the types of pain arising from the esophagus (peptic esophagitis) and dissection of the aorta. Their patterns and intensity help to distinguish them from respiratory pain. Esophageal disease is typically accompanied by a burning pain, frequently after eating. Acid reflux may worsen with recumbency. Aortic dissection is often described with a sharp, tearing sensation of acute onset, with radiation to the shoulder; these are often signs of impending cardiovascular collapse.

Arthritis of the cervical spine is a common cause of thoracic pain. Usually the cause is quite clear because of the characteristic distribution of the pain. Cervical spondylosis occasionally causes severe pain in the chest and arms, but it is more apt to mimic myocardial infarction than is respiratory pain. A metastatic tumor to the thoracic spine often causes bilateral symmetric pain; there is often discomfort to palpation over the affected area. Unilateral pain, along the distribution of an intercostal nerve, is characteristic of herpes zoster before the appearance of the skin eruption and is often described as an intense burning sensation.

Anxiety may produce or intensify chest pain. Usually, pain related to anxiety is accompanied by dyspnea and hyperventilation. Manifestations of vasomotor instability, such as excessive palmar sweating, flushing, and tachycardia, may accompany the complaint of chest pain due to anxiety. Rarely does the pain conform to a characteristic or consistent pattern. Anxiety also interferes with the quantification of pain originating in a somatic lesion and with its management.

FEVER

In the patient with lung disease, fever usually, but not invariably, signifies infection. When the lung disease is chronic, as in bronchitis and emphysema, a bout of acute bronchitis usually elicits only a modest fever, even though the sputum turns purulent. In contrast, an acute pneumonia or lung abscess may be associated with high fever.

The possibility that fever is due to infection lends urgency to the situation. The wide range of pulmonary infections is considered elsewhere in this book. Often overlooked at the outset is miliary tuberculosis, which occasionally escapes detection on the initial chest radiograph. Favoring this diagnosis is a history of recent contact with a patient with active tuberculosis, general malaise, easy fatigability, and anorexia during the previous few weeks. This insidious onset differs strikingly from the more sudden onset of acute pneumonia.

Neoplasms are also associated with fever. In certain neoplasms, such as carcinoma within a bronchus, the fever is generally a secondary effect attributable to infection distal to obstruction; necrosis within the tumor is a less common cause. In others, such as hypernephroma, fever and chills are striking, even though evidence of infection is absent. A mesothelioma of the pleura is often associated with fever. Presumably, in patients with neoplasms who have no evidence of infection, necrosis within the tumor leads to the elaboration of fever-producing factors within and around the tumor.

Acute hypersensitivity pneumonitis (extrinsic allergic alveolitis) is sometimes accompanied by fever.

In contrast to the pulmonary disorders in which fever is a characteristic feature, pulmonary sarcoidosis is uncommonly associated with fever unless there is extrapulmonary involvement, such as lymphadenopathy or EN. Nor is pneumoconiosis associated with fever unless complicated by necrosis in the midst of conglomerate fibrosis or by superimposed tuberculosis. Among the other many disorders of the lungs that cause no fever (and few systemic complaints) are idiopathic pulmonary fibrosis, lymphangitic carcinomatosis, multiple pulmonary metastases, alveolar proteinosis, idiopathic pulmonary hemosiderosis, and alveolar microlithiasis.

PULMONARY-CUTANEOUS SYNDROMES

Examination of the skin may provide important clues in the diagnosis and treatment of patients with pulmonary disease. Some skin lesions either accompany pulmonary disease or complicate its treatment; occasionally, systemic diseases that affect both skin and lung first manifest themselves in the skin.

This section focuses on processes in which there is prominence of cutaneous manifestations that might impact the care of the patient with pulmonary disease. The diagnosis and development of a differential diagnosis of cutaneous lesions is beyond the scope of this chapter and can be found in general dermatology textbooks.[51-53]

■ ATOPIC DERMATITIS

Atopy refers to a group of disorders, including asthma, allergic rhinitis, and atopic dermatitis, in which immune and pharmacologic responses are abnormal. The atopic person usually has a family history of one or more of these disorders. Atopic dermatitis is a common disorder, affecting 1% to 3% of the population in the United States. In 85% of affected subjects, the skin lesions appear before 5 years of age.[54] The dermatitis may resolve as the patient reaches adulthood; in the adult, either the skin lesions or respiratory systems may predominate although there is a wide range of individual variability.

In infants, the skin lesions often begin as dry, erythematous plaques on the cheeks; excoriations and scaling may be prominent. In older children, the lesions localize in flexures; lichenification and excoriated papules are prominent features (Fig. 29-20). In adults, the lesions favor the hands and extremities. Atopic subjects also manifest prominent folds of the lower eyelids, periorbital hyperpigmentation with facial pallor, generalized dry skin, and white dermatographism. At any age, pruritus may be prominent, leading to secondary bacterial infection (bacterial impetigo) within the lesions.

The cause of atopic dermatitis is unknown. In all likelihood, the pathogenesis is multifactorial, probably including disordered immune regulation as a causative factor. Patients with atopic dermatitis often have elevated levels of IgE; may have abnormalities of CD30, macrophage-derived chemoattractant, interleukins (IL)-12, -16, -18, and -31, and thymus and activation-regulated chemokine; and have mutations of the filaggrin gene. The use of any of these biomarkers has not yet been demonstrated to be diagnostic or of prognostic value.[54] In persons with atopic dermatitis, abnormalities in cell-mediated immunity and lymphocyte function increase the risk of disseminated viral disease, particularly herpes simplex. The role of food or environmental antigenic challenge in flares of atopic dermatitis is unsettled, but it is known that asthma can be precipitated by such challenges.

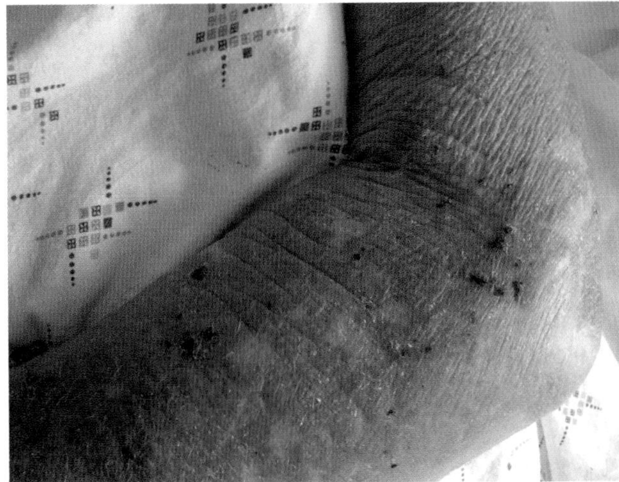

Figure 29-20 Atopic dermatitis is characterized by lichenification, excoriations, and slight scale.

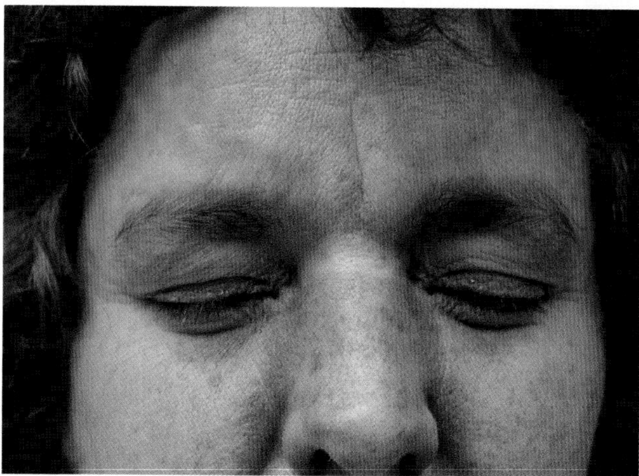

Figure 29-21 Heliotrope eruption of dermatomyositis.

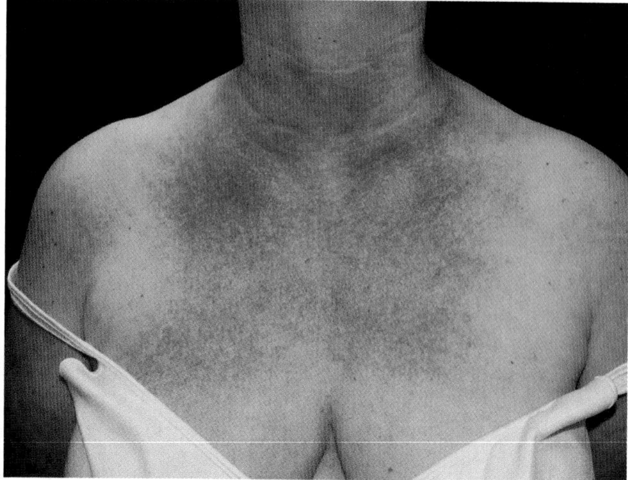

Figure 29-23 Photodistributed poikiloderma in a patient with dermatomyositis.

The relationship between atopic dermatitis and lung disease is imperfect. Although hyposensitization is useful for asthma, it is either not helpful or is detrimental in atopic dermatitis. In addition, the use of omalizumab, while beneficial for asthma, has demonstrated mixed results for patients with atopic dermatitis. Recent evidence suggests that the use of dupilumab, an IL-4, IL-13 antagonist might be useful for atopic dermatitis, as well as for the associated asthma[55]

■ COLLAGEN VASCULAR DISORDERS

Common collagen vascular disorders warrant discussion in relation to possible coexisting pulmonary manifestations, especially dermatomyositis (DM) and scleroderma.

■ DERMATOMYOSITIS

DM is an idiopathic inflammatory myopathy characterized by proximal, symmetrical, slowly progressive muscle weakness, and characteristic cutaneous lesions.[56,57] The pathognomonic skin lesions include a heliotrope eruption, which consists of erythematous-to-violaceous periorbital changes that may be accompanied by edema (Fig. 29-21), and Gottron papules, which consist of erythematous papules over the bony prominences on the dorsal hands (Fig. 29-22). Patients may also manifest a photodistributed poikiloderma (Fig. 29-23), nail-fold changes, and an erythematous-to-violaceous scaly alopecia. Patients with DM frequently complain of marked itching.

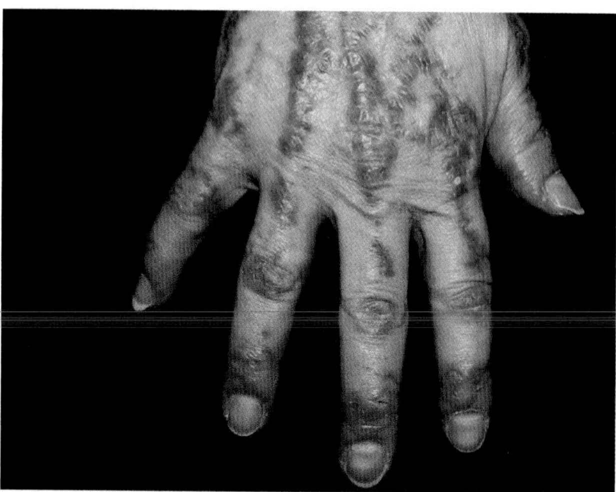

Figure 29-22 Gottron papules in dermatomyositis: Erythematous to violaceous lesions are most prominent over the joints. In addition, this patient demonstrates cuticular and periungual changes that are frequent in dermatomyositis.

Patients with DM may also have other systemic manifestations, including arthritis, esophageal disease, and cardiopulmonary disease; some have a malignancy. Others with the characteristic cutaneous lesions of DM are not weak and do not have an increase in muscle-derived enzymes. These patients are said to have amyopathic dermatomyositis if they have skin lesions with normal strength, and normal muscle-derived enzyme assessments for a period of 2 or more years without having been treated with systemic immunosuppressives or corticosteroids for more than a month.

Pulmonary disease occurs in classic dermatomyositis and in amyopathic dermatomyositis in approximately 15% to 65% of patients. Interstitial pneumonitis is a primary process in DM/polymyositis. Interstitial lung disease also occurs in patients with amyopathic dermatomyositis; in this subset of patients, survival is poor.

Pulmonary involvement is more frequent in patients with esophageal dysfunction. Lung disease may also occur as a direct complication of the muscle disease, for example, hypoventilation or aspiration in patients with dysphagia, or may be a result of treatment, such as opportunistic infections or drug-induced hypersensitivity pneumonitis.

Pulmonary disease appears to be more prominent in patients in southeast Asia, China, and Japan; however, there are many reports of patients in the United States with varying ethnicities who have developed pulmonary disease, particularly interstitial fibrosis, as well as rapidly progressive and, at times, fatal disease.[58] Patients with polymyositis and lung disease tend to have antisynthetase antibodies, particularly the Jo-1 antibody. However, Jo-1 is rarely found in patients with dermatomyositis. Recently, the anti-melanoma-differentiation gene 5 antibodies appeare to be associated with an increased risk of pulmonary disease.

Treatment of interstitial lung disease in patients with dermatomyositis is often difficult. Several recent studies have suggested that Mycophenolate mofetil is useful for these patients.[59,60]

■ SCLERODERMA

Scleroderma refers to hard skin. This process may be localized to the skin or may be part of a systemic disease.[61,62] Localized cutaneous scleroderma may occur as limited plaques of morphea, generalized morphea, deep morphea, or linear scleroderma. Interstitial pneumonitis is a rare complication of morphea or linear scleroderma.

Two principal forms of progressive systemic sclerosis (PSS) have been described: limited scleroderma (acrosclerosis) and diffuse scleroderma. Acrosclerosis is the more common of the two and is characterized by sclerosis of the skin of the fingers (sclerodactyly) (Fig. 29-24) and Raynaud's phenomenon (Fig. 29-25).

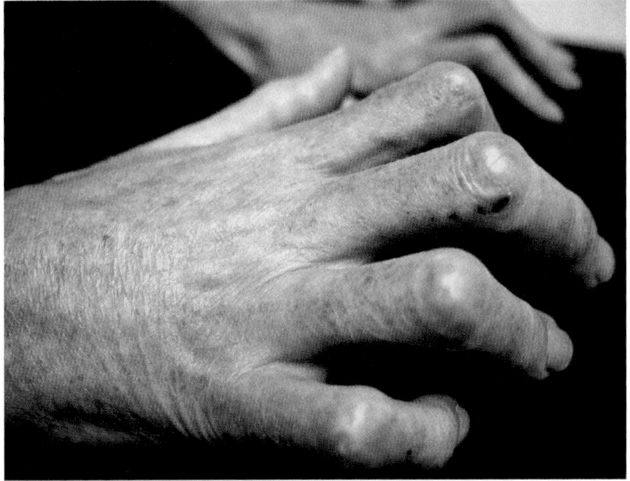

Figure 29-24 Acrosclerosis characterized by marked contractures and sclerodactyly.

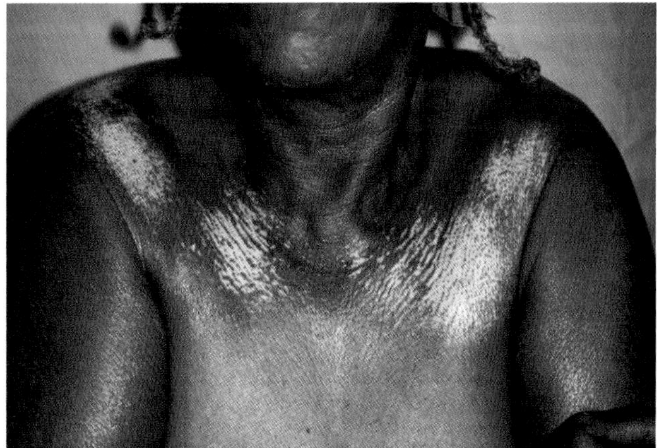

Figure 29-26 Vitiligo-like dyspigmentation associated with progressive systemic sclerosis.

A variant (CREST syndrome) includes calcinosis, Raynaud's syndrome, esophageal dysmotility, sclerodactyly, and telangiectasia.

In contrast, patients with diffuse scleroderma have widespread sclerosis beyond the acral areas of sclerodactyly. The prognosis for diffuse scleroderma is much worse than for acrosclerosis. Both types of scleroderma are often preceded by Raynaud's phenomenon, diffuse arthralgias, or arthritis. The skin manifestations begin with transient, recurrent swelling of the hands, and progress to tapered fingers with shiny, hidebound skin (sclerodactyly). The feet, chest, face, and scalp are often involved in the sclerotic process. In time, the skin becomes taut, leading to contractures of the large and small joints that culminate in a claw-like deformity of the hand.

A variety of pigmentary disturbances may occur in scleroderma, including generalized hyperpigmentation that resembles adrenal insufficiency, focal hyperpigmentation or hypopigmentation, and areas of perifollicular pigmentation that resemble vitiligo (Fig. 29-26). Raynaud's phenomenon leads to small pitted scars at the fingertips or frank ulceration, with or without gangrene of the fingertips, toes, knuckles, and ankles, especially the malleoli.

The face often undergoes distinctive changes, leading to a fixed stare and inability to wrinkle the forehead. As the facial tissues shrink, the nose becomes pinched, the cheeks sunken, the mouth narrowed, and the lips thinned. In diffuse scleroderma, cutaneous sclerosis, accompanied by a yellowish-brown hue, spreads from the chest to the head and extremities. Sharply delineated, broad telangiectatic macules appear on the face, buccal mucosa, lips, and hands.

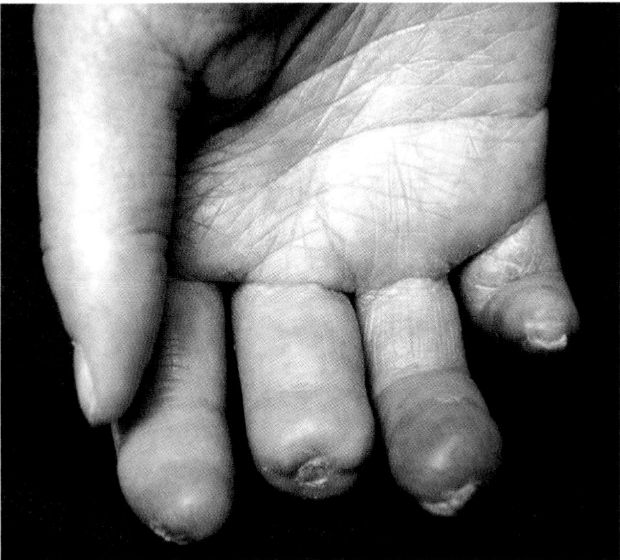

Figure 29-25 Raynaud's phenomenon in this patient was so severe that autoamputation of the distal digits occurred.

PSS is associated with interstitial pneumonitis. This is more common in patients with diffuse disease than in patients with limited disease. Pulmonary hypertension has been reported to occur in patients with CREST syndrome (see Chapter 72).

■ INFECTIONS

A variety of infections involving the lungs may have cutaneous involvement.[63] Prototypical examples are described below.

Blastomycosis

Skin lesions are as common as pulmonary lesions in patients with blastomycosis. Cutaneous disease usually represents dissemination from a pulmonary focus that is often small and may be inapparent. The typical presentation is as a solitary nodule or multiple papules or nodules on the face, wrists, hands, or feet, which subsequently ulcerate and discharge pus (Fig. 29-27). The lesions grow eccentrically at the periphery and atrophy centrally over a period of months, eventually forming an arciform or serpiginous contour with sharply elevated and verrucous borders. Miliary abscesses occur along the borders of the lesions. In addition to the cutaneous involvement, osteolytic lesions may occur.

Coccidioidomycosis

Coccidioidomycosis is usually manifest as a pulmonary infection. In its acute form, it is often associated with cutaneous symptoms; roughly 20% of patients develop erythema nodosum (EN). EN is often accompanied by fever, arthritis, and eosinophilia. In patients with progressive pulmonary disease and eventual disseminated disease, the skin may be affected; subcutaneous granulomatous eruptions form and undergo necrosis and ulceration. After several months, the lesions tend to become verrucous. A third form is primary cutaneous disease, which occurs in farmers and laboratory workers as a chancriform lesion with sporotrichotic spread. This variant is extremely rare.

Actinomycosis

The thoracic form of this disease presents as a pulmonary parenchymal process that sometimes forms multiple draining sinus tracts.[64] Diagnosis is often difficult, but identification of sulfur granules in the draining exudates is helpful.

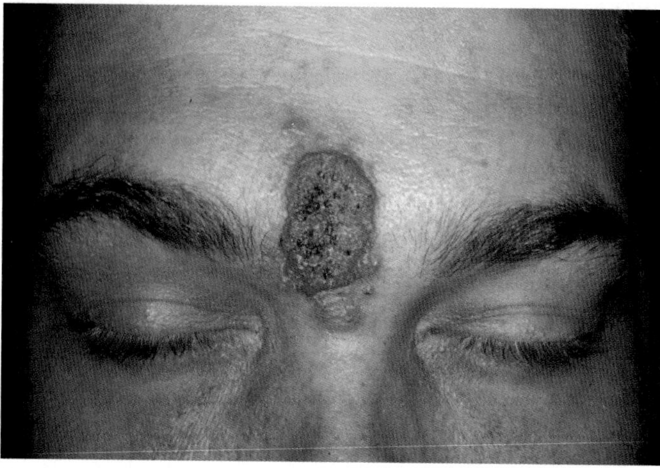

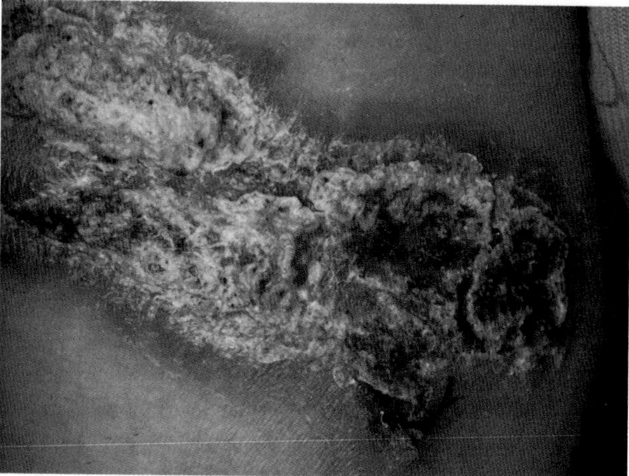

Figure 29-27 **A, B.** Blastomycosis: verrucous lesions on the face (**A**) and trunk (**B**).

Tuberculosis

Cutaneous involvement results from direct inoculation with the tubercle bacillus via either the skin or mucus membranes, or as a consequence of widespread organ involvement that begins in the respiratory tract.

When the tubercle is introduced via the skin or mucus membranes by a contaminated syringe or a wound in a previously unexposed host, a nodule usually develops at the site of injury. Within several weeks, the nodule evolves into a chancre, a well-circumscribed ulcer. Particularly if host defenses are impaired, these chancriform lesions, which are typically located on the extremities, develop associated regional lymphadenitis, followed by systemic dissemination of the organism.

A person who was previously infected with *Mycobacterium tuberculosis* is apt to develop *tuberculosis verrucosa cutis* after receiving a cutaneous inoculation. The characteristic lesion in a sensitized person is a papule or a pustule, which becomes verrucous. On occasion, this disorder produces plaque-like lesions of the extremities, consisting of verrucoid–indurated papules surrounded by an erythematous halo.

Lupus vulgaris is the most common form of cutaneous postprimary tuberculosis that follows inoculation or lymphatic or hematogenous spread of *M. tuberculosis.*[65] Patients with this disorder typically present with reddish-brown plaques surrounded peripherally by yellowish nodules, especially on the neck or extremities. The skin lesions tend to spread centrifugally as the center becomes atrophic. Papillary growths also occur in the nasal, buccal, and conjunctival mucosa. Histologically, lupus vulgaris generally shows epithelioid tubercles with caseation necrosis. Chronic cutaneous eruptions tend to involute, leaving considerable scarring. Treatment with antituberculosis drugs is effective in treating these skin manifestations.

Disseminated miliary tuberculosis may result in macules, papules, or vesicles. In children, especially those who are debilitated, subcutaneous nodules or gummas appear, ulcerate, and eventually develop draining sinus tracts, especially in the extremities and trunk. *Scrofuloderma,* which occurs following the necrosis of cervical nodules, is associated with fistula and sinus tract formation in the overlying cutaneous tissues.

Tuberculids are skin lesions that are considered to represent either a hypersensitivity reaction to *M. tuberculosis* or an embolic response to atypical *Mycobacteria.* EN also occurs in association with primary tuberculosis.

HIV Infection

Early in the epidemic of HIV infection, the incidence of Kaposi's sarcoma (KS) increased. However, since the advent of HAART therapy, KS has become less common.[66,67] KS can occur in any immune-suppressed individual, whether the immune dysfunction is due to HIV infection, age, or iatrogenic immunosuppression in transplant recipients.

Human herpesvirus-8 (HHV-8) has been identified and linked to all forms of KS. In addition, HHV-8 viremia is associated with progression on KS in both classic and endemic forms. In the elderly population, KS has an indolent course and occurs primarily on the lower extremities. At the outset, the lesions are dark-blue, purplish, or reddish papules, macules, and nodules (Fig. 29-28). After months to years, plaques evolve in association with thickening of the skin from midtibia to ankle and lymphedema. In patients with immune dysfunction, including AIDS, KS is more aggressive and is often widespread in its cutaneous manifestations.

The respiratory tract is second only to the gastrointestinal tract in frequency of systemic involvement. Tumors may involve the larynx, trachea, bronchi, pulmonary parenchyma, and pleura. Accordingly, local manifestations of respiratory tract involvement range from hoarseness, signs of airway obstruction, cough, and hemoptysis, to dyspnea. When the parenchyma of the lung is affected, chest radiographs usually show many small nodules; occasionally, parenchymal infiltration of the lung is massive. On bronchoscopic examination, bronchial and tracheal lesions appear as small bluish nodules. Bloody pleural effusions are rare.

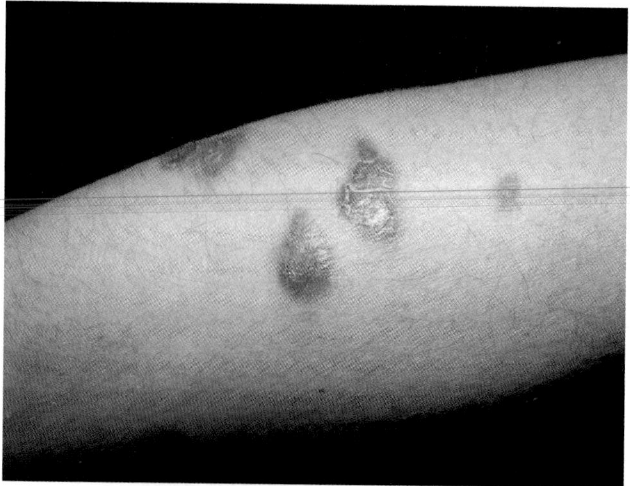

Figure 29-28 Kaposi's sarcoma in an HIV-positive patient.

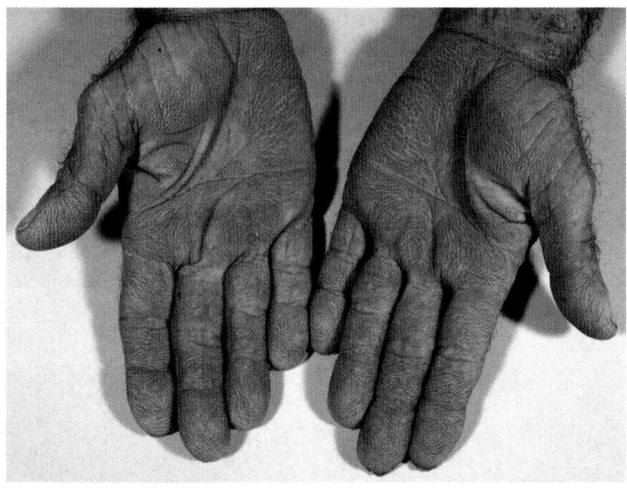

Figure 29-29 Tripe palms. *(Used with permission of Dr. Jon Dyer.)*

LUNG CANCER

Several paraneoplastic syndromes may occur in patients with lung cancer.[68] In most instances the dermatosis is not specific for lung cancer; other sites may be involved. The following are some of the more ominous manifestations of potential pulmonary malignancy.

Tripe palms is a paraneoplastic condition that is manifest as rugose thickening of the palms and, occasionally, the soles (Fig. 29-29).[69] Patients often have coexistent acanthosis nigricans (AN). Patients with tripe palms and AN usually have adenocarcinomas of the gastrointestinal tract; however, when tripe palms occur in the absence of AN, patients often have squamous cell carcinoma of the lung.

Patients with *Bazex syndrome (acrokeratosis paraneoplastica)* develop an erythematous-to-violaceous psoriasiform eruption primarily on acral surfaces.[70] (Fig. 29-30). The ears, nose, cheeks, hands, feet, and knees are most often affected, but the nails may become dystrophic, and the palms and soles may develop a keratoderma in later stages of the disease. The disorder may develop in stages, and is associated primarily with carcinomas of the upper respiratory and digestive tracts (larynx, pharynx, trachea, bronchus, and/or upper esophagus); the malignancy is often detected concurrently. If the tumor is effectively treated the eruption may resolve, but it may return with tumor recurrence.

Ectopic ACTH-producing tumors cause many of the typical signs and symptoms of Cushing syndrome. Intense hyperpigmentation, present in only 6% to 10% of patients with Cushing disease, is especially common in association with ectopic ACTH production and should alert the clinician to the possibility of a hormone-secreting tumor. Although the cause of the hyperpigmentation is unclear, it may be related to tumor production of the peptide β-lipotropin, which contains within its sequence of 91 amino acids the 22–amino acid sequence of β-MSH. A myasthenia gravis–like syndrome, including profound proximal muscle weakness, may be a striking clinical feature and may reflect either underlying hypokalemia or polymyositis. Small cell carcinoma of the lung is the tumor most often associated with ectopic ACTH production, although other malignancies have been reported.

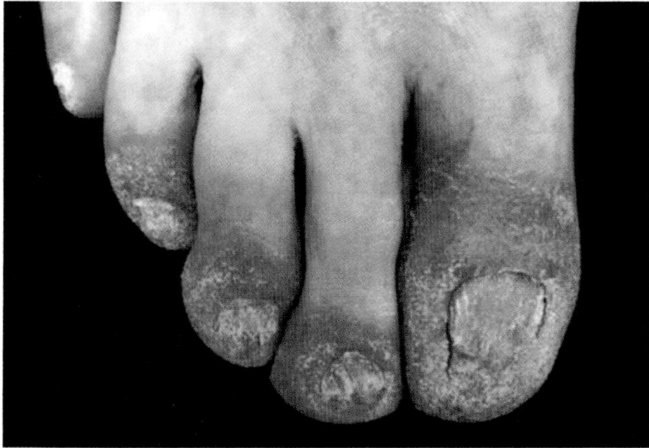

Figure 29-30 Acrokeratosis paraneoplastica (Bazex syndrome). This patient was thought to have psoriasis prior to the diagnosis of a squamous cell carcinoma of the tonsillar pillar.

The *carcinoid syndrome* is another example of a hormonal syndrome associated with a nonendocrine tumor. The disorder is probably most often caused by the release of the enzyme kallikrein from tumor cells, with subsequent conversion of kininogen to vasoactive kinin peptides, including bradykinin; in addition, increased blood levels of histamine may be important in the rare metastatic gastric carcinoid. The most striking cutaneous manifestations are episodes of flushing, initially lasting 10 to 30 minutes and involving only the upper half of the body; as the flush resolves, gyrate and serpiginous patterns may be noted. With successive attacks more extensive areas may be affected and the redness takes on a cyanotic quality, eventually leading to a more permanent facial cyanotic flush with associated telangiectasia, resembling rosacea. Persistent edema and erythema of the face may result in leonine facies. A pellagra-like picture, which has been noted in some patients, may be due to abnormal tryptophan metabolism. Systemic symptoms associated with the cutaneous flushing include abdominal pain with explosive watery diarrhea, shortness of breath, and hypertension.

Carcinoid tumors are usually found in the appendix or small intestine; extraintestinal carcinoid tumors may arise in the bile ducts, pancreas, stomach, ovaries, or bronchi.[71] The carcinoid syndrome occurs primarily when an intestinal carcinoid tumor metastasizes to the liver or with extraintestinal tumors; flushing attacks can be provoked by palpation of hepatic or abdominal metastases or by alcohol ingestion, enemas, emotional stress, or sudden changes in body temperature. When the syndrome is associated with bronchial adenomas of the carcinoid variety, the flushing is more prolonged and often associated with fever, marked anxiety, disorientation, sweating, salivation, and lacrimation.

Migratory superficial thrombophlebitis and multiple deep venous thromboses have been noted in patients with cancer, especially those with tumors arising in the pancreas, lung, stomach, prostate, or hematopoietic system. The neck, chest, abdominal wall, pelvis, and limbs are most frequently affected.

LYMPHOMATOID GRANULOMATOSIS

Lymphomatoid granulomatosis is classified as a B cell lymphoproliferative disorder of uncertain malignant potential. It has been associated with Epstein–Barr Virus infection and may occur more frequently in patients with immunologic diseases undergoing therapy with immunosuppressive agents, particularly thiopurines and methotrexate. The skin is the most commonly affected extrapulmonary site, occurring in 40% to 50% of patients.[72]

In 10% to 25% of patients, the skin lesions are the first clinical evidence of the disorder; the skin lesions precede involvement of the lungs by 2 weeks to 9 years. Because of the frequent occurrence of skin lesions, ease of performing a skin biopsy, and characteristic histology of the disease, careful dermatologic examination should be carried out in patients suspected of having lymphomatoid granulomatosis.

The characteristic cutaneous lesions are 1- to 4-cm erythematous-to-purplish dermal papules, or subcutaneous nodules, with or without ulceration.[73]

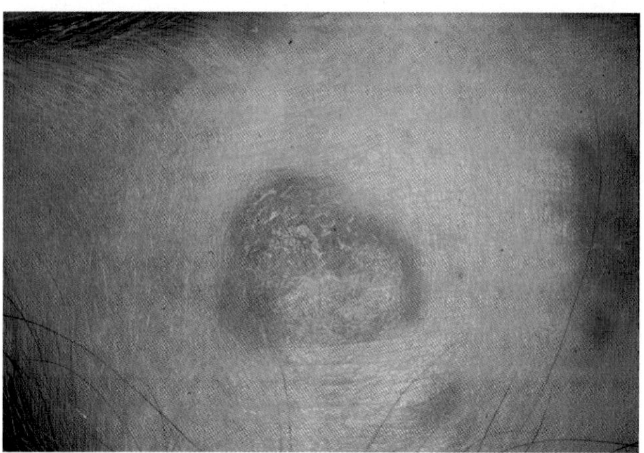

Figure 29-31 Lymphomatoid granulomatosis. This young woman developed the acute onset of multiple erythematous plaques on her face, accompanied by dyspnea and fever. She died within a month from pulmonary disease.

The lesions generally occur over the buttocks, thighs, and lower extremities (Fig. 29-31), but they may occur anywhere. Healing is often accompanied by scarring and hyperpigmentation.

The skin histopathology is similar to that observed in the lungs and is characterized by a marked angiocentric and angiodestructive lymphohistiocytic infiltrate composed predominantly of CD4-positive T cells. EBV-positive B cells are often present.

REACTIVE DERMATOSES

Two disorders in this category warrant mention: pachydermoperiostosis and EN.

Pachydermoperiostosis is a syndrome in which HOA is associated with cutaneous changes of the face and extremities that are similar to those that occur in patients with acromegaly. Although this disorder is generally benign, it is occasionally associated with bronchogenic carcinoma.

EN is a relatively common process and is usually acute and self-limited.[74] The typical clinical presentation is the sudden onset of one or more, tender, erythematous nodules on the anterior legs, which are more easily palpated than visualized (Fig. 29-32). The eruption is often preceded by a prodrome of fever, malaise, or arthralgias. As the lesions age, they may develop an ecchymotic appearance. They heal over a 4- to 6-week period, usually without scar formation. Ulceration of the primary process is rare. Although EN is usually acute, patients with chronic or recurrent disease have been described using such terms as "chronic EN," "EN migrans," "subacute nodular migratory panniculitis" (Vilanova's disease), or "septal granulomatous panniculitis." Chronic or recurrent EN most commonly occurs in middle-aged women. The disease is often present for several years and is most common on the legs.

Etiologic or associated conditions are present in about 50% of patients with EN. The associated conditions can be divided into three broad categories: infections, drugs, or systemic diseases (usually inflammatory disorders). The infectious agents associated with EN tend to primarily affect the respiratory or gastrointestinal tract and are most often bacterial or fungal in origin. The most common drugs are antibiotics and oral contraceptives. Pregnancy, particularly in its second trimester, is a known association, and the EN will recur with subsequent pregnancies or with the administration of oral contraceptives. EN-like lesions may occur in Behçet disease and are accompanied by oral and genital ulcerations, pathergy, uveitis, or CNS disease or other systemic manifestations.

A specific variant of sarcoidosis associated with EN is known as Löfgren syndrome.[75] This is an acute, self-resolving process in which EN occurs with bilateral hilar lymphadenopathy, arthritis, and anterior uveitis. Granulomatous colitis (Crohn disease), regional enteritis, and ulcerative colitis have been associated with EN. In patients with inflammatory bowel disease, it appears that the EN parallels the activity of the bowel disease. At least half of the cases of EN are not found to have an associated or underlying process.

NEUTROPHILIC DERMATOSES: SWEET SYNDROME AND PYODERMA GANGRENOSUM

Sweet syndrome (Fig. 29-33) and pyoderma gangrenosum (Fig. 29-34) are distinct dermatoses, but they share common associations and are often managed using similar therapies.[76,77] In addition, a condition known as neutrophilic dermatosis of the dorsal hands (Fig. 29-35) often has characteristics that overlap between a superficial variant of pyoderma gangrenosum (also termed atypical pyoderma gangrenosum) and Sweet syndrome.[77] The associated diseases include inflammatory bowel disease, rheumatoid arthritis, and myelogenous malignancy and premalignancy. Extracutaneous neutrophilic inflammation has been reported in multiple organs, but the lungs are most frequently involved. The inflammatory reaction may cause pulmonary infiltrates, including cavitary disease. It is critical that infectious diseases be excluded with appropriate cultures before initiating therapy with corticosteroids or other immunosuppressive therapy.

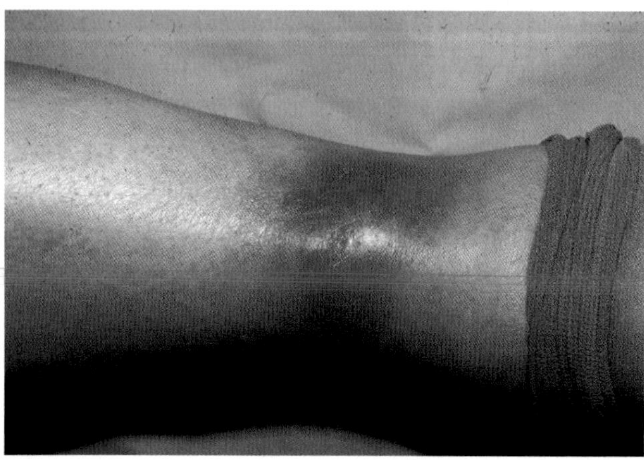

Figure 29-32 Erythema nodosum. Red tender subcutaneous nodule on the leg.

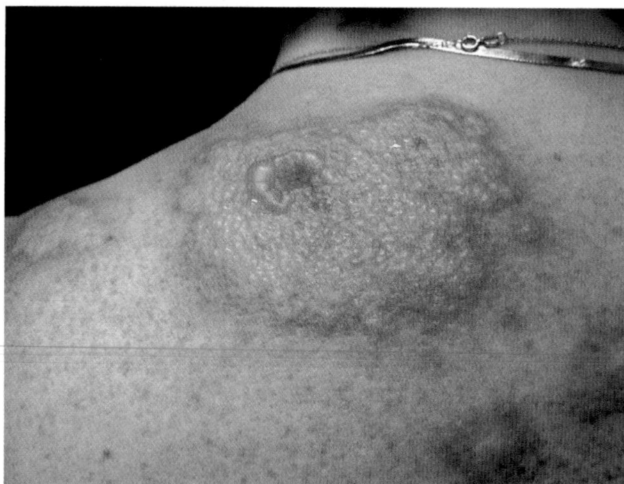

Figure 29-33 Acute febrile neutrophilic dermatosis (Sweet syndrome): erythematous plaque with what appears to be vesiculation on the surface.

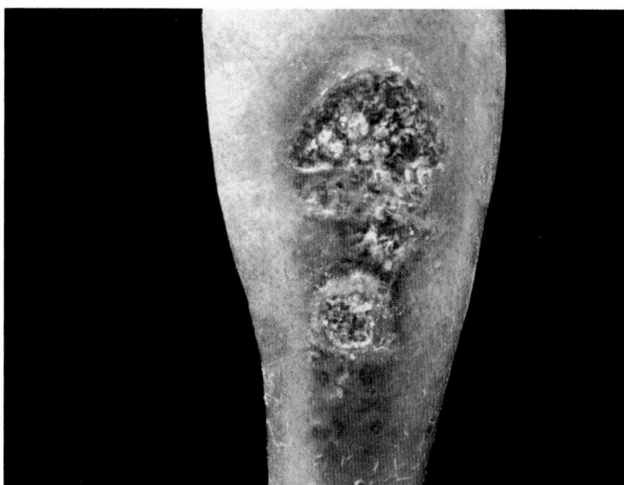

Figure 29-34 Pyoderma gangrenosum: large ulceration on the leg with a violaceous, undermined border. This patient had active Crohn's disease.

PRURITUS

Pruritus is a symptom that accompanies many dermatoses, but it may also accompany systemic diseases.[78] Patients without an obvious cause for their itching require a systemic evaluation, which usually includes a chest x-ray. Causes for pruritus are not commonly found, but Hodgkin disease and other malignancies might be uncovered during the evaluation. Effective treatment of an underlying malignancy will result in a disappearance of the pruritus.

URTICARIA

Urticaria is a reactive cutaneous disease manifested by transient urticarial skin lesions. Acute urticaria is almost always due to the ingestion of a food or medication and usually subsides within several days. The presence of chronic urticaria requires a thorough evaluation and, at times, pulmonary evaluation may reveal an infectious, inflammatory, or neoplastic cause (<25% of patients).

VASCULITIC SYNDROMES

Important vasculitic syndromes with cutaneous and pulmonary (Chapter 60) involvement are discussed below: Churg–Strauss syndrome, granulomatosis with polyangiitis (formerly known as Wegener granulomatosis), polyarteritis nodosa, and urticarial vasculitis.

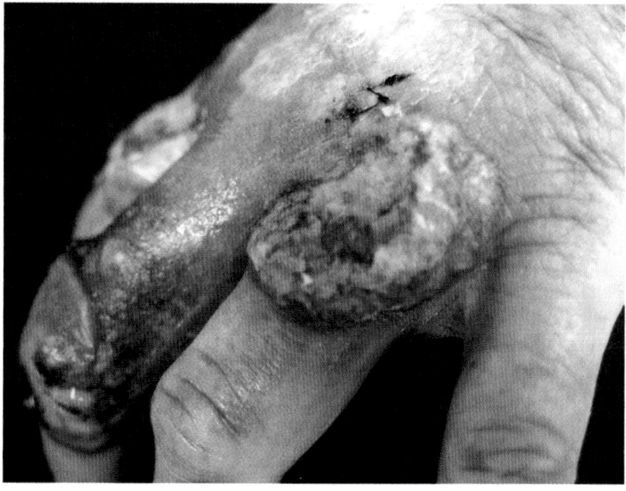

Figure 29-35 Neutrophilic dermatosis of the dorsal hands (also known as atypical pyoderma gangrenosum). Such patients often have a hematologic malignancy or premalignant process.

Churg–Strauss Syndrome

The clinical picture of allergic rhinitis, asthma, peripheral eosinophilia, and pulmonary infiltrates occurring with systemic vasculitis has been designated the Churg–Strauss syndrome.[79] However, the histologic finding of necrotizing granulomas and tissue eosinophilia is not unique to this clinical syndrome. Indeed, the same histologic appearance may be seen in a wide variety of systemic diseases, including allergic granulomatosis, granulomatosis with polyangiitis (see below), rheumatoid arthritis, and lymphoproliferative disease.

One or more types of skin lesions develop in 70% of patients with Churg–Strauss syndrome. Most common is palpable purpura of the extremities; histologically, the lesions show necrotizing vasculitis without granuloma formation. In one-third of patients, the cutaneous lesions are nonspecific—that is, erythematous and urticarial. In another one-third, however, the skin lesions are distinctive—that is, tender, red-to-violaceous, indurated nodules, measuring 0.5 to 2 cm, which develop central crusting or become infarcted. These nodules occur most often over the scalp or symmetrically over the extensor surfaces of the extremities. These nodules are the ones most likely to have the histologic picture of necrotizing granulomatous vasculitis and eosinophilic infiltration; immunofluorescence staining may show vascular deposition of fibrin and complement.

Granulomatosis with Polyangiitis

About 45% of patients with granulomatosis with polyangiitis have cutaneous manifestations, most often small vessel vasculitis.[80] Occasionally, biopsy of the skin lesions reveals a granulomatous vasculitis. In addition, the presence of cutaneous disease is usually indicative of active systemic involvement; therefore, such patients should be carefully evaluated and aggressively treated.

Polyarteritis Nodosa

Patients with polyarteritis nodosa frequently have cutaneous lesions. The skin disease may represent small vessel vasculitis as in granulomatosis with polyangiitis or may represent medium-sized vessel involvement. In the latter case, the manifestation is livedo reticularis or ulceration.

Urticarial Vasculitis

Urticarial lesions may occur in patients as a manifestation of small vessel vasculitis. Urticarial vasculitis was first described in four patients with recurrent attacks of erythematous urticarial and hemorrhagic skin lesions associated with synovitis and, sometimes, abdominal distress. The patients did not have systemic lupus erythematosus or paraproteinemia, but they did have hypocomplementemia; two had nephritis.

Urticarial lesions may also be an early clinical manifestation of lesions that become typical palpable purpura. The spectrum of urticarial vasculitis has also grown in recent years to include the presence of lung disease, characterized by asthma or obstructive lung disease. Patients with hypocomplementemic urticarial vasculitis often have or develop obstructive pulmonary disease, whereas most patients with normal complement levels, chronic urticarial, and vasculitis have little or no systemic involvement.[81]

Patients are often treated with corticosteroids or other immunosuppressive drugs. Although these agents are useful in controlling the cutaneous lesions, they do not appear to have any impact on progression of the pulmonary disease.

TOXIC EPIDERMAL NECROLYSIS

Toxic epidermal necrolysis (TEN) is one of the true dermatologic emergencies.[82] This disorder is most often due to drug administration and develops acutely. Patients often have a prodrome followed shortly by widespread skin involvement with a superficial blistering

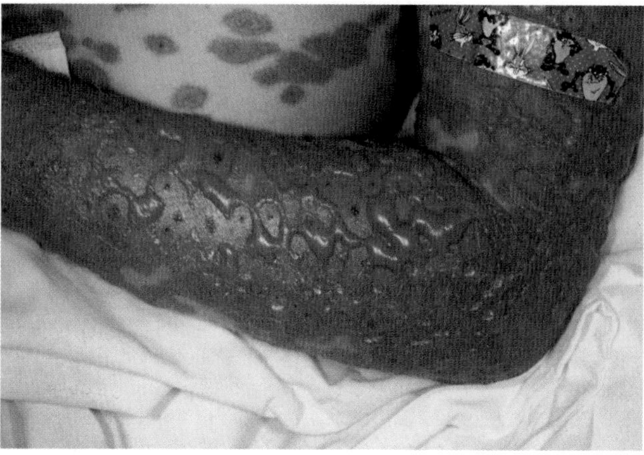

Figure 29-36 Stevens–Johnson syndrome/toxic epidermal necrolysis.

(Fig. 29-36). Multiple mucosal surfaces are affected (Fig. 29-37). Prognosis is dependent upon the extent of the blistering, age, and the presence of comorbid diseases.

Lung involvement in TEN is unusual, but affected patients often are treated in an intensive care unit or burn unit and frequently become ventilator-dependent. Infections, particularly pneumonia, are a frequent complication and may result in death.

YELLOW NAIL SYNDROME

Thick, yellow discoloration of all 20 nails occurs in the yellow nail syndrome[83] (Fig. 29-38). The nails are thick, but there is no onycholysis and no subungual debris, allowing clinical differentiation from onychomycosis. The nails are not clubbed, and there are no underlying bony abnormalities. This disorder is almost always associated with pulmonary abnormalities, including pleural effusions, lymphoma, and sleep apnea. There is no known therapy for the nail changes in this disorder, but improvement of the associated pulmonary disease may result in improvement of the nails.

MISCELLANEOUS DISORDERS

Pulmonary-cutaneous syndromes include a number of inherited congenital and developmental disorders.

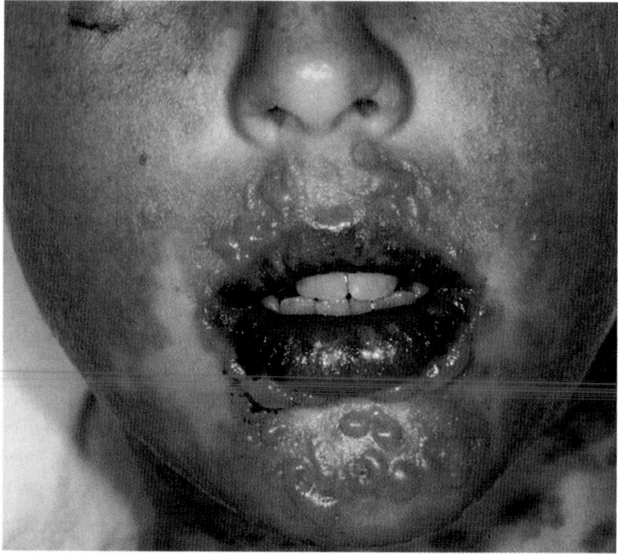

Figure 29-37 Mucosal lesions of Stevens–Johnson syndrome/toxic epidermal necrolysis.

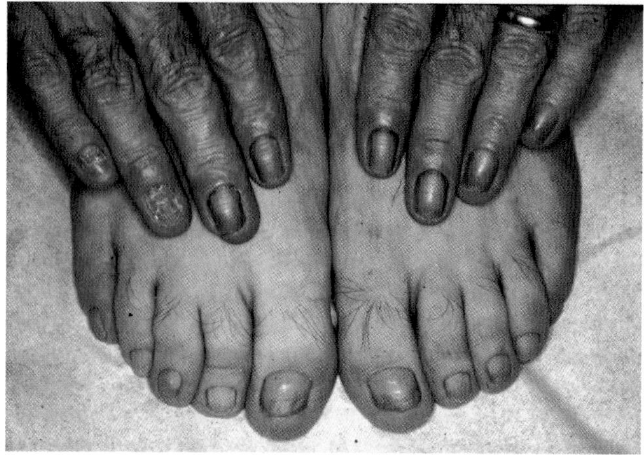

Figure 29-38 Yellow nail syndrome. All 20 nails were affected in this patient.

α_1-Antitrypsin Deficiency

α_1-Antitrypsin deficiency is regularly associated with pulmonary (Chapters 39 and 40) or hepatic disease. Cutaneous manifestations may also occur in some patients with this inherited disorder and most commonly manifest as panniculitis or, rarely, as a cutaneous vasculitis.[84,85] Although the panniculitis is a lobular panniculitis, in contrast to the septal panniculitis that is found in EN, the clinical disease is similar except that these patients' lesions may ulcerate.

Cutis Laxa

Cutis laxa is caused by a disorder in the formation of elastin that is transmitted as a dominant hereditary trait.[86] In children with this disorder, skinfolds of the abdomen and face are large and pendulous. The pulmonary manifestations of cutis laxa include emphysema and pulmonary artery stenosis.

Cystic Fibrosis and the Skin

CF is an inherited disorder that frequently affects the lungs and results in premature death (Chapter 50). Some patients with CF have skin disease.[87] Specifically, cutaneous vasculitis seems to be more frequent in CF patients, probably due to the frequent formation of circulating immune complexes.

Ehlers–Danlos Syndrome

The most important disorder of collagen affecting the skin and lungs is Ehlers–Danlos syndrome (cutis hyperelastica), a hereditary disorder of collagen in which the skin and blood vessels are unduly elastic and fragile and the joints are hyperextensible. The skin is smooth, rubbery, and bruisable; the joints are hypermobile. Associated systemic abnormalities include megaesophagus, megacolon, dissecting aortic aneurysm, and diaphragmatic and inguinal hernias. Among the pulmonary disorders are spontaneous pneumothorax, arteriovenous fistulas, megatrachea, and bronchial ectasia.[88]

Birt–Hogg–Dubé Syndrome

Birt, Hogg, and Dubé described an autosomal dominant condition that is manifested by multiple facial flesh-colored papules characterized histologically as trichodiscomas.[89] BHD is due to heterozygous mutations in the folliculin (FLCN) gene located on chromosome 17, which encodes a highly conserved tumor suppressor protein. (Fig. 29-39) Affected patients frequently develop renal cell carcinomas, particularly oncocytomas. In addition, multiple lung cysts and development of spontaneous pneumothorax at a young age are common. Although there is no known therapy, recognition of affected patients may lead to discovery of renal tumors prior to metastasis and assessment of family members.

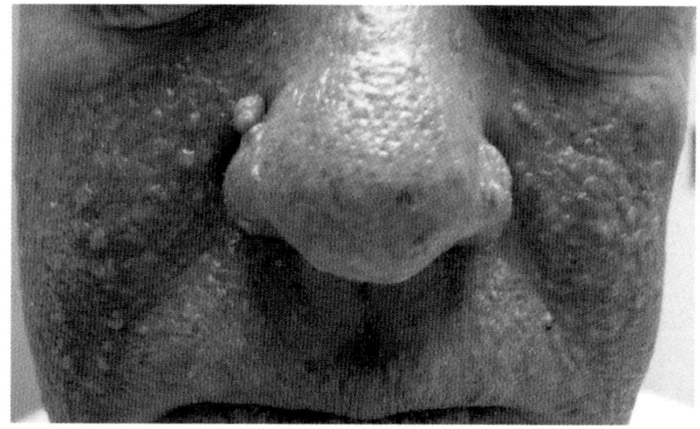

Figure 29-39 Flesh-colored central facial papules in a patient with Birt–Hogg–Dubé syndrome.

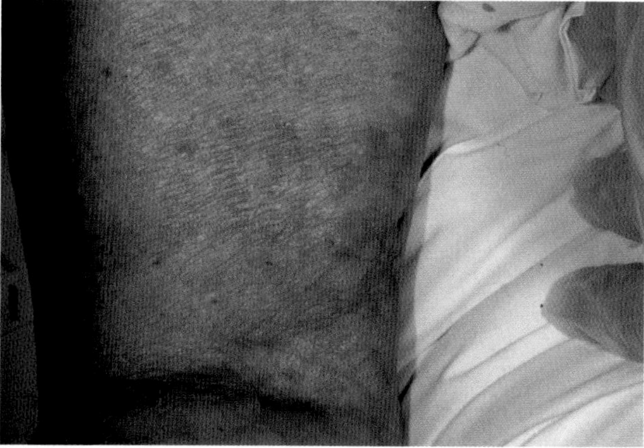

Figure 29-41 Peau 'd orange changes in a patient with nephrogenic systemic fibrosis.

Hemorrhagic Telangiectasia

Hereditary hemorrhagic telangiectasia (HHT), also known as Osler–Rendu–Weber syndrome, is an autosomal dominant disorder that is manifested by vascular ectasia in various organs, including the skin and mucus membranes (Fig. 29-40). HHT often is first manifested as nosebleeds. Eventually lesions affect the lips, tongue, nasal mucosa, palate, and palms. Patients with HHT may have arteriovenous malformations in the lungs or CNS. Epistaxis, melena, and hemoptysis are common in adults.

Nephrogenic Systemic Fibrosis

Nephrogenic systemic fibrosis is a disorder of the skin in which a rapid onset of skin hardening (Fig. 29-41) occurs in patients with some form of renal disease.[90] Often the onset of the fibrosis is preceded by anasarca. The disease has been linked to gadolinium deposition in tissue following its use for MRI or MRA. Initial descriptions of the disease focused on the cutaneous findings, but it has become evident that patients may also have systemic fibrosis, including pulmonary fibrosis. There is no known effective therapy for these patients, but with time the fibrosis does seem to lessen.

Paraneoplastic Pemphigus

Paraneoplastic pemphigus (PNP) is a severe mucocutaneous disease with a specific pattern of immunofluorescence. It is a rare vesiculobullous disorder. Patients with PNP often present with severe oral erosions and polymorphous cutaneous lesions, including targetoid lesions, bullae, and erosions (Fig. 29-42). Patients with PNP often have a lymphoproliferative disorder with a high prevalence of Castleman disease. In addition to the mucocutaneous disease, these patients frequently have bronchiolitis obliterans.[68]

Sarcoidosis

Sarcoidosis is a multisystem disorder with protean manifestations (Chapter 55). Skin lesions occur in about 25% of patients and may be "histopathologically specific" or "nonspecific." The most common nonspecific manifestation is EN. Histopathologically specific lesions are manifestations of granulomatous inflammation in the skin. Although associated with chronic disease in the past, it now appears that there are many patients with self-limiting granulomatous disease of the skin. Skin lesions are most commonly papules, plaques, or nodules. Rarely is there a great deal of surface change, and ulceration is uncommon.

Several clinical variants are worth noting. Papular lesions on the knees (Fig. 29-43) are commonly associated with EN and are self-limiting. Lesions on the nasal ala (Fig. 29-44) are frequently associated with sarcoidosis of the upper respiratory tract (SURT), and a thorough otolaryngologic evaluation is indicated. Erythematous-to-violaceous plaques on the face are known as lupus pernio (Fig. 29-45); residual scarring in this disorder is possible. In addition, patients tend to have accompanying chronic disease in the lungs. Finally, lesions of sarcoidosis frequently occur within scars or tattoos (Fig. 29-46). In this circumstance it may be difficult to distinguish sarcoidosis from foreign body granulomas.

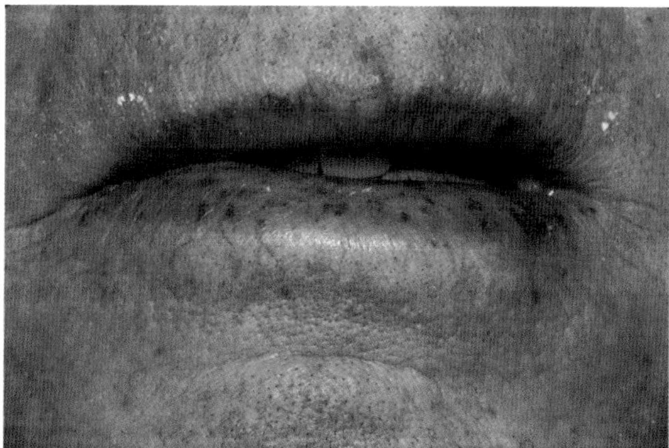

Figure 29-40 Mucosal telangiectasia in a patient with hereditary hemorrhagic telangiectasia.

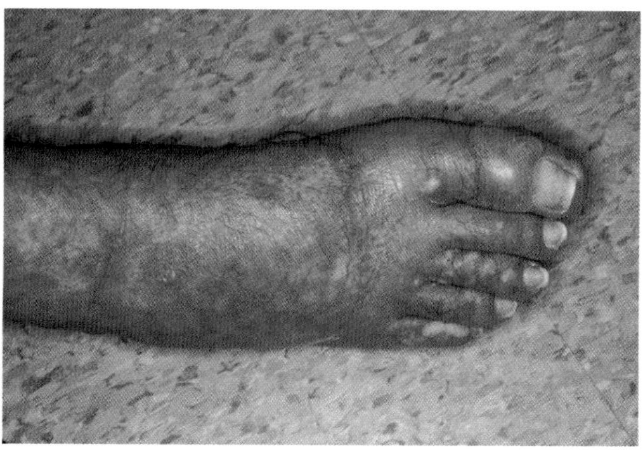

Figure 29-42 Paraneoplastic pemphigus.

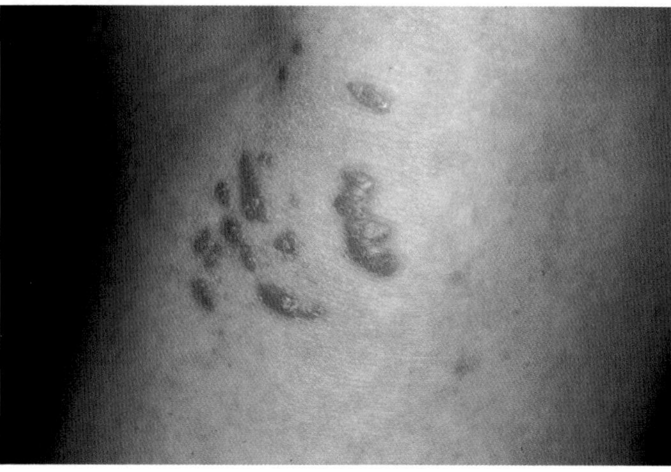

A

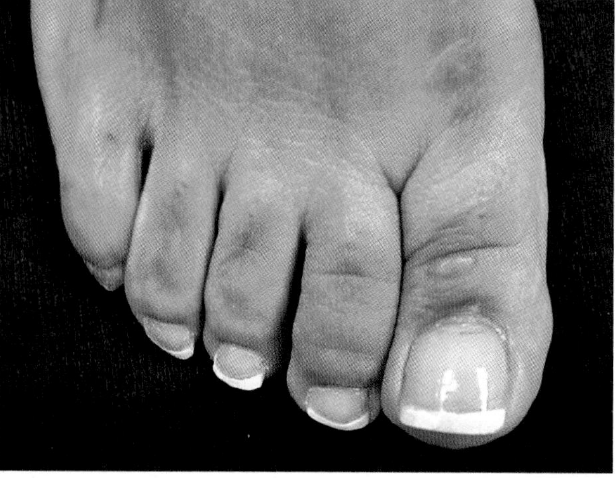

B

Figure 29-43 **A, B.** Sarcoidosis: acute onset of papular lesions (**A**) on the knees and feet (**B**) were associated with a self-limited course in these patients.

Tuberous Sclerosis

Tuberous sclerosis is a hereditary disorder characterized by mental retardation, epilepsy, and skin lesions, including adenoma sebaceum, Shagreen patches, and ash leaf macules. Also seen as part of this disorder are retinal phakomas, calcification of basal ganglia, and ungual fibromas. Approximately 9% of patients with visceral tuberous sclerosis have pulmonary manifestations; some of the pulmonary lesions are cystic and may be associated with recurrent spontaneous pneumothorax and hamartomas. Certain poorly understood diseases, such as fibrocystic pulmonary dysplasia, may represent a forme fruste of tuberous sclerosis.

MEDICATION TOXICITY

Cutaneous toxicity may arise from therapy given for pulmonary disease. In addition, pulmonary toxicity may develop in the setting of treatment of dermatologic disorders.

■ DERMATOLOGIC TOXICITY FROM AGENTS USED TO TREAT PULMONARY DISEASE

Two examples of dermatologic injury from agents used to treat lung disease are described below: epidermal growth factor receptor inhibitors and immunosuppressive agents.

Epidermal Growth Factor Receptor Inhibitors

Epidermal growth factor receptor inhibitors are now being used for the treatment of solid tumors, including lung cancers. These agents are regularly associated with development of an acneiform eruption on the face.[91] The presence and severity of the eruption appear to correlate with survival.

Immunosuppressive Therapy in Lung Transplant Recipients

Patients who are organ recipients are regularly treated with corticosteroids in combination with various immunosuppressive agents. Therapy with corticosteroids has well-known dermatologic consequences, including striae, steroid-acne, or folliculitis, and an increased risk of superficial fungal infections. The intensity of the immunosuppression and duration of therapy are associated with increasing risk of cutaneous malignancy, specifically nonmelanoma skin cancer (NMSC) and KS. Squamous cell carcinoma is overrepresented in comparison to basal cell carcinoma; in addition, the tumors appear to be more aggressive in the presence of immunosuppressive therapy. Therefore, in patients who develop multiple squamous cell carcinomas immunosuppressive therapy should be less intense, if possible, or substitution of cyclosporin and azathioprine by other "less" toxic agents should be considered.

Figure 29-44 Sarcoidosis affecting the nasal ala is regularly associated with granulomatous disease in the upper respiratory tract (SURT).

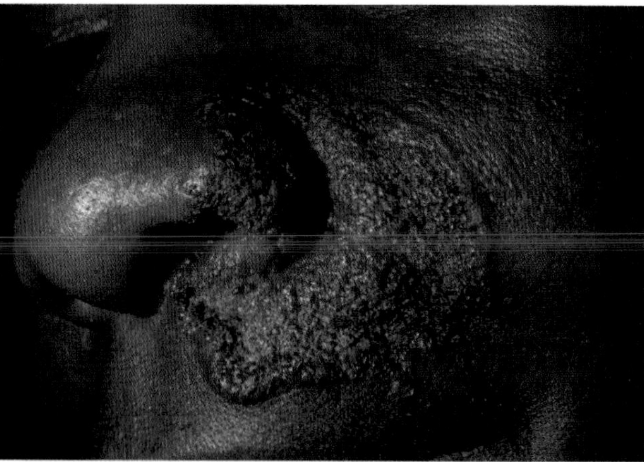

Figure 29-45 Lupus pernio (sarcoidosis).

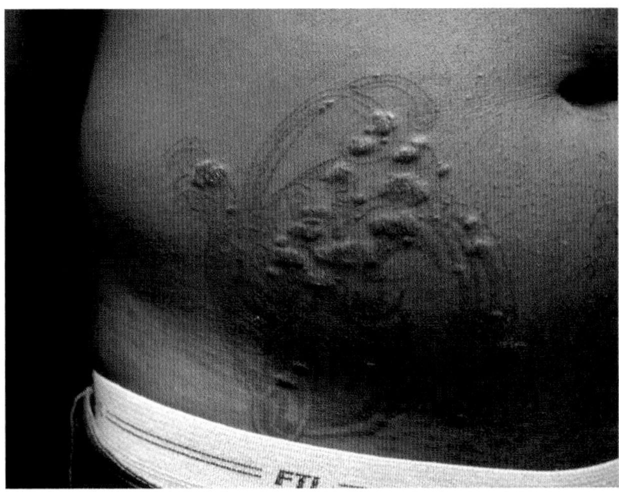

Figure 29-46 Sarcoidosis within tattoos.

PULMONARY TOXICITY FROM DERMATOLOGIC THERAPIES

Two examples of pulmonary toxicity arising from agents used to treat dermatologic disorders are described below: methotrexate and tumor necrosis factor-α inhibitors.

Methotrexate

Methotrexate is a common systemic therapy for patients with psoriasis. In addition, it is regularly used for cutaneous dermatomyositis, cutaneous sarcoidosis, and cutaneous lymphomas. Pulmonary toxicity is not common and is believed to be idiosyncratic. Most of the dermatologic use is for psoriasis vulgaris and psoriatic arthritis; fortunately, pulmonary disease appears to be quite rare in these patients. No specific monitoring is recommended.

Tumor Necrosis Factor-α Inhibitors

A growing number of tumor necrosis factor (TNF) antagonists are available, including infliximab, etanercept, and adalimumab. These therapies have revolutionized our approach to psoriasis, psoriatic arthritis, inflammatory bowel disease, and rheumatoid arthritis. All have been associated with an increased risk of infection, particularly pneumonia and tuberculosis.

SUMMARY

The diagnostic approach to a patient with suspected pulmonary disease begins with a thorough history and physical examination. Elements of the family history, along with determination of work and other environmental exposures, are important components of the history. Many times, characteristic cutaneous findings shed light on an underlying pulmonary diagnosis. The clinical examination is complemented by radiographic studies, assessment of pulmonary and cardiac function, and routine and specialized laboratory studies, as warranted.

ACKNOWLEDGMENTS

The authors acknowledge that a portion of the content of this chapter is based on a chapter from the prior edition: Darren B. Taichman and Alfred P. Fishman, Approach to the Patient with Respiratory Symptoms.

REFERENCES

1. Aberle DR, Adams AM, Berg CD, et al. Reduced lung-cancer mortality with low-dose computed tomographic screening. National Lung Screening Trial Research Team. *N Engl J Med*. 365: 395–409, 2011.
2. Doyle TJ. Subclinical interstitial lung disease: why you should care. *Am J Resp Crit Care Med*. 2012;185:1147–1153.
3. Loudon R, Murray JF. History and Physical Examination. *Clin Chest Med*. 1987;8:265–272.
4. Schraufnagel DE. In: Mason RJ, Broaddus VC, Martin TR, et al., eds. *Textbook of Respiratory Medicine*. 5th ed. Philadelphia, PA: Saunders; 2010:349–367.
5. Ayo DS, Aughenbaugh GL, Yi ES, Hand JL, Ryu JH. Cystic lung disease in Birt-Hogg-Dube syndrome. *Chest*. 2007;132:679–684.
6. Vandemergel X, Renneboog B. Prevalence, aetiologies and significance of clubbing in a department of general internal medicine. *Eur J Intern Med*. 2008;19:325–329.
7. Roussos C, Macklem PT. The respiratory muscles. *N Engl J Med*. 1982;307:786–797.
8. Markel H. The stethoscope and the art of listening. *N Engl J Med*. 2006;354:551–553.
9. Bohadana A, Izbicki G, Kraman SS. Fundamentals of Lung Auscultation. *N Engl J Med*. 2014;370:744–751. doi:10.1056/NEJMra1302901.
10. Pasterkamp H, Kraman SS, Wodicka GR. Respiratory sounds. Advances beyond the stethoscope. *Am J Respir Crit Care Med*. 1997; 156(3 Pt 1):974–987.
11. Dellinger RP, Parrillo JE, Kushnir A, Rossi M, Kushnir I. Dynamic visualization of lung sounds with a vibration response device: a case series. *Respiration*. 2008;75:60–72.
12. Web site: www.easyauscultation.com/lung-sounds.aspx. Assessed August 25, 2014.
13. Kraman SS. Transmission of lung sounds through light clothing. *Respiration*. 2008;75:85–88.
14. Sapira JD. About egophony. *Chest*. 1995;108:865–7. Erratum in: Chest 108:1776, 1995.
15. Forgacs P. Breath sounds. *Thorax*. 1978;33:681–683.
16. Piirila P, Sovijarvi AR, Kaisla T, Rajala HM, Katila T. Crackles in patients with fibrosing alveolitis, bronchiectasis, COPD, and heart failure. *Chest*. 1991;99:1076–1083.
17. Schwartzstein RM. Physiology of dyspnea. In: Rose B, ed. UpToDate. Wellesley, MA: 2006.
18. Parshall MB, Schwartzstein RM, Adams L, et al.; American Thoracic Society Committee on Dyspnea. An official American Thoracic Society statement: update on the mechanisms, assessment, and management of dyspnea. *Am J Respir Crit Care Med*. 2012;185:435–452.
19. Simon PM, Schwartzstein RM, Weiss JW, et al. Distinguishable sensations of breathlessness induced in normal volunteers. *Am Rev Respir Dis*. 1989;140:1021–1027.
20. Simon PM, Schwartzstein RM, Weiss JW, et al. Distinguishable types of dyspnea in patients with shortness of breath. *Am Rev Respir Dis*. 142:1009–1014.
21. Elliott MW, Adams L, Cockcroft A, MacRae KD, Murphy K, Guz A. The language of breathlessness. Use of verbal descriptors by patients with cardiopulmonary disease. *Am Rev Respir Dis*. 1991;144:826–832.
22. Mahler DA, Harver A, Lentine T, Scott JA, Beck K, Schwartzstein RM. Descriptors of breathlessness in cardiorespiratory diseases. *Am J Respir Crit Care Med*. 1996;154:1357–1363.
23. O'Donnell DE, Bertley JC, Chau LK, Webb KA. Qualitative aspects of exertional breathlessness in chronic airflow limitation: pathophysiologic mechanisms. *Am J Respir Crit Care Med*. 1997; 155:109–115.

24. Moy ML, Woodrow Weiss J, Sparrow D, Israel E, Schwartzstein RM. Quality of dyspnea in bronchoconstriction differs from external resistive loads. *Am J Respir Crit Care Med.* 2000; 162(2 Pt 1):451–455.
25. Schwartzstein R. In: Mahler D, O'Donnell DE, eds. *Dyspnea: Mechanisms, Measurement, and Management.* New York, NY: Marcel Dekker, Inc; 2005:115–146.
26. Scano G, Stendardi L, Grazzini M. Understanding dyspnoea by its language. *Eur Respir J.* 2005;25:380–385.
27. Binks AP, Moosavi SH, Banzett RB, Schwartzstein RM. "Tightness" sensation of asthma does not arise from the work of breathing. *Am J Respir Crit Care Med.* 2002;165:78–82.
28. Banzett RB, Pedersen SH, Schwartzstein RM, Lansing RW. The affective dimension of laboratory dyspnea: air hunger is more unpleasant than work/effort. *Am J Respir Crit Care Med.* 2008;177: 1384–1390.
29. Hardie GE, Janson S, Gold WM, Carrieri-Kohlman V, Boushey HA. Ethnic differences: word descriptors used by African-American and white asthma patients during induced bronchoconstriction. *Chest.* 2000;117:935–943.
30. Gui P, Ebihara S, Kanezaki M, et al. Gender differences in perceptions of urge to cough and dyspnea induced by citric acid in healthy never smokers. *Chest.* 2010;138:1166–1172.
31. Killian KJ, Gandevia SC, Summers E, Campbell EJ. Effect of increased lung volume on perception of breathlessness, effort, and tension. *J Appl Physiol Respir Environ Exerc Physiol.* 1984; 57:686–691.
32. Yorke J, Moosavi SH, Shuldham C, Jones PW. Quantification of dyspnoea using descriptors: development and initial testing of the Dyspnoea-12. *Thorax.* 2010;65:21–26.
33. Cheng TO. Platypnea-orthodeoxia syndrome: etiology, differential diagnosis, and management. *Catheter Cardiovasc Interv.* 1999;47:64–66.
34. Mahler D, Horowitz MB. Clinical evaluation of exertional dyspnea. *Clin Chest Med.* 1994;15:259–269.
35. Maisel AS, Krishnaswamy P, Nowak RM, et al. Rapid measurement of B-type natriuretic peptide in the emergency diagnosis of heart failure. *N Engl J Med.* 2002;347:161–167.
36. Irwin RS, Baumann MH, Bolser DC, et al. Diagnosis and management of cough executive summary: ACCP evidence-based clinical practice guidelines. *Chest.* 2006;129(1 Suppl): 1S–23S.
37. Silvestri RC. In: Barnes PJ, King TE Jr, eds. *Evaluation Of Subacute And Chronic Cough In Adults.* UpToDate, Wellesley, MA: 2012.
38. Jegoux F, Legent F, Beauvillain de Montreuil C. Chronic cough and ear wax. *Lancet.* 2002;360:618
39. Irwin RS, Glomb WB, Chang AB. Habit cough, tic cough, and psychogenic cough in adult and pediatric populations: ACCP evidence-based clinical practice guidelines. *Chest.* 2006;129 (1 Suppl):174S–179S.
40. Smyrnios NA, Irwin RS, Curley FJ. Chronic cough with a history of excessive sputum production. The spectrum and frequency of causes, key components of the diagnostic evaluation, and outcome of specific therapy. *Chest.* 1995;108:991–997.
41. Tseng DS, Kwong J, Rezvani F, Coates AO. Angiotensin-converting enzyme-related cough among Chinese-Americans. *Am J Med.* 2010;123:183. e11–e15.
42. Weinberger SE. Etiology and evaluation of hemoptysis in adults. In: Mathur PN, ed. UpToDate. Wellesley, MA: 2013.
43. Kolb T, Gilbert C, Fishman EK, Terry P, Pearse D, Feller-Kopman D, et al. Dieulafoy's disease of the bronchus. *Am J Respir Crit Care Med.* 2012;186:1191.
44. Delage A, Tillie-Leblond I, Cavestri B, Wallaert B, Marquette CH. Cryptogenic hemoptysis in chronic obstructive pulmonary disease: characteristics and outcome. *Respiration.* 2010;80: 387–392.
45. Cahill BC, Ingbar DH. Massive hemoptysis. Assessment and management. *Clin Chest Med.* 1994;15:147–167.
46. Meisel J, Cottrell D. Differential diagnosis of chest pain in adults. In: Aronson MD, ed. UpToDate. Wellesley, MA: 2013.
47. Bonica J. In: *The Management of Pain.* Philadelphia, PA: Lea & Febiger; 1990:1043–1061.
48. Richter JE. Gastroesophageal reflux disease as a cause of chest pain. *Med Clin North Am.* 1991;75:1065–1080.
49. Martina B, Bucheli B, Stotz M, Battegay E, Gyr N. First clinical judgment by primary care physicians distinguishes well between nonorganic and organic causes of abdominal or chest pain. *J Gen Intern Med.* 1997;12:459–465.
50. Bösner S, Becker A, Haasenritter J, et al. Chest pain in primary care: epidemiology and pre-work-up probabilities. *Eur J Gen Pract.* 2009;15:141–146.
51. Bolognia JL. *Dermatology.* Edinburgh: Mosby; 2003.
52. Callen JP. *Dermatological Signs of Internal Disease.* 3rd ed. London: Saunders; 2003.
53. Freedberg IM. *Fitzpatrick's Dermatology in General Medicine.* 6th ed. New York, NY: McGraw-Hill; 2003.
54. Eichenfield L, Tom WL, Chamlin SL, et al. Guidelines of care for the management of atopic dermatitis: section 1. Diagnosis and assessment of atopic dermatitis. *J Am Acad Dermatol.* 2014;70(2): 338–351. In press.
55. Beck LA, Thaçi D, Hamilton JD, et al. Dupilumab treatment in adults with moderate-to-severe atopic dermatitis.
56. Femia AN, Vleugels RA, Callen JP. Cutaneous dermatomyositis: an updated review of treatment options and internal associations. *Am J Clin Dermatol.* 2013;14:291–313.
57. Chen Z, Cao M, Plana MN, et al. Utility of anti-melanoma differentiation-associated gene 5 antibody measurement in identifying patients with dermatomyositis and a high risk for developing rapidly progressive interstitial lung disease: a review of the literature and a meta-analysis. *Arthritis Care Res (Hoboken).* 2013;62:1316–1324.
58. Morganroth PA, Kreider ME, Okawa J, Taylor L, Werth VP. Interstitial lung disease in classic and skin-predominant dermatomyositis: a retrospective study with screening recommendations. *Arch Dermatol.* 2010;146:729–738.
59. Morganroth PA, Kreider ME, Werth VP. Mycophenolate mofetil for interstitial lung disease in dermatomyositis. *Arthritis Care Res (Hoboken).* 2010;62:1496–1501.
60. Saketkoo LA, Espinoza LR. Experience of mycophenolate mofetil in 10 patients with autoimmune-related interstitial lung disease demonstrates promising effects. *Am J Med Sci.* 2009;337: 329–335.
61. Zulian F, Vallongo C, Woo P, et al. Localized scleroderma in childhood is not just a skin disease. *Arthritis Rheum.* 2005;52: 2873–2881.
62. Steen VD. The lung in systemic sclerosis. *J Clin Rheumatol.* 2005;11: 40–46.
63. Trent JT, Kirsner RS. Identifying and treating mycotic skin infections. *Adv Skin Wound Care.* 2003;16:122–129.

64. Fazeli MS, Bateni H. Actinomycosis: a rare soft tissue infection. *Dermatol Online J.* 2005;11:18.

65. Akoglu G, Karaduman A, Boztepe G, et al. A case of lupus vulgaris successfully treated with antituberculous therapy despite negative PCR and culture. *Dermatology.* 2005;211:290–292.

66. Serraino D, Angeletti C, Carrieri MP, et al. Kaposi's sarcoma in transplant and HIV-infected patients: an epidemiologic study in Italy and France. *Transplantation.* 2005;80:1699–1704.

67. Pellet C, Kerob D, Dupuy A, et al. Kaposi's sarcoma-associated herpesvirus viremia is associated with the progression of classic and endemic Kaposi's sarcoma. *J Invest Dermatol.* 2006;126: 621–627.

68. Wang J, Zhu X, Li R, et al. Paraneoplastic pemphigus associated with Castleman tumor: a commonly reported subtype of paraneoplastic pemphigus in China. *Arch Dermatol.* 2005;141: 1285–1293.

69. Patel A, Teixeira F, Redington AE. Palmoplantar keratoderma ("tripe palms") associated with primary pulmonary adenocarcinoma. *Thorax.* 2005;60:976.

70. Webb KG, Malone JC, Callen JP. Acral psoriasiform eruption in a man with squamous cell carcinoma of the tonsillar pillar. *Arch Dermatol.* 2005;141:389–394.

71. Scnirer II, Yao JC, Ajani JA. Carcinoid: a comprehensive review. *Acta Oncol.* 2003;42:672–692.

72. Katzenstein AL, Doxtader E, Narendra S. Lymphomatoid granulomatosis: insights gained over 4 decades. *Am J Surg Pathol.* 2010;34:e35–e48.

73. Beaty MW, Toro J, Sorbara L, et al. Cutaneous lymphomatoid granulomatosis: correlation of clinical and biologic features. *Am J Surg Pathol.* 2001;25:1111–1120.

74. Requena L, Yus ES. Erythema nodosum. *Dermatol Clin.* 2008;26: 425–438 .

75. English JC 3rd, Patel PJ, Greer KE. Sarcoidosis. *J Am Acad Dermatol.* 2001;44:725–743.

76. Brown TS, Marshall G, Callen JP. Cavitating pulmonary infiltrate in an adolescent with pyoderma gangrenosum: a rarely recognized extracutaneous manifestation of a neutrophilic dermatosis. *J Am Acad Dermatol.* 2000;43:108–112.

77. Schadt CR, Callen JP. Management of neutrophilic dermatoses. *Dermatol Ther.* 2012;25:158–172.

78. Yosipovitch G, Bernhard JD. Clinical practice. Chronic pruritus. *N Engl J Med.* 2013;368:1625–1634.

79. Guillevin L, Pagnoux C, Mouthon L. Churg-strauss syndrome. *Semin Respir Crit Care Med.* 2004;25:535–545.

80. Lynch JP 3rd, White E, Tazelaar H, Langford CA. Wegener's granulomatosis: evolving concepts in treatment. *Semin Respir Crit Care Med.* 2004;25:491–522.

81. McDuffie FC, Sams WM Jr, Maldonado JE, Andreini PH, Conn DL, Samayoa EA. Hypocomplementemia with cutaneous vasculitis and arthritis. Possible immune complex syndrome. *Mayo Clin Proc.* 1973;48:340–348.

82. Sekula P, Dunant A, Mockenhaupt M, et al; RegiSCAR study group. Comprehensive survival analysis of a cohort of patients with Stevens-Johnson syndrome and toxic epidermal necrolysis. *J Invest Dermatol.* 2013;133:1197–1204.

83. Piraccini BM, Urciuoli B, Starace M, Tosti A, Balestri R. Yellow nail syndrome: clinical experience in a series of 21 patients. *J Dtsch Dermatol Ges.* 2014;12(2):131–137.

84. Patterson CC, Ross P Jr, Pope-Harman AL, Knight DA, Magro CM. Alpha-1 anti-trypsin deficiency and Henoch-Schönlein purpura associated with anti-neutrophil cytoplasmic and anti-endothelial cell antibodies of immunoglobulin-A isotype. *J Cutan Pathol.* 2005;32:300–306.

85. Ortiz PG, Skov BG, Benfeldt E. Alpha-1-antitrypsin deficiency-associated panniculitis: case report and review of treatment options. *J Eur Acad Dermatol Venereol.* 2005;19:487–490.

86. Harris RB, Heaphy MR, Perry HO. Generalized elastolysis (cutis laxa). *Am J Med.* 1978;65:815–822.

87. Fradin MS, Kalb RE, Grossman ME. Recurrent cutaneous vasculitis in cystic fibrosis. *Pediatr Dermatol.* 1987;4:108–111.

88. Safdar Z, O'Sullivan M, Shapiro JM. Emergent bullectomy for acute respiratory failure in Ehlers-Danlos syndrome. *J Int Care Med.* 2004;19:349–351.

89. Gupta N, Seyama K, McCormack FX. Pulmonary manifestations of Birt-Hogg-Dubé syndrome. *Fam Cancer.* 2013;12:387–396.

90. Cowper SE, Boyer PJ. Nephrogenic systemic fibrosis: an update. *Curr Rheumatol Rep.* 2006;8:151–157.

91. Molinari E, De Quatrebarbes J, Andre T, Aractingi S. Cetuximab-induced acne. *Dermatology.* 2005;211:330–333.

CHAPTER 30

Modern Approach to Thoracic Imaging Diagnosis

Eduardo J. Mortani Barbosa Jr.
Warren B. Gefter

INTRODUCTION

This chapter is not intended to provide a comprehensive review of the entire scope of thoracic imaging; dedicated textbooks in radiology serve this purpose well. Moreover, the chapter does not provide a comprehensive guide to the interpretation of thoracic imaging studies. Rather, the focus is on what modern thoracic imaging can provide to empower clinicians to diagnose and manage common clinical scenarios in the second decade of the 21st century. The goal is to present a strategic approach to thoracic imaging, which starts with broad clinical categories of disease and addresses the following central clinical questions: What is the differential diagnosis and how can a specific diagnosis be confirmed? What is the prognosis and how can disease progression and therapeutic effectiveness best be monitored?

In each subsection, organized initially by imaging technique, and subsequently, by broad diagnostic categories, the authors aim to answer these questions by providing a practical, logical, and evidence-based approach that emphasizes which imaging tests to order and what to expect from each test. Oftentimes, imaging findings are either pathognomonic or highly characteristic of a diagnosis in the appropriate clinical context and, therefore, will suffice for clinical diagnosis and management. However, when this is not the case, tissue sampling or additional laboratory tests may be required for diagnostic confirmation; these scenarios are outlined and options discussed for tissue sampling, including image-guided percutaneous biopsy, bronchoscopy, and surgical biopsy. In addition, the ways in which modern functional and quantitative radiographic techniques may impact the field of thoracic imaging in the near future will be considered, and validated clinical applications differentiated from promising research applications that may evolve into useful clinical tools in the next several decades.

Finally, since radiology and, in particular, thoracic imaging, play such a major and central role in modern medicine, our ultimate goal is to enable the practicing pulmonologist to use imaging resources consistently, wisely, efficiently, and effectively.

SUMMARY OF TECHNIQUES: DIAGNOSTIC AND INTERVENTIONAL

The inception of the field of radiology dates back to 1895 with Wilhelm Röentgen's serendipitous discovery of x-rays and subsequent production of the first radiograph. Within only a few years, radiology became established as a new medical field. Chest radiography, although one of the first clinical applications and currently over 100 years old, is still the most frequently performed imaging test worldwide and the cornerstone of initial imaging assessment of most patients with thoracic diseases. Nonetheless, over the last four decades we have witnessed an explosion of technical innovation and developments, with the introduction of ultrasound (US), computed tomography (CT), magnetic resonance imaging (MR), positron emission tomography (PET), and hybrid scanners (PET/CT and PET/MR), which have greatly expanded the ability of modern imaging to accurately diagnose even the smallest or earliest disease processes and revolutionized the practice of medicine.

More recently, the widespread impact that computers have made on the acquisition, distribution, visualization, and postacquisition processing of medical images have consolidated the central role of radiology. In the future, we hypothesize that major trends will include quantitative imaging, functional imaging, molecular diagnosis, and value assessment with regard to generating better patient outcomes. In the following sections we present current clinical applications, advantages, and disadvantages of each modality, as well as appropriateness criteria for ordering each test, according to the clinical scenario.

CHEST RADIOGRAPHY

Two basic types of chest radiographic examinations are available—bedside portable AP (anteroposterior) and the combination of PA (posteroanterior) and lateral projections. Supplementary views include oblique, lordotic, lateral decubitus, and expiratory radiographs. For most clinical scenarios, the evaluation should begin with a chest radiograph, as this study remains the most cost-effective imaging test for diagnosing a variety of common clinical conditions. Moreover, chest radiographs are universally available and can be obtained even in patients who cannot be moved to an advanced scanner (e.g., patients in the ICU setting). Nonetheless, in many clinical scenarios, additional advanced imaging will be required to clarify radiographic findings or obtain more accurate characterization of disease pattern and severity (Figs. 30-1–30-4).

Whereas the basic physical principles of radiography have not changed in over a century, the quality and clinical availability of chest radiographs have been greatly enhanced in recent decades due to the transition from analog to digital technology. Digital imaging provides better image contrast, reduces the number of suboptimal or nondiagnostic examinations, and permits more immediate examination availability using image transfer and display software.

Currently, two standards for digital radiography exist: computed radiography (CR) and digital radiography (DR), which differ in the process of imaging acquisition. CR utilizes a photostimulable phosphor cassette, just as does the film-screen analog technique; however, the latent image is read by a laser and converted from an analog to digital signal, rather than being transferred to film. DR bypasses this step and utilizes flat panel detectors that directly transform the x-ray signal to a digital image via integrated, thin-film, transistor readout systems. From a practical perspective, DR images are often sharper, with better spatial resolution and, consequently, better visualization of detail. In addition, DR streamlines workflow for routine images and offers the possibility of tailoring the radiation dose.

Most modern facilities use a combination of CR and DR units, due to cost considerations. The principal benefit of CR and DR technology is the ability to process the acquired images to emphasize specific anatomical areas (e.g., lung parenchyma, soft tissues, bones), thereby greatly reducing the need to repeat examinations due to over- or underpenetration by the x-ray beam.[1] Digital methods to "remove" the ribs from the image are now available using either postprocessing bone-suppression software or dual-energy

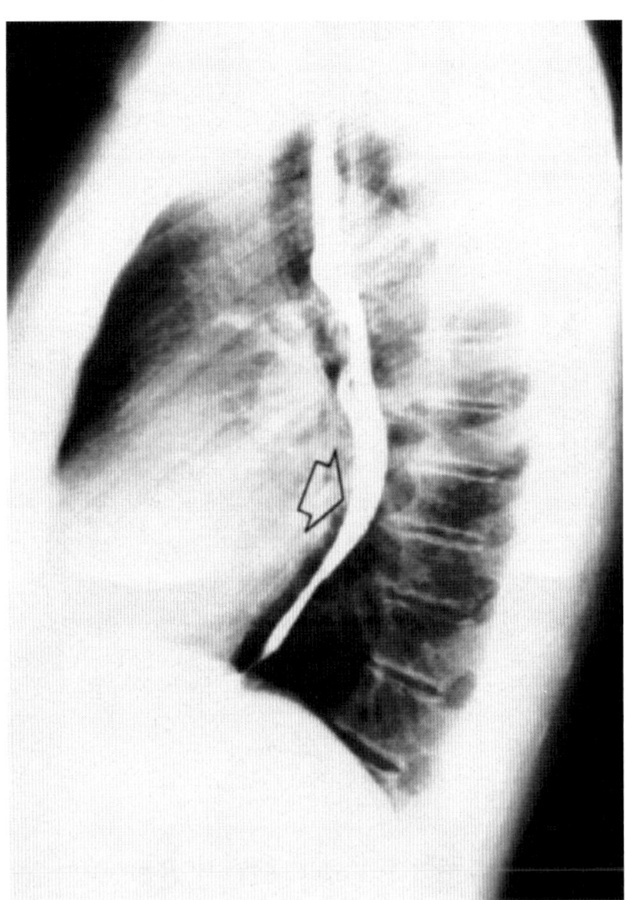

Figure 30-1 Lateral chest radiograph following barium contrast swallow. Not only is this technique very useful for evaluating the esophagus, it is also able to demonstrate left atrial enlargement, with consequent posterior displacement of the contrast column *(arrow)*.

acquisition techniques. These approaches can provide an unobstructed view of the lungs for improved detection of nodules and other pulmonary findings. In addition, computer-aided diagnostic techniques may now assist the radiologist in the detection of subtle lung lesions.

The PA view obtained in the erect position is the standard radiographic examination and demonstrates the anatomy and most thoracic pathologic processes. In particular, the PA view allows evaluation of pulmonary masses and consolidation, diffuse lung disease, pleural effusion, pneumothorax, mediastinal abnormalities, and disorders of the rib cage and scapular girdle.

The lateral view provides additional information by better depicting the posterior diaphragms and posterior lung bases, retrocardiac left lung base, anterior mediastinum, and thoracic spine.

The AP view provides similar information to the PA view, but it is limited by lower spatial and contrast resolution and by magnification of the mediastinal structures. In addition, it is less sensitive for detection of small pneumothoraces and pleural effusions. The AP view is often performed in the supine position in bedridden patients, particularly those who are postoperative or in the ICU. AP portable chest radiographs can be very helpful in assessing the position of support lines, tubes, and medical devices. Medical devices can also be enhanced using newer digital image-processing algorithms.

Supplementary views are not routinely performed, unless there is a specific clinical question. In the past, lordotic views were obtained to better visualize the lung apices by displacing the clavicle and first rib shadows superiorly. However, their role has been largely replaced by CT. Expiratory views may be more sensitive in detecting small pneumothoraces, particularly in the setting of recent lung interventional procedures. Lateral decubitus views, although used less frequently than in the past, may be helpful in determining if a pleural opacity seen on standard views is a freely mobile effusion or a loculated effusion or pleural mass. When the patient is imaged with the pleural opacity on the dependent side, a freely mobile pleural effusion conforms to the most dependent region of the hemithorax and a sharp horizontal level demonstrated due to gravity. If a nondependent lucency is seen in the chest or abdomen, in conjunction with a sharp horizontal level delineating it from normal anatomical structures, the diagnosis of a small pneumothorax or pneumoperitoneum may be made. Finally, oblique views are helpful in determining if a questionable radiographic abnormality seen on the frontal view is real or artifactual, as well as in determining its location in the thorax. Performed properly, supplementary views can increase the diagnostic accuracy and clinical utility of chest radiography, sometimes obviating the need for chest CT with its attendant higher cost and radiation exposure.

Many radiographic techniques that were widely used in the past (e.g., laminography, bronchography, air contrast studies, and fluoroscopy) have been made obsolete by other techniques and are of historical interest only. The exception is focused fluoroscopy for evaluation of diaphragmatic motion ("sniff test"), in which the patient is imaged during quiet breathing, deep breathing, and forceful inspiration ("sniff"). A paralyzed hemidiaphragm moves paradoxically upward with forceful inspiration. Fluoroscopy in conjunction with barium swallow may also be used to assess esophageal diseases.

CHEST CT

CT is the current cornerstone of advanced thoracic imaging. It is a digital cross-sectional imaging technique that utilizes a rotating x-ray source around the patient, coupled to diametrically positioned sodium iodide detectors in a circular configuration. As the scanner gantry rotates, multiple projections are generated at different angles with different x-ray beam attenuations, depending on which part of the patient's anatomy was traversed. Following scan acquisition, through a mathematical procedure (filtered back projection or, more recently, iterative reconstruction), the sum of projections is transformed into an image in which the relative density of each small volume of the patient's anatomy (voxel) is proportional to its x-ray absorption coefficient, and normalized from a scale of −1000 to > +1000 HU (Hounsfield units, zero representing the absorption coefficient of water, −1000 of air). Because it eliminates the main drawback of radiographic techniques, that is, the projection of a three-dimensional (3D) structure into a two-dimensional image, CT allows very accurate localization of pathologic processes. Moreover, the superior contrast resolution of CT allows detailed evaluation of mediastinal and chest wall soft tissue attenuation structures, which are poorly assessed radiographically. CT is also superior to chest radiographs for detection of small pulmonary lesions, as well as for their characterization (Figs. 30-5 and 30-6).

Early CT scanners had a single row of detectors and a single x-ray source, acquiring one axial image at a time before the scanner table was moved to acquire the next image. This process could take more than 30 minutes for a single thoracic CT examination. Most modern scanners have between 64 and 320 rows of detectors, one or two x-ray tubes, extremely fast and continuous gantry rotation, and simultaneous table translation, resulting in helical image acquisition and the ability to scan the entire chest in less than 1 second. Modern CT scanners are able to produce high-quality, submillimeter, isotropic resolution images that can be reconstructed in any arbitrary plane without loss of detail. Postprocessing techniques utilizing computational algorithms also allow 3D reconstructions,

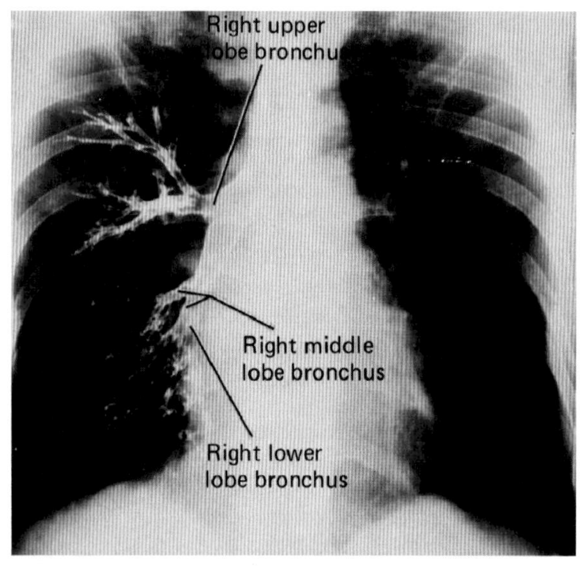

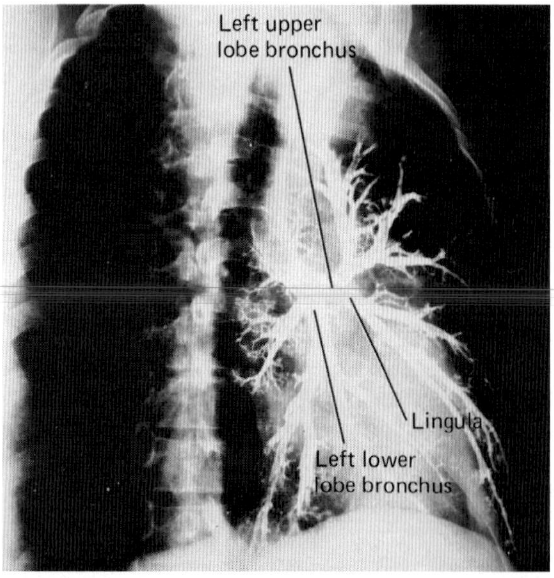

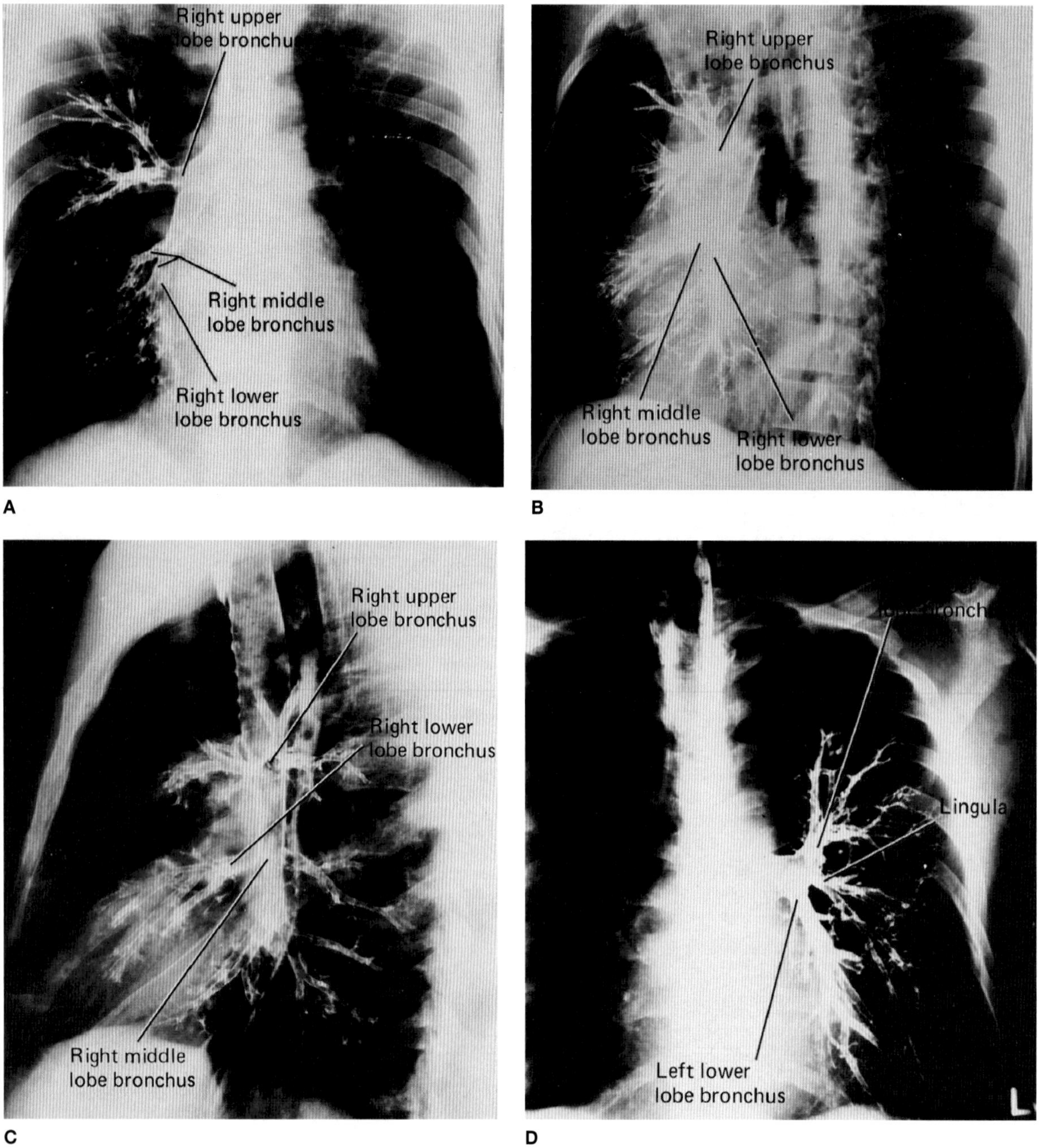

A

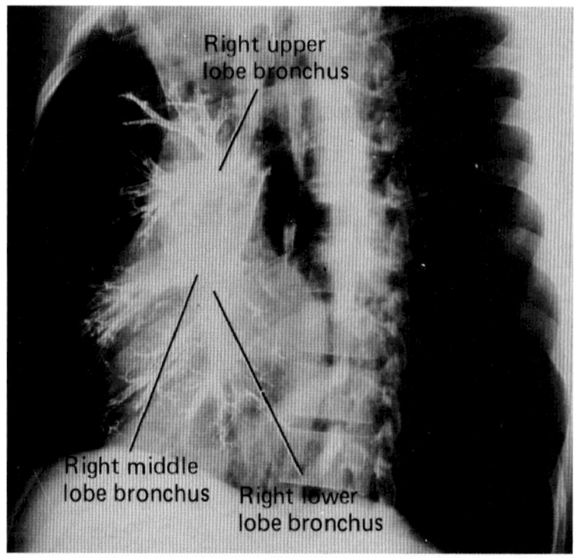

B

C

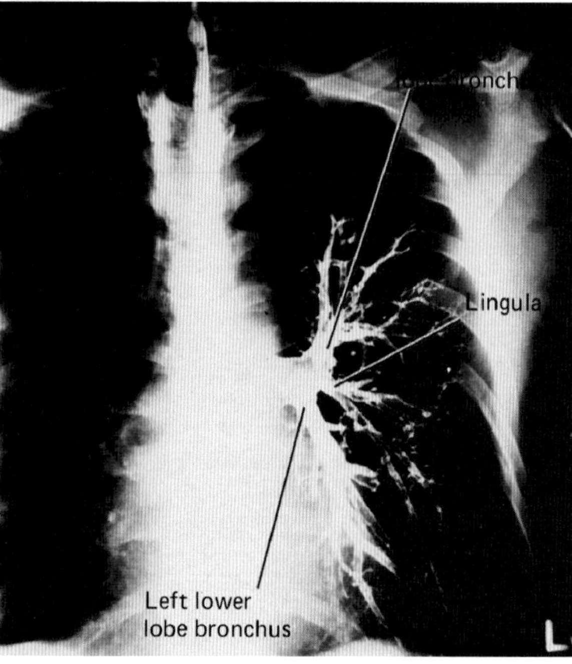

D

E

Figure 30-2 Normal bronchogram. The normal bronchial anatomy of the right lung is shown in the PA (**A**), oblique (**B**), and lateral (**C**) projections. The corresponding anatomy of the left lung is demonstrated in the PA (**D**) and oblique (**E**) projections; the latter also illustrates bronchiectasis. Although valuable to demonstrate bronchial anatomy and pathology, the bronchogram is an obsolete examination, having been replaced by CT and airway reconstruction techniques.

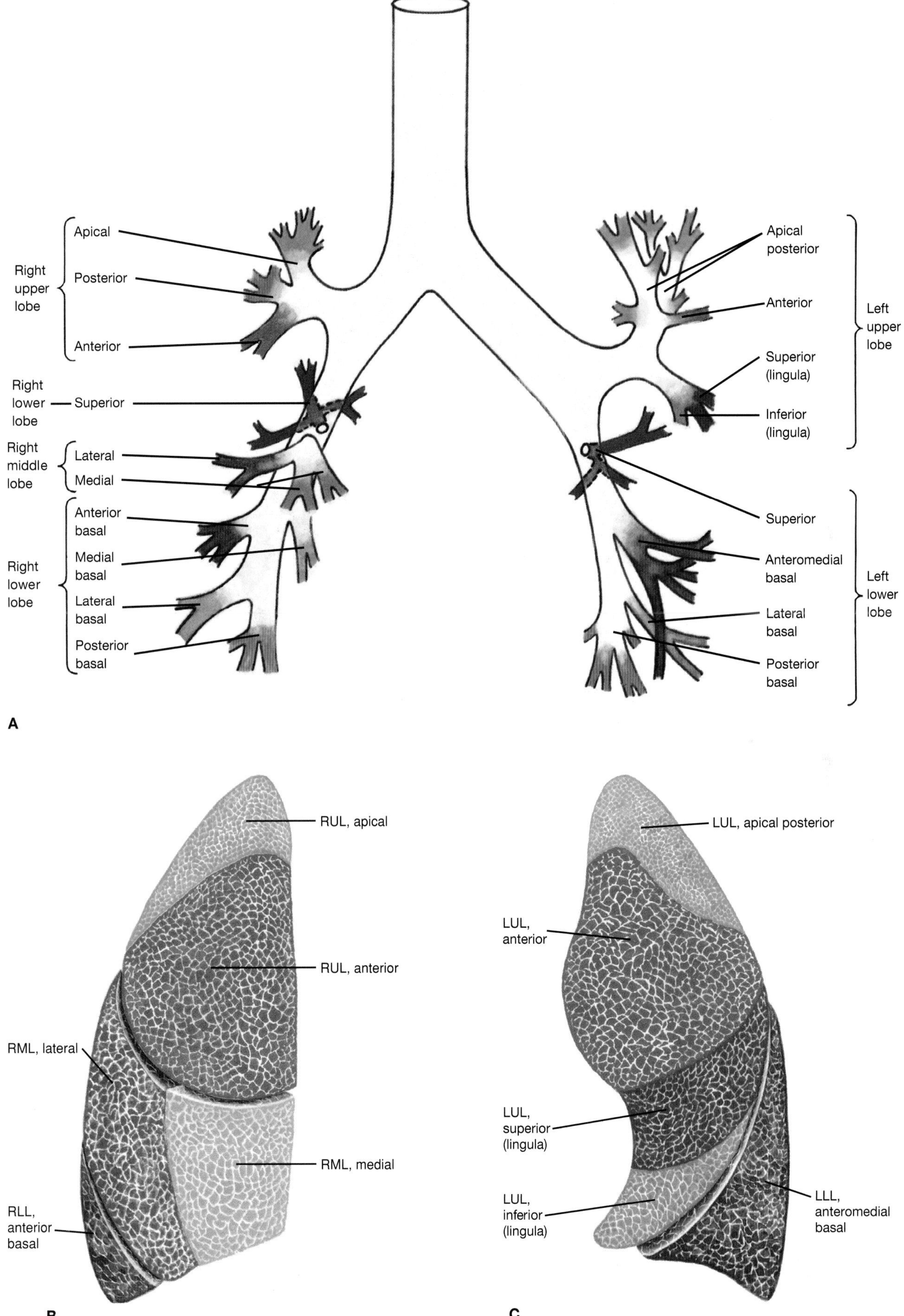

Figure 30-3 Topographic anatomy of the tracheobronchial tree and respective pulmonary subsegments. **A.** Tracheobronchial tree. **B.** Right lung segments. **C.** Left lung segments. Currently, CT is the best modality for accurate anatomical delineation of pulmonary airway segmentation. RUL, right upper lobe; RML, right middle lobe; RLL, right lower lobe; LUL, left upper lobe; LLL, left lower lobe.

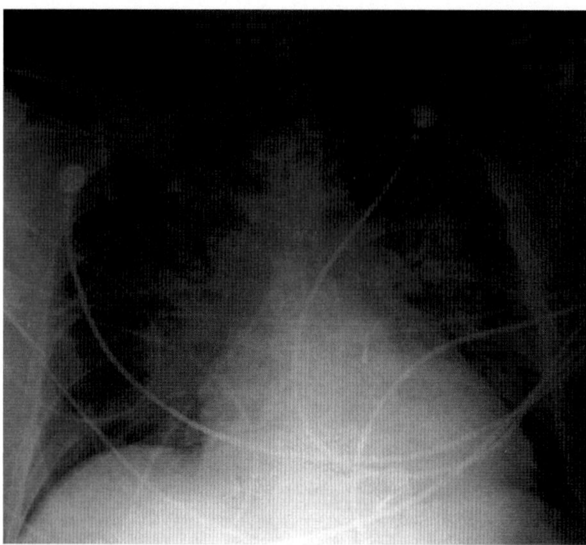

Figure 30-4 Portable AP (anteroposterior) projection chest radiograph, in a patient in the ICU, demonstrating multiple support tubes and lines and the typical configuration of cardiogenic pulmonary edema, with symmetrical bilateral consolidations with perihilar predominance.

such as volume rendering and maximal intensity projection images, which can be utilized to demonstrate complex 3D vascular or airway anatomy and pathology.

An important concept is that of high-resolution CT ("HRCT") of the thorax. Historically, when early CT scanners were limited to the acquisition of relatively thick axial slices (7 to 10 mm) in the thorax, the only way to adequately assess lung parenchymal detail was to acquire serial thin (1 mm) anatomic images utilizing an axial, rather than helical mode; this required noncontiguous (i.e., slices with an interslice gap, typically 20 mm wide), rather than contiguous, slices. These images were also reconstructed using a high spatial frequency algorithm, sharpening edges and allowing improved visualization of fine detail. The result was a set of higher spatial resolution, thin-section images that sampled the lung parenchyma and provided excellent insight into certain pulmonary disorders. This was termed "high-resolution CT" or "HRCT" of the chest, differentiating it from the "standard" chest CT scan, in which thicker sections were acquired through the entire chest in a contiguous helical mode (i.e., without interslice gaps). Generally, a choice had to be made as to which of these two types of scans to perform, since both studies could not be performed simultaneously. Standard CTs were ordered for a general assessment of larger pulmonary lesions, as well as mediastinal, bone, and chest

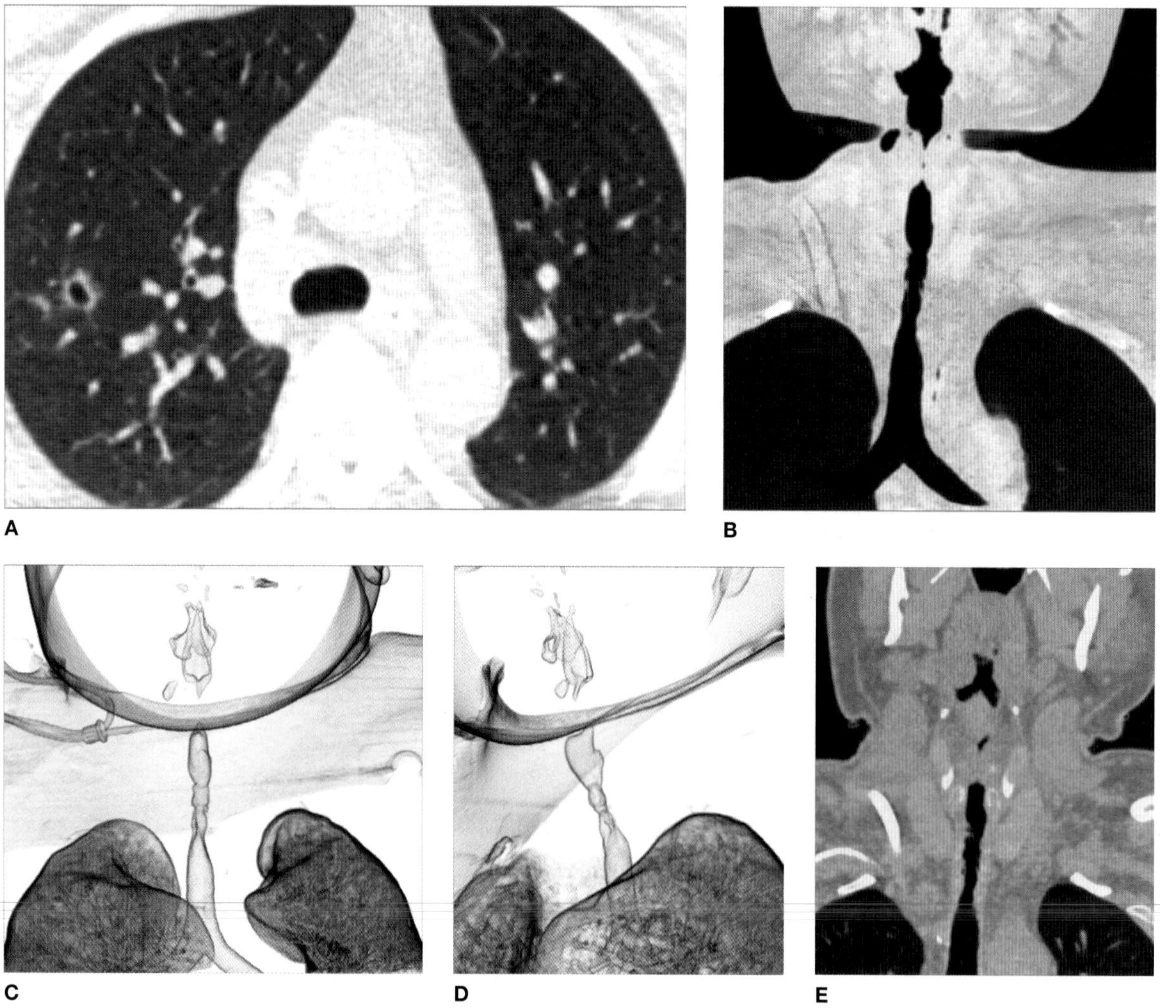

Figure 30-5 CT offers the best imaging evaluation of the pulmonary parenchyma and airways, and advanced postprocessing techniques can provide exquisite views of disease distribution and extension. Granulomatosis with polyangiitis (formerly known as Wegener granulomatosis) affecting the lung and airways. **A.** Cavitary nodule in the right upper lobe; (**B**) minimum intensity projection image demonstrating irregular, long segment narrowing of the upper and middle trachea; (**C**) and (**D**) two different projections of a 3D volume rendering airway reconstruction demonstrating the complex configuration of the stenotic tracheal segment; (**E**) coronal reformatted image depicting tracheal wall thickening associated with stenosis.

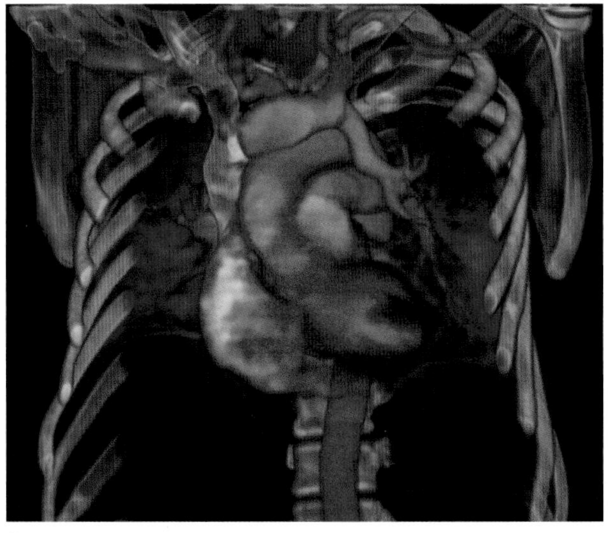
A

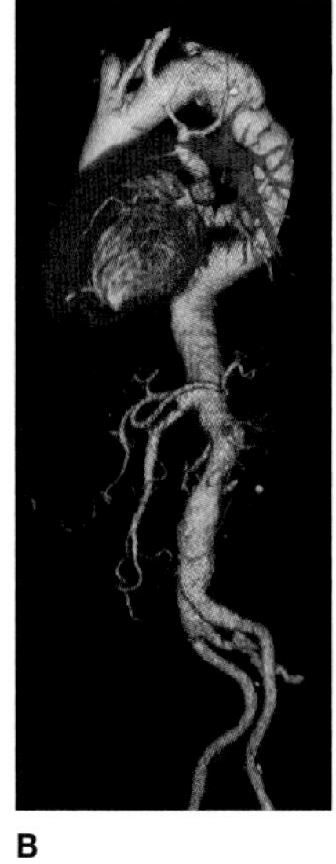
B

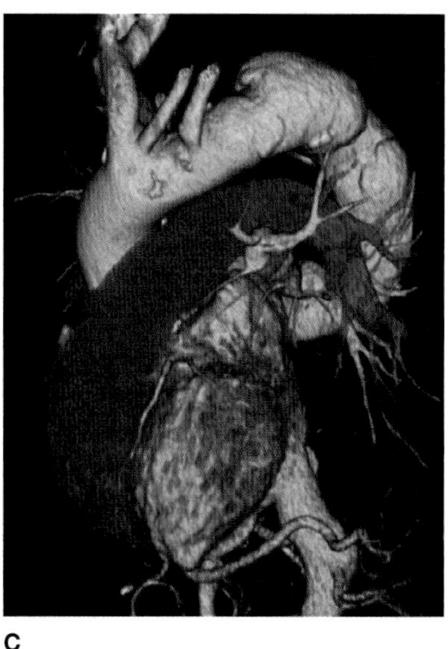
C

Figure 30-6 CT allows acquisition of isotropic volumetric images, in which advanced 3D postprocessing can be performed to demonstrate complex disease processes with a high level of detail. **A.** VR (volume rendering) reconstruction demonstrating partial anomalous pulmonary venous connection of the left upper lobe to the left brachiocephalic vein; (**B**) and (**C**) VR reconstructions at different degrees of rotation, demonstrating the complex configuration of a thoracic aortic aneurysm. These images are invaluable for treatment planning.

wall pathology. High-resolution chest CTs were ordered to assess pulmonary parenchymal disease, such as bronchiectasis, interstitial diseases, and micronodular diseases.

With advances in CT technology, however, it is currently feasible to acquire volumetric, isotropic thin-section (1 mm) images throughout the entire thorax in a single breath-hold, and to reconstruct them in any arbitrary plane (typically axial, sagittal, and coronal) using soft tissue and high-resolution algorithms. Consequently, every chest CT is now effectively both a standard, as well as a high-resolution CT, combining the advantages of each in a single study. This simplifies the ordering process for clinicians. Currently, when ordering a chest CT, there are only two decisions that the clinician needs to make: (1) whether to include expiratory imaging; and (2) whether to perform the study with or without intravenous contrast (these are discussed in detail below).

The first important decision is whether to perform expiratory images, noting that normally, a chest CT is acquired in full inspiration. The reason to avoid performing expiratory images for every patient is to decrease medically unnecessary radiation exposure. Typically, an expiratory CT is ordered if there is a clinical concern for an obstructive lung disease (e.g., asthma, COPD, or small airway disease) or if there is a risk of developing bronchiolitis obliterans (e.g., related to lung or bone marrow transplantation) (Video 30-1A,B). Expiratory CT may also be ordered to assess for large airway diseases, such as tracheobronchomalacia. Expiratory CT is currently the best imaging test to demonstrate small airway air trapping and, therefore, it is a very useful tool to evaluate potential causes of a "mosaic attenuation pattern" on CT (as discussed in detail in the following sections addressing specific diseases).

The second important decision is whether to perform the study with or without intravenous contrast administration. For the sake of decreasing medically unnecessary radiation exposure, there are very few indications for combined chest CT (i.e., with and without intravenous contrast); these are discussed below. The vast majority of chest CT is performed either with or without intravenous contrast. Generally, to assess the lung parenchyma and airways, no intravenous contrast is required. Assessment of bone lesions also usually does not benefit from intravenous contrast administration. On the other hand, vascular and cardiac assessment is greatly enhanced by intravenous contrast. Moreover, mediastinal and hilar pathology (including lymphadenopathy) and cervical and chest wall masses are more conspicuous and better evaluated using intravenous contrast. For certain thoracic neoplasms, the enhancement pattern adds information to their diagnostic characterization. Finally, assessment of pleural diseases also is enhanced using intravenous contrast administration.

It is important to emphasize that since iodinated CT intravenous contrast is excreted primarily by the kidneys, substantially impaired renal function may preclude intravenous contrast administration and may increase the risk of nephrotoxicity. Additional risks associated with intravenous contrast administration include local effects related to contrast extravasation at the injection site and anaphylactoid reactions, ranging from clinically insignificant symptoms to life-threatening airway or cardiovascular collapse; the latter is very rare with the low osmolar contrast material currently utilized.

When performing chest CT with intravenous contrast, it is important to inform the radiologist of the clinical indication. Broadly, three different basic protocols can be utilized: (1) standard contrast-enhanced CT; (2) CT angiography (CTA) for visualization of the aorta or coronary arteries; and (3) CTA for visualization of the pulmonary arteries ("pulmonary embolism [PE] protocol").

Video 30-1 **A.** Axial cine images using lung window and inspiratory acquisition. This CT airway examination demonstrates bronchiectasis, mosaic attenuation, and faint peribronchial opacities, compatible with a diagnosis of bronchiolitis obliterans. Inspiratory acquisitions should ideally reflect the lung appearance at TLC (total lung capacity). **B.** Same patient as in Video 30.1A. Axial cine images on lung window/level, expiratory acquisition, in this CT airway examination, demonstrating same findings earlier, plus dynamic partial collapse of the trachea and central bronchi, compatible with tracheobronchomalacia superimposed on bronchiolitis obliterans. Note the value of expiratory imaging to establish the diagnosis of tracheobronchomalacia and to increase the conspicuity of the mosaic attenuation pattern reflecting small airway disease. Expiratory acquisitions should ideally reflect residual volume (RV). *Access at www.fishmansonline.com*

Video 30-2 **A.** Axial cine images using soft tissue window, demonstrating a massive saddle embolus straddling the bifurcation of the main pulmonary artery. Note that the clot extends to the bilateral lower lobes; oligemia of the right lower lobe is demonstrated. Also note right ventricular enlargement and leftward deviation of the interventricular septum, findings compatible with right ventricular strain. **B.** Same patient as in Video 30.2A. Full-color, coronal, 3D VR (volume rendering) thick slab cine (anterior to posterior), emphasizing cardiovascular structures. This type of reconstruction provides exquisite detail of vascular anatomy and extent of massive pulmonary embolism. *Access at www.fishmansonline.com*

Video 30-3 Full-color, coronal 3D VR (volume rendering) with 360 degrees of rotation about the long axis of the trachea, emphasizing central airways. **A.** Lower magnification with vertical and horizontal axis for spatial orientation. **B.** Higher magnification without axis. The images demonstrate an irregular, long region of segmental stenosis involving the upper trachea. The patient also presented with multiple pulmonary nodules, at least one of which was cavitary. A diagnosis of granulomatosis with polyangiitis or GPA (previously known as Wegener granulomatosis) was established on tracheal biopsy. *Access at www.fishmansonline.com*

For a standard contrast-enhanced CT, the injection rate and imaging acquisition relative to the contrast injection are tailored for maximum enhancement of parenchymal organs and soft tissues; consequently the images are acquired during the venous or equilibrium phase of contrast distribution. This is the standard approach for routine, contrast-enhanced chest CT.

CTA of the aorta and CTA of the coronary arteries are dedicated examinations that are tailored for maximum enhancement of these systemic vessels and are not covered further in this chapter. In particular, cardiac CTA is a thriving application that is usually performed in conjunction with ECG gating to compensate for cardiac motion. CTA of the pulmonary arteries is a well-established application and the current reference standard for the diagnosis of PE (Video 30-2A,B). With this CT technique, contrast injection and imaging acquisition are optimized for maximum enhancement of the pulmonary arteries. This requires a high rate of injection (4–6 mL/s, as opposed to 2 mL/s for regular contrast-enhanced CT) through a large-caliber peripheral IV access (ideally larger than 20G) and very fast volumetric imaging acquisition, usually using contrast bolus tracking to maximize the probability of scanning the patient at the peak of opacification of the pulmonary arteries. When optimally performed, this study allows confident diagnosis of PE in even small subsegmental vessels via direct visualization of vascular filling defects. It also allows accurate assessment of pulmonary vascular caliber and distribution to diagnose pulmonary hypertension, chronic thromboembolic disease, and vasculitides.

CTA of the pulmonary arteries has supplanted conventional pulmonary angiography (except for therapeutic applications) and largely supplanted ventilation–perfusion scanning, although the latter still has an important role in specific clinical settings, such as pregnancy, young patients with normal chest radiographs, or in patients with renal insufficiency. This advanced CTA technique not only allows the diagnosis of PE and possible complications, such as pulmonary infarcts, but also accurately reflects the overall clot burden and signs of right ventricular strain, both important prognostic indicators.[2]

An additional, specific advanced application of CT in the chest is the evaluation of the airways. The imaging protocol for CT of the airways utilizes thin-section (1 mm), volumetric, isotropic images, both in full inspiration and end expiration. The images are acquired from the base of the tongue to the basilar segmental bronchi to include the entire tracheobronchial tree and larynx. Postprocessing 3D techniques are routinely utilized—that is, volume rendering, minimal intensity projections, and virtual bronchoscopy (Video 30-3A,B). The result is accurate depiction of global, regional, and local large airway disorders, including tracheobronchomalacia, airway stenoses, infiltrative and obstructive neoplasms, and inflammatory conditions.

An important consideration recently receiving much attention is the issue of medical radiation exposure in CT. CT, as any imaging modality that utilizes x-rays, exposes the patient to ionizing radiation, which is a known carcinogen due to stochastic effects and which, at very high doses, can have deterministic detrimental effects. To understand the true magnitude of the risks associated with radiation exposure related to diagnostic chest CT, it is critical to have a basic understanding of the ways in which radiation dose is measured, as well as how to quantitatively estimate risk based on best available evidence.

Ionizing radiation dose equivalent (which takes into account energy absorbed (J/kg) and the biologic effects of the specific type of radiation) is measured in Sieverts (Sv). Every human is exposed to approximately 3 mSv/yr of background radiation from natural and man-made sources. In contrast, a chest radiograph delivers 0.1 to 0.2 mSv, whereas a chest CT performed using standard protocols delivers between 5 to 20 mSv. Deterministic effects are extremely rare below 2000 mSv of acute exposure. Although it is difficult to quantify the magnitude of stochastic effects, the International Commission of Radiological Protection (ICRP) estimates the risk coefficient (additional cancers due to radiation exposure) as 0.00005 per mSv of exposure (i.e., ~5% per 1000 mSv). In summary, CT delivers a low, but nonnegligible, radiation dose that is unlikely to cause detrimental biologic effects if used in a prudent and medically justifiable manner.

Notwithstanding the relative small risks, radiologists, engineers, and physicists have made substantial strides to develop reconstruction algorithms and protocol optimization techniques that decrease the radiation dose of thoracic CT to the lowest attainable level and that allows diagnostic-quality images. Among the recent dose-reduction methods that have become widely available are iterative reconstruction techniques, combined with tube current and voltage modulation. The combined effects can generate markedly reduced radiation dose, down to sub-mSv (<1 mSv) levels. This is particularly useful for low-dose screening CT, which is discussed in detail later (see Lung Cancer Evaluation).[3,4]

Finally, CT has a major role for guidance of thoracic interventional procedures, which is described in detail below.

CHEST MR

MR is another advanced cross-sectional technique utilized in thoracic imaging. The physics behind MR is complex and beyond the scope of this chapter. Fundamentally, MR uses a very strong static magnetic field (main field) generated by superconducting coils in combination with a radiofrequency radiation pulse sequence and variable magnetic field (gradients) to cause oscillation of hydrogen proton nuclear spins. The result is generation of a radiofrequency signal, which is detected and measured. The signal can be also spatially localized to generate an image that can be obtained in any arbitrary plane. Image contrast with MR depends on the physical properties of the tissue being imaged, as well as on the specific pulse sequence utilized (Fig. 30-7).

MR has advantages and disadvantages with respect to CT. The main advantage of MR is the lack of ionizing radiation. CT utilizes high-energy x-rays, whereas MR utilizes low-energy radiofrequency

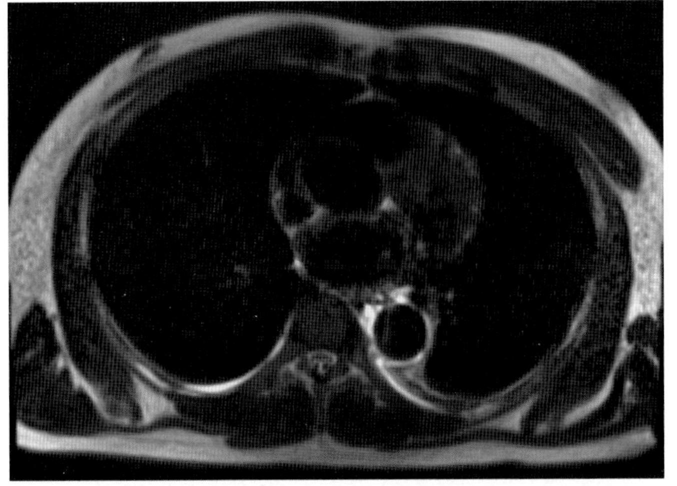

A

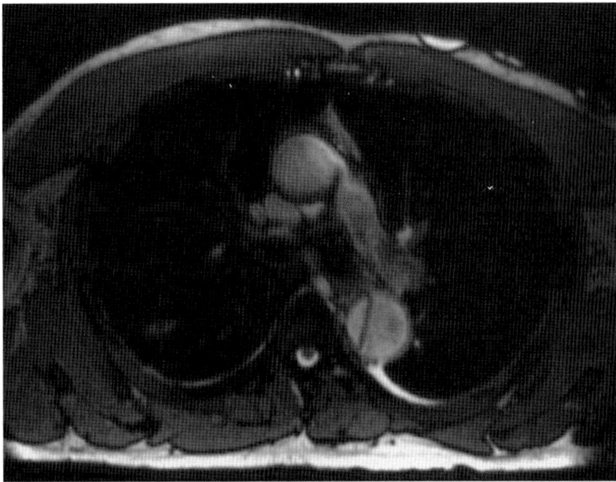

B

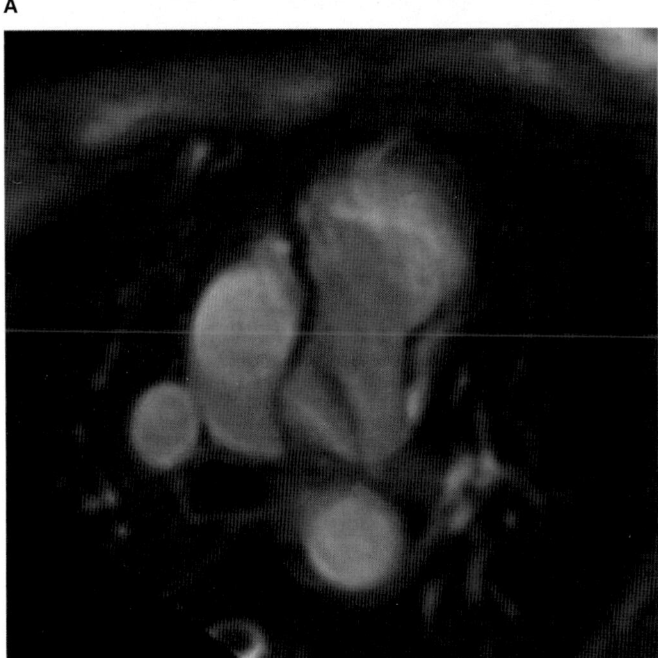

C

Figure 30-7 MR offers lower spatial resolution than CT; however, it allows better contrast resolution and tissue characterization through utilization of varied pulse sequences that emphasize specific aspects of tissue composition. For example, (**A**) and (**B**) demonstrate a dissection of the descending thoracic aorta. **A.** The blood pool appears black and this is, therefore, termed a "black blood" sequence (typically, spin echo sequence). In contrast (**B**) demonstrates the blood pool to be bright and is, therefore, termed a "bright blood" sequence (typically, steady-state free precession gradient echo sequence). **C.** Different patient with a patent ductus arteriosus (PDA), which causes a linear flow artifact (dark band from the aorta to the left PA).

radiation which has minimal biologic effects and no ionization potential. MR also has better contrast resolution than CT and is exquisitely sensitive in the detection of water and fat. MR thus provides a greater degree of soft tissue characterization than is possible with CT. Examples of this greater resolution of soft tissue densities include identification of proteinaceous fluid in bronchogenic cysts, which can appear solid on CT, and the presence of fat in confirming thymic hyperplasia as a cause for an anterior mediastinal mass, thereby enabling differentiation from lymphoma. Another advantage of MR over CT is that iodinated contrast material is not used, obviating the potential problem of CT contrast allergy. In the past, MR also had the advantage of intrinsic multiplanar imaging, but modern multidetector-based CT now demonstrates similar capability.

The disadvantages of MR include longer examination time, greater susceptibility to artifacts, lower spatial resolution, and generally very low signal-to-noise ratio in the lung parenchyma, making it unsuitable for optimal pulmonary parenchymal evaluation. However, it should be noted that recently developed fast-proton MR sequences appear promising for the evaluation of patients who need to undergo multiple serial imaging studies and in whom cumulative radiation exposure is of particular concern, such as in young patients with cystic fibrosis.

From a clinical perspective, MR is not the first-line advanced modality for assessment of pulmonary diseases, but it is a very valuable technique for evaluation of the heart and great vessels, for tissue characterization of mediastinal and chest wall masses, and for dynamic assessment of thoracic wall and diaphragmatic motion. Current applications of MR, in addition to those mentioned earlier, include evaluation of the brachial plexus, local staging of superior sulcus tumors, evaluation of neurogenic tumors and lesions involving the thoracic spine, and cardiac or paracardiac masses.[5,6]

Recently considerable interest has arisen in the use of hyperpolarized gases, including helium-3 and xenon-129, for MR imaging of the lungs. Hyperpolarized gas MR can provide detailed images of pulmonary ventilation, as well as information on lung microstructure, beyond the resolution of CT. The latter includes measurements of alveolar size and alveolar–capillary membrane thickness. Nonetheless, to date, hyperpolarized gas MR remains investigational.

PET, PET/CT, AND PET/MR

PET is a nuclear medicine emission tomographic technique (see Chapter 32), in which an intravenously administered radionuclide that decays via positron emission (most often ^{18}F coupled

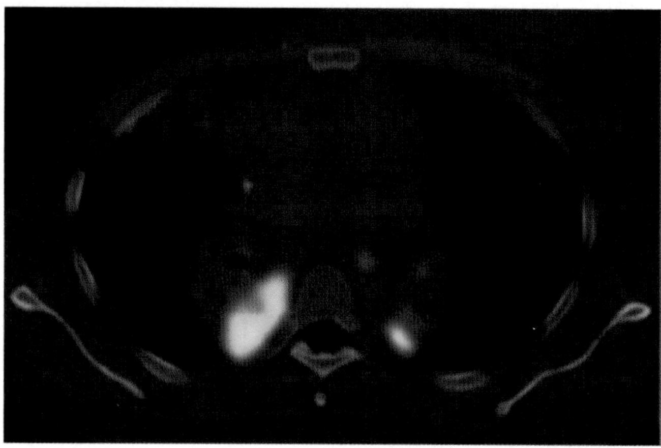

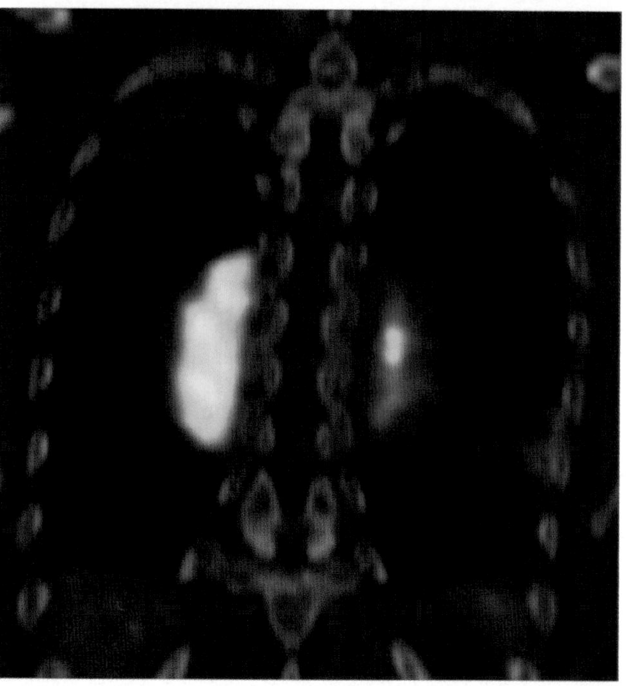

Figure 30-8 Fusion images combining CT and PET data in a patient with multifocal MALT pulmonary lymphoma. (**A**) Axial and (**B**) coronal images demonstrate that the areas of consolidation in the posterior medial lungs also demonstrate high FDG uptake, thus appearing bright yellow in this color scheme, a typical feature of metabolically active lymphomas.

to deoxyglucose [FDG]), generates an annihilation event (when a positron collides with an electron and two antiparallel 511-keV photons are simultaneously generated). The event is registered by coincidence detectors, allowing localization of the origin inside the body. Because FDG is very similar to glucose in biodistribution and pharmacokinetics, it effectively concentrates in tissues that have a high metabolic rate and therefore increased glucose uptake—namely, the brain, heart (in the nonfasting state), and many neoplasms; in addition, FDG is concentrated where it is metabolized and excreted: the liver, kidneys, and urinary collecting system. FDG-PET images essentially map the biodistribution of glucose in the body. CT and MR may be performed almost simultaneously with PET in dedicated hybrid scanners (PET/CT and, more recently, PET/MR). The higher spatial resolution of these modalities is helpful for localization of the abnormal PET signals in fused imaging analysis (Fig. 30-8).

It is a common misconception that PET/CT is specific for cancer diagnosis. In reality, it is not. Many normal tissues and inflammatory or infectious processes have a high metabolic rate and high glucose uptake and, therefore, are also bright on PET images. Moreover, many cancers are not highly metabolically active or are not FDG avid, and these may not be detectable by PET imaging. A typical example in the chest is an indolent adenocarcinoma in situ (AIS), formerly called bronchioloalveolar cell carcinoma (BAC).

The strength of PET/CT relies on its ability to accurately stage malignancy if the primary neoplasm is FDG avid. In this context, it is superior to CT or MR because it may demonstrate small metastases in normal-sized structures, particularly lymph nodes, which would not be detectable by CT or MR. PET/CT is, therefore, routinely employed for staging of malignancies such as lung cancer, lymphoma, head and neck carcinoma, and esophageal carcinoma.[7]

ULTRASOUND

US has a more limited application to thoracic imaging. The primary reason is that both the thoracic cage and the lungs act as reflecting interfaces that block penetration of the US mechanical wave. However, US has been shown to be useful for specific applications, such as detection of pneumothorax or pneumonia, as well as in evaluation of pleural effusions and chest wall pathology. In addition, it is useful in guiding imaging interventions. Thoracic US is discussed in detail in Chapter 31.

IMAGE-GUIDED INTERVENTIONS

Image-guided interventions have dramatically changed the diagnosis of thoracic diseases that require tissue sampling for pathologic confirmation. They have also impacted the treatment of many benign and malignant diseases. Increasingly, image-guided biopsy procedures are being performed for tumor genotyping to guide more targeted, personalized therapies. Half a century ago, surgical procedures were necessary to obtain tissue from the lungs, mediastinum, or chest wall. Surgical biopsies may require hospitalization, are costlier, and carry small, but measurable rates of morbidity and mortality. Currently, most diagnostic procedures can be performed percutaneously or via bronchoscopy in a minimally invasive fashion. Bronchoscopy and endobronchial interventions are described in Chapters 35 and 36 (Fig. 30-9).

Percutaneous transthoracic biopsies (PTBs) may be performed via a variety of imaging guidance systems, most commonly CT, but also fluoroscopy or US (Videos 30-4 and 30-5A,B). Different needle types, lengths, and calibers may be chosen according to the clinical question and lesion characteristics. As a general rule,

Video 30-4 4D cine using custom window. The images are acquired sequentially at the same level and used for guidance in performing a transthoracic fine-needle aspiration (TTNA). The needle was advanced to perfectly engage a small RUL nodule (9 × 7 mm). Final diagnosis was primary adenocarcinoma. *Access at www.fishmansonline.com*

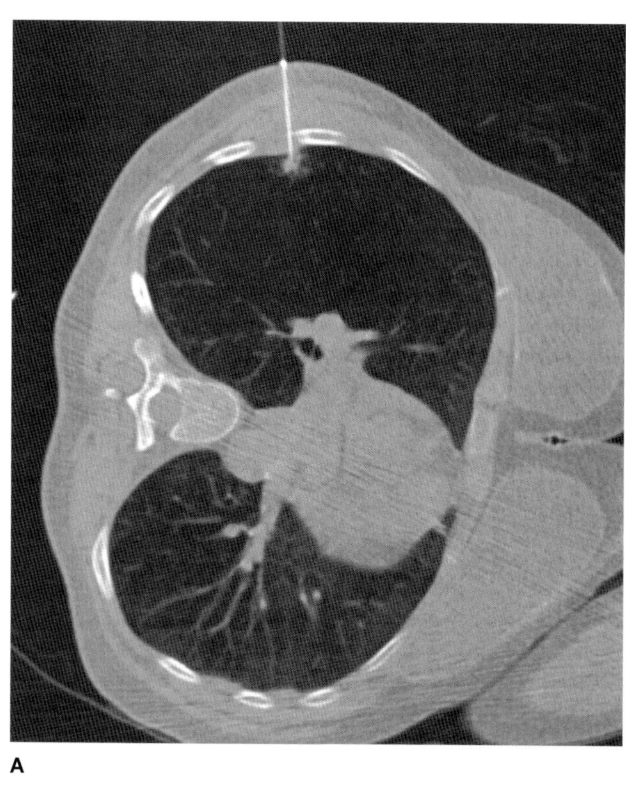

A

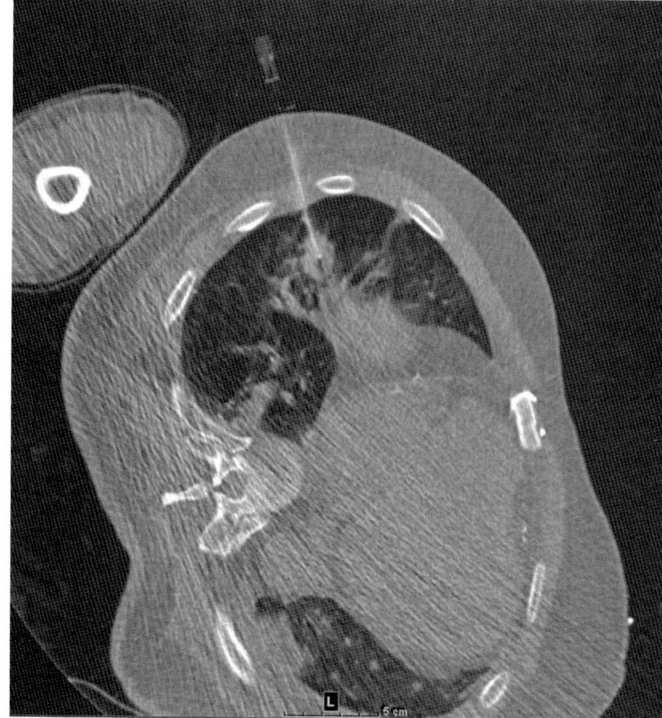

B

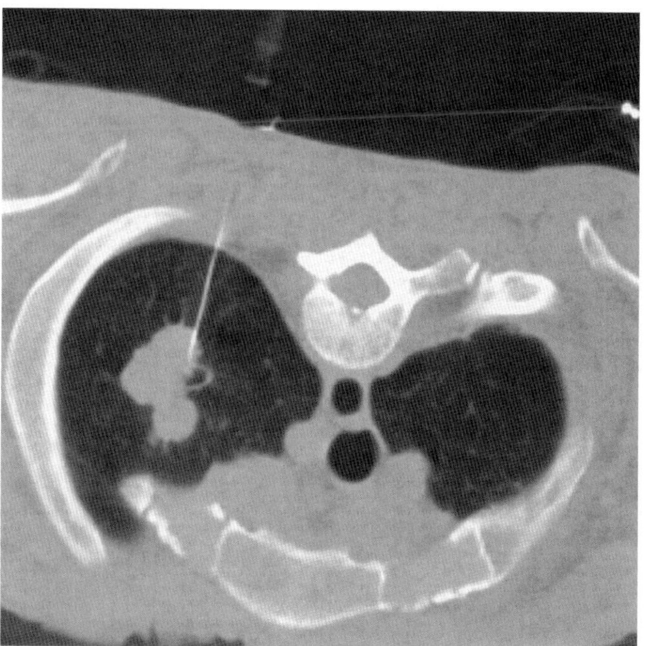

C

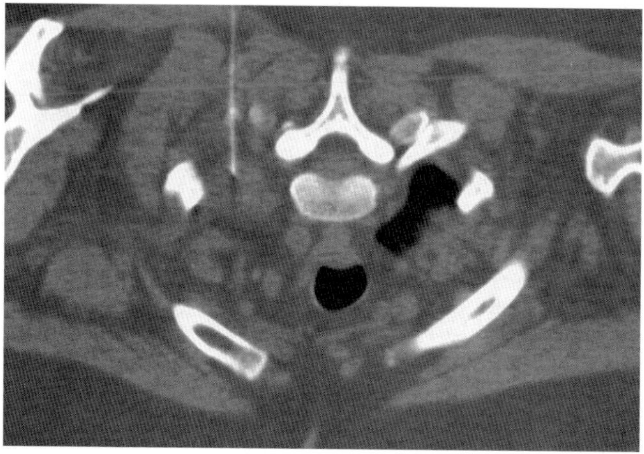

D

Figure 30-9 CT offers accurate, near–real-time localization of lesions for image-guided percutaneous small-needle biopsy. **A.** CT-guided biopsy of a small (0.8 cm) RUL spiculated nodule, a biopsy-proved adenocarcinoma; (**B**) CT-guided biopsy of a larger (1.8 × 2.2 cm) RML nodule, biopsy-proved small cell carcinoma; (**C**) CT-guided biopsy of a lobulated LUL mass (3.0 × 4.2 cm), biopsy-proved adenocarcinoma; (**D**) CT-guided biopsy of a soft tissue mass in the left superior sulcus, biopsy-proved malignant neurogenic neoplasm.

Video 30-5 4D cine using custom window. **A.** Lung window. **B.** Reversed lung window. The images are acquired sequentially at the same level and used for guidance in performing a transthoracic fine-needle aspiration (TTNA). The needle was advanced to perfectly engage a 14- × 13-mm LUL nodule. Final diagnosis was metastasis from RCC (renal cell carcinoma). *Access at www.fishmansonline.com*

superficial chest wall lesions can be accessed via US or CT; pleural, pulmonary, and anterior mediastinal lesions are accessed via CT; central hilar lesions and deep mediastinal masses are not accessible via PTB.

There are two basic types of PTB: fine-needle aspiration (FNA) and automated core needle biopsies (CNBs). In FNA, a small-caliber needle (25–22G) is inserted through the chest wall into the lesion via CT guidance. The tip of the needle is positioned inside the lesion. Negative pressure (suction) is applied via a syringe, and fluid or clusters of cells are aspirated. The material obtained via FNA is processed using cytopathology techniques, and specific stains and molecular tests can be performed.

In contradistinction, CNB uses a larger coaxial system in which a 19G introducer (outer core) hollow needle is advanced to the pleura or close to the edge of the lesion, followed by introduction of a 20G automated inner core biopsy needle, which is advanced to the lesion. An automated mechanism is then activated, rapidly moving the needle forward and filling the needle trough, or shallow receptacle, with cylindrical "cores" of tissue. The outer sheath instantly moves forward to cut the tissue and keep it in the trough. This process is repeated several times as multiple tissue cores are obtained. The material obtained via CNB is processed using surgical pathology techniques. Both FNA and CNB provide material for microbiology studies, including stains and cultures.

From a diagnostic perspective, FNA is almost equally accurate to CNB for diagnosis of malignant diseases, although CNB is superior for diagnosis of benign diseases. FNA sensitivity for diagnosis of lung cancer is 80% to 95%, and the rate is higher if onsite cytopathology is available and the procedure is approved and performed by experienced radiologists. Limitations of FNA include diagnosis of indolent or low-grade malignancies (for which more tissue or histoarchitecture is required for confident pathologic diagnosis) and inflammatory or infectious diseases—scenarios in which CNB is superior. The advantage of FNA over CNB is a lower complication rate and the capacity to engage and sample very small lesions that would otherwise be inaccessible.

Lesion location, lesion size, and patient body habitus are major determinants utilized by the radiologist in deciding the optimal biopsy technique. All other factors being equal, large pulmonary masses (>3 cm), pleural masses, chest wall masses, and large anterior mediastinal masses are best sampled via CNB. On the other hand, small pulmonary nodules (as small as 0.8 cm), pulmonary nodules in highly mobile regions (posterior or anterior lung bases), and small lymph nodes are best approached using FNA.

Complications related to PTB are relatively infrequent, but occasionally they can be life-threatening. For mediastinal, chest wall, and pleural biopsies, the major risk is hemorrhage, with infection and postprocedural pain following in incidence. Major vascular injury is rare, but it has been reported following biopsies of mediastinal masses. For lung biopsies, the major risk is pneumothorax, followed by hemorrhage, infection, and, rarely, air embolism. While air embolism is the rarest complication, with reported frequency of 0.05% to 0.10%, it is potentially the most life-threatening, due to its unpredictable nature and difficult treatment. Pneumothorax rate varies widely according to institution, and estimates from 5% to 50% have been reported. Most postprocedural pneumothoraces are small and not clinically significant; however, in up to 5% to 10% of patients, a large or symptomatic pneumothorax requires chest tube placement.

The following precautions are advised to minimize the risks associated with PTB: (1) critical appraisal of the clinical need for biopsy and whether PTB is the best approach; (2) thorough preprocedural laboratory assessment to ensure normal platelet count and function and normal coagulation profile. Anticoagulants and antiplatelet medications should be discontinued after conferring with the referring physician; (3) performance or supervision of the procedure by an experienced radiologist; (4) careful preprocedural planning, choosing a patient position and needle trajectory that minimizes the risk of vascular injury and decreases the distance to the lesion; (5) proper biopsy technique with purposeful, fast, accurate needle motion, confirming with imaging the needle location, depth, and relationship to the lesion prior to, and after, each needle movement; and (6) minimization of the effects of patient motion by tracking chest wall movement and advancing the needle in a consistent phase of the respiratory cycle.[8,9]

Therapeutic, percutaneous, image-guided techniques have also been increasingly accepted and utilized. These range from percutaneous chest tube or drain placement to ablation of neoplasms utilizing microwave or cryoablation techniques. The same principles of imaging guidance described for PTB apply for percutaneous therapeutic interventions. Given their complexity and the availability of alternative treatment options (such as surgery or radiation therapy), their use is best reserved for selected patients following discussion with multidisciplinary healthcare teams.

OBSTRUCTIVE LUNG DISEASES, WITH EMPHASIS ON COPD

Pulmonary ventilation, as is the case for pulmonary perfusion, is not homogeneous; it is affected by gravity, airway caliber, and chest wall mechanics. Ventilation is greater at the bases in the erect position due to greater regional changes in lung volume with inspiration, but the apical–basal ventilation gradient is smaller than the perfusion gradient (noting that perfusion is also greater at the bases). Therefore, the ventilation–perfusion ratio (V/Q) is greater at the apices in the erect patient. A similar pattern occurs in the supine patient between the dependent posterior and the nondependent anterior lungs, albeit to a lesser extent. Changes in relative ventilation affect the relative volume and average density of the lung parenchyma and, therefore, can be depicted by imaging.

Chronic obstructive pulmonary disease (COPD) is a complex group of disorders characterized by chronic, progressive airflow limitation that is not fully reversible and is associated with a range of pathologic changes in the lungs (Chapters 39 and 40). In addition, significant extrapulmonary effects caused by chronic inflammation and structural changes are observed. The chronic airflow limitation is caused by a mixture of small airway disease (obstructive bronchiolitis) and parenchymal destruction (emphysema). In addition, large airway inflammation, with increased sputum production and cough, is the hallmark of chronic bronchitis, part of the spectrum of COPD. The relative contributions of these components vary substantially from patient to patient. The presence and extent of each component has the potential to affect clinical presentation, disease severity, prognosis, and therapeutic response. COPD is strongly related to smoking. It has emerged as the third leading cause of death in the United States.

Another clinically prevalent obstructive lung disease is asthma, which is an inflammatory condition affecting mainly small airways, with increased mucus production, airway wall inflammation, and reduced luminal caliber (Chapters 44–46). Asthma differs from COPD from an imaging standpoint in that the clinical manifestations are usually intermittent and reversible, and the degree of hyperinflation tends to be mild, except in severe, longstanding disease.[10,11]

Chest radiographs are not particularly useful in diagnosing obstructive lung disease. In early disease, these are generally normal, as is the case with most asthmatic patients. In more severe or advanced disease, hyperinflation ensues and can be detected radiographically. The classic radiographic appearance of hyperinflation is manifested by increased radiolucency of the lungs; low, flat diaphragms; exaggerated verticality of the heart; increased AP diameter of the chest; and widening of the retrosternal lucent space. Of all these criteria, diaphragmatic flattening is probably the most reliable in supporting a diagnosis of COPD, as it is likely associated with severe emphysema. Care must be taken in making a diagnosis, however, as hyperinflation can be simulated radiographically when a healthy person exerts a maximal inspiratory effort. The lungs also appear hyperinflated in very slender persons. Therefore, it is unwise to make the diagnosis of emphysema solely on the basis of the radiographic finding of hyperinflation (Figs. 30-10 and 30-11).

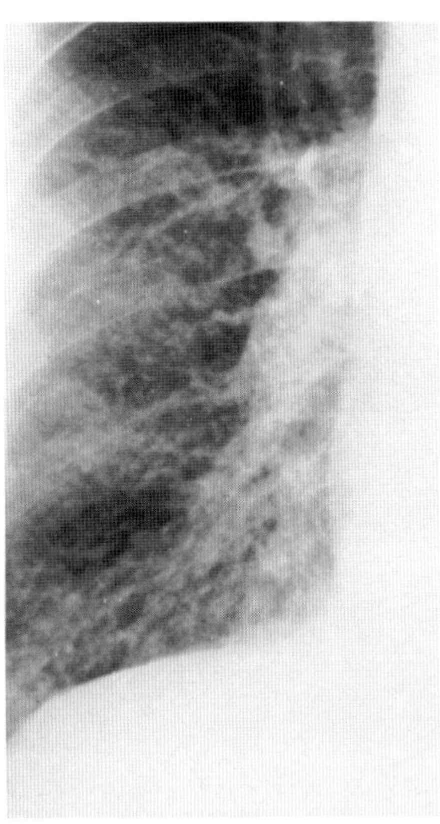

Figure 30-10 Detail view of the lung parenchyma in a PA radiograph, demonstrating increased bronchovascular markings, which are particularly prominent throughout the central lung fields. The patient has COPD with predominant chronic bronchitis. Hyperaeration is minimal.

Radiographic evaluation of the pulmonary vessels may also support a diagnosis of emphysema. Two distinctly different vascular patterns have been identified in patients with chronic bronchitis and emphysema: arterial deficiency and increased lung markings. Patients who show the arterial deficiency pattern often have panlobular emphysema and manifest the clinical syndrome of the "pink puffer." Those who have the pattern of increased lung markings often have centrilobular emphysema and manifest the "blue bloater" syndrome. Notably, these radiographic findings occur relatively late in the clinical course of emphysema. Moreover, these findings are not specific and must be considered in the clinical context provided.

Similarly, the diagnosis of chronic bronchitis is a clinical one, based upon a history of chronic cough and sputum production and supplemented by characteristic abnormalities in pulmonary function tests. The radiograph rarely provides substantive help. Vascular markings throughout the lung fields are sometimes prominent, but this finding is nonspecific.

CT, on the other hand, is capable of demonstrating the pathologic changes associated with COPD, including large and small airway inflammation and parenchymal destruction (emphysema). Three basic types of emphysema can be detected by CT—centrilobular, paraseptal, and panlobular.

Centrilobular emphysema is characterized by focal areas of lucency within the centers of secondary pulmonary lobules and without perceptible walls. The lobular arteries and bronchi are maintained, appearing as small dots within the involved secondary lobules. These features help to differentiate the holes of centrilobular emphysema from the cysts of cystic lung disease, as the latter have thin walls and are devoid of internal structure.

Paraseptal emphysema occurs peripherally, adjacent to the visceral pleura, and adjacent to the bronchovascular interstitium. Centrilobular and paraseptal emphysema are both associated with

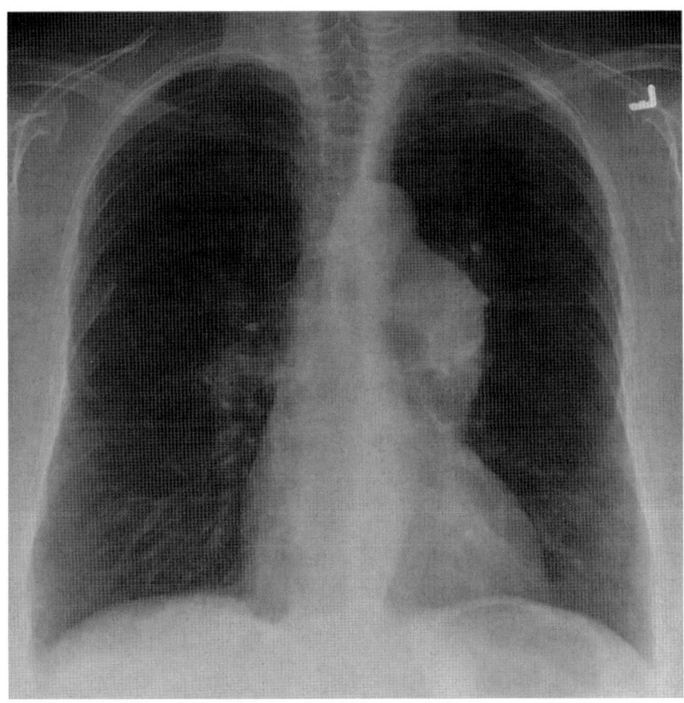

A

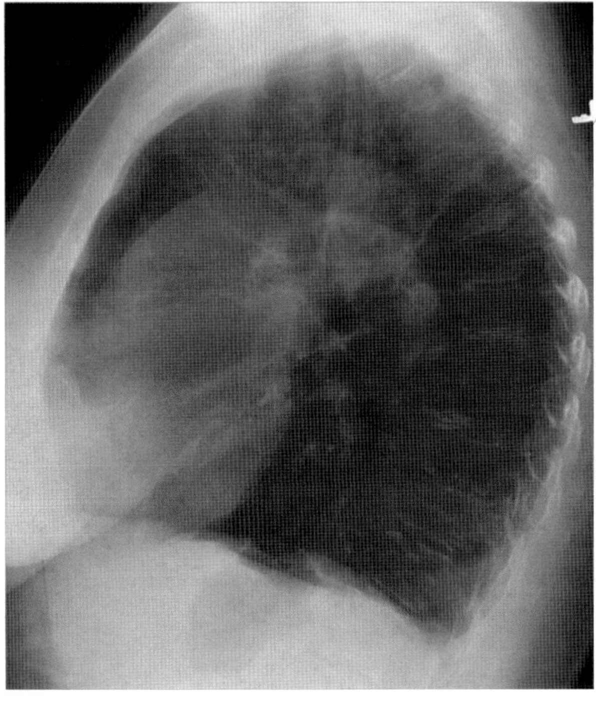

B

Figure 30-11 (**A**) PA and (**B**) lateral of a patient with severe emphysema-predominant COPD. Salient features are hyperinflation (denoted by flattening of the diaphragms and increased craniocaudal and anteroposterior diameters of the chest) and hyperlucency of the parenchyma. Also note prominence of the central pulmonary arteries, compatible with pulmonary hypertension.

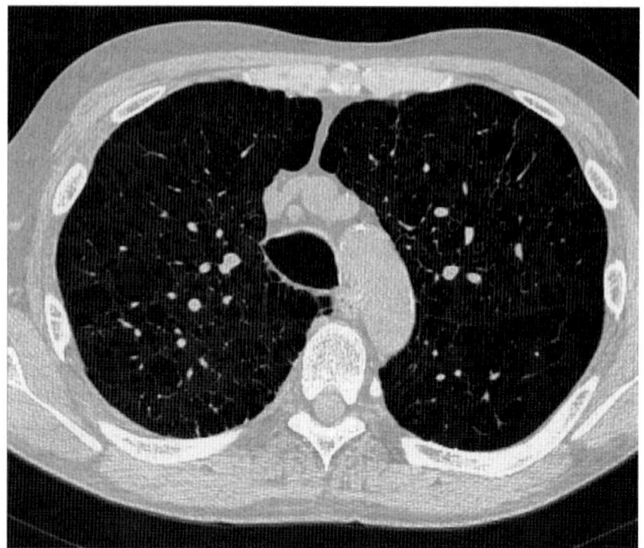

A

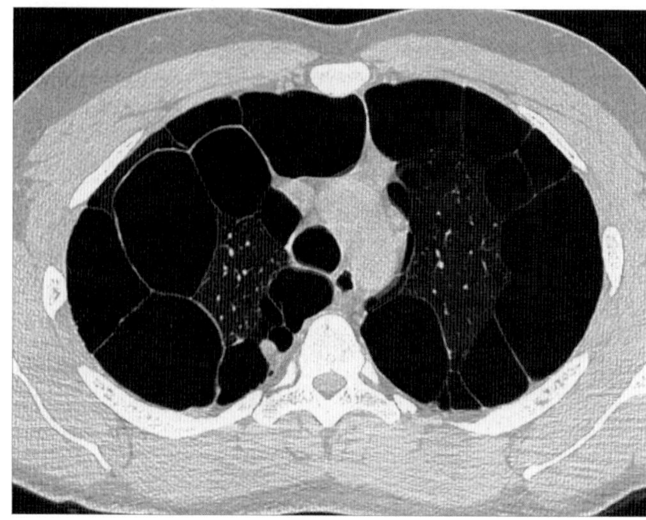

B

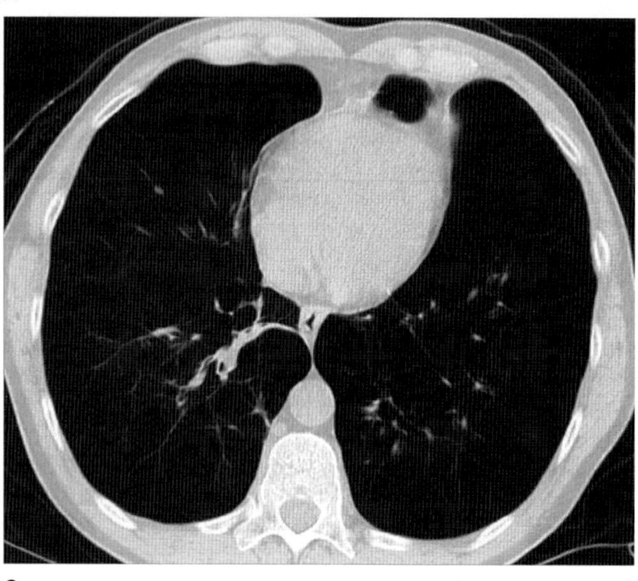

C

Figure 30-12 Three different phenotypes of emphysema. **A.** Centrilobular. **B.** Paraseptal. **C.** Panlobular. The images demonstrate different configurations and anatomical distribution of parenchymal destruction. (**A**) and (**B**) are typically smoking-related, whereas the patient in (**C**) had α1-antitrypsin deficiency.

smoking and, therefore, tend to coexist, although the contribution of each form for the total amount of emphysema varies substantially. There is generally upper lung predominance, except in very severe disease. The extreme form of paraseptal emphysema is evident as bullous disease, in which the cystic spaces may become large enough to compromise lung mechanics due to their mass effect.

Finally, panlobular emphysema is a distinct entity in which there is diffuse hyperlucency, hypovascularity, and a paucity of interstitial markings, often with a basilar predominance. These important findings can be overlooked even in patients with marked panlobular emphysema, since there are no discrete holes, as is the case in centrilobular emphysema. This form of emphysema is less likely associated with smoking, and more likely associated with α1-antitrypsin deficiency, a genetic condition that can be exacerbated by smoking (Figs. 30-12 and 30-13).[12–14]

Large airway inflammation as a manifestation of chronic bronchitis may be suggested by the presence of airway wall thickening, the diagnosis of which is somewhat subjective, although several studies have described computer-assisted quantitative measurement methods. Mucoid impaction is a reliable indicator of airway inflammation, but it is not specific for COPD, as it can be seen in the setting of asthma, acute bronchitis, or bronchopneumonia.

Small airway inflammation was previously the most difficult component of COPD to diagnose by imaging. While it is still not possible to directly image inflammation of the very distal airways, expiratory CT now provides the best technique to indirectly diagnose small airway disease. The presence of small airway disease may be inferred by the presence of expiratory air trapping. Normally, the average CT attenuation of aerated lung parenchyma increases in expiration due to volume averaging of voxels that contain less air. In contrast, with air trapping, the increased lung attenuation with expiration is not observed. Thus, in the presence of small airway disease a "mosaic attenuation pattern" is demonstrated on CT images obtained in end expiration, with the darker (lower attenuation) areas corresponding to areas of regional air trapping. Up to 25% of the lung may show air trapping in healthy subjects (typically at the lung bases); higher degrees of air trapping correlate with decreases in functional parameters assessed with pulmonary function testing, such as residual volume (RV) or functional residual capacity (FRC) (Figs. 30-14 and 30-15).

The major future trend in the imaging of COPD is the development of computer-assisted quantification techniques for disease phenotyping, namely, detecting and measuring the severity and

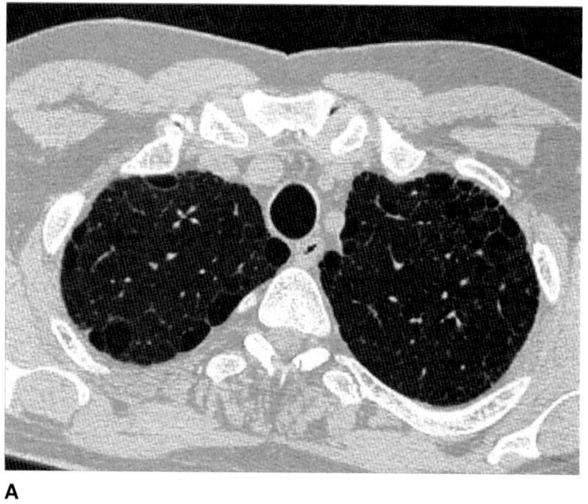

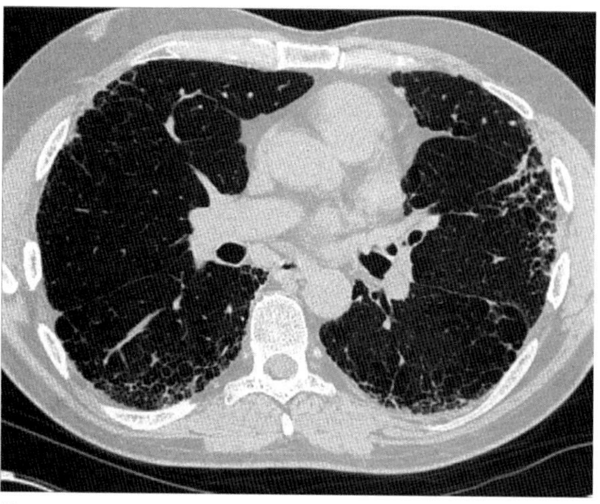

Figure 30-13 Severe emphysema and pulmonary fibrosis in a long-term smoker. **A.** Paraseptal and centrilobular emphysema involving the upper lung fields; (**B**) Additional presence of traction bronchiectasis, peripheral reticulation and honeycombing—features of fibrosis. Smoking-related pulmonary fibrosis is associated with COPD and resembles UIP from an imaging standpoint.

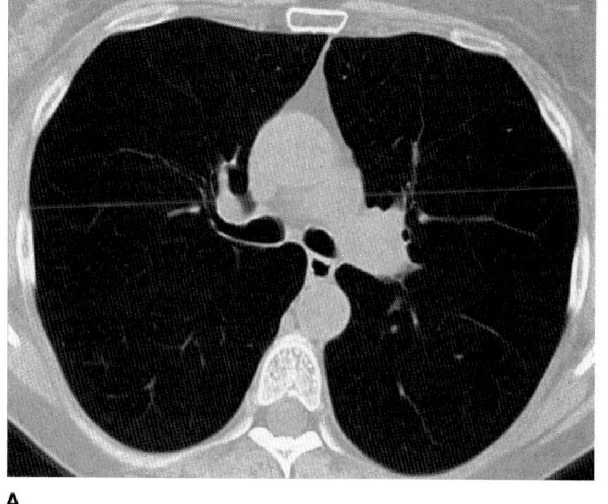

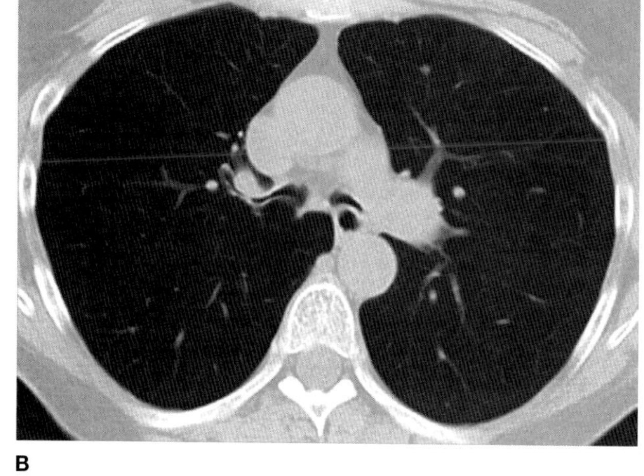

Figure 30-14 (**A**) Inspiratory and (**B**) expiratory CT images at the level of the mainstem bronchi, demonstrating dynamic expiratory collapse of the central airways, indicative of bronchomalacia, a common association with COPD.

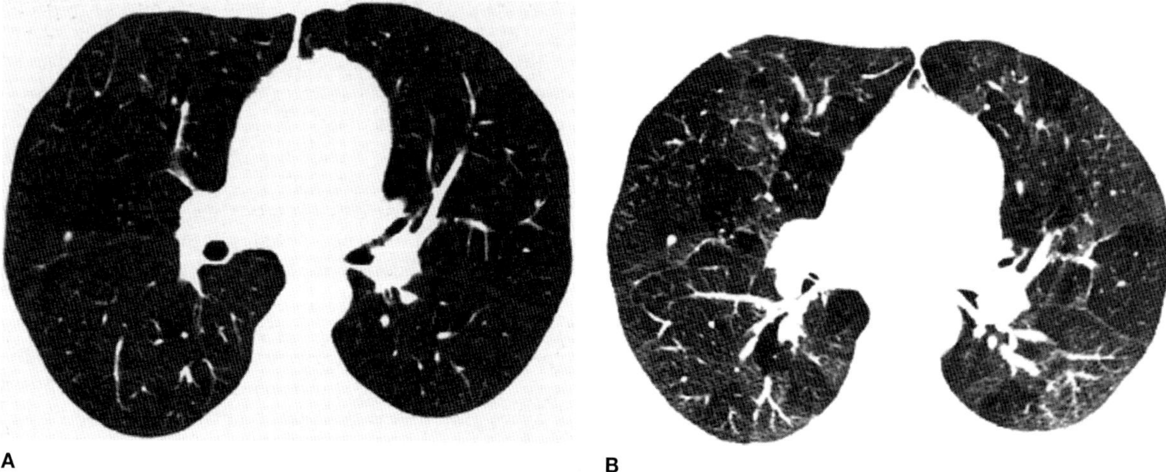

Figure 30-15 (**A**) Inspiratory and (**B**) expiratory CT images demonstrate the presence of mosaic attenuation (i.e., geographic areas of low parenchymal attenuation interspersed within normal, higher-attenuation areas in expiration), characteristic of air trapping. This patient had a diagnosis of bronchiolitis obliterans.

relative contributions of emphysema and large and small airway diseases to the overall clinical presentation and functional status. Many studies have been published on this subject in the last decade. For quantitative imaging, strict standardization of the scanning technique is required. Sophisticated computer algorithms are also required to accurately separate the lung parenchyma, central airways, central vasculature, mediastinum, and chest wall structures based upon attenuation characteristics and geometric constraints using thin-section, isotropic volumetric data sets primarily obtained using CT. A variety of computational methods can then be applied to detect several disease patterns and characterize their extent and distribution, for both diagnosis and disease quantification as a means of better assessing prognosis and response to therapies.[15,16]

It has been established that "attenuation masks" that separate all low attenuation voxels in the segmented lung parenchyma (e.g., areas of <-950 HU), not including central airways, can accurately quantify the volume of emphysema compared with the reference standard of pathologic assessment. Such CT measures of emphysema demonstrate strong correlation with functional metrics that denote obstruction (e.g., FEV1/FVC,%). Moreover, it is possible to measure the thickness of the central airways (to the fifth or sixth generation) as a quantitative metric in chronic bronchitis. In addition, small airway disease can be indirectly measured using quantification of expiratory air trapping, which can be accomplished via several different techniques. The simplest method uses attenuation masks in expiration. Voxels measuring less than -856 HU on expiratory CT are considered areas of air trapping. This attenuation threshold has been validated in multiple publications. More sophisticated techniques take into account how much each voxel varies in attenuation between full inspiration and end expiration (at FRC). The latter approach requires mathematical, nonrigid registration techniques that track individual voxel motion and regional volume changes between data acquired at two different time points, allowing for a one-on-one correspondence between lung voxels in inspiration and expiration.[17,18]

While these sophisticated quantitative applications are still largely investigational, they will likely reach the clinical realm within this decade. Studies continue to validate the superiority of quantitative imaging over standard qualitative assessment of thoracic imaging studies, demonstrating improved correlations with disease severity and functional impairment. Such quantitative imaging will ultimately provide better tools to estimate prognosis and monitor the efficacy of therapy.

INTERSTITIAL LUNG DISEASE

Interstitial lung disease (ILD) is a broad and complex topic, with many distinct and unrelated clinical entities potentially contributing to a single imaging pattern. Their detailed pathophysiology is described elsewhere. The focus of this discussion is the contribution of imaging to the differential diagnosis of ILD, emphasizing the most common and clinically relevant diseases.

The chest radiographic pattern of interstitial disease differs from the pattern of alveolar disease in that with interstitial disease the imaging pattern tends to be discrete and sharp, rather than fluffy and irregular; the lesions tend to be diffused, rather than localized. In addition, coalescence is not a typical feature in ILD, and the small opacities are characteristically nodular, reticular, or linear. Large masses or consolidations are not characteristic of the interstitial pattern (Fig. 30-16).

In and of itself, the recognition of an interstitial pattern on chest radiographs is not specific for a particular diagnosis. Most often a CT is necessary for further characterization. However, two observations that may provide useful insight into the likely diagnosis are the temporal course and distribution of disease.

Most interstitial diseases have a chronic, progressive course. Therefore, recognition of an acute interstitial pattern, that is, development and rapid evolution over hours or a few days, is strongly suggestive of interstitial pulmonary edema. This is even more likely if ancillary findings indicative of congestive heart failure or volume overload are present, such as cardiomegaly, pleural effusions, and widening of the vascular pedicle in the mediastinum. Occasionally, a rapidly changing interstitial pattern represents atypical pneumonia due to *Pneumocystis jiroveci*, cytomegalovirus, or mycoplasma. The acute interstitial disorders typically cause a radiographic linear or reticular pattern, which is characterized by prominent Kerley lines throughout the lungs.

In his original description in 1951, Kerley associated thin, radiographic parenchymal opacities with left ventricular failure. Initially, Kerley lines were thought to represent swollen pulmonary lymphatics. It is now recognized that Kerley lines usually represent edematous septae within the pulmonary interstitium. Three patterns exist. Kerley type B lines are the most familiar and are particularly prominent at the lung bases, where they appear as straight, thin, peripheral lines approximately 1 cm long and oriented parallel to the diaphragm. Kerley type A lines represent septae deep within the substance of the lungs; they radiate from the hili, but they are thinner than central vessels. Kerley type C lines probably represent coalescence of A and B lines and are difficult to recognize.

Chronic ILDs may be caused by a wide variety of diseases, including idiopathic interstitial pneumonias, connective tissue diseases, pneumoconiosis, sarcoidosis, lymphangitic spread of malignancy, infections, Langerhans cell histiocytosis (LCH), and lymphangioleiomyomatosis (LAM). Of note, LCH and LAM are not interstitial diseases per se, but rather cystic lung diseases that can present as an interstitial pattern on chest radiography; they are better characterized as cystic diseases on CT.

Characterization of the pattern of interstitial disease as nodular, reticular, or linear on chest radiograph may help in differential diagnosis, since many of the ILDs have a predilection for one of these three patterns. However, beyond that, the radiographic findings are not sufficient for a specific diagnosis. Nonetheless, separation of the distribution of disease into two broad categories can be helpful—upper lung predominant versus basilar predominant.

Upper lung–predominant distribution favors airway-related pathology, with inhalational diseases such as infections, LCH, and pneumoconiosis predominating in this group. Moreover, sarcoidosis is also typically upper lung predominant, a finding compatible with the hypothesis that the disease is triggered by an inhaled agent, although its exact cause remains elusive. On the other hand, basilar-predominant distribution favors idiopathic interstitial pneumonias and connective tissue diseases, in which increased blood flow and greater regional volume changes may play a role in explaining the lower lung predominance. Following such radiographic assessment, CT is generally the next diagnostic step.[19,20]

CT has been validated as the optimal imaging technique for evaluating chronic ILDs. CT can often identify interstitial disease that is not seen on chest radiography, and it provides better disease pattern characterization to enable identification of the underlying etiology, as well as better qualitative or quantitative assessment of severity. CT patterns of ILD follow, to some degree, the patterns seen on the chest radiograph; however, CT allows distinction of reticular, linear, and nodular patterns much more confidently. In addition, it permits evaluation of ancillary findings, such as honeycombing, traction bronchiectasis, ground-glass opacities, and cystic changes, all of which may be very challenging or impossible

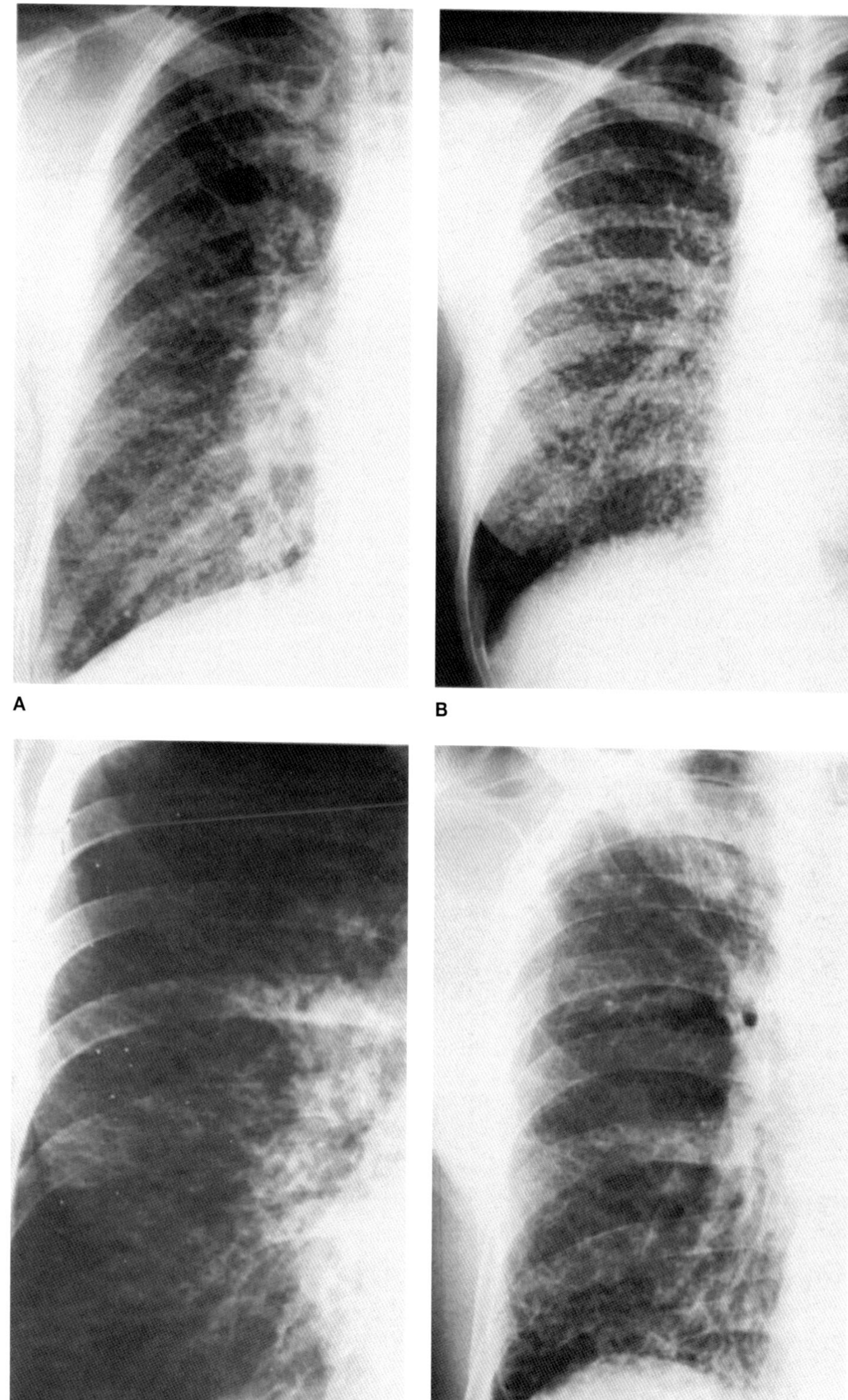

Figure 30-16 Radiographic patterns of interstitial disease. **A.** Linear interstitial pattern produced by interstitial pulmonary edema. The pattern is caused by fluid in the axial and septal interstitial spaces of the lungs, particularly in interlobar septae. **B.** Nodular interstitial pattern due to sarcoidosis. Multiple small, discrete nodules involve both lung fields diffusely. Adenopathy is absent. **C.** Lymphangitic spread of neoplasm. The linear interstitial pattern was caused by metastatic carcinoma of the pancreas. **D.** Reticular interstitial lung pattern. The pattern is most marked at the bases and is characteristic of idiopathic pulmonary fibrosis or collagen vascular disease, particularly scleroderma (as in this patient).

to recognize on chest radiographs. Important to emphasize is that, as previously discussed, every chest CT performed using current protocols on modern scanners may serve as a high-resolution examination. Therefore, the distinction between standard and high-resolution chest CT is obsolete, and detailed interstitial disease characterization can be performed on all current chest CT studies.[21]

Careful analysis of the CT in evaluating ILD can be described as comprising three steps.

The first step in the diagnostic approach of ILD on CT is to exclude interstitial pulmonary edema as the cause. An acute course and ancillary findings of cardiomegaly, bilateral pleural effusions, and central vascular engorgement strongly suggest interstitial pulmonary edema. CT findings include symmetric

Video 30-6 Axial cine images using lung window, demonstrating a typical usual interstitial pneumonia (UIP) pattern of fibrosing interstitial lung disease—in this case, idiopathic (and, therefore, classified as IPF, or idiopathic pulmonary fibrosis). *Access at www.fishmansonline.com*

Video 30-7 Axial cine images using lung window, demonstrating mild interstitial lung disease characterized by basilar-predominant ground-glass opacities without overt fibrotic features, likely reflecting cellular nonspecific interstitial pneumonia (NSIP). In this case, the findings were attributed to connective tissue disease (likely due to scleroderma). *Access at www.fishmansonline.com*

bilateral axial (peribronchovascular) and interlobular septal thickening, with central and basilar predominance. Ground-glass opacities may be present, denoting concomitant alveolar edema. It is important to remember that lymphangitic spread of neoplasm may present with a similar CT pattern; however, the temporal course is not acute and the findings are often asymmetric and more nodular, with additional features of malignancy present, such as pulmonary masses and hilar or mediastinal lymphadenopathy.[22,23]

The second step is to decide whether usual interstitial pneumonia (UIP) is the most likely cause of the pattern. UIP is the pathologic correlate of idiopathic pulmonary fibrosis, although it may also be associated with connective tissue disorders and asbestosis, as well. The latter should be considered if other findings that correlate with asbestos exposure, such as pleural plaques, are present. It is important to recognize UIP because it generally has a much worse prognosis than other causes of ILD and because typical CT features may be sufficient for diagnosis and obviate the need for surgical lung biopsy. CT imaging findings of UIP include symmetric, basilar-predominant reticular opacities, peripheral stacked layers of small cysts (honeycombing), and traction bronchiectasis (Video 30-6). Honeycombing, in particular, is the imaging finding most suggestive of, and specific for, UIP. If this constellation of findings is present, the pattern can be confidently diagnosed as typical UIP and a surgical biopsy avoided.[22]

The third step is to ascertain whether there are features that suggest fibrosis but which are not typical of UIP. In the absence of honeycombing, the combination of reticulation, architectural distortion, and traction bronchiectasis indicates the presence of fibrosis. If fibrosis is present, the differential diagnosis is relatively limited, including atypical UIP, fibrotic nonspecific interstitial pneumonia (NSIP), end-stage sarcoidosis, and chronic hypersensitivity pneumonitis (CHP). Fibrotic NSIP is favored over atypical UIP if there is central, rather than peripheral, predominance, and honeycombing and associated ground-glass opacities are absent. Moreover, the early phase of NSIP may manifest as multifocal bilaterally symmetric ground-glass opacities without fibrotic features or consolidation, denoting early inflammatory changes (cellular NSIP) (Video 30-7). Untreated cellular NSIP generally progresses to fibrotic NSIP, though cellular NSIP tends to respond to anti-inflammatory drugs such as steroids. Nonetheless, significant overlap occurs between fibrotic NSIP and atypical UIP. Both may be idiopathic or associated with connective tissue disorders. Clinical correlation and laboratory tests usually are required to exclude a connective tissue disorder. Of note, the presence of a patulous esophagus may be a clue to the diagnosis of CREST syndrome or systemic sclerosis (Figs. 30-17 and 30-18).[24]

Sarcoidosis is suspected when there is a combination of upper lung–predominant disease that is bilaterally symmetric, axial and interlobular septal interstitial thickening, multiple diminutive nodules with perilymphatic distribution (see section on Pulmonary Nodules and Lung Cancer, below), and associated mediastinal and hilar lymphadenopathy. Mosaic air trapping may also be present. The presence of fibrotic features denotes end-stage disease (radiographic Stage IV). The differential diagnosis includes interstitial pulmonary edema and lymphangitic spread of neoplasm, with interlobular septal thickening as the unifying theme for these three entities.[25]

CHP frequently is associated with a mosaic attenuation pattern that is accentuated on expiratory imaging, denoting heterogeneous small airway air trapping. In addition, CHP tends to show upper zone predominance and may cause multiple tiny nodules. The presence of air trapping is somewhat specific for CHP in the setting of pulmonary fibrosis that does not conform to typical UIP or show features of sarcoidosis, unless the patient has superimposed asthma or COPD (Figs. 30-19–30-21).[26]

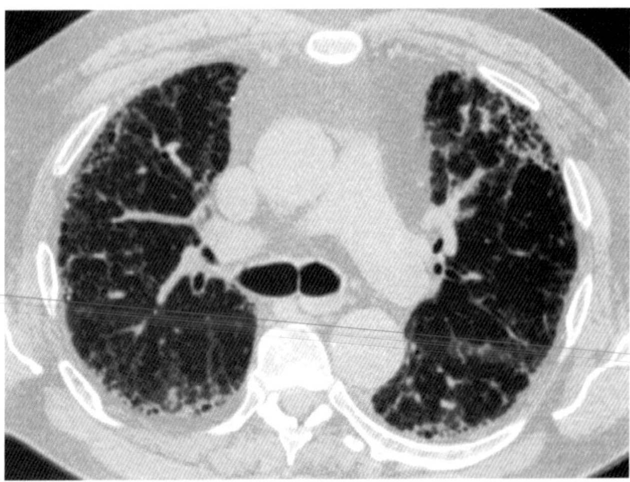

A

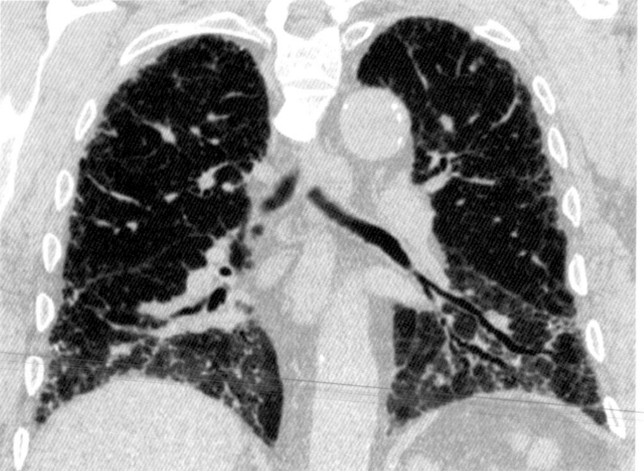

B

Figure 30-17 (**A**) Axial and (**B**) coronal CT images demonstrate a classic usual interstitial pneumonia (UIP) pattern, depicting symmetric, basilar- and peripheral-predominant reticulation, traction bronchiectasis and honeycombing. A UIP pattern confers the worst prognosis among interstitial diseases and is associated with the clinical diagnosis of idiopathic pulmonary fibrosis (IPF).

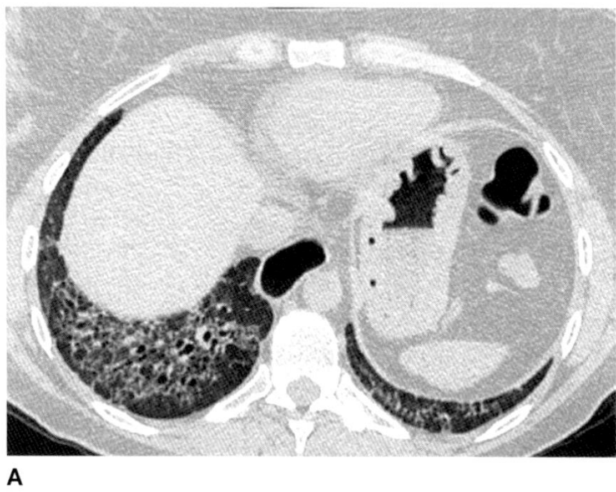

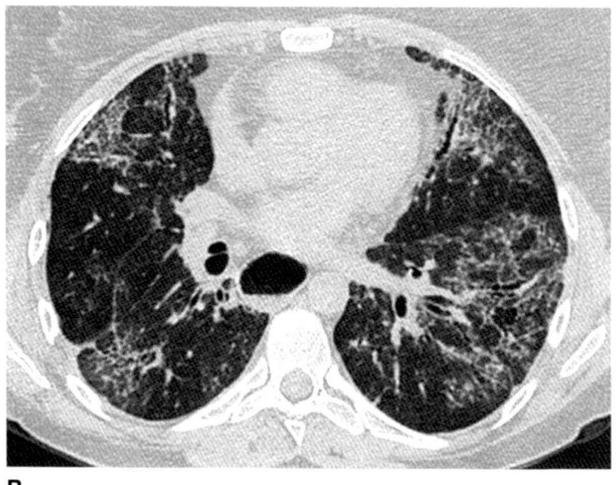

Figure 30-18 (**A**) Axial basilar and (**B**) axial midlung CT images in a patient with nonspecific interstitial pneumonia (NSIP) pattern. This pattern is distinguished from UIP by the absence of honeycombing and the more central (or peribronchovascular) distribution of reticulation denoting fibrosis. Traction bronchiectasis is also noted. The patient had a clinical diagnosis of scleroderma.

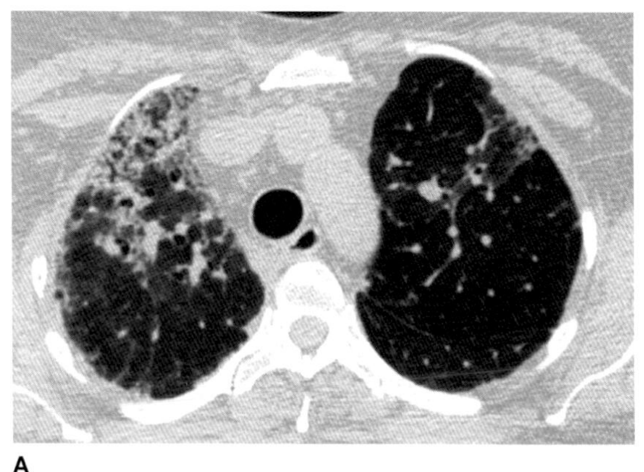

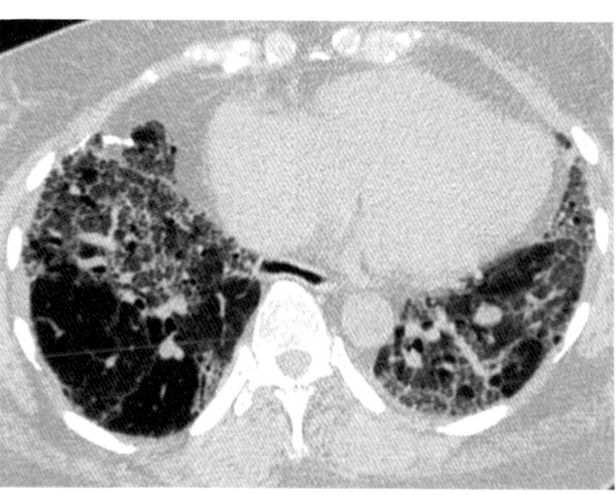

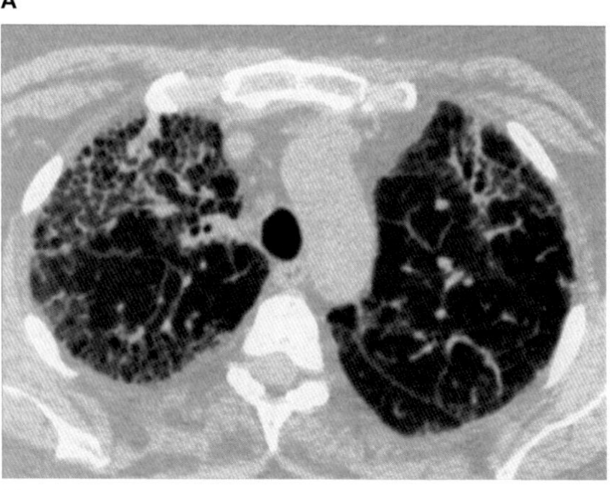

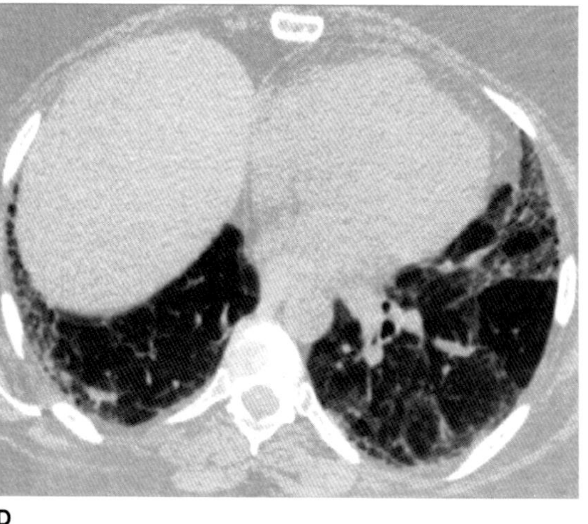

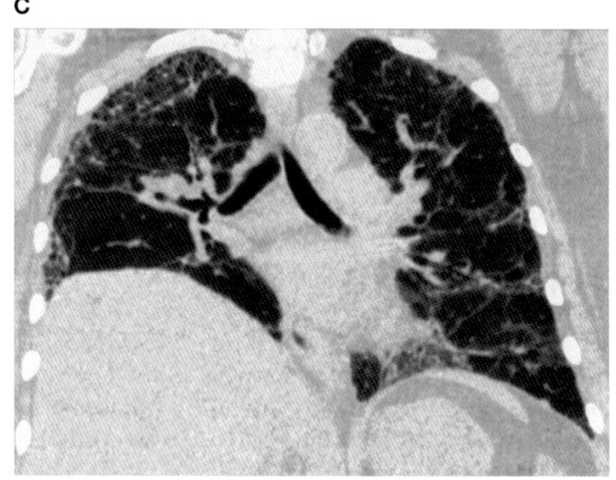

Figure 30-19 (**A**) and (**B**) are axial apical and axial basilar CT images in a patient with biopsy-proved CHP (chronic hypersensitivity pneumonitis); (**C**), (**D**), and (**E**) are axial apical, axial basilar, and coronal CT images in another patient with the same diagnosis, but with a more severe presentation. CHP is a differential diagnosis of fibrosing interstitial disease. It differs from UIP and NSIP by the upper lung predominance, patchy (or nonhomogeneous) distribution, and presence of air trapping (noting mosaic attenuation).

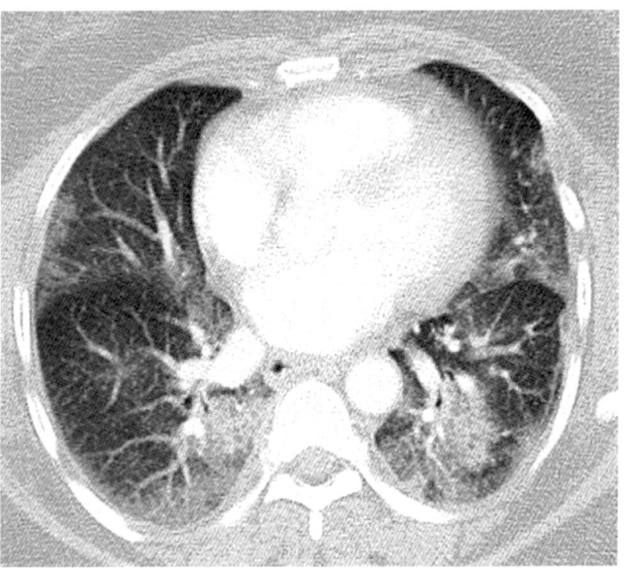

Figure 30-20 Multifocal airspace consolidation and ground-glass opacities in a patient with cryptogenic organizing pneumonia (COP). Infection is the most common differential diagnosis.

Pneumoconioses, particularly silicosis and berylliosis, may present with interstitial interlobular septal and axial thickening, as well as with perilympathic nodules—a pattern that can be indistinguishable from sarcoidosis. The presence of calcified nodules and mediastinal or hilar lymph nodes support the diagnosis of pneumoconiosis, but these findings may also be seen with sarcoidosis. Specific environmental exposure history is, of course, central in suggesting the diagnosis of pneumoconioses.

Currently, severity of ILD is assessed routinely via subjective analysis of disease extent on CT, along with evaluation of the degree of restriction on pulmonary function testing. Ongoing research has shown the promise of computational quantitative imaging techniques, which allow not only accurate diagnosis based upon pattern, but also quantification of the individual contributions of each pattern feature (e.g., ground-glass opacities and septal thickening) to the overall disease extent. This approach offers the potential for better tools for monitoring disease progression, predicting prognosis, and development of quantitative, surrogate imaging biomarkers for future medication trials.[27]

PULMONARY NODULES AND LUNG CANCER

Pulmonary nodules are exceedingly common and may be noted in up to 50% of CT examinations performed in hospital settings. Furthermore, the differential diagnosis is extremely broad and the imaging findings often nonspecific. Therefore, management of pulmonary nodules can be very challenging. We aim here to present a practical, evidence-based approach that is centered on answering four key questions: (1) Is the nodule likely malignant? If so, what is the best approach to tissue sampling? (2) If not, does the nodule need to be followed? If so, how often and for how long? (3) If it is not likely malignant, is the nodule likely to be manifestation of an infectious or inflammatory process that requires pathologic confirmation for proper management? (4) Does the nodule have any features that allow either a specific diagnosis or a confident diagnosis of benignity? The reader is also referred to Chapter 110 for further discussion.

The discussion of pulmonary nodules starts with their definition, which is not always straightforward. While there is no question that well-circumscribed round or ovoid opacities should be characterized as nodules, the distinction of nodules from focal consolidations and interstitial opacities can sometimes be cloudy, particularly when ill-defined or ground-glass nodules are taken into account. As a general rule, any opacity that has mostly convex borders and a shape that can be described as round or ovoid should be classified as a nodule. This has implications for differential diagnosis (Figs. 30-22 and 30-23).

From an imaging perspective, the following descriptors are important in assigning a nodule to a particular differential diagnostic category: number (solitary versus multiple), size, border, CT attenuation, and distribution (if multiple). Below each category is described and a strategic approach to diagnosis and management discussed, emphasizing a combination of clinical and CT findings.[28,29]

To answer the first question, that is, the nodule likely to be malignant, one must be cognizant of the pretest clinical probability. Age is important; the older the patient, the more likely that a lung nodule is malignant. Smoking history and COPD are major risk factors for lung cancer and should be taken into account. A known diagnosis

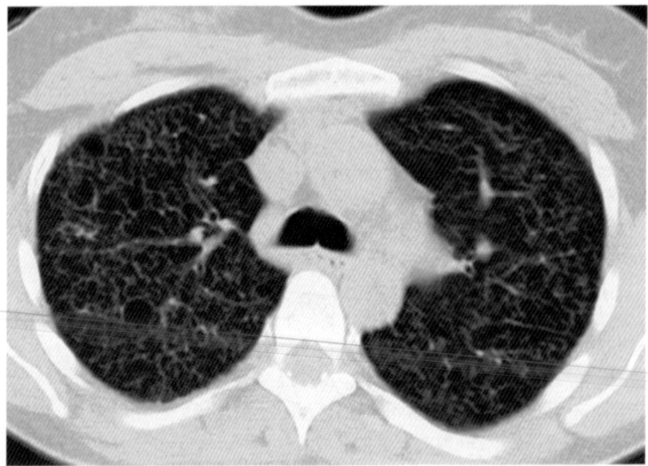

A

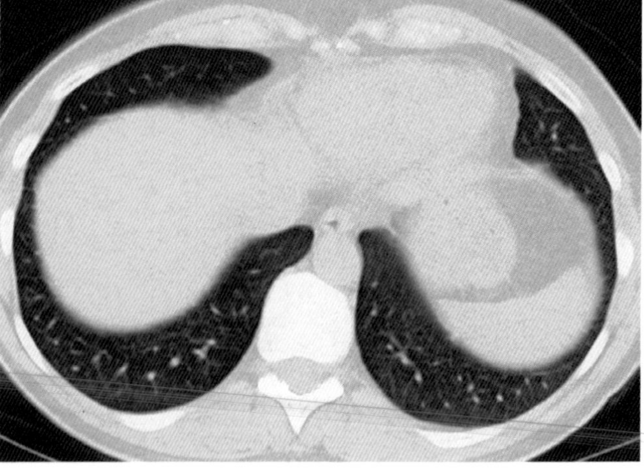

B

Figure 30-21 (**A**) and (**B**) are axial apical and axial basilar CT images in a patient with Langerhans cell histiocytosis (LCH). Although LCH is not considered an interstitial lung disease proper (instead, it is classified as a cystic lung disease), this disease does cause an interstitial pattern on chest radiographs. Key features are cysts with upper lung predominance, occasional nodules, and associated hyperinflation. A strong smoking history is often elicited.

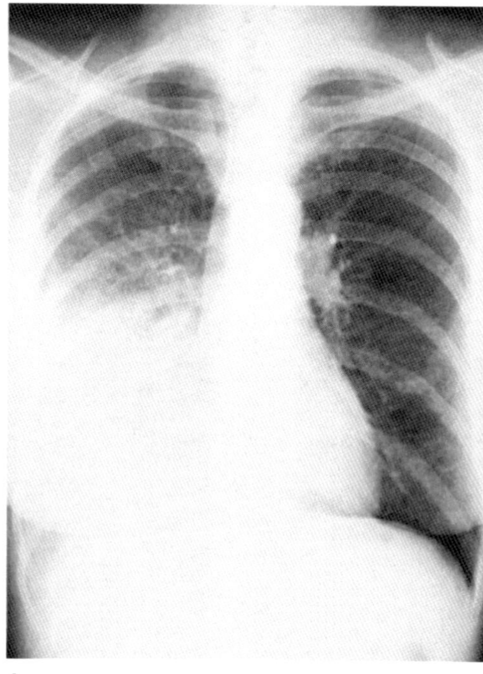

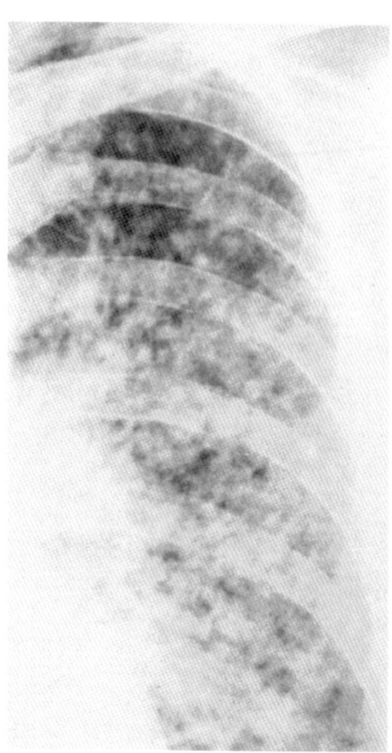

Figure 30-22 Radiographic patterns of adenocarcinoma. **A.** Large area of consolidation in the right lower lobe. The alveolar pattern suggests pneumonia, but it failed to improve with antibiotic treatment and was discovered to be an adenocarcinoma. **B.** Multiple ill-defined nodules. The nodules have irregular or fuzzy margins that are characteristic of alveolar, rather than interstitial, nodulation, in this patient with metastatic adenocarcinoma.

of malignancy also places the patient at a higher risk of pulmonary metastases.

Nodule features on CT are of considerable importance in suggesting malignancy. For a solitary nodule, the larger its size, the more likely it is malignant and represents a primary bronchogenic carcinoma. Ill-defined borders are also more highly associated with primary bronchogenic carcinoma than benign etiologies, although infectious processes, such as fungal pneumonia, also have to be considered in the proper clinical setting. Mixed attenuation nodules, that is, subsolid nodules with coexistence of solid and ground-glass components, are highly associated with a diagnosis of primary bronchogenic carcinoma. Multiple nodules that are well circumscribed, vary in size, and are basilar predominant are strongly suggestive of metastatic disease (Figs. 30-24–30-32).

The best evidence-based guidelines for management of solid pulmonary nodules are those published by the Fleischner Society.[30] Although originally described only for solitary nodules, the guidelines are oftentimes applied to multiple nodules.

The Fleischner Society guidelines stratify the risk of malignancy and recommend imaging follow-up intervals according to nodule size and clinical risk factors (Table 30-1). Nodules measuring <4 mm in a low-risk patient do not require follow-up, whereas larger nodules in higher-risk patients require follow-up at progressively shorter intervals (between a maximum of 12 months and a minimum of 3 months). Most nodules measuring more than 8 mm and lacking definitive benign imaging characteristics or confirmation of temporal stability are potentially malignant and, therefore, require more aggressive evaluation. Evaluation may include short-term interval CT follow-up, PET imaging, and often tissue sampling, which can be accomplished via minimally invasive transthoracic CT-guided or bronchoscopic techniques, or rarely, via surgical biopsy. As a general rule, peripheral and smaller nodules are more accurately sampled using transthoracic CT-guided techniques, whereas central or larger masses are more safely approached via bronchoscopic techniques.

It has been shown that only two CT features generally allow confident diagnosis of benignity for solid nodules: a benign pattern of calcification and absence of growth for at least 2 years.

A benign pattern of calcification includes any of the following: central, concentric, diffuse, or coarse ("popcorn" calcification). On the other hand, punctuate or eccentric calcifications are considered indeterminate, as both benign and malignant nodules may demonstrate these findings. Recognition of a benign pattern of calcification is, therefore, very important, as it may obviate the need for imaging follow-up or intervention, alleviating patient and clinician anxiety.

As noted, the second benign feature is interval stability for 2 years as measured by CT, following the Fleischner Society guidelines. The feature is based on the concept of doubling time, which is the time required for a nodule to double in volume. Very fast doubling time (<1 month) is most characteristic of inflammatory or infectious nodules. Extremely slow doubling time (>24 months) is more typical of benign processes, such as granulomas, hamartomas, intraparenchymal lymph nodes, or pulmonary arteriovenous malformations. Intermediate doubling times (>1 month but <24 months) are observed with most malignancies, as well as some indolent infections. In this indeterminate range of growth rate, tissue sampling should be strongly considered to exclude primary or metastatic malignancy.[31]

A CT finding of low-attenuation areas compatible with macroscopic fat in an otherwise well-circumscribed pulmonary nodule is strongly suggestive of a benign pulmonary hamartoma and can obviate the need for more aggressive workup. Care must be taken, however, in differentiating true fat from noise on thin-section CT performed with high-resolution ("HRCT") reconstruction kernels. The use of soft tissue kernels may help in making a more confident diagnosis of fat.

Cavitation is a useful finding in narrowing the differential diagnosis, although it is not specific for malignancy. A cavitary nodule suggests a necrotizing malignancy, particularly primary or metastatic squamous cell carcinoma. However, a number of benign entities may present with cavitary nodules, most typically septic emboli if multiple, granulomatous infections (including mycobacterial and fungal), bacterial abscesses, and granulomatosis with polyangiitis (GPA, formerly known as Wegener granulomatosis).

Ancillary findings on chest CT that support a diagnosis of malignancy include hilar and mediastinal lymphadenopathy, unilateral

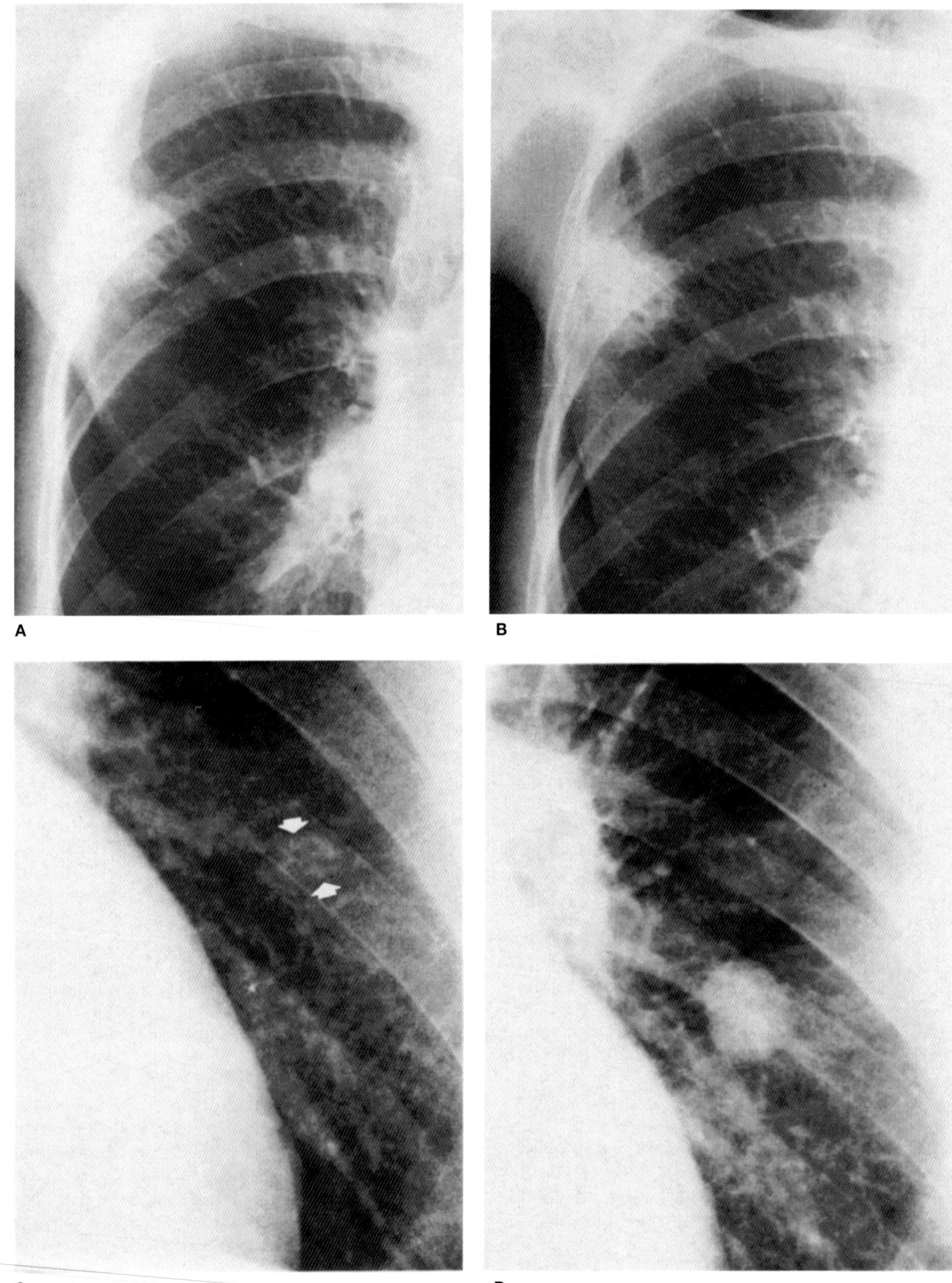

Figure 30-23 *Top:* Carcinoma of the lung with a long doubling time. An interval of 18 months elapsed between (**A**) and (**B**). The right upper lobe lesion, which enlarged minimally during that time, proved to be primary squamous cell. *Bottom:* Carcinoma of the lung with a short doubling time. An interval of 4 months elapsed between (**C**) and (**D**). The nodule was not detected on the first radiograph (**C**). It proved to be a primary small cell carcinoma.

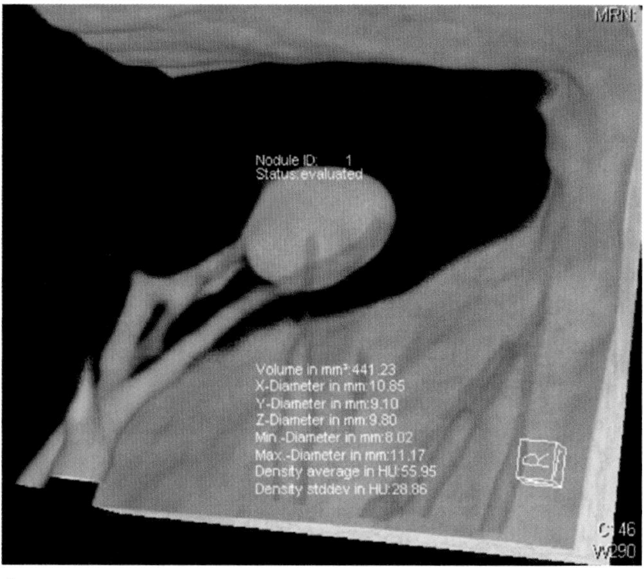

A

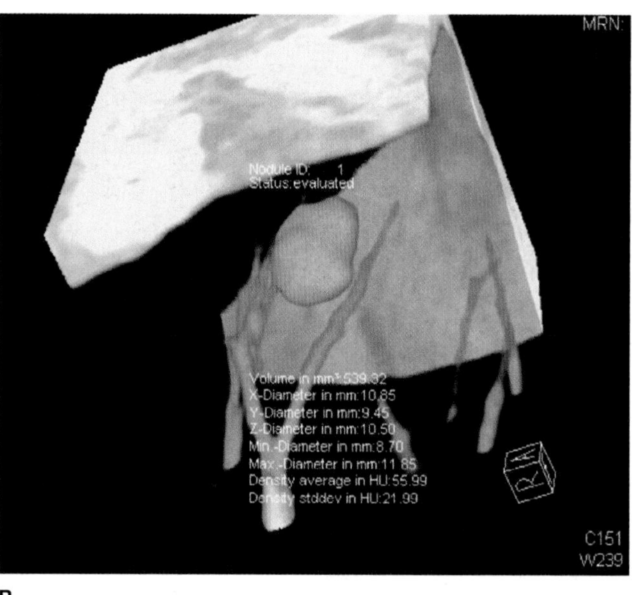

B

Figure 30-24 CT allows accurate volumetric measurement, which is not possible with chest radiographs, with the use of postprocessing software for nodule segmentation and volume calculation. This nodule grew from 441 mm³ (**A**) to 539 mm³ (**B**) in 7 months, an increase of 19%; it was later confirmed as metastasis from colon cancer.

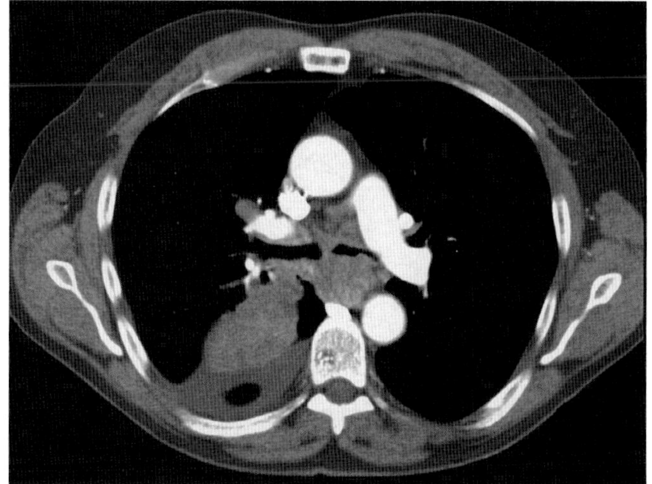

A

B

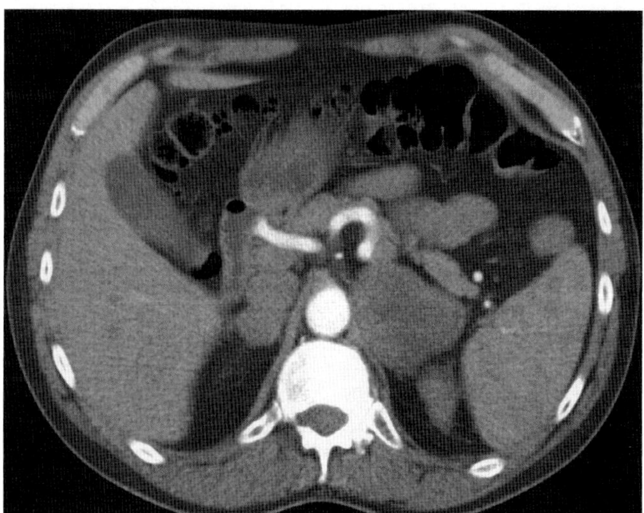

C

Figure 30-25 Advanced-stage lung cancer. The right lower lobe mass was proved to represent a small cell carcinoma. **A.** Axial CT on soft tissue window demonstrates the primary RLL mass, a malignant right pleural effusion, and mediastinal lymphadenopathy. **B.** Axial CT on lung window demonstrates multiple metastatic nodules in the left lung. **C.** Axial CT on soft tissue window demonstrates bilateral adrenal metastasis. The constellation of findings indicates Stage IV disease.

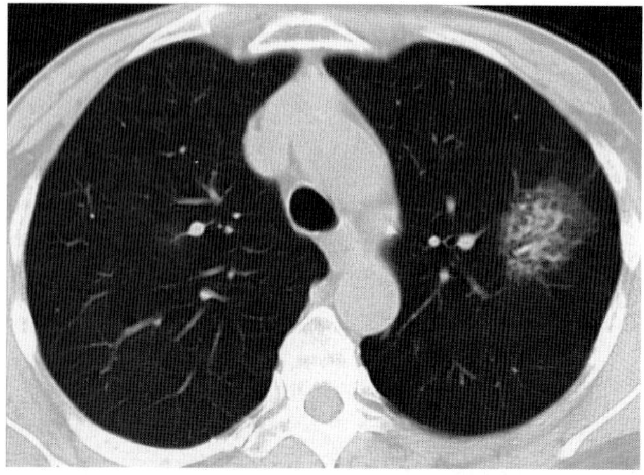

A

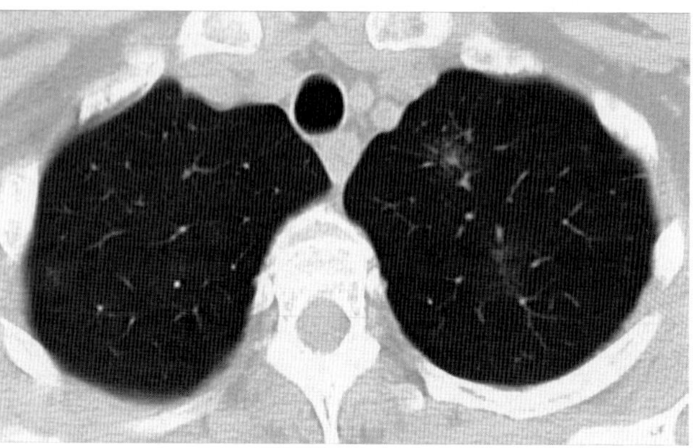

B

Figure 30-26 Spectrum of pulmonary adenocarcinoma. **A.** Axial CT image demonstrates a dominant, mixed-attenuation left upper lobe nodule, with solid and ground-glass components, which was resected and characterized as an adenocarcinoma. **B.** Axial CT image at a higher level demonstrates multiple smaller nodules, some of them mixed, most of purely ground-glass attenuation, which are compatible with multiple lesions in the spectrum of atypical adenomatous hyperplasia (AAH), adenocarcinoma in situ (AIS), and minimally invasive adenocarcinoma (MIA). In the past, all of these lesions would have been classified as BACs (bronchoalveolar carcinomas), a terminology that should no longer be utilized, as discussed in the text.

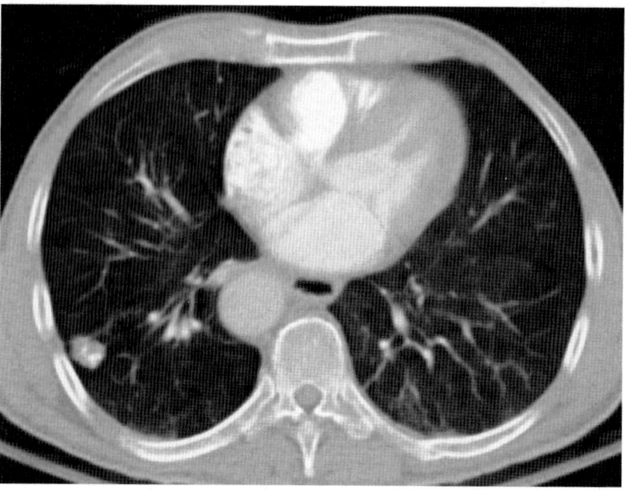

Figure 30-28 Right lower lobe nodule with coarse calcification, typical of a benign pulmonary hamartoma. Incidentally noted is a right-sided descending thoracic aorta.

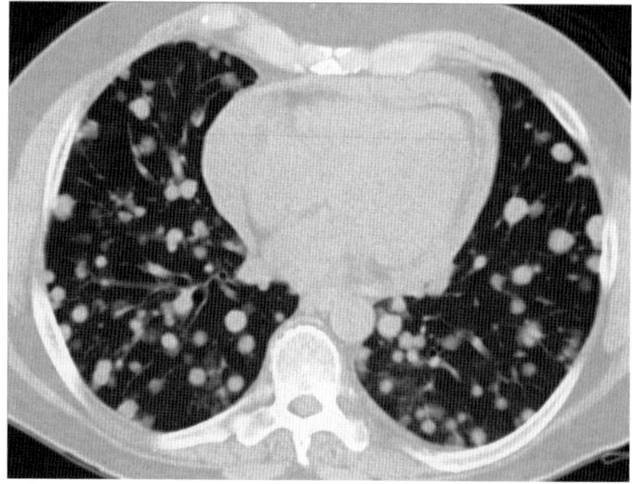

Figure 30-29 Differential diagnosis of multiple pulmonary nodules: axial CT image showing multiple well-circumscribed nodules, of varying size, characteristic of pulmonary metastases, in this case from renal cell carcinoma.

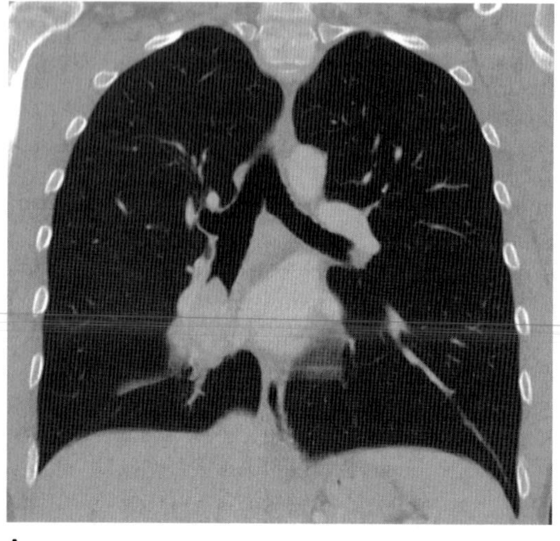

A

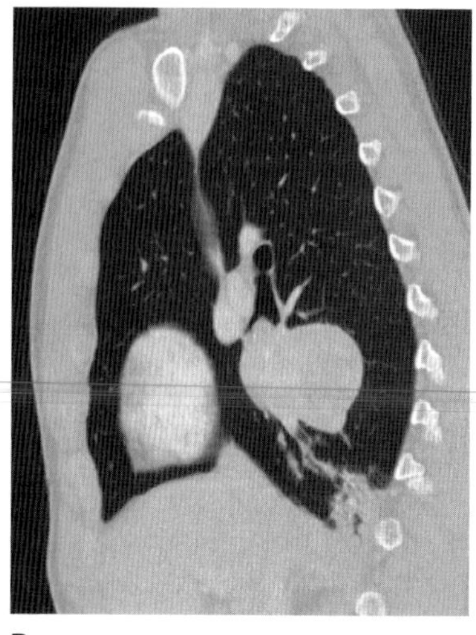

B

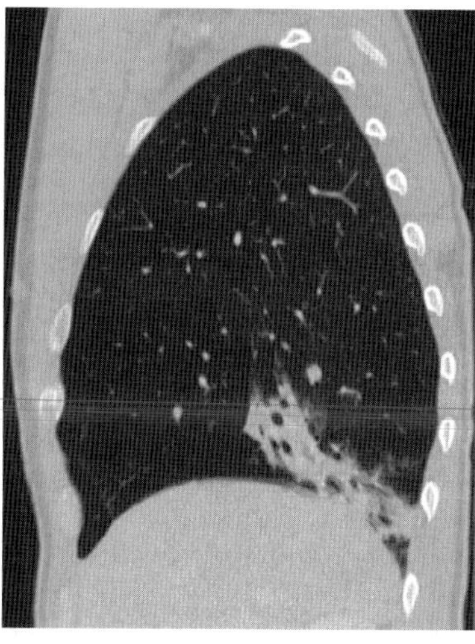

C

Figure 30-27 Coronal (**A**) and two sagittal CT images (**B**) and (**C**) showing a large endobronchial mass obstructing the RLL and growing concentrically into the lung parenchyma, with well-circumscribed borders. Note the associated atelectasis of the RLL basilar posterior segment. This mass was a carcinoid neoplasm.

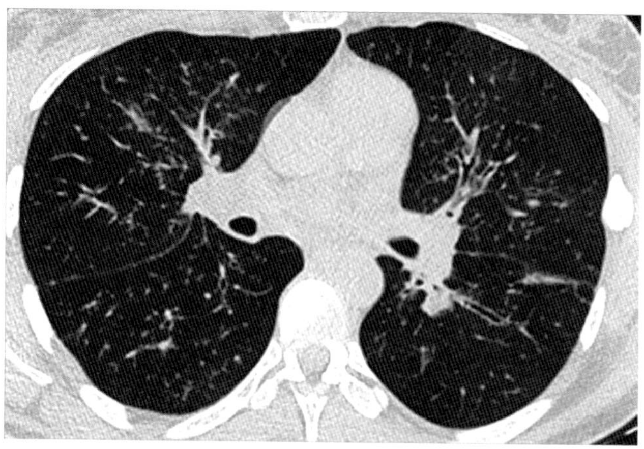

Figure 30-30 Differential diagnosis of multiple pulmonary nodules: axial CT image demonstrating very numerous, very small (1–2 mm) pulmonary nodules with a perilymphatic distribution (along the septal and axial interstitial compartments), typical of sarcoidosis—the diagnosis in this patient. This pattern can also be seen in lymphangitic carcinomatosis.

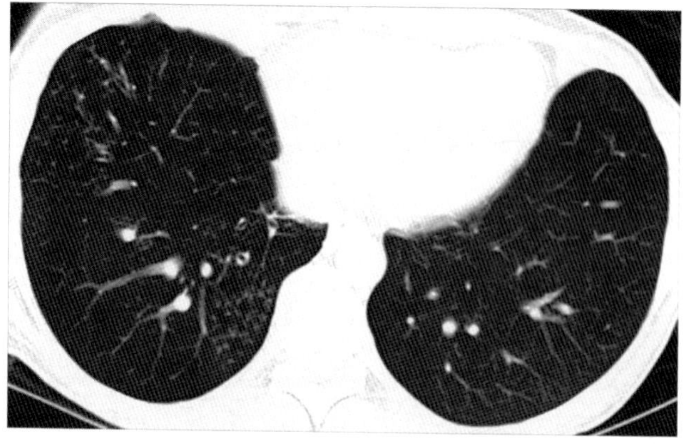

Figure 30-31 Differential diagnosis of multiple pulmonary nodules: axial CT images demonstrating multiple clusters of small nodules (measuring <2–3 mm each) in the RLL and RML, with centrilobular distribution and tree-in-bud configuration. This pattern is typical of infection and usually represents bronchiolitis. In this case, it was due to nontuberculous mycobacterial infection.

pleural effusion, pleural nodules, and hepatic, osseous, or adrenal metastases.

MULTIPLE PULMONARY NODULES

Most of the previously mentioned discussion applies to solitary or few pulmonary nodules, which should be approached similarly. In the setting of numerous, usually small (subcentimeter) pulmonary nodules, a different diagnostic approach must be utilized, emphasizing the distribution of the nodules. Two characteristics of the spatial distribution are relevant: (1) upper lung–predominant versus basilar predominant versus widespread; and (2) centrilobular versus perilymphatic versus random. The otherwise very long list of differential diagnoses can be substantially narrowed by correctly recognizing the distribution.

As discussed previously, an upper lung–predominant distribution suggests inflammatory or infectious etiologies, in which the inciting factor is inhaled; the exception is primary bronchogenic carcinomas that are more likely in the upper lungs, but uncommonly multiple. A lower lung–predominant distribution suggests hematogenously disseminated processes, such as hematogenous metastasis or hematogenous infectious processes. Diffuse distribution comprises a combination of both differential diagnoses and is the least specific.

The centrilobular distribution implies that the majority of nodules are in or near the center of the secondary pulmonary lobule. Such a distribution suggests small airway and acinar disease, indicative of endobronchial spread. This distribution can be further subclassified into two groups: (1) centrilobular nodules in which

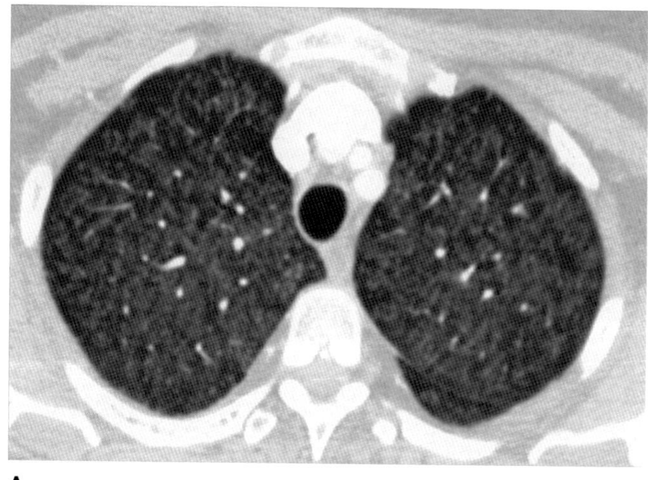

A

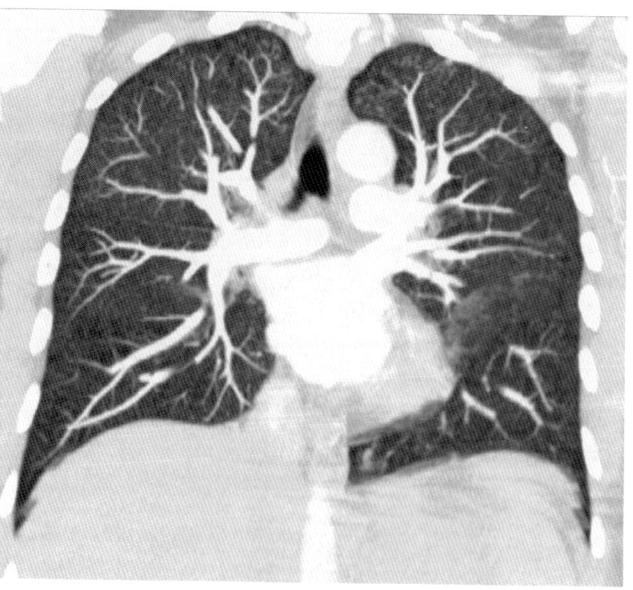

B

Figure 30-32 Differential diagnosis of multiple pulmonary nodules: (**A**) axial and (**B**) coronal MIP (maximum intensity projection) images demonstrate very numerous, very small (1–2 mm) pulmonary nodules with centrilobular distribution, low attenuation, and indistinct contours. Also noted is symmetric upper lung field predominance. The diagnosis is acute hypersensitivity pneumonitis. In a smoker, the differential diagnosis includes respiratory bronchiolitis.

TABLE 30-1 Fleischner Society Recommendations for Follow-Up and Management of Nodules Smaller than 8 mm Detected Incidentally at Nonscreening CT

Nodule Size (mm)	Low-Risk Patient	High-Risk Patient
≤4	No follow-up needed	Follow up CT at 12 mo; if stable, stop
>4–6	Follow up CT at 12 mo; if stable, stop	Initial follow-up at 6–12 mo, then at 18–24 mo if stable
>6–8	Initial follow-up at 6–12 mo, then at 18–24 mo if stable	Initial follow-up at 3–6 mo, then at 9–12 mo and at 24 mo if stable
>8	Follow-up at around 3, 9, and 24 mo, CT, PET/CT, and/or biopsy[a]	Same as for low risk[a]

Notes:
These recommendations apply for solid, noncalcified nodules—see Table 30-2 for ground-glass nodules.
Size is measured as an average of length and width (axial), for nonspherical nodules.
High-risk patient has a more than minimal history of smoking, and/or other risk factors such as prior or known malignancy, and/or increased risk for metastatic disease. A low-risk patient does not have any known risk factors for primary or metastatic lung cancer.
The higher the risk and the bigger the nodule, the shorter the follow-up interval is and the longer the period of follow-up is, up to 24 months if there is continued stability.
[a]Nodules measuring >8 mm generally require tissue diagnosis via CT-guided percutaneous biopsy, bronchoscopy, or surgical resection, depending on clinical and technical considerations.
Source: Adapted with permission from MacMahon H, Austin JH, Gamsu G, et al. Guidelines for management of small pulmonary nodules detected on CT scans: a statement from the Fleischner Society, Radiology. 2005;237(2):395–400.

the nodules are fuzzy, ill-defined, and often of ground-glass attenuation—findings indicative of small airway inflammatory diseases, as can be seen with respiratory bronchiolitis–interstitial lung disease (RB-ILD) and subacute hypersensitivity pneumonitis; and (2) centrilobular nodules in which the nodules are sharp, well defined, and measure less than 2 mm—findings associated with distal bronchiolar filling, a pattern referred to as, "tree-in-bud." A tree-in-bud pattern strongly suggests infectious bronchiolitis of bacterial, viral, or mycobacterial etiology. Least commonly, the centrilobular distribution may indicate small vessel disease, such as pulmonary vasculitides or capillary hemangiomatosis. Among the vasculitides, Churg–Strauss syndrome and microscopic polyangiitis are primary considerations.

The perilymphatic distribution implies that the majority of nodules are within the septal and bronchovascular interstitial compartments. A perilymphatic distribution is associated with diseases with lymphatic system involvement. Such a distribution suggests a narrow differential diagnosis, including pulmonary interstitial edema, sarcoidosis, or lymphangitic spread of neoplasm ("lymphangitic carcinomatosis"). The latter two diagnoses are more likely if there is nodular interstitial thickening.

A random distribution usually implies hematogenous dissemination of metastases or infection. The archetypal infectious process with numerous random nodules is miliary tuberculosis, although miliary fungal infections can be indistinguishable. Patients with miliary infectious are often immunocompromised and may present with bacteremia or fungemia.

GROUND-GLASS PULMONARY NODULES

Ground-glass nodules deserve separate consideration, as their pathophysiology, differential diagnosis, biologic behavior, and management strategies differ considerably from solid pulmonary nodules.

Ground-glass attenuation is defined as increased attenuation of the lung parenchyma, although the attenuation is not as high as soft tissue attenuation and, therefore, is insufficient to obscure adjacent pulmonary vessels. From a pathology perspective, ground-glass attenuation implies partial filling of the distal airspaces (acini) at a scale below the spatial resolution of CT, causing volume averaging of gas, acinar structures, and material partially filling the alveoli. It is often associated with the lepidic growth pattern, that is, cellular proliferation along the walls of the alveoli, rather than the more common hilic (radial) growth pattern characteristic of most neoplasms.

Multiple ground-glass nodules were described previously, and the rationale for their imaging assessment is included in the description of multiple pulmonary nodules.

Solitary or few ground-glass attenuation nodules carry a different implication from solid nodules. The differential diagnosis is essentially limited to nonspecific infectious or inflammatory processes versus indolent primary bronchogenic adenocarcinoma or premalignant lesions. Therefore, these lesions must be followed to assess their persistence and chronicity. Most nonspecific infectious or inflammatory processes resolve spontaneously within 3 months. Therefore, lesions that persist on a 3-month follow-up chest CT are suspicious for malignancy.

Ground-glass nodules include a spectrum of premalignant to low-grade malignant diseases, which correlate pathologically with the diagnoses of atypical adenomatous hyperplasia (AAH) (a premalignant precursor to adenocarcinomas), AIS, and minimally invasive adenocarcinoma (MIA). These specific diagnoses cannot be differentiated accurately by CT imaging findings or by small biopsies; surgical biopsy is generally necessary. Nonetheless, CT features suggest a specific diagnosis. Namely, smaller lesions (particularly those ≤5 mm) with pure ground-glass attenuation are more likely AAH, whereas the larger the lesion and the more complex its structure (particularly if solid or cystic areas are noted), the more likely it represents AIS (formerly called bronchioloalveolar carcinoma, BAC) or MIA. Large (≥5 mm) or progressive solid components are strongly associated with invasive adenocarcinomas.

The Fleischner Society has published a statement with evidence-based recommendations for management of ground-glass (subsolid) nodules.[32] The statement is mostly based on the revised classification of pulmonary adenocarcinoma proposed in 2011 by the International Association for the Study of Lung Cancer (IASLC), the American Thoracic Society (ATS), and the European Respiratory Society (ERS).[33] In the same spirit as the original recommendations for solid nodules, subsolid nodules are stratified according to size, and different follow-up intervals are proposed. However, unlike the guidelines for solid nodules, those for ground-glass nodules do not differentiate between low- and high-risk

TABLE 30-2 Fleischner Society Recommendations for the Management of Subsolid Pulmonary Nodules Detected at CT

Nodule Size (mm)	Management Recommendations	Additional Remarks
Solitary pure GGNs		
≤5 mm	No CT follow-up required	Obtain contiguous 1-mm-thick sections to confirm that nodule is truly a pure GGN
>5 mm	Initial follow-up CT at 3 mo to confirm persistence, then annual surveillance CT for a minimum of 3 yr	FDG PET is of limited value, potentially misleading, and therefore not recommended
Solitary part-solid nodules	Initial follow-up CT at 3 mo to confirm persistence. If persistent and solid component <5 mm, then yearly surveillance CT for a minimum of 3 yr. If persistent and solid component ≥5 mm, then biopsy or surgical resection[a]	Consider PET/CT for part-solid nodules >10 mm
Multiple subsolid nodules		
Pure GGNs ≤5 mm	Obtain follow-up CT at 2 and 4 yr	Consider alternate causes for multiple GGNs ≤5 mm
Pure GGNs >5 mm without dominant lesions	Initial follow-up CT at 3 mo to confirm persistence and then annual surveillance CT for a minimum of 3 yr	FDG PET is of limited value, potentially misleading, and therefore not recommended
Dominant nodule(s) with part-solid or solid component	Initial follow-up CT at 3 mo to confirm persistence. If persistent, biopsy or surgical resection is recommended, especially for lesions with >5-mm solid component[a]	Consider lung-sparing surgery for patients with dominant lesion(s) suspicious for lung cancer

Notes:
These guidelines assume meticulous evaluation, optimally with contiguous thin sections (1 mm) reconstructed with narrow and/or mediastinal windows to evaluate the solid component and wide and/or lung windows to evaluate the nonsolid component of nodules, if indicated. When electronic calipers are used, bidimensional measurements of both the solid and ground-glass components of lesions should be obtained as necessary. The use of a consistent low-dose technique is recommended, especially in cases for which prolonged follow-up is recommended, particularly in younger patients. With serial scans, always compare with the original baseline study to detect subtle indolent growth.
[a]Small biopsies (CT-guided percutaneous biopsy vs. transbronchial biopsies) may be limited to establish a diagnosis of adenocarcinoma in situ or minimally invasive adenocarcinoma. Consider surgical resection for a complete pathologic analysis of the lesion.
Source: Reproduced with permission from Naidich DP, Bankier AA, MacMahon H, et al. Recommendations for the management of subsolid pulmonary nodules detected at CT: a statement from the Fleischner Society. Radiology. 2013;266(1):304–317.

groups because of the incidence of subsolid lesions in younger and nonsmoking patients.

The algorithm for subsolid lesions is more involved, also accounting for multiplicity of nodules and the fact that many subsolid nodules are inflammatory (Table 30-2). For example, a subsolid nodule measuring <5 mm does not need any follow-up. If it is >5 mm, then an initial follow-up chest CT should be obtained at 3 months to determine persistence. If persistent, then yearly surveillance is recommended for a minimum of 3 years (Many institutions, including our own, pursue longer surveillance.). If a subsolid nodule >5 mm demonstrates a solid component measuring more than 5 mm and is persistent after 3 months, then tissue sampling and/or resection is emphasized, as these nodules have a very high probability of representing AIS or MIA. The size of the solid component correlates with the likelihood of an invasive component being present.

For multiple ground-glass opacities, the algorithm is similar and the management dictated by the CT characteristics of the most suspicious nodule; the only difference is that if all nodules measure <5 mm, a longer initial follow-up interval (2–4 years) is suggested, as infectious or inflammatory etiologies become far more likely in that setting. Important caveats are the limited usefulness of PET/CT for evaluation of subsolid nodules, since most are not substantially metabolically active (therefore, a negative PET/CT can be misleading), the need to obtain clinical correlation, and the requirement for a meticulous evaluation protocol that includes thin-section (1 mm) volumetric images and consistent use of low radiation dose CT technique.[32]

A comprehensive management algorithm for both solid and subsolid pulmonary nodules was recently published by the American College of Chest Physicians.[34] The algorithm commences with identification of a new nodule on chest CT and proceeds with follow-up recommendations according to size, risk factors for malignancy, and surgical risk. The recommendations emphasize the need for tissue sampling for most nodules larger than 8 mm and compare the advantages and disadvantages of surgical biopsy, CT-guided percutaneous biopsy, and bronchoscopy with biopsy. The specific recommendations for nodules measuring <8 mm are in line with the Fleischner Society guidelines.

LUNG CANCER

The classification, pathophysiology, epidemiology, and management of lung cancer are described elsewhere (Chapters 112–118). This chapter focuses on the contributions of imaging to lung cancer screening, initial diagnosis, and staging.

Lung cancers are typically initially identified on chest radiography or are noted incidentally on chest CT performed for another clinical indication (except in the context of lung cancer screening). Most lung cancers present as pulmonary nodules or masses. Hilar or mediastinal lymphadenopathy and overt signs of metastatic disease are indicative of more advanced stages of disease. Central masses may cause obstructive atelectasis or consolidation.

At initial presentation, the clinical aim is to confirm the diagnosis pathologically, for which tissue sampling is required. In the past, surgical biopsies were the only available options, but in the last two decades, minimally invasive biopsies performed either percutaneously using CT guidance, or transbronchially with bronchoscopic techniques, have been strongly favored for their better risk/benefit ratio, lower complication rate, faster patient recovery, and good diagnostic accuracy. As a general rule, most peripheral lesions (i.e., within 3 cm of a costal pleural surface) are better accessed percutaneously using CT guidance, whereas central lesions, particularly if an airway visible on CT leads to the lesion, are better accessed via bronchoscopy.[33,35]

Once the diagnosis of lung cancer is pathologically confirmed and fully characterized, staging is of paramount importance to determine the extent of disease and, therefore, the management approach. The most current staging system for lung cancer is the seventh edition of the TNM classification, which was published in 2010. Several references depict visual maps of the T, N, and M criteria and tables with the detailed revised classification.[36,37] In summary, the most important aspects of staging are the size and location of the primary tumor (T), the presence of abnormally enlarged lymph nodes and their location and distribution (N), and the presence of distant metastasis (M). By combining the T, N and M scores, a specific stage from I to IV is obtained, and management strategies are tailored for the type of cancer (histology and genotypic profile) and the staging classification. It cannot be overemphasized that imaging, particularly CT, plays an overarching role not only in tumor detection, but also in tumor staging. It is the primary method for obtaining TNM staging information. PET/CT is also valuable, particularly for nodal staging and identification of distant metastasis. Finally, nodal metastasis may be evaluated using endobronchial US combined with transbronchial biopsies of suspicious lymph nodes.

LUNG CANCER SCREENING

A discussion of the role of modern imaging in the diagnosis of lung cancer would not be complete without mention of the current status of lung cancer CT screening.

Several major prospective multicenter trials using low-dose CT to screen for lung cancer are currently underway. The two largest trials are the National Lung Screening Trial (NLST) in the United States and the Nederlands-Leuvens Longkanker Screenings Onderzoek (NELSON) in the Netherlands and Belgium. Many additional smaller prospective trials (including the DANTE trial in Italy and Danish Randomized Lung Cancer CT Screening Trial in Denmark) are also ongoing.

The NLST, launched in 2002, has published promising initial results. This trial compared the performance of low-dose chest CT versus single, frontal view chest radiographs. In the low-dose CT arm there was a statistically significant lung cancer–specific mortality reduction of 20.0% (95% CI: 3.8–26.7), far greater than that expected by chance. A lower, but still statistically significant decrease in all-cause mortality of 6.7% was also observed in the low-dose CT cohort.[38,39]

The NELSON trial, launched in 2003, compared low-dose CT against no screening. In addition, NELSON differed from the NLST in many important aspects, including serial imaging protocol and patient selection criteria. Final results are not available at the time of this writing, but partial results from the NELSON and other European trials did not demonstrate a significant difference in lung cancer mortality (RR 1.37, 95% CI: 0.63–2.97) or all-cause mortality (1.46, 95% CI: 0.99–2.15); these results are from the Danish trial, which is coordinated with the NELSON trial. The reasons for the discrepant results between the North American and European trials are being actively investigated and may be at least partially related to patient selection criteria and management protocols.[40,41]

In summary, while the NLST provides compelling evidence of the mortality benefit from low-dose CT screening in high-risk patients and demonstrates its superiority to radiographic screening, many important questions remain regarding cost-effectiveness of screening, as well as optimal management of false-positive results. Modeling studies are currently underway and recommendations based on cost-effective analysis are expected in the future.

PULMONARY INFECTIONS

Pulmonary infections comprise a very broad group of diseases caused by a wide variety of viruses, bacteria, and fungi. The imaging findings are helpful to establish a diagnosis of pneumonia, but they are virtually never specific as to etiology. Therefore, most patients with suspected pulmonary infections are treated empirically, based upon epidemiologic considerations. Subgroups of vulnerable patients (particularly very ill or immunocompromised patients) may require etiologic confirmation, which can be obtained by sampling the abnormalities via percutaneous or bronchoscopic techniques and requesting microbiologic testing of the material.

The imaging approach to a suspected pulmonary infection involves identifying the imaging patterns that are more likely associated with an infectious etiology, as well as recognizing the more likely associations with a specific pattern. The most typical pattern of pneumonia is focal or multifocal consolidation, denoted by dense, conspicuous alveolar opacities that obscure vascular contours on CT and which may or may not be associated with air bronchograms. Other patterns include focal or multifocal ground-glass opacities (which can be difficult to recognize on chest radiographs and require CT for adequate evaluation); peribronchovascular patchy opacities (bronchopneumonia pattern); centrilobular nodules with tree-in-bud configuration (bronchiolitis pattern); multiple nodules or masses (cavitary or not); solitary cavitary nodule or mass; and nodules or masses associated with calcifications or ground-glass halo. None of these patterns is specific for infection; they are even less specific for a particular infectious etiology. Nonetheless, some imaging patterns allow a narrower differential diagnosis in the proper clinical setting and are worth recognizing.[42–49]

Notable radiographic patterns include: (1) focal or multifocal consolidation, which favors typical bacterial infection (e.g., *Streptococcus pneumoniae*). A bronchopneumonia pattern can be seen in a variety of bacterial and viral infections. (2) Focal or multifocal ground-glass opacities favor atypical infections, including *Pneumocystis jiroveci* and hematogenously disseminated bacterial and viral infections (e.g., CMV pneumonitis).[50,51] (3) A bronchiolitis pattern may be seen in community-acquired viral infections, including influenza, parainfluenza, and adenovirus. If associated with air trapping, respiratory syncytial virus (RSV) should be considered. (4) Multiple cavitary nodules or masses suggest septic emboli or virulent infections, such as those due to *Staphylococcus aureus*. (5) A solitary cavitary mass suggests a pulmonary abscess; anaerobic infections related to aspiration are primary considerations, although if in the upper lobes, reactivation tuberculosis must be excluded.[52] (6) Calcified nodules or masses suggest granulomatous infectious, typically chronic, and favor mycobacterial (tuberculous and nontuberculous) or fungal etiologies.[53,54] (7) Nodules or masses with ground-glass halo are suggestive of opportunistic fungal infection, particularly invasive aspergillosis, in the setting of immunocompromised hosts who are neutropenic.

With regard to localized alveolar disease, the very important distinction between atelectasis and consolidation needs to be clarified. Patchy opacification of airspaces without a decrease in the volume of the affected area suggests consolidation, while opacification of airspaces associated with a decrease in the volume of the affected area suggests atelectasis. The differential diagnosis depends largely on the extent to which lung volume is decreased. However, assessment of the magnitude of volume loss is not always useful. For example, while pneumonia usually is associated with minimal or no volume loss, occasionally, volume loss is considerable. On the other hand, atelectasis usually has moderate or severe loss of volume, but in some instances, there may be little volume loss (Figs. 30-33–30-37).

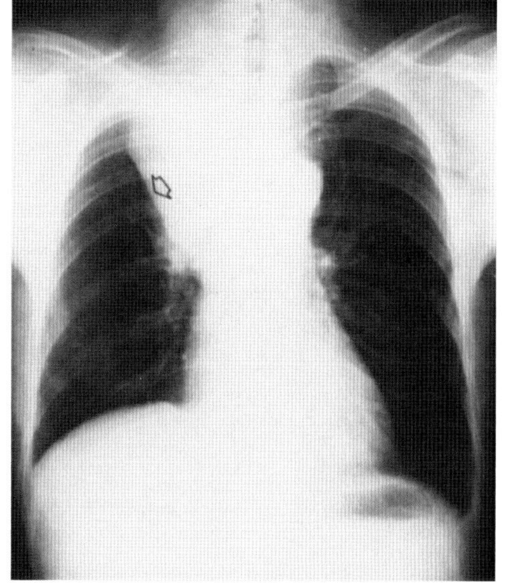

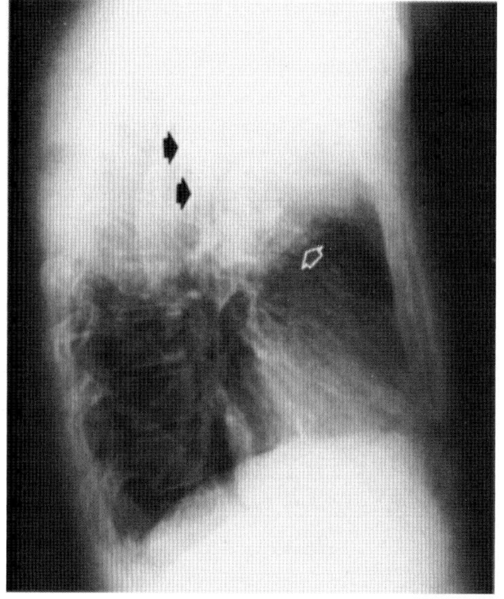

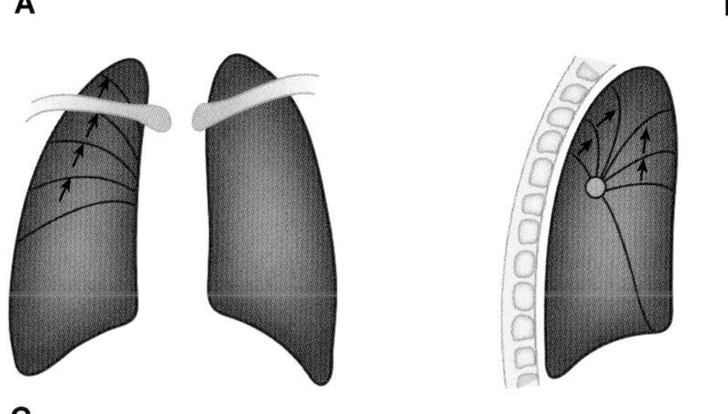

Figure 30-33 Right upper lobe atelectasis secondary to bronchogenic carcinoma. **A.** PA view. The minor fissure is elevated *(arrow)*. **B.** Lateral view. The minor fissure is displaced upward *(open arrow)*, and the major fissure is displaced anteriorly *(closed arrows)*. **C.** Schematic representation of atelectasis of the right upper lobe.

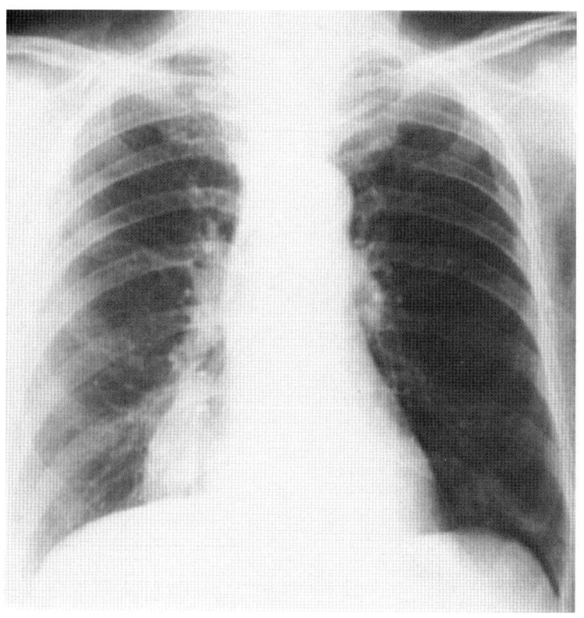

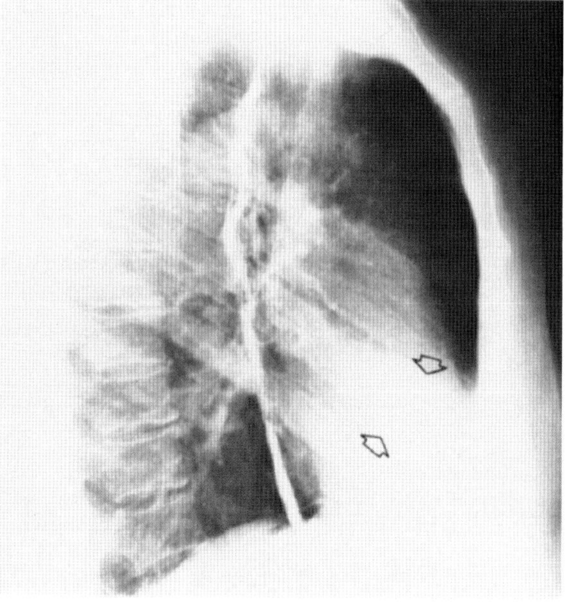

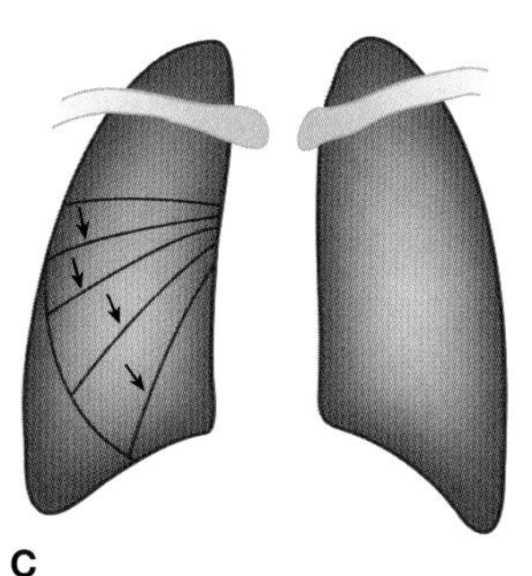

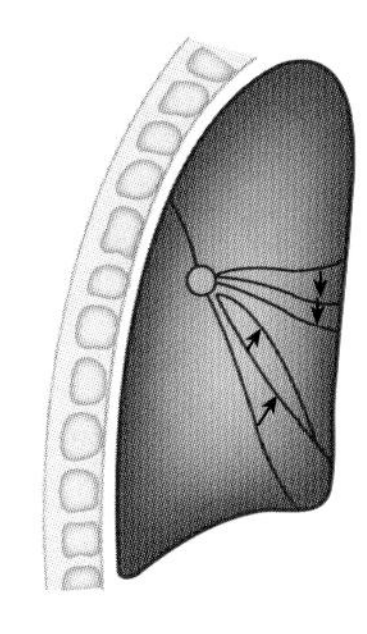

Figure 30-34 Right middle lobe atelectasis secondary to right middle lobe syndrome. **A.** PA view. The middle lobe is collapsed against the right side of the heart. **B.** Lateral view. The major and minor fissures are drawn together *(arrows)*, creating an opacity that overlies the cardiac shadow. **C.** Schematic representation of right middle lobe atelectasis.

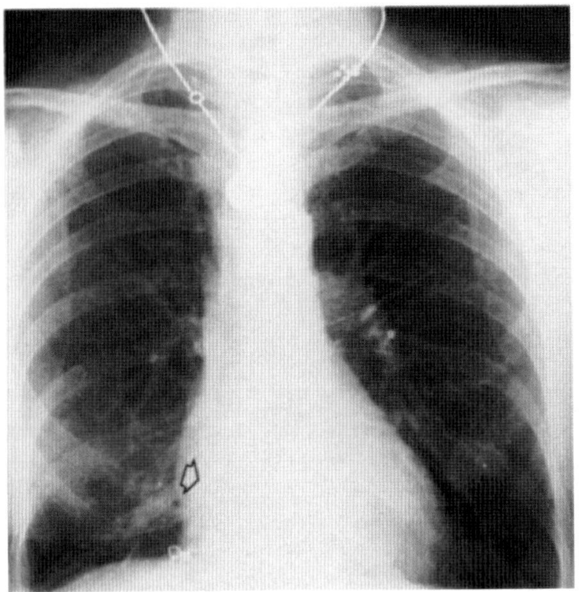
A

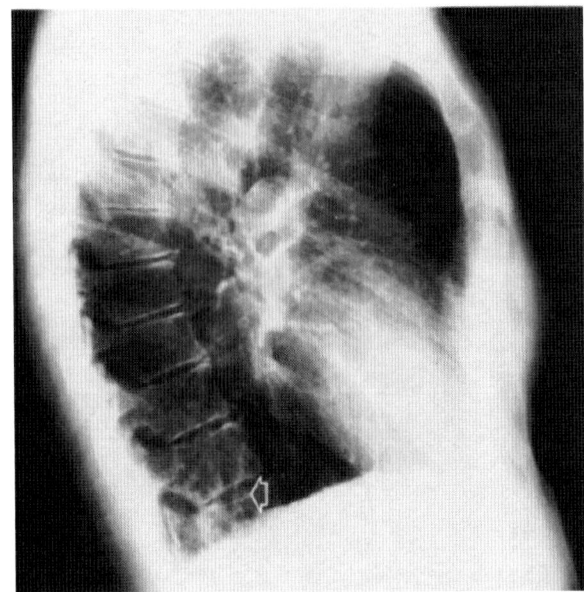
B

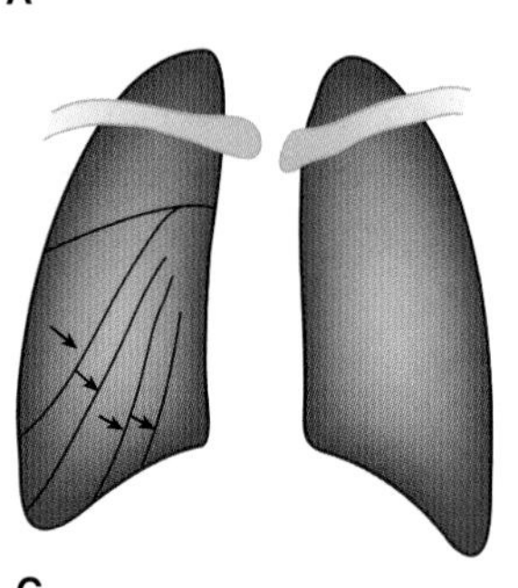
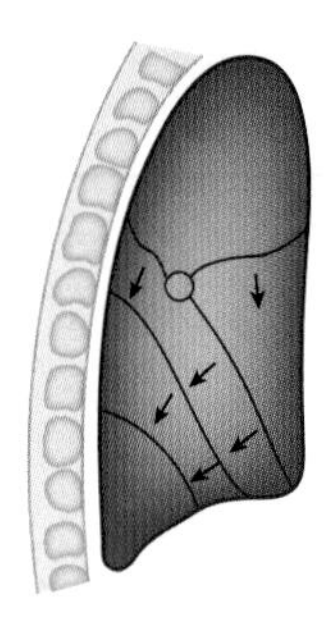
C

Figure 30-35 Atelectasis (severe) of the right lower lobe due to chronic inflammatory disease. **A.** PA view. Secondary signs of atelectasis are present in the right lung: small hemithorax, stretching of the pulmonary vessels, hyperlucent lung, and small hilus. In this instance, these secondary signs are important in suspecting atelectasis. In addition, there is downward displacement of the right hilus, and the collapsed lower lobe can be seen (poorly) through the right heart border *(arrow)*. **B.** Lateral view. The entire right lower lobe appears only as a diffuse opacity overlying the spine *(arrow)*. The posterior portion of the right hemidiaphragm cannot be identified (silhouette sign). **C.** Schematic representation of collapse of right lower lobe.

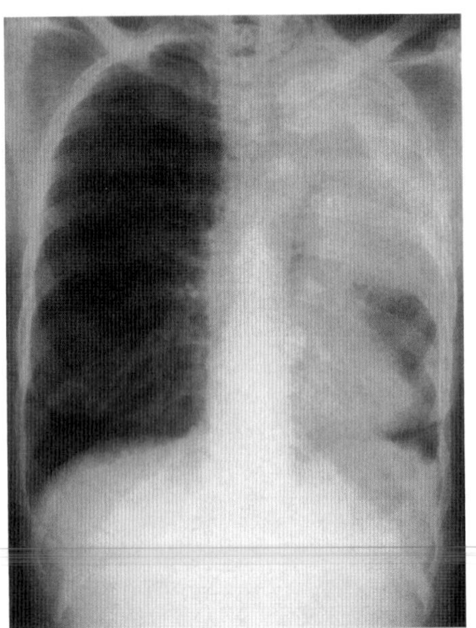
A

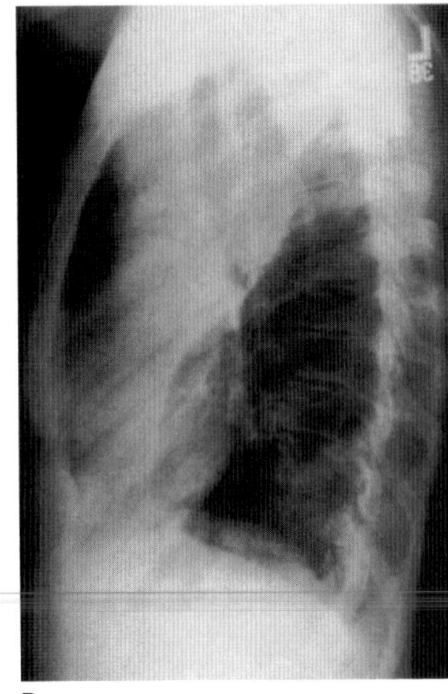
B

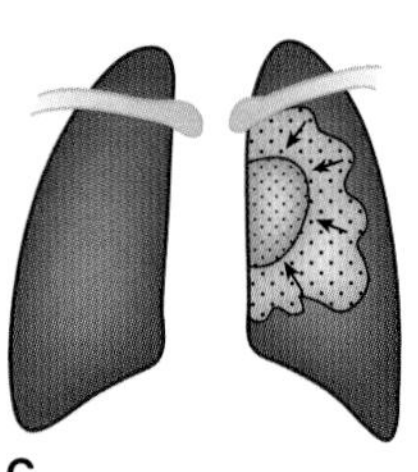
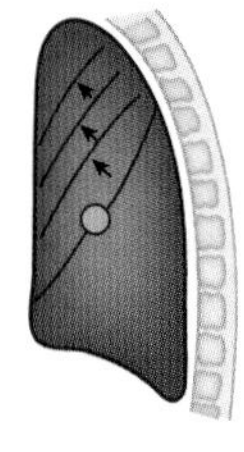
C

Figure 30-36 Left upper lobe atelectasis secondary to bronchogenic. **A.** PA view. The left superior mediastinum and left side of the heart are indistinct, due to collapse of the left upper lobe medially. **B.** Lateral view. The collapsed lung is seen as an opacity anterior to the major fissure, which is displaced anteriorly. **C.** Schematic representation of collapse of left upper lobe.

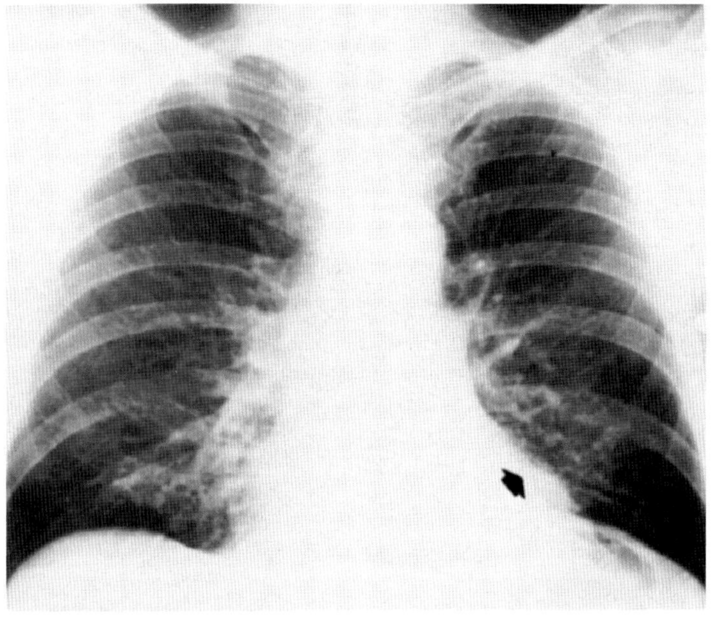

A

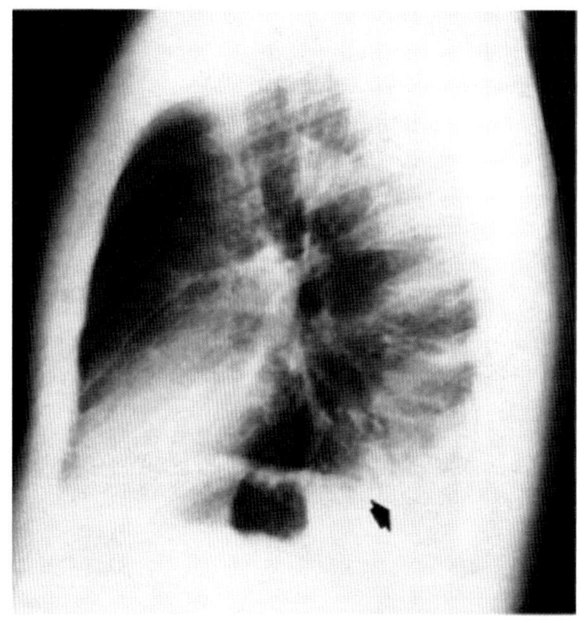

B

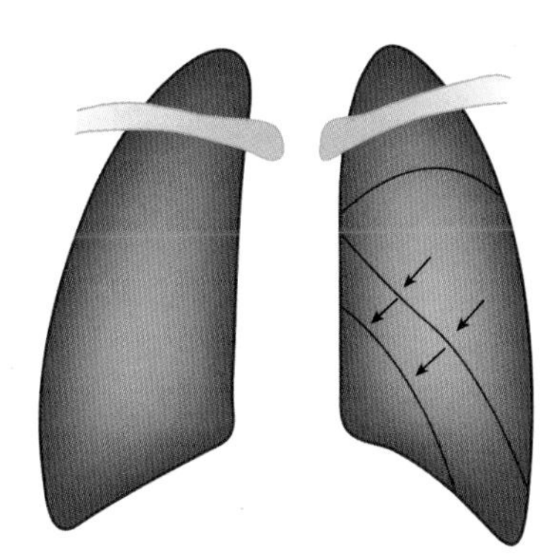

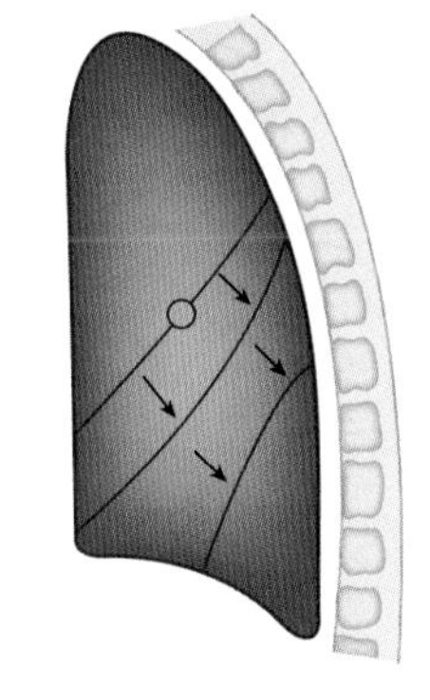

C

Figure 30-37 Left lower lobe atelectasis (postoperative). **A.** PA view. The collapsed left lower lobe is seen as a straight line *(arrow)* behind the left heart border. No vasculature can be seen through the heart shadow, and the medial border of the left hemidiaphragm is obscured by the collapsed left lower lobe *(arrow)*. **B.** Lateral view. Opacity over the spine and absence of left posterior diaphragm. This is difficult to differentiate from a pleural effusion. **C.** Schematic representation of collapsed left lower lobe.

Consolidations are statistically likely to represent pneumonias, especially in the acute setting, whereas atelectasis indicates airway obstruction (obstructive atelectasis), adjacent mass effect (compressive atelectasis), or, more rarely, surfactant deficiency or scarring (adhesive atelectasis). For practical purposes, focal airspace opacities, particularly if lobar, are considered consolidations if the degree of volume loss is negligible or mild, and atelectasis if the degree of volume loss is substantial. The various patterns of lobar atelectasis are important to recognize, since this radiographic finding is a very common manifestation of carcinoma of the lung or, occasionally, some other endobronchial neoplasm.

Atelectasis is also common in the postoperative patient (the so-called, "dependent atelectasis"), presumably because of hypoventilation of dependent parts of the lungs and inadequate clearing of respiratory secretions. In this instance, loss of volume may be mild or absent. Atelectasis may also occur as a consequence of inflammatory disease of the airways or aspiration of a foreign body. Atelectasis also invariably accompanies pleural effusions and pneumothorax. With pleural effusions, atelectasis is greatest in the vicinity of the pleural effusion. Rounded atelectasis is a subtype characterized by ovoid peripheral opacity, associated with underlying chronic pleural disease (manifested by loculated effusion or pleural thickening). There is architectural distortion and convergence of the bronchovascular structures supplying the area of rounded atelectasis ("comet tail sign"). It is important to recognize the typical features of rounded atelectasis, as it can be confused with pulmonary neoplasms.

In nonimmunocompromised hosts, most acute consolidations reflect bacterial pneumonias and should improve to complete resolution with treatment, generally within 4 to 6 weeks; radiographic clearance lags a few weeks behind clinical improvement. Therefore, in adult patients it is important to obtain chest radiographs at the end of this time frame to demonstrate complete resolution of the consolidation. Any consolidation that persists (>1 month) in spite of optimal empirical treatment should be considered potentially neoplastic; the differential diagnosis includes pulmonary mucinous adenocarcinoma (formerly classified as BAC), pulmonary lymphoma (of the MALT type, denoting low-grade extranodal lymphomas), or hemorrhagic metastasis (such as from breast, renal cell carcinoma, or melanoma primaries). In addition, atypical infectious processes (such as fungal or mycobacterial infection) may present as persistent consolidations, as well as several noninfectious or inflammatory processes, such as cryptogenic organizing pneumonia (COP), eosinophilic pneumonia, and granulomatous vasculitides (e.g., granulomatosis with polyangiitis). Most chronic consolidations ultimately require chest CT and tissue sampling (via transthoracic or bronchoscopic approaches) for final diagnosis (Figs. 30-38–30-43).

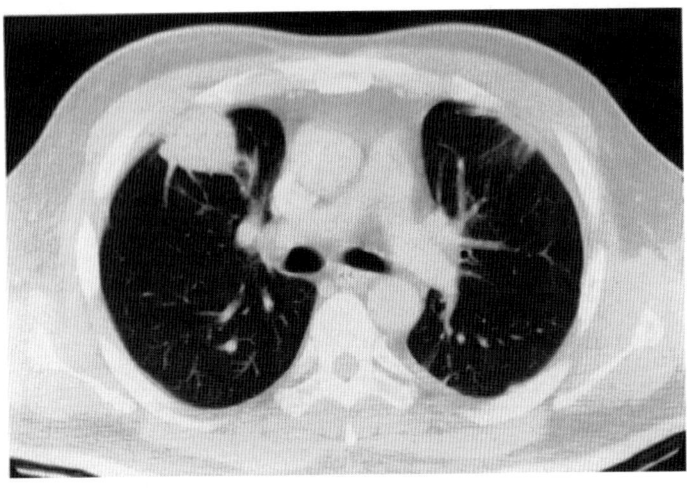

Figure 30-38 Axial CT image showing rounded atelectasis. A mass with a "tail" can be seen in the anterior segment of the right upper lobe. Pleural thickening is seen on the left side, with transpulmonary bands extending into the left upper lobe. The mass on the right represents rounded atelectasis, a finding usually associated with asbestos exposure or chronic pleural disease. The changes on the left probably represent an early stage in the development of rounded atelectasis.

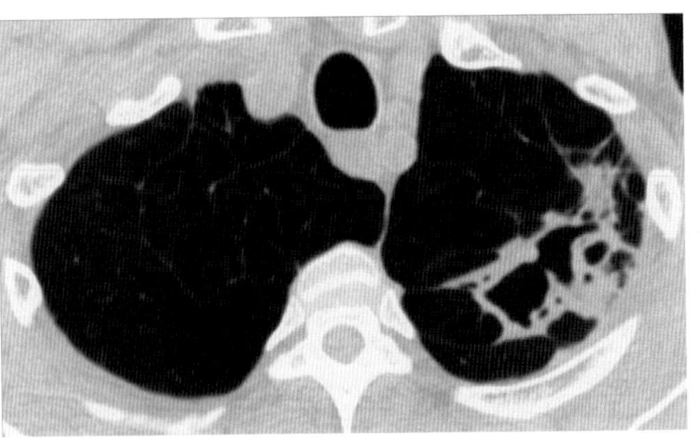

A

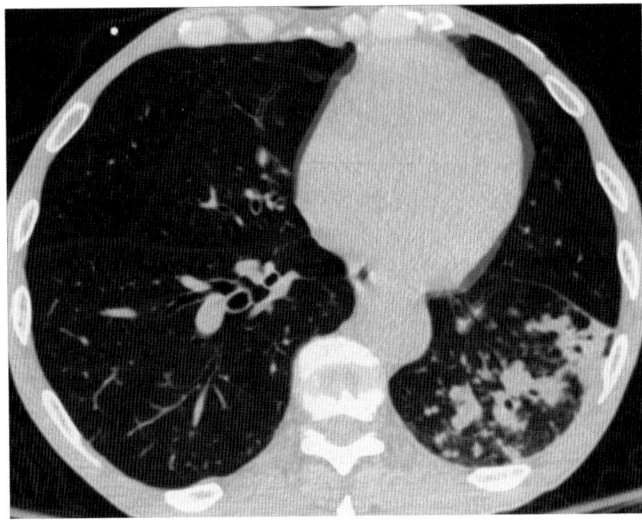

B

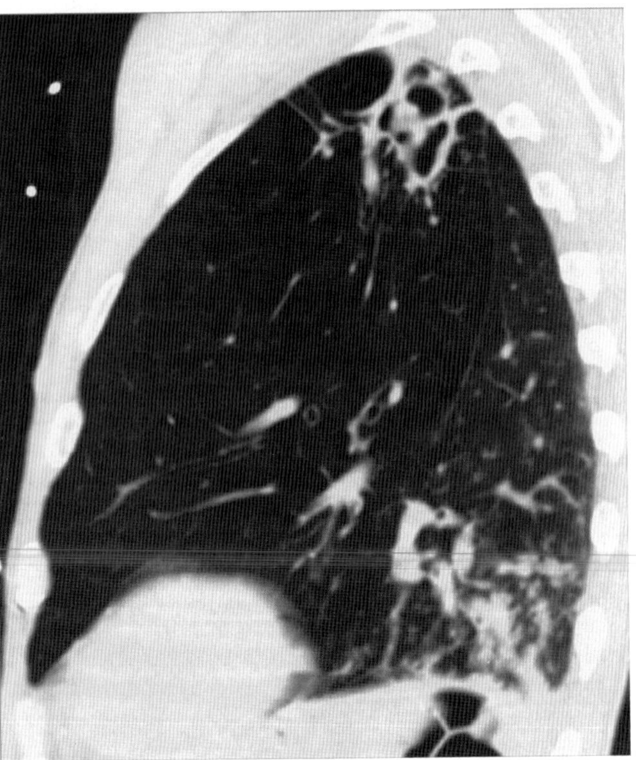

C

Figure 30-39 **A.** Axial CT image shows an irregular cavity in the left upper lobe, with architectural distortion of the surrounding parenchyma. **B.** Axial CT at a lower level demonstrates bronchiectasis, mucoid impaction and peribronchial consolidations in the left lower lobe, as well as a few centrilobular nodules. **C.** Sagittal CT at the median left lung demonstrates both disease processes. This constellation of findings is very characteristic of reactivation tuberculosis and is highly suggestive of the diagnosis, which was confirmed in this case. The left lower lobe opacities reflect endobronchial spread of the mycobacteria from the left upper lobe cavity.

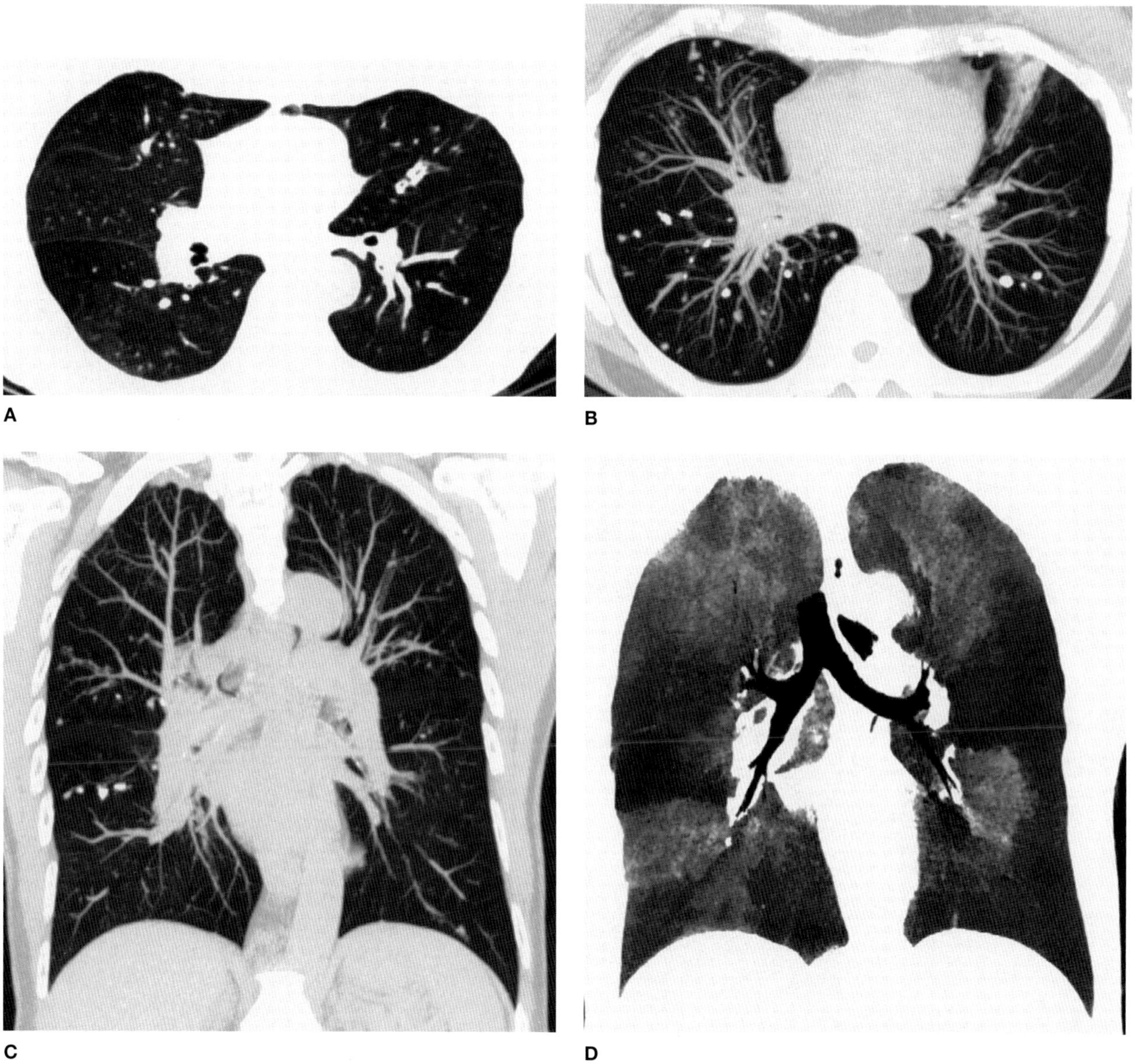

A

B

C

D

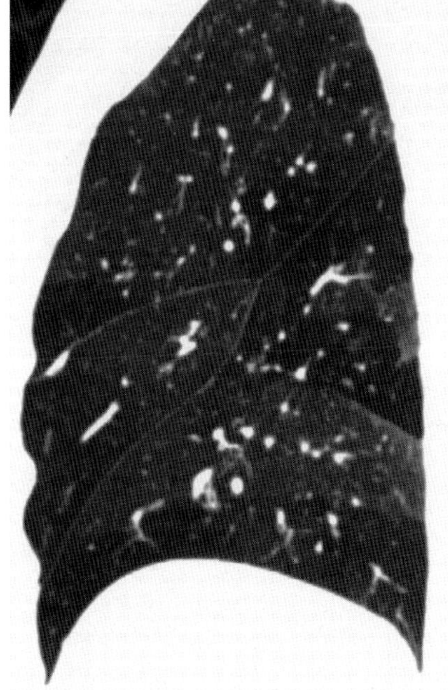

E

Figure 30-40 A. Axial CT image showing left upper lobe bronchiectasis with wall thickening, as well as a striking mosaic attenuation pattern suggestive of air trapping. **B.** Axial CT MIP (maximum intensity projection) reconstruction and (**C**) coronal CT MIP reconstruction demonstrate multiple calcified and noncalcified small nodules. **D.** Coronal CT MinIP (minimum intensity projection) reconstruction clearly shows the mosaic attenuation pattern, which is also notable in (**E**), a sagittal image. This constellation of findings was due to nontuberculous mycobacterial infection, specifically MAI *(Mycobacterium avium-intracellulare)*.

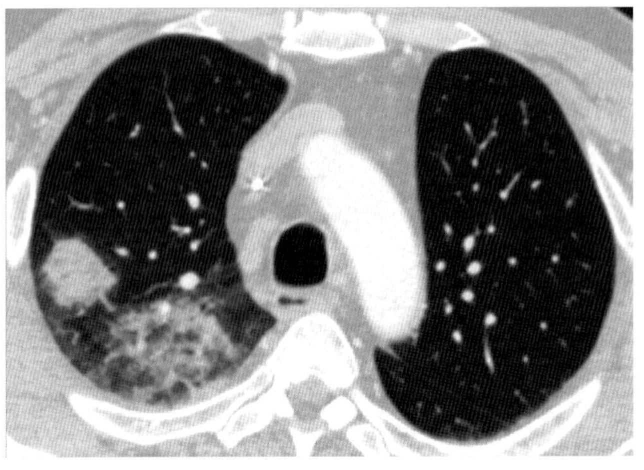

A

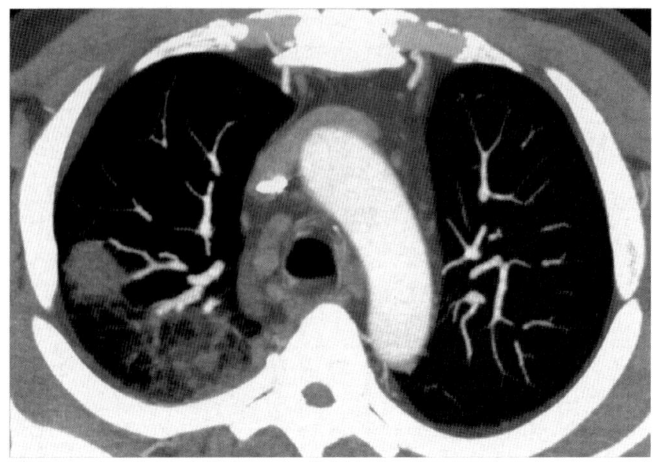

B

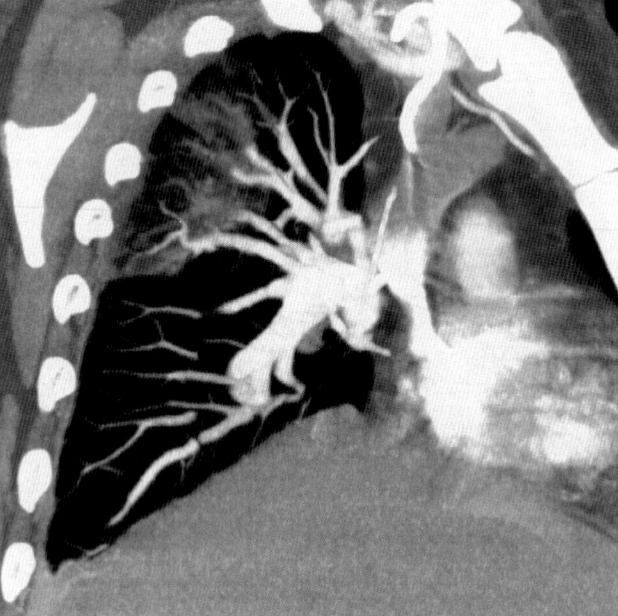

C

Figure 30-41 Immunocompromised patient (post-bone marrow transplant) with neutropenia and fever. **A.** Axial CT shows consolidation and ground-glass opacity in the RUL. (**B**) Axial MIP reconstruction and (**C**) curved MIP reconstruction, contrast-enhanced CT, demonstrate that several right upper lobe arteries are "amputated" at the areas of consolidation in the RUL, a finding that is indicative of angioinvasive aspergillosis, given the clinical setting.

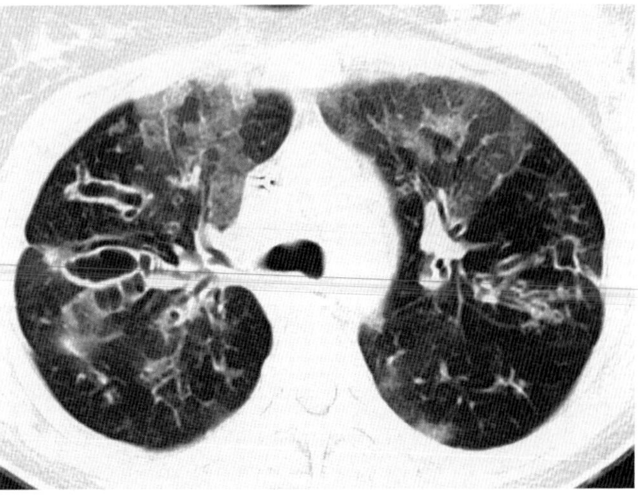

A

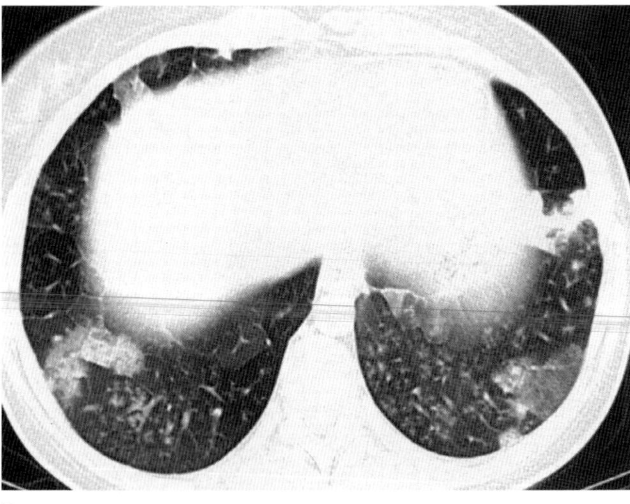

B

Figure 30-42 **A.** Axial CT through the level of the carina demonstrates extensive bronchiectasis. **B.** Axial CT at a lower level demonstrates multiple areas of consolidation and numerous centrilobular nodules. This patient had a diagnosis of cystic fibrosis, complicated by superinfection by *Pseudomonas aeruginosa*.

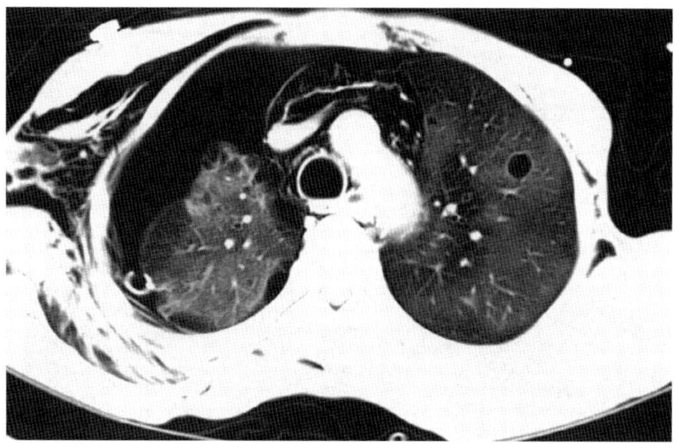

A

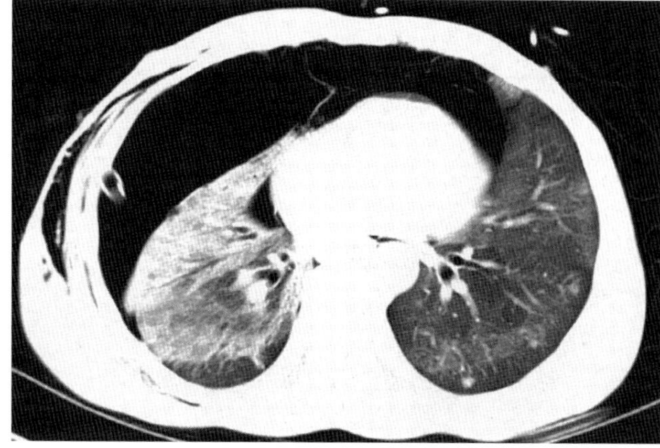

B

Figure 30-43 **A.** Axial CT through the upper lung fields demonstrates a large right-side pneumothorax with a chest tube partially visualized. The lung parenchyma demonstrates diffuse, but nonhomogeneous, ground-glass opacities, as well as scattered cysts. **B.** Axial CT at a lower level demonstrates diffuse ground-glass opacities, small nodules, and patchy areas of consolidation. This patient had AIDS complicated by *Pneumocystis jiroveci* pneumonia. Spontaneous pneumothorax is a known complication of this disease.

PULMONARY EDEMA: CARDIOGENIC AND NONCARDIOGENIC

Imaging offers a comprehensive display of the anatomy of the cardiopulmonary system and its function. Chest radiographs can demonstrate the heart size and configuration, the width of the vascular pedicle, as well as the caliber and distribution of the pulmonary arteries and veins. Pulmonary arteries and veins can generally be distinguished on chest radiographs by their anatomical location, with the pulmonary veins more horizontal, more inferior, and more lateral to the pulmonary arteries in relationship to the hila. The distinction is, nonetheless, seldom useful radiographically and, therefore, the generic terms *pulmonary vessels* and *pulmonary vasculature* are used. CT and MRI more readily depict the pulmonary arteries and veins. The pulmonary arteries arise from the main pulmonary artery trunk, while the pulmonary veins enter the left atrium and are readily distinguished on cross-sectional imaging even without intravenous contrast. Moreover, CT and MRI can accurately evaluate cardiac structure and function, particularly cardiac MRI, providing quantitative metrics to assess ventricular and valvular function.

Congestive heart failure is a common clinical condition characterized by systolic and/or diastolic dysfunction of the left ventricle, leading to increasing diastolic filling pressure, increasing left atrial pressure, and fluid retention. Ultimately, left ventricular failure leads to right ventricular failure. The heart is almost invariably enlarged, and the central pulmonary vasculature appears prominent and indistinct. These changes are easier to recognize on PA and lateral views than on portable chest radiographs.

A rational progression of chest radiographic findings in congestive heart failure can be fully appreciated on PA, erect radiographs and is strongly correlated with increases in pulmonary capillary wedge pressure (PCWP, reflecting left atrial pressure), indicating progressive pulmonary venous congestion.

The first stage is correlated with a PCWP of 13 to 18 mm Hg and is characterized by increased width of the vascular pedicle and vascular redistribution in the erect patient; the caliber of the upper lung vessels is increased relative to the lower lung vessels (cephalization), and cardiomegaly is present.

The second stage is correlated with PCWP of 18 to 25 mm Hg and is characterized additionally by the presence of pulmonary interstitial edema—which is manifested on chest radiography as Kerley lines, thickened fissures, and peribronchial cuffing with indistinct contour of the central vessels. Kerley B lines, as previously described, represent small (1–2 cm), thin, linear opacities that are seen peripherally perpendicular to a pleural surface, reflecting edema involving interlobular septae.

Finally, the third stage is correlated with PCWP >25 mm Hg and is characterized by the additional presence of alveolar edema, manifested as fluffy (cotton-wool appearance), symmetric airspace consolidation with mid and lower lung field predominance. Pleural effusions are often present in stages II or III and may be present earlier if there is a substantial component of right ventricular dysfunction or central volume overload, such as in patients with pulmonary hypertension or superimposed chronic renal or liver disease.

Pleural effusions often accompany biventricular heart failure. However, while the pulmonary congestion usually clears rapidly in response to therapy, the pleural effusions often remain after the pulmonary vessels have returned to normal size and require a longer time to resolve. Pleural effusions in congestive heart failure may be unilateral or bilateral, although they are most often bilateral. The effusions are nearly always transudates. Therefore, the presence of a unilateral effusion, particularly an isolated left effusion, should prompt consideration of a diagnostic thoracentesis. If the effusion is an exudate, an alternate cause, such as malignancy or infection, should be considered (Figs. 30-44 and 30-45).

CT may demonstrate the same findings and the same pattern of progression according to the degree of left heart dysfunction and PCWP increase. Nonetheless, it allows better assessment of cardiac chamber size, vascular caliber, and presence of pulmonary interstitial or alveolar edema. Nonetheless, because the combination of clinical, laboratory, and radiographic findings generally suffices for the diagnosis of congestive heart failure, CT is not routinely obtained in patients in this setting, although it is not uncommon to establish the diagnosis on CT studies performed for other reasons.

As previously discussed, pulmonary interstitial edema presents on CT as axial (peribronchovascular) and septal interstitial thickening (interlobular and intralobular); the findings are usually symmetric, smooth, and lower lung field predominant. The differential diagnosis, especially if the pattern of interstitial thickening is nodular, upper lung predominant, or asymmetric, includes sarcoidosis and lymphangitic spread of neoplasm. Pulmonary

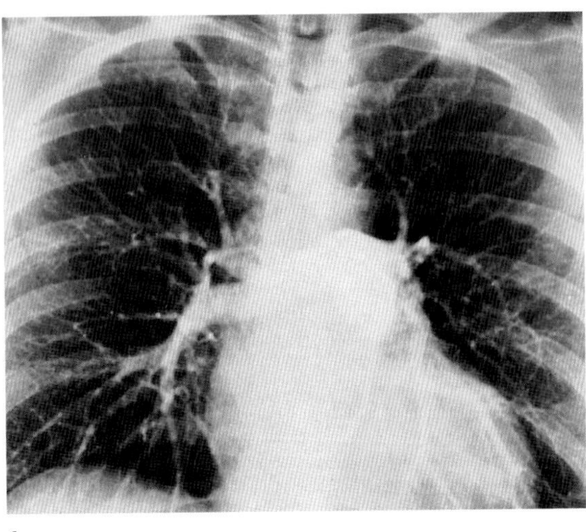

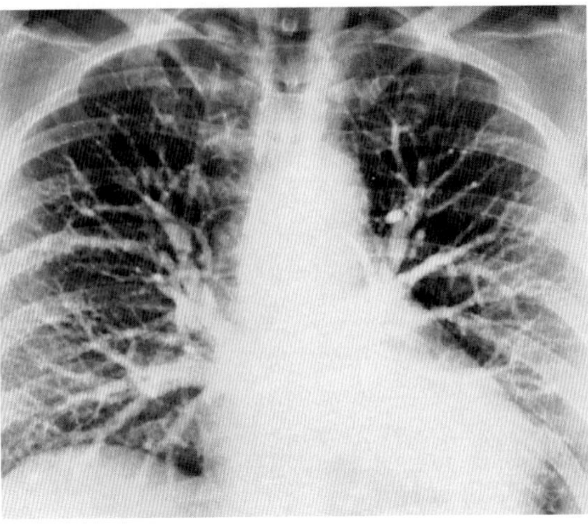

Figure 30-44 Pulmonary arteries and veins: **A.** The early phase of the pulmonary angiogram depicts the normal course and caliber of the pulmonary arteries. **B.** The late phase shows the normal course and caliber of the pulmonary veins. The veins have a more horizontal course than the arteries and enter the hila below the arteries.

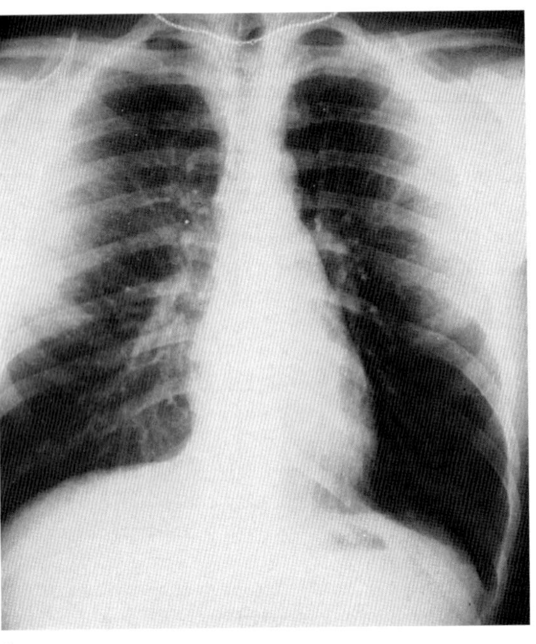

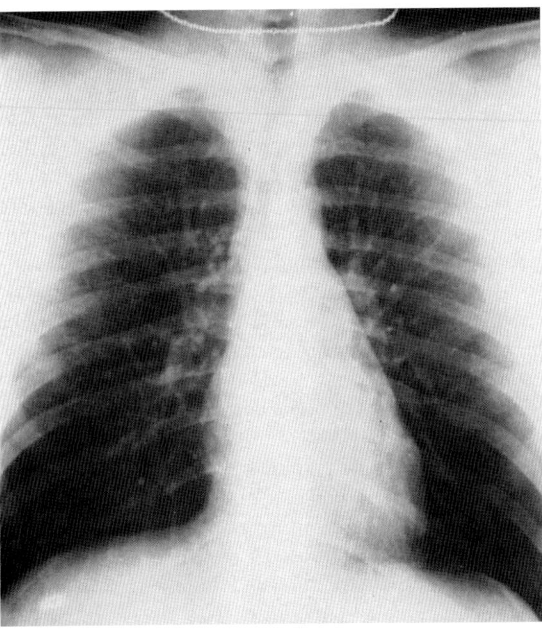

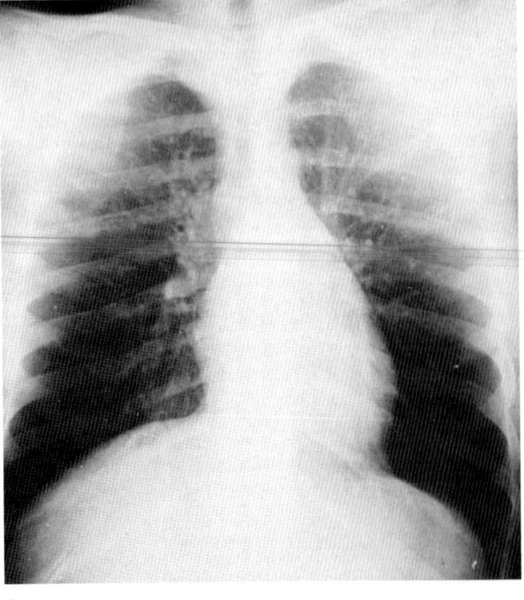

Figure 30-45 Effect of gravity on the pulmonary vasculature. Vascular patterns are compared in a normal subject in the erect, supine, and upside-down positions. **A.** Erect posture. The vascular pattern is more prominent at the bases. **B.** Supine position. The vascular pattern is more uniform. **C.** Upside-down position. The vascular pattern is more marked at the apices.

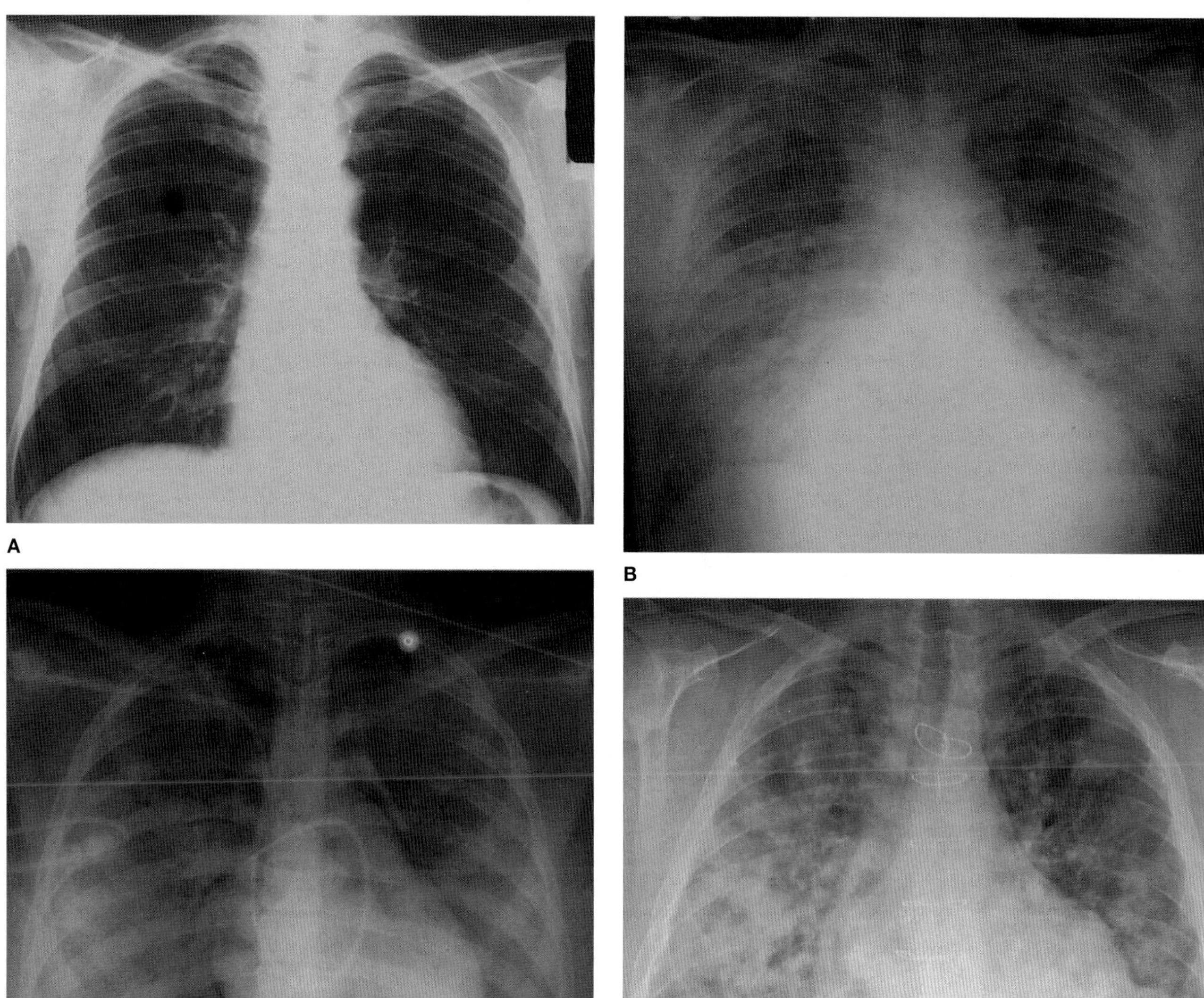

Figure 30-46 Patterns of diffuse alveolar disease. **A.** Normal PA chest radiograph, for comparison. **B.** Cardiogenic edema, with severe, symmetric, basilar-predominant airspace opacities, associated with cardiomegaly and likely small effusions. **C.** Noncardiogenic edema, with severe, symmetric, more diffuse airspace opacities; however, the cardiac size is normal and no pleural effusions are present. This patient has ARDS. **D.** Diffuse alveolar hemorrhage (DAH)—patchy, but fairly diffuse, airspace opacities are noted, with borderline heart size. This patient had systemic lupus erythematosus. Note that this pattern can be difficult to distinguish from diffuse pneumonia or pulmonary edema – clinical correlation is often needed.

alveolar edema is demonstrated as airspace opacities (ground-glass or consolidation), with fluid-filled acinar structures; the opacities are symmetric, ill-defined, confluent, and central and lower lung field predominant. Findings of pulmonary alveolar edema often coexist with pulmonary interstitial edema, but not vice versa. The exception is flash pulmonary edema, in which alveolar edema develops so rapidly that there is not enough time for interstitial edema to manifest. Flash pulmonary edema may occur with sudden changes in intravascular volume, such as following resuscitation in trauma patients or with sudden changes in cardiac function, as occurring with cardiac arrhythmias or myocardial infarction.

Pulmonary edema is the prototype of diffuse lung disease. Etiologically, it can be broadly separated into cardiogenic and noncardiogenic causes. Cardiogenic edema is caused by congestive heart failure.[55,56] Noncardiogenic edema is a manifestation of increased permeability of the pulmonary capillaries in which cardiac function is relatively preserved. Major differential diagnoses include acute hypersensitivity reactions, inhaled toxins, near-drowning, sepsis, and several processes that lead to the pathologic diagnosis of diffuse alveolar damage (DAD), most notably acute respiratory distress syndrome (ARDS).[57–61] From an imaging perspective, cardiogenic edema is more likely associated with cardiomegaly and functional impairment of the ventricles and tends to clear rapidly following administration of diuretics and drugs that optimize cardiovascular status. Noncardiogenic edema tends to resolve slowly and often requires clinical and laboratory correlation for etiologic characterization (Figs. 30-46–30-48).

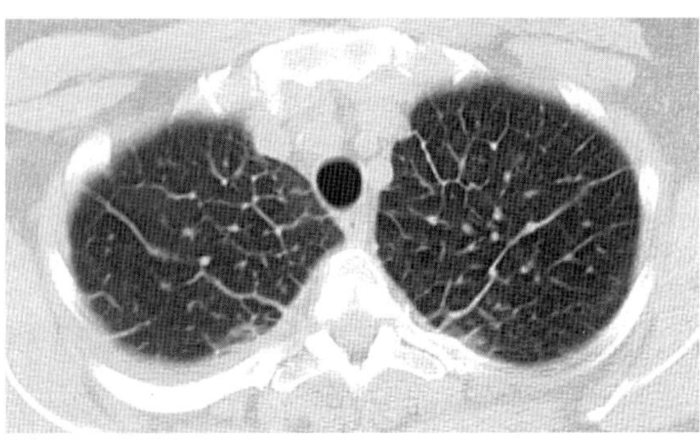

A

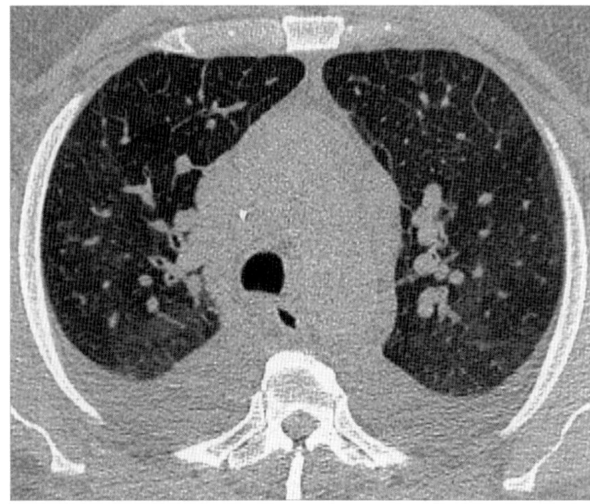

B

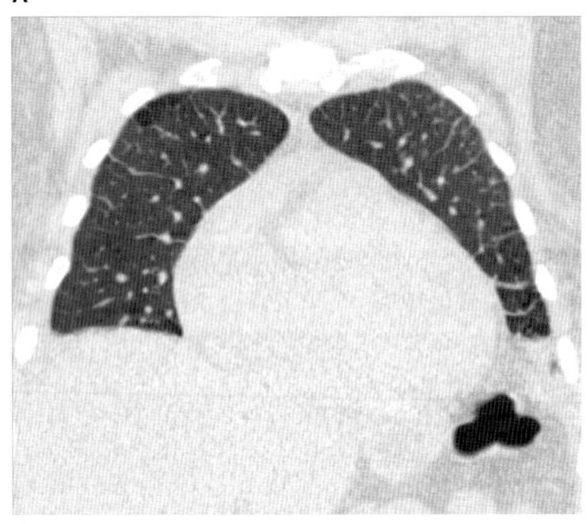

C

Figure 30-47 CT findings of pulmonary interstitial edema. **A.** Axial CT at the lung apices demonstrates classic smooth interlobular septal thickening, the hallmark of interstitial edema. **B.** Axial CT at the level of the carina demonstrates additional axial (peribronchial) interstitial thickening and vascular engorgement, indicating interstitial edema. Also note bilateral pleural effusions, in keeping with cardiogenic failure and volume overload. **C.** Coronal CT clearly demonstrates smooth interlobular septal thickening, which is diffuse, due to interstitial edema.

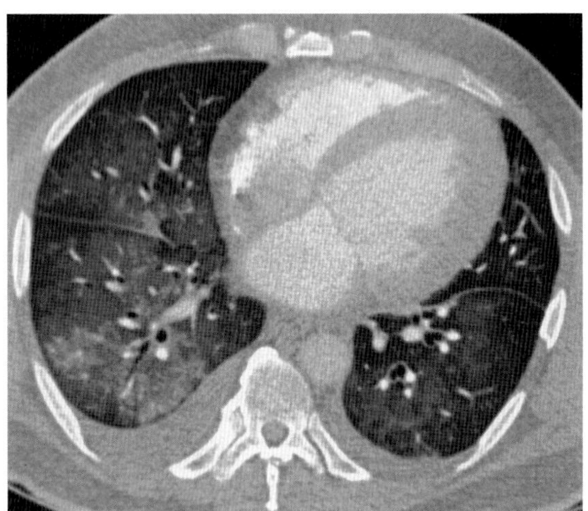

A

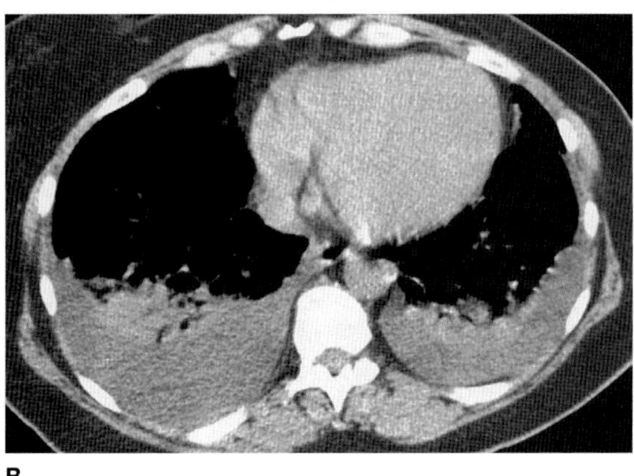

B

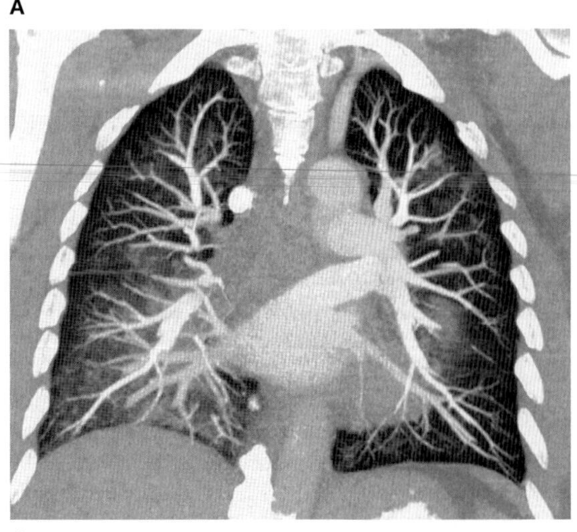

C

Figure 30-48 CT findings of pulmonary alveolar edema. **A.** Axial CT at the lung bases demonstrates diffuse ground-glass opacities, reflecting alveolar edema. Note left ventricular dilatation. **B.** Axial CT at the same level on mediastinal window demonstrates bilateral pleural effusions, in keeping with cardiogenic failure. **C.** Coronal MIP CT reconstruction clearly demonstrates diffuse ground-glass opacities more prominent along the bronchovascular bundles, characteristic of alveolar edema.

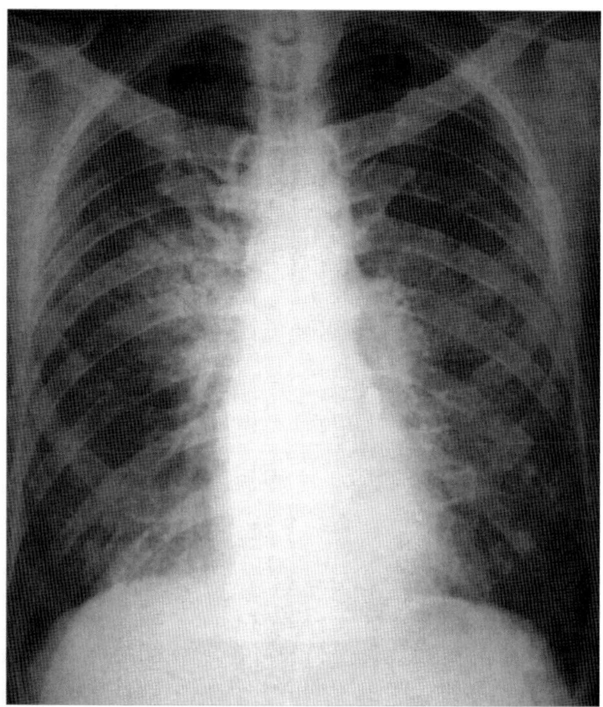

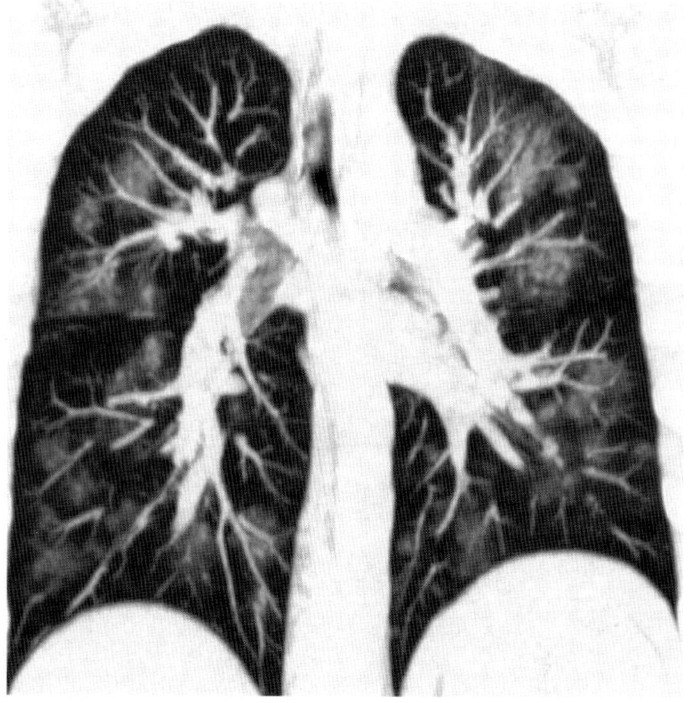

Figure 30-49 CT findings of diffuse alveolar hemorrhage (DAH). **A.** PA chest radiograph demonstrates patchy, but predominantly perihilar, alveolar opacities. **B.** Coronal MIP CT reconstruction better demonstrates the patchy, but widespread, ground-glass opacities, more prominent along the bronchovascular bundles. This patient had a diagnosis of DAH due to Goodpasture syndrome. This pattern can be indistinguishable from pulmonary edema or diffuse infection. Clinical correlation is often needed to narrow the differential diagnosis.

In the proper clinical setting, diffuse alveolar opacities represent pulmonary edema until proved otherwise. If standard therapy for congestive heart failure fails to clear the opacities, and if clinical and laboratory findings exclude noncardiogenic pulmonary edema, other diagnostic entities must be considered. The most important is a diffuse pneumonia, which can be caused by several bacterial and viral agents, including, most notably, influenza. Other differential diagnostic considerations for diffuse lung disease include diffuse alveolar hemorrhage, pulmonary alveolar proteinosis, extensive multifocal mucinous adenocarcinoma, acute hypersensitivity pneumonitis, for example, that due to drug toxicity,[62] sarcoidosis, NSIP, and desquamative interstitial pneumonia (DIP). These entities are described elsewhere in Chapters 54–66 (Fig. 30-49).

PULMONARY EMBOLISM AND PULMONARY HYPERTENSION

Two critically important clinical entities involving the pulmonary vasculature can be assessed using CT: PE and pulmonary hypertension. Each is discussed subsequently.

■ PULMONARY EMBOLISM

Contrast-enhanced, multidetector chest CT provides a powerful and readily available technique for the evaluation of PE and has become the current reference standard for the diagnosis of acute and chronic pulmonary thromboembolic disease. Not only does CT enable direct visualization of clots, it also can provide alternative diagnoses to explain symptoms in the many patients who do not prove to have PE. Moreover, CT may facilitate diagnosis of associated right heart strain when present, a finding of prognostic importance. While CT may be limited in detecting small, peripheral, subsegmental clots, particularly if the study is not of optimal quality, it has a very high negative predictive value for PE. CT may also be combined with CT venography of the pelvis and lower extremities in selected cases, when clinically indicated.

The major disadvantage of CT relative to ventilation–perfusion scanning is the breast radiation dose, which is of concern in young women and pregnant patients. The problem is further heightened by the current overutilization of CT PE studies, manifested by a yield of positive cases that is generally under 10%. Technical methods to reduce the CT radiation dose continue to be introduced. However, the best approach to radiation dose reduction is to improve the appropriate utilization of CT. Better clinical pretest assessment of risk factors for PE is required. Such assessment using the Wells, Simplified Geneva, and PERC scores are frequently not used. Other more objective and easily implemented scoring systems have been advocated.

D-dimer measurement is a very useful screening test that carries a high negative predictive value for PE; measurement is particularly useful in the emergency room setting. A negative D-dimer in combination with a low or intermediate clinical suspicion for PE may obviate the need for CT in approximately 50% of outpatients and 20% of inpatients.

Young patients with normal chest radiographs (and without a history of asthma or COPD) can undergo radionuclide perfusion scans as an alternative to CT; the diagnostic yield of perfusion scans in this setting is high and the breast dose significantly lower than with CT. Patients with coexisting symptoms and/or signs of DVT should have Doppler US of their lower extremities as the initial test.[63–65]

The imaging workup of suspected PE in pregnancy presents several unique challenges, as both fetal and maternal breast radiation doses must be considered. Moreover, D-dimer is generally positive in pregnancy and, thus, not of value. In addition, there

Video 30-8 **A.** Full-color, coronal 3D VR (volume rendering) thick slab cine (anterior to posterior) emphasizing cardiovascular and pulmonary parenchymal structures and demonstrating marked ectasia of the central pulmonary arteries, compatible with pulmonary hypertension (in this patient, mean pulmonary artery pressure was 100 mm Hg). Also note asymmetry of arterial caliber, with relative oligemia of the left lower lobe and ectatic right upper lobe arteries, attributed to chronic thromboembolic pulmonary hypertension. **B.** Same patient as in Video 30.8A. Coronal, minimum intensity projection (minIP) thick slab cine (anterior to posterior). This type of reconstruction provides excellent assessment of mosaic attenuation, which, in this case is due to mosaic perfusion secondary to chronic thromboembolic pulmonary hypertension. The brighter areas of the lung parenchyma are relatively hyperperfused, whereas the darker areas are oligemic, and correlate with areas of diminished regional vascular caliber. *Access at www.fishmansonline.com*

are no useful pretest clinical risk assessment scoring systems for pregnancy. Recently published national guidelines recommend the use of ventilation–perfusion scans in pregnant women with normal chest radiographs (and without COPD or recently active asthma) and CT in the setting of chest radiographic abnormalities that do not provide an alternative diagnosis to PE.[66]

Acute and chronic pulmonary thromboembolic disease can be distinguished on CT imaging by the morphology of the pulmonary arterial filling defects. Acute emboli are usually more centrally located within the vessel lumen and may be occlusive. The nonopacified pulmonary arterial branches tend to be dilated in the setting of acute thromboembolic disease. In contrast, chronic clots are more likely eccentric along the vessel wall, nonocclusive, and sometimes calcified (if long-standing). The involved vessels tend to be smaller than normal. Moreover, chronic thromboembolic disease tends to present with associated dilated central pulmonary arteries, indicating pulmonary hypertension, whereas acute emboli generally present with normal caliber central pulmonary arteries, unless there is pre-existing pulmonary hypertension (Video 30-8A). Other findings suggesting chronic thromboembolic disease include a mosaic perfusion pattern and the presence of dilated bronchial or other systemic collateral vessels (Video 30-8B).

Given the immense functional reserve of the normal pulmonary vasculature, it is uncommon for acute PE to cause pulmonary hypertension and right ventricular dysfunction. Nonetheless, in the setting of large embolic burden, as measured by an obstruction index of the pulmonary arterial circulation of 40% or higher on helical chest CT, poor clinical outcomes are associated with right ventricular dysfunction. This situation generally only occurs with massive saddle emboli in the large proximal pulmonary arteries, or with a large number of relatively smaller emboli occluding the more distal segmental or subsegmental arteries. Chronic pulmonary thromboembolism, on the other hand, is far more prone to be associated with pulmonary hypertension, even in the absence of a substantial thromboembolic burden, due to molecular adaptation mechanisms that lead to remodeling of the pulmonary vasculature, including medial hypertrophy and in situ small vessel thrombosis.[67–69]

More recently, dual-energy CT has been proposed as a method for the combined assessment of acute and chronic emboli, pulmonary vascular anatomy, pulmonary parenchymal abnormalities, and pulmonary perfusion. Pulmonary perfusion, in particular, is obtained via dual-energy CT's ability to derive iodine maps. Identification of pulmonary perfusion defects can increase the sensitivity and specificity of CT for clot detection. Dual-energy CT has also been used for quantitative perfusion in chronic thromboembolic PE, given the strong correlation of dual-energy CT derived perfusion parameters with subjective assessment of a mosaic attenuation pattern. Consequently, contrast-enhanced chest CT is the most useful

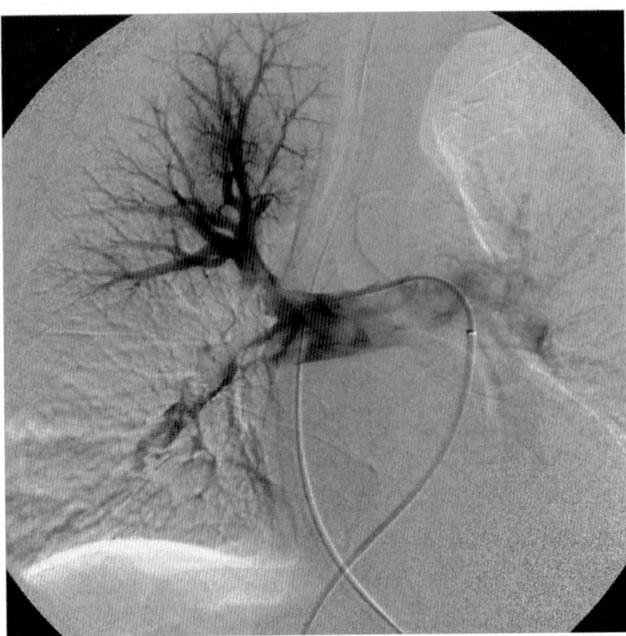

Figure 30-50 Pulmonary angiogram, arterial phase. Note normal caliber of the pulmonary arteries, with multiple filling defects in the right main, right interlobar, and proximal right upper lobar arteries, diagnostic of acute pulmonary embolism.

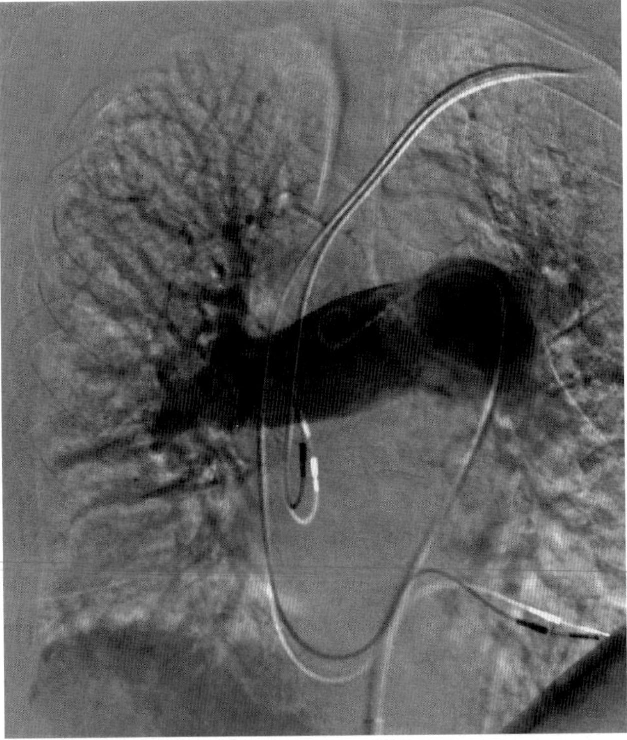

Figure 30-51 Pulmonary angiogram, arterial phase. Note marked dilatation of the pulmonary arteries, without occlusive filling defects, but with overall poor delineation of the arteries, suggesting semiocclusive defects and increased contrast transit time. The constellation of findings indicates chronic thromboembolic pulmonary hypertension (CTEPH).

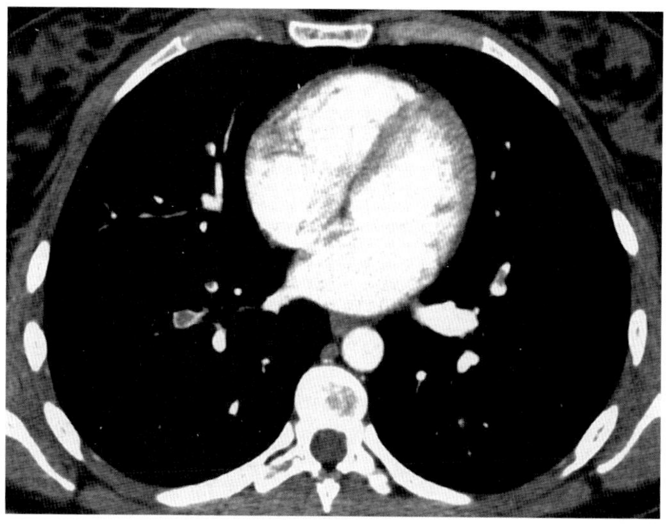

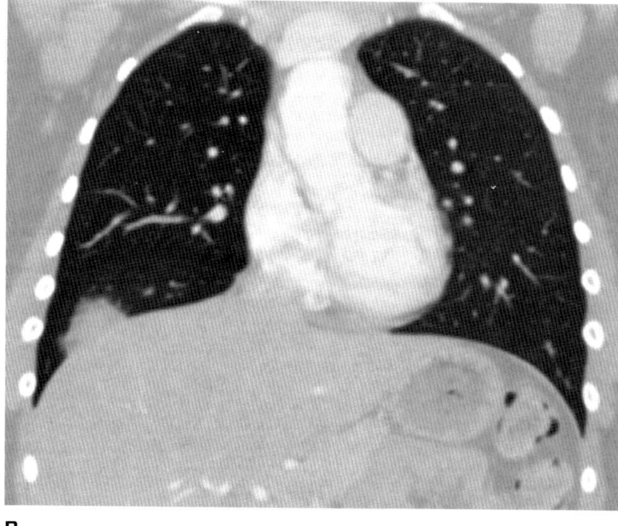

Figure 30-52 Acute pulmonary embolism. **A.** Axial CT at the lung bases demonstrates filling defects in the right lower lobe segmental arteries and left lower lobe anterior segmental artery, compatible with acute PE. **B.** Coronal CT image demonstrates a peripheral RLL consolidation, compatible with pulmonary infarct.

diagnostic modality for diagnosing chronic thromboembolic pulmonary hypertension (Figs. 30-50–30-53).[70–72]

PULMONARY HYPERTENSION

Because of its dual vascular supply (systemic and pulmonary, in series), the lungs effectively receive slightly greater than 100% of the cardiac output (100% via the pulmonary circulation and 1%–2% via the systemic bronchial circulation arising from the aorta), far more than the brain, heart, liver, or kidneys (which comprise the group of highly perfused organs). In addition, the pulmonary circulation is a low-pressure, low-impedance, high-flow system that demonstrates some remarkable physiologic adaptations, such as vasoconstriction whenever there is tissue hypoxia (the opposite response of arteries elsewhere in the body, which normally vasodilate in response to hypoxia), and the ability to adapt to major changes in flow with minimal changes in pressure. Inasmuch as the caliber and distribution of pulmonary vessels provide insight into the pathophysiology of the cardiopulmonary system, imaging methods can be used to study pulmonary vascular diseases.

Pulmonary blood flow is not uniform in the normal, upright human. Moreover, the blood flow pattern shifts with changes in posture, during exercise, and in a variety of heart and lung diseases. In the normal pulmonary circulation, gravity and distance from the heart are the predominant determinants of the pattern of

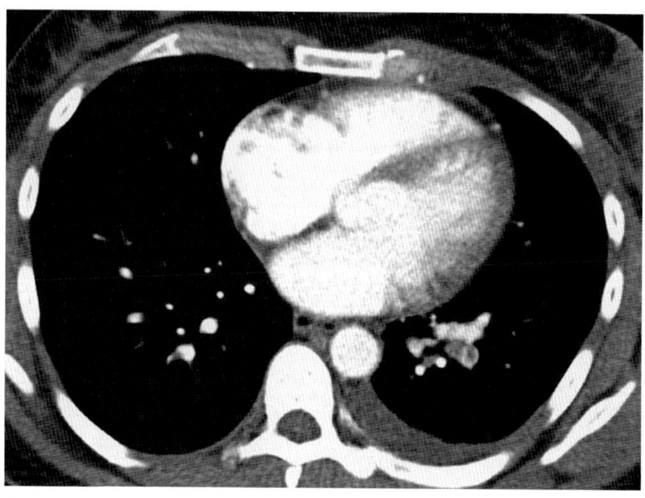

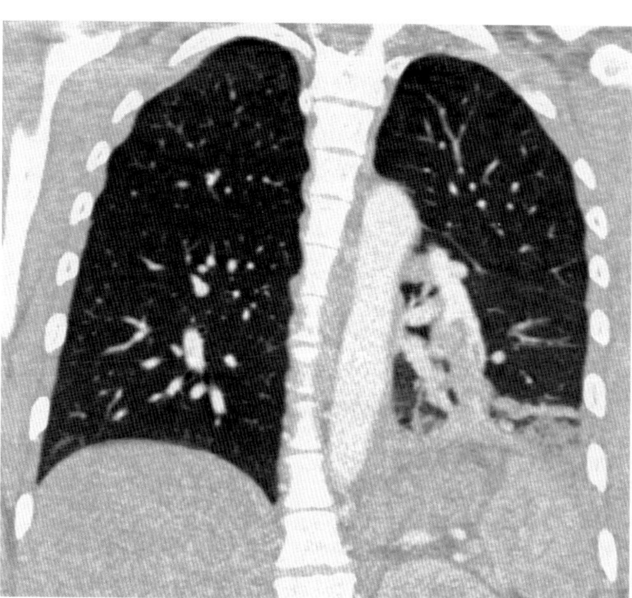

Figure 30-53 Acute pulmonary embolism. **A.** Axial CT at the lung bases demonstrates filling defects in the left lower lobe segmental arteries, compatible with acute PE. Note small left pleural effusion. **B.** Coronal CT image demonstrates a peripheral LLL consolidation, compatible with pulmonary infarct.

blood flow, given that pulmonary vascular impedance is relatively uniform throughout the lungs (1/10 of average systemic vascular impedance). Assuming a normal average pulmonary arterial pressure of 15 mm Hg, in an adult patient in the erect position a gradient of 22 to 23 mm Hg exists between the apex (2–3 mm Hg) and the bases (25 mm Hg). Given that vascular impedance in the lungs is uniformly low, flow to the bases is approximately 10 times greater than flow to the apices. These differences are greatly reduced in supine position, in which there is a much smaller pressure gradient between the posterior and anterior lungs; consequently, flow is far more uniform in the supine position. In the healthy patient, exercise may increase cardiac output and pulmonary blood flow fivefold, with minimal changes in pressure due to decreased pulmonary vascular impedance. The decline in pulmonary vascular impedance is secondary to capillary recruitment and increased vascular distension.

In pathologic conditions in which pulmonary arterial or venous pressures are increased, or in which alveolar pressure is elevated, the importance of gravity as the major determinant of pulmonary flow is diminished. Furthermore, impaired gas exchange and ventilation may cause alveolar hypoxia that further interferes with pulmonary blood flow via hypoxic vasoconstriction of small arterioles.

The concept of lung "perfusion zones" is based on functional compartmentalization of the lung into three zones according to the relationships among pulmonary arterial, pulmonary venous, and alveolar pressures. In Zone 1, average alveolar pressure > arterial pressure > venous pressure, such that perfusion is minimal. In Zone 2, average arterial pressure > alveolar pressure > venous pressure, such that perfusion is pulsatile. In Zone 3, average arterial pressure > venous pressure > alveolar pressure, such that perfusion is continuous. Normal healthy subjects do not manifest Zone 1 physiology; however, patients on mechanical ventilation with high positive end-expiratory pressure (PEEP) or patients with COPD and air trapping may develop large areas of Zone 1 physiology. Moreover, heart diseases characterized by left ventricular dysfunction demonstrate increased left atrial and, consequently, increased pulmonary venous pressure. In the short term, this may cause vascular redistribution (with cephalization of the pulmonary vasculature) or pulmonary edema (if acute and more severe). In the long term, adaptation mechanisms of the pulmonary arterial circulation and right ventricle, including increased vascular impedance and right ventricular hypertrophy and dilatation, ultimately result in increased pulmonary arterial pressure; pulmonary hypertension ensues. Understanding the underlying pathophysiology is important for interpreting the imaging findings of pulmonary hypertension.

In its broadest sense, pulmonary hypertension is a pathophysiologic condition in which pulmonary hemodynamics are altered, including an increase in pulmonary vascular impedance and a consequent increase in mean pulmonary arterial pressure above 25 mm Hg (current diagnostic criteria). The pathophysiology, current WHO classification, and treatment of pulmonary hypertension are described in Chapter 72.

The reference standard for diagnosis of pulmonary hypertension is right heart catheterization, an invasive diagnostic modality which allows direct measurement of right ventricular pressure and pulmonary arterial pressure, as well as indirect measurement of pulmonary venous pressure throughout the cardiac cycle. Noninvasive imaging tests cannot measure pressure directly, although echocardiography can be used to estimate pulmonary arterial pressure via Doppler techniques that measure the velocity of the regurgitant jet through the tricuspid valve during systole. The right atrial pressure is usually assumed to be 7 to 8 mm Hg plus the central venous pressure, as estimated by physical evaluation of neck veins distention. These pressures cannot be directly measured by Doppler ultrasonography.

From a diagnostic standpoint, imaging tests may, nonetheless, provide important insight into the possible presence and potential etiology of pulmonary hypertension. The hemodynamic distinction between precapillary pulmonary hypertension (defined by mean pulmonary arterial pressure >25 mm Hg and PCWP <15 mm Hg) and postcapillary pulmonary hypertension (defined by mean pulmonary arterial pressure >25 mm Hg and PCWP >15 mm Hg) can generally be made by advanced imaging. Precapillary pulmonary hypertension includes pulmonary arterial hypertension, pulmonary hypertension due to lung parenchymal diseases, chronic thromboembolic pulmonary hypertension, and miscellaneous causes (WHO Classes I, III, IV, and V). Postcapillary pulmonary hypertension includes pulmonary venous hypertension associated with left heart disease (WHO Class II).

Imaging studies are important in separating pulmonary arterial hypertension from pulmonary hypertension related to pulmonary parenchymal diseases, left ventricular failure, and chronic thromboembolic pulmonary disease, since the management of these entities differs substantially.

Chest radiographs are helpful in the initial assessment of suspected pulmonary hypertension, although they are not sensitive for early diagnosis. Given their low cost and universal availability, chest radiographs can provide an assessment of cardiac size and pulmonary vasculature caliber and distribution, as well as suggest findings of congestive heart failure or diffuse lung parenchymal disease. Published studies suggest that on erect PA examinations, if PCWP is greater 13 but less than 18 mm Hg, there is usually vascular redistribution with relative hypervascularity of the upper lung fields; if between 18 and 25 mm Hg, there is also interstitial pulmonary edema; if greater than 25 mm Hg, there is usually alveolar edema and often pleural effusions. If pulmonary hypertension is present in these clinical settings, strong consideration should be given to left ventricular failure as a causal factor.

Chest CT and, increasingly, MRI have been proposed as diagnostic tests that can provide pertinent detailed information regarding the pulmonary parenchyma, cardiac anatomy and function, and the status of the pulmonary vasculature, with minimum patient risk.

Chest CT has a major role in evaluating patients with suspected pulmonary hypertension. It is the best imaging test to demonstrate lung parenchymal disease. A normal appearance of the lung parenchyma on chest CT in the setting of pulmonary hypertension effectively eliminates the possibility of COPD or ILD significantly contributing to the pulmonary hypertension and should prompt search for alternative etiologies.

Furthermore, chest CT is also useful for direct assessment of the pulmonary arteries in the setting of suspected pulmonary arterial hypertension. It has been reported that a main pulmonary artery caliber >29 mm, when measured 2 cm from the pulmonary valve, has a sensitivity of 84%, a specificity of 75%, and a positive predictive value of 97% for the presence of pulmonary arterial hypertension, as confirmed by invasive imaging. Moreover, if the main pulmonary artery has a maximum transverse diameter greater than that of the proximal ascending thoracic aorta, there is a sensitivity of 70%, specificity of 92%, and positive predictive value of 96% for the presence of pulmonary arterial hypertension. One should be mindful to first determine that the ascending aorta is not aneurysmal when performing these measurements.

An additional chest CT finding suggesting pulmonary arterial hypertension is enlargement of the segmental arteries greater than 1.25 times the caliber of the adjacent bronchus. A combination of positive findings increases diagnostic confidence. For instance, the presence of enlarged main pulmonary artery (>29 mm) and concomitant enlargement of three out of four segmental arteries (arterial/bronchial diameter > 1.25) provides a very high specificity (100%) for the diagnosis of pulmonary arterial hypertension. However, if pulmonary fibrosis or emphysema is present, the correlation between pulmonary artery dimension and severity of pulmonary hypertension is substantially weaker. In these clinical settings, a combination of findings is warranted to suggest the diagnosis.

A prospective study comparing right heart catheterization and chest CT demonstrated that CT-derived measurement of the main pulmonary artery diameter (MPAD) correlates more strongly with the presence of pulmonary hypertension in patients without ILD (MPAD >31.6 mm associated with a PPV of 90.0% and a NPV of 58.3%) than in patients with ILD (MPAD >25 mm associated with a PPV of 46.3% and a NPV of 83.8%), although in both groups the MPAD was significantly greater in patients with pulmonary hypertension than in those without. One conclusion is that pulmonary hypertension is more likely to be present even with normal caliber pulmonary arteries if the underlying diagnosis is ILD. The presence of bronchial artery hypertrophy >1.5 mm has also been implicated in pulmonary arterial hypertension, although this sign is probably far more common in chronic pulmonary thromboembolic disease.

Several pulmonary parenchymal findings are associated with pulmonary arterial hypertension, although they are not individually sensitive or specific enough to warrant the diagnosis. The first is mosaic attenuation, which is more commonly seen in the setting of pulmonary hypertension due to chronic pulmonary thromboembolic disease, but which can also be seen in the presence of small airway disease without pulmonary hypertension, among other possibilities. Widespread tiny centrilobular ground-glass nodules may also be present, similar to those observed in hypersensitivity pneumonitis, but pathologically deemed to represent cholesterol granulomas or large plexogenic arterial lesions, which have been described in 7% to 47% of patients with pulmonary arterial hypertension.[73–75]

MRI is currently the reference standard for assessment of congenital heart diseases, as it accurately delineates structural changes, cardiac situs, intracardiac shunts, atrial–ventricular and ventriculoarterial relationships, and vascular dimensions, along with wall motion and valvular abnormalities. It is the most useful modality for assessing right ventricular anatomy and function, which is a critical prognostic determinant in pulmonary hypertension. Furthermore, contrast-enhanced MRI, through demonstration of delayed enhancement, uniquely enables detection of the presence and extent of myocardial scarring related to prior infarction, myocarditis, or infiltrative disease in the myocardium—findings that may be associated with left ventricular dysfunction and pulmonary venous hypertension. MRI, similar to Doppler echocardiography, can be used to quantitatively measure flow velocity using phase contrast imaging, allowing for estimation of arterial and intracardiac pressures. However, a major strength of MRI when compared with echocardiography is that arbitrary planes can be set without limitation by available acoustic windows, providing for greater accuracy and reproducibility. Further developments in MRI techniques will increase the clinical usefulness of this modality. In the future, it is conceivable that the combination of advanced CT and MRI techniques will be able to provide a thorough anatomical and functional assessment of the heart–lung unit in patients with suspected pulmonary hypertension, obviating the need for invasive right heart catheterization in selected patients (Figs. 30-54–30-56).[76–78]

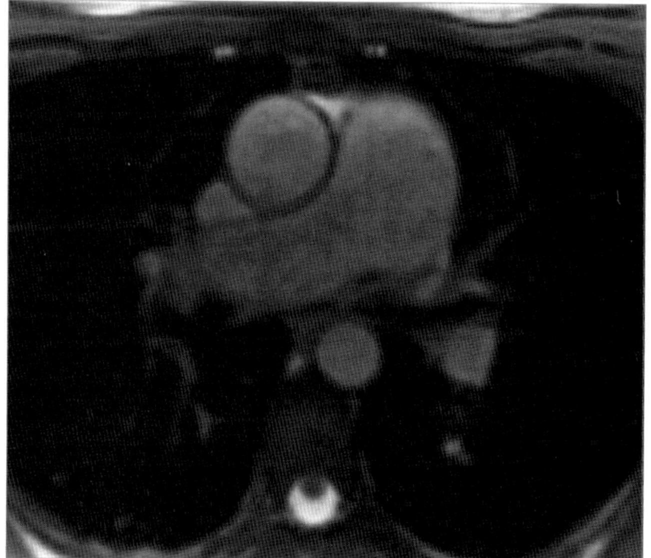

A

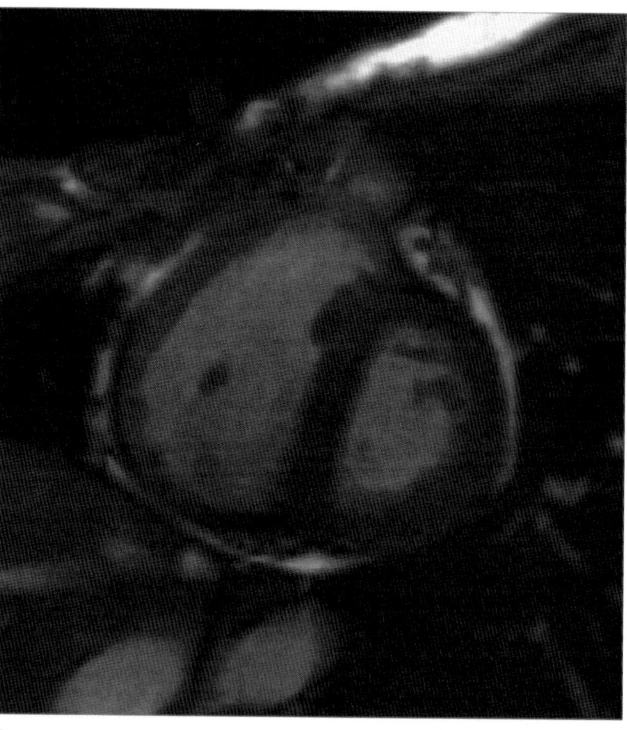

B

Figure 30-54 Pulmonary hypertension and right ventricular strain. **A.** Steady-state, free precession axial (SSFP) MR image ("bright blood") demonstrates dilatation of the central pulmonary arteries, with the main PA larger than the ascending aorta, compatible with pulmonary arterial hypertension. **B.** SSFP MR image, short axis of the heart, demonstrates right ventricular dilatation and straightening of the interventricular septum, indicative of right ventricular strain. The septum is normally convex toward the RV, due to normally higher LV pressure.

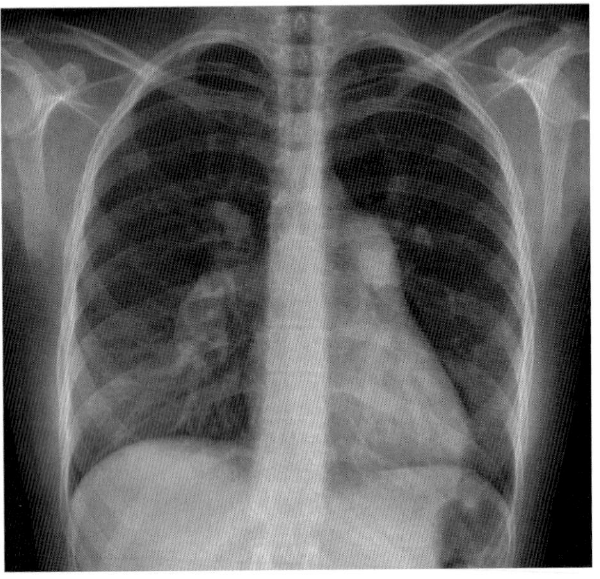

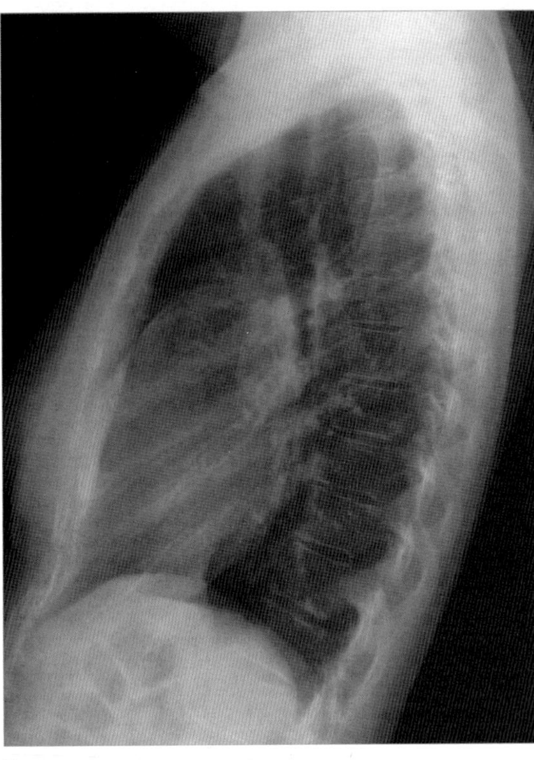

Figure 30-55 Pulmonary hypertension due to cardiac shunt. (**A**) PA, (**B**) lateral chest radiographs demonstrate moderate dilatation of the central pulmonary arteries, secondary to a long-standing uncorrected atrial septal defect (ASD).

PLEURAL, DIAPHRAGMATIC, AND CHEST WALL DISEASES

Radiographic imaging of the pleural space, diaphragm, and chest wall plays an important role in the diagnosis and evaluation of common, clinically important disorders involving these structures.

PLEURAL DISEASES

Pleural pathology can be broadly classified, for imaging purposes, into three major categories: pneumothoraces; pleural effusions; and pleural thickening, nodules, or masses. These are described in the subsections that follow.

Pneumothorax

Even though generally placed within the subgroup of pleural pathology, pneumothorax, characterized as the presence of gas within the pleural cavity separating the parietal from the visceral pleura, is rarely related to a disease process of the pleura itself (see also Chapter 31). Rather, it is associated with pulmonary or chest wall lesions. Nonetheless, pneumothorax is a very important clinical diagnosis, since it can lead to substantial morbidity or mortality if undetected or not properly treated.

Imaging is generally extremely accurate in the diagnosis of pneumothorax. The only exception is a portable chest radiograph obtained

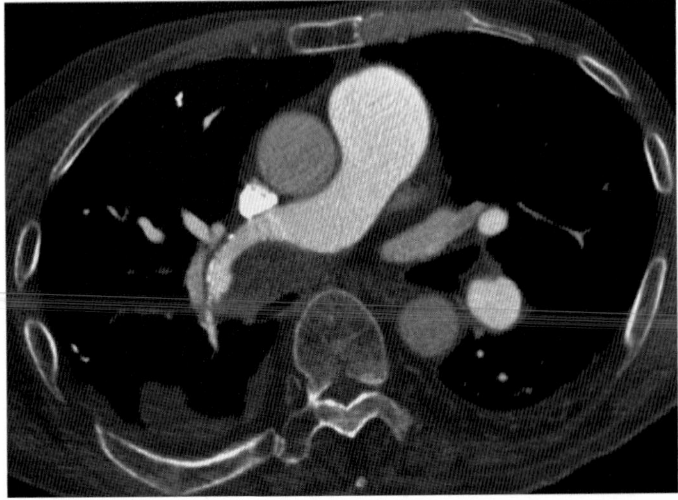

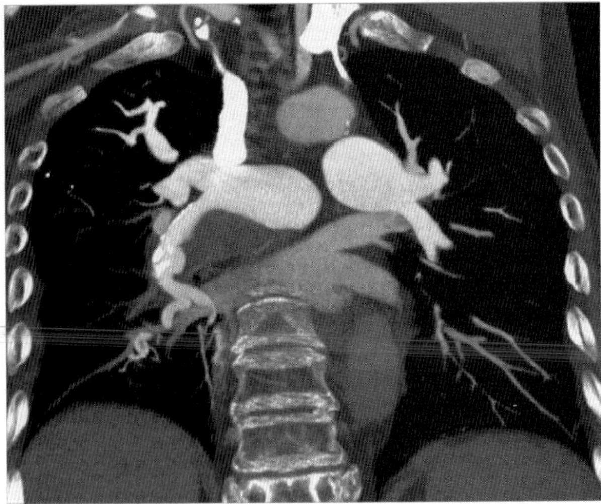

Figure 30-56 Chronic thromboembolic pulmonary hypertension (CTEPH): (**A**) axial CT image and (**B**) coronal MIP CT image demonstrating marked dilatation of the central pulmonary arteries, partially occlusive filling defect in the right main pulmonary artery, and tortuosity of the pulmonary arteries, with asymmetric vascular caliber. The constellation of findings reflects CTEPH.

in a supine position, which is relatively insensitive for detection of small pneumothoraces. In this scenario a pneumothorax should be suspected if there is increased lucency in the least dependent portion of the hemithorax (the anterolateral costophrenic angle in supine position), known as the "deep sulcus sign." This finding should prompt a lateral decubitus film, with the patient positioned with the suspected pneumothorax in the nondependent side; findings include a sharply marginated lucency along the lateral nondependent hemithorax.

On the other hand, erect PA radiographs are very sensitive and can detect even very small pneumothoraces, which are identified as crescentic-shaped lucencies lateral and superior to the apex of the lung and delineated from the lung parenchyma by a thin visceral pleural line. If there is doubt regarding the presence of a very small pneumothorax, an expiratory view may help by increasing the conspicuity of the pneumothorax, as the lung volumes will be reduced while the pneumothorax volume remains constant, resulting in an increase in the percent volume of the hemithorax occupied by the pneumothorax. In addition, lung parenchymal attenuation will be slightly increased relative to the pneumothorax.

Finally, CT is the most accurate modality for detecting pneumothorax and can demonstrate even minuscule pneumothoraces (<1%) that cannot be detected by standard radiographic techniques.

Special cases include tension and loculated pneumothoraces. Tension pneumothorax is a critical diagnosis that requires emergent treatment. A tension pneumothorax manifests on imaging as substantial lung collapse, contralateral mediastinal shift, and downward ipsilateral diaphragmatic displacement. It is generally associated with respiratory and cardiovascular compromise and requires prompt decompression. Loculated pneumothorax occurs when there are inflammatory or neoplastic adhesions between the parietal and visceral pleura, causing gas to accumulate in the pleural space in unusual locations and geometric configurations that do not respect gravitational gradients.

Imaging can also be performed to monitor a pneumothorax, for example, to decide if and when to place a chest tube, and also to investigate the etiology. Most pneumothoraces are either traumatic (in the setting of rib fractures or pulmonary lacerations) or iatrogenic (in the setting of pulmonary, mediastinal, or chest wall interventional procedures, which may be percutaneous, bronchoscopic, or surgical). CT is the best imaging modality to demonstrate rib fractures and pulmonary lacerations. Occasionally, a patient presents with a spontaneous pneumothorax. Most often these are related to rupture of pulmonary blebs or bullae, which may occur in patients with COPD or cystic lung diseases; in some cases, no specific cause can be demonstrated.[79]

A chronic pneumothorax usually occurs in association with pleural effusion, resulting in a hydropneumothorax. Hydropneumothoraces are generally associated with surgical procedures, malignancy, or severe infections, such as empyema. A chronic pneumothorax strongly suggests the presence of a bronchopleural fistula, as gas-forming infection in the pleural space is rare (Figs. 30-57 and 30-58).[80]

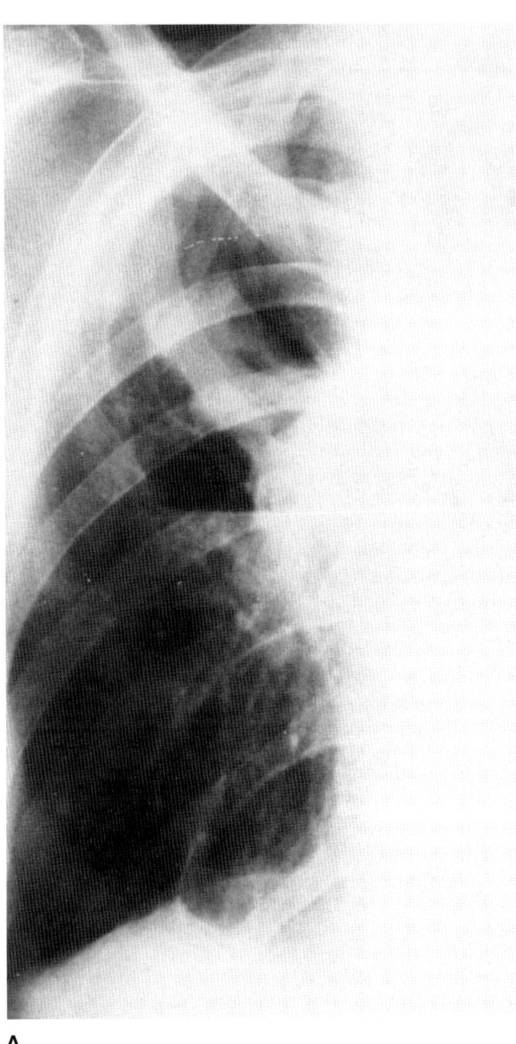
A

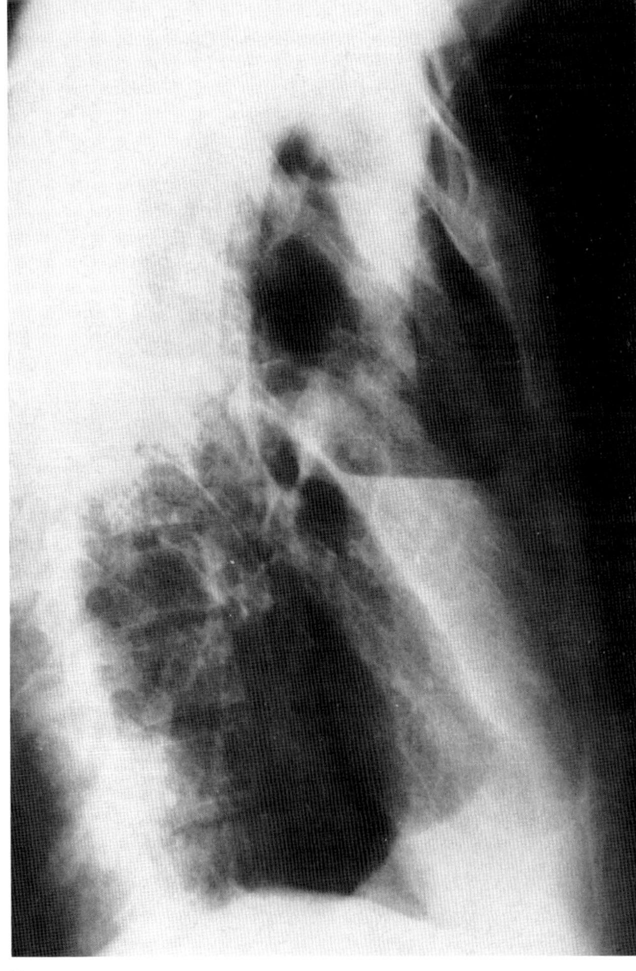
B

Figure 30-57 Hydropneumothorax. **A.** PA view. A distinct air–fluid level is seen overlying the right hilus. **B.** Lateral view. The fluid and air are anterior to the hilus. The findings are difficult to differentiate from a lung cavity, but the very thin edge suggests localization in the pleural space. This was a hydropneumothorax and was secondary to a postoperative bronchopleural fistula.

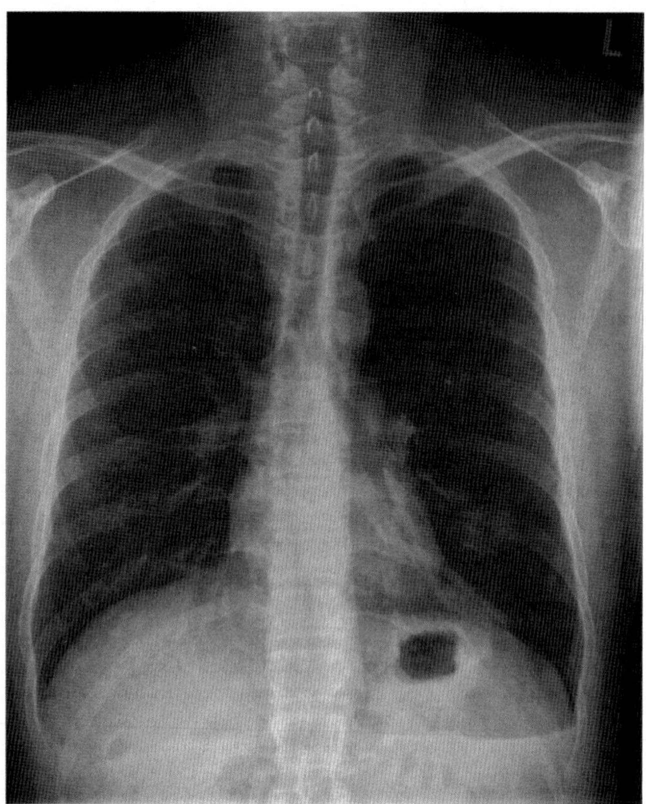

A

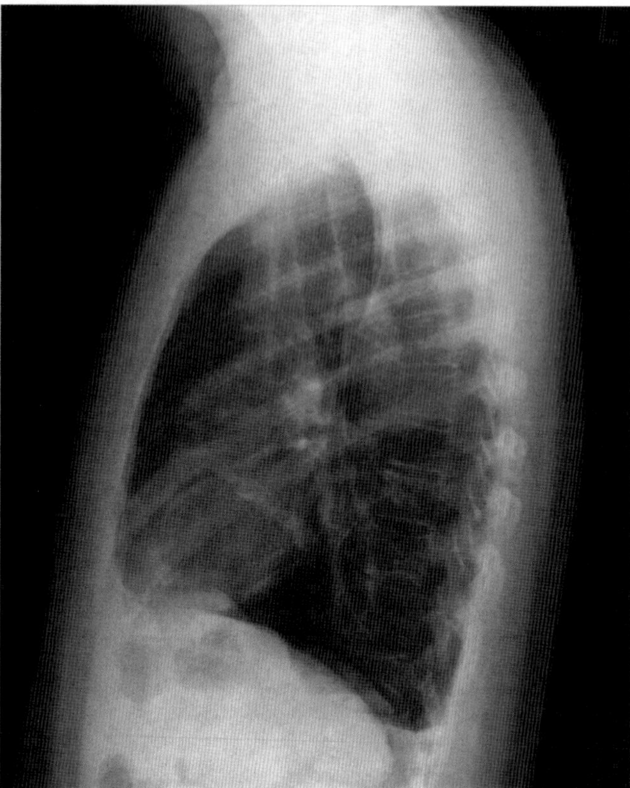

B

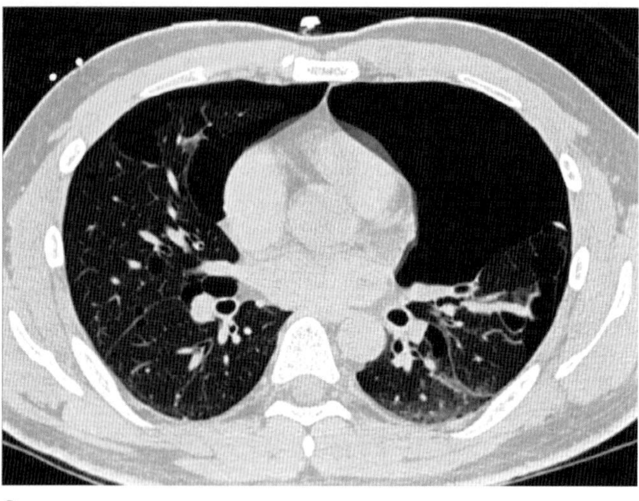

C

Figure 30-58 Bilateral pneumothoraces. (**A**) PA and (**B**) lateral chest radiographs demonstrate bilateral pneumothoraces, approximately 20% on the right and 40% on the left. The patient presented with spontaneous pneumothoraces. **C.** Axial CT at the lung bases confirms bilateral pneumothoraces and also indicates the etiology, demonstrating multiple pulmonary cysts. The patient was found to have Birt–Hogg–Dubé syndrome, a genetic disease that causes pulmonary cysts and predisposes the patient to recurrent spontaneous pneumothorax.

Pleural Effusions

Fluid in the pleural cavity appears radiographically as a homogeneous opacity that generally occupies a dependent position. A small pleural effusion that is barely perceptible or is overlooked on the PA view is often readily apparent on the lateral radiograph as blunting of the posterior costophrenic sulcus. The best non-CT radiographic study for demonstrating small quantities of pleural fluid is the lateral decubitus view, with the suspected pleural effusion on the dependent side. Using this technique, as little as 25 mL of fluid can be detected. Larger pleural effusions usually blunt the lateral costophrenic sulcus on the PA radiograph as well.

Occasionally, pleural fluid remains between the diaphragm and the lung, that is, infrapulmonary or subpulmonic, displacing the lung upward so that the lateral costophrenic angle remains sharp. The presence of a subpulmonic accumulation of fluid should be suspected if the diaphragm appears elevated, particularly along its lateral aspect on the frontal radiograph; if the costophrenic sulcus is blunted posteriorly; or if the gastric gas bubble is separated from the dome of the apparent left hemidiaphragm by more than a few millimeters (The last finding is frequently normal, however). CT is especially sensitive in identifying even the smallest of pleural effusions, which may be undetectable on chest radiographs. In the intensive care unit, where many portable radiographs are obtained in supine patients, CT imaging is particularly helpful in the diagnosis of pleural effusions, often revealing sizable effusions that are unsuspected.

Pleural effusions can be classified into two major categories: transudates and exudates. Transudates are characterized by low protein concentration relative to the plasma, and very low cellularity; exudates are characterized by higher protein concentration and cellularity, as discussed in detail elsewhere (Chapters 76 and 77). Transudative pleural effusions are commonly caused by congestive

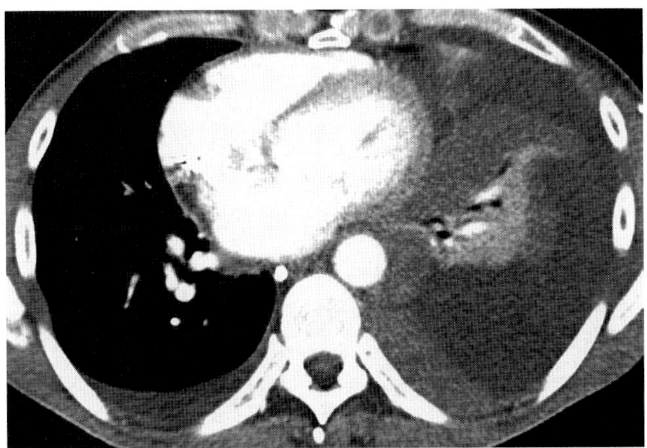

Figure 30-59 Malignant pleural effusion. Axial CT image demonstrates bilateral pleural effusions. The left effusion is associated with enhancing pleural masses, better visualized at the posterior medial costophrenic angle and adjacent to the descending thoracic aorta. This is characteristic of a malignant effusion. The patient was later diagnosed with mesothelioma.

heart failure, volume overload in the setting of renal dysfunction, or ascites in the setting of hepatic failure. Rarely, they are due to connective tissue disease or metastatic neoplasm. Broad causes of exudative effusions include parapneumonic collections, pulmonary infarction, malignancy (metastatic or due to primary pleural neoplasms), connective tissue disorders, subdiaphragmatic inflammatory processes, and infections (including empyema). Obtaining a specific diagnosis usually requires extensive evaluation that includes CT or MR, thoracentesis, and, possibly, pleural biopsy (Fig. 30-59).

Imaging modalities, particularly CT, may suggest, but not confirm, that an effusion is more likely a transudate or an exudate, thereby guiding patient management. Most transudates are bilateral, simple, nonloculated effusions occurring in dependent locations. Many exudates are unilateral, loculated effusions. A loculated effusion usually conforms to an unusual shape, commonly ovoid or with geometric edges, and sometimes along the fissures. Loculated effusions may resemble pulmonary masses on chest radiographs, although the pleural location can be readily ascertained on CT. The differential diagnosis of pleural effusions is one scenario in which US can be used to provide additional information beyond CT. For example, US may demonstrate internal septations within an effusion, a finding that can be difficult to demonstrate using CT and which is highly associated with exudative effusions. Furthermore, US can be used therapeutically to provide real-time guidance for thoracentesis and chest tube placement.[81–83] Conversely, US may occasionally fail to detect exudative pleural effusions, including empyemas, which are echogenic and which are readily detected by CT.

Pleural Thickening, Nodules, and Masses

Pleural diseases that cause diffuse thickening or localized nodularity may be separated into three broad etiologic categories: inflammatory, infectious, and neoplastic (both benign and malignant). Specific subgroups that are commonly encountered, but rarely clinically relevant, include apical pleural thickening (apical capping), which is usually bilateral and age-related and usually idiopathic (attributed to age-related ischemic changes); however, apical capping may potentially be associated with sequelae of granulomatous infections, particularly if accompanied by apical parenchymal scarring. Blunting of the lateral costophrenic angle on the PA view with sparing the posterior costophrenic angle on the lateral may be attributed to postinflammatory pleural thickening. Radiographic follow-up is helpful in excluding a focal mass. Multifocal pleural plaques, which are smoothly marginated, localized areas of pleural thickening, and which are often associated with calcifications, are common late manifestations of prior asbestos exposure. Frequently, they are the sole imaging manifestation of past asbestos exposure. CT is the optimal modality for their detection and characterization.

Diffuse pleural thickening involving both hemithoraces is more likely of inflammatory etiology, although bilateral pleural metastases can definitely occur and should be considered. Unilateral, extensive pleural thickening is more suspicious for a malignant etiology, either pleural metastases or primary malignancy, such as pleural mesothelioma. Nodular thickening of the mediastinal pleura and involvement of the interlobar fissures are particularly correlated with a malignant etiology; as a rule, the more nodular the pleural thickening appears, the more likely a malignant process is its cause. The differential diagnosis includes empyema, particularly tuberculous empyema, which may be indistinguishable from mesothelioma based on imaging appearance. Imaging cannot distinguish mesothelioma, pleural metastases, and tuberculous empyema; tissue sampling and correlation with other clinical and laboratory findings is required.[84–86]

A special case to consider is extensive pleural thickening associated with calcifications and diminished volume of the adjacent lung parenchyma—a fibrothorax. Most fibrothoraces reflect sequelae of prior substantial pleural inflammation caused by empyema or hemothorax, and their clinical significance is due to their potential to impair chest wall mechanics and restrict lung expansion.

A localized pleural nodule suggests a benign pleural neoplasm, such as a solitary fibrous tumor of the pleura or lipoma. The nodule may be difficult to distinguish from a localized area of pleural thickening, but generally it is larger and more symmetric in contour. On CT, these nodules usually have a characteristic appearance: Their shape is ovoid with their largest diameter parallel to the chest wall, and their edges are flat and tapering. The appearance is similar to the extrapleural sign on chest radiographs, which is defined as a shadow that has smooth margins, tapering edges with obtuse angles with the chest wall, and is generally seen well in only one of the two standard views of the chest. Occasionally, a peripheral nerve sheath tumor (e.g., schwannoma or neurofibroma) arising from an intercostal nerve may mimic a pleural nodule. These lesions, however, tend to cause indentation of adjacent ribs due to long standing mass effect, helping to suggest the diagnosis.

Rarely, solitary or multiple pleural nodules without associated effusion may represent a malignant process; the classic example is the so-called "drop" metastases from thymic neoplasms.

DIAPHRAGMATIC DISEASES

Diaphragmatic evaluation can be performed initially via chest radiographs, ideally PA and lateral views. The normal hemidiaphragm has smooth contours and gentle curvature, with its dome near its center and no focal protrusions, with the left hemidiaphragm slightly lower than the right. The most common diaphragmatic abnormality is an eventration, in which there is focal weakness of the muscle, correlated with focal protrusion or bulge. Diaphragmatic paralysis should be suspected when an entire hemidiaphragm is elevated, typically more than 2 cm in comparison to the normal side. To confirm diaphragmatic paralysis, the standard test is a fluoroscopic dynamic evaluation ("sniff test"), in which the patient is imaged during shallow breathing, deep breathing, and forceful inspiration ("sniff"). The normal hemidiaphragm moves downward with the sniff maneuver, while a paralyzed hemidiaphragm will demonstrate paradoxical upward motion.

Diaphragmatic hernias can be classified into three broad categories: hiatal, congenital, and traumatic. Hiatal hernias occurring

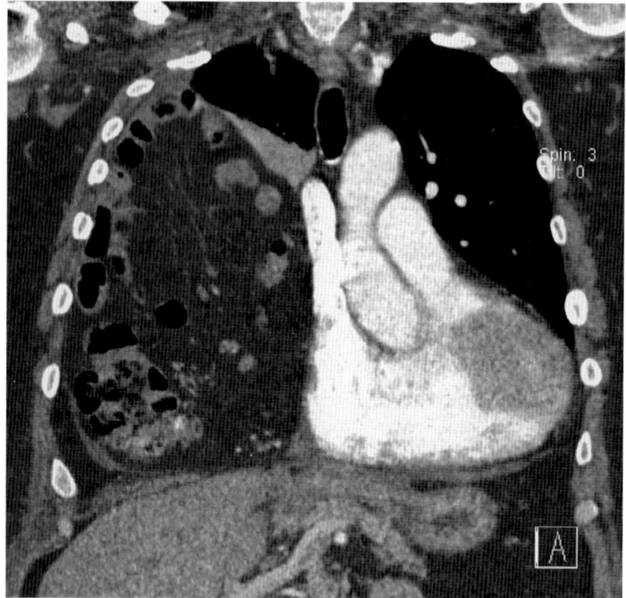

Figure 30-60 Diaphragmatic hernia. Coronal CT image demonstrates a wide defect in the right hemidiaphragm. The right lung is nearly completely collapsed, and the right hemithorax is nearly completely occupied by small and large bowel loops with associated mesenteric fat. This is diagnostic of diaphragmatic hernia, in this case due to blunt trauma to the abdomen.

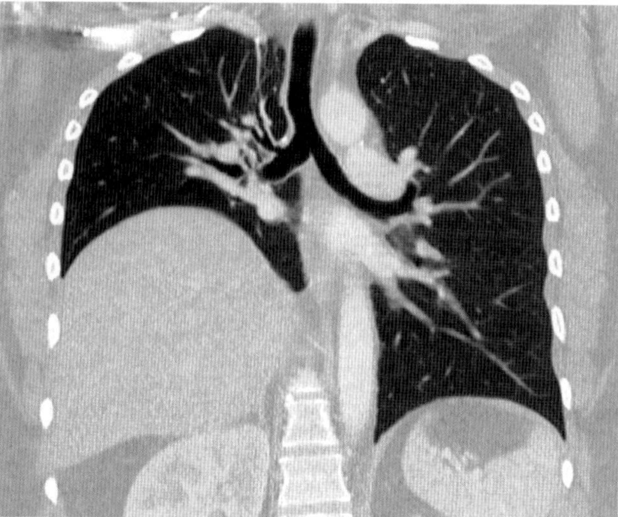

Figure 30-61 Diaphragmatic paralysis. Coronal CT image shows marked elevation of the right hemidiaphragm. Fluoroscopic examination confirmed a paralyzed right hemidiaphragm.

through the centrally placed esophageal hiatus are the most common, and usually contain a portion of the stomach, although very large hernias can contain small or large bowel loops as well. Congenital hernias are usually through the paired foramina of Morgagni (anterior and medial) or the paired foramina of Bochdalek (posterior and central). The latter are more frequent and are usually small, incidental hernias containing fat. When large, these congenital hernias can contain viscera, either bowel loops (Morgagni) or retroperitoneal structures such as the kidney (Bochdalek), but these are virtually always diagnosed in infancy. Traumatic hernias should be suspected in patients who had blunt trauma and present with a newly elevated hemidiaphragm. These are more common on the left, as the liver usually prevents herniation on the right except in very large defects. Traumatic diaphragmatic ruptures may occur in the setting of trauma without detectable herniation, and the actual herniation of abdominal viscera into the thorax may occur days, months, or even years later. Inquiry regarding a history of remote trauma is thus important in the evaluation of diaphragmatic hernias. Multiplanar coronal and sagittal CT or MR images allow accurate assessment of diaphragmatic contour abnormalities, and are the reference standard for the diagnosis of diaphragmatic rupture. MR offers the additional advantage of functional assessment with fast gradient echo cine sequences (Figs. 30-60 and 30-61).[87–89]

CHEST WALL MASSES

Chest wall masses may extend into the pleura and cause pleural nodularity or masses. These are very difficult to detect radiographically unless causing bone destruction or substantial mass effect. CT or MR associated with tissue sampling is generally necessary for accurate diagnosis. The differential diagnosis of chest wall masses includes soft tissue infection (cellulitis, phlegmon, abscess), which is generally associated with trauma and surgical procedures; hematoma, also often associated with trauma or surgical procedures; extension of infection arising from the lung, with the prototype disease being actinomycosis; and rarely neoplasms, such as soft tissue sarcomas, metastatic disease, and malignant nerve sheath tumors.

MEDIASTINAL DISEASES

Mediastinal diseases encompass multiple systems, organs, and a vast array of differential diagnoses. Before discussing mediastinal diseases, it is necessary to define the contents of the mediastinum and its boundaries.

The anatomic delineations of "compartments" of the mediastinum are not defined consistently throughout the medical literature. For radiographic diagnosis, a simple classification has been employed: (1) The *anterior compartment*, which extends from the sternum anteriorly to the heart, aorta, and brachiocephalic vessels posteriorly, comprises only the thymus, fat tissue, and a few lymph nodes. (2) The *middle* or *visceral compartment* contains the heart, great vessels, trachea and its branches, esophagus, and descending aorta. It extends from the posterior border of the anterior compartment to the anterior border of the vertebral column. These boundaries differ from the anatomist's classification, which relegates portions of the esophagus and the descending aorta to the posterior mediastinum. (3) The *posterior compartment* contains the vertebrae and paravertebral sulci.

Application of this classification to the lateral chest radiograph facilitates generation of a relevant differential diagnosis. However, with modern modalities such as CT or MR, one is able to accurately categorize mediastinal masses according to their exact location within the mediastinum, obviating the need for compartmental localization. For example, instead of categorizing a mass as in the posterior mediastinum, CT or MR often allows accurate differentiation among different etiologies, such as paraspinal masses, neurogenic neoplasms, vascular lesions, and esophageal masses (Figs. 30-62 and 30-63).[90]

This section focuses on diseases of the lymph nodes and thymus. Cardiac and systemic vascular diseases are beyond the scope of this textbook and will be mentioned only briefly. Pulmonary vascular diseases have been described previously. Esophageal diseases and spinal or paraspinal diseases are discussed briefly (Fig. 30-64).

Before a discussion on mediastinal neoplasms, it is important to emphasize the role of CT for evaluation of suspected mediastinal infections in the postoperative patient.

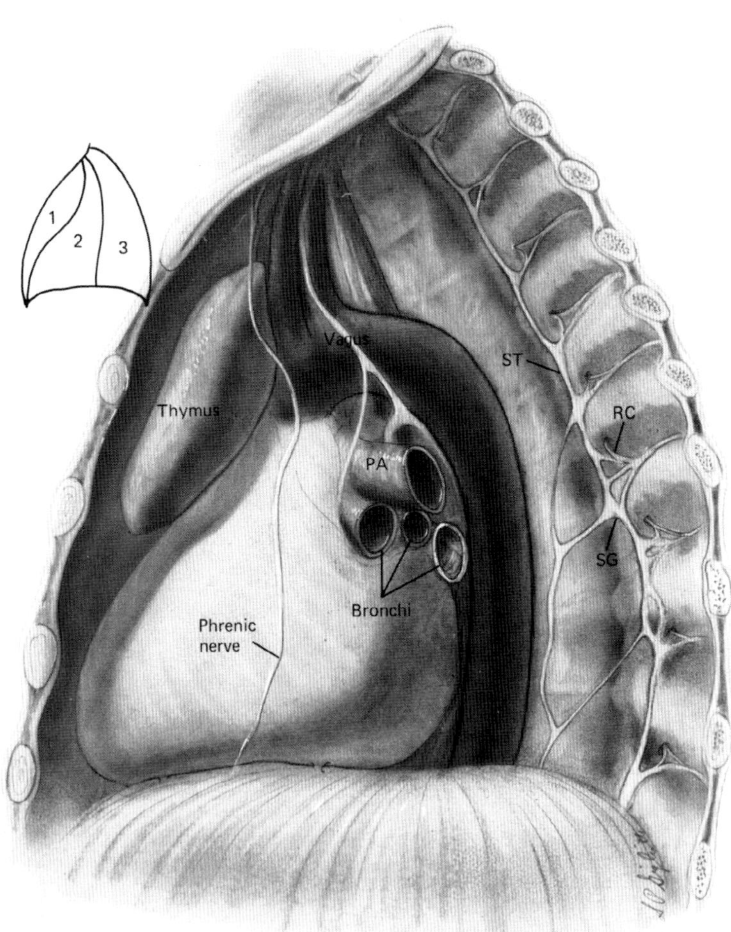

A

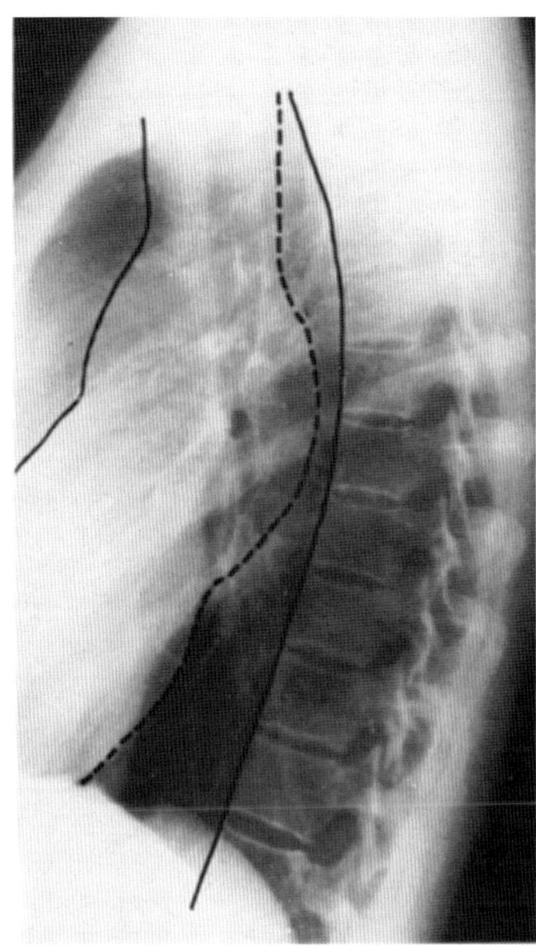

B

Figure 30-62 Compartments of the mediastinum: **A.** Anatomic view of the compartments of the mediastinum. The subdivisions (1, anterior; 2, middle; 3, posterior) in the small schematic *(top left)* correspond to those designated by the *solid black lines* in **B.** PA, pulmonary artery; ST; sympathetic trunk; SG, sympathetic ganglion; RC, ramus communicans. **B.** Radiographic division of the mediastinum. The *closed lines* delineate the anterior, middle, and posterior compartments. The *dashed line* represents the division of the middle and posterior mediastinum that is conventionally used by anatomists. *(**A:** Reproduced with permission from Jones KW, Pietra GG, Sabiston DC. Primary Neoplasms and Cysts of the Mediastinum, in Fishman AP (ed). Pulmonary Diseases and Disorders. New York: McGraw-Hill; 1980:1490–1521.)*

Mediastinitis is a catastrophic complication of multiple types of cardiothoracic surgeries and, if unrecognized and not treated aggressively, it often leads to a fatal outcome. In the immediate postoperative period in a patient status, post cardiac, central vascular, major pulmonary, or esophageal surgery, the presence of a small amount of gas and fluid in the mediastinum is an expected occurrence. The findings tend to subside within hours or a few days. While there is no absolute rule to apply to the time frame over which a pneumomediastinum or mediastinal fluid collection becomes clearly pathologic, some general guidelines are helpful in guiding management decisions: (1) It is expected that any postoperative fluid or gas collection will decrease in size over time, and any increase in size is suspicious for an evolving mediastinitis. (2) Large fluid and gas collections (those measuring >2 cm in the smallest diameter) are almost always pathologic. (3) Any persistent mediastinal fluid or gas collection more than 1 week following surgery is suspicious, and the index of suspicion rises if the patient is clinically worsening, if there are laboratory signs to support infection (e.g., leukocytosis with a left shift), and if there are CT features suggesting active inflammation, such as rim enhancement in the boundaries of the collection. Any of these findings should prompt aggressive management with percutaneous or surgical drainage of the collection and institution of broad-spectrum antibiotics.

A spontaneous pneumomediastinum has different clinical implications, as it may be a sign of an ominous condition, such as esophageal perforation (which warrants urgent surgical treatment), or a relatively benign condition when associated with barotrauma and tear of the distal airways or acini. Clinical correlation and careful clinical observation are very important to distinguish these etiologies (Fig. 30-65).[91,92]

The classical differential diagnosis of masses in the anterior compartment includes enlarged lymph nodes, substernal goiter or thyroid neoplasm, thymic hyperplasia and thymic neoplasms, and germ cell neoplasms. Distinction among these can be made on the basis of the patient's age and clinical presentation, their position within the anterior mediastinum, and the appearance on CT or MR.

Thyroid masses invariably lie high in the anterior mediastinum and often displace or compress the trachea and esophagus. On CT, the thyroid has characteristic high attenuation on unenhanced images due to its iodine content, and multinodular goiter often presents with a very heterogeneous texture containing cystic and calcified opacities within a background of dense thyroid parenchyma. Ultimately, any high anterior mediastinal mass with these imaging characteristics and unequivocal contiguity with the thyroid gland on CT or MR is deemed to represent a thyroid neoplasm or multinodular goiter, until proved otherwise.[93]

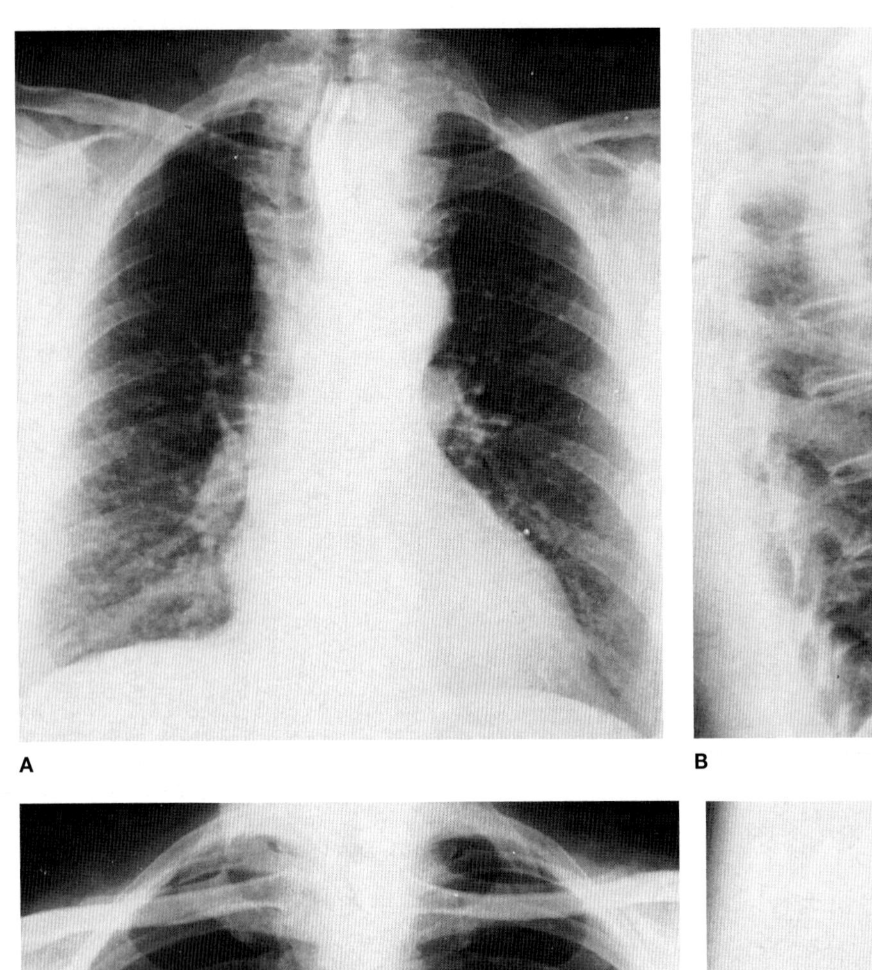

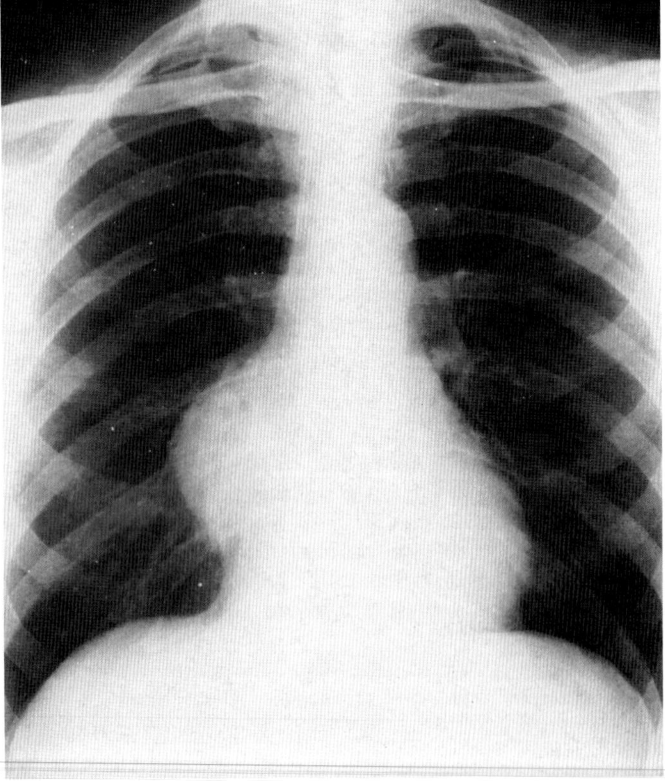

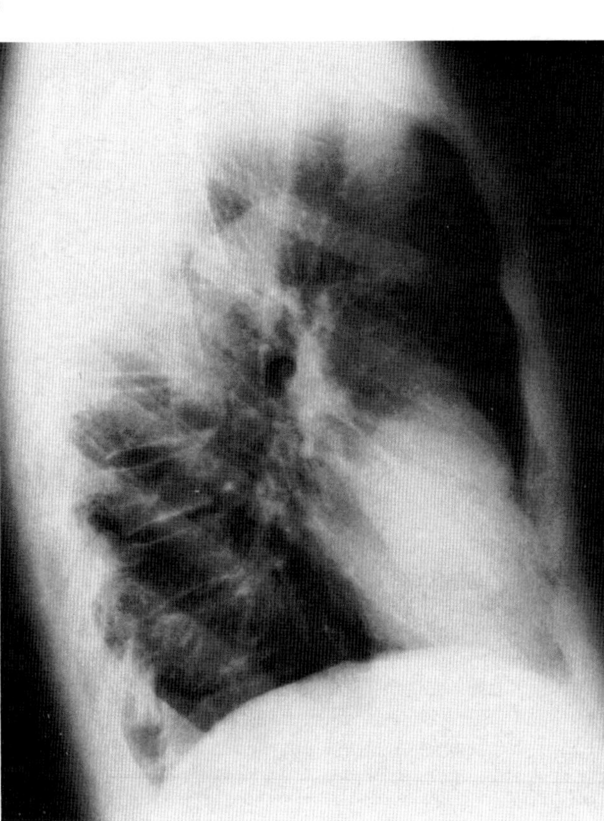

Figure 30-63 Radiographic spectrum of mediastinal masses: Substernal thyroid. **A.** PA view. A large mass in the neck extends below the clavicle. The trachea and esophagus are displaced to the right. **B.** Lateral view. The trachea and esophagus are also displaced posteriorly. Several calcifications are present within the mass. **C.** PA view. A discrete mass (thymoma) lies along the right heart border. **D.** Lateral view. The mass also overlies the anterior portion of the cardiac shadow. Despite being radiographically well circumscribed, the mass may be either invasive or noninvasive thymoma. CT is required for further characterization.

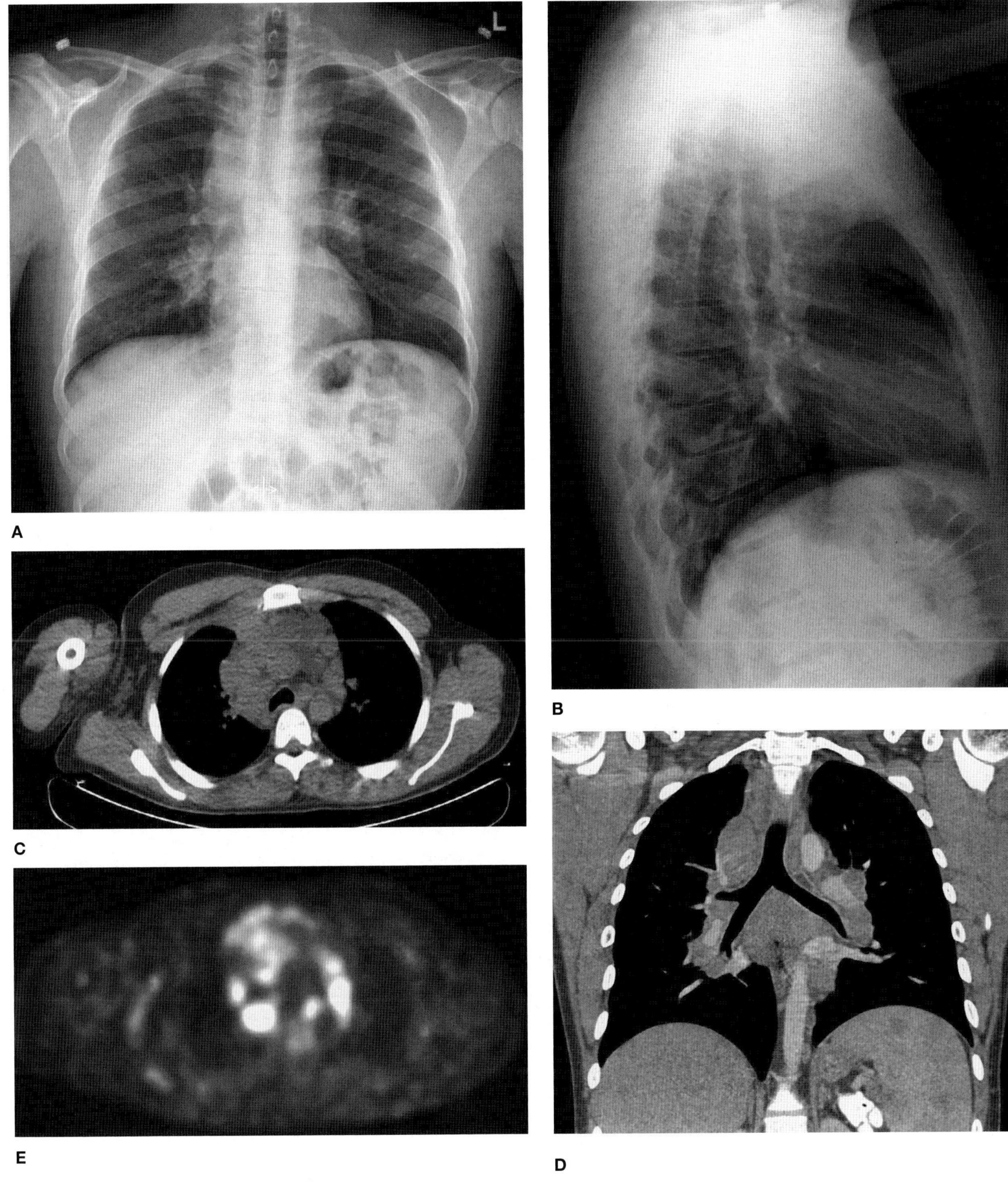

Figure 30-64 Lymphadenopathy: (**A**) PA and (**B**) lateral chest radiographs demonstrate marked widening of the bilateral paratracheal stripes and mild prominence of the bilateral pulmonary hila, compatible with mediastinal and hilar lymphadenopathy. (**C**) Axial noncontrast CT and (**D**) Coronal contrast-enhanced CT better demonstrate the extent of mediastinal and hilar lymphadenopathy. Pathology confirmed a large B-cell lymphoma. **E.** Axial FDG-PET at the level of the upper lung fields demonstrates increased glucose uptake within the enlarged mediastinal lymph nodes, indicative of increased metabolic activity. This study can be performed to monitor treatment response.

If an anterior mediastinal mass does not arise from the thyroid, the differential diagnosis of germ cell neoplasm, thymoma, and lymphoma can be challenging using imaging; tissue sampling is almost always necessary. Nonetheless, some clinical and imaging features may suggest a specific diagnosis. For example, germ cell neoplasms tend to occur in younger patients and are often heterogeneous—in particular, CT demonstration of fat and calcification within an anterior mediastinal mass is diagnostic of a teratoma.[94] Teratomas may also contain cystic components. Thymic hyperplasia or neoplasms tend to conform to the triangular shape of the thymus (particularly benign thymomas, although invasive thymomas and thymic carcinomas may have a more irregular configuration). Thymomas tend to occur in older patients and may be associated with the diagnosis of myasthenia gravis. Because of the presence of intracellular

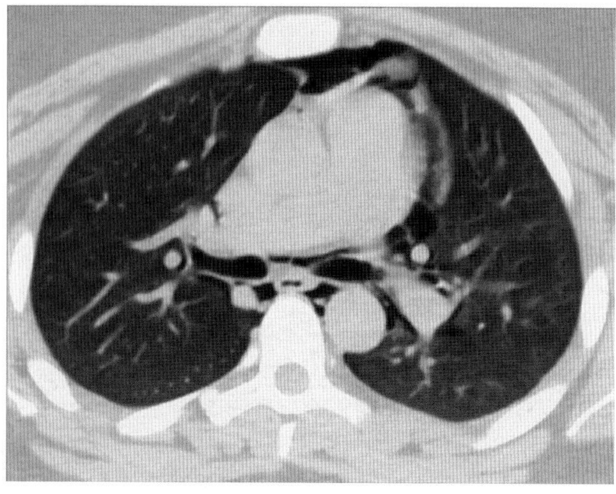

A B

Figure 30-65 Pneumomediastinum. **A.** Axial CT at the level of the mainstem bronchi demonstrates gas within the anterior, middle, and posterior mediastinal compartments, compatible with pneumomediastinum. **B.** Coronal CT demonstrates the full extent of the pneumomediastinum. Note absence of pneumothorax. There is also subtle pulmonary interstitial emphysema, denoted by linear lucencies parallel to the proximal airways. This patient had barotrauma related to a severe asthma exacerbation.

lipids in the normal thymus, thymic hyperplasia can be distinguished from thymomas and infiltration by lymphoma using proton chemical shift MR; signal loss is noted in out-of-phase sequences. Finally, lymphomas occur over a wide age range (with Hodgkin disease having a bimodal distribution) and are generally homogeneous on CT and MR, unless treated (Figs. 30-66 and 30-67).[95]

Lymphadenopathy in the thorax has an extremely broad differential diagnosis, and it is best assessed using CT or MR. Anatomically, the largest lymph nodal chains in the thorax can be divided in axillary, supraclavicular (which includes lower cervical chains), mediastinal, and bilateral hilar. Smaller chains include internal thoracic (mammary), anterior cardiophrenic (or paracardiac), and

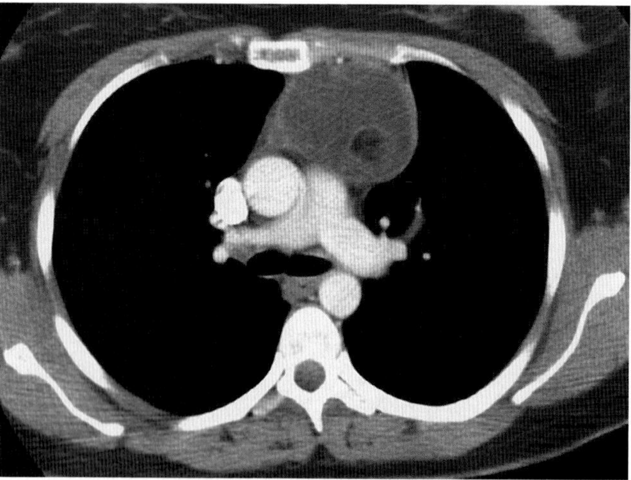

A

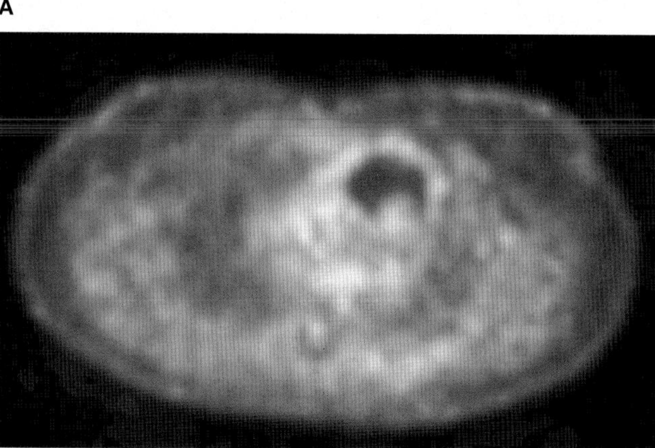

C

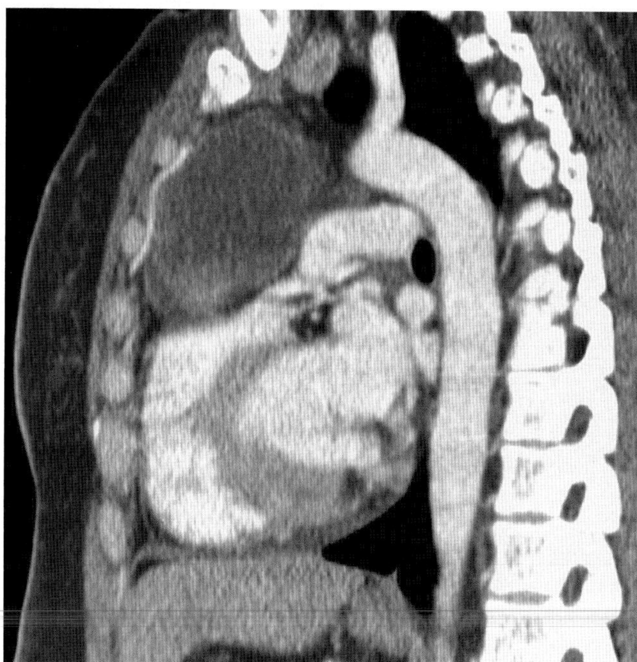

B

Figure 30-66 Anterior mediastinal mass. (**A**) Axial contrast-enhanced CT and (**B**) Sagittal contrast-enhanced CT show a heterogeneous, well-circumscribed anterior mediastinal mass. The mass is mostly cystic, with a nodular component that measures fat attenuation. Enhancing components are also noted. **C.** Axial FDG-PET through the mass demonstrates lack of glucose uptake. The constellation of findings is diagnostic of a mature teratoma, a benign germ cell neoplasm.

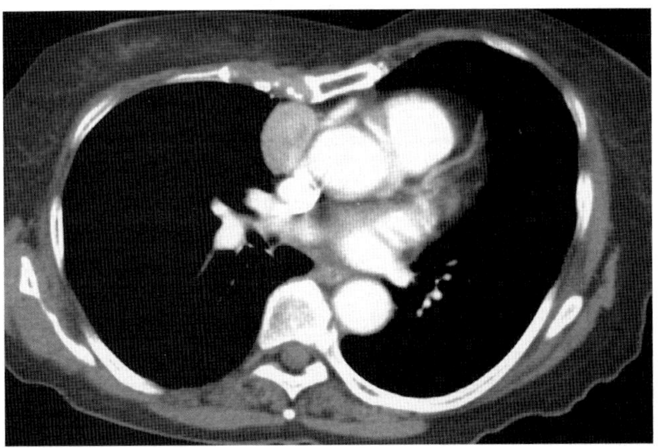

Figure 30-67 Anterior mediastinal mass. Axial contrast-enhanced CT demonstrates a homogeneous, enhancing, well-circumscribed anterior mediastinal mass along the anterior right heart border. Pathology confirmed a thymoma.

retrocrural. Mediastinal lymph node stations are further subdivided into prevascular, paratracheal (upper and lower, right and left), subaortic (or AP window), subcarinal, para-aortic, and paraesophageal.

A normal lymph node on CT or MR has an ovoid, reniform shape ("kidney shape") and a fatty hilum and measures less than 1 cm in its smallest diameter. An abnormal lymph node is frequently rounded, loses the delineation of the hilum, and measures more than 1 cm in its smallest diameter. It is important to emphasize that early neoplastic or infectious disease may be associated with "normal" lymph nodes on CT or MR, but "abnormal" lymph nodes on CT or MR are virtually never normal from a pathologic standpoint, even if the diagnosis is not clinically significant.

From an imaging perspective, establishing the etiology of mediastinal lymphadenopathy implies assessing the size, configuration, number, and location of the enlarged lymph nodes. Enhancement patterns on CT or MR have a limited role, although FDG uptake on PET/CT may be helpful. The presence of calcification is also an important sign in narrowing the differential diagnosis.

The following guidelines should be utilized in the general assessment of mediastinal and thoracic lymphadenopathy.[96–98]

Very large (measuring >2–3 cm), confluent, conglomerate lymphadenopathy is malignant until proven otherwise. Considerations include nodal metastasis and lymphoma, particularly high-grade, large B-cell lymphomas or Hodgkin disease. An anterior mediastinal, prevascular location favors lymphoma. Distribution of disease may help elucidate the origin of the primary neoplasm, in case the diagnosis is not obvious or previously established if one is cognizant of the typical lymphatic drainage pathways. For example, lung carcinomas present more frequently with ipsilateral hilar, subcarinal, and paratracheal lymphadenopathy; head and neck squamous cell carcinomas more often involve supraclavicular lymph nodes; breast carcinomas frequently involve ipsilateral axillary and internal thoracic lymph nodes; hepatocellular carcinomas usually involve anterior cardiophrenic lymph nodes (paracardiac nodes).

An increased number of nodes in disseminated lymphadenopathy, symmetric distribution involving multiple nodal stations, and moderately or substantially enlarged nodes suggest a low-grade lymphoproliferative disease, particularly chronic lymphocytic leukemia/small lymphocytic lymphomas (CLL/SLL). Note that early disease may present with only mildly enlarged lymph nodes.

Mild or moderately enlarged lymph nodes with a bilateral hilar and lower paratracheal distribution suggests the diagnosis of sarcoidosis.

Mild, bilateral, predominantly axillary lymphadenopathy can be seen in the setting of connective tissue diseases, such as systemic lupus erythematosus.

Mild disseminated lymphadenopathy can be seen in systemic infections, particularly "mono-like" syndromes caused by mononucleosis, CMV, and related infections.

Necrotizing lymphadenopathy may be seen in the setting of infectious lymphadenitis (particularly mycobacterial), but is also commonly seen in nodal metastasis.

Coarsely calcified lymph nodes, particularly mediastinal and hilar, suggest sequelae of granulomatous inflammation, including sarcoidosis and mycobacterial or fungal infection; however, treated malignancy and pneumoconiosis should also be considered in the differential diagnosis in the proper clinical setting.

Mild lymphadenopathy can be ascribed to a "reactive" etiology, including prior infections, congestive heart failure, or ILDs. Reactive lymphadenopathy is a diagnosis of exclusion.

Additional structures of the middle mediastinal compartment are the heart and central vessels. Aortic or aortic branch aneurysms can be suggested on chest radiographs by the presence of mediastinal widening and prominence of the aortic contours. Diagnostic confirmation and full characterization require CT or MR, typically with intravenous contrast. Duplication cysts of the foregut may arise from the esophagus or tracheobronchial tree and are also common in the middle compartment. These localized masses are smooth and well circumscribed; generally, they do not contain air, and their attenuation is low on CT (generally of simple fluid density) without contrast enhancement. However, duplication cysts containing highly proteinaceous fluid may have CT densities comparable to soft tissue, thus mimicking solid masses. As indicated earlier, MRI is useful in characterizing proteinaceous fluid and, thus, may be diagnostic in these cases. Bronchogenic cysts commonly occur at the tracheal carina or paratracheal region, whereas esophageal duplication cysts are characteristically located near the distal esophagus. However, esophageal and bronchogenic cysts may occur anywhere within the middle compartment.

A dilated (patulous) esophagus is sometimes seen on the chest radiograph as a long tubular mass in the middle compartment and is readily identified by CT. The significance of a patulous esophagus is its association with dysmotility disorders, such as achalasia, CREST syndrome, and presbyesophagus. Neoplasms of the esophagus or trachea may also present as more localized mediastinal masses by chest radiograph; usually, CT is required for recognition. Early esophageal neoplasms may involve primarily the mucosa and may not be well seen on the CT, even if clearly demonstrated on a barium swallow study or endoscopy. Hiatal hernias are readily diagnosed using CT. The presence of esophageal wall thickening is usually clinically relevant. Smooth and concentric wall thickening favors esophagitis, particularly reflux esophagitis; irregular and eccentric wall thickening is concerning for esophageal carcinoma.[99]

In the posterior (paraspinal) compartment, the most common radiographic abnormalities are neurogenic neoplasms. However, neoplasms or infections of the vertebral column may also present as masses in the posterior compartment. CT or MR usually distinguishes between a neurogenic neoplasm, which is unilateral and paraspinal in location, and lesions which erode or destroy the vertebrae and are generally present on both sides of the vertebral column. MR is the best modality to diagnose a neurogenic neoplasm (Figs. 30-68 and 30-69).[100,101] Other considerations in the posterior compartment include paraspinal hematoma in the setting of trauma, and rarely, extramedullary hematopoiesis in patients with hemoglobinopathies, myeloproliferative disorders, or bone marrow infiltration.

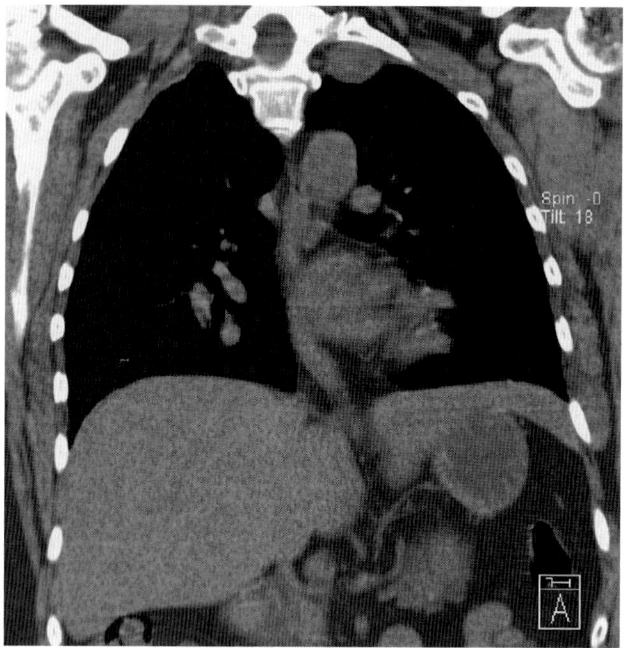

Figure 30-68 Posterior mediastinal mass. Coronal noncontrast CT shows a homogeneous, well-circumscribed posterior mediastinal mass in the left superior sulcus medially. Note absence of aggressive features by CT. Pathology confirmed a neurogenic neoplasm (schwannoma).

OUTLOOK FOR THE FUTURE

This chapter provides a modern, evidence-based overview of the wide scope and central role imaging plays in the diagnosis and management of thoracic diseases. Currently, it is inconceivable to imagine practicing thoracic medicine and surgery without the constant support of radiologist consultants and their armamentarium of basic and advanced imaging modalities.

Predicting the long-term future is most often a futile endeavor. However, there are clear trends that allow us to attempt to forecast likely innovations and changes in the field of thoracic imaging over the next decade.

The most important trend is demonstrating that imaging-based diagnostic and therapeutic approaches are beneficial to patient care, improving morbidity and mortality, and decreasing the overall cost of care. This trend is imposed by the current global economic environment and the mandate to increase the efficiency of healthcare systems by diminishing waste and redundancy and eliminating procedures that do not positively impact patient outcomes. Future clinical trials will emphasize what imaging can offer to empower practitioners to diagnose thoracic diseases earlier, faster, and in a less invasive manner. In addition, studies will address delivery of therapeutic approaches that will be more effective and less costly and contribute to better patient outcomes and quality of life.

Another important trend is combining functional and anatomical information within a single imaging modality. PET/CT already offers this capability by coupling anatomic and metabolic imaging. MR and CT, when performed with 4D cine sequences, may provide insight into chest wall, central airway, and lung mechanics, as well as detect air trapping related to small airway disease. MR performed with specific pulse sequences may provide surrogates of tissue characterization. Thoracic oncology will greatly benefit from new molecular imaging agents that target important cellular and subcellular biochemical pathways associated with carcinogenesis. Furthermore, molecular imaging will allow in vivo real-time assessment of the genetic and epigenetic processes underlying a number of pathologic conditions in the heart, lungs, and mediastinum, leading to more targeted, individualized, and, ultimately, more effective therapeutics.

Quantitative imaging will be another trend, which will aim to provide a much better assessment of disease severity, particularly for diffuse lung diseases, such as COPD and ILD. Instead of simply reporting the presence of a specific disease and, at most, subjectively classifying the severity of the disease, radiologists will utilize computational image analysis tools to provide accurate disease quantification that reflects, and highly correlates with, physiologic metrics. Quantitative imaging utilizing computer-assisted detection and quantification of disease-specific imaging patterns on CT, MR, and PET/CT will, therefore, allow development of biomarkers that will reflect disease prognosis and response to therapies far more accurately and earlier then currently possible. Future drug trials will particularly benefit from this approach.

More distant on the horizon is computer-assisted diagnosis utilizing pattern recognition and classification. Its development will allow radiologists and clinicians to improve diagnostic accuracy, particularly in complex diffuse diseases or in the setting of coexisting diseases.

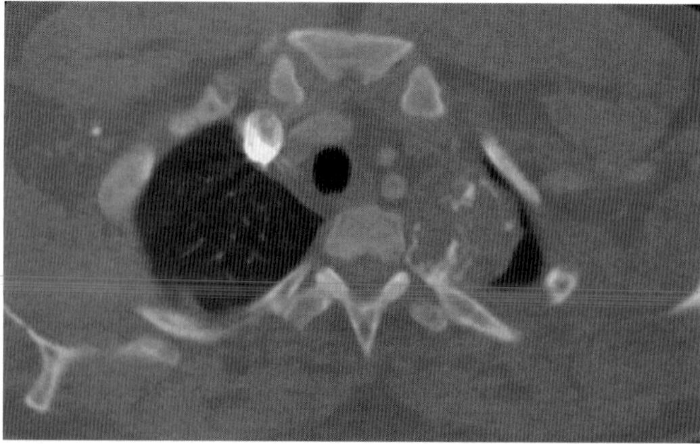

A

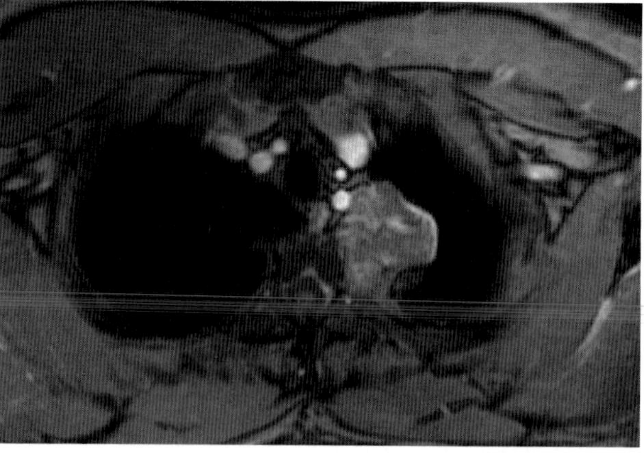

B

Figure 30-69 Posterior mediastinal mass. **A.** Axial noncontrast CT demonstrates a large left posterior mediastinal mass that appears to arise from the left posterior second rib, which demonstrates expansion and cortical destruction. Note irregular calcifications within the mass. **B.** Axial T1-weighted postcontrast MR shows moderate enhancement throughout the lesion. The constellation of findings suggests a primary bone neoplasm with chondroid differentiation. Pathology confirmed a chondrosarcoma.

Finally, it is of interest to consider what role plain chest radiography will play in the future, if any. Practical and economic considerations imply that chest radiographs will not disappear soon, given their low cost, very low radiation dose, universal availability, portability, and capacity to address basic clinical questions. Nevertheless, we hypothesize that this century-old technique will not last another century; rather, it will be replaced in the next decades by newer generations of CT scanners that will offer similar qualities of portability and ultralow radiation dose, along with vastly improved diagnostic accuracy and 4D capabilities.

Irrespective of the many uncertainties, challenges, and exciting prospects for the future, it is undeniable that thoracic imaging will continue to be an indispensable companion to the practicing physician caring for patients with thoracic disorders and a central component of modern pulmonary medicine.

ACKNOWLEDGMENT

The authors dedicate this chapter to the memory of the late Wallace Miller, Sr., MD, who authored the previous version. Dr. Miller was an enlightening presence and a major source of inspiration to generations of thoracic radiologists and pulmonologists.

REFERENCES

1. Schaefer-Prokop C, Neitzel U, Venema HW, Uffmann M, Prokop M. Digital chest radiography: An update on modern technology, dose containment and control of image quality. *Eur Radiol.* 2008;18(9):1818–1830.
2. Bae KT. Optimization of contrast enhancement in thoracic MDCT. *Radiol Clin North Am.* 2010;48(1):9–29.
3. Hamberg LM, Rhea JT, Hunter GJ, Thrall JH. Multi-detector row CT: radiation dose characteristics. *Radiology.* 2003;226(3):762–772.
4. Wallace AB, Goergen SK, Schick D, Soblusky T, Jolley D. Multidetector CT dose: clinical practice improvement strategies from a successful optimization program. *J Am Coll Radiol.* 2010;7(8):614–624.
5. Van Beek EJ, Hoffman EA. Functional imaging: CT and MRI. *Clin Chest Med.* 2008;29(1):195–216.
6. Wielpütz M, Kauczor HU. MRI of the lung: state of the art. *Diagn Interv Radiol.* 2012;18(4):344–353.
7. Mawlawi O, Pan T, Macapinlac HA. PET/CT imaging techniques, considerations, and artifacts. *J Thorac Imaging.* 2006;21(2):99–91.
8. Lal H, Neyaz Z, Nath A, Borah S. CT-guided percutaneous biopsy of intrathoracic lesions. *Korean J Radiol.* 2012;13(2):210–226.
9. Wu CC, Maher MM, Shepard JA. CT-guided percutaneous needle biopsy of the chest: preprocedural evaluation and technique. *AJR Am J Roentgenol.* 2011;196(5):W511–W514.
10. Rodrigo GJ, Rodrigo C, Hall JB. Acute asthma in adults: a review. *Chest.* 2004;125:1081–1102.
11. Silva CI, Colby TV, Müller NL. Asthma and associated conditions: high-resolution CT and pathologic findings. *AJR Am J Roentgenol.* 2004;183:817–824.
12. Thurlbeck WM, Müller NL. Emphysema: definition, imaging, and quantification. *AJR Am J Roentgenol.* 1994;163:1017–1025.
13. Goldin JG. Imaging the lungs in patients with pulmonary emphysema. *J Thorac Imaging.* 2009;24:163–170.
14. Litmanovich D, Boiselle PM, Bankier AA. CT of pulmonary emphysema—current status, challenges, and future directions. *Eur Radiol.* 2009;19:537–551.
15. Madani A, De Maertelaer V, Zanen J, Gevenois PA. Pulmonary emphysema: radiation dose and section thickness at multidetector CT quantification–comparison with macroscopic and microscopic morphometry. *Radiology.* 2007;243:250–257.
16. Mannino DM. COPD: epidemiology, prevalence, morbidity and mortality, and disease heterogeneity. *Chest.* 2002;121:121S–126S.
17. Matsuoka S, Yamashiro T, Washko GR, Kurihara Y, Nakajima Y, Hatabu H. Quantitative CT assessment of chronic obstructive pulmonary disease. *Radiographics.* 2010;30(1):55–66.
18. Barbosa EM Jr, Song G, Tustison N, et al. Computational analysis of thoracic multidetector row HRCT for segmentation and quantification of small airway air trapping and emphysema in obstructive pulmonary disease. *Acad Radiol.* 2011;18(10):1258–1269.
19. Webb WR. Thin-section CT of the secondary pulmonary lobule: anatomy and the image–the 2004 Fleischner lecture. *Radiology.* 2006;239(2):322–338.
20. Hansell DM, Bankier AA, MacMahon H, McLoud TC, Müller NL, Remy J. Fleischner Society: glossary of terms for thoracic imaging. *Radiology.* 2008;246(3):697–722.
21. American Thoracic Society; European Respiratory Society. American Thoracic Society/European Respiratory Society International Multidisciplinary Consensus Classification of the idiopathic interstitial pneumonias. This joint statement of the American Thoracic Society (ATS), and the European Respiratory Society (ERS) was adopted by the ATS board of directors, June 2001 and by the ERS Executive Committee, June 2001. *Am J Respir Crit Care Med.* 2002;165:277–304.
22. Churg A, Müller NL. Cellular vs fibrosing interstitial pneumonias and prognosis: a practical classification of the idiopathic interstitial pneumonias and pathologically/radiologically similar conditions. *Chest.* 2006;130:1566–1570.
23. Kim DS, Collard HR, King TE Jr. Classification and natural history of the idiopathic interstitial pneumonias. *Proc Am Thorac Soc.* 2006;3:285–292.
24. Capobianco J, Grimberg A, Thompson BM, Antunes VB, Jasinowodolinski D, Meirelles GS. Thoracic manifestations of collagen vascular diseases. *Radiographics.* 2012;32(1):33–50.
25. Criado E, Sánchez M, Ramírez J, et al. Pulmonary sarcoidosis: typical and atypical manifestations at high-resolution CT with pathologic correlation. *Radiographics.* 2010;30(6):1567–1586.
26. Silva CI, Müller NL, Lynch DA, et al. Chronic hypersensitivity pneumonitis: Differentiation from idiopathic pulmonary fibrosis and nonspecific interstitial pneumonia by using thin-section CT. *Radiology.* 2008;246:288–297.
27. Mueller-Mang C, Grosse C, Schmid K, Stiebellehner L, Bankier AA. What every radiologist should know about idiopathic interstitial pneumonias. *Radiographics.* 2007;27(3):595–615.
28. Edey AJ, Hansell DM. Incidentally detected small pulmonary nodules on CT. *Clin Radiol.* 2009;64(9):872–884.
29. Khan A. ACR Appropriateness criteria on solitary pulmonary nodule. *J Am Coll Radiol.* 2007;4(3):152–155.
30. MacMahon H, Austin JH, Gamsu G, et al. Guidelines for management of small pulmonary nodules detected on CT scans: a statement from the Fleischner Society. *Radiology.* 2005;237(2):395–400
31. Austin JH. The incidental small pulmonary nodule and the Fleischner criteria 5 years later: have we learned anything more? *J Thorac Imaging.* 2011;26(2):88–89.
32. Naidich DP, Bankier AA, MacMahon H, et al. Recommendations for the management of subsolid pulmonary nodules detected

at CT: a statement from the Fleischner Society. *Radiology.* 2013;266(1):304–317.

33. Travis WD, Brambilla E, Noguchi M, et al. International association for the study of lung cancer/American thoracic society/European respiratory society international multidisciplinary classification of lung adenocarcinoma. *J Thorac Oncol.* 2011;6(2):244–285.
34. Gould MK, Donington J, Lynch WR, et al. Evaluation of individuals with pulmonary nodules: when is it lung cancer? Diagnosis and management of lung cancer, 3rd ed: American College of Chest Physicians evidence-based clinical practice guidelines. *Chest.* 2013;143(5 Suppl):e93S–e120S.
35. Pelosi G. The new taxonomy of lung adenocarcinoma stemming from a multidisciplinary integrated approach: novel pathology concepts and perspectives. *J Thorac Oncol.* 2011;6(2):241–243.
36. Lababede O, Meziane M, Rice T. Seventh edition of the cancer staging manual and stage grouping of lung cancer: quick reference chart and diagrams. *Chest.* 2011;139(1):183–189.
37. UyBico SJ, Wu CC, Suh RD, Le NH, Brown K, Krishnam MS. Lung cancer staging essentials: the new TNM staging system and potential imaging pitfalls. *Radiographics.* 2010; 30(5):1163–1181.
38. The National Lung Screening Trial Research Team, Aberle DR, Adams AM, Berg CD, et al. Reduced lung-cancer mortality with low-dose computed tomographic screening. *N Engl J Med.* 2011;365:395–409.
39. The National Lung Screening Trial Research Team, Church TR, Black WC, Aberle DR, et al. Results of initial low-dose computed tomographic screening for lung cancer. *N Engl J Med.* 2013;368:1980–1991.
40. Nair A, Hansell D. European and North American lung cancer screening experience and implications for pulmonary nodule management. *Eur Radiol.* 2011;21:2445–2454.
41. Boiselle P. Computed tomography screening for lung cancer. *JAMA.* 2013;309(11):1163–1170.
42. Reynolds JH, McDonald G, Alton H, Gordon SB. Pneumonia in the immunocompetent patient. *Br J Radiol.* 2010;83(996): 998–1009.
43. Herold CJ, Sailer JG. Community-acquired and nosocomial pneumonia. *Eur Radiol.* 2004;14(Suppl 3):E2–E20.
44. Lutfiyya MN, Henley E, Chang LF, Reyburn SW. Diagnosis and treatment of community-acquired pneumonia. *Am Fam Physician.* 2006;73:442–450.
45. Sharma S, Maycher B, Eschun G. Radiological imaging in pneumonia: recent innovations. *Curr Opin Pulm Med.* 2007;13:159–169.
46. Washington L, Palacio D. Imaging of bacterial pulmonary infection in the immunocompetent patient. *Semin Roentgenol.* 2007;42:122–145.
47. Ostendorf U, Ewig S, Torres A. Nosocomial pneumonia. *Curr Opin Infect Dis.* 2006;19:327–338.
48. Porzecanski I, Bowton DL. Diagnosis and treatment of ventilator-associated pneumonia. *Chest.* 2006;130:597–604.
49. Heussel CP, Kauczor HU, Ullmann AJ. Pneumonia in neutropenic patients. *Eur Radiol.* 2004;14:256–271.
50. Maki DD. Pulmonary infections in HIV/AIDS. *Semin Roentgenol.* 2002;35:124–139.
51. Oh YW, Effman EL, Godwin JD. Pulmonary infections in immunocompromised hosts: the importance of correlating the conventional radiologic appearance with the clinical setting. *Radiology.* 2000;217:647–656.
52. Harisinghani MG, McLoud TC, Shepard JA, Ko JP, Shroff MM, Mueller PR. Tuberculosis from head to toe. *Radiographics.* 2000;20(2):449–470.
53. Erasmus JJ, McAdams HP, Farrell MA, Patz EF Jr. Pulmonary nontuberculous mycobacterial infection: radiologic manifestations. *Radiographics.* 1999;19(6):1487–1505.
54. Chong S, Lee KS, Yi CA, et al. Pulmonary fungal infection: imaging findings in immunocompetent and immunocompromised patients. *Eur J Radiol.* 2006;59:371–383.
55. Gluecker T, Capasso P, Schnyder P, et al. Clinical and radiologic features of pulmonary edema. *Radiographics.* 1999;19(6):1507–1531; discussion 1532–1533.
56. Ware LB, Matthay MA. Clinical practice: acute pulmonary edema. *N Engl J Med.* 2005;353:2788–2796.
57. Bernard GR. Acute respiratory distress syndrome: a historical perspective. *Am J Respir Crit Care Med.* 2005;172:798–806.
58. Desai SR. Acute respiratory distress syndrome: imaging of the injured lung. *Clin Radiol.* 2002;57:8–17.
59. Fan E, Needham DM, Stewart TE. Ventilatory management of acute lung injury and acute respiratory distress syndrome. *JAMA.* 2005;294:2889–2896.
60. Gattinoni L, Caironi P, Pelosi P, Goodman LR. What has computed tomography taught us about the acute respiratory distress syndrome? *Am J Respir Crit Care Med.* 2001;164:1701–1711.
61. Rubenfeld GD, Caldwell E, Peabody E, et al. Incidence and outcomes of acute lung injury. *N Engl J Med.* 2005;353:1685–1693.
62. Rossi SE, Erasmus JJ, McAdams HP, Sporn TA, Goodman PC. Pulmonary drug toxicity: radiologic and pathologic manifestations. *Radiographics.* 2000;20(5):1245–1259.
63. Mamlouk MD, vanSonnenberg E, Gosalia R, et al. Pulmonary embolism at CT angiography: implications for appropriateness, cost, and radiation exposure in 2003 patients. *Radiology.* 2010;256(2):625–632.
64. Agnell G, Becattini C. Acute pulmonary embolism. *N Engl J Med.* 2010 ;363(3):266–274.
65. Anderson DR, Kahn SR, Rodger MA, et al. Computed tomographic pulmonary angiography vs ventilation-perfusion lung scanning in patients with suspected pulmonary embolism: a randomized controlled trial. *JAMA.* 2007;298:2743–2753.
66. Leung AN, Bull TM, Jaeschke R, et al. An official American Thoracic Society/Society of Thoracic Radiology clinical practice guideline: evaluation of suspected pulmonary embolism in pregnancy. *Am J Respir Crit Care Med.* 2011;184(10):1200–1208.
67. Wood KE. Major pulmonary embolism: review of pathophysiologic approach to the golden hour of hemodynamically significant pulmonary embolism. *Chest.* 2002;121:877–905.
68. Van der Meer RW, Pattynama PM, van Strijen MJ, et al. Right ventricular dysfunction and pulmonary obstruction index at helical CT: prediction of clinical outcome during 3-month follow-up in patients with acute pulmonary embolism. *Radiology.* 2005;235:798–780.
69. Nural MS, Elmali M, Findik S, et al. Computed tomographic pulmonary angiography in the assessment of severity of acute pulmonary embolism and right ventricular dysfunction. *Acta Radiol.* 2009;50:629–637.
70. Araoz PA, Haramati LB, Mayo JR, Barbosa EJ Jr, Rybicki FJ, Colletti PM. Panel discussion: pulmonary embolism imaging and outcomes. *AJR Am J Roentgenol.* 2012;198(6):1313–1319.

71. Ghaye B, Ghuysen A, Bruyere PJ, D'Orio V, Dondelinger RF. Can CT pulmonary angiography allow assessment of severity and prognosis in patients presenting with pulmonary embolism? What the radiologist needs to know. *RadioGraphics.* 2006;26:23–40.

72. Remy-Jardin M, Pistolesi M, Goodman LR, et al. Management of suspected acute pulmonary embolism in the era of CT angiography: a statement from the Fleischner Society. *Radiology.* 2007;245(2):315–329.

73. Tan RT, Kuzo R, Goodman LR, Siegel R, Haasler GB, Presberg KW. Utility of CT scan evaluation for predicting pulmonary hypertension in patients with parenchymal lung disease. *Chest.* 1998;113:1250–1256.

74. Alhamad EH, Al-Boukai AA, Al-Kassimi FA, et al. Prediction of pulmonary hypertension in patients with or without interstitial lung disease: reliability of CT findings. *Radiology.* 2011;260:875–883.

75. Hoey ET, Mirsadraee S, Pepke-Zaba J, Jenkins DP, Gopalan D, Screaton NJ. Dual-energy CT angiography for assessment of regional pulmonary perfusion in patients with chronic thromboembolic pulmonary hypertension: initial experience. *AJR Am J Roentgenol.* 2011;196:524–553.

76. Champion HC, Michelakis ED, Hassoun PM. Comprehensive invasive and non-invasive approach to the right ventricle-pulmonary circulation unit: state of the art and clinical and research implications. *Circulation.* 2009;120:992–1007.

77. Barbosa EJ Jr, Gupta NK, Torigian DA, Gefter WB. Current Role of Imaging in the diagnosis and management of pulmonary hypertension. *AJR Am J Roentgenol.* 2012;198(6):1320–1331.

78. Auger WR, Kim NH, Trow TK. Chronic thromboembolic pulmonary hypertension. *Clin Chest Med.* 2010;31:741–758.

79. Baumann MH, Strange C, Heffner JE, et al. Management of spontaneous pneumothorax: an American College of Chest Physicians Delphi consensus statement. *Chest.* 2001;119:590–602.

80. O'Connor AR, Morgan WE. Radiological review of pneumothorax. *BMJ.* 2005;330(7506):1493–1497.

81. English JC, Leslie KO. Pathology of the pleura. *Clin Chest Med.* 2006;27:157–180.

82. Qureshi NR, Gleeson FV. Imaging of pleural disease. *Clin Chest Med.* 2006;27:193–213.

83. Porcel JM, Light RW. Diagnostic approach to pleural effusion in adults. *Am Fam Physician.* 2006;73:1211–1220.

84. Bonomo L, Feragalli B, Sacco R, Merlino B, Storto ML. Malignant pleural disease. *Eur J Radiol.* 2000;34:98–118.

85. Wang ZJ, Reddy GP, Gotway MB, et al. Malignant pleural mesothelioma: evaluation with CT, MR imaging, and PET. *RadioGraphics.* 2004;24:105–119.

86. Aquino SL. Imaging of metastatic disease to the thorax. *Radiol Clin North Am.* 2005;43:481–495.

87. Gierada DS, Slone RM, Fleishman MJ. Imaging evaluation of the diaphragm. *Chest Surg Clin North Am.* 1998;8:237–280.

88. Eren S, Ciris F. Diaphragmatic hernia: diagnostic approaches with review of the literature. *Eur J Radiol.* 2005;54:448–459.

89. Verhey PT, Gosselin MV, Primack SL, Kraemer AC. Differentiating diaphragmatic paralysis and eventration. *Acad Radiol.* 2007;14:420–425.

90. Gibbs JM, Chandrasekhar CA, Ferguson EC, Oldham SA. Lines and stripes: where did they go?—From conventional radiography to CT. *RadioGraphics.* 2007;27:33–48.

91. Zylak CM, Standen JR, Barnes GR, Zylak CJ. Pneumomediastinum revisited. *RadioGraphics.* 2000;20:1043–1057.

92. Exarhos DN, Malagari K, Tsatalou EG, et al. Acute mediastinitis: spectrum of computed tomography findings. *Eur Radiol.* 2005;15:1569–1574.

93. Weber AL, Randolph G, Aksoy FG. The thyroid and parathyroid glands: CT and MR imaging and correlation with pathology and clinical findings. *Radiol Clin North Am.* 2000;38:1105–1129.

94. Drevelegas A, Palladas P, Scordalaki A. Mediastinal germ cell tumors: a radiologic-pathologic review. *Eur Radiol.* 2001;11:1925–1932.

95. Nishino M, Ashiku SK, Kocher ON, Thurer RL, Boiselle PM, Hatabu H. The thymus: a comprehensive review. *Radiographics.* 2006;26(2):335–348.

96. Sharma A, Fidias P, Hayman LA, Loomis SL, Taber KH, Aquino SL. Patterns of lymphadenopathy in thoracic malignancies. *Radiographics.* 2004;24(2):419–434.

97. Boiselle PM, Patz EF Jr, Vining DJ, Weissleder R, Shepard JA, McLoud TC. Imaging of mediastinal lymph nodes: CT, MR, and FDG PET. *RadioGraphics.* 1998;18:1061–1069.

98. de Langen AJ, Raijmakers P, Riphagen I, Paul MA, Hoekstra OS. The size of mediastinal lymph nodes and its relation with metastatic involvement: a meta-analysis. *Eur J Cardiothorac Surg.* 2006;29:26–29.

99. Korst RJ, Altorki NK. Imaging for esophageal tumors. *Thorac Surg Clin.* 2004;14:61–69.

100. Lee JY, Lee KS, Han J, et al. Spectrum of neurogenic tumors in the thorax: CT and pathologic findings. *J Comput Assist Tomogr.* 1999;23:399–406.

101. Tanaka O, Kiryu T, Hirose Y, Iwata H, Hoshi H. Neurogenic tumors of the mediastinum and chest wall: MR imaging appearance. *J Thorac Imaging.* 2005;20:316–320.

CHAPTER 31

Thoracic Ultrasonography

Lisa Chen
Paul H. Mayo

INTRODUCTION

Thoracic ultrasonography is a readily available, noninvasive imaging method that has proved particularly useful for pulmonary and critical care specialists. The technique is easy to learn and engenders multiple applications related to lung and pleural disease. The ease of use and portability of ultrasonography allows physicians to perform point-of-care imaging and reduce dependence on traditional thoracic imaging techniques, such as chest computerized tomography (CT) and standard radiography (CXR).

This chapter focuses on use of ultrasonography for diagnosis and management of pleural and lung diseases and emphasizes those areas that are of particular interest to the pulmonary specialist. Many elements of thoracic ultrasonography that have utility for the pulmonary consultant are also germane to critical care medicine. However, this chapter focuses on the broad context of pulmonary medicine, rather than the elements of thoracic ultrasonography that are specific to critical care. Furthermore, the chapter is written with the assumption that the pulmonary consultant will personally perform image acquisition, interpret the image, and apply results at the bedside—a paradigm that is different from the standard one of thoracic imaging requiring reliance on a radiologist's acquisition and interpretation of the image. While this approach is advantageous with regard to cost and clinical efficiency, it requires technical and cognitive skills. An additional advantage of clinician-performed, point-of-care thoracic ultrasonography is that it couples imaging results with the clinician's overall knowledge of the case. Indeed, thoracic ultrasonography is not performed in vacuo, rather, it is always combined with other key elements of clinical evaluation, such as the history, physical examination, and laboratory analysis. Ultrasonography is an *additional* tool in the diagnosis and management of pleuropulmonary disease.

TRAINING IN THORACIC ULTRASONOGRAPHY

The goal of training in thoracic ultrasonography is, of course, to enable clinical competence in performing the procedure. "Competence" must be defined to facilitate development of specific learning objectives as the goals of training. One pragmatic approach is to establish a reasonable minimum standard for competence. The Statement of Critical Care Ultrasonography provides a well-defined description of training goals in pleural and lung ultrasonography.[1] The statement is a good starting point for pulmonary specialists who seek training in the field, and the competencies outlined should constitute the initial learning objectives.

No definitive literature is available to guide the optimal duration of training or the minimal number of studies to be performed and interpreted. No widely accepted course of study for the cognitive elements of the field exists, and, at present there is no formal certification process.

Despite these limitations, many clinicians are competent in thoracic ultrasonography. Compared with the training required in the complex fields of cardiac and abdominal ultrasonography, training in thoracic ultrasonography is straightforward. The authors have considerable experience in training many fellows and attending physicians in thoracic ultrasonography and have found that a motivated learner will achieve skill in the basic elements of pleural and lung ultrasonography within several hours of formal teaching. Training should include practicing image acquisition, initially on normal human models and then on patients at the bedside. In addition, training should include a review of a comprehensive image set of normal and abnormal findings, enabling the learner to recognize a wide range of findings during their initial encounter at the bedside. The cognitive elements of the field may be learned through reading chapters or review articles.[2–4] For more advanced training, comprehensive textbooks are available.[5,6] Formal courses on thoracic ultrasonography are offered. In addition, the learner may choose to develop a local training resource, which requires identification of a local expert who is able to help with bedside training.

EQUIPMENT NEEDS

Thoracic ultrasonography may be performed using a wide variety of ultrasound machines. Virtually any machine that is used for or cardiac or abdominal ultrasonography will generally yield adequate image quality. A probe designed for cardiac ultrasonography, employing a frequency range of 3.5 to 5.0 MHz works well, as the small footprint of the probe allows for easy placement between rib interspaces; frequency selection allows for adequate penetration to enable imaging the deeper structures of the thorax. A larger, curvilinear abdominal probe gives serviceable images as well. A linear vascular probe using a frequency range of 7.5 to 10.0 MHz is required for detailed imaging of the pleural surface; the higher frequency improves the resolution, but at the sacrifice of signal penetration.

Every machine has its own design characteristics, so that the operator must adapt machine setup to optimize image quality. What works well using one machine may not translate into the same effectiveness when using another. Some machines have presets for thoracic ultrasonography, but they may not necessarily be the optimal setup for thoracic imaging. Consequently, the operator must be prepared to alter machine settings from standard cardiac, abdominal, or thoracic presets. Machines from the 1990s that lack extensive postimage processing often give excellent results. Modern, high-end cardiac echocardiography machines give excellent cardiac image quality, but they often yield poor near-field images. Many modern portable machines have acceptable thoracic imaging capability and provide the additional advantage that they are designed specifically for point-of-care scanning.

SCANNING TECHNIQUE

For the pulmonary specialist, thoracic ultrasonography may be performed with the patient in a seated position. The supine scanning position is more typical for the critically ill patient, but it has the disadvantage that it is difficult to scan the posterior chest. The standard transducer orientation is the transducer indicator oriented in a cephalad position, defining the primary scanning plane in a longitudinal axis. With the screen indicator placed to the left of the screen, images on the left side of the screen represent cephalad structures.

Machine control is integral to good quality image acquisition; hence, total, near, and far field gains must be adjusted for optimization. Depth should be set to place the target structure in the middle of the screen, and the focal point should be adjusted for optimal image quality of the target structure. Using adequate ultrasound coupling gel and application of firm pressure, the transducer is applied perpendicular to the chest wall and adjusted to examine the rib interspace. Adjacent interspaces are examined by sliding the transducer to the next interspace. In this way, the examiner performs a scan line while the transducer is moved over the chest wall. In an orderly fashion, multiple adjacent scan lines are performed so that the entire chest wall can be imaged. Using this approach, the examiner obtains multiple, two-dimensional, tomographic ultrasound planes of the thorax, in effect, developing a three-dimensional model. If a focal abnormality is identified, the examiner may then perform a more detailed ultrasonographic examination of the area.

Aerated lung blocks ultrasound, whereas the liver and spleen do not. Consequently, to visualize the peridiaphragmatic area, the transducer may be angled such that the scanning plane passes through the liver or spleen to obtain an adequate image window. In addition, bone also blocks ultrasound. So, when an abnormality lies deep to a rib, the transducer may need to be angled to look over or under the rib. Conversely, pleural effusion and consolidated lung each transmit ultrasound. Their presence may yield a window for examination of the heart, mediastinum, or, in the case of pleural effusion, the lung. While the standard scanning plane is longitudinal, a transverse plane may be utilized on occasion. This may be required when examining for a "lung point" or to establish an optimal angle for needle insertion for access to a lung mass. Most thoracic ultrasonography is performed using a cardiac or abdominal transducer. A vascular transducer is preferred if detailed examination of pleural anatomy is required.

PLEURAL ULTRASONOGRAPHY

Ultrasonography is particularly effective for identifying pleural fluid, since fluid is either anechoic or hypoechoic relative to adjacent soft tissue. While physical examination is neither specific nor sensitive for detection of pleural effusion,[7] a pleural effusion as small as 5 cc may be identified with ultrasonography.[8] Pleural ultrasonography is superior to standard chest radiography in identifying pleural effusions and in differentiating a pleural effusion from pleural thickening or atelectasis.[7,9] Compared with chest CT, pleural ultrasound demonstrates 93% sensitivity and specificity for identification of pleural effusion.[10] When a patient has complete hemithoracic opacification on CXR, ultrasound has 95% sensitivity for identification of pleural effusion.[9]

IDENTIFICATION OF PLEURAL FLUID

The pulmonary specialist will generally examine the patient in the seated position. Pleural fluid, unless loculated, distributes by gravitational effect to the most dependent part of the thorax. Therefore, the ultrasonography examination focuses on the lower, dependent area of the posterior thorax.

The examiner seeks to identify three characteristic findings indicating the presence of a pleural effusion: (1) An anechoic or hypoechoic space that is surrounded by typical anatomic boundaries. This space represents the pleural effusion. Diagnosis requires definitive identification of a relatively echo-free space surrounded by the typical anatomic boundaries (Fig. 31-1; Video 31-1). (2) Typical anatomic boundaries. This element requires definitive identification of the chest wall, lung surface, and diaphragm. The heart may form an anatomic boundary on the left side. Recognition of the diaphragm requires definitive identification of the subdiaphragmatic organs (including liver, spleen, and kidneys) (Fig. 31-2; Video 31-2). (3) Dynamic changes typical of a pleural effusion, as described later) (Video 31-3).

Usually, pleural fluid is hypoechoic relative to the liver or spleen. However, complex pleural effusions may demonstrate echogenicity similar to these organs. The chest wall, as a "stationary" structure, does not show dynamic changes with respiration. Lung that is adjacent to, or surrounded by, pleural fluid is compressed by the pleural effusion and, consequently, is airless. The atelectatic lung, which is of tissue density and presents a pattern of alveolar consolidation on ultrasonography examination, is visualized as "floating" in the pleural fluid. It moves in both cardiac- and respiratory-phasic fashion—one of the typical dynamic changes required for identification of pleural effusion. Other typical dynamic changes include those of swirling debris or fibrin strands agitated by respiratory

Video 31-1 Typical anatomic boundaries that surround a hypoechoic pleural effusion: chest wall, surface of lung, and diaphragm. The image was obtained using a 3.5-MHz transducer. The transducer was in longitudinal orientation and placed perpendicular to the chest wall to scan through the seventh intercostal space in the right midaxillary line. *Access at www.fishmansonline.com*

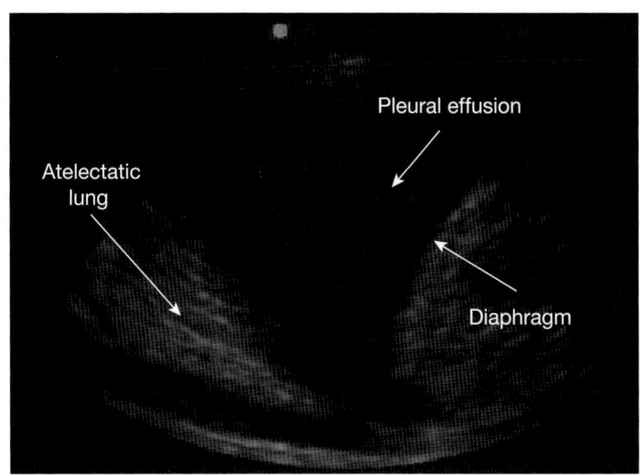

Figure 31-1 Typical anatomic boundaries that surround a hypoechoic pleural effusion. The image was obtained using a 3.5-MHz transducer. The transducer was in longitudinal orientation and placed perpendicular to the chest wall to scan through the seventh intercostal space in the right midaxillary line.

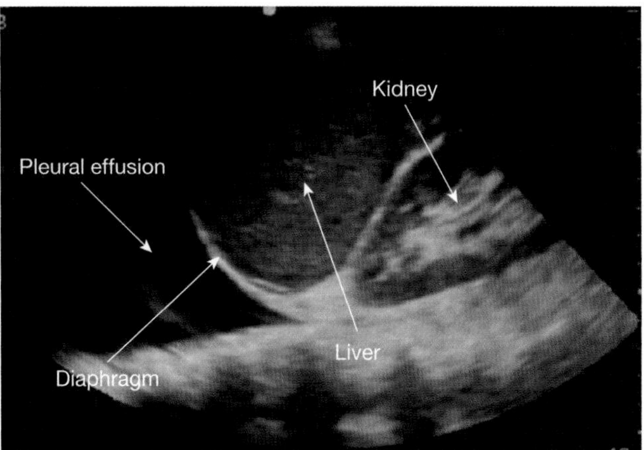

Figure 31-2 Pleural effusion above the diaphragm, liver, hepatorenal space, and kidney. These structures must be positively identified before thoracentesis to avoid inadvertent subdiaphragmatic device insertion. The image was obtained using a 3.5-MHz transducer. The transducer was in longitudinal orientation and placed perpendicular to the chest wall to scan through the eighth intercostal space in the right midaxillary line.

Video 31-2 Pleural effusion above the diaphragm, liver, hepatorenal space, and kidney. These structures must be positively identified before thoracentesis to avoid inadvertent subdiaphragmatic device insertion. The image was obtained using a 3.5-MHz transducer. The transducer was in longitudinal orientation and placed perpendicular to the chest wall to scan through the eighth intercostal space in the right midaxillary line. *Access at www.fishmansonline.com*

or cardiac motion. On occasion, a highly cellular pleural effusion forms a layer because of gravitational effects if the patient is immobile for a period of time; patient movement disrupts the fluid-to-cell interface.

Identification of the diaphragm is imperative for localizing a pleural effusion and enabling safe performance of thoracentesis. Subdiaphragmatic device insertion is a serious complication of thoracentesis.

The diaphragm is a curvilinear structure lying above the spleen and liver, which demonstrates respirophasic movement. The inexperienced operator may mistake the hepatorenal or splenorenal space for the diaphragm, as they appear as curvilinear structures that resemble the diaphragm. The overlying spleen or liver may then be mistaken for an echo-dense pleural effusion. This may result in inadvertent subdiaphragmatic device insertion while attempting a thoracentesis with potentially catastrophic consequence to the patient (Fig. 31-2; Video 31-2). It is helpful to identify the kidney when scanning below the diaphragm to avoid this dangerous pitfall. Identification of the chest wall allows measurement of the depth required for needle penetration when planning thoracentesis. Identification of the underlying lung allows the operator to limit the depth of needle insertion to avoid visceral pleural laceration.

CHARACTERIZATION OF THE PLEURAL EFFUSION

Ultrasound examination can be helpful in distinguishing transudative from exudative effusions. Transudates lack constituents that are ultrasound reflectors and are, therefore, echo-free (anechoic) (Fig. 31-3; Video 31-4). An anechoic pleural effusion is very likely to be transudative, although some may have a complex, nonseptated pattern.[11] Slow flowing movement of ill-defined heterogeneous elements within a hypoechoic effusion, referred to as swirling, may be observed with a transudate, but its presence suggests an exudative cellular effusion, such as that associated with malignancy.[12]

A heterogeneously echogenic pattern, with swirling echoes, septations, fronds, or strands is typically observed with exudates. However, very cellular exudates, such as empyema or hemothorax, may demonstrate homogeneous echogenicity (Fig. 31-4; Video 31-5).[13] Exudates are usually echogenic, but are occasionally anechoic. The presence of strands, debris, or septations is characteristic of a parapneumonic effusion or empyema.[14]

The presence of a septated effusion on ultrasonography suggests the need for fibrinolytic therapy or surgical intervention, prolonged chest tube drainage, and longer hospital stay when compared with effusions lacking ultrasound complexity (Fig. 31-5; Video 31-6).[15] Pleural ultrasound is superior to CT scanning in detecting pleural fluid complexity.[16]

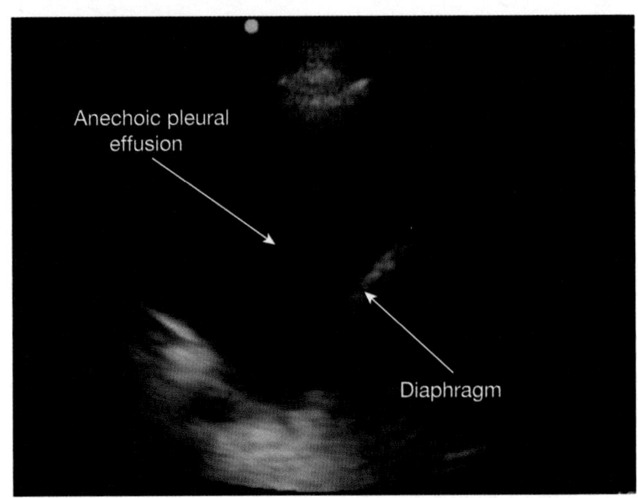

Figure 31-3 Anechoic pleural effusion, likely a transudate. The image was obtained using a 3.5-MHz transducer. The transducer was in longitudinal orientation and placed perpendicular to the chest wall to scan through the sixth intercostal space in the right midaxillary line.

By making a number of defined measurements, the volume of a pleural effusion may be reasonably estimated using ultrasonography.[17] For clinical purposes, it generally suffices to characterize the effusion as small, moderate, or large. Finally, pleural effusions may become loculated collections, which characteristically develop in nondependent positions and fail to move with changes in body position. The loculum may be thick-walled and often has internal hyperechoic complexity.

PERFORMANCE OF THORACENTESIS

Pleural ultrasonography facilitates performance of thoracentesis. When compared with physical examination combined with standard chest radiography, ultrasonography is superior in identifying a safe site for needle insertion.[7] A meta-analysis supports the use of ultrasonography to guide thoracentesis to reduce the risk of pneumothorax.[18] As needle insertion is required not only for simple thoracentesis, but also for a wide variety of pleural procedures requiring use of guidewires and device placement, pleural ultrasonography is an essential component of interventional practice.

Thoracic ultrasonography allows for identification of a safe site, depth, and angle for needle insertion. Using the technique of scan lines described previously, the operator identifies the pleural effusion and establishes the best site and trajectory for needle insertion and, hopefully, avoiding any injury to structures that surround the fluid collection. The site is marked by indenting the skin with a needle cap. Just prior to sterile skin preparation, the operator rescans to confirm site selection, depth of needle penetration required,

Video 31-3 Dynamic findings typical of a pleural effusion, including movement of atelectatic lung, movement of the diaphragm, and movement of echogenic elements within the effusion (plankton sign). The image was obtained using a 3.5-MHz transducer. The transducer was in longitudinal orientation and placed perpendicular to the chest wall to scan through the sixth intercostal space in the right midaxillary line. *Access at www.fishmansonline.com*

Video 31-4 Anechoic pleural effusion, likely a transudate. The image was obtained using a 3.5-MHz transducer. The transducer was in longitudinal orientation and placed perpendicular to the chest wall to scan through the sixth intercostal space in the right midaxillary line. *Access at www.fishmansonline.com*

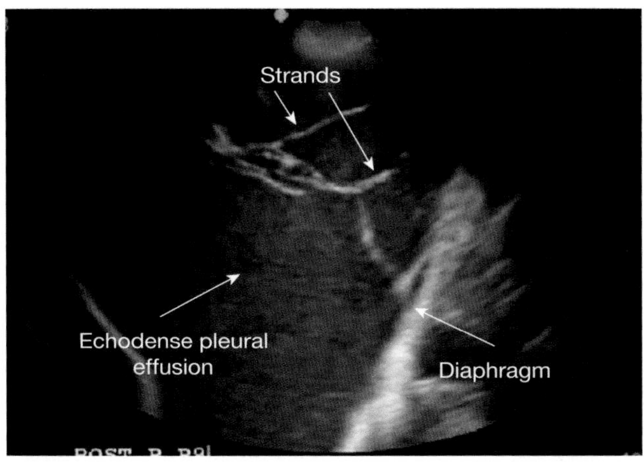

Figure 31-4 Pleural effusion with a homogeneously echogenic pattern and mobile strands suggestive of an exudate. Thoracentesis showed a hemothorax. The image was obtained using a 3.5-MHz transducer. The transducer was in longitudinal orientation and placed perpendicular to the chest wall to scan through the sixth intercostal space in the right midaxillary line.

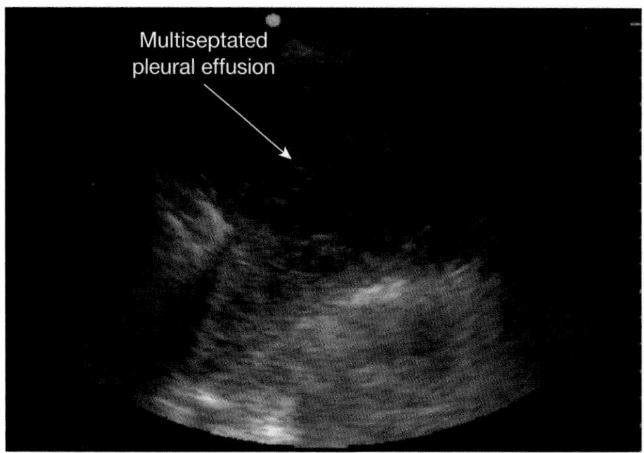

Figure 31-5 Multiseptated pleural effusion. The pattern is consistent with a complex parapneumonic effusion or empyema that will likely require fibrinolytic treatment or surgical drainage. The image was obtained using a 3.5-MHz transducer. The transducer was in longitudinal orientation and placed perpendicular to the chest wall to scan through the fourth intercostal space in the left midaxillary line.

and the angle of insertion. The procedure is then performed using an angle of insertion of the needle and syringe assembly that duplicates the angle of the transducer employed at the time of the final scan. No patient movement is permitted between the final scan and needle insertion, as this may cause movement of the fluid within the thorax.

For the pulmonary specialist, thoracentesis is usually performed with the patient in the seated position. For more complex procedures requiring tunneling of a catheter or chest tube insertion, the patient may be supine or in lateral decubitus position. Using the same scan line technique as utilized for the upright patient, the operator identifies the pleural effusion based on the previously described ultrasound criteria; once again, the site, angle, and depth for safe needle insertion are determined. Immediately before final skin preparation, the operator rescans to confirm that it is a safe site for device insertion and, without patient movement, proceeds with device insertion.

While ultrasonography facilitates pleural access, pitfalls exist. Although pneumothorax is a rare occurrence with ultrasound-assisted thoracentesis, the operator should always check for pneumothorax before and after the procedure by examining the anterior chest for lung sliding (see Lung Ultrasonography). The presence of sliding lung rules out pneumothorax. The most common cause of pneumothorax following ultrasound-assisted thoracentesis is the presence of nonexpandable lung, rather than visceral pleural laceration.[19]

In selecting a site, the operator needs to be aware that the lung may move in a respirophasic fashion. Safe site selection is predicated on the absence of intermittent respirophasic movement of lung into the needle path. When such movement is observed, constituting the so-called "curtain sign," needle insertion is contraindicated at that point.

In performing ultrasound-assisted thoracentesis, several causes may account for failure of fluid return, despite good site selection.

In edematous or obese patients, the operator may press the probe into the skin surface with some force, causing a compression artifact. As the measurement for depth of needle penetration is made when the skin is indented by the probe, if the skin has rebounded, the distance of needle penetration required may be greater than that predicted during initial measurement.

In performing the procedure in patients who lack subcutaneous tissue, the operator may place tension on the skin at the time of mark placement, displacing the skin from the underlying soft tissue. When the tension is released, the mark may rebound to a new position on the chest wall that is not optimal for needle insertion.

While it is not necessary to use real-time needle guidance in performing ultrasound-assisted thoracentesis, failure of needle insertion to yield fluid may warrant rescanning to confirm appropriate site selection. Occasionally, a "dry" tap results from tissue impaction in the needle during insertion or as a result of septations occluding the needle.

PLEURAL PATHOLOGY

In addition to identification of pleural fluid, ultrasonography allows visualization of a variety of pleural pathologies.

A number of pleural diseases cause echogenic abnormalities within the pleural space. Some of these solid pleural abnormalities may coexist with pleural effusions. For example, metastatic pleural disease often occurs with a coexisting pleural effusion, such that the pleural effusion acts as an acoustic window that allows ready observation of the metastatic disease. Metastatic tumors are usually hyperechoic and are often multiple (Fig. 31-6; Video 31-7). They may demonstrate a variety of different sizes and shapes, such as nodular, hemispheric, or circular. The tumors may be broad-based

Video 31-5 Pleural effusion with homogeneous echogenic pattern and mobile strands, suggestive of an exudate. Thoracentesis showed a hemothorax. The image was obtained using a 3.5-MHz transducer. The transducer was in longitudinal orientation and placed perpendicular to the chest wall to scan through the sixth intercostal space in the right midaxillary line. *Access at www.fishmansonline.com*

Video 31-6 Multiseptated pleural effusion. This pattern is consistent with a complex parapneumonic effusion or empyema that will likely require fibrinolytic treatment or surgical drainage. The image was obtained using a 3.5-MHz transducer. The transducer was in longitudinal orientation and placed perpendicular to the chest wall to scan through the fourth intercostal space in the left midaxillary line. *Access at www.fishmansonline.com*

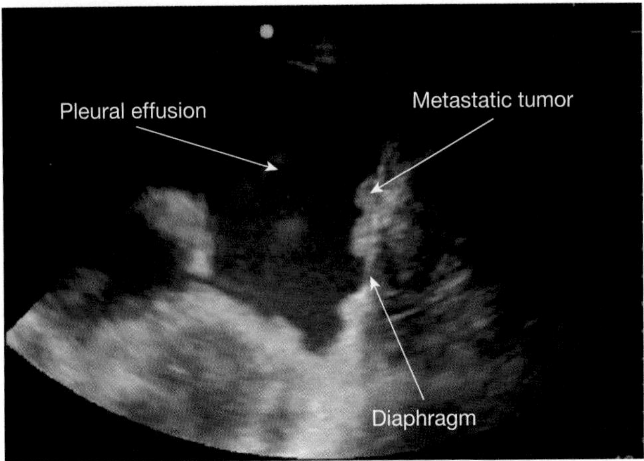

Figure 31-6 Pleural effusion with pleural masses on the diaphragm caused by metastatic breast cancer in the pleural space. The image was obtained using a 3.5-MHz transducer. The transducer was in longitudinal orientation and placed perpendicular to the chest wall to scan through the fifth intercostal space in the left midaxillary line.

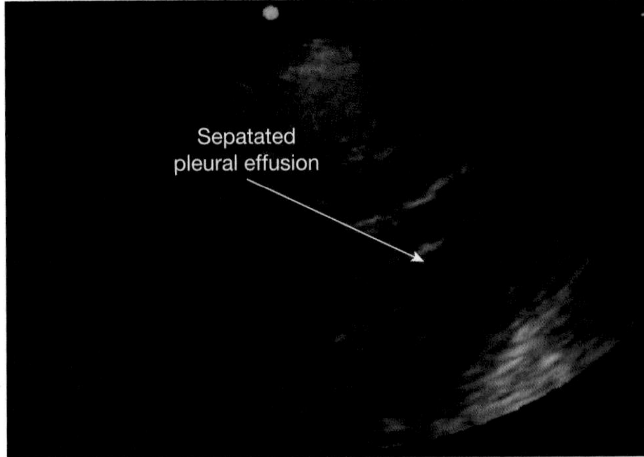

Figure 31-7 Complex, multiloculated pleural effusion with thick septations caused by an empyema. The transducer was in longitudinal orientation and placed perpendicular to the chest wall to scan through the sixth intercostal space in the right midaxillary line.

or have frond-like protrusions. Chest wall or diaphragmatic invasion may cause disruption of normal tissue interfaces and direct extension of tumor into adjacent structures, each of which is visible with ultrasonography. Ultrasonography is superior to chest CT for the diagnosis of transpleural chest wall invasion.[20]

Benign pleural tumors, such as benign mesothelioma, chondroma, lipoma, or thoracic sclerosis are very uncommonly found during pleural ultrasonography. They are usually hyperechoic, have a distinct capsule, and do not demonstrate invasion through adjacent tissue planes. Ultrasonographic morphology is not sufficiently diagnostic, but the technique may be used to guide biopsy.

Primary pleural malignancy, such as malignant mesothelioma, has ultrasonographic features that include pleural thickening with unclear and irregular borders, nodularity, and evidence of chest wall or diaphragmatic invasion.

Inflammatory diseases that involve the pleural space are characteristically caused by infection. Both parietal and visceral pleurae are thickened and hyperechoic, while the underlying lung may demonstrate an alveolar consolidation pattern. Within the pleural fluid collection, linear mobile echogenic elements float freely. Over time, the elements may thicken and divide the effusion into multiple fluid-filled cavities that have variable echogenicity. Eventually, the infected space becomes a multiseptated conglomerate of thick-walled cavities (Fig. 31-7; Video 31-8). A homogeneously echogenic empyema may be so dense that no dynamic findings are discernible within the pleural collection. This makes differentiation from the underlying liver or spleen difficult and may even complicate delineation of the diaphragm, which is a key element in identifying a safe site for device insertion.

Pleural fibrosis shows variable echogenicity, so it may be difficult to differentiate fibrosis from an adjacent pleural effusion. Color-flow Doppler is helpful in distinguishing between the two.[21] Color-flow Doppler signals are generally absent from areas of fibrosis but are present in pleural effusions due to small ultrasound reflectors moving within the fluid.

LUNG ULTRASONOGRAPHY

Lung ultrasonography is performed using the same equipment and scanning techniques as used for pleural ultrasonography. As with pleural ultrasonography, the results are immediately available for integration into the standard tools of patient evaluation, including the history, physical examination, and laboratory analysis. Lung ultrasonography is designed to be used in a goal-directed fashion at the point of care.

In a series of landmark articles, Daniel Lichtenstein described and validated the important elements of the field of lung ultrasonography, the clinical utility of which is now supported by a growing literature. The following discussion is based on Lichtenstein's terminology.[5]

BASIC FINDINGS OF LUNG ULTRASONOGRAPHY

Several basic findings are central to the diagnostic application of ultrasonography to lung diseases. These include lung sliding, lung pulse, A lines, B lines, and consolidation. Each is discussed in subsequent sections.

Lung Sliding

When the transducer is placed perpendicular to the chest wall and orientated to enable imaging through rib interspaces, the pleural line is visualized approximately 5 mm deep to the rib periosteum. Normally, examination of the pleural line demonstrates a shimmering to-and-fro movement that is respirophasic—the so called "lung sliding," which is caused by movement of the visceral pleura against the parietal pleura during breathing (Fig. 31-8; Video 31-9).

The presence of lung sliding indicates that, at that point of examination, no pneumothorax is present; that is, the lung is fully

Video 31-7 Pleural effusion with pleural masses on the diaphragm. The patient had metastatic breast cancer in the pleural space. The image was obtained using a 3.5-MHz transducer. The transducer was in longitudinal orientation and placed perpendicular to the chest wall to scan through the sixth intercostal space in the left midaxillary line. *Access at www.fishmansonline.com*

Video 31-8 Complex multiloculated pleural effusion with thick septations caused by an empyema. The transducer was in longitudinal orientation and placed perpendicular to the chest wall. The examiner moved the transducer over several intercostal spaces to show the extent of the fluid collection. The scan line is in right midaxillary line. *Access at www.fishmansonline.com*

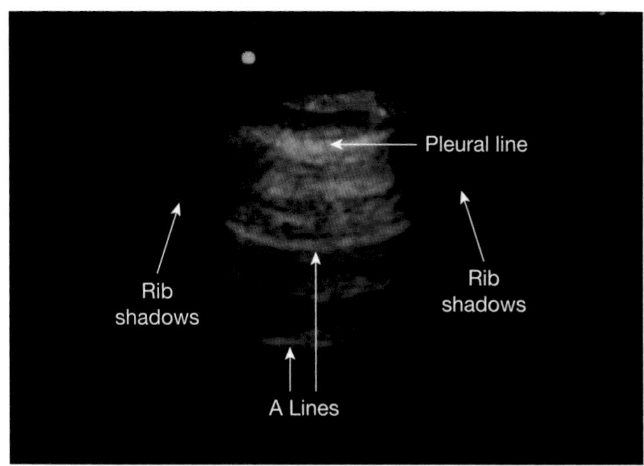

Figure 31-8 Pleural line, A lines, and adjacent rib shadows. The image was obtained using a 3.5-MHz transducer. The transducer was in longitudinal orientation and placed perpendicular to the chest wall to scan through the second intercostal space in the midclavicular line.

Video 31-10 Absence of lung sliding. The image was obtained using a 7.5-MHz vascular transducer. The transducer was in longitudinal orientation and placed perpendicular to the chest wall to scan through the second intercostal space in the midclavicular line. The resolution of the 7.5-MHz transducer is superior to that of the 3.5-MHz transducer, although depth of penetration is reduced (See also Video 78-2). *Access at www.fishmansonline.com*

inflated against the inside of the chest wall.[22] Lung sliding can be detected rapidly over the anterior upper chest by moving the probe over multiple interspaces. Since a loculated pneumothorax is very uncommon, in the supine or upright patient, examination of several anterior interspaces suffices to rule out pneumothorax. Free air in the pleural space rises to the nondependent part of the thorax, unlike fluid, which gravitates to the dependent position. Lung sliding is generally more prominent at the base of the lung as a result of the effect of diaphragmatic movement on lung inflation; lung sliding may be more difficult to detect at the lung apex. To optimize visualization of lung sliding, the ultrasound machine gain should be decreased and depth adjusted to place the pleural line in center of the screen.

A finding related to lung sliding is lung pulse. If a normal subject suspends respiration, lung sliding is temporarily absent; however, cardiophasic movement of the pleural line continues due to the lung movement that derives from transmission of cardiac contraction. The finding of lung pulse has the same implication as lung sliding; when noted, there is no pneumothorax at the site of the examination.

While lung sliding and lung pulse, when present, rule out pneumothorax, their absence is less helpful (Video 31-10). The absence of lung sliding indicates the *possibility* of pneumothorax. Other causes for absence of lung sliding include pleurodesis, apnea, mainstem bronchial obstruction, giant lung bullae, and severe parenchymal lung disease. The absence of lung sliding should be correlated with the clinical context. For example, if a patient demonstrates lung sliding before an ipsilateral thoracentesis or central-line insertion, the absence of lung sliding following the procedure suggests a very high probability of a procedure-related pneumothorax. On the other hand, the patient who has had prior chemical pleurodesis will lack lung sliding upon initial ultrasonographic evaluation.

While the absence of lung sliding is only indicative of the possibility of pneumothorax, it is still feasible to diagnose the disorder using lung ultrasonography, based on identification of a so-called "lung point."[23]

Most pneumothoraces result in only partial collapse of the affected lung; hence, the partially deflated lung is, at some point, still apposed to the chest wall. Under these circumstances, when the transducer is placed into an anterior interspace, no lung sliding will be noted, as the lung is not inflated against the inside of the chest wall. More laterally, lung sliding may become apparent if there is partial collapse of the lung. At the interface between the aerated lung and the pneumothorax space, the lung will be seen to enter the scanning plane in respirophasic manner (Video 31-11). This interface is called the *lung point*. Identification of a lung point is diagnostic of pneumothorax and allows for an estimate of pneumothorax size. While a lung point is 100% specific for pneumothorax, its sensitivity depends on the skill of the examiner; furthermore, a very large pneumothorax will not have a lung point. High-frequency vascular probes are useful in examining for lung point.

A Lines

Once the pleural line has been examined, the depth setting on the machine is increased to examine deeper structures within the thorax. The normal lung reveals *A lines,* which are one or more horizontally orientated lines visible deep to the pleural line (Fig. 31-8; Video 31-9). When multiple, they are equidistant; their separation distance corresponds to the distance between the chest wall and pleural line. A lines are reverberations of the pleural line caused by echoes reflecting off the air just deep to the pleural line, which then reflect off of the probe face. When this reflection returns to the probe, it appears on the screen as an ultrasound interface similar to the pleural line, but twice as far away. A lines may be single or multiple, but they are always separated by the same distance. In the presence of sliding lung, A lines indicate normally aerated lung. When present without lung sliding, they suggest the possibility of a pneumothorax. A lines correlate with a normal aeration pattern seen on a CT scan.[24]

B Lines

Using standard scanning technique and a depth set to visualize deeper structures, B lines may be observed instead of A lines. B lines have several distinct characteristics: (1) They are vertical in orientation; (2) one or more per field may be seen; (3) they extend to bottom of the device screen; (4) they originate at the pleural interface; (5) they move with the pleural interface (if it is mobile); and (6) they efface A lines where A lines and B lines intersect (Fig. 31-9; Video 31-12). The presence of B lines correlates with an interstitial

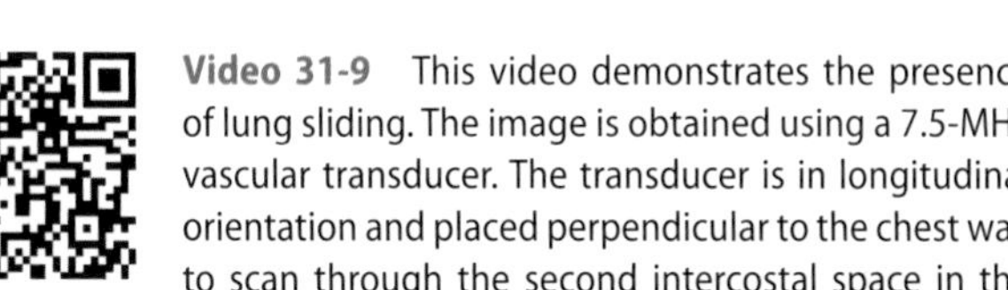

Video 31-9 This video demonstrates the presence of lung sliding. The image is obtained using a 7.5-MHz vascular transducer. The transducer is in longitudinal orientation and placed perpendicular to the chest wall to scan through the second intercostal space in the midclavicular line. The resolution of the 7.5-MHz transducer is superior to that of the 3.5-MHz transducer at the expense of reduced penetration (See also Video 78-1). *Access at www.fishmansonline.com*

Video 31-11 Lung point. A pneumothorax has caused partial deflation of the lung. Respirophasic movement of the partially deflated lung into the pneumothorax space is seen. The image was obtained using a 7.5-MHz vascular transducer. The transducer was in transverse orientation and placed perpendicular to the chest wall to scan through the fifth intercostal space in the right anterior axillary line (See also Video 78-4). *Access at www.fishmansonline.com*

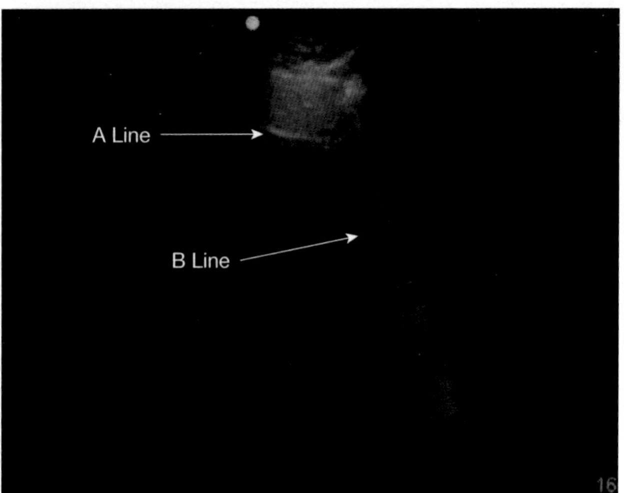

Figure 31-9 B lines. The image was obtained using a 3.5-MHz transducer. The transducer was in longitudinal orientation and placed perpendicular to the chest wall to scan through the second intercostal space in the midclavicular line.

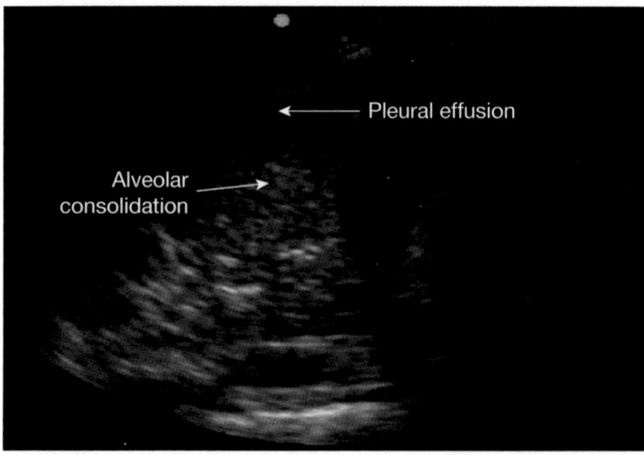

Figure 31-10 Alveolar consolidation of the left lower lobe and pleural effusion. The image was obtained using a 3.5-MHz transducer. The transducer was in longitudinal orientation and placed perpendicular to the chest wall to scan through the sixth intercostal space in the left posterior axillary line.

pattern or alveolar abnormalities noted on CT scanning (reticular pattern or ground glass abnormality).[25]

B lines result from of any interstitial infiltrative process, such as inflammation, neoplasm, fibrosis, or edema.[26–30] B lines may be focal, scattered, or profuse in distribution, based on the underlying disease process. Disorders associated with a granular pattern on standard chest radiography or with ground glass opacification on chest CT are associated with B lines.

As with any radiographic abnormality, clinical correlation is required to determine the cause of B lines. For example, normal individuals often have one or two inconsequential B lines on examination of the lateral lower rib interspaces. More than two B lines in a single field is considered significant. Pneumonia may be manifest with focal B lines detected over the involved lobe or segment. Pulmonary fibrosis results in scattered B lines, whereas cardiogenic pulmonary edema yields profuse bilateral B lines. Pleural morphology may be useful in distinguishing B lines related to elevation of left atrial pressure from those caused by a primary lung process. Typically, the B lines noted in cardiogenic pulmonary edema are associated with a smooth pleural surface, while those seen in primary lung injury manifest an irregular pleural surface.[30] As B lines originate from the area of the visceral pleura, their presence rules out pneumothorax.

Consolidation

Consolidated lung is manifest as tissue density on ultrasound.[31] Its echogenicity is similar to that of the liver (sonographic hepatization of lung) (Fig. 31-10; Video 31-13). Consolidation may be localized to a specific lobe or segment of the lung and may also be observed in the lung periphery as a subpleural consolidation pattern. Within the consolidated lung, punctate, hyperechoic foci are often visible. These foci represent air retained within the bronchi. If they move in respirophasic manner, the finding indicates patency of the bronchus supplying that portion of the lung (Video 31-14).[32] Demonstration of consolidation on lung ultrasonography correlates strongly with results of chest CT scanning.[25]

As with chest radiography and CT scanning, the finding of alveolar consolidation on lung ultrasonography is not diagnostic. While pneumonia may result in alveolar consolidation, so will atelectasis (compressive, resorptive, or cicatricial). Severe pulmonary edema, with complete filling of the alveolar compartment, and infiltrative processes, such as tumor, may result in the ultrasonographic finding of lung consolidation. While lung ultrasonography identifies consolidation, the pulmonary specialist determines its cause.

■ ADVANCED LUNG ULTRASONOGRAPHY

A wide variety of additional lung ultrasound findings have been described. Mastery of the basic findings is the first step of training for the pulmonary specialist. The reader is referred to standard texts for a complete review of the subject.[5]

■ LIMITATIONS OF LUNG ULTRASONOGRAPHY

Any disease process resulting in focal abnormality surrounded by aerated lung, for example, a solitary pulmonary nodule with normal surrounding lung, will not be visible with ultrasonography. Similarly, mediastinal structures are not visible using surface ultrasonography unless there is a convenient acoustic window related to lung consolidation or pleural effusion.

Documentation of the results of lung ultrasonography is challenging compared with CXR and chest CT scanning, in which results can be stored indefinitely in a durable format and serial studies compared. While a written report of lung ultrasonography is important and can be generated in a durable format, comparison of serial studies is difficult.

Video 31-12 B lines. The image was obtained using a 3.5-MHz transducer. The transducer was in longitudinal orientation and placed perpendicular to the chest wall to scan through the second intercostal space in the midclavicular line (See also Video 78-5). *Access at www.fishmansonline.com*

Video 31-13 Alveolar consolidation of the left lower lobe and pleural effusion. The image was obtained using a 3.5-MHz transducer. The transducer was in longitudinal orientation and placed perpendicular to the chest wall to scan through the sixth intercostal space in the left posterior axillary line. *Access at www.fishmansonline.com*

Video 31-14 Mobile air bronchograms in an area of alveolar consolidation. The gain was turned down to bring out the punctate hyperechoic mobile foci that have respirophasic movement. The foci represent air within the bronchi surrounded by alveolar consolidation. The image was obtained using a 3.5-MHz transducer. The transducer was in longitudinal orientation and placed perpendicular to the chest wall to scan through the sixth intercostal space in the right midaxillary line. *Access at www.fishmansonline.com*

CLINICAL APPLICATIONS

With development of high-quality, portable ultrasound machines, it is now feasible to integrate lung ultrasonography into both hospital- and office-based pulmonary practice. Ultrasonography will never completely replace CXR or chest CT, and it should be viewed as a complementary imaging modality. Its utility has been well characterized for critical care applications, and it is being increasingly utilized in pulmonary medicine.

PROCEDURES

In addition to its utility in performing pleural procedures, ultrasonography may be used to guide other transthoracic interventions. For example, thoracic ultrasonography is useful in localizing masses abutting the pleural surface. As noted previously, although a lung mass that is entirely surrounded by aerated lung is not visible with ultrasonography, if part of the mass abuts the pleural surface, it may be visualized, and its size and pattern of echogenicity characterized (Fig. 31-11; Video 31-15). While lung ultrasonography has limited utility in establishing etiology of masses, localization of the abnormality and delineation of a safe path for needle insertion may be helpful. Furthermore, ultrasonography may be used as an alternative to CT to guide transthoracic needle insertion.[33]

Pneumothorax is a complication of a variety of pulmonary procedures, including bronchoscopy, thoracentesis, and transthoracic needle insertion. Ultrasonography is superior to CXR in the detection of pneumothorax and can be used in place of radiography for postprocedure evaluation.[34,35]

Following pleural drain insertion, ultrasound may be useful in determining whether the lung is expanded. In addition, ultrasound may assist in determination of when to remove the chest drain following tube clamping and may be used to rapidly ascertain whether there is continued leakage of air into the pleural space.[36]

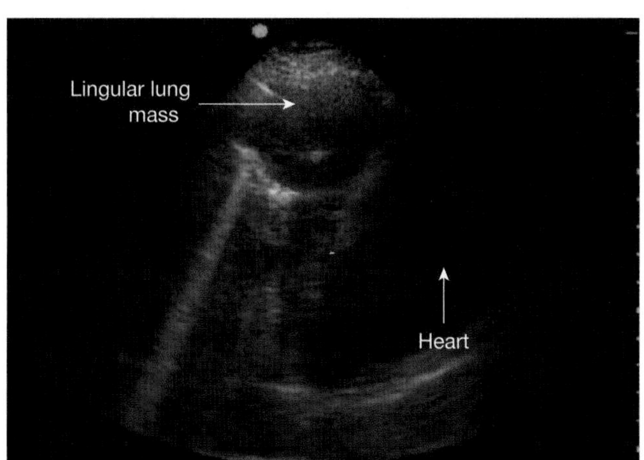

Figure 31-11 Lingular lung mass adjacent to the chest wall and heart. The image was obtained using a 3.5-MHz transducer. The transducer was in longitudinal orientation and placed perpendicular to the chest wall to scan through the fifth intercostal space in the left anterior axillary line.

Video 31-15 Lingular lung mass adjacent to the chest wall and heart. The image was obtained using a 3.5-MHz transducer. The transducer was in longitudinal orientation and placed perpendicular to the chest wall to scan through the fifth intercostal space in the left anterior axillary line. *Access at www.fishmansonline.com*

ASSESSMENT OF DIAPHRAGMATIC FUNCTION

Thoracic ultrasonography is useful in assessing diaphragmatic function.[37] The diaphragm is easy to identify with ultrasonography, and characteristics of diaphragmatic function, such as velocity, force, and amplitude of contraction can be readily assessed.

DIAGNOSIS OF SPECIFIC DISEASES

Lung ultrasonography is useful for the diagnosis and follow-up of community-acquired pneumonia.[38] It also has utility in the diagnosis of pulmonary embolism.[39,40] Thoracic ultrasonography may be useful in the evaluation of dyspnea in the critical care setting and may be helpful in assessing dyspnea in less acute settings.[30,41]

REDUCTION IN USE OF CHEST RADIOGRAPHY AND CHEST CT SCANNING

Thoracic ultrasonography has been compared with both CXR and chest CT scanning. For many indications, it is superior to CXR and similar to chest CT.[24,42,43]

CONCLUSION

Thoracic ultrasonography is a useful imaging modality for the pulmonary consultant. Thoracic ultrasonography is easy to learn and has multiple applications as a point-of-care tool. The technique may allow the pulmonary consultant to reduce the use of CXR and chest CT while providing information of immediate clinical relevance.

REFERENCES

1. Mayo PH, Beaulieu Y, Doelken P, et al. American college of chest physicians/la société de réanimation de langue française statement on competence in critical care ultrasonography. *Chest*. 2009;135:1050–1060.
2. Mayo PH. Ultrasound evaluation of the lung. In: Levitov AB, Mayo PH, Slonim AD, eds. *Critical Care Ultrasonography*. New York, NY: McGraw Hill; 2009: 251–258.
3. Koenig SJ, Narasimhan M, Mayo PH. Thoracic ultrasonography for the pulmonary specialist. *Chest*. 2011;140:1332–1341.
4. Mayo PH, Doelken P. Pleural ultrasonography. *Clin Chest Med*. 2006;27:215–227.
5. Lichtenstein DA. *Whole Body Ultrasonography in the Critically Ill*. Berlin, Germany: Springer-Verlag; 2010:117–208.
6. Mathis G. *Chest Sonography*. Berlin, Germany: Springer-Verlag; 2011.
7. Diacon AH, Brutsche MH, Soler M. Accuracy of pleural puncture site: a prospective comparison of clinical examination with ultrasound. *Chest*. 2003;123:436–441.
8. Gryminski J, Krakowka P, Lypaceqicq G. The diagnosis of pleural effusion by ultrasonic and radiologic techniques. *Chest*. 1976;70:33–37.
9. Kelbel C, Borner N, Schadmand S, et al. Diagnosis of pleural effusions and atelectasis: sonography and radiology compared. *Rofo*. 1991;154:159–163.
10. Lichtenstein D, Goldstein I, Mourgeon E, et al. Comparative diagnostic performances of auscultation, chest radiography, and

lung ultrasonography in acute respiratory distress syndrome. *Anesthesiology*. 2004;100:9–15.

11. Chen HJ, Tu CY, Ling SJ. Sonographic appearances in transudative pleural effusions: not always an anechoic pattern. *Ultrasound Med Biol*. 2008;34:362–369.
12. Chian CF, Su WL, Soh LH, et al. Echogenic swirling pattern as a predictor of malignant pleural effusions in patients with malignancies. *Chest*. 2004;126:129–134.
13. Yang PC, Luh KT, Chang DB, et al. Value of sonography in determining the nature of pleural effusion: analysis of 320 cases. *AJR Am J Roentgenol*. 1992;159:29–33.
14. Tu CY, Hsu WH, Hsia TC, et al. Pleural effusions in febrile medical ICU patients chest ultrasound study. *Chest*. 2004;126:1274–1280.
15. Chen KY, Liaw YS, Wang HC, Luh KT, Yang PC. Sonographic septation: a useful prognostic indicator of acute thoracic empyema. *JIUM*. 2000;19:837–843.
16. McLoud TC, Flower CD. Imaging the pleura: sonography, CT, and MR imaging. *AJR Am J Roentgenol*. 1991;156:1145–1153.
17. Vignon P, Chastagner C, Berkane V, et al. Quantitative assessment of pleural effusion in critically ill patients by means of ultrasonography. *Crit Care Med*. 2005;33(8):1757–1763.
18. Gordon CE, Feller-Kopman D, Balk EM, Smetana GW. Pneumothorax following thoracentesis: a systematic review and meta-analysis. *Arch Intern Med*. 2010;170:332–339.
19. Heidecker J, Huggins JT, Sahn SA, Doelken P. Pathophysiology of pneumothorax following ultrasound-guided thoracentesis. *Chest*. 2006;130:1173–1184.
20. Bandi V, Lunn W, Ernst A, Eberhardt R, Hoffmann H, Herth FJ. Ultrasound vs. CT in detecting chest wall invasion by tumor: a prospective study. *Chest*. 2008;133:881–886.
21. Wu RG, Yuan A, Liaw YS, et al. Image comparison of real-time gray-scale ultrasound and color Doppler ultrasound for use in diagnosis of minimal pleural effusion. *Am J Respir Crit Care Med*. 1994;150:510–514.
22. Lichtenstein DA, Menu Y. A bedside ultrasound sign ruling out pneumothorax in the critically ill. Lung sliding. *Chest*. 1995;108: 1345–1348.
23. Lichtenstein D, Mezière G, Biderman P, Gepner A. The "lung point": an ultrasound sign specific to pneumothorax. *Intensive Care Med*. 2000;26:1434–1440.
24. Lichtenstein D, Goldstein I, Mourgeon E, Cluzel P, Grenier P, Rouby JJ. Comparative diagnostic performances of auscultation, chest radiography, and lung ultrasonography in acute respiratory distress syndrome. *Anesthesiology*. 2004;100:9–15.
25. Lichtenstein D, Mezière G. A lung ultrasound sign allowing bedside distinction between pulmonary edema and COPD: the comet-tail artifact. *Intensive Care Med*. 1998;24:1331–1334.
26. Lichtenstein D, Mézière G, Biderman P, Gepner A, Barré O. The comet-tail artifact. An ultrasound sign of alveolar-interstitial syndrome. *Am J Respir Crit Care Med*. 1997;156:1640–1646.
27. Agricola E, Bove T, Oppizzi M, et al. "Ultrasound comet-tail images": a marker of pulmonary edema: a comparative study with wedge pressure and extravascular lung water. *Chest*. 2005;127: 1690–1695.
28. Agricola E, Picano E, Oppizzi M, et al. Assessment of stress-induced pulmonary interstitial edema by chest ultrasound during exercise echocardiography and its correlation with left ventricular function. *J Am Soc Echocardiogr*. 2006;19: 457–463.
29. Jambrik Z, Monti S, Coppola V, et al. Usefulness of ultrasound lung comets as a nonradiologic sign of extravascular lung water. *Am J Cardiol*. 2004;93:1265–1270.
30. Copetti R, Soldati G, Copetti P. Chest sonography: a useful tool to differentiate acute cardiogenic pulmonary edema from acute respiratory distress syndrome. *Cardiovasc Ultrasound*. 2008; 6:1–10.
31. Lichtenstein DA, Lascols N, Mezière G, Gepner A. Ultra-sound diagnosis of alveolar consolidation in the critically ill. *Intensive Care Med*. 2004;30:276–281.
32. Lichtenstein D, Mezière G, Seitz J. The dynamic air bronchogram. A lung ultrasound sign of alveolar consolidation ruling out atelectasis. *Chest*. 2009;135:1421–1425.
33. Sheth S, Hamper UM, Stanley DB, Wheeler JH, Smith PA. US guidance for thoracic biopsy: a valuable alternative to CT. *Radiology*. 1999;210:721–726.
34. Kreuter M, Eberhardt R, Wenz H, Schmitteckert H, Heussel CP, Herth F. Diagnostic value of transthoracic ultrasound compared to chest radiography in the detection of a post-interventional pneumothorax. *Ultraschall Med*. 2011;32(Suppl 2):E20–E23.
35. Lichtenstein DA, Mezière G, Lascols N, et al. Ultra-sound diagnosis of occult pneumothorax. *Crit Care Med*. 2005;33:1231–1238.
36. Galbois A, Ait-Oufella H, Baudel JL, et al. Pleural ultrasound compared with chest radiographic detection of pneumothorax resolution after drainage. *Chest*. 2010;138:648–655.
37. Matamis D, Soilemezi E, Tsagourias M, et al. Sonographic evaluation of the diaphragm in critically ill patients. Technique and clinical applications. *Intensive Care Med*. 2013;39:801–810.
38. Reissig A, Copetti R, Mathis G, et al. Lung ultrasound in the diagnosis and follow-up of community-acquired pneumonia: a prospective, multicenter, diagnostic accuracy study. *Chest*. 2012;142: 965–972.
39. Pfeil A, Reissig A, Heyne JP, et al. Transthoracic sonography in comparison to multislice computed tomography in detection of peripheral pulmonary embolism. *Lung*. 2010;188:43–50.
40. Mathis G, Blank W, Reissig A, Lechleitner P, Reuss J, Schuler A, Beckh S. Thoracic ultrasound for diagnosing pulmonary embolism: a prospective multicenter study of 352 patients. *Chest*. 2005;128:1531–1538.
41. Lichtenstein DA, Meziere GA. Relevance of lung ultrasound in the diagnosis of acute respiratory failure. *Crit Care Med*. 2008;134: 117–125.
42. Zanobetti M, Poggioni C, Pini R. Can chest ultrasonography replace standard chest radiography for evaluation of acute dyspnea in the ed? *Chest*. 2011;139:1140–1147.
43. Xirouchaki N, Magkanas E, Vaporidi K, et al. Lung ultrasound in critically ill patients: comparison with bedside chest radiography. *Intensive Care Med*. 2011;37:1488–1493.

CHAPTER 32

Physiologic and Metabolic Study of Pulmonary Disorders Using Conventional Imaging Techniques and Positron Emission Tomography

Ghassan El-Haddad
Søren Hess
Daniel Worsley
Abass Alavi

INTRODUCTION

Since the mid-1950s, the use of radiopharmaceuticals has made it possible to assess a variety of pulmonary disorders. In 1955, ^{133}Xe was introduced for the study of regional pulmonary ventilation.[1] Shortly thereafter, it became possible to evaluate regional pulmonary blood flow using inhaled carbon dioxide containing radioactive $^{15}O_2$ or intravenous injection of ^{133}Xe dissolved in saline solution.[3] In 1964, intravenous injection of ^{131}I-macroaggregated albumin made it feasible to obtain perfusion scans of the lungs.[4] Although these techniques rapidly gained wide acceptance as tests of regional abnormalities in ventilation and pulmonary blood flow, the main practical application has been in the diagnostic evaluation of patients with suspected pulmonary embolism (PE). Increasingly, the role of nuclear medicine in respiratory medicine has been expanded to include disorders such as preoperative assessment of lung function, inflammatory lung disease, and lung cancer. The more widespread availability of positron emission tomography (PET) and integrated PET/CT (computed tomography) has provided powerful tools to aid in the diagnosis, staging, and management of patients with lung cancer.

RADIOPHARMACEUTICALS AND TECHNIQUES IN VENTILATION–PERFUSION LUNG SCANNING

Radiopharmaceuticals commonly utilized in both perfusion and ventilation studies, as well as the techniques employed are discussed in subsequent sections.

■ PERFUSION AGENTS AND TECHNIQUES

Clinical application of perfusion lung scanning was first described in 1964, when iodine 131–labeled macroaggregates of albumin was utilized in the evaluation of pulmonary perfusion.[4] Currently, the two agents used for pulmonary perfusion imaging are technetium 99m–labeled human albumin microspheres (^{99m}Tc HAM) and macroaggregated albumin (^{99m}Tc MAA). ^{99m}Tc MAA particles range in size from 10 to 150 μm; more than 90% of injected particles measure between 10 and 90 μm. ^{99m}Tc HAM particles are relatively uniform in size and range between 35 and 60 μm. However, ^{99m}Tc MAA is considered the agent of choice for routine perfusion lung scanning because of its availability, short residence time in the lungs, and relatively low cost.

Radiolabeled particles are injected intravenously while the patient is in the supine position, thereby limiting the effect of gravity on regional pulmonary arterial blood flow. Following the administration of ^{99m}Tc MAA, particles mix uniformly with venous blood flowing to the heart; the particles lodge in precapillary arterioles of the lungs, obstructing approximately 0.1% of their total number. The usual administered dose of radioactivity is between 74 and 185 MBq (2–5 mCi) (typically, 200,000 to 500,000 particles are injected during clinical perfusion scan). The usual pediatric-administered activity is 0.5 to 2.0 MBq/kg (20–80 mCi/kg), with a minimum of 7 to 8 MBq (approximately 200 mCi).

The blockage of pulmonary precapillary arterioles by ^{99m}Tc MAA is transient; the biologic half-life in the lung ranges between 2 and 8 hours. The physical half-life of ^{99m}Tc is 6 hours. The MAA particles are cleared by enzymatic hydrolysis, forming smaller particles that are phagocytized by reticuloendothelial cells. In pediatric patients and patients with suspected or known right-to-left shunts, severe pulmonary hypertension, poor respiratory function, pregnancy, prior pneumonectomy, or a single lung transplant, the number of particles injected should be reduced. In infants and children, the use of low number of particles can be calculated based on weight.[5] The distribution of particles in the lungs is proportional to regional pulmonary blood flow at the time of injection.[6] A routine perfusion scan should include at least six views of the lungs: Anterior, posterior, right and left lateral, and right and left posterior oblique views, using large field of view high-resolution gamma camera. Right and left anterior oblique views may be helpful in selected cases. In spite of imaging in multiple projections, the perfusion scan may underestimate perfusion abnormalities. A solitary segmental perfusion defect within the medial basal segment of the right lower lobe is completely surrounded by normal lung. Consequently, a perfusion defect in this segment will not be detected on planar perfusion imaging.

Perfusion lung scans are routinely utilized to examine patients with suspected PE. Unfortunately, perfusion imaging is sensitive, but not specific, for diagnosing PE. Virtually all lung diseases (including tumors, infections, asthma, and chronic obstructive pulmonary disease [COPD]) may cause decreased pulmonary arterial blood flow in the affected lung zones. Therefore, combined use of perfusion and ventilation studies improves the diagnostic specificity of lung scanning for PE (Fig. 32-1). PE almost always causes abnormal perfusion, while ventilation is preserved (mismatched defects) (Fig. 32-2). In contrast, in parenchymal pulmonary disorders, decreased ventilation and perfusion are noted in the same lung region (matched defects). Conditions in which the ventilation abnormality may appear larger than the perfusion abnormality (reverse mismatch), indicating a functional right-to-left shunt, include airway obstruction, mucus plug, atelectasis, and pneumonia.[7] Reverse mismatch may be exacerbated in patients on positive end-expiratory pressure (PEEP)[8] as PEEP is less efficiently transmitted to obstructed, well-perfused areas, in patients with metabolic alkalosis,[9] or in patients treated with inhaled albuterol.

■ VENTILATION AGENTS AND TECHNIQUES

Historically, ^{133}Xe has been the agent used to determine regional ventilation.[1,10] ^{133}Xe has a physical half-life of 5.24 days and a low gamma energy emission of 81 keV compared to 140 keV for ^{99m}Tc. The examination is somewhat laborious and encompasses three phases. Thus, other tracers, such as ^{81m}Kr, and, the ^{99m}Tc-labeled aerosols – Technegas and Pertechnegas – are now replacing it.

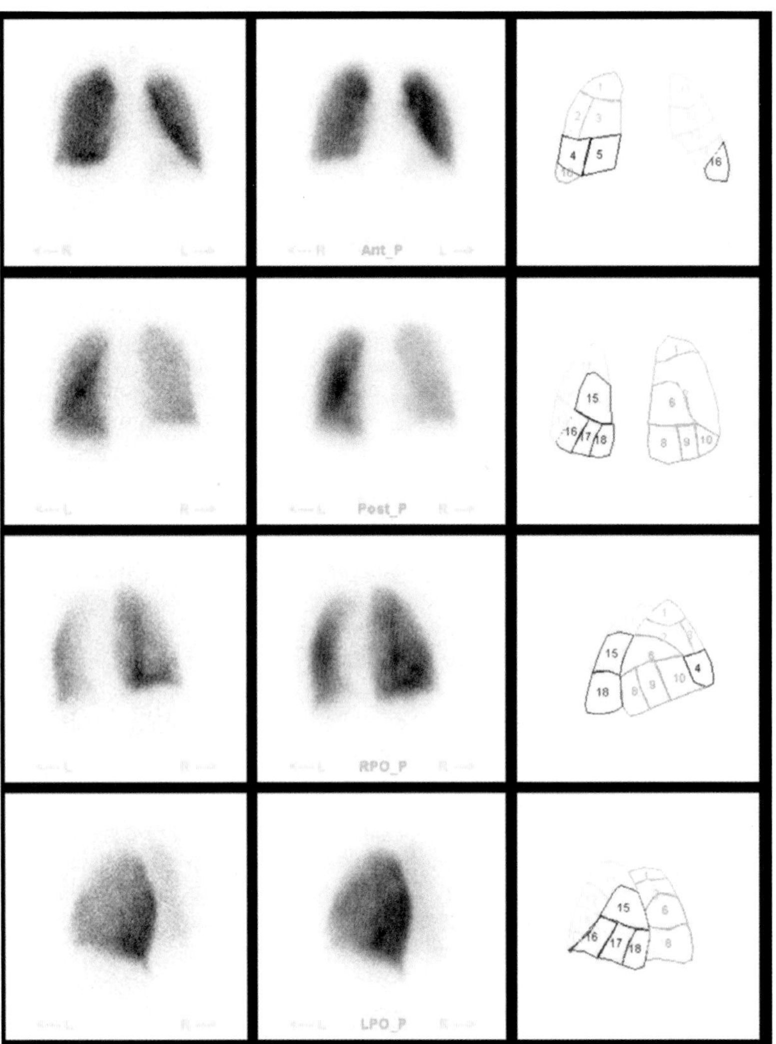

Figure 32-1 Normal ventilation–perfusion lung scanning. Ventilation scan using ^{99m}Tc Technegas® aerosol *(left column)*: Uniform distribution of the aerosol throughout both lungs. Perfusion scan using ^{99m}Tc MAA *(middle column)*: Uniform distribution of particles throughout both lungs.

^{81m}Kr is a noble gas that has a very short physical half-life (13 seconds). Therefore, images acquired using this agent reveal ventilation to major airway systems only. However, the short physical half-life of ^{81m}Kr allows generation of lung images in multiple projections that can be matched with perfusion images. ^{81m}Kr is produced from a rubidium-81 generator. The parent radionuclide has a physical half-life of 4.7 hours, which limits the useful lifetime of the generator to only 1 day. Imaging with ^{81m}Kr is generally performed following the perfusion scan due to its higher energy than ^{99m}Tc.

A radioaerosol is produced by nebulizing the radiopharmaceutical into a fine mist, which is subsequently inhaled. ^{99m}Tc-labeled aerosol studies can be performed following the inhalation of several preparations; ^{99m}Tc DTPA (diethylene triamine penta-acetic acid) is the most popular and commonly used worldwide. The advantages of ^{99m}Tc aerosols are that they are widely available, inexpensive, and have a 140-keV energy photopeak, which is ideal for gamma camera imaging. One limitation of this agent is its relatively rapid absorption across the pulmonary capillaries into the blood in the presence of inflammation, including that caused by smoking (typical ^{99m}Tc DTPA aerosol biologic half-life is about 80 minutes compared to ~20 to 30 minutes in smokers).[11,12] Since ^{99m}Tc DTPA aerosol is cleared from the alveoli by transepithelial diffusion, the clearance rate may be used as an index of alveolar–epithelial membrane integrity.[11]

^{99m}Tc-labeled radioaerosols have particles between 0.5 and 2 μm in size and are produced by utilizing commercially available nebulizers.[13] The patient generally breathes from the nebulizer (with oxygen at 8 to 10 L/min) for 3 to 5 minutes or until 37 MBq (1 mCi) of radioactivity is deposited in the lungs. Only 2% to 10% of administered radioactivity goes to the lungs. The regional distribution of radioactivity in the lungs is proportional to local ventilation. ^{99m}Tc-labeled radioaerosol studies are generally performed before perfusion imaging. Although less preferred, the ventilation study can be performed following the perfusion scan, but the dose placed in the nebulizer should be increased to at least 1665 MBq (45 mCi), instead of the usually used 1110 MBq (30 mCi) to overwhelm the activity present in the lungs from ^{99m}Tc MAA.

The lungs are imaged in multiple projections, which correspond to those obtained during the subsequent perfusion study. Ventilation studies using ^{99m}Tc-labeled radioaerosols require minimal patient cooperation and can be performed at the bedside and on patients who are on ventilators. Disadvantages of ^{99m}Tc-labeled radioaerosols include the central deposition of radioactivity in patients on PEEP, patients with COPD or airway obstruction, and the need to dispose of the substantial unused amount of radioactivity that is deposited in the nebulizer. Indeed, the central deposition of ^{99m}Tc-labeled radioaerosol in patients with COPD is a major drawback to the use of aerosol agents, and newer agents have been developed to overcome this deficiency, including ^{99m}Tc Technegas and ^{99m}Tc Pertechnegas.[14]

LUNG SCANNING IN THE DIAGNOSIS OF ACUTE PULMONARY EMBOLISM

PE is a common and potentially fatal disorder for which treatment is highly effective in decreasing mortality and morbidity if initiated soon after the event.[15] The accurate and expeditious diagnosis of acute PE can be difficult because of the nonspecificity of clinical, laboratory, and radiographic findings. Despite diagnostic advances, delays in diagnosis of PE are still common and represent an important clinical issue.[16]

Venous thromboembolism (VTE) and PE are no longer considered a one-time only event, as they have a high recurrence and mortality rate.[17] Although the incidence of PE has not significantly changed over the past three decades,[18] the overall mortality rate from PE has decreased substantially (by roughly 30% from 1998 to 2009),[19] which has been attributed to better detection and treatment of deep venous thrombosis (DVT), risk factor modification, and improvement in PE diagnostic tests.[19–21] Although prompt anticoagulation therapy remains the cornerstone of PE treatment, as it is effective and reduces mortality, it is not without risks, including hemorrhagic complications.[22] Therefore, accurate diagnosis of PE is essential, not only to prevent death from recurrent embolism but also to avoid complications related to unnecessary anticoagulant therapy.

Ventilation–perfusion (V/Q) lung imaging has been shown to be a safe, noninvasive technique in evaluating regional pulmonary function undertaken for a variety of purposes. The technique has been widely used in the assessment of patients with suspected PE.

The first major study that utilized perfusion lung scanning as a screening test for the diagnosis of PE was the Urokinase Pulmonary Embolism Trial (UPET).[23] In more than 90% of patients enrolled in the trial, perfusion lung scanning was performed following intravenous administration of ^{131}I-labeled MAA. Lung imaging was

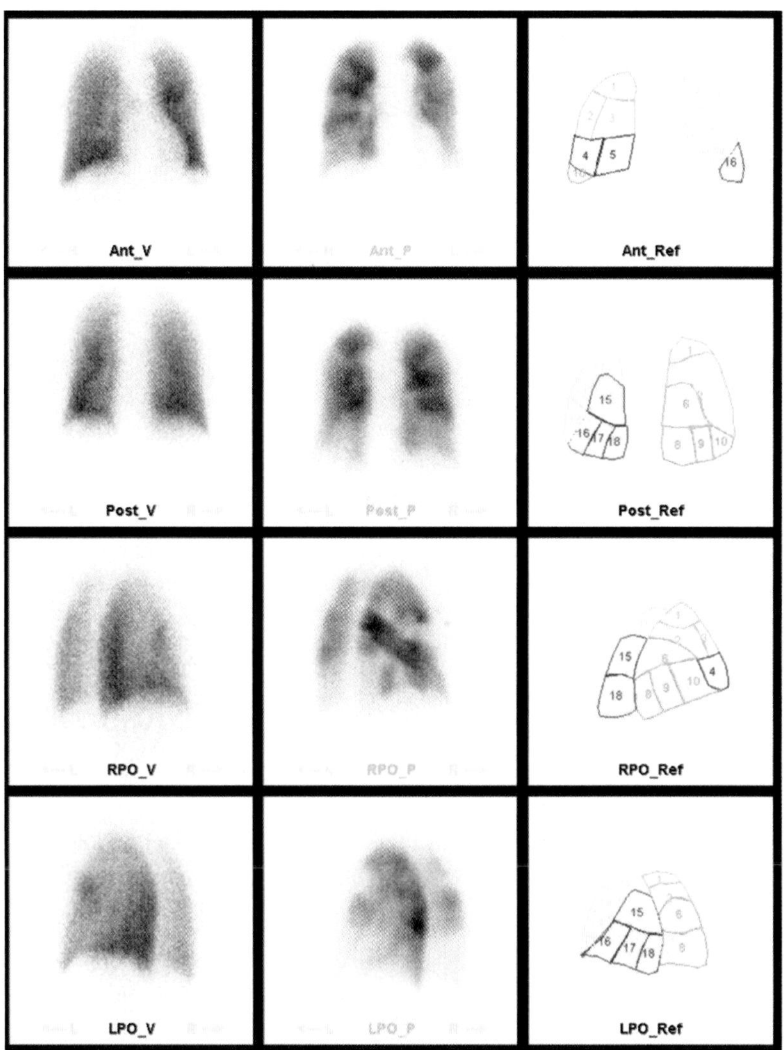

Figure 32-2 High probability scan for pulmonary embolism. Ventilation scan using ^{99m}Tc Technegas® aerosol *(left column)* is within normal limits. Perfusion scan using ^{99m}Tc MAA *(middle column)* shows large segmental defects in both lungs. This combination of findings (mismatch) is consistent with pulmonary embolism.

carried out using rectilinear scanners; ventilation studies were not performed. Despite utilizing a suboptimal radiopharmaceutical and imaging equipment, the UPET study established perfusion lung scanning as an effective technique in both screening for PE and assessing restoration of pulmonary blood flow following an embolic event. Approximately 75% to 80% of perfusion defects resolved by 3 months; those that did not, persisted after 1 year, indicating that most patients with acute PE either completely lyse the thrombi or partially recanalize the pulmonary artery.

Data from prospective, large, outcome-based studies have reported on the important diagnostic information provided by V/Q scanning in patients suspected of having acute PE when coupled with clinical assessment and noninvasive leg testing.[24,25] In patients with suspected PE who had a non–high probability or nondiagnostic V/Q scan, normal cardiorespiratory reserve, and negative serial noninvasive leg tests for proximal venous thrombosis (as determined by serial impedance plethysmography [IPG]), PE at 3 months of follow-up occurred in only 0.6% of cases while the patients were not on anticoagulation.[24] Among patients with suspected PE, but who had a low probability clinical assessment and negative serial noninvasive leg tests, as well as a nondiagnostic V/Q scan, PE at 3 months follow-up occurred in 0.5% of patients.[25] When the probability for clinical assessment was intermediate, PE occurred in only 0.4% of patients.[25]

These studies demonstrated that anticoagulation could be safely withheld in patients with adequate cardiorespiratory reserve who did not have high probability V/Q scans or proximal venous thrombosis, since the incidence of recurrent PE is very low. Unfortunately, the criteria used in the studies to categorize the probability of PE ("normal," "nondiagnostic," or "high") were different than those used in the Prospective Investigation of Pulmonary Embolism Diagnosis (PIOPED), and direct comparison is not possible. In the Prospective Investigative Study of Acute Pulmonary Embolism Diagnosis (PISA-PED),[26] which utilized perfusion scanning alone in conjunction with the chest radiograph, the sensitivity and specificity of scintigraphy were 92% and 87%, respectively. The prevalence of PE was high (39%). When considered in conjunction with clinical assessment of the likelihood of PE ("very likely," "possible," or "unlikely"), the positive predictive value (PPV) of a perfusion scan was 99%; the combination of a near-normal or abnormal perfusion scan without segmental defects and low clinical likelihood of PE had a negative predictive value (NPV) of 97%. Using standardized clinical assessment and perfusion lung scanning, the authors were able to accurately diagnose or exclude PE (PPV, 96%; NPV, 98%). CT angiography (CTA) was required in only a minority of cases having discordant clinical and scintigraphic findings.

■ PROSPECTIVE INVESTIGATION OF PULMONARY EMBOLISM DIAGNOSIS STUDY

To date, the most comprehensive prospective investigation addressing the role of V/Q scanning in the diagnosis of PE has been the PIOPED study. This multi-institutional study was designed to evaluate the efficacy of various conventional methods for diagnosing acute PE. In particular, PIOPED focused on the sensitivity and specificity of lung scans in the diagnosis of acute PE. Although the clinical diagnosis of PE is not definitive, results from PIOPED emphasize the importance of incorporating clinical assessment in evaluating patients suspected of having acute PE. As expected, combining clinical assessment with lung scan interpretation improves diagnostic accuracy of the imaging technique.

Ninety-two percent of patients with PE in PIOPED had at least one of the following risk factors: Immobilization and recent surgery (two most common risks), underlying malignancy, history of DVT or PE, estrogen use, or pre-existing cardiac disease. Of patients diagnosed with PE in PIOPED, >90% had dyspnea, tachycardia, or pleuritic chest pain. Similarly, although chest radiographic findings alone are not sensitive or specific for PE, they are essential for diagnosing conditions that can mimic PE clinically. The most common radiographic findings in patients with PE were atelectasis or parenchymal opacity. Furthermore, chest radiographic findings heavily influence the criteria utilized for estimating the probability of PE based on lung scan patterns. For example, in patients with COPD, the sensitivity of a high probability V/Q scan is significantly lower than in patients with no cardiopulmonary disease. The more severe the underlying cardiopulmonary disease, the higher the likelihood of the scan will be of intermediate probability. Intermediate probability occurred in 60% of patients with COPD in PIOPED, compared with only 13% of patients with a normal chest x-ray.[27]

The sensitivity, specificity, and PPV from PIOPED of V/Q lung scans in detecting acute PE are presented in Table 32-1.

TABLE 32-1 Sensitivity, Specificity, and Positive Predictive Value of Lung Scans in Detecting Pulmonary Embolism in Patients Enrolled in PIOPED

Lung Scan Interpretation (Probability)	Sensitivity (%)	Specificity (%)	Positive Predictive Value (%)
High[a]	40	98	87
High, intermediate[b]	82	64	49
High, intermediate, low[c]	98	12	32

[a]*Only high-probability scans considered indicative of PE; all other classifications considered negative for PE.*
[b]*High- and intermediate- probability scans considered indicative of PE; all other classifications considered negative for PE.*
[c]*High-, intermediate-, and low- probability scans considered indicative of PE; normal or near-normal scans considered negative for PE.*

All patients enrolled in PIOPED were to undergo a V/Q scan and pulmonary arteriogram. However, a large number of patients with low probability or normal V/Q scans did not undergo pulmonary arteriography to avoid additional risks. Therefore, there was a selection bias toward patients with intermediate or high probability scans, leading to an overestimation of the sensitivity, but underestimation of the specificity of V/Q scanning. In an analysis of the angiography results in PIOPED, PE occurred more frequently on the right than on the left, and more commonly in the lower lung zones. One of the limitations of V/Q scanning in PIOPED was the interobserver variability in scan interpretation. As expected, agreement among readers was excellent for normal, high, and very low probability V/Q scans (92%–95%). However, it was not as good for intermediate and low probability studies.[27]

Use of anatomic lung segment reference charts has been shown to reduce interobserver disagreement when interpreting scans. Other interpretative pitfalls include false-negative and -positive readings. False-negative interpretations (i.e., low probability read with PE present) do occur, and patients who have a recent history of immobilization (bed rest for 3 days), recent surgery, trauma to the lower extremities, or central venous instrumentation are particularly at risk. In patients with low or very low probability scans who have none of the aforementioned risk factors, the prevalence of PE is only 4.5%. Conversely, in patients with low or very low probability scans and one or more of the risk factors, the prevalence of PE is 12% and 21%, respectively (Table 32-2).

TABLE 32-2 Risk Factors and Prevalence of Pulmonary Embolism in Patients with Low Probability and Very Low Probability Lung Scans Enrolled in PIOPED

	Patients with 0 Risk Factor[a]	Patients with 1 Risk Factor[a]	Patients with ≥2 Risk Factors[a]	Total
PE positive	14 (2.2%)	19 (2.9%)	37 (5.7%)	70
PE negative	301 (46.4%)	136 (21.0%)	142 (21.9%)	579
Prevalence of PE	4.5%	12.2%	20.7%	10.8%

[a]*Risk factors include immobilization, trauma to lower extremities, surgery, and central venous instrumentation within 3 months of enrollment.*

Patients with false-negative lung scans tend to have nonocclusive subsegmental thrombi and a low pulmonary clot burden. The prognostic value of a low probability scan is excellent, particularly in patients with a low clinical pretest likelihood of disease or negative lower leg ultrasound.[28] The most common cause of V/Q mismatch in patients who do not have acute PE is chronic or unresolved PE. Other causes include compression of the pulmonary vasculature (e.g., from mass lesions, lymphadenopathy, or mediastinal fibrosis), vessel wall abnormalities (e.g., pulmonary artery tumors or vasculitis), nonthromboembolic intraluminal obstruction (e.g., tumor emboli or foreign body emboli), and congenital vascular abnormalities (e.g., pulmonary artery agenesis or hypoplasia).

In patients who have unilateral V/Q mismatch (hypoperfusion or absent perfusion) within an entire lung or in multiple contiguous segments and normal perfusion in the contralateral lung, extrinsic compression of the pulmonary vasculature, congenital abnormalities, or proximal PE should be considered. Patients with a suspected false-positive scan or unilateral V/Q mismatch often require further imaging using CTA, even though emboli are frequently multiple (in 90%) and bilateral (in 85% of cases), and unilateral decreased or absent perfusion to one lung is uncommonly the result of PE.

Shortly after the PIOPED study, helical CTA was introduced.[29] This led to PIOPED II, which is the largest multicentered, prospective, outcome-based study to date designed to assess the accuracy of CTAin evaluation of acute PE in comparison to the composite reference standard.[30]

In PIOPED II, CTA had a sensitivity, specificity, PPV, and NPV of 83%, 96%, 86%, and 95%, respectively, in detecting acute PE.[30] Study results suggested that the predictive value of CTA is highly concordant with the pretest clinical probability of PE using Wells' criteria.[25] The PPV of PE with a positive CTA was 97% for a main or lobar artery, 68% for a segmental vessel, and 25% for a subsegmental branch. The probability of a false-negative chest CTA is minimal in large PE, but false-negative findings may occur in the small group of patients with clot limited to subsegmental arteries. The PPV of PE in patients with positive CTA and high, intermediate, or low clinical probability was 96%, 92%, 58%, respectively. NPV of PE in patients with negative CTA and low, intermediate, or high clinical probability was 96%, 89%, and 60%, respectively.

The limitations of the study included use of 4- to 16-slice multidetector CT (mostly 4-detector) and use of noninvasive diagnostic test in the reference standard. In contrast to original PIOPED population, of whom 68% were inpatients, PIOPED II included only 11% inpatients. Inpatients are more likely to have abnormalities on chest radiographs, which would potentially interfere with optimal V/Q scan reading.[31] Also, the accuracy of CTA would be lower if patients with inconclusive interpretations of CT (51 patients or 6%) were included, giving an overall sensitivity and specificity of 78% and 90%, respectively. The overall PPV of 86% and NPV of 95% are comparable to V/Q performance parameters. The combination of CT venography and CTA increased the sensitivity from 83% to 90% when using CTA alone. CT venography, however, showed similar results in diagnosing or excluding DVT as compression ultrasound.[32]

Finally, PIOPED III, a multicenter collaborative investigative trial was designed to determine the diagnostic accuracy of gadolinium-enhanced magnetic resonance angiography (Gd-MRA) of the pulmonary arteries in combination with magnetic resonance venography (MRV) of the veins of the thighs in patients with clinically suspected acute PE. In PIOPED III, most centers had difficulty in obtaining MR pulmonary angiograms of adequate quality; indeed, studies were deemed inadequate in 25% of patients.[33] Adequacy of the studies varied between 11% and 52% among centers. Adequate quality images were obtained in assessing the main or lobar pulmonary arteries in 91% of patients, segmental pulmonary arteries in 87%, and subsegmental branches in 73%. A technically adequate

MRA had a sensitivity of 78% and specificity of 99%. These findings led the PIOPED III investigators to conclude that MRA should only be considered at centers that routinely perform it well, and for patients who have contraindications to other standard tests.

V/Q SCAN INTERPRETATION AND MODIFICATIONS TO ORIGINAL PIOPED CRITERIA

Several diagnostic schemes have been suggested for interpretation of V/Q scans. The original PIOPED criteria were developed to interpret scans generated from the study based upon experience gathered over the preceding decade. A PE is characterized by V/Q mismatch, which is an area of normal ventilation corresponding to a segmental, wedge-shaped area of decreased or absent perfusion extending to the pleural surface. The segmental defect should correspond to vascular anatomy. Due to the high proportion (44%) of intermediate probability V/Q scans in PIOPED[34] and interobserver disagreements, several revisions and modifications have been made to the original criteria.

One nuance in V/Q scan interpretation is the so-called "gestalt interpretation," which is based on an experienced nuclear medicine physician's subjective estimate of the likelihood of PE (without using specific interpretation criteria). This interpretation takes into account various published lung image interpretation algorithms, clinical data, ancillary findings, and pathophysiologic features of PE, which are integrated with the individual case presentation. The gestalt interpretation has been shown to correlate well with the fraction of patients with angiographic evidence of PE in the PIOPED study, with good-to-excellent intra- and interobserver variability.[35,36] Thus, experienced readers (such as the PIOPED investigators) can provide an accurate estimate of the probability of PE based on clinical, radiographic, and scintigraphic findings.

Another nuance is the "triple match," which is a reference to matching perfusion, ventilation, and chest radiographic abnormality. Based on the PIOPED data, in the presence of a triple match, the prevalence of PE varies depending on the location of the abnormality. A triple match in the upper (prevalence of PE, 11%) or middle lung (prevalence of PE, 12%) zones is considered low probability for PE, but a triple match in the lower lung zones should be interpreted as intermediate probability (prevalence of PE, 33%).[37]

Yet another nuance is the "stripe sign," which describes a rim of perfused lung tissue between the perfusion defect and adjacent pleural surface.[38] In PIOPED, this sign excluded the diagnosis of PE within the affected zone in 93% of cases. Hence, in the absence of other perfusion abnormalities, a V/Q scan with a stripe sign should be considered very low probability for PE. A single, moderate-sized V/Q mismatch was found to harbor PE in 36% of cases in PIOPED[39]; if present, the V/Q scan should be described as intermediate probability for PE. A single matched V/Q defect (of any size) was found to correspond to PE in 26% of cases in PIOPED; such a finding should be classified as intermediate probability.[39]

The limitations in original PIOPED led the investigators to revise the original interpretation criteria for easier application and better integration of clinical pretest probability of PE. Modifications to the original PIOPED interpretation criteria were used in the PIOPED II trial (Table 32-3),[40] which decreased the number of intermediate scan readings (73.5% of patients had V/Q scans with definitive interpretation) and provided a more accurate assessment of angiographically proven PE than the original criteria (sensitivity increased to 83%; specificity essentially unchanged at 96%).

On the other hand, the PISA-PED[26] criteria (Table 32-4) for interpretation of perfusion lung scans were based on diagnosing PE when there was one or more wedge-shaped perfusion defects. PE was considered absent when there was normal or near-normal perfusion or a nonsegmental, non–wedge-shaped perfusion defect.[41] All other scans were called nondiagnostic.

TABLE 32-3 Revised PIOPED Criteria for Interpretation of Lung Scans[a]

High probability (≥80%)
≥2 Large segmental perfusion defects (>75% of a segment) without corresponding ventilation or radiographic abnormalities
One large segmental perfusion defect and ≥2 moderate segmental perfusion defects (25–75% of a segment) without corresponding ventilation or radiographic abnormalities
≥4 Moderate segmental perfusion defects without corresponding ventilation or radiographic abnormalities
Intermediate probability (20–79%)
One moderate to <2 large segmental perfusion defects without corresponding ventilation or radiographic abnormalities
Corresponding ventilation–perfusion defects and radiographic parenchymal opacity in lower lung zone
Single, moderate, matched ventilation–perfusion defects with normal radiographic findings
Corresponding ventilation–perfusion defects and small pleural effusion
Difficult to categorize as normal, low, or high probability
Low probability (<19%)
Multiple matched ventilation–perfusion defects, regardless of size, with normal radiographic findings
Corresponding ventilation–perfusion defects and radiographic parenchymal opacity in upper or middle lung zone
Corresponding ventilation–perfusion defects and large pleural effusion
Any perfusion defects with substantially larger radiographic abnormality
Defects surrounded by normally perfused lung (stripe sign)
>3 Small segmental perfusion defects (<25% of a segment) with a normal radiograph
Nonsegmental perfusion defects (cardiomegaly, aortic impression, enlarged hilum)
Very low probability
≥3 Small segmental perfusion defects (<25% of a segment) with a normal radiograph
Normal scan
No perfusion defects; perfusion outlines the shape of the lung seen on the radiograph

[a]*Criteria generated after completion of prospective study.*

According to modified PIOPED II criteria (Table 32-4) established in 2008, PE was diagnosed when there were equivalent of two large, segmental perfusion scan–chest radiograph mismatches (which may include one large and two moderate segmental mismatches, or four moderate segmental mismatches).[41] PE was considered absent when there was normal perfusion. PE was deemed very low probability when there was a nonsegmental perfusion defect smaller than the corresponding radiographic lesion, one to three small segmental defects, a solitary matched chest x-ray abnormality and perfusion defect in the mid or upper lung zones, a stripe sign, or a pleural effusion ≥1/3 of the pleural cavity with no other perfusion defect in either lung. The scan was considered nondiagnostic with all other findings.

When perfusion scans obtained in PIOPED II were reinterpreted using a composite reference standard (all PIOPED II patients were eligible for this study if they had a diagnosis based on CTA or digital subtraction angiography [DSA], an interpretable perfusion scan and chest radiograph, and a positive Wells' score), investigators

TABLE 32-4 Modified PIOPED II and PISA-PED Criteria for Interpretation of Perfusion Scans

	Modified PIOPED II	PISA-PED
PE present	• High probability (≥2 segments of perfusion scan—chest radiograph mismatch. May be ≥2 large segmental mismatches, or 1 large and 2 moderate mismatches, or 4 moderate segmental mismatches)	• ≥1wedge-shaped perfusion defects

PE absent	• Normal perfusion
	• Very low probability
	  • Nonsegmental lesion (eg, prominent hilum, cardiomegaly, elevated diaphragm, linear atelectasis, costophrenic angle effusion with no other perfusion defect in either lung)
	  • Perfusion defect smaller than radiographic lesion
	  • 1–3 small segmental defects
	  • Solitary CXR-Q matched defect in the mid or upper lung zone confined to a single segment
	  • Stripe sign present around the perfusion defect (best tangential view)
	  • Pleural effusion ≥1/3rd the pleural cavity with no other perfusion defect in either lung
		• Normal perfusion
		• Near normal
		  • Contour defect (caused by enlarged heart, mediastinum, or diaphragm)
		• Perfusion defect, not wedge-shaped

Not diagnostic	• All other findings	• Cannot classify as PE-positive or PE-negative

Source: Data from Miniati, M, Pistolesi, M, Marini, C, et al. Value of perfusion lung scan in the diagnosis of pulmonary embolism: results of the Prospective Investigative Study of Acute Pulmonary Embolism Diagnosis (PISA-PED). Am J Respir Crit Care Med. 1996;154(5):1387–1393; and Sostman, HD, Miniati, M, Gottschalk, A, et al. Sensitivity and specificity of perfusion scintigraphy combined with chest radiography for acute pulmonary embolism in PIOPED II. J Nucl Med. 2008;49(11):741–748.

found only 21% of patients with nondiagnostic results using revised PIOPED II criteria.[41] Only 11% patients had nondiagnostic perfusion scans among the 72% of patients with normal or near-normal chest radiographs. The prevalence of PE in the sample was 19%. Using the modified PIOPED II criteria, and after excluding nondiagnostic perfusion scans, the sensitivity of "PE present" reached 85%, and the specificity of "PE absent" reached 93%. When using PISA-PED criteria, none had nondiagnostic perfusion scans; the sensitivity of a "PE present" scan was 80% and the specificity of "PE absent" scan was 97%. Based on these findings, it was postulated that perfusion scintigraphy combined with chest radiography can provide diagnostic accuracy similar to CTA at a lower cost and, most importantly, with a lower radiation dose.[41]

■ SPECT V/Q IMAGING FOR THE EVALUATION OF PULMONARY EMBOLISM

Single-photon emission tomography (SPECT) V/Q imaging has several advantages over planar imaging, including higher contrast resolution and avoidance of overlapping small perfusion defects by normal tissue, particularly at the lung bases.[42] In the last two decades, technologic advances have been made with SPECT and new radiopharmaceuticals developed for SPECT ventilation studies, such as ^{99m}Tc Technegas.[43] Due to the availability of Technegas outside the United States, most SPECT V/Q scanning is performed in Australia and Europe (Figs. 32-3 and 32-4).

Total acquisition time for the SPECT V/Q examination is between 20 and 30 minutes for a dual-headed camera.[44] The advantages of SPECT over planar imaging in the evaluation for PE have been reported in several studies.[45–48] Importantly, SPECT V/Q scans have been reported by most investigators to be ≤3% nondiagnostic.[44] When compared to planar V/Q scans, SPECT V/Q scans show more and better delineated mismatched defects, better quantification, and less interobserver variation.[46]

In most studies, sensitivity (80%–100%) of SPECT V/Q scanning is higher than planar V/Q scan, but the specificity (93%–100%) is not always higher.[44] Some investigators have also suggested the

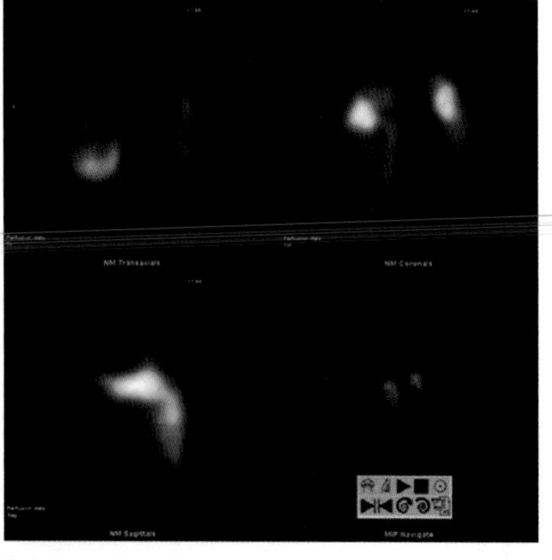
A

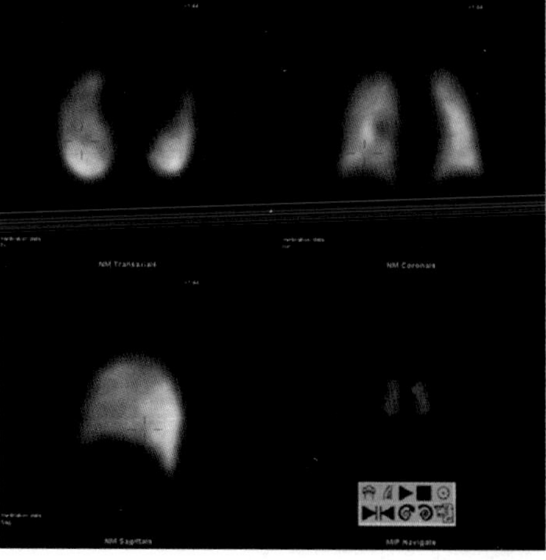
B

Figure 32-3 High probability V/Q SPECT scan for pulmonary embolism. Perfusion scan using ^{99m}Tc MAA in transaxial, coronal, and sagittal views (**A**) shows large segmental defects in both lungs. Ventilation scan using ^{99m}Tc Technegas® aerosol in transaxial, coronal, and sagittal views (**B**) is within normal limits. This combination of findings (mismatch) is consistent with pulmonary embolism.

Figure 32-4 V/Q SPECT scan for pulmonary embolism. Perfusion scan using ^{99m}Tc MAA in transaxial, coronal, and sagittal views (**A**) and ventilation scan using ^{99m}Tc Technegas® aerosol in transaxial, coronal, and sagittal views (**B**) show matched defects.

A

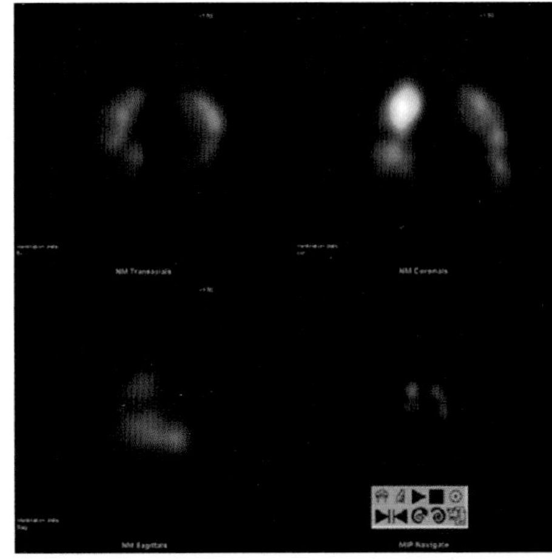

B

use of combined SPECT V/Q scan and low-dose CT scanning to improve accuracy in diagnosing PE.[49] The interpretation criteria, however, for SPECT V/Q scanning are not yet clearly defined or universal (i.e., it remains unclear whether modified PIOPED or PISA-PED criteria can be simply transposed from planar to SPECT V/Q scanning). Despite the many advantages of SPECT, substitution of planar V/Q by SPECT V/Q scan in patients with suspected PE remains controversial.[31,50,51]

There is a growing interest in "positive" imaging based on the use of antibody fragments and radiolabeled peptides directed against components of thromboemboli and glycoprotein IIb/IIIa receptors on the surface of activated platelets. ^{99m}Tc-labeled apcitide is a synthetic peptide that binds with high affinity and specificity to the glycoprotein IIb/IIIa receptor on the membrane of activated platelets.[52] The main advantage of the agent is its ability to distinguish between acute and chronic DVT.

Several ^{99m}Tc-labeled peptides directed against activated platelets are currently under investigation in the evaluation of patients with suspected PE. Radiolabeled peptide imaging has the potential to serve as a single, comprehensive modality in the evaluation of patients with VTE.

Finally, another agent under investigation is ^{99m}Tc-labeled anti–D-dimer (DI-80 B3) monoclonal antibody Fab′ fragment that binds specifically to thromboemboli. In a recent prospective, multicenter study to investigate the sensitivity and specificity of ^{99m}Tc DI-80 B3/SPECT in patients with suspected acute PE, ^{99m}Tc-DI-80 B3/SPECT had a sensitivity of 76.2% and a specificity of 90.5%.[53] At the current time, further studies and development of newer radiopharmaceuticals are required to fully realize this potential.

RECOMMENDATIONS FOR THE USE OF V/Q SCANNING AND CT ANGIOGRAPHY IN SUSPECTED PULMONARY EMBOLISM

Over the past decade, significant technical improvements have occurred in both CTA and V/Q scanning. However, use of CTA of the chest in patients with suspected PE has increased significantly and has markedly surpassed use of V/Q scanning.[54] Although studies show equivalent outcome-based results, the ready availability of CTA, particularly after hours, and the bias toward anatomic, rather than functional imaging, has made CTA the favored diagnostic test for PE.[55]

In a recent large prospective randomized study with high pretest probability and/or positive D-dimer levels, the false-negative rates for V/Q scan and CTA were very close at 1% and 0.4%, respectively.[56] Despite the fact that CTA can detect more small emboli than V/Q scan,[56] the risk of recurrent PE and death have not decreased during the CTA era.[57] In fact the ability of sophisticated new multidetector CT scans to detect emboli in subsegmental branches of the pulmonary arteries has created a healthcare challenge, pushing clinicians to now treat patients who have incidental, asymptomatic pulmonary emboli, whose natural history and optimal management are currently unknown (except in cancer patients in whom these emboli carry a poor prognosis).[58,59] These scans are usually ordered in the emergency department with no particular pretest diagnosis. The same logic will probably be true with SPECT V/Q scan, as it is not yet clear whether treating small, peripheral PE will confer a benefit unless the patients have significant clot burden and limited cardiovascular reserve.[34]

In patients with a normal chest radiograph, the V/Q lung scan is an effective, noninvasive initial study. However, in patients with significant chest radiographic abnormalities, CTA is more likely to provide a definitive diagnosis of PE or an alternative diagnosis, as well as a risk assessment of PE based on the evaluation of right ventricular size and function.[60,61] Furthermore, the combination of CTA and CT venography has the potential to provide a single, comprehensive evaluation of patients with suspected VTE, albeit with increased radiation exposure. V/Q scan remains an important alternative to CT in patients with contrast allergy or renal failure.

V/Q scan may be the modality of choice to evaluate patients with chronic thromboembolic disease and in providing follow-up of PE after therapy.[31] There is concern regarding the high radiation exposure, particularly to the female breast, associated with chest CTA.[62,63] CTA delivers a minimum radiation dose of 20 mGy (2.0 rad) to the breasts of an average-sized woman,[64] whereas breast irradiation with V/Q scan is approximately 0.28 to 0.9 mGy.[65] Furthermore, concern exists that increasing use of CTA may result in an increased incidence of radiation-related cancer in the future.[62] The potential latent carcinogenic effects of such radiation exposure at this time remain unknown.

As part of the American Board of Internal Medicine's *Choosing Wisely* campaign, which focused on potentially unnecessary or harmful medical tests and procedures, the Society of Nuclear Medicine recommended avoiding CTA to diagnose PE in young women with a normal chest radiograph, and consideration of a V/Q study instead.[66] Considerable debate exists regarding fetal radiation doses from pulmonary CTA versus V/Q scanning.[67] During pregnancy, when only a perfusion scan with 50 MBq of ^{99m}Tc MAA is used, the fetal absorbed dose is 0.1 to 0.2 mGy. It is estimated that a 16-slice MDCT scan gives an absorbed fetal dose of 0.24 to 0.66 mGy during the first trimester.[68] A comparison between CTA and V/Q scan for the evaluation of PE is summarized in Table 32-5.

In summary, based upon results from prospective and outcome-based studies, the following conclusions can be drawn regarding the use of V/Q scan and CTA in evaluating patients with suspected PE:

TABLE 32-5 Comparison of CTA and V/Q Scan in the Evaluation of PE

	Advantages	Disadvantages
CTA	- Accuracy - Interobserver agreement - Provides alternative diagnosis, and risk assessment based on the evaluation of right ventricular size and function - After hours availability - High speed in image acquisition - Suitable for unstable patients - Binary reports ("PE" or "no PE")	- Radiation exposure - Contrast allergy - Nephrotoxicity - Relative cost - Potential overdiagnosis of nonclinically relevant peripheral PE
V/Q scan	- High NPV in low pretest probability - High PPV in high pretest probability - Low radiation - Relative cost - Serial follow-up	- Low overall specificity - Low interobserver agreement - After hours availability - Slower speed in image acquisition - Unsuitable for unstable patients - Limited in providing alternative diagnosis - Unpopular probabilistic reports

Source: Data from Reid, JH, Coche, EE, Inoue, T, et al. Is the lung scan alive and well? Facts and controversies in defining the role of lung scintigraphy for the diagnosis of pulmonary embolism in the era of MDCT. Eur J Nucl Med Mol Imaging. 2009;36(3):505–521.

1. Proper pretest clinical probability scoring is important irrespective of the modality used. When imaging results for either V/Q scan or CTA are discordant with the pretest probability, the alternative test should be recommended.
2. A normal V/Q scan excludes the diagnosis of clinically significant PE.
3. Patients with very low or low probability scans and a low clinical likelihood of PE have a low (<5%) prevalence of PE and generally do not require pulmonary angiography or anticoagulation.
4. Patients with very low or low probability scans, intermediate or high clinical likelihood of PE, and negative serial noninvasive venous studies of the lower extremities generally do not require anticoagulation. In selected cases, CTA is helpful in excluding PE and providing an alternative diagnosis.
5. Clinically stable patients with intermediate probability scans require noninvasive venous studies of the legs; if negative, CTA is required for definite diagnosis of PE.
6. A clinically stable patient with a high probability scan and high clinical likelihood of PE, or a patient suspected of having a false-positive scan, requires treatment; no further diagnostic tests are required to confirm the diagnosis.
7. Clinically stable patients with high probability scans and a low clinical likelihood of PE require noninvasive venous studies of the legs; if negative, CTA may be required for definitive diagnosis.
8. V/Q scintigraphy has a high NPV and should be used particularly where low radiation dose is desirable, such as in young female with normal chest radiograph, in an outpatient with low clinical probability plus normal chest radiograph, a patient with high clinical probability plus normal chest radiograph, a patient with prior contrast anaphylaxis and strong allergic history, and a patient with renal failure or multiple myeloma. Since, in most patients, PE can be excluded on the basis of a normal perfusion pattern, to minimize radiation to the fetus in a pregnant patient, a 1- to 2-day protocol is suggested. Perfusion-only scans should be performed on day 1, using a reduced dose of ^{99m}Tc MAA.
9. V/Q scan is preferred over pulmonary CTA for follow-up of PE and investigation of the etiology of pulmonary hypertension.
10. If after-hours imaging is not available and a patient has a high clinical suspicion of PE, a reasonable approach includes administering a single dose of low–molecular-weight heparin and imaging the patient the next morning. This strategy may be particularly advisable for performing V/Q scintigraphy in young women to avoid the excessive breast radiation exposure associated with CTA.
11. If there is a contraindication to V/Q scan or CTA, MRA of the pulmonary artery may be performed in centers that perform it well. There is always concern about nephrogenic systemic fibrosis/nephrogenic fibrosing dermopathy, which occurs rarely in patients with poor renal function who receive gadolinium-containing contrast material.[69,70]
12. Whenever possible V/Q scintigraphy should be interpreted as either "positive for PE," "nondiagnostic," or "no evidence of PE."

EVALUATION OF CHRONIC THROMBOEMBOLIC PULMONARY HYPERTENSION

Chronic thromboembolic pulmonary hypertension (CTEPH) is defined as the persistence of pulmonary hypertension (defined as a mean pulmonary artery pressure >25 mm Hg) after a single or recurrent PE (see Chapter 73). CTEPH is a serious, underdiagnosed disease and the only cause of pulmonary hypertension that can be potentially cured by pulmonary endarterectomy (PEA). Estimates are that between 0.5% and 3.8% of patients eventually develop CTEPH after an acute PE; CTEPH may develop in up to 10% of those with a history of recurrent PE.[71,72]

It is not entirely clear why some patients with a history of acute PE go on to develop CTEPH. The risk of developing CTEPH increases in patients with a history of prior PE, presentation at a younger age, larger perfusion defects, and idiopathic PE at presentation.[71] Diagnosis is the key to survival in CTEPH, as without appropriate treatment long-term prognosis is poor. There is positive correlation between increased mean pulmonary artery pressure and mortality.[73] Unfortunately, the clinical features, laboratory studies, chest radiograph, electrocardiogram, and echocardiogram are often unreliable in distinguishing CTEPH from primary and nonthromboembolic secondary pulmonary hypertension.

In most centers, conventional pulmonary angiography remains the gold standard imaging study to confirm the diagnosis of CTEPH and determine whether surgical intervention is indicated; chest CTA and MRA provide complementary information, if needed.

V/Q lung scanning is a safe, noninvasive technique that facilitates selection of patients with pulmonary hypertension for pulmonary angiography to confirm the diagnosis of chronic PE. V/Q scanning remains one of the most important diagnostic tests to help distinguish CTEPH from other forms of pulmonary hypertension. In a retrospective analysis, V/Q scanning had a sensitivity of 97.4% for detection of chronic thromboembolic disease, while that for CTA was only 51%.[74]

Patients with CTEPH usually have at least one, and often several, segmental or larger, mismatched perfusion defects.[75] To prevent potential adverse hemodynamic effects when performing V/Q scans in patients with pulmonary hypertension, the number of ^{99m}Tc MAA particles administered should be reduced. V/Q scanning may underestimate the magnitude of central vascular occlusion by chronic emboli, as determined at conventional pulmonary angiography or thromboendarterectomy.[76]

Most patients with primary or secondary nonthromboembolic pulmonary hypertension have low probability scans. The distribution of ^{99m}Tc MAA particles within the lungs is diffuse and nonhomogenous. Patients with CTEPH rarely, if ever, have normal or very low probability scans. Thus, a low probability V/Q scan effectively excludes chronic thromboembolism as the cause of pulmonary hypertension. In patients with primary pulmonary hypertension, areas of reverse mismatch on the V/Q scan have been shown to correlate with areas of mosaic-increased attenuation on high-resolution CT scans.[77] In a small study of 55 patients suspected of having CTEPH, the detection rates for central emboli with CTA were similar to conventional pulmonary angiography, although detection of segmental disease was superior with conventional pulmonary angiography.[78]

Even though SPECT is more sensitive than planar perfusion lung scanning for identifying obstructed segments in CTEPH, the technique still underrepresents the true extent of the vascular occlusions in CTEPH.[79] Although CTA and MRA may provide complementary information, they often miss the eccentric lesions of CTEPH. Accordingly, the V/Q scan remains the screening study of choice for CTEPH. Any patient with unexplained pulmonary hypertension should be evaluated for the presence of CTEPH; a V/Q scan is recommended as screening method of choice.[80]

QUANTITATIVE VENTILATION–PERFUSION LUNG SCANNING

In patients undergoing pulmonary resection, bronchoscopic lung volume reduction, or lung transplantation, quantitative V/Q lung scanning is a useful method for determining regional lung function and, thus, predicting postoperative pulmonary function (see Chapter 103).[81–83]

Currently, the presurgical assessment to predict response to lung volume reduction surgery (LVRS) in patients with emphysema is mainly performed using chest CT scanning,[84] which provides an anatomic diagnosis of emphysema, delineates its extent and distribution, and detects any other incidental findings that may represent a contraindication to the procedure. A V/Q scan can provide additional information concerning the heterogeneity and distribution of the functional disruption caused by emphysema.[84] Patients with advanced, upper lobe–predominant emphysema derive the most benefit from LVRS,[85] and perfusion scintigraphy is a commonly available test for assessing the distribution of emphysema by reflecting regional lung function.[86] Rectangular regions of interest over the anterior and posterior scintigraphic images of each lung are divided into upper, middle, and lower zones of equal craniocaudal height, and the geometric mean for a given zone is obtained and presented as the percent perfusion to that zone.[87]

In patients being considered for lung cancer surgical resection, a V/Q scan can predict postoperative pulmonary function and enable assessment of the risk of surgery for patients with borderline pulmonary function.[88] The predicted postoperative forced expiratory volume in 1 second (ppo FEV_1) is calculated by multiplying the preoperative value by the ratio of the counts in the remaining lung to total lung activity (Fig. 32-5).[89,90]

Lung perfusion scintigraphy can be used to quantify the degree of right-to-left shunting due to patent foramen ovale, atrial septal defect, elevated right heart pressures, or hepatopulmonary syndrome (HPS).[91,92] The number of injected ^{99m}Tc MAA particles should be reduced in patients with suspected right-to-left shunt. Normally, $<5\%$ of ^{99m}Tc MAA is taken up in the brain, but in HPS, fewer MAA particles are entrapped in pulmonary vasculature and are able to enter the systemic circulation and lodge in different organs (thyroid, spleen, liver, kidneys, and brain), leading to $>6\%$ uptake in the brain (Fig. 32-6). The major disadvantage of perfusion scintigraphy is that it cannot distinguish intracardiac from intrapulmonary right-to-left shunt. Estimation of the right-to-left shunt fraction is calculated using the following equation: $100 \times (\text{TBC} - \text{TLC})/(\text{TBC})$, where TBC is total body count and TLC is total lung count. A less precise alternative method of right-to-left shunt quantification derives an estimate of total body counts from the measurement of renal and/or cerebral activity.

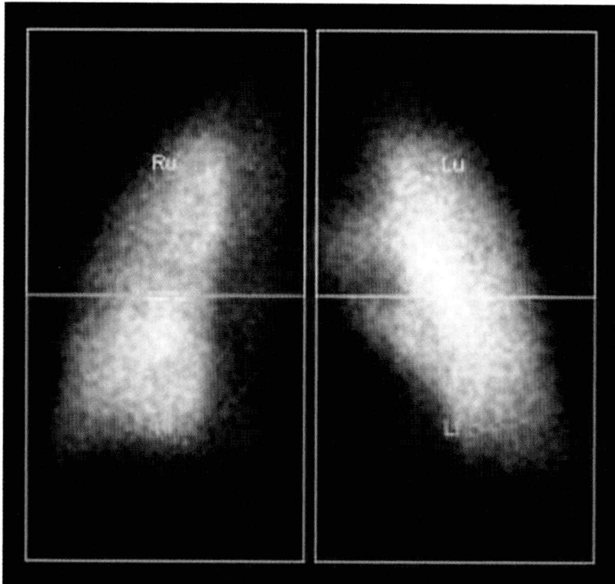

Figure 32-5 Quantitative perfusion lung scan. Regional perfusion can be quantified by outlining regular or irregular regions of interest and generating ratios that correspond to percent of total pulmonary function. Images shown were analyzed by dividing each lung into two equal rectangles.

ASSESSMENT OF ALVEOLAR–CAPILLARY MEMBRANE PERMEABILITY AND MUCOCILIARY CLEARANCE

The clearance rate of inhaled ^{99m}Tc DTPA aerosol from the lungs can be measured using a gamma camera and provides an index of lung epithelial permeability.[11] Aerosols of relatively small aerodynamic diameter (e.g., ^{99m}Tc DTPA) are deposited largely within the small airways and alveoli; the normal half time of ^{99m}Tc DTPA wash out from the lungs is about 80 minutes.[12] In the presence of epithelial

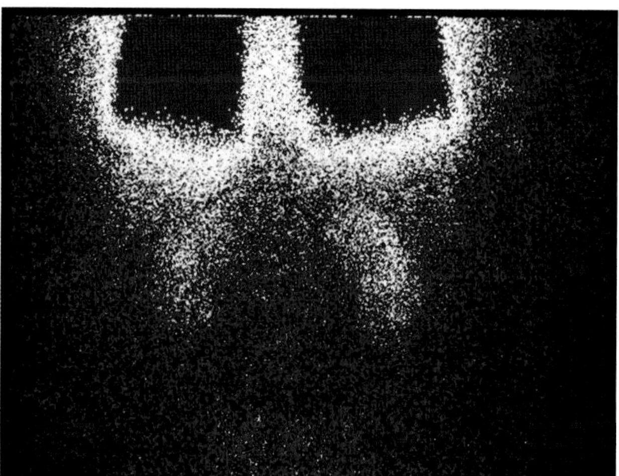

Figure 32-6 Right-to-left shunt in a patient with hepatopulmonary syndrome. Perfusion scan using ^{99m}Tc MAA is showing particles in the systemic circulation lodged in the kidneys.

alveolar damage, the clearance of ^{99m}Tc DTPA is accelerated.[11] Examples of such injuries include amiodarone toxicity, inhalation damage in fire victims, pneumoconiosis, idiopathic pulmonary fibrosis, collagen vascular diseases, sarcoidosis, acute respiratory distress syndrome, and pneumocystis pneumonia.[11,93] Cigarette smoking or physiologic factors, such as posture and exercise, also influence epithelial lung clearance.[11,94] Since increased alveolar–capillary membrane permeability is relatively nonspecific, ^{99m}Tc DTPA aerosol clearance studies have been utilized only to assess the effects of therapy in patients with known pulmonary diseases.

Mucociliary clearance is a primary physiologic defense mechanism, protecting the lungs from damage caused by inhaled particles and microorganisms. Determination of mucociliary clearance may be obtained after the inhalation of relatively large aerosolized particles, followed by measurement of the rate of clearance using a gamma camera. The rate of mucociliary clearance depends on several factors, including ciliary activity and mucus production. Inhaled particles, such as ^{99m}Tc MAA or ^{99m}Tc sulfur colloid, tend to be deposited within the proximal airways.[95] The normal mucociliary clearance half time is approximately 24 hours. Delayed mucociliary clearance is seen in patients with airway inflammation (e.g., cystic fibrosis, COPD, asthma, or viral respiratory tract infections), following bronchial surgery, or after irradiation.

Scintigraphic assessment of alveolar–capillary membrane integrity and mucociliary clearance has not gained wide clinical use,[93] but it is employed in the development of orally inhaled drugs that are administered by inhalation by assessing their deposition patterns, extent of delivery, and depth of penetration into the lungs.[96] In addition, the technique is applicable in quantification of the impact of new drugs on the rate of mucociliary clearance—a key biomarker for products in development for the treatment of respiratory diseases.[97]

POSITRON EMISSION TOMOGRAPHY

PET is used in assessing nonmalignant thoracic disease, as well as pulmonary nodules and known or suspected malignancy. Following are considered basic principles and the role of PET in evaluating inflammatory lung diseases in the overall population, and infections in immunocompromised hosts. Comparison is made with other diagnostic tests, including ^{67}Ga-citrate scanning. The role of PET in assessment of lung nodules and cancer is discussed in a separate section (see Role of Positron Emission Tomography in the Assessment of the Solitary Pulmonary Nodule and Lung Cancer).

BASIC PRINCIPLES

PET is a nuclear medicine imaging modality that provides a 3D image of molecular processes in the body. A PET scan detects gamma rays emitted by positron-emitting tracers. The most commonly used radiopharmaceutical in clinical PET is 2-[^{18}F] fluorodeoxy-D-glucose (FDG), a fluorine-labeled glucose analog with a favorable, 110-minute half-life. FDG competes with glucose for transport into cells and for enzymatic phosphorylation by hexokinase. Unlike glucose, once phosphorylated to FDG-6-phosphate, FDG does not undergo further metabolism; rather, it is trapped inside the cell, and its net accumulation allows for detection by PET.[98]

FDG uptake is proportional to the metabolic activity of the cells that have undergone malignant transformation and, as such, have increased glucose transport and metabolism and increased hexokinase activity. FDG accumulation also depends on various factors, including cellular mitotic rates, level of hypoxia (hypoxia-inducible factor-1-alpha upregulates glucose transport receptors), and degree of cell differentiation (well-differentiated tumors have low FDG uptake).[99] In addition, inflammatory cells share many of the same features as malignant cells; therefore, FDG-PET imaging can be employed to assess infectious and inflammatory processes and diseases. FDG-PET imaging is performed in the fasting state to minimize competitive inhibition of FDG uptake by circulating glucose in the plasma (hyperglycemia may result in decreased FDG accumulation in either malignant or inflammatory cells).

A key advantage of PET over conventional imaging techniques is the possibility of accurate quantification of the ongoing metabolic activities in normal or diseased states. The most common means used for this purpose is measurement of the standardized uptake value (SUV), a semiquantitative expression of the intensity of FDG accumulation in a region of interest (ROI) assigned on the PET scan. SUV normalizes the amount of FDG accumulation in an ROI to the total injected dose and the patient's body weight. It is calculated by dividing the mean activity within a selected region (or volume) of interest (in mCi/mL) by the injected dose (in mCi/kg). SUVmax is derived from the single voxel showing the highest uptake within a defined ROI, which typically represents the most metabolically active part of a tumor or inflammatory process.[100,101] However, it is important to note that several factors can impact SUV, including extravasation of the compound administered, hyperglycemia, respiratory motion, time from injection, and size of ROI.

Today, the mainstay for PET imaging is integrated PET/CT scanners, which allow combining metabolic and structural imaging modalities into a single device. Based on existing data from the past decade, PET/CT scans have been shown to be superior to images generated from separate PET and CT studies for assessing a multitude of disorders.[102] The newest generation of PET/CT scanners contain a state-of-the-art multidetector CT machine that provides up to 128 slices, and time-of-flight PET technologies that reconstruct high-quality images using low FDG doses and short scan times, especially in large patients.[103] PET/CT has some limitations related to attenuation artifacts, leading to false-positive results on corrected images. In addition, motion and misregistration between PET and CT images can also result in major artifacts in regions adjacent to the heart and diaphragm.[104] Combined PET/MRI systems are now commercially available, but their added potential clinical benefit has not yet been validated.[105] This is particularly true in thoracic disorders.

ROLE OF POSITRON EMISSION TOMOGRAPHY IN PULMONARY INFLAMMATION AND INFECTION

FDG-PET has been used in the evaluation of patients with a variety of inflammatory disorders, including venous thromboembolic disease, infections in immunocompromised hosts, and other noninfectious inflammatory conditions. Each of these entities is discussed in subsequent sections.

Potential Role for FDG-PET in Evaluating Suspected Venous Thromboembolism

In recent years, FDG-PET/CT has been explored in many inflammatory conditions. Activated inflammatory cells demonstrate increased FDG uptake due to increased numbers of cell surface glucose transporters following cellular stimulation by various cytokines.[106] Similar biochemical changes are also seen with VTE.

Based on our own experience and that reported in the literature,[107] the potential value of PET in assessing VTE is clear for several reasons. Current imaging techniques, which are based on structural detection of thrombi, are limited; DVT and PE are only two manifestations of VTE, which may occur in parts of the venous system (e.g., within the pelvis) that are not easily accessible by conventional methods. This limitation also applies to the detection of occult disease (e.g., cancer), which is often a key factor in developing VTE (Fig. 32-7). Furthermore, structural imaging techniques cannot differentiate among different phases of thrombus formation, which may hold therapeutic implications.

We believe that many of these shortcomings will be overcome by using FDG-PET/CT. Several case reports have addressed the incidental detection of VTE with FDG-PET/CT in patients with

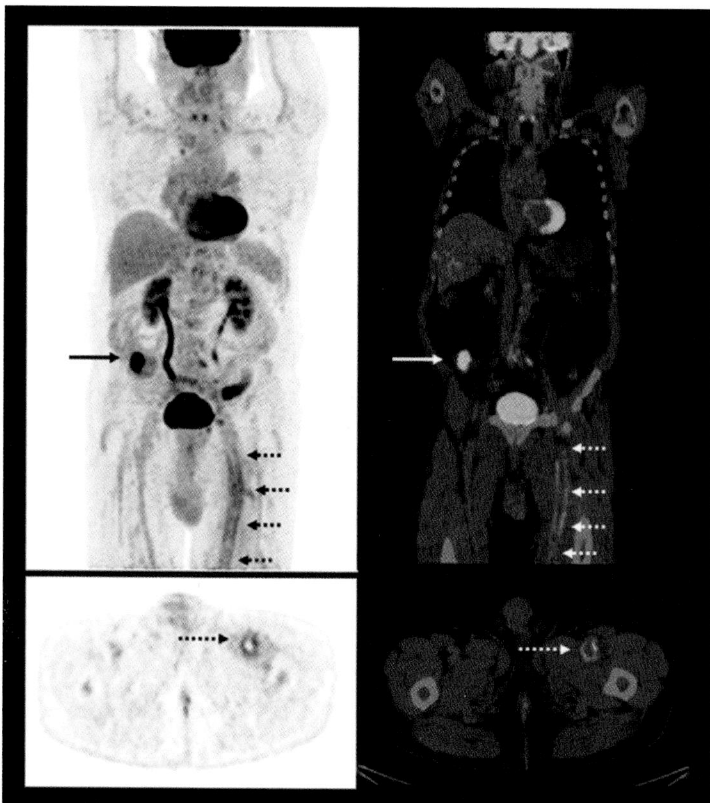

Figure 32-7 Left femoral thrombosis on FDG-PET/CT scan. Maximum intensity projection PET scan (**top left**), transaxial PET scan (**bottom left**), fused coronal PET/CT scan (**top right**), and fused transaxial PET/CT scan (**bottom right**) in a patient with venous thromboembolism having a FDG-PET/CT in search of underlying malignancy. Increased FDG uptake is seen along the acutely thrombosed vein *(interrupted arrows)*, and focally increased FDG uptake is seen in the cecum *(solid arrows)* corresponding to a biopsy-proven colon cancer.

cancer or bacteremia.[108,109] Inflammatory processes also play a key role in nonmalignant, noninfectious VTE, that is, local vessel wall inflammation and inflammatory components, including activated leukocytes in the thrombus itself.

In a small, prospective, proof-of-concept series,[110] both DVT and PE were shown to be visible on FDG-PET/CT. All patients with proved acute lower extremity DVT had marked FDG uptake along the venous wall at the site of thrombus. Diagnosis was established by positive compression ultrasound in patients with symptoms less than a week; no history of cancer, infection, or prior DVT; and a high clinical probability by Wells' DVT score. Conversely, none of the control patients with suspected, but disproved, DVT had FDG uptake in any part of the venous vasculature. The diagnosis was disproved by negative compression ultrasound in patients with symptoms less than a week; no history of cancer, infection, or prior DVT; and a low clinical probability by Wells' DVT score. Results were more equivocal in PE with some patients with high probability V/Q scans showing no FDG uptake in the pulmonary arteries. However, this may be attributed to significantly longer symptom duration (i.e., months) in some patients. It may, in fact, be that FDG-PET/CT was truly negative for active thrombi, since recent data suggest a significant decrease in FDG avidity over time.

In a pivotal study of 12 patients with confirmed proximal thrombosis in the lower extremity, the authors not only found a specificity of 87.5% to 100% and sensitivity of 87.5% to 100% (depending on SUVmax threshold used), but also a steady decrease in SUVmax and possible complete normalization within 3 months.[111] These findings are in accordance with VTE pathophysiology: The thrombus may be classified as acute when inflammatory cells and mediators are abundant, subacute with subsiding inflammation and increasing fibrosis, and finally, chronic with recanalization and loss of inflammation. This pathophysiology will have significant clinical implications, since active thrombi need therapy, while unresolved old clots require no treatment. However, a substantial fraction of patients with VTE experience symptoms of recurrence, and in as many as half the morphologic features suggestive of the diagnosis remain for years after the first event.[107] FDG-PET/CT likely will differentiate new, active clots from old, inactive ones and facilitate an individualized therapeutic approach.

Although the literature is still sparse, the role of FDG-PET/CT imaging appears to be very promising in VTE and may contribute significantly by detecting clots at any location throughout the body, by early diagnosis of underlying malignancy, and by differentiating acute from chronic thrombi.

Imaging of the Thorax in the Immunocompromised Host

In the last three decades, ^{67}Ga-citrate and white blood cells labeled with ^{111}In or ^{99m}Tc were considered as appropriate agents for imaging pulmonary infection and inflammation. However, due to poor image quality, laborious labeling techniques, and the requirement for imaging several days after injection, imaging with either ^{67}Ga-citrate or radiolabeled white blood cells is now considered obsolete. In recent years these methods have been largely replaced by FDG-PET/CT in the evaluation of suspected infection or inflammation in many anatomic locations. This is also the case in the lungs, where FDG-PET/CT is employed for evaluating suspected pulmonary infections, fever of unknown origin in the immunocompromised host (Fig. 32-8), opportunistic infections in patients infected with

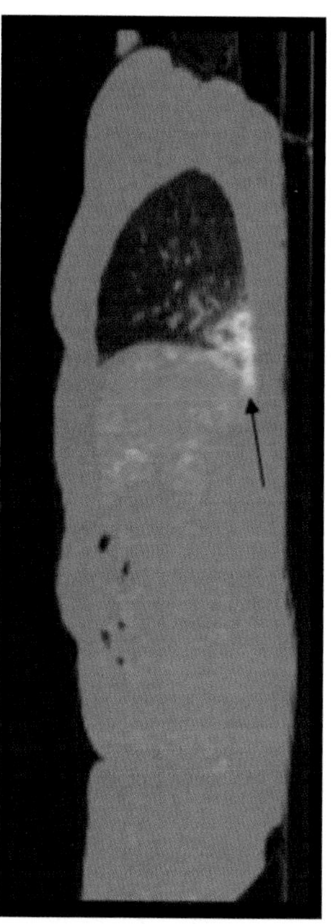

Figure 32-8 Fever of unknown origin in an immunocompromised patient with a kidney transplant. Conventional chest x-ray was normal. Fused sagittal FDG-PET/CT image shows characteristically increased FDG uptake in the right lower lung *(arrow)* consistent with lobar pneumonia.

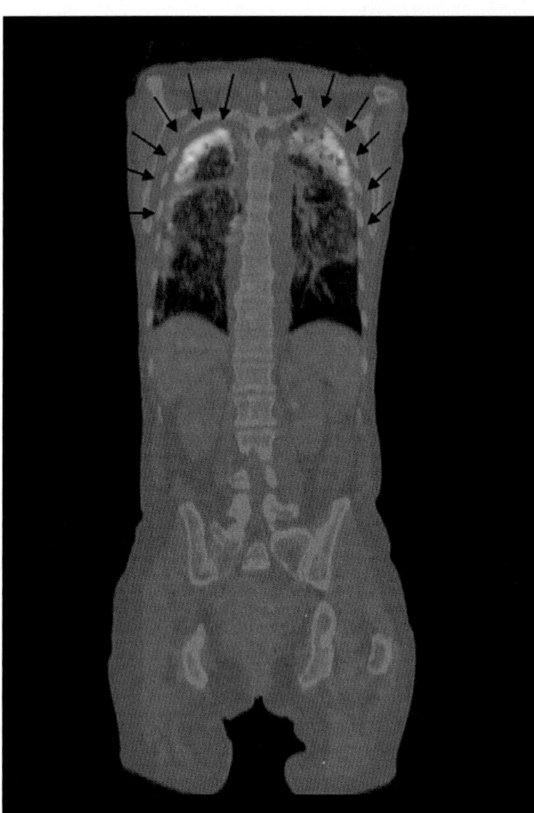

Figure 32-9 *Pneumocystis jirovecii* pneumonia. Diffuse, markedly increased FDG lung uptake bilaterally *(arrows)* in a patient with human immunodeficiency virus.

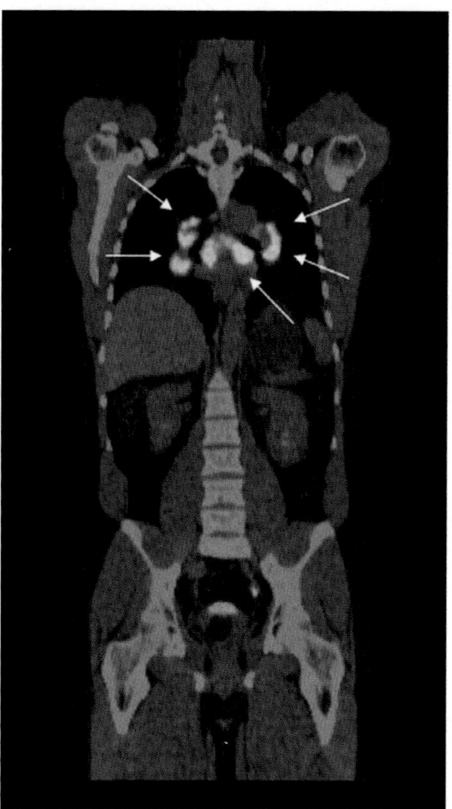

Figure 32-10 Sarcoidosis. Typical presentation of sarcoidosis on FDG-PET/CT with markedly increased FDG uptake in mediastinal and hilar lymph nodes *(arrows)*. Similar patterns are seen in patients with lymphoma.

HIV (Fig. 32-9), and a multitude of inflammatory disorders.[112] In spite of limited data, an early pilot study also suggested that FDG-PET might be helpful in determining treatment response in patients with tuberculosis.[113]

Noninfectious Inflammatory Lung Disease

^{67}Ga-citrate lung imaging has been used to quantify the degree of alveolitis in various interstitial lung diseases, particularly sarcoidosis and idiopathic pulmonary fibrosis. Unfortunately, pulmonary accumulation of ^{67}Ga in idiopathic pulmonary fibrosis was found not to be reliable in predicting the response to treatment or prognosis.[114] Also, in these settings, FDG-PET/CT appears to be substantially superior to ^{67}Ga. A novel potential indication is the assessment of inflammatory disease activity in COPD using FDG-PET/CT. Even with sparse reports in the literature, the evidence points toward a correlation between the distribution and severity of emphysema and the degree of FDG uptake, which may have significant implications for managing patients with this serious disorder.

Sarcoidosis is a multisystem inflammatory granulomatous disease, which involves the lungs in 90% of patients; it may affect any organ in the body. Scintigraphy with ^{67}Ga-citrate has been advocated for assessment of disease activity, but in recent years, this technique has been overshadowed by FDG-PET, which has several technical advantages, including lower radiation exposure, shorter time interval between injection and imaging, and higher quality images. Hilar and mediastinal lymph nodes (as well as any other soft tissues) harboring active granulomas due to sarcoidosis accumulate FDG (Fig. 32-10). Although FDG-PET cannot distinguish sarcoidosis from other diseases, such as Hodgkin or non-Hodgkin lymphomas, the technique is quite effective in assessing the extent of disease after an initial diagnosis, thereby selecting the appropriate site for a successful biopsy. FDG-PET can also provide a means for assessing response to treatment (Fig. 32-11).

FDG-PET has been found to be more sensitive (97%) than ^{67}Ga-citrate scintigraphy (88%) in detecting active sarcoidosis.[115] Comparative studies have shown that FDG-PET can detect more intra- and extrathoracic lesions than ^{67}Ga scintigraphy, with better interobserver agreement.[115–118] High FDG uptake in the involved lung parenchyma correlates with disease severity as revealed by bronchoalveolar lavage.[119] FDG-PET will likely have an increasing role in evaluating the efficacy of therapeutic interventions in this serious disease.[118] In a recent study of 90 patients with chronic sarcoidosis and persistent symptoms, FDG-PET/CT proved helpful in detecting active inflammatory sites, especially in patients with normal ACE levels, thereby influencing adjustment of therapy.[120]

Pneumoconioses may be progressive, even after dust exposure has ceased. The inhaled particles activate pulmonary macrophages that secrete cytokines that mediate an inflammatory reaction, inducing fibroblast proliferation and collagen deposition. FDG is taken up by both fibroblasts and alveolar inflammatory cells. The intensity of pulmonary FDG uptake in pneumoconioses depends on whether active inflammation (increased uptake) or end-stage fibrosis (reduced uptake) predominates at the time of the scan.[121] In addition, progressive massive fibrosis has been shown to be associated with increased FDG accumulation.[122] The findings from FDG-PET have direct clinical implications, as therapeutic interventions are ineffective in end-stage fibrosis.

Interstitial lung disease may also be FDG-avid, but there is limited data on the use of FDG-PET in this setting (Fig. 32-12). In a small prospective study of 21 patients, FDG-PET did not allow differentiation of idiopathic from nonidiopathic pulmonary fibrosis.[123] However, dual–time point FDG-PET imaging holds promise in differential diagnosis and prediction of disease progression in patients with idiopathic interstitial pneumonia.[124]

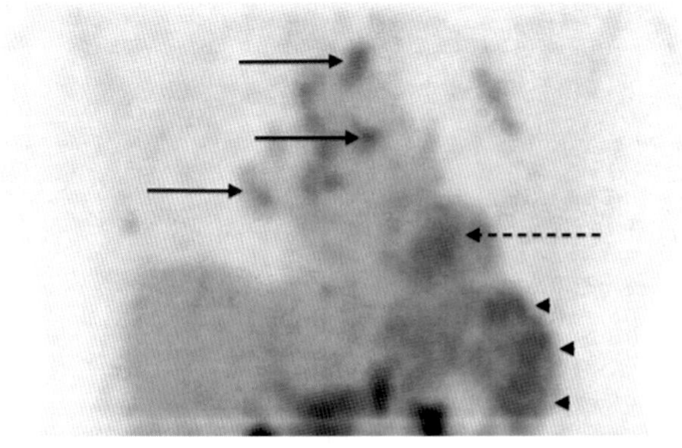

A

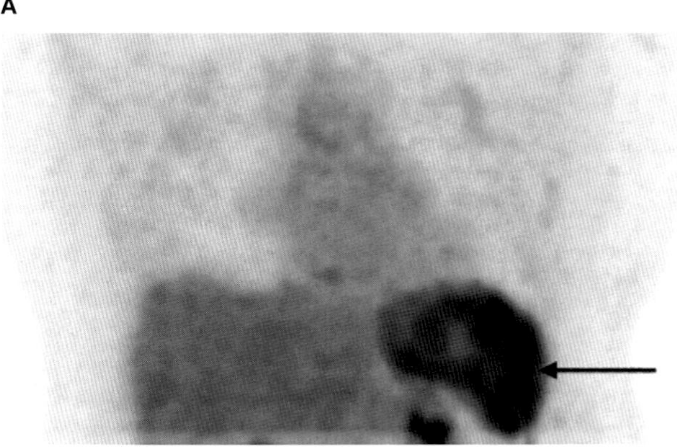

B

Figure 32-11 **A.** FDG-PET/CT images of the thorax and upper abdomen reveal significant disease activity in mediastinal and hilar lymph nodes *(solid arrows)*, the myocardium *(interrupted arrow)*, and the spleen *(arrow heads)*. **B.** Following successful treatment, there is substantial response in the affected site in the heart and the lymph nodes. However, there is significantly increased uptake of FDG in the splenic lesions *(solid arrow)*, which demonstrates the complexity of the biologic behavior of sarcoidosis in various organs during the course of the disease.

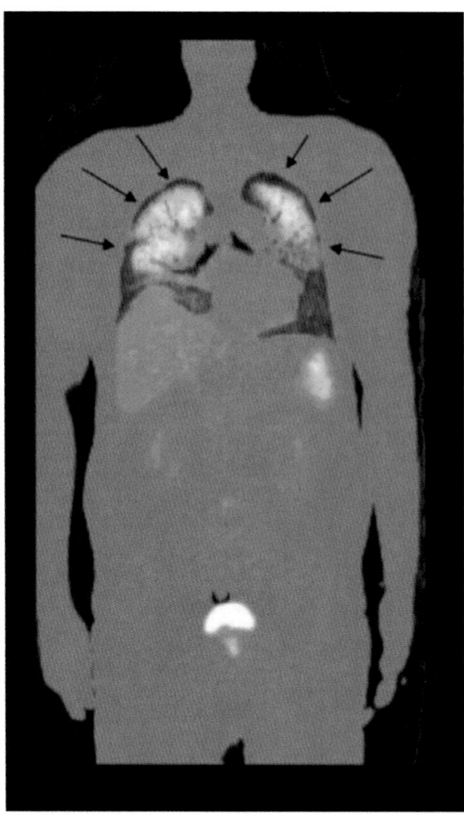

Figure 32-12 Interstitial lung disease. The patient presented with dyspnea and intermittent fever and the PET/CT showed diffusely increased FDG uptake in both lungs *(arrows)*.

ROLE OF POSITRON EMISSION TOMOGRAPHY IN ASSESSMENT OF THE SOLITARY PULMONARY NODULE AND LUNG CANCER

Current clinical indications for FDG-PET imaging in malignant lung disease include evaluation of the solitary pulmonary nodule (SPN), staging of lung cancer (nonsmall cell, small cell, mesothelioma), and planning and monitoring the response to therapy.

EVALUATION OF THE SOLITARY PULMONARY NODULE

An SPN is defined as a round or oval radiographic opacity in the lung parenchyma that measures up to 3 cm in size and is not associated with mediastinal adenopathy or atelectasis (see Chapter 110).[125] An SPN is commonly identified on chest radiographs or CT scans. In the United States, approximately 150,000 new SPNs are diagnosed per year; 30% to 50% of such lesions are malignant and may represent a potentially curable stage of bronchogenic carcinoma.[126] Therefore, early and accurate diagnosis is essential for timely intervention, as lung cancer remains, by far, the leading cause of cancer death among both men and women in the world. Importantly, survival depends on the stage of the cancer when diagnosed.[127]

The most common type of lung cancer is nonsmall cell lung cancer (NSCLC) (adenocarcinoma, squamous cell carcinoma, and large cell carcinoma), which accounts for about 85% of lung cancers.[127] About 10% to 15% of lung cancers are small cell carcinoma, which tend to spread quickly; fewer than 5% of lung cancers are neuroendocrine (carcinoid) tumors, which tend to grow slowly and rarely spread.[127] Most malignant SPNs are adenocarcinoma (47%), followed by squamous cell carcinoma (22%), and small cell lung cancer.[126] Of benign SPNs, about 80% are caused by infectious granulomas.[125]

While a number of benign etiologies for SPNs may have a characteristic appearance on CT, many cannot be characterized accurately using CT and often require further invasive assessment for accurate diagnosis. Certain factors, including smoking history, characteristics of the nodule (size, edge irregularity, and spiculation, pure ground-glass opacity, and absence of calcification), and the age when such lesions are detected are features that determine the probability of malignancy. Despite application of radiographic and other clinical criteria employed for distinguishing benign from malignant lesions, considerable overlap exists.[128] CXRs and CT scans are not accurate in differentiating benign from malignant noncalcified pulmonary nodules that range from 1 to 3 cm in diameter. However, benign patterns of calcification and morphologic stability over 2 years are the most reliable signs of benignity.[128] Bayesian analysis can be used to stratify risk (based on clinical information and imaging characteristics) and guide management of SPN.[129]

FDG-PET provides an accurate, noninvasive diagnostic assessment of SPNs, without the morbidity and costs associated with invasive tissue sampling.[130] In a prospective multicenter trial designed to determine the utility of FDG-PET in discriminating between benign and malignant pulmonary nodules, the sensitivity and specificity of FDG-PET ranged from 92% to 98% and 69% to 100%, respectively (Table 32-6).[130] False-positive studies are seen with active granulomas due to aspergillosis, tuberculosis, or sarcoidosis.[106] False-positive findings may also be related to injection technique (Fig. 32-13). False-negative results are noted with hyperglycemia, malignancies that have a low metabolic activity (e.g., adenocarcinoma *in situ*, previously known as bronchoalveolar cell carncinoma, or carcinoid tumors),[131] and nodules that are <8 mm in diameter.

TABLE 32-6 FDG-PET in Evaluation of Solitary Pulmonary Nodules

Nodule Size (cm)	Type of Analysis	Sensitivity %	Sensitivity 95% Confidence Interval	Specificity %	Specificity 95% Confidence Interval	Accuracy (%)
≤1.5	SUV	80	60–100	95	85–100	88
	Visual	100	100–100	74	55–93	
>1.5	SUV	96	90–100	80	55–100	93
	Visual	98	94–100	60	45–74	91
≤3	SUV	90	82–98	92	85–99	91
	Visual	98	94–100	69	56–82	88
All sizes	SUV	92	82–100	90	79–100	91
	Visual	98	82–100	69	57–81	89

Source: Adapted with permission from Lowe VJ, Fletcher JW, Gobar L, et al. Prospective investigation of positron emission tomography in lung nodules. J Clin Oncol. 1998;16(3):1075–1084.

In one meta-analysis of 40 studies that included 1474 pulmonary lesions evaluated using FDG-PET (including dedicated and gamma camera-based PET), the technique had an average sensitivity of 97% and specificity of 78%.[132]

In general, SUVmax >2.5 has been shown to be very sensitive and specific for differentiating malignant lesions from benign ones.[133] Several studies have shown that no significant differences are noted between results using a semiquantitative analysis of FDG uptake with SUV and those based on qualitative visual assessment.[132,134,135] FDG uptake greater than that in the liver or mediastinum (which typically have an SUV of about 2.0) is considered indicative of malignancy.[130] Visual analysis may be more sensitive for nodules that are smaller than 1.5 cm in diameter, but it carries a lower specificity.[130] Lesions that have no visually detectable FDG uptake have a very low probability for malignancy.[136]

The low accuracy of FDG-PET in assessing nodules having a "ground-glass" or "mixed" appearance on CT scanning is likely related to the cell types that predominate in these lesions, including pure adenocarcinoma *in situ* (bronchioloalveolar cell cancer) or adenocarcinomas with bronchioloalveolar features.[137] In a study of 344 patients in whom a definitive diagnosis was known (prevalence of malignancy: 53%, average size of nodule: 16 mm), FDG-PET had a sensitivity of 92% compared with 96% for CT, but the specificity of PET was markedly better than that of CT, at 82% versus 41%.[138]

As noted previously, the sensitivity of FDG-PET is a function of lesion size and the degree of respiratory motion. In one study addressing the issue of size, the technique's sensitivity in detecting malignancy was 69% for nodules ranging from 5 to 10 mm in diameter and 95% for nodules >10 mm in diameter.[139] The lower limit of spatial resolution of PET, which is about 5 to 6 mm, is lower than

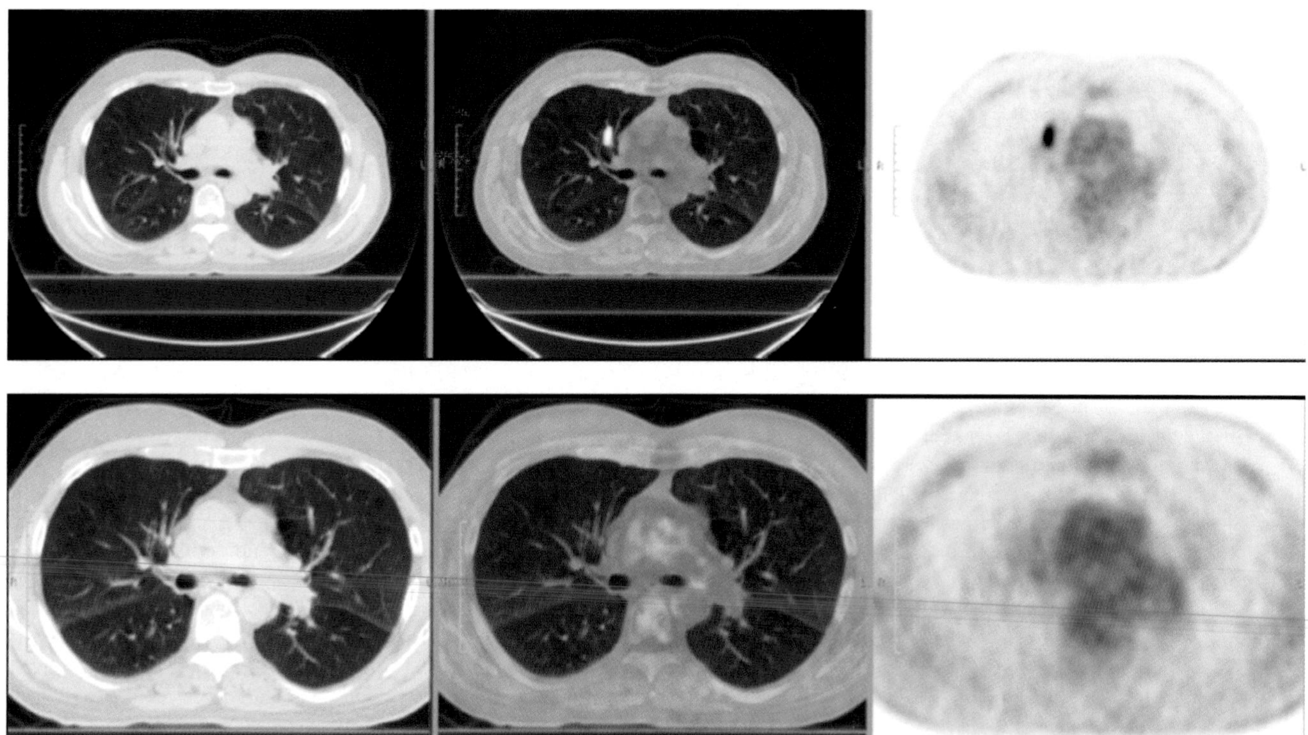

Figure 32-13 A patient referred for characterization of the right upper lobe pulmonary nodule. Transaxial CT, fused PET/CT, and PET images at baseline (**top row**) show solitary, intense focal uptake in the right upper lope. The intense focal uptake was not present in a repeat scan one week later (**bottom row**). This is an example of a false positive finding related to injection technique.

that of CT or MRI. Therefore, PET is not recommended for SPN <8 mm.[140] One method aimed at compensating for this limitation is based on using lesion size measured on CT imaging to correct the underestimated SUV with conventional measurements.

Lung cancers have a wide range of FDG uptake. Furthermore, while most infectious or inflammatory pulmonary disorders generally have a lower FDG uptake than malignancies, overlap exists. An SUV threshold of 2.5, measured at a single point in time, has been proposed to separate malignant (higher SUV) from benign (lower SUV) disorders. Based on the observation in animal and human studies that FDG uptake by malignant tumors increases over time, while that of inflammatory tissue decreases, dual–time point FDG-PET scanning has been proposed as a potentially useful means of improving discrimination between benign and malignant diseases.

Using dual–time point FDG-PET scanning, images are obtained 1 hour and a later time point after administration of FDG. In one study in which an SUV cutoff value of 2.5 and a 10% increase in SUV were used to indicate malignancy, the sensitivity and specificity of FDG-PET were 80% and 94%, respectively, for the single–time point method, and 100% and 89%, respectively, for the dual–time point technique.[141] Recent meta-analysis comparing diagnostic performance of integrated PET/CT scanners showed that dual–time point FDG-PET/CT is more specific than single–time point FDG-PET/CT.[142] Dual time imaging is not required in lesions with a baseline SUV of <1.0, since these lesions have a very high likelihood of being benign, and dual time imaging may result in false-positive examinations.[141] Even for nodules with SUVmax of <2.5, dual time imaging technique may not discriminate accurately between benign and malignant lesions, particularly in areas with a high incidence of granulomatous disease, since false-positive examinations have been reported in association with granulomatous inflammation.[143]

In a study comparing the accuracy of integrated FDG-PET/CT scanning with dynamic CT scanning for pulmonary nodule characterization, FDG-PET/CT scanning was found to be more sensitive and accurate than dynamic CT scanning. The sensitivity, specificity, and accuracy for malignancy with dynamic CT scanning were 81%, 93%, and 85%, respectively, whereas the values for PET/CT scanning were 96%, 88%, and 93%, respectively.[144] Assessment of multiple pulmonary nodules using FDG-PET is limited because of false-positive findings in instances of active granulomatous disease, such as tuberculosis, fungal disease, sarcoidosis, or rheumatoid lesions. In this setting, pattern recognition on CT, in combination with FDG-PET, may improve characterization of the lesions.

Guidelines from the American College of Chest Physicians (ACCP) recommend use of FDG-PET in patients where the probability of cancer is low or moderate (5%–60%) and an indeterminate nodule measures at least 8 to 10 mm.[140] Current National Comprehensive Cancer Network (NCCN) guidelines version 4.2014 recommend FDG-PET for the diagnosis of suspected NSCLC in solid, noncalcified pulmonary nodules >8 mm in diameter.[145] PET/CT scan is not recommended as a screening tool for healthy individuals, since the likelihood of finding cancer is extremely low and the risk increased with detecting harmless findings that may lead to more tests or invasive procedures.[66]

We wish to point out that the data in the literature are based on assigning standard ROIs to the lesions visualized by FDG-PET. Unfortunately, because of the limited spatial resolution of PET imaging, along with respiratory motion of pulmonary lesions, the SUVs generated by this approach result in substantial underestimation of values; the degree of underestimation is proportional to the size of the lesion and the degree of respiratory motion. The physical factors described are known as the "partial volume effect" and, as such, introduce substantial errors to the quantitative data from PET studies, particularly those performed in the evaluation of pulmonary nodules.[146] Therefore, methodologies that can correct for partial volume effects should be employed for accurate measurement of metabolic activity of the lesions assessed. By adopting this approach, significant changes will be noted in the SUVs in most clinical settings. Therefore, total reliance on what has been described in the literature will result in significant mismanagement of patients with SPNs.[147] In particular, adopting an SUV of 2.5 as a threshold for separating malignant and benign lesions is fraught with error and should be abandoned. Many lesions that are smaller than 3 or 4 cm will be prone to such errors.

USE OF POSITRON EMISSION TOMOGRAPHY IN LUNG CANCER

The application of FDG-PET in assessing NSCLC is considered later, followed by a discussion of FDG-PET in small cell lung cancer.

Nonsmall Cell Lung Carcinoma

A major role of FDG-PET is in the staging of NSCLC. Correct lung cancer staging is important because treatment options and prognosis vary significantly by stage. FDG-PET imaging may have a significant impact on patient management by identifying unsuspected sites of disease and by guiding selection of a biopsy site (Fig. 32-14). Similarly, a negative PET scan indicates a low likelihood for malignancy and supports use of conservative management and follow-up (Fig. 32-15). Patients with stage I or II NSCLC are typically referred for surgical resection, while those with stage III or stage IV disease are almost never surgical candidates; in these advanced stages, chemotherapy, radiation therapy, or both may be offered.

The basis for staging NSCLC is the TNM system. For T (tumor) staging, CT and MRI remain the best imaging modalities to demonstrate the local extent of the tumor and its relationship to adjacent organs and vessels. FDG-PET is limited for T staging due to its inability to accurately define the tumor limits. However, FDG-PET/CT has demonstrated a clear advantage in T staging of certain cases, especially in areas of postobstructive atelectasis[148] or low CT density variation and may in the future replace CT and MRI alone for this purpose.[149,150]

In a prospective study of 50 patients with NSCLC, integrated FDG-PET/CT provided additional diagnostic information in 41% of patients and was significantly more accurate in TNM disease staging than either PET or CT alone.[151] Integrated PET/CT provides important clinical information by virtue of accurate localization of known disease and identification of lesions that do not consistently accumulate FDG, such as carcinoid tumors and adenocarcinoma *in situ* (bronchioloalveolar cell carcinoma).[151] PET/CT without contrast-enhanced CT is unable to distinguish confined, centrally located tumors from those producing direct invasion of mediastinal structures. Therefore, clinicians may still rely on contrast-enhanced CT scans to help define mediastinal vascular invasion. From a prognostic point of view, FDG uptake in NSCLC has been correlated with tumor growth rate, aggressiveness, and proliferation capacity, and it has been found to be an independent prognostic factor correlated with survival in patients with NSCLC, especially early-stage disease.[152]

Mediastinal nodal staging most often determines appropriateness for surgical resection. Mediastinal staging using CT scanning is based primarily on assessment of lymph node size; nodes <1 cm in their short axis are considered benign, while those >1 cm are considered potentially malignant. Unfortunately, up to 21% of nodes <1 cm are malignant, and up to 40% of nodes >1 cm are benign.[153,154] A systematic review of the medical literature relating to the accuracy of CT scanning for noninvasive staging of the mediastinum in patients with lung cancer showed a sensitivity and specificity of 51% and 86%, respectively.[155] A large meta-analysis reported the median sensitivity and specificity of CT scanning for identifying malignant mediastinal nodes as 61% and 79%, respectively.[156] These results were similar to an earlier meta-analysis that reported an average sensitivity and specificity of 60% and 77% for CT scanning, respectively (using a transaxial short axis >1.0 cm).[157] In that same meta-analysis of 14 studies (514 patients) for FDG-PET and 29 studies (2,226 patients) for FDG-PET/CT, sensitivity and

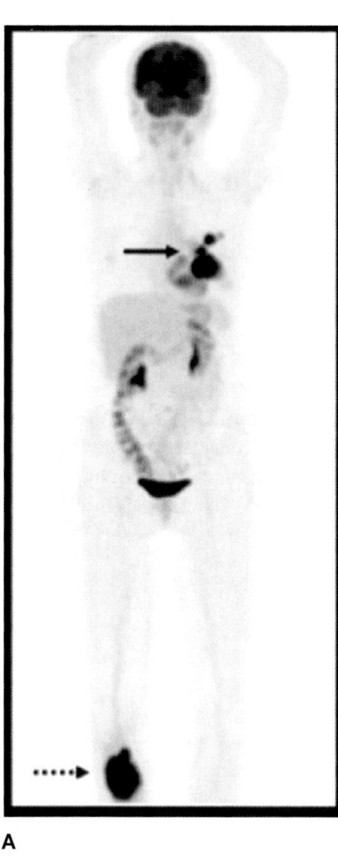

A

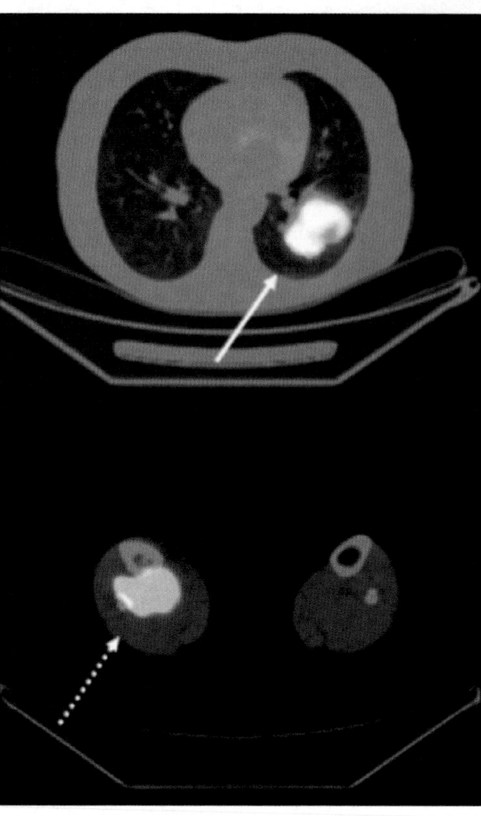

B

Figure 32-14 Lung cancer. Preoperative evaluation of a patient with a lung cancer in the left lower lobe intended for curative surgery. Whole-body maximum intensity projection PET (**A**) and fused transaxial PET/CT (**B**) show increased FDG uptake in the lung tumor *(solid arrows)*, and unexpected focal FDG uptake in a soft tissue mass in the left proximal tibia *(interrupted arrows)*. Biopsy showed metastasis from the lung cancer obviating surgery.

specificity were higher for determining nodal status in patients with NSCLC (sensitivity and specificity of 79% and 91%, respectively).[157]

The accuracy of FDG-PET in the evaluation of mediastinal lymph nodes depends on the size of the nodes. As reported in a large meta-analysis of 39 studies, the sensitivity and specificity of FDG-PET was 100% and 78%, respectively, in patients with enlarged mediastinal lymph nodes.[156] Sensitivity and specificity were 82% and 93%, respectively, for normal-sized nodes.[156] Positive PET findings in this situation should be confirmed by directed biopsy, as inflammatory or infectious processes can lead to false-positive results. Absence of tissue diagnosis could result in patients with surgically resectable disease being denied curative surgery.

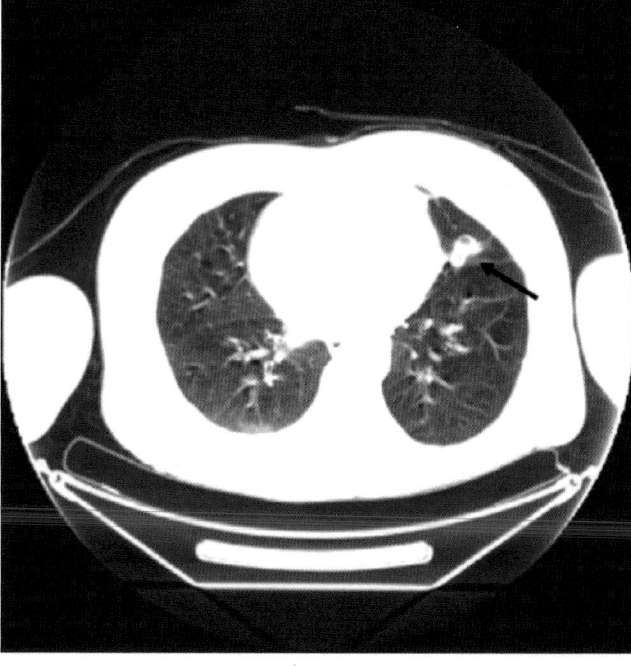

A

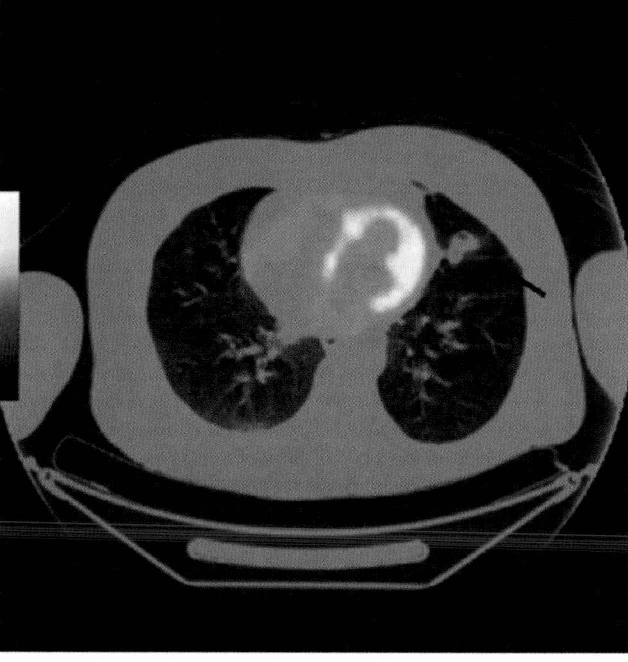

B

Figure 32-15 Suspected lung cancer. CT scan (**A**) shows a mass suspected of malignancy *(arrow)*. Transaxial fused PET/CT (**B**) shows no abnormal FDG uptake in the mass *(arrow)* consistent with benign process. There is slight misalignment between CT and PET images, but this had no bearing on the interpretation.

Exact classification as N1 or N2 disease is somewhat difficult using FDG-PET alone; anatomic information provided by a CT scan as part of combined FDG-PET/CT imaging is important for this purpose. Integrated PET/CT scanners combine the advantages of both studies, but there are as yet few studies addressing the accuracy of this modality. In one study, the accuracy of mediastinal lymph node staging increased from 89% with FDG-PET alone to 93% with FDG-PET/CT, compared to 63% with CT; a change in the planned treatment was noted in up to 15% of patients.[154] In another study, FDG-PET/CT was significantly better than CT alone for nodal staging: Sensitivity rose from 70% for CT to 85% for FDG-PET/CT; specificity rose from 69% to 84%; and accuracy rose from 69% to 84%.[158] FDG-PET is the best modality to detect tumor in normal-size lymph nodes.

Using an SUVmax of 2.5 is a reasonable threshold for distinguishing between benignity and malignancy, but SUV may be falsely low in lymph node <1 cm due to partial volume effect, and visual assessment is generally accurate.[159] Lymph nodes containing calcification are more likely to be benign, even if they accumulate FDG.[160] Interestingly, studies have shown that FDG-PET/CT has a lower specificity and accuracy for nodes >1 cm compared with those <1 cm, but it still performs better for large lymph nodes than does CT alone.[161,162] The incidence of false-positive nodes is generally larger than that of true-negative nodes as staged by FDG-PET.[162] For patients with stage II or III disease, the incidence of false-negative results is higher with PET than with mediastinoscopy (11.7% and 3%, respectively).[163] These studies illustrate an important limitation of FDG-PET. Therefore, this modality is not currently considered the "gold standard" for confirmation or exclusion of N2/N3 disease in patients with NSCLC.

The variability in false-positive examinations suggests that FDG-PET results should not replace histologic confirmation for suspected mediastinal nodal metastases.[164] FDG-PET–positive lymph nodes still require pathologic confirmation, usually by mediastinoscopy. Other choices of nodal sampling include transbronchial, transthoracic, or transesophageal needle aspiration, or more extensive surgery. These invasive procedures may be guided by the PET findings, as mediastinoscopy is limited to the anterior mediastinum; in addition, approximately 15% of patients may still be found to have N2 disease at thoracotomy.[165] The use of intraoperative FDG-sensitive gamma probes to guide lymph node sampling following the injection of FDG may be helpful.[166]

While studies have demonstrated that patients with metastases detected at mediastinoscopy have a worse prognosis than patients in whom N2 disease is found only at surgery,[167,168] no prospective studies have yet been conducted to determine whether patients with negative mediastinal nodes on preoperative FDG-PET have a similar prognosis to those in whom N2 disease is found at thoracotomy following a negative mediastinoscopy. Therefore, mediastinoscopy still remains part of the standard protocol for mediastinal staging.[163] Guidelines from the ACCP recommend the use of FDG-PET to evaluate for mediastinal and extrathoracic disease in the staging of patients with clinical IA, IB to IIIB lung cancer being treated with curative intent.[140] Patients with abnormal FDG-PET scan need sampling of abnormal lymph nodes prior to surgical resection of the primary tumor.[140]

In addition to being the most accurate noninvasive imaging modality available to evaluate the mediastinum in patients with lung cancer, whole-body FDG-PET imaging is useful in evaluating extrathoracic sites for possible metastatic disease. FDG-PET is superior to conventional imaging in detecting distant metastases. In one prospective study, FDG-PET showed a high sensitivity and specificity in the detection of distant metastases alone (92% and 83%, respectively); 11% of patients had distant metastases detected by FDG-PET that other modalities had failed to detect.[164] Detection of unsuspected extrathoracic metastases may be identified in 6% to 24% of patients (mean frequency of about 13%), and the likelihood for detecting unsuspected metastases increases with the patient's stage.[163] This is particularly important in patients with locally advanced stage III lung cancer.[169] In one multicenter trial, addition of FDG-PET to the conventional workup prevented unnecessary surgery in one out of five patients with suspected NSCLC, with a 50% decrease in futile thoracotomy in comparison to a conventional workup.[170] The likelihood for occult metastatic disease at presentation can be found in up to 30% of patients with adenocarcinoma or large cell carcinoma, but is less common with squamous cell carcinoma (under 15% of patients).[163]

The two most common sites for NSCLC metastases are the adrenal glands and bone marrow. Studies have shown that FDG-PET has a sensitivity of 93% to 100% for the characterization of metastatic adrenal lesions in patients with bronchogenic carcinoma (specificity, 80%–100% and accuracy, 92%–100%).[171–173] Necrotic or hemorrhagic adrenal metastases and small lesions can lead to false-negative FDG-PET.[173] Despite the fact that benign adrenal adenomas generally demonstrate mild FDG uptake that is less than the liver, false-positive studies may still occur.[172] FDG-PET/CT can improve characterization of adrenal masses by improving the specificity based on the combination of SUV and CT attenuation.[174] A Hounsfield Unit (HU) measurement of <10 is indicative of a benign adrenal lesion, even if the SUV measurement is >3.1.[174]

In detecting bone marrow metastases, a comparison of ^{99m}Tc methylene diphosphonate (^{99m}Tc MDP) standard bone scintigraphy to FDG-PET showed a higher accuracy with FDG-PET, (96% vs. 66%).[175] FDG-PET may detect bone marrow metastases before reactive bone formation takes place or prior to development of gross anatomic abnormalities. In a comparison of FDG-PET/CT to ^{99m}Tc MDP and ^{18}F-fluorine PET (F-PET), FDG-PET/CT had a lower sensitivity than F-PET, but was superior to ^{99m}Tc MDP. However, FDG-PET/CT had a higher specificity.[176]

Numerous benign skeletal conditions (including trauma, infection, and physiologic variants) may cause a false-positive FDG-PET. A recent meta-analysis of 17 studies addressed this issue comparing FDG-PET/CT, FDG-PET, MRI, and ^{99m}Tc MDP. The pooled sensitivity of each modality in the detection of bone marrow metastases was 92%, 87%, 77%, and 86%; the specificity was 98%, 94%, 92%, and 88%, respectively.[177]

In the initial evaluation for brain metastases in patients with NSCLC, FDG-PET brain imaging does not provide additional clinical information.[178] Current ACCP recommendations for patients with clinical stage IIIA and IIIB NSCLC are to obtain routine imaging for extrathoracic metastases, including a head CT scan or MRI, plus either whole-body FDG-PET or bone scan plus abdominal imaging.[140]

Until recently, radiation therapy planning has been based on CT imaging because of its excellent delineation of structures in attaining precise assignments of the radiation portals. However, a number of studies have demonstrated the added benefit of PET in defining and refining radiation treatment volumes, thereby reducing (or increasing) the radiation portal and allowing an increase in dose delivery to target tissues, as well as eliminating exposure to normal tissues to avoid toxicity from this therapy.[179] PET/CT is particularly helpful in planning radiation therapy for patients with lung cancer associated with atelectasis. In a prospective study of 76 patients, 34% of patients eligible for radical radiation therapy after conventional staging received palliative therapies instead because of FDG-PET/CT-based detection of advanced disease.[180] FDG-PET/CT frequently changed the planning target volume, which was associated with excellent survival.[180]

FDG-PET imaging may allow for better evaluation of the response to treatment than anatomic imaging, and it may also provide prognostic information that correlates strongly with survival rate following initiation of therapy (Fig. 32-16).[181] Assessment of prognosis can be improved with early FDG-PET imaging, as a 50% decrease in SUV between scans performed at 1 and 3 weeks following initiation of chemotherapy was shown to predict a favorable response.[182]

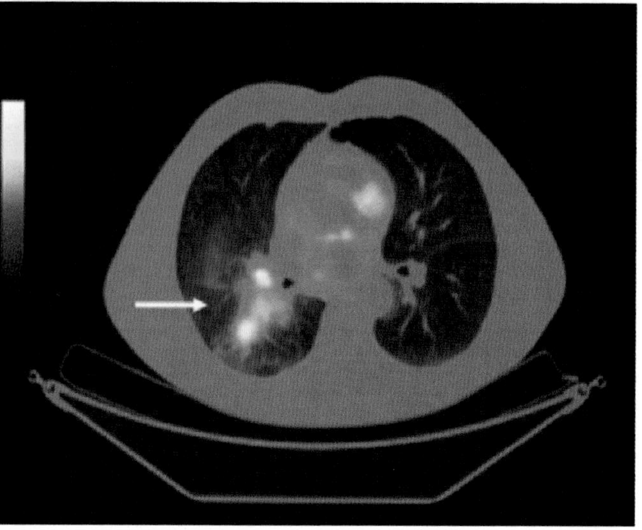

A

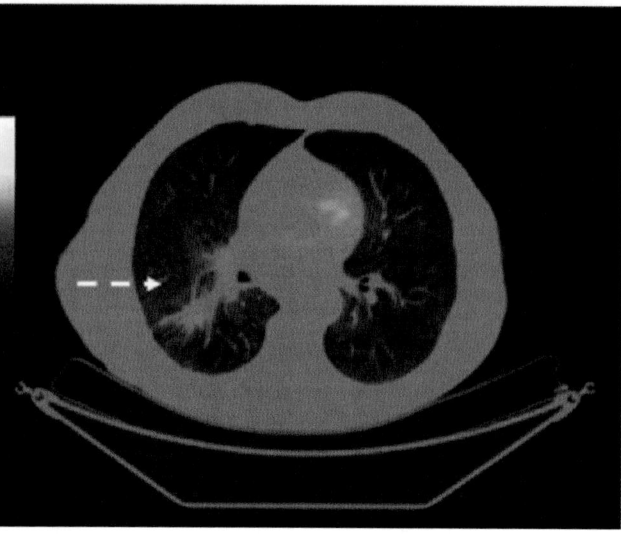

B

Figure 32-16 Treatment response in lung cancer. Fused transaxial PET/CT scan at baseline (**A**) showed marked FDG uptake in a tumor in the right lung hilum and mediastinal lymph nodes *(solid arrow)*. Repeat scan (**B**) after three cycles of chemotherapy reveals marked response to treatment *(interrupted arrow)*.

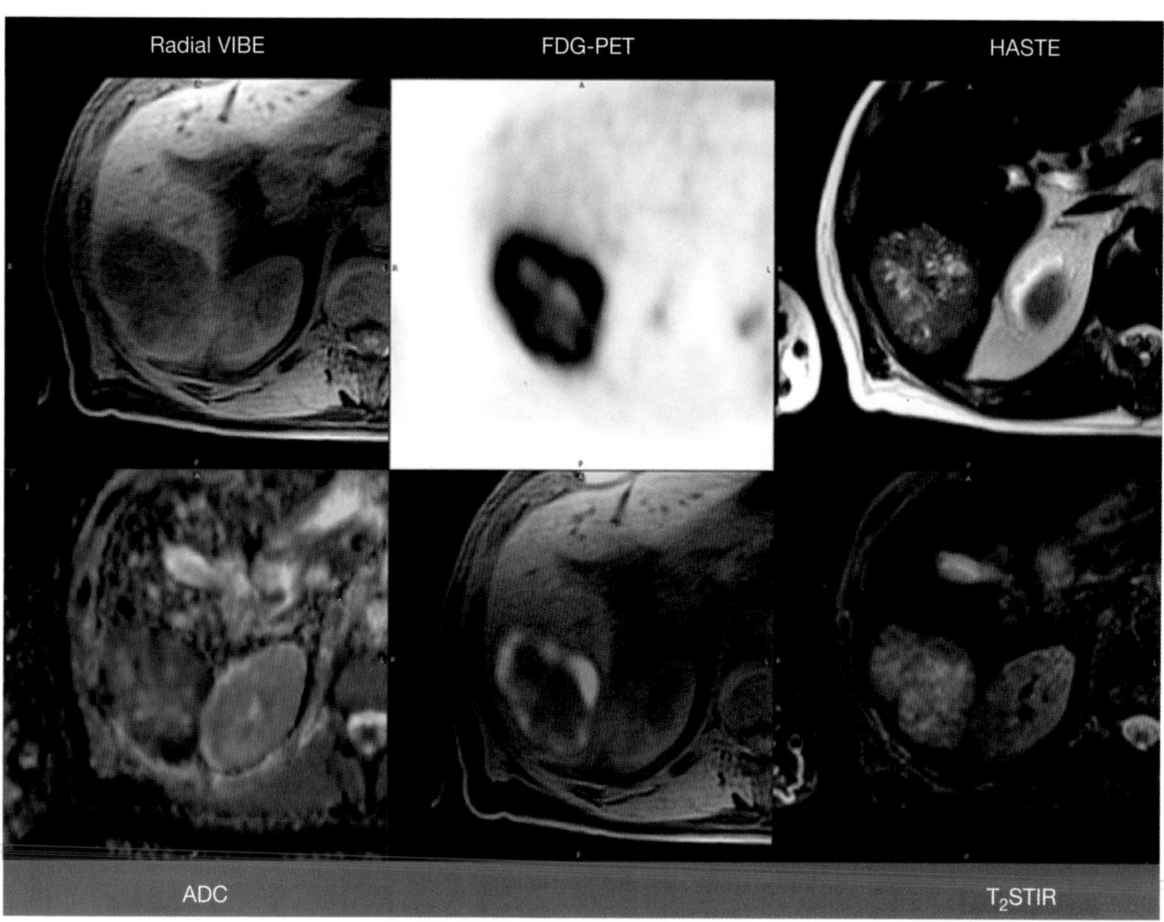

Figure 32-17 A 72-year-old male with lung cancer and liver metastases. Multisequence PET/MR of the liver demonstrates excellent co-registration of PET and multiple MRI sequences. Simultaneous acquisition maximizes accuracy of image registration and facilitates voxel-to-voxel correlations to support quantitative imaging. *(Used with permission of Dr. Kent Friedman. Department of Radiology. Nuclear Medicine Section. New York University School of Medicine, New York, USA.)*

In patients with residual parenchymal abnormalities following radiotherapy for lung cancer, FDG-PET scanning can be used to distinguish between persistent or recurrent cancer and radiation fibrosis.[183] In a study evaluating changes in FDG uptake following definitive radiation therapy, the higher the residual SUVmax in the primary tumor (cutoff, 3.7) or lymph nodes (cutoff, 3.1), the worse was the prognosis.[183] FDG-PET is also useful in assessing response to percutaneous radiofrequency ablation of NSCLC.[184] The novel hybrid method PET/MRI is emerging and shows great potential in lung cancer management (Fig. 32-17).

Small Cell Lung Carcinoma

Small cell lung carcinoma (SCLC) accounts for 18% to 25% of cases of lung cancer. SCLC has a high proliferation rate that results in avid FDG uptake.[185] At presentation, patients are either considered to have limited disease (LD), in which tumor is confined to unilateral chest, or extensive disease (ED), in which tumor has spread to contralateral chest or distant sites. Approximately 60% to 70% of patients present with ED, while 30% to 40% of patients have LD. Except in rare cases of surgically operable, limited-stage SCLC, patients with LD receive chemotherapy and radiation; those with ED are treated with chemotherapy alone. The role of FDG-PET in the staging of SCLC remains controversial, but it may change management in up to 37% of patients for initial staging, and in up to 15% of patients for restaging.[185] Complete metabolic response on posttherapeutic FDG-PET/CT in patients with SCLC is an important prognostic factor, as overall survival is significantly longer compared with that for patients who do not have a complete response.[186]

Mesothelioma

Benign fibrous mesothelioma is a rare, nonmalignant, localized tumor of the pleura that is unrelated to asbestos exposure. The tumor can be cured by excisional surgery. In contrast, malignant pleural mesothelioma (MPM), which is a rare cancer, is the most common primary pleural neoplasm. Affected patients have a median survival of 12 to 18 months. Thus, it is important to differentiate between benign pleural lesions and MPM. The radiologic appearances of benign and malignant pleural diseases are very similar. More than 50% of patients have a pleural effusion at the time of diagnosis; however, pleural fluid cytology is positive in only approximately 25%.[187] Reverse bevel needle biopsy and CT-guided percutaneous needle biopsy of the pleura have low sensitivities of about 21% to 43% and 25% to 60%, respectively.[187] Distinction based on histopathologic criteria is also difficult.

Currently, definitive diagnosis is based on video-assisted thoracoscopic surgery (VATS) (sensitivity, 90%), which, for MPM, carries the risk of tumor seeding along the operative tract. Therefore, radiation therapy is performed to all entry ports following the procedure. CT scan and MRI cannot always differentiate between benign and malignant pleural processes and are of limited value in staging of MPM.[188] Findings from CT and MRI studies can be used in tandem with those from FDG-PET in managing these difficult patients (Fig. 32-18).

Use of FDG-PET in mesothelioma in the mid-90s provided a paradigm shift in the management of patients with this serious cancer.[189] Because of the rarity of this disease, only limited studies have been performed, but FDG-PET has shown promising results in differentiating MPM from benign pleural disease. FDG uptake in MPM is significantly greater in benign pleural disease.[190] For the first time, this approach allowed separating malignant transformations from those that were purely related to inflammatory reactions. This significantly improved the clinician's ability to determine the sites of biopsy in this population. The degree of metabolic activity of the lesion has been shown to correlate with survival[191]; higher FDG uptake in MPM is associated with significantly shorter survival.[188] Using the single SUV cutoff technique, however, may not be the optimal approach. Dual-time point imaging and SUVmax on FDG-PET/CT in the delayed phase (120 minutes) have been found to be more reliable, diagnostic, and prognostic factors than that in the early phase (60 minutes)[192]; dual-time point imaging enhances the role of FDG-PET in this population.[193] This approach allows separation of malignant from inflammatory lesions. While malignant lesions show increasing activity over time, inflammatory lesions show a decline. In recent years, global disease assessment has become feasible using modern quantitative techniques. In general, it provides a single number expressing the disease activity in the entire body as one summed score, "the global disease burden," instead of assessing the parameters independently on a per-lesion basis.[194] The so-called "image segmentation methodologies" permit better definition of the boundaries of malignant lesions based on PET images and determination of lesional and whole-body metabolic burden.[194]

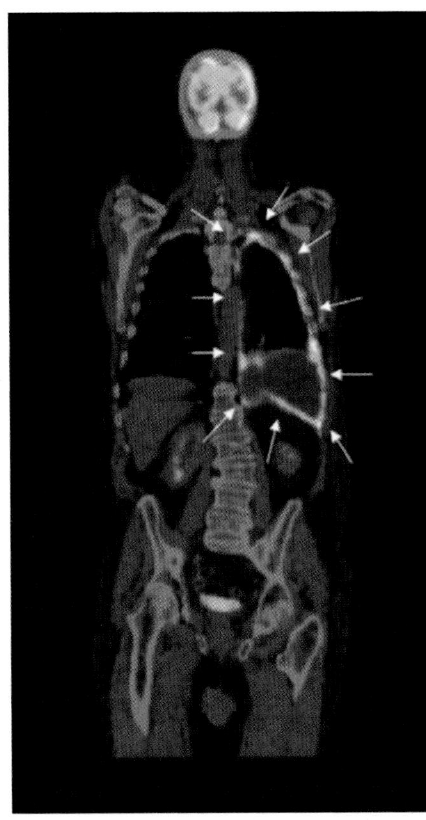

Figure 32-18 Transaxial coronal view of FDG-PET/CT scan demonstrating diffusely increased FDG activity throughout the diaphragmatic, mediastinal, and lateral left pleura, consistent with malignant mesothelioma.

In addition to differentiating benign from malignant pleural disease and facilitating assessment of prognosis in MPM, FDG-PET has shown good results in staging, planning of radiotherapy, evaluation of therapy response, and posttreatment surveillance.[194] In a study of 15 patients, FDG-PET upstaged 13% of patients, downstaged 27% of patients, and changed management in 20% of cases.[195] In another study of 29 patients, FDG-PET/CT had a major impact on increasing the accuracy of MPM-TNM staging and determining appropriate therapy.[196]

Finally, FDG-PET is useful in identifying the extent of disease locally and in the mediastinum. In addition, it is helpful in evaluating abnormal findings in the contralateral lung, and in detecting occult extrathoracic metastases. The metabolic response after neoadjuvant chemotherapy, as determined by FDG-PET, was found to be an independent prognostic factor for patients with resectable MPM, thereby helping to determine which patients are good candidates for extrapleural pneumonectomy.[197]

REFERENCES

1. Knipping HW, Bolt W, Venrath H, Valentin H, Ludes H, Endler P. [A new method of heart and lung function testing, the regional functional analysis in the lung and heart clinic by the radioactive noble gas xenon 133 (isotope thoracography)]. *Dtsch Med Wochenschr.* 1955;80(31-32):1146–1147.
2. West JB, Dollery CT. Distribution of blood flow and ventilation-perfusion ratio in the lung, measured with radioactive carbon dioxide. *J Appl Physiol.* 1960;15:405–410.
3. Newhouse MT, Wright FJ, Ingham GK, Archer NP, Hughes LB, Hopkins OL. Use of scintillation camera and 133-xenon for study of topographic pulmonary function. *Respir Physiol.* 1968;4(2):141–153.
4. Ueda H, Iio M, Kaihara S. Determination of regional pulmonary blood flow in various cardiopulmonary disorders. Study and application of macroaggregated albumin (Maa) labelled with I-131 (I). *Jpn Heart J.* 1964;190:431–444.
5. Ciofetta G, Piepsz A, Roca I, et al. Guidelines for lung scintigraphy in children. *Eur J Nucl Med Mol Imaging.* 2007;34(9): 1518–1526.
6. Melsom MN, Flatebo T, Kramer-Johansen J, et al. Both gravity and non-gravity dependent factors determine regional blood flow within the goat lung. *Acta Physiol Scand.* 1995;153(4): 343–353.
7. Carvalho P, Lavender JP. The incidence and etiology of the ventilation/perfusion reverse mismatch defect. *Clin Nucl Med.* 1989;14(8):571–576.
8. Hawker FH, Torzillo PJ, Southee AE. PEEP and "reverse mismatch". A case where less PEEP is best. *Chest.* 1991;99(4): 1034–1036.
9. Palmaz JC, Barnett CA, Reich SB, Krumpe PE, Farrer PA. Reverse ventilation–perfusion mismatch. *Clin Nucl Med.* 1984;9(1):6–9.
10. Dollery CT, Gillam PM. The distribution of blood and gas within the lungs measured by scanning after administration of 133xe. *Thorax.* 1963;18:316–325.
11. Coates G, O'Brodovich H. Measurement of pulmonary epithelial permeability with 99mTc-DTPA aerosol. *Semin Nucl Med.* 1986;16(4):275–284.
12. Sundram FX. Clinical studies of alveolar-capillary permeability using technetium-99m DTPA aerosol. *Ann Nucl Med.* 1995;9(4):171–178.
13. Jogi J, Jonson B, Ekberg M, Bajc M. Ventilation-perfusion SPECT with 99mTc-DTPA versus Technegas: a head-to-head study in obstructive and nonobstructive disease. *J Nucl Med.* 2010;51(5):735–741.
14. Scalzetti EM, Gagne GM. The transition from technegas to pertechnegas. *J Nucl Med.* 1995;36(2):267–269.
15. Worsley DF, Alavi A. Radionuclide imaging of acute pulmonary embolism. *Semin Nucl Med.* 2003;33(4):259–278.
16. Ozsu S, Oztuna F, Bulbul Y, et al. The role of risk factors in delayed diagnosis of pulmonary embolism. *Am J Emerg Med.* 2011;29(1):26–32.
17. Goldhaber SZ, Bounameaux H. Pulmonary embolism and deep vein thrombosis. *Lancet.* 2012;379(9828):1835–1846.
18. Heit JA. The epidemiology of venous thromboembolism in the community: implications for prevention and management. *J Thromb Thrombolysis.* 2006;21(1):23–29.
19. Park B, Messina L, Dargon P, Huang W, Ciocca R, Anderson FA. Recent trends in clinical outcomes and resource utilization for pulmonary embolism in the United States: findings from the nationwide inpatient sample. *Chest.* 2009;136(4):983–990.
20. Silverstein MD, Heit JA, Mohr DN, Petterson TM, O'Fallon WM, Melton LJ 3rd. Trends in the incidence of deep vein thrombosis and pulmonary embolism: a 25-year population-based study. *Arch Intern Med.* 1998;158(6):585–593.
21. Skaf E, Stein PD, Beemath A, Sanchez J, Olson RE. Fatal pulmonary embolism and stroke. *Am J Cardiol.* 2006;97(12): 1776–1777.
22. Hunt JM, Bull TM. Clinical review of pulmonary embolism: diagnosis, prognosis, and treatment. *Med Clin North Am.* 2011;95(6): 1203–1222.
23. The urokinase pulmonary embolism trial. A national cooperative study. *Circulation.* 1973;47(2 suppl):II1–II108.
24. Hull RD, Raskob GE, Ginsberg JS, et al. A noninvasive strategy for the treatment of patients with suspected pulmonary embolism. *Arch Intern Med.* 1994;154(3):289–297.
25. Wells PS, Ginsberg JS, Anderson DR, et al. Use of a clinical model for safe management of patients with suspected pulmonary embolism. *Ann Intern Med.* 1998;129(12):997–1005.
26. Miniati M, Pistolesi M, Marini C, et al. Value of perfusion lung scan in the diagnosis of pulmonary embolism: results of the Prospective Investigative Study of Acute Pulmonary Embolism Diagnosis (PISA-PED). *Am J Respir Crit Care Med.* 1996;154(5):1387–1393.
27. Stein PD, Gottschalk A. Critical review of ventilation/perfusion lung scans in acute pulmonary embolism. *Prog Cardiovasc Dis.* 1994;37(1):13–24.
28. Rajendran JG, Jacobson AF. Review of 6-month mortality following low-probability lung scans. *Arch Intern Med.* 1999;159(4): 349–352.
29. Remy-Jardin M, Remy J, Wattinne L, Giraud F. Central pulmonary thromboembolism: diagnosis with spiral volumetric CT with the single-breath-hold technique–comparison with pulmonary angiography. *Radiology.* 1992;185(2):381–387.
30. Stein PD, Fowler SE, Goodman LR, et al. Multidetector computed tomography for acute pulmonary embolism. *N Engl J Med.* 2006;354(22):2317–2327.
31. Freeman LM, Haramati LB. V/Q scintigraphy: alive, well and equal to the challenge of CT angiography. *Eur J Nucl Med Mol Imaging.* 2009;36(3):499–504.
32. Goodman LR, Stein PD, Matta F, et al. CT venography and compression sonography are diagnostically equivalent: data from PIOPED II. *AJR Am J Roentgenol.* 2007;189(5): 1071–1076.
33. Stein PD, Chenevert TL, Fowler SE, et al. Gadolinium-enhanced magnetic resonance angiography for pulmonary embolism: a multicenter prospective study (PIOPED III). *Ann Intern Med.* 2010;152(7):434–443, W142–W143.
34. The PIOPED Investigators. Value of the ventilation/perfusion scan in acute pulmonary embolism. Results of the prospective investigation of pulmonary embolism diagnosis (PIOPED). *JAMA.* 1990;263(20):2753–2759.

35. Hagen PJ, Hartmann IJ, Hoekstra OS, Stokkel MP, Teule GJ, Prins MH. How to use a gestalt interpretation for ventilation-perfusion lung scintigraphy. *J Nucl Med.* 2002;43(10):1317–1323.

36. Hagen PJ, Hartmann IJ, Hoekstra OS, et al. Comparison of observer variability and accuracy of different criteria for lung scan interpretation. *J Nucl Med.* 2003;44(5):739–744.

37. Worsley DF, Kim CK, Alavi A, et al. Detailed analysis of patients with matched ventilation-perfusion defects and chest radiographic opacities. *J Nucl Med.* 1993;34(11):1851–1853.

38. Sostman HD, Gottschalk A. Prospective validation of the stripe sign in ventilation-perfusion scintigraphy. *Radiology.* 1992;184(2):455–459.

39. Gottschalk A, Sostman HD, Coleman RE, et al. Ventilation-perfusion scintigraphy in the PIOPED study. Part II. Evaluation of the scintigraphic criteria and interpretations. *J Nucl Med.* 1993;34(7):1119–1126.

40. Sostman HD, Stein PD, Gottschalk A, et al. Acute pulmonary embolism: sensitivity and specificity of ventilation-perfusion scintigraphy in PIOPED II study. *Radiology.* 2008;246(3):941–946.

41. Sostman HD, Miniati M, Gottschalk A, Matta F, Stein PD, Pistolesi M. Sensitivity and specificity of perfusion scintigraphy combined with chest radiography for acute pulmonary embolism in PIOPED II. *J Nucl Med.* 2008;49(11):1741–1748.

42. Reid JH, Coche EE, Inoue T, et al. Is the lung scan alive and well? Facts and controversies in defining the role of lung scintigraphy for the diagnosis of pulmonary embolism in the era of MDCT. *Eur J Nucl Med Mol Imaging.* 2009;36(3):505–521.

43. Leblanc M, Leveillee F, Turcotte E. Prospective evaluation of the negative predictive value of V/Q SPECT using 99mTc-Technegas. *Nucl Med Commun.* 2007;28(8):667–672.

44. Stein PD, Freeman LM, Sostman HD, et al. SPECT in acute pulmonary embolism. *J Nucl Med.* 2009;50(12):1999–2007.

45. Collart JP, Roelants V, Vanpee D, et al. Is a lung perfusion scan obtained by using single photon emission computed tomography able to improve the radionuclide diagnosis of pulmonary embolism? *Nucl Med Commun.* 2002;23(11):1107–1113.

46. Bajc M, Olsson CG, Olsson B, et al. Diagnostic evaluation of planar and tomographic ventilation/perfusion lung images in patients with suspected pulmonary emboli. *Clin Physiol Funct Imaging.* 2004;24(5):249–256.

47. Reinartz P, Wildberger JE, Schaefer W, Nowak B, Mahnken AH, Buell U. Tomographic imaging in the diagnosis of pulmonary embolism: a comparison between V/Q lung scintigraphy in SPECT technique and multislice spiral CT. *J Nucl Med.* 2004;45(9):1501–1508.

48. Miles S, Rogers KM, Thomas P, et al. A comparison of single-photon emission CT lung scintigraphy and CT pulmonary angiography for the diagnosis of pulmonary embolism. *Chest.* 2009;136(6):1546–1553.

49. Gutte H, Mortensen J, Jensen CV, et al. Detection of pulmonary embolism with combined ventilation-perfusion SPECT and low-dose CT: head-to-head comparison with multidetector CT angiography. *J Nucl Med.* 2009;50(12):1987–1992.

50. Bajc M, Jonson B. Ventilation/perfusion SPECT–an essential but underrated method for diagnosis of pulmonary embolism and other diseases. *Eur J Nucl Med Mol Imaging.* 2009;36(5):875–878.

51. Stein PD, Sostman HD, Dalen JE, et al. Controversies in diagnosis of pulmonary embolism. *Clin Appl Thromb Hemost.* 2011;17(2):140–149.

52. Taillefer R. Radiolabeled peptides in the detection of deep venous thrombosis. *Semin Nucl Med.* 2001;31(2):102–123.

53. Morris TA, Gerometta M, Yusen RD, et al. Detection of pulmonary emboli with 99mTc-labeled anti-D-dimer (DI-80B3)Fab' fragments (ThromboView). *Am J Respir Crit Care Med.* 2011;184(6):708–714.

54. Schoepf UJ. Diagnosing pulmonary embolism: time to rewrite the textbooks. *Int J Cardiovasc Imaging.* 2005;21(1):155–163.

55. Remy-Jardin M, Pistolesi M, Goodman LR, et al. Management of suspected acute pulmonary embolism in the era of CT angiography: a statement from the Fleischner Society. *Radiology.* 2007;245(2):315–329.

56. Anderson DR, Kahn SR, Rodger MA, et al. Computed tomographic pulmonary angiography vs ventilation-perfusion lung scanning in patients with suspected pulmonary embolism: a randomized controlled trial. *JAMA.* 2007;298(23):2743–2753.

57. Burge AJ, Freeman KD, Klapper PJ, Haramati LB. Increased diagnosis of pulmonary embolism without a corresponding decline in mortality during the CT era. *Clin Radiol.* 2008;63(4):381–386.

58. Dentali F, Ageno W, Becattini C, et al. Prevalence and clinical history of incidental, asymptomatic pulmonary embolism: a meta-analysis. *Thromb Res.* 2010;125(6):518–522.

59. O'Connell CL, Razavi PA, Liebman HA. Symptoms adversely impact survival among patients with cancer and unsuspected pulmonary embolism. *J Clin Oncol.* 2011;29(31):4208–4209; author reply 4209–4210.

60. Hall WB, Truitt SG, Scheunemann LP, et al. The prevalence of clinically relevant incidental findings on chest computed tomographic angiograms ordered to diagnose pulmonary embolism. *Arch Intern Med.* 2009;169(21):1961–1965.

61. Becattini C, Agnelli G, Vedovati MC, et al. Multidetector computed tomography for acute pulmonary embolism: diagnosis and risk stratification in a single test. *Eur Heart J.* 2011;32(13):1657–1663.

62. Brenner DJ, Hall EJ. Computed tomography–an increasing source of radiation exposure. *N Engl J Med.* 2007;357(22):2277–2284.

63. Einstein AJ, Henzlova MJ, Rajagopalan S. Estimating risk of cancer associated with radiation exposure from 64-slice computed tomography coronary angiography. *JAMA.* 2007;298(3):317–323.

64. Parker MS, Hui FK, Camacho MA, Chung JK, Broga DW, Sethi NN. Female breast radiation exposure during CT pulmonary angiography. *AJR Am J Roentgenol.* 2005;185(5):1228–1233.

65. Radiation dose to patients from radiopharmaceuticals (addendum 2 to ICRP publication 53). *Ann ICRP.* 1998;28(3):1–126.

66. The Society of Nuclear Medicine and Molecular Imaging. SNMMI Participates in Choosing Wisely Campaign. http://www.snmmi.org/ClinicalPractice/content.aspx?ItemNumber=9914. Accessed September 2, 2014. Reston, VA: 2013.

67. Scarsbrook AF, Gleeson FV. Investigating suspected pulmonary embolism in pregnancy. *BMJ.* 2007;334(7590):418–419.

68. Hurwitz LM, Yoshizumi T, Reiman RE, et al. Radiation dose to the fetus from body MDCT during early gestation. *AJR Am J Roentgenol.* 2006;186(3):871–876.

69. Kanal E, Barkovich AJ, Bell C, et al. ACR guidance document for safe MR practices. *AJR Am J Roentgenol.* 2007;188(6): 1447–1474.

70. Chrysochou C, Power A, Shurrab AE, et al. Low risk for nephrogenic systemic fibrosis in nondialysis patients who have chronic kidney disease and are investigated with gadolinium-enhanced magnetic resonance imaging. *Clin J Am Soc Nephrol.* 2010;5(3):484–489.

71. Pengo V, Lensing AW, Prins MH, et al. Incidence of chronic thromboembolic pulmonary hypertension after pulmonary embolism. *N Engl J Med.* 2004;350(22):2257–2264.

72. Miniati M, Monti S, Bottai M, et al. Survival and restoration of pulmonary perfusion in a long-term follow-up of patients after acute pulmonary embolism. *Medicine (Baltimore).* 2006; 85(5):253–262.

73. Riedel M, Stanek V, Widimsky J, Prerovsky I. Long term follow-up of patients with pulmonary thromboembolism. Late prognosis and evolution of hemodynamic and respiratory data. *Chest.* 1982;81(2):151–158.

74. Tunariu N, Gibbs SJ, Win Z, et al. Ventilation-perfusion scintigraphy is more sensitive than multidetector CTPA in detecting chronic thromboembolic pulmonary disease as a treatable cause of pulmonary hypertension. *J Nucl Med.* 2007;48(5):680–684.

75. Fedullo P, Kerr KM, Kim NH, Auger WR. Chronic thromboembolic pulmonary hypertension. *Am J Respir Crit Care Med.* 2011;183(12):1605–1613.

76. Ryan KL, Fedullo PF, Davis GB, Vasquez TE, Moser KM. Perfusion scan findings understate the severity of angiographic and hemodynamic compromise in chronic thromboembolic pulmonary hypertension. *Chest.* 1988;93(6):1180–1185.

77. Engeler CE, Kuni CC, Tashjian JH, Engeler CM, du Cret RP. Regional alterations in lung ventilation in end-stage primary pulmonary hypertension: correlation between CT and scintigraphy. *AJR Am J Roentgenol.* 1995;164(4):831–835.

78. Bergin CJ, Sirlin CB, Hauschildt JP, et al. Chronic thromboembolism: diagnosis with helical CT and MR imaging with angiographic and surgical correlation. *Radiology.* 1997;204(3): 695–702.

79. Soler X, Hoh CK, Test VJ, Kerr KM, Marsh JJ, Morris TA. Single photon emission computed tomography in chronic thromboembolic pulmonary hypertension. *Respirology.* 2011;16(1): 131–137.

80. Wilkens H, Lang I, Behr J, et al. Chronic thromboembolic pulmonary hypertension (CTEPH): updated Recommendations of the Cologne Consensus Conference 2011. *Int J Cardiol.* 2011; 154(suppl 1):S54–S60.

81. Wang SC, Fischer KC, Slone RM, et al. Perfusion scintigraphy in the evaluation for lung volume reduction surgery: correlation with clinical outcome. *Radiology.* 1997;205(1):243–248.

82. Jamadar DA, Kazerooni EA, Martinez FJ, Wahl RL. Semi-quantitative ventilation/perfusion scintigraphy and single-photon emission tomography for evaluation of lung volume reduction surgery candidates: description and prediction of clinical outcome. *Eur J Nucl Med.* 1999;26(7):734–742.

83. Wilson H, Carby M, Beddow E. Lung volume reduction surgery for native lung hyperinflation following single-lung transplantation for emphysema: which patients? *Eur J Cardiothorac Surg.* 2012;42(3):410–413.

84. Washko GR, Hoffman E, Reilly JJ. Radiographic evaluation of the potential lung volume reduction surgery candidate. *Proc Am Thorac Soc.* 2008;5(4):421–426.

85. Fishman A, Martinez F, Naunheim K, et al. A randomized trial comparing lung-volume-reduction surgery with medical therapy for severe emphysema. *N Engl J Med.* 2003;348(21): 2059–2073.

86. Chenuel B, Haouzi P, Olivier P, Marie PY, Chalon B, Borrelly J. Effect of exercise on lung-perfusion scanning in patients with bronchogenic carcinoma. *Eur Respir J.* 2002;20(3):710–716.

87. Kotloff RM, Hansen-Flaschen J, Lipson DA, et al. Apical perfusion fraction as a predictor of short-term functional outcome following bilateral lung volume reduction surgery. *Chest.* 2001;120(5):1609–1615.

88. Zhu X, Zhao M, Liu C, Zhou J. Prediction of the postoperative pulmonary function in lung cancer patients with borderline function using ventilation-perfusion scintigraphy. *Nucl Med Commun.* 2012;33(3):283–287.

89. Wernly JA, DeMeester TR, Kirchner PT, Myerowitz PD, Oxford DE, Golomb HM. Clinical value of quantitative ventilation-perfusion lung scans in the surgical management of bronchogenic carcinoma. *J Thorac Cardiovasc Surg.* 1980; 80(4):535–543.

90. British Thoracic, Society, Society of Cardiothoracic Surgeons of Great Britain and Ireland Working Party. BTS guidelines: guidelines on the selection of patients with lung cancer for surgery. *Thorax.* 2001;56(2):89–108.

91. Krowka MJ, Wiseman GA, Burnett OL, et al. Hepatopulmonary syndrome: a prospective study of relationships between severity of liver disease, PaO(2) response to 100% oxygen, and brain uptake after (99 m)Tc MAA lung scanning. *Chest.* 2000;118(3): 615–624.

92. Madsen PH, Hess S, Madsen HD. A case of unexplained hypoxemia. *Respir Care.* 2012;57(11):1963–1966.

93. O'Doherty MJ, Peters AM. Pulmonary technetium-99m diethylene triamine penta-acetic acid aerosol clearance as an index of lung injury. *Eur J Nucl Med.* 1997;24(1):81–87.

94. Beadsmoore C, Cheow HK, Szczepura K, Szczepura K, Ruparelia P, Peters AM. Healthy passive cigarette smokers have increased pulmonary alveolar permeability. *Nucl Med Commun.* 2007; 28(2):75–77.

95. Regnis JA, Robinson M, Bailey DL, et al. Mucociliary clearance in patients with cystic fibrosis and in normal subjects. *Am J Respir Crit Care Med.* 1994;150(1):66–71.

96. Newman SP, Wilding IR, Hirst PH. Human lung deposition data: the bridge between in vitro and clinical evaluations for inhaled drug products? *Int J Pharm.* 2000;208(1–2):49–60.

97. Pavia D, Sutton PP, Lopez-Vidriero MT, Agnew JE, Clarke SW. Drug effects on mucociliary function. *Eur J Respir Dis Suppl.* 1983;128(Pt 1):304–317.

98. Delbeke D. Oncological applications of FDG PET imaging. *J Nucl Med.* 1999;40(10):1706–1715.

99. Bos R, van Der Hoeven JJ, van Der Wall E, et al. Biologic correlates of (18)fluorodeoxyglucose uptake in human breast cancer measured by positron emission tomography. *J Clin Oncol.* 2002; 20(2):379–387.

100. Benz MR, Evilevitch V, Allen-Auerbach MS, et al. Treatment monitoring by 18 F-FDG PET/CT in patients with sarcomas: interobserver variability of quantitative parameters in treatment-induced changes in histopathologically responding and nonresponding tumors. *J Nucl Med.* 2008;49(7):1038–1046.

101. Lodge MA, Chaudhry MA, Wahl RL. Noise considerations for PET quantification using maximum and peak standardized uptake value. *J Nucl Med.* 2012;53(7):1041–1047.

102. Brink JA. PET/CT unplugged: the merging technologies of PET and CT imaging. *AJR Am J Roentgenol*. 2005;184(5 suppl):S135–S137.

103. El Fakhri G, Surti S, Trott CM, Scheuermann J, Karp JS. Improvement in lesion detection with whole-body oncologic time-of-flight PET. *J Nucl Med*. 2011;52(3):347–353.

104. Osman MM, Cohade C, Nakamoto Y, Marshall LT, Leal JP, Wahl RL. Clinically significant inaccurate localization of lesions with PET/CT: frequency in 300 patients. *J Nucl Med*. 2003;44(2):240–243.

105. Kjaer A, Loft A, Law I, et al. PET/MRI in cancer patients: first experiences and vision from Copenhagen. *MAGMA*. 2013;26(1): 37–47.

106. El-Haddad G, Zhuang H, Gupta N, Alavi A. Evolving role of positron emission tomography in the management of patients with inflammatory and other benign disorders. *Semin Nucl Med*. 2004;34(4):313–329.

107. Hess S, Madsen PH, Basu S, Høilund-Carlsen PF, Alavi A. Potential role of FDG PET/CT imaging for assessing venous thromboembolic disorders. *Clin Nucl Med*. 2012;37(12): 1170–1172.

108. Nielsen AL, Thomassen A, Hess S, Alavi A, Høilund-Carlsen PF. Deep venous thrombosis and pulmonary embolism detected by FDG PET/CT in a patient with bacteremia. *Clin Nucl Med*. 2013;38(4):276–277.

109. Khandelwal AR, Li G, Takalkar AM. Incidental detection of unsuspected pulmonary embolism on oncologic FDG PET/CT imaging. *Clin Nucl Med*. 2011;36(8):720–722.

110. Hess S, Madsen PH, Iversen ED, Frifelt JJ, Hoilund-Carlsen PF, Alavi A. FDG-PET/CT for venous thromboembolic disorders: Preliminary results. *J Nucl Med*. 2013;54(suppl 2):2017.

111. Rondina MT, Lam UT, Pendleton RC, et al. (18)F-FDG PET in the evaluation of acuity of deep vein thrombosis. *Clin Nucl Med*. 2012;37(12):1139–1145.

112. Kwee TC, Torigian DA, Alavi A. Nononcological applications of positron emission tomography for evaluation of the thorax. *J Thorac Imaging*. 2013;28(1):25–39.

113. Sathekge M, Maes A, Kgomo M, Stoltz A, Van de Wiele C. Use of 18 F-FDG PET to predict response to first-line tuberculostatics in HIV-associated tuberculosis. *J Nucl Med*. 2011;52(6):880–885.

114. Grijm K, Verberne HJ, Krouwels FH, Weller FR, Jansen HM, Bresser P. Semiquantitative 67 Ga scintigraphy as an indicator of response to and prognosis after corticosteroid treatment in idiopathic interstitial pneumonia. *J Nucl Med*. 2005;46(9):1421–1426.

115. Keijsers RG, Grutters JC, Thomeer M, et al. Imaging the inflammatory activity of sarcoidosis: sensitivity and inter observer agreement of (67)Ga imaging and (18)F-FDG PET. *Q J Nucl Med Mol Imaging*. 2011;55(1):66–71.

116. Nishiyama Y, Yamamoto Y, Fukunaga K, et al. Comparative evaluation of 18 F-FDG PET and 67 Ga scintigraphy in patients with sarcoidosis. *J Nucl Med*. 2006;47(10):1571–1576.

117. Prager E, Wehrschuetz M, Bisail B, et al. Comparison of 18F-FDG and 67Ga-citrate in sarcoidosis imaging. *Nuklearmedizin*. 2008;47(1):18–23.

118. Braun JJ, Kessler R, Constantinesco A, Imperiale A. 18 F-FDG PET/CT in sarcoidosis management: review and report of 20 cases. *Eur J Nucl Med Mol Imaging*. 2008;35(8): 1537–1543.

119. Keijsers RG, Grutters JC, van Velzen-Blad H, van den Bosch JM, Oyen WJ, Verzijlbergen FJ. (18)F-FDG PET patterns and BAL cell profiles in pulmonary sarcoidosis. *Eur J Nucl Med Mol Imaging*. 2010;37(6):1181–1188.

120. Sobic-Saranovic D, Grozdic I, Videnovic-Ivanov J, et al. The utility of 18 F-FDG PET/CT for diagnosis and adjustment of therapy in patients with active chronic sarcoidosis. *J Nucl Med*. 2012;53(10):1543–1549.

121. Alavi A, Gupta N, Alberini JL, et al. Positron emission tomography imaging in nonmalignant thoracic disorders. *Semin Nucl Med*. 2002;32(4):293–321.

122. Chung SY, Lee JH, Kim TH, Kim SJ, Kim HJ, Ryu YH. 18 F-FDG PET imaging of progressive massive fibrosis. *Ann Nucl Med*. 2010;24(1):21–27.

123. Nusair S, Rubinstein R, Freedman NM, et al. Positron emission tomography in interstitial lung disease. *Respirology*. 2007;12(6):843–847.

124. Umeda Y, Demura Y, Ishizaki T, et al. Dual-time-point 18 F-FDG PET imaging for diagnosis of disease type and disease activity in patients with idiopathic interstitial pneumonia. *Eur J Nucl Med Mol Imaging*. 2009;36(7):1121–1130.

125. Ost D, Fein AM, Feinsilver SH. Clinical practice. The solitary pulmonary nodule. *N Engl J Med*. 2003;348(25):2535–2542.

126. Gould MK, Fletcher J, Iannettoni MD, et al. Evaluation of patients with pulmonary nodules: when is it lung cancer?: ACCP evidence-based clinical practice guidelines (2nd edition). *Chest*. 2007;132(3 suppl):108S–130S.

127. American Cancer Society. Lung cancer (non-mall cell). http://www.cancer.org/cancer/lungcancer-non-smallcell/detailedguide/non-small-cell-lung-cancer-key-statistics. Accessed September 2, 2014. Atlanta, GA: 2013.

128. Winer-Muram HT. The solitary pulmonary nodule. *Radiology*. 2006;239(1):34–49.

129. Gurney JW. Determining the likelihood of malignancy in solitary pulmonary nodules with Bayesian analysis. Part I. Theory. *Radiology*. 1993;186(2):405–413.

130. Lowe VJ, Fletcher JW, Gobar L, et al. Prospective investigation of positron emission tomography in lung nodules. *J Clin Oncol*. 1998;16(3):1075–1084.

131. Daniels CE, Lowe VJ, Aubry MC, Allen MS, Jett JR. The utility of fluorodeoxyglucose positron emission tomography in the evaluation of carcinoid tumors presenting as pulmonary nodules. *Chest*. 2007;131(1):255–260.

132. Gould MK, Maclean CC, Kuschner WG, et al. Accuracy of positron emission tomography for diagnosis of pulmonary nodules and mass lesions: a meta-analysis. *JAMA*. 2001;285(7): 914–924.

133. Erasmus JJ, McAdams HP, Patz EF Jr, Goodman PC, Coleman RE. Thoracic FDG PET: State of the art. *Radiographics*. 1998;18(1):5–20.

134. Lowe VJ, Hoffman JM, DeLong DM, Patz EF, Coleman RE. Semiquantitative and visual analysis of FDG-PET images in pulmonary abnormalities. *J Nucl Med*. 1994;35(11): 1771–1176.

135. Nomori H, Watanabe K, Ohtsuka T, Naruke T, Suemasu K, Uno K. Visual and semiquantitative analyses for F-18 fluorodeoxyglucose PET scanning in pulmonary nodules 1 cm to 3 cm in size. *Ann Thorac Surg*. 2005;79(3):984–988; discussion 989.

136. Hashimoto Y, Tsujikawa T, Kondo C, et al. Accuracy of PET for diagnosis of solid pulmonary lesions with 18 F-FDG uptake below the standardized uptake value of 2.5. *J Nucl Med*. 2006; 47(3):426–431.

137. Lee KS, Kim Y, Han J, Ko EJ, Park CK, Primack SL. Bronchioloalveolar carcinoma: clinical, histopathologic, and radiologic findings. *Radiographics.* 1997;17(6):1345–1357.

138. Fletcher JW, Kymes SM, Gould M, et al. A comparison of the diagnostic accuracy of 18 F-FDG PET and CT in the characterization of solitary pulmonary nodules. *J Nucl Med.* 2008;49(2):179–185.

139. Bastarrika G, Garcia-Velloso MJ, Lozano MD, et al. Early lung cancer detection using spiral computed tomography and positron emission tomography. *Am J Respir Crit Care Med.* 2005;171(12):1378–1383.

140. Silvestri GA, Gould MK, Margolis ML, et al. Noninvasive staging of non-small cell lung cancer: ACCP evidenced-based clinical practice guidelines (2nd edition). *Chest.* 2007;132(3 suppl): 178S–201S.

141. Matthies A, Hickeson M, Cuchiara A, Alavi A. Dual time point 18 F-FDG PET for the evaluation of pulmonary nodules. *J Nucl Med.* 2002;43(7):871–875.

142. Zhang L, Wang Y, Lei J, Tian J, Zhai Y. Dual time point 18FDG-PET/CT versus single time point 18FDG-PET/CT for the differential diagnosis of pulmonary nodules: a meta-analysis. *Acta Radiol.* 2013;54(7):770–777.

143. Chen CJ, Lee BF, Yao WJ, et al. Dual-phase 18 F-FDG PET in the diagnosis of pulmonary nodules with an initial standard uptake value less than 2.5. *AJR Am J Roentgenol.* 2008;191(2):475–479.

144. Yi CA, Lee KS, Kim BT, et al. Tissue characterization of solitary pulmonary nodule: comparative study between helical dynamic CT and integrated PET/CT. *J Nucl Med.* 2006;47(3):443–450.

145. National Comprehensive Cancer Network. NCCN Guidelines. http://www.nccn.org/professionals/physician_gls/f_guidelines.asp. Accessed September 2, 2014. Site Fort Washington, PA: 2013.

146. Hickeson M, Yun M, Matthies A, et al. Use of a corrected standardized uptake value based on the lesion size on CT permits accurate characterization of lung nodules on FDG-PET. *Eur J Nucl Med Mol Imaging.* 2002;29(12):1639–1647.

147. Kwee TC, Cheng G, Lam MG, Basu S, Alavi A. SUV of 2.5 should not be embraced as a magic threshold for separating benign from malignant lesions. *Eur J Nucl Med Mol Imaging.* 2013;40(10):1475–1477.

148. Cho A, Hur J, Kang WJ, et al. Usefulness of FDG PET/CT in determining benign from malignant endobronchial obstruction. *Eur Radiol.* 2011;21(5):1077–1087.

149. Yi CA, Shin KM, Lee KS, et al. Non-small cell lung cancer staging: efficacy comparison of integrated PET/CT versus 3.0-T whole-body MR imaging. *Radiology.* 2008;248(2):632–642.

150. Cuaron J, Dunphy M, Rimner A. Role of FDG-PET scans in staging, response assessment, and follow-up care for non-small cell lung cancer. *Front Oncol.* 2012;2:208.

151. Lardinois D, Weder W, Hany TF, et al. Staging of non-small-cell lung cancer with integrated positron-emission tomography and computed tomography. *N Engl J Med.* 2003;348(25):2500–2507.

152. Higashi K, Ueda Y, Arisaka Y, et al. 18 F-FDG uptake as a biologic prognostic factor for recurrence in patients with surgically resected non-small cell lung cancer. *J Nucl Med.* 2002;43(1):39–45.

153. De Leyn P, Vansteenkiste J, Cuypers P, et al. Role of cervical mediastinoscopy in staging of non-small cell lung cancer without enlarged mediastinal lymph nodes on CT scan. *Eur J Cardiothorac Surg.* 1997;12(5):706–712.

154. Antoch G, Stattaus J, Nemat AT, et al. Non-small cell lung cancer: dual-modality PET/CT in preoperative staging. *Radiology.* 2003;229(2):526–533.

155. Toloza EM, Harpole L, McCrory DC. Noninvasive staging of non-small cell lung cancer: a review of the current evidence. *Chest.* 2003;123(1 suppl):137S–146S.

156. Gould MK, Kuschner WG, Rydzak CE, et al. Test performance of positron emission tomography and computed tomography for mediastinal staging in patients with non-small-cell lung cancer: a meta-analysis. *Ann Intern Med.* 2003;139(11):879–892.

157. Dwamena BA, Sonnad SS, Angobaldo JO, Wahl RL. Metastases from non-small cell lung cancer: mediastinal staging in the 1990s–meta-analytic comparison of PET and CT. *Radiology.* 1999;213(2):530–536.

158. Shim SS, Lee KS, Kim BT, et al. Non-small cell lung cancer: prospective comparison of integrated FDG PET/CT and CT alone for preoperative staging. *Radiology.* 2005;236(3):1011–1019.

159. Hellwig D, Graeter TP, Ukena D, et al. 18 F-FDG PET for mediastinal staging of lung cancer: which SUV threshold makes sense? *J Nucl Med.* 2007;48(11):1761–1766.

160. Kim BT, Lee KS, Shim SS, et al. Stage T1 non-small cell lung cancer: preoperative mediastinal nodal staging with integrated FDG PET/CT–a prospective study. *Radiology.* 2006;241(2):501–509.

161. Al-Sarraf N, Gately K, Lucey J, Wilson L, McGovern E, Young V. Lymph node staging by means of positron emission tomography is less accurate in non-small cell lung cancer patients with enlarged lymph nodes: analysis of 1,145 lymph nodes. *Lung Cancer.* 2008;60(1):62–68.

162. Shiraki N, Hara M, Ogino H, et al. False-positive and true-negative hilar and mediastinal lymph nodes on FDG-PET–radiological-pathological correlation. *Ann Nucl Med.* 2004; 18(1):23–28.

163. Bunyaviroch T, Coleman RE. PET evaluation of lung cancer. *J Nucl Med.* 2006;47(3):451–469.

164. Pieterman RM, van Putten JW, Meuzelaar JJ, et al. Preoperative staging of non-small-cell lung cancer with positron-emission tomography. *N Engl J Med.* 2000;343(4):254–261.

165. De Leyn P, Schoonooghe P, Deneffe G, et al. Surgery for non-small cell lung cancer with unsuspected metastasis to ipsilateral mediastinal or subcarinal nodes (N2 disease). *Eur J Cardiothorac Surg.* 1996;10(8):649–654; discussion 654–655.

166. Nwogu C, Fischer G, Tan D, Glinianski M, Lamonica D, Demmy T. Radioguided detection of lymph node metastasis in non-small cell lung cancer. *Ann Thorac Surg.* 2006;82(5): 1815–1820; discussion 1820.

167. Vansteenkiste JF, De Leyn PR, Deneffe GJ, et al. Survival and prognostic factors in resected N2 non-small cell lung cancer: a study of 140 cases. Leuven Lung Cancer Group. *Ann Thorac Surg.* 1997;63(5):1441–1450.

168. Nakanishi R, Osaki T, Nakanishi K, et al. Treatment strategy for patients with surgically discovered N2 stage IIIA non-small cell lung cancer. *Ann Thorac Surg.* 1997;64(2):342–348.

169. MacManus MP, Hicks RJ, Matthews JP, et al. High rate of detection of unsuspected distant metastases by pet in apparent stage III non-small-cell lung cancer: implications for radical radiation therapy. *Int J Radiat Oncol Biol Phys.* 2001;50(2):287–293.

170. Van Tinteren H, Hoekstra OS, Smit EF, et al. Effectiveness of positron emission tomography in the preoperative assessment of patients with suspected non-small-cell lung cancer: the PLUS multicentre randomised trial. *Lancet.* 2002;359(9315): 1388–1393.

171. Erasmus JJ, Patz EF Jr, McAdams HP, et al. Evaluation of adrenal masses in patients with bronchogenic carcinoma using 18

F-fluorodeoxyglucose positron emission tomography. *AJR Am J Roentgenol.* 1997;168(5):1357–1360.

172. Yun M, Kim W, Alnafisi N, Lacorte L, Jang S, Alavi A. 18 F-FDG PET in characterizing adrenal lesions detected on CT or MRI. *J Nucl Med.* 2001;42(12):1795–1799.

173. Kumar R, Xiu Y, Yu JQ, et al. 18 F-FDG PET in evaluation of adrenal lesions in patients with lung cancer. *J Nucl Med.* 2004;45(12):2058–2062.

174. Brady MJ, Thomas J, Wong TZ, Franklin KM, Ho LM, Paulson EK. Adrenal nodules at FDG PET/CT in patients known to have or suspected of having lung cancer: a proposal for an efficient diagnostic algorithm. *Radiology.* 2009;250(2):523–530.

175. Bury T, Barreto A, Daenen F, Barthelemy N, Ghaye B, Rigo P. Fluorine-18 deoxyglucose positron emission tomography for the detection of bone metastases in patients with non-small cell lung cancer. *Eur J Nucl Med.* 1998;25(9):1244–1247.

176. Kruger S, Buck AK, Mottaghy FM, et al. Detection of bone metastases in patients with lung cancer: 99mTc-MDP planar bone scintigraphy, 18 F-fluoride PET or 18 F-FDG PET/CT. *Eur J Nucl Med Mol Imaging.* 2009;36(11):1807–1812.

177. Qu X, Huang X, Yan W, Wu L, Dai K. A meta-analysis of (1)(8)FDG-PET-CT, (1)(8)FDG-PET, MRI and bone scintigraphy for diagnosis of bone metastases in patients with lung cancer. *Eur J Radiol.* 2012;81(5):1007–1015.

178. Posther KE, McCall LM, Harpole DH Jr, et al. Yield of brain 18 F-FDG PET in evaluating patients with potentially operable non-small cell lung cancer. *J Nucl Med.* 2006;47(10):1607–1611.

179. Bradley JD, Perez CA, Dehdashti F, Siegel BA. Implementing biologic target volumes in radiation treatment planning for non-small cell lung cancer. *J Nucl Med.* 2004;45(suppl 1):96S–101S.

180. Mac Manus MP, Everitt S, Bayne M, et al. The use of fused PET/CT images for patient selection and radical radiotherapy target volume definition in patients with non-small cell lung cancer: Results of a prospective study with mature survival data. *Radiother Oncol.* 2013;106(3):292–298.

181. Patz EF Jr, Connolly J, Herndon J. Prognostic value of thoracic FDG PET imaging after treatment for non-small cell lung cancer. *AJR Am J Roentgenol.* 2000;174(3):769–774.

182. Nahmias C, Hanna WT, Wahl LM, Long MJ, Hubner KF, Townsend DW. Time course of early response to chemotherapy in non-small cell lung cancer patients with 18 F-FDG PET/CT. *J Nucl Med.* 2007;48(5):744–751.

183. Lopez Guerra JL, Gladish G, Komaki R, Gomez D, Zhuang Y, Liao Z. Large decreases in standardized uptake values after definitive radiation are associated with better survival of patients with locally advanced non-small cell lung cancer. *J Nucl Med.* 2012;53(2):225–233.

184. Singnurkar A, Solomon SB, Gonen M, Larson SM, Schöder H. 18 F-FDG PET/CT for the prediction and detection of local recurrence after radiofrequency ablation of malignant lung lesions. *J Nucl Med.* 2010;51(12):1833–1840.

185. Kamel EM, Zwahlen D, Wyss MT, Stumpe KD, von Schulthess GK, Steinert HC. Whole-body (18)F-FDG PET improves the management of patients with small cell lung cancer. *J Nucl Med.* 2003;44(12):1911–1917.

186. Ziai D, Wagner T, El Badaoui A, et al. Therapy response evaluation with FDG-PET/CT in small cell lung cancer: a prognostic and comparison study of the PERCIST and EORTC criteria. *Cancer Imaging.* 2013;13:73–80.

187. Adams RF, Gleeson FV. Percutaneous image-guided cutting-needle biopsy of the pleura in the presence of a suspected malignant effusion. *Radiology.* 2001;219(2):510–514.

188. Wang ZJ, Reddy GP, Gotway MB, et al. Malignant pleural mesothelioma: evaluation with CT, MR imaging, and PET. *Radiographics.* 2004;24(1):105–119.

189. Benard F, Sterman D, Smith RJ, Kaiser LR, Albelda SM, Alavi A. Metabolic imaging of malignant pleural mesothelioma with fluorodeoxyglucose positron emission tomography. *Chest.* 1998;114(3):713–722.

190. Kramer H, Pieterman RM, Slebos DJ, et al. PET for the evaluation of pleural thickening observed on CT. *J Nucl Med.* 2004;45(6):995–998.

191. Benard F, Sterman D, Smith RJ, et al. Prognostic value of FDG PET imaging in malignant pleural mesothelioma. *J Nucl Med.* 1999;40(8):1241–1245.

192. Abe Y, Tamura K, Sakata I, et al. Clinical implications of 18 F-fluorodeoxyglucose positron emission tomography/computed tomography at delayed phase for diagnosis and prognosis of malignant pleural mesothelioma. *Oncol Rep.* 2012;27(2):333–338.

193. Mavi A, Basu S, Cermik TF, et al. Potential of dual time point FDG-PET imaging in differentiating malignant from benign pleural disease. *Mol Imaging Biol.* 2009;11(5):369–378.

194. Basu S, Saboury B, Torigian DA, Alavi A. Current evidence base of FDG-PET/CT imaging in the clinical management of malignant pleural mesothelioma: emerging significance of image segmentation and global disease assessment. *Mol Imaging Biol.* 2011;13(5):801–811.

195. Nanni C, Castellucci P, Farsad M, et al. Role of 18 F-FDG PET for evaluating malignant pleural mesothelioma. *Cancer Biother Radiopharm.* 2004;19(2):149–154.

196. Erasmus JJ, Truong MT, Smythe WR, et al. Integrated computed tomography-positron emission tomography in patients with potentially resectable malignant pleural mesothelioma: staging implications. *J Thorac Cardiovasc Surg.* 2005;129(6):1364–1370.

197. Tsutani Y, Takuwa T, Miyata Y, et al. Prognostic significance of metabolic response by positron emission tomography after neoadjuvant chemotherapy for resectable malignant pleural mesothelioma. *Ann Oncol.* 2013;24(4):1005–1010.

CHAPTER 33

Pulmonary Function Testing

Michael A. Grippi
Gregory Tino

INTRODUCTION

The assessment of human pulmonary function dates back to the seventeenth century, when the earliest measurements of tidal volume were noted. In 1800, Humphry Davy employed a hydrogen dilution technique to measure his own residual volume (RV).[1] Subsequently, John Hutchinson, in his treatise, *On the Capacity of the Lungs and on Respiratory Functions,* defined the functional subdivisions of lung volume and reported the results of vital capacity measurements performed in more than 1800 subjects. He related these measurements to the subjects' height, age, and weight, thereby establishing a basis for determining normal values.[2,3]

Progress in development of techniques for pulmonary function testing progressed slowly over the next century. However, in the 1950s, pulmonary physiologists made use of the tools provided by the evolving fields of electronics and computer science. Currently, many techniques exist for assessing both the integrated performance of the cardiovascular and respiratory systems and their individual components. This chapter focuses on commonly used tests of pulmonary function.[4] Detailed assessment of integrated pulmonary and cardiovascular function is described in Chapter 34. Additional tests that have not yet been validated or are not routinely available for clinical purposes[5] are not included in the discussion.

LUNG VOLUMES AND SUBDIVISIONS

Important quantitative aspects of respiratory function are the changes in lung volume with inspiration and expiration and the absolute volume of air that the lungs hold at various times during the respiratory cycle. These volumes and changes in volume are described in subsequent sections.

DEFINITIONS AND ASSESSMENT

For purposes of quantification and comparison, the total volume of gas in the lungs is conventionally subdivided into compartments (volumes) and combinations of two or more volumes (capacities). For many of these subdivisions, the end-expiratory volume – the volume of gas remaining in the lungs at the end of normal expiration – is the point of reference. Lung volumes and capacities are defined in Table 33-1 and are depicted schematically in the tracing shown in Figure 33-1, which was obtained using a device called a spirometer. The relationships between the volumes recorded directly by the spirometer and the other lung volumes and capacities – including total lung capacity (TLC), functional residual capacity (FRC), RV, and inspiratory capacity (IC) – are highlighted in the figure.

Spirometers that measure volume or change in volume versus time have been used extensively in pulmonary function laboratories. Previously, through manual calculations, or, in modern times, through application of microprocessors, the relationships among volume, flow, and time are generated to provide a measure of the respiratory system's ability to move air. Two examples of volume-type spirometers of historical note are shown in Figure 33-2. They are discussed briefly to highlight the ingenuity behind their use in determining clinically important physiologic measurements.

In the water-sealed spirometer (Fig. 33-2A), a mouthpiece is attached to a tube through which air passes into a lightweight bell that is inverted over a water bath. Air movement through the mouthpiece into the bell during expiration causes the bell to rise; conversely, as air is withdrawn from the system during inspiration, the bell falls. The change in volume with time can be recorded on a calibrated rotating drum or digitally noted by a computer and displayed on a screen in both graphic and numeric formats.

In the dry, rolling-seal spirometer (Fig. 33-2B), a cylinder with a rolling plastic seal is substituted for the spirometer bell and its water seal. Movement of air through the mouthpiece effects a change in the position of the piston, which is attached to a variable resistor. The resistor, in turn, generates voltage signals proportional to volume changes reflected in displacement of the piston. These signals are processed by a computer to generate graphic and numeric outputs similar to those of the water-sealed spirometer.

Currently, most pulmonary function laboratories utilize flow-type spirometers using pneumotachographs or rotating turbines to determine airflow. Two types of pneumotachographs are in general use: hot wire and flow resistive. In the hot-wire type, air flowing past

TABLE 33-1 Glossary for Static Lung Volumes and Capacities

Term	Symbol	Definition
Volumes		
Residual volume	RV	Volume of air remaining in the lungs after maximal expiration
Expiratory reserve volume	ERV	Maximal volume of air expired from the resting end-expiratory level
Tidal volume	TV[a]	Volume of air inspired or expired with each breath during quiet breathing
Inspiratory reserve volume	IRV	Maximal volume of air inspired from the resting end-inspiratory level
Capacities		
Inspiratory capacity	IC	Maximal volume of air inspired from the end-expiratory level (the sum of IRV and TV)
Vital capacity	VC	Maximal volume of air expired form the maximal inspiratory level
Inspiratory vital capacity	IVC	Maximal volume of air inspired form the maximal expiratory level
Functional residual capacity	FRC	Volume of air remaining in the lungs at the end-expiratory level (the sum of RV and ERV)
Total lung capacity	TLC	Volume of air in the lungs after maximal inspiration (the sum of all volume compartments)

[a]*The symbol TV is traditionally used for tidal volume to indicate a subdivision of static lung volumes. However, the symbol* V_T *is used for tidal volume in formulas for gas exchange.*

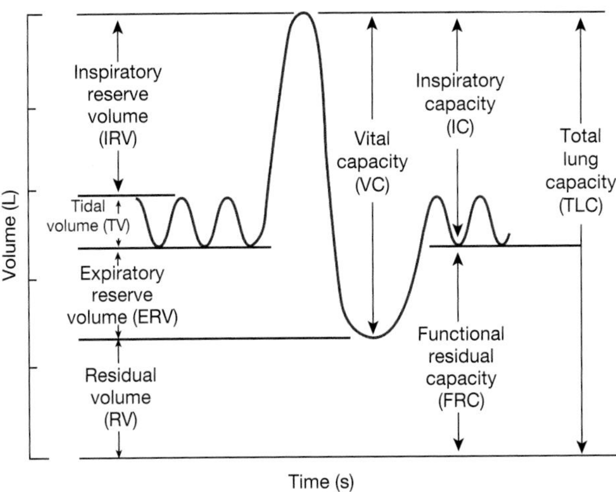

Figure 33-1 The subdivisions of lung volume as recorded by a spirometer. The record is generated on paper calibrated for volume in the vertical direction and time in the horizontal. The term *capacity* is applied to a subdivision composed of two or more *volumes*. The definitions of these subdivisions are found in Table 33-1.

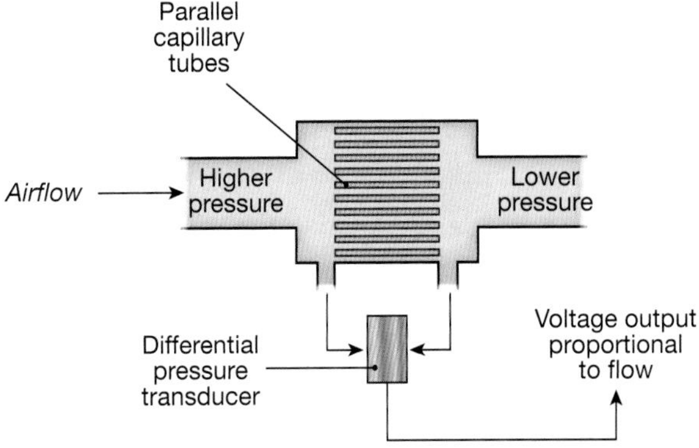

Figure 33-3 Principle of pneumotachography. During unidirectional airflow, a pressure drop is created across a resistive element made up of an array of parallel capillary tubes. The magnitude of the pressure drop is related to airflow, as described by Poiseuille's law for a laminar flow system. The pressure drop is transduced to a proportional voltage output, which can be recorded. A heating element (not shown) maintains the temperature of the expired gas near body temperature.

a heated wire cools the wire, thereby altering its resistance in proportion to changes in airflow. Flow-resistive pneumotachographs contain a resistive element composed of parallel tubes (Fig. 33-3), a wire mesh, or a fibrous, paperlike element. Airflow through the resistive element results in a pressure gradient across the device, which can be measured by a very sensitive differential pressure gauge. In the model depicted in Figure 33-3, the array of parallel,

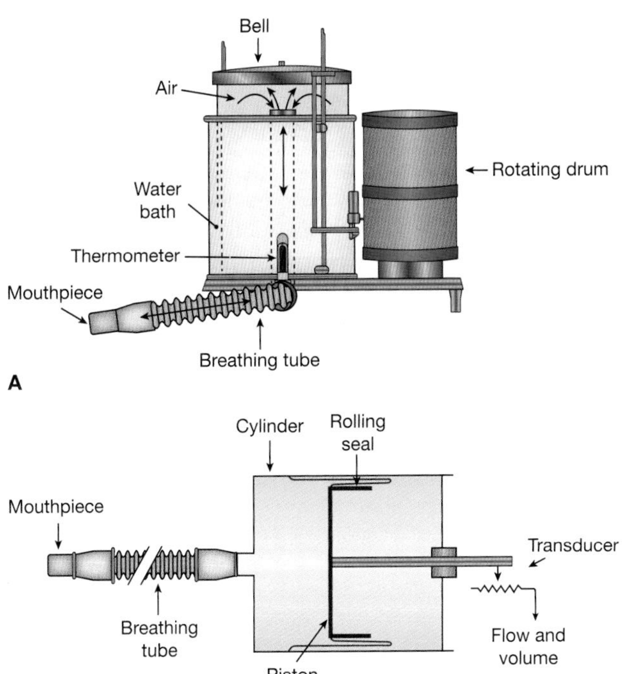

Figure 33-2 Two types of spirometers: water sealed (**A**) and dry rolling seal (**B**). Movement of air through the breathing tube results in movement of the bell (**A**) or piston (**B**). The output signal is either mechanical (pen on rotating drum) or electrical (flow and volume as voltage changes). The primary design criteria for these instruments are that inertia and resistance to airflow must be held to negligible levels, and the calibration must be accurate and stable.

small-bore tubes maintains a laminar gas flow pattern through the pneumotachograph. As a result, the pressure–flow characteristics of the system can be described by Poiseuille's law:

$$\Delta P = \dot{V}\frac{8\eta l}{\pi r^4}$$

where

ΔP = pressure drop across the resistive element, dyn/cm^2
$\dot{V}$ = gas flow, cm^3/s
η = viscosity of gas, dyn s/cm^2
l = length of resistive element, cm
r = radius of resistive element, cm

Hence, under laminar flow conditions, the flow of gas in each tube is proportional to the pressure drop across the tube. The calculation for the overall pressure drop across the entire resistive element is based on the parallel arrangement of the array of tubes. The pressure drop across the resistive element is sensed by a pressure transducer and converted to a voltage output that is proportional to flow. The flow signal can be integrated electronically to yield volume. The output signals for flow and volume are displayed on a monitor and recorded. Minimal standards have been established by the American Thoracic Society (ATS) and the European Respiratory Society (ERS) (Table 33-2) for spirometers used either for diagnostic purposes or patient monitoring.[6–8]

In a diagnostic setting, spirometers are used to (1) evaluate symptoms, signs, or abnormal laboratory tests; (2) measure the effect of disease on pulmonary function; (3) screen persons at risk of having pulmonary disease; (4) assess preoperative risk; (5) assess prognosis; and (6) assess health status before enrollment in strenuous physical activity programs.

On the other hand, spirometers used for patient monitoring are used to (1) assess therapeutic interventions, including bronchodilator therapy, management of congestive heart failure, etc.; (2) characterize the course of diseases affecting lung function (e.g., obstructive or interstitial lung diseases, congestive heart failure, or neuromuscular diseases); (3) track pulmonary function in persons working in occupations or receiving medications known to affect the lung; (4) evaluate large numbers of people in disability assessments; and (5) provide data as part of epidemiologic surveys.[8]

In general, the diagnostic spirometer is used to assess a patient's lung function for purposes of comparison with values expected in a

TABLE 33-2 Minimal Recommendations for Diagnostic Spirometry

Test	Range/Accuracy (BTPS)	Flow Range (L/s)	Time(s)	Resistance and Back Pressure	Test Signal
VC	0.5–8 L ± 3% of reading or ± 0.050 L, whichever is greater	0–14	30		3-L cal syringe
FVC	0.5–8 L ± 3% of reading or ± 0.050 L, whichever is greater	0–14	15	<1.5 $cmH_2O/L/s$	24 standard waveforms 3-L cal syringe
FEV_1	0.5–8 L ± 3% of reading or ± 0.050 L, whichever is greater	0–14	1	<1.5 $cmH_2O/L/s$	24 standard waveforms
Time zero	The time point from which all FEV_t measurements are taken			Back extrapolation	
PEF	Accuracy: ± 10% of reading or ± 0.30 L/s, whichever is greater Precision: ± 5% of reading or ± 0.15 L/s, whichever is greater	0–14		Mean resistance at 200, 400, 600 L/s must be <2.5 $cmH_2O/L/s$	26 flow standard waveforms
$FEF_{25-75\%}$	7.0 L/s ± 5% of reading or ± 0.200 L/s, whichever is even greater	±14	15	Same as FEV_1	24 standard waveforms
Instantaneous flows	±5% of reading or 0.200 L/s, whichever is greater	0–14		<1.5 $cmH_2O/L/s$	Proof from manufacturer
MVV	250 L/min at TV of 2 L within ± 10% of reading or ± 15 L/min, whichever is greater	±14 ± 3%	12–15	<1.5 $cmH_2O/L/s$	Sine wave pump

Note: BTPS, body temperature and pressure, saturated with water vapor; VC, vital capacity; FVC, forced expiratory vital capacity; FEV_1, forced expiratory volume in 1 s; PEF, peak expiratory flow; $FEF_{25-75\%}$, forced expiratory flow, 25–75%; MVV, maximal voluntary ventilation; TV, tidal volume.
Source: Reproduced with permission of Miller MR1, Hankinson J, Brusasco V, et al. Standardisation of spirometry. Eur Respir J. 2005;26(2):319–338.

normal population. The monitoring spirometer, which is less expensive and more portable, is used to evaluate a patient's performance over time and to study large numbers of people for epidemiologic or other purposes.

THE VITAL CAPACITY AND ITS SUBDIVISIONS

Two methods of performing a vital capacity maneuver can be used: closed-circuit and open-circuit methods. In the closed-circuit method, the seated patient, with nose clip in place, breathes quietly into the apparatus. After several breaths to establish the resting end-expiratory level, which serves as a point of reference for all subsequent measurements, the patient is urged to inspire fully and then, after reaching a plateau at maximal inspiration, to expire maximally. This expiration must be performed slowly and evenly; attempts by the patient with obstructive pulmonary disease to maximize flow often reduce expiratory volumes because of dynamic compression of the airways caused by high positive pleural pressures (see Chapter 10). Figure 33-1 illustrates schematically this relaxed or "slow" vital capacity maneuver. From the record, tidal volume, inspiratory reserve volume, expiratory reserve volume (ERV), vital capacity, and IC are calculated. A similar maneuver in which the subject breathes out as rapidly and forcefully as possible after a maximal inspiration provides a measure of the forced vital capacity (FVC). Other timed measurements of expiratory airflow (e.g., the forced expiratory volume in 1 second, or FEV_1) are also determined from this type of record (see Dynamic Mechanical Properties of the Respiratory System).

In the open-circuit method of determining vital capacity, the patient inspires maximally, inserts the mouthpiece, and then exhales with a slow, constant effort to the point of maximal expiration. With this technique, the resting end-expiratory position is not recorded. Thus, only the vital capacity, not its component volumes, can be measured. The open-circuit technique offers some advantages. Since the patient inspires from room air before expiring into the apparatus, concern over acquisition of infection from contaminated inspired air is minimized. In addition, the open-circuit method is generally completed in a shorter time, providing a major advantage when epidemiologic studies are being performed on large numbers of subjects.

FUNCTIONAL RESIDUAL CAPACITY AND RESIDUAL VOLUME

One compartment of the TLC that cannot be measured by spirometry is RV, the volume of air remaining in the lungs at the end of a maximal expiration. RV is determined indirectly in three steps: (1) FRC is typically measured using one of the three techniques: closed-circuit helium, open-circuit nitrogen, or total-body plethysmograph. (2) ERV is determined spirometrically. (3) RV is calculated as the difference between FRC and ERV. In principle, it is possible to determine the RV using a dilution technique or body plethysmography after maximal expiration. In practice, however, the resting end-expiratory level is a more reproducible starting point for determining FRC than is the maximal end-expiratory level for determining RV.

Closed-Circuit Helium Method

The closed-circuit helium dilution method for determining FRC is a variation of the hydrogen dilution method first used in the early 19th century. Both methods take advantage of the virtual insolubility of the test gas in body tissues and the law of conservation of mass. The development and simplification of this test were accomplished over a 20-year span in the mid-20th century. Schematic depictions of the principle upon which the technique is based and the apparatus used are shown in Figure 33-4.

When a fully manual device is used for measuring FRC, the system is prepared by the addition of about 2 L of air and sufficient helium to achieve an initial helium concentration of approximately 10% in the apparatus. The patient, with nose clip in place, then breathes room air through the mouthpiece (Fig. 33-4A). After a preliminary period of quiet breathing to familiarize the patient with the mouthpiece, apparatus, and environment, and after the baseline resting end-expiratory level is established, the test begins.

At the end of a normal expiration, the valve at the mouthpiece is turned to connect the patient to the spirometer system

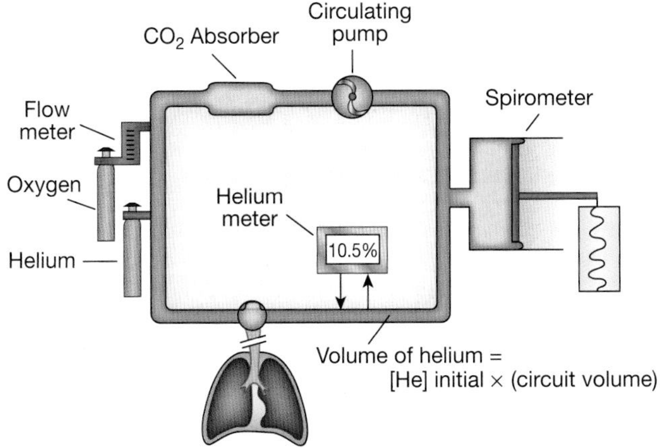

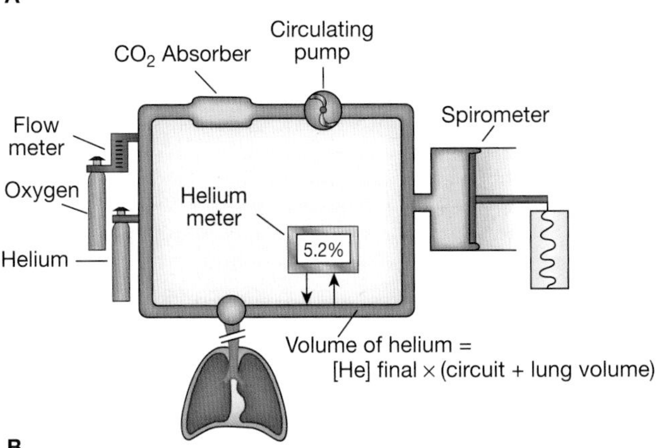

Figure 33-4 Closed-circuit helium dilution method for measurement of FRC. **A.** Spirometer and tubing system with helium before subject begins breathing through the circuit. At the end of an expiration, the mouthpiece valve is turned and the patient rebreathes through the circuit. Expired CO_2 is "scrubbed" out of the system, and O_2 is added to compensate for continued O_2 uptake in the lungs. **B.** During equilibration, the measured helium concentration falls, reflecting a dilutional effect of the additional volume (FRC) on the spirometer circuit.

(Fig. 33-4B). As the patient rebreathes from the closed circuit, the blower circulates the gas mixture. The CO_2 is absorbed by soda lime (CO_2 absorber), while O_2 is added through a valve and flowmeter at a rate corresponding to the subject's O_2 consumption. As the helium, which was at first contained entirely within the apparatus, mixes with air contained in the lungs, its concentration, as monitored by the helium analyzer, falls. Stabilization of the helium concentration, indicated by a rate of change in concentration of less than 0.02% over a 30-second interval, signals the point at which the helium concentration has equilibrated throughout the lung-breathing circuit system; equilibration, the end-point of the test, occurs within 7 minutes in normal persons. However, in patients in whom the distribution of ventilation is abnormal – for example, those with chronic obstructive pulmonary disease (COPD)– equilibration may take much longer. Upon equilibration, the following equation, based on the law of conservation of mass, is applied:

$$F_{0He} \times V_0 = F_{F_{He}} \times V_F$$

where

F_{0He} = initial concentration of helium
V_0 = initial volume of system, L
$F_{F_{He}}$ = final concentration of helium
V_F = final volume of system, L

The initial volume of the system is the volume of the spirometer and circuit tubing, whereas the final volume consists of the initial volume plus FRC. The latter value is the only unknown in the preceding equation. Corrections are usually made for the small amount of helium dissolved in body tissues during the test and for slight volume changes caused by a respiratory exchange ratio that is not equal to 1.0.[9] Although the method described here is based on a manually operated device, the same principles hold when all the mechanical and computational steps are accomplished with a computer-controlled system.

Nitrogen Washout Method

Conceptually, the nitrogen washout method is similar to the helium dilution method described previously; however, it relies on an open circuit rather than the closed circuit used in the helium dilution method. The open-circuit nitrogen washout method for determining FRC.[10] requires that the subject breathe 100% O_2 for 7 minutes; during this period, the concentration of N_2 in expired gas is monitored. When the expired N_2 concentration falls to zero, all the N_2 present in the lungs at the start of O_2 breathing has been "washed out." The total volume of gas expired and the concentration of N_2 in the expired gas are measured.

The calculation of FRC is based on the reasonable assumption that the volume of N_2 in the lungs at the start of the test (i.e., the product of lung volume and the concentration of N_2 in the lungs) is the same as the total volume of N_2 expired and collected during the period of the test – that is, the product of the total volume of gas expired and the concentration of N_2 in the expired gas:

$$F_{0_{N_2}} \times V_0 = F_{E_{N_2}} \times V_E$$

where

$F_{0_{N_2}}$ = concentration of N_2 in the lungs
V_0 = volume of gas in the lungs, L
$F_{E_{N_2}}$ = concentration of N_2 in the expired gas
V_E = volume of expired gas, L

Since the test is started at the end of a quiet expiration, the volume of gas in the lungs is FRC. This volume is calculated by substituting into the above equation the initial concentration of N_2 in the lungs, estimated at 0.81 in fasting and 0.79 to 0.80 in nonfasting subjects, and the measured values for volume and N_2 concentration of expired gas.

Body Plethysmography

The word plethysmography is derived from the Greek plethysmos, meaning "enlargement." Although the concept of measuring FRC by recording changes in the volume of the body during "enlargement" of the chest was described in 1882, not until 1956 did DuBois and coworkers introduce a practical plethysmographic technique, based on Boyle's law, for determining thoracic gas volume (TGV).[11]

Any of three types of body plethysmographs can be used: (1) the *pressure plethysmograph,* in which pressure during breathing varies while volume remains constant; (2) the *volume plethysmograph,* in which volume varies during breathing while pressure remains constant; and (3) the *pressure-corrected flow plethysmograph,* which couples the pressure plethysmograph's fidelity of response to high-speed events with the volume plethysmograph's ability to follow large changes in volume. Since the conceptual basis for all three devices is similar, only the most popular one – the pressure plethysmograph – will be described.

The pressure plethysmograph (Fig. 33-5) contains a pneumotachograph and transducer for measuring flow and volume, and two strain-gauge transducers, one for sensing pressure at the mouth (Pm) and the other for sensing pressure in the box (Pbx). A solenoid-operated shutter mechanism is situated between the mouthpiece and the pneumotachograph. The three transducers are connected to

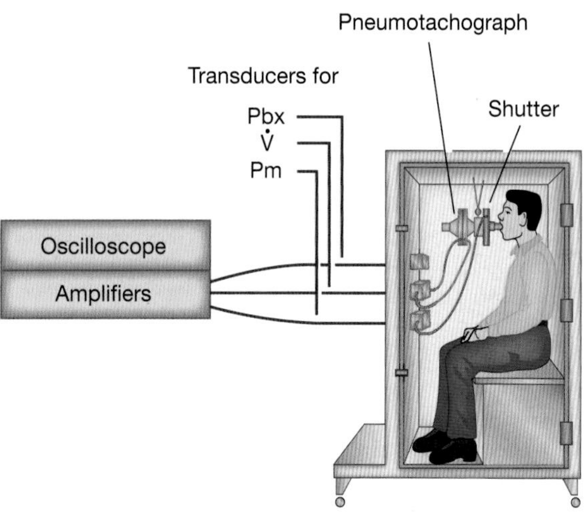

Figure 33-5 Constant-volume, variable-pressure plethysmograph used for measuring functional residual capacity and airway resistance. The device has a fixed volume. Thoracic gas volume changes associated with changes in alveolar pressure are reflected as changes in pressure within the plethysmograph.

an amplifying and monitoring system so that box pressure (or lung volume) and mouth pressure are displayed simultaneously on the X and Y axes, respectively, of an oscilloscope (Fig. 33-6).

In order to determine FRC, the patient, seated comfortably within the box with nose clip in place, is asked to breathe quietly through the mouthpiece. At the end of a quiet expiration, the shutter is closed and the patient is instructed to pant gently against it. The panting movements cause both mouth pressure and box pressure to change. With each inspiratory effort, as mouth pressure falls and gas in the lungs is rarefied, lung volume increases. Because the plethysmograph is a closed box, the increase in lung volume produces a corresponding increase in box pressure. With each expiratory effort, as lung volume decreases, box pressure falls. Because the shutter is closed while the measurements are made, mouth pressure equals alveolar pressure (PA). These oscillations in mouth pressure and box pressure or lung volume appear on the oscilloscope as a closed loop (Fig. 33-6). Measurement of the slope of this loop is used to determine the volume of gas in the lungs at the time of shutter closure – that is, TGV or V_{TG}. When the occlusion occurs at resting, end-expiratory lung volume, the measurement yields FRC (see below).

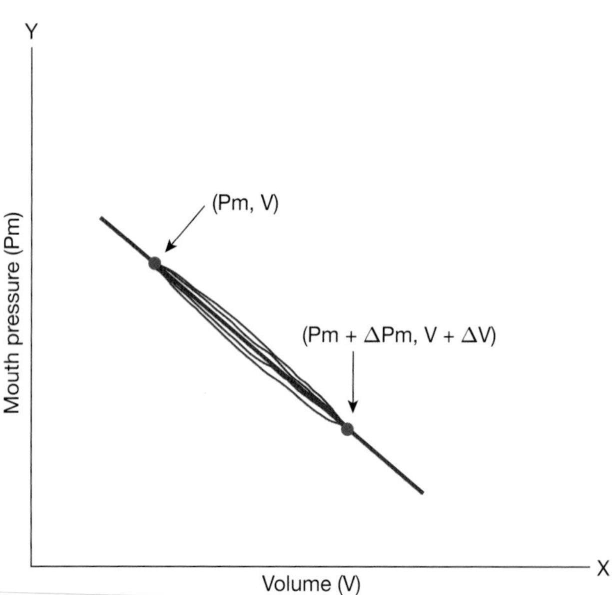

Figure 33-6 Pressure–volume loop obtained from a person seated in a body plethysmograph. Pressure at the mouth represents alveolar pressure; pressure in the box represents thoracic gas volume. After the shutter has closed at end-expiration (Pm, V), the subject attempts to inspire. Pm falls, and the pressure in the box increases. This increase in box pressure is calibrated in terms of an equivalent volume change. The new position of the trace at the end of the inspiratory effort is (Pm + ΔPm, V + ΔV). The slope of the loop depends on the volume of gas in the lungs when the shutter is closed (FRC).

Applying Boyle's law to the plethysmographic determination of lung volume,

$$PV = (P + \Delta P)(V + \Delta V)$$

where

P = pressure in the lungs at end-expiration (atmospheric pressure), cmH_2O
ΔP = change in pulmonary pressure produced by respiratory efforts, cmH_2O
V = volume of gas in the lungs at end expiration (FRC), L
ΔV = change in gas volume in the lungs produced by compression (during expiration) and rarefaction (during inspiration) secondary to respiratory efforts, L

In the pressure plethysmograph, ΔV is sensed as a change in pressure within the box, and ΔP is determined from the change in mouth pressure during breathing efforts against the closed shutter.

Rearranging the above equation and solving for V yield

$$V = \frac{\Delta V}{\Delta P}(P + \Delta P)$$

However, since ΔP is small compared to P (atmospheric pressure), it may be disregarded. The equation then becomes

$$V = P \times \frac{\Delta V}{\Delta P}$$

where

V = functional residual capacity, L
P = atmospheric pressure, cmH_2O
ΔV/ΔP = inverse of slope of the loop on the oscilloscope

Therefore, the only unknown in this equation is V, which can be calculated by incorporating values for barometric pressure and the inverse of the slope of the plot of mouth pressure versus box pressure (ΔP/ΔV).

Two methods for measuring static lung volumes using plethysmography have been standardized by the ATS and ERS. One entails shutter closure at FRC, followed by expiration to RV, and then an IC maneuver to TLC; the other method is shutter closure at FRC, followed by an IC maneuver to TLC, and then an expiratory vital capacity maneuver to RV.[12] Application of each method may yield different calculations of lung volumes.[13]

Comparison of Methods

Compared to the dilution and washout techniques, body plethysmography is, by far, the fastest method available for determining FRC. Indeed, it enables several determinations to be made per minute. Although the equipment required for body plethysmography is more expensive than that required for the other methods, in a busy laboratory this technique generally proves to be more economical because of the time saved and the additional uses to which the equipment can be put (e.g., measurement of airway resistance; see Airway Resistance). Technically, the test is only slightly more difficult than the inert gas dilution method.

Sources of error inherent in the use of body plethysmography and discrepancies between results obtained by body plethysmography and the inert gas techniques should be noted. In patients with COPD[14] or asthma,[15] values for FRC obtained by body plethysmography may be artifactually high because of pressure differences between the mouth and alveoli generated during panting across narrowed airways. Consequently, pressures recorded at the mouth during shutter occlusion of the airway underestimate changes in alveolar pressure. Overestimation of TLC using body plethysmography appears to be greatest in patients whose FEV_1 (see below) is less than 30% predicted.[16]

The inert gas dilution and washout methods are similar both in principle and in results. The values for FRC with these techniques match those from the body plethysmograph except in persons in whom considerable areas of the lungs are poorly ventilated, usually due to obstructive airway disease. In these individuals, complete mixing or washout of the indicator gas is very slow, at times requiring 45 minutes or longer. Because of the slow equilibration of gas concentrations in the poorly ventilated areas, the usual time allotted for the test is inadequate, resulting in a lower value for FRC by the washout methods than by body plethysmography. One strategy commonly used to deal with this problem is to prolong the washout time. The primary advantage of these techniques over body plethysmography is that they can be used in persons for whom the plethysmograph is impractical – for example, those with marked obesity, skeletal abnormalities, or claustrophobia.

TEMPERATURE CORRECTION FACTORS

By convention, all lung volumes described above and airflows (see below) are expressed in terms of body temperature and pressure, saturated with water vapor (BTPS). This practice enables direct comparison of pulmonary function data from laboratories operating at different ambient temperatures and altitudes. To convert the volume of gas collected in a volume-type spirometer under ambient conditions (i.e., ambient temperature and pressure, saturated with water vapor, or ATPS) to BTPS, a conversion factor is applied (Table 33-3). Previously, it was presupposed that air entering a spirometer was cooled *immediately* to ambient temperature and remained saturated with water vapor (ATPS). Under this assumption, only ambient temperature was considered in determining the appropriate correction factor. However, studies have addressed the assumption that expired gas is immediately cooled,[17,18] as well as the practical consequences of temperature correction errors. The ATS recommends temperature correction of results from volume-type spirometers based on *measured* gas temperature at the time of testing.

TABLE 33-3 Factors for Converting Volumes from ATPS to BTPS at Barometric Pressure of 760 mm Hg[a]

Ambient Temperature (°C)	Multiplier to Convert Volumes to BTPS[b]
20	1.101
21	1.096
22	1.091
23	1.085
24	1.080
25	1.074
26	1.069
27	1.062

[a]*Based on Boyle's, Charles's, and Dalton's laws.*
[b]*Volume at ATPS × multiplier = volume at BTPS.*
Note: ATPS, ambient temperature and pressure, saturated with water vapor; BTPS, body temperature and pressure, saturated with water vapor.

RADIOGRAPHIC ASSESSMENT OF LUNG VOLUME

Although initial reports describing use of radiographic techniques to measure lung volumes date back over 40 years, these methods have not found widespread use in adult populations. More sophisticated computerized tomographic (CT) applications have demonstrated good correlation with plethysmographic and gas dilution techniques in normals. However, significant differences may be observed in patients with COPD,[19] in whom TLC determinations using plethysmography may be up to 2 L greater than TLC assessed with CT scanning.[20]

STATIC MECHANICAL PROPERTIES OF THE RESPIRATORY SYSTEM

Exploration of the elastic properties of the respiratory system and their effect on lung volumes and work of breathing began in earnest during the earlier part of the 20th century. Although the groundwork had been laid centuries before (by Robert Hooke's *The Theory of Springs* in 1678), between 1923 and 1956 investigators provided a wealth of information about the elastic properties of the respiratory system and its components and the work done in overcoming these elastic forces during breathing.

STATIC COMPLIANCE OF THE LUNGS

The elastic properties of the lungs are determined by relating the change in the volume of air contained in the lungs to the corresponding change in the recoil force of the lungs. Change in lung volume is most easily measured by determining the volume of gas inspired or expired at the mouth. Although expedient, this approach to determining the elastic properties of the lungs can underestimate the change in lung volume when incorporated into techniques (see below) that require the subject to expire gently against a closed shutter, a maneuver that compresses thoracic gas. However, the problem can be circumvented by placing the subject in a volume plethysmograph that uses a spirometer attached to the plethysmograph to record changes in TGV due to gas compression.

The recoil force of the lungs, measured as the transpulmonary pressure (Fig. 33-7), is the difference between the alveolar and pleural pressures (PA and Ppl, respectively). Alveolar pressure is determined as the pressure at the airway opening (Pao) – that is, the mouth – when airflow is arrested and the glottis is open. The pleural pressure is determined indirectly by measuring the pressure in the esophagus using an esophageal balloon catheter. This technique, first introduced in 1949, has been improved over the years and provides accurate reflections of changes in pleural pressure at all lung volumes except those below FRC.[21]

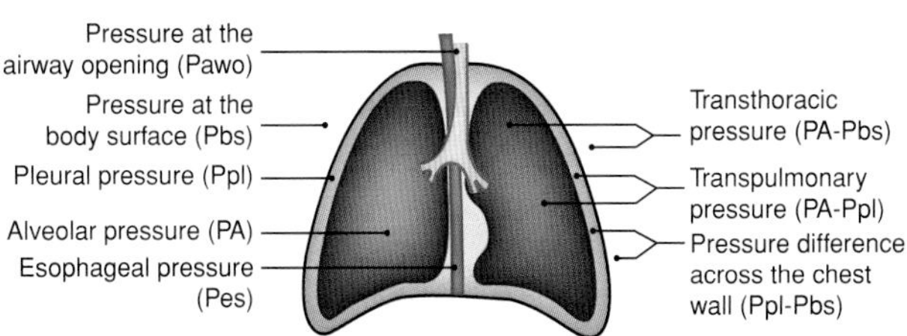

Figure 33-7 Schematic representation of the chest depicting pressure terms and gradients used in analysis of the mechanics of breathing. The expressions for individual pressure measurements on the left are relative to atmospheric pressure. Pleural pressure (Ppl) is not routinely measured directly but is approximated by esophageal pressure (Pes) measured with a balloon catheter.

A thin rubber balloon, about 10 cm long, is placed over a small-diameter polyethylene catheter. Several holes in the terminal portion of the catheter allow pressure to be transmitted from the balloon, through the catheter, to a transducer. The balloon is positioned in the lower third of the esophagus, where esophageal pressure and, therefore, balloon pressure accurately reflect the pressure acting on the lung surface (pleural pressure). Use of an elongated balloon of low volume helps to minimize changes in pressure due to esophageal contractions. By conveying mouth pressure and esophageal pressure to opposite sides of a differential pressure transducer, an output signal is generated that is proportional to the difference between these two pressures – that is, the transpulmonary pressure (PA − Ppl).

To determine the elastic properties of the lungs, the patient, with esophageal balloon in place, is seated in a closed body plethysmograph. The patient then breathes ambient air through a tube to the outside until the volume trace, inscribed by the plethysmograph spirometer, indicates that the end-expiratory level is stable. At this juncture, the patient is instructed to first inspire slowly to TLC and then to expire slowly to the resting end-expiratory level (FRC). This maneuver is then repeated; during the second expiration, the shutter is activated to occlude the airway intermittently. Since each closure of the shutter interrupts the expiration briefly, the recorded trace of expiratory volume versus time displays a staircase pattern (Fig. 33-8A). The plateau resulting from each closure of the shutter marks a finite period of zero change in lung volume as the lungs empty during expiration. Associated with each plateau is a corresponding plateau in transpulmonary pressure.

The relationship between the change in volume and the change in pressure is a measure of the *recoil force* of the lungs at each of the lung volumes that are registered (Fig. 33-8B). The resulting curve provides several useful indices of the elastic behavior of the lungs. The slope of the curve over the range corresponding to the tidal volume is the *static lung compliance.* The transpulmonary pressure attained at TLC is the *maximal static recoil pressure.* The ratio of the maximal static recoil pressure to the corresponding maximal lung volume is the *coefficient of retraction.* However, since these values are derived from only small segments of the curve, inspection of the total static pressure–volume curve remains the most comprehensive means of assessing the elastic properties of the lungs.

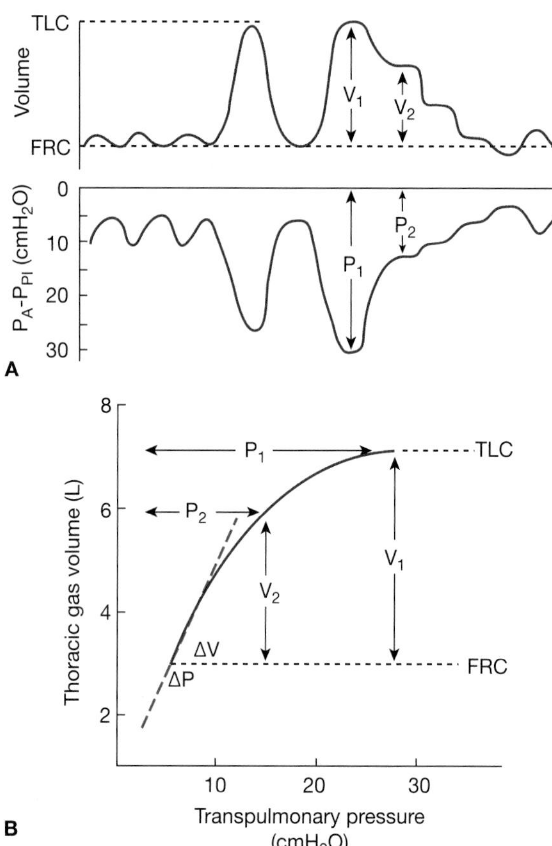

Figure 33-8 Measurement of the elastic properties of the lungs. **A.** Recordings of changes in lung volume and transpulmonary pressure (PA − Ppl) using the esophageal balloon technique described in the text. Simultaneous measurements of volume and pressure are obtained during periods of arrested airflow at lung volumes ranging from TLC to just below FRC. **B.** Thoracic gas volume is plotted on the ordinate and transpulmonary pressure on the abscissa. The curve formed by the plot using values from **A** describes the elastic properties of the lungs. The slope of the line, ΔV/ΔP, over the range of the tidal volume is the static compliance of the lungs.

STATIC COMPLIANCE OF THE CHEST WALL

Functionally, the chest wall includes the bony thorax, intercostal muscles, overlying soft tissue, pleura, and diaphragm. The chest wall is distensible and has its own distinctive elastic properties. In the normal, end-expiratory, resting position of the respiratory system (FRC), the inward recoil of the lung is balanced by the outward recoil of the chest wall (Fig. 33-9B). As the volume of the thoracic cavity enlarges progressively during inspiration from FRC to TLC, the outward recoil pressure of the chest wall lessens, becoming zero at approximately 70% of TLC; beyond this point, the chest wall begins to recoil inwardly (Fig. 33-9C). Conversely, as the chest wall is compressed below FRC by the action of the expiratory muscles, the natural outward recoil tendency is increased (Fig. 33-9A).

In practice, assessment of the elastic properties of the chest wall is accomplished by first determining the compliance curve of the respiratory system as a whole and then subtracting the contribution of the lungs. For a given lung volume, the pressure across the chest wall, Ppl − Pbs (Fig. 33-7), is simply the difference between the transthoracic (PA − Pbs) and transpulmonary (PA − Ppl) pressures. As indicated above, Ppl is determined using an esophageal balloon catheter.

ELASTIC PROPERTIES OF THE RESPIRATORY SYSTEM AS A WHOLE

The elasticity of the respiratory system as a whole is determined by measuring the change in volume resulting from a change in pressure applied to the system – that is, the transthoracic pressure (PA − Pbs) – *while the respiratory muscles are completely relaxed.*

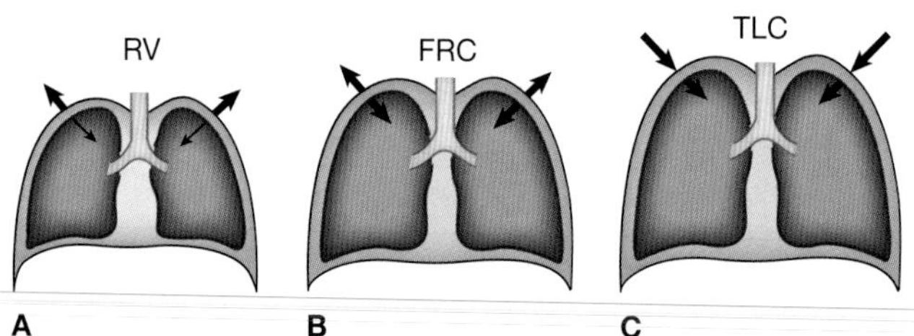

Figure 33-9 Schematic depiction of elastic recoil vectors across the lung and chest wall as determined by the level of inflation. **A.** At RV, the outwardly directed recoil pressure of the chest wall is large and the inwardly directed recoil pressure of the lung is small. **B.** At FRC, the recoil pressures of the lung and chest wall are equal and in opposite directions. **C.** At TLC, both recoil pressures are directed inward, and each contributes substantially to the overall recoil pressure of the respiratory system.

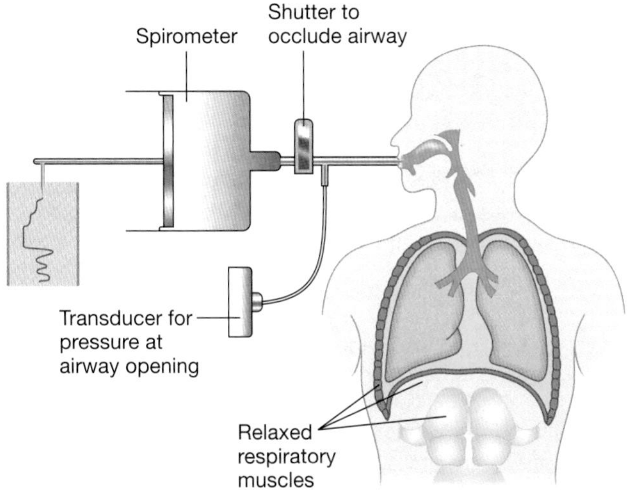

Figure 33-10 Relaxation technique for measurement of elastic recoil pressure of the respiratory system. After a period of normal tidal volume breathing, the subject inspires to TLC. A shutter in the airway is closed, and the subject relaxes his or her respiratory muscles. The shutter is periodically opened, permitting exhalation of a small volume of air measured by the spirometer. Airway pressures are recorded at times of shutter closure (i.e., during no airflow, when mouth pressure equals alveolar pressure). A pressure–volume curve is then constructed from the simultaneously recorded values for pressure and volume.

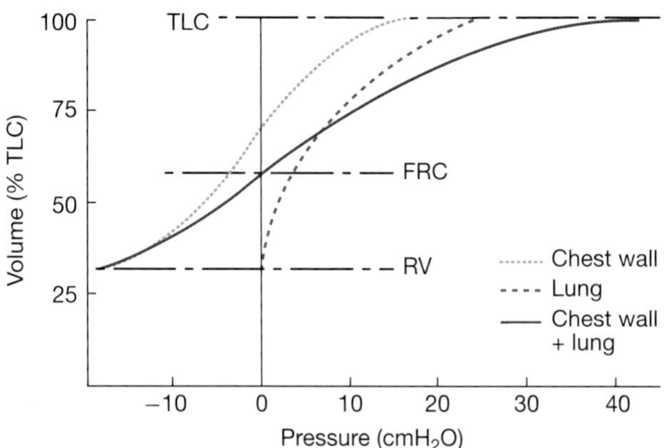

Figure 33-11 The pressure–volume curves of the respiratory system and its components. The elastic recoil pressures of the total respiratory system *(solid line)* over the vital capacity range are the sum of the recoil pressures of the lung *(dashed line)* and chest wall *(dotted line)*. At FRC, the chest wall recoil pressure is counterbalanced by the lung recoil pressure. The net result is a total system recoil pressure of 0. The total system recoil pressure is obtained by relaxation pressure or continuous positive-pressure breathing techniques. The chest wall recoil pressure is calculated as the difference between the recoil pressure of the entire respiratory system and the recoil pressure of the lungs.

The first method used for this evaluation employed the relaxation technique described by Rahn and associates.[22] The subject breathes quietly into an apparatus consisting of a spirometer, a shutter, and a pressure transducer connected to the subject's side of the shutter (Fig. 33-10). After a period of quiet breathing, the subject is instructed to inspire maximally; the shutter is closed at peak inspiration, and the subject is then asked to relax the respiratory muscles completely while keeping the glottis open. Periodically, the shutter is opened, allowing a small volume of air to move from the subject into the spirometer; the shutter is then closed again. This maneuver is repeated until FRC is reached. During the periods of arrested airflow, pressure at the mouth (Pao) is equal to the pressure in the alveoli (PA). Provided the pressure at the body surface is atmospheric and the respiratory muscles are completely at rest, this value represents transthoracic pressure. In practice, however, full relaxation of the respiratory muscles is difficult, and a contribution by them to the pressure at the airway opening is frequently unavoidable.

A more practical technique entails the application of continuous positive pressure to the airways during spontaneous breathing. The subject breathes quietly into a water-sealed spirometer until a constant end-tidal level is achieved. A weight is then placed on the spirometer bell to increase the pressure in the respiratory system and, thereby, to raise the resting end-expiratory lung volume. This procedure is repeated using several different weights so that a pressure–volume curve of the total respiratory system can be constructed.

The individual pressure–volume curves for the lungs and chest wall and the composite curve for the intact respiratory system are shown in Figure 33-11. As illustrated, the elastic recoil of the chest wall alone is determined by subtracting the recoil pressure of the lung from that of the total respiratory system. Chest wall elasticity is an important determinant of the subdivisions of lung volume and the overall compliance of the respiratory system; the latter is, in turn, an important determinant of the work of breathing.

Several features of the pressure–volume relationships shown in Figure 33-11 are worth emphasizing. As lung volume approaches RV, the elastic recoil pressure of the respiratory system is largely due to the outwardly directed recoil pressure of the chest wall. At RV, the contribution of the lung to the recoil pressure of the respiratory system is minimal. At the other extreme of lung volume, TLC, elastic recoil pressure is high and directed inwardly, due to the combined elastic recoils of the lung and chest wall. At FRC, the outwardly directed recoil of the chest wall balances the inwardly directed recoil of the lung, and the transthoracic pressure is zero (i.e., PA − Pbs = 0). Indeed, the system "comes to rest" at FRC because of the counterbalancing of these forces at that volume. Since alveolar pressure at FRC is zero, no pressure gradient exists for airflow. Therefore, the system remains stationary until acted upon by the muscles of inspiration or expiration.

■ ELASTIC PROPERTIES OF THE RESPIRATORY SYSTEM IN HEALTH AND DISEASE

The elastic properties of the respiratory system are altered by a wide variety of diseases that can affect the lung parenchyma or chest wall, either selectively or in concert. Most instances of clinically significant reductions in static compliance are due to abnormalities in the lung. The two standard clinical measures of the elastic properties of the lung are static lung compliance and maximal static recoil pressure.

Static lung compliance, Cst,L, is determined over the linear portion of the pressure–volume curve, between FRC and a lung volume corresponding to FRC plus 0.5 L. Normal values vary among laboratories, ranging from 0.147 to 0.375 L/cmH_2 O, with a mean of 0.262 L/cmH_2O. Some variability is related to age and sex; Cst,L decreases with age and is higher in males than in females.

Maximal static recoil pressure is the recoil pressure at TLC. Once again, normal values vary. Data from one series of 51 normal subjects.[23] are shown in Table 33-4.

In disease states characterized by an increased elastic recoil pressure, such as diffuse interstitial fibrosis, the pressure–volume curve is shifted to the right and the static lung compliance decreases (Fig. 33-12A and B). The increased elastic recoil pressure contributes to a

TABLE 33-4 Normal Maximal Static Recoil Pressures for Adults (cmH_2O)

	Male Age (Yr)			Female Age (Yr)		
	25–35	36–64	65–75	25–35	36–64	65–75
Mean ± SD	35.9 ± 8.5	33.0 ± 8.7	33.0 ± 2.9	36.4 ± 5.8	25.7 ± 4.0	23.7 ± 3.9
Range	24.0–48.0	21.5–48.0	17.0–42.2	21.0–48.0	20.0–30.0	18.0–31.6

Source: Data from Knudson RJ, Clark DF, Kennedy TC, et al. Effect of aging alone on mechanical properties of the normal adult human lung. J Appl Physiol. 1977;43:1054–1062.

decrease in FRC and TLC. By expressing the volume axis of the pressure–volume curve in terms of *percent predicted TLC* (Fig. 33-12B), instead of *absolute TLC* (Fig. 33-12A), the reduction in maximal lung volume is clearly evident; that is, maximal recoil pressure is increased, despite the reduced TLC.

In contrast to the effects of fibrosis, emphysema, which destroys alveolar walls and enlarges alveolar spaces, reduces lung elastic recoil pressure (Pel). This change increases both TLC and FRC. The shift of the pressure–volume curve upward and to the left (Fig. 33-12A and B) indicates that lung compliance increases and that the maximal recoil pressure decreases. If the volume axis is expressed as percent predicted TLC (Fig. 33-12B), the increase in lung volume is more clearly demonstrated.

As noted previously, disorders affecting primarily the chest wall can also significantly alter the elastic properties of the respiratory system. Among these are obesity, kyphoscoliosis, and fibrothorax. These disorders limit chest wall excursion and lung expansion and reduce FRC. In addition, they produce decreases in static compliance of the lung and chest wall and maximal recoil pressure.

RESPIRATORY MUSCLE STRENGTH

Ventilatory performance depends not only on the mechanical properties of the lungs and chest wall, but also on the strength of the respiratory muscles. Evaluation of respiratory muscle strength was undertaken as early as the mid-19th century. Subsequently, using simplified methods of measurement, Black and Hyatt established normal values (Table 33-5).[24]

The maximal pressure generated by an isometric contraction varies directly with the resting length of the muscle. Consequently, values for maximal inspiratory and expiratory pressures depend on the lung volume at which the tests are performed (Fig. 33-13).[25] When TLC is less than 70% of the predicted value, the maximal expiratory pressure will be low. Similarly, when RV exceeds 40% of the predicted TLC, the maximal inspiratory pressure will be low.

The only equipment required for measurement of maximal inspiratory or expiratory pressure is an aneroid vacuum and pressure gauge. To determine maximal expiratory pressure, the patient is urged to inspire fully to TLC and then to expire as forcefully as possible into the gauge. The highest pressure attained and held for at least 1 second is the *maximal expiratory pressure* (PE_{max}). The *maximal inspiratory pressure* (PI_{max}) is determined by having the patient inspire maximally from the gauge after having expired completely to RV. The value recorded is the lowest pressure attained and held for at least 1 second.

Measurement of maximal static respiratory pressures is particularly important in evaluating respiratory muscle weakness in patients with neuromuscular disease, as described in Chapters 84 and 85 . In such patients, spirometric tests are often normal, despite respiratory muscle weakness, because maximal pressures are not required to achieve maximal expiratory flow rates (see Flow–Volume Curves).

Another useful function of these measurements is in examining patients whose coordination in performing spirometry or whose degree of motivation is suspicious In such patients, determination of maximal pressures is often helpful in determining whether optimal efforts are being expended during pulmonary function testing (see Approach to Interpreting Commonly Performed Pulmonary Function Tests).

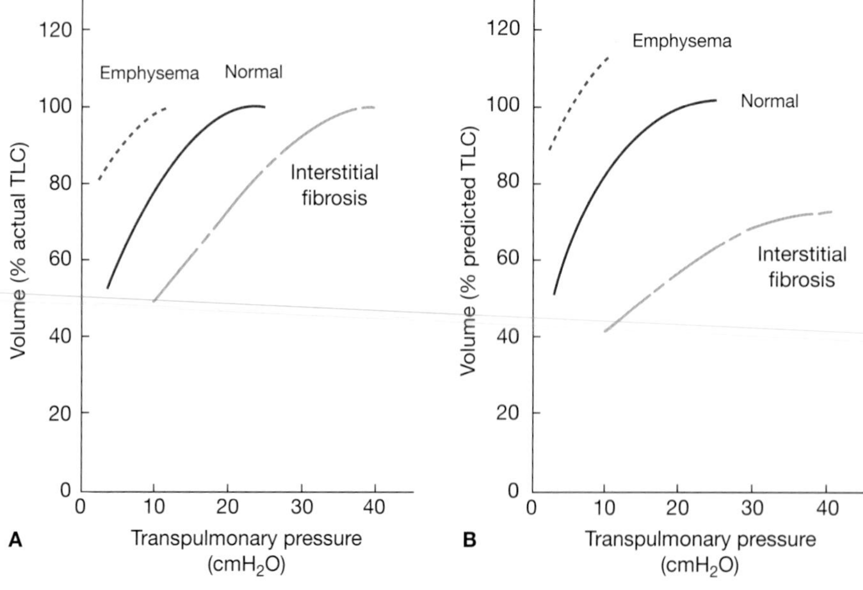

Figure 33-12 Pressure–volume curves of the lungs in health and disease. **A.** Volume expressed as percent of actual TLC. Differences in transpulmonary pressures in normal and diseases states are evident. Changes in lung volume that occur with disease are demonstrated on the plots. **B.** Volume expressed as percent of predicted TLC. In addition to the differences in transpulmonary pressures, alterations in lung volumes in the disease states are evident.

PART 3 Symptoms and Signs of Respiratory Disease

TABLE 33-5 Prediction Equations and Lower Limits of Normal for Maximal Inspiratory (PI_{max}) and Maximal Expiratory (PE_{max}) Pressures (cmH_2O)[a]

	PI_{max}		PE_{max}	
	Predicted Mean (cmH_2O)	Lower Limit of Normal	Predicted Mean (cmH_2O)	Lower Limit of Normal[b]
Male	143 – (0.55 × age)	71	268 – (1.03 × age)	111
Female	104 – (0.51 × age)	39	170 – (0.53 × age)	88

[a]*Age range = 20–86 yr.*
[b]*Independent of age.*
Source: Data from Black LF, Hyatt RE. Maximal respiratory pressures: Normal values and relationship to age and sex. Am Rev Respir Dis. 1969;99(5):696–702.

DYNAMIC MECHANICAL PROPERTIES OF THE RESPIRATORY SYSTEM

The static tests of pulmonary function described in the previous section are based on measurements of volume and pressure made while airflow is arrested. These static tests are particularly useful in defining the elastic properties of the respiratory system. Considerable additional information can be gained from tests done during airflow – that is, under "dynamic" conditions.

Although measurements of static lung volumes began about 300 years ago, the assessment of pulmonary function during airflow began in 1933, when the test now known as the *maximal voluntary ventilation* (MVV) was first proposed. This test did not become popular until a few years later, when Cournand and Richards developed regression equations to determine normal values. Subsequently, investigators proposed that the volume of air expired during specific time intervals be determined. In 1955, determination of the average airflow during the middle half of a forced expiratory vital capacity was described. Determination of these indices of dynamic lung function is now generally part of the battery of tests, both static and dynamic, included under the designation *spirometry.*

The more practical tests of dynamic function can, for convenience, be divided into four categories: FVC, flow–volume curves, MVV, and airway resistance. Other dynamic tests, including assessment of airway reactivity and the function of small airways, will be considered separately.

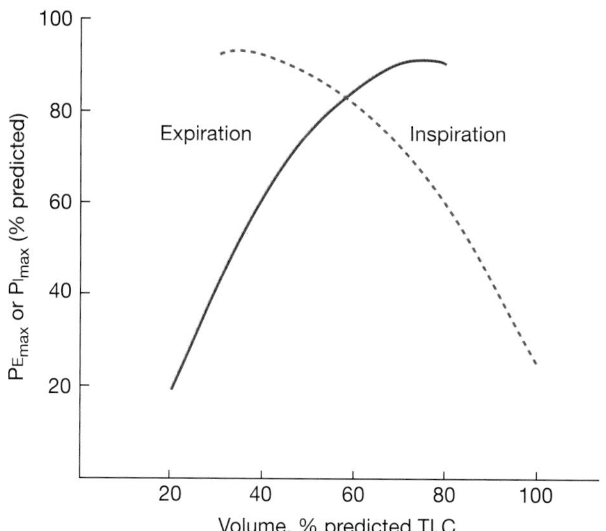

Figure 33-13 Effect of lung volume on maximal inspiratory *(dashed line)* and maximal expiratory *(solid line)* pressures. See text for discussion.

■ FORCED VITAL CAPACITY

Both expiratory and inspiratory measurements of the FVC are routinely made in pulmonary function laboratories. Unless otherwise specified, FVC refers to the forced *expiratory* maneuver.

Forced Expiratory Vital Capacity

The forced expiratory vital capacity is measured during expiration. The maneuver entails two steps: a full inspiration to TLC, followed by a rapid, forceful, maximal expiration (to RV) into a spirometer. The forced expiratory vital capacity (FVC) is normally equal to the relaxed or slow vital capacity (VC). However, a discrepancy between FVC and VC appears in obstructive disease of the airways: the FVC is less than the VC.

The relationship between expired volume and time during an FVC maneuver is used to determine airflow during expiration and the volume of air expired within designated intervals; these values provide an indirect measure of the flow-resistive properties of the lung. The FVC is displayed in one of the two ways: expired volume plotted against time (Fig. 33-14) or airflow plotted against lung volume – that is, an expiratory "flow–volume curve" (see below). The normal volume–time display of the FVC consists of a smooth curve with a gradually and progressively decreasing slope. Irregularities in the curve suggest either a failure of coordination or a suboptimal

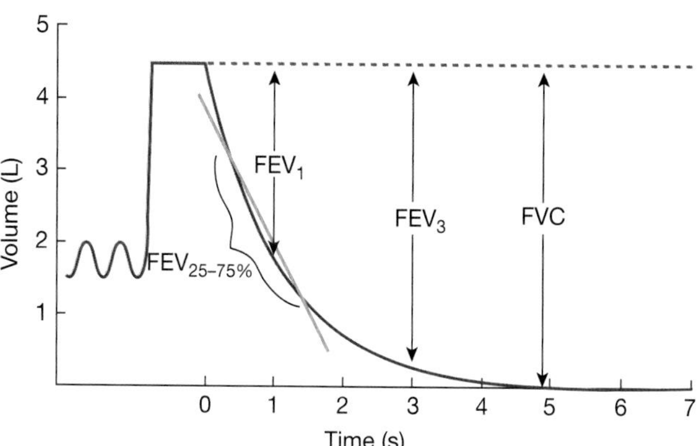

Figure 33-14 Forced expiratory vital capacity maneuver. After an initial period of tidal volume breathing, the patient inspires maximally to TLC and then exhales as rapidly and as forcefully as possible into a spirometer. Shown on the left of the tracing are a series of tidal volume breaths and the maximal inspiration to TLC. The forced expiration begins at time 0. Nearly all the volume is exhaled in the first 3 seconds of the maneuver. The values for FVC, FEV_1, and FEV_3 are measured from the maximal inspiratory level. The $FEF_{25-75\%}$ is the slope of the line connecting the points on the volume–time trace that correspond to 25% and 75% of the FVC.

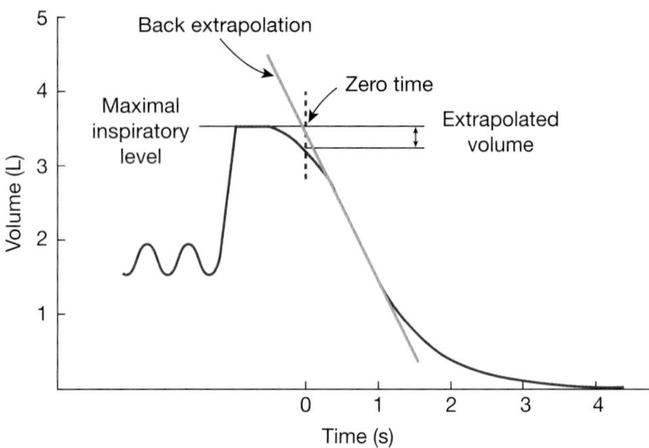

Figure 33-15 Technique of back extrapolation for determining the zero time in calculation of FEV_1. Zero time is determined as the point of intersection of a tangent drawn through the steepest portion of the spirogram and a line drawn horizontally through the maximal inspiratory level.

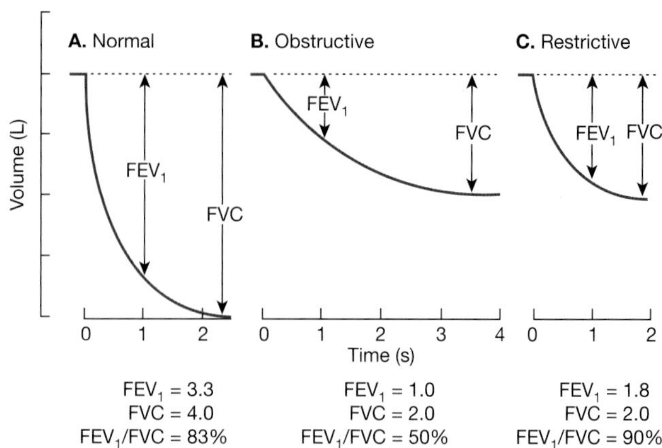

Figure 33-16 Representative spirograms from a normal subject (**A**), a patient with obstructive lung disease (**B**), and a patient with restrictive lung disease (**C**), obtained during a forced expiratory vital capacity maneuver. In the normal subject, expiration is completed within 3 seconds, and 83% of the volume is expired in the first second (FEV_1/FVC% = 83). In the patient with obstructive disease, expiration is prolonged, and only half the volume is expired in the first second (FEV_1/FVC% = 50). In the patient with restrictive disease, although the magnitude of the reduction in exhaled volume is the same as in the obstructed patient, most of the volume is exhaled within the first second (FEV_1/FVC% = 90).

effort. At times, the onset of the forced expiration is unclear (Fig. 33-15) because of hesitation on the part of the patient. When this occurs, the start of expiration ("zero time") is determined with the "back extrapolation" method (Fig. 33-15).[8] A tangent taken through the part of the curve with the steepest slope is extrapolated back to the maximal inspiratory volume; the point of intersection is considered to be the time of onset of expiration.

Several values are commonly determined from the volume–time plot of the FVC (Table 33-6, Fig. 33-14): (1) the *volume expired in the first second,* expressed either as an absolute volume (FEV_1) or as a percentage of the FVC (FEV_1/FVC%); (2) *the volume expired in the first 3 seconds,* expressed either as an absolute volume (FEV_3) or as a percentage of the FVC (FEV_3/FVC%); and (3) *the forced midexpiratory flow rate* ($FEF_{25-75\%}$). The $FEF_{25-75\%}$ is determined by locating the points on the volume–time curve corresponding to 25% and 75% of the FVC and then calculating the slope of a straight line passing through those two points. The slope of this line represents the average airflow over the midportion of the FVC.

Although the *relaxed* or *slow vital capacity* (VC) may be normal or only modestly reduced in patients with obstructive disease of the airways, the volume–time relationship of the FVC maneuver is usually distinctly abnormal in such patients (Fig. 33-16A and B). Most obvious is a flattening of the slope of the curve at any given lung volume, reflecting the reduced airflow. In addition, the duration of the forced expiratory maneuver is prolonged. Normally, expiration is complete within 6 seconds; in obstructive airway disease, expiratory airflow may continue for 10 to 12 seconds. These changes in the expiratory airflow reduce the FEV_1 and FEV_3, the FEV_1/FVC%, the FEV_3/FVC%, and the $FEF_{25-75\%}$.

Restrictive lung disorders reduce the slow vital capacity. However, the *configuration* of the volume–time relationship may not be abnormal (Fig. 33-16C). Although the FEV_1 and FEV_3 are reduced because of the reduced vital capacity, the FEV_1/FVC% and FEV_3/FVC% remain normal or even exceed normal values. Often, because of the reduced vital capacity, the $FEF_{25-75\%}$ is also less than predicted.

TABLE 33-6 Values Obtained from Forced Expiratory Volume–Time Curves

FVC (BTPS) (L)	Forced vital capacity; the total volume expired
FEV_1 (BTPS) (L)	Volume of air expired in the first second
FEV_1/FVC%	Volume of air expired in the first second, expressed as percent of the FVC
FEV_3/FVC%	Volume of air expired in the first 3 s, expressed as percent of the FVC
$FEF_{25-75\%}$ (BTPS) (L/s)	Forced midexpiratory airflow

Note: BTPS, body temperature and pressure, saturated with water vapor.

Forced Inspiratory Vital Capacity

Measurement of the forced inspiratory vital capacity (FIVC) consists of two steps: (1) full expiration to RV, followed by (2) a rapid maximal inspiratory effort (Fig. 33-17). The rate of airflow over the middle half of the forced inspiratory vital capacity ($FIF_{25-75\%}$) is determined using a procedure similar to that described previously for the $FEF_{25-75\%}$.

In normal subjects, the $FIF_{25-75\%}$ is greater than the $FEF_{25-75\%}$. Since inspiratory flow is more dependent on effort than is expiratory

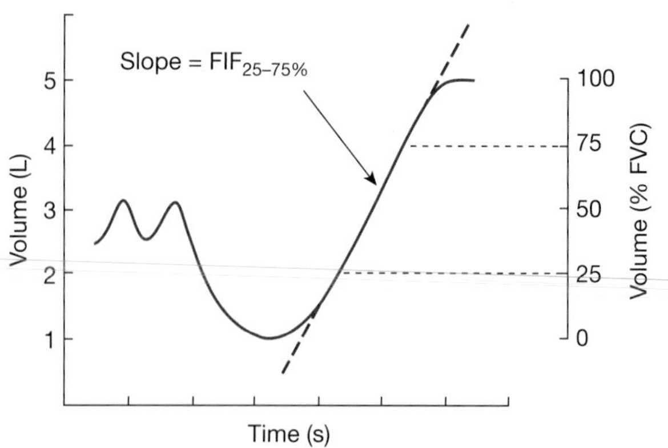

Figure 33-17 Forced inspiratory volume–time curve. The $FIF_{25-75\%}$ is the slope of a line between the points on the trace corresponding to 25% and 75% of the inspired volume.

flow, a fall in the $FIF_{25-75\%}$ is usually a more sensitive indicator of respiratory muscle dysfunction or a suboptimal effort than is the $FEF_{25-75\%}$. When airway resistance is high, a disproportionate fall in $FIF_{25-75\%}$ relative to $FEF_{25-75\%}$ suggests an extrathoracic site of airway obstruction (see Approach to Interpreting Commonly Performed Pulmonary Function Tests).

FLOW–VOLUME RELATIONSHIPS

In addition to analysis of the relationship between volume and time depicted on a spirogram, examination of the relationship between flow and volume provides useful information about lung function. A flow–volume curve, which shows the relationship between lung volume and maximal airflow as lung volume changes during a forced expiration, is shown in Figure 33-18. The test comprises four phases of breathing into a spirometer: (1) tidal breathing for several breaths, (2) a maximal inspiratory effort to TLC, followed by (3) a maximal expiration to RV done as forcefully and quickly as possible, and (4) another maximal inspiratory effort to TLC. Volume is displayed on the horizontal axis and airflow on the vertical axis. Airflow is measured at the mouth using a pneumotachograph; volume is measured either by integrating the pneumotachographic record during expiration or as a change in TGV, determined by a pressure-corrected flow plethysmograph. The records obtained by the two techniques for determining volume differ because the body plethysmograph senses compression of intrathoracic gas during a forced expiration, whereas measurements of volume made at the mouth do not (Fig. 33-19). Differences between curves obtained with the two techniques for measuring volume are most marked in patients with airway obstruction in whom considerable gas compression occurs during a forced expiration.

For the sake of comparison, tracings of flow versus volume and volume versus time, recorded during the same FVC maneuver and aligned by using a common volume axis as the abscissa, are shown in Figure 33-20. Selected measurements are more evident in one tracing or the other – for example, maximal expiratory flow in the flow–volume curve and volume expired in 1 second (FEV_1) in the volume–time curve.

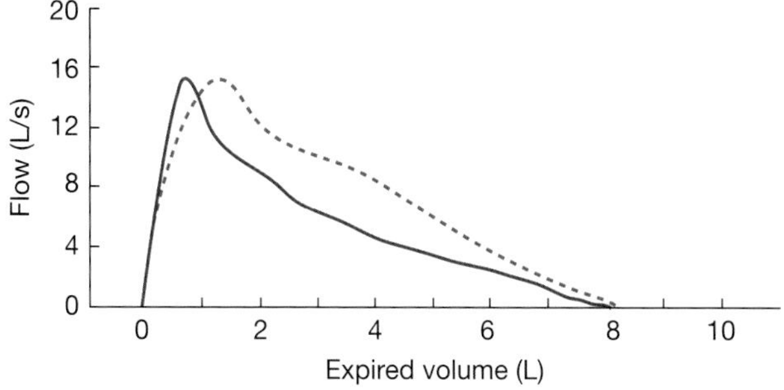

Figure 33-19 Comparison of the flow–expired-volume curve *(solid line)* with a simultaneously recorded flow–thoracic-gas-volume curve *(dashed line)*. The difference between the two curves results from the compression of gas in the lungs during a forced expiration.

Comparison of serial curves from a single person or curves from different subjects requires that the curves be aligned on the volume (horizontal) axis so that points of maximal inspiration or maximal expiration coincide. As may be seen in Figure 33-21A, which illustrates typical curves from a normal subject and two patients, one with pulmonary fibrosis and the other with obstructive airway disease, the information provided by this form of representation is limited; that is, the vital capacities and airflows from the patients are abnormally low. The limitation stems from the fact that the change in volume during expiration is shown relative to the *maximal inspiratory level* rather than to an *absolute volume* of gas in the lungs – that is, RV or TLC. When RV or TLC is known so that absolute volumes can be plotted on the horizontal axis (Fig. 33-21B), additional insight is gained into the flow–volume relationship depicted in Figure 33-21A. The patient with obstructive disease of the airways manifests a reduction in expiratory airflow at elevated lung volumes,

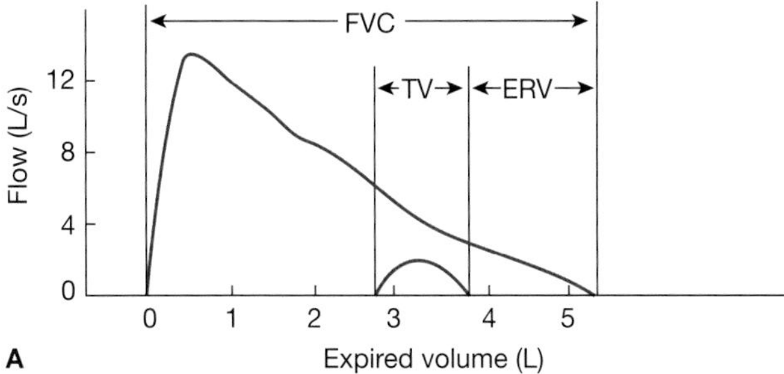

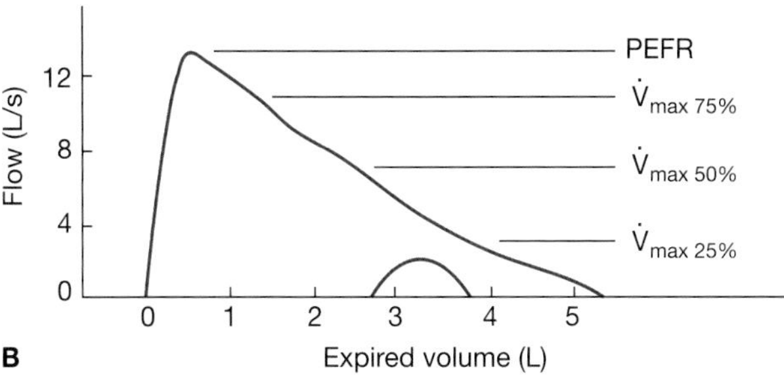

Figure 33-18 Flow–volume plots during forced expiration *(outer trace)* and quiet expiration *(inner trace)*. **A.** The subdivisions of lung volume. **B.** The common flow measurements. PEFR = peak expiratory flow rate; $\dot{V}_{max,75\%}$, $\dot{V}_{max,50\%}$, and $\dot{V}_{max,25\%}$ = flows at 75%, 50%, and 25% of the vital capacity, respectively.

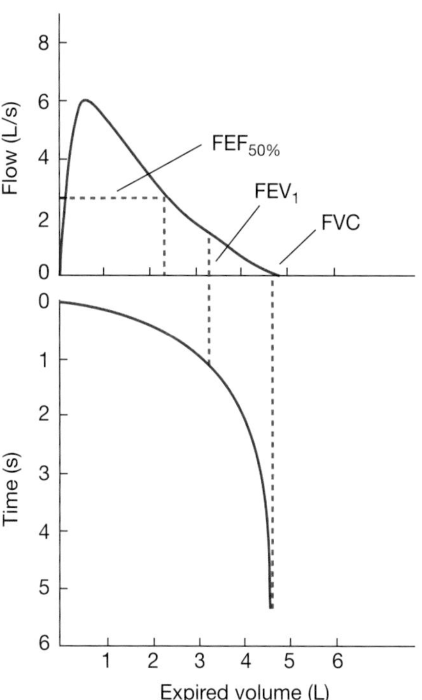

Figure 33-20 Flow–volume and volume–time curves depicting the same forced expiration aligned along a common volume axis (abscissa). Points corresponding to the FEV_1, FVC, and $FEF_{50\%}$ obtained from the volume–time plot are shown on the flow–volume curve.

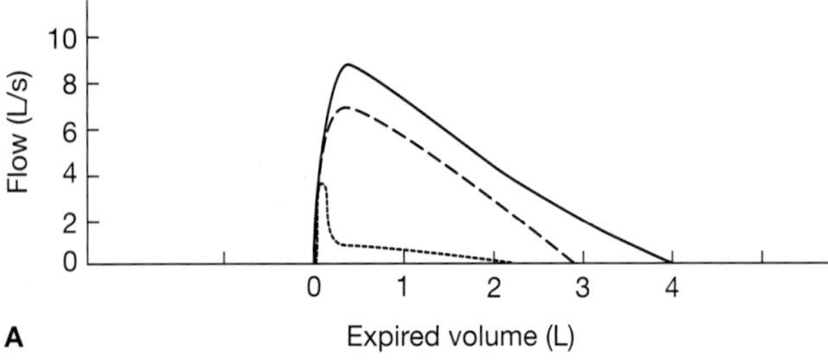

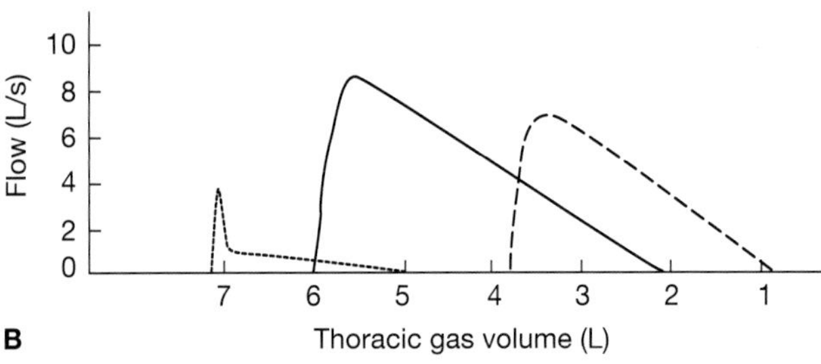

Figure 33-21 Airflow at different lung volumes. **A.** Flow–volume curves aligned at TLC. **B.** Flow–volume curves displayed relative to thoracic gas volume. Although the curves aligned at TLC (**A**) show striking differences in the pattern of airflow, they provide no insight into the relationship between lung volumes and airflow. See text for discussion.

which should enhance airflow. In contrast, the reduced rate of airflow in the patient with pulmonary fibrosis is normal, or even supranormal, when the lung volume at which the airflow occurs is taken into account; that is, the reduced airflow is primarily a function of the reduced lung volume, rather than of airway obstruction.

MAXIMAL VOLUNTARY VENTILATION

The previous considerations of dynamic lung function focus on a single timed maximal expiratory or inspiratory maneuver. In contrast, the MVV depends on the movement of air into and out of the lungs during continued maximal effort throughout a preset interval (Fig. 33-22). The MVV is a simple, informative test that provides an overall assessment of effort, coordination, and the elastic and flow-resistive properties of the respiratory system.[26,27]

In performing the test, the patient is urged to breathe as hard and as fast as possible. As a rule, the patient automatically adjusts

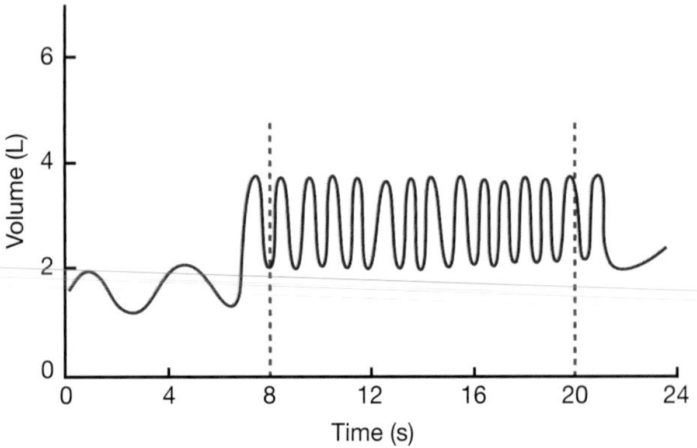

Figure 33-22 Maximal voluntary ventilation (MVV). After a period of relaxed breathing, the subject breathes rapidly and as forcefully as possible. The total volume of air inspired over 12 seconds and expressed in L/min is the MVV.

frequency and tidal volume for optimal performance. However, extremes of frequency or tidal volume are to be avoided, since neither panting nor slow deep breathing leads to the highest possible values. The total volume that is expired during a 12-second interval, expressed in liters per minute (BTPS), is the MVV. In some patients the test cannot be done because of an inability to continue the necessary effort for 12 seconds.

A normal value for MVV indicates that the overall integrated performance of the respiratory system is intact, thereby excluding moderate to severe restrictive or obstructive disease. In addition, a normal value suggests that the elastic and flow-resistive properties of the respiratory system, respiratory muscle strength, coordination of respiratory performance, and motivation of the patient are all normal. Although this test is very useful in detecting overall disturbances in integrated performance and diffuse tracheobronchial and pulmonary parenchymal diseases, other tests are required to pinpoint specific disorders.

The difference between the MVV and the resting minute ventilation is the *breathing reserve.* At one time, a low breathing reserve was correlated with the breathlessness in lung diseases. However, this determination is now primarily of historical interest.

RESPIRATORY RESISTANCE

Total respiratory resistance (Rrs) is the resistance to airflow and chest expansion offered by the airways (Raw), chest wall (Rw), and lung tissue (Rti):

$$\text{Rrs} = \text{Raw} + \text{Rw} + \text{Rti}$$

The overall resistance of the respiratory system can be determined with a technique employing forced oscillation (see Small-Airway Function). However, further methodologic refinements permitting determination of *pulmonary resistance* – the sum of airway and tissue resistances (Raw + Rti) – have not proved to be worthwhile clinically, particularly since measurement of transpulmonary pressure with an esophageal balloon is necessary. Other variations of the determination of resistance measurements have also been explored. However, the only clinically useful measurement of resistance is airway resistance, which is now routinely determined in pulmonary function laboratories.

AIRWAY RESISTANCE

Airway resistance (Raw) is defined as the ratio of the driving pressure (P) for flow to the actual rate of airflow ($\dot{V}$) along the airways – that is, the mouth, nasopharynx, larynx, and central and peripheral airways:

$$\text{Raw} = \frac{\Delta P}{\dot{V}}$$

where ΔP, the drop in pressure over the entire length of the airways, is determined as the difference between alveolar pressure (P_A) and pressure at the mouth (Pm) or airway opening (Pao).

Although airflow and pressure at the airway opening are easily measured, the difficulty in measuring alveolar pressure prevented the routine determination of airway resistance until DuBois and colleagues introduced the plethysmographic technique in 1956.[28]

With this technique, the patient, seated in the body plethysmograph, pants at a rate of about two breaths per second while airflow is measured using a pneumotachograph. During inspiration and expiration, gas in the alveoli is alternately rarefied and compressed, causing changes in pressure within the sealed plethysmograph. The relationship between plethysmograph pressure and airflow during the panting maneuver is displayed on the X and Y axes of an oscilloscope (Fig. 33-23).

While the panting continues, a shutter at the airway opening is closed so that airflow is transiently interrupted. Using the

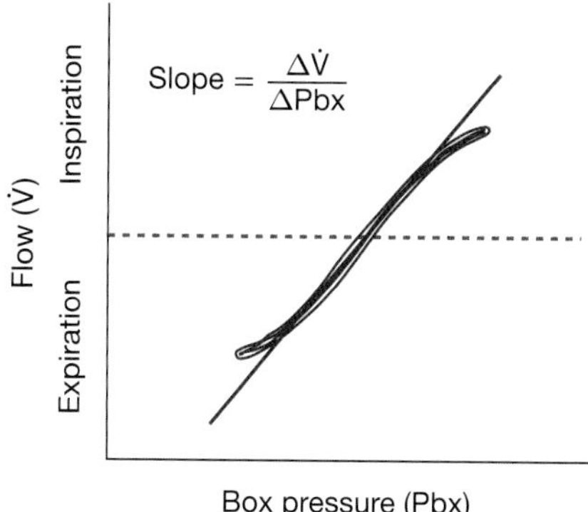

Figure 33-23 Plot of airflow ($\dot{V}$) versus body plethysmograph pressure (Pbx). The slope of this curve, in the range of 0 to 0.5 L/s of inspiratory flow, divided into the slope of the loop obtained when the shutter is closed (see Fig. 33-7) provides a measure of airway resistance (Raw).

technique employed in the determination of FRC, changes in pressure in the plethysmograph (equivalent to changes in lung volume) and at the mouth are displayed on the X and Y axes, respectively, of the oscilloscope (Fig. 33-6). However, since airflow is zero while the shutter is closed, the pressure at the mouth equals alveolar pressure (Pao = P_A).

Panting while the shutter is open allows the determination of the relationship between airflow ($\dot{V}$) and plethysmograph pressure (Pbx) – that is, $\dot{V}$/Pbx. Similarly, panting against a closed shutter enables the determination of the relationship between alveolar pressure (P_A) and plethysmograph pressure – that is, P_A/Pbx. Airway resistance is calculated by dividing the slope of the loop obtained by plotting P_A versus Pbx while the shutter is closed by the slope obtained by plotting $\dot{V}$ versus Pbx while the shutter is open:

$$Raw = \frac{P_A/Pbx}{\dot{V}/Pbx} = \frac{P_A}{\dot{V}}$$

where

Raw = airway resistance, $cmH_2O/L/s$
P_A = alveolar pressure, cmH_2O
$\dot{V}$ = airflow, L/s

Raw is measured during a panting maneuver for several reasons:[29] (1) The rapid respiratory frequency in panting circumvents the poor low-frequency response characteristics of many plethysmographs. (2) The small inspired and expired volumes minimize temperature fluctuations in the plethysmograph that would otherwise occur as tidal breaths of air at body temperature are exchanged with breaths of air at room temperature. (3) During panting, the glottis remains open, thereby minimizing its contribution to overall airway resistance. Use of plethysmographs linked to microprocessors that automatically correct for temperature-related volume differences has made possible the determination of airway resistance during quiet breathing instead of during panting.

Airway resistance varies inversely with lung volume; it is low at large lung volumes and increases curvilinearly as lung volume and, consequently, airway diameters are reduced (Fig. 33-24A).[30] In contrast, the inverse of airway resistance, airway *conductance,* is linearly related to lung volume (Fig. 33-24B). Interpretation of a given value for airway resistance or airway conductance requires that the lung volume at which the measurement is made be taken into account. *Specific conductance* (SGaw) is calculated by dividing airway conductance by the lung volume.

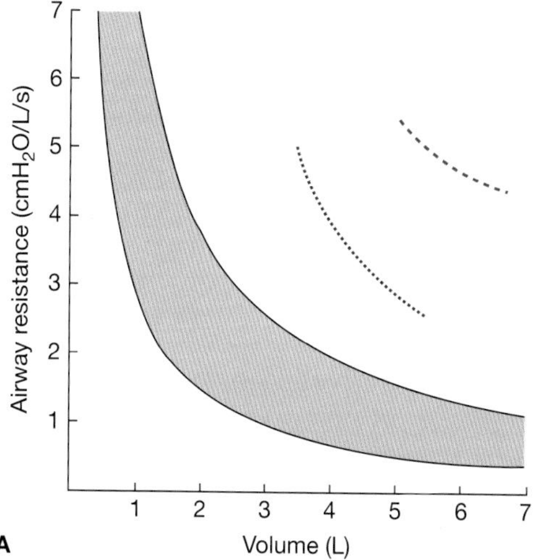

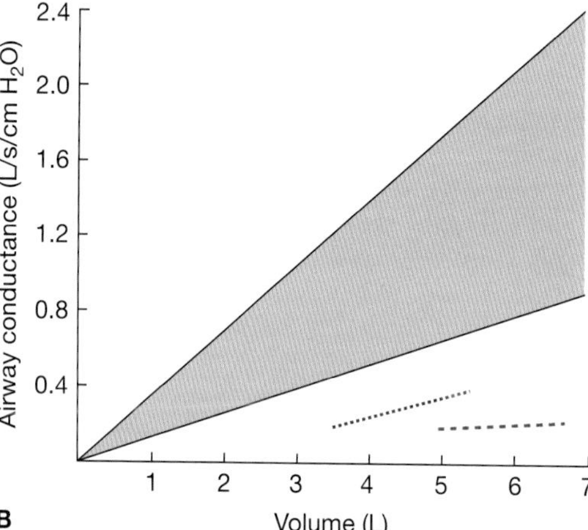

Figure 33-24 The relationship between airway resistance (**A**) and airway conductance (**B**). The shaded area represents the predicted normal range. Values are shown for an asthmatic patient before *(dashed line)* and after *(dotted line)* bronchodilator therapy. Airway resistance increases as lung volume decreases. Conversely, airway conductance, the inverse of resistance, decreases as lung volume decreases.

Defining the range of normal for Raw is difficult because of the lack of data obtained from populations sorted into smoking and nonsmoking groups and because of the inter- and intraindividual variations of Raw with lung volume. One classification scheme proposed for defining normal and abnormal Raw in adults in whom FRC exceeds 2 L is given in Table 33-7.

At times, an apparent discrepancy occurs between forced expiratory flow rates and values for airway resistance. For example,

TABLE 33-7 Categorization of Increased Airway Resistance (Raw)

Category	Raw ($cmH_2O/L/s$)
Mild	2.8–4.5
Moderate	4.54–8.0
Severe	>8.0

Source: Data from Ries A and Clausen JT: In Wilson AF (ed). Pulmonary Function Testing. Indications and Interpretations, Orlando, FL, Grune and Stratton; 1985.

although the FEV_1 and $FEF_{25-75\%}$ may be abnormally low (suggesting some degree of airway obstruction), Raw may be within normal limits (arguing against appreciable airway obstruction). This apparent contradiction arises because Raw is determined during *inspiration,* when airways are enlarged because of surrounding negative pleural pressure, whereas FEV_1 and $FEF_{25-75\%}$ are determined during a forceful *expiration,* when airways are compressed by high positive pleural pressures. Therefore, the discrepancy is simply a manifestation of dynamic airway obstruction in which the narrowing is confined to expiration.

MEASUREMENT OF EXHALED NITRIC OXIDE

Over the last two decades, the important role of nitric oxide (NO) in a variety of biologic processes has been described.[31] The concept that NO is a marker of airway inflammation, and, hence, has a potential role as a measure of airway function in the setting of inflammatory airway diseases, has been investigated.[32,33] Studies have demonstrated that, at least in asthma, levels of exhaled NO are elevated during exacerbations (when other measures of airway inflammation show activity), even in the absence of symptoms or changes in spirometry.[34,35] Exhaled levels of NO may also be helpful in classifying the severity of asthma.[36] Levels of NO decrease with inhaled corticosteroid use and rise with corticosteroid tapering. Some advocate measurement of exhaled NO as part of routine chronic asthma management.[31]

Standards have been developed for measuring exhaled NO levels.[31] While exhaled NO measurement has not yet assumed the status of a "standard" pulmonary function test, pulmonary function laboratories will likely soon add the test to their repertoires.

AIRWAY REACTIVITY

The dynamic tests of airway function described previously are designed to determine intrinsic properties of the airways in a subject breathing room air at rest. In many clinical situations, such as evaluation of chronic cough, assessment of airway hyperresponsiveness is desirable. This section reviews *bronchoprovocation testing* (BPT),[37,38] which assesses reactivity of the airways to selected pharmacologic or environmental agents.

BACKGROUND

One test of bronchial reactivity that has been incorporated into routine pulmonary function testing is determination of the effect on airflow of administration of a nebulized bronchodilator agent. However, bronchoprovocation tests are designed to quantify the degree of bronchoconstriction following the application of a particular stimulus. A number of tests of bronchial reactivity are currently in clinical use (Table 33-8). Among the agents used for inhalation challenges are methacholine, histamine, carbacholine, and specific antigens chosen in accord with the patient's history. In addition to the inhalation challenge tests in which pharmacologic agents are used, tests of bronchial reactivity may be based on inhalation of cold or dry air, isocapnic hyperventilation, or exercise.

INDICATIONS FOR BRONCHOPROVOCATION TESTING

The principal indication for BPT is a history suggestive of bronchospasm induced by an environmental or occupational agent, generally in the setting of normal pulmonary function tests (including determination of airflow before and after administration of an inhaled bronchodilator). For example, comparison of FEV_1 before and after administration of a pharmacologic agent such as methacholine or histamine can be useful in establishing the diagnosis of asthma. Also, inhalation of a suspected specific antigen may be useful in uncovering asthma when skin tests are equivocal, or in proving that asthma is occupation related. In some instances, exercise testing may disclose airway hyperreactivity in persons who are free of bronchoconstriction while at rest. Airway hyperresponsiveness to methacholine may presage an accelerated decline in pulmonary function.[39] However, the impact of therapy with agents like inhaled bronchodilators or corticosteroids in preventing progression is unclear.

TABLE 33-8 Tests of Bronchial Reactivity

Test	Reference
Inhalational challenges	
Pharmacologic agents	
Methacholine	Chai et al. *J Allergy Clin Immunol.* 1975;56:323–327
Histamine	Chai et al. *J Allergy Clin Immunol.* 1975;56:323–327
Carbocholine	Orehek et al. *Br Med J.* 1975;1:123–125
Specific antigens	
Toluene diisocyanate	Salvaggio. *J Allergy Clin Immunol.* 1979;64:646–649
Bacillus subtilis	Salvaggio. *J Allergy Clin Immunol.* 1979;64:646–649
Pollen	Spector. *J Allergy Clin Immunol.* 1979;64:580–586
Molds	Spector. *J Allergy Clin Immunol.* 1979;64:580–586
House dust	Spector. *J Allergy Clin Immunol.* 1979;64:580–586
Exercise-induced asthma	
Cold-air challenge	Strauss et al. *N Engl J Med.* 1977;297:743–747
Dry-air challenge	Hahn et al. *Am Rev Respir Dis.* 1984;130:575–579
Isocapnic hyperventilation	Eschenbacher et al. *Am Rev Respir Dis.* 1985;131:894–901

METHODS OF BRONCHOPROVOCATION TESTING

Several methods of BPT are in general clinical use. These include methacholine challenge, exercise challenge, and antigen challenge, each of which is described briefly in subsequent sections.

Inhalation Challenge: Methacholine

Inhalation challenge using methacholine has become popular because of standardization of the technique, ease and safety of performing the test, and high sensitivity of the test in detecting asthma.[40,41] Methacholine is a synthetic cholinergic agent that evokes airway smooth muscle constriction. Because baseline pulmonary function and breathing pattern influence the site of deposition of the inhaled methacholine particles and, thereby, the response, a standard method for aerosolizing the agent is used to ensure reproducible results.[42]

One method in common use is that of intermittent aerosol generation. Standardization entails the delivery of a 0.6-second pulse of airflow at 20 lb/in.^{2} to a nebulizer, which, in turn, discharges particles that range from 0.3 to 4 μm in diameter into the airways. Methacholine for delivery by aerosol is prepared in concentrations ranging from 0.1 to 25 mg/mL using bicarbonate-buffered isotonic saline (containing 0.4% phenol) as the diluent. The cumulative dose delivered is expressed in inhalation units. One inhalation unit is equivalent to the single inhalation of a solution containing 1 mg of methacholine per milliliter (Table 33-9).

TABLE 33-9 Concentrations and Cumulative Doses of Methacholine Employed in the Methacholine Challenge Test

Methacholine Concentration (mg/mL)	Cumulative Dose (Inhalation Units)[a]
0.1	0.5
0.5	3
1.0	8
2.0	18
5.0	43
10.0	93
25.0	218

[a]*After five inhalations of a nebulized solution containing methacholine in a concentration of 1 mg/mL.*

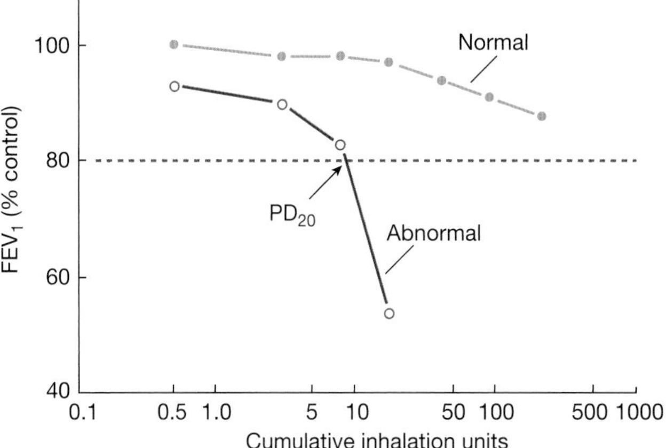

Figure 33-25 Plot of FEV_1,% control versus cumulative dose of methacholine administered by inhalation (logarithmic scale), to a normal subject and a subject with hyperreactive airways. The PD_{20} is the cumulative dose, which results in a 20% drop in the FEV_1 from the baseline measurement (after inhalation of diluent alone). In the subject with normal airway reactivity, the maximal cumulative dose of methacholine administered fails to elicit a 20% drop in FEV_1.

At the outset, the patient is challenged with five inhalations containing only aerosolized diluent. The necessity of the diluent step has been recently questioned. In addition to adding time and expense, it may force a greater absolute drop in FEV_1 needed to prove bronchial hyperreactivity. A fall in FEV_1 below 90% of the baseline value (i.e., the prechallenge control FEV_1) establishes that the airways are hyperreactive, and therefore, the test is terminated. However, if the FEV_1 does not fall below 90% of the control value, increasing concentrations of methacholine are given in stepwise increments of five-breath inhalations. The breaths are taken slowly from FRC to TLC. Then, 1 to 1.5 minutes after each dose, an FVC maneuver is performed. The interval between each increase in concentration is kept to a minimum because the response is judged in terms of the *cumulative* dose. However, the deep inspiration that immediately precedes the expiratory portion of the FVC maneuver may decrease bronchomotor tone in airways narrowed by methacholine. This effect lasts up to 6 minutes, thus limiting the shortest acceptable interval between dosage steps.[43] If the postchallenge FEV_1 falls below 80% of the control FEV_1, or if the patient experiences cough or chest tightness at any step, the test is stopped. The magnitude of the bronchoconstrictor response to inhalational challenge is related to the control FEV_1. A lower baseline FEV_1 (even in the normal range) correlates with increased bronchial reactivity.[44–47] Additional measurements of dynamic airway function (e.g., specific conductance) may provide supplemental data but also prolong the study. Another dosing option in use is the 2-minute tidal breathing protocol. This protocol typically yields results similar to the one described previously.

The results are plotted on four-cycle semilog graph paper: the number of cumulative inhalation units, expressed logarithmically, against the FEV_1, as percent of control (Fig. 33-25). A curve is constructed through the points; the dose corresponding to the point at which the FEV_1 is 80% of the control FEV_1 is designated as the *provocation dose,* or PD_{20} FEV_1.

Exercise Challenge

Persons without a history of asthma who develop cough, wheezing, or dyspnea after exercise may have exercise-induced bronchospasm (EIB). In these individuals, an exercise test may prove useful in establishing the diagnosis. Such exercise testing in asthmatics can be useful to assess the degree of impairment during exercise, or the impact of therapies.

Several factors that may influence the outcome of the test should be kept in mind. The temperature and humidity of the laboratory should be tightly controlled. Some centers use dry air inhalation during exercise. In addition, the duration of the test needs to be monitored. The goal of testing for EIB is to produce at least 4 minutes of exercise at the target heart rate and ventilation. Exercise should not continue for more than 6 to 8 minutes, in order to avoid "run-through" of the bronchospasm – that is, reversal at the end of the test.

The type of exercise also influences the outcome. As a rule, the more intense the exercise, the more likely is bronchoconstriction to occur. Free-range running provides the most potent stimulus for bronchoconstriction, followed by treadmill running, bicycle ergometry, swimming, and walking. An asthmatic may swim comfortably at a level of exercise that is incapacitating on the treadmill. The motor-driven treadmill or electromagnetically braked cycle ergometer are the preferred modes of exercise for formal testing.

The FEV_1 is the most useful measurement made during testing for EIB. Measurements are made just before and immediately after the exercise and at 5-minute intervals for the following 30 minutes. A decrease in FEV_1 of 10% or more below the pre-exercise value constitutes a positive test. Some have suggested that a decrement of 15% is of greater diagnostic value. False-positive responses can occur in patients with vocal cord dysfunction or abnormal posterior arytenoid motion.

Inhalation Challenge: Antigen

Compared with the relatively safe methacholine challenge test, BPT using a specific antigen is unpredictable and potentially hazardous. Since establishing the minimum dose required to induce bronchoconstriction is difficult, too much of the antigen may be given. A late response, far more severe than the initial one, often develops about 6 hours after the challenge. Despite these reservations about antigen challenge, testing is warranted under certain circumstances: to uncover a particular agent in the environment that causes bronchoconstriction, to establish the diagnosis of occupational asthma, to prove that bronchoconstriction is caused by a particular antigen after routine skin tests have failed to support the clinical suspicion, and to convince a skeptical patient about the cause of his or her asthma. Recommendations for preparing concentrations of antigens and the technique of antigen challenge testing are specific to the antigen in question and may be found in the literature. These tests should only be performed in laboratories which have considerable experience in BPT.

TABLE 33-10 Bronchoprovocation Testing: Precautions and Contraindications

- Baseline FEV_1/FVC% <60 (relative) or <50 (absolute)
- Recent upper respiratory tract infection
- Recent influenza vaccination
- Recent administration of bronchodilator
- Ingestion of caffeine within 6 h before testing
- Cold-air breathing, hyperventilation, exercise within 6 h before testing
- Recent acute myocardial infarction or cerebrovascular accident, uncontrolled hypertension, or known aortic aneurysm

PRECAUTIONS AND CONTRAINDICATIONS

Although the overall risk of serious complications is low, bronchoprovocation tests may be unnecessary, invalid, or even dangerous in some circumstances (Table 33-10). For example, the patient who manifests appreciable airway obstruction by conventional testing may develop life-threatening airway narrowing during a bronchoprovocation test. In such a patient, a simple bronchodilator study would be more appropriate and informative. If bronchodilators fail to reverse the increase in airway resistance, and if it is important to prove that bronchial hyperreactivity does exist, BPT is sometimes done, with extreme caution, on another day, as antigen dosages are titrated carefully and details of the procedure monitored closely.

Absolute contraindications include severe airways obstruction (FEV_1 <50% predicted), myocardial infarction or stroke in the preceding 3 months, uncontrolled hypertension, or known aortic aneurysm. Moderate airflow limitation, pregnancy, lactation, and concurrent use of cholinesterase inhibitor medication represent relative contraindications.

A recent viral upper respiratory tract infection can cause airway hyperreactivity for up to 6 weeks in normal subjects. Similarly, influenza vaccination increases responsiveness to inhalation challenges in asthmatics for a few days to a week. In these conditions, BPT should not be undertaken until the sensitization effects of the infection or vaccination have worn off. Also, bronchodilators, including caffeine, should be withheld for at least 6 hours before a bronchoprovocation test, if possible, in order to prevent blunting of the bronchoconstrictor response. Finally, cold air, hyperventilation, and exercise should be avoided for at least 6 hours before testing in order to prevent the induction of a refractory period or late response that would overlap the test results.

SMALL-AIRWAY FUNCTION

Up to this point, discussion of tests of dynamic lung function has addressed the tracheobronchial tree as a unit. However, in a variety of common clinical settings, including asthma, COPD, cigarette smoking, lung transplantation complicated by bronchiolitis obliterans syndrome, ARDS, and cystic fibrosis,[48–52] structural (and functional) abnormalities of the airways may be centered primarily in the small, peripheral airways – that is, those 2 mm or smaller in diameter. Because of their small contribution to airway resistance, estimated to be about 10% to 38% (at a lung volume equivalent to 50% of VC), the small airways can undergo considerable damage before the usual tests of either static or dynamic lung function become abnormal.[53,54] Consequently, efforts have been made to utilize tests aimed at early detection of small-airway disease in the hope of early intervention to limit progression of the disease.

Once obstructive disease of the peripheral airways arises, the small airways' contribution to overall resistance increases, and abnormalities in their function may be detected using specialized tests (see below), or, in some cases, analysis of selected aspects of the expiratory VC maneuver. In particular, abnormal values for $FEF_{25-75\%}$, in conjunction with normal values for FVC and FEV_1, are often useful in identifying small-airway disease. The basis for this approach is that $FEF_{25-75\%}$ measures airflow during the effort independent part of the FVC, when the small airways contribute substantially to the limitation of airflow.

A number of specialized tests of small airways' function have been developed over the last several decades, and some have found resurgent use in evaluating selected patient populations.[48] Several, along with their underlying physiologic basis, are described in subsequent sections.

FORCED OSCILLATION TECHNIQUE AND IMPULSE OSCILLOMETRY

The forced oscillation technique (FOT) and a variation of FOT, impulse oscillometry, are based on assessment of airway impedance and a component of airway impedance, airway resistance. Using a loudspeaker applied to the airway opening and measuring pressure and flow over a range of oscillation frequencies, airway resistance can be measured and compartmentalized into segments reflecting resistance in medium-to-large and small airways. In normals, over an oscillatory range of 5 to 25 Hz, respiratory resistance and its major component, airways resistance, are frequency independent. With development of airways obstruction, respiratory resistance becomes frequency-dependent. Furthermore, as small airways narrow or close, a component of impedance distinct from resistance – reactance (a concept which refers to the "out-of-phase" relationship between pressure and flow during oscillation and which is ascribed to energy storage, as determined by the elastic properties of the respiratory system) – is significantly affected, particularly when measured during the expiratory phase of respiration.[48,51,52,55]

DYNAMIC COMPLIANCE

Dynamic compliance, defined as the change in lung volume during airflow produced by a given change in transpulmonary pressure, is normally independent of breathing frequency. However, under conditions of nonuniformity of ventilation throughout the lung, increases in breathing frequency are associated with a fall in dynamic compliance. This frequency dependence of compliance was first noted in a patient with emphysema.[56,57]

During the test, the patient, with an esophageal balloon in place, first inspires maximally to TLC and then expires to the resting end-expiratory position (FRC); the patient then breathes at a normal tidal volume and respiratory rate (15 breaths per minute). In order to enable the patient to monitor these parameters, tidal volume and the resting end-expiratory level are displayed on an oscilloscope within sight of the patient. At the same time, changes in tidal volume and transpulmonary pressure are displayed on another oscilloscope (Fig. 33-26). The slope of the line connecting the end-inspiratory and end-expiratory points on the pressure–volume loop – that is, the points of zero airflow – is the dynamic compliance. This procedure is repeated with breathing frequencies of 30 and 60 breaths per minute. Values for dynamic compliance (Cdyn,L) at the various frequencies are expressed as a ratio of the dynamic compliance to the static inspiratory compliance (Cst,L) or as a percentage of Cst,L (Fig. 33-27) for the same range of tidal volumes.

In normal subjects, Cdyn,L/Cst,L remains above 0.8, even at frequencies greater than 60 breaths per minute. However, in the presence of obstructive disease of the small airways, Cdyn,L/Cst,L falls progressively to values below 0.8 as breathing frequency increases. It is worth emphasizing that interpretation of frequency dependence of compliance with regard to small-airway disease is valid only if the static compliance and overall airway resistance are normal. Abnormalities in these other measurements indicate

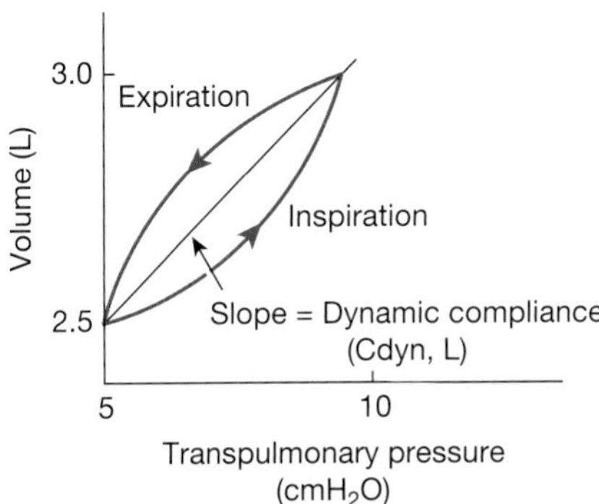

Figure 33-26 Measurement of dynamic lung compliance (Cdyn,L). During the inspiratory and expiratory phases of the respiratory cycle, a loop relating volume to transpulmonary pressure is generated. The slope of a line drawn through the points of zero airflow (at end inspiration and end expiration) is the dynamic compliance. Determination of Cdyn,L can be done at a variety of respiratory frequencies to assess the frequency dependence of compliance (Fig. 36-27).

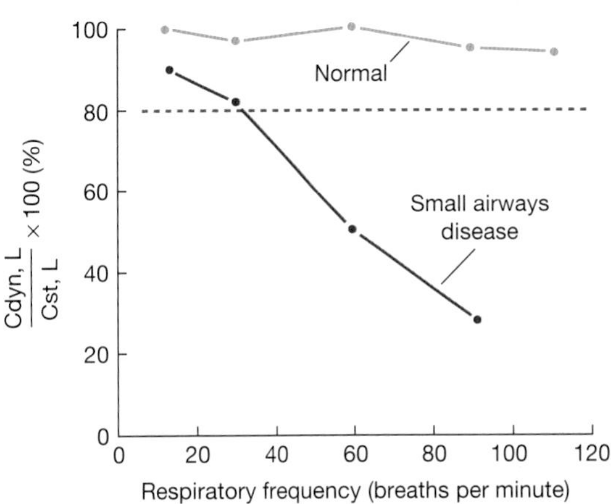

Figure 33-27 Determination of frequency dependence of dynamic compliance. Dynamic compliance is determined as shown in Figure 36-26 and is expressed as a percentage of static lung compliance (Cdyn, L/Cst, L × 100,%) at a variety of respiratory frequencies. Normally, Cdyn,L is ≥80% of Cst,L and is independent of respiratory frequency. In patients with obstructive airway disease, including those with disease limited to the small airways, Cdyn,L falls relative to Cst,L as respiratory frequency increases.

disease that is not likely to be confined to the small airways and for which frequency dependence of dynamic compliance is another manifestation. The physiologic basis for the fall in Cdyn,L/Cst,L as respiratory frequency increases is the presence of unequal time constants throughout the lung (see above).

SINGLE-BREATH NITROGEN WASHOUT, MULTIPLE BREATH NITROGEN WASHOUT, AND CLOSING VOLUME

In 1949, Fowler described the single-breath nitrogen washout test for assessing the uniformity of ventilation throughout the lungs. In performing this test, the patient first expires maximally to RV before filling his or her lungs by taking a maximal breath of 100% O_2. During the subsequent expiration, the concentration of nitrogen at the mouth is continuously recorded and plotted against the volume of expired gas. Originally, interest focused on the initial part of the tracing that depicts the changing concentration in expired nitrogen as the first 750 to 1200 mL of gas is exhaled. Over this range, the change in nitrogen concentration in persons with normal lungs is less than 2.5%. In contrast, when disease of the lungs or tracheobronchial tree results in abnormal intrapulmonary distribution of inspired gas, the change in nitrogen concentration exceeds 2.5%.

Almost 20 years later, Fowler's test was modified to include a bolus of xenon at the beginning of inspiration and to record the concentration of xenon during the following expiration.[58] Abrupt changes in the concentration of expired xenon as RV was approached suggested that important information about the small airways could be obtained from the terminal portion of the curve.

These observations with xenon rekindled interest in Fowler's original technique and also directed attention to the terminal portion of expiration. The procedure is depicted in Figure 33-28. To perform the maneuver for this measurement, the seated patient

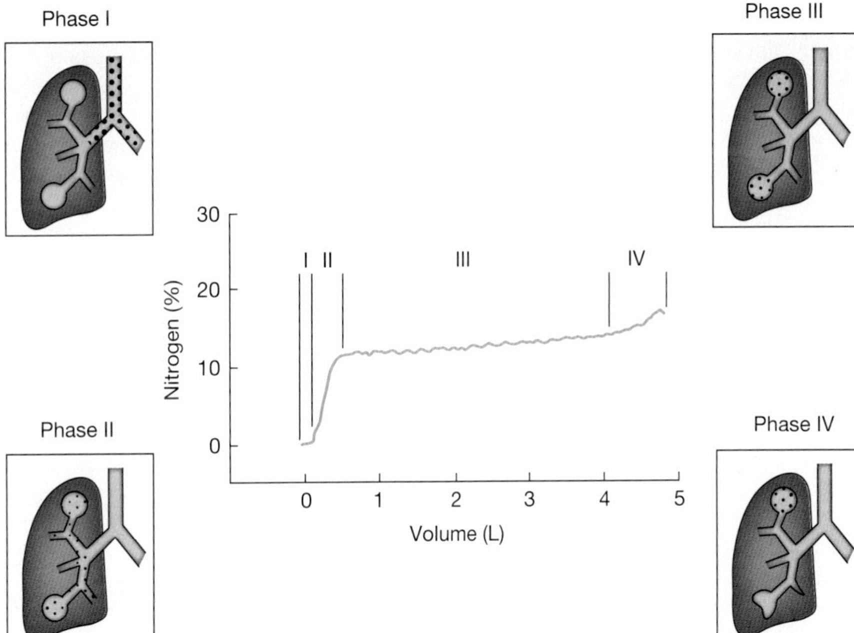

Figure 33-28 Contributions of different lung regions to the nitrogen concentration–volume curve obtained during the single-breath nitrogen washout test. See text for discussion.

takes two deep breaths of air and then expires to RV. At the end of this maximal expiration, a valve is opened so that the patient can take a full breath of 100% O_2 to TLC. The patient then expires slowly to RV while N_2 concentration and expired volume are recorded continuously.

Four distinct phases can be identified in the continuous record relating N_2 concentration to expired volume. Phase I, the initial expirate, contains virtually no N_2, since it derives from the O_2-containing dead space. Phase II represents a mixture of gases from the dead space and the alveoli. Phase III is due to a mixture of gases from alveoli located at the apices, midlung fields, and bases. Phase IV, characterized by an upward shift in N_2 concentration, is caused by closure of alveoli in the dependent parts of the lungs at low lung volumes. This final expirate derives from alveoli in the middle and upper regions of the lungs, where N_2 concentrations are higher than at the bases.

The explanation for these phases resides in the intrapulmonary distribution of gases during the respiratory maneuvers used in performing the test. In the normal upright person, a gradient of pleural pressures exists from apex to base, so that pleural pressure is more negative at the apices than at the bases. Because the alveoli at the bases operate on a lower portion of their pressure–volume curve (Fig. 33-11), they expand more than do apical alveoli per unit change in pleural pressure. However, the less negative pleural pressures and decrease in elastic recoil pressure at the bases also cause small airways to close during expiration as lung volume approaches RV. Thus, the pleural pressure gradient from top to bottom of the chest causes nonuniform distribution of gas within the normal upright lungs.

In the single-breath nitrogen washout test, a breath of 100% O_2 is taken, starting from RV. At RV, small basal airways are closed. Therefore, at the start of the O_2 breath, the N_2-containing air remaining in the dead space is preferentially drawn into the middle and apical lung zones as 100% O_2 gradually replaces air in the dead space. As the inspiration continues, the small airways at the bases open. Since their compliances are greater than those in the middle or at the top of the upright lungs, the inspired O_2 is then preferentially distributed to the bases.

During the expiration from TLC, the four phases then represent, as indicated above, the sequential emptying of dead-space gas and a mixture of dead-space and alveolar gas, followed by mixtures of alveolar gases from different parts of the lungs, as determined by the preceding intrapulmonary distribution of inspired O_2.[59]

The volume from the onset of phase IV to the completion of the full expiratory maneuver is termed the *closing volume* (CV). In healthy young adults, the normal closing volume averages about 10% of the VC. Narrowing or obstruction of small peripheral airways causes closing volume to enlarge. The closing volume also increases progressively as people grow older, so that by the age of 50, the closing volume sometimes reaches 25% of the VC. Cigarette smokers consistently experience an increase in closing volume. In both aging normal persons and cigarette smokers at any age, a decrease in pulmonary elasticity seems to be responsible for the increase in closing volume.

■ HELIUM–OXYGEN FLOW–VOLUME CURVES

In 1963, the effects of changes in gas density and viscosity on maximal expiratory flow throughout the vital capacity range were described.[60] Almost 10 years later, gas-density-related and viscosity-related concepts were applied to determine the site of airway obstruction in asthma. These principles were then applied for the specific purpose of detecting obstruction of small airways when other tests of pulmonary function were within normal limits.[61] While application of helium–oxygen flow–volume curves in the assessment of small airways function is physiologically elegant, the test is rarely performed in clinical practice.

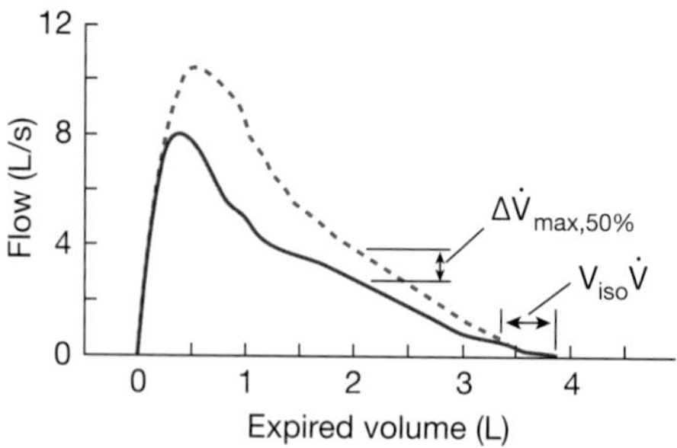

Figure 33-29 Maximal expiratory flow–volume curves generated in breathing room air *(solid line)* and breathing a helium–oxygen mixture *(dashed line)*. The airflows achieved with the less dense helium mixture are higher than those with air at all but the lowest lung volumes. The point of first intersection of these two curves demarcates the volume of isoflow ($V_{iso}\dot{V}$). The difference between the flows achieved when 50% of the vital capacity has been expired is the $\Delta\dot{V}_{max,50\%}$. The use of these measurements as indicators of small-airway disease is described in the text.

The use of a helium–oxygen mixture to detect small-airway disease requires comparison of two maximal expiratory flow–volume curves, one that is generated while the patient breathes air and the other while the patient breathes helium and oxygen (Fig. 33-29). At least three maximal expiratory flow curves are obtained with room air and three with helium–oxygen.[29]

In normal subjects, at lung volumes greater than 10% of the VC, the primary site of resistance to airflow is in the larger airways, where flow is turbulent and, therefore, density dependent. At these lung volumes, the flow attained with the helium–oxygen mixture will be higher than that attained with air. At lung volumes less than 10% of the VC, the primary site of resistance is in the smaller airways, where flow is laminar and, therefore, not density dependent. In this circumstance, the less dense helium mixture has no effect on flow (Fig. 33-29). In disease of the small airways, the primary site of resistance shifts at large volumes from the larger to the smaller airways. As a result, the flow-enhancing effect of the less dense gas disappears at volumes well above 10% of the VC.

In practice, two sets of maximal expiratory flow–volume curves are obtained, one while the subject is breathing air and the other after three VC breaths of the helium–oxygen mixture to replace at least 95% of the alveolar N_2. Comparisons are then made of the superimposed curves (Fig. 33-29). One comparison is made at 50% of the VC in order to compare maximal expiratory flows (i.e., the $\Delta\dot{V}_{max,50\%}$); the other is at the volume at which the flows become identical – that is, the *volume of isoflow* ($V_{iso}\dot{V}$).[62] The curves are superimposed at RV or TLC, as long as the vital capacities of each curve are within 2.5% to 5.0% of the largest VC recorded.[29]

The percentage change in expiratory flow while breathing helium–oxygen compared to air at 50% of the VC, $\Delta\dot{V}E_{max,50\%}$, is calculated as

$$\Delta\dot{V}E_{max,50\%} = \frac{\dot{V}E_{max,50\%}(\text{helium–oxygen}) - \dot{V}E_{max,50\%}(\text{air})}{\dot{V}E_{max,50\%}(\text{air})} \times 100$$

where $\dot{V}E_{max,50\%}$ (helium–oxygen) and $\dot{V}E_{max,50\%}$ (air) are the expiratory flows at 50% of the VC during helium–oxygen and air breathing, respectively. As noted previously, the volume of isoflow is normally less than 10% of the VC; when it is increased, it indicates small-airway obstruction. The $\Delta\dot{V}E_{max,50\%}$ is also specific for small-airway disease, and unlike the closing volume, it is considered to be unaffected by changes in the elastic properties of the lung. Questions remain, however, about the validity and sensitivity of tests of density dependence of flow in assessing small-airway disease. Although they are conceptually attractive, the practical value of helium–oxygen flow–volume curves in detecting small-airway disease is debatable.

GAS EXCHANGE FUNCTIONS

Traditional measurements of the gas exchange functions of the lung include oxygen uptake ($\dot{V}_{O_2}$), carbon dioxide elimination ($\dot{V}_{CO_2}$), respiratory dead space (VD), alveolar gas composition (PA_{O_2} and PA_{CO_2}), diffusing capacity for carbon monoxide (DL_{CO}), and arterial blood gas tensions (Pa_{O_2} and Pa_{CO_2}). These determinations require a steady state of the ventilation and circulation and constant body stores of O_2 and CO_2. A steady state with respect to O_2 implies that O_2 uptake measured at the mouth equals the rate of O_2 transport across the alveolar membrane, and that, in turn, both rates are equal to O_2 consumption by the tissues. The same type of definition applies to CO_2 exchange in the tissues, in the alveolar capillaries, and at the mouth.

VENTILATION, OXYGEN UPTAKE, AND CARBON DIOXIDE ELIMINATION

The total volume of air breathed per minute ($\dot{V}E$) is the *minute ventilation*. It is equal to the product of the tidal volume (VT) and the breathing frequency (f). As a rule, minute ventilation is determined by measuring the volume of expired gas relative to time. When the measurement is performed manually, the necessary equipment includes gas-collecting bags, low-resistance directional valves, a stopwatch, and a device for measuring gas volume. In practice, the patient, with nose clip in place, breathes through a mouthpiece for at least 3 to 5 minutes while expired gas is vented to the atmosphere. This preliminary period is intended to put the patient at ease and to achieve a steady state of respiration and circulation. When a steady heart rate and breathing pattern are achieved, a valve is turned without the patient's knowledge, and expired gas is collected for 3 minutes.

The minute ventilation is determined by dividing the total volume of expired gas collected in the spirometer by the time of collection (3 minutes). The average tidal volume is obtained by dividing $\dot{V}E$ by the number of breaths per minute. Values for minute ventilation and tidal volume are expressed in terms of body conditions (BTPS). In the resting adult, the minute ventilation is typically 6 to 8 L/min; the corresponding tidal volume is 0.4 to 0.6 L.

The quantity of CO_2 in inspired air is negligible. Consequently, the amount of CO_2 produced per minute ($\dot{V}_{CO_2}$) can be calculated as the product of the expired volume of ventilation ($\dot{V}E$) and the concentration of CO_2 in the expired air (FE_{CO_2}):

$$\dot{V}_{CO_2} = \dot{V}E \times FE_{CO_2}$$

Oxygen uptake ($\dot{V}O_2$) is calculated as the difference between the amounts of O_2 in inspired and expired air:

$$\dot{V}O_2 = (\dot{V}I \times FI_{O_2}) - (\dot{V}E \times FE_{O_2})$$

where

$\dot{V}I$ = inspired volume of ventilation, L/min
FI_{O_2} = concentration of O_2 in the inspired air
FE_{O_2} = concentration of O_2 in the expired air

In the steady state, O_2 uptake by alveolar capillary blood exceeds CO_2 output from alveolar capillary blood. As a result, the expired volume of gas is less than the corresponding inspired volume. Since N_2 does not undergo exchange in the lungs, the difference between CO_2 output and O_2 uptake results in a higher concentration of N_2 in expired air than in inspired air. Based on the change in nitrogen concentration, the inspired volume of ventilation can be calculated from the expired volume of ventilation:

$$\dot{V}_I = \dot{V}_E \frac{F_{E_{N_2}}}{F_{I_{N_2}}}$$

where

FE_{N_2} = concentration of N_2 in expired air
FI_{N_2} = concentration of N_2 in inspired air

In the normal, resting subject who is tested after several hours of fasting, the ratio of CO_2 output to O_2 uptake, the *respiratory exchange ratio* (R), is about 0.8. The respiratory exchange ratio at any instant is calculated by simultaneously determining the P_{O_2} and P_{CO_2} in an alveolar gas sample. As indicated above, in the steady state, the R determined by sampling alveolar gas equals the R of alveolar capillary blood, which, in turn, equals the R of the tissues. The steady-state R, when alveolar gas, blood, and tissue are all in dynamic equilibrium, is the *respiratory quotient* (RQ). Hence, in the steady state, when the O_2 and CO_2 stores of the body are not changing, the RQ, reflecting cellular metabolism, can be determined by analyzing alveolar gas for O_2 and CO_2.

Unlike tidal volume and ventilation, which are expressed in terms of BTPS, $\dot{V}_{O_2}$ and $\dot{V}_{CO_2}$ are given in terms of standard temperature and pressure, dry (STPD).

DEAD SPACE

Not all of the air breathed participates in gas exchange. Part of each breath remains in the mouth, nose, pharynx, larynx, trachea, bronchi, and bronchioles. This volume, the *anatomic dead space,* is about equal, in milliliters, to the subject's ideal body weight, in pounds (e.g., about 150 mL in a typical adult male). Inspired air reaching alveoli that are not exposed to pulmonary capillary blood also does not participate in gas exchange. This volume plus the anatomic dead space equals the *physiologic dead space.* In a normal person, the anatomic and physiologic dead spaces are virtually identical and constitute about one-third of the tidal volume.

Determination of the physiologic dead space has proved to be of practical importance in a variety of clinical conditions. It is calculated by considering each breath (VT) to consist of dead space (VD) and an alveolar volume that participates in gas exchange (VA):

$$VT = VD + VA$$

Physiologic dead space can be calculated using a modification of the *Bohr equation,* which recognizes that all of the test gas expired derives from two sources: the physiologic dead space and the alveolar gas-exchanging volume. If we use CO_2 as the marker gas, the total amount of CO_2 eliminated per minute equals the sum of the CO_2 coming from the dead space per minute and from the alveolar compartment per minute:

$$\dot{V}E \times FE_{CO_2} = (\dot{V}D \times FI_{CO_2}) + (\dot{V}A \times FA_{CO_2})$$

where

$\dot{V}E$ = minute ventilation, L/min
FE_{CO_2} = fractional concentration of CO_2 in expired gas
$\dot{V}D$ = minute dead space ventilation, L/min
FI_{CO_2} = fractional concentration of CO_2 in inspired gas
$\dot{V}A$ = minute alveolar ventilation, L/min
FA_{CO_2} = fractional concentration of CO_2 in alveolar gas.

Since, in a subject breathing room air, FI_{CO_2} is practically zero, the last equation is generally simplified as follows.

$$VE \times FE_{CO_2} = VA \times FA_{CO_2}$$

where VE and VA represent volumes of ventilation, rather than rates.

Recalling that VA = VT − VD and substituting partial pressures for the fractional concentration terms, the relationship becomes

$$VE \times PE_{CO_2} = (VT - VD)\ PA_{CO_2}$$

where $P_{E_{CO_2}}$ and $P_{A_{CO_2}}$ are the partial pressures of CO_2 in mixed expired gas and alveolar gas, respectively.

Assuming that arterial blood and alveolar gas are in equilibrium with respect to CO_2, when Pa_{CO_2} is substituted for $P_{A_{CO_2}}$ and the equation rearranged, it becomes

$$V_D = V_T \frac{Pa_{CO_2} - P_{E_{CO_2}}}{Pa_{CO_2}}$$

Thus, if arterial blood is sampled during collection of expired gas, and if the partial pressures of CO_2 in expired gas and arterial blood are determined, the physiologic dead space can be calculated. In order for the physiologic dead space to be separated from the total dead space determined by the above equation, the dead space of the apparatus is subtracted from the value for total dead space.

ALVEOLAR GAS COMPOSITION

In normal subjects, values for Po_2 and P_{CO_2} in an end-tidal sample approximate mean alveolar values. However, when imbalances exist in alveolar ventilation and blood flow because of lung disease, inhomogeneity in alveolar gas composition often invalidates the use of end-tidal gas tensions as a measure of mean alveolar gas composition.

In practice, mean alveolar P_{O_2} ($\bar{P}_{A_{O_2}}$) and mean alveolar P_{CO_2} ($\bar{P}_{A_{CO_2}}$) are often determined indirectly. Arterial P_{CO_2} is assumed to equal mean alveolar P_{CO_2} on the grounds of the narrow arteriovenous difference for P_{CO_2} across the lungs, the high solubility of CO_2, and the presumed role of pulmonary capillary blood as a tonometer. Mean alveolar P_{O_2} is calculated using the alveolar gas equation:

$$\bar{P}_{A_{CO_2}} = \bar{P}_{I_{O_2}} - \bar{P}_{A_{CO_2}} \left[F_{I_{O_2}} + \frac{1 + F_{I_{O_2}}}{R} \right]$$

The alveolar gas equation takes advantage of the fact that the total pressure of gases in the alveoli is equal to the sum of the partial pressures of the individual gases. This equation simply states that the mean alveolar P_{O_2} is the difference between inspired P_{O_2} and mean alveolar P_{CO_2}, allowing for a correction factor when the respiratory exchange ratio differs from 1.0.

DIFFUSING CAPACITY

The diffusing capacity of the lung for carbon monoxide ($D_{L_{CO}}$) can be determined by steady-state, rebreathing, and single-breath methods. The most frequently used method is a modification of the single-breath method first described in 1915 and subsequently modified in 1957.[63] Although the single-breath test has been shown to exhibit a large interlaboratory variation, it has proved to be a valuable measure of lung function in a wide variety of disease states. In fact, with continuing refinement of the standards,[6,64,65] the variability, which may be as much as 12% or greater, is likely to decrease; however, the variability will probably not be reduced to the range for vital capacity measurements (about 4%).

The diffusing capacity is intended to provide an estimate of the rate at which test molecules – usually CO – move by diffusion from alveolar gas to pulmonary capillary blood. Factors that influence the measurement are the physicochemical properties of the test gas, the extent and thickness of the alveolar capillary barrier, the resistance to diffusion offered by the red blood cell membrane, and the reaction rates of the test gas and hemoglobin, and pulmonary capillary blood volume. As a rule, the diffusing capacity is interpreted as an index of the surface area engaged in alveolar capillary diffusion. Clinical entities that can reduce the diffusing capacity include parenchymal lung diseases, particularly interstitial lung disease, emphysema, pulmonary hypertension, and anemia. Polycythemia and alveolar hemorrhage syndromes, on the other hand, may increase the diffusing capacity.

Carbon monoxide has emerged as the most practical test gas because of its affinity for hemoglobin. The diffusing capacity for CO is defined as the amount of CO transferred per minute per mm Hg of driving pressure:

$$D_{L_{CO}} = \frac{\dot{V}_{CO}}{\bar{P}_{A_{CO}} - \bar{P}_{C_{CO}}}$$

where

$D_{L_{CO}}$ = the diffusing capacity of the lung for CO, mL/min/mm Hg (STPD)
$\dot{V}_{CO}$ = the amount of CO transferred, mL/min
$\bar{P}_{A_{CO}}$ = the mean alveolar PCO, mm Hg
$\bar{P}_{C_{CO}}$ = the mean capillary PCO, mm Hg.

Since the blood Pco in nonsmokers is essentially zero, the term $\bar{P}_{C_{CO}}$ is customarily neglected. In practice, $D_{L_{CO}}$ is determined by calculating $\dot{V}_{CO}$ as the difference between inspired and expired samples and estimating the mean alveolar Pco. Generally, one of the two techniques is used to determine $D_{L_{CO}}$: the single-breath or the steady-state technique.

The Single-Breath Method

The breathing maneuvers required for the single-breath method consist of tidal breathing for a few breaths, unforced expiration to RV, and then a single full, rapid inspiration of a gas mixture containing approximately 0.3% CO and an inert gas – traditionally, 10% helium (some newer systems use methane). The breath is held for 10 ± 2 seconds and then rapidly expired. An inspiratory time of less than 4 seconds, and a sample collection of no more than 3 seconds are required. Longer expiratory times and sample collection time greater than 3 seconds should be noted in the test report. The initial portion of the expirate containing dead-space gas is discarded; the remainder is collected, and the concentrations of CO and helium are measured.[63] A variety of automated systems are commercially available for performing the single-breath diffusing capacity. However, the essential components in all systems are a source of the special inspired gas mixture, a device for measuring the volume of gas inspired and expired, rapid response analyzers to measure the concentration of gases (see below), a timer, and appropriate valving and collection devices to trap the desired portion of the expirate.

The diffusing capacity of the lung for CO is calculated according to the following equation.

$$D_{L_{CO}} = \frac{V_A \times 60}{(\text{barometric perssure} - 47)} \times \text{time} \times \text{In} \frac{F_{A_{CO}}, \text{initial}}{F_{A_{CO}}, \text{final}}$$

where

V_A = alveolar volume
$F_{A_{CO}}$, initial = alveolar concentration of CO at the start of breath hold
$F_{A_{CO}}$, final = alveolar concentration of CO at the end of breath hold.

The concentration of CO in the alveoli at the start of the period of breath holding ($F_{A_{CO}}$, initial) is calculated from the inspired concentration of CO and, for helium-based systems, the inspired concentration of helium and the expired concentration of helium, according to the equation

$$F_{A_{CO}}, \text{initial} = \frac{F_{E_{He}}}{F_{I_{He}}} \times F_{I_{CO}}$$

where

$F_{E_{He}}$ = expired concentration of helium
$F_{I_{He}}$ = inspired concentration of helium
$F_{I_{CO}}$ = inspired concentration of CO

The concentration of CO in the alveoli at the end of the breath-holding period (FA_{CO}, final) is equal to the concentration of CO in the expired gas. The alveolar volume (VA) is determined in one of two ways. Originally, VA was calculated as the sum of the RV, determined by the closed-circuit helium or body plethysmograph techniques described previously, and the volume of inspired gas, as recorded on the spirometer. Later, VA came to be calculated from the single-breath dilution of helium that occurs during the determination of DL_{CO}. Finally, the time of breath holding is measured (in seconds) from the spirometer recording of the maneuver.

Although the single-breath method is relatively simple and has the advantage of requiring no blood samples, breath holding is clearly artificial, and the maneuver is difficult for dyspneic patients. Therefore, a steady-state method is sometimes used.

The Steady-State Method

In the steady-state method, a gas mixture containing 0.1% carbon monoxide is breathed until the rate of CO uptake from the lung is constant.[66] CO uptake ($\dot{V}_{CO}$) is determined from the difference between the amount of CO in the inspired and expired gas using an equation similar to that presented previously for calculation of O_2 consumption.

Comparison of Single-Breath and Steady-State Methods

Certain differences between the single-breath and steady-state techniques merit special mention.[29] The single-breath method is more popular because it is relatively easy to perform; it is well standardized, and it is less effected by nonuniformity of ventilation in comparison to the steady-state method. However, one drawback is that the patient is required to perform an inspiratory vital capacity maneuver of at least 88% of the VC and to hold his or her breath for 10 seconds. Another is that the test is extremely difficult to perform during exercise. The steady-state method is more attractive intrinsically than the single-breath method, since it requires no respiratory maneuvers and can be done during exercise. However, it does require an arterial blood sample (for determination of P_{CO_2}), and it is technically more difficult to perform.

The steady-state method for determining diffusing capacity tends to give lower values for the resting subject than does the single-breath method. The discrepancy is generally attributed to the fact that the surface area for diffusion is smaller during the quiet tidal breathing employed in the steady-state method than during the full inspiration to TLC, as required in the single-breath method. Also, during quiet breathing, some areas of the lung receive considerably less ventilation than during a breath hold at TLC.

Factors Other than Diffusion that Influence Test Results

A low DL_{CO} need not indicate a diffusion defect. A number of additional respiratory and nonrespiratory factors may reduce or increase the DL_{CO}. A reduction in the lung volume alone can reduce the DL_{CO}. Therefore, some laboratories "normalize" the diffusing capacity for lung volume by dividing DL_{CO} by alveolar volume – a manipulation that assumes a linear relationship between DL_{CO} and VA, which is not the case.

Anemia artificially decreases the DL_{CO} as determined by either method, but the effect of low hemoglobin concentration can be adjusted by application of a correction factor.[67] Conversely, polycythemia and intrapulmonary hemorrhage tend to increase the value for DL_{CO}. In fact, an unexpectedly high value for DL_{CO} may be a helpful clinical clue in detecting radiographically occult pulmonary hemorrhage.

Although the equation for DL_{CO} assumes that the CO back pressure in blood is negligible, the blood of a heavy smoker sometimes contains as much as 10% carboxyhemoglobin. Such levels of carboxyhemoglobin will be accompanied by appreciable concentrations of dissolved CO in the plasma. The resulting back pressure of CO will reduce the DL_{CO}. A correction equation may be applied to adjust the DL_{CO} for this effect.

Altitude also affects the DL_{CO}.[6] Pa_{O_2} falls with increasing altitude above sea level. The reduction in Pa_{O_2} allows CO to diffuse more rapidly into the blood. A specific adjustment should be made for inspired oxygen partial pressure.

Measurement of diffusing capacity is quite useful in the evaluation of patients with a number of pulmonary conditions. Decrement in DL_{CO} has been shown to predict exertional hypoxemia. In addition, DL_{CO} levels have been correlated with disease severity and prognosis in primary pulmonary hypertension, idiopathic pulmonary fibrosis, and alveolitis associated with systemic sclerosis.

ARTERIAL BLOOD GAS COMPOSITION

The determination of arterial P_{O_2} and P_{CO_2} provides useful information about the overall efficiency of external gas exchange. Heavy reliance is placed upon them for this purpose in managing acute respiratory failure, particularly in intensive care units. Less dramatic, but important, is their use in a variety of other settings (e.g., exercise testing) and for assorted calculations (e.g., the alveolar–arterial O_2 gradient and respiratory dead space).

Technique for Sampling Arterial Blood

Arterial blood is sampled either through an indwelling arterial catheter or by percutaneous arterial puncture. Sampling through an indwelling catheter avoids the acute changes in ventilation that sometimes result from apprehension and pain associated with percutaneous puncture.

Three anatomic sites are generally used for obtaining arterial blood samples: the radial, brachial, and femoral arteries. For several reasons, the radial artery is the preferred sampling site. Because of its superficial location at the wrist, the radial artery is easy to palpate and easy to compress by direct pressure, facilitating hemostasis when sampling is complete. In addition, no large veins lie in its immediate vicinity. Furthermore, the ulnar artery usually provides an adequate collateral circulation to the hand in the rare instance of postsampling thrombosis of the radial artery.

Arterial blood samples are drawn anaerobically into plastic or glass syringes coated with heparin. Because room air at sea level has a P_{O_2} of approximately 150 mm Hg and a P_{CO_2} of approximately zero mm Hg, air bubbles in the syringe will artificially increase the arterial P_{O_2} and reduce the arterial P_{CO_2}. The sample either is immediately analyzed or is placed on ice in order to minimize the metabolism of blood cells, particularly the white cells. If the icing precaution is neglected and the analysis is delayed, the Pa_{CO_2} of the sample will increase and the Pa_{O_2} and pH will decrease; the rate of change depends on the temperature of the sample and the elapsed time before analysis (Table 33-11).[68]

TABLE 33-11 In vitro Changes in Arterial Blood Gas Values at 37°C

Measurement	Change Over 10 min
pH (units)	−0.01
P_{CO_2} (mm Hg)	+1.000
O_2 content (vol%)	−0.001

Source: Data from Kelman GR, Nunn JF. Nomograms for correction of blood P_{O_2}, P_{CO_2}, pH, and base excess for time and temperature. J Appl Physiol. 1966;21: 1484–1490.

TABLE 33-12 Effect of Altitude on Mean Alveolar and Arterial O_2 Pressures

Altitude (Feet)	Barometric Pressure (mm Hg)	Ambient P_{O_2} (mm Hg)	Alveolar P_{CO_2} (mm Hg)
0	760	159	103
1000	733	154	98
2000	707	148	94
3000	681	143	90
4000	656	138	85
5000	632	133	81
6000	609	128	77
8000	565	118	69
10,000	523	110	61
12,000	484	101	54

Source: Data from Wasserman K. Cardiovascular manifestations of respiratory insufficiency. Clin Notes Respir Dis. Fall; 1973;12(2):3–10.

TABLE 33-13 Classification of Primary Respiratory Disorders of Acid–Base Balance

Disorder	Definition
Acute respiratory alkalosis (acute alveolar hyperventilation)	Pa_{CO_2} below lower limit of normal (<36 mm Hg), with accompanying alkalemia (pH >7.44)
Chronic respiratory alkalosis (chronic alveolar hyperventilation)	Pa_{CO_2} below lower limit of normal, with pH normal (or near normal) due to renal compensation and lowered serum bicarbonate concentration (<19 mEq/L)
Acute respiratory acidosis (acute alveolar hypoventilation	Pa_{CO_2} above upper limit of normal (>44 mm Hg), with accompanying acidemia (pH <7.36)
Chronic respiratory acidosis (chronic alveolar hypoventilation)	Pa_{CO_2} above upper limit of normal, with pH normal (or near normal) due to renal compensation and elevated serum bicarbonate concentration (>30 mEq/L)

Interpretations

Analysis of arterial blood gases as part of pulmonary function testing is based primarily on determination of Pa_{O_2}, Pa_{CO_2}, and pH. As a rule, these parameters are measured directly. Other values, including O_2 saturation, bicarbonate concentration, and base excess (or deficit), are usually calculated. This section deals with the interpretation of Pa_{O_2}, Pa_{CO_2}, and pH. Additional consideration of arterial blood gases, with particular reference to acid–base balance, is found in Chapter 17.

Arterial P_{O_2} (Pa_{O_2}) The physiologic determinants of normal Pa_{O_2} have been described elsewhere. For example, normal values for arterial P_{O_2} depend on altitude (Table 33-12). Therefore, normal values for arterial P_{O_2} in Denver (altitude of approximately 1500 m) are less than those at sea level by about 20 mm Hg.

Arterial P_{O_2} also decreases with age. A regression equation can be used to predict the decrease:[69]

$$Pa_{O_2} = 109 - 0.43\ (\text{age in years})$$

The standard deviation of this relationship is ±4.10 mm Hg.

A third physiologic influence is body position. Assumption of the supine position causes abdominal contents to displace the diaphragm cephalad, thereby closing small airways at the lung bases and creating ventilation-perfusion inhomogeneities that decrease Pa_{O_2}.

Many more pathologic conditions than physiologic states can lower Pa_{O_2}. In each instance, however, arterial hypoxemia may be attributed to one or more of the following generic mechanisms: alveolar hypoventilation, ventilation-perfusion mismatch, diffusion impairment, and venous admixture ("shunt"). Considerations of the individual disorders within these categories and the mechanisms leading to hypoxemia are found throughout this book.

Arterial P_{CO_2} (Pa_{CO_2}) and pH In a steady state, the level of Pa_{CO_2} reflects the level of alveolar ventilation. In the absence of a disorder in metabolic acid–base balance, an increase or decrease in Pa_{CO_2} beyond normal limits indicates a primary disorder in alveolar ventilation. A summary of these disorders and useful criteria for distinguishing among them, based on arterial blood gas composition, are given in Table 33-13.

Acute *respiratory alkalosis,* produced by alveolar hyperventilation, is characterized by hypocapnia (Pa_{CO_2} < 36 mm Hg) and an appropriately elevated pH (>7.44). In time (e.g., 24 hours or more), renal compensation occurs, and the concentration of bicarbonate in serum decreases. If alveolar hyperventilation continues, a chronic respiratory alkalosis, partly or completely "compensated," ensues.

A low Pa_{CO_2} is not necessarily indicative of a primary disturbance in alveolar ventilation. Instead, it may be a consequence of respiratory compensation (partial or complete) for metabolic acidosis; this possibility is signaled by the coexistence of hypocapnia and a low pH (<7.36). Since the kidney and respiratory system do not overcompensate for acid–base derangements, the coexistence of hypocapnia and acidemia suggest the presence of two primary disturbances.

Acute respiratory acidosis, caused by alveolar hypoventilation, is characterized by an abnormally high Pa_{CO_2} (>44 mm Hg) and a subnormal pH (<7.36). Again, in time (24 hours or more), renal compensation for the primary respiratory disorder restores the serum bicarbonate concentration and blood pH toward normal. A high value for Pa_{CO_2} may also reflect respiratory compensation for a primary metabolic alkalosis ($[HCO_3^-] > 30$ mEq/L). In this circumstance, however, blood pH will be abnormally high (pH > 7.44), rather than low. In general, the elevation in Pa_{CO_2} in compensation for metabolic alkalosis does not exceed about 55 mm Hg. A Pa_{CO_2} exceeding this value in the setting of a metabolic alkalosis suggests the likely coexistence of a primary respiratory acidosis.

This discussion has been limited primarily to alterations in arterial blood gas values in primary respiratory acidosis or alkalosis. Metabolic derangements often complicate the picture. These disorders are considered elsewhere (Chapter 17).

■ TESTING FOR AIR-TRAVEL-RELATED HYPOXEMIA

Travel in commercial jet airliners typically results in exposure of passengers and crew to conditions equivalent to about 6000 to 8000 ft above sea level. For individuals with normal pulmonary gas exchange, the resulting Pa_{O_2} falls within a clinically acceptable range. However, for many patients with lung disease, the resulting Pa_{O_2} may well be problematic, even in those patients who do not require supplemental oxygen at sea level. Consequently, assessment of patients with chronic lung diseases, particularly COPD and interstitial lung diseases, has become part of the repertoire of tests offered by many pulmonary function laboratories.[70–74] One approach to estimating the resultant Pa_{O_2} during air travel is based upon use of regression equations (Fig. 33-30). Using the patient's resting Pa_{O_2} at

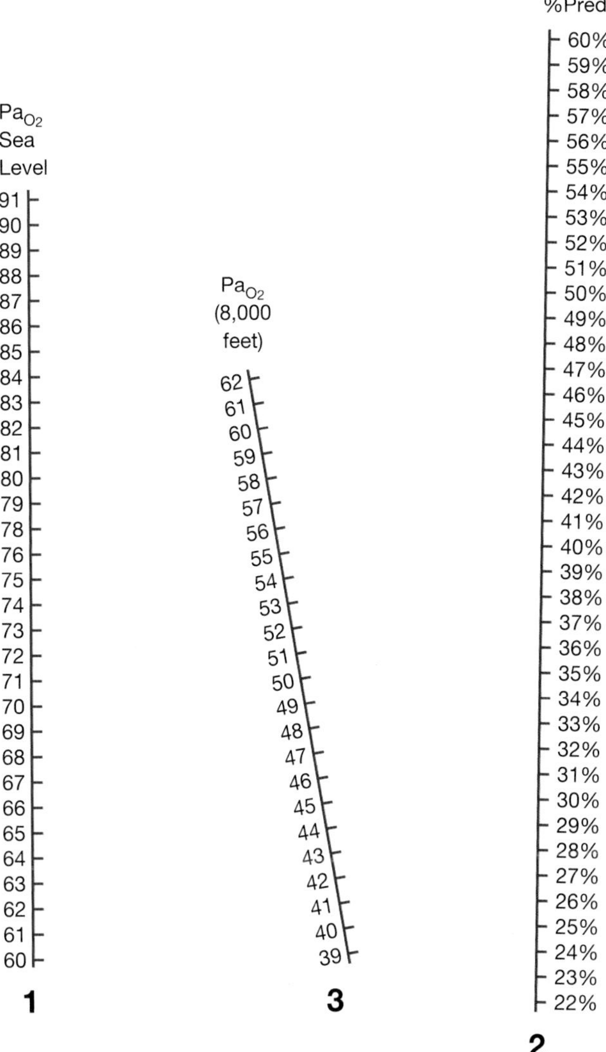

Figure 33-30 Nomogram for predicting in-flight oxygen tension. Using a straight edge, the patient's resting Pa_{O_2} at sea level (*Column 1*) is aligned with his or her FEV_1 percent of predicted (*Column 2*). The expected in-flight Pa_{O_2} (*Column 3*) is estimated as the value where the line crosses the center scale. *(Data from Dillard TA, Berg BW, Rajagopal KR, et al. Hypoxemia during air travel in patients with chronic obstructive pulmonary disease. Ann Intern Med. 1989;111:362–367; and Knudson RJ, Slatin RC, Lebowitz MD, et al. The maximum expiratory flow-volume curve: Normal standards, variability, and effects of age. Am Rev Respir Dis. 1976;113:587–600.)*

sea level and his or her FEV_1 percent of predicted, the expected in-flight Pa_{O_2} can be estimated. Some experts advocate use of the nomogram for determining which patients ought to undergo hypoxia inhalation testing (HIT), while others advocate performance of HIT for all traveling patients at risk for in-flight hypoxemia.

HIT is based on the observation that exposure to hypoxic gas mixtures can reproducibly mimic the Pa_{O_2} arising under true hypobaric conditions. Exposure to 15.1% oxygen for 20 minutes reliably duplicates the resultant Pa_{O_2} at 8000 ft. During performance of the test, the patient, with nose clips in place, breathes from a reservoir though a mouthpiece. The electrocardiogram is monitored, and arterial blood gases are obtained at the conclusion of the test. Supplemental oxygen can then be titrated and prescribed according to the findings.

The British Thoracic Society (BTS) has published recommendations for use of supplemental oxygen during air travel, based on the patient's oxygen saturation at sea level and the presence or absence of risk factors.[71]

The BTS recommends no in-flight supplemental oxygen if the oxygen saturation at sea level is >95%; if the oxygen saturation is 92% to95%, supplemental oxygen is recommended if additional risk factors are present, including: hypercapnia, FEV_1 <50% predicted, lung cancer, interstitial lung disease with fibrosis, chest wall or respiratory muscle disorders, need for mechanical ventilation, cardiac or cerebrovascular disease, or travel within 6 weeks of hospital discharge following an acute exacerbation of chronic lung or heart disease. Supplemental oxygen is also recommended if oxygen saturation is <92% or if the patient uses supplemental oxygen at sea level, for whom an increase in oxygen flow during flight is advised.

The BTS also recommends supplemental oxygen for patients whose Pa_{O_2} on challenge testing (using an FI_{O_2} of 15% for 20 minutes) is <50 mm Hg and, possibly, for those whose Pa_{O_2} is between 50 and 55 mm Hg; in the latter group, a walk test may be helpful.[71]

CONTROL OF BREATHING

The rate, depth, and pattern of breathing reflect a complex interplay of neurohumoral and chemical regulatory mechanisms that drive the respiratory apparatus. Tests used to evaluate the control of breathing, based on assessment of the ventilatory response to controlled hypercapnia or hypoxia, are uncommonly performed in the clinical setting. However, since these tests highlight important physiologic mechanisms that affect the level and pattern of ventilation, they are summarized in subsequent sections.

■ VENTILATORY RESPONSE TO CO_2

The ventilatory response to changes in Pa_{CO_2} is linear over a broad range (Fig. 33-31). Determination of the ventilatory response to controlled hypercapnia generally is based on one of the two methods: the steady-state method[75] or the rebreathing method.[76]

Steady-State Method

After a control period in which CO_2-free air is breathed to establish a baseline, the patient is subjected to two or more periods of breathing CO_2-enriched air. Care is taken to achieve a steady state of ventilation and circulation during each exposure. Especially at the higher concentrations of inspired CO_2, at least 10 to 20 minutes is required for a steady state to be reached in alveoli, arterial blood, cerebrospinal fluid, and the chemosensitive areas of the brain. The ventilatory response to CO_2 is then determined from a plot of $\dot{V}_E$ versus Pa_{CO_2}. In patients without underlying lung disease, end-tidal CO_2 concentration is often substituted for Pa_{CO_2}. In addition, in order to eliminate the influence of variations in arterial PO_2 on the

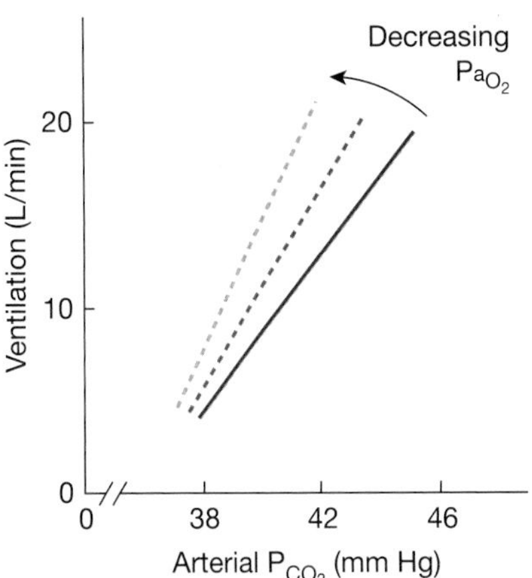

Figure 33-31 Linear relationship between minute ventilation ($\dot{V}_E$) and arterial P_{CO_2}. The dashed lines show the increased slope of the relationship of $\dot{V}_E$ versus P_{CO_2} as Pa_{O_2} decreases.

ventilatory response to CO_2, the inspired gas is enriched with O_2 during the control and test periods.

Rebreathing Method

This method entails rebreathing a CO_2-enriched gas mixture from a bag for approximately 4 minutes. The validity of the approach requires rapid equilibration of CO_2 among alveolar gas, arterial and mixed venous blood, and the chemosensitive areas of the brain. The bag is filled at the outset with a mixture of 7% CO_2 in O_2; O_2 is substituted for air in this mixture to avoid the ambiguity of a hypoxic stimulus to ventilatory drive.

The result of the CO_2 rebreathing test is described by the use of two terms: (1) the *slope* of the line relating change in ventilation response to change in end-tidal P_{CO_2} ($\Delta\dot{V}_E/P_{CO_2}$), determined by using the method of least squares linear regression analysis, and (2) the *x-intercept* of the relationship between $\dot{V}_E$ and end-tidal P_{CO_2}.

Normal Response to CO_2 and Modifying Influences

As indicated above, the normal increase in ventilatory response to increasing concentrations of inspired CO_2 is linear. Normal responses are categorized as low (<1.5 L/min/mm Hg), intermediate (1.5–5.0 L/min/mm Hg), or high (>5.0 L/min/mm Hg). Most normal persons (about 80%) have an intermediate ventilatory response. A variety of factors, both genetic and environmental, seem to influence the ventilatory response to CO_2 (Table 33-14).

■ VENTILATORY RESPONSE TO HYPOXIA

The response to acute hypoxia in normal persons is largely determined by the peripheral arterial chemoreceptors, as long as the level of hypoxia is mild to moderate. Even at sea level, the level of arterial P_{O_2} in normal persons provides an appreciable chemoreceptor drive, accounting for about 10% of the minute ventilation. Unlike the linear response of $\dot{V}_E$ to progressive hypercapnia, the response to hypoxemia is curvilinear (Fig. 33-32). The magnitude of the ventilatory response to a decrease in arterial P_{O_2} depends on the Pa_{CO_2}, increasing as the concentration of CO_2 in arterial blood is increased.

As may be seen from the hyperbolic curves in Figure 33-32, the rate of change in ventilation is greater over the lower range of oxygenation (when Pa_{O_2} falls below 60 mm Hg). Not shown in Figure 33-32 is the depression of ventilation brought about by severe hypoxemia, presumably because of the central depressing effect of severe hypoxia on respiratory neurons.

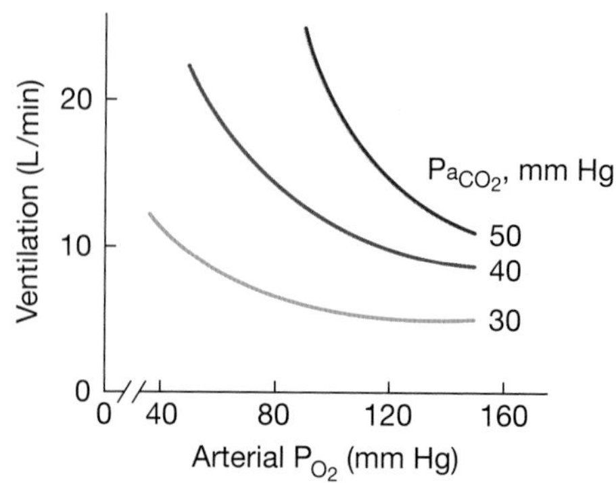

Figure 33-32 The curvilinear relationship between ventilation and arterial P_{O_2} at various levels of arterial P_{CO_2}. The rate of change of ventilation as P_{O_2} falls (slope) increases precipitously at a P_{O_2} of approximately 60 mm Hg when P_{CO_2} is 40 mm Hg. The abrupt increase in ventilation occurs at a higher P_{O_2} when the level of P_{CO_2} is elevated, and at a lower P_{O_2} when the prevailing P_{CO_2} is lower.

Although tests for assessing the ventilatory response to hypoxia are less well standardized than those for measuring the hypercapnic response, they, too, may be conveniently categorized into steady-state and nonsteady-state methods. In one steady-state method,[75] successive ventilatory responses are determined to a series of increasingly severe hypoxic gas mixtures, each administered for at least 10 minutes; Pa_{CO_2} is kept constant by the addition of CO_2 to the inspired gas mixture as hypoxia-induced hyperventilation develops. In another, the effect of hypoxia on the slope of the plot of $\dot{V}_E$ versus P_{CO_2} as P_{O_2} is lowered from hyperoxic (at least 200 mm Hg) to hypoxic (40 mm Hg) levels is determined. The normal response to diminished inspired oxygen concentrations is characterized by an increase in sensitivity (slope) without a change in the CO_2 threshold.

TABLE 33-14 Factors Associated with an Altered Ventilatory Response to CO_2

Factor	Reference
Depressed Response	
Endurance training	Byrne-Quinn et al. *J Appl Physiol.* 1971;30:91–98
Aging	Peterson et al. *Am Rev Respir Dis.* 1981;124:387–391
Genetic/racial predilection	Beral et al. *Lancet.* 1971;2:1290–1294
Metabolic alkalosis	Koboyashi et al. *Am Rev Respir Dis.* 1993;147:1192–1198
	Heinemann and Goldring. *Am J Med.* 1974;57:361–370
Narcotics, barbiturates, and other CNS depressants	Lambertsen. *Handbook of Physiology.* Section 3: Respiration, vol I. Washington, DC: American Physiological Society; 1964: 545–555
Neurologic disorders (encephalitis, brain stem disease)	Plum, Brown. *Ann NY Acad Sci.* 1963;109:915–931
Myxedema	Zwillich et al. *N Engl J Med.* 1975;292:662–665
	Duranti et al. *Am J Med.* 1993;95:29–37
Obesity-hypoventilation syndrome	Zwillich et al. *Am J Med.* 1975;59:343–348
Chronic obstructive pulmonary disease (COPD)	Flenley, Millar. *Clin Sci.* 1967;33:319–334
Accentuated Response	
Metabolic acidosis	Heinemann, Goldring. *Am J Med.* 1974;57:361–370
Drugs (e.g., aminophylline, salicylates, thyroxine, progesterone)	Lambertsen. *Handbook of Physiology.* Section 3: Respiration, vol I. Washington, DC: American Physiological Society; 1964: 545–555

Three nonsteady-state techniques are currently in use. In the hypoxic rebreathing test,[77] the subject rebreathes a hypoxic gas mixture containing 7% CO_2. As arterial hypoxemia intensifies, causing an increase in ventilation and in CO_2 elimination into the closed circuit, the P_{CO_2} in the system is held constant at a predetermined level by the diversion of a fraction of the expired gas through a CO_2 absorber. The ventilatory response is determined at two or more levels of P_{CO_2}, since the hypoxic response is influenced by P_{CO_2}. An alternative rebreathing test[78] induces progressive hypoxemia by adding N_2 to the inspired gas mixture over a 20-minute period. Finally, in a relatively simple test, the patient induces a transient drop in arterial P_{O_2} by inhaling pure N_2 for a few breaths. The relationship between $\dot{V}_E$ and Pa_{O_2} is plotted; the slope of the relationship is the sensitivity to hypoxia. Because the duration of the hypoxia is brief, presumably only the peripheral chemoreceptors are stimulated. No adjustment is made for the drop in P_{CO_2} that occurs during the hypoxia-stimulated increase in ventilation.

Finally, in a relatively simple test,[79] a transient drop in arterial P_{O_2} is induced by having the patient inhale pure N_2 for a few breaths. The relationship between $\dot{V}_E$ and Pa_{O_2} is plotted; the slope of the relationship is the sensitivity to hypoxia. Because the duration of the hypoxia is brief, presumably only the peripheral chemoreceptors are stimulated.

Normal Responses to Hypoxia and Modifying Influences

The normal ventilatory response to acute hypoxia varies among individuals. Several factors may influence the relationship (Table 33-15). A high ventilatory response to CO_2 may be associated with a high sensitivity to hypoxia; in addition, higher levels of arterial P_{CO_2} are associated with a higher ventilatory response to hypoxia. Interestingly, a long duration of hypoxia before the test period, as is the case for example, in native residents at high altitude and persons with cyanotic congenital heart disease, a blunted response to acute hypoxia is observed. Finally, a variety of other clinical disorders, including myxedema and hypothyroidism, autonomic nervous system dysfunction, chronic narcotic addiction, and the chronic use of methadone, are characterized by a reduced hypoxic response.

TABLE 33-15 Factors Associated with an Altered Ventilatory Response to Hypoxia

Factor	Reference
Depressed Response	
Long-standing hypoxia	
High-altitude dwelling	Severinghaus et al. *Respir Physiol.* 1966;1: 308–334
Congenital cyanotic heart disease	Blesa et al. *N Engl J Med.* 1977;296: 237–241
Aging	Kronenberg et al. *J Clin Invest.* 1973;52: 1812–1819
Hypothyroidism	Zwillich et al. *N Engl J Med.* 1975;292:662–665
Riley–Day syndrome	Edelman et al. *J Clin Invest.* 1970;49:1153–1165
Chronic use of methadone	Marks. *Am Rev Respir Dis.* 1970;108:1088–1093
Following carotid endarterectomy	Wade et al. *N Engl J Med.* 1970;282: 823–829
Accentuated Response	
Heightened CO_2 response	Rebuketal. *J Appl Physiol.* 1973;35: 173–177
Hypercapnia	Rebuck, Woodley. *J Appl Physiol.* 1975;38: 16–19

NONVENTILATORY MEASURES OF VENTILATORY DRIVE

Measurement of ventilation in response to acute hypoxia or hypercapnia provides a useful index of respiratory output when the ventilatory apparatus (thorax, diaphragm, abdominal muscles, lung, and airways) is normal. This situation obviously does not apply in certain neuromuscular disorders in which the thorax and diaphragm behave abnormally. In addition, it does not apply in some instances of pulmonary disease, notably obstructive airway disease, in which the respiratory apparatus may not be capable of responding normally, even though it is intact and chemosensitivity is normal. In this instance, a decrease in ventilatory response may be attributable to the excessive mechanical load placed on the muscles of respiration.

When ventilation fails to provide a reliable measure of the ventilatory drive (efferent discharge from the respiratory neurons), the diaphragmatic electromyograph (EMG) or the pressure generated by the inspiratory muscles during the first 0.1 second of an occluded inspiration (the $P_{0.1}$)[80] has been used for the clinical assessment of the control of breathing.

The electrical activity of the diaphragm is directly related to neural activity of the phrenic nerve. Therefore, it provides a measure of efferent neural traffic to the diaphragm. The diaphragmatic EMG may be recorded in patients by placing the tip of an esophageal catheter, containing bipolar electrodes, at the level of the diaphragm.

The second approach to obtaining a nonventilatory measure of ventilatory drive is the determination of $P_{0.1}$, which is the negative pressure generated by the inspiratory muscles during the first 100 milliseconds of an inspiratory effort made against an occluded airway. During this brief period, contraction of the respiratory muscles is virtually isometric, and the force generated correlates with activity recorded by the diaphragmatic EMG.

In performing the test, airflow in the inspiratory line of the breathing circuit is randomly interrupted during the preceding expiration. The 100-millisecond period has proved to be so brief as to be imperceptible, thereby obviating any corrective action by the subject during the breath against the occlusion. However, the $P_{0.1}$ is far from foolproof. A major concern is that $P_{0.1}$ is affected by resting lung volume: $P_{0.1}$ is reduced when FRC is abnormally high, a common occurrence in obstructive disease of the airways.

ASSESSMENT OF INTEGRATED FUNCTIONS: 6-MINUTE WALK TEST

A complete evaluation of a patient with respiratory symptoms often requires assessment of exercise capacity, in addition to traditional pulmonary function tests and radiographic studies. A number of exercise studies can be employed, including cardiopulmonary exercise tests (Chapter 34), cardiac stress tests, and exercise-induced bronchospasm protocols. One of the most widely used, practical modalities is the 6-minute walk test (6MWT). Despite its simplicity, the 6MWT has become a powerful tool in the evaluation of functional status and prognosis of patients with a variety of functional impairments.

TECHNICAL ASPECTS

The 6MWT is performed indoors. There is an initial period of rest in a chair for at least 10 minutes, during which baseline vital signs are taken. The patient then stands and is asked to rate baseline dyspnea and overall fatigue using the Borg scale (from 1 to 10). The patient, walking at a comfortable pace, completes 60-m laps on a walking course which is 30 m in length. Cones are used to mark the turnaround points. For patients using supplemental oxygen, the oxygen is delivered at standard rate, or as prescribed by a physician, or as determined by protocol. The patient should not carry or push the oxygen source during testing. The number of laps and a postwalk Borg scale assessment are recorded, as is the total distance walked over 6 minutes (6MWD).

Although pulse oximetry during the 6MWT is considered optional, it has become standard at many institutions. In some cases, pulse oximetry can be used to titrate levels of oxygen supplementation. Obtaining a high-quality oximeter signal is imperative.

A number of sources of variability are inherent in 6MWT. A modest training effect has been reported when two studies are performed within 1 week. Concomitant medication use can also impact the 6MWT. Improved test performance, for example, occurs after bronchodilator use in patients with COPD. Shorter height, female sex, and higher body weight are associated with reduced performance.[81] Despite these factors, the 6MWT has been found to have excellent reproducibility, especially when performed in evaluation of specific clinical entities, such as idiopathic pulmonary fibrosis.[82]

Several modifications of the 6MWT are in clinical use. During a *shuttle-walking test*, the patient walks on a 10 m course while the walking speed is increased every minute until the patient cannot reach the turnaround point within the set time. The *timed walk test (TWT)*, which has been designed for patients with idiopathic pulmonary fibrosis, has three stopping criteria based on changes in oxyhemoglobin saturation.

Absolute contraindications to performing the 6MWT include unstable angina or myocardial infarction within 1 month of the study. Resting tachycardia of greater than 120 beats per minute, systolic blood pressure greater than 180 mm Hg, or diastolic blood pressure greater than 100 mm Hg are relative contraindications. The study should be terminated if the patient develops chest pain, severe dyspnea, leg cramps, diaphoresis, or profound oxyhemoglobin saturation.

INTERPRETATION

Although the 6MWT is limited in its inability to provide objective measures of functional capacity, such as oxygen uptake, the test provides very useful clinical information. In addition, it realistically represents the patient's functional capacity during physical effort that more closely reflects his or her daily activity. Reliable reference equations establishing standard performance during a 6MWT in healthy patients are not currently available.

The 6MWT has several indications, including, most notably, measurement of the response to a number of medical and surgical interventions. Pulmonary rehabilitation clearly improves 6MWT performance in patients with COPD, while pharmacologic interventions for pulmonary arterial hypertension and heart failure, among other disorders, have also been shown to favorably affect test results. Lung transplantation (unilateral and bilateral) and lung volume reduction surgery for emphysema have been shown to significantly improve results of the 6MWT.

6MWT also has been used to assess functional status in patients with COPD, cystic fibrosis,[83] heart failure, and peripheral vascular disease, and in determining eligibility for, and timing of, lung transplantation. In the absence of well-established reference standards, the clinical value of performing a single test in these patient groups is limited. Serial studies are likely to be more useful than a single 6MWT.

Recently, a number of publications have established the value of the 6MWT in predicting morbidity and mortality from heart and lung disease. Results from the test have been shown to have an inverse relationship with mortality in severe COPD. Walk distance and velocity, as well as magnitude of oxyhemoglobin desaturation, are correlated with survival in idiopathic pulmonary fibrosis. Similar correlations have been made in heart failure and primary pulmonary hypertension.

Finally, at some institutions, results of the 6MWT are utilized to not only establish the presence of exertional hypoxemia, but also to titrate supplemental oxygen with activity.

QUALITY CONTROL IN THE PULMONARY FUNCTION LABORATORY

Meaningful interpretation of pulmonary function tests requires confidence in the accuracy and reproducibility of results provided by the pulmonary function laboratory. Previously, it was tacitly assumed that all data from all laboratories, especially when reported as "percent predicted," were equally reliable. In recent years, the fallacy of this assumption has been explicitly recognized, and steps have been taken to standardize equipment and procedures and to ensure accuracy, reproducibility, and uniformity in testing and reporting.[6,8] To accomplish this goal, both analytical and nonanalytical factors must be taken into account.

NONANALYTICAL FACTORS IN QUALITY CONTROL

A familiar example of a confounding influence that may distort test results is the anxious patient who pauses outside the laboratory door to "calm the nerves" by smoking one or more cigarettes before undergoing pulmonary function testing. Cigarette smoking before the diffusing capacity of the lungs is determined can generate enough carboxyhemoglobin to reduce a normal value to subnormal levels.

Another example of a nonanalytical factor is the failure to achieve patient understanding and comfort for tests that usually require patient cooperation. Unfortunately, a preliminary explanation before the patient arrives at the laboratory or prior exposure of the patient to the laboratory and its personnel is usually impractical. Use of explanatory sheets or descriptive brochures may prove helpful. If such materials are not available, laboratory personnel are obligated to make the patient comfortable and even perform "practice runs" before undertaking final testing.

When the patient arrives at the pulmonary function laboratory, an assessment should be made of his or her prior experiences. Did the patient undergo other tests or procedures that could alter the outcome of the pulmonary function tests in question? Is the patient fatigued or in pain? Should a period of rest precede the tests in order to ensure optimal performance? If delay is impractical, the test report should include the fact that the patient was fatigued or in pain.

Medication use before pulmonary function testing can seriously affect the results. For example, self-administration of bronchodilators before testing can artificially enhance tests of airflow. If medications have been taken before the patient arrives at the laboratory, the time of administration should be part of the record. Also, a request for pulmonary function test results for patients who regularly take bronchodilators should indicate whether the tests are to be done without interruption of the regular schedule of medications, whether bronchodilators are to be discontinued before the test is done, or whether regular bronchodilators are to be discontinued so that the effects of bronchodilation can be tested. Appropriate comments about bronchodilators are part of the report.

A major nonanalytical cause of misinterpreting results is the inappropriate application of predicted normal values to the patient population by the laboratory (see Approach to Interpreting Commonly Performed Pulmonary Function Tests). For example, normal values based on data obtained using physically fit hospital personnel do not necessarily apply to those who have a sedentary existence. Noncomparable race, as well as lifestyle, may complicate comparisons. Anthropologic differences among control and test populations are not easily reconciled. Extraordinary height, weight, or age cannot be easily extrapolated if corresponding subjects are not represented in the control group. Using patient-reported height, rather than making measurement of patient height, may introduce an error in the selection of appropriate normal values.[84] Comparison of control and test results at different altitudes can be invalid if due regard is not paid to the influence of hypoxia on certain measurements (e.g., diffusing capacity).

ANALYTICAL FACTORS IN QUALITY CONTROL

Performance of pulmonary function tests is replete with opportunities for error. The equipment, techniques, use of control values, and calculations are potential sources of error. In an attempt to minimize errors, standardization of techniques has been advocated. For example, with respect to performing the FVC maneuver, guidelines have been established for the number of attempts required, acceptable variability between efforts, and methods for selecting test data in order to arrive at acceptable results. To avoid misuse of spirometers, criteria have been set for minimal performance with respect to capacity, accuracy, and frequency response of various spirometers; in addition, standards have been developed for determining the single-breath diffusing capacity. Potential sources of discrepancies – such as breath-holding time, concentration of hemoglobin, dead space of the equipment and the patient, F_{IO_2}, volume of the alveolar sample, number of tests, and acceptable variability in results – are taken into account.

QUALITY CONTROL OF TEST RESULTS

Guidelines for standardization play a major role in reducing discrepancies between laboratories. However, measures are also required to ensure accuracy and reproducibility within any given laboratory. Among the elements of control that merit consideration are calibration, validation of calibration, and performance of a control measurement. *Calibration* is the adjustment of an instrument's output so that it validly reflects a known input. *Verification of calibration* entails introduction of the same known input and demonstration that the correct output is reproduced. *Performance of a control measurement* refers to the testing of a substrate that has known properties, similar to those usually tested, to prove the accuracy of the instrumentation.

One example of the application of these principles is blood gas analysis. Use of control measurements derived from tonometered blood or commercially prepared buffer solutions is now widespread. Another example is assessment of diffusing capacity[85] and routine incorporation of simulator testing in its measurement.[86]

Unfortunately, similar controls do not exist for pulmonary function tests. Therefore, laboratory technologists have the responsibility for continuing to be alert, not only with respect to faithful observance of guidelines for standardization, but also to detect in-house sources of error – for example, a leak in the system, malfunction of gas analyzers, faulty analog-to-digital converters, and faulty electronics that reduce frequency response.

RESPONSIBILITY AND COST IN QUALITY CONTROL

All who work in the laboratory must be concerned with quality control[87] and resist the frequent temptation to cut corners. Time has to be set aside for the technologist to care for and calibrate equipment, to establish proper control values for the laboratory, to search for inconsistencies in the data and interpretation, and to keep up with changing standards. Also, equipment and supplies, including calibrating syringes and calibrating gases, are expensive. However, when put into the balance, the cost and waste of producing erroneous results exceed, by far, the expense of practicing quality control.

INFECTION CONTROL

Given the relatively close contact between patients and technical staff during performance of pulmonary function tests, the issue of infection control is one that must be carefully considered. To date, the role of pulmonary function equipment in transmission of disease appears to be minimal. Although the presence of potential pathogens on laboratory mouthpieces, valves, and tubing has been well documented, implication of these organisms in the transmission of disease has not been established. Nevertheless, the potential hazards should be recognized and appropriate care exercised.

Infection control begins with practice of the basic principles of hygiene. Hand washing between patients and use of protective gloves by staff when they are handling potentially contaminated equipment are important considerations. Care must be taken in working with mouthpieces, nose clips, and any other implements that come in contact with mucosal surfaces. These devices, if reused, should be disinfected or sterilized after each use. Other equipment – manifolds, tubing, etc. – should be sterilized on a regular basis. In fact, guidelines from the ATS call for the disinfection or sterilization before reuse of any equipment surface with visible condensation from expired air.[6,88]

Because of recent growing concern over cross-contamination among patients and laboratory personnel, manufacturers now produce a variety of in-line filters and disposable pneumotachographs. Care should be taken, however, to assure that response characteristics of the test equipment are not driven to unacceptable levels by use of these devices. Current literature on this topic should be consulted regularly.

APPROACH TO INTERPRETING COMMONLY PERFORMED PULMONARY FUNCTION TESTS

A standard battery of pulmonary function tests is commonly used to identify and quantify abnormalities in the performance of the respiratory system. An organized approach to interpreting these studies is critical. Once a patient's baseline values are established, the tests are valuable in tracking the course of the disorder and its response to treatment.

Results of pulmonary function tests are interpreted by comparing individual patient data with reference or predicted values for normal subjects.[89,90] Ideally, predicted values should be generated from large groups of well-defined, normal or healthy subjects with proper distribution of anthropometric characteristics such as sex, age and height, and ethnic background. Despite dedicated attempts to improve prediction formulas, however, many still fail to take into account important sources of discrepancy, such as the racial and ethnic backgrounds of the patients and the control population, the effects of altitude and exposure to air pollution, and effects of inordinate body size or old age. As a result, not all sets of predicted normals are applicable in pulmonary function laboratories outside the immediate vicinity of the patient populations from whom the data were collected.[91] Extrapolation beyond the characteristics of the reference population should be avoided.

Published guidelines from a joint Task Force of the ATS and ERS recommended that in the United States, ethnically appropriate reference equations from the National Health and Nutrition Examination Survey (NHANES) III be used for individuals aged 8 to 80 years. The Task Force did not recommend any specific set of reference equations for laboratories in Europe, but it suggested the need for an investigation conducted throughout Europe to derive contemporary equations for prediction of normal lung function.

The same ATS/ERS Task Force recommended that each pulmonary function test result falling below the fifth percentile of the frequency distribution of values measured in the reference population be considered abnormal. If normal test results fall in a normal distribution, values below the fifth percentile can be estimated using Gaussian statistics. If the distribution of normal values is non-Gaussian, the lower limit of normal is estimated using a nonparametric technique, for example, the 95th percentile method. Traditionally, but without a sound statistical basis, most laboratories have used an arbitrary cut-off of 80% predicted to define normal. While this method may be reasonable in children, errors may arise if it is applied to adult test results.

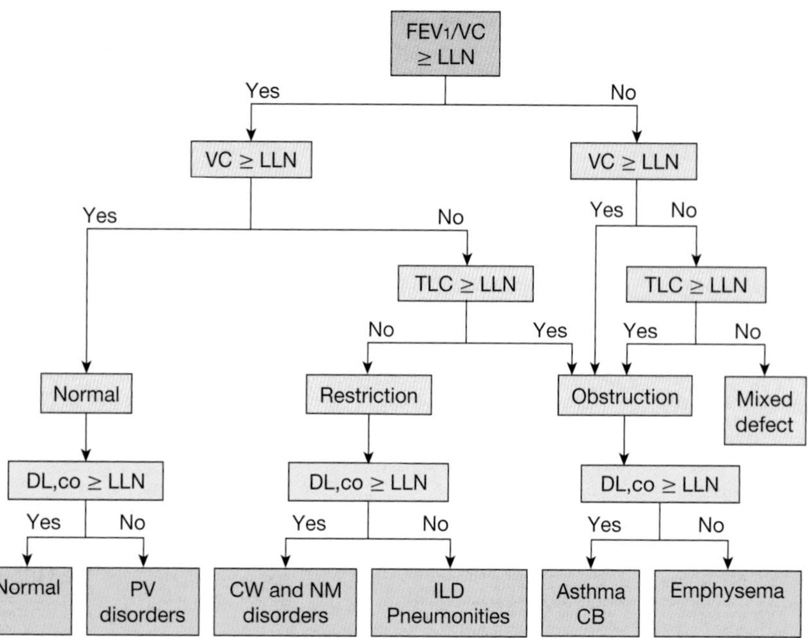

Figure 33-33 Proposed sequence of test review in the interpretation of pulmonary function tests. See text for discussion. LLN, lower limit of normal; PV, pulmonary vascular; CW, chest wall; NM, neuromuscular; ILD, interstitial lung disease; CB, chronic bronchitis. *(Reproduced with permission from Pellegrino R, Viegi G, Brusasco V, et al. Interpretive strategies for lung function tests. Eur Respir J. 2005;26(5):948–968.)*

■ INTERPRETATION SCHEME AND CLASSIFICATION OF ABNORMAL PATTERNS

A variety of schemes have been proposed for sorting out abnormalities in pulmonary function test results. Many are based on initial categorization of findings reflective of one of the four basic patterns described in the following paragraphs.

An *obstructive* pattern stems from narrowing of any portion of the airways – from upper airway to bronchioles less than 2 mm in diameter – that results in a reduction of maximal airflow in relation to maximal volume.

A *restrictive* pattern is elicited by diseases of the lung, chest wall, pleural space, or neuromuscular respiratory apparatus that reduce lung volumes, particularly TLC, and vital capacity.

A *combined obstructive–restrictive* pattern results from pathologic processes that reduce lung volumes, vital capacity, and airflow, and that also include an element of airway narrowing.

Finally, *abnormal gas transfer* may be noted as part of one of the aforementioned patterns or in isolation and reflects an abnormality in the alveolar capillary membrane, impairing oxygen uptake from alveolar gas to pulmonary capillary blood.

Overlap among categories is not uncommon. For example, widespread interstitial disease, as in idiopathic pulmonary fibrosis, often shows a pattern that indicates important components of both restrictive disease and abnormal gas transfer.

One useful sequence recommended by the ATS/ERS Task Force for analyzing a conventional battery of pulmonary function test results is illustrated in Figure 33-33.

Analysis begins with evaluation of the ratio of FEV_1 to VC. While, historically, the ratio of FEV_1 to FVC (FEV_1/FVC%) served as the basis for distinguishing obstructive disorders from normality or restrictive disease, the ATS/ERS Task Force currently recommends using as the denominator the FVC, *or* the VC ("slow" VC or SVC), *or* the FIVC, whichever is greatest. If the ratio is less than the lower limit of normal (i.e., below the fifth percentile) and the VC (defining VC as any of the three previously noted vital capacity measurements) is at or above the lower limit of normal, the pattern is obstructive. If TLC is not at or above the lower limit of normal, a mixed obstructive–restrictive pattern is suggested. Distinction between asthma and chronic bronchitis on the one hand, and emphysema on the other, is based upon whether the D_{LCO} is normal (asthma or chronic bronchitis) or reduced (emphysema). The previous practice of using a value for FEV_1/FVC% of less than 70% to define obstruction results in misdiagnosis of airway obstruction in men over 40 years and women over 50 years of age, as well as overdiagnosis of COPD in elderly, asymptomatic nonsmokers.

If FEV_1/VC and VC are each equal to or greater than the respective lower limits of normal, spirometry is considered normal; measurement of the D_{LCO} can then help distinguish between normal pulmonary function and pulmonary vascular disorders. If VC is below the lower limit of normal, a reduced TLC supports a diagnosis of restriction, while a normal TLC indicates an obstructive pattern. Once again, in the setting of a restrictive pattern, measurement of D_{LCO} can be used to distinguish between pulmonary parenchymal disorders and disorders of the chest wall or respiratory muscles. Note that according to these guidelines, an obstructive pattern may be diagnosed in the setting of a *normal* FEV_1/VC, if VC is reduced and TLC is normal or elevated.

Once the predominant abnormality is defined with initial pulmonary function testing, the whole battery may not be necessary in following the course of the disease or in assessing its response to treatment. For example, particular determinations, such as spirometry, may suffice in patients with airway diseases. Notably, according to the ATS/ERS guidelines, the severity of the abnormality in each of the obstructive, restrictive, or mixed patterns is expressed on the basis of the FEV_1 (Table 33-16). Standards have been established for

TABLE 33-16 Grading of Severity of Abnormal Spirometry Based on FEV_1

Severity	FEV_1 Percent Predicted
Mild	>70
Moderate	60–69
Moderately severe	50–59
Severe	35–49
Very severe	<35

Source: Modified with permission from Pellegrino R, Viegi G, Brusasco V, et al. Interpretive strategies for lung function tests. Eur Respir J. 2005;26(5):948–968.

TABLE 33-17 Conditions Associated with Reduced Peak Inspiratory ($P_{I_{max}}$) and Expiratory ($P_{E_{max}}$) Pressures

Condition	$P_{I_{max}}$	$P_{E_{max}}$
Poor effort	↓	↓
Fatigue	↓	↓
Neuromuscular disease	↓	↓
Increased lung volume	↓	N
Decreased lung volume	N	↓

Note: ↓, decreased; N, normal.

defining significant changes in results over time: A 15% or greater change in FVC or in FEV_1, or a greater than 10% change in DL_{CO} is considered significant.

ASSESSING RESPIRATORY MUSCLE STRENGTH AND EFFORT

One additional measurement that is frequently useful in assessing results of routine spirometry is assessment of respiratory muscle strength. Respiratory muscle strength is expressed in terms of peak inspiratory (PI_{max}) and peak expiratory (PE_{max}) pressures, determined under static conditions.[24] The technique was outlined in a previous section. Any of a number of factors may be responsible for low peak inspiratory or expiratory pressures (Table 33-17): suboptimal effort, fatigue, weakness of the respiratory muscles, deformity of the chest wall, or intrinsic diseases of the lungs or chest wall. Although the first three factors characteristically reduce both peak inspiratory and expiratory pressures, disease of the lungs or chest wall often reduces, selectively, one or the other peak pressure. Thus, diseases that reduce lung volumes (e.g., widespread interstitial fibrosis) and shorten the length of the expiratory muscles at the end-inspiratory position generally reduce maximal expiratory pressure. Conversely, diseases that increase lung volume, such as obstructive airway disease, by decreasing the inspiratory muscle length at end-expiration generally reduce maximal inspiratory pressure.

If airflow during spirometry is reduced, determination of the peak inspiratory and expiratory pressures may be helpful in suggesting the mechanism. Many pulmonary function tests depend on the cooperation of the patient. Poorly reproducible peak flows that are consistently subnormal raise the question of poor effort. Conversely, consistently low values that occur despite maximal effort may signal neuromuscular disease.

ADDITIONAL DETAILS OF PULMONARY FUNCTION TEST RESULTS IN AN OBSTRUCTIVE PATTERN

Included in the obstructive pulmonary disorders (Table 33-18) are chronic obstructive diseases of the airways (chronic bronchitis and emphysema), bronchiectasis, asthma, small-airway disease, and upper-airway obstruction.

Except for diseases confined to the small airways, as noted previously, the hallmark of the obstructive pattern is a reduction in the FEV_1/VC%. Notably, some healthy subjects have a reduced FEV_1/FVC% and an FEV_1 in the normal range. The clinical significance of these findings is unclear. Results of additional tests (e.g., lung volumes, DL_{CO}, assessment of bronchodilator responsiveness) may help distinguish those with airway obstruction from true normals.[92] Measurement of airway resistance (Raw) or specific airway conductance (SGaw) may be useful in assessing airway obstruction in subjects unable to perform a maximal forced expiratory maneuver.

Changes in lung volume commonly accompany the abnormal findings on spirometry, but, as indicated in Figure 33-33, lung volume measurement is not mandatory in establishing the presence of obstruction. Frequently, but not invariably, lung volumes are abnormally high. Typically, all three lung volumes – RV, FRC, and TLC – are increased.

In addition to uncovering the pattern of chronic obstructive airway disease described above, certain additional tests provide insight into the sites and mechanisms of obstructive airway disease.

Reversible Versus Irreversible Obstructive Airway Disease

The response to inhaled bronchodilators traditionally has been used to help distinguish between chronic obstructive airway disease (chronic bronchitis and emphysema), in which airway resistance is virtually fixed, and asthma, in which bronchoconstriction is a prominent feature. This is an oversimplification, since a sizable minority of patients with COPD manifest a bronchodilator response. Furthermore, the absence of a bronchodilator response in a laboratory setting does not necessarily predict lack of a clinical response.

A universally agreed upon definition of reversibility is lacking. Expressing change in FEV_1 or FVC as percent of predicted values may be more advantageous than expression of changes in the values relative to baseline. In general, an increase in FEV_1 or FVC of at least 12% above baseline *and* an absolute increment of at least 200 mL is considered evidence of significant bronchodilation. If the increase in spirometric values is not significant, a decrease in lung volumes toward normal may be an indication of bronchodilator responsiveness.

TABLE 33-18 Causes of an Obstructive Pattern

Disease Process	Anatomic Location of Lesion	Cause of Reduced Airflow
Chronic obstructive pulmonary disease (COPD)		
Chronic bronchitis	Large and small (<2-mm diameter) airways	Narrowing of airways by fibrosis, secretions, edema
Emphysema	Lung parenchyma	Loss of lung elastic recoil
Cystic fibrosis	Large and small airways	Narrowing of airway by fibrosis, retained secretions, edema Loss of elastic recoil
Asthma	Large and small airways	Narrowing of airways by smooth muscle contraction, edema, retained secretions
Small-airway disease	Small airways	Narrowing, stenosis of small airways
Upper-airway obstruction	Major, central airways (trachea, main bronchi)	Anatomic or functional narrowing of upper airway

Chronic Bronchitis Versus Emphysema

Although chronic bronchitis and emphysema usually coexist, occasionally one or the other exists in virtually pure form. Two pulmonary function tests have proved valuable in distinguishing between the two – diffusing capacity (DL_{CO}), which is routinely measured, and static lung compliance (Cst,L), which is uncommonly measured clinically. Emphysema, characterized by a loss of alveolar units and a decrease in alveolar surface area, is associated with a low DL_{CO}, whereas the DL_{CO} in chronic bronchitis is usually normal or near normal.

The loss of alveolar units in emphysema also causes a decrease in the elastic recoil pressure of the lungs. As a result, Cst,L is increased in emphysema, whereas it is usually not appreciably altered in chronic bronchitis.

Small-Airway Disease

In obstructive disease of the small airways (i.e., those less than 2 mm in diameter), expiratory flow is usually normal, except at low lung volumes; that is, the FEV_3 and $FEF_{25-75\%}$ are abnormally low. Other, uncommonly performed tests for isolated, small-airway disease, including the helium–oxygen flow–volume loop, nitrogen washout test, and frequency dependence of dynamic compliance, would also be anticipated to be abnormal. Lung volumes and DL_{CO} are normal. Bronchodilators are virtually without effect.

The practical value of tests of small-airway function is problematic. At one time, high hopes were held that early detection of small-airway disease might reinforce measures, such as cessation of smoking, that would prevent or arrest progression to irreversible obstructive disease of the airways. However, enthusiasm for testing for small-airway disease has waned, since it is still unclear if small-airway disease is a reversible phase in the evolution of clinically significant obstructive airway disease that affects larger bronchi.

Upper-Airway Obstruction

The designation *upper-airway obstruction* is an umbrella for anatomic or functional narrowing of the large upper airways – the larynx, extra- and intrathoracic trachea, and lobar bronchi. Although upper-airway obstruction of any cause may reduce expiratory or inspiratory airflow, an alteration in the contour of the flow–volume loop has proved to be the most reliable abnormality in conventional pulmonary function testing. The observation from routine spirometry that the ratio of FEV_1 to peak expiratory flow rate (PEFR) exceeds 8 mL/L/min should prompt careful performance and review of the flow–volume loop, as described later.

Upper-airway obstruction can be divided into three major types: (1) fixed obstruction, (2) variable extrathoracic obstruction, and (3) variable intrathoracic obstruction.[93]

A *fixed obstruction*, such as tracheal narrowing by scar tissue at the site of a previous tracheotomy, is one in which the geometry and cross-sectional area of the lesion do not change during the respiratory cycle. Characteristically, both inspiratory and expiratory flows are affected about equally (Fig. 33-34A).

A *variable obstruction* is one in which the configuration of the obstructive lesion changes with the phases of respiration. Depending on its location in the tracheobronchial tree (extra- or intrathoracic), this type of lesion usually affects predominantly either inspiration or expiration.

The inspiratory arm of the flow–volume loop is primarily affected by a *variable extrathoracic* obstruction, leaving the expiratory limb relatively unaffected (Fig. 33-34B). The abnormal configuration of the flow–volume loop is attributable to the following sequence: during forced expiration, tracheal pressure exceeds atmospheric, so that the degree of obstruction decreases; conversely, during forced inspiration, intratracheal pressure becomes less than atmospheric and the trachea tends to collapse.

The expiratory arm of the flow–volume loop is primarily affected by a *variable intrathoracic* obstruction (Fig. 33-34C). The following sequence is responsible for producing this abnormality in the flow–volume loop: during forced expiration, as pleural pressure reaches and then exceeds intratracheal pressure downstream from the lesion (i.e., toward the mouth), the obstruction tends to increase; conversely, during a forced inspiration, as intratracheal pressure exceeds pleural pressure, the intrathoracic obstruction decreases.

Variable intrathoracic lesions often coexist with obstructive airway disease. In considering a variable intrathoracic lesion, the respective roles played by obstructive disease of the airways (i.e., chronic bronchitis, emphysema, and asthma) and an obstructive upper-airway lesion (anatomic or functional) in deforming the flow–volume loop must be determined. Fortunately, this distinction is often possible. Although both upper-airway obstruction and obstructive airway disease (reversible and irreversible) do decrease maximal expiratory flow, the shapes of the flow–volume cures are frequently quite distinctive (Fig. 33-34C and D). Thus, in obstructive airway disease, despite a decrease in airflow, the

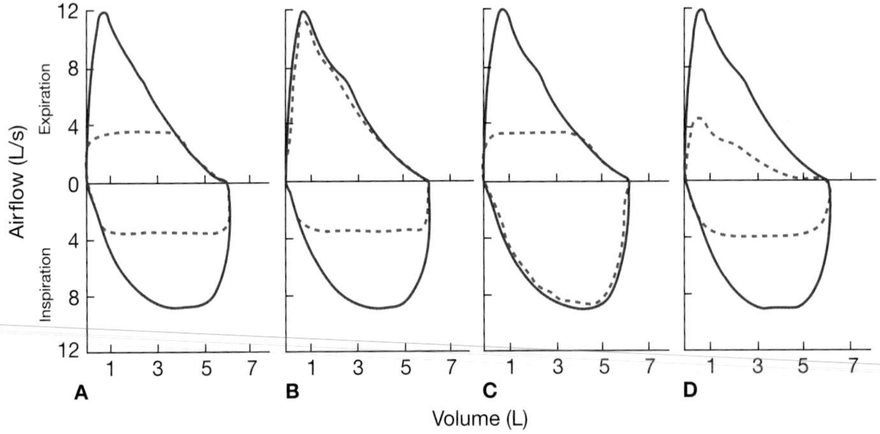

Figure 33-34 Schematic flow–volume loops in four pathologic conditions. **A.** In a fixed upper-airway obstruction, both inspiratory and expiratory limbs are truncated. **B.** In a variable extrathoracic obstruction, the inspiratory limb is flattened while the expiratory limb is not altered. **C.** In a variable intrathoracic obstruction, the expiratory limb is flattened while the inspiratory portion is unchanged. **D.** In chronic obstructive airway disease, although expiratory airflow is reduced, the tapering in airflow during expiration is generally maintained so that the configuration of the loop is different from that in variable intrathoracic obstruction.

TABLE 33-19 Distinguishing Features of Disorders Producing an Obstructive Pattern

Disorder	FEV_1	FVC	FEV_1/VC%	Response of FEV_1 to Administration of Bronchodilator	Tests of Small-Airway Function	Lung Volumes	DL_{CO}	Flow–Volume Loop
COPD								
Chronic bronchitis	↓	↓	↓	NC	ABN	↑	NL	ABN
Emphysema	↓	↓	↓	NC	ABN	↑	↓	ABN
Asthma	↓	↓	↓	↑	ABN	↑	NL	ABN
Small-airway disease	NL	NL	NL	NC	ABN	NL	NL	NL
Upper-airway obstruction	↓	↓	↓	NC	NL or ABN	NL or ↑	NL	ABN[a]

[a]Configuration frequently characteristic for upper-airway obstruction.
Note: ↓, decrease; ↑, increase, NC, no significant change; NL, normal; ABN, abnormal.

expiratory limb of the loop generally retains its normal configuration (Fig. 33-34D) – that is, an early peak in flow, followed by gradual tapering. In contrast, in upper-airway obstruction (fixed and variable intrathoracic), the expiratory limb is flat and flow is decreased throughout most of expiration (Fig. 33-34C).

In addition to changes in the shape of the flow–volume loop, clues from routine pulmonary function tests often alert the clinician to the possibility of upper-airway obstruction. As noted previously, when FEV_1/PEFR >8, the possibility of upper-airway obstruction should be considered. Finally, the presence of any of the following may also provide clues: $FEF_{50\%}/FIF_{50\%}$ of at least 1, where $FEF_{50\%}$ and $FIF_{50\%}$ are the forced expiratory flow at 50% of FVC and the forced inspiratory flow at 50% of FIVC, respectively; $FIF_{50\%}$ less than 100 L/min; and $FEV_1/FEV_{0.5}$ at least 1.5.

Distinguishing test features of disorders producing an obstructive pattern are summarized in Table 33-19.

ADDITIONAL DETAILS OF PULMONARY FUNCTION TEST RESULTS IN A RESTRICTIVE PATTERN

The restrictive pattern (Table 33-20) characteristically occurs in several groups of disorders including: (1) a primary disorder of the lung parenchyma in which functional tissue is lost through disease (e.g., an alveolar filling process, such as pneumonia, tumor, atelectasis, or fibrosis); (2) surgical removal of lung tissue (e.g., lobectomy); (3) constrictive disease of the pleura and chest wall (e.g., extensive pleural fibrosis, large pleural effusion or pleural mass, kyphoscoliosis, obesity); and (4) neuromuscular diseases, notably those in which the generation of respiratory force is reduced (e.g., disorders of the spinal cord, peripheral nerves, neuromuscular junction, and muscle).

The diagnosis of restriction is based upon the finding of a normal FEV_1/VC and reduced VC in the setting of a decreased TLC. While TLC generally is reduced in most disorders producing a restrictive pattern, FRC is usually preserved in disorders characterized by decreased respiratory force (e.g., the neuromuscular disorders) and is reduced in the others. In neuromuscular disorders, ERV is decreased because of loss of expiratory force, so that RV is often increased. In the other types of restrictive disorders, RV is usually reduced.

Whether or not the DL_{CO} is reduced in the restrictive disorders depends on the underlying disease process. Primary parenchymal disorders and removal of lung tissue decrease the diffusing surface area and reduce DL_{CO}. Diseases of the pleura and chest wall that limit thoracic excursion during the inspiratory vital capacity maneuver, which is part of the technique for determining DL_{CO}, also reduce this measurement.

ADDITIONAL DETAILS OF PULMONARY FUNCTION TEST RESULTS IN A MIXED OBSTRUCTIVE–RESTRICTIVE PATTERN

Occasionally, a battery of pulmonary function tests demonstrates features of both obstructive and restrictive patterns. Most often, the mixed pattern is characterized by a low FEV_1/VC% (indicating obstructive airway disease) and VC and reduced TLC (indicating coexisting restrictive disease).

A number of disorders can produce the mixed obstructive/restrictive pattern. Sarcoidosis and interstitial fibrosis, when severe, generally result in this pattern because the parenchymal disease causes restriction and narrowing of the airways by adjacent fibrosis, evoking signs of airway obstruction. The mixed pattern also occurs in complicated situations when there is more than one cause – for example, a lobar pneumonia or large pleural effusion occurring in a patient with underlying chronic bronchitis or emphysema.

ISOLATED DECREASE IN THE EFFICIENCY OF GAS TRANSFER

An isolated reduction in the DL_{CO} suggests one of the two possible abnormalities: (1) interstitial lung disease that is so mild as not to affect measurements of airflow or lung volume, or (2) widespread occlusive disease of the pulmonary microcirculation (e.g., due to an inflammatory process or multiple small emboli). In occlusive vascular disorders, tests of airflow and lung volume are usually normal.

TABLE 33-20 Causes of a Restrictive Pattern

Disease Process	Anatomic Location of Lesion	Cause of Pulmonary Function Test Abnormality
Primary parenchymal disease	Lung parenchyma	Loss of lung tissue ⟶ reduced volumes and flows
Surgical removal of lung tissue	Lung parenchyma	Loss of lung tissue ⟶ reduced volumes and flows
Diseases of pleura and chest wall	Pleura, chest wall	Limited expansion of thoracic cavity ⟶ reduced volumes and flows
Reduced generation of expiratory force	Central nervous system, peripheral nerves, neuromuscular junction, muscles of respiration	Reduced muscle tension ⟶ reduced expiratory flow, atelectasis

TABLE 33-21 Categorization of Reduction in Efficiency of Gas Transfer: Measurement of $D_{L_{CO}}$

Severity	$D_{L_{CO}}$, Percent Predicted
Mild	>60, but less than lower limit of normal
Moderate	40–60
Severe	<40

Source: Modified with permission from Pellegrino R, Viegi G, Brusasco V, et al. Interpretive strategies for lung function tests. Eur Respir J. 2005;26(5):948–968.

Although other disorders can also decrease $D_{L_{CO}}$, almost invariably they also reduce airflow, lung volumes, or both. Quantification of the degree to which the $D_{L_{CO}}$ is reduced by any of these processes is indicated in Table 33-21. Notably, interlaboratory differences are substantial for measurements of $D_{L_{CO}}$.

SUMMARY OF APPROACH TO INTERPRETATION

Pulmonary function tests are designed to detect common disorders. Test interpretation relies heavily on recognition of major patterns of abnormality (Table 33-22). These patterns often suggest pathogenetic mechanisms and are helpful to the clinician in arriving at a diagnosis. The degree of abnormality provides a quantitative measure of the extent of involvement at a particular time. Moreover, repeated testing makes it possible to pace and quantify the course of the illness and to assess the effects of therapeutic interventions.

TABLE 33-22 Characteristic Alterations in Pulmonary Function Tests According to the Major Patterns of Abnormality

Pattern	Airflow (FEV_1/VC%)	Airflow Response to Bronchodilators	Volumes	Lung $D_{L_{CO}}$
Obstructive				
Irreversible	↓	↔	↑	↔ or ↓
Reversible	↓	↑	↑	↔
Small-airway disease	↓	↔	↔	↔
Upper-airway obstruction	↓	↔	↔ or ↑	↔
Restrictive				
Parenchymal disease	↔ or ↑	↔	↓	↓
Surgical resection	↔	↔	↓	↓
Pleural, chest wall disease	↔	↔	↓	↔
Reduced expiratory force generation	↔	↔	↓	↔
Mixed obstructive–restrictive	↓	↔ or ↑	↓	↓
Isolated reduction in efficiency of gas transfer	↔	↔	↔	↓

Note: ↓, decreased; ↑, increased; ↔, no change or normal.

REFERENCES

1. Davy H. *Researches, Chemical and Philosophical; Chiefly Concerning Nitrous Oxide, or Dephlogisticated Nitrous Air, and its Respiration*. London. *Johnson*. 1800;400–410.
2. Hutchinson J. On the capacity of the lungs, and on the respiratory functions, with a view of establishing a precise and easy method of detecting disease by the spirometer. *Med Chir Trans*. 1846;29:137–252.
3. Yemault JC, Pride N, Laszlo G. How the measurement of residual volume developed after Davy (1800). *Eur Respir J*. 2000;16:561–564.
4. Ruppel GL, Enright PL. Pulmonary function testing. *Respir Care*. 2012;57:165–175.
5. MacIntyre NR. The future of pulmonary function testing. *Respir Care*. 2012;57:154–161.
6. ATS Statement: single breath carbon monoxide diffusing capacity (transfer factor): Recommendations for a standard technique—1995 update. *Am J Respir Crit Care Med*. 1995;152:2185–2198.
7. Hankinson JL, Das MK: Frequency response of portable PEF meters. *Am J Respir Crit Care Med*. 1995;152:702–706.
8. ATS Statement: Standardization of spirometry—1994 update. *Am J Respir Crit Care Med*. 1995;152:1107–1136.
9. Clausen JL (ed): *Pulmonary Function Testing: Guidelines and Controversies*. New York, NY: Academic Press; 1982.
10. Darling RC, Cournand A, Richards DW Jr: Studies on the intrapulmonary mixture of gases: III. An open circuit method for measuring residual air. *J Clin Invest*. 1940;19:609–618.
11. DuBois AB, Botelho SY, Bedell GN, et al. A rapid plethysmograph method for measuring thoracic gas volume: A comparison with a nitrogen washout method for measuring functional residual capacity in normal subjects. *J Clin Invest*. 1956;35:322–326.
12. Wanger J, Clausen JL, Coates A, et al. ATS/ERS Task Force. Standardisation of lung function testing. Standardisation of the measurement of lung volumes. *Eur Respir J*. 2005;26:511–522.
13. Borg BM, Thompson BR: The measurement of lung volumes using body plethysmography: A comparison of methodologies. *Respir Care*. 2012;57:1076–1083.
14. Rodenstein DO, Stanescu DC: Reassessment of lung volume measurement by helium dilution and by body plethysmography in chronic airflow obstruction. *Am Rev Respir Dis*. 1982;126:1040–1044.
15. Shore S, Milic-Emili J, Martin JG. Reassessment of body plethysmographic technique for the measurement of thoracic gas volume in asthmatics. *Am Rev Respir Dis*. 1982;126:515–520.
16. O'Donnell CR, Bankier AA, Stiebellehner L, et al. Comparison of plethysmographic and helium dilution lung volumes: which is best for COPD? *Chest*. 2010;137:1108–1115.
17. Hankinson JL, Viola JO. Dynamic BTPS correction factors for spirometric data. *J Appl Physiol*. 1983;55:1354–1360.
18. Pincock AC, Miller MR. The effect of temperature on recording spirograms. *Am Rev Respir Dis*. 1983;128:894–898.
19. Heussel CP, Herth FJF, Kappes J, et al. Fully automatic quantitative assessment of emphysema in computed tomography: Comparison with pulmonary function testing and normal values. *Eur Radiol*. 2009;19:2391–2402.
20. Garfield JL, Marchetti N, Gaughan JP, Steiner RM, Criner GJ. Total lung capacity by plethysmography and high-resolution computed tomography in COPD. *Int J Chron Obstruct Pulmon Dis*. 2012;7:119–126.

21. Milic-Emili J, Mead J, Turner JM, Glauser EM. Improved technique for estimating pleural pressure from esophageal balloons. *J Appl Physiol.* 1964;19:207–211.

22. Rahn H, Otis AB, Chadwick LE, Fenn WO. The pressure volume diagram of the thorax and lung. *Am J Physiol.* 1946;146: 161–178.

23. Knudson RJ, Clark DF, Kennedy TC, Knudson DE. Effect of aging alone on mechanical properties of the normal adult human lung. *J Appl Physiol.* 1977;43:1054–1062.

24. Black LF, Hyatt RE: Maximal respiratory pressures: Normal values and relationship to age and sex. *Am Rev Respir Dis.* 1969;99:696–702.

25. Ringqvist T: The ventilatory capacity in healthy subjects: An analysis of causal factors with special reference to the respiratory forces. *Scand J Clin Lab Invest.* 1966;18(Suppl 88):5–179.

26. Dawson A. Spirometry. In: Wilson AF, ed. *Pulmonary Function Testing Indications and Interpretations: A Project of the California Thoracic Society.* Orlando, FL: Grune & Stratton; 1985;9–31.

27. Gandevia B, Hugh-Jones P: Terminology for measurements of ventilator capacity. *Thorax.* 1957;12:290–293.

28. DuBois AB, Botelho SY, Comroe JH Jr. A new method for measuring airway resistance in man using a body plethysmograph: Values in normal subjects and in patients with respiratory disease. *J Clin Invest.* 1956;35:327–335.

29. Wilson AF (ed): *Pulmonary Function Testing: Indications and Interpretations.* Orlando, FL: Grune and Stratton; 1985.

30. Briscoe WA, DuBois AB: The relationship between airway resistance, airway conductance, and lung volume in subjects of different age and body size. *J Clin Invest.* 1958;37:1279–1285.

31. Dweik RA, Boggs PB, Erzurum SC, et al. An official ATS clinical practice guideline: interpretation of exhaled nitric oxide levels (FE_{NO}) for clinical applications. *Am J Respir Crit Care Med.* 2011; 184:602–615.

32. Dummer JF, Epton MJ, Cowan JO, et al. Predicting corticosteroid response in chronic obstructive pulmonary disease using exhaled nitric oxide. *Am J Respir Crit Care Med.* 2009;180:846–852.

33. Olin AC, Rosengren A, Thelle DS, et al. Increased fraction of exhaled nitric oxide predicts new-onset wheeze in a general population. *Am J Respir Crit Care Med.* 2010;181:324–327.

34. Michils A, Baldassarre S, Van Muylem A. Exhaled nitric oxide and asthma control: A longitudinal study in unselected patients. *Eur Respir J.* 2008;31:539–546.

35. van Veen IH, ten Brinke A, Sterk PJ, et al. Exhaled nitric oxide predicts lung function decline in difficult-to-treat asthma. *Eur Respir J.* 2008;32:344–349.

36. Dweik RA, Sorkness RL, Wenzel S, et al. Use of exhaled nitric oxide measurement to identify a reactive, at-risk phenotype among patients with asthma. *Am J Respir Crit Care Med.* 2010;181: 1033–1041.

37. Smith L, McFadden ER Jr. Bronchial hyperreactivity revisited. *Ann Allergy Asthma Immunol.* 1995;74:454–470.

38. Reddy C. Bronchoprovocation testing. *Clinic Rev Allerg Immunol.* 2009;37:167–172.

39. O'Connor GT, Sparrow D, Weiss ST. A prospective longitudinal study of methacholine airway responsiveness as a predictor of pulmonary-function decline: the normative aging study. *Am J Respir Crit Care Med.* 1995;152:87–92.

40. Birnbaum S, Barreiro TJ. Methacholine challenge testing: Identifying its diagnostic role, testing, coding and reimbursement. *Chest.* 2007;131:1932–1935.

41. Katial RK, Covar RA. Bronchoprovocation testing in asthma. *Immunol Allergy Clin N Am.* 2012;32:413–431.

42. Townley RG, Bewtra AK, Nair NM, et al. Methacholine inhalation challenge studies. *J Allergy Clin Immunol.* 1979;64: 569–574.

43. Malmberg P, Larsson K, Sundblad BM, Zhiping W. Importance of the time interval between FEV1 measurements in a methacholine provocation test. *Eur Respir J.* 1993;6:680–686.

44. Britton J, Pavord I, Richards K, et al. Factors influencing the occurrence of airway hyperreactivity in the general population: the importance of atopy and airway calibre. *Eur Respir J.* 1994;7:881–887.

45. Horsley JR, Sterling IJ, Waters WE, Howell JB. How common is increased airway reactivity amongst the elderly? *Gerontology.* 1993;39:38–48.

46. Paoletti P, Carrozzi L, Viegi G, et al. Distribution of bronchial responsiveness in a general population: Effect of sex, age, smoking, and level of pulmonary function. *Am J Respir Crit Care Med.* 1995;151:1770–1777.

47. Ulrik CS. Bronchial responsiveness to inhaled histamine in both adults with intrinsic and extrinsic asthma: the importance of prechallenge forced expiratory volume in 1 second. *J Allergy Clin Immunol.* 1993;91:120–126.

48. Verbanck S. Physiologic measurement of the small airways. *Respiration.* 2012;84:177–188.

49. Burgel P-R: The role of small airways in obstructive airway disease. *Eur Respir Rev.* 2011;20:23–33.

50. Downie SR, Salome CM, Verbanck S, et al. Ventilation heterogeneity is a major determinant of airway hyperresponsiveness in asthma, independent of airway inflammation. *Thorax.* 2007;62:684–689.

51. Oostveen E, MacLeod D, Lorino H, et al. The forced oscillation technique in clinical practice: methodology, recommendations and future developments. *Eur Respir J.* 2003;22:1026–1041.

52. Williamson PA, Clearie K, Menzed D, et al. Assessment of small airways disease using alveolar nitric oxide and impulse oscillometry in asthma and COPD. *Lung.* 2011;189:121–129.

53. Cosio M, Ghezzo H, Hogg JC, et al. The relations between structural changes in small airways and pulmonary-function tests. *New Engl J Med.* 1978;298:1277–1281.

54. Hoppin FC, Green M, Morgan MS: Relationship of central and peripheral airway resistance to lung volume in dogs. *J Appl Physiol.* 1978;44:728–737, .

55. Williamson PA, Clearie K, Menzed D, et al. Assessment of small airways disease using alveolar nitric oxide and impulse oscillometry in asthma and COPD. *Lung.* 2011;189:121–129.

56. Mead J, Lindgren I, Gaensler EA. The mechanical properties of the lungs in emphysema. *J Clin Invest.* 1955;34:1005–1016.

57. Woolcock AJ, Vincent NJ, Macklem PT. Frequency dependence of compliance as a test for obstruction in the small airways. *J Clin Invest.* 1969;48:1097–1106.

58. Dollfuss RE, Milic-Emili J, Bates DV. Regional ventilation of the lung, studied with boluses of 133xenon. *Respir Physiol.* 1967;2:234–246.

59. Sandqvist L, Kjellmer I. Normal values for the single breath nitrogen elimination test in different age groups. *Scand J Clin Lab Invest.* 1960;12:131–135.

60. Schilder DP, Roberts A, Fry DL. Effect of gas density and viscosity on the maximal expiratory flow-volume relationship. *J Clin Invest.* 1963;42:1705–1713.

61. Hutcheon M, Griffin P, Levison H, Zamel N. Volume of isoflow: a new test in the detection of mild abnormalities of lung mechanics. *Am Rev Respir Dis.* 1974;110:458–465.
62. Dosman J, Bode F, Urbanetti J, et al. The use of a helium-oxygen mixture during maximum expiratory flow to demonstrate obstruction in small airways in smokers. *J Clin Invest.* 1975;55:1090–1099.
63. Ogilvie CM, Forster RE, Blakemore WS, Morton JW. A standardized breath holding technique for the clinical measurement of the diffusing capacity of the lung for carbon monoxide. *J Clin Invest.* 1957;36:1–17.
64. Huang YCT, MacIntyre NR. Real-time gas analysis improves the measurement of single-breath diffusing capacity. *Am Rev Respir Dis.* 1992;146:946–950.
65. Neas LM, Schwartz J: the determinants of pulmonary diffusing capacity in a national sample of U.S. adults. *Am J Respir Crit Care Med.* 1996;153:656–664.
66. Filley GF, MacIntosh DJ, Wright GW: Carbon monoxide uptake and pulmonary diffusing capacity in normal subjects at rest and during exercise. *J Clin Invest.* 1954;33:530–539.
67. Cotes JE, Dabbs JM, Elwood PC, et al. Iron deficiency anaemia: its effect on transfer factor for the lung (diffusing capacity) and ventilation and cardiac frequency during sub-maximal exercise. *Clin Sci.* 1972;42:325–335.
68. Kelman GR, Nunn JF: Nomograms for correction of blood P_{O_2}, P_{CO_2} pH, and base excess for time and temperature. *J Appl Physiol.* 1966;21:1484–1490.
69. Sorbini CA, Grassi V, Solinas E, Muiesan G. Arterial oxygen tension in relation to age in healthy subjects. *Respiration.* 1968;25:3–13.
70. Dine CJ, Kreider ME: Hypoxia altitude simulation test. *Chest.* 2008;133:1002–1005.
71. British Thoracic Society Standards of Care Committee. Managing passengers with respiratory disease planning air travel: British Thoracic Society recommendations. *Thorax.* 2002;57:289–304.
72. Mortazavi A, Eisenberg MJ, Langleben D, et al. Altitude-related hypoxia: risk assessment and management for passengers on commercial aircraft. *Aviat Space Environ Med.* 2003;74:922–927.
73. Gong H, Tashkin DP, Lee EY, et al. Hypoxia-altitude simulation test: Evaluation of patients with chronic airway obstruction. *Am Rev Respir Dis.* 1994;130:980–986.
74. Dillard TA, Moores LK, Bilello KL, et al. The preflight evaluation. *Chest.* 1995;107:352–357.
75. Lloyd BB, Cunningham DJC. A quantitative approach to the regulation of human respiration. In: Cunningham DJC, Lloyd BB, eds. *The Regulation of Human Respiration.* Oxford, Blackwell; 1963: 331–349.
76. Read DJC. A clinical method for assessing the ventilatory response to carbon dioxide. *Aust Ann Med.* 1966;16:20–32.
77. Rebuck AS, Campbell EJM: A clinical method for assessing the ventilatory response to hypoxia. *Am Rev Respir Dis.* 1974;109: 345–350.
78. Weil JV, Byrne-Quinn E, Sodal IE, et al. Hypoxic ventilatory drive in normal man. *J Clin Invest.* 1970;49:1061–1072.
79. Edelman NH, Epstein PE, Lahiri S, Cherniack NS. Ventilatory response to transient hypoxia and hypercapnia in man. *Respir Physiol.* 1973;17:302–314.
80. Whitelaw WA, Derenne JP, Milic-Emili J. Occlusion pressure as a measure of respiratory center output in conscious man. *Respir Physiol.* 1975;23:181–199.
81. Casanova C, Celli BR, Barria P, et al. The 6-min walk distance in healthy subjects: reference standards from seven countries. *Eur Respir J.* 2011;37:150–156.
82. du Bois RM, Weycker D, Albera C, et al. Six-minute-walk test in Idiopathic Pulmonary Fibrosis: test validation and minimal clinically important difference. *Am J Respir Crit Care Med.* 2011;183:1231–1237.
83. Ketchell RI, Roughton M, Agent P, et al. Predicting survival in end-stage cystic fibrosis. *Resp Med.* 2009;103:1441–1447.
84. Parker JM, Dillard TA, Phillips YY. Impact of using stated instead of measured height upon screening spirometry. *Am J Respir Crit Care Med.* 1994;150:1705–1708.
85. McCormack MC. Facing the noise: Addressing the endemic variability in DL_{CO} testing. *Respir Care.* 2012;57:17–23.
86. Jensen R, Crapo R, Muchmore D, et al. Quality control of DL,CO instruments in global clinical trials. *Eur Respir J.* 2009;33:828–834.
87. Haynes JM. Quality assurance of the pulmonary function technologist. *Respir Care.* 2012;57:114–122.
88. Tablan OC, Williams WW, Martone WJ. Infection control in pulmonary function laboratories. *Infect Control.* 1985;6: 442–444.
89. Knudson RJ, Lebowitz MD, Holberg CJ, Burrows B. Changes in the normal maximal expiratory flow-volume curve with growth and aging. *Am Rev Respir Dis.* 1983;127:725–734.
90. Morris AH, Kanner RE, Crapo RO, Gardner RM (eds). *Clinical Pulmonary Function Testing: A Manual of Uniform Laboratory Procedures.* 2nd ed. Salt Lake City, UT, Intermountain Thoracic Society; 1984.
91. Rubin BK, Enger M, Dhand R, et al. Respiratory care year in review 2010: Part 1. Asthma, COPD, Pulmonary function testing, ventilator-associated pneumonia. *Respir Care.* 2011;56: 488–502.
92. Barisione G, Crimi E, Bartolini S, et al. How to interpret reduced forced expiratory volume in 1 s (FEV1)/vital capacity ratio with normal FEV1. *Eur Resp J.* 2009;33:1396–1402.
93. Kryger M, Bode F, Antic R, Anthonisen N. Diagnosis of obstruction of the central and upper airways. *Am J Med.* 1976;61: 85-93.

CHAPTER 34

Principles and Applications of Cardiopulmonary Exercise Testing

Karl T. Weber
Kevin P. Newman

INTRODUCTION

Cardiopulmonary exercise (CPX) testing draws on the recognition that the thorax represents a metabolic gas transport unit, the function of whose requisite components – diaphragm, heart, lungs, rib cage, and corresponding skeletal muscles – is to transport O_2 to and CO_2 from metabolizing tissues. Unit O_2 and CO_2 transport must adjust to physiological and pathophysiological stresses that augment the body's consumption of oxygen ($\dot{V}_{O_2}$) and carbon dioxide production ($\dot{V}_{CO_2}$). During strenuous levels of muscular work, for example, $\dot{V}_{O_2}$ may rise eightfold, accompanied by increased $\dot{V}_{CO_2}$. Cardiovascular or ventilatory disease can disrupt the unit's functional integrity. With severe disease, an abnormality in respiratory gas transport may be apparent at rest, when the body's O_2 requirements are modest. Resting function is preserved with less severe expressions of disease, but abnormal respiratory gas transport becomes apparent when the unit is stressed by an elevation in $\dot{V}_{O_2}$.

CPX testing includes the monitoring of respiratory gas exchange ($\dot{V}_{O_2}$ and $\dot{V}_{CO_2}$), minute ventilation ($\dot{V}_E$), and its components, tidal volume and respiratory rate, together with blood pressure, heart rate, and the electrocardiogram. CPX testing represents a useful approach in the clinical evaluation of a whole host of disorders and circumstances. This chapter addresses physiological principles and the clinical application of CPX testing in the evaluation of major disorders that impair heart or lung function. The chapter is by no means an exhaustive review. For a more detailed discussion of specific entities, the interested reader is referred to several other textbooks.[1,2]

PRINCIPLES, DEFINITIONS, AND CLINICAL APPLICATION OF CARDIOPULMONARY EXERCISE TESTING

The metabolic gas transport unit, also referred to as the "cardiopulmonary unit," links metabolizing tissues to the atmosphere and its supply of O_2. O_2 transport to tissues must be precise and based upon prevailing need. CO_2 produced by tissues must be eliminated into the atmosphere in an equally efficient manner.

RESTING OXYGEN UPTAKE AND TRANSPORT

Concepts and calculations pertaining to $\dot{V}_{O_2}$ and O_2 content, transport, and extraction are reviewed in Table 34-1. The heart and lungs accommodate to the metabolic requirements of tissues; they must do so on a moment-to-moment basis, according to physiological priorities. Tissue requirements for O_2 dictate a certain $\dot{V}_E$ and cardiac output. In an average-sized person, resting $\dot{V}_{O_2}$ averages 250 mL/min or 3.5 mL/min/kg body weight (one metabolic equivalent) and is associated with a $\dot{V}_E$ of 8 to 10 L/min and cardiac output of 4 to 6 L/min. O_2 transport, also termed O_2 delivery, ranges between 730 and 1040 mL/min and is more than adequate to satisfy resting $\dot{V}_{O_2}$. On average, 25% of arterial O_2 content is extracted by tissues. O_2 delivery and extraction each increase during physiological stress in proportion to the elevation in O_2 demand. Factors that normally determine O_2 availability at rest and during exercise include cardiac output, hemoglobin concentration and its percent saturation, and O_2 extraction.

EXERCISE OXYGEN UPTAKE AND TRANSPORT

$\dot{V}_E$ and O_2 delivery must each rise during exercise. Strenuous work can raise $\dot{V}_E$ 8 to 10 times its resting level. Ventilation normally poses no limitation on the ability of tissues to carry out aerobic work. By contrast, the extent to which cardiac output rises during progressive work is less dramatic. In untrained subjects, cardiac output increases four to five times its resting value. Cardiac output rises 600 mL/min for every 100 mL/min increment in $\dot{V}_{O_2}$. This is considered the normal "gain" setting between the heart and its cardiac output and $\dot{V}_{O_2}$. O_2 availability during physical activity is further ensured by enhanced O_2 extraction and circulatory autoregulation. Reflexive and humoral influences produce vasoconstriction in less

TABLE 34-1 Oxygen Utilization, Content, Transport, and Extraction

O_2 utilization 250 mL/min	= Cardiac output · (arterial O_2 content – venous O_2 content) = 5000 mL/min · (19 mL/dL – 14 mL/dL)
Arterial O_2 content 19 mL/dL	= Hemoglobin · % saturation · O_2 combining capacity = 14 g/dL · 0.96 · 1.34 mL/g
Venous O_2 content 14 mL/dL	= 14 g/dL · 0.96 · 1.34 mL/g
Arteriovenous O_2 difference 5 mL/dL	= Arterial O_2 content – venous O_2 content = 19 mL/dL – 14 mL/dL
O_2 transport 950 mL/min	= Cardiac output · arterial O_2 content = 5000 mL/min · 19 mL/dL
O_2 extraction 25%	$= \frac{\text{Arteriovenous } O_2 \text{ difference}}{\text{Arterial } O_2 \text{ content}} \cdot 100\%$ $= \frac{19-14}{19} \cdot 100\%$

Source: Reproduced with permission from Weber KT. Gas transport and the cardiopulmonary unit. In: Weber KT, Janicki JS, eds. Cardiopulmonary Exercise Testing: Physiologic Principles and Clinical Applications. Philadelphia, PA: Saunders; 1986.

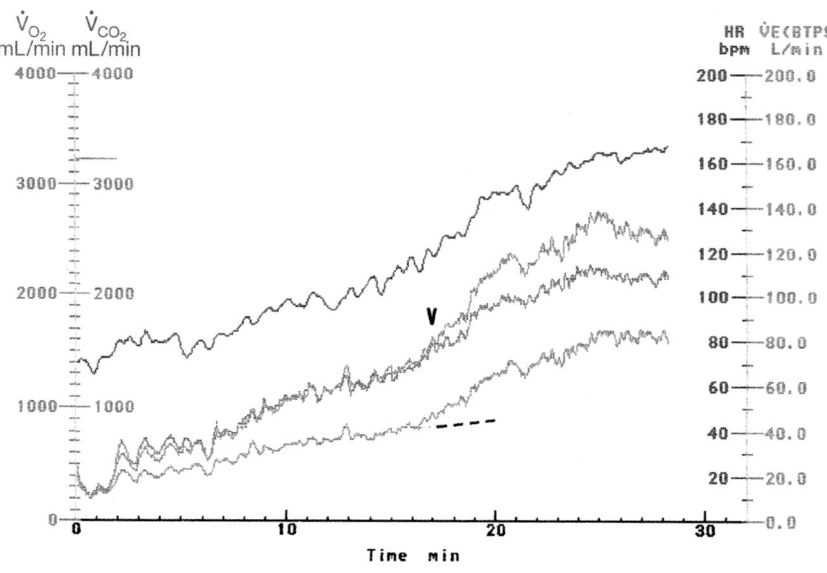

Figure 34-1 Cardiopulmonary exercise response in a 40-year-old man without heart or lung disease. Shown are 2 minutes of standing rest, followed by incremental treadmill exercise. Individual responses *(color coded)* include oxygen uptake ($\dot{V}_{O_2}$), carbon dioxide production ($\dot{V}_{CO_2}$), minute ventilation ($\dot{V}_E$), and heart rate (HR). Maximal O_2 uptake, a plateau in $\dot{V}_{O_2}$ was attained after the crossover of $\dot{V}_{CO_2}$ and $\dot{V}_{O_2}$ *(arrowhead)*, representing the AT and accompanied by a disproportionate (broken line) rise in $\dot{V}_E$.

metabolically active tissues, permitting a greater apportionment of blood flow to exercising muscle.

Physiological limits to the elevation in cardiac output (i.e., cardiac reserve) and O_2 extraction (approximately 75%–80% of arterial O_2 content) determine aerobic capacity of untrained subjects to incremental exercise. Beyond these physiological limits, any additional increment in work is not accompanied by an elevation in O_2; a plateau in $\dot{V}_{O_2}$ is attained and is termed the *maximal oxygen uptake* ($\dot{V}_{O_2max}$). CPX test results, including $\dot{V}_{O_2max}$, are shown in Figure 34-1 for a 40-year-old man without clinically apparent heart or lung disease. Shown are individual responses in $\dot{V}_{O_2}$, $\dot{V}_{CO_2}$, $\dot{V}_E$, and heart rate during progressive increments in treadmill work. A $\dot{V}_{O_2max}$ of 2198 mL/min (27.2 mL/min/kg) was attained. This is a true plateau in $\dot{V}_{O_2}$, with $\dot{V}_{O_2}$ remaining invariant for 2.5 stages (5 minutes) of exercise.

$\dot{V}_{O_2max}$ should not be equated or used synonymously with peak $\dot{V}_{O_2}$ achieved during symptom-limited exercise. $\dot{V}_{O_2max}$ reflects a person's aerobic capacity—a physiological capacity of the cardiovascular system. In an average-sized, untrained person whose maximum cardiac output and arteriovenous oxygen difference are 20 L/min and 12 mL/dL, respectively, a $\dot{V}_{O_2max}$ of 2400 mL/min is expected. In athletes, a greater cardiac reserve and enhanced capacity for oxidative metabolism by trained skeletal muscle are available, providing for greater aerobic capacity. In patients with heart disease, whose ability to raise cardiac output during exercise is impaired, $\dot{V}_{O_2max}$ is proportionally reduced (see above).

■ CARBON DIOXIDE PRODUCTION

The right heart "accepts" metabolically produced CO_2, and the alveolar exchange surface expels CO_2 into the atmosphere. CO_2 is a major respiratory stimulant that maintains eucapnia. Seventy-five to 80% of O_2 is converted to CO_2. Accordingly, resting $\dot{V}_{CO_2}$ averages 190 mL/min and represents a *metabolic source* of CO_2. The resting $\dot{V}_{CO_2}/\dot{V}_{O_2}$ ratio, or respiratory gas exchange ratio (R), typically ranges between 0.75 and 0.85. The absolute value of R depends on the proportion of carbohydrates and fats available from the diet. $\dot{V}_{O_2}$ and $\dot{V}_{CO_2}$ rise in proportion to one another during physical activity as long as an adequate amount of O_2 is available to sustain oxidative metabolism.

With strenuous levels of muscular work, $\dot{V}_{O_2}$ rises to a level where the heart is unable to provide O_2 at a commensurate rate. Consequently, tissue O_2 availability becomes inadequate. Working skeletal muscle enhances its use of less efficient anaerobic metabolism to derive energy. This leads to lactate production from working muscle beyond that normally produced. This *nonmetabolic source* of CO_2 is derived from rapid buffering of the lactate by bicarbonate; the CO_2 generated serves as a respiratory stimulant. The accompanying increase in $\dot{V}_E$ maintains eucapnia and raises the respiratory gas exchange ratio above that associated with aerobic metabolism. Anaerobic metabolism during a progressive exercise test is heralded by this disproportionate rise in $\dot{V}_E$ and $\dot{V}_{CO_2}$ relative to $\dot{V}_{O_2}$. The corresponding level of $\dot{V}_{O_2}$ at which anaerobic metabolism occurs is termed the *anaerobic threshold* (AT).[1] The point during exercise at which $\dot{V}_{CO_2}$ exceeds $\dot{V}_{O_2}$ and $\dot{V}_E$ rises disproportionately is shown in Figure 34-1. Anaerobiosis normally occurs when 60% or more of a person's aerobic capacity has been attained. For the 40-year-old man whose exercise response is shown in Figure 34-1, the AT occurred at a $\dot{V}_{O_2}$ of 18.8 mL/min/kg, or 69% of his $\dot{V}_{O_2max}$.

■ CLINICAL APPLICATION OF CARDIOPULMONARY EXERCISE TESTING

Patients with cardiovascular or respiratory disease of mild-to-moderate severity frequently note limiting symptoms of fatigue or breathlessness during physical activity. Because their quality of life is compromised, they seek or are referred for medical evaluation. Re-creating muscular work in a monitored setting permits an evaluation of the nature and severity of such symptoms and the relative importance of abnormal heart or lung function. This strategy provides information surpassing that available from static measures of heart and lung function, such as ejection fraction, lung volumes, or airflows, determined at rest. The continuous monitoring of $\dot{V}_{O_2}$, $\dot{V}_{CO_2}$, $\dot{V}_E$, respiratory rate, and tidal volume during incremental exercise can be performed simply and on a breath-by-breath basis. Data shown in Figure 34-1 are displayed throughout the test. The choice of a particular CPX test (see above) depends on the nature and expression of the clinical disorder and the particular problem to be addressed. For most clinical evaluations, isotonic forms of exercise are used. Isotonic work is an acceptable, negotiable, and reproducible form of exercise for patients with heart or lung disease.

It should be noted, however, that while noninvasive CPX testing may help determine the impairment in aerobic capacity, abnormalities in ventilation with exercise, and their severity in patients with lung disease, these parameters are not necessarily diagnostic. For example, $\dot{V}_{O_2max}$, AT, or exercise $\dot{V}_E$ do not identify the underlying structural defect responsible for a patient's abnormal response. This may require invasive monitoring during CPX testing to identify specific hemodynamic abnormalities. Echocardiography and specialized pulmonary function studies may be required. The physician must draw upon sound clinical judgment and complementary laboratory tests to derive an understanding of the nature and severity of the heart or lung disease.

NONINVASIVE TREADMILL EXERCISE

Walking represents a common daily exercise rather than a specialized skill. A patient who walks into the physician's office or down a hospital corridor can walk on a treadmill at 1.0 or 1.5 mph, zero grade. Treadmills are programmable. The Bruce protocol, which employs marked increments in treadmill speed and slope over short periods in the evaluation of myocardial ischemia, may not be useful for patients with limited exercise tolerance. A modified Naughton protocol of gradually progressive exercise (Table 34-2) serves to stress the cardiopulmonary unit for patients with heart or lung disease who have a wide range of exercise tolerance. In this protocol, the first two stages of exercise represent very low workloads and are a warmup for patients with heart or lung disease of minor severity; the stages represent near-maximal exercise for patients with more advanced disease.

$\dot{V}_{O_2max}$ is defined as $\dot{V}_{O_2}$ that remains invariant (<1 mL/min/kg for 30 seconds or more) despite an increment in workload. An invariant $\dot{V}_{O_2}$ for at least two stages of exercise is preferred (Fig. 34-1). $\dot{V}_{O_2max}$ follows the AT, and this definition of $\dot{V}_{O_2max}$ presumes that the AT has already been achieved. The AT generally occurs at 60% of a patient's aerobic capacity. $\dot{V}_{O_2max}$ associated with incremental treadmill exercise provides a greater aerobic capacity than does cycle ergometry because it works a larger group of muscles.[3] A patient's aerobic capacity to incremental treadmill exercise is used to grade the functional impairment (Table 34-3). $\dot{V}_{O_2max}$ is an objective measure of functional status—in contradistinction to the New York Heart Association classification, which is based on perceptions and biases of the patient and physician. Treadmill O_2max determination is reproducible in patients with a wide variety of cardiovascular disorders.[2] A $\dot{V}_{O_2max}$ of under 20 mL/min/kg has been selected as the cutoff for grading impaired aerobic capacity; adult men and women, including the elderly (over 65 years of age), have an expected $\dot{V}_{O_2max}$ of more than 20 mL/min/kg.[4]

TABLE 34-2 Modified Naughton Treadmill Exercise Protocol

Stage	Speed	Grade	Physical Activities
1	1.0	0	Driving a car Sitting and writing or eating
2	1.5	0	Dressing; knitting Walking to bathroom Light auto repair
3	2.0	3.5	Shave self in bathroom Wash entire body Food shopping
4	2.0	7.0	Sexual activity Raking leaves Plastering
5	2.0	10.5	Stacking firewood Mowing lawn (powered) Walking downstairs
6	3.0	7.5	Scrubbing floors Gardening Walking upstairs
7	3.0	10.0	Lifting and carrying 65–80 lb Carpentry Climbing hills (no load)
8	3.0	12.5	Digging Snow shoveling Climbing stairs (20-lb load)
9	3.0	15.0	Beyond this level, work loads are equal to very vigorous exercise (e.g., skiing, basketball)
10	3.4	14.0	
11	3.4	16.0	
12	3.4	18.0	
13	3.4	20.0	
14	3.4	22.0	

Source: Reproduced with permission from Weber KT, Janicki JS, McElroy PA. Cardiopulmonary exercise (CPX) testing. In: Weber KT, Janicki JS, eds. Cardiopulmonary Exercise Testing: Physiologic Principles and Clinical Applications. Philadelphia, PA: Saunders; 1986.

TABLE 34-3 Classification of Cardiac and Circulatory Failure

Class	Severity	$\dot{V}_{O_2max}$ (mL/kg/min)	Anerobic Threshold (mL/kg/min)	Predicted Cardiac Index (L/m²/min)
A	Mild to none	>20	>14	>8
B	Mild to moderate	16–20	11–14	6–8
C	Moderate to severe	10–16	8–11	4–6
D	Severe	6–10	5–8	<4

Source: Adapted with permission from Weber KT, Janicki JS, McElroy PA. Pulmonary hypertension. In: Weber KT, Janicki JS, eds. Cardiopulmonary Exercise Testing: Physiologic Principles and Clinical Applications. Philadelphia, PA: Saunders; 1986.

The duration of symptom-free treadmill exercise should not be equated with $\dot{V}_{O_2max}$. Treadmill time suffers from not having an objective, quantitative end-point. Differences in gait and body weight create different levels of work for equivalent stages of treadmill exercise. Symptom-limited exercise time is subject to patient motivation and physician bias.[5] Peak heart rate attained with exercise is also a less precise measure of $\dot{V}_{O_2max}$. This is particularly true in patients with atrial fibrillation.

Determination of the AT can be defined according to one or more criteria.[1] These include (1) a disproportionate rise in $\dot{V}_{CO_2}$, $\dot{V}_E$, or R relative to $\dot{V}_{O_2}$ and (2) a disproportionate rise in end-tidal CO_2 relative to end-tidal O_2. These criteria can best be applied to breath-by-breath respiratory gas exchange data. In our laboratory, a simpler strategy is used. The AT is identified as the level of $\dot{V}_{O_2}$ attained during treadmill work after the plots of $\dot{V}_{O_2}$ and $\dot{V}_{CO_2}$ cross, when R exceeds 1.0. Figure 34-1 depicts the crossover in $\dot{V}_{CO_2}$ and $\dot{V}_{O_2}$ from breath-by-breath gas exchange data monitored throughout incremental treadmill exercise. It also demonstrates the point at which $\dot{V}_E$ rises disproportionately. Measured days or weeks apart, this noninvasive determination of the AT is reproducible in a wide range of patients with cardiac or circulatory failure and correlates with lactate threshold (see above).[2,6,7]

The normal ventilatory response to incremental treadmill exercise consists of an increase in $\dot{V}_E$ created by an increase in respiratory rate and tidal volume. Ventilatory reserves, represented by maximal voluntary ventilation (MVV) and vital capacity determined during routine pulmonary function testing, are only partly utilized during light, moderate, and maximal exercise by normal persons. The ratio of maximal exercise $\dot{V}_E$ to MVV reflects use of this ventilatory reserve. Exercise $\dot{V}_E$ in normal subjects and patients with predominant cardiovascular disease rarely exceeds 50% of MVV.[8] The same is true of the ratio between maximal exercise tidal volume and vital capacity. These limitations in ventilatory responses are consistent with a ventilatory effort that can be voluntarily sustained at rest without the appearance of fatigue or breathlessness.

An oximeter, worn on either an earlobe or a finger, provides noninvasive monitoring of arterial O_2 saturation during exercise. This is a useful screening procedure in patients in whom O_2 desaturation might be anticipated (e.g., those with congenital heart disease with right-to-left shunt, restrictive or obstructive lung disease, or pulmonary vascular disease). Normal subjects and patients with chronic cardiac or circulatory failure do not develop arterial hypoxemia (arterial O_2 saturation under 90%) during exercise. In patients in whom O_2 desaturation is evident from oximetry, confirmatory evidence from direct measurement of arterial blood gases during repeat exercise may be advisable.

Thus, incremental treadmill exercise can be used to determine the following: the AT with a submaximal test, the AT and $\dot{V}_{O_2max}$ with a maximal test, the ventilatory response to submaximal or maximal exercise, and arterial O_2 desaturation during submaximal or maximal exercise.

INVASIVE TREADMILL EXERCISE

Invasive hemodynamic monitoring may be necessary to better define the nature and severity of an underlying cardiopulmonary disorder.[2] A triple-lumen flotation catheter can be safely used for hemodynamic monitoring during upright exercise. The hemodynamic response to incremental treadmill exercise in normal subjects is characterized by a progressive rise in cardiac output, accomplished with minimal elevations in left and right ventricular filling pressures. The rise in cardiac output occurs because of an increment in stroke volume, which is most apparent at low and moderate workloads, and because of an elevation in heart rate, which accompanies the entire exercise response. Systemic O_2 extraction rises progressively with incremental exercise to exceed 70% at maximal workloads. A rise in mixed venous lactate concentration, as observed with pulmonary arterial blood sampling, occurs when O_2 extraction exceeds 60% and when the subject is working at greater than 60% of $\dot{V}_{O_2max}$.

Systolic and mean arterial pressures rise during upright exercise. Because of skeletal muscle vasodilatation, arterial diastolic pressure remains essentially invariant during exercise. Systemic vascular resistance falls by 50% to approximately 600 dynes·s·cm^{-5} during incremental, isotonic treadmill exercise. In normal persons, pulmonary artery systolic, mean, and diastolic pressures rise only minimally with exercise and only with higher workloads. Pulmonary vascular resistance, like systemic vascular resistance, falls 50% to about 60 dynes·s·cm^{-5} during incremental isotonic exercise.

CHRONIC CARDIAC FAILURE

In physiological terms, *cardiac failure* is defined as an impairment in cardiac output secondary to a disease process affecting the myocardium. Ischemic heart disease and dilated cardiomyopathies are examples of disease entities that can result in chronic cardiac failure. $\dot{V}_{O_2max}$ and the AT each predict cardiac reserve and, thereby, the severity of cardiac failure. These parameters further serve to objectively demonstrate a patient's functional capacity, which is not predicted from the cardiac ejection fraction. Patients with an ejection fraction under 20% may still be able to swim.

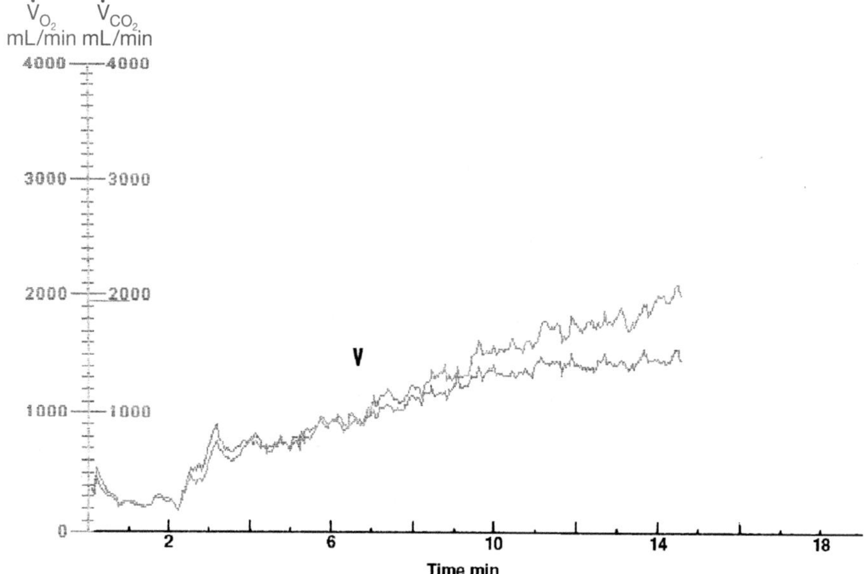

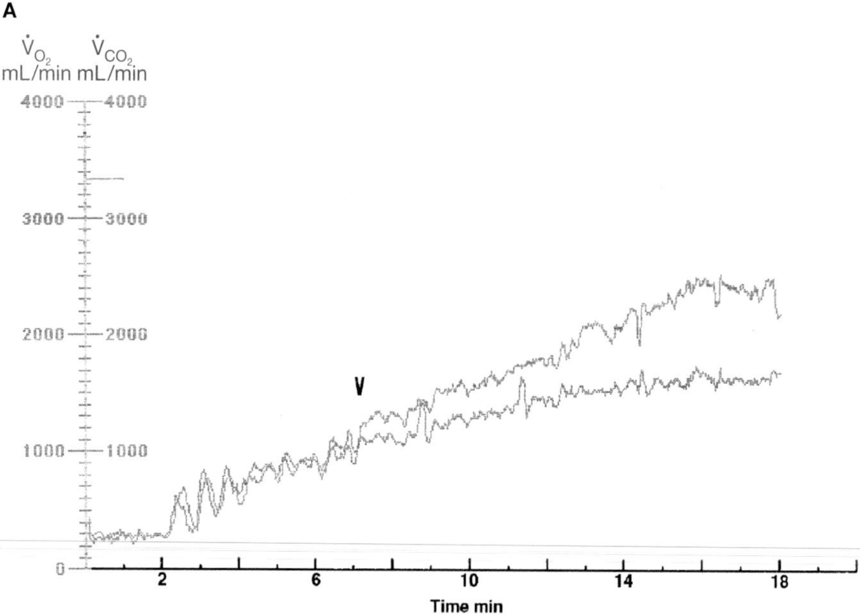

Figure 34-2 Cardiopulmonary exercise test results for a 45-year-old woman (**A**) and a 40-year-old man *(right panel)*, each with ischemic heart disease and chronic cardiac failure. Only $\dot{V}_{O_2}$ and $\dot{V}_{CO_2}$ are shown, to better demonstrate the anaerobic threshold (AT) and $\dot{V}_{O_2max}$ attained by each patient. On the left, the AT was seen with a $\dot{V}_{O_2}$ of 11.6 mL/min/kg and a $\dot{V}_{O_2max}$ of 16.5 mL/min/kg. This represents a functional class B response. The AT and $\dot{V}_{O_2max}$ are 8.5 and 13.7 mL/min/kg, respectively (**B**). This corresponds to functional class C.

SYSTOLIC DYSFUNCTION

In patients with chronic cardiac failure, $\dot{V}_{O_2max}$ attained during incremental treadmill exercise is primarily a function of maximal cardiac output.[8,9] This conclusion has been confirmed by numerous studies.[10–14] An impairment in aerobic capacity is gauged according to the exercise AT and $\dot{V}_{O_2max}$ and assigned a functional class as reviewed in Table 34-3. These parameters are, in turn, used to predict maximal exercise cardiac index (or cardiac reserve). Examples of $\dot{V}_{O_2max}$ and the AT attained by two patients with chronic cardiac

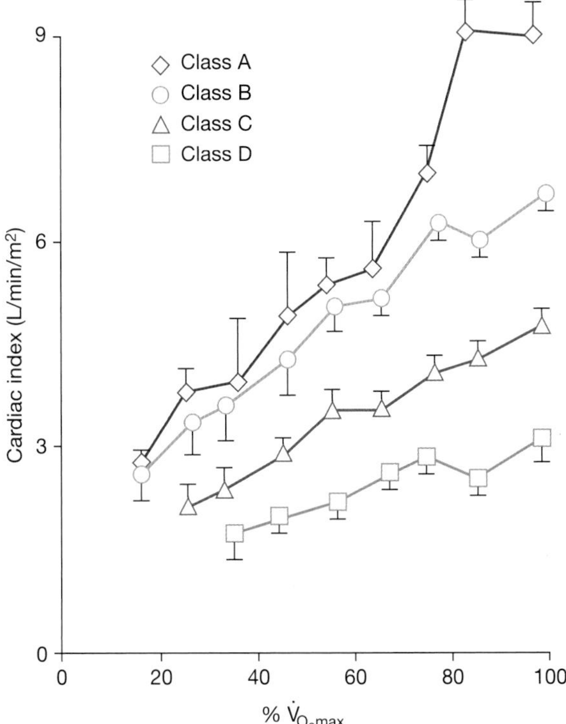

Figure 34-3 Relationship between treadmill exercise cardiac index and normalized aerobic capacity for patients with chronic cardiac failure of diverse origin and severity, subdivided according to each functional class. *(Reproduced with permission from Weber KT, Janicki JS. Cardiopulmonary exercise testing for evaluation of chronic cardiac failure. Am J Cardiol. 1985;55(2):22A–31A.)*

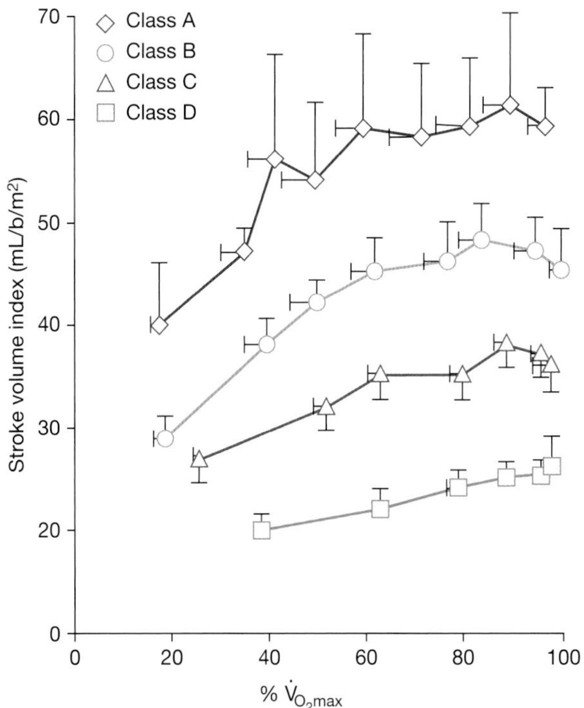

Figure 34-4 Relationship between treadmill exercise stroke volume index and normalized aerobic capacity for patients with chronic cardiac failure of varying severity, as expressed by each functional class. *(Reproduced with permission from Weber KT, Janicki JS. Cardiopulmonary exercise testing for evaluation of chronic cardiac failure. Am J Cardiol. 1986;55(2):22A–31A.)*

failure (one class B, the other class C) are given in Figure 34-2. To measure $\dot{V}_{O_2max}$ in such patients, they must be exercised to exhaustion. The AT is achieved at submaximal workloads short of exhaustion; it, too, stratifies the degree of cardiac dysfunction.

Validation of these concepts was obtained during treadmill exercise using invasive measures of cardiac output and mixed venous lactate concentration.[15,16] Patients had chronic cardiac failure of varying severity (classes A to D), due to either ischemic or myopathic heart disease. In each exercise class, the arteriovenous O_2 difference rose to 12 mL/dL or more at maximum exercise, corresponding to a systemic O_2 extraction in excess of 70%, suggesting that O_2 extraction reached maximal physiological levels. The reduction in aerobic capacity of a patient with chronic cardiac failure is, therefore, due primarily to impaired cardiac reserve. The cardiac output–O_2 relation to progressive treadmill exercise for these patients is given in Figure 34-3. For each exercise class, cardiac output is presented as a percentage of $\dot{V}_{O_2max}$ (set equal to 100%) that existed at rest and throughout each stage of exercise. Cardiac output rose by 600 mL/min/m^2 for each dL/min/m^2 increase in $\dot{V}_{O_2}$ in each class. This indicates that the heart responds to tissue O_2 requirements irrespective of the severity of heart failure, but it is limited by the maximal cardiac output it can attain. Differences in cardiac output achieved at peak exercise are seen between classes. Progressive reductions in cardiac reserve are responsible for different aerobic capacities observed in these patients. $\dot{V}_{O_2max}$, therefore, serves as a noninvasive measure of peak exercise cardiac output and is given for each functional class in Table 34-3.

The cardiac output response to exercise is a function of the rises in stroke volume and heart rate. Responses in stroke volume for patients with chronic cardiac failure are shown in Figure 34-4 for each exercise class. In class A and B patients, stroke volume rises 50% during lighter workloads that represent less than 60% of $\dot{V}_{O_2max}$; at larger workloads, further increments in stroke volume are less apparent. A 25% rise in stroke volume occurs at submaximal exercise in class C patients, whereas in class D patients, exercise stroke volume is no different from its resting value. Exercise stroke volume is a result of several factors, including systolic wall stress, mitral or tricuspid regurgitation that may appear during exercise, and depressed myocardial contractility.

For each functional class of chronic cardiac failure, the heart rate–$\dot{V}_{O_2}$ response to upright incremental exercise is represented by a common slope.[17] The average slope is 3.6 beats/min for every 1-mL/min/kg increment in $\dot{V}_{O_2}$. Peak heart rate achieved is a function of maximal workload performed. Maximal exercise heart rate is, therefore, different for each class. In class D patients, the elevation in heart rate is the sole mechanism by which cardiac output rises during exercise.

Some patients with chronic cardiac failure deviate from this heart rate– $\dot{V}_{O_2}$ relation by having an inappropriate sinus tachycardia, either at rest and throughout exercise or simply during exercise. In the presence of a reduced ejection fraction and ventricular dilation, this inappropriately rapid heart rate further compromises exercise cardiac output and reduces aerobic capacity. β-Adrenergic receptor blockade is useful in attenuating resting or exercise heart rate under these circumstances.[18] Such chronotropic dysfunction (see below) to exercise may also apply to patients with chronic atrial fibrillation. An example of an inappropriate rapid heart rate relative to incremental treadmill exercise (Naughton protocol) is given in Figure 34-5 for a patient with atrial fibrillation and dilated cardiomyopathy of uncertain origin.

As in normal persons, lactate production appears in patients with chronic cardiac failure when systemic O_2 extraction exceeds 60%. Mixed venous lactate concentration during exercise rises above resting values when 60% or more of $\dot{V}_{O_2max}$ is attained.[7,16] Given

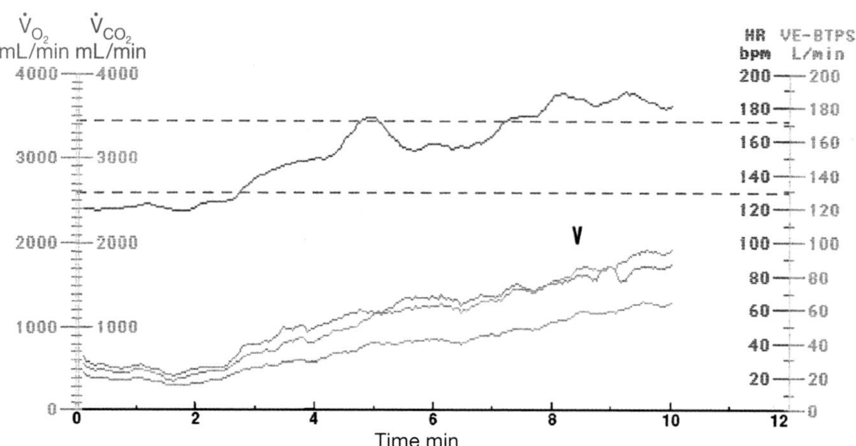

Figure 34-5 Cardiopulmonary exercise test results in a 48-year-old man with atrial fibrillation and dilated (idiopathic) cardiomyopathy. Note the rapid heart rate at rest and throughout incremental treadmill exercise. Predicted maximum heart rate range in this patient is shown by the broken lines. He achieved this rate during the first stage of exercise and exceeded it during the last stage of exercise. This is an inappropriate heart rate response. The AT is 13 mL/min/kg *(arrow)*, in keeping with functional class B. He did not achieve $\dot{V}_{O_2max}$ and, therefore, had a peak $\dot{V}_{O_2}$ of 15 mL/min/kg.

differences in aerobic capacity between exercise classes, different workloads are associated with this lactate threshold (Fig. 34-6). In class D patients whose cardiac output response is limited, the lactate threshold occurs at very light workloads ($\dot{V}_{O_2}$ of 5–8 mL/min/kg). Corresponding values for class C, B, and A patients are 8 to 11 mL/min/kg, 11 to 14 mL/min/kg, and more than 14 mL/min/kg, respectively. Thus, lactate threshold and $\dot{V}_{O_2max}$ reflect the severity of chronic cardiac failure as given in Table 34-3. A noninvasively determined AT based on measurements of respiratory gas exchange, as discussed previously, corresponds to the invasively measured lactate threshold.[7,12,16,19]

Exercise left ventricular filling pressure, as gauged from an occlusive wedge pressure recording, rises to a different degree in each exercise class with chronic cardiac failure (Fig. 34-7). In class A patients, the rise in wedge pressure during isotonic exercise rarely exceeds 18 mm Hg. This resembles a normal response. In class B patients, more dramatic elevations in exercise wedge pressure – to 25 mm Hg or higher – are frequently noted. Resting filling pressure is increased in class C and D patients; a further rise may be seen during upright exercise, often to levels in excess of 30 mm Hg. Despite these marked levels of pulmonary venous pressure, patients do not develop evidence of pulmonary congestion after exercise. Moreover, elevations in wedge pressure neither would predict exercise cardiac reserve and aerobic capacity nor are responsible for exertional dyspnea in these patients. Dyspnea corresponds with the lactate threshold and a disproportionate rise in $\dot{V}_E$ relative to $\dot{V}_{O_2}$.[8,16,20,21] Patients can be encouraged to exercise to exhaustion, attaining $\dot{V}_{O_2max}$ in the presence of dyspnea. In patients with acute cardiac failure, pulmonary congestion and dyspnea correlate with the elevation in wedge pressure; pulmonary edema occurs when hydrostatic pressure exceeds the colloidal osmotic pressure of 25 mm Hg and these patients should not be exercised.

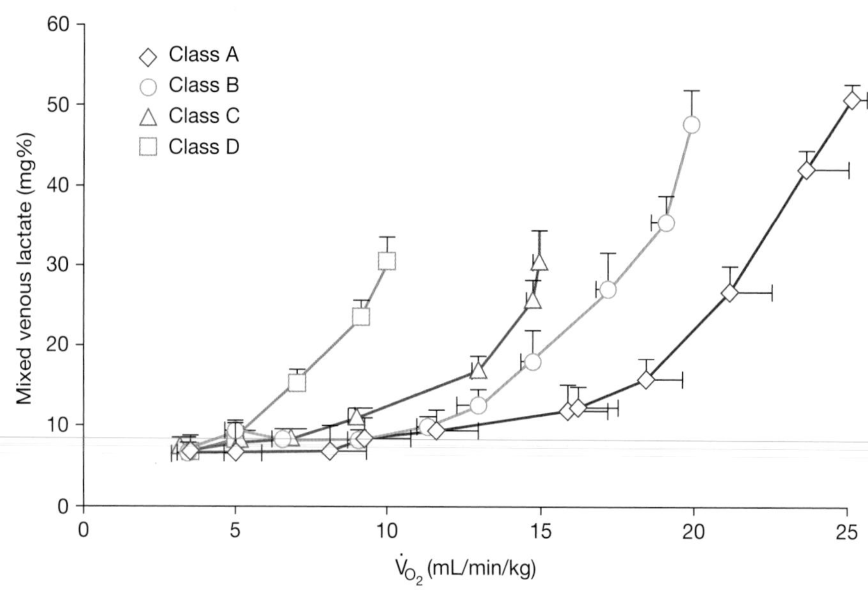

Figure 34-6 Relationship between mixed venous lactate concentration and $\dot{V}_{O_2}$ to incremental treadmill exercise for patients with chronic cardiac failure of varying severity, as expressed by each functional class. *(Reproduced with permission from Weber KT, Janicki JS. Cardiopulmonary exercise testing for evaluation of chronic cardiac failure. Am J Cardiol. 1987;55(2):22A–31A.)*

$\dot{V}_E$ rises appropriately during incremental exercise in patients with chronic cardiac failure. The response in $\dot{V}_E$ most closely corresponds to $\dot{V}_{CO_2}$ throughout exercise (aerobic and anaerobic work) and is sufficient to sustain alveolar ventilation, thereby preventing hypoxemia and hypercapnia. Maximum $\dot{V}_E$ attained with exercise is less than 50% of MVV. Thus, these patients do not exhaust their ventilatory reserve in responding to exercise, even when their pulmonary compliance may be adversely elevated as a result of chronic pulmonary congestion and elevations in pulmonary venous pressure that appear with exercise. To minimize the work of breathing during exercise, class C and D patients use a pattern of rapid, shallow breathing to increase $\dot{V}_E$. Thus, the rise in tidal volume during exercise above its resting value is modest and compatible with a substantial portion of each breath being wasted in ventilation of anatomic dead space.[8] The response of class A and B patients more closely approximates that of healthy persons, in whom respiratory rate rises progressively during incremental exercise and the rise in tidal volume occurs early during the transition from rest to low-level exercise.

DIASTOLIC DYSFUNCTION

In 30% or more of patients with symptomatic heart failure, primary diastolic dysfunction is held responsible. The ejection fraction is normal or only minimally impaired in these patients. Diastolic dysfunction relates to an inability of the left ventricle to accommodate left atrial and pulmonary venous blood flow during diastole without a marked increase in filling pressure. Abnormal diastolic relaxation and filling typically appear in patients with chronic ischemic heart disease (with previous myocardial infarction), in those with hypertensive heart disease, and especially in elderly women. Responsible mechanisms are thought to include abnormal tissue structure, as occurs with

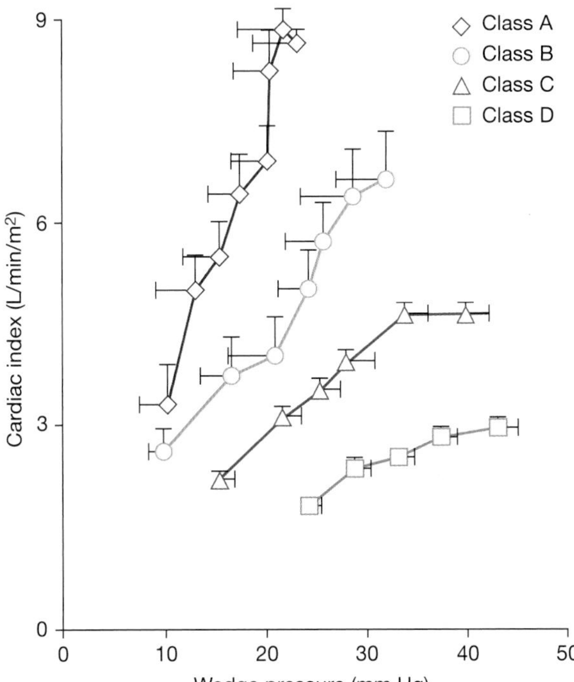

Figure 34-7 Relationship between treadmill exercise cardiac index and occlusion wedge pressure in patients with chronic cardiac failure, subdivided according to functional class. *(Reproduced with permission from Weber KT, Janicki JS. Cardiopulmonary exercise testing for evaluation of chronic cardiac failure. Am J Cardiol. 1988;55(2):22A–31A.)*

fibrous tissue accumulation or amyloid infiltration and abnormal calcium handling by sarcoplasmic reticulum. Factors extrinsic to the myocardium may also be contributory. Examples include the interaction between the pressure- or volume-overloaded right ventricle with the left ventricle and leftward shift of the interventricular septum and the interplay between the heart and pericardium.

Invasive CPX testing, together with incremental bicycle exercise, has been used to address the hemodynamic response of patients with primary diastolic dysfunction.[22] Most patients studied had systemic hypertension, and many were elderly; all had a clinical history of pulmonary congestion. Peak exercise $\dot{V}_{O_2}$ was reduced, owing to a reduction in exercise cardiac output and stroke volume responses; arteriovenous O_2 difference rose above 10 mL/dL. The level of $\dot{V}_{O_2}$ achieved with exercise correlated with peak cardiac output response. In comparison to age-matched controls, expected exercise-associated increments in left ventricular end-diastolic volume were not seen and were accompanied by increased left ventricular filling pressure. Thus, abnormalities in diastolic filling abrogated the Frank–Starling mechanism, thereby restricting the rise in exercise cardiac output; this finding may serve to explain symptoms of fatigue and breathlessness that these patients experience on exertion.

Primary diastolic dysfunction has been observed in patients following cardiac transplantation[23] in whom there is an abnormal blunting of stroke volume and heart rate responses to exercise. Despite the slower exercise heart rate in the transplanted, denervated heart, in which diastolic filling periods would accordingly be longer, diastolic dysfunction is present, limiting the exercise cardiac output response. Abnormal diastolic function has also been observed in the elderly and contributes to impaired exercise cardiac output response.[24]

CHRONOTROPIC DYSFUNCTION

Cardiac reserve in exercise depends not only on systolic and diastolic functions but also on heart rate and rhythm, including a coordinated contraction of the atria and ventricles. CPX testing has been used to address the contribution of abnormal heart rate and rhythm on the AT and $\dot{V}_{O_2max}$, broadly categorized here as chronotropic dysfunction. This includes abnormal sinus tachycardia, bradyarrhythmias, atrioventricular dissociation, and atrial fibrillation. CPX testing has proved useful in the evaluation of pacemaker function and technique.[25] Improvements in the AT at submaximal levels of work have been demonstrated for single-chamber, activity-triggered pacing compared with fixed-rate atrial or ventricular pacing. It too can help determine the optimum upper rate limit in heart failure patients with pacemakers. This can be determined by the highest pacing rate which still produces an increase in oxygen consumption.[26] With recent advancements in pacemaker technology, cardiac resynchronization therapy (CRT) is being increasingly offered to patients with heart failure. In a study involving CRT patients undergoing CPX testing, significant increments in peak $\dot{V}_{O_2}$, $\dot{V}_{O_2}$ at AT and all ventilation and metabolic parameters were noted. Patients with baseline $\dot{V}_{O_2}$ of less than 14 mL/min/kg had the most benefit.[27] Similarly, patients with severe heart failure and atrial fibrillation had better hemodynamic performance with chronic biventricular pacing than left ventricular pacing alone.[28]

Some patients with chronic cardiac failure deviate from this heart rate– $\dot{V}_{O_2}$ relation by having inappropriate sinus tachycardia, either at rest and throughout exercise, or simply during exercise. In the presence of reduced ejection fraction and ventricular dilation, this inappropriately rapid heart rate further compromises exercise cardiac output and reduces aerobic capacity. Under these circumstances, β-adrenergic receptor blockade is useful in attenuating the resting or exercise heart rate. Such chronotropic dysfunction (see below) to exercise may also apply to patients with chronic atrial fibrillation. An example of an inappropriate rapid heart rate during incremental treadmill exercise (Naughton protocol) is given in Figure 34-5 for a patient with atrial fibrillation and dilated cardiomyopathy of uncertain origin.[29]

SURVIVAL AND PROGNOSIS

Various gas exchange parameters have been used to assess prognosis in patients with heart failure, including AT, peak $\dot{V}_{O_2}$, and $\dot{V}_E/\dot{V}_{CO_2}$ slope (a marker of ventilatory efficiency).[13,30–33] $\dot{V}_{O_2}$ at AT and $\dot{V}_{CO_2}$ slope are less subject to patient motivation or premature cessation of exercise and hence are more useful parameters. Class D patients with little or no exercise cardiac reserve (see Table 34-3) with AT <8 mL/min/kg have a marked reduction in 1- and 2-year survival as contrasted to Class A and B patients with respective exercise cardiac index responses of >8 and 6 to 8 L/min/m^2.[13,30,31] $\dot{V}_{O_2}$ at AT combined with $\dot{V}_E/\dot{V}_{CO_2}$ is a better prognostic indicator than peak $\dot{V}_{O_2}$ alone.[34] A low peak Pa_{CO_2} with exercise is responsible for the prognostic power of $\dot{V}_E/\dot{V}_{CO_2}$ slope and by itself is also an independent predictor of prognosis.[35] Resting end-tidal CO_2 has been shown to be a predictor of cardiac-related events.[36] Another $\dot{V}_{O_2}$ kinetics parameter that is a strong predictor of survival and less dependent on motivation is the mean response time ($\dot{V}_{O_2}$ deficit/Δ $\dot{V}_{O_2}$).[37] In the recovery period, slow normalization of $\dot{V}_{O_2}$ is associated with poor prognosis.[38]

The fluctuations in breathing patterns and its association with prognosis have also been studied in heart failure. Cyclic fluctuations in $\dot{V}_E$ at rest that persist during effort (external oscillatory ventilation) are associated with poor prognosis, whereas oscillations at rest alone are not.[39–41]

EFFICACY OF MEDICATIONS

The response to various heart failure medications on gas exchange and hemodynamics has been studied. Patients with heart failure taking spironolactone had a significant increase in peak oxygen consumption, DL_{CO}, and membrane diffusing capacity.[42,43] In a study in which losartan was added to an ACE inhibitor, there was a significant increase in peak $\dot{V}_{O_2}$ and exercise capacity;[44] however, in another study in which candesartan was added, there was no increase in the peak $\dot{V}_{O_2}$ or exercise capacity.[45] Peak $\dot{V}_{O_2}$ has been used as a prognostic marker in heart failure, but in a study involving patients with chronic heart failure taking carvedilol, peak $\dot{V}_{O_2}$ was not found to be a useful prognostic marker.[46]

EXERCISE TRAINING

Exercise training leads to an improvement in exercise tolerance and peak $\dot{V}_{O_2}$ in patients with heart failure who have left ventricular dysfunction.[47] Exercise training in moderate stable heart failure results in favorable qualitative, rather than quantitative, changes in skeletal muscle.[48] Correction of maximum oxygen uptake for skeletal muscle mass, rather than total body mass, is a more sensitive measure of changes associated with exercise training.[48] Only progressive/increasing workload seems to markedly improve oxygen uptake.[49]

ISCHEMIC HEART DISEASE

Ischemia can be diagnosed with the help of ST segment changes during incremental exercise on treadmill or an ergometer during CPX testing. The sensitivity and specificity of ST changes for ischemia is not high. Parameters of gas exchange on CPX testing can be used to improve the diagnostic ability of the exercise-induced ST changes. Using O_2 pulse flattening duration and $\Delta \dot{V}_{O_2}/\Delta$ work rate slope with ST changes, the sensitivity and specificity for diagnosing ischemia improved from 46% to 66%, respectively, to 87% and 74%, respectively.[50] Myocardial stress/rest scintigraphy was used as the standard for detecting ischemia in this study. In another study, exercise cardiac output estimated from $\dot{V}_{O_2}$ at AT correlated with multivessel coronary artery disease, adverse cardiac events and clinically driven revascularization.[51] In postmyocardial infarction patients undergoing 3 weeks of exercise training, a significant improvement in $\dot{V}_{O_2}$ was found.[52]

Parameters of gas exchange measured during CPX testing have proven useful in the diagnosis of ischemia. Myocardial ischemia produces transient depression of left ventricular systolic function and, consequently, a reduction in stroke volume and cardiac output. Graphically, this decline in cardiac output should be reflected in a decline in the rate of increase in oxygen consumption per workload ($\Delta \dot{V}_{O_2}/\Delta$ Work Rate [WR] in watts). Thus, a blunted slope of $\Delta \dot{V}_{O_2}/\Delta$ WR should reflect myocardial ischemia. This analysis of gas exchange has been compared to SPECT myocardial scintigraphy. CPX testing demonstrates improved sensitivity and specificity in the detection of myocardial ischemia. Another valid parameter for the detection of myocardial ischemia is a flattening of the graph of O_2 pulse (mL/beat).[50] As is the case with heart failure, peak $\dot{V}_{O_2}$ and AT are prognosticators of adverse prognosis in patients with ischemic heart disease.

CPX testing has been utilized to assess the presence of right ventricular dysfunction in patients following an inferior myocardial infarction. Right ventricular dysfunction was analyzed utilizing echocardiographic parameters. Patients with right ventricular infarction had significantly lower oxygen consumption than those who had suffered an inferior infarction without right ventricular involvement.[53]

CHRONIC CIRCULATORY FAILURE

Circulatory failure, in physiological terms, refers to an inability of the heart to raise its cardiac output in a manner commensurate with prevailing $\dot{V}_{O_2}$. Responsible factors are extrinsic to the myocardium and include such entities as valvular heart disease, intrinsic pulmonary vascular disease, pericardial disease, and anemia.

VALVULAR HEART DISEASE

Mitral or aortic valve disease may alter the functional integrity of the cardiopulmonary unit by impairing the heart's ability to increase cardiac output in accordance with $\dot{V}_{O_2}$. Pathophysiological alterations within the unit that result from chronic valvular disease and that determine the clinical course and outcome following valve replacement include right heart overload and structural remodeling of the pulmonary vasculature and lung interstitium. The more marked the preoperative impairment in cardiac reserve, the poorer the long-term prognosis. Similarly, the greater the elevation in pulmonary vascular resistance, the more delayed is its return to normal levels and the slower the postoperative abatement of symptoms. The decision for surgical intervention requires an assessment of cardiopulmonary status—one that can be assessed noninvasively and monitored over time to detect a decline in cardiac reserve. Noninvasive CPX testing serves this purpose. Because of the heightened risk of syncope and the myocardial ischemia and arrhythmias that can occur during exercise in patients with aortic valvular stenosis, these patients should exercise with extreme caution, if at all.

Incompetence of the mitral and aortic valves is an example of a disorder that can result in chronic circulatory failure. Each creates a volume overload on the left ventricle. The onset of ventricular dysfunction is generally unpredictable and may initially appear only during vigorous levels of physical activity. As dysfunction progresses, symptoms appear at lower levels of activity and, finally, at rest.

Resting cardiac output is often not distinguishable among class A, B, C, or D patients with mitral or aortic regurgitation. Cardiac reserve is reduced, however, and, accordingly, so is aerobic capacity.[2] No impairment in systemic O_2 extraction has been reported. Thus, as in chronic cardiac failure, any observed decrease in aerobic capacity must be due to a decline in maximal forward cardiac output. To the extent that cardiac output can rise, the exercise cardiac output– $\dot{V}_{O_2}$ relation is preserved among these classes, averaging 600 mL/min/m^2 for every dL/min/m^2 rise in $\dot{V}_{O_2}$. Responses in cardiac output and wedge pressure for each exercise class are given in Figure 34-8. As in chronic cardiac failure, marked elevations in wedge pressure are seen in class C and D patients; this is also true for class B patients with mitral or aortic regurgitation. However, these

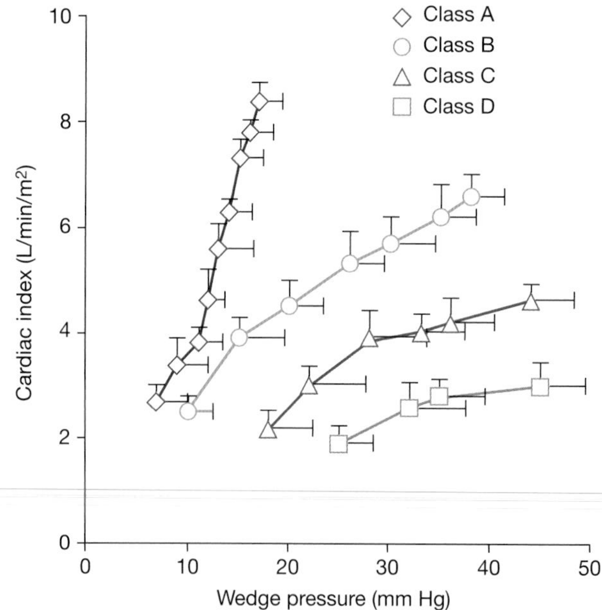

Figure 34-8 Relationship between treadmill exercise cardiac index and wedge pressure in patients with chronic mitral or aortic regurgitation, divided according to functional class. *(Reproduced with permission from Weber KT, Janicki JS (eds). Cardiopulmonary Exercise Testing: Physiologic Principles and Clinical Applications. Philadelphia: WB Saunders; 1986.)*

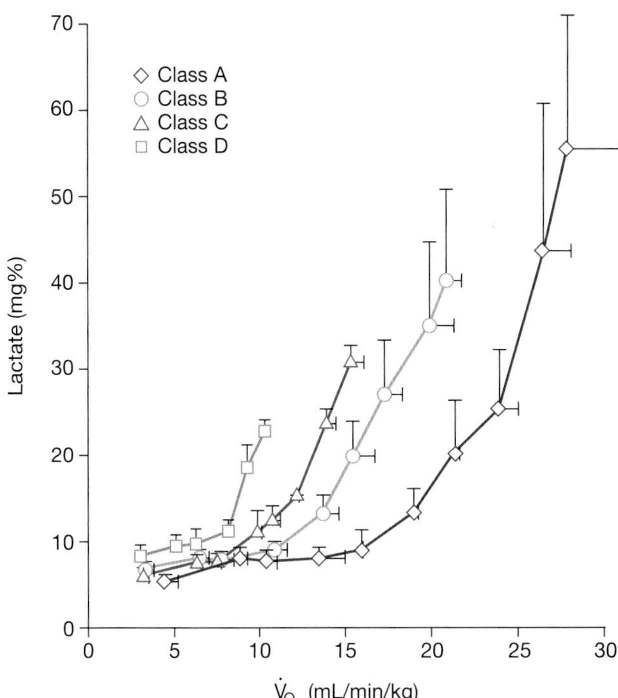

Figure 34-9 Relationship between mixed venous lactate concentration and $\dot{V}_{O_2}$ observed during incremental treadmill exercise in patients with chronic mitral or aortic regurgitation. As in chronic cardiac failure, the lactate threshold (lactate >12 mg/dL) occurs at different levels of $\dot{V}_{O_2}$, depending on functional class. *(Reproduced with permission from Weber KT, Janicki JS (eds). Cardiopulmonary Exercise Testing: Physiologic Principles and Clinical Applications. Philadelphia: WB Saunders; 1986.)*

patients do not develop clinical evidence of pulmonary congestion following exercise, and dyspnea correlates with the lactate threshold. Exercise wedge pressure does not presage aerobic capacity or functional class in these patients.

AT can be used as an alternative measure in patients with valvular incompetence who are unable to attain $\dot{V}_{O_2max}$. The lactate threshold occurs at 60% to 70% of the patient's aerobic capacity and corresponds to a level of systemic O_2 extraction of 60% or more. Figure 34-9 depicts the response in mixed venous lactate concentration as a function of O_2 for each exercise class with mitral or aortic regurgitation. As in patients with chronic cardiac failure, the lactate threshold occurs at progressively lower levels of work as the severity of valvular disease increases.[2] The invasively measured lactate threshold correlates well with the valve obtained using noninvasive respiratory gas exchange measurements (see above).

The reduced mitral valve orifice that accompanies rheumatic mitral valvular stenosis leads to left atrial chamber enlargement, pulmonary venous hypertension, and right heart pressure overload. Pulmonary vascular resistance in most patients ranges between 200 and 600 dynes·s·cm^{-5}. Mitral stenosis is responsible for reduced left ventricular filling at rest and during exercise. An exercise-associated rise in heart rate reduces the diastolic filling period to further curtail left ventricular filling.

Cardiac output fails to rise appropriately with exercise in patients with chronic circulatory failure due to mitral stenosis.[2] For most symptomatic patients, cardiac output fails to rise appropriately during symptom-limited exercise because of a limited stroke volume response. Systemic O_2 extraction increases markedly with exercise, as do pulmonary capillary wedge and mean pulmonary artery pressures. Preoperative assessment of mitral stenosis should include not only calculation of mitral valve area but also exercise test-determined cardiac reserve and functional status. A decision regarding surgery should be based on these objective measures and clinical judgment, not simply on a laboratory-based calculation of reduced valve area.

A preoperative assessment of valvular surgery patients by CPX testing can help predict the degree of postoperative recovery. Preoperative peak $\dot{V}_{O_2}$ of 19 mL/min/kg and greater in patients undergoing surgery for mitral and aortic regurgitation correlates with higher percentage of patients attaining NYHA Functional Class I at 1 year after surgery.[54,55] $\dot{V}_{O_2max}$ along with AT has been used to follow progress of postoperative rehabilitation and training in valve surgery patients.[56,57] Exercise parameters can be helpful in assessing patients with valvular disease patients in whom there is a discrepancy between symptoms and echocardiographic data. A $\dot{V}_{O_2max}$ less than 75% predicted in moderate-to-severe mitral stenosis correlates with higher transvalvular gradients and higher pulmonary artery pressures at the end of exercise than does a $\dot{V}_{O_2max}$ greater than 75% of max predicted.[58]

In the absence of pulmonary arterial hypertension in patients undergoing mitral valve replacement, the presence of significant tricuspid regurgitation is associated with lower $\dot{V}_{O_2max}$ and AT and steeper $\dot{V}_E/\dot{V}_{CO_2}$ than when significant tricuspid regurgitation is absent.[59]

■ HYPERTROPHIC CARDIOMYOPATHY

Hypertrophic cardiomyopathy, the best known genetically determined cardiovascular condition, is marked by significant left ventricular hypertrophy, which may be asymmetric, concentric, or localized (apical). Two major clinical concerns in the disorder are the risk of sudden death and the difficulty in making the diagnosis when the classic asymmetric septal hypertrophy and the classic hemodynamic findings are absent. Exercise testing, in general, is a simple, but imprecise, method to screen for malignant dysrhythmias. CPX testing has been useful in distinguishing the physiologic left ventricular hypertrophy of athletes from hypertrophic cardiomyopathy.[60] Peak $\dot{V}_{O_2}$ is significantly higher in the athletes. A peak $\dot{V}_{O_2}$ 20% above predicted $\dot{V}_{O_2max}$ separates this group from those with genetically proven hypertrophic cardiomyopathy. A number of patients with hypertrophic cardiomyopathy experience symptoms of fatigue and dyspnea which do not correlate with hemodynamic findings. CPX testing can separate real from perceived symptoms. The percent predicted peak $\dot{V}_{O_2}$, combined with a quality of life questionnaire, appears to be helpful in making this distinction.[61]

■ OBSTRUCTIVE SLEEP APNEA

CPX testing can safely be performed in patients with sleep apnea to evaluate abnormalities in gas exchange and the response to continuous positive airway pressure therapy. Patients with moderate or severe obstructive sleep apnea have impaired exercise capacity, low peak $\dot{V}_{O_2}$, and low AT.[62] The abnormal parameters on CPX testing can be improved with continuous positive airway pressure therapy. In one study involving severe sleep apnea, 2 months of nasal continuous positive airway pressure treatment resulted in higher right ventricular ejection fraction, peak $\dot{V}_{O_2}$, peak $\dot{V}_{O_2}$, AT, and oxygen pulse.[63]

Patients with heart failure who have central sleep apnea have an increased mortality rate compared to those without it. Patients with heart failure often lack the classical symptoms of central sleep apnea and, hence, its presence may be underestimated. Treating central sleep apnea in heart failure has beneficial effects on cardiac function. Patients with heart failure with central sleep apnea have a highly augmented ventilatory response to exercise. This is manifested by a significantly increased slope of $\dot{V}_E/\dot{V}_{CO_2}$, which correlates with the severity of sleep apnea. Thus, patients with heart failure who have an increased $\dot{V}_E/\dot{V}_{CO_2}$ slope should be considered for a full sleep study to confirm the presence of sleep apnea.[64]

■ CONGENITAL HEART DISEASE

Patients with cyanotic congenital heart disease have limitations in exercise tolerance. CPX testing can be used to objectively assess their exercise limitation and ventilatory efficiency.

In a study of 25 adults with uncorrected cyanotic congenital heart disease, peak oxygen uptake and Pa_{O_2} were significantly reduced compared with normal subjects, while Pa_{CO_2} was only slightly reduced. Ventilatory efficiency, expressed as $\dot{V}_E/\dot{V}_{CO_2}$, was found to be markedly impaired at rest and during exercise. $\dot{V}_E/\dot{V}_{CO_2}$ correlated more strongly with patients' symptoms than hypoxemia and peak oxygen uptake.[65] For the corresponding NYHA class, patients with adult congenital heart disease and patients with heart failure had no significant differences in peak $\dot{V}_{O_2}$.[66]

CPX testing has also been used for assessing the response to transcatheter closure of atrial septal defect in adult patients. Improved peak oxygen uptake, peak oxygen pulse, and vital capacity have been reported following closure.[67] In one study, improvements in the prolonged $\dot{V}_{O_2}$ slope and $\dot{V}_{CO_2}$ slope were noted, reflecting improvement in recovery from maximal exercise.[68]

Tricuspid valve surgery in patients with Ebstein's anomaly produces reduced right ventricular volumes, increased pulmonary blood flow, and increased left ventricular filling and cardiac output. This is reflected by an increased $\dot{V}_{O_2max}$.[69]

■ PULMONARY HYPERTENSION

Pulmonary hypertension is expressed as an abnormal elevation in resting or exercise pulmonary artery pressure (see Chapter 72). Chronic left heart failure with attendant elevated left atrial pressure remains the most common cause of pulmonary *venous* hypertension. Pulmonary *arterial* hypertension (PAH) accompanies intrinsic pulmonary vascular disease or arteriolar vasoconstriction associated with hypoxemia due to intrinsic lung disease. PAH creates right ventricular pressure overload and an impediment to left ventricular filling. Accordingly, exercise cardiac output is compromised and aerobic capacity declines. PAH represents an example of chronic circulatory failure.

Patients with PAH have been studied with elective right heart catheterization using a triple-lumen flotation catheter and subsequent exercise testing.[2] Resting and peak treadmill exercise hemodynamic responses are given in Table 34-4. At rest, right heart and pulmonary arterial pressures exceeded the normal range. Right ventricular systolic pressure at rest was in excess of 50 mm Hg, and in one-quarter of patients it approximated or exceeded left ventricular (and systemic arterial) systolic pressure. Resting wedge pressure was normal in these patients. Calculated pulmonary vascular resistance exceeded the upper range of normal (170 dynes·s·cm^{-5}) in all patients; in more than one-third, it was above 1000 dynes·s·cm^{-5}, approximating systemic vascular resistance.

TABLE 34-4 Resting and Peak Exercise Hemodynamics for Patients with Nonhypoxic Pulmonary Vascular Disease and Pulmonary Hypertension

		Resting	Exercise
PA	(mm Hg)	29 ± 9	47 ± 20
RVSP	(mm Hg)	52 ± 30	86 ± 37
RVDP	(mm Hg)	7 ± 4	16 ± 10
PCW	(mm Hg)	10 ± 3	22 ± 14
PVR	(dynes · s · cm^{-5})	412 ± 319	302 ± 331
CO	(L/m^2/min)	2.8 ± 1.6	5.3 ± 2.2
AP	(mm Hg)	106 ± 6	130 ± 8
Art O_2 sat	(%)	97 ± 2	96 ± 2

PA, mean pulmonary artery pressure; RVSP and RVDP, right ventricular systolic and diastolic pressures, respectively; PCW, wedge pressure; PVR, pulmonary vascular resistance; CO, cardiac output; AP, mean arterial pressure.

Source: Adapted with permission from Weber KT, Janicki JS. Pulmonary Hypertension. In: Weber KT, Janicki JS, eds. Cardiopulmonary Exercise Testing: Physiologic Principles and Clinical Applications. Philadelphia, PA: Saunders; 1986.

Peak cardiac output attained with maximal exercise for each functional class (Table 34-3) is similar to that observed for chronic cardiac failure and valvular heart disease. The impairment in exercise cardiac output is related to the extent to which pulmonary vascular resistance is elevated. Patients with a markedly elevated resting pulmonary vascular resistance (above 1000 dynes·s·cm^{-5}) proved to be functional class D. In this group of patients with intrinsic pulmonary vascular disease, arterial O_2 desaturation during exercise was not observed, emphasizing the importance of compromised cardiac reserve—a function of the inability of the right ventricle to generate sufficient pulmonary blood flow to sustain left ventricular filling and, thereby, systemic blood flow. Patients with PAH stopped exercising because of breathlessness or fatigue or both; none experienced retrosternal chest pain, light-headedness, or syncope; none developed arrhythmias. In most, it was possible to determine the $\dot{V}_{O_2max}$; in all, the AT could be attained (see above). CPX test results for a 42-year-old woman with PAH are shown in Figure 34-10.

Patients with PAH have significant ventilation–perfusion mismatch; during exercise ventilation is increased. This abnormality in ventilatory inefficiency is reflected by the reduction in end-tidal CO_2 (pET_{CO_2}). The reduction in end-tidal CO_2 is proportional to the decrease in percent predicted $\dot{V}_{O_2}$ and increase in the mean pulmonary artery pressure. In normal subjects, the pET_{CO_2} increases from rest to AT, whereas in patients with PAH, the pET_{CO_2} decreases from rest to AT.[70] On CPX testing the slope of regression between CO_2 production and minute ventilation can also be used to assess the ventilation–perfusion mismatch. The $\dot{V}_E/\dot{V}_{CO_2}$ slope is greater in patients with PAH compared with cardiac dysfunction and the same peak $\dot{V}_{O_2}$. Conversely, for the same $\dot{V}_E/\dot{V}_{CO_2}$ slope, patients with LV dysfunction have a lower peak $\dot{V}_{O_2}$.[71]

Measurement of CPX testing-based parameters in PAH is reliable and reproducible, even in patients with limited exercise tolerance. The parameters correlate well with the decrease in DL_{CO} and NYHA class.[72,73] Even in children with pulmonary hypertension, peak $\dot{V}_{O_2}$ strongly correlates with pulmonary vascular index.[74] CPX testing can be used for the objective assessment of safety and efficacy of treatment strategies in patients with PAH.[75–77] Peak $\dot{V}_{O_2}$ is an independent, strong predictor of survival in these patients.[78]

CHRONIC LUNG DISEASES

In a normal subject performing maximal exercise, minute ventilation rarely exceeds 50% of MVV; in addition, tidal volume uncommonly exceeds 50% of vital capacity. Given this large ventilatory reserve, exercise is normally not limited by ventilation. This is not the case in patients with lung disease, in whom ventilatory reserve is reduced. A number of factors may limit exercise in patients with lung disease, including altered lung mechanics, impaired gas exchange and resultant hypoxemia, pulmonary hypertension, or respiratory muscle fatigue.

■ OBSTRUCTIVE LUNG DISEASE

Exercise intolerance commonly accompanies chronic obstructive pulmonary disease (COPD), with dyspnea limiting physical activity to modest levels of work. Patients with COPD have a higher $\dot{V}_E$ for any given workload; this is largely due to increased dead space ventilation. Given their reduction in MVV and greater exercise $\dot{V}_E$, these patients often exercise with a $\dot{V}_E$/MVV ratio that exceeds 75%.

Use of such a large portion of the ventilatory reserve cannot be sustained, accounting for breathlessness and termination of exercise. In patients with moderate or severe COPD, this generally occurs before they reach their AT, implying a ventilatory, rather than cardiac, limitation to exercise. The workload at which patients terminate exercise represents a peak $\dot{V}_{O_2}$; it is not their $\dot{V}_{O_2max}$, as can be attained in patients with chronic cardiac or circulatory failure in whom ventilatory responses pose no limitation to exercise.

In severe emphysema, DL_{CO} is reduced, in keeping with alveolar capillary destruction. In such patients, a significant fall in arterial O_2 saturation often appears during exercise. This is in contrast to patients with chronic bronchitis, in whom O_2 saturation may actually increase. The improvement in oxygenation in these patients is a result of improved ventilation in areas with low ventilation–perfusion ratios. DL_{CO} portends exercise-induced arterial O_2 desaturation. Patients with a DL_{CO} less than 55% of predicted are most likely to experience hypoxemia with exercise. Arterial hypoxemia limits effort tolerance, for several reasons: (1) reduced O_2 delivery to exercising muscle, including those associated with respiration; (2) increased chemical drive to respiration, with a corresponding inappropriate $\dot{V}_E$ for a given level of work; and (3) secondary pulmonary vasoconstriction.

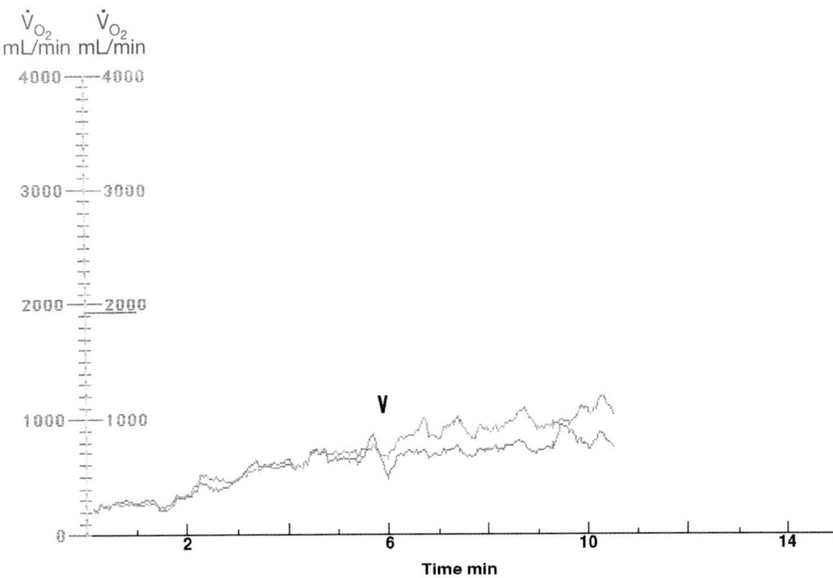

Figure 34-10 Cardiopulmonary exercise test results for a 42-year-old woman with pulmonary arterial hypertension of uncertain origin. The first 2 minutes represent standing rest. The patient attained the AT (7 mL/min/kg) during stage 2 of exercise (1.5 mph, 0 grade) and a $\dot{V}_{O_2max}$ of 10 mL/min/kg, corresponding to functional class D.

By measuring $\dot{V}_{O_2}$ peak in patients with COPD undergoing CPX testing, an objective assessment of exercise capacity can be made. Peak $\dot{V}_{O_2}$ in severe COPD correlates with resting FEV_1% predicted, total treadmill time, and total metabolic equivalent values.[79] CPX testing can better define respiratory limitations than pulmonary function testing alone in patients with COPD filing for disability due to shortness of breath.[80]

The increase in breathing capacity with exercise in COPD, measured by the ratio of $\dot{V}_E$/MVV, correlates with peak $\dot{V}_{O_2}$ and can be predicted by FEV_1/FVC measured during resting pulmonary function testing.[81] In chronic COPD, peak $\dot{V}_{O_2}$ can be estimated by equations that take into account the distance walked by the patient and the lung function tests. However, the correlation between measured and estimated peak $\dot{V}_{O_2}$ is not strong enough to predict exercise capacity. If peak $\dot{V}_{O_2}$ has to be used for clinical decision making, it should be measured, rather than estimated.[82] In COPD, skeletal muscle abnormalities have been described and contribute to reduced exercise capacity. Peak $\dot{V}_{O_2}$ in COPD correlates well with fat-free mass, a bioimpedance index of muscle mass.[83] In patients with COPD, physiologic parameters measured by CPX testing have prognostic implications as well. Based on multivariate analysis the Pa_{O_2} slope ($\Delta Pa_{O_2}/\Delta \dot{V}_{O_2}$) is most closely associated with survival.[84] Similarly, Pa_{O_2max}, along with FEV_1, has been found to independently predict mortality.[85] Overall, a linear relationship exists between peak $\dot{V}_{O_2}$ and pulmonary function testing parameters in COPD.[86]

RESTRICTIVE LUNG DISEASE

Patients with known interstitial lung disease, a diverse group of disease entities, experience limiting dyspnea on exertion. This may be secondary to reduced ventilatory reserve or development of arterial O_2 desaturation. The evaluation of exercise performance may also be useful in patients who complain of dyspnea out of proportion to their pulmonary function studies. Dyspnea on exertion may appear in a patient with an abnormal chest radiograph before pulmonary function studies are abnormal. Exercise testing may be indicated in these patients to detect abnormal ventilatory reserve and its response over time. Patients with interstitial lung disease tend to breathe at a higher respiratory rate and lower tidal volume than do normal subjects for any given $\dot{V}_{O_2}$. Because they have a reduced MVV, their ability to exercise is limited by nearly full utilization of their reduced ventilatory reserve.

As in patients with airway disease, the DL_{CO} is a good predictor of arterial O_2 desaturation during exercise in patients with interstitial lung disease. Most patients with a DL_{CO} below 60% develop desaturation. If a patient has a normal DL_{CO}, he or she is unlikely to develop exercise-induced arterial O_2 desaturation. Measurement of DL_{CO} can be used to screen patients for exercise studies. Finally, the degree of arterial O_2 desaturation during exercise correlates with the reduction in DL_{CO}.

CPX testing is a sensitive test for gas exchange abnormalities. In one study involving biopsy-proven sarcoidosis, CPX testing predicted pulmonary dysfunction earlier than did physical examination, chest radiography, and spirometry.[87,88] In another study involving survivors of severe acute respiratory distress syndrome, aerobic capacity using CPX testing was found to be below normal in 41% of patients in whom mild pulmonary function abnormalities were not enough to explain low exercise tolerance.[89] CPX testing has been used for procuring prognostic information in patients with interstitial lung disease. Peak $\dot{V}_{O_2}$ in patients with parenchymal lung disease awaiting transplant, along with Pa_{O_2} slope, has been used to predict survival.[90,91] In other parenchymal lung diseases, such as cystic fibrosis, breathing reserve index at AT has been used to distinguish ventilatory-limited patients from those without ventilatory limitations.[92]

EVALUATION OF EXERTIONAL DYSPNEA

Normally, a person is unaware of the act of breathing and the fact that 500 to 750 mL of air enters and leaves the lungs 10 to 15 times each minute. $\dot{V}_{O_2}$ increases secondary to normal or abnormal chemical stimuli (e.g., hypercapnia, hypoxemia, acidemia) or anxiety. When breathing is perceived to be inappropriate relative to the level of physical activity, it is considered an abnormal awareness of breathing that is termed breathlessness, shortness of breath, or dyspnea.[2] Dyspnea on exertion is common in patients with heart disease, pulmonary parenchymal or airway disease, and pulmonary vascular disease. Deformities of the chest wall and diseases associated with weakness of the respiratory muscles are also accompanied by exertional breathlessness. Dyspnea may seriously hinder a patient's ability to carry out muscular work, thereby compromising quality of life. The evaluation of dyspnea includes requisite historical information that characterizes its nature, onset, severity, relationship to exercise, and the patient's underlying physical condition and customary daily activity. Other associated symptoms – such as palpitations, anginal chest pain, and lightheadedness – must be taken into consideration.

An objective and reliable estimate of dyspnea on exertion and its severity can be gauged from exercise testing. Dyspnea occurs when $\dot{V}_E$ is excessive relative to $\dot{V}_{O_2}$ and when $\dot{V}_E$ is driven by chemical stimuli or altered lung mechanics. Dyspnea with exercise can appear when $\dot{V}_E$ occupies an excessive proportion of MVV. An estimation of MVV can be derived by multiplying the patient's FEV_1 by 35. As a corollary, maximal encroachment on the vital capacity by exercise tidal volume cannot be sustained for long. Such ventilatory effort poses a substantial workload on respiratory muscles. An MVV maneuver during pulmonary function testing cannot be sustained for more than a few seconds, while more than 70% of the MVV cannot be sustained by normal subjects for more than several minutes. Hence, the ventilatory response to exercise that is associated with dyspnea in patients with heart or lung disease follows a similar pattern of short-lived, near-maximal ventilation.

The patient with pulmonary vascular disease or advanced interstitial lung disease may be unable to sustain alveolar ventilation during exercise at a level commensurate with that required for adequate arterial O_2 saturation. Consequently, hypoxemia may compound the patient's exercise response and be responsible for a heightened chemical drive to respiration. In the case of COPD, the need to move air through a partly obstructed tracheobronchial tree creates an added workload on respiratory muscles. Air flows in these patients are already compromised at rest and must increase with exercise; they may approach peak expiratory flows observed with maximal effort during pulmonary function testing.

Patients with mild, moderate, or severe cardiac or circulatory failure rarely use more than 50% of their ventilatory reserve at maximal exercise, and they do not experience arterial O_2 desaturation during exercise. If one estimates MVV from the FEV_1 (as noted earlier), for an FEV_1 of 1, 2, or 3 L, MVV is expected to equal 35, 70, or 105 L, respectively. In patients with chronic cardiac or circulatory failure, exercise maximum $\dot{V}_E$ has been found to range between 62 and 29 L/min for class A through D patients, respectively. Hence, unless there is a major reduction in MVV (or in FEV_1 to <3 L), these patients will not have a ventilatory limitation to exercise. Finally, patients are able to cross their AT and, if encouraged, may reach their point of exhaustion attaining $\dot{V}_{O_2max}$. By monitoring the breath-by-breath response in $\dot{V}_{O_2}$ and $\dot{V}_{CO_2}$ during exercise, the physician can immediately determine when the patient has achieved the AT and $\dot{V}_{O_2max}$. These end-points are not attained in the patients with lung disease or those with coexistent heart and lung disease in whom the respiratory system is the primary limitation to exercise. Table 34-5 summarizes the salient features used to differentiate primary ventilatory from cardiac or circulatory failure as the cause of exertional dyspnea, as detected by exercise testing.

OTHER APPLICATIONS OF CARDIOPULMONARY EXERCISE TESTING

CPX testing, with its ability to foretell cardiac and ventilatory reserves, has proved useful in clinical decision making in a variety of circumstances, including assessment of a patient's candidacy for cardiac transplantation and preoperative assessment of risk.

TABLE 34-5 Ventilatory versus Cardiac/Circulatory Failure as the Predominant Cause of Exertional Dyspnea

Ventilatory Failure
1. Exercise maximum $\dot{V}_E$ utilizes >70% of MVV
2. Exercise-associated arterial hypoxemia
3. Failure to cross AT and to achieve $\dot{V}_{O_2max}$
Cardiac/Circulatory Failure
1. Cross AT and can achieve $\dot{V}_{O_2max}$
2. Maximum exercise $\dot{V}_E$ does not exceed 50% of MVV
3. Does not develop arterial hypoxemia with exercise

MVV, maximal voluntary ventilation; AT, anaerobic threshold.

CARDIAC TRANSPLANTATION

The severity of chronic cardiac and circulatory failure is gauged according to $\dot{V}_{O_2max}$ and the AT (Table 34-3) and is used to predict exercise cardiac reserve. This approach has been applied to patients with systolic dysfunction secondary to chronic ischemic heart disease or dilated (idiopathic) cardiomyopathy, who are considered potential candidates for cardiac transplantation. The ejection fraction or resting hemodynamic parameters (e.g., resting cardiac index or wedge pressure) do not help predict the severity of cardiac failure or functional capacity and are no longer a mainstay in decision making. The same is true for subjective evaluation of functional status using the New York Heart Association criteria. Incremental exercise testing, with identification of AT and peak $\dot{V}_{O_2}$ achieved thereafter, has emerged as a valuable tool to objectively address cardiac reserve and functional capacity and which predicts survival.[30,31,93–95] In fact, consensus has been reached on recommending transplantation based on clinical criteria, in combination with functional stratification based on exercise test results.[96] Class D patients, having little or no cardiac reserve, have a marked reduction in 1- and 2-year survival and, therefore, are candidates for urgent transplantation. Class C patients with a modest increment in exercise cardiac output are probable candidates. On the other hand, class A patients in whom cardiac reserve remains intact, or class B patients in whom cardiac reserve is only minimally impaired, do not have an adequate indication for transplantation. Decision is deferred, and serial exercise studies are used to assess recovery or deterioration in the setting of optimal medical therapy.

Incremental exercise testing may also provide useful information after cardiac transplantation, including recovery of cardiac and ventilatory reserves. The importance of diastolic dysfunction in limiting exercise tolerance following cardiac transplantation was reviewed earlier. A blunted heart rate response to exercise is expected in these patients owing to cardiac denervation. Such chronotropic incompetence is demonstrated in Figure 34-11, along with exercise test results.

Recipients of lung or heart/lung transplant do not experience the degree of return in cardiac reserve and gas exchange as do patients with heart transplant alone. These patients experience considerable exercise limitation and reduced maximum oxygen uptake despite normalization of resting cardiopulmonary function. Such limitation may be a function of peripheral factors, such as abnormalities in the peripheral circulation and peripheral neuromuscular function.[97] CPX testing may be utilized to predict survival in lung transplant recipients. Lower exercise capacity as defined by lower percent predicted peak $\dot{V}_{O_2}$ appears to have prognostic value.[98]

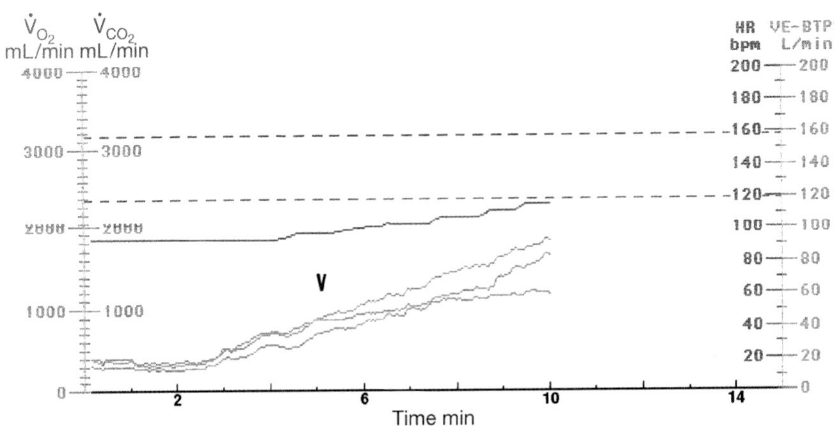

Figure 34-11 Cardiopulmonary exercise test results for a 62-year-old male cardiac transplant recipient. During this incremental treadmill test he attained an AT and $\dot{V}_{O_2max}$ of 8 and 11 mL/min/kg, respectively. Note the blunted heart rate response (predicted peak heart rate range shown as *broken lines*).

■ SURGICAL RISK ASSESSMENT

Preoperative incremental exercise testing has proved useful in assessing postoperative morbidity and mortality in the elderly and patients with underlying heart or lung disease who are scheduled for major intrathoracic or intra-abdominal surgery. The premise underlying this approach is based on recognition that during and after surgery, there may be a need to call on cardiac and ventilatory reserves—namely, the ability to increase cardiac output and maintain O_2 delivery, and to increase $\dot{V}_E$ and prevent hypoxemia. Several studies have demonstrated the utility of measuring the AT and peak $\dot{V}_{O_2}$, using exercise testing, in addressing these reserves and in identifying patients prone to postoperative complications.[99-101] Pulmonary function testing proved insensitive in forecasting postoperative course. Class C and D patients, with little or no cardiac reserve, had a greater number of morbid and mortal events following surgical interventions than did class A or B patients. Class A patients had few, if any, postoperative complications and no mortality. The risk of complications could, therefore, be gauged best by a patient's preoperative aerobic capacity.[99-102] The direct assessment of the AT or $\dot{V}_{O_2max}$ and prediction of cardiac reserve, and, by inference, ventilatory reserve supersede the value of an age-determined impairment in aerobic capacity.

AT is a particularly important parameter in assessing preoperative risk. It gives an objective assessment independent of patient motivation and does not require excessive amounts of exercise. In a large study of elderly patients undergoing major intro-abdominal surgery, an AT of less than 11 mL/min/kg along with preoperative ischemia was associated with high mortality.[100] Patients evaluated by CPX testing with unfavorable AT can be electively admitted to intensive care units and their hemodynamics optimized before major surgery.[100,103] Risk stratifying based on AT is even better at predicting patients who are not at risk for adverse events.[100,103]

Patients undergoing other major surgeries, such as radical esophagectomy with three-field lymphadenectomy, have also been risk stratified by CPX testing. Extensive fluid shifts are expected in the postoperative period with surgical interventions on the lymphatic system. CPX testing can provide a thorough assessment of the cardiopulmonary reserve in such patients. In a study involving such patients, a peak $\dot{V}_{O_2}$ of 800 mL/min/m^2 was associated with low risk of complications.[104] In another study involving patients with abdominal aortic aneurysm repair. a higher percentage of patients with adverse complications had a peak $\dot{V}_{O_2}$ less than 20 mL/min/kg.[105] Peak $\dot{V}_{O_2}$ has also been used to risk stratify liver transplant patients. Patients dying within 100 days of transplantation are more likely to have peak $\dot{V}_{O_2}$ <60% of predicted and AT <50% of predicted peak $\dot{V}_{O_2}$ compared with survivors.[106]

Patients with lung cancer have a high likelihood of concomitant COPD and coronary artery disease due to the common risk factor of smoking. Surgery might offer the only chance of cure in these patients and often implies resection of a variable portion of the lung tissue surrounding the cancer to ensure eradication. Removal of functional lung tissue in an already compromised cardiopulmonary system resection can be risky. It is imperative that a preoperative assessment of cardiopulmonary reserve be made before such a surgery (see Chapter 103). By performing preoperative CPX testing in patients being considered for lung cancer resection surgery, an objective assessment of the cardiopulmonary reserve can be made. Peak $\dot{V}_{O_2}$ has been used to risk stratify these patients, along with FEV_1 and DL_{CO}.[107] Correcting peak $\dot{V}_{O_2}$ for weight and expressing it as a percentage of predicted improves the predictive power of peak $\dot{V}_{O_2}$. Elderly patients, female patients, and patients with short stature may have a peak $\dot{V}_{O_2}$ below the absolute cutoff value, but they may still be eligible for surgery when peak $\dot{V}_{O_2}$ is expressed as percentage predicted.[108]

The predictive value of peak $\dot{V}_{O_2}$ is greater in patients with a FEV_1 <70%.[109] Peak $\dot{V}_{O_2}$ <50% of predicted is associated with a high complication rate. Patients with peak $\dot{V}_{O_2}$ >50% predicted can undergo surgery without excess mortality.[108] A peak $\dot{V}_{O_2}$ <10 mL/min/kg is generally considered prohibitive for surgery.[110] Risk stratification based upon peak $\dot{V}_{O_2}$ is particularly useful in assessing patients for lung resection who have borderline pulmonary function (predicted postoperative FEV_1 or DL_{CO} <40%). In these patients, a peak $\dot{V}_{O_2}$ <15 mL/min/kg is associated with an increased risk, and peak $\dot{V}_{O_2}$ <10 mL/min/kg carries a very high risk of postoperative complications.[111]

SUMMARY

CPX testing provides for an extensive evaluation of patients having diseases and disorders of the cardiorespiratory unit. The diagnostic information provided extends far beyond that obtained by testing of heart and lung function measured at rest, or by standard exercise testing with electrocardiographic monitoring. Position papers on CPX testing should be consulted for further diagnostic and prognostic stratification.[112,113]

REFERENCES

1. Wasserman K, ed. *Exercise Gas Exchange in Heart Disease.* Armonk, NY: Futura; 1996.
2. Weber KT, Janicki JS, eds. *Cardiopulmonary Exercise Testing: Physiologic Principles and Clinical Applications.* Philadelphia, PA: W.B. Saunders; 1986.
3. Page E, Cohen-Solal A, Jondeau G, et al. Comparison of treadmill and bicycle exercise in patients with chronic heart failure. *Chest.* 1994;106:1002–1006.
4. Pollock ML, Wilmore JH, Fox SM. *Health and Fitness Through Physical Activity.* New York, NY: Wiley; 1978.
5. Clark AL, Poole-Wilson PA, Coats AJS. Effects of motivation of the patient on indices of exercise capacity in chronic heart failure. *Br Heart J.* 1994;71:162–165.

6. Dickstein K, Barvik S, Aarsland T, Snapinn S. Reproducibility of cardiopulmonary exercise testing in men following myocardial infarction. *Eur Heart J.* 1985;9:948–954.

7. Matsumura N, Nishijima H, Kojima S, Hashimoto F, Minami M, Yasuda H. Determination of anaerobic threshold for assessment of functional state in patients with chronic heart failure. *Circulation.* 1983;68:360–367.

8. Weber KT, Kinasewitz GT, Janicki JS, Fishman AP. Oxygen utilization and ventilation during exercise in patients with chronic cardiac failure. *Circulation.* 1982;65:1213–1223.

9. Weber KT, Kinasewitz GT, West JS, Janicki JS, Reichek N, Fishman AP. Long-term vasodilation therapy with trimazosin in chronic cardiac failure. *N Engl J Med.* 1980;303: 242–250.

10. Cohen-Solal A. Cardiopulmonary exercise testing in chronic heart failure. In: Wasserman K, ed. *Exercise Gas Exchange in Heart Disease.* Armonk, NY: Futura; 1996:17–38.

11. Franciosa JA, Leddy CL, Wilen M, Schwartz DE. Relation between hemodynamic and ventilatory responses in determining exercise capacity in severe congestive heart failure. *Am J Cardiol.* 1984;53:127–134.

12. Metra M, Raddino R, Dei Cas L, Visioli O. Assessment of peak oxygen consumption, lactate and ventilatory thresholds and correlation with resting and exercise hemodynamic data in chronic congestive heart failure. *Am J Cardiol.* 1990;65: 1127–1133.

13. Szlachcic J, Massie BM, Kramer BL, Topic N, Tubau J. Correlates and prognostic implication of exercise capacity in chronic congestive heart failure. *Am J Cardiol.* 1985;55:1037–1042.

14. Wilson JR, Ferraro N. Exercise intolerance in patients with chronic left heart failure: relation to oxygen transport and ventilatory abnormalities. *Am J Cardiol.* 1983;51:1358–1363.

15. Weber KT, Janicki JS. Cardiopulmonary exercise testing for evaluation of chronic cardiac failure. *Am J Cardiol.* 1985;55: 22A–31A.

16. Weber KT, Janicki JS. Lactate production during maximal and submaximal exercise in patients with chronic heart failure. *J Am Coll Cardiol.* 1985;6:717–724.

17. McElroy PA, Janicki JS, Weber KT. Physiological correlates of the heart rate response to upright isotonic exercise: relevance to rate-responsive pacemakers. *J Am Coll Cardiol.* 1988;11:94–99.

18. Weber KT, Likoff MJ, McCarthy D. Low dose beta blockade in the treatment of chronic cardiac failure. *Am Heart J.* 1982; 104:877–879.

19. Sullivan MJ, Knight JD, Higginbotham MB, Cobb FR. Relation between central and peripheral hemodynamics during exercise in patients with chronic heart failure. Muscle blood flow is reduced with maintenance of arterial perfusion pressure. *Circulation.* 1989;80:769–781.

20. Lipkin DP, Canepa-Anson R, Stephens MR, Poole-Wilson PA. Factors determining symptoms in heart failure: comparison of fast and slow exercise tests. *Br Heart J.* 1986;55: 439–445.

21. Sullivan MJ, Higginbotham MB, Cobb FR. Increased exercise ventilation in patients with chronic heart failure: intact ventilatory control despite hemodynamic and pulmonary abnormalities. *Circulation.* 1988;77:552–559.

22. Kitzman DW, Sheikh KH, Beere PA, Philips JL, Higginbotham MB. Age-related alterations of Doppler left ventricular filling indexes in normal subjects are independent of left ventricular mass, heart rate, contractility and loading conditions. *J Am Coll Cardiol.* 1991;18:1243–1250.

23. Kao AC, Van Trigt P III, Shaeffer-McCall GS, et al. Central and peripheral limitations to upright exercise in untrained cardiac transplant recipients. *Circulation.* 1994;89:2605–2615.

24. Higginbotham MB. Diastolic dysfunction and exercise gas exchange. In: Wasserman K, ed. *Exercise Gas Exchange in Heart Disease.* Armonk, NY: Futura; 1996:39–54.

25. Treese N. Exercise gas exchange to evaluate cardiac pacemaker function. In: Wasserman K, ed. *Exercise Gas Exchange in Heart Disease.* Armonk, NY: Futura; 1996:257–270.

26. Kindermann M, Schwaab B, Finkler N, Schaller S, Bohm M, Frohlig G. Defining the optimum upper heart rate limit during exercise: a study in pacemaker patients with heart failure. *Eur Heart J.* 2002;23:1301–1308.

27. Auricchio A, Kloss M, Trautmann SI, Rodner S, Klein H. Exercise performance following cardiac resynchronization therapy in patients with heart failure and ventricular conduction delay. *Am J Cardiol.* 2002;89:198–203.

28. Garrigue S, Bordachar P, Reuter S, et al. Comparison of permanent left ventricular and biventricular pacing in patients with heart failure and chronic atrial fibrillation: prospective haemodynamic study. *Heart.* 2002;87:529–534.

29. Guazzi M, Arena R. The impact of pharmacotherapy on the cardiopulmonary exercise test response in patients with heart failure: a mini review. *Curr Vasc Pharmacol.* 2009;7: 557–569.

30. Likoff MJ, Chandler SL, Kay HR. Clinical determinants of mortality in chronic congestive heart failure secondary to idiopathic dilated or to ischemic cardiomyopathy. *Am J Cardiol.* 1987;59:634–638.

31. van den Broek SAJ, van Veldhuisen DJ, de Graeff PA, Landsman MLJ, Hillege H, Lie KI. Comparison between New York Heart Association classification and peak oxygen consumption in the assessment of functional status and prognosis in patients with mild to moderate chronic congestive heart failure secondary to either ischemic or idiopathic dilated cardiomyopathy. *Am J Cardiol.* 1992;70:359–363.

32. Mejhert M, Linder-Klingsell E, Edner M, Kahan T, Persson H. Ventilatory variables are strong prognostic markers in elderly patients with heart failure. *Heart.* 2002;88:239–243.

33. Arena R, Myers J, Aslam SS, Varughese EB, Peberdy MA. Peak V_{O_2} and VE/V_{CO_2} slope in patients with heart failure: a prognostic comparison. *Am Heart J.* 2004;147:354–360.

34. Gitt AK, Wasserman K, Kilkowski C, et al. Exercise anaerobic threshold and ventilatory efficiency identify heart failure patients for high risk of early death. *Circulation.* 2002;106:3079–3084.

35. Guazzi M, Reina G, Tumminello G, Guazzi MD. Exercise ventilation inefficiency and cardiovascular mortality in heart failure: the critical independent prognostic value of the arterial CO_2 partial pressure. *Eur Heart J.* 2005;26:472–480.

36. Arena R, Peberdy MA, Myers J, Guazzi M, Tevald M. Prognostic value of resting end-tidal carbon dioxide in patients with heart failure. *Int J Cardiol.* 2006;109:351–358.

37. Schalcher C, Rickli H, Brehm M, et al. Prolonged oxygen uptake kinetics during low-intensity exercise are related to poor prognosis in patients with mild-to-moderate congestive heart failure. *Chest.* 2003;124:580–586.

38. Queiros MC, Mendes DE, Ribeiro MA, Mendes M, Rebocho MJ, Seabra-Gomes R. Recovery kinetics of oxygen uptake after cardiopulmonary exercise test and prognosis in patients with left ventricular dysfunction. *Rev Port Cardiol.* 2002;21:383–398.
39. Corrà U, Giordano A, Bosimini E, et al. Oscillatory ventilation during exercise in patients with chronic heart failure: clinical correlates and prognostic implications. *Chest.* 2002;121:1572–1580.
40. Koike A, Shimizu N, Tajima A, et al. Relation between oscillatory ventilation at rest before cardiopulmonary exercise testing and prognosis in patients with left ventricular dysfunction. *Chest.* 2003;123:372–379.
41. Leite JJ, Mansur AJ, de Freitas HF, et al. Periodic breathing during incremental exercise predicts mortality in patients with chronic heart failure evaluated for cardiac transplantation. *J Am Coll Cardiol.* 2003;41:2175–2181.
42. Cicoira M, Zanolla L, Rossi A, et al. Long-term, dose-dependent effects of spironolactone on left ventricular function and exercise tolerance in patients with chronic heart failure. *J Am Coll Cardiol.* 2002;40:304–310.
43. Agostoni P, Magini A, Andreini D, et al. Spironolactone improves lung diffusion in chronic heart failure. *Eur Heart J.* 2005;26:159–164.
44. Dayi SU, Akbulut T, Akgoz H, et al. Long-term combined therapy with losartan and an angiotensin-converting enzyme inhibitor improves functional capacity in patients with left ventricular dysfunction. *Acta Cardiol.* 2005;60:373–377.
45. Ellis GR, Nightingale AK, Blackman DJ, et al. Addition of candesartan to angiotensin converting enzyme inhibitor therapy in patients with chronic heart failure does not reduce levels of oxidative stress. *Eur J Heart Fail.* 2002;4:193–199.
46. Corrà U, Mezzani A, Bosimini E, et al. Limited predictive value of cardiopulmonary exercise indices in patients with moderate chronic heart failure treated with carvedilol. *Am Heart J.* 2004;147:553–560.
47. Toda G, Shibata S, Nakamizo R, Seto S, Yano K. Effect of physical exercise training on health-related quality of life and exercise tolerance in patients with left ventricular dysfunction. *J Cardiol.* 2004;44:179–187.
48. Lemaitre JP, Harris S, Hannan J, Fox KA, Denvir MA. Maximum oxygen uptake corrected for skeletal muscle mass accurately predicts functional improvements following exercise training in chronic heart failure. *Eur J Heart Fail.* 2006;8:243–248.
49. Klocek M, Kubinyi A, Bacior B, Kawecka-Jaszcz K. Effect of physical training on quality of life and oxygen consumption in patients with congestive heart failure. *Int J Cardiol.* 2005;103:323–329.
50. Belardinelli R, Lacalaprice F, Carle F, et al. Exercise-induced myocardial ischaemia detected by cardiopulmonary exercise testing. *Eur Heart J.* 2003;24:1304–1313.
51. Bigi R, Desideri A, Rambaldi R, Cortigiani L, Sponzilli C, Fiorentini C. Angiographic and prognostic correlates of cardiac output by cardiopulmonary exercise testing in patients with anterior myocardial infarction. *Chest.* 2001;120:825–833.
52. Motohiro M, Yuasa F, Hattori T, et al. Cardiovascular adaptations to exercise training after uncomplicated acute myocardial infarction. *Am J Phys Med Rehabil.* 2005;84:684–691.
53. Smarz K, Zaborska B, Jaxa-Chamiec T, Maciejewski P, Budaj A. Right ventricular dysfunction and exercise capacity after inferior (posterior) wall acute myocardial infarction. *Am J Cardiol.* 2012;110:784–789.
54. Kim HJ, Ahn SJ, Park SW, et al. Cardiopulmonary exercise testing before and one year after mitral valve repair for severe mitral regurgitation. *Am J Cardiol.* 2004;93:1187–1189.
55. Kim HJ, Park SW, Cho BR, Hong SH, Park PW, Hong KP. The role of cardiopulmonary exercise test in mitral and aortic regurgitation: it can predict post-operative results. *Korean J Intern Med.* 2003;18:35–39.
56. Yuda S, Nakatani S, Kosakai Y, et al. Mechanism of improvement in exercise capacity after the maze procedure combined with mitral valve surgery. *Heart.* 2004;90:64–69.
57. Ueshima K, Kamata J, Kobayashi N, et al. Effects of exercise training after open heart surgery on quality of life and exercise tolerance in patients with mitral regurgitation or aortic regurgitation. *Jpn Heart J.* 2004;45:789–797.
58. Omede P, Bucca C, Rolla G, et al. Cardiopulmonary exercise testing and exhaled nitric oxide in the assessment of patients with mitral stenosis. *Minerva Cardioangiol.* 2004;52:29–35.
59. Groves PH, Lewis NP, Ikram S, Maire R, Hall RJ. Reduced exercise capacity in patients with tricuspid regurgitation after successful mitral valve replacement for rheumatic mitral valve disease. *Br Heart J.* 1991;66:295–301.
60. Sharma S, Elliott PM, Whyte G, et al. Utility of metabolic exercise testing in distinguishing hypertrophic cardiomyopathy from physiologic left ventricular hypertrophy in athletes. *J Am Coll Cardiol.* 2000;36:864–870.
61. Huff CM, Turer AT, Wang A. Correlations between physician-perceived functional status, patient-perceived health status, and cardiopulmonary exercise results in hypertrophic cardiomyopathy. *Qual Life Res.* 2013;22:647–652.
62. Ozturk LM, Metin G, Cuhadaroglu C, Utkusavas A, Tutluoglu B. Cardiopulmonary responses to exercise in moderate-to-severe obstructive sleep apnea. *Tuberk Toraks.* 2005;53:10–19.
63. Lin CC, Lin CK, Wu KM, Chou CS. Effect of treatment by nasal CPAP on cardiopulmonary exercise test in obstructive sleep apnea syndrome. *Lung.* 2004;182:199–212.
64. Arzt M, Harth M, Luchner A, et al. Enhanced ventilatory response to exercise in patients with chronic heart failure and central sleep apnea. *Circulation.* 2003;107:1998–2003.
65. Glaser S, Opitz CF, Bauer U, et al. Assessment of symptoms and exercise capacity in cyanotic patients with congenital heart disease. *Chest.* 2004;125:368–376.
66. Diller GP, Dimopoulos K, Okonko D, et al. Exercise intolerance in adult congenital heart disease: comparative severity, correlates, and prognostic implication. *Circulation.* 2005;112:828–835.
67. Giardini A, Donti A, Formigari R, et al. Determinants of cardiopulmonary functional improvement after transcatheter atrial septal defect closure in asymptomatic adults. *J Am Coll Cardiol.* 2004;43:1886–1891.
68. Giardini A, Donti A, Specchia S, et al. Recovery kinetics of oxygen uptake is prolonged in adults with an atrial septal defect and improves after transcatheter closure. *Am Heart J.* 2004;147:910–914.
69. Kühn A, De Pasquale Meyer G, Müller J, et al. Tricuspid valve surgery improves cardiac output and exercise performance

in patients with Ebstein's anomaly. *Int J Cardiol.* 2011;166(2): 494–498.

70. Yasunobu Y, Oudiz RJ, Sun XG, Hansen JE, Wasserman K. End-tidal P_{CO_2} abnormality and exercise limitation in patients with primary pulmonary hypertension. *Chest.* 2005;127:1637–1646.
71. Mitani R, Haraguchi M, Takata S, et al. Excessive ventilatory response during exercise in patients with non-hypoxic pulmonary hypertension. *Circ J.* 2002;66:453–456.
72. Hansen JE, Sun XG, Yasunobu Y, et al. Reproducibility of cardiopulmonary exercise measurements in patients with pulmonary arterial hypertension. *Chest.* 2004;126:816–824.
73. Sun XG, Hansen JE, Oudiz RJ, Wasserman K. Exercise pathophysiology in patients with primary pulmonary hypertension. *Circulation.* 2001;104:429–435.
74. Yetman AT, Taylor AL, Doran A, Ivy DD. Utility of cardiopulmonary stress testing in assessing disease severity in children with pulmonary arterial hypertension. *Am J Cardiol.* 2005;95:697–699.
75. Hoeper MM, Faulenbach C, Golpon H, Winkler J, Welte T, Niedermeyer J. Combination therapy with bosentan and sildenafil in idiopathic pulmonary arterial hypertension. *Eur Respir J.* 2004;24:1007–1010.
76. Hoeper MM, Halank M, Marx C, et al. Bosentan therapy for portopulmonary hypertension. *Eur Respir J.* 2005;25: 502–508.
77. Wonisch M, Fruhwald FM, Maier R, et al. Continuous haemodynamic monitoring during exercise in patients with pulmonary hypertension. *Int J Cardiol.* 2005;101:415–420.
78. Wensel R, Opitz CF, Anker SD, et al. Assessment of survival in patients with primary pulmonary hypertension: importance of cardiopulmonary exercise testing. *Circulation.* 2002;106: 319–324.
79. Yazici M, Arbak P, Balbay O, et al. Relationship between arterial blood gas values, pulmonary function tests and treadmill exercise testing parameters in patients with COPD. *Respirology.* 2004;9:320–325.
80. Fink G, Moshe S, Goshen J, et al. Functional evaluation in patients with chronic obstructive pulmonary disease: pulmonary function test versus cardiopulmonary exercise test. *J Occup Environ Med.* 2002;44:54–58.
81. Ong KC, Wang YT. Factors associated with improvement in breathing capacity during exercise in patients with chronic obstructive pulmonary disease. *Respirology.* 2003;8:332–338.
82. Chuang ML, Lin IF, Vintch JR. Comparison of estimated and measured maximal oxygen uptake during exercise testing in patients with chronic obstructive pulmonary disease. *Intern Med J.* 2004;34:469–474.
83. Gosker HR, Lencer NH, Franssen FM, van der Vusse GJ, Wouters EF, Schols AM. Striking similarities in systemic factors contributing to decreased exercise capacity in patients with severe chronic heart failure or COPD. *Chest.* 2003;123:1416–1424.
84. Hiraga T, Maekura R, Okuda Y, et al. Prognostic predictors for survival in patients with COPD using cardiopulmonary exercise testing. *Clin Physiol Funct Imaging.* 2003;23: 324–331.
85. Tojo N, Ichioka M, Chida M, Miyazato I, Yoshizawa Y, Miyasaka N. Pulmonary exercise testing predicts prognosis in patients with chronic obstructive pulmonary disease. *Intern Med.* 2005;44:20–25.
86. Efremidis G, Tsiamita M, Manolis A, Spiropoulos K. Accuracy of pulmonary function tests in predicted exercise capacity in COPD patients. *Respir Med.* 2005;99:609–614.
87. Mascolo MC, Truwit JD. Role of exercise evaluation in restrictive lung disease: new insights between March 2001 and February 2003. *Curr Opin Pulm Med.* 2003;9:408–410.
88. Akkoca O, Celik G, Ulger F, et al. Exercise capacity in sarcoidosis. Study of 29 patients. *Med Clin (Barc).* 2005;124: 686–689.
89. Ong KC, Ng AW, Lee LS, et al. Pulmonary function and exercise capacity in survivors of severe acute respiratory syndrome. *Eur Respir J.* 2004;24:436–442.
90. Miki K, Maekura R, Hiraga T, et al. Impairments and prognostic factors for survival in patients with idiopathic pulmonary fibrosis. *Respir Med.* 2003;97:482–490.
91. Kawut SM, O'Shea MK, Bartels MN, Wilt JS, Sonett JR, Arcasoy SM. Exercise testing determines survival in patients with diffuse parenchymal lung disease evaluated for lung transplantation. *Respir Med.* 2005;99:1431–1439.
92. Sexauer WP, Cheng HK, Fiel SB. Utility of the breathing reserve index at the anaerobic threshold in determining ventilatory-limited exercise in adult cystic fibrosis patients. *Chest.* 2003;124:1469–1475.
93. Cohn JN, Rector TS. Prognosis of congestive heart failure and predictors of mortality. *Am J Cardiol.* 1988;62:25A–30A.
94. Mancini DM, Eisen H, Kussmaul W, Mull R, Edmunds LH Jr, Wilson JR. Value of peak exercise oxygen consumption for optimal timing of cardiac transplantation in ambulatory patients with heart failure. *Circulation.* 1991;83:778–786.
95. Stevenson LW. Role of exercise testing in the evaluation of candidates for cardiac transplantation. In: Wasserman K, ed. *Exercise Gas Exchange in Heart Disease.* Armonk, NY: Futura; 1996: 271–286.
96. Mudge GH, Goldstein S, Addonizio LJ, et al. 24th Bethesda conference: cardiac transplantation. Task Force 3: recipient guidelines/prioritization. *J Am Coll Cardiol.* 1993;22:21–31.
97. Schwaiblmair M, Reichenspurner H, Müller C, et al. Cardiopulmonary exercise testing before and after lung and heart-lung transplantation. *Am J Respir Crit Care Med.* 1999; 159:1277–1283.
98. Armstrong HF, Garber CE, Bartels MN. Exercise testing parameters associated with post lung transplant mortality. *Respir Physiol Neurobiol.* 2012;181:118–122.
99. Bechard D, Wetstein L. Assessment of oxygen consumption as a preoperative criterion for lung resection. *Ann Thorac Surg.* 1987;44:344–349.
100. Older P, Smith R, Courtney P, Hone R. Preoperative evaluation of cardiac failure and ischemia in elderly patients by cardiopulmonary exercise testing. *Chest.* 1993;104:701–704.
101. Smith TP, Kinasewitz GT, Tucker WY, Spillers WP, George RB. Exercise capacity as a predictor of post-thoracotomy morbidity. *Am Rev Respir Dis.* 1984;129:730–734.
102. Gilbreth EM, Weisman IM. Role of exercise stress testing in preoperative evaluation of patients for lung resection. *Clin Chest Med.* 1994;15:389–403.
103. Older P, Hall A, Hader R. Cardiopulmonary exercise testing as a screening test for perioperative management of major surgery in the elderly. *Chest.* 1999;116:355–362.
104. Nagamatsu Y, Shima I, Yamana H, Fujita H, Shirouzu K, Ishitake T. Preoperative evaluation of cardiopulmonary

reserve with the use of expired gas analysis during exercise testing in patients with squamous cell carcinoma of the thoracic esophagus. *J Thorac Cardiovasc Surg.* 2001;121: 1064–1068.

105. Nugent AM, Riley M, Megarry J, O'Reilly MJ, MacMahon J, Lowry R. Cardiopulmonary exercise testing in the pre-operative assessment of patients for repair of abdominal aortic aneurysm. *Ir J Med Sci.* 1998;167:238–241.
106. Epstein SK, Freeman RB, Khayat A, Unterborn JN, Pratt DS, Kaplan MM. Aerobic capacity is associated with 100-day outcome after hepatic transplantation. *Liver Transpl.* 2004;10: 418–424.
107. Bolliger CT. Evaluation of operability before lung resection. *Curr Opin Pulm Med.* 2003;9:321–326.
108. Win T, Jackson A, Sharples L, et al. Cardiopulmonary exercise tests and lung cancer surgical outcome. *Chest.* 2005;127: 1159–1165.
109. Villani F, De Maria P, Busia A. Exercise testing as a predictor of surgical risk after pneumonectomy for bronchogenic carcinoma. *Respir Med.* 2003;97:1296–1298.
110. Schuurmans MM, Diacon AH, Bolliger CT. Functional evaluation before lung resection. *Clin Chest Med.* 2002;23:159–172.
111. Beckles MA, Spiro SG, Colice GL, Rudd RM; American College of Chest Physicians. The physiologic evaluation of patients with lung cancer being considered for resectional surgery. *Chest.* 2003;123(1 Suppl):105S–114S.
112. Balady GJ, Arena R, Sietsema K, et al. Clinician's Guide to cardiopulmonary exercise testing in adults: a scientific statement from the American Heart Association. *Circulation.* 2010;122:191–225.
113. Guazzi M, Adams V, Conraads V, et al. EACPR/AHA Scientific Statement. Clinical recommendations for cardiopulmonary exercise testing data assessment in specific patient populations. *Circulation.* 2012;126:2261–2274.

CHAPTER 35

Diagnostic Bronchoscopy, Transthoracic Needle Biopsy, and Related Procedures

Anil Vachani

Daniel H. Sterman

INTRODUCTION

Gustav Killian reported his experience with the first bronchoscopy in 1898. Technological advances during the next century facilitated development of bronchoscopy as a pivotal diagnostic and therapeutic tool in pulmonary medicine. Although a number of bronchoesophagologists contributed to refinement of the technique based upon use of a rigid instrument, the advent of flexible fiberoptic bronchoscopy, pioneered by Ikeda in 1967, opened new horizons to clinicians. More recently, transthoracic needle biopsy (TTNB) has been added to the pulmonologist's diagnostic armamentarium, although it is now most frequently performed by radiologists under CT guidance.

This chapter comprises an overview of bronchoscopy, TTNB, and related techniques. Following a general discussion of bronchoscopy and associated general instrumentation, indications for the technique and patient preparation are considered. Specific applications of diagnostic bronchoscopy are discussed. Subsequently, safety factors related to bronchoscopy and complications of the technique are reviewed. Finally, TTNB is described.

GENERAL INSTRUMENTATION

The initial bronchoscope, developed by Killian in Europe and further perfected by Chevalier Jackson in the United States, was a rigid metal tube that permitted either spontaneous or mechanical ventilation. With development of fiberoptic and advanced electronic technology, the flexible bronchoscope has, to a large extent, replaced the rigid bronchoscope for most diagnostic and some therapeutic indications. Therapeutic interventional bronchoscopy, including the use of rigid bronchoscopes, is discussed in Chapter 36.

■ FLEXIBLE FIBEROPTIC AND VIDEOBRONCHOSCOPY

Although the optical resolution of early fiberoptic bronchoscopes was inferior to that of rigid devices, their flexibility, ease of manipulation, and simplicity of use, which permit rapid examination under topical anesthesia, have made flexible bronchoscopy the primary endoscopic procedure in pulmonary diseases.

Unlike the larger-bore rigid bronchoscope, the flexible bronchoscope varies from ultrathin – allowing for neonatal endoscopy – to larger, adult size therapeutic devices. The diameter of the working channel permits aspiration of secretions or introduction of accessories required for diagnostic purposes (see Bronchoscopy Technique). With flexible bronchoscopy, the patient's ventilation is assured by airflow around the bronchoscope, between the external wall of the device and the tracheobronchial tree. Thus, the appropriate selection of bronchoscope size is crucial.

Fiberoptic systems have largely been replaced by videobronchoscopes, which utilize a miniaturized CCD camera at the tip of the scope that provides electronic transmission of images to a television monitor. Flexible bronchoscopes are more fragile and more prone to damage than are rigid metal instruments. Appropriate care and adherence to safety techniques during procedures, as well as during routine cleaning and maintenance of the instruments, help assure extended instrument life and reduce repair costs.

■ ULTRATHIN BRONCHOSCOPES

Ultrathin bronchoscopes, flexible scopes with external diameters ≤3 mm, were initially developed for pediatric applications; however, these have now incorporated larger working channels, allowing for their use in the diagnosis of peripheral pulmonary lesions in adults.[1,2] Ultrathin bronchoscopes can be advanced to more peripheral bronchi than conventional bronchoscopes under direct observation, allowing for examination of sixth- to eighth-generation bronchi. Ultrathin scopes may be particularly useful when combined with additional diagnostic tools, such as navigational bronchoscopy and radial ultrasound probes (see Ultraminiature Radial Probes and Navigational Bronchoscopy).

DIAGNOSTIC BRONCHOSCOPY ACCESSORIES

The working channel of the fiberoptic or videobronchoscope, although of relatively small diameter, allows the insertion of various diagnostic and therapeutic accessories.

■ BIOPSY FORCEPS

Simple visualization of lesions is usually not sufficient to determine a precise diagnosis and to guide management. Pathological confirmation through biopsy is frequently required. A variety of instruments with improved distal control (i.e., control beyond the tip of the bronchoscope) have been developed that permit tissue cutting and retrieval of biopsy specimens.

The cutting cups of biopsy forceps may be round or elliptic and may have smooth or jagged edges. The use of nonserrated edges, however, seems to reduce tissue trauma and the concomitant risk of bleeding. The biopsy procedure is simple and generally associated with only minimal complications in the case of a visible lesion. Even peripheral lesions, which are not visible through the bronchoscope, may be biopsied. With diffuse parenchymal or interstitial lung disease, specimens may be obtained without fluoroscopic guidance. With smaller or focal lesions, however, the diagnostic yield of biopsies increases when fluoroscopy is used. The development of new electromagnetic and remote guidance systems suggests that further improvement in the diagnostic yield of bronchoscopic biopsies can be expected.

■ BRONCHIAL BRUSHES

Lesions not accessible to direct biopsy with a forceps can at times be approached with a bronchial brush. This device consists of a rigid central wire surrounded by brushes of various sizes and shapes. To-and-fro movement of the brush against the adjacent tissue produces minor trauma but enables collection of ample specimens for cytological or microbiological analysis.

In some clinical circumstances, there is a need to obtain an uncontaminated specimen from the lower respiratory tract for microbiological studies. A brush protected by an additional sheath and tip may be passed through the working channel of the bronchoscope (protected brush specimen, as discussed later). In these cases, special attention is needed not to use an excessive amount of local anesthetic or saline lavage, since these solutions contain bacteriostatic material that may inhibit microbial growth. The diagnostic yield depends on use of proper technique, appropriate choice of brush, and careful collection and preservation of the specimen.

■ NEEDLES FOR ASPIRATION AND BIOPSY

The first performance of a transbronchoscopic needle aspiration (TBNA) through a rigid bronchoscope was reported by Schieppati in 1958. Wang et al.[3] then developed a flexible needle technique using a fiberoptic bronchoscope in 1978. Initially, several models of needles were designed to obtain cytological material; subsequently, histological specimens from peribronchial mediastinal and hilar lymph nodes were obtained with larger-bore needles. These biopsy needles are also useful in the diagnosis of endobronchial and submucosal lesions and can serve as a complementary technique to percutaneous needle aspiration of peripheral pulmonary nodules or masses.

The tip of the needle is protected by a metal hub during the insertion and withdrawal to avoid damage to the flexible scope. Perforation of the working channel of the scope may occur if the needle is advanced in an exposed position. The diagnostic yield depends on two factors: Optimization of the bend of the tip of the bronchoscope and proper performance of bronchial wall puncture by the needle through the intercartilaginous space. Familiarity with the type of needle used increases the success rate.

TBNA is generally safe, although pneumothorax and hemomediastinum can occur. Clinically significant bleeding is extremely rare, particularly when a 22-gauge needle is used, even if a major vessel is inadvertently punctured or if the patient suffers from superior vena cava syndrome.

ENDOBRONCHIAL ULTRASOUND

Among the new diagnostic modalities available to chest physicians, endobronchial ultrasound (EBUS) has unquestionably had the most profound impact.[4] Two major barriers to EBUS development existed: Ultrasound probe size and sound wave transmission in air-filled structures. Ultrasound engineering advances allowed the former barrier to be overcome. The latter was surmounted by developing an integrated, fluid-filled balloon surrounding the EBUS probe, thereby allowing for a sound wave–transducing medium interface to exist between the ultrasound probe and airway wall (i.e., ultrasonographic coupling).

Ultrasound frequency is an important consideration for EBUS application. Lower frequencies give better penetration depth with less resolution; higher frequencies provide better spatial resolution, but less penetration depth. For EBUS applications, the frequencies range from 7.5 to 30 MHz. Currently, there are three EBUS probes available for different applications: (1) Ultraminiature radial probes (20 and 30 MHz), (2) radial balloon probes (20 MHz), and (3) convex probe or curvilinear EBUS (CP-EBUS). Each of these is discussed in greater detail later.

■ ULTRAMINIATURE RADIAL PROBES

Ultraminiature EBUS (UM-EBUS) was developed to allow for improved assessment and sampling of peripheral pulmonary lesions (Fig. 35-1A). There are two ultraminiature radial probes currently available, with diameters of 1.4 and 2.0 mm, allowing insertion into bronchoscopes with working channels of 2.0 and 2.6 mm, respectively. When a lesion is reached with the probe, the usual normal lung "snowstorm" appearance is replaced by a focal ultrasound alteration that can be marked by fluoroscopy, a guide sheath (GS), or both fluoroscopy and GS (Fig. 35-1B and Video 35-1). After the lesion is localized, the GS can be left in place, allowing for guided biopsies of the lung using forceps, brush, or needle biopsy.

■ RADIAL BALLOON PROBE

To overcome the ultrasonographic coupling problem with UM-EBUS probes in the central airways, a radial EBUS probe was developed; the probe is inserted into an outer sheath with a distal tip balloon. The balloon is filled with saline to provide a fluid medium to allow for sound wave transmission from the probe to the airway wall. The radial balloon EBUS (RB-EBUS; Olympus Corporation, Tokyo, Japan) probe provides <1-mm resolution with a 360-degree visualization of paratracheal and peribronchial structures (Fig. 35-1). Five to seven layers of the tracheal and proximal bronchial wall have been described using RB-EBUS.[5]

■ CONVEX PROBE EBUS

The convex probe EBUS (CP-EBUS) bronchoscope, introduced in 2005, has a built-in curvilinear ultrasound transducer with a

Video 35-1 The ultraminiature (UM)-EBUS probe is used via the working channel of a fiberoptic bronchoscope to identify a focal lung lesion. When the lesion is reached with the probe, there is an alteration in the ultrasound image, with replacement of the usual normal lung "snowstorm" appearance by the presence of a denser focal lesion that surrounds the centrally located probe. *Access at www.fishmansonline.com*

PART 3 Symptoms and Signs of Respiratory Disease

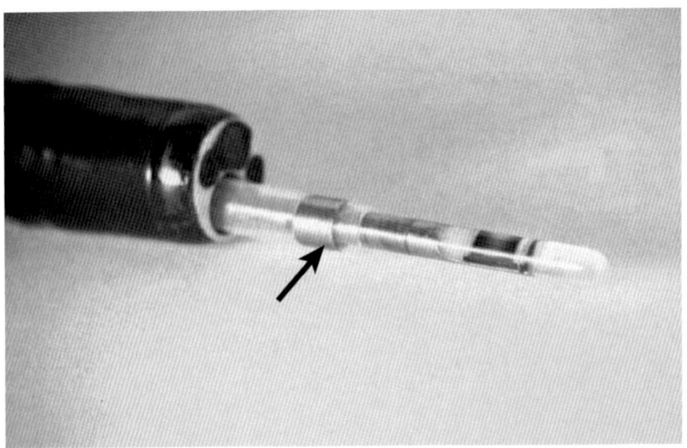

A

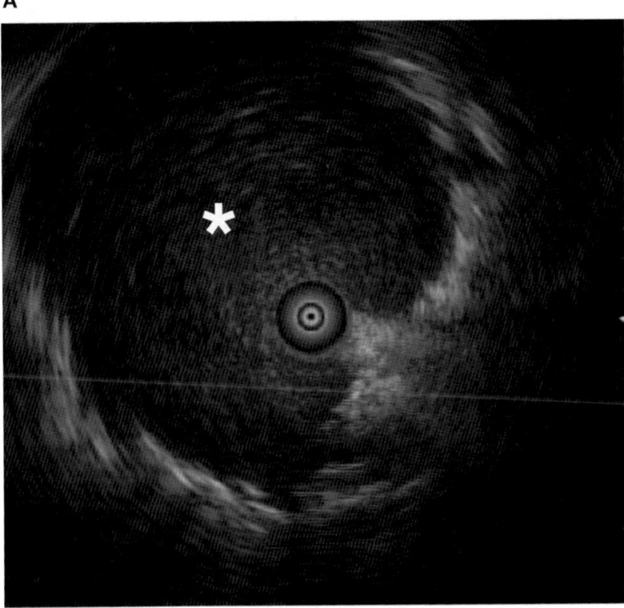

B

Figure 35-1 **A.** The ultraminiature (UM)-EBUS probe contains a circulating ultrasound crystal that provides a 360-degree view of the surrounding structures when full airway ultrasonographic coupling occurs. The probe is inserted through a guide sheath (*arrow*; Olympus Corporation, Tokyo, Japan), which can remain in the airway on UM-EBUS probe removal to allow for instrument guidance for biopsy. **B.** This UM-EBUS image demonstrates a focal lung lesion (*asterisk*) surrounding the probe.

larger distal diameter (6.9 mm) compared with a standard bronchoscope. White light videobronchoscopy occurs at a 35-degree oblique angle with EBUS at 90 degrees from the longitudinal axis. Dedicated biopsy needles (21 or 22 gauge) are inserted through the 2-mm working channel to perform aspirations of the target lesion (Fig. 35-2A). Real-time EBUS imaging displays needle penetration through the tracheobronchial wall into the target during the biopsy maneuver (Fig. 35-2B). If there is difficulty in achieving adequate EBUS images because of poor ultrasonographic coupling, a saline-filled balloon surrounding the transducer can be used to improve image quality. In addition, Doppler capabilities allow vascular structure differentiation, which minimizes the risk of unintended vascular puncture.

NAVIGATIONAL BRONCHOSCOPY

A recent advance in the evaluation of peripheral pulmonary lesions and mediastinal and hilar adenopathy has been the development of navigational approaches, such as electromagnetic navigational bronchoscopy (EMB) and virtual bronchoscopy (VB) (Fig. 35-3).[6–9]

EMB utilizes an electromagnetic board to generate a magnetic field around the patient, a magnetic sensor probe, an extended working channel, and three-dimensional integration of CT scan reconstruction and bronchoscopy position. In essence, this system works on the same triangulation principle as a global positioning system and allows the bronchoscopist to direct the FB through the airways to the target.

VB-based approaches utilize virtual navigation by creating a CT scan–based "road map" that can be overlaid onto real-time endoscopic images. Navigational systems can be used in conjunction with ultrathin bronchoscopies combined with radial EBUS probes and GSs to confirm that a lesion has been reached and to maintain the position for acquisition of diagnostic material. The role of navigational bronchoscopy in the evaluation of peripheral pulmonary nodules is discussed later.

In addition to diagnostic indications, navigational bronchoscopy is increasingly used for targeted cancer therapeutic delivery, including guided stereotactic radiosurgery, fiducial placement, or implantation of radiotherapy monitoring devices.[10,11]

Navigational bronchoscopy systems may be limited in general application by their high capital cost and training necessary for optimal system utilization. At the current time, the greatest experience and yield with these technologies has occurred in centers of excellence, with results unlikely to be reproducible in less experienced centers.

PATIENT PREPARATION AND MONITORING DURING BRONCHOSCOPY

Success of bronchoscopy, whether diagnostic or therapeutic, depends, in large part, on proper preparation of the patient, including relief of anxiety, muscle relaxation, cough suppression, and adequate anesthesia. Time spent in achieving these goals will be well worth it in reducing the risks of complications and in increasing the ease of performance of the procedure. As with any other procedure, analysis of the risk–benefit ratio helps reduce the complication rate. During and shortly after the procedure, appropriate monitoring of hemodynamic parameters (heart rate, rhythm, and blood pressure), oxygenation, and ventilation contributes to the safety of bronchoscopy.

Most flexible bronchoscopies are performed after patient premedication with sedative agents and the use of bronchoscopically instilled lidocaine for local anesthesia of the upper airway, larynx, and tracheobronchial tree. Most frequently, moderate sedation is achieved using a combination of a short-acting benzodiazepine (e.g., midazolam) and a narcotic agent (e.g., fentanyl). Intravenous propofol may also be used to provide moderate sedation and appears to provide similar results in terms of patient satisfaction and degree of hypoxia, with the advantage of a faster recovery time.[12] Because the use of propofol can lead to deep sedation, it is important that these patients receive careful monitoring. Deep sedation (i.e., a deeper state of depressed consciousness with potential for compromised airway function and spontaneous respiration) and general anesthesia are increasingly being employed given the shift of diagnostic and therapeutic bronchoscopy toward more complex and lengthier diagnostic procedures.

Anticholinergic medication (e.g., atropine or glycopyrrolate) has been advocated by some to reduce the risk of vasovagal reactions and to minimize airway secretions, thereby allowing for better examinations of the tracheobronchial tree. However, in a large randomized trial comparing these two drugs with placebo, glycopyrrolate, but not atropine, led to a reduction in airway secretions.[13] There was no significant reduction in cough, patient discomfort, oxygen desaturation, or procedure time with either drug. Current recommendations discourage the use of these agents during bronchoscopy.[12]

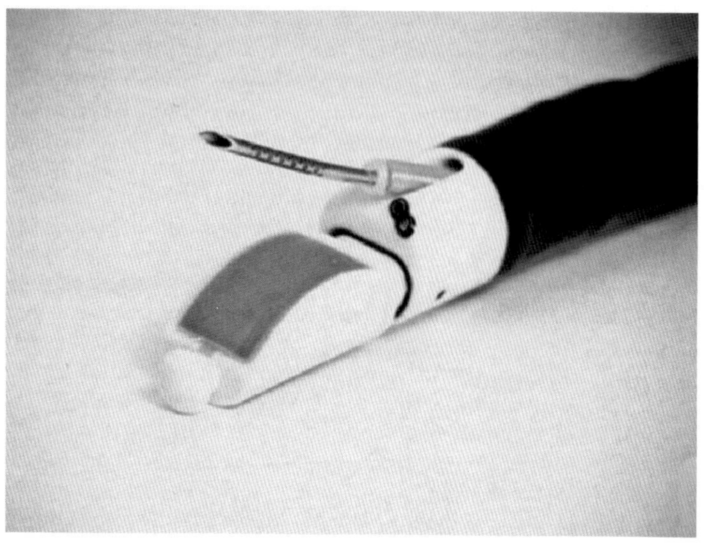
A

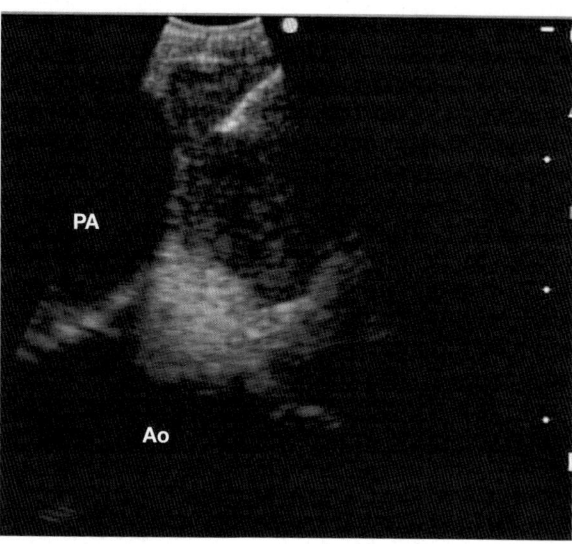

B

Figure 35-2 **A.** The convex probe (CP)-EBUS TBNA (BF-UC160 F-OL8; Olympus Corporation, Tokyo, Japan) videobronchoscope has an integrated ultrasound probe that scans 90 degrees perpendicular from the longitudinal axis, a 35-degree forward oblique video view, and a 2.0-mm working channel through which a dedicated biopsy needle can be passed. Distal tip dimples on the needle provide an echogenic surface to reflect ultrasound waves to allow needle visualization. **B.** This CP-EBUS image demonstrates a left paratracheal lymph node with the ascending aorta (Ao), the pulmonary artery (PA), and the needle present in the lymph node.

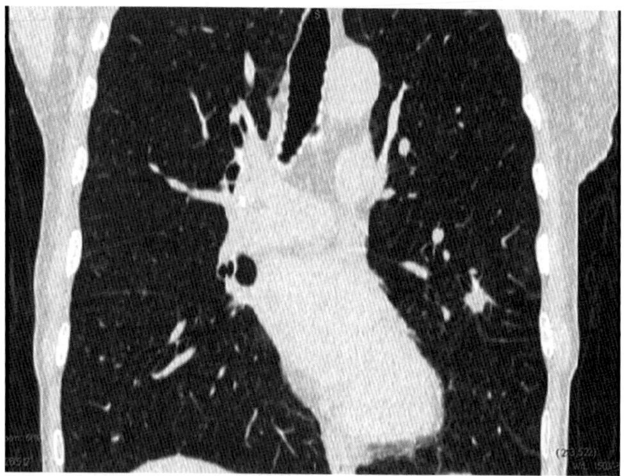
A

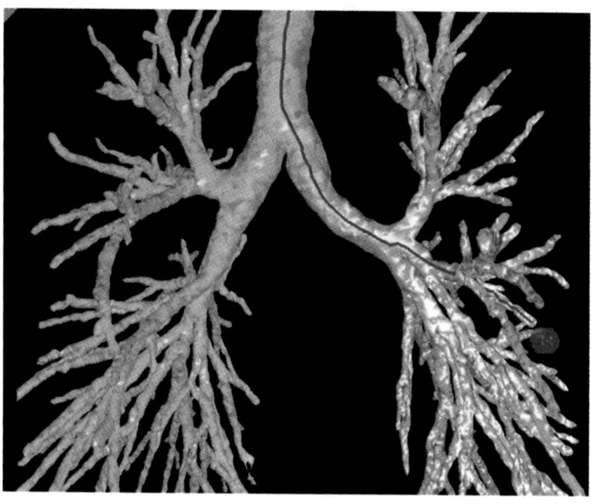
B

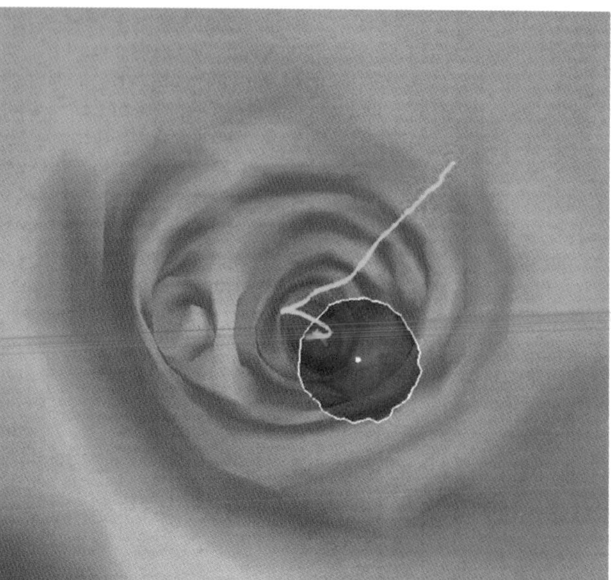
C

Figure 35-3 Use of a virtual bronchoscopy–based system for navigation. **A.** Chest CT image of a spiculated left upper lobe pulmonary nodule. **B.** Three-dimensional reconstruction of the tracheobronchial tree with the nodule identified. **C.** Virtual bronchoscopic image demonstrating the pathway to the peripheral nodule.

BRONCHOSCOPY TECHNIQUE

Central components of the routine bronchoscopic technique are discussed later.

ASSESSMENT OF AIRWAY ANATOMY AND FUNCTION

Thorough bronchoscopic evaluation begins with examination of the upper airways. Special attention should be paid to the integrity of air passages and the function of the nasopharynx and larynx. The vocal cords should be examined for the presence of polyps and tumors and for evidence of cord paralysis.

Once upper airway inspection is completed, a systematic evaluation of the lower respiratory tract should be performed. Critically important is the distinction among normal anatomy, anatomic variations without clinical significance, and frankly pathological conditions. These considerations have important implications regarding potential diagnostic and therapeutic approaches. For example, finding an abnormal branching of a bronchus may be of no clinical significance. On the other hand, such an abnormality could explain symptoms of frequent infections due to impaired ventilation and drainage of the affected area. Special skills and observational experience are required for bronchoscopic examination after surgery, especially following creative bronchoplastic procedures or lung transplantation.

Assessment of airway integrity, with special attention to dynamic changes in airway caliber during either relaxed breathing or forced expiration and coughing, may be crucial in determining appropriate therapeutic maneuvers. Flexible bronchoscopy is superior to rigid bronchoscopy for this assessment. Relaxation and prolapse of the membranous portion of the trachea and main bronchi secondary to destruction of elastic connective tissue may account for exacerbations of expiratory airflow obstruction. On the other hand, finding localized, posttraumatic chondromalacia has very different therapeutic implications. On the basis of these bronchoscopic determinations, the choice of performing an open surgical approach or bronchoscopic therapeutic correction may be made.

Bronchoscopic examination generally permits evaluation and localization of congenital or postsurgical pathological changes in bronchial integrity, such as tracheoesophageal or bronchopleural fistulas. Bronchoscopic observation and early diagnosis of bronchial rupture after chest trauma also greatly influence further therapy and prognosis. The same is true for evaluation of postsurgical anastomoses following reconstructive surgery or lung transplantation.

Advances in airway management of critically ill patients who require prolonged intubation or tracheotomy have resulted in a lower incidence of tracheal injuries. Tracheal injuries documented by bronchoscopy are not rare, however. Important complications of tracheotomy include tracheal stenosis, tracheomalacia, and tracheoinnominate artery fistula. Complications specific to the use of percutaneous tracheotomy, which is increasingly used in the intensive care unit, include flaps of cartilage protruding into the tracheal lumen and extraluminal placement of the tracheostomy tube. Such complications can have significant bearing on clinical outcome.

EVALUATION OF TRACHEOBRONCHIAL MUCOSA

Careful examination of the mucosal surface is crucial in the formulation of differential diagnosis. Rapid development of granulation tissue is frequently associated with reaction to a foreign body. Inflammatory mucosal reactions, although not very characteristic, should raise the possibility of mycobacterial infection, nonspecific viral and nonviral infections, and other granulomatous diseases, such as sarcoidosis.

The distinction between normal, pale-pink mucosa and hypervascular areas in the tracheobronchial tree may provide important diagnostic clues. Most frequently, changes in mucosal coloration are associated with an inflammatory reaction due to bronchitis. These findings are, however, very distinctive from small hemangiomas or vascular

Video 35-2 White light and autofluorescence bronchoscopy (AFB) demonstrating a focal airway lesion at the carina between the lingua and superior division of the left upper lobe. The lesion demonstrates abnormal autofluorescence, manifested by a brownish color on AFB. The remainder of the airway examination demonstrates normal green fluorescence. *Access at www.fishmansonline.com*

distentions due to compression by enlarged, neoplastic lymph nodes. Similarly, a network of small mucosal lymphatics may be visible, with lymphatic interruption due to surgery, radiation therapy, fibrosis, or malignancy. This is most frequently associated with local edema, which contributes to airflow obstruction. In addition, distinct and characteristic mucosal discoloration can be observed in Kaposi sarcoma.[14–16]

Ulcerations of the mucosa are more characteristic of Wegener granulomatosis or malignancy. Loss of the usual mucosal luster and presence of a roughened surface may alert the expert bronchoscopist to an early infiltrative or neoplastic process. Previously sustained injuries are characterized by the formation of mucosal and submucosal fibrosis, resulting in airway retraction or distortion.

Autofluorescence bronchoscopy (AFB) permits observation and analysis of tracheobronchial mucosal surfaces using the discriminant characteristic of tissue autofluorescence (Video 35-2). It is well known that when stimulated with light of a specific wavelength, normal tissues emit specific fluorescence. Changes in the structural integrity of the same tissues due to pathological processes modify or suppress the autofluorescence. The fluorescent emissions are too low in intensity to be seen by the human eye. With the use of a monochromatic light source, computer-controlled image analysis, and a sophisticated camera attached to a fiberoptic bronchoscope, the airways can be examined for varying degrees of autofluorescence as an indicator of early-stage malignant changes. The acquisition of images is obtained in real time and helps in the detection of minute areas of change in normal tracheobronchial mucosal fluorescence. Biopsies from areas of abnormal fluorescence increase the rate of detection of small, premalignant (dysplasia) or early malignant (carcinoma in situ) lesions in the tracheobronchial tree. Confirmation is provided by biopsy of the suspect or abnormal areas under direct bronchoscopic control, followed by pathological review.

Although AFB may provide the ability to localize these early lesions with greater sensitivity than white light bronchoscopy (WLB),[17–20] longitudinal studies demonstrate that only 0% to 9% of moderate dysplastic foci and 0% to 32% of severe dysplastic foci progress to CIS or invasive cancer,[21–23] and 60% to 65% of moderate/severe dysplastic lesions regress or resolve spontaneously.[21] The uncertainty of the natural history of central airway dysplastic lesions, combined with the increasing incidence of peripheral adenocarcinomas not accessible to bronchoscopic visualization, makes it unlikely that AFB will find a role as a routine screening tool for lung cancer in large populations.

Narrow band imaging (NBI) uses a unique filter to select light wavelengths that preferentially are absorbed by hemoglobin, thereby permitting superior microvasculature detection. Because angiogenesis occurs preferentially in dysplastic and neoplastic lesions, NBI may identify early dysplastic lesions better than WLB or AFB. Early studies with NBI in high-risk patients demonstrated its ability to detect lesions that could not be visualized by WLB, with a similar sensitivity to AFB.[24,25] A recent study compared WLB, AFB, and NBI in the same patients who presented for airway surveillance and revealed similar sensitivity for AFB and NBI, but improved specificity with NBI for detecting abnormal lesions.[24] Although current clinical applications for AFB and NBI are limited, they may play a role in future risk stratification, prognostication, or chemoprevention trials in high-risk patients.

Video 35-3 This video demonstrates the findings on "alveoloscopy" using a confocal microscopy probe (Cellvizio™, Mauna Kea Technologies, Paris, France). A thin probe is advanced into the distal lung parenchyma through the working channel of a flexible bronchoscope and is able to image autofluorescence of structures of the lung. In particularly, elastin in the alveolar wall is readily detected, and therefore allows for visualization of the architecture of the alveolus, including areas of breakdown in the alveolar wall as may be seen in emphysema. In addition, intra-alveolar macrophages emit significant autofluorescence and are therefore readily visualized with the Cellvizio™ probe. These are the cells seen to be mobile within the elastin-containing alveolar walls on the video. Type I and type II pneumocytes are not readily visualized with this technology. *Access at www.fishmansonline.com*

Another promising technique, optical coherence tomography (OCT), is analogous to ultrasound imaging except that infrared light waves, rather than acoustic waves, are used.[26–31] By using light instead of sound waves, OCT overcomes the major limitations of ultrasound in the lung: The inability to image through air and its poor spatial resolution. At present, OCT can resolve structures as small as 3 μm, rendering this imaging technique superior to conventional CT or magnetic resonance imaging for detecting microscopic airway abnormalities. The ability to acquire such precise views in real time may have important clinical implications in the near future.[32,33] A similar modality, fibered confocal fluorescence microscopy (FCFM) is based on confocal microscopy that allows thin section imaging via use of a flexible fiberoptic miniprobe that can be introduced through a fiberoptic bronchoscope. This technology does not rely on light reflectance as in OCT, but rather cellular and tissue autofluorescence upon laser excitation. This technique may offer the possibility of an "optical biopsy" of peripheral lung lesions in the future (Video 35-3).

■ EVALUATION OF PERIBRONCHIAL STRUCTURES

The trachea and bronchi are surrounded by mediastinal and parenchymal structures. Developmental or pathological changes in these organs may be noted during bronchoscopic evaluation. An enlarged goiter or thymus can compress upper airways, resulting in airflow obstruction. Lymphadenopathy may produce structural changes, including widening of the carina due to subcarinal involvement and compression of other bronchi—as, for example, in the right middle lobe syndrome. Calcification of peribronchial lymph nodes may result in erosion of the bronchial wall and formation of a broncholith. These lesions are potential sources of obstruction, infection, or dangerous hemoptysis.

Development of the techniques of standard TBNA and EBUS-TBNA provide diagnostic options for the evaluation of peribronchial structures that pose much less risk and a lower complication rate than mediastinoscopy; in addition, they are less costly.

■ PERFORMANCE OF BRONCHIAL AND PARENCHYMAL BIOPSIES

Improvements in bronchoscopic instrumentation since the days of Chevalier Jackson have permitted performance of endobronchial biopsies, as well as biopsy of peripheral lung lesions. Knowledge of the underlying disease process has a significant influence on the choice of specific diagnostic procedures and risk of complications. In the case of diffuse lung diseases, such as sarcoidosis, use of fluoroscopy has not been demonstrated to improve the diagnostic yield of transbronchial biopsies (TBBs). Fluoroscopy is useful, however, in providing information regarding the proximity of the forceps to the pleura and in more rapidly establishing the diagnosis of complications (e.g., pneumothorax).

Bronchoscopically visible lesions are generally biopsied with minimal risk; if bleeding occurs, it can usually be controlled easily

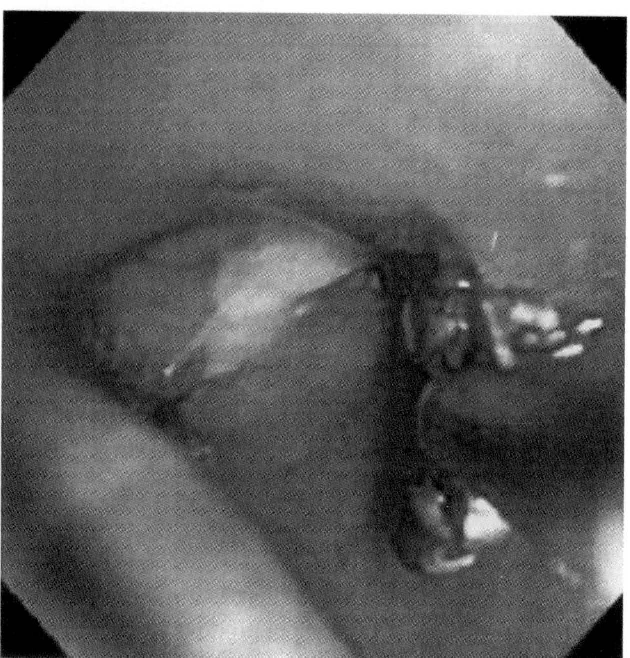

Figure 35-4 "Hot" forceps biopsy of a vascular endobronchial lesion. Use of the electrocautery forceps allows for safe, hemostatic biopsy of friable or vascularized endobronchial lesions (such as bronchial carcinoids), while obtaining pathologically interpretable tissue biopsy specimens.

(Fig. 35-4). The diagnostic yield of bronchoscopy for peripheral lesions depends on a number of factors, including lesion size, its location in the lung, and on the relationship between the lesion and bronchus. The presence of a bronchus sign on chest CT predicts a much higher yield of bronchoscopy for peripheral lung lesions. In these cases, fluoroscopy is mandatory to assure proper positioning of the cytology brush, biopsy forceps, or needle. An exciting new area is the potential application of radial EBUS in evaluation of peripheral pulmonary nodules. Radial probe EBUS allows for acquisition of diagnostic tissue via TBB performed with fewer passes; it may permit differentiation between benign and malignant nodules based entirely on nodule architecture. In the future, peripheral EBUS nodule characterization may even obviate the need for pathological diagnosis in certain patients with suspicious nodules.

The diagnosis of various infectious diseases can be established using a variety of transbronchoscopic sampling techniques. The role of bronchoscopic biopsy has been reaffirmed in immunocompromised hosts, in whom documentation of the precise pathogen is crucial for appropriate therapy. For example, while the presence of cytomegalovirus (CMV) in bronchoalveolar lavage (BAL) fluid may not be diagnostic, documentation of intracellular inclusion bodies on a biopsy specimen is practically pathognomonic. Simple, cost-effective transbronchoscopic tissue sampling can obviate much more complicated, expensive, and higher-risk thoracic surgical procedures.

■ SAMPLING OF AIRWAY AND ALVEOLAR CONSTITUENTS

Bronchoscopy provides easy and relatively safe access to material in the tracheobronchial tree and distal alveolar spaces. A variety of studies are routinely performed on specimens obtained from the airways and alveolar spaces using several techniques. For example, aspirated secretions can be sent for microscopy and culture to determine the offending organism in cases of infection or suspected infection. Cytological analysis of bronchoscopically obtained materials can provide proof of malignancy. With the advent of lung transplantation, the success of the procedure depends, in large measure, on the early diagnosis of rejection or infection in these immunocompromised

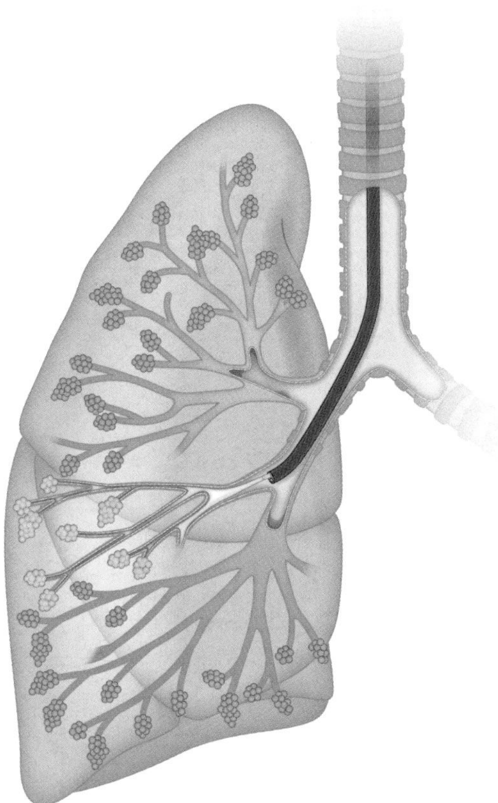

Figure 35-5 Bronchoalveolar lavage is performed by wedging the tip of bronchoscope in the segmental bronchus of interest. Normal saline is instilled into the distal air spaces, and then collected by suctioning back into a sterile container.

subjects. The most commonly employed bronchoscopic techniques for sampling the airways and alveolar spaces include "bronchial washing," bronchial brushing, and BAL.

BRONCHOALVEOLAR LAVAGE

A very useful bronchoscopic technique is BAL.[34,35] BAL is safe, even in critically ill patients, when biopsy or brushings may be contraindicated because of the risk of bleeding. Normal saline solution, devoid of any bacteriostatic material, is instilled into distal air spaces through the "wedged" bronchoscope and then aspirated through the instrument's suction channel (Fig. 35-5). The fluid collected in this manner is analyzed for gross appearance to detect possible alveolar hemorrhage. The fluid may also be subjected to a variety of tests, depending on the clinical circumstances: Microbiological testing, specific cytological analysis and cell count, immunological parameters, presence of various biochemical mediators related to pathological processes, tissue markers, polymerase chain reaction, electron microscopy, flow cytometry, and DNA probes.

Overall, the diagnostic yield of BAL is very much dependent on specific patient characteristics, underlying pathological process, and many technical factors.

INDICATIONS FOR DIAGNOSTIC BRONCHOSCOPY

Although there are several indications for diagnostic bronchoscopy (Table 35-1), evaluation of a lung nodule or mass and mediastinal staging of a lung cancer are the most common. There are many other potential indications, some of which are discussed subsequently.[36]

BRONCHOGENIC CARCINOMA

Bronchoscopy plays a central role in the evaluation of lung masses and nodules, including those suspicious for bronchogenic carcinoma.

TABLE 35-1 Indications for Diagnostic Flexible Bronchoscopy

Signs and symptoms
Hemoptysis
Stridor
Unilateral wheezing
Hoarseness
Unexplained chronic cough
Infections
Pneumonia in immunocompromised host
Nonresolving pneumonia
Cavitary lesion
Diffuse lung disease
Interstitial lung disease
Diffuse alveolar damage and hemorrhage
Drug-induced lung disease
Malignancy
Lung nodule or mass
Endobronchial tumor
Suspected airway invasion by adjacent malignancies (e.g., esophagus or thyroid)
Early detection (positive sputum cytology/negative CT scan)
Mediastinal or hilar lymphadenopathy or mass
Mediastinal staging or restaging
Other airway disorders
Mucus plugging
Foreign body aspiration
Benign airway stricture (e.g., idiopathic, granulomatosis with polyangiitis [formerly known as Wegener granulomatosis], sarcoidosis, or tuberculosis)
Intensive care
Bronchoscopy-guided intubation (difficult airway)
Endotracheal tube position
Miscellaneous
Lung transplant
Bronchopleural fistula
Aerodigestive fistula
Chest trauma
Chemical/thermal injury of airways
Preoperative and postoperative for lung resection surgery

Source: Reproduced with permission from Casal RF, DE Ost, GA Eapen. Flexible Bronchoscopy. Clin Chest Med. 2013;34(3):341–352.

Diagnosis

Bronchoscopy most commonly is performed in the evaluation of patients with suspected lung cancer. It remains the most commonly used modality for the diagnosis of bronchogenic carcinoma and plays an important role in staging of the disease, as well. Centrally located lesions generally may be approached using flexible bronchoscopy with minimal risk. Bronchogenic carcinoma of the central airways may manifest as exophytic mass lesions with partial or total bronchial lumen occlusion, as peribronchial tumors with extrinsic compression of the airway, with submucosal tumor infiltration, or with some combination of these entities. The mucosal abnormalities seen with peribronchial tumors or with submucosal infiltration often are subtle—the airways should be examined closely for

Video 35-4 Demonstrated in this video is the utilization of a standard 22-gauge Wang™ transbronchial aspiration needle (MW-122, ConMed, Utica, NY) for sampling of a partially necrotic endobronchial lesion in the right main stem bronchus. The advantages of bronchoscopic needle aspiration of endobronchial lesions include decreased bleeding risk compared to endobronchial biopsy or brushing; facilitation of sampling of material from the center of the lesion avoiding necrotic surface; and the ability to obtain real-time feedback through rapid on-site evaluation (ROSE) of aspirates by cytopathology. *Access at www.fishmansonline.com*

characteristic changes such as erythema, loss of bronchial markings, and nodularity of the mucosal surface.

Central lesions usually are sampled using a combination of bronchial washes, bronchial brushings, and endobronchial biopsies. The yield of bronchoscopy is highest for endoscopically visible lesions, with a diagnostic yield of approximately 90%.[37] Attempts should be made to obtain biopsy specimens from areas of the lesion that seem viable. Endobronchial needle aspiration (EBNA) to obtain a "core" biopsy from centrally located tumors should be considered, particularly if the lesion appears necrotic (Video 35-4). For submucosal lesions, EBNA can be performed by inserting the needle into the submucosal plane at an oblique angle; in patients with peribronchial disease causing extrinsic compression, the needle should be passed through the bronchial wall into the lesion. For all of these indications, EBNA has been shown to increase the diagnostic yield over conventional sampling methods.

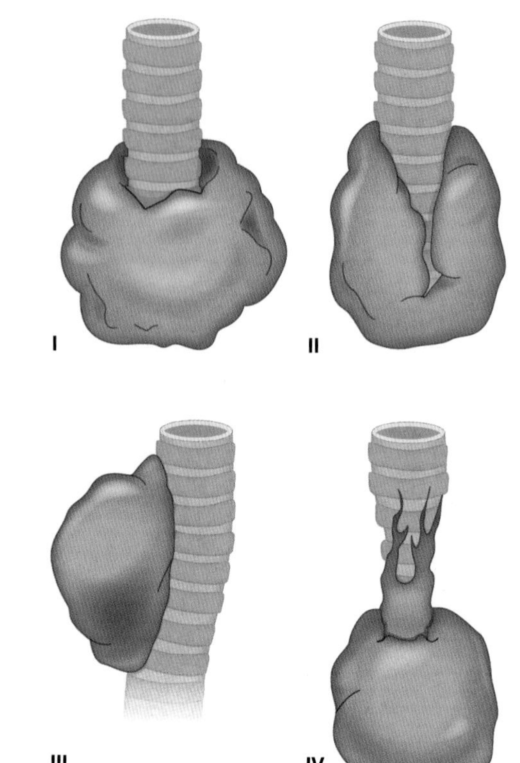

Figure 35-6 Tsuboi classification of tumor–bronchus relationship. (see text for details)

Evaluation of Peripheral Lesions and Lung Nodules

The evaluation of peripheral lesions or lung nodules remains a common dilemma for chest physicians. A balance between pretest probability of a specific diagnosis and the complication risk associated with a biopsy method must be assessed.[38] Surgical biopsy offers a superior yield at the cost of increased cost and morbidity. TTNB has a high yield, but it carries a 15% to 25% risk of pneumothorax.[39–41] Although bronchoscopy has the advantage of a low complication risk, it has been hampered by a significantly lower diagnostic yield than these other modalities.

The yield of flexible bronchoscopy for peripheral pulmonary lesions, defined as lesions that are not visible beyond the segmental bronchi, is significantly lower than for central lesions. The overall sensitivity of standard bronchoscopy, based on studies that used a combination of TBB, cytology brush, BAL, and TBNA is 78% for peripheral disease.[42–58] Success depends on several factors, including lesion size, distance from the proximal airways, and the presence of a bronchus sign. The bronchus sign on CT may reflect the relationship of a tumor with the airway, and it has been categorized into four patterns by Tsuboi[59]: type I, in which the bronchial lumen is patent up to the tumor; type II, in which the bronchus is contained in the tumor mass; type III, in which the bronchus is compressed, narrowed, and displaced by the tumor, but the bronchial mucosa is intact; and type IV, in which the proximal bronchus is narrowed by the submucosal and peribronchial spread or tumor or by the enlarged lymph nodes (Fig. 35-6). TBB has the lowest diagnostic yield for lesions with a type III or IV tumor–bronchus pattern. In these cases, the use of peripheral TBNA may improve the overall diagnostic yield of bronchoscopy.

A recent study evaluating the use of conventional diagnostic bronchoscopy for screen-detected nodules demonstrated a diagnostic yield of only 13.5%, with a negative predictive value of 47.6%.[60] Given this poor performance, conventional bronchoscopy should not be performed in the evaluation of small, peripheral pulmonary nodules.[39,54] The use of guided bronchoscopic approaches (e.g., navigational bronchoscopy, UM-EBUS, or ultrathin bronchoscopy) has significantly improved the diagnostic yield of small, peripheral pulmonary lesions. In a randomized comparison of traditional, fluoroscopically guided TBBs versus UM-EBUS–guided TBB, no statistical difference was found in establishing a diagnosis for lesions greater than 3 cm; however, for lesions smaller than 3 cm and for lesions smaller than 2 cm, the sensitivity of EBUS-guided TBB remained at 75% and 71%, whereas that of standard TBB fell dramatically to 31% and 23%, respectively.[61] Similar improvements have also been reported with the use of EMB- or VB-based systems for peripheral pulmonary lesions.

A recent meta-analysis of 30 studies with >3000 nodules reported a combined diagnostic yield of 70% for all available guided bronchoscopic techniques.[62] The diagnostic yield was influenced by the size of the primary lesion, with a yield of 61% for lesions <2 cm and 82% for lesions >2 cm.[62] Several other factors have also been described that impact the likelihood of obtaining diagnostic tissue using guided bronchoscopy: Ability to place UM-EBUS probe completely within a lesion (as opposed to adjacent to it), presence of a bronchus sign on CT scan, location in the middle lobe or lingula, and distance from the visceral pleura.[63–66] The use of TBNA in addition to conventional diagnostic procedures (TBB and BAL) in UM-EBUS–localized lesions also significantly improves diagnostic yield.[67]

Although it is increasingly clear that guided approaches are better than conventional bronchoscopy for smaller lesions, there are few comparative studies guiding the selection of a particular modality. In one randomized study of EMB alone, UM-EBUS alone, or EMB followed by confirmatory UM-EBUS, there was a significantly higher yield with the combined approach (combination, 88%; UM-EBUS, 69%; EMN, 59%),[68] suggesting that the highest yield may come from combined diagnostic modalities. However, a recent randomized study comparing ultrathin bronchoscopy with and without VB did not demonstrate any significant difference in the overall diagnostic yield (67% vs. 60%), although VB-assisted bronchoscopy was better for lesions in the RUL, lesions invisible on plain films, and lesions in the peripheral third of the lung.[69] Further studies are needed to help define the utility and specific indications for combination approaches for the diagnosis of peripheral lung lesions.

Video 35-5 This video demonstrates use of a 22-gauge EBUS-TBNA aspiration needle (Olympus, Center Valley, PA) to sample a left hilar node. The convex probe-EBUS scope is used to identify the left hilar node, allowing visualization of the TBNA needle entering the node in real time. The TBNA needle can be seen entering the left hilar node from the upper left portion of the video. The to-and-fro needle movement allows for collection of lymph node aspirate material. *Access at www.fishmansonline.com*

Staging

Bronchoscopy is an important modality for establishing lung cancer stage. In patients with potentially resectable tumors, a thorough airway examination helps confirm the absence of a concomitant, radiographically occult lesion. For lesions that involve the central airways, it is important to document the extent of disease and the degree of involvement of the main stem bronchi and main carina.

The use of CP-EBUS allows for real-time visualization and TBNA of hilar and mediastinal lymph nodes (Video 35-5). Sampling of lymph nodes using EBUS-TBNA is now commonly performed for nodal staging in patients with lung cancer. This technique frequently allows the establishment of both diagnosis and nodal stage, obviating the need for, and avoiding the risks associated with, sampling of the primary parenchymal lesion. TBNA has proved particularly useful with the employment of rapid on-site evaluation (ROSE), in which a cytopathologist present in or near the bronchoscopy suite can evaluate specimens in real time.

In general, patients with lung cancer may be separated into four categories with respect to intrathoracic radiographic characteristics, as suggested by the American College of Chest Physicians (ACCP) guidelines on lung cancer staging (Fig. 35-7).[70] In radiographic pattern A, mediastinal infiltration is extensive, with encircling of vessels and airways. In this case, the risk of malignant involvement can be assumed, and biopsy to establish diagnosis should be performed by the safest method available for that particular case. In pattern B, there is discrete lymph node enlargement that can be measured by CT, which may also be FDG-avid. In this case, sampling is recommended as the likelihood of mediastinal involvement is high and requires confirmation. In radiographic pattern C, the presence of a central tumor or suspected N1 disease makes the likelihood of mediastinal node involvement relatively high (20%–25%), necessitating invasive sampling. In the final group (i.e., those with a

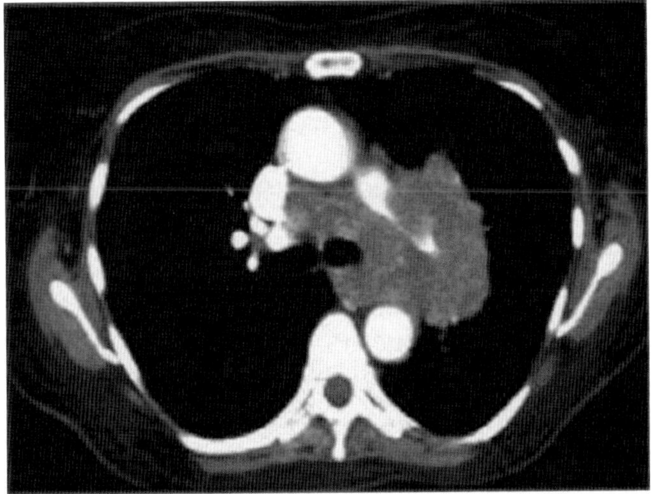

A

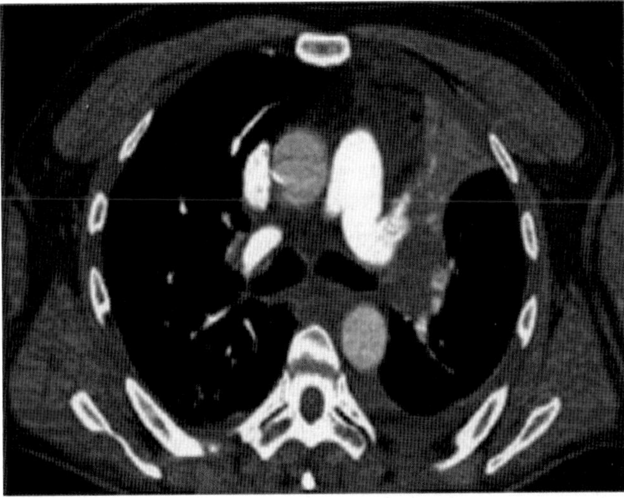

B

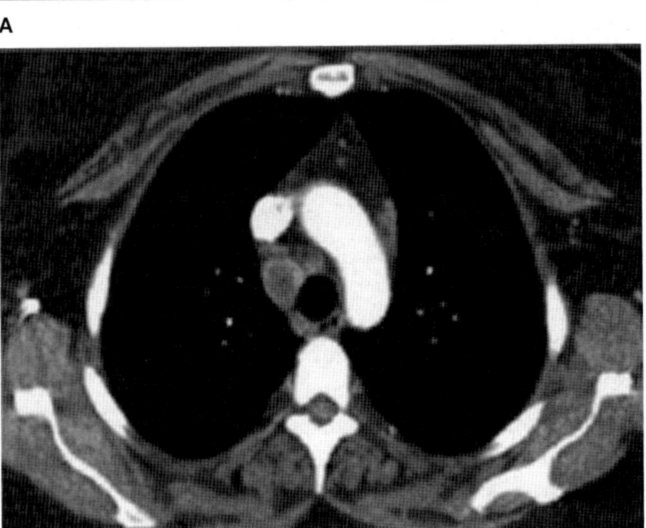

C

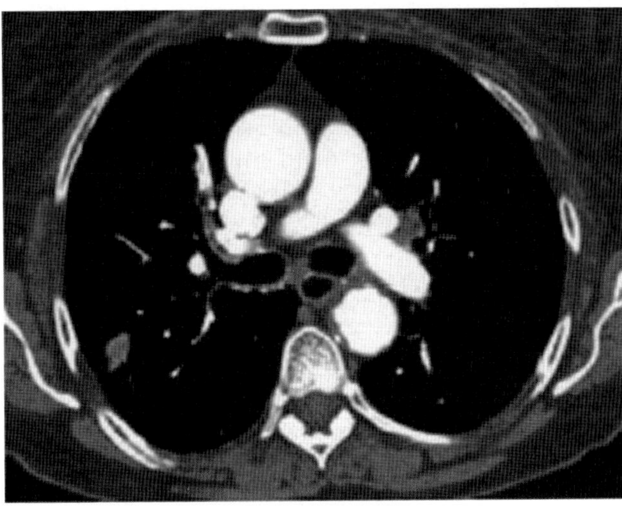

D

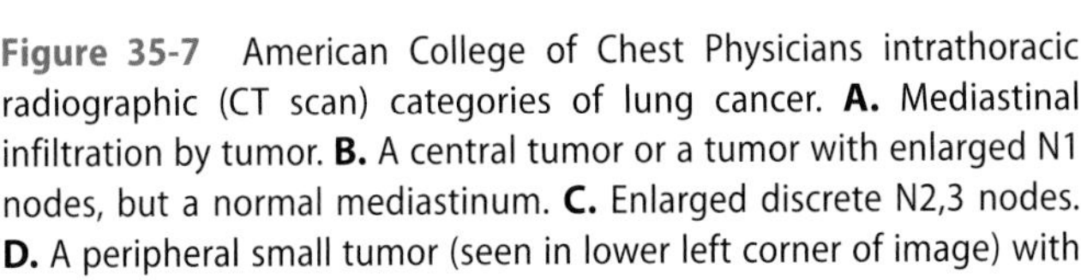

Figure 35-7 American College of Chest Physicians intrathoracic radiographic (CT scan) categories of lung cancer. **A.** Mediastinal infiltration by tumor. **B.** A central tumor or a tumor with enlarged N1 nodes, but a normal mediastinum. **C.** Enlarged discrete N2,3 nodes. **D.** A peripheral small tumor (seen in lower left corner of image) with normal-sized lymph nodes. *(Reproduced with permission from Silvestri GA, Gonzalez AV, Jantz MA, et al. Methods for staging non-small cell lung cancer: Diagnosis and management of lung cancer, 3rd ed. American College of Chest Physicians evidence-based clinical practice guidelines. Chest. 2013;143(5 Suppl):e211S–250S.)*

peripheral clinical stage I tumor), the chance of either distant metastases or mediastinal involvement is quite low (radiographic group D), especially if the mediastinum is also normal by positron emission tomography (PET) scan. The decision to pursue invasive staging should be considered on an individual case basis.

Several systematic reviews have confirmed that the sensitivity of EBUS-TBNA is equivalent to that of mediastinoscopy.[70–73] A recent randomized study of 241 patients with potentially resectable NSCLC compared mediastinoscopy alone to a combined approach of EBUS-TBNA and EUS-FNA, followed by surgical staging if the needle technique did not identify nodal metastases.[74] The needle approach followed by mediastinoscopy resulted in a significantly greater sensitivity (94%) compared to the other approaches and resulted in fewer unnecessary thoracotomies. One limitation to this approach has been the difficulty in many centers to operationalize a combined EBUS-TBNA and endoscopic ultrasound (EUS)-FNA procedure. Interestingly, recent studies have shown that the EBUS-TBNA scope can be used through both the airway and the esophagus, resulting in similar results.[75,76] The ACCP guidelines now recommend that a needle approach should be used first when performing mediastinal staging. However, because of a relatively high false-negative rate, a negative result with a needle technique should prompt consideration of surgical staging methods.

EVALUATION OF HEMOPTYSIS

One of the most frequent indications for bronchoscopy is hemoptysis. Bronchoscopic evaluation can be of help in determining the precise location and source of bleeding. The choice of instrument (rigid vs. flexible scope) and timing of the procedure are dictated by clinical circumstances.[77] Studies have shown that active bleeding and its site are visualized more commonly with early bronchoscopy (within 48 hours) than with more delayed examination.[77–79] In the case of a normal chest radiograph and hemoptysis, trace signs of bleeding are commonly seen, but not the site of origin.[80] In these circumstances, examination using an ultrathin flexible instrument may be beneficial in identifying the source of bleeding in a peripheral airway once the more proximal airways have been cleared of blood by a therapeutic scope. In some instances, bronchoscopy is useful not only as a diagnostic method, but also to perform therapeutic maneuvers (see Chapter 36, Interventional Bronchoscopy).

PULMONARY INFECTIONS

Bronchoscopy is a useful technique in the diagnosis of pulmonary infections, allowing for the collection of respiratory samples for evaluation with special stains and culture. Several common clinical areas in which bronchoscopy may play an important diagnostic role are described subsequently.

Pneumonia

In general, bronchoscopy is not indicated for the diagnosis of community-acquired pneumonia, which is currently treated empirically with appropriate antibiotic therapy; however, bronchoscopy is likely to be useful in cases of nonresolving pneumonia,[81,82] defined as a lack of improvement or worsening of symptoms despite a minimum of 10 days of antibiotic therapy or failure of radiographic abnormalities to resolve after 2 to 3 months. The causes of nonresolving pneumonia are myriad and include inadequate antibiotic therapy, resistant or highly virulent organisms, impaired host defenses, obstructing endobronchial lesions, or a noninfectious cause. Although controversial, bronchoscopy should be considered in these patients.

Ventilator-Associated Pneumonia

Ventilator-associated pneumonia (VAP) is defined as a pneumonia occurring more than 48 hours after intubation and initiation of mechanical ventilation.[83,84] VAP is usually suspected when an intubated, mechanically ventilated patient has signs of infection and an abnormal chest radiograph. Intubated patients experience colonization of their upper and lower airways with nosocomial organisms; because of an abnormal mucociliary clearance mechanism, these patients are at greater risk for developing pulmonary infections. In addition, mechanically ventilated patients are often treated empirically with broad-spectrum antibiotics and, therefore, are at greater risk for infection with resistant organisms and unusual lower respiratory tract pathogens. Guidelines support the use of either a quantitative or semiquantitative strategy in the diagnosis of VAP.[83] Quantitative sampling can be performed using endotracheal aspirates, or BAL or protected specimen brush (PSB) collected with or without a bronchoscope.[83,85]

Quantitative BAL entails the performance of a standardized BAL, with infusion of at least 120 mL of saline for adequate sampling of a pulmonary subsegment. Quantitative culture of the aspirated material is performed to determine the number of colony-forming units (CFUs) recovered.

PSB uses a double catheter system in which an outer cannula and distal, biodegradable plug protect the bronchoscopic brush within the inner cannula from contamination with secretions in the upper airway and suction channel of the bronchoscope. When the bronchoscope is positioned proximal to the segmental orifice of interest, the PSB inner cannula is advanced into a subsegment and the protective distal plug ejected. The brush is then advanced peripherally, rotated gently, and retracted into the inner cannula. The inner cannula is subsequently retracted into the outer cannula and the bronchoscope removed from the airway. The distal portion of the catheter is cleaned with 70% alcohol and the brush clipped into saline solution under sterile conditions. The PSB is then submitted for quantitative bacterial culture within 15 minutes of performance of the procedure.

The threshold for diagnosis of VAP using PSB is 10^3 CFU/mL. PSB has higher specificity than sensitivity for the presence of VAP—a positive result greatly increases the likelihood that pneumonia is present. For quantitative BAL, a threshold of 10^4 or 10^5 CFU/mL is used for diagnosis of VAP.[86] The detection of VAP by quantitative BAL culture has a sensitivity of 40% to 90% and a specificity of 45% to 100%.[86] Because a larger proportion of lung parenchyma is sampled with BAL, this may be a better method than PSB for VAP diagnosis. However, samples contaminated by upper airway secretions (based on a high percentage of squamous epithelial cells) should be interpreted with caution. There are likely a number of factors that affect the diagnostic yield of the bronchoscopic methods, such as a change in antibiotics before sampling, inadequate technique in sampling, and lack of a gold standard for comparison.

Infections in Immunocompromised Patients

Pulmonary infections in immunocompromised patients constitute the most common complication in this population and represent an important contributor to mortality. Such infections are increasingly common, reflecting the expanding use of aggressive chemotherapeutic regimens and the ever increasing number of solid organ and hematopoietic stem cell transplantations. The differential diagnosis of pulmonary infiltrates is broad in scope; however, most cases are caused by infectious agents, including bacterial, fungal, viral, and mycobacterial pathogens.[87] Bronchoscopy is the most commonly used diagnostic procedure in these patients and should be performed as early as possible, because a delay in diagnosis of longer than 5 days has been shown to significantly increase mortality.

The sensitivity of bronchoscopy varies, depending on the immunocompromised population studied and the specific etiological disorder. In non–human immunodeficiency virus (HIV)-infected patients, the yield of BAL for *Pneumocystis jirovecii* pneumonia (known previously as *Pneumocystis carinii* pneumonia [PCP]) is approximately 80%, compared with a greater than 90% yield observed in HIV-seropositive patients.[88,89] This difference is due to the much lower organism load present in non–HIV-seropositive subjects. Although empirical therapy often is initiated in patients suspected of having PCP infection, bronchoscopy should be performed in most cases to confirm the diagnosis. Bronchoscopic lung biopsy may increase the diagnostic yield of BAL for diagnosis of PCP infection, particularly in the non–HIV-infected population.[88] Bronchoscopy also has a high diagnostic yield for CMV; however, because CMV cultures from BAL are not specific, the diagnosis of CMV pneumonia should be limited to patients with pathological evidence of CMV infection demonstrated by the presence of CMV inclusion bodies on BAL or biopsy. Although bronchoscopy also is useful for the diagnosis of aspergillosis – the sensitivity is approximately 50% – the disease often is peripheral and patchy and, thus, is not easily diagnosed by BAL or bronchoscopic biopsy. Overall, in immunocompromised patients with infiltrates, the diagnostic yield of bronchoscopy varies from 30% to 80% and is impacted by factors such as the prevalence of an infectious etiology, timing of bronchoscopy, and use of prophylactic antibiotics.[90–97]

Mycobacterial Infections

In cases in which pulmonary tuberculosis is suspected, the initial diagnostic evaluation should consist of serial examination of sputum for the presence of acid-fast bacilli in stained smears. Ideally, induced sputum samples should be obtained. If sputum study results are negative, or if a patient is unable to produce sputum and tuberculosis is still suspected, bronchoscopy with BAL and biopsy should be performed. The use of bronchoscopy allows for the opportunity to establish a rapid diagnosis (by positive smear or histopathology), providing the potential for earlier intervention and treatment while awaiting culture results. Bronchoscopy should be performed with appropriate infection control precautions to minimize the risk of nosocomial transmission. A bronchoscopy may cause the patient to produce sputum for several days afterward; these specimens also should be collected and analyzed, if possible.

The utility of bronchoscopy in establishing a rapid diagnosis varies widely in the literature, with reported diagnostic yields of 30% to 70%, although the overall yield of culture is considerably higher.[98] One study has shown an improvement in diagnostic yield from 58% to 81% with use of UM-EBUS–guided biopsy and washings.[99] The yield in patients with miliary tuberculosis, in whom sputum smears frequently are negative, is approximately 70%. Bronchoscopy also is useful in tuberculosis manifesting as an endobronchial lesion or with mediastinal and hilar adenopathy, in which case, diagnostic tissue may be obtained with TBNA.

Human Immunodeficiency Virus Syndrome

The introduction of highly active antiretroviral therapy (HAART) has resulted in a sharp decline in the incidence of opportunistic infections in HIV-infected patients. Nevertheless, infectious complications remain one of the most common indications for bronchoscopy in this population. PCP remains the most frequent serious opportunistic infection in HIV-seropositive patients. Bronchoscopy with BAL remains the preferred diagnostic procedure for this disease, although in select centers, use of sputum induction has had a relatively high diagnostic yield and may mitigate the need for bronchoscopy. As previously mentioned, bronchoscopic lung biopsy may increase the diagnostic yield of BAL.[88] Empirical therapy often is initiated in patients with suspected Pneumocystis infection; such therapy can impair the diagnostic yield of BAL if the procedure is not performed within 24 hours. In patients receiving pentamidine prophylaxis, the diagnostic yield is decreased unless the upper lobes are sampled.[100–102] Several PCR assays have been tested on BAL fluid, induced sputum, and oral wash specimens; these generally have been more sensitive, but less specific, than traditional microbiological methods.

Bronchoscopy also plays an important diagnostic role in HIV-positive patients with infections caused by mycobacteria, including tuberculosis, atypical bacterial pneumonias, and various fungal infections. Kaposi sarcoma, caused by human herpesvirus type 8 (HHV8), can manifest with violaceous endobronchial plaques that typically occur at airway bifurcations; pulmonary parenchymal involvement is characterized by lymphangitic infiltration of tumor, leading to the development of nodules and masses.

■ DIFFUSE LUNG DISEASES

A wide range of acute and chronic pulmonary disorders are capable of causing a diffuse interstitial lung disease pattern of injury. These processes include infection, neoplasm, pulmonary edema, alveolar hemorrhage, alveolar proteinosis, occupational lung diseases, drug-induced disease, and various types of idiopathic or collagen vascular disease–associated interstitial lung disease. The pattern of lung injury should first be evaluated using high-resolution chest CT imaging, which helps to narrow the differential diagnosis and, in some cases, is virtually diagnostic of certain disorders. In many cases, it is still necessary to obtain samples for cytological and histological evaluation to confirm a specific diagnosis and to help exclude other possible disorders.

The most common bronchoscopic procedures used to help establish the diagnosis in diffuse lung disease are BAL and TBB. The findings on high-resolution CT (HRCT) can be used to determine the best location for BAL or TBB. In truly diffuse disease, the right middle lobe and the lingula are the best locations for BAL; with these sites, ease of access and good fluid retrieval are typical. BAL should be performed using a total of 100 to 200 mL of saline instilled in multiple aliquots. It is important to obtain a reasonable sampling of the alveolar spaces for the necessary cellular analysis.

The value of BAL is well documented in the diagnosis of diffuse parenchymal diseases, and findings may be diagnostic in eosinophilic pneumonia, eosinophilic granuloma, and pulmonary alveolar proteinosis.[36] In most other diffuse disorders, BAL findings are mostly supportive of a suspected diagnosis (Table 35-2) and helps to rule out potential infectious etiologies. In disorders such as sarcoidosis, hypersensitivity pneumonitis, and organizing pneumonia, the use of BAL in combination with bronchoscopic lung biopsy can often establish the diagnosis and avoid the need for surgical lung biopsy. For example, with pulmonary sarcoidosis, the diagnosis usually is established by a combination of BAL and biopsy findings. The BAL can be used to exclude the presence of tuberculosis and fungal infections and may demonstrate the characteristic high CD4+/CD8+ ratio seen in sarcoidosis, whereas bronchoscopic biopsy specimens may demonstrate the classic finding of noncaseating granulomas. In general, TBB should be performed in several affected areas, and at least five or six specimens should be taken. The sensitivity of TBB for diagnosis of sarcoidosis is only approximately 60% to 70%, and many patients require further invasive testing, such as surgical lung biopsy.[103,104]

In patients with mediastinal and hilar adenopathy, needle techniques for lymph node sampling should also be considered, as this can provide diagnostic evidence of noncaseating granulomas in 80% to 90% of cases.[105–110] A recent randomized study showed endosonographic needle approaches to have a greater diagnostic yield when compared with bronchoscopic lung biopsy.[111] The addition of TBNA to TBB results in an improved overall diagnostic yield in suspected cases of sarcoidosis.[105] At present, the data suggest that all patients with suspected sarcoidosis should undergo a needle technique for lymph node sampling, but it is unclear if bronchoscopic biopsy should be performed in all cases, given the added risk of pneumothorax and hemorrhage. The presence of mediastinal and hilar adenopathy, with or without parenchymal lung changes, also

TABLE 35-2 BAL Findings in Diffuse Lung Disease

Diffuse Lung Disease	Typical BAL Cellular Pattern	T lymphocyte CD4/CD8 Ratio	Other Relevant BAL Findings
Sarcoidosis	↑ Total cell count ↑ Lymphocytes	↑	-
Hypersensitivity pneumonitis	↑ Total cell count ↑ Lymphocytes	↓	Neutrophils can be increased with recent exposure to antigen
Chronic beryllium disease	↑ Total cell count ↑ Lymphocytes	↑	BAL lymphocyte proliferation with beryllium salts
Asbestosis	↑ Neutrophils	↑	Ferruginous bodies
Idiopathic pulmonary fibrosis	↑ Neutrophils ↓ Lymphocytes	-	-
Cryptogenic organizing pneumonia	↑ Neutrophils ↑ Lymphocytes	↓	Foamy macrophages
Pulmonary alveolar proteinosis	Variable	-	Milky fluid and foamy macrophages with PAS-positive material
Drug-induced lung disease	Variable	↓	Foamy macrophages with amiodarone exposure
Pulmonary Langerhans cell histiocytosis	↑ Total cell count Variable differential	-	CD1+ Langerhans cells
Eosinophilic pneumonia	↑↑ Eosinophils	-	Eosinophil counts greater in acute than in chronic pneumonia

Source: Reproduced with permission from Casal RF, DE Ost, GA Eapen. Flexible Bronchoscopy. Clin Chest Med. 2013;34(3):341–352.

raises the possibility of lymphoma. In these cases, TBNA samples should also be evaluated with flow cytometry for evidence of clonal proliferation to exclude the possibility of lymphoma.

Bronchoscopy has a limited role in the diagnosis of idiopathic pulmonary fibrosis (IPF).[112] A nonspecific increase in levels of neutrophils, eosinophils, and, less commonly, lymphocytes has been documented in BAL fluid. Histological evidence of IPF generally requires documentation of a number of pathological changes consistent with usual interstitial pneumonia. This is often difficult with bronchoscopic biopsies, which are frequently limited by the small size of the specimen obtained and lack of histological preservation because of mechanical crushing of the tissue. Cryobiopsy may improve the yield of bronchoscopy in IPF, as it allows for increased size of the obtained specimens with increased amounts of alveolated lung parenchyma. In cases in which the diagnosis of IPF is probable or definite on the basis of clinical and HRCT criteria, bronchoscopy (and surgical lung biopsy) is not required. In situations in which the HRCT findings are not atypical for IPF, bronchoscopy can be performed to evaluate for the presence of other potential etiological disorders. If the specific diagnosis cannot be established on the basis of BAL and TBB findings, surgical lung biopsy should be considered.

COMPLICATIONS OF BRONCHOSCOPY

Bronchoscopy is a potentially hazardous procedure. Complications are generally due to inappropriate preparation of patients before bronchoscopy, effects of local or general anesthesia, and manipulation of various instruments. Appropriate training and experience of the bronchoscopist and supporting team are crucial in reducing the rate of complications.

Any diagnostic or therapeutic manipulation should be considered in relation to the underlying condition of the patient, localization of the area of investigation, and other surrounding structures in the thorax. It is essential to develop good communication between the bronchoscopist and other members of the team. While the bronchoscopist concentrates on the field of work – which, as seen through the bronchoscope, is two-dimensional – other team members are responsible for monitoring the patient (oxygen saturation, blood pressure, heart rhythm, etc.) and checking and maintaining the adequacy of ancillary equipment (suction, oxygenation, and accessories such as forceps, balloons, catheters, and laser light guides). Risks are decreased if, for example, special attention is paid to the control of accessories during their manipulation beyond the tip of the bronchoscope. Premature deployment of the needle biopsy device or inappropriate bending of the bronchoscope while an instrument is inside the flexible portion can result in perforation of the bronchoscope. Activation of the laser with a broken light guide inside the bronchoscope or inadequate protrusion of the tip of the fiber beyond the bronchoscope may result in airway fires or severe burns to the patient. Attention to details and proper maintenance of the equipment, including accessories, enhance safety for the patient and staff. Diagnostic yield and therapeutic results are also improved. Overall, when bronchoscopy is performed by an experienced endoscopist, backed up by a well-trained team and appropriate facilities, mortality and morbidity are very low.

ANESTHESIA AND RELATED BLOOD GAS ABNORMALITIES

Approximately half of the life-threatening complications of diagnostic bronchoscopy are associated with the risk of topical anesthesia and sedation. Risk is significantly increased in the elderly, and in those with serious concomitant illnesses. Predisposing factors include cardiovascular disease, chronic pulmonary disease, renal and hepatic dysfunction, seizures, and altered mental status. Mild sedation, anxiolysis, muscular relaxation, and anterograde amnesia increase patient cooperation and permit quicker and less traumatic procedures. Doses of benzodiazepines, opiates, propofol, and topical anesthetics must be adjusted if there is underlying organ dysfunction. In the event of severe respiratory depression from excess sedation, flumazenil and naloxone can be administered to reverse the effects of benzodiazepines and narcotics.

Inadequate topical anesthesia potentiates coughing, gagging, and patient discomfort and increases the risk of injury during bronchoscopy. However, topical anesthetics such as lidocaine, the most frequently used agent, are absorbed systemically through the respiratory mucosa, increasing the risk of cardiac or central nervous system toxicity. Although rare, these complications are more likely to occur in patients with underlying low cardiac output, hepatic dysfunction, and oropharyngeal candidiasis.

Another, less frequent complication of excessive lidocaine use is methemoglobinemia and resultant tissue hypoxia. This condition should be suspected when cyanosis occurs following the procedure in combination with low oxygen saturation, but a higher than expected Pa_{O_2} for the degree of cyanosis, and low oxygen saturation. Sampling of arterial blood reveals chocolate-brown blood. Methemoglobinemia occurs because lidocaine causes the rate of hemoglobin oxidation to exceed the reductive capacity of erythrocytes, leading to accumulation of methemoglobin. The diagnosis of this disorder can be made using co-oximetry. Treatment with methylene blue (1–2 mg/kg body weight) should be administered to symptomatic patients or when methemoglobin levels exceed 30%.

Introduction of the bronchoscope under general anesthesia or under conscious sedation with topical anesthesia frequently results in a decrease in oxygenation and in hypoventilation, with demonstrable increases in Pa_{CO_2}. The mechanism responsible for hypoxemia include acute upper airway obstruction, hypoventilation, and ventilation–perfusion mismatching. In patients with underlying chronic lung disease, severe hypoxemia may occur, triggering life-threatening cardiac arrhythmias. Skillful manipulation of rigid and flexible bronchoscopes reduces the risk of injury to the upper airways, which can result in life-threatening laryngospasm during or after completion of the procedure. Particular caution must be exercised in patients with underlying bronchospastic disorders, superior vena cava syndrome, or history of angioedema.

All patients undergoing bronchoscopic procedures should be monitored continuously (electrocardiogram, blood pressure, O_2 saturation, and, if indicated, expiratory CO_2 concentration). Use of supplemental oxygen during the procedure should be routine. Bronchoscopy probably should not be performed in patients who are unable to maintain adequate oxygenation on full ventilator support with high levels of supplemental oxygen.

Significant oxygen desaturation may occur during BAL. The degree of desaturation is directly related to the duration of the procedure and the volume of lavage fluid used. Return to the prebronchoscopy level of O_2 saturation may be prolonged after removal of the bronchoscope, and supplemental O_2 should be continued throughout the procedure and during the postbronchoscopy observation period.

FEVER AND INFECTION

Appearance of transient fever after bronchoscopy, reported in 5% to 30% of procedures, generally does not require any therapy. The incidence of fever is increased in the elderly, in those with underlying chronic pulmonary disease or documented endobronchial obstruction, and in those with bronchoscopic interventions for malignancy. The incidence of fever and extension of pulmonary infiltrates increase with the volume of BAL fluid and the total number of pulmonary segments lavaged. In most cases, these complications resolve spontaneously within 24 hours. However, persistent fever in the setting of progressive radiographic infiltrates suggests postprocedure pneumonia and necessitates antibiotic therapy. The incidence of postbronchoscopic infections is higher in immunocompromised hosts and those with chronic suppurative lung disease (e.g., cystic fibrosis). There have also been reports of purulent pericarditis and mediastinitis following TBNA of mediastinal nodes or masses.[113,114]

In high-risk cardiac patients, including those with prosthetic valves, prior endocarditis, complicated cyanotic heart disease, or surgically constructed systemic-pulmonary shunts, American Heart Association guidelines indicate that prophylactic antibiotics are optional prior to flexible bronchoscopy.

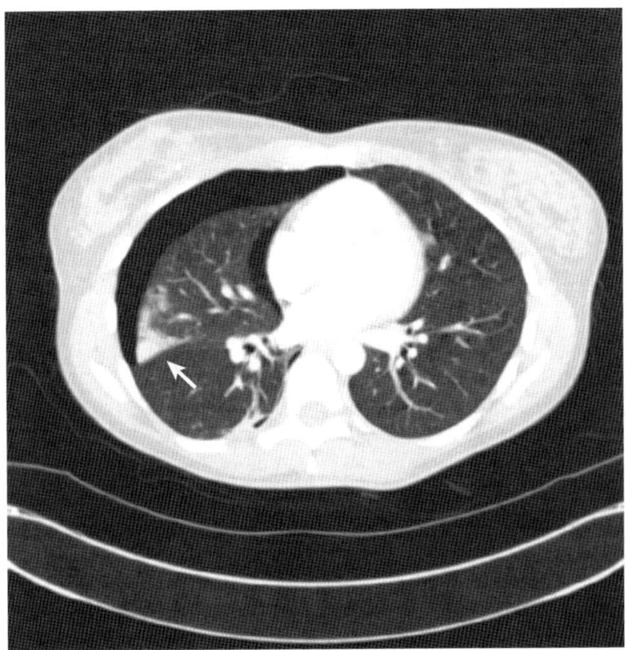

Figure 35-8 CT image demonstrating a pneumothorax of the right lung following transbronchial lung biopsy. An area of focal hemorrhage in the lateral right upper lobe *(white arrow)* as a result of biopsy can also be seen.

PNEUMOTHORAX

Most of the serious complications related to diagnostic bronchoscopy have been reported in association with performance of TBBs. Pneumothorax following TBB occurs in 4% to 5% of cases, (Fig. 35-8) although a recent population-based study suggested pneumothorax rates of approximately 1%.[115-124] The impact of fluoroscopy on the incidence of pneumothorax remains controversial. Uncontrolled studies have not found a difference in the incidence of pneumothorax following TBB when performed with and without fluoroscopy.[125]

The risk of pneumothorax is not related to the size of the bronchoscopic biopsy forceps. The incidence of pneumothorax is increased, however, in immunocompromised hosts. This is likely due to the increased risk of pneumothorax associated with PCP. The risk is also elevated in mechanically ventilated patients, with peripheral lung biopsies, and in the presence of bullous lung disease. For these reasons, a postbronchoscopic expiratory chest radiograph is routinely performed. In rare cases, the development of pneumothorax can be delayed, with patients developing the complication after discharge. In case of a significant pneumothorax, a chest tube should be inserted immediately to avoid oxygen desaturation or tension physiology.

HEMORRHAGE

One of the most frequently reported complications related to bronchoscopy is hemorrhage. Clinically significant bleeding as a consequence of diagnostic bronchoscopy is reported to occur in 1% to 4% of cases, but it is more likely to occur after TBB and brushings.[123,124,126,127] Although hemorrhage may also occur from inadvertent perforation of pulmonary vessels during TBNA, this is a very rare complication. Bleeding is more common in patients with immunosuppressed state, thrombocytopenia, uremia, liver disease, pulmonary hypertension, concurrent anticoagulation, and those on positive pressure ventilation.

The incidence of postbronchoscopy hemorrhage in uremic patients is reported as high as 45%. Consequently, a blood urea nitrogen (BUN) level above 30 mg/dL or a creatinine level above

3 mg/dL should be considered relative contraindications to bronchoscopy. TBB or brushing should not be performed if the platelet count is below 50,000/mm^3. Thrombocytopenic patients may receive platelet transfusions if biopsy is necessary. Similarly, coagulopathic patients should receive vitamin K, fresh frozen plasma, or cryoprecipitate prior to the procedure and biopsy.

Increasingly, patients referred for bronchoscopy are receiving antiplatelet therapy. Importantly, aspirin use has not been shown to increase hemorrhage risk, and it generally does not require discontinuation prior to diagnostic bronchoscopy.[128] In contrast, the risk of bleeding from clopidogrel therapy is very high following TBB.[129] If TBBs are necessary, clopidogrel should be discontinued 5 to 7 days prior to the procedure. We also recommend discontinuation prior to TBNA, although the risk of major bleeding is lower, and successful TBNA can be performed without discontinuation. In cases where clopidogrel therapy cannot be discontinued (e.g., recent coronary artery stenting), careful assessment of the goals of bronchoscopy should be considered and the need for TBB should be clearly defined.

TRANSTHORACIC NEEDLE BIOPSY

TTNB has proved a valuable diagnostic procedure in patients with a variety of thoracic radiographic abnormalities.

INDICATIONS AND CONTRAINDICATIONS

TTNB was first used for the diagnosis of pulmonary disease in 1883, when Leyden performed the procedure on three patients with pneumonia. Since that time, many published series have described the use of TTNB for the diagnosis of a variety of benign and malignant thoracic lesions.[130–139] The approach to biopsy may employ either an aspiration approach or an approach based on procuring histological samples with use of cutting needles. The use of histological samples provides improved diagnostic accuracy in lymphoma, both Hodgkin and non-Hodgkin varieties, in which anatomic structure is important in delineating the type of lymphoma, and in distinguishing between clonal, neoplastic processes, and inflammatory conglomerations of lymphocytes. Histological specimens may also improve the yield in the diagnosis of pulmonary hamartomas, characterized by the presence of cartilage or adipose tissue.

The major indications for TTNB include evaluation of solitary lung nodules and masses, (Fig. 35-9) mediastinal and hilar lesions, metastatic disease to the lung from a known extrathoracic malignancy, chest wall invasion by lung carcinoma, and pulmonary consolidation or infiltrates that are likely to be of infectious origin.

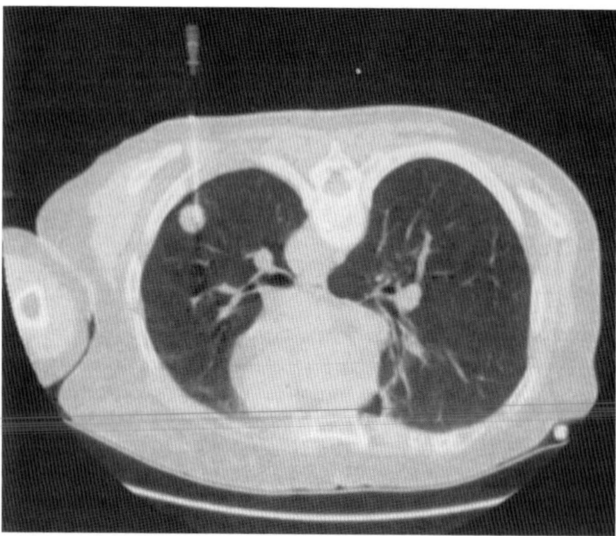

Figure 35-9 Transthoracic needle aspiration of pulmonary nodule. CT scan image of TTNA performed for a 2-cm right lower lobe nodule using a 22-gauge Westcott needle (Becton Dickinson & Co, Franklin Lakes, NJ). The needle can be seen entering the nodule. *(Used with permission of Ana Kolansky, MD.)*

With the "reemergence" of thoracoscopy and development of video-assisted and robotic-assisted thoracic surgical techniques, patients can more easily undergo complete excision of pulmonary nodules. In the past, many pulmonologists performed TTNB as the initial diagnostic procedure for intrapulmonary lesions, especially those in the lung periphery. Physicians are now faced with the dilemma of whether to send patients directly to thoracoscopic biopsy for a definitive answer. Two commonly used strategies – the use of PET or serial CT scanning – can be used to obtain additional evidence regarding the likelihood of malignancy. In appropriately selected patients, the presence of a PET-positive lesion or a lesion increasing in size on serial CT scans may obviate the need for TTNB.

Few absolute contraindications to TTNB exist. These include an uncooperative patient or one with an intractable cough, as patients must be able to suspend respirations for 5 to 10 seconds while the needle crosses the pleura. In addition, TTNB is absolutely contraindicated in patients with a suspected pulmonary hydatid cyst because of the risk of capsule rupture and systemic dissemination. Relative contraindications include bullous emphysema, pulmonary arterial hypertension, and coagulation or platelet disorders. Patients with bullous emphysema are at increased risk of developing symptomatic or tension pneumothoraces after biopsy, although most induced pneumothoraces are small and can be treated conservatively. Those with pulmonary hypertension who undergo TTNB have a higher chance of developing pulmonary hemorrhage and significant hemoptysis.

TECHNIQUE

Proper technique in performing TTNB is critical in obtaining adequate material for reliable interpretation. In addition to the mechanics of needle insertion and aspiration, the choice of needle type and careful specimen processing are important aspects of the procedure.

Choice of Needle

Many needle types are available for TTNB.[140,141] They vary in both length and width. In the early 1960s, TTNA was performed using large-bore cutting needles; significant hemorrhagic complications were reported. More recently, thin-needle aspiration has become standard, with devices ranging in size from 18 to 22 gauge. Coaxial needle systems have been introduced for the purpose of obtaining multiple samples from a single pleural penetration. These systems are also useful for procuring specimens for histological evaluation.

Radiographic Guidance and Biopsy Planning

Although TTNB can be performed under fluoroscopic or ultrasound guidance, CT is now the most commonly used image guidance approach for this procedure. CT can be used either intermittently during the procedure to guide needle placement, or with CT fluoroscopy (CTF), which allows for near real-time acquisition of images to guide needle adjustments. The diagnostic yield from either of these CT-based approaches appears to be similar.

Ultrasound-guided biopsies should be considered for peripheral lung lesions that extend to the pleural edge, or for the diagnosis of mediastinal masses. Ultrasound guidance also offers the advantage of real-time lesion imaging, easy portability, and absence of exposure to ionizing radiation for both the clinician and the patient.

Biopsy planning is an important step and should be performed prior to the procedure. Considerations include choosing a needle path that avoids traversal of bullae, vessels, and bronchi. Crossing of interlobular fissures should also be avoided, as this increases the risk of pneumothorax.[142] In cases with more than one lesion, a more peripheral lesion is preferred to decrease the amount of lung traversed during needle insertion. In addition, upper lobe lesions are preferred over the lower lobe because of less respiratory motion in the upper lobes.

There are a number of different biopsy needles available for use, varying in length, gauge, and sampling mechanism. In general, needles can be divided into those used for aspiration, cutting needles for histological evaluation, and automatic core biopsy needles. The choice of biopsy needle depends on various factors, including characteristics of the lesion, amount of tissue desired, and operator preference.

Needle Insertion

The lesion is localized using CT guidance, and the overlying skin is marked and anesthetized with 1% or 2% lidocaine. The needle is first inserted through the skin into the subcutaneous tissues. The needle is then advanced to the level of the pleura, followed by verification of the needle position and angle by CT. The needle is then advanced in one motion through the pleura to the prescribed length. The needle position can be confirmed prior to biopsy.

Ideal aspiration technique necessitates having the tip of the needle as close to the center of the lesion as possible. If an aspiration or cutting needle is used, the inner stylet should be removed. A syringe is attached to the needle hub. While suction is applied, the needle tip is advanced and withdrawn about 0.5 to 1 cm within the lesion. The needle is then removed from the chest, suction is released, and the aspirated material is flushed into a specimen container. Several samples should be obtained to increase the diagnostic yield. With a necrotic mass, aspiration should also be performed in peripheral locations of the lesion to obtain viable cells and to decrease the risk of false-negative results.

A coaxial technique can also be employed using a larger entry needle, which is advanced into the lesion, followed by a smaller biopsy needle that can be passed through the lumen of the larger needle into the lesion. This approach allows multiple passes into the lesion without repositioning of the needle with each pass.

RESULTS

TTNB has an excellent success rate in the diagnosis of primary or metastatic pulmonary malignancies, with meta-analyses demonstrating pooled sensitivity of 90% (95% CI, 88%–91%);[54] lower yields are seen for lesions smaller than 1.5 cm.[135,139,143] CT guidance yields better performance when compared with fluoroscopy.[144] Aspiration biopsies have similar sensitivity to biopsies performed with cutting needles, but a poorer ability to determine a specific diagnosis from benign lesions. There is also concern that aspiration samples provide a lower likelihood of yielding sufficient tissue for molecular analysis, which is increasingly required in patients diagnosed with lung cancer.

Major causes of false-negative results in malignant disease are inadequate sampling of the lesion and aspiration in an area of necrosis or postobstructive pneumonia. In addition, small, central malignant lesions may be difficult to diagnose accurately. Aspiration of vascular tumors, such as angiosarcoma, carcinoid, or metastatic renal cell carcinoma, may yield a bloody aspirate with few, if any, malignant cells. False-positive results are extremely rare (1%–2%) and are typically reported in the setting of inflammatory processes, such as tuberculosis, radiation fibrosis, organizing pneumonia, and pulmonary infarction.

In the absence of a specific benign diagnosis, a lung biopsy that is negative for malignancy does not rule out the presence of neoplastic disease, especially if the biopsy was unsatisfactory. The degree of suspicion of malignancy in a particular clinical situation becomes extremely important in dictating the next step following a negative TTNB. For a smoker with a high risk of bronchogenic carcinoma, the proper course may lead to videothoracoscopic biopsy of the lesion, whereas in a young, otherwise healthy nonsmoker, close observation with serial CT scans may be the preferred option.

COMPLICATIONS

As mentioned previously, the most common complication of TTNB is pneumothorax; incidence rates reported in the literature vary from 8% to 61%. A recent population-based analysis reported a rate of pneumothorax of 15%, with 7% of all biopsies resulting in a pneumothorax requiring management with a chest tube.[40] Preexisting lung disease – in particular, bullous emphysema – is the most significant predisposing factor to development of pneumothorax after TTNB.[142,145–148] The vast majority of patients who develop clinically significant pneumothoraces after the procedure have an underlying diagnosis of chronic obstructive pulmonary disease. Other risk factors are smaller nodule size, crossing more than one pleural surface with the needle, needle size, and increased patient age.[142,145–148] Factors such as depth of lesion and increased number of transthoracic passes are controversial.[145,149]

Uncommon complications of TTNB include hemorrhage and hemoptysis, reported in approximately 1% of all biopsies. Although these are typically minor, one large study reported a transfusion requirement in 18% of cases with hemorrhage.[40] Cases of fatal hemorrhage from tracheobronchial obstruction from clot and subsequent asphyxia after use of large-bore (18-gauge) cutting needles have been reported.

Air embolism is a rare complication caused by creation of a communication between atmospheric air and a pulmonary vein. To minimize this risk, the needle should never be left open to air while in the chest, and the patient should be discouraged from deep breathing, straining, or coughing during the procedure. The procedure should be halted and the needle withdrawn if the patient is actively coughing. If an air embolism is suspected, 100% oxygen should be administered through a nonrebreather face mask and the patient placed in the left lateral decubitus position, with the head down: This position optimizes capture of air in the right heart. The patient should be transferred immediately to a hyperbaric chamber.

SUMMARY

Technological advances in diagnostic bronchoscopy continue to improve our ability to perform minimally invasive, accurate evaluations of the tracheobronchial tree and to perform an ever increasing array of diagnostic procedures. The continued development of imaging technologies and ancillary tools will certainly provide improvements in many of the modalities described earlier. Future improvements will include refinements in video and ultrasound imaging technology and the development of newer modalities, such as molecular imaging. This will be accompanied by further improvements in the ancillary tools, such as miniaturization of diagnostic accessories and further refinements in steerable probes that will allow improved access to peripheral regions of the lung. These opportunities will need to be accompanied by well-designed studies to delineate the appropriate use of these techniques in clinical practice.

REFERENCES

1. Rooney CP, Wolf K, McLennan G. Ultrathin bronchoscopy as an adjunct to standard bronchoscopy in the diagnosis of peripheral lung lesions. A preliminary report. *Respiration*. 2002;69(1):63–68.
2. Yamamoto S, Ueno K, Imamura F, et al. Usefulness of ultrathin bronchoscopy in diagnosis of lung cancer. *Lung Cancer*. 2004;46(1):43–48.
3. Wang KP, Terry P, Marsh B. Bronchoscopic needle aspiration biopsy of paratracheal tumors. *Am Rev Respir Dis*. 1978;118(1):17–21.
4. Haas AR, Vachani A, Sterman DH. Advances in diagnostic bronchoscopy. *Am J Respir Crit Care Med*. 2010;182(5):589–597.
5. Kurimoto N, Murayama M, Yoshioka S, Nishisaka T, Inai K, Dohi K. Assessment of usefulness of endobronchial ultrasonography

in determination of depth of tracheobronchial tumor invasion. *Chest*. 1999;115(6):1500–1506.

6. Eberhardt R, Gompelmann D, Herth FJ. Electromagnetic navigation in lung cancer: research update. *Expert Rev Respir Med*. 2009;3(5):469–473.
7. Eberhardt R, Kahn N, Gompelmann D, Schumann M, Heussel CP, Herth FJ. LungPoint–a new approach to peripheral lesions. *J Thorac Oncol*. 2010;5(10):1559–1563.
8. Gildea TR, Mazzone PJ, Karnak D, Meziane M, Mehta AC. Electromagnetic navigation diagnostic bronchoscopy: a prospective study. *Am J Respir Crit Care Med*. 2006;174(9):982–989.
9. Makris D, Scherpereel A, Leroy S, et al. Electromagnetic navigation diagnostic bronchoscopy for small peripheral lung lesions. *Eur Respir J*. 2007;29(6):1187–1192.
10. Anantham D, Feller-Kopman D, Shanmugham LN, et al. Electromagnetic navigation bronchoscopy-guided fiducial placement for robotic stereotactic radiosurgery of lung tumors: a feasibility study. *Chest*. 2007;132(3):930–935.
11. McGuire FR, Liming J, Ochran T, Kerley JM, McLemore TL. Real-time endobronchial ultrasound guided implantation of radiotherapy monitoring devices. *J Bronchology*. 2007;14(1):42–45.
12. Wahidi MM, Jain P, Jantz M, et al. American College of Chest Physicians consensus statement on the use of topical anesthesia, analgesia, and sedation during flexible bronchoscopy in adult patients. *Chest*. 2011;140(5):1342–1350.
13. Malik JA, Gupta D, Agarwal AN, Jindal SK. Anticholinergic premedication for flexible bronchoscopy: a randomized, double-blind, placebo-controlled study of atropine and glycopyrrolate. *Chest*. 2009;136(2):347–354.
14. Gruden JF, Huang L, Webb WR, Gamsu G, Hopewell PC, Sides DM. AIDS-related Kaposi sarcoma of the lung: radiographic findings and staging system with bronchoscopic correlation. *Radiology*. 1995;195(2):545–552.
15. Hanson PJ, Harcourt-Webster JN, Gazzard BG, Collins JV. Fibreoptic bronchoscopy in diagnosis of bronchopulmonary Kaposi's sarcoma. *Thorax*. 1987;42(4):269–271.
16. Stover DE, White DA, Romano PA, Gellene RA. Diagnosis of pulmonary disease in acquired immune deficiency syndrome (AIDS). Role of bronchoscopy and bronchoalveolar lavage. *Am Rev Respir Dis*. 1984;130(4):659–662.
17. Chhajed PN, Shibuya K, Hoshino H, et al. A comparison of video and autofluorescence bronchoscopy in patients at high risk of lung cancer. *Eur Respir J*. 2005;25(6):951–955.
18. Edell E, Lam S, Pass H, et al. Detection and localization of intraepithelial neoplasia and invasive carcinoma using fluorescence-reflectance bronchoscopy: an international, multicenter clinical trial. *J Thorac Oncol*. 2009;4(1):49–54.
19. Haussinger K, Becker H, Stanzel F, et al. Autofluorescence bronchoscopy with white light bronchoscopy compared with white light bronchoscopy alone for the detection of precancerous lesions: a European randomised controlled multicentre trial. *Thorax*. 2005;60(6):496–503.
20. Ueno K, Kusunoki Y, Imamura F, et al. Clinical experience with autofluorescence imaging system in patients with lung cancers and precancerous lesions. *Respiration*. 2007;74(3):304–308.
21. Bota S, Auliac JB, Paris C, et al. Follow-up of bronchial precancerous lesions and carcinoma in situ using fluorescence endoscopy. *Am J Respir Crit Care Med*. 2001;164(9):1688–1693.
22. Breuer RH, Pasic A, Smit EF, et al. The natural course of preneoplastic lesions in bronchial epithelium. *Clin Cancer Res*. 2005;11(2 Pt 1):537–543.
23. Hoshino H, Shibuya K, Chiyo M, et al. Biological features of bronchial squamous dysplasia followed up by autofluorescence bronchoscopy. *Lung Cancer*. 2004;46(2):187–196.
24. Herth FJ, Eberhardt R, Anantham D, Gompelmann D, Zakaria MW, Ernst A. Narrow-band imaging bronchoscopy increases the specificity of bronchoscopic early lung cancer detection. *J Thorac Oncol*. 2009;4(9):1060–1065.
25. Vincent BD, Fraig M, Silvestri GA. A pilot study of narrow-band imaging compared to white light bronchoscopy for evaluation of normal airways and premalignant and malignant airways disease. *Chest*. 2007;131(6):1794–1799.
26. Coxson HO, Quiney B, Sin DD, et al. Airway wall thickness assessed using computed tomography and optical coherence tomography. *Am J Respir Crit Care Med*. 2008;177(11):1201–1206.
27. Han S, El-Abbadi NH, Hanna N, et al. Evaluation of tracheal imaging by optical coherence tomography. *Respiration*. 2005;72(5):537–541.
28. Lam S, Standish B, Baldwin C, et al. In vivo optical coherence tomography imaging of preinvasive bronchial lesions. *Clin Cancer Res*. 2008;14(7):2006–2011.
29. Tsuboi M, Hayashi A, Ikeda N, et al. Optical coherence tomography in the diagnosis of bronchial lesions. *Lung Cancer*. 2005;49(3):387–394.
30. Whiteman SC, Yang Y, Gey van Pittius D, Stephens M, Parmer J, Spiteri MA. Optical coherence tomography: real-time imaging of bronchial airways microstructure and detection of inflammatory/neoplastic morphologic changes. *Clin Cancer Res*. 2006;12(3 Pt 1):813–818.
31. Williamson JP, McLaughlin RA, Phillips MJ, et al. Using optical coherence tomography to improve diagnostic and therapeutic bronchoscopy. *Chest*. 2009;136(1):272–276.
32. Hariri LP, Mino-Kenudson M, Applegate MB, et al. Towards the guidance of transbronchial biopsy: identifying pulmonary nodules with optical coherence tomography. *Chest*. 2013;144(4):1261–1268.
33. Michel RG, Kinasewitz GT, Fung KM, Keddissi JI. Optical coherence tomography as an adjunct to flexible bronchoscopy in the diagnosis of lung cancer: a pilot study. *Chest*. 2010;138(4):984–988.
34. Meyer KC. Bronchoalveolar lavage as a diagnostic tool. *Semin Respir Crit Care Med*. 2007;28(5):546–560.
35. Turner-Warwick M, Haslam PL. Clinical applications of bronchoalveolar lavage. *Clin Chest Med*. 1987;8(1):15–26.
36. Casal RF, Ost DE, Eapen GA. Flexible bronchoscopy. *Clin Chest Med*. 2013;34(3):341–352.
37. Mazzone P, Jain P, Arroliga AC, Matthay RA. Bronchoscopy and needle biopsy techniques for diagnosis and staging of lung cancer. *Clin Chest Med*. 2002;23(1):137–158, ix.
38. Ost DE, Gould MK. Decision making in patients with pulmonary nodules. *Am J Respir Crit Care Med*. 2012;185(4):363–372.
39. Gould MK, Donington J, Lynch WR, et al. Evaluation of individuals with pulmonary nodules: when is it lung cancer? Diagnosis and management of lung cancer, 3rd ed: American College of Chest Physicians evidence-based clinical practice guidelines. *Chest*. 2013;143(5 Suppl):e93S–e120S.
40. Wiener RS, Schwartz LM, Woloshin S, Welch HG. Population-based risk for complications after transthoracic needle lung biopsy of a pulmonary nodule: an analysis of discharge records. *Ann Intern Med*. 2011;155(3):137–144.
41. Wiener RS, Wiener DC, Gould MK. Risks of transthoracic needle biopsy: how high? *Clin Pulm Med*. 2013;20(1):29–35.

42. Baaklini WA, Reinoso MA, Gorin AB, Sharafkaneh A, Manian P. Diagnostic yield of fiberoptic bronchoscopy in evaluating solitary pulmonary nodules. *Chest*. 2000;117(4):1049–1054.

43. Baba M, Iyoda A, Yasufuku K, et al. Preoperative cytodiagnosis of very small-sized peripheral-type primary lung cancer. *Lung Cancer*. 2002;37(3):277–280.

44. Bandoh S, Fujita J, Tojo Y, et al. Diagnostic accuracy and safety of flexible bronchoscopy with multiplanar reconstruction images and ultrafast Papanicolaou stain: evaluating solitary pulmonary nodules. *Chest*. 2003;124(5):1985–1992.

45. Bilaceroglu S, Kumcuoglu Z, Alper H, et al. CT bronchus sign-guided bronchoscopic multiple diagnostic procedures in carcinomatous solitary pulmonary nodules and masses. *Respiration*. 1998;65(1):49–55.

46. Cox ID, Bagg LR, Russell NJ, Turner MJ. Relationship of radiologic position to the diagnostic yield of fiberoptic bronchoscopy in bronchial carcinoma. *Chest*. 1984;85(4):519–522.

47. Gasparini S, Zuccatosta L, Zitti P, Bichi Secchi E, Ferretti M, Gusella P. Integration of TBNA and TCNA in the diagnosis of peripheral lung nodules. Influence on staging. *Ann Ital Chir*. 1999;70(6):851–855.

48. Kawaraya M, Gemba K, Ueoka H, et al. Evaluation of various cytological examinations by bronchoscopy in the diagnosis of peripheral lung cancer. *Br J Cancer*. 2003;89(10):1885–1888.

49. Lam WK, So SY, Hsu C, Yu DY. Fibreoptic bronchoscopy in the diagnosis of bronchial cancer: comparison of washings, brushings and biopsies in central and peripheral tumours. *Clin Oncol*. 1983;9(1):35–42.

50. Mak VH, Johnston ID, Hetzel MR, Grubb C. Value of washings and brushings at fibreoptic bronchoscopy in the diagnosis of lung cancer. *Thorax*. 1990;45(5):373–376.

51. Mori K, Yanase N, Kaneko M, Ono R, Ikeda S. Diagnosis of peripheral lung cancer in cases of tumors 2 cm or less in size. *Chest*. 1989;95(2):304–308.

52. Naidich DP, Sussman R, Kutcher WL, Aranda CP, Garay SM, Ettenger NA. Solitary pulmonary nodules. CT-bronchoscopic correlation. *Chest*. 1988;93(3):595–598.

53. Radke JR, Conway WA, Eyler WR, Kvale PA. Diagnostic accuracy in peripheral lung lesions. Factors predicting success with flexible fiberoptic bronchoscopy. *Chest*. 1979;76(2):176–179.

54. Rivera MP, Mehta AC, Wahidi MM. Establishing the diagnosis of lung cancer: diagnosis and management of lung cancer, 3rd ed: American College of Chest Physicians evidence-based clinical practice guidelines. *Chest*. 2013;143(5 Suppl):e142S–e165S.

55. Trkanjec JT, Peros-Golubicic T, Grozdek D, Ivicevic A, Alilovic M. The role of transbronchial lung biopsy in the diagnosis of solitary pulmonary nodule. *Coll Antropol*. 2003;27(2):669–675.

56. Wongsurakiat P, Wongbunnate S, Dejsomritrutai W, et al. Diagnostic value of bronchoalveolar lavage and postbronchoscopic sputum cytology in peripheral lung cancer. *Respirology*. 1998;3(2):131–137.

57. Zavala DC. Diagnostic fiberoptic bronchoscopy: techniques and results of biopsy in 600 patients. *Chest*. 1975;68(1):12–19.

58. Cortese DA, McDougall JC. Bronchoscopic biopsy and brushing with fluoroscopic guidance in nodular metastatic lung cancer. *Chest*. 1981;79(5):610–611.

59. Tsuboi E, Ikeda S, Tajima M, Shimosato Y, Ishikawa S. Transbronchial biopsy smear for diagnosis of peripheral pulmonary carcinomas. *Cancer*. 1967;20(5):687–698.

60. van 't Westeinde SC, Horeweg N, Vernhout RM, et al. The role of conventional bronchoscopy in the workup of suspicious CT scan screen-detected pulmonary nodules. *Chest*. 2012;142(2):377–384.

61. Paone G, Nicastri E, Lucantoni G, et al. Endobronchial ultrasound-driven biopsy in the diagnosis of peripheral lung lesions. *Chest*. 2005;128(5):3551–3557.

62. Wang Memoli JS, Nietert PJ, Silvestri GA. Meta-analysis of guided bronchoscopy for the evaluation of the pulmonary nodule. *Chest*. 2012;142(2):385–393.

63. Fielding DI, Robinson PJ, Kurimoto N. Biopsy site selection for endobronchial ultrasound guide-sheath transbronchial biopsy of peripheral lung lesions. *Intern Med J*. 2008;38(2):77–84.

64. Kurimoto N, Miyazawa T, Okimasa S, et al. Endobronchial ultrasonography using a guide sheath increases the ability to diagnose peripheral pulmonary lesions endoscopically. *Chest*. 2004;126(3):959–965.

65. Yamada N, Yamazaki K, Kurimoto N, et al. Factors related to diagnostic yield of transbronchial biopsy using endobronchial ultrasonography with a guide sheath in small peripheral pulmonary lesions. *Chest*. 2007;132(2):603–608.

66. Yoshikawa M, Sukoh N, Yamazaki K, et al. Diagnostic value of endobronchial ultrasonography with a guide sheath for peripheral pulmonary lesions without X-ray fluoroscopy. *Chest*. 2007; 131(6):1788–1793.

67. Chao TY, Chien MT, Lie CH, Chung YH, Wang JL, Lin MC. Endobronchial ultrasonography-guided transbronchial needle aspiration increases the diagnostic yield of peripheral pulmonary lesions: a randomized trial. *Chest*. 2009;136(1):229–236.

68. Eberhardt R, Anantham D, Ernst A, Feller-Kopman D, Herth F. Multimodality bronchoscopic diagnosis of peripheral lung lesions: a randomized controlled trial. *Am J Respir Crit Care Med*. 2007;176(1):36–41.

69. Asano F, Shinagawa N, Ishida T, et al. Virtual bronchoscopic navigation combined with ultrathin bronchoscopy: a randomized clinical trial. *Am J Respir Crit Care Med*. 2013;188(3):327–333.

70. Silvestri GA, Gonzalez AV, Jantz MA, et al. Methods for staging non-small cell lung cancer: diagnosis and management of lung cancer, 3rd ed: American College of Chest Physicians evidence-based clinical practice guidelines. *Chest*. 2013;143(5 Suppl):e211S–e250S.

71. Adams K, Shah PL, Edmonds L, Lim E. Test performance of endobronchial ultrasound and transbronchial needle aspiration biopsy for mediastinal staging in patients with lung cancer: systematic review and meta-analysis. *Thorax*. 2009;64(9):757–762.

72. Gu P, Zhao YZ, Jiang LY, Zhang W, Xin Y, Han BH. Endobronchial ultrasound-guided transbronchial needle aspiration for staging of lung cancer: a systematic review and meta-analysis. *Eur J Cancer*. 2009;45(8):1389–1396.

73. Varela-Lema L, Fernandez-Villar A, Ruano-Ravina A. Effectiveness and safety of endobronchial ultrasound-transbronchial needle aspiration: a systematic review. *Eur Respir J*. 2009; 33(5):1156–1164.

74. Annema JT, van Meerbeeck JP, Rintoul RC, et al. Mediastinoscopy vs endosonography for mediastinal nodal staging of lung cancer: a randomized trial. *JAMA*. 2010;304(20):2245–2252.

75. Herth FJ, Krasnik M, Kahn N, Eberhardt R, Ernst A. Combined endoscopic-endobronchial ultrasound-guided fine-needle aspiration of mediastinal lymph nodes through a single bronchoscope in 150 patients with suspected lung cancer. *Chest*. 2010; 138(4):790–794.

76. Hwangbo B, Lee GK, Lee HS, et al. Transbronchial and transesophageal fine-needle aspiration using an ultrasound bronchoscope in mediastinal staging of potentially operable lung cancer. *Chest*. 2010;138(4):795–802.

77. Dweik RA, Stoller JK. Role of bronchoscopy in massive hemoptysis. *Clin Chest Med.* 1999;20(1):89–105.

78. Gong H Jr, Salvatierra C. Clinical efficacy of early and delayed fiberoptic bronchoscopy in patients with hemoptysis. *Am Rev Respir Dis.* 1981;124(3):221–225.

79. Sakr L, Dutau H. Massive hemoptysis: an update on the role of bronchoscopy in diagnosis and management. *Respiration.* 2010;80(1):38–58.

80. Jackson CV, Savage PJ, Quinn DL. Role of fiberoptic bronchoscopy in patients with hemoptysis and a normal chest roentgenogram. *Chest.* 1985;87(2):142–144.

81. Feinsilver SH, Fein AM, Niederman MS, Schultz DE, Faegenburg DH. Utility of fiberoptic bronchoscopy in nonresolving pneumonia. *Chest.* 1990;98(6):1322–1326.

82. Kuru T, Lynch JP 3rd. Nonresolving or slowly resolving pneumonia. *Clin Chest Med.* 1999;20(3):623–651.

83. American Thoracic Society, Infectious Diseases Society of America. Guidelines for the management of adults with hospital-acquired, ventilator-associated, and healthcare-associated pneumonia. *Am J Respir Crit Care Med.* 2005;171(4): 388–416.

84. Chastre J, Fagon JY. Ventilator-associated pneumonia. *Am J Respir Crit Care Med.* 2002;165(7):867–903.

85. Koenig SM, Truwit JD. Ventilator-associated pneumonia: diagnosis, treatment, and prevention. *Clin Microbiol Rev.* 2006;19(4): 637–657.

86. Torres A, El-Ebiary M. Bronchoscopic BAL in the diagnosis of ventilator-associated pneumonia. *Chest.* 2000;117(4 Suppl 2): 198S–202S.

87. Kotloff RM, Ahya VN, Crawford SW. Pulmonary complications of solid organ and hematopoietic stem cell transplantation. *Am J Respir Crit Care Med.* 2004;170(1):22–48.

88. Broaddus C, Dake MD, Stulbarg MS, et al. Bronchoalveolar lavage and transbronchial biopsy for the diagnosis of pulmonary infections in the acquired immunodeficiency syndrome. *Ann Intern Med.* 1985;102(6):747–752.

89. Stover DE, Zaman MB, Hajdu SI, Lange M, Gold J, Armstrong D. Bronchoalveolar lavage in the diagnosis of diffuse pulmonary infiltrates in the immunosuppressed host. *Ann Intern Med.* 1984;101(1):1–7.

90. Campbell JH, Blessing N, Burnett AK, Stevenson RD. Investigation and management of pulmonary infiltrates following bone marrow transplantation: an eight year review. *Thorax.* 1993;48(12):1248–1251.

91. Dunagan DP, Baker AM, Hurd DD, Haponik EF. Bronchoscopic evaluation of pulmonary infiltrates following bone marrow transplantation. *Chest.* 1997;111(1):135–141.

92. Feinstein MB, Mokhtari M, Ferreiro R, Stover DE, Jakubowski A. Fiberoptic bronchoscopy in allogeneic bone marrow transplantation: findings in the era of serum cytomegalovirus antigen surveillance. *Chest.* 2001;120(4):1094–1100.

93. Milburn HJ, Prentice HG, du Bois RM. Role of bronchoalveolar lavage in the evaluation of interstitial pneumonitis in recipients of bone marrow transplants. *Thorax.* 1987;42(10):766–772.

94. Patel NR, Lee PS, Kim JH, Weinhouse GL, Koziel H. The influence of diagnostic bronchoscopy on clinical outcomes comparing adult autologous and allogeneic bone marrow transplant patients. *Chest.* 2005;127(4):1388–1396.

95. White P, Bonacum JT, Miller CB. Utility of fiberoptic bronchoscopy in bone marrow transplant patients. *Bone Marrow Transplant.* 1997;20(8):681–687.

96. Rano A, Agusti C, Jimenez P, et al. Pulmonary infiltrates in non-HIV immunocompromised patients: a diagnostic approach using non-invasive and bronchoscopic procedures. *Thorax.* 2001;56(5):379–387.

97. Jain P, Sandur S, Meli Y, Arroliga AC, Stoller JK, Mehta AC. Role of flexible bronchoscopy in immunocompromised patients with lung infiltrates. *Chest.* 2004;125(2):712–722.

98. Brodie D, Schluger NW. The diagnosis of tuberculosis. *Clin Chest Med.* 2005;26(2):247–271, vi.

99. Lin SM, Chung FT, Huang CD, et al. Diagnostic value of endobronchial ultrasonography for pulmonary tuberculosis. *J Thoracic Cardiovasc Surg.* 2009;138(1):179–184.

100. Jules-Elysee KM, Stover DE, Zaman MB, Bernard EM, White DA. Aerosolized pentamidine: effect on diagnosis and presentation of Pneumocystis carinii pneumonia. *Ann Intern Med.* 1990;112(10):750–757.

101. Read CA, Cerrone F, Busseniers AE, Waldhorn RE, Lavelle JP, Pierce PF. Differential lobe lavage for diagnosis of acute Pneumocystis carinii pneumonia in patients receiving prophylactic aerosolized pentamidine therapy. *Chest.* 1993;103(5): 1520–1523.

102. Baughman RP, Dohn MN, Shipley R, Buchsbaum JA, Frame PT. Increased Pneumocystis carinii recovery from the upper lobes in Pneumocystis pneumonia. The effect of aerosol pentamidine prophylaxis. *Chest.* 1993;103(2):426–432.

103. Costabel U, Ohshimo S, Guzman J. Diagnosis of sarcoidosis. *Curr Opin Pulm Med.* 2008;14(5):455–461.

104. Tournoy KG, Bolly A, Aerts JG, et al. The value of endoscopic ultrasound after bronchoscopy to diagnose thoracic sarcoidosis. *Eur Respir J.* 2010;35(6):1329–1335.

105. Agarwal R, Aggarwal AN, Gupta D. Efficacy and safety of conventional TBNA in sarcoidosis: a systematic review and meta-analysis. *Respir Care.* 2012;58(4):683–693.

106. Garwood S, Judson MA, Silvestri G, Hoda R, Fraig M, Doelken P. Endobronchial ultrasound for the diagnosis of pulmonary sarcoidosis. *Chest.* 2007;132(4):1298–1304.

107. Iwashita T, Yasuda I, Doi S, et al. The yield of endoscopic ultrasound-guided fine needle aspiration for histological diagnosis in patients suspected of stage I sarcoidosis. *Endoscopy.* 2008;40(5):400–405.

108. Oki M, Saka H, Kitagawa C, et al. Real-time endobronchial ultrasound-guided transbronchial needle aspiration is useful for diagnosing sarcoidosis. *Respirology.* 2007;12(6):863–868.

109. Tournoy KG, Annema JT, Krasnik M, Herth FJ, van Meerbeeck JP. Endoscopic and endobronchial ultrasonography according to the proposed lymph node map definition in the seventh edition of the tumor, node, metastasis classification for lung cancer. *J Thorac Oncol.* 2009;4(12):1576–1584.

110. Wong M, Yasufuku K, Nakajima T, et al. Endobronchial ultrasound: new insight for the diagnosis of sarcoidosis. *Eur Respir J.* 2007;29(6):1182–1186.

111. von Bartheld MB, Dekkers OM, Szlubowski A, et al. Endosonography vs conventional bronchoscopy for the diagnosis of sarcoidosis: the GRANULOMA randomized clinical trial. *JAMA.* 2013;309(23):2457–2464.

112. Raghu G, Collard HR, Egan JJ, et al. An official ATS/ERS/JRS/ALAT statement: idiopathic pulmonary fibrosis: evidence-based guidelines for diagnosis and management. *Am J Respir Crit Care Med.* 2011;183(6):788–824.

113. Epstein SK, Winslow CJ, Brecher SM, Faling LJ. Polymicrobial bacterial pericarditis after transbronchial needle aspiration.

Case report with an investigation on the risk of bacterial contamination during fiberoptic bronchoscopy. *Am Rev Respir Disease*. 1992;146(2):523–525.

114. Haas AR. Infectious complications from full extension endobronchial ultrasound transbronchial needle aspiration. *Eur Respir J*. 2009;33(4):935–938.

115. Andersen HA. Transbronchoscopic lung biopsy for diffuse pulmonary diseases. Results in 939 patients. *Chest*. 1978;73(5 Suppl):734–736.

116. Asano F, Aoe M, Ohsaki Y, et al. Deaths and complications associated with respiratory endoscopy: a survey by the Japan Society for Respiratory Endoscopy in 2010. *Respirology*. 2012;17(3):478–485.

117. Herf SM, Suratt PM. Complications of transbronchial lung biopsies. *Chest*. 1978;73(5 Suppl):759–760.

118. Hernandez Blasco L, Sanchez Hernandez IM, Villena Garrido V, de Miguel Poch E, Nunez Delgado M, Alfaro Abreu J. Safety of the transbronchial biopsy in outpatients. *Chest*. 1991;99(3):562–565.

119. Hopkins PM, Aboyoun CL, Chhajed PN, et al. Prospective analysis of 1,235 transbronchial lung biopsies in lung transplant recipients. *J Heart Lung Transplant*. 2002;21(10):1062–1067.

120. Izbicki G, Shitrit D, Yarmolovsky A, et al. Is routine chest radiography after transbronchial biopsy necessary?: A prospective study of 350 cases. *Chest*. 2006;129(6):1561–1564.

121. O'Brien JD, Ettinger NA, Shevlin D, Kollef MH. Safety and yield of transbronchial biopsy in mechanically ventilated patients. *Crit Care Med*. 1997;25(3):440–446.

122. Simpson FG, Arnold AG, Purvis A, Belfield PW, Muers MF, Cooke NJ. Postal survey of bronchoscopic practice by physicians in the United Kingdom. *Thorax*. 1986;41(4):311–317.

123. Facciolongo N, Patelli M, Gasparini S, et al. Incidence of complications in bronchoscopy. Multicentre prospective study of 20,986 bronchoscopies. *Monaldi Arch Chest Dis*. 2009;71(1):8–14.

124. Tukey MH, Wiener RS. Population-based estimates of transbronchial lung biopsy utilization and complications. *Respir Med*. 2012;106(11):1559–1565.

125. Anders GT, Johnson JE, Bush BA, Matthews JI. Transbronchial biopsy without fluoroscopy. A seven-year perspective. *Chest*. 1988;94(3):557–560.

126. Cordasco EM Jr, Mehta AC, Ahmad M. Bronchoscopically induced bleeding. A summary of nine years' Cleveland clinic experience and review of the literature. *Chest*. 1991;100(4):1141–1147.

127. Wahidi MM, Rocha AT, Hollingsworth JW, Govert JA, Feller-Kopman D, Ernst A. Contraindications and safety of transbronchial lung biopsy via flexible bronchoscopy. A survey of pulmonologists and review of the literature. *Respiration*. 2005;72(3):285–295.

128. Herth FJ, Becker HD, Ernst A. Aspirin does not increase bleeding complications after transbronchial biopsy. *Chest*. 2002;122(4):1461–1464.

129. Ernst A, Eberhardt R, Wahidi M, Becker HD, Herth FJ. Effect of routine clopidogrel use on bleeding complications after transbronchial biopsy in humans. *Chest*. 2006;129(3):734–737.

130. Chang YC, Yu CJ, Lee WJ, et al. Imprint cytology improves accuracy of computed tomography-guided percutaneous transthoracic needle biopsy. *Eur Respir J*. 2008;31(1):54–61.

131. De Filippo M, Onniboni M, Rusca M, et al. Advantages of multidetector-row CT with multiplanar reformation in guiding percutaneous lung biopsies. *Radiol Med*. 2008;113(7):945–953.

132. Gupta S, Krishnamurthy S, Broemeling LD, et al. Small (</ = 2-cm) subpleural pulmonary lesions: short- versus long-needle-path CT-guided Biopsy–comparison of diagnostic yields and complications. *Radiology*. 2005;234(2):631–637.

133. Hiraki T, Mimura H, Gobara H, et al. Incidence of and risk factors for pneumothorax and chest tube placement after CT fluoroscopy-guided percutaneous lung biopsy: retrospective analysis of the procedures conducted over a 9-year period. *AJR Am J Roentgenol*. 2010;194(3):809–814.

134. Khan MF, Straub R, Moghaddam SR, et al. Variables affecting the risk of pneumothorax and intrapulmonal hemorrhage in CT-guided transthoracic biopsy. *Eur Radiol*. 2008;18(7):1356–1363.

135. Kothary N, Lock L, Sze DY, Hofmann LV. Computed tomography-guided percutaneous needle biopsy of pulmonary nodules: impact of nodule size on diagnostic accuracy. *Clin Lung Cancer*. 2009;10(5):360–363.

136. Satoh S, Ohdama S, Matsubara O, Okochi Y, Tanaka R, Kimula Y. CT-guided automated cutting needle biopsy by a combined method for accurate specific diagnosis of focal lung lesions. *Radiat Med*. 2005;23(1):30–36.

137. Schaefer PJ, Schaefer FK, Heller M, Jahnke T. CT fluoroscopy guided biopsy of small pulmonary and upper abdominal lesions: efficacy with a modified breathing technique. *J Vasc Interv Radiol*. 2007;18(10):1241–1248.

138. Yoshimatsu R, Yamagami T, Kato T, et al. Percutaneous needle biopsy of lung nodules under CT fluoroscopic guidance with use of the "I-I device." *Br J Radiol*. 2008;81(962):107–112.

139. Ng YL, Patsios D, Roberts H, et al. CT-guided percutaneous fine-needle aspiration biopsy of pulmonary nodules measuring 10 mm or less. *Clin Radiol*. 2008;63(3):272–277.

140. Birchard KR. Transthoracic needle biopsy. *Semin Intervent Radiol*. 2011;28(1):87–97.

141. Cham MD, Lane ME, Henschke CI, Yankelevitz DF. Lung biopsy: special techniques. *Semin Respir Crit Care Med*. 2008;29(4):335–349.

142. Kazerooni EA, Lim FT, Mikhail A, Martinez FJ. Risk of pneumothorax in CT-guided transthoracic needle aspiration biopsy of the lung. *Radiology*. 1996;198(2):371–375.

143. Li H, Boiselle PM, Shepard JO, Trotman-Dickenson B, McLoud TC. Diagnostic accuracy and safety of CT-guided percutaneous needle aspiration biopsy of the lung: comparison of small and large pulmonary nodules. *AJR Am J Roentgenol*. 1996;167(1):105–109.

144. Schreiber G, McCrory DC. Performance characteristics of different modalities for diagnosis of suspected lung cancer: summary of published evidence. *Chest*. 2003;123(1 Suppl):115S–128S.

145. Geraghty PR, Kee ST, McFarlane G, Razavi MK, Sze DY, Dake MD. CT-guided transthoracic needle aspiration biopsy of pulmonary nodules: needle size and pneumothorax rate. *Radiology*. 2003;229(2):475–481.

146. Ko JP, Shepard JO, Drucker EA, et al. Factors influencing pneumothorax rate at lung biopsy: are dwell time and angle of pleural puncture contributing factors? *Radiology*. 2001;218(2):491–496.

147. Laurent F, Michel P, Latrabe V, Tunon de Lara M, Marthan R. Pneumothoraces and chest tube placement after CT-guided transthoracic lung biopsy using a coaxial technique: incidence and risk factors. *AJR Am J Roentgenol*. 1999;172(4):1049–1053.

148. Poe RH, Kallay MC, Wicks CM, Odoroff CL. Predicting risk of pneumothorax in needle biopsy of the lung. *Chest*. 1984;85(2):232–235.

149. Cox JE, Chiles C, McManus CM, Aquino SL, Choplin RH. Transthoracic needle aspiration biopsy: variables that affect risk of pneumothorax. *Radiology*. 1999;212(1):165–168.

CHAPTER 36

Interventional Bronchoscopy

Andrew R. Haas
Daniel H. Sterman

INTRODUCTION

The first interventional bronchoscopy (also referred to as therapeutic bronchoscopy throughout this chapter) was performed by Gustav Killian in 1897 when he removed a pork bone from the right mainstem bronchus of a patient. For nearly 70 years bronchoscopy was predominantly a therapeutic procedure performed for foreign body extraction. Two events shifted the landscape of bronchoscopy—the lung cancer epidemic and the development of flexible bronchoscopy by Shigeto Ikeda in 1967. Following an escalation in lung cancer incidence, malignant airway obstruction requiring therapeutic intervention became much more common than foreign body extraction. As a result, new tools were developed to address malignant airway obstruction based upon a minimally invasive bronchoscopic approach. In addition, bronchoscopy-based technology has been developed to address chronic obstructive pulmonary disease (COPD) and asthma. Application of the technology has entered clinical trials and may alter the therapeutic options for these diseases processes. This chapter presents an overview of interventional bronchoscopy modalities that can be utilized for benign and malignant airway obstruction, COPD, and asthma.

INDICATIONS FOR INTERVENTIONAL BRONCHOSCOPY

Many potential indications for interventional bronchoscopy have been recognized, including malignant airway obstruction, benign airway obstruction, and foreign body extraction, among others. (Table 36-1). The majority of therapeutic bronchoscopies performed today are undertaken for management of malignant airway obstruction, most commonly from lung cancer. It is estimated that up to 40% of patients with lung cancer develop symptomatic airway obstruction at some point during their disease process. Although lung cancer is the most common source of malignant airway obstruction, any primary thoracic malignancy, or any malignancy with pulmonary metastases, may result in symptomatic airway obstruction. Regaining airway patency to palliate symptomatic dyspnea and other respiratory symptoms may have significant impact on the quality of life of patients with advanced malignancy.

Benign airway obstruction etiologies are listed in Table 36-2 and consist of a variety of localized inflammatory and systemic conditions. Although the etiologic airway process is benign and not malignant, the interventions and management of these complex processes is far from benign to the patient. Interventional bronchoscopy techniques can often correct the presenting symptoms; however, the stenosis and symptoms often recur and patients may require repeat procedures to maintain airway patency. Selected patients may need to proceed with airway resection of the benign stenotic airway segment.[1]

Most patients with airway obstruction have clinical symptoms; dyspnea as the most common patient complaint. Depending on the rapidity of airway obstruction, dyspnea may have a rapid onset, or more commonly, an insidious evolution that gradually limits the patient activities. It is not uncommon for a family member to recognize this limitation more readily than the patient. As the airway obstruction worsens, the patient may begin to have orthopnea, which is a harbinger of an evolving critical airway obstruction. Other symptoms, such as cough, inability to clear secretions, chest discomfort, or fever from post obstructive pneumonia may develop. Early intervention is important to prevent worsening respiratory compromise or death.

SPECIAL CONSIDERATIONS FOR PATIENT PREPARATION, SEDATION, AND MONITORING

All patients undergoing bronchoscopy should undergo a complete pre-bronchoscopy evaluation, including a medical history, physical examination, and chest imaging. Although routine laboratory tests are not required, each evaluation should be individualized on the basis of patients' underlying conditions and therapeutic procedures planned. CT scan is important to assess the degree of airway involvement and to plan interventions to be undertaken.

Sedation and analgesia for patients undergoing interventional bronchoscopy must be considered carefully. Stable patients who can lay flat without distress can undergo bronchoscopy with moderate sedation. Should the patient have moderate or severe respiratory distress or be unable to lay flat, strong consideration should be given to additional monitoring or anesthesiology procedural assistance. Patients with high oxygen requirements may require endotracheal intubation to reduce the risk of developing hypoxemic respiratory failure during moderate sedation. Moreover, if patients are unable to lie flat, they may require an initial upright bronchoscopy under minimal sedation to temporize luminal diameter before undergoing general anesthesia and more definitive interventional bronchoscopy.

Similar to diagnostic bronchoscopy, if a patient is stable for moderate sedation, topical analgesia of the oropharynx and airways should be achieved with lidocaine, followed by administration of a combination of a short-acting benzodiazepine (e.g., midazolam) and a narcotic (e.g., fentanyl).[2] Rigid bronchoscopy is most safely

TABLE 36-1 Indications for Interventional Bronchoscopy

Hemoptysis
Atelectasis from inspissated secretions
Foreign body removal
Tracheobronchial tree neoplasms (primary or metastatic)
Direct bronchoscopic debulking
Laser therapy
Electrocautery/Argon plasma coagulation
Cryotherapy
Brachytherapy
Photodynamic therapy
Stent placement
Airway strictures and stenoses
Rigid bronchoscopic dilation
Stricture/stenosis incision
Balloon tracheobronchoplasty dilation
Stent replacement
Lung lavage (pulmonary alveolar proteinosis)
Bronchoscopic drainage—lung abscess
Endotracheal tube and percutaneous tracheostomy placement
Treatment of persistent air leak
Evolving therapies for emphysema
Bronchial thermoplasty in severe asthma

TABLE 36-2 Etiologies of Benign Tracheobronchial Stenosis

Endotracheal intubation
Tracheostomy tube
Granulomatosis with polyangiitis (formerly known as Wegener granulomatosis)
Amyloidosis
Sarcoidosis
Tuberculosis
Inflammatory bowel disease
Idiopathic
Trauma
Lung transplantation
Post resection or airway repair
Trauma
Recurrent stenosis after prior stenosis resection
Sleeve resection
External beam radiotherapy or high dose-rate brachytherapy (HDRB)
Photodynamic therapy
Thermal injury from fire exposure
Tracheobronchopathia osteochondroplastica
Postpneumonectomy syndrome
Fibrosing mediastinitis
Large vascular aneurysms

performed with a patient receiving general anesthesia and breathing spontaneously or being ventilated with a jet ventilator.[3] General anesthesia with inhaled anesthetics (e.g., sevoflurane) should be avoided in favor of total intravenous anesthesia in order to avoid exposure of the bronchoscopist to inhaled anesthetics when the ventilator circuit is open. With appropriate planning and monitoring, the vast majority of patients can undergo interventional bronchoscopy with low complication rates.

TYPES OF AIRWAY OBSTRUCTION

Figure 36-1 demonstrates the three main types of airway obstruction that may be encountered: purely intrinsic (A), purely extrinsic (B), or a combination of both intrinsic and extrinsic airway obstruction (C). Attention to preprocedural CT scan imaging allows fairly accurate assessment of these components and permits the therapeutic bronchoscopist to plan an approach. For lesions that are purely intrinsic, direct bronchoscopic debulking with rigid bronchoscopy, thermal ablation, or snare extraction, with or without stent placement, is appropriate. For purely extrinsic lesions, no tumor is present to debulk, and modalities used in purely intrinsic disease cannot be employed because of the risk of airway perforation. Extrinsic lesions are most amenable to balloon bronchoplastic dilatation and endoluminal stent placement. For mixed intrinsic–extrinsic lesions, all tumor removal modalities, as well as dilatation and stent placement, are feasible.

ENDOLUMINAL AIRWAY OBSTRUCTION

Endoluminal obstruction of the tracheobronchial tree may result from various benign and malignant processes. The most common cause of endobronchial obstruction is advanced lung carcinoma. In patients with inoperable central airway tumors, restoration of airway patency may provide palliation and may even prolong life, particularly in the case of impending respiratory failure or postobstructive pneumonia.

Signs and symptoms of central malignant airway obstruction vary, but often include progressive dyspnea and functional limitation, wheezing, cough, stridor, hoarseness, hemoptysis, and chest pain. A careful pretreatment evaluation should be performed to distinguish symptoms attributable to focal tracheobronchial lesions from those related to underlying obstructive lung disease, parenchymal lung disease, or both. Although pulmonary function testing and thoracic imaging techniques, such as chest CT, may be useful in the evaluation of a patient with suspected malignant airway obstruction, bronchoscopy, either rigid or flexible, remains the diagnostic and therapeutic "gold standard." Increasingly, however, three-dimensional reconstruction CT imaging, so-called "virtual bronchoscopy," is being applied as a reliable noninvasive method of assessing the nature and extent of malignant airway obstruction, thereby allowing preprocedural intervention planning.

The bronchoscopic approach to management of malignant airway obstruction depends on the lesion location, presence or absence of associated extrinsic compression, and degree of clinical urgency. Rigid bronchoscopic debulking using adjunctive thermal ablation is recommended when airway recanalization must be performed on an emergency basis. If endobronchial obstruction is accompanied by marked extrinsic compression, stent placement may be beneficial.

The complexity of a lesion is equally important in determining the best approach to therapeutic bronchoscopy. Benign tracheal webs often are managed using laser or electrocautery-mediated resection alone, whereas complex fibrotic strictures may warrant the combination of rigid bronchoscopic or balloon dilation, thermal incision, and stent placement. For focal tracheal stenosis in patients at low risk for complications, surgical resection with primary reanastomosis should remain the treatment of choice.

EXTRINSIC AIRWAY COMPRESSION

Extrinsic airway compression usually results from malignant involvement of structures adjacent to the central airways, such as mediastinal lymph nodes or the esophagus, but it may be associated with a benign process, such as fibrosing mediastinitis, tuberculosis, aneurysmal dilatation of the aorta, or sarcoidosis. The clinical signs and symptoms of extrinsic airway compression often mimic those of endobronchial obstruction. The diagnosis is established on the basis of bronchoscopic detection of marked airway narrowing in the absence of an endoluminal mass.

Therapeutic options in the management of extrinsic airway compression are limited. Ablative endoscopic approaches, such as laser therapy, cryotherapy, PDT, and electrocautery are contraindicated because of the lack of demonstrable benefit and risk of airway perforation. Although some patients with malignant disease may benefit from endobronchial brachytherapy, tracheobronchial stent placement is the palliative treatment of choice for patients with symptomatic extrinsic airway compression.

TYPES OF THERAPEUTIC BRONCHOSCOPY INTERVENTIONS

A wide variety of therapeutic bronchoscopic interventions may be offered. Each is described in subsequent sections.

RIGID BRONCHOSCOPY

The initial bronchoscope, developed by Killian, and further optimized by Chevalier Jackson, was a rigid metal tube that permitted either spontaneous or mechanical ventilation.[4] Over the decades, rigid bronchoscopes of various lengths and sizes that are adaptable for diverse applications in children and adults have become available. Although the flexible bronchoscope has, to a large extent, replaced the rigid scope for most diagnostic and some therapeutic indications, rigid bronchoscopy still has vital therapeutic applications.

Modern rigid bronchoscopy systems are equipped with optical capabilities to allow better direct, magnified, circumferential

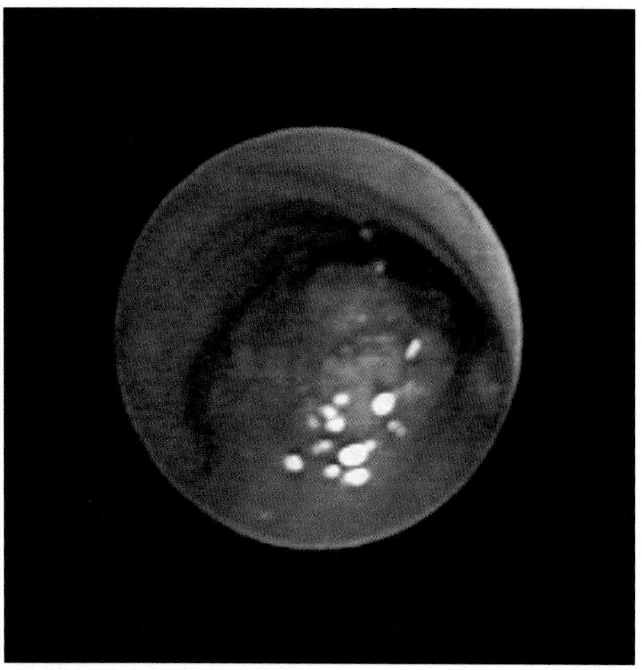
A

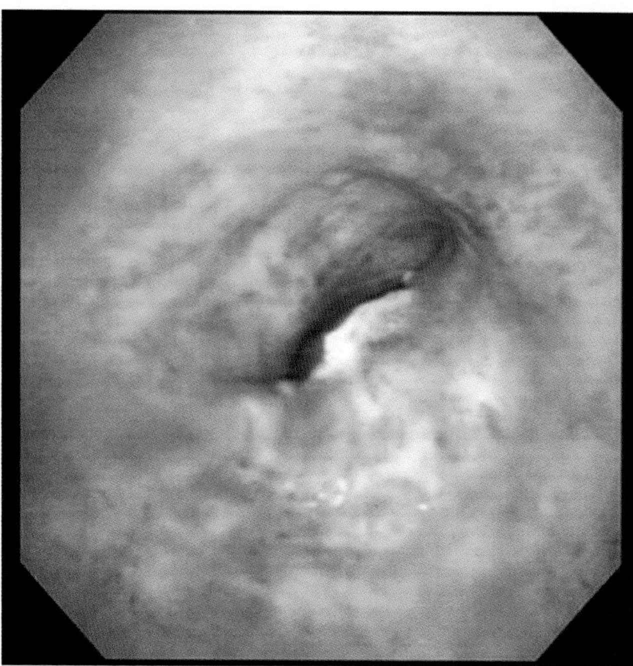
B

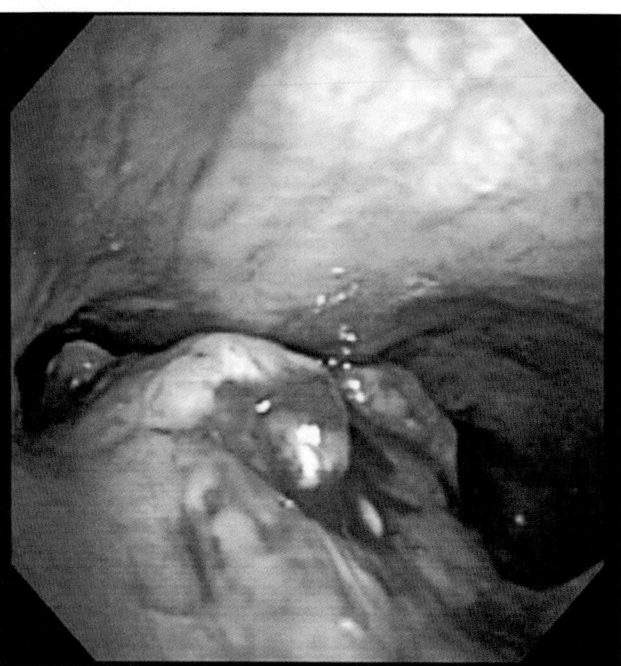
C

Figure 36-1 Types of airway compression. Intrinsic (**A**). Extrinsic (**B**). Mixed intrinsic and extrinsic (**C**).

illumination and visualization. The main advantage of rigid bronchoscopy over flexible bronchoscopy is its luminal working diameter, which allows multiple therapeutic instruments to be utilized simultaneously while ventilating the patient. Rigid bronchoscopy allows a number of therapies, such as laser photocoagulation, placement of endobronchial stents, balloon dilation, electrocautery, argon beam coagulation, and cryotherapy to be performed safely and effectively. Perhaps most importantly, in the setting of malignant airway disease or obstruction, a rigid bronchoscope can be used to "core out" large bulky airway tumors more efficiently and effectively than any thermal modalities (Video 36-1). Initial rigid bronchoscopic debulking, followed by thermal modality ablation to cauterize remaining tumor is common.[5] For benign, fibrotic airway stenosis, the rigid bronchoscope becomes a very effective modality to partially debulk stenotic tissue and to dilate the stenosis.[6] In experienced centers, rigid bronchoscopic airway recanalization remains the treatment of choice for serious or life-threatening tracheobronchial obstruction.

The main complication from rigid bronchoscopy is dental injury from the scope cracking or fracturing teeth. Other complications, such as oropharyngeal laceration, arytenoid cartilage disarticulation, or vocal cord injury, are possible. Meticulous care upon rigid

Video 36-1 A patient with a right paratracheal mass who underwent diagnostic and therapeutic bronchoscopy. Endoluminal tumor growth was present along the right lateral tracheal wall. The video demonstrates effective and efficient use of rigid bronchoscopy to mechanically debride tumor. *Access at www.fishmansonline.com*

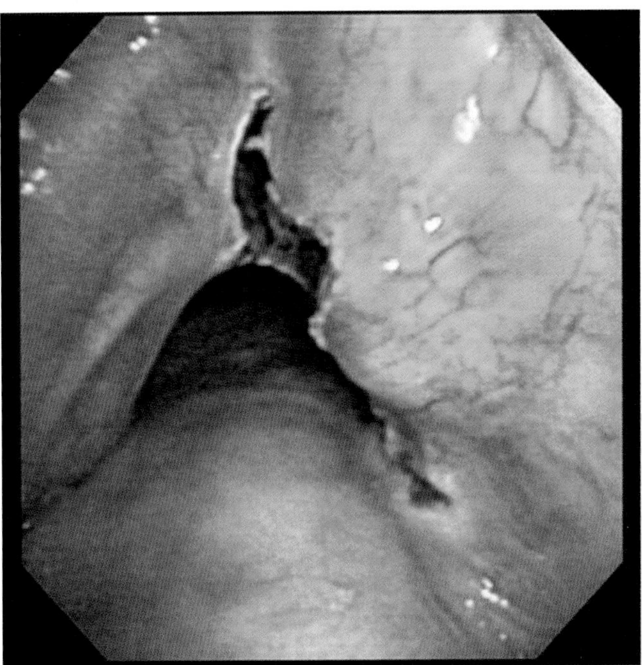

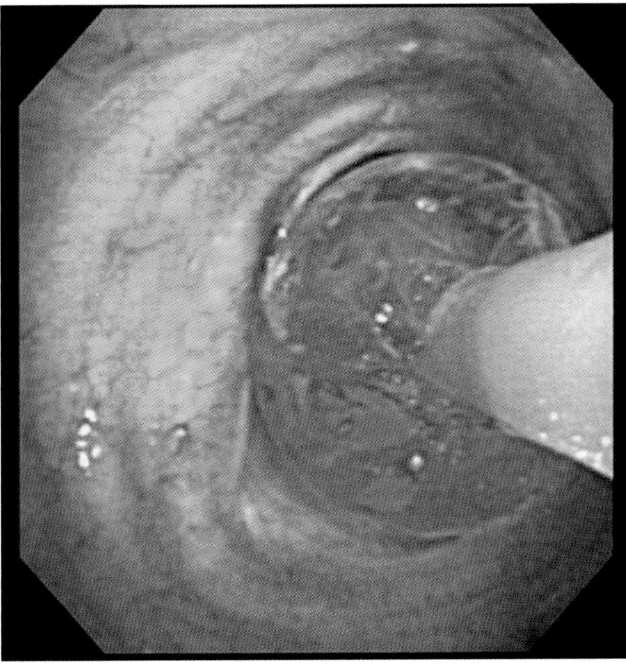

A B

Figure 36-2 Electrocautery incisions were made into the benign stenotic lesion (**A**). Following incision, balloon bronchoplasty dilatation was performed (**B**).

bronchoscope intubation is critical to avoid these possible complications. Intrathoracic complications, such as airway perforation, major bleeding from tumor debulking, and pneumothorax or pneumomediastinum are also possible but are infrequent in experienced hands.

BALLOON TRACHEOBRONCHOPLASTY

Balloon dilatation has become an attractive alternative to rigid bronchoscopy for management of airway obstruction in benign and malignant airway obstruction, especially in anatomic locations where a rigid bronchoscope cannot enter or the luminal diameter is too narrow to allow safe rigid bronchoscope passage. High-pressure balloons of various lengths and diameters specifically designed for the tracheobronchial tree are readily available. These balloons are filled with saline or radio-opaque contrast media, advanced to the site of interest through the bronchoscope, and inflated until the desired diameter is attained.

In the setting of benign stenosis, an initial defect in the stenosis is often made with a thermal modality so as to control the stenotic release point (Fig. 36-2). This approach has been used successfully in benign stenoses from endobronchial tuberculosis, idiopathic subglottic stenosis, and post-transplant anastomotic strictures.[7] It is less successful when used alone to treat airway compromise accompanied by extrinsic airway compression, as the initial bronchoscopic improvement often rapidly returns to its original position as the extrinsic process persists. Complications of balloon tracheobronchoplasty include bronchospasm, chest pain, mucosal laceration, airway perforation, bleeding, postprocedure airway edema, pneumothorax, and pneumomediastinum.

BRONCHOSCOPIC LASER THERAPY

Perhaps the most widely known technique in therapeutic bronchoscopy is laser photocoagulation or photoablation. Table 36-3

TABLE 36-3 Therapeutic Bronchoscopy Ablation Modalities

Therapy	Type of Lesion Therapy	Type of Bronchoscope	Rapidity of Positive Result	Repeatability
Mechanical debridement	Endoluminal or submucosal	Rigid or flexible (rigid preferable)	++++	+
Laser	Endoluminal	Rigid or flexible (rigid preferable)	++++	++++
Argon plasma	Endoluminal	Rigid or flexible	++++	++++
Brachytherapy	Endoluminal or submucosal	Flexible	+	+
Cryotherapy	Endoluminal	Rigid or flexible	++	+++
Balloon dilation	Endoluminal or submucosal with extraluminal compression	Rigid or flexible (rigid preferable)	++++	++++
Photodynamic therapy	Endoluminal	Flexible	++	+++
Electrocautery	Endoluminal	Rigid or flexible	+++	++++
Stent	Endoluminal with extraluminal compression	Rigid or flexible (Dumon stent requires rigid bronchoscope; Wall stents and Gianturco stents require fluoroscopy)	++++	+++

Video 36-2 A patient who presented with a new right mainstem obstruction from lung cancer. The video shows Nd:YAG tumor coagulation and debulking. *Access at www.fishmansonline.com*

Video 36-3 A patient with a history of renal cell carcinoma who presented with dyspnea and left lung atelectasis. CT scan demonstrated left mainstem bronchus obstruction. The video shows a rigid bronchoscopy with electrocautery snare excision and removal of a large polypoid renal carcinoma metastasis. The point of airway attachment was then cauterized using electrocautery. *Access at www.fishmansonline.com*

compares characteristics of the laser modality compared with other modalities to be presented later. Lasers produce a beam of monochromatic, coherent light that induces tissue vaporization, coagulation, hemostasis, and necrosis. Although primarily useful in endoluminal malignant tumor ablation, bronchoscopic laser therapy also is beneficial in other tracheobronchial disorders, including inflammatory strictures, obstructive granulation tissue, amyloidosis, and benign tumors, such as hamartomas and lipomas.

Since the initial report of endobronchial laser ablation of an obstructive neoplasm by Laforet in 1976, several types of lasers have become available for management of tracheobronchial obstruction.[8] The carbon dioxide (CO_2) laser, used primarily by otolaryngologists, allows shallow tissue penetration (to a depth of 0.1–0.5 mm) and very precise cutting, but it has minimal hemostatic properties. With the development of other laser modalities, the CO_2 laser has minimal current application in endobronchial tumor ablation, and its role remains primarily in management of laryngeal lesions.

For therapeutic bronchoscopy, neodymium:yttrium-aluminum-garnet (Nd:YAG) laser ablation is most commonly used (Video 36-2). It provides tissue penetration to a depth of 3 to 5 mm, superior coagulation and improved hemostasis, but at the cost of less cutting precision. Nd:YAG laser procedures may be performed through a rigid or flexible bronchoscope. Success rates and complications directly related to laser therapy are not different when the procedure is performed through a rigid bronchoscope with the patient under general anesthesia, or through a flexible bronchoscope with use of topical anesthesia and moderate sedation.

Use of Nd:YAG laser photoablation therapy as a single modality is associated with a recanalization rate >90% for endobronchial obstruction of large central airways; however, it is less successful in treating peripheral lesions or extrinsic airway compression.[9,10] Nd:YAG laser photocoagulation may be an important treatment tool for patients with airway obstruction caused by benign endoluminal tumors. The Nd:Yap (yttrium-aluminum-perovskite) laser, with a patented wavelength of 1.34 μ wavelength, is purported to have better water absorption at that wavelength, improving the power-to-effective ratio compared with traditional Nd:YAG laser and carrying a lower complication risk.

Although endobronchial laser therapy generally is safe and well tolerated, it may be complicated by cardiac arrhythmias, airway perforation, pneumothorax, hemorrhage, hypoxemia, or endobronchial fire.[11,12] Endoluminal laser utilization requires careful consideration of the lesion anatomic location and configuration relative to vital intrathoracic structures. If the lesion is in close proximity to the esophagus or pulmonary artery, endobronchial laser therapy carries risk for fistula formation. Laser therapy in a patient with tracheobronchial narrowing caused by extrinsic compression may result in airway perforation. In rare cases, pulmonary edema or fatal pulmonary venous gas embolism have been reported.[13] Patients with standard silicone endotracheal tubes or silicone tracheobronchial stents, and those who require high concentrations of supplemental oxygen, are at increased risk for endobronchial fire. The bronchoscopist needs to ensure the inspired oxygen level is, ideally, <40%, especially if the patient is receiving mechanical ventilator support during the procedure. Fortunately, the overall risk of endobronchial fire is <0.1%.

ENDOBRONCHIAL ELECTROCAUTERY AND CRYOTHERAPY

Electrocautery and cryotherapy are cost-effective alternatives to laser therapy for the management of tracheobronchial lesions and obstruction, as equipment expenses are substantially less compared to laser therapy. Penetration depth and per treatment effectiveness may be less than with laser therapy.

As with the Nd:YAG laser, both electrocautery and cryotherapy may be administered through either a rigid or flexible bronchoscope. Electrocautery effects on tissue are similar to those of Nd:YAG laser, with tissue destruction induced by coagulative necrosis (Video 36-3). Argon plasma coagulation (APC) is similar to electrocautery except that it uses argon gas to conduct the electrical current rather than a contact probe. Electrocautery and APC have a 1- to 3-mm penetration depth and are, therefore, more suitable for the treatment of superficial and spreading lesions (Video 36-4).

In contrast with electrocautery or APC, cryotherapy induces tissue necrosis through hypothermic intracellular crystallization and microthrombosis. Specially designed cryoprobes are inserted through the bronchoscope until they contact target tissue. Cryoprobe activation introduces liquid nitrous oxide or liquid nitrogen through a small orifice in the probe under pressure, resulting in rapid cryoprobe cooling with creation of an "ice ball" (approximate temperature, 20°C) at the probe tip on target tissue. This freezing effect is maintained for approximately 20 seconds; the area is then allowed to thaw, and freezing is repeated 2 to 3 times to achieve necrosis by cellular rupture from repeated cycles of intracellular micro-crystallization.

Electrocautery, APC, and cryotherapy have been used successfully to relieve airway obstruction and treat hemoptysis caused by benign and malignant tracheobronchial tumors, polyps, and granulation tissue.[5,9,14-19] These modalities have been used effectively in radiographically occult mucosal lung cancer, carcinoma in situ, and mucosal dysplasia. Cryotherapy may be advantageous in cryoextraction of foreign bodies that can be frozen to the probe and removed.[20] This technique works very well for mucoid plugs or blood clots in large airways where other modalities may be associated with some difficulty in successful removal. Due to the repeat treatment cycles needed to achieve effect, cryotherapy is not ideal for efficient relief of symptomatic airway obstruction.

Although the range of complications from electrocautery and cryotherapy are the same as those discussed for laser therapy, the most common complication of each is bleeding secondary to disruption of endobronchial tumor without full-tissue coagulation. The estimated incidence of clinically significant bleeding in patients treated with electrocautery is 2.5%. Rarely, gas embolism can occur with APC.[21,22]

ENDOBRONCHIAL BRACHYTHERAPY

Endobronchial brachytherapy refers to bronchoscopic radiation delivery to a localized airway lesion; it is often referred to as high dose-rate brachytherapy (HDRB) due to high radiation dosage delivery to a focused area. The technique aims to delivery therapeutic radiation to localized lesions while minimizing risk to nontarget tissues.

Video 36-4 This patient had a prior bronchoscopy for minor hemoptysis; endobronchial biopsies demonstrated carcinoma in situ. The video demonstrates argon plasma coagulation ablation of the involved sites from prior biopsies. *Access at www.fishmansonline.com*

Endobronchial brachytherapy involves the bronchoscopic insertion of a thin, hollow "afterloading" catheter across an area of interest (usually malignant) under direct bronchoscopic and fluoroscopic guidance. The catheter is left in place and the patient travels to a radiation oncology department where radioactive beads are inserted into the catheter at the desired location for a predetermined period, depending on the dose rate.

Relief of airway obstruction is the primary goal of HDRB, although curative treatment may be attempted in more advanced lesions by combining HDRB with external beam irradiation in selected patients. HDRB is not effective for rapid airway recanalization due to its delay in response of 14 to 21 days. It is best used as an adjunct to rigid bronchoscopy with or without thermal tumor ablation, endobronchial stent placement, or conventional external beam irradiation to recanalize an obstructed airway. HDRB appears safest and most effective for management of central airway lesions. Among patients with malignant airway obstruction, recanalization rates range from 60% to 90%, with decreased dyspnea, cessation of hemoptysis, and relief of cough in most cases.[16,23,24] HDRB has also been shown to be effective for radiographically occult, minimally invasive cancer in central airways, CIS, or mucosal dysplasia. Moreover, reports of the utility of HDRB in management of benign granulation tissue in lung transplant recipients or patients with or subglottic stenosis have been reported.[25–27]

Serious complications of HDRB can occur, particularly massive hemoptysis, from bronchovascular fistula formation secondary to necrosis of the airway wall and adjacent vascular structures. Because of the risk of fatal hemorrhage, every effort should be made to rule out central vascular tumor involvement before application of HDRB.

■ PHOTODYNAMIC THERAPY

Photodynamic therapy (PDT) currently is FDA-approved for palliation of malignant airway obstruction and as an alternative to surgery in selected patients with minimally invasive central lung cancer or CIS. PDT works on the principle that certain compounds, such as hematoporphyrin derivatives or aminolevulinic acid (ALA), function as photosensitizing agents, rendering malignant cells susceptible to damage from monochromatic light. Tumor necrosis occurs as a result of oxygen free radical formation and ischemic vasculature necrosis mediated by thromboxane A_2 release.

The selective PDT effect on malignant cells is thought to be due to greater photosensitizing agent uptake and retention in neoplastic cells compared with normal cells; the exception is reticuloendothelial cells, particularly those in the skin. The relative tumor selectivity is most pronounced within 24 to 48 hours after photosensitizing agent infusion; therefore, treatment of the bronchoscopically targeted lesion should be performed within that time frame. Maximal tissue necrosis occurs 24 to 48 hours after light administration and requires repeat bronchoscopy to debride the necrotic and sloughed area treated. Due to the delayed onset of PDT action, it is not useful in patients with acute respiratory distress from evolving airway obstruction.

Ideal candidates for PDT include patients with airway obstruction caused by malignant endobronchial masses with minimal extrinsic airway compression, and patients with minimally invasive central airway tumors. Although surgical resection remains the treatment of choice for early lung cancer, some patients refuse surgery or have tumors that are deemed inoperable because of high surgical risk. In these cases, PDT may represent an appropriate alternative. Response rates are highest in patients with small tumors and minimal airway penetration depth.[28,29] In patients with bulky tumors, endobronchial PDT may substantially reduce the obstruction, with objective increases in spirometric measurements and subjective improvement in dyspnea and quality of life; however, treatment is not curative.[30] Endoluminal metastatic tumors may also be treated successfully with PDT.

Complications of PDT include increased skin photosensitivity and hemoptysis resulting from extensive tumor necrosis into a vascular structure. Cutaneous photosensitivity, similar to a sunburn, occurs in up to 20% of patients in various reported series; it may be obviated by adequate sunlight precautions. Sensitivity to sunlight after photosensitizer administration may persist for 6 weeks or longer.

■ TRACHEOBRONCHIAL STENTING

The medical term, "stent" refers to any device designed to maintain the integrity of hollow tubular structures, such as the airways, coronary arteries, or esophagus. Anecdotal reports of attempts to implant stents in the tracheobronchial tree date back to 1915. The Montgomery T-tube, designed in the 1960s, was the first reliable, dedicated airway stent.[31] However, stent implantation in the lower trachea and bronchi did not become standard medical practice until 1990, when Jean Francois Dumon reported the safety and ease of placement of a dedicated silicone airway stent.[32]

Two main types of endobronchial stents are in use today—silicone or self-expanding metal (SEMS). Silicone stents generally are placed by rigid bronchoscopy with the patient under general anesthesia. Silicone stents are relatively inexpensive (~$500 USD) compared with SEMSs (~$2000 USD). Bifurcated silicone stents also are available and have been effectively used in the management of carinal compression associated with malignant tumors, tracheoesophageal fistulas, and tracheobronchomalacia.

Unlike silicone stents, SEMSs may be placed using flexible bronchoscopy and require less technical rigor than silicone stent placement. The main limitation with SEMS is that uncovered varieties may induce mucosal inflammation and granulation tissue formation which may require repeat endoscopic intervention to maintain airway patency.[33–35] For this reason, SEMSs have an FDA black-box warning against their utilization in *benign* airway stenosis, unless all other treatment options, including silicone stenting, have been explored and failed. An exception to this warning applies in bronchial anastomotic dehiscence in lung transplantation. In this setting, insertion of a temporary uncovered SEMS across the dehiscence exploits the fact that focal granulation tissue may develop and promote dehiscence closure.[36]

Endobronchial stents have a critical role in multimodality bronchoscopic approaches to both benign and malignant airway obstruction. Airway obstruction caused by locally advanced lung carcinoma may be treated with a combination of thermal tumor ablation and stent implantation to regain and preserve airway lumen diameter by preventing tumor ingrowth (Fig. 36-3). Stent placement may be combined with balloon dilatation in the endoscopic management of benign fibrotic strictures. Most large studies of endobronchial stent placement have demonstrated impressive efficacy.

Dumon and colleagues reported excellent clinical outcomes and few complications with silicone stent placement in patients with malignant airway obstruction; a lower success rate was noted among patients with tracheal stenosis caused by other disorders.[32] Success, broadly defined as symptomatic relief, in limited studies has been reported to be achieved in between 78% and 98%, although none of the early trials used objective measures to determine efficacy.[37–39] In a small study in patients who were intubated because of respiratory failure secondary to unresectable tracheobronchial and mediastinal disease, stent placement facilitated extubation in most.[40] Stent placement benefits seem to persist in patients who survive for a period of several months or years after stent implantation. Long-term follow-up data are derived from patients with benign disease, since the mean follow-up period in patients with malignant airway obstruction usually does not exceed 3 to 4 months.

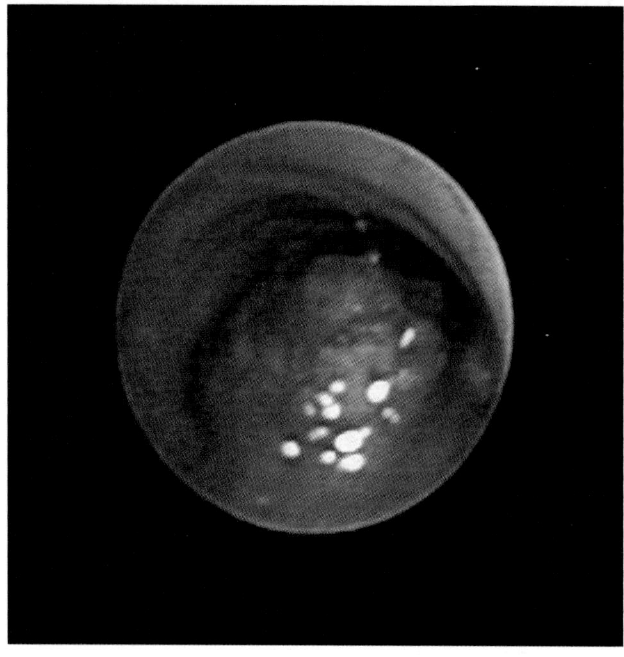

A

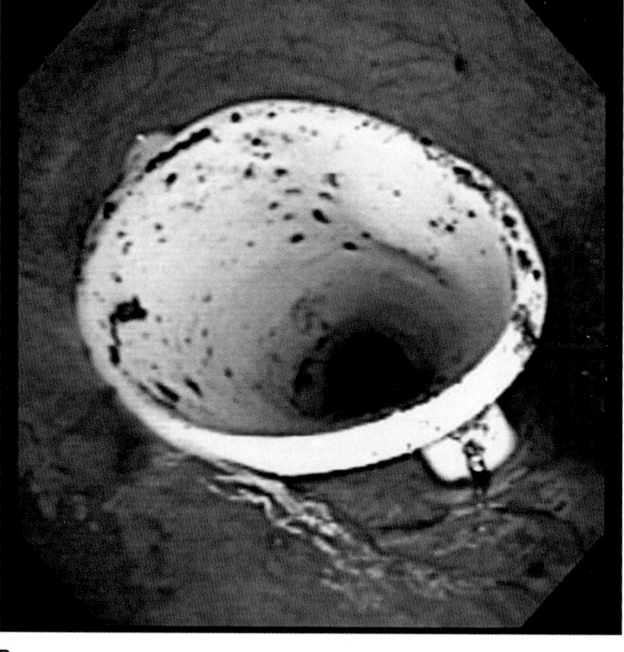

B

Figure 36-3 A large tumor nearly completely obstructs the tracheal lumen (**A**). Manual debulking using a rigid bronchoscope dramatically improved airway luminal diameter. An endotracheal silicone stent was placed to prevent tracheal re-occlusion (**B**).

Complications from endobronchial stents include stent migration, granulation tissue formation, tumor overgrowth, stent bacterial colonization and recurring infection, stent fracture, and inspissated secretions clogging the stent. In addition, massive and fatal hemorrhage associated with stent erosion into central vascular structures can occur.

Stenting for Tracheobronchomalacia

Diffuse or focal tracheobronchomalacia is, perhaps, the most challenging disorder encountered by the therapeutic bronchoscopist. Cartilaginous tracheobronchomalacia reflects tracheal or main bronchi circumferential exhalation airway collapse due to loss of structural integrity of the airway cartilaginous rings. Membranous, or crescentic, tracheobronchomalacia, also known as excessive dynamic airway collapse (EDAC), is manifested by intact cartilaginous rings, but anterior displacement of the posterior membrane during exhalation to variable degree as a result of posterior membrane laxity. This condition is commonly seen with COPD, asthma, obesity, and chronic cough. Dynamic CT scanning may suggest tracheobronchomalacia or EDAC, but the gold standard remains flexible bronchoscopy performed to assess airway collapse with the patient breathing spontaneously.[41] Focal airway malacia may be a complication of long-standing intubation or an anastomotic complication after lung transplantation.[42]

The endoscopist must maintain restraint in therapeutic interventions for patients with tracheobronchomalacia or EDAC. Management of diffuse tracheobronchomalacia should focus on identifying and treating any underlying conditions that may perpetuate cartilaginous inflammation (e.g., relapsing polychondritis) and airway collapse. If the tracheobronchomalacia is symptomatic and progressive despite systemic therapy, initial consideration for tracheostomy should be entertained. If symptoms are not resolved with tracheostomy, or if they recur or progress after an initial improvement, evaluation for placement of a silicone bifurcation Y stent should be undertaken. These patients may also require nighttime ventilator support. Patients with EDAC may benefit from a trial of silicone stent placement as well, but this should not be considered definitive therapy.[43,44] For those who benefit in terms of decreased respiratory symptoms and improved pulmonary function, silicone stent removal, followed by surgical plication or buttressing of the posterior membrane, can be performed with acceptable clinical outcomes.[43,45] For many patients with focal tracheomalacia, particularly from postintubation injury, surgical resection with primary reanastomosis may be the best therapeutic option. If patients are not surgical candidates or prefer to avoid surgery, silicone stent placement often will provide the structural integrity necessary to obviate patient symptoms, but at the risk of long-term stent complications.

■ MANAGEMENT OF HEMOPTYSIS

Bronchoscopy may be of value in hemoptysis for several reasons: to identify site of bleeding, to provide endobronchial therapy to reduce or stop bleeding, to clear blood clots that might impair gas exchange, or to place an endoluminal blocking device to prevent further airway occlusion with blood. Because of visualization difficulties during active bleeding, instruments with large and maximally effective suction channels should be used. Rigid bronchoscopy generally is preferred with massive bleeding or when the need to remove large clots is anticipated.

In attempts to cease bleeding, iced saline or an epinephrine solution can be instilled into a bleeding airway or applied topically onto a proximal bleeding site in attempt to induce vasoconstriction. In addition, balloon catheters can be placed into the bleeding airway to tamponade bleeding and prevent proximal airway soilage in hope of generating a hemostatic clot. Large endobronchial blockers are available to occlude the entire right or left mainstem bronchus to control bleeding. Other effective methods for control of proximal visible bleeding sources, particularly from endobronchial neoplasms, are thermal modalities, such as Nd:YAG laser or APC photocoagulation.[46] Recent reports have demonstrated the benefit from endobronchial packing accomplished with either flexible or rigid bronchoscopy using oxidized regenerated cellulose, which isolates the segmental or subsegmental bleeding site and promotes endobronchial clot formation by induction of fibrin polymerization.[47,48] Frequently, these procedures are temporizing, while definitive management with surgery or bronchial artery embolization is considered.[49]

■ FOREIGN BODY REMOVAL

Bronchoscopy was developed primarily for foreign body removal; prior to the lung cancer epidemic, foreign body removal represented the overwhelming indication for bronchoscopy for decades.

Foreign body aspiration is more likely to occur in children than in adults, with most foreign bodies occurring in children younger than 3 years. In children, the foreign body most often lodges in a mainstem bronchus, whereas in adults foreign bodies usually are wedged distally, most commonly in the right lower lobe. Before bronchoscopic extraction was possible, most foreign body aspirations resulted in high morbidity and mortality, commonly from postobstructive pneumonia. Today, foreign bodies can be removed with either flexible or rigid bronchoscopy, depending on local expertise and foreign body size and composition. If available, rigid bronchoscopy remains the tool of choice for foreign body removal due to several factors: a larger access channel, which permits use of larger and more adaptable retrieval tools; protection of the vocal cords from trauma upon (foreign body) removal; and ability to provide and maintain ventilation.

Various instruments have been developed for use with bronchoscopy for foreign body removal, including grasping forceps, balloon catheters, retrieval baskets, snares, and magnetic extractors. The instrument choice depends on the foreign body material composition, size, shape, and location in the tracheobronchial tree. Grasping forceps may be helpful in the retrieval of hard objects with an irregular surface. Smooth objects or organic material (e.g., nuts, food particles) may require use of expandable baskets or a combination of balloon catheters, suction devices, and grasping forceps. Balloon catheters frequently are used to dislodge a foreign body and bring it proximally into a larger airway before its removal with other instruments.

■ SECRETION ASPIRATION

According to a survey of bronchoscopists in the United States, removal of retained secretions is cited as a leading indication for therapeutic bronchoscopy. Aspiration of bronchoscopic secretions may be indicated in patients with respiratory muscle weakness (e.g., due to underlying neuromuscular disease or the postoperative state) who cannot generate adequate cough for secretion clearance. In critically ill or mechanically ventilated patients, removal of secretions and mucus plugs usually can be rapidly achieved with flexible bronchoscopy. For ease of secretion removal, a flexible scope with a large diameter suction channel is ideal. The secretion volume and viscosity may dictate the interval necessary for bronchoscopy procedures to relieve segmental or lobar atelectasis from inspissated mucus plugs. Bronchoscopic secretion aspiration should not be considered "routine" in the postoperative period or in other conditions in which good chest physiotherapy and maintenance of adequate pulmonary toilet may be more effective.

Two specific disorders are worth highlighting in the context of therapeutic bronchoscopy: pulmonary alveolar proteinosis (PAP) and allergic bronchopulmonary aspergillosis (ABPA). In PAP, large-volume repeated bronchoalveolar lavage has been used for therapeutic clearance of alveolar material composed predominantly of surfactant.[50,51] For patients with more extensive disease or impaired gas exchange, the standard approach is sequential whole-lung lavage.[52] In ABPA, lavage with saline solution may be insufficient to remove tenacious secretion impactions (described as "plastic bronchitis"), and use of bronchoscopic forceps or snare may prove helpful.

■ CLOSURE OF BRONCHOPLEURAL FISTULA

Prolonged air leaks may be encountered following primary or secondary spontaneous pneumothorax, particularly in the setting of underlying parenchymal lung disease; however, they are more commonly seen pulmonary resection. Current management for prolonged air leaks usually includes prolonged chest tube drainage using a Heimlich valve, attempts at surgical repair, pleural blood patch, or pleurodesis.

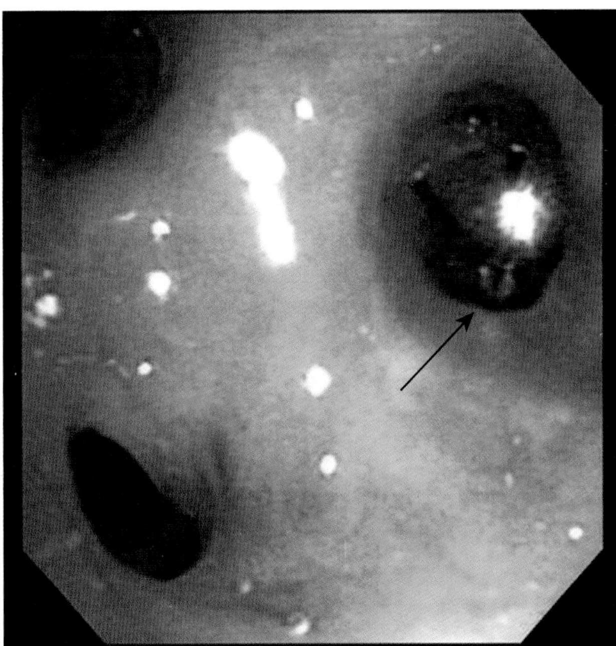

Figure 36-4 A patient presented with a spontaneous pneumothorax from severe emphysema. A chest tube was placed in the left chest and a persistent air leak was noted. Balloon occlusion localized the leak to the left upper lobe anterior segment. A one way endobronchial valve was placed *(arrow)* with complete air leak resolution.

Therapeutic bronchoscopy may be a useful adjunct to prolonged air-leak intervention in confirming suspected bronchopleural or alveolopleural fistulae and in specifying their precise location. The most common approach is to perform selective balloon catheter airway occlusion while observing the chest tube air-leak rate and volume. Depending on the fistula location and size, bronchoscopic procedures can be attempted with the goal of occluding and sealing the bronchopleural fistula. It is much more difficult to achieve fistula obliteration in an area of infected lung or recurrent malignancy. Many different techniques for permanent closure have been reported. Several potentially useful agents have been described, including surgical gel, autologous airway blood patch, and thrombin injection to create fibrin clot, among a variety of others.[53–55] In addition, laser photocoagulation or hypertonic saline injection surrounding small, proximal bronchopleural fistulas has been reported to be beneficial. Recent reports suggest that the placement of one-way endobronchial valves may effectively lead to complete or partial resolution in the large majority of patients with prolonged air leaks from diverse causes (Fig. 36-4).[56–59]

BRONCHOSCOPIC TREATMENTS FOR COMMON BENIGN LUNG CONDITIONS

One of the major advances in therapeutic bronchoscopic use over the past decade has been the development of experimental bronchoscopic interventions for highly prevalent lung diseases, such as asthma and emphysema.

■ BRONCHOSCOPIC EMPHYSEMA TREATMENT

The National Emphysema Treatment Trial (NETT) demonstrated the role of lung volume reduction surgery (LVRS) as the first major surgical intervention for emphysema to improve patient symptoms, as well as mortality, in certain patient subsets.[60] Unfortunately, these benefits were associated with an approximate 5% procedural mortality and substantial perioperative morbidity, including prolong air leaks and cardiac arrhythmias. These factors have spurred

Video 36-5 The video demonstrates fluoroscopic deployment of an investigational endobronchial coil for treatment of emphysema. *Access at www.fishmansonline.com*

development of minimally invasive, bronchoscopic approaches to achieve similar outcomes as the NETT trial, but without the considerable morbidity observed.

The bronchoscopic lung volume reduction (BLVR) approaches under ongoing evaluation utilize a range of techniques, including airway occlusion using silicone plugs (the Endobronchial Watanabe Spigot); insertion of one-way bronchial valves; creation of artificial noncompressible communications ("bypass tracts") between cartilaginous airways and emphysematous parenchyma,[61] injection of a biologic glue to promote scarring,[62] treatment of affected lung segments with steam,[63,64] and placement of endobronchial coils (Video 36-5).[65]

Endobronchial valves have been studied most extensively and are designed to limit ventilation to the most severely involved lung regions in emphysema in an effort to reduce total lung volume, residual volume, and dynamic hyperinflation.[66,67] When placed correctly, the valves allow one-way flow of secretions and air out of the occluded pulmonary segment but prevent air entry beyond the valve (Video 36-6). The major advantage of the bronchial valves is reversibility; that is, the valves generally are removable with minimal risk to the patient. Preliminary studies have suggested that collateral ventilation across incomplete fissures may reduce bronchial valve effectiveness.[68]

Results from the first randomized study of endobronchial valves, a double-blinded, sham-controlled multicenter trial of the Zephyr endobronchial valve, demonstrated modest increases in forced expiratory ventilation in 1 second (FEV_1) and 6-minute walk distance at 6 months; unfortunately, there was an increased rate of complications, including COPD exacerbations and hemoptysis.[69] This valve is available for placement in Europe and Asia, but it is not approved in the United States at this time. One of the major downsides of the biologic approaches to induce scarring and atelectasis is development of permanent lung tissue destruction, with no option for reversibility in the event of worsening lung function or development of cancer. These approaches remain under investigation. Selecting the best technology for use in appropriate patients will be key; it is unlikely that a single approach will apply to all patients with emphysema.

BRONCHIAL THERMOPLASTY

Chronic asthma is a major cause of morbidity, increased health care utilization and cost, and death. Bronchial thermoplasty (BT) is a new bronchoscopic procedure that delivers controlled radiofrequency energy to the bronchial wall of conducting airways with the intent of inhibiting airway smooth muscle contractile function and attenuating bronchoconstriction during asthma exacerbations.

BT is performed using a radiofrequency device that delivers thermal energy to the bronchial wall during an outpatient bronchoscopic procedure. Three separate procedures are performed in order to treat all accessible upper and lower lobe airways ranging from 3 to 10 mm in diameter (Fig. 36-5). The initial randomized, multicenter Airway Intervention with Radiofrequency (AIR) trial in patients with moderate-to-severe disease demonstrated decreased asthma exacerbations in the group undergoing BT compared with patients on standard medical treatment alone.[70] This study was followed by a randomized, sham-controlled, multicenter trial (AIR2) which demonstrated significant improvement in the primary end point—asthma-related quality of life.[71] Although an increase was noted in early post-treatment asthma exacerbations requiring emergency department visits and hospitalizations, long-term follow-up data showed decreased asthma-related health care utilization for patients undergoing BT compared with those undergoing the sham procedure.[72] Based on these data, BT received FDA approval for patients with severe asthma in April 2010, but procedural reimbursement remains problematic with most private insurers. Studies are ongoing to collect additional safety data and to assess the durability of the treatment effect.

Video 36-6 A patient with severe, heterogeneous, upper lobe-predominant emphysema who was enrolled in a clinical trial of endobronchial valves. The video demonstrates valve deployment device positioning and valve deployment. *Access at www.fishmansonline.com*

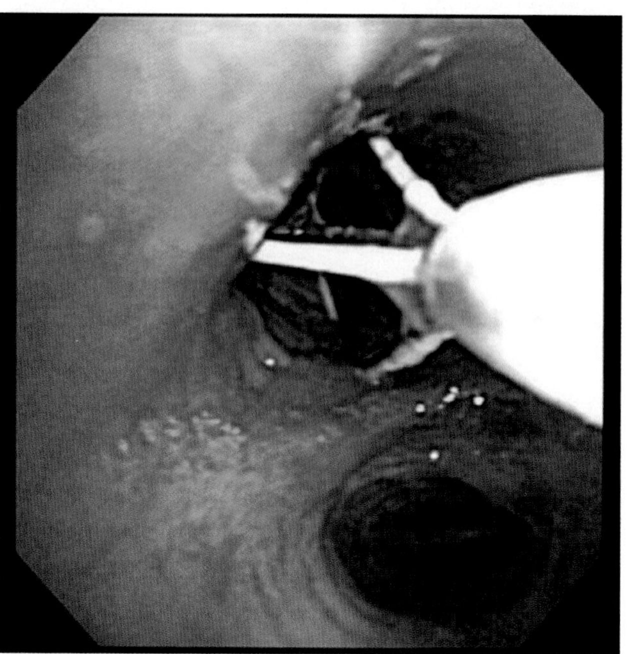

Figure 36-5 Radiofrequency array used in the airway for bronchial thermoplasty in patients with severe asthma.

SUMMARY

Technologic advances in bronchoscopy continue to improve the pulmonologist's ability to perform minimally invasive, accurate evaluations of the tracheobronchial tree and to implement an ever-increasing array of therapeutic and palliative airway interventions. The role of therapeutic bronchoscopy will continue to evolve as further improvements are made in bronchoscopes, accessory equipment, imaging techniques, and novel technologies to treat lung diseases in which bronchoscopy was once thought to have no role. Therapeutic bronchoscopy may soon be used to provide treatment for conditions that traditionally have been treated with surgery. The major challenges in adopting many new bronchoscopic techniques into routine clinical practice will be ensuring adequate procedural competence and having well-designed studies to delineate the appropriate use of the interventions.

REFERENCES

1. D'Andrilli A, Ciccone AM, Venuta F, et al. Long-term results of laryngotracheal resection for benign stenosis. *Eur J Cardiothorac Surg.* 2008;33(3):440–443.
2. Pawlowski J. Moderate and deep sedation techniques. In: Ernst A, Herth FJF, eds. *Principles and Practice of Interventional Pulmonology*. New York, NY: Springer; 2013:63.

3. Perrin G, Colt HG, Martin C, Mak MA, Dumon JF, Gouin F. Safety of interventional rigid bronchoscopy using intravenous anesthesia and spontaneous assisted ventilation. A prospective study. *Chest*. 1992;102(5):1526–1530.
4. Marsh BR. Historic development of bronchoesophagology. *Otolaryngol Head Neck Surg*. 1996;114(6):689–716.
5. Bolliger CT, Sutedja TG, Strausz J, Freitag L. Therapeutic bronchoscopy with immediate effect: laser, electrocautery, argon plasma coagulation and stents. *Eur Respir J*. 2006;27(6):1258–1271.
6. Schokkenbroek AA, Franssen CF, Dikkers FG. Dilatation tracheoscopy for laryngeal and tracheal stenosis in patients with wegener's granulomatosis. *Eur Arch Otorhinolaryngol*. 2008;265(5):549–555.
7. Mayse ML, Greenheck J, Friedman M, Kovitz KL. Successful bronchoscopic balloon dilation of nonmalignant tracheobronchial obstruction without fluoroscopy. *Chest*. 2004;126(2): 634–637.
8. Laforet EG, Berger RL, Vaughan CW. Carcinoma obstructing the trachea Treatment by laser resection. *N Engl J Med*. 1976; 294(17):941.
9. Boxem T, Muller M, Venmans B, Postmus P, Sutedja T. Nd-YAG laser vs bronchoscopic electrocautery for palliation of symptomatic airway obstruction: a cost-effectiveness study. *Chest*. 1999;116(4):1108–1112.
10. Ramser ER, Beamis JF Jr. Laser bronchoscopy. *Clin Chest Med*. 1995;16(3):415–426.
11. D'Aloia A, Faggiano P, Fiorina C, et al. Cardiac arrest due to ventricular fibrillation as a complication occurring during rigid bronchoscopic laser therapy. *Monaldi Arch Chest Dis*. 2003;59(1): 88–90.
12. Iacono AT, Masciangelo TN, Grgurich WF, et al. A new complication related to laser bronchoscopy in a single lung transplant recipient. *Chest*. 1994;106(1):311–313.
13. Peachey T, Eason J, Moxham J, Jarvis D, Driver M. Systemic air embolism during laser bronchoscopy. *Anaesthesia*. 1988;43(10): 872–875.
14. Choi HS, Kim SY, Choi CW, You JH, Kang HM, Park MJ. Use of bronchoscopic electrocautery in removing an endotracheal metastasis. *Lung Cancer*. 2007;58(2):286–290.
15. Asimakopoulos G, Beeson J, Evans J, Maiwand MO. Cryosurgery for malignant endobronchial tumors: analysis of outcome. *Chest*. 2005;127(6):2007–2014.
16. Lee P, Kupeli E, Mehta AC. Therapeutic bronchoscopy in lung cancer. Laser therapy, electrocautery, brachytherapy, stents, and photodynamic therapy. *Clin Chest Med*. 2002;23(1):241–256.
17. Au JT, Carson J, Monette S, Finley DJ. Spray cryotherapy is effective for bronchoscopic, endoscopic and open ablation of thoracic tissues. *Interact Cardiovasc Thorac Surg*. 2012;15(4):580–584.
18. Noppen M, Meysman M, Van Herreweghe R, Lamote J, D'Haese J, Vincken W. Bronchoscopic cryotherapy: preliminary experience. *Acta Clin Belg*. 2001;56(2):73–77.
19. Mathur PN, Wolf KM, Busk MF, Briete WM, Datzman M. Fiberoptic bronchoscopic cryotherapy in the management of tracheobronchial obstruction. *Chest*. 1996;110(3):718–723.
20. Reddy AJ, Govert JA, Sporn TA, Wahidi MM. Broncholith removal using cryotherapy during flexible bronchoscopy: a case report. *Chest*. 2007;132(5):1661–1663.
21. Feller-Kopman D, Lukanich JM, Shapira G, et al. Gas flow during bronchoscopic ablation therapy causes gas emboli to the heart: a comparative animal study. *Chest*. 2008;133(4):892–896. doi: 10.1378/chest.07-2266.
22. Reddy C, Majid A, Michaud G, et al. Gas embolism following bronchoscopic argon plasma coagulation: a case series. *Chest*. 2008;134(5):1066–1069.
23. Chella A, Ambrogi MC, Ribechini A, et al. Combined nd-YAG laser/HDR brachytherapy versus nd-YAG laser only in malignant central airway involvement: a prospective randomized study. *Lung Cancer*. 2000;27(3):169–175.
24. Sutedja G, Baris G, Schaake-Koning C, van Zandwijk N. High dose rate brachytherapy in patients with local recurrences after radiotherapy of non-small cell lung cancer. *Int J Radiat Oncol Biol Phys*. 1992;24(3):551–553.
25. Tendulkar RD, Fleming PA, Reddy CA, Gildea TR, Machuzak M, Mehta AC. High-dose-rate endobronchial brachytherapy for recurrent airway obstruction from hyperplastic granulation tissue. *Int J Radiat Oncol Biol Phys*. 2008;70(3):701–706.
26. Madu CN, Machuzak MS, Sterman DH, et al. High-dose-rate (HDR) brachytherapy for the treatment of benign obstructive endobronchial granulation tissue. *Int J Radiat Oncol Biol Phys*. 2006;66(5):1450–1456.
27. Halkos ME, Godette KD, Lawrence EC, Miller JI Jr. High dose rate brachytherapy in the management of lung transplant airway stenosis. *Ann Thorac Surg*. 2003;76(2):381–384.
28. Moghissi K, Dixon K, Thorpe JA, Stringer M, Oxtoby C. Photodynamic therapy (PDT) in early central lung cancer: a treatment option for patients ineligible for surgical resection. *Thorax*. 2007;62(5):391–395.
29. Freitag L, Ernst A, Thomas M, Prenzel R, Wahlers B, Macha HN. Sequential photodynamic therapy (PDT) and high dose brachytherapy for endobronchial tumour control in patients with limited bronchogenic carcinoma. *Thorax*. 2004;59(9):790–793.
30. Minnich DJ, Bryant AS, Dooley A, Cerfolio RJ. Photodynamic laser therapy for lesions in the airway. *Ann Thorac Surg*. 2010;89(6):1744–1748. doi: 10.1016/j.athoracsur.2010.02.025.
31. Montgomery WW, Montgomery SK. Manual for use of montgomery laryngeal, tracheal, and esophageal prostheses. *Ann Otol Rhinol Laryngol Suppl*. 1986;125:1–16.
32. Dumon JF. A dedicated tracheobronchial stent. *Chest*. 1990;97(2): 328–332.
33. Choudhary C, Gildea TR, Salman R, Guzman ED, Mehta AC. Management of tracheomediastinal fistula using self-expanding metallic stents. *Ann Thorac Surg*. 2008;85(5):1800–1802.
34. Husain SA, Finch D, Ahmed M, Morgan A, Hetzel MR. Long-term follow-up of ultraflex metallic stents in benign and malignant central airway obstruction. *Ann Thorac Surg*. 2007;83(4): 1251–1256.
35. Saad CP, Murthy S, Krizmanich G, Mehta AC. Self-expandable metallic airway stents and flexible bronchoscopy: long-term outcomes analysis. *Chest*. 2003;124(5):1993–1999.
36. Mughal MM, Gildea TR, Murthy S, Pettersson G, DeCamp M, Mehta AC. Short-term deployment of self-expanding metallic stents facilitates healing of bronchial dehiscence. *Am J Respir Crit Care Med*. 2005;172(6):768–771.
37. Saji H, Furukawa K, Tsutsui H, et al. Outcomes of airway stenting for advanced lung cancer with central airway obstruction. *Interact Cardiovasc Thorac Surg*. 2010;11(4):425–428. doi: 10.1510/icvts.2010.238196.
38. Amjadi K, Voduc N, Cruysberghs Y, et al. Impact of interventional bronchoscopy on quality of life in malignant airway obstruction. *Respiration*. 2008;76(4):421–428. doi: 10.1159/000152832.
39. Ernst A, Simoff M, Ost D, Goldman Y, Herth FJ. Prospective risk-adjusted morbidity and mortality outcome analysis after

therapeutic bronchoscopic procedures: results of a multi-institutional outcomes database. *Chest.* 2008;134(3):514–519.

40. Noppen M, Stratakos G, Amjadi K, et al. Stenting allows weaning and extubation in ventilator- or tracheostomy dependency secondary to benign airway disease. *Respir Med.* 2007;101(1):139–145.

41. Lee KS, Sun MR, Ernst A, Feller-Kopman D, Majid A, Boiselle PM. Comparison of dynamic expiratory CT with bronchoscopy for diagnosing airway malacia: a pilot evaluation. *Chest.* 2007;131(3):758–764.

42. Carden KA, Boiselle PM, Waltz DA, Ernst A. Tracheomalacia and tracheobronchomalacia in children and adults: an in-depth review.. *Chest.* 2005;127(3):984–1005.

43. Ernst A, Odell DD, Michaud G, Majid A, Herth FF, Gangadharan SP. Central airway stabilization for tracheobronchomalacia improves quality of life in patients with COPD. *Chest.* 2011;140(5): 1162–1168. doi: 10.1378/chest.10-3051.

44. Ernst A, Majid A, Feller-Kopman D, et al. Airway stabilization with silicone stents for treating adult tracheobronchomalacia: a prospective observational study. *Chest.* 2007;132(2):609–616.

45. Majid A, Guerrero J, Gangadharan S, et al. Tracheobronchoplasty for severe tracheobronchomalacia: a prospective outcome analysis. *Chest.* 2008;134(4):801–807.

46. Morice RC, Ece T, Ece F, Keus L. Endobronchial argon plasma coagulation for treatment of hemoptysis and neoplastic airway obstruction. *Chest.* 2001;119(3):781–787.

47. Reisz G. Topical hemostatic tamponade: another tool in the treatment of massive hemoptysis. *Chest.* 2005;127(6):1888–1889.

48. Nogueira CC, Ferreira S, Oliveira A, et al. Bronchoscopic hemostatic tamponade with oxidized regenerated cellulose for major hemoptysis control: two case reports. *Rev Port Pneumol.* 2010;16(6):917–920.

49. Shigemura N, Wan IY, Yu SC, et al. Multidisciplinary management of life-threatening massive hemoptysis: a 10-year experience. *Ann Thorac Surg.* 2009;87(3):849–853. doi: 10.1016/j.athoracsur.2008.11.010.

50. Cheng SL, Chang HT, Lau HP, Lee LN, Yang PC. Pulmonary alveolar proteinosis: treatment by bronchofiberscopic lobar lavage. *Chest.* 2002;122(4):1480–1485.

51. Udwadia ZF, Patel DB, Kapadia FN, Gandhe UM, Butani M. Pulmonary alveolar proteinosis with respiratory failure–therapeutic role of bronchoscopic and whole lung lavage. *J Assoc Physicians India.* 1998;46(8):738–739.

52. Kavuru MS, Popovich M. Therapeutic whole lung lavage: a stop-gap therapy for alveolar proteinosis. *Chest.* 2002;122(4): 1123–1124.

53. Andreetti C, D'Andrilli A, Ibrahim M, et al. Submucosal injection of the silver–human albumin complex for the treatment of bronchopleural fistula. *Eur J Cardiothorac Surg.* 2010;37(1):40–43. doi: 10.1016/j.ejcts.2009.07.006.

54. Kodama H, Yamakado K, Murashima S, et al. Intractable bronchopleural fistula caused by radiofrequency ablation: endoscopic bronchial occlusion with silicone embolic material. *Br J Radiol.* 2009;82(983):e225–e227. doi: 10.1259/bjr/23975691.

55. Tedde ML, Scordamaglio PR, Minamoto H, Figueiredo VR, Pedra CC, Jatene FB. Endobronchial closure of total bronchopleural fistula with occlutech figulla ASD N device. *Ann Thorac Surg.* 2009;88(3):e25–e26. doi: 10.1016/j.athoracsur.2009.06.069.

56. Gillespie CT, Sterman DH, Cerfolio RJ, et al. Endobronchial valve treatment for prolonged air leaks of the lung: a case series. *Ann Thorac Surg.* 2011;91(1):270–273.

57. Alexander ES, Healey TT, Martin DW, Dupuy DE. Use of endobronchial valves for the treatment of bronchopleural fistulas after thermal ablation of lung neoplasms. *J Vasc Interv Radiol.* 2012;23(9):1236–1240. doi: 10.1016/j.jvir.2012.06.009.

58. Ferguson JS, Sprenger K, Van Natta T. Closure of a bronchopleural fistula using bronchoscopic placement of an endobronchial valve designed for the treatment of emphysema. *Chest.* 2006;129(2):479–481.

59. Travaline JM, McKenna RJ Jr, De Giacomo T, et al; Endobronchial Valve for Persistent Air Leak Group. Treatment of persistent pulmonary air leaks using endobronchial valves. *Chest.* 2009;136(2):355–360. doi: 10.1378/chest.08-2389.

60. Fishman A1, Martinez F, Naunheim K, et al; National Emphysema Treatment Trial Research Group. A randomized trial comparing lung-volume–reduction surgery with medical therapy for severe emphysema. *N Engl J Med.* 2003;348(21):2059–2073. doi: 10.1056/NEJMoa030287.

61. Rendina EA, De Giacomo T, Venuta F, et al. Feasibility and safety of the airway bypass procedure for patients with emphysema. *J Thorac Cardiovasc Surg.* 2003;125(6):1294–1299.

62. Herth FJ, Eberhardt R, Ingenito EP, Gompelmann D. Assessment of a novel lung sealant for performing endoscopic volume reduction therapy in patients with advanced emphysema. *Expert Rev Med Devices.* 2011;8(3):307–312. doi: 10.1586/erd.11.10.

63. Snell GI, Hopkins P, Westall G, Holsworth L, Carle A, Williams TJ. A feasibility and safety study of bronchoscopic thermal vapor ablation: a novel emphysema therapy. *Ann Thorac Surg.* 2009;88(6):1993–1998. doi: 10.1016/j.athoracsur.2009.06.038.

64. Snell G, Herth FJ, Hopkins P, et al. Bronchoscopic thermal vapour ablation therapy in the management of heterogeneous emphysema. *Eur Respir J.* 2012;39(6):1326–1333. doi: 10.1183/09031936.00092411.

65. Slebos DJ, Klooster K, Ernst A, Herth FJ, Kerstjens HA. Bronchoscopic lung volume reduction coil treatment of patients with severe heterogeneous emphysema. *Chest.* 2012;142(3):574–582.

66. Wood DE, McKenna RJ Jr, Yusen RD, et al. A multicenter trial of an intrabronchial valve for treatment of severe emphysema. *J Thorac Cardiovasc Surg.* 2007;133(1):65–73.

67. Wan IY, Toma TP, Geddes DM, et al. Bronchoscopic lung volume reduction for end-stage emphysema: report on the first 98 patients. *Chest.* 2006;129(3):518–526.

68. Fessler HE. Collateral ventilation, the bane of bronchoscopic volume reduction. *Am J Respir Crit Care Med.* 2005;171(5):423–424.

69. Sciurba FC, Ernst A, Herth FJ, et al; VENT Study Research Group. A randomized study of endobronchial valves for advanced emphysema. *N Engl J Med.* 2010;363(13):1233–1244. doi: 10.1056/NEJMoa0900928.

70. Cox G, Thomson NC, Rubin AS, et al; AIR Trial Study Group. Asthma control during the year after bronchial thermoplasty. *N Engl J Med.* 2007;356(13):1327–1337.

71. Castro M, Rubin AS, Laviolette M, et al. Effectiveness and safety of bronchial thermoplasty in the treatment of severe asthma: a multicenter, randomized, double-blind, sham-controlled clinical trial. *Am J Respir Crit Care Med.* 2010;181(2):116–124. doi: 10.1164/rccm.200903-0354 OC.

72. Castro M, Rubin A, Laviolette M, et al; AIR2 Trial Study Group Persistence of effectiveness of bronchial thermoplasty in patients with severe asthma. *Ann Allergy Asthma Immunol.* 2011;107(1):65–70. doi: 10.1016/j.anai.2011.03.005.

CHAPTER 37

Diagnostic Thoracic Surgical Procedures: Thoracoscopy, VATS, and Thoracotomy

Robert E. Merritt

INTRODUCTION

Thoracoscopy, video-assisted thoracic surgery (VATS), and thoracotomy are well-established surgical techniques used by thoracic surgeons to diagnose benign and malignant diseases involving the thorax.

Thoracoscopy first emerged as a diagnostic tool in the early 20th century when therapeutic pneumothorax became the surgical treatment of choice for tuberculosis. In 1910, Hans Christian Jacobaeus performed the first thoracoscopic intrapleural pneumolysis for collapse therapy in the treatment of tuberculosis.[1–3] He used a rigid cystoscope with a light source to access the pleural cavity and perform a pneumolysis. After development of effective antimicrobial therapy for tuberculosis, thoracoscopy evolved as an effective diagnostic procedure to evaluate pleural effusions and pleural disease.[4] During direct diagnostic thoracoscopy, a fiberoptic mediastinoscope or bronchoscope was placed through a small intercostal incision; pleural fluid could be aspirated and sent for analysis (Fig. 37-1). In addition, the parietal pleura, visceral pleura, fissures, hilum, and diaphragm could be inspected directly.[5]

By 1990, thoracoscopy evolved into VATS. Development of high-resolution video cameras and endoscopic linear mechanical stapling devices allowed the expansion of application of VATS into the diagnosis and treatment of pulmonary nodules and interstitial lung diseases (ILDs).[6,7] The use of diagnostic thoracotomy has declined significantly since the emergence of VATS; however, the diagnostic thoracotomy may be necessary in cases in which VATS is not feasible (Table 37-1).

TECHNICAL CONSIDERATIONS

VATS is performed in the operating room under general anesthesia. A double-lumen tube is placed to isolate the lungs to enable establishment of one-lung ventilation, which is essential for performing the procedure. The use of one-lung ventilation creates sufficient space for maneuvering within the hemithorax to perform the planned procedure. Carbon dioxide (CO_2) insufflation can also be used to provide additional working space within the chest cavity by lowering the position of the diaphragm. The more inferiorly located diaphragm provides better exposure of the costophrenic sulci and lower lobes. When CO_2 is used, the maximum insufflation pressure is maintained below 6 mm Hg to avoid decreased venous return to the right heart and associated hypotension.

The typical VATS procedure utilizes three to four incisions that range from 5 to 12 mm in size. The incisions are usually arranged in a triangular configuration, with the area of interest located in the center of the triangle. (Fig. 37-2) A 5- or 10-mm fiberoptic thoracoscope is connected to a video camera and is most commonly inserted into the most inferiorly placed VATS incision (Fig. 37-3). The chest cavity is clearly visualized on a video monitor and the parietal pleura, visceral pleura, hilum, diaphragm, and mediastinum can be directly inspected. Upon completion of the procedure, a chest tube is inserted under direct visualization through one of the VATS incisions to evacuate air and pleural fluid during the early postoperative period. Simple diagnostic VATS procedures are typically well tolerated, and patients can be discharged after 1 to 2 days in the hospital. Currently, the disease processes assessed using VATS are listed in Table 37-2.

■ MANAGEMENT OF PLEURAL DISEASE

Both malignant and benign diseases of the pleura may be diagnosed and managed with VATS. Although thoracentesis (including pleural fluid cytology analysis) is the initial diagnostic tool of choice for an undiagnosed pleural effusion, VATS procedures provide a higher diagnostic yield: 90% to 100% compared to 60% to 80% for thoracentesis.[8–10] When the diagnosis of a pleural effusion is not determined following thoracentesis, VATS can be utilized to obtained pleural fluid and pleural biopsies for definitive diagnosis.

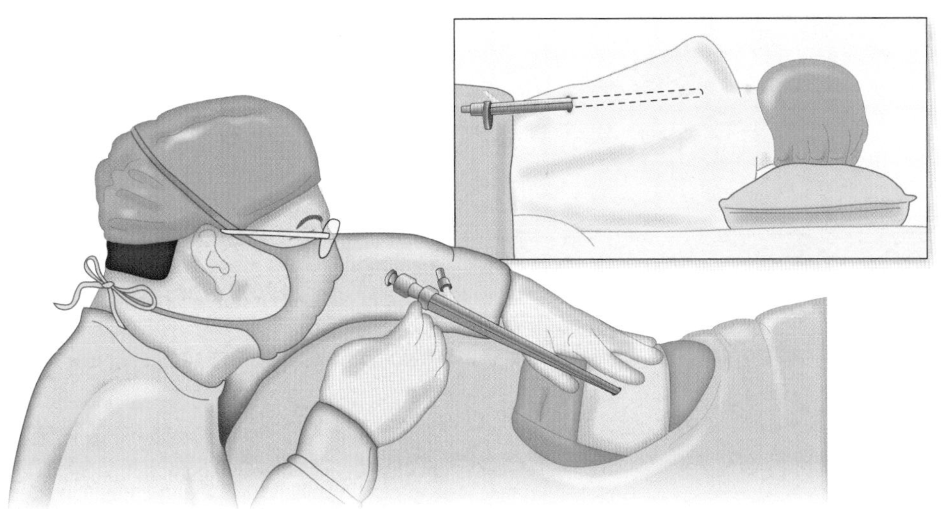

Figure 37-1 Use of a rigid bronchoscope as a thoracoscope.

TABLE 37-1 Contraindications to Video-Assisted Thoracic Surgery (VATS)

Severe hypoxia
Previous pneumonectomy or bilobectomy
Mechanical ventilator dependence
Severe chronic obstructive pulmonary disease
Pleural adhesions
Previous pleurodesis procedure
Coagulopathy
Recent acute myocardial infarction
Severe pulmonary hypertension

Malignant pleural effusions usually present as a result of an obstruction of subpleural lymphatics and are associated with advanced primary lung cancer or metastatic epithelial carcinomas that involve the lung. VATS may provide both diagnostic and therapeutic value in the management of malignant pleural effusions. A pleurodesis can be achieved by instilling chemical agents, such as talc, doxycycline, bleomycin, or tetracycline into the pleural cavity to promote pleural adhesion formation. The process obliterates the potential space between the parietal pleura and visceral pleura, thus preventing accumulation of pleural fluid. Efficacy rates in the range of 94% to 96% for VATS pleurodesis for malignant pleural effusions have been reported,[11,12] along with a morbidity rate of 2.6%.[12] In essence, the VATS approach for diagnosis and management of malignant pleural effusions is highly effective because it provides minimally invasive access to the thoracic cavity for sampling of fluid and pleural tissue, and it enables lysis of loculated adhesions and instillation of a chemical pleurodesis agent.

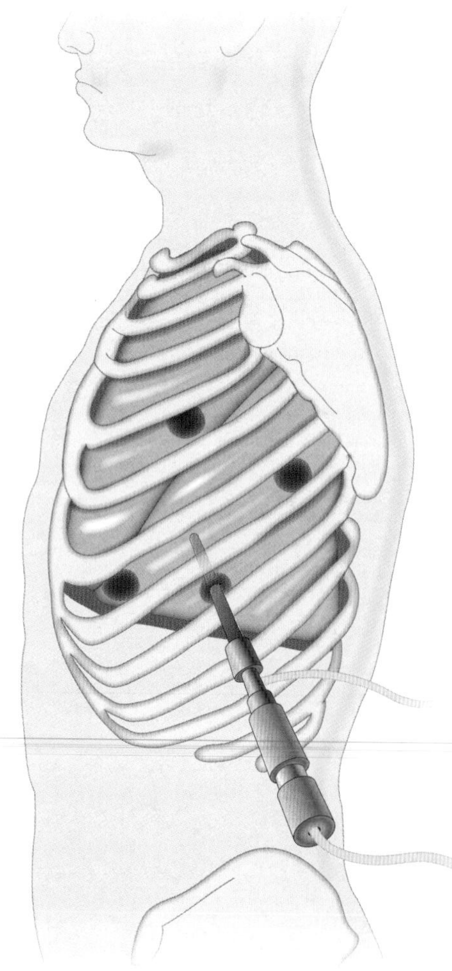

Figure 37-2 Placement of VATS incisions.

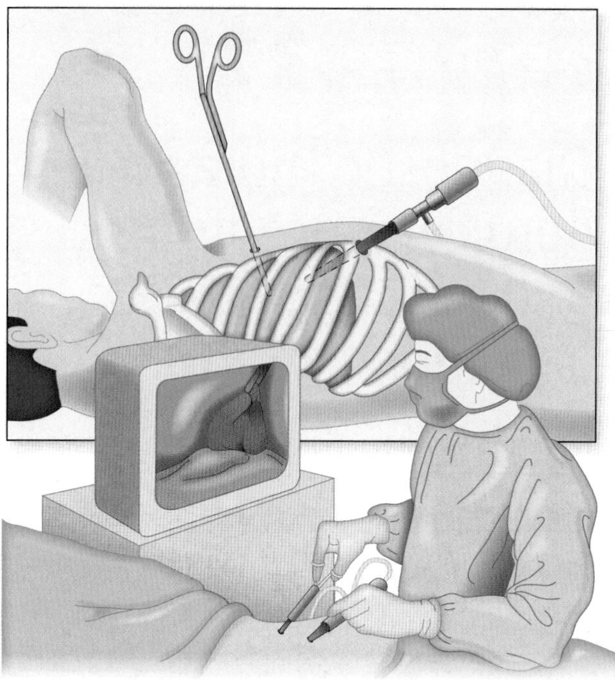

Figure 37-3 Placement of the thoracoscope through the most inferior of the VATS incisions. A video camera is connected to the thoracoscope and the image displayed on a video monitor.

The most common benign condition involving the pleura is an infection of the pleural space or empyema. Patients who present with pneumonia often have associated pleural effusions, which may be either a parapneumonic effusion or an empyema (see Chapter 76). The pleural fluid should be sampled with thoracentesis to enable the distinction between parapneumonic effusion and empyema. If the pleural fluid Gram stain or culture is positive for a pathogen, or if the fluid pH is less than 7.1, an empyema is diagnosed.

The classification of empyema is based on the temporal evolution of the pleural space infection and dictates the optimal management.

TABLE 37-2 Current Indications for Video-Assisted Thoracic Surgery (VATS)

Diagnosis of pleural effusion
Drainage of empyema
Pleurodesis
Diagnosis of a suspicious pulmonary nodule
Biopsy of the pleura
Lung biopsy for diagnosis of interstitial lung disease
Resection of pulmonary metastatic nodules
Resection of primary lung carcinoma
Biopsy of mediastinal lymph nodes
Resection of blebs or bullae for treatment of spontaneous pneumothorax
Drainage of pericardial effusion

Video 37-1 Use of VATS in drainage of empyema. *Access at www.fishmansonline.com*

Video 37-2 Use of VATS in evaluation of indeterminate pulmonary nodule. *Access at www.fishmansonline.com*

Three phases of empyema have been described: (1) The *exudative phase*, an initial phase characterized by free-flowing purulent fluid within the pleural space. Simple drainage with chest tube thoracostomy and intravenous antibiotics are usually sufficient to manage the pleural effusion. (2) The *fibropurulent phase*, characterized by loculated pleural fluid collections and fibrinous exudative deposits on the visceral pleural surfaces. In this phase, the empyema often requires a VATS or thoracotomy to lyse adhesions, break up loculations, and promote drainage of the purulent pleural fluid (Video 37-1). (3) The *fibrous phase*, characterized by formation of a thick, fibrous rind on the visceral pleural surface of the lung. A thoracotomy is usually required to achieve a complete decortication.

Early decortication using a VATS-based approach during the fibropurulent phase is highly effective and may significantly decrease morbidity associated with empyema.[13] VATS offers a decided advantage over simple chest tube thoracostomy because of multiple factors: (1) Loculated purulent fluid may be completely drained, since adhesions are directly visualized and lysed during VATS. (2) Atelectatic lung may be reexpanded under direct vision. (3) Chest tubes can be placed in the appropriate position for optimal drainage in the postoperative period.

The definitive drainage of purulent fluid associated with empyema using VATS can significantly improve patient outcomes and prevent progression to a fibrothorax, which often requires an open thoracotomy.

■ EVALUATION OF LUNG PARENCHYMAL DISEASE

Diagnosis of the solitary pulmonary nodule remains one of the most common indications for VATS. A widely cited, multi-institution, randomized study demonstrating a 20% reduction in lung cancer mortality using low-dose computed tomography (CT) to screen for lung nodules in patients at risk for lung cancer[14] will certainly increase enthusiasm for screening programs and enhance detection of indeterminate pulmonary nodules.

Currently available modalities for the diagnosis of indeterminate solitary pulmonary nodules include high-resolution CT, positron emission tomography (PET), CT-guided fine-needle aspiration (FNA), and VATS. In a randomized trial for evaluation of solitary lung nodules, CT scans performed with intravenous contrast administration have been shown to have an overall accuracy rate of 77%, sensitivity of 98%, and specificity of 58%.[15] The coupling of PET scan-based images with CT scans is often useful to determine if a lung nodule is hypermetabolic, which increases the probability of malignancy (see Chapter 32). In cases of granulomatous diseases, PET scans may generate false-positive results, as inflammatory cells readily accumulate the tracer employed, 18-fluorodeoxyglucose (18F-FDG). The sensitivity and specificity of PET–CT scanning in the evaluation of indeterminate solitary pulmonary nodules have been reported at 92% and 90%, respectively.[16]

Development of VATS has improved the diagnostic yield in evaluation of indeterminate solitary pulmonary nodules. This minimally invasive technique is well tolerated. Patients experience less postoperative pain and recover more quickly compared with patients who undergo conventional open thoracotomy.

Pulmonary nodules located in the outer third of the lung parenchyma are ideally suited for VATS wedge excisional biopsy. For lung lesions smaller than 10 mm, localization can be facilitated using transthoracic wire placement into the area of the lesion under CT guidance prior to the VATS procedure. In addition, the technique of navigational bronchoscopy (see Chapter 36, Sterman) can be employed to inject dye or place fiducial markers in close proximity to small nodules that might be difficult to locate during VATS. The diagnostic yield for VATS using wedge excision of a pulmonary nodule approaches 100%. Furthermore, since morbidity and mortality rates are exceedingly low, the VATS technique is ideal for evaluation of indeterminate pulmonary nodules (Video 37-2).

Although diffuse ILDs often present with characteristic patterns on CT scanning, histologic confirmation is often necessary to determine appropriate treatment. Reports indicate that in as many as 84% of cases of ILD evaluated with surgical lung biopsy, the course of therapy is altered by the biopsy findings.[17]

The VATS technique has been shown to result in less postoperative pain and lower morbidity compared with thoracotomy performed for purposes of lung biopsy.[18,19] Furthermore, in a randomized, controlled clinical trial, VATS and thoracotomy appear equivalent in postoperative outcomes when performed for diagnosis of ILD.[20]Given this diagnostic equivalency, and, in the author's experience, reduced postoperative pain, shorter hospital stay, and faster recovery associated with VATS, it remains the preferred diagnostic technique for patients with ILD who are ambulatory and have sufficient pulmonary reserve to tolerate one-lung ventilation. Thoracotomy is reserved for patients who are ventilator-dependent and too hypoxic to tolerate one-lung ventilation.

SUMMARY

Thoracoscopy, VATS, and thoracotomy are valuable diagnostic tools employed in the evaluation of benign and malignant diseases of the pleura and lung. VATS has emerged as a primary diagnostic method for diagnosis and treatment of malignant pleural effusions and empyema. In addition, VATS has improved the diagnostic yield in evaluation of indeterminate solitary pulmonary nodules. VATS has largely replaced diagnostic thoracotomy for ILD, since VATS results in less postoperative pain, shorter hospital stay, and faster postoperative recovery.

REFERENCES

1. Bloomberg AE. Thoracoscopy in perspective. *Surg Gynecol Obstet*. 1978;147:433–443.
2. Jacobaeus HC. The cauterization of adhesions in artificial pneumothorax treatment of pulmonary tuberculosis under thoracoscopic control. *Arch Radiol Electrotherapy*. 1923;28:136–146.
3. Jacobaeus HC. The cauterization of adhesions in artificial pneumothorax treatment of tuberculosis. *Surg Gynecol Obstet*. 1921;32:493–500.
4. Braimbridge MV. The history of thoracoscopic surgery. *Ann Thorac Surg*. 1993;56:610–614.
5. Lewis RJ, Kunderman PJ, Sisler GE, Mackenzie JW. Direct Diagnostic Thoracoscopy. *Ann Thorac Surg*. 1976;21:536–539.
6. Mack MJ, Aronoff RJ, Acuff TE, Douthit MB, Bowman RT, Ryan WH. Present role of thorscoscopy in the diagnosis and treatment of diseases of the chest. *Ann Thorac Surg*. 1992;54:403–409.
7. Hazelrigg SR, Nunchuck SK, LoCicero J. Video assisted thoracic surgery study group data. *Ann Thorac Surg*. 1993;56:1039–1044.

8. Collins TR, Sahn SA. Thoracentesis: clinical value, complications, technical problems, and patient experience. *Chest*. 1987;91:817–822.
9. Baumgartner WA, Mark JB. The use of thoracoscopy in the diagnosis of pleural disease. *Arch Surg*. 1980;115:420–421.
10. Kohman LJ. Thoracoscopy for the evaluation and treatment of pleural space disease. *Chest Surg Clin North Am*. 1994;4:467–479.
11. Yim AP, Chung SS, Lee TW, Lam CK, Ho JK. Thoracoscopic management of malignant pleural effusions. *Chest*. 1996;109:1234–1238.
12. Marrazz A, Noto A, Casa L, et al. Video-thoracoscopic surgical pleurodesis in the management of malignant pleural effusion: the importance of an early intervention. *J Pain Symptom Manage*. 2005;30:75–79.
13. Landreneau RJ, Keenan RJ, Hazelrigg SR, Mack MJ, Naunheim KS. Thoracoscopy for empyema and hemothorax. *Chest*. 1996;109:18–24.
14. The national lung screening trial research team. Reduced lung-cancer mortality with low-dose computed tomographic screening. *N Engl Med*. 2011;365:395–409.
15. Swensen SJ, Viggiano RW, Midthun DE, et al. Lung nodule enhancement at CT: multicenter study. *Radiology*. 2000;214:73–80.
16. Lowe VJ, Fletcher JW, Gobar L, et al. Prospective investigation of positron emission tomography in lung nodules. *J Clin Oncol*. 1998;16:1075–1084.
17. Lee YC, Wu CT, Hsu HH, Huang PM, Chang YL. Surgical lung biopsy for diffuse pulmonary disease: experience of 196 patients. *J Thorac Cardiovasc Surg*. 2005;129:984–990.
18. Chang AC, Yee J, Orringer MB, Iannettoni MD. Diagnostic thoracoscopic lung biopsy: an outpatient experience. *Ann Thorac Surg*. 2002;74:1942–1946.
19. Ferson PF, Landreneau RJ, Dowling RD, et al. Comparison of open versus thoracoscopic lung biopsy for diffuse infiltrative pulmonary disease. *J Thorac Cardiovasc Surg*. 1993;106:194–199.
20. Miller JD, Urschel JD, Cox G. A randomized, controlled trial comparing thorcoscopy and limited thoracotomy for lung biopsy in interstitial lung disease. *Ann Thorac Surg*. 2000;70:1647–1650.

CHAPTER 38

Evaluation of Respiratory Impairment and Disability

Akshay Sood

INTRODUCTION

Management of a patient with chronic lung disease does not end with its treatment. Those with chronic pulmonary disorders need additional assistance and guidance on issues related to respiratory impairment, including causation or attribution; apportionment; eligibility for, and access to, various compensation systems; workplace modifications or removal from the workplace; and vocational and other forms of rehabilitation. Unfortunately, most physicians avoid providing these services, often with disastrous socioeconomic and medical consequences for the patient.

Multiple reasons underlie the general attitude of physician reluctance in addressing impairment. These include a fear and poor understanding of the legal system as it relates to work-related diseases, pervasive confusion about various compensation systems, a mistaken notion that those who seek impairment assistance are usually malingerers, lack of training in impairment evaluation, and a desire to avoid uncompensated efforts in the context of an already burdensome clinical schedule. This chapter provides an understanding of this complex, but ignored, area in clinical pulmonary medicine.

TERMINOLOGY

This field of impairment and disability evaluation bridges medicine and law; hence, its terminology, drawn from both fields, can be confusing. The terms, impairment and disability, are often used interchangeably, but they are not synonymous. In 1980, the World Health Organization issued a statement defining *impairment* as, "any loss or abnormality of psychological, physiologic, or anatomical structure or function," and *disability* as, "any restriction or lack, resulting from impairment, of ability to perform an activity within the range considered normal for a human being."[1] The resulting social and occupational disadvantage is designated as handicap.

For a patient with chronic lung disease, the goal of respiratory impairment evaluation is objective measurement of the extent of loss of function, primarily through application of pulmonary function or exercise testing. The physician plays a key role in impairment evaluation. On the other hand, the impact of the respiratory impairment on a person's ability to perform day-to-day activities is called disability, which is typically determined through application of administrative and legal instruments by experts in these areas. The experts not only rely upon the evaluation of impairment provided by the physician, but also take into consideration other social and legal issues, as well as the energy requirements of the occupation. Impairment may occur without disability, and disability may occur without measurable impairment. Furthermore, two individuals with exactly the same respiratory impairment may suffer differing impacts on their lives, and consequently, have different levels of disability.

Respiratory impairment may be *temporary* or *permanent*. In contrast to temporary impairment, permanent impairment is not expected to improve with time or treatment. Disability may be *partial* or *total*. Total disability implies that an individual is unable to perform any work of the kind that he or she has the skills and qualifications to perform. Partial disability implies that an individual is able to perform some, but not all, of the work.

Causation or *attribution* refers to whether an exposure has been a "substantial" contributing factor in either causing or exacerbating lung disease. The level of certainty required in determining causation for occupational lung disease is different from the usual standard of 95% certainty used in medical research. The commonly accepted standard of certainty for occupational cases is that the illness is substantially caused, or exacerbated by, an occupational exposure on a "more probable than not" basis, or a level of certainty greater than 50%.

Apportionment describes the relative contribution of multiple factors to the total respiratory impairment. For instance, both chronic inhalational asbestos exposure and cigarette smoking may be contributory factors to lung cancer. From a scientific perspective, it is usually difficult, if not impossible, to "apportion" the relative roles of multiple exposures in causation of an individual's complex, multifactorial disease. Physicians are often asked to state their opinion on apportionment in the context of the body of available knowledge in that area.

IMPAIRMENT SYSTEMS COMMONLY USED IN THE UNITED STATES

Patients seeking an impairment evaluation can be usually classified into three general types: (1) Those with advanced lung disease who apply for disability benefits under the Social Security Impairment program, (2) those with work-related lung disease who apply under the Workers' Compensation System (but also other programs, such as the Black Lung Benefits Act for coal mine workers), and (3) those who develop lung disease while working for certain employers, such as the Veterans Administration. The most commonly used impairment guidelines in the United States are the Social Security Impairment program and the Workers' Compensation System. Each are discussed in greater detail in subsequent sections.

■ SOCIAL SECURITY IMPAIRMENT

The US Social Security Administration incorporates two programs that provide financial and rehabilitative benefits to disabled individuals. Both require objective demonstration of disability using medical standards set forth in the Social Security Act.

The first program is orchestrated through Title II of the Act, known as Social Security Disability Insurance. The program is available to individuals who are insured as a result of their contributions to the Social Security trust fund (through federal taxes paid on employment earnings during their work careers). The second is orchestrated through Title XVI of the Act, known as supplemental security income, or SSI. This program is available to disabled individuals who have limited income or resources and who are not covered by contributions to the Social Security trust fund. For adults, the definition of disability is the same whether application for benefits is made under Title II or Title XVI of the Social Security Act. The Social Security Administration defines disability as, "the inability to engage in any substantial gainful activity by reason of any medically determinable physical or mental impairment(s) which can be expected to result in death or which has lasted or can be expected to last for a continuous period of not less than 12 months." The methods used for disability evaluation under Social Security are important for the physician to understand for two reasons: (1) Disability designation under Social Security is a common and important source of financial support for many patients who are under the care of pulmonary physicians and (2) the pulmonary physician often takes an active role in helping determine eligibility under this program.

Evaluation of disability under Social Security is a staged process, beginning with application to a local Social Security field office or the Office of Disability Determination Services (DDS). The Office of DDS gathers objective medical information primarily from the treating physician, who is the preferred source of medical evaluation. If the available information is insufficient to make a determination of disability, the DDS may purchase additional testing and/or request examination from a consultant, such as a pulmonary physician.

The Social Security Administration has decided that certain specific impairments of each major body system are severe enough to prevent a person from engaging in any gainful employment and, therefore, serve as prima facie evidence that disability exists. These impairments have been codified as the Listings of Impairments.[2] Listings under the respiratory system include specific categories of disease severity, including chronic respiratory disorders; asthma; cystic fibrosis; pneumoconiosis; bronchiectasis; mycobacterial, mycotic, and other chronic persistent infections of the lung; cor pulmonale due to chronic pulmonary vascular hypertension; sleep-related breathing disorders; and lung transplant.

If a claimant cannot meet the severity criteria of the Listings, the claimant may still receive an award of benefits by presenting pertinent medical information to the DDS. An initial judgment may then be made by the DDS, but the claimant has the right to challenge an unfavorable decision and to have it reviewed by other members of the DDS staff. If the decision is still unfavorable, the claimant may appeal to the Office of Hearings and Appeals for review by an administrative law judge, who may request expert physician testimony before making a decision. Once again, the claimant may request that an unfavorable decision be reviewed by an appeals council.

The Social Security program has some unusual requirements that distinguish it from other compensation programs: (1) The program requires a "hard copy" of the volume–time curve of a recent spirogram obtained following administration of inhaled bronchodilator when obstruction is present. (2) The program incorporates arbitrary, height-specific cut points for spirometric lung function for deciding impairment status; these cut points are not determined by race, ethnicity, age, or gender. (3) The program accepts an arterial blood gas measured during steady-state *submaximal* exercise at a work rate of 5 metabolic equivalents (METs) for rating impairment in gas exchange. (4) The program denotes the patient as either impaired or not impaired, rather than specifying a percent impairment. In this setting of binary categorization, those considered impaired under Social Security criteria are expected to have a level of impairment sufficient to prevent working for a period of 1 year or longer. (5) Unlike Workers' Compensation programs, the Social Security program does not focus on occupational causation. The sole criterion for granting benefits is whether or not the claimant is able to participate in gainful employment. (6) The Social Security program also takes into account impairment from coexisting nonpulmonary conditions, such as substance abuse.

A major revision to the Social Security impairment criteria was proposed in February 2013.[3] Although the revision has not yet been approved, it is expected that the program will drop its requirements for hard copy spirometric tracings, add age and gender to the spirometric criteria, and add height and gender to the diffusing capacity criteria. If approved, it is also expected to be the first major impairment program to accept graphical printouts of pulse oximetry on room air at rest or after a 6-minute walk test for evaluating gas exchange impairment.

■ WORKERS' COMPENSATION SYSTEM

The Workers' Compensation system is a "no-fault" system of medical care and disability insurance in which private insurers or self-insured employers pay benefits to an employee sustaining an injury or illness due to workplace exposure. Under Workers' Compensation rules, workers cannot sue their employer for injury or illness.

The rules for the Workers' Compensation system vary from one state to another, but they usually follow one of the six editions of the American Medical Association (AMA) Guides to the Evaluation of Permanent Impairment.[4] The various editions of the AMA Guides contain markedly different sets of recommendations on impairment evaluation, so one must choose the right edition for the purpose. Use of the wrong edition may result in an erroneous impairment rating. While other guidelines are available on the Internet without charge, use of web-based AMA Guides carries a fee.

The sixth edition of the AMA Guides uses a standardized grid that incorporates five classes of impairment severity.[4] The grids incorporate objective, test-based key criteria for defining the impairment class, along with other criteria for fine-tuning the severity grade within a given class. Among the various objective tests, *the most severely affected test result is used to define the impairment class.*

Although the American Thoracic Society (ATS) has also developed consensus guidelines for rating impairment from chronic respiratory conditions and asthma,[5,6] these guidelines may not be accepted by a specific compensation program. While the AMA Guides generally follow the ATS schema, there exist substantial differences between the two guidelines.

FIVE GENERAL STEPS FOR IMPAIRMENT RATING

Five steps constitute the process of completing a respiratory impairment evaluation.

The first step is confirmation of the diagnosis of lung disease. Because of the medicolegal nature of the evaluation, the physician should have greater certainty of the medical diagnosis than is sometimes used in clinical practice. In other words, objective confirmation of the diagnosis is preferable.

The second step is defining maximal medical improvement (MMI). MMI occurs at the point when, following maximal therapy, no further clinical or physiologic improvement is expected to occur (although deterioration might). If therapy has not been maximized, the physician should either delay impairment evaluation or give a temporary rating. A permanent impairment evaluation should be performed only at, or after, MMI has been reached.

The third step is identifying the correct guideline for rating impairment. As discussed previously, several compensation systems exist, each with its own unique guideline. Therefore, identification of the compensation system for which the patient is eligible is essential, and the evaluating physician must be familiar with the specific guideline to be used. Of course, some patients may be eligible for more than one compensation program and may apply for more than one program contemporaneously.

The fourth step is to supplement the history and physical examination findings with appropriate objective tests. Performance of these tests should strictly adhere to standards of the ATS.[7–10]

The fifth and final step requires writing a comprehensive report of the patient's history, physical examination, and review of objective tests. The assessment should provide clear and accurate answers, in lay terms, to the questions asked. The evaluation should state the diagnosis and whether MMI has been reached, and it should make note of the presence and degree of respiratory impairment. The specific impairment scheme used, including the specific page and table of the guideline used, should be referenced. In work-related respiratory disorders, causation, apportionment, and work restrictions should also be addressed, as requested.

GENERAL APPROACH FOR EVALUATING RESPIRATORY IMPAIRMENT

After determining patient eligibility for a specific compensation system, as described previously, the physician gathers data that is relevant to rating respiratory impairment. In general, impairment criteria are based upon history, physical examination, and objective test results.

The medical history focuses on detailed past and present occupational history, tobacco use and environmental exposures, presence and severity of respiratory symptoms, such as dyspnea, cough, sputum production, and wheezing, and medication history. Relevant features in the physical examination include breathing pattern, shape of chest wall, adventitious lung sounds, cyanosis, digital clubbing, and evidence of cor pulmonale.

RESTING PULMONARY FUNCTION TESTS

Pulmonary function tests (PFTs) (Chapter 33) are the cornerstone for rating respiratory impairment and should be performed according to the most recent ATS standards.[7–10] Spirometry and diffusing capacity are the key PFTs for assessing respiratory impairment for chronic respiratory conditions. Postbronchodilator spirometry is used when airflow limitation is present. Methacholine challenge tests are used for rating impairment for asthma under the AMA Guides.[4]

Resting and exercise-related hypoxemia, derived from arterial blood gas results and adjusted for altitude and arterial P_{CO_2} level, may be used under the Social Security impairment system to classify gas exchange abnormalities. However, arterial blood gas sampling needs to be repeated within 3 weeks to 6 months of the first sample.[3] Although the presence of hypoxemia was previously used to rate impairment as severe under the fifth edition of the AMA Guides, the sixth edition does not include hypoxemia in the rating of respiratory impairment since it is considered invasive and difficult to standardize.[4]

Adjustment of PFTs for race, ethnicity, and gender is recommended by most impairment guidelines, with the notable exception of the Social Security impairment system, which currently uses uniform height-specific cut points for all individuals, irrespective of race, ethnicity, and gender.[2] Thus, under this system, older women are more likely to be rated as disabled than are younger men.

According to the sixth edition of the AMA Guides, specific NHANES III reference standards for spirometry should be used for Caucasian Americans, Mexican Americans, and African Americans.[4,11] For the remaining population subgroups, no clear guidelines are provided. Corrected single-breath carbon monoxide diffusing capacity (DL_{CO}) is used under the AMA Guides, ATS guidelines, and Social Security Impairment guidelines for impairment rating, but it is not used under the Veterans Administration guidelines. Crapo's reference standards for DL_{CO} are used for comparison with measured values.

The cut points for impairment classification, as suggested by the various impairment guidelines (Tables 38-1–38-3) are set arbitrarily and may differ from those recommended for assessing degree of lung disease severity by other professional organizations, such as the 2005 ATS statement[8] or by the Global Initiative for Chronic Obstructive Lung Disease (GOLD).[13] Some investigators have suggested that lung function thresholds should be expressed as a z-score, which converts a raw measurement on a test to a standardized score expressed in units of standard deviations.[14,15] This strategy, although scientifically valid, is not currently used for impairment evaluation.

Methacholine bronchoprovocation tests are useful for assessing bronchial hyperresponsiveness and in rating impairment from asthma under the AMA Guide and ATS guidelines (Tables 38-1 and 38-2).[4,6] The methacholine PC_{20} (provocative concentration of methacholine, expressed as mg/mL that results in at least 20% drop in FEV_1 compared to the pretest baseline) is a key parameter for rating asthma impairment under the sixth edition of the AMA Guides.[4] The performance of methacholine bronchoprovocation tests should also strictly adhere to the ATS guidelines.[16]

TABLE 38-1 Classification of Respiratory Impairment from Chronic Lung Diseases, Using the Sixth Edition of the American Medical Association (AMA) Guides to the Evaluation of Permanent Impairment

American Medical Association Class	Class 0	Class 1: 2–10% impairment of the whole person	Class 2: 11–23% impairment of the whole person	Class 3: 24–40% impairment of the whole person	Class 4: 45–65% impairment of the whole person
Severity grade (%)		A (2%), B (4%), C (6%), D (8%), E (10%)	A (11%), B (14%), C (17%), D (20%), E (23%)	A (24%), B (28%), C (32%), D (36%), E (40%)	A (45%), B (50%), C (55%), D (60%), E (65%)
Objective Tests					
FVC (% predicted)	≥80% predicted and	70–79% predicted or	60–69% predicted or	50–59% or	<50% or
FEV_1 (% predicted)	≥80% predicted and	65–79% predicted or	64–55% predicted or	45–54% or	<45% or
FEV_1/FVC%	>Lower limit of normal and/or >75% predicted) and	N/A	N/A	N/A	N/A
D_{LCO} (% predicted)	≥75% predicted	65–74% predicted	55–64% predicted	45–54%	<45%
$\dot{V}_{O_2max}$					
mL/kg/min	>25 or	22–25 or	21–18 or	15–17 or	<15 or
METs	>7.1	6.1–7.1	5.1–6.0	4.3–5.0	<4.3
History	No current symptoms and/or intermittent dyspnea that does not require treatment	Dyspnea controlled with intermittent or continuous treatment or intermittent mild dyspnea despite continuous treatment	Constant mild dyspnea despite continuous treatment or intermittent moderate dyspnea despite continuous treatment	Constant moderate dyspnea despite continuous treatment or intermittent severe dyspnea despite continuous treatment	Constant severe dyspnea despite continuous treatment or intermittent extreme dyspnea despite continuous treatment
Physical Findings	No current signs of disease	Physical findings not present with continuous treatment or intermittent mild physical findings	Constant mild physical findings despite continuous treatment or intermittent moderate physical findings	Constant moderate physical findings despite continuous treatment or intermittent severe physical findings	Constant severe physical findings despite continuous treatment or intermittent extreme physical findings

FVC, forced vital capacity; FEV_1, forced expiratory volume in the first second; D_{LCO}, diffusing capacity of carbon monoxide; $\dot{V}_{O_2max}$, measured maximal exercise capacity; MET or metabolic equivalent is the multiple of basal oxygen consumption, approximately 3.5 mL/kg/min; N/A, not applicable.

Source: Reproduced with permission from American Medical Association. The pulmonary system. In: Rondinelli RD, ed. Guides to the Evaluation of Permanent Impairment. 6th ed. American Medical Association; 2008:77–99.

EXERCISE TESTS

Maximal cardiopulmonary exercise tests are difficult to perform due to need for specialized equipment and trained personnel, are expensive and not readily available, and carry a risk to the patient. Test performance should strictly adhere to the ATS guidelines.[17] Clear agreement on the role of exercise tests in the evaluation of respiratory impairment is lacking. Generally, in cases in which subjective dyspnea is disproportionate to the resting PFT results,

TABLE 38-2 American Thoracic Society's (ATS) Classification of Respiratory Impairment[5]

Impairment Class	Normal	Mildly Impaired	Moderately Impaired	Severely Impaired
Work ability		Usually able to perform most jobs	Diminished ability to perform many jobs	Unable to meet physical demands of most jobs including travel to work
FVC (% predicted)	≥80%	60–79%	51-59%	≤50%
FEV_1 (% predicted)	≥80%	60–79%	41-59%	≤40%
FEV_1/FVC	≥75%	60–74%	41-59%	≤40%
D_{LCO} (% predicted)	≥80%	60–79%	41-59%	≤40%
$\dot{V}_{O_2max}$ (mL/kg/min)	≥25 (or 7.1 METs)			≤15 (or 4.3 METs)

FVC, forced vital capacity; FEV_1, forced expiratory volume in the first second; D_{LCO}, diffusing capacity of carbon monoxide; $\dot{V}_{O_2max}$, measured maximal exercise capacity; MET or metabolic equivalent is the multiple of basal oxygen consumption, approximately 3.5 mL/kg/min.

Source: Data from Evaluation of impairment/disability secondary to respiratory disorders. American Thoracic Society. Am Rev Respir Dis. 1986;133(6):1205–1209. This document was published in 1986 and is currently in revision. Certain aspects of this document may be out of date and caution should be used when applying these in clinical practice or other usages.

TABLE 38-3 Impairment Rating Guidelines for Chronic Obstructive Lung Diseases using the Social Security, Veterans Administration, American Medical Association (AMA) Guides, and American Thoracic Society (ATS) Guidelines

(A) SOCIAL SECURITY

Height without Shoes (cm)	Height without Shoes (in)	FEV_1 Equal to or Less than (L, BTPS)
≤154	≤60	1.05
155–160	61–63	1.15
161–165	64–65	1.25
166–170	66–67	1.35
171–175	68–69	1.45
176–180	70–71	1.55
≥181	≥72	1.65

(B) VETERANS ADMINISTRATION

Chronic Bronchitis

Pronounced (100% rating): with copious productive cough and dyspnea at rest; PFTs showing a severe degree of chronic airway obstruction with symptoms of associated severe emphysema or cyanosis and findings of right-sided heart involvement

Severe (60% rating): with severe productive cough and dyspnea on slight exertion and PFTs indicative of severe ventilatory impairment

Moderately severe (30% rating): persistent cough at intervals throughout the day, considerable expectoration, considerable dyspnea on exercise, rales throughout chest, beginning chronic airway obstruction

Moderate (10% rating): considerable night or morning cough, slight dyspnea on exercise, scattered bilateral rales

Mild (0% rating): slight cough, no dyspnea, few rales

Emphysema

Pronounced (100% rating): intractable and totally incapacitating; with dyspnea at rest, or marked dyspnea and cyanosis on mild exertion; severity of emphysema confirmed by CXR and PFTs

Severe (60% rating): exertional dyspnea sufficient to prevent climbing one flight of steps or walking one block without stopping; ventilatory impairment of severe degree confirmed by PFTs with marked impairment of health

Moderate (30% rating): with moderate dyspnea occurring after climbing one flight of steps or walking more than one block on a level surface; PFTs consistent with findings of moderate emphysema

Mild (10% rating): with evidence of ventilatory impairment on PFTs and/or definite dyspnea on prolonged exertion

(C) AMA GUIDES AND ATS GUIDELINES

Use criteria outlined in Tables A and B respectively in the text

FEV_1, forced expiratory volume in the first second; BTPS, body temperature and pressure saturated with water vapor.
For mixed obstructive and restrictive lung diseases with gas exchange impairment, evaluate under any of the criteria listed in Tables 38-3(A), 38-6(A), or 38-7.
Social Security impairment system has separate guidelines for patients with bronchiectasis.
Source: Data from Social Security Administration and Veterans Administration.[2,12]

or when PFTs are difficult to interpret because of submaximal performance, cardiopulmonary exercise tests may be considered. Such tests may also help identify unanticipated coexisting conditions, such as cardiovascular or pulmonary vascular disease, as the cause of exercise limitation.

Exercise testing may also be useful in determining whether an individual can perform a specific job with a known energy requirement. Under the ATS guidelines, the estimation of impairment from oxygen consumption at peak exercise ($\dot{V}_{O_2peak}$) is based on the widely held, but untested, assumptions that a worker involved in manual labor can comfortably work at 40% of $\dot{V}_{O_2peak}$ (corresponding to lower limit of generally accepted normal values for anaerobic threshold) for prolonged periods,[5] and that $\dot{V}_{O_2}$ requirements can be assigned to specific occupations. Individuals whose $\dot{V}_{O_2peak}$ is ≤15 mL/kg/min would be uncomfortable performing most jobs because they would find it difficult to travel back and forth to their place of employment (Table 38-2).[5] Unfortunately, data on $\dot{V}_{O_2}$ requirements of most jobs in modern workplaces are not currently available. Furthermore, jobs with the same title may vary considerably in their $\dot{V}_{O_2}$ requirements from one work site to another.

Submaximal exercise tests at a workload of approximately 17 mL O_2/kg/min (5 METs) or less of exercise can be performed at steady state to obtain arterial blood gases, which are then used to evaluate impairment of gas exchange under the Social Security impairment system when criteria for neither obstructive nor restrictive disorders are met. Use of submaximal exercise tests is however not currently recommended by any other impairment guideline.

IMAGING

Imaging studies are primarily useful for confirming the diagnosis of lung disease. They are less useful in rating respiratory impairment, since the correlation between radiographic abnormality and physiologic dysfunction is imperfect.

Chest radiographic evidence of pneumoconiosis is rated according to the 2011 International Labor Organization's (ILO) International Classification of Radiographs of Pneumoconiosis scheme (also called "B-reading"). The 2011 standards extended the applicability of the Classification to digital chest radiographs. The extent or profusion of small-sized parenchymal opacities is rated as 0, 1, 2, or 3. An intermediate score of 1/0 (i.e., profusion of small opacities greater than 0 but less than 1 profusion score) is often used to confirm the presence of pneumoconiosis.

Some determinations of respiratory impairment are not dependent on PFTs. They are based on environment-related diagnoses (e.g., occupational asthma or hypersensitivity pneumonitis) and warrant proscription of continuing exposure to inciting agents). In addition, impairment may be based upon prognosis (e.g., unresectable lung cancer) or public health considerations (e.g., pulmonary tuberculosis).

SCIENTIFIC RATIONALE FOR CHOICE OF TESTS USED FOR IMPAIRMENT EVALUATION FOR CHRONIC RESPIRATORY DISORDERS

Impairment evaluation for chronic respiratory conditions is based upon PFT values at rest and with exercise. The premise for these tests is that $\dot{V}_{O_2peak}$ reasonably measures ability to work, and that resting PFTs, such as forced expiratory volume in 1 second (FEV_1) and DL_{CO}, reasonably predict $\dot{V}_{O_2peak}$ values.

OXYGEN CONSUMPTION AT PEAK EXERCISE AS THE GOLD STANDARD FOR MEASURING ABILITY TO WORK

Most of the available medical literature appears to support the view that $\dot{V}_{O_2peak}$ value, expressed as mL/kg/min, is the gold standard for assessing impairment.[18,19] With exercise on a cycle ergometer, $\dot{V}_{O_2}$ increases linearly with external work,[17] and $\dot{V}_{O_2peak}$ represents the maximal work an individual can perform during a short burst of activity. Some have advocated use of percent predicted $\dot{V}_{O_2peak}$ values (i.e., loss of aerobic capacity), instead of $\dot{V}_{O_2peak}$ expressed in mL/kg/min (i.e., remaining aerobic ability) for evaluating impairment in patients with respiratory disease, since the latter approach overestimates impairment in older and obese subjects Fig. 38-1.[20,21] In addition, some consider the value for $\dot{V}_{O_2}$ at anaerobic threshold ($\dot{V}_{O_2}AT$) as a better index for work ability than $\dot{V}_{O_2peak}$.[21] Individuals are unable to sustain work rates above anaerobic threshold values. However, no major guidelines currently use percent predicted $\dot{V}_{O_2peak}$ values or $\dot{V}_{O_2}AT$ to rate impairment.

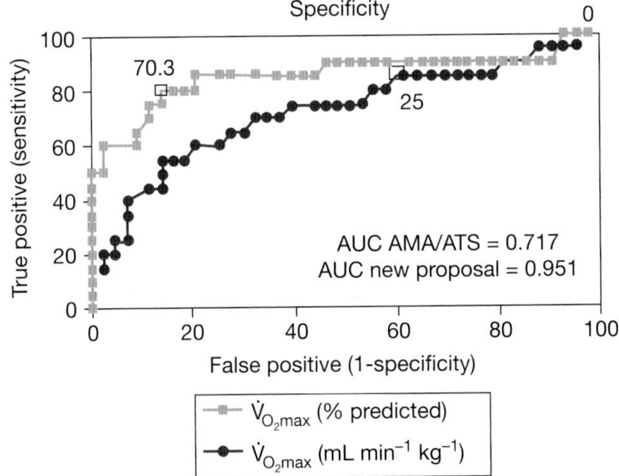

Figure 38-1 Receiver operating characteristics (ROC) curves of two classifications (AMA/ATS vs. new classification proposed by Neder et al.), using the $\dot{V}_{O_2}$ at anaerobic threshold ($\dot{V}_{O_2}AT$) as the "gold standard." The *open squares* represent the cutoffs for normality for $\dot{V}_{O_2peak}$ using the two classification schema. Neder et al. have advocated the use of percent predicted $\dot{V}_{O_2peak}$ values (i.e., loss of aerobic capacity) instead of $\dot{V}_{O_2peak}$ in mL/kg/min (i.e., remaining aerobic ability) for the evaluation of impairment in patients with respiratory disease since the latter approach overestimates impairment in older and obese subjects. AMA, American Medical Association; ATS, American Thoracic Society; AUC, area under the ROC curve; $\dot{V}_{O_2}$, oxygen consumption. *(Reproduced with permission from Neder JA, Nery LE, Bagatin E, Lucas SR, Ancao MS, Sue DY. Differences between remaining ability and loss of capacity in maximum aerobic impairment. Braz J Med Biol Res. 1998;31(5):639–646.)*

COMPARISON OF RESTING PULMONARY FUNCTION TESTS WITH OXYGEN CONSUMPTION AT PEAK EXERCISE

Low values for resting PFTs (i.e., FEV_1 or DL_{CO}) predict low $\dot{V}_{O_2peak}$ levels; poor scores on the Short Physical Performance Battery (tests that assess lower extremity function); less distance walked during the 6-minute walk test; and a greater risk of self-reported functional limitation.[22,23]

FEV_1 is linearly correlated with $\dot{V}_{O_2peak}$ levels,[23] but the reported correlations vary widely between studies, resulting in variance values ranging from 0.25 to 0.71.[23–28] Use of absolute versus percent predicted values largely yield similar correlation measures.[27] Although some studies demonstrate that FEV_1 and forced vital capacity (FVC) have similar predictive value for $\dot{V}_{O_2peak}$ levels,[27] most report FEV_1 to be a stronger predictor than FVC. A 2005 ATS statement indicated that percent predicted FEV_1, rather than FVC, should be used to categorize severity of impairment for all respiratory diseases.[8] The predictive ability of FEV_1 for $\dot{V}_{O_2peak}$ increases if it is used in combination with another variable, such as DL_{CO}, minute ventilation ($\dot{V}_E$), or dead space ventilation measure during exercise (V_D/V_T).[27] DL_{CO} does not predict $\dot{V}_{O_2peak}$ among healthy controls,[24] but it does so among subjects with COPD and those with occupational lung diseases, where it may account for a variance of 0.25 to 0.76 in various studies.[26,27,29]

Despite the previously noted correlations in population studies, resting PFTs cannot accurately predict $\dot{V}_{O_2peak}$ values among individuals, particularly those with occupational lung diseases. In a comparison study of impairment ratings obtained using simultaneous resting PFTs and cardiopulmonary exercise tests conducted in 216 ambulatory patients with COPD, the two methods resulted in similar impairment rating in only 30.1%. Ratings were similar between the two methods in the extreme subgroups of normal or severely impaired individuals. 61.1% were found to be less impaired according to exercise testing than according to resting PFTs, and 8.8% were more impaired according to exercise testing than resting PFTs (Table 38-4). These data suggest that use of resting PFTs and exercise testing for rating impairment often yields discrepant results.

TABLE 38-4 Degree of Impairment, as Assessed by Resting Pulmonary Function Tests and Cardiopulmonary Exercise Tests[a19]

Degree of Impairment	Resting PFT (%)	CPET (%)
None	6	28
Mild	26	36
Moderate	38	20
Severe	30	16

PFT, pulmonary function test; CPET, cardiopulmonary exercise test; FEV_1, Forced expiratory volume in 1 second.

[a]Among 216 ambulatory patients with COPD with mean percent predicted FEV_1 of 54.1 ± 16.8% and mean age of 57.9 ± 6.9 years

Source: Reproduced with permission from Fink G, Moshe S, Goshen J, et al. Functional evaluation in patients with chronic obstructive pulmonary disease: pulmonary function test versus cardiopulmonary exercise test. J Occup Environ Med. 2002;44(1):54–58.

PFTs other than FEV_1 and DL_{CO} may also help predict $\dot{V}_{O_2peak}$ values. These include inspiratory capacity in flow-limited obstructive diseases;[30] peak inspiratory pressure in chronic obstructive diseases;[26] exercise ventilation ($\dot{V}_E$) in both obstructive and restrictive lung diseases;[27] and submaximal exercise tests, including 6-minute walk test duration.[20] Use of these tests is however not currently recommended by any impairment guideline. Performance of maximal voluntary ventilation (MVV) is not recommended except under the Black Lung Benefits Act.[31] MVV is markedly effort dependent and bears a fixed relationship with FEV_1;[32] therefore, it is of limited value.

Further, both baseline oxygen saturation and the lowest oxygen saturation measured with a finger oximeter probe during a submaximal test correlate with $\dot{V}_{O_2peak}$ in patients with idiopathic pulmonary fibrosis,[20] but not in those with COPD.[33]

ASTHMA

Unlike most chronic respiratory conditions, asthma is an episodic disease, and impairment evaluation for asthma is particularly difficult. Therefore, most impairment rating schemes incorporate separate guidelines for rating asthma impairment.

■ DETERMINANTS OF WORK ABILITY IN ASTHMA

Among subjects with methacholine-confirmed asthma, a lower self-reported work ability is associated with lower PC_{20} value (i.e., higher degree of airway hyperresponsiveness), greater clinical severity of disease (based on minimum medication need to maintain asthma control), and the presence of respiratory symptoms in the workplace.[34] However, no relationships are evident with regard to baseline FEV_1 or FVC in both unadjusted and adjusted analyses.[34] Although controversial, methacholine PC_{20} (see Chapter 33) has been accepted as the key parameter for rating asthma impairment under the sixth edition of the AMA Guides.[4]

■ COMPARISON BETWEEN RESPIRATORY SYMPTOMS AND PC_{20}

For most subjects with asthma, greater breathlessness perceived during asthma attacks is not correlated with greater decline in peak expiratory flow rate [35] or with a lower PC_{20}.[36]

■ COMPARISON BETWEEN MINIMUM MEDICATION NEED AND PC_{20}

Almost all medications used to treat asthma improve PC_{20} values, that is, decrease bronchial hyperresponsiveness.[37–49] In one study, patients with asthma with the minimum medication needed to control symptoms were divided into four groups: (1) those who required no medication; (2) those who required short-acting β_2-agonist occasionally, but not daily; (3) those who required daily short-acting β_2-agonist; and (4) those who required additional inhaled corticosteroid dosing. The mean PC_{20} value was highest in group 1 and lowest in group 4; the differences between each group were significant.[50] Minimum medication need is, therefore, an important predictor for both work ability and airway hyperresponsiveness in asthma.

■ COMPARISON BETWEEN PERCENT PREDICTED FEV_1 AND PC_{20}

In a small clinical population of smokers and nonsmokers, as well as in a population of subjects with asthma with concomitant stable bronchiectasis, baseline FEV_1 has been shown to correlate with methacholine PC_{20} values.[51]

■ IMPAIRMENT RATING FOR ASTHMA

Impairment ratings for episodic diseases like asthma are problematic; the rating schemes differ dramatically as well (Tables 38-5A–38-5C).

The methacholine PC_{20} is the key parameter for rating asthma impairment under the sixth edition of the AMA Guides (Table 38-5B).[4] On the other hand, PC_{20} and extent of FEV_1 reversibility are given less weight than are either minimum medication need or postbronchodilator FEV_1 in the multicomponent asthma impairment scoring scheme recommended by the 1993 ATS guidelines (Table 38-5C).[6] Under Social Security impairment criteria, patients with asthma may be rated by FEV_1 or by a clinical history of frequent, severe exacerbations, despite maximal asthma therapy; a methacholine PC_{20} measurement is not required (Table 38-5A). On the contrary, AMA Guides and ATS guidelines do not

TABLE 38-5A Impairment Rating Guidelines for Asthma Using the Social Security, Veterans Administration, American Medical Association (AMA) Guides, and American Thoracic Society (ATS) Guidelines

(A) SOCIAL SECURITY
(1) Asthma with chronic asthmatic bronchitis: evaluate under the criteria for chronic obstructive airway disease (Table 38-3A)
(2) Attacks, in spite of prescribed treatment and requiring physician intervention, occurring at least once every 2 mo, or at least 6 times a year. Each in-patient hospitalization >24 h for control of asthma counts as two attacks. An evaluation period of at least 12 consecutive months must be used to determine the frequency of attacks
(B) VETERANS ADMINISTRATION[a]
Pronounced (100% rating): asthmatic attacks very frequently with severe dyspnea on slight exertion between attacks and with marked loss of weight or other evidence of severe impairment of health
Severe (60% rating): frequent attacks of asthma (one or more attacks weekly), marked dyspnea on exertion between attacks with only temporary relief by medication; more than light manual labor precluded
Moderate (30% rating): asthmatic attacks rather frequent (separated by only 10–14-d intervals) with moderate dyspnea on exertion between attacks
Mild (10% rating): paroxysms of asthmatic type breathing (high-pitched expiratory wheezing and dyspnea) occurring several times a year with no clinical findings between attacks
(C) AMA GUIDES AND ATS GUIDELINES
Use scoring criteria in Tables 38-5B and 38-5C, respectively

[a]*In the absence of clinical findings of asthma at time of examination, a verified history of asthmatic attacks must be on record.*
Source: Data from Social Security Administration and Veterans Administration.[2,12]

TABLE 38-5B Classification of Respiratory Impairment from Asthma, using the Sixth Edition of the American Medical Association (AMA) Guides to the Evaluation of Permanent Impairment

Class	Class 0	Class 1	Class 2	Class 3	Class 4
Whole person impairment rating (%)	0	2–10%	11–23%	24–40%	45–65%
Severity grade (%)		A (2%), B (4%), C (6%), D (8%), E (10%) (minimal)	A (11%), B (14%), C (17%), D (20%), E (23%) (mild)	A (24%), B (28%), C (32%), D (36%), E (40%) (moderate)	A (45%), B (50%), C (55%), D (60%), E (65%) (severe)
Clinical parameters (minimum medication need)	No medication required	Occasional bronchodilator, not daily	Daily low-dose inhaled steroid (<500 μg beclomethasone or equivalent)	Daily medium or high-dose inhaled steroids (500–1000 μg beclomethasone or equivalent) and/or short periods of systemic steroids and a long-acting bronchodilator. Daily use of steroids (systemic and inhaled) and daily use of maximum bronchodilators	Asthma not controlled by treatment
Maximum postbronchodilator percent predicted FEV_1	>80%	70–80%	60–69%	50–59%	<50%
PC_{20} (key factor)[a]	6–8 mg/mL	3–5 mg/mL	>0.5–3 mg/mL	0.25–0.5 mg/mL	0.125–0.24 mg/mL

FEV_1, forced expiratory volume in the first second; PC_{20}, provocative concentration of methacholine associated with 20% decrease in FEV_1 from baseline.

[a]The methacholine PC_{20} is the key parameter for rating asthma impairment. If PC_{20} cannot be obtained, postbronchodilator percent predicted FEV_1 is used as the key factor.

Source: Reproduced with permission from American Medical Association. The pulmonary system. In: Rondinelli RD, ed. Guides to the Evaluation of Permanent Impairment. 6th ed. American Medical Association; 2008.

incorporate frequency of acute exacerbations in the impairment rating for asthma. Given the efficacy of currently recommended asthma therapies, frequent emergency room visits or hospitalizations generally reflect inadequate treatment and failure to achieve the objectives of treatment. The AMA Guides and ATS guidelines instead use minimum medication need for asthma control as a better reflection of the severity of disease for the purpose of impairment assessment than frequency of asthma exacerbations. Hence, it is easy to see why impairment ratings for the same patient with asthma might vary widely among various compensation systems.

Impairment rating for occupational asthma is even more problematic. In these cases, both temporary and long-term impairment evaluation should be performed.[6] Temporary impairment for patients with sensitizer-induced occupational asthma should be performed after removing the worker from exposure. Early cessation of exposure improves prognosis in sensitizer-induced occupational asthma. Sometimes, physiologic tests may be normal, and symptoms and need for treatment may subside after early cessation of exposure, resulting in 0% measureable impairment. However, such an individual should be considered as100% disabled on a permanent basis from working in a job that exposes him or her to the specific sensitizing agent.[6] It is not necessary to wait for long-term impairment rating to initiate vocational rehabilitation in such a case.[6] The long-term impairment evaluation is performed using the rating systems devised for nonoccupational asthma at least 2 years after cessation of exposure, when improvement has been shown to plateau.[52]

PNEUMOCONIOSES

According to the AMA Guides, those who develop pneumoconiosis should limit further exposure to the offending agent, "particularly if radiographic changes have occurred at a relatively young age or if there is associated physiologic impairment."[4] It follows that an older patient who is nearing retirement, with minimal radiographic change after a long history of exposure, could elect to continue in the workplace under the assumption of a lower risk of developing future disabling disease. Such discretionary decisions should be made based on a discussion between the patient and physician.[4] While the Veterans Administration has specific guidelines for impairment ratings for pneumoconiosis, the Social Security construct is based upon standard criteria for assessing impairment from any chronic respiratory disorder, as listed in Tables 38-3(A), 38-6(A), and 38-7.[2]

COAL WORKERS' PNEUMOCONIOSIS

In 1972, the Black Lung Benefits Act set eligibility criteria for the awarding of benefits to coal miners and their survivors in the United States. The Act defines pneumoconiosis as, "a chronic dust disease of the lung and its sequelae, including respiratory and pulmonary impairments arising out of coal mine employment." This definition encompasses two classes of coal dust–related lung diseases: medical or "clinical" pneumoconioses and statutory or legal pneumoconioses. Medical or "clinical" pneumoconioses include diseases that pulmonologists usually consider as pneumoconioses (such as coal workers' pneumoconiosis, anthracosis, anthracosilicosis, massive pulmonary fibrosis, silicosis, or silicotuberculosis). Statutory or legal pneumoconioses include any chronic restrictive or obstructive pulmonary disease arising out of coal mine employment, including chronic bronchitis and emphysema.

A coal miner applying for Black Lung benefits must show that he or she has pneumoconiosis, that the pneumoconiosis resulted from coal mine employment, and that it has resulted in "total disability," defined as inability to perform usual coal mine work. The miner must supply medical evidence of pneumoconiosis that includes (1) a chest radiograph, along with a report of the findings using the ILO classification system; (2) a physician report detailing the occupational, medical, and smoking history, as well as all manifestations of chronic respiratory disease; (3) spirometric results (including MVV); (4) altitude-adjusted arterial blood gas results; and (5) biopsy or autopsy evidence, if available.

TABLE 38-5C American Thoracic Society's (ATS) Asthma Impairment Rating Guideline

(A) POST-BRONCHODILATOR FEV_1	
Score	FEV_1 (%Predicted)
0	>lower limit of normal
1	70–lower limit of normal
2	60–69
3	50–59
4	<50

(B) REVERSIBILITY OF FEV_1 OR DEGREE OF AIRWAY HYPERRESPONSIVENESS[a]		
Score	%FEV_1 Change	PC_{20} (mg/mL)
0	<10	>8
1	10–19	8–>0.5
2	20–29	0.5–>0.125
3	≥30	≤0.125

(C) MINIMUM MEDICATION NEEDS[b]	
Score	Medication
0	No medication
1	Occasional bronchodilator, not daily, and/or occasional cromolyn, not daily
2	Daily bronchodilator and/or daily cromolyn and/or daily inhaled low-dose inhaled steroid (<800 μg beclomethasone or equivalent)
3	Bronchodilator on demand and daily high-dose inhaled steroid (>800 μg beclomethasone or equivalent) or occasional course (1–3/y) of systemic steroid
4	Bronchodilator on demand and daily high-dose inhaled steroid (>1000 μg beclomethasone or equivalent) and daily systemic steroid

(D) SUMMARY OF IMPAIRMENT RATING CLASSES	
Impairment Rating	Sum of Scores from Sections A, B, and C
0	0
I	1–3
II	4–6
III	7–9
IV	10–11
V	Asthma not controlled despite maximal treatment, i.e., FEV_1 remaining <50% despite use of ≥20 mg Prednisone per day

FEV_1, forced expiratory volume in the first second; PC_{20}, provocative concentration of methacholine associated with 20% decrease in FEV_1 from baseline.

[a]When the postbronchodilator FEV_1 value is above the lower limit of normal, the PC_{20} value should be determined and used for rating of impairment; when the post-bronchodilator FEV_1 value is <70% of the predicted value, the degree of reversibility is used; when the FEV_1 value is between 70% of the predicted value and the lower limit of normal, either the degree of reversibility of FEV_1 or the PC_{20} can be used.

[b]The need for minimum medication should be demonstrated by the treating physician, for example, previous records of exacerbations when medications have been reduced.

Source: Adapted with permission of the American Thoracic Society. Copyright © 2013 American Thoracic Society. Guidelines for the evaluation of impairment/disability in patients with asthma. American Thoracic Society. Medical Section of the American Lung Association. Am Rev Respir Dis. 1993;147(4):1056–1061. Official journal of the American Thoracic Society. This document was published in 1993 and is currently in revision. Certain aspects of this document may be out of date and caution should be used when applying these in clinical practice or other usages.

Chest radiographic findings are accepted to show pneumoconioses if they demonstrate the presence of either small parenchymal opacities of at least category 1/0 profusion or large opacities. The absence of radiographic evidence of pneumoconioses makes medical or clinical pneumoconioses unlikely, but it may be noted in patients with statutory or legal pneumoconiosis.[31] Spirometry must meet the 1979 ATS repeatability criteria that require the maximum FVC and FEV_1 be within 5% or 100 mL, whichever is greater.[53] The arterial blood gas analysis may be performed at rest or with exercise. The Department of Labor has published detailed tables of FEV_1, FVC, and MVV, as well as arterial blood gas values delineating criteria for "total disability."[31]

■ UNITED STATES DEPARTMENT OF ENERGY EMPLOYEES IN NUCLEAR WEAPONS FACTORIES

The US Energy Employees' Occupational Illness Compensation Program Act (EEOICPA) was enacted to provide compensation and medical benefits to workers who acquired disease in the course of their work in the nuclear defense industry. Those eligible include employees and former employees of the Department of Energy at nuclear weapons factories, as well as private contractors and subcontractors at those locations. In addition to exposure to silica, asbestos, or mixed dusts that occurred during uranium ore extraction, many workers were also exposed to beryllium (used in the manufacture of ballistic missile nose cones) and radiation.

TABLE 38-6 Impairment Rating Guidelines for Restrictive Lung Diseases using the Social Security, Veterans Administration, American Medical Association (AMA) Guides, and American Thoracic Society (ATS) Guidelines

(A) SOCIAL SECURITY		
Height without Shoes (cm)	**Height without Shoes (in)**	**Vital Capacity Equal to or Less than (L, BTPS)**
≤154	≤60	1.25
155–160	61–63	1.35
161–165	64–65	1.45
166–170	66–67	1.55
171–175	68–69	1.65
176–180	70–71	1.75
≥181	≥72	1.85
(B) VETERANS ADMINISTRATION		
Leaves the rating to the judgment of the physician, according to symptoms, anatomical extent, pulmonary functions and complications.		
(C) AMA GUIDES AND ATS GUIDELINES		
Use criteria outlined in Tables 38-6A and B, respectively		

BTPS, body temperature and pressure saturated with water vapor.
In severe kyphoscoliosis, the measured span between the fingertips when the upper extremities are abducted 90 degrees should be substituted for height.
For mixed obstructive and restrictive lung diseases with gas exchange impairment, evaluate under any of the criteria listed in Tables 38-3A,38-6A, or 7.
Source: Data from Social Security Administration and Veterans Administration.[2,12]

In contradistinction to Black Lung evaluation, the Part E of the EEOICPA has adopted the standards of the fifth edition of AMA Guides to the Evaluation of Permanent Impairment as the method of rating impairment.

LUNG CANCER

According to the AMA Guides, lung cancer is a cause of severe impairment for the period extending from the time of diagnosis to 1 year, thereafter. If no evidence of tumor is found at reevaluation at 1 year, then impairment is recalculated on the basis of the degree of physiologic impairment present at that time. On the other hand, if there is evidence of tumor, the patient remains classified as severely impaired.

Under the Social Security system, lung cancer produces impairment if it is unresectable, is incompletely resected, is recurrent or metastatic, is of small cell histology, is a squamous cell cancer with

TABLE 38-7 Social Security Impairment Criteria for Evaluating Chronic Impairments of Gas Exchange due to Clinically Documented Pulmonary Disease

(1) Arterial blood gases demonstrating values of Pa_{O_2} and simultaneously determined Pa_{CO_2} measured while at rest (breathing room air, awake and sitting, or standing), in a clinically stable condition on at least two occasions, 3 or more weeks apart within a 6-mo period, equal to or less than the values specified below or arterial blood gas values during steady-state exercise breathing room air (level of exercise equivalent to or less than 17.5 mL O_2 consumption/kg/min or 5 METs), equal to or less than the values specified below.

Pa_{CO_2} (in mm Hg) and	At test sites <3000 ft above sea level, $Pa_{O_2} \leq$ (in mm Hg)	At test sites 3000–6000 ft above sea level, $Pa_{O_2} \leq$ (in mm Hg)	At test sites >6000 ft above sea level, $Pa_{O_2} \leq$ (in mm Hg)
≤ 30	65	60	55
31	64	59	54
32	63	58	53
33	62	57	52
34	61	56	51
35	60	55	50
36	59	54	49
37	58	53	48
38	57	52	47
39	56	51	46
≥40	55	50	45
Or			

(2) Diffusing capacity for carbon monoxide less than 10.5 mL/mm Hg/min (single-breath method) or less than 40% of predicted normal. (All methods, actual values and predicted normal values and the sources of the predicted value should be reported).

Source: Data from Social Security Administration.[2]

metastasis beyond hilar nodes, or is one of other histologic types with metastasis to hilar lymph nodes. Under the Veterans Administration system, degree of impairment is not categorized clearly, but rather, is left to the judgment of the physician.

SLEEP APNEA

Impairment ratings for sleep apnea are problematic and vary widely among compensation systems. Resting and exercise PFTs are not useful for rating impairment related to sleep apnea. Therefore, the AMA Guides recommend assessment of complications of sleep apnea, such as the presence of cor pulmonale or polycythemia, and rate the complications according to the appropriate organ systems. Any "add-on" for strictly defining respiratory impairment must be determined by a sleep specialist and should not exceed 3% of total impairment.[4] Under the Social Security system, sleep apnea is rated according to criteria for cor pulmonale, obesity, or organic mental disorders.[2]

AMERICANS WITH DISABILITIES ACT

Although many physicians think of impairment assessment as an evaluation that follows injury, or termination of employment, or is undertaken at an advanced stage of lung disease, in reality, important assessments are also made prior to the start of a job. Until recently, people with physical impairment were excluded from employment because of an unreasonable fear that an impaired employee would be a detriment at the workplace. The Americans with Disabilities Act (ADA), which was enacted by the United States in 1992, produced a fundamental change in the way in which physical impairments are viewed at the workplace.

Many of the regulations established by the ADA deal with removal of physical barriers that prevent impaired workers from entering and functioning within the workplace. Others are specifically directed at removing bias and prejudice from the opportunity to enter the workforce. While the ADA has not altered the methods of impairment evaluation used by physicians, it does have a substantial impact on the timing of evaluations and the way the evaluations are reported and used. For instance, while preemployment physical examinations were commonly requested by employers prior to enactment of the ADA, they are no longer allowed, due to the perceived risk that a qualified individual might be excluded from employment because of an impairment that has little or nothing to do with the job requirements. Before making a job offer, employers are no longer allowed to ask if a prospective employee has a physical impairment, although they may ask if he or she can perform the duties of the job. Once a job offer is made and accepted, physical examination is permissible to confirm that the job can be performed in a safe and acceptable manner. In fact, the employer is legally permitted to make a job offer conditional on the applicant passing a physical examination, as long as the same physical requirements are required for every employee in the same job category. These examinations, known as preplacement physicals, must deal only with job-related issues and must be consistent with business necessity.

The other major change in the determination of work-related physical fitness is that businesses are required to make "reasonable" accommodations for physical impairments, as long as the impairments do not interfere with the essential requirements of the job. Employers are not, however, required to make unreasonably extensive changes to a work area or to undertake "action requiring significant difficulty or expense" to accommodate an otherwise qualified applicant.

REFERENCES

1. Wood PH. Appreciating the consequences of disease: the international classification of impairments, disabilities, and handicaps. *WHO Chron.* 1980;34(10):376–380.
2. United States Department of Health and Human Services. *Social Security Administration: Disability Evaluation under Social Security*. Vol HHS Publication No SSA Publication No 64-039. Baltimore, MD: United States Government Printing Office; 2001. http://www.ssa.gov/disability/professionals/bluebook/3.00-Respiratory-Adult.htm. Accessed April 16, 2013.
3. Social Security Administration. 20 CFR Parts 404 and 416. Revised Medical Criteria for Evaluating Respiratory System Disorders; Proposed Rule. *Federal Register.* 2013;78(23):7968–7985.
4. American Medical Association. The pulmonary system. In: Rondinelli RD, ed. *Guides to the Evaluation of Permanent Impairment.* 6th ed. American Medical Association; 2008: 77–99.
5. Evaluation of impairment/disability secondary to respiratory disorders. American Thoracic Society. *Am Rev Respir Dis.* 1986;133(6):1205–1209.
6. Guidelines for the evaluation of impairment/disability in patients with asthma. American Thoracic Society. Medical Section of the American Lung Association. *Am Rev Respir Dis.* 1993;147(4):1056–1061.
7. Miller MR, Crapo R, Hankinson J, et al. General considerations for lung function testing. *Eur Respir J.* 2005;26(1):153–161.
8. Pellegrino R, Viegi G, Brusasco V, et al. Interpretative strategies for lung function tests. *Eur Respir J.* 2005;26(5):948–968.
9. Macintyre N, Crapo RO, Viegi G, et al. Standardisation of the single-breath determination of carbon monoxide uptake in the lung. *Eur Respir J.* 2005;26(4):720–735.
10. Miller MR, Hankinson J, Brusasco V, et al. Standardisation of spirometry. *Eur Respir J.* 2005;26(2):319–338.
11. Hankinson JL, Odencrantz JR, Fedan KB. Spirometric reference values from a sample of the general U.S. population. *Am J Respir Crit Care Med.* 1999;159(1):179–187.
12. Veterans Administration DoMaS. Chapter 5: Pulmonary diseases. *Physician's Guide for Disability Evaluation Examinations*, Volumes 11–56 of Veterans Admin. information bulletin, Veterans Administration; 1985:5-1 to 5-7.
13. Rabe KF, Hurd S, Anzueto A, et al; Global Initiative for Chronic Obstructive Lung Disease. Global strategy for the diagnosis, management, and prevention of chronic obstructive pulmonary disease: GOLD executive summary. *Am J Respir Crit Care Med.* 2007;176(6):532–555.
14. Miller MR, Pincock AC. Predicted values: how should we use them? *Thorax.* 1988;43(4):265–267.
15. Vaz Fragoso CA, Gill TM. Respiratory impairment and the aging lung: a novel paradigm for assessing pulmonary function. *J GerontolA Biol Sci Med Sci.* 2012;67(3):264–275.
16. Crapo RO, Casaburi R, Coates AL, et al. Guidelines for methacholine and exercise challenge testing-1999. This official statement of the American Thoracic Society was adopted by the ATS Board of Directors. 1999. *Am J Respir Crit Care Med.* 2000;161(1):309–329.
17. American Thoracic Society, American College of Chest Physicians. ATS/ACCP Statement on cardiopulmonary exercise testing. *Am J Respir Crit Care Med.* 2003;167(2):211–277.
18. Pichurko BM. Exercising your patient: which test(s) and when? *Respir Care.* 2012;57(1):100–110; discussion 110–103.
19. Fink G, Moshe S, Goshen J, et al. Functional evaluation in patients with chronic obstructive pulmonary disease: pulmonary function test versus cardiopulmonary exercise test. *J Occup Environ Med.* 2002;44(1):54–58.

20. Rusanov V, Shitrit D, Fox B, Amital A, Peled N, Kramer MR. Use of the 15-steps climbing exercise oximetry test in patients with idiopathic pulmonary fibrosis. *Respir Med.* 2008;102(7):1080–1088.
21. Neder JA, Nery LE, Bagatin E, Lucas SR, Ancao MS, Sue DY. Differences between remaining ability and loss of capacity in maximum aerobic impairment. *Braz J Med Biol Res.* 1998;31(5):639–646.
22. Eisner MD, Iribarren C, Yelin EH, et al. Pulmonary function and the risk of functional limitation in chronic obstructive pulmonary disease. *Am J Epidemiol.* 2008;167(9):1090–1101.
23. Pineda H, Haas F, Axen K, Haas A. Accuracy of pulmonary function tests in predicting exercise tolerance in chronic obstructive pulmonary disease. *Chest.* 1984;86(4):564–567.
24. Bogaard HJ, Woltjer HH, van Keimpema AR, Postmus PE, de Vries PM. Prediction of peak oxygen uptake in men using pulmonary and hemodynamic variables during exercise. *Med Sci Sports Exerc.* 2000;32(3):701–705.
25. Ong KC, Ong YY. Cardiopulmonary exercise testing in patients with chronic obstructive pulmonary disease. *Ann Acad Med Singapore.* 2000;29(5):648–652.
26. Dillard TA, Piantadosi S, Rajagopal KR. Determinants of maximum exercise capacity in patients with chronic airflow obstruction. *Chest.* 1989;96(2):267–271.
27. Cotes JE, Zejda J, King B. Lung function impairment as a guide to exercise limitation in work-related lung disorders. *Am Rev Respir Dis.* 1988;137(5):1089–1093.
28. Dimopoulou I, Tsintzas OK, Daganou M, Cokkinos DV, Tzelepis GE. Contribution of lung function to exercise capacity in patients with chronic heart failure. *Respiration.* 1999;66(2):144–149.
29. Carlson DJ, Ries AL, Kaplan RM. Prediction of maximum exercise tolerance in patients with COPD. *Chest.* 1991;100(2):307–311.
30. Diaz O, Villafranca C, Ghezzo H, et al. Role of inspiratory capacity on exercise tolerance in COPD patients with and without tidal expiratory flow limitation at rest. *Eur Respir J.* 2000;16(2):269–275.
31. United States Government Printing Office. Part 718 - Standards for determining coal miners' total disability or death due to pneumoconiosis. http://www.ecfr.gov/cgi-bin/retrieveECFR?gp=1&SID=5c92730f5b89d3c7474009fc8605a504&ty=HTML&h=L&n=20y4.0.2.2.5&r=PART. Accessed April 16, 2013.
32. Ferris BG. Epidemiology Standardization Project (American Thoracic Society). *Am Rev Respir Dis.* 1978;118(6Pt 2):1–120.
33. Fukushima T, Ohrui T, Itabashi S, et al. Prolonged hypoxemia after 10 min walking exercise in aged patients with chronic obstructive pulmonary disease. *Tohoku J Exp Med.* 1990;162(4):345–353.
34. Balder B, Lindholm NB, Lowhagen O, et al. Predictors of self-assessed work ability among subjects with recent-onset asthma. *Respir Med.* 1998;92(5):729–734.
35. Boudreau D, Styhler A, Gray-Donald K, Martin JG. A comparison of breathlessness during spontaneous asthma and histamine-induced bronchoconstriction. *Clin Invest Med.* 1995;18(1):25–32.
36. Boulet LP, Leblanc P, Turcotte H. Perception scoring of induced bronchoconstriction as an index of awareness of asthma symptoms. *Chest.* 1994;105(5):1430–1433.
37. Page CP, Cotter T, Kilfeather S, Sullivan P, Spina D, Costello JF. Effect of chronic theophylline treatment on the methacholine dose-response curve in allergic asthmatic subjects. *Eur Respir J.* 1998;12(1):24–29.
38. Perng DW, Huang HY, Lee YC, Perng RP. Leukotriene modifier vs inhaled corticosteroid in mild-to-moderate asthma: clinical and anti-inflammatory effects. *Chest.* 2004;125(5):1693–1699.
39. Svendsen UG, Frolund L, Madsen F, Nielsen NH. A comparison of the effects of nedocromil sodium and beclomethasone dipropionate on pulmonary function, symptoms, and bronchial responsiveness in patients with asthma. *J Allergy Clin Immunol.* 1989;84(2):224–231.
40. Kanniess F, Richter K, Bohme S, Jorres RA, Magnussen H. Montelukast versus fluticasone: effects on lung function, airway responsiveness and inflammation in moderate asthma. *Eur Respir J.* 2002;20(4):853–858.
41. Berkman N, Avital A, Bardach E, Springer C, Breuer R, Godfrey S. The effect of montelukast on bronchial provocation tests and exhaled nitric oxide levels in asthmatic patients. *Isr Med Assoc J.* 2003;5(11):778–781.
42. O'Connor BJ, Towse LJ, Barnes PJ. Prolonged effect of tiotropium bromide on methacholine-induced bronchoconstriction in asthma. *Am J Respir Crit Care Med.* 1996;154(4Pt 1):876–880.
43. Overbeek SE, Rijnbeek PR, Vons C, Mulder PG, Hoogsteden HC, Bogaard JM. Effects of fluticasone propionate on methacholine dose-response curves in nonsmoking atopic asthmatics. *Eur Respir J.* 1996;9(11):2256–2262.
44. Silkoff PE, McClean PA, Slutsky AS, et al. Exhaled nitric oxide and bronchial reactivity during and after inhaled beclomethasone in mild asthma. *J Asthma.* 1998;35(6):473–479.
45. Derom EY, Pauwels RA, Van der Straeten ME. The effect of inhaled salmeterol on methacholine responsiveness in subjects with asthma up to 12 hours. *J Allergy Clin Immunol.* 1992;89(4):811–815.
46. Yates DH, Sussman HS, Shaw MJ, Barnes PJ, Chung KF. Regular formoterol treatment in mild asthma. Effect on bronchial responsiveness during and after treatment. *Am J Respir Crit Care Med.* 1995;152(4Pt 1):1170–1174.
47. Zu Wallack RL, Kass J, Shiue ST, et al. Effect of inhaled triamcinolone on bronchial hyperreactivity and airways obstruction in asthma. *Ann Allergy.* 1990;64(2Pt 2):207–212.
48. van Rensen EL, Straathof KC, Veselic-Charvat MA, Zwinderman AH, Bel EH, Sterk PJ. Effect of inhaled steroids on airway hyperresponsiveness, sputum eosinophils, and exhaled nitric oxide levels in patients with asthma. *Thorax.* 1999;54(5):403–408.
49. Bel EH, Zwinderman AH, Timmers MC, Dijkman JH, Sterk PJ. The protective effect of a beta 2 agonist against excessive airway narrowing in response to bronchoconstrictor stimuli in asthma and chronic obstructive lung disease. *Thorax.* 1991;46(1):9–14.
50. Juniper EF, Frith PA, Hargreave FE. Airway responsiveness to histamine and methacholine: relationship to minimum treatment to control symptoms of asthma. *Thorax.* 1981;36(8):575–579.
51. Ip M, Lam WK, So SY, Liong E, Chan CY, Tse KM. Analysis of factors associated with bronchial hyperreactivity to methacholine in bronchiectasis. *Lung.* 1991;169(1):43–51.
52. Malo JL, Cartier A, Ghezzo H, Lafrance M, McCants M, Lehrer SB. Patterns of improvement in spirometry, bronchial hyperresponsiveness, and specific IgE antibody levels after cessation of exposure in occupational asthma caused by snow-crab processing. *Am Rev Respir Dis.* 1988;138(4):807–812.
53. ATS statement–Snowbird workshop on standardization of spirometry. *Am Rev Respir Dis.* 1979;119(5):831–838.

PART 4

Obstructive Lung Diseases

CHAPTER 39

Pathology of Chronic Obstructive Pulmonary Disease: Diagnostic Features and Differential Diagnosis

Joanne L. Wright
Andrew Churg

Chronic obstructive pulmonary disease (COPD) is a general name for the chronic airflow obstruction that develops most often as a result of chronic tobacco smoking, but also after exposure to biomass fuels. The pathology of COPD encompasses a variety of pathologic lesions in the airways, lung parenchyma, and pulmonary vasculature, and these lesions can be correlated, to a greater or lesser degree, with changes in pulmonary function tests and clinical appearances. In general, although the mechanisms involved are complex, airflow obstruction can be attributed largely to a marked increase in airway resistance secondary to a variable mix of structural abnormalities involving all or many of the compartments of the airway. However, in individual cases, it may be difficult to prove associations between physiologic abnormalities and pathologic changes. The Global Initiative on Obstructive Lung Disease (GOLD), recently revised,[1] classifies patients with COPD purely upon indices of airflow and thus far there is only limited integration with pathologic findings.

This chapter presents the pathologic features of COPD and how these findings can be differentiated from other lesions associated with airflow obstruction.

HISTORY OF PATHOLOGIC DESCRIPTIONS OF COPD

The word emphysema is derived from Greek and means "to blow into," hence "air-containing" or "inflated." Although "voluminous lungs" and lungs "turgid particularly from air" were described respectively by Bonet in 1679[2] and Morgagni in 1769,[3] the first description of enlarged airspaces in emphysema in the human, together with illustrations, was furnished by Ruysh in 1721,[4] followed by Matthew Baillie in 1807, who not only clearly recognized and illustrated emphysema, but also pointed out its essentially destructive character.[5,6]

Laennec,[7] writing in the early 1800s, made a number of seminal contributions to the basic descriptions of pathologic changes in COPD. He was the first to make a clear-cut distinction between interstitial emphysema and emphysema proper, and related the enlarged airspaces to the clinical syndrome of emphysema. He also recognized that air trapping and increased collateral ventilation were features of emphysematous lungs, and that the peripheral airways were the primary site of obstruction in emphysema. Furthermore, he noted that airspaces enlarged with increasing age, and he distinguished these changes from emphysema. He was the first to describe an association of emphysema with chronic bronchitis and to clearly describe the pathology of bronchiectasis.

Little of major importance was added to the gross descriptive morphology of emphysema for almost the next 150 years. The foundation of modern knowledge of the pathologic anatomy of pulmonary emphysema was laid by J. Gough in 1952[8] when he described centrilobular emphysema and distinguished it from panlobular emphysema. The paper section technique developed by Gough and Wentworth[9] was largely responsible for this advance, as it made examinations of sections of entire inflated lungs possible and simple (Fig. 39-1). A comprehensive microscopic description of emphysema was then provided by McLean,[10,11] who demonstrated the relationship of destruction to inflammatory alterations of the bronchioles, and also discussed alterations of the vasculature.

LESIONS OF THE LUNG PARENCHYMA IN COPD: EMPHYSEMA

A major problem in describing the pathologic features of emphysema has been the lack of a generally accepted and easy to apply definition. In 1959, a Ciba Guest Symposium defined emphysema in anatomic terms as "a condition of the lung characterized by increase beyond the normal of airspaces, distal to the terminal bronchiole, either from dilatation or from destruction of their walls."[12] Subsequent definitions differed in that destruction of respiratory tissue became a requirement[13–15]: "Emphysema is a condition of the lung characterized by abnormal, permanent enlargement of the airspaces distal to the terminal bronchiole, accompanied by destruction of their walls." This requirement separates emphysema from enlargement of airspaces unaccompanied by destruction, the latter now being termed overinflation.

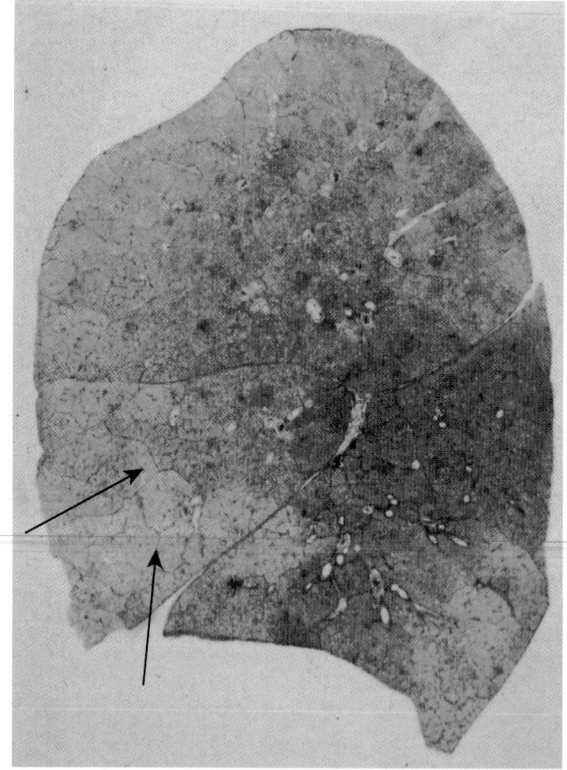

Figure 39-1 Gough sagittal section. Paper mount. Normal lung.

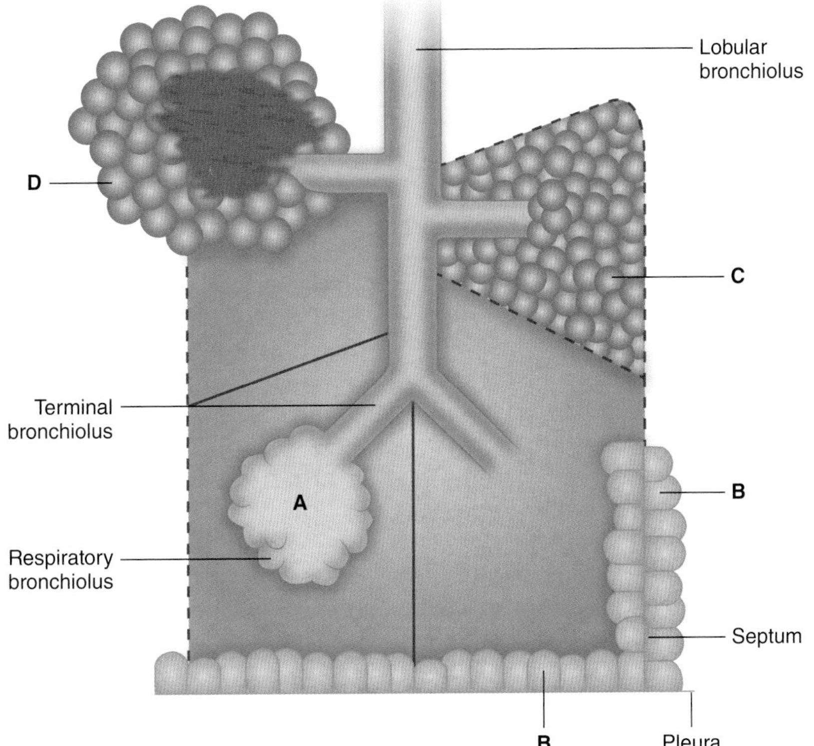

Figure 39-2 Anatomic varieties of emphysema. **A.** Centriacinar (centrilobular). **B.** Paraseptal (distal acinar). **C.** Panacinar (panlobular). **D.** Irregular (scar). The *dashed lines* mark the edge of the acinus. Only centriacinar and panacinar emphysema are commonly observed in COPD, although paraseptal emphysema often can be found in focal areas in lungs with centriacinar emphysema.

Destruction has been similarly difficult to define in an unambiguous way. A committee of the National Institutes of Health[16] proposed that destruction was present when "there was nonuniformity in the pattern of respiratory airspace enlargement so that the orderly appearance of the acinus and its components is disturbed and may be lost." They recognized that emphysema was a subset of airspace enlargement defined as "an increase in airspace size as compared with the airspace of normal lungs. The term applies to all varieties of airspace enlargement distal to the terminal bronchioles, whether occurring with or without fibrosis or destruction." While these definitions, when strictly applied, would eliminate airspace enlargement due to overinflation or failure of septation, they would not eliminate airspace enlargement due to reorganization of the airspaces, such as is found in honeycomb lung. This may be part of the confusion when combined emphysema and fibrosis is considered (see the section below).

CLASSIFICATION OF EMPHYSEMA

Not only is emphysema defined in terms of lung structure, it is also classified in similar terms; therefore, several anatomic definitions are important. The part of the lung involved in emphysema is the acinus, which is defined as the unit of lung structure distal to the terminal bronchiole (final generation membranous bronchiole) and that consists of three orders of respiratory bronchioles: a single order of alveolar ducts, followed by the alveolar sacs, and finally the alveoli. Alveolar ducts are entirely alveolated and characteristically contain smooth muscle around the mouths of their alveoli. While the walls of alveolar sacs are also formed entirely by alveoli, muscle is absent. Alveolar pores of Kohn (also known as vents, stomata, or fenestrae) are normal components of adult alveoli, responsible for collateral ventilation. However, they may also be an initial site of destruction in the development of emphysema, particularly centriacinar emphysema.

The acinus is a three-dimensional anatomic structure, but it cannot be easily identified by gross examination. What can be seen instead on the surface of lung slices is the secondary lobule of Miller, defined as the tissue bounded on four sides by interlobular septa or pleura (see Fig. 39-1). Lobules vary tremendously in size, but are generally 2 to 4 cm on a side, and contain between three to five acini. The terminal bronchiole and subtending respiratory bronchioles tend to be situated in the center of the lobule. For this reason "centrilobular" emphysema and "panlobular" emphysema are reasonable and widely used approximations for the more accurate "centriacinar" and "panacinar" emphysema (see below).

The ways in which the acini are involved determine the classification of emphysema. There are four recognized patterns (Fig. 39-2). The acinus (and lobule) may be more or less uniformly involved; this is panacinar (panlobular) emphysema. The proximal portion of the acinus (center of the lobule) may be dominantly involved; the best term for this lesion is proximal acinar emphysema, although the usual term is centrilobular or centriacinar emphysema. Alternately, the proximal portion of the acinus may be normal, and the distal part (alveolar sacs and ducts) may be dominantly involved. This is distal acinar emphysema, more commonly referred to as paraseptal emphysema since the lesion is accentuated along lobular septa where the peripheral parts of the acini lie. Finally, the acinus may be irregularly involved, producing irregular emphysema or paracicatricial emphysema, so called because it is usually associated with obvious adjacent scarring.

MORPHOLOGY OF EMPHYSEMA

■ CENTRILOBULAR EMPHYSEMA

This destructive lesion of the respiratory bronchioles has a number of characteristic features on gross examination of the lung. In the *classical* lesion, the enlarged, destroyed respiratory bronchioles coalesce in series and in parallel to produce sharply demarcated

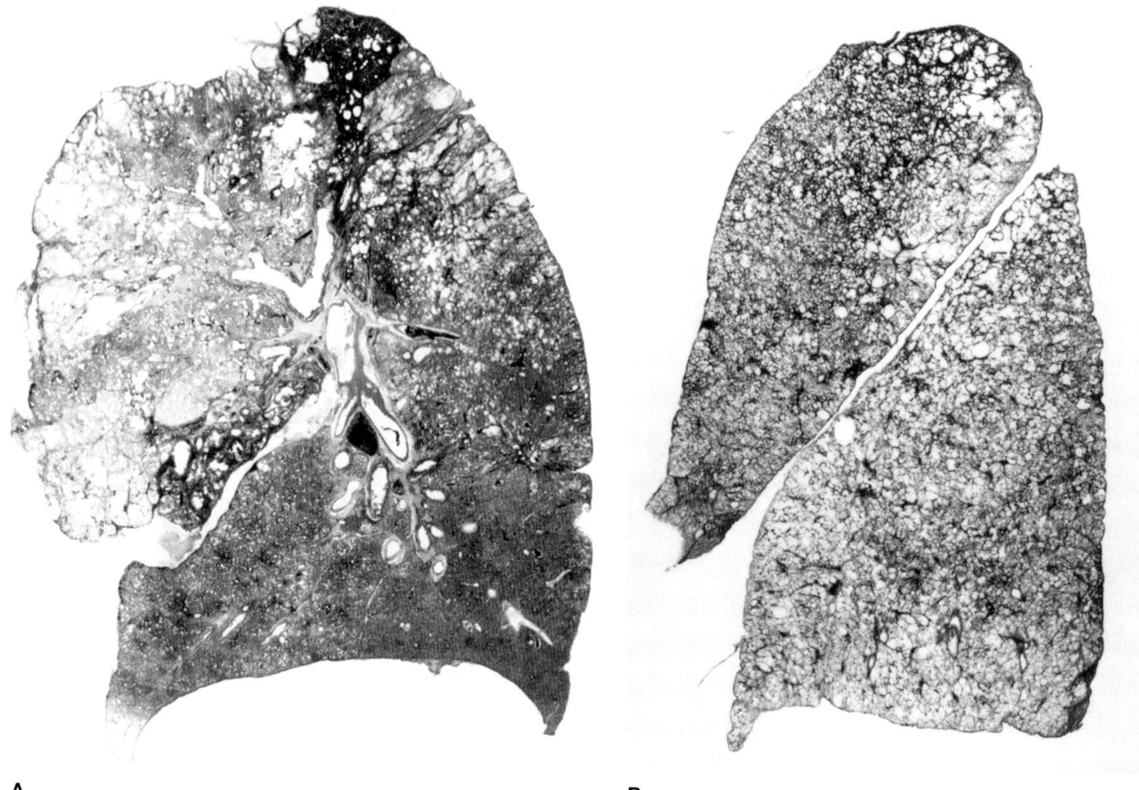

Figure 39-3 Pathologic subtypes of emphysema. **A.** Predominantly centriacinar emphysema. Emphysema is more severe in upper lobes. **B.** Predominant panacinar emphysema. Emphysema is more severe in the lower lobes.

emphysematous spaces, separated from the acinar periphery (the lobular septa), by intact alveolar ducts and sacs of normal size. The walls of the emphysematous spaces and adjacent tissue characteristically contain variable amounts of black pigment.

The lesions vary qualitatively as well as quantitatively even within the same lung. There is striking irregularity of involvement of lobules, and even within the same lobule.[17,18] The lesions are usually more common and become more severe in the upper than in the lower zones of the lung (Figs. 39-3A and 39-4A,B).[19–24] Most affected are the upper lobe, particularly the posterior and apical segments, and the superior segment of the lower lobe. In cases of severe CLE, the destruction proceeds toward the periphery of the lobule, and the distinction between CLE and PLE becomes blurred.

In CLE, alveolar pores are abnormal in size and shape, and occasionally contain epithelial debris and macrophages. Although there are numerous pores of variable size in the emphysematous areas,[25] there are also increased numbers of pores in the grossly normal areas, and accentuation of these changes in the center of the lobule.[26] Thus, it appears that in CLE the pores of Kohn are possibly the initial site of destruction.

There is increased cellularity in the alveolar walls of cigarette smokers,[27] and when this has been quantified, the parenchyma in severe emphysema has increased numbers of neutrophils, macrophages, eosinophils, and both CD4 and CD8 T lymphocytes.[28] There is also a significant inflammatory cell infiltrate in the airspaces in severe emphysema, with the same cell types increased.[28] Although not readily apparent grossly or on standard histologic stains, use of histochemical stains or biochemical analysis demonstrates that collagen is increased in both centrilobular and panlobular emphysema.[29–31]

PANLOBULAR EMPHYSEMA

The recognition of mild panlobular emphysema is very difficult. The normal lung has a very characteristic appearance when seen through a dissecting microscope: The multifaceted alveoli form a contrast to the larger, cylindrical conducting structures that are alveolar ducts and respiratory bronchioles. In panlobular emphysema the distinction between alveolar ducts and alveoli becomes lost as alveoli lose their sharp angles, enlarge, and then lose their contrast in size and shape with the ducts, resulting in simplification of the lung architecture, with formation of small box-like structures. As the process becomes worse, the architectural derangement becomes more obvious, with progressive effacement and loss of the orderly arrangement of the lung until little remains other than the supporting framework of vessels, septa, and bronchi. The best way to see panlobular emphysema grossly is to examine lung slices immersed in a water or fixative bath and then immediately after removal from the bath. The immersed specimen shows enlarged airspaces and, when the slices are lifted from the bath, panlobular emphysema can be suspected because the lung parenchyma "falls away" from the supporting structures and protrudes slightly above them. In contrast to centrilobular emphysema, panlobular emphysema is usually worse in the lower lobes (Fig. 39-3B).

Histologic examination is a sensitive method of recognizing panlobular emphysema. The pattern is again one of simplification with diminishing contrast between alveoli and alveolar ducts (Fig. 39-4C,D). Despite the greater extent of tissue destruction, in panlobular emphysema the pores of Kohn are more uniform and inconspicuous than those found in centrilobular emphysema.[32]

Panlobular emphysema is the characteristic lung lesion seen in α1-antitrypsin deficiency,[33] but may also occur as a consequence of permanent obliteration of airways (obliterative bronchiolitis, constrictive bronchiolitis). Most often, obliteration of airways results in collapse of the distal lung parenchyma and dilatation of the bronchi proximal to the obliterated airways. This is the sequence of events in postinfective bronchiectasis. In some instances, however, the lung parenchyma does not collapse, but remains fully expanded or

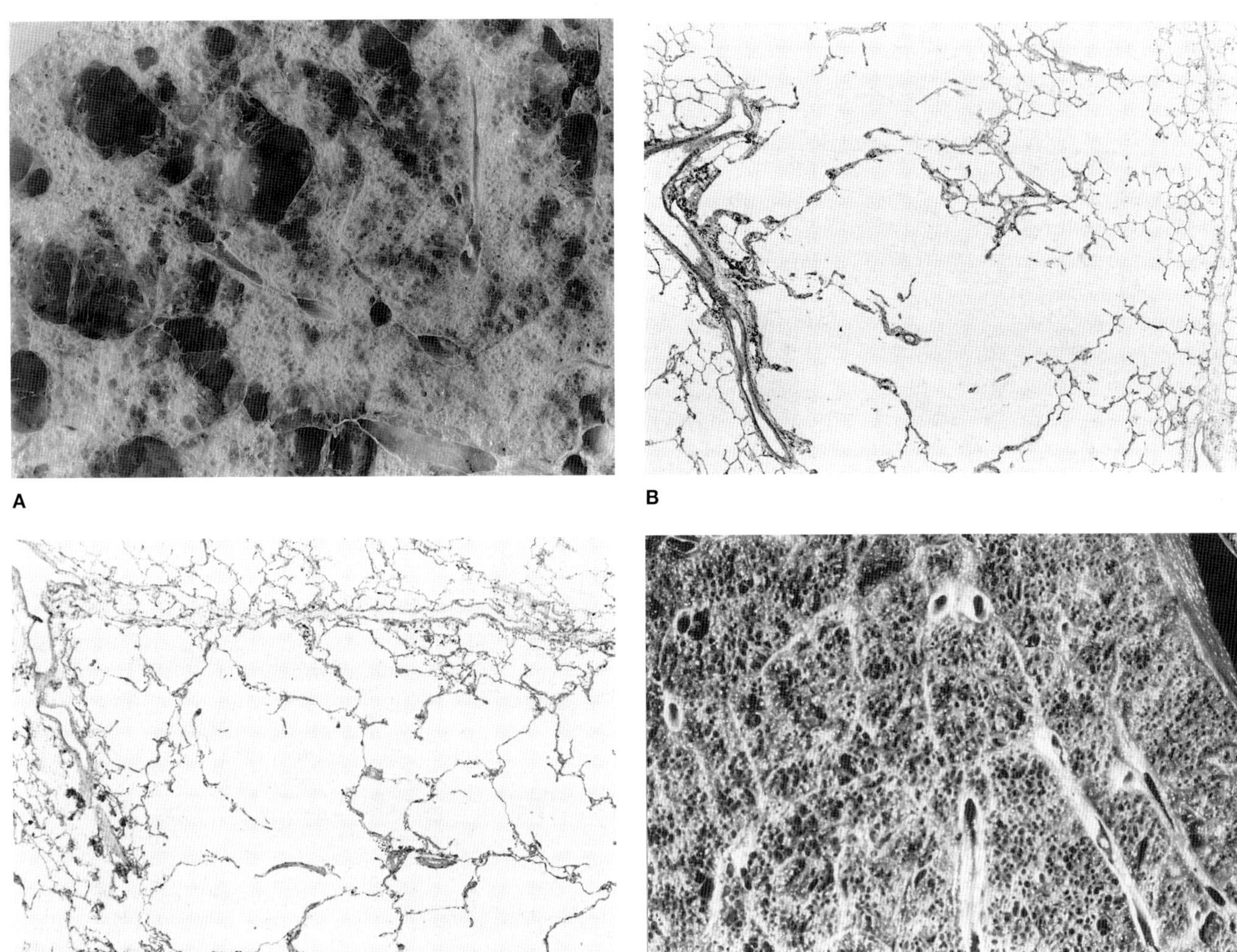

Figure 39-4 **A, B.** Gross and histologic sections illustrating centriacinar; and (**C, D**) panacinar emphysema. **A.** Cut surface from a lung with centriacinar emphysema showing holes in the center of lobules surrounded by relatively normal parenchyma. The severity varies among lobules. **B.** Microscopic section showing that the airspace enlargement in centriacinar emphysema is most marked adjacent to the abnormal respiratory bronchiole, corresponding to the center of the lobule. Also, some of the alveolar walls of the abnormal airspaces are thickened and fibrotic (H&E, ×16). **C.** Cut surface of a lung slice showing how the entire lobule is uniformly affected in panacinar emphysema. **D.** Microscopic section demonstrating that in panacinar emphysema, the airspaces adjacent to the lobular septa are enlarged to the same degree as those in the center of the lobule (H&E, ×16).

becomes emphysematous. The parenchymal sequel to bronchial and bronchiolar obliteration depends on the extent of the obliteration and the amount of collateral ventilation between adjacent airspaces distal to unobstructed airways. If collateral ventilation is present, then the units distal to the obliterated airways will remain expanded by virtue of the air reaching them by collateral ventilation, producing overexpansion and destruction of lung parenchyma beyond the obliterated airways. The terms Swyer–James or MacLeod syndrome are applied when this process affects most of one lung but spares the other.

DISTAL ACINAR EMPHYSEMA: PARASEPTAL EMPHYSEMA

The original description of distal acinar emphysema is generally credited to Loeschcke,[34] who described collections of subpleural bullae. It was Heard,[24,35] however, who first noted that the lesions could extend into the substance of the lung, where they lay along the septa, and coined the term "paraseptal" emphysema. Since the distal part of the acinus (alveolar sacs and ducts) is dominantly involved, emphysema is most striking adjacent to the pleura (superficial emphysema or mantel emphysema), along lobular septa (paraseptal emphysema), at the margins of lobules and acini (periacinar emphysema), and along vessels and airways, which, when cut longitudinally, display a linear pattern. The characteristic morphology is that of multiple contiguous, enlarged airspaces, varying from <0.5 mm to >2 cm in diameter.

Paraseptal emphysema is usually limited in extent, and is found most commonly along the anterior and posterior parts of the upper lobe and along the posterior surface of the lower lobe. When extensive, it is usually more severe in the upper half of the lung. Gough has stressed that it is associated with fibrosis of the tissue between the enlarged airspaces, and this is certainly a common finding.[36] Paraseptal emphysema is frequently found in association with centriacinar emphysema,[20] but it is most known for its association with spontaneous pneumothoraces in young thin adults.[37]

IRREGULAR EMPHYSEMA

Irregular emphysema is logically named, because the acinus is indeed irregularly involved in it. Irregular emphysema is almost invariably

TABLE 39-1 Differential Diagnosis of Airspace Enlargement

	Distribution	Enlarged Structure
Centrilobular emphysema	Upper lobes, center of lobule	Alveolar ducts, alveoli
Panlobular emphysema	Lower lobe, uniform in lobule	Alveoli
Paraseptal emphysema	Apical, adjacent to septum	Alveoli
Irregular emphysema	No typical site, adjacent to scars	Alveoli
Aging	Uniform in lung	Alveolar ducts
Compensatory alterations	Uniform in lung	Alveoli
Obstructive alterations	Affected area	Alveoli
Genetic alterations	Uniform in lung	Lack of septation
Asthma	During acute attack	Alveoli
Honeycomb lung	Variable—often subpleural	Total remodeling

adjacent to a scar, giving name to the synonyms scar or paracicatricial emphysema. Most scars within the lung are usually small and the emphysema is limited in extent. The severity of irregular emphysema depends on the extent of damage to lung tissue, and multiple scars through the lung may lead to multiple foci of irregular emphysema.

DIFFERENTIAL DIAGNOSIS OF EMPHYSEMA

GAS TRAPPING

The lungs of an asthmatic who has succumbed during an attack are usually characterized by gas trapping, and thus remain inflated, with focal areas of atelectasis (Table 39-1). In a patient with long-standing asthma who has died from other causes, or has had a lung resection, there may still be areas of atelectasis. Focal bronchiectasis can be found also, particularly in the anterior segment of the upper lobe. However, parenchymal destruction is not a feature of asthma, and thus gross, microscopic, and morphometric analyses will all be normal in the chronic asthmatic.

NONEMPHYSEMATOUS AIRSPACE ENLARGEMENT

Although not part of the differential diagnosis of COPD, nonemphysematous airspace enlargement also occurs in infancy. In congenital lobar hyperinflation (emphysema), the lobes are overinflated rather than emphysematous, but in some instances they may be polyalveolar.[38,39] Some other genetic abnormalities will also give enlarged airspaces, but this is due to failure of septation with a simplified rather than a destroyed alveolar framework.

At the other side of the age spectrum, the term senile emphysema was once used to describe the enlarged airspaces found in the aged. On gross examination, lungs round out with increasing age. An analysis of Gough sections showed increases in anteroposterior distance, height, perimeter, and area of the lung up to the age of 59 years. After this age, only the anteroposterior diameter continued to increase significantly, thus "rounding" the lung dimensions.[40] This change is due to an increase in the volume proportion of alveolar duct air,[41] with shallower and flatter alveoli,[42] a process termed ductectasia. There is no evidence of lung destruction; thus, the condition does not fulfill the criteria for emphysema.

If a part of the lung collapses or is removed, the remaining lung can expand to fill the increased amount of space available, a process known as compensatory overinflation. The exact way that this happens and the limits of the process are unknown. However, no tissue destruction has occurred and, by definition, this is not emphysema. It is not clear how much larger the overinflated lung can become, or how it expands to reach the new and larger volume. It is generally thought that the possible extent of overinflation is modest and that all the parts of the acinus are equally expanded.

Obstructive overinflation can occur in adults, and two mechanisms may be involved. In one, the obstruction in the bronchus may act as a ball valve, so that air enters on inspiration but does not leave on expiration. Alternatively, the bronchus may be completely obstructed and air may be trapped behind channels of collateral ventilation. Whatever the mechanism, the affected part of the lung can expand considerably. Obstructive overinflation differs in a number of ways from compensatory overinflation, although, in both, the lung contains too much air per unit of lung and lung tissue.

HONEYCOMB LUNG

The airspace enlargement that occurs in cryptogenic fibrosing alveolitis (usual interstitial pneumonia [UIP]) and other fibrotic lung diseases could possibly be confused with emphysema. While honeycomb spaces are enlarged airspaces, they are the result of parenchymal remodeling with formation of new airspaces, rather than destruction of normal airspaces, and thus have thickened and irregular walls with none of the structure of an acinus. They are lined by bronchiolar epithelium, and often contain mucus; the walls have abundant and well-collagenized connective tissue, which may also contain impressive amounts of muscle and sometimes fat. There is usually interstitial inflammation in the form of varying degrees of lymphocytic and plasma cell infiltration.

COMBINED EMPHYSEMA AND FIBROSIS

Despite the definition of emphysema, which limits fibrosis, the significance of a mixture of fibrosis and emphysema has recently been reevaluated in relationship to its clinical, radiologic, and pathologic components.[43] The problem is that people who smoke cigarettes not only can develop respiratory bronchiolitis-interstitial lung disease (RB-ILD), but also have a higher incidence of developing UIP (idiopathic interstitial fibrosis), and mixtures of these with emphysema are not uncommon. When the combination of emphysema and UIP occurs, lung volumes can be preserved, but the diffusing capacity becomes markedly decreased, and pulmonary hypertension develops, with its associated significant negative prognosis. CT scans generally show centrilobular or mixed centrilobular and paraseptal emphysema in the upper lobes, with increased reticular markings and honeycomb remodeling in the lower lobes. Pathologically, there is both gross and microscopic emphysema and interstitial fibrosis with fibroblast foci in the areas of active fibrosis.[44] We have recently reviewed this topic with a focus on the pathologic differential diagnosis (Fig. 39-5A–D).[45]

LESIONS OF THE LARGE AIRWAYS IN COPD

The majority of studies in this area have focused upon the lesions present when the clinical signs and symptoms of chronic bronchitis are also present.

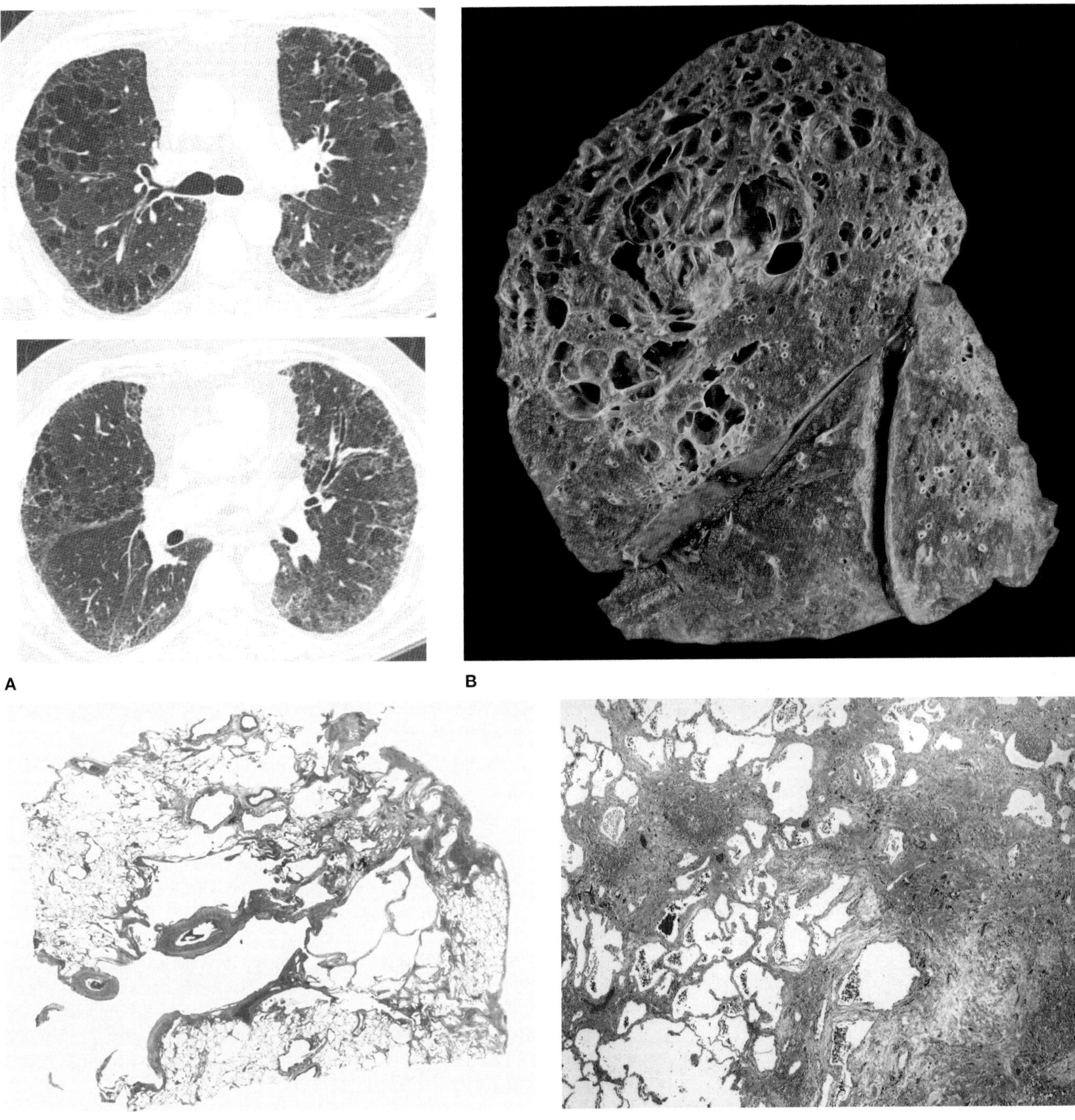

Figure 39-5 Combined fibrosis and emphysema in a case of chronic (fibrotic) hypersensitivity pneumonitis. **A.** Computed tomography scan from upper zone *(top)* shows emphysema and a suggestive of reticulation; lower image from midlung zone shows extensive reticulation indicating the presence of underlying fibrosis. **B.** Gross photo (sagittal slice) from this case showing marked upper zone emphysema, with fibrosis evident in the most posterior portion of the upper lobe, and the posterior portions of the lower lobe. **C.** Whole mount from the upper lobe. There are large emphysematous spaces, several with extensive surrounding fibrosis; at higher magnification, many of these fibrotic rims had fibroblast foci (not shown), indicating that this process is really interstitial fibrosis stretched around pre-existing emphysema. **D.** Image from lower lobe showing a UIP-like area, a common finding in chronic hypersensitivity pneumonitis. Elsewhere there were noncaseating granulomas (not shown). *(Reproduced with permission from Wright JL, Tazelaar H, Churg A. Fibrosis with Emphysema. Histopathology. 2011;58(4):517–524 (This document was published in 1993. Certain aspects of this document may be out of date and caution should be used when applying the information in clinical practice and other usages).)*

■ GROSS FINDINGS

Gross lesions in the large airways are few and subtle. Bronchial pits are the dilated openings of one or more mucus glands into the epithelium. They are most often found along the margins of the cartilaginous rings and at the bifurcations of the airways. In nonbronchitis the pits can be seen using a hand lens or a dissecting microscope, but in chronic bronchitis, the ducts may be distended with mucus and the mucus may protrude into the lumen of the bronchus and be visible grossly. It is not correct to refer to these as diverticula. First, these are protrusions of normal ducts; and second, they do not extend through all of the muscle coats of the bronchial wall.

While enlarged bronchial pits are the most obvious gross lesions in COPD, careful examination of lung specimens will show that the bronchi do not taper progressively as they approach the pleura,[46] and they also display prominent circular ridges, probably due to bands

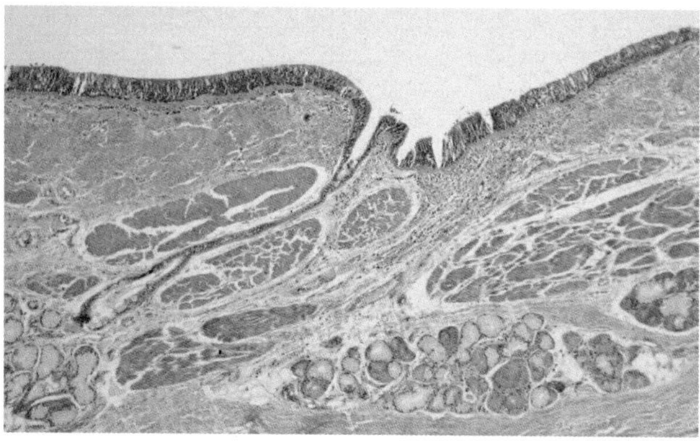

Figure 39-6 Large airway from a subject with chronic bronchitis. The overall wall is thickened with inflammation and fibrosis, and there is prominence of the smooth muscle in addition to the bronchial mucus glands.

of hypertrophic smooth muscle.[47,48] Gross mucus may be present in the airway lumen, particularly in subjects with chronic bronchitis.[49]

MICROSCOPIC FINDINGS

The intraluminal mucus found in the airways of subjects with COPD contains a mixed population of epithelial cells and acute and chronic inflammatory cells; large numbers of neutrophils can be found during an exacerbation.

Detailed microscopic analysis of the large airways in COPD reveals alterations in the entire airway wall (Fig. 39-6). Epithelial changes are mild in degree and are not necessarily consistent from patient to patient. Epithelial sloughing can occur, but in most instances the epithelium is generally intact and shows only mild goblet cell or squamous cell metaplasia, both of which appear to be more marked if the subject has symptoms of chronic bronchitis.[50,51] The reticular basement membrane thickness is within the normal range.

The thickness or area of mucus glands in subjects with COPD in general, or chronic bronchitis in particular, is increased over a population mean, but has a distribution that extensively overlaps that of normals and asthmatics.[52–55] Interestingly, there appears to be a decreased percentage of serous acini in these glands, a feature that apparently does not occur in asthma (discussed below).[56]

Thickening of the inner wall (area internal to the muscular layer) appears to be the most consistent component of airway wall thickening in the large airways of subjects with COPD, and appears to be generalized.[57,58] This increase in thickness can be partially attributed to edema and hyperemia of the bronchi,[59] but is also due to an increase in fibrous tissue or other matrix proteins.

In the large airways of subjects with COPD, increases in the thickness of the muscular layer have not been consistently identified. Although some studies[60] have found that the average proportion of muscle in main, lobar, and segmental bronchi was approximately doubled in patients with chronic bronchitis and airflow obstruction, others have found that a substantial number of patients fell within the normal range.[54,55,61]

Alteration in the amount of cartilage in COPD does not appear to be a consistent finding. While some studies[59,62,63] described cartilage atrophy in chronic bronchitis and/or emphysema, or circumferentially arranged cartilage that extended farther distally in nonbronchitis than bronchitis,[64] this was not supported by other reports.[54,65] However, histologic signs of cartilage damage, as judged by loss of cellular or pericellular metachromasia and vacuolated or empty lacunae can be consistently identified.[66]

The large airways in COPD show a mild, usually mixed, inflammatory infiltrate. Bronchus-associated lymphoid tissues (BALT) is not consistently found, but its frequency appears to be considerably higher (82%) in smokers than nonsmokers (14%).[67] Bronchial biopsy analysis consistently shows an increase in CD8 T cells, with eosinophils and neutrophils found during exacerbations (reviewed in Refs.[50,68]). Chronic inflammation can also be found around the bronchial glands, particularly in subjects with chronic bronchitis.[69]

DIFFERENTIAL DIAGNOSIS

ASTHMA

In asthma the large airways are not dilated, but mucus plugs are classically identified in the large airways of subjects with fatal or near-fatal asthma,[70] and the mucus may be continuous with that present in the ducts of the mucus glands (Table 39-2). Visible bronchial pits are not a standard feature of asthma, and although the airway wall may be thickened, this is usually not apparent grossly.

In the large airways of subjects with asthma, desquamation of the epithelium is a common feature,[71,72] and this may be worse in people who have persistent rather than intermittent activity. Sloughing of cohesive epithelial clusters produces the creola bodies found in cytology specimens. Goblet cell metaplasia can be marked in both asthma and bronchiectasis,[73] but there is a considerable degree of variability, so that this feature cannot be used in isolation to distinguish among

TABLE 39-2 Pathologic Differential Diagnosis of Large Airway Lesions in COPD

	Dilatation	Structural Distortion	Pits	Glands	Submucosal Fibrosis	Basement Membrane	Epithelium	Lumenal Mucus	Cartilage	Muscles
Chronic bronchitis	✓	Fibrosis and inflammation	✓	✓	✓	X	Goblet cell metaplasia	✓	✓	✓/X
Asthma	Focal	Focal	X	✓	✓	✓	Goblet cell metaplasia	✓	X	✓
Bronchiectasis	✓	Fibrosis and inflammation	✓	✓/X	✓	X	Focal goblet cell metaplasia	✓	✓	X
Tracheobronchopathia osteoplastica	✓	Bony nodules	X	X	X	X	X	X	✓	X
Tracheomegaly	✓	X	Diverticula	X	X	X	X	X	X	X
Relapsing polychondritis	✓	✓	X	X	X	X	X	X	✓	X

Check mark indicates that the feature is present; X indicates that the feature is absent.

the airways of subjects with COPD, asthma, and bronchiectasis. These epithelial cell changes result in an overall thickening of the epithelium in asthma, but not in COPD.[58] In asthma, the reticular basement membrane (lamina reticularis) is characteristically thickened. This alteration occurs early in the course of disease, and remains even when the asthma is mild or well controlled (reviewed in Ref.[56]).

The airways of asthmatics demonstrate a greater severity of inner wall thickening, with values double those found in patients with COPD.[58] The increase in thickness is due to variable increases in fibrous tissue, inflammatory cells, edema fluid, and vascular prominence.[50,56] Analysis of the muscular wall in subjects with severe or fatal asthma compared with normals or those with COPD shows a marked increase in amount of muscle, with a lesser increase in asthmatics who died with rather than from their asthma (discussed in Ref.[74]). There has also been a suggestion that the increase in muscle mass may occur relatively early during childhood.[56]

Neutrophils are the predominant cells present in the mucus of patients with bronchiectasis, while eosinophils and accompanying Charcot Leyden crystals are the hallmark of asthmatic mucus. As noted, the cartilaginous destruction present in polychondritis is severe and associated with chronic inflammation, thus easily distinguishing the two processes. Depending upon the severity of the inflammation in bronchiectasis, there may be significant cartilaginous destruction.

Airways from fatal and near-fatal asthma also contain isolated aggregates of lymphoid cells, roughly in the same proportion as that present in COPD.[75] However, in asthma, by contrast to COPD, there is an inflammatory infiltrate consisting of activated eosinophils, and activated CD4 T cells in the submucosa,[76] and both mast cells and neutrophils within the glands.[70] There is little in the literature regarding the inflammatory cell infiltrates present in the airway walls in bronchiectasis. Compared with asthma, there appear to be fewer eosinophils, but a similar population of CD45 (as opposed to any specific subtype) lymphocytes, with both cell types having a greater density in the inner, as opposed to the outer aspect of the airway.[77]

BRONCHIECTASIS

In bronchiectasis, there is by definition an abnormal and permanent dilatation of the bronchi, and this is usually present to a much greater degree than is found in COPD, and is often accompanied by airway distortion. There is exaggeration of the muscular ridges and the presence of multiple bronchial gland–based pits. The large airway walls can be thickened and/or irregularly thinned as a result of inflammation and fibrosis, and there is often inspissated mucus or actual purulent material.

MISCELLANEOUS CONDITIONS

Tracheobronchomegaly (Mounier-Kuhn syndrome) is characterized by a marked dilatation of the trachea and major bronchi, with diameters 5 to 10 cm above normal values.[78] In this condition there are multiple true diverticula, with out-pouchings formed of membranous tracheal tissue between the cartilaginous rings,[79] with atrophy or absence of elastic fibers.[80]

Patients with tracheobronchopathia osteoplastica have an obstructive pulmonary function pattern[81]; however, unlike the trachea and large airways in COPD, cartilaginous and bony nodules are present in the subepithelial space (submucosa). Relapsing polychondritis[82,83] shows variable dynamic expiratory and/or inspiratory obstruction depending on the size and location of the airways involved. In this disease, however, the obstruction is due to impaired airway clearance of inflammatory debris, and an ineffective cough because of dynamic upper airway collapse. The airways are dilated and the walls are thickened because of the extensive fibrosis and chronic inflammation due to the immunologic nature of this condition. In particular, the cartilaginous plates show extensive destruction.

LESIONS OF THE SMALL AIRWAYS IN COPD

In the context of COPD, small airways refer to airways with an internal diameter of 2 mm or less. In COPD, intraluminal mucus can be found in the small airways, and there appears to be an overall relationship between the degree to which the airways are occluded by mucus and the FEV_1.[84] Goblet cells are rare in normal small airways, but goblet cell metaplasia is a frequent finding in the airways of patients with COPD.[85–87]

Similar to the large airways, there is alteration of all of the small airway wall compartments in patients with COPD (Fig. 39-7). These changes result in an overall decrease in the internal bronchiolar diameter and, as assessed by a conformity index, produce significant deformity. Similar results are obtained from three-dimensional reconstructions.[74] Detailed measurements of the airway walls show that the increased wall thickness is due to increases in the epithelium, subepithelial fibrous tissue compartment (submucosa, lamina propria), smooth muscle, and adventitia.[58,84] While there is no direct evidence, it seems appropriate that these changes would result in airway obliteration, a process which appears to happen relatively early in airflow obstruction, with the number of airways in patients with severe airflow obstruction reduced to one-tenth of the numbers calculated in the normal lung (see Fig. 39-8A,B).[88] Although the adventitia is thickened, there is a loss of alveolar attachments to the airway wall,[89] an important process because it allows early airway collapse on expiration.

One of the earliest histologic abnormalities that can be detected in cigarette smokers is the presence of macrophages in the lumen of the respiratory bronchioles.[90] However, an inflammatory infiltrate can also be identified within the walls of both membranous and respiratory bronchioles in subjects with COPD. When examined in conjunction with the GOLD (Global Strategy for the Diagnosis, Management, and Prevention of COPD) stage, the proportion of airways which had measurable neutrophils appear to be increased in GOLD stages 2 to 4, and airways with measurable macrophages show a progressive increase from GOLD stage 0 to 4, while there does not seem to be any alteration in the percentage of airways that contain eosinophils among the GOLD stages.[91] The percentage of airways with CD4, CD8, and B cells also increase with GOLD stage, but when these data are expressed as total accumulated volume, only the B cells and CD8 cells show progressive increases. The presence of lymphoid follicles is markedly increased in GOLD stages 3 and 4. Interestingly, histone deacetylase 2 (HDAC2) appears to be downregulated in the

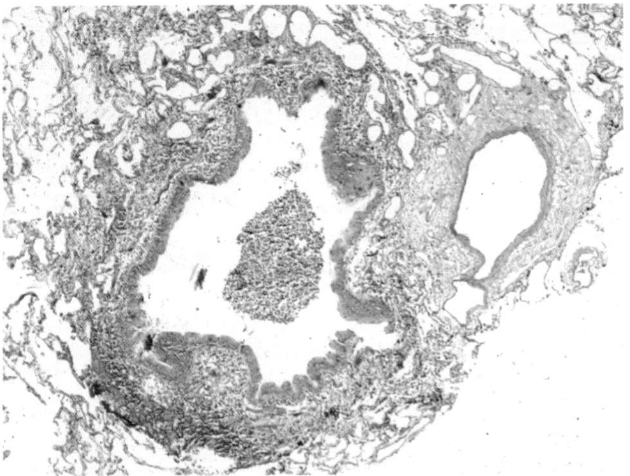

Figure 39-7 A small airway from a subject with COPD. The lumen contains mucus and inflammatory debris. There is goblet cell metaplasia of the epithelium. The subepithelial (submucosal) layer is increased in thickness due to an increase in fibrous tissue and inflammatory cells.

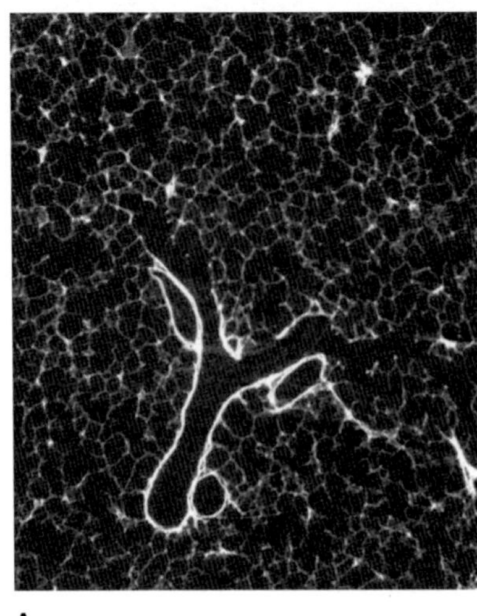
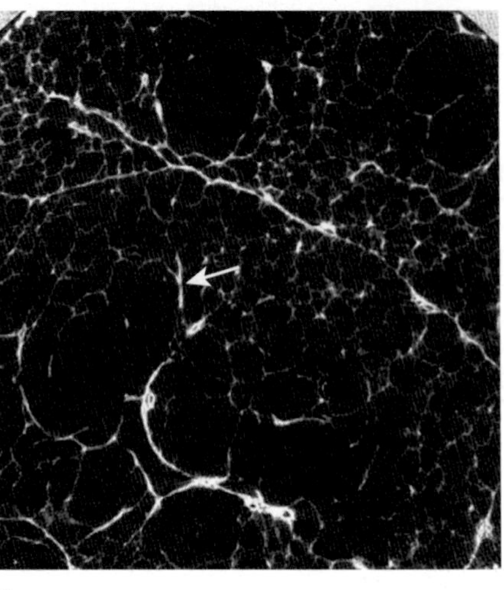

A B

Figure 39-8 **A.** Micro-CT scan image of an airway from a normal lung. Note the regular progression from membranous bronchiole to respiratory bronchiole to alveolar duct. **B.** Micro-CT scan image of an airway from a lung with centrilobular emphysema. Note the irregular airway emptying into a centrilobular hole. Partially obliterated airway is seen at the *arrow*. *(Figures used with permission of Dr. James C Hogg.)*

small airways of smokers with COPD,[92] a finding which may be of considerable importance since downregulation of the HDAC system is associated with a pro-inflammatory cytokine profile.

DIFFERENTIAL DIAGNOSIS

ASTHMA

Mucus plugs and goblet cell hyperplasia are markedly increased in the small airways of asthmatics[73,93] and this increase is generally much greater than that seen in COPD. In addition, the basement membrane thickness is approximately 20% greater than that found in either normals or patients with COPD.[73] The peripheral airways of asthmatics have an inflammatory infiltrate that features lymphocytes and eosinophils,[73,77,94] with many of the inflammatory cells in the adventitial, as opposed to the submucosal compartment. The data regarding the vessels in the submucosa are controversial, with some studies suggesting that they are congested, but not increased in number, in asthmatics compared with COPD (discussed in Ref.[74]), and others demonstrating an increased number of vessels, but a lesser total area in asthma compared with COPD.[95] Although smooth muscle is increased in asthmatics, the increase is not as great as that present in the large airways.[96] Moreover, the distribution of smooth muscle increase in the bronchial tree may be quite different, with some patients displaying a generalized increase, while in others the increase is restricted to the larger airways.[97] Overall, the small airways in asthmatic subjects who have died because of their disease have a greater area of subepithelial fibrous tissue, smooth muscle, and adventitial fibrous tissue than do subjects who died with their disease, which in turn have a greater area than do the airways of subjects with COPD.[98] Thus, although the same qualitative changes are present in both asthmatics and COPD, they are more severe in asthmatics and most severe in cases of fatal asthma. Interestingly, there appears to be a loss of alveolar attachments in cases of fatal asthma,[99] although this is less than that present in the airways of patients with COPD.

FOLLICULAR BRONCHIOLITIS

Follicular bronchiolitis is characterized by narrowing of the bronchioles due to adventitial and subepithelial lymphoid follicles, and accompanied by a lymphoplasmacytic inflammatory infiltrate.[100] The condition is classically found in patients with rheumatoid arthritis or those with IgA deficiency. This process can mimic severe COPD small airway disease, but the inflammatory infiltrate is generally magnified compared to COPD, while there is little goblet cell metaplasia in the airway epithelium.

PANBRONCHIOLITIS

The presence of foamy macrophages in the airway wall and lumen and extending down into the alveolar ducts and alveoli is a feature of the condition known as panbronchiolitis, originally described in Japan but now known to occur worldwide.[101,102] Follicular hyperplasia of the peribronchiolar lymphoid tissue is frequent, and bronchiolectasis is found in the more advanced lesions.

CONSTRICTIVE BRONCHIOLITIS

The term constrictive bronchiolitis appears to have been coined by Gosink et al.[103] In constrictive bronchiolitis, the airway lumen is occluded by a progressive thickening of the subepithelial (submucosal) space. Both the membranous and respiratory bronchioles are involved, and show transmural inflammatory cell infiltrates, occasionally with epithelial necrosis. Mucus plugs can also be identified. As the process evolves, the inflammatory infiltrate wanes, and greater amounts of fibrous tissue can be demonstrated both in the peribronchial and subepithelial portions of the airway, acting to narrow or obliterate the airway lumen.[104] Lesions of constrictive bronchiolitis, particularly in the organized phase, may be difficult to demonstrate, and may require elastic stains to outline the obliterated airway. Thus, the lesions in COPD differ from constrictive bronchiolitis only in degree.

Mineral dust–induced airway disease is a distinctive type of constrictive bronchiolitis, characterized by a stereotypic response of the small airways to high doses of particulate, regardless of the specific mineral dust involved. The lesions consist of fibrosis and thickening of the walls of both the membranous and respiratory bronchioles, sometimes extending down the alveolar ducts, the latter finding providing diagnostic discrimination from tobacco smoke–induced airway disease, which tends not to involve the alveolar ducts. Pigment deposition is highly variable, and is not a diagnostic feature.[105] Other forms of constrictive bronchiolitis may be related to ingestion of toxic compounds such as *Sauropus androgynus* ingestion,[106–109] *or* related to diffuse neuroendocrine cell hyperplasia.[110–113]

PROLIFERATIVE BRONCHIOLITIS

The lesions of proliferative bronchiolitis have been elegantly described and illustrated.[114–116] Within the lumens of the membranous and respiratory bronchioles are plugs of organizing fibroblastic (granulation) tissue. Occasionally, ulceration of the epithelium can be seen, and early lesions may have fibrin. The granulation tissue is formed of a pale matrix with proliferating spindle cells, accompanied by chronic inflammatory cells. As the lesions age, the granulation tissue usually shrinks and contracts. However, in a certain proportion of cases, the bronchiolar cells proliferate over the granulation tissue, and incorporate it into the subepithelial space, leaving an irregular airway lumen.

Although acute bronchiolitis, be it bacterial or viral in nature, is usually easily distinguished from the lesions of COPD by the presence of extensive epithelial damage, healed lesions may

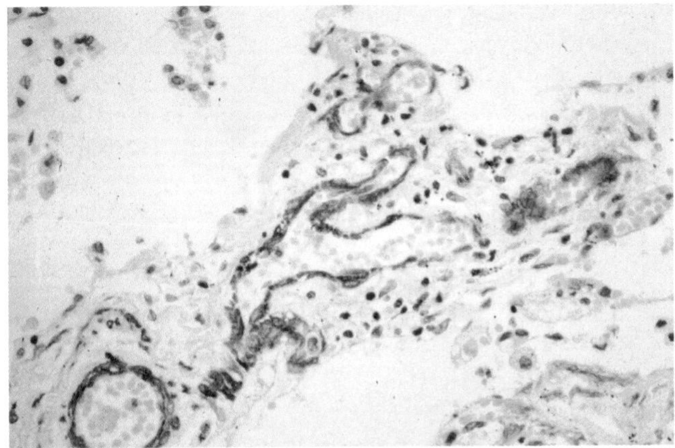

Figure 39-9 A small pulmonary artery from a subject with COPD. These vessels, situated adjacent to the alveolar ducts, are normally poorly muscularized, but in this case, the vessel has a distinct circumferential muscular layer.

show nonspecific airway fibrosis and chronic inflammation, or the residua of proliferative bronchiolitis. Interestingly, latent adenoviral infection has been suggested as a contributor to airflow obstruction in adults by amplifying the inflammatory response in the bronchioles of cigarette smokers.[117] Airway disease complicating other diseases may also need to be distinguished from that of COPD. For example, posttransplant bronchiolitis[115,118] or airway disease in patients with inflammatory bowel disease (both Crohn disease and ulcerative colitis)[119] include both proliferative and constrictive bronchiolitis. Inflammatory bowel disease may also have large airway involvement.

LESIONS OF THE VESSELS IN COPD

There are no consistent alterations in the large elastic pulmonary arteries of subjects with COPD. Atheromata can be found,[120] but unless there is pulmonary hypertension, the incidence is probably not greater than that found in a carefully matched population.

Cigarette smokers, with or without pulmonary hypertension, have an increase in arterial muscle media thickness as well as intimal fibrosis in the muscular arteries, and progressive muscularization of the small arterioles (reviewed in Ref.[121]). Increases in intimal thickness with longitudinal muscle formation are a common feature in lungs of patients with COPD (Fig. 39-9).[11,122,123] There appears to be a progressive increase in the numbers of smaller muscularized arteries, percent medial thickness, and percent intimal thickness of muscularized arteries from nonsmokers, to smokers without obstruction, to smokers with airflow obstruction.[124]

The lesions of primary pulmonary hypertension and hypertension secondary to vascular shunting also include intimal fibrosis and increased muscular media thickness. Intimal fibrosis is often cellular in its early phases, but progresses to concentric laminar fibrosis, which can almost totally obliterate the vessel lumen. These changes are of much greater severity than those identified secondary to COPD. Vasculitis, fibrinoid necrosis, and plexiform lesions are never found in COPD. Lesions of chronic thromboembolic disease include eccentric intimal thickening, and the occasional formation of webs due to recanalization of the thrombi.

NONPATHOLOGIC, CT SCAN–BASED, EVALUATION OF TISSUE COMPARTMENTS IN COPD

CT scanning has provided useful information on the lung parenchyma, airways, and pulmonary vasculature in patients with COPD.

EMPHYSEMA

The advent of high-resolution CT scanners has allowed identification of even mild emphysema, and can distinguish between emphysema and senile lung airspace enlargement. When combined with general morphometric principles, emphysema can be quantified, and emphysema progression can be monitored.[125–128]

AIRWAYS

Evaluation of this compartment is in its developmental phase, with much of the work being performed on phantom airways or in large animals. In humans, thin-section CT scans are able to demonstrate evidence of airway wall remodeling in the more proximal airways (first- to sixth-generation airways) of subjects with COPD or asthma, and it has been suggested that changes in these airways can be extrapolated to the smaller airways.[129] Certainly, the data do suggest that these measurements correlate with lung physiology, independent from emphysema.[130]

PULMONARY ARTERIES

Measurements of the mainstem pulmonary artery are easily performed on CT scans using contrast, and these data have shown prognostic significance. Evaluation of the smaller vessels is much more difficult, but initial work has found that determination of the total cross-sectional area of the vessels which have an individual cross-sectional area of less than 5 mm^2 have a significant negative correlation with pulmonary arterial pressure, at least in patients with severe emphysema.[131,132]

SUMMARY

There are a number of pathologic alterations of the lung in COPD. These involve almost all of the lung compartments, including the parenchyma, vasculature, and large and small airways. These changes can overlap the pathologic findings present in other diseases associated with airflow obstruction, or other diseases that are manifested in the lung. It is important to be able to make the distinction among these diseases. Although the pathologic alterations roughly correlate to alterations in pulmonary function, it is important to remember that their individual contributions are not well worked out. Thus, it may be difficult on an individual patient basis to proceed from a clinical classification such as the GOLD classification to a mechanistic/pathologic explanation of the airflow obstruction. Advances in CT scanning technology have allowed evaluation and quantification of emphysema, and there is developing work suggesting that evaluation of the airways and pulmonary arterial system may also be possible.

REFERENCES

1. *Global Strategy for the Diagnosis, Management and Prevention of COPD*, Global Initiative for Chronic Obstructive Lung Disease (GOLD) 2014. http://www.goldcopd.org/.
2. Bonet T. *Sepulchretum Sive Anatomia Practica ex Cadaveribus morbo denatis, proponens historias observationes omnium pene humani corporis affectuum, ipsorumoue causas reconditas revelans*. Geneva; 1679.
3. Morgagni GB. *The Seats and Causes of Disease. Investigated by Anatomy; in Five Books, Containing a Great Variety of Dissections, with Remarks*. London: Johnson and Payne; 1769.
4. Ruysh F. *Observationes Anatomica-Chirurgicae. Tractatio Anatomica*. Amsterdam: 1721.
5. Baillie M. *A Series of Engravings, Accompanied with Explanations Which are Intended to Illustrate the Morbid Anatomy of Some of*

the Most Important Parts of the Human Body Divided into 10 Fascicule. London: W. Bulmer and Co; 1799.

6. Baillie M. *The Morbid Anatomy of Some of the Most Important Parts of the Human Body*. 3rd ed. London: W. Bulmer and Co; 1807.
7. Laennec RTH. *A Treatise on the Diseases of the Chest and on Mediate Auscultation*. London: T. and G. Underwood; 1834.
8. Gough J. The pathological diagnosis of emphysema. *Proc R Soc Med*. 1952;45:576–577.
9. Gough J, Wentworth JE. The use of thin sections of entire organs in morbid anatomical studies. *J R Microsc Soc*. 1949;69: 231–235.
10. McLean KH. The histology of generalized pulmonary emphysema. I. The genesis of the early centrolobular lesion: focal emphysema. *Australas Ann Med*. 1957;6:124–140.
11. McLean KH. The significance of pulmonary vascular changes in emphysema. *Australas Ann Med*. 1958;7:69–84.
12. Ciba Guest Symposium. Terminology, definitions, and classification of chronic pulmonary emphysema and related conditions. *Thorax*. 1959;14:286–299.
13. World Health Organization. Chronic cor pulmonale: report of an expert committee: technical Report Series. *Circulation*. 1963; 27:594–615.
14. American Thoracic Society. Chronic bronchitis, asthma, and pulmonary emphysema: A statement by the committee on diagnostic standards for nontuberculous respiratory diseases. *Am Rev Respir Dis*. 1962;85:762–768.
15. Medical Research Council. Definition and classification of chronic bronchitis for clinical and epidemiological purposes. *Lancet*.1965;1:775–779.
16. Snider GL, Thurlbeck WM, Bengali ZH. The definition of emphysema. Report of a national heart lung and blood institute division of lung diseases workshop. *Am Rev Respir Dis*. 1985;132:182–185.
17. Leopold JG, Gough J. The centrilobular form of hypertrophic emphysema and its relation to chronic bronchitis. *Thorax*. 1957;12:219–235.
18. Wyatt JP, Fischer VW, Sweet H. Centrilobular emphysema. *Lab Invest*. 1961;10:159–177.
19. Snider GL, Brody JS, Doctor L. Subclinical pulmonary emphysema - Incidence and anatomic patterns. *Am Rev Respir Dis*. 1966;21:155–166.
20. Thurlbeck WM. The incidence of pulmonary emphysema with observations on the relative incidence and spatial distribution of various types of emphysema. *Am Rev Respir Dis*. 1963;87:206–215.
21. Hernandez JA, Anderson AE Jr, Holmes WL, Foraker AG. Macroscopic relations in emphysematous and aging lungs. *Geriatrics*. 1966;21:155–166.
22. Bignon J, Andre-Bougaran J, Brouet G. Parenchymal, bronchiolar and bronchial measurements in centrilobular emphysema. Relation to weight of right ventricle. *Thorax*. 1970;25: 556–567.
23. Mitchell RS, Silvers GW, Goodman N, Dart G, Maisel JC. Are centrilobular emphysema and panlobular emphysema two different diseases? *Hum Pathol*. 1970;1:433–441.
24. Heard BE. Further observations on the pathology of pulmonary emphysema in chronic bronchitis. *Thorax*. 1959;14:58–70.
25. Cosio MG, Shiner RJ, Saetta M, et al. Alveolar fenestrae in smokers. *Am Rev Respir Dis*. 1986;133:126–131.
26. Nagai A, Inano H, Matsuba K, Thurlbeck WM. Scanning electronmicroscopic morphometry of emphysema in humans. *Am J Respir Crit Care Med*. 1994;150:1411–1415.
27. Eidelman D, Saetta M, Ghezzo H, et al. Cellularity of the alveolar walls in smokers and its relation to alveolar destruction. *Am Rev Respir Dis*. 1990;141:1547–1552.
28. Retamales I, Elliott WM, Meshi B, et al. Amplification of inflammation in emphysema and its association with latent adenoviral infection. *Am J Respir Crit Care Med*. 2001;164:469–473.
29. Cardoso WV, Sekhon HS, Hyde DM, Thurlbeck WM. Collagen and elastin in human pulmonary emphysema. *Am Rev Respir Dis*. 1993;147:975–981.
30. Lang MR, Fiaux GW, Gillooly M, Stewart JA, Hulmes DJ, Lamb D. Collagen content of alveolar wall tissue in emphysematous and non-emphysematous lungs. *Thorax*. 1994;49:319–326.
31. Lang MR, Fiaux GW, Hulmes DJ, Lamb D, Miller A. Quantitative studies of human lung airspace wall in relation to collagen and elastin content. *Matrix*. 1993;13:471–480.
32. Kuhn C 3rd, Tavassoli F. The scanning electron microscopy of elastase-induced emphysema. *Lab Invest*. 1976;34:2–9.
33. Laurell CB, Eriksson S. The electrophoretic a1-globulin pattern of serum in a1-antitrypsin deficiency. *Scand J Clin Lab Invest*. 1963;15:132–140.
34. Loeschcke H. Sotrungen des Luftgehalts. In: Henke F, Lubarsch O, eds. *Atmungswege und Lugen: Handbuch der speziellen Pathologische anatomie und Histologie*. Berlin: Springer-Verlag; 1928:640–641.
35. Heard BE. A pathological study of emphysema of the lungs with chronic bronchitis. *Thorax*. 1958;13:136–149.
36. Gough J. The pathogenesis of emphysema. In: Liebow AA, Smith DE, eds. *The Lung*. Baltimore, MD: Williams and Wilkins; 1968:109–133.
37. Lindskog GE, Halasz NA. Spontaneous pneumothorax: a consideration of pathogenesis and management with review of seventy-two hospitalized cases. *AMA Arch Surg*. 1957;75:693–698.
38. Tapper D, Schuster S, McBride J, et al. Polyalveolar lobe: anatomic and physiologic parameters and their relationship to congenital lobar emphysema. *J Pediatr Surg*. 1980;15:931–937.
39. Hislop A, Reid LM. New pathological findings in emphysema of childhood. 2. Overinflation of a normal lobe. *Thorax*. 1971;26:190–194.
40. Anderson WF, Anderson AE, Hernandez JA, Foraker AG. Topography of aging and emphysematous lungs. *Am Rev Respir Dis*. 1964;90: 411–423.
41. Angus GE, Thurlbeck WM. Number of alveoli in the human lung. *J Appl Physiol*. 1972;32:483–485.
42. Ryan SF, Vincent TN, Mitchell RS, Filley GF, Dart G. Ductectasia; an asymptomatic pulmonary change related to age. *Med Thorac*. 1965;22:181–187.
43. Cottin V, Nunes H, Brillet PY, et al. Combined pulmonary fibrosis and emphysema: a distinct underrecognised entity. *Eur Respir J*. 2005;26:586–593.
44. Kawabata Y, Hoshi E, Murai K, et al. Smoking-related changes in the background lung of specimens resected for lung cancer: a semiquantitative study with correlation to postoperative course. *Histopathology*. 2008;53:707–714.
45. Wright JL, Tazelaar H, Churg A. Fibrosis with Emphysema. *Histopathology*. 2011;58:517–524.
46. Restrepo GL, Heard BE. Air trapping in chronic bronchitis and emphysema. Measurements of the bronchial cartilage. *Am Rev Respir Dis*. 1964;90:395–400.

47. Wang NS, Ying WL. The pattern of goblet cell hyperplasia in human airways. *Hum Pathol.* 1977;8:301–311.

48. Wang NS, Ying WL. Morphogenesis of human bronchial diverticulum. A scanning electron microscopic study. *Chest.* 1976; 69:201–204.

49. Aikawa T, Shimura S, Sasaki H, Takishima T, Yaegashi H, Takahashi T. Morphometric analysis of intraluminal mucus in airways in chronic obstructive pulmonary disease. *Am Rev Respir Dis.* 1989;140:477–482.

50. Jeffery PK. Comparison of the structural and inflammatory features of COPD and asthma. Giles F. Filley Lecture. *Chest.* 2000; 117:251S–260S.

51. Trevisani L, Sartori S, Bovolenta MR, et al. Structural characterization of the bronchial epithelium of subjects with chronic bronchitis and in asymptomatic smokers. *Respiration.* 1992;59:136–141.

52. Thurlbeck WM, Angus GE. A distribution curve for chronic bronchitis. *Thorax.* 1964;19:436–442.

53. Thurlbeck WM, Angus GE, Pare JP. Mucous gland hypertrophy in chronic bronchitis, and its occurrence in smokers. *Br J Dis Chest.* 1963;57:73–78.

54. Takizawa T, Thurlbeck WM. Muscle and mucous gland size in the major bronchi of patients with chronic bronchitis, asthma and asthmatic bronchitis. *Am Rev Respir Dis.* 1971;104: 331–336.

55. Dunnill MS, Massarella GR, Anderson JA. A comparison of the quantitative anatomy of the bronchi in normal subjects in status asthmaticus in chronic bronchitis and in emphysema. *Thorax.* 1969;24: 176–179.

56. Jeffery PK. Remodeling in asthma and chronic obstructive lung disease. *Am J Respir Crit Care Med.* 2001;164: 528–538.

57. Tiddens HA, Pare PD, Hogg JC, Hop WC, Lambert R, De Jongste JC. Cartilaginous airway dimensions and airflow obstruction in human lungs. *Am J Respir Crit Care Med.* 1995;152: 260–266.

58. Pare PD, Wiggs BR, James A, Hogg JC, Bosken CH. The comparative mechanics and morphology of airways in asthma and in chronic obstructive pulmonary disease. *Am Rev Respir Dis.* 1991;143:1189–1193.

59. Wright RR, Stuart CM. Chronic bronchitis with emphysema: a pathological study of the bronchi. *Med Thorac.* 1965;22:210–218.

60. Carlile A, Edwards C. Structural variation in the named bronchi of the left lung: a morphometric study. *Br J Dis Chest.* 1983; 77:344–348.

61. Nagai A, West WW, Paul JL, Thurlbeck WM. The National Institutes of Health intermittent positive pressure breathing trails: pathology studies. I. Interrelationship between morphologic lesions. *Am Rev Respir Dis.* 1985;132:937–945.

62. Wright RR. Bronchial atrophy and collapse in chronic obstructive pulmonary emphysema. *Am J Pathol.* 1960;37:63–77.

63. Thurlbeck WM, Pun R, Toth J, Fraser RG. Bronchial cartilage in chronic obstructive lung disease. *Am Rev Respir Dis.* 1974;109:73–80.

64. Tandon MK, Campbell AH. Bronchial cartilage in chronic bronchitis. *Thorax.* 1969;27:607–612.

65. Greenberg SD, Boushy SF, Jenkins DE. Chronic bronchitis and emphysema: correlation of pathologic findings. *Am Rev Respir Dis.* 1967;96:918–928.

66. Haraguchi M, Shimura S, Shirato K. Morphometric analysis of bronchial cartilage in chronic obstructive pulmonary disease and bronchial asthma. *Am J Respir Crit Care Med.* 1999;159: 1005–1013.

67. Richmond I, Pritchard GE, Ashcroft T, Avery A, Corris PA, Walters EH. Bronchus associated lymphoid tissue (BALT) in human lung: its distribution in smokers and non smokers. *Thorax.* 1993;48:1130–1134.

68. Turato G, Zuin R, Saetta M. Pathogenesis and pathology of COPD. *Respiration.* 2001;68:117–128.

69. Mullen JB, Wright JL, Wiggs BR, Pare PD, Hogg JC. Reassessment of inflammation of airways in chronic bronchitis. *Br Med J (Clin Res Ed).* 1985;291:1235–1239.

70. Carroll NG, Mutavdzic S, James AL. Increased mast cells and neutrophils in submucosal mucous glands and mucus plugging in patients with asthma. *Thorax.* 2002;57:677–682.

71. Jeffery PK, Wardlaw AJ, Nelson FC, Collins JV, Kay AB. Bronchial biopsies in asthma. An ultrastructural, quantitative study and correlation with hyperreactivity. *Am Rev Respir Dis.* 1989;140:1745–1753.

72. Laitinen A, Laitinen LA. Airway morphology: epithelium/ basement membrane. *Am J Respir Crit Care Med.* 1994;150: S14–S17.

73. Haraguchi M, Shimura S, Shirato K. Morphologic aspects of airways of patients with pulmonary emphysema followed by bronchial asthma-like attack. *Am J Respir Crit Care Med.* 1996;153:638–643.

74. Thurlbeck WM, Wright JL. *Thurlbeck's Chronic Airflow Obstruction.* 2nd ed. Hamilton, ON: B.C. Decker; 1999.

75. Elliot JG, Jensen CM, Mutavdzic S, Lamb JP, Carroll NG, James AL. Aggregations of lymphoid cells in the airways of nonsmokers, smokers, and subjects with asthma. *Am J Respir Crit Care Med.* 2004;169:712–718.

76. Fabbri LM, Romagnoli M, Corbetta L, et al. Differences in airway inflammation in patients with fixed airflow obstruction due to asthma or chronic obstructive pulmonary disease. *Am J Respir Crit Care Med.* 2003;167:418–424.

77. Haley KJ, Sunday ME, Wiggs BR, et al. Inflammatory cell distribution within and along asthmatic airways. *Am J Respir Crit Care Med.* 1998;158:565–572.

78. Katz I, LeVine M, Herman P. Tracheobronchiomegaly: the Mounier-Kuhn syndrome. *Am J Roentgenol Radium Ther Nucl Med.* 1962;88:1084–1094.

79. Woodring JH, Howard RS 2nd, Rehm SR. Congenital tracheobronchomegaly (Mounier-Kuhn syndrome): a report of 10 cases and review of the literature. *J Thorac Imaging.* 1991;6:1–10.

80. Van Schoor J, Joos G, Pauwels R. Tracheobronchomegaly: the Mounier-Kuhn syndrome. *Eur Respir J.* 1991;4:1303–1306.

81. Lundgren R, Stjernberg NL. Tracheobronchopathia osteochondroplastica. A clinical bronchoscopic and spirometric study. *Chest.* 1981;80:706–709.

82. Littlewood JM. Update on the United States epidemiology study. *Postgrad Med J.* 1996;72:S6.

83. Mohsenifar Z, Tashkin DP, Carson SA, Bellamy PE. Pulmonary function in patients with relapsing polychondritis. *Chest.* 1982;81:711–717.

84. Hogg JC, Chu F, Utokaparch S, et al. The nature of small-airway obstruction in chronic obstructive pulmonary disease. *N Engl J Med.* 2004;350:2645–2653.

85. Wright JL, Lawson LM, Paré PD, Kennedy S, Wiggs B, Hogg JC. The detection of small airways disease. *Am Rev Respir Dis.* 1984;129:989–994.

86. Wright JL, Lawson LM, Pare PD, Wiggs BR, Kennedy S, Hogg JC. Morphology of peripheral airways in current smokers and ex-smokers. *Am Rev Respir Dis.* 1983;127:474–477.

87. Saetta M, Turato G, Baraldo S, et al. Goblet cell hyperplasia and epithelial inflammation in peripheral airways of smokers with both symptoms of chronic bronchitis and chronic airflow limitation. *Am J Respir Crit Care Med.* 2000;161:1016–1021.

88. McDonough JE, Yuan R, Suzuki M, et al. Small-airway obstruction and emphysema in chronic obstructive pulmonary disease. *N Engl J Med.* 2011;365:1567–1575.

89. Saetta M, Ghezzo H, King M, Angus GE, Wang N-S, Cosio MG. Loss of alveolar attachments in smokers. A morphometric correlate of lung function impairment. *Am Rev Respir Dis.* 1985;132:894–900.

90. Niewoehner DE, Kleinerman J, Rice DB. Pathologic changes in the peripheral airways of young cigarette smokers. *N Engl J Med.* 1974;291:755–758.

91. National Heart Lung and Blood Institute, World Health Organization. Global Strategy for the Diagnosis, Management, and Prevention of Chronic Obstructive Pulmonary Disease: NHLBI/WHO Workshop. 2001.

92. Isajevs S, Taivans I, Svirina D, Strazda G, Kopeika U. Patterns of inflammatory responses in large and small airways in smokers with and without chronic obstructive pulmonary disease. *Respiration.* 2011;81:362–371.

93. Aikawa T, Shimura S, Sasaki H, Ebina M, Takishima T. Marked goblet cell hyperplasia with mucus accumulation in the airways of patients who died of severe acute asthma attack. *Chest.* 1992;101:916–921.

94. Carroll N, Cooke C, James A. The distribution of eosinophils and lymphocytes in the large and small airways of asthmatics. *Eur Respir J.* 1997;10:292–300.

95. Hashimoto M, Tanaka H, Abe S. Quantitative analysis of bronchial wall vascularity in the medium and small airways of patients with asthma and COPD. *Chest.* 2005;127:965–968.

96. Carroll NG, Elliot J, Morton A, James A. The structure of large and small airways in nonfatal and fatal asthma. *Am Rev Respir Dis.* 1993;147:405–410.

97. Ebina M, Yaegashi H, Chiba R, Takahashi T, Motomiya M, Tanemura M. Hyperreactive site in the airway tree of asthmatic patients revealed by thickening of bronchial muscles. *Am Rev Respir Dis.* 1990;141:1327–1332.

98. Kuwano K, Bosken CH, Pare PD, Bai TR, Wiggs BR, Hogg JC. Small airways dimensions in asthma and in chronic obstructive pulmonary disease. *Am Rev Respir Dis.* 1993;148:1220–1225.

99. Mauad T, Silva LF, Santos MA, et al. Abnormal alveolar attachments with decreased elastic fiber content in distal lung in fatal asthma. *Am J Respir Crit Care Med.* 2004;170:857–862.

100. Wells AU, deBois RM. Bronchiolitis in association with connective tissue disorders. In: King TE, ed. *Bronchiolitis.* Philadelphia, PA: W.B. Saunders; 1993:655–666.

101. Iwata M, Sato A, Colby TV. Diffuse panbronchiolitis. In: Epler GR, ed. *Diseases of the Bronchioles.* New York, NY: Raven; 1994:153–180.

102. Kitaichi M. Comparative pathology of inflammatory airways disease: a report made after the 1987 Milan congress. *Sarcoidosis.* 1992;9:625–628.

103. Gosink BB, Friedman PJ, Liebow AA. Bronchiolitis obliterans. Roentgenologic pathologic correlation. *Am J Roentgenol Radium Ther Nucl Med.* 1973;117:816–832.

104. Colby TV, Myers JL. Clinical and histologic spectrum of bronchiolitis obliterans, including bronchiolitis obliterans organizing pneumonia. *Sem Respir Med.* 1992;13:119–133.

105. Churg A, Wright JL. Small airways disease caused by mineral dusts. *Appl Occup Environ Hyg.* 1998;13:617–620.

106. Lai RS, Chiang AA, Wu MT, et al. Outbreak of bronchiolitis obliterans associated with consumption of Sauropus androgynus in Taiwan. *Lancet.* 1996;348:83–85.

107. Lin TJ, Lu CC, Chen KW, Deng JF. Outbreak of obstructive ventilatory impairment associated with consumption of Sauropus androgynus vegetable. *J Toxicol Clin Toxicol.* 1996;34:1–8.

108. Ger LP, Chiang AA, Lai RS, Chen SM, Tseng CJ. Association of *Sauropus androgynus* and bronchiolitis obliterans syndrome: a hospital-based case-control study. *Am J Epidemiol.* 1997;145:842–849.

109. Hsiue TR, Guo YL, Chen KW, Chen CW, Lee CH, Chang HY. Dose-response relationship and irreversible obstructive ventilatory defect in patients with consumption of *Sauropus androgynus. Chest.* 1998;113:71–76.

110. Davies S, Gosney J, Hansell D, et al. Diffuse idiopathic pulmonary neuroendocrine cell hyperplasia: an under-recognised spectrum of disease. *Thorax.* 2007;62:248–252.

111. Aguayo SM, Miller YE, Waldron JA, et al. Brief report: idiopathic diffuse hyperplasia of pulmonary neuroendocrine cells and airways disease. *N Engl J Med.* 1992;327:1285–1288.

112. Armas OA, White DA, Erlandson RA, Rosai J. Diffuse idiopathic pulmonary neuroendocrine cell proliferation presenting as interstitial lung disease. *Am J Surg Pathol.* 1995;19:963–970.

113. Miller RR, Muller NL. Neuroendocrine cell hyperplasia and obliterative bronchiolitis in patients with peripheral carcinoid tumors. *Am J Surg Pathol.* 1995;19:653–658.

114. Myers JL, Colby TV. Pathologic manifestations of bronchiolitis, constrictive bronchiolitis, cryptogenic organizing pneumonia, and diffuse panbronchiolitis. In: King TE, ed. *Bronchiolitis.* Philadelphia, PA: W.B. Saunders; 1993:611–622.

115. Wright JL, Cagle P, Churg A, Colby TV, Myers J. Diseases of the small airways. *Am Rev Respir Dis.* 1992;146:240–262.

116. Colby TV. Bronchiolar pathology. In: Epler GR, ed. *Diseases of the Bronchioles.* New York, NY: Raven; 1994:77–100.

117. Matsuse T, Hayashi S, Kuwano K, Keunecke H, Jefferies WA, Hogg JC. Latent adenoviral infection in the pathogenesis of chronic airways obstruction. *Am Rev Respir Dis.* 1992;146:177–184.

118. Paradis I, Yousem S, Griffith B. Airway obstruction and bronchiolitis obliterans after lung transplantation. In: King TE, ed. *Bronchiolitis.* Philadelphia, PA: W.B. Saunders; 1993:750–764.

119. Camus P, Piard F, Ashcroft T, Gal AA, Colby TV. The lung in inflammatory bowel disease. *Medicine (Baltimore).* 1993;72:151–183.

120. Dunnill MS. An assessment of the anatomical factor in cor pulmonale in emphysema. *J Clin Pathol.* 1961;14:246–258.

121. Wright JL, Levy RD, Churg A. Pulmonary hypertension in chronic obstructive pulmonary disease: current theories of pathogenesis and their implications for treatment. *Thorax.* 2005;60:605–609.

122. Naeye RL, Greenberg D, Valdivia E. Small pulmonary vessels in advanced pulmonary emphysema. *Arch Pathol Lab Med.* 1974;97:216–220.

123. Hicken P, Heath D, Brewer DB, Whitaker W. The small pulmonary arteries in emphysema. *J Pathol Bacteriol.* 1965;90:107–114.

124. Hale KA, Ewing SL, Gosnell BA, Niewoehner DE. Lung disease in long-term cigarette smokers with and without chronic airflow obstruction. *Am Rev Respir Dis.* 1984;130: 716–721.

125. Gorbunova V, Jacobs SS, Lo P, et al. Early detection of emphysema progression. *Med Image Comput Comput Assist Interv.* 2010;13: 193–200.

126. Gierada DS, Bierhals AJ, Choong CK, et al. Effects of CT section thickness and reconstruction kernel on emphysema quantification relationship to the magnitude of the CT emphysema index. *Acad Radiol.* 2010;17:146–156.

127. Bellia M, Benfante A, Menozzii M, et al. Validation of lung densitometry threshold at CT for the distinction between senile lung and emphysema in elderly subjects. *Monaldi Arch Chest Dis.* 2011;75:162–166.

128. Yuan R, Nagao T, Pare PD, et al. Quantification of lung surface area using computed tomography. *Respir Res.* 2010;11:153.

129. Nakano Y, Muro S, Sakai H, et al. Computed tomographic measurements of airway dimensions and emphysema in smokers. Correlation with lung function. *Am J Respir Crit Care Med.* 2000;162:1102–1108.

130. Mair G, Maclay J, Miller JJ, et al. Airway dimensions in COPD: relationships with clinical variables. *Respir Med.* 2010;104: 1683–1690.

131. Matsuoka S, Washko GR, Yamashiro T, et al. Pulmonary hypertension and computed tomography measurement of small pulmonary vessels in severe emphysema. *Am J Respir Crit Care Med.* 2010;181:218–225.

132. Matsuoka S, Washko GR, Dransfield MT, et al. Quantitative CT measurement of cross-sectional area of small pulmonary vessel in COPD: correlations with emphysema and airflow limitation. *Acad Radiol.* 2012;17:93–99.

CHAPTER 40

Chronic Obstructive Pulmonary Disease: Epidemiology, Pathophysiology, Pathogenesis, and α1-Antitrypsin Deficiency

Robert M. Senior
Richard A. Pierce
Jeffrey J. Atkinson

Chronic obstructive pulmonary disease (COPD) is defined as a disease state characterized by airflow obstruction that is not fully reversible and for which there is no other explanation for the obstruction. The obstruction is usually progressive and associated with an abnormal inflammatory response of the lungs to noxious particles and gas. Unlike earlier definitions, this definition does not mention emphysema or chronic bronchitis. According to criteria set by the Global Initiative for Obstructive Lung Disease,[1] airflow obstruction is present when there is a reduction of the postbronchodilator FEV_1/FVC ratio below 0.7 and its severity is graded by the percentage of the postbronchodilator FEV_1 of the predicted normal FEV_1 (Table 40-1). However, 0.7 as the cutoff value for the FEV_1/FVC ratio has been controversial as it may be too high for all age groups and lead to misdiagnosis of COPD in healthy middle-aged and older individuals.[2] Alternatively, use of the lower limit of normal (LLN) for the FEV_1/FVC ratio has been recommended,[3] but it is uncertain whether this criterion improves the detection of clinically significant COPD or prognosis in elderly individuals.[4,5] Classification of COPD by GOLD has undergone further refinement recently with addition of self-reported severity of dyspnea and history of COPD exacerbations.[1] Chapter 42 comments further about risk stratification.[6]

EPIDEMIOLOGY

COPD is a major health problem worldwide.[7,8] Its prevalence is being recognized increasingly in countries at all levels of development.[9] An ever-increasing number of smokers and an expanding number of elderly people are major factors in the surge in the worldwide prevalence of COPD. In a study from Canada, 27.6% of individuals reaching the age of 80 were diagnosed with COPD by a physician over the preceding 14 years.[10] In large areas of the world where indoor air pollution is generated by burning biomass for heating and cooking, COPD is prevalent among nonsmokers, especially women.[11] Moreover, COPD is not restricted to smokers in developed countries. Of 4291 never-smokers over age 40, involving 14 developed countries, 5.6% met criteria for moderate to severe COPD, of whom 81.2% were undiagnosed.[12]

At present, COPD is the third most common cause of death in the United States.[13,14] As might be expected from the mortality figures, surveys indicate a high prevalence of COPD. The 2011 Behavioral Risk Factor Surveillance System (BRFSS), which is a state-based telephone survey of the US civilian adult population aged >18 years, found that 6.3% of US adults (an estimated 15 million nationwide) were told that they have COPD by a healthcare provider and a large percentage of these individuals reported having had spirometry.[15] Another survey, the 2010 National Health Interview Survey of approximately 27,000 adults in US households, yielded an estimate of 5 million adults in the United States with emphysema and

TABLE 40-1 Classification of Airflow Limitation in Patients with FEV_1/FVC < 0.7

Severity Stage	Postbronchodilator FEV_1
1: Mild	$FEV_1 \geq 80\%$ predicted
2: Moderate	$50\% \geq FEV_1 < 80\%$ predicted
3: Severe	$30\% \geq FEV_1 < 50\%$ predicted
4: Very severe	$FEV_1 < 30\%$ predicted

Source: Modified with permission from Vestbo J, Hurd SS, Augusti AG, et al. Global strategy for the diagnosis, management, and prevention of chronic obstructive pulmonary disease. Am J Respir Crit Care Med. 2013;187(4):347–365.

TABLE 40-2 Risk Factors for COPD

Environmental	Host-based
Smoking	Genetic
Indoor air pollution	Airway hyperreactivity
Occupation	
Low socioeconomic status	

10 million with chronic bronchitis, not all of whom may have airflow obstruction.[16] Although these figures are impressive, they may be an underestimate, since COPD is likely to be unrecognized in some groups such as elderly persons living in poverty. Other statistics support these national surveys. Among 1575 cigarette smokers, aged 30 or older, with a 10 or more pack-year smoking history, approximately 20% met spirometric criteria for COPD.[17]

The number of deaths due to COPD in the United States has been rising. In 2008, COPD was the primary cause of death in 141,090 Americans.[14] and was a comorbidity in many other deaths. The number of women dying of COPD now exceeds men and has more than doubled in recent decades. Based on the Third National Health and Nutrition Examination Survey (NHANES III), life expectancy is shortened by 5.8 years for men aged 65 with GOLD stage 4 COPD and by an additional 3.5 years if smoking has continued.[18]

ETIOLOGY

Risk factors for the development of COPD are environmental and host based (Table 40-2). In developed countries, smoking tobacco is the predominant risk factor. However, as noted above, never-smokers also develop COPD and women predominate in this cohort.[11,12] In places where solid fuels are burned, indoor air pollution is probably the dominant risk factor. Other factors associated with COPD include second-hand tobacco exposure, age, level of education, tuberculosis, hospitalization for respiratory illness before the age of 10 years (see further comment below), a family history of COPD, and the number of years worked in dusty jobs.[19] Clearly, multiple risk factors may be present in a single individual.

ENVIRONMENTAL

Smoking

A history of smoking is present in 80% to 90% of the individuals with COPD in developed countries. In the United States an impressive level of overlap exists between the geographic distribution of smokers and the geographic distribution of individuals who have been told they have COPD (Fig. 40-1). In a European study involving 6836 individuals with normal spirometry, age 20 to 44, smoking was the most commonly recognized risk factor for the development of new COPD over a decade.[20] Deterioration of FEV_1 correlates with pack-years of smoking, but the relationship between amount of smoking and risk of COPD is unpredictable on an individual basis (Fig. 40-2), In the Million Women Study conducted in the United Kingdom, that involved 232,461 current, 328,417 former smokers, and 619,774 never-smokers at baseline, the relative risk of death from chronic lung disease, presumably mostly COPD, over a 12-year follow-up was increased about 35-fold among middle-aged women who smoked.[21] Among former smokers, the age at smoking cessation affects the subsequent rate of deterioration of lung function. The rate is closest to never smokers for those who quit prior to age 30, but even for those who quit after age 40, deterioration is less than in continued smokers (Fig. 40-3).

The effects of gender on the risk of developing COPD from smoking are unclear. Women may be more susceptible to lung injury from smoking than men as they show more lung function reduction in association with lower total exposure and they predominate among individuals with early onset of COPD[22] and never-smokers with COPD. However, among individuals with advanced COPD treated with long-term oxygen therapy, men have a higher mortality rate than women, a difference that cannot be explained by comorbidities.[23] Some data indicate racial disparities in the risk of developing COPD, with African Americans showing similar severity of COPD to whites with lesser pack-years of smoking.[24,25] Hispanic ethnicity appears to confer protection from the risk of COPD and a reduced risk of accelerated decline in lung function due to smoking.[26]

According to statistics from the Center for Disease Control and Prevention (CDC), in 2010 there were an estimated 45.3 million smokers in the United States representing 19.3% of all adults over age 18.[27] The percentage was similar in African Americans and whites. Smoking was present in 21% of men and 17% of women. Hispanics and Asians had the lowest percentage of smokers at 12% and 9%, respectively, while the percentage was highest at 27% among American Indian/Alaska Natives. Beyond age 65 the incidence of smoking was 9.5%. The number of smokers worldwide is predicted to be 1.5 to 1.9 billion in 2025.[28] Thus, COPD will continue to be a profound health problem well into the future.

Among smokers who have already sustained reductions in FEV_1, the consequences of continued smoking on ventilatory function are more impressive than when all smokers are grouped together.[29] The Lung Health Study, which followed middle-aged smokers for 11 years, found accelerated decline in those who already had a reduced FEV_1 at the start.[30] Despite these findings, progressive decline in the FEV_1 is not inevitable among individuals with COPD (Fig. 40-4).[31,32]

Environmental Tobacco Smoke Exposure or Second-Hand Smoke

Environmental tobacco smoke exposure (ETS) is implicated in loss of many years of life of adults and children in the United States, with notable sensitivity among African Americans,[33] but COPD, specifically, as a cause of the life shortening due to ETS is not clear[34] Controlled experimental studies with normal volunteers indicate that short-term exposures to ETS at levels comparable to those in real-life situations have effects on serum cytokine levels and pulmonary function that if recurrent or chronic might translate into COPD.[35,36] However, when smoking and other risk factors are controlled both workplace and home ETS but not prenatal ETS increase the risk of development of COPD.[37] Data regarding in utero effects of maternal smoking on lung growth and subsequent risk of childhood wheezing or asthma are becoming evident. However, doubt exists regarding the quantitative impact on the development of COPD in individuals with only prenatal exposure. It seems likely that similar to cystic fibrosis, individuals with enhanced genetic risk factors could be adversely modulated by ETS,[38] but to date no definitive proof of gene-by-environment interactions for ETS have been demonstrated. The data does not suggest that ETS is harmless but rather it is less definitively causal of COPD as an independent risk than chronic smoking or occupational exposures.[37] Avoidance in individuals with existing lung disease is clearly indicated given the association with exacerbation. The attitude that there is no risk-free dose of ETS, is likely the safest approach; this applies to all ETS-related diseases and not just COPD.[34]

Indoor Air Pollution

As stated above, indoor air pollution from burning solid fuels such as wood and animal dung for cooking and heating is widespread in parts of the world. This practice exposes women and children to high concentrations of smoke containing respirable particles and complex gas mixtures for many hours daily and thus the risk of COPD. It compounds the risk of COPD in smokers who are more likely to be men in these settings. Cough and sputum occur among those

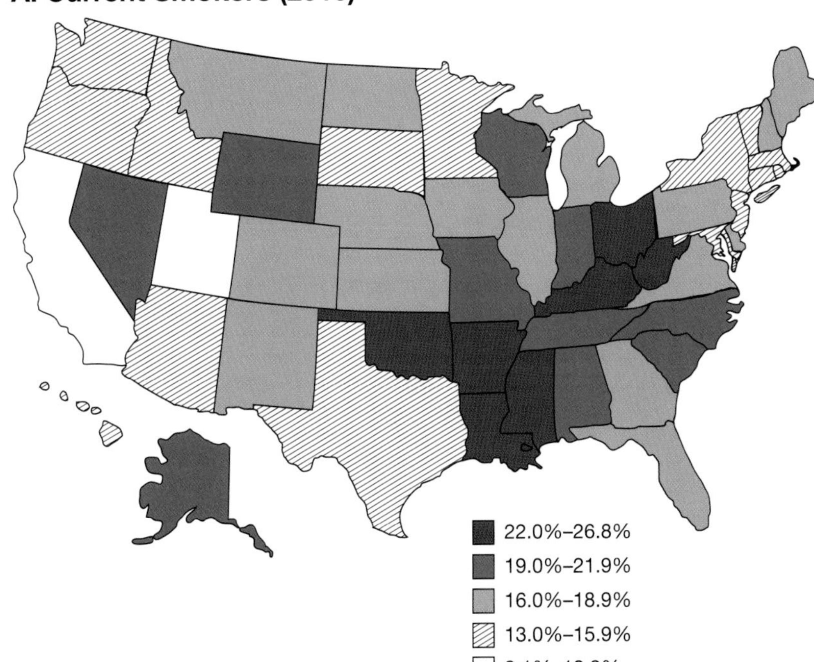

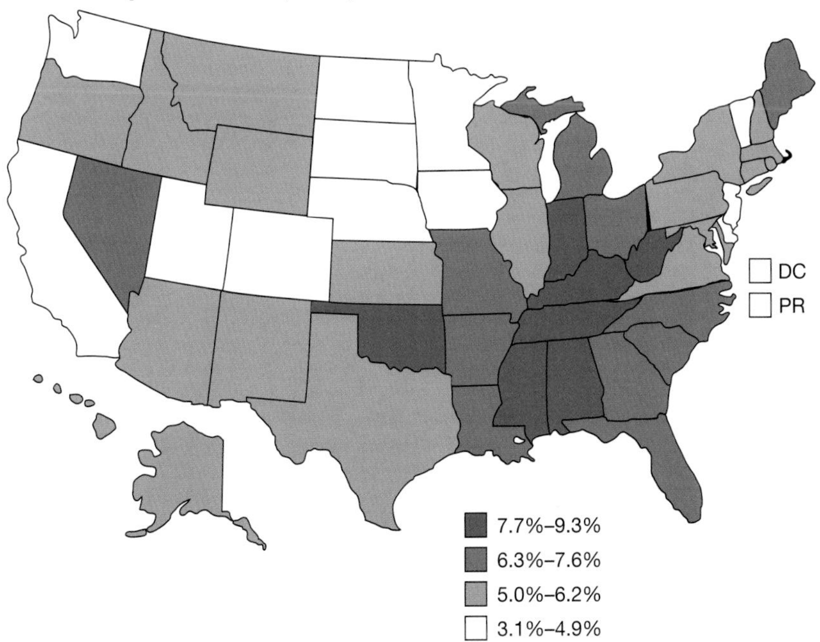

Figure 40-1 **A.** Percentage of persons aged ≥18 years who were current cigarette smokers, by state. Behavioral Risk Factor Surveillance System, United States, 2010. Persons who reported smoking at least 100 cigarettes during their lifetime and who, at the time of the survey, reported smoking cigarettes every day or some days. **B.** Age-adjusted prevalence of chronic obstructive pulmonary disease (COPD) among adults—Behavioral Risk Factor Surveillance System, United States, 2011. Based on an affirmative response to the question, "Has a doctor, nurse, or other health professional ever told you that you have COPD, emphysema, or chronic bronchitis?" *(**A.** Reproduced with permission from Vital Signs. Current Cigarette Smoking Among Adults Aged ≥18 Years—United States, 2005–2010. Morbidity and Mortality Weekly Report. 2011;60(35):1207–1212. **B.** Reproduced with permission from Chronic Obstructive Pulmonary Disease Among Adults—United States, 2011. Morbidity and Mortality Weekly Report. 2012;61(46):938–943.)*

exposed to indoor air pollution and an association with COPD is evident.[39,40] Abatement of bronchitic symptoms coincident with measures that reduce the levels of smoke strongly implicates the indoor air pollution.[41] The World Health Organization estimates that more than 1 million people a year die of COPD precipitated by indoor air pollution.[42] International advocacy organizations such as the Global Alliance for Clean Cook-stoves seek to curb indoor air pollution.

Occupation

The possibility that occupation-related inhalation of particulates and gases carries a risk for COPD was slow in gaining acceptance, but acceptance is widespread now.[43,44] The delay was understandable since smoking among workers in certain occupations was a confounding factor. Also, workers beginning jobs with a high risk of causing lung disease typically have better lung function than normal (the "healthy worker" phenomenon), obscuring work-related effects among relatively young workers. In addition, among cohorts of workers, those with COPD may drop out, causing an underestimate of risk in follow-up studies of individuals still working.

Despite these problems, studies from different groups around the world, urban and rural, workforce-based and community-based, clearly implicate occupations producing exposures to dusts, gases, and fumes as risk factors for COPD.[44] The American Thoracic Society has estimated that the occupational contribution to the population burden of COPD is 15%.[45] Apart from the well-recognized risk of occupations involving exposure to organic and inorganic dusts, less obviously "risky" occupations, such as construction, plastics manufacturing, and utility work may carry an increased risk of COPD.[46] The risk of adverse occupational exposure is particularly

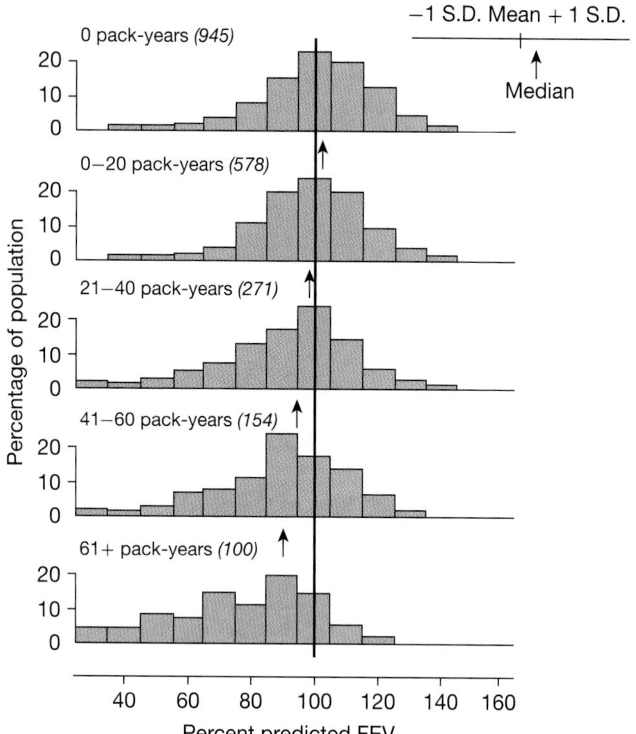

Figure 40-2 Distribution of percent predicted FEV_1 in adults with varying pack-years of smoking. Subjects with "respiratory trouble" before age 16 are excluded. The proportion of smokers with normal expiratory airflow decreases with increasing pack-years. Nevertheless, many smokers have a normal FEV_1 despite large cigarette-smoking histories. Means, medians, and ± standard deviation of the data for each group are shown in the abscissas. The numbers in parentheses are the numbers of subjects. *(Reproduced with permission from Burrows B, Knudson RJ, Cline M, et al. Quantitative relationships between cigarette smoking and ventilatory function. Am Rev Respir Dis. 1977;115:195–205.)*

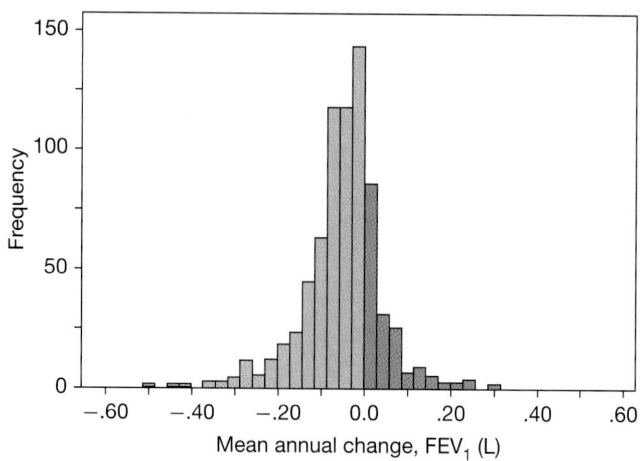

Figure 40-3 Histogram of the mean annual FEV_1 decline (L) for 751 patients with COPD followed for a median of 64 months and up to 10 years, having an average of 5.44 annual measurements, average age 66 years, 92% male, stratified by ATS/ERS and GOLD severity classification as follows: 32 (4%) mild ($FEV_1\% \geq 80$); 256 (34%) moderate ($FEV_1\%$ 50–79); 245 (33%) severe ($FEV_1\%$ 30–49); and 218 (29%) very severe ($FEV_1\% < 30$). *(Reproduced with permission from Casanova C, de Torres JP, Aguirre-Jaíme A, et al. The progression of chronic obstructive pulmonary disease is heterogeneous: the experience of the BODE cohort. Am J Respir Crit Care Med. 2011;184(9):1015–1021.)*

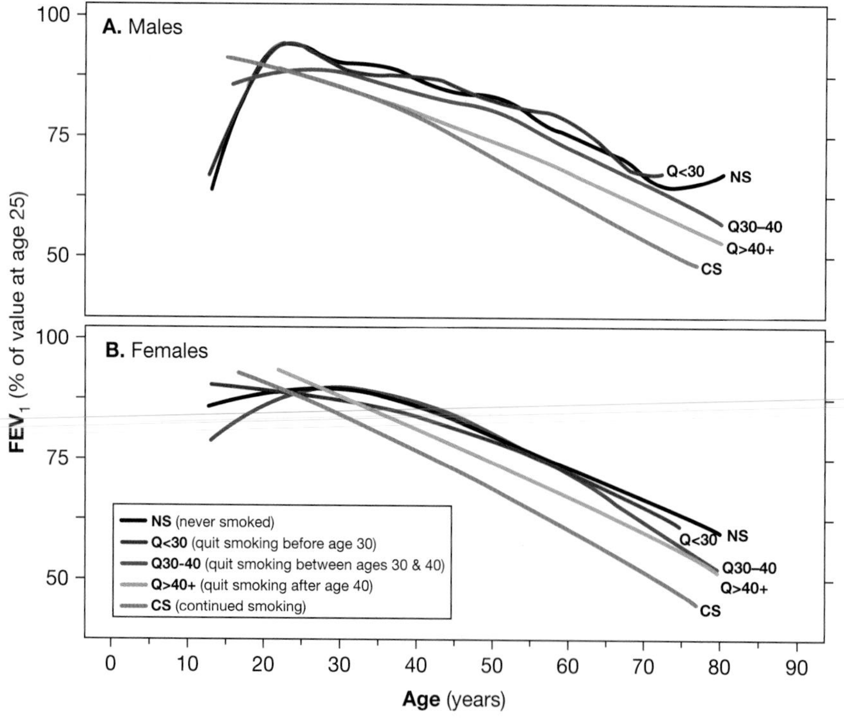

Figure 40-4 The effect of age of quitting smoking on FEV_1. Mean FEV_1 values (expressed as percent of its value at age 25) in smokers who quit smoking before the age 30 (Q < 30), between 30 and 40 years of age (Q30–40) and after age 40 (Q40+). Curves from healthy never smokers (NS) and continuous smokers (CS) are included for comparison. **A.** Males. **B.** Females. The mean annual FEV_1 decline for males was 15.5 mL in quitters before age 30, 24.0 mL in quitters 30 to 40 years of age, and 28.9 mL in quitters after age 40; for females, the values were 10.4 mL quitting before age 30, 16.5 mL in quitters between 30 and 40 years of age, and 21.0 mL in quitters after the age of 40. *(Reproduced with permission from Kohansal R, Martinez-Camblor P, Agustí A, et al. The natural history of chronic airflow obstruction revisited: an analysis of the Framingham offspring cohort. Am J Respir Crit Care Med. 2009;180(1):3–10.)*

important in workers who smoke or have other factors that raise their risk for COPD, such as α1-antitrypsin deficiency.[47]

Childhood Lower Respiratory Tract Infections

Since the status of lung function in very early childhood predicts ventilatory function many years later,[48] it is plausible that lower respiratory tract infections (LRIs) during childhood might adversely affect lung development and increase the risk of developing COPD later in life. However, lung function in children who had pneumonia up to age 2 infrequently had reduced lung function 10 years after the infection.[49] If there was a ventilatory defect, it was most often restrictive. Where reduced airflow was observed, an adenovirus was the predominant class of pathogens responsible for the pneumonia. It is notable that COPD exacerbations may leave only a minor lasting effect on airflow. Continued smokers enrolled in the Lung Health Study had only an additional loss of 7 mL of FEV_1 per year for those having one exacerbation per year, while among those who had quit smoking, exacerbations had no permanent effect on the FEV_1.[50]

LOW SOCIOECONOMIC STATUS

A low socioeconomic status is a risk factor for COPD. The relationship may be linked to an increased amount of smoking and other factors, including deficient medical care for respiratory infections, occupational exposure to inhaled particulates, and increased exposure to household allergens. The importance of smoking is evident. In the United States in 2011, 45% of adults with a General Education Diploma (GED) were smokers compared to 10% of individuals with a college degree, and among adults living below the poverty level, 33% were smokers in contrast to 20% of individuals living above the poverty level.[51]

HUMAN IMMUNODEFICIENCY VIRUS INFECTION

Individuals with human immunodeficiency virus (HIV) who smoke have an increased risk of COPD or more specifically emphysema development.[52–54] The risk appears to be modulated by activation of alveolar macrophages with evidence of enhanced production of matrix metalloproteinases (MMPs) in these individuals.[55] Although HIV can infect macrophages,[56] it is unclear if this is a direct alteration due to HIV infection or a response to some downstream alteration of the suppression of innate immune responses, like chronic *Pneumocystis* infection.[57] The occurrence of COPD and pulmonary hypertension in smokers with HIV appears to be more common in individuals with a high viral load and lower CD4 cell counts and not an adverse consequence of antiretroviral therapy.[58] However, emphysema is not reversible and relation to viral load or recovery of CD4 cell counts is not straightforward. Other health issues like malnutrition may contribute. A multicenter study about the lung in HIV supported by the National Insitutes of Health is underway.

HOST BASED

Genetics

The field of COPD genetics is moving rapidly so that capturing this subject is aiming at a moving target. Aggregation of COPD in families and concordance of pulmonary function in twin studies have established a role for genetic predisposition to COPD.[59–61] Moreover, the occurrence of reduced maximal expiratory airflow among nonsmoking first-degree relatives of individuals with early-onset COPD provides further support.[62] Perhaps most compelling is the marked variability in development of COPD among smokers. Dissecting specific genetic factors that increase the risk of COPD has proven difficult. α_1-AT deficiency illustrates this difficulty,[63] where even among individuals with an identified genetic risk factor, wide, unexplained variability in the occurrence of COPD exists.[64]

However, deficiency of functional α_1-AT represents the best-known genetic risk for COPD (see below). In this example genetic mutations discovered in small initial sample sizes can be replicated in larger analysis despite a significant gene-by-environment interaction. To this end, very rare mutations in the coding sequence of elastin cause cutus laxa and can also lead to COPD.[65–67] Although Marfan and Ehler–Danlos syndromes cause lung parenchymal blebs[68] and in mouse models demonstrate developmental of airspace enlargement,[69,70] no human cohort has demonstrated clear penetration of a fixed obstructive lung disease phenotype.[71]

Polymorphisms of genes involved in protease–antiprotease balance, antioxidant function, inflammation, and immune responses have been implicated in COPD in studies utilizing candidate gene approaches (Table 40-3).[72–74] However, none of these polymorphisms are consistently confirmed in other cohorts or large genome-wide association studies of lung function or COPD (Table 40-4).[75–78] Failure of confirmation may indicate flaws in previous studies, but differences in COPD phenotypes, ethnic background, or other factors might explain discrepancies between previous studies and subsequent data. Despite misgivings of reproducibility in candidate gene studies it should be noted a minor allele frequency (MAF) of less than 5% typically excludes rare polymorphisms from GWAS style studies. Rare alleles may be quite important if the effect is large as demonstrated by α_1-AT (SerpinA1) (Table 40-3).

TABLE 40-3 Examples of COPD-Related Genes from Candidate Approach Studies

Gene Symbol	Functional Category	Locus	Polymorphism	MAF[a]
SERPINA1	Antiprotease	14q32	rs28929474=A	0.01
MMP12	Protease	11q22	rs2276109=G	0.07
MMP1	Protease	11q22	rs1799750=del	0.45
SOD3	Antioxidant	4p15	rs1799895=G	0.02
HMOX1	Antioxidant	22q13	rs3074372 $(GT)_n$>33	0.13[b]
EPHX1	Detoxifying	1q42	rs2234922=G	0.19
GSTM1	Detoxifying	1p13	rs366631=T	0.19
ADRB2	Adrenergic	5q32	rs1800888=T	0.01
TGFB1	Cytokine	19q13	rs2241712=A	0.35

SERPINA1 (α1-antitrypsin) included for appreciation of allelic frequency of genes discovered by candidate gene approach or meta-analysis of candidate genes.
[a]Minor allele frequency (MAF) from 1000 Genomes or from [b]study when not available.

TABLE 40-4 Examples of COPD-Related Genes from Genome Wide Association Studies of Spirometry (prebronchodilator)

Gene Symbol	Functional Category	Locus	Polymorphism	MAF[a]	Association
TNS1	Cell adhesion to matrix	2q35	rs2571445=G	0.33	FEV_1
FAM13A	Signal transduction	4q22	rs7671167=T	0.48	COPD, FEV_1/FVC
HHIP	Lung development	4q31	rs11100860=G	0.39	COPD, FEV_1/FVC
HTR4	Serotonin receptor	5q33	rs3995090=C	0.47	COPD, FEV_1
AGER	Glycosylation receptor	6p21	rs2070600=T	0.07	FEV_1/FVC
THSD4	TGFβ signaling	15q23	rs12899618=G	0.12	FEV_1/FVC
CHRNA3/5[b]	Nicotine addiction	15q25	rs8034191=T	0.21	COPD, FEV_1/FVC
IREB2[b]	Iron homeostasis	15q25	rs2568594=G	0.32	FEV_1/FVC
BICD1	Telomere/senescence	12p11	rs10844154=A	0.38	Emphysema
TMEM26	Transmembrane protein	10q21	10761570=T	0.44	Decline in FEV_1

[a]*Minor allele frequency (MAF) from 1000 Genomes, Polymorphism studied is not always minor allele.*
[b]*Polymorphism no longer significant for association with physiology measures when only nonsmokers evaluated.*

Traits like emphysema quantified by CT lung density, subjective dyspnea, and 6-minute walk distance can also be utilized as each trait has been independently associated with prognosis in COPD. Of note, analysis based on radiographic emphysema characterization does not seem to reveal the same genetic locations as airway physiology-based phenotyping (Table 40-4),[79] possibly reflecting the advantage of extending genetic evaluation to other reproducible quantitative phenotypes, as differential genetic susceptibility to disease characteristics may reveal distinct independent pathways within the larger COPD population.

Very large GWAS studies of physiologic traits used to define COPD (FEV_1, FEV_1/FVC ratio) in populations that include nonsmokers and individuals too young to have COPD increase the understanding of how genetic factors interact with the environmental etiologic factors. For example, lung development and smoking habit may be teased out by examining COPD-susceptibility loci for association with the same traits in nonsmokers or younger individuals. This is important, as polymorphisms related to nicotine addiction[80] (e.g., CHRNA3/5) need to be separated from polymorphisms that mark susceptibility to smoke exposure given the difficulty with quantifying lifetime smoke exposure. On the other hand, polymorphisms related to genes involved predominantly in lung development (e.g., HHIP) will result in alterations of the physiologic traits even in never-smokers, but may also augment increased susceptibility to smoking.[81] It is notable that the different approaches of genetic analysis have not yielded as much cross-confirmation in COPD as has been seen in other diseases, despite the fairly large size of recent GWAS studies. In addition, although the same approaches have been utilized in asthma, a diagnosis that relies on the same physiologic traits, the polymorphisms discovered in asthma do not overlap COPD associated pathways.[82–84] This distinct genetic framework of COPD versus asthma supports many years of work in mouse models defining divergent immune pathways in these two common airway diseases.[85]

Airway Hyperresponsiveness

Airway hyperresponsiveness (AHR) is present when there is an acute, temporary decline in maximal expiratory airflow in response to inhaling potential bronchoconstricting agents such as methacholine or histamine. In individuals with COPD, AHR is associated with accelerated decline of FEV_1 and therefore is a negative prognostic marker.[86] In the Lung Health Study, AHR was second to smoking as an important determinant of decline in FEV_1 and was not related to the initial level of obstruction. AHR was greater in women smokers than men smokers.[86] Although AHR decreased after smoking cessation and bronchodilator responsiveness improved, bronchodilator responsiveness did not correlate with the rate of FEV_1 decline.[87]

A major question about the relationship of AHR to COPD involves consideration of the so-called "Dutch hypothesis," which ascribes a role of allergy to the development of COPD. Observations that argue against AHR as a cause of COPD are that smokers typically do not show AHR until their FEV_1 is already reduced and that experimental induction of emphysema can lead to AHR.[88] It is plausible that AHR may be a consequence of emphysema, as airway wall stiffness and parenchymal tethering are affected by the extracellular matrix.[89] If unmeasured emphysema is also connected to AHR, this may contribute to the gender bias and decline rate findings as emphysema presence may predict accelerated future decline regardless of smoking habit.[90] As noted, the genetic distinction of asthma and COPD polymorphisms would also favor a great proportion of COPD having a nonasthmatic origin.

PATHOPHYSIOLOGY

A persistent reduction in FEV_1/FVC is the defining physiological feature of COPD. Increased airway resistance, increased residual volume (RV), increased RV/total lung capacity ratio (RV/TLC), decreased inspiratory capacity, decreased maximum voluntary ventilation (MVV), abnormal distribution of ventilation, and ventilation–perfusion mismatching are also typical physiological features.

AIRFLOW OBSTRUCTION

The low FEV_1 and low FEV_1/FVC in COPD are not reversible with inhaled bronchodilators, although small improvements are common, especially if responsiveness is tested with both ipratropium and albuterol.[91] Thus, COPD differs from asthma, in which inhaled bronchodilators can produce large improvements in FEV_1. Maximal inspiratory flow may be relatively well preserved in the presence of a low FEV_1/FVC and a low FEV_1. A reduced FEV_1 with a normal FEV_1/FVC and normal TLC should not be interpreted as an obstructive ventilatory defect. This pulmonary function pattern is called nonspecific and infrequently progresses to COPD.[92]

The FEV_1 is the result of the balance between the elastic recoil of the lungs promoting expiratory flow and the resistance of the airways that limits flow during performance of an FVC. In normal lungs, as well as in lungs affected by COPD, maximal expiratory flow diminishes as the lungs empty because the lung parenchyma provides progressively less elastic recoil and the cross-sectional area of the airways falls leading to an increase in airway resistance. The decrease in

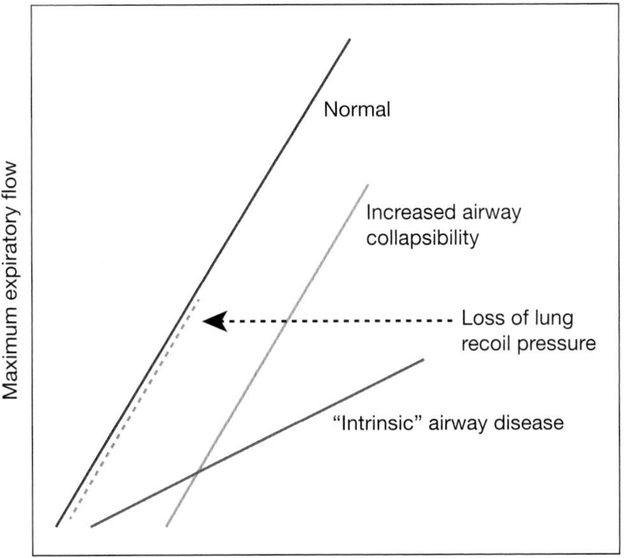

Figure 40-5 Analysis of reduced maximum expiratory flow in COPD from maximum expiratory flow versus lung recoil pressure curves. With loss of lung recoil pressure – that is, "emphysema" (heavy interrupted line) – the slope of the flow–pressure curve remains normal, but the curve terminates at lower pressure than normal. With intrinsic airway obstruction – that is, "bronchitis" – the slope is reduced. Increased airway collapsibility, which may be a result of decreased elastic recoil, causes the curve to be displaced to the right. Commonly in COPD, the flow–pressure curve has premature termination and a decreased slope and is shifted rightward, indicating that decreased elastic recoil, increased airway resistance, and increased airway collapsibility are all involved in causing the reduced maximum expiratory flow. *(From Pride NB, Milic-Emili J. Lung mechanics, in Calverley PMA, Pride NB [eds]. Chronic Obstructive Pulmonary Disease. London, Chapman & Hall; 1995.)*

flow coincident with the decrease in lung volume is apparent on the expiratory limb of the flow–volume curve (Fig. 40-5). In mild COPD the abnormality in airflow is evident only at lung volumes at or below functional residual capacity, appearing as a "scooped out" lower part of the descending limb of the flow–volume curve. In advanced COPD, the entire curve demonstrates decreased expiratory flow. By measuring pressure–volume and pressure–flow relationships it is theoretically possible to assess the relative importance of decreased elastic recoil ("emphysema") from increased airway resistance ("small airway disease") as the cause for the reduced FEV_1 As discussed below, the correlation between FEV_1 and small airway pathology is strong and likely contributes to the reduction independent of the correlation of FEV_1 with emphysema.

There is wide variability in COPD in the relationships between FEV_1, exercise tolerance, and quality of life.[93] Variability also extends to the relationship between the FEV_1 and alveolar gas exchange. However, the Pa_{O_2} and oxygen saturation usually remain near normal until the FEV_1 has decreased to about half of the predicted normal while elevation of the Pa_{CO_2} seldom occurs until the FEV_1 is less than about one-fourth of the predicted.[94] Thus, other causes of hypoxemia or an elevated Pa_{CO_2}, such as the obesity hypoventilation syndrome, should be considered in patients with abnormal arterial blood gases and only mild to moderate COPD. Similarly, pulmonary hypertension and right ventricular failure do not occur unless COPD is severe and associated with chronic hypoxemia (Pa_{O_2} <55 mm Hg). Diastolic dysfunction is common in the general population, where COPD is prevalent, and should be considered when pulmonary hypertension is discrepant with COPD severity.

ABNORMAL DISTRIBUTION OF VENTILATION AND VENTILATION–PERFUSION MISMATCHING

Abnormal distribution of ventilation results from the heterogeneity of the pathologic process affecting airways and lung parenchyma. This heterogeneous ventilation results in ventilation–perfusion mismatching that is characteristic of COPD. Abnormality in the distribution of ventilation is evident in the pattern of nitrogen washout during breathing of 100% oxygen. The nitrogen washout is delayed because of regions that are poorly ventilated, and the shape of the nitrogen washout curve reflects compartments with different washout rates due to regional differences in compliance and airway resistance. Radioisotopic ventilation scanning with ^{133}xenon also reveals regional heterogeneity of ventilation in COPD, but can also demonstrate the ability of airway mucus to trap xenon tracer.

The multiple inert gas elimination technique (MIGET), which enables quantification of the ventilation–perfusion profile, has demonstrated different ventilation–perfusion patterns among patients with advanced COPD (Fig. 40-6). In one pattern, the

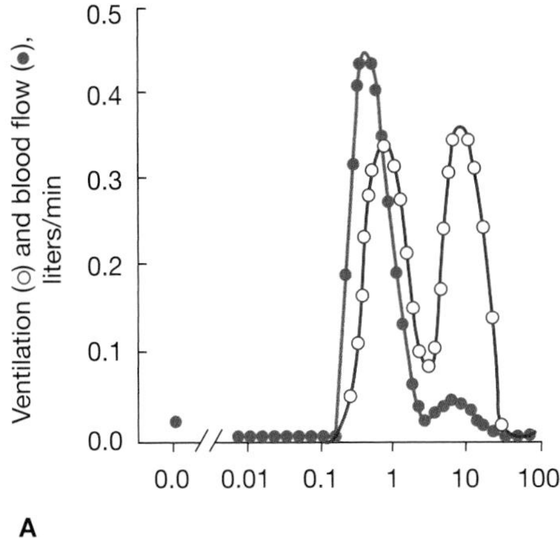

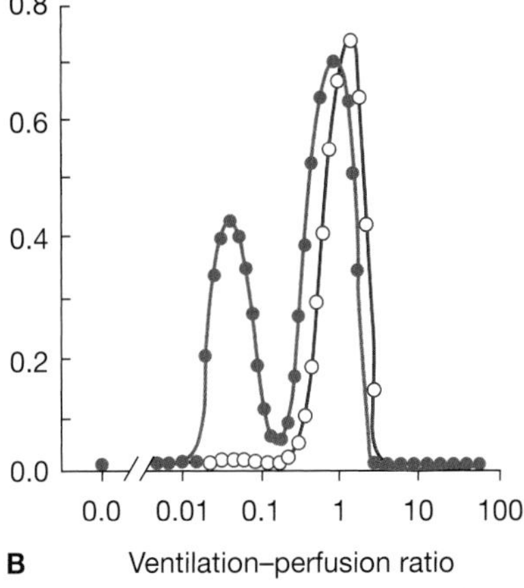

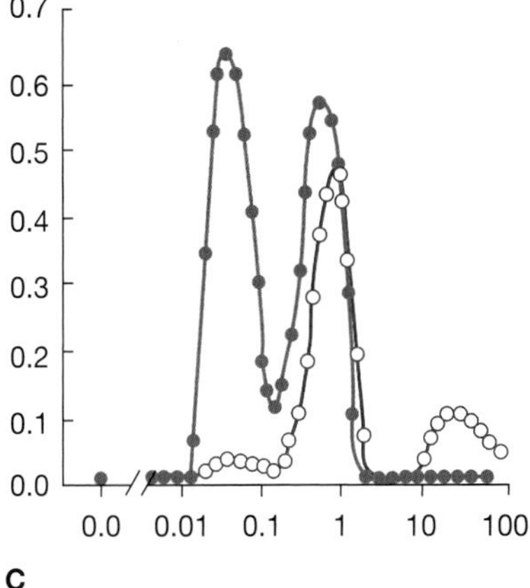

Figure 40-6 Ventilation–perfusion distributions in three persons with COPD determined by the multiple inert gas elimination technique (MIGET). **A.** Regions of high ventilation–perfusion characteristic of "emphysematous," type A COPD. **B.** Regions of low ventilation–perfusion characteristic of "chronic bronchitis," type B COPD. **C.** Regions of both high and low ventilation–perfusion characteristic of many people with COPD. In the normal person, not shown, ventilation–perfusion virtually overlaps and peaks at about a ventilation–perfusion ratio of 1. *(Reproduced with permission from Wagner PD, Dantzker DR, Dueck R, et al. Ventilation-perfusion inequality in chronic obstructive pulmonary disease. J Clin Invest. 1977;59(2):203–216.)*

so-called type A ("pink puffer") COPD, there is a substantial amount of ventilation distributed to high ventilation–perfusion regions. This likely reflects actual loss of vascular elements in conjunction with the pathologic changes of the gas exchange parenchyma. In a second pattern, called type B ("blue bloater") COPD, there is a substantial amount of pulmonary blood flow perfusing low ventilation regions. This simple classification was important historically in the development of understanding COPD pathophysiology, but has fallen out of use because most people with COPD are not easily classified as either type A or type B. They have both high and low ventilation–perfusion regions.

Ventilation–perfusion mismatching accounts for essentially all of the reduction in Pa_{O_2} that occurs in COPD, so modest elevations of the inspired oxygen concentration are effective in treating hypoxemia. If hypoxemia is difficult to correct, other problems such as right- to left-sided intracardiac or intrapulmonary shunting need to be considered in addition to COPD.

HYPERINFLATION

Increases in total lung capacity, functional residual capacity (FRC), residual volume, and the residual volume to total lung capacity ratio (RV/TLC) are common in COPD. These abnormalities may be beneficial in that they help to preserve expiratory airflow by increasing lung elastic recoil and the cross-sectional areas of airway lumens. However, they have adverse effects. They displace the diaphragm into a flattened position causing a number of adverse effects (Fig. 40-7). In addition, they put the thoracic cage at a mechanical disadvantage so that inspiration requires work rather than being passively assisted by the elastic recoil of the chest wall. These abnormalities of increased lung volume may increase further with exertion because reductions in airflow in diseased lungs reduce expiratory volume during rapid breathing. This phenomenon, called dynamic hyperinflation, adds to the workload on the inspiratory muscles while further reducing their mechanical advantage. Dynamic hyperinflation is an important mechanism of dyspnea with exertion in COPD.[95]

Hyperinflation of the residual volume and FRC reduce the inspiratory capacity, which has prognostic significance that is independent of FEV_1. In one study of individuals with moderate to severe COPD, those whose ratio of inspiratory capacity to total lung capacity was less than 25% had a much shorter life span than those with a ratio greater than 25%, even though the two groups had comparable percent predicted FEV_1.[96]

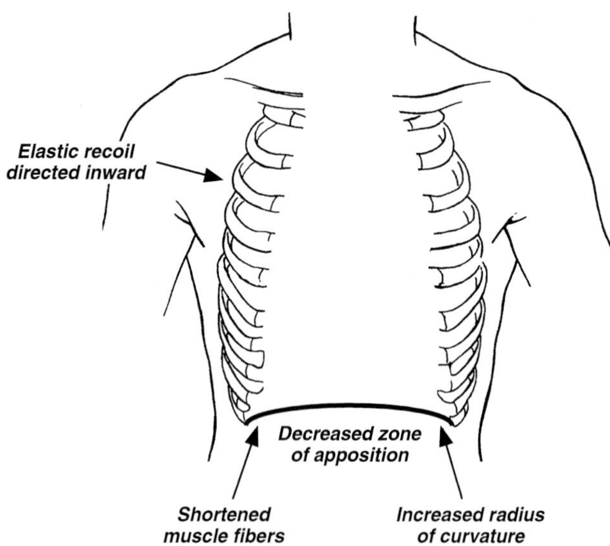

Figure 40-7 Detrimental effects of hyperinflation on diaphragmatic function. Hyperinflation causes flattening of the diaphragm, which (1) decreases the zone of apposition between the diaphragm and the abdominal wall, hindering rib cage movement; (2) shortens diaphragmatic muscle fiber length, decreasing the force that can be generated by the diaphragm; (3) increases the radius of curvature of the diaphragm, thereby decreasing transpulmonary pressure (at constant tension); and (4) directs diaphragmatic muscle fibers medially, impairing inflation with diaphragmatic contraction. In addition, hyperinflation prevents the thorax from assisting inspiration during tidal breathing because the resting volume of the thorax is above the volume at which the rib cage recoils outward during inspiration. *(Reproduced with permission from Yusen RD, Lefrak SS. Evaluation of patients with emphysema for lung volume reduction surgery. Washington University Emphysema Surgery Group, Semin Thorac Cardiovasc Surg. 1996;8(1):83–93.)*

DYSPNEA

People with COPD typically seek medical care because shortness of breath limits their activities and quality of life. Dyspnea is seldom a complaint until the FEV_1 has fallen below about 60% of predicted. However, the correlation between FEV_1 and exercise limitation is not strong. Some individuals are relatively free of dyspnea despite a severely reduced FEV_1. Commonly, the discomfort associated with breathing is associated with inspiration rather than expiration.[97] Measurement of dyspnea has proven complicated.[98] A number of indices are in use.

An increased sense of effort relating to the pressures needed from the respiratory muscles relative to their maximum pressure-generating capacity is thought to be an important factor in causing the dyspnea associated with COPD. Signals of "length-tension inappropriateness" from the respiratory muscles due to hyperinflation are another factor. Dynamic hyperinflation, as described above, exaggerates these problems for respiratory muscles. Also, impulses from airways undergoing abnormal dynamic compression during exhalation have been described. Hypoxemia and hypercapnia play only a small role during periods of clinical stability. Oxygen administration may decrease breathlessness by reducing ventilation during exertion and through poorly understood direct effects not associated with changes in ventilation.

PHYSIOLOGICAL–PATHOLOGICAL CORRELATIONS

In 1968, Hogg and colleagues observed that airways 2 mm or less in internal diameter normally contribute only a minor part of the total airway resistance, but that these airways are the principal sites of increased airway resistance in COPD.[99] For many years, the physical basis for small airway resistance in COPD was considered to be a combined result of emphysema causing small airway instability and collapse along with multiple anatomic abnormalities narrowing the lumens of small airways. Because emphysema and small airway pathology are both common in individuals with COPD their relative contributions to airflow obstruction have been difficult to discern.

Fixed reduction in airflow is associated with several specific pathologic findings in the small airways of advanced COPD (Fig. 40-8). Small airways in the lungs of individuals with COPD typically show goblet cell metaplasia, replacement of Clara cells with mucus-secreting cells, and infiltration of the airway walls by inflammatory cells that, in severe disease, include an increased surface area of lymphoid follicles.[100] The cellular changes are accompanied by increased connective tissue in the subepithelial and adventitial compartments of the airway walls.[100] Alveolar tissue surrounding small airways normally provides radial traction on bronchioles at points where alveolar septa attach. Loss of these bronchiolar attachments as a result of proteolytic destruction may contribute to airway distortion, narrowing, and instability.

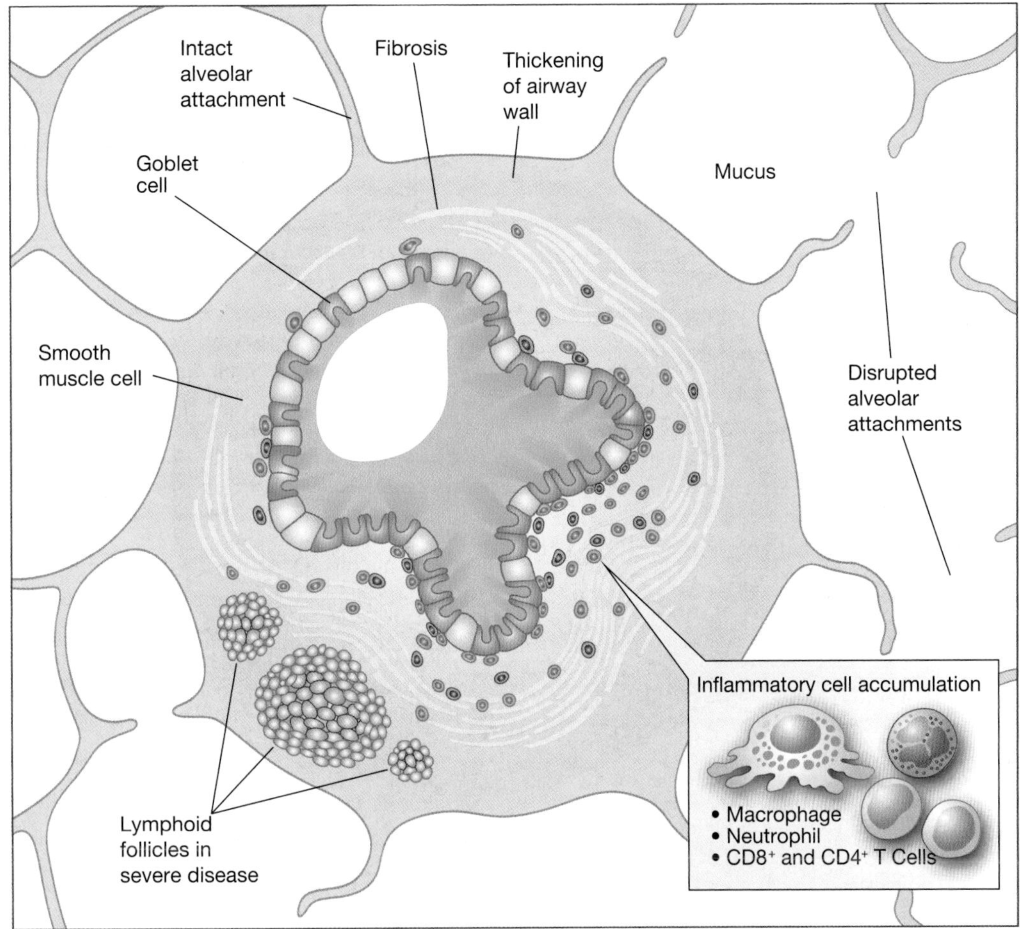

Figure 40-8 Pathologic lesions in small airways in COPD. Multiple abnormalities lead to partial obstruction of the lumen and altered shape and mechanical properties of the airways. *(Reproduced with permission from Senior RM, Silverman EK. Chronic obstructive pulmonary disease. In: Nabel EG, ed. ACP Medicine: Pulmonary, Hamilton, Ontario. Canada: Decker Publishing; 2011.)*

Although pathologic studies suggested the numeric loss of very small airways seen at autopsy is insufficient to produce the degree of airway resistance increases seen early in COPD, recent radiologic studies have confirmed there is a significant loss of visible (2–2.5-mm diameter) airways before radiographic emphysema is present.[101] Indeed, the loss of small airways can be impressive, reaching 90% in severe COPD. The large-scale pathologic loss of terminal airways in advanced disease will contribute significantly to the small airway resistance[101] but whether radiographic loss of small airway surface area in early disease is pathologic destruction, severe wall thickening or mucus plugging that obscures the lumen below the radiographic resolution is not yet clear. However, more severe airflow obstruction is clearly associated with increases in thickness of all components of the airway wall.[100] The greatest relative increase in components of the airway wall is in the connective tissue–rich adventitial layer but the epithelial layer, the lamina propria, and the smooth muscle–containing layer all demonstrate significant increases in advanced disease and small airway mucus plugs have been demonstrated to be significantly associated with airflow limitation in severe disease. Thus, overall, compared to small airway pathology and radiologic loss of small airways, emphysema occurs late in the development of COPD and appears to have a limited role in causing the airflow obstruction in early COPD.[102]

PATHOGENETIC MECHANISMS

COPD represents the clinical expression of complex alterations in structure and function of alveolar tissue and small airways. Many processes at the tissue and cellular levels can be implicated, including inflammation, cell proliferation, apoptosis, altered phenotype of lung cells, and remodeling of the extracellular matrix (Fig. 40-9). Numerous mediators, most notably proteinases, oxidants, and cytokines, are involved in these processes. Studies in genetically altered mice have proven invaluable in helping to elucidate the pathogenesis of COPD, especially emphysema.

■ INFLAMMATION

Innate Immune Responses

As reflected in the definition of COPD, inflammation occupies a central role in current thinking about the pathogenesis of COPD. The inflammation paradigm is that smoking and other types of inhaled irritants lead to recruitment of innate inflammatory cells to the lungs and airways and that products of these recruited cells injure lung tissue and disrupt normal mechanisms of lung repair. Indeed, inflammation is prominent in airways and lung parenchyma in biopsies, surgical specimens, and postmortem material from individuals with COPD.[100,103–105] Other indicators of inflammation are increased inflammatory cells in bronchoalveolar lavage fluid (BALF)[106–108] and sputum[109–111] and increased volatile products of inflammatory cells in exhaled breath.[112,113] Systemic inflammation is also present in current smokers, with elevations in white blood cell counts, neutrophil subsets, or liver-derived acute phase reactants.[114–116] Inflammatory cells associated with COPD in the lung include predominantly neutrophils,

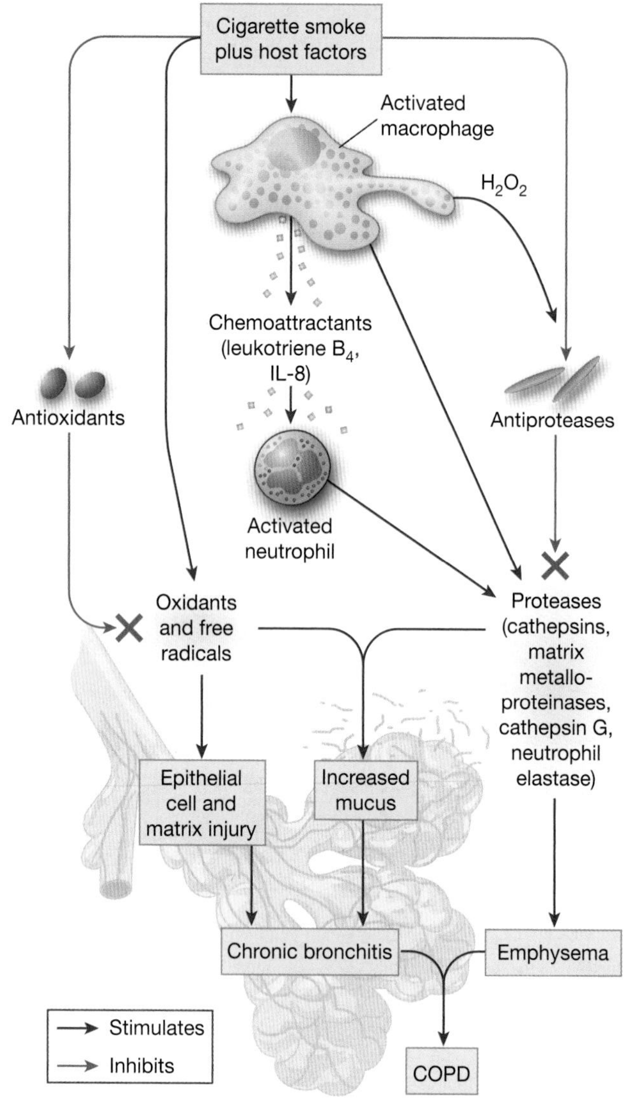

FIGURE 40-9 The pathogenesis of COPD from smoking. Smoking stimulates resident cells to release factors that recruit inflammatory cells to the lungs. The various inflammatory cells that accumulate in the peripheral tissues of the lungs release proteinases and oxidants that damage or degrade extracellular matrix in the walls of alveoli, alveolar ducts, and respiratory bronchioles. In addition, agents in smoke and those released by inflammatory cells inactivate proteinase inhibitors such as α1-antitrypsin, and cause senescence and apoptosis of lung cells that produce extracellular matrix. Products of the damaged extracellular matrix, such as peptides of degraded elastin, are chemotactic for inflammatory cells; thus degradation of the extracellular matrix may lead to a feedback loop that perpetuates inflammation. These matrix-derived products may also elicit immune responses that lead to destruction of extracellular matrix. Not shown are the role of mechanical forces that may also promote deformation of lung tissue. *(Reproduced with permission from Senior RM, Silverman EK. Chronic obstructive pulmonary disease. In: Nabel EG, ed. ACP Medicine: Pulmonary, Hamilton, Ontario. Canada: Decker Publishing; 2011.)*

macrophages, and sometimes eosinophils, but also dendritic cells and lymphocytes (see Acquired Immune Responses). Once the inflammatory process is initiated by smoking the process may persist long after smoking has stopped.[117] Systemic neutrophil counts generally decrease within weeks but activated alveolar macrophages may be present even years after smoking cessation.[117–119]

Unlike nonsmokers, macrophage accumulations are found specifically in respiratory bronchioles, even in young smokers, and BALF from smokers contains many fold increases in macrophages compared to the numbers in BALF from nonsmokers.[120,121] Besides releasing proteinases that might degrade the extracellular matrix of the lung,[122] alveolar macrophages in COPD make chemotactic factors that recruit other inflammatory cells to the lungs. Likewise, structural cells of the lungs in COPD produce proteinases and chemotactic factors for inflammatory cells.[123,124] Expression of interleukin-8 (IL-8), macrophage inflammatory protein-1α (MIP-1α), and monocyte chemoattractant protein-1 (MCP-1), for example, are upregulated in bronchiolar epithelium in COPD.[125,126] Peptides of elastin are chemotactic for inflammatory cells and may act as epitopes for T-cell responses.[127–129] In mice, genetically induced overexpression of cytokines, such as IL-13 or γ-interferon by lung cells leads to emphysema via a robust innate immune response, with inflammatory cell proteinases being integral in emphysema pathogenesis.[130–132]

Acquired Immune Responses

Cellular and humoral immunity may also be involved in emphysema pathogenesis or the continued progression after smoking cessation. CD4+ and CD8+ T cells and B cells accumulate in alveolar and airway tissue in COPD and form bronchus-associated lymphoid tissue (BALT) in the walls of small airways.[100] The increasing BALT presence in small airways correlates with severity of GOLD stage.[100] In mice, exposure to antibodies directed at endothelial cells alone elicits alveolar septal cell destruction and emphysema.[133] Speculation about antigens for immunologically driven emphysema in patients include microbial pathogens, peptides altered by tobacco smoke, and peptides released from lung extracellular matrix.[128,129,134] Difficulties in distinguishing cellular and humoral responses to microbial colonization of advanced airway disease in COPD from pathologic self-directed immune responses will require further study,[135] but more targeted immunosuppresion in treating advanced COPD has not yet shown benefit.[136,137] Intrinsic in this issue is the accelerated emphysema in smokers with HIV, but that may be complicated by direct virus infection inducing macrophage alterations, rather than suppression of acquired immune responses.[55,56]

■ PROTEINASE–ANTIPROTEINASE IMBALANCE

The discovery in the 1960s of α_1-AT deficiency associated early-onset emphysema and the production of emphysema in experimental animal models with elastolytic enzymes have promoted the imbalance of proteinases relative to their inhibitors as a key factor in emphysema development.[138,139] Although additional mechanisms, like apoptosis and oxidant stress, have been uncovered in recent years, the importance of proteinase excess continues to prevail as an important mechanism in emphysema development.

Proteinases of several biochemical classes, and different specific inhibitors, are implicated in the pathogenesis of emphysema. Serine proteinases, especially neutrophil elastase, and several matrix metalloproteinases, have been the proteinases for which there are the most data.[140–143] It is notable that both neutrophils, which are the source of neutrophil elastase and MMP-12 from alveolar macrophages are largely related to continued smoking. Progression after smoking cessation may follow different pathways. As discussed in the genetics section many of these genes have been implicated in candidate gene studies but not genome-wide association studies (Tables 40-4 and 40-5).[144–146] Although neutrophil elastase and its main inhibitor α_1-AT have predominated the proteinase–antiproteinase imbalance hypothesis, MMPs appear prominent in mouse models and in samples from smokers and individuals with COPD. It is likely a combination of many local imbalances involving different proteinases and antiproteinases contribute to the progressive lung destruction.

TABLE 40-5 Proteinases That May Affect the Lung Parenchyma

Proteinase	Cell of Origin
Neutrophil elastase	Neutrophil (monocyte)
Proteinase 3	Neutrophil (monocyte)
Cathepsin G	Neutrophil (monocyte, mast cell)
MMP-1[a]	Macrophage, epithelial cell
MMP-9 (Gelatinase B)	Macrophage, neutrophil, eosinophil, fibroblast, epithelial cell
MMP-12 (Macrophage elastase)	Macrophage
Cathepsin L	Macrophage
Cathepsin S	Macrophage

Note: Parentheses denote minor cellular sources.
[a]Lacks elastase activity.

Several aspects of proteinases in COPD should be noted, as a straightforward destructive mechanism only is likely an oversimplification. In addition to destruction of lung elastin and other matrix components, proteinases process cytokines and surface receptors involved in the inflammatory and immune responses.[147–151] Inflammatory cells may not be the exclusive sources of the proteinases as structural cells also produce matrix-degrading proteinases.[152] Even the apparently simple emphysema model of placing elastases in the lungs of experimental animals results in complex responses that can be altered by nonproteinase-related mechanisms including stem cell and immunologic responses.[153,154] It must also be emphasized that little is known about proteinases in the pathogenesis of the small airway pathology of COPD. Virtually all of the information about proteinases in COPD pertains to emphysema pathogenesis despite clear evidence of small airway obliteration in advanced disease.

OXIDANT–ANTIOXIDANT IMBALANCE

Reactive oxygen species in cigarette smoke or released by inflammatory cells and structural cells of the lungs in response to smoke may lead to lung injury (see Chapter 41). Up to 20 mg of tar may be deposited in a smoker's lung per cigarette smoked. This tar contains more than 10^{17} stable, long-lived radicals per gram. The gas phase of tobacco smoke contains 10^{15} organic radicals per puff of smoke, although in general these small oxygen- and carbon-centered species are more short-lived and reactive than the radicals in the particulate phase. In addition, tobacco smoke appears to "prime" neutrophils and alveolar macrophages to generate elevated amounts of reactive oxygen species, such as hydrogen peroxide, hydroxyl radicals, and superoxide radicals. The lung tissue of smokers contains significantly more iron than that of nonsmokers,[155] providing a catalyst for the production of hydroxyl radicals from H_2O_2. This is of interest given the finding of an iron-binding protein polymorphism in the genome wide association studies of smokers with COPD, IREB2 (Table 40-4). Smokers also demonstrate increased production of neutrophil myeloperoxidase,[106,112] which is capable of yielding oxidized halogens such as hypochlorous acid (HOCl). Oxidants modify and inactivate proteins, such as protease inhibitors (α_1-AT and secretory leukoprotease inhibitor), and histone deacetylase 2 (HDAC2), which is involved in glucocorticoid mediated anti-inflammatory responses. Oxidants can affect lipids, DNA, and some specific end products, such as 4-hydroxy-2-nonenal (4-HNE) and 8-hydroxy-2′-deoxyguanosine (8-OHdG), may be markers of COPD.[156,157]

Oxidants can promote inflammation and proteinase expression, facilitate proteinase-mediated extracellular matrix degradation by enhancing matrix molecule susceptibility to proteolytic cleavage, and participate in nonenzymatic degradation of matrix molecules like type I collagen. In experimental animals the combination of cigarette smoke and elastase leads to greater emphysema than either insult alone, suggesting that these insults do not elicit identical responses.[158] Animal models of antioxidant deficiency result in increased susceptibility to both cigarette smoke and direct elastase-induced disease.[159–161]

APOPTOSIS AND SENESCENCE

Emphysematous human lung specimens demonstrate increased apoptotic and senescent cells compared to healthy lung specimens.[162,163] An early theory of emphysema development was that alveolar vascular destruction preceded loss of alveolar tissue. Consistent with this early theory, the blockade of vascular endothelial growth factor (VEGF) signaling in alveolar endothelial cells or genetic downregulation of VEGF production in alveolar epithelium produces apoptosis and noninflammatory emphysema in rodents.[164] In vitro, cigarette smoke induces apoptosis of several lung cell types.[157,165,166] An important feature of experimental models of emphysema due to apoptosis is that there is minimal inflammation.[167] Of interest, the BICD1 gene polymorphism linked to emphysema (Table 40-4) encodes for a protein in the apoptosis pathway.[79] In contrast to the expanding body of information linking emphysema to apoptosis, there is only scant information about apoptosis of the cells of small airways in COPD.[168] Much remains to be learned about apoptosis in the context of COPD airway disease.

Senescence of lung cells as a cause of emphysema stems from the knowledge of alveolar loss with aging and animal models[169,170] where accelerated aging results in emphysematous changes. Lung fibroblasts isolated from human lungs with COPD demonstrate increased markers of senescence and senescent fibroblasts do not maintain the extracellular matrix.[171] However, much of the information regarding telomeres in human COPD relates to inflammatory cell telomere shortening, with telomere length being a biomarker of chronic lifelong inflammatory excess present in individuals with COPD.[172] Whether lung epithelial cells are driven to an injury-related replicative senescence is unknown, but human diseases of telomere deficiency and excess alveolar epithelial apoptosis tend to result in pulmonary fibrosis and not COPD.[173,174]

MUCUS HYPERSECRETION

Airway mucus is a normal protective barrier that is constantly replenished and cleared in health (see Chapter 6). Mucin glycoproteins, the main components of mucus, have a core protein rich in serine and threonine, to which carbohydrates and cysteine residues are attached. Mucus is secreted from submucosal glands and airway goblet cells. In COPD there is hyperplasia of goblet cells and hypertrophy of glands with an increase in the ratio of glandular mucus cells to serous cells. The changes in COPD are associated with an alteration of the mucus proteins (MUCs) to favor a predominance of MUC5B over the typical MUC5AC form, and an increase in the MUC2 form, which is uncommon in normal lung mucus.[175,176] Other alterations in the mucus layer in COPD include greater acidity, less mucin glycosylation, and decreased antimicrobial peptides. Mediators responsible for mucus hypersecretion include proteinases, cytokines, oxidants, and epidermal growth factor receptor (EGFR) ligands.[177,178] The negative charge of mucus glycoproteins results in sequestration of proteases, volatile hydrocarbons and possibly preservation of the hydration of the ciliated layer, resulting in protection of the underlying lung and likely improved carcinogen clearance. However, the symptoms of mucus hypersecretion are common complaints in individuals with COPD; quantity and location of mucus may be particularly important in symptomantic COPD.

Determining the relationship between chronic cough and sputum in patients with COPD and the natural history of COPD has been elusive.[179] Reports vary from finding weak to strong correlations between cough and sputum production and COPD progression, COPD exacerbations, and mortality.[180–182] A relationship between chronic mucus hypersecretion in small airways and adverse outcomes is plausible as histological analysis of small airway pathology in COPD demonstrated that the extent of small airway luminal obstruction by mucus correlated with the GOLD stage and was inversely correlated with survival after lung volume reduction surgery.[104] Whether the mucus glycoproteins are a beneficial factor that mark the degree of inflammation (e.g., a biomarker of inflammation) or are themselves a pathologic factor in the severity of symptoms or progression of disease is an important question, as treatment of mucus hypersecretion without adequate suppression of the inciting inflammation may result in undesired consequences.[182,183]

PATHOGENESIS OF EMPHYSEMA

■ GENERAL CONCEPTS

Emphysema is defined as "a condition of the lung characterized by abnormal, permanent enlargement of airspaces distal to the terminal bronchiole, accompanied by destruction of their walls, and without obvious fibrosis."[184] However, studies since this definition was enunciated indicate increased collagen per unit volume of airspace wall in emphysematous tissue[185] and active expression of elastin production (Fig. 40-10).[186] Thus, emphysematous lung tissue should be viewed as actively undergoing remodeling rather than as inert. Further indications of activity in emphysematous lung tissue include the presence of many inflammatory cells[103] and cellular changes of apoptosis and senescence.[187]

Degradation of lung elastin by elastase activity from inflammatory cells is probably the predominant mechanism for emphysema in most smokers. However, the biology of emphysema is clearly complex and still incompletely understood. It includes inflammatory cell recruitment, proteinase–antiproteinase imbalance, oxidant–antioxidant imbalance, and responses of lung cells to proteinases and oxidants from inflammatory cells and to constituents of tobacco smoke. It may also involve humoral and cellular immunity. Degradation of extracellular matrix components besides elastin, particularly collagens, may be an important feature. In some situations, apoptosis of lung cells may precede degradation of extracellular matrix. Senescence of lung cells, a recently identified phenomenon in emphysema, has unclear implications, but suggests that lung repair mechanisms are depressed.

According to the proteinase–antiproteinase hypothesis, there is a constant or episodic release of proteinases, active at neutral pH, into the lung parenchyma. These proteinases come principally from inflammatory cells (Table 40-5). Under normal conditions circulating proteinase inhibitors, especially α_1-AT, and inhibitors produced locally in the lungs, permeate lung tissue and prevent these proteinases from digesting the structural proteins of the lungs (Table 40-6). Emphysema results when the balance between proteinases and

TABLE 40-6 Proteinase Inhibitors in the Lung

Inhibitor	Cell of Origin	Class of Proteinases Inhibited
α1-antitrypsin	Hepatocyte (mononuclear phagocyte)	Serine[a]
α2-macroglobulin	Hepatocyte, lung fibroblast (macrophage)	Serine, MMP[b], Cysteine
TIMPs (1,2,3,4)[c]	Resident lung cell	MMP
SLPI[d]	Resident lung cell (macrophage)	Serine[e]
Elafin	Large-airway epithelial cell	Serine
Cystatin C	Bronchial epithelial cell (macrophage)	Cysteine

Note: Parentheses denote minor cellular sources.
[a]α1-antitrypsin has its greatest affinity for neutrophil elastase.
[b]Matrix metalloproteinase.
[c]Tissue inhibitors of metalloproteinases.
[d]Secretory leukocyte protease inhibitor.
[e]SLPI does not inhibit proteinase 3 (PR3).

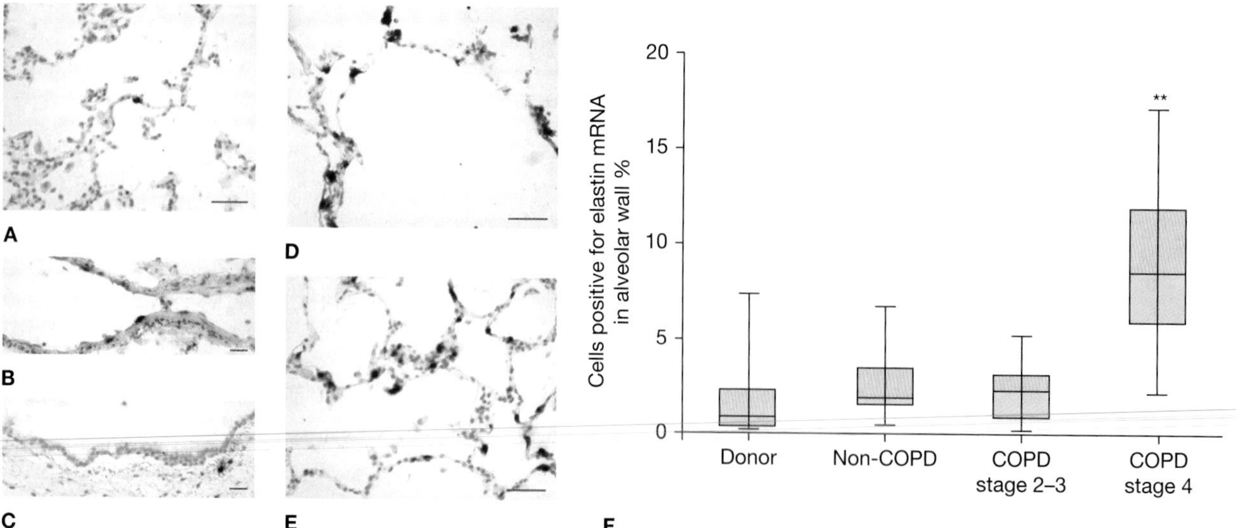

Figure 40-10 Active expression of elastin production in severely emphysematous lung removed for lung transplantation. Elastin mRNA *(blue signal)* as detected by in situ hybridization is rarely detected in donor lungs in (**A**) parenchyma, (**B**) intralobal pulmonary arteries or (**C**) airways, but is prevalent in parenchyma of GOLD 4 COPD lungs in regions with moderate (**D**) and severe (**E**) alveolar enlargement. Quantification of cells positive for elastin mRNA (**F**) reveals significantly higher elastin expression in alveolar walls of GOLD 4 COPD lungs compared to donor lungs or less severe COPD lungs. *(Reproduced with permission Deslee G, Woods JC, Moore CM, et al. Elastin expression in very severe human COPD. Eur Respir J. 2009;34(2):324–331.)*

antiproteinases in lung tissue tilts in favor of proteinases due to increased proteinase release into the tissue and/or a reduction in the antiproteinase content in the tissue. The proteolytic events leading to emphysema occur in microenvironments adjacent to lung cells; proteinase–antiproteinase balance may not be reflected in measurements of large samples of emphysematous lung tissue.

An important addition to ideas about proteinases and destruction of lung extracellular matrix has come from studies linking mechanical stresses on lung tissue and proteolytic events. Proteolytic damage resulting in local loss of structural integrity of lung tissue increases tissue susceptibility to proteinases.[187] As some fibers are lost, the load on remaining fibers increases, propagating mechanical failure analogous to mechanical failure of a partially cut rope under strain.[188] Biochemically, when lung tissue is overstretched new binding sites for proteases are exposed, increasing the rate of proteolysis.[189] Accordingly, a vicious cycle linking proteinases and tissue destruction may exist.

LUNG ELASTIC FIBERS

Because α_1-AT inhibits neutrophil elastase and papain is a potent elastase, the original observations linking proteinases to emphysema led to the concept that destruction of alveolar elastic fibers is key to emphysema development.[139] Indeed the proteinase–antiproteinase hypothesis of emphysema pathogenesis was originally the "elastase–antielastase hypothesis."

Structurally, the extracellular matrix of the lung is organized into three interdependent cable systems: (1) an axial system that extends from the central airways through the peripheral airways to the alveolar ducts; (2) a parenchymal system that comprises the matrix of the alveolar septae; and (3) a peripheral system that arises from the visceral pleura and extends into the interlobular septae, forming a fibrous sac around the lung. Distal to the respiratory bronchioles, the axial system forms a helix encircling the alveolar ducts, extending into the interstitium of alveolar walls. Elastic fibers, of which elastin is the main component, loop around alveolar ducts, form rings at the mouths of the alveoli, and penetrate as wisps into the alveolar septae, where they are concentrated at bends and junctions (Fig. 40-11). Elastic fibers, which possess rubberlike reversible extensibility, come under tension and provide elastic recoil throughout the respiratory cycle. Unlike elastic fibers, the interstitial collagen fibers in alveolar septa are nondistensible and have high tensile strength. They can be thought of as relaxed ropes that straighten during inspiration and become taut at total lung capacity.

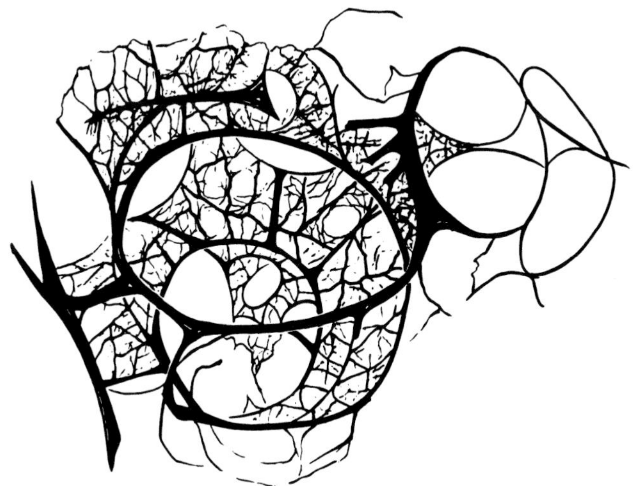

Figure 40-11 Alveolar elastic fiber network. Artist's sketch of the elastic fibers in the parenchyma of human lung showing how elastic fibers form a helix encircling the alveolar ducts and penetrate into alveolar septae. *(Reproduced with permission from Pierce JA, Ebert RV. Fibrous network of the lung and its change with age. Thorax. 1965;20(5):469–476.)*

Elastin is resistant to many proteinases, most notably the collagenases that cleave interstitial collagens. However, there are a number of enzymes that may come into contact with the lung that can degrade elastin (Table 40-5). Elastic fibers in the lung normally last a full human life span.[190] Histological studies of emphysematous lung tissue support the hypothesis that elastic fibers are perturbed in emphysema. There are fragmented elastic fibers in α_1-AT deficiency and poorly formed elastic fibers and clumps of elastin in smokers with centriacinar emphysema.[191] The latter changes appear to be from aberrant synthesis of new elastin and resemble the findings in the lungs in emphysema induced experimentally with elastase.

Animal models employing elastase-induced emphysema have shown acute depletion of elastin following an intratracheal injection of human neutrophil elastase, followed by a burst of synthesis of extracellular matrix including elastin.[192] Over a few weeks, the elastin content of the lungs returns to normal, although the lungs still display emphysema. The elastic fibers, like the elastic fibers in human emphysema, appear disorganized. New elastin gene expression occurs even in severe emphysema in humans (Fig. 40-10). However, there are significant barriers to effective repair of damaged elastic fibers in the mature lung. When elastic fibers are damaged enough to fail under load, there is no mechanism for cells to recreate a structure with a length many times the size of each cell. The injured adult lung lacks the mechanical and morphogen gradients that initiate alveolar formation during development, and may also be unable to coordinate the expression of the many components necessary for functional elastic fiber synthesis.

LUNG COLLAGEN TURNOVER

Although elastic fiber destruction dominates thinking about the proteolytic basis for the pathogenesis of emphysema, degradation of alveolar wall collagen and aberrant collagen deposition in alveolar tissue may also be involved. Indeed, in some forms of experimental emphysema collagen destruction appears to be the critical event. Mice genetically engineered to harbor a transgene that leads to expression of human MMP-1 (collagenase) in lung tissue develop structural changes typical of emphysema.[140] and these changes are due to destruction of alveolar type III collagen.[193] In these models, emphysema occurs without obvious disruption and faulty resynthesis of elastic fibers as the elastic fibers in these lungs look normal. Expression of MMP-1 by alveolar epithelial cells in human emphysematous tissue fits with the idea that collagenolytic activity plays a role in emphysema.[152]

Analogous to elastin peptides promoting emphysema in mice exposed to cigarette smoke (128), a peptide derived from collagen, proline-glycine-proline (PGP), is a neutrophil chemoattractant, associated with COPD and experimental emphysema.[194] PGP is generated by the sequential breakdown of collagen by MMPs 8 and 9 and prolyl endopopetidase.[195] Blocking PGP reduces emphysema in mice exposed to cigarette smoke.[196]

In emphysematous lungs the pores of Kohn are larger and more numerous than in normal lungs (Fig. 40-12). Because interstitial collagens and basement membrane collagens are prominent in alveolar walls, it is plausible that collagenous structures undergo degradation in the process of generating of these interalveolar pores.

ALPHA 1-ANTITRYPSIN DEFICIENCY

In 1963 Laurell and Erikson described α_1-AT deficiency and its association with COPD.[197] Ever since then, α_1-AT deficiency has played an important role in the clinical and basic science aspects of COPD.[198]

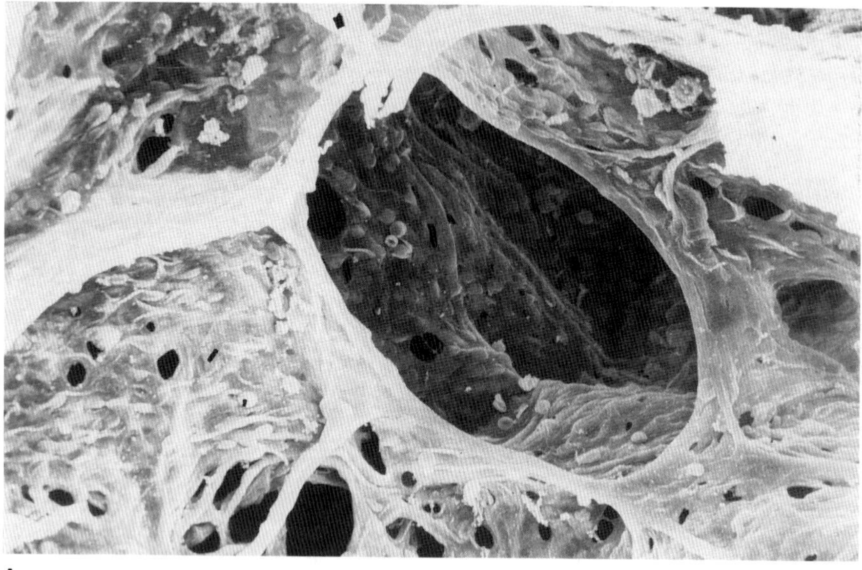

A

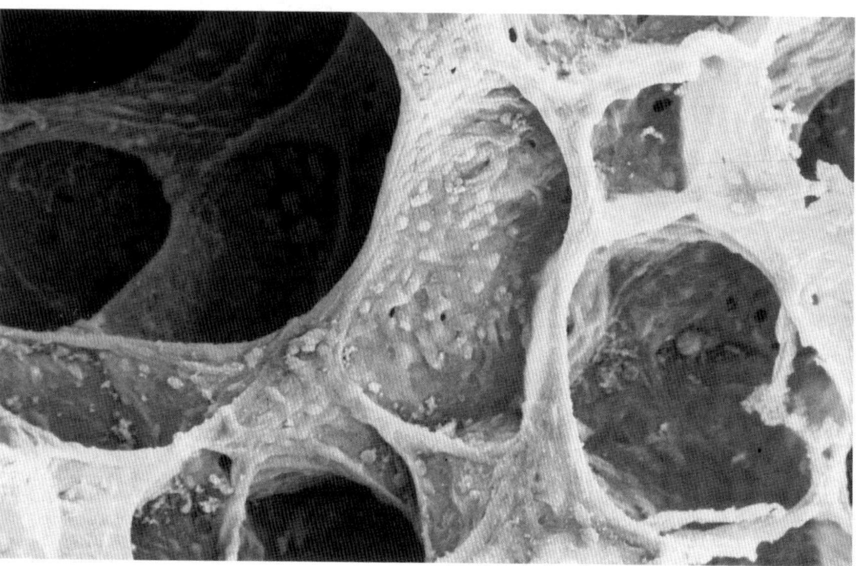

B

Figure 40-12 Holes in alveolar walls in early emphysema. Scanning electron micrographs of alveolar walls from surgically resected specimens: lung with mild emphysema (**A**) and nonemphysematous lung (**B**). Holes are more numerous in alveolar walls in the emphysematous lung than in the normal lung. Original magnification ×250. *(Reproduced with permission from Nagai A, Inano H, Matsuba K, et al. Scanning electron microscopic morphometry of emphysema in humans. Am J Respir Crit Care Med. 1994;150 (5 Pt 1):1411–1415.)*

BACKGROUND

Human plasma contains at least six proteins that function as proteinase inhibitors. Together, they make up about 10% of the total plasma protein. At a concentration of 100 to 273 mg/dL (~18–50 μmol/L) in adults with a normal phenotype, Pi MM,[199] α_1-AT has the highest concentration of all of the plasma proteinase inhibitors. α_1-AT is a member of a family of serine proteinase inhibitors called serpins (SERPINA1).

α_1-AT is a glycoprotein of 52 kDa synthesized primarily by hepatocytes. Mononuclear phagocytes and bronchial epithelial cells are other less abundant cellular sources. α_1-AT consists of a single polypeptide chain of 394 amino acids. Carbohydrate side chains account for 12% of the α_1-AT molecular mass. The 12.2-kb gene, *SERPINA1*, that encodes α_1-AT is on the proteinase inhibitor (PI) locus on chromosome 14. The α_1-AT gene has seven exons and six introns. Exons four through seven code for the mature protein. The first two exons and a segment of the third exon are encoded in the transcript expressed in macrophages, but not in hepatocytes. α_1-AT is an acute-phase reactant. Plasma levels rise with trauma, estrogen therapy, use of birth-control pills, and during pregnancy, however the levels do not rise to normal among individuals with severe deficiency.

Inhibition of neutrophil elastase and other serine proteinases by α_1-AT involves cleavage by the proteinase of the reactive site of α_1-AT between methionine[358] and serine[359] and formation of an enzyme-inhibitor complex that renders the proteinase inactive. Because the complex is quite stable, inactivation is essentially permanent. α_1-AT has a higher affinity for neutrophil elastase than trypsin or other serine proteinases. It is notable that oxidation of the critical methionine residue results in a 2000-fold reduction in the rate of association with neutrophil elastase.[200] The capacity of α_1-AT to inhibit serine proteinases besides trypsin has led some authors to call the protein α_1-PI or α_1-antiproteinase, but the name α_1-AT has become a fixture.

Apart from inhibition of serine proteinases, α_1-AT has numerous other activities. These include promoting immune tolerance, reducing production of proinflammmatory cytokines, and protecting various cell types from cell death through inhibition of caspases.[201–207]

From the genetic standpoint, α_1-AT disease is an autosomal recessive disorder, which means that one mutated α_1-AT allele from each parent must be transmitted to the affected offspring. Thus, for example, on average if MZ parents have four children, there will be two that are MZ and one each will be MM and ZZ. More than 120 different α_1-AT alleles are known,[208] most of which are single nucleotide polymorphisms (SNPs) that do not alter expression of the protein or its function and so have no clinical significance. Letters are used to specify the allelic variants. The original letters were chosen to reflect electrophoretic mobility: F = fast, M = medium, S = slow, and Z = ultraslow. Homozygosity for the M allele, Pi MM, is present in about 95% of adults in the United States. Homozygosity for the Z allele, Pi ZZ, is associated with severe deficiency of α_1-AT (<15% of normal) and accounts for virtually all of the individuals with severe α_1-AT deficiency. In the United States, the prevalence of the Pi ZZ phenotype is about 1 in 3000 people; worldwide, it is estimated that there are 3.4 million persons with severe α_1-AT deficiency, mainly Pi ZZ.[209]

Heterozygosity of the M allele with an S or Z allele is very common. In the United States, 3% to 8% of the adult population are Pi MS heterozygotes and 2% to 4% are Pi MZ heterozygotes. Pi MS and Pi MZ individuals have mean blood α_1-AT levels 75% and 57% of normal, respectively. Pi MS heterozygosity does not carry an increased risk of COPD.[210] The relationship of Pi MZ heterozygosity to the risk of COPD has been controversial, but recent studies indicate that Pi MZ individuals have slightly impaired air flow, measured as FEV_1/FVC or FEV_1/VC ratios, and slightly more emphysema on CT scans than matched Pi MM individuals.[211]

The abnormality in the Z α_1-AT protein is a point mutation in a single nucleotide at codon 342 that results in coding for lysine instead of glutamic acid. This amino acid substitution changes the charge attraction between the amino acids normally present in positions 342 and 290 in α_1-AT and prevents the formation of a fold in the molecule. With this change in tertiary structure, the molecule is susceptible to dimerization with another α_1-AT molecule that can result in polymerization of α_1-AT in the endoplasmic reticulum. Polymerization impedes secretion of the protein from hepatocytes and explains the low levels of α_1-AT in plasma and other body fluids. In contrast to the Z variant, the S variant of α_1-AT, which involves a single nucleotide substitution of glutamic acid[264] with valine, polymerizes more slowly than the Z protein and does not accumulate in the liver.

Polymers of Z type α_1-AT are chemotactic and recruit neutrophils to the lungs.[212,213] Oxidation of α_1-AT, as occurs with exposure to cigarette smoke, promotes polymerization of Z type α_1-AT.[214] Together, these findings suggest a pathway for the increased risk of COPD in Pi ZZ smokers. An unfolded protein response (UPR) in monocytes and other cell types may be another pathway for increasing the risk of COPD associated with Pi ZZ. According to this paradigm, activation of a UPR occurs in cells that make ZZ α_1-AT which leads to an inflammatory phenotype of increased cytokine production and activation of the NF-kB pathway.[215] Thus, in both of these pathways, a key feature is increased inflammation, which leads to increased proteinase and oxidant stress burdens in tissues. Moreover, compared to M α_1-AT, Z type α_1-AT has a slower rate of association with neutrophil elastase than does M α_1-AT.[216] The net result is that the α_1-AT produced by Pi ZZ individuals is less effective than M protein.

Quantification of serum α_1-AT is done routinely by immunoassay. To confirm an immunoassay showing severe deficiency, specialized laboratories use isoelectric focusing to phenotype α_1-AT (Fig. 40-13). To definitively identify α_1-AT genotypes, analysis is performed with molecular probes.[217]

CLINICAL ASPECTS

Severe α_1-AT deficiency may present in adults as chronic respiratory symptoms (COPD, unremitting asthma, and bronchiectasis), liver disease, (chronic virus–negative hepatitis, cirrhosis, and hepatoma) or skin disease (panniculitis).[198] In practice, however, about 80% of patients are discovered because of respiratory symptoms and most of the rest are detected by screening for α_1-AT deficiency prompted by finding the deficiency in a family member with lung disease. In middle-aged and older individuals with chronic respiratory symptoms, the disease is often not diagnosed for more than 5 years after the onset of the symptoms.[218]

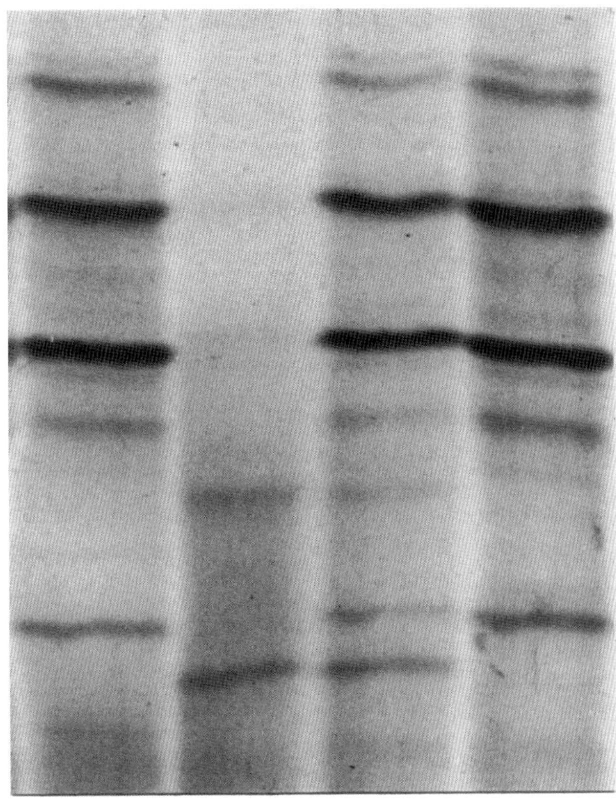

Figure 40-13 Patterns of Pi M, Pi Z, and Pi MZ α_1-AT on isoelectric focus. By this analysis, α_1-AT has microheterogeneity and thus appears as multiple bands. Pi M and Pi Z have distinctly different band patterns, while Pi MZ has a pattern that combines the patterns of both Pi M and Pi Z. *(Used with permission of John A. Pierce, MD.)*

Lung Disease

The classic patient with Pi Z α_1-AT deficiency presents with the typical symptoms of COPD, but is younger than usual, often around age 40. The patient has an increased total lung capacity, a decreased DL_{CO} and radiographic studies show hyperlucent lower lung fields reflecting the predominance of emphysema in those regions (Fig. 40-14). This classic patient reports a mild smoking history relative to the severity of COPD and a family history of chronic respiratory symptoms in parents, siblings, and other close relatives.

In fact, however, there are many exceptions to this classic clinical picture of Pi Z α_1-AT deficiency. Wheezing, cough and sputum mimicking asthma, or chronic bronchitis, that are poorly responsive to standard therapy may be the predominant symptoms. Radiographic emphysema may be modest relative to the severity of the airflow obstruction and may have upper lobe predominance of emphysema,[219] and no other family members may have chronic respiratory symptoms, including siblings who are discovered to have the same level of deficiency as the patient. Discovery of SNPs in genes associated with COPD indicate that modifier genes may account for the differences in COPD occurrence between individuals who share the PiZ phenotype.[220] Because the pulmonary presentation of α_1-AT deficiency often deviates from the classic presentation, experts in this field have advised that everyone diagnosed with COPD be screened for α_1-AT deficiency and that screening be extended to people with certain other conditions (Table 40-7).[221]

About 10,000 individuals in the United States are recognized to have severe α_1-AT deficiency, but estimates from gene frequency

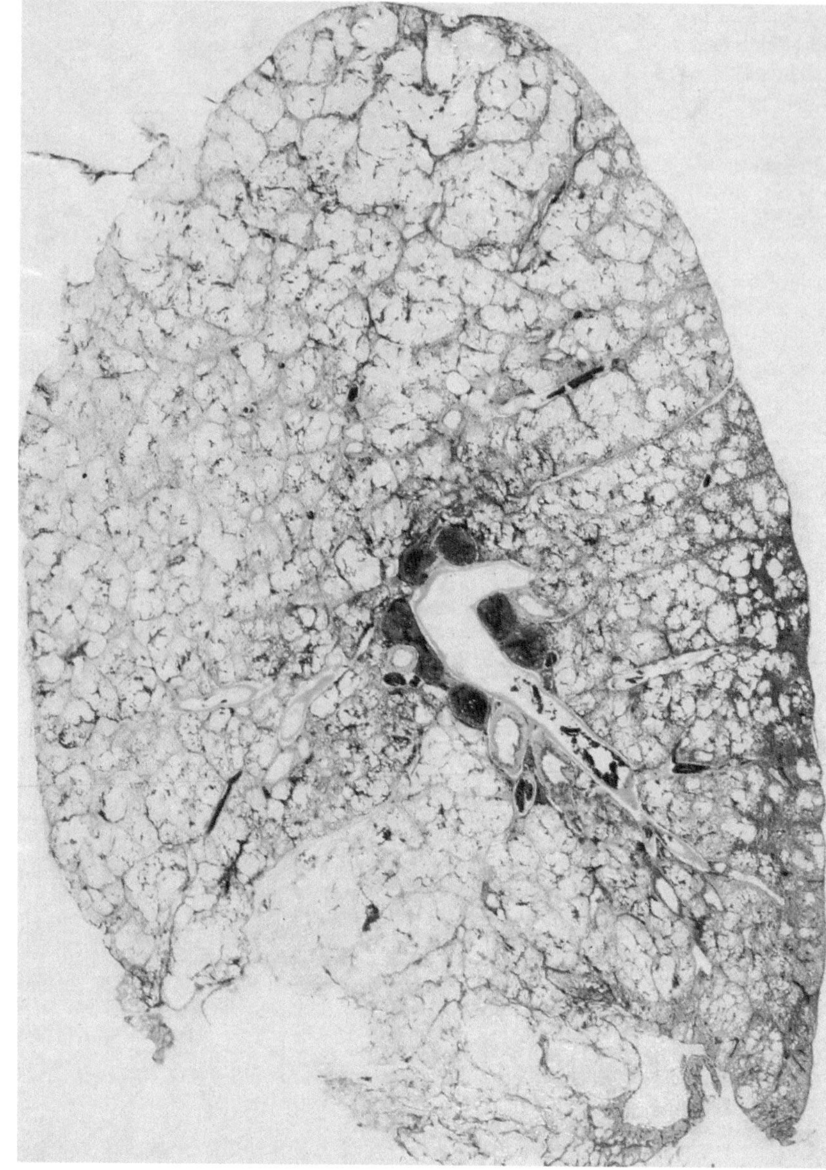

Figure 40-14 Lung pathology of Pi Z-type α_1-AT deficiency. Panacinar emphysema that is worst in the lung base. Paper-mounted whole lung section.

TABLE 40-7 Clinical Situations for Assessment of α_1-AT Status

Early-onset COPD (age of 45 yr or less)
Early-onset emphysema (age 45 yr or less)
Emphysema in the absence of a recognized risk factor (smoking, occupational dust exposure, etc.)
Emphysema with prominent basilar hyperlucency
Asthma with airflow obstruction that is incompletely reversed after aggressive treatment
Bronchiectasis without evident etiology
Otherwise unexplained liver disease
Necrotizing panniculitis
Antiproteinase 3-positive vasculitis (C-ANCA [antineutrophil cytoplasmic antibody] positive vasculitis)
Family history of any of the following: emphysema, bronchiectasis, liver disease, panniculitis

Source: Data from American Thoracic Society; European Respiratory Society. American Thoracic Society/European Respiratory Society Statement: standards for the diagnosis and management of individuals with alpha-1 antitrypsin deficiency. Am J Respir Crit Care Med. 2003;168(7):818–900.

calculations suggest a much larger number, at least 100,000. The discrepancy between known and unknown individuals reflects the fact that many severely deficient individuals are clinically well and, as noted above, clinicians commonly do not consider the diagnosis even among symptomatic individuals. Irrespective of the precise number, the point is that unrecognized deficiency is common. In a recent study involving 3457 individuals with moderate or more severe fixed airflow obstruction undergoing routine pulmonary function testing at 19 US medical centers, 0.63% had severe α_1-AT deficiency (ZZ and SZ) and 10.88% were MS or MZ heterozygotes.[222] Extrapolating these figures to the large number of people with COPD countrywide yields a large number of severely deficient people.

Smoking hastens the development of COPD in most people with severe α_1-AT deficiency. The typical Pi Z individual who smokes has respiratory symptoms by age 40. Besides smoking, male gender and a history of asthma are also associated with worse lung function among deficient individuals.[223] Specific occupational exposures may also impart increased risk of disease,[224–226] but studies of nonindex cases and screened individuals confirm that smoking is the predominant risk factor associated with increased mortality.[227]

Although emphysema is the predominant lung pathology associated with Pi Z α_1-AT, bronchiectasis has been reported to be common.[228] However, this finding has not been universal and it remains unknown whether bronchiectasis is more prevalent in these individuals than among individuals with comparable COPD and a normal α_1-AT phenotype.[229] Among patients with bronchiectasis due to nontubercluous mycobacterial (ATM) pulmonary infections, heterozygous α_1-AT abnormalities are common, but the basis for this association is obscure as most of the affected individuals do not have severe α_1-AT deficiency.[230]

Liver Disease

Pi Z α_1-AT deficiency can present as liver dysfunction in infancy ranging from asymptomatic jaundice to liver failure. In most instances, the clinical manifestations are mild and resolve spontaneously, but α_1-AT deficiency represents one of the main indications for liver transplantation in children. In adults, liver abnormalities may be limited to tests of liver function. However, among Pi Z individuals who live beyond age 60, liver abnormalities are common and may overshadow respiratory symptoms. Indeed, among those individuals who have not smoked and for other unexplained reasons have avoided significant pulmonary function deterioration, hepatic cirrhosis and associated complications is the predominant terminal illness. In such individuals there is also a high incidence of hepatic cell carcinoma.[231]

THERAPY

Therapy for COPD associated with α_1-AT deficiency includes the standard measures for COPD—cessation of smoking, inhaled bronchodilators and inhaled corticosteroids, pulmonary rehabilitation, pneumococcal and influenza vaccinations, and supplemental oxygen (see Chapter 42). Lung volume reduction surgery has not proven as successful as in individuals with normal α_1-AT.[232] Because progression of disease tends to be slow, qualifying for lung transplantation seldom has urgency.

Up to the present time, the only specific treatment has been the so-called augmentation therapy that consists of weekly intravenous administration of α_1-AT isolated from pooled plasma obtained from healthy individuals, of which several preparations are commercially available. This therapy should be limited to individuals with severe α_1-AT deficiency; for lack of need and expense it is not recommended for MZ heterozygotes.[233] The effectiveness of augmentation therapy has been most evident in individuals with reductions in FEV1 of 30% to 65% predicted.[221] Delivery of α_1-AT by inhalation may improve the convenience of augmentation in the future. Safe and effective genetic approaches to achieve permanent correction of α_1-AT deficiency have not yet been developed, despite efforts with α_1-AT–carrying vectors and transplantation with stem cell–derived hepatocytes that carry normal genes.[234–237]

From the standpoint of liver disease, α_1-AT antitrypsin deficiency is a paradoxical situation in that there is a severe systemic deficiency of α_1-AT despite substantial production of α_1-AT by the liver. The distinction between what is happening in the liver and what is happening systemically is clinically important. Infusions of α_1-AT, or other techniques under investigation for boosting systemic α_1-AT levels, can compensate for severe systemic α_1-AT deficiency and so help protect the lung, but these approaches do not correct or ameliorate problems associated with the accumulation of abnormal α_1-AT in liver cells. At present, liver transplantation is the only treatment for the liver defect. Drugs to promote degradation of hepatocyte accumulations of Z antitrypsin, presumably the underlying mechanisms for liver injury,[238,239] or to prevent α_1-AT polymerization in the liver are under investigation.[240]

CONCLUDING COMMENT

Better understanding of COPD is imperative. This potentially disabling and fatal disease is already epidemic in many countries and appears destined to become a worldwide epidemic in coming decades due to indoor air pollution from use of solid fuels and trends of smoking prevalence.

REFERENCES

1. Vestbo J, Hurd SS, Agusti AG, et al. Global strategy for the diagnosis, management, and prevention of chronic obstructive pulmonary disease: GOLD executive summary. *Am J Respir Crit Care Med.* 2013;187:347–365.
2. Hardie JA, Buist AS, Vollmer WM, Ellingsen I, Bakke PS, Mørkve O. Risk of over-diagnosis of COPD in asymptomatic elderly never-smokers. *Eur Respir J.* 2002;20:1117–1122.
3. Swanney MP, Ruppel G, Enright PL, et al. Using the lower limit of normal for the FEV1/FVC ratio reduces the misclassification of airway obstruction. *Thorax.* 2008;63:1046–1151.
4. Roberts SD, Farber MO, Knox KS, et al. FEV1/FVC ratio of 70% misclassifies patients with obstruction at the extremes of age. *Chest.* 2006;130:200.
5. Guder G, Brenner S, Angermann CE, et al. GOLD or lower limit of normal definition? A comparison with expert-based diagnosis of chronic obstructive pulmonary disease in a prospective cohort-study. *Respir Res.* 2012;13:13.
6. Lange P, Marott JL, Vestbo J, et al. Prediction of the clinical course of chronic obstructive pulmonary disease, using the new GOLD classification: a study of the general population. *Am J Respir Crit Care Med.* 2012;186:975.
7. Buist AS, McBurnie MA, Vollmer WM, et al. International variation in the prevalence of COPD (the BOLD Study): a population-based prevalence study. *Lancet.* 2007;370:741.
8. Mannino DM, Buist AS. Global burden of COPD: risk factors, prevalence, and future trends. *Lancet.* 2007;370:765.
9. Kurmi OP, Lam KB, Ayres JG. Indoor air pollution and the lung in low- and medium-income countries. *Eur Respir J.* 2012;40:239.
10. Gershon AS, Warner L, Cascagnette P, Victor JC, To T. Lifetime risk of developing chronic obstructive pulmonary disease: a longitudinal population study. *Lancet.* 2011;378:991.
11. Salvi SS, Barnes PJ. Chronic obstructive pulmonary disease in non-smokers. *Lancet.* 2009;374:733.
12. Lamprecht B, McBurnie MA, Vollmer WM, et al. COPD in never smokers: results from the population-based burden of obstructive lung disease study. *Chest.* 2011;139:752.
13. Minino AM. Death in the United States, 2009. *NCHS Data Brief.* 2011;(64):1.
14. Minino AM, Murphy SL, Xu J, Kochanek KD. Deaths: final data for 2008. *Natl Vital Stat Rep.* 2011;59:1.
15. Centers for Disease Control and Prevention (CDC). Chronic obstructive pulmonary disease among adults–United States, 2011. *MMWR Morb Mortal Wkly Rep.* 2012;61:938.
16. Schiller JS, Lucas JW, Ward BW, Peregoy JA. Summary health statistics for U.S. adults: National Health Interview Survey, 2010. *Vital Health Stat 10.* 2012;1.
17. Mintz ML, Yawn BP, Mannino DM, et al. Prevalence of airway obstruction assessed by lung function questionnaire. *Mayo Clin Proc.* 2011;86:375.
18. Shavelle RM, Paculdo DR, Kush SJ, Mannino DM, Strauss DJ. Life expectancy and years of life lost in chronic obstructive pulmonary disease: findings from the NHANES III Follow-up Study. *Int J Chron Obstruct Pulmon Dis.* 2009;4:137.
19. Hooper R, Burney P, Vollmer WM, et al. Risk factors for COPD spirometrically defined from the lower limit of normal in the BOLD project. *Eur Respir J.* 2012;39:1343.
20. de Marco R, Accordini S, Anto JM, et al. Long-term outcomes in mild/moderate chronic obstructive pulmonary disease in

the European community respiratory health survey. *Am J Respir Crit Care Med.* 2009;180:956.

21. Pirie K, Peto R, Reeves GK, Green J, Beral V; Million Women Study Collaborators. The 21st century hazards of smoking and benefits of stopping: a prospective study of one million women in the UK. *Lancet.* 2013;381:133.
22. Sorheim IC, Johannessen A, Gulsvik A, Bakke PS, Silverman EK, DeMeo DL. Gender differences in COPD: are women more susceptible to smoking effects than men? *Thorax.* 2010;65:480.
23. Ekstrom MP, Jogreus C, Strom KE. Comorbidity and sex-related differences in mortality in oxygen-dependent chronic obstructive pulmonary disease. *PLoS One.* 2012;7:e35806.
24. Chatila WM, Wynkoop WA, Vance G, Criner GJ. Smoking patterns in African Americans and whites with advanced COPD. *Chest.* 2004;125:15.
25. Dransfield MT, Bailey WC. COPD: racial disparities in susceptibility, treatment, and outcomes. *Clin Chest Med.* 2006; 27:463.
26. Bruse S, Sood A, Petersen H, et al. New Mexican Hispanic smokers have lower odds of chronic obstructive pulmonary disease and less decline in lung function than non-Hispanic whites. *Am J Respir Crit Care Med.* 2011;184:1254.
27. Centers for Disease Control and Prevention (CDC). Vital signs: current cigarette smoking among adults aged >/= 18 years–United States, 2005–2010. *MMWR Morb Mortal Wkly Rep.* 2011;60:1207.
28. Guindon GE, Boisclair D. Past, Current and Future Trends in Tobacco Use. WHO Tobacco Control Papers, Center for Tobacco Control Research and Education 63, 2003.
29. Drummond MB, Hansel NN, Connett JE, Scanlon PD, Tashkin DP, Wise RA. Spirometric predictors of lung function decline and mortality in early chronic obstructive pulmonary disease. *Am J Respir Crit Care Med.* 2012;185:1301.
30. Anthonisen NR, Connett JE, Murray RP. Smoking and lung function of Lung Health Study participants after 11 years. *Am J Respir Crit Care Med.* 2002;166:675.
31. Vestbo J, Edwards LD, Scanlon PD, et al. Changes in forced expiratory volume in 1 second over time in COPD. *N Engl J Med.* 2011;365:1184.
32. Casanova C, de Torres JP, Aguirre-Jaime A, et al. The progression of chronic obstructive pulmonary disease is heterogeneous: the experience of the BODE cohort. *Am J Respir Crit Care Med.* 2011;184:1015.
33. Max W, Sung HY, Shi Y. Deaths from secondhand smoke exposure in the United States: economic implications. *Am J Public Health.* 2012;102:2173.
34. United States Department of Health and Human Services. The Health Consequences of Involuntary Exposure to Tobacco Smoke: a report of the surgeon general. www.surgeongeneral.gov/library/reports/secondhandsmoke/fullreport.pdf 2006.
35. Flouris AD, Metsios GS, Carrillo AE, et al. Acute and short-term effects of secondhand smoke on lung function and cytokine production. *Am J Respir Crit Care Med.* 2009;179:1029.
36. Eisner MD, Anthonisen N, Coultas D, et al. An official American Thoracic Society public policy statement: novel risk factors and the global burden of chronic obstructive pulmonary disease. *Am J Respir Crit Care Med.* 2010;182:693.
37. Eisner MD, Balmes J, Katz PP, Trupin L, Yelin EH, Blanc PD. Lifetime environmental tobacco smoke exposure and the risk of chronic obstructive pulmonary disease. *Environ Health.* 2005;4:7.
38. Collaco JM, Vanscoy L, Bremer L, et al. Interactions between secondhand smoke and genes that affect cystic fibrosis lung disease. *JAMA.* 2008;299:417.
39. Hu G, Zhou Y, Tian J, et al. Risk of COPD from exposure to biomass smoke: a metaanalysis. *Chest.* 2010;138:20.
40. Kurmi OP, Semple S, Simkhada P, Smith WC, Ayres JG. COPD and chronic bronchitis risk of indoor air pollution from solid fuel: a systematic review and meta-analysis. *Thorax.* 2010;65:221.
41. Smith-Sivertsen T, Diaz E, Pope D, et al. Effect of reducing indoor air pollution on women's respiratory symptoms and lung function: the RESPIRE Randomized Trial, Guatemala. *Am J Epidemiol.* 2009;170:211.
42. World Health Organization. Fact sheet No292: indoor air pollution and health. http://www.who.int/mediacentre/factsheets/fs292/en/ 1. 2011.
43. Naidoo RN. Occupational exposures and chronic obstructive pulmonary disease: incontrovertible evidence for causality? *Am J Respir Crit Care Med.* 2012;185:1252.
44. Mehta AJ, Miedinger D, Keidel D, et al. Occupational exposure to dusts, gases, and fumes and incidence of chronic obstructive pulmonary disease in the Swiss Cohort Study on Air Pollution and Lung and Heart Diseases in Adults. *Am J Respir Crit Care Med.* 2011;185:1292.
45. Balmes J, Becklake M, Blanc P, et al. American Thoracic Society Statement: occupational contribution to the burden of airway disease. *Am J Respir Crit Care Med.* 2003;167:787.
46. Hnizdo E, Sullivan PA, Bang KM, Wagner G. Association between chronic obstructive pulmonary disease and employment by industry and occupation in the US population: a study of data from the Third National Health and Nutrition Examination Survey. *Am J Epidemiol.* 2002;156:738.
47. Mayer AS, Stoller JK, Bucher Bartelson B, James Ruttenber A, Sandhaus RA, Newman LS. Occupational exposure risks in individuals with PI*Z alpha(1)-antitrypsin deficiency. *Am J Respir Crit Care Med.* 2000;162:553.
48. Stern DA, Morgan WJ, Wright AL, Guerra S, Martinez FD. Poor airway function in early infancy and lung function by age 22 years: a non-selective longitudinal cohort study. *Lancet.* 2007;370:758.
49. Edmond K, Scott S, Korczak V, et al. Long term sequelae from childhood pneumonia; systematic review and meta-analysis. *PLoS One.* 2012;7:e31239.
50. Kanner RE, Anthonisen NR, Connett JE. Lower respiratory illnesses promote FEV(1) decline in current smokers but not ex-smokers with mild chronic obstructive pulmonary disease: results from the lung health study. *Am J Respir Crit Care Med.* 2001;164:358.
51. Centers for Disease Control and Prevention (CDC). Current cigarette smoking among adults - United States, 2011. *MMWR Morb Mortal Wkly Rep.* 2012;61:889.
52. Gingo MR, He J, Wittman C, et al. Contributors to diffusion impairment in HIV-infected persons. *Eur Respir J.* 2013;43(1): 195–203.
53. Sigel K, Wisnivesky J, Gordon K, et al. HIV as an independent risk factor for incident lung cancer. *AIDS.* 2012;26:1017.
54. Crothers K, Huang L, Goulet JL, et al. HIV infection and risk for incident pulmonary diseases in the combination antiretroviral therapy era. *Am J Respir Crit Care Med.* 2011;183:388.
55. Kaner RJ, Santiago F, Crystal RG. Up-regulation of alveolar macrophage matrix metalloproteinases in HIV1(+) smokers with early emphysema. *J Leukoc Biol.* 2009;86:913.

56. Yearsley MM, Diaz PT, Knoell D, Nuovo GJ. Correlation of HIV-1 detection and histology in AIDS-associated emphysema. *Diagn Mol Pathol.* 2005;14:48.

57. Morris A, Sciurba FC, Lebedeva IP, et al. Association of chronic obstructive pulmonary disease severity and Pneumocystis colonization. *Am J Respir Crit Care Med.* 2004;170:408.

58. Morris A, Gingo MR, George MP, et al. Cardiopulmonary function in individuals with HIV infection in the antiretroviral therapy era. *AIDS.* 2012;26:731.

59. Larson RK, Barman ML. The familial occurrence of chronic obstructive pulmonary disease. *Ann Intern Med.* 1965;63:1001.

60. Lebowitz MD, Knudson RJ, Burrows B. Family aggregation of pulmonary function measurements. *Am Rev Respir Dis.* 1984;129:8.

61. Gottlieb DJ, Wilk JB, Harmon M, et al. Heritability of longitudinal change in lung function. The Framingham study. *Am J Respir Crit Care Med.* 2001;164:1655.

62. DeMeo DL, Carey VJ, Chapman HA, et al. Familial aggregation of FEF(25–75) and FEF(25–75)/FVC in families with severe, early onset COPD. *Thorax.* 2004;59:396.

63. DeMeo DL, Campbell EJ, Brantly ML, et al. Heritability of lung function in severe alpha-1 antitrypsin deficiency. *Hum Hered.* 2009;67:38.

64. Castaldi PJ, Demeo DL, Hersh CP, et al. Impact of non-linear smoking effects on the identification of gene-by-smoking interactions in COPD genetics studies. *Thorax.* 2011;66:903.

65. Van Maldergem L, Vamos E, Liebaers I, et al. Severe congenital cutis laxa with pulmonary emphysema: a family with three affected sibs. *Am J Med Genet.* 1988;31:455.

66. Corbett E, Glaisyer H, Chan C, Madden B, Khaghani A, Yacoub M. Congenital cutis laxa with a dominant inheritance and early onset emphysema. *Thorax.* 1994;49:836.

67. Hadj-Rabia S, Callewaert BL, Bourrat E, et al. Twenty patients including 7 probands with autosomal dominant cutis laxa confirm clinical and molecular homogeneity. *Orphanet J Rare Dis.* 2013; 8:36.

68. Dyhdalo K, Farver C. Pulmonary histologic changes in Marfan syndrome: a case series and literature review. *Am J Clin Pathol.* 2011;136:857.

69. Lima BL, Santos EJ, Fernandes GR, et al. A new mouse model for marfan syndrome presents phenotypic variability associated with the genetic background and overall levels of Fbn1 expression. *PLoS One.* 2010;5:e14136.

70. Neptune ER, Frischmeyer PA, Arking DE, et al. Dysregulation of TGF-beta activation contributes to pathogenesis in Marfan syndrome. *Nat Genet.* 2003;33:407.

71. Morgan AW, Pearson SB, Davies S, Gooi HC, Bird HA. Asthma and airways collapse in two heritable disorders of connective tissue. *Ann Rheum Dis.* 2007;66:1369.

72. Smolonska J, Wijmenga C, Postma DS, Boezen HM. Meta-analyses on suspected chronic obstructive pulmonary disease genes: a summary of 20 years' research. *Am J Respir Crit Care Med.* 2009;180:618.

73. Castaldi PJ, Cho MH, Cohn M, et al. The COPD genetic association compendium: a comprehensive online database of COPD genetic associations. *Hum Mol Genet.* 2010;19:526.

74. Brogger J, Steen VM, Eiken HG, Gulsvik A, Bakke P. Genetic association between COPD and polymorphisms in TNF, ADRB2 and EPHX1. *Eur Respir J.* 2006;27:682.

75. Wilk JB, Shrine NR, Loehr LR, et al. Genome-wide association studies identify CHRNA5/3 and HTR4 in the development of airflow obstruction. *Am J Respir Crit Care Med.* 2012;186:622.

76. Cho MH, Boutaoui N, Klanderman BJ, et al. Variants in FAM13 A are associated with chronic obstructive pulmonary disease. *Nat Genet.* 2010;42:200.

77. Hansel NN, Ruczinski I, Rafaels N, et al. Genome-wide study identifies two loci associated with lung function decline in mild to moderate COPD. *Hum Genet.* 2013;132:79.

78. Soler Artigas M, Loth DW, Wain LV, et al. Genome-wide association and large-scale follow up identifies 16 new loci influencing lung function. *Nat Genet.* 2011;43:1082.

79. Kong X, Cho MH, Anderson W, et al. Genome-wide association study identifies BICD1 as a susceptibility gene for emphysema. *Am J Respir Crit Care Med.* 2011;183:43.

80. Harari O, Wang JC, Bucholz K, et al. Pathway analysis of smoking quantity in multiple GWAS identifies cholinergic and sensory pathways. *PLoS One.* 2012;7:e50913.

81. Soler Artigas M, Wain LV, Repapi E, et al. Effect of five genetic variants associated with lung function on the risk of chronic obstructive lung disease, and their joint effects on lung function. *Am J Respir Crit Care Med.* 2011;184:786.

82. Myers RA, Himes BE, Gignoux CR, et al. Further replication studies of the EVE Consortium meta-analysis identifies 2 asthma risk loci in European Americans. *J Allergy Clin Immunol.* 2012;130:1294.

83. Sleiman PM, Flory J, Imielinski M, et al. Variants of DENND1B associated with asthma in children. *N Engl J Med.* 2010;362:36.

84. Wan YI, Shrine NR, Soler Artigas M, et al. Genome-wide association study to identify genetic determinants of severe asthma. *Thorax.* 2012;67:762.

85. Himes BE, Sheppard K, Berndt A, et al. Integration of Mouse and Human Genome-Wide Association Data Identifies KCNIP4 as an Asthma Gene. *PLoS One.* 2013;8:e56179.

86. Tashkin DP, Altose MD, Connett JE, Kanner RE, Lee WW, Wise RA. Methacholine reactivity predicts changes in lung function over time in smokers with early chronic obstructive pulmonary disease. The Lung Health Study Research Group. *Am J Respir Crit Care Med.* 1996;153:1802.

87. Anthonisen NR, Lindgren PG, Tashkin DP, Kanner RE, Scanlon PD, Connett JE; Lung Health Study Research Group. Bronchodilator response in the lung health study over 11 yrs. *Eur Respir J.* 2005;26:45.

88. Bellofiore S, Eidelman DH, Macklem PT, Martin JG. Effects of elastase-induced emphysema on airway responsiveness to methacholine in rats. *J Appl Physiol.* 1989;66:606.

89. Khan MA, Ellis R, Inman MD, Bates JH, Sanderson MJ, Janssen LJ. Influence of airway wall stiffness and parenchymal tethering on the dynamics of bronchoconstriction. *Am J Physiol Lung Cell Mol Physiol.* 2010;299:L98.

90. Nishimura M, Makita H, Nagai K, et al. Annual change in pulmonary function and clinical phenotype in chronic obstructive pulmonary disease. *Am J Respir Crit Care Med.* 2012;185:44.

91. Hanania NA, Sharafkhaneh A, Celli B, et al. Acute bronchodilator responsiveness and health outcomes in COPD patients in the UPLIFT trial. *Respir Res.* 2011;12:6.

92. Iyer VN, Schroeder DR, Parker KO, Hyatt RE, Scanlon PD. The nonspecific pulmonary function test: longitudinal follow-up and outcomes. *Chest.* 2011;139:878.

93. Jones PW, Agusti AG. Outcomes and markers in the assessment of chronic obstructive pulmonary disease. *Eur Respir J.* 2006;27:822.

94. Rodriguez DA, Jover L, Drakulovic MB, et al. Below what FEV1 should arterial blood be routinely taken to detect chronic respiratory failure in COPD? *Arch Bronconeumol.* 2011;47:325.

95. O'Donnell DE, Revill SM, Webb KA. Dynamic hyperinflation and exercise intolerance in chronic obstructive pulmonary disease. *Am J Respir Crit Care Med.* 2001;164:770.
96. Casanova C, Cote C, de Torres JP, et al. Inspiratory-to-total lung capacity ratio predicts mortality in patients with chronic obstructive pulmonary disease. *Am J Respir Crit Care Med.* 2005;171:591.
97. Mahler DA, Harver A, Lentine T, Scott JA, Beck K, Schwartzstein RM. Descriptors of breathlessness in cardiorespiratory diseases. *Am J Respir Crit Care Med.* 1996;154:1357.
98. Mahler DA. Mechanisms and measurement of dyspnea in chronic obstructive pulmonary disease. *Proc Am Thorac Soc* 2006;3:234.
99. Hogg JC, Macklem PT, Thurlbeck WM. Site and nature of airway obstruction in chronic obstructive lung disease. *N Engl J Med.* 1968;278:1355.
100. Hogg JC, Chu F, Utokaparch S, et al. The nature of small-airway obstruction in chronic obstructive pulmonary disease. *N Engl J Med.* 2004;350:2645.
101. McDonough JE, Yuan R, Suzuki M, et al. Small-airway obstruction and emphysema in chronic obstructive pulmonary disease. *N Engl J Med.* 2011;365:1567.
102. Mitzner W. Emphysema–a disease of small airways or lung parenchyma? *N Engl J Med.* 2011;365:1637.
103. Retamales I, Elliott WM, Meshi B, et al. Amplification of inflammation in emphysema and its association with latent adenoviral infection. *Am J Respir Crit Care Med.* 2001;164:469.
104. Hogg JC, Chu FS, Tan WC, et al. Survival after lung volume reduction in chronic obstructive pulmonary disease: insights from small airway pathology. *Am J Respir Crit Care Med.* 2007;176:454.
105. Lapperre TS, Willems LN, Timens W, et al. Small airways dysfunction and neutrophilic inflammation in bronchial biopsies and BAL in COPD. *Chest.* 2007;131:53.
106. Linden M, Rasmussen JB, Piitulainen E, et al. Airway inflammation in smokers with nonobstructive and obstructive chronic bronchitis. *Am Rev Respir Dis.* 1993;148:1226.
107. Soler N, Ewig S, Torres A, Filella X, Gonzalez J, Zaubet A. Airway inflammation and bronchial microbial patterns in patients with stable chronic obstructive pulmonary disease. *Eur Respir J.* 1999;14:1015.
108. Sethi S, Maloney J, Grove L, Wrona C, Berenson CS. Airway inflammation and bronchial bacterial colonization in chronic obstructive pulmonary disease. *Am J Respir Crit Care Med.* 2006; 173:991.
109. Rutgers SR, Timens W, Kaufmann HF, van der Mark TW, Koëter GH, Postma DS. Comparison of induced sputum with bronchial wash, bronchoalveolar lavage and bronchial biopsies in COPD. *Eur Respir J.* 2000;15:109.
110. Ropcke S, Holz O, Lauer G, et al. Repeatability of and relationship between potential COPD biomarkers in bronchoalveolar lavage, bronchial biopsies, serum, and induced sputum. *PLoS One.* 2012;7:e46207.
111. Singh D, Edwards L, Tal-Singer R, Rennard S. Sputum neutrophils as a biomarker in COPD: findings from the ECLIPSE study. *Respir Res.* 2010;11:77.
112. Fens N, de Nijs SB, Peters S, et al. Exhaled air molecular profiling in relation to inflammatory subtype and activity in COPD. *Eur Respir J.* 2011;38:1301.
113. Kostikas K, Papatheodorou G, Psathakis K, Panagou P, Loukides S. Oxidative stress in expired breath condensate of patients with COPD. *Chest.* 2003;124:1373.
114. Cockayne DA, Cheng DT, Waschki B, et al. Systemic biomarkers of neutrophilic inflammation, tissue injury and repair in COPD patients with differing levels of disease severity. *PLoS One.* 2012;7:e38629.
115. Eagan TM, Ueland T, Wagner PD, et al. Systemic inflammatory markers in COPD: results from the Bergen COPD Cohort Study. *Eur Respir J.* 2010;35:540.
116. Fontes JD, Yamamoto JF, Larson MG, et al. Clinical correlates of change in inflammatory biomarkers: The Framingham Heart Study. *Atherosclerosis.* 2013;228(1):217–223.
117. Marques LJ, Teschler H, Guzman J, Costabel U. Smoker's lung transplanted to a nonsmoker. Long-term detection of smoker's macrophages. *Am J Respir Crit Care Med.* 1997;156:1700.
118. Asthana A, Johnson HM, Piper ME, Fiore MC, Baker TB, Stein JH. Effects of smoking intensity and cessation on inflammatory markers in a large cohort of active smokers. *Am Heart J.* 2010;160:458.
119. Frohlich M, Sund M, Lowel H, Imhof A, Hoffmeister A, Koenig W.. Independent association of various smoking characteristics with markers of systemic inflammation in men. Results from a representative sample of the general population (MONICA Augsburg Survey 1994/95). *Eur Heart J.* 2003;24:1365.
120. Matsuba K, Shirakusa T, Kuwano K, Hayashi S, Shigematsu N. Small airways disease in patients without chronic air-flow limitation. *Am Rev Respir Dis.* 1987;136:1106.
121. Crapo JD, Barry BE, Gehr P, Bachofen M, Weibel ER. Cell number and cell characteristics of the normal human lung. *Am Rev Respir Dis.* 1982;126:332.
122. Russell RE, Thorley A, Culpitt SV, et al. Alveolar macrophage-mediated elastolysis: roles of matrix metalloproteinases, cysteine, and serine proteases. *Am J Physiol Lung Cell Mol Physiol.* 2002;283:L867.
123. Heguy A, O'Connor TP, Luettich K, et al. Gene expression profiling of human alveolar macrophages of phenotypically normal smokers and nonsmokers reveals a previously unrecognized subset of genes modulated by cigarette smoking. *J Mol Med (Berl).* 2006;84:318.
124. Poliska S, Csanky E, Szanto A, et al. Chronic obstructive pulmonary disease-specific gene expression signatures of alveolar macrophages as well as peripheral blood monocytes overlap and correlate with lung function. *Respiration.* 2011; 81:499.
125. Fuke S, Betsuyaku T, Nasuhara Y, et al. Chemokines in bronchiolar epithelium in the development of chronic obstructive pulmonary disease. *Am J Respir Cell Mol Biol.* 2004;31:405.
126. Witherden IR, Vanden Bon EJ, Goldstraw P, et al. Primary human alveolar type II epithelial cell chemokine release: effects of cigarette smoke and neutrophil elastase. *Am J Respir Cell Mol Biol.* 2004;30:500.
127. Senior RM, Griffin GL, Mecham RP. Chemotactic activity of elastin-derived peptides. *J Clin Invest.* 1980;66:859.
128. Houghton AM, Quintero PA, Perkins DL, et al. Elastin fragments drive disease progression in a murine model of emphysema. *J Clin Invest.* 2006;116:753.
129. Grumelli S, Corry DB, Song LZ, et al. An immune basis for lung parenchymal destruction in chronic obstructive pulmonary disease and emphysema. *PLoS Med.* 2004;1:e8.
130. Zhu Z, Homer RJ, Wang Z, et al. Pulmonary expression of interleukin-13 causes inflammation, mucus hypersecretion, subepithelial fibrosis, physiologic abnormalities, and eotaxin production. *J Clin Invest.* 1999;103:779.

131. Wang Z, Zheng T, Zhu Z, et al. Interferon gamma induction of pulmonary emphysema in the adult murine lung. *J Exp Med.* 2000;192:1587.

132. Ma B, Kang MJ, Lee CG, et al. Role of CCR5 in IFN-gamma-induced and cigarette smoke-induced emphysema. *J Clin Invest.* 2005;115:3460.

133. Taraseviciene-Stewart L, Scerbavicius R, Choe KH, et al. An animal model of autoimmune emphysema. *Am J Respir Crit Care Med.* 2005;171:734.

134. Greene CM, Low TB, O'Neill SJ, et al. Anti-proline-glycine-proline or antielastin autoantibodies are not evident in chronic inflammatory lung disease. *Am J Respir Crit Care Med.* 2010; 181:31.

135. Brusselle GG, Demoor T, Bracke KR, Brandsma CA, Timens W. Lymphoid follicles in (very) severe COPD: beneficial or harmful? *Eur Respir J.* 2009;34:219.

136. Aaron SD, Vandemheen KL, Maltais F, et al. TNFalpha antagonists for acute exacerbations of COPD: a randomised double-blind controlled trial. *Thorax.* 2013;68:142.

137. Rennard SI, Fogarty C, Kelsen S, et al. The safety and efficacy of infliximab in moderate to severe chronic obstructive pulmonary disease. *Am J Respir Crit Care Med.* 2007;175:926.

138. Eriksson S. Pulmonary emphysema and alpha1-antitrypsin deficiency. *Acta Med Scand.* 1964;175:197.

139. Goldring IP, Greenburg L, Ratner IM. On the production of emphysema in Syrian hamsters by aerosol inhalation of papain. *Arch Environ Health.* 1968;16:59.

140. Foronjy RF, Okada Y, Cole R, D'Armiento J. Progressive adult-onset emphysema in transgenic mice expressing human MMP-1 in the lung. *Am J Physiol Lung Cell Mol Physiol.* 2003;284:L727.

141. Foronjy R, Nkyimbeng T, Wallace A, et al. Transgenic expression of matrix metalloproteinase-9 causes adult-onset emphysema in mice associated with the loss of alveolar elastin. *Am J Physiol Lung Cell Mol Physiol.* 2008;294:L1149.

142. Hautamaki RD, Kobayashi DK, Senior RM, Shapiro SD. Requirement for macrophage elastase for cigarette smoke-induced emphysema in mice. *Science.* 2007;277:2002.

143. Shapiro SD, Goldstein NM, Houghton AM, Kobayashi DK, Kelley D, Belaaouaj A. Neutrophil elastase contributes to cigarette smoke-induced emphysema in mice. *Am J Pathol.* 2003;163:2329.

144. Hunninghake GM, Cho MH, Tesfaigzi Y, et al. MMP12, lung function, and COPD in high-risk populations. *N Engl J Med.* 2009;361:2599.

145. DeMeo DL, Hersh CP, Hoffman EA, et al. Genetic determinants of emphysema distribution in the national emphysema treatment trial. *Am J Respir Crit Care Med.* 2007;176:42.

146. Ito I, Nagai S, Handa T, et al. Matrix metalloproteinase-9 promoter polymorphism associated with upper lung dominant emphysema. *Am J Respir Crit Care Med.* 2005;172:1378.

147. Gearing AJ, Beckett P, Christodoulou M, et al. Matrix metalloproteinases and processing of pro-TNF-alpha. *J Leukoc Biol.* 1995;57:774.

148. Schonbeck U, Mach F, Libby P. Generation of biologically active IL-1 beta by matrix metalloproteinases: a novel caspase-1-independent pathway of IL-1 beta processing. *J Immunol.* 1998;161:3340.

149. Van den Steen PE, Proost P, Wuyts A, Van Damme J, Opdenakker G. Neutrophil gelatinase B potentiates interleukin-8 tenfold by aminoterminal processing, whereas it degrades CTAP-III, PF-4, and GRO-alpha and leaves RANTES and MCP-2 intact. *Blood.* 2000;96:2673.

150. McQuibban GA, Gong JH, Wong JP, Wallace JL, Clark-Lewis I, Overall CM. Matrix metalloproteinase processing of monocyte chemoattractant proteins generates CC chemokine receptor antagonists with anti-inflammatory properties in vivo. *Blood.* 2002;100:1160.

151. Liu Z, Zhou X, Shapiro SD, et al. The serpin alpha1-proteinase inhibitor is a critical substrate for gelatinase B/MMP-9 in vivo. *Cell.* 2000;102:647.

152. Imai K, Dalal SS, Chen ES, et al. Human collagenase (matrix metalloproteinase-1) expression in the lungs of patients with emphysema. *Am J Respir Crit Care Med.* 2001;163:786.

153. Kuhn C 3rd, Starcher BC. The effect of lathyrogens on the evolution of elastase-induced emphysema. *Am Rev Respir Dis.* 1980;122:453.

154. Ishii Y, Itoh K, Morishima Y, et al. Transcription factor Nrf2 plays a pivotal role in protection against elastase-induced pulmonary inflammation and emphysema. *J Immunol.* 2005;175:6968.

155. Ghio AJ, Hilborn ED, Stonehuerner JG, et al. Particulate matter in cigarette smoke alters iron homeostasis to produce a biological effect. *Am J Respir Crit Care Med.* 2008;178:1130.

156. Deslee G, Woods JC, Moore C, et al. Oxidative damage to nucleic acids in severe emphysema. *Chest.* 2009;135:965.

157. Deslee G, Adair-Kirk TL, Betsuyaku T, et al. Cigarette smoke induces nucleic-acid oxidation in lung fibroblasts. *Am J Respir Cell Mol Biol.* 2010;43:576.

158. Yao H, Arunachalam G, Hwang JW, et al. Extracellular superoxide dismutase protects against pulmonary emphysema by attenuating oxidative fragmentation of ECM. *Proc Natl Acad Sci U S A.* 2010;107:15571.

159. Foronjy RF, Mirochnitchenko O, Propokenko O, et al. Superoxide dismutase expression attenuates cigarette smoke- or elastase-generated emphysema in mice. *Am J Respir Crit Care Med.* 2006;173:623.

160. Potts-Kant EN, Li Z, Tighe RM, et al. NAD(P)H:quinone oxidoreductase 1 protects lungs from oxidant-induced emphysema in mice. *Free Radic Biol Med.* 2012;52:705.

161. Rangasamy T, Cho CY, Thimmulappa RK, et al. Genetic ablation of Nrf2 enhances susceptibility to cigarette smoke-induced emphysema in mice. *J Clin Invest.* 2004;114:1248.

162. Tsuji T, Aoshiba K, Nagai A. Alveolar cell senescence in patients with pulmonary emphysema. *Am J Respir Crit Care Med.* 2006;174:886.

163. Tsuji T, Aoshiba K, Nagai A. Cigarette smoke induces senescence in alveolar epithelial cells. *Am J Respir Cell Mol Biol.* 2004;31:643.

164. Kasahara Y, Tuder RM, Taraseviciene-Stewart L, et al. Inhibition of VEGF receptors causes lung cell apoptosis and emphysema. *J Clin Invest.* 2000;106:1311.

165. Green LA, Petrusca D, Rajashekhar G, et al. Cigarette smoke-induced CXCR3 receptor up-regulation mediates endothelial apoptosis. *Am J Respir Cell Mol Biol.* 2012;47:807.

166. Kosmider B, Messier EM, Chu HW, Mason RJ. Human alveolar epithelial cell injury induced by cigarette smoke. *PLoS One.* 2011;6:e26059.

167. Tang K, Rossiter HB, Wagner PD, Breen EC. Lung-targeted VEGF inactivation leads to an emphysema phenotype in mice. *J Appl Physiol.* 2004;97:1559.

168. Mebratu YA, Schwalm K, Smith KR, Schuyler M, Tesfaigzi Y. Cigarette smoke suppresses Bik to cause epithelial cell hyperplasia and mucous cell metaplasia. *Am J Respir Crit Care Med.* 2011;183:1531.

169. Aoshiba K, Nagai A. Senescence hypothesis for the pathogenetic mechanism of chronic obstructive pulmonary disease. *Proc Am Thorac Soc.* 2009;6:596.

170. Calvi CL, Podowski M, D'Alessio FR, et al. Critical transition in tissue homeostasis accompanies murine lung senescence. *PLoS One.* 2011;6:e20712.

171. Togo S, Holz O, Liu X, et al. Lung fibroblast repair functions in patients with chronic obstructive pulmonary disease are altered by multiple mechanisms. *Am J Respir Crit Care Med.* 2008;178:248.

172. Lee J, Sandford AJ, Connett JE, et al. The relationship between telomere length and mortality in chronic obstructive pulmonary disease (COPD). *PLoS One.* 2012;7:e35567.

173. Fernandez BA, Fox G, Bhatia R, et al. A Newfoundland cohort of familial and sporadic idiopathic pulmonary fibrosis patients: clinical and genetic features. *Respir Res.* 2012;13:64.

174. Young LR, Gulleman PM, Bridges JP, et al. The alveolar epithelium determines susceptibility to lung fibrosis in Hermansky-Pudlak syndrome. *Am J Respir Crit Care Med.* 2012;186:1014.

175. Innes AL, Woodruff PG, Ferrando RE, et al. Epithelial mucin stores are increased in the large airways of smokers with airflow obstruction. *Chest.* 2006;130:1102.

176. Fahy JV, Dickey BF. Airway mucus function and dysfunction. *N Engl J Med.* 2010;363:2233.

177. Hewson CA, Edbrooke MR, Johnston SL. PMA induces the MUC5AC respiratory mucin in human bronchial epithelial cells, via PKC, EGF/TGF-alpha, Ras/Raf, MEK, ERK and Sp1-dependent mechanisms. *J Mol Biol.* 2004;344:683.

178. Shao MX, Nakanaga T, Nadel JA. Cigarette smoke induces MUC5AC mucin overproduction via tumor necrosis factor-alpha-converting enzyme in human airway epithelial (NCI-H292) cells. *Am J Physiol Lung Cell Mol Physiol.* 2004;287:L420.

179. Nadel JA. Mucous hypersecretion and relationship to cough. *Pulm Pharmacol Ther.* 2013;26(5):510–513.

180. Kim V, Han MK, Vance GB, et al. The chronic bronchitic phenotype of COPD: an analysis of the COPDGene Study. *Chest.* 2011;140:626.

181. Forey BA, Thornton AJ, Lee PN. Systematic review with meta-analysis of the epidemiological evidence relating smoking to COPD, chronic bronchitis and emphysema. *BMC Pulm Med.* 2011;11:36.

182. Guerra S, Sherrill DL, Venker C, Ceccato CM, Halonen M, Martinez FD. Chronic bronchitis before age 50 years predicts incident airflow limitation and mortality risk. *Thorax.* 2009;64:894.

183. Poole P, Black PN, Cates CJ. Mucolytic agents for chronic bronchitis or chronic obstructive pulmonary disease. *Cochrane Database Syst Rev.* 2012;8:CD001287.

184. Snider GL. Chronic obstructive pulmonary disease: a definition and implications of structural determinants of airflow obstruction for epidemiology. *Am Rev Respir Dis.* 1989;140:S3.

185. Vlahovic G, Russell ML, Mercer RR, Crapo JD. Cellular and connective tissue changes in alveolar septal walls in emphysema. *Am J Respir Crit Care Med.* 1999;160:2086.

186. Deslee G, Woods JC, Moore CM, et al. Elastin expression in very severe human COPD. *Eur Respir J.* 2009;34:324.

187. Tuder RM, Kern JA, Miller YE. Senescence in chronic obstructive pulmonary disease. *Proc Am Thorac Soc.* 2012;9:62.

188. Szabari MV, Parameswaran H, Sato S, Hantos Z, Bartolák-Suki E, Suki B. Acute mechanical forces cause deterioration in lung structure and function in elastase-induced emphysema. *Am J Physiol Lung Cell Mol Physiol.* 2012;303:L567.

189. Jesudason R, Sato S, Parameswaran H, et al. Mechanical forces regulate elastase activity and binding site availability in lung elastin. *Biophys J.* 2010;99:3076.

190. Shapiro SD, Endicott SK, Province MA, Pierce JA, Campbell EJ. Marked longevity of human lung parenchymal elastic fibers deduced from prevalence of D-aspartate and nuclear weapons-related radiocarbon. *J Clin Invest.* 1991;87:1828.

191. Fukuda Y, Masuda Y, Ishizaki M, Masugi Y, Ferrans VJ. Morphogenesis of abnormal elastic fibers in lungs of patients with panacinar and centriacinar emphysema. *Hum Pathol.* 1989;20:652.

192. Kuhn C, Yu SY, Chraplyvy M, Linder HE, Senior RM. The induction of emphysema with elastase. II. Changes in connective tissue. *Lab Invest.* 1976;34:372.

193. Shiomi T, Okada Y, Foronjy R, et al. Emphysematous changes are caused by degradation of type III collagen in transgenic mice expressing MMP-1. *Exp Lung Res.* 2003;29:1.

194. Weathington NM, van Houwelingen AH, Noerager BD, et al. A novel peptide CXCR ligand derived from extracellular matrix degradation during airway inflammation. *Nat Med.* 2006;12:317–323.

195. Braber S, Koelink PJ, Henricks PA, et al. Cigarette smoke-induced lung emphysema in mice is associated with prolyl endopeptidase, an enzyme involved in collagen breakdown. *Am J Physiol Lung Cell Mol Physiol.* 2011;300:L255–L265.

196. van Houwelingen AH, Weathington NM, Verweij V, Blalock JE, Nijkamp FP, Folkerts G. Induction of lung emphysema is prevented by l-arginine-threonine-arginine. *FASEB J.* 2008;22:3403–3408.

197. Laurell CB, Eriksson S. The electrophoretic alpha1-1 globulin pattern of serum in alpha1-antitrypsin deficiency. *Scand J Clin Lab Invest.* 1963;15:132.

198. Stoller JK, Aboussouan LS. A review of alpha1-antitrypsin deficiency. *Am J Respir Crit Care Med.* 2012;185:246.

199. Donato LJ, Jenkins SM, Smith C, Katzmann JA, Snyder MR. Reference and interpretive ranges for alpha(1)-antitrypsin quantitation by phenotype in adult and pediatric populations. *Am J Clin Pathol.* 2012;138:398.

200. Beatty K, Bieth J, Travis J. Kinetics of association of serine proteinases with native and oxidized alpha-1-proteinase inhibitor and alpha-1-antichymotrypsin. *J Biol Chem.* 1980;255:3931.

201. Petrache I, Fijalkowska I, Zhen L, et al. A novel antiapoptotic role for alpha1-antitrypsin in the prevention of pulmonary emphysema. *Am J Respir Crit Care Med.* 2006;173:1222.

202. Churg A, Wang X, Wang RD, Meixner SC, Pryzdial EL, Wright JL. Alpha1-antitrypsin suppresses TNF-alpha and MMP-12 production by cigarette smoke-stimulated macrophages. *Am J Respir Cell Mol Biol.* 2007;37:144.

203. Pott GB, Chan ED, Dinarello CA, Shapiro L. Alpha-1-antitrypsin is an endogenous inhibitor of proinflammatory cytokine production in whole blood. *J Leukoc Biol.* 2009;85:886.

204. Greene CM, Miller SD, Carroll TP, et al. Anti-apoptotic effects of Z alpha1-antitrypsin in human bronchial epithelial cells. *Eur Respir J.* 2010;35:1155.

205. Marcondes AM, Li X, Tabellini L, et al. Inhibition of IL-32 activation by alpha-1 antitrypsin suppresses alloreactivity and increases survival in an allogeneic murine marrow transplantation model. *Blood*. 2011;118:5031.

206. Ozeri E, Mizrahi M, Shahaf G, Lewis EC. alpha-1 antitrypsin promotes semimature, IL-10-producing and readily migrating tolerogenic dendritic cells. *J Immunol*. 2012;189:146.

207. Tawara I, Sun Y, Lewis EC, et al. Alpha-1-antitrypsin monotherapy reduces graft-versus-host disease after experimental allogeneic bone marrow transplantation. *Proc Natl Acad Sci U S A*. 2012;109:564.

208. DeMeo DL, Silverman EK. Alpha1-antitrypsin deficiency. 2: genetic aspects of alpha(1)-antitrypsin deficiency: phenotypes and genetic modifiers of emphysema risk. *Thorax*. 2004;59:259.

209. de Serres FJ. Worldwide racial and ethnic distribution of alpha1-antitrypsin deficiency: summary of an analysis of published genetic epidemiologic surveys. *Chest*. 2002;122:1818.

210. Sandford AJ, Weir TD, Spinelli JJ, Paré PD. Z and S mutations of the alpha1-antitrypsin gene and the risk of chronic obstructive pulmonary disease. *Am J Respir Cell Mol Biol*. 1999;20:287.

211. Sorheim IC, Bakke P, Gulsvik A, et al. alpha(1)-Antitrypsin protease inhibitor MZ heterozygosity is associated with airflow obstruction in two large cohorts. *Chest*. 2010;138:1125.

212. Mulgrew AT, Taggart CC, Lawless MW, et al. Z alpha1-antitrypsin polymerizes in the lung and acts as a neutrophil chemoattractant. *Chest*. 2004;125:1952.

213. Mahadeva R, Atkinson C, Li Z, et al. Polymers of Z alpha1-antitrypsin co-localize with neutrophils in emphysematous alveoli and are chemotactic in vivo. *Am J Pathol*. 2005;166:377.

214. Alam S, Li Z, Janciauskiene S, Mahadeva R. Oxidation of Z alpha1-antitrypsin by cigarette smoke induces polymerization: a novel mechanism of early-onset emphysema. *Am J Respir Cell Mol Biol*. 2011;45:261.

215. Carroll TP, Greene CM, O'Connor CA, Nolan AM, O'Neill SJ, McElvaney NG. Evidence for unfolded protein response activation in monocytes from individuals with alpha-1 antitrypsin deficiency. *J Immunol*. 2010;184:4538.

216. Ogushi F, Fells GA, Hubbard RC, Straus SD, Crystal RG. Z-type alpha 1-antitrypsin is less competent than M1-type alpha 1-antitrypsin as an inhibitor of neutrophil elastase. *J Clin Invest*. 1987;80:1366.

217. Silverman EK, Sandhaus RA. Clinical practice. Alpha1-antitrypsin deficiency. *N Engl J Med*. 2009;360:2749.

218. Stoller JK, Sandhaus RA, Turino G, Dickson R, Rodgers K, Strange C. Delay in diagnosis of alpha1-antitrypsin deficiency: a continuing problem. *Chest*. 2005;128:1989.

219. Parr DG, Stoel BC, Stolk J, Stockley RA. Pattern of emphysema distribution in alpha1-antitrypsin deficiency influences lung function impairment. *Am J Respir Crit Care Med*. 2004;170:1172.

220. Kim WJ, Wood AM, Barker AF, et al. Association of IREB2 and CHRNA3 polymorphisms with airflow obstruction in severe alpha-1 antitrypsin deficiency. *Respir Res*. 2012;13:16.

221. American Thoracic Society/European Respiratory Society statement: standards for the diagnosis and management of individuals with alpha-1 antitrypsin deficiency. *Am J Respir Crit Care Med*. 2003;168:818.

222. Rahaghi FF, Sandhaus RA, Strange C, et al. The prevalence of alpha-1 antitrypsin deficiency among patients found to have airflow obstruction. *COPD*. 2012;9:352.

223. Demeo DL, Sandhaus RA, Barker AF, et al. Determinants of airflow obstruction in severe alpha-1-antitrypsin deficiency. *Thorax*. 2007;62:806.

224. Sigsgaard T, Brandslund I, Omland O, et al. S and Z alpha1-antitrypsin alleles are risk factors for bronchial hyperresponsiveness in young farmers: an example of gene/environment interaction. *Eur Respir J*. 2000;16:50.

225. Banauch GI, Brantly M, Izbicki G, et al. Accelerated spirometric decline in New York City firefighters with alpha(1)-antitrypsin deficiency. *Chest*. 2010;138:1116.

226. Wood AM, Harrison RM, Semple S, Ayres JG, Stockley RA. Outdoor air pollution is associated with rapid decline of lung function in alpha-1-antitrypsin deficiency. *Occup Environ Med*. 2010;67:556.

227. Tanash HA, Nilsson PM, Nilsson JA, Piitulainen E. Survival in severe alpha-1-antitrypsin deficiency (PiZZ). *Respir Res*. 2010;11:44.

228. Parr DG, Guest PG, Reynolds JH, Dowson LJ, Stockley RA. Prevalence and impact of bronchiectasis in alpha1-antitrypsin deficiency. *Am J Respir Crit Care Med*. 2007;176:1215.

229. Chan ED, Iseman MD. Significance of bronchiectasis in patients with alpha1-antitrypsin deficiency. *Am J Respir Crit Care Med*. 2008;178:208; author reply 208.

230. Chan ED, Kaminska AM, Gill W, et al. Alpha-1-antitrypsin (AAT) anomalies are associated with lung disease due to rapidly growing mycobacteria and AAT inhibits Mycobacterium abscessus infection of macrophages. *Scand J Infect Dis*. 2007;39:690.

231. Lewis EC. Expanding the clinical indications for alpha(1)-antitrypsin therapy. *Mol Med*. 2012;18:957.

232. Stoller JK, Gildea TR, Ries AL, Meli YM, Karafa MT; National Emphysema Treatment Trial Research Group. Lung volume reduction surgery in patients with emphysema and alpha-1 antitrypsin deficiency. *Ann Thorac Surg*. 2007;83:241.

233. Sandhaus RA, Turino G, Stocks J, et al. alpha1-Antitrypsin augmentation therapy for PI*MZ heterozygotes: a cautionary note. *Chest*. 2008;134:831.

234. Brantly ML, Chulay JD, Wang L, et al. Sustained transgene expression despite T lymphocyte responses in a clinical trial of rAAV1-AAT gene therapy. *Proc Natl Acad Sci U S A*. 2009;106:16363.

235. Yusa K, Rashid ST, Strick-Marchand H, et al. Targeted gene correction of alpha1-antitrypsin deficiency in induced pluripotent stem cells. *Nature*. 2011;478:391.

236. Flotte TR, Trapnell BC, Humphries M, et al. Phase 2 clinical trial of a recombinant adeno-associated viral vector expressing alpha1-antitrypsin: interim results. *Hum Gene Ther*. 2011;22:1239.

237. Sandhaus RA. Gene therapy meets stem cells. *N Engl J Med*. 2012;366:567.

238. Hidvegi T, Ewing M, Hale P, et al. An autophagy-enhancing drug promotes degradation of mutant alpha1-antitrypsin Z and reduces hepatic fibrosis. *Science*. 2010;329:229.

239. Marciniak SJ, Lomas DA. Alpha1-antitrypsin deficiency and autophagy. *N Engl J Med*. 2010;363:1863.

240. Chang YP, Mahadeva R, Chang WS, Lin SC, Chu YH. Small-molecule peptides inhibit Z alpha1-antitrypsin polymerization. *J Cell Mol Med*. 2009;13:2304.

CHAPTER 41

Cigarette Smoking and Smoking Cessation

Stephen I. Rennard
David M. Daughton

GENERAL BACKGROUND

Native Americans discovered the use of the tobacco plant, *Nicotiana tabacum*, during antiquity. By the time Columbus arrived in America, tobacco use was widespread throughout the Western Hemisphere and was well integrated into Native American cultures. Production of tobacco and its trade represented a major economic activity in the pre-Columbian Americas. Early European explorers learned of the tobacco plant from Native Americans, and by the mid-17th century tobacco was widely used in Europe.

The most important, but not the only, active psychopharmaceutical drug contained in the leaves of the tobacco plant is nicotine.[1,2] Nicotine is a major metabolic product of the tobacco plant, and it is likely that it evolved as a protection against insect predators, as nicotine is a potent insect neurotoxin.[3] Interestingly, nicotine has been exploited in this regard as a commercial insecticide. Nicotine, however, is the major addicting substance in tobacco, although the addiction to tobacco is more complex than addiction to nicotine alone. Other psychoactive compounds are also present in tobacco smoke, including monoamine oxidase inhibitors.[4] These may have either direct effects or interact with other psychoactive drugs.[1,2] In addition, conditioned behavior and social interactions are important drivers of smoking.[5–8]

Nicotine is a potent euphoriant. On a molar basis, nicotine is more active than such euphoria-inducing drugs as cocaine, amphetamine, or morphine.[9] Nicotine elicits complex effects on the central nervous system (CNS), which are discussed in more detail below. Many of these effects, however, are perceived as desirable, accounting for the popularity of smoking. For example, nicotine ameliorates anxiety, reduces perception of pain,[10] mitigates symptoms of depression,[11] and induces a sense of well-being[9] while causing a state of arousal.[12] In contrast to many euphoriants that impair cognition, nicotine can improve task performance and attention time by measurable degrees in nonhabituated individuals and may have beneficial effects on cognition.[12]

Despite its perceived benefits, smoking of tobacco has long been controversial. King James of England wrote in 1604 "[Smoking is] a custom loathsome to the eye, hateful to the nose, harmful to the brain, dangerous to the lungs, and in the black stinking fume thereof, nearest resembling the horrible Stygian smoke of the pit that is bottomless.[13]" The Surgeon General's Report of 1964 outlined the convincing evidence for the health consequences of smoking.[14] Since that time there has been a gradual increase in efforts to control tobacco use and the associated health consequences. Changes in social attitude, public health efforts, and both pharmacologic and nonpharmacologic approaches have been developed that have meaningful benefits. The current chapter will focus on treatment designed to help a smoker achieve abstinence.

NICOTINE ADDICTION

Nicotine exerts its biologic effects on "nicotinic" receptors, a subset of cholinergic receptors, whose endogenous ligand is acetylcholine.[15,16] Nicotinic receptors are homo- or heteropentamers that bind two ligand molecules and form an ion channel.[17] In man, 17 genes code for distinct component chains, resulting in a very large number of potential pentamers, although only a relatively few are believed to have a biologic role. In the brain, nine alpha and three beta receptors are expressed. However the major receptors are composed of complexes (alpha4)(beta2), (alpha3)(beta4), and (alpha7). The (alpha4)(beta2) complex incorporates other subunits, particularly (alpha5), (alpha6), or (beta3), and these may modulate the effects of ligands, including nicotine.[17] The $(alpha4)_3(beta2)_2$ receptor is believed to be particularly important in the addicting effects of nicotine. Deleting the (beta2) receptor in mice eliminates behavioral responses to nicotine, while mutations in the gene can result in markedly increased sensitivity to nicotine.[18] The $(alpha7)_5$ receptor, for example, is believed to mediate some of the cognitive effects of nicotine, including sensory gating and learning.[18,19] In contrast the muscarinic receptors, the other major class of cholinergic receptors, are single chain G-protein–coupled receptors. Nicotine has no effect on these receptors.

Nicotinic receptors are ion channels and upon binding of nicotine, permeability of the channel is increased.[15–18] For example, binding of nicotine to the $(alpha4)_3(beta2)_2$ allows influx of calcium. This, in turn, modulates release of neurotransmitters. It is likely that the behavioral responses to nicotine result from the actions of many neurotransmitters, but dopamine is believed to be a major mediator of nicotine effects. In this context, dopamine is a key mediator of pleasure and reward and is required for the reinforcing effects that lead to drug self-administration in animal models.[20] As such, dopaminergic signaling is believed to be key in the pathogenesis of many addictions and compulsive behaviors. Nicotine also modulates the release of other neurotransmitters, including glutamate and gamma-amino butyric acid (GABA). Interestingly, chronic administration of nicotine desensitizes neurons that release GABA, which inhibits dopamine release. In contrast, there is no desensitization of glutamate release, which augments dopamine release. Chronic nicotine exposure, therefore, can lead to further augmentation, nicotine-induced dopamine release.[21,22] Moreover, the CNS alterations that occur following nicotine administration can be very long lasting; for example, alterations in nicotine receptor levels in rats exposed in utero persist until adult life.[23] The adolescent brain may be particularly sensitive to long-term alterations induced by nicotine.[24] This may account for the sensitivity of adolescents to addiction. Persistent changes in the brain may also account for the observation that, even after achieving abstinence, a smoker is at risk for relapse and if relapse occurs, the smoker reverts to the previous "steady-state" habit much more rapidly than that habit developed initially.

Nicotine is contained in the leaves of the tobacco plant. Nicotine is a weak base and as a result will be charged in acidic environments. Many forms of tobacco, such as cigars and chewing tobacco, are alkalinized, which results in uncharged nicotine that can be more readily absorbed through the buccal mucosa. Thus, cigar smokers do not have to inhale to achieve desired blood nicotine levels. The process of smoking a cigarette is more complex.[25] Air sucked through the burning end of a cigarette becomes heated. As the hot air passes down the bole of a cigarette, it causes the nicotine in the tobacco to volatilize. As the mixture cools, the nicotine condenses on smoke particles resulting in a nicotine aerosol. Conventional cigarettes have been designed so that the resulting particle size is ideal to reach the alveolar structures of the lung. Uncharged nicotine is lipid soluble and is rapidly absorbed from the alveolar gas into the pulmonary capillary blood and then into the arterial circulation. Inhaled nicotine, therefore, reaches the brain in about ½ a circulation time or about 15 to 20 seconds. In its neutral form, nicotine readily crosses the blood–brain barrier and exerts its psychoactive effects. A cigarette, therefore, is a very effective means of delivering nicotine to the brain. It also allows a smoker to control the dose of delivered drug with considerable precision.

After absorption, nicotine distributes into various body pools. This results in a marked difference between arterial and venous nicotine levels and a rapid drop in nicotine levels upon completion of a cigarette.[26] Nicotine is then catabolized by several enzymes. The most important of these is CYP2A6 which oxidizes nicotine to cotinine and cotinine to hydroxycotinine.[27] Nicotine can also be oxidized by alternative CYP450 enzymes and may be inactivated and excreted by glucuronidation. Genetic variants in nicotine metabolizing enzymes can influence smoking behavior. In normal metabolizers, nicotine is cleared with a half-life of about 2 hours. As a result, nicotine levels increase throughout the day for individuals who smoke steadily. The increase in nicotine levels can result in levels believed to fully saturate all nicotinic receptors.[1,2] In this setting, it is likely that smoking behavior is more dependent on conditioned responses than on psychopharmacologic effects of nicotine. Conversely, nicotine levels fall at night. The drop in nicotine levels is thought to initiate the early stages of withdrawal. Importantly, the lower levels allow for nicotinic receptors to be in the unbound state. As a result, the first cigarette in the morning can have a large psychodynamic effect. This is well recognized by smokers who will often report that the "most enjoyable" cigarette is the first one smoked in the morning. In addition, the drop in nicotine levels is thought to initiate the early stages of withdrawal. How long it takes a smoker to smoke the first cigarette of the day, therefore, serves as a gauge of addiction, with short times indicating stronger addiction. Smoking within 30 minutes of awakening is a key question in the Fagerstrom test for nicotine dependence.[28]

Several lines of evidence support genetic influences on smoking behavior.[29–32] Twin studies suggest that genetics accounts for about 50% of the variance in smoking. Interestingly, there appears to be a genetic basis for withdrawal symptoms.[33] A number of genes have been suggested to play a role in both candidate gene and in genome-wide association studies. Although many of the candidate genes have been difficult to reproduce, an extremely strong signal has been consistently observed in a region of chromosome 15 that includes the genes for three nicotinic receptors.[34] Among COPD patients, this region is also associated with intensity of smoking assessed by cigarettes smoked per day, suggesting it may be related to intensity of addiction.[35] As might be expected of a gene related to smoking behavior, this region has also been strongly linked to the risk for several smoking-related diseases.[36–39] Candidate genes include not only genes in the dopamine pathway, but also other neurotransmitter pathways as well as cell adhesion molecules that are thought to contribute to long-term memory and neural adaptation.

Genetic variation in nicotine metabolizing enzymes has received particular attention.[31] Many, but not all studies have demonstrated that individuals with variants in CYP2A6 who metabolize nicotine slowly smoke fewer cigarettes and maintain lower cotinine and carbon monoxide levels consistent with their requiring less total intake.[35,40,41] Consistent with a reduced level of smoking, some studies have shown reduced risk for cancer in slow metabolizers.[42,43] Similarly, better lung function has been reported among individuals with haplotypes associated with slow metabolism compared to those with genes associated with rapid metabolism who smoke the same number of cigarettes.[44]

It is plausible that the slower decline in blood nicotine levels associated with slow nicotine metabolism makes these individuals less likely to experience withdrawal. In addition, the persistence of nicotine may decrease the "reward" of smoking. Both of these effects may contribute to increased likelihood that a slow metabolizer can achieve abstinence from smoking[40] and better quit rates have been observed among slow metabolizers in clinical trials.[31,45] On the other hand, slow metabolizers who are experimenting with smoking may have higher and more sustained nicotine levels. Consistent with this, a prospective study of adolescents observed a threefold risk of becoming a regular smoker among slow metabolizers.[46]

Smoking cigarettes is more complex than nicotine addiction. Conditioned behaviors also play a key role.[1,2] In this context, a smoker typically inhales 10 puffs per cigarette. This would be 300 puffs for a 1½ pack per day smoker or more than 100,000 puffs annually. In addition, smoking frequently occurs in recurrent settings: after eating, when irritated, when bored, when sad, in specific social settings, etc. As such, smoking becomes associated with these settings which serve as operant cues to induce smoking behavior. Nicotine, moreover, has been demonstrated to increase both the intensity of operant conditioning as well as its persistence.[6,47] The development of addiction to tobacco, therefore, involves not only development of addiction to nicotine, but also acquisition of conditioned behaviors, which nicotine facilitates. Because these cue-mediated behaviors can be very persistent, they are major causes of relapse.

Tobacco addiction most commonly begins in late childhood or adolescence,[48–51] although smoking can begin in young adulthood.[52,53] Historically, in the United States, the peak incidence for developing a regular tobacco habit is in adolescence. Individuals who do not acquire a habit prior to age 20 were unlikely to do so as adults.[48] The demographics of smoking initiation were well known to the tobacco industry. Marketing campaigns designed to promote the image of specific brands of cigarettes were carefully designed and were exceedingly effective in leading to logo recognition among children as young as kindergartners[51,54] and contributed to brand selection among American adolescents. The susceptibility of children to these campaigns was a major driver in leading to the current ban on tobacco advertising in media likely to be seen by children. Importantly, since most exploratory smoking occurs in peer-related social settings, the social context of smoking is a crucial variable in determining smoking initiation.[51,55,56]

Most children who begin to smoke do so on an occasional basis. Within a few years, however, a regular habit may develop. Most often this habit is characterized by smoking only a few cigarettes daily. As noted above, slow metabolizers may be particularly susceptible to addiction due to higher nicotine levels and longer persistence.[46] The number of cigarettes smoked, however, generally increases for the first 8 to 10 years. Important variations on this pattern exist, suggesting biologic differences among smokers. Some smokers achieve a "mature addiction" very rapidly. In contrast, as many as 15% of smokers, termed "chippers," may continue to smoke episodically and may not be fully addicted.[57,58]

Smoking is more common among those with psychiatric disorders.[59–61] This includes individuals with depression, anxiety disorders, and cognitive disorders such as schizophrenia as well as other drug dependencies. The basis for this relationship is unclear. Nicotine has modest antidepressant and antianxiety effects, and the suggestion has been made that some individuals with mood disorders may smoke to "auto-medicate." Alternatively, it has been suggested that smoking and psychiatric disorders may share common genetic risk factors. Another possibility is that smoking early in life may lead to alterations in the CNS that may lead, in turn, to psychiatric disorders. In support of this, smoking more commonly precedes first psychotic episodes.[61] Whatever the mechanisms, the concurrent presence of psychiatric disorders can complicate efforts to achieve smoking abstinence.

Once a smoker achieves a "mature" addiction, cigarette consumption typically remains very constant. Interestingly, the smoker appears to adjust both nicotine intake and number of cigarettes smoked independently. If supplemental nicotine is administered, smokers will often reduce their nicotine consumption.[62] Alternatively, if smoking is restricted, for example, by decreasing the number of cigarettes available, smokers will alter their smoking strategy, for example, by smoking each cigarette more deeply, to maintain a relatively constant nicotine intake.[63] Similarly, acidification of the urine increases while alkalinization slows nicotine clearance, and there are corresponding increases and decreases in nicotine intake that are achieved with no change in the number of cigarettes smoked.[64] Rather, smokers alter the way in which individual cigarettes are smoked, that is, the depth and duration of inhalation and the number of puffs, thus modifying the nicotine absorbed. Consistent with self-regulation of nicotine administration, low–nicotine-content cigarettes do not result in lower nicotine consumption.[65] This illustrates the complexity of smoking where both nicotine addiction and conditioned behaviors contribute.

While the pathogenetic mechanisms underlying withdrawal symptoms are incompletely understood, it is generally believed that some withdrawal symptoms are related to decreases in nicotine blood levels below certain thresholds. Variations in nicotine metabolism would be expected to affect the timing of symptom onset. Some smokers, for example, may experience nicotine withdrawal at night when sleep interferes with nicotine intake.[66] The concept that nicotine replacement can help ameliorate withdrawal symptoms by maintaining nicotine blood levels is also an important concept underlying nicotine replacement as an aid to smoking cessation. In addition, susceptibility to specific symptoms may be genetically determined.[67,68]

SMOKING AS A PUBLIC HEALTH PROBLEM

Cigarette smoking is a major public health problem and is perhaps the most important cause of preventable disease. The number of deaths attributed to cigarette smoking in the United States has been estimated to be well in excess of 400,000 annually and has been for many years.[69,70] This exceeds deaths attributed to other specific causes.[71] The health burden attributable to smoking parallels smoking prevalence. As a result, smoking-induced disease is becoming more common in the developing world where smoking prevalence has been increasing, particularly in specific subpopulations such as young and middle-aged males.[72] In the United States, where comprehensive tobacco control programs have reduced smoking prevalence, the burden of tobacco-related disease has begun to decrease.[73–75] Smoking can cause disease through a variety of mechanisms, which are reviewed in other chapters. However, some pathophysiologic effects persist after cessation. Smoking-related disease, therefore, will continue to be a major health problem for many decades.

Since Dr. Luther Terry released the first Surgeon General's report on smoking and health in 1964,[14] the prevalence of adult smokers in the United States has dropped from 40% to under 20%.[75] Antismoking awareness has increased worldwide to the extent that smoking bans have become commonplace in public buildings, workplaces, and public transportation. In 1984, Surgeon General C. Everett Koop[76] proclaimed that the United States' number one health goal was to achieve a smoke-free society by the year 2000." Unfortunately, this goal was not achieved, but the importance of the public health initiatives that followed, evidenced by the overall incidence of smokers in the adult population in the United States, continues to decrease.[73–75] A more realistic goal of adult smoking reduction to 12% in the United States was put into place through the Healthy People 2010.[77] Whether this goal will be obtained remains to be determined; however, it still highlights the importance of a smoke-free society. The greatest reductions in smoking have been in states with the most comprehensive tobacco control programs, supporting the effectiveness of currently available interventions.

Public health approaches to control smoking-related disease begin with the social factors that are key in initiating and maintaining smoking.[51] The experience a child has with the initial attempts at smoking appear to be important as is an individual's attitude toward smoking, that is, the "image" of the smoker, peer pressure, parental cigarette use, and availability.[51,78,79] Social attitudes can account for very low smoking prevalence in some groups. These observations support attempts to place restrictions on smoking in public places and other efforts to "de-normalize" smoking.[51]

As in ancient America, the use of tobacco products has become well integrated into modern cultures worldwide. Tobacco is a multibillion dollar industry. In some regions, tobacco is a crucial cash crop in an agricultural economy. In addition, the manufacturing, distribution, marketing, and sale of tobacco products employ many individuals worldwide. Taxation on tobacco products has become an important means for the support of many governments. Thus, any changes in tobacco usage are likely to have economic impacts well beyond any health effects.

The use of tobacco not only has an economic role, but a cultural one as well. In some societies, for example, certain Native American tribes, tobacco usage has religious significance. In other groups, tobacco usage is associated with a strong cultural "image." Often this image may have been created through direct efforts of the tobacco industry to market their product. In this regard, advertising messages promoting the image of the cigarette smoker as rugged, independent, and masculine or as sophisticated, independent, and feminine have been developed.[80,81] While these images of cigarette smoking have their origins in advertising campaigns, the effectiveness of such marketing programs cannot be underestimated.[51,79] The portrayal of these images in media, such as film, may help promote smoking, which supports restrictions on advertisements as part of public health initiatives directed at tobacco control.[51,82,83] Whatever the reasons, cigarettes clearly have a cultural significance. The social and economic impact of tobacco usage, therefore, must be considered when attempting to deal with smoking as a public health problem.

In an effort to combat the public health ramifications of tobacco usage in the United States, the Master Settlement Agreement was signed into effect in 1998.[84] It served as a measure to recoup what states had lost through Medicaid expenditures due to smoking-related illnesses and as a measure to fine the tobacco industry for deceitful actions. Four major United States tobacco companies awarded 46 states $206 billion to be paid over 25 years and to be utilized as the states saw fit. Four states had previously settled separately. Unfortunately, since its inception, many states have failed to use the funding for tobacco control causes, instead using it to fill budget deficits or to support other state programs. Among many other actions, the agreement also prohibited advertisements targeted at youth and permitted access to tobacco industry documents. Based on current understanding of the complex factors that interact to cause tobacco addiction, these approaches are rational. The issues are also complex and controversial. It is likely that social and public health interventions will continue to evolve and be part of ongoing political debate.

Smoking prevention. As noted above, smoking initiation is generally a pediatric problem.[51] Precisely why some children begin smoking is not fully understood, although both social and genetic factors contribute as discussed above.[51] Currently as many as 40% of American children will experiment with cigarettes, of whom one-fourth will eventually smoke by the twelfth grade.[85] A number of factors are believed to contribute, including the child's social environment and the child's attitude toward smoking, which appears to be based, in large part, on the smoking behavior of parents, friends, and peer group role models.[51,78,79] Attitudes toward smoking appear to be important factors leading to smoking initiation, which may depend, at least in part, on advertising and marketing programs, hence the effectiveness of bans on advertising. The reasons for initiating smoking, however, are not entirely environmental, as several lines of investigation (see above) suggest a genetic basis for smoking as well. These concepts support the basis for interventions to reduce smoking initiation. Interventions aimed at altering the social milieu have benefit.[86] Participation in sporting activities is associated with lower rates of smoking initiation.[48,87]

A second approach to limiting smoking initiation is to restrict the sale of tobacco products to minors. Many states have legal restrictions on such sales. In many cases, however, these laws are not enforced. Active enforcement, however, can lead to a decrease in sales to minors[88] and a decrease in both experimental smoking and in regular cigarette use among younger smokers,[89] although the general effectiveness of these measures is unclear.[90] For such measures to be effective, they must be uniformly enforced in the community, and vending machines must be made inaccessible to minors.[91,92] Another approach to restrict tobacco usage by minors is taxation.[93] While there is controversy over how "elastic" purchase of tobacco is,[94] increasing price decreases use, and this effect may be particularly prominent among less addicted smokers.[93] Inasmuch as adolescents may have less disposable income, the effect may be even greater among adolescents. Some analyses support an association between higher price, particularly through taxation and lower smoking initiation and prevalence.[95] However assessment of the specific effectiveness is difficult methodologically.

Measures aimed at restricting tobacco sales to minors may lead to a deferral for smoking initiation, as young adults remain at risk for[52,53] smoking initiation. Thus, if measures are effective at delaying smoking initiation among children, parallel measures may also be required to affect smoking initiation among older adolescents and young adults. Currently available data suggest that smoking behavior among high school students decreased steadily since the initiation of efforts designed to reduce initiation (Fig. 41-1). There does not appear to be a corresponding increase in smoking among older individuals, which supports the concept that smoking prevention is a legitimate and achievable public health goal. While it is difficult to determine the effectiveness of specific public health initiatives,[96] the evidence is clear that smoking rates can be decreased by population-based measures and that states with the most comprehensive programs have achieved the greatest gains.[51,73–75]

SMOKING CESSATION

BACKGROUND AND GENERAL APPROACH

Smoking should be regarded as a primary addictive disorder.[97] This contrasts with the "classic" view of smoking as a "habit" or "life style choice." An estimated 75% of Americans wish to quit but only 3% are able to achieve prolonged abstinence in any year, which indicates the involuntary nature of the established addiction.[98] In addition, current concepts suggest smoking should be regarded as a chronic relapsing disorder. In this context, a "cessation attempt" should be regarded as an attempt to induce a remission. The abstinent smoker, moreover, should always be viewed as at risk for relapse. The goal for therapy is to induce a remission that is as durable as possible. However, the clinician needs to be prepared to reinduce remission in the event that relapse occurs. In this context, smokers who are "quit" should remain in active surveillance, and relapses should not be regarded as "failures." In this model, the health consequences of smoking should be regarded as secondary effects. Importantly, there are health benefits of cessation that are well established. These are the subject of the Surgeon General's Report (2014).

Current recommendations are to assess smoking and willingness to quit at every visit.[97,99,100] Interestingly, success in quitting may be related to acute problems that may have motivated a patient to be willing to consider quitting (see Stages of Change).[101] This acute motivation may be present even if the acute event is not directly related to smoking, and the clinician should be ready to utilize these windows of opportunity. In contrast, not inquiring about smoking can have adverse effects. Not asking is thought to send three messages: (1) that the physician does not care if the patient smokes; (2) that the physician does not have an effective intervention to offer; and/or (3) that the physician does not think that the patient will be able to quit. All of these "nonmessages" have negative effects, particularly as smokers gradually make the decision to quit. A sense of empowerment and control over the behavior is believed to be key to making and succeeding in a quit attempt[102] and to subsequent risk of relapse.[103] Inadvertently eroding a patient's sense of mastery is an unanticipated adverse consequence of not asking about smoking. In addition, many patients are unaware of the potential available therapies; appropriate information can increase motivation to engage in quit attempts. Smokers unwilling to make a quit attempt should be encouraged as much as possible, provided with specific information if desired and reminded that the issue will be brought up again in the future.

Approach to a Quit Attempt

A smoking quit attempt should be approached in a similar way to induction of remission from cancer. As with cancer, each patient should be given the best chance of achieving remission. In general this will require two classes of intervention: nonpharmacologic approaches and pharmacotherapy, which should be used together to optimize success.

Evaluation

As with the management of any complex disease, smokers should undergo an initial organized assessment.[97,100] Motivation or reason to

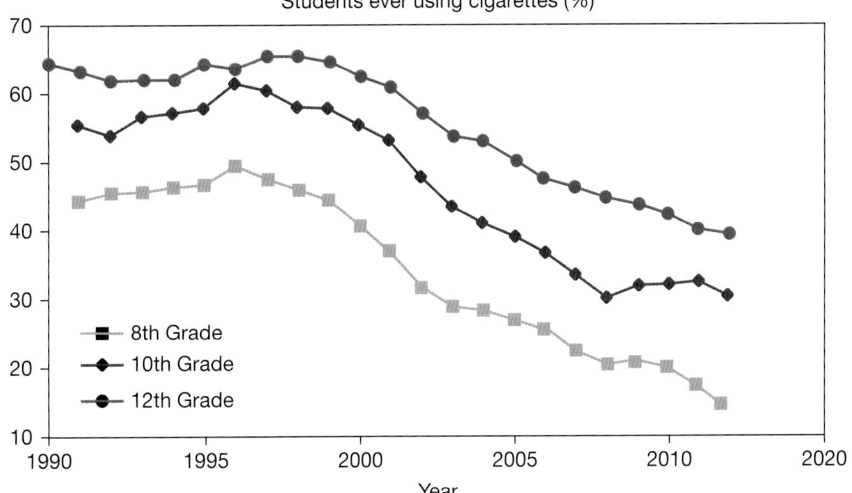

Figure 41-1 Prevalence of ever smoking among American Youth. *(Data from Johnston LD, O'Malley PM, Bachman JG, Schulenberg JE. Decline in teen smoking continues into 2012. Monitoring the Future Press Release. University of Michigan News Service, Ann Arbor.)*

TABLE 41-1 Items and Scoring for Fagerstrom Test for Nicotine Dependence

Questions	Answers	Points
1. How soon after you wake up do you smoke your first cigarette?	Within 5 min	3
	6–30 min	2
	31–60 min	1
	After 60 min	0
2. Do you find it difficult to refrain from smoking in places where it is forbidden, e.g., in church, at the library, in cinema, etc.?	Yes	1
	No	0
3. Which cigarette would you hate most to give up?	The first one in the morning	1
	All others	0
4. How many cigarettes/day do you smoke?	10 or less	0
	11–20	1
	21–30	2
	31 or more	3
5. Do you smoke more frequently during the first hours after waking than during the rest of the day?	Yes	1
	No	0
6. Do you smoke if you are so ill that you are in bed most of the day?	Yes	1
	No	0

Source: Used with permission of K.O. Fagerstrom.

quit and the patient's confidence in their ability to stop smoking, that is, self-efficacy, should be assessed. For patients who indicate they are not currently interested in quitting, the goal is simple: to move them through the stages of change[104] so a quit attempt will be made. For some, this may be as simple as providing information about health risks. For others, it may be information about effective interventions.

The intensity of addiction can be assessed with the Fagerstrom test for nicotine dependence (Table 41-1).[28] The most important question is time to first cigarette, and smokers who smoke within 30 minutes of awakening are usually heavily addicted to nicotine. These patients and those with Fagerstrom scores ≥7 comprise a group of individuals likely to benefit from nicotine replacement therapy (NRT) or varenicline. In contrast, patients with low Fagerstrom scores who are able to cope with smoke-free environments for an extended time period (>4 hours) without developing discomforting withdrawal symptoms, may not require NRT. For these individuals, the benefit of pharmacologic support is unknown.

Past experience with quit attempts should be reviewed. Many patients will have a number of prior tries. Individuals who had particular difficulty with withdrawal symptoms should be prepared for this, and medications can be gauged to attempt to mitigate their intensity. Approaches that achieved abstinence, but were followed by relapse, should be considered as they are likely to succeed again. In these cases, interventions should be guided by reducing risks of relapse.

NONPHARMACOLOGIC APPROACHES

Nonpharmacologic approaches provide the smoker with guidance and support as progress is made through a quit attempt.[97,99,100] It is likely that effective support improves adherence with pharmacotherapy and results in therapeutic synergy. In addition, conditioned responses, that is, cue-driven behaviors, are largely dealt with thorough behavioral strategies. This generally requires individual interviews to define individual smoking patterns. These patterns can also help identify situations that increase risk of relapse. In general, success increases with the intensity of support,[97,99,100] but most smokers will decline referral to intensive programs and will receive only the support provided in the office setting. The remainder of this section summarizes commonly used approaches.[97,99,100,105]

Stages of Change and Smoking Cessation

The Stages of Change model has been very useful to guide behavioral support. Prochaska and DiClemente[104] described the smoking cessation process as involving five stages: precontemplation, contemplation, preparation, action, and maintenance. These stages are viewed as a continuum with smokers progressing sequentially through each stage. In the precontemplation stage, smokers are not interested in quitting smoking and will likely be nonresponsive to direct intervention. Smokers in the contemplation stage are considering quitting smoking and may be receptive to a physician's advice about the risks and benefits of quitting. In the preparation stage, smokers are actively preparing to quit. The action stage encompasses both initial abstinence and the 6-month postcessation period. The maintenance period commences after the 6-month abstinence period. It is rare for a smoker to progress successfully through these stages in the initial quit attempt. The cycle will likely be repeated several times before smoking a prolonged abstinence, that is remission, is achieved. Thus the clinician must be encouraging and willing to support repeated attempts.

The National Cancer Institute's (NCI) recommended model for smoking intervention is based, in part, on five NCI supported trials involving more than 30,000 patients and was later expanded by the Public Health Service.[97,99,100] This approach, popularly referred to as "the five A's," emphasizes the role of medical professionals to ask patients about their smoking status, assess their willingness to make a quit attempt, advise smokers to stop, assist them in their stop smoking efforts, and arrange for follow-up visits to support the patient's efforts. This approach utilizes brief intervention techniques and emphasizes the role of physicians as facilitators in the quitting process.

Simple advice has been assessed in a number of studies, and meta-analysis suggests a small but significant benefit of these limited interventions.[100] Physician advice is effective both in the outpatient and hospital setting and may also be effective when given by letter, email, or telephone.[106–108]

Group Counseling

Group counseling programs for smoking cessation are offered by several commercial and voluntary health organizations. These programs are similar in content and typically include lectures, group interactions, exercises on self-recognition of one's habit, some form of tapering method leading to a quit day, development of coping skills, and suggestions for relapse prevention. Group counseling programs sponsored by voluntary health organizations are generally the best cost value for smokers.[97,99,100] However, these programs are generally limited to large metropolitan areas and are offered on a sporadic basis. One-year success rates associated with group counseling programs are typically in the 15% to 35% range.[97,99,100] The high success rates are likely affected by selection bias, that is, participants may be more motivated to quit.

Gradual Reduction Versus Abrupt Abstinence

Gradual reduction or tapering intuitively appears to offer smokers the least abrasive way to stop smoking, and may be effective for some.[109–111] However, gradually cutting down can be stressful when smokers attempt to reduce their cigarette use below their critical blood nicotine threshold. At this stage, smokers may begin to experience tobacco withdrawal symptoms. Rather than suffer prolonged discomfort, many taperers will gradually return to their customary cigarette levels and will not succeed in quitting. One of the negative consequences of tapering is that this method can strongly reinforce the smoker's belief of their underlying need for cigarettes, that is, it can undermine self-efficacy. Combining tapering with pharmacotherapy to prevent withdrawal may be useful in this setting,[110] but this is not an FDA-approved use for any medication. Abrupt abstinence is often stressful and can lead to tobacco withdrawal symptoms. However, within a few weeks of total abstinence, complete abstainers experience less frequent cigarette cravings than taperers and are less prone to relapse. Cigarette tapering is often a component of many group programs in which gradual cigarette reduction is used as a preparatory stage leading toward a target quit day.

Educational Techniques

For years, cigarette smoking was viewed as largely a social or psychological habit. As such, the ability to quit was viewed as a measure of personal motivation and psychological willpower. Motivation to stop smoking, combined with sufficient psychological resources, was seen as a driving force behind successful cigarette abstinence. Thus, if smokers could be educated about the health risks of cigarette smoking, they could theoretically become sufficiently motivated and psychologically empowered to quit. Unfortunately, anticipated benefits of the smoking cessation value of educational awareness messages were overly optimistic and simplistic. Educational programs to aid smoking cessation have produced disappointing results with high long-term failure rates.[97,99,100] Nevertheless, education about smoking is still regarded as a useful activity, particularly when the information can address problems of specific interest to individual patients. In this regard, as noted above, a major predictor of success is "self-efficacy," which is the patient's sense that they are likely to succeed. Education that improves self-efficacy should be a therapeutic goal.

Other Modes

The goal of hypnosis in smoking cessation is to enable the smoker to achieve an altered state of consciousness to enhance the ability to quit. Controlled trials of hypnosis have generally been unable to document long-term smoking cessation efficacy. While one meta-analysis suggested the possibility of a treatment effect,[112] this was not supported in another meta-analysis.[113] Aversive conditioning is based on the premise that smoking is a learned response that can be extinguished by creating an association between smoking and a negative sensation. By design, adversive conditioning techniques can produce smoker discomfort and are now rarely employed. However, there are few recent studies, and a treatment benefit cannot be excluded.[112] Acupuncture has been advocated, but controlled trials with "sham" acupuncture have not clearly demonstrated an effect. Meta-analyses have not been conclusive, but suggest the possibility of an effect.[112,114]

Resources Available

The resources available to support smoking cessation vary among communities. Some have readily available and affordable group programs, while these may be unavailable in other places. Toll-free tobacco quit lines are currently provided by many countries, including the United States and Canada. Telephone counseling is an effective smoking intervention.[108] Thus, clinicians should encourage every smoker who wishes to quit to utilize a National Quit Line (e.g., in the United States: 1-800-Quit-Now). Additional support can be found via the internet using smokefree.gov. Using this approach, a smoker can choose to talk with a telephone specialist with either internet instant messaging or telephone support. Both methods are designed to provide smokers with a personalized quit plan that would be available in most clinical settings.

PHARMACOLOGIC TREATMENT

Three classes of agents, nicotine replacement, bupropion, and varenicline, are approved to aid smoking cessation.[115] In addition, two other agents, clonidine and nortriptyline are supported by guidelines for "off-label" use as secondary agents. In addition, several other agents are under active investigation and have shown promise.[97,99,100] As noted above, combination of nonpharmacologic support and pharmacotherapy optimizes success in achieving abstinence.[97,99,100] The remainder of this section summarizes currently available pharmacotherapy.

Nicotine Replacement Therapies

Five nicotine replacement therapies are approved for use to aid in smoking cessation. Lozenges, polacrilex (gum), and transdermal systems are available over the counter (OTC). Nasal spray and a nicotine inhaler are available with a prescription. Other nicotine preparations, including nicotine toothpicks and e-cigarettes, have been developed and marketed as consumer products. Their efficacy and safety in smoking cessation remains undetermined. Initial concerns about potential hazards of concurrent smoking while using NRT led to warnings against this practice. However, the Food and Drug Administration recently (April, 2013) removed this warning from the OTC formulations, as the benefits of smoking cessation greatly exceed any potential hazards.

NRT is usually started on the scheduled quit day. The concept is to replace nicotine that would be absorbed from cigarettes and thereby reduce the intensity of withdrawal. Smokers will, however, experience withdrawal symptoms albeit with less intensity. In clinical trials, the five approved formulations have demonstrated about twofold increases in quit rates above placebo when used alone[97,99,100] and one trial comparing gum, inhaler, and nasal spray found no difference in efficacy.[116] They differ, however, in their pharmacokinetics.[117] The transdermal systems provide the slowest delivery of nicotine, but maintain steady-state levels throughout the day. The other formulations allow episodic dosing. A common practice is to combine a transdermal system with another formulation, a "patch-plus" regimen.[118,119] This allows a smoker to increase nicotine delivery at times of urges. Clinical trial data supports better success with combined NRT compared to monotherapy.[97,99,100]

Nicotine Polacrilex Gum Nicotine polacrilex gum was the first NRT to gain FDA approval. It is now commercially available OTC in 2 and 4-mg forms. In nicotine polacrilex, nicotine is bound to a resin that contains a buffering agent to improve delivery of nicotine through the buccal mucosa. The rate of chewing can influence the rate of nicotine release. In addition, acid foods or drinks convert nicotine base to its salt, which, because of its charge, does not cross the buccal mucosa. To be absorbed into the venous circulation, the nicotine-containing saliva must be retained in the mouth as long as possible. If swallowed, the nicotine can cause local irritation of the stomach. When absorbed into the portal circulation, high first-pass metabolism in the liver limits blood nicotine levels. If chewed properly, absorption takes place gradually, and blood levels peak after about 30 minutes.[117] Ad lib use of 2-mg nicotine polacrilex is associated with blood nicotine levels less than 40% of customary smoking. The 4-mg dose is recommended for individuals who are heavier smokers or who have had discomforting tobacco withdrawal symptoms on the 2-mg dose.[97] A fixed dosage regimen rather than ad lib usage may have better success,[120] perhaps because it can produce higher blood nicotine levels. A common recommendation is that a smoker use one piece of gum every 1 to 2 hours for the first 6 weeks after quitting followed by gradual reduction over 6 weeks. Many smokers continue to use gum at times of craving for an extended time and some can use sufficient gum to sustain nicotine addiction without smoking.

Although effective in clinical trials, less successful results have been observed with nicotine gum in general practice and unsupervised settings. This may be due, in part, to requirement that the gum be chewed properly. Adverse effects from the gum include exacerbation of local effects: temporomandibular joint (TMJ) disease, trauma to dental appliances, sore jaw, oral irritation or ulcers, and excess salivation; effects from swallowed nicotine: hiccups; and effects from systemic absorption of nicotine: nausea, vomiting, abdominal pain, constipation, diarrhea, palpitations, and headache. Use of the gum is not recommended in individuals with poor dentition or who have dental appliances.[115]

Nicotine Polacrilex Lozenge A nicotine polacrilex lozenge is also available "over the counter." Chewing is not required, but acid food and/or beverages will impair absorption as with gum. Dosing, absorption, and duration of therapy with the lozenge are similar to those for the gum.[121] Because it is not chewed, the lozenge does not share the problems of exacerbating TMJ disease or damaging dental appliances. Other side effects are similar to those of the gum.

Transdermal Nicotine The primary advantage of transdermal patch delivery systems are ease of use and controlled drug delivery. Several formulations are available "over the counter." In general, they achieve nicotine blood levels roughly 40% to 50% of that achieved by customary smoking of about 30 cigarettes daily.[117] Transdermal nicotine systems have been repeatedly found to reduce tobacco withdrawal symptoms and significantly enhance smoking cessation rates.[97,99,100] Unlike nicotine polacrilex gum, transdermal nicotine systems and the nicotine lozenge have improved quit rates in primary care settings.[101,122] This difference is likely due to the ease of patch use in this setting. The recommended use period for patches varies according to product, but a minimum of 4 weeks of therapy is probably required to help achieve long-term abstinence.

Patches are most commonly worn at night, which provides a level of nicotine when a smoker awakes. Often this is a time when the individual is at risk to relapse, since the low nicotine levels are associated both with withdrawal and with increased effect of the smoked cigarette. On the other hand, delivery of nicotine at night may disturb sleep, particularly through vivid dreams or insomnia. Spontaneous long-term use of the patch has not been observed, suggesting that the very slow kinetics of nicotine delivery with this system is insufficient to sustain addiction effectively.[123] In addition, perhaps due to the partial replacement of nicotine, most smokers on patches will still experience some tobacco withdrawal symptoms during the first few days of quitting. While these symptoms will likely be less severe compared to quitting cold turkey, some patients will be tempted to smoke and wear patches. Early concerns about increased cardiac risk among individuals who smoked while wearing the patch have not been substantiated. In fact, reduced smoking may decrease cardiac events.[124–126]

Nicotine Inhaler The nicotine inhaler is a plastic nicotine-containing cartridge that fits on a mouthpiece. Nicotine is released when air is inhaled through the device, which is similar in size to a cigarette. The nicotine is not effectively delivered to the lungs as the particle size is too large. Rather, it is deposited and absorbed through the buccal mucosa, which results in pharmacokinetics that resemble nicotine polacrilex. Blood levels depend on the frequency of inhalations but can be about one-third of conventional smoking. Usual dosing is 6 to 16 cartridges per day for 6 to 12 weeks followed by gradual reduction over 6 to 12 weeks. Because the use of the inhaler recapitulates many of the actions associated with smoking: preparation of the device, oral stimulation, inhalation, etc.; it may be particularly effective in smokers for whom these behaviors are particularly strongly conditioned. In addition to the adverse effects described for the lozenge, the inhaler may cause irritation of the throat and mouth and may precipitate bronchospasm in individuals with reactive airways.

Nicotine Nasal Spray The nasal spray delivers nicotine to the nasal mucosa through which it is absorbed. It has the most rapid pharmacokinetics of the currently available nicotine replacement formulations but does not reproduce that of a cigarette.[117] Nasal irritation is very common, particularly when initiating therapy. The recommended dose is one to two sprays per hour for 3 months with a maximum of 80 sprays per day. Because the spray can deliver large amounts of nicotine, it may be particularly effective for heavily addicted smokers. It also likely has a greater risk of nicotine overdose and may have a greater potential to sustain a long-term addiction.

Combination Therapy Although not approved by drug regulatory agencies, various combinations of nicotine replacement may have utility for selected individuals who need higher doses. In particular, combination of a transdermal system with an ad lib modality has been demonstrated to increase quit rates.[97,99,100,122,127] Because of its increased success, it is recommended by some as initial therapy.[115]

Bupropion

Bupropion is approved as an antidepressant, and it is also effective as an aid for smoking cessation.[97,99,100,128] It is believed to act by potentiating dopaminergic and noradrenergic signaling. The formulations for depression and for smoking cessation have different trade names, which has clinical relevance. First, an appropriate diagnosis is often required for reimbursement. Second, care is needed not to prescribe bupropion under one name to an individual already taking it under its other name, as over dosage can result.

In clinical trials, bupropion approximately doubles quit rates compared to placebo. Subjects with a history of depression, however, appeared to benefit from bupropion but did not with nicotine replacement, suggesting that bupropion may be a superior initial choice in such individuals. Combination of nicotine replacement with bupropion has been assessed and appears more effective than either agent alone.

The currently recommended dose is 150-mg daily for 3 days followed by 150-mg twice daily. Because the drug is excreted slowly, steady state-levels are achieved after 6 to 7 days. For this reason, the quit date should be scheduled after a week of therapy so that blood levels are established. As the 150-mg once daily dose was nearly as effective as the 150-mg twice daily,[129,130] many practitioners use the lower dose routinely. The appropriate duration of therapy is not established. Clinical trials that formed the basis for approval treated for 7 weeks, although a 12-week course is commonly recommended. With prolonged therapy, there is an increase in secondary quits, and therapy for 1 year resulted in more quits than therapy for 7 weeks.

The drug is generally well tolerated. The most common adverse effects are dry mouth, insomnia, agitation, and headache. In combination with nicotine replacement, an increase in blood pressure may also occur. Bupropion reduces seizure threshold and a seizure risk of 0.1% has been reported. Because of its reduction in seizure threshold, bupropion is contraindicated among those predisposed to seizures, or with anorexia nervosa or bulimia.

In 2008, the FDA first noted that both bupropion and varenicline (see below) had a "possible association (with) suicidal events."[131] The benefits of smoking cessation were felt to outweigh any potential risks, and the medicines were not withdrawn from the market. However, both labels now contain a black box warning, suggesting that patients and their caregivers should be alerted to the possibility of neuropsychiatric symptoms, and patients should be monitored for changes in behavior, hostility, agitation, depressed mood, suicidal ideation, and suicide attempts. Most practitioners make a routine practice of reassessing patients 3 to 7 days after the quit day to both monitor for adverse effects and to provide additional support for the quit attempt. In this context, a second visit has been demonstrated to greatly improve success.[97,99,100]

Varenicline

Varenicline is a partial agonist at the (alpha4)(beta2) nicotinic receptor.[132] As such, it can partially activate the receptor thereby mitigating withdrawal symptoms. In addition, by occupying the receptor, it can prevent nicotine from acting, and thus can reduce the rewarding and reinforcement effects associated with nicotine. This may be particularly important in preventing a lapse from becoming a full relapse once abstinence has been achieved. Both of these effects are supported by evidence from clinical trials.[133–136] Varenicline consistently improves success in quitting compared to placebo by an effect of two- to fourfold.[97,136] In addition, head-to-head trials have demonstrated superiority compared to bupropion.[133,134] Fewer data compare varenicline to NRT, and a recent meta-analysis failed to show a difference, though superiority of varenicline could not be excluded.[136]

Varenicline is given orally. Usually medicine is started at 0.5-mg once daily for 3 days followed by 0.5-mg twice daily for 4 days and then 1-mg twice daily for 3 months. Individuals who have achieved abstinence at 3 months may have less relapse if therapy is continued for an additional 3 months. A quit date is usually recommended for 1 week after starting medication, but success has been reported with a broader window of quit dates from 1 to 5 weeks that was comparable to a fixed quit rate.[137,138] This increased flexibility may be an advantage in starting a quit attempt when patients are seen for problems other than smoking cessation.

The most common adverse reactions are nausea, insomnia, visual disturbances, syncope, and skin reactions. The incidence of nausea is reduced with the dose titration described above.[139] The most serious concerns with varenicline have been with psychiatric and cardiovascular side effects. Varenicline has the same boxed warning as bupropion, indicating that patients and their caregivers should be alerted to the possibility of neuropsychiatric symptoms, and patients should be monitored for changes in behavior, hostility, agitation, depressed mood, suicidal ideation, and suicide attempts.[131] However, clinical trials have failed to confirm psychiatric adverse effects, although they cannot be fully excluded.[140] A meta-analysis that reported significant increase in cardiovascular events[141] was felt to be methodologically flawed as it excluded studies with no events.[142] A subsequent meta-analysis that included all available studies found no difference between varenicline and placebo, although a small difference may be present.[142] Currently the FDA recommends that patients taking varenicline be alert for development of new or worsening symptoms of cardiovascular disease.[143] Varenicline has also been associated with accidental injuries from falls and vehicular accidents.[144] This has resulted in an FDA advisory regarding operating heavy machinery while using varenicline.[145]

Off-Label Agents

Clonidine Clonidine is an α-adrenergic agonist active in the CNS that is used to treat hypertension. A number of clinical trials have evaluated its efficacy in smoking cessation and have generally shown a trend toward benefit, although individual trials have generally not been statistically significant, and its use is supported by a meta-analysis.[146] The Department of Health and Human Services (DHHS) guidelines suggest it can be used by experienced practitioners comfortable with the drug.[97,99,100] Major adverse effects of clonidine are drowsiness, fatigue, dry mouth, and postural hypotension.

Nortriptyline Nortriptyline is a tricyclic antidepressant that has been evaluated for efficacy in smoking cessation in several studies. Both individual studies and meta-analyses support its benefit as an aid to smoking cessation,[128,147] and it is also recommended as a possible second-line agent for practitioners comfortable with its use by the DHHS guidelines.[97,99,100] Major adverse effects of nortriptyline include drowsiness and dry mouth. As with other tricyclics, CNS and cardiovascular effects, including arrhythmias, may occur.

Investigational Drugs

A number of other agents approved for other uses have also been assessed for smoking cessation. None are currently recommended off-label by established guidelines, although several are under investigation. These include topiramate, an antiseizure medication that has been evaluated for several addictions, including combined alcohol and tobacco addiction, and selegiline, an agent used as an adjunct in the treatment of Parkinson disease that has also shown promise in smoking cessation.[148] Several other agents have been assessed. Selective serotonin reuptake inhibitor (SSRI) antidepressants have been demonstrated to be without benefit.[128] Opiate antagonists and anxiolytics have generally been without benefit,[97,99,100,149] but buspirone remains controversial as studies have been mixed.

Nicotine vaccines are also under investigation. Antibodies can be made to nicotine, if it is presented bound to an appropriate carrier.[150,151] The antibodies then bind nicotine reversibly. By slowing the delivery of nicotine to the brain, the vaccine would distort the pharmacokinetics of a cigarette. These investigational agents may have utility for long-term relapse prevention or for prevention of smoking initiation. However, phase 3 trials have not shown clinical benefits to date.[150]

PRACTICAL CONCERNS DURING THE QUIT ATTEMPT

Approach

As noted above, the first step is to have a patient willing to make a quit attempt. Current practice is to optimize the chance for success with each attempt. In general this will be achieved with nonpharmacologic support combined with pharmacotherapy. The more active the nonpharmacologic support the greater the likelihood of success. Patients will vary, however, in the type of support they will accept. It is also important to select an appropriate pharmacotherapy. Many practitioners initiate treatment with NRT, because of greater experience and reduced potential for adverse effects. The "patch-plus" regimen that combines a transdermal system with an ad lib formulation is often recommended.[97,99,100,115] Bupropion may be more appropriate for individuals with a history of depression.[152] Varenicline has the greatest efficacy, but is often reserved for secondary attempts to induce a remission from smoking.[115] The quit date should be linked to the pharmacotherapy: generally this is 1 week after initiating bupropion or varenicline and on the same day as initiating NRT. Varenicline may offer some flexibility, with a quit date 1 to 5 weeks after starting treatment.[138] A follow-up visit should be scheduled about 10 days after initiating bupropion or varenicline to check for side effects. A follow-up in the immediate postquitting period is associated with improved success. This may be particularly important for cessation attempts that begin in hospital.[153]

Withdrawal Symptoms

The first 3 days of abstinence are usually the most difficult. Tobacco withdrawal symptoms (Table 41-2) generally peak during the first 72 hours then gradually subside over a 3- to 4-week period. These symptoms can include restlessness, anxiety, difficulty concentrating, irritability, frustration, depression, and an almost unrelenting craving for cigarettes. Common suggestions to help smokers cope with these

TABLE 41-2 Nicotine Withdrawal Symptoms (DSM-IV)

Dysphoric or depressed mood
Insomnia
Irritability, frustration, or anger
Anxiety
Difficulty concentrating
Restlessness
Decreased heart rate
Increased appetite or weight gain

early withdrawal symptoms in addition to NRT can include: (1) Be active. Increased activity may curtail some of the drive to smoke. (2) Use deep breathing exercises. The simplest breathing exercise involves nothing more than extended breath holding followed by slow exhalation through pursed lips. (3) Avoid high-risk situations for smoking during the first 3 weeks of quitting. (4) Use plenty of cinnamon gum or chewable candies. (5) Combat strong urges to smoke: The urge to smoke will go away whether one smokes or not.

Cravings

Of all the symptoms associated with nicotine withdrawal, cravings to smoke are the most persistent. Unlike the other symptoms, cravings can also recur long after abstinence is achieved. During the second and third weeks of abstinence, the craving waves usually occur less frequently, but can sometimes catch smokers off guard because of their unexpected intensity. The decrease in frequency is greater than the decrease in intensity, and cravings can be precipitated months and years after abstinence if precipitated by specific cues. In this context, cravings recapitulate, in some ways, the grief response. Relapse is commonly associated with concurrent alcohol consumption. It is likely that alcohol, and the associated situations in which it is consumed, serves both as a cue leading to craving and decreases the inhibitions that may prevent smoking. Ex-smokers should be aware of these moments of hazard.

Depression

At some time during the first 3 months of abstinence, some smokers may experience depression. For many this depression is mild and transient. For a small minority of smokers, quitting smoking may produce a clinical depression that may require antidepressant therapy, counseling, or return to smoking. Depressive symptoms are associated with relapse.[154]

Weight Gain

One of the most disheartening components of quitting smoking is weight gain.[97,99,100] Rapid weight gain is common during the first 6 to 8 weeks of cigarette abstinence. This is followed by a more gradual increase in weight to roughly 4-kg at 6 months. Average weight gain at 10 years following cessation is 4.4 and 5.0-kg for males and females, respectively. The health risks associated with postcessation weight gain are unknown but are likely surpassed by the health benefits of stopping smoking.

RISKS OF SMOKING CESSATION

Smoking cessation may be associated with some hazards in selected cases. Nicotine and other components of cigarette smoke may have a significant antidepressant effect, and many endogenously depressed individuals may have empirically found smoking helped alleviate their symptoms. Depression is a well-recognized manifestation of the nicotine withdrawal syndrome. At times, this depression can be of major clinical importance. Exacerbations of ulcerative colitis are more common in former smokers and may develop at times long after smoking cessation.[155] These potential adverse effects should not minimize the importance of smoking cessation, but the clinician should be prepared to address them when necessary. Anecdotal reports have suggested that asthma may worsen following cessation. However, smoking generally makes asthmatics worse[156] and induces resistance to the therapeutic effects of inhaled glucocorticoids. Thus, asthma symptoms generally improve with smoking cessation.[157] Some smokers report an increase in cough in the weeks following cessation. However, among individuals with chronic bronchitis, symptoms of cough and sputum production decrease dramatically in the months following cessation.[158,159]

SPECIAL POPULATIONS

Smoking cessation approaches for special populations are generally the same as for the general population.[97,99,100] Smoking cessation treatment can be started in hospital at the time of acute illness.[153] Success will be dependent on adequate follow-up and support. Interestingly, withdrawal symptoms may be particularly mild in hospital, perhaps because there are few options to smoke. Concurrent treatment of individuals hospitalized with psychiatric illness for smoking cessation can be successful and does not compromise treatment of the comorbid psychiatric problem.[97,99,100] Treatment of pregnant smokers has been extensively reviewed.[97,99,100]

Smoking is a major risk factor for COPD. All three approved forms of pharmacotherapy: NRT,[160] bupropion,[161] and varenicline[162] have demonstrated efficacy in the COPD population.

HARM REDUCTION

A more controversial approach for smokers who are unwilling or unable to quit at all, is that the health consequences may be partially addressed by reducing the exposure to smoke-derived toxins. This approach, termed "harm reduction," has been the subject of several reviews, including an Institute of Medicine report.[163,164] Four general categories of harm reduction are theoretically possible: (1) administration of agents to counteract the effects of cigarette smoking; (2) smoking reduction; (3) development of less toxic tobacco products; and (4) alternate nicotine delivery systems. It is important to recognize that clear health benefits have not been established for any of these approaches, however.

Since cigarette smoking is thought to cause its effects through pathogenetic mechanisms that are at least partially defined, it is appealing to use such mechanisms as targets for therapeutic intervention. In this regard, antioxidants to ameliorate the oxidant-induced injury caused by cigarette smoke, and protease inhibitors to bolster the antiprotease defenses are both potential therapies. While conceptually appealing, no data exist to suggest that any such approach is of benefit in continuing smokers.

Pharmacologic support may facilitate reduction in smoking. The observation that most smokers maintain a relatively constant nicotine intake creates the possibility that nicotine replacement can help sustain smoking reduction. Smoking reduction has also been achieved with several formulations of nicotine replacement, and there is some evidence for physiologic benefit. Short-term smoking reduction, facilitated with the use of nicotine polacrilex gum, was associated with improvements in lower respiratory tract inflammation assessed by bronchoscopy and bronchoalveolar lavage in a group of heavy smokers.[165,166] In patients with cardiac disease who reduced smoking, there were measurable improvements in cardiac function that were associated with improved oxygen delivery to the heart due to reduced carbon monoxide.[125]

Reducing the delivery of cigarette smoke toxins while still providing the smoker with a satisfactory cigarette has been pursued by some tobacco companies. This was a major motivation in the development of filtered cigarettes and of low-tar, low-nicotine cigarettes. Unfortunately these approaches do not reduce, and may actually increase, exposure to smoke-derived toxins. As most smokers maintain constant nicotine intake, many smokers compensate for altered smoke composition by simply smoking more or by changing the way in which they smoke each cigarette.[167,168] By causing an altered smoking strategy, filtered and low-yield cigarettes may actually deliver more toxins.

Many of the cigarette-derived toxins are generated as a result of pyrolysis.[25] As a result, tobacco products that do not burn have the promise to yield fewer toxins. Several cigarette-like devices have been developed with similar goals. Some burn small amounts of processed tobacco together with a carbon heat source to have a taste that more closely resembles a cigarette.[169] Others electrically heat the tobacco.

Whether the electronic cigarette will be effective as an alternative to smoking at present remains to be determined.[164] Because of its widespread use, the electronic cigarette has become particularly controversial. This has led to reviews and position statements relating to these products.[170,171] Potential harm-reduction products appear to deliver less toxins in standardized smoking regimes. However, limited data are available on physiologic effects. In one study, a reduction in lower respiratory tract inflammation and airway metaplasia was observed among heavy smokers who switched to a harm-reduction product.[172] Whether such products are associated with health benefits, however, remains to be determined.

Nonburned tobacco products may also have advantages. Moist snuff, which has low nitrosamine content due to its processing, has been widely used for several decades in Sweden. It has been associated with a measurable decrease in a number of tobacco-related diseases among Swedish men compared to cigarettes, but not compared to abstinence.[173–176]

Harm-reduction strategies may have unforeseen problems. Reduced-risk products, or smoking reduction strategies may encourage smokers to continue and thus discourage quit attempts. Available data, however, suggest the opposite. Smokers who switch to harm-reduction products or who reduce with pharmacologic support appear to have an increased rate of subsequent quits. It may be that the sense of mastery that comes with the reduction effort helps make smokers "able" to quit. There are other potential hazards. Reduced-risk products, for example, might be particularly appealing for individuals beginning smoking both because they may be easier to smoke and because they are not perceived as having significant risks. Finally, if use of reduced-risk products erodes the social climate that discourages smoking, such products could increase use of conventional cigarettes.

CONCLUSION

Cigarette smoking is a complex social and medical issue. The physician has a particularly important role in curbing smoking. Not only must the physician participate in efforts to reduce smoking as a citizen, but as a protector of public health and a possessor of specific expertise in healthcare matters, the physician must take an active role in health promotion. Such a role includes discouraging smoking initiation among younger patients, encouraging and assisting smoking patients to quit, and participating in social efforts designed to reduce smoking at various levels.

For individuals who are smokers, the clinician needs to approach smoking as a chronic relapsing disorder for which a range of effective treatments are available. These include nonpharmacologic and pharmacologic therapies and optimal results from a combined approach.

ACKNOWLEDGMENTS

The authors thank Ms. Lisa Hepp for assistance with prior drafts, Ms. Deborah A. R. Rennard for assistance in preparing this draft and Ms. Lillian Richards for secretarial support.

REFERENCES

1. Benowitz NL. Pharmacology of nicotine: addiction, smoking-induced disease, and therapeutics. Annu Rev Pharmacol Toxicol. 2009;49:57–71.
2. Benowitz NL. Nicotine addiction. N Engl J Med. 2010;362: 2295–2303.
3. Baldwin IT. An ecologically motivated analysis of plant-herbivore interactions in native tobacco. Plant Physiol. 2001;127: 1449–1458.
4. Fowler JS, Logan J, Wang GJ, Volkow ND. Monoamine oxidase and cigarette smoking. Neurotoxicology. 2003;24:75–82.
5. Chaudhri N, Caggiula AR, Donny EC, Palmatier MI, Liu X, Sved AF. Complex interactions between nicotine and nonpharmacological stimuli reveal multiple roles for nicotine in reinforcement. Psychopharmacology. 2006;184:353–366.
6. Davis JA, Gould TJ. Associative learning, the hippocampus, and nicotine addiction. *Curr Drug Abuse Rev.* 2008;1:9–19.
7. Myers MG, Gwaltney CJ, Strong DR, et al. Adolescent first lapse following smoking cessation: situation characteristics, precipitants and proximal influences. *Addict Behav.* 2011;36:1253–1260.
8. Mills AL, Messer K, Gilpin EA, Pierce JP. The effect of smoke-free homes on adult smoking behavior: a review. *Nicotine Tob Res.* 2009;11:1131–1141.
9. Henningfield JE, Miyasato K, Jasinski DR. Abuse liability and pharmacodynamic characteristics of intravenous and inhaled nicotine. *J Pharmacol Exp Ther.* 1985;234:1–12.
10. Pomerleau OF. Nicotine as a psychoactive drug: anxiety and pain reduction. *Psychopharmacol Bull.* 1986;22:865–869.
11. McClernon FJ, Hiott FB, Westman EC, Rose JE, Levin ED. Transdermal nicotine attenuates depression symptoms in nonsmokers: a double-blind, placebo-controlled trial. *Psychopharmacology.* 2006;189:125–133.
12. Heishman SJ, Kleykamp BA, Singleton EG. Meta-analysis of the acute effects of nicotine and smoking on human performance. *Psychopharmacology*. 2010;210:453–469.
13. Robert Barker, London, was the original publisher in 1604. The citation was found on line at the folloiwng URL www.laits.utexas.edu/poltheory/james/blaste/blaste.html.
14. U.S. Department of Health EaW. Smoking and health. Report of the advisory committee to the surgeon general of the public health service. 1964.
15. Gotti C, Clementi F. Neuronal nicotinic receptors: from structure to pathology. *Prog Neurobiol.* 2004;74:363–396.
16. Drenan RM, Lester HA. Insights into the neurobiology of the nicotinic cholinergic system and nicotine addiction from mice expressing nicotinic receptors harboring gain-of-function mutations. *Pharmacol Rev.* 2012;64:869–879.
17. Gotti C, Clementi F, Fornari A, et al. Structural and functional diversity of native brain neuronal nicotinic receptors. *Biochem Pharmacol.* 2009;78:703–711.
18. Changeux JP. Nicotine addiction and nicotinic receptors: lessons from genetically modified mice. *Nat Rev Neurosci.* 2010;11: 389–401.
19. Hajos M, Hurst RS, Hoffmann WE, et al. The selective alpha7 nicotinic acetylcholine receptor agonist pnu-282987 [n-[(3 r)-1-azabicyclo[2.2.2]oct-3-yl]-4-chlorobenzamide hydrochloride] enhances gabaergic synaptic activity in brain slices and restores auditory gating deficits in anesthetized rats. *J Pharmacol Exp Ther.* 2005;312:1213–1222.
20. Leslie FM, Mojica CY, Reynaga DD. Nicotinic receptors in addiction pathways. *Mol Pharmacol.* 2013;83:753–758.
21. Mansvelder HD, McGehee DS. Cellular and synaptic mechanisms of nicotine addiction. *J Neurobiol.* 2002;53:606–617.
22. Mansvelder HD, McGehee DS. Long-term potentiation of excitatory inputs to brain reward areas by nicotine. *Neuron.* 2000;27:349–357.
23. Slotkin TA, Ryde IT, Seidler FJ. Additive and synergistic effects of fetal nicotine and dexamethasone exposure on cholinergic synaptic function in adolescence and adulthood: implications for the adverse consequences of maternal smoking and pharmacotherapy of preterm delivery. *Brain Res Bull.* 2010;81:552–560.
24. Goriounova NA, Mansvelder HD. Short- and long-term consequences of nicotine exposure during adolescence for prefrontal

cortex neuronal network function. *Cold Spring Harb Perspect Med.* 2012;2:a012120.

25. Borgerding M, Klus H. Analysis of complex mixtures–cigarette smoke. *Exp Toxicol Pathol.* 2005;57(Suppl 1):43–73.
26. Henningfield JE, London ED, Benowitz NL. Arterial-venous differences in plasma concentrations of nicotine after cigarette smoking. *JAMA.* 1990;263:2049–2050.
27. Hukkanen J, Jacob P III, Benowitz NL. Metabolism and disposition kinetics of nicotine. *Pharmacol Rev.* 2005;57:79–115.
28. Heatherton TF, Kozlowski LT, Frecker RC, Fagerstrom K-O. The Fagerström Test for Nicotine Dependence: a revision of the Fagerström Tolerance Questionnaire. *Br J Addict.* 1991;86: 1119–1127.
29. Lessov-Schlaggar CN, Pergadia ML, Khroyan TV, Swan GE. Genetics of nicotine dependence and pharmacotherapy. *Biochem Pharmacol.* 2008;75:178–195.
30. Schnoll RA, Johnson TA, Lerman C. Genetics and smoking behavior. *Curr Psychiatry Rep.* 2007;9:349–357.
31. Ray R, Tyndale RF, Lerman C. Nicotine dependence pharmacogenetics: role of genetic variation in nicotine-metabolizing enzymes. *J Neurogenet.* 2009;23:252–261.
32. Tobacco and Genetics Consortium. Genome-wide meta-analyses identify multiple loci associated with smoking behavior. *Nat Genet.* 2010;42:441–447.
33. Pergadia ML, Agrawal A, Loukola A, et al. Genetic linkage findings for DSM-IV nicotine withdrawal in two populations. *Am J Med Genet B Neuropsychiatr Genet.* 2009;150B:950–959.
34. Liu JZ, Tozzi F, Waterworth DM, et al. Meta-analysis and imputation refines the association of 15q25 with smoking quantity. *Nat Genet.* 2010;42:436–440.
35. Siedlinski M, Cho MH, Bakke P, et al. Genome-wide association study of smoking behaviours in patients with COPD. *Thorax.* 2011;66:894–902.
36. Thorgeirsson TE, Geller F, Sulem P, et al. A variant associated with nicotine dependence, lung cancer and peripheral arterial disease. *Nature.* 2008;452:638–642.
37. Hung RJ, McKay JD, Gaborieau V, et al. A susceptibility locus for lung cancer maps to nicotinic acetylcholine receptor subunit genes on 15q25. *Nature.* 2008;452:633–637.
38. Amos CI, Wu X, Broderick P, et al. Genome-wide association scan of tag SNPs identifies a susceptibility locus for lung cancer at 15q25.1. *Nat Genet.* 2008;40:616–622.
39. Pillai SG, Ge D, Zhu G, et al. A genome-wide association study in chronic obstructive pulmonary disease (COPD): identification of two major susceptibility loci. *PLoS Genet.* 2009;5: e1000421.
40. Malaiyandi V, Sellers EM, Tyndale RF. Implications of cyp2a6 genetic variation for smoking behaviors and nicotine dependence. *Clin Pharmacol Ther.* 2005;77:145–158.
41. Carter B, Long T, Cinciripini P. A meta-analytic review of the cyp2a6 genotype and smoking behavior. *Nicotine Tob Res.* 2004;6: 221–227.
42. Fujieda M, Yamazaki H, Saito T, et al. Evaluation of cyp2a6 genetic polymorphisms as determinants of smoking behavior and tobacco-related lung cancer risk in male Japanese smokers. *Carcinogenesis.* 2004;25:2451–2458.
43. Kamataki T, Fujieda M, Kiyotani K, Iwano S, Kunitoh H. Genetic polymorphism of cyp2a6 as one of the potential determinants of tobacco-related cancer risk. *Biochem Biophys Res Commun.* 2005;338:306–310.
44. Minematsu N, Nakamura H, Iwata M, et al. Association of cyp2a6 deletion polymorphism with smoking habit and development of pulmonary emphysema. *Thorax.* 2003;58: 623–628.
45. Lerman C, Tyndale R, Patterson F, et al. Nicotine metabolite ratio predicts efficacy of transdermal nicotine for smoking cessation. *Clin Pharmacol Ther.* 2006;79:600–608.
46. O'Loughlin J, Paradis G, Kim W, et al. Genetically decreased cyp2a6 and the risk of tobacco dependence: a prospective study of novice smokers. *Tob Control.* 2004;13:422–428.
47. Guy EG, Fletcher PJ. Nicotine-induced enhancement of responding for conditioned reinforcement in rats: role of prior nicotine exposure and alpha4beta2 nicotinic receptors. *Psychopharmacology.* 2013;225:429–440.
48. Escobedo LG, Anda RF, Smith PF, Remington PL, Mast EE. Sociodemographic characteristics of cigarette smoking initiation in the United States. *JAMA.* 1990;264:1550–1555.
49. Dierker L, Swendsen J, Rose J, He J, Merikangas K. Transitions to regular smoking and nicotine dependence in the adolescent national comorbidity survey (ncs-a). *Ann Behav Med.* 2012;43: 394–401.
50. Gilpin EA, Lee L, Evans N, Pierce JP. Smoking initiation rates in adults and minors: United States, 1944–1988. *Am J Epidemiol.* 1994;140:535–543.
51. National Center for Chronic Disease Prevention and Health Promotion (US) Office on Smoking and Health. *Preventing Tobacco Use Among Youth and Young Adults: A Report of the Surgeon General.* Atlanta, GA: Centers for Disease Control and Prevention (US); 2012.
52. Freedman KS, Nelson NM, Feldman LL. Smoking initiation among young adults in the United States and Canada, 1998–2010: a systematic review. *Prev Chronic Dis.* 2012;9:E05.
53. Bernat DH, Klein EG, Forster JL. Smoking initiation during young adulthood: a longitudinal study of a population-based cohort. *J Adolesc Health.* 2012;51:497–502.
54. Fischer PM, Schwartz MP, Richards JW, Goldstein AO, Rojas TH. Brand logo recognition by children aged 3 to 6 years. *JAMA.* 1991;266:3145–3148.
55. Pierce JP, White VM, Emery SL. What public health strategies are needed to reduce smoking initiation? *Tob Control.* 2012;21:258–264.
56. Headen SW, Bauman KE, Deane GD, Koch GG. Are the correlates of cigarette smoking initiation different for black and white adolescents? *Am J Pub Health.* 1991;81:854–858.
57. Shiffman S. Tobacco "chippers"–individual differences in tobacco dependence. *Psychopharmacology.* 1989;97:539–547.
58. Shiffman S, Paty JA, Gnys M, Kassel JD, Elash C. Nicotine withdrawal in chippers and regular smokers: subjective and cognitive effects. *Health Psychol.* 1995;14:301–309.
59. Lasser K, Boyd JW, Woolhandler S, Himmelstein DU, McCormick D, Bor DH. Smoking and mental illness: a population-based prevalence study. *JAMA.* 2000;284:2606–2610.
60. Kalman D, Morissette SB, George TP. Co-morbidity of smoking in patients with psychiatric and substance use disorders. *Am J Addict.* 2005;14:106–123.
61. Myles N, Newall HD, Curtis J, Nielssen O, Shiers D, Large M. Tobacco use before, at, and after first-episode psychosis: a systematic meta-analysis. *J Clin Psychiatry.* 2012;73:468–475.
62. Benowitz NL, Jacob P III. Intravenous nicotine replacement suppresses nicotine intake from cigarette smoking. *J Pharmacol Exp Ther.* 1990;254:1000–1005.

63. Benowitz NL, Jacob P III, Kozlowski LT, Yu L. Influence of smoking fewer cigarettes on exposure to tar, nicotine, and carbon monoxide. *N Engl J Med.* 1986;315:1310–1313.

64. Benowitz NL, Jacob P III. Nicotine renal excretion rate influences nicotine intake during cigarette smoking. *J Pharmacol Exp Ther.* 1985;234:153–155.

65. Benowitz NL, Hall SM, Herning RI, Jacob PI, Jones RT, Osman AL. Smokers of low yield cigarettes do not consume less nicotine. *N Eng J Med.* 1983;309:139–142.

66. Daughton DM, Fix AJ, Roberts DE, Rennard SI. Sleep disturbance smoking: a tobacco addiction syndrome? *Am Rev Respir Dis.* 1988;137:A464.

67. Xian H, Scherrer JF, Madden PA, et al. Latent class typology of nicotine withdrawal: genetic contributions and association with failed smoking cessation and psychiatric disorders. *Psychol Med.* 2005;35:409–419.

68. Xian H, Scherrer JF, Madden PA, et al. The heritability of failed smoking cessation and nicotine withdrawal in twins who smoked and attempted to quit. *Nicotine Tob Res.* 2003;5:245–254.

69. Rostron B. Smoking-attributable mortality in the United States. *Epidemiology.* 2011;22:350–355.

70. Fenelon A, Preston SH. Estimating smoking-attributable mortality in the United States. *Demography.* 2012;49:797–818.

71. Mokdad AH, Marks JS, Stroup DF, Gerberding JL. Actual causes of death in the United States, 2000. *JAMA.* 2004;291:1238–1245.

72. Ezzati M, Lopez AD. Measuring the accumulated hazards of smoking: global and regional estimates for 2000. *Tob Control.* 2003;12:79–85.

73. Centers for Disease Control and Prevention (CDC). Consumption of cigarettes and combustible tobacco–United States, 2000–2011. *MMWR Morb Mortal Wkly Rep.* 2012;61:565–569.

74. Centers for Disease Control and Prevention (CDC). Current tobacco use among middle and high school students–United States, 2011. *MMWR Morb Mortal Wkly Rep.* 2012;61:581–585.

75. Centers for Disease Control and Prevention (CDC). Current cigarette smoking among adults - United States, 2011. *MMWR Morb Mortal Wkly Rep.* 2012;61:889–894.

76. Koop CE. A smoke-free society by the year 2000. *N Y State J Med.* 1985;85:290–292.

77. Centers for Disease Control. Healthy People 2010. 2011. http://www.cdc.gov/nchs/healthy_people/hp2010.htm.

78. Santi S, Best JA, Brown KS, Cargo M. Social environment and smoking initiation. *Int J Addict.* 1991;25:881–903.

79. Pierce JP, Lee L, Gilpin EA. Smoking initiation by adolescent girls, 1944 through 1988. *JAMA.* 1994;271:608–611.

80. Toll BA, Ling PM. The Virginia Slims identity crisis: an inside look at tobacco industry marketing to women. *Tob Control.* 2005;14:172–180.

81. Braun S, Mejia R, Ling PM, Perez-Stable EJ. Tobacco industry targeting youth in Argentina. *Tob Control.* 2008;17:111–117.

82. Gendall P, Hoek J, Thomson G, et al. Young adults' interpretations of tobacco brands: implications for tobacco control. *Nicotine Tob Res.* 2011;13:911–918.

83. Aloise-Young PA, Slater MD, Cruickshank CC. Mediators and moderators of magazine advertisement effects on adolescent cigarette smoking. *J Health Commun.* 2006;11:281–300.

84. Wiki. *Tobacco Master Settlement Agreement.* Wikipedia; 2013.

85. Johnston LD, O'Malley PM, Bachman JG, Schulenberg JE. *Monitoring the future national survey results on drug use.* University of Michigan; 2013;1975–2012.

86. Mercken L, Moore L, Crone MR, et al. The effectiveness of school-based smoking prevention interventions among low- and high-SES European teenagers. *Health Educ Res.* 2012;27: 459–469.

87. Aaron DJ, Dearwater SR, Anderson R, Olsen T, Kriska AM, Laporte RE. Physical activity and the initiation of high-risk health behaviors in adolescents. *Med Sci Sports Exerc.* 1995;27: 1639–1645.

88. Centers for Disease Control and Prevention (CDC). Estimates of retailers willing to sell tobacco to minors–California, August-September 1995 and June-July 1996. *MMWR Morb Mortal Wkly Rep.* 1996;45:1095–1099.

89. Jason LA, Ji PY, Anes MD, Birkhead SH. Active enforcement of cigarette control laws in the prevention of cigarette sales to minors. *JAMA.* 1991;266:3159–3161.

90. Fichtenberg CM, Glantz SA. Youth access interventions do not affect youth smoking. *Pediatrics.* 2002;109:1088–1092.

91. Rigotti NA, DiFranza JR, Chang Y, Tisdale T, Kemp B, Singer DE. The effect of enforcing tobacco-sales law on adolescents' access to tobacco and smoking behavior. *N Engl J Med.* 1997;337:1044–1051.

92. Bierer MF, Rigotti NA. Public policy for the control of tobacco-related disease. *Med Clin North Am.* 1992;76:515–539.

93. Chaloupka FJ, Straif K, Leon ME. Effectiveness of tax and price policies in tobacco control. *Tob Control.* 2011;20:235–238.

94. Sen A, Wirjanto T. Estimating the impacts of cigarette taxes on youth smoking participation, initiation, and persistence: empirical evidence from Canada. *Health Econ.* 2010;19:1264–1280.

95. Zhang B, Cohen J, Ferrence R, Rehm J. The impact of tobacco tax cuts on smoking initiation among Canadian young adults. *Am J Prev Med.* 2006;30:474–479.

96. Wilson LM, Avila Tang E, Chander G, et al. Impact of tobacco control interventions on smoking initiation, cessation, and prevalence: a systematic review. *J Environ Public Health.* 2012;2012:961724.

97. Fiore MC, Jae'n CR, Baker TB, et al. *Treating Tobacco Use and Dependence: 2008 Update. Clinical Practice Guideline.* Rockville, MD: US Department of Health and Human Services, Public Health Service; 2008.

98. Centers for Disease Control and Prevention (CDC). Cigarette smoking among adults and trends in smoking cessation – United States, 2008. *MMWR Morb Mortal Wkly Rep.* 2009;58:1227–1232.

99. Fiore MC, Bailey WC, Cohen SJ. *Smoking Cessation.* Guideline technical report no. 18. Rockville, MD: U.S. Department of health and human services, public health service, agency for health care policy and research. *Publication No AHCPR 97-Noo4, October 1997.* 1997.

100. Fiore M, Bailey W, Cohen S, et al. *Treating Tobacco Use and Dependence.* Rockville, MD: U.S. Department Of Health and Human Services; 2000.

101. Daughton DM, Susman J, Sitorius M, et al. Transdermal nicotine therapy and primary care: importance of counseling, demographic and patient selection factors on one-year quit rates. *Arch Fam Med.* 1998;7:425–430.

102. Gwaltney CJ, Metrik J, Kahler CW, Shiffman S. Self-efficacy and smoking cessation: a meta-analysis. *Psychol Addict Behav.* 2009;23:56–66.

103. Gulliver SB, Hughes JR, Solomon LJ, Dey AN. An investigation of self-efficacy, partner support and daily stresses as predictors of relapse to smoking in self-quitters. *Addiction.* 1995;90:767–772.

104. Prochaska JO, DiClemente CC. Stages of change in the modification of problem behaviors. *Prog Behav Modif.* 1992;28:183–218.

105. Niaura R. Nonpharmacologic therapy for smoking cessation: characteristics and efficacy of current approaches. *Am J Med.* 2008;121:S11–S19.

106. Borland R, Balmford J, Hunt D. The effectiveness of personally tailored computer-generated advice letters for smoking cessation. *Addiction.* 2004;99:369–377.

107. Houston TK, Coley HL, Sadasivam RS, et al. Impact of content-specific email reminders on provider participation in an online intervention: a dental PBRN study. *Stud Health Technol Inform.* 2010;160:801–805.

108. Stead LF, Perera R, Lancaster T. A systematic review of interventions for smokers who contact quitlines. *Tob Control.* 2007;16(Suppl 1):i3–i8.

109. Cinciripini PM, Wetter DW, McClure JB. Scheduled reduced smoking: effects on smoking abstinence and potential mechanisms of action. *Addict Behav.* 1997;22:759–767.

110. Hughes JR, Solomon LJ, Livingston AE, Callas PW, Peters EN. A randomized, controlled trial of NRT-aided gradual vs. abrupt cessation in smokers actively trying to quit. *Drug Alcohol Depend.* 2010;111:105–113.

111. Lindson-Hawley N, Aveyard P, Hughes JR. Reduction versus abrupt cessation in smokers who want to quit. *Cochrane Database Syst Rev.* 2012;11:CD008033.

112. Tahiri M, Mottillo S, Joseph L, Pilote L, Eisenberg MJ. Alternative smoking cessation aids: a meta-analysis of randomized controlled trials. *Am J Med.* 2012;125: 576–584.

113. Barnes J, Dong CY, McRobbie H, Walker N, Mehta M, Stead LF. Hypnotherapy for smoking cessation. *Cochrane Database Syst Rev.* 2010;(10):CD001008.

114. White AR, Rampes H, Liu JP, Stead LF, Campbell J. Acupuncture and related interventions for smoking cessation. *Cochrane Database Syst Rev.* 2011;(1):CD000009.

115. Rennard SI, Rigotti NA, Daughton DM. Pharmacotherapy for smoking cessation in adults. *UpToDate*; 2013.

116. Hajek P, West R, Foulds J, Nilsson F, Burrows S, Meadow A. Randomized comparative trial of nicotine polacrilex, a transdermal patch, nasal spray, and an inhaler. *Arch Intern Med.* 1999;159:2033–2038.

117. Rigotti NA. Clinical practice. Treatment of tobacco use and dependence. *N Engl J Med.* 2002;346:506–512.

118. Bohadana A, Nilsson F, Rasmussen T, Martinet Y. Nicotine inhaler and nicotine patch as a combination therapy for smoking cessation: a randomized, double-blind, placebo-controlled trial. *Arch Intern Med.* 2000;160:3128–3134.

119. Schneider NG, Cortner C, Gould JL, Koury MA, Olmstead RE. Comparison of craving and withdrawal among four combination nicotine treatments. *Human Psychopharmacol.* 2008;23:513–517.

120. Killen JD, Fortmann SP, Newman B, Varady A. Evaluation of a treatment approach combining nicotine gum with self-guided behavioral treatments for smoking relapse prevention. *J Consult Clin Psychol.* 1990;58:85–92.

121. Dautzenberg B, Nides M, Kienzler JL, Callens A. Pharmacokinetics, safety and efficacy from randomized controlled trials of 1 and 2 mg nicotine bitartrate lozenges (nicotinell). *BMC Clin Pharmacol.* 2007;7:11.

122. Smith SS, McCarthy DE, Japuntich SJ, et al. Comparative effectiveness of 5 smoking cessation pharmacotherapies in primary care clinics. *Arch Intern Med.* 2009;169:2148–2155.

123. Pickworth WB, Bunker EB, Henningfield JE. Transdermal nicotine: reduction of smoking with minimal abuse liability. *Psychoparmacology.* 1994;115:9–14.

124. Nicotine replacement therapy for patients with coronary artery disease. Working group for the study of transdermal nicotine in patients with coronary artery disease. *Arch Intern Med.* 1994;154: 989–995.

125. Mahmarian JJ, Moye LA, Nasser GA. Nicotine patch therapy in smoking cessation reduces the extent of exercise-induced myocardial ischemia. *J Am Coll Cardiol.* 1997;30:125–130.

126. Joseph AM, Norma SM, Ferry LH. The safety of transdermal nicotine as an aid to smoking cessation in patients with cardiac disease. *N Engl J Med.* 1996;335:1792–1798.

127. Piper ME, Smith SS, Schlam TR, Fiore MC, Jorenby DE, Fraser D, Baker TB. A randomized placebo-controlled clinical trial of 5 smoking cessation pharmacotherapies. *Arch Gen Psychiatry.* 2009;66:1253–1262.

128. Hughes JR, Stead LF, Lancaster T. Antidepressants for smoking cessation. *Cochrane Database Syst Rev.* 2007(1):CD000031.

129. Hurt RD, Sachs DP, Glover ED, et al. A comparison of sustained-release bupropion and placebo for smoking cessation. *N Engl J Med.* 1997;337:1195–1202.

130. Swan GE, McAfee T, Curry SJ, et al. Effectiveness of bupropion sustained release for smoking cessation in a health care setting: a randomized trial. *Arch Intern Med.* 2003;163:2337–2344.

131. US Food and Drug Administration. The smoking cessation aids varenicline (marketed as chantix) and bupropion (marketed as zyban and generics): suicidal ideation and behavior. *FDA Drug Saf Newslett.* 2009;2:1–4. http://www.fda.gov/downloads/Drugs/DrugSafety/DrugSafetyNewsletter/ucm107318.pdf.

132. Coe JW, Brooks PR, Vetelino MG, et al. Varenicline: an alpha-4beta2 nicotinic receptor partial agonist for smoking cessation. *J Med Chem.* 2005;48:3474–3477.

133. Gonzales D, Rennard SI, Nides M, et al. Varenicline, an alpha-4beta2 nicotinic acetylcholine receptor partial agonist, vs sustained-release bupropion and placebo for smoking cessation: a randomized controlled trial. *JAMA.* 2006;296:47–55.

134. Jorenby DE, Hays JT, Rigotti NA, et al. Efficacy of varenicline, an alpha4beta2 nicotinic acetylcholine receptor partial agonist, vs placebo or sustained-release bupropion for smoking cessation: a randomized controlled trial. *JAMA.* 2006;296:56–63.

135. Tonstad S, Tonnesen P, Hajek P, Williams KE, Billing CB, Reeves KR. Effect of maintenance therapy with varenicline on smoking cessation: a randomized controlled trial. *JAMA.* 2006;296:64–71.

136. Cahill K, Stead LF, Lancaster T. Nicotine receptor partial agonists for smoking cessation. *Cochrane Database Syst Rev.* 2012;4:CD006103.

137. Hughes JR, Russ CI, Arteaga CE, Rennard SI. Efficacy of a flexible quit date versus an a priori quit date approach to smoking cessation: a cross-study analysis. *Addict Behav.* 2011;36:1288–1291.

138. Rennard S, Hughes J, Cinciripini PM, et al. A randomized placebo-controlled trial of varenicline for smoking cessation allowing flexible quit dates. *Nicotine Tobacco Res.* 2012;14:343–350.

139. Oncken C, Gonzales D, Nides M, et al. Efficacy and safety of the novel selective nicotinic acetylcholine receptor partial agonist, varenicline, for smoking cessation. *Arch Intern Med.* 2006;166:1571–1577.

140. Gunnell D, Irvine D, Wise L, Davies C, Martin RM. Varenicline and suicidal behaviour: a cohort study based on data from the general practice research database. *BMJ.* 2009;339:b3805.

141. Singh S, Loke YK, Spangler JG, Furberg CD. Risk of serious adverse cardiovascular events associated with varenicline: a systematic review and meta-analysis. *CMAJ*. 2011;183:1359–1366.

142. Prochaska JJ, Hilton JF. Risk of cardiovascular serious adverse events associated with varenicline use for tobacco cessation: systematic review and meta-analysis. *BMJ*. 2012;344:e2856.

143. FDA. *FDA Drug Safety Communication: Safety Review Update of Chantix (varenicline) and Risk of Cardiovascular Adverse Events*. Rockville, MD: US Food and Drug Administration; 2012. http://www.fda.gov/Drugs/DrugSafety/ucm330367.htm.

144. Moore TJ, Cohen MR, Furberg CD. *Strong Safety Signal Seen for New Varenicline Risks*. Institute for Safe Medicine Practices; Horsham, PA 2008.

145. FDA. Http://www.Fda.Gov/drugs/drugsafety/drugsafetypodcasts/ucm077547.Htm. 2008, accessed June 30, 2013.

146. Gourlay SG, Stead LF, Benowitz NL. Clonidine for smoking cessation. *Cochrane Database Syst Rev*. 2004;(3):CD000058.

147. Stead LF, Lancaster T. Combined pharmacotherapy and behavioural interventions for smoking cessation. *Cochrane Database Syst Rev*. 2012;10:CD008286.

148. Anthenelli RM, Blom TJ, McElroy SL, Keck PE Jr. Preliminary evidence for gender-specific effects of topiramate as a potential aid to smoking cessation. *Addiction*. 2008;103:687–694.

149. David S, Lancaster T, Stead LF, Evins AE. Opioid antagonists for smoking cessation. *Cochrane Database Syst Rev*. 2006;(4):CD003086.

150. Hatsukami DK, Jorenby DE, Gonzales D, et al. Immunogenicity and smoking-cessation outcomes for a novel nicotine immunotherapeutic. *Clin Pharmacol Ther*. 2011;89:392–399.

151. Fahim RE, Kessler PD, Kalnik MW. Therapeutic vaccines against tobacco addiction. *Expert Rev Vaccines*. 2013;12: 333–342.

152. Jorenby DE, Leischow SJ, Nides MA, et al. A controlled trial of sustained-release bupropion, a nicotine patch, or both for smoking cessation. *New Engl J Med*. 1999;340:685–691.

153. Rigotti NA, Clair C, Munafo MR, Stead LF. Interventions for smoking cessation in hospitalised patients. *Cochrane Database Syst Rev*. 2012;5:CD001837.

154. Allen SS, Hatsukami DK, Christianson D. Nicotine withdrawal and depressive symptomatology during short-term smoking abstinence: a comparison of postmenopausal women using and not using hormone replacement therapy. *Nicotine Tob Res*. 2003;5:49–59.

155. Higuchi LM, Khalili H, Chan AT, Richter JM, Bousvaros A, Fuchs CS. A prospective study of cigarette smoking and the risk of inflammatory bowel disease in women. *Am J Gastroenterol*. 2012;107:1399–1406.

156. Broekema M, ten Hacken NH, Volbeda F, et al. Airway epithelial changes in smokers but not in ex-smokers with asthma. *Am J Respir Crit Care Med*. 2009;180:1170–1178.

157. Polosa R, Thomson NC. Smoking and asthma: dangerous liaisons. *Eur Respir J*. 2013;41:716–726.

158. Buist AS, Sexton GJ, Nagy JM, Ross BB. The effect of smoking cessation and modification on lung function. *Am Rev Respir Dis*. 1976;114:115–122.

159. Swan GE, Hodgkin JE, Roby T, Mittman C, Jacobo N, Peters J. Reversibility of airways injury over a 12-month period following smoking cessation. *Chest*. 1992;101:607–612.

160. Anthonisen NR, Connett JE, Kiley JP, et al. Effects of smoking intervention and the use of an inhaled anticholinergic bronchodilator on the rate of decline of FEV1. The Lung Health Study. *JAMA*. 1994;272:1497–1505.

161. Tashkin D, Kanner R, Bailey W, et al. Smoking cessation in patients with chronic obstructive pulmonary disease: a double-blind, placebo-controlled, randomised trial. *Lancet*. 2001;357:1571–1575.

162. Tashkin DP, Rennard S, Hays JT, Ma W, Lawrence D, Lee TC. Effects of varenicline on smoking cessation in patients with mild to moderate COPD: a randomized controlled trial. *Chest*. 2011;139:591–599.

163. Clearing. *Clearing the Smoke: Assessing the Science Base for Tobacco Harm Reduction*. Washington, D.C.: National Academy Press; 2001.

164. Rodu B. The scientific foundation for tobacco harm reduction, 2006–2011. *Harm Reduct J*. 2011;8:19.

165. Rennard SI, Daughton D, Fujita J, et al. Short-term smoking reduction is associated with reduction in measures of lower respiratory tract inflammation in heavy smokers. *Eur Respir J*. 1990;3:752–759.

166. Millatmal T, Daughton D, Thompson AB, et al. Smoking reduction: an alternative approach for smokers who cannot quit. *Monaldi Arch Chest Dis*. 1994;49:421–424.

167. Jarvis MJ, Boreham R, Primatesta P, Feyerabend C, Bryant A. Nicotine yield from machine-smoked cigarettes and nicotine intakes in smokers: evidence from a representative population survey. *J Natl Cancer Inst*. 2001;93:134–138.

168. Strasser AA, Lerman C, Sanborn PM, Pickworth WB, Feldman EA. New lower nicotine cigarettes can produce compensatory smoking and increased carbon monoxide exposure. *Drug Alcohol Depend*. 2007;86:294–300.

169. RJ Reynolds Tobacco Company. *New Cigarette Prototypes that Heat Instead of Burn Tobacco*. Winston-Salem, NC: RJ Reynolds Tobacco Company; 1988.

170. Schraufnagel DE, Blasi F, Drummond MB, Lam DC, Latif E, Rosen MJ, Sansores R, Van Zyl-Smit R. Electronic cigarettes. A position statement of the forum of international respiratory societies. *Am J Respir Crit Care Med*. 2014;190:611–618.

171. Drummond MB, Upson D. Electronic cigarettes. Potential harms and benefits. *Annals of the American Thoracic Society*. 2014;11:236–242.

172. Rennard SI, Umino T, Millatmal T, et al. Evaluation of subclinical respiratory tract inflammation in heavy smokers who switch to a cigarette-like nicotine delivery device that primarily heats tobacco. *Nicotine Tob Res*. 2002;4:467–476.

173. Hansson J, Galanti MR, Hergens MP, et al. Use of snus and acute myocardial infarction: pooled analysis of eight prospective observational studies. *Eur J Epidemiol*. 2012;27: 771–779.

174. Nordenvall C, Nilsson PJ, Ye W, Andersson TM, Nyren O. Tobacco use and cancer survival: a cohort study of 40,230 Swedish male construction workers with incident cancer. *Int J Cancer*. 2013;132:155–161.

175. Arefalk G, Hergens MP, Ingelsson E, et al. Smokeless tobacco (snus) and risk of heart failure: results from two Swedish cohorts. *Eur J Prev Cardiol*. 2012;19:1120–1127.

176. Lee PN. Summary of the epidemiological evidence relating snus to health. *Regul Toxicol Pharmacol*. 2011;59:197–214.

CHAPTER 42

Course and Treatment of Chronic Obstructive Pulmonary Disease

M. Bradley Drummond
Robert A. Wise

In past decades, the treatment of chronic obstructive pulmonary disease (COPD) has been approached by many physicians and patients alike with a nihilistic attitude, assuming that the disease was progressive, incurable, and untreatable. More recently, as our understanding of the clinical epidemiology and value of therapy of COPD has improved, this attitude has changed. Physicians have come to approach COPD in the same way as other chronic diseases, such as diabetes, rheumatoid arthritis, and coronary artery disease. With modern comprehensive treatment, the diagnosis of COPD is compatible with prolonged survival, good quality of life, and independent functional status for many who have this illness. The purpose of this chapter is to summarize the current understanding of the course of COPD and best approaches to treatment.

OVERVIEW OF COPD

COPD is a disorder that is characterized by slow emptying of the lung during a forced expiration. In practice, this is measured as the forced expiratory volume in 1 second/forced vital capacity (FEV_1/FVC) ratio, and the arbitrary definition of airflow obstruction is generally taken to be an FEV_1/FVC ratio lower than 0.70.[1] Because the rate of emptying of the lung falls with advancing age, many elderly individuals demonstrate airflow obstruction even in the absence of a clinical diagnosis of COPD. For this reason, an alternative criterion to define airflow obstruction incorporates lower limit of normal thresholds instead of the fixed ratio criteria.[2] Several disorders cause chronic airflow obstruction—long-standing asthma, cystic fibrosis, bronchiectasis, bronchiolitis obliterans, lymphangioleiomyomatosis, panbronchiolitis, silicosis, Sjögren syndrome, and diffuse interstitial processes such as eosinophilic granuloma and sarcoidosis. The diagnosis of COPD is usually limited to individuals who have chronic airflow obstruction associated with tobacco smoke or some other noxious inhalant, and it is usually not difficult to distinguish it from other causes of chronic airflow obstruction. The most commonly associated clinical disorders associated with COPD are emphysema and chronic bronchitis. *Emphysema* is defined anatomically by airspace enlargement due to disappearance of alveolar septae (see Chapter 39). This leads to the characteristic loss of elastic recoil, which, in turn, causes slowing of airflow from the lungs, hyperinflation, and air trapping (see Chapter 40). *Chronic bronchitis* is characterized by chronic cough and sputum production, which is present in about one out of three people with early COPD. Chronic cough and sputum production in cigarette smokers is often, but not always, associated with chronic airflow obstruction. When chronic mucus hypersecretion is associated with airflow obstruction, it is often called *chronic obstructive bronchitis*. The anatomic correlates of chronic bronchitis are mucus gland hyperplasia and goblet cell metaplasia in large- and medium-sized airways.[3] Patients with COPD also have *small- and medium-sized airway involvement* with inflammation, narrowing, tortuosity, mucus plugging, and fibrosis that contributes to the airflow limitation. As the disease evolves, there is obliteration of small airways. Some patients with a long-standing history of asthma develop airflow obstruction that is not completely reversible, episodes of cough and wheeze, and chronic sputum production. These individuals are often classified as having *chronic asthmatic bronchitis* and tend to have a somewhat better prognosis for survival than those with typical tobacco-related COPD. Physicians have a tendency to classify women as having asthma and men as having COPD despite similar medical histories.

NATURAL HISTORY OF COPD

COPD results from an increase in the rate of decline in lung function over time. Normal nonsmoking adults lose FEV_1 at a rate of 30 mL/yr, thought to be the consequence of the aging-related loss of elastic recoil of the lung. Persons who develop COPD may start in early adulthood with lower levels of lung function and also have increased rates of decline.[4,5] Studies of patients with COPD show an average annual decline in FEV_1 of 45 to 69 mL/yr (Fig. 42-1A). However, there may be considerable heterogeneity between patients and over time.[6,7] This leads to the insidious loss of ventilatory reserve capacity that often is asymptomatic and unrecognized by patients and physicians alike. Chronic bronchitis may be dismissed as an innocent "smoker's cough" because patients fail to understand that it is abnormal to produce daily sputum. As ventilatory reserve decreases, people with mild COPD tend to limit strenuous activities, so breathlessness with activities of daily living is not ordinarily an early symptom of the disease. When the ventilatory reserve decreases to the extent that mild exertion such as climbing stairs, bed making, or carrying groceries is limited, patients tend to seek medical advice. In some cases, the first clinical presentation of disease is an acute episode of bronchospasm, dyspnea, or even respiratory failure in association with a respiratory infection or exposure to respiratory irritants. Thus, the onset of COPD may appear precipitous even though it is the cumulative result of decades of progression.

People who discontinue smoking with mild to moderate degrees of airflow obstruction cease the rapid decline in FEV_1, and have better survival (Fig. 42-1B).[8] The improvement in survival depends largely upon the stage of disease. Persons who quit smoking with earlier disease have better outcomes compared with those who continue to smoke or those who quit smoking later in the disease. Once the disease is advanced, the inflammatory response persists and the proportional loss of lung function tends to progress. Because there are many years of asymptomatic decline in lung function, it is possible to diagnose COPD with forced expiratory spirometry before the disease is apparent and implement aggressive smoking intervention programs. There is a consensus that smokers with respiratory symptoms should be tested for COPD with spirometry. However, there is debate whether it is of value to screen for COPD among all cigarette smokers.[9] Opponents of using spirometry for case-finding argue that the finding of a normal test would not alter physician behavior because all smokers should be encouraged to quit. It has also been argued that a normal spirometry test might provide a false sense of complacency for active smokers. Those who support the use of spirometry for COPD case-finding argue that early detection and aggressive smoking intervention have been proved to halt disease progression and improve survival, and the finding of abnormal spirometry may encourage patients and healthcare professionals to be more aggressive with smoking cessation. Moreover, some evidence points to the benefits of drug therapy in terms of lung function decline and survival in patients with mild to moderate airflow obstruction.[10–12] While these data arise from post hoc analysis, the findings are promising.

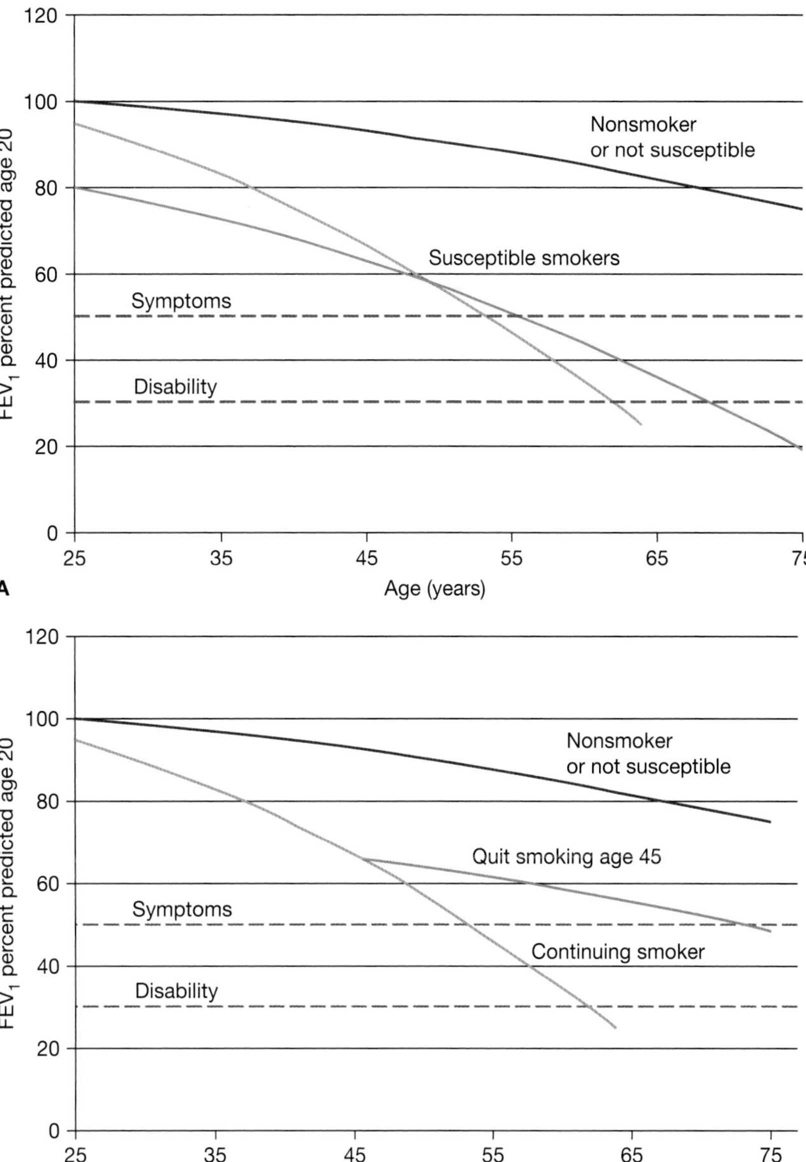

Figure 42-1 **A.** The natural history of COPD is presented for three hypothetical individuals. Pulmonary function is plotted as the percent of predicted lung function for a young adult who has attained maximal lung growth. Those who do not smoke, or are not susceptible to cigarette smoke typically lose about 25% of their young adult lung function throughout life. Individuals are susceptible to the adverse effects of smoking because of increased decline of lung function, or low lung function in young adult life. Although the abnormality of lung function is detectable for many years, symptoms do not develop until there is loss of approximately 50% of lung function *(upper dashed line)*, which occurs in middle age or later. If the disease progresses, it may lead to substantial disability within a decade of the onset of symptoms *(lower dashed line)*. **B.** The natural history of COPD is displayed for a hypothetical continuing smoker, and an individual who quit smoking at age 45. The axes are identical to those in (**A**). If an individual ceases smoking in the asymptomatic phase of COPD, the rate of decline of lung function reverts toward normal. In this example, the detection of abnormal lung function and cessation of smoking has a substantial effect of delaying the onset of respiratory symptoms. This plot is modified from the work of Fletcher and Peto and is commonly referred to as Fletcher curves. *(Reproduced with permission from Fletcher C, Peto R. The natural history of chronic airflow obstruction. Br Med J. 1977;1(6077):1645–1648.)*

With the progression of COPD comes progressive exercise limitation.[13] This is due to the increased work of breathing as ventilation increases with exercise. With increased respiratory rate, patients develop dynamic hyperinflation—a condition in which the end-expiratory lung volume does not return to the static end-expiratory volume of functional residual capacity (FRC). The hyperinflation that occurs causes increased work of breathing and exacerbates dyspnea. An indicator of dynamic hyperinflation is the inspiratory capacity (IC), which progressively falls with increasing ventilation. Measures that reduce dynamic hyperinflation, increasing IC, can improve exercise capacity. These include alterations in breathing pattern, oxygen supplementation, and use of inhaled bronchodilators.

As COPD progresses, ventilation–perfusion inhomogeneity causes an increase in the alveolar–arterial oxygen difference. Eventually, alveolar hypoxemia leads to pulmonary hypertension, which becomes manifested as cor pulmonale. The alveolar hypoxemia may be compounded by alveolar hypoventilation—manifested by arterial hypercapnia. Physical findings indicative of cor pulmonale are venous engorgement, edema, and physical findings of pulmonary hypertension and right ventricular failure including accentuated pulmonic second heart sound, right ventricular heave, tricuspid regurgitation murmur, hepatojugular reflux, and ascites. Chest imaging shows central enlargement of the pulmonary arteries. Once cor pulmonale is clinically apparent, survival is markedly reduced in proportion to the elevation of pulmonary artery pressure. Chronic respiratory failure is defined by chronic hypoxemia (sea-level resting Pa_{O_2} ≤60 mm Hg or 8 kPa) with or without attendant hypercapnia (Pa_{CO_2} >45 mm Hg).

Patients with advanced COPD may restrict their activities to a bed-and-chair lifestyle because of severe exercise incapacitation. This limitation can lead to social isolation, depression, and skeletal muscle deconditioning, which, in turn, further restrict activity and impair quality of life. Protein and calorie malnutrition occurs as the consequence of impaired nutritional intake caused by dyspnea.[14] Malnutrition is augmented by increased metabolic demands caused by increased basal oxygen consumption, inefficient skeletal muscle oxygen utilization, and cachexia-producing cytokines such as tumor necrosis factor-α (TNF-α).[15]

DIAGNOSIS OF COPD

Physical examination and chest imaging are insensitive methods for diagnosis of COPD. Physical findings of hyperinflated lungs such as low-lying diaphragm, decreased breath sounds, and hyperresonant chest percussion are highly specific for COPD, but usually only in

TABLE 42-1 Conditions Suggesting α1-Antitrypsin Deficiency

Early-onset emphysema (age under 45 yr)
Emphysema in a nonsmoker
Emphysema predominantly in lung bases (panacinar)
Necrotizing panniculitis (Weber–Christian disease)
c-ANCA positive vasculitis (e.g., Wegener granulomatosis)
Family history of early-onset emphysema or non–smoking-related emphysema
Bronchiectasis without other etiology

advanced disease.[16] One study has suggested that a distance between the thyroid cartilage and the sternal notch less than 4 cm in a smoker older than age 45 is highly indicative of the presence of COPD.[17] Clubbing of the fingers is rare in COPD and, if present, suggests another diagnosis such as bronchiectasis, asbestosis, or lung cancer. High-resolution computed tomography (HRCT) of the lung is useful in establishing the presence of emphysema. Quantitative analysis of HRCT is a promising technique for early detection of emphysema. α_1-Antitrypsin deficiency is an uncommon, but not rare, condition associated with premature emphysema. Testing for α_1-antitrypsin deficiency is indicated in those most likely to have the disorder (see Chapter 40 and Table 42-1). Some experts advise that all patients with COPD should be tested for α_1-antitrypsin deficiency because treatments are available for those with the most severe form of deficiency.[18] HIV/AIDS is also associated with premature emphysema and accelerated lung function decline,[19,20] and screening for HIV should be performed for persons with emphysema and HIV risk factors such as intravenous drug use or high-risk sexual activity.

The diagnosis of COPD, classification of its severity, and progression of the disease can be monitored with spirometry, a simple, noninvasive, and inexpensive test. The FEV_1/FVC ratio, reflecting the rate of emptying of the lung, is used to define the presence of an obstructive ventilatory defect, commonly defined as a ratio less than 0.70 or below the lower limit of normal. Once airflow obstruction is established, the severity of the airflow limitation is classified by the reduction of FEV_1 compared with a healthy reference population. Table 42-2 shows the widely used GOLD classification of severity based on the FEV_1. Lung volume measurements, by plethysmography, helium dilution, nitrogen washout, or single-breath methods typically show hyperinflation (elevated TLC) and air trapping (elevated residual volume [RV]), and thus are useful to exclude restrictive lung diseases. The carbon

TABLE 42-2 Classification of Severity of Airflow Limitation in COPD

GOLD Classification	Characteristics
I Mild COPD[a]	$FEV_1 \geq 80\%$ predicted
II Moderate COPD[a]	FEV_1 50–79% predicted
III Severe COPD[a]	FEV_1 30–49% predicted
IV Very severe COPD[a]	$FEV_1 < 30\%$ predicted or $< 50\%$ predicted with room air Pa_{O_2} < 60 mm Hg (8.0 kPa)

[a]*Postbronchodilator FEV_1/FVC less than or equal to 0.70.*
Source: Data from the 2011GOLD COPD guidelines, www.goldcopd.com; Celli BR, MacNee W. ATS/ERS Task Force. Standards for the diagnosis and treatment of patients with COPD: A summary of the ATS/ERS position paper. Eur Respir J. 2004;23(6):932–946.

TABLE 42-3 Modified Medical Research Council Dyspnea Scale (mMRC Scale)

Grade	Description
0	Not troubled with breathlessness except with strenuous exercise
1	Troubled by shortness of breath when hurrying on the level or walking up a slight hill
2	Walks slower than people of the same age on the level because of breathlessness or has to stop for breath when walking at own pace on the level
3	Stops for breath after walking about 100 yards or after a few minutes on the level
4	Too breathless to leave the house or breathless when dressing or undressing

Source: Data from Celli BR, MacNee W. ATS/ERS Task Force. Standards for the diagnosis and treatment of patients with COPD: A summary of the ATS/ERS position paper. Eur Respir J. 2004;23(6):932–946.

monoxide diffusing capacity (D_{CO}) is an indicator of emphysema and is roughly inversely correlated with the anatomic extent of emphysema in patients who have an FEV_1 greater than 1.0 L.

CLASSIFICATION OF COPD

Classification of COPD involves determination of symptoms and assessment of risk. Symptoms are determined using standardized questionnaires (**see** Table 42-3 and **www.catsonline.org**), while risk assessment is defined by severity of ventilatory limitation and exacerbation history. Based on symptoms and risk of exacerbations, individuals are grouped into one of four different patient categories (see Fig. 42-2). The categories are informative for determining prognosis and treatment of COPD. Additional instruments are available for quantifying the impact of COPD.[21]

PROGNOSIS OF COPD

The prognosis in COPD may vary widely. Physicians are poor prognosticators of survival in COPD.[22] In part, this is because the disease is one of widely varying rates of progression, and, in part because death is often due to susceptibility to intercurrent illness and other smoking-related illness such as lung cancer rather than progressive respiratory failure. Recent studies have demonstrated heterogeneity in lung function decline, with some patients with COPD having little or no decline in FEV_1 over time.[6,7]

Several factors have been identified that predict poor survival in COPD. These include low FEV_1, active smoking status, hypoxemia, poor nutrition, the presence of cor pulmonale, resting tachycardia, low exercise capacity, severe dyspnea, poor health–related quality of life, anemia, frequent exacerbations, comorbid illnesses, and low D_{CO}.[23] Patients with an FEV_1 less than 35% predicted have about 10% mortality per year.[24] If a patient reports that they are unable to walk 100 m without stopping because of breathlessness, the 5-year survival is only 30%.[25] A multidimensional prognostic index that takes into account several indicators of COPD prognosis is the BODE index (*b*ody mass index [BMI], *o*bstructive ventilatory defect severity, *d*yspnea severity, and *e*xercise capacity).[26] See Table 42-4 for calculation of the BODE prognostic score. The components are derived from measures of the BMI (weight in kg/height m^2), FEV_1 percent predicted, and the modified Medical Research Council dyspnea score (Table 42-3). A BODE score greater than 7 is associated with a 30% 2-year mortality; whereas a score of 5 to 6 is associated with 15% 2-year mortality. If the BODE score is less than 5, the 2-year mortality is less than 10%. In settings where the 6-minute

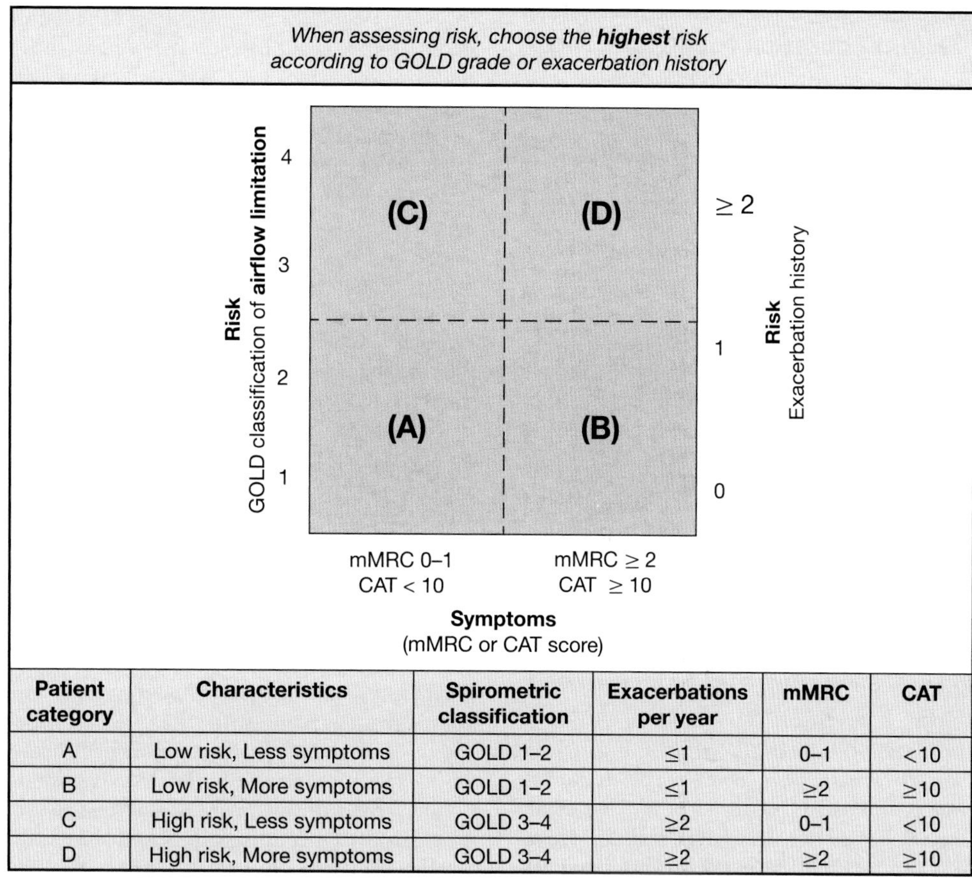

Patient category	Characteristics	Spirometric classification	Exacerbations per year	mMRC	CAT
A	Low risk, Less symptoms	GOLD 1–2	≤1	0–1	<10
B	Low risk, More symptoms	GOLD 1–2	≤1	≥2	≥10
C	High risk, Less symptoms	GOLD 3–4	≥2	0–1	<10
D	High risk, More symptoms	GOLD 3–4	≥2	≥2	≥10

Figure 42-2 Combined COPD assessment. An understanding of the impact of COPD on an individual patient combines assessment of symptoms and future risk of exacerbation. To use this figure, first assess symptoms with the modified medical research council (mMRC) or COPD assessment test (CAT) scale and determine if the patient has less symptoms (mMRC <2 or CAT <10) or more symptoms (mMRC ≥2 or CAT ≥10). Next, assess the risk of future exacerbation by determining prior exacerbation history and severity of airflow limitation with high risk of future exacerbation in individuals with GOLD airflow classification 3 to 4 or ≥2 exacerbations in the prior year (future risk should be determined by the method indicating higher risk). With this figure, individuals are stratified into one of four categories (A, B, C, D). which helps describe the burden of disease and informs potential treatments. *(Reproduced with permission from Global Strategy for the Diagnosis, Management, Prevention of COPD, © Global Initiative for Chronic Obstructive Lung Disease (GOLD), all rights reserved. Available from http://www.goldcopd.org.)*

walk test is not available, the ADO index (*a*ge, *d*yspnea and *o*bstruction) also provides useful prognostic information (Table 42-5).[27] The ADO index ranges from 0 to 10 points, with each point increase in the index associated with a 42% increase in odds of death at 3 years for patients with longstanding and severe COPD.

TREATMENT OF STABLE COPD

The goals of treatment of COPD are to prevent progression and complications of the disease, relieve symptoms, improve exercise capacity, improve quality of life, treat exacerbations, and improve survival.[28,29] Efforts are being made to standardize the most optimal treatment guidelines for COPD.[30]

EDUCATION

The diagnosis of COPD can be a life-changing event for people, so understanding the nature and prognosis of the disease is an important and underemphasized aspect of care. There is a wide divergence of understanding of the implications of having COPD, and many patients do not understand that COPD comprises both the diagnoses of emphysema and chronic bronchitis. Table 42-6 lists

TABLE 42-4 Calculation of the BODE Index[a]

Variable	Points on the BODE Index: 0	1	2	3
FEV_1 (% predicted)	≥65	50–64	36–49	≤35
Distance walked in 6 min (m)	≥350	250–349	150–249	≤149
mMRC dyspnea scale	0–1	2	3	4
Body mass index (kg/m^2)	>21	<=21		

[a]*The BODE index is calculated as the sum of points from each row.*
Source: Adapted with permission from Celli BR, Cote CG, Marin JM, et al. The body-mass index, airflow obstruction, dyspnea, and exercise capacity index in chronic obstructive pulmonary disease. N Engl J Med. 2004;350(10):1005–1012.

TABLE 42-5 Calculation of the ADO Index[a]

Variable	Points on the ADO Index: 0	1	2	3	4	5
FEV_1 (% predicted)	≥65	36–64	≤35	–	–	–
mMRC dyspnea scale	0–1	2	3	4	–	–
Age (yr)	40–49	50–59	60–69	70–79	80–89	≥90

[a]*The ADO index is calculated as the sum of points from each row.*
Source: Adapted with permission from Puhan MA, Garcia-Aymerich J, Frey M, et al. Expansion of the prognostic assessment of patients with chronic obstructive pulmonary disease: the updated BODE index and the ADO index. Lancet. 2009;374(9691):704–711.

TABLE 42-6 Patient Education Topics for Office Management of COPD

Risk factors for COPD
Smoking cessation advice and instruction
Reduction of noxious environmental exposures
Immunization for influenza and pneumococcus
Respiratory hygiene and avoidance of infections
Nature and prognosis of COPD
Indications, dose, benefits, and adverse effects of medications
Proper inhaler and nebulizer use
Strategies to improve adherence with prescribed treatment
Pacing, arm support, and other strategies to minimize dyspnea
Importance of regular exercise and social interaction
Options for pulmonary rehabilitation programs
Recognition and early treatment of exacerbations
Indications for and proper use of supplemental oxygen
Options for surgical management if indicated
Advanced directives for end-of-life care

topics that should be discussed with COPD patients. It is neither possible nor effective to cover all of these topics in a single session, so several sessions with repetition and expansion of the educational messages are necessary. Supplemental written materials or referral to a health educator is also necessary for many patients. Local and national volunteer health organizations provide useful educational materials and group educational sessions (e.g., www.copdfoundation.org, www.lung.org). Special counseling is needed for patients with α_1-antitrypsin deficiency and their family members to determine whether genetic testing is necessary or desired. In patients with advanced disease, discussions about end-of-life planning and advance directives regarding life support are often welcomed by patients and initiate discussions between the patient and family. Patients should be encouraged to discuss information that they obtain from newspapers or the Internet, as some may be instructive, but others are incorrect. Physicians should be prepared to deal with patients' sense of guilt, as many view COPD as a self-induced disease. Caregivers need to address the reality that COPD is often stigmatized by patients, their families, and other healthcare providers. The physician should let the patient understand that nicotine dependence is a strong physical addiction and difficulty quitting smoking is not a measure of moral weakness or lack of will. The general message provided should be realistic, but positive. Current treatments for COPD can usually improve quality of life, restore activity levels, maintain social interactions, and reduce the frequency of complications.

PREVENTION OF COPD PROGRESSION AND COMPLICATIONS

Presently, there are no proven treatments that prevent the progression of COPD in patients who continue to smoke cigarettes. *Smoking cessation*, however, does prevent the excessive decline in lung function and should be a primary goal for physicians caring for COPD patients. Patients with mild or moderate COPD may not know that they have underlying lung disease that can be halted by smoking cessation,[4] or may adopt a fatalistic attitude that it is too late for help. Even severely impaired patients who are dyspneic at rest or use continuous oxygen may continue to smoke cigarettes or relapse after quitting. A smoking history should be obtained at each patient encounter because many patients fail to volunteer the extent of their smoking or report a smoking relapse following cessation. In patients who do smoke, achieving cessation should be a primary and persistent goal of treatment.[31] Approaches to smoking cessation are given in detail in Chapter 41. For patients who do smoke, a direct, unambiguous, and personalized smoking cessation message should be given by the physician. The message should emphasize the harm of continued smoking, the benefits of cessation in terms of activities that are meaningful for the individual, and the understanding that smoking cessation is a realistic and achievable goal. Techniques of motivational interviewing are readily learned and are effective in changing health behaviors.[32] Assistance with pharmacologic adjuncts such as nicotine replacement therapy, varenicline, or bupropion and referral to smoking cessation groups should be offered. Follow-up of smoking status and repeated smoking cessation messages should be performed at each encounter.

Exposure to respiratory irritants should be avoided in the workplace as well as the home. Although heavy occupational dust exposure rarely is the primary cause of COPD, exposure to dusty occupational jobs in smokers can increase the lung function deterioration from smoking and increase symptoms of cough and sputum.[33] In developing countries, heavy exposure to particulates from burning of biomass fuels is associated with COPD, even in the absence of cigarette smoking.[34] Efforts to improve indoor air quality may be effective in reducing symptoms and disease progression. Respiratory protective equipment should be worn by COPD patients exposed to heavy dust concentrations. There is no level of FEV_1 that absolutely prohibits the use of respiratory protective equipment, but patients with COPD often experience untoward breathlessness with these masks because of the increased dead space and increased inspiratory resistance. Thus, many COPD patients need to change their work environment if they cannot tolerate protective devices. If COPD is complicated by allergy or overlaps with allergic asthma, environmental control measures should be instituted to the extent that these strategies are helpful. Smoking of marijuana and cocaine may cause airway irritation, and although there is no convincing evidence that they contribute to progression of COPD, their use ought to be discouraged.[35]

Pneumococcal vaccination is recommended, although the evidence of its particular efficacy in COPD is lacking.[36] Annual *influenza immunization* can prevent or attenuate this potentially fatal infection. The killed vaccine is preferred, as cold-attenuated live influenza vaccines have not been approved for use in older patients and those with underlying lung disease. High-potency influenza immunization is recommended for older patients who may have an impaired immune response to the vaccine. During influenza epidemics, the use of neuraminidase inhibitors such as zanamivir and oseltamivir can minimize severity of infection if taken within 48 hours of onset of illness and are useful against both influenza A and B, and may limit the spread of infection. Peramivir, an injectable form of neuraminidase inhibitor, is now available for treatment of individuals with respiratory failure.

Replacement therapy with α_1-antitrypsin should be considered for those individuals with severe deficiency. Observational studies suggest that individuals with moderate degrees of impairment (FEV_1 35%–65% predicted) appear to benefit most in terms of preservation of lung function and improved survival.[37] The human plasma–derived preparation of α_1-antitrypsin is administered intravenously in a dose of 60 mg/kg weekly. Although the replacement treatment is derived from pooled human plasma, the risk of viral transmission is low and immunization for hepatitis B is not mandatory before initiating therapy.

DRUG THERAPY

Over the past several decades, the evidence base for use of drug therapy in COPD has expanded, and provides an objective and generally optimistic picture that such treatment is effective. Bronchodilators and anti-inflammatory agents are used to reverse bronchoconstriction, improve lung function, improve quality of life, exercise capacity, and prevent exacerbations. Recent evidence however suggests that a combination of inhaled steroids and long-acting bronchodilators may improve survival as well as reduce exacerbations.[38–40] Proposed future drug treatments that might alter progression of COPD are under active investigation, including inhibitors of cytokines, proteases, and oxidative stress. There is a poor correlation between the effect of bronchodilating drugs on lung function and symptom relief, so monitoring of treatment requires attention to patient-centered outcomes as well as lung function. Small amounts of bronchodilation can cause considerable improvement in functional capacity through decrease in dynamic exercise hyperinflation; and reduction in days of exacerbation can make considerable improvement in patients' quality of life.

The usual approach to drug treatment for COPD is to sequentially add agents using the minimum number of agents and the most convenient dosing schedule, starting with the agents having the greatest benefit, best tolerance, and lowest cost. One approach to step-up therapy is provided in Figure 42-3. Inhaled bronchodilators are the foundation of treatment for COPD. They are given on a regular basis to maintain bronchodilation and on an as needed basis for relief of symptoms.[41,42] Most breathless patients benefit from regular use of a maintenance bronchodilator. Both β-agonist and anticholinergic classes are available in short-duration (4–6 hours) and long-duration (12–24 hours) forms (Table 42-7). The choice of bronchodilator class and duration of effect depends upon the preference of the patient and the cost of the preparation. Combination of different classes of bronchodilators is often more effective than increasing the dose of a single agent, and combination inhalers can simplify treatment regimens. Patients with advanced COPD often use a combination of bronchodilators, including long-acting maintenance anticholinergics and β-agonists as well as symptomatic use of shorter-acting bronchodilators. Individuals with exacerbations may benefit from a combination inhaler of corticosteroids and long-acting bronchodilator. Long-acting oral preparations of theophylline are useful adjuncts in cases in which inhaled medication is too expensive or not acceptable for the patient. Chronic use of systemic corticosteroids should be reserved for individuals with very frequent or life-threatening exacerbations in those cases where discontinuation of steroids

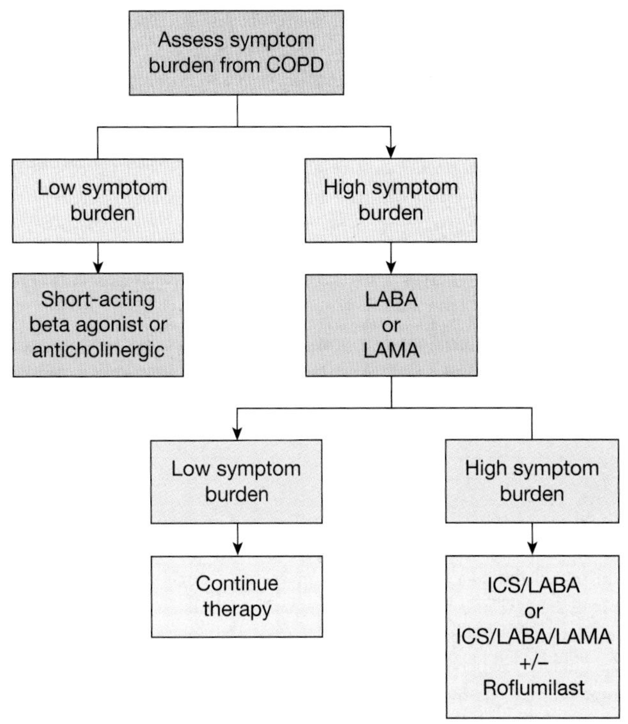

Figure 42-3 Decision tree for pharmacologic treatment of COPD. Treatments are determined by symptom burden, which is determined by assessment of dyspnea and COPD exacerbation risk. If patients are stable for 6 to 12 months, consideration should be given to trial reductions of treatment. In addition to pharmacologic interventions described here, treatment should also include preventative measures, smoking cessation counseling, pulmonary rehabilitation, and advanced therapies. LABA, long-acting beta agonist; LAMA, long-acting muscarinic antagonist; ICS, inhaled corticosteroid.

TABLE 42-7 Inhaled Bronchodilators

Drug Name	Dosage/Frequency	Formulation
β-Sympathomimetics		
Olodaterol		Soft Mist inhaler, 5 μg
Albuterol	2 inhalations q4–6h	Metered-dose inhaler, 90 μg/puff
	3 mL nebulized q4–6h	Nebulized solution 1.25–2.5 mg/3 mL
Levalbuterol	2 inhalations q4–6h	Metered-dose inhaler, 45 μg/puff
	3 mL nebulized TID	Nebulized solution 0.63–1.25 mg/3 mL
Salmeterol	1 inhalation BID	Dry powder inhaler, 50 μg/dose
Formoterol	1 capsule inhaled BID	Dry powder inhaler, 12 μg/capsule
	2 mL nebulized BID	Nebulized solution 20 μg/2 mL
Arformoterol	2 mL nebulized BID	Nebulized solution 15 μg/2 mL
Indacaterol	1 capsule daily	Dry powder inhaler, 75 μg/capsule
Anticholinergic Bronchodilators		
Ipratropium	2 puffs q4–6h	Metered-dose inhaler, 17 μg/puff
	2.5 mL nebulized q6–8h	Nebulized solution 0.5 mg/2.5 mL
Tiotropium	1 inhalation daily	Dry powder inhaler 18 μg/dose
Aclidinium	1 inhalation BID	Dry powder inhaler 400 μg/dose
Combination Therapies		
Ipratropium/albuterol	1 puff q6h	Soft Mist inhaler, 20 μg ipratropium and 100 μg albuterol
Umeclidinium/vilanterol		Dry powder inhaler, 62.5 μg/25 μg

cannot be tolerated. Response to treatment is judged by symptomatic improvement, functional status, frequency of exacerbations, and spirometry. If patients are doing well for 6 to 12 months on a stable treatment regimen, then it is reasonable to see if a trial withdrawal of one of the drug components can be tolerated.

Inhaled corticosteroids do not effectively alter the progression of COPD in those who continue to smoke. Inhaled corticosteroids are most useful in patients who have an overlap between asthma and COPD and those who have frequent exacerbations. Inhaled corticosteroids can reduce the frequency of exacerbations and slow the decline in quality of life.[39] In patients with chronic bronchitis and obstructive lung disease, inhaled corticosteroids improve pulmonary function, and the results are additive to those achieved with long-acting bronchodilators.[39,43] The efficacy of inhaled corticosteroids cannot be predicted based on the response to oral corticosteroids, so it is not necessary to conduct an oral steroid trial before initiating this treatment. Combined corticosteroid and long-acting bronchodilator inhalers are available in the United States and throughout the rest of the world and can simplify the treatment regimen. Inhaled corticosteroids, although poorly absorbed, probably do contribute to steroid side effects such as cataracts, capillary fragility, and osteoporosis in susceptible individuals. High doses of inhaled corticosteroids are associated with increased risk of pneumonia.[44] In most cases, the risk is low compared to the benefit of treatment, but it is prudent to prescribe the lowest effective dose. In patients who are at risk for osteoporosis (i.e., older age, cigarette smoking, low exercise) as most patients with COPD are, it is prudent to recommend prophylactic treatment such as calcium supplements and vitamin D. In those with established osteoporosis, bisphosphonates are advised. Monitoring for osteoporosis with DEXA bone scans is guided by the overall clinical situation and is not required for all patients using inhaled corticosteroids.

Adverse effects of inhaled therapy can occur. Inhaled anticholinergic agents are generally very safe. They may lead to an increased frequency of supraventricular arrhythmias, acute urinary retention in those with bladder outlet obstruction, or acute narrow-angle glaucoma if sprayed in the eye. β-Agonists, both short acting and long acting, may lead to side effects such as tremor, tachycardia, or hypokalemia.

Inhaled agents are administered by metered-dose inhaler (MDI), dry powder inhaler (DPI), or as a nebulized solution. The selection of route of administration is made by cost and convenience of the device because all are similarly effective if used properly. Many patients find that it is difficult to coordinate an MDI, and addition of a spacer device is helpful. There are many forms of DPI, some more intuitive to use than others, so specific instruction and demonstration is required by most patients. Nebulizers are easier for patients to coordinate, but each treatment takes longer to complete, and they require additional effort to maintain cleanliness. Although nebulized medications are more expensive overall, the cost of the medication is often covered by insurance, so many patients prefer nebulizers for financial considerations.

Adherence with inhaled medication, particularly when it does not provide immediate symptom relief is poor. Typically about half of patients do not take their medication in the dose or quantity prescribed. Reasons for this include a lack of understanding of the role of the medication, failure of the medication to provide meaningful benefit, complexity of the treatment program, and expense of the treatment. Many patients do not want to confide poor adherence to their physician, so it is important for the physician to ascertain this information in a way that does not interfere with the relationship with the patient. For example, a physician could inquire, "It is often difficult for patients to remember to take all of their medications. Has this been a problem for you?" or "Are you able to afford all your medication?" or "Do you think that your medicines are working for you?" If nonadherence is a problem, the treating physician can undertake actions to improve adherence, such as simplification of the medication program, education about the benefits of treatment, linking drug use to established habits such as meals or tooth brushing, or prescribing less costly drugs.

Proper use of MDIs is difficult for many patients to learn and retain. Repeated review and training of patients in MDI use is an important component of treatment of COPD and asthma. The inhaler should be held about 4 cm from the mouth to minimize deposition of larger droplets in the mouth. The patient should exhale to FRC and take a slow inhalation to TLC over about 5 seconds. The slow inhalation diminishes impaction of particles in the mouth and larynx. At the initiation of inspiration the patient should actuate the MDI one time. After full inspiration, the patient should hold the breath for about 10 seconds to permit settling of particles in the distal airspaces. If the patient finds that hoarseness or mouth irritation occurs with inhaler use, this can often be corrected by use of a spacer, slowing the rate of inspiration, and rinsing the mouth after each inhaler use. Although waiting a period of time between inhalations or between different MDIs is sometimes recommended for optimal effect, the benefit is small compared with the inconvenience and risk of worsening adherence. Therefore, it is usually appropriate to permit the patient to take additional inhalations as soon as he or she has rested a few seconds.

If the patient has difficulty coordinating the actuation of the MDI with inspiration, a spacer device or holding chamber can be used. This device is placed directly in the mouth and the MDI can be actuated prior to inspiration. DPIs usually require less coordination than MDIs, but there are many different devices, some rather complicated to use. Very frail patients may not have adequate inspiratory flow to effectively use a DPI. Therefore, each device requires individual instruction and review of technique. (For a compendium of patient instructions, see http://www.ginasthma.com/OtherResources.asp.)

Theophylline is taken as a long-acting oral preparation once or twice daily. Although it is possible to monitor blood levels, because the drug is protein bound there is a poor correlation between efficacy or adverse effects and serum levels. Theophylline is a bronchodilator; it improves arterial oxygenation and exercise tolerance.[45] If typical side effects such as nausea, vomiting, tremor, or tachyarrhythmias occur, the dose should be adjusted irrespective of serum levels. Prescriptions for theophylline to treat COPD have diminished in recent years because of the availability of long-acting inhaled agents. However, theophylline is still an effective second-line drug for patients who show benefit or prefer inexpensive oral medications. Theophylline has other putative pharmacologic actions that might be beneficial for the COPD patient: improvement in diaphragm contractility, prevention of respiratory muscle fatigue, increased ventilatory drive, potentiation of catecholamine function, prevention of microvascular permeability, increased mucociliary clearance, prevention of late-phase antigen responses, inhibition of mast cell histamine release, and suppression of leukocyte activation. Evidence has suggested that the anti-inflammatory effect of theophylline is mediated by augmentation of steroid effects through activation of histone deacetylase (HDAC), an effect that is of particular importance in COPD patients who have lower HDAC activity.[46]

Roflumilast is a more specific inhibitor of phosphodiesterase-4, which is a mild bronchodilator with anti-inflammatory properties. It is marketed in the United States for reduction of exacerbations of COPD in individuals with chronic bronchitis.[47]

Oral corticosteroids are effective for treatment of COPD exacerbations. About 10% to 20% of chronic symptomatic patients show substantial short-term improvement in pulmonary function, but it is not possible to identify these patients based on clinical characteristics alone. Because of the well-defined long-term adverse effects of systemic corticosteroids, and the ill-defined long-term benefits, most patients should not be maintained on long-term oral or systemic corticosteroids. Patients with COPD who are on chronic corticosteroids can most often taper the dose at the equivalent of 5 mg of prednisone per week, and exclusively reserve their use for exacerbations. Long-term low doses of oral corticosteroids are occasionally needed by patients who cannot afford or tolerate inhaled agents, and who suffer frequent exacerbations. Patients on long-term systemic steroids should receive prophylaxis for osteoporosis with calcium and vitamin D or bisphosphonates, and should be instructed about the need for stress-dose steroids for acute illnesses.

Long-term macrolide antibiotics should be used sparingly in patients with COPD who do not have symptomatic bronchiectasis. Macrolides, which have immunomodulatory properties, have been demonstrated to reduce the frequency of exacerbations in patients susceptible to frequent exacerbations.[48] Thus, the use of long-term antibiotics may have a role in those susceptible to frequent, severe exacerbations.

Mucolytic agents to control mucus hypersecretion with the use of expectorants and physical means such as high-frequency chest wall oscillation is not of proven benefit in improving lung function, although symptoms are sometimes improved. N-acetylcysteine is a mucolytic with antioxidant properties does not prevent exacerbations, nor does it alter the decline in FEV_1. The role of antioxidant mucolytics such as N-acetylcysteine or carbocysteine is unclear but may have a role in reducing exacerbations.[49,50]

Opiates can be effective in the management of severe dyspnea related to COPD. Given differential response to these therapies, as well as the associated potential for respiratory depression, short acting and low-dose preparations should be initially used. While typically associated with severe, end-stage management in the hospice setting, short-acting opiates can be considered in patients with less severe lung impairment but symptomatic dyspnea refractory to pharmacotherapy, oxygen supplementation, and rehabilitation.

■ EXERCISE AND REHABILITATION

Regular prudent self-directed exercise is recommended for all individuals with COPD to prevent the muscle deconditioning that often accompanies the disorder. Individuals should be encouraged to perform at least 20 to 30 minutes of constant low-intensity aerobic exercise such as walking at least three times per week. Even the most severely impaired patients with COPD can usually attain an exercise regimen of 30 minutes of walking at 1 mph (i.e., one-half mile in 30 minutes). It is important to instruct patients that they should exercise to a level of dyspnea that is tolerable for the entire exercise period. Patients should understand that dyspnea, by itself, is not injurious to the heart or lungs, but patients should pace themselves to avoid severe dyspnea that disrupts activity, can lead to panic reactions, and is distressing to onlookers. Patients who demonstrate desaturation with exertion may be prescribed supplemental oxygen for exercise. Some may benefit in terms of exercise capacity and training effect even if they do not have demonstrable oxygen desaturation.[51] Many patients, particularly those with marked hyperinflation, find that they can ambulate better with the use of a rolling walker that supports the arms, improving the mechanical advantage of the accessory muscles in the neck.

Formal rehabilitation programs offer a comprehensive approach to exercise training, patient education, nutritional counseling, group support, and psychological support that cannot be efficiently provided in the physician's office. Rehabilitation programs are established as an effective component of COPD management and should be offered to patients who have substantial limitation in daily activities. A detailed discussion of rehabilitation is provided in Chapter 43.

■ NUTRITIONAL SUPPORT

In patients with very severe COPD (FEV_1 less than 35% predicted) about half show protein–calorie malnutrition.[52] Reasons for this include increased resting metabolic demands, inadequate caloric intake due to dyspnea and anorexia, and possibly elaboration of cachexia-associated inflammatory cytokines such as TNF-α, IL-1, and IL-6. Patients with a BMI of less than 90% of normal have increased mortality and decreased exercise capacity. Muscle wasting and loss of bone mass may be present even in patients who have normal BMI.[53] Although clinical trials of nutritional supplementation have been disappointing, it is prudent to monitor body weight in COPD patients and encourage caloric supplementation as needed since those patients who do gain weight show improved survival.[54] High-fat diets have the theoretical advantage of offering higher caloric content with lower CO_2 production than high carbohydrate diets, but there is no convincing evidence that this strategy is clinically superior to a well-balanced diet. For patients with less advanced disease, a balanced diet with avoidance of overweight or underweight is a rational goal. In particular, patients with mild to moderate disease who quit smoking tend to gain excessive weight, which might adversely affect lung function.[55]

■ SLEEP DISORDERS IN COPD

Sleep disturbances, including insomnia and daytime hypersomnolence, are common symptoms in patients with COPD,[56,57] and are often overlooked because of the focus on breathlessness and exercise intolerance. The causes for sleep symptoms are multifactorial and include anxiety, depression, resting hypoxemia, nocturnal bronchospasm, sleep apnea, and nocturnal oxygen desaturation (NOD). Patients with COPD often relate insomnia to a fear of suffocation or death during sleep, a situation that may respond to repeated reassurance, cognitive therapy, or small doses of anxiolytics or antidepressants. Patients with resting hypoxemia treated with low-flow nasal oxygen often report improved sleep quality. Nocturnal bronchospasm, more common among those with an asthmatic component to their disease, may respond to longer-acting bronchodilators, or rearrangement of the dosing schedule to provide nocturnal coverage. In some cases, treatment for gastroesophageal reflux by elevation of the head of the bed and prescription of acid suppressant drugs can help. Sleep apnea syndrome, probably not more common in COPD patients than the general community, has particularly severe complications in COPD. Patients with COPD and sleep apnea, the so-called "overlap syndrome" are prone to develop pulmonary hypertension and daytime hypercapnia.[58] Accordingly, symptoms of sleep apnea such as snoring, intermittent nocturnal breathing, and daytime hypersomnolence should be sought in patients with COPD. If present, then formal sleep studies and treatment with continuous positive airway pressure (CPAP) are indicated. NOD is common during rapid eye movement sleep in patients with COPD. The causes are not entirely understood, but contributing factors include hypoventilation, ventilation–perfusion mismatch, respiratory muscle dysfunction, and increases in upper airway resistance. NOD is thought to be associated with poorer sleep quality and pulmonary hypertension. It is controversial whether NOD is associated with poorer survival. However, small studies have shown inconclusive results about the utility of treating NOD.

Current guidelines do not recommend that all patients with COPD have nocturnal oxygen monitoring, nor do they recommend treatment with supplemental oxygen or nocturnal ventilation if NOD is found. Many physicians, though, will prescribe these diagnostic studies and treatments for selected symptomatic patients, and most insurance companies will provide reimbursement for such treatment. Patients who have resting room air daytime hypoxemia should be prescribed nocturnal oxygen at the same flow rate as used during the day, and it is usually not necessary to monitor nocturnal oxygen saturation in such patients.

■ MANAGEMENT OF DEPRESSION

Depression is a common comorbidity in individuals with COPD. The recognition and treatment of depression is important as this comorbidity is associated with poorer prognosis, increased risk of exacerbations, and poor health status. While there is little evidence to suggest that depression should be treated differently in COPD patients, pulmonary rehabilitation has been shown to reduce depression with COPD.

■ AIR TRAVEL

Patients with COPD should not avoid air travel, but must be aware of the medical and regulatory issues that are involved.[59] Modern airplanes are pressurized to an equivalent altitude of approximately 5000 to 8000 ft, but may, on occasion, pressurize to an equivalent altitude of 10,000 ft without providing emergency oxygen. Many patients with COPD who do not use sea-level oxygen can tolerate short flights without supplemental oxygen. As flight distance becomes longer, the flying altitude becomes higher and the cabin pressure becomes lower, so transcontinental or transoceanic flights should prompt medical advice. The general rule of thumb used by the commercial airline industry is that patients who can ambulate 50 m without stopping are safe for air travel. A more conservative approach is to estimate the Pa_{O_2} during air travel by performing a high altitude simulation test. High altitude simulation can be performed by administering 15% oxygen via a face mask or by using 100% nitrogen in a 40% Venturi mask.[60] If the oxygen saturation falls below 86% or 50 mm Hg, then supplemental oxygen is recommended. Formulas are available to estimate altitude hypoxemia from sea-level room-air blood gases. Figure 42-4 provides a nomogram for estimating altitude Pa_{O_2} from sea-level room-air arterial oxygen tensions.[61] If estimated altitude Pa_{O_2} is used, it is prudent to prescribe oxygen for estimated altitude Pa_{O_2} of 54 mm Hg or lower. Patients who use oxygen supplementation at sea level should increase their resting oxygen prescription by a flow rate of 2 L/min. For patients with COPD who travel by air frequently, low-cost finger pulse-oximeters that are marketed to airplane pilots can be used to adjust their oxygen flow.

Airlines have inconsistent policies with respect to providing supplemental oxygen for travelers, so it is important to check with the airline service desk before booking travel. The United States Federal Aviation Administration has promulgated regulations that permit some approved portable oxygen concentrators to be carried on board by passengers as personal luggage with a physician's statement of need. These may be rented from oxygen supply companies or specialized websites.

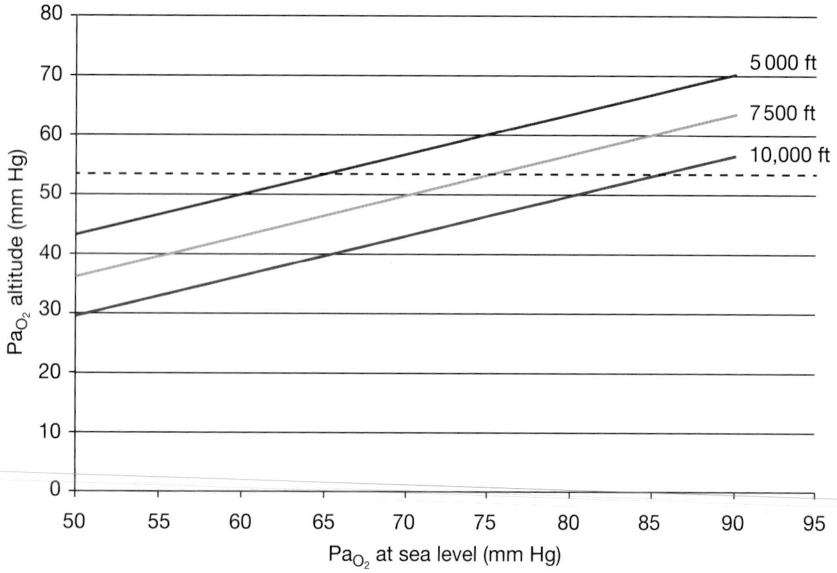

■ LONG-TERM OXYGEN THERAPY

In addition to smoking intervention in early COPD, treatment of resting daytime hypoxemia with oxygen is a treatment that prolongs survival.[62–64] The two strongest indications for prescription of long-term oxygen therapy are (1) resting room-air Pa_{O_2} ≤55 mm Hg or oxygen saturation ≤88% while a person is in usual state of health; and (2) resting room-air Pa_{O_2} 56 to 60 mm Hg or oxygen saturation 88% to 89% with supporting evidence of chronic hypoxemia such as polycythemia, pulmonary hypertension, cor pulmonale, or psychological impairment. Oxygen is usually administered by nasal cannula, with the flow rate adjusted to maintain a resting saturation greater than 90%. The usual starting flow rate is 2 L/min, although some patients with severe hypercapnia require lower flows. A few patients, particularly those with concomitant interstitial pulmonary disease or cardiac disorders, require higher flow rates.

The most convenient and cost-effective oxygen source at home is usually a concentrator device that uses a molecular sieve to extract oxygen from room air. For ambulation, small compressed air cylinders, portable concentrators, or liquid oxygen reservoirs that can be carried provide patients with the ability to leave their homes. Conserving devices such as reservoirs or demand valves permit portable ambulatory oxygen tanks to last up to 10 hours. Compressed oxygen cylinders or liquid oxygen reservoirs should be provided to patients who use electrically driven oxygen concentrators for emergency use in the event of a power failure. Ideally, oxygen should be used constantly 24 hours per day. At least 18 hours of oxygen per day, however, has been shown to have substantial benefit over 12 hours per day. If continuous oxygen supplementation is prescribed following an exacerbation of COPD, it is recommended to check arterial oxygen levels in 6 weeks, as many patients will no longer require oxygen.

Nasal drying or congestion is a common symptom for those who use continuous oxygen. This may be alleviated to some extent by alternating the nasal cannula from one nostril to the other or placing it in the mouth for periods. Copious watery nasal secretions often respond well to ipratropium nasal spray, and dry, crusted nasal mucosa is treated with hourly instillations of saline nasal spray.

Smoking or exposure to any open flame is prohibited by the danger of fire and airway burns in those who use oxygen. This is a surprisingly common cause of burns in the United States, with estimates that up to 50% of patients on oxygen continue to smoke to some extent.[65] Accordingly, it is safer to counsel patients to discontinue oxygen while smoking or cooking over an open flame if they insist on doing these activities. Patients at particular risk are those who live alone, have cognitive impairment, and do not have functioning smoke detectors.

Oxygen delivery via a transtracheal catheter is an option for selected patients who cannot tolerate other oxygen delivery methods, and who can attend to the regular maintenance of the catheter. High-flow humidified nasal cannulas are also an option for individuals who need high concentrations of oxygen but who cannot tolerate a facemask.

Figure 42-4 Estimated Pa_{O_2} at altitude based on resting sea-level arterial oxygen tension. Isopleths are drawn for the range of cabin pressures that occur on commercial aircraft. The dashed line is drawn at 54 mm Hg, which indicates a threshold for prescribing supplemental oxygen for air travel. *(Data of Gong H Jr, Tashkin DP, Lee EY, et al. Hypoxia-altitude simulation test. Evaluation of patients with chronic airway obstruction. Am Rev Respir Dis. 1984;130:980–986.)*

Ambulatory oxygen, although not shown to improve survival, may be provided for patients who desaturate with exertion. Some, but not all, patients show improved exercise capacity and reduced breathlessness. There is a growing body of evidence that suggests that oxygen supplementation may also benefit COPD patients who do not have exercise desaturation by reduction in minute ventilation and diminution of dynamic hyperinflation.[51] Because it permits greater exercise intensity, oxygen supplementation is also a useful adjunct for aerobic conditioning during pulmonary rehabilitation.

COMPLICATIONS

■ COPD EXACERBATIONS

Exacerbations are characterized by worsening cough, dyspnea, and sputum production beyond normal day-to-day variation. These exacerbations are associated with acute deterioration of lung function during the exacerbation and may also accelerate the longitudinal loss of lung function. Acute exacerbations of COPD are a major cause of hospitalization, healthcare costs, morbidity, and mortality in COPD. Exacerbations have been associated with respiratory viral infections including rhinovirus, respiratory syncytial virus, influenza, adenovirus, and metapneumovirus. Bacterial infections or superinfections are also associated with COPD exacerbations. The most frequent pathogens are *Haemophilus influenzae, Moraxella catarrhalis,* and *Streptoccous pneumoniae*. In patients who have been treated with antibiotics, gram-negative bacteria may also be present. Severe air pollution, especially particulates, sulfur dioxide, ozone, and nitrogen dioxide have been associated with elevated risk for hospitalization due to COPD. On average, patients with COPD have two to three exacerbations per year, but there is wide variation, and the frequency of exacerbations is only roughly correlated with severity of airflow obstruction. The best predictor of future exacerbations is a past history of frequent exacerbations,[66] and these are more common in patients with chronic cough and sputum production. Only half of COPD exacerbations come to the attention of treating physicians, and many of these eventually resolve without specific treatment. The management of these exacerbations depends upon the severity. Indications for hospital evaluation or hospitalization are listed in Table 42-8. Arterial blood gas studies and chest radiographs are useful for evaluating etiology and severity of acutely ill patients. Spirometry during the acute exacerbation is usually not helpful in predicting the severity or duration of the exacerbation.

For patients treated at home, increasing the frequency and intensity of inhaled short-acting bronchodilators for several days is effective in mild exacerbations. A hand-held inhaler and spacer are usually effective, but a nebulizer may be needed for those who cannot coordinate well or who have severe dyspnea. Increasing dyspnea accompanied by a change in the quantity or color of phlegm is usually an indication of bacterial infection and should prompt initiation of antibiotics. The choice of antibiotic is determined by severity of the underlying disease, resistance patterns of likely pathogens, and likelihood of treatment failure (Table 42-9). After initiation of therapy, the antibiotic treatment should be tailored based on sputum cultures.

A course of corticosteroids, equivalent to 30 to 60 mg of prednisone for 7 to 14 days, will shorten the duration of symptoms for patients with exacerbations managed as outpatients.[67,68]

For patients admitted to the hospital, intensification of inhaled bronchodilator treatment, systemic corticosteroids, and antibiotics are administered.[69] Controlled oxygen supplementation should be provided at the lowest level needed to reverse hypoxemia and minimize the induction of hypercapnia. The selection of the oral or intravenous route for antibiotics and corticosteroids is determined by the severity of the illness and the ability of the patient to tolerate oral medication. Evaluation for the cause of the exacerbation does not have to be extensive if it responds to initial treatment and conforms to the patient's usual exacerbation pattern. Sputum culture for resistant bacterial strains, a chest radiograph for exclusion of pneumonia and pneumothorax, and an electrocardiogram for exclusion of myocardial ischemia and arrhythmia are useful tests in all hospitalized patients. Echocardiography for assessment of ventricular function, and Doppler venous flow studies, radionuclide, or computed tomographic lung imaging for evaluation of pulmonary thromboembolism need to be performed in selected cases. Usually a 2-week course of steroids is sufficient for hospitalized patients.

Treatment in an intensive care setting should be undertaken for patients with severe exacerbations or those who require more constant attention (Table 42-8). For patients with respiratory failure,

TABLE 42-8 Indications for Hospitalization in COPD

Indications for Hospital Assessment or Admission for COPD Exacerbation
Sudden onset of new or severe symptoms (e.g., dyspnea)
Inability to sleep or eat because of dyspnea
Severe or very severe underlying COPD
Onset of new physical findings (e.g., edema, cyanosis, change in mental status)
Failure to respond to initial medical treatment
Associated comorbidities (e.g., cardiac, renal, hepatic failure, or diabetes)
Diagnostic uncertainty (e.g., suspected pneumonia or pulmonary embolism)
Unusual presenting symptoms
Older age or frailty
Inadequate home or social support
History of poor adherence with treatment
Indications for ICU Admission for COPD Exacerbation
Severe dyspnea unresponsive to initial treatment
Change in mental status (e.g., confusion, lethargy, coma)
Persistent or worsening hypoxemia, hypercapnia, or respiratory acidosis
Need for sedation or narcotic pain control

Source: Data from 2011 GOLD COPD guidelines (www.goldcopd.com) and 2004 ATS/ERS Standards for treatment of COPD.

TABLE 42-9 Antimicrobial Treatment of COPD Exacerbations

First Line
Amoxicillin 500–875 mg PO TID
Doxycycline 100 mg PO BID
Alternatives
Amoxicillin/clavulanate 875 mg PO BID
Azithromycin 500 mg, then 250 mg PO QD × 4 d
Clarithromycin 500 mg PO BID
Second-generation cephalosporins
Severe COPD or previous antibiotics
Levofloxacin 500–750 mg PO QD × 7 d
Ciprofloxacin 500 mg PO QD × 7 d

noninvasive mask ventilation has proved to be an effective strategy to avert endotracheal intubation, shorten duration of illness, and improve outcomes.[70] Attention needs to be paid to selecting and fitting a comfortable well-sealed mask, and providing a ventilator that minimizes the patient's work of breathing and triggering effort. When noninvasive mask ventilation is not successful in sustaining ventilation, or the patient is too ill to use the mask, endotracheal intubation and mechanical ventilation are needed to treat respiratory failure. The mechanical ventilator should be set to provide minute ventilation that does not overventilate the patient and cause alkalemia, which may ultimately impede liberation from the ventilator. The inspiratory flow rates and inspiratory to expiratory time ratios should be adjusted to provide a prolonged duration of expiration to minimize dynamic hyperinflation (auto-PEEP), which can lead to dyspnea, discoordination, and barotrauma. Weaning and liberation from mechanical ventilation can be hindered by anxiety, oversedation, mucus secretions, intravascular volume overload, myocardial ischemia, or respiratory muscle deconditioning. Survival after an episode of acute respiratory failure for COPD patient with hypercarbia is about 50% at 2 years after discharge, with about half of the patients being readmitted to the hospital within 6 months.[71]

PNEUMOTHORAX

COPD is thought to be the most common cause for secondary spontaneous pneumothorax. A pneumothorax can either cause an acute symptomatic exacerbation of COPD from rupture of a bleb, or may occur during the course of an exacerbation as a consequence of hyperinflation or mechanical ventilation. Because this is a life-threatening but quickly treatable cause for worsening respiratory failure in COPD, it should always be considered in the differential diagnosis for worsening dyspnea in COPD. The physical examination can be misleading because diminished breath sounds are a component of the underlying disease. Imaging studies are usually diagnostic, but at times it can be difficult to distinguish a pneumothorax from an over-distended bulla. If the patient's clinical situation can tolerate it, imaging with inspiratory and expiratory views, or chest computed tomograms can be helpful. In the intensive care unit, upright and cross-table lateral views sometimes show mobility of the pleural air.

Urgent treatment for the patient in extremis is performed by aspirating the pleural space at the second intercostal space anteriorly in the midclavicular line. Definitive emergency treatment is placement of a thoracostomy tube, which should be done with care to avoid laceration of a bulla and creation of a bronchopleural fistula. In patients with advanced COPD, recurrence of a pneumothorax can be life-threatening, so definitive pleural sclerosis with surgical or medical thoracoscopy should be considered.

COR PULMONALE

Pulmonary hypertension and consequent right ventricular failure, *cor pulmonale*, are usually the consequence of chronic alveolar hypoxia, with secondary contributions from destruction of the alveolar capillary bed, lung hyperinflation, and increased blood viscosity.[72] Diagnosis of pulmonary hypertension and right ventricular failure can be difficult, as physical findings of venous engorgement, and right ventricular hypertrophy and dilatation are late signs. Peripheral edema is poorly correlated with resting right atrial pressure and may reflect fluid retention from activation of the renin–angiotensin–aldosterone system. Functional imaging studies including echocardiography or radionuclide ventriculography are more probative for evaluation of right ventricular function. Doppler echocardiographic measures of pulmonary artery systolic pressure correlate weakly with severity of pulmonary hypertension by right heart catheterization.[73] Once cor pulmonale is present, survival is diminished. If the pulmonary artery pressure exceeds 25 mm Hg, the average 5-year survival is diminished by 50%.[74]

The primary treatment of cor pulmonale consists of continuous oxygen to overcome hypoxemia and diuretic to optimize volume status. Calcium channel blockers and other vasodilators can dilate the pulmonary circulation, but they worsen hypoxemia and their benefit is not established. Phlebotomy increases exercise capacity when the hematocrit exceeds 55%, but persistent erythrocytosis suggests inadequate oxygen supplementation or another cause. Anticoagulation, which is considered beneficial in severe pulmonary vascular hypertension of other causes, is of uncertain benefit in patients with pulmonary hypertension caused by COPD.

SUPRAVENTRICULAR ARRHYTHMIAS

Supraventricular tachyarrhythmias are common in patients with COPD, as a consequence of right atrial enlargement, increased endogenous adrenergic tone, hypoxemia, and drug treatment—specifically theophylline and anticholinergic bronchodilators. Treatment is similar to that in nonpulmonary patients; however, the presence of COPD should not prevent evaluation for treatable causes of arrhythmias such as pulmonary embolism, hyperthyroidism, or valvular heart disease, which may be difficult to diagnose in COPD patients.

HYPERCAPNIA

Chronic hypercapnia secondary to alveolar hypoventilation can be considered an adaptive response to obstructive lung disease by decreasing the work of breathing, preventing respiratory muscle fatigue, and allowing a diminished sensation of dyspnea. The adverse effect of chronic hypercapnia is the development of alveolar hypoxia and consequent pulmonary hypertension. Accordingly, the approach to chronic hypercapnia is the use of supplemental oxygen in controlled concentrations. In patients who are very sensitive to oxygen, it is preferable to provide oxygen in controlled concentrations with Venturi masks rather than nasal cannula.

Nocturnal ventilation has been effective in reducing daytime hypercapnia in patients with neuromuscular disease and kyphoscoliosis. Short-term trials have shown divergent effects of nocturnal ventilation in patients with COPD. A 2-year controlled long-term trial of nocturnal ventilation in hypercapnic patients with COPD has shown modest improvement in symptoms and quality of life, and a trend toward reduced hospitalization, but only small improvements in daytime hypercapnia.[75] Thus, based on our current state of knowledge, long-term nocturnal ventilation ought to be reserved for selected symptomatic patients with frequent hospitalizations who can tolerate the treatment.

ADVANCED TREATMENTS

For patients who have far-advanced disease evidenced either by severe breathlessness or short life expectancy, more aggressive treatments should be considered. Undertaking these treatments requires thoughtful consideration by patients and their families, and frank discussion of the risks and benefits by the medical caregivers.

LUNG VOLUME REDUCTION SURGERY

Lung volume reduction surgery (LVRS) is a surgical procedure that involves stapled resection of 20% to 30% of the lung bilaterally, usually from the apices. The procedure is equally safe and effective, done by median sternotomy or video-assisted thoracoscopy (VATS). The theory behind this procedure is that the remaining lung expands to fill the thorax, thereby increasing its elastic recoil pressure, which improves expiratory airflow. The reduction of lung volume permits the diaphragm to attain a more normal, domed configuration, which improves its mechanical efficiency. Moreover, the preferential removal of unventilated bullae reduces residual volume, permitting an increase in the vital capacity. While some patients show substantial

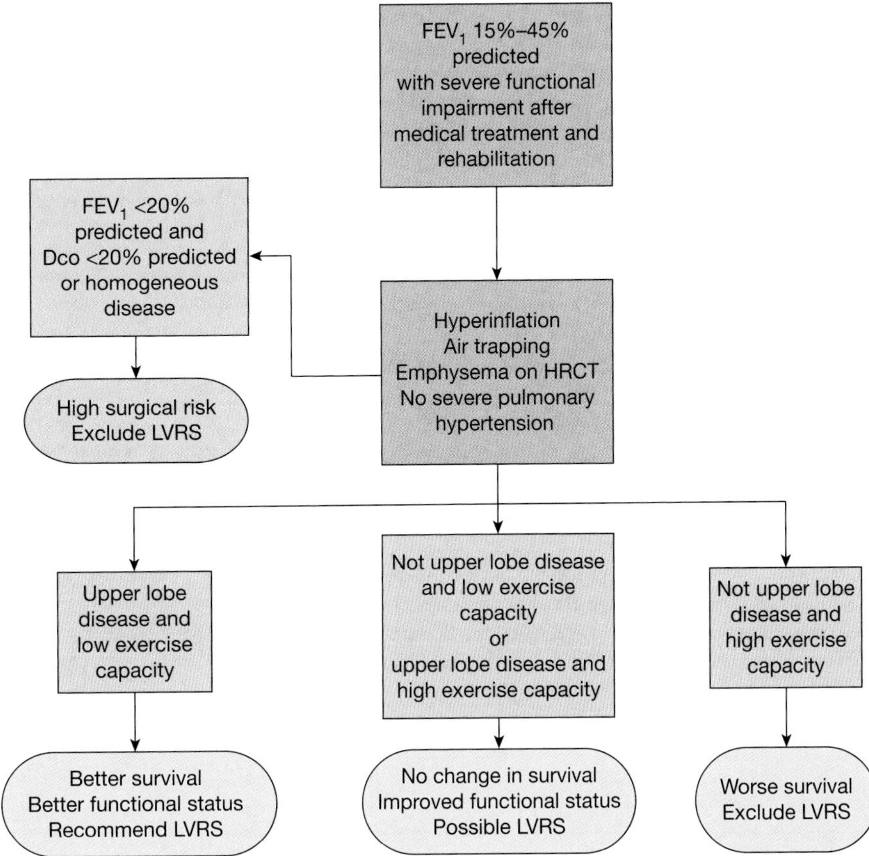

Figure 42-5 Decision tree for selection of candidates for lung volume reduction surgery (LVRS) based on distribution of emphysema on high-resolution computed tomogram (HRCT) and functional impairments.

physiological and symptomatic improvement following LVRS, many do not.[76] An algorithm for selection of patients for LVRS, based on distribution of emphysema and functional measures, is presented in Figure 42-5. Generally, LVRS should not be done on patients with an FEV_1 less than 20% predicted and either diffusing capacity less than 20% predicted or diffuse homogeneous emphysema on HRCT, because these patients have high surgical mortality. The group of patients who fare best with LVRS are those who have emphysema predominantly in the upper lung zones and low exercise capacity despite pulmonary rehabilitation. These patients have improved survival after LVRS and show improved functional status and quality of life. Conversely, patients without upper lobe predominance (i.e., lower lobe emphysema or homogeneous emphysema) and who have adequate exercise capacity after rehabilitation, have worse outcomes after LVRS. In selected cases, resection of a pulmonary nodule may be accompanied by LVRS as an attempt to improve postoperative functional status. Although LVRS was originally proposed as a temporizing measure while patients were awaiting lung transplantation, most LVRS candidates are not suitable candidates for lung transplantation. However, prior LVRS does not alter the outcome of subsequent lung transplantation.

Surgical resection of a single large bulla is rarely indicated for treatment of COPD. Isolated giant bullae are usually the result of an expanding congenital cyst. The generally accepted indication for resection of a single large bulla is that it occupies more than one-third of the hemithorax and causes compression of normal lung. Some believe that a preserved D_{CO} is an indicator of those most likely to improve following a bullectomy.

Preliminary studies with nonsurgical approaches to lung volume reduction using a variety of techniques to induce atelectasis of a target lobe are under investigation. In a study of COPD patients with severe airflow obstruction, hyperinflation and heterogeneous emphysema, placement of endobronchial valves for a bronchoscopic LVRS was associated with modest improvements in relevant clinical outcomes, although these results are balanced by an increased risk of infection and COPD exacerbation.[77,78] Selection of patients with proper anatomy appears to be important predictors of success to these nonsurgical approaches. These methods may ultimately provide an alternative approach to surgical LVRS for patients with severe COPD.

LUNG TRANSPLANTATION

In younger patients with advanced disease, lung transplantation should be a treatment consideration. Criteria for lung transplantation referral in patients with COPD are an FEV_1 below 25% predicted, BODE index greater than 5, hypercapnia, resting hypoxemia, secondary pulmonary hypertension, and accelerated decline in FEV_1 in patients under the age of 60 to 65 years.[79] For additional information see Chapter 107 (lung transplantation).

CHRONIC VENTILATOR SUPPORT

Some patients remain on long-term ventilator support following an episode of acute respiratory failure. Most often these patients are treated in a long-term ventilator unit, but some can be managed at home with adequate support. In some cases, the goal of long-term ventilator support is to provide rehabilitation via respiratory care, nutrition, and exercise to eventually be liberated from the ventilator entirely or for substantial portions of the day. In other cases, the goal of care is to provide comfort and support for terminal care without attempts at rehabilitation. Whatever the goal, a coordinated team of physicians, respiratory therapists, physical therapists, nutritionists, social workers, psychologists, and nurses are needed to undertake the care of these patients. The treatment of long-term ventilator patients differs from the treatment of acute respiratory failure in the intensive care unit. Ventilators are less sophisticated in terms of modes of ventilation and monitoring, but more portable. Ventilation is often performed with an uncuffed tracheostomy with an air leak to avoid complications at the cuff site. Sufficiency of ventilation is judged by noninvasive measures of oxygenation and patient comfort. Narcotics in small doses are administered for relief of dyspnea. Diagnostic studies and invasive testing are performed less frequently than in critical care units. Although the care in long-term ventilator units is complex and expensive, the quality of life experienced by patients in chronic ventilator units is similar to that of patients confined to a bed-and-chair existence by other chronic maladies. The survival of COPD patients on long-term mechanical ventilation is less than those on such treatment for neuromuscular diseases, in part, because of their older age and comorbidities.[80]

CONCLUSIONS

COPD develops insidiously. However, the disease can be easily detected with simple spirometric testing before symptoms occur, and cessation of smoking can slow or even halt the disease progression and prolong survival. Once the disease is symptomatic, a coordinated, comprehensive, and individualized approach to treatment, both pharmacologic and nonpharmacologic, can increase functional status, prevent complications, and improve the quality of life. Exacerbations of COPD can range from those that are nuisances to those that are life-threatening, but treatment can shorten the duration of illness and improve outcomes. In advanced disease, treatments including surgical approaches are directed toward relief of symptoms and prolongation of survival. Thus, although there is certainly need for improvement in our treatment of symptomatic COPD, current treatments are effective and a nihilistic attitude is not warranted.

DISCLOSURES

Disclosure of financial conflicts: During the preceding 5 years, Dr. Wise has received fees for consultation or support of research from the following companies: Astra-Zeneca, Boehringer-Ingelheim, GlaxoSmithKline, InterMune, Merck, MedImmune, Mylan, Novartis, Pfizer, Pulmonx, Sunovion, Spiration. Financial conflicts of interest are managed by the Johns Hopkins University School of Medicine.

During the preceding 5 years, Dr. Drummond has received fees for consultation from Boehringer-Ingelheim and Lupin Pharmaceuticals.

REFERENCES

1. From the Global Strategy for the Diagnosis, Management and Prevention of COPD, Global Initiative for Chronic Obstructive Lung Disease (GOLD). 2011. http://www.goldcopd.org/. Accessed July 20, 2013.
2. Pellegrino R, Viegi G, Brusasco V, et al. Interpretative strategies for lung function tests. *Eur Respir J.* 2005;26(5):948–968.
3. Hogg JC, Chu F, Utokaparch S, et al. The nature of small-airway obstruction in chronic obstructive pulmonary disease. *N Engl J Med.* 2004;350(26):2645–2653.
4. Anthonisen NR, Connett JE, Murray RP. Smoking and lung function of Lung Health Study participants after 11 years. *Am J Respir Crit Care Med.* 2002;166(5):675–679.
5. Anthonisen NR, Connett JE, Kiley JP, et al. Effects of smoking intervention and the use of an inhaled anticholinergic bronchodilator on the rate of decline of FEV1. The Lung Health Study. *JAMA.* 1994;272(19):1497–1505.
6. Vestbo J, Edwards LD, Scanlon PD, et al. Changes in forced expiratory volume in 1 second over time in COPD. *N Engl J Med.* 2011;365(13):1184–1192.
7. Drummond MB, Hansel NN, Connett JE, Scanlon PD, Tashkin DP, Wise RA. Spirometric predictors of lung function decline and mortality in early chronic obstructive pulmonary disease. *Am J Respir Crit Care Med.* 2012;185(12):1301–1306.
8. Anthonisen NR, Skeans MA, Wise RA, Manfreda J, Kanner RE, Connett JE. The effects of a smoking cessation intervention on 14.5-year mortality: a randomized clinical trial. *Ann Intern Med.* 2005;142(4):233–239.
9. U.S. Preventive Services Task Force. Screening for chronic obstructive pulmonary disease using spirometry: U.S. Preventive Services Task Force recommendation statement. *Ann Intern Med.* 2008;148(7):529–534.
10. Jenkins CR, Jones PW, Calverley PM, et al. Efficacy of salmeterol/fluticasone propionate by GOLD stage of chronic obstructive pulmonary disease: analysis from the randomised, placebo-controlled TORCH study. *Respir Res.* 2009;10:59.
11. Decramer M, Celli B, Kesten S, Lystig T, Mehra S, Tashkin DP. Effect of tiotropium on outcomes in patients with moderate chronic obstructive pulmonary disease (UPLIFT): a prespecified subgroup analysis of a randomised controlled trial. *Lancet.* 2009; 374(9696):1171–1178.
12. Dusser D, Bravo ML, Iacono P. The effect of tiotropium on exacerbations and airflow in patients with COPD. *Eur Respir J.* 2006;27(3):547–555.
13. O'Donnell DE. Hyperinflation, dyspnea, and exercise intolerance in chronic obstructive pulmonary disease. *Proc Am Thorac Soc.* 2006;3(2):180–184.
14. Ezzell L, Jensen GL. Malnutrition in chronic obstructive pulmonary disease. *Am J Clin Nutr.* 2000;72(6):1415–1416.
15. Donahoe M, Rogers RM, Wilson DO, Pennock BE. Oxygen consumption of the respiratory muscles in normal and in malnourished patients with chronic obstructive pulmonary disease. *Am Rev Respir Dis.* 1989;140(2):385–391.
16. Badgett RG, Tanaka DJ, Hunt DK, et al. Can moderate chronic obstructive pulmonary disease be diagnosed by historical and physical findings alone? *Am J Med.* 1993;94(2):188–196.
17. Straus SE, McAlister FA, Sackett DL, Deeks JJ. Accuracy of history, wheezing, and forced expiratory time in the diagnosis of chronic obstructive pulmonary disease. *J Gen Intern Med.* 2002;17(9):684–688.
18. American Thoracic Society, European Respiratory Society. American Thoracic Society/European Respiratory Society statement: standards for the diagnosis and management of individuals with alpha-1 antitrypsin deficiency. *Am J Respir Crit Care Med.* 2003;168(7):818–900.
19. Morris A, Crothers K, Beck JM, Huang L. An official ATS workshop report: emerging issues and current controversies in HIV-associated pulmonary diseases. *Proc Am Thorac Soc.* 2011;8(1):17–26.
20. Drummond MB, Kirk GD, Astemborski J, et al. Association between obstructive lung disease and markers of HIV infection in a high-risk cohort. *Thorax.* 2012;67(4):309–314.
21. Jones PW, Harding G, Berry P, Wiklund I, Chen WH, Kline Leidy N. Development and first validation of the COPD Assessment Test. *Eur Respir J.* 2009;34(3):648–654.
22. Christakis NA, Escarce JJ. Survival of Medicare patients after enrollment in hospice programs. *N Engl J Med.* 1996;335(3): 172–178.
23. Berry CE, Wise RA. Mortality in COPD: causes, risk factors, and prevention. *COPD.* 2010;7(5):375–382.
24. Anthonisen NR, Wright EC, Hodgkin JE. Prognosis in chronic obstructive pulmonary disease. *Am Rev Respir Dis.* 1986;133(1): 14–20.
25. Nishimura K, Izumi T, Tsukino M, Oga T. Dyspnea is a better predictor of 5-year survival than airway obstruction in patients with COPD. *Chest.* 2002;121(5):1434–1440.

26. Celli BR, Cote CG, Marin JM, et al. The body-mass index, airflow obstruction, dyspnea, and exercise capacity index in chronic obstructive pulmonary disease. *N Engl J Med*. 2004;350(10):1005–1012.

27. Puhan MA, Garcia-Aymerich J, Frey M, et al. Expansion of the prognostic assessment of patients with chronic obstructive pulmonary disease: the updated BODE index and the ADO index. *Lancet*. 2009;374(9691):704–711.

28. Sin DD, McAlister FA, Man SF, Anthonisen NR. Contemporary management of chronic obstructive pulmonary disease: scientific review. *JAMA*. 2003;290(17):2301–2312.

29. Sutherland ER, Cherniack RM. Management of chronic obstructive pulmonary disease. *N Engl J Med*. 2004;350(26):2689–2697.

30. Schunemann HJ, Woodhead M, Anzueto A, et al. A guide to guidelines for professional societies and other developers of recommendations: introduction to integrating and coordinating efforts in COPD guideline development. An official ATS/ERS workshop report. *Proc Am Thorac Soc*. 2012;9(5):215–218.

31. A clinical practice guideline for treating tobacco use and dependence: A US Public Health Service report. The Tobacco Use and Dependence Clinical Practice Guideline Panel, Staff, and Consortium Representatives. *JAMA*. 2000;283(24):3244–3254.

32. Lai DT, Cahill K, Qin Y, Tang JL. Motivational interviewing for smoking cessation. *Cochrane Database Syst Rev*. 2010;(1):CD006936.

33. Coggon D, Newman Taylor A. Coal mining and chronic obstructive pulmonary disease: a review of the evidence. *Thorax*. 1998;53(5):398–407.

34. Salvi SS, Barnes PJ. Chronic obstructive pulmonary disease in non-smokers. *Lancet*. 2009;374(9691):733–743.

35. Johnson MK, Smith RP, Morrison D, Laszlo G, White RJ. Large lung bullae in marijuana smokers. *Thorax*. 2000;55(4):340–342.

36. Varkey JB, Varkey AB, Varkey B. Prophylactic vaccinations in chronic obstructive pulmonary disease: current status. *Curr Opin Pulm Med*. 2009;15(2):90–99.

37. Survival and FEV1 decline in individuals with severe deficiency of alpha1-antitrypsin. The Alpha-1-Antitrypsin Deficiency Registry Study Group. *Am J Respir Crit Care Med*. 1998;158(1):49–59.

38. Nannini L, Cates CJ, Lasserson TJ, Poole P. Combined corticosteroid and long acting beta-agonist in one inhaler for chronic obstructive pulmonary disease. *Cochrane Database Syst Rev*. 2004;(3):CD003794.

39. Calverley PM, Anderson JA, Celli B, et al; TORCH investigators. Salmeterol and fluticasone propionate and survival in chronic obstructive pulmonary disease. *N Engl J Med*. 2007;356(8):775–789.

40. Tashkin DP, Celli B, Senn S, et al. A 4-year trial of tiotropium in chronic obstructive pulmonary disease. *N Engl J Med*. 2008;359(15):1543–1554.

41. Ram FS, Sestini P. Regular inhaled short acting beta2 agonists for the management of stable chronic obstructive pulmonary disease: Cochrane systematic review and meta-analysis. *Thorax*. 2003;58(7):580–584.

42. Appleton S, Poole P, Smith B, Veale A, Bara A. Long-acting beta2-agonists for chronic obstructive pulmonary disease patients with poorly reversible airflow limitation. *Cochrane Database Syst Rev*. 2002;(3):CD001104.

43. Rennard SI, Tashkin DP, McElhattan J, et al. Efficacy and tolerability of budesonide/formoterol in one hydrofluoroalkane pressurized metered-dose inhaler in patients with chronic obstructive pulmonary disease: results from a 1-year randomized controlled clinical trial. *Drugs*. 2009;69(5):549–565.

44. Drummond MB, Dasenbrook EC, Pitz MW, Murphy DJ, Fan E. Inhaled corticosteroids in patients with stable chronic obstructive pulmonary disease: a systematic review and meta-analysis. *JAMA*. 2008;300(20):2407–2416.

45. Ram FS, Jones PW, Castro AA, et al. Oral theophylline for chronic obstructive pulmonary disease. *Cochrane Database Syst Rev*. 2002;(4):CD003902.

46. Ito K, Ito M, Elliott WM, et al. Decreased histone deacetylase activity in chronic obstructive pulmonary disease. *N Engl J Med*. 2005;352(19):1967–1976.

47. Calverley PM, Rabe KF, Goehring UM, Kristiansen S, Fabbri LM, Martinez FJ. Roflumilast in symptomatic chronic obstructive pulmonary disease: two randomised clinical trials. *Lancet*. 2009;374(9691):685–694.

48. Albert RK, Connett J, Bailey WC, et al.; COPD Clinical Research Network. Azithromycin for prevention of exacerbations of COPD. *N Engl J Med*. 2011;365(8):689–698.

49. Zheng JP, Kang J, Huang SG, et al. Effect of carbocisteine on acute exacerbation of chronic obstructive pulmonary disease (PEACE Study): a randomised placebo-controlled study. *Lancet*. 2008;371(9629):2013–2018.

50. Decramer M, Rutten-van Molken M, Dekhuijzen PN, et al. Effects of N-acetylcysteine on outcomes in chronic obstructive pulmonary disease (Bronchitis Randomized on NAC Cost-Utility Study, BRONCUS): a randomised placebo-controlled trial. *Lancet*. 2005;365(9470):1552–1560.

51. Emtner M, Porszasz J, Burns M, Somfay A, Casaburi R. Benefits of supplemental oxygen in exercise training in nonhypoxemic chronic obstructive pulmonary disease patients. *Am J Respir Crit Care Med*. 2003;168(9):1034–1042.

52. Cano NJ, Roth H, Court-Ortune I, et al. Nutritional depletion in patients on long-term oxygen therapy and/or home mechanical ventilation. *Eur Respir J*. 2002;20(1):30–37.

53. Schols AM, Wouters EF. Nutritional abnormalities and supplementation in chronic obstructive pulmonary disease. *Clin Chest Med*. 2000;21(4):753–762.

54. Ferreira I, Brooks D, Lacasse Y, Goldstein R. Nutritional intervention in COPD: a systematic overview. *Chest*. 2001;119(2):353–363.

55. Wise RA, Enright PL, Connett JE, et al. Effect of weight gain on pulmonary function after smoking cessation in the Lung Health Study. *Am J Respir Crit Care Med*. 1998;157(3 Pt 1):866–872.

56. Collop N. Sleep and sleep disorders in chronic obstructive pulmonary disease. *Respiration*. 2010;80(1):78–86.

57. Weitzenblum E, Chaouat A. Sleep and chronic obstructive pulmonary disease. *Sleep Med Rev*. 2004;8(4):281–294.

58. Owens RL, Malhotra A. Sleep-disordered breathing and COPD: the overlap syndrome. *Respir Care*. 2010;55(10):1333–1344; discussion 1344–1336.

59. Shrikrishna D, Coker RK. Managing passengers with stable respiratory disease planning air travel: British Thoracic Society recommendations. *Thorax*. 2011;66(9):831–833.

60. Vohra KP, Klocke RA. Detection and correction of hypoxemia associated with air travel. *Am Rev Respir Dis*. 1993;148(5):1215–1219.

61. Gong H Jr, Tashkin DP, Lee EY, Simmons MS. Hypoxia-altitude simulation test. Evaluation of patients with chronic airway obstruction. *Am Rev Respir Dis*. 1984;130(6):980–986.

62. Long term domiciliary oxygen therapy in chronic hypoxic cor pulmonale complicating chronic bronchitis and emphysema. Report of the Medical Research Council Working Party. *Lancet.* 1981;1(8222):681–686.

63. Crockett AJ, Cranston JM, Moss JR, Alpers JH. Domiciliary oxygen for chronic obstructive pulmonary disease. *Cochrane Database Syst Rev.* 2000;(4):CD001744.

64. Continuous or nocturnal oxygen therapy in hypoxemic chronic obstructive lung disease: a clinical trial. Nocturnal Oxygen Therapy Trial Group. *Ann Intern Med.* 1980;93(3):391–398.

65. Cooper CB, Waterhouse J, Howard P. Twelve year clinical study of patients with hypoxic cor pulmonale given long term domiciliary oxygen therapy. *Thorax.* 1987;42(2):105–110.

66. Hurst JR, Vestbo J, Anzueto A, et al. Susceptibility to exacerbation in chronic obstructive pulmonary disease. *N Engl J Med.* 2010;363(12):1128–1138.

67. Niewoehner DE, Erbland ML, Deupree RH, et al. Effect of systemic glucocorticoids on exacerbations of chronic obstructive pulmonary disease. Department of Veterans Affairs Cooperative Study Group. *N Engl J Med.* 1999;340(25):1941–1947.

68. Singh JM, Palda VA, Stanbrook MB, Chapman KR. Corticosteroid therapy for patients with acute exacerbations of chronic obstructive pulmonary disease: a systematic review. *Arch Intern Med.* 2002;162(22):2527–2536.

69. McCrory DC, Brown CD. Anti-cholinergic bronchodilators versus beta2-sympathomimetic agents for acute exacerbations of chronic obstructive pulmonary disease. *Cochrane Database Syst Rev.* 2002;(4):CD003900.

70. Ram FS, Picot J, Lightowler J, Wedzicha JA. Non-invasive positive pressure ventilation for treatment of respiratory failure due to exacerbations of chronic obstructive pulmonary disease. *Cochrane Database Syst Rev.* 2004;(3):CD004104.

71. Connors AF Jr, Dawson NV, Thomas C, et al. Outcomes following acute exacerbation of severe chronic obstructive lung disease. The SUPPORT investigators (Study to Understand Prognoses and Preferences for Outcomes and Risks of Treatments). *Am J Respir Crit Care Med.* 1996;154(4 Pt 1):959–967.

72. Naeije R. Pulmonary hypertension and right heart failure in chronic obstructive pulmonary disease. *Proc Am Thorac Soc.* 2005;2(1):20–22.

73. Fisher MR, Criner GJ, Fishman AP, et al. Estimating pulmonary artery pressures by echocardiography in patients with emphysema. *Eur Respir J.* 2007;30(5):914–921.

74. Chaouat A, Naeije R, Weitzenblum E. Pulmonary hypertension in COPD. *Eur Respir J.* 2008;32(5):1371–1385.

75. Duiverman ML, Wempe JB, Bladder G, et al. Two-year home-based nocturnal noninvasive ventilation added to rehabilitation in chronic obstructive pulmonary disease patients: a randomized controlled trial. *Respir Res.* 2011;12:112.

76. Fishman A, Martinez F, Naunheim K, et al. A randomized trial comparing lung-volume-reduction surgery with medical therapy for severe emphysema. *N Engl J Med.* 2003;348(21):2059–2073.

77. Sciurba FC, Ernst A, Herth FJ, et al. A randomized study of endobronchial valves for advanced emphysema. *N Engl J Med.* 2010;363(13):1233–1244.

78. Ingenito EP, Wood DE, Utz JP. Bronchoscopic lung volume reduction in severe emphysema. *Proc Am Thorac Soc.* 2008;5(4):454–460.

79. Orens JB, Estenne M, Arcasoy S, et al. International guidelines for the selection of lung transplant candidates: 2006 update–a consensus report from the Pulmonary Scientific Council of the International Society for Heart and Lung Transplantation. *J Heart Lung Transplant.* 2006;25(7):745–755.

80. Schonhofer B, Euteneuer S, Nava S, Suchi S, Kohler D. Survival of mechanically ventilated patients admitted to a specialised weaning centre. *Intensive Care Med.* 2002;28(7):908–916.

CHAPTER 43

Rehabilitation in Chronic Obstructive Pulmonary Disease and Other Respiratory Disorders

Andrew L. Ries

Rehabilitation for patients with chronic lung diseases is well established as a means of enhancing standard pharmacologic and other therapies in controlling and alleviating symptoms and optimizing functional capacity.[1–4] The primary goal of any rehabilitation program is to restore the patient to the highest possible level of independent function. This goal is accomplished by helping patients and significant others learn more about the underlying disease, treatment options, and coping strategies. Patients are encouraged to participate actively in providing their own health care, become more independent in daily activities, and be less dependent on health professionals and expensive medical resources. Rather than addressing solely reversal of the disease process, rehabilitation focuses on improving disability from disease.

Historically, pulmonary rehabilitation strategies were developed and have been used primarily for patients with chronic obstructive pulmonary disease (COPD). However, pulmonary rehabilitation has also been applied successfully to patients with other chronic lung conditions, including interstitial diseases, cystic fibrosis, bronchiectasis, and thoracic cage abnormalities.[3,5–7] It has been used successfully in the evaluation and preparation of patients for surgery, such as lung transplantation and volume reduction lung surgery, and in maximizing recovery after surgery.[8–11] Pulmonary rehabilitation has been used to facilitate patient recovery from acute processes such as acute lung injury, or exacerbations of chronic lung disease requiring mechanical ventilation or acute hospital care. Pulmonary rehabilitation is appropriate for any patient with stable lung disease who is disabled by respiratory symptoms. Even patients with advanced disease may benefit if they are selected appropriately and realistic goals are set.

This chapter defines pulmonary rehabilitation and outlines issues related to patient selection and evaluation. Key components of a pulmonary rehabilitation program are described and results of rehabilitation programs reviewed. Finally, the role of rehabilitation prior to and following lung surgery is reviewed.

DEFINITION

In 2006, the American Thoracic Society and European Respiratory Society adopted the following definition:

> Pulmonary rehabilitation is an evidence-based, multidisciplinary, and comprehensive intervention for patients with chronic respiratory diseases who are symptomatic and often have decreased daily life activities. Integrated into the individualized treatment of the patient, pulmonary rehabilitation is designed to reduce symptoms, optimize functional status, increase participation, and reduce healthcare costs through stabilizing or reversing systemic manifestations of the disease.[2]

This definition focuses on three important features of successful rehabilitation. First, the program is *multidisciplinary.* Pulmonary rehabilitation programs utilize expertise from various healthcare disciplines that is integrated into a comprehensive, cohesive program tailored to the needs of each patient. Second, the program is tailored to the *individual.* Patients with disabling lung disease require individual assessment of needs, individual attention, and a program designed to meet realistic individual goals. Third, the program addresses *multidimensional outcomes* that include physical, psychological, and social function as well as healthcare utilization.

The interdisciplinary team of healthcare professionals in pulmonary rehabilitation may include physicians, nurses, respiratory and physical therapists, psychologists, exercise specialists, and others with appropriate expertise. The specific team make up depends upon the resources and expertise available, but it usually includes at least one full-time staff member. Responsibilities of team members generally cross disciplines.[12]

Within this general framework, successful pulmonary rehabilitation programs have been established in both outpatient and inpatient settings and with different formats. A key to success is a dedicated, enthusiastic staff that is familiar with respiratory problems and can relate well to pulmonary patients and motivate them.

PATIENT SELECTION

Any patient with symptomatic chronic lung disease is a candidate for pulmonary rehabilitation (Table 43-1). Appropriate patients are aware of disability from their disease and are motivated to participate actively in their own care to improve their health status. Patients with mild chronic disease may not perceive their symptoms to be severe enough to warrant a comprehensive care program. On the other hand, patients with severe disease who are bed bound may be too limited to benefit greatly.

Criteria based on arbitrary lung function parameters or age alone should not be used in selecting patients.[1] Pulmonary function is not a good predictor of symptoms, function, or improvement after rehabilitation.[13] Chronic lung disease is commonly associated with systemic features that contribute to functional limitations and may benefit from rehabilitation.[14] In general, selection should be based upon a person's disability from their disease, potential for improvement, and motivation to participate actively in a comprehensive self-care program. Also, pulmonary rehabilitation is not a primary mode of therapy. Patients should be stabilized on standard medical therapy and should not have other disabling or unstable conditions that might limit their ability to participate fully in the program and to concentrate on the necessary tasks.

The ideal patient for pulmonary rehabilitation, then, is one with functional limitation from moderate to severe lung disease who is stable on standard therapy, not distracted or limited by other serious or unstable medical conditions, willing and able to learn about his or her disease, and motivated to devote the time and effort necessary to benefit from a comprehensive care program.

TABLE 43-1 Patient Selection Criteria for Pulmonary Rehabilitation

Symptomatic chronic lung disease
Stable on standard therapy
Functional limitation from disease
Relationship with primary care provider
Motivated to be actively involved in and take responsibility for own health care
No other interfering or unstable medical conditions
No arbitrary lung function or age criteria

PATIENT EVALUATION

The initial step is screening patients to ensure appropriate selection and to set realistic individual and program goals. The evaluation process includes the following components: interview, medical evaluation, psychosocial assessment, diagnostic testing, and goal setting (Table 43-2).

INTERVIEW

The screening interview is an important first step. It serves to introduce the patient to the program, review the medical history, and identify psychosocial problems and needs. Family members and significant others should be included. Communication with the primary care provider is important to establish the vital link for the rehabilitation staff to clarify medical questions prior to the program and facilitate subsequent recommendations. Care and attention in this initial evaluation helps in setting goals compatible with everyone's expectations as well as appropriate programmatic objectives.

MEDICAL EVALUATION

Reviewing medical history helps to identify the patient's lung disease and assess its severity. Other medical problems that might preclude or delay participation may be identified. Available laboratory data should be reviewed, including pulmonary function and exercise tests, rest and exercise arterial blood gas measurements, chest radiographs, electrocardiogram, and pertinent blood tests. Program

TABLE 43-2 Components of a Comprehensive Pulmonary Rehabilitation Program

- Patient evaluation
  - Interview
  - Medical evaluation
  - Psychosocial assessment
  - Diagnostic testing
    - Pulmonary function
    - Exercise
    - Arterial blood gases/oximetry
  - Goal setting
- Program content
  - Education
  - Respiratory and chest physiotherapy instruction
    - Bronchial hygiene
    - Breathing retraining techniques
    - Oxygen
  - Exercise
  - Psychosocial support

staff can then determine the need for any additional information or action before the program begins.

PSYCHOSOCIAL ASSESSMENT

Successful rehabilitation requires attention not only to the patient's physical problems but also to psychological, emotional, and social issues. Patients with chronic illnesses experience psychosocial difficulties as they struggle to deal with symptoms they may not fully understand.[15]

Neuropsychological impairment is common in patients with chronic lung diseases and cannot be accounted for solely on the basis of age, depression, or organic disease. Commonly, such patients become depressed, frightened, anxious, and more dependent on others to care for their needs. Progressive dyspnea is a frightening symptom and may lead to a vicious "fear–dyspnea" cycle: With progressive disease, less exertion results in more dyspnea, which produces more fear and anxiety, which, in turn, lead to more dyspnea. Ultimately, the patient avoids any physical activity associated with both of these unpleasant symptoms.

In addressing these problems, the initial evaluation should assess the patient's psychological state and pay attention to "psychosocial clues" that may be apparent during the screening interview (e.g., level of family and social support, the patient's living arrangement, activities of daily living, hobbies, and employment potential). Important clues in initial interviews to the patient's emotional state may be evident in nonverbal communication, such as facial expression, physical appearance, handshake, and personal space (distance between individuals when conversing). Cognitive impairment that may limit the patient's ability to participate fully in the rehabilitation program may be identified. Family members and significant others may provide valuable insight and should be included in the screening process and program whenever possible.

DIAGNOSTIC TESTING

Planning an appropriate rehabilitation program requires accurate, current information. The complexity of the testing procedures performed depends upon individual patient and program goals as well as the facilities and expertise available.

Pulmonary function testing is used to characterize lung disease and quantify impairment. Spirometry and lung volume measurements are most useful. Other tests (e.g., diffusing capacity, maximal respiratory pressures to assess muscle strength) can be added as needed.

Exercise testing helps to assess the patient's exercise tolerance and to evaluate changes in arterial blood gases (e.g., hypoxemia or hypercapnia) with exercise.[16,17] This may also uncover coexisting diseases (e.g., heart disease). The exercise test is also used to establish a safe and appropriate prescription for subsequent training.

Maximal exercise of patients with chronic lung disease is limited largely by their breathing reserve, though chronic lung diseases are increasingly recognized as being associated with systemic effects that may also contribute to exertional symptoms (e.g., muscle fatigue). Simple pulmonary function tests such as spirometry can be used to estimate a patient's capacity for sustained breathing (maximal ventilation) during exercise. The forced expiratory volume in 1 second (FEV_1) is most useful in this regard. However, lung function only provides an estimate of an individual patient's maximum work capacity. Exercise tolerance depends also on the patient's perception and tolerance of the subjective symptom of breathlessness. Therefore, it is important to exercise patients to assess their physical function and symptom tolerance.

Exercise evaluation for rehabilitation is most easily performed with the type of activity planned for training (e.g., treadmill for a walking training program). Laboratory exercise testing is most commonly performed using either (1) rapid, progressive, incremental levels to a symptom-limited maximum or (2) defined steady-state levels.[16,18] The former is most useful for determining exercise tolerance and the limitations to maximum performance. The latter may be preferred for assessing training prescriptions. Simpler exercise tests, such as the 6-minute walk test, have been used increasingly in recent years to measure exercise tolerance outside of a laboratory setting.[19] These timed distance walk tests measure the maximum distance a person can walk within a defined period (e.g., 6 minutes). Such tests have the advantage of requiring less equipment and technical expertise; however, attention must be paid to the details of testing procedures because variations in factors such as the walking course, patient instructions, encouragement during tests, use of oxygen or monitoring devices, and number of tests performed will influence the results. Also, these tests do not provide the detailed physiologic data typically included in more formal laboratory exercise tests.

Measurement of arterial blood gases at rest and during exercise is important because of the frequent but unpredictable occurrence of exercise-induced hypoxemia.[20] Arterial blood gas sampling during exercise makes testing more complex. The noninvasive estimate of arterial oxygen saturation by cutaneous (e.g., pulse) oximetry is useful for continuous monitoring, but it has limited accuracy (95% confidence limits, ±4–5%).[21]

GOALS

After a patient's medical, physiologic, and psychosocial state have been evaluated, specific goals should be set that are compatible with his or her disease, needs, and expectations. Goals should be realistic in light of the objectives of the program. Family members and significant others should be included in this process so that everyone understands what can and cannot be achieved. Programs should evaluate individual patients to document changes before and after pulmonary rehabilitation with standardized outcome measures of exercise tolerance (e.g., 6-minute walk distance) and symptoms (e.g., dyspnea) or health status (e.g., health-related quality of life).

PROGRAM CONTENT

Comprehensive pulmonary rehabilitation programs typically include several key components: education, instruction in respiratory and chest physiotherapy, psychosocial support, and exercise training (Table 43-2). Often, the various components are provided simultaneously; for example, during an exercise session, a patient may learn and practice breathing techniques for symptom control while being encouraged and supported by staff or other patients. Although there is no consensus regarding the optimal duration of a pulmonary rehabilitation intervention, typical programs last 6 to 12 weeks with 2 to 3 sessions per week, each session including several hours of supervised exercise training and individual or group education and psychosocial interventions.

EDUCATION

Successful pulmonary rehabilitation depends upon an understanding of lung disease and active involvement by patients and important others in providing social support. Education is an integral component; even patients with severe disease can gain a better understanding of their disease and learn specific means to deal with problems. Instruction can be provided individually or in small groups, but it should be adapted to different learning abilities. Topics discussed commonly include normal lung function, chronic lung disease, medications, nutrition, travel, stress reduction and relaxation, reasons to call the physician, and planning a daily schedule. Individual instruction and coaching may be provided on the use of respiratory therapy equipment and supplemental oxygen, breathing techniques, bronchial drainage, chest percussion, energy-saving techniques, and self-care tips. The general philosophy is to encourage patients to assume responsibility for their own care and become partners with their physician in providing the care.[22]

Despite the importance of education, it is unlikely that increased patient knowledge alone will lead to improved health status. It is more difficult to change patient attitudes and behaviors. Patients require specific, individualized treatment strategies, instruction, and reinforcement. Thus, education is a necessary but not sufficient component of pulmonary rehabilitation.

RESPIRATORY AND CHEST PHYSIOTHERAPY TECHNIQUES

Patients with chronic lung disease use, abuse, and are confused about respiratory and chest physiotherapy techniques. In pulmonary rehabilitation, each patient's needs for respiratory care techniques should be assessed and instruction provided in proper use. These techniques may include chest physiotherapy to control secretions; breathing retraining techniques to relieve and control dyspnea and improve ventilatory function; and proper use and care of respiratory equipment, including nebulizers, metered dose inhalers, and supplemental oxygen.[23]

BRONCHIAL HYGIENE

Patients with chronic lung diseases frequently have abnormal lung clearance mechanisms that increase problems with retained secretions and infection. Therefore, rehabilitation programs teach a variety of chest physiotherapy techniques for secretion control (e.g., coughing, postural drainage, chest vibration, and percussion). These are important for patients who experience excess mucus production during exacerbations as well as for those with chronic sputum production. The use of mucolytic agents to reduce viscosity of secretions is of questionable benefit.[24,25]

BREATHING RETRAINING TECHNIQUES

Pulmonary rehabilitation typically includes instruction in breathing techniques, such as diaphragmatic and pursed lips breathing—techniques aimed at helping patients relieve and control breathlessness, improve their ventilatory pattern (i.e., slower respiratory rate and increased tidal volume), prevent dynamic airway compression, improve respiratory synchrony of the abdominal and thoracic musculature, and improve gas exchange.[26] Review of studies evaluating these techniques indicates that improvement in symptoms (e.g., dyspnea) is a more consistent finding than are measurable changes in physiological parameters. The diaphragmatic breathing technique is a maneuver in which the patient consciously coordinates abdominal wall expansion with inspiration and slows expiration through pursed lips. The primary effect is to slow respiratory rate and increase tidal volume. Pursed lips breathing is commonly taught to pulmonary patients, particularly those with COPD. This technique was observed by Laennec as early as 1830 and was advocated as a physical exercise for pulmonary patients in the early part of the twentieth century. As a maneuver assumed naturally by many patients with respiratory disease, pursed lips breathing is characterized by tensing the lips and narrowing the mouth opening during expiration. The aim is to slow expiration and maintain positive airway pressure to "stent the airways open" and prevent collapse.[27]

OXYGEN

When chronic oxygen therapy is required, available delivery methods should be reviewed to help select the best system for the patient's needs. Supplemental oxygen is beneficial for patients with severe resting hypoxemia. Long-term continuous oxygen therapy has been clearly shown to improve survival and reduce mortality and morbidity in hypoxemic patients with COPD.[28,29] The benefits of supplemental oxygen for nonhypoxemic patients or those with intermittent hypoxemia (e.g., during exercise or sleep) are less clearly defined. Although continuous oxygen therapy is feasible and safe, maintaining patients on supplemental oxygen presents several challenges. Handling equipment is particularly difficult for physically disabled and frail patients. Therefore, it is important to assess each person's oxygen needs and provide appropriate instruction.[30]

Several new developments have improved the efficiency of gas delivery systems and patient compliance with continuous oxygen therapy. Liquid oxygen provides more gas with less weight than tanks of compressed gas, particularly in portable systems. Oxygen conserving devices may increase the efficiency of delivery, reducing flow requirements and prolonging the life span of portable gas sources. Transtracheal oxygen delivery may help to improve compliance and avoid problems with nasal catheters; however, patients must be instructed carefully in caring for the catheter.[31]

EXERCISE

Exercise is important in pulmonary rehabilitation.[32,33] Considerable evidence supports favorable responses to exercise training in patients with chronic lung diseases.[3] Benefits are both physiological and psychological. Patients may increase their maximum capacity and endurance for physical activity, even though objective measures of lung function do not usually change. Patients may also benefit from learning to perform physical tasks more efficiently. Exercise training provides an ideal opportunity for patients to learn their capacity for physical work and use and practice methods for controlling dyspnea (e.g., breathing and relaxation techniques). Of all the components in a comprehensive pulmonary rehabilitation program, exercise is probably the most costly and labor-intensive, considering the personnel, equipment, and expertise required. Principles of exercise for patients with lung disease differ from those based on normals or other patient populations because of differences in the limitations to exercise and the problems encountered in training.

Many approaches have been used to train the person with chronic lung disease. To be successful, the program should be tailored to the individual's physical abilities, interests, resources, and environment. For general application, techniques should be simple and inexpensive. As in normals and other patients, benefits are largely specific to the muscles and tasks involved in training. Patients tend to do best with activities and exercises for which they are trained. Walking programs are particularly useful. They have the added benefit of encouraging patients to expand social horizons. In inclement weather, many can walk indoors (e.g., at shopping malls). Other types of exercise (e.g., cycling, swimming) are also effective. Patients should be encouraged to incorporate regular exercise into daily activities they enjoy (e.g., golf, gardening). Since many persons with chronic lung disease have limited exercise tolerance, emphasis during training should be placed on increasing endurance. Changes in endurance with rehabilitation are often greater than changes in maximal exercise tolerance and allow patients to become more functional within their physical limits. Increase in maximum exercise is also possible as patients gain experience and confidence. Resistive training is also used commonly in rehabilitation and can lead to significant increases in muscle strength that are important for many activities of daily living.[34]

EXERCISE PRESCRIPTION

Selecting a training target based upon a predetermined percentage of predicted maximal heart rate or ($\dot{V}_{O_2}$) is a well-established practice for normals or patients without underlying pulmonary disease. However, in patients with chronic lung diseases, the best method of choosing an appropriate training prescription is less clearly defined. Exercise tolerance in pulmonary patients is typically limited by maximal achievable ventilation and breathlessness. Such patients frequently do not reach their limits of cardiac or peripheral muscle performance.

Much controversy exists regarding the appropriate training intensity target for patients with chronic lung disease. Use of a target heart rate has been advocated by some, although it is recognized that such a target may not be reliable for patients with more severe disease.

Many patients with lung disease can be trained at a high percentage of maximal exercise tolerance, with work levels approaching or even exceeding the maximal level reached on the initial exercise test. In a study of 52 patients with moderate to severe COPD, patients were able to perform endurance exercise testing at an average workload of 95% of their baseline maximum.[35] After 8 weeks of training, these patients were training at 86% of the baseline maximum. In fact, many patients with severe COPD were exercising at levels exceeding their baseline maximum. In another study that examined 59 patients with moderate to severe COPD who trained at levels near their ventilatory limits, a mean peak exercise ventilation of 100% of measured maximal voluntary ventilation was achieved after 12 days of training and at 3 months of follow-up.[36] These findings suggest that even patients with advanced disease can be trained successfully at or near maximal exercise levels.

Based on the findings noted previously, some pulmonary rehabilitation programs define exercise targets and progression during training more by symptom tolerance than heart rate, work level, or other physiological measurements. Ratings of perceived symptoms (e.g., breathlessness) help teach patients to exercise to "target" levels of breathing discomfort. A typical approach is to begin training at a level that the patient can sustain with reasonable comfort for several minutes and then to increase the time or exercise level according to symptom tolerance. Patients are encouraged to exercise daily and increase exercise duration up to 15 to 30 minutes of continuous activity. This graduated program helps patients to achieve a goal of improved tolerance for tasks of daily living, which often require a period of sustained activity.

BLOOD GAS CHANGES

A major problem in planning a safe exercise program for patients with lung disease is the potential for worsening of hypoxemia with exercise. Patients who are not hypoxemic at rest may develop changes in arterial oxygenation that cannot be predicted reliably from resting measurements of pulmonary function or gas exchange.[20] Normal individuals do not become hypoxemic with exercise. In patients with obstructive lung disease, Pa_{O_2} changes unpredictably during exercise. In patients with mild COPD, Pa_{O_2} typically does not change with exercise; in fact, it may even improve. However, in patients with moderate to severe COPD, Pa_{O_2} may increase, decrease, or remain the same. Patients with interstitial lung disease commonly develop worsening oxygenation with exercise.

Based on these observations, it is important to evaluate a patient's oxygenation status both at rest and during exercise. Such testing is also used to prescribe oxygen therapy at rest and with physical activity. With the availability of convenient, portable systems for ambulatory oxygen delivery, hypoxemia is not a contraindication to safe exercise training.

OTHER TYPES OF EXERCISE

Exercise programs for pulmonary patients typically emphasize lower extremity training (e.g., walking or cycling). Since exercise conditioning is largely specific to the muscles and tasks involved in training other forms of exercise may be particularly valuable for persons with chronic lung diseases.

Upper Extremity Training

Many patients with chronic lung disease report disabling dyspnea with daily activities involving the upper extremities (e.g., lifting, grooming) at much lower work levels than with the lower extremities. Upper extremity exercise is accompanied by a higher ventilatory demand for a given level of work than is lower extremity exercise. Given the aforementioned muscle specificity of training, upper extremity exercises may be important in helping pulmonary patients cope better with common daily activities.[37]

Ventilatory Muscle Training

The potential role of ventilatory muscle fatigue as a cause of respiratory failure and ventilatory limitation in patients with chronic lung disease has stimulated attempts to train the ventilatory muscles. Techniques of isocapnic hyperventilation, inspiratory resistive loading, and inspiratory threshold loading have been shown to improve function of the respiratory muscles in both normals and patients. In normals, respiratory muscle function does not limit exercise tolerance; therefore, specific respiratory muscle training is unlikely to be of clinical benefit. In patients with COPD, the patient group most extensively studied, improvement in general exercise performance from ventilatory muscle training alone has not been demonstrated consistently. Thus, the role of respiratory muscle training as a routine component of pulmonary rehabilitation has not been clearly established.

PSYCHOSOCIAL SUPPORT

An essential component of pulmonary rehabilitation is psychosocial support, the goal of which is to help patients combat progressive feelings of hopelessness and an inability to cope with chronic, progressive disease.[15] Depression is common in patients with chronic pulmonary disorders, as are anxiety (especially anxiety over dyspnea), denial, anger, and isolation. Patients become sedentary and dependent upon family members, friends, and medical services to provide for their needs. Excessive concern over other physical problems and psychosomatic complaints arise. Sexual dysfunction and fear are common and represent often unspoken consequences of chronic lung disease. Patients may also demonstrate cognitive and neuropsychological dysfunction, possibly related to or exacerbated by the effects of hypoxemia on the brain.

Psychosocial support is provided best by a warm and enthusiastic staff who can communicate effectively with patients and devote the time and effort necessary to understand and motivate them. Family members and significant others should be included in activities so that they can understand the disease and help the patient cope. Support groups are also effective. Patients with severe psychological disorders may benefit from individual counseling and therapy. Psychotropic drugs should generally be reserved for patients with more severe psychological dysfunction.

BENEFITS OF PULMONARY REHABILITATION

A growing body of evidence supports the expected results and benefits of pulmonary rehabilitation in the management of patients with chronic lung disease (Table 43-3). Evidence-based guidelines were

TABLE 43-3 Results of Pulmonary Rehabilitation

Decreases in
Medical resource utilization (e.g., hospitalizations, emergency room visits)
Respiratory symptoms (e.g., breathlessness)
Psychological symptoms (e.g., depression, fear)
Increases in
Quality of life
Physical activity
Exercise tolerance (endurance, maximal level of activities of daily living, strength)
Knowledge
Independence
Return to work possible
No change in lung function
Possible prolonged survival

published by a joint effort of the American College of Chest Physicians (ACCP) and the American Association of Cardiovascular and Pulmonary Rehabilitation (AACVPR) in 1997 and updated in 2007.[3,38] The 2007 ACCP/AACVPR Panel made and rated 26 recommendations and statements regarding pulmonary rehabilitation. Of these, seven were given the highest rating representing strong evidence and documented benefits. These included improvements in lower extremity exercise training, dyspnea, and health-related quality of life and the decline in benefits over 12 to 18 months from a 6- to 12-week intervention. They also felt that there was high-quality evidence supporting exercise in pulmonary rehabilitation regarding both high and low intensity training, increase in muscle strength and muscle mass from strength training, and upper extremity training. Other benefits with moderate level evidence included greater physiologic benefits from higher exercise training intensity, incorporation of education in pulmonary rehabilitation, and benefits for some patients with chronic respiratory diseases other than COPD. It should be noted that once a patient is stabilized on a standard drug treatment regimen, lung function (e.g., spirometric flow rates, lung volumes) does not change after pulmonary rehabilitation.

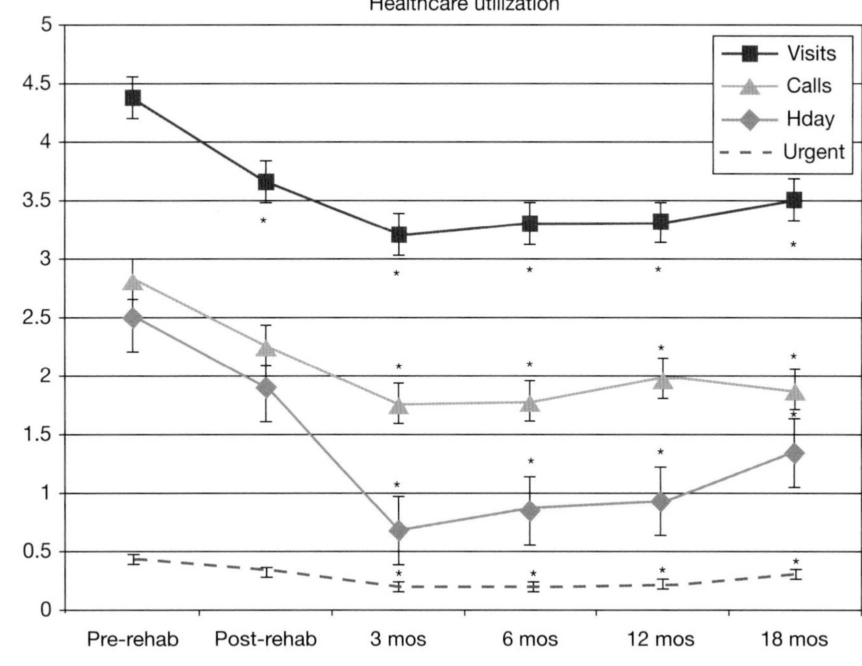

Figure 43-1 Changes in healthcare utilization over 18 months after pulmonary rehabilitation in a collaborative study of 647 patients in 10 centers in California. Results are presented as mean ± SE. *(Reproduced with permission from California Pulmonary Rehabflitation Collaborative Group: Effects of pulmonary rehabfl itation on dyspnea, quality of life and health care costs in California. J Cardiopulmonary Rehabfl. 2004;24:52–62.)*

In addition to the ACCP/AACVPR Guidelines, several other reviews support the benefits of pulmonary rehabilitation. The ATS/ERS Statement of Pulmonary Rehabilitation provides a systematic review and concludes that there is strong and growing evidence for improvement in exercise endurance, dyspnea, functional capacity, and quality of life and reduced healthcare utilization from pulmonary rehabilitation.[2] In a 2006 Cochrane Review, Lacasse et al.[39] analyzed 31 randomized trials in patients with COPD and concluded that rehabilitation forms an important component of the management of COPD. They reported statistically and clinically significant improvement in important domains of quality of life (dyspnea, fatigue, emotions, and patients' control over disease). Improvement in measures of exercise capacity was slightly below the threshold for clinical significance.

Benefits and cost savings associated with pulmonary rehabilitation have been demonstrated not only in highly specialized centers, but also in community-based practice settings.[3,40] A collaborative study of 647 patients in 10 centers in California reported significant improvements in dyspnea and health-related quality of life along with substantial reduction in measures of healthcare utilization over 18 months of follow-up.[41] (Fig. 43-1). Similar findings with a reduction in hospital and intensive care unit days in the year after compared with the year before pulmonary rehabilitation were reported by a consortium of 11 centers in Connecticut and New York in 128 patients.[42] In addition, pulmonary rehabilitation following a hospital admission for acute exacerbation may reduce subsequent hospital admission and mortality.[43]

PULMONARY REHABILITATION AND LUNG SURGERY

In recent years, surgical options for patients with severe, disabling lung disease have been used more frequently. Lung surgery in these patients represents new challenges and may further compromise already reduced lung function. Pulmonary rehabilitation has been found to be a valuable adjunct in preparing the patient for surgery or in postsurgery recovery.

LUNG TRANSPLANTATION

Pulmonary rehabilitation is recommended and used commonly in both the preoperative and postoperative phases of lung transplantation programs.[8,9,44] Although the general strategies of rehabilitation may be similar, the individual and program goals and specific program components differ (Table 43-4).

TABLE 43-4 Goals of Pulmonary Rehabilitation in Lung Transplantation

Pretransplant
Maintain and increase mobility and exercise tolerance
Monitor disease progression
Prevent complications
Provide education about
Underlying disease
Transplantation procedures
Self-care and self-assessment
Provide psychosocial support during waiting period for patients and families
Posttransplant
Improve physical work tolerance
Monitor clinical status and assess symptoms and oxygenation
Prevent complications
Reinforce self-care and self-assessment
Encourage compliance with medical regimen
Provide psychosocial support for adaptation to new demands and expectations

PRETRANSPLANT REHABILITATION

Patients with advanced lung disease who are candidates for lung transplantation are usually evaluated by the transplant team and then referred for pulmonary rehabilitation after their transplant candidacy is approved. Rehabilitation staff evaluate the patient to assess needs and plan an appropriate program that can be maintained throughout a waiting period, which may last months to years. Since these patients have advanced disease with limited life expectancy, the goals in the preoperative period differ from those that typically apply to rehabilitation in chronic lung disease.

The overall goals of pretransplant pulmonary rehabilitation are to maintain function, monitor disease progression, prevent complications, provide education about the underlying lung disease and lung transplantation, and offer psychosocial support for patients and families in coping with the stresses of waiting for a potentially life-saving procedure. Although patients may have some initial improvement in exercise tolerance or endurance as they begin rehabilitation, the primary goal for these patients is to maintain mobility and exercise capacity. Exercise sessions also provide an excellent means to monitor disease progression and to detect, at an earlier stage, problems that commonly occur (e.g., increased breathlessness or reduced arterial oxygenation with exercise).

The goals of education in the pretransplant period are to teach patients about their underlying lung disease, the transplant procedure itself, and expectations following transplantation. Patients can also be taught techniques for self-care and self-assessment that will be useful before and after surgery. The psychosocial stresses of waiting for transplantation are considerable. Many patients feel as though their lives are "on hold." Some may have moved away from family and social support networks to live close to the transplant center. Providing support for patients and families during this time, whether through formal group support sessions or informal contact with supportive staff and other patients, helps patients cope better with these problems.

POSTTRANSPLANT REHABILITATION

After lung transplantation, patients must learn to cope with a new level of function, new expectations, and a new set of problems. Rehabilitation for patients in this phase can facilitate physical reconditioning, help implement self-care and assessment techniques, and facilitate coping with the psychosocial adaptations to a new life-style.

Goals of exercise training after rehabilitation are improved physical work tolerance and continued assessment of symptoms and oxygenation as early warning signs of complications, including rejection and infection. Educational goals are focused on self-care and assessment and the importance of compliance with a new medical regimen. Psychosocial support can assist with adaptation to a new set of stresses related to additional demands and expectations from both patients for themselves and significant others. Patients who are used to being sick, disabled, and cared for by others may now be expected to be well, independent, return to work, and provide support for others.

LUNG VOLUME REDUCTION SURGERY

Pulmonary rehabilitation has been recommended as an important modality in the evaluation for and preparation of patients for this procedure as well as in the postoperative recovery phase.[11,45] Since these patients have severe, disabling chronic lung disease, they are typically good candidates for pulmonary rehabilitation. Enrolling patients in rehabilitation prior to surgery has the advantage of optimizing their functional status, improving physical and psychological symptoms, helping them learn more about their disease and alternative treatment options, and improving their skills for coping and actively co-managing their disease. Patients can then make an informed decision about surgical treatment based upon their optimal level of baseline function. After surgery, similar to the posttransplant period, rehabilitation helps patients to adapt to new levels of function and to reassess symptoms and oxygenation needs.

REHABILITATION AFTER LUNG RESECTION

Patients who undergo pulmonary resection frequently experience a significant increase in symptoms and reduced functional status. This is particularly true for patients with underlying chronic lung disease. Most commonly, surgery is used to treat patients with thoracic neoplasms who are deemed to have resectable disease and are operative candidates. Following resection, these patients with already limited lung function have to learn to adapt to a new, lower level of function.[46,47]

Similar changes may be observed in patients who undergo radiation therapy. Patients in a stable phase of their treatment or in remission may be appropriate candidates for pulmonary rehabilitation. Improvement in health status, physical and psychological symptoms, exercise tolerance, and quality of life – as well as reduced healthcare burdens – are potential benefits. These patients' survival may be as limited by their underlying lung disease as by their treated malignancy.

SUMMARY AND FUTURE OF PULMONARY REHABILITATION

Pulmonary rehabilitation has been well established as a means of improving functional status and reducing the disability and economic burden of the growing number of patients with chronic lung diseases. In adopting a broad rehabilitation medicine perspective, such programs provide interdisciplinary expertise directed toward the needs of the individual disabled patient.

Much of the experience in pulmonary rehabilitation has been in patients with COPD. However, it is clear that similar benefits can result for patients with other disabling pulmonary conditions. Pulmonary rehabilitation may also play an important role in the preoperative evaluation, preparation, and postoperative recovery of patients undergoing surgical procedures, including lung transplantation, lung volume reduction surgery, and lung resection. In many parts of the world, a major challenge for the widespread application of pulmonary rehabilitation to the large number of patients with chronic lung diseases relates to acceptance by health policy makers and health insurers about the benefits and cost savings associated with this treatment. In the United States, for instance, Medicare, the major government sponsored health insurance program that sets standards for many health insurers, recently implemented a national coverage policy for pulmonary rehabilitation.[48] This is a major step forward; however, the current relatively low reimbursement rates have threatened the financial viability of many existing programs. It is hoped that, with time and experience, the benefits of pulmonary rehabilitation as an effective, preventive health intervention that can improve patient outcomes and reduce healthcare costs will be better recognized.

REFERENCES

1. American Association of Cardiovascular and Pulmonary Rehabilitation. *Guidelines for Pulmonary Rehabilitation Programs.* 4th ed. Champaign, IL: Human Kinetics; 2011.
2. American Thoracic Society, European Respiratory Society. ATS/ERS statement on pulmonary rehabilitation. *Am J Respir Crit Care Med.* 2006;173:1390–1413.
3. Ries AL, Bauldoff GS, Carlin BW, et al. Pulmonary rehabilitation: joint ACCP/AACVPR evidence-based clinical practice guidelines. *Chest.* 2007;131(suppl5):4S–42S.
4. Qaseem A, Wilt TJ, Weinberger SE, et al. Diagnosis and management of stable chronic obstructive pulmonary disease: a

clinical practice guideline update from the American College of Physicians, American College of Chest Physicians, American Thoracic Society, and European Respiratory Society. *Ann Intern Med*. 2011;155:179–191.

5. Ferreira A, Garvey C, Connors GL, et al. Pulmonary rehabilitation in interstitial lung disease: benefits and predictors of response. *Chest*. 2009;135:442–447.
6. Naji NA, Connor MC, Donnelly SC, McDonnell TJ. Effectiveness of pulmonary rehabilitation in restrictive lung disease. *J Cardiopulm Rehabil*. 2006;26:237–243.
7. Salhi B, Troosters T, Behaeqel M, Joos G, Derom E. Effects of pulmonary rehabilitation in patients with restrictive lung diseases. *Chest*. 2010;137(2):273–279.
8. Palmer SM, Tapson VF. Pulmonary rehabilitation in the surgical patient: lung transplantation and lung volume reduction surgery. *Respir Care Clin N Am*. 1998;4(1):71–83.
9. Biggar DG, Malen JF, Trulock EP, Cooper JD. Pulmonary rehabilitation before and after lung transplantation. In: Casaburi R, Petty TL, eds. *Principles and Practice of Pulmonary Rehabilitation*. Vol 1. Philadelphia, PA: WB Saunders; 1993:459–467.
10. Ries AL. Pulmonary rehabilitation and lung volume reduction surgery. In: Fessler HE, Reilly JJ Jr, Sugarbaker DJ, eds. *Lung Volume Reduction Surgery for Emphysema*. New York, NY: Marcel Dekker; 2004:123–148.
11. Ries AL, Make BJ, Lee SM, et al. The effects of pulmonary rehabilitation in the National Emphysema Treatment Trial. *Chest*. 2005; 128:3799–3809.
12. Ries AL, Squier HC. The team concept in pulmonary rehabilitation. In: Fishman AP, ed. *Pulmonary Rehabilitation*. New York, NY: Marcel Dekker; 1996:55–65.
13. Niederman MS, Clemente PH, Fein AM, et al. Benefits of a multidisciplinary pulmonary rehabilitation program: improvements are independent of lung function. *Chest*. 1991;99:798–804.
14. Spruit MA, Pennings HJ, Janssen PP, et al. Extra-pulmonary features in COPD patients entering rehabilitation after stratification for MRC dyspnea grade. *Respir Med*. 2007;101:2454–2463.
15. Emery CF, Huffman MJ, Busby AK. Behavioral medicine in pulmonary rehabilitation: psychological, cognitive, and social factors. In: Hodgkin JE, Celli BR, Connors GL, eds. *Pulmonary Rehabilitation: Guidelines to Success*. St. Louis, MO: Mosby; 2009: 269–284.
16. American Thoracic Society, American College of Chest Physicians. ATS/ACCP statement on cardiopulmonary exercise testing. *Am J Respir Crit Care Med*. 2003;167:211–277.
17. Ries AL. The role of exercise testing in pulmonary diagnosis. *Clin Chest Med*. 1987;8:81–89.
18. Wasserman K, Hansen JE, Sue DY, et al. *Principles of Exercise Testing and Interpretation*. 15th ed. Philadelphia, PA: Lippincott Williams & Wilkins; 2012.
19. American Thoracic Society. ATS Statement: guidelines for the Six-Minute Walk Test. *Am J Respir Crit Care Med*. 2002;166:111–117.
20. Ries AL, Farrow JT, Clausen JL. Pulmonary function tests cannot predict exercise-induced hypoxemia in chronic obstructive pulmonary disease. *Chest*. 1988;93:454–459.
21. Ries AL, Farrow JT, Clausen JL. Accuracy of two ear oximeters at rest and during exercise in pulmonary patients. *Am Rev Respir Dis*. 1985;132:685–689.
22. Ries AL, Bullock PJ, Larsen CA, et al. *Shortness of Breath, A Guide to Better Living and Breathing*. 6th ed. St. Louis, MO: Mosby; 2001.
23. Rochester DF, Goldberg SK. Techniques of respiratory physical therapy. *Am Rev Respir Dis*. 1980;122(suppl):133–146.
24. Jones AP, Rowe BH. Bronchopulmonary hygiene physical therapy for chronic obstructive pulmonary disease and bronchiectasis. *Cochrane Database Syst Rev*. 2000;2:CD000045.
25. Poole P, Black PN, Cates CJ. Mucolytic agents for chronic bronchitis or chronic obstructive pulmonary disease. *Cochrane Database Syst Rev*. 2012;8:CD001287.
26. Breslin E. Breathing retraining in chronic obstructive pulmonary disease. *J Cardiopulmonary Rehabil*. 1995;15(1):25–33.
27. Gosselink R. Breathing techniques in patients with chronic obstructive pulmonary disease (COPD). *Chron Respir Dis*. 2004; 1(3):163–172.
28. Nocturnal Oxygen Therapy Trial Group. Continuous or nocturnal oxygen therapy in hypoxemic chronic obstructive lung disease: a clinical trial. *Ann Intern Med*. 1980;93:391–398.
29. Medical Research Council Working Party. Long-term domiciliary oxygen therapy in chronic hypoxic cor pulmonale complicating chronic bronchitis and emphysema. *Lancet*. 1981;1: 681–686.
30. Stoller JK, Panos RJ, Krachman S, Doherty DE, Make B, Long-term Oxygen Therapy Trial Group. Oxygen therapy for patients with COPD: current evidence and the Long-Term Oxygen Treatment Trial. *Chest*. 2010;138(1):179–187.
31. Tiep B, Carter R. Oxygen conserving devices and methodologies. *Chron Respir Dis*. 2008;5:109–114.
32. Ries AL. The importance of exercise in pulmonary rehabilitation. *Clin Chest Med*. 1994;15(2):327–337.
33. Casaburi R. Exercise training in chronic obstructive lung disease. In: Casaburi R, Petty TL, eds. *Principles and Practice of Pulmonary Rehabilitation*. 1st ed. Philadelphia, PA: WB Saunders; 1993:204–224.
34. O'Shea SD, Taylor NF, Paratz JD. Progressive resistance exercise improves muscle strength and may improve elements of performance of daily activities for people with COPD: a systematic review. *Chest*. 2009;136:1269–1283.
35. Punzal PA, Ries AL, Kaplan RM, Prewitt LM. Maximum intensity exercise training in patients with chronic obstructive pulmonary disease. *Chest*. 1991;100:618–623.
36. Carter R, Nicotra B, Clark L, et al. Exercise conditioning in the rehabilitation of patients with chronic obstructive pulmonary disease. *Arch Phys Med Rehabil*. 1988;69:118–122.
37. Costi S, Crisafulli E, Antoni FD, et al. Effects of unsupported upper extremity exercise training in patients with COPD. *Chest*. 2009;136:387–395.
38. ACCP-AACVPR Pulmonary Rehabilitation Guidelines Panel. Pulmonary rehabilitation: joint ACCP/AACVPR evidence based guidelines. *Chest*. 1997;112:1363–1396.
39. Lacasse Y. Pulmonary rehabilitation for chronic obstructive pulmonary disease. *Cochrane Database Syst Rev*. 2006;(suppl 4): CD003793. doi:10.1002/14651858.CD003793.pub2
40. Griffiths TL, Phillips CJ, Davies S, Burr ML, Campbell IA. Cost effectiveness of an outpatient multidisciplinary pulmonary rehabilitation programme. *Thorax*. 2001;56:779–784.
41. California Pulmonary Rehabilitation Collaborative Group. Effects of pulmonary rehabilitation on dyspnea, quality of life and health care costs in California. *J Cardiopulmonary Rehabil*. 2004; 24:52–62.
42. Raskin J, Spiegler P, McCusker C, et al. The effect of pulmonary rehabilitation on healthcare utilization in chronic obstructive

pulmonary disease: the Northeast Pulmonary Rehabilitation Consortium. *J Cardiopulmonary Rehabil.* 2006;26:231–236.

43. Puhan MA, Gimeno-Santos E, Scharplatz M, Troosters T, Walters EH, Steurer J. Pulmonary rehabilitation following exacerbations of chronic obstructive pulmonary disease. *Cochrane Database Syst Rev.* 2011 Oct 5;(10):CD005305. doi: 10.1002/14651858.CD005305.pub3.
44. Mathur S, Hornblower E, Levy RD. Exercise training before and after lung transplantation. *Phys Sportsmed.* 2009;37(3):78–87.
45. National Emphysema Treatment Trial Research Group. A randomized trial comparing lung-volume-reduction surgery with medical therapy for severe emphysema. *New Engl J Med.* 2003;348:2059–2073.
46. Granger CL, McDonald CF, Berney S, Chao C, Denehy L. Exercise intervention to improve exercise capacity and health related quality of life for patients with non-small cell lung cancer: a systematic review. *Lung Cancer.* 2011;72(2):139–153.
47. Benzo RP. Pulmonary rehabilitation in lung cancer. *J Cardiopulm Rehabil.* 2007;27:61–64.
48. Birnbaum S. Pulmonary rehabilitation: a classic tune with a new beat, but is anyone listening? *Chest.* 2011;139:1498–1502.

CHAPTER 44

The Biology of Asthma

Matthew C. Bell
William W. Busse

Asthma is characterized by recurrent attacks of breathlessness and wheezing, which vary in severity and frequency from person to person.[1] More than 18 million adults and 7 million children are affected in the United States alone, making asthma one of the most common chronic diseases in this country.[2] Attempts to elucidate the underlying pathophysiology of the disease have led to the realization that asthma truly is a protean disease with various cell types and mechanisms playing variable but important roles in each patient. This degree of mechanistic variation explains the numerous phenotypes of this disease as well as the differences in response to treatment.

By the simplest definition, the pathogenesis of asthma involves bronchoconstriction, airway inflammation, and airway hyperresponsiveness.[3] It is, however, the complex interplay between these factors that defines the disease in general and specifically in an individual patient. A closer examination of the factors involved in each of these components allows a better understanding of this complex disease.

THE ACUTE INFLAMMATORY RESPONSE IN ASTHMA

Perhaps the best illustration of the features of the acute inflammatory response, that is central to the pathogenesis of asthma, is the reaction to the initial and then subsequent exposures to inhaled antigen. While important cellular and molecular mediators will be described later in greater detail, a brief review of the acute inflammatory response serves as a foundation upon which further concepts can be introduced to illustrate the variable but persistent changes that occur in the airway in asthma. When a novel antigen is introduced to the airway of an at-risk individual, it initially becomes trapped in the mucus lining the airway. Here it can be taken up by antigen presenting cells, most notably dendritic cells, which are distributed through the epithelium of the airways.[4,5] After the uptake of allergen, the dendritic cells travel to pulmonary lymph nodes whereby the antigen is presented to naïve $CD4^+$ T cells.[5] Signals derived from the dendritic cell determine which type of $CD4^+$ T cell will be produced. Prior to this event, the dendritic cell is influenced by a complex network of molecular signals that are derived from airway epithelial cells and other local cell types. In allergic inflammation, for example, thymic stromal lymphopoietin (TSLP) and granulocyte–monocyte colony stimulating factor (GM-CSF), which are derived from bronchial epithelial cells, and induce the dendritic cell to promote T_H2 differentiation of naïve $CD4^+$ T cells, thus setting up an environment favorable to the eventual development of allergic inflammation.[5] Upon rechallenge with the sensitizing antigen, these now T_H2 differentiated $CD4^+$ T cells are recruited back to the airway by other signals, such as the chemokines CCL17 and CCL22, secreted by dendritic cells.[6] Upon arrival in the airway, the $CD4^+$ T_H2 cells become key sources of the T_H2 cytokines, namely IL-4, IL-5, and IL-13, which serve as the molecular catalysts to establish a framework for acute allergic inflammation.[6]

After rechallenge with antigen, the local environment of the airways is now rich with T_H2 cytokines, which act on other cell types, either present or recruited to the airway, to propagate the acute allergic inflammatory response. B cells, in the presence of IL-4 and IL-13, are influenced to produce antigen-specific IgE, which binds to high-affinity IgE receptors (FcεRI) on mast cells (MC). When inhaled antigen cross-links the membrane-bound IgE on the mast cells, a variety of preformed and synthesized meditators are released to cause bronchoconstriction, airway edema, and local tissue damage.[7] Mast cells also release chemoattractants such as leukotrienes and cytokines, to recruit a variety of other cells, including eosinophils, basophils, neutrophils, and lymphocytes, which then contribute to the late phase inflammatory response.[7] The eosinophil appears to be, in most cases, the most important and abundant inflammatory cell associated with the late phase response and possibly contributes to the subsequent airflow obstruction.[8] The vast numbers of mediators the eosinophil produces are reviewed later in the chapter. Eosinophil products can cause local tissue damage, mucus hypersecretion, increased vascular permeability, smooth muscle contraction, and a sustained inflammatory response whereby other cell types are recruited to the site of inflammation to perpetuate the reaction.[7,8] The roles of neutrophils and basophils in the pathogenesis of the acute and late-phase allergic inflammatory responses are less well defined.

While the acute allergic response to allergen illustrates the pattern of inflammation seen in asthma, it should be noted that other forms of inflammation can and do play important roles in asthma. Viral respiratory infections, especially with human rhinovirus (HRV), are important triggers for asthma exacerbations.[9] The response to HRV is a primarily T_H1 driven response with increased production of IL-8 and IL-1β and the appearance of airway neutrophilia, as opposed to the strong T_H2 response seen after allergen exposure.[9,10] In asthma, there is evidence that diminished production of the type I and III interferons, antiviral cytokines, may be deficient in some patients with asthma thus leading to increased risk for viral respiratory infections and a greater susceptibility to exacerbations of asthma.[9,10]

This pattern of acute- and late-phase inflammatory response to antigen is, however, a central component of asthma. Chronic inflammation is a later development of the disease and will be described later. Many of the cell types and inflammatory mediators seen in asthma were briefly touched upon in the preceding paragraphs and will now be further developed.

CELL TYPES IN ASTHMA

A study of the pathogenesis of any complex disease begins at the cellular level. The importance of cells of the immune system, including mast cells, basophils, $CD4^+$ T cells, eosinophils, neutrophils, macrophages, dendritic cells, and T lymphocytes, as well as their molecular mediators has long been recognized and appreciated in the development and regulation of inflammation. The contribution of airway smooth muscle cells, especially in relationship to the acute asthmatic response, has also been well documented. More recently, epithelial cells of the airway have become the focus of intense research and emerging importance to both acute and chronic inflammation in asthma. Their role in airway inflammation, and especially in the airway remodeling as is seen in the chronic forms of asthma, is being increasingly cited as a major contributor to the severity of this disease.

■ CELLS OF THE IMMUNE SYSTEM IN ASTHMA

The contributions of each of the aforementioned immune system cell types in the pathogenesis of asthma are considered below.

Mast Cells

Human mast cells are derived from the same $CD34^+$/$cKit^+$ hematopoietic stem cell population that also gives rises to eosinophils, basophils, neutrophils, and monocytes.[11] They are resident cells in most tissues of the body and are commonly found in association with blood vessels, nerves, and surfaces that have contact with the external environment.[12] Mast cells exist in two types in humans and are differentiated by their immunohistochemical staining properties.[13] MC_T mast cells contain only the neutral protease tryptase, while MC_{TC} mast cells contain chymase, carboxypeptidase A_3, and cathepsin G-like protease in addition to tryptase.[13–15] In normal lung tissue, mast cells are located in the subepithelium of the bronchi, bronchioles, and alveolar walls and are almost exclusively of the MC_T type.[13] This distribution of mast cell types is also seen in mild asthma. In severe asthma, however, mast cells in the submucosa are decreased in number and are primarily of the MC_{TC} type.[16] MC_{TC} mast cells are also seen in the airway epithelium of severe asthma, a finding not seen in normal lungs or in milder disease.[16] Mast cells increasingly infiltrate airway smooth muscle bundles in asthma where they likely contribute to ongoing bronchoconstriction through release of their mediators.[17]

While mast cells appear to have some importance in nonallergic asthma as well, they are essential components of the allergic (IgE-mediated) response seen in many asthma patients.[18] Antigen-specific IgE molecules bind allergen and cross-link high-affinity IgE receptors (FcεRI) present on the mast cell surface. This results in the release of preformed mediators, such as histamine, tryptase, chymase, and heparin, as well as tumor necrosis factor-alpha (TNF-α) and vascular endothelial growth factor (VEGF) in some cases (Fig. 44-1).[19] Upon activation, mast cells also generate and release newly synthesized mediators, which contribute to the ongoing inflammatory milieu. These include leukotrienes (predominantly LTC_4), prostaglandins (predominantly PGD_2), thromboxane A_2, platelet activating factor (PAF), growth factors including GM-CSF, fibroblast growth factor-2, and VEGF, and various other cytokines including TNF-α, IL-4, IL-5, IL-8, and IL-13 (Fig. 44-1).[19,20]

The effect of mast cell mediator release contributes to numerous features in the asthmatic response.[7] Histamine, leukotrienes, and the various proteases increase mucus production. Prostaglandins, leukotrienes, thromboxane A_2, and histamine cause bronchoconstriction and increase vascular permeability. The various proteases cause local tissue damage and are important in the activation of various protein precursors. Finally, synthesized cytokines contribute to the recruitment, differentiation, and activation of other inflammatory cells, resulting in the propagation of the inflammatory response.

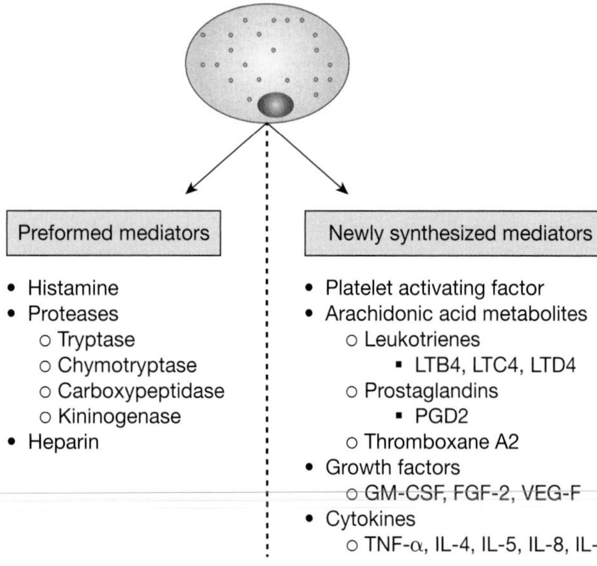

Figure 44-1 The mast cell and its mediators. GM-CSF, granulocyte-monocyte colony stimulating factor; FGF-2, fibroblast growth factor 2; VEGF, vascular endothelial growth factor; TNF-α, tumor necrosis factor alpha.

Basophils

In addition to sharing a common progenitor cell, basophils share many similarities with mast cells, with the exception that basophils are present primarily in the peripheral circulation. Both cells express FcεRI on their cell surface and release both preformed, as well as newly synthesized mediators and cytokines, upon cross-linking by IgE–antigen complexes. The major preformed mediator released from basophils is histamine. Preformed heparin and tryptase are also released, albeit at lower concentrations than mast cells.[21] Basophils synthesize and release LTC_4 upon activation, but unlike mast cells, they do not produce PGD_2.[21] Upon activation, basophils produce large quantities of IL-4 and IL-13, cytokines that play an important role in the T_H2 differentiation, which will be discussed later.[21] More recently, two other roles of basophils in the pathogenesis of asthma have been discovered, both of which also play important roles in T_H2 differentiation. First, basophils can act as antigen presenting cells via their expression of major histocompatibility complex (MHC) class II and co-stimulatory molecules.[22] Second, basophils, along with eosinophils, are also the primary target of IL-33, a potent promoter of allergic inflammation and T_H2 polarization.[23]

Eosinophils

Eosinophils, like basophils and mast cells, are granulocytes derived from $CD34^+$ hematopoietic stem cells. Early eosinophil production is highly dependent upon the presence of GM-CSF and IL-3.[24] Eosinophil precursors are recruited to the airway in asthma as the result of cytokine and chemokine signaling, which involves IL-5, eotaxins, RANTES, macrophage inflammatory protein (MIP)-1α, and macrophage chemotactic factors 2,3, and 4 (MCP-2,3,4).[25] IL-5 is critically important for the terminal differentiation of eosinophils and release from the bone marrow.[24]

Once in the airway, eosinophils are activated and contribute to the inflammatory response through releasing a wide variety of mediators including cytokines (IL-1, IL-2, IL-3, IL-4, IL-5, IL-6, IL-8, IL-10, IL-12, IL-13, IL-16, IL-18, tumor necrosis factor-α [TNF-α] and transforming growth factor-α and β [TGF-α and TGF-β]), chemokines (MIP-1, MCP-2, RANTES and eotaxin), and lipid mediators (PGE_1, PGE_2, thromboxane B_2, PAF, LTC_4) (Fig. 44-2).[26,27] Eosinophils secrete granule proteins, which are important in the eosinophil's primordial role as the primary defender against parasites, as well as in the pathogenesis of asthma.[26,28] Eosinophils contain both primary and secondary granules. The primary granules contain Charcot–Leyden crystal protein, while the secondary granules contain the four principal cationic proteins: major basic protein (MBP), eosinophil cationic protein (ECP), eosinophil-derived neurotoxin (EDN), and eosinophil peroxidase (EPO).[26] These cationic proteins play various roles in the pathogenesis of asthma including the induction of mast cell and basophil degranulation (ECP and MBP), increasing airway mucus production (ECP), and formation of reactive oxygen species (EPO) (Fig. 44-2).[26]

Over the past 30 years, the role of the eosinophil in asthma has undergone considerable re-evaluation. Since the discovery of the eosinophil by Ehrlich in 1879 and the later discovery that Ehrlich's cells were present in the sputum of asthmatic patients, the eosinophil has been viewed as the primary effector cell in asthma.[29] Studies have noted that peripheral blood eosinophilia is a characteristic of asthma and often in relationship to disease severity, and that eosinophilic infiltrates were found in the airways of asthma patients at autopsy, regardless of whether asthma was the primary cause of death.[30,31] Later studies detected increased eosinophils and eosinophil products

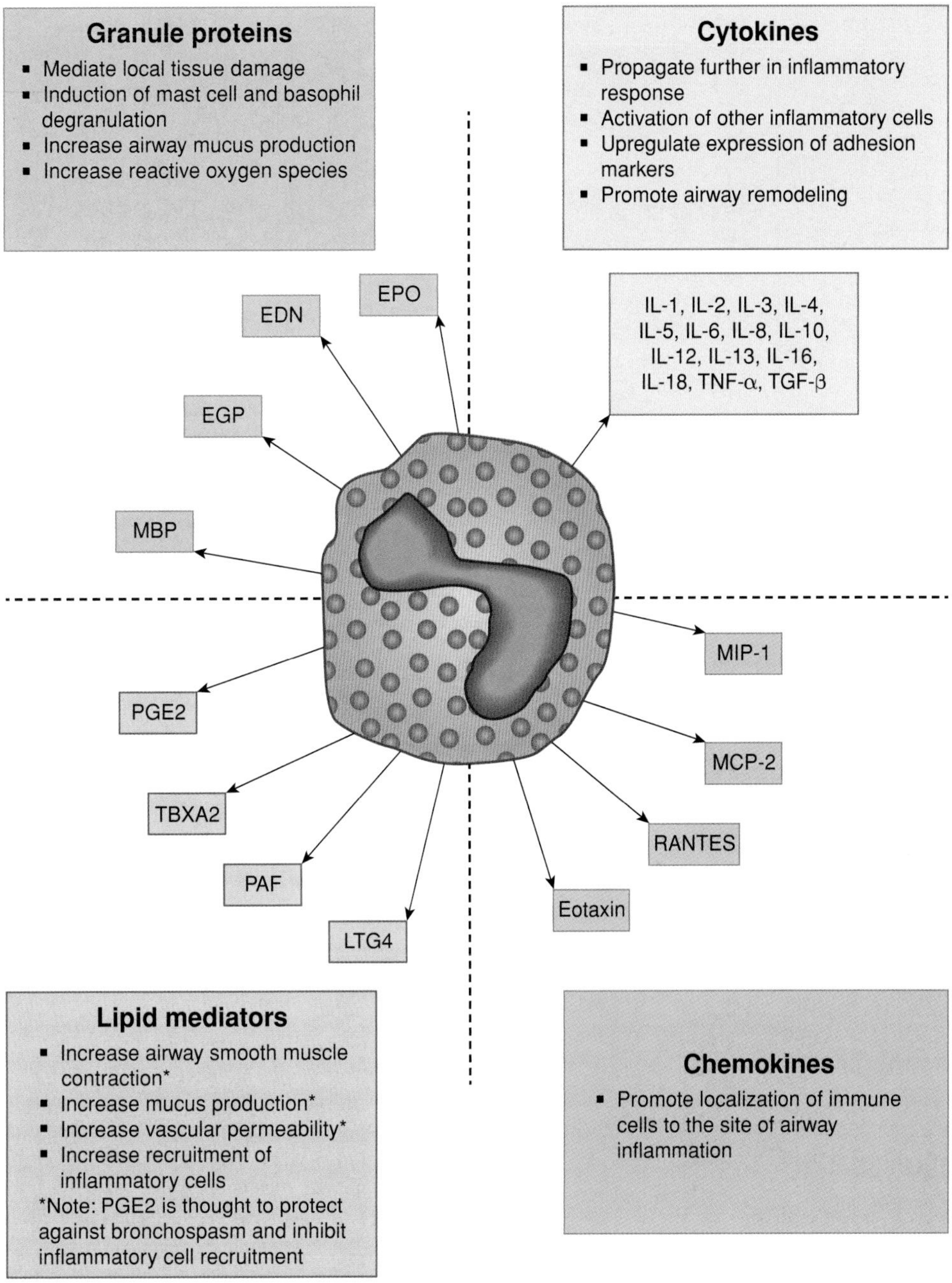

Figure 44-2 Eosinophil products in asthma. EPO, eosinophil peroxidase; EDN, eosinophil-derived neurotoxin; ECP, eosinophil cationic protein; MBP, major basic protein; PGE_2, prostaglandin E2; $TBXA_2$, thromboxane A_2; PAF, platelet activating factor; LTC_4, leukotriene C4; RANTES, regulated upon activation normal T cell expressed and secreted; MCP-2, monocyte chemotactic protein 2; MIP-1, macrophage inhibitory protein 1; TNF-α, tumor necrosis factor alpha; TGF-β, transforming growth factor beta.

in bronchoalveolar lavage (BAL) fluid after antigen challenge.[32] The view that the eosinophil was the principal effector of asthma was largely unchallenged until the new millennium brought new therapies, including monoclonal antibodies to IL-5, into evaluation.

The importance of IL-5 to the differentiation and survival of the eosinophil has been previously noted. Initial studies with monoclonal antibodies to IL-5 in asthma showed a decrease in sputum and peripheral blood eosinophilia, as expected, but failed to demonstrate significant benefit in a wide variety of clinical outcome measures, that is, symptoms or improved airflow obstruction.[33,34] Although this lack of effect on parameters of clinical asthma was a surprise, it led to an increasing interest in the heterogeneity of asthma with the realization that eosinophils may play greater or lesser roles in different patients.

Later studies with anti-IL-5 were conducted in patients who had persistent eosinophilia despite treatment with inhaled corticosteroids (ICS), and in these patients were noted clinical outcomes, the prevention of exacerbations.[35,36] Eosinophils play an important role in a certain subset of asthma, but the contribution of their role appears to be defined by phenotypes and is not necessarily generalizable to the entire asthmatic population. Finally, eosinophils are likely a prime contributor to airway remodeling seen in chronic asthma, and will be discussed in this capacity later in the chapter.

Neutrophils

Neutrophils are granulocytes derived from $CD34^+$ hematopoietic stem cells and are normally present in the bloodstream, as well as in various tissues, including the lung. They contain primary (azurophilic) and secondary (specific) granules, which contain a variety of antimicrobial enzymes, neutral proteases, and acid hydrolases.[37] Neutrophils are attracted to the airway by various cytokines and

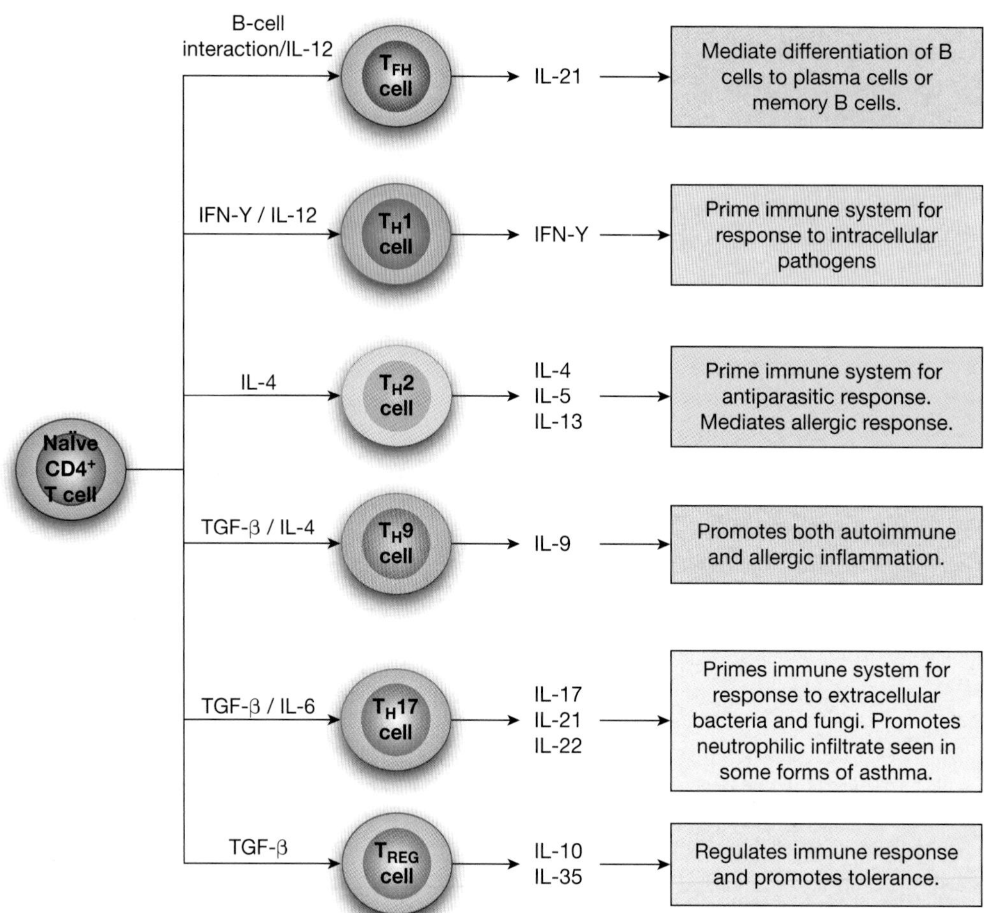

Figure 44-3 $CD4^+$ T Lymphocyte subsets. IFN-γ, interferon gamma; TGF-β, transforming growth factor beta; TFH cell, T follicular helper cell; T_{REG} cell, regulatory T cell.

chemokines including IL-8, IL-17, and granulocyte colony stimulating factor (G-CSF).[38,39] Airway neutrophilia can be seen in many respiratory conditions, viral respiratory infections, COPD, and asthma.[10,39]

The role of neutrophils in response to viral respiratory infections was introduced previously. In response to inoculation with a respiratory virus, such as HRV, dendritic cells, and other mononuclear cells produce proinflammatory cytokines and chemokines, which recruit neutrophils to the airway.[10] Neutrophils contribute to the inflammatory milieu by secreting cytokines such as TNF-α, IL-1, IL-8, and IL-18, to attract other inflammatory cells, upregulate cytokine production, and produce airway inflammation and enhance bronchial hyperresponsiveness.[40] Neutrophil products, such as elastase, can have more direct effects on the airway and cause mucus production.[10] In addition, because neutrophils are found in severe asthma, they are proposed to play a more prominent role in this phenotype.[41] Prominent neutrophilic inflammation has been noted in the sputum of patients with severe asthma exacerbations, in BAL fluid from patients with noninfectious status asthma, and in autopsy specimens from the airway in patients with acute, fatal asthma.[42–44] Other studies have demonstrated subgroups of patients with chronic asthma in whom the primary inflammatory cell type is neutrophils rather than eosinophils.[45,46] These patients are often more difficult to treat and less responsive to treatment with corticosteroids.

Lymphocytes

Unlike the previously discussed cell types, T cells are lymphocytes and derived from the common lymphoid progenitor. Numerous subsets of T cells have been identified and are important contributors to asthma, including $CD4^+$ helper T cells and their subsets (T_H1, T_H2, T_H9, and T_H17), $CD8^+$ cytotoxic T cells, and regulatory T cells (T_{REG}).

$CD4^+$ helper T cells recognize antigens presented to them by antigen presenting cells (APCs) and, in turn, secrete cytokines to influence the inflammatory response. In the airway, the dendritic cell is the most important APC and its role will be described later. A complex series of events involving cytokines and various transcription factors determines whether $CD4^+$ T cells will differentiate into T_H1 cells, T_H2 cells, T_H9 cells, or T_H17 cells (Fig. 44-3).[47]

T_H2 cells are recognized as the primary drivers of inflammation in asthma and allergic disease. When T_H2 cells encounter antigen presented by dendritic cells, they produce IL-4, IL-5, and IL-13, all of which play critical roles in the pathogenesis of asthma and are part of the clinical disease as demonstrated by detection of increased levels of these cytokines in the BAL fluid of patients with asthma.[48,49] IL-4 increases IgE production by plasma cells. As mentioned previously, IL-5 is critical in the terminal differentiation and homing of eosinophils to the airway. IL-13 also increases IgE production and plays a prominent role in airway hyperresponsiveness and tissue remodeling.[50]

The role of T_H1 cells in asthma is not as well defined as T_H2 cells. Although it has been presumed that T_H1 cells counteract the asthma-inducing effects of T_H2 cells, this likely is an over-simplification. T_H1 products have been shown to be increased during asthma exacerbation.[51] Some studies have also suggested that T_H1 cells may play a more prominent role in chronic severe asthma as evidenced by increased levels of the primary T_H1 cytokine, interferon-γ (IFN-γ), in the BAL fluid of patients with severe asthma.[52]

T_H9 cells are a relatively newly defined cell population whose primary cytokine is generation of IL-9. T_H9 cells function similarly to T_H2 cells in that they increase allergic inflammation. Mast cells are the primary IL-9 receptor-bearing cell, and T_H9 cells are important contributors to the previously described increased mast cell activation seen in asthma.[20] Because mast cells also produce VEGF and fibroblast growth factor-2, T_H9 cells likely contribute to airway remodeling seen in chronic asthma.[20]

The role of T_H17 cells in asthma is an area of intense research. With the identification of subphenotypes of asthma patients with primarily neutrophilic inflammation, the role of IL-17 (the primary cytokine produced by T_H17 cells) in asthma has become of considerable interest. Although IL-17 is found to be increasingly expressed in patients with severe asthma,[53] it is, however, also found in high concentrations in patients with mild asthma (FEV_1 >70% predicted) and these values correlate negatively with the PC_{20}.[54] Thus, while T_H17 cells most certainly play a role in patients with primarily neutrophilic asthma, they are also likely important in milder forms of disease as well.

The primary function of $CD8^+$ cytotoxic T cells is the destruction of human cells that are infected with viruses or other intracellular pathogens. $CD8^+$ T cells also likely play a role in asthma, though the extent of their contribution has yet to be fully elucidated.[50] IL-4 and IL-5 producing $CD8^+$ T cells are present in the airways of asthmatic patients.[55] IL-5 production by $CD8^+$ T cells is increased in the presence of a viral respiratory infection, and the overall cytokine production by $CD8^+$ T cells correlates with asthma severity.[56,57] Whether $CD8^+$ T cells function as direct contributors or bystanders in the worsening of asthma has yet to be determined.[50]

T_{REG} cells also appear to play a critical role in asthma development. T_{REG} cells serve to limit inflammatory responses and promote immune tolerance through the production of IL-10 and TGF-β.[50,58] In patients with asthma and other allergic disorders, T_{REG} cells appear to be less effective in limiting T_H2 inflammation.[59,60] However, after allergen immunotherapy, for example, T_{REG} cells increase in the nasal mucosa and may act to promote allergen tolerance.[61] Interestingly, farm exposure early in life is associated with a decreased incidence of allergic disease and asthma, a fact that may be related to increased numbers and function of T_{REG} cells in infants living in this environment.[62]

Natural killer cells (NK cells) are members of the innate immune system and serve as a first line of defense against infections. Their role in the pathogenesis of asthma has yet to be fully elucidated. They obviously appear in response to viral respiratory infections, and NK cells increase during asthma exacerbations.[63] NK cells are capable of producing numerous cytokines including IFN-γ, IL-4, IL-5, and IL-13.[64] NK cells from patients with atopic asthma are skewed toward the production of IL-4 as opposed to IFN-γ upon activation.[64] IFN-γ production by NK cells is also inhibited by prostaglandin D2, a T_H2-promoting lipid mediator produced by mast cells.[65] NK cells may also play a role in "dendritic cell editing" by killing immature dendritic cells, which might influence a certain type of T_H response.[66]

Macrophages and Dendritic Cells

Macrophages and dendritic cells are descendants from the $CD34^+$ hematopoietic stem cell and arise from a common committed precursor cell.[67] Macrophages arise from circulating monocytes and function, primarily, to clear debris and microbes from the airway. They may also function as antigen presenting cells, although this role is likely less important than that of the dendritic cell.[68] Alveolar macrophages may further differentiate into M1 or M2 subsets based on exposure to various cytokines and toll like receptor (TLR) agonists.[67] M1 macrophages are "classic" macrophages, and clear microbes from the airway. They also produce cytokines, such as IL-12, IL-6, and TNF-α, as well as high levels of nitric oxide (NO).[67] M1 macrophages have traditionally been described as suppressing allergic inflammation, primarily through their secretion of T_H1 cytokines such as IL-12; this is not fully resolved.[67]

Differentiation into M2 macrophages is influenced by an environment rich in T_H2 cytokines such as IL-4 and IL-13, thus implicating their role in asthma. When compared with M1 macrophages, M2 macrophages are poor at clearing intracellular pathogens.[67] They release cytokines such as IL-13 and thus are likely contribute to the airway hyperresponsiveness.[67]

Dendritic cells are the lung's primary presenter of antigen to T cells. Their role as the primary APC places the dendritic cell at a critical junction in determining what type of T cell response will be directed toward the antigen (i.e., T_H1, T_H2). Dendritic cells in humans exist in two broad categories: the myeloid dendritic cell (mDC) and the plasmacytoid dendritic cell (pDC). While both types of dendritic cells are present in the human lung, their anatomic localization within the lung is poorly understood. [5] Upon encountering antigen in the airway, dendritic cells migrate to local lymph nodes where they present antigen to T lymphocytes. Both pDC and mDC levels increase in the airway (and coincidently decrease in the blood) after exposure to inhaled allergen.[69–71] Because dendritic cells lie close to the epithelial barrier, they receive numerous signals from epithelial cells, which can influence their effect on T cells. TSLP is produced by epithelial cells and promotes dendritic cells to direct T_H2 differentiation and recruit T_H2 cells to the airway.[5] Other epithelial cell–derived factors, such as GM-CSF, TNF-α, CCL-20, IL-1β, and TNF-related apoptosis-inducing ligand (TRAIL), have similar T_H2 promoting effects.[5] pDC represent the lung's primary source of IFN-α, a potent antiviral cytokine, and they are recruited to the lung during times of viral infections.[72] As viral infections commonly precede asthma exacerbations and may predispose infants to develop asthma, this role of the pDC cannot be understated.[73] The importance of pDC to the development of asthma was illustrated by a recent study which showed that decreased pDC levels in childhood was directly correlated to increased number and severity of viral respiratory infections, increased episodes of wheeze, and increased asthma diagnosis.[74] The function of mDC is not as well known in human asthma, but the role of both dendritic cell types in contributing to the development and propagation of the disease will continue to be an important area of asthma research.

RESIDENT CELLS OF THE AIRWAY

The roles of airway smooth muscle cells and airway epithelial cells in the biology of asthma are considered below.

Airway Smooth Muscle

Given that bronchospasm and bronchial constriction are critical components of asthma, it is intuitive that the cell type responsible for this component, the airway smooth muscle cell, would be a key factor in asthma pathogenesis and pathophysiology. While its importance seems obvious, the details of why airway smooth muscle function is so different in the asthmatic airway compared with the normal airway have been elusive. It has been well documented that the smooth muscle layer surrounding the airway is thicker in asthma compared to nonasthmatic controls. These difference are due to both smooth muscle hypertrophy and hyperplasia.[75] Increased inflammatory cells, including mast cells, can be found within the smooth muscle bundles of asthmatic airways, and the interplay between these cells, the airway epithelium, and the smooth muscle layer, is an important determinant of the asthmatic response.[17] Numerous cytokines, chemokines, and growth factors are involved in this interaction including those produced by the airway smooth muscle cell itself and those produced by other cell types with which the airway smooth muscle cell communicates. Airway smooth muscle cells in asthma are more prolific producers of these cytokines, and this function likely plays a role in their ability to proliferate more rapidly than those of nonasthmatic subjects.[76]

The treatment of asthma has long focused on preventing or reversing contraction of bronchial smooth muscles. β2-agonists, both short and long acting, have long been key to the treatment of asthma, and these medications act directly on the airway smooth muscle. More recently, debulking of airway smooth muscle, with the use of bronchial thermoplasty, has shown improvement in asthma control, which, in theory, further supports the role that airway smooth muscle plays in asthma pathophysiology.[77,78]

Airway Epithelial Cells

The epithelial lining of the airway is an area of intense research, and its importance, beyond being a simple anatomic barrier, is being increasingly recognized and appreciated. The airway epithelium represents a vast surface area (100 m^2) that is in contact with some 10,000 L of inhaled air daily.[79] As the area of initial contact between the lung and the external airborne environment, functions of the airway epithelium are likely key to determine the body's response to airborne substances.

The airway epithelium is composed of three major cell types: the ciliated columnar epithelial cell, the mucus-secreting goblet cell, and the surfactant secreting Clara cell.[79] Both overproduction of mucus by goblet cells and underproduction of important anti-inflammatory peptides by Clara cells have been noted in patients with asthma.[80,81] The tight junctions between epithelial cells have also been noted to be defective in patients with asthma, which can serve to decrease the ability of the airway epithelium to act as a protective barrier.[79] The airway epithelium in asthma is also less capable of defending itself against reactive oxygen species, a defect that leads to further damage to this airway barrier.[82] Epithelial cells in asthma produce lower amounts of Type I interferon in response to respiratory viruses, which can increase the severity to respiratory infections and promote asthma exacerbations.[83] TSLP promotes T_H2-driven inflammation and is overproduced by epithelial cells in asthmatic patients, thus providing a crucial link between the airway epithelium and the T_H2 type inflammation seen in asthma.[84,85] Finally, epithelial cells are capable of secreting endothelins, which are peptides with significant bronchoconstrictive activity.[86]

MOLECULAR MEDIATORS IN ASTHMA

The above-mentioned cells are able to initiate, perpetuate, coordinate, and regulate the inflammatory process with the synthesis and secretion of several different classes of molecular mediators. These mediators have a variety of functions, as discussed below.

CYTOKINES

Cytokines are small-molecular-weight glycosylated signaling molecules that are secreted by a number of different cell types with autocrine, paracrine, or endocrine directive activities.[87] Cytokine is a broad term and includes many subcategories including interleukins, interferons, and growth factors.[87] Cytokine secretion is usually a brief, self-limited event. It may, however, require new mRNA and protein synthesis, which takes place over a matter of hours rather than seconds or minutes.[88] A variety of cytokines have been implicated in the regulation of airway inflammation and thus in the pathogenesis of asthma (Table 44-1).[89] The support for cytokine involvement in inflammation was first obtained by the detection of these mediators in the airways of patients with asthma, particularly in bronchoalveolar lavage fluid after allergen challenge and in situ hybridization of retrieved cells or biopsy materials.[90,91]

The overall effect of the complex cytokine network in the airway depends on a number of factors, including the relative abundance of the various cytokines, their ability to recruit and perpetuate the actions of inflammatory cells such as eosinophils and lymphocytes, and their ability to amplify or suppress inflammation by interacting with structural cells such as fibroblasts, endothelial cells, and epithelial cells. There is no question, however, that cytokines are key mediators in the pathogenesis of the chronic inflammation characteristic of asthma.

CHEMOKINES

The chemokines are small-molecular-weight proteins, 8 to 12 kD, that are classified into four categories based on the organization of specific cysteine residues in their protein sequence: XC, CC, CXC, CX_3C.[92] The predominant function of chemokines is the recruitment or chemotaxis of inflammatory cells.[92] Some chemokines also have additional signaling function. There are corresponding families of chemokine receptors for each class of chemokines. Notably, there is considerable overlap and redundancy in the chemokines and their target receptors.

Since the localization of inflammatory cells into the airway is dependent to a large extent on chemotaxis via chemokine signaling, the chemokine receptors have become an attractive target for asthma therapy. There are currently chemokine receptor inhibitors for CCR5 as well as others in development as potential therapy for asthma.[93,94]

IgE

The initial association of IgE with asthma was based on several epidemiological studies.[95–97] With the increased understanding of the role of mast cell mediators in the pathogenesis of asthma, the importance of IgE in triggering mast cell activation and the resulting airway inflammation has been underscored. This relationship between IgE levels and asthma, and its function, led to the development of a humanized monoclonal antibody directed to IgE for asthma therapy.[98] This antibody (omalizumab, Xolair®) has been shown to be effective in the treatment of severe asthma, specifically allowing a significant reduction in dosage of corticosteroids and prevention of asthma exacerbation, further supporting a key role of IgE in asthma.[99]

LEUKOTRIENES

The leukotrienes (LT) are a family of lipid compounds generated from the metabolism of arachidonic acid via the lipoxygenase pathway (Fig. 44-4).[100] These compounds are typically not preformed

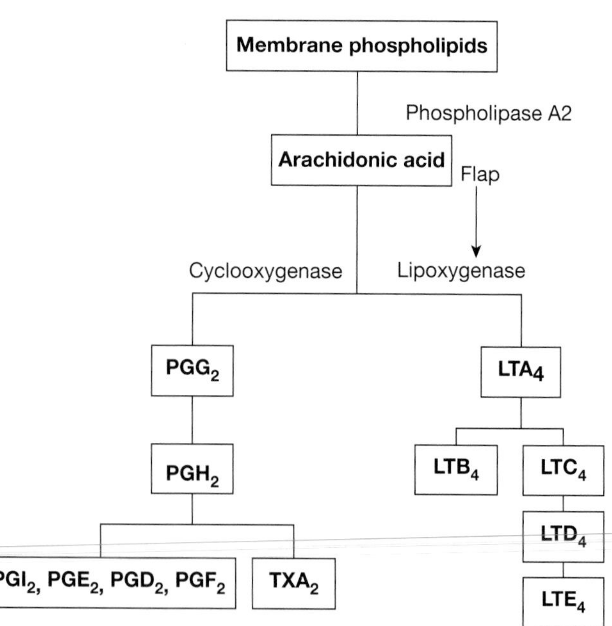

Figure 44-4 Formation of arachidonic acid metabolites. PG, prostaglandin; TXA_2, thromboxane A_2; LT, leukotriene; FLAP, 5-lipoxygenase activating protein.

TABLE 44-1 Cytokines and Lipid Mediators in Asthma

Cytokines		
Cytokine	**Cell Sources**	**Proposed Cell Targets/Functions in Asthma**
Interleukins		
IL-1	DCs, monocytes, macrophages, mast cells, B and T cells, neutrophils, endothelial cells, airway epithelial cells	*Basophils*: Increased production of cytokines and histamine *DCs*: Increased cytokine production, upregulation of MHC and co-stimulatory molecules *Macrophages*: Increased cytokine production *Mast cells*: Increased cytokine production, degranulation, and survival *Neutrophils*: Increased survival and release of proteases *B cells*: Increased antibody production *T cells*: Increased proliferation—especially for T_H2 and T_H17 cells
IL-2	$CD4^+$ T Cells	*T cells*: Increased survival and proliferation, increased T_H2 cytokine production
IL-3	T Cells, mast cells	*Basophils*: Increased survival and release of IL-4, IL-6, and histamine *Eosinophils*: Increased degranulation *Mast cells*: Increased survival and histamine release *Hematopoietic stem cells*: Increased production of mast cells, basophils, neutrophils, eosinophils, macrophages, erythrocytes, megakaryocytes, and dendritic cells
IL-4	T cells, mast cells, basophils, eosinophils	*Airway smooth muscle cells*: Increased airway hyperresponsiveness *Basophils*: Increased recruitment *Eosinophils*: Increased recruitment *Goblet cells*: Increased mucus production *Mast cells*: Increased recruitment, upregulation of FCεRI *B cells*: Increased class switching to IgE, upregulation of FCεRII *T cells*: Increased recruitment, increased T_H2 differentiation, increased production of T_H2 cytokines, decreased differentiation of T_H1 cells, decreased IFN-γ production by T_H1 cells
IL-5	T cells, mast cells	*Basophils*: Increased proliferation, maturation, and functional activation *Eosinophils*: Increased proliferation, chemoattraction, maturation, functional activation, and degranulation
IL-6	Macrophages, DCs, mast cells, neutrophils, B and T cells, endothelial cells, airway epithelial cells	*T cells*: Increased production of T_H2 cytokines, decreased differentiation of T_H1 cells, decreased IFN-γ production by T_H1 cells, promotes differentiation of T_H17 cells, downregulation of T_{REG} cells
IL-7	Bone marrow stromal cells	*Eosinophils:* Increased activation and survival *B cells:* Increased proliferation and survival *T cells:* Increased maturation and survival
IL-8	Airway epithelial cells, neutrophils, eosinophils, monocytes/macrophages	*Eosinophils*: Chemoattraction *Neutrophils*: Chemoattraction
IL-9	T cells	*Mast cells*: Increased recruitment and maturation, increased expression of proteases, upregulation of FCεRI *T cells*: Increased growth and proliferation
IL-10	Monocytes/macrophages, B cells, T cells (specifically T_{REG} cells)	*DCs*: Inhibits expression of co-stimulatory molecules thus inhibiting T_H cell activation *Eosinophils*: Inhibits survival, recruitment, and maturation *Monocytes/macrophages*: Downregulates MHC Class II expression, downregulates inflammatory cytokine production *T cells*: Downregulates IFN-γ and IL-2 production by T_H1 cells and IL-4 and IL-5 production by T_H2 cells
IL-11	Airway epithelial cells, eosinophils, airway smooth muscle cells	*Airway epithelial cells:* Regulate proliferation *Macrophages:* Inhibit production of TNF-α, IL-1, IL-12 *B cells:* Increases immunoglobulin production *T cells:* Inhibits production of TH1 cytokines, Increases IL-4 and IL-10 production
IL-12	Dendritic cells, B cells, macrophages	*NK cells*: Increased IFN-γ production *T cells*: Increased IFN-γ production, increased TH1 differentiation, decreased T_H2 and T_H17 differentiation

(continued)

TABLE 44-1 Cytokines and Lipid Mediators in Asthma *(Continued)*

Cytokines		
Cytokine	**Cell Sources**	**Proposed Cell Targets/Functions in Asthma**
IL-13	Mast cells, T cells	*Airway epithelial cells*: Increased permeability, increased mucus production, production of inducible nitric oxide synthase *Airway smooth muscle cells*: Increased airway hyperreactivity *Eosinophils*: Promotes migration and survival *Macrophages*: Activation and enhanced MHC Class II expression *B cells*: Increased class switching to IgE and production of IgE
IL-14	T cells	*B cells*: Increased proliferation, suppression of Ig secretion
IL-15	Monocytes/macrophages, DCs	*DCs*: Increased activation and survival, increased production of IFN-γ *Mast cells*: Increased survival *Monocytes/macrophages*: Increased phagocytic activity, increased production of IL-8, IL-12, MCP-1 *Neutrophils:* Increased survival and phagocytic activity, increased IL-8 production *NK cells*: Increased maturation and survival, increased production of IFN-γ, TNF-α, and GM-CSF *T cells*: Increased proliferation of memory CD8$^+$ T cells, Increased proliferation of T_H17 cells
IL-16	T cells, airway epithelial cells, DCs, eosinophils, mast cells	*DCs:* Increased chemoattraction *Eosinophils*: Increased chemoattraction *Monocytes/macrophages*: Increased chemoattraction, upregulation of MHC class II expression *T cells:* Increased migration, maturation, and proliferation
IL-17	T cells, NK cells	*Airway epithelial cells:* Increased production of IL-6, IL-8, G-CSF, PGE_2 *Eosinophils*: Increased chemoattraction *Neutrophils*: Increased production from stem cells, increased chemoattraction
IL-18	DCs, monocytes, macrophages, neutrophils, airway epithelial cells	*Basophils*: Increased production of cytokines and histamine *DCs*: Increased cytokine production, upregulation of MHC and costimulatory molecules *Macrophages*: Increased cytokine production *Mast cells*: Increased cytokine production, degranulation, and survival *Neutrophils*: Increased survival and release of proteases *NK cells*: Increased IFN-γ production. *T cells*: Promotes T_H1 differentiation.
IL-19	Monocytes	*T cells*: Increased production of T_H2 cytokines and downregulation of IFN-γ production
IL-20	Monocytes	Unclear
IL-21	T cells	*B cells*: Increased proliferation of IgA, IgG, IgM producing plasma cells and decrease in IgE producing plasma cells *T cells*: Increased differentiation into T_H17 cells, upregulation of T_H1 cytokine production
IL-22	T cells, NK cells	*Respiratory epithelial cells*: Increased production of antimicrobial peptides
IL-23	DCs	*Macrophages*: Increased TNF-α production *T cells*: Increased IL-17 production, promotion of T_H17 differentiation
IL-24	Monocytes, T cells	Unclear
IL-25	Airway epithelial cells, eosinophils, mast cells	*T cells*: Increased production of T_H2 cytokines
IL-26	Monocytes, T cells	Unclear
IL-27	Macrophages, DCs	*T cells*: Increased differentiation into IL-10 producing T_{REG} and T_H1 cells, decreased development of T_H2 and T_H17 cells
IL-28 (IFN-λ2,λ3)	DCs	Inhibits viral replication *DCs:* Increase ability to stimulate production of T_{REG} cells
IL-29 (IFN-λ1)	DCs	Inhibits viral replication *DCs*: Increase ability to stimulate production of T_{REG} cells
IL-31	T cells	*Airway epithelial cells*: Attenuate proliferation of epithelial cells
IL-32	NK cells, Airway epithelial cells, T cells	*Macrophages*: Upregulation of proinflammatory cytokines *Airway epithelial cells*: Decreased production of proangiogenic factors

TABLE 44-1 Cytokines and Lipid Mediators in Asthma *(Continued)*

Cytokines		
Cytokine	**Cell Sources**	**Proposed Cell Targets/Functions in Asthma**
IL-33	Endothelial cells, airway epithelial cells, dying cells	*Basophils*: Increased production of cytokines and histamine *DCs*: Increased cytokine production, upregulation of MHC and co-stimulatory molecules *Eosinophils:* Increased proliferation, survival, and chemokine production *Macrophages:* Increased cytokine production *Mast cells*: Increased cytokine production, degranulation, and survival *Neutrophils*: Increased survival and release of proteases *NK cells*: Increased IFN-γ and T_H2 cytokines *T cells*: Promotes T_H2 differentiation, enhances release of T_H2 cytokines
IL-35	T_{REG} cells	*T cells*: Decreased production of T_H2 cytokines, suppression of T cell proliferation
IL-36	Airway epithelial cells	*T cells*: Increased T_H1 differentiation
IL-37	Hematopoietic cells	*Macrophages*: Decreased secretion of proinflammatory cytokines *Airway epithelial cells*: Decreased secretion of proinflammatory cytokines
Interferons		
IFN-α	Monocytes/macrophages	*Virus infected cells*: Inhibition of viral replication
IFN-β	Monocytes/macrophages	*Virus infected cells*: Inhibition of viral replication
IFN-γ	T cells, NK cells	*Macrophages*: Differentiation, activation, and expression of Fcγ receptor. Increased cytokine production *T cells*: Increased differentiation to T_H1 cells, increased cytotoxicity of $CD8^+$ T cells
IFN-λ	See above	See above
Growth factors		
bFGF	Endothelial cells	*Fibroblasts*: Proliferation and extracellular matrix formation
G-CSF	Monocytes, fibroblasts, airway epithelial cells	*Neutrophils*: Proliferation and differentiation
GM-CSF	T cells, airway epithelial cells, macrophages	*DCs:* Maturation *Eosinophils:* Increased survival, degranulation *Macrophages*: Differentiation, increased survival, increased cytokine production *Neutrophils*: Increased chemotaxis and survival
M-CSF	Fibroblasts, endothelial cells, macrophages, airway smooth muscle cells	*Hematopoietic stem cells*: Differentiation of monocytes
PDGF	Platelets, monocytes, macrophages	*Fibroblasts*: Proliferation and chemoattraction
SCF	Bone marrow stromal cells, fibroblasts	*Mast cells*: Chemoattraction, induction of histamine release, differentiation, proliferation
TGF-β	Eosinophils, T cells, macrophages, airway epithelial cells, endothelial cells, airway smooth muscle cells	*Fibroblasts*: Chemoattraction and increased conversion to myofibroblasts, increased synthesis of collagen *Macrophages:* Chemoattraction *Neutrophils*: Chemoattraction *T cells:* Increased differentiation of T_{REG}, T_H9, and T_H17 cells, inhibition of T_H1 and T_H2 differentiation
VEGF	Macrophages, airway epithelial cells, T cells, eosinophils	*Airway smooth muscle cells*: Hyperplasia and increased airway hyperresponsiveness *DCs:* Increased proliferation and activation *Endothelial cells*: Increased angiogenesis and vascular permeability *Airway epithelial cells:* Increased proliferation, mucus production *Fibroblasts*: Promotion of subepithelial fibrosis
Other		
TNF-α	Monocytes/macrophages, DCs, mast cells, eosinophils, neutrophils, B and T cells, airway epithelial cells, airway smooth muscle cells, fibroblasts	*Airway epithelial cells*: Upregulation of adhesion molecules *Airway smooth muscle cells*: Increased airway hyperresponsiveness *Endothelial cells*: Upregulation of adhesion molecules *Eosinophils*: Chemoattraction, increased activation *Fibroblasts*: Increased conversion to myofibroblasts *Macrophages*: Chemoattraction *Mast cells*: Increased histamine release *Neutrophils*: Chemoattraction *T cells*: Increased activation and cytokine release

(continued)

TABLE 44-1 Cytokines and Lipid Mediators in Asthma (Continued)

Cytokines		
Cytokine	Cell Sources	Proposed Cell Targets/Functions in Asthma
TSLP	Airway epithelial cells	*DCs*: Increased ability to attract T_H2 cells *Eosinophils*: Induced release of proinflammatory cytokines and chemokines *Mast cells*: Increased production of T_H2 cytokines *T cells*: Increased differentiation to T_H2 cells

Lipid Mediators		
Mediator	Cell Sources	Proposed Cell Targets/Functions in Asthma
Leukotrienes		
Dihydroxy acid leukotriene (LTB4)	DCs, monocytes/macrophages, neutrophils	*B lymphocytes*: Increased expression of CD23, CD54, and CD105 *DCs*: Recruitment, increased skewing of T_H0 cells to T_H1 type *Eosinophils*: Recruitment *Mast cells*: Recruitment *Monocytes/macrophages*: Increased production of IL-6, TNF-α, MCP-1 *Neutrophils*: Recruitment and activation *Airway smooth muscle cells*: Increased proliferation *T lymphocytes:* Recruitment
Cysteinyl leukotrienes (LTC_4, LTD_4, LTE_4)	DCs, eosinophils, mast cells, monocytes/macrophages	*Airway smooth muscle cells*: Bronchoconstriction *DCs*: Increased migration to lymph nodes *Endothelial cells*: Increased vascular permeability and upregulation of adhesion molecules *Eosinophils*: Recruitment *Goblet cells*: Increased mucus production *Mast cells*: Increased production of IL-5, IL-8, TNF-α, and MIP-1β *Monocytes/macrophages*: Increased production of MCP-1, TNF-α, and MMP-9 *T lymphocytes*: Increased T_H2 immune response
Prostanoids		
PGD_2	Mast cells	*Airway smooth muscle cells*: Bronchoconstriction *Eosinophils*: Recruitment, increased degranulation *Monocytes/macrophages*: Increased cytokine production *Neutrophils*: Inhibition of activation *T lymphocytes*: Recruitment, increased production of T_H2 cytokines, inhibition of IFN-γ production
PGE_2	Airway smooth muscle cells, airway epithelial cells, endothelial cells, macrophages	*Airway smooth muscle cells*: Inhibition of allergen-induced bronchoconstriction *Eosinophils*: Inhibits recruitment *Monocytes/macrophages*: Decreased cytokine production, downregulation of MHC Class II expression *T cells*: Decreased proliferation, decreased T_H2 cytokine production
PGI2 (Prostacyclin)	Endothelial cells, monocyte/macrophages	*Endothelial cells*: Vasodilatation *Eosinophils*: Inhibition of recruitment *T cells*: Increased IL-10 production
Thromboxane A_2	Platelets, endothelial cells, monocyte/macrophages	*Airway smooth muscle cells*: Bronchoconstriction *Eosinophils*: Recruitment

and stored in cells for release upon activation; rather, they are rapidly synthesized following activation of the source cell. LTC_4, LTD_4, and LTE_4 are potent bronchoconstrictors that are produced by several cell types, including eosinophils and mast cells, whereas LTB_4 is a neutrophil attractant.[100] The leukotrienes are also able to increase mucus secretion in the airway and facilitate a plasma leak generating edema in the airway.[100,101] Leukotriene receptor antagonists (e.g., montelukast, Singulair®) are currently used in the treatment of asthma.[102] Although effective in some patients, the leukotriene modifiers have limitations as regards overall potency, thus raising questions as to what are the conditions, or phenotypes, in which leukotrienes dominate.[103]

Prostanoids

The prostanoids (PG) are a family of lipid compounds generated from the metabolism of arachidonic acid via the cyclooxygenase pathway (Fig. 44-4).[104] Most of the prostanoids, that is, PGD_2, PGF_2, and TXA_2, are potent bronchoconstrictors and products of several cell types including eosinophils and mast cells.[104] However, another prostanoid, PGE_2, has bronchodilatory and anti-inflammatory activity.[105,106] The use of nonsteroidal anti-inflammatory medications to inhibit cyclooxygenase activity has not been shown to have an appreciable effect on airway inflammation. It has been observed that PGD_2 is the predominant prostanoid involved in asthma.[107] Therefore, specific PGD_2 receptor antagonists are currently being considered to ameliorate some of the bronchoconstriction in asthma.[108–110]

NITRIC OXIDE

The role of nitric oxide (NO) in the pathogenesis of asthma remains unclear. NO is continually synthesized at low levels in the airways of normal subjects. Sources of NO in the respiratory tract include airway epithelial cells, smooth muscle cells, sensory nerves, endothelial cells, and macrophages.[111] At low levels, NO is a bronchodilator and vasodilator that antagonizes endothelin and has protective effects in the airway.[111] Higher levels of NO are found in asthma, secondary to increased inducible NO synthase expression, and may be detrimental to airway epithelium.[112] This may be mediated by the ability of NO to react with superoxide anion in inflamed tissue to produce biologic oxidants that contribute to ongoing tissue damage and chronic asthmatic inflammation.[111] The production of NO is also thought to reflect the level or severity of airway inflammation. Thus, exhaled NO measurement has been utilized successfully as a tool to reflect the extent of airway inflammation as a measure of asthma control.[112]

GRANULE PROTEINS

Granulocytes, that is, mast cells, basophils, eosinophils, and neutrophils, are capable of releasing granule proteins, many of which has been proposed to play significant roles in the pathogenesis of asthma.

Insights into the kinetics and importance of mast cell mediators have been obtained from measurements of BAL histamine and tryptase.[113] These studies have demonstrated that mast cell activation is an early event, with elevated BAL histamine and tryptase levels being seen 12 minutes after endobronchial antigen challenge; the levels of tryptase returning to normal 48 hours after antigen challenge.[113] The levels of histamine remain elevated after 48 hours, raising the possibility that non-mast cells (e.g., basophils) are subsequently recruited and activated to produce histamine at these later points or that mast cells generate and continue to release histamine over time following an initial activation.[113] Furthermore, BAL of allergic asthmatic subjects had only moderately elevated levels of tryptase at baseline but higher concentrations of tryptase following antigen challenge.[113]

Histamine is capable of inducing bronchoconstriction, increasing vascular permeability to cause edema, and increasing mucus secretion.[114] The role of tryptase is not well established, although there are data to suggest that it can activate inflammatory cells such as eosinophils, mast cells, and epithelial cells by cleaving a family of protease activated receptors (PARs) on their cell surfaces.

Major basic protein (MBP) is the principal protein constituent of eosinophil granules. It is toxic to epithelial tissues, induces airway hyperresponsiveness, and causes histamine release from basophils.[115] ECP is more cytotoxic to the epithelium than MBP and damages target cells by membrane pore formation.[116] Eosinophil-derived neurotoxin (EDN), as the name implies, damages myelinated neurons.[117] EPO differs from neutrophil and monocyte myeloperoxidases (MPOs); it causes LTC_4 and LTD_4 degradation and causes histamine release from mast cells.[118]

Neutrophil release of MPO and neutrophil elastase enhances host defense functions but is also potentially injurious to normal tissues, including airway epithelium.[119] The primary granules of neutrophils contain MPO and lysozyme as well as hydrolases and proteinases, which are important in tissue penetration by neutrophils.[119] Secondary granules contain lysozyme and collagenases, which can also potentially damage airway tissue.[119] Neutrophil granule proteins are considered toxic to airway epithelium and tissue.

REMODELING IN ASTHMA

As occurs in most chronic inflammatory disorders in which there is an "injury–repair" cycle, tissue remodeling is a key component of asthma. Airway remodeling in asthma involves epithelial changes, increases in smooth muscle mass, increased angiogenesis, increased fibroblast/myofibroblast activity, increased fibrosis, and many other important changes that affect the structure and function of the large and small airways of the lung.[120] Prolonged infiltration of inflammatory cells and the cytokines, chemokines, and growth factors, which they generate, contribute to these structural changes, which help define the features of asthma in some patients.

As mentioned previously, airway epithelium serves not only as an anatomic barrier, but also as a key player in asthma pathogenesis. Defects in airway epithelium are ubiquitous in human asthma and, when injury occurs, the repair process has been likened to a chronic wound, which may not heal normally as a result of repetitive and ongoing insults.[121] As with other types of chronic wounds, the body attempts to heal the epithelial damage by promoting the release of growth factors from the underlying mesenchyme. This, in turn, leads to increased extracellular matrix deposition, fibrosis, and size and number of airway smooth muscle cells.[122] These even have been likened to the function of the epithelial–mesangial trophic unit (EMTU), a key component of early lung morphogenesis, which, in a sense, becomes reactivated in chronic asthma.[122] The consequence of prolonged epithelial injury is a protracted release of proinflammatory cytokines and profibrogenic growth factors such as TGF-β. When these reactions are combined with the inflammatory milieu derived from the immune cells recruited to the airway by this long-term damage, the effects of these morphologic changes are manifested in chronic airflow obstruction, which is often resistant to pharmacologic treatment, and results in permanent airflow obstruction.

PHENOTYPIC CLUSTERS IN ASTHMA

Several recent studies have begun to identify phenotypes, or subphenotypes, of asthma. These studies have confirmed that asthma is a very heterogeneous disease.[123,124] Specifically, studies by Haldar and colleagues in the United Kingdom used sputum eosinophilia, in addition to measurements of atopic status and other characteristics, to identify these subphenotypes.[123] Interestingly, they identified a cluster of patients with symptomatic disease who had very little eosinophilic involvement and lacked evidence of atopic sensitization. Other groups fit a more "classic" pattern of asthma with evidence of eosinophilic involvement and atopic sensitization. Other clusters fell somewhere between the two. This study, and others, are probing the heterogeneity of the disease and discovering the reasons behind differences in disease course and response to conventional asthma therapy.

CONCLUSION

Asthma is a complex disease in which the contributions of many different immune cells, structural cells, molecular mediators, and external factors combine to produce acute and chronic inflammation and airflow obstruction. The study of these different factors has led to a greater understanding and appreciation of the breadth of this disease and a recognition of its complexity and heterogeneity. It has also led to the realization that different phenotypes of asthma exist and treatment of asthma based on the specific phenotype represents an emerging, potentially more specific and effective possibility. Over the last decade, many new advances in therapy have been made that target specific inflammatory mediators in asthma. The fact that these have not been universally successful speaks to the heterogeneity and redundancy of asthma. As research delves further into the pathogenesis and pathophysiology of asthma, many more targets will emerge, which will hopefully lead to novel therapies to improve the lives of asthmatic patients and with these interventions greater insight into the effects of individual mediators and in whom they may be relevant.

REFERENCES

1. World Health Organization. Office of Health Communications and Public Relations. *Asthma*. Geneva: World Health Organization; 2006.
2. Akinbami LJ, Moorman JE, Bailey C, et al. Trends in asthma prevalence, health care use, and mortality in the United States, 2001–2010. *NCHS Data Brief.* 2012;(94):1–8.
3. National Asthma Education and Prevention Program. Expert Panel Report 3 (EPR-3): Guidelines for the Diagnosis and Management of Asthma-Summary Report 2007. *J Allergy Clin Immunol.* 2007;120(5 Suppl):S94–S138.
4. Vermaelen KY, Carro-Muino I, Lambrecht BN, Pauwels RA. Specific migratory dendritic cells rapidly transport antigen from the airways to the thoracic lymph nodes. *J Exp Med.* 2001; 193(1):51–60.
5. Gill MA. The role of dendritic cells in asthma. *J Allergy Clin Immunol.* 2012;129(4):889–901.
6. Lambrecht BN, Hammad H. The role of dendritic and epithelial cells as master regulators of allergic airway inflammation. *Lancet.* 2010;376(9743):835–843.
7. Pearlman DS. Pathophysiology of the inflammatory response. *J Allergy Clin Immunol.* 1999;104(4 Pt 1):S132–S137.
8. Busse WW, Calhoun WF, Sedgwick JD. Mechanism of airway inflammation in asthma. *Am Rev Respir Dis.* 1993;147(6 Pt 2): S20–S24.
9. Brooks GD, Buchta KA, Swenson CA, Gern JE, Busse WW. Rhinovirus-induced interferon-gamma and airway responsiveness in asthma. *Am J Respir Crit Care Med.* 2003;168(9): 1091–1094.
10. Gern JE. Viral respiratory infection and the link to asthma. *Pediatr Infect Dis J.* 2008;27(10 Suppl):S97–S103.
11. Kirshenbaum AS, Goff JP, Semere T, Foster B, Scott LM, Metcalfe DD. Demonstration that human mast cells arise from a progenitor cell population that is CD34(+), c-kit(+), and expresses aminopeptidase N (CD13). *Blood.* 1999;94(7):2333–2342.
12. Metcalfe DD, Baram D, Mekori YA. Mast cells. *Physiol Rev.* 1997;77(4):1033–1079.
13. Irani AA, Schechter NM, Craig SS, DeBlois G, Schwartz LB. Two types of human mast cells that have distinct neutral protease compositions. *Proc Natl Acad Sci U S A.* 1986;83(12): 4464–4468.
14. Irani AM, Goldstein SM, Wintroub BU, Bradford T, Schwartz LB. Human mast cell carboxypeptidase. Selective localization to MCTC cells. *J Immunol.* 1991;147(1):247–253.
15. Schechter NM, Irani AM, Sprows JL, Abernethy J, Wintroub B, Schwartz LB. Identification of a cathepsin G-like proteinase in the MCTC type of human mast cell. *J Immunol.* 1990;145(8):2652–2661.
16. Balzar S, Fajt ML, Comhair SA, et al. Mast cell phenotype, location, and activation in severe asthma. Data from the Severe Asthma Research Program. *Am J Respir Crit Care Med.* 2011; 183(3):299–309.
17. Brightling CE, Bradding P, Symon FA, Holgate ST, Wardlaw AJ, Pavord ID. Mast-cell infiltration of airway smooth muscle in asthma. *N Engl J Med.* 2002;346(22):1699–1705.
18. Robinson DS. The role of the mast cell in asthma: induction of airway hyperresponsiveness by interaction with smooth muscle? *J Allergy Clin Immunol.* 2004;114(1):58–65.
19. Williams CM, Galli SJ. The diverse potential effector and immunoregulatory roles of mast cells in allergic disease. *J Allergy Clin Immunol.* 2000;105(5):847–859.
20. Kearley J, Erjefalt JS, Andersson C, et al. IL-9 governs allergen-induced mast cell numbers in the lung and chronic remodeling of the airways. *Am J Respir Crit Care Med.* 2011;183(7):865–875.
21. Stone KD, Prussin C, Metcalfe DD. IgE, mast cells, basophils, and eosinophils. *J Allergy Clin Immunol.* 2010;125(2 Suppl 2): S73–S80.
22. Sokol CL, Chu NQ, Yu S, Nish SA, Laufer TM, Medzhitov R. Basophils function as antigen-presenting cells for an allergen-induced T helper type 2 response. *Nat Immunol.* 2009;10(7): 713–720.
23. Pecaric-Petkovic T, Didichenko SA, Kaempfer S, Spiegl N, Dahinden CA. Human basophils and eosinophils are the direct target leukocytes of the novel IL-1 family member IL-33. *Blood.* 2009;113(7):1526–1534.
24. Sanderson CJ. Interleukin-5, eosinophils, and disease. *Blood.* 1992;79(12):3101–3109.
25. Wardlaw AJ. Molecular basis for selective eosinophil trafficking in asthma: a multistep paradigm. *J Allergy Clin Immunol.* 1999;104(5):917–926.
26. Rothenberg ME, Hogan SP. The eosinophil. *Annu Rev Immunol.* 2006;24:147–174.
27. Gleich GJ. Mechanisms of eosinophil-associated inflammation. *J Allergy Clin Immunol.* 2000;105(4):651–663.
28. Abu-Ghazaleh RI, Dunnette SL, Loegering DA, et al. Eosinophil granule proteins in peripheral blood granulocytes. *J Leukoc Biol.* 1992;52(6):611–618.
29. Wenzel SE. Eosinophils in asthma–closing the loop or opening the door? *N Engl J Med.* 2009;360(10):1026–1028.
30. Horn BR, Robin ED, Theodore J, Van Kessel A. Total eosinophil counts in the management of bronchial asthma. *N Engl J Med.* 1975;292(22):1152–1155.
31. Filley WV, Holley KE, Kephart GM, Gleich GJ. Identification by immunofluorescence of eosinophil granule major basic protein in lung tissues of patients with bronchial asthma. *Lancet.* 1982;2(8288):11–16.
32. Woolley KL, Adelroth E, Woolley MJ, Ellis R, Jordana M, O'Byrne PM. Effects of allergen challenge on eosinophils, eosinophil cationic protein, and granulocyte-macrophage colony-stimulating factor in mild asthma. *Am J Respir Crit Care Med.* 1995;151(6):1915–1924.
33. Leckie MJ, ten Brinke A, Khan J, et al. Effects of an interleukin-5 blocking monoclonal antibody on eosinophils, airway hyper-responsiveness, and the late asthmatic response. *Lancet.* 2000;356(9248):2144–2148.
34. Flood-Page P, Swenson C, Faiferman I, et al. A study to evaluate safety and efficacy of mepolizumab in patients with moderate persistent asthma. *Am J Respir Crit Care Med* 2007;176(11):1062–1071.
35. Haldar P, Brightling CE, Hargadon B, et al. Mepolizumab and exacerbations of refractory eosinophilic asthma. *N Engl J Med.* 2009;360(10):973–984.
36. Nair P, Pizzichini MM, Kjarsgaard M, et al. Mepolizumab for prednisone-dependent asthma with sputum eosinophilia. *N Engl J Med.* 2009;360(10):985–993.

37. Bainton DF, Ullyot JL, Farquhar MG. The development of neutrophilic polymorphonuclear leukocytes in human bone marrow. *J Exp Med.* 1971;134(4):907–934.

38. Kelly JT, Busse WW. Host immune responses to rhinovirus: mechanisms in asthma. *J Allergy Clin Immunol.* 2008;122(4): 671–682; quiz 683–674.

39. Linden A, Hoshino H, Laan M. Airway neutrophils and interleukin-17. *Eur Respir J.* 2000;15(5):973–977.

40. Sims JE, Smith DE. The IL-1 family: regulators of immunity. *Nat Rev Immunol.* 2010;10(2):89–102.

41. Jatakanon A, Uasuf C, Maziak W, Lim S, Chung KF, Barnes PJ. Neutrophilic inflammation in severe persistent asthma. *Am J Respir Crit Care Med.* 1999;160(5 Pt 1):1532–1539.

42. Fahy JV, Kim KW, Liu J, Boushey HA. Prominent neutrophilic inflammation in sputum from subjects with asthma exacerbation. *J Allergy Clin Immunol.* 1995;95(4):843–852.

43. Lamblin C, Gosset P, Tillie-Leblond I, et al. Bronchial neutrophilia in patients with noninfectious status asthmaticus. *Am J Respir Crit Care Med.* 1998;157(2):394–402.

44. Sur S, Crotty TB, Kephart GM, et al. Sudden-onset fatal asthma. A distinct entity with few eosinophils and relatively more neutrophils in the airway submucosa? *Am Rev Respir Dis.* 1993;148(3):713–719.

45. Green RH, Brightling CE, Woltmann G, Parker D, Wardlaw AJ, Pavord ID. Analysis of induced sputum in adults with asthma: identification of subgroup with isolated sputum neutrophilia and poor response to inhaled corticosteroids. *Thorax.* 2002;57(10):875–879.

46. Simpson JL, Scott R, Boyle MJ, Gibson PG. Inflammatory subtypes in asthma: assessment and identification using induced sputum. *Respirology.* 2006;11(1):54–61.

47. Zhou L, Chong MM, Littman DR. Plasticity of CD4+ T cell lineage differentiation. *Immunity.* 2009;30(5):646–655.

48. Robinson DS, Hamid Q, Ying S, et al. Predominant TH2-like bronchoalveolar T-lymphocyte population in atopic asthma. *N Engl J Med.* 1992;326(5):298–304.

49. Prieto J, Lensmar C, Roquet A, et al. Increased interleukin-13 mRNA expression in bronchoalveolar lavage cells of atopic patients with mild asthma after repeated low-dose allergen provocations. *Respir Med.* Aug 2000;94(8):806–814.

50. Lloyd CM, Hessel EM. Functions of T cells in asthma: more than just T(H)2 cells. *Nat Rev Immunol.* 2010;10(12): 838–848.

51. Corrigan CJ, Kay AB. CD4 T lymphocyte activation in acute severe asthma. *Int Arch Allergy Appl Immunol.* 1991;94(1–4): 270–271.

52. Shannon J, Ernst P, Yamauchi Y, et al. Differences in airway cytokine profile in severe asthma compared to moderate asthma. *Chest.* 2008;133(2):420–426.

53. Chang Y, Al-Alwan L, Risse PA, et al. Th17-associated cytokines promote human airway smooth muscle cell proliferation. *Faseb J.* 2012;26(12):5152–5160.

54. Barczyk A, Pierzchala W, Sozanska E. Interleukin-17 in sputum correlates with airway hyperresponsiveness to methacholine. *Respir Med.* 2003;97(6):726–733.

55. Ying S, Humbert M, Barkans J, et al. Expression of IL-4 and IL-5 mRNA and protein product by CD4 +and CD8+ T cells, eosinophils, and mast cells in bronchial biopsies obtained from atopic and nonatopic (intrinsic) asthmatics. *J Immunol.* 1997; 158(7):3539–3544.

56. Thurau AM, Streckert HJ, Rieger CH, Schauer U. Increased number of T cells committed to IL-5 production after respiratory syncytial virus (RSV) infection of human mononuclear cells in vitro. *Clin Exp Immunol.* 1998;113(3):450–455.

57. Cho SH, Stanciu LA, Holgate ST, Johnston SL. Increased interleukin-4, interleukin-5, and interferon-gamma in airway CD4+ and CD8+ T cells in atopic asthma. *Am J Respir Crit Care Med.* 2005;171(3):224–230.

58. Seroogy CM, Gern JE. The role of T regulatory cells in asthma. *J Allergy Clin Immunol.* 2005;116(5):996–999.

59. Ling EM, Smith T, Nguyen XD, et al. Relation of CD4+CD25+ regulatory T-cell suppression of allergen-driven T-cell activation to atopic status and expression of allergic disease. *Lancet.* 2004;363(9409):608–615.

60. Grindebacke H, Wing K, Andersson AC, Suri-Payer E, Rak S, Rudin A. Defective suppression of Th2 cytokines by CD4CD25 regulatory T cells in birch allergies during birch pollen season. *Clin Exp Allergy.* 2004;34(9):1364–1372.

61. Radulovic S, Jacobson MR, Durham SR, Nouri-Aria KT. Grass pollen immunotherapy induces Foxp3-expressing CD4+ CD25+ cells in the nasal mucosa. *J Allergy Clin Immunol.* 2008;121(6):1467–1472, 1472.e1.

62. Schaub B, Liu J, Hoppler S, et al. Maternal farm exposure modulates neonatal immune mechanisms through regulatory T cells. *J Allergy Clin Immunol.* 2009;123(4):774–782, e775.

63. Lin SJ, Chang LY, Yan DC, Huang YJ, Lin TJ, Lin TY. Decreased intercellular adhesion molecule-1 (CD54) and L-selectin (CD62 L) expression on peripheral blood natural killer cells in asthmatic children with acute exacerbation. *Allergy.* 2003;58(1):67–71.

64. Culley FJ. Natural killer cells in infection and inflammation of the lung. *Immunology.* 2009;128(2):151–163.

65. Chen Y, Perussia B, Campbell KS. Prostaglandin D2 suppresses human NK cell function via signaling through D prostanoid receptor. *J Immunol.* 2007;179(5):2766–2773.

66. Moretta A. Natural killer cells and dendritic cells: rendezvous in abused tissues. *Nat Rev Immunol.* 2002;2(12):957–964.

67. Moreira AP, Hogaboam CM. Macrophages in allergic asthma: fine-tuning their pro- and anti-inflammatory actions for disease resolution. *J Interferon Cytokine Res.* 2011;31(6):485–491.

68. Kugathasan K, Roediger EK, Small CL, McCormick S, Yang P, Xing Z. CD11 c +antigen presenting cells from the alveolar space, lung parenchyma and spleen differ in their phenotype and capabilities to activate naive and antigen-primed T cells. *BMC Immunol.* 2008;9:48.

69. Bratke K, Lommatzsch M, Julius P, et al. Dendritic cell subsets in human bronchoalveolar lavage fluid after segmental allergen challenge. *Thorax.* 2007;62(2):168–175.

70. Upham JW, Denburg JA, O'Byrne PM. Rapid response of circulating myeloid dendritic cells to inhaled allergen in asthmatic subjects. *Clin Exp Allergy.* 2002;32(6):818–823.

71. Jahnsen FL, Moloney ED, Hogan T, Upham JW, Burke CM, Holt PG. Rapid dendritic cell recruitment to the bronchial mucosa of patients with atopic asthma in response to local allergen challenge. *Thorax.* 2001;56(11):823–826.

72. Gill MA, Palucka AK, Barton T, et al. Mobilization of plasmacytoid and myeloid dendritic cells to mucosal sites in children with respiratory syncytial virus and other viral respiratory infections. *J Infect Dis.* 2005;191(7):1105–1115.

73. Gern JE, Rosenthal LA, Sorkness RL, Lemanske RF Jr. Effects of viral respiratory infections on lung development and

childhood asthma. *J Allergy Clin Immunol.* 2005;115(4):668–674; quiz 675.

74. Upham JW, Zhang G, Rate A, et al. Plasmacytoid dendritic cells during infancy are inversely associated with childhood respiratory tract infections and wheezing. *J Allergy Clin Immunol.* 2009;124(4):707–713.
75. James AL, Elliot JG, Jones RL, et al. Airway smooth muscle hypertrophy and hyperplasia in asthma. *Am J Respir Crit Care Med.* 2012;185(10):1058–1064.
76. Borger P, Tamm M, Black JL, Roth M. Asthma: is it due to an abnormal airway smooth muscle cell? *Am J Respir Crit Care Med.* 2006;174(4):367–372.
77. Castro M, Rubin AS, Laviolette M, et al. Effectiveness and safety of bronchial thermoplasty in the treatment of severe asthma: a multicenter, randomized, double-blind, sham-controlled clinical trial. *Am J Respir Crit Care Med* 2010;181(2):116–124.
78. Pavord ID, Cox G, Thomson NC, et al. Safety and efficacy of bronchial thermoplasty in symptomatic, severe asthma. *Am J Respir Crit Care Med.* 2007;176(12):1185–1191.
79. Holgate ST. Epithelium dysfunction in asthma. *J Allergy Clin Immunol.* 2007;120(6):1233–1244; quiz 1245–1236.
80. Shijubo N, Itoh Y, Yamaguchi T, et al. Serum levels of Clara cell 10-kDa protein are decreased in patients with asthma. *Lung.* 1999;177(1):45–52.
81. Hauber HP, Foley SC, Hamid Q. Mucin overproduction in chronic inflammatory lung disease. *Can Respir J.* 2006;13(6): 327–335.
82. Bucchieri F, Puddicombe SM, Lordan JL, et al. Asthmatic bronchial epithelium is more susceptible to oxidant-induced apoptosis. *Am J Respir Cell Mol Biol.* 2002;27(2):179–185.
83. Wark PA, Johnston SL, Bucchieri F, et al. Asthmatic bronchial epithelial cells have a deficient innate immune response to infection with rhinovirus. *J Exp Med.* 2005;201(6):937–947.
84. Soumelis V, Reche PA, Kanzler H, et al. Human epithelial cells trigger dendritic cell mediated allergic inflammation by producing TSLP. *Nat Immunol.* 2002;3(7):673–680.
85. Ying S, O'Connor B, Ratoff J, et al. Thymic stromal lymphopoietin expression is increased in asthmatic airways and correlates with expression of Th2-attracting chemokines and disease severity. *J Immunol.* 2005;174(12):8183–8190.
86. Goldie RG, Henry PJ. Endothelins and asthma. *Life Sci.* 1999; 65(1):1–15.
87. O'Shea JJ. Jaks, STATs, cytokine signal transduction, and immunoregulation: are we there yet? *Immunity.* 1997;7(1):1–11.
88. Schena FP, Gesualdo L, Grandaliano G, Montinaro V. Progression of renal damage in human glomerulonephritides: is there sleight of hand in winning the game? *Kidney Int.* 1997;52(6):1439–1457.
89. Mathur SK, Busse WW. The biology of asthma, in *Fishman's Pulmonary Diseases and Disorders*, vol 1, Fourth Edition. In: Fishman AP, Elias JA, Fishman JA, Grippi MA, Senior RM, Pack AL, eds. New York, NY: McGraw Hill; 2008, 773–785.
90. Batra V, Khurana S, Musani AI, et al. Concentration of cytokines and growth factors in BAL fluid after allergen challenge in asthmatics and their effect on alpha-smooth muscle actin and collagen III synthesis by human lung fibroblasts. *Chest.* 2003;123(3 Suppl):398S–399S.
91. Kuperman DA, Huang X, Koth LL, et al. Direct effects of interleukin-13 on epithelial cells cause airway hyperreactivity and mucus overproduction in asthma. *Nat Med.* 2002;8(8):885–889.
92. Garrood T, Lee L, Pitzalis C. Molecular mechanisms of cell recruitment to inflammatory sites: general and tissue-specific pathways. *Rheumatology (Oxford).* 2006;45(3):250–260.
93. Suzaki Y, Hamada K, Nomi T, et al. A small-molecule compound targeting CCR5 and CXCR3 prevents airway hyperresponsiveness and inflammation. *Eur Respir J.* 2008;31(4):783–789.
94. Fryer AD, Stein LH, Nie Z, et al. Neuronal eotaxin and the effects of CCR3 antagonist on airway hyperreactivity and M2 receptor dysfunction. *J Clin Invest.* 2006;116(1):228–236.
95. Turner KJ, Rosman DL, O'Mahony J. Prevalence and familial association of atopic disease and its relationship to serum IgE levels in 1,061 school children and their families. *Int Arch Allergy Appl Immunol.* 1974;47(5):650–664.
96. Burrows B, Martinez FD, Halonen M, Barbee RA, Cline MG. Association of asthma with serum IgE levels and skin-test reactivity to allergens. *N Engl J Med.* 1989;320(5):271–277.
97. Sears MR, Burrows B, Flannery EM, Herbison GP, Hewitt CJ, Holdaway MD. Relation between airway responsiveness and serum IgE in children with asthma and in apparently normal children. *N Engl J Med.* 1991;325(15):1067–1071.
98. Presta LG, Lahr SJ, Shields RL, et al. Humanization of an antibody directed against IgE. *J Immunol.* 1993;151(5):2623–2632.
99. Busse W, Corren J, Lanier BQ, et al. Omalizumab, anti-IgE recombinant humanized monoclonal antibody, for the treatment of severe allergic asthma. *J Allergy Clin Immunol.* 2001;108(2):184–190.
100. Busse WW. The role of leukotrienes in asthma and allergic rhinitis. *Clin Exp Allergy.* 1996;26(8):868–879.
101. Wenzel SE. The role of leukotrienes in asthma. *Prostaglandins Leukot Essent Fatty Acids.* 2003;69(2–3):145–155.
102. Horwitz RJ, McGill KA, Busse WW. The role of leukotriene modifiers in the treatment of asthma. *Am J Respir Crit Care Med.* 1998;157(5 Pt 1):1363–1371.
103. O'Byrne PM, Gauvreau GM, Murphy DM. Efficacy of leukotriene receptor antagonists and synthesis inhibitors in asthma. *J Allergy Clin Immunol.* 2009;124(3):397–403.
104. Chung KF, Barnes PJ. Role of inflammatory mediators in asthma. *Br Med Bull.* 1992;48(1):135–148.
105. Main IH. The Inhibitory actions of prostaglandins on respiratory smooth muscle. *Br J Pharmacol Chemother.* 1964;22:511–519.
106. Mathe AA, Hedqvist P. Effect of prostaglandins F2 alpha and E2 on airway conductance in healthy subjects and asthmatic patients. *Am Rev Respir Dis.* 1975;111(3):313–320.
107. Robinson C, Hardy CC, Holgate ST. Pulmonary synthesis, release, and metabolism of prostaglandins. *J Allergy Clin Immunol.* 1985;76(2 Pt 2):265–271.
108. Schmidt J, Bell F, Akam E, et al. Biochemical and pharmacological characterization of AZD1981, an orally available selective DP2 antagonist in clinical development for asthma. *Br J Pharmacol.* 2013;168(7):1626–1638.
109. Singh D, Cadden P, Hunter M, et al. Inhibition of the asthmatic allergen challenge response by the CRTH2 antagonist OC000459. *Eur Respir J.* 2013;41(1):46–52.
110. Busse WW, Wenzel SE, Meltzer EO, et al. Safety and efficacy of the prostaglandin D2 receptor antagonist AMG 853 in asthmatic patients. *J Allergy Clin Immunol.* 2013;131(2):339–345.
111. Ricciardolo FL. Multiple roles of nitric oxide in the airways. *Thorax.* 2003;58(2):175–182.
112. Barnes PJ, Dweik RA, Gelb AF, et al. Exhaled nitric oxide in pulmonary diseases: a comprehensive review. *Chest.* 2010; 138(3):682–692.

113. Sedgwick JB, Calhoun WJ, Gleich GJ, et al. Immediate and late airway response of allergic rhinitis patients to segmental antigen challenge. Characterization of eosinophil and mast cell mediators. *Am Rev Respir Dis.* 1991;144(6):1274–1281.

114. White MV. The role of histamine in allergic diseases. *J Allergy Clin Immunol.* 1990;86(4 Pt 2):599–605.

115. Gundel RH, Letts LG, Gleich GJ. Human eosinophil major basic protein induces airway constriction and airway hyperresponsiveness in primates. *J Clin Invest.* 1991;87(4):1470–1473.

116. Motojima S, Frigas E, Loegering DA, Gleich GJ. Toxicity of eosinophil cationic proteins for guinea pig tracheal epithelium in vitro. *Am Rev Respir Dis.* 1989;139(3):801–805.

117. Durack DT, Sumi SM, Klebanoff SJ. Neurotoxicity of human eosinophils. *Proc Natl Acad Sci U S A.* 1979;76(3):1443–1447.

118. Everse J, Everse KE, Grisham MB. *Peroxidases in Chemistry and Biology.* Boca Raton, FL: CRC Press; 1991.

119. Monteseirin J. Neutrophils and asthma. *J Investig Allergol Clin Immunol.* 2009;19(5):340–354.

120. Al-Muhsen S, Johnson JR, Hamid Q. Remodeling in asthma. *J Allergy Clin Immunol.* 2011;128(3):451–462; quiz 463–454.

121. Davies DE, Wicks J, Powell RM, Puddicombe SM, Holgate ST. Airway remodeling in asthma: new insights. *J Allergy Clin Immunol.* 2003;111(2):215–225; quiz 226.

122. Knight DA, Holgate ST. The airway epithelium: structural and functional properties in health and disease. *Respirology.* 2003;8(4):432–446.

123. Haldar P, Pavord ID, Shaw DE, et al. Cluster analysis and clinical asthma phenotypes. *Am J Respir Crit Care Med.* 2008; 178(3):218–224.

124. Moore WC, Meyers DA, Wenzel SE, et al. Identification of asthma phenotypes using cluster analysis in the Severe Asthma Research Program. *Am J Respir Crit Care Med.* 2010; 181(4):315–323.

CHAPTER **45**

Asthma: Epidemiology

Augusto A. Litonjua
Andrea J. Apter
Scott T. Weiss

Asthma is a clinical syndrome that affects 25 million Americans and accounts for 12.7 million medical visits yearly. One-third of those afflicted with asthma are children under the age of 18 years. It is estimated that roughly half of these children received their diagnosis prior to the age of 6 years. As a result, the origins of asthma are believed to have a clear genomic component that is often manifested in early childhood. The clinical course of this illness is influenced greatly by exposures, including respiratory viruses, indoor allergens, maternal tobacco smoke, and other physical and social aspects of the environment. Thus, this clinical disease has important consequences in childhood and may have important consequences for adult obstructive lung disease.

Asthma is an extremely common clinical problem and the most common cause of hospitalization for children in the United States. The estimated total annual costs of asthma care is rising dramatically and totaled approximately $56 billion in 2007 in the United States,[1] representing a $3 billion increase since 2002. These costs include $50.1 billion per year in medical expenses, $3.8 billion per year in missed school or lost work days, and $2.1 billion per year in premature deaths. The paradox of this illness is that despite important strides in understanding etiologic environmental factors and mechanisms of airway inflammation characteristic of the syndrome, its prevalence and morbidity remain unacceptably high. Although asthma morbidity and mortality rates have been steady over the last few years, the rates are dramatically higher than 25 years ago and continue to be very significant, particularly for urban minority groups, low-income populations, and children.

The purpose of this chapter is to describe trends in asthma epidemiology, specifically prevalence, hospitalization, and mortality. In so doing, we examine potential reasons for these trends, and the recent research on the interactions of genes and environment. We also examine the relationship of the intermediate phenotypes of airway hyperresponsiveness and allergy to the asthma syndrome and consider a variety of risk factors for asthma occurrence. We conclude with a review of asthma natural history and the implications of the current trends.

DEFINITIONS AND PREVALENCE

In 2007, the National Asthma Education and Prevention Program Expert Panel Report 3 (NAEPPR3)[2] defined asthma as

> a chronic inflammatory disorder of the airways in which many cells and cellular elements play a role: in particular, mast cells, eosinophils, neutrophils (especially in sudden onset, fatal exacerbations, occupational asthma, and patients who smoke), T lymphocytes, macrophages, and epithelial cells. In susceptible individuals, this inflammation causes recurrent episodes of coughing (particularly at night or early in the morning), wheezing, breathlessness, and chest tightness. These episodes are usually associated with widespread but variable airflow obstruction that is often reversible either spontaneously or with treatment.

Because asthma is a clinical syndrome, there is no gold standard for its diagnosis. As such, physicians employ nonstandardized algorithms for making the diagnosis, such as a history of wheezing or a parental history of asthma in conjunction with a favorable response to a bronchodilator to identify the asthmatic patient. Frequently, age, gender, and other patient characteristics such as smoking status or response to allergen may influence a physician's diagnosis. Rarely are tests of airway responsiveness used to investigate symptomatic patients in the clinical setting.

In general, epidemiologic surveys have tended to rely on historical or questionnaire sources to identify patients with asthma. Asthma cases have been identified, either by physicians or surveys of population groups in whom the definition of who is asthmatic has been left to the patients themselves, surrogates, or the report of the diagnosis having been made by the patient's physician. Clearly, each of these methods of identifying asthma patients has inherent weaknesses. One must, therefore, assume that some bias in the reporting of cases is present and that the biases in each method of gathering data are different.

The National Health Interview Survey (NHIS) is an annual random population household interview survey that provides information on asthma prevalence in the United States. Its data demonstrate an almost doubling of asthma prevalence over the last quarter century,

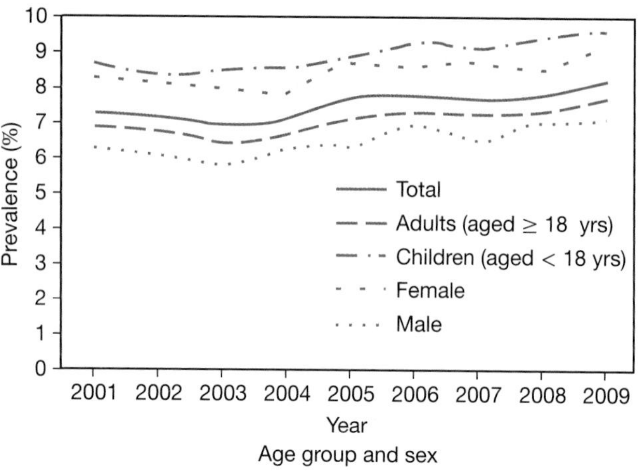

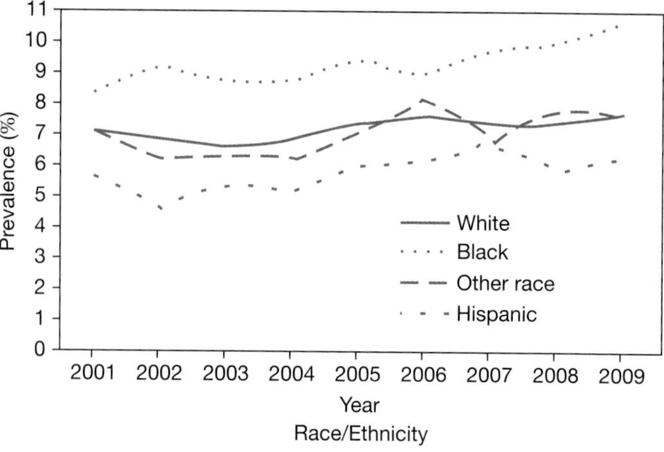

Figure 45-1 Current asthma prevalence figures from the National Health Interview Survey (NHIS), United States, by age group, sex, and race/ethnicity. Prevalence measures include persons who answered "yes" to the questions: "Have you ever been told by a doctor or other health professional that [you/your child] had asthma?" and "Do [you/your child] still have asthma?" *(Reproduced with permission from Vital signs: asthma prevalence, disease characteristics, and self-management education. United States, 2001–2009. MMWR Morb Mortal Wkly Rep. 2011;60(17):547–552.)*

from 3.2 per 100 population in 1981 to 5.5% per 100 in 1996.[3] In 1997 the NHIS questions and methodology were modified, limiting comparisons of prevalence before and after 1997. Instead of asking whether the respondent or a family member had had asthma over the past 12 months the newer version asks, "Have you ever been told by a doctor or other health professional that you had asthma?" (lifetime prevalence). Information about adults can no longer be obtained from a family member or proxy. If the response is affirmative, an "attack" question is asked, "During the past 12 months have you had an episode of asthma or asthma attack?" Beginning in 2001, if the lifetime prevalence response was positive, a point prevalence or "Current" measure was added asking, "Do you still have asthma?" The data from the "Current" question, is most comparable with previous data, but not exactly the same. Most recent data from the CDC, which analyzed data from the NHIS, indicated a plateau in asthma prevalence from 2001 through 2003, but prevalence has continued to rise since then (Fig. 45-1).[4] The prevalence in children under 18 years remains higher than adults, for example, in 2009, 9.6 per 100 compared with 7.7 (Fig. 45-1).

There is a difference in prevalence by racial/ethnic groups. Until 1997 racial groups were classified as black or white with black population having slightly higher 12-month prevalence. Beginning in 2003, racial and ethnic classification was expanded to include Hispanics. The most recent data from 2009 shows that prevalence was 11.1 for black non-Hispanics, 6.3 for Hispanics, and 8.1 per 100 for white non-Hispanics.[4] It is noteworthy that the rate for Hispanics of Puerto Rican descent was 14.2 per 100.[5]

The current data show a significant modification of prevalence by gender, in that males tend to predominate in the younger age group, whereas gender ratios equalize in the pubertal years, and females predominate throughout the rest of the adult life. For example, the current prevalence for males less than 18 years in 2009 was 11.3 per 100 compared with 7.9 for females, but in adults 18 years and older female prevalence (9.7 per 100) is almost twice that for males (5.5 per 100).[4] Thus, age and gender play an important role in modifying disease prevalence. In addition, there also appears to be some regional variation in asthma prevalence rates. Asthma prevalence was highest in the Northeast (9.3%), followed by the Midwest (8.8%), the West (7.7%), and the South (7.5%).[4]

ASTHMA HEALTHCARE USE

Drawing from data from multiple national surveys, the analyses performed by the CDC suggest that hospitalization and emergency

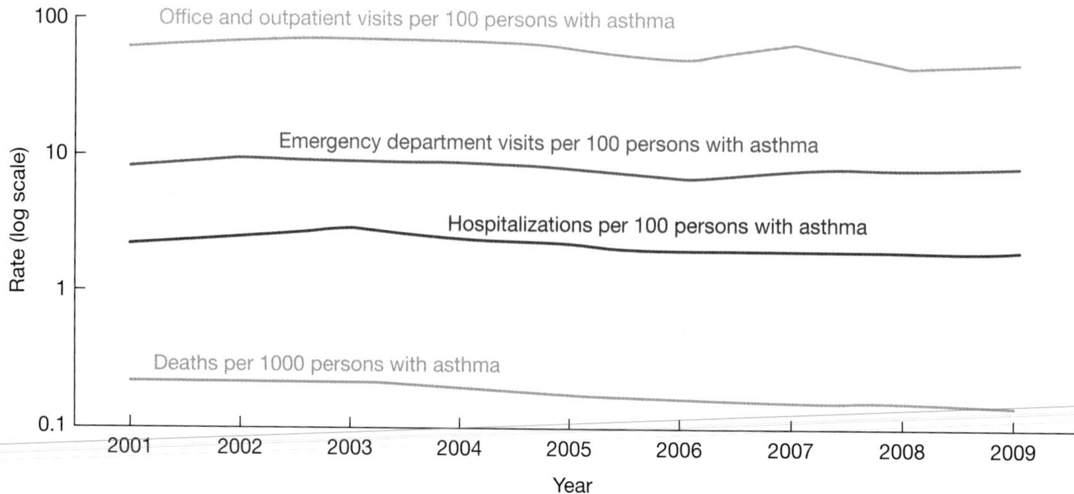

Figure 45-2 Asthma healthcare encounters per 100 persons with asthma, and asthma deaths per 1000 persons with asthma: United States, 2001 to 2009. *(Reproduced with permission from Akinbami LJ, Moorman JE, Bailey C, et al. Trends in asthma prevalence, health care use, and mortality in the United States, 2001–2010. NCHS Data Brief. 2012;(94):1–8.)*

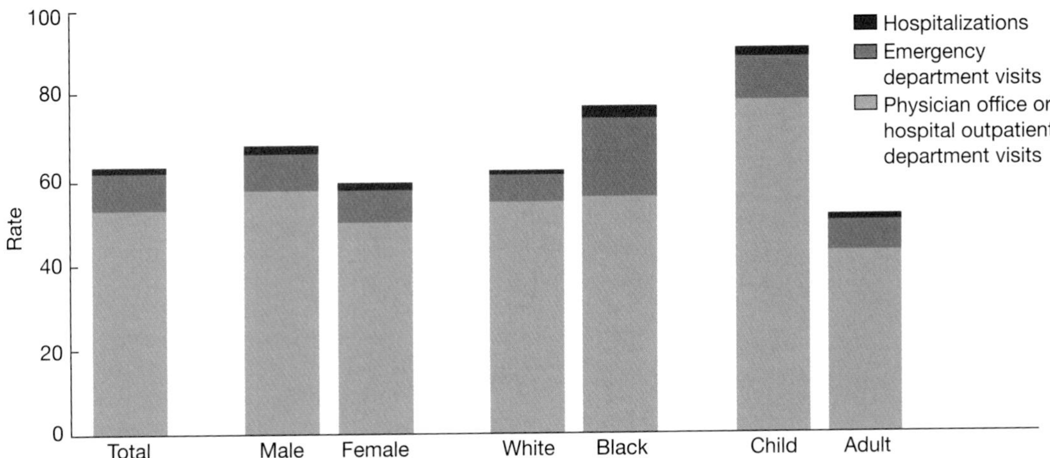

Figure 45-3 Asthma healthcare encounters per 100 persons with asthma: United States, 2001 to 2009. Hospitalizations are three times more frequent and emergency department visits almost five times more frequent among blacks. Healthcare utilization is more frequent in children than adults. *(Reproduced with permission from Akinbami LJ, Moorman JE, Bailey C, et al. Trends in asthma prevalence, health care use, and mortality in the United States, 2001–2010. NCHS Data Brief. 2012;(94):1–8.)*

department (ED) visit rates for asthma have remained stable from 2001 to 2009, a period of rising prevalence (Fig. 45-2).[6] Asthma visits in primary care settings (defined as physician offices and hospital outpatient departments) declined during this period. Asthma healthcare use is known to vary by demographic characteristics. For the period 2007 to 2009, asthma healthcare use across all healthcare settings was greater for children than for adults (Fig. 45-3): outpatient visit rates for children (0–17 years) averaged 78.7 per 100 persons with asthma versus 42.5 for adults; ED visits for children averaged 10.7 per 100 persons with asthma versus 7.0; while hospitalization rates were similar for both groups (2.1 per 100 persons with asthma for children vs. 1.9 for adults).[6] With respect to gender, for the 2007 to 2009 period, males had higher annual average outpatient visit rates than women (57.6 per 100 persons with asthma for men vs. 49.8 for women), while ED visit and hospitalization rates were about the same for both sexes (8.7 ED visits per 100 persons with asthma for males vs. 7.6 for women, and 1.8 hospitalizations per 100 persons with asthma for males vs. 2.0 for women). With respect to race, asthma outpatient visits per 100 persons with asthma were similar for black (54.9) and white (56.0) persons, but ED visits were three times higher in blacks (18.4 per 100 persons with asthma) than whites (6.1 per 100 persons with asthma), and hospitalizations were two times higher in blacks (2.8 per 100 persons) than whites (1.3 per 100 persons).

TRENDS IN ASTHMA MORTALITY

Asthma mortality rates in the United States are quite low. Recent data show that for the period 2007 to 2009, the asthma death rate per 100 persons with asthma was 0.015.[6] Figure 45-4 shows the trends in asthma mortality in the United States between 1980 and 2004.[7] There is an overall decline in deaths since 1998, although 11% of that decline can be attributed to the new coding instituted in 1999. As seen in Figure 45-2, the decline in death rates for asthma has continued through 2009. However, the downward trend in countrywide asthma mortality belies pockets of very high prevalence, morbidity, and mortality in urban minority populations. For instance, in 2009, blacks had a greater likelihood of dying from asthma than whites (Rate ratio = 1.93).[8]

These mortality rates do not represent a public health concern in an absolute sense, as the number of deaths is still very low. However, the rates do represent a clear public health concern because almost all asthma deaths are preventable, and certain urban and minority areas have extremely high mortality rates, suggesting inadequate care practices.

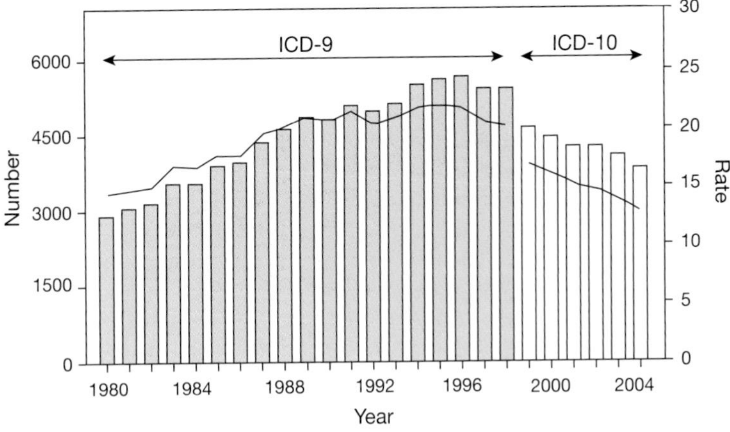

Figure 45-4 Asthma mortality trends, by year and International Classification of Diseases (ICD), United States, 1980 to 2004. Since1980, deaths from asthma rose. Beginning in 1998, both the overall number of deaths and the rate have clearly declined. However, a new mortality coding scheme was implemented in 1999. About 11% of the decline in asthma deaths can be attributed to the new coding scheme. *(Reproduced with permission from Moorman JE, Rudd RA, Johnson CA, et al. National surveillance for asthma–United States, 1980–2004. MMWR Surveill Summ. 2007;56(8):1–54.)*

INTERMEDIATE PHENOTYPES

There are two intermediate phenotypes that contribute to the asthmatic syndrome: airway responsiveness and allergy. Both have a genetic component, and both are influenced by environmental factors. We will discuss these phenotypes and their interrelationship to each other and to asthma.

AIRWAY RESPONSIVENESS

Airway responsiveness is measured by quantifying decline in lung function caused by using increasing doses of a bronchoconstrictive stimulus, such as histamine or methacholine (see Chapter 33). When the patient's FEV_1 decreases by 20% from its initial value, or after a maximum stimulus dose has been administered, the test is terminated. The dose at which this drop occurs is called the *provocative dose* (PD_{20}). Individuals who manifest a PD_{20} at a low dose of

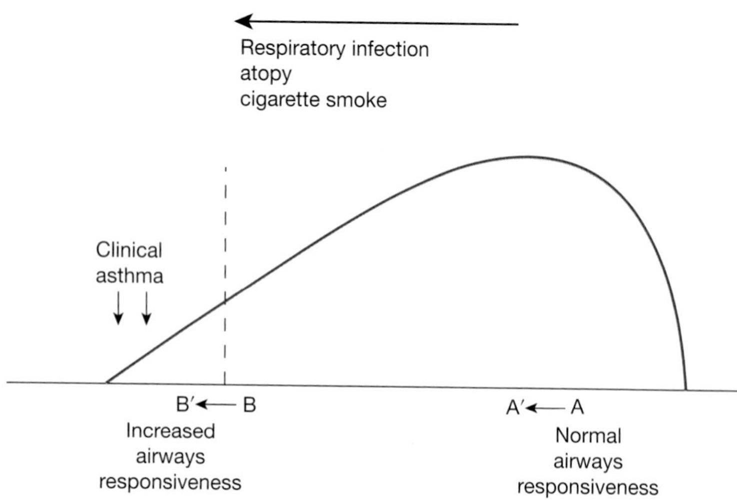

Figure 45-5 The effect of environmental exposures on the population distribution of airway responsiveness acting to move people in a more responsive direction. *(Reproduced with permission from Brown RW, Weiss ST. The influence of lower respiratory illness on childhood asthma: defining risk and susceptibility. Semin Respir Infect. 1991;6(4):225–234.)*

stimulus are said to have increased airway responsiveness and are hyperresponsive to the inhaled agent.

Cross-sectional population-based surveys of children and adults conducted in many different countries and using a variety of techniques for measuring airway responsiveness have shown that the prevalence of airway hyperresponsiveness is upward of 20% in the general population,[9–11] with women having a higher prevalence than men The prevalence of increased airway responsiveness exceeds the prevalence of asthma by two- to fivefold.

These studies have also demonstrated that airway responsiveness is log normally distributed in the general population. An example of this is given in Figure 45-5. In this population-based study of the distribution of histamine airway responsiveness, symptomatic or asthmatic subjects appear at the more responsive end of the distribution, but there is considerable overlap with asymptomatic subjects.[8] Other population-based studies have confirmed that a large number of asymptomatic subjects manifest increased airway hyperresponsiveness to this agent.

It has been well demonstrated in studies of both children and adults that airway hyperresponsiveness antedates and predicts the development of asthma.[12–16] Increased airway responsiveness carries at least twice the risk for the development of asthma in children and young adults. However, increased airway responsiveness is a necessary, but not a sufficient condition for the development of asthma. In all likelihood, subjects who are genetically predisposed have increased airway responsiveness.[15] They then encounter environmental stimuli that generate airway inflammation. The inflammation then moves them in the direction of greater responsiveness and the development of respiratory symptoms. This theoretical paradigm is graphically depicted in Figure 45-5.[17]

A variety of mechanical factors influence airway responsiveness. First, and most important, is the level of lung function. Individuals with lower levels of lung function are more likely to have increased airway responsiveness.[18–20] In part, this is simply a mathematical phenomenon. Since airway responsiveness is expressed as a percent change from baseline, the baseline value will obviously be important in determining the level at which an individual would be considered responsive (i.e., have a PD_{20}). This can be best understood with a simple mathematical example. A man with a 5-L FEV_1 would be required to drop his prechallenge level of lung function by 1 L to achieve a PD_{20} for FEV_1. In contrast, a man with a 500-mL FEV_1 will only need to drop his FEV_1 by 100 mL to achieve a comparable PD_{20} for FEV_1. Other factors, such as the central deposition and distribution of the inhaled aerosol, the fact that airflow is inversely proportional to the fourth power of the airway radius, and baseline bronchomotor tone all contribute to the relationship of lung function to airway responsiveness. For this reason, airway responsiveness is likely to be increased at the extremes of age (i.e., in children and older adults) and reduced in young adults between the ages of 15 and 45 years.[19]

■ ALLERGY

Allergy refers to immediate (Type 1) hypersensitivity to environmental antigens. It is characterized by wheal and flare reactions to skin testing with common environmental antigens, usually with appropriate clinical history. Atopy is the demonstration of allergy and familial aggregation of this trait.

Initially described over 20 years ago by Mosmann and colleagues,[21–23] the Th1–Th2 dichotomy has been helpful in explaining the pathophysiology of the allergic response. This model is also the basis for clinical research seeking to understand the development of asthma. Antigen presenting cells (APCs) display peptide antigens, either allergenic or infectious, on their cell surfaces for recognition by naïve T cells (Th0).[24] Th0 differentiate into Th1 or Th2 cells, depending on the nature of the antigen, the characteristics of the APC, local concentration of cytokines, and other cofactors not fully understood.[25] Th1 cells secrete IFN-γ, while Th2 cells secrete IL-4 and IL-5. (see Chapter 44). For example, activation of APC by microbial products results in production of IL-12 and Th0 cells differentiate into Th1 cells. The presence of IL-4 results in differentiation of Th0 cells into Th2 cells. Th2 cells promote allergic inflammation through the production of cytokines including IL-4, IL-5, and IL-13. IL-4 and IL-13 induce B lymphocytes to differentiate into IgE-producing plasma cells. IL-5 secreted by Th2 cells results in eosinophil production and resistance to apoptosis.[26] A Th1 response results in activation of macrophages and natural killer cells and production of IgG1, which plays a role in complement binding and opsonization. Th1 and Th2 cells cross-regulate each other. That is, IFN-γ inhibits Th2 proliferation and IL-4 inhibits IFN-γ–induced macrophage activation. T-regulatory (Treg) cells are recently characterized cells that inhibit Th1 and Th2 cells.[27] These cells are characterized by their secretion of IL-10 and transforming growth factor (TGF)-β, and, via the expression of Foxp3, lead to suppression or proliferation of other T cells.[28,29] Tregs also suppress effector cells of allergic inflammation (e.g., basophils, eosinophils, and mast cells),[30,31] and regulate IgE production.[32] Thus, it is likely that Tregs play a role in airway tolerance in the prevention of asthma.[33]

Since the initial description of the Th1/Th2 dichotomy, it has become clear that mechanisms involved in asthma and the allergic response are much more complicated. The role of the epithelium and upstream pathways has become clearer (as reviewed in Williams et al.[34]). Initial activation occurs in the epithelium, upon interaction of allergen and/or pathogen (damage)-associated molecular patterns and toll-like receptors. Early response cytokines, including thymic stromal lymphopoietin (TSLP), IL-33, and IL-25 (previously termed IL-17E) are released in the local tissue environment. These set off a cascade of events that include dendritic cell skewing to a phenotype that supports differentiation of Th2 cells, and also expansion of innate immune effector leukocytes secreting IL-4, IL-5, and IL-13 leading to a Th2 inflammatory response. Other cytokines are now recognized to play a role in the acute response and chronic inflammation characteristic of asthma and allergies, including IL-9, IL-17, IL-22, among many others.[26,35]

CLINICAL MARKERS OF ALLERGY

Many clinical allergy markers have been utilized in epidemiologic studies of asthma. Total or allergen-specific IgE, measured by serologic testing, or specific allergen skin testing, assess sensitization as well as exposure to environmental antigens and frequently are used to determine the prevalence of allergic responsiveness. Skin test reactivity depends on at least three separate factors: (1) an intact immune system; (2) the presence of IgE-sensitized mast cells that release mediators when exposed to antigen; (3) and skin that can respond to histamine with the development of an inflammatory response, including erythema and induration. Although these manifestations of an allergic response depend on prior exposure to an environmental antigen, they do not measure or take into account the level of exposure in the environment.

Total serum IgE, although used in epidemiologic studies, has relatively limited value in the diagnoses of atopic diseases, with the exception of allergic bronchopulmonary aspergillosis. Total and specific IgE levels correlate with each other and with skin test results, but no level of total IgE avoids misclassifying a significant proportion of those with and without allergic diseases. The limitations in clinical information imposed by these tests reduce their utility when they are used in epidemiologic studies.

Total and specific IgE measurements appear to be comparable in males and females. Both increase with age and peak approximately at the age of 15 years. After this time, there is a progressive decline, although the decline in skin test reactivity exceeds the reduction in total serum IgE, perhaps related to local factors in the skin.

It is believed that IgE responses to inhalant allergens are commonly set in early childhood. In early life, the immune system is characterized by immature humoral and cellular responses. Initially thought to be unresponsive, in fact, the neonatal response is strongly biased toward a Th2 function.[36–38] As the neonate grows and the immune system matures, there is a shift toward a more balanced immune response in healthy individuals. The process by which this shift comes about is the object of intense research. For example, it is known that potent neonatal Th1 responses can be induced under specific circumstances (e.g., infections).[39–42] Immunomodulatory agents that can promote neonatal Th1 immunity are the subject of current research.[43,44] Thus, sensitization, that is, production of IgE directed at environmental antigens, is not only a function of genetic susceptibility, dose, timing, and duration of allergen exposure, but likely reflects early exposure to other environmental antigens, particularly microbial or viral organisms. One hypothesis of the development of atopic disease, the "hygiene hypothesis," states that the prevention of Th2-mediated disorders is dependent upon early exposure to infectious agents. That is, respiratory or gastrointestinal infections may stimulate macrophages to produce interferon-α and IL-12 that stimulate NK cells to produce IFN-γ, which would inhibit the development of a Th2-type response. The Tucson Children's Respiratory Study, a birth cohort of 1246 subjects, noted that children who had a nonwheezing lower respiratory tract illness before 9 months of age had lower total IgE levels at 9 months and 6 years of age when compared with children who had no lower respiratory illnesses before 9 months of age.[45,46] These children were also less likely to be atopic than those who had no lower respiratory tract illnesses. These investigators also found that children exposed to more siblings at home or to day care in the first 6 months of life, presumably exposed to more infections, were protected from the development of asthma between ages 6 and 13 years.[47] Findings from some other cohorts have shown similar effects of early life exposure to day care or more siblings on asthma risk.[48–50] On the other hand, several other birth cohorts have found either that early day care exposure had no effect on asthma development or that it increased the risk for asthma and asthma-like symptoms in children.[51–54] This research confirms the complexity of environmental influences on the immune system.

RELATIONSHIP OF AIRWAY RESPONSIVENESS AND ALLERGY TO ASTHMA

Atopy and increased airway responsiveness are independent factors, both of which are related to the asthma phenotype. While the prevalence of atopy is higher among asthmatics than nonasthmatics, the association may not be causal. Systematic reviews have shown that at a population level, there is no correlation between the prevalence of atopy and the prevalence of asthma.[55–57] It is likely that there are common factors that raise the risk of both conditions. Studies that have investigated phenotypes of asthma using clustering methods have shown that there are asthma cases that are predominantly atopic with positive skin test reactivity, eosinophilia, and a younger age of onset, whereas there are other clusters that are predominantly nonatopic with neutrophilia and an older age of onset.[58,59]

Atopy and airway responsiveness may also occur together. Studies have shown that individuals who are sensitized to an allergen have bronchospasm when exposed to that allergen,[60,61] but individuals may have airway hyperresponsiveness without atopic manifestations. The introduction of omalizumab, a recombinant, humanized anti-IgE antibody, is helping to elucidate the relationship of airway responsiveness and allergy. Omalizumab lowers total serum IgE and reduces eosinophils in sputum.[62–64] In some studies it has allowed reduction of corticosteroid therapy, but in others it has failed to show reduction in airway hyperresponsiveness, supporting the notion that airway hyperreactivity and allergy have other separate influences.

Since the first report of a longitudinal relationship between exposure to higher levels of dust mite allergen and the development of asthma,[65] researchers have explored the relationship between exposure to allergen and the subsequent development of asthma. A birth cohort design has been used to examine this relationship. Preventing loss of participants to follow-up makes these studies difficult to conduct. It is also difficult to measure exposure to allergen, that is, to quantify inhalation by subjects, while accounting for intermittent and varying exposure over time and place. Nevertheless, most studies have investigated exposure to allergens in house dust early in life. Furthermore, there is an imperfect correlation among skin test reactivity, total serum IgE level, and peripheral blood eosinophil count, such that no single phenotypic marker completely defines the atopic state. These longitudinal studies have shown that exposure to high levels of allergens early in life increases the risk for sensitization and atopy.[66,67] However, the effect on asthma appears to depend on the atopic status of the parents. In children of atopic parents, exposure to high levels of allergen in early life increased the risk of asthma in childhood,[66] whereas in studies where cohorts were not selected for parental atopy, there was no significant effect of exposure to allergens in early life and asthma risk in childhood.[67,68] These studies suggest the theme that asthma and allergies have some common determinants but are likely separate entities, and that genetic susceptibility likely interacts with environmental exposures in determining risk for the development of asthma.

GENETIC SUSCEPTIBILITY AND GENE–ENVIRONMENT INTERACTIONS

Geneticists describe asthma as a complex disease, a disease in which many genes influence the development and phenotype of asthma, each having only a small influence. Since the human genome project was completed in 2000, remarkable advances have been made in identifying asthma genes.

There are two main types of genetic studies: linkage studies and association studies. In an association study, candidate genes are examined to determine a statistical association between polymorphism in the gene and asthma phenotypes; either cases and controls or trios can be used. These studies focus on known pathophysiology. An extension of the candidate gene association study is the genome-wide association study (GWAS). In this case, a panel of markers, commonly single nucleotide polymorphisms (SNPs) and numbering 500,000 to over 2 million, are genotyped and association analysis is conducted to find associations with asthma phenotypes. This type of association study is hypothesis free and does not focus on known pathophysiology.

Linkage studies start with families with well-characterized phenotypes such as asthma. Genes within families are examined for linkage, the sharing of genes markers that may be located near or at the disease gene. Association studies are then used to follow-up and "fine map" the linkage peak. These studies focus on novel genes.

To date, five genes *ADAM 33*,[69] *DPP10*,[70] *PHF11*,[71] *NPSR1*,[72] and *HLA-G*,[73] have been identified by linkage and fine mapping. One gene *ORMDL3*[74] has been identified by GWAS. Two large meta-analyses of asthma GWAS have been conducted in European and ethnically diverse US populations,[75,76] with surprising consistency in results. In both of these studies, SNPs at or near four loci achieved genome-wide levels of significance in their *p*-values: the 17q21 locus (*ORMDL3/GSDML*), the *IL1RL1/IL18R1* locus, *TSLP*, and *IL33*.

ENVIRONMENTAL RISK FACTORS

Below we present some of the most important environmental risk factors for the development or exacerbation of asthma not discussed earlier.

PERINATAL FACTORS

Prematurity carries an increased risk for the development of asthma. A recent review and meta-analysis showed that infants born at less than 37 weeks' gestation are at greater risk for developing asthma than term infants.[77] Prematurity also is associated with bronchopulmonary dysplasia,[78] a disease characterized by increased airway responsiveness and asthma symptoms. Some investigators have found that low birth weight independent of prematurity has been associated with asthma risk.[79,80] The strength of the association between prematurity and/or low birth weight on asthma or asthma symptoms appears be greatest in very young children, but the effects decrease over time.[81,82] Note that blacks have higher rates of prematurity than whites; thus, prematurity may contribute to racial differences in asthma prevalence and morbidity. Young maternal age (i.e., <20 years) has not been shown to have a consistent independent association with the development of asthma. Despite much research, there is no conclusive evidence that breastfeeding influences atopic sensitization or the development of asthma.[83,84]

Recent studies have focused on maternal diet during pregnancy and its effect on the development of asthma and allergies, with the hypothesis that nutritional deficiency or excess may lead to programming of the fetus for adult disease.[85] These studies have mostly used nutrient intake estimates derived from food frequency questionnaires that assess how often a particular standard serving of a food or drink is eaten. The responses to the questionnaire, in conjunction with a database of nutrient composition of foods, are then used to calculate the amount of a particular nutrient over a specified time period.[86] A few studies have measured the particular nutrient in either maternal or cord blood samples. A meta-analysis found that there was weak support for protective effects of higher maternal intakes of vitamin A, E, and zinc for the prevention of asthma in children.[87]

VITAMIN D

In the strict sense of the word, vitamin D is not a vitamin, since humans are able to produce the compound in the skin upon exposure to the UVA rays from the sun. While the first report of an effect of vitamin D on asthma and allergies appeared in 1934,[88] research into the effects of vitamin D did not begin in earnest until the last decade. There are two opposing hypotheses regarding the role of vitamin D in asthma. Wjst and Dold[89] suggested that fortification of food with vitamin D and the widespread use of multivitamins in childhood contributed to the rise in asthma and allergies. On the other hand, given the documented decrease in the levels of the circulating form of vitamin D in population studies,[90] Litonjua and Weiss hypothesized that the increasing prevalence of vitamin D deficiency led to the increase in asthma prevalence worldwide.[91]

With regard to the development of asthma and allergies, four cohort studies have reported beneficial effects of a higher maternal intake of vitamin D in pregnancy on outcomes in their children.[92–95] However, other studies have not replicated these findings.[96–99] More consistent results have been found with regard to the role of vitamin D in disease severity or treatment. These studies have shown that asthmatics with higher circulating vitamin D levels have greater lung function,[100,101] lower risks for exacerbations,[102,103] and generally more severe indices of disease.[104] Clinical trials of vitamin D supplementation to prevent asthma development and to prevent exacerbations are ongoing.

INDOOR AND OUTDOOR ALLERGENS

Indoor allergen sources include animals (cats, dogs, rodents), insects (mites, cockroaches), and fungi. Allergens are well-known precipitants of asthma exacerbations and increased morbidity.[105,106] There has been some recent investigation as to whether exposure to pets early in life would be useful in preventing asthma,[107–109] but a recent pooled analysis of 11 European birth cohorts did not find any effect of pet ownership on asthma and allergic rhinitis in school age children.[110] It is noteworthy that animal allergens, particularly cat allergen, can be found in settled dust and in circulating air in homes, school classrooms, and other buildings that never housed a cat.[111–113]

House dust mites are ubiquitous in all but very dry climates and exposure and sensitization to mite body and fecal allergens is associated with asthma.[65,66] Mites infest fabrics, including mattresses, bedding, floor coverings, and upholstered furniture. The use of wall-to-wall carpets has increased exposure to mites. Covering mattresses and pillows with vapor-permeable fine weave materials, washing bedding in hot (>30°F) water, vacuuming weekly, and removing carpets, especially from the bedroom, reduce mite levels.[114,115]

Whether reducing exposure results in improvement in asthma outcome has been the focus of several studies,[116,117] with inconsistent results. A Cochrane meta-analysis of 54 trials using varying methods of mite-allergen reduction (physical methods, chemical methods, and a combination) concluded that there was no clinical benefit of dust mite allergen reduction.[118] Adherence to the demanding protocols for control of mite exposure is difficult and may not always result in sufficient reduction in personal aeroallergen exposure. More recent studies have focused on multifaceted intervention programs that target other environmental exposures (e.g., environmental tobacco smoke [ETS]) in addition to allergen avoidance, and may have more promise than single allergen avoidance.[119–123]

Sensitization to cockroach has been shown to be associated with the development of asthma and asthma morbidity.[106,124] Although the presence of this allergen is not limited to low-income homes, it has not been studied in more affluent settings. Removal of this allergen is difficult and more research is needed to evaluate the impact on asthma of allergen removal.[125–127]

Home, school, and workplace dampness and the presence of fungi have been associated with reports of respiratory symptoms.[128] Sensitization to molds has also been shown to be associated with greater asthma morbidity.[129]

Day care establishments may be sources of indoor allergens, including pets, insects, and fungi.[130] They also may be sources of gram-negative bacterial endotoxin and lipopolysaccharides, which induce Th1 activity and have been hypothesized to be protective against the development of allergy and asthma. However, longitudinal studies have not consistently supported this notion. A recent study of 3963 children found no effect of early day care attendance on the development of asthma symptoms, airway hyperresponsiveness, and allergic sensitization at 8 years of age.[51]

Outdoor allergens include trees, grass, and weed pollen constituents. Susceptible individuals may have increased asthma symptoms at times of pollination.[131] For example, in the Northeast and Midwest grass pollinates in May and June and ragweed in late August and September. Pollens most closely linked to exacerbations of asthma in at-risk individuals are trees such as birch, oak, and Western red cedar; grasses; and ragweed. A recent study, however, suggests that asthmatics react to airborne allergens regardless of their sensitization status.[132] This will require further study.

■ SMOKING AND ENVIRONMENTAL TOBACCO SMOKE

Maternal cigarette smoking is a major risk factor for the development of asthma in the first year of life. Both a meta-analysis[133] and a pooled analysis[134] showed that the risk of developing asthma ranges from around 40% to 85% greater among children born to mothers who smoked during pregnancy compared to children born to mothers who did not smoke. This effect appears to be strongest in children who developed asthma before 2 years of age.[133]

ETS exacerbates asthma in children of all ages.[135] Wilson and coworkers[136] evaluated a cotinine-feedback behavioral intervention administered to caregivers that successfully reduced ETS exposure and healthcare utilization by children with asthma at 1-year follow-up. However, in a follow-up study, the effect was only seen in children at highest risk for exacerbation.[137] In adults, cigarette smoking is associated with the development of airway hyperreactivity.[138] Whether this hyperreactivity represents asthma or COPD can be difficult to determine. Cigarette smoking in asthma produce a synergistic and accelerated decline in lung function.[139,140] In addition, the response to corticosteroid therapy used for asthma is reduced in active smokers.[139]

■ OTHER POLLUTANTS

Outdoor pollutants implicated in the development or exacerbations of asthma include ozone, sulfur dioxide, particulate matter, and components of motor vehicle exhaust.[141,142] Measuring exposure to potential pollutants is difficult and correlating exposure with symptoms and exacerbations of disease is very expensive. Most monitoring of pollutants is from fixed external stations. Sometimes proxy measures of pollutant exposure, such as traffic counts, are used. Although potentially more accurate, monitoring of personal exposures is particularly difficult and expensive.[143] Assessing which of the many possible simultaneous outdoor inhalants affects asthma morbidity is also a formidable task. Conclusions drawn from such data may be indirect. An example is the observation that asthma morbidity is highest among low-income individuals who tend to live in less desirable areas, which are frequently those with high traffic volumes and pollution.

There has been much interest in indoor environmental pollutants, such as nitrogen dioxide, sulfur dioxide, volatile organic compounds, and particulate matter, and their possible association with asthma, particularly in inner city homes.[144,145] As with studies of outdoor pollution difficulties in measurement over time, controlling for other exposures such as allergens, infectious agents, and social determinants of health, while linking exposures to symptoms and physical findings makes research challenging.

■ RACE/ETHNICITY AND SOCIOECONOMIC STATUS

As discussed at the beginning of this chapter, asthma prevalence and especially morbidity and mortality are higher in blacks than whites. Whether these racial differences in asthma prevalence, hospitalization, and mortality are solely due to inadequate treatment and access to medical care remains unclear, but there is indisputable evidence of unequal treatment of minority and low-income groups by health professionals.[146] In addition, environmental factors that are the products of poverty, such as urban crowding, exposure to tobacco smoke or other pollutants or allergens contribute to these findings.[147] A recent line of research to explain some of the racial and socioeconomic disparities in asthma has focused on the effect of stress and violence in the pathogenesis of asthma and morbidity related to asthma.[148,149] These studies have shown that exposure to stress or violence is related to asthma in children, even after adjusting for socioeconomic status.

There is much current debate about the relative importance of social and genetic effects and/or gene–environment interactions that might account for the health disparity seen in asthma and other diseases. In most studies race and ethnicity are not well defined and socioeconomic factors tend to be inseparably linked to ethnicity and race. Perceptions of a person's race influence social experiences including those with the health system. In a recent survey, black and Hispanic women were more likely to report a doctor's diagnosis of asthma and less likely to report a diagnosis of hay fever or eczema. However, these women had higher mean total IgE levels and were more likely to be sensitized to aeroallergens.[150] The investigators concluded that these findings could represent either underdiagnosis by medical personnel (e.g., fewer referrals to an allergist or other specialist) or underreporting of symptoms by patients. They also concluded that it was unlikely that genetics alone could explain the differences in sensitization and that these differences more likely were related to differences in housing and community environmental exposures.

As our cultural and ethnic diversity increases, communication between patient and healthcare provider becomes more complicated and miscommunication more likely. In addition, prior experiences of discrimination or perceived discrimination contribute to distrust of the health system.[151,152] These may result in mistrust of the medical advice, or refusal of treatment and poor adherence and thus contribute to health disparities. One study found patients' beliefs in the risks over the benefits of inhaled steroids to be associated with lower adherence.[153] In focus groups, blacks with moderate or severe asthma who reported their adherence was influenced by reliance on their own assessment of asthma control over that of the health provider. They expressed concern about adverse effects of inhaled steroid therapy and several had misperceptions of their risks. Such misperceptions can be addressed in the patient–provider encounter. Adherence was also adversely affected by the cost of the medication or its copay and insurers' approval policies and restricted formularies.

■ OBESITY

Obesity has reached epidemic proportions in the United States and has been related to asthma in cross-sectional and longitudinal studies. A number of mechanisms for this relationship have been proposed.[154,155] Some of these mechanisms may begin early in life to confer risk for both disorders.[156,157] A mechanical effect is postulated to be the result of decreased tidal volume and decreased functional residual capacity leading to reduced ability of the smooth muscles to stretch and thus respond to changes in respiration with exercise. Obesity enhances gastroesophageal reflux, a condition associated with asthma. Immune effects also have been postulated. For example, certain inflammatory cytokines such as tumor necrosis factor-α (TNF-α) and IL-6 are expressed by adipocytes. TNF expression is increased in asthma exacerbations and may have a role in amplifying the inflammatory response of asthma. IL-6 stimulates a Th1 response, which may contribute to the inflammation of severe asthma. Leptin, a product of adipocytes, is a member of the IL-6 cytokine family. Whether or not leptin plays a role in asthma is unknown. Because asthma in adults is more common in women and because estrogen is increased in obesity, estrogen has been hypothesized to play a role in a link between asthma and obesity but no such role has been demonstrated.

Since asthma and obesity are both complex diseases, it is possible that some genetic susceptibilities are shared (pleiotropy).[157] There is some evidence for this in that there are regions of the human genome important for both asthma and obesity, such as chromosome 6p, which contains the gene for TNF. Alternatively, it is possible that obesity is related to asthma as an epiphenomenon; that is, there are shared lifestyle or social exposures, for example, physical exercise or diet, that influence both obesity and asthma. Obesity is more prevalent in the same socioeconomic groups in which asthma is more prevalent. No randomized interventional studies have been completed showing that weight reduction ameliorates asthma. Clearly, more research is needed.

■ ACETAMINOPHEN

It has been postulated that acetaminophen use may increase the risk of developing asthma due to its pro-oxidant effects (by depletion of the antioxidant glutathione in lung tissue).[158] Several studies have reported on the association of acetaminophen use, either in pregnancy, in early life, and in adulthood, and the development of asthma.[159-162] However, the issue with studies that investigate over-the-counter medications such as acetaminophen is the possibility of confounding by indication, meaning that these individuals have comorbidities (e.g., respiratory infections) for which they may take the acetaminophen for its antipyretic or analgesic effects. To address this, investigators of the Melbourne Atopy Cohort Study found that when they adjusted for the frequency of respiratory infections, the association between acetaminophen use and asthma at age 6 or 7 years disappeared.[163] Therefore, while more studies need to be done, it is not likely that taking acetaminophen in usual doses is a cause of asthma.

■ RESPIRATORY ILLNESS

Many epidemiologic studies have shown a prominent association between lower respiratory tract viral infections and wheezing illnesses in infancy and increased risk of chronic childhood asthma.[164,165] Respiratory syncytial virus (RSV) has drawn particular attention, since it is the major cause of bronchiolitis in children and RSV infection is associated with IgE production, airway inflammation, and increased airway responsiveness. Human rhinoviruses (HRVs) which are a more common cause of upper and lower respiratory infections than RSV, may also cause bronchiolitis,[166] and have also been associated with asthma onset.[167] This is particularly true of the newly identified type C rhinoviruses. Respiratory tract infections by parainfluenza viruses, influenza virus, and human metapneumovirus during infancy are all associated with childhood wheezing.

It is hypothesized that susceptibility to asthma associated with viral infection in early life results from the interaction of developmental, genetic, and environmental factors. Developmentally, infancy is a time of pulmonary alveolarization and a time when the immune system has not reached full maturity. Several studies have now documented the synergy of allergen sensitization and respiratory infections in the risk for developing asthma. Kusel et al.[168] showed that among sensitized children, the risk for developing asthma by the age of 6 years was almost double that of children who were not sensitized. Jackson and colleagues[167] showed that while HRV was the dominant factor in developing asthma by the age of 6 years, the risk was highest when concomitant allergen sensitization was present.

Atopic status and airway hyperresponsiveness may be important genetically determined characteristics that influence whether RSV, HRV, or other respiratory viral infections increase the risk of developing asthma. Most children who wheezed only during the first 2 years of life had lower levels of lung function when evaluated at the age of 2 and 6 years. In contrast, children who wheezed early in life and who were still wheezing at the age of 6 years had normal lung function, but statistically elevated serum total IgE levels when studied during the first year of life. When restudied at the age of 6 years, they had elevated IgE, but lung function had deteriorated and was below that of individuals who had never wheezed.[45] This has led to the hypothesis that there are two wheezing syndromes associated with lower respiratory tract infection in young children. One occurs in children with small airway caliber who lack airway hyperresponsiveness, and have excellent prognosis. The other syndrome, which represents early-onset asthma, is associated with increased prevalence of allergic markers, bronchial hyperreactivity, and a significant decrease in lung function over the first 6 years of life.

Viral respiratory illnesses trigger asthmatic exacerbations. A number of studies have demonstrated a close temporal relationship at the individual and population levels, between virus infection and asthma exacerbations. These studies have also demonstrated that (1) asthmatics may be more susceptible than normal subjects to viral lower respiratory infections;[169-171] for example, in a surveillance study of 5.3 million children aged 17 years or younger during the 2003 to 2009 influenza seasons and the 2009 pandemic, Dawood and colleagues[170] found that 32% and 44%, respectively, of the children hospitalized had asthma; (2) in contrast to viral infections, bacterial infections are not associated with asthmatic exacerbations, although agents such as *Mycoplasma* and *Chlamydia* may be involved with persistence of asthma;[172] (3) viruses precipitate a high percentage of severe (vs. mild) asthmatic exacerbations; during the 2009 influenza pandemic, a greater proportion of asthmatics required intensive care;[170] and (4) viral infections can induce nonspecific increases in airway responsiveness and airway obstruction.[173-175]

PROGNOSIS

The prognosis of asthma in early childhood has been clarified substantially by data from the Tucson Children's Respiratory Study.[45,46] These investigators followed a cohort of children through the first 6 years of life. They characterized four groups of children: "persistent wheezers," who wheezed both before and after the age of 3 years; "transient early wheezers," who wheezed before the age of 3 years and then stopped; "transient late wheezers," who wheezed after the age of 3 years but not before; and "never wheezers." Totally 40% of all children in the Tucson Children's Respiratory Study cohort wheezed in the first year of life.

Significant predictors of persistent wheezing, and hence children at greatest risk for developing chronic asthma were young maternal age, IgE level at 9 months, parents with asthma, maternal cigarette smoke exposure in utero, abnormal lung function at birth, and male gender. It is likely that early-life wheezing is predominantly a mechanical factor and less due to severe and chronic airway inflammation. It also seems unlikely that allergen exposure predominates as a factor in early childhood.

The characteristics of older children who wheeze are atopy, female gender, and active and passive cigarette smoking. By preadolescence, atopy and environmental allergen exposure are important risk factors for wheezing in children.

In roughly half of all childhood asthmatics, symptoms decrease or disappear by late adolescence and early adulthood. Characteristics that suggest a good prognosis include male gender, precipitation of attacks by viral respiratory illness, and children with airway parenchymal desynapsis (i.e., large lungs but small airways). These children are predominantly male, and, although often atopic, still are likely to outgrow their asthma. In a longitudinal study of children from East Boston, initially 5 to 9 years of age followed over a 13-year period, the effect of asthma on lung growth was different for boys than girls.[176] Boys with asthma had larger growth in vital capacity than boys without asthma and tended to have mild disease. This was associated with fewer hospitalizations for asthma, despite somewhat greater prevalence than in girls. Asthmatic girls, however, had persistent reductions in FEV_1 and were more likely to be hospitalized for asthma, despite an initially reduced prevalence relative to the boys. These data are consistent with asthma being milder in boys in that the boys are more likely to "outgrow" their asthma. In contrast, the Childhood Asthma Management Program (CAMP) followed lung function of 1041 children (420 girls and 621 boys) with mild to moderate persistent asthma, who participated in a clinical trial of asthma treatment.[177] The authors used lung function data of 5415 nonasthmatic children from the Harvard Six Cities Study for comparison. In children of both sexes aged 6 to 18 years, the FEV_1/FVC ratio was significantly lower and FVC was significantly higher for asthmatic children, compared to nonasthmatic children. In contrast to the East Boston study, boys had lower FEV_1 between the ages of 10 to 18, whereas there were no significant differences in girls. Taken together, these studies suggest that asthma that starts in early life (i.e., by the age of 6 years) leads to decrements in lung function that are persistent through adolescence. These patterns have been borne out in other longitudinal studies (reviewed by Grad and Morgan[178]).

In both adolescents and adults, airway responsiveness predicts the development of asthma[12-16] and antedates and predicts accelerated decline in lung function.[179,180] Both persistent symptoms[181] and active smoking[140] conferred more rapid rates of lung function decline in longitudinal studies. The severity of adult asthma is clearly predicted by the severity of childhood asthma, and the persistence of symptoms in childhood and early adulthood is associated with reduced lung function and more severe disease later in adult life.

IMPLICATIONS OF CURRENT TRENDS IN PREVALENCE, MORBIDITY, HOSPITALIZATIONS, AND MORTALITY

Although prevalence, morbidity, and hospitalizations have remained stable recently, these absolute levels remain unacceptably high, particularly for certain minority groups and low-income populations. Risk factors such as obesity, prematurity, young maternal age, and cigarette smoking are all associated with these same patient groups, speaking about social and healthcare disparities. There are many vulnerable groups for which no data on asthma prevalence and morbidity yet exist. Certainly, genetic differences exist from patient to patient. These differences must be better characterized. Understanding the influence of gene-gene and gene-environment interactions is crucial. Gene-environmental interactions must be carefully studied for all exposures, and particularly for the exposure of socioeconomic status and cultural groups.

REFERENCES

1. Barnett SB, Nurmagambetov TA. Costs of asthma in the United States: 2002–2007. *J Allergy Clin Immunol.* 2011;127(1):145–152.
2. National Asthma Education and Prevention Program. Expert Panel Report 3 (EPR-3): guidelines for the Diagnosis and Management of Asthma-Summary Report 2007. *J Allergy Clin Immunol.* 2007;120(5 Suppl):S94–S138.
3. Mannino DM, Homa DM, Akinbami LJ, Moorman JE, Gwynn C, Redd SC. Surveillance for asthma–United States, 1980–1999. *MMWR Surveill Summ.* 2002;51(1):1–13.
4. Centers for Disease Control and Prevention (CDC). Vital signs: asthma prevalence, disease characteristics, and self-management education: United States, 2001–2009. *MMWR Morb Mortal Wkly Rep.* 2011;60(17):547–552.
5. Moorman JE, Zahran H, Truman BI, Molla MT. Current asthma prevalence—United States, 2006–2008. *MMWR Surveill Summ.* 2011;60 (Suppl):84–86.
6. Akinbami LJ, Moorman JE, Bailey C, et al. Trends in asthma prevalence, health care use, and mortality in the United States, 2001–2010. *NCHS Data Brief.* 2012;(94):1–8.
7. Moorman JE, Rudd RA, Johnson CA, et al. National surveillance for asthma–United States, 1980–2004. *MMWR Surveill Summ.* 2007;56(8):1–54.
8. Rijcken B, Schouten JP, Weiss ST, Meinesz AF, de Vries K, van der Lende R. The distribution of bronchial responsiveness to histamine in symptomatic and in asymptomatic subjects. A population-based analysis of various indices of responsiveness. *Am Rev Respir Dis.* 1989;140(3):615–623.
9. Paoletti P, Carrozzi L, Viegi G, et al. Distribution of bronchial responsiveness in a general population: effect of sex, age, smoking, and level of pulmonary function. *Am J Respir Crit Care Med.* 1995;151(6):1770–1777.
10. Rijcken B, Schouten JP, Weiss ST, Speizer FE, van der Lende R. The relationship between airway responsiveness to histamine and pulmonary function level in a random population sample. *Am Rev Respir Dis.* 1988;137(4):826–832.
11. Wassmer G, Jörres RA, Heinrich J, Wjst M, Reitmeir P, Wichmann HE. The association between baseline lung function and bronchial responsiveness to methacholine. *Eur J Med Res.* 1997;2(2):47–54.
12. Carey VJ, Weiss ST, Tager IB, Leeder SR, Speizer FE. Airways responsiveness, wheeze onset, and recurrent asthma episodes in young adolescents. The East Boston Childhood Respiratory Disease Cohort. *Am J Respir Crit Care Med.* 1996;153(1): 356–361.
13. Porsbjerg C, von Linstow ML, Ulrik CS, Nepper-Christensen S, Backer V. Risk factors for onset of asthma: a 12-year prospective follow-up study. *Chest.* 2006;129(2):309–316.
14. Porsbjerg C, von Linstow ML, Ulrik CS, Nepper-Christensen SC, Backer V. Outcome in adulthood of asymptomatic airway hyperresponsiveness to histamine and exercise-induced bronchospasm in childhood. *Ann Allergy Asthma Immunol.* 2005;95(2):137–142.
15. Rasmussen F, Taylor DR, Flannery EM, et al. Outcome in adulthood of asymptomatic airway hyperresponsiveness in childhood: a longitudinal population study. *Pediatr Pulmonol.* 2002;34(3):164–171.
16. Zhong NS, Chen RC, Yang MO, Wu ZY, Zheng JP, Li YF. Is asymptomatic bronchial hyperresponsiveness an indication of potential asthma? A two-year follow-up of young students with bronchial hyperresponsiveness. *Chest.* 1992;102(4): 1104–1109.
17. Brown RW, Weiss ST. The influence of lower respiratory illness on childhood asthma: defining risk and susceptibility. *Semin Respir Infect.* 1991;6(4):225–234.
18. Short PM, Lipworth SI, Lipworth BJ. Relationships between airway hyperresponsiveness, inflammation, and calibre in asthma. *Lung.* 2011;189(6):493–497.
19. Sparrow D, O'Connor GT, Rosner B, Segal MR, Weiss ST. The influence of age and level of pulmonary function on nonspecific airway responsiveness. The Normative Aging Study. *Am Rev Respir Dis.* 1991;143(5 Pt 1):978–982.
20. Suh DI, Choi SH, Lee JK, Kim JT, Koh YY. Relationships of methacholine and adenosine 5'-monophosphate (AMP) responsiveness to the postbronchodilator FEV(1)/FVC ratio in children with asthma. *J Asthma.* 2011;48(4):345–350.
21. Mosmann TR, Bond MW, Coffman RL, Ohara J, Paul WE. T-cell and mast cell lines respond to B-cell stimulatory factor 1. *Proc Natl Acad Sci U S A.* 1986;83(15):5654–5658.
22. Mosmann TR, Cherwinski H, Bond MW, Giedlin MA, Coffman RL. Two types of murine helper T cell clone. I.

Definition according to profiles of lymphokine activities and secreted proteins. *J Immunol.* 1986;136(7):2348–2357.

23. Mosmann TR, Coffman RL. TH1 and TH2 cells: different patterns of lymphokine secretion lead to different functional properties. *Annu Rev Immunol.* 1989;7:145–173.
24. Goldberg AL, Rock KL. Proteolysis, proteasomes and antigen presentation. *Nature.* 1992;357(6377):375–379.
25. Akdis CA, Akdis M. Mechanisms and treatment of allergic disease in the big picture of regulatory T cells. *J Allergy Clin Immunol.* 2009;123(4):735–746; quiz 747–738.
26. Jutel M, Akdis CA. T-cell subset regulation in atopy. *Curr Allergy Asthma Rep.* 2011;11(2):139–145.
27. Sakaguchi S. Regulatory T cells: key controllers of immunologic self-tolerance. *Cell.* 2000;101(5):455–458.
28. Baecher-Allan C, Brown JA, Freeman GJ, Hafler DA. CD4+CD25high regulatory cells in human peripheral blood. *J Immunol.* 2001;167(3):1245–1253.
29. Campbell DJ, Ziegler SF. FOXP3 modifies the phenotypic and functional properties of regulatory T cells. *Nat Rev Immunol.* 2007;7(4):305–310.
30. Xystrakis E, Boswell SE, Hawrylowicz CM. T regulatory cells and the control of allergic disease. *Expert Opin Biol Ther.* 2006;6(2):121–133.
31. Jutel M, Akdis CA. T-cell regulatory mechanisms in specific immunotherapy. *Chem Immunol Allergy.* 2008;94:158–177.
32. Meiler F, Klunker S, Zimmermann M, Akdis CA, Akdis M. Distinct regulation of IgE, IgG4 and IgA by T regulatory cells and toll-like receptors. *Allergy.* 2008;63(11):1455–1463.
33. Lloyd CM, Hawrylowicz CM. Regulatory T cells in asthma. *Immunity.* 2009;31(3):438–449.
34. Williams CM, Rahman S, Hubeau C, Ma HL. Cytokine pathways in allergic disease. *Toxicol Pathol.* 2012;40(2):205–215.
35. Wisniewski JA, Borish L. Novel cytokines and cytokine-producing T cells in allergic disorders. *Allergy Asthma Proc.* 2011;32(2):83–94.
36. Chen N, Field EH. Enhanced type 2 and diminished type 1 cytokines in neonatal tolerance. *Transplantation.* 1995;59(7):933–941.
37. Forsthuber T, Yip HC, Lehmann PV. Induction of TH1 and TH2 immunity in neonatal mice. *Science.* 1996;271(5256):1728–1730.
38. Powell TJ Jr, Streilein JW. Neonatal tolerance induction by class II alloantigens activates IL-4-secreting, tolerogen-responsive T cells. *J Immunol.* 1990;144(3):854–859.
39. Fadel SA, Ozaki DA, Sarzotti M. Enhanced type 1 immunity after secondary viral challenge in mice primed as neonates. *J Immunol.* 2002;169(6):3293–3300.
40. Jupelli M, Guentzel MN, Meier PA, Zhong G, Murthy AK, Arulanandam BP. Endogenous IFN-gamma production is induced and required for protective immunity against pulmonary chlamydial infection in neonatal mice. *J Immunol.* 2008;180(6):4148–4155.
41. Mor G, Yamshchikov G, Sedegah M, et al. Induction of neonatal tolerance by plasmid DNA vaccination of mice. *J Clin Invest.* 1996;98(12):2700–2705.
42. Sarzotti M, Robbins DS, Hoffman PM. Induction of protective CTL responses in newborn mice by a murine retrovirus. *Science.* 1996;271(5256):1726–1728.
43. Diesner SC, Forster-Waldl E, Olivera A, Pollak A, Jensen-Jarolim E, Untersmayr E. Perspectives on immunomodulation early in life. *Pediatr Allergy Immunol.* 2012;23(3):210–223.
44. Zaghouani H, Hoeman CM, Adkins B. Neonatal immunity: faulty T-helpers and the shortcomings of dendritic cells. *Trends Immunol.* 2009;30(12):585–591.
45. Martinez FD, Wright AL, Taussig LM, Holberg CJ, Halonen M, Morgan WJ. Asthma and wheezing in the first six years of life. The Group Health Medical Associates. *New Engl J Med.* 1995;332(3):133–138.
46. Taussig LM, Wright AL, Holberg CJ, Halonen M, Morgan WJ, Martinez FD. Tucson Children's Respiratory Study: 1980 to present. *J Allergy Clin Immunol.* 2003;111(4):661–675; quiz 676.
47. Ball TM, Castro-Rodriguez JA, Griffith KA, Holberg CJ, Martinez FD, Wright AL. Siblings, day-care attendance, and the risk of asthma and wheezing during childhood. *N Engl J Med.* 2000;343(8):538–543.
48. Celedon JC, Wright RJ, Litonjua AA, et al. Day care attendance in early life, maternal history of asthma, and asthma at the age of 6 years. *Am J Respir Crit Care Med.* 2003;167(9):1239–1243.
49. Midodzi WK, Rowe BH, Majaesic CM, Saunders LD, Senthilselvan A. Early life factors associated with incidence of physician-diagnosed asthma in preschool children: results from the Canadian Early Childhood Development cohort study. *J Asthma.* 2010;47(1):7–13.
50. Nicolaou NC, Simpson A, Lowe LA, Murray CS, Woodcock A, Custovic A. Day-care attendance, position in sibship, and early childhood wheezing: a population-based birth cohort study. *J Allergy Clin Immunol.* 2008;122(3):500–506. e505.
51. Caudri D, Wijga A, Scholtens S, et al. Early daycare is associated with an increase in airway symptoms in early childhood but is no protection against asthma or atopy at 8 years. *Am J Respir Crit Care Med.* 2009;180(6):491–498.
52. Hagerhed-Engman L, Bornehag CG, Sundell J, Aberg N. Day-care attendance and increased risk for respiratory and allergic symptoms in preschool age. *Allergy.* 2006;61(4):447–453.
53. Nafstad P, Brunekreef B, Skrondal A, Nystad W. Early respiratory infections, asthma, and allergy: 10-year follow-up of the Oslo Birth Cohort. *Pediatrics.* 2005;116(2):e255–e262.
54. Svanes C, Jarvis D, Chinn S, Omenaas E, Gulsvik A, Burney P. Early exposure to children in family and day care as related to adult asthma and hay fever: results from the European Community Respiratory Health Survey. *Thorax.* 2002;57(11):945–950.
55. Pearce N, Pekkanen J, Beasley R. How much asthma is really attributable to atopy? *Thorax.* 1999;54(3):268–272.
56. Ronchetti R, Rennerova Z, Barreto M, Villa MP. The prevalence of atopy in asthmatic children correlates strictly with the prevalence of atopy among nonasthmatic children. *Int Arch Allergy Immunol.* 2007;142(1):79–85.
57. Ronchetti R, Jesenak M, Rennerova Z, Barreto M, Ronchetti F, Villa MP. Relationship between atopic asthma and the population prevalence rates for asthma or atopy in children: atopic and nonatopic asthma in epidemiology. *Allergy Asthma Proc.* 2009;30(1):55–63.
58. Haldar P, Pavord ID, Shaw DE, et al. Cluster analysis and clinical asthma phenotypes. *Am J Respir Crit Care Med.* 2008;178(3):218–224.
59. Moore WC, Meyers DA, Wenzel SE, et al. Identification of asthma phenotypes using cluster analysis in the Severe Asthma Research Program. *Am J Respir Crit Care Med.* 2010;181(4):315–323.
60. Fernandez C, Cardenas R, Martin D, et al. Analysis of skin testing and serum-specific immunoglobulin E to predict airway reactivity to cat allergens. *Clin Exp Allergy.* 2007;37(3):391–399.

61. Langley SJ, Goldthorpe S, Craven M, Morris J, Woodcock A, Custovic A. Exposure and sensitization to indoor allergens: association with lung function, bronchial reactivity, and exhaled nitric oxide measures in asthma. *J Allergy Clin Immunol*. 2003;112(2):362–368.

62. Kuhl K, Hanania NA. Targeting IgE in asthma. *Curr Opin Pulm Med*. 2012;18(1):1–5.

63. Tan R, Corren J. Omalizumab in the treatment of asthma. *Expert Rev Respir Med*. 2011;5(6):747–756.

64. Walker S, Burch J, McKenna C, Wright K, Griffin S, Woolacott N. Omalizumab for the treatment of severe persistent allergic asthma in children aged 6–11 years. *Health Technol Assess*. 2011;15(Suppl 1):13–21.

65. Sporik R, Holgate ST, Platts-Mills TA, Cogswell JJ. Exposure to house-dust mite allergen (Der p I) and the development of asthma in childhood. A prospective study. *N Engl J Med*. 1990;323(8):502–507.

66. Celedon JC, Milton DK, Ramsey CD, et al. Exposure to dust mite allergen and endotoxin in early life and asthma and atopy in childhood. *J Allergy Clin Immunol*. 2007;120(1):144–149.

67. Lau S, Illi S, Sommerfeld C, et al. Early exposure to house-dust mite and cat allergens and development of childhood asthma: a cohort study. Multicentre Allergy Study Group. *Lancet*. 2000;356(9239):1392–1397.

68. Cole Johnson C, Ownby DR, Havstad SL, Peterson EL. Family history, dust mite exposure in early childhood, and risk for pediatric atopy and asthma. *J Allergy Clin Immunol*. 2004;114(1):105–110.

69. Van Eerdewegh P, Little RD, Dupuis J, et al. Association of the ADAM33 gene with asthma and bronchial hyperresponsiveness. *Nature*. 2002;418(6896):426–430.

70. Allen M, Heinzmann A, Noguchi E, et al. Positional cloning of a novel gene influencing asthma from chromosome 2q14. *Nat Genet*. 2003;35(3):258–263.

71. Zhang Y, Leaves NI, Anderson GG, et al. Positional cloning of a quantitative trait locus on chromosome 13q14 that influences immunoglobulin E levels and asthma. *Nat Genet*. 2003;34(2):181–186.

72. Laitinen T, Polvi A, Rydman P, et al. Characterization of a common susceptibility locus for asthma-related traits. *Science*. 2004;304(5668):300–304.

73. Nicolae D, Cox NJ, Lester LA, et al. Fine mapping and positional candidate studies identify HLA-G as an asthma susceptibility gene on chromosome 6p21. *Am J Hum Genet*. 2005;76(2):349–357.

74. Moffatt MF, Kabesch M, Liang L, et al. Genetic variants regulating ORMDL3 expression contribute to the risk of childhood asthma. *Nature*. 2007;448(7152):470–473.

75. Moffatt MF, Gut IG, Demenais F, et al. A large-scale, consortium-based genomewide association study of asthma. *N Engl J Med*. 2010;363(13):1211–1221.

76. Torgerson DG, Ampleford EJ, Chiu GY, et al. Meta-analysis of genome-wide association studies of asthma in ethnically diverse North American populations. *Nat Genet*. 2011;43(9):887–892.

77. Jaakkola JJ, Ahmed P, Ieromnimon A, et al. Preterm delivery and asthma: a systematic review and meta-analysis. *J Allergy Clin Immunol*. 2006;118(4):823–830.

78. Trembath A, Laughon MM. Predictors of bronchopulmonary dysplasia. *Clin Perinatol*. 2012;39(3):585–601.

79. Gold DR, Burge HA, Carey V, Milton DK, Platts-Mills T, Weiss ST. Predictors of repeated wheeze in the first year of life: the relative roles of cockroach, birth weight, acute lower respiratory illness, and maternal smoking. *Am J Respir Crit Care Med*. 1999;160(1):227–236.

80. Raby BA, Celedon JC, Litonjua AA, et al. Low-normal gestational age as a predictor of asthma at 6 years of age. *Pediatrics*. 2004;114(3):e327–e332.

81. Caudri D, Wijga A, Gehring U, et al. Respiratory symptoms in the first 7 years of life and birth weight at term: the PIAMA Birth Cohort. *Am J Respir Crit Care Med*. 2007;175(10):1078–1085.

82. Edwards CA, Osman LM, Godden DJ, Campbell DM, Douglas JG. Relationship between birth weight and adult lung function: controlling for maternal factors. *Thorax*. 2003;58(12): 1061–1065.

83. Brew BK, Allen CW, Toelle BG, Marks GB. Systematic review and meta-analysis investigating breast feeding and childhood wheezing illness. *Paediatr Perinat Epidemiol*. 2011;25(6):507–518.

84. Matheson MC, Allen KJ, Tang ML. Understanding the evidence for and against the role of breastfeeding in allergy prevention. *Clin Exp Allergy*. 2012;42(6):827–851.

85. Barouki R, Gluckman PD, Grandjean P, Hanson M, Heindel JJ. Developmental origins of non-communicable disease: implications for research and public health. *Environ Health*. 2012;11:42.

86. Willett W. Food frequency methods. In: Willett W, ed. *Nutritional Epidemiology*. 2nd ed. New York, NY: Oxford University Press; 1998.

87. Nurmatov U, Devereux G, Sheikh A. Nutrients and foods for the primary prevention of asthma and allergy: systematic review and meta-analysis. *J Allergy Clin Immunol*. 2011;127(3):724–733. e1–e30.

88. Rappaport BZ, Reed CI, Hathaway ML, Struck HC. The treatment of hay fever and asthma with viosterol of high potency. *J Allergy*. 1934;5(6):541–553.

89. Wjst M, Dold S. Genes, factor X, and allergens: what causes allergic diseases? *Allergy*. 1999;54(7):757–759.

90. Ginde AA, Liu MC, Camargo CA Jr. Demographic differences and trends of vitamin D insufficiency in the US population, 1988–2004. *Arch Intern Med*. 2009;169(6):626–632.

91. Litonjua AA, Weiss ST. Is vitamin D deficiency to blame for the asthma epidemic? *J Allergy Clin Immunol*. 2007;120(5): 1031–1035.

92. Camargo CA Jr, Rifas-Shiman SL, Litonjua AA, et al. Maternal intake of vitamin D during pregnancy and risk of recurrent wheeze in children at age 3 years. *Am J Clin Nutr*. 2007;85: 788–795.

93. Devereux G, Litonjua AA, Turner S, et al. Maternal vitamin D intake during pregnancy and early childhood wheezing. *Am J Clin Nutr*. 2007;85:853–859.

94. Erkkola M, Kaila M, Nwaru BI, et al. Maternal vitamin D intake during pregnancy is inversely associated with asthma and allergic rhinitis in 5-year-old children. *Clin Exp Allergy*. 2009;39(6):875–882.

95. Miyake Y, Sasaki S, Tanaka K, Hirota Y. Dairy food, calcium and vitamin D intake in pregnancy, and wheeze and eczema in infants. *Eur Respir J*. 2010;35(6):1228–1234.

96. Camargo CA Jr, Ingham T, Wickens K, et al. Cord-blood 25-hydroxyvitamin D levels and risk of respiratory infection, wheezing, and asthma. *Pediatrics*. 2011;127(1):e180–e187.

97. Gale CR, Robinson SM, Harvey NC, et al. Maternal vitamin D status during pregnancy and child outcomes. *Eur J Clin Nutr*. 2008;62(1):68–77.

98. Morales E, Romieu I, Guerra S, et al. Maternal vitamin D status in pregnancy and risk of lower respiratory tract infections, wheezing, and asthma in offspring. *Epidemiology*. 2012;23(1):64–71.
99. Rothers J, Wright AL, Stern DA, Halonen M, Camargo CA Jr. Cord blood 25-hydroxyvitamin D levels are associated with aeroallergen sensitization in children from Tucson, Arizona. *J Allergy Clin Immunol*. 2011;128(5):1093–1099. e1–e5.
100. Chinellato I, Piazza M, Sandri M, et al. Serum vitamin D levels and exercise-induced bronchoconstriction in children with asthma. *Eur Respir J*. 2011;37(6):1366–1370.
101. Li F, Peng M, Jiang L, et al. Vitamin D deficiency is associated with decreased lung function in Chinese adults with asthma. *Respiration*. 2011;81(6):469–475.
102. Brehm JM, Acosta-Perez E, Klei L, et al. Vitamin D insufficiency and severe asthma exacerbations in Puerto Rican children. *Am J Respir Crit Care Med*. 2012;186(2):140–146.
103. Brehm JM, Schuemann B, Fuhlbrigge AL, et al. Serum vitamin D levels and severe asthma exacerbations in the Childhood Asthma Management Program study. *J Allergy Clin Immunol*. 2010;126(1):52–58. e5.
104. Brehm JM, Celedon JC, Soto-Quiros ME, et al. Serum vitamin D levels and markers of severity of childhood asthma in Costa Rica. *Am J Respir Crit Care Med*. 2009;179(9):765–771.
105. Phipatanakul W, Celedon JC, Hoffman EB, Abdulkerim H, Ryan LM, Gold DR. Mouse allergen exposure, wheeze and atopy in the first seven years of life. *Allergy*. 2008;63(11):1512–1518.
106. Rosenstreich DL, Eggleston P, Kattan M, et al. The role of cockroach allergy and exposure to cockroach allergen in causing morbidity among inner-city children with asthma. *N Engl J Med*. 1997;336(19):1356–1363.
107. Celedon JC, Litonjua AA, Ryan L, Platts-Mills T, Weiss ST, Gold DR. Exposure to cat allergen, maternal history of asthma, and wheezing in first 5 years of life. *Lancet*. 2002;360(9335):781–782.
108. Litonjua AA, Milton DK, Celedon JC, Ryan L, Weiss ST, Gold DR. A longitudinal analysis of wheezing in young children: the independent effects of early life exposure to house dust endotoxin, allergens, and pets. *J Allergy Clin Immunol*. 2002;110(5):736–742.
109. Remes ST, Castro-Rodriguez JA, Holberg CJ, Martinez FD, Wright AL. Dog exposure in infancy decreases the subsequent risk of frequent wheeze but not of atopy. *J Allergy Clin Immunol*. 2001;108(4):509–515.
110. Lodrup Carlsen KC, Roll S, Carlsen KH, et al. Does pet ownership in infancy lead to asthma or allergy at school age? Pooled analysis of individual participant data from 11 European birth cohorts. *PLoS One*. 2012;7(8):e43214.
111. Permaul P, Hoffman E, Fu C, et al. Allergens in urban schools and homes of children with asthma. *Pediatr Allergy Immunol*. 2012;23(6):543–549.
112. Abramson SL, Turner-Henson A, Anderson L, et al. Allergens in school settings: results of environmental assessments in 3 city school systems. *J Sch Health*. 2006;76(6):246–249.
113. Tranter DC, Wobbema AT, Norlien K, Dorschner DF. Indoor allergens in Minnesota schools and child care centers. *J Occup Environ Hyg*. 2009;6(9):582–591.
114. Custovic A, Simpson A. The role of inhalant allergens in allergic airways disease. *J Investig Allergol Clin Immunol*. 2012;22(6):393–401; quiz follow 401.
115. Fernandez-Caldas E. Dust mite allergens: mitigation and control. *Curr Allergy Asthma Rep*. 2002;2(5):424–431.
116. Halken S, Host A, Niklassen U, et al. Effect of mattress and pillow encasings on children with asthma and house dust mite allergy. *J Allergy Clin Immunol*. 2003;111(1):169–176.
117. Horak F Jr, Matthews S, Ihorst G, et al. Effect of mite-impermeable mattress encasings and an educational package on the development of allergies in a multinational randomized, controlled birth-cohort study – 24 months results of the Study of Prevention of Allergy in Children in Europe. *Clin Exp Allergy*. 2004;34(8):1220–1225.
118. Gotzsche PC, Johansen HK. House dust mite control measures for asthma: systematic review. *Allergy*. 2008;63(6):646–659.
119. Klinnert MD, Liu AH, Pearson MR, et al. Outcome of a randomized multifaceted intervention with low-income families of wheezing infants. *Arch Pediatr Adolesc Med*. 2007;161(8):783–790.
120. Maas T, Dompeling E, Muris JW, Wesseling G, Knottnerus JA, van Schayck OC. Prevention of asthma in genetically susceptible children: a multifaceted intervention trial focussed on feasibility in general practice. *Pediatr Allergy Immunol*. 2011;22(8):794–802.
121. Maas T, Kaper J, Sheikh A, et al. Mono and multifaceted inhalant and/or food allergen reduction interventions for preventing asthma in children at high risk of developing asthma. *Cochrane Database Syst Rev*. 2009(3):CD006480.
122. Scott M, Roberts G, Kurukulaaratchy RJ, Matthews S, Nove A, Arshad SH. Multifaceted allergen avoidance during infancy reduces asthma during childhood with the effect persisting until age 18 years. *Thorax*. 2012;67(12):1046–1051.
123. Morgan WJ, Crain EF, Gruchalla RS, et al. Results of a home-based environmental intervention among urban children with asthma. *N Engl J Med*. 2004;351(11):1068–1080.
124. Litonjua AA, Carey VJ, Burge HA, Weiss ST, Gold DR. Exposure to cockroach allergen in the home is associated with incident doctor-diagnosed asthma and recurrent wheezing. *J Allergy Clin Immunol*. 2001;107(1):41–47.
125. Eggleston PA, Wood RA, Rand C, Nixon WJ, Chen PH, Lukk P. Removal of cockroach allergen from inner-city homes. *J Allergy Clin Immunol*. 1999;104(4 Pt 1):842–846.
126. Gergen PJ, Mortimer KM, Eggleston PA, et al. Results of the National Cooperative Inner-City Asthma Study (NCICAS) environmental intervention to reduce cockroach allergen exposure in inner-city homes. *J Allergy Clin Immunol*. 1999;103(3 Pt 1):501–506.
127. Sever ML, Arbes SJ Jr, Gore JC, et al. Cockroach allergen reduction by cockroach control alone in low-income urban homes: a randomized control trial. *J Allergy Clin Immunol*. 2007;120(4):849–855.
128. Quansah R, Jaakkola MS, Hugg TT, Heikkinen SA, Jaakkola JJ. Residential dampness and molds and the risk of developing asthma: a systematic review and meta-analysis. *PLoS One*. 2012;7(11):e47526.
129. Gent JF, Kezik JM, Hill ME, Tsai E, Li DW, Leaderer BP. Household mold and dust allergens: exposure, sensitization and childhood asthma morbidity. *Environ Res*. 2012;118:86–93.
130. Salo PM, Sever ML, Zeldin DC. Indoor allergens in school and day care environments. *J Allergy Clin Immunol*. 2009;124(2):185–192, 192 e181–e189; quiz 193–184.
131. Canova C, Heinrich J, Anto JM, et al. The influence of sensitisation to pollens and moulds on seasonal variations in asthma attacks. *Eur Respir J*. 2013;42(4):935–945.

132. Burney PG, Newson RB, Burrows MS, Wheeler DM. The effects of allergens in outdoor air on both atopic and nonatopic subjects with airway disease. *Allergy.* 2008;63(5):542–546.

133. Burke H, Leonardi-Bee J, Hashim A, et al. Prenatal and passive smoke exposure and incidence of asthma and wheeze: systematic review and meta-analysis. *Pediatrics.* 2012;129(4):735–744.

134. Neuman A, Hohmann C, Orsini N, et al. Maternal smoking in pregnancy and asthma in preschool children: a pooled analysis of eight birth cohorts. *Am J Respir Crit Care Med.* 2012; 186(10):1037–1043.

135. Gold DR. Environmental tobacco smoke, indoor allergens, and childhood asthma. *Environ Health Perspect.* 2000;108(Suppl 4): 643–651.

136. Wilson SR, Yamada EG, Sudhakar R, et al. A controlled trial of an environmental tobacco smoke reduction intervention in low-income children with asthma. *Chest.* 2001;120(5):1709–1722.

137. Wilson SR, Farber HJ, Knowles SB, Lavori PW. A randomized trial of parental behavioral counseling and cotinine feedback for lowering environmental tobacco smoke exposure in children with asthma: results of the LET'S Manage Asthma trial. *Chest.* 2011;139(3):581–590.

138. Weiss ST, Utell MJ, Samet JM. Environmental tobacco smoke exposure and asthma in adults. *Environ Health Perspect.* 1999; 107(Suppl 6):891–895.

139. James AL, Palmer LJ, Kicic E, et al. Decline in lung function in the Busselton Health Study: the effects of asthma and cigarette smoking. *Am J Respir Crit Care Med.* 2005;171(2):109–114.

140. Lange P, Parner J, Vestbo J, Schnohr P, Jensen G. A 15-year follow-up study of ventilatory function in adults with asthma. *N Engl J Med.* 1998;339(17):1194–1200.

141. Gowers AM, Cullinan P, Ayres JG, et al. Does outdoor air pollution induce new cases of asthma? Biological plausibility and evidence; a review. *Respirology.* 2012;17(6):887–898.

142. Jacquemin B, Schikowski T, Carsin AE, et al. The role of air pollution in adult-onset asthma: a review of the current evidence. *Semin Respir Crit Care Med.* 2012;33(6):606–619.

143. Brauer M. How much, how long, what, and where: air pollution exposure assessment for epidemiologic studies of respiratory disease. *Proc Am Thorac Soc.* 2010;7(2):111–115.

144. Breysse PN, Diette GB, Matsui EC, Butz AM, Hansel NN, McCormack MC. Indoor air pollution and asthma in children. *Proc Am Thorac Soc.* 2010;7(2):102–106.

145. Hulin M, Simoni M, Viegi G, Annesi-Maesano I. Respiratory health and indoor air pollutants based on quantitative exposure assessments. *Eur Respir J.* 2012;40(4):1033–1045.

146. Institute of Medicine. *Unequal Treatment: Confronting Racial and Ethnic Disparities in Health Care.* Washington, DC: National Academy Press; 2002.

147. Forno E, Celedon JC. Asthma and ethnic minorities: socioeconomic status and beyond. *Curr Opin Allergy Clin Immunol.* 2009;9(2):154–160.

148. Wright RJ. Epidemiology of stress and asthma: from constricting communities and fragile families to epigenetics. *Immunol Allergy Clin North Am.* 2011;31(1):19–39.

149. Yonas MA, Lange NE, Celedon JC. Psychosocial stress and asthma morbidity. *Curr Opin Allergy Clin Immunol.* 2012;12 (2):202–210.

150. Litonjua AA, Celedon JC, Hausmann J, et al. Variation in total and specific IgE: effects of ethnicity and socioeconomic status. *J Allergy Clin Immunol.* 2005;115(4):751–757.

151. Armstrong K, Putt M, Halbert CH, et al. Prior experiences of racial discrimination and racial differences in health care system distrust. *Med Care.* 2013;51(2):144–150.

152. Shoff C, Yang TC. Untangling the associations among distrust, race, and neighborhood social environment: a social disorganization perspective. *Soc Sci Med.* 2012;74(9):1342–1352.

153. Apter AJ, Boston RC, George M, et al. Modifiable barriers to adherence to inhaled steroids among adults with asthma: it's not just black and white. *J Allergy Clin Immunol.* 2003;111(6):1219–1226.

154. Shore SA. Obesity and asthma: possible mechanisms. *J Allergy Clin Immunol.* 2008;121(5):1087–1093; quiz 1094–1085.

155. Farah CS, Salome CM. Asthma and obesity: a known association but unknown mechanism. *Respirology.* 2012;17(3): 412–421.

156. Jensen ME, Wood LG, Gibson PG. Obesity and childhood asthma—mechanisms and manifestations. *Curr Opin Allergy Clin Immunol.* 2012;12(2):186–192.

157. Litonjua AA, Gold DR. Asthma and obesity: common early-life influences in the inception of disease. *J Allergy Clin Immunol.* 2008;121(5):1075–1084; quiz 1085–1076.

158. Micheli L, Cerretani D, Fiaschi AI, Giorgi G, Romeo MR, Runci FM. Effect of acetaminophen on glutathione levels in rat testis and lung. *Environ Health Perspect.* 1994;102(Suppl 9):63–64.

159. McKeever TM, Lewis SA, Smit HA, Burney P, Britton JR, Cassano PA. The association of acetaminophen, aspirin, and ibuprofen with respiratory disease and lung function. *Am J Respir Crit Care Med.* 2005;171(9):966–971.

160. Shaheen S, Potts J, Gnatiuc L, et al. The relation between paracetamol use and asthma: a GA2LEN European case-control study. *Eur Respir J.* 2008;32(5):1231–1236.

161. Shaheen SO, Newson RB, Sherriff A, et al. Paracetamol use in pregnancy and wheezing in early childhood. *Thorax.* 2002;57(11):958–963.

162. Shaheen SO, Sterne JA, Songhurst CE, Burney PG. Frequent paracetamol use and asthma in adults. *Thorax.* 2000;55(4): 266–270.

163. Lowe AJ, Carlin JB, Bennett CM, et al. Paracetamol use in early life and asthma: prospective birth cohort study. *BMJ.* 2010;341:c4616.

164. Busse WW, Lemanske RF Jr, Gern JE. Role of viral respiratory infections in asthma and asthma exacerbations. *Lancet.* 2010;376(9743):826–834.

165. Holt PG, Strickland DH, Sly PD. Virus infection and allergy in the development of asthma: what is the connection? *Curr Opin Allergy Clin Immunol.* 2012;12(2):151–157.

166. Miller EK, Lu X, Erdman DD, et al. Rhinovirus-associated hospitalizations in young children. *J Infect Dis.* 2007;195(6): 773–781.

167. Jackson DJ, Gangnon RE, Evans MD, et al. Wheezing rhinovirus illnesses in early life predict asthma development in high-risk children. *Am J Respir Crit Care Med.* 2008;178(7):667–672.

168. Kusel MM, de Klerk NH, Kebadze T, et al. Early-life respiratory viral infections, atopic sensitization, and risk of subsequent development of persistent asthma. *J Allergy Clin Immunol.* 2007;119(5):1105–1110.

169. Corne JM, Marshall C, Smith S, et al. Frequency, severity, and duration of rhinovirus infections in asthmatic and non-asthmatic individuals: a longitudinal cohort study. *Lancet.* 2002;359(9309): 831–834.

170. Dawood FS, Kamimoto L, D'Mello TA, et al. Children with asthma hospitalized with seasonal or pandemic influenza, 2003–2009. *Pediatrics.* 2011;128(1):e27–e32.

171. Miller EK, Griffin MR, Edwards KM, et al. Influenza burden for children with asthma. *Pediatrics.* 2008;121(1):1–8.

172. Papadopoulos NG, Christodoulou I, Rohde G, et al. Viruses and bacteria in acute asthma exacerbations–a GA(2) LEN-DARE systematic review. *Allergy.* 2011;66(4):458–468.

173. Cheung D, Dick EC, Timmers MC, de Klerk EP, Spaan WJ, Sterk PJ. Rhinovirus inhalation causes long-lasting excessive airway narrowing in response to methacholine in asthmatic subjects in vivo. *Am J Respir Crit Care Med.* 1995;152(5 Pt 1):1490–1496.

174. Gern JE, Calhoun W, Swenson C, Shen G, Busse WW. Rhinovirus infection preferentially increases lower airway responsiveness in allergic subjects. *Am J Respir Crit Care Med.* 1997;155(6):1872–1876.

175. Xepapadaki P, Papadopoulos NG, Bossios A, Manoussakis E, Manousakas T, Saxoni-Papageorgiou P. Duration of postviral airway hyperresponsiveness in children with asthma: effect of atopy. *J Allergy Clin Immunol.* 2005;116(2):299–304.

176. Weiss ST, Tosteson TD, Segal MR, Tager IB, Redline S, Speizer FE. Effects of asthma on pulmonary function in children. A longitudinal population-based study. *Am Rev Respir Dis.* 1992;145(1):58–64.

177. Strunk RC, Weiss ST, Yates KP, Tonascia J, Zeiger RS, Szefler SJ. Mild to moderate asthma affects lung growth in children and adolescents. *J Allergy Clin Immunol.* 2006;118(5):1040–1047.

178. Grad R, Morgan WJ. Long-term outcomes of early-onset wheeze and asthma. *J Allergy Clin Immunol.* 2012;130(2):299–307.

179. Peat JK, Woolcock AJ, Cullen K. Rate of decline of lung function in subjects with asthma. *Eur J Respir Dis.* 1987;70(3):171–179.

180. Ulrik CS, Lange P. Decline of lung function in adults with bronchial asthma. *Am J Respir Crit Care Med.* 1994;150(3):629–634.

181. Kelly WJ, Hudson I, Raven J, Phelan PD, Pain MC, Olinsky A. Childhood asthma and adult lung function. *Am Rev Respir Dis.* 1988;138(1):26–30.

CHAPTER 46

Asthma: Clinical Presentation and Management

Omar S. Usmani

Peter J. Barnes

ASTHMA—A HETEROGENEOUS DISEASE

Asthma is a chronic inflammatory disorder of the airways characterized by marked variability in airflow obstruction that is often reversible, either spontaneously or with treatment.[1] This inflammation presents clinically in susceptible patients with recurrent symptoms of wheezing, chest tightness, cough, and, occasionally, dyspnea and contributes to the heightened airway hyperresponsiveness to specific and nonspecific stimuli; a pathognomonic feature of asthma. Increased airway hyperresponsiveness manifests in patients as intolerance to smoke, dust, air pollution, and strong odors, where exposure to such agents in healthy individuals does not induce such symptoms. Asthma is not a single disease entity with a unique pathogenesis, but rather recognized to be a clinical syndrome and heterogeneous disease;[2] that is, asthma comprises multiple endotypes that manifest common symptoms, but have distinct and probably different pathophysiologic and etiologic mechanisms with an interplay between genetic and environmental factors. This phenotypic heterogeneity in the expression of asthma is multidimensional and includes variability in pathologic, clinical, and physiologic parameters among different patients.[3]

RISK FACTORS FOR ASTHMA

Several risk factors for asthma are considered below.

■ ATOPY AND ALLERGENS

The most important factor predisposing to asthma is atopy (Table 46-1). Asthma has been classified as *atopic* (extrinsic) *or nonatopic* (intrinsic) depending on the suspected role of allergens as etiologic factors. Atopic asthma involves an exaggerated immune response characterized by immunoglobulin E (Ig-E) activation and mast cell degradation. Atopy can be clinically elicited with a positive skin prick test or specific antibodies to IgE in serum against common aeroallergens such as house dust mite, grass and tree pollens, cat and dog fur, rodents (in laboratory workers), and cockroaches (in inner city populations). House dust mite is recognized as a significant cause of asthma throughout the developed world, although the relative importance of different indoor allergens may vary among populations. Patients with atopic asthma commonly suffer

TABLE 46-1 Risk Factors and Triggers Involved in Asthma

Endogenous Factors	Environmental Factors	Triggers
Atopy	Allergens–indoor	Allergens (especially house dust mite, animal dander, cockroach, indoor fungi, perennial allergens, and seasonal pollens)
Airway hyperresponsiveness	Allergens–outdoor (fungi, pollens)	Changes in the weather (cold air, thunderstorms)
Ethnicity	Obesity	Drugs (angiotensin-converting enzyme inhibitors, aspirin, β-blockers, NSAIDs)
Gender	Occupational sensitizers	Exercise and hyperventilation
Genetic predisposition	Parasitic infections	Extreme emotional expression (laughing, stress)
	Respiratory infections (early childhood, viral)	Irritants (household sprays, paint fumes)
	Socioeconomic status	Respiratory infections
	Tobacco smoking (active and passive)	Sulfur dioxide and pollutant gases
		Tobacco smoking

from other atopic diseases, including allergic rhinitis that may be seasonal (hayfever), and may be found in over 80% of asthmatic patients; allergic conjunctivitis; and atopic dermatitis (eczema). Nonatopic asthmatic patients (approximately 10%) have a negative skin prick test, normal serum IgE concentrations, and usually show later onset of disease (adult-onset asthma). In this group, their asthma is more severe, persistent, there is more sensitivity to aspirin and commonly they have concomitant nasal polyps. This classification, although appropriate from a pathologic perspective, does not readily help clinicians as it does not aid in establishing an etiologic diagnosis nor does it help in defining treatment strategies.[4] There is a high prevalence of atopy among nonasthmatics and a large percentage of skin prick sensitive persons report no allergic symptoms. Around 50% of asthma can be attributed to atopy in the developed world and the prevalence of atopy among asthmatics is mainly determined by the general prevalence of atopy in the population.[5,6] In addition, the immunopathology in bronchial biopsies and sputum in patients with nonatopic asthma appear to be identical to that found in atopic asthmatic patients. Therefore, the finding that an asthmatic is atopic does not imply that the disease is allergic in nature or, that atopy is causing asthma. Moreover, respiratory tract viruses have emerged as the most frequent triggers for exacerbations in both children and adults and may play a more prominent role than allergens as triggers of acute exacerbations in most patients.[7] House dust mites are the most common indoor allergen, where particles excreted from the digestive tract contain the principal allergen *Dermatophagoides pteronyssinus*. Other main sources of inhaled indoor allergen are cat and dog fur, and cockroaches (Table 46-1). Although asthmatic symptoms often improve when the allergen is removed, rigorous allergen avoidance has not shown any evidence for a reduced risk of developing asthma.

Although allergens are often triggers of acute exacerbations of asthma, allergens themselves may induce subclinical airway inflammation that may lead to enhanced airway responsiveness and greater susceptibility to the provocative effects of other triggers such as respiratory viral infections and exercise. In this regard, it is important to understand the distinction between triggers and etiologic risk factors. A trigger is any agent capable of inducing or exacerbating asthma and whereas triggers may lead to symptoms, they do so only in susceptible persons who already possess the underlying asthmatic diathesis.

VIRAL INFECTIONS

Acute upper respiratory tract viral infections are the commonest triggers of exacerbations of asthma and most are due to rhinovirus infections. Viral infections not only give symptoms of the common cold and cause acute inflammatory rhinitis, but may also play a role in asthma development and potentially, airway remodeling through increasing inflammation in the lower airways.[8] Asthma is recognized to be more common in children who have had croup or lower respiratory tract infections in early life, although viral infections in the absence of atopy do not appear to be risk factors for the development of asthma.[9] Other viruses commonly implicated in acute exacerbations of asthma are respiratory syncytial virus, influenza virus, and parainfluenza virus. Bacterial infection with species of *Mycoplasma* and *Chlamydia* are also associated with exacerbations of asthma, whereas other bacterial infections are not.

OCCUPATIONAL EXPOSURE

Occupational asthma accounts for approximately 5% of all adult cases of asthma, and the disease can often be classified according to its etiology. In these circumstances, not only is the specific agent that triggers the symptoms known, but the same agent is usually the underlying cause of asthma.

EXERCISE-INDUCED ASTHMA

Many asthma patients have worsening of symptoms on or after physical exercise and another category of asthma is exercise-induced, where exercise per se is not the cause of, but rather one of many nonimmunologic triggers that produce symptoms in patients who already have the disease. In this condition, the trigger is thought to be the drying of the airway mucosa as a result of hyperventilation that leads to osmotically induced mast cell mediator release and bronchospasm.

OBESITY

Obesity is a major risk factor for asthma where abdominal obesity (waist circumference) and general obesity (BMI) both show a strong correlation with the risk of new-onset asthma.[10]

DRUGS

Drugs that may worsen asthma control include β-blockers, occasionally angiotensin-converting enzyme (ACE) inhibitors, aspirin, and nonsteroidal anti-inflammatory drugs (NSAIDs).

CLINICAL PRESENTATION AND DIAGNOSIS

Asthma is a clinical diagnosis made on the basis of a medical history of typical symptoms, consideration to provocative factors, and supported with objective confirmation of variable airflow obstruction. As the disease is heterogeneous in its presentation and severity, the clinical features of asthma show great variability both between individual asthmatics, and also within the same patient over time. It is also important to recognize that asthma is often associated with different comorbidities including allergic rhinitis, atopic dermatitis, rhinosinusitis, gastroesophageal reflux disease, diabetes, depression, obesity, all of which may affect the clinical expression and severity of the disease.[11] The following clinical features and laboratory assessments are important in the consideration of the diagnosis of asthma.

MEDICAL HISTORY

The typical symptoms of asthma are paroxysmal wheezing, cough, breathlessness, and chest tightness, which may temporally be related to exposure to triggers or exercise. Cough may be productive of clear or yellow/green discolored sputum, where the latter may be tenacious and difficult to expectorate and reflect the underlying airway inflammation rather than a respiratory infection. Indeed, cough may be present in isolation to other symptoms and as the sole manifestation of an episode of asthma.[12] Breathlessness may occur as a result of the dynamic lung hyperinflation that accompanies acute asthma episodes and patients may report the sensation of difficulty in "getting air in" their lungs. Exertional symptoms may not be apparent if the patient's ability to exert themselves is limited by other health conditions such as rheumatologic or cardiac disease and, therefore, asthma may be underdiagnosed in the elderly. No single symptom is specific or more significant for asthma, although wheezing is a useful sign, as nonasthmatics rarely report frequent wheezing. In younger patients, the symptom of chest tightness is helpful, since it occurs more often in association with asthma than with other pulmonary or cardiac disorders. The pattern of symptom occurrence, the precipitating or aggravating factors, and the profile of a typical exacerbation are important elements in the clinical evaluation.

In patients with poorly controlled asthma, symptoms may temporally evolve slowly over days or weeks, or present abruptly. The severity and frequency with which symptoms occur varies greatly within the asthmatic population. The recurrent paroxysmal nature of symptom presentation is characteristic of asthma and symptoms improve, sometimes rather spontaneously, although usually with treatment. Nocturnal episodes are common in adult asthmatics and typically patients awake in the early hours of the morning with symptoms.

Distinguishing whether nocturnal symptoms are due to asthma, angina, or gastroesophageal reflux may be difficult, but early-morning asthma symptoms are usually relieved with administration of inhaled bronchodilators, in contrast to cardiovascular symptoms which occur at any time during the night and, gastroesophageal reflux which tends to usually cause symptoms soon after the patient reclines at night.

Chest symptoms that vary by season and are accompanied by symptoms of irritation of other mucus membranes, such as conjunctivitis and rhinitis, are typical of allergic asthma. Triggers such as indoor allergens of house dust mite, cockroach, and animal dander proteins are more likely to result in perennial symptoms, whereas pollens and some mold spores are likely to provoke seasonal symptoms. The presence of rhinosinusitis, nasal polyps, conjunctivitis, or eczema, coupled with a family history of asthma or atopy, may further support the diagnosis of asthma. Symptoms after heavy exertion, especially in the cold air, are highly suggestive of exercise-induced asthma and typically, patients experience symptoms at the end of exercise, rather than during its performance. Excessive coughing after exercise in the absence of wheeze may also be a sign of asthma. Premenopausal women with asthma may experience a deterioration of asthma control perimenstrually.[13] The medical history should elicit risk factors for asthma (Table 46-1), and special consideration should address symptoms induced by aspirin or those associated with the patient's occupation.

■ ASTHMA AND ASPIRIN SENSITIVITY

The association of asthma and sensitivity to aspirin or other NSAIDs is well established.[14] Aspirin-sensitive asthma affects approximately 5% of all asthmatics, although it is more common in patients with severe asthma (~20%) and in those frequently hospitalized for their asthma. This subtype of asthma is usually characterized by a tetrad of asthma, nasal polyps, chronic hypertrophic eosinophilic sinusitis, and aspirin intolerance. Classically, perennial rhinitis is the first symptom in this syndrome, preceding the development of aspirin sensitivity, and then followed much later by nasal polyps that are usually bilateral and originate from the turbinates and the paranasal sinuses. Even in small doses, aspirin typically causes wheezing, facial flushing, rhinorrhea, and conjunctival irritation. Although aspirin-induced asthmatic episodes often resemble allergic reactions, there is no evidence that immunolglobulin (Ig)-E–related mechanisms are at work. Aspirin-induced asthma is due to blockade of cyclooxygenase 1 by nonsteroidal anti-inflammatory drugs and has been associated with enhanced leukotriene production and mast cell activation, but the cellular pathways responsible for these events remain unclear. The diagnosis of aspirin sensitivity is made on the basis of the clinical history and can be confirmed by a provocative aspirin challenge, although this test carries a potential health risk of anaphylaxis for the patient.

Aspirin-sensitive asthma usually responds to standard therapy with inhaled corticosteroids (ICSs), although the condition is associated with severe asthma, who are a group of patients often refractory to treatment with inhaled and oral CS. Potentially, antileukotriene therapy should be efficacious in these patients, but have been found to be no more effective compared to their use in patients with allergic asthma. Aspirin desensitization may sometimes be needed, and should only be performed in specialized centers. In all asthmatic patients with aspirin sensitivity, the nonselective cyclooxygenase (COX) inhibitors should be avoided, but when an anti-inflammatory analgesic is needed, the selective COX-2 inhibitors are usually safe to use.

Occupational Asthma

Occupational asthma is asthma arising de novo that is initiated as a consequence of exposure to a specific etiologic agent in people without prior asthma. In contrast, work-exacerbated asthma is defined as the worsening of asthma, that is already pre-existing or concurrent, triggered by nonspecific irritants in the workplace.[15] Occupational asthma may be classified into (i) that caused by a sensitizing agent in the workplace (sensitizer-induced asthma) where the specific sensitizing agent causes asthma through an identified underlying immunologic mechanism and (ii) asthma caused by exposure to irritant compounds (irritant-induced asthma) where the exposure agent is not considered to be sensitizing.[16] Table 46-2 highlights the causes of both sensitizer-induced occupational asthma and the common agents responsible for irritant-induced occupational asthma. The diagnosis of occupational asthma is based on a demonstrable link between asthma symptoms and workplace exposure, showing work-related variability in measurements of lung function made serially.[16] Classically, a typical history of asthma-like symptoms during the working week and improvement over the weekend or on vacation are elicited and symptoms may occur either during exposure to the etiologic substance, or they may be delayed until the evening or night after the work day. Early detection and avoidance of occupational asthma is important where, if the patient is removed from exposure within the first 6 months of symptoms, there is usually complete recovery.

TABLE 46-2 Causes of Occupational Asthma

Sensitizing Agent-Induced Asthma	
Agent	**Workers at Risk**
Acrylate	Dental workers; adhesive handlers
Anhydrides	Workers using epoxy resin for plastics
Animal protein allergens	Veterinary workers; animal handlers
Cereals (grains)	Bakery workers; grain workers; farmers
Dyes	Textile workers
Enzymes	Pharmaceutical workers; bakery workers; laboratory workers
Formaldehyde, glutaraldehyde	Hospital and healthcare workers
Gums	Carpet makers
Isocyanates	Installers of insulation; manufacturers of plastics; rubbers and foam; spray painters
Latex	Healthcare workers; rubber workers
Persulfate	Hairdressers
Seafoods	Seafood handlers and processors
Wood dusts	Forestry workers; sawmill workers; carpenters
Common Agents Responsible for Irritant-Induced Asthma	
Acids (acetic, hydrochloric, sulfuric)	
Alkaline dust	
Ammonia	
Bleach	
Chlorine	
Cleaning agents	
Diesel exhaust	
Endotoxins	
Formalin	
Mustard	
Oxide (calcium)	
Paints (heated)	

■ PHYSICAL EXAMINATION

The most typical physical finding in asthma is wheezing on auscultation, which is usually caused by turbulent airflow through narrowed airways. Wheezing may be heard throughout the chest and is classically polyphonic, present to a greater extent during expiration, although it may also be heard during inspiration. The quality and character of wheezing is not specific to asthma or to the severity of the underlying disease. There may be no abnormal physical findings when asthma is under control yet conversely, in cases of very severe airway obstruction, breath sounds and wheezing may be absent. Examination of the upper respiratory tract may reveal clinical signs of rhinitis, sinusitis, or nasal polyps.

During an acute exacerbation of disease, physical signs of increased ventilation may be observed with the use of accessory muscles of respiration and chest signs of hyperinflation. A sign of severe airway obstruction is pulsus paradoxus, which is the exaggerated decrease in systolic blood pressure during inspiration by >10 mm Hg. As ventilatory effort can be diminished with respiratory muscle fatigue, pulsus paradoxus may be absent, but its absence does not preclude severe airway obstruction. Stridor is a high-pitched inspiratory sound and indicates airflow turbulence in the upper airways. In the acute setting, stridor should prompt a review of causes such as epiglottitis or foreign body, and in chronic presentation conditions such as upper airway tumors, tracheal–bronchial stenosis, vocal cord dysfunction/paralysis, and airway narrowing due to thyroid enlargement should be excluded.

LABORATORY INVESTIGATION

The diagnosis of asthma is usually apparent from the medical history with symptoms of variable and intermittent airway obstruction and objective measurements of lung function and spirometry support the diagnostic process. Similarly, the clinical history provides relevant information regarding the relationship between symptoms and allergen exposure, but skin prick testing and serology may be useful in identifying specific allergic triggers of asthma. Radiologic examination of the thorax, blood tests, and body plethysmography are not routinely indicated, unless there is some uncertainty in the diagnosis, where these tests may be used to exclude other conditions that may mimic asthma or complicate its clinical presentation.

■ LUNG FUNCTION TESTS

Peak flow meters are portable devices, readily available for patient use, that measure the peak expiratory flow (PEF). Serial readings of PEF that vary by more than 20% either spontaneously or in response to treatment are supportive of a diagnosis of asthma. Twice-daily PEF measurements, morning and evening, may also demonstrate diurnal variation, which is a typical feature of asthmatic patients.

Spirometry measures the expiratory volume and flow of air using forced maneuvers from full lung inflation, as a function of time. Simple spirometry is important for objectively demonstrating airflow obstruction, confirming the diagnosis of asthma, establishing the severity of the disease, and monitoring the response to therapy. Patients with asthma typically show a reduced forced expiratory flow in 1 second (FEV_1), reduced PEF, preserved forced vital capacity (FVC), and an FEV_1/FVC ratio of 0.7 or greater, but with worsening disease, FEV_1 less than 60% predicted the FEV_1/FVC ratio is more usually <0.7.[17] Home PEF monitoring may be of diagnostic use, confirming the diurnal variations in airflow obstruction, especially in patients who demonstrate normal spirometry during clinic visits. Spirometry also allows the assessment of the flow–volume loop, which shows a reduced maximum expiratory flow.

Bronchodilator reversibility is a measure of the magnitude of airway smooth muscle relaxation. A postbronchodilator increase in FEV_1 of >12% and 200 mL is often considered evidence of reversible airway obstruction, where measures are taken 15 minutes after an inhaled short-acting β_2-agonist (SABA). However, this level of increase is arbitrary and lacks sensitivity or specificity for detecting asthma. In addition, bronchodilator reversibility is diminished in well-controlled asthmatic patients, so it is not a good measure of asthma severity or response to therapy. In some patients, bronchodilator reversibility may be demonstrated by a 2- to 4-week trial of oral corticosteroids (prednisone or prednisolone 30–40 mg daily). Bronchodilator reversibility may also occur in patients with chronic obstructive pulmonary disease (COPD), and although asthma and COPD are distinct diseases, an "overlap syndrome" is described between the two conditions.[18–20]

■ BODY PLETHYSMOGRAPHY

Whole-body plethysmography is rarely required to establish a diagnosis of asthma in family practice, but may help in patients where there is diagnostic uncertainty. In stable asthma, measurement of the lung volumes may reveal an increase in residual volume, which reflects airway closure at a lung volume that is higher than normal. Air trapping is typically seen in patients with severe asthma. Airway resistance is characteristically increased and, during acute episodes of disease exacerbation, functional residual capacity and total lung capacity may also be observed to be increased. Measurement of the diffusing capacity of the lung (DL_{CO}) may also differentiate patients with COPD from those with asthma. In stable asthma, DL_{CO} is usually normal, but there may be a small increase in some patients. In contrast, patients with COPD typically have a reduced DL_{CO}, which reflects alveolar septal destruction and loss of pulmonary capillary volume—characteristic features of emphysematous patients.

■ BRONCHIAL CHALLENGE TESTING

Assessing bronchial hyperresponsiveness (BHR) is a sensitive tool that, although not routinely undertaken in clinical practice, may be helpful in diagnosing asthma, particularly when there is diagnostic uncertainty in the context of normal pulmonary function tests and unexplained chest symptoms (see Chapter 33).[21] Bronchial challenge tests assess the abnormally increased airway hyperresponsiveness observed in patients with asthma, by detecting the exaggerated response to inhaled bronchoprovocative agents. The provocation agents can be classified into two categories: direct and indirect. Direct stimuli such as histamine and methacholine, which are normally used in the clinic, act on airway smooth muscle receptors, whereas indirect stimuli act through intermediate pathways that include the release of mast cell mediators, and/or through local and central neurologic reflexes. Indirect stimuli include adenosine monophosphate (AMP), mannitol, exercise, hypertonic saline, and isocapnic hyperventilation.

Increased BHR is typically defined as the inhaled concentration of the bronchoprovocative agent that reduces FEV_1 by 20% (PC_{20}). This criterion for the test has maximal sensitivity but not maximal specificity and thus, when a diagnostic PC_{20} threshold of ≤8 mg/mL is used, pharmacologic challenges are sensitive tests with a high negative predictive value, that is, a PC_{20} >8 mg/mL excludes a diagnosis of asthma with a high degree of accuracy. Similarly, a positive result, although consistent with is not diagnostic for asthma. False-negative results can be obtained in patients who experience only intermittent symptoms and are tested when they are asymptomatic. The prevalence of abnormal responsiveness in nonatopic, nonasthmatic subjects who have no history of prior respiratory problems ranges between 5% and 10%. Knowledge of family history, personal atopy, and comorbidities clearly improves the prediction that abnormal airway responsiveness predisposes to the subsequent development of asthma.[22]

Technical factors related to the test procedure must be strictly controlled and follow standard operating procedures that include: the aerosol generation, the method of inhalation (intermittent versus continuous), and the measurement and calculation of the response. Medications such as β_2-agonists, theophylline, long-acting muscarinic antagonists, and CSs may influence the test and decrease airway responsiveness. Measuring BHR may have additional utility in the management of asthma. Patients whose disease is considered to be clinically controlled, may still have BHR and underlying airway inflammation and studies have shown that using AHR to guide treatment with ICSs, leads to an additional improvement in symptoms, lung function, and airway biopsy findings, compared with conventional assessment.[23]

Exercise testing of patients using cycle, treadmill, or free running challenges is occasionally undertaken to show postexercise bronchoconstriction if there is a suggestive history of exercise-induced asthma.[24] In professional athletes, asthma may be both under- or overdiagnosed and objective confirmation by appropriate lung function testing with bronchodilator or exercise challenge is often needed. Allergen challenge is rarely utilized in the routine management of patients with asthma and should only be undertaken by a specialist center if a specific causative or occupational agent is to be identified, such as aspirin.

■ BLOOD TESTS

Blood tests are usually not helpful in establishing the diagnosis of asthma. The eosinophil count in the peripheral blood film may be raised in atopic conditions and eosinophilia may support a diagnosis of asthma; however, a normal level does not rule out atopy or exclude asthma. In patients receiving CSs, eosinophilic counts may be normal or low. Because of their poor sensitivity and specificity, blood eosinophil counts are not recommended in the routine monitoring of asthma severity or as a barometer of airway inflammation. Markedly high levels may be present in disorders such as tropical parasitic eosinophilia, allergic bronchopulmonary aspergillosis (ABPA), Churg–Strauss syndrome, and Loeffler's syndrome as discussed elsewhere in this volume. In these hypereosinophilic conditions, clinical suspicion may warrant additional blood tests directed to ruling out vasculitis or ABPA, which are uncommon causes of asthma symptoms.

Total serum immunoglobulin E (IgE) may be measured in patients. Epidemiologic studies demonstrate an association between asthma and total serum IgE levels, standardized for sex and age. There is also a relationship between total serum IgE and asthma in patients with negative skin tests. Importantly, total IgE levels are used to calculate the dose of the anti-IgE antibody therapy, omalizumab, when it is used for asthma treatment as discussed below in Anti-IgE Monoclonal Antibodies. Blood tests of specific IgE to inhaled allergens, radioallergosorbent testing (RAST), and immunoCAP may help identify or confirm allergy to specific allergens, such as house dust mite, cockroach, *Aspergillus* species, pollens, or animal dander.

In acute exacerbations of disease, arterial blood gases may reveal hypoxemia and the arterial Pa_{CO_2} may be reduced due to hyperventilation. With a severe exacerbation, the arterial Pa_{CO_2} may rise due to respiratory muscle fatigue and an inability to maintain the required alveolar ventilation.

■ SKIN TESTS

If the clinical history suggests specific aeroallergens are important triggers or when asthma symptoms in a patient are accompanied by other symptoms typical of allergic disease, such as conjunctivitis or rhinitis, skin prick tests may be helpful to determine whether the patient is allergic, and to investigate the role of specific allergens as a cause of asthma. Sensitivity to a particular allergen such as house dust mite, cockroach, *Aspergillus* species or animal dander can be verified by skin tests or in vitro serum antibody studies (see above). Antihistamines and antidepressants should be avoided when undertaking testing as these drugs can interfere with the response. Positive responses on skin prick testing may help encourage patients to undertake allergen avoidance measures or, in selected cases, may help develop immunotherapy regimens.

■ CHEST IMAGING

Chest radiography is usually unremarkable and normal in patients with mild-to-moderate asthma; however, in more severe disease, nonspecific findings such as hyperinflation, prominent hilar vessels, and bronchial wall thickening may be seen. In patients with an exacerbation of their symptoms, chest radiography may be useful to exclude a pneumothorax. Consolidation shadowing in the lung usually indicates pneumonia or eosinophilic infiltrates in patients with ABPA. High-resolution computed tomography (HRCT) of the chest may identify atelectasis, bronchial wall thickening, or areas of bronchiectasis in patients with severe asthma, but these changes are not diagnostic of asthma. Emphysema is absent. Multidetector computed tomography (MDCT) undertaken in inspiration and expiration provides additional information concerning the tracheobronchial tree during the entire respiratory cycle.

■ EXHALED NITRIC OXIDE

The measurement of fractional nitric oxide gas in the exhaled breath (FeNO) of patients is being utilized as a noninvasive test to assess intrapulmonary eosinophilic inflammation.[25] Portable, compact hand-held devices allow FeNO measurements to be undertaken at the bedside and in family practice. Typically, asthmatic patients have elevated FeNO levels compared with healthy subjects, which correlate with the amount of eosinophils in sputum. ICSs and oral leukotriene receptor antagonists have been shown to decrease FeNO levels. These observations suggest a possible role for FeNO as an index of asthma disease severity, as a test of treatment efficacy and, in the assessment of patient adherence with asthma therapy. Measurements of FeNO have also been used successfully to titrate inhaled steroids without any loss of asthma control; thus, FeNO may be used as a tool in conjunction with other clinical measures to optimize asthma management as recommended by guidelines, that is, achieving disease control using the lowest doses of medications possible. In the research environment, FeNO can be partitioned into that arising from the central bronchial/conducting airways, or to that generated in peripheral alveolar regions, allowing an assessment of the site of intrapulmonary inflammation.[26,27] Patients with severe refractory asthma have shown greater alveolar NO concentrations compared to those with mild asthma.

■ SPUTUM EXAMINATION

The sputum differential count may be helpful. Induced sputum eosinophil counts have been used as an endpoint in clinical trials of therapeutic agents targeted at patients with eosinophilic lung diseases like asthma.[28] Research studies have shown sputum eosinophilia predicts clinical outcomes, particularly asthma exacerbations, when CSs are withdrawn. Induced sputum eosinophil counts have also been shown to guide anti-inflammatory treatment in patients with asthma in a management strategy that minimizes eosinophilic inflammation.[23] However, induced sputum remains a research tool as it is rather an unpleasant procedure for the patient and further studies are needed before measurement of sputum eosinophils can be widely used as a biomarker to monitor patients in clinical practice.

DIFFERENTIAL DIAGNOSIS

There are a number of conditions to consider in the differential diagnosis of asthma and these are listed in Table 46-3. Usually, it is not difficult to differentiate asthma from other conditions causing wheeze and dyspnea. The degree of diagnostic accuracy is probably dependent on the age of the patient, where the diagnosis in young adults is usually not difficult since there are few other conditions that mimic asthma or confound its clinical presentation. With increasing age, cardiovascular disease and other forms of chronic lung disease are more common, and the differential diagnosis of episodic chest symptoms is broader.

TABLE 46-3 Differential Diagnosis of Asthma

Upper Airway	Pulmonary	Cardiac	Other
Foreign body	Allergic bronchopulmonary aspergillosis (ABPA)	Angina	Anemia
Postnasal drip	Bronchiectasis	Left ventricular failure	Carcinoid
Upper airway obstruction	Churg–Strauss syndrome	Mitral valve disease	Functional
Vocal cord dysfunction	COPD		Gastroesophageal reflux
Tracheobroncho-malacia	Cystic fibrosis		Hyperventilation
	Interstitial lung disease		Mastocytosis
	Lung cancer		Obesity
	Pneumonia		
	Pneumothorax		
	Sarcoidosis		

Patients with upper airway obstruction can mimic severe asthma, and typically these patients present with localized wheeze and stridor of the large airways. Assessing the flow–volume loop in such patients will reveal a reduction in inspiratory flow as well as expiratory flow, and bronchoscopy can demonstrate the site of narrowing in the upper airways. Vocal cord dysfunction can be assessed using nasoendoscopy, which allows the observation of abnormalities in the movement of the vocal cords, and is most helpful when adduction of the cords is detected in the presence of the patient's symptoms.[29] Persistent wheezing auscultated in a localized area of the chest wall may indicate endobronchial obstruction due to lung cancer or a foreign body. Eosinophilic pneumonias and systemic vasculitis, including the Churg–Strauss syndrome and polyarteritis nodosa may be associated with wheezing and their systemic clinical manifestations may help in their identification.

COPD is usually easy to differentiate from asthma. The symptoms in patients with COPD are more persistent, show less variability, are progressive, and usually exhibit minimal reversibility to bronchodilator agents. The literature highlights an "overlap syndrome," where COPD patients have features of asthma with increased sputum eosinophils and a response to oral corticosteroids; these patients probably have both diseases concomitantly.[20] Important cardiologic causes to consider include left ventricular failure, where usually bibasal lung crackles are present in contrast to the scattered polyphonic wheeze in asthma. Anemia should always be thought of as a cause of dyspnea, especially in elderly patients. The symptoms of gastroesophageal reflux disease (GERD) may be mistaken for those of asthma; however, it is important to recognize that GERD is common in patients with asthma and has been identified as a potential trigger for asthma symptoms.[30]

TREATMENT OF ASTHMA

Treating asthmatic patients is generally straightforward; with effective and safe drugs, most asthmatics are now managed by family doctors. The successful management of asthma requires an appreciation of the heterogeneity of the disease with respect to etiology, clinical presentation, severity, natural history, and response to therapy. It is unlikely that a single management approach will work for all patients and hence, treatment should be tailored to the individual patient. It will also be recognized that symptom severity in patients varies over time with periods of remission that are interspersed with acute exacerbations, and thus the patient should be monitored regularly and treatment should be modified on an ongoing basis to meet the patient's current needs. There are several aims in the management of patients with asthma (Table 46-4) and although prominence has been placed on drug therapy, there are important patient-orientated approaches that focus on correct inhaler usage, emphasize self-management action plans, and address environmental control.

TABLE 46-4 Aims of Asthma Therapy

Control symptoms
Prevent (or minimize risk of) exacerbations
Eliminate emergency visits
Maintain lung function as close to as normal levels as possible
Decrease diurnal variation, especially nocturnal
Maintain normal levels of daily activities, including exercise
Eliminate or minimize adverse effects from medicine

INHALER DEVICES

Drug delivery to the lungs via the inhaled route remains the cornerstone of therapy for patients with asthma. Inhaled therapy targets drug directly to the lungs and allows a distinct therapeutic advantage over systemic therapy with the use of smaller drug doses, a more rapid onset of therapeutic action, and decreased adverse effects. There are several types of inhaler device and drug delivery systems used in clinical practice for the management of asthma and these include the pressurized metered-dose inhaler (pMDI), spacers, dry powder inhalers (DPIs), and nebulizers.[31] There are potentially over 250 device drug combinations available and this leads to confusion in prescribing among healthcare practitioners. Indeed, studies have shown that not just patients, but healthcare workers are uncertain about the correct use of inhaler devices and physician's knowledge, in particular, remains poor and may be related to a lack of education and instruction about inhaler usage during their training.[32] It has been shown that training and counseling patients in their inhalation technique can increase their adherence to device usage, and patients may be assessed with respect to their suitability for a particular inhaler device by using portable handheld meters that assess inhalation flows. Evidence-based guidelines from the American College of Chest Physicians,[33] recommend the following points for healthcare practitioners to consider when choosing an inhaler for their patient; the clinical condition and disease severity; availability of the inhaler device for the drug prescription; the patient's ability to use the selected device correctly; consideration given to using the same device type for all drugs; the setting and convenience of outpatient and inpatient use; the time required for drug administration; cost and reimbursement; and the inhaler preference of the patient as well as the prescriber. The advantages and disadvantage of the common inhaler device types are shown in Table 46-5.

PRESSURIZED METERED-DOSE INHALERS

The pMDIs contain the drug as a liquid suspension or solution with propellant in a sealed canister and, other formulation ingredients may be present such as ethanol, chemical preservatives, flavoring agents, and surfactant. Most inhaler therapies are now free of chlorofluorocarbon (CFC) propellants having being replaced by non–ozone-depleting propellants such as hydrofluorocarbons (HFCs). Upon actuation of the pMDI canister, there is quick vaporization of the propellant and this provides the force to aerosolize and propel the liquid drug out of the canister at high velocity. Vaporization of the

TABLE 46-5 Advantages and Disadvantages of Inhalation Devices

	Advantages	Disadvantages
Pressurized metered-dose inhaler (pMDI)	Compact and portable Multi-dose Quick treatment time Drug in sealed canister Inexpensive	High oropharyngeal deposition Difficulty in hand–mouth coordination Propellants may cause "cold Freon" effect and affect climate change Difficult to assess empty canister
Dry powder inhaler (DPI)	Compact and portable Quick treatment time Breath-actuated function removes need for coordination	Need adequate inhalation flow to disperse drug High oropharyngeal deposition Humidity can cause drug degradation Patients may be intolerant to additives, e.g., lactose
Nebulizers	Large doses of drug can be given Can be used with relaxed tidal breathing Suitable for young, old, and acutely ill patients Many drug solutions can be aerosolized	Bulky, cumbersome, and expensive Wasted drug in nebulizer reservoir Variation in aerosol output performance between models Time consuming Need for power source Regular cleaning and maintenance

propellant also causes cooling of the drug aerosol which can sometimes give rise to the "cold Freon effect," which is the sensation experienced by some patients of cold aerosol hitting the back of their oropharynx, which can stop them from inhaling the drug and sometimes cause paradoxical bronchospasm. Some of the formulation ingredients added to pMDIs described above, have been shown to cause bronchospasm, wheeze, and cough in asthmatic patients. pMDIs are compact, portable, and inexpensive devices. Recent advances in the technologic design of pMDIs include the addition of a dose counter.

Optimal clinical efficacy with a pMDI is obtained when the device is actuated at the start of a deep and slow inhalation lasting for 5 seconds followed, at the end of inspiration, by a breath-hold pause of 10 seconds. Failure to inhale slowly and deeply with pMDIs is a more common mistake than the actual patient coordination between inhalation and actuation. However, the latter problem is more pertinent in elderly patients and add-on spacer attachments, device-holding adaptors, and breath-actuated pMDIs have been developed to overcome this. Breath-actuated metered-dose inhalers utilize the patient's inspiratory force to trigger and activate the inhaler device, although it has been shown breath-actuated pMDIs offer no advantage over patients with good conventional pMDI inhaler technique. In contrast, breath- "coordinated" devices are different from breath-"actuated" metered-dose inhalers in that they do not depend upon the patient's inspiratory flow for actuation and help patients achieve coordination with aerosol inhalation.

■ SPACERS

Spacer devices are used with pMDIs and are designed to assist in the delivery of inhaled drug to the lungs by promoting ease of pMDI use, and reduce oropharyngeal deposition by slowing the high velocity of the emitted aerosol cloud. The plastic walls of the spacer trap the large dug particles and this decreases oropharyngeal impaction, which may lead to a decrease in local unwanted side effects, particularly with CSs, and also a reduction in systemic adverse effects by minimizing the amount of drug absorbed via the gastrointestinal tract. In addition, increasing the distance the aerosolized drug travels (by using the spacer as an extension attachment to the pMDI device), slows the emitted aerosol cloud and allows more evaporation of the propellant, leading to relatively smaller drug particles that have a greater potential to deposit within the lungs. Spacers include valve-holding reservoir chambers with a one-way inhalation valve in the mouthpiece only allowing airflow through the chamber when the patient inhales; simple extension devices that are nonvalved add-on products that require a reasonably good amount of coordination; and reverse-flow devices where the aerosol spray is actuated away from the patient into a collapsible reservoir chamber or bag through which outside air is entrained to provide the airflow stream for inhalation.

Spacer devices each differ in their design characteristics and should be prescribed only with the pMDI they are compatible with, as each spacer–inhaler combination has distinct aerosol output characteristics.[34] To reduce the electrostatic charge in spacers which can significantly contribute to decreased drug available to be delivered to the lungs, spacers should be primed with the pMDI prior to use, and one-dose actuation at a time from a pMDI into the spacer device should be employed as opposed to simultaneous multiple-dose administrations. Spacers should be washed with ionic detergent and air dried. Antistatic spacer devices are available and can be used.

■ DRY POWDER INHALERS

DPIs are propellant-free devices that contain finely milled powdered drug particles bound into loose aggregates or, drug particles associated with larger carrier molecules such as lactose. DPI devices are breath-actuated in their operation, and critically rely on the patient's inspiratory effort to deaggregate the drug from its carrier particle to achieve optimal delivery and deposition within the lungs. Studies have shown that DPIs are highly dependent on the patient's inspiratory flow for therapeutic success, and have observed that patients with asthma and those with COPD use suboptimal inspiratory flows from DPIs leading to low pulmonary deposition.[35]

DPIs can be classified into single-dose delivery systems that either require drug to be individually loaded into the inhaler prior to use or where individual doses are dispensed from punctured gelatin capsules. In contrast, multiple-dosing delivery DPIs avoid the inconvenience associated with repeated drug loading and can be divided into "multi-dose" or "multi–unit-dose" systems. Multi-dose systems deliver drug that is metered from a powder reservoir, whereas multiple–unit-dose devices either contain drug sealed in individual foil blisters, or drug sealed in pockets on a moving strip. Deterioration of the drug may occur in damp and humid conditions, and so all these devices should be stored in a dry environment.

A newer generation of DPIs have been developed that rely less on the patient's inspiratory effort, requiring either lower inhalation flows to aerosolize the drug or, in some circumstances, deliver the drug wholly independent of the patient's breathing maneuver.

NEBULIZERS

The main types of nebulizer commonly used in clinical practice can be divided into two categories: ultrasonic and jet nebulizers.[36] Ultrasonic nebulizers utilize the vibration from a piezoelectric crystal at a high frequency to produce aerosol clouds for inhalation from the liquid drug. Ultrasonic nebulizers are smaller and less noisy compared to jet nebulizers, but are usually less robust, more expensive, and not as effective in nebulizing liquid suspensions of drug. Jet nebulizers use either compressed gas or an electrical compressor to generate aerosolized particles. High-velocity air streams are generated and directed through a narrow Venturi opening, across the liquid drug solution/suspension, to produce aerosolized droplets within the nebulizing chamber.

Nebulizers require tidal breathing at rest for effective use and do not require much patient coordination. However, it is recognized that there is great variation in the aerosol output generated from each of the different nebulizer devices, and the inhalation maneuver will affect drug delivery to the lungs that can be greatly reduced with crying, as may occur with children, or when there are shallow and rapid inhalations.[37] Consideration should be given to the nebulizer–face-mask combination as incorrect mask insertion into the nebulizer may give rise to unwanted deposition of drug onto the face and eyes, particularly in children. Generally, nebulizer devices are large, lack portability, and have a longer treatment time than conventional inhalers.

There are now a newer generation of nebulizer devices that offer a marked improvement in the efficiency and precision of pulmonary drug delivery.[38] These devices are more costly as units compared to conventional nebulizers, but may be cost-effective by decreasing drug loss from the nebulizer chamber particularly during exhalation, and overall by delivering a reduced drug dose to the lungs but more effectively. Nebulizer systems have also been developed that control the patient's inhalation maneuver so as to minimize the variability in dose delivery that occurs during use, and there are systems that provide feedback to the patient and allow an assessment of patient compliance.

THERAPEUTIC DRUGS

A wide variety of agents are used in the management of asthma.

BRONCHODILATORS

Bronchodilators reverse the bronchoconstriction of asthma, principally by acting to relax airway smooth muscle, and this results in the rapid relief of symptoms. Bronchodilators are not adequate enough to control asthma in patients with persistent symptoms, as they have little effect on the underlying airway inflammation. The classes of bronchodilators in current clinical use include β_2-adrenergic agonists, anticholinergics, and theophylline, where β_2-agonists are the most efficacious.

β_2-Adrenergic Agonists

Inhaled β_2-adrenergic agonists are the drugs of choice for relief of respiratory symptoms due to acute airway obstruction.

Mode of Action β_2-Agonists activate β_2-adrenergic receptors resulting in an increase in intracellular cyclic AMP, which leads to relaxation of airway smooth muscle cells. β_2-Agonists act as functional antagonists; that is, they prevent and reverse the contraction of airway smooth muscle cells by bronchoconstrictors, and it is this action that mainly accounts for their efficacy as bronchodilators in asthma. These drugs also have nonbronchodilator effects that include the inhibition of mast cell mediator release, the inhibition of sensory nerve activation, and a reduction in plasma exudation, which may be clinically useful.[39]

Clinical Use SABAs, such as albuterol and terbutaline, have a rapid onset of action and a 3- to 6-hour duration of activity. This pharmacodynamic characteristic of a rapid onset of bronchodilation allows these drugs to be used as quick-relief medications or "relievers" on an as-needed basis. As a matter of caution, increasing use of SABA indicates that asthma is not controlled and patients should be reviewed. At recommended doses, inhaled β-agonists have few adverse effects, although when used at higher doses by nebulizer, patients may experience short-lived side effect. Long-acting β_2-agonists (LABAs) include formoterol and salmeterol. Both drugs are given twice daily by the inhaled route and have a duration of action of over 12 hours. In particular, formoterol has an onset of action as rapid as albuterol and can be used as a "reliever" component in fixed-dose combinations of LABA with ICS medication. LABA should not be used as monotherapy for the control of asthma of any severity and should not be given in the absence of ICS therapy as they do not control the underlying inflammation. However, fixed-dose combinations of LABA with ICS are now increasingly used in the management of asthma and have proved to be highly effective in improving the control of asthmatic patients, reducing disease exacerbations, and allowing asthma to be controlled using lower doses of CSs.[40] Studies have also shown the clinical benefits of LABA/ICS fixed combinations compared with the monocomponents administered using two separate inhalers. Interestingly, the combination of formoterol and budesonide, and recently formoterol and beclomethasone dipropionate, have been demonstrated to be effective when used as both a controller and reliever agent, and thus provides the advantage of a single device used for both purposes.[41]

Adverse Effects The commonest adverse effects of β_2-agonists are palpitations and muscle tremors, which are unusual with the inhaled route and seen more commonly with high-dose nebulizer therapy and in elderly patients. The safety of β_2-agonists has been an issue of concern. An association has been demonstrated between the amount of SABA used and asthma deaths, but thorough analyses demonstrate that the increased use of rescue SABA implies poor asthma control, which itself is a risk factor for asthma death. A slight increase in deaths from asthma has been observed with the use of LABA, but this is most likely related to the lack of use of parallel ICS, as the LABA therapy on its own fails to suppress the asthmatic airway inflammation, and this highlights the need to always use ICS when LABA are given which can most suitably be achieved by using a combination ICS/LABA inhaler.[42] Patients should also be reminded to avoid β-adrenergic receptor–blocking drugs, including those contained in topical ophthalmic preparations, as they can precipitate severe and sometimes life-threatening asthmatic episodes. Accordingly, β-blockers are contraindicated during acute asthma exacerbations and the risk–benefit ratio should be considered before they are used in stable patients with asthma. Some patients experience deterioration in their asthma control following inhaled β-agonist treatment and possible mechanisms and contributory factors include paradoxical bronchospasm, increased BHR, and tolerance to the drug. With prolonged exposure to a drug, down-regulation of the β-receptor may occur and this can limit therapeutic efficacy; that is, lead to tachyphylaxis to treatment. Indeed, β-receptor mutations and gene polymorphisms have been implicated in influencing the response to inhaled β-agonists.[43]

Anticholinergics

Anticholinergic agents are another class of drugs to be considered in asthma management.

Mode of Action Muscarinic receptor antagonists, such as ipratropium bromide, induce airway smooth-muscle relaxation by blocking muscarinic receptors on airway smooth muscle, inhibiting vagally mediated cholinergic tone and preventing mucus secretion.[39]

Clinical Use In general, the anticholinergic drugs are not as efficacious compared to the β_2-agonists as bronchodilator agents. Anticholinergics prevent the cholinergic reflex component of bronchoconstriction, whereas in contrast, β_2-agonists inhibit all bronchoconstrictor mechanisms. Hence, anticholinergics tend only to be used as add-on bronchodilator treatment in asthmatics who remain uncontrolled on other inhaled therapy. In the treatment of acute severe asthma, high doses of anticholinergic therapy may be given by nebulizer, but should only be given following β_2-agonist treatment as anticholinergics do not have such a fast onset of bronchodilation. A combination preparation of albuterol and ipratropium bromide is available for nebulization therapy. It has recently been shown that the long-acting anticholinergic drug tiotropium may be as useful as an asthma treatment, as it is in patients with COPD, although the drug is currently not licensed for the treatment of patients with asthma.

Adverse Effects Adverse effects are usually not a concern with anticholinergics as there is minimal absorption into the systemic circulation, but the most commonly experienced side effect is dry mouth, and in elderly patients, glaucoma and urinary retention can occur.

Theophylline

Oral theophylline was primarily used as an adjunct bronchodilator treatment, but due to its narrow therapeutic index and adverse effect profile, together with the availability of safer and more effective alternatives, theophylline is now infrequently used in patients with asthma.[44]

Mode of Action Theophylline inhibits phosphodiesterases in airway smooth muscle cells, which increases intracellular cyclic AMP and this leads to a bronchodilator effect. However, the doses required for bronchodilator activity commonly cause adverse effects, which are mainly a consequence of direct phosphodiesterase inhibition. Theophylline has been shown to exhibit anti-inflammatory effects, which are likely to arise through different molecular pathways; for example, theophylline has been shown to stimulate a key nuclear enzyme, histone deacetylase-2, which is an important intracellular mechanism for switching off inflammatory genes that have been activated.

Clinical Use Theophylline is normally administered as an oral slow-release formulation either once or twice a day, as this results in more steady plasma concentrations compared to standard theophylline tablets. In severe asthmatic patients, theophylline may be used as an add-on bronchodilator treatment, although plasma concentrations of 10 to 20 mg/L are typically needed, and these levels are usually associated with adverse effects. In contrast, the anti-inflammatory effects of theophylline seem to occur at plasma levels below the traditional therapeutic range of 10 to 20 mg/L, and at low doses, the drug is better tolerated. Low-dose theophylline has additive effects to ICS and is particularly helpful in severe asthmatic patients, where withdrawal of theophylline may result in clear worsening of asthma control. Intravenous aminophylline is now seldom used for the treatment of asthmatic patients, only very rarely in those with acute severe asthma exacerbations.

Adverse Effects The adverse effects of theophylline are directly related to drug levels in the plasma and are infrequently observed at concentrations below 10 mg/L. The measurement of plasma theophylline may be useful in determining and guiding the correct clinical dose. Headaches, nausea, and vomiting are the commonest adverse effects, which arise from the inhibition of phosphodiesterase. Palpitations and diuresis may be troublesome, and with higher plasma concentrations, epileptic seizures, cardiac arrhythmias, and death may occur due to adenosine A_1-receptor antagonism. Oral theophylline is well absorbed through the gastrointestinal route and is largely inactivated in the liver by the enzyme CYP450 and so, drugs that inhibit CYP450 activity such as allopurinol and erythromycin may increase plasma levels of theophylline with consequently, a greater potential for adverse effects.

CORTICOSTEROIDS

Corticosteroids (CSs) are potent anti-inflammatory agents and when administered by the inhaled route are the most effective therapy available for treating and controlling asthma, and have greatly contributed to a reduction in asthma mortality in the Western world.[45]

Mode of Action

CSs reduce the number and activation of inflammatory cells in the airways. The reduction in eosinophils, activated T lymphocytes, and surface mast cells in the airways contribute to the lessening in the airway hyperresponsiveness that is seen with CS therapy. There are several molecular mechanisms underlying the action of CS on airway inflammation and the main pathways center on the inhibition of transcription factors NF-κB and AP-1, which switch off the transcription of multiple activated genes encoding inflammatory proteins such as cytokines, chemokines, inflammatory enzymes, and adhesion molecules. Another key mechanism in the action of CS is the inhibition of the recruitment of histone deacetylase-2 to the inflammatory gene complex, which reverses the histone acetylation associated with increased gene transcription. CSs increase the expression of β_2-receptors and this may contribute to the complementary clinical effects observed when CS are combined with LABA.[46] Transcriptional activation is responsible for most of the endocrine and metabolic adverse effects of CS.

Clinical Use—Inhaled Corticosteroids

CSs are usually administered by the inhaled route for maintenance controller therapy in patients with asthma. ICS have been shown to prevent the symptoms of asthma, reduce severe exacerbations rates, improve lung function, and reduce airway hyperresponsiveness. Early and timely treatment with ICS appears to avert the irreversible changes in airway function that occur with chronic asthma. Patients with persistent asthma stabilized on ICS experience increased exacerbations when treatment is withdrawn, indicating that ICS suppress symptoms and inflammation, but do not cure the underlying disease. ICS are beneficial in treating asthmatic patients of any age and at any stage of disease severity. They are first-line therapy for patients with persistent asthma and are usually administered twice a day, although ICS may be effective given once a day in some patients with mild symptoms. The dose–response curve of ICS is relatively flat, meaning that higher doses are only incrementally better than low-to-medium doses. If low-to-medium doses of ICS do not control persistent asthma symptoms, it is usual practice now to add a LABA, preferably as a combination of the two drugs delivered from a single inhaler device.

Clinical Use—Systemic Corticosteroids

Oral CSs are reserved to treat acute exacerbations of asthma. Typically prednisolone or prednisone 30 to 45 mg is given once daily for 5 to 10 days and on finishing the course of treatment, no tapering of the dose is required. Some asthmatic patients, especially those with more severe disease, require maintenance treatment with oral CS and in these patients it is important to determine the lowest dose necessary to maintain asthma control in light of the greater potential for adverse effects with higher doses. CSs may also be administered intravenously (methylprednisolone or hydrocortisone) for the treatment of acute severe asthma, although studies show oral CSs are as equally efficacious and easier to take.

Adverse Effects

ICS may give rise to local oropharyngeal adverse effects such as oral candidiasis, dysphonia, and hoarseness, but these may be lessened with the use of a spacer device. There exist concerns about the systemic adverse effects of ICS from swallowing of the oropharyngeal dose and lung absorption, but these depend upon the individual pharmacokinetic properties of the different CS and overall, studies show that ICS have minimal systemic adverse effects.[47] At higher drug doses, ICS may suppress plasma and urinary cortisol levels, and in prepubertal children it has been shown that the initial decrease in attained height from ICS persists as a reduction in adult height, but is not progressive or cumulative and is approximately a loss of 1 cm. Most importantly, ICS allow the effective control of asthma symptoms and disease, and maintenance therapy may decrease the need and number of prescribed courses of oral CS, and thus, reduce the total-body systemic exposure to CS in general.

Oral CS gives rise to greater systemic adverse effects than ICS, with a greater potential in those on chronic maintenance therapy. Adverse effects include bruising, diabetes, truncal obesity, osteoporosis, duodenal and gastric ulceration, hypertension, mood and behavioral changes, proximal myopathy, and cataracts. It is important to assess and monitor bone density if patients are administered chronic oral CS therapy so that preventive treatment for osteoporosis with bisphosphonates or estrogen in postmenopausal women may be initiated if levels of bone density are borderline or low. If CS adverse effects are a considerable problem, steroid-sparing agents may occasionally be considered.

ANTILEUKOTRIENES

Leukotriene pathway inhibitors are a group of compounds that alter the pathophysiologic effects of leukotrienes derived from the 5-lipoxygenation of arachidonic acid. Two classes of agents are available: inhibitors of the 5-lipoxygenase enzyme (zileuton) and cysteinyl-leukotriene receptor type-1 antagonists (montelukast, zafirlukast, and pranlukast).[48]

Mode of Action

Cysteinyl-leukotriene receptor type-1 antagonists inhibit the smooth muscle bronchoconstriction, microvascular leakage, and eosinophilic airway inflammation that occur through activation of cys-LT_1-receptors. These agents predominantly act on the inflammatory mediators produced by mast cells in asthma, and also to a lesser extent on mediators produced by eosinophils.

Clinical Use

Antileukotrienes have less effect on airway inflammation and provide modest clinical benefit compared to ICS. ICSs are more effective anti-inflammatory agents and clinically superior in controlling asthma than antileukotrienes. Antileukotriene treatments may be useful as add-on therapy to selected mild asthmatic patients on low-dose ICS, although these agents are less efficacious than add-on therapy with LABA. Antileukotrienes may be helpful when CS use is poorly tolerated or not desired by the patient, or there is concomitant rhinosinusitis. These drugs are usually given orally once or twice a day.

Adverse Effects

Antileukotrienes are usually well tolerated, but can sometimes give rise to gastrointestinal upset, hepatotoxicity, and hypersensitivity reactions including anaphylaxis and angioedema.

CROMONES

Cromolyn sodium and nedocromil sodium are classified as asthma-controller drugs. Their main mechanisms of action seem to be to inhibit sensory nerve and mast cell activation, and therefore they are effective in blocking trigger-induced asthma such as allergen- or exercise-induced symptoms. However, these drugs have a short duration of action, requiring up to four times a day inhalation, and consequently have somewhat little benefit in the long-term control of asthma. They are popular in the treatment of children with asthma because they are remarkably safe, although they are inferior to ICS with respect to most relevant clinical outcomes, and low-dose ICSs are now favored in children as they are more efficacious and have an established safety profile.

CORTICOSTEROID-SPARING TREATMENTS

Some patients experience serious adverse effects with CS therapy, especially oral CS therapy in those with severe asthma, and in an attempt to minimize CS exposure and reduce patient requirement, various immunomodulatory treatments have been tried. Many agents have been utilized as steroid-sparing therapies including azathioprine, colchicine, cyclosporin A, gold, methotrexate, and intravenous gamma globulin; but none of these treatments have shown long-term efficacy and importantly, each has been associated with a high-risk adverse effect profile and cannot be recommended to be used in lieu of CSs.

ANTI-IGE MONOCLONAL ANTIBODIES

Omalizumab is a monoclonal antibody to IgE that inhibits IgE-mediated reactions by neutralizing serum IgE without binding to cell-bound IgE. It is used as an adjunctive agent for atopic asthmatic patients who are dependent on CS therapy.[49] Studies in patients with moderate-to-severe CS-dependent asthma show an improvement in asthma control, a reduction in the number of disease exacerbations, and a significant steroid-sparing effect. However, anti-IgE treatment is very expensive and appropriate only for specific patients who have a high circulating IgE within a precise range and are not controlled on maximal doses of inhaled and/or oral CS therapy. Omalizumab is usually given as a subcutaneous injection every 2 to 4 weeks and is relatively safe with few significant adverse effects, although anaphylaxis has occasionally been reported. A 3- to 4-month trial of therapy should be undertaken to ascertain any objective benefit with this treatment.

IMMUNOTHERAPY

Allergen immunotherapy is of benefit in highly selected patients with defined allergic triggers.[50] Asthmatic patients with a single specific allergic trigger and concomitant nasal symptoms derive the greatest benefit than patients with multiple allergic triggers. Allergen-specific immunotherapy (ASIT) involves the repeated administration of allergen products to induce immunologic and clinical tolerance to the specific allergen. ASIT may be given subcutaneously and studies have supported efficacy by this route of administration, but there is a risk of adverse effects including anaphylaxis. In contrast, sublingual ASIT has recently been shown to be an effective and safe alternative in patients with seasonal allergy, although data for perennial allergies related to asthma is lacking.

NONPHARMACOLOGIC MANAGEMENT

Alternative therapies may be popular and more acceptable with some patients and include acupuncture, breathing control, chiropraxy, homeopathy, hypnotherapy, and yoga; but placebo-controlled studies show these treatments lack efficacy and they should not be clinically recommended.[51] The concern with these therapies is that they may lead to discontinuation of effective drug therapy and destabilize asthma control in patients. However, as these therapies are considered not to be harmful, patients may utilize them as an adjunct to their conventional pharmacotherapy.

FUTURE TREATMENTS

Although current asthma therapy with CSs and β_2-agonists are effective in controlling disease symptoms in the majority of patients, poorly controlled asthma still remains a problem in a considerable proportion of patients.[52] Poor adherence to prescribed controller therapy contributes to poor asthma control, and the use of combination LABA/ICS therapy delivered by a single inhaler device and/or the use of combination LABA/ICS therapy as both a controller and reliever agent, may partly address this problem. Indeed, the majority of current inhaler devices target their treatment to the large airways of the lung and research is ongoing to assess the clinical implications of targeting inhaled therapy to the peripheral lung regions, where they may be ongoing untreated inflammation additionally contributing to the patient's clinical state.[53] Asthma continues to remain an unmet need as the life-long treatments currently used only address the clinical symptoms and have little effect on the underlying structural alterations associated with asthma. There is also pressing need for the development of novel therapies for patients who have side effects with systemic CSs.[54]

Ultra–long-acting bronchodilators with once-daily dosing have been approved for COPD but not for asthma, and these treatments have allowed the production of several combination therapies incorporated with once-daily CS are in development.

CS resistance is a particular problem in patients with severe asthma, and several molecular mechanisms have been elucidated that may lead to novel therapeutic approaches, including the reversal of this resistance by drugs such as theophylline and nortriptyline. New treatments have been developed to control disease in very select groups of asthmatic patients. In patients with severe eosinophilic asthma (<5% of all asthmatic patients) despite treatment with high doses of CSs, blocking antibodies against interleukin-5 have been shown to reduce disease exacerbations. In contrast, anti–TNF-α antibodies have not been shown to be effective in patients with severe asthma. Several other blockers of specific mediators such as prostaglandin D(2), IL-9, and IL-13 are in clinical trials in patients with subtypes of severe asthma. New broad-spectrum anti-inflammatory treatments are in clinical development and include phosphodiesterase-4, NF-κB, and p38 MAP kinase inhibitors, but these drugs act on signal transduction pathways that are common to many immune cells, and present the risk of troublesome adverse effects particularly by the parenteral route and hence, there is ongoing research into their delivery by the inhaled route.

Studies of the steroid-sparing effects of macrolide antibiotics in asthma management have yielded discordant results. Macrolides might benefit some patients with infection by atypical bacteria, but recent results are not encouraging, although there could be an effect in patients with predominant neutrophilic asthma.

Bronchial thermoplasty has recently been advocated in selected patients with severe asthma and may be of benefit, and clinical studies although limited have demonstrated improved outcomes.[55]

MANAGEMENT OF CHRONIC ASTHMA

Management guidelines in asthma now focus on the control of asthma symptoms using a stepwise approach to drug therapy.[1] There has been a shift away from treatment based on disease severity with the realization that asthma does not necessarily remain in the same category permanently, but may change over months or years and that patients may move up or down in their asthma severity based on factors such as the presence of allergens, the incorrect/correct use of medications and treatments, and lack of adherence to the prescribed treatment regimen. If control at a particular step is not adequate, then treatment should be increased to the next level. The principles of therapy embody the fact that effective treatment should lead to better asthma control and allow the patient to move to a less severe category, and therefore for ongoing management of asthma, classification by level of control may be more relevant and useful. The aims of chronic therapy in asthma are highlighted in Table 46-2.

The Global Initiative for Asthma (GINA) stratifies patients into four categories of the level of asthma control; controlled (where therapy is maintained or stepped down); partly controlled (where consideration is given to stepping up therapy); uncontrolled (where treatment is stepped up until symptom control is achieved); and exacerbation (where patients are treated according to the exacerbation algorithms).[1] The characteristics that contribute to determining the level of control involve an assessment of the following: daytime symptoms experienced in the last week; limitations in activities of daily living; nocturnal symptoms or awakenings the need for rescue reliever medication during the week; lung function; and the number of exacerbations (if any) in the last week and last year.

STEPWISE TREATMENT

The stepwise approach to asthma management is a description of the levels of treatment required to achieve good asthma control.[1] Some patients may experience acute worsening of asthma control, such as those with a concomitant upper respiratory tract infection, and may need to step up more than one step at a time.

Step 1

For all asthma patients, a SABA delivered by a metered-dose inhaler is all that is required and gives relief of acute symptoms. The increasing use of a reliever medication more than three times a week, or triggering of symptoms from exercise, provide an indication that controller therapy is needed. An important, but often overlooked part of asthma management relates to measures to control environmental triggers. Recognized triggers that worsen asthma control in the patient such as aeroallergens or occupational agents should be avoided, although this is not always possible. Patients with asthma may also have several triggers; therefore the impact of avoiding a single trigger will vary considerably between patients. However, complete removal from exposure to house dust mite has been shown to reduce asthma severity and airway hyperresponsiveness.

Guidelines recommend that influenza vaccination should be administered in adult asthmatics. However, where studies suggest it is unlikely to induce asthma exacerbations, there is no conclusive evidence regarding the efficacy of vaccination on influenza-related asthma complications or a reduction in exacerbations of asthma. Asthmatic patients, especially the elderly or those with comorbid conditions that increase the risk of death from influenza infection, should receive inactivated influenza vaccine if there are no other contraindications. The CDC recommends a single dose of Pneumovax for adults from 19 to 64 who have chronic illnesses, including asthma.

Steps 2–3

When patient symptoms are no longer intermittent, the addition of a long-term controller medication on a scheduled daily basis is recommended, and the treatment of choice for all patients is an ICS to alleviate the underlying airway inflammation. It is usual to start with a low-to-intermediate dose of ICS twice daily (e.g., 200 μg beclomethasone dipropionate (BDP) or equivalent BID) and if symptoms are controlled after 3 months the dose should be stepped down. However, if symptoms persist and are not controlled, a LABA should be added as a fixed combination drug with an ICS delivered from a single inhaler device, as studies show a clinical advantage compared with the monocomponents administered using two separate inhalers. Indeed, low-dose ICS with LABA therapy has been shown to be as efficacious at high-dose ICS treatment.[56] The dose of the ICS should be adjusted up or down accordingly to the need for rescue inhaler treatment and to the control of the patient symptoms. Alternative add-on therapies to ICS that can be considered include low doses of slow-release oral theophylline or an antileukotriene, but these are less effective than the LABA/ICS combination.

Step 4–5

In patients with worsening symptoms, the addition of low-dose slow-release oral theophylline to high-dose LABA/ICS may be helpful. Recently, it has been shown that the addition of the inhaled long-acting anticholinergic tiotropium bromide to LABA/ICS treatment in patients with poorly controlled asthma, significantly decreases asthma exacerbations and improves bronchodilator lung function.[57] In patients with severe asthma who fail to achieve symptom control, maintenance therapy with systemic oral CSs may be indicated, and there should always be an aim to titrate down to the lowest possible daily (or every other day) dose that maintains asthma control. Occasionally, anti-IgE therapy with omalizumab may be tried in patients who are CS dependent and continue to remain uncontrolled, but this treatment is only suitable for highly selected patients. Allergen-specific immunotherapy may be considered in this group; however, the risk of severe events including death is highest in patients with severe asthma.

STEP-DOWN TREATMENT

Once asthma patients achieve stable symptoms and have stable peak flow readings, it is important to slowly decrease therapy to find the optimal dose to control symptoms. Indeed, asthma severity may fluctuate and improve with time, owing to improved disease management, changes in environmental exposure, or because of the natural history of the disease, and most asthma guidelines recommend a step-down approach once patients are controlled.[1] Overtreatment of patients, particularly with ICS, can cause significant morbidity and adverse effects, especially in moderate-to-severe asthmatics. It may also be unnecessarily costly. Unfortunately, in such patients there is a tendency to maintain a static treatment regimen, even after symptoms are controlled and clinical stability is achieved. Studies have now supported the notion that stable asthmatic patients on high-dose ICS may be overtreated and that reductions in the inhaled dose can be achieved without significant increases in asthma exacerbations, visits to the family practitioner, or recourse to oral CS use.[58] A gradual reduction in medications starting with the treatment with the greatest toxicity should be attempted once stability is achieved and sustained for several months, and symptoms should be monitored on a long-term basis using both objective lung function and subjective symptom measures. Most patients should be maintained on an ICS, and this treatment should not be stopped as this provides anti-inflammatory protection. In those asthmatic patients that needed admission to hospital and/or ventilatory support, a longer period of stability on maintenance therapy may be justified before consideration of a step-down treatment approach.

MANAGEMENT OF REFRACTORY ASTHMA

Most asthmatic patients are controlled with appropriate stepwise therapy, but approximately 5% of asthmatics are difficult to control, do not remain symptom free despite maximal inhaled therapy, and may require maintenance treatment with oral CSs. In this group of patients, a thorough investigation of factors aggravating or contributing to poor asthma control should be undertaken. It is important to check adherence with medication and inhaler technique, particularly if the patient's disease is unstable despite the maximal recommended dose of therapy. Nonadherence with medication remains an important factor for the poor control of asthma and may be particularly manifest with ICS, as patients may be concerned about adverse effects or describe lack of immediate clinical benefit from this treatment. Monitoring adherence to ICS therapy in the clinic is difficult as there are no useful plasma measurements that can be made, however in contrast, the measurement of plasma cortisol suppression and absolute plasma drug concentrations may be useful in monitoring adherence to oral CSs. Evidence suggests nonadherence may be commoner in those with psychosocial problems or depression and these conditions should be actively sought and addressed during the clinical assessment. A detailed review of factors such as exposure to environmental allergens, unidentified occupational agents, or drugs that worsen asthma control such as aspirin or β-blockers should also be undertaken. Asthma may coexist with a number of disorders that can affect lung function, and the successful management of asthma often requires treatment of these associated conditions that are thought to aggravate asthmatic symptoms. Rhinosinusitis and gastroesophageal reflux disease are the most common of the disorders associated with poorly controlled asthma.

The relationship between rhinosinusitis and asthma is well established as described in the "united airway disease hypothesis," where treating the inflammation of allergic rhinitis in the upper airways has been shown to translate into improved asthma control.[59,60] It has also been postulated that poor asthma control may arise as a result of the inability of current inhaler devices to target drug therapy to the ongoing inflammation in the peripheral lung regions, and possibly treatment of this lung compartment with targeted anti-inflammatory therapy may result in improved symptoms.[53] In spite of the lack of data from meta-analyses which fail to show a consistent effect of antireflux therapy on asthma symptoms and lung function, many clinicians will assess and treat the possibility that gastroesophageal reflux disease may be aggravating asthma.[61]

As discussed earlier, patients with vocal cord dysfunction may present with wheeze and stridor and an escalation in asthma therapy. This disorder can be assessed using nasoendoscopy to observe abnormalities in the movement of the vocal cords, and if confirmed patients should be weaned off CSs. Speech therapy intervention may be helpful. Bronchoscopy or MDCT to exclude tracheobronchomalacia may be considered. A reconsideration of the potential differential diagnoses should be explored in the refractory asthmatic patient and this may require specialist referral (Table 46-3).

Patients who require high doses of oral CSs to maintain asthma control are referred to as CS-"dependent" asthmatics. In contrast, patients with complete CS-"resistant" asthma show a failure to respond to high-dose oral CS therapy, but this is very uncommon affecting less than 1 in 1000 patients. Several molecular mechanisms have been implicated in CS resistance and the impairment of their anti-inflammatory action, and this has led to the identification of new drug targets for future therapies.[62] There is evidence that in asthmatic patients who smoke (approximately 20% of the population), smoking itself hinders the anti-inflammatory action of CSs leading to relative CS resistance with the need for higher drug doses to achieve asthma control. It is recognized that smoking asthmatics compared to nonsmoking asthmatics have a faster decline in lung function, more severe asthma, more frequent hospital admissions, and a higher risk of death. Smoking cessation should be strongly pursued in this group as this intervention has been shown to reduce CS resistance and improve lung function.

Some asthmatic patients have unstable disease with rapid variations in lung function that may lead to recurrent and severe attacks of asthma, despite appropriate treatment for the disease.[63] These patients may be divided into type I brittle asthma, where there is a sustained pattern of chaotic peak flow variability on a daily basis or; type II brittle asthma, where asthma symptoms and lung function are well controlled, but there are abrupt and unpredictable falls in peak flow that may be catastrophic and result in sudden death. These patients are difficult to treat as they do not usually respond to maximal high-dose CS therapy but rely and need subcutaneous epinephrine injections. The assessment of treatment adherence and education on allergen avoidance is particularly important in these patients and they should wear an identification bracelet of their condition. The importance of carrying a portable epinephrine autoinjector at all times and being taught to self-administer this treatment should be a central part of their management.

ASTHMA EDUCATION AND MONITORING

Asthma education and training is important as patients need to understand the disease, its management, how to use inhalers properly, adverse effects of treatment, and importantly when to use reliever and controller treatments. Education may improve adherence to treatment recommendations and also engage the patient in self-management strategies particularly in terms of recognizing their symptoms, identifying and avoiding asthma triggers, objectively measuring any deterioration in their asthma control, and treating exacerbations of asthma at their earliest stages by stepping up their therapy. Educating the patient in the self-administration of oral CSs and access to healthcare advice are also important elements in a management program, which are designed to reduce emergency hospitalizations and patient morbidity. Studies have shown that written personal patient action plans result in better asthma control, reduced emergency room visits and hospitalizations, and decreased morbidity in both adults and children. Written plans are particularly useful and recommended in patients with unstable disease who have frequent exacerbations. The additional provision of a program of educational sessions (one-to-one or in small groups) with a knowledgeable healthcare professional has been shown to be more effective than written materials alone. Like drug therapy, the educational program and the method and frequency of reinforcement should be tailored to the patient's individual needs. Patients should be reassured that with proper treatment, their symptoms and occasional exacerbations can be minimized, and in most cases a normal lifestyle and life expectancy can be anticipated.

Home monitoring of asthma symptoms and control is an important aspect of self-management programmers. PEF measurements allow patients to be monitored on a long-term basis with relative ease using hand-held, compact, portable devices. Asthma treatment guidelines recommend patients use PEF measurements not only to monitor the course of the disease, but also to dictate self-administered treatment regimens.[1] Indeed, studies show improvements in measures of asthma control when peak flow measurements are used by patients (in relation to their personal best peak flow) to adjust medication usage. However, despite the advantages of written plans highlighted above, the US Centers for Disease Control and Prevention (CDC) analyzed asthma data from adults and children between 2001 and 2009 in a national health interview survey and showed that only one-third of patients with asthma reported being given a written asthma action plan, and just over two-thirds of patients had been taught the appropriate response to symptoms of an asthma attack.[64] It should be recognized that not all patients are capable of comprehending and executing complicated treatment plans. There are also concerns that peak flow–guided self-management may lead to overtreatment with medication, and hence the potential for increased morbidity due to adverse effects. Similarly, patients with severe asthma in whom self-management plans are more readily recommended, may tend to use more oral CSs where it may be unclear whether the increased use is appropriate or medically warranted (although the increase in medication may be initially viewed as a potential benefit of peak flow monitoring). Action plans should be written using clear, simple language and individualized based on patients' understanding of their asthma, its severity, and their demonstrated ability to comply with instructions.

MANAGEMENT OF ACUTE SEVERE ASTHMA

Asthma is characterized by exacerbations of disease, which can lead to substantial morbidity, occasional mortality, and considerable medical and economic costs. Patients with asthma fear disease exacerbations as they can be life-threatening and exacerbation-prone patients seem to be at increased risk for attacks of near-fatal asthma. Analysis of asthma mortality data identifies that patients experience worsening symptoms and deterioration in asthma control of a period of several hours to several days, before the event.[65] Indeed, life-threatening episodes can develop in any asthmatic patient, but particularly those patients with severe and poorly controlled disease; those who frequently access the emergency room; or patients who are hospitalized, are all recognized to be at high risk of life-threatening events. The importance of educating all patients with asthma should not be underestimated, as well as their carers, and in particular healthcare professional should identify and closely monitor such at-risk patients.

CLINICAL FEATURES

Patients with a moderate exacerbation of their disease notice a deterioration in their asthma control by an increase in daytime and nocturnal symptoms of cough, chest tightness, wheeze, and dyspnea, that do not respond to their usual maintenance therapy and require more reliever drug. A history of prodromal symptoms may be elicited that precede an asthma attack, such as itching under the chin, discomfort between the scapulae, or inexplicable fear (impending doom). A fall in home peak flow recordings also signify a worsening of asthma and the GINA guidelines classify exacerbations based on the peak flow into mild (PEF >80% predicted), moderate (PEF between >60% and 80% predicted), and acute severe (PEF between <60% predicted).[1] Patients may become so breathless in acute severe exacerbations that they become exhausted, unable to talk freely in complete sentences, and show life-threatening features of confusion, agitation, and cyanosis. Clinical examination usually shows an increased respiratory rate, hyperinflation, and tachycardia. In acute severe asthma, pulsus paradoxus (the accentuated decrease in systolic blood pressure [>10 mm Hg] during inspiration), may be present. Life-threatening signs are a silent chest, bradycardia, and hypotension. Investigations will show a marked fall in PEF and spirometric values; hypoxemic saturations on air and arterial blood gases may reveal a low Pa_{O_2}, and initially a low Pa_{CO_2} usually due to hyperventilation. In life-threatening situations the PEF will be <30% of predicted, oxygen saturation (Sa_{O_2}) measured by pulse oximetry <92% and, arterial blood gases on air will show a Pa_{O_2} <60 mm Hg (8 kPa) and a rising Pa_{CO_2} will indicate impending respiratory failure and requires immediate monitoring and therapy. A chest radiograph is not routinely recommended in the absence of a suspected pneumothorax, pulmonary consolidation, failure to respond to treatment satisfactorily, or a requirement for ventilation.

PHARMACOLOGIC TREATMENT

The cornerstone of therapy for worsening asthma control requires the escalation of both ICSs and quick-relief inhaled β_2-agonists.[1] Exacerbations of asthma should never be treated by escalating bronchodilators alone and asthma fatalities usually result when patients fail to promptly seek medical attention. Studies have shown patients dying from asthma commonly self-medicate with escalating doses of reliever bronchodilator medication in the preceding days to an asthma attack. A short course of oral CS therapy for at least several days may be needed to control and prevent a mild–moderate exacerbation and tapering of the dose should be undertaken with close outpatient follow-up. Very mild or subacute exacerbations in asthmatics with mild persistent disease may be managed in some cases by escalating the dose of ICSs in cases in which patients are taking low-doseCS. In less severe exacerbations, patients who promptly respond to treatment in the emergency department may be discharged but close outpatient follow-up is essential.

In patients with an acute severe exacerbation presenting to the emergency department, oxygen at high concentrations and high flows should be given continuously by face mask to achieve oxygen saturations (Sp_{O_2}) of between 94% and 98%. Hypoxemia is to be avoided at all costs, as patients die from hypoxemia in acute asthma and oxygen therapy is critical to prevent death in severe acute asthma, so continuous monitoring of oxygen saturation is needed until there is a meaningful response to treatment.

High doses of inhaled SABA given either by nebulizer (oxygen-driven) or via a pMDI with a spacer should be the first-line agents in acute asthma and be administered as early as possible. While generally well tolerated, occasionally nebulized bronchodilators cause arrhythmia and continuous electrocardiogram monitoring is required. In those patients in whom inhaled therapy cannot be used reliably, or in severely ill patients with impending respiratory failure, intravenous β_2-agonists may be given. In patients not responding, nebulized anticholinergic treatment (ipratropium bromide) may be added as they provide additional bronchodilation. Systemic CSs should be given in adequate doses in all cases of acute severe asthma for at least 5 days or until recovery and should be tapered after this response over a 2-week period, particularly in cases of severe asthma exacerbations. In patients unable to take oral CSs, intravenous therapy (e.g., hydrocortisone) should be administered in the emergency department.

A single dose of intravenous magnesium sulfate for patients has been shown to be effective when added to inhaled β_2-agonists. It is relatively well tolerated and can be considered in patients with acute severe asthma who have not had an initial good response to inhaled bronchodilator therapy, or in those with life-threatening features.

Patients should be referred to the intensive care unit for intubation and ventilation if they have acute severe or life-threatening asthma that is failing to respond to therapy indicated by: a deteriorating PEF, worsening hypoxemia, a normal or rising Pa_{CO_2}, poor respiratory effort, and exhaustion or confusion. Intravenous aminophylline may be used, but the risks of toxicity are much greater than when inhaled β_2-adrenergic agonists are used. Sedatives should never be given as they may depress ventilation, and antibiotics should not be routinely administered, unless there are clinical or radiologic signs of pneumonia.

ACKNOWLEDGMENT

Dr. Omar Usmani is a recipient of a UK National Institute for Health Research (NIHR) Career Development Fellowship.

REFERENCES

1. Global Strategy for Asthma Management and Prevention, Global Initiative for Asthma (GINA). 2012. Available at: http://www.ginasthma.org/. Accessed February 10, 2013.
2. Borish L, Culp JA. Asthma: a syndrome composed of heterogeneous diseases. *Ann Allergy Asthma Immunol.* 2008;101(1):1–8.
3. Haldar P, Pavord ID, Shaw DE, et al. Cluster analysis and clinical asthma phenotypes. *Am J Respir Crit Care Med.* 2008;178:218–224.
4. Pekkanen J, Lampi J, Genuneit J, Hartikainen AL, Järvelin MR. Analyzing atopic and non-atopic asthma. *Eur J Epidemiol.* 2012; 27:281–286.
5. Pearce N, Pekkanen J, Beasley R. How much asthma is really attributable to atopy? *Thorax.* 1999;54:268–272.
6. Ronchetti R, Jesenak M, Rennerova Z, Barreto M, Ronchetti F, Villa MP. Relationship between atopic asthma and the population prevalence rates for asthma or atopy in children: atopic and nonatopic asthma in epidemiology. *Allergy Asthma Proc.* 2009; 30:55–63.
7. Jackson DJ, Sykes A, Mallia P, Johnston SL. Asthma exacerbations: origin, effect, and prevention. *J Allergy Clin Immunol.* 2011; 128:1165–1174.
8. Proud D. Role of rhinovirus infections in asthma. *Asian Pac J Allergy Immunol.* 2011;29:201–208.
9. Holt PG, Sly PD. Viral infections and atopy in asthma pathogenesis: new rationales for asthma prevention and treatment. *Nat Med.* 2012;18:726–735.
10. Shore S. Obesity and asthma: location, location, location. *Eur Respir J.* 2013;41:253–254.
11. Ledford DK, Lockey RF. Asthma and comorbidities. *Curr Opin Allergy Clin Immunol.* 2013;13:78–86.
12. Niimi A. Cough and asthma. *Curr Respir Med Rev.* 2011;7: 47–54.
13. Thornton J, Lewis J, Lebrun CM, Licskai CJ. Clinical characteristics of women with menstrual-linked asthma. *Respir Med.* 2012;106:1236–1243.
14. Velazquez JR, Teran LM. Aspirin-intolerant asthma: a comprehensive review of biomarkers and pathophysiology. *Clin Rev Allergy Immunol.*2013;45(1):75–86.
15. Henneberger PK, Redlich CA, Callahan DB, et al. An official American Thoracic Society statement: work-exacerbated asthma. *Am J Respir Crit Care Med.* 2011;184:368–378.
16. Tarlo SM, Lemiere C. Occupational asthma. *N Engl J Med.* 2014; 370:640–649.
17. Sorkness RL, Bleeker ER, Busse W, et al. Lung function in adults with stable but severe asthma: air trapping and incomplete reversal of obstruction with bronchodilation. *J Appl Physiol.* 2008; 104(2):394–403.
18. Hanania NA, Celli BR, Donohue JF, Martin UJ. Bronchodilator reversibility in COPD. *Chest.* 2011;140:1055–1063.
19. Barnes PJ. Against the Dutch hypothesis: asthma and chronic obstructive pulmonary disease are distinct diseases. *Am J Respir Crit Care Med.* 2006;174:240–243.
20. Gibson PG, Simpson JL. The overlap syndrome of asthma and COPD: what are its features and how important is it? *Thorax.* 2009;64:728–735.
21. Anderson SD, Brannan JD. Bronchial provocation testing: the future. *Curr Opin Allergy Clin Immunol.* 2011;11:46–52.
22. Sears MR. Predicting new and persistent asthma. *Am J Respir Crit Care Med.* 2012;186:469–470.
23. Green RH, Brightling CE, McKenna S, et al. Asthma exacerbations and sputum eosinophil counts: a randomised controlled trial. *Lancet.* 2002;360:1715–1721.
24. Randolph C. Diagnostic exercise challenge testing. *Curr Allergy Asthma Rep.* 2011;11:482–490.
25. Barnes PJ, Dweik RA, Gelb AF, et al. Exhaled nitric oxide in pulmonary diseases: a comprehensive review. *Chest.* 2010;138: 682–692.
26. Usmani OS, Barnes PJ. Assessing and treating small airways disease in asthma and chronic obstructive pulmonary disease. *Ann Med.* 2012;44:146–156.
27. Paredi P, Kharitonov SA, Meah S, Barnes PJ, Usmani OS. A novel approach to partition central and peripheral airway nitric oxide. *Chest.* 2014;145:113–119.
28. Reddel HK, Taylor DR, Bateman ED, et al. An official American Thoracic Society/European Respiratory Society statement: asthma control and exacerbations: standardizing endpoints for clinical asthma trials and clinical practice. *Am J Respir Crit Care Med.* 2009;180:59–99.

29. Balkissoon R, Kenn K. Asthma: vocal cord dysfunction (VCD) and other dysfunctional breathing disorders. *Semin Respir Crit Care Med.* 2012;33:595–605.
30. Pacheco-Galván A, Hart SP, Morice AH. Relationship between gastro-oesophageal reflux and airway diseases: the airway reflux paradigm. *Arch Bronconeumol.* 2011;47:195–203.
31. Berger W. Aerosol devices and asthma therapy. *Curr Drug Deliv.* 2009;6:38–49.
32. Plaza V, Sanchis J, Roura P, et al. Physicians' knowledge of inhaler devices and inhalation techniques remains poor in Spain. *J Aerosol Med Pulm Drug Deliv.* 2012;25:16–22.
33. Dolovich MB, Ahrens RC, Hess DR, et al. Device selection and outcomes of aerosol therapy: evidence-based guidelines: American College of Chest Physicians/American College of Asthma, Allergy, and Immunology. *Chest.* 2005;127:335–371.
34. Wilkes W, Fink J, Dhand R. Selecting an accessory device with a metered-dose inhaler: variable influence of accessory devices on fine particle dose, throat deposition, and drug delivery with asynchronous actuation from a metered-dose inhaler. *J Aerosol Med.* 2001;14:351–360.
35. Azouz W, Chrystyn H. Clarifying the dilemmas about inhalation techniques for dry powder inhalers: integrating science with clinical practice. *Prim Care Respir J.* 2012;21:208–213.
36. Muers MF. Overview of nebulizer treatment. *Thorax.* 1997;52:S25–S30.
37. Dolovich M. Aerosol delivery to children: what to use, how to choose. *Pediatr Pulmonol Suppl.* 1999;18:79–82.
38. Smaldone GC. Smart nebulizers. *Respir Care.* 2002;47:1434–1441.
39. Barnes PJ. Distribution of receptor targets in the lung. *Proc Am Thorac Soc.* 2004;1:345–351.
40. Barnes PJ. Scientific rationale for inhaled combination therapy with long-acting beta2-agonists and corticosteroids. *Eur Respir J.* 2002;19:182–191.
41. Chapman KR, Barnes NC, Greening AP, Jones PW, Pedersen S. Single maintenance and reliever therapy (SMART) of asthma: a critical appraisal. *Thorax.* 2010;65:747–752.
42. Chowdhury BA, Dal Pan G. The FDA and safe use of long-acting beta-agonists in the treatment of asthma. *N Engl J Med.* 2010;362:1169–1171.
43. Morrow T. Implications of pharmacogenomics in the current and future treatment of asthma. *J Manag Care Pharm.* 2007;13:497–505.
44. Barnes PJ. Theophylline. *Am J Respir Crit Care Med.* 2013;188:901–906.
45. Louis R, Schleich F, Barnes PJ. Corticosteroids: still at the frontline in asthma treatment? *Clin Chest Med.* 2012;33:531–541.
46. Adcock IM, Maneechotesuwan K, Usmani O. Molecular interactions between glucocorticoids and long-acting beta2-agonists. *J Allergy Clin Immunol.* 2002;110:S261–S268.
47. Derendorf H, Nave R, Drollmann A, Cerasoli F, Wurst W. Relevance of pharmacokinetics and pharmacodynamics of inhaled corticosteroids to asthma. *Eur Respir J.* 2006;28:1042–1050.
48. Polosa R. Critical appraisal of antileukotriene use in asthma management. *Curr Opin Pulm Med.* 2007;13:24–30.
49. Kuhl K, Hanania NA. Targeting IgE in asthma. *Curr Opin Pulm Med.* 2012;18:1–5.
50. Cappella A, Durham SR. Allergen immunotherapy for allergic respiratory diseases. *Hum Vaccin Immunother.* 2012;8:1499–1512.
51. Huntley A, White AR, Ernst E. Relaxation therapies for asthma: a systematic review. *Thorax.* 2002;57:127–131.
52. Demoly P, Annunziata K, Gubba E, Adamek L. Repeated cross-sectional survey of patient-reported asthma control in Europe in the past 5 years. *Eur Respir Rev.* 2012;21:66–74.
53. Usmani OS. Treating the small airways. *Respiration.* 2012;84:441–453.
54. Barnes PJ. Severe asthma: advances in current management and future therapy. *J Allergy Clin Immunol.* 2012;129:48–59.
55. Wechsler ME, Laviolette M, Rubin AS, et al. Bronchial thermoplasty: long-term safety and effectiveness in patients with severe persistent asthma. *J Allergy Clin Immunol.* 2013;132:1295–1302.
56. Usmani OS, Ito K, Maneechotesuwan K, et al. Glucocorticoid receptor nuclear translocation in airway cells after inhaled combination therapy. *Am J Respir Crit Care Med.* 2005;172:704–712.
57. Kerstjens HA, Engel M, Dahl R, et al. Tiotropium in asthma poorly controlled with standard combination therapy. *N Engl J Med.* 2012;367:1198–1207.
58. Hawkins G, McMahon AD, Twaddle S, Wood SF, Ford I, Thomson NC. Stepping down inhaled corticosteroids in asthma: randomised controlled trial. *BMJ.* 2003;326:1115–1118.
59. Compalati E, Ridolo E, Passalacqua G, Braido F, Villa E, Canonica GW. The link between allergic rhinitis and asthma: the united airways disease. *Expert Rev Clin Immunol.* 2010;6:413–423.
60. Corren J, Manning BE, Thompson SF, Hennessy S, Strom BL. Rhinitis therapy and the prevention of hospital care for asthma: a case-control study. *J Allergy Clin Immunol.* 2004;113:415–419.
61. Chan WW, Chiou E, Obstein KL, Tignor AS, Whitlock TL. The efficacy of proton pump inhibitors for the treatment of asthma in adults: a meta-analysis. *Arch Intern Med.* 2011;171:620–629.
62. Barnes PJ. Corticosteroid resistance in patients with asthma and chronic obstructive pulmonary disease. *J Allergy Clin Immunol.* 2013;131:636–645.
63. Toungoussova O, Foschino Barbaro MP, Esposito LM, et al. Brittle asthma. *Monaldi Arch Chest Dis.* 2007;67:102–105.
64. Centers for Disease Control and Prevention Vital Signs - Asthma in the US. http://www.cdc.gov/vitalsigns/Asthma/. Accessed February 10, 2013.
65. Tattersfield AE, Postma DS, Barnes PJ, et al. Exacerbations of asthma: a descriptive study of 425 severe exacerbations. The FACET International Study Group. *Am J Respir Crit Care Med.* 1999;160:594–599.

CHAPTER 47

Aspirin- and Exercise-Induced Asthma

Jose L. Gomez
Geoffrey L. Chupp
Gregory P. Geba

Asthma is well known to be triggered by specific immune factors such as aeroallergen exposures. There are, however, several important nonallergic triggers for the development of asthmatic bronchial obstruction. Two of the most important are aspirin and related nonsteroidal anti-inflammatory drugs (NSAIDS) and exercise. Both can provoke airway responses in the setting of established symptomatic aeroallergen-induced asthma or in isolation. These two nonspecific triggers may also share pathophysiologic mechanisms, including mast cell and leukotriene-related pathways, and may be related to vascular response–mediated airway narrowing.

ASPIRIN-INDUCED ASTHMA

The first report of aspirin-induced asthma (AIA) was that of Hirschberg in 1902. Six decades later, the association between aspirin sensitivity, asthma, and nasal polyps was documented in a classic paper by Samter and Beer.[1] In 1928, the clinical importance of sensitivity to aspirin was highlighted by van Leewen, who challenged 100 asthmatics with aspirin, provoking bronchoconstriction in 16. Several others[2,3] have made similar observations, documenting a prevalence of aspirin sensitivity in asthmatics that ranges from 5% to as high as 30%, depending on the characteristics of the asthmatics studied (severity increases risk) and the criteria applied to make the diagnosis.

Aspirin was originally recognized as the first drug capable of precipitating asthma. With the development of chemically related analgesic and nonsteroidal anti-inflammatory drugs (NSAIDs) after 1950, other agents were found to exacerbate asthma. In a study of 781 asthmatics observed over a period of 2 years, drugs were noted to provoke asthmatic airway responses in 10.5% of patients.[4] Reactions to NSAIDs were thought to be responsible for 77% of all cases, with aspirin accounting for two-thirds of the reactions to NSAIDs, or nearly 50% of all cases of drug-induced asthma. Therefore, although aspirin is the most common drug to induce asthma and the most common NSAID to cause asthma, other NSAIDs are responsible for an important number of these reactions.

■ CLINICAL PRESENTATION

Reactions to aspirin take two distinct forms: Cutaneous—most commonly characterized by urticaria and angioedema,[5] and respiratory—characterized by rhinoconjunctivitis and bronchospasm.[6] The cutaneous reactions that develop after the ingestion of NSAIDs include hives with or without angioedema, may develop in individuals with a history of chronic urticaria or healthy individuals, and are the result of exposure to a single drug in this class or to one of multiple NSAIDs.[5] The wide spectrum of underlying variables suggests that the pathogenic processes leading to these clinical presentations are diverse. The fact that a great majority of patients were able to tolerate the same NSAIDs before the development of the urticarial process, suggests that the NSAIDs interact with an underlying urticarial tendency but do not directly and independently cause the hives. This explains why the avoidance of NSAIDs does not eliminate the urticarial symptoms in all patients. However, the identification of the reaction as one provoked by a single or by multiple NSAIDs is fundamental to develop a therapeutic plan in these subjects, to provide guidance with respect to the restriction of exposure to the inciting agent in this therapeutic class.

The respiratory manifestations of aspirin sensitivity involve both the upper (nasal) and lower airway (asthma), and are generally temporally linked. Sometimes, upper respiratory symptoms, typically rhinitis, precede the development of lower respiratory reactions to these agents. AIA can occur on a background of established asthma or can appear de novo without previous asthma symptoms. This observation has led to the use of more accurate descriptors for this condition including, aspirin-induced asthma (AIA) or aspirin-exacerbated respiratory disease (AERD), the latter a more inclusive term that extends beyond the lower airway manifestations (asthma), to include the upper airway (nasal and sinus mucosa).

The typical presentation of this syndrome is characterized by an initial complaint of upper respiratory symptoms, similar to those caused by a viral illness. The syndrome peaks in the third decade of life. Upper respiratory symptoms become persistent and extend to involve the nasal mucosa and paranasal sinuses. Marked eosinophilia is often observed in the setting of chronic rhinitis, and nasal polyps. A detailed history documenting a relationship between the ingestion of aspirin and/or NSAIDs and the upper and lower respiratory symptoms helps to establish the connection between these agents and the development of nasal polyps. Typically, though symptoms may improve, the inflammation persists despite substantially reduced or absent exposure to aspirin or NSAIDs.

In addition to Samter's classical description of nasal polyps, asthma, and aspirin sensitivity,[1] the documentation of sinusitis involving one or several paranasal sinuses at some point in the disease in almost all patients is an additional feature of the syndrome.[7] The nasal and sinus inflammation is often accompanied by anosmia, recurrent sinus infections often leading to recurrent surgeries to remove polyps to provide relief for the chronic sinus congestion. Opacification of one or more sinuses on plain radiographs can be seen in 90% of these patients, while sinus CT has a higher sensitivity to detect mucosal thickening resulting from chronic hyperplastic eosinophilic sinusitis, and air fluid levels.

Atopy does not seem to be the main pathogenic mechanism in AIA. This observation is based on evidence from multiple sources and includes the observation that many patients with AIA are not atopic; with a rate of positive aeroallergen skin testing between 30% and 60%, a substantial proportion exhibit negative skin tests and IgE levels in the normal range. The documentation of NSAID-specific IgEs has not been successful, and the peripheral blood eosinophilia, complement activation, and serum histamine elevation seen after acute aeroallergen challenge of atopic asthmatics, are absent after acute aspirin challenge. Thus, the term, pseudoallergy has been used to describe some of the AIA reactions.

In contrast, the typical reaction after aspirin ingestion in these patients is the slow development (within ½ to 4 hours, mean 50 minutes) of nasal congestion with profuse rhinorrhea, cutaneous flushing involving the head and neck, conjunctivitis, and bronchial obstruction, the latter usually manifested as wheezing. A typical reaction provoked by an oral challenge under laboratory conditions is illustrated in Figure 47-1. In severe reactions, headache, nausea and vomiting, and acute hypercarbic respiratory failure culminating in death can occur. Life-threatening responses with faster kinetics have also been reported with systemically administered NSAIDs such as ketorolac.[8]

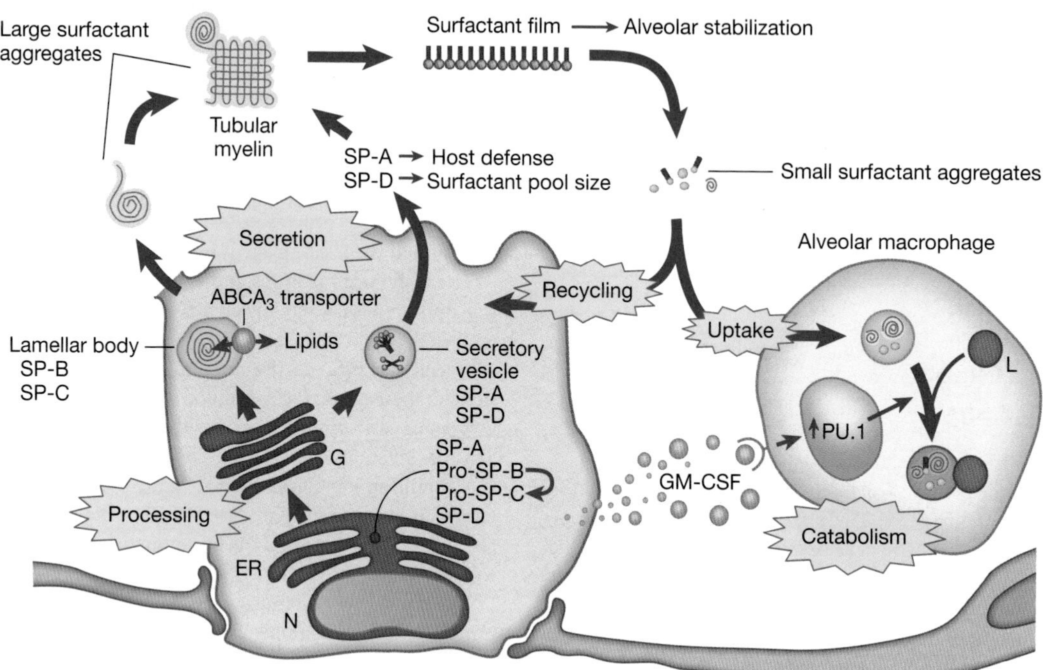

Figure 47-1 Typical reaction to aspirin in AIA. The timeline illustrates the kinetics of respiratory compromise and nasoocular symptoms after graded aspirin or placebo challenge. IPPB, intermittent positive-pressure ventilation with β-adrenergic agonist bronchodilator. *(Data from Stevenson DD, Simon RA. Aspirin sensitivity: Respiratory and cutaneous manifestations, in Middleton E Jr, et al (eds). Allergy: Principles and Practice. St. Louis, CV Mosby. 1993;1747–1767.)*

Combined cutaneous and respiratory reactions (i.e., true urticarial eruptions in association with asthma) occur in <3% of cases.[9]

GENETICS

In contrast to classic atopic asthma, which patients develop during childhood and adolescence, AIA typically occurs in individuals in the third to fourth decade of life. An original report by Lockey describing a consanguineous family suggested an autosomal recessive pattern.[10] However, a subsequent report by Von Maur indicated an autosomal dominant pattern.[11] The late onset of the disease points to important environmental influences that may play a significant role in the development of the syndrome. Both genders are affected by the disease; however, the prevalence is higher in women than men.

Notwithstanding the lack of familial association in most cases, one study did show an increase in the expression of *HLA-DQW2* in a group of patients.[12] A later study showed increased expression of *HLA-DPB1*0301* (Odds ratios: 4.4 and 5.3) and decreased expression of *DPB1*0401* (OR: 0.42 and 0.48) in AIA versus normals and nonaspirin-sensitive asthmatics, respectively, among Europeans.[13] Korean investigators confirmed a higher risk of AIA in patients carrying *HLA-DPB1*0301*, while those carrying *HLA-DRB1*1302* and or *DQB1*0609* exhibited a higher risk of aspirin-induced urticaria.[14]

Several genes in the arachidonic acid pathway have been associated with molecular defects responsible for aspects of the pathogenesis of the disease. The single nucleotide polymorphism (SNP) rs730012 (A-444C) in the Leukotriene C4 synthase *(LTC4S)* gene was associated with higher gene expression in blood eosinophils and higher relative risk of AIA (2.62; 95% CI: 1.38, 4.98) in Europeans with AIA.[15] An additional study from the same group showed a functional and gender association of the rs20417 SNP (G-765C) in the *COX-2* promoter region in AIA patients with more severe disease.[16] A Japanese group found an association between the rs4794067 SNP in the *TBX21* gene, the human analogue for the *T-bet* gene in mice, that, when absent, had previously been shown to result in airway eosinophilia and hyperresponsiveness. The rs4794067 polymorphism was in linkage disequilibrium with a synonymous coding 390A-G SNP in exon 1 and was significantly associated with AIA.[17] Another study showed heightened transcription or polymorphisms in the 5-lipooxygenase activating protein *(ALOX5AP)* gene in AIA.[18] New insight may result from the recent observation of selective expression in AIA patients of cysteinyl leukotriene type 2 receptor, but not type 1 receptor, expressed by infiltrating inflammatory cells of the upper airway, not observed in aspirin-sensitive patients with chronic allergic rhinitis and normal controls.[19]

The number of genetic studies in AIA has increased significantly over the last decade, with the advent of high throughput technologies. The majority of studies have used a candidate gene approach, with some positive associations. The interpretation of the evidence suggests that the development of AIA is the result of the interaction between multiple polymorphisms and the environment; however, some of these findings in specific populations may not be generalizable to all individuals with disease due to different allelic frequencies and individual environmental risk factors that modify the AIA phenotype.

Gene expression profiling of nasal polyps of individuals with AIA has shown higher levels of periostin expression;[20] this observation is particularly relevant for both the upper and lower airway, since periostin is also secreted by bronchial epithelial cells and is associated with TGF-β stimulation and increased extracellular matrix deposition in the airway of asthmatics.[21]

CROSS-REACTIVITY

Cross-reactivity of aspirin with other NSAIDs was first recognized in 1967 by Vanselow and Smith.[22] This report was followed by others of reactions to structurally unrelated NSAIDs, which suggested that these reactions were not atopic in nature. It was subsequently shown that the ability of these drugs to provoke asthma in susceptible patients was related to their ability to inhibit cyclooxygenase (COX), and that the degree of cross-reactivity with aspirin was related to the degree to which these agents inhibited COX in vitro.[23,24] Subsequently, the discovery of isoforms of COX has revealed that the dominant form that is inhibited by low doses of aspirin and is capable of eliciting airways responses in AIA is COX-1. Drugs that are less potent inhibitors of COX-1, but are structurally related to aspirin (e.g., sodium salicylate), at clinical doses, do not provoke AIA.

The association of AIA with the COX-1 isoform of the enzyme has been strengthened by studies with specific inhibitors of COX-2, which, at clinical doses, nearly completely spare inhibition of COX-1. Two separate studies have shown convincingly that selective inhibitors of COX-2 (celecoxib and rofecoxib) do not provoke airway changes typical of AIA in patients known to have the disorder, or in those who were challenged in the laboratory de novo in the process of diagnosing the disease.[25,26] In individuals challenged with celecoxib, including high doses, no reaction was seen (Fig. 47-2).[27,28] The increased risk of thrombotic cardiovascular events with rofecoxib and celecoxib, has limited the evaluation of these effects in larger populations of individuals with AIA. A list of NSAIDs reported to provoke AIA and those not associated with AIA is given in Table 47-1.

Curiously, although at least two studies involving nearly 100 subjects showed that a later generation, highly specific COX-2

TABLE 47-1 NSAIDs in Aspirin-Induced Asthma (AIA)

NSAIDs that Can Provoke Airway Narrowing in AIA
Carboxylic acids
Salicylates
Acetylsalicylic acid (aspirin, Easpirin, Zorpin)
Acetic acids
Indomethacin (Indocin)
Sulindac (Clinoril)
Tolmetin (Tolectin)
Diclofenac (Voltaren)
Ketorolac (Toradol)
Zomepirac (Zomax)
Propionic acids
Ibuprofen (Motrin, Advil, Nuprin)
Naproxen (Naprosyn)
Fenamates
Meclofenamate (Meclomen)
Mefenamic acid (Ponstel)
Enolic acids
Piroxicam (Feldene)
NSAIDs and Analgesics that Appear to Be Well Tolerated in AIA
Sodium salicylate
Choline salicylate
Salicylamide
Dextropropoxyphene
Acetaminophen in low doses
Selective COX-2 inhibitors

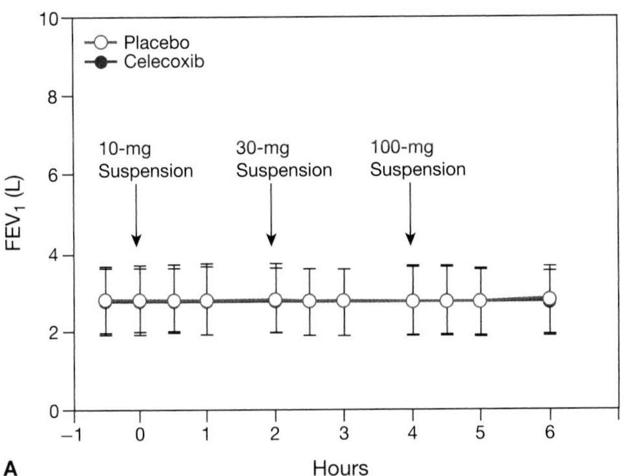

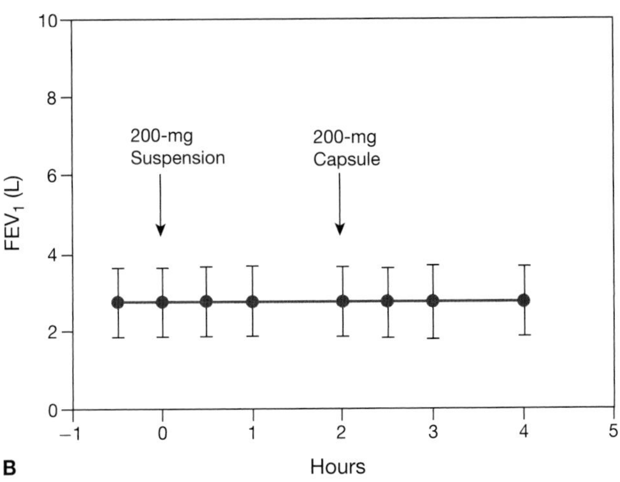

Figure 47-2 Lack of airway bronchoconstriction to increasing doses of a COX-2 inhibitor in aspirin-sensitive asthmatics. FEV_1 measured before and after oral challenge. **A.** Double-blind crossover challenge. **B.** Open label challenge. *(Reproduced with permission from Gyllfors P, et al. Biochemical and clinical evidence that aspirin-intolerant asthmatic subjects tolerate the cyclo-oxygenase 2-selective drug celecoxib. J Allergy Clin Immunol. 2003;111(5):1116–1121.)*

inhibitor, etoricoxib, did not provoke acute responses with doses up to 120 mg,[29,30] another study showed a small, though detectable risk of cutaneous reactions after challenge with etoricoxib.[31] In one case report involving a single patient, challenge with etoricoxib was associated with a reduction of FEV_1 and development of rhinorrhea 30 minutes after a 60 mg dose. Thus, although the vast majority of patients with ASA may not develop symptoms when administered COX-2 inhibitors, confirmation of ability to tolerate these agents with formal testing may be the most conservative approach.

A number of other analgesics have long been considered to be well tolerated in patients with AIA. They are also listed in Table 47-1. However, some analgesics, formerly considered safe for use by these patients, were subsequently shown to be capable of provoking bronchospasm if given in large doses. For example, doses generally greater than 1000 mg of acetaminophen, and salicylate, at doses of 2000 mg or greater, can provoke significant declines in FEV_1 in some aspirin-sensitive asthmatics. Reactions to high doses of these drugs, when they occur, tend to be milder than those seen with aspirin. A similar phenomenon has been observed with meloxicam and nimesulide, drugs that inhibit COX-2 somewhat more than COX-1. At typical clinical doses they are generally well tolerated in patients with AIA; however, at high doses, cross-reactions may be observed.

The documentation of NSAID-specific IgE antibodies and anaphylactic reactions to NSAID after a period of sensitization is much less common than non–IgE-mediated reactions, which tend to occur after first exposure. However they must be considered in the differential diagnosis in the appropriate clinical situation. Avoidance of the specific NSAID involved prevents relapses.[32]

An interesting association of AIA with sensitivity to hydrocortisone has been made. After several case reports of the association, two studies[33] demonstrated that a small percentage of patients with aspirin-induced asthma may experience acute bronchospasm (15–30 minutes) after the intravenous or intramuscular injection of hydrocortisone. The vehicles and diluents used in the hydrocortisone preparations could not be linked to the reactivity. One of these studies showed no bronchoconstrictor response to methylprednisolone, dexamethasone, or betamethasone when given intravenously, indicating that these potent anti-inflammatory steroid preparations, related to hydrocortisone but with different side chain chemical structure, could be used safely.[34] The mechanism of this reaction is not known, though corticosteroids can reduce phospholipase PLA2 activity (generally decreasing eicosanoid production) and broadly inhibit isoforms of COX, especially COX-2.[35]

PATHOGENESIS

The combination of epidemiologic data, genetic and genomic information, with the observation that COX-2 inhibitors exhibit a relatively safe profile in individuals with AIA has pointed to key aspects of the pathophysiology of AIA. The main theory supports an alteration in the balance between leukotrienes and prostaglandins generated by the lipooxygenase- and COX-dependent pathways of arachidonic acid metabolism (Fig. 47-3). Other attempts to explain the spectrum of symptoms are based on the release of other mediators, most likely from mast cells, basophils, or platelets. These theories include upregulation of mast cell–basophil mediator release by substances not yet identified that affect mast cell membranes, increased histamine production by basophils of patients with aspirin-induced asthma in comparison to normal subjects, decreased production of prostaglandin E2 (PGE2) with enhanced production of leukotriene B4 (LTB4) by AIA basophils, and enhanced aspirin-induced release of serotonin and other mediators by AIA platelets.[9,36] It has been proposed that complement activation may be important in these processes.[37] However, the role of complement activation in AIA has been questioned by data showing no significant changes in CH50 and C4 levels in patients experiencing an asthma exacerbation after acute oral aspirin challenge.[38]

Alterations in arachidonic acid metabolism appear to play a central role in AIA. The major pathways of COX and lipooxygenase metabolism of arachidonic acid are illustrated in Figure 47-3. Arachidonic acid is derived from membrane phospholipid by phospholipase A2. It is then metabolized via the COX pathway to prostaglandins (COX-2 > COX-1) and thromboxanes (COX-1 > COX-2) or via the lipooxygenase pathway to sulfidopeptide (cysteinyl) leukotrienes. The leukotrienes have a variety of effects, including the induction of contraction of bronchial smooth muscle. In contrast, the prostaglandins, in particular PGE2, act as bronchodilators and may inhibit T cell–mediated inflammatory responses in the lung. Aspirin and the other NSAIDs that cause AIA inhibit COX-1 activity. A shift occurs after the administration of aspirin or appropriate doses of these other agents, shunting approximately 90% of the arachidonic acid metabolism to the 5-lipooxygenase pathway, decreasing prostaglandin and thromboxane production, and increasing leukotriene generation. In comparison to normal controls, patients with AIA generate leukotrienes in exaggerated quantities after aspirin challenge. Discovery that AIA patients produce less of the anti-inflammatory mediators lipoxins and 15-epimer lipoxin might enhance effects of this shift.[39] AIA patients may also be more sensitive than normal subjects to the bronchoconstrictor properties of leukotrienes (particularly LTE4) and more susceptible to the loss of the bronchodilating and potentially anti-inflammatory effects of PGE2. The data supporting these conclusions are briefly summarized below.

Several groups have analyzed the nasal lavage fluid from aspirin-sensitive and control patients and found inducible levels of cysteinyl leukotrienes and plasma proteins when patients with AIA received oral or nasal aspirin challenges.[40,41] One study found that LTC4 and LTD4 levels were not significantly induced in normal subjects, but could be induced to some degree in patients with allergic rhinitis and in those with isolated nasal polyps (rising 93% and 69% above baseline levels, respectively).[41] Similarly, although histamine levels rose significantly in the AIA group (greater than threefold increase in total protein) they did not rise significantly in the control groups. Analysis of the nasal lavage fluids showed impressive increases in lactoferrin and lysozyme, suggesting that submucosal glands are stimulated in this process.

In a follow-up study, the cellular source of these nasal abnormalities was investigated by analysis of nasal lavage fluid after induction by aspirin challenge for the presence of mast cell tryptase and eosinophil cationic protein (ECP).[40] Significant increases in nasal tryptase, histamine, and cysteinyl leukotrienes were observed after AIA was provoked in these patients. ECP levels at baseline were variable and did not

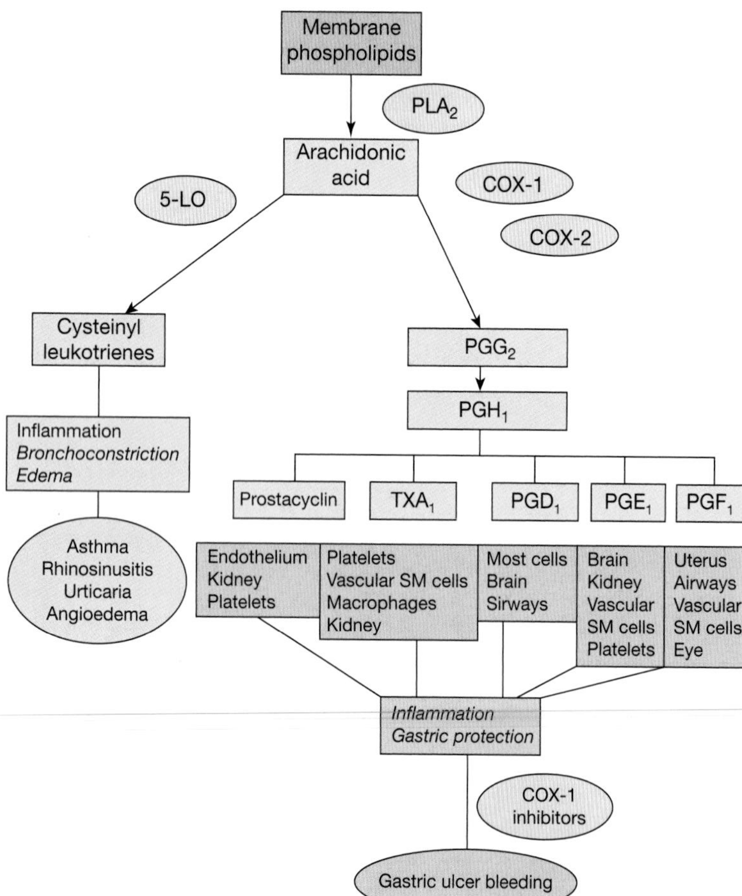

Figure 47-3 Enzymatic pathways of arachidonic acid metabolism. *(Reproduced with permission from Sanchez-Borges M, et al. Cutaneous reactions to aspirin and nonsteroidal anti-inflammatory drugs. Clin Rev Allergy Immunol. 2003;24(2):125–135.)*

increase significantly after challenge. A similar study before and after intranasal challenge with aspirin revealed changes in the vascular permeability of patients with AIA, an associated influx of eosinophils coupled with increased ECP, and an associated increase in tryptase suggestive of mast cell activation.[42] These findings are consistent with earlier work[8] that documented similar increases in blood tryptase (4 hours) and urinary LTE4 levels (6 hours); the decreases in blood eosinophil counts demonstrated could be associated with eosinophil recruitment at the tissue level after aspirin challenge.

The metabolism of arachidonic acid in the lung has not been studied as extensively. The available data show both similarities and differences with findings in the nose and circulation. For example, bronchoalveolar lavage fluid (BALF) obtained 30 minutes after inhalation of threshold doses of lysine–aspirin contained decreased levels of COX-dependent mediators (PGE2, PGD2, thromboxane B2 [TXB2], and PGF2α). However, only small increases in LTE4 and 5-hydroxyeicosatetraenoic acid (HETE) levels were noted. Lysine–aspirin inhalation also did not produce a significant rise in tryptase levels in BALF and led to a significant fall in ECP levels despite baseline eosinophil and ECP levels, which were higher in the AIA group than in placebo-treated nonasthmatic individuals.[43] The authors postulated that the altered pulmonary eicosanoid production might be related to eosinophilic inflammation in the airways of patients with AIA.

Additional understanding of the mechanism of bronchospasm in AIA has been gained by other investigators who used inhibitors of leukotriene effector function. One study administered a specific sulfidopeptide leukotriene receptor antagonist via inhalation and noted that it attenuated aspirin-induced asthma in five of six subjects by 43% to 74%.[44] This was followed by a double-blind, placebo-controlled, crossover study that showed that a specific leukotriene receptor antagonist given as a single oral dose 1 hour before perithreshold lysine–aspirin inhalant provocative challenge could almost completely block the development of aspirin-induced bronchospasm.[45] This was achieved without evidence of any direct bronchodilatory effect of the drug before lysine–aspirin challenge, confirming that leukotriene receptor antagonist was effective in preventing analgesic-induced (dipyrone) bronchospasm.

The effects of leukotrienes in the lung can also be modulated by blocking 5-lipooxygenase activation. The efficacy of this approach was demonstrated in a randomized, double-blind, crossover study in which the 5-lypooxygenase inhibitor zileuton (600 mg orally, four times a day, for 6–8 days before aspirin challenge) led to a greater than 70% reduction in baseline urinary LTE4 excretion, a greater than 60% reduction in mean maximal urinary concentration of LTE4 after aspirin challenge, and almost complete suppression of subthreshold and threshold oral aspirin-induced bronchospasm.[46] In addition, nasoocular, gastrointestinal, and cutaneous manifestations were reduced to the levels of symptoms produced by placebo challenge. Similar data have been generated with the cysteinyl leukotriene receptor antagonists montelukast and zafirlukast.[44,45,47]

Analysis of mast cells isolated from patients with AIA shows that the overproduction of cysteinyl leukotrienes by these cells is very sensitive to the regulatory role of PGE2, suggesting an additional molecular mechanism to account for the excess sensitivity to the COX inhibition associated with NSAIDS in AIA.[48] Altered cellular cross talk involving platelets and leukocytes has been recently recognized as a potential source of excess cysteinyl leukotrienes in individuals with AIA through a biologic mechanism known as transcellular biosynthesis.[49]

In summary, although the mechanism of AIA remains incompletely understood, there appears to be a clear role for lipooxygenase products in the pathogenesis of the disorder. The available data also suggest that mast cells, stimulated by aspirin directly or indirectly, discharge their leukotriene mediators in large amounts into nasal secretions, but may not play the same role in the lung. The presence of increased numbers of eosinophils and altered eosinophil phenotype may be more relevant to the pathophysiology in the lung and may be linked to the airway inflammation that characterizes this disorder. This probably reflects their recruitment secondary to the release of mast cell–derived mediators, including leukotrienes and cytokines.

DIAGNOSIS

Despite the characteristic clinical features of AIA, diagnostic evaluation is fundamental, given the presence of false positive and negative diagnosis based on clinical history alone.[27] Several *in vitro* assays have been described in individuals with AIA; however, their standardization and availability as diagnostic tests has not materialized. This ranges from cellular assays, to biomarkers in serum, induced sputum, and exhaled condensate, to assays performed on saliva and on urine.[36,50] The use of provocation tests with aspirin or NSAIDS for persons suspected to have this disorder (Table 47-2) is used in the diagnosis of AIA employing protocols using single-blind or double-blind approaches.

A traditional protocol begins with a 3 mg dose of aspirin, although higher initial doses (30 mg) have been recently advocated.

TABLE 47-2 Diagnosis of Aspirin-Induced Asthma (AIA): Aspirin Challenge Protocols

Single-Blind Oral 3-Day Aspirin Challenge			
	Test Days		
Time	1	2	3
0	Placebo	ASA 30 mg	ASA 100–150 mg
3 h	Placebo	ASA 45–60 mg	ASA 150–325 mg
6 h	Placebo	ASA 60–100 mg	ASA 325–650 mg

Double-Blind Oral Aspirin Challenge

Both tester and patient are blinded to eliminate potential bias.

Bronchial Challenge with Lysine–Aspirin	
Time (min)	Challenge (Lysine–Aspirin in mg/mL)
0	Placebo
45	Placebo
90	11.25
135	22.5
180	45
225	90
270	180
315	360
350	360 (10 breaths)

Patients receive four breaths of all doses of lysine–aspirin unless otherwise indicated.

Source: Data from DD Stevenson. Aspirin and NSAID sensitivity. Immunol Allergy Clin N Am. 2004;24:491–505; Stevenson DD, Simon RA. Sensitivity to aspirin and nonsteroidal antiinflammatory drugs, in Middleton E Jr, Reed CE, Ellis EF (eds). Allergy: Principles and Practice. St. Louis, CV Mosby, 1993; Phillips GD, Foord R, Holgate ST. Inhaled lysine-apirin as a bronchoprovocation procedure in aspirin-sensitive asthma: Its repeatibility, absence of a late-phase reaction, and the role of histamine. J Allergy Clin Immunol. 1989;84:232–241.

If reactions occur at this dose, patients are easily treated. The dosage is then increased to a maximum of 650 mg over a 3-day period. Due to concerns regarding the safety of the protocol, the use of leukotriene antagonists to decrease the rates of severe lower respiratory tract reactions during provocation tests has gained popularity.[51] The improvement in the safety profile for the oral aspirin challenge has also allowed reduction in the time needed to complete the protocol from 3 to 2 days. Spirometric pulmonary function is monitored serially during the challenge to assess the degree of bronchial obstruction. Airway reactivity to methacholine is not a viable surrogate for spirometry, since aspirin does not consistently alter methacholine sensitivity. Aspirin challenge should probably be reserved for use in centers experienced in its application and adverse effects. An alternative to oral challenge, used in some centers in Europe and elsewhere for the diagnosis of AIA, is the inhalation of stabilized lysine–aspirin, followed by serial lung function measurements, or nasal provocation with aspirin or lysine–aspirin followed by serial rhinomanometry or acoustic rhinometry.[52] Since lysine–aspirin is not available for clinical use in the United States, intranasal ketorolac challenge has been advocated as an alternative.[53]

■ TREATMENT

Given the particular pathophysiologic characteristics of AIA, optimal treatment of patients with AIA requires knowledge of the best approaches to treat acute aspirin-induced bronchial symptoms and associated nasal and sinus pathology. No specific therapy has emerged which can be recommended for the routine treatment of acute bronchospasm provoked by NSAIDs. Corticosteroids are not effective after acute aspirin ingestion, and theophylline and cromolyn sodium play no definite role.[9] Treatment of symptoms after acute ingestion, therefore, relies mainly on β-adrenergic agonists to reverse bronchospasm, and topical vasoconstrictors for both nasal congestion and eye symptoms. Frequent applications of these agents usually are necessary to maintain nasal and airway potency over the 2- to 6-hour reaction duration. On a chronic basis, the treatment of AIA depends on the correct diagnosis and avoidance of aspirin and other COX inhibitors that could cross-react to induce acute bronchospasm. Patients should be instructed that many over-the-counter medications contain aspirin or other NSAIDs, and they should carefully read package inserts before using any medication.

Drug treatment of AIA should focus on treating the underlying asthma and the strict avoidance of aspirin and cross-reacting NSAIDs. Currently, there also appears to be no role for systemic corticosteroids or theophylline in the prevention of AIA. Some investigators have found that antihistamines such as clemastine and mast cell stabilizers such as ketotifen, cromolyn, and nedocromil can have prophylactic efficacy.[54–56] However, not all subjects on these drugs are protected against bronchoconstriction after aspirin challenge. 5-lipooxygenase inhibitor zileuton was not found to be effective in preventing FEV_1 decline or nasoocular reactions to direct aspirin challenge,[57] although it had been previously shown to improve chronic asthma symptoms when added to conventional therapy in another study.[58] In contrast, experience with the cysteinyl leukotriene receptor antagonists has been variable, but mostly positive[56,59,60] and may be more effective in those who carry the variant C allele of LTC4S than in noncarriers.[61] Pretreatment with inhaled or systemic steroids or long-acting β-agonist (salmeterol) was shown to at least partially attenuate aspirin-induced respiratory lung function declines. The failure of tacrolimus (0.1 mg/kg), (a drug which could potentially affect both T cell generated cytokine responses and prevent release of mast cell histamine and leukotrienes) to prevent aspirin-induced respiratory reactions in patients with AERD on aspirin challenge in another study[62] suggests that this agent cannot be relied upon to prevent reactions from aspirin and cannot be used to facilitate "silent" aspirin desensitization of the patient with AERD.

In cases in which aspirin (or cross-reacting NSAIDs) cannot be avoided (i.e., in the setting of cardiovascular prophylaxis) or the efficacy of prophylactic measures cannot be assured, aspirin "desensitization" can be considered. Protocols are available for selected patients (Fig. 47-4).[63] These methods can effectively protect many from experiencing symptoms on exposure to aspirin or NSAIDs and will maintain this level of desensitization as long as aspirin is ingested indefinitely at doses of 325 to 650 mg a day. In a study of 25 aspirin-sensitive asthmatics, such therapy was shown to reduce nasal symptoms by 67% and asthma severity by 48%.[63,64] In the largest study of its kind, 172 patients with AERD were desensitized,

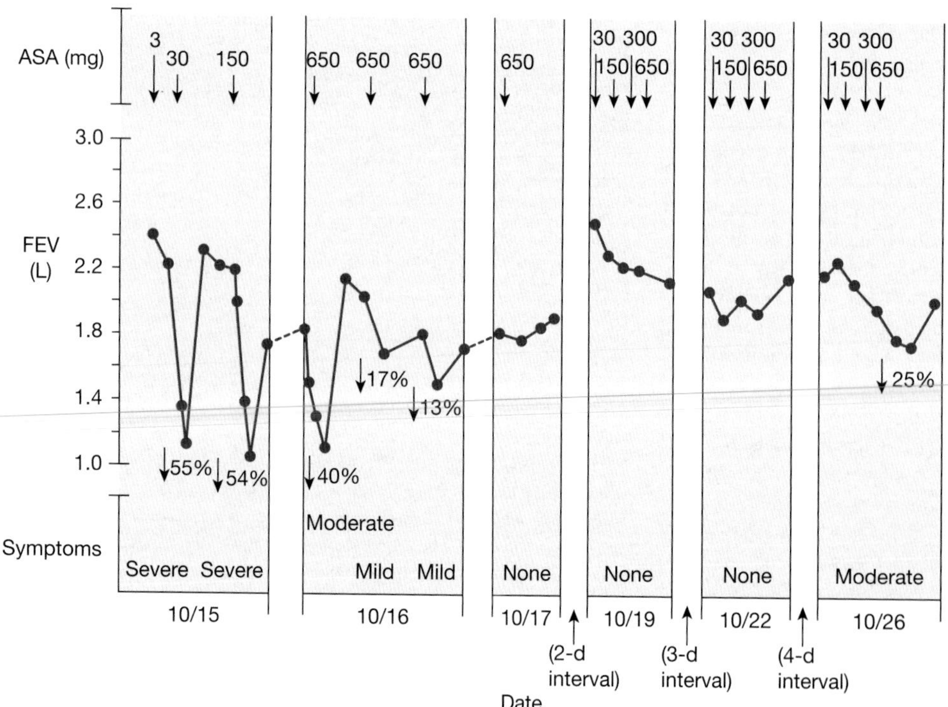

Figure 47-4 Airway desensitization to aspirin challenge in AIA. Timeline of respiratory function and overall symptoms after serial aspirin dosing. The reappearance of respiratory compromise and symptoms after 4 days without aspirin shows the need for continuous aspirin administration to maintain desensitized state. *(Data from Pleskow WW, et al. Aspirin desensitization in aspirin-sensitive asthmatic patients: Clinical manifestations and characterization of the refractory period. J Allergy Clin Immunol. 1982;69:11–19.)*

treated with 1300 mg of aspirin each day and followed for 1 to 5 years.[65] Clinical improvements were noted over the first 6 months, including reduction in dose of systemic corticosteroid and improvement in global assessments, which were maintained, but not further enhanced, during the remainder of the study. Approximately 67% (115 of 172) improved, 16 failed to improve, 24 discontinued because of aspirin-related side effects, and another 17 dropped out for other reasons.

It is interesting to note that although there are some reports of increased methacholine reactivity developing in patients soon after aspirin challenge,[44] baseline methacholine responsiveness does not seem to be successfully downregulated by aspirin desensitization. Also, there is no firm evidence that aspirin desensitization leads to abatement in skin disease in those with aspirin–urticaria syndrome.

Inhaled PGE2 was shown to prevent bronchoconstriction in a high proportion of patients challenged with inhaled L-lysine–aspirin in two small studies. In two studies[66] using misoprostol, a stable analogue of PGE1, prior to challenge with L-lysine–aspirin (400 μg 1 hour before) or predetermined threshold dose of aspirin (400 before, followed by then 200 μg with the provocative dose of aspirin), evidence was provided of some protection in 7 of 11 patients ($p = 0.024$) and in 6 of 7 patients (statistically only significant at time points 3 hours after challenge), respectively. To test whether asthma symptoms might improve on treatment with misoprostol, another group performed a double blind crossover study that showed that misoprostol, given for a period of 6 weeks (at dose of 800–1600 μg per day) led to a small improvement in nasal symptomatology without any effect on asthma control in 17 patients with proven AIA.[66] Thus, evidence of a specific method to control AIA apart from desensitization methods described above, has not been proven to be reliable. Fortunately, for those who require aspirin to prevent disease, such as those on low-dose aspirin, given for cardiovascular prophylaxis, the threshold needed to provoke airway and skin reactions is above that of the dose required for cardiovascular prophylaxis.

The potential contribution of chronic sinusitis to asthma exacerbations is well established. Aspirin sensitivity, chronic sinusitis, and nasal polyposis are well documented to coexist in AIA. Thus, the presence of these upper airway disorders must be considered in patients with AIA and effective treatment instituted if they are identified. High-dose topical intranasal corticosteroids can shrink polyp tissue and prevent obstruction of nasal passageways. In the setting of chronic sinusitis, standard approaches – including topical vasoconstrictors, antihistamines, and antibiotics – should also be utilized. Surgery to drain sinuses and remove polyps has been shown to be effective in the short term; however, polyps can regrow and the sinusitis often recurs.[2] The initial approach to nasal polyps in AIA is medical management, with aspirin desensitization playing an important role to decrease symptoms and improve postoperative outcomes in those requiring endoscopic sinus surgery, however, there is limited data on long-term follow-up in patients with nasal polyposis and AIA.[67] In selected cases where aspirin predominantly provokes nasal symptoms, administration of intranasal lysine–aspirin at increasing weekly doses successfully desensitized such patients and prevented regrowth of polyps.[68] A more recent and larger (though, due to drop-outs, under-powered randomized clinical trial) employed a crossover design after withdrawal of intranasal steroids. Lower doses of lysine–aspirin were administered more frequently (16 mg intranasally every 48 hours).[69] Results showed encouraging immunohistochemical changes characterized by a decreased expression of CysLT1 receptor on nasal submucosal inflammatory cells from turbinate tissue, but no clinical (diary scores of nasal and chest symptoms) or objective improvement on rhinometry. Two US studies that piloted the use of intranasal ketorolac administration with a modified aspirin challenge have shown the ability of ketorolac to induce nasal and lower respiratory reactions as part of the diagnostic element of the challenge. In addition, the administration of ketorolac prior to the modified aspirin challenge has the ability to decrease the severity of the FEV_1 decline, the frequency of laryngospasm and other extrapulmonary reactions. The rate of partial to complete desensitization was estimated at 77% for the intranasal portion of the protocol.[53] An additional advantage was the shortening in the duration of the desensitization.[70]

Despite aspirin desensitization and careful treatment of commonly associated sinusitis, a significant proportion of AIA patients do not achieve complete control of asthma or nasal symptoms. It is postulated that this may reflect permanently remodeled airways or residual allergic triggers that require specific allergy control measures and anti-inflammatory therapy. Evaluation of the effect of strict allergen avoidance, specific allergen immunotherapy, more intensive local management of the inflamed nasal mucosa and anti-IgE treatment in this scenario may better clarify the role of atopy in persistence of symptoms after aspirin desensitization.

EXERCISE-INDUCED ASTHMA

The first report of exercise-induced asthma (EIA) is attributed to John Floyer in 1698.[71] Nearly 300 years later, interest in this subject grew when it was recognized that exercise or hyperventilation could provoke asthma attacks. EIA can be defined as a condition in which vigorous physical activity triggers acute airway narrowing in persons with heightened airway reactivity.[72] It appears that EIA is always associated with the asthmatic diathesis, although EIA can be seen before other characteristic features of asthma emerge. Various reports indicate that EIA is common, affecting between 50% and 90% of all asthmatics[73] and 40% of patients with allergic rhinitis without known asthma.[74] Some have suggested that all asthmatics can be shown to manifest airway narrowing to thermal provocations of sufficient intensity, whether induced by exercise or hyperventilation. Other susceptible persons are first degree relatives of asthmatics, atopic "nonasthmatics," and patients with cystic fibrosis. Approximately 10% of pediatric patients can be found to have EIA, a higher prevalence than that of clinical asthma.

Elite athletes may be more predisposed to developing EIA.[75] Surveys conducted of athletes at the Atlanta (summer) and Nagano (winter) Olympic Games, showed a prevalence of 16% to 17%. The prevalence may actually be higher in those who are regularly exposed to high minute ventilation of cold, dry air typical of winter sports. In some studies the prevalence of EIA reported in figure skating (35%), and ice hockey (35%)[75] may be responsible for driving the overall incidence of EIA in winter sports to as high an estimate as 23%.[76]

CLINICAL PRESENTATION

Several societies have adopted a definition of EIA as clinical asthma where exercise triggers symptoms.[77] This is important given the recognition of exercise-induced bronchoconstriction (EIB) in individuals without asthma. Patients with EIA generally manifest a series of fairly predictable symptoms and alterations in pulmonary function that can be assessed by laboratory testing (Fig. 47-5). Normal persons and asthmatics generally first respond to exercise with bronchodilation, probably mediated by the release of catecholamines.[78,79] This response is short-lived, peaking at midexercise, and is followed by return of normal baseline airway tone at the end of exercise. In patients with EIA, the transient bronchodilation and reversal are followed by bronchoconstriction coincident with

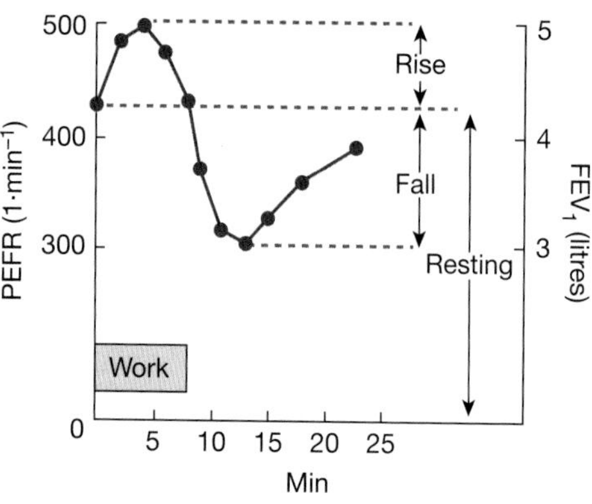

Figure 47-5 Typical pulmonary function changes induced by exercise in EIA. Transient bronchodilation during exercise and bronchospasm after exercise are noted. *(Data from Anderson SD. Is there a unifying hypothesis for exercise-induced asthma? J Allergy Clin Immunol. 1984;73:660–665.)*

symptoms of cough, wheezing, dyspnea, and chest tightness typical of asthmatic attacks. Typically, when they are provoked with a brief, intense exercise period in the laboratory, maximal bronchoconstriction occurs 5 to 10 minutes after the cessation of exercise and lasts for 30 to 60 minutes (Fig. 47-4). Rarely does this form of bronchoconstriction result in ventilatory failure, although it can limit the performance of trained athletes.

In addition to asthma after exercise, many athletes describe dyspnea during exercise. If these athletes are able to continue to exercise despite the initial airway obstruction and increase their level of activity, relief of bronchoconstriction often occurs. This is associated with symptomatic improvement that is described as "running through the attack." The development of dyspnea during exercise is ostensibly related to the development of bronchoconstriction at lower work intensities (simulating a postexercise state), which is reversed by interval training at higher intensities (simulating an exercise state). This has been taken as evidence that airway function during exercise reflects a balance between bronchoconstrictor and protective bronchodilator influences, and that this balance can be influenced by rapid changes in exercise intensity.[75,78]

The reproducibility of EIA is highly dependent on the specific characteristics of the stimulus- and patient-related factors. The net influence of exercise intensity, the temperature and humidity of the inspired air, the presence of allergens and pollutants in the environment, and the patient's baseline airway reactivity are fundamental in determining whether exercise will lead to bronchoconstriction. If asthma is better controlled at baseline, EIA may be more difficult to provoke. If climatic conditions vary, even though asthma is not well controlled, EIA may fail to develop. Classic work has shown that for a fixed minute ventilation, cold, dry air inspired during exercise is more likely to provoke EIA than warm, humid air.[79,80] Thus, EIA is more likely to occur with jogging outdoors during the winter than with swimming indoors. A recent study in children showed that exercise-induced wheeze was associated with an increased rate of urgent medical visits independently of asthma severity or socioeconomic factors, suggesting that EIB may be a surrogate marker of poorly controlled asthma rather than a distinct asthma phenotype.[81]

It is interesting to note that about 50% of patients with EIA will not manifest a bronchoconstrictive response if rechallenged with the same stimulus within 60 minutes and thus appear to be in a "refractory state." Neither baseline airway obstruction nor the degree of obstruction provoked by exercise can be used to determine who will be refractory to repeated exercise challenges. Furthermore, after 3 hours, even patients who were refractory to repeated challenge will regain ability to bronchoconstrict with exercise.

PATHOPHYSIOLOGY

The heterogeneity of responses present in EIA and bronchoconstriction, are influenced by the fundamental differences in the types of exercise and the environmental aspects of specific disciplines. Despite the attempt to categorize EIA as a unique entity the truth is that this is almost impossible. Two pathogenic schemas have been proposed for the bronchoconstriction seen in EIA. The two theories focus on the roles of (1) heat exchange, water loss, and airway rewarming; and (2) airway inflammation. The role of inflammation as a reaction to these stimuli or as an enhancer of the effects of these two pathophysiologic pathways is likely tied to leukotrienes and related lipooxygenase products.

Heat Exchange and Water Loss

During tidal breathing, heat (via conduction and evaporation) and water (via evaporation) are transferred from the mucosa of the upper airways to the entering air. Since exercise requires marked increases in minute ventilation, surpassing the volume of air that can be inspired through nasal structures, air enters directly through the mouth, bypassing the normal warming and conditioning function of the nose. The lower respiratory mucosa then attempts to compensate for the function of the bypassed nose. Heat and water fluxes first occur. The lower airways are cooled and dried and are subject to rewarming by warm blood carried by the bronchial circulation.

In the late 1970s, a number of investigators postulated that EIA was the result of increased heat loss in the airway. This was based on the observation that cold, dry air caused a greater fall in FEV_1 than did hot, dry air[82] and on correlations between heat exchange and the degree of bronchoconstriction. Others, however, showed that the temperature of the inspired air was not crucial to inducing bronchoconstriction, and that temperatures of dry inspired air that varied by as much as 60 degrees could still provoke airway narrowing.[80,83] This suggested that airway evaporative water loss might be more important than airway cooling. The water loss was predicted to change the osmolarity of the cellular and extracellular components of the airway wall, stimulating increased bronchial blood flow to increase the delivery of water.[80] In addition, bronchial wall hyperosmolarity was hypothesized to increase the release of proinflammatory mediators from resident airway immune cells such as mast cells.[82] This concept was supported by work that demonstrated that changes in the humidity of inspired air, and not temperature, determine the magnitude of EIA. Further support for this construct came from studies using cold gas mixtures with different water-carrying capacities, which showed a significant correlation between evaporative heat loss but not total heat loss or temperature gradient on the airway response.[84]

In apparent contrast to these data is the considerable body of work that does not support the concept that osmolar changes precipitate EIA. The most important of these showed that increasing minute ventilation at constant humidity increases the severity of EIA.[74] The combination of overlapping mechanisms including airway cooling, airway dehydration and osmolar changes account for the pathogenic features responsible for EIA, rather than a single mechanism.[114]

Airway Rewarming

An important theory that also remains to be unequivocally proven is that offered by McFadden, who proposed that the process of airway rewarming is active in the pathogenesis of the airway narrowing that occurs in EIA.[85] This theory postulates that loss of heat associated with exercise transiently leads to decreased bronchial blood flow.

At the end of exercise, the bronchi undergo reactive hyperemia characterized by vascular engorgement. This leads to airway caliber compromise and airway wall edema. The strongest support for this theory arises from studies showing that the severity of EIA could be controlled by regulation of the thermal gradient during exercise and the rate of rewarming after exercise. The presence of an elevated airway permeability index in individuals with EIA is associated with the severity of EIB,[86] suggests that individuals with abnormal vascular permeability may be more susceptible to larger fluid shifts and airway physiologic changes associated with exercise. Sodium ingestion also seems to affect vascular volume and increase airway inflammation in the setting of exercise.[87]

In summary, there is evidence that associates exercise-induced bronchoconstriction with a sequence of events that includes heat loss, water loss, and airway rewarming. The degree to which these temperature and water alterations contribute to the pathogenesis of EIA is still, however, a topic of debate and investigation.

Inflammation and EIA

Theories postulating a role for inflammatory mediators in the pathogenesis of EIA have recently received new support and are being harmonized with the already considerable evidence supporting a role for inflammation in the pathogenesis of other forms of asthma. New information in exercise suggests that those predisposed to EIA, specifically elite athletes, may manifest a degree of airway inflammation that had not been previously appreciated. Instead of demonstrating a lower rate of EIA, allowing a potentially higher level of exercise performance, which might be expected on the basis of selection of those best equipped to excel in sports, elite athletes appear to exhibit a paradoxically higher incidence of EIA and a higher degree of airway inflammation without necessarily manifesting a higher prevalence of underlying clinical asthma.

Older data on the role of inflammation in EIA did not necessarily support this link. One study analyzing the characteristics of bronchoalveolar lavage (BAL) fluid from patients with EIA 12 minutes after exercise failed to find evidence for mast cell mediator release since BAL histamine, tryptase, LTC4, and PGD2 levels were not altered. Similarly, studies performed 1 hour and 25 hours after exercise did not reveal significant differences in BAL cellularity or in histamine or tryptase levels.

In contrast, one group studying elite cross-country skiers, found elevated airway T lymphocytes and eosinophils compared to controls.[88] Several others have demonstrated changes in exhaled NO, which generally decreased with exercise, suggesting a high basal level and ventilatory clearance of this gas associated with airway inflammation,[75] while another observed increases in plasma adenosine after exercise.[89] A different group documented the presence of a late phase airway response after exercise that was demonstrable in 50% of competitive athletes studied.[90] Most importantly, the new concept that these changes might be provoked by exercise, rather than be a reflection of underlying inflammation in those who manifest EIA, is supported by Helenius,[91] who showed that athletes who stopped high-level training and modulated the amount of exercise they subsequently pursued, experienced reduced asthma symptoms and diminished bronchial responsiveness to histamine. Additional observations using exhaled breath condensate (EBC) have shown elevations of cysteinyl leukotrienes,[92] RANTES and eotaxin,[93,94] after exercise. RANTES has also been found to be elevated in the EBC of asthmatic children with EIB after exercise challenge.

Leukotrienes in EIA To determine whether leukotrienes play a role in the pathogenesis of EIA, LTD4 receptor antagonists and 5-lipooxygenase inhibitors have been employed. Studies using an intravenous LTD4 receptor antagonist 20 minutes before exercise demonstrated significant attenuation of the maximal provoked bronchoconstriction and mean time to recover from bronchoconstriction (8 minutes for the treatment group vs. 33 minutes for placebo).[95] Similar results were noted by others using oral or inhaled leukotriene antagonists. In general, although the protection was relatively small, it was significant and equivalent in potency to inhaled cromolyn.

The results obtained with peptidoleukotriene antagonists are consistent with those obtained when the effects of a 5-lipooxygenase inhibitor on bronchoconstriction induced by cold, dry air were evaluated. In the most important study of this kind,[96] a 5-lipooxygenase antagonist was an effective as cromolyn or terbutaline in augmenting respiratory heat exchange. Thus, leukotrienes may well mediate the airway inflammation and contribute to the pathogenesis of EIA.

■ GENETICS AND GENOMICS

Little information is available on the potential genetic underpinnings of EIA, however, some of the observations from genetic and genomic studies are summarized here. Using microarray analysis, a group demonstrated enhanced transcription of 5-lipooxygenase (ALOX5) and 5-lipooxygenase activating protein (ALOX5AP) genes.[18] A more recent study examined the transcriptional profile of induced sputum after an exercise challenge and identified the upregulation of transglutaminase 2 (TGM2), a molecule associated with an increase in the activity of secreted phospholipase A2, the rate-limiting step on eicosanoid formation.[97] The same investigators described the predominant role of airway MUC5AC expression during exercise challenge in a similar setting.[98]

Other investigators have provided evidence of leukotriene C4 synthase (A-444C) promoter polymorphisms in association with greater severity of EIA in studies conducted in a large cohort of Korean children with asthma.[99] However, these polymorphisms are not associated with montelukast responsiveness in a subsequent pharmacogenomics study of the same population.[100] These observations suggest the potential existence of disease-modifying genes in exercise-induced bronchospasm.

■ DIFFERENTIAL DIAGNOSIS

The diagnosis of EIA is most accurately established by employing validated exercise protocols coupled with pulmonary function testing. However, patients are commonly given a presumptive diagnosis based on their history and physical examination. Important points in the clinical history include the level and type of exercise that provokes asthma, the timing of symptom onset, situations that modify symptom onset, environmental conditions and the precise symptoms experienced. Many of the symptoms of EIA can mimic other conditions that would require an entirely different therapeutic approach (Table 47-3). For example, chest

TABLE 47-3 Differential Diagnosis of Exercise-Induced Asthma

Cardiac Disease	Functional Abnormalities
Coronary ischemia	Vocal cord dysfunction
Mitral valve prolapse	Panic disorders
Atrial myxoma	General
Cardiomyopathy	Deconditioning
Arrhythmias	Anemia
Lung Disease	
Fixed airway obstruction	
Interstitial lung disease	
Exercise-induced cough	

tightness with exercise should be unequivocally distinguished from coronary ischemia. Other cardiac disorders that can mimic EIA are arrhythmias, cardiomyopathies, atrial myxoma, and mitral valve prolapse, all of which can manifest with dyspnea and wheezing. The presence of a murmur, click, or other findings on physical examination should help to identify patients with these conditions. Exercise-induced anaphylaxis can also mimic EIA but will generally exhibit skin manifestations (urticaria), and respiratory symptoms will be less prominent. Two other conditions that have been reported to mimic EIA are fixed glottal and tracheal obstruction, which become noticeable with the increased ventilation of exercise and exercise-induced vocal cord/arytenoids dysfunction, not present at rest. Some have also suggested that panic disorders and the excessive tachypnea associated with deconditioning can be confused with EIA. Symptoms due to these other conditions generally are greatest during exercise provocation rather than afterward, when airflow limitation due to EIA usually reaches its peak.

Exercise-induced cough is another phenomenon that can mimic EIA. Both may be induced by changes in the osmolarity of the airways reflecting water loss from the respiratory tract during exercise, the inhalation of humid air also prevents both phenomena. However, EIA and exercise-induced cough respond differently to β-adrenergic agonists, suggesting that they are mediated by different underlying mechanisms. It is postulated that exercise-induced cough is the direct result of the osmolarity changes provoked by airway drying, whereas EIA is due to the mediator release that results from the process of airway drying. Therefore, although nearly all patients with EIA cough with exercise provocation, there are patients who have exercise-induced cough without bronchospasm, and thus do not have EIA.

PHYSIOLOGIC DOCUMENTATION

Because a simple history or cough or wheezing may not reliably predict EIA, especially in those in whom a trial of preventive measures has not been successful, formal exercise testing may be required.[75] The clinician needs to document airflow obstruction that reaches a peak just after provocation, during the recovery period. In athletes, the presence of EIA and EIB has major implications in their exercise performance and management. In addition, societies and committees have created practice guidelines to assist in the documentation of EIA.[77,101,102] Bronchial provocation tests (BPT) are used to identify airway hyperresponsiveness and they can be classified as indirect and direct. Indirect tests include exercise, the inhalation of dry air (isocapnic hyperventilation [ISH], also known as eucapnic voluntary hyperpnea), hypertonic saline, and mannitol. The direct methods include methacholine, histamine, carbachol and AMP inhalation.

Indirect methods trigger airway hyperreactivity through different mechanisms that affect the release of inflammatory mediators and cause bronchoconstriction. Exercise provocation, whether performed on an ergometer or a treadmill, leads to significantly greater increases in heart rate, metabolic rate, and oxygen consumption. Exercise, but not ISH, is accompanied by increased numbers of circulating basophils and increased circulating catecholamines and cAMP. The differences in the last two parameters probably explain why the bronchodilatory response that characterizes exercise is not provoked by ISH. The bronchoconstriction induced by ISH is similar to that induced by exercise in terms of magnitude, time course, and refractory period. Two main advantages over exercise include the ease with which the ISH protocol can be standardized and the finding that oxygen consumption and heart rate are not increased with ISH. As a result, ISH is useful in differentiating EIA from occult cardiac disease and is especially valuable when elderly or cardiac patients are being evaluated.

The most commonly used ISH protocol for the diagnosis of EIA in the United States is that published by O'Byrne et al.[103] and modified by Philips et al. (Fig. 47-6).[104] This is accomplished by registering changes in pulmonary function in response to varying rates of ventilation using dry air with a fixed CO_2 content of 4.9% to maintain isocapnia. Each ventilatory challenge is performed for 3 minutes, with spirometry performed at intervals thereafter (usually 2, 5, and 10 minutes after the end of hyperventilation). Serial increase in hyperventilation is performed until maximal voluntary ventilation is reached. If the FEV_1 falls greater than 10% after provocation, the test is considered positive, confirming the diagnosis of EIA. Although some have pointed out that it is not necessary to condition air to subfreezing temperatures to perform the test, Scandinavian investigators showed that assessing bronchoconstrictor responses to whole-body exposure to very cold air significantly increased the number of asthmatic patients who experienced bronchoconstriction. Others have pointed out the need to assess athletes in the field performing in the sport in which they compete, since they may not have a significant drop in FEV_1 symptoms during in the laboratory during challenge.[75]

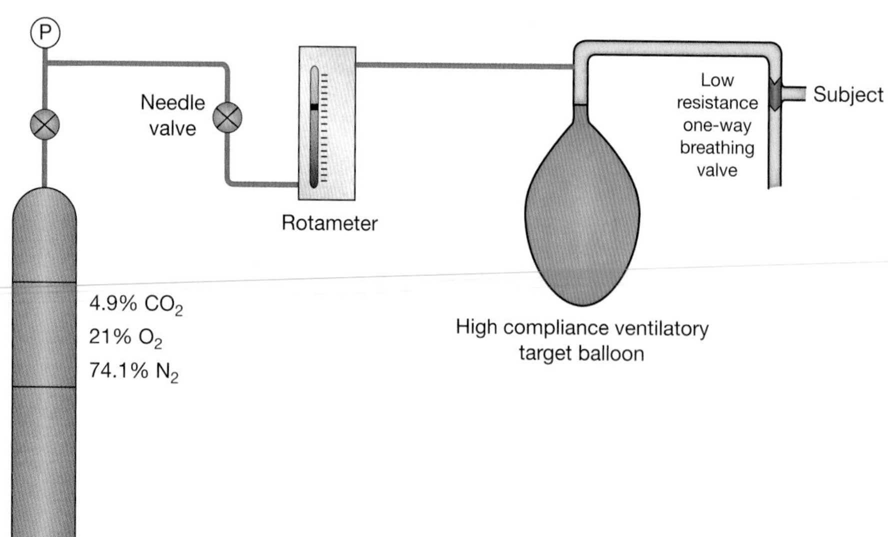

Figure 47-6 Apparatus for isocapnic hyperventilation challenge to diagnose EIA. *(Data from Phillips YY, et al. Eucapnic voluntary hyperventilation of compressed gas mixture: A simple method for bronchial challenge by respiratory heat loss. Am Rev Respir Dis. 1985;131:31–35.)*

To optimize the validity, repeatability and practicality of exercise testing for the diagnosis of EIA, a variety of testing protocols have been pursued. Unfortunately, the criteria used to define a positive test in these studies are different, making standardization difficult. Although the optimal diagnostic algorithm for the assessment of EIA is still lacking,[72,75] data reported on athletes from the 2002 Olympic Winter Games,[105] compared eucapnic voluntary hyperventilation (EVH) with exercise testing outdoors in the cold (20°C and 45% humidity). The EVH test for 6 minutes with cold dry air was determined to perform best in assessing the presence of EIA.

The mannitol inhalation test relies on the airway fluid changes to incremental doses of this hyperosmolar dry powder. This bronchial provocation agent was approved by the FDA in 2010 and is available for adults and children older than 6 years of age. A decline in FEV_1 equal to or larger than 10% is considered positive. In a similar fashion, the inhalation of hypertonic saline (4.5%) takes advantage of the same physiologic principle to evaluate for the presence of bronchoconstriction. The most popular direct challenge method is the methacholine challenge test, supported by its standardization and reproducibility; it has been approved by the International Olympic Committee Medical Commission.

In addition to the difficulties inherent in the standardization of the challenge protocol, the clinician must be aware of situations that can lead to false-negative evaluations. Specifically, it is important that all drugs that can potentially attenuate bronchoconstrictor responses – such as calcium channel blockers, methylxanthines, cromolyn, and β-adrenergic agonists – be discontinued for a sufficient period before the evaluation.

TREATMENT

A variety of nonpharmacologic and pharmacologic approaches have been employed in treatment of EIA.

Nonpharmacologic Treatments

The treatment of EIA is influenced by the underlying process driving this response. In patients with asthma who experience EIA, optimization of the asthma therapy is the first step. Inhaled steroids attenuate the development of EIA during laboratory provocation and increase the threshold for the development of EIA clinically. Prophylactic measures to prevent EIA include avoiding exercises that expose the patient to cold, dry air and favoring those in which the patient breathes humid air during exercise. Patients can reduce the severity of their EIA by breathing through the nose rather than through the mouth during exercise. Face masks (e.g., 3M Cold Weather Mask) can be effectively used by the many people who find it impossible to breathe through the nose during intense exercise.

It is still unclear whether physical training and improvement in work capacity can relieve symptoms of EIA. Training ought to be useful, at least theoretically, since a better-trained athlete may require a lower mandatory minute volume—which may lead to less water loss from the airways and less severe EIA. Pre-exposure of patients with EIA to air high in ozone in two studies performed in Los Angeles and Toronto showed that EIA was not enhanced. This suggests that choosing a day to exercise on the basis of ozone will not help prevent EIA. A series of repeated short sprints has been shown to be effective in inducing the refractory state, which might then allow the athlete to maximally exercise without developing EIA.[106] A warm up period to induce the refractory period has been advocated by some to improve performance in the competitive athlete.[107] A high-intensity interval warm-up in recreational athletes prior to an exercise challenge resulted in improved FEV_1, and this protective effect was increased when used in combination with salbutamol.[108] A systematic review of the effect of warming-up prior to exercise found that interval and variable-intensity protocols are effective short-term strategies to prevent EIB.[109]

TABLE 47-4 Treatment of Exercise-Induced Asthma (EIA)

Treatment Immediately Before Exercise (10–20 min before)	Treatment of Underlying Disease (Days Before)
β-Adrenergic agonists	Goal: Improved asthma control
Cromolyn sodium	Inhaled corticosteroids
Nedocromil	Systemic corticosteroids
? Anticholinergics	? Theophylline
? Inhaled furosemide	
Leukotriene receptor antagonists	

A low sodium diet has also been advocated as a nonpharmacologic intervention in individuals with EIA, based on the observation that those with a low sodium diet had smaller declines in FEV_1 with exercise compared to those ingesting normal or high amounts of sodium.[110]

Pharmacologic Treatment

Several classes of drugs have been shown to prevent EIA if administered just before (10–15 minutes) exercise. The list includes β-adrenergic agonists, cromolyn sodium, anticholinergics, and possibly rapid-release theophylline (Table 47-4).[75,103] β-Adrenergic agonists are the most effective drugs for use against EIA and, therefore, are the mainstay of therapy. They have a rapid onset of action and are 90% effective in preventing EIA when used just before exercise. They are especially useful if the patient has some reversible airway obstruction, since they also improve lung function before exercise. Long-acting β-adrenergic agonists (LABA) have also been found to be effective in preventing EIA. The duration of protection they confer may approach 10 hours or more. It is interesting to note that the cough so often associated with EIA appears to occur independent of the bronchospasm provoked by exercise. Although exercise-induced airway narrowing is prevented by the inhalation of β-adrenergic agonists before exercise, the cough is not.

Cromolyn sodium also has been shown to attenuate bronchoconstriction in most patients with EIA. This medication is not a bronchodilator and, therefore, does not reverse bronchoconstriction. Cromolyn does, however, have two advantages over other agents. First, it does not contribute to tachycardia and is therefore useful in elderly patients or patients with cardiac compromise. In addition, cromolyn has been shown to prevent the late bronchoconstrictor response to exercise. Related drugs (including nedocromil, minocromil, and oxatomide, but not ketotifen) have been shown to be similarly effective against EIA. Anticholinergics, such as ipratropium bromide, prevent airway narrowing after exercise in a high percentage of patients with EIA. They are especially useful in those who experience a rapid bronchodilating effect of the drug. The slower onset of action for most patients, however, limits their utility after bronchodilation has occurred.

Theophylline has weak bronchodilatory effects, high side-effect profile, and slow onset of action and is not recommended for routine use as pretreatment for EIA. However, it has been shown to confer protection against EIA if 100 to 200 mg is taken 2 hours before exercise. Other orally administered drugs that are not commonly used, but have the potential to be helpful in preventing EIA, are terbutaline, albuterol (2 hours before exercise), some alpha adrenergic agonists, and verapamil if taken 1½ hour before exercise as well as the inhaled antihistamine clemastine.[78] In addition, terfenadine was shown by one group to prevent EIA.[111]

For athletes, organizations including the World Anti-Doping Association and International Olympic Committee, have developed standards that incorporate physiologic documentation of bronchial hyperresponsiveness, including bronchoprovocation tests, permitting use of certain medications, particularly short acting β-agonists.[112] Due to concerns related to doping, all practitioners involved in the management of athletes should review the specific guidelines developed by the appropriate governing bodies. Some of these agencies include the World Anti-Doping Agency (WADA; http://www.wada-ama.org/), International Olympic Committee (IOC; http://www.olympic.org/ioc), National Collegiate Athletic Association (NCAA; http://www.ncaa.org/), and US Anti-Doping Agency (www.usantidoping.org), among others.

Despite the observation that inhaled furosemide can prevent EIA in adults and children, their use for this indication has not evolved as standard therapy. Leukotriene antagonists have been advocated by some and shown to be effective, especially if treatment with short acting β-agonists in insufficient.[75] Because of their low side-effect profile, leukotriene antagonists would appear to be well suited as single agents for use against EIA. However, additional head-to-head studies showing efficacy during exercise need to be conducted before these agents can be recommended over inhaled β-adrenergic agonists in routine prophylaxis against EIA. A recent study showed that the combination of inhaled budesonide and montelukast, was superior to either agent alone, shortening the duration of EIB.[113]

Management needs to be tailored to individual needs and response to therapy. Despite the mechanistic differences seen in EIA and EIB, an approach that optimizes underlying asthma control is key, since the two syndromes are associated with impaired airway function. In individuals with chronic asthma, EIB seems to be a marker of suboptimal control, and an increase of controlling agents is advocated.[77,114]

REFERENCES

1. Samter M, Beers RF. Intolerance to aspirin. Clinical studies and consideration of its pathogenesis. *Ann Intern Med.* 1968;68(5):975–983.
2. Slavin RG. Nasal polyps and sinusitis. In: Middleton E, Reed C, Ellis EF, Adkinson EF, Yunginger JW, Busse WW, eds. *Allergy, Principles, and Practice.* 4th ed. St. Louis, MO: Mosby-Year Book; 1993:1455–1470.
3. Weber RW, Hoffman M, Raine DA, Nelson HS. Incidence of bronchoconstriction due to aspirin, azo dyes, non-azo dyes, and preservatives in a population of perennial asthmatics. *J Allergy Clin Immunol.* 1979;64(1):32–37.
4. Iamandescu IB. NSAIDs-induced asthma: peculiarities related to background and association with other drug or non-drugs etiological agents. *Allergol Immunopathol (Madr).* 1989;17(6): 285–290.
5. Sánchez-Borges M, Capriles-Hulett A, Caballero-Fonseca F. Cutaneous reactions to aspirin and nonsteroidal anti-inflammatory drugs. *Clin Rev Allergy Immunol.* 2003;24(2):125–136.
6. Stevenson DD, Zuraw BL. Pathogenesis of aspirin-exacerbated respiratory disease. *Clin Rev Allergy Immunol.* 2003;24(2): 169–188.
7. Berges-Gimeno MP, Simon RA, Stevenson DD. The natural history and clinical characteristics of aspirin-exacerbated respiratory disease. *Ann Allergy Asthma Immunol.* 2002;89(5): 474–478.
8. Hebert WG, Scopelitis E. Ketorolac-precipitated asthma. *South Med J.* 1994;87(2):282–283.
9. Stevenson DD, Settipane RA. *Aspirin Sensitivity: Respiratory and Cutaneous Manifestations.* 4th ed. St. Louis, MO: Mosby; 1993.
10. Lockey RF, Rucknagel DL, Vanselow NA. Familial occurrence of asthma, nasal polyps and aspirin intolerance. *Ann Intern Med.* 1973;78(1):57–63.
11. Von Maur K Jr, Adkinson NF Jr, Van Metrer TE, Marsh DG, Norman PS. Aspirin intolerance in a family. *J Allergy Clin Immun.* 1974;54:380–395.
12. Mullarkey MF, Thomas PS, Hansen JA, Webb DR, Nisperos B. Association of aspirin-sensitive asthma with HLA-DQw2. *Am Rev Respir Dis.* 1986;133(2):261–263.
13. Dekker JW, Nizankowska E, Schmitz-Schumann M, et al. Aspirin-induced asthma and HLA-DRB1 and HLA-DPB1 genotypes. *Clin Exp Allergy.* 1997;27(5):574–577.
14. Kim SH, Choi JH, Lee KW, et al. The human leucocyte antigen-DRB1*1302-DQB1*0609-DPB1*0201 haplotype may be a strong genetic marker for aspirin-induced urticaria. *Clin Exp Allergy.* 2005;35(3):339–344.
15. Sanak M, Pierzchalska M, Bazan-Socha S, Szczeklik A. Enhanced expression of the leukotriene C(4) synthase due to overactive transcription of an allelic variant associated with aspirin-intolerant asthma. *Am J Respir Cell Mol Biol.* 2000;23(3):290–296.
16. Szczeklik W, Sanak M, Szczeklik A. Functional effects and gender association of COX-2 gene polymorphism G-765 C in bronchial asthma. *J Allergy Clin Immunol.* 2004;114(2): 248–253.
17. Akahoshi M, Obara K, Hirota T, et al. Functional promoter polymorphism in the TBX21 gene associated with aspirin-induced asthma. *Hum Genet.* 2005;117(1):16–26.
18. Hilberg T, Deigner HP, Möller E, et al. Transcription in response to physical stress–clues to the molecular mechanisms of exercise-induced asthma. *FASEB J.* 2005;19(11):1492–1494.
19. Corrigan C, Mallett K, Ying S, et al. Expression of the cysteinyl leukotriene receptors cysLT(1) and cysLT(2) in aspirin-sensitive and aspirin-tolerant chronic rhinosinusitis. *J Allergy Clin Immunol.* 2005;115(2):316–322.
20. Stankovic KM, Goldsztein H, Reh DD, Platt MP, Metson R. Gene expression profiling of nasal polyps associated with chronic sinusitis and aspirin-sensitive asthma. *Laryngoscope.* 2008;118(5):881–889.
21. Sidhu SS, Yuan S, Innes AL, et al. Roles of epithelial cell-derived periostin in TGF-beta activation, collagen production, and collagen gel elasticity in asthma. *Proc Natl Acad Sci U S A.* 2010;107(32):14170–14175.
22. Vanselow NA, Smith JR. Bronchial asthma induced by indomethacin. *Ann Intern Med.* 1967;66(3):568–572.
23. Szczeklik A, Gryglewski RJ, Czerniawska-Mysik G. Relationship of inhibition of prostaglandin biosynthesis by analgesics to asthma attacks in aspirin-sensitive patients. *Br Med J.* 1975;1(5949):67–69.
24. Szczeklik A, Gryglewski RJ, Czerniawska-Mysik G. Clinical patterns of hypersensitivity to nonsteroidal anti-inflammatory drugs and their pathogenesis. *J Allergy Clin Immunol.* 1977;60(5):276–284.
25. Stevenson DD, Simon RA. Lack of cross-reactivity between rofecoxib and aspirin in aspirin-sensitive patients with asthma. *J Allergy Clin Immunol.* 2001;108(1):47–51.

26. Szczeklik A, Nizankowska E, Bochenek G, Nagraba K, Mejza F, Swierczynska M. Safety of a specific COX-2 inhibitor in aspirin-induced asthma. *Clin Exp Allergy.* 2001;31(2): 219–225.

27. Melillo G, Balzano G, Bianco S, et al. Report of the INTERASMA Working Group on Standardization of Inhalation Provocation Tests in Aspirin-induced Asthma. Oral and inhalation provocation tests for the diagnosis of aspirin-induced asthma. *Allergy.* 2001;56(9):899–911.

28. Gyllfors P, Bochenek G, Overholt J, et al. Biochemical and clinical evidence that aspirin-intolerant asthmatic subjects tolerate the cyclooxygenase 2-selective analgesic drug celecoxib. *J Allergy Clin Immunol.* 2003;111(5):1116–1121.

29. Viola M, Quaratino D, Gaeta F, Caruso C, Valluzzi R, Romano A. Etoricoxib tolerability in patients with hypersensitivity to nonsteroidal anti-inflammatory drugs. *Int Arch Allergy Immunol.* 2007;143(2):103–108.

30. El Miedany Y, Youssef S, Ahmed I, El Gaafary M. Safety of etoricoxib, a specific cyclooxygenase-2 inhibitor, in asthmatic patients with aspirin-exacerbated respiratory disease. *Ann Allergy Asthma Immunol.* 2006;97(1):105–109.

31. Sánchez-Borges M, Caballero-Fonseca F, Capriles-Hulett A. Safety of etoricoxib, a new cyclooxygenase 2 inhibitor, in patients with nonsteroidal anti-inflammatory drug-induced urticaria and angioedema. *Ann Allergy Asthma Immunol.* 2005;95(2): 154–158.

32. Simon RA, Namazy J. Adverse reactions to aspirin and nonsteroidal antiinflammatory drugs (NSAIDs). *Clin Rev Allergy Immunol.* 2003;24(3):239–252.

33. Dajani BM, Sliman NA, Shubair KS, Hamzeh YS. Bronchospasm caused by intravenous hydrocortisone sodium succinate (Solu-Cortef) in aspirin-sensitive asthmatics. *J Allergy Clin Immunol.* 1981;68(3):201–204.

34. Szczeklik A, Nizankowska E, Czerniawska-Mysik G, Sek S. Hydrocortisone and airflow impairment in aspirin-induced asthma. *J Allergy Clin Immunol.* 1985;76(4):530–536.

35. Aksoy MO, Li X, Borenstein M, Yi Y, Kelsen SG. Effects of topical corticosteroids on inflammatory mediator-induced eicosanoid release by human airway epithelial cells. *J Allergy Clin Immunol.* 1999;103(6):1081–1091.

36. Ameisen JC, Capron A, Joseph M, et al. Aspirin-sensitive asthma: abnormal platelet response to drugs inducing asthmatic attacks. Diagnostic and physiopathological implications. *Int Arch Allergy Appl Immunol.* 1985;78(4):438–448.

37. van OSS C, Friedmann JC, Fontaine M. Anticomplementary action of aspirin. *Nature.* 1961;189:147.

38. Pleskow WW, Chenoweth DE, Simon RA, Stevenson DD, Curd JG. The absence of detectable complement activation in aspirin-sensitive asthmatic patients during aspirin challenge. *J Allergy Clin Immunol.* 1983;72(5 Pt 1):462–468.

39. Sanak M, Levy BD, Clish CB, et al. Aspirin-tolerant asthmatics generate more lipoxins than aspirin-intolerant asthmatics. *Eur Respir J.* 2000;16(1):44–49.

40. Fischer AR, Rosenberg MA, Lilly CM, et al. Direct evidence for a role of the mast cell in the nasal response to aspirin in aspirin-sensitive asthma. *J Allergy Clin Immunol.* 1994;94(6 Pt 1): 1046–1056.

41. Kowalski ML, Sliwinska-Kowalska M, Igarashi Y, et al. Nasal secretions in response to acetylsalicylic acid. *J Allergy Clin Immunol.* 1993;91(2):580–598.

42. Kowalski ML, Grzegorczyk J, Wojciechowska B, Poniatowska M. Intranasal challenge with aspirin induces cell influx and activation of eosinophils and mast cells in nasal secretions of ASA-sensitive patients. *Clin Exp Allergy.* 1996;26(7): 807–814.

43. Sladek K, Dworski R, Soja J, et al. Eicosanoids in bronchoalveolar lavage fluid of aspirin-intolerant patients with asthma after aspirin challenge. *Am J Respir Crit Care Med.* 1994;149 (4 Pt 1):940–946.

44. Christie PE, Smith CM, Lee TH. The potent and selective sulfidopeptide leukotriene antagonist, SK&F 104353, inhibits aspirin-induced asthma. *Am Rev Respir Dis.* 1991;144(4): 957–958.

45. Dahlén B, Kumlin M, Margolskee DJ, et al. The leukotriene-receptor antagonist MK-0679 blocks airway obstruction induced by inhaled lysine-aspirin in aspirin-sensitive asthmatics. *Eur Respir J.* 1993;6(7):1018–1026.

46. Israel E, Fischer AR, Rosenberg MA, et al. The pivotal role of 5-lipoxygenase products in the reaction of aspirin-sensitive asthmatics to aspirin. *Am Rev Respir Dis.* 1993;148(6 Pt 1): 1447–1451.

47. Berges-Gimeno MP, Simon RA, Stevenson DD. The effect of leukotriene-modifier drugs on aspirin-induced asthma and rhinitis reactions. *Clin Exp Allergy.* 2002;32(10):1491–1496.

48. Wang XS, Wu AY, Leung PS, Lau HY. PGE suppresses excessive anti-IgE induced cysteinyl leucotrienes production in mast cells of patients with aspirin exacerbated respiratory disease. *Allergy.* 2007;62(6):620–627.

49. Laidlaw TM, Kidder MS, Bhattacharyya N, et al. Cysteinyl leukotriene overproduction in aspirin-exacerbated respiratory disease is driven by platelet-adherent leukocytes. *Blood.* 2012;119(16):3790–3798.

50. Gaber F, Daham K, Higashi A, et al. Increased levels of cysteinyl-leukotrienes in saliva, induced sputum, urine and blood from patients with aspirin-intolerant asthma. *Thorax.* 2008;63(12):1076–1082.

51. White A, Ludington E, Mehra P, Stevenson DD, Simon RA. Effect of leukotriene modifier drugs on the safety of oral aspirin challenges. *Ann Allergy Asthma Immunol.* 2006;97(5): 688–693.

52. Casadevall J, Ventura PJ, Mullol J, Picado C. Intranasal challenge with aspirin in the diagnosis of aspirin intolerant asthma: evaluation of nasal response by acoustic rhinometry. *Thorax.* 2000;55(11):921–924.

53. Lee RU, White AA, Ding D, et al. Use of intranasal ketorolac and modified oral aspirin challenge for desensitization of aspirin-exacerbated respiratory disease. *Ann Allergy Asthma Immunol.* 2010;105(2):130–135.

54. Szczeklik A, Serwonska M. Inhibition of idiosyncratic reactions to aspirin in asthmatic patients by clemastine. *Thorax.* 1979;34(5):654–657.

55. Szczeklik A, Czerniawska-Mysik G, Serwonska M, Kuklinski P. Inhibition by ketotifen of idiosyncratic reactions to aspirin. *Allergy.* 1980;35(5):421–424.

56. Yoshida S, Sakamoto H, Ishizaki Y, et al. Efficacy of leukotriene receptor antagonist in bronchial hyperresponsiveness and hypersensitivity to analgesic in aspirin-intolerant asthma. *Clin Exp Allergy.* 2000;30(1):64–70.

57. Pauls JD, Simon RA, Daffern PJ, Stevenson DD. Lack of effect of the 5-lipoxygenase inhibitor zileuton in blocking oral

aspirin challenges in aspirin-sensitive asthmatics. *Ann Allergy Asthma Immunol.* 2000;85(1):40–45.

58. Dahlén B, Nizankowska E, Szczeklik A, et al. Benefits from adding the 5-lipoxygenase inhibitor zileuton to conventional therapy in aspirin-intolerant asthmatics. *Am J Respir Crit Care Med.* 1998;157(4 Pt 1):1187–1194.
59. Dahlén SE, Malmström K, Nizankowska E, et al. Improvement of aspirin-intolerant asthma by montelukast, a leukotriene antagonist: a randomized, double-blind, placebo-controlled trial. *Am J Respir Crit Care Med.* 2002;165(1):9–14.
60. Stevenson DD, Simon RA, Mathison DA, Christiansen SC. Montelukast is only partially effective in inhibiting aspirin responses in aspirin-sensitive asthmatics. *Ann Allergy Asthma Immunol.* 2000;85(6 Pt 1):477–482.
61. Asano K, Shiomi T, Hasegawa N, et al. Leukotriene C4 synthase gene A(-444)C polymorphism and clinical response to a CYS-LT(1) antagonist, pranlukast, in Japanese patients with moderate asthma. *Pharmacogenetics.* 2002;12(7):565–570.
62. Stevenson DD, Mehra PK, White AA, Gupta S, Woessner KM, Simon RA. Failure of tacrolimus to prevent aspirin-induced respiratory reactions in patients with aspirin-exacerbated respiratory disease. *J Allergy Clin Immunol.* 2005;116(4):755–760.
63. Pleskow WW, Stevenson DD, Mathison DA, Simon RA, Schatz M, Zeiger RS. Aspirin desensitization in aspirin-sensitive asthmatic patients: clinical manifestations and characterization of the refractory period. *J Allergy Clin Immunol.* 1982;69(1 Pt 1):11–19.
64. Stevenson DD, Pleskow WW, Simon RA, et al. Aspirin-sensitive rhinosinusitis asthma: a double-blind crossover study of treatment with aspirin. *J Allergy Clin Immunol.* 1984;73(4):500–507.
65. Berges-Gimeno MP, Simon RA, Stevenson DD. Long-term treatment with aspirin desensitization in asthmatic patients with aspirin-exacerbated respiratory disease. *J Allergy Clin Immunol.* 2003;111(1):180–186.
66. Wasiak W, Szmidt M. A six week double blind, placebo controlled, crossover study of the effect of misoprostol in the treatment of aspirin sensitive asthma. *Thorax.* 1999;54(10):900–904.
67. Kamani T, Sama A. Management of nasal polyps in 'aspirin sensitive asthma' triad. *Curr Opin Otolaryngol Head Neck Surg.* 2011;19(1):6–10.
68. Patriarca G, Bellioni P, Nucera E, et al. Intranasal treatment with lysine acetylsalicylate in patients with nasal polyposis. *Ann Allergy.* 1991;67(6):588–592.
69. Parikh AA, Scadding GK. Intranasal lysine-aspirin in aspirin-sensitive nasal polyposis: a controlled trial. *Laryngoscope.* 2005;115(8):1385–1390.
70. White A, Bigby T, Stevenson D. Intranasal ketorolac challenge for the diagnosis of aspirin-exacerbated respiratory disease. *Ann Allergy Asthma Immunol.* 2006;97(2):190–195.
71. Floyer J. *A Treatise of the Asthma.* London: R. Wilkin and J. Innys; 1698.
72. McFadden ER. Exercise-induced airway obstruction. *Clin Chest Med.* 1995;16(4):671–682.
73. Kawabori I, Pierson WE, Conquest LL, Bierman CW. Incidence of exercise-induced asthma in children. *J Allergy Clin Immunol.* 1976;58(4):447–455.
74. Cypcar D, Lemanske RF. Asthma and exercise. *Clin Chest Med.* 1994;15(2):351–368.
75. Storms WW. Asthma associated with exercise. *Immunol Allergy Clin North Am.* 2005;25(1):31–43.
76. Wilber RL, Rundell KW, Szmedra L, Jenkinson DM, Im J, Drake SD. Incidence of exercise-induced bronchospasm in Olympic winter sport athletes. *Med Sci Sports Exerc.* 2000;32(4):732–737.
77. Weiler JM, Bonini S, Coifman R, et al. American Academy of Allergy, Asthma & Immunology Work Group report: exercise-induced asthma. *J Allergy Clin Immunol.* 2007;119(6):1349–1358.
78. Anderson SD. *Exercise-Induced Asthma.* 4th ed. St. Louis, MO: Mosby; 1993.
79. Anderson SD, Schoeffel RE, Black JL, Daviskas E. Airway cooling as the stimulus to exercise-induced asthma–a re-evaluation. *Eur J Respir Dis.* 1985;67(1):20–30.
80. Anderson SD. Is there a unifying hypothesis for exercise-induced asthma? *J Allergy Clin Immunol.* 1984;73(5 Pt 2):660–665.
81. Mainardi TR, Mellins RB, Miller RL, et al. Exercise-induced wheeze, urgent medical visits, and neighborhood asthma prevalence. *Pediatrics.* 2013;131(1):e127–e135.
82. Deal EC, McFadden ER, Ingram RH, Strauss RH, Jaeger JJ. Role of respiratory heat exchange in production of exercise-induced asthma. *J Appl Physiol.* 1979;46(3):467–475.
83. Hahn A, Anderson SD, Morton AR, Black JL, Fitch KD. A reinterpretation of the effect of temperature and water content of the inspired air in exercise-induced asthma. *Am Rev Respir Dis.* 1984;130(4):575–579.
84. Ingenito E, Solway J, Lafleur J, Lombardo A, Drazen JM, Pichurko B. Dissociation of temperature-gradient and evaporative heat loss during cold gas hyperventilation in cold-induced asthma. *Am Rev Respir Dis.* 1988;138(3):540–546.
85. McFadden ER. Exercise-induced asthma. Assessment of current etiologic concepts. *Chest.* 1987;91(6 Suppl):151S–157S.
86. Otani K, Kanazawa H, Fujiwara H, Hirata K, Fujimoto S, Yoshikawa J. Determinants of the severity of exercise-induced bronchoconstriction in patients with asthma. *J Asthma.* 2004;41(3):271–278.
87. Mickleborough TD, Lindley MR, Ray S. Dietary salt, airway inflammation, and diffusion capacity in exercise-induced asthma. *Med Sci Sports Exerc.* 2005;37(6):904–914.
88. Karjalainen EM, Laitinen A, Sue-Chu M, Altraja A, Bjermer L, Laitinen LA. Evidence of airway inflammation and remodeling in ski athletes with and without bronchial hyperresponsiveness to methacholine. *Am J Respir Crit Care Med.* 2000;161(6):2086–2091.
89. Vizi E, Huszár E, Csoma Z, et al. Plasma adenosine concentration increases during exercise: a possible contributing factor in exercise-induced bronchoconstriction in asthma. *J Allergy Clin Immunol.* 2002;109(3):446–448.
90. Chhabra SK, Ojha UC. Late asthmatic response in exercise-induced asthma. *Ann Allergy Asthma Immunol.* 1998;80(4):323–327.
91. Helenius I, Rytilä P, Sarna S, et al. Effect of continuing or finishing high-level sports on airway inflammation, bronchial hyperresponsiveness, and asthma: a 5-year prospective follow-up study of 42 highly trained swimmers. *J Allergy Clin Immunol.* 2002;109(6):962–968.
92. Bikov A, Gajdócsi R, Huszár É, et al. Exercise increases exhaled breath condensate cysteinyl leukotriene concentration in asthmatic patients. *J Asthma.* 2010;47(9):1057–1062.

93. Zietkowski Z, Skiepko R, Tomasiak-Lozowska MM, Mroczko B, Szmitkowski M, Bodzenta-Lukaszyk A. RANTES in exhaled breath condensate of allergic asthma patients with exercise-induced bronchoconstriction. *Respiration.* 2010;80(6): 463–471.

94. Zietkowski Z, Skiepko R, Tomasiak-Lozowska MM, Zietkowska E, Bodzenta-Lukaszyk A. Eotaxin in exhaled breath condensate of allergic asthma patients with exercise-induced bronchoconstriction. *Respiration.* 2011;82(2):169–176.

95. Manning PJ, Watson RM, Margolskee DJ, Williams VC, Schwartz JI, O'Byrne PM. Inhibition of exercise-induced bronchoconstriction by MK-571, a potent leukotriene D4-receptor antagonist. *N Engl J Med.* 1990;323(25):1736–1739.

96. Israel E, Dermarkarian R, Rosenberg M, et al. The effects of a 5-lipoxygenase inhibitor on asthma induced by cold, dry air. *N Engl J Med.* 1990;323(25):1740–1744.

97. Hallstrand TS, Wurfel MM, Lai Y, et al. Transglutaminase 2, a novel regulator of eicosanoid production in asthma revealed by genome-wide expression profiling of distinct asthma phenotypes. *PLoS One.* 2010;5(1):e8583.

98. Hallstrand TS, Debley JS, Farin FM, Henderson WR. Role of MUC5AC in the pathogenesis of exercise-induced bronchoconstriction. *J Allergy Clin Immunol.* 2007;119(5): 1092–1098.

99. Kim HB, Lee SY, Shim JY, Kim JH, Kang MJ, Hong SJ. The leukotriene C4 synthase (A-444C) promoter polymorphism is associated with the severity of exercise-induced asthma in Korean children. *J Allergy Clin Immunol.* 2006;117(5): 1191–1192.

100. Lee SY, Kim HB, Kim JH, et al. Responsiveness to montelukast is associated with bronchial hyperresponsiveness and total immunoglobulin E but not polymorphisms in the leukotriene C4 synthase and cysteinyl leukotriene receptor 1 genes in Korean children with exercise-induced asthma (EIA). *Clin Exp Allergy.* 2007;37(10):1487–1493.

101. Carlsen KH, Anderson SD, Bjermer L, et al. Exercise-induced asthma, respiratory and allergic disorders in elite athletes: epidemiology, mechanisms and diagnosis: part I of the report from the Joint Task Force of the European Respiratory Society (ERS) and the European Academy of Allergy and Clinical Immunology (EAACI) in cooperation with GA2LEN. *Allergy.* 2008;63(4):387–403.

102. Fitch KD, Sue-Chu M, Anderson SD, et al. Asthma and the elite athlete: summary of the International Olympic Committee's consensus conference, Lausanne, Switzerland, January 22–24, 2008. *J Allergy Clin Immunol.* 2008;122(2):254–260, 260.e1–e7.

103. O'Byrne PM, Ramsdale EH, Hargreave FE. Isocapnic hyperventilation for measuring airway hyperresponsiveness in asthma and in chronic obstructive pulmonary disease. *Am Rev Respir Dis.* 1991;143(6):1444–1445.

104. Phillips YY, Jaeger JJ, Laube BL, Rosenthal RR. Eucapnic voluntary hyperventilation of compressed gas mixture. A simple system for bronchial challenge by respiratory heat loss. *Am Rev Respir Dis.* 1985;131(1):31–35.

105. Rundell KW, Anderson SD, Spiering BA, Judelson DA. Field exercise vs laboratory eucapnic voluntary hyperventilation to identify airway hyperresponsiveness in elite cold weather athletes. *Chest.* 2004;125(3):909–915.

106. Schnall RP, Landau LI. Protective effects of repeated short sprints in exercise-induced asthma. *Thorax.* 1980;35(11):828–832.

107. Eggleston PA. *Exercise-Induced Asthma.* St. Louis, MO: Mosby; 1996.

108. Mickleborough TD, Lindley MR, Turner LA. Comparative effects of a high-intensity interval warm-up and salbutamol on the bronchoconstrictor response to exercise in asthmatic athletes. *Int J Sports Med.* 2007;28(6):456–462.

109. Stickland MK, Rowe BH, Spooner CH, Vandermeer B, Dryden DM. Effect of warm-up exercise on exercise-induced bronchoconstriction. *Med Sci Sports Exerc.* 2012;44(3):383–391.

110. Gotshall RW, Mickleborough TD, Cordain L. Dietary salt restriction improves pulmonary function in exercise-induced asthma. *Med Sci Sports Exerc.* 2000;32(11):1815–1819.

111. Finnerty JP, Harvey A, Holgate ST. The relative contributions of histamine and prostanoids to bronchoconstriction provoked by isocapnic hyperventilation in asthma. *Eur Respir J.* 1992;5(3): 323–330.

112. Carlsen KH, Anderson SD, Bjermer L, et al. Treatment of exercise-induced asthma, respiratory and allergic disorders in sports and the relationship to doping: part II of the report from the Joint Task Force of European Respiratory Society (ERS) and European Academy of Allergy and Clinical Immunology (EAACI) in cooperation with GA(2)LEN. *Allergy.* 2008;63(5):492–505.

113. Duong M, Amin R, Baatjes AJ, et al. The effect of montelukast, budesonide alone, and in combination on exercise-induced bronchoconstriction. *J Allergy Clin Immunol.* 2012;130(2): 535–539.e533.

114. Morton AR, Fitch KD. Australian association for exercise and sports science position statement on exercise and asthma. *J Sci Med Sport.* 2011;14(4):312–316.

115. Anderson SD, Daviskas E. The mechanism of exercise-induced asthma is . . . *J Allergy Clin Immunol.* 2000;106(3):453–459.

CHAPTER 48

Allergic Bronchopulmonary Aspergillosis (Mycosis) and Severe Asthma with Fungal Sensitivity

Geoffrey L. Chupp

INTRODUCTION

Allergic bronchopulmonary aspergillosis (ABPA) is an idiopathic inflammatory disease of the lung, characterized by an allergic inflammatory response to colonization of the airways by *Aspergillus fumigatus* or other fungi. The entity was first described in 1952 by Hinson et al., and then again in 1967, when Scadding recognized an association between the disease and proximal bronchiectasis in areas previously affected by infiltrates (predominantly in the upper lobes).[1,2] The first adult case of ABPA was reported in the United States in 1968.[3] Although most cases entail hypersensitivity to *Aspergillus* spp. (especially *A. fumigatus*), the finding of a virtually identical clinical syndrome associated with immune sensitivity to *Candida albicans* (most commonly), *Helminthosporium, Alternaria, Curvularia lunata, Drechslera hawaiiensis, Stemphylium languinosum, Saccharomyces cerevisiae*, or *Pseudallescheria boydii* has led some to use the term *allergic bronchopulmonary mycosis* to describe the syndrome.[4] However, since the predominant causative organism is *A. fumigatus* and the commercially available laboratory testing is for this organism, ABPA is primarily designated as the diagnosis. In addition, a new entity has been recently recognized that appears to be on the continuum between fungal allergy, at one end, and ABPA at the other: severe asthma with fungal sensitivity (SAFS).[5]

The precise prevalence of ABPA is unknown, in part due to variability in diagnostic criteria used in various studies, the lack of distinction between ABPA and mold-sensitive asthma, and delays in the diagnosis of patients with long-standing disease; however, it is clear that ABPA is a relatively common entity. Estimates are that true ABPA complicates approximately 7% to 14% of cases of chronic steroid-dependent asthma and approximately 7% to 15% of cases of cystic fibrosis (CF).

Most cases of ABPA are recognized in the third to fifth decade of life, but they may present during childhood. In some patients, it is likely that ABPA starts early in life and continues, unrecognized, until adulthood. Interestingly, familial cases have been reported, suggesting that genetic factors underlie development of ABPA.[6,7] The spectrum of disease is broad. Patients may be asymptomatic, have mild-to-moderate asthma, or have severe and debilitating disease, leading to lung transplantation. However, if recognized early and managed aggressively, ABPA is treatable and may remit indefinitely; progressive lung damage can be avoided.

For the purposes of this discussion, the focus is on ABPA. However, clinicians should be cognizant that diagnostic testing for other fungi needs to be pursued when organisms other than *Aspergillus* spp. are suspected. In addition, the newly defined form of asthma noted previously, SAFS, is discussed and differentiated from ABPA.

PATHOGENESIS

Although the pathogenesis of ABPA is poorly understood, it is believed to be the result of an exaggerated immunologic reaction to chronic airway colonization by *Aspergillus* (or other relevant fungal) species.[8] *Aspergillus* spp. are globally ubiquitous, thermotolerant fungi that reside in decaying organic matter and colonize most domestic environments, including carpets and air duct systems.

In humans, airborn *Aspergillus* spores or conidia that are inhaled are immunologically inert, and in normal individuals are cleared by innate immune system mechanisms to maintain airway homeostasis. However, in susceptible individuals, conidia colonize airways, germinate into somatic hyphae that stimulate a chronic allergic inflammatory response that results in tissue injury and, ultimately, dictates the clinical features of ABPA. In contrast to a true infection in which fungal hyphae invade the lung parenchyma, colonization of the airways with germinating fungal spores represents an abnormal state that contributes to the exaggerated Th2 inflammatory response without clear tissue invasion. While a detailed understanding of the mechanisms that drive this process remains poorly understood, it appears that susceptibility to *Aspergillus* colonization and development of clinical disease depend on host factors, such as genetic background, T-cell responsiveness to *Aspergillus* antigens, the magnitude of tissue response to *Aspergillus*, and the level of environmental exposure to this ubiquitous fungus.

Investigations into the genetic risk factors associated with ABPA have identified several candidate genes, suggesting that the pathogenesis of ABPA requires both host and environmental factors.[9] Best characterized is the association between gene mutations in the CF transmembrane conductance regulator (CFTR) and the pathogenesis of ABPA.[10,11] CFTR mutations are more common among patients with ABPA compared with the general population or with individuals with severe asthma without sensitivity to *A. fumigatus*. Another genetic link to ABPA is that Th2-type T-cell reactivity to selected *Aspergillus* antigens is determined by the presence of MHC Class II DR2 or DR5 alleles, which may predispose patients to the disease, whereas the MHC DQ2 allele may be protective.[12,13] In addition, investigators have determined that there is an increased prevalence of polymorphisms in the promoter region of the pathogen associated molecular pattern receptor, Toll (TLR) 9, in individuals with ABPA compared with controls or patients with SAFS.[14] We recently determined that children with severe asthma and ABPA are more likely to carry the Chitotriosidase 1 (CHIT1) exon 10 mutation.[15,16] Individuals with the exon 10 mutation have lower levels of, or lack, chitinase activity in serum and are unable to degrade chitin, a structural polysaccharide in the cell wall of lower life forms such as *A. fumigatus*.[17–19]

At the microscopic level, ABPA is characterized by an intense eosinophilic and mononuclear cell inflammatory response, leading into areas of parenchymal scarring, airway remodeling, and bronchiectasis.[20,21] Immunologic studies demonstrate the presence of a type I hypersensitivity reaction, with elevated serum levels of total IgE and *A. fumigatus*-specific IgE in individuals with ABPA. In addition, patients have evidence of an exaggerated Type III hypersensitivity reaction, indicated by the presence of *A. fumigatus-specific* IgG antibodies (classically called "precipitins" or precipitating antibodies) and circulating immune complexes during disease exacerbations. A type IV cell-mediated immune reaction may also be at work, based on the finding of dual (immediate and delayed) cutaneous reactions and *in vitro* lymphocyte transformation to *A. fumigatus* antigen stimulation in some patients.[22,23]

A substantial amount of work has been done on the immune response in ABPA, demonstrating that several cell types and pathways are involved in the pathogenesis of this destructive variant of asthma.[17,18] A pathogenetic role for helper T lymphocytes is suggested by a number of findings, including the presence of increased numbers of airway Th2 cells and elevated levels of soluble interleukin 2 receptors (suggesting T-cell activation) in the circulation of persons with active ABPA[24]; the derivation of *A. fumigatus*-specific T-cell clones with T helper–2 (Th2) patterns of cytokine production from the blood of patients with ABPA[25,26]; positive correlations between activated T-cell number, levels of the T-cell–derived cytokines IL-4 and IL-5, and number of airway eosinophils in the disease; the critical role IL-5 plays in murine models of ABPA[27–34]; and increased reactivity of Th2 cells to *A. fumigatus* antigens among patients with ABPA as compared with patients with asthma and skin reactivity to *Aspergillus*.

In addition to lymphocytes, eosinophils and basophils may contribute to local airway injury, and neutrophils likely play a role in airway inflammation and tissue damage in ABPA, as evidenced by the fact that sputum IL-8 levels correlate with sputum neutrophilia, matrix metalloproteinase levels, and FEV_1 among patients with ABPA.[35,36]

It is also clear that the fungus itself contributes substantially to the pathogenesis of disease. *A. fumigatus*-derived proteases likely cause epithelial cell injury and protective barrier disruption, triggering immune hypersensitivity by inducing inflammation or by allowing increased penetration of fungal antigens into the airway wall.[37] *Aspergillus*-derived proteases may also stimulate proinflammatory cytokines, such as IL-8, and release of growth factors; proteases may also cause tissue damage, leading to bronchiectasis.[36]

A variety of other *Aspergillus*-derived antigens (including cytotoxins and heat shock proteins) with demonstrated ability to bind IgE and IgG derived from the blood of patients with ABPA have also been shown to drive both the IgE (hypersensitivity) and IgG immune responses. *A. fumigatus*-derived proteases with antibody-binding capacity may also amplify the inflammatory response. *A. fumigatus* antigens, such as Aspf1 (a cytotoxic protein), Aspf2 (a fibrinogen binding protein), Aspf5 (a metalloprotease), Aspf6 (manganese superoxide dismutase), Aspf8 (a ribosomal protein), Aspf13 and Aspf18 (serine proteases), as well as Aspf3 and Aspf4, have all been implicated in these processes. Finally, host response to *Aspergillus fumigatus* antigens includes surfactant proteins (SP) A and D, which may play a protective role against ABPA by interfering with binding between *A. fumigatus* antigens and IgE. Notably, however, SPD levels do not correlate with acute exacerbations of ABPA in humans.[38–40]

CLINICAL FEATURES

Although ABPA typically presents in patients with a history of difficult-to-control asthma, the spectrum of presentation is highly variable and should be considered in any patient with difficult-to-control asthma and hypersensitivity to *A. fumigatus* (Table 48-1).[40] Typical presenting complaints are often nonspecific and include dyspnea, wheezing, poor asthma control, cough (sometimes productive of thick, brown mucus plugs), malaise, low-grade fever, and occasionally, hemoptysis. There may be an antecedent history of recurrent asthma exacerbations in conjunction with pneumonias without a culture-identified bacterial source. In addition, atopy with rhinitis, drug allergy, and/or allergic conjunctivitis are also common. It is often not until a patient has been repeatedly ill over weeks to months and unresponsive to standard treatments that the diagnosis is considered.[41] As patients with SAFS have the same clinical presentation, differentiation from ABPA is based on interpretation of laboratory testing and radiographic studies.[40]

DIAGNOSTIC GUIDELINES

In general, the diagnosis of ABPA is based on appropriate clinical features in combination with supporting radiologic and serologic findings. While there are no absolutely specific diagnostic criteria, similar guidelines have been proposed by multiple expert panels to aid clinicians in the diagnosis of ABPA (Table 48-1).[20,42] These guidelines have evolved over time and have been recently updated by several societies. Although there is no agreement on clinical criteria that should trigger screening for ABPA, in most asthma centers, all asthmatics with difficult-to-control asthma are screened by checking an eosinophil count, total IgE, and radioallergosorbent test for 22 aeroallergens, including *A. fumigatus and Alternaria.*

TABLE 48-1 Criteria for the Diagnosis of ABPA

Seropositive ABPA (ABPA-S)
History of asthma (almost always difficult to control)
Elevated total serum IgE (usually >1000 IU/mL)
Immediate skin test reactivity to *Aspergillus fumigatus* OR elevated specific serum IgE to *A. fumigatus*
Presence of serum precipitins (by gel diffusion) or elevated specific serum IgG to *A. fumigatus*
ABPA central bronchiectasis (ABPA-CB)
Above criteria are positive
Central bronchiectasis by high-resolution CT scan or CXR
Other supportive clinical findings
Peripheral blood eosinophilia (often absent, especially if patient is on oral or inhaled corticosteroids)
Patchy, fleeting infiltrates (often absent, especially if patient is on oral corticosteroids)
Expectoration of brown mucus plugs
Mucoid-impacted bronchi evident on radiographic studies
Sputum culture positive for *A. fumigatus*

Using the Patterson criteria (Table 48-1), ABPA may be considered to exist in two different forms: ABPA-seropositive (S) and ABPA-central bronchiectasis (CB).

Patients with ABPA-S usually display all of the following diagnostic criteria proposed by Greenberger and Patterson: (1) history of asthma; (2) total IgE >1000 IU/mL; (3) elevated serum anti-*AF* IgE and IgG (twofold higher than *A. fumigatus* allergic asthma controls); (4) positive immediate hypersensitivity skin test to *A. fumigatus*; and/or (5) serum anti-*A. fumigatus* IgG antibodies to *A. fumigatus*. The last criterion is considered positive when either the double gel diffusion, enzyme-linked immunoassay (ELISA), or fluorescent enzyme immunoassay (FEIA) are positive for anti-*AF* IgG antibodies.[43]

Patients with ABPA-S have normal chest radiographic studies, with no evidence of bronchiectasis. In contrast, patients with ABPA-CB have the classic features of advanced disease (expectoration of mucus plugs or sputum culture positive for *A. fumigatus*) and are positive for all of the criteria of ABPA-S listed earlier. Patients with ABPA-CB also have central bronchiectasis on high-resolution CT scanning or chest X-ray.[44,45] Patients with ABPA-S tend to have fewer symptoms, lower IgE levels, less severe airflow obstruction, and fewer exacerbations than do persons with ABPA-CB. Although IgE levels fluctuate with disease activity, a normal IgE level in a symptomatic, untreated patient with asthma virtually excludes the diagnosis.[46] It remains unclear whether ABPA-S is a milder form of the disease (e.g., representing a different host response) or an earlier stage of illness. Identification of *Aspergillus* (or other relevant fungus) in the sputum and dual (immediate and delayed) cutaneous reactions to challenge with *Aspergillus* (by prick test or intradermal) are also common clinical features of ABPA. Rare cases lacking a history of asthma, but meeting the other major diagnostic criteria, have been reported.[41]

TABLE 48-2 Criteria for the Diagnosis of Severe Asthma with Fungal Sensitivity (SAFS)

1. History of poorly controlled asthma (>500 μg/d of fluticasone or the equivalent, near continuous oral corticosteroids for >6 mo, or >2 oral steroid tapers per year)
2. Total serum IgE <1000 IU/mL
3. Positive immediate skin test reactivity to *Aspergillus fumigatus* OR elevated specific serum IgE to *A. fumigatus*
4. Absence of serum precipitins (by gel diffusion) and elevated specific serum IgG to *A. fumigatus*
5. No radiographic evidence of bronchiectasis or infiltrates

SEVERE ASTHMA WITH FUNGAL SENSITIVITY

The broad spectrum of clinical, laboratory, and radiographic abnormalities evident in patients with asthma with fungal allergy has led to the description of additional diagnostic categories of allergic fungal disease. The most relevant of these diagnoses is based on studies that demonstrate that antifungal therapies are effective in patients with poorly controlled asthma that have some of the criteria for ABPA-S, but do not reach the threshold for diagnosis. These patients have been designated as having SAFS.

Whether SAFS is a unique disease or is on the continuum from asthma to ABPA remains unclear. However, the primary distinction is that patients with SAFS have a milder allergic reaction and lack the exaggerated IgG response that is typical of patients with ABPA. Therefore, patients with SAFS are difficult to distinguish from patients with ABPA, and especially ABPA-S, as the clinical features are identical between the two entities and both lack radiographic abnormalities.

The diagnosis of SAFS is based on the interpretation of *Aspergillus*-specific immunologic studies. The diagnostic criteria for SAFS (Table 48-2) overlap substantially with ABPA-S and include: (1) severe uncontrolled asthma (treatment requirement of >500 μg/d of fluticasone or the equivalent, need for near continuous oral corticosteroids for 6 months or >2 oral steroid tapers per year); (2) positive skin prick test or RAST for *A. fumigatus* or other fungi; (3) total serum IgE (<417 IU/mL or <1000 ng/mL)); and (4) absence of IgG against *A. fumigatus* (by ELISA, gel diffusion, or FEIA).

In general, patients with SAFS typically have normal radiographic studies and a milder immunologic response that may be identified in patients with milder asthma. Although it remains unclear whether these patients are on the continuum from asthma to ABPA or are at risk of progressing to frank ABPA, the importance of identifying such patients is based on several studies indicating that antifungal therapies may significantly improve asthma control and reduce oral corticosteroid exposure.[47–49]

The differential diagnosis of ABPA is broad and includes corticosteroid-dependent asthma without ABPA, SAFS, chronic obstructive pulmonary disease (COPD), chronic necrotizing aspergillosis, tuberculosis, parasitic infections, hypersensitivity pneumonitis, Churg–Strauss syndrome, acute eosinophilic pneumonia (including drug-induced pneumonitis), chronic eosinophilic pneumonia, lymphoma, idiopathic hypereosinophilic syndrome, autoimmune disease, crack cocaine use, CF, and other causes of bronchiectasis. In addition, the diagnosis of ABPA in patients with mold-sensitive asthma and CF poses particular diagnostic challenge. This is especially true in asthmatics, since, by definition, bronchiectasis is absent; furthermore, serum precipitins to *Aspergillus* spp. may be present in up to 10% of patients with positive immediate skin tests to *Aspergillus* and in up to 25% of asthmatics, making distinction from ABPA-S difficult.

Persons with mold-sensitive asthma or ABPA may have peripheral blood eosinophilia and/or elevated serum total IgE levels. However, most persons with ABPA have 2- to 20-fold higher serum levels of *Aspergillus*-specific IgE and total IgE than do mold-sensitive asthmatics without ABPA. A more confusing diagnostic conundrum occurs when considering the diagnosis of ABPA in patients with CF, because patients with CF alone may manifest chronic airflow obstruction, recurrent exacerbations with infections and/or bronchoconstriction, underlying bronchiectasis, pulmonary infiltrates, chronic sputum production, *Aspergillus* colonization of the airways, and positive serum precipitins.

Distinguishing ABPA in patients with CF is critical, because infectious CF exacerbations and the presence of ABPA require different treatments. The steroid treatment required for ABPA may be detrimental in the setting of infection, yet antibiotics alone given for infection may be inadequate to control the inflammation associated with ABPA. Among patients with CF, factors associated with the risk of ABPA include adolescent age, atopy, severe lung disease, and colonization with *Pseudomonas aeruginosa*. ABPA should be suspected in patients with CF who develop clinical deterioration, exhibit a greater than fourfold increase in total serum IgE (especially >1000 IU/mL), have immediate cutaneous reactivity to *Aspergillus* or increased *Aspergillus*-specific IgE or IgG, and show a change in baseline CXR. Annual screening of total serum IgE is recommended; if the level rises >500 IU/mL, immediate cutaneous hypersensitivity testing for reactivity to *A. fumigatus* or testing for serum anti-*A. fumigatus* IgE is recommended.[11,50] The presence

TABLE 48-3 Clinical Stages of ABPA

Stage I: Acute
- Acute asthma symptoms
- Elevated serum IgE (>1000 IU/mL)
- Peripheral blood eosinophilia (may be absent in patients treated with oral corticosteroids)
- Fleeting infiltrates on chest X-ray (may be absent in patients treated with oral corticosteroids)
- Positive specific IgE, IgG, skin test reactivity, or precipitins to *Aspergillus fumigatus*
- Responds to steroids/antifungal therapy

Stage II: Remission
- Resolution of symptoms
- Resolution of pulmonary infiltrates
- Improvement in eosinophilia and *A. fumigatus* specific blood abnormalities

Stage III: Exacerbation/Recurrence
- Recurrence/worsening of clinical symptoms
- Recurrent pulmonary infiltrates
- Rising IgE levels

Stage IV: Steroid-Dependent Asthma
- Refractory steroid-dependent asthma
- Persistently elevated serum IgE levels
- Persistently elevated *A. fumigatus*–specific blood abnormalities

Stage V: Fibrotic Lung Disease
- Refractory steroid-dependent asthma
- Fibrotic lung disease (irreversible obstructive and restrictive defects with impaired diffusing capacity)
- Chronic bronchiectasis symptoms (sputum production, frequent infections)

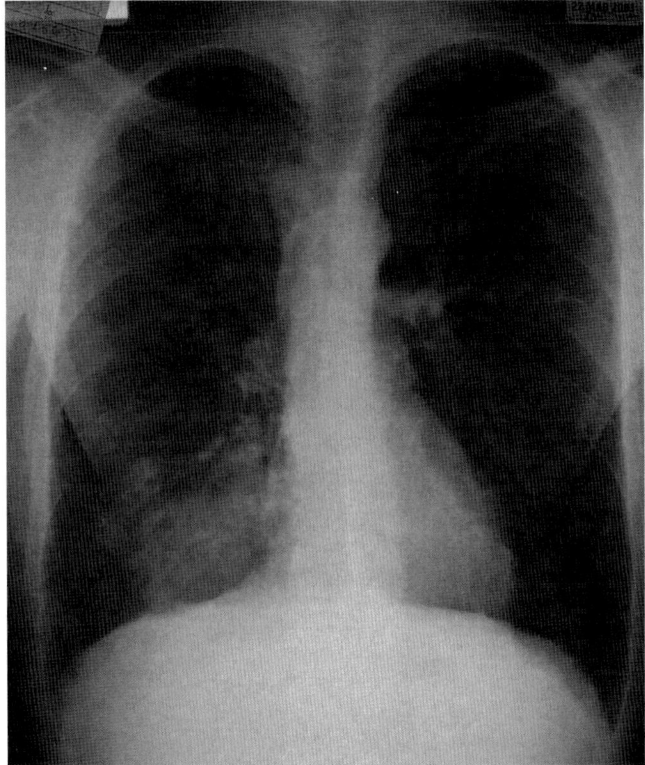
A

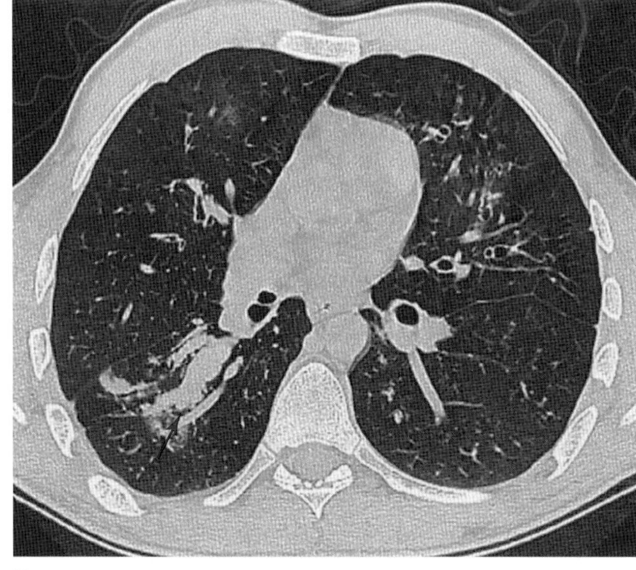
B

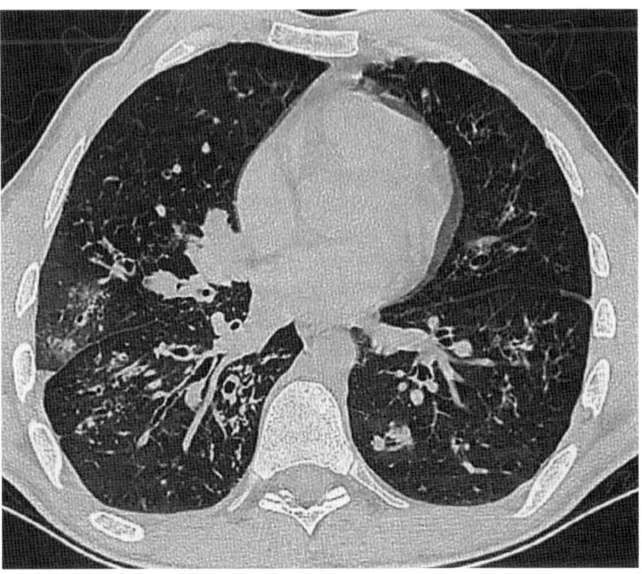
C

Figure 48-1 A 27-year-old man with a history of moderate asthma, recurrent bronchitis, and mild hemoptysis. Serologic studies were consistent with ABPA (IgE, 9490 IU/mL) and radiographic studies were consistent with bronchiectasis. **A.** PA chest X-ray shows hyperinflated lungs, bronchial dilatation, and right lower lobe opacity consistent with mucoid impaction. **B.** High-resolution CT scan image of impacted bronchus *(arrow)* and chronic inflammatory changes. **C.** Dilated central bronchus consistent with cylindrical/central bronchiectasis.

of IgE reactive against the purified *Aspergillus* allergens Aspf3 and Aspf4 may be useful in distinguishing patients with ABPA and CF or *Aspergillus*-sensitive asthma from patients without ABPA.[10]

CLINICAL STAGING OF ABPA

Five clinical stages of ABPA have been recognized, based on clinical, serologic, and radiographic characteristics (Table 48-3). A modified version proposed by the International Society for Human and Animal Mycology (ISHAM) has not been widely adopted.[20,51]

Using the classic staging system, Stage I, the *acute* stage, is characterized by symptoms of moderate-to-severe asthma, elevated total IgE (typically >1000 IU/mL), elevated anti-*A. fumigatus* IgE or hypersensitivity skin test to *A. fumigatus*, infiltrates on chest radiograph (with or without proximal bronchiectasis), peripheral blood eosinophilia (frequently >2000/mm^3), and positive precipitating or anti-IgG antibodies to *A. fumigatus* (up to fivefold concentration of serum may be required for detection of the precipitating antibodies).

Patients with stage II ABPA have disease that is in *remission.* This stage is characterized by the resolution of symptoms, radiographic clearing, and decreased stabilization of total IgE levels. Remissions are of varying length, may last several months to years, or may be permanent, allowing corticosteroid treatment to be tapered or discontinued.

Patients with stage III ABPA have *recurrent* disease or disease *exacerbations* (Fig. 48-1). This stage of ABPA is common and is characterized by development of new pulmonary infiltrates and, usually, a substantial increase in total IgE. Elevation of IgE may precede clinical or radiologic worsening during this stage; an isolated increase in the severity of bronchospasm does not constitute an exacerbation

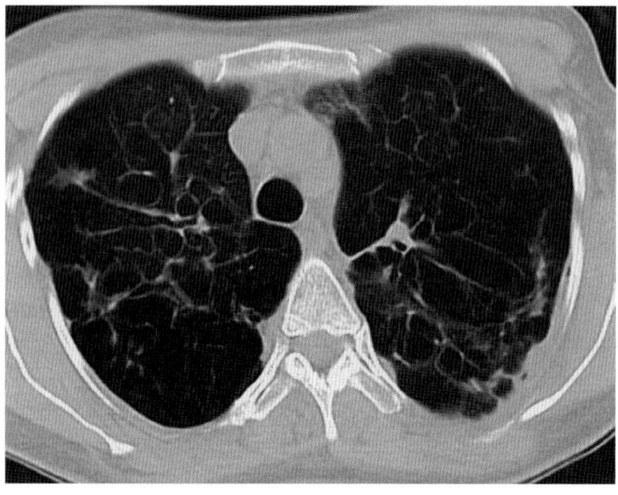

Figure 48-2 Representative CT image of the lungs of a 41-year-old woman who presented with Stage-V ABPA after a long history of mild asthma (IgE, 1500 IU/mL). Pulmonary function studies demonstrated severe combined obstructive and restrictive defects. CT shows bilateral upper lobe scarring and emphysematous changes.

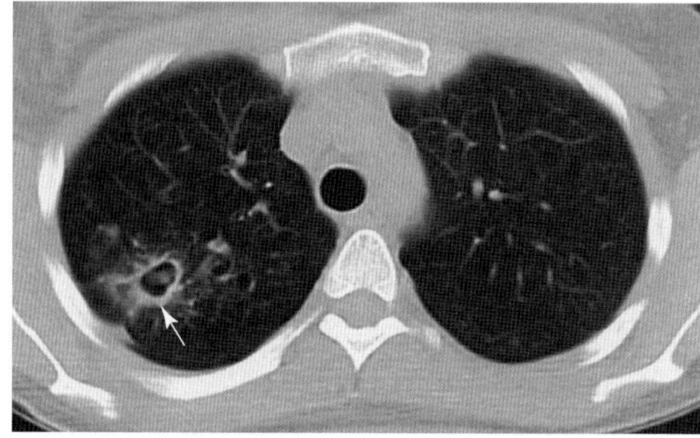

Figure 48-3 A 21-year-old woman with ABPA, who responded to treatment with oral corticosteroids and chronic antifungal therapy, developed an aspergilloma and hemoptysis *(arrow)*. Amphotericin paste injection failed and the patient ultimately underwent a right upper lobe lobectomy.

in the absence of a change in biomarkers. Although a majority of disease exacerbations are associated with a concomitant increase in symptoms, exacerbations may occur in the absence of any increase in symptoms. Indeed, since up to one-third of patients with radiographic infiltrates may be asymptomatic, evolving progressive lung damage may remain unrecognized. Total serum IgE levels should be monitored every 1 to 2 months for at least a year after diagnosis, and chest radiographs should be performed intermittently. *Aspergillus*-specific IgA levels may also be elevated in the acute or exacerbation stages of disease. Exacerbations are more likely to occur during seasons or in environments when mold counts are high.

Stage IV ABPA is defined as *steroid-dependent asthma*. In stage IV disease, total IgE, *Aspergillus* precipitins, and *Aspergillus*-specific IgE and IgG typically remain elevated, despite chronic steroid therapy. The frequency of exacerbations may increase.

Stage V is defined as *pulmonary fibrosis*. Stage V patients have prominent symptoms of dyspnea; are often steroid dependent because of persistent bronchospasm; frequently have chronic sputum production, recurrent respiratory infections, and irreversible pulmonary function abnormalities (obstruction, restriction, and/or gas exchange abnormalities), and may have cyanosis or clubbing. The serologic profile of patients with stage IV disease persists during stage V. Stage V disease is generally thought to be the consequence of longstanding, often unrecognized, disease, but it may occur occasionally among patients with little prior clinical evidence to suggest the diagnosis (Fig. 48-2).

DIAGNOSTIC STUDIES

In addition to the blood abnormalities described earlier, analysis of BAL fluid from patients with ABPA often reveals a moderate eosinophilia (especially in steroid-naive patients) and increased levels of *Aspergillus*-specific IgE and IgA, but not IgG. On bronchoscopy, mucoid impaction may be evident, and bronchial brushings may reveal mucus that contains aggregates of eosinophils, fungal hyphae, and eosinophil-derived Charcot–Leyden crystals. The finding of hyphae-filled mucus plugs is considered pathognomonic for ABPA. Pulmonary function tests typically reveal an obstructive ventilatory defect (due to bronchospasm or mucus impaction of the bronchi) during Stages I, III, IV, and often, V and may not correlate with the duration of ABPA or asthma. Patients with Stage V disease typically also have a restrictive ventilatory defect and a reduced DLCO (Fig. 48-2).

The typical radiographic manifestations of ABPA include parenchymal infiltrates and bronchiectasis (Figs. 48-1–48-3). The infiltrates are often irregular and transient (1–6 weeks). They have a predilection for upper lobes, although all lobes may be affected. The bronchiectasis is classically cylindric and proximal (central), occurring within the proximal two-thirds of the lung (Fig. 48-1B). Mucoid impaction in dilated bronchi leads to a characteristic (but nonspecific) radiographic appearance of ABPA termed the "finger in glove" opacity. "Tramline shadows" (parallel linear shadows extending from the hilum in bronchial distribution and reflecting longitudinal views of inflamed, edematous bronchi), "toothpaste shadows" (representing mucoid impaction of the bronchi), "ring shadows" (dilated bronchi with inflamed bronchial walls seen on end), local consolidation, or lobar collapse are also common features. Involvement of the small airways may lead to centrilobular nodules and branching tree-in-bud opacities (Fig. 48-1). Less common radiographic findings include bullous changes, pneumothorax, pleural effusion, cavitating nodular lesions, aspergilloma (Figs. 48-2 and 48-3) and migratory parenchymal opacities, some of which have a ground-glass appearance. High-resolution CT scanning is the most reliable noninvasive means of detecting proximal bronchiectasis.

Open-lung biopsy is usually not required to establish the diagnosis of ABPA. Histopathologic findings include intense bronchocentric inflammation with prominent eosinophilia, as well as lymphocytes, plasma cells, and monocytes. Bronchi may be filled and/or impacted with copious mucus plugs containing fibrin, Charcot–Leyden crystals, Curschmann spirals, and fungal hyphae. Bronchiectasis of segmental and subsegmental bronchi may be evident. Regions of bronchocentric granulomatosis, eosinophilic pneumonia, eosinophilic microabscess, lymphocytic or desquamative interstitial pneumonitis, proliferative or obliterative bronchiolitis, lipoid pneumonia, or interstitial fibrosis may also be seen.

TREATMENT

The goals of treatment for individuals with ABPA consist of controlling symptoms, preventing exacerbations, and preserving normal lung function.

Systemic corticosteroids are the mainstay of therapy for ABPA. Without treatment, ABPA may cause significant irreversible lung damage due to bronchiectasis and pulmonary fibrosis. Therefore, initiation of appropriate treatment early in the course of disease is essential. Although most data are derived from small uncontrolled trials, and definitive proof that corticosteroid therapy prevents the development of central bronchiectasis is lacking, retrospective studies suggest that early therapeutic intervention using corticosteroids may prevent progression to lung fibrosis.

Therapy for Stage I or III disease should include prednisone, 0.5 to 1 mg/kg a day for 2 weeks, followed by 0.5 mg/kg every other day for 6 to 8 weeks. A subsequent taper (by 5–10 mg every 2 weeks) over the ensuing 3 months may then be tried. The duration of treatment must be guided by activity and severity of disease, with an aim of minimizing cumulative exposure to systemic corticosteroids. A low maintenance dose (e.g., 5.0–7.5 mg/d) may be required long term to control the disease and prevent recurrence in some patients.

Corticosteroid therapy leads to relief of symptoms and decreases in airflow obstruction, decreases (>35%) in serum IgE, reductions in peripheral blood eosinophils, and resolution of pulmonary inflammation and infiltrates. IgE levels should be monitored within a few months of an acute episode or exacerbation and should be followed every 2 months thereafter since levels may rise, reflecting disease activity, prior to an exacerbation or in the absence of clinical symptoms. Escalation of steroid therapy should be considered if IgE levels rise more than 100%. The CXR should be monitored within the first year of an acute episode or exacerbation and may be followed yearly thereafter if the disease is quiescent. Pulmonary function testing should be followed closely as well.

Although treatment of acute exacerbations is believed to be helpful in preventing fibrotic complications of ABPA, it is not known if early detection and treatment of disease flares has any effect on disease progression. Therefore, high-dose systemic corticosteroid treatment of asymptomatic individuals is not recommended. Patients with CF and ABPA flares may derive symptomatic or functional improvement from steroid treatment. However, patients with CF who are on steroids should be followed closely for development of invasive aspergillosis. It is unclear whether development of ABPA alters the course of CF disease progression.

Although not advocated as primary treatment, inhaled corticosteroids are useful for control of bronchospasm and may help minimize the dose of systemic steroid necessary to control wheezing. They have been used occasionally as a steroid-sparing agent for the treatment of symptomatic exacerbations and pulmonary infiltrates, and they may help maintain stability of lung function. In addition, adjuvant treatment with bronchodilators and antibiotics also helps control bronchospasm and secondary respiratory infections.

In the last decade, development of oral antifungal agents has brought new hope to patients with ABPA.[52,53] Even though the current concept is that ABPA is not a classic "infection," evidence is mounting to support use of the antifungal agent, itraconazole, in patients with ABPA. Presumably, the agent minimizes the degree of fungal colonization.

In one randomized controlled study, itraconazole (200 mg twice daily for 16 weeks) led to significant reductions in corticosteroid dose, decreased IgE levels, greater resolution of pulmonary infiltrates, and gains in exercise tolerance or pulmonary function.[54] Several clinical studies have demonstrated that treatment with itraconazole also reduces *Aspergillus* antibody titers and eosinophilia compared with placebo.

Itraconazole treatment (200 mg/d or every other day) is generally recommended for patients with ABPA who are steroid dependent, have frequent relapses, and in whom the cost and risks are thought not to outweigh the potential benefits. Itraconazole also has demonstrated utility in ABPA associated with CF. If itraconazole is used, steady-state blood levels can be checked after 1 to 2 weeks, 4 hours after the dose is given, to assess drug absorption.[55]

Since itraconazole interferes with the hepatic metabolism of several medications, including cyclosporine, oral hypoglycemics, tacrolimus, terfenadine, cisapride, and midazolam, particular caution should be exercised with its use among patients taking any of these medications. In addition, physicians must be mindful of adrenal insufficiency associated with itraconazole treatment among patients with ABPA using inhaled corticosteroids, as itraconazole may cause reduced steroid clearance and/or possible direct suppression of adrenal steroid production. Interval screening for adrenal insufficiency should be considered among such persons. In contrast, the efficacy of itraconazole in ABPA may be less among persons taking agents that raise gastric pH, as an elevated gastric pH may dramatically reduce drug absorption.

Other antifungal agents, including nystatin, amphotericin B, miconazole, clotrimazole, and natamycin, are generally ineffective in controlling ABPA. Ketoconazole may be effective, but its utility is limited by hepatotoxicity. Efficacy of voriconazole has not yet been studied in ABPA, but anecdotal reports from our center and others suggest similar results to itraconazole.[56–59]

Finally, the new biologically engineered antibody directed against IgE, omalizumab, is an intriguing consideration for use in ABPA, but the agent has not been extensively studied in large randomized trials. Given that the recommended dosing of this biologic is based on patient weight and serum IgE level, many patients with ABPA are outside of the dosing nomogram. However, multiple case reports and small series indicate that at conventional doses (up to 375 mg subcutaneously every 2 weeks), administration may improve disease activity and spare oral corticosteroid dosing.[60–69]

In addition to medical therapy, all patients with ABPA-related bronchiectasis should be prescribed standard airway clearance treatments, including hypertonic saline and mucus clearance valves or percussion vests, depending on the severity of disease. In addition, patients with ABPA should avoid areas and environmental conditions associated with high mold counts, such as decomposing organic materials and moldy indoor environments. One should consider the use of HEPA filters if such exposures are unavoidable.

PROGNOSIS

With appropriate treatment, long-term control of ABPA is feasible, and durable remissions are common. Treatment of Stage I disease using corticosteroids typically results in decreased sputum production, improved control of bronchospasm, >35% reduction in total IgE within 8 weeks, clearing of precipitating antibodies, and resolution of radiographic infiltrates. IgE levels typically do not completely normalize, but rather, they decrease by approximately one-half of peak levels seen in the acute stage. Progression of Stage IV disease to pulmonary fibrosis may be prevented if patients are maintained on low-dose steroids; most patients with Stage V disease have a stable course over several years. Persons with an FEV_1 persistently <0.8 L have a worse prognosis.

In addition to severe airflow obstruction and pulmonary fibrosis, long-term complications of ABPA occasionally include the development of an aspergilloma (Fig. 48-3), chronic or recurrent lobar atelectasis, allergic *Aspergillus* sinusitis, or *Aspergillus* tissue invasion and semi-invasive *Aspergillosis*. Transplantation has been undertaken successfully among patients with ABPA. However, post-transplant recurrence of ABPA has been reported.

REFERENCES

1. Hinson KF, Moon AJ, Plummer NS. Broncho-pulmonary aspergillosis; a review and a report of eight new cases. *Thorax.* 1952; 7:317–333.
2. McCarthy DS. Bronchiectasis in allergic bronchopulmonary aspergillosis. *Proc R Soc Med.* 1968;61:503–506.
3. Patterson R, Greenberger PA, Lee TM, et al. Prolonged evaluation of patients with corticosteroid-dependent asthma stage of allergic bronchopulmonary aspergillosis. *J Allergy Clin Immunol.* 1987;80:663–668.

4. Chowdhary A, Agarwal K, Kathuria S, Gaur SN, Randhawa HS, Meis JF. Allergic bronchopulmonary mycosis due to fungi other than Aspergillus: a global overview. *Crit Rev Microbiol.* 2013; 40(1):30–48.
5. Antoniu S. Itraconazole for severe asthma with fungal sensitivity. *Expert Opin Pharmacother.* 2009;10:1231–1233.
6. Shah A, Kala J, Sahay S, Panjabi C. Frequency of familial occurrence in 164 patients with allergic bronchopulmonary aspergillosis. *Ann Allergy Asthma Immunol.* 2008;101:363–369.
7. Shah A, Khan ZU, Chaturvedi S, Malik GB, Randhawa HS. Concomitant allergic Aspergillus sinusitis and allergic bronchopulmonary aspergillosis associated with familial occurrence of allergic bronchopulmonary aspergillosis. *Ann Allergy.* 1990; 64:507–512.
8. Wark P. Pathogenesis of allergic bronchopulmonary aspergillosis and an evidence-based review of azoles in treatment. *Respir Med.* 2004;98:915–923.
9. Agarwal R. Allergic bronchopulmonary aspergillosis: lessons learnt from genetics. *Indian J Chest Dis Allied Sci.* 2011;53: 137–140.
10. Rapaka RR, Kolls JK. Pathogenesis of allergic bronchopulmonary aspergillosis in cystic fibrosis: current understanding and future directions. *Med Mycol.* 2009;47(Suppl 1):S331–S337.
11. Knutsen AP, Slavin RG. Allergic bronchopulmonary aspergillosis in asthma and cystic fibrosis. *Clin Dev Immunol.* 2011; 2011:843763.
12. Chauhan B, Santiago L, Kirschmann DA, et al. The association of HLA-DR alleles and T cell activation with allergic bronchopulmonary aspergillosis. *J Immunol.* 1997;159:4072–4076.
13. Chauhan B, Hutcheson PS, Slavin RG, Bellone CJ. MHC restriction in allergic bronchopulmonary aspergillosis. *Front Biosci.* 2003;8:s140–s148.
14. Carvalho A, Pasqualotto AC, Pitzurra L, Romani L, Denning DW, Rodrigues F. Polymorphisms in toll-like receptor genes and susceptibility to pulmonary aspergillosis. *J Infect Dis.* 2008; 197:618–621.
15. Vicencio AG, Chupp GL, Tsirilakis K, et al. CHIT1 mutations: genetic risk factor for severe asthma with fungal sensitization? *Pediatrics.* 2010;126:e982–e985.
16. Ober C, Chupp GL. The chitinase and chitinase-like proteins: a review of genetic and functional studies in asthma and immune-mediated diseases. *Curr Opin Allergy Clin Immunol.* 2009;9:401–408.
17. Ober C, Tan Z, Sun Y, et al. Effect of variation in CHI3L1 on serum YKL-40 level, risk of asthma, and lung function. *N Engl J Med.* 2008;358:1682–1691.
18. Chupp GL, Lee CG, Jarjour N, et al. A chitinase-like protein in the lung and circulation of patients with severe asthma. *N Engl J Med.* 2007;357:2016–2027.
19. Dickey BF. Exoskeletons and exhalation. *N Engl J Med.* 2007; 357:2082–2084.
20. Agarwal R, Chakrabarti A, Shah A, et al. ABPA complicating asthma ISHAM working group. Allergic bronchopulmonary aspergillosis: review of literature and proposal of new diagnostic and classification criteria. *Clin Exp Allergy.* 2013;43:850–873.
21. Knutsen AP. Immunopathology and immunogenetics of allergic bronchopulmonary aspergillosis. *J Allergy.* 2011;2011:785983.
22. Slavin RG, Hutcheson PS, Chauhan B, Bellone CJ. An overview of allergic bronchopulmonary aspergillosis with some new insights. *Allergy Asthma Proc.* 2004;25:395–399.
23. Arora S, Hernandez Y, Erb-Downward JR, McDonald RA, Toews GB, Huffnagle GB. Role of IFN-gamma in regulating T2 immunity and the development of alternatively activated macrophages during allergic bronchopulmonary mycosis. *J Immunol.* 2005;174:6346–6356.
24. Brown JE, Greenberger PA, Yarnold PR. Soluble serum interleukin 2 receptors in patients with asthma and allergic bronchopulmonary aspergillosis. *Ann Allergy Asthma Immunol.* 1995;74: 484–488.
25. Rathore VB, Johnson B, Fink JN, Kelly KJ, Greenberger PA, Kurup VP. T cell proliferation and cytokine secretion to T cell epitopes of Asp f 2 in ABPA patients. *Clin Immunol.* 2001;100: 228–235.
26. Banerjee B, Kurup VP, Greenberger PA, Johnson BD, Fink JN. Cloning and expression of *Aspergillus fumigatus* allergen Aspf 16 mediating both humoral and cell-mediated immunity in allergic bronchopulmonary aspergillosis (ABPA). *Clin Exp Allergy.* 2001;31:761–770.
27. Kurup VP, Raju R, Manickam P. Profile of gene expression in a murine model of allergic bronchopulmonary aspergillosis. *Infect Immun.* 2005;73:4381–4384.
28. Hogaboam CM, Gallinat CS, Taub DD, Strieter RM, Kunkel SL, Lukacs NW. Immunomodulatory role of C10 chemokine in a murine model of allergic bronchopulmonary aspergillosis. *J Immunol.* 1999;162:6071–6079.
29. Grunig G, Corry DB, Leach MW, Seymour BW, Kurup VP, Rennick DM. Interleukin-10 is a natural suppressor of cytokine production and inflammation in a murine model of allergic bronchopulmonary aspergillosis. *J Exp Med.* 1997;185:1089–1099.
30. Wang JM, Chu HW, Bosse M, St-Pierre J, Boutet M, Laviolette M. Dexamethasone and cyclosporin A modulation of cytokine expression and specific antibody synthesis in an allergic bronchopulmonary aspergillosis murine model. *Eur J Clin Invest.* 1996;26: 951–959.
31. Chu HW, Wang JM, Boutet M, Boulet LP, Laviolette M. Immunohistochemical detection of GM-CSF, IL-4 and IL-5 in a murine model of allergic bronchopulmonary aspergillosis. *Clin Exp Allergy.* 1996;26:461–468.
32. Chu HW, Wang JM, Boutet M, Laviolette M. Tumor necrosis factor-alpha and interleukin-1 alpha expression in a murine model of allergic bronchopulmonary aspergillosis. *Lab Anim Sci.* 1996;46:42–47.
33. Kurup VP, Mauze S, Choi H, Seymour BW, Coffman RL. A murine model of allergic bronchopulmonary aspergillosis with elevated eosinophils and IgE. *J Immunol.* 1992;148: 3783–3788.
34. Kurup VP. Murine monoclonal antibodies binding to the specific antigens of Aspergillus fumigatus associated with allergic bronchopulmonary aspergillosis. *J Clin Lab Anal.* 1989;3:116–121.
35. Hernandez Y, Arora S, Erb-Downward JR, McDonald RA, Toews GB, Huffnagle GB. Distinct roles for IL-4 and IL-10 in regulating T2 immunity during allergic bronchopulmonary mycosis. *J Immunol.* 2005;174:1027–1036.
36. Chen GH, Olszewski MA, McDonald RA, et al. Role of granulocyte macrophage colony-stimulating factor in host defense against pulmonary *Cryptococcus neoformans* infection during murine allergic bronchopulmonary mycosis. *Am J Pathol.* 2007;170: 1028–1040.
37. Arora S, Huffnagle GB. Immune regulation during allergic bronchopulmonary mycosis: lessons taught by two fungi. *Immunol Res.* 2005;33:53–68.

38. Monod M, Jaton-Ogay K, Reichard U. Aspergillus fumigatus-secreted proteases as antigenic molecules and virulence factors. *Contrib Microbiol.* 1999;2:182–192.

39. Vaid M, Kaur S, Sambatakou H, Madan T, Denning DW, Sarma PU. Distinct alleles of mannose-binding lectin (MBL) and surfactant proteins A (SP-A) in patients with chronic cavitary pulmonary aspergillosis and allergic bronchopulmonary aspergillosis. *Clin Chem Lab Med.* 2007;45:183–186.

40. Greenberger PA. When to suspect and work up allergic bronchopulmonary aspergillosis. *Ann Allergy Asthma Immunol.* 2013;111:1–4.

41. Ricketti AJ, Greenberger PA, Patterson R. Varying presentations of allergic bronchopulmonary aspergillosis. *Int Arch Allergy Appl Immunol.* 1984;73:283–285.

42. Knutsen AP, Bush RK, Demain JG, et al. Fungi and allergic lower respiratory tract diseases. *J Allergy Clin Immunol.* 2012;129:280–291; quiz 292–293.

43. Patterson R, Greenberger PA, Halwig JM, Liotta JL, Roberts M. Allergic bronchopulmonary aspergillosis. Natural history and classification of early disease by serologic and roentgenographic studies. *Arch Intern Med.* 1986;146:916–918.

44. Greenberger PA. Aspergillosis–clinical aspects. *Zentralbl Bakteriol Mikrobiol Hyg A.* 1986;261:487–495.

45. Mendelson EB, Fisher MR, Mintzer RA, Halwig JM, Greenberger PA. Roentgenographic and clinical staging of allergic bronchopulmonary aspergillosis. *Chest.* 1985;87:334–339.

46. Ricketti AJ, Greenberger PA, Patterson R. Serum IgE as an important aid in management of allergic bronchopulmonary aspergillosis. *J Allergy Clin Immunol.* 1984;74:68–71.

47. Denning DW, O'Driscoll BR, Powell G, et al. Randomized controlled trial of oral antifungal treatment for severe asthma with fungal sensitization: the Fungal Asthma Sensitization Trial (FAST) study. *Am J Respir Crit Care Med.* 2009;179:11–18.

48. Agarwal R. What is the current place of azoles in allergic bronchopulmonary aspergillosis and severe asthma with fungal sensitization. *Expert Rev Respir Med.* 2012;6:363–371.

49. Pasqualotto AC, Powell G, Niven R, Denning DW. The effects of antifungal therapy on severe asthma with fungal sensitization and allergic bronchopulmonary aspergillosis. *Respirology.* 2009;14:1121–1127.

50. Knutsen A, Slavin RG. Allergic bronchopulmonary mycosis complicating cystic fibrosis. *Semin Respir Infect.* 1992;7:179–192.

51. Greenberger PA. Chapter 18: allergic bronchopulmonary aspergillosis. *Allergy Asthma Proc.* 2012;33(1):S61–S63.

52. Wark PA, Hensley MJ, Saltos N, et al. Anti-inflammatory effect of itraconazole in stable allergic bronchopulmonary aspergillosis: a randomized controlled trial. *J Allergy Clin Immunol.* 2003;111:952–957.

53. Denning DW, Van Wye JE, Lewiston NJ, Stevens DA. Adjunctive therapy of allergic bronchopulmonary aspergillosis with itraconazole. *Chest.* 1991;100:813–819.

54. Stevens DA, Schwartz HJ, Lee JY, et al. A randomized trial of itraconazole in allergic bronchopulmonary aspergillosis. *N Engl J Med.* 2000;342:756–762.

55. Redmann S, Charles BG. A rapid HPLC method with fluorometric detection for determination of plasma itraconazole and hydroxy-itraconazole concentrations in cystic fibrosis children with allergic bronchopulmonary aspergillosis. *Biomed Chromatogr.* 2006;20:343–348.

56. Chishimba L, Niven RM, Cooley J, Denning DW. Voriconazole and posaconazole improve asthma severity in allergic bronchopulmonary aspergillosis and severe asthma with fungal sensitization. *J Asthma.* 2012;49:423–433.

57. Glackin L, Leen G, Elnazir B, Greally P. Voriconazole in the treatment of allergic bronchopulmonary aspergillosis in cystic fibrosis. *Ir Med J.* 2009;102:29.

58. Erwin GE, Fitzgerald JE. Case report: allergic bronchopulmonary aspergillosis and allergic fungal sinusitis successfully treated with voriconazole. *J Asthma.* 2007;44:891–895.

59. Bandres Gimeno R, Munoz Martinez MJ. Prolonged therapeutic response to voriconazole in a case of allergic bronchopulmonary aspergillosis. *Archi Bronconeumol.* 2007;43:49–51.

60. Wong R, Wong M, Robinson PD, Fitzgerald DA. Omalizumab in the management of steroid dependent allergic bronchopulmonary aspergillosis (ABPA) complicating cystic fibrosis. *Paediatr Respir Rev.* 2013;14:22–24.

61. Collins J, Devos G, Hudes G, Rosenstreich D. Allergic bronchopulmonary aspergillosis treated successfully for one year with omalizumab. *J Asthma Allergy.* 2012;5:65–70.

62. Elmallah MK, Hendeles L, Hamilton RG, Capen C, Schuler PM. Management of patients with cystic fibrosis and allergic bronchopulmonary aspergillosis using anti-immunoglobulin e therapy (omalizumab). *J Pediatric Pharmacol Ther.* 2012;17: 88–92.

63. Sastre I, Blanco J, Mata H, Garcia F. A case of allergic bronchopulmonary aspergillosis treated with omalizumab. *J Investig Allergol Clin Immunol.* 2012;22:145–147.

64. Tillie-Leblond I, Germaud P, Leroyer C, et al. Allergic bronchopulmonary aspergillosis and omalizumab. *Allergy.* 2011;66: 1254–1256.

65. Lin RY, Sethi S, Bhargave GA. Measured immunoglobulin E in allergic bronchopulmonary aspergillosis treated with omalizumab. *J Asthma.* 2010;47:942–945.

66. Randhawa I, Chin T, Nussbaum E. Resolution of corticosteroid-induced diabetes in allergic bronchopulmonary aspergillosis with omalizumab therapy: a novel approach. *J Asthma.* 2009;46: 445–457.

67. Lebecque P, Leonard A, Argaz M, Godding V, Pilette C. Omalizumab for exacerbations of allergic bronchopulmonary aspergillosis in patients with cystic fibrosis. *BMJ Case Rep.* 2009; 2009.

68. Kanu A, Patel K. Treatment of allergic bronchopulmonary aspergillosis (ABPA) in CF with anti-IgE antibody (omalizumab). *Pediatr Pulmonol.* 2008;43:1249–1251.

69. Zirbes JM, Milla CE. Steroid-sparing effect of omalizumab for allergic bronchopulmonary aspergillosis and cystic fibrosis. *Pediatr Pulmonol.* 2008;43:607–610.

CHAPTER 49

Upper Airway Obstruction in Adults

Christine Won
Gaetane Michaud
Meir H. Kryger

INTRODUCTION

The upper airway is conventionally described as being made up of all the structures that conduct air between the carina and the nares and includes the trachea, larynx, pharynx, nasal airway, and oral airway. Upper airway structures may change their physiologic function in response to pressures around them, and anatomic structures near them. Thus, physiologically, the segments of the upper airway behave differently when they are subject to pleural pressures (anatomically intrathoracic) or ambient pressures (anatomically extrathoracic). Furthermore we now know that extrathoracic airway function may change with posture, sleep/wake state, and the function and anatomy of tissues surrounding the airway.

The upper airway evolved anatomically in humans to subserve several important functions including swallowing, breathing, and vocalization.[1] The multifunctionality of the upper airway increases the risk of certain diseases (e.g., aspiration and sleep apnea).[2] These functions require that different segments of the airway have differing properties. The trachea receives some support by the tracheal rings, the nasal airway is surrounded by rigid structures, and the oral airway has a rigid boney roof, the hard palate. On the other hand, the pharyngeal airway does not have rigid structures supporting it. It is a collapsible tube whose patency is maintained by muscles whose function is affected by arousal state (sleep/wake, and more specifically during sleep, the stage of sleep), the structures around it, and posture. Thus, the pharyngeal airway is divided anatomically and physiologically into the nasopharynx, retropalatal oropharynx, retroglossal oropharynx, and hypopharynx.

Clinically significant obstruction in adults may occur anywhere within the upper airway. Common etiologies of upper airway obstruction (UAO) include neoplasia, scar formation, skeletal facial malformations, infection, inflammatory disorders, trauma, extrinsic compression related to pathology of adjacent structures, and functional changes related to posture and sleep/wake state. Airway obstruction may be classified as extrinsic, intrinsic, or mixed (Fig. 49-1).

UAO can be acute and life-threatening, or chronic and resulting in significant symptoms, some of which may not even relate to the respiratory system. Initial management of acute UAO focuses on securing the airway and stabilizing the patient. Often the intervention is surgical. Some diseases require bypassing the obstruction using translaryngeal intubation or tracheostomy. Definitive long-term management depends on the underlying etiology and physiology, and may include both medical and surgical interventions. The still evolving fields of imaging and interventional pulmonology offer new diagnostic and management modalities. This chapter provides an overview of acute and chronic UAO in adults and focuses on clinical presentation, assessment, etiology, and management. Obstructive sleep apnea is covered in Chapter 99 of this volume.

HISTORICAL PERSPECTIVE

Acute UAO can be so distressing to the patient and to those around him/her that it is not surprising that tracheostomy has been used as a treatment for at least 3000 years, as described in ancient Egyptian tablets and Greek and Roman writings.[3] Tracheostomy was considered dangerous because it might lead to catastrophes (e.g., laceration of the carotid artery) or infections that may not be controlled. Even Hippocrates warned about the dangers of tracheostomy. By the mid-16th century, the tracheostomy had been performed to relieve UAO caused by a pharyngeal abscess.

Although the procedure was already widely known within the medical profession in the 18th century, it was seen as potentially very dangerous. The first president of the United States, George Washington, died of acute UAO likely caused by epiglottis while his doctors (who were familiar with tracheostomy) treated him with blood letting.[4] During the 19th century, the procedure was used to treat UAO caused by croup and diphtheria.

By the early 20th century, nonsurgical treatments were used to treat UAO; for example, rigid bronchoscopy was used to remove foreign bodies from the trachea.[5] The flexible fiberoptic bronchoscope was introduced in 1966, and the next four decades saw the introduction of many diagnostic and therapeutic modalities including: Nd:YAG laser, video

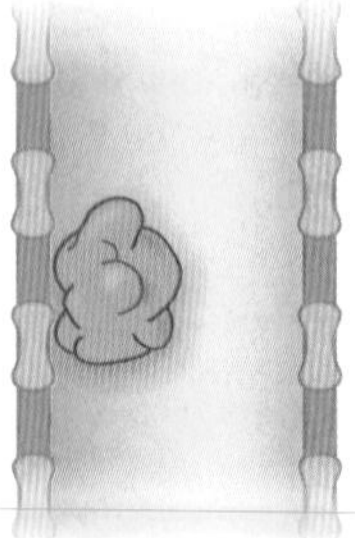

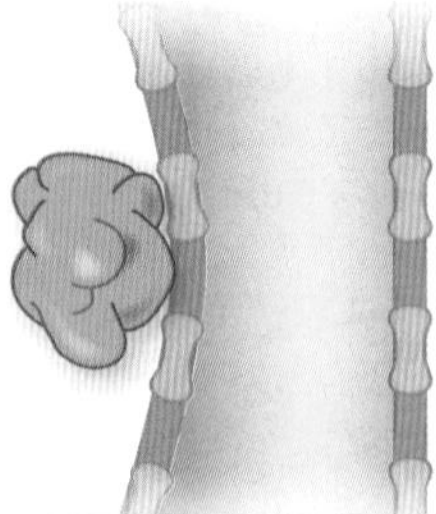

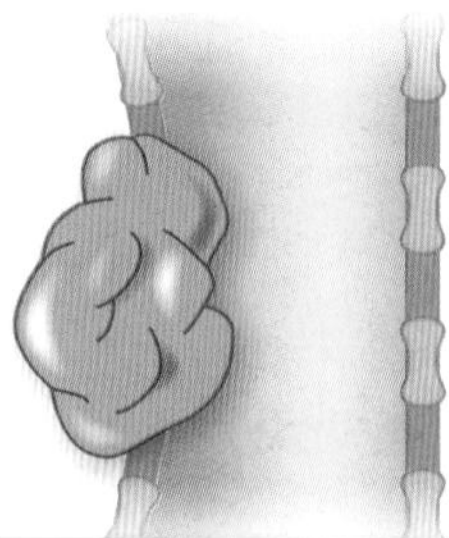

Figure 49-1 Classification of airway tumor involvement. **A.** Intrinsic stenosis. Purely endoluminal tumor without breech of the cartilage. **B.** Extrinsic stenosis. Extraluminal tumor causing mass effect but no endoluminal involvement. **C.** Mixed stenosis. Extraluminal tumor causing mass effect and endoluminal involvement.

bronchoscopy, airway stenting, endobronchial ultrasonography, endobronchial electrocautery, cryotherapy, argon laser coagulation, thermal laser therapy, photodynamic therapy (PDT), brachytherapy, and percutaneous tracheostomy.[6]

There are newly described causes of UAO and novel imaging techniques, both radiographic and endoscopic, which are in evolution to detect and quantify UAO. Treatment strategies are continuously advancing. The incidence of malignancy and related obstruction of the upper airway has increased due in part to tobacco use and exposure to modern environmental toxins. It is estimated that 20% to 30% of lung cancer patients present with symptomatic airway obstruction. The exact prevalence, however, is unknown as a result of the nihilistic view of lung cancer, particularly in the setting of advanced disease. Complications of endotracheal intubation and tracheostomy have become well-recognized causes of benign upper airway stenosis and malacia. Again, it is likely that this pathology is underreported and many people are inappropriately treated for asthma or other chronic peripheral airway diseases. Improvement in pharmacologic agents to treat infectious, inflammatory, and malignant etiologies, as well as developments in radiation oncology, have influenced the management of UAO. More recently, advances involving anesthetic agents and anesthesia techniques, along with development of sophisticated surgical procedures for reconstruction of the larynx, trachea, and bronchi, have had a considerable impact on the management of this condition. Development of new endoscopic and imaging techniques and introduction of interventional pulmonology also have proved useful in the management of UAO.

In the mid-1960s it became apparent that UAO occurred in some patients only during sleep and until the mid-1980s the only effective treatment was tracheostomy, which was used to bypass the segment of the airway obstructing during sleep.[7] Up to that era, the main focus of the laboratory diagnosis of pulmonary disease was for patients with obstructive intrathoracic disease and soon the importance of being able to diagnose UAO became apparent.[8] Soon the notion of using positive airway pressure to overcome UAO was established.[9]

CLINICAL FEATURES

Upper and lower airway obstruction may present with similar symptoms (e.g., shortness of breath, noisy breathing) and physical findings (e.g., wheezing, diminished breath sounds). Asthma and chronic obstructive pulmonary disease, common causes of lower airway obstruction, are often incorrectly assumed to be causing the patient's symptoms.

Significant UAO may be asymptomatic for a prolonged period of time, resulting in delayed presentation, diagnosis and possibly a catastrophic outcome. When UAO develops or worsens acutely, asphyxia and death may result within minutes to hours. When UAO develops slowly, diagnoses may be delayed or incorrect, and, in the case of malignancy in the upper airway, may lead to incurable disease.

Dyspnea and noisy breathing, the most common symptoms of UAO, are often prominent during exercise and also may be intensified or relieved by a change in body position. The patient may indicate that breathing is labored while supine and may experience sleep disordered breathing in the forms of obstructive sleep apnea or upper airway resistance syndrome (see Chapter 99). Therefore, daytime somnolence may be a prominent feature of UAO. In severely affected patients, peripheral edema as a result of cor pulmonale may be present as a consequence of chronic hypoxemia and hypercarbia during sleep and wakefulness.

In most cases, significant anatomic obstruction precedes the development of symptoms. By the time dyspnea on exertion occurs, the airway diameter at the site of obstruction is likely to be reduced to about 8 mm. Shortness of breath at rest often develops when the airway diameter is about 5 mm, and stridor is now often present. Stridor is a loud, musical sound of constant pitch that usually indicates the presence extrathoracic airway obstruction most often affecting the larynx or upper trachea.

Unlike wheezing, which is a feature of diffuse peripheral airway obstruction and occurs primarily during expiration, stridor usually occurs during inspiration and is loudest in the neck. The sound can usually be appreciated without using a stethoscope. Although one would expect to be able to distinguish stridor from wheezing coming from lower airways, sound recordings from the neck and chest have shown that the sounds from the asthmatic wheeze and stridor have similar frequencies. Hence there may be errors in diagnosis and a UAO caused by a tumor or foreign body may be mistakenly treated as asthma.

Breathing maneuvers that increase inspiratory airflow, such as forced inspiration or voluntary hyperventilation, accentuate the intensity of stridor. Neck flexion may change the loudness of stridor. When the obstructing lesion is fixed, both inspiratory and expiratory stridorous sounds may be heard. At times, the character of a patient's voice may be a clue to the presence of UAO. Hoarseness may be a sign of a laryngeal abnormality. Muffling of the voice may be present when vocal cords are paralyzed.

LABORATORY ASSESSMENT

Just as UAO must be quite advanced before development of symptoms, physiologic abnormalities do not become apparent on lung function testing until severe obstruction occurs. Studies of subjects breathing through tubes of varying diameters suggest that UAO must narrow the airway lumen to less than 8 mm in diameter to produce abnormalities on a flow–volume loop. This corresponds to an obstruction of more than 80% of the normal median diameter of the tracheal lumen. The forced expiratory volume in 1 second (FEV_1) remains above 90% of control until a 6-mm orifice is created. Therefore, spirometry, which is often the first screening test for pulmonary symptoms, may not be an effective way to detect upper airway abnormalities. The peak expiratory flow rate (PEFR) and maximal voluntary ventilation (MVV) are more sensitive than the FEV_1 in detecting UAO. Of note, a noncritical airway may become so with a lesser degree of obstruction in the context of airway secretions, edema, or bleeding.[10]

The flow–volume loop, which is a recording of maximal inspiratory and expiratory flows at various lung volumes, is an important tool for the diagnosis of UAO. The configuration of the normal flow–volume loop is shown in Figure 49-2. During a forced expiratory maneuver from total lung capacity (TLC), the maximal flow achieved during the first 25% of the forced vital capacity is dependent on effort, that is, an increase in driving pressure (effort) may result in increased flow. During the remaining 75% of the forced vital capacity maneuver, flow is determined by the mechanical properties of the lungs and is not effort dependent. During this portion of forced exhalation, a linear deceleration of flow is caused by dynamic compression of the intrathoracic airways (Fig. 49-3A). An increase in effort and therefore pleural pressure causes further compression of the intrathoracic airways and a further limitation of airflow. At higher lung volumes, flow may be limited by a UAO. At low lung volumes, flow may not be affected by a UAO, since measurement of flow in this effort-independent portion of the curve represents the function of the peripheral airways. Since the FEV_1 reflects a large portion of flow at these lower lung volumes, it is not a sensitive test for UAO. Because the PEFR reflects flow at higher lung volumes, it may be abnormal when the FEV_1 is not.

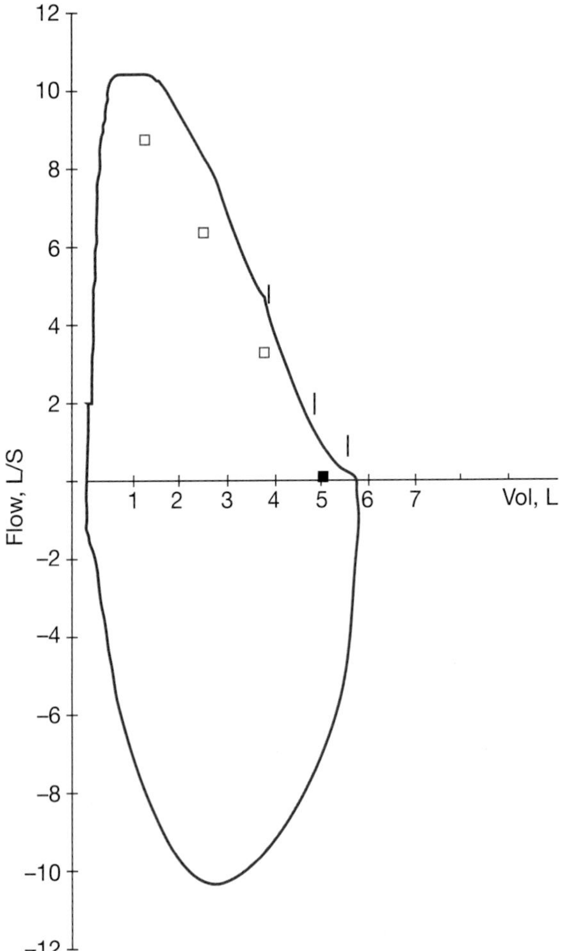

Figure 49-2 Normal flow–volume loop following maximal expiratory *(above)* and inspiratory *(below)* effort. Small vertical lines denote seconds.

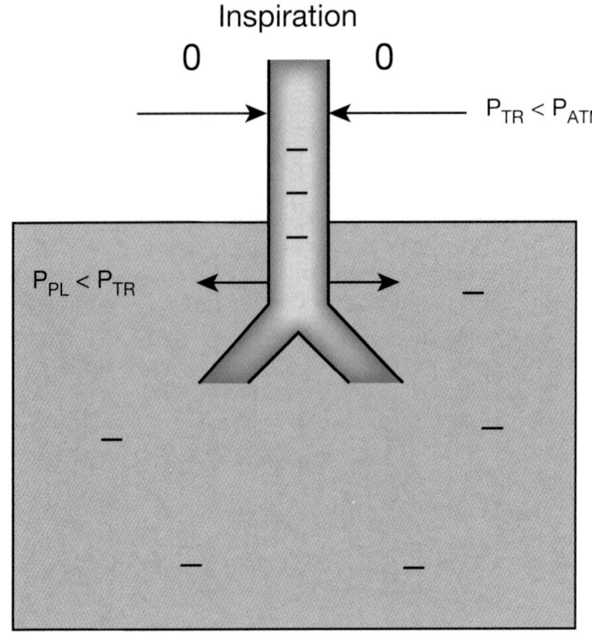

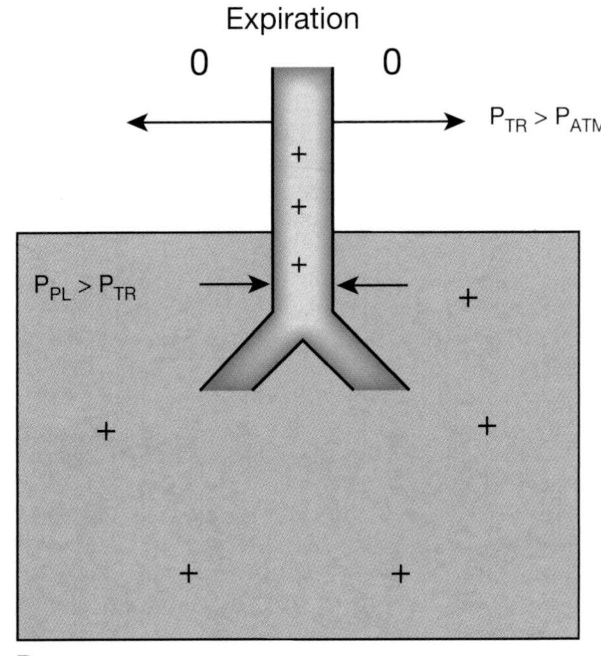

Figure 49-3 Forces acting on intra- and extrathoracic airway walls during inspiration and expiration. 0, atmospheric pressure; +, positive pressure; −, negative pressure. **A.** During inspiration, extrathoracic tracheal pressure (P_{TR}) falls below atmospheric pressure (P_{ATM}), favoring narrowing of the lumen *(arrows)*. Intrapleural pressure (P_{PL}) becomes negative, favoring airway enlargement *(arrows)*. **B.** During expiration, the extrathoracic tracheal pressure (P_{TR}) becomes positive and, therefore, greater than P_{ATM}, favoring enlargement of the lumen *(arrows)*. Intrapleural pressure (P_{PL}) is positive, causing dynamic compression of the intrathoracic trachea *(arrows)*.

In generating the flow–volume loop, forced inspiratory flow is limited by effort during the entire inspiratory maneuver. Flow increases from residual volume to near the midportion of the curve, where it becomes maximal at the peak inspiratory flow rate. Flow then declines until TLC is reached. The pressure surrounding the extrathoracic portion of the upper airway is atmospheric. The turbulent nonlaminar airflow, which occurs during forced inspiration and causes airway pressure to fall in this portion of the airway, favors slight narrowing of the extrathoracic airway (Fig. 49-3B). Peak inspiratory flow, therefore, is less than peak expiratory flow in normal subjects. Because of the dynamic compression of the intrathoracic airways that occurs during exhalation, flow during the middle of inspiration, that is, the forced inspiratory flow at 50% of the forced vital capacity ($FIF_{50\%}$), is usually greater than flow during the middle of forced expiration, that is, the forced expiratory flow at 50% of the forced vital capacity ($FEF_{50\%}$). Typical patterns of the flow–volume loop may be seen, depending on whether the obstruction to flow is "fixed" or "variable," and whether the site of the obstruction is above or below the thoracic outlet or suprasternal notch.

Fixed obstructions of the upper airway are those in which the cross-sectional area does not change in response to transmural pressure differences during inspiration or expiration. A fixed obstruction may occur in either the intrathoracic or extrathoracic airways. Irrespective of the site of the obstruction, a fixed lesion results in the flattening of the inspiratory and expiratory phases of the flow–volume loop. A *variable obstruction* is one that responds to transmural pressure changes, eliciting varying degrees of obstruction during the respiratory cycle. Since the stresses on the intrathoracic and extrathoracic airways are different, changes seen in the flow–volume loop vary according to the site of the obstruction.

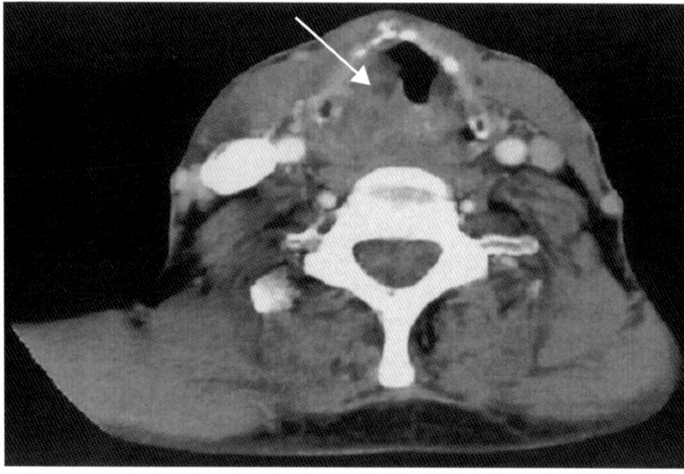

A

B

Figure 49-4 **A, B.** Flow–volume loop in fixed upper airway obstruction due to laryngeal abscess in a 56-year-old man who developed persistent wheezing, hoarseness of voice, and intermittent stridor for 3 months after a brief intubation for asthma exacerbation. Computed tomography scan of the neck (**A**) shows a laryngeal abscess with significant impingement on the laryngeal inlet. The flow–volume loop (**B**) demonstrates a plateau of flow during inspiration and expiration; the $FEF_{50\%}/FIF_{50\%}$ ratio is near 1.

A number of conditions have been associated with nondistensible narrowing of the upper airway and fixed airway obstruction. Benign strictures and malignancy are common examples. Maximal inspiratory and expiratory flow–volume loops with fixed obstruction show constant flow, represented by a plateau during both inspiration and expiration (Fig. 49-4A,B). On the expiratory curve, the plateau effect is seen in the effort-dependent portion of the curve near TLC; very little change is noted in the effort-dependent portion near residual volume. Since the inspiratory curve is similar in appearance, the ratio of $FEF_{50\%}$ to $FIF_{50\%}$ is normal (close to 1). The forced inspiratory volume in 1 second (FIV_1) and FEV_1 are nearly the same in fixed UAO.

Unilateral vocal cord paralysis is a common cause of variable extrathoracic obstruction. A variable extrathoracic airway obstruction increases the turbulence of inspiratory flow, and intraluminal pressure falls markedly below atmospheric pressure. This leads to partial collapse of an already narrowed airway and a plateau in the inspiratory flow loop (Fig. 49-5A,B). Expiratory flow is not significantly affected, since the markedly positive pressure in the airway tends to decrease the obstruction. The ratio of $FEF_{50\%}$ to $FIF_{50\%}$ is high (usually greater than 2). Similarly, the FEV_1 is greater than the FIV_1.

A variable obstruction in the intrathoracic airways reverses the situation. A predominant reduction in maximal expiratory flow is associated with a relative preservation of maximal inspiratory flow. This association occurs because intrapleural pressure becomes decidedly positive during forced expiration and causes dynamic compression of the intrathoracic airways. The obstruction caused by an intrathoracic lesion is accentuated and a plateau in expiratory flow occurs on the flow–volume loop (Fig. 49-6A,B). A plateau of flow suggests that the lesion has caused the airway lumen to reach its minimal size. A flow peak may precede the plateau, suggesting that the obstruction may not affect flow until a certain lung volume is reached. During inspiration, intrapleural pressure is markedly negative; therefore, the obstruction is decreased. The ratio of $FEF_{50\%}$ to $FIF_{50\%}$ is very low and may approach 0.3. Similarly, the FEV_1 is considerably lower than the FIV_1. Although the flow ratios are similar to those seen in patients with COPD and chronic asthma, these disorders are distinguished from UAO by the appearance of the flow–volume loop. Thus, the expiratory curve in patients with COPD and asthma is primarily altered in the effort-independent portion of the curve, leading to a characteristic shape unlike the plateau configuration of a UAO (Fig. 49-7).

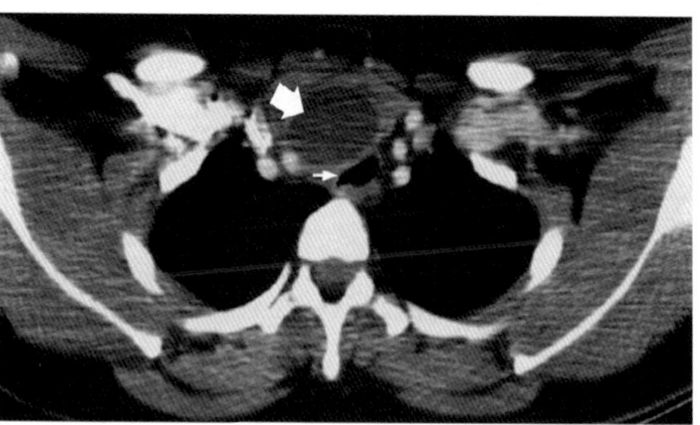

A

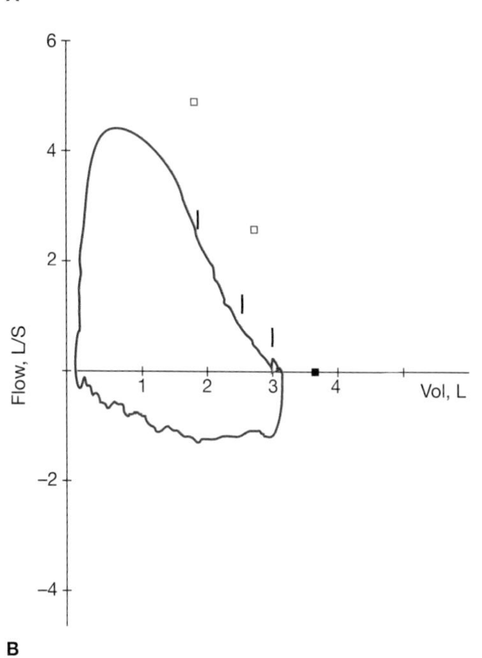

B

Figure 49-5 Variable extrathoracic obstruction due to thyroid cyst in a 32-year-old woman with dyspnea on exertion. **A.** Computed tomography of the neck shows a 10- × 4-cm cystic mass *(large arrow)* in the thyroid gland compressing the trachea *(small arrow)*. **B.** Flow–volume loop shows inspiratory obstruction. $FEF_{50\%}/FIF_{50\%}$ is very high, and the inspiratory curve is flattened.

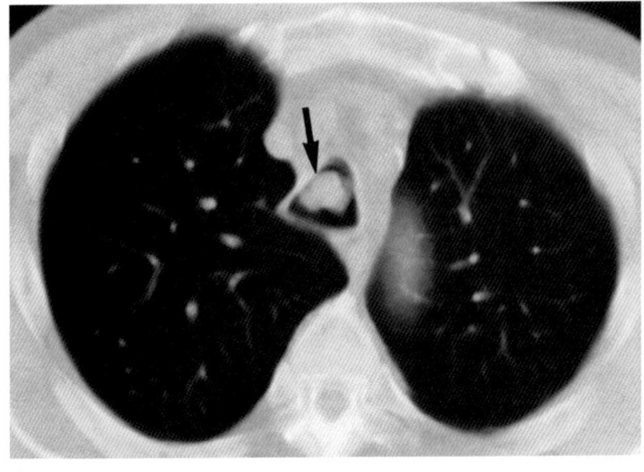

A

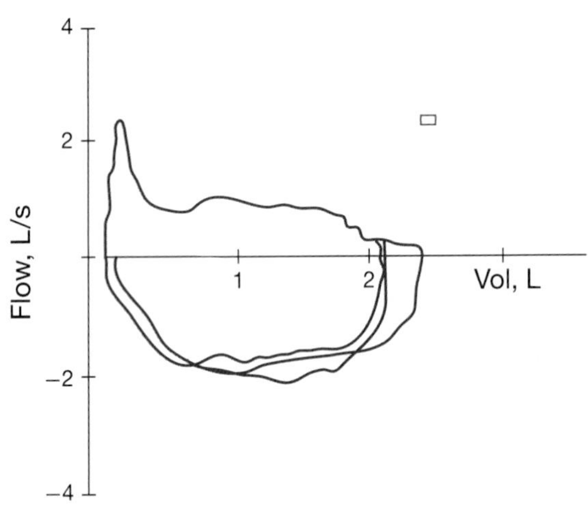

B

Figure 49-6 Variable intrathoracic obstruction due to squamous cell carcinoma of the trachea. **A.** Computed tomography of the chest shows a tracheal lesion *(arrow)*, which was not readily apparent on plain chest radiograph. **B.** Superimposed flow–volume loops show a plateau of expiratory flow preceded by a peak of flow at higher lung volumes. The forced inspiratory flow is preserved in comparison to expiratory flow, but it is also reduced. $FEF_{50\%}/FIF_{50\%}$ is 0.4.

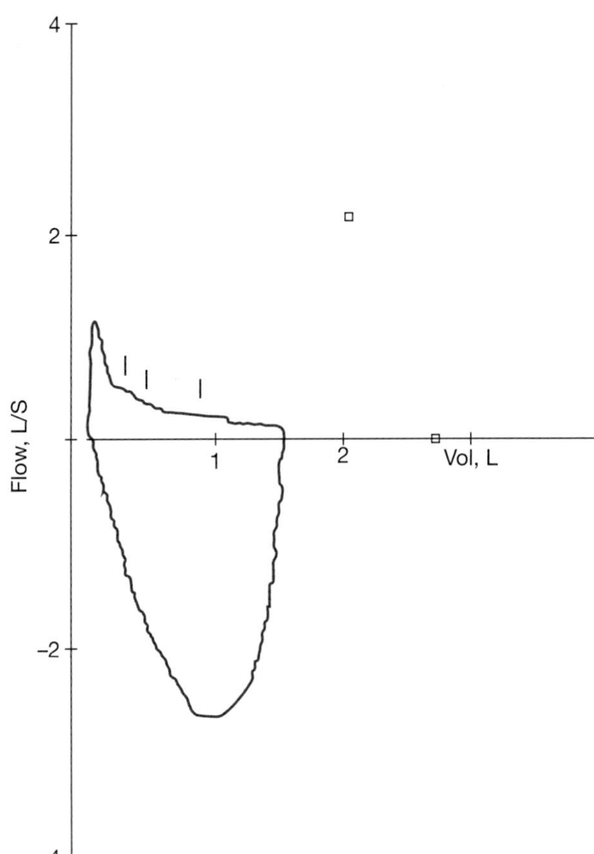

Figure 49-7 Flow–volume loop typical of chronic obstructive lung disease. Very low $FEF_{50\%}/FIF_{50\%}$ and typical curvilinear shape are noted.

When a hospital laboratory or physician's office is not equipped to perform flow–volume loops, results of other tests, such as routine spirometry, may be helpful. If the forced spirogram shows that the PEFR is reduced disproportionately to the reduction in FEV_1, a UAO should be suspected. Other findings that suggest the diagnosis include a ratio of less than 1.0 for the inspiratory flow between 25% and 75% of the inspired vital capacity ($FIF_{25-75\%}$) and a value of less than 1.0 for the expiratory flow between 25% and 75% of the expired vital capacity ($FEF_{25-75\%}$). Another indication is an FEV_1 that is decreased to the same degree as the $FEF_{25-75\%}$. The MVV may also be a useful test, since it measures both inspiratory and expiratory flows. A ratio of MVV to FEV_1 of less than 25% is often found with UAO. Whenever the MVV is reduced in association with a normal FEV_1, a diagnosis of UAO should be considered.

In contrast to the situation in patients with diffuse obstructive disease of the lower airways (e.g., COPD, asthma), the distribution of ventilation in the lungs is normal, and ventilation–perfusion mismatch does not occur. Hypercarbia is not seen unless the degree of obstruction is very severe, although nocturnal hypercarbia may occur while daytime levels of P_{CO_2} are normal. Hypoxemia is also not present except during exercise and with severe airflow limitation, when it may accompany increases in the level of P_{CO_2}. In contrast to asthma and many instances of COPD, the airflow obstruction caused by an upper airway lesion does not resolve following the inhalation of a bronchodilator unless there is also a component of small airway disease that is often the case.

IMAGING

When acute airflow obstruction occurs as a result of an abnormality of the extrathoracic airway, roentgenographic studies of the soft tissues of the upper chest and neck in the emergency setting may be helpful (Fig. 49-8). However, computed tomography (CT) has afforded the most important approach to imaging of the extrathoracic airways (Fig. 49-9). The standard chest roentgenogram is often not helpful in detecting the presence, or the cause, of UAO. Occasionally, in patients with chronic airway obstruction, generalized hyperinflation of the lungs may occur; in the absence of asthma or COPD this finding may raise suspicion of occult disease in the central airways. The trachea is usually well visualized on the posteroanterior (PA) and lateral views in chest roentgenograms of good quality. It is located in the midline and is moderately deviated at the level of the aortic arch. However, many standard roentgenograms are underpenetrated so that the trachea may become a "blind spot." In one study, only 13 of 53 tracheal tumors were evident to the radiologist on the standard PA roentgenogram. The use of digital imaging techniques may avoid such pitfalls. However, thoracic CT studies have become the procedure of choice for imaging the upper airway.

The sensitivity of CT scanning for detecting upper airway disease surpasses that of the routine chest roentgenogram (97% vs. 66%, respectively). Helical CT (HCT) scanning minimizes artifacts due to respiratory motion and provides imaging of the whole thoracic volume during a single breathhold.[11] The technique represents

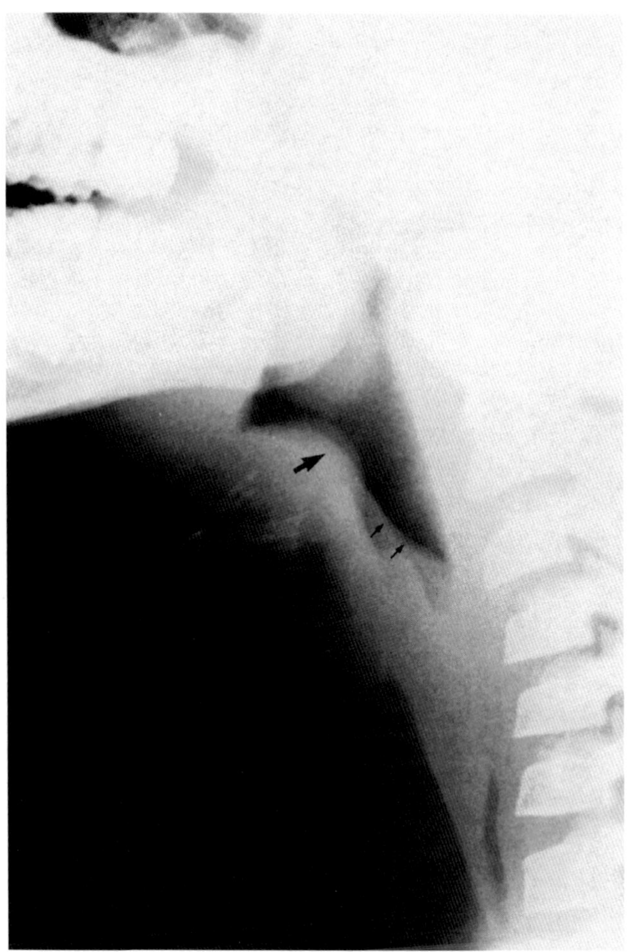

Figure 49-8 Acute epiglottitis. Lateral soft tissue radiograph of the neck of a patient with stridor shows swelling of the epiglottis *(large arrow)* and loss of normal convexity of the edematous aryepiglottic folds *(small arrows)*.

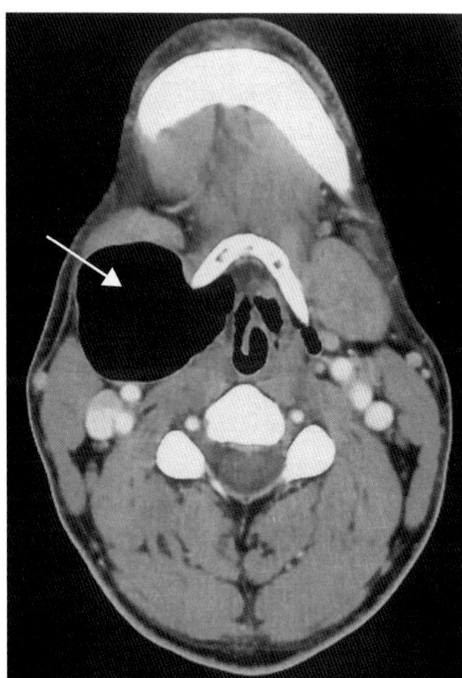

Figure 49-9 Computed tomography scan of the neck demonstrating a large laryngocele compressing the lateral wall of the larynx *(arrow)* causing positional air flow obstruction.

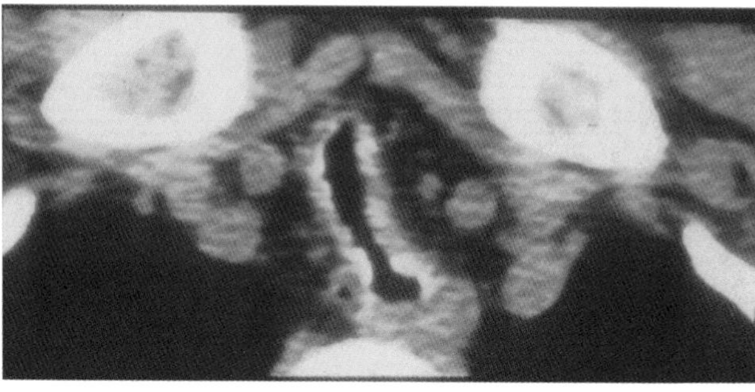

A

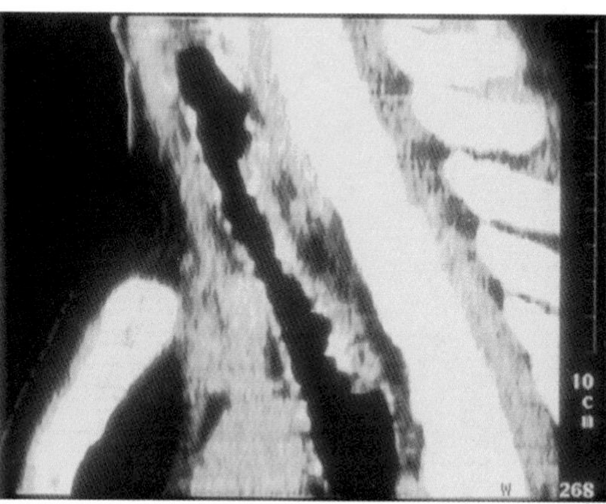

B

Figure 49-10 **A.** Computed tomography scan of the chest demonstrating marked narrowing of the trachea with intraluminal calcified nodular projections in a patient with tracheopathia osteoplastica. **B.** Computed tomography scan of the chest demonstrating multiplanar reformation of the trachea in the sagittal plane of the same patient.

an improvement over conventional CT scanning in that it allows detection of intraluminal, submucosal, and extraluminal lesions (Figs. 49-10A,B and 49-11). Since the early 1990s, HCT has become the preferred noninvasive modality for evaluation of the central airways. The use of HCT using multidetector technology and thin collimation provides high-resolution images of the entire thorax, improved special resolution, greater speed of image acquisition, and

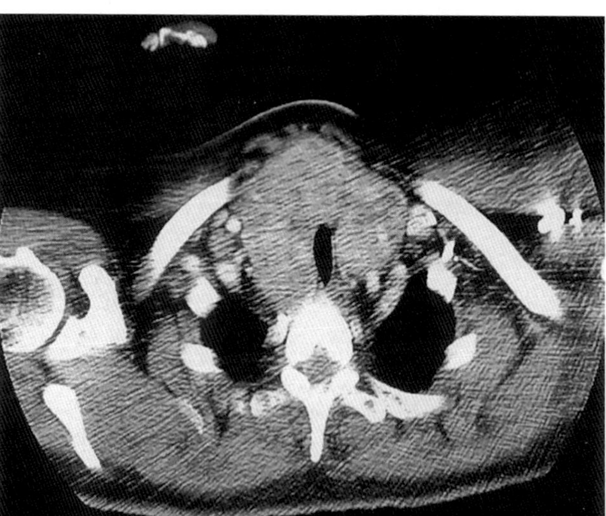

Figure 49-11 Computed tomography scan of the chest demonstrating marked extraluminal compression of the trachea caused by intrathoracic goiter.

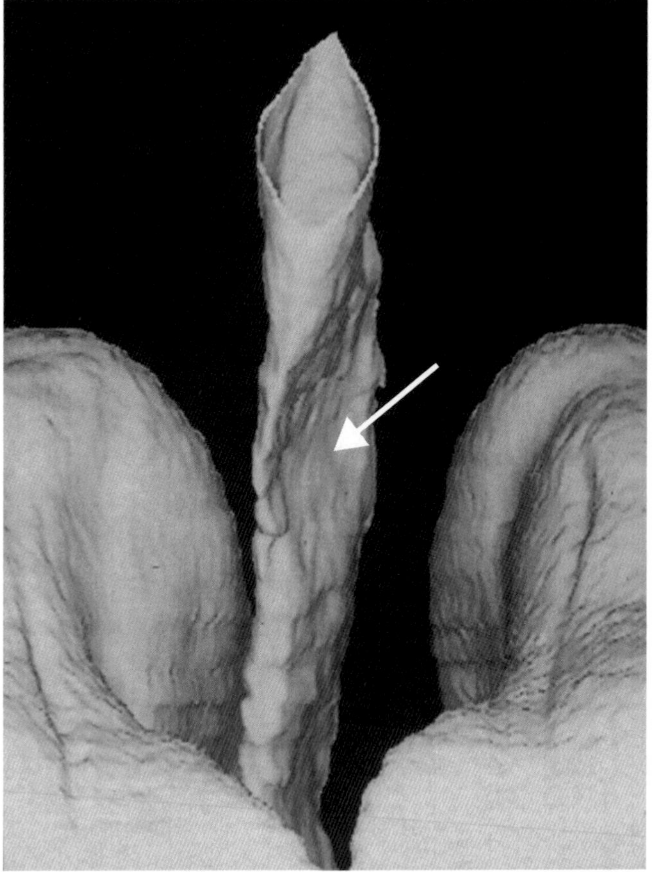

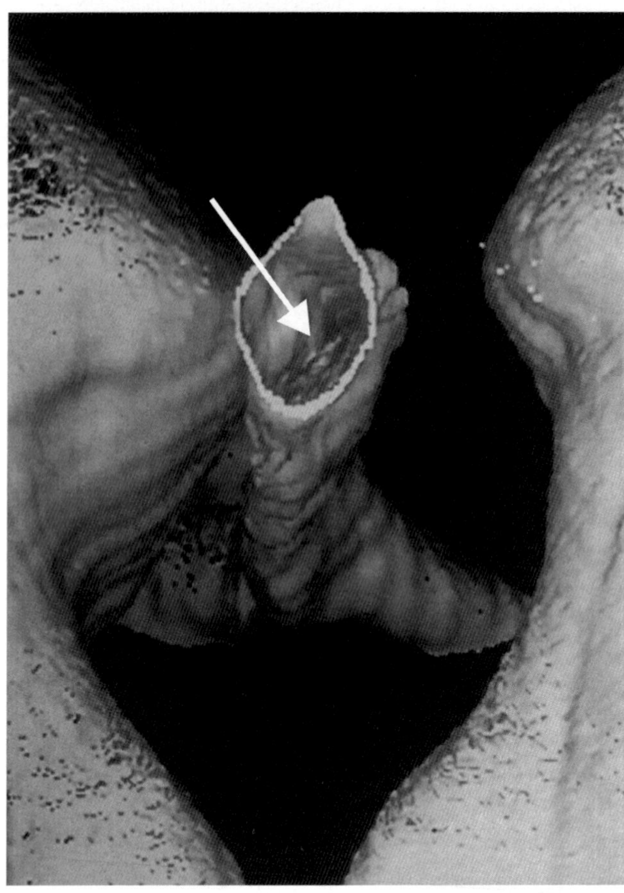

Figure 49-12 Helical computed tomography scan of the chest with three-dimensional reconstruction of the upper airway showing focal tracheal compression *(arrows)* (**A, B.**)

excellent contrast enhancement. HCT techniques using multiplanar and three-dimensional reconstruction can provide virtual images of the thorax that enhance the perception of local and diffuse anatomic lesions of the upper airways (Fig. 49-12). The images may demonstrate the degree of tracheal widening or narrowing, show the location and longitudinal extent of abnormalities, assess tracheal wall thickness, and demonstrate associated extratracheal diseases.

The use of paired inspiratory dynamic and expiratory multislice HCT has proved helpful for the diagnosis of tracheomalacia. Because the maximal degree of collapse in tracheomalacia usually occurs during exhalation rather than at end expiration, dynamic expiratory imaging is preferable to end-expiratory imaging. If complete collapse is not demonstrated during expiration, then one should confirm the diagnosis by quantitatively measuring the degree of airway luminal narrowing during expiration. Tracheomalacia is generally defined as a reduction in cross-sectional area of greater than 50% on expiratory images; however, this cut point may not be discriminatory enough to detect clinically significant tracheomalacia.[12]

Another novel CT-based imaging technique is virtual bronchoscopy. The use of volumetric imaging allows for an intraluminal three-dimensional reconstruction of the airways and surrounding tissues. The technique has been used with a high degree of accuracy in assessing the width, length, and contour of fixed airway lesions, but it has not been effective in defining dynamic airway lesions, such as excessive dynamic airway collapse.

Magnetic resonance imaging (MRI) is another modality that may be used to assess the central airways and surrounding mediastinal structures. MRI provides a multiplane image of the chest without the need for contrast material. However, the technique is best used to investigate vascular structures surrounding central airways, such as vascular rings or aneurysms that may compress the trachea, rather than the airways themselves, which are better visualized using CT scanning.

ENDOSCOPY

Bronchoscopy and direct laryngoscopy provide a real-time morphologic and functional evaluation of the upper airway. Imaging techniques are often limited by their inability to document the dynamic nature of many airway lesions and may underestimate the extent of an obstruction.

With respect to laryngeal disease, endoscopy allows the operator to determine whether the vocal cords are mobile or fixed in abduction or adduction or alternatively moving paradoxically. This valuable information can help guide management. In cases of traumatic or thermal injury to the airways, edema, laryngeal fracture, or carbonaceous materials can be readily identified.

CAUSES OF UPPER AIRWAY OBSTRUCTION

UAO may be observed in a wide variety of settings, including infections, trauma (including iatrogenic), vascular disorders, and a wide variety of benign and malignant tumors. Each is discussed below.

■ INFECTION

A broad variety of infections may eventuate in UAO.

Deep Cervical Space Infections

Deep cervical space infections occur in potential spaces bounded by the deep cervical fascia. The cervical fascia is divided into a superficial and, a more complex, deep layer. This configuration and complexity divides the neck into functional units. Infection can spread along the planes formed by the cervical fascia. Infections affecting the deep neck tissues may result in life-threatening UAO.

Patients with deep cervical space infections may present with sore throat, odynophagia, neck swelling, pain, fever, and dyspnea. Stridor and profound respiratory difficulty are signs of significant UAO. Parapharyngeal, peritonsillar, submandibular, and retropharyngeal abscesses appear to be common locations in adults. The bacteriology and initiating event of deep cervical infections appear to have changed over time.

Mixed infections caused by aerobic and anaerobic infections are common and have been reported in up to two-thirds of cases.[13] *Streptococcus viridans* and *Klebsiella pneumonia* are common pathogens. *Staphylococcus aureus, Staphylococcus epidermidis, Streptococcus pneumoniae, Escherichia coli*, and *Haemophilus influenzae* are other agents that are commonly reported. Alpha and beta hemolytic *streptococci* appear to have significantly declined in frequency. Overall, an odontogenic origin is probably most common, with upper respiratory tract infections as an important etiology in children. Intravenous drug abuse, mandibular fractures, iatrogenic and noniatrogenic traumatic injury to the upper airway, underlying malignancy, and poor underlying immune status are associated conditions. Ludwig's angina – an infection of the submandibular space and the floor of the mouth – is potentially lethal and is commonly associated with significant UAO. This entity is usually a cellulitic process and can affect the submandibular spaces bilaterally. Many cases with true Ludwig's angina require tracheostomy.

Treatment of deep cervical infections involves maintenance of oxygenation and ventilation by securing an adequate airway, administration of appropriate antibiotics, and when indicated, use of surgical drainage. Complications of deep cervical infections include UAO, Lemierre's syndrome (see next paragraph), distant infection, septic embolization, carotid artery rupture, pulmonary embolism, direct extension of infection resulting in mediastinitis and empyema, and rupture of the abscess during intubation or other interventions.[14]

One particularly virulent cervical infection, known as Lemierre's syndrome, arises from a nasopharyngitis or peritonsillar abscess. This lateral pharyngeal space infection results in suppurative thrombophlebitis of the internal jugular vein, septicemia, and metastatic abscess formation, particularly in the lungs and joints. *Fusobacterium necrophorum* is usually the causative agent and has been cultured from blood in over 80% of cases. Symptoms begin with a sore throat, fever, and painful swelling in the neck, followed by tender lymphadenopathy and tenderness along the sternocleidomastoid muscle (representing thrombophlebitis of the internal jugular vein). Dysphagia, trismus, and UAO may occur as a result of swelling of the lateral pharyngeal space. Contrast-enhanced CT scan of the neck is most useful in establishing the diagnosis of thrombosis of the internal jugular vein and may demonstrate soft tissue abscesses, fasciitis, and myositis, which may require extensive surgical debridement. Without the use of early and appropriate antibiotics, such as high-dose penicillin with metronidazole, or monotherapy with clindamycin, the mortality rate approaches 100%.

Epiglottitis

Epiglottitis is an infectious process that causes variable degrees of inflammation and edema of the epiglottis and supraglottic structures. Supraglottitis may be more appropriate term in adults, since the supraglottic structures usually are involved with variable involvement of the epiglottis. This condition can be life-threatening. Its prevalence is 0.18 to 9.7 cases per million adults; the mortality rate may be as high as 7.1%. Clinical presentation includes odynophagia, with inability to swallow secretions, sore throat, dyspnea, hoarseness, fever, tachycardia, and stridor. In one review, 44% of the patients had a normal routine oropharyngeal examination.[15]

Fiberoptic laryngoscopy is necessary to make the diagnosis. The procedure is safe in adults with suspected epiglottitis and should be done without delay. Radiographic studies can be helpful in ruling out other etiologies with similar presentations and in evaluating potential complications. However, the airway must be secured, and radiographic studies should not delay diagnosis or management.

Supraglottitis may involve the base of the tongue, uvula, pharynx, and false vocal cords. The disease may be increasing in prevalence among adults and declining in children, perhaps, reflecting introduction of *Haemophilus b* conjugate vaccines. Young adult males are commonly affected. The disorder appears to be more prevalent in colder, winter months and in smokers. Blood cultures are positive in less than one-third of cases. Although *Haemophilus influenzae* is the most common organism isolated in children, adult supraglottitis may be caused by a variety of organisms, including *Haemophilus influenzae, pneumococci*, group A *streptococci, S. aureus, Streptococcus viridans*, a variety of anaerobic organisms, mycobacteria, fungi, and viruses. Throat cultures can be helpful in diagnosis and management; however, treatment should not be delayed while awaiting culture results.

Illicit drug use may be associated with epiglottitis, with inhalation of heated objects (e.g., metal pieces from a crack cocaine pipe or the tip of a marijuana cigarette) causing thermal injury to supraglottic structures. Signs, symptoms, and roentgenographic and laryngoscopic findings are similar to infectious epiglottitis.

Initial antibiotic therapy using a third-generation cephalosporin or extended-spectrum penicillin is reasonable. The prevalence of resistant organisms should be taken into account when choosing empiric antibiotic coverage. Corticosteroids often are used in management of acute epiglottitis despite lack of evidence to support their use. Based on anecdotal case reports, epinephrine is also used.

Patients should be observed closely and experienced staff should be available immediately to secure the airway by intubation or surgical approach, if needed. Securing the airway is extremely important in patients who develop stridor and other signs of significant airway obstruction. Mortality in this group has been reported to be as high as 17.6%.[16]

Laryngotracheobronchitis and Bacterial Tracheitis

Laryngotracheobronchitis, often called croup, is commonly seen in children who present with hoarseness, barking cough, shortness of breath, and stridor. This is an acute viral illness characterized by narrowing of the subglottic area. Adult croup is a rare condition. Rare instances of diphtheric croup have been described in adults. Noninfectious membranous tracheitis related to trauma also has been reported.

Acute bacterial tracheitis refers to involvement of the subglottic trachea by bacterial infection and usually follows an episode of viral laryngotracheobronchitis. Thick, purulent exudates and mucosal edema may cause symptoms of UAO. *S. aureus* appears to be the predominant organism. Prompt antibiotic therapy, close observation with attention to airway compromise, and frequent suctioning are important. Data to suggest effectiveness of steroids or epinephrine in adults are lacking.

Rhinoscleroma is a chronic, progressive granulomatous infection of the upper airway that may cause airflow obstruction. This disorder affects primarily the nose and paranasal sinuses, but also may involve the nasopharynx, larynx, trachea, and bronchi. The causative organism is *Klebsiella rhinoscleromatis*. Rhinoscleroma is endemic in Africa, Asia, and South America and is rare in North America. About 5% of patients have diffuse narrowing of the trachea.[17] Prolonged antibiotic therapy with trimethoprim/sulfamethoxazole is effective.

Tuberculosis

The incidence of laryngeal tuberculosis may be on the rise due to the epidemic caused by the human immune deficiency virus. This form of the infection is relatively uncommon, accounting for less than 1% of tuberculosis cases. Laryngeal tuberculosis may present as progressive hoarseness and ulceration or a laryngeal mass. In the appropriate clinical context, a positive purified protein derivative (PPD) skin test and acid-fast bacilli in sputum may suggest the diagnosis. However, a biopsy from the laryngeal abnormality usually is required. Biopsy features include granulomatous inflammation, caseating granulomas, and acid-fast bacilli. The true vocal cords and epiglottis are the areas most affected. Treatment with antituberculous medications is usually adequate and should be instituted promptly, since the disease is highly contagious. Surgical interventions, including tracheostomy, are reserved for airway obstruction and long-term complications and, in one report, were required in 12% of the cases.[18]

Endobronchial tuberculosis may result in significant airflow limitation that is related to the initial lesion or subsequent stricture formation. A barking cough and sputum production are common findings. The diagnosis of tuberculosis can be delayed while the diagnosis of malignancy is being entertained. Early diagnosis and treatment with antituberculous medications should decrease the development of fibrostenosis and resultant airflow limitation. The role of steroids in reducing the incidence of fibrostenotic complications remains unclear and controversial. Management may require endoscopic or surgical approaches.

UPPER AIRWAY TUMORS

Both head and neck cancers and tracheal tumors may cause UAO.

Head and Neck Cancer

The great majority of cancers that impact the upper airway are squamous cell carcinomas, and the incidence of oropharyngeal cancer appears to be increasing in some countries (Fig. 49-13).[19] Other less common cancers occurring in the oropharynx include salivary gland carcinomas, lymphomas, and lymphoepitheliomas. Tobacco and alcohol abuse represent the most significant risk factor for the development of head and neck cancers. Other risk factors may include a diet poor in fruits and vegetables,[20] and infection with the human papillomavirus (HPV), especially HPV-type-16.[21–23] A 23% decline in head and neck cancers has been observed in the United States over the last three decades. The reported incidence was 10.8 cases per 100,000 per year from 2005 to 2009, as compared with 14.6 cases per 100,000 per year from 1976 to 1983.[24,25]

The clinical manifestations of head and neck cancer depend on the location and stage. Cancers at the base of the tongue and pharyngeal walls are insidious. These cancers grow either in an infiltrative or exophytic pattern. Because of the lack of pain fibers at the base of the tongue, these tumors are often asymptomatic until they are far advanced. The most common location of a primary tumor of the oropharynx is the anterior tonsillar pillar or tonsil. Symptoms of these cancers include hoarseness, hemoptysis, sore throat, dysphagia, referred otalgia due to cranial nerve involvement, and trismus due to pterygoid muscle involvement. Life-threatening UAO may be seen. Five percent of newly undiagnosed laryngeal cancers (a subcategory of head and neck cancers) present with severe dyspnea or stridor and may require emergency laryngectomy or tracheostomy. Patients who have had head and neck surgery for cancer have a very high prevalence of obstructive sleep apnea.[26]

TRACHEAL TUMORS

Tumors that originate in the trachea are uncommon, and make up only about 2% of all tumors that form in the upper airway. Although rare, when they do occur, approximately 80% of tracheal tumors are malignant. Primary tracheal cancers are rare with a reported incidence of 0.1 per 100,000 per year.[27] Adenoid cystic carcinoma and squamous cell carcinoma comprise the majority of primary malignant tracheal tumors. Squamous cell carcinoma is almost always associated with cigarette smoking. These tumors grow quickly, and in nearly half of cases, they are often too large to be removed by the time they are discovered. Adenoid cystic carcinoma grows much more slowly, and has not been found to be related to smoking. Men and women have the same risk for this type of cancer, and it is commonly diagnosed around the age of 40 years. Dyspnea, cough, hemoptysis, wheeze, and stridor are frequent presenting symptoms. Surgery remains the most effective management. Emergency treatment with procedures to recannulize the airway, including airway stenting, may be necessary pending definitive surgery. Postoperative radiation therapy appears useful for primary tracheal malignancies, particularly when surgical margins are positive. Palliative radiation is used for local control when surgery is contraindicated. Five-year survivals for adenoid cystic and squamous cell carcinomas are reported at 52% and 39%, respectively.[28] Favorable prognostic factors include negative airway margins at the time of resection and adenoid cystic histology.

More commonly, malignancies found in the trachea result from direct extension of primary lung cancer or regional extension to the lymph nodes (Fig. 49-14). Metastases to central airways

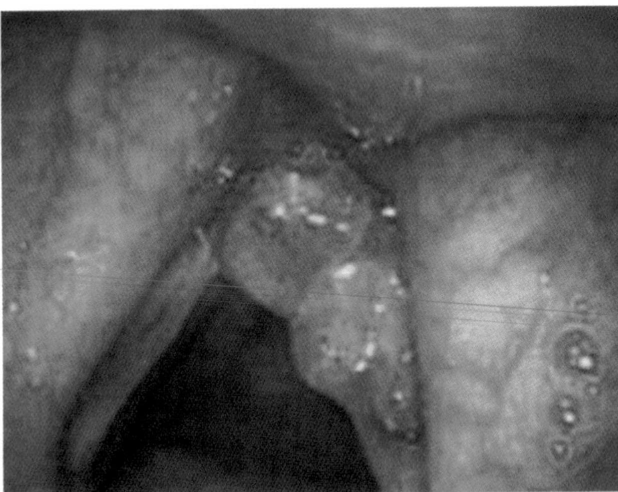

Figure 49-13 Laryngeal squamous cell carcinoma.

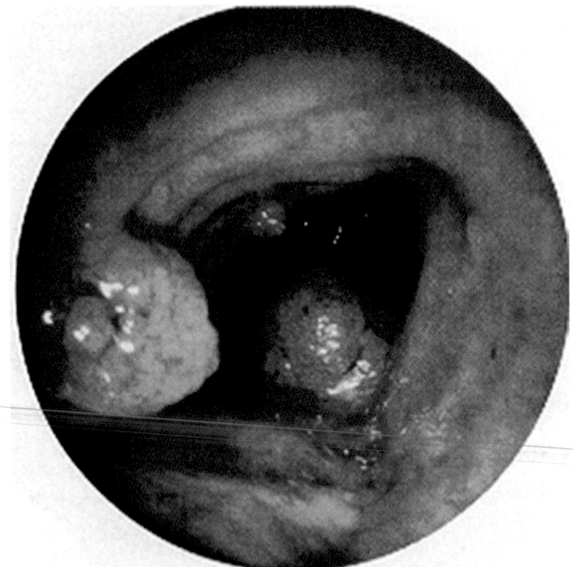

Figure 49-14 Squamous cell carcinoma of the lung.

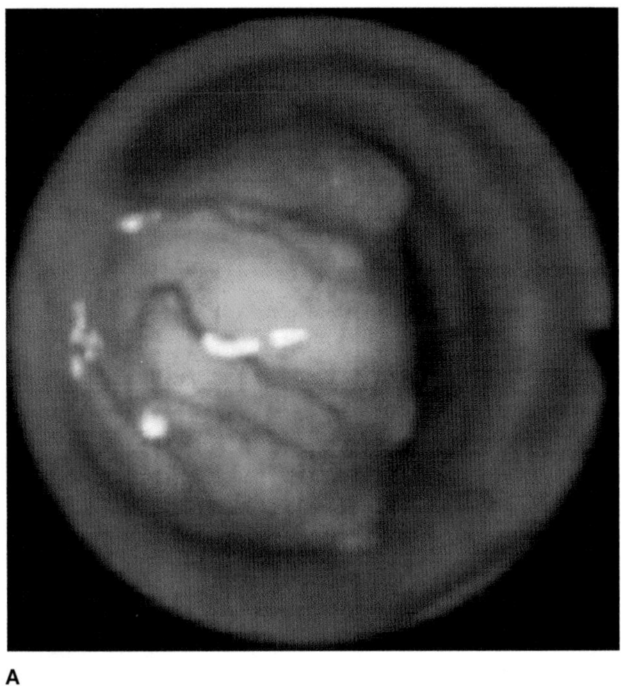

A

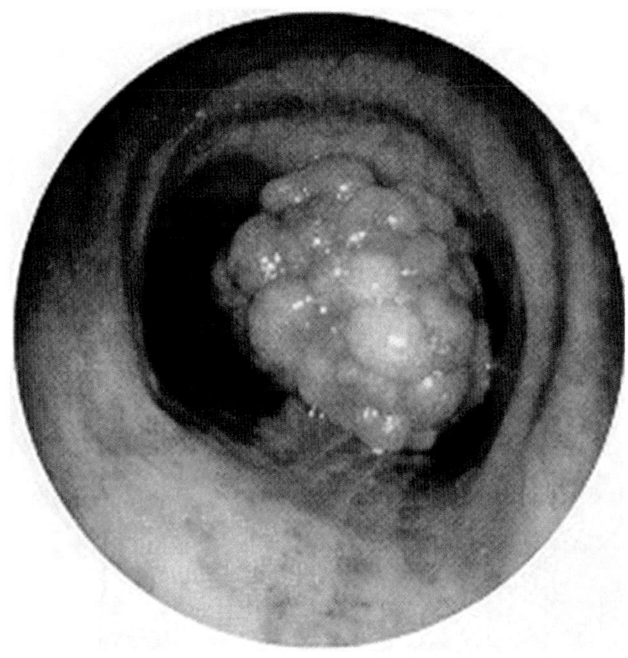

B

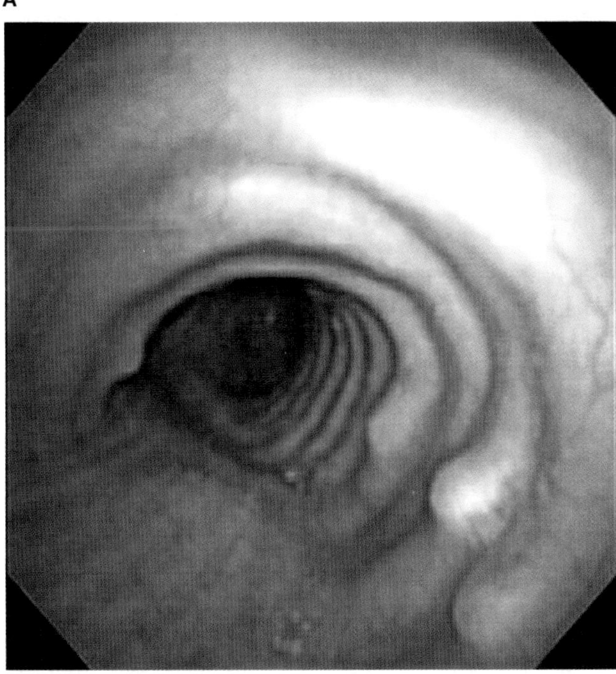

C

Figure 49-15 Nonmalignant tracheal tumors. **A.** Harmatoma. **B.** Papillomatosis. **C.** Chondromas.

from nonpulmonary malignancies are uncommon, although endobronchial metastases from breast, colorectal, renal, ovarian, thyroid, uterine, testicular, nasopharyngeal, and adrenal carcinomas, as well as sarcomas, melanomas, and plasmacytomas have been described. In an autopsy series of over 1300 patients with solid tumors, metastatic disease to central airways occurred in 2%.[29] The mediastinal lymph nodes are also a common site for disease involvement from hematologic malignancies such as lymphoma.

Nonmalignant tracheal tumors include papillomas, chondromas, and hemangiomas (Fig. 49-15). Chondromas are the most common type of benign tracheal tumor. It is formed from the cartilage rings of the trachea, and has the potential to become malignant over time. Recurrent respiratory papillomatosis in adults, caused by human papilloma virus types 6 or 11 (or, much less commonly, types 16 or 18) may result in UAO and death. Although the larynx is most commonly affected (Fig. 49-16), the tracheobronchial tree may be involved, with a predilection toward areas with prior mucosal injury, including tracheostomy sites and tracheal injuries. Lesions tend to progress down through the tracheobronchial tree. Pulmonary parenchymal involvement is rare, but it may be severe, and bronchiectasis, pulmonary nodules, and abscess formation may occur. Malignant transformation is also possible. The course of the disease is difficult to predict. Recurrent endoscopic interventions (debulking), with attendant risk of airway stenosis, are often required. It is important to minimize intervention unless clinically relevant obstruction exists due to concerns regarding extension secondary to airway injury. No controlled trials on the role of antiviral therapy have been conducted. Available data suggest beneficial effects of intralesional cidofovir. Favorable effects also have been reported with the use of interferon-A. Chemotherapy, radiation therapy, and

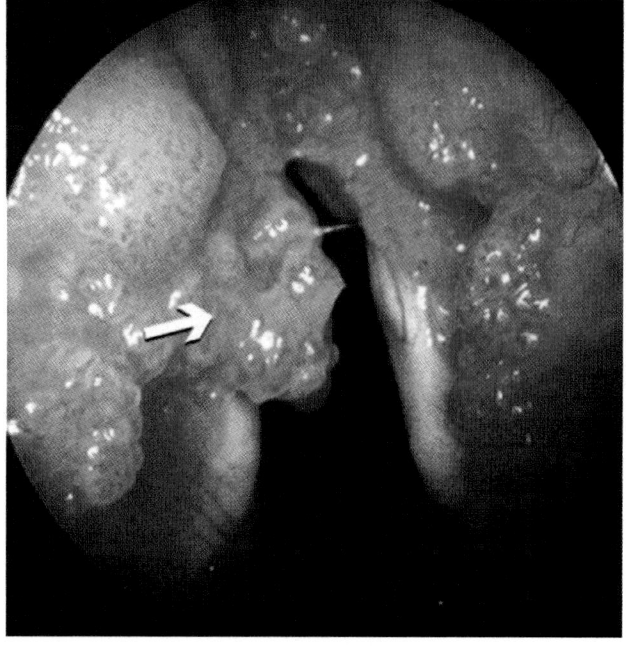

Figure 49-16 Recurrent laryngeal papillomatosis *(arrow)*.

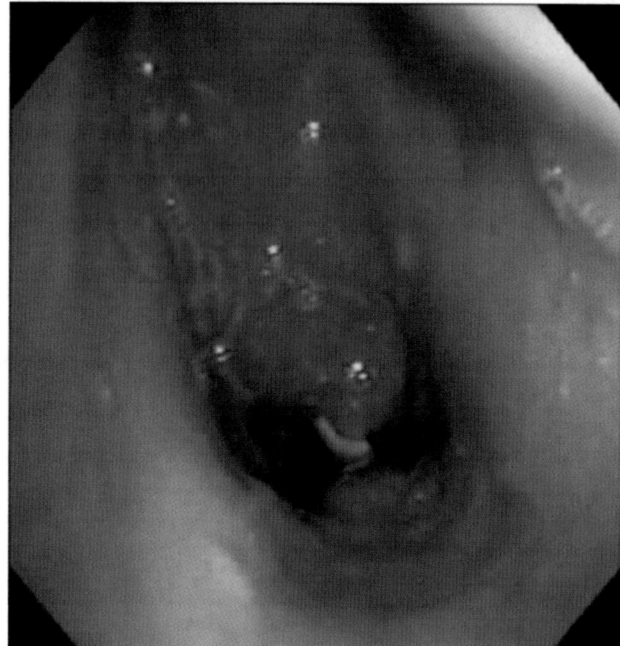

Figure 49-17 Posttracheostomy stenosis.

targeted surgical resection are utilized for confirmed malignant transformation.

■ LARYNGEAL AND TRACHEAL STENOSIS

Common causes of laryngeal and tracheal stenosis include prior intubation and tracheotomy. However, many other causes have been reported.

Postintubation and Posttracheotomy

Concentric scar formation in the larynx or trachea may lead to narrowing and obstruction to airflow. Significant stenosis, defined as obstruction exceeding 50% of the lumen, can lead to serious symptoms and functional limitations.

Endotracheal intubation, tracheostomy, and prior laryngotracheal instrumentation account for most cases of laryngotracheal stenosis. The reported frequencies of tracheal stenosis following tracheostomy or laryngotracheal intubation vary widely (0.6–65%) (Figs. 49-17 and 49-18).[30,31] Although injury to the laryngotracheal airway is common following intubation or tracheostomy, the incidence of symptomatic stenosis, demonstrated by radiographs or bronchoscopy, appears to be much lower (<2%). A recent 8-year retrospective review from Lahey Clinic identified certain patient demographics associated with an increased incidence of postintubation and posttracheostomy stenosis. These included female gender (75%), obesity (66%), diabetes mellitus (35.4%), hypertension (51.6%), and cardiovascular disease (45.1%) and current smoker (38.7%).[32]

Tracheal stenosis in the region of the tube cuff is related to pressure-induced ischemic injury of the mucosa and cartilage and its risk can be minimized by use of large-volume, low-pressure cuffs. The duration of translaryngeal intubation also affects the frequency and severity of laryngotracheal stenosis.

Stenosis following tracheostomy may be above the stoma, at the level of the stoma, at the cuff site, or at the tip of the cannula. Damage to the cartilage above the stoma is a common cause of tracheal stenosis after tracheostomy. In addition to ischemic mucosal injury and ischemic chondritis, anterior and lateral tracheal wall damage, with "buckling in" fractures of the cartilage, is an important factor. The fractures can be minimized by avoiding excessive pressure on the cartilage during the procedure, selecting the appropriate size and length of the tracheostomy tube, avoiding infection, and using the lowest possible cuff pressure.

Percutaneous tracheostomy is growing in popularity as an alternative to the standard procedure. The ideal anatomic site for percutaneous tracheostomy is between the second and third, or the first and second, tracheal rings (not the subglottic space). The incidence of symptomatic tracheal stenosis following percutaneous tracheostomy is comparable to the incidence that occurs after open techniques. When symptomatic tracheal stenosis and tracheomalacia are included as long-term complications, the incidence has been reported to be less than 2.5%.[33]

Other Causes of Tracheal Stenosis

Other causes of laryngeal and tracheal stenosis are uncommon. They include airway trauma, including external injury; inhalational burns, irradiation; tracheal infections, including bacterial tracheitis, tuberculosis, and diphtheria; granulomatosis with polyangiitis

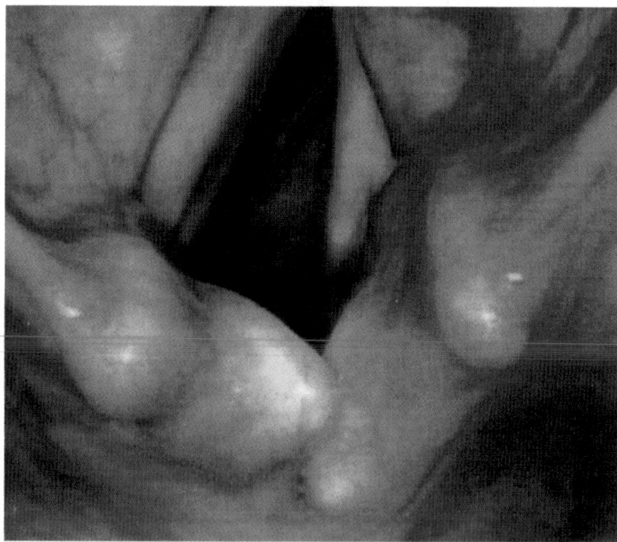

Figure 49-18 Postintubation trauma.

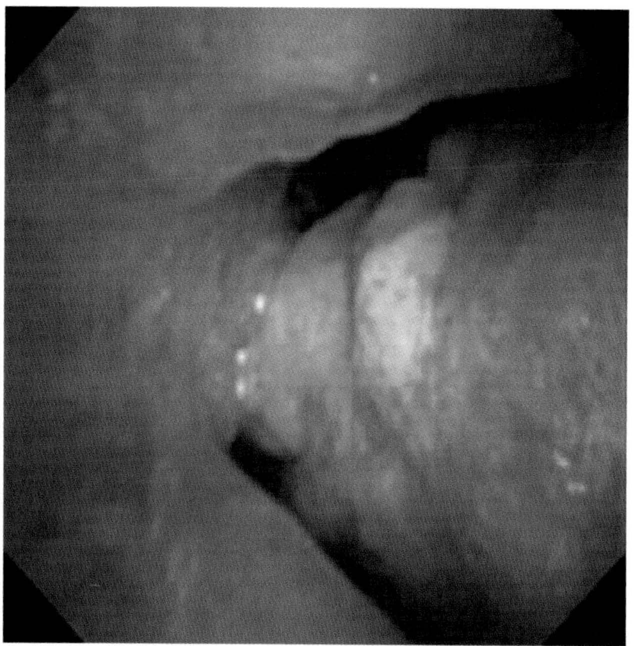

Figure 49-19 Airway sarcoid.

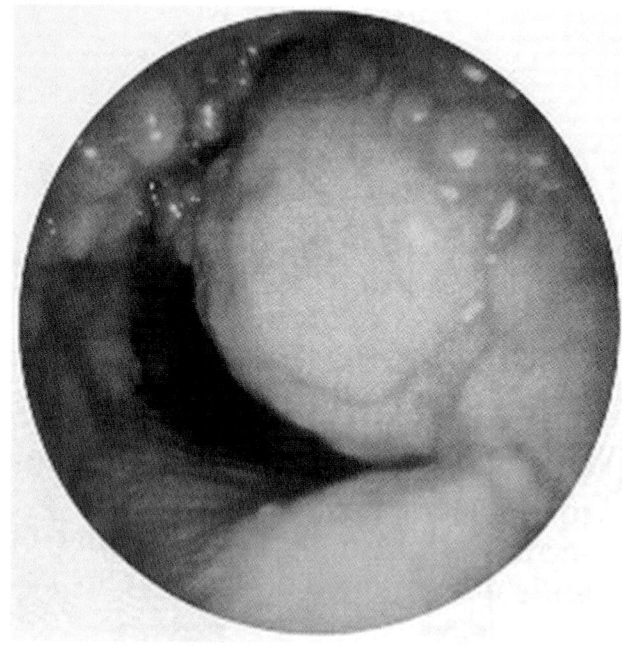

Figure 49-20 Amyloid pseudotumor.

(formerly known as Wegener granulomatosis); sarcoidosis; amyloidosis; collagen vascular diseases, including relapsing polychondritis, polyarteritis; inflammatory bowel disease; and congenital disorders.

Granulomatosis with polyangiitis may present with significant subglottic stenosis, a complication reported in 16% to 23% of patients. Subglottic stenosis may be the only manifestation of Wegener's granulomatosis and have a clinical course distinct from other manifestations of the disease. Endoscopic biopsy of suspected sites of involvement is positive in only 5% to 15% of cases.

Sarcoidosis may be associated with granulomatous infiltration and obstruction of the upper airways (Fig. 49-19). Laryngeal involvement is more common, but tracheal stenosis has been described. Radiographs may show diffuse tracheal stenosis, which progresses despite corticosteroid therapy. Bronchoscopy may reveal extensive tracheal narrowing.

Pulmonary amyloidosis includes tracheobronchial manifestations. The chest roentgenogram may show diffuse narrowing and wall thickening involving a long tracheal segment. Involvement is diffuse and circumferential, often with ossification of the amyloid deposits (Fig. 49-20). Bronchoscopy demonstrates multiple plaques on tracheal walls or localized tumor-like masses.

Relapsing polychondritis is a rare systemic disease characterized by recurrent episodes of inflammation of cartilaginous structures. Respiratory manifestations are often severe and may be life-threatening. Inflammation occurs in all cartilage types, including the elastic cartilage of the ears and nose, hyaline cartilage of all peripheral joints, and axial fibrocartilage. The most common presenting symptom is pain in the external ear due to auricular chondritis. Respiratory tract involvement may develop years after the first occurrence of auricular chondritis. Symptoms include hoarseness, aphonia, and choking. Tenderness over the thyroid and laryngeal cartilages may be present. When the trachea is involved, endoscopic examination shows inflammation and stenosis. CT demonstrates major airway collapse caused by destruction of cartilaginous rings or airway narrowing due to inflammatory edema and fibrosis. CT findings also include diffuse, smooth thickening of the trachea and proximal bronchi; thickened, densely calcified cartilaginous rings; tracheal wall nodularity; and diffuse narrowing of the tracheobronchial lumen. The posterior tracheal membrane is spared.[34]

Tracheopathia osteoplastica is a rare, benign disease of the trachea and major bronchi in which cartilaginous or osseous nodules project into the airway lumen, often causing considerable airway deformity. The posterior membranous portion of the tracheal wall is spared. The disorder may begin just below the larynx, but most often it affects the lower two-thirds of the trachea. Extension into the proximal portions of the major bronchi may be noted. The condition usually occurs over the age of 50 years and may cause severe airflow obstruction. Its etiology is unknown.

On rare occasion, inflammatory bowel disease produces tracheobronchial stenosis and severe airflow obstruction. The associated airway mucosal inflammation may be steroid responsive early in the course of illness. If fibrosis ensues, medical management has limited success.

Laryngopharyngeal reflux may contribute to subglottic stenosis and, when documented, merits treatment.

Idiopathic progressive subglottic stenosis may be diagnosed in the absence of a clear, underlying etiology. Since most affected patients are females, a hormonal etiology has been proposed. However, estrogen receptors have not been demonstrated in specimens studied.[35]

In addition to medical management, repeated rigid and flexible bronchoscopy-based interventions aimed at reestablishing airway patency may be necessary, particularly in those who are not considered to be surgical candidates or in those with simple web-like stenoses. In cases of web-like stenosis, radial incisions sparing the posterior membrane are made and then the airway dilated either using a balloon or the rigid bronchoscope barrel. With respect to more complex stenosis, endoscopic intervention is generally considered a bridge in patients considered good operative candidates with potentially resectable disease. There exists concern on the part of many experts that repeated endoscopic intervention may result in extension of the area of scar rendering potentially resectable stenoses no longer amenable to surgical intervention.[36] Unfortunately resection and reanastomosis is limited by the length of trachea to be resected.[37,38] A multidisciplinary approach incorporating medical and surgical specialists as described by Brichet is utilized in many centers.[39]

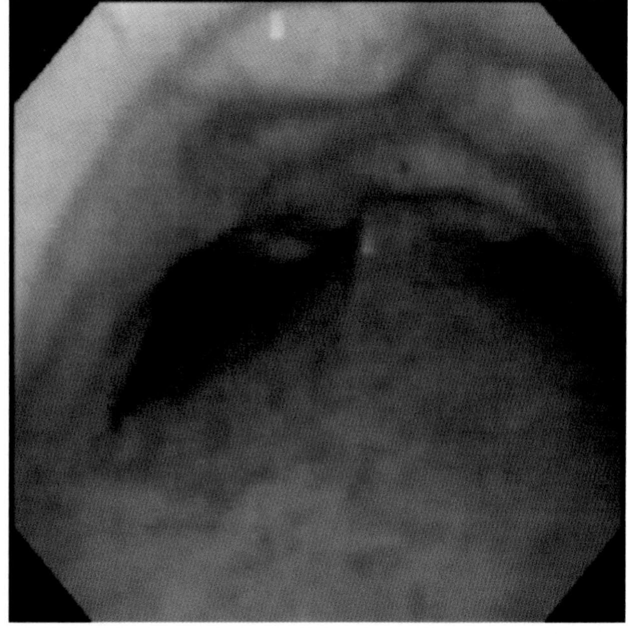

Figure 49-21 Bronchoscopic view of tracheomegaly or Mounier-Kuhn syndrome.

■ TRACHEOMALACIA

Tracheomalacia refers to loss of tracheal rigidity and resulting susceptibility to collapse. Tracheomalacia may be diffuse or localized to a tracheal segment. The affected portion may be intrathoracic, in which airway obstruction is accentuated during expiration. Less common is extrathoracic obstruction resulting from cervical malacia, in which airway obstruction is most marked during inspiration. Tracheobronchomalacia is the term used to describe the condition when the mainstem bronchi are involved.

Tracheomalacia in adults may be classified as congenital or acquired. The congenital form, described more extensively in children, is related to a variety of congenital disorders and associated syndromes. The disorder may persist into adult life and is referred to as "idiopathic giant trachea," "tracheomegaly," or the "Mounier-Kuhn syndrome" (Fig. 49-21). Bronchiectasis and recurrent respiratory infections are common. Tracheal diverticuli have been reported in more advanced disease. Although atrophy of the longitudinal elastic fibers and muscularis layer has been described, the etiology of these changes is unclear. The diagnosis is made when the diameters of the trachea or right or left mainstem bronchi exceed the upper limits of normal by 3 or more standard deviations. In a recent article by O'Dell, patients with tracheobronchomalacia attributable to Mounier-Kuhn were found to benefit symptomatically from airway stenting and tracheobronchoplasty.[40]

Acquired or secondary tracheomalacia in adults may be related to a variety of conditions.[41] Tracheostomy and endotracheal intubation are probably the most common etiologies. Usually, limited, focal weakness of the trachea and excessive dynamic airway collapse are present. Tracheomalacia may be caused by conditions that are associated with chronic pressure on the tracheal wall, inflammation of the cartilaginous support or mucosa, interference with tracheal blood flow, or chronic infection. Traumatic injury to the central airways or surgical interventions also may lead to tracheomalacia.

Symptoms of tracheomalacia include dyspnea, a seal-barking paroxysmal cough, recurrent pulmonary infections, and respiratory failure in a small subset.[42] Many of these patients will also have decreased exercise tolerance and in severe cases impaired quality of life.

Tracheomalacia is diagnosed by using direct bronchoscopic visualization to confirm significant narrowing of the tracheal lumen during regular, forced expiration. Assessment of the central airways using end-expiratory, dynamic, three-dimensional CT images is useful. Application of continuous positive airway pressure (CPAP) has been reported as beneficial as pneumatic splint for the airways. Tracheobronchoplasty may be useful in selected patients and has been shown to improve quality of life and exercise tolerance.[42] Optimal medical management includes treatment of associated infections and of distal airway disease.

■ EXTRINSIC COMPRESSION OF THE CENTRAL AIRWAY

The upper airway is subject to extrinsic compression by a variety of pathologies that involve adjacent structures. The compression may affect the intrathoracic trachea or extrathoracic trachea and upper airway.

Mediastinal Masses and Lymphadenopathy

Rarely, mediastinal masses present with serious limitation to airflow that develop either acutely or indolently. Common symptoms include chest pain, fever, dyspnea, and cough. Based on one large series, approximately 40% of mediastinal masses are malignant; 25% are cystic. The anterosuperior compartment is the most common site of mediastinal malignancies. Thymic neoplasms and lymphoma are the most common malignancies, followed by neurogenic tumors and teratomas. Both Hodgkin and non-Hodgkin lymphomas may be manifested by severe respiratory compromise due to airway compression. A similar syndrome may be due to a metastatic tumor to the mediastinal lymph nodes arising from bronchogenic or other carcinomas.

Patients with large mediastinal masses present a challenge during the perioperative period because of the potential for development of acute UAO and other respiratory complications. In adults, complete airway obstruction during induction of anesthesia is rare. Serious pulmonary complications develop intra- and postoperatively in about 4% and 7% of patients, respectively. Complications may occur while the patient is placed in the supine position, during induction, or following extubation. Patients with severe symptoms, including stridor, and those with greater than 50% airway obstruction appear at high risk for respiratory complications; asymptomatic patients are at significantly less risk. Patients with reduced peak expiratory flow and mixed obstructive–restrictive patterns on pulmonary function testing also appear to be at increased risk for postoperative complications.

Middle mediastinal masses include benign cysts that are bronchogenic, enterogenous (duplication), pericardial, pleural, and thymic in origin. Most bronchogenic cysts are asymptomatic. However, some evoke cough, chest pain, and dyspnea. Severe respiratory distress and compressive symptoms can occur. Usually, cyst contents appear to have the density of water on CT or MRI. Mucoid contents may give the impression of solid appearance on CT. Surgical resection and transthoracic or transbronchial drainage are options for management. Surgical intervention appears to be the preferred treatment in patients who are symptomatic. The role of interventions, including surgery, in asymptomatic patients is controversial. Enterogenous cysts are usually removed surgically.

Enlarged mediastinal lymph nodes that compress the airway may arise from infectious and noninfectious benign etiologies. One notable example is fibrosing mediastinitis, defined as the presence of excessive mediastinal fibrous tissue that tends to invade and destroy normal structures. The entity is thought to represent a reaction to an infectious granulomatous disease, especially histoplasmosis. The incidence in populations exposed to histoplasmosis remains low. Constriction of the central airways and vessels and the resulting cardiopulmonary limitations may develop several years after the initial infection. Hemoptysis is common, as are cough, dyspnea, and chest pain. CT imaging shows mediastinal fibrosis, calcification, and compression of mediastinal structures. Bronchoscopic findings include concentric airway narrowing and mucosal edema with hyperemia. Unfortunately, hemoptysis tends to be recurrent, and the disease does not respond to corticosteroids or antifungal agents. Surgical intervention is generally ineffective and may be hazardous.

Neck and Thyroid-Related Causes

Retrosternal extension of a diffuse goiter may cause extrathoracic or intrathoracic airway obstruction. Up to 90% of patients with substernal goiter report respiratory symptoms. A choking sensation occurs in about one-third of patients with diffuse thyroid enlargement and 14% in patients with solitary thyroid nodules. Orthopnea is prevalent when the goiter is intrathoracic and may be enhanced by obesity. Flow–volume loops show evidence of UAO in one-third of patients. Lack of correlation has been reported between symptomatic obstruction and CT findings.[43]

Laryngoceles and saccular cysts, which are abnormal dilatations of the laryngeal saccule (ventricle), are uncommon. Saccular cysts usually are filled with mucus. Laryngoceles communicate with the laryngeal lumen, resulting in air-filled structures noted on radiographic studies. Laryngoceles may be internal (i.e., confined to the larynx), external (i.e., extending into the thyrohyoid membrane superiorly), or combined. Most are asymptomatic. Hoarseness, dysphagia, pain, or signs of airway obstruction or infection may occur. A neck mass during the valsalva maneuver may be detectable. Pyocele formation (i.e., infection in the laryngocele) may result in airway obstruction, aspiration pneumonia, or infection of the lateral pharyngeal space. The incidence of laryngeal carcinoma in association with laryngoceles makes close evaluation necessary. Endoscopic and surgical approaches may be employed in management.

Parathyroid cysts may be located in the neck or mediastinum. Fifty percent are accompanied by clinical hyperparathyroidism. Paroxysmal symptoms of airway obstruction can develop. Surgical excision is the treatment of choice; results are generally good.

Cervical osteophytes, common in the elderly, are related to either degenerative spinal arthritis or more generalized idiopathic skeletal hyperostosis; the osteophytes may be associated with dysphagia. In addition, airway narrowing and ulcerations due to osteophytes have been reported. The airway compression may make even elective endotracheal intubation difficult, despite adequate preoperative evaluation.

Finally, significant upper airway compression may arise from cervical lymph node involvement with infectious or malignant disorders, hematomas or pseudoaneurysms (related to trauma, surgical interventions, central line placement, or coagulation abnormalities), abscess formation, or other expanding lesions in the soft tissue of the neck.

Diseases of the Esophagus

Involvement of the trachea, glottis, or vocal cords by advanced esophageal cancer is common and associated with a poor prognosis; estimated 1-year survival is less than 10%. Airway obstruction requiring stent placement is associated with a median survival of 1 to 4 months after the placement. Tracheal obstruction may develop if an esophageal stent is placed in the setting of significant tracheal compromise. Development of tracheoesophageal fistula represents a devastating complication.

Placement of stents simultaneously in the trachea and esophagus is effective palliation for a tracheoesophageal fistula.[44] If such double stenting is anticipated for a fistula or for simultaneous esophageal and tracheal obstructions, the tracheal stent is placed first to ensure patency of the airway, followed by the esophageal stent. Palliative external or local radiation therapy, chemotherapy, or other treatment modalities (e.g., PDT) may be effective with or without accompanying airway interventions. The risk of esophageal disruption and rupture should be considered if stenting is performed after these local measures are employed.

Achalasia may cause a variety of pulmonary complications, including cough, aspiration with pneumonia or abscess formation, and rarely UAO. Tracheal compression by a dilated megaesophagus is the usual etiology. Ensuring patency of the airway and decompressing the esophagus are necessary in urgent management.

Vascular Abnormalities

Vascular rings, defined as anomalies of the aortic arch or its branches that compress the trachea or esophagus, are rare in adults (incidence <0.2%). Respiratory symptoms are common.

Right-sided aortic arch occurs in less than 0.1% in adults and may be associated with complete vascular rings, while double aortic arch and right-sided aortic arch with aberrant left subclavian artery appear to be the most common etiologies of vascular rings in adults.

The right-sided aortic arch usually crosses over the right main-stem bronchus and descends on either the right or the left side. The vascular ring is usually completed by the ligamentum arteriosum arising from the descending aorta, an aberrant left subclavian artery, or an aortic diverticulum. With a double aortic arch, the left arch crosses over the left main-stem bronchus and joins the descending aorta to complete the ring; the ligamentum arteriosum does not contribute to the vascular ring. Symptoms, resulting from malacia of the compressed airway and resultant dynamic airway obstruction, may be misdiagnosed as exercise-induced asthma. An increase in aortic diameter due to rising blood pressure during exercise, intravenous fluid administration, or anatomic changes with aging may contribute to symptoms. Surgical intervention is indicated in symptomatic patients.

Pulmonary artery sling with anomalous origin of the left pulmonary artery from the right pulmonary artery is very rare in adults. In neonates, the condition is symptomatic and can be fatal without surgical intervention. However, in adults the condition is usually diagnosed incidentally on imaging a patient who has no significant symptoms. This disorder may be associated with a complete tracheal ring, forming the "sling-ring" complex. This condition may present with a right paratracheal mass noted on the chest radiograph.

Compression of the trachea by large aortic or innominate artery aneurysms or pseudoaneurysms may occur and complicate management in the perioperative period. Surgical repair is indicated to relieve symptoms.

■ FOREIGN BODY ASPIRATION

Foreign body aspiration, more common in children than adults (in whom the peak incidence is in the sixth decade), is usually recognized from the patient's history. Foreign bodies commonly lodge in the bronchi after migrating through the trachea. In adults, food products are the most commonly aspirated material. The penetration syndrome, defined as the sudden onset of choking and intractable cough after aspirating a foreign body, with or without vomiting, is often followed by persistent cough, fever, chest pain, dyspnea, and wheezing. Impairment of the normal protective airway mechanisms is common; among the frequent associations are neurologic disorders, trauma with loss of consciousness, sedative or alcohol use, poor dentition, and advanced age. Emergency measures, entailing a food extractor or the Heimlich maneuver, can be life-saving. Flexible bronchoscopy is usually successful in removing foreign bodies, although back-up rigid bronchoscopy should be available and is preferred as the primary procedure at some centers. A complicating chemical bronchitis from aspiration of vegetables or nuts may affect visualization and management of the foreign body. Certain nut oils also cause a significant foreign body mucosal reaction resulting in the development of granulation tissue that may be misdiagnosed as endobronchial tumor.

TRAUMA

A variety of traumatic injuries may eventuate in UAO.

Facial Trauma

Emergency access to the airway is necessary in up to 6% of cases of facial trauma complicating motor vehicle accidents and other causes of crush injuries. If intubation is difficult or impossible due to the injury or related airway obstruction, emergency cricothyroidotomy or tracheostomy must be considered.

Laryngotracheal Injuries

Blunt and penetrating injuries to the laryngotracheal airway are rare. Without a high index of suspicion, clinicians may miss the diagnosis. The incidence of penetrating injuries appears to be increasing.

Stridor, wheezing, dysphonia, hemoptysis, and general neurologic deficits are common. Cervical crepitus and subcutaneous emphysema also may be present. Cervical ecchymoses and hematomas, pneumomediastinum, and pneumothorax should prompt consideration of a laryngotracheal injury.

Management includes prompt securing of the airway, but blind endotracheal intubation should be avoided, since it carries the risk of complete airway obstruction. Some experts recommend tracheostomy as the primary airway management strategy. Awake fiberoptic intubation can be useful. Flexible fiberoptic laryngoscopy, rigid or flexible bronchoscopy, and CT imaging may be helpful in assessing the degree of injury. Unfortunately, the mortality of laryngotracheal injuries remains high (20%–40%). Thoracic injuries and closed head injuries are commonly associated pathologies that can influence management and prognosis.

Inhalation Injuries

Thermal and chemical injuries to the upper respiratory tract may lead to serious consequences, including airway obstruction. Unfortunately, the mortality rate increases significantly when burns are accompanied by inhalational injury. Symptoms can be delayed in becoming manifest, making early recognition and intervention vital in the management of patients with inhalational injuries. The presence of cough, dyspnea, hoarseness, or loss of consciousness, or the findings of singed nasal hairs, carbonaceous sputum, or burns involving the face indicate a high likelihood of inhalation injury.

Early flexible bronchoscopy remains important in evaluation and management of patients with inhalation injuries, enabling the assessment of the extent and severity of the injury, procurement of samples for bacteriologic studies, and bronchoscopic intubation, as necessary. Translaryngeal intubation is the standard method of securing the airway in inhalation injury; early tracheostomy is used in some centers. A role for prophylactic corticosteroids or antibiotics is currently not supported by published reports. Significant tracheal stenosis may develop in patients who survive the initial insult, especially when translaryngeal intubation or tracheostomy is necessary.

ENDOTRACHEAL TUBE–RELATED TRAUMA

Postextubation stridor due to glottic edema, laryngospasm, or laryngotracheal stenosis is a serious event. Reintubation rates for UAO due to endotracheal tube–related trauma in critically ill patients have been reported to range from 4% to 33%. An "acceptable" rate is considered to be 5% to 15%. The cuff leak test does not accurately predict success or failure of extubation. Although the efficacy of corticosteroids or racemic epinephrine in the management of postextubation stridor is not substantiated, both are used extensively in clinical practice.

Translaryngeal intubation may also produce vocal cord paralysis, accounting for 10% to 15% of all cases. Paralysis may be unilateral or bilateral. Affected patients may present with hoarseness or airway obstruction. Findings may occur immediately after extubation or be delayed. Prolonged intubation, use of a large endotracheal tube (number 8 or larger), placement of the tube cuff close to the vocal cords, or use of excessive cuff pressure are risk factors. The condition usually resolves spontaneously within 10 weeks.

Vocal cord (contact) granuloma may develop 4 to 6 weeks after intubation. Symptoms include prolonged hoarseness, exertional dyspnea, and stridor. Management, using antireflux medications, inhaled and systemic corticosteroids, antibiotics, botulinum toxin injection, speech therapy, smoking cessation, and rest of the voice are usually successful. Surgical intervention is reserved for cases that fail conservative management.

On occasion, dislocation of the arytenoid cartilages occurs during intubation. Rheumatoid arthritis that affects the cricoarytenoid cartilage is a risk factor for this condition. Rigid bronchoscopy or surgical interventions may be needed to reduce the dislocation. Other disorders that may cause complications during intubation include hyperostosis of the cervical spine due to ankylosing spondylitis and cricoarytenoid joint disease due to systemic lupus erythematosus.

NEUROMUSCULAR DISORDERS

Neuromuscular disorders may affect the bulbar muscles, many of which surround the upper airway (Fig. 49-22). When this occurs, resistance to airflow is increased, and the flow–volume loop often shows an inspiratory flow plateau typical of variable extrathoracic UAO. In addition, a pattern of flow oscillations during inspiration ("sawtooth pattern") may be seen.[45] The abnormal flow pattern, first noted in patients with sleep apnea,[46] is commonly seen in extrapyramidal disorders, myasthenia gravis, and motor neuron disease; it may also be seen in patients who have functional stridor and wheezing (see Vocal Cord Dysfunction section). In extrapyramidal disorders, the flow oscillations correspond to vocal cord tremor. In motor neuron diseases, muscle denervation causes irregular muscle fasciculation, resulting in tremor of upper airway muscles.

Upper airway symptoms may be seen in Shy–Drager syndrome with extrapyramidal involvement and in Parkinson disease.[47,48] Patients may present with symptoms of chronic dyspnea or with stridor and respiratory failure relieved by endotracheal intubation or tracheostomy. Bilateral vocal cord paralysis may also occur with familial bulbar spinal muscle atrophy, postpoliomyelitis syndrome,

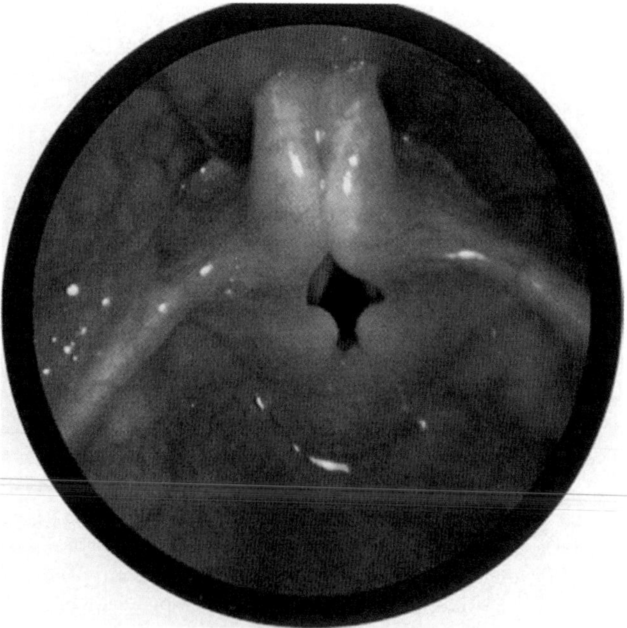

Figure 49-22 Laryngomalacia.

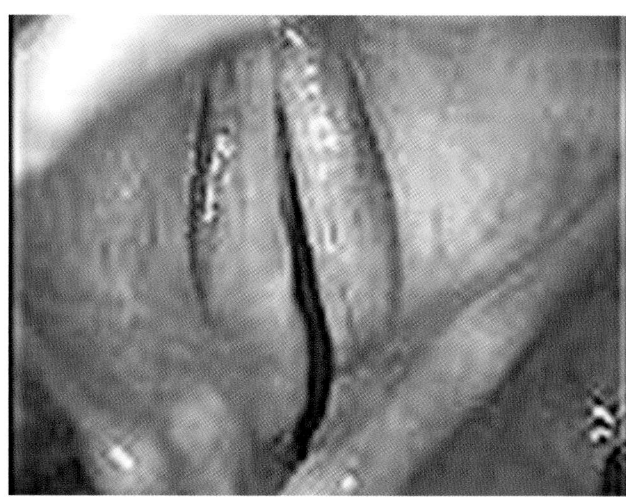

Figure 49-23 Bilateral vocal cord paralysis.

Parkinson disease, multiple sclerosis, acute poliomyelitis, amyotrophic lateral sclerosis, Guillain–Barré syndrome, brain stem stroke, and large cerebral hemisphere stroke. Dystonic extrapyramidal reactions due to neuroleptic medications (e.g., haloperidol) may cause significant UAO. The usual reactions to these medications are akathisia, dyskinesia, dysarthria, and dystonic reactions, such as torticollis. Laryngeal–pharyngeal dystonia may cause severe upper airway dysfunction, and if not reversed, symptoms can last for days or lead to respiratory arrest.

BILATERAL VOCAL CORD PARALYSIS

Bilateral vocal cord paralysis is a serious condition resulting in nocturnal stridor, oxygen desaturation, sleep disruption or, in extreme cases, acute respiratory failure (Fig. 49-23). Thyroidectomy is the most common cause of bilateral recurrent laryngeal nerve injury, with its consequent bilateral vocal cord paralysis.[49] As mentioned earlier, bilateral vocal cord paralysis may occur with numerous neurologic conditions. Nonneurologic causes include endotracheal intubation injury, laryngeal trauma, infection, and thoracic aortic aneurysm. Bilateral vocal cord paralysis results in abnormalities of inspiratory flow and a distinctive flow–volume loop.

Spontaneous recovery of vocal cord motility is rare after surgical injury of the recurrent laryngeal nerve. For those patients showing no spontaneous functional recovery, several surgical techniques to achieve a glottic space enlargement are available. CO_2 laser endoscopic surgery has led to shorter hospitalization and higher patient compliance.[50,51] Endoscopic surgeries include arytenoidectomy with or without posterior true and false cord cordectomy. Surgeries aim to improve breathing with minimal deglutition impairment and improve quality of voice. Restenosis of the glottis space is the main problem that leads patients to reoperations.

VOCAL CORD DYSFUNCTION

The glottis plays an active role in adjusting airflow, both voluntarily and through reflex control from laryngeal and lung receptors. During a normal respiratory cycle, the vocal folds widely abduct during inspiration and slightly adduct during expiration. Occasionally, the glottis can become dysfunctional in the absence of organic disease. The disorder, most commonly called vocal cord dysfunction or paradoxical vocal fold motion, is characterized by paradoxical closure of the vocal cords intermittently during inspiration. The glottis angle formed by the true vocal folds can become acute and cause airflow obstruction during inspiration and/or expiration. The mechanism is unknown, but likely multifactorial. Laryngeal hypersensitivity has been associated with reflux, upper respiratory tract infections, postnasal drip, irritants, exercise, as well as psychogenic factors.

Signs and symptoms of vocal cord dysfunction resemble those of laryngeal edema, laryngospasm, vocal cord paralysis, or asthma. Wheezing or stridor and shortness of breath are typical and are often so dramatic that they suggest acute asphyxia and respiratory failure. Intubation and other emergency measures are used frequently. However, symptoms are often brief and may remit without intervention. Distinguishing physical examination findings include tracheal localization of wheezing or stridor with absent peripheral airway expiratory wheezing; however, it should be understood that this might also occur during severe asthma attacks.

On pulmonary function testing, patients with vocal cord dysfunction typically have normal spirometry without evidence of obstructive ventilatory defect. Some may demonstrate a pattern of variable extrathoracic airway obstruction, resulting in an increase in the ratio of $FEF_{50\%}$ to $FIF_{50\%}$. Some patients show a pattern of "sawtoothing," or fluttering of the inspiratory limb of the flow–volume loop, representing fluctuations in the abnormal cord motion (Fig. 49-24). Often, attempts to perform the flow–volume loop maneuver generate variable results from test to test. A normal alveolar–arterial oxygen gradient and absence of bronchial hyperresponsiveness are other clues to the diagnosis.

The diagnosis of vocal cord dysfunction is confirmed during direct visualization of the vocal cords during an attack. The anterior

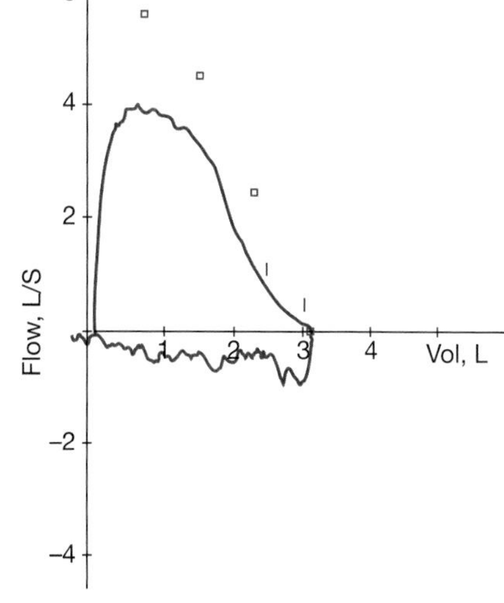

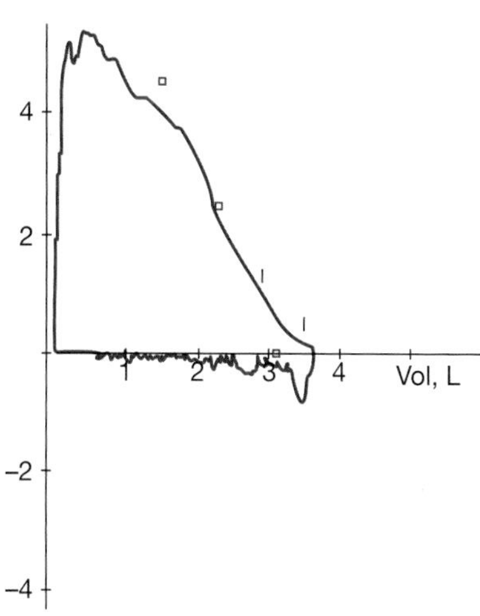

Figure 49-24 Variable extrathoracic obstruction due to vocal cord dysfunction. Two consecutive flow–volume loops from a young woman with inspiratory stridor. Variable effort accounts for the differences in configuration. $FEF_{50\%}/FIF_{50\%}$ in each is very high. The inspiratory loop is flat and demonstrates a sawtooth pattern. This pattern has also been associated with sleep apnea syndrome and various neuromuscular disorders.

two-thirds of the vocal folds adduct and give the presence of a posterior diamond-shaped chink in the folds during inspiration.[52]

The true prevalence of the disorder is unknown because it is often mistakenly diagnosed as asthma, and many patients in fact have both vocal cord dysfunction and asthma. Patients without asthma are predominantly women who have been misdiagnosed as having asthma for an average of 5 years. Typically, patients have been treated with large doses of oral corticosteroids, and have experienced frequent emergency room visits, hospitalizations, and endotracheal intubations.

Psychiatric disorders are common in these patients. Major psychiatric disorders, personality disorders, and sexual and physical abuse are commonly uncovered. Whereas many patients are unaware of their self-induced wheeze or stridor, others appear to derive secondary gain from their symptoms and manifest factitious illness. A high index of suspicion is warranted when the adventitious sounds are loudest over the neck in a patient who presents with wheezing, stridor, or both. Despite their respiratory distress, patients often have little difficulty completing full sentences and can hold their breath; the laryngeal-induced sounds disappear during a panting maneuver.

Treatment includes discussion of the diagnosis with the patient, discontinuation of unnecessary medications, and referral to a speech therapist or psychotherapist. The response to bronchodilator therapy is usually poor. Administration of an inhaled helium–oxygen mixture may alleviate symptoms during an acute attack.

ANGIOEDEMA

Angioedema is characterized by well-demarcated swelling of the face, lips, tongue, and mucus membranes of the nose, mouth, and throat. When the larynx is involved, UAO may occur and is fatal in as many as 25% of patients. In most instances, the cause of angioedema is unclear; prior exposure to common allergens, such as drugs, chemical additives, and insect bites should be suspected.

Contrary to what might be thought, the most common causes of angioedema are not IgE initiated. They include reactions to histamine-releasing drugs, such as narcotics and radiocontrast materials, to aspirin and other nonsteroidal anti-inflammatory drugs, and to angiotensin-converting enzyme inhibitors. Hereditary angioedema, a rare cause of UAO, is an autosomal-dominant trait that occurs in all races. The underlying mechanism is a deficiency in production or function of C1 esterase inhibitor, a serum protease inhibitor that regulates the complement, fibrinolytic, and kinin pathways. Hereditary angioedema is characterized by painless nonpitting edema of the face and upper airway. The disorder usually begins in childhood and becomes more prominent in adolescence. Swelling progresses over many hours and then resolves spontaneously over 1 to 3 days. Despite the slow progression, death may occur from laryngeal obstruction. Physical stimuli (cold, heat, stress) and circulating immune complex diseases (e.g., due to serum sickness or systemic lupus erythematosus) are also known to cause angioedema.

Emergency management includes foremost securing the airway. Epinephrine is used for allergic angioedema. Administration of corticosteroids and antihistamines are often used, although current evidence suggests that such a therapy is rather ineffective in kinin-induced angioedema.[53] Thus, symptom-related medical care should be provided until the swellings have disappeared. Approaches targeting the kallikrein–kinin system, such as kallikrein inhibitors[54] and bradykinin type-2 receptor antagonists[55] may improve pharmacotherapy. It is probable that these drugs may also be beneficial in patients with bradykinin-mediated drug-induced angioedema.

MISCELLANEOUS ETIOLOGIES

Postpneumonectomy syndrome refers to compression of the left main bronchus between the aortic arch and left pulmonary artery following a right pneumonectomy. The syndrome also may be seen following a left pneumonectomy, sometimes in the setting of a right-sided aortic arch. Mediastinal repositioning prostheses, with or without additional fixation methods, may be useful in selected patients.

Mucus ball formation related to transtracheal oxygen catheters has been described. Although transtracheal oxygen delivery decreases supplemental oxygen flow requirements by approximately 50% during rest and 30% during activity, development of symptomatic mucus balls (occurring in up to one-third of patients) remains a major disadvantage of the technique. Death and life-threatening events secondary to airway obstruction have been reported.

MANAGEMENT OF UPPER AIRWAY OBSTRUCTION

Key elements in the management of UAO include general principles, securing the airway, and specific interventions.

GENERAL MANAGEMENT

The primary goals in management of any patient with UAO are assurance of adequate oxygenation and ventilation and management of the underlying condition. If airway obstruction is partial, and the patient's condition is stable, close monitoring and diagnostic studies are appropriate. Depending upon the underlying etiology, temporary measures may include close observation in an intensive care unit, elevation of the head of the bed, administration of humidified oxygen, use of a helium–oxygen inhalation mixture (see next paragraph), systemic corticosteroids, and inhaled racemic epinephrine, pending definitive medical or surgical management.

A helium–oxygen gas mixture (heliox) may be useful in management of UAO when the obstruction is temporary and reversible. The physiologic rationale for heliox is based upon a reduction in work of breathing achieved through administration of a low-density gas. In particular, heliox has a lower density than does oxygen, room air, or a mixture of the two, resulting in conversion of the predominantly turbulent flow at the site of obstruction to a more laminar pattern. Furthermore, since laminar flow requires a smaller pressure gradient than turbulent flow to achieve the same flow rate, the accompanying work of breathing is less (see Chapter 10). The major limitation of the modality is an inability to deliver gas with an inspiratory fraction of oxygen ($F_{I_{O_2}}$) of more than 40%. Despite physiologic evidence and clinical reports of efficacy, prospective, randomized studies demonstrating improved outcome in patients receiving heliox are lacking, as are data supporting use of corticosteroids or inhaled epinephrine in airway obstruction from a variety of causes.

SECURING THE AIRWAY

Although under controlled circumstances, a significant portion of the so-called difficult airways and intubations may be identified in the course of a thorough preoperative assessment, the patient with impending airway obstruction presents a challenge. Under such circumstances, a critical first concern is deciding whether an artificial airway is needed emergently.[56] Regardless of the airway utilized, emphasis is placed on ensuring adequate oxygenation and ventilation.

Airways judged unsafe for routine management may be addressed according to the "difficult airway algorithm" recommended by the American Society of Anesthesiologists (see also Chapter 146).[57] A difficult airway is defined as a clinical circumstance in which a conventionally trained anesthesiologist experiences difficulty using face mask ventilation, endotracheal intubation, or both.

Airway access in emergency situations may be challenging because the patient frequently is critically ill and can deteriorate quickly. The likelihood of a difficult intubation can be estimated by using the Mallampati score or a modification of the score to assess potential laryngeal exposure and prospects for adequate airway visualization.

A number of parameters, such as mouth opening distance, jaw size, thyromental distance, and cervical range of motion, have been incorporated into airway assessment scoring systems; each parameter has limited sensitivity and specificity. Combining scoring systems provides better accuracy of prediction. The "rule of threes," which is a useful, simple bedside tool, predicts successful direct laryngoscopy if the examiner can place three finger breadths (~6 to 7 cm) between the upper and lower teeth, the mandible and hyoid bones, and the thyroid cartilage and sternal notch. In the emergency setting of UAO, the most experienced physician available should secure the airway. Appropriate equipment and monitoring, along with back-up resources for alternative and invasive airway management, should be available.

A variety of invasive and noninvasive techniques are available as alternatives to standard, laryngoscopy-guided orotracheal intubation. Invasive methods include surgical and/or percutaneous tracheostomy, surgical and percutaneous transtracheal (needle) cricothyrotomy, translaryngeal guided or "retrograde" intubation, fiberoptic endotracheal intubation, and use of a rigid ventilating bronchoscope. Noninvasive techniques include use of specialized laryngoscope blades, Glidescope™, guiding and lighted stylets, directional tip control tubes, and esophageal–tracheal (Combitube) or laryngeal mask airways. In selected circumstances, tactile intubation, nasotracheal intubation, or blind orotracheal intubation may be employed.

CRICOTHYROIDOTOMY

Cricothyroidotomy (either surgical or based on Seldinger technique) has a long history of use in emergency access to the airway when more conservative approaches fail or are contraindicated. Currently, surgical cricothyroidotomy is performed by surgeons, anesthesiologists, and intensive care specialists. In early reports, a high incidence of laryngeal stenosis during intermediate and long-term follow-up was noted, perhaps related to the presence of infectious laryngeal disease or the use of large-bore tubes. In addition, the risk of subglottic stenosis also appears high in patients with prolonged prior intubation. Hence, although the procedure is useful for short-term airway control, tracheostomy should be considered if prolonged airway access is required.

TRACHEOSTOMY

Most tracheostomies are performed on intubated patients in the intensive care unit. Percutaneous tracheostomy is rapidly becoming the method of choice in the intensive care unit and is associated with acceptable intraoperative and postoperative complication rates. Advantages of the technique over the traditional procedure include low cost, short procedure time, low complication rate, and elimination of the need to transport critically ill patients to the operating room. Adaptation of percutaneous techniques for emergency situations also has been described.

In a review of over 1100 patients who underwent tracheostomy, 76% were performed in patients who required prolonged ventilation, 6% for UAO, 7% for extensive maxillofacial trauma, and 11% as an adjunct for head and neck or chest surgeries; only 0.26% were performed as emergency procedures. Overall mortality was 0.7%.[58]

INTERVENTIONAL BRONCHOSCOPIC TECHNIQUES

Interventional bronchoscopy is discussed in chapter 36. Use of these techniques for managing UAO is well established and is briefly summarized in the following paragraphs.

Rigid bronchoscopy allows oxygenation, ventilation, and application of various diagnostic and therapeutic interventions, including debridement of obstructing lesions, control of bleeding, and removal of foreign bodies. Complications include anesthetic risks, barotrauma, damage to teeth, lips or gums, airway perforation, bleeding, and mucosal injury.

Thermal modalities may be used to devitalize tissue prior to mechanical debridement or to cauterize the base of lesions following debulking. Electrocautery, laser (Nd-Yag, CO_2, i.e., Yap), argon plasma coagulation, and cryotherapy can be applied through rigid or flexible bronchoscopy. Side effects include bleeding, perforation, airway fire and damage to cartilage.

Photodynamic therapy is based on the principle of targeted tissue apoptosis after local activation of a systemically injected photosensitive chemotherapeutic agent. In essence, PDT creates a phototoxic cell reaction when nonthermal laser light is applied by bronchoscopy and activates a drug trapped in these target cells. The major disadvantage of this technique is that the tissue necrosis occurs within 48 to 72 hours and as such the ability to debride the airway is delayed for several days. Bleeding and obstruction from necrotic tumor and edema are potential immediate complications. PDT may also result in airway perforation.

Standard cryotherapy, based on repeated freeze–thaw cycles to achieve cell necrosis and tissue damage is used in benign and malignant disorders of the upper airway. Cryotherapy has excellent hemostatic effects; the incidence of perforation or bleeding is low. Due to the delayed beneficial effect, cryotherapy is not usually used under emergent conditions. In recent years a cryobiopsy technique has been developed in which the tissue is simply frozen to the probe and then sheared from the surface, obviating the thaw cycle. Applied in this fashion, cryotherapy can be used for the immediate treatment of airway obstruction. In addition, cryotherapy has the advantage over other thermal modalities in that cartilage is cryoresistant.

Finally, external beam radiation and brachytherapy are useful modalities for palliative management of airway obstruction and hemoptysis. For external beam radiation, unwanted exposure of adjacent structures is a limiting factor, while hemorrhage, radiation bronchitis, and fistulae with surrounding structures are known complications of radiotherapy. The maximal effect of all radiation techniques is delayed days to weeks and there is a risk of worsening of obstruction during therapy due to airway edema.

AIRWAY STENTS

Airway stents are used in the palliative management of both benign and malignant airway obstruction.[59] Available tracheal stents include expandable metal, silicone, and hybrid prostheses. Major complications include stent migration, granulation tissue formation, and stent interference with mucociliary clearance. In a series of over 1500 patients who had stents placed for UAO due to benign or malignant disorders, stent migration was reported in 9.5%, granulation tissue formation in 7.9% and obstruction in 3.6%. Due to concerns regarding stent fracture, the FDA posed a warning on the use of metallic airway stents for benign disease. Currently, metallic stents are only recommended in benign disease for patients who are not candidates for or have failed a trial of silicone stent placement.

REFERENCES

1. Davidson TM, Sedgh J, Tran D, Stepnowsky CJ Jr. The anatomic basis for the acquisition of speech and obstructive sleep apnea: evidence from cephalometric analysis supports The Great Leap Forward hypothesis. *Sleep Med.* 2005;6(6):497–505.
2. Yamashiro Y, Kryger M. Is laryngeal descent associated with increased risk for obstructive sleep apnea? *Chest.* 2012; 141(6):1407–1413.
3. Carroll CM, Pahor A. The history of tracheotomy. *J Ir Coll Physicians Surg.* 2001;30(4):237–238.
4. Morens DM. Death of a president. *N Engl J Med.* 1999;341 (24):1845–1849.
5. Ayers ML, Beamis JF Jr. Rigid bronchoscopy in the twenty-first century. *Clin Chest Med.* 2001;22(2):355–364.
6. Du Rand IA, Barber PV, Goldring J, et al. British Thoracic Society guideline for advanced diagnostic and therapeutic flexible bronchoscopy in adults. *Thorax.* 2011;66 Suppl 3:iii1–iii21.

7. Kryger M, Quesney LF, Holder D, Gloor P, MacLeod P. The sleep deprivation syndrome of the obese patient. A problem of periodic nocturnal upper airway obstruction. *Am J Med.* 1974;56(4):530–539.
8. Kryger M, Bode F, Antic R, Anthonisen N. Diagnosis of obstruction of the upper and central airways. *Am J Med.* 1976;61(1):85–93.
9. Sullivan CE, Issa FG, Berthon-Jones M, Eves L. Reversal of obstructive sleep apnoea by continuous positive airway pressure applied through the nares. *Lancet.* 1981;1(8225):862–865.
10. Owens GR, Murphy DM. Spirometric diagnosis of upper airway obstruction. *Arch InternMed.* 1983;143(7):1331–1334.
11. Boiselle PM, Feller-Kopman D, Ashiku S, Weeks D, Ernst A. Tracheobronchomalacia: evolving role of dynamic multislice helical CT. *Radiol Clin North Am.* 2003;41(3):627–636.
12. Boiselle PM, O'Donnell CR, Bankier AA, et al. Tracheal collapsibility in healthy volunteers during forced expiration: assessment with multidetector CT. *Radiology.* 2009;252(1): 255–262.
13. Wang LF, Kuo WR, Tsai SM, Huang KJ. Characterizations of life-threatening deep cervical space infections: a review of one hundred ninety-six cases. *Am J Otolaryngol.* 2003;24(2): 111–117.
14. Riordan T, Wilson M. Lemierre's syndrome: more than a historical curiosa. *Postgrad Med J.* 2004;80(944):328–334.
15. Ames WA, Ward VM, Tranter RM, Street M. Adult epiglottitis: an under-recognized, life-threatening condition. *Br J Anaesth.* 2000;85(5):795–797.
16. Mayo-Smith MF, Spinale JW, Donskey CJ, Yukawa M, Li RH, Schiffman FJ. Acute epiglottitis. An 18-year experience in Rhode Island. *Chest.* 1995;108(6):1640–1647.
17. Gaafar HA, Gaafar AH, Nour YA. Rhinoscleroma: an updated experience through the last 10 years. *Acta Otolaryngol.* 2011;131(4):440–446.
18. Yencha MW, Linfesty R, Blackmon A. Laryngeal tuberculosis. *Am J Otolaryngol.* 2000;21(2):122–126.
19. de Souza DL, de Camargo Cancela M, Perez MM, Curado MP. Trends in the incidence of oral cavity and oropharyngeal cancers in Spain. *Head Neck.* 2012;34(5):649–654.
20. Sanchez MJ, Martinez C, Nieto A, et al. Oral and oropharyngeal cancer in Spain: influence of dietary patterns. *Eur J Cancer Prev.* 2003;12(1):49–56.
21. D'Souza G, Kreimer AR, Viscidi R, et al. Case-control study of human papillomavirus and oropharyngeal cancer. *N Engl J Med.* 2007;356(19):1944–1956.
22. Gillison ML, Koch WM, Capone RB, et al. Evidence for a causal association between human papillomavirus and a subset of head and neck cancers. *J Natl Cancer Inst.* 2000;92(9):709–720.
23. Mork J, Lie AK, Glattre E, et al. Human papillomavirus infection as a risk factor for squamous-cell carcinoma of the head and neck. *N Engl J Med.* 2001;344(15):1125–1131.
24. Carvalho AL, Nishimoto IN, Califano JA, Kowalski LP. Trends in incidence and prognosis for head and neck cancer in the United States: a site-specific analysis of the SEER database. *Int J Cancer.* 2005;114(5):806–816.
25. Sikora AG, Toniolo P, DeLacure MD. The changing demographics of head and neck squamous cell carcinoma in the United States. *Laryngoscope.* 2004;114(11):1915–1923.
26. Steffen A, Graefe H, Gehrking E, Konig IR, Wollenberg B. Sleep apnoea in patients after treatment of head neck cancer. *Acta Otolaryngol.* 2009;129(11):1300–1305.
27. Honings J, van Dijck JA, Verhagen AF, van der Heijden HF, Marres HA. Incidence and treatment of tracheal cancer: a nationwide study in the Netherlands. *Ann Surg Oncol.* 2007;14(2):968–976.
28. Gaissert HA, Grillo HC, Shadmehr MB, et al. Long-term survival after resection of primary adenoid cystic and squamous cell carcinoma of the trachea and carina. *Ann Thorac Surg.* 2004;78(6):1889–1896; discussion 1896–1887.
29. Berkman N, Breuer R, Kramer MR, Polliack A. Pulmonary involvement in lymphoma. *Leuk Lymphoma.* 1996;20(3–4):229–237.
30. Lorenz RR. Adult laryngotracheal stenosis: etiology and surgical management. *Curr Opin Otolaryngol Head Neck Surg.* 2003;11(6):467–472.
31. Goldenberg D, Ari EG, Golz A, Danino J, Netzer A, Joachims HZ. Tracheotomy complications: a retrospective study of 1130 cases. *Otolaryngol Head Neck Surg.* 2000;123(4):495–500.
32. Zias N, Chroneou A, Tabba MK, et al. Post tracheostomy and post intubation tracheal stenosis: report of 31 cases and review of the literature. *BMC Pulm Med.* 2008;8:18.
33. Kost KM. Endoscopic percutaneous dilatational tracheotomy: a prospective evaluation of 500 consecutive cases. *Laryngoscope.* 2005;115(10 Pt 2):1–30.
34. Ernst A, Rafeq S, Boiselle P, et al. Relapsing polychondritis and airway involvement. *Chest.* 2009;135(4):1024–1030.
35. Perotin JM, Jeanfaivre T, Thibout Y, et al. Endoscopic management of idiopathic tracheal stenosis. *Ann Thorac Surg.* 2011;92(1): 297–301.
36. Ashiku SK, Kuzucu A, Grillo HC, et al. Idiopathic laryngotracheal stenosis: effective definitive treatment with laryngotracheal resection. *J Thorac Cardiovasc Surg.* 2004;127(1):99–107.
37. Grillo HC. Development of tracheal surgery: a historical review. Part 2: Treatment of tracheal diseases. *Ann Thorac Surg.* 2003;75(3):1039–1047.
38. Ernst A, Feller-Kopman D, Becker HD, Mehta AC. Central airway obstruction. *Am J Respir Crit Care Med.* 2004;169(12): 1278–1297.
39. Brichet A, Verkindre C, Dupont J, et al. Multidisciplinary approach to management of postintubation tracheal stenoses. *Eur Respir J.* 1999;13(4):888–893.
40. Odell DD, Shah A, Gangadharan SP, et al. Airway stenting and tracheobronchoplasty improve respiratory symptoms in Mounier-Kuhn syndrome. *Chest.* 2011;140(4):867–873.
41. Carden KA, Boiselle PM, Waltz DA, Ernst A. Tracheomalacia and tracheobronchomalacia in children and adults: an in-depth review. *Chest.* 2005;127(3):984–1005.
42. Majid A, Guerrero J, Gangadharan S, et al. Tracheobronchoplasty for severe tracheobronchomalacia: a prospective outcome analysis. *Chest.* 2008;134(4):801–807.
43. Torchio R, Gulotta C, Perboni A, et al. Orthopnea and tidal expiratory flow limitation in patients with euthyroid goiter. *Chest.* 2003;124(1):133–140.
44. Freitag L, Tekolf E, Steveling H, Donovan TJ, Stamatis G. Management of malignant esophagotracheal fistulas with airway stenting and double stenting. *Chest.* 1996;110(5):1155–1160.
45. Levent E, Sariman N. Analysis of obstructive sleep apnea patients with "sawtooth sign" on the flow-volume curve. *Sleep Breath.* 2011;15(3):357–365.
46. Shore ET, Millman RP. Abnormalities in the flow-volume loop in obstructive sleep apnoea sitting and supine. *Thorax.* 1984;39(10):775–779.

47. Mu L, Sobotka S, Chen J, et al. Alpha-synuclein pathology and axonal degeneration of the peripheral motor nerves innervating pharyngeal muscles in parkinson disease. *J Neuropathol Exp Neurol.* 2013;72(2):119–129.

48. Alfonsi E, Versino M, Merlo IM, et al. Electrophysiologic patterns of oral-pharyngeal swallowing in parkinsonian syndromes. *Neurology.* 2007;68(8):583–589.

49. Yumoto E, Minoda R, Hyodo M, Yamagata T. Causes of recurrent laryngeal nerve paralysis. *Auris Nasus Larynx.* 2002; 29(1):41–45.

50. Maurizi M, Paludetti G, Galli J, Cosenza A, Di Girolamo S, Ottaviani F. CO_2 laser subtotal arytenoidectomy and posterior true and false cordotomy in the treatment of post-thyroidectomy bilateral laryngeal fixation in adduction. *Eur Arch Otorhinolaryngol.* 1999;256(6):291–295.

51. Rovo L, Jori J, Brzozka M, Czigner J. Airway complication after thyroid surgery: minimally invasive management of bilateral recurrent nerve injury. *Laryngoscope.* 2000;110(1):140–144.

52. Christopher KL, Wood RP 2nd, Eckert RC, Blager FB, Raney RA, Souhrada JF. Vocal-cord dysfunction presenting as asthma. *N Engl J Med.* 1983;308(26):1566–1570.

53. Agostoni A, Cicardi M. Hereditary and acquired C1-inhibitor deficiency: biological and clinical characteristics in 235 patients. *Medicine.* 1992;71(4):206–215.

54. Tanaka KA, Szlam F, Katori N, Vega JD, Levy JH. Evaluation of a novel kallikrein inhibitor on hemostatic activation in vitro. *Thromb Res.* 2004;113(5):333–339.

55. Icatibant: HOE 140, JE 049, JE049. *Drugs R D.* 2005;6(4): 239–244.

56. Sue RD, Susanto I. Long-term complications of artificial airways. *Clin Chest Med.* 2003;24(3):457–471.

57. American Society of Anesthesiologists Task Force on Management of the Difficult Airway. Practice guidelines for management of the difficult airway: an updated report by the American Society of Anesthesiologists Task Force on Management of the Difficult Airway. *Anesthesiology.* 2003;98(5):1269–1277.

58. Lim JW, Friedman M, Tanyeri H, Lazar A, Caldarelli DD. Experience with percutaneous dilational tracheostomy. *Ann Otol Rhinol Laryngol.* 2000;109(9):791–796.

59. Chan KP, Eng P, Hsu AA, Huat GM, Chow M. Rigid bronchoscopy and stenting for esophageal cancer causing airway obstruction. *Chest.* 2002;122(3):1069–1072.

CHAPTER 50

Cystic Fibrosis

Judith A. Voynow
Maria Mascarenhas
Andrea Kelly
Thomas F. Scanlin

Cystic fibrosis (CF) is a common inherited disease that has a high frequency in Caucasians. The disorder affects all exocrine glands, with symptoms involving the lungs and pancreas usually dominating the clinical picture. Even though the gene responsible for CF and its gene product, an integral membrane glycoprotein, have been identified, two aspects of the disease make CF particularly difficult to both diagnose and manage. First, there is tremendous variability in the degree and pattern of involvement of organs in different persons. In addition, we lack information about the precise details of the molecular and cellular pathogenesis of the disease. This chapter focuses on the pathophysiology and management of CF. Our current understanding of the genetics and underlying molecular biology is highlighted. Complications of the disorder are addressed, and a brief discussion of relevant psychosocial and reproductive issues is provided. Finally, potential future directions in treatment are described.

GENETICS

CF demonstrates an autosomal-recessive pattern of inheritance. In the United States, the incidence of the disease is approximately 1 in 3000 in Caucasians, 1 in 6000 in Hispanics, and 1 in 10,000 in African Americans. The frequency of unaffected heterozygote carriers of a CF mutation is estimated to be 1 in 26 in persons of Northern European ancestry.

CF is caused by mutations in a single gene named the *cystic fibrosis transmembrane conductance regulator* (CFTR). This gene was identified with an approach known as positional cloning, which permitted mapping of the gene, without prior knowledge of the biochemical defect, through use of polymorphic DNA markers. The first genetic marker that was found to be linked to CF was paraoxonase. In 1985, the demonstration of the linkage of CF to two DNA markers, D7S15 and D7S8, and to the *met* oncogene established the localization of the CF gene to the long arm of chromosome 7. Following a series of molecular cloning experiments, which included "chromosome walking" and "jumping," a candidate gene was identified. This was proved to be the CF gene in 1989, largely through the discovery of a frequent mutation.[1,2]

The CF gene spans approximately 230 kb of DNA and contains 27 exons. The mRNA is 6.5 kb and is detected in a variety of tissues, including lungs, pancreas, and sweat glands, which are predominantly affected in pathogenesis of the disease. The deduced polypeptide was predicted to be an integral membrane glycoprotein containing 1480 amino acids (Fig. 50-1) (see "Pathogenesis" below). Several major and minor splicing variants in the transcripts have been described in individuals with and without CF. In most cases, however, the significance of the alternative splicings is not clear.

The most common CF mutation, and the first to be described, is a three-base deletion in exon 10 that causes a deletion of phenylalanine from position 508 (ΔF508 or F508del) of the CFTR glycoprotein. This mutation accounts for 66% of CF mutations.[3] However, more than 1900 CF mutations have now been reported, and the list continues to grow. In addition, a number of benign sequence variations have been described. A listing of the most common mutations and their relative frequency is included in Table 50-1. The large number of mutations makes accurate detection of a satisfactory percentage of carriers extremely difficult, and carrier screening for the general population has not been recommended or implemented. Testing for 32 of the most common mutations is widely available; such testing will detect approximately 90% of the carriers in Caucasians of Northern European descent. In families with an affected individual and known mutations, prenatal diagnosis and

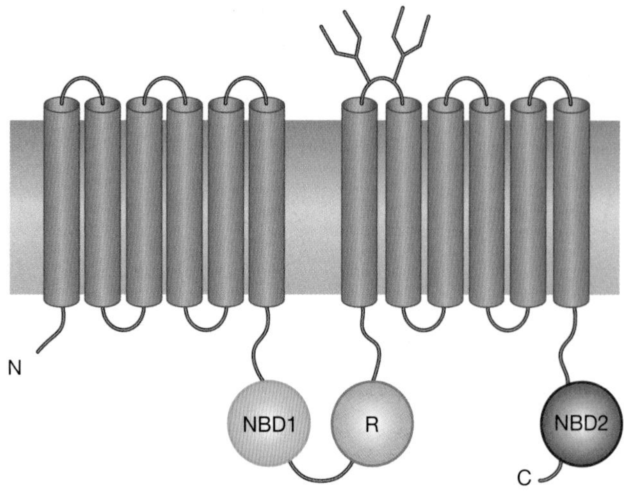

Figure 50-1 Domain model of the cystic fibrosis transmembrane conductance regulator (CFTR). Based on hydrophobicity plots, CFTR has 12 transmembrane-spanning domains, two nucleotide (N) binding domains (NBD 1 and NBD 2), and a regulatory (R) domain. The 12 transmembrane domains form the ion channel "pore." In the closed state, the "R" domain is believed to obstruct the channel. Channel opening requires binding of two adenosine triphosphates (ATPs) to the nucleotide binding domains. This model is similar to other ATP-binding cassette transporter proteins that bind ATP and transport ions or micronutrients. *(Modified with permission from Riordan J, Rommens JM, Kerem B, et al. Identification of the cystic fibrosis gene: Cloning and characterization of complementary DNA. Science; 245(4922):1066–1073.)*

carrier testing using direct detection of mutations is accurate and available. In families with a member diagnosed as having CF, but with undetected mutations, sequencing of the complete CFTR coding region and critical intronic regions is now also available to detect rare mutations.

PATHOGENESIS

Discovery of the gene responsible for CF and description of its product, CFTR, have provided the necessary foundation for understanding the pathogenesis of the disorder at the molecular and cellular levels. CFTR is an integral membrane glycoprotein of approximately 170 kD that is expressed in epithelial cells of affected organs. CFTR contains 1480 amino acids, which are arranged in 12 transmembrane domains, two nucleotide binding domains, and a putative regulatory domain (Fig. 50-1). The most common mutation, F508del, is a three-base deletion that causes deletion of phenylalanine from position 508, located in the proposed first nucleotide-binding domain. The original structural model, which was based on hydrophobicity plots, has proved to be essentially correct in its main features. CFTR shares many structural features with the "adenosine triphosphate (ATP)-binding cassette" transporter family, which includes P glycoproteins, as well as a number of bacterial transporters. CFTR has been clearly shown to function as an apical chloride channel in airway epithelial cells.

The localization of CFTR to the apical aspect of airway epithelial cells, to the ciliated duct of submucosal gland cells, and to submucosal serous cells, and the role of CFTR as an apical chloride channel fits nicely with the simplest hypothesis to account for the pathogenesis of pulmonary disease in CF. Decreased secretion of chloride and water by airway epithelial cells results in dehydrated mucus (Fig. 50-2). However, CFTR may have other functions, such as regulation of other ion channels, including the epithelial sodium channel. Loss of CFTR causes increased reabsorption of sodium; increased epithelium sodium channel activity alone alters regulation of ions and water, resulting in mucus obstruction of airways. CFTR transports bicarbonate; loss of CFTR function may result in acidification of the small intestinal lumen and, possibly, the airway lining fluid. Alternatively, CFTR may also function in *intracellular* membranes (e.g., endoplasmic reticulum, endosomes, phagosomes, and clathrin-coated vesicles). A consequence of the altered function of CFTR in intracellular membranes may explain abnormalities of CF glycoproteins: Increased sulfation of respiratory mucins, with decreased sialylation and increased fucosylation of both secreted and membrane glycoproteins. Altered glycosylation of airway glycoproteins may significantly impact

TABLE 50-1 Most Common CFTR Mutations in the United States

Name of Mutation	Frequency (%)	Population with High Prevalence
ΔF508	66	
G542X	2.4	Spanish
G551D	2.1	English
3120+1G→A	1.5	African American, Arabian
W1282X	1.4	Jewish-Ashkenazi
N1303K	1.3	Italian
R553X	0.9	Hispanic
621+1G→T	0.9	Multiethnic
1717−1G→A	0.7	Italian
3849+10kbC→T	0.7	Hispanic
R117H	0.7	
1898+1G→T	0.4	East Asian
ΔI507	0.3	Hispanic
2789+5G→A	0.3	
G85E	0.3	
R347P	0.2	
R334W	0.2	Multiethnic
R1162X	0.2	Multiethnic
R560T	0.2	
3659delC	0.2	
A455E	0.2	
2184delA	0.1	
S549N	0.1	Multiethnic
711+1G→T	0.1	
R75X	0.2	Hispanic
406−1G→A	0.2	Hispanic
I148T	0.2	Hispanic/French
2307insA	0.2	African American
A559T	0.2	African American
ΔF311	0.2	African American
G480 C	0.2	African American
405+3A→C	0.2	African American
S1255X	0.2	African American

Data based on the most frequent mutations found overall in the United States. Source: Adapted with permission from Bobadilla JL, Macek M Jr., Fine JP, et al. Cystic fibrosis: A worldwide analysis of CFTR mutations-correlation with incidence data and application to screening. Hum Mutat. 2002;19(6):575–606.

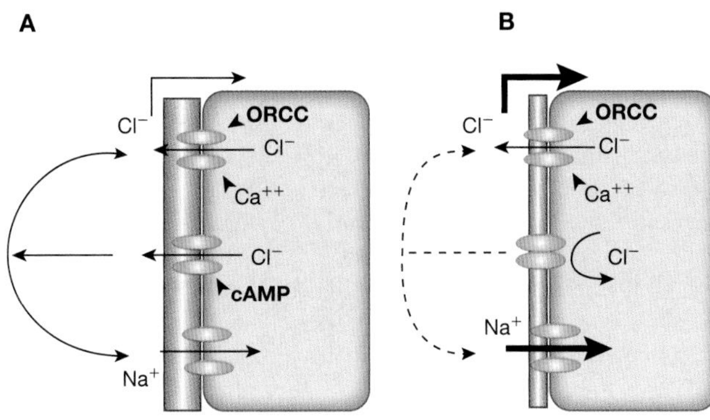

Figure 50-2 Simplified model of ion transport in airway epithelium. **A.** Normal airway cell with multiple apical ion channels. At the top, two different chloride channels are represented, the outwardly rectifying chloride channel (ORCC) and the Ca^{++}-gated chloride channel. In the center, cyclic adenosine monophosphate (cAMP)-gated cystic fibrosis transmembrane conductance regulator (CFTR) is shown. The apical sodium channel is depicted at the bottom. Experimental data suggest that CFTR interacts with the other channels, although the type of interaction is not clear *(solid arcs)*. **B.** CF cell with nonfunctioning cAMP-gated apical chloride transport. The function of the other channels is affected in an unknown manner *(dashed arc)*. The net result of ion channel activity on the pericellular fluid composition *(hatched area)* is under investigation. Many questions remain concerning the function of CFTR and ion transport in the airway.

bacterial–epithelial interactions and innate immune functions in the lung.[4]

In addition to the effect of CFTR on epithelial ion channels and glycoprotein processing, loss of CFTR function negatively impacts innate immunity and accentuates inflammation. Absence of CFTR function is associated with impaired bacterial killing in vitro and defective function of antimicrobials including human β-defensin 1 and lysozyme. Absence of CFTR is also associated with increased interleukin-8 (IL-8) production and decreased IL-10 in vitro. In the CF airway, excessive neutrophil elastase cleaves complement and immunoglobulins, interfering with bacterial opsonization. CF airways have increased oxidant stress due to neutrophilic inflammation and reduced antioxidants such as glutathione. Together, these factors synergistically increase the inflammatory milieu in the airways in CF.

A long-standing impediment to progress has been the absence of a completely suitable animal model. A number of mouse models of CF have been developed and while these have been useful in understanding some features of the disease such as the regulation of inflammation, a drawback has been the absence of spontaneous development of lung disease.[5] Two recently developed animal models in the ferret[6] and pig[7] have shown promise in developing some features of the early lung disease of CF.

CFTR mutations have been grouped into five classes,[8] depending on the effect of the mutation on the expression, processing, and function of the protein (Fig. 50-3). The most common mutation, F508del, is a processing mutation in which very little of the mutant protein reaches the apical surface. If the mutant protein escapes normal intracellular processing, however, F508del protein functions normally in the apical membrane. Furthermore, only 25% of normal CFTR transcripts are properly processed and transported to the cell surface. The remaining 75% are degraded before being processed. These data suggest that one therapeutic strategy to overcome the defect in CF is to disrupt normal intracellular processing mechanisms. A phase III clinical trial is in progress to test a therapeutic small molecule which is based on this concept.

PATHOPHYSIOLOGY

In CF, all exocrine glands appear to be affected primarily, albeit to varying degrees. Because exocrine glands perform highly specialized functions in a variety of organs – for example, in the skin, respiratory tract, gastrointestinal tract, and reproductive system – the number of possible symptoms and complications in CF is large. Table 50-2 highlights the complications and symptoms of CF according to the age groups in which they most often occur.[9] Obstruction of exocrine ducts by viscous secretions appears to play a cardinal role in the pathogenesis of almost all manifestations of the disease. In 10% to 20% of patients, the initial manifestation is often *meconium ileus* – that is, obstruction of the intestine by thick, viscous meconium stool. Chronic pulmonary disease, pancreatic insufficiency, and focal biliary cirrhosis progress gradually throughout the course of the disease, albeit at different rates in different patients. Progressive obstruction of exocrine ducts is a regular feature of the disease except in sweat glands, where obstruction of ducts has not been implicated in pathogenesis.

■ RESPIRATORY TRACT

In the lungs, hypersecretion of viscid mucus and chronic bacterial infection combine to produce a progressive and distinctive type of

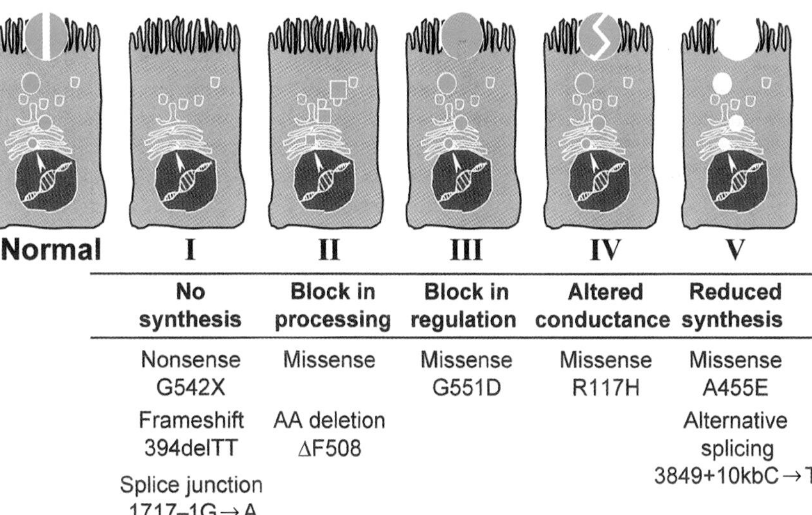

Figure 50-3 Classification of cystic fibrosis transmembrane conductance regulator (CFTR) mutations by molecular and biochemical abnormalities. This schematic depicts the effect of different classes of CFTR mutations on expression and function in the cell. Class I mutations block mRNA transcription. Class II mutations prevent normal CFTR protein processing and localization. Class III mutations permit CFTR localization at the apical membrane but inhibit chloride channel conductance. Class IV mutations result in partial chloride channel conductance. Class V mutations affect transcription, translation, or protein processing resulting in reduced CFTR expression at the apical membrane. Examples of mutations in each class are depicted below the cell models. Epithelial cell models with finger-like projections depict cilia at the apical surface. Fully processed CFTR protein is depicted by the *gray circles* embedded among the cilia at the apical surface of the cells. *(Adapted with permission from Zielenski J1, Tsui LC. Cystic fibrosis: genotypic and phenotypic variations. Annu Rev Genet. 1995;29:777–807.)*

TABLE 50-2 Presenting Signs and Symptoms of CF

Infancy	Childhood	Adolescence/Adult
Positive prenatal test for CF mutations or hyperechoic bowel on ultrasound	Pulmonary infection with *Staphylococcus* and *Pseudomonas*	Chronic bronchitis with bronchiectasis
Positive CF newborn screen	Malnutrition with steatorrhea and pancreatic insufficiency	Pansinusitis
Meconium ileus	Heat prostration with hypoelectrolytemia and metabolic alkalosis	Hemoptysis
Obstructive jaundice	Atypical asthma with clubbing and/or bronchiectasis	Recurrent pancreatitis
Edema with hypoproteinemia and hypothrombinemia	Esophageal varices and/or hyperplenism	Cholelithiasis
Failure to thrive	Nasal polyps	Chronic abdominal pain and constipation
Salty taste and/or salt loss syndrome		Obstructive apnea
Rectal prolapse		CF-related diabetes
Intestinal obstruction with or without intussusceptions/volvulus		Osteopenia
Recurrent pneumonia/bronchiolitis		Chronic respiratory failure

chronic obstructive airway disease that eventually leads to diffuse, severe bronchiectasis. The earliest pathologic lesions are found in the distal bronchioles. Whether the viscid secretions are primary or are secondary to chronic bacterial infections remain unsettled. In favor of a primary disturbance is the demonstration of mucus obstructing submucosal gland ducts in the airways of neonates with CF, who have not yet developed any evidence of bacterial infection or chronic colonization of the airways. With the use of sophisticated culture methods, bacterial pathogens can almost invariably be isolated from the respiratory tract of patients with CF. The most common pathogens isolated from sputum cultures are *Staphylococcus aureus* and *Pseudomonas aeruginosa*. Less commonly found are *Escherichia coli, Klebsiella*, and *Haemophilus influenzae*. In later stages of the disease, *Pseudomonas* usually predominates. By adulthood, more than 80% of patients are colonized with *P. aeruginosa*. Chronic infection with *P. aeruginosa* elicits an anaerobic milieu within mucus plugs in the CF airway.[10] Using anaerobic culture conditions, large numbers of anaerobes, particularly *Prevotella, Veillonella*, and *Propionibacterium*, were detected in CF sputum but not in induced sputum from healthy volunteers.[11] There is a correlation between *P. aeruginosa*–positive cultures and presence of the anaerobes. Multidrug-resistant organisms (MDROs) are detected in CF sputum cultures with higher prevalence and chronicity apparently associated with acute and chronic administration of antibiotics to suppress *P. aeruginosa*. These pathogens include *Stenotrophomonas maltophilia, Achromobacter xylosoxidans*, and *Burkholderia cepacia complex*. Other opportunistic pathogens including *Aspergillus* and nontuberculous mycobacteria have also been detected more commonly in CF sputum cultures. There is still controversy concerning whether these MDRO are actively contributing to CF lung disease or are commensal pathogens present in bronchiectatic airways.

Neutrophil-dominated lower airway inflammation also plays a primary role in the pathogenesis of the characteristic central bronchiectasis of CF.[12] Bronchoalveolar lavage fluid (BALF) demonstrates increased neutrophils and various cytokines, especially IL-8, even in infants whose BALF is sterile.[13,14]

Typically, respiratory secretions increase when a patient with CF, already chronically colonized with *Pseudomonas,* develops a viral respiratory tract infection. In turn, the increase in secretions leads to a gradual increase in cough and sputum production and then to an exacerbation of the pulmonary disease, usually manifested by increase in respiratory rate; retraction of the chest during inspiration; and diffuse, coarse inspiratory crackles. Leukocytosis is common. The chest radiograph demonstrates worsening hyperinflation. Both peribronchial thickening and nodular or cystic densities are more marked than usual. Pulmonary function tests show a worsening over baseline. Usually, residual volume (RV) increases; forced vital capacity (FVC) and forced expiratory volume in 1 second (FEV_1) decrease; the forced expiratory flow between 25% and 75% of the exhaled vital capacity ($FEF_{25-75\%}$) also decreases. Treatment using antibiotics and chest physiotherapy generally succeed in restoring most indices of pulmonary function to, or almost to, baseline. However, *Pseudomonas* and *Staphylococcus* persist in sputum cultures.

The most attractive hypothesis to account for the pattern of response to treatment is that therapy reduces the number and, probably, virulence of organisms. Despite the virtual return to baseline after an exacerbation, however, the cumulative effect of repeated episodes is progressive bronchiectasis or atelectasis, or a combination of the two, accompanied by a gradual and irreversible decrease in pulmonary function. The striking degree of airway destruction and relative sparing of the pulmonary parenchyma at autopsy are shown in Figure 50-4. A simplified scheme illustrating the evolution of the process is shown in Figure 50-5.

GASTROINTESTINAL TRACT

Although pancreatic function may be either normal or abnormal at birth, it gradually becomes increasingly abnormal in most patients with CF as the pancreatic ducts become progressively obstructed by thick, viscous secretions from the exocrine portion of the organ; pancreatic enzymes that are trapped within the ducts lead to autodestruction of the pancreas. A cycle of destruction and obliteration of the ducts is set into motion, leading to cystic dilatation of ducts proximal to sites of obstruction and fibrosis of the body of the pancreas. In advanced stages of the disease, pancreatic fibrosis sometimes causes obliteration of the islets of Langerhans and, consequently, diabetes. This concept has been challenged by the notion that CFTR may have a direct effect on β-cell dysfunction as, discussed in the next section.

The liver and biliary tract are also affected in CF. Here too, the primary mechanism appears to be obstruction of small intrahepatic bile ducts by abnormally viscid secretions, leading to accumulation of toxic bile acids, depletion of hepatic antioxidants, and subsequent liver injury. CFTR is localized to the apical surface of the bile duct epithelium and not in the hepatocytes. Risk factors for liver disease appear to be male sex, meconium ileus, PiZ heterozygous state, and transforming growth factor-β1 (TGF-β1) polymorphisms. Elevated liver enzymes can be seen intermittently in 40% to 50% of patients with CF. Hepatic steatosis is frequently seen and may be related to malnutrition, essential fatty acid, choline and carnitine deficiency. Focal biliary cirrhosis, multilobular cirrhosis, and portal hypertension are also seen. Some newborn infants with CF develop the *inspissated bile syndrome,* characterized by prolonged obstructive jaundice starting at 2 to 8 weeks of age. The jaundice often clears

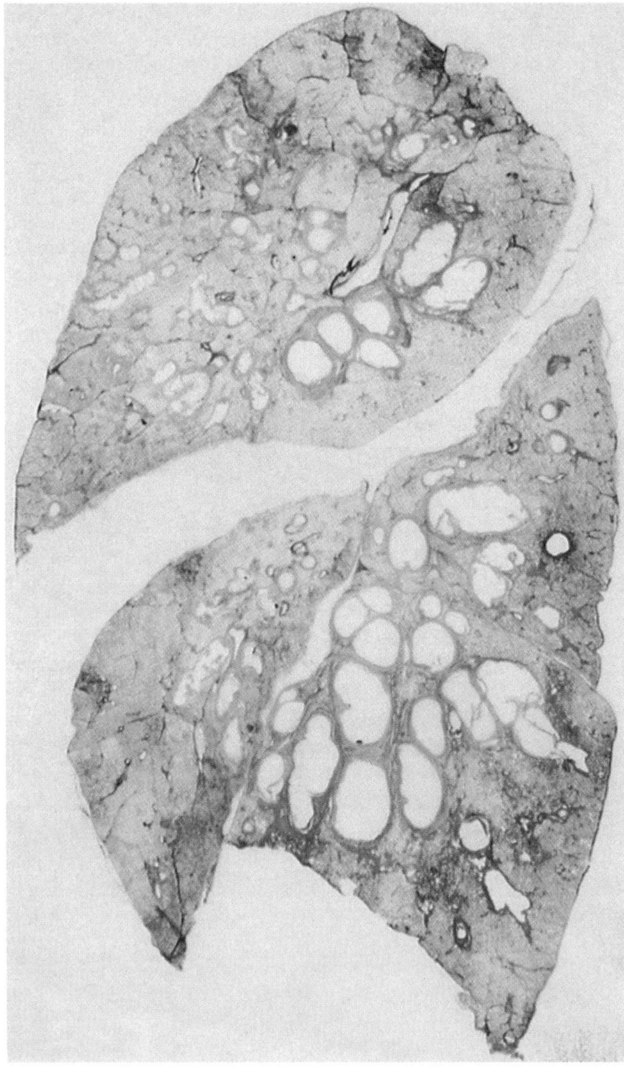

Figure 50-4 Section of lung from autopsy of a patient with CF, demonstrating remarkable dilation of large airways and preservation of intervening pulmonary parenchyma. *(Used with permission of Dr. S. Moolten.)*

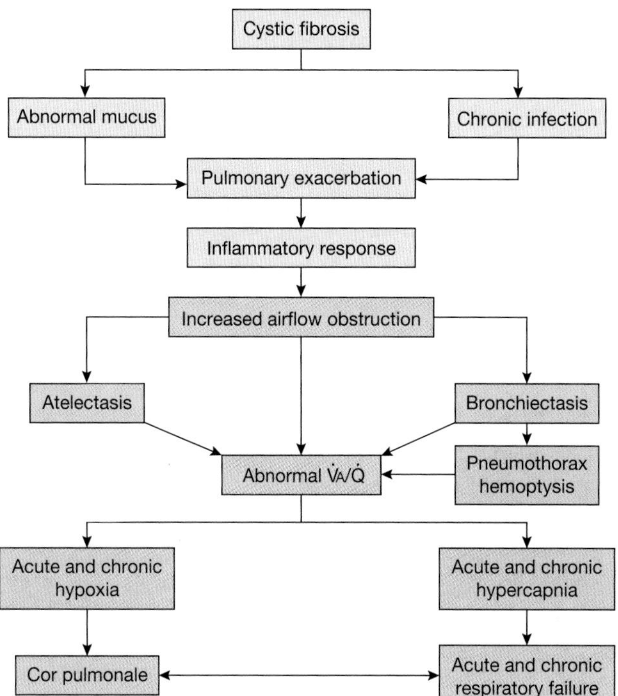

Figure 50-5 Simplified scheme for pathogenesis and progression of pulmonary disease in CF.

without therapy. Gall bladder anomalies may be seen in about 24% to 50% of patients and include microgall bladder, gall stones, and gall bladder dysfunction.[15] The most striking pathologic change in the intestines is hyperplasia of the mucus glands and goblet cells. Biochemical abnormalities in intestinal mucins may contribute to malabsorption of specific nutrients and bile acids. Much of the malabsorption in CF can be corrected by administration of pancreatic enzyme replacement therapy (PERT). However, the abnormal mucins may lead to slowing of intestinal transit time; the slowing, combined with maldigestion of food substances, sometimes causes fecal impaction in the terminal ileum and ileocecal area, a condition referred to as *meconium ileus equivalent* or distal intestinal obstruction syndrome. The fecal impaction, in turn, occasionally causes volvulus or intussusception of the bowel (Fig. 50-6).

■ ENDOCRINE INSUFFICIENCIES

Important CF-associated endocrine disorders are discussed below.

Cystic Fibrosis–Related Diabetes

Diabetes mellitus is a common comorbidity in CF and increases in frequency with increasing age. According to data from University of Minnesota where annual cystic fibrosis–related diabetes (CFRD) screening is recommended for all patients ≥6 years, CFRD affects 2% of children, 19% of adolescents, and 40% to 50% of adults.[16] Similarly, CFRD was found in over a third of 775 patients of age ≥6 years undergoing CFRD screening over a 15-year period.[17]

Underscoring its relevance, CFRD has been associated with decreased survival,[18–24] worse pulmonary function, and lower BMI.[23] Declines in pulmonary function and nutritional status have been observed even prior to the CFRD onset.[22,25] Moreover, less significant glucose impairments are associated with greater declines in nutritional status over the previous year in children[25]; these findings suggest more subtle glucose abnormalities may be clinically relevant in CF. Microvascular complications, such as retinopathy, nephropathy, and neuropathy also occur in CFRD but may be limited to those individuals with fasting hyperglycemia (FH).[17]

Fortunately, early identification and treatment of CFRD appear to curb the impact of CFRD upon survival.[16] Insulin treatment of adults with CFRD without FH improves BMI,[26] and small studies have found insulin treatment improves weight in children even prior to development of CFRD.[27–29]

As described above, CFRD is considered an insulin-deficient state. In fact, delayed and blunted insulin secretion in response to a glucose load or meal prevails even in the setting of "normal" glucose tolerance in CF,[30–32] and these abnormalities progress with worsening glucose intolerance.[30,32,33] This progressive decline in insulin secretion has traditionally been considered a product of "collateral damage" extending from obstructive damage to the exocrine pancreas.

This "bystander" model has been challenged in more recent years. Animal models suggest CFTR may play a direct role in β-cell dysfunction.[34,35] For instance, CFTR knockout ferrets demonstrate glucose abnormalities and insulin secretion defects as newborns.[35] Moreover, the T2DM GWAS-implicated gene, *TCF7L2*, which may contribute to the defective insulin secretion that underlies T2DM, confers an even stronger risk of CFRD. In addition, disturbances in secretion/function of incretins, gut-secreted hormones that potentiate insulin secretion, have been described in CF[36] and in T2DM.[37–40,44–47]

Osteoporosis/Vitamin D Deficiency

Low bone mineral density occurs in as many as 85% of adults with CF. The origin of osteoporosis in CF is multifactorial and is attributed to

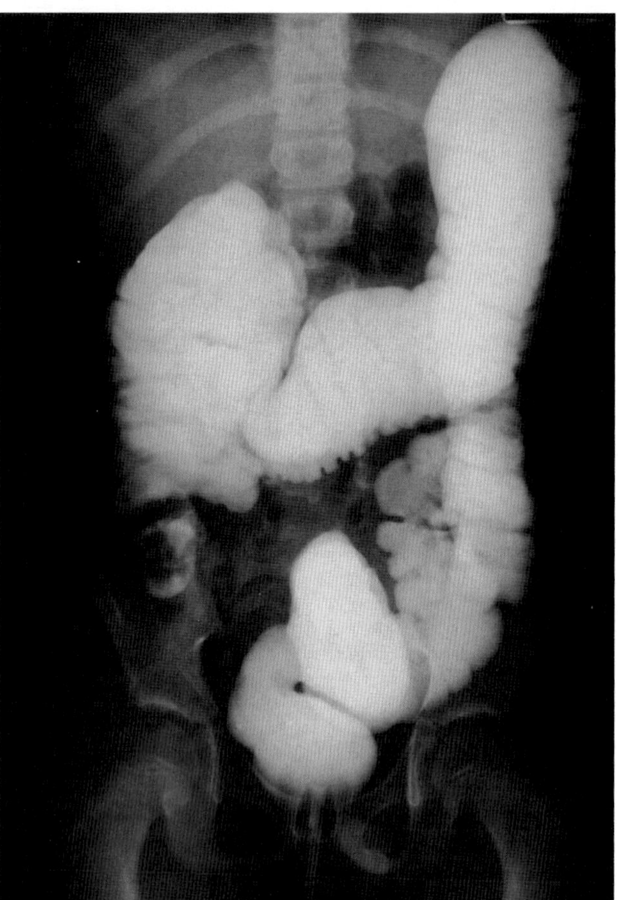

A

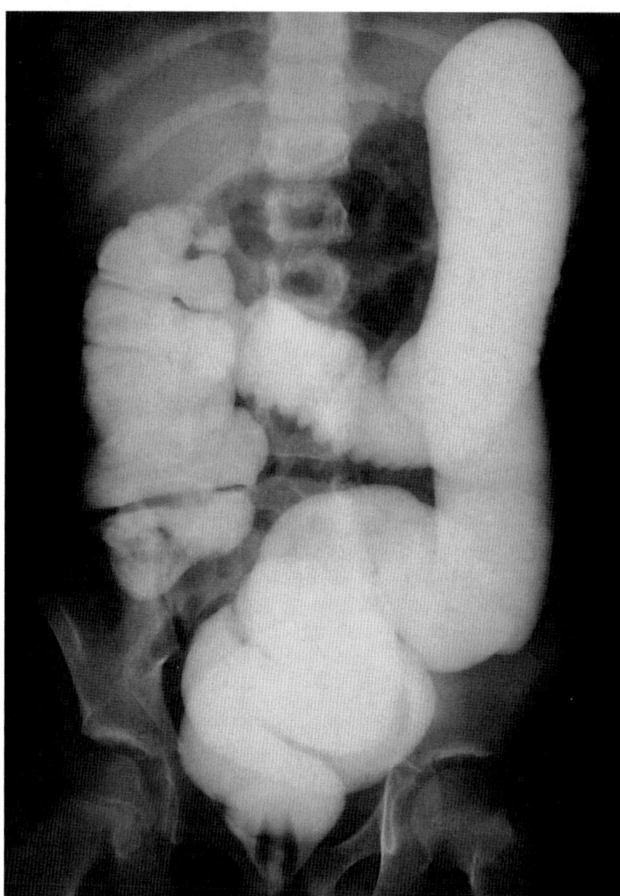

B

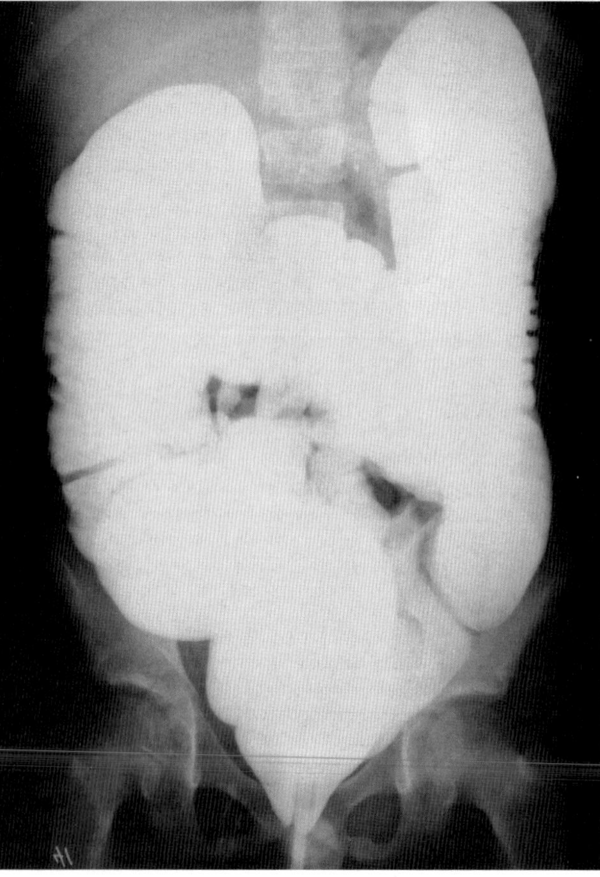

C

Figure 50-6 Distal intestinal obstruction syndrome (DIOS). **A.** Presenting Gastrografin enema of a child who had crampy abdominal pain and a right lower–quadrant mass. Fecal impaction with intussusception is demonstrated. **B.** Partial resolution of the obstruction following Gastrografin administration. **C.** Complete resolution of the intussusception and fecal impaction.

pancreatic insufficiency and malnutrition and poor growth, CFRD, deficiencies in vitamin D, vitamin K, and calcium levels, elevated inflammatory cytokines, pubertal delay, diabetes, and exposure to glucocorticoids.[41] Bone histology in clinically stable CF adults is significant for decreased cancellous bone volume and decreased connectivity.[42] Importantly, the sequelae of low bone density in CF patients include increased risk of vertebral and rib fractures, approximately twice as great as the general population, and increased risk of kyphosis.

■ REPRODUCTIVE ORGANS

Except for an increase in viscosity and an abnormal midcycle ferning pattern in cervical mucus, no consistent pathologic changes occur in the female reproductive tract in patients with CF. In the male reproductive tract, however, the vas deferens is either atretic or absent at birth. Although the pathogenesis of this lesion is not certain, viscous secretions may contribute to obstruction in utero, followed by failure of development of the vas deferens. Spermatogenesis and testicular development are otherwise normal. Because of either partial or complete obstruction of the vas deferens, approximately 98% of males with CF are aspermic.

■ SWEAT GLANDS

The sweat glands of patients with CF manifest no distinctive histologic changes. Nonetheless, their function is abnormal. Micropuncture experiments have shown that the precursor solution secreted by the sweat glands is isotonic to plasma, both in CF patients and in normal subjects. In normal persons, as the sweat flows along the duct of the gland, sodium and chloride are reabsorbed, so that by the time the opening at the skin surface is reached, sweat is hypotonic to plasma with respect to both sodium and chloride concentrations. In CF, the relative impermeability to chloride ions is thought to be responsible for the elevated chloride and sodium concentrations which are the basis for the diagnostic test, the quantitative pilocarpine iontophoresis sweat test, and are also responsible for the characteristic increase in potential differences across isolated, perfused sweat glands from CF patients.

DIAGNOSIS

The diagnosis of CF requires the demonstration of abnormally high concentrations of sodium and chloride in the sweat of a person who has the characteristic history and symptoms of CF. The most prominent clinical features are chronic pulmonary disease and pancreatic insufficiency. The most compelling family history for the diagnosis is CF in a sibling. If the clinical picture and/or the family history support the diagnosis, and if two sweat tests using the quantitative pilocarpine iontophoresis method are clearly positive, the diagnosis of CF can be made with assurance. Identification of two pathologic mutations, in addition to the characteristic clinical picture, is accepted as a criterion for the diagnosis. However, CF is a complex syndrome (Table 50-2) whose clinical manifestations are sometimes subtle. In addition, the family history is not always straightforward. Therefore, a high index of suspicion, coupled with a battery of clinical tests, is sometimes required to establish the diagnosis, especially in adolescents or young adults.

Since CF occurs with a high frequency in the general population, the diagnosis should be considered routinely in a broad array of differential diagnoses. Although Table 50-2 categorizes symptoms according to the age at which they most often occur, symptoms at any age should prompt consideration of the diagnosis of CF.

The most consistent feature of CF is an abnormally high concentration of sodium and chloride in sweat. Measurement of the chloride concentration is recommended for clinical testing. The only reliable sweat test is based on iontophoresis of pilocarpine, followed by quantitative determination of the concentration of chloride in an adequate, measured volume of sweat. Guidelines for the proper performance of a sweat test have been published.[43] In children, concentrations of chloride of less than 40 mEq/L are usually regarded as normal. However, the average of values for sodium and chloride concentrations is about 20 mEq/L for normal subjects and 95 mEq/L for those with CF. In children, values between 40 and 60 mEq/L are traditionally considered borderline elevated; such values call for further evaluation. As a result of recent experience with CF newborn screening, it has been suggested that sweat chloride values above 30 mEq/L may be diagnostic in the first few months of life.

The concentration of sodium and chloride in sweat increases gradually with age. Conditions other than CF in which the concentrations of sodium and chloride in sweat are abnormally high include malnutrition, adrenal insufficiency, hereditary nephrogenic diabetes insipidus, ectodermal dysplasia, and fucosidosis. Except in some instances of malnutrition, these conditions are readily distinguished from CF.[44] The finding of abnormal concentrations of sodium and chloride in sweat should automatically prompt evaluation of the patient to determine if, and to what extent, other organs are affected.

Genetic analysis can be used to confirm the diagnosis of CF. In patients with minimal symptoms, the diagnosis of CF can be made with certainty if two CF-associated alleles are present. As mentioned previously, screening for 32 of the most common alleles yields an overall sensitivity of 90% due to undetected alleles. Therefore, a negative mutation analysis does not rule out a diagnosis of CF, and atypical patients should be followed carefully.

Newborn screening is now standard practice in the United States.[45] The initial stage of screening often uses the neonatal blood spot to determine the concentration of immunoreactive trypsinogen. If this is elevated, secondary screens vary in individual states from repeat immunotrypsinogen determination to F508del or 25 to 32 mutation screen. The screening programs have a sensitivity ranging from 87% to 99%. Risks versus benefits and the relative costs of the screening programs are being evaluated to determine the best approach. Infants with positive newborn screens for CF are referred to CF centers for sweat test confirmation. It has been proposed that infants who have a positive newborn screen, but do not otherwise fulfill the criteria for a diagnosis of CF,[45] should be termed as having "CFTR metabolic syndrome"[46,53] and at a minimum they should be followed in a CF center until their status can be clarified.

CLINICAL EVALUATION

The evaluation of patients with CF includes chest radiography, tests of pulmonary performance, sputum culture, and assessment of pancreatic, endocrine, hepatic, and reproductive functions. Each is described below.

■ PULMONARY ASSESSMENT

Pulmonary assessment includes chest radiography; measurement of pulmonary function, including that of small airways; and evaluation of gas exchange.

Chest Radiography

Rarely is the chest radiograph completely normal in CF. In the person with minor pulmonary symptoms, the manifestations may be questionable (e.g., mild hyperinflation and minimal peribronchial thickening). However, the radiographic findings become more distinctly abnormal as the disease increases in severity. Peribronchial thickening, which is often most prominent in the upper lobes of the lungs early in the course of the disease, usually progresses to affect all lobes. In the advanced stage of pulmonary involvement, ring shadows, cystic lesions, and nodular densities are increasingly apparent, as are areas of bronchiectasis and atelectasis. The central pulmonary artery often enlarges in the middle stages of the disease, but the cardiac silhouette remains within normal limits until the disease is far advanced. The variability in the chest radiograph is illustrated in Figure 50-7 for three siblings with CF when each was 17 years old.

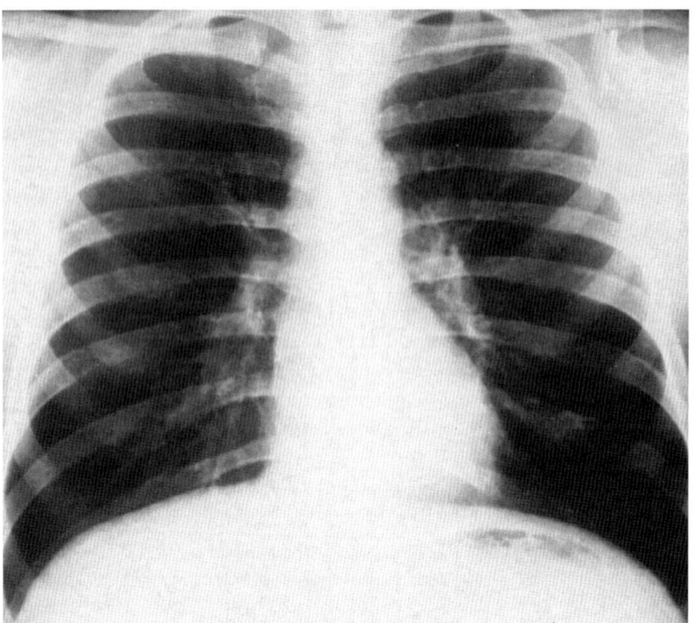

A

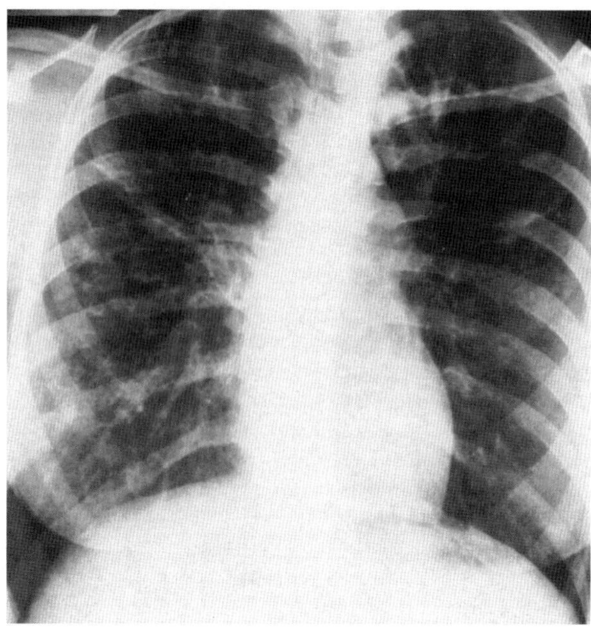

B

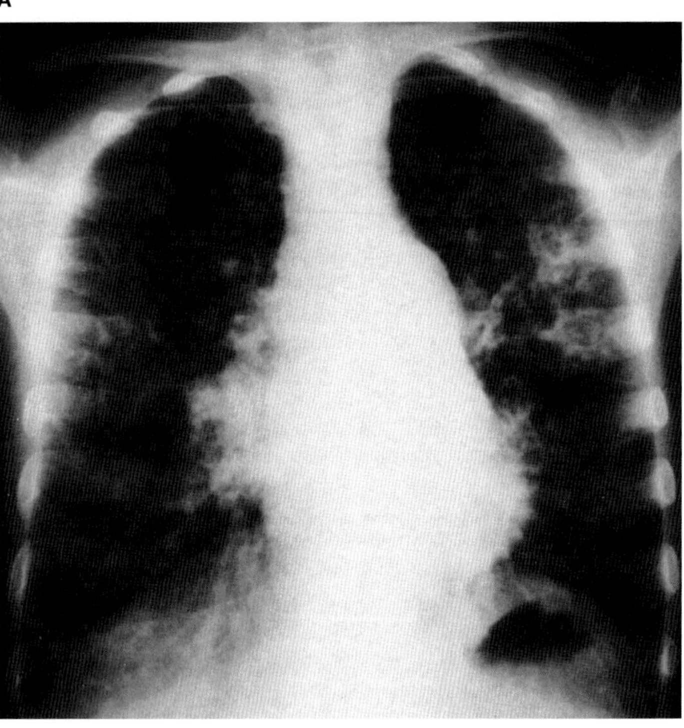

C

Figure 50-7 Chest radiographs of three siblings with CF taken when the patients were 17 years of age. **A.** Mild hyperinflation; otherwise normal. Patient is now 32 years old and has been hospitalized once for treatment of electrolyte depletion. **B.** Diffuse peribronchial thickening, mild hyperinflation, and cystic changes in both upper lobes. The patient was hospitalized seven times for pulmonary exacerbations, once for diabetes, and once for hemoptysis. She died at age 34 following complications from lung transplantation. **C.** Severe hyperinflation, diffuse peribronchial thickening, multiple infiltrates, and increased pulmonary vascular markings and heart size. The patient died 1 month later from respiratory failure complicated by congestive heart failure.

High-resolution computed tomography (HRCT) scans are more sensitive than plain radiographs. The most common abnormalities described are bronchiectasis, peribronchial thickening, mosaic perfusion, air trapping, and mucus plugging.[47] Early bronchiectasis is easily detected on the CT scan, even when routine chest radiographs are normal, as seen in Figure 50-8. CT scan abnormalities may be detected prior to a change in pulmonary function tests. Chest CT scan abnormalities have been detected in asymptomatic newborn infants diagnosed by newborn screening.[48] Currently, there are no standard recommendations for CT use due to the radiation exposure incurred by these studies.

Pulmonary Performance

The lungs of patients with CF are usually morphologically and functionally normal at birth. Over time, accumulation of tracheobronchial secretions and recurrent infections progressively impair pulmonary function in almost all patients. In the fully developed clinical syndrome, all the pulmonary function abnormalities seen in chronic bronchitis, emphysema, and asthma may occur. However, one complicating regular feature of CF – bronchiectasis – modifies pulmonary performance. Chronic, local infection and airway damage increase the compliance of bronchiectatic airways, resulting in airway collapse during rapid expirations or cough. The usefulness of pulmonary function testing in CF is twofold: Tracing the natural history of the disease and assessing the value of therapeutic interventions.

The earliest stages of the pulmonary disorder are the most difficult to quantify. In infants, tests are limited almost entirely to those that do not depend on the patient's understanding and cooperation. A variety of methods to measure infant pulmonary function have been devised; one method, the raised volume rapid thoracoabdominal compression technique, requires sedation of infants but provides values most similar to standard spirometric values, and has detected reduced

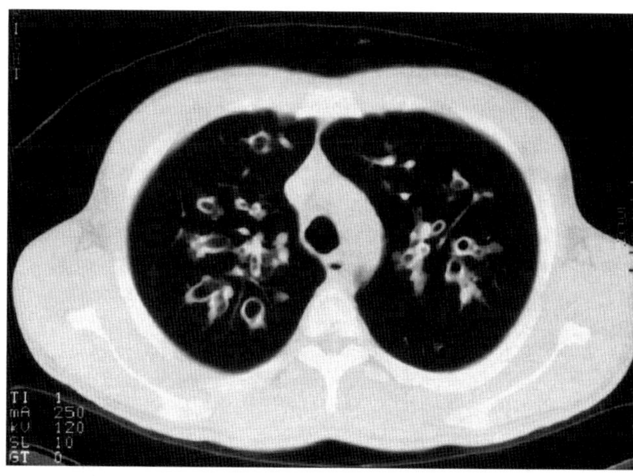

Figure 50-8 High-resolution chest computed tomography scan from a patient with CF. Marked bronchiectasis with peribronchial thickening is shown in the upper lobes.

pulmonary function in infants with CF[49] Nitrogen multiple breath washout or lung clearance index, can be performed in preschool age children and detects early ventilation inhomogeneity that correlates with airflow obstruction by spirometry.[50] After age 6, pulmonary function tests originally designed for adults may be performed quite readily on children. Changes in pulmonary performance throughout the natural history of CF can be described with confidence.

Obstruction in Small Airways

The small airways – that is, the bronchioles – are vulnerable to obstruction early in the course of CF. At this stage, as in cigarette smokers, results of tests for small airway disease are apt to be abnormal, while those of tests for obstruction of large airways are still normal. Three factors interact in causing the obstruction: (1) Intrinsic disease of the smaller airways, often in association with bronchiectasis in the proximal, larger airways; (2) viscid secretions, impaired ciliary action, and impaired cough; and (3) progressive decrease in lung elastic recoil.

The progressive reduction in lung elastic recoil in CF is predominantly a function of overinflation due to intrinsic airway disease, rather than loss of pulmonary parenchyma. This mechanism differs from that in chronic bronchitis and emphysema, in which the combined effects of parenchymal destruction and overinflation are responsible for the decrease in elastic recoil. Emphysema is not a regular feature of CF. In some patients, emphysema occurs only late in the course of the disease (Fig. 50-4).

Airway smooth muscle tone increases only slightly in CF. Exercise elicits bronchodilation, followed shortly thereafter by bronchoconstriction. Both the bronchodilation and bronchoconstriction are far less impressive in CF than in asthma. Indeed, exaggerated bronchomotor responses in CF raise the possibility of superimposed asthma. In distinguishing between contributions to airway obstruction by intrinsic airway disease caused by CF and asthma, maximal expiratory flow–volume curves are sometimes helpful.

Because of the bronchiolar locus of the early lesions in CF, abnormalities in breathing frequency–dependent tests (e.g., dynamic lung compliance), in volume-dependent tests (e.g., closing volume), and in maximal expiratory flow ($\dot{V}E_{max}$) at low lung volumes are demonstrable, even though results of tests of large airway function (e.g., FEV_1 and airway resistance) are still normal.

Change in Lung Volumes

As with chronic bronchitis, emphysema, and asthma, RV in CF increases. Thereafter, an increase in functional residual capacity and, sometimes, in total lung capacity is seen. As CF lung disease progresses, air trapping increases in severity and is manifest as an elevated ratio of RV to total lung capacity. This change decreases the compliance of the lung and increases the work of breathing.

Abnormalities in Gas Exchange

Early in the evolution of the pulmonary abnormalities in CF – that is, when tests of small airway function alone are abnormal – ventilation–perfusion abnormalities usually result in widening of the alveolar–arterial oxygen gradient and an increase in the ratio of dead space to tidal volume (V_D/V_T). These abnormalities portend increasing inhomogeneities in alveolar ventilation and blood flow as the affected child grows to adulthood. The diffusing capacity for carbon monoxide ($D_{L_{CO}}$) is low at rest and does not increase normally during exercise. This observation is difficult to reconcile with the preservation of the gas-exchanging surface of the lungs (in the absence of emphysema) until late in the course of the disease (Fig. 50-4).

As obstructive disease of the airways progresses and exaggerates the imbalances between alveolar ventilation and blood flow, arterial hypoxemia develops; pulmonary hypertension, cor pulmonale, and right ventricular failure follow, in turn. Late in the course of the disease, hypercapnia and respiratory acidosis contribute to the final picture of respiratory failure. At this juncture, the ventilatory response to inhaled CO_2 is depressed. Bouts of infection punctuate the course of the illness; during each episode, pulmonary function deteriorates, but it usually returns toward baseline, except in the preterminal stages of the disorder.

SPUTUM CULTURE

The unique respiratory flora isolated from sputum or oropharyngeal cultures from patients with CF is helpful in establishing the diagnosis and in guiding the antimicrobial therapy for acute exacerbations. In many patients with CF, *P. aeruginosa* and *S. aureus* are found alone, or in combination with other organisms, in the sputum. There is growing evidence of correlations between different organisms and CF lung disease progression. The presence of mucoid *Pseudomonas* is important because acquisition of mucoid *Pseudomonas* predicts more rapid progression of CF lung disease.[51] Similarly, acquisition of methicillin-resistant *S. aureus* is associated with a decline in pulmonary function[52] and worse survival.[53] Infection with *B. cepacia complex* organisms may be aggressive with rapid deterioration of clinical status or may have an indolent course; the presence of mucoid-positive organisms appears to be protective.[54] Chronic antibiotic therapy to suppress *Pseudomonas* has improved clinical outcomes but has also led to a greater number of MDROs identified in sputum, including *S. maltophilia* and *A. xylosoxidans*. Chronic colonization with *S. maltophilia*, induces a serologic response and independently correlates with progression in airflow obstruction.[55]

In addition to bacteria, sputum cultures for detection of molds and nontuberculous mycobacteria are helpful to guide therapy for patients with acute exacerbations unresponsive to antibiotic therapy, or for patients with unexplained progression of lung disease. Allergic bronchopulmonary aspergillosis (ABPA) complicates CF lung disease,[56] and recent evidence suggests that *Aspergillus fumigatus* may also be associated with airway infection or allergy-triggered asthma in the absence of ABPA.[57] The prevalence of nontuberculous mycobacteria ranges from 7% to 24% with the most frequent species identified as *Mycobacterium avium complex* and *Mycobacterium abscessus*.[58]

PANCREATIC FUNCTION

The evaluation of pancreatic function is an important part of establishing the diagnosis of CF, since almost 90% of patients have pancreatic insufficiency. Infants with pancreatic insufficiency due to CF can present with failure to thrive and loose or frequent stools.

However, visual appearance does not always correlate with the degree or presence of fat malabsorption. Currently the diagnosis of pancreatic insufficiency can be made by measuring fecal elastase (FE)-1 levels and assessment of the degree of malabsorption is best accomplished by the determination of the coefficient of fat malabsorption. The FE-1 test is performed on a random single stool sample. It is easy to obtain and in patients with CF, a human enzyme-linked immunosorbent assay (ELISA) for FE has a sensitivity of 98% to 100% and a specificity of 93% to 100%, even while patients are taking pancreatic enzyme supplements.[59] Also available is a polyclonal assay that detects human as well as porcine elastase and should not be used to diagnose pancreatic insufficiency in patients already on pancreatic enzyme supplementation. There is some debate as to the value used for the diagnosis of pancreatic insufficiency.[60] The coefficient of fat absorption is performed by collecting stools for 72 hours while the patient is ingesting a high-fat diet (documented on a 3-day diet record) and analyzing the stool fat content. A malabsorption coefficient of greater than 7% is usually considered abnormal. Patients with CF usually have a malabsorption coefficient around 20% to 30%. The test is not popular with families who find the stool collections very unappealing. Pancreatic stimulation tests are the most accurate measurement of pancreatic function but are invasive, cumbersome, and at this time are not clinically available.

Cystic Fibrosis–Related Diabetes

Because the onset of CFRD is generally insidious, and FH tends to be a late manifestation, annual CFRD screening with an oral glucose tolerance test (OGTT) starting by age 10 is recommended.[61,62] Based upon the fasting, 1-hour, and 2-hour plasma glucose (PG0, PG1, and PG2) during the OGTT, the following glucose tolerance categories are defined.

- Normal glucose tolerance (NGT) = PG1 <200 mg/dL and PG2 <140 mg/dL
- Indeterminate = PG1 ≥200 mg/dL but PG2 <140 mg/dL
- Impaired glucose tolerance (IGT) = PG2 ≥140 and <200 mg/dL
- CFRD = PG2 ≥200 mg/dL
  Without FH = PG0 <126 mg/dL
  With FH = PG0 ≥126 mg/dL

Contrary to what one might expect, isolated impaired fasting glucose (PG0 100–125 mg/dL) is not associated with worse survival, nutritional status, pulmonary function, or progression to CFRD.[63] Over 10 years, FH occurs in 60% of patients with CFRD without FH at baseline.[17] At least in children, increased plasma glucose at 1 hour during the OGTT predicts increased risk of progression to CFRD.[64]

Additional CFRD screening measures include fasting and postprandial glucose measurements during hospitalizations for acute illness.[61,62] Home glucose monitoring should also occur periodically during and after continuous overnight enteral feeds as well as during intercurrent illnesses, intravenous antibiotic therapy, and glucocorticoid treatment.[65] While an elevated hemoglobin A1C (>6.5%) is consistent with CFRD, the HbA1C tends to underestimate overall glucose intolerance in CF patients and is not generally recommended for CFRD screening.

Osteoporosis/Vitamin D Deficiency

Patients with CF are at risk for vitamin D deficiency and osteoporosis. Annual serum 25-hydroxy vitamin D levels should be monitored. In addition, in all adults and children greater than 8 years with risk factors for osteopenia including malnutrition, chronic glucocorticoid use, moderate-to-severe airway obstruction (FEV_1 <50% predicted), or history of fracture or delayed puberty, a DXA scan should be obtained to monitor bone mineral density.[41]

LIVER FUNCTION

Evaluation of liver function (transaminases, bilirubin, gamma glutamyl transferase [GGT]) is an important part of the evaluation of CF. Transient elevations of serum transaminases can be often seen and may be related to intercurrent illnesses and medications. However, these tests can often be relatively normal, even in patients with mild or moderate focal biliary cirrhosis. The prothrombin time is sometimes prolonged, owing to a combination of malabsorption and decreased synthesis of clotting factors by the liver. Obtaining a level of protein induced by vitamin K absence-II (PIVKA-II) to assess vitamin K status can be helpful in these instances. A liver ultrasound with Doppler should be performed in patients with persistently elevated liver function tests. Fatty liver, cirrhosis, splenomegaly, varices, and reversal of portal blood flow can be seen on ultrasound. Occasionally, patients present with bleeding esophageal varices from advanced cirrhosis and an upper endoscopy is helpful diagnostically and therapeutically.

SEMEN ANALYSIS

Occasionally, a man who is found to have aspermia during the course of an evaluation for infertility is found to have CF. In men with CF, a complete semen analysis is part of the evaluation. Azoospermia is found in more than 98% of men with the disorder.

MUTATION ANALYSIS

There are currently over 1900 mutations associated with CF (http://www.genet.sickkids.on.ca/cftr/). A new initiative, The Clinical and Functional TRanslation of CFTR (CFTR2) (www.cftr2.org), funded by NIH, the US CFF, and Sequenom, is a website dedicated to publishing the functional implications of CFTR mutations. Patients homozygous for the most common mutation, F508del have pancreatic insufficiency; patients with CF who have pancreatic insufficiency tend to have a worse prognosis. F508del is one of the major mutations classified as disease causing; other mutations are associated with CF-related disorders, and yet other mutations have no known clinical importance or unknown significance. Several mutations, including R117H, are associated with pancreatic sufficiency and a mild phenotype. Interestingly, the phenotype of R117H is linked to the expression of the polyT and polyTG intronic domains found 5' to exon 9. A T5 polymorphism expressed with R117H results in congenital bilateral absence of the vas deferens (CBAVD) or idiopathic pancreatitis, and may be complicated by mild lung disease. In contrast, R117H associated with T7 or T9 may have no manifestations of CF or CF-related disease.[66]

Certain alleles associated with CF (e.g., 3849+10kbC→T) are associated with nasal polyposis and bronchiectasis but normal sweat test results. The diagnosis of CF can be made with confidence in these patients. More problematic are persons with atypical presentations, normal sweat test results, and at least one CF-associated mutation. More extensive genotyping should be attempted for all patients with a high clinical suspicion for CF (see "Genetics") because mutation analyses will be used to determine eligibility for mutation-specific protein-correcting therapies. For example, therapy for CF patients with the G551D mutation with the CFTR potentiator ivacaftor® results in astonishing improvements in respiratory tract symptoms, weight gain, and shift from positive to borderline sweat chloride values (see "Therapy," "Genetics," and "Future Directions").[67]

Patients with the same genotype may have dramatically different phenotypes, supporting the concept that modifier genes play an important role in determining the CF phenotype. Three large GWAS consortia are collaborating to define modifier genes associated with lung disease severity[68] and with specific disease manifestations such as CFRD,[69] liver disease,[70] and meconium ileus.[71] Investigations using these large well-characterized cohorts recruited by the consortia have identified chromosomal regions of interest but have not yet confirmed gene targets or polymorphisms that confer increased risk of severe lung disease. Using a hypothesis-driven approach, several potential candidate modifier genes for severity of lung disease were identified, including α_1-antitrypsin, HLA antigens, nitric oxide synthase, mannose-binding lectin, TGF-β, tumor necrosis factor-α (TNF-α), and β_2-adrenergic receptor. However, none of these genetic polymorphisms were validated as gene modifiers by GWAS analysis in the combined consortia.

ATYPICAL CLINICAL PRESENTATIONS

Atypical clinical presentations confound the diagnosis of CF in adults; a high index of suspicion is required to establish the diagnosis. Approximately 6% of all CF is diagnosed after age 18. Late presentations of CF tend to occur in persons with pancreatic sufficiency; indeed, overweight or well-nourished persons may have CF. Recovery of unusual gram-negative organisms, mucoid *Pseudomonas* species, or *S. aureus* from sputum of asthmatics with persistent sputum production, chest radiographic abnormalities, or clubbing should prompt referral for sweat testing. Recurrent sinusitis and nasal polyposis may be the only manifestations of CF in a mildly affected person. Isolation of *P. aeruginosa* from deep nasal cultures should raise the suspicion of CF. Frequently, the sinus findings on CT mimic fungal sinusitis, demonstrating concentric, inhomogeneous material. Occasionally, persistent inflammation produces bony destruction that is mistaken for previous surgical intervention. Sweat testing and referral to a CF center should be considered for men with azoospermia or CBAVD. The clinical entity, "CFTR-related disease" has recently been defined by an international working group. CFTR-related disease encompasses patients with evidence of CFTR dysfunction who do not meet the criteria for CF disease (e.g., only one CFTR mutation, a normal sweat test, and single organ involvement). CFTR-related diseases include CBAVD, idiopathic pancreatitis, and diffuse bronchiectasis.[72]

TREATMENT

Intensive, comprehensive CF treatment programs designed to deal with particular symptoms, correct deficiencies, and prevent progression and complications of the disease have led to a dramatic increase in the median age of survival. Although the value of comprehensive treatment is beyond question, far less certain are the utility of each component of the treatment plan and the level of each component necessary in a given patient. At present, the best approach still appears to be determination of the type and degree of abnormality in individual patients and design of a treatment program that will improve or maintain function of the organ systems affected. Two recent reviews highlight the evidence supporting each component of CF therapy.[73,74] To ensure that the treatment regimen meets the needs of the individual patient, that necessary treatment is not omitted, or that side effects of prescribed treatments do not go unnoticed, it is often desirable to hospitalize the patient for diagnosis and evaluation. Hospitalization also provides an excellent opportunity for counseling the patient, parents, and family about the diverse aspects of the diagnosis, treatment, prognosis, and inheritance pattern of CF. Hospitalization provides the opportunity to monitor the response of individual patients to each component of the therapeutic program.

An important aspect of the care of patients with CF is the network of more than 100 CF centers that exist throughout the United States and the larger network throughout the world. CF centers use a team approach to the care of patients. A CF care team usually includes physicians, nurses, respiratory therapists, physical therapists, nutritionists, social workers, and genetic counselors.

MANAGEMENT OF PULMONARY DISEASE

Management of CF-related pulmonary disease focuses on chronic respiratory management and treatment of acute exacerbations.

Chronic Maintenance Therapy

More than 90% of the patients with CF die from respiratory failure or pulmonary complications. The goals of treating the pulmonary disorder in CF are to prevent and treat the complications of airway obstruction and infection. Although management of the pulmonary disorder consists of many components applied in combination,[75] the individual components of therapy are discussed separately below.

Chest Physiotherapy

Almost all treatment programs for CF include a strategy intended to clear pulmonary secretions to prevent complications arising from airway plugging by viscous secretions. Chest physiotherapy – that is, "percussion and postural drainage" – performed regularly, is the most widely prescribed method. In infants and young children, chest physiotherapy is generally performed routinely, twice daily. Percussion and postural drainage technique has been modified to exclude head-down positioning which increased the risk of GE reflux and increased the duration of acute exacerbations of cough in infants.[76] In addition to manual chest percussion and postural drainage, there are several other effective modalities for chest physiotherapy. These alternative measures include the high-frequency chest-wall oscillation (HFCWO) vest; the flutter device, a small pipe-like device that produces an oscillating resistance during a forced expiratory maneuver; the acapella device that produces both positive expiratory pressure (PEP) and an oscillating resistance during forced expiratory maneuver; PEP mask; intrapulmonary percussive ventilation; autogenic drainage and active cycle of breathing; and exercise.[77]

Overall, due to the difficulty in designing unbiased, well-controlled trials with sufficient power to unequivocally distinguish efficacy between treatments, evidence does not exist to demonstrate superiority of one airway clearance mechanism over another. Therefore, the recommendations based on expert opinion are that airway clearance should be initiated in asymptomatic infants because they develop signs of lung disease within the first few months of life, and that patients should be offered and instructed in a variety of methods so that they can select the methods that they deem provides the most subjective benefit.[78] Some form of physiotherapy that is effective in mucus clearance is required daily because without chest physiotherapy, pulmonary function deteriorates.[79] At present, most CF centers recommend that all patients with CF attempt to maintain clearance of pulmonary secretions with a method that is applied regularly (e.g., twice daily). An additional recommendation is that chest physiotherapy be applied more often during an exacerbation of the chronic pulmonary infection. Unfortunately, the recommendation of chest physiotherapy on a regular basis – a time-consuming and often arduous form of treatment – is difficult to implement without considerable support and encouragement from family and health professionals.

Mucolytics and Inhaled Hypertonic Saline

A number of mucolytic agents have been tried over the years. One that has endured is *N*-acetylcysteine. In the test tube, this agent is quite effective in dissolving mucin components and in decreasing the viscosity of sputum from patients with CF.[80–82] Although some centers who have outstanding pulmonary outcomes, have used this agent as a standard part of the chronic regimen as an adjunct to airway clearance therapy in CF, others have been reluctant to use it because of a lack of randomized controlled trials.[83] One CF center which has a track record of outstanding CF outcomes recommended using *N*-acetylcysteine in combination with sodium cromolyn and albuterol (W. Warwick, personal communication). We continue to recommend its use to our CF patients. Interestingly, *N*-acetylcysteine was found to activate CFTR Cl^- conductance in cultured epithelial cells.[84]

In 1994, Pulmozyme, a DNA-cleaving enzyme, was approved for use in patients with CF following a large phase III multicenter trial.[85] More than 900 patients were enrolled for a 6-month period. Three dosing regimens were employed: Placebo, 2.5 mg inhaled once daily, and 2.5 mg inhaled twice daily. The treatment groups showed a 5% improvement in FEV_1 over placebo, as well as a slightly lower relative risk of exacerbation of lower respiratory tract infection after 6 months. There was no difference between the once- and twice-daily treatment groups. A second study revealed that Pulmozyme, inhaled once daily over 96 weeks, maintained pulmonary function and decreased the relative risk of respiratory tract exacerbations in young CF patients with normal FEV_1 (≥85%).[86] Currently, this drug is in fairly widespread use for CF. However, questions regarding patient selection and timing and duration of use of this expensive drug remain unanswered.

Abnormal homeostasis of airway surface fluid results in dehydrated secretions and impaired mucociliary clearance. As a strategy to improve airway surface hydration and airway clearance, inhaled hypertonic therapy was evaluated. Patients with CF, age 6 years and older, inhaled 7% hypertonic saline twice daily following a bronchodilator for 48 weeks; results revealed only a modest improvement in FEV_1, but a significant reduction in the number of pulmonary exacerbations and days lost from school or work.[87] Inhaled 7% hypertonic saline did not decrease the frequency of pulmonary exacerbations in CF infants and children less than 6 years of age,[88] and therefore did not meet the primary outcome for approval as a maintenance therapy in this age group. However, in a subset of infants tested, infant pulmonary function testing revealed an improvement in $FEV_{0.5}$ in the hypertonic saline group suggesting that this therapy may be useful and considered on an individual basis.

Bronchodilators and Anti-Inflammatory Agents

Bronchodilators are often used in treating the pulmonary manifestations of CF. Their use should be individualized. For example, in many patients, bronchospasm that is reversible with bronchodilators at one point in the course of the illness may prove refractory a short time later. Some patients undergo deterioration in pulmonary function following use of bronchodilators. In infants who are audibly wheezing, a bronchodilator can be tried. In older patients, pulmonary function testing provides a more objective and quantitative measure of bronchodilator effectiveness.

Corticosteroids have been used with good results in infants with severe obstructive airway disease that does not respond to antibiotics and bronchodilators and in patients with CF in whom the pulmonary disease is complicated by severe asthma or allergic bronchopulmonary aspergillosis (ABPA). Preliminary observations initially suggested that patients with CF would benefit from long-term administration of alternate-day corticosteroids, based on the presumption that corticosteroids would decrease the airway inflammatory response. However, in a large, placebo-controlled, multicenter trial of alternate-day corticosteroids administered in two dosage regimens (1 mg/kg and 2 mg/kg), the development of many side effects precluded a general recommendation for long-term corticosteroid treatment in CF.[89] Subgroup analysis led to the suggestion that patients with moderately severe obstructive airway disease and those with chronic *Pseudomonas* infection might benefit from treatment for periods of less than 1 year. Beneficial effects were sufficient to prompt further studies of anti-inflammatory agents in CF. A controlled 4-year trial of high doses of ibuprofen in 40 patients with CF showed improvement in the rate of decline of pulmonary function in children.[90] Questions remain whether side effects that might accrue with continued therapy will justify the gains. In concert, these two studies suggest that future development of a lung-specific anti-inflammatory agent with fewer systemic side effects may offer a promising approach.

Antibiotics

Two major innovations using antibiotics have been implemented as part of the regimen of maintenance therapy for CF. First, inhaled therapies have been demonstrated to successfully eradicate initial *Pseudomonas* infection and postpone chronic colonization in three large prospective trials of patients with CF in North America and in Europe.[91–93] Second, chronic inhaled and/or oral antibiotic therapies successfully decrease the progression of lung disease related to chronic *Pseudomonas* infection. In addition to these therapies, it is important to emphasize that person-to-person transmission of *P. aeruginosa* and other opportunistic microbes is another source for chronic colonization. In healthcare facilities for CF patients, contact isolation precautions are recommended.[94]

Chronic airway colonization/infection with *P. aeruginosa* promotes progression of lung disease. Hoiby et al. championed early treatment of *P. aeruginosa*–positive sputum cultures with inhaled colistin and oral ciprofloxacin, even in the absence of symptoms, as a modality to prevent chronic colonization.[95] The EPIC trial[91] tested four randomized regimens: Cycled therapy versus culture-driven therapy; and 28 days of inhaled tobramycin inhalation solution (TIS) in the presence or absence of 14 days of oral ciprofloxacin. Approximately 80% of patients remained free of *P. aeruginosa* for the duration of the study (18 months) with no difference concerning time to first pulmonary exacerbation attributed to regularly cycled therapy or the addition of ciprofloxacin. The ELITE study[92] was an open label randomized study comparing 28 to 56 days of inhaled TIS which revealed approximately 90% eradication at the end of therapy with 66% to 69% of patients having *Pseudomonas*-free cultures at the end of the 27-month study. In addition, a trial comparing inhaled colistin and oral ciprofloxacin to inhaled TIS and oral ciprofloxacin showed no difference between regimens in eradication with approximately 62% to 65% of patients with *Pseudomonas*-free cultures at 6 months.[93] Therefore, although the evidence from these three studies supports antibiotic eradication of new *Pseudomonas* infection, there is no consensus yet for a specific therapeutic regimen.

Another approach that has been advocated is suppression of chronic *Pseudomonas* colonization by alternating monthly cycles of inhaled antibiotics. Inhaled, preservative-free TIS, 300 mg twice daily for 28 days on and 28 days off, improved pulmonary function (FEV_1 increased by 10%) at the end of the third treatment cycle (20 weeks) compared to placebo.[96] Recently, inhaled aztreonam, 75 mg three times per day, was tested in an open label study of cycling monthly regimen for patients with chronic *P. aeruginosa* infection.[97] Patients reported improved symptoms and pulmonary function during on-therapy months with sustained weight gain over the 18-month duration of the study. Currently, prospective clinical trials are evaluating the efficacy of continuous alternating inhaled antibiotics compared to on–off cycling inhaled antibiotics.

Another antibiotic which has been studied as a chronic therapy in CF is azithromycin. Azithromycin, 250 mg or 500 mg thrice weekly, was evaluated in CF patients colonized with *P. aeruginosa*. After 6 months of therapy, patients on azithromycin had a modest improvement in FEV_1 (6.2%), increased weight gain, and decreased rates of pulmonary exacerbations.[98] Although macrolide antibiotics have been reported to have anti-inflammatory properties,[99] there is no direct evidence of azithromycin-induced anti-inflammatory activity in CF. One concern about inhaled tobramycin, inhaled aztreonam, and oral azithromycin as chronic therapies is the risk of bacterial resistance and selection for growth of MDRO. In addition, questions regarding selection of patients and timing and duration of treatment remain unanswered.

CFTR Potentiators and Correctors

The most exciting breakthrough in CF therapies was announced in 2011 with the proof-of-concept demonstration that an oral drug, ivacaftor®, corrected the physiologic impact of a CFTR mutation, G551D. The G551D mutant CFTR protein is expressed at the cell surface but does not conduct chloride or regulate other ion channels. Ivacaftor® was discovered using a high throughput screening approach.[100] In a phase III randomized, placebo-controlled, double-blind trial for CF patients with at least one copy of G551D mutation, ivacaftor®, administered orally, 150 mg twice per day for 48 weeks, increased FEV_1 percent predicted by 10.6%, decreased risk of pulmonary exacerbations by 55%, improved CF quality of life (CFQL) respiratory symptom scores by 8.6 points, decreased sweat chloride values by 48 mmol/L, and was associated with an average 2.7-kg weight gain.[67] Currently, other mutations similar to G551D are being tested as potential ivacaftor® targets. Importantly, other compounds that potentially correct F508del CFTR are being tested. One lead compound, VX-809 has been reported to decrease sweat chloride values in a dose-dependent manner.[101] VX-809 will be combined with ivacaftor® for complementary combined therapy to enhance both processing and functioning of F508del-CFTR in homozygous patients.

Management of Acute Exacerbations of CF Bronchitis

During the past few decades of treatment of CF, antibiotics have proven to be the key element responsible for increased survival. A reasonable approach balances the dangers of overzealous administration of antibiotics against progressive airway damage and bronchiectasis resulting from untreated infection. The approach is based on sputum culture at the time of diagnosis and at regular intervals thereafter.

When signs and symptoms herald an exacerbation of pulmonary infection (i.e., increased cough or sputum production, dyspnea, decreased exercise tolerance, decreased appetite) or new abnormalities on the physical examination (i.e., increased respiratory rate, use of accessory muscles, changes on auscultation of the chest including decreased breath sounds, new crackles or wheezes, weight loss), new abnormalities on the chest radiograph, or a decline in pulmonary function tests, chest physiotherapy is increased and appropriate antibiotics are given orally, or for severe exacerbations, intravenously.

Currently useful agents for treating staphylococcal infections include dicloxacillin, cephalexin, the third-generation penicillin–clavulanic acid combinations, and macrolides. Early in the course of the pulmonary disease, a small fraction of *Pseudomonas* strains may be sensitive to tetracycline, trimethoprim/sulfamethoxazole, or chloramphenicol. Occasionally, even *Pseudomonas* strains considered resistant according to laboratory sensitivity tests apparently respond to these antibiotics. A mechanism that has been proposed to account for this phenomenon is that even though the antibiotic is not bactericidal, it may inhibit either growth of the organism or its production of exotoxin and proteases. Ciprofloxacin, a quinolone derivative that can be given orally, is initially effective against many strains of *Pseudomonas* and has gained widespread use in the outpatient management of CF. A major disadvantage in its use is that resistance often develops after a few courses of treatment.

For treatment of a severe pulmonary exacerbation of CF caused by methicillin-resistant *Staphylococcus*, vancomycin or linezolid are indicated. For *Pseudomonas,* a combination of an aminoglycoside given intravenously and a semisynthetic penicillin is generally used. This combination is presumed to act synergistically on *Pseudomonas*, and the *Pseudomonas* is less likely to become resistant to either antibiotic.

The most popular antibiotic combination currently in use is tobramycin and ceftazidime. To achieve high levels of antibiotics in the airways and in secretions, the aminoglycoside is generally administered in higher doses, 10 mg/kg/d instead of 7.5 mg/kg/d. A recent randomized trial comparing once-daily versus three-times–daily regimens of tobramycin revealed that once-daily IV therapy provided equivalent efficacy with less nephrotoxicity in children.[102] Dosing should be titrated for serum peak levels of 20 to 30 mg/L and trough levels of 1 mg/L or less.

Third-generation penicillins and cephalosporins, piperacillin, and ceftazidime; carbapenems, imipenem and meropenem; and the latest β-lactam, aztreonam, are also quite effective against *Pseudomonas.* When given alone, resistance often develops quickly. Usually, these agents are used in combination with an aminoglycoside. Because the sensitivity and resistance patterns of the *Pseudomonas* often change, various combinations are tried at different times, with clinicians relying on sensitivities from recent isolates to determine which is most effective for the particular strain of *Pseudomonas.* For other resistant gram-negative organisms, such as *B. cepacia, S. maltophilia,* and *Achromobacter xylosoxidans,* other antibiotic combinations are indicated, including ceftazidime, meropenem, ciprofloxacin, minocycline, aztreonam, chloramphenicol, or trimethoprim/sulfamethoxazole.

Staphylococcus, Pseudomonas, and other gram-negative organisms, such as *B. cepacia, A. xylosoxidans,* and *S. maltophilia,* once found in the sputum, are rarely eradicated. However, most other manifestations of an exacerbation of pulmonary disease abate during a 2-week course of antibiotics administered intravenously; for example, the densities seen on the chest radiograph decrease, the white blood cell count decreases, fever and respiratory rate decrease, and pulmonary function test results, which often deteriorate at the start of an exacerbation, return to their previous baseline. Although many patients begin to show improvement after 5 to 7 days, most CF centers continue antibiotics intravenously for at least 2 weeks to decrease the relapse rate and to avoid a decrease in the interval between exacerbations. Indeed, some centers routinely recommend a 3- to 4-week course of intravenous antibiotics to treat an exacerbation of a pulmonary infection. In the occasional-hospitalized patient who experiences a relapse or manifests an increase in symptoms shortly after administration of intravenous antibiotics is stopped, long-term intravenous administration of an aminoglycoside can be continued with use of a heparin lock. This technique may be helpful in allowing the patient to return home while still receiving effective doses of aminoglycosides.

Nutritional Support

Patients with CF should have a detailed nutrition assessment at diagnosis and annually as per the CFF guidelines.[60] Nutritional status should be screened at every visit. Patients are prescribed a high-calorie balanced diet. The CFF recommends that for infants and young children (0–2 years) weight for length be maintained at the 50th percentile and that children and adolescents (2–20 years of age) have their BMI percentile at the 50th percentile. Although it is true that pulmonary function is the predominant factor in determining morbidity and mortality in CF, it is becoming increasingly clear that overall patient status is closely tied to nutritional status. Importantly, achieving and maintaining normal nutritional status is associated with maintenance of lung function in young children and adults. Calorie goals are often 110% to 120% of usual calorie requirements. At these caloric intakes, protein intake is often adequate to meet needs. Patients are encouraged to achieve calorie goals by the ingestion of calorically dense foods. If this is hard to achieve, calorie boosters (vegetable oils, butter, and cheese) are recommended followed by the use of high-calorie supplements (shakes). Calorie needs may be increased in patients with chronic lung disease, malabsorption, and chronic liver disease. Nocturnal nasogastric feeds may be used in the short term for aggressive nutritional rehabilitation, and patients who need long-term support have placement of a gastrostomy tube for ease of care. Typically standard formulas are used but some patients with feeding intolerance and poor weight gain benefit from hydrolyzed formulas. Intravenous or parenteral nutrition is rarely used, but may be required in patients who have had GI surgery.

Pancreatic status (insufficiency or sufficiency) should be determined and monitored as needed. The mainstay in managing the pancreatic insufficiency of CF is PERT which consists of enteric-coated capsules containing amylases, proteases, and lipases. PERT should be ingested before meals that contain protein, fat, or complex carbohydrates. Dosing guidelines have been developed by the CFF. Fibrosing colonopathy or the development of colonic strictures is a complication that appears to be related to high PERT doses exceeding 10,000 lipase units/kg/d and was first noted following the introduction of high-potency pancreatic enzymes.[103] Most patients can be managed with pancreatic enzyme doses within the published guidelines. Patients who require higher pancreatic enzyme doses should be evaluated by a dietitian and a pediatric gastroenterologist.

Patients with pancreatic insufficiency are at risk for fat-soluble vitamin deficiency. Guidelines also exist for vitamin supplementation and CF-specific vitamin products are available.[60] It is recommended that fat-soluble vitamin status be monitored annually and additional supplements (Vitamin D) may be required if levels are still low. It is very unusual for patients with CF to be vitamin A deficient if they are on a CF-specific vitamin preparation. Supplemental salt is needed by patients to prevent salt depletion. Salt is added to infant formula and children and adults are encouraged to salt their foods liberally and to take salt-containing liquids and snacks during hot weather and periods of increased physical activity.

MANAGEMENT OF CYSTIC FIBROSIS–RELATED DIABETES

Insulin is the treatment of choice for CFRD, and ideally the regimen is customized to fit the needs of the individual patient. Combinations of basal (long-acting) and bolus (rapid-acting) insulins are used in the treatment of CFRD with FH. In the absence of FH, premeal rapid-acting insulin is the main treatment approach. Frequent meals, snacking, and "grazing" are not uncommon in CF, and the requirement of multiple daily injections can be prohibitive for some individuals. The insulin pump offers flexibility and can negate the need for frequent injections.[104] Moreover, calories are not restricted in CFRD although either avoidance of foods of low nutritional value (sugared soda or confection) or their consumption in combination with complex carbohydrates, protein, and fats is useful in avoiding excessive hyperglycemia. Pancreatic enzyme replacement also appears to improve meal-related glucose excursion.[36] The role of treatment of prediabetes and early insulin deficiency in preserving pancreatic β-cell function, pulmonary function, and nutritional status has yet to be defined.

NATURAL HISTORY AND PROGNOSIS

A comprehensive treatment program for CF has unequivocally improved overall survival of patients. Fifty years ago, the median survival was only a few years of age. For the 5-year period from 2007 to 2011 the median predicted survival was 36.8 years of age (CF Foundation Patient Registry, 2011 Annual Data Report, Bethesda, MD). However, because CF is a complex disorder that affects different organs to different degrees, it is difficult to describe a "typical course" for a patient with CF. Some patients die in childhood or adolescence, while others survive well beyond age 40.

An important determinant of the natural history of CF is the severity of the pulmonary disease and the rate at which it progresses. Although most patients' condition improves in response to therapy, skillful management does less to influence the course of the severely affected than that of the mildly affected patient.

A variety of scoring systems have been devised for CF. The clinical scoring system devised by Shwachman and Kulczycki and the chest radiograph scoring system devised by Brasfield and associates are widely used. However, although these and more elaborate scoring systems are useful in categorizing patients according to the severity of illness, none has proved useful in prognosticating the course of an individual patient.

Because CF is a genetic disease, the question of a familial pattern of severity is often raised. Figure 50-7 shows chest radiographs of three siblings with CF; the radiographs demonstrate mild, moderate, and severe disease in individuals in the same family. The capsule histories, which are included in the figure legend, also illustrate the variability in courses experienced.

Patients with CF can be categorized not only with respect to severity of illness, but also with regard to survival. For example, more than half of patients with CF who underwent surgery for meconium ileus before 1965 died in the first 2 months of life. Although this situation had improved markedly by 1976, the survival rate for patients with meconium ileus was still not as good as for all other patients with CF. In addition, the survival rate was much lower for females than for males, especially in adolescents. In recent years, differences between the patients in these groups have declined or disappeared. Because of improvements in the collection of mortality statistics, comparison of current data with those from previous years may be somewhat misleading, but 50% survival age has not been increasing as rapidly in recent years as in the 1970s and 1980s. Furthermore, there is a difference in outcomes among individual CF centers.

COMPLICATIONS

The course of CF is often characterized by a gradual decrease in pulmonary function, punctuated by further abrupt declines during exacerbations. Malnutrition, when present despite therapy, usually correlates best with the severity of the pulmonary disease. However, the course of CF may be suddenly altered by certain complications of the disease.

HYPOELECTROLYTEMIA AND METABOLIC ALKALOSIS

Hypoelectrolytemia and metabolic alkalosis are serious complications that are especially apt to occur during periods of hot weather, when losses of sodium and chloride increase. Electrolyte depletion may be life-threatening, especially in infants and young children (Table 50-3). Prompt fluid replacement with isotonic saline is critical.

INTESTINAL OBSTRUCTION

Intestinal obstruction in patients with CF may be related to distal intestinal obstructive syndrome (DIOS), volvulus, intussusception, and adhesions from prior surgery. Acute or chronic crampy abdominal pain can be seen in patients with CF with pancreatic insufficiency and pancreatic sufficiency. This is most often due to DIOS which is related to intestinal dysmotility, poor hydration of intestinal contents, and malabsorption. Typically the pain is in the right lower quadrant of the abdomen and is related to a buildup of stool in the terminal ileum, cecum, and ascending colon. Treatment consists of adequate fluid and electrolyte intake, use of polyethylene glycol solutions, and treatment of malabsorption. If the obstruction is incomplete and manifested solely by a tender right lower–quadrant mass, then the above-described measures are used. Nasogastric infusion of polyethylene glycol solutions is also used successfully in the hospitalized patient. If these measures are unsuccessful or the patient has an obstruction, then hyperosmolar contrast enemas are administered by a radiologist

TABLE 50-3 Hypoelectrolytemia and Metabolic Alkalosis in Two Cystic Fibrosis Patients

	Serum Electrolytes, mEq/L				
Patient	Na	K	Cl	CO_2	Serum pH
No. 1	123	2.2	49	48	7.60
No. 2	125	2.4	55	41	7.63

Source: Modified with permission from Scanlin TF. Cystic fibrosis, in Fleisher G, Ludwig S (eds). Textbook of Pediatric Emergency Medicine. Baltimore: Williams & Wilkins; 1983.

after hospitalization is required. It is important that patients are well hydrated, that the terminal ileum is cleared of stool and that an abdominal x-ray is performed to document clearance of stool prior to the patient being discharged from the hospital. Adherent stool/mucus may serve as the leading edge for a volvulus or intussusception (Fig. 50-6) and surgical consultation may be required. Careful pre- and postoperative management is essential to avoid the deterioration in pulmonary function that may follow the use of anesthesia.

LIVER DISEASE

Liver disease is often asymptomatic and can be detected by evaluation of liver function tests on routine yearly studies. Assessment of liver status (synthetic function) and anatomy (abdominal ultrasound with Doppler) are important in the diagnosis of cirrhosis and portal hypertension. Only a small percentage of patients with significant liver disease will need liver transplantations unlike other chronic liver diseases seen in children. Liver biopsy is recommended in patients in whom an etiology other than CF liver disease needs to be established.[105] It is recommended that other causes of liver disease be ruled out and that patients receive hepatitis A and B immunizations. There is a paucity of data to support the routine use of ursodeoxycholic acid in patients with CF-related liver disease. However, this medication is often used in doses of 10 to 20 mg/kg/d as a choleretic agent to improve bile flow.[59] Persistent hepatomegaly or splenomegaly, or complications of portal hypertension establish significant liver involvement. Patients may develop esophageal varices as a result of portal hypertension and present with upper gastrointestinal bleeding. Once bleeding has been identified as due to varices and hemoptysis has been excluded, therapeutic endoscopy (sclerotherapy or band ligation) is required. For patients with complications of portal hypertension, transjugular intrahepatic portosystemic shunting or surgical portosystemic shunts can effectively decompress esophageal varices by decreasing portal pressure as a bridge to liver transplantation.

Liver transplantation is another option for many patients with CF who have end-stage liver disease. Indications include significant synthetic dysfunction, unresponsive or recurrent esophageal varices with recurrent upper GI bleeding, ascites, and encephalopathy. Patients need to be evaluated by a hepatologist. Ideal candidates are those with an FEV_1 of at least 50% of predicted. Colonization with a multidrug-resistant or panresistant strain of *Pseudomonas* is a relative contraindication to transplantation. In patients in whom poor pulmonary function or drug-resistant pulmonary infection is an issue, double organ (liver and lung) transplantation may be considered. Despite concerns about worsening airway infection during transplant-associated immunosuppression, liver transplantation in patients with CF does not worsen their pulmonary status.[106]

ATELECTASIS

Atelectasis of a lung segment or lobe sometimes occurs in CF. Acute atelectasis is generally associated with few symptoms (Fig. 50-9A). If it is untreated, however, the end result of atelectasis is a severely bronchiectatic segment or lobe (Fig. 50-9B). Vigorous chest physiotherapy, in conjunction with antibiotics, is often successful in reexpanding the affected lung region. Bronchoscopy is occasionally helpful. As a rule, however, bronchoscopy is no more effective than chest physiotherapy and pulmonary pharmacotherapy. Resection of a persistently atelectatic or bronchiectatic lobe is undertaken only when the remaining areas of the lung are in relatively good condition, overall pulmonary function is good, and the evidence convincing that the affected segment is responsible for intolerable symptoms (fever, cough, or sputum production).

PNEUMOTHORAX

Recurrent pneumothorax is common in CF, particularly in older patients (Fig. 50-9C). Tension pneumothorax occurs in up to 30% of patients with CF who develop pneumothorax. Tube thoracostomy is indicated when the pneumothorax occupies more than 10% of the area of the hemithorax seen on the posteroanterior chest radiograph. Because the frequency of recurrence of pneumothorax is high, attempts are often made at the time of the initial event to achieve chemical or surgical pleurodesis. Surgical pleurodesis is more effective at preventing recurrence of a pneumothorax and is no longer considered a contraindication to lung transplantation.

HEMOPTYSIS

Expectoration of a small amount of blood-streaked sputum is a fairly common occurrence in CF and is generally managed by intensifying home therapy for pulmonary infection. In contrast, hemoptysis (the expectoration of at least 30–60 mL of fresh blood) requires hospitalization, even with a chest radiograph that is virtually unchanged (Fig. 50-9D). The probable mechanism underlying most instances of hemoptysis in CF is the erosion of an area of localized infection into a bronchial vessel. Massive hemoptysis (blood loss of 240 mL) is uncommon in CF. However, it represents a potentially life-threatening situation. Bronchoscopy, and sometimes thoracic surgery, may be required to control the hemorrhage. Bronchial artery embolization has been used successfully in patients with CF and is now the treatment of choice when a physician experienced in the procedure is available.[107]

INFECTION WITH UNUSUAL ORGANISMS

CF produces central bronchiectasis, even though the disease initially is in the small bronchioles. Bronchiectatic airways are frequently colonized with unusual organisms, including *Aspergillus* and atypical mycobacteria. As is the case with pathogenic bacteria, eradication of these organisms from the airways is virtually impossible. The focus of therapy is directed toward verifying that the organisms are resulting in worsening of the disease and controlling the infection, rather than effecting a microbiologic cure.

Mycobacteria

The prevalence of infection with atypical mycobacteria in CF mandates surveillance for these organisms in sputum cultures at least annually.[108] When atypical mycobacteria are cultured, antimicrobial sensitivities should be obtained. A decision about therapy for isolation of atypical mycobacteria is based on the likelihood that the organism is contributing to airway infection and a decline in pulmonary function. Isolation of the same organism on several occasions, positive smears, presence of progressive chest radiographic changes, further decline in pulmonary status despite vigorous antipseudomonal (or antistaphylococcal) therapy, persistent night sweats, and fever are clinical clues that the atypical mycobacteria are contributing to disease. Demonstration of tissue infection with transbronchial lung biopsy is rarely recommended. A clinical database has been established by the CF Foundation to track results of treatment for atypical mycobacterial infections in patients with CF. The current standard for therapy is treatment with several antimicrobials for synergy and to prevent development of resistance.

Aspergillus

In an analogous fashion, molds, especially *Aspergillus,* are occasionally isolated from patients with CF. Approximately 5% to 15% of patients have ABPA. The diagnosis of ABPA in CF is difficult because of overlapping symptoms between the two disorders. Diagnostic criteria for ABPA are (1) reversible airway obstruction, (2) proximal bronchiectasis, (3) history of pulmonary infiltrates, (4) skin test positivity to aspergillus antigens, (5) precipitating serum antibodies to *A. fumigatus,* (6) elevated total serum immunoglobulin E (IgE), (7) elevated specific serum IgE and serum immunoglobin G (IgG) to *Aspergillus,* and (8) peripheral eosinophilia. A negative skin test for *Aspergillus* effectively rules out the diagnosis of ABPA. During the

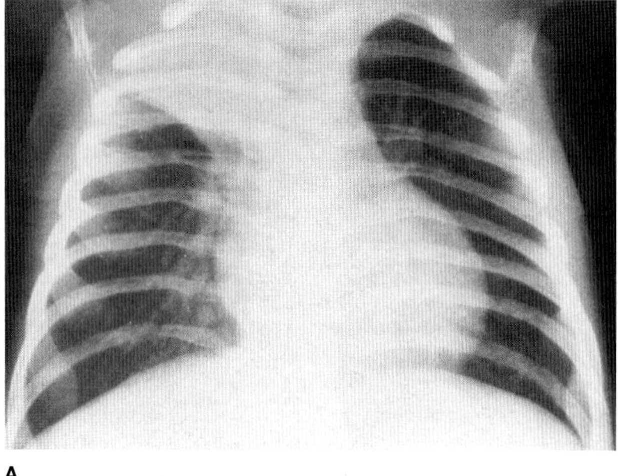
A

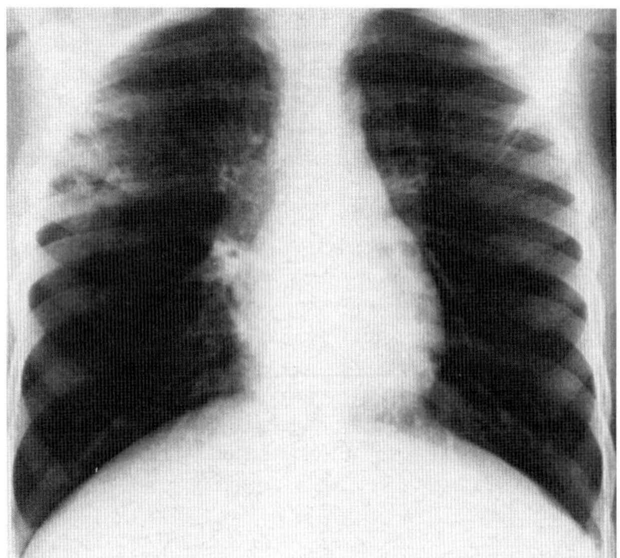
B

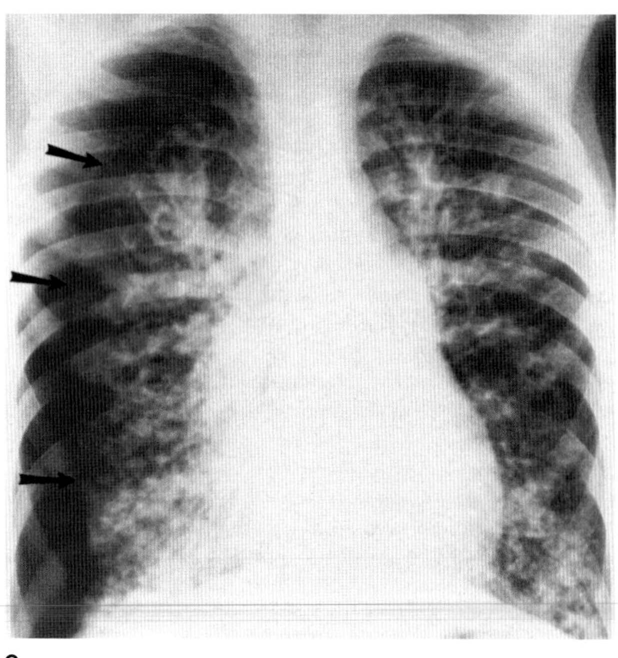
C

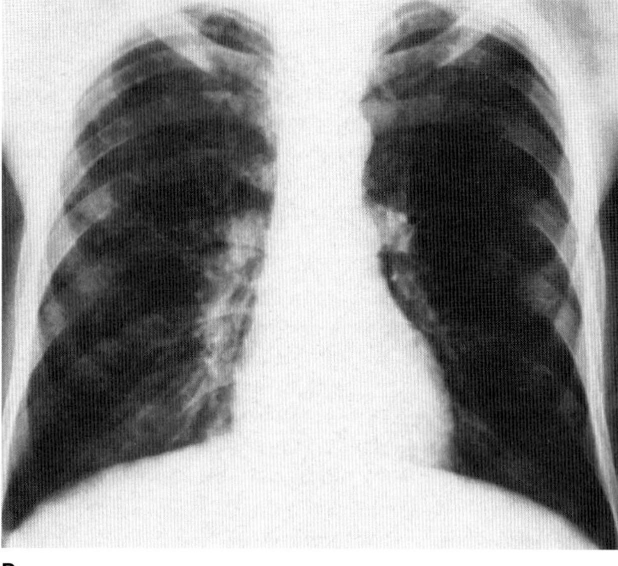
D

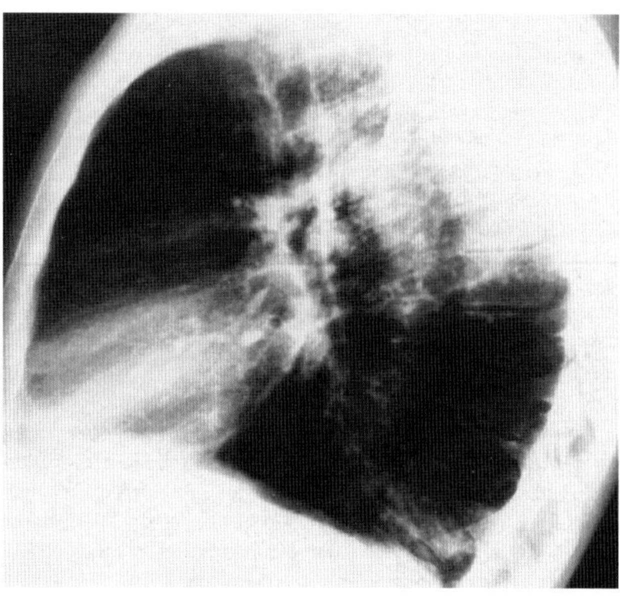
E

Figure 50-9 Chest radiographs of patients with pulmonary complications of CF. **A.** Atelectasis of the right upper lobe in a 4-month-old boy. The atelectasis resolved with antibiotics and chest physiotherapy. **B.** The same patient at 9 years of age with mild hyperinflation, central bronchiectasis, resolving right upper lobe infiltrate. The diagnosis of allergic bronchopulmonary aspergillosis was made, and the patient improved after treatment with prednisone. **C.** Pneumothorax of the right lung *(arrows)* in a 13-year-old boy. The pneumothorax resolved after tube thoracostomy and tetracycline sclerosis. The patient died 3 years later from respiratory failure with congestive heart failure. There were no recurrences of the pneumothorax. **D, E.** A 43-year-old man showing hyperinflation and diffuse peribronchial thickening. The radiograph was taken during an episode of significant hemoptysis, and no acute changes were seen on the radiograph.

active phase of ABPA, elevations in total IgE and eosinophil count are seen. Rises in *Aspergillus*-specific titers (IgE and IgG) are more specific for ABPA than are serum precipitins. ABPA in patients with CF is treated with corticosteroids and itraconazole. The level of total IgE is used to follow the activity of the disease.

Gram-Negative Bacteria

In the late 1970s and early 1980s, the importance of *B. cepacia* (formerly *Pseudomonas cepacia* [PC]) was recognized. *B. cepacia* is a gram-negative, oxidase-positive rod that is uniformly resistant to polymyxin and, frequently, panresistant. Isolation of *B. cepacia* requires plating on special oxidative fermentive polymyxin B bacitracin lactose (OFPBL) or PC agar plates to retard growth of other gram-negative rods and enhance growth of *B. cepacia.* The plates must be maintained for a minimum of 4 days. *B. cepacia* colonization has been associated with septicemia, which is very rarely seen with *P. aeruginosa.* The clinical course after acquisition of *B. cepacia* may be fulminant, with death occurring in a matter of months. However, most patients' disease follows a more benign course. Carefully controlled epidemiologic studies are needed to better define risk factors and to establish the true virulence of *B. cepacia.* Experimental evidence exists that at least one strain of *B. cepacia* may be transmitted in an epidemic fashion. The combination of a poor clinical course after acquisition of *B. cepacia* and the evidence supporting epidemic transmission has led to cohorting or isolation of patients with CF infected with *B. cepacia,* as recommended by the CF Foundation and the Centers for Disease Control (CDC).

In addition to being colonized with *Pseudomonas* and *Burkholderia* species, patients with CF may be colonized with other gram-negative, oxidase-positive organisms, such as *S. maltophilia, Pseudomonas oryzihabitans,* and *A. xylosoxidans.* These are pathogenic organisms, similar in importance to *P. aeruginosa.* Antibiotic therapy should be directed toward these bacteria when they are isolated from the patient with CF who is experiencing an acute exacerbation. The prolonged, prophylactic, aggressive use of antibiotics in CF has led to emergence of resistant organisms. A multiply resistant *Pseudomonas* is an organism that is resistant to all agents in at least two different classes of antibiotics. Resistance to oral fluoroquinolones occurs after about 3 weeks of therapy; if the agent is withheld, the organism occasionally becomes sensitive again.

RESPIRATORY FAILURE

As the pulmonary disease of CF progresses and the degree of hypoxia increases, patients are at risk to develop pulmonary hypertension and cor pulmonale. An increase in hypoxia often occurs during exacerbations of the pulmonary disease. During the acute episode, antibiotic treatment for the underlying pulmonary disorder is intensified and supplemental oxygen is added. Expectant monitoring and aggressive treatment of nocturnal hypoxemia (maintaining Sa_{O_2} ≥95%) prevent the onset of cor pulmonale. When respiratory failure develops in CF, that is, hypercarbia (Pa_{CO_2} at least 55 mm Hg) in addition to hypoxemia, management becomes extremely difficult. Noninvasive mechanical ventilation using bilevel positive airway pressure has been used successfully in patients with end-stage CF awaiting lung transplant; it improved oxygenation, reduced respiratory rate, and was successfully transitioned to home nocturnal use.

Mechanical ventilation is generally instituted when an acute episode, such as viral pneumonia or status asthmaticus, thrusts the patient into acute respiratory failure. This approach is particularly indicated in the patient who has had good pulmonary function before the acute episode. Mechanical ventilation is less apt to be successful if the patient has previously experienced a bout of respiratory failure. When respiratory failure marks the end of a chronic course of progressive pulmonary insufficiency despite adequate medical therapy, mechanical ventilation is usually unhelpful. None of the indications or contraindications for mechanical ventilation is absolute; however, and the clinical outcome depends, to a large extent, on the availability of a dedicated and skilled intensive care team experienced in caring for patients with CF.

COMPLICATIONS RELATED TO LUNG TRANSPLANTATION

Lung transplantation has emerged as an option for patients with end-stage CF.[109] Despite initial concerns about immunosuppression in patients with suppurative lung disease, the outcome for those with CF who undergo lung transplantation is among the best reported for this procedure. Timing for lung transplantation has changed with the adoption of a Lung Allocation Score (LAS) which takes into consideration parameters to predict 1-year survival, with a transplant versus without a transplant, and medical urgency. The impact of this organ allocation system is a dramatic decrease in the number of patients on the waiting list for transplantation and a significant shortening of wait times for transplantation.

One major complication postlung transplantation for CF patients is the risk of infection due to resistant organisms. Colonization with *B. cepacia complex*, or rapidly growing mycobacteria such as *M. abscessus*, has been reported to negatively impact survival.[110] *Aspergillus* may cause invasive infections in the parenchyma or the anastomosis site. Other complications, not specific to CF patients, include acute and chronic graft rejection. Acute graft rejection is associated with a humoral immune response to donor HLA antigens and complement activation.[111] Importantly, acute graft rejection is a negative prognostic factor for chronic graft rejection. Chronic allograft rejection is characterized by obliterative bronchiolitis following transplantation. Obliterative bronchiolitis is a progressive occlusion of the bronchiolar lumina by inflammatory cells and submucosal fibrosis. Transient improvement in airflow is seen following augmentation of immunosuppression. About 50% of transplant patients develop obliterative bronchiolitis after the second year following the procedure. The disease pursues a relentless downhill course, with a median survival of about 2 years following the initial diagnosis.

The poor prognosis associated with obliterative bronchiolitis has several important implications for patient selection and timing of referral for transplantation. First, the main reason for seeking lung transplant is to improve the quality of life, rather than to improve survival. Second, the timing of referral for lung transplantation needs to be calculated to optimize the candidate's fitness for transplant yet delay transplant until absolutely necessary considering the risk of developing obliterative bronchiolitis.

Results from clinical studies may aid with proper timing of referral for lung transplantation in CF. CF patients with severe airflow obstruction as indicated by FEV_1 less than 30% of predicted have a 50% 2-year mortality. Other important clinical parameters useful in determining the timing of transplantation are the presence of hypoxemia (Pa_{O_2} under 55) and hypercarbia (Pa_{CO_2} above 50). Of interest, in both single and multivariate analyses, female gender is associated with an increased relative risk, suggesting that for female patients, referral for lung transplantation should be considered at an even earlier stage.

Because CF is a multisystem disorder, both management and proper selection of patients are more complicated than for other diseases managed with lung transplantation. Among the most difficult challenges presented by patients with CF before transplantation is the microbiology of their lower airways. As discussed previously, colonization with multidrug-resistant *B. cepacia*, specifically the genotype, genomovar III, has been associated with a poor clinical outcome. For poorly understood reasons, patients with CF metabolize drugs differently from those without CF, complicating the dosing of medications, including cyclosporine. The difficulties in achieving an optimal drug dose may be related to malabsorption or enhanced excretion of the drug. Nutritional issues also complicate the posttransplantation management of patients with CF. About

50% of all patients with CF over 30 years of age are overtly diabetic, and administration of corticosteroids induces diabetes in another 10%. Maintenance of proper nutrition is important in CF, especially for rapid postoperative recovery. Finally, gastroesophageal reflux may negatively impact pulmonary outcomes following transplantation. Despite all the special challenges to successful lung transplantation posed by patients with CF, their actuarial survival is quite good. The median survival is 7.1 years, reinforcing the tenet that lung transplantation is done principally to improve quality of life.

PSYCHOSOCIAL ISSUES

A number of psychosocial issues are important in the management of patients with CF. Special circumstances should be recognized for adults with the disorder.

■ GENERAL

Careful attention to the emotional, social, and financial well-being of the patient with CF and his or her family has considerable value in favorably influencing the course of the disease. At the time of diagnosis, it is important to strike an optimistic note while educating the patient about the illness and its management. As part of the early encounter with the patient, the importance of identifying and reinforcing the emotional and financial strengths of the family, as well as weaknesses that will need buttressing, should be recognized. Medical care for CF patients is costly, especially if hospital admissions are required. Many states have programs for children with disabilities that provide support for patients and families. Several states have also established special programs for adults with CF.

As the disease runs its course, counseling and feedback about disease progression are essential. As the patient and family go about setting educational, career, and family goals, they need guidance in realistic planning. It is vital that the physician develop and maintain a positive attitude. The patient who gives up hope is liable to undergo rapid deterioration. Conversely, even patients with severe pulmonary disease can continue to function well and be productive. At the stage when medical therapy is of no further avail, however, the patient and family require considerable emotional support to accept the inevitable. In recent years, many CF centers have allowed patients to die at home, rather than in the hospital. The family requires specific instructions about how to provide physical and emotional comfort for the patient in the home. Usually, home visits by some members of the CF team are required. Not all families have the strength or resources to care for the patient dying at home.

■ SPECIAL CONSIDERATIONS IN ADULT PATIENTS

In the 5-year period spanning 2007 to 2011, the median life expectancy for patients with CF was about 37 years (CF Foundation Patient Registry, 2011 Annual Data Report, Bethesda, MD). Managing a chronic illness becomes more complicated when patients must also begin to manage their independence and make life decisions regarding education, marriage, children, careers, insurance, and self-care. Intense support for both patients and their families is required. Patients with a relatively mild clinical course of disease form healthy and satisfying relationships in a manner similar to that of their healthy, age-matched peers. With advanced disease, patients with CF have more difficulty in forming intimate relationships. Disturbances in body image, decreased mobility, and lack of opportunity to meet suitable partners are cited as reasons for the decreased ability to form intimate relationships in the severely affected young adult with CF.

The adult patient with CF faces unique problems with self-care. Families of patients with CF provide a tremendous amount of care that is expensive and time-consuming to replace for the independently living adult. When the disease flares, patients must "step up" their level of care at precisely the time when they are least able to do so. Judicious use of hospitalization and home care must be provided if the patient is to recover. The trend toward home management of a pulmonary exacerbation using intravenous antibiotics alone ignores the obvious contributions of nutrition, airway clearance, and rest toward resolution of the problem.

REPRODUCTIVE ISSUES

More than 98% of male patients with CF are sterile, secondary to bilateral absence of the vas deferens. Microsurgical epididymal sperm aspiration (MESA), coupled with in vitro fertilization, has been successful in producing pregnancies in a few carefully selected patients. Not all males with CF are sterile, however. In addition to counseling, these men should be offered semen analysis.

Pregnancy for women with CF is increasingly common, and several important issues remain unsolved. In 2004, 191 women with CF were pregnant (CF Foundation Patient Registry, 2004 Annual Data Report, Bethesda, MD). This stands in marked contrast to the total of 13 pregnancies in 10 patients recorded from 1960 to 1966 (data from the 1994 CF Foundation Data Registry).

Maternal clinical status before pregnancy is the most important prognostic factor of maternal outcome. In a study of 25 women with 38 pregnancies, no significant difference was seen between pre- and postgravid gas exchange or nutritional status. A small, but statistically significant, decline in spirometry was noted. However, the decline was not outside the range of expected decline for the natural progression of the disease. More severely affected women suffered an irreversible decline in clinical status during pregnancy. Without an appropriately matched control group of nongravid women with CF, it was not possible to determine whether pregnancy per se was responsible for the decline or whether the decline is a reflection of the natural history of the disease. Comparison of matched groups of pregnant and nonpregnant and CF women from a registry suggested that there was no difference in the rate of decline between these groups. However, the pregnant women received a greater number of therapies and more intense monitoring of their health.[112]

Recommendations about pregnancy for women who are either mildly affected or severely affected is straightforward. For the woman with moderately compromised pulmonary status (i.e., FVC under 50%–60% of predicted), an overall assessment of the clinical situation is recommended, although no firm guidelines can be given. Increased incidence of fetal prematurity is noted in women with a pregravid FVC below 50% of predicted, lending additional weight against recommending pregnancy to women with moderate-to-severe airflow obstruction. In any woman with CF who is contemplating pregnancy, thorough evaluation and treatment of nutritional deficiencies and pulmonary exacerbations are required. Frequent use of antibiotics is unavoidable, and the teratogenic risk of many antibiotics is unknown. Despite this theoretical risk, good maternal and fetal health depends on aggressive management of pulmonary exacerbations, including use of antibiotics. Management of the gravid patient with CF is best accomplished in a CF center that has a program in high-risk obstetrics. A European consensus panel has published detailed guidelines for the management of pregnancy in women with CF.[113]

For men with CF who opt for MESA and for women with CF who are contemplating pregnancy, all offspring are obligate heterozygotes for CF. These offspring need to be counseled that their risk of having a child with CF is about 1 in 50 if the genotype of the spouse is not known. Although genetic testing of children from affected parents is not recommended, they should receive genetic counseling on reaching adolescence. Parents with CF also need to consider the ethical issues of a premature parental death and its effect on the family. If the spouse of an individual with CF is a known carrier of a CF mutation, the availability of in vitro fertilization with preimplantation genetic testing provides a method to avoid having a child who is affected with CF.

Discovery of the CF gene in 1989 led to the hope that prenatal diagnosis might eventually decrease the incidence of the disease. There is a suggestion that this may in fact be occurring.[114]

FUTURE DIRECTIONS

To further enhance survival in CF, physicians must look into insights gained from basic research. Although much work needs to be done, much has already been accomplished, warranting a realistic expectation that major breakthroughs will soon occur in the treatment of the disorder.

Progress toward cure of CF will require a multidisciplinary approach. Management of the lung disease in CF will probably be based on combined methods. However, the momentum gained from recent improvements in our understanding of the molecular details of CFTR structure and function provides a basis for realistic optimism that specific therapy will result in better outcomes for patients with CF. As described above, specific single molecule therapy has already become a reality for CF patients who have the G551D mutation. A phase III trial of the combination of two small molecules for the most common CF mutation, F508del, is underway. Newer compounds that are based on a better understanding of the structure and function of CFTR[115–117] are already progressing from the bench to bedside.

REFERENCES

1. Riordan JR, Rommens JM, Kerem B, et al. Identification of the cystic fibrosis gene: cloning and characterization of complementary DNA. *Science.* 1989;245:1066–1073; erratum 1437.
2. Rommens JM, Iannuzzi MC, Kerem B, et al. Identification of the cystic fibrosis gene: chromosome walking and jumping. *Science.* 1989;245(4922):1059–1065.
3. Bobadilla JL, Macek M Jr, Fine JP, Farrell PM. Cystic fibrosis: a worldwide analysis of CFTR mutations-correlation with incidence data and application to screening. *Hum Mutat.* 2002;19: 575–606.
4. Stoykova LI, Scanlin TF. Cystic Fibrosis (CF), *Pseudomonas Aeruginosa*, CFTR and the CF Glycosylation Phenotype: A Review and Update. *Curr Org Chem.* 2008;12:900–910.
5. Bruscia EM, Zhang PX, Ferreira E, et al. Macrophages directly contribute to the exaggerated inflammatory response in cystic fibrosis transmembrane conductance regulator-/- mice. *Am J Respir Cell Mol Biol.* 2009;40(3):295–304.
6. Sun X, Sui H, Fisher JT, et al. Disease phenotype of a ferret CFTR-knockout model of cystic fibrosis. *J Clin Invest.* 2010;120(9): 3149–3160.
7. Stoltz DA, Meyerholz DK, Pezzulo AA, et al. Cystic fibrosis pigs develop lung disease and exhibit defective bacterial eradication at birth. *Sci Transl Med.* 2010;2(29):29ra31.
8. Welsh MJ, Smith AE. Molecular mechanisms of CFTR chloride channel dysfunction in cystic fibrosis. *Cell.* 1993;73:1251–1254.
9. Voynow JA, Scanlin TF. Cystic fibrosis. In: Fishman AP, Elias JA, Fishman JA, Grippi MA, Senior RM, Pack AI, eds. *Fishman's Pulmonary Diseases and Disorders.* Vol 1. 4th ed. New York, NY: McGraw Hill Medical; 2008:863–885.
10. Worlitzsch D, Tarran R, Ulrich M, et al. Effects of reduced mucus oxygen concentration in airway Pseudomonas infections of cystic fibrosis patients. *J Clin Invest.* 2002;109(3):317–325.
11. Tunney MM, Field TR, Moriarty TF, et al. Detection of anaerobic bacteria in high numbers in sputum from patients with cystic fibrosis. *Am J Respir Crit Care Med.* 2008;177(9):995–1001.
12. Konstan MW, Hilliard KA, Norvell TM, Berger M. Bronchoalveolar lavage findings in cystic fibrosis patients with stable, clinically mild lung disease suggest ongoing infection and inflammation. *Am J Respir Crit Care Med.* 1994;150: 448–454.
13. Khan TZ, Wagener JS, Bost T, Martinez J, Accurso F, Riches DW. Early pulmonary inflammation in infants with cystic fibrosis. *Am J Respir Crit Care Med.* 1995;151:1075–1082.
14. Armstrong DS, Grimwood K, Carlin JB, et al. Lower airway inflammation in infants and young children with cystic fibrosis. *Am J Respir Crit Care Med.* 1997;156:1197–1204.
15. Flass T, Narkewicz MR. Cirrhosis and other liver disease in cystic fibrosis. *J Cyst Fibros.* 2012. S1569–S1993(12)00227-5.
16. Moran A, Dunitz J, Nathan B, Saeed A, Holme B, Thomas W. Cystic fibrosis-related diabetes: current trends in prevalence, incidence, and mortality. *Diabetes Care.* 2009;32(9):1626–1631.
17. Schwarzenberg SJ, Thomas W, Olsen TW, et al. Microvascular complications in cystic fibrosis-related diabetes. *Diabetes Care.* 2007;30(5):1056–1061.
18. Moran A, Hardin D, Rodman D, et al. Diagnosis, screening and management of cystic fibrosis related diabetes mellitus: a consensus conference report. *Diabetes Res Clin Pract.* 1999;45(1):61–73.
19. Finkelstein SM, Wielinski CL, Elliott GR, et al. Diabetes mellitus associated with cystic fibrosis. *J Pediatr.* 1988;112(3):373–377.
20. Marshall BC, Butler SM, Stoddard M, Moran AM, Liou TG, Morgan WJ. Epidemiology of cystic fibrosis-related diabetes. *J Pediatr.* 2005;146(5):681–687.
21. Milla CE, Warwick WJ, Moran A. Trends in pulmonary function in patients with cystic fibrosis correlate with the degree of glucose intolerance at baseline. *Am J Respir Crit Care Med.* 2000;162(3 Pt 1):891–895.
22. Lanng S, Thorsteinsson B, Nerup J, Koch C. Influence of the development of diabetes mellitus on clinical status in patients with cystic fibrosis. *Eur J Pediatr.* 1992;151(9):684–687.
23. Koch C, Rainisio M, Madessani U, et al. Presence of cystic fibrosis-related diabetes mellitus is tightly linked to poor lung function in patients with cystic fibrosis: data from the European Epidemiologic Registry of Cystic Fibrosis. *Pediatr Pulmonol.* 2001;32(5):343–350.
24. Rosenecker J, Hofler R, Steinkamp G, et al. Diabetes mellitus in patients with cystic fibrosis: the impact of diabetes mellitus on pulmonary function and clinical outcome. *Eur J Med Res.* 2001;6(8):345–350.
25. Hameed S, Morton JR, Jaffe A, et al. Early glucose abnormalities in cystic fibrosis are preceded by poor weight gain. *Diabetes Care.* 2010;33(2):221–226.
26. Moran A, Pekow P, Grover P, et al. Insulin therapy to improve BMI in cystic fibrosis-related diabetes without fasting hyperglycemia: results of the cystic fibrosis related diabetes therapy trial. *Diabetes Care.* 2009;32(10):1783–1788.
27. Hameed S, Morton JR, Field PI, et al. Once daily insulin detemir in cystic fibrosis with insulin deficiency. *Arch Dis Child.* 2012;97(5):464–467.
28. Bizzarri C, Lucidi V, Ciampalini P, Bella S, Russo B, Cappa M. Clinical effects of early treatment with insulin glargine in patients with cystic fibrosis and impaired glucose tolerance. *J Endocrinol Invest.* 2006;29(3):RC1–RC4.
29. Mozzillo E, Franzese A, Valerio G, et al. One-year glargine treatment can improve the course of lung disease in children and adolescents with cystic fibrosis and early glucose derangements. *Pediatr Diabetes.* 2009;10(3):162–167.
30. Lanng S, Thorsteinsson B, Roder ME, et al. Pancreas and gut hormone responses to oral glucose and intravenous glucagon

in cystic fibrosis patients with normal, impaired, and diabetic glucose tolerance. *Acta Endocrinol.* 1993;128(3):207–214.

31. Mohan V, Alagappan V, Snehalatha C, Ramachandran A, Thiruvengadam KV, Viswanathan M. Insulin and C-peptide responses to glucose load in cystic fibrosis. *Diabete Metab.* 1985;11(6):376–379.
32. Moran A, Diem P, Klein DJ, Levitt MD, Robertson RP. Pancreatic endocrine function in cystic fibrosis. *J Pediatr.* 1991;118(5):715–723.
33. Yung B, Noormohamed FH, Kemp M, Hooper J, Lant AF, Hodson ME. Cystic fibrosis-related diabetes: the role of peripheral insulin resistance and beta-cell dysfunction. *Diabet Med.* 2002;19(3):221–226.
34. Stalvey MS, Muller C, Schatz DA, et al. Cystic fibrosis transmembrane conductance regulator deficiency exacerbates islet cell dysfunction after beta-cell injury. *Diabetes.* 2006;55(7):1939–1945.
35. Olivier AK, Yi Y, Sun X, et al. Abnormal endocrine pancreas function at birth in cystic fibrosis ferrets. *J Clin Invest.* 2012;122(10):3755–3768.
36. Kuo P, Stevens JE, Russo A, et al. Gastric emptying, incretin hormone secretion, and postprandial glycemia in cystic fibrosis–effects of pancreatic enzyme supplementation. *J Clin Endocrinol Metab.* 2011;96(5):E851–E855.
37. Nauck M, Stockmann F, Ebert R, Creutzfeldt W. Reduced incretin effect in type 2 (non-insulin-dependent) diabetes. *Diabetologia.* 1986;29(1):46–52.
38. Vilsboll T, Krarup T, Deacon CF, Madsbad S, Holst JJ. Reduced postprandial concentrations of intact biologically active glucagon-like peptide 1 in type 2 diabetic patients. *Diabetes.* 2001; 50(3):609–613.
39. Kjems LL, Holst JJ, Volund A, Madsbad S. The influence of GLP-1 on glucose-stimulated insulin secretion: effects on beta-cell sensitivity in type 2 and nondiabetic subjects. *Diabetes.* 2003;52(2):380–386.
40. Nauck MA, Heimesaat MM, Orskov C, Holst JJ, Ebert R, Creutzfeldt W. Preserved incretin activity of glucagon-like peptide 1 [7–36 amide] but not of synthetic human gastric inhibitory polypeptide in patients with type-2 diabetes mellitus. *J Clin Invest.* 1993;91(1):301–307.
41. Aris RM, Merkel PA, Bachrach LK, et al. Guide to bone health and disease in cystic fibrosis. *J Clin Endocrinol Metab.* 2005;90(3):1888–1896.
42. Elkin SL, Vedi S, Bord S, Garrahan NJ, Hodson ME, Compston JE. Histomorphometric analysis of bone biopsies from the iliac crest of adults with cystic fibrosis. *Am J Respir Crit Care Med.* 2002;166(11):1470–1474.
43. LeGrys VA, Yankaskas JR, Quittell LM, Marshall BC, Mogayzel PJ Jr, Cystic Fibrosis Foundation. Diagnostic sweat testing: the Cystic Fibrosis Foundation guidelines. *J Pediatr.* 2007; 151(1):85–89.
44. Ruddy RM, Scanlin TF. Abnormal sweat electrolytes in a case of celiac disease and a case of psychosocial failure to thrive. Review of other reported causes. *Clin Pediatr.* 1987;26(2):83–89.
45. Farrell PM, Rosenstein BJ, White TB, et al. Guidelines for diagnosis of cystic fibrosis in newborns through older adults: Cystic Fibrosis Foundation consensus report. *J Pediatr.* 2008; 153(2):S4–S14.
46. Borowitz D, Parad RB, Sharp JK, et al. Cystic Fibrosis Foundation practice guidelines for the management of infants with cystic fibrosis transmembrane conductance regulator-related metabolic syndrome during the first two years of life and beyond. *J Pediatr.* 2009;155(6 Suppl):S106–S116.
47. Brody AS, Tiddens HA, Castile RG, et al. Computed tomography in the evaluation of cystic fibrosis lung disease. *Am J Respir Crit Care Med.* 2005;172(10):1246–1252.
48. Sly PD, Brennan S, Gangell C, et al. Lung disease at diagnosis in infants with cystic fibrosis detected by newborn screening. *Am J Respir Crit Care Med.* 2009;180(2):146–152.
49. Linnane BM, Hall GL, Nolan G, et al. Lung function in infants with cystic fibrosis diagnosed by newborn screening. *Am J Respir Crit Care Med.* 2008;178(12):1238–1244.
50. Jensen R, Stanojevic S, Gibney K, et al. Multiple breath nitrogen washout: a feasible alternative to mass spectrometry. *PLoS One.* 2013;8(2):e56868.
51. Li Z, Kosorok MR, Farrell PM, et al. Longitudinal development of mucoid Pseudomonas aeruginosa infection and lung disease progression in children with cystic fibrosis. *JAMA.* 2005; 293(5):581–588.
52. Dasenbrook EC, Merlo CA, Diener-West M, Lechtzin N, Boyle MP. Persistent methicillin-resistant Staphylococcus aureus and rate of FEV1 decline in cystic fibrosis. *Am J Respir Crit Care Med.* 2008;178(8):814–821.
53. Dasenbrook EC, Checkley W, Merlo CA, Konstan MW, Lechtzin N, Boyle MP. Association between respiratory tract methicillin-resistant Staphylococcus aureus and survival in cystic fibrosis. *JAMA.* 2010;303(23):2386–2392.
54. Zlosnik JE, Costa PS, Brant R, et al. Mucoid and nonmucoid Burkholderia cepacia complex bacteria in cystic fibrosis infections. *Am J Respir Crit Care Med.* 2011;183(1):67–72.
55. Waters V, Yau Y, Prasad S, et al. Stenotrophomonas maltophilia in cystic fibrosis: serologic response and effect on lung disease. *Am J Respir Crit Care Med.* 2011;183(5):635–640.
56. Mroueh S, Spock A. Allergic bronchopulmonary aspergillosis in patients with cystic fibrosis. *Chest.* 1994;105(1):32–36.
57. Moss RB. Allergic bronchopulmonary aspergillosis and Aspergillus infection in cystic fibrosis. *Curr Opin Pulm Med.* 2010;16(6):598–603.
58. Olivier KN, Weber DJ, Wallace RJ Jr, et al. Nontuberculous mycobacteria. I: multicenter prevalence study in cystic fibrosis. *Am J Respir Crit Care Med.* 2003;167(6):828–834.
59. Gelfond D, Borowitz D. Gastrointestinal complications of cystic fibrosis. *Clin Gastroenterol Hepatol.* 2013;11(4):333–342.
60. Kalnins D, Wilschanski M. Maintenance of nutritional status in patients with cystic fibrosis: new and emerging therapies. *Drug Des Devel Ther.* 2012;6:151–161.
61. Moran A, Brunzell C, Cohen RC, et al. Clinical care guidelines for cystic fibrosis-related diabetes: a position statement of the American Diabetes Association and a clinical practice guideline of the Cystic Fibrosis Foundation, endorsed by the Pediatric Endocrine Society. *Diabetes Care.* 2010;33(12): 2697–2708.
62. O'Riordan SM, Robinson PD, Donaghue KC, Moran A. Management of cystic fibrosis-related diabetes in children and adolescents. *Pediatr Diabetes.* 2009;10(Suppl 12):43–50.
63. Frohnert BI, Ode KL, Moran A, et al. Impaired fasting glucose in cystic fibrosis. *Diabetes Care.* 2010;33(12):2660–2664.
64. Ode KL, Frohnert B, Laguna T, et al. Oral glucose tolerance testing in children with cystic fibrosis. *Pediatr Diabetes.* 2010;11(7):487–492.

65. O'Riordan SM, Robinson PD, Donaghue KC, Moran A. Management of cystic fibrosis-related diabetes. *Pediatr Diabetes.* 2008;9(4 Pt 1):338–344.

66. Castellani C, Cuppens H, Macek M Jr, et al. Consensus on the use and interpretation of cystic fibrosis mutation analysis in clinical practice. *J Cyst Fibros.* 2008;7(3):179–196.

67. Ramsey BW, Davies J, McElvaney NG, et al. A CFTR potentiator in patients with cystic fibrosis and the G551D mutation. *N Engl J Med.* 2011;365(18):1663–1672.

68. Wright FA, Strug LJ, Doshi VK, et al. Genome-wide association and linkage identify modifier loci of lung disease severity in cystic fibrosis at 11p13 and 20q13.2. *Nat Genet.* 2011;43(6):539–546.

69. Blackman SM, Hsu S, Ritter SE, et al. A susceptibility gene for type 2 diabetes confers substantial risk for diabetes complicating cystic fibrosis. *Diabetologia.* 2009;52(9):1858–1865.

70. Bartlett JR, Friedman KJ, Ling SC, et al. Genetic modifiers of liver disease in cystic fibrosis. *JAMA.* 2009;302(10):1076–1083.

71. Sun L, Rommens JM, Corvol H, et al. Multiple apical plasma membrane constituents are associated with susceptibility to meconium ileus in individuals with cystic fibrosis. *Nat Genet.* 2012;44(5):562–569.

72. Bombieri C, Claustres M, De Boeck K, et al. Recommendations for the classification of diseases as CFTR-related disorders. *J Cyst Fibros.* 2011;10(Suppl 2):S86–102.

73. Cohen-Cymberknoh M, Shoseyov D, Kerem E. Managing cystic fibrosis: strategies that increase life expectancy and improve quality of life. *Am J Respir Crit Care Med.* 2011;183(11):1463–1471.

74. Flume PA, O'Sullivan BP, Robinson KA, et al. Cystic fibrosis pulmonary guidelines: chronic medications for maintenance of lung health. *Am J Respir Crit Care Med.* 2007;176(10):957–969.

75. Mogayzel PJ Jr, Naureckas ET, Robinson KA, et al. Cystic fibrosis pulmonary guidelines. Chronic medications for maintenance of lung health. *Am J Respir Crit Care Med.* 2013;187(7):680–689.

76. Button BM, Heine RG, Catto-Smith AG, et al. Chest physiotherapy in infants with cystic fibrosis: to tip or not? A five-year study. *Pediatr Pulmonol.* 2003;35(3):208–213.

77. Flume PA, Robinson KA, O'Sullivan BP, et al. Cystic fibrosis pulmonary guidelines: airway clearance therapies. *Respir Care.* 2009;54(4):522–537.

78. Schechter MS. Evaluating the evidence for airway-clearance therapy in cystic fibrosis. *Respir Care.* 2009;54(4):458–460.

79. Reisman JJ, Rivington-Law B, Corey M, et al. Role of conventional physiotherapy in cystic fibrosis. *J Pediatr.* 1988;113:632–636.

80. Reas HW. The effect of N-acetylcysteine on the viscosity of tracheobronchial secretions in cystic fibrosis of the pancreas. *J Pediatr.* 1963;62:31–35.

81. Suk JS, Boylan NJ, Trehan K, et al. N-acetylcysteine enhances cystic fibrosis sputum penetration and airway gene transfer by highly compacted DNA nanoparticles. *Mol Ther.* 2011;19(11):1981–1989.

82. Bear CE. 50 years ago in the Journal of Pediatrics: the effect of N-acetylcysteine on the viscosity of tracheobronchial secretions in cystic fibrosis of the pancreas. *J Pediatr.* 2013;162(1):85.

83. Nash EF, Stephenson A, Ratjen F, Tullis E. Nebulized and oral thiol derivatives for pulmonary disease in cystic fibrosis. *Cochrane Database Syst Rev.* 2009(1):CD007168.

84. Varelogianni G, Oliynyk I, Roomans GM, Johannesson M. The effect of N-acetylcysteine on chloride efflux from airway epithelial cells. *Cell Biol Int.* 2010;34(3):245–252.

85. Fuchs HJ, Borowitz DS, Christiansen DH, et al. Effect of aerosolized recombinant human DNase on exacerbations of respiratory symptoms and on pulmonary function in patients with cystic fibrosis. *N Engl J Med.* 1994;331:637–642.

86. Quan JM, Tiddens HA, Sy JP, et al. A two-year randomized, placebo-controlled trial of dornase alfa in young patients with cystic fibrosis with mild lung function abnormalities. *J Pediatr.* 2001;139:813–820.

87. Elkins MR, Robinson M, Rose BR, et al. A controlled trial of long-term inhaled hypertonic saline in patients with cystic fibrosis. *N Engl J Med.* 2006;354(3):229–240.

88. Rosenfeld M, Ratjen F, Brumback L, et al. Inhaled hypertonic saline in infants and children younger than 6 years with cystic fibrosis: the ISIS randomized controlled trial. *JAMA.* 2012; 307(21):2269–2277.

89. Eigen H, Rosenstein BJ, FitzSimmons S, Schidlow DV. A multicenter study of alternate-day prednisone therapy in patients with cystic fibrosis. Cystic Fibrosis Foundation Prednisone Trial Group. *J Pediatr.* 1995;126(4):515–523.

90. Konstan MW, Byard PJ, Hoppel CL, Davis PB. Effect of high-dose ibuprofen in patients with cystic fibrosis. *N Engl J Med.* 1995;332(13):848–854.

91. Treggiari MM, Retsch-Bogart G, Mayer-Hamblett N, et al. Comparative efficacy and safety of 4 randomized regimens to treat early Pseudomonas aeruginosa infection in children with cystic fibrosis. *Arch Pediatr Adolesc Med.* 2011;165(9): 847–856.

92. Ratjen F, Munck A, Kho P, Angyalosi G. Treatment of early Pseudomonas aeruginosa infection in patients with cystic fibrosis: the ELITE trial. *Thorax.* 2010;65(4):286–291.

93. Taccetti G, Bianchini E, Cariani L, et al. Early antibiotic treatment for Pseudomonas aeruginosa eradication in patients with cystic fibrosis: a randomised multicentre study comparing two different protocols. *Thorax.* 2012;67(10):853–859.

94. Saiman L, Siegel J, Cystic Fibrosis Foundation Consensus Conference on Infection Control Participants. Infection control recommendations for patients with cystic fibrosis: microbiology, important pathogens, and infection control practices to prevent patient-to-patient transmission. *Am J Infect Control.* 2003;31(3 Suppl):S1–S62.

95. Hoiby N., Frederiksen B., Pressler T. Eradication of early *Pseudomonas aeruginosa* infection. *J Cyst Fibros.* 2005;4:49–54.

96. Ramsey BW, Pepe MS, Quan JM, et al. Intermittent administration of inhaled tobramycin in patients with cystic fibrosis. Cystic Fibrosis Inhaled Tobramycin Study Group. *N Engl J Med.* 1999;340(1):23–30.

97. Oermann CM, Retsch-Bogart GZ, Quittner AL, et al. An 18-month study of the safety and efficacy of repeated courses of inhaled aztreonam lysine in cystic fibrosis. *Pediatr Pulmonol.* 2010;45(11):1121–1134.

98. Saiman L, Marshall BC, Mayer-Hamblett N, et al. Azithromycin in patients with cystic fibrosis chronically infected with Pseudomonas aeruginosa: a randomized controlled trial. *JAMA.* 2003;290(13):1749–1756.

99. Shinkai M, Henke MO, Rubin BK. Macrolide antibiotics as immunomodulatory medications: proposed mechanisms of action. *Pharmacol Ther.* 2008;117(3):393–405.

100. Rogan MP, Stoltz DA, Hornick DB. Cystic fibrosis transmembrane conductance regulator intracellular processing, trafficking, and opportunities for mutation-specific treatment. *Chest.* 2011;139(6):1480–1490.

101. Clancy JP, Rowe SM, Accurso FJ, et al. Results of a phase IIa study of VX-809, an investigational CFTR corrector compound, in subjects with cystic fibrosis homozygous for the F508del-CFTR mutation. *Thorax.* 2012;67(1):12–18.
102. Smyth A, Tan KH, Hyman-Taylor P, et al. Once versus three-times daily regimens of tobramycin treatment for pulmonary exacerbations of cystic fibrosis–the TOPIC study: a randomised controlled trial. *Lancet.* 2005;365(9459):573–578.
103. FitzSimmons SC, Burkhart GA, Borowitz D, et al. High-dose pancreatic-enzyme supplements and fibrosing colonopathy in children with cystic fibrosis. *N Engl J Med.* 1997;336(18):1283–1289.
104. Sulli N, Bertasi S, Zullo S, Shashaj B. Use of continuous subcutaneous insulin infusion in patients with cystic fibrosis related diabetes: three case reports. *J Cyst Fibros.* 2007;6(3):237–240.
105. Debray D, Kelly D, Houwen R, Strandvik B, Colombo C. Best practice guidance for the diagnosis and management of cystic fibrosis-associated liver disease. *J Cyst Fibros.* 2011;10(Suppl 2):S29–S36.
106. Dowman JK, Watson D, Loganathan S, et al. Long-term impact of liver transplantation on respiratory function and nutritional status in children and adults with cystic fibrosis. *Am J Transplant.* 2012;12(4):954–964.
107. Hurt K, Simmonds NJ. Cystic fibrosis: management of haemoptysis. *Paediatr Respir Rev.* 2012;13(4):200–205.
108. Leung JM, Olivier KN. Nontuberculous mycobacteria in patients with cystic fibrosis. *Semin Respir Crit Care Med.* 2013;34(1):124–134.
109. Kotloff RM, Thabut G. Lung transplantation. *Am J Respir Crit Care Med.* 2011;184(2):159–171.
110. Hadjiliadis D. Special considerations for patients with cystic fibrosis undergoing lung transplantation. *Chest.* 2007;131(4): 1224–1231.
111. Martinu T, Pavlisko EN, Chen DF, Palmer SM. Acute allograft rejection: cellular and humoral processes. *Clin Chest Med.* 2011;32(2):295–310.
112. McMullen AH, Pasta DJ, Frederick PD, et al. Impact of pregnancy on women with cystic fibrosis. *Chest.* 2006;129(3): 706–711.
113. Edenborough FP, Borgo G, Knoop C, et al. Guidelines for the management of pregnancy in women with cystic fibrosis. *J Cyst Fibros.* 2008;7(Suppl 1):S2–S32.
114. Massie J, Curnow L, Gaffney L, Carlin J, Francis I. Declining prevalence of cystic fibrosis since the introduction of newborn screening. *Arch Dis Child.* 2010;95(7):531–533.
115. Amaral MD, Kunzelmann K. Molecular targeting of CFTR as a therapeutic approach to cystic fibrosis. *Trends Pharmacol Sci.* 2007;28(7):334–341.
116. Rabeh WM, Bossard F, Xu H, et al. Correction of both NBD1 energetics and domain interface is required to restore DeltaF508 CFTR folding and function. *Cell.* 2012;148(1-2): 150–163.
117. Mendoza JL, Schmidt A, Li Q, et al. Requirements for efficient correction of DeltaF508 CFTR revealed by analyses of evolved sequences. *Cell.* 2012;148(1–2):164–174.

CHAPTER 51

Bronchiolitis

Gary R. Epler

DISEASES OF THE BRONCHIOLES

Diseases of the bronchioles occur throughout the bronchiolar structures, from bronchiolar airways to alveolar ducts and alveoli (Table 51-1). Acute and chronic bronchiolitis are seen from near the bronchi, all the way to the respiratory bronchioles; constrictive bronchiolitis is seen in the midbronchioles, while diffuse panbronchiolitis occurs from the distal bronchioles to the respiratory bronchioles, and smoker's bronchiolitis involves the respiratory bronchioles. Bronchiolitis obliterans organizing pneumonia (BOOP) includes both the terminal bronchioles and alveoli and is discussed in Chapter 57.

New bronchiolar disorders continue to be described, including diffuse panbronchiolitis and smoker's bronchiolitis. New causes of bronchiolitis obliterans have also been described, including lung transplantation, pulmonary microcarcinoids, *Sauropus androgynous* vegetable drink, and food-flavoring. This chapter includes a discussion of the pathological, clinical, radiographic findings, and treatment of the bronchiolar airway disorders.

BRONCHIOLAR ANATOMY

Bronchioles are noncartilagenous small airways which are usually 1 mm or less in diameter; they have been called the bridge between the bronchi and alveoli.[1] The bronchioles have cartilage and mucus glands that are commonly found in the bronchi, but bronchioles also contain ciliated epithelium, smooth muscle, and Clara cells.[2] Clara cells are columnar cells with apical surfaces capable of secreting proteins and surfactant. Neuroendocrine cells are common in the proximal bronchioles.

More distal in the airways are approximately 30,000 terminal bronchioles that have an average diameter of about 0.6 mm. These bronchioles have circular smooth muscles in the their walls; the surface cilia gradually disappear distally. Terminal bronchioles branch into 224,000 respiratory bronchioles that differ from the bronchioles: respiratory bronchioles have two to three alveolar structures in the walls containing columnar cells with cuboidal type II cells and squamous type I cells. These structures terminate in 13.8 million alveolar ducts and 300 million alveoli.

TABLE 51-1 Clinical Classification of the Bronchiolar Diseases

Airway diseases

- Acute and chronic bronchiolitis
- Respiratory bronchiolitis
- Follicular bronchiolitis
- Diffuse panbronchiolitis
- Bronchiolitis obliterans

Interstitial diseases

- Respiratory bronchiolitis-interstitial lung disease (RB-ILD)
- Bronchiolitis obliterans organizing pneumonia (BOOP)

THE CLINICAL SPECTRUM OF THE BRONCHIOLAR DISEASES

The wide variety of bronchiolar diseases that may be seen in clinical practice are discussed below.

ACUTE AND CHRONIC CELLULAR BRONCHIOLITIS

Acute and chronic cellular bronchiolitis is characterized pathologically as acute or chronic inflammation of the bronchioles without a fibrotic component.[3] The inflammation may be submucosal, mural, or peribronchiolar. Clinically, this is a common respiratory illness in children that is caused by several infectious agents, including *Mycoplasma*, adenovirus, influenza, parainfluenza, herpes virus, and adenoviruses. In the adult, bronchiolitis is rare and caused by similar viruses. Symptoms include a flu-like illness with persistent nonproductive cough of several weeks duration. There is generally no wheezing and no airflow obstruction. The chest x-ray is normal. The illness usually subsides over time. Cough suppressants may be utilized. Sometimes, a brief course of corticosteroid therapy is given for a severe, relentless cough. If symptoms are not responsive to corticosteroid therapy or if symptoms worsen, the illness may be fibrotic constrictive bronchiolitis – a disorder with a different clinical course and prognosis.

RESPIRATORY BRONCHIOLITIS

Respiratory bronchiolitis is sometimes called smoker's bronchiolitis, as cigarette smoking is almost always the cause of this lesion.[3] The characteristic histological feature is the accumulation of tan-brown macrophages in the lumens of respiratory bronchioles and adjacent alveoli-often seen as an incidental finding in cigarette smokers. For example, respiratory bronchiolitis was found in 70 of 79 (88.6%) smokers who underwent surgery for spontaneous pneumothorax.[4] There are usually no clinical symptoms associated with this type of respiratory bronchiolitis. Treatment is smoking cessation.

In some situations, respiratory bronchiolitis may extend into the interstitium and is referred to as respiratory bronchiolitis-interstitial lung disease (RB-ILD). Affected individuals have shortness of breath, bilateral crackles, reticulonodular opacities on chest radiography, decreased vital capacity, and decreased diffusing capacity. Treatment is smoking cessation, but often a course of corticosteroid therapy is needed for resolution.

FOLLICULAR BRONCHIOLITIS

Follicular bronchiolitis is characterized by hyperplastic lymphoid aggregates forming 1- to 2-mm peribronchiolar nodules.[3] Follicular bronchiolitis is often limited to a pathological description with no clinical counterpart. It occurs in the connective tissue disorders, such as rheumatoid arthritis. In some patients, there may be cough, sputum production, and small linear radiographic opacities.[5]

DIFFUSE PANBRONCHIOLITIS

Diffuse panbronchiolitis was first described in the 1960s and is characterized by chronic inflammation and lymphofollicles of the respiratory bronchioles and adjacent centrilobular regions, with infiltration of histiocytosis, plasma cells, and lymphocytes.[6] There is also an interstitial accumulation of foam cells in the walls of respiratory bronchioles and adjacent alveolar ducts and alveoli (Fig. 51-1). The disorder is largely restricted to the Asian countries, but diffuse panbronchiolitis has been reported in the United States, Australia, Canada, and Spain.[7-10] The disorder has been reported in Kartagener syndrome.[11] In recent years, there appears to be a major decrease in the incidence and prevalence of diffuse panbronchiolitis in Japan.[12]

Symptoms include chronic cough, sputum production, shortness of breath, and almost all individuals have chronic paranasal sinusitis. Rhonchi and crackles are common. Radiographic findings show hyperinflation and diffuse small nodular opacities bilaterally. Pulmonary function testing shows airflow obstruction with decreased forced expired volume in one second (FEV_1) and FEV_1 to forced vital capacity (FEV_1/FVC) ratio. Hypercapnia and cor pulmonale occur late. There is often an associated increase in the cold-hemagglutinin titer. There appears to be a major susceptibility gene located between the HLA-A and HLA-B loci on the short arm of chromosome six.[13]

The disorder is progressive. In the past, diffuse panbronchiolitis was a fatal disease with a 10-year survival of less than 20% in patients with *Pseudomonas aeruginosa* infection. However, the introduction of low-dose, long-term erythromycin and other macrolides has resulted in a dramatic improvement in survival. Among Chinese patients, Li et al.[14] showed azithromycin, 500 mg once daily, for 3 months and 500 mg three times weekly for 6 to 12 months, resulted in complete cure in 27.5% of patients, elimination of symptoms in 70.6%, and a 5-year survival of 94.1%. The macrolides may prevent influx of neutrophils into the alveoli, decrease interleukin-8, and interfere with the pathological potency of *P. aeruginosa*.[15]

BRONCHIOLITIS OBLITERANS

Bronchiolitis obliterans is an important lesion because it can be severely disabling and deadly. Traditionally, bronchiolitis obliterans

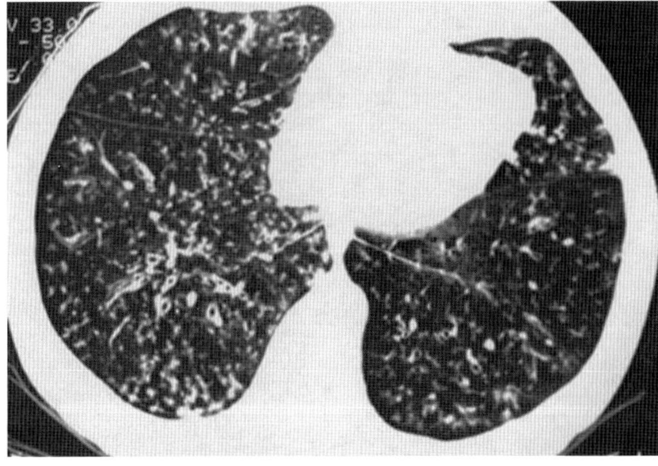

A

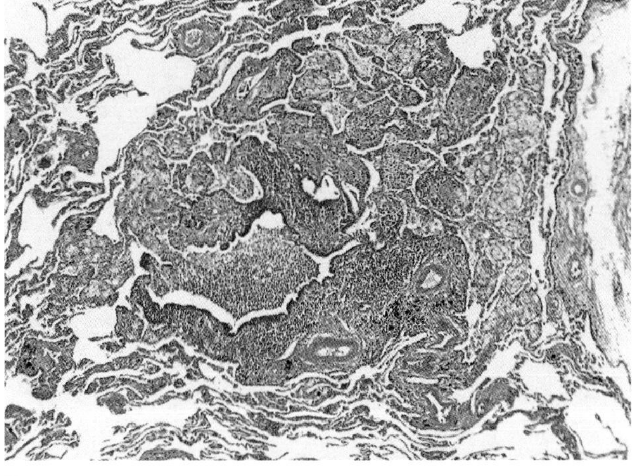

B

Figure 51-1 Diffuse panbronchiolitis. **A.** The chest CT scan shows bilateral centrilobular nodules with branching showing "tree-in-bud" pattern. **B.** The pathology micrograph shows chronic inflammation of the respiratory bronchioles, with interstitial accumulation of foam cells in the walls of the respiratory bronchioles, adjacent alveolar ducts, and alveoli. *(Used with permission of Dr. Kenneth W. Tsang, Queen Mary Hospital, Hong Kong, China; and Dr. Thomas V. Colby, Lung Pathology, Mayo Clinic Scottsdale.)*

TABLE 51-2 Pathological Findings of Bronchiolitis Obliterans

Constrictive bronchiolitis
• Concentric fibrotic lesion of the mid to distal bronchioles
• The lesion surrounds the lumen, causing extrinsic narrowing and obliteration
• Distortion of the lumen and mucostasis
• Muscle layer hypertrophic early, atrophic late, and replaced by fibrotic tissue in end-stage disease
• May be patchy and focal
• Late stage includes traction bronchiectasis and bronchiolectasis
Proliferative bronchiolitis
• Intraluminal polypoid myxoid fibroblastic tissue arising with the bronchiole wall.
• May be organized polypoid granulation tissue from the bronchioles to the respiratory bronchioles including the alveoli
• No disruption of the lung architecture
• No traction bronchiectasis

has been used as a clinical term to describe irreversible fibrosis of the bronchiolar airway that is idiopathic or occurs after accidental toxic fume inhalation or a viral pneumonia. However, pathologists may see two distinctive lesions that, in turn, have a different clinical course and response to treatment.

Histologically, the two lesions are *proliferative bronchiolitis* and *constrictive bronchiolitis* (Table 51-2). Depending on severity, obliteration of the bronchioles, the obliterans term, may or may not occur with these lesions. The histological distinction between these two lesions is that constrictive bronchiolitis arises in a concentric fashion outside the bronchiole walls as a fibrotic lesion, and proliferative bronchiolitis arises from within the bronchiole walls as an inflammatory lesion.

The term *bronchiolitis obliterans* is used in this chapter, as it has been used by clinicians for more than a hundred years and almost always reflects the fibrosing, constrictive, pathological lesion.[16] The proliferative lesion is often self-limiting and less severe, or responds to corticosteroid therapy with complete resolution; it usually does not result in the clinical label of bronchiolitis obliterans.

Proliferative bronchiolitis is an inflammatory bronchiolitis characterized by intraluminal polypoid connective tissue masses of myxoid fibroblastic tissue which resembles granulation tissue that arises from within the bronchioles.[1] Central clusters of mononuclear inflammatory cells may be found in these polypoid masses. This type of bronchiolitis includes organized polypoid granulation inflammatory tissue in the distal bronchiole airways, respiratory bronchioles, alveolar ducts, and alveoli in the form of BOOP[17] Additional distinctive histological findings with proliferative bronchiolitis associated with BOOP include no disruption in the lung architecture, interstitial fibrosis, absence of traction bronchiectasis, or histological honeycombing (Fig. 51-2).

Constrictive bronchiolitis is a fibrotic, concentric bronchiolitis lesion with or without complete obliteration (Fig. 51-3). This lesion is usually seen in the mid to distal area of bronchioles and does not extend into the respiratory bronchioles or alveoli. The lesion is characterized by a peribronchiolar fibrotic process that surrounds, rather than fills, the lumen, resulting in extrinsic compression and obliteration of the airway.[3] There is mural thickening by submucosal collagenous fibrosis with progressive concentric narrowing associated with luminal distortion, mucus stasis, and chronic inflammation.[18]

Constrictive bronchiolitis was called "fibrosing bronchiolitis" in the German pathology literature.[19] The lesion preferentially involves membranous bronchioles and is characterized by fibrosis of the stroma and narrowing the lumen in a concentric fashion. The muscle layer may be hypertrophic in early lesions, atrophic in late stages, and replaced by fibrotic tissue at the end stage. Visscher and Myers noted that constrictive bronchiolitis is often patchy and focal, making the diagnosis difficult from a transbronchial biopsy; advanced cases may be especially inconspicuous because of lack of active inflammation and disappearance of bronchioles.[20]

There are several causes of bronchiolitis obliterans and associated systemic disorders (Table 51-3).

Idiopathic Bronchiolitis Obliterans

Idiopathic bronchiolitis obliterans occurs among individuals who have no obvious inciting agent or associated systemic disorder,

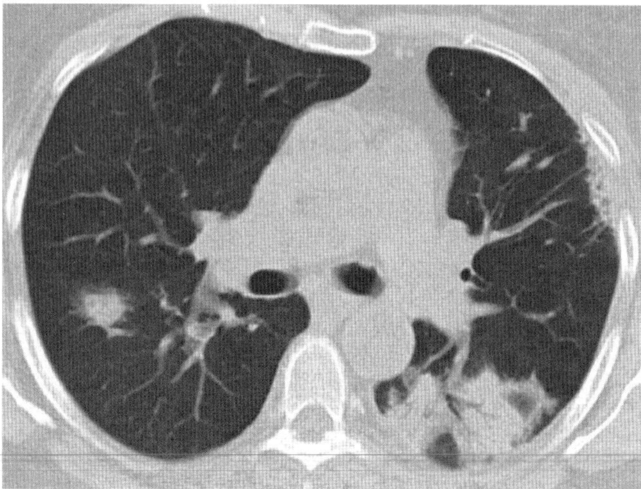
A

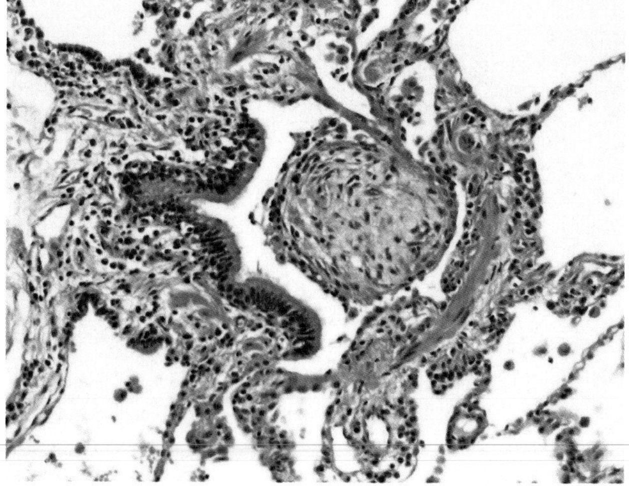
B

Figure 51-2 Bronchiolitis obliterans organizing pneumonia. **A.** The chest CT scan shows bilateral patchy ground-glass opacities, air bronchograms, and peripheral-based triangular infiltrates. **B.** The pathology micrograph shows organized polypoid granulation tissue filling the distal bronchiole and extending into the alveoli. *(Used with permission of Dr. Ritu R. Gill, Chest Radiology, Brigham and Women's Hospital, Boston, and Dr. Thomas V. Colby, Lung Pathology, Mayo Clinic Scottsdale.)*

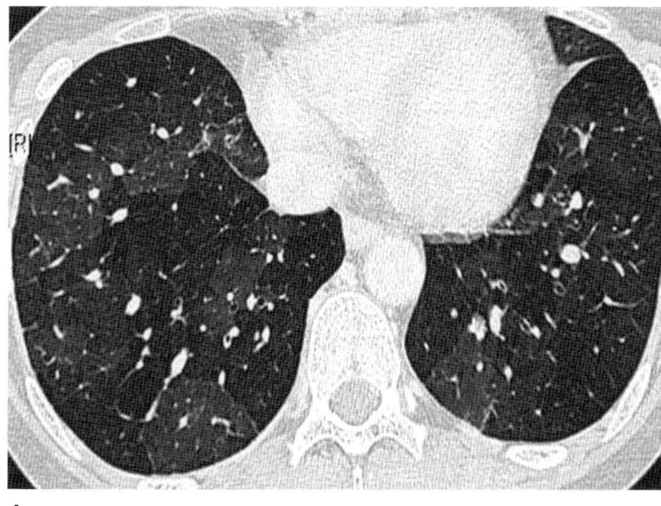

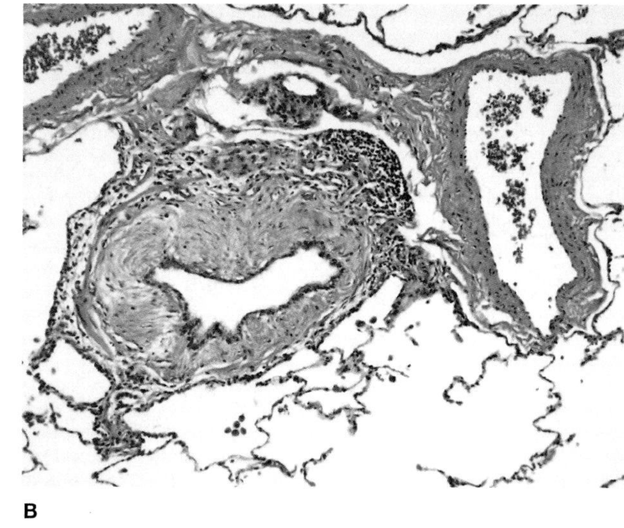

A B

Figure 51-3 Constrictive bronchiolitis. **A.** The expiratory chest CT scan shows the mosaic pattern of air trapping seen from obliterated bronchioles. **B.** The pathology micrograph shows extrinsic fibrosis of the bronchiolar wall in a concentric manner constricting and obliterating the bronchiolar lumen. *(Used with permission of Dr. Ritu R. Gill, Chest Radiology, Brigham and Women's Hospital, Boston, and Dr. Thomas V. Colby, Lung Pathology, Mayo Clinic Scottsdale.)*

and who have airflow obstruction and constrictive bronchiolitis histologically. This disorder continues to be exceedingly rare. Symptoms begin with a nonproductive cough, and shortness of breath develops later. Physical examination shows no wheezing but may demonstrate an unusual finding of early inspiratory crackles. The crackles occur early because of the scarring around the mid-bronchiole airways, causing snapping closure of the airways and resultant crackling sound.

TABLE 51-3 Clinical Classification of Bronchiolitis Obliterans

Idiopathic
Toxic fumes
Post-respiratory infections
Connective tissue disorders
Drug-related
Organ transplantation
• Lung
• Bone marrow and stem cell
Aspiration
Neuroendocrine hyperplasia
Microcarcinoids
Sauropus androgynous
Stevens-Johnson Syndrome
Primary biliary cirrhosis
Miscellaneous diseases
• Ataxia-telangiectasia
• IgA nephropathy
• HIV
• Paraneoplastic pemphigus and paraneoplastic autoimmune multi-organ syndrome (PAMS)
• Swyer–James syndrome
• Inflammatory bowel disease

Pulmonary function studies show irreversible decrease in the FEV_1 and FEV_1/FVC with no improvement after bronchodilator inhalation. The diffusing capacity is highly variable, from increased, to normal, to markedly decreased.

The chest roentgenogram is often normal or shows hyperinflation. High-resolution chest CT scans during inspiration and expiration can be helpful for establishing a diagnosis (Fig. 51-1). For example, a 65-year-old woman with idiopathic bronchiolitis obliterans had a normal chest CT scan in the inspiratory study, but the expiratory study showed extensive lobular air trapping.[21] These expiratory images show low-attenuation areas in the secondary pulmonary lobules, resulting in a typical mosaic pattern with scattered areas of low attenuation. Additional thin-section CT findings include constriction of the pulmonary vessels within the low-attenuation areas, expiratory air trapping, bronchial dilation, and sometimes, centrilobular nodules or branching linear densities.[22]

Treatment consists of high-dose corticosteroids such as prednisone with an initial dose of 60 mg daily, followed by lower-dose therapy for usually one year in patients who respond. For those who do not respond by three months, corticosteroids are discontinued and employed for life-threatening exacerbations. Immune-suppression treatment can be utilized and lung transplantation for individuals with life-threatening and severe disease.

Patients who survive the initial episode may stabilize for several years or progress to end-stage airflow disease and cor pulmonale.[23] For example, a 43-year-old woman had idiopathic bronchiolitis obliterans for 24 years and showed relentless progression of airway obstruction with 19 admissions for respiratory failure.[24] The autopsy in this patient showed complete obliteration of smaller airways. The FEV_1 decreased from 1.06 L to 0.40 L terminally.

Myong et al.[25] described three women aged 41 to 54 who developed cough and progressive shortness of breath during 6 months to 10 years; lung tissue showed constrictive bronchiolitis with bronchiolar airway obliteration. The thin-section CT scans showed low-attenuation changes of the mosaic pattern. None responded to corticosteroid treatment. One woman died 8 months after the diagnosis from lymphoma and the other two were stable.

Toxic Fume Bronchiolitis Obliterans

Toxic fume bronchiolitis obliterans is a three-phase response disease. The exposure usually occurs from an accidental explosion resulting in nose, throat, and eye irritation with no major respiratory symptoms. Phase one is an asymptomatic latency period of 6 to 12 hours after exposure. Phase two begins suddenly with acute-onset respiratory failure and acute respiratory distress syndrome. Successful treatment results in another asymptomatic latency period of 7 to 10 days. Phase three then occurs as constrictive bronchiolitis with irreversible airflow obstruction, progressive shortness of breath, and chronic respiratory failure.

This disorder occurs after accidental exposures to sulfur dioxide fumes, nitric acid fumes, and nitrogen dioxide in freshly filled corn silos. Unusual accidental exposures to toxic fumes may cause this lesion. For example, two workers in a lithium battery factory were accidentally exposed to thionyl chloride, and one of them developed findings consistent with bronchiolitis obliterans.[26] This acidic compound is used in the manufacturing process and produces sulfur dioxide and hydrochloric acid fumes when in contact with water.

Smoke inhalation bronchiolitis obliterans was described in a 23-year-old man who was in a fire while sleeping in his newly constructed house.[27] He was unconscious when rescued. There was cough and mild dyspnea after recovery. He returned 3 years later because of persistent dyspnea. He had finger clubbing, an FEV_1 of 0.90 L, and an FEV_1/FVC of 34%. The burning synthetic structural materials used to build his house produced gases containing acrolein, formaldehyde, acetaldehyde, nitrogen dioxide, and sulfur dioxide.

There has been a report of bronchiolitis obliterans from mustard gas occurring from a chemical warfare attack in a 37-year-old man who had cough, sputum production, shortness of breath, and airflow obstruction for 14 years after the exposure.[28] Later, investigators[29] used high-resolution chest CT scan findings for the diagnosis of bronchiolitis obliterans in a group of individuals exposed to the same mustard gas attack. They treated 18 individuals with bronchodilator treatment and 18 with interferon gamma-1b and 7.5 mg of prednisolone. Patients had baseline FEV_1 values of 49.3% and 48.7% predicted, respectively. Both groups improved after 6 months of treatment; however, the group treated with interferon gamma had a significantly higher posttreatment FEV_1 of 66.3% compared to 57.3% for the group treated with bronchodilators ($p = 0.001$).

King et al.[30] reported constrictive bronchiolitis among 38 US soldiers returning from Iraq and Afghanistan and found a common exposure to a sulfur-mine fire in 2003 among 28 of them.

A 42-year-old police officer exposed to the dust in the cloud from the New York City World Trade Center disaster of September 11, 2001 developed decreased FEV_1 and FEV_1/FVC in April 2002.[31] The lung biopsy showed regions of constrictive bronchiolitis. He was treated with oral corticosteroid therapy and azithromycin. By April 2003, pulmonary function studies had returned to normal values.

An unusual radiographic appearance of scattered lung cysts has been reported in a 49-year-old woman with severe airflow obstruction and constrictive bronchiolitis.[32]

Diacetyl appears to be a common exposure among artificial butter flavoring workers who developed constrictive bronchiolitis. A report of nine microwave popcorn factory workers showed airflow obstruction among the mixers, and biopsy of some individuals showed constrictive bronchiolitis.[33] Investigators[34] have reported that four workers at a cookie factory who were exposed to diacetyl developed severe and persistent airflow obstruction, with FEV_1 ranging from 25% to 44%. Lung biopsy showed constrictive bronchiolitis and bronchiolar airway distortion.

Post-Respiratory Infection Bronchiolitis Obliterans

Post-respiratory infection bronchiolitis obliterans may occur after adenovirus pneumonia, influenza or parainfluenza pneumonia, or after *Mycoplasma* pneumonia.[35] Cough develops several days after the initial infection. Chest radiographs may show diffuse reticulonodular opacities early but are normal or show hyperinflation late. Expiratory, high-resolution chest CT scans show low-attenuation mosaic pattern. Tissue shows constrictive bronchiolitis with extensive scarring that obliterates many of the bronchioles, corresponding clinically with severe airflow obstruction. At this stage, the lesion is not responsive to corticosteroid medication. Lung transplantation has been utilized for severe post-*Mycoplasma* pneumonia bronchiolitis obliterans.[36]

Connective Tissue Bronchiolitis Obliterans

Connective tissue bronchiolitis obliterans occurs most commonly in rheumatoid arthritis and has been reported in scleroderma, lupus erythematosus, and Sjögren's syndrome.[37,38]

Rheumatoid arthritis-related constrictive bronchiolitis often has a poor prognosis. Among 25 individuals with rheumatoid arthritis and bronchiolitis obliterans, most had severe airflow obstruction, often with an FEV_1 less than 1 L, and the process was not responsive to corticosteroids.[39] The outcome was poor, as chronic respiratory failure occurred in 40% of the patients; four patients died.

Drug-Related Bronchiolitis Obliterans

Drug-related bronchiolitis obliterans has been reported with penicillamine and gold used for treatment of rheumatoid arthritis. The penicillamine-related bronchiolitis obliterans has a poor prognosis, sometimes requiring lung transplantation for management.[40] Fatal bronchiolitis obliterans has been reported in a 12-year-old girl with juvenile rheumatoid arthritis after a 6-month course of intramuscular gold.[41] Although cause and effect are difficult to confirm for both of these agents, patients receiving these medications who develop unexplained cough or dyspnea need to be evaluated for the possibility of bronchiolitis obliterans.

Bone-Marrow Transplantation Bronchiolitis Obliterans

Bone-marrow transplantation bronchiolitis obliterans occurs much less frequently as allogeneic stem-cell transplantation has become so common; however, bronchiolitis obliterans may occur in up to 9% of allogeneic bone-marrow recipients.[42] Bronchiolitis obliterans occurs only after graft-versus-host reaction, and therefore, is rarely seen after autologous bone-marrow transplantation. As complications of chronic graft-versus-host develop after 100 days, bronchiolitis obliterans is usually seen 6 to 12 months after transplantation. Donor type-2 T-helper lymphocytes appear to be the primary mediators. The pathological lesion is concentric bronchiolar fibrosis typical of constrictive bronchiolitis. There is generally a poor response to corticosteroid therapy; mortality ranges from 40% to 100%.[42] Living donor lobar lung transplantation has been used successfully for bone-marrow transplant-related bronchiolitis obliterans.[43]

Stem-Cell Transplant Bronchiolitis Obliterans

Stem-cell transplant bronchiolitis obliterans has replaced bone-marrow transplantation-associated bronchiolitis obliterans as allogeneic hematopoietic stem-cell transplantation has become more widespread (see Chapter 95). The prevalence of bronchiolitis obliterans ranges from 2% to 3% among all allogeneic recipients to 6% among those who develop chronic graft-versus-host disease (cGVHD).[44] These data underestimate the incidence of bronchiolitis obliterans (26%) when using an annualized rate of decline in FEV1 of 5%. Those with cGVHD had a rate of 30%, but more importantly, they had a mortality rate of 40% at 10 years. cGVHD is the major risk factor for bronchiolitis obliterans, as high as 80% of patients with bronchiolitis obliterans are preceded with cGVHD. Other risk factors include low IgG levels, use of peripheral blood stem cells, poor pretransplant lung function, and respiratory infection during the first 100 days. Biopsy specimens performed early show bronchiolitis, fibrous obliteration of the respiratory bronchioles, and inflammatory cell infiltrates; later lesions show constrictive bronchiolitis with circumferential fibrosis. The mechanism of bronchiolitis obliterans is based on chronic rejection that may involve donor cytotoxic T cells.

Preventive treatment of stem-cell transplantation bronchiolitis obliterans consists of early and aggressive treatment of respiratory infections and cGVHD. Treatment includes high-dose systemic corticosteroids and immunosuppression with calcineurin inhibitors, sirolimus, azathioprine, and anti-thymocyte globulin. Prognosis continues to be poor despite treatment and supportive care, with an overall survival rate of 44% at 2 years and 13% at 5 years.[44]

In a study of 2087 allogeneic stem-cell transplantation recipients from 1994 to 2005, there were 57 (2.8%) who developed bronchiolitis obliterans.[45] The time interval between transplantation and bronchiolitis obliterans ranged from 83 days to 907 days with a median time of 335 days. Acute graft-versus-host disease was not found to be a risk factor, whereas cGVHD was a significant risk factor. The development of bronchiolitis obliterans was related to the stem-cell source, with related peripheral blood stem-cell transplantation (3.83%) the highest. Unrelated bone-marrow transplantation (2.91%) and cord-blood transplantation (2.65%) were lower, with related bone-marrow transplantation (1.62%) the lowest. The outcome among these 57 patients showed that 8 (16.7%) improved, 10 (21.7%) showed no change, and 28 (60.9%) died; the cause of death was respiratory failure in 17 (60.7%).

The high-resolution chest CT findings in bronchiolitis obliterans among patients receiving allogeneic stem-cell transplantation shows geographic hypoattenuation and air trapping with subpleural predominance.[46] In some patients, the geographic hypoattenuation involved more than half of both lungs.

Extracorporeal photodynamic therapy has been used for the treatment of cGVHD and bronchiolitis obliterans.[47] The role of this treatment in the management of bronchiolitis obliterans in stem-cell transplantation recipients has not yet been established. Some patients have improved pulmonary function.

Mesenchymal stem-cell treatment was used for one patient. A 38-year-old patient received peripheral blood stem cells from her sibling and developed bronchiolitis obliterans 8 months later with an FEV_1 <0.7 L.[48] She was treated experimentally with human bone marrow–derived mesenchymal stem cells from her sister on day 275 and on day 305, resulting in disappearance of symptoms and improved pulmonary function. This may be an effective treatment on a case-by-case basis, but at this time, there are too many unknown variables involved to advocate its use (e.g., absence of large scale studies, availability of a standardized source of mesenchymal cells, and an understanding of potential carcinogenic effects).

Lung Transplant Bronchiolitis Obliterans

Lung transplant bronchiolitis obliterans has emerged as the most important clinical complication among lung transplant recipients since the mid-1980s and has continued to plague thoracic surgeons and patients, with minimal change in occurrence and mortality (see Chapter 107).

The terminology has become the bronchiolitis obliterans syndrome (BOS), which is a clinical classification based on FEV_1. The classification was developed because BOS is a common problem among lung transplantation recipients. The approach eliminates the need for low-yield transbronchial biopsy or other invasive procedure to establish a definitive diagnosis of bronchiolitis obliterans. A clinical severity classification has been used.[49] A National Institutes of Health (NIH) diagnostic classification of BOS in cGVHD[50] has also been developed (Table 51-4).

Many years after the initial description of bronchiolitis obliterans occurring in lung transplant recipients, BOS remains a common process with devastating consequences.[51] At least one-half of lung transplantation recipients surviving 5 years will develop airflow obstruction. BOS has not declined significantly in incidence, and no totally effective treatment is available.

TABLE 51-4 Bronchiolitis Obliterans Syndrome (BOS) Classifications

BOS clinical severity classification	
BOS 0	FEV_1 >90% of baseline and FEF_{25-75} >75% baseline
BOS 0-p	FEV_1 81–90% of baseline and/or FEF_{25-75} ≤75%
BOS 1	FEV_1 66–80% of baseline
BOS 2	FEV_1 51–65% of baseline
BOS 3	FEV_1 50% or less of baseline
NIH chronic graft-versus-host BOS classification	
1. FEV_1 <70% predicted or FEV_1/FVC <70%	
2. Expiratory HRCT showing air trapping, small airway thickening or bronchiectasis, residual volume >120% predicted, or constrictive bronchiolitis by pathology	
3. Absence of respiratory infection	

The frequency and severity of acute cellular rejection continues to be the major risk factor. For example, a study showed that lung transplant recipients who had more than three episodes of acute rejection in any 12-month period eventually had a 100% incidence of bronchiolitis obliterans.[52] Both types of acute rejection are involved, including acute vascular rejection and lymphocytic bronchiolitis.

Primary graft dysfunction (PGD) is a term used for a process that occurs during the initial postoperative phase characterized by pulmonary edema and acute respiratory failure. This process has been associated with high perioperative mortality and is a risk factor for the subsequent severity of bronchiolitis obliterans.[53]

A classification system for PGD (Table 51-5) has been established based on oxygenation and the presence of pulmonary edema.[54]

Daud et al.[55] found that among 334 lung transplant recipients, 130 (39%) had grade-one PGD, 69 (20%) had grade-two, and 70 (21%) had grade-three. All grades were associated with increased risk of bronchiolitis obliterans, with a risk ratio ranging from 1.73 for grade-one to 2.53 for grade-three. This risk was independent of acute rejection.

Innate immunity may play a role in development of postlung transplant bronchiolitis obliterans. There are several risk factors that activate this innate system, including prolonged ischemic time, cytomegalovirus (CMV) pneumonia, *Aspergillus* colonization, PGD, gastroesophageal reflux disease (GERD), and community respiratory virus infections.[51]

Autoimmunity as a mediator in BOS has been proposed as a biphasic rejection.[56] The first phase is recurrent tissue injury from airway insults, and the second phase is sequestered self-antigens and fragments released into the lung, triggering autoreactive T-cell proliferation and autoantibody production.

TABLE 51-5 Classification of Primary Graft Dysfunction (PGD)

PGD grade 0: Pa_{O_2}/FI_{O_2} >300 mm Hg
PGD grade 1: Pa_{O_2}/FI_{O_2} >300 mm Hg and pulmonary edema
PGD grade 2: Pa_{O_2}/FI_{O_2} 200–300 mm Hg and pulmonary edema
PGD grade 3: Pa_{O_2}/FI_{O_2} <200 mm Hg and pulmonary edema

Pa_{O_2}/FI_{O_2}: Arterial oxygen (mm Hg) to the fraction of inspired oxygen.

Eberlein et al.[57] found that an oversized allograft can be associated with improvement, including higher expiratory airflows, and less frequent occurrence of BOS. Circulating fibrocyte levels correlated with BOS after lung transplantation.[58] Levels of KL-6, a high–molecular-weight human MUC1 gene mucin, are increased and correlated with the level of FEV_1 decline in lung transplantation recipients.[59] Bourdin et al.[60] showed that donor Clara cell secretory protein polymorphism is a risk factor for BOS. Gastroesophageal reflux, a cause of bronchiolitis obliterans, occurs in as many as 50% of lung transplant recipients, and early fundoplication may improve rates of bronchiolitis obliterans and survival.[61]

Chronic productive cough and shortness of breath were commonly reported as symptoms in early reports, but bronchiolitis obliterans is now diagnosed earlier than in the past, and these symptoms may not be present. Gradual onset of progressive shortness of breath is the most common symptom. Early inspiratory crackles may be heard. The decreases in FEV_1 may be mild to severe and life-threatening.

The chest x-ray is often normal; however, the combination of newly decreased FEV_1 and the expiratory high-resolution chest CT scan showing mosaic pattern have virtually become diagnostic.[62]

Management of lung transplantation bronchiolitis obliterans begins with early and aggressive treatment of acute organ rejection, including both the acute vascular rejection and lymphocytic bronchiolitis. Treatment of bronchiolitis obliterans generally includes a calcineurin inhibitor, a purine synthesis inhibitor, and a corticosteroid.

The calcineurin inhibitor tacrolimus has become an alternative to cyclosporine, with evidence for similar survival and a decrease in episodes of acute rejection with use of tacrolimus.[63] In addition, compliance with tacrolimus appears to be better than cyclosporine. New-onset diabetes after transplantation is a major complication of tacrolimus, and there is an increased risk of infections.

Mycophenolate mofetil (MMF) has generally replaced azathioprine[64] as the purine synthesis inhibitor. Both alloimmune and nonalloimmune mechanisms are involved in development of bronchiolitis obliterans; therefore, vigorous treatment of infections is needed at all times during the posttransplant period.

Extracorporeal photopheresis (ECP) appears to be effective for early treatment of BOS. It consists of the patient's white blood cells being exposed to ultraviolet light in the presence of 8-methoxypsoralen in a photoactivation chamber.[65,66] In a study of 60 lung transplant recipients, ECP treatment decreased the rate of the FEV_1 decline and improved FEV_1 actual value by 25% in patients. In addition, the rate of decline in lung function was sustained over both the 6- and 12-month period.[65] In a study of 1012 lung transplant recipients, 194 developed BOS and 51 received ECP.[66] There were 31 (61%) who responded to the therapy and showed sustained stabilization of the FEV_1 for at least 6 months. Responders showed significantly greater survival and less need for re-transplantation. Treatment was more effective when given soon after the diagnosis of BOOP.

The macrolides, such as erythromycin, appear to be an effective treatment in a subset of patients with BOS. The finding of bronchoalveolar lavage neutrophils may distinguish responders from nonresponders.[67] The process in the responders is referred to as neutrophilic reversible allograft airway dysfunction (NRAD).[68] An additional important finding about azithromycin is that this agent may reduce gastroesophageal reflux in lung transplant recipients, further decreasing the risk of constrictive bronchiolitis.[67] Early treatment resulted in responders having more lower-grade BOS.[69] A thin-section CT study showed patients with NRAD had more centrilobular nodularity at the beginning of treatment, and they had improved bronchus dilation, consolidation, and air trapping.[70]

The six-minute walk test can be useful for monitoring lung transplant recipients with bronchiolitis obliterans. In a 2009 study, patients who walked farther than 330 m had a median survival of 1178 days, compared to 263 days for lung recipients who walked less.[71]

A 2011 study of traffic air pollution as estimated by the proximity of the home to a major road showed that lung transplant recipients living near a major road within 171 m were 2.06 times more likely to develop BOS and 2.20 times more likely to die than patients living far away.[72]

Aspiration Bronchiolitis Obliterans

Aspiration bronchiolitis obliterans was first reported in 1908 occurring in a 2.5-year-old child who aspirated a prune pit that eventually caused respiratory failure and death.[73] Activated charcoal used for management of a medication-related suicide attempts has been reported as a cause of bronchiolitis obliterans.[74] Massive gastroesophageal reflux has been reported as a cause of bronchiolitis obliterans in a patient who later underwent a gastrojejunostomy that relieved the symptoms and prevented recurrent aspiration, accompanied by a corresponding improvement in the FEV_1.[75]

Neuroendocrine Hyperplasia-Related Bronchiolitis Obliterans

Neuroendocrine hyperplasia-related bronchiolitis obliterans has been reported to occur among six patients who developed shortness of breath and fibrotic bronchioles.[76] In a case report of a 65-year-old man who had 20 years of shortness of breath and a severely decreased FEV_1 of 19% predicted, neuroendocrine hyperplasia with fibrotic narrowed bronchioles was observed.[77] In addition, in another report of two women who had airflow obstruction and unexplained cystic lung disease, biopsies showed showed diffuse idiopathic neuroendocrine cell hyperplasia.[78]

Carcinoid-Related Bronchiolitis Obliterans

Carcinoid-related bronchiolitis obliterans has occurred in patients with multiple tumorlets and microcarcinoids located within the bronchioles, resulting in bronchiolitis obliterans and airflow obstruction.[38,79]

Sauropus Androgynus Bronchiolitis Obliterans

Sauropus androgynus bronchiolitis obliterans has been reported among women who consume this leafy vegetable. It is cultivated in India, Malaysia, Indonesia, China, and Vietnam. The leaves are boiled and blended with pineapples or guavas to make a mixed vegetable-fruit juice which is consumed for its alleged effects of body weight reduction and blood pressure control. The leaves contain the alkaloid papaverine. Among 194 patients in Taiwan, the obstructive ventilatory defect was irreversible and resulted in progressive deterioration in some patients resulting in lung transplantation.[80] In a report of five patients in Japan, the illness occurred 6 months after ingestion; four were mothers and daughters, and none improved with corticosteroid treatment.[81]

Stevens–Johnson-Related Bronchiolitis Obliterans

Stevens–Johnson-related bronchiolitis obliterans has been described in a woman who developed progressive dyspnea 12 days after developing diffuse oral erythematous lesions and blisters after antibiotic therapy.[82] She developed progressive respiratory failure and died 2 months later. Autopsy showed constrictive bronchiolitis with obliterated bronchioles.

Primary Biliary Cirrhosis Bronchiolitis Obliterans

Primary biliary cirrhosis bronchiolitis obliterans has been reported in a 39-year-old woman.[83] Early there was improvement from corticosteroid therapy, but later deterioration and death. Lung tissue showed concentric submucosal fibrosis and scarring, constricting the lumen of the airway, consistent with constrictive bronchiolitis and bronchiolar airway obliteration.

Paraneoplastic Autoimmune Multi-Organ Syndrome Bronchiolitis Obliterans

Paraneoplastic autoimmune multi-organ syndrome bronchiolitis obliterans, also referred to as paraneoplastic pemphigus-related bronchiolitis obliterans, has been reported in several patients.[38,84–86] A patient with myasthenia gravis died from bronchiolitis obliterans after surgical resection of a Castleman tumor.[84] Another patient had this paraneoplastic syndrome and developed constrictive bronchiolitis.[85] In a 2009 report from Mayo Clinic of three patients, all had severe airflow obstruction, with FEV_1 <1 L.[86] Two of them died and the third had stable chronic respiratory failure. A case report describes a 44-year-old woman with Castleman tumor and paraneoplastic syndrome; autopsy showed partial obliteration of the bronchiolar lumen by fibrolymphocytic tissue and dense inflammatory infiltrates surrounding the bronchioles. The oral mucosa, skin and bronchioles showed similar immunophenotypes.[87]

Swyer–James Syndrome Bronchiolitis Obliterans

Swyer–James syndrome bronchiolitis obliterans is not congenital in origin but is secondary to respiratory infection occurring during infancy.[38,88] Respiratory infections that can cause this syndrome include measles, whooping cough, tuberculosis, *Mycoplasma* pneumonia, influenza A, and adenovirus types 3, 7, and 21.

Miscellaneous Systemic Disorders Associated with Bronchiolitis Obliterans

Bronchiolitis obliterans has been reported in four patients with *ataxia-telangiectasia* who died from respiratory failure secondary to bronchiolitis obliterans.[89] Another report describes an elderly man with renal failure from *IgA nephropathy* characterized by diffuse crescentic glomerulonephritis who died from progressive respiratory failure and bronchiolitis obliterans.[90] *HIV-related bronchiolitis obliterans and* [91] *inflammatory bowel disease bronchiolitis obliterans* have been reported.[38]

SUMMARY

In summary, the bronchiolar airway diseases include acute and chronic bronchiolitis, follicular bronchiolitis, diffuse panbronchiolitis, and bronchiolitis obliterans. Acute bronchiolitis is usually transient, whereas diffuse panbronchiolitis responds to macrolide therapy. Postlung transplantation bronchiolitis obliterans continues to be a major problem, with minimal change in frequency or response to treatment.

REFERENCES

1. Colby TV. Bronchiolitis. Pathologic considerations. *Am J Clin Pathol.* 1998;109(1):101–109.
2. Plopper CG, Have-Opbroek AW. Chapter 2: Anatomical and histological classification of the bronchioles. In: Epler GR, ed. *Diseases of the Bronchioles.* New York, NY: Raven Press; 1994:15–25.
3. Ryu JH, Myers JL, Swensen SJ. Bronchiolar disorders. *Am J Respir Crit Care Med.* 2003;168:1277–1292.
4. Cottin V, Streichenberger N, Gamondes JP, Thevenet F, Loire R, Cordier JF. Respiratory bronchiolitis in smokers with spontaneous pneumothorax. *Eur Resp J.* 1998;12:702–704.
5. Terada T. Follicular bronchiolitis and lymphocytic interstitial pneumonia in a Japanese man. *Diagn Pathol.* 2011;6:85.
6. Azuma A, Kudoh S. Diffuse panbronchiolitis in East Asia. *Respirology.* 2006;11(3):249–261.
7. Krishnan P, Thachil R, Gillego V. Diffuse panbronchiolitis: a treatable sinobronchial disease in need of recognition in the United States. *Chest.* 2002;121(2):659–661.
8. Sandrini A, Balter MS, Chapman KR. Diffuse panbronchiolitis in a Caucasian man in Canada. *Can Respir J.* 2003;10(8):449–451.
9. Anthony M, Singham S, Soans B, Tyler G. Diffuse panbronchiolitis: not just an Asian disease: Australian case series and review of the literature. *Biomed Imaging Interv J.* 2009;5(4):1–4.
10. Urbano Aranda Y, García San José I, López Gabaldón E. Diffuse panbronchiolitis: a very rare disease in Western countries. *Arch Bronconeumol.* 2012;48(5):184–185.
11. Mittal V, Shah A. Situs inversus totalis: the association of Kartagener's syndrome with diffuse bronchiolitis and azoospermia. *Arch Bronconeumol.* 2012;48(5):179–182.
12. Kono C, Yamaguchi T, Yamada Y, et al. Historical changes in epidemiology of diffuse panbronchiolitis. *Sarcoidosis Vasc Diffuse Lung Dis.* 2012;29(1):19–25.
13. Keicho N, Hijikata M. Genetic predisposition to diffuse panbronchiolitis. *Respirology.* 2011;16(4):581–588.
14. Li H, Zhou Y, Fan F, et al. Effect of azithromycin on patients with diffuse panbronchiolitis: retrospective study of 51 cases. *Intern Med.* 2011;50(16):1663–1669.
15. Cameron EJ, McSharry C, Chaudhuri R, Farrow S, Thomson NC. Long-term macrolide treatment of chronic inflammatory airway disease. *Clin Exp Allergy.* 2012;42(9):1302–1312.
16. Epler GR. Constrictive bronchiolitis obliterans: the fibrotic airway disorder. *Expert Rev Resp Med.* 2007;1(1):139–147.
17. Epler GR. Bronchiolitis obliterans organizing pneumonia (BOOP), 25 years. *Expert Rev Respir Med.* 2011;5(3):353–361.
18. Couture C, Colby TV. Histopathology of bronchiolar disorders. *Semin Respir Crit Care Med.* 2003;24(5):489–498.
19. Popper HH. Bronchiolitis, an update. *Virchows Arch.* 2000; 437(5):471–481.
20. Visscher DW, Myers JL. Bronchiolitis. The pathologist's perspective. *Proc Am Thorac Soc.* 2006;3:41–47.
21. Stern EJ, Frank MS. Small-airway diseases of the lungs: Findings at expiratory CT. *AJR Am J Roentgenol.* 1994;163:37–41.
22. Kang EY, Woo OH, Shin BK, Yong HS, Oh YW, Kim HK. Bronchiolitis: classification, computed tomographic and histopathologic features, and radiologic approach. *J Comput Assist Tomogr.* 2009;33(1):32–41.
23. Kraft M, Mortenson RL, Colby TV, Newman L, Waldron JA Jr, King TE Jr. Cryptogenic constrictive bronchiolitis. *Am Rev Respir Dis.* 1993;148:1093–1101.
24. Noble MI, Fox B, Horsfield K, et al. Obliterative bronchiolitis with atypical features: CT scan and necropsy findings. *Eur Respir J.* 1993;6(8):1221–1225.
25. Myong NH, Shin DH, Lee KY. A clinicopathologic study on three cases of constrictive bronchiolitis. *J Korean Med Sci.* 2001; 16(2):150–154.
26. Konichezky S, Schattner A, Ezri T, et al. Thionyl-chloride-induced lung injury and bronchiolitis obliterans. *Chest.* 1993; 104:971–973.
27. Tasaka S, Kanazawa M, Mori M, et al. Long-term course of bronchiectasis and bronchiolitis obliterans as late complication of smoke inhalation. *Respiration.* 1995;62:40–42.
28. Thomason JW, Rice TW, Milstone AP. Bronchiolitis obliterans in a survivor of a chemical weapons attack. *JAMA.* 2003; 290(5):598–599.
29. Ghanei M, Panahi Y, Mojtahedzadeh M, Khalili AH, Aslani J. Effect of gamma interferon on lung function of mustard gas exposed patients, after 15 years. *Pulm Pharmacol Ther.* 2006; 19:148–153.

30. King MS, Eisenberg R, Newman JH, et al. Constrictive bronchiolitis in soldiers returning from Iraq and Afghanistan. *N Engl J Med.* 2011;365(3):222–230.
31. Mann JM, Sha KK, Kline G, Breuer FU, Miller A. World Trade Center Dyspnea: bronchiolitis obliterans with functional improvement. *Am J Ind Med.* 2005;48:225–229.
32. Kawano-Dourado L, Baldi BG, Dias OM, et al. Scattered lung cysts as the main radiographic finding of constrictive bronchiolitis. *Am J Respir Crit Care Med.* 2012;186(3):294–295.
33. Akpinar-Elci M, Travis WD, Lynch DA, Kreiss K. Bronchiolitis obliterans syndrome in popcorn production plant workers. *Eur Respir J.* 2004;24:298–302.
34. Cavalcanti Zdo R, Albuquerque Filho AP, Pereira CA, Coletta EN. Bronchiolitis associated with exposure to artificial butter flavoring in workers at a cookie factory in Brazil. *J Bras Pneumol.* 2012;38(3):395–399.
35. Penn CC, Liu C. Bronchiolitis following infection in adults and children. *Clin Chest Med.* 1993;14:645–654.
36. Daxböck F, Brunner G, Popper H, et al. A case of lung transplantation following Mycoplasma pneumoniae infection. *Eur J Clin Microbiol Infect Dis.* 2002;21(4):318–322.
37. White ES, Tazelaar HD, Lynch JP. Bronchiolar complications of connective tissue diseases. *Sem Resp Crit Care Med.* 2003;24(5):547–565.
38. Parambil JG, Yi ES, Ryu JH. Obstructive bronchiolar disease identified in the non-transplant population. *Respirology.* 2009;14:443–448.
39. Devouassoux G, Cottin V, Lioté H, et al. Characterisation of severe obliterative bronchiolitis in rheumatoid arthritis. *Eur Respir J.* 2009;33:1053–1061.
40. Boehler A, Vogt P, Speich R, Weder W, Russi EW. Bronchiolitis obliterans in a patient with localized scleroderma treated with D-penicillamine. *Eur Respir J.* 1996;9:1317–1319.
41. Pegg SJ, Lang BA, Mikhail EL, Hughes DM. Fatal bronchiolitis obliterans in a patient with juvenile rheumatoid arthritis receiving chrysotherapy. *J Rheumatol.* 1994;21:549–551.
42. Marras TK, Chan CK. Obliterative bronchiolitis complication bone marrow transplantation. *Sem Resp Crit Care Med.* 2003;24(5):531–542.
43. Sano Y, Date H, Nagahiro I, Aoe M, Shimizu N. Living-donor lobar lung transplantation for bronchiolitis obliterans after bone marrow transplantation. *Ann Thorac Surg.* 2005;79:1051–1052.
44. Chien JW, Duncan S, Williams KM, Pavletic SZ. Bronchiolitis obliterans syndrome after allogeneic hematopoietic stem cell transplantation– an increasingly recognized manifestation of chronic graft-versus-host disease. *Biol Blood Marrow Transplant.* 2010;16(1 Suppl):S106-S114.
45. Nakaseko C, Ozawa S, Sakaida E, et al. Incidence, risk factors and outcomes of bronchiolitis obliterans after allogeneic stem cell transplantation. *Int J Hematol.* 2011;93(3):375–382.
46. Song I, Yi CA, Han J, et al. CT findings of late-onset noninfectious pulmonary complications in patients with pathologically proven graft-versus-host disease after allogeneic stem cell transplant. *AJR Am J Roentgenol.* 2012;199(3):581–587.
47. Pandya CM, Soubani AO. Bronchiolitis obliterans following hematopoietic stem cell transplantation: a clinical update. *Clin Transplant.* 2010;24(3):291–306.
48. Liang W, Xia H, Wang Y, Zhao RC. Allogeneic mesenchymal stem cell injections for the treatment of bronchiolitis obliterans syndrome following allogeneic hematopoietic stem cell transplantation. *J Cancer Sci Ther.* 2012;4(7):185–187.
49. Estenne M, Hertz MI. Bronchiolitis obliterans after human lung transplantation. *Am J Respir Crit Care Med.* 2002;166(4):440–444.
50. Filipovich AH, Weisdorf D, Pavletic S, et al. National Institutes of Health consensus development project on criteria for clinical trials in chronic graft-versus-host disease: I. Diagnosis and staging working group report. *Biol Blood Marrow Transplant.* 2005;11(12):945–956.
51. Todd JL, Palmer SM. Bronchiolitis obliterans syndrome. *Chest.* 2011;140(2):502–508.
52. Keller CA, Cagle PT, Brown RW, Noon G, Frost AE. Bronchiolitis obliterans in recipients of single, double, and heart-lung transplantation. *Chest.* 1995;107:973–980.
53. Burton CM, Iversen M, Milman N, et al. Outcome of lung transplanted patients with primary graft dysfunction. *Eur J Cardiothorac Surg.* 2007;31(1):75–82.
54. Christie JD, Carby M, Bag R, Corris P, Hertz M, Weill D. Report of the ISHLT Working Group on Primary Lung Graft Dysfunction Part II: Definition. A consensus statement of the International Society for Heart and Lung Transplantation. *J Heart Lung Transplant.* 2005;24:1454–1459.
55. Daud SA, Yusen RD, Meyers B, et al. Impact of immediate primary lung allograft dysfunction on bronchiolitis obliterans syndrome. *Am J Respir Crit Care Med.* 2007;175:507–513.
56. Sumpter TL, Wilkes DS. Role of autoimmunity in organ allograft rejection: a focus on immunity to type V collagen in the pathogenesis of lung transplant rejection. *Am J Physiol Lung Cell Mol Physiol.* 2004;286(6):L1129–L1139.
57. Eberlein M, Permutt S, Chahla MF, et al. Lung size mismatch in bilateral lung transplantation is associated with allograft function and bronchiolitis obliterans syndrome. *Chest.* 2012;141(2):451–460.
58. LaPar DJ, Burdick MD, Emaminia A, et al. Circulating fibrocytes correlate with bronchiolitis obliterans syndrome development after lung transplantation: a novel clinical biomarker. *Ann Thorac Surg.* 2011;92:470–477.
59. Ohshimo S, Bonella F, Sommerwerck U, et al. Comparison of serum KL-6 versus bronchoalveolar lavage neutrophilia for the diagnosis of bronchiolitis obliterans in lung transplantation. *J Heart Lung Transplant.* 2011;30:1374–1380.
60. Bourdin A, Mifsud NA, Chanez B, et al. Donor clara cell secretory protein polymorphism is a risk factor for bronchiolitis obliterans syndrome after lung transplantation. *Transplantation.* 2012;94:652–658.
61. Cantu E, Appel JZ, Hartwig MG, et al. Early fundoplication prevents chronic allograft dysfunction in patients with gastroesophageal reflux disease. *Ann Thorac Surg.* 2004;78:1142–1151.
62. Knollmann FD, Kapell S, Lehmkuhl H, et al. Dynamic high-resolution electron-beam CT scanning for the diagnosis of bronchiolitis obliterans syndrome after lung transplantation. *Chest.* 2004;126:447–456.
63. Fan Y, Xiao YB, Weng YG. Tacrolimus versus cyclosporine for adult lung transplant recipients. *Transplant Proc.* 2009;41:1821–1824.
64. Celik MR, Lederer DJ, Wilt J, et al. Tacrolimus and azathioprine versus cyclosporine and mycophenolate mofetil after lung transplantation. *J Heart Lung Transplant.* 2009;28:697–703.
65. Morrell MR, Despotis GJ, Lublin DM, Patterson GA, Trulock EP, Hachem RR. The Efficacy of photopheresis for bronchiolitis obliterans syndrome after lung transplantation. *J Heart Lung Transplant.* 2010;29:242–431.

66. Jaksch P, Scheed A, Keplinger M, et al. A prospective interventional study on the use of extracorporeal photopheresis in patients with bronchiolitis obliterans syndrome after lung transplantation. *J Heart Lung Transplant.* 2012;31:950–957.
67. Verleden GM, Vos R, De Vleeschauwer SI, et al. Obliterative bronchiolitis following lung transplantation. *Eur Soc Organ Transplant.* 2009;22:773–779.
68. Verleden GM, Vos R, De Vleeschauwer S, et al. Neutrophilic reversible airways dysfunction after liver transplantation. *Transplant Proc.* 2011;43:2078–2081.
69. Federica M, Nadia S, Monica M, et al. Clinical and immunological evaluation of 12-month azithromycin therapy in chronic lung allograft rejection. *Clin Transplant.* 2011;25:E381–E389.
70. De Jong PA, Vos R, Verleden GM, Vanaudenaerde BM, Verschakelen JA. Thin-section computed tomography findings before and after azithromycin treatment of neutrophilic reversible lung allograft dysfunction. *Eur Radiol.* 2011;21:2466–2474.
71. Nathan SD, Shlobin OA, Reese E, et al. Prognostic value of the 6 min walk test in bronchiolitis obliterans syndrome. *Respir Med.* 2009,103(12):1816–1821.
72. Nawrot TS, Vos R, Jacobs L, et al. The impact of traffic air pollution on bronchiolitis obliterans syndrome and mortality after lung transplantation. *Thorax.* 2011;66:748–754.
73. Epler GR. Miscellaneous causes of bronchiolitis obliterans. In: Epler GR, ed. *Diseases of the Bronchioles.* New York, NY:Raven Press; 1994; 15–25.
74. Elliott CG, Colby TV, Kelly TM, Hicks HG. Charcoal lung: bronchiolitis obliterans after aspiration of activated charcoal. *Chest.* 1989;96(3):672–674.
75. Rinaldi M, Martinelli L, Volpato G, et al. Gastro-esophageal reflux as cause of obliterative bronchiolitis: a case report. *Transplant Proc.* 1995;27(3):2006–2007.
76. Miller RR, Müller NL. Neuroendocrine cell hyperplasia and obliterative bronchiolitis in patients with peripheral carcinoid tumors. *Am J Surg Pathol.* 1995;19:653–658.
77. Brown MJ, English J, Müller NL. Bronchiolitis obliterans due to neuroendocrine hyperplasia. *AJR Am J Roentgenol.* 1997;168:1561–1562.
78. Rowan C, Hansell DM, Renzoni E, et al. Diffuse cystic lung disease of unexplained cause with coexistent small airway disease. *Am J Surg Pathol.* 2012;36:228–234.
79. Sheerin N, Harrison NK, Sheppard MN, Hansell DM, Yacoub M, Clark TJ. obliterative bronchiolitis caused by multiple tumourlets and microcarcinoids successfully treated by single lung transplantation. *Thorax.* 1995;50:207–209.
80. Hsiue TR, Guo YL, Chen KW, Chen CW, Lee CH, Chang HY. Dose-response relationship and irreversible obstructive ventilatory defect in patients with consumption of Sauropus androgynus. *Chest.* 1998;113(1):71–76.
81. Oonakahara K, Matsuyama W, Higashimoto I, et al. Outbreak of bronchiolitis obliterans associated with consumption of Sauropus androgynus in Japan. *Respiration.* 2005;72:221.
82. Tsunoda N, Iwanaga T, Saito T, Kitamura S, Saito K. Rapidly progressive bronchiolitis obliterans associated with Stevens-Johnson syndrome. *Chest.* 1990;98(1):243–245.
83. Chatte G, Streichenberger N, Boillot O, Gille D, Loire R, Cordier JF. Lymphocytic bronchitis/bronchiolitis in a patient with primary biliary cirrhosis. *Eur Respir J.* 1995;8:176–179.
84. Chorzelski T, Hashimoto T, Maciejewska B, Amagai M, Anhalt GJ, Jablonska S. Paraneoplastic pemphigus associated with Castleman tumor, myasthenia gravis and bronchiolitis obliterans. *J Am Acad Derm.* 1999;41:393–400.
85. Hasegawa Y, Shimokata K, Ichiyama S, Saito H. Constrictive bronchiolitis obliterans and paraneoplastic pemphigus. *Eur Resp J.* 1999;13:934–937.
86. Maldonado F, Pittelkow MR, Ryu JH. Constrictive bronchiolitis associated with paraneoplastic autoimmune multi-organ syndrome. *Respirology.* 2009;14:129–133.
87. Iida K, Yamaguchi F, Hibi K, Tate G, et al. Characterisation of inflammatory infiltrates in lesions of the oral mucosa, skin, and bronchioles in a case of paraneoplastic pemphigus. *Eur J Dermatol.* 2012;22(1):154–155.
88. Sulaiman A, Cavaille A, Vaunois B, Tiffet O. Swyer-James-MacLeod syndrome; repeated chest drainages in a patient misdiagnosed with pneumothorax. *Interact Cardiovasc Thorac Surg.* 2009;8:482–484.
89. Ito M, Nakagawa A, Hirabayashi N, Asai J. Bronchiolitis obliterans in ataxia-telangiectasia. *Virchows Arch.* 1997;430(2):131–137.
90. Hernandez JL, Gomez-Roman J, Rodrigo E, et al. Bronchiolitis obliterans and IgA nephropathy. *Am J Respir Crit Care Med.* 1997;156:665–668.
91. Diaz F, Collazos J, Martinez E, Mayo J. Bronchiolitis obliterans in a patient with HIV infection. *Resp Med.* 1997;91:171–173.

CHAPTER 52

Bullous Disease of the Lung

Fernando J. Martinez

DEFINITION

A *bulla* is an air-containing space within the lung parenchyma that arises from destruction, dilatation, and confluence of airspaces distal to terminal bronchioles and is larger than 1 cm in diameter (Fig. 52-1).[1] Its walls are composed of attenuated and compressed parenchyma. Bullae occur in various clinical contexts: (1) with emphysema ("bullous emphysema"); (2) with pulmonary fibrosis, as in the late stages of sarcoidosis or complicated pneumoconiosis; (3) in so-called "vanishing lung," in which the parenchyma is rapidly replaced by multiple bullae; and (4) in lungs that are otherwise normal ("bullous lung disease") and, therefore, likely secondary to a mechanism different from that of bullae occurring in conjunction with emphysema (Table 52-1).[2,3]

Distinctions are drawn between bullae, blebs, and cysts (Table 52-2).[2] A *bleb* is an accumulation of air between the two layers of the visceral pleura that arises when the thin covering of the bleb ruptures and permits entry of air (Fig. 52-1). *Cysts* are epithelial-lined cavities that may resemble bullae on radiographs.[3] Many fall into the category of developmental anomalies and include mixtures of mesenchymal and epithelial components that are normally present in the lung. The pathologic nature of these cystic lesions is reflected

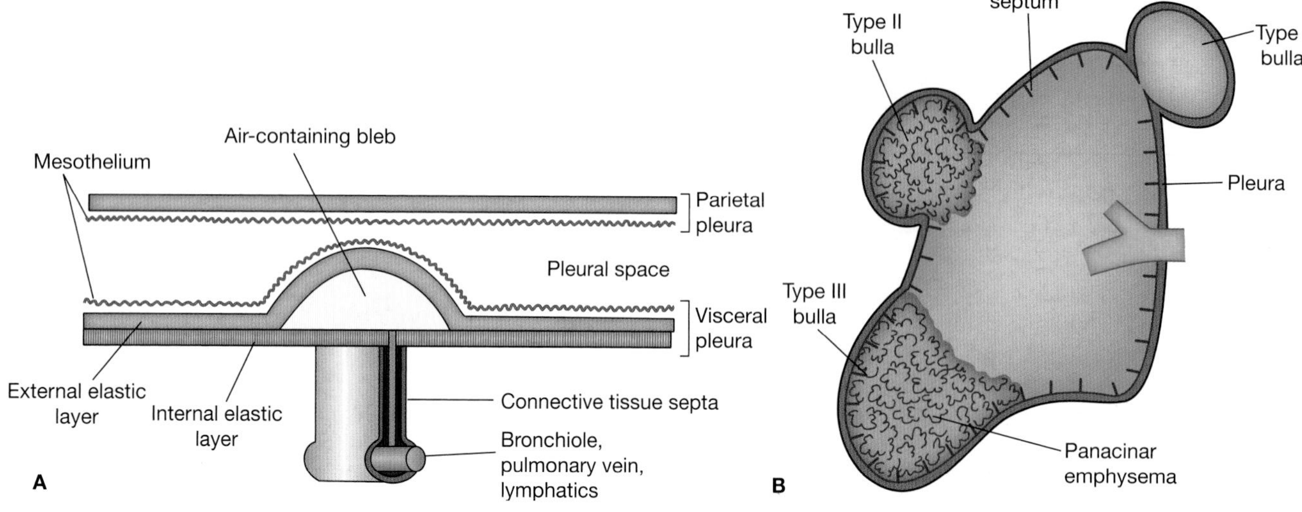

Figure 52-1 Blebs and bullae. **A.** Development of a bleb. A bleb is an accumulation of air within the pleura that is not confined by connective tissue septa within the lung. Air that escapes within the substance of the lungs makes its way to the surface, separating the internal from the external elastic layers on the visceral pleura. **B.** Different types of bullae. In contrast to a bleb, a bulla is confined by connective tissue septa of the lung and is deep to the internal elastic layer of the visceral pleura. Three different types of bullae are shown arising from a lung that has been removed from within the chest wall. A type I bulla is shown at the apex, a type II is in the middle zone, and a type III is arising at the base. The short *dark lines* denote connective tissue septa. Panacinar emphysematous parenchyma is present within the types II and III bullae. *(Adapted with permission from Reid L. The Pathology of Emphysema. Chicago: Year Book; 1967:211–240.)*

in their names: "cystic adenomatoid malformations," "peripheral bronchogenic cysts," "congenital polycystic disease," and "atypical bronchopulmonary sequestration."[1]

The term *bullous disease* is reserved for multiple bullae in lungs that are otherwise normal.[2] This entity is different in etiology and pathogenesis from that in which bullae occur in conjunction with underlying chronic obstructive pulmonary disease (COPD). Confusion occasionally arises between the two entities because some pathologists regard bullous disease as a subset of panacinar emphysema.[1] However, this view is not useful as (1) panacinar emphysema tends to occur in the lower lobes, whereas bullous disease favors the upper lobes; (2) the natural history of the two disorders is quite different; and (3) panacinar emphysema has certain distinctive features not shared by bullous disease. Bullae may occur not only as part of obstructive lung disease, but also as a complication of fibrotic lung disease (Table 52-1).

TABLE 52-1 Classification of Bullae

Primary
Vanishing lung syndrome
Single giant bulla
Bullous lung disease
Secondary
Emphysema
Paraseptal
Panacinar
Centriacinar
Pulmonary fibrosis
Sarcoidosis
Idiopathic pulmonary fibrosis
Progressive massive fibrosis
Conglomerate silicosis
Fibrotic tuberculosis
Other fibrotic lung disorders
Familial disorders
α_1-antitrypsin deficiency
Ehlers–Danlos syndrome
Salla disease
Marfan syndrome
Fabry disease
Cutis laxa

ETIOLOGY

Bullae may originate in a variety of clinical and pathogenetic settings: (1) with emphysema of distal acini; (2) in the setting of cigarette smoking; (3) in conjunction with scar tissue formation, which "traps" areas of normal lung, enlarges airspaces by traction on surrounding intact alveoli, or produces retraction or shrinkage of intact walls of adherent alveoli; (4) in the setting of intravenous drug abuse; (5) as a result of chronic inflammation and destructive

TABLE 52-2 Characteristics of Blebs, Bullae, and Cysts

	Bleb	Bulla	Cyst
Site	Within visceral pleura	Arises within secondary lobule	Lung parenchyma or mediastinum
Size	1–2 cm	1 cm to 75% of a lung	2–10 cm
Lining	Elastic laminae of the pleura	Connective tissue septa	Epithelium
Associated condition	Spontaneous pneumothorax	Bronchogenic carcinoma	Respiratory infection

changes in terminal and first-order respiratory bronchioles, resulting in airspace distention from delayed emptying; and (6) with α_1-antitrypsin deficiency.[2,4,5]

CLASSIFICATION

Bullae are classified anatomically into three main types (Fig. 52-1B).[1,2] Type I bullae are characterized by a narrow neck that connects the bullae with the pulmonary parenchyma. This type of bulla may be caused by overinflation of a volume of flawed lung tissue. The walls of type I bullae are thin, and their interiors are empty. Type I bullae are usually found at the lung apices and along the edges of the lingula and middle lobes. They often occur in association with paraseptal emphysema. Scanning electron microscopy has demonstrated that the thin neck is a consistent feature and that pleural mesothelial cells on the external surface are either reduced in number or completely absent; bundles of collagen fibers lie naked and separated from one other by small pores or crevices.

Type II bullae arise from the subpleural parenchyma and are characterized by a neck of panacinar emphysematous lung tissue. The interior of these airspaces consists of emphysematous lung in which blood vessels are still present. In contrast to type I bullae, the outer wall is formed by pleura covered with intact mesothelial cells. Although connective tissue septae are present within the bullae, they are not found in the wall. Type II bullae may occur anywhere in the lung, but they are most frequent in the upper lobe, at the anterior surface of the middle lobe, and over the diaphragm.

Type III bullae consist of slightly hyperinflated lung connected to the rest of the lung by a broad base extending deep into the parenchyma. This type is believed to represent an atrophic form of emphysema.

PATHOGENESIS

Several hypotheses have been proposed over the years for how bullae develop, although none have been proved.[1,2,3,6] These include (1) weakness of the alveolar walls predisposes to the formation of bullae, particularly at the apices of the lungs, where pleural pressures are most negative. This theory underscores the proclivity of bullae for the upper lobes and stresses the influence of mechanical forces acting upon flawed tissue. (2) Inflammatory disease of a bronchiole leads to progressive air trapping and "tension airspaces." (3) Disordered collateral ventilation produces the findings. (4) The same mechanisms responsible for generalized emphysema are operative in the formation of bullae. (5) Underlying paraseptal emphysema produces bullous disease.

Of all the hypotheses, that of underlying paraseptal emphysema is the most popular.[1,2] The hypothesis envisages destruction of alveoli adjacent to connective septae or the pleura. The pattern relates to the fact that capillaries in alveolar walls that abut connective tissue septa are less numerous than elsewhere because of a sparse network of arterioles and arteries in peripheral alveoli. Consequently, these regions of the acinus have less vascularity and greater compliance.

Dynamic computerized tomography and intrabulla pressure measurements have raised questions about the theory that bullae are formed by positive pressure within the airspace.[1,7] The lung surrounding a bulla is less compliant than the bulla itself; accordingly, the pressure necessary to inflate the surrounding lung is greater than that necessary to inflate the bulla. The pressure within a giant bulla has been found to be the same as pleural pressure. Therefore, when a bulla and its surrounding lung are exposed to the same negative pleural pressure, the bulla fills preferentially and completely like an inflated paper bag, prior to the surrounding lung inflating. Further inspiration increases the elastic recoil pressure, thereby exerting a greater retractive force on the lung parenchyma and enlarging the airspace. Nevertheless, bullae can be removed from within the lung while still maintaining their volume, indicating a positive intrabulla pressure.

Bullae within the intact chest are molded and compressed to fit adjacent anatomic configurations. However, if the lung is released from these constraints (e.g., when removed from the chest cavity), bullae project as shiny bubbles at the lung surface (Fig. 52-2).

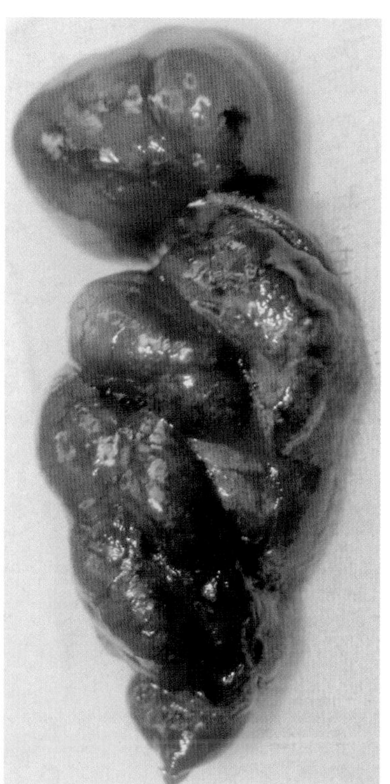

A

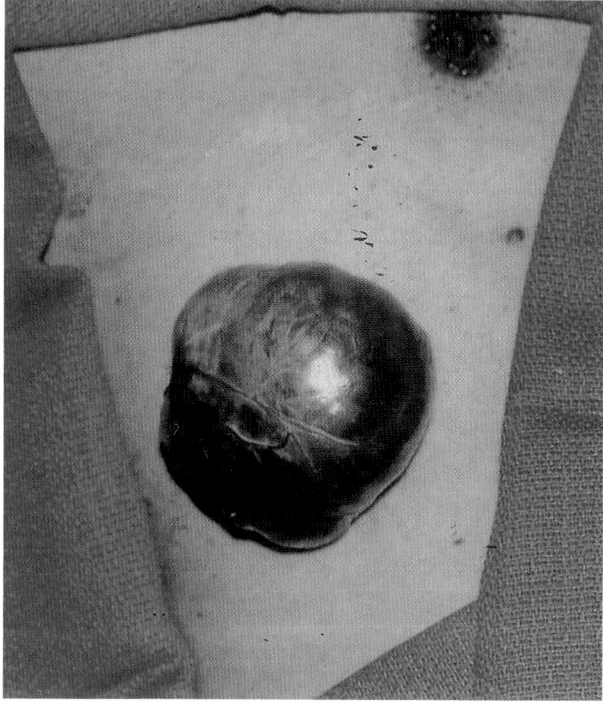

B

Figure 52-2 **A.** Surgically resected specimen with a bulla projecting from the lung surface. **B.** A bulla is shown projecting through a previous chest tube insertion site onto the surface of the skin.

Within the thoracic cavity, large bullae cause crowding of adjacent lung parenchyma, and structures such as bronchi are displaced, stretched, and narrowed over the bullae surfaces. Very large airspaces can expand across the midline or even extend into the neck. Bullae represent more than just overexpanded alveoli, because the remnants of bronchioles and their accompanying vessels sometimes persist as trabeculae within the bullae. Interlobular septae can be incorporated into the wall as the airspace expands from within the secondary lobule.

Two important risk factors for bullous emphysema are cigarette smoking and α_1-antitrypsin deficiency. Many patients with bullous emphysema are cigarette smokers, and most bullous lesions are associated with paraseptal or centriacinar emphysema. Although bullous emphysema is typically found in young males, elderly patients with α_1-antitrypsin deficiency who are lifelong nonsmokers may develop bullous changes in later life. A hereditary predisposition to bullous emphysema is also suggested by its association with a variety of rare familial disorders, including Fabry disease, Salla disease, cutis laxa, Ehlers–Danlos syndrome, and Marfan syndrome.[1] Giant bullous emphysema has also been reported with histologic changes of placental transmogrification—a rare, benign lung disease of unknown etiology in which the lung shows bullous changes or, rarely, cysts or nodules.[8,9] Lung pathology demonstrates papillary structures similar to placental villi surrounding the pulmonary epithelium. The tight skin mouse, which has a dominant mutation for the elastase gene and is characterized by multiple connective tissue abnormalities, serves as a unique model for bullous emphysema.[10]

DISTRIBUTION OF BULLAE

As noted previously, the tendency for bullae to occur in the upper lobes is usually attributed to the greater mechanical stresses imposed on the lung apices than bases. Because intrapleural pressure near the lung apices is more negative than at the bases, apical alveoli are subjected to greater expanding stresses than are basal alveoli. Radioactive gas studies and in situ freezing techniques have demonstrated that alveoli in the upper lung zones are considerably larger than those in the lower zones. Gravity also plays a role, as the upright lung behaves like a coiled spring, which, when allowed to dangle in the upright position, shows larger gaps between coils at the top than the bottom.

Engineering techniques used to study the distribution of stresses in aircraft have been applied to the analysis of stresses on the lung.[1] These have shown that the larger expanding stresses at the apices are directed primarily in a vertical direction, and to a lesser extent, laterally. The stresses tend to increase with expansion of the lung, but they are present also when the lung volume decreases below functional residual capacity (FRC). The increase in apical stress at low lung volumes has been attributed to an increase in the rigidity of the lungs as residual volume is approached.

EVALUATION AND DIAGNOSIS

In asymptomatic individuals, bullae may be detected in the course of routine chest radiography. Small bullae rarely become visible on the chest radiograph but are usually easily visible by computed tomography (CT). As a rule, small bullae usually produce no symptoms, signs, or discernible alterations in pulmonary function.[11] However, rupture of one or more bullae may lead to spontaneous pneumothorax (see below). In some patients bullae give rise to progressive dyspnea or chest pain (Fig. 52-3A,B).[12] On occasion, a patient with bullous lung disease develops sudden, severe breathlessness secondary to development of a spontaneous pneumothorax[13] or sudden increase in bulla size due to air trapping. In patients with known bullous disease infection in a bulla can occur (see below). Radiographically, infection is usually identified by the appearance of an air–fluid level (Fig. 52-4A).[4–6] The physical findings in a patient with one or more bullae usually reflect the overall state of the lungs. Only infrequently do giant bullae reach a size sufficient to cause a localized decrease in regional air entry, with absent breath sounds and increased resonance to percussion.

LABORATORY

Routine laboratory testing in the evaluation of bullae includes the measurement of hemoglobin and hematocrit to identify if anemia is contributing to respiratory symptoms and to assess for possible secondary polycythemia due to chronic hypoxemia.[1,12] Measuring an α_1-antitrypsin level should be obtained to diagnose α_1-antitrypsin deficiency.[14] Finally evaluation of arterial blood gases, performed while the patient is breathing room air if possible, is generally indicated in patients with severe respiratory insufficiency and those being evaluated for possible bullectomy.[12] As noted in Table 52-3, a Pa_{CO_2} greater than 45 mm Hg is considered a relative contraindication for bullectomy.[15]

IMAGING

Imaging techniques used in the evaluation of bullous lung disease include chest radiography, computed tomography, and nuclear medicine-based studies.

Chest Radiography

Although routine chest radiography is the most practical method for identifying the presence of bullae, the technique generally discloses less than 50% of bullae identified on CT.[16,17] In a given patient, serial radiographs taken over years are invaluable in tracing evolution of the disease.[11] The presence of the condition is suggested by areas of increased radiolucency that are sharply delineated by fine radiopaque lines representing the walls of the bullae. These lines, or "hairline shadows," are composed of compressed and fused interlobular septae or pleura.[10,18] Because the hairline shadows appear incomplete on the chest radiograph, they delineate only segments of the bulla wall (Fig. 52-3A). Distinction between hairline shadows produced by a bulla, and thicker, sometimes irregular, walls of a cavity is usually not difficult. More difficult is distinguishing bullae from cysts. The presence of other radiologic signs of emphysema or fibrotic lung disorders suggests that the cystic structure is a bulla.[13] Similarly, distinguishing between a large bulla and pneumothorax may be challenging.[12,19] In general, the pleural line associated with a large bulla is usually concave relative to the lateral chest wall, whereas the pleural line associated with a pneumothorax is convex relative to the lateral chest wall.[12] Similarly observation of "the double-wall sign" (i.e., the presence of air on both sides of the bulla wall) may be helpful in identifying the findings as due to a bulla.[18]

A chest radiograph obtained after forced expiration is sometimes helpful in demonstrating the presence of bullae: air trapping during the expiratory maneuver accentuates their outline by preventing a decrease in their size as the surrounding lung empties.[3] Large bullae sometimes displace the mediastinum contralaterally and may even compress the opposite lung.

Computed Tomography

CT provides valuable anatomic information about the size, number, and relationships of bullae, as well as crowding of adjacent lung and disposition of the pulmonary vasculature (Fig. 52-3B).[20–22] Bullae are identified as areas of radiolucency that usually do not contain blood vessels and that are confined by visible walls. High-resolution computed tomography (HRCT) shows that large bullae are frequently associated not only with distal acinar (paraseptal) emphysema, but also with centriacinar emphysema—the type of emphysema usually associated with cigarette smoking.[20]

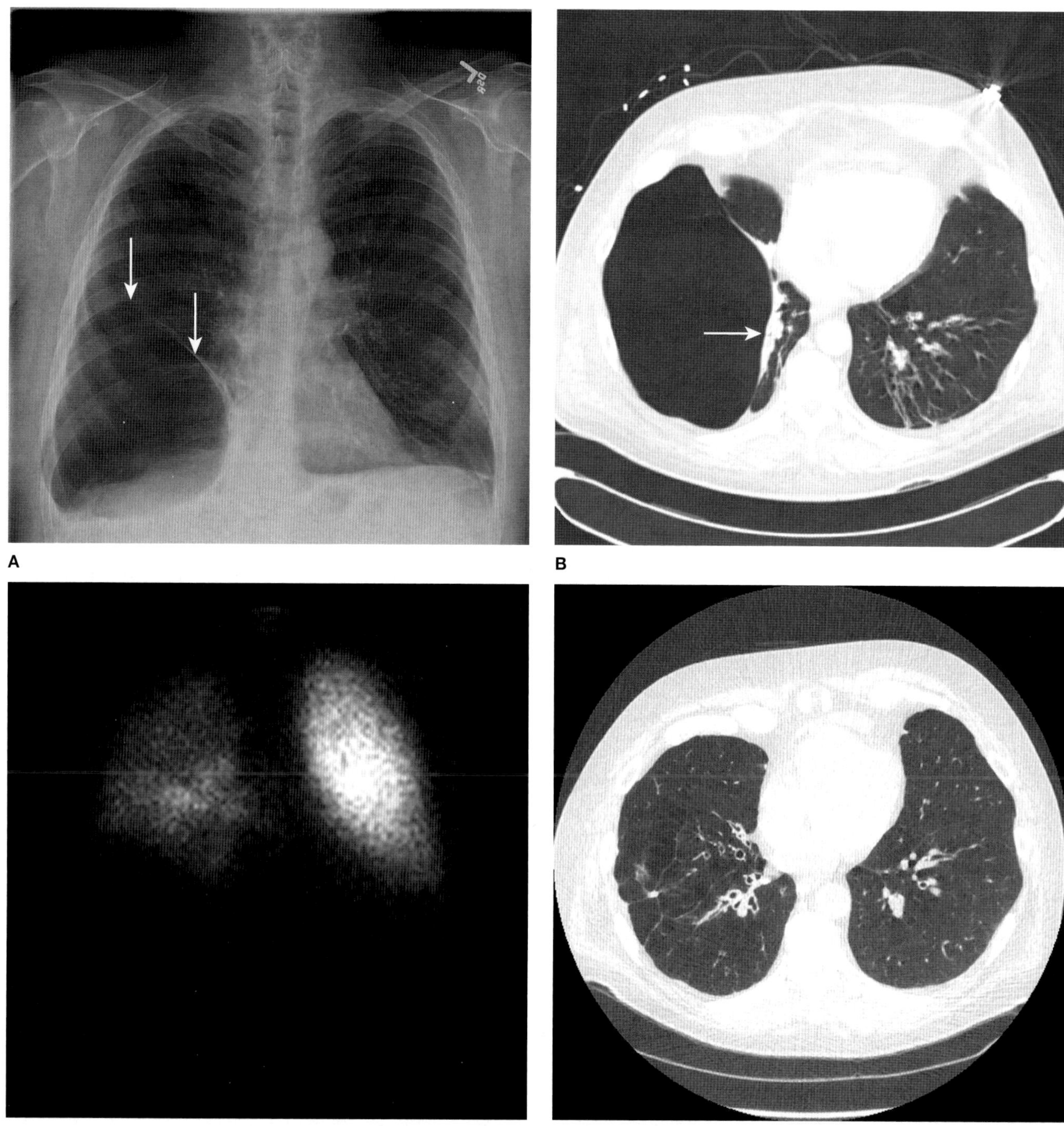

Figure 52-3 **A.** Chest radiograph demonstrating a right lower lobe bulla. Note the demarcating lines, or "hairline shadows" *(arrows)*. **B.** CT image of the lungs demonstrating the right lower lobe bulla with compressed lung *(arrow)*. **C.** Perfusion scintigraphy demonstrating decreased perfusion to the right lower lung zone. **D.** CT image of the lung following surgical resection of the right lower lobe bulla.

These observations are consistent with the hypothesis that peripheral airspaces in paraseptal emphysema may coalesce to form larger bullae that may crowd normal adjacent lung. In addition, CT has shown that when bullae occur in the context of generalized emphysema, the extent of bullous emphysema correlates poorly with measurements of pulmonary function, and that the main determinant of respiratory function is the severity of emphysema in the bullous-free parts of the lung.[23]

On chest CT, giant bullae are predominantly located in the upper lobes and are generally subpleural.[12] However, in patients with α_1-antitrypsin deficiency, bullae are most commonly located at the lung bases. Approximately half of the patients have bilateral bullae (Fig. 52-4), and, occasionally, deviation of the mediastinal structures to the contralateral side may be noted.[12] CT has been used to create three-dimensional reconstructions of bullae, which can then be used to calculate bullae volumes (Fig. 52-5).

Nuclear Imaging

Lung scanning using radionuclide-based techniques may provide useful preoperative information in evaluating patients with bullous lung disease.[24] A lung perfusion scan provides a semiquantitative assessment of regional blood flow (Fig. 52-3C); results of ventilation

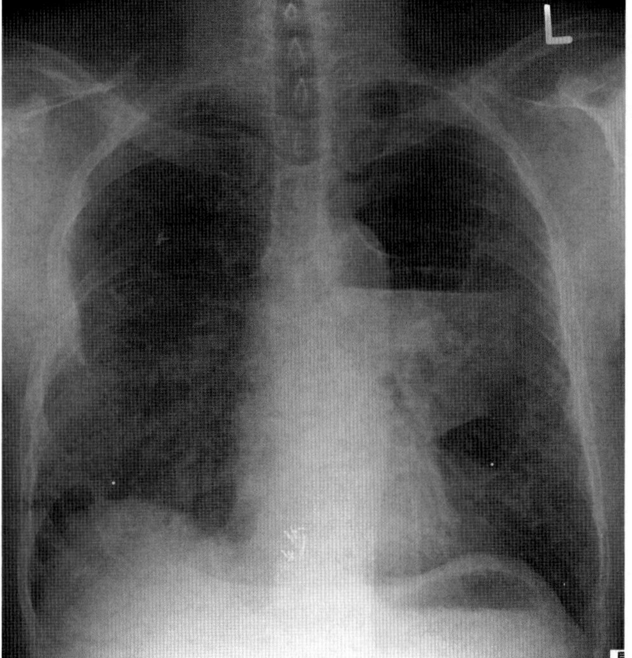

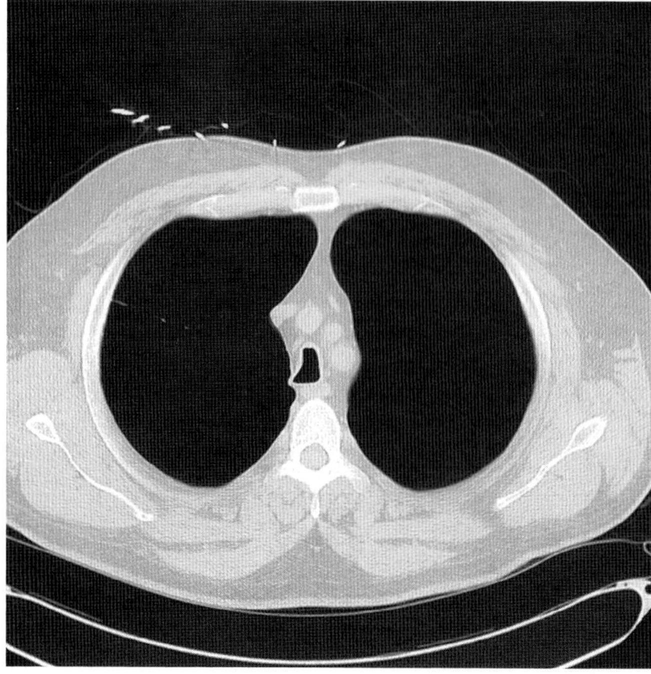

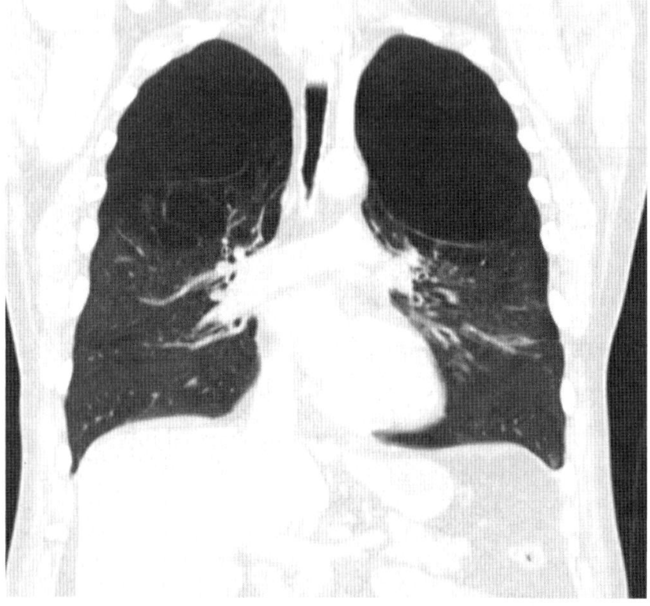

Figure 52-4 **A.** Chest radiograph *(PA view)* showing bilateral upper zonal areas of increased radiolucency and an air-fluid level in the left upper lobe bulla. **B.** Chest CT scan *(axial view)* demonstrating bilateral upper lobe bullae. **C.** Chest CT scan *(coronal view)* demonstrating bilateral upper lobe bullae.

scans vary with the technique. A single-breath scan using ^{133}xenon often fails to demonstrate ventilation of a bulla, whereas a continuous ventilation scan often shows slow filling and emptying of the structure.[24,25] Complete lack of communication between the airways and bulla is reflected in the absence of filling during all phases of the continuous ventilation scan.

PULMONARY PHYSIOLOGY

Clinical evaluation of bullous lung disease is aided by assessment of pulmonary function, pulmonary mechanics, exercise performance, and the pulmonary circulation.

Pulmonary Function Tests

Pulmonary function tests have considerable practical value in distinguishing between individuals with localized bullae in whom intervening lung is normal (bullous disease), and those in whom localized bullae are part of obstructive airways disease (bullous emphysema) (Table 52-4).[12] The distinction is important, since those with obstructive airways disease are generally poor surgical candidates because of impaired pulmonary function.

In individuals with bullous disease, the volume of air in the lungs can be estimated using plain radiography, CT, body plethysmography, or other pulmonary function test methods for determining lung volume, including closed circuit (helium dilution) and open circuit (nitrogen washout) techniques.[12,15] The volume of air trapped in a bulla can be determined as the difference between the functional residual capacities determined plethysmographically and by open or closed circuit methods (Table 52-4). This difference is due to the relative inability of the inert gas used in the circuit methods to enter the bulla.

Pulmonary Mechanics

Distinction between widespread obstructive airways disease with concomitant bullae and bullous lung disease has practical

TABLE 52-3 Potential Indications and Contraindications for Classical Bullectomy[a]

Parameter	Indications	Contraindications
Clinical	Young age (<50 y)	Age >50 y
	Rapid progressive dyspnea despite maximal medical therapy	Comorbid illness
	Ex-smoker	Cardiac disease
		Pulmonary hypertension
		>10% weight loss
		Frequent respiratory infections—chronic bronchitis
		Ongoing tobacco use
Physiologic	Normal or slightly ↓ FVC	FEV_1 <35% predicted
	FEV_1 >40% predicted	"Low" trapped gas volume
	Little bronchoreversibility	Decreased DL_{CO}
	"High" trapped lung volume	
	Normal or near-normal DL_{CO}	
	Normal Pa_{O_2} and Pa_{CO_2}	
Imaging	*CXR*—bulla >1/3 hemithorax	*CXR*—vanishing lung syndrome
	CT—large and localized bulla with vascular crowding and normal, compressed pulmonary parenchyma around bulla	Poorly defined bullae
		CT—multiple ill-defined bullae in underlying lung
	Angiography—vascular crowding with preserved distal vascular branching	*Angiography*—vague bullae; disrupted vasculature elsewhere
	Isotope scan—well-localized matching defect with normal uptake and washout for underlying lung	*Isotope scan*—absence of target zones, poor washout in remaining lung

[a]*Data from www.thoracic.org/copd.*

significance, since surgical lung resection in generalized emphysema offers a less certain therapeutic response than does resection of giant bullae in the absence of widespread obstructive lung disease (Table 52-3).[12] As large bullae expand, they initially cause relaxation of adjacent elastic lung tissue; with continued expansion, adjacent lung is compressed. Relaxation of the surrounding pulmonary parenchyma results in a decrease in radial traction on airways, thereby increasing airflow resistance. The effects of bullectomy on respiratory mechanics are inconsistent. Generally, resection of a large bulla increases lung static elastic recoil (by allowing for decompression of elastic lung parenchyma) and decreases airways resistance.

The diffusing capacity (DL_{CO}), rather than lung elastic recoil, is usually determined to aid in distinguishing between widespread emphysema and localized bullae, as more widespread loss of alveolar surface area in emphysema reduces the DL_{CO}; indeed, the DL_{CO} correlates better with morphologic estimates of emphysema than do most other tests.[12,15] Although the combination of a decreased DL_{CO} and reduced static elastic recoil pressure favors the diagnosis of widespread emphysema rather than localized bullae, both measurements may also be decreased by bullae that compress adjacent normal lung (Table 52-3).[3] Respiratory muscle strength, assessed by measurements of maximal inspiratory and transdiaphragmatic pressures, improves after bullectomy in some patients with bullous emphysema.[26]

Exercise Testing

In patients with a few circumscribed bullae and otherwise normal lungs, exercise testing reveals that the alveolar–arterial difference in Pa_{O_2}, ratio of dead space to tidal volume, DL_{CO}, and arterial oxygenation remain normal or near normal with exercise.[11] On the other hand, in patients in whom bullae are associated with panacinar emphysema, the alveolar–arterial difference in Pa_{O_2} is widened at rest and during exercise.[27] The latter group of patients also may develop arterial hypoxemia during exercise. The Pa_{O_2} tends to hover around the upper limit of normal at rest and during exercise, and the ratio of dead space to tidal volume is higher than in patients with normal intervening lung. The steady-state DL_{CO} is also reduced and fails to increase normally during exercise.

Patients in whom bullae are associated with chronic bronchitis also show a widened alveolar–arterial difference in Pa_{O_2} and an increase in the ratio of dead space to tidal volume at rest. However, in these patients the decrease in Pa_{O_2} during exercise is modest, even though the Pa_{O_2} at rest is abnormally high and increases further during exercise (indicating progressive alveolar hypoventilation).[2]

Pulmonary Circulation

In general, resting pulmonary arterial pressure and blood flow are within normal limits in patients with bullous lung disease (i.e., the bullae act like "amputated" segments of lung); the volume of the vascular bed available for recruitment as cardiac output increases is limited.[1,2] However, in patients in whom bullous disease has severely reduced the extent of the pulmonary vascular bed, pulmonary arterial pressure may be elevated at rest and during exercise; in a few instances, pulmonary and cor pulmonale may be observed.[1,2] Exercise in bullous lung disease is generally associated with an excessive increase in pulmonary arterial pressure as increases in pulmonary blood flow are not effectively accommodated by the restricted vascular bed.[2] Underlying pulmonary disease further exaggerates the increase in pulmonary artery pressure during exercise.

COMPLICATIONS

The major complications of bullous lung disease are fluid accumulation (including infection) in the bulla, spontaneous pneumothorax, bronchogenic cancer, chest pain, and hemoptysis.

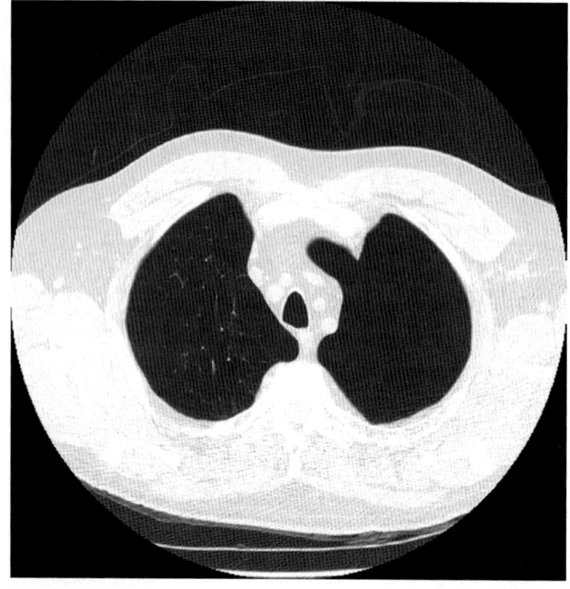

A

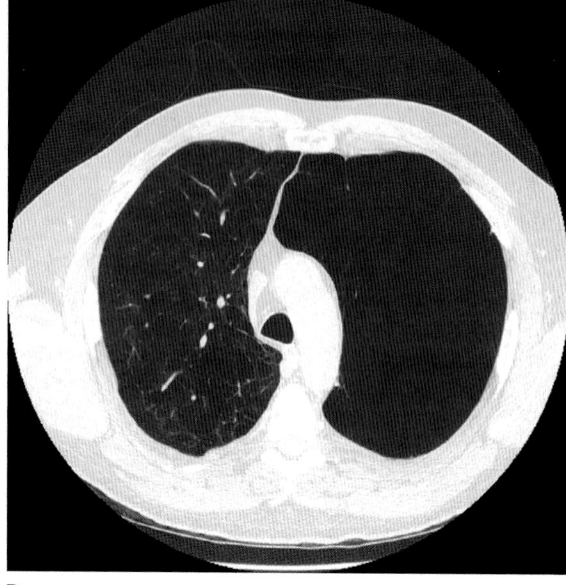

B

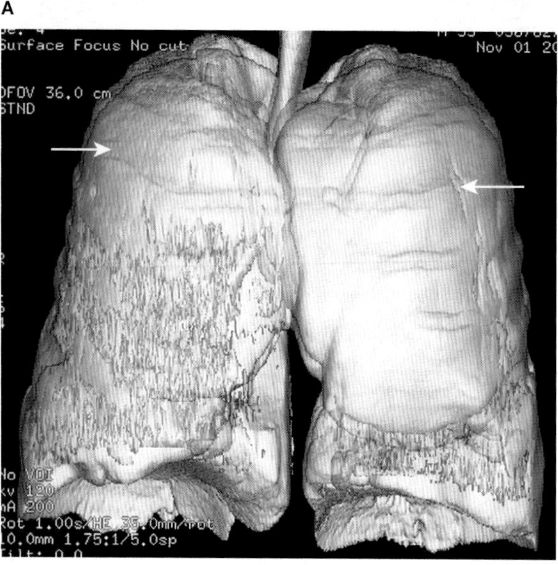

C

Figure 52-5 **A.** Chest CT *(axial view)* showing bilateral upper lobe bullae. **B.** Chest CT *(axial view)* demonstrating larger left upper lobe compared to right upper bulla. **C.** Chest CT (*coronal view;* three-dimensional reconstruction) demonstrating bilateral upper lobe bullae *(arrows)*.

TABLE 52-4 Pulmonary Function Tests

Test	Bullous Disease	Obstructive Airways Disease and Bullae
TLC, L	N	N ↑
RV, L	N	↑
FRC, L	N	↑
FRC,[a] L	↑	↑
RV/TLC%	N	↑
FEV$_1$, L	N ↓	↓
FVC, L	N ↓	↓
FEV$_1$/FVC%	N	↓
MVV, L/min	N	↓
DL$_{CO}$/V$_A$, (mL/min/mm Hg)/L	N	↓
Raw, cm H$_2$O/L/s	N ↑	↑
Cst, exp, L/cm H$_2$O	N ↑	↑
Pst, TLC, cm H$_2$O	N ↓	↓

Note: N, normal; ↑, increased; ↓, decreased.
[a]FRC determined by body plethysmography.

FLUID ACCUMULATION

The determination that an air–fluid level is within a bulla and not in a newly formed cyst or cavity is generally based on the new appearance of fluid in a previously known bulla or the presence of other bullae (Fig. 52-6).[12] CT of the chest is indicated to assure that the air–fluid level is within a bulla and to identify any surrounding pneumonia, adjacent pulmonary nodule, or an increase in wall thickness of the bulla. The latter aids in differentiating an air–fluid level within a bulla from other disorders such as tuberculosis, fungal disease, lung abscess, or cavitary bronchogenic lung cancer. These processes typically have substantially thicker cavity walls.

The presence of a fluid level within a bulla, especially if the bulla is located subpleurally, occasionally prompts the mistaken diagnosis of a loculated hydropneumothorax. CT is helpful in separating these two conditions.

Benign, Sterile Bullous Fluid

Benign, sterile fluid accumulations in a bulla can result from adjacent pneumonia or from poorly functioning bronchial communications with inadequate drainage of normally accumulating fluid.[28] In asymptomatic patients who have a thin-walled bulla without

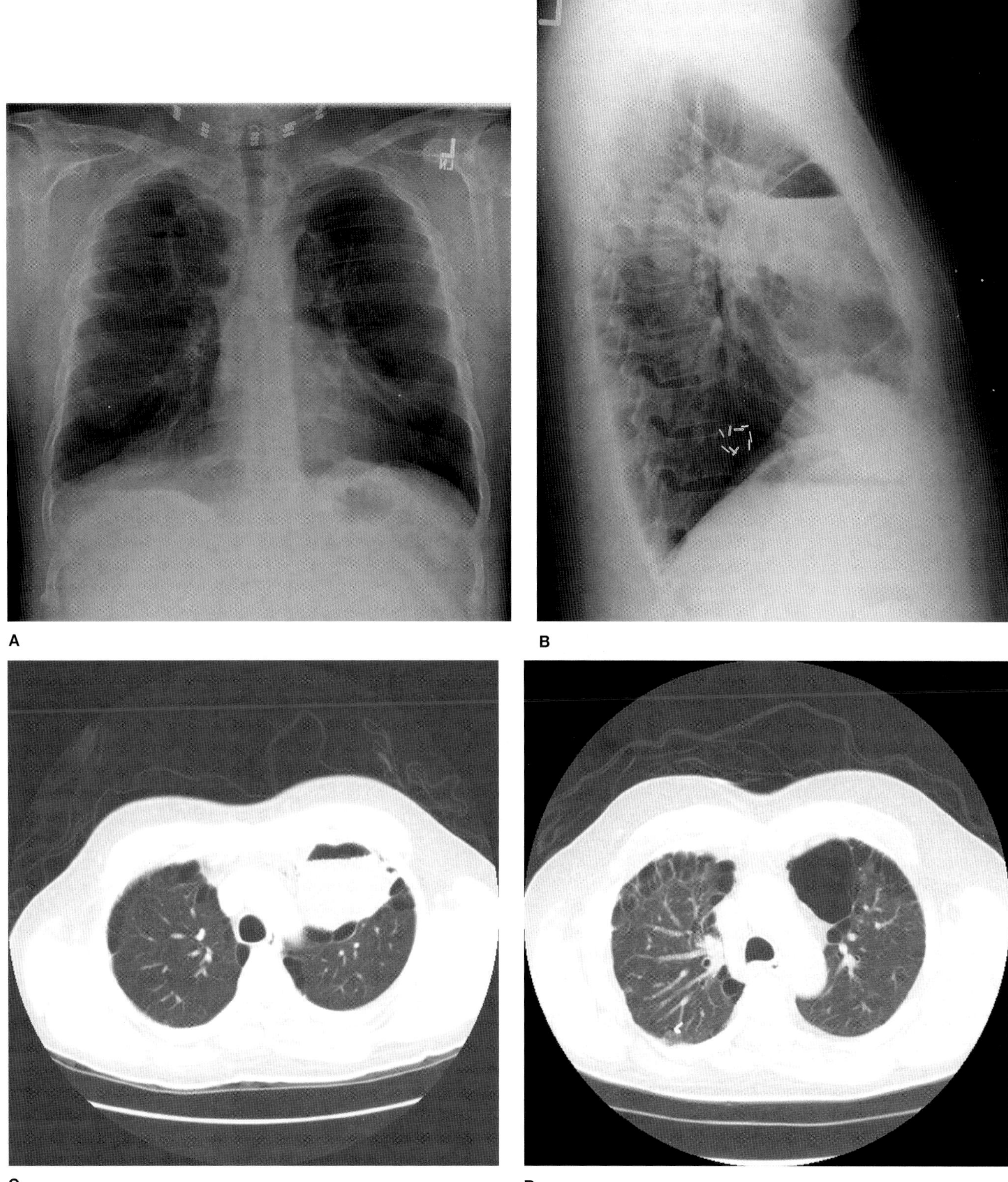

Figure 52-6 **A.** AP chest radiograph demonstrating an air–fluid level in a left upper lung bulla. **B.** Lateral chest radiograph demonstrating air–fluid level in a left upper lung bulla. **C.** CT image of the infected left upper lobe bulla. **D.** CT image of the same bulla after a prolonged course of antibiotics.

chest CT evidence of an adjacent pneumonitis or nodule, continued observation without specific therapy is appropriate.[4] Close radiologic evaluation is typically performed at 6- to 12-week intervals to ensure that an infection or bronchogenic carcinoma is not present. In patients with clinical and radiographic evidence of adjacent pneumonia antibiotic therapy is indicated.[29] The air–fluid level may persist for weeks to months after resolution of active infection.

Infected Bulla

A superinfection within a bulla can occur with clinical manifestations including fever, cough, purulent sputum production, dyspnea, and pleuritic chest pain. Laboratory findings may include leukocytosis and positive sputum cultures. When clinical and radiographic findings suggest an infected bulla, empiric antibiotics should be initiated based on a regimen similar to that used for community-acquired pneumonia in a patient with COPD.[4,12] Bacterial species that have been identified from infected bullae include methicillin-resistant *Staphylococcus aureus* (MRSA), Bacteroides, *Pseudomonas aeruginosa*, and mycobacteria.[30–32] Treatment is sometimes prolonged and may require parenteral or intrabulla administration, since poor drainage of the bulla inevitably slows resolution of the disease process.[33] The course of the infection should be followed by interval chest radiographs, in part as bulla infection has been associated with bronchogenic cancer.[34] If a patient does not improve with empiric antibiotics percutaneous aspiration of bullous fluid can be performed under CT guidance to confirm the presence of infection and to identify the antibiotic sensitivities of the infecting organism.[4,30] It should be recognized that percutaneous aspiration carries an increased risk of pneumothorax and empyema.[12] Tube thoracostomy[35] and endoscopic drainage have also been utilized.[36]

■ PNEUMOTHORAX

Spontaneous pneumothorax may be a complication of paraseptal emphysema, particularly in patients who continue to smoke. The typical presentation is a sudden onset or worsening of dyspnea with or without pleuritic chest pain. Ultrastructural assessments suggest the possibility of air leaking through the wall of the bullae with sloughling of mesothelial cells,[37] while lung density measures suggest a valve like effect with air trapping.[38] A few case reports have described a pneumothorax occurring when a bronchogenic carcinoma eroded through the wall of a bulla.[39]

Tube thoracostomy drainage of pleural air is often required; this depends on the size of the pneumothorax and the degree of respiratory impairment.[12,40,41] Patients with ruptured bullae also tend to have prolonged air leaks, along with pleural and parenchymal infections. Subsequent management is directed at preventing recurrence. For patients with a bulla and a secondary spontaneous pneumothorax, pleurodesis using mechanical abrasion of the pleura via video-assisted thoracoscopic surgery (VATS) can be considered.[39,41,42] For patients with minimal surrounding diffuse emphysema, a bullectomy can be performed at the time of pleurodesis; for those with diffuse bullous emphysema, pleurodesis is often performed without bullectomy.[12]

■ BRONCHOGENIC CANCER

Primary lung cancer has been reported to be associated with bullous lung disease.[43–46] Presenting manifestations include pneumothorax and hemoptysis.[46] The increased incidence of lung cancer may be due to the fact that lung cancer occurs more frequently in fibrotic lungs that are, themselves, predisposed to development of bullae.[1] Other explanations for the increased incidence of malignancy include dystrophic changes in lung parenchyma caused by bullous disease or persistence of carcinogens in poorly ventilated bullae.[1] The CT appearances for bronchogenic cancer complicating bullae include a nodule or mass extruding from the wall of the bulla, a nodule or mass confined within the lumen, a soft tissue density thickening the wall of the bulla, a pneumothorax, and an air–fluid level.[37,47–50]

■ CHEST PAIN AND HEMOPTYSIS

Chest pain may occur with a bulla and is attributed to overdistention of the structure.[12] The pain is angina-like and located retrosternally. The symptom is sometimes so severe as to constitute an indication for surgical intervention. Hemoptysis, which is occasionally massive, can result from rupture of blood vessels within the walls of bullae.[51]

TREATMENT

Many patients with bullous lung disease can be managed medically.[52] Because the natural history of a bulla is unpredictable, patients with bullous disease should be monitored by chest radiography at regular intervals to ensure that the disease is stable. Occasionally, bullae enlarge suddenly and rapidly for no apparent reason; alternatively, they may shrink or disappear.[50,53,54]

■ MEDICAL MANAGEMENT

The finding of a bulla in an asymptomatic patient calls for reassurance, a recommendation for annual chest radiography, advice to stop smoking, and an alert to the need for a prompt visit to a physician should symptoms develop. Activities that promote rupture of bullae (e.g., contact sports and scuba diving) should be proscribed.[1,14] Chronic bronchitis, asthma, or emphysema associated with bullae require treatment in their own right. For patients with α_1-antitrypsin deficiency augmentation therapy with antiproteases may be appropriate.[14] Endobronchial therapy with endobronchial valves (see Chapter 36) has been recently reported.[55–57]

■ SURGICAL MANAGEMENT

Although randomized trials of giant bullectomy have not been performed, the potential benefits of elective bullectomy have been described in a number of case series.[15,58,59] In general, significant symptomatic and functional improvements have been reported for 5 or more years in 60% to 90% of patients.[15,58,59] Patients with diffuse emphysema tend to deteriorate faster than patients without diffuse emphysema.[59] A systematic review of bullectomy reported that hypoxemia was more likely to improve compared with spirometric parameters or D_{LCO}.[59] Patients with radiographic evidence of compressed lung were the most to likely experience improved oxygenation.[59] Perioperative mortality ranges from 0% to 7% for bullectomy via open thoracotomy; patients with diffuse emphysema seem to experience a higher mortality rate.[59] Causes of death include pneumonia, respiratory failure, pulmonary embolism, and cardiovascular complications.

■ INDICATIONS

The most common indication for bullectomy is severe dyspnea due to a bulla occupying 30% or more of the hemithorax or spontaneous secondary pneumothorax.[22,60,61] A key challenge for the clinician is selecting the optimal patient for bullectomy. A key factor suggesting that bullectomy may be beneficial is a bulla that occupies greater than 50% of the hemithorax with radiographic evidence that the bulla is compressing adjacent normal pulmonary parenchyma (Table 52-3; Fig. 52-3A,B).[15,58] An overall enumeration of criteria reported to define patients who are most likely to benefit from bullectomy is presented in Table 52-3.

As noted in Table 52-3 physiologic data have been reported to provide valuable information in guiding the decision to perform bullectomy. The majority of patients who undergo bullectomy have an FEV_1 less than 80% predicted but greater than or equal to 40% predicted; these thresholds have been supported by case series.[60]

Similarly, patients likely to benefit have physiologic evidence of air trapping (e.g., total lung capacity [TLC] >100% predicted, residual volume [RV] >150% predicted).[62] Some have suggested that the difference in lung volume measured by body plethysmography versus helium dilution techniques can be compared to estimate the volume of nonventilated lung. A larger nonventilated volume suggests a more favorable response to bullectomy.[15,58]

CONTRAINDICATIONS

As noted in Table 52-3 features associated with a less favorable result following bullectomy include older age, ongoing cigarette smoking, significant comorbid disease, lower pulmonary function (FEV_1 and DL_{CO}), hypercapnia, poorly defined bullae on chest imaging, and pulmonary hypertension.[59,60,62–68] Similarly, patients with chronic sputum production or frequent lung infections have been suggested to be less likely to improve.[58,59]

PREOPERATIVE EVALUATION AND MANAGEMENT

The preoperative evaluation for bullectomy includes pulmonary function testing and imaging as noted earlier. Underlying COPD should be treated aggressively with an appropriate combination of inhaled medications and pulmonary rehabilitation.[58] Preoperative cardiac evaluation is appropriate given the increased risk of cardiovascular comorbidity among patients with COPD.[69]

ANESTHETIC MANAGEMENT

Standard monitoring during the procedure includes blood pressure, pulse oximetry, capnography, core temperature, and continuous electrocardiography.[70] Arterial and central venous pressure monitoring are not mandatory but frequently utilized.[58] Bullectomy is typically performed under general anesthesia.[70] Short-acting anesthetic agents are preferred over longer-acting agents to facilitate early extubation.[70] Intravenous agents are typically used for induction of anesthesia, as severe bullous disease may make the uptake and distribution of inhalational agents erratic.[70] A thoracic epidural catheter is usually placed for administration of epidural anesthetic agents during and/or after surgery.[70]

After anesthetic induction, appropriate positioning, and sterile draping, an endotracheal tube that allows isolation of ventilation to one lung is placed to administer single lung ventilation to the nonoperative lung and to enable deflation of the operative lung.[70] Immediately postoperatively patients are assessed for anemia, cardiac ischemia, electrolyte abnormalities, hypercapnia, hypoxemia, and inadequate lung reexpansion.[70] If these factors are acceptable, the patient may be extubated; in the majority of cases this occurs in the operating room.[71]

OPERATIVE APPROACH AND TECHNIQUES

Although many surgeons prefer an open approach for bullectomy there is increasing application of VATS techniques.[62,72–74] When an open thoracotomy is performed, the posterolateral approach is generally used for unilateral bullous disease, while median sternotomy is often utilized for resection of bilateral bullae.[62] The amount of lung resected in addition to the main bulla is dependent on a balance between removing diseased tissue to optimize reexpansion of compressed tissue while avoiding resecting healthy lung tissue and minimizing prolonged air leak around the suture line.[22,59] For a single bulla that is well-demarcated and has a clear, narrow pedicle, a simple stapled excision is adequate. When the bulla is broad based or when numerous bullae merge indistinctly, a broad stapled wedge resection is usually necessary.[71] Lobectomy and segmentectomy may be utilized in unusual settings.[61,62,75]

Ablation or excision of bullae can be achieved by a variety of surgical methods, including plication, laser ablation, and excision with a stapler.[22,58] The latter is the most frequently utilized. Numerous approaches are utilized to minimize postoperative air leaks, including applying exogenous materials to buttress staple sutures (e.g., bovine pericardial or polytetrafluoroethylene strips), fibrin sealant to areas of air leak intraoperatively, and creating a "pleural tent."[76–80] The Brompton technique, or modified Monaldi procedure, utilizes a limited thoracotomy to visualize the bulla, insufflation of the bulla with iodized talc, and drainage of the bulla for several days with a Foley catheter under water seal.[66,81,82] Talc is subsequently instilled into the pleural cavity to achieve pleurodesis.

The postoperative approach includes careful attention to respiratory status, pain control, minimizing bronchoconstriction and hyperinflation, monitoring for development or worsening of a pneumothorax, and prevention of thromboembolic disease.[58] Attention to the proper function of chest tubes is key to minimize the negative implications of pneumothorax. Thoracostomy tubes are generally left in place until the lung is fully expanded and there is no evidence of air leak. In those patients with persistent slow air leaks a minichest tube with a unidirectional flutter valve (e.g., Heimlich valve) can be used to facilitate discharge of the patient. The management of postoperative pain to ensure early mobilization of the patient and effective cough is crucial to minimize complications.[71]

SUMMARY

Recognition of bullous lung disease and its causes, classification, and underlying pathophysiology have important clinical implications. Careful clinical, radiographic, and physiologic assessment allows identification of patients whose dyspnea may be substantially improved through a variety of medical, surgical, and bronchoscopic interventions.

REFERENCES

1. Murphy DM, Fishman AP. Bullous disease of the lung. In: Fishman AP, ed. *Fishman's Pulmonary Diseases and Disorders*. 4th ed. New York, NY: McGraw-Hill; 2008.
2. Laurenzi GA, Turino GM, Fishman AP. Bullous disease of the lung. *Am J Med*. 1962;32:361–378.
3. Gaensler E, Jederlinic P, FitzGerald M. Patient work-up for bullectomy. *J Thorac Imaging*. 1986;1:75–93.
4. Chandra D, Rose SR, Carter RB, Musher DM, Hamill RJ. Fluid-containing emphysematous bullae: a spectrum of illness. *Eur Respir J*. 2008;32(2):303–306.
5. Leatherman JW, McDonald FM, Niewohner DE. Fluid-containing bullae in the lung. *South Med J*. 1985;78(6):708–710.
6. Richardson MS, Reddy VD, Read CA. New air-fluid levels in bullous lung disease: a reevaluation. *J Natl Med Assoc*. 1996; 88(3):185–187.
7. Morgan MD, Edwards CW, Morris J, Matthews HR. Origin and behaviour of emphysematous bullae. *Thorax*. 1989;44(7):533–538.
8. McChesney T. Placental transmogrification of the lung: a unique case with remarkable histopathologic features. *Lab Invest*. 1979;40:245–246.
9. Horsley WS, Gal AA, Mansour KA. Unilateral giant bullous emphysema with placental transmogrification of the lung. *Ann Thorac Surg*. 1997;64:226–228.
10. Ito S, Bartolak-Suki E, Shipley JM, Parameswaran H, Majumdar A, Suki B. Early emphysema in the tight skin and pallid mice: roles of microfibril-associated glycoproteins, collagen, and mechanical forces. *Am J Respir Cell Mol Biol*. 2006;34(6): 688–694.
11. Boushy SF, Kohen R, Billig DM, Heiman MJ. Bullous emphysema: clinical, roentgenologic and physiologic study of 49 patients. *Dis. Chest*. 1968;54(4):17–24.

12. Martinez F. Evaluation and medical management of giant bullae in COPD. In: Rose B, ed. *UpToDate*. Waltham, MA: UpToDate; 2013.
13. Mireles-Cabodevila E, Sahi H, Farver C, Mohammed TL, Culver DA. A young patient with a minimal smoking history presents with bullous emphysema and recurrent pneumothorax. *Chest*. 2007;132(1):338–343.
14. Stoller JK, Aboussouan LS. A review of α1-antitrypsin deficiency. *Am J Resp Crit Care Med*. 2012;185(3):246–259.
15. Martinez F, Chang A. Surgical therapy for chronic obstructive pulmonary disease. *Sem Respir Crit Care Med*. 2005;26(2):167–191.
16. Mitlehner W, Friedrich M, Dissmann W. Value of computed tomography in the detection of bullae and blebs in patients with primary spontaneous pneumothorax. *Respiration*. 1992;59: 221–227.
17. Mostafa M, Mostafa S. Role of the chest radiography, spirometry, and high resolution computed tomography in the early diagnosis of emphysema. *Egypt J Radiol Nuc Med*. 2919;41:509–515.
18. Waitches GM, Stern EJ, Dubinsky TJ. Usefulness of the double-wall sign in detecting pneumothorax in patients with giant bullous emphysema. *AJR Am J Roentgenol*. 2000;174(6):1765–1768.
19. Waseem M, Jones J, Brutus S, Munyak J, Kapoor R, Gernsheimer J. Giant bulla mimicking pneumothorax. *J Emerg Med*. 2005;29(2):155–158.
20. Sharma N, Justaniah AM, Kanne JP, Gurney JW, Mohammed TL. Vanishing lung syndrome (giant bullous emphysema): CT findings in 7 patients and a literature review. *J Thorac Imaging*. 2009;24(3):227–230.
21. Marti-Bonmati L, Catala FJ, Ruiz Perales F. Computed tomography differentiation between cystic bronchiectasis and bullae. *J Thorac Imaging*. 1991;7(1):83–85.
22. Meyers B, Patterson G. Chronic obstructive pulmonary disease. 10: bullectomy, lung volume reduction surgery, and transplantation for patients with chronic obstructive pulmonary disease. *Thorax*. 2003;58:634–638.
23. Gould GA, Redpath AT, Ryan M, et al. Parenchymal emphysema measured by CT lung density correlates with lung function in patients with bullous disease. *Eur Respir J*. 1993;6:698–704.
24. Suga K, Iwanaga H, Tokuda O, Okada M, Matsunaga N. Intrabullous ventilation in pulmonary emphysema: assessment with dynamic xenon-133 gas SPECT. *Nucl Med Commun*. 2012;33(4):371–378.
25. Nakahara K, Nakaoka K, Ohno K, et al. Functional indications for bullectomy of giant bulla. *Ann Thorac Surg*. 1983;35(5):480–487.
26. Travaline JM, Addonizio VP, Criner GJ. Effect of bullectomy on diaphragm strength. *Am J Respir Crit Care Med*. 1995;152: 1697–1701.
27. Wade JF 3rd, Mortenson R, Irvin CG. Physiologic evaluation of bullous emphysema. *Chest*. 1991;100(4):1151–1154.
28. Henao-Martinez AF, Fernandez JF, Adams SG, Restrepo C. Lung bullae with air-fluid levels: what is the appropriate therapeutic approach? *Respir Care*. 2012;57(4):642–645.
29. Mahler DA, Gerstenhaber BJ, D'Esopo ND. Air-fluid levels within lung bullae associated with pneumonitis. *Lung*. 1981; 159(3):163–171.
30. Peters JI, Kubitschek KR, Gotlieb MS, Awe RJ. Lung bullae with air-fluid levels. *Am J Med*. 1987;82(4):759–763.
31. Chandra D, Soubra SH, Musher DM. A 57-year-old man with a fluid-containing lung cavity: infection of an emphysematous bulla with methicillin-resistant Staphylococcus aureus. *Chest*. 2006;130(6):1942–1946.
32. Kobashi Y, Yoshida K, Miyashita N, Niki Y, Oka M. Infectious bulla of the lung caused by Mycobacterium intracellulare. *J Infect Chemother*. 2005;11(6):293–296.
33. Chon SH, Shinn SH, Lee CB. Giant fluid-filled bulla treated by instillation of antibiotics after percutaneous drainage. *Thorac Cardiovasc Surg*. 2010;58(2):122–124.
34. Asai N, Ohkuni Y, Matsunuma R, Nakashima K, Iwasaki T, Kaneko N. Infectious giant bulla associated with lung cancer. *J Bras Pneumol*. 2011;37(3):404–408.
35. Kirschner LS, Stauffer W, Krenzel C, Duane PG. Management of a giant fluid-filled bulla by closed-chest thoracostomy tube drainage. *Chest*. 1997;111(6):1772–1774.
36. Takanami I. Endoscopic drainage of an infected giant bulla. *Interact Cardiovasc Thorac Surg*. 2006;5(6):794–795.
37. Ohata M, Suzuki H. Pathogenesis of spontaneous pneumothorax. With special reference to the ultrastructure of emphysematous bullae. *Chest*. 1980;77(6):771–776.
38. Smit HJ, Golding RP, Schramel FM, Deville WL, Manoliu RA, Postmus PE. Lung density measurements in spontaneous pneumothorax demonstrate airtrapping. *Chest*. 2004;125(6): 2083–2090.
39. Okada D, Koizumi K, Haraguchi S, Kawamoto M, Mikami I, Tanaka S. Pneumothorax manifesting primary lung cancer. *Jpn J Thorac Cardiovasc Surg*. 2002;50(3):133–136.
40. Tschopp JM, Rami-Porta R, Noppen M, Astoul P. Management of spontaneous pneumothorax: state of the art. *Eur Respir J*. 2006;28(3):637–650.
41. Baumann MH, Strange C, Heffner JE, et al. Management of spontaneous pneumothorax: an American College of Chest Physicians Delphi consensus statement. *Chest*. 2001;119(2): 590–602.
42. Isaka M, Asai K, Urabe N. Surgery for secondary spontaneous pneumothorax: risk factors for recurrence and morbidity. *Interact Cardiovasc Thorac Surg*. 2013;17(2):247–252.
43. Farooqi AO, Cham M, Zhang L, et al. Lung cancer associated with cystic airspaces. *Am J Roentgenol*. 2012;199(4):781–786.
44. Hirai S, Hamanaka Y, Mitsui N, Morifuji K, Sutoh M. Primary lung cancer arising from the wall of a giant bulla. *Ann Thorac Cardiovasc Surg*. 2005;11(2):109–113.
45. Arab WA, Echave V, Sirois M, Gomes MM. Incidental carcinoma in bullous emphysema. *Can J Surg*. 2009;52(3): E56–E57.
46. Erne BV, Graff M, Klemm W, Danzl JG, Leschber G. Bulla in the lung. *Lancet*. 2012;380(9849):1280.
47. Tsutsui M, Araki Y, Shirakusa T, Inutsuka S. Characteristic radiographic features of pulmonary carcinoma associated with large bulla. *Ann Thorac Surg*. 1988;46(6):679–683.
48. Maki D, Takahashi M, Murata K, Sawai S, Fujino S, Inoue S. Computed tomography appearances of bronchogenic carcinoma associated with bullous lung disease. *J Comput Assist Tomogr*. 2006;30(3):447–452.
49. Kaneda M, Tarukawa T, Watanabe F, Adachi K, Sakai T, Nakabayashi H. Clinical features of primary lung cancer adjoining pulmonary bulla. *Interact Cardiovasc Thorac Surg*. 2010;10(6):940–944.
50. Park HY, Lim SY, Park HK, Park SY, Kim TS, Suh GY. Regression of giant bullous emphysema. *Intern Med*. 2010;49(1):55–57.
51. Chen CW, Perng WC, Li MH, Yan HC, Wu CP. Hemorrhage from an enlarged emphysematous bulla during commercial air travel. *Aviat Space Environ Med*. 2006;77(12):1275–1277.

52. Byrd RP Jr, Roy TM. Spontaneous resolution of a giant pulmonary bulla: what is the role of bronchodilator and anti-inflammatory therapy? *Tenn Med.* 2013;106(1):39–42.

53. Shanthaveerappa HN, Mathai MG, Byrd RP Jr, Fields CL, Roy TM. Spontaneous resolution of a giant pulmonary bulla. *J Ky Med Assoc.* 2001;99(12):533–536.

54. Stanescu D, Veriter CL. Spontaneous regression of a giant pulmonary bulla. *Thorax.* 1996;51(12):1283.

55. Santini M, Fiorello A, Di Crescenzo VG, Vicidomini G, Busiello L, Laperuta P. Use of unidirectional endobronchial valves for the treatment of giant emphysematous bulla. *J Thorac Cardiovasc Surg.* 2010;139(1):224–226.

56. Santini M, Fiorelli A, Vicidomini G, Di Crescenzo VG, Messina G, Laperuta P. Endobronchial treatment of giant emphysematous bullae with one-way valves: a new approach for surgically unfit patients. *Eur J Cardiothorac Surg.* 2011;40(6):1425–1431.

57. Noppen M, Tellings JC, Dekeukeleire T, et al. Successful treatment of a giant emphysematous bulla by bronchoscopic placement of endobronchial valves. *Chest.* 2006;130(5):1563–1565.

58. Martinez F. Bullectomy for giant bullae in COPD. In: Rose B, ed. *UpToDate.* Waltham, MA: UpToDate; 2013.

59. Snider GL. Reduction pneumoplasty for giant bullous emphysema. Implications for surgical treatment of nonbullous emphysema. *Chest.* 1996;109(2):540–548.

60. Palla A, Desideri M, Rossi G, et al. Elective surgery for giant bullous emphysema. A 5-year clinical and functional follow-up. *Chest.* 2005;128:2043–2050.

61. Neviere R, Catto M, Bautin N, et al. Longitudinal changes in hyperinflation parameters and exercise capacity after giant bullous emphysema surgery. *J Thorac Cardiovasc Surg.* 2006; 132: 1203–1207.

62. Schipper P, Meyers B, Battafarano R, Guthrie T, Patterson G, Cooper J. Outcomes after resection of giant emphysematous bullae. *Ann Thorac Surg.* 2004;78:976–982.

63. Fitzgerald M, Keelan P, Angell D. Long-term results of surgery for bullous emphysema. *Surgery.* 1974;68:566–582.

64. Laros C, Gellisen H, Bergstein P, et al. Bullectomy for giant bullae in emphysema. *J Thorac Cardiovasc Surg.* 1986;91:63–70.

65. Kinnear W, Tatterfield A. Emphysematous bullae: surgery is best for large bullae and moderately impaired lung function. *BMJ.* 1990;300:208–209.

66. Shah SS, Goldstraw P. Surgical treatment of bullous emphysema: experience with the Brompton technique. *Ann Thorac Surg.* 1994;58(5):1452–1456.

67. Gunstensen J, McCormack RJ. The surgical management of bullous emphysema. *J Thor Cardiovas Surg.* 1973;65(6):920–929.

68. Nickoladze G. Functional results of surgery for bullous emphysema. *Chest.* 1992;101:119–122.

69. Augoustides JG, Neuman MD, Al-Ghofaily L, Silvay G. Preoperative cardiac risk assessment for noncardiac surgery: defining costs and risks. *J Cardiothorac Vasc Anesth.* 2013; 27(2):395–399.

70. Brister NW, Barnette RE, Kim V, Keresztury M. Anesthetic considerations in candidates for lung volume reduction surgery. *Proc Am Thorac Soc.* 2008;5(4):432–437.

71. Boasquevisque CH, Yildirim E, Waddel TK, Keshavjee S. Surgical techniques: lung transplant and lung volume reduction. *Proc Am Thorac Soc.* 2009;6(1):66–78.

72. Greenberg JA, Singhal S, Kaiser LR. Giant bullous lung disease: evaluation, selection, techniques, and outcomes. *Chest Surg Clin N Am.* 2003;13(4):631–649.

73. Tsuchida M, Nakayama K, Shinonaga M, Tatebe S, Yamaguchi A. Video-assisted thoracic surgery for thorascopic resection of giant bulla. *Surg Today.* 1996;26(5):349–352.

74. Menconi GF, Melfi FM, Mussi A, Palla A, Ambrogi MC, Angeletti CA. Treatment by VATS of giant bullous emphysema: results. *Eur J Cardiothorac Surg.* 1998;13(1):66–70.

75. FitzPatrick MJ, Kittle CF, Lin TK, Dowell JC. Some physiologic changes associated with surgical excision of emphysematous bullae. *Am J Med.* 1957;22:534–548.

76. Cho S, Huh DM, Kim BH, et al. Staple line covering procedure after thoracoscopic bullectomy for the management of primary spontaneous pneumothorax. *Thorac Cardiovasc Surg.* 2008;56(4):217–220.

77. Moser C, Opitz I, Zhai W, et al. Autologous fibrin sealant reduces the incidence of prolonged air leak and duration of chest tube drainage after lung volume reduction surgery: a prospective randomized blinded study. *J Thorac Cardiovasc Surg.* 2008; 136(4):843–849.

78. Brunelli A, Al Refai M, Muti M, Sabbatini A, Fianchini A. Pleural tent after upper lobectomy: a prospective randomized study. *Ann Thorac Surg.* 2000;69(6):1722–1724.

79. Venuta F, De Giacomo T, Rendina EA, Ricci C, Coloni GF. Thoracoscopic pleural tent. *Ann Thorac Surg.* 1998;66(5): 1833–1834.

80. Cooper JD. Technique to reduce air leaks after resection of emphysematous lung. *Ann Thorac Surg.* 1994;57(4):1038–1039.

81. Wang H, Xu Z, Gao W. A modified Brompton technique for the treatment of giant bulla in patients with diffuse emphysema. *Thorac Cardiovasc Surg.* 2012;60(2):161–163.

82. Goldstraw P, Petrou M. The surgical treatment of emphysema. The Brompton approach. *Chest Surg Clin N Am.* 1995;5(4):777–796.

CHAPTER 53 Bronchiectasis

Alan F. Barker
Steven L. Brody

Bronchiectasis (*broncos,* airways; *ectasia,* dilatation) is a morphologic term used to describe abnormal, irreversibly dilated and thick-walled bronchi. This is an anatomic definition that evolved from Laennec's original description in 1819 of ectatic bronchi in pathologic specimens. Bronchiectasis represents the end stage of a variety of pathologic processes that cause destruction of the bronchial wall and its surrounding supporting tissues. Etiologies include prior lung infection, systemic inflammatory disorders, and genetic disorders of host defense, however, bronchiectasis is considered to be idiopathic in up to half of the affected individuals. The clinical manifestations include chronic cough and copious mucopurulent expectoration.[1] Bronchiectasis shares many features with chronic bronchitis, including inflamed and easily collapsible airways, airflow obstruction on spirometry, and frequent exacerbations.

PREVALENCE

Bronchiectasis was a common disabling and fatal condition in the pre-antibiotic era and remains more common in medically underserved regions of the world. Overall, it is an important cause of suppurative lung disease with a significant impact on the quality of life of affected individuals and on the health system as patients utilize many medical care resources including frequent clinic visits, hospitalizations, diagnostic imaging such as high-resolution computed tomography scan (HRCT) of the chest and parenteral antibiotics.[2] In the United States, the overall prevalence has been estimated to be 52 per 100,000, but varies by age. In persons aged 18 to 34 years the prevalence is approximately 4.2 per 100,000 but in those who are 75 years old or it is estimated to be greater than 272 per 100,000. There are an estimated 110,000 affected individuals in the United States.[3] In most series, 60% of affected individuals are women. The incidence is higher in some ethnic groups living in isolated regions including the native peoples in Alaska, Maori populations in New Zealand and the Pacific, and Aboriginal groups in Central Australia. In North America and Europe, improved health care has decreased the incidence, thus bronchiectasis due to cystic fibrosis (CF) and other genetic diseases now significantly contribute to the fraction of affected adults.

PATHOPHYSIOLOGY

The pathogenesis of bronchiectasis is not known in many cases, and in others may vary with etiology, so that the pathophysiology often remains descriptive. Gross pathology reflects chronic changes so that initial changes of injury proposed to lead to initial airway obstruction are not often observed. The abnormal bronchial dilatation in bronchiectasis principally affects the medium-sized bronchi, but typically extends to the distal bronchi and bronchioles. On gross examination of surgically resected or autopsied lungs, the affected bronchi and bronchioles are so prominent as to be visible all the way to the pleural surface. These dilated and ectatic bronchi are commonly filled with purulent secretions. The affected bronchi show transmural inflammation, mucosal edema, cratering, ulceration, and neovascularization. The bronchial epithelium may show a polypoidal appearance due to underlying granuloma formation and lymphoid aggregates, ridging due to bronchial smooth muscle hypertrophy, and pitting due to the dilated bronchial mucus glands. Severe cases may show denudation of epithelial lining, with destruction of underlying elastic laminae, smooth muscle, and cartilage with fibrotic changes replacing these structures. Dilated and tortuous bronchial arteries may be seen secondary to the development of extensive bronchial-pulmonary anastomoses.

Microscopically, bronchiectasis is associated with airway epithelial remodeling characterized by mucus cell metaplasia, and decrease in ciliated cells. In other regions, cuboidal and squamous metaplasia predominate. Intense infiltration of the bronchial wall with neutrophils, lymphocytes, and monocytes is common. Hypertrophy of bronchial glands, and lymphoid hyperplasia are also seen.

Various explanations have been advanced for the phenomenon of bronchiectasis after bronchial obstruction. Following bronchial obstruction, airways proximal to the collapse are exposed to strong dilating forces caused by the difference in the atmospheric pressure in the bronchi and the negative pressure in the pleural space. Over time, these forces acting on weakened, inflamed airways may result in permanent and pathologic airway dilatation. The presence of surrounding lung fibrosis, atelectasis, and loss of lung volume leading to regional increases in local retractile lung forces may also play a role. Animal experiments suggest that obstruction may facilitate the development of bronchiectasis by interfering with bronchial clearance and promoting bacterial infection, bronchial wall inflammation, and weakening.

It has long been recognized that the pathologic changes are associated with chronic bacterial infection, independent of the initial cause of bronchiectasis. The concept of the "vicious cycle" of recurrent infectious and inflammatory insults proposed by Peter Cole et al.,[4] 37 years ago has largely been accepted. The cycle is initiated by an infection and an airway insult in a host at genetic risk. This vicious cycle theory proposed that chronic bacterial endobronchial infection and inflammation damage or destroy mucociliary defenses, leading to secretion stasis, which in turn propagates furthers bacterial infection, and increases airway inflammation and bronchial dilatation. Specific primary defects in innate host defense (e.g., IgG deficiency) have been identified as causative.[5] Furthermore, acute bacterial infection and chronic biofilm formation in the airways alone are not sufficient to produce true bronchiectasis. Impaired airway epithelial cell function, immune response, or other systemic inflammatory conditions resulting in insufficient airway clearance are additionally required. Once injury ensues, the appearance of *Pseudomonas aeruginosa* in the respiratory tract of bronchiectasis patients on a chronic or recurring basis has been associated with worsening airway clearance and airway obstruction, resulting in impaired health-related quality of life (HQOL) and worsened lung function.[6] This may be due to the ability of this organism to release virulent exotoxins, form biofilms on tissue surfaces, and easily develop hypermutable *P. aeruginosa* strains resistant to antibiotics, all factors perpetuating and propagating bronchial damage.

Specificity biochemical and molecular markers of non-CF bronchiectasis are not established and robust animal models of bronchiectasis have not been developed. Early biochemical changes are proposed related to infection and reflect a stereotyped host immune response. Later in disease, neutrophils, macrophages, and monocytes, along with their products are abundant. At both stages, cytokines such as tumor necrosis factor-a (TNF-a) and interleukin-8 may be elevated, providing a sustained signal for inflammatory cell recruitment.[7] Neutrophil- and macrophage-derived elastases and proteases isolated in large quantities in sputum have been proposed to contribute to airway injury and subsequent chronic bronchiectasis pathology.[8]

CLINICAL FEATURES

The classic clinical manifestations of bronchiectasis are daily cough and mucopurulent sputum production. Cough is invariably present and often may be the only symptom for years. Purulent, tenacious sputum production, frequently worse in the morning (having accumulated during recumbency in sleep) is present in most patients. Sputum production may be intermittent, being affected by recurrent infections, bronchial plugging, and antibiotic therapy. "Dry bronchiectasis" presenting as cough, minimal sputum expectoration, and/or hemoptysis is occasionally described. Hemoptysis may be seen in 40% to 70% of patients and may vary from blood streaks to large clots. Increasing cough, dyspnea, and volume and darkening of sputum color, fever, hemoptysis, and chest pain are hallmarks of acute exacerbations. Often patients give a history of recurrent chest infections, although single episodes of severe pneumonia, tuberculosis, or pertussis with secondary pneumonia may also result in bronchiectasis.

On physical examination chest auscultation usually reveals findings of early and midinspiratory crackles as well as diffuse rhonchi and prolonged expiration. Bronchial breath sounds may be heard in severe cases or patients with a complicating pneumonia. Digital clubbing and hypertrophic pulmonary osteoarthropathy, although common in the pre-antibiotic era, are rarely seen now. In advanced cases, there may be evidence of respiratory insufficiency and cor pulmonale.[9]

PREDISPOSING OR ASSOCIATED CONDITIONS

Previously bronchial damage secondary to childhood respiratory tract infections such as pneumonia, pertussis, complicated measles, and tuberculosis were implicated as common causes of bronchiectasis. However, with the early use of antibiotics and childhood immunizations, the focus has shifted from postinfectious to intrinsic host defense causes. Often regarded as a condition in which extensive investigation is unlikely to yield treatable causes, recent studies have shown results to the contrary (Table 53-1). Most series from referral centers identified an association or contributing cause in approximately 50% of patients. Careful investigation and the identification of the genetic basis for immune and other disorders of innate airway defense have reduced the number of idiopathic cases and increased the number of individuals that may considered for specific therapy. The overall impact of these efforts is a bimodal distribution in the age of adult patients with bronchiectasis composed of those with genetic causes first presenting in childhood and an elderly population, typically composing the idiopathic group.

INFECTION

A number of pulmonary infections have been associated with the development of bronchiectasis. Complicating secondary infections with adenovirus, herpesvirus, and bacteria such as *Staphylococcus aureus*, *Klebsiella pneumoniae*, and *Pseudomonas aeruginosa* contribute to the severity of a necrotizing bronchopneumonia. *Streptococcus pneumoniae*, *Haemophilus influenzae*, and *Moraxella* infections typically do not cause bronchiectasis, but may be chronically present within bronchiectatic airways. Necrotizing pneumonias secondary to chronic aspiration or bronchial obstruction are often complicated by parenchymal destruction and bronchiectasis. Tuberculosis can result in bronchiectasis by several mechanisms. Bronchiectasis may be a consequence of tuberculous bronchitis, postobstructive bronchial damage secondary to posttuberculous bronchial wall stenosis, and extraluminal bronchial obstruction by enlarged tuberculous lymph nodes.

The association of nontuberculous *Mycobacterium (NTM)* with bronchiectasis is well documented. CT scan of the chest in such cases is relatively specific, showing small irregular nodules in the middle lobe or lingula, but other parts of the lung may be affected. While traditionally considered a secondary pathogen in an abnormal host or a colonizer in damaged lungs (bullous emphysema, cavitary lung disease) it is now recognized that NTM can cause bronchiectasis in apparently normal hosts. A recent study of individuals with idiopathic bronchiectasis infected with NTM demonstrated shared features with primary ciliary dyskinesia (PCD) (slow cilia beat frequency, low nasal nitric oxide) suggesting the presence of either an underlying genetic or acquired defect.[14] One phenotype for NTM-associated bronchiectasis seems to involve predominantly slender white women 50 to 70 years old with kyphoscoliosis. An underlying primary lung disease or immune defect has not been identified in this subpopulation.[15]

BRONCHIAL OBSTRUCTION

Localized bronchiectasis may also been seen in middle-lobe syndrome, and is usually caused by intraluminal or extraluminal obstruction

TABLE 53-1 Associated Factors and Etiologies of Bronchiectasis

Author, Year	Anwar et al., 2013[10]	Altenburg et al., 2013[11]	McShane et al., 2012[5]	Li et al., 2005[12]	Pasteur, 2000[13]
Patients (*n*)	**189**	**83**	**106**	**136**	**150**
Age (mean)	**66**	**62**	**61**	**12**	**53**
Etiology or Association					
Immunodeficiency	2	2	18	52	12
Postinfection	46	28	10	5	44
Aspiration	2	1	12	25	6
Primary ciliary dyskinesia	2	1	3	20	4
Alpha-1 antitrypsin deficiency	2	1	12	0	0
Congenital structural malformation	0	1	1	5	1
Allergic bronchopulmonary aspergillosis	7	2	1	0	11
Asthma	6	14	0	0	0
Rheumatoid arthritis	9	0	13	0	6
Hematologic (Stem-cell transplant)	0	0	15	0	1
Inflammatory bowel disease	5	0	3	0	2
Idiopathic (%)	82(43)	27(17)	7(6)	35(26)	80 (53)

secondary to tumor, enlarged lymph nodes, or abnormalities of bronchial structure and branching. Endobronchial adenomas, fibromas, chondromas, and lower respiratory tract papillomatosis causing partial airway obstruction and bronchiectasis have been described.

ASPIRATION/INHALATION AIRWAY INJURY

Aspiration or inhalation of foreign matter, such as noxious fumes or particulates into the airways, may result in bronchiectasis. This may involve aspiration of oropharyngeal secretions containing microaerophilic and anaerobic bacteria, leading to a necrotizing pneumonia. Refluxed material from the esophagus or stomach containing food particles, gastric, biliary, and pancreatic secretions, and gut microbes may enter and damage airways, especially if the aspiration events are large and repeated. Depressed sensorium (stroke, alcohol and drug use, seizure, postanesthetic), neuronal or spinal cord dysfunction (amyotrophic lateral sclerosis, multiple sclerosis, syringomyelia), defective laryngeal function (postsurgery, postirradiation), esophageal disorders (dysmotility, achalasia, tracheoesophageal fistula), and gastric disorders (gastric outlet obstruction) influence the likelihood and frequency of aspiration. Bronchiectasis may present years after foreign body aspiration (aspiration is often unrecognized), although bronchiectasis has been seen to occur in animals as soon as 2 to 8 weeks after experimental foreign body introduction into the bronchial tree. GERD is the most common condition in this category contributing to the risk of bronchiectasis CCDC.

CYSTIC FIBROSIS

CF is a common cause of bronchiectasis in the United States and other developed countries (see Chapter 50). This is an autosomal recessive, monogenic disorder that presents most commonly in childhood as a multisystem disease. However, 3% to 7% of patients with CF are diagnosed in adulthood, and due to improvements in therapy, there are now more adults over 18 years old with CF than younger individuals. CF is caused by a genetic deficiency in the Cystic fibrosis transmembrane conductance regulator (CFTR). Approximately 2000 mutations in the CF gene have been identified. Clues suggesting CF as a cause of bronchiectasis include upper lobe radiographic involvement and sputum cultures showing mucoid *P. aeruginosa* or *S. aureus*. The diagnosis of CF rests on a combination of clinical criteria accompanied by sweat chloride values above 40 to 60 mmol/L. However, intermediate or normal sweat chloride values may be seen in patients with clinical manifestations of CF and genetically confirmed CF. Screening for other mutations in the CFTR gene may be necessary in these circumstances. Measurement of the electrical potential difference across the nasal epithelium, available in specialized centers, is sometimes used to corroborate the diagnosis.

PRIMARY CILIARY DYSKINESIA

PCD is a genetically heterogeneous syndrome caused by defect in motile cilia. The true prevalence is unknown but estimated to affect 1:20,000 to 1:100,000 people.[16] The tissue-specific location of cells with motile cilia reflects the clinical features including chronic otitis media, rhinosinusitis, bronchiectasis, infertility, and laterality defects including situs inversus. PCD has an autosomal-recessive inheritance pattern and has been ascribed to mutations in over 30 genes to date that are estimated to account for approximately 60% of all cases. The involvement of many genes in this syndrome is consistent with the knowledge that over 2000 proteins are involved with cilia assembly, structure and function. The ciliary axoneme contains nine outer and two inner pairs of microtubules that are connected to dynein motor proteins forming characteristic structures of motor complexes called inner and outer dynein arms that can be observed by transmission electron microscopy of preparations of cilia from respiratory epithelial cells. Known causative genes in PCD encode proteins for dynein motors (e.g., DNAI1, DNAI2, DNAH5, DNAH11), cilia motor regulation and structural assembly (e.g., RSPH4 A, RSPH9, CCDC39, CCDC40) and motor complex preassembly (e.g., DNAAF1, DNAAF2, HEATR2).[16]

In 1933 Kartagener described the PCD syndrome, as the triad of situs inversus, bronchiectasis, and either nasal polyps or recurrent sinusitis, while the description by Afzelius in 1976 of the defects in the ultrastructure of ciliary dynein arms revealed the basis of this condition.[17,18]Thus, clinical findings include, respiratory distress in neonates, recurrent respiratory tract infections, bronchiectasis, situs inversus, infertility, and heterotaxy in approximately 50%. Laterality defects are the result of motile cilia defects in the embryonic node, a midline structure transiently present during early development that contains cilia. Directional movement of fluid in the node activates downstream programs that establish left and right sidedness of organs. In the absence of flow, *situs solitus* (normal left-right), *situs inversus* (fully reversed right-left, functional organs), or intermediate states may occur resulting in cardiac defects. Thus, individuals with congenital heart disease may also have cilia dysfunction, complicating exacerbation of pulmonary disease in heart failure.[19] Hydrocephalus due to dysfunction of the motile cilia of the brain ventricles is exceedingly rare.

In a study of 94 patients from 68 families, Noone et al.[20] showed that cough was seen in 100% of patients, bronchiectasis (98%), sinusitis (47%), otitis media (92%), and situs inversus (46%). Although most patients with PCD are identified in childhood, this disorder may not be accurately diagnosed until adulthood. Like CF, bronchiectasis occurs in children and is progressive, however in contrast to CF, lung disease is not as severe and lifespan is usually normal.

Accurate testing for PCD is technically demanding and should be performed in specialized centers.[21] Nasal nitric oxide (NO) is emerging as the most sensitive screening test, with levels of NO being characteristically low, a feature that can be shared with CF.[20] Once CF is excluded (e.g., by sweat test), then nasal NO together with clinical features provides high specificity for diagnosis. Ciliated epithelial cells obtained from the inferior or middle turbinate using a sterile cytology brush may be studied for ciliary beat pattern and frequency using digital high-speed video imaging. This requires experienced observers. Abnormalities in ciliary beat have been correlated to ultrastructural defects, but normal ciliary motion cannot fully exclude PCD since some mutations are associated with near normal beat frequencies. Axonemal structure of respiratory cilia may be visualized by transmission electron microscopy and defects in dynein arms, peripheral and central tubules, radial spokes, and basal bodies may be seen. These studies are technically challenging and no structural abnormalities may be found in cases of PCD,[22] particularly when mutations involve regulatory proteins. Genetic testing is available in some research centers.

COPD AND BRONCHIECTASIS

Cigarette smoking causes COPD but is probably not an etiology for bronchiectasis although there is overlap in clinical characteristics that have prognostic and management implications. The phenotype includes frequent exacerbations requiring medical attention in an urgent care setting,[23] HRCT scans that have both emphysema and bronchiectasis portend a reduced prognosis,[24] obstructive impairment on pulmonary function, and sputum microbiology that contains *P. aeruginosa*.[6,25,26]

ALPHA-1 ANTITRYPSIN DEFICIENCY (AATD)

Unimpeded neutrophil elastase contributes to the alveolar destruction of emphysema in AATD. Abundant elastin in airways could also be subject to destruction. There may be a spectrum of disease with heterogeneous lung conditions rather than simply pure emphysema in patients with AATD. Small case series have identified bronchiectatic changes in patients with AATD. Cuvelier et al. measured AAT alleles in patients with known bronchiectasis and healthy blood donors. They did not find any significant differences in AAT alleles between patients with bronchiectasis and control individuals except in those patients with both emphysema and bronchiectasis. There were more abnormal alpha-1 alleles in those patients with coexisting emphysema and bronchiectasis. They concluded that bronchiectasis might be a consequence of emphysema.[27] In a study of 74 patients by Parr et al. with AATD (PiZ phenotype), 70 out of 74 were found to have bronchiectasis on HRCT scan. They defined clinically significant bronchiectasis as patients with regular sputum production and HRCT findings of bronchiectasis affecting four or more lobes.[28] Fifty-seven patients had bronchiectasis in four or more bronchopulmonary segments. Twenty (27%) met the criteria for clinically significant bronchiectasis. In general, those with more severe bronchiectasis had more severe emphysema. Whether there is a common pathway that contributes to both emphysema and bronchiectasis in patients with AATD or whether emphysema predisposes to bronchiectasis is still unknown.[28]

■ ALLERGIC BRONCHOPULMONARY ASPERGILLOSIS

Allergic bronchopulmonary aspergillosis (ABPA) is a hypersensitivity lung disease caused by the ubiquitous fungus *Aspergillus fumigatus* and usually occurs as a complication of persistent asthma or CF. The excessive mucus production and impaired mucociliary clearance in these conditions allow the inhaled conidia of *Aspergillus* to persist and germinate, releasing exoproteases and other fungal products that further compromise clearance, breach epithelium, and activate immune responses. ABPA is characterized by a marked local and systemic eosinophilia, an elevated level of *A. fumigatus*—specific IgG and IgE antibodies, as well as a nonspecific elevation of total IgE. Clinically, ABPA manifests as difficult-to-control or recurring episodes of asthma, pulmonary infiltrates, and central bronchiectasis that may progress to fibrosis. Criteria have been established for the diagnosis of ABPA in the non-CF as well as the CF population.[29]

■ INFLAMMATORY DISORDERS

Inflammatory and fibrotic processes affecting large and small airways may be seen in several rheumatic diseases and autoimmune states. Significantly higher frequencies of bronchiectasis (20%–35%) have been found in *rheumatoid arthritis* (RA) patients undergoing HRCT, both in symptomatic (30%) and asymptomatic (8%) patients, and was independent of smoking status. Bronchiectasis may precede or follow the development of RA, and the coexistence of both conditions is considered to portend a reduced survival.[30] *Sjögren syndrome* may also be complicated by bronchiectasis presumed to be secondary to the effects of inspissated bronchial secretions causing atelectasis and bronchial wall destruction.[31] *Relapsing polychondritis* may be complicated by bronchiectasis in regions of recurring pneumonia as well as regions free of infection. It is not clear whether the chondritis itself or the recurrent infections predispose to bronchiectasis. Inflammatory bowel disease such as *chronic ulcerative colitis* is associated with bronchiectasis. The pathogenesis remains unknown, although autoimmune and immune complex deposition theories have been proposed. This variant of bronchiectasis does not respond to colectomy and has been known to appear and progress after colectomy. Bronchiectasis seen in sarcoidosis is usually traction bronchiectasis secondary to parenchymal and peribronchial fibrosis. Endobronchial sarcoid may result in localized bronchiectasis secondary to obstruction, atelectasis, and bronchial wall destruction.[32]

■ IMMUNE DEFICIENCIES

Bronchiectasis is associated with defects in both cellular and humoral immunity. Bronchiectasis is found in HIV and HTLV-1 infected individuals.[33] It is also associated with acquired immunodeficiencies associated with stem-cell transplant and chemotherapy.[5,12] Recurrent sinopulmonary infections and bronchiectasis are associated with defects in humoral immunity and hypogammaglobulinemia. Several forms of antibody deficiency have been linked with the development of bronchiectasis, including X-linked agammaglobulinemia, common variable immunodeficiency, IgA deficiency, and IgG subclass deficiency (usually IgG-G2 and IgG-G4).[34] The issue of subclass deficiency (in the presence of normal or near-normal levels of total IgG) as a cause of bronchiectasis is controversial due to the wide range of values in normal individuals and the difficulties involved in accurately measuring these levels. An immunizing challenge with common humoral bacterial antigens, such as capsular polysaccharides of *H. influenzae* and *S. pneumoniae* followed by measurement of antibody titers 4 to 6 weeks later, may help establish the presence of such a deficiency. The lack of an antibody response is suggestive that humoral deficiency is present.[35] Early diagnosis of these conditions and replacement with intravenous immunoglobulin significantly reduces infections and prevents bronchiectasis, although the efficacy of this treatment in patients with selective IgM, IgA, and IgG subclass deficiency remains controversial. Standard doses in adults of 300 mg/kg by intravenous infusion every 4 weeks have been proved to reduce rates and severity of respiratory infections, but higher doses of 600 mg/kg appear more efficacious in reducing respiratory exacerbations and preserving pulmonary function in some patients.[36] Hyper-IgE syndrome is accompanied by recurrent lower respiratory infections leading to bronchiectasis and cystic lung destruction. Respiratory infection with *Pseudomonas* is a contributor to mortality.[37]

DIAGNOSIS OF BRONCHIECTASIS

The diagnosis of bronchiectasis is based on history, clinical features, and radiologic demonstration of bronchiectatic airways. The diagnostic evaluation in these patients is largely aimed at identifying potentially treatable underlying causes of bronchiectasis (Table 53-2). After confirming the diagnosis with chest imaging, CBC with differential

TABLE 53-2 Clinical Approach to the Patient with Suspected Bronchiectasis

History	Recurrent lower and/or upper respiratory tract infections, pneumonia
	Daily mucopurulent sputum production
Initial studies	CBC with differential
	Chest x-ray
	Immunoglobulins IgG, IgM, IgA
	Sputum: bacterial culture and sensitivity, mycobacteria, fungi
Confirms diagnosis	Chest CT (non-contrast)
Other studies	Sweat chloride and/or genetic panel for CFTR alleles
	Allergic bronchopulmonary aspergillus panel (IgE, precipitins, or skin test)
	Bronchoscopy (for cultures, obstruction)
	Nasal nitric oxide
	Alpha-1 antitrypsin level; phenotype
	Pulmonary function (spirometry pre- and postbronchodilator)
	Serum antibody response to bacterial antigen challenge, e.g., pneumococcal vaccine

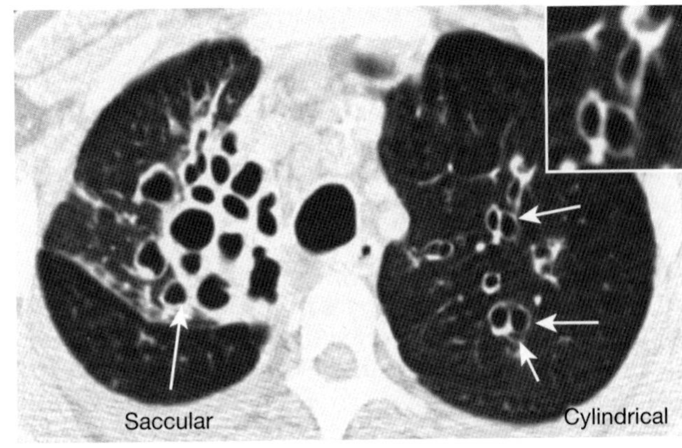

Figure 53-1 Chest computed tomography. *(Left chest) Cylindrical* bronchiectasis: dilated and thickened airways *(arrows and insert). (Right chest) Saccular* or cystic bronchiectasis: very dilated airways clustered into saccules, cysts, or grapelike clusters *(arrow).*

for eosinophils, serum immunoglobulins IgG, IgA, and gM, sweat chloride or genetic CF testing, sputum culture for bacteria, mycobacteria, and fungi are productive starting tests. Subsequent testing will depend on clues from the history and likelihood of other conditions.

CHEST RADIOGRAPH

The chest x-ray may be abnormal and show the presence of increased pulmonary markings, ring-like structures, atelectasis, dilated and thickened airways (tram lines), and mucus plugging (finger-in-glove) appearance; however, the chest radiograph may be normal even in the presence of bronchiectasis.

HIGH-RESOLUTION COMPUTED TOMOGRAPHY

HRCT is now the defining test for the diagnosis of bronchiectasis. HRCT can accurately diagnose bronchiectasis, localize, and describe areas of parenchymal abnormality, and identify bronchiolar abnormalities and mucus plugging. It also can identify focal areas of air trapping as an indicator of small airway disease (mosaic attenuation).

Airway dilatation can be gauged when seen in cross section. A luminal diameter more than 1.5 times the adjacent vessel is indicative of bronchiectasis (Figs. 53-1 and 53-2). Other findings include bronchial wall thickening and small airway plugging with debris (tree-in-bud) (Figs. 53-2 and 53-3). The distribution and pattern of

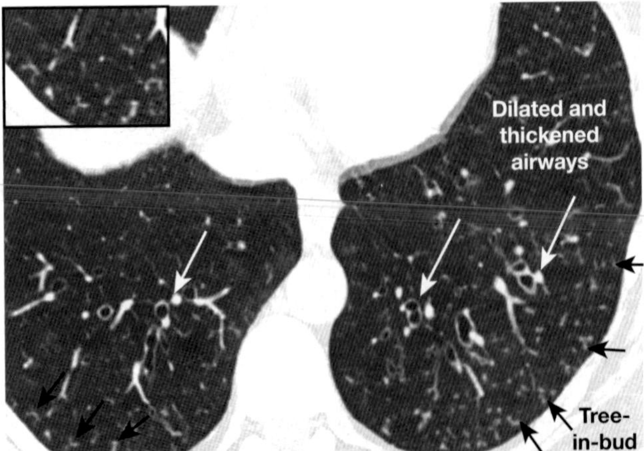

Figure 53-2 Chest computed tomography. Extensive peripheral branching opacities of tree-in-bud *(black arrows)*. Dilated and thickened airways *(white arrows).*

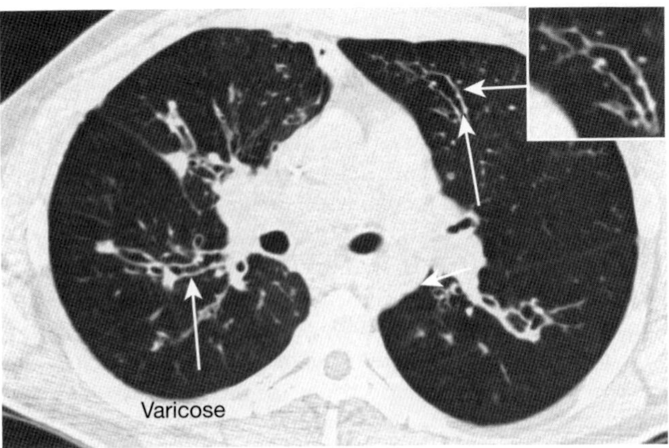

Figure 53-3 Chest computed tomography shows *varicose* bronchiectasis: dilated airways with irregular thickened mucosa *(arrows).*

bronchiectasis may implicate a specific cause. Cartier et al.[38] found that bilateral predominantly upper lobe bronchiectasis is seen most commonly in CF, ABPA, and sequelae of tuberculosis. A middle-lobe distribution with irregular ground glass nodules is very characteristic of NTM.[15] A lower lobe predominance is seen in most other causes. HRCT scoring systems for CF have been developed to identify disease at an early stage, grade severity, monitor disease progression, and utilize as endpoints in clinical trials. With similar CT findings in bronchiectasis, these scoring systems may be applicable for non-CF bronchiectasis.[39] PCD children have been assessed with one of these scoring systems and correlated with pulmonary function and compared to age and gender-matched CF children and adults.[40]

Bronchiectasis may be classified by pathologic features and radiographic appearance. Reid[41] described a correlation between pathologic and bronchographic findings in bronchiectasis; since then, this has been the most widely used classification. In *cylindrical* bronchiectasis, the bronchi are regularly outlined (tubular), dilated in diameter, with straight walls, often coming to a straight abrupt end instead of a tapering end due to obstruction of the peripheral bronchial tree by secretions, casts, and inflammatory wall edema. *Varicose* bronchiectasis (illusion to varicose veins) is marked by the presence of irregular dilatations, outpouchings, and tortuosity of the airways. *Saccular* (cystic) bronchiectasis is characterized by the presence of cystic distortion of the distal airways that may be focal or more generalized, resulting in saccules that appear as a cluster of grapes (Fig. 53-1 *arrows and inset*). Traction bronchiectasis, a term used to describe the dilated airways seen in diffuse pulmonary fibrosis secondary to fibrous tissue traction and elevated negative intrathoracic pressure, should be distinguished from usual bronchiectasis, because of the lack of intrinsic airway pathology and paucity of sputum expectoration. Congenital bronchial cysts (central and peripheral) are developmentally abnormal cystic bronchial structures, often filled with mucus and lined with respiratory epithelium. While usually lacking connection with the parent bronchus and distal alveoli, if infected they may communicate and mimic localized bronchiectasis. Intralobar bronchopulmonary sequestration too may become infected and communicate with the bronchial tree, mimicking localized bronchiectasis.

PULMONARY FUNCTION

Pulmonary function is usually abnormal. The degree of impairment depends not only on the nature and extent of the morphologic abnormalities of bronchiectasis, but also on the presence or absence of associated COPD. Thus, patients with mild localized bronchiectasis and no chronic bronchitis may have normal lung function tests. Spirometry will often show a pattern of airflow obstruction, with normal or reduced forced vital capacity (FVC), reduced forced

TABLE 53-3 Microbiology in Bronchiectasis

Author, Year	Li et al., 2005[12]	Angrill et al., 2002[7]	Pasteur et al., 2000[13]	Nicotra et al., 1995[45]
Mean age (y)	**12**	**53**	**58**	**57**
Patients (*n*)	**136**	**42**	**150**	**123**
Microbiologic Flora (%)				
Haemophilus influenzae	53(40)	11(26)	52(35)	37(30)
Pseudomonas aeruginosa	15(11)	4(9)	46(31)	38(31)
Streptococcus pneumoniae	23(18)	6(14)	20(13)	13(11)
Staphylococcus aureus	5(4)	NA	NA	9(7)
Moraxella catarrhalis	3(2)	2(5)	30(20)	3(2)
Nocardia	0	NA	NA	4(3)
Anaerobes	1(1)	NA	NA	2(1)
Mycobacteria	0	NA	NA	49(40)
Aspergillus	1(1)	1(2)	3(2)	6(5)
Two or more organisms	21	NA	NA	60

expiratory volume in 1 second (FEV_1), and reduced FEV_1/FVC ratio. In some patients with accompanying atelectasis and/or parenchymal and pleural scarring, restrictive or mixed/obstructive and restrictive physiology may be seen with reduced FVC and normal FEV_1/FVC ratios. The Lung Clearance Index (LCI; multiple breath nitrogen washout) is another method to detect airflow obstruction. The LCI has been used to detect early airflow obstruction in CF and may be more sensitive than changes in spirometry. In bronchiectasis the LCI is reproducible and correlates better with abnormalities on chest CT than FEV1.[42]The diffusing capacity for carbon monoxide is initially normal but may decrease with progressive disease. Impaired oxygenation is highly variable, most likely due to heterogeneity among patients in anatomic disease distribution.

MICROBIOLOGY

The sputum of patients with bronchiectasis is frequently found to be colonized with potentially pathogenic microorganisms (Table 53-3). The most frequent microorganisms isolated are *H. influenzae*, *S. pneumoniae*, and *P. aeruginosa* and are often implicated as the cause of exacerbations. Sequencing of lung microbiota in patients with bronchiectasis demonstrates both diversity of communities and a predominance of *Haemophilus*, *Pseudomonas*, and *Streptococci* in stable patients and during exacerbations.[43,44] Colonization with *P. aeruginosa*, in particular, has been associated with more severe impairment of lung function, more intense inflammatory response, and more extensive lung disease independent of the cause of bronchiectasis.[6] Instances of airway colonization with other potential pathogens that may require specific treatment include *Nocardia asteroides*, *A. fumigatus*, and nontuberculous mycobacteria. Anaerobic bacteria are identified in genomic surveys of airway microbiota of individuals with non-CF bronchiectasis; however, there is no direct implication for therapy.[43,44]

TREATMENT

The management of bronchiectasis is aimed at treating underlying conditions, controlling infection, reducing inflammation, improving bronchial hygiene, and surgical resection of focal bronchiectasis or severely affected segments or lobes. With few quality clinical trials for guidance, treatment often has to be tailored to the specific needs, tolerances, and preferences of individual patients.

■ CONTROL OF INFECTION

Since infection plays a major role in the causation and perpetuation of bronchiectasis, reducing the microbial load and associated inflammatory mediators remains a cornerstone of therapy. Antibiotics are indicated to treat an acute exacerbation. Antibiotics are directed at commonly isolated pathogens such as *H. influenzae* and *P. aeruginosa*. Oral fluoroquinolones are often used as initial antibiotic choices for treatment durations of 10 to 14 days. In the face of failure to respond to treatment or the occurrence of frequent exacerbations over short periods of time, sputum cultures and sensitivity tests should be performed to help define antibiotic selection and/or aid in alternative diagnoses, for example, atypical mycobacteria or fungus. Severe exacerbations due to *P. aeruginosa* require the intravenous administration of antipseudomonal antibiotics and potential hospitalization.

The role of prophylactic/suppressive antibiotics remains controversial. Several approaches to the prescription of suppressive antibiotics exist, including daily antibiotics, antibiotics given for 1 to 2 weeks each month, as well as more prolonged courses lasting weeks to months.

The use of daily, twice weekly, and thrice weekly macrolides (erythromycin, azithromycin) as biologic response modifiers in CF and diffuse panbronchiolitis has generated considerable interest regarding a role in the treatment of bronchiectasis. In the EMBRACE and BAT trials, azithromycin was associated with a decrease in exacerbations compared with placebo. However, no significant difference was noted in lung function.[11,46] In the BAT trial gastrointestinal intolerance and macrolide resistance was common. Similarly, in the BLESS study, erythromycin decreased the number of exacerbations and ameliorated the decline in lung function but with a consequential development of macrolide resistance.[47] Macrolides have been shown to have several biologic effects not related to their antibacterial properties. These include effects on nuclear transcription factors with downregulation of proinflammatory cytokines, suppression of iNOS, reduced adhesion molecule expression, reduced neutrophil chemotaxis and degranulation, cytoprotection against phospholipids, improvement in mucus rheology, reduction in bronchial hyperreactivity, effects on *Pseudomonas* biofilm production, and quorum sensing function.[48]

Administration of antibiotic aerosols (chiefly tobramycin 300 mg nebulized twice daily and aztreonam 75 mg three times daily) are effective in CF. Pilot studies of non-CF bronchiectasis have demonstrated a reduction in *Pseudomonas* density and even eradication of *Pseudomonas* in some patients, although side effects were also noticed, including increased cough, wheezing, dyspnea, tinnitus, voice alteration, and tobramycin resistance.[49] The effects of other aerosolized antibiotics, such as colistin, ciprofloxacin,[50] and gentamicin[51] alone, or in rotation with tobramycin need to be assessed for efficacy and side effects.

NTM-associated bronchiectasis should be considered in patients not responding to antibacterial therapy. The diagnosis requires two or more separate expectorated sputum collections with positive cultures for NTM or one positive culture from a bronchial wash and radiologic evidence of progressive infiltrates, multiple nodules, or cavitation on chest imaging. American Thoracic Society guidelines provide treatment guidance for the individual NTM species.[52]

ABPA responds to oral prednisone in doses of 0.5 to 1 mg/kg per day. The addition of antifungal azoles (itraconazole 400 mg/day for 2 months; then 200 mg/day; or voriconazole 300 mg twice daily)[53] may confer additional benefits in terms of reducing fungal burden, steroid dose, and exacerbations. Early and appropriate therapy for ABPA may prevent or delay permanent airway destruction. Because of its relapsing course, monitoring of clinical, radiographic, and serologic responses (IgE) is necessary.

BRONCHIAL HYGIENE

Airway mucus clearance is a problem in bronchiectasis. Chest percussion and postural drainage have been the traditional method of facilitating mucus clearance. The onerous and labor-intensive nature of physical therapy procedures such as chest wall percussion and postural drainage, and potential issues of hypoxemia and chest discomfort may result in poor patient compliance. These issues have led to a search for alternative therapies. Autogenic drainage, mechanical vibration with ultrasonic devices, positive expiratory pressure, and flutter valve devices have been shown to achieve good airway clearance provided the patient has motivation, breath control, and the neuromuscular function to perform. An intrapulmonary percussive ventilation device and vibratory vest help provide mucus clearance in patients unable to perform the other techniques.[54] Studies document increased sputum expectoration using all these methods, with no method being demonstrably more effective or preferred. Thus, it is recommended that patients should choose their modality based on ability, motivation, preference, needs, and resources.

MUCUS CLEARANCE

Mucus hypersecretion is a prominent feature of bronchiectasis and little is known about the effects of current therapies, because of the difficulties in quantifying mucus hypersecretion in clinical studies, both at baseline and in response to treatment. Maintenance of hydration with oral and/or intravenous fluids is considered useful in preventing inspissated sputum retention. Humidification of inhaled air or oxygen as an adjunct to airway clearance techniques has been shown to significantly increase the wet weight of sputum produced. The use of nebulized normal or hypertonic saline may be considered as adjuncts to bronchial hygiene, although bronchospasm may be associated with the use of these agents. A randomized multicenter study evaluating the efficacy of aerosolized DNAse in non-CF bronchiectasis did not find it efficacious in this group of patients.[55] Rather it was associated with increased pulmonary exacerbation rates, hospitalizations, antibiotic use, and a fall in FEV_1 and FVC. The anti-osmolar agent, mannitol, has shown efficacy to stabilize pulmonary function and reduce exacerbations.[56]

BRONCHODILATORS

Bronchodilators, such as beta agonists or anticholinergics, are used in patients with bronchiectasis, since these patients show signs of airflow obstruction and hyperreactivity. Formoterol in addition to budesonide has been shown to reduce symptoms and improve scoring on an HQOL questionnaire as compared to budesonide alone.[24]

Anti-inflammatory Therapy Persistent endobronchial inflammation is known to play a significant role in the pathogenesis of bronchiectasis, and anti-inflammatory therapy may be beneficial. The role of inhaled steroids (fluticasone) in bronchiectasis was evaluated by Tsang et al.,[57] who found reduced sputum volume and purulence, and reduced rates of exacerbations.

SURGERY

Bronchiectasis is usually a diffuse disease and surgical extirpation of affected areas is often not feasible. However, in selected cases surgical resection of the most severely affected segments, bleeding segments, or areas harboring resistant tuberculosis or atypical mycobacteria may confer significant benefits in terms of symptom control, reduction of tenacious sputum production, elimination of large-volume bronchial bleeding, reduction of acute infective episodes, and improved quality of life. The surgical approach varies according to the centers offering this treatment, with some preferring a video-assisted thoracoscopy approach, while others recommend the lateral thoracotomy approach. The complications associated with surgery include spread of infection, bleeding, prolonged air leak, and poor lung expansion following surgery.[58]

Lung transplantation is now considered a viable option in advanced cases, when earlier the risks of persistence of infection in the face of prolonged immunosuppression seemed prohibitive. The outcomes of patients receiving lung transplantation in non-CF bronchiectasis were reported from the United Kingdom. Fifty-four patients underwent bilateral lung transplantation between 1997 and 2007. The mean age was 54 and the median transplant list waiting time was 309 days. The median survival time for transplant recipients was 8 years.[59]

MISCELLANEOUS

While not evaluated specifically for bronchiectasis, vaccinations against *S. pneumoniae* and influenza should be considered in these patients. Smoking cessation should be emphasized as a matter of routine. Patients with advanced bronchiectasis with evidence of exercise and/or nocturnal desaturation should be considered for oxygen supplementation to delay the onset of pulmonary hypertension and cor pulmonale and improve exercise tolerance. Pulmonary rehabilitation and inspiratory muscle training may be considered, as these modalities have been documented to improve exercise tolerance.[60]

REFERENCES

1. King PT, Holdsworth SR, Freezer NJ, Villanueva E, Holmes PW. Characterisation of the onset and presenting clinical features of adult bronchiectasis. *Respir Med.* 2006;100:2183–2189.
2. Seitz AE, Olivier KN, Adjemian J, Holland SM, Prevots R. Trends in bronchiectasis among medicare beneficiaries in the United States, 2000 to 2007. *Chest.* 2012;142:432–439.
3. Weycker D, Edelsberg J, Oster G, Tino G. Prevalence and economic burden of bronchiectasis. *Clin Pulm Med.* 2005;12:205–209.
4. Cole PJ. Inflammation: a two-edged sword–the model of bronchiectasis. *Eur J Respir Dis Suppl.* 1986;147:6–15.
5. McShane PJ, Naureckas ET, Strek ME. Bronchiectasis in a diverse US population: effects of ethnicity on etiology and sputum culture. *Chest.* 2012;142:159–167.
6. Wilson CB, Jones PW, O'Leary CJ, Hansell DM, Cole PJ, Wilson R. Effect of sputum bacteriology on the quality of life of patients with bronchiectasis. *Eur Respir J.* 1997;10:1754–1760.
7. Angrill J, Agusti C, de Celis R, et al. Bacterial colonisation in patients with bronchiectasis: microbiological pattern and risk factors. *Thorax.* 2002;57:15–19.
8. Chan SC, Shum DK, Ip MS. Sputum sol neutrophil elastase activity in bronchiectasis: differential modulation by syndecan-1. *Am J Respir Crit Care Med.* 2003;168:192–198.

9. Alzeer AH, Al-Mobeirek AF, Al-Otair HA, Elzamzamy UA, Joherjy IA, Shaffi AS. Right and left ventricular function and pulmonary artery pressure in patients with bronchiectasis. *Chest.* 2008;133:468–473.
10. Anwar GA, McDonnell MJ, Worthy SA, et al. Phenotyping adults with non-cystic fibrosis bronchiectasis: a prospective observational cohort study. *Respir Med.* 2013;107:1001–1007.
11. Altenburg J, de Graaff CS, Stienstra Y, et al. Effect of azithromycin maintenance treatment on infectious exacerbations among patients with non-cystic fibrosis bronchiectasis: the BAT randomized controlled trial. *JAMA.* 2013;309:1251–1259.
12. Li AM, Sonnappa S, Lex C, et al. Non-CF bronchiectasis: does knowing the aetiology lead to changes in management? *Eur Respir J.* 2005;26:8–14.
13. Pasteur MC, Helliwell SM, Houghton SJ, et al. An investigation into causative factors in patients with bronchiectasis. *Am J Respir Crit Care Med.* 2000;162:1277–1284.
14. Fowler CJ, Olivier KN, Leung JM, et al. Abnormal nasal nitric oxide production, ciliary beat frequency and Toll-like receptor response in pulmonary nontuberculous mycobacterial disease epithelium. *Am J Respir Crit Care Med.* 2013;187(12):1374–1381.
15. Glassroth J. Pulmonary disease due to nontuberculous mycobacteria. *Chest.* 2008;133:243–251.
16. Leigh MW, Pittman JE, Carson JL, et al. Clinical and genetic aspects of primary ciliary dyskinesia/Kartagener syndrome. *Genet Med.* 2009;11:473–487.
17. Afzelius BA. A human syndrome caused by immotile cilia. *Science.* 1976;193:317–319.
18. Eliasson R, Mossberg B, Camner P, Afzelius BA. The immotile-cilia syndrome. A congenital ciliary abnormality as an etiologic factor in chronic airway infections and male sterility. *N Engl J Med.* 1977;297:1–6.
19. Nakhleh N, Francis R, Giese RA, et al. High prevalence of respiratory ciliary dysfunction in congenital heart disease patients with heterotaxy. *Circulation.* 2012;125:2232–2242.
20. Noone PG, Leigh MW, Sannuti A, et al. Primary ciliary dyskinesia: diagnostic and phenotypic features. *Am J Respir Crit Care Med.* 2004;169:459–467.
21. Stannard WA, Chilvers MA, Rutman AR, Williams CD, O'Callaghan C. Diagnostic testing of patients suspected of primary ciliary dyskinesia. *Am J Respir Crit Care Med.* 2010;181: 307–314.
22. Olin JT, Burns K, Carson JL, et al.; for the Genetic Disorders of Mucociliary Clearance Consortium. Diagnostic yield of nasal scrape biopsies in primary ciliary dyskinesia: a multicenter experience. *Pediatr Pulmonol.* 2011;46:483–488.
23. Hurst JR, Vestbo J, Anzueto A, et al.; Evaluation of COPD Longitudinally to Identify Predictive Surrogate Endpoints (ECLIPSE) Investigators. Susceptibility to exacerbation in chronic obstructive pulmonary disease. *N Engl J Med.* 2010;363: 1128–1138.
24. Martinez-Garcia MA, Soler-Cataluna JJ, Catalan-Serra P, Roman-Sanchez P, Tordera MP. Clinical efficacy and safety of budesonide-formoterol in non-cystic fibrosis bronchiectasis. *Chest.* 2012;141:461–468.
25. Almagro P, Salvado M, Garcia-Vidal C, et al. *Pseudomonas aeruginosa* and mortality after hospital admission for chronic obstructive pulmonary disease. *Respiration.* 2012;84:36–43.
26. Murphy TF, Brauer AL, Eschberger K, et al. *Pseudomonas aeruginosa* in chronic obstructive pulmonary disease. *Am J Respir Crit Care Med.* 2008;177:853–860.
27. Cuvelier A, Muir JF, Hellot MF, et al. Distribution of alpha(1)-antitrypsin alleles in patients with bronchiectasis. *Chest.* 2000;117:415–419.
28. Parr DG, Guest PG, Reynolds JH, Dowson LJ, Stockley RA. Prevalence and impact of bronchiectasis in alpha1-antitrypsin deficiency. *Am J Respir Crit Care Med.* 2007;176:1215–1221.
29. Agarwal R. Allergic bronchopulmonary aspergillosis. *Chest.* 2009; 135:805–826.
30. Demoruelle MK, Weisman MH, Simonian PL, et al. Brief report: airways abnormalities and rheumatoid arthritis-related autoantibodies in subjects without arthritis: early injury or initiating site of autoimmunity? *Arthritis Rheum.* 2012;64:1756–1761.
31. Soto-Cardenas MJ, Perez-De-Lis M, Bove A, et al. Bronchiectasis in primary Sjogren's syndrome: prevalence and clinical significance. *Clin Exp Rheumatol.* 2010;28:647–653.
32. Cohen M, Sahn SA. Bronchiectasis in systemic diseases. *Chest.* 1999;116:1063–1074.
33. Verghese A, al-Samman M, Nabhan D, Naylor AD, Rivera M. Bacterial bronchitis and bronchiectasis in human immunodeficiency virus infection. *Arch Intern Med.* 1994;154:2086–2091.
34. Tarzi MD, Grigoriadou S, Carr SB, Kuitert LM, Longhurst HJ. Clinical immunology review series: an approach to the management of pulmonary disease in primary antibody deficiency. *Clin Exp Immunol.* 2009;155:147–155.
35. Vendrell M, de Gracia J, Rodrigo MJ, et al. Antibody production deficiency with normal IgG levels in bronchiectasis of unknown etiology. *Chest.* 2005;127:197–204.
36. Eijkhout HW, van Der Meer JW, Kallenberg CG, et al.; Inter-University Working Party for the Study of Immune Deficiencies. The effect of two different dosages of intravenous immunoglobulin on the incidence of recurrent infections in patients with primary hypogammaglobulinemia. A randomized, double-blind, multicenter crossover trial. *Ann Intern Med.* 2001;135:165–174.
37. Freeman AF, Kleiner DE, Nadiminti H, et al. Causes of death in hyper-IgE syndrome. *J Allergy Clin Immunol.* 2007;119:1234–1240.
38. Cartier Y, Kavanagh PV, Johkoh T, Mason AC, Muller NL. Bronchiectasis: accuracy of high-resolution CT in the differentiation of specific diseases. *AJR Am J Roentgenol.* 1999;173:47–52.
39. de Jong PA, Ottink MD, Robben SG, et al. Pulmonary disease assessment in cystic fibrosis: comparison of CT scoring systems and value of bronchial and arterial dimension measurements. *Radiology.* 2004;231:434–439.
40. Santamaria F, Montella S, Tiddens HA, et al. Structural and functional lung disease in primary ciliary dyskinesia. *Chest.* 2008;134:351–357.
41. Reid LM. Reduction in bronchial subdivision in bronchiectasis. *Thorax.* 1950;5:233–247.
42. Rowan SA, Bradley JM, Bradbury I, et al. Lung clearance index is a repeatable and sensitive indicator of radiological changes in bronchiectasis. *Am J Respir Crit Care Med.* 2014;189: 586–592.
43. Rogers GB, van der Gast CJ, Cuthbertson L, et al. Clinical measures of disease in adult non-CF bronchiectasis correlate with airway microbiota composition. *Thorax.* 2013;68(8):731–737.
44. Tunney MM, Einarsson GG, Wei L, et al. Lung microbiota and bacterial abundance in patients with bronchiectasis when clinically stable and during exacerbation. *Am J Respir Crit Care Med.* 2013;187:1118–1126.
45. Nicotra MB, Rivera M, Dale AM, Shepherd R, Carter R. Clinical, pathophysiologic, and microbiologic characterization of bronchiectasis in an aging cohort. *Chest.* 1995;108:955–961.

46. Wong C, Jayaram L, Karalus N, et al. Azithromycin for prevention of exacerbations in non-cystic fibrosis bronchiectasis (EMBRACE): a randomised, double-blind, placebo-controlled trial. *Lancet.* 2012;380:660–667.

47. Serisier DJ, Martin ML, McGuckin MA, et al. Effect of long-term, low-dose erythromycin on pulmonary exacerbations among patients with non-cystic fibrosis bronchiectasis: the BLESS randomized controlled trial. *JAMA.* 2013;309:1260–1267.

48. Rubin BK, Henke MO. Immunomodulatory activity and effectiveness of macrolides in chronic airway disease. *Chest.* 2004;125:70S–78S.

49. Barker AF, Couch L, Fiel SB, et al. Tobramycin solution for inhalation reduces sputum *Pseudomonas aeruginosa* density in bronchiectasis. *Am J Respir Crit Care Med.* 2000;162:481–485.

50. Wilson R, Welte T, Polverino E, et al. Ciprofloxacin dry powder for inhalation in non-cystic fibrosis bronchiectasis: a phase II randomised study. *Eur Respir J.* 2013;41:1107–1115.

51. Murray MP, Govan JR, Doherty CJ, et al. A randomized controlled trial of nebulized gentamicin in non-cystic fibrosis bronchiectasis. *Am J Respir Crit Care Med.* 2011;183:491–499.

52. Griffith DE, Aksamit T, Brown-Elliott BA, et al. An official ATS/IDSA statement: diagnosis, treatment, and prevention of nontuberculous mycobacterial diseases. *Am J Respir Crit Care Med.* 2007;175:367–416.

53. Wark PA, Hensley MJ, Saltos N, et al. Anti-inflammatory effect of itraconazole in stable allergic bronchopulmonary aspergillosis: a randomized controlled trial. *J Allergy Clin Immunol.* 2003;111:952–957.

54. Hess DR. Airway clearance: physiology, pharmacology, techniques, and practice. *Respir Care.* 2007;52:1392–1396.

55. O'Donnell AE, Barker AF, Ilowite JS, Fick RB. Treatment of idiopathic bronchiectasis with aerosolized recombinant human DNase I. rhDNase Study Group. *Chest.* 1998;113:1329–1334.

56. Gjoerup J, Hilberg O, Bendstrup E. Inhaled mannitol in the treatment of non-cystic fibrosis bronchiectasis in adults. *Respirology.* 2012;17:927–932.

57. Tsang KW, Tan KC, Ho PL, et al. Inhaled fluticasone in bronchiectasis: a 12 month study. *Thorax.* 2005;60:239–243.

58. Zhang P, Jiang G, Ding J, Zhou X, Gao W. Surgical treatment of bronchiectasis: a retrospective analysis of 790 patients. *Ann Thorac Surg.* 2010;90:246–250.

59. Titman A, Rogers CA, Bonser RS, Banner NR, Sharples LD. Disease-specific survival benefit of lung transplantation in adults: a national cohort study. *Am J Transplant.* 2009;9:1640–1649.

60. Newall C, Stockley RA, Hill SL. Exercise training and inspiratory muscle training in patients with bronchiectasis. *Thorax.* 2005;60:943–948.

PART 5

Interstitial and Inflammatory Lung Diseases

SECTION 11 Immunologic and Interstitial Diseases

CHAPTER 54

Interstitial Lung Disease: A Clinical Overview and General Approach

Danielle Antin-Ozerkis

INTRODUCTION

Commonly, interstitial lung disease (ILD) presents with dyspnea on exertion, diffuse bilateral infiltrates on chest imaging, and restriction with diffusion impairment on physiologic testing. When tissue is obtained, the lung parenchyma may contain any combination of abnormalities, including inflammation, fibrosis, and granulomas. While many forms of ILD are extremely rare, there are some, such as idiopathic pulmonary fibrosis (IPF) and sarcoidosis that are seen commonly in general pulmonary practice. Masqueraders of ILD such as infection, pulmonary edema, and malignancy will be encountered in the assessment of an abnormal chest radiograph, and distinguishing these from true ILD is crucial.

ILD refers to a heterogeneous collection of more than one hundred distinct lung disorders that tend to be grouped together because they share clinical, radiographic, and pathologic features. These disorders are sometimes called diffuse parenchymal lung disease (DPLD) to make the point that the interstitium is not the only compartment of the lung affected. Entities such as organizing pneumonia or pulmonary alveolar proteinosis may cause an alveolar filling process. Respiratory bronchiolitis and chronic hypersensitivity pneumonitis may center on the airway, involving this compartment as well. Occasionally, purely airway-centered diseases like bronchiolitis obliterans may be initially identified as an ILD because of overlapping radiographic findings. A structured approach is necessary since treatments may vary considerably depending on the diagnosis.

Diagnosis is based upon a comprehensive history, a careful physical examination, as well as review of laboratory data, physiologic studies, radiography, and in some cases, pathologic tissue obtained from lung biopsy. Multidisciplinary review is an important part of the process and can have a significant impact on diagnostic and management decisions. For each patient, decisions regarding diagnostic approach and therapy must be individualized based upon the patient's respiratory status, comorbid medical conditions, and personal approach to medical care.

DIAGNOSTIC APPROACH TO ILD

Several classification schemes for ILD have been proposed, which include histopathologic and clinical characteristics.[1] The American Thoracic Society (ATS)/European Respiratory Society (ERS) consensus panel classification system was published in 2001 and has recently been revised.[2] One approach is given in Figure 54-1.

It is often helpful in the case of any individual patient to incorporate a combination of historical, clinical, radiographic, and pathologic features. Distinguishing those patients who have a known cause for their ILD (e.g., connective tissue disease, occupational or environmental exposure, or drug toxicity) from those who do not (e.g., IPF, sarcoidosis) is an important first step. Clinical features, such as acuity of onset, may help to classify disease as well. For example, the subacute time course of a patient with organizing pneumonia will be quite different than the insidious onset of dyspnea in IPF. The radiographic pattern of IPF will be characterized by bibasilar traction bronchiectasis and honeycombing, while sarcoidosis may demonstrate upper lobe-predominant nodular opacities with retraction and volume loss. Histopathologic characterization may range from acute inflammation to granulomatous involvement, or fixed fibrosis and collagen deposition.

It is important to note that the names used to describe the clinical entities themselves must be distinguished from the radiographic and

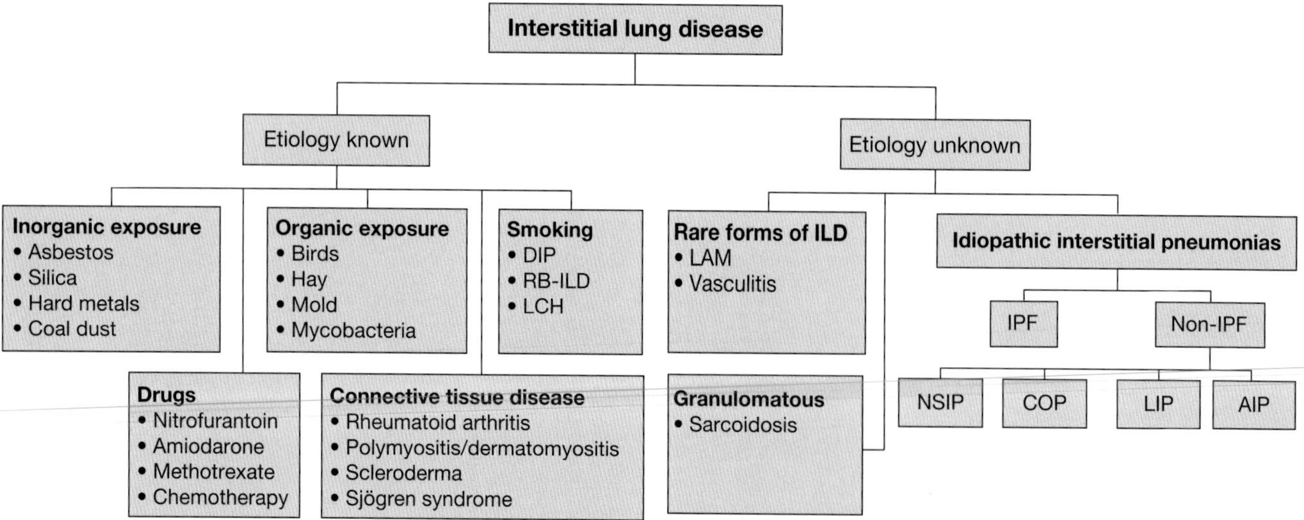

Figure 54-1 An overview of ILD classification. DIP, desquamative interstitial pneumonia; RB-ILD, respiratory bronchiolitis interstitial lung disease; LCH, Langerhans cell histiocytosis; LAM, lymphangioleiomyomatosis; IPF, idiopathic pulmonary fibrosis; NSIP, nonspecific interstitial pneumonia; COP, cryptogenic organizing pneumonia; LIP, lymphocytic interstitial pneumonia; AIP, acute interstitial pneumonia. *(Data from ATS/ERS classification, 2001.)*

TABLE 54-1 Time Course of Disease Onset

Acute
Cryptogenic organizing pneumonia
Acute eosinophilic pneumonia
Acute hypersensitivity pneumonitis
Diffuse alveolar hemorrhage
Acute interstitial pneumonia
Acute exacerbation of idiopathic pulmonary fibrosis or other ILDs
Subacute to Chronic
Connective tissue disease–associated ILD
Idiopathic pulmonary fibrosis
Sarcoidosis
Chronic hypersensitivity pneumonitis
Occupational lung disease
Nonspecific interstitial pneumonia
Desquamative interstitial pneumonitis
Respiratory bronchiolitis interstitial lung disease
Lymphocytic interstitial pneumonia
Chronic eosinophilic pneumonia

pathological terms used to describe the findings. For example, IPF is the clinical entity associated with a usual interstitial pneumonia (UIP) pattern on chest CT and on pathology. However, the finding of a UIP pattern alone does not ensure a diagnosis of IPF, as this may also be seen in other entities, such as the connective tissue diseases.

CLINICAL HISTORY

The typical presentation of ILD is nonspecific and may include vague pulmonary complaints, such as dyspnea on exertion or cough, and an abnormal radiograph. In some cases the time course of the disease may suggest certain forms of ILD (Table 54-1). The acute forms of ILD must be distinguished from respiratory infections and pulmonary edema due to congestive heart failure.

It is important to consider key features of the patient. For example, the differential diagnosis for dyspnea and diffuse infiltrates on chest radiograph will vary markedly between immunocompetent patients and those who have undergone organ or bone marrow transplantation, are neutropenic from recent chemotherapy, or who have advanced HIV disease. In the immunocompetent host, it is often after a lack of response to antibiotics or diuretics that ILD is suspected. Other clinical features may affect the presentation as well. In elderly or disabled patients, musculoskeletal issues may limit mobility and dyspnea may be a late symptom. In a patient with other cardiopulmonary disease, relatively minor ILD may cause an earlier onset of disabling dyspnea and the discovery of ILD for this reason. It is helpful to attempt an objective quantification of the degree of dyspnea, such as the distance the patient walks before becoming breathless or the number of steps climbed before a rest must be taken.

Often a persistent cough after a respiratory infection leads to the initial chest radiograph. While other respiratory symptoms are less common, they may help focus the differential diagnosis. For example, a history of wheezing may suggest an airway-centered process such as hypersensitivity pneumonitis, eosinophilic pneumonia, or sarcoidosis.[3] Substernal chest pain is commonly described by patients with sarcoidosis.[4] Pleuritic chest pain may herald serositis in a patient with connective tissue disease, or pneumothorax in cystic lung diseases such as lymphangioleiomyomatosis (LAM) and Langerhans cell histiocytosis (LCH).[5–7] Hemoptysis may suggest diffuse alveolar hemorrhage, though it is not present in most cases.[8]

SYSTEMIC SYMPTOMS

Connective tissue disease is a frequent cause of ILD, and patients may come with a pre-existing diagnosis. However, most will not and it is incumbent on the physician to search carefully for suggestions of underlying autoimmune disease, as the pulmonologist may be the first to make such a diagnosis, prompted by the onset of ILD. In some cases, nonspecific systemic symptoms such as night sweats, fever, fatigue, or weight loss suggest an underlying inflammatory condition. In others, one can arrive at a specific diagnosis by merely performing a thorough review of systems. For example, careful questioning regarding dermatologic symptoms may lead to the discovery of dermatomyositis as demonstrated by a heliotrope rash, Gottron's papules, or "mechanic's hands," all of which may be relatively specific features that do not bother the patient. Patients with underlying systemic sclerosis (scleroderma) may give a history of skin tightness and thickening, telangiectasias, Raynaud's phenomenon, or digital pitting. Papular eruptions, lupus pernio, and erythema nodosum may be seen in sarcoidosis.[9] Patients with systemic lupus erythematosus (SLE) may describe malar rash, photosensitivity skin reaction, or hair loss.

Gastrointestinal symptoms may be indicative of underlying esophageal motility problems related to connective tissue disease such as systemic sclerosis and polymyositis, or may be the root cause of the ILD itself. In particular, symptoms suggestive of acid reflux (chest burning or pressure, cough after meals, regurgitation of food) should be sought. Chronic, intermittent aspiration can lead to progressive fibrotic lung disease from recurrent lung injury. Patient descriptions of coughing or choking while eating or noting food "going down the wrong pipe" are suggestive of frank aspiration and could lead to a discovery of progressive neuromuscular diseases such as amyotrophic lateral sclerosis (ALS), cerebrovascular accidents, or other causes of oropharyngeal and laryngeal dysfunction.[10] Other gastrointestinal complaints, such as bloating and diarrhea, may suggest inflammatory bowel disease or bacterial overgrowth due to bowel dysmotility in systemic sclerosis.

Musculoskeletal complaints can be helpful in identifying underlying connective tissue disease as well. In particular, arthralgias, morning stiffness, joint swelling and erythema, and deformities may be evidence of an underlying inflammatory disorder such as rheumatoid arthritis, Sjögren syndrome, or mixed connective tissue disorder. Swollen fingers ("sausage digits") may be observed in systemic sclerosis and polymyositis. Raynaud's phenomenon manifests as either blue/purple discoloration or whiteness of the digits (fingers or toes) in the cold. In some cases this may be quite profound and can even be associated with digital ulcerations and, rarely, digital gangrene. This finding is most suggestive of underlying scleroderma, mixed connective tissue disease, SLE, and antisynthetase syndrome.[11]

Ophthalmologic symptoms may direct the clinician toward particular clinical entities. Inquiries regarding dry eyes or the use of eye drops may uncover sicca syndrome, as seen in Sjögren syndrome and overlap connective tissue diseases. Patients with a history of uveitis may have underlying SLE or sarcoidosis. Neurologic symptoms may suggest vasculitis or sarcoidosis.

A detailed review of systems may uncover sequelae of longstanding ILD. Increasing edema, syncopal events, or exertional chest discomfort may indicate severe pulmonary hypertension and *cor pulmonale* in the patient with advanced fibrotic lung disease and hypoxemia. Alternatively, in a patient with systemic sclerosis, these findings might indicate a second primary problem such as pulmonary arterial hypertension. The presence of palpitations or syncope in a patient with sarcoidosis can lead to a diagnosis of cardiac sarcoidosis.

The review of systems will sometimes also lead to a related secondary diagnosis. For example, more typical causes of exertional chest discomfort, such as cardiac ischemia, may be truly present and may be exacerbated by exertional desaturation. This is particularly important to remember, as patients with underlying immune-related diseases appear to be at increased risk for coronary artery disease.[12]

In addition, pleuritic chest pain, leg swelling, and increasing dyspnea should prompt consideration of acute pulmonary embolism, as patients with ILD are at increased risk for this complication.[13,14]

PAST MEDICAL HISTORY

As mentioned, a prior diagnosis of connective tissue disease (systemic sclerosis, rheumatoid arthritis, SLE) is extremely pertinent for patients with ILD. In the case of HIV disease, specific forms of lung disease such as lymphocytic interstitial pneumonia (LIP) are more commonly observed. A prior history of acute or chronic kidney disease might suggest underlying vasculitis, pulmonary–renal syndromes, or connective tissue disease. A history of liver disease could suggest sarcoidosis, primary biliary cirrhosis, or underlying genetic abnormalities resulting in short telomere length.[15–17] A history of facial nerve paralysis (Bell's palsy) might represent unrecognized sarcoidosis.[18]

OCCUPATIONAL HISTORY

The occupational history should be thorough, including a review of all jobs held in the past. In particular, attention should be paid to any occupation in which a history of exposure to organic or inorganic products was present (Table 54-2). Specific inquiries may be made regarding a history of construction work, including demolition, plumbing, and electrical work. The patient should be questioned about employment in factories and manufacturing plants, the electronics industry, metal working, stone cutting, and mining. The clinician should specifically inquire about exposure to asbestos, silica, hard metals, and beryllium, as workers often know when these have been present in their work environment.[19,20] Inquiries may additionally be made regarding the jobs held by the household contacts of patients. For example, spouses may have been subjected to significant levels of dust inhalation via clothing worn by the worker.[21] In cases where a relevant exposure has occurred, details should be obtained regarding the worker's specific duties, the typical proximity to the exposure of interest and any use of respiratory protection. In some cases, related respiratory illnesses in coworkers can raise suspicion. There may be a long latency period between the exposure and the onset of symptoms and radiographic changes, so the occupational history must explore jobs held many years in the past. A history of farm work or other agricultural employment should raise suspicion for an environmental cause of ILD. Exposure to moldy hay, bird feathers and droppings, and a variety of organic products can lead to chronic hypersensitivity pneumonitis.

TABLE 54-2 Occupational Interstitial Lung Disease

Occupation	Type of ILD	Exposure
Electrician Plumber Pipe fitter Construction worker Ship builder Insulation installer	Asbestosis	Asbestos
Stone cutter Miner Sand blaster	Silicosis	Crystalline silica dust
Metal grinder	Giant cell interstitial pneumonia Hard metal lung disease	Hard metals Cobalt Tungsten carbide
Metal worker Factory workers Nuclear weapons Aircrafts Electronics Ceramics Golf clubs Bicycle frames	Berylliosis	Beryllium
Coal worker	Coal worker's pneumoconiosis	Coal dust
Paint sprayer Plastic worker	Chemical worker's lung	Isocyanates
Bird breeder	Bird breeder's lung	Bird droppings Bird feathers
Farm worker Haying Mushroom compost	Farmer's lung Mushroom worker's lung	Thermophilic bacteria
Office worker	Humidifier lung Ventilation pneumonitis	Fungi/Molds
Lifeguard	"Hot tub" hypersensitivity pneumonitis	*Mycobacteria*

ENVIRONMENTAL HISTORY

Organic exposures are also frequently encountered in household and office settings. For example, humidification systems may be contaminated with mold.[22] Hot tubs and other aerosolized water sources have led to lung disease related to the growth of *Mycobacterium avium*.[23] The exposure history should include a thorough inquiry regarding the home heating and humidification system, a history of water damage, or visible evidence of significant mold growth on walls. An assessment of the timing of any water damage relative to the onset of the lung disease can be helpful. Domestic birds are a common source of feathers and dropping antigen. Bird owners often have multiple birds and have owned birds for many years. Frequently, these pets are considered to be cherished members of the family, residing in bedrooms and main living spaces. A history of hobbies and materials used should also be obtained.

Cigarette smoke is one of the most common environmental exposures and is strongly linked with several forms of ILD, including desquamative interstitial pneumonitis (DIP), respiratory bronchiolitis-ILD, and LCH. Cigarette smoking has been identified as a risk factor for IPF.

MEDICATION HISTORY

Numerous drugs have been implicated in the development of ILD, ranging from acute pneumonitis to chronic fibrotic lung disease (Table 54-3). The use of several commonly prescribed drugs should be sought. Nitrofurantoin, used for suppression of recurrent urinary tract infections, may lead to severe ILD.[24] Amiodarone, used for management of atrial and ventricular arrhythmias, is known to lead to lung toxicity.[25] Nonsteroidal anti-inflammatory drugs (NSAIDs) are commonly used and may lead to eosinophilic and other inflammatory lung disease.[26] While less frequently used in the general population, a history of recent chemotherapy should trigger suspicion for drug-related lung disease.[27] Similarly, a history of immune-modulating drug use, such as in the treatment of rheumatoid arthritis or Crohn's disease is suspicious.[24,25,28] So many drugs have been reported in association with ILD that it is recommended to review the patient's entire medication history thoroughly with this in mind. A helpful online source of information is: http://www.pneumotox.com. This independent resource is compiled and regularly updated by members of the University Hospital in Dijon, France, and the GEPPI (Groupe d'Etudes de la Pathologie Pulmonaire Iatrogène). It lists all reports of suspected drug-induced lung disease, categorizes the radiographic patterns observed, and gives an assessment of the quality of the compiled information.

TABLE 54-3 Drugs Implicated in Interstitial Lung Disease

Antibiotics	**Chemotherapeutic**
Nitrofurantoin	All-trans retinoic acid (ATRA)
Minocycline	Alpha-interferon
Cephalosporins	Antithymocyte globulin
Antiarrhythmic	Bleomycin
Amiodarone	Busulfan
Tocainide	Carmustine (BCNU)
Anti-inflammatory	Chlorambucil
Azathioprine	Colony-stimulating factors (GM-CSF)
Etanercept	Cyclophosphamide
Gold salts	Cytosine arabinoside
Infliximab	Docetaxel
Methotrexate	Geftinib
NSAIDs	Gemcitabine
Penicillamine	Interleukin-2
Sulfasalazine	Irinotecan
Neurologic/Psychiatric	Melphalan
Carbamazepine	Mitomycin C
Phenytoin	Paclitaxel
Drugs of Abuse	Procarbazine
Cocaine	Vinorelbine
Heroin	**Other**
Talc	Bacille Calmette-Guérin (BCG)
	Mineral oil
	Radiation

Source: Data from Camus. Drug-induced and iatrogenic infiltrative lung disease. Clinics in Chest Med. 2004;25:479–519.

FAMILY HISTORY

Most forms of ILD are not heritable, though several do have a genetic component. When heritable disease is suspected, it is important to consider both systemic disorders as well as those that primarily affect the lung. In particular, by considering a patient's concomitant medical history or the history of family members, specific diagnoses may be uncovered. Several inborn errors of metabolism (Gaucher disease and Niemann-Pick, for example) are inherited in an autosomal recessive fashion. Other rare diseases such as Hermansky–Pudlak syndrome, Burt–Hogg–Dubé syndrome, and neurofibromatosis type I are autosomal dominant disorders.[29] The cystic lung disease, LAM may be associated with mutations in the tuberous sclerosis complex (TSC) genes, in which systemic hamartomas are present, including a high incidence of renal angiomyolipomas.[29]

The telomere shortening syndromes that lead to dyskeratosis congenita may lead to a phenomenon known as genetic anticipation, in which telomere lengths are progressively shortened in subsequent generations. This leads to the earlier onset of more severe disease in each subsequent generation. In the case of IPF, mutations in the telomerase genes have been demonstrated among 8% to 15% of familial cases and among 1% to 3% of patients with sporadic disease.[17] Several other genes have been linked with the onset of IPF, including those involved in the regulation of surfactant protein C and MUC5B.[30,31] There may be familial predisposition to sarcoidosis, but inheritance is more complex, involving an interaction of genetic and environmental factors.[32]

PHYSICAL EXAMINATION

Most patients with pulmonary fibrosis have lung findings characterized by fine, inspiratory, basilar "Velcro" crackles and many will have digital clubbing. In contrast, patients with nonfibrotic lung disease may have clear lung fields on auscultation. The location of the abnormal breath sounds may be suggestive of the underlying diagnosis, such as the upper lobe findings in silicosis and sarcoidosis in contrast to the lower lobe abnormalities in IPF. Additional breath sounds such as wheezing and inspiratory squeaks can indicate airway disease, which may focus the examiner's differential diagnosis on airway-centered diseases such as bronchiolitis, sarcoidosis, and hypersensitivity pneumonitis. These additional sounds should not be present in a patient with IPF.

Other cardiopulmonary manifestations of disease should also be sought. Signs of pulmonary hypertension and right heart failure include an increased P2 component, a right ventricular heave, elevated jugular venous pressure, and lower extremity edema.

Dermatologic and musculoskeletal signs of connective tissue disease, including skin rashes, sclerodactyly, skin thickening, digital ulceration, "mechanic's hands," synovitis, joint deformities, Raynaud's phenomenon, and telangiectasias, may be extremely helpful in narrowing the differential diagnosis. Less common findings such as cutaneous neurofibromas or café-au-lait spots in neurofibromatosis, albinism in Hermansky–Pudlak syndrome, and facial angiofibromas, periungual fibromas, and Shagreen patch in TSC may all be key features only recognized through a careful and focused search.

CHEST IMAGING

Findings on chest radiography and high-resoluaion computed tomography are discussed below.

CHEST RADIOGRAPH

An abnormal chest radiograph is often the first indication of underlying ILD. The pattern and distribution of abnormalities often help in formulating a differential diagnosis (Table 54-4). For example, sarcoidosis, silicosis, and LCH are among the diseases with an upper lobe predominance, while IPF, connective tissue disease–associated ILD, and asbestosis are all lower lobe predominant. Peripheral alveolar opacities are typical findings in organizing pneumonia and chronic eosinophilic pneumonia. The chest radiograph is also helpful for assessing lung volumes. In particular, fibrotic lung disease such as IPF leads to small lung fields whereas lung volumes are maintained and may even demonstrate hyperinflation in diseases such as LAM and LCH. In many cases, the presence of lymphadenopathy, with hilar fullness observed on chest radiograph, is the feature that leads to an accurate diagnosis, such as in sarcoidosis.

HIGH-RESOLUTION CHEST COMPUTED TOMOGRAPHY

High-resolution computed tomography (HRCT) of the chest is significantly more sensitive than chest radiograph for abnormalities in ILD. Characteristic patterns observed on HRCT can be quite specific in some cases. For example, the characteristic radiographic features of IPF are collectively known as the "UIP pattern," since these features have been demonstrated to confidently predict the presence of pathologic UIP when surgical biopsy is obtained (Table 54-5).[33,34] This pattern consists of peripheral, subpleural, basilar-predominant reticular opacities in combination with basilar honeycombing and without features, such as ground-glass opacities, cysts or nodules, to suggest another form of ILD.[35] When these features are accurately recognized, patients can be spared a surgical biopsy for diagnosis (Fig. 54-2).

Several radiographic patterns have been identified that help to focus the differential diagnosis (Table 54-4). In particular, a peripheral reticular pattern, that is basilar predominant may be seen in IPF, NSIP, and connective tissue disease–associated ILD (Fig. 54-3). Nodular infiltrates may suggest sarcoidosis, hypersensitivity pneumonitis, and LCH, though the nature of the nodules

TABLE 54-4

Distribution of ILD	
Upper lung zone	**Lower lung zone**
Sarcoidosis	Usual interstitial pneumonia (UIP/IPF)
Silicosis	Nonspecific interstitial pneumonia (NSIP)
Coal worker's pneumoconiosis	Connective tissue disease–associated ILD
Hypersensitivity pneumonitis	Asbestosis
Langerhans cell histiocytosis	Desquamative interstitial pneumonia (DIP)
Berylliosis	
Chronic eosinophilic pneumonia	
Pattern of ILD	
Peripheral reticular	**Ground glass**
Idiopathic pulmonary fibrosis/usual interstitial pneumonia	NSIP
Nonspecific interstitial pneumonia	Cryptogenic organizing pneumonia
	Eosinophilic pneumonia (chronic or acute)
	Pulmonary edema
Nodular	Infection (opportunistic or viral)
Sarcoidosis	Alveolar hemorrhage
Berylliosis	Hypersensitivity pneumonitis
Hypersensitivity pneumonitis	Desquamative interstitial pneumonia
Langerhans cell histiocytosis	Sarcoidosis
Silicosis	Pulmonary alveolar proteinosis
Metastatic disease	
Talcosis	**Cystic**
Granulomatous polyangiitis (formerly known as Wegener's granulomatosis)	Lymphangioleiomyomatosis
Respiratory bronchiolitis ILD	Langerhans cell histiocytosis
	Lymphocytic interstitial pneumonia
	Pneumocystis jiroveci pneumonia (PCP)

Source: Data from Diagnostic Thoracic Imaging, Miller W. McGraw Hill; 2006.

and their location may make one or another diagnosis more likely (Fig. 54-4). The finding of diffuse cystic abnormalities leads to a specific differential diagnosis, including LAM, LCH, and LIP. The term "ground glass" refers to areas of lung tissues with increased attenuation, but not enough to obscure or distort lung architecture, blood vessels, and lymphatics. Alveolar opacities are a related finding and reflect more dense attenuation of lung tissue, sometimes containing air bronchograms. Many forms of ILD are characterized by ground-glass and alveolar opacities. When observed in characteristic distributions, such as the peripheral, patchy alveolar opacities in cryptogenic organizing pneumonia (COP) and chronic eosinophilic pneumonia, they are quite suggestive of an underlying pathologic pattern (Fig. 54-5).[36] However, the radiographic appearance in such cases is nonspecific and other testing, including lung biopsy, may be required for diagnosis.

TABLE 54-5 Radiographic Characteristics of the UIP Pattern

"Definite UIP"
Peripheral, subpleural distribution
Basilar predominance
Reticular markings and traction bronchiectasis
Honeycombing
Absence of inconsistent features
Atypical for a "Definite UIP"
Upper or mid lung predominance
Peribronchovascular distribution
Ground-glass abnormality (out of proportion to reticulation)
Profuse micronodules
Multiple, bilateral, discrete cysts
Diffuse, bilateral, mosaic attenuation or air trapping
Consolidation

Source: Data from Schmidt. Respirology. 2009;14(7):934–939.

LABORATORY TESTING

Routine laboratory testing, while often normal, may lead to the diagnosis of a previously unrecognized systemic disease, or may be suggestive of the underlying lung disease. Its importance may also lie in the discovery of associated conditions, such as elevated liver enzymes or hypercalcemia in sarcoidosis, or renal insufficiency in pulmonary renal syndromes and other connective tissue disease with renal involvement. Other examples include the presence of peripheral eosinophilia in chronic eosinophilic pneumonia, Churg–Strauss syndrome, drug reaction, and other forms of vasculitis. Anemia may worsen symptoms of dyspnea in the setting of ILD and may reflect an underlying hemolytic condition, or chronic gastrointestinal blood loss in inflammatory bowel disease. In addition to eliciting causes for the ILD, recognition of underlying chronic organ dysfunction will also help determine the ability of the patient to tolerate treatment.

More advanced testing is often necessary, including serologic testing for underlying connective tissue disease (Table 54-6). Many of the tests listed here are employed by ILD centers in the evaluation of patients newly presenting with diffuse lung disease, though no clear standard exists. Importantly, ILD can be the sole manifestation or the presenting feature of a connective tissue disease, making a careful evaluation for previously unrecognized autoimmune disease essential.[37]

PULMONARY FUNCTION TESTS

Pulmonary function tests (PFTs) are a mainstay in the pulmonologist's armamentarium in the evaluation and management of ILD. Importantly, they assist in assessing the severity of disease and help determine prognosis in many forms of disease.[38,39] They are a relatively noninvasive method to gauge disease progression and measure response to therapy.[40] The testing typically include spirometry, measurement of lung volumes, and diffusing capacity. Exercise testing, such as the 6-minute walk test, is particularly important for patients with ILD.

Typically, spirometry in most forms of ILD demonstrates a restrictive ventilatory defect due to decreased compliance and increased recoil of the lung parenchyma.[41] The presence of obstruction suggests either concomitant obstructive lung disease, often from prior smoking exposure, or the presence of an airway-centered lung ILD such as LCH, LAM, or sarcoidosis. Decreased static lung volumes confirm the presence of restriction. In the case of airway-centered

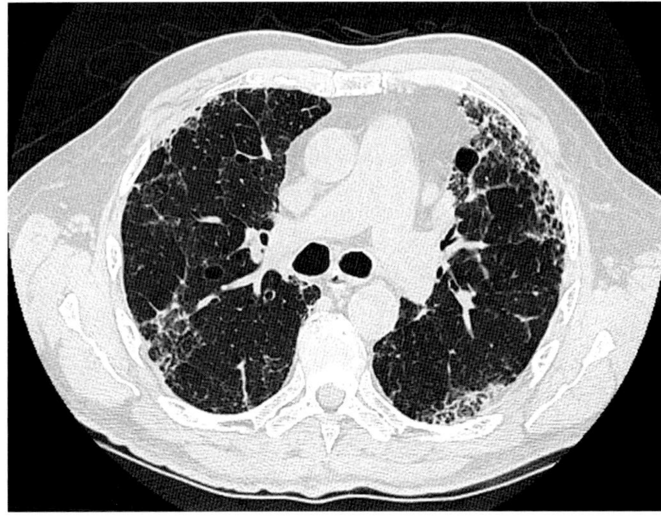

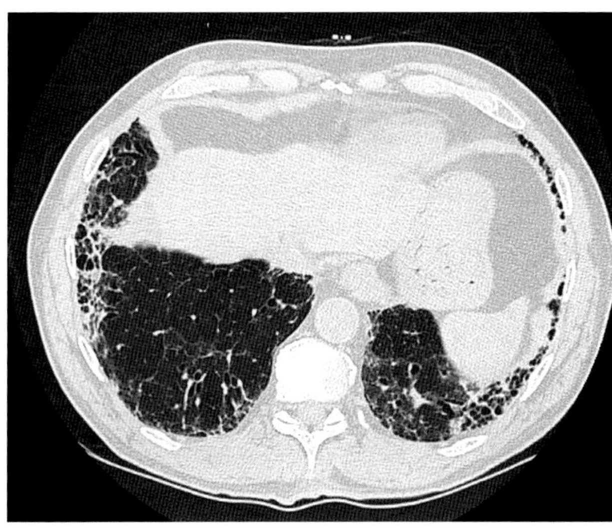

Figure 54-2 An 82-year-old man with progressive dyspnea and a usual interstitial pneumonia (UIP) radiographic pattern. High-resolution (1.25-mm thick sections) CT images at the level of the midthorax (**A**) and lower thorax (**B**) show peripheral reticular markings with architectural distortion and small subpleural cysts/honeycombing. Ground-glass opacities and other features atypical for IPF are absent. The patient had no exposures and no clinical evidence of connective tissue disease. The final diagnosis was idiopathic pulmonary fibrosis (IPF). No lung biopsy was performed, as a diagnosis was made based upon CT criteria alone.

diseases, the lung volume measurements may indicate unrecognized air trapping and hyperinflation.

Diffusion impairment, demonstrated by a decrement in the diffusing capacity (DL_{CO}), is frequently observed in ILD and is often the earliest physiologic abnormality.[42] The decreased DL_{CO} reflects the presence of either fibrotic tissue or inflammatory cells (or both) in the interstitium of the lung, leading to a defect at the level of the alveolar–capillary membrane. The diffusion impairment is typically lower than predicted by alveolar volume.[41] With activity, exertional desaturation is a frequent occurrence among patients with ILD, and which may predict prognosis in certain forms of ILD.[43–45] Formal 6-minute walk testing is quite useful, additionally offering an assessment of exercise capacity in terms of distance walked, heart rate response, and causes for exercise discontinuation (including leg discomfort or chest pain). However, if this is not available, measurement of pulse oximetry with ambulation in the hallway or with stair climbing can offer important information, including an understanding of reasons for the patient's dyspnea as well as a marker of disease severity.

BRONCHOSCOPY

Bronchoscopy is a generally well-tolerated procedure that can be quite useful in the diagnosis of DPLD. It allows inspection of the upper and lower airways, bronchoalveolar lavage (BAL), and the performance of transbronchial lung biopsy. All may be completed as an outpatient procedure, with relatively minimal sedation.

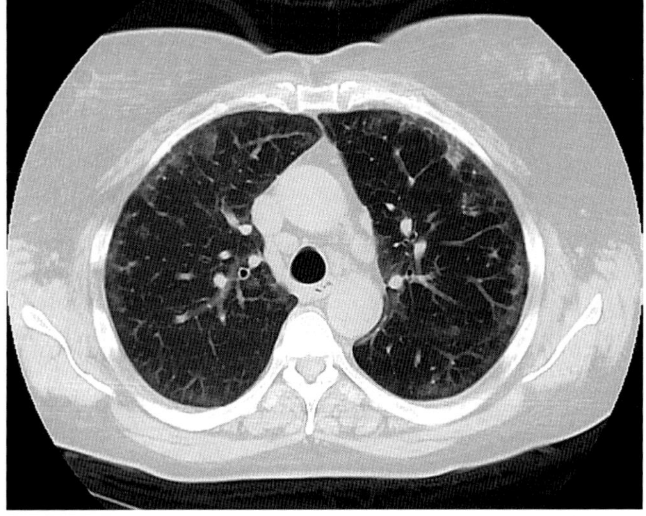

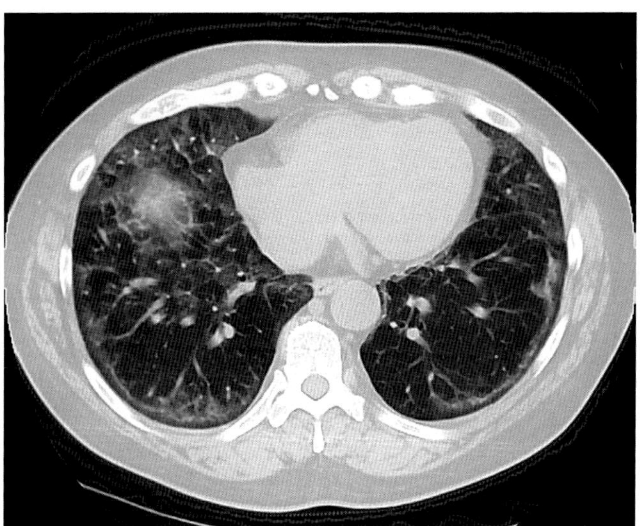

Figure 54-3 A 55-year-old woman with progressive dyspnea on exertion. She had finger swelling and Raynaud phenomenon, with an antinuclear antibody titer of 1:2560 (nucleolar). Axial CT image through the midthorax (**A**) and lower thorax (**B**) show ground-glass opacities in a peripheral distribution, reticular markings, and mild architectural distortion. Subpleural sparing is evident. These findings are all compatible with a nonspecific interstitial pneumonia (NSIP) pattern. The final diagnosis was scleroderma lung disease.

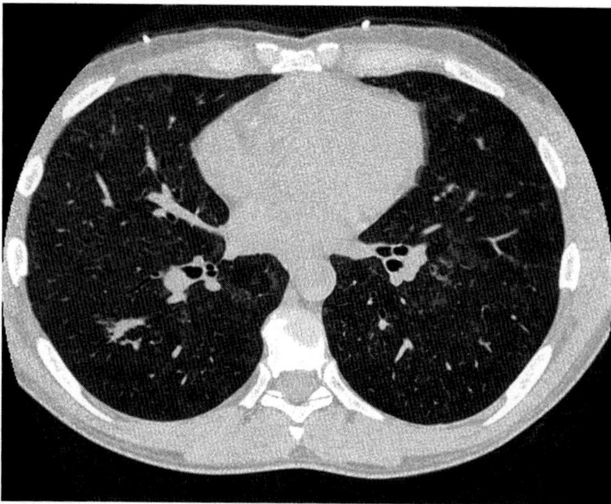

Figure 54-4 A 47-year-old man who enjoyed soaking in the hot tub after exercising at the gym developed dyspnea and hypoxemia. He improved clinically with removal from the presumed source of exposure. High-resolution CT images at the level of the midthorax demonstrate diffuse centrilobular ground-glass nodules as well as areas of lobular lucency, consistent with air trapping. These findings are consistent with subacute hypersensitivity pneumonitis.

TABLE 54-6

Serologic Testing in ILD	
Test	**Disease**
ANA	Scleroderma, SLE, MCTD
SSA	Sjögren syndrome, Polymyositis
SSB	Sjögren syndrome
CK Aldolase Jo-1 Myositis-associated antibodies	Polymyositis, dermatomyositis
Jo-1 Myositis-associated antibodies	Antisynthetase syndrome
Scl-70 Anticentromere antibody	Scleroderma
RF CCP	Rheumatoid arthritis
RNP Antihistone antibody	Mixed connective tissue disease
p-ANCA, c-ANCA	ANCA-associated vasculitis

ANA, antinuclear antibody; CK, creatine kinase; ESR, erythrocyte sedimentation rate; SSA, anti-Ro antibody; SSB, anti-La antibody; RF, rheumatoid actor; CCP, cyclic citrullinated peptide; RNP, ribonucleoprotein; CRP, C-reactive protein; ANCA, antineutrophil cytoplasmic antibody.

BAL allows the sampling of the protein and cellular components of the lung fluid. Tests typically performed on this fluid include cell count and differential, cytology, and a variety of viral assays and microbiologic cultures, depending on the clinical scenario. In some cases, the BAL fluid appearance itself may be diagnostic, for example with the finding of progressively bloody lavage specimens in diffuse alveolar hemorrhage.[46] Similarly, the presence of milky white or tan BAL fluid–containing debris that settles out suggests pulmonary alveolar proteinosis. Periodic acid–Schiff (PAS) staining confirms the diagnosis.

Specific testing on BAL fluid, including cell count and differential, can be diagnostic in the correct clinical context. BAL eosinophilia (>25%) indicates an eosinophilic process, and in combination with the clinical scenario of acute respiratory failure with bilateral alveolar opacities on chest radiograph suggests acute eosinophilic pneumonia. Significant BAL lymphocytosis suggests the presence of a granulomatous ILD, suggestive of hypersensitivity pneumonitis, drug reaction, or cellular NSIP when greater than 50%.[46] A high ratio of CD4+/CD8+ T lymphocytes may be specific, not sensitive for sarcoidosis, though this is not considered a diagnostic test.[46,47] BAL neutrophilia has not been shown to be helpful in distinguishing among the idiopathic ILDs.[48] Notably, increasing patient age may shift the cellular composition of BAL fluid toward lymphocytes and neutrophils so results should be interpreted cautiously.[49]

Specialty testing on BAL fluid may also be important to consider. BAL can accurately confirm a work exposure, for example a positive

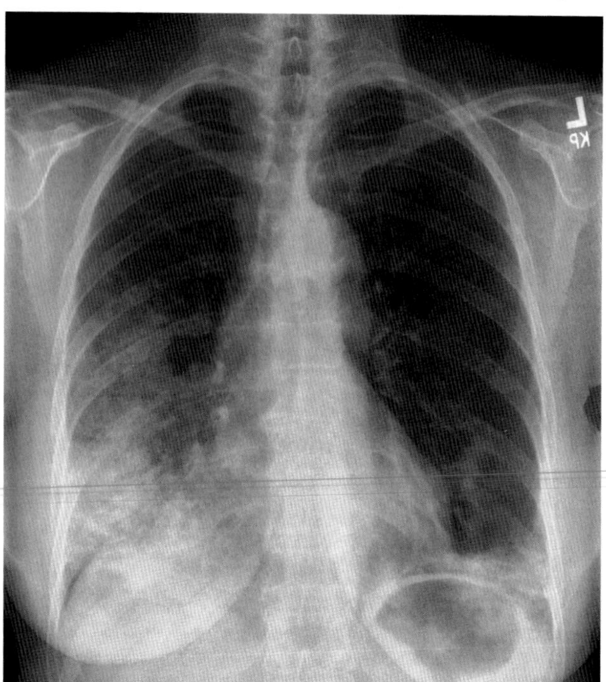

A

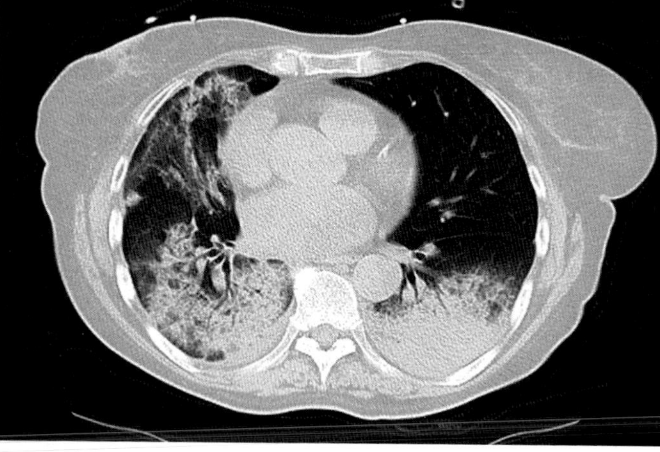

B

Figure 54-5 A 58-year-old woman with organizing pneumonia (OP) secondary to radiation for breast cancer. Frontal chest radiograph (**A**) demonstrates ground-glass and alveolar opacities. High-resolution CT images at the level of the midthorax (**B**) demonstrate both ground-glass opacities and areas of consolidation. She had complete response to corticosteroid therapy.

lymphocyte proliferation assay in chronic beryllium disease or the presence of asbestos bodies in asbestosis.[50] The demonstration of CD1a positive cells on flow cytometry may lead to a diagnosis of LCH, and clonal cell populations may be demonstrated in the BAL fluid of patients with pulmonary lymphoid malignancies.[46,51] Much research has focused on identifying molecular and cellular profiles to predict prognosis and response to therapy, however BAL is not widely used for this purpose outside the research setting.[52]

One of the major reasons to obtain BAL fluid in the diagnosis and treatment of ILD is to rule out infection, either as a primary cause of the diffuse lung disease, or as a secondary complication of immunosuppressive therapy. In the immunocompromised host, BAL fluid is highly sensitive for the diagnosis of bacterial, viral, fungal, and mycobacterial diseases.[53] Specialized staining may identify *Pneumocystis jiroveci* infection, endemic fungi, and mycobacterial disease. Immunofluorescent antibody and polymerase chain reaction (PCR) assays are now commonly utilized, and significantly increase yield.[46,54,55]

Transbronchial biopsy is safe, with risk for pneumothorax of approximately 1% and significant bleeding less than 2%.[56,57] Biopsy forceps are introduced via the flexible bronchoscope and tissue samples are obtained with fluoroscopic guidance. Multiple passes are made, with yield improving when more than four specimens are obtained.[58] Despite the relatively small size of these specimens as compared with surgical lung biopsy, diagnostic information in certain forms of ILD are particularly amenable to diagnosis by bronchoscopy, especially granulomatous diseases such as sarcoidosis, hypersensitivity pneumonitis, and drug toxicity.[59]

SURGICAL LUNG BIOPSY

Despite a high yield in certain forms of lung disease, the utility of transbronchial biopsy for most of the idiopathic interstitial pneumonias (such as IPF, NSIP, and LIP) is low and surgical biopsy is often required for accurate diagnosis.[60] The usual technique is video-assisted thoracoscopic surgery (VATS) that has a low morbidity and mortality in selected populations.[61] VATS biopsy should be performed by surgeons familiar with the techniques needed for ILD diagnosis. Wedge biopsies are taken from three separate lobes, and include areas of normal appearing lung; when only the most affected areas are sampled, specimens demonstrate end-stage honeycomb lung and the procedure may be nondiagnostic. Risks of VATS include prolonged air leak, bleeding, infection, and incisional site pain.[62] Generally, the length of hospital stay after a VATS procedure is 2 to 3 days, though a few centers perform VATS biopsy as an outpatient procedure in selected patients.[63] For most patients, there is no significant loss of lung function; however, cases of acute exacerbation of IPF following biopsy have been reported.[62,64] Patients must be able to tolerate general anesthesia with single lung ventilation.[62] Risk factors for complications and mortality include advanced respiratory failure as indicated by high P_{CO_2} and/or severe hypoxemia, significant pulmonary hypertension, problems with clotting, and immunosuppression.[65,66] Patients older than 65 years of age have morbidity and mortality rates no different than younger patients, though those over 75 may have higher rates of air leak.[67,68] Preoperative cardiac evaluation should be considered since many patients undergoing biopsy for ILD are older, or have a significant smoking history.[69]

A comprehensive approach including the clinical history, laboratory testing, and radiographic appearance can help assess if pathologic information is needed for accurate diagnosis. If a specific cause for the ILD can be identified, such as underlying connective tissue disease or a temporally correlated drug or environmental exposure, pathologic tissue may not change management and may not be worth the operative risk. When no etiology of the lung disease can be found, the radiographic appearance is crucial to help determine if surgical biopsy is needed. The most important question to be answered with biopsy is whether the patient has IPF or some other form of idiopathic interstitial pneumonia.[70] Specific features on HRCT are highly predictive of the histopathologic finding of UIP, the histologic correlate of IPF (Table 54-5).[33,34] An assessment of the HRCT as "definite UIP" by an experienced observer can spare some patients a surgical biopsy in the correct clinical setting.[35] When most features are present, but honeycombing is not, the pattern is called "possible UIP" and it is this group in which surgical biopsy is the most helpful. The differential diagnosis in these cases includes NSIP, UIP, and chronic hypersensitivity pneumonitis and radiographic appearance alone cannot be used to make an accurate diagnosis.[71,72] Each case should be assessed individually before a decision to pursue biopsy is made. In some, it may not be necessary and in others, though potentially helpful, the risk of the procedure outweighs the benefit of the information gained.

PATHOLOGY AND MULTIDISCIPLINARY REVIEW

Several major pathologic patterns are described in the idiopathic interstitial pneumonias, including granulomatous ILD, UIP, NSIP, and organizing pneumonia. However, these same patterns may be observed in patients with systemic diseases and other causes for ILD and therefore the pathology must be interpreted within the context of the clinical scenario and radiographic studies. It has been demonstrated that the final diagnosis will often change after a group discussion involving clinicians, radiologists, and pathologists.[73] The diagnosis also frequently differs between academic and community-based physicians, with academic physicians being less likely to arrive at a diagnosis of IPF.[74]

The UIP pattern is the histologic correlate of IPF and has specific features, including a heterogeneous appearance in which areas of fibrosis and honeycombing are interspersed with areas of normal lung. The changes are most pronounced in the periphery of the lung and should not predominantly involve the airways. Fibroblastic foci should be present and atypical features should be absent. The most recent guidelines offer categories in which the pathologist may interpret the pattern as "UIP," "Probable UIP," "Possible UIP," "Unclassifiable fibrosis," and "Not UIP."[75] These, in combination with the HRCT and clinical features, will lead to a definite, probable, possible IPF diagnosis, or one of "Not IPF." However, the clinical context must always be considered as a UIP pattern is not completely specific for IPF. For example, a patient with a history of bird exposure, whose HRCT demonstrates upper lobe predominance with lobular areas of air trapping, may have UIP on biopsy, but the final diagnosis will be chronic hypersensitivity pneumonitis. A patient with morning stiffness, deforming arthritis, positive serology for anti-CCP antibodies and UIP will be given a diagnosis of rheumatoid arthritis–associated ILD.

Granulomatous histology may be observed in idiopathic disease such as sarcoidosis, but may be present in many other forms of ILD, including drug toxicity and hypersensitivity pneumonitis. In addition to ILD, the possibility of diffuse infections, including mycobacterial disease, must always be kept in mind. The morphology and location of the granulomas, as well as the appearance of the surrounding tissue, must be considered in combination with the clinical features.[76] For example, a history of beryllium exposure in combination with sarcoidal granulomas on pathology will change the diagnosis to chronic beryllium disease. A patient with diffuse centrilobular ground-glass nodules, a history of humidifier use, and loosely formed granulomas on histology most likely carries a diagnosis of subacute hypersensitivity pneumonitis.

Nonspecific interstitial pneumonia is characterized by interstitial inflammation and fibrosis in a homogeneous pattern, as opposed to the heterogeneity of UIP. It may range from predominantly cellular to fibrotic in nature, with interstitial thickening but without significant honeycomb change (Fig. 54-6).[77] While this pattern may be idiopathic, it is much more commonly associated with connective

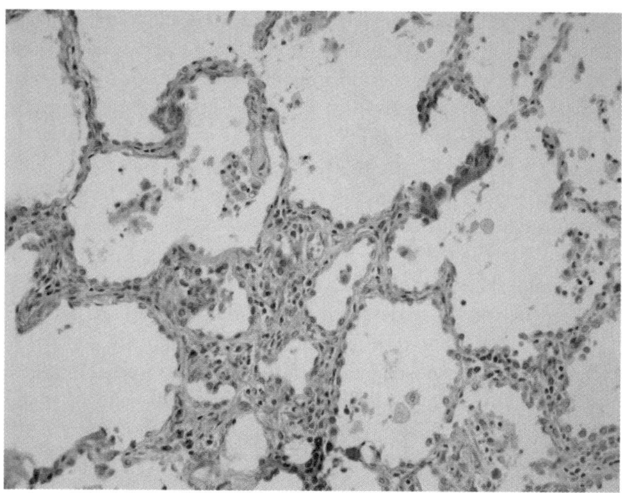

Figure 54-6 Nonspecific interstitial pneumonia (NSIP). There is diffuse, homogeneous septal fibrosis with a mild mononuclear infiltrate, as well as mild diffuse type II cell hypertrophy. No organizing pneumonitis, fibroblast foci, granulomas, or eosinophilic infiltrate are seen. Honeycombing is absent. There is a very mild accumulation of alveolar macrophages in the alveoli. 20× objective. *(Used with permission of Robert Homer, MD, PhD, Yale School of Medicine.)*

tissue disease. For example, a patient with a history of Raynaud's syndrome, skin thickening, diffuse ground-glass opacities on HRCT, and pathologic NSIP is likely to have underlying systemic sclerosis.

Organizing pneumonia is characterized histopathologically by intra-alveolar granulation tissue containing myofibroblasts and connective tissue (Fig. 54-7). The finding of organizing pneumonia on histopathology should prompt an exhaustive search for a cause before being called COP, which is idiopathic. For example, a patient with peripheral alveolar opacities on chest imaging and features of OP on biopsy who is found to have taken chronic nitrofurantoin as suppressive therapy for urinary infections may be suffering from drug toxicity. Likewise, a patient with OP who has muscle weakness, papular lesions on the hands, and heliotrope rash likely carries a diagnosis of dermatomyositis.

TREATMENT

Approach to treatment includes general and specific measures, as discussed below.

REMOVAL FROM EXPOSURES

The treatment of ILD varies with the specific diagnosis. Importantly, if any causative exposure can be identified, this should be eliminated. For example, if a drug reaction is suspected, that drug should be discontinued. For environmental exposures, the situation may require more extensive remediation. For example, in addition to removal of birds from the home, extensive cleaning of upholstery, window coverings, and ventilation systems may be required. The cleaning should not be performed by the patient. Even these measures may not remove all residual antigen, and removal of the patient from the location may be necessary.[78] In the case of extensive water damage and mold growth, significant demolition and reconstruction may be necessary. In the case of occupational exposures, some situations may be addressed by altering the particular job being done by the patient, changing the substances used, or using protective respiratory equipment, but others may require complete removal from the suspected exposure.[79] In many cases, patients' livelihoods may be at stake, involving severe financial consequences, disability, and workers' compensation. Identification of a workplace hazard for a patient may lead to the discovery of a public health issue or one that affects

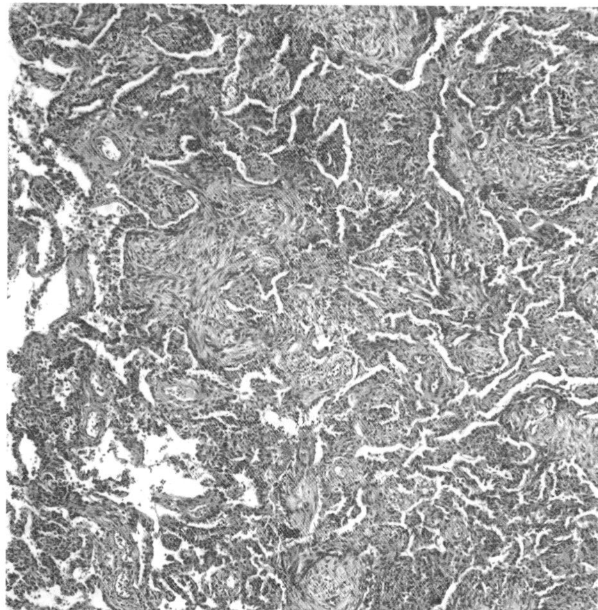

Figure 54-7 Organizing pneumonia (OP). There is fibromyxoid granulation tissue within alveolar ducts accompanied by a lymphoplasmacytic infiltrate. Notable is the absence of hyaline membranes, necrosis, neutrophilic or eosinophilic infiltrate, granulomas, and established fibrosis. 10× objective. *(Used with permission of Robert Homer, MD, PhD, Yale School of Medicine.)*

the health of coworkers.[80] Referral to and coordination with an Occupational Medicine specialist may be necessary to appropriately assess and remediate home and workplace exposures.

IMMUNOSUPPRESSIVE THERAPY

Some forms of ILD, including COP, connective tissue disease–associated ILD, and sarcoidosis, may demonstrate a favorable response to corticosteroids and other immunosuppressive agents.[81] However, in diseases such as IPF, what was once thought to be standard of care (prednisone plus azathioprine) has been demonstrated to carry harm without potential for benefit.[82] When considering the use of these drugs, an assessment should be made regarding the likelihood of response as well as the relative risks and benefits of the therapy.

The many side effects of corticosteroids include glucose intolerance, bone loss, cataract development, and mood instability.[83] Increased risk for infection may be substantial.[84] Some inflammatory diseases such as COP, CEP, and sarcoidosis can be quite sensitive to corticosteroids and relatively quick weaning to low dosages may be feasible and effective. In disorders such as connective tissue disease–associated ILD, when a more prolonged course of therapy is anticipated, the early addition of steroid sparing medications, such as azathioprine or mycophenolate mofetil, can permit lower doses of corticosteroids to be used. Certain forms of ILD, including scleroderma lung disease, vasculitis with alveolar hemorrhage, and severe cases of connective tissue disease–associated ILD may require drugs such as cyclophosphamide, which carry increased risk for severe side effects. Such medications should only be prescribed by practitioners familiar with the use and toxicities of these agents.

When actively treating ILD, objective measures of improvement, including PFTs, exercise oximetry, and chest radiography should be employed to avoid the unnecessary continuation of therapy. In particular, when corticosteroids are used, there is often an initial boost in mood and energy level that may not correspond to actual improvements in lung function. If no clinical improvement is seen after 3 to 6 months of therapy, discontinuation of immunosuppressive therapy should be strongly considered.

ANTIFIBROTIC DRUGS

For progressive fibrotic lung diseases, particularly IPF, the lack of adequate treatment options has led to a search for new therapies. In particular, pirfenidone, a small-molecule drug which appears to have antifibrotic properties, may stabilize lung function and is approved for use in Japan, Europe, and Canada and is currently being evaluated for approval in the United States. Multiple phase II and III studies of novel agents for IPF and for scleroderma-ILD are ongoing.

SUPPORTIVE THERAPY

Supportive therapy directed at improving quality of life and decreasing respiratory symptoms should be a part of the approach to care of all patients with ILD. Formal exercise testing in the PFT laboratory offers a standardized approach to the assessment of oxygen needs. However, a check of oximetry with simple ambulation in the hallway or with stair climbing can uncover the need for oxygen supplementation. The use of oxygen for patients with ILD is encouraged to maintain saturations >90% both at rest and with exercise.[85] No data exist regarding the impact of nocturnal oxygen use on mortality in ILD, but this is often utilized based upon data suggesting that nocturnal hypoxemia has a significant negative impact on quality of life.[86] Home and portable systems should be used to encourage ease of use and mobility. Collaboration among physicians, patients, and oxygen providers can help identify the ideal system for each patient.

The role of pulmonary rehabilitation has been studied in chronic obstructive lung disease and leads to increased muscle strength and improved endurance.[87] Similar improvements may be evident in the fibrotic lung diseases.[88,89] In addition to the potential benefits of improved muscle strength and stamina, patients with ILD may also benefit from the ongoing education regarding oxygen use, breathing and pacing techniques, and social support.[90] As patients with chronic lung disease frequently suffer from anxiety and depression, pulmonary rehabilitation may benefit patients by identifying these issues, leading to appropriate specialist referrals.[91]

TREATMENT OF COMORBIDITIES

Several common comorbidities should be sought among patients with ILD. In particular, an assessment for underlying coronary artery disease should be undertaken when dyspnea on exertion is present, as the risk for ischemic heart disease is increased among patients with IPF.[92,93] Due in part to prior tobacco exposure, patients with IPF have an increased risk of developing lung cancer.[85] Nodules should be individually assessed based on size, appearance, and growth. No specific screening recommendations for this patient population exist. The prevalence of obstructive sleep apnea appears to be quite high among patients with ILD, even in the absence of excessive sleepiness or large body habitus, although these features are important to assess.[94–96] There is a high prevalence of gastroesophageal reflux (GERD) among patients with IPF, though only a minority have symptoms.[97,98] Studies have suggested that GERD may be intimately involved in the pathogenesis of IPF and be linked with progression of disease.[99] The evaluation and treatment of GERD in patients with ILD is an evolving field. Based on existing data, it is not clear how aggressive therapy should be. If symptoms exist, therapy is typically utilized. However, whether to seek evidence of asymptomatic GERD through more invasive testing and whether to treat such patients is not clear.[85]

In addition to native comorbidities, side effects from therapy should be assessed. In particular, the use of corticosteroids can lead to weight gain, fluid retention, diabetes, and osteoporosis. Glucocorticoid-induced osteoporosis may be prevented by the use of calcium and vitamin D supplementation early in the course of steroid use.[100] Fracture risk assessment can identify patients in whom bisphosphonate therapy is indicated.[100]

Pulmonary hypertension develops in a significant number of patients with ILD and may be due to the effects of chronic hypoxia and the focal destruction of capillaries in fibrotic lung tissue.[101] Pulmonary hypertension contributes to progressive diffusion impairment and may contribute to progressive respiratory failure. It is important to ensure that no other cause for the pulmonary hypertension can be identified. For example, a concomitant pulmonary arterial vasculopathy, such as seen in scleroderma or MCTD should be sought, as specific therapy for the pulmonary arterial hypertension may be indicated in those circumstances.[102] In addition, common causes of pulmonary hypertension, such as left-sided systolic or diastolic cardiac dysfunction may be present.[103] Right heart catheterization can distinguish between the various etiologies of pulmonary hypertension and is often required, as echocardiogram has limited sensitivity and specificity in this population.[101] Whether to utilize pulmonary vasodilator therapy in patients with PH secondary to ILD is uncertain at this time. There is concern that use of these medications may worsen ventilation–perfusion matching, however some patients may have symptomatic and functional improvement.[104]

PALLIATIVE CARE

Symptom control is particularly important for patients with all stages of ILD. Pulmonary rehabilitation is encouraged to improve dyspnea in all symptomatic patients. The breathlessness due to advanced ILD may be treated with oxygen supplementation, low-dose opiates and anxiolytics.[105] Cough can be quite problematic and difficult to control; low-dose opiates may be of some benefit and low dose corticosteroids are occasionally used, understanding their long-term risk.[85] Evaluation for acid and nonacid reflux should be considered whenever intractable cough persists.

Palliative care services and hospice referral are appropriate for advanced ILD to maintain a focus on the physical, psychological and spiritual needs of patients and their families.[106] Prognosis in ILD may be uncertain, depending upon the specific diagnosis, the severity of disease, and progressiveness already demonstrated.[107] Particularly in IPF, the likelihood of either progressive respiratory failure or acute decline due to exacerbation should be discussed. End-of-life discussions and advanced directives regarding mechanical ventilation should be broached.[106]

LUNG TRANSPLANTATION

Although lung transplantation has significant associated morbidity and mortality, it is an important and potentially life-extending alternative for patients with progressive fibrotic lung disease. Most patients with ILD referred for lung transplantation have IPF, and for those with advanced disease, survival after lung transplantation is superior to the natural history of their disease.[108] Patients must have a strong social support system as well as the emotional and physical ability to tolerate a complex medical regimen of immunosuppressive therapy.[109]

The timing of listing is complicated in ILD, since the rate of progression is difficult to predict, and abrupt exacerbation of disease may occur.[110] Historically, patients with IPF had high mortality while on lung transplant waiting lists. With newer systems of prioritization, patients with severe IPF are often transplanted quickly, making the correct timing of listing important.[111] In general, a severely impaired D_{LCO} (<39%) as well as advanced fibrosis on HRCT predict poor survival and are considered to be triggers for active listing.[112] Regardless of ILD diagnosis, severe and progressive impairments in pulmonary function predict earlier mortality.[113] Early referral to a lung transplant center is useful as it allows full evaluation and education earlier in the disease course.

CONCLUSION

The approach to ILD includes a careful history and physical examination, with a focus on identifying an etiology for the ILD. Important considerations include a complete investigation of environmental, occupational, and drug exposures as well as a thorough search for underlying connective tissue disease. Laboratory tests, pulmonary physiologic studies, radiography, and biopsy of lung tissue may be necessary. Multidisciplinary review is an essential part of the diagnostic evaluation. Decisions regarding diagnostic and therapeutic approach must be individualized.

REFERENCES

1. Nicholson AG. Classification of idiopathic interstitial pneumonias: making sense of the alphabet soup. *Histopathology.* 2002;41(5):381–391.
2. Travis WD, Costabel U, Hansell DM, et al. An Official American Thoracic Society/European Respiratory Society Statement: Update of the International Multidisciplinary Classification of the Idiopathic Interstitial Pneumonias. *American Journal of Respiratory and Critical Care Medicine.* 2013;188(6):733–748.
3. Schwarz MI. Approach to the evaluation and diagnosis of interstitial lung disease. In: Schwarz MI, King TE, eds. *Interstitial Lung Disease.* 4th ed. London: BC Decker Inc; 2003:1–30.
4. James D. Sarcoidosis of the respiratory system. *Semin Respir Med.* 1986;8:1–111.
5. Leslie KO, Trahan S, Gruden J. Pulmonary pathology of the rheumatic diseases. *Semin Respir Crit Care Med.* 2007;28(4):369–378.
6. Franquet T, Gimenez A, Torrubia S, Sabate JM, Rodriguez-Arias JM. Spontaneous pneumothorax and pneumomediastinum in IPF. *Eur Radiol.* 2000;10(1):108–113.
7. Mendez JL, Nadrous HF, Vassallo R, Decker PA, Ryu JH. Pneumothorax in pulmonary Langerhans cell histiocytosis. *Chest.* 2004;125(3):1028–1032.
8. Lara AR, Schwarz MI. Diffuse alveolar hemorrhage. *Chest.* 2010;137(5):1164–1171.
9. Marchell RM, Judson MA. Cutaneous sarcoidosis. *Semin Respir Crit Care Med.* 2007;31(4):442–451.
10. Sorenson EJ, Crum B, Stevens JC. Incidence of aspiration pneumonia in ALS in Olmsted County, MN. *Amyotroph Lateral Scler.* 2007;8(2):87–89.
11. Chatterjee S. Q: when do Raynaud symptoms merit a workup for autoimmune rheumatic disease? *Cleve Clin J Med.* 2013;80(1):22–25.
12. Zoller B, Li X, Sundquist J, Sundquist K. Risk of subsequent coronary heart disease in patients hospitalized for immune-mediated diseases: a nationwide follow-up study from Sweden. *PLoS One.* 2012;7(3):e33442.
13. Sode BF, Dahl M, Nielsen SF, Nordestgaard BG. Venous thromboembolism and risk of idiopathic interstitial pneumonia: a nationwide study. *Am J Respir Crit Care Med.* 2010;181(10):1085–1092.
14. Swigris JJ, Olson AL, Huie TJ, et al. Increased risk of pulmonary embolism among US decedents with sarcoidosis from 1988 to 2007. *Chest.* 2011;140(5):1261–1266.
15. Kochar R, Fallon MB. Pulmonary diseases and the liver. *Clin Liver Dis.* 2011;15(1):21–37.
16. Hamburg BJ, Schneider F, Woodske ME. A 48-year-old woman with prior liver disease presenting with dyspnea and ground glass opacities. *Chest.* 2012;141(5):1351–1355.
17. Armanios M, Blackburn EH. The telomere syndromes. *Nat Rev Genet.* 2012;13(10):693–704.
18. Papadimitraki ED, Kyrmizakis DE, Kritikos I, Boumpas DT. Ear-nose-throat manifestations of autoimmune rheumatic diseases. *Clin Exp Rheumatol.* 2004;22(4):485–494.
19. Kradin RL, Digumarthy SR, Baggish AL, Mark EJ. Case records of the Massachusetts General Hospital. Case 12-2010. An 89-year-old man with progressive dyspnea. *N Engl J Med.* 2010;362(16):1522–1531.
20. Fontenot AP, Amicosante M. Metal-induced diffuse lung disease. *Semin Respir Crit Care Med.* 2008;29(6):662–669.
21. Rake C, Gilham C, Hatch J, Darnton A, Hodgson J, Peto J. Occupational, domestic and environmental mesothelioma risks in the British population: a case-control study. *Br J Cancer.* 2009;100(7):1175–1183.
22. Greenberger PA. Mold-induced hypersensitivity pneumonitis. *Allergy Asthma Proc.* 2004;25(4):219–223.
23. Embil J, Warren P, Yakrus M, et al. Pulmonary illness associated with exposure to Mycobacterium avium complex in hot tub water. Hypersensitivity pneumonitis or infection? *Chest.* 1997;111(3):813–816.
24. Hardak E, Berger G, Krivoy N, Solomonov A, Yigla M. Nitrofurantoin pulmonary toxicity: neglected threat. *Curr Drug Saf.* 2010;5(2):125–128.
25. Camus P, Martin WJ 2nd, Rosenow EC 3rd. Amiodarone pulmonary toxicity. *Clin Chest Med.* 2004;25(1):65–75.
26. Goodwin SD, Glenny RW. Nonsteroidal anti-inflammatory drug-associated pulmonary infiltrates with eosinophilia. Review of the literature and Food and Drug Administration Adverse Drug Reaction reports. *Arch Intern Med.* 1992;152(7):1521–1524.
27. Camus P, Kudoh S, Ebina M. Interstitial lung disease associated with drug therapy. *Br J Cancer.* 2004;91(Suppl 2):S18–S23.
28. Camus P, Bonniaud P, Fanton A, Camus C, Baudaun N, Foucher P. Drug-induced and iatrogenic infiltrative lung disease. *Clin Chest Med.* 2004;25(3):479–519, vi.
29. Devine MS, Garcia CK. Genetic interstitial lung disease. *Clin Chest Med.* 2012;33(1):95–110.
30. van Moorsel CH, van Oosterhout MF, Barlo NP, et al. Surfactant protein C mutations are the basis of a significant portion of adult familial pulmonary fibrosis in a Dutch cohort. *Am J Respir Crit Care Med.* 2010;182(11):1419–1425.
31. Seibold MA, Wise AL, Speer MC, et al. A common MUC5B promoter polymorphism and pulmonary fibrosis. *N Engl J Med.* 2011;364(16):1503–1512.
32. Rybicki BA, Iannuzzi MC, Frederick MM, et al. Familial aggregation of sarcoidosis. A case-control etiologic study of sarcoidosis (ACCESS). *Am J Respir Crit Care Med.* 2001;164(11):2085–2091.
33. Hunninghake GW, Lynch DA, Galvin JR, et al. Radiologic findings are strongly associated with a pathologic diagnosis of usual interstitial pneumonia. *Chest.* 2003;124(4):1215–1223.
34. Flaherty KR, Toews GB, Travis WD, et al. Clinical significance of histological classification of idiopathic interstitial pneumonia. *Eur Respir J.* 2002;19(2):275–283.
35. Schmidt SL, Sundaram B, Flaherty KR. Diagnosing fibrotic lung disease: when is high-resolution computed tomography sufficient to make a diagnosis of idiopathic pulmonary fibrosis? *Respirology.* 2009;14(7):934–939.
36. Lynch DA, Travis WD, Muller NL, et al. Idiopathic interstitial pneumonias: CT features. *Radiology.* 2005;236(1):10–21.

37. Strange C, Highland KB. Interstitial lung disease in the patient who has connective tissue disease. *Clin Chest Med.* 2004;25(3): 549–559, vii.

38. Egan JJ, Martinez FJ, Wells AU, Williams T. Lung function estimates in idiopathic pulmonary fibrosis: the potential for a simple classification. *Thorax.* 2005;60(4):270–273.

39. Jegal Y, Kim DS, Shim TS, et al. Physiology is a stronger predictor of survival than pathology in fibrotic interstitial pneumonia. *Am J Respir Crit Care Med.* 2005;171(6):639–644.

40. Flaherty KR, Mumford JA, Murray S, et al. Prognostic implications of physiologic and radiographic changes in idiopathic interstitial pneumonia. *Am J Respir Crit Care Med.* 2003;168(5) 543–548.

41. Martinez FJ, Flaherty K. Pulmonary function testing in idiopathic interstitial pneumonias. *Proc Am Thorac Soc.* 2006;3(4):315–321.

42. Hegewald MJ. Diffusing capacity. *Clin Rev Allergy Immunol.* 2009;37(3):159–166.

43. Lama VN, Flaherty KR, Toews GB, et al. Prognostic value of desaturation during a 6-minute walk test in idiopathic interstitial pneumonia. *Am J Respir Crit Care Med.* 2003;168(9): 1084–1090.

44. Villalba WO, Sampaio-Barros PD, Pereira MC, et al. Six-minute walk test for the evaluation of pulmonary disease severity in scleroderma patients. *Chest.* 2007;131(1):217–222.

45. Caminati A, Harari S. IPF: New insight in diagnosis and prognosis. *Respir Med.*104(Suppl 1):S2–S10.

46. Meyer KC. Bronchoalveolar lavage as a diagnostic tool. *Semin Respir Crit Care Med.* 2007;28(5):546–560.

47. Kantrow SP, Meyer KC, Kidd P, Raghu G. The CD4/CD8 ratio in BAL fluid is highly variable in sarcoidosis. *Eur Respir J.* 1997; 10(12):2716–2721.

48. Welker L, Jorres RA, Costabel U, Magnussen H. Predictive value of BAL cell differentials in the diagnosis of interstitial lung diseases. *Eur Respir J.* 2004;24(6):1000–1006.

49. Meyer KC, Rosenthal NS, Soergel P, Peterson K. Neutrophils and low-grade inflammation in the seemingly normal aging human lung. *Mech Ageing Dev.* 1998;104(2):169–181.

50. Cordeiro CR, Jones JC, Alfaro T, Ferreira AJ. Bronchoalveolar lavage in occupational lung diseases. *Semin Respir Crit Care Med.* 2007;28(5):504–513.

51. Auerswald U, Barth J, Magnussen H. Value of CD-1-positive cells in bronchoalveolar lavage fluid for the diagnosis of pulmonary histiocytosis X. *Lung.* 1991;169(6):305–309.

52. Meyer KC. The role of bronchoalveolar lavage in interstitial lung disease. *Clin Chest Med.* 2004;25(4):637–649, v.

53. Ramirez P, Valencia M, Torres A. Bronchoalveolar lavage to diagnose respiratory infections. *Semin Respir Crit Care Med.* 2007;28(5):525–533.

54. Lee BE, Robinson JL, Khurana V, Pang XL, Preiksaitis JK, Fox JD. Enhanced identification of viral and atypical bacterial pathogens in lower respiratory tract samples with nucleic acid amplification tests. *J Med Virol.* 2006;78(5):702–710.

55. Azoulay E, Bergeron A, Chevret S, Bele N, Schlemmer B, Menotti J. Polymerase chain reaction for diagnosing pneumocystis pneumonia in non-HIV immunocompromised patients with pulmonary infiltrates. *Chest.* 2009;135(3):655–661.

56. Hernandez Blasco L, Sanchez Hernandez IM, Villena Garrido V, de Miguel Poch E, Nunez Delgado M, Alfaro Abreu J. Safety of the transbronchial biopsy in outpatients. *Chest.* 1991;99(3): 562–565.

57. Alzeer AH, Al-Otair HA, Al-Hajjaj MS. Yield and complications of flexible fiberoptic bronchoscopy in a teaching hospital. *Saudi Med J.* 2008;29(1):55–59.

58. Descombes E, Gardiol D, Leuenberger P. Transbronchial lung biopsy: an analysis of 530 cases with reference to the number of samples. *Monaldi Arch Chest Dis.* 1997;52(4):324–329.

59. Leslie KO, Gruden JF, Parish JM, Scholand MB. Transbronchial biopsy interpretation in the patient with diffuse parenchymal lung disease. *Arch Pathol Lab Med.* 2007;131(3):407–423.

60. Wall CP, Gaensler EA, Carrington CB, Hayes JA. Comparison of transbronchial and open biopsies in chronic infiltrative lung diseases. *Am Rev Respir Dis.* 1981;123(3):280–285.

61. Hunninghake GW, Zimmerman MB, Schwartz DA, et al. Utility of a lung biopsy for the diagnosis of idiopathic pulmonary fibrosis. *Am J Respir Crit Care Med.* 2001;164(2): 193–196.

62. Riley DJ, Costanzo EJ. Surgical biopsy: its appropriateness in diagnosing interstitial lung disease. *Curr Opin Pulm Med.* 2006;12(5):331–336.

63. Chang AC, Yee J, Orringer MB, Iannettoni MD. Diagnostic thoracoscopic lung biopsy: an outpatient experience. *Ann Thorac Surg.* 2002;74(6):1942–1946; discussion 1946–1947.

64. Kreider ME, Hansen-Flaschen J, Ahmad NN, et al. Complications of video-assisted thoracoscopic lung biopsy in patients with interstitial lung disease. *Ann Thorac Surg.* 2007;83(3): 1140–1144.

65. Carrillo G, Estrada A, Pedroza J, et al. Preoperative risk factors associated with mortality in lung biopsy patients with interstitial lung disease. *J Invest Surg.* 2005;18(1):39–45.

66. Lettieri CJ, Veerappan GR, Helman DL, Mulligan CR, Shorr AF. Outcomes and safety of surgical lung biopsy for interstitial lung disease. *Chest.* 2005;127(5):1600–1605.

67. Hazelrigg SR, Nunchuck SK, LoCicero J 3rd. Video Assisted Thoracic Surgery Study Group data. *Ann Thorac Surg.* 1993;56(5): 1039–1043; discussion 1043–1034.

68. Jaklitsch MT, DeCamp MM Jr, Liptay MJ, et al. Video-assisted thoracic surgery in the elderly. A review of 307 cases. *Chest.* 1996;110(3):751–758.

69. Jaklitsch M, Billmeier S. Preoperative evaluation and risk assessment for elderly thoracic surgery patients. *Thorac Surg Clin.* 2009;19(3):301–312.

70. Katzenstein AL, Mukhopadhyay S, Myers JL. Diagnosis of usual interstitial pneumonia and distinction from other fibrosing interstitial lung diseases. *Hum Pathol.* 2008;39(9):12751294.

71. Flaherty KR, Thwaite EL, Kazerooni EA, et al. Radiological versus histological diagnosis in UIP and NSIP: survival implications. *Thorax.* 2003;58(2):143–148.

72. Sumikawa H, Johkoh T, Colby TV, et al. Computed tomography findings in pathological usual interstitial pneumonia: relationship to survival. *Am J Respir Crit Care Med.* 2008; 177(4):433–439.

73. Flaherty KR, King TE Jr, Raghu G, et al. Idiopathic interstitial pneumonia: what is the effect of a multidisciplinary approach to diagnosis? *Am J Respir Crit Care Med.* 2004;170(8):904–910.

74. Flaherty KR, Andrei AC, King TE Jr, et al. Idiopathic interstitial pneumonia: do community and academic physicians agree on diagnosis? *Am J Respir Crit Care Med.* 2007;175(10): 1054–1060.

75. Raghu G, Collard HR, Egan JJ, et al. An official ATS/ERS/JRS/ALAT statement: idiopathic pulmonary fibrosis:

evidence-based guidelines for diagnosis and management. *Am J Respir Crit Care Med.* 2011;183(6):788–824.

76. Cheung OY, Muhm JR, Helmers RA, et al. Surgical pathology of granulomatous interstitial pneumonia. *Ann Diagn Pathol.* 2003;7(2):127–138.
77. Travis WD, Hunninghake G, King TE Jr, et al. Idiopathic nonspecific interstitial pneumonia: report of an American Thoracic Society project. *Am J Respir Crit Care Med.* 2008;177(12):1338–1347.
78. Craig TJ, Hershey J, Engler RJ, Davis W, Carpenter GB, Salata K. Bird antigen persistence in the home environment after removal of the bird. *Ann Allergy.* 1992;69(6):510–512.
79. Girard M, Lacasse Y, Cormier Y. Hypersensitivity pneumonitis. *Allergy.* 2009;64(3):322–334.
80. Glazer CS, Rose CS, Lynch DA. Clinical and radiologic manifestations of hypersensitivity pneumonitis. *J Thorac Imaging.* 2002; 17(4):261–272.
81. Gogali A, Wells AU. New pharmacological strategies for the treatment of pulmonary fibrosis. *Ther Adv Respir Dis.* 2010;4(6): 353–366.
82. Idiopathic Pulmonary Fibrosis Clinical Research Network, Raghu G, Anstrom KJ, King TE Jr, Lasky JA, Martinez FJ. Prednisone, azathioprine, and N-acetylcysteine for pulmonary fibrosis. *N Engl J Med.* 2012;366(21):1968–1977.
83. Moghadam-Kia S, Werth VP. Prevention and treatment of systemic glucocorticoid side effects. *Int J Dermatol.* 2010;49(3): 239–248.
84. Cutolo M, Seriolo B, Pizzorni C, et al. Use of glucocorticoids and risk of infections. *Autoimmun Rev.* 2008;8(2):153–155.
85. Bradley B, Branley HM, Egan JJ, et al. Interstitial lung disease guideline: the British Thoracic Society in collaboration with the Thoracic Society of Australia and New Zealand and the Irish Thoracic Society. *Thorax.* 2008;63(Suppl 5):v1–58.
86. Clark M, Cooper B, Singh S, Cooper M, Carr A, Hubbard R. A survey of nocturnal hypoxaemia and health related quality of life in patients with cryptogenic fibrosing alveolitis. *Thorax.* 2001;56(6):482–486.
87. Laviolette L, Bourbeau J, Bernard S, et al. Assessing the impact of pulmonary rehabilitation on functional status in COPD. *Thorax.* 2008;63(2):115–121.
88. Swigris JJ, Brown KK, Make BJ, Wamboldt FS. Pulmonary rehabilitation in idiopathic pulmonary fibrosis: a call for continued investigation. *Respir Med.* 2008;102(12):1675–1680.
89. Holland A, Hill C. Physical training for interstitial lung disease. *Cochrane Database Syst Rev.* 2008;(4):CD006322.
90. Nici L, Donner C, Wouters E, et al. American Thoracic Society/ European Respiratory Society statement on pulmonary rehabilitation. *Am J Respir Crit Care Med.* 2006;173(12):1390–1413.
91. Singer HK, Ruchinskas RA, Riley KC, Broshek DK, Barth JT. The psychological impact of end-stage lung disease. *Chest.* 2001;120(4):1246–1252.
92. Ponnuswamy A, Manikandan R, Sabetpour A, Keeping IM, Finnerty JP. Association between ischaemic heart disease and interstitial lung disease: a case-control study. *Respir Med.* 2009;103(4):503–507.
93. Nathan SD, Basavaraj A, Reichner C, et al. Prevalence and impact of coronary artery disease in idiopathic pulmonary fibrosis. *Respir Med.* 2010;104(7):1035–1041.
94. Lancaster LH, Mason WR, Parnell JA, et al. Obstructive sleep apnea is common in idiopathic pulmonary fibrosis. *Chest.* 2009;136(3):772–778.
95. Mermigkis C, Stagaki E, Tryfon S, et al. How common is sleep-disordered breathing in patients with idiopathic pulmonary fibrosis? *Sleep Breath.* 2010;14(4):387–390.
96. Rasche K, Orth M. Sleep and breathing in idiopathic pulmonary fibrosis. *J Physiol Pharmacol.* 2009;60(Suppl 5):13–14.
97. Tobin RW, Pope CE 2nd, Pellegrini CA, Emond MJ, Sillery J, Raghu G. Increased prevalence of gastroesophageal reflux in patients with idiopathic pulmonary fibrosis. *Am J Respir Crit Care Med.* 1998;158(6):1804–1808.
98. Raghu G, Freudenberger TD, Yang S, et al. High prevalence of abnormal acid gastro-oesophageal reflux in idiopathic pulmonary fibrosis. *Eur Respir J.* 2006;27(1):136–142.
99. Raghu G, Yang ST, Spada C, Hayes J, Pellegrini CA. Sole treatment of acid gastroesophageal reflux in idiopathic pulmonary fibrosis: a case series. *Chest.* 2006;129(3):794–800.
100. Maricic M. Update on glucocorticoid-induced osteoporosis. *Rheum Dis Clin North Am.* 2011;37(3):415–431, vi.
101. Patel NM, Lederer DJ, Borczuk AC, Kawut SM. Pulmonary hypertension in idiopathic pulmonary fibrosis. *Chest.* 2007;132(3):998–1006.
102. Hassoun PM. Pulmonary arterial hypertension complicating connective tissue diseases. *Semin Respir Crit Care Med.* 2009;30(4):429–439.
103. Corte TJ, Wort SJ, Wells AU. Pulmonary hypertension in idiopathic pulmonary fibrosis: a review. *Sarcoidosis Vasc Diffuse Lung Dis.* 2009;26(1):7–19.
104. Poor HD, Girgis R, Studer SM. World Health Organization Group III pulmonary hypertension. *Prog Cardiovasc Dis.* 2012;55(2):119–127.
105. Mahler DA, Selecky PA, Harrod CG, et al. American College of Chest Physicians consensus statement on the management of dyspnea in patients with advanced lung or heart disease. *Chest.* 2010;137(3):674–691.
106. Lanken PN, Terry PB, Delisser HM, et al. An official American Thoracic Society clinical policy statement: palliative care for patients with respiratory diseases and critical illnesses. *Am J Respir Crit Care Med.* 2008;177(8):912–927.
107. Nathan SD, Shlobin OA, Weir N, et al. Long-term course and prognosis of idiopathic pulmonary fibrosis in the new millennium. *Chest.* 2011;140(1):221–229.
108. George TJ, Arnaoutakis GJ, Shah AS. Lung transplant in idiopathic pulmonary fibrosis. *Arch Surg.* 2011;146(10):1204–1209.
109. Merlo CA, Orens JB. Candidate selection, overall results, and choosing the right operation. *Semin Respir Crit Care Med.* 2010;31(2):99–107.
110. Martinez FJ, Safrin S, Weycker D, et al. The clinical course of patients with idiopathic pulmonary fibrosis. *Ann Intern Med.* 2005;142(12 Pt 1):963–967.
111. O'Beirne S, Counihan IP, Keane MP. Interstitial lung disease and lung transplantation. *Semin Respir Crit Care Med.* 2010;31(2):139–146.
112. Mogulkoc N, Brutsche MH, Bishop PW, Greaves SM, Horrocks AW, Egan JJ. Pulmonary function in idiopathic pulmonary fibrosis and referral for lung transplantation. *Am J Respir Crit Care Med.* 2001;164(1):103–108.
113. Latsi PI, du Bois RM, Nicholson AG, et al. Fibrotic idiopathic interstitial pneumonia: the prognostic value of longitudinal functional trends. *Am J Respir Crit Care Med.* 2003;168(5): 531–537.

CHAPTER 55
Systemic Sarcoidosis

David R. Moller
Edward S. Chen

Sarcoidosis is a multisystem disorder characterized by noncaseating granulomatous inflammation at sites of disease.[1] Although any organ can be involved, the disease most commonly affects the lungs and intrathoracic lymph nodes. A diagnosis of sarcoidosis is most securely established from compatible clinical and radiologic findings, confirmed by a biopsy showing noncaseating epithelioid granulomas in more than one organ and the exclusion of granulomatous disorders of known cause. Clinical, epidemiologic, and family studies support the hypothesis that sarcoidosis is triggered by exposure to microbial agents in individuals with a genetic susceptibility to the disease. The clinical course is highly variable, with a mortality rate of <1% to 5%. Corticosteroids remain the mainstay of treatment for patients with threatened organ failure or progressive disease.

HISTORICAL PERSPECTIVE

Jonathan Hutchinson was the first to describe a case of sarcoidosis in 1887; he called it Mortimer's malady, after one of his patients who presented with face and limb skin lesions. In 1889, Besnier of Paris described a 34-year-old man with violaceous skin lesions of the nose, ear lobules, and central face; he proposed that the lesions were a variant of lupus erythematosus leading to its designation as "lupus pernio." In 1899, Caesar Boeck first described the characteristic noncaseating granulomas in a patient with peripheral lymphadenopathy and skin nodules. He proposed the term *multiple benign sarcoids of the skin* because he thought the granulomatous changes resembled sarcomatous tissue. Subsequently, descriptions of sarcoid-type lesions in the eyes, bones, lungs, and salivary glands were made, but the systemic and unifying nature of sarcoidosis was not recognized for almost 20 years.

The view that sarcoidosis is a systemic disorder is largely based on the work of Jorgen Schaumann, a Swedish dermatologist, who in 1914 presented the view that Besnier lupus pernio and Boeck's multiple sarcoids were manifestations of the same disease termed "lymphogranulomatose benigne," thought to represent a variant of tuberculosis. In 1935, Williams and Nickerson reported that intradermal inoculation of a suspension of sarcoidosis tissue resulted in firm papules in patients with suspected sarcoidosis. Ansgar Kveim demonstrated that these papules contained sarcoidosis-like granulomas on biopsy. Louis Siltzbach and others would demonstrate in worldwide studies that this "Kveim" reaction was positive (showed granulomas) in up to 80% of sarcoidosis and was highly specific for the disease. Sven Löfgren of Sweden in the 1940s noted that sarcoidosis frequently begins with asymptomatic bilateral hilar adenopathy or with acute erythema nodosum. In the 1950s, corticosteroids were reported to be successful in treating sarcoidosis. More recently, the tools of cell and molecular biology have advanced our understanding of the immunologic, genetic, and etiologic basis of sarcoidosis, but have not yet led to breakthroughs in the development of safe, effective therapies or cure.

EPIDEMIOLOGY

Sarcoidosis is found worldwide, although the frequency of the disease varies among different geographic regions. Accurate measurements of disease prevalence are unknown, because many people with sarcoidosis are asymptomatic and there is neither sensitive nor specific diagnostic tests. Estimated prevalence rates between 10 and 40 cases per 100,000 population are reported in North America, southern Europe, and Japan.[2] Higher prevalence rates are noted in Sweden, Denmark, and US Blacks. More than 80% of cases occur in persons between 20 and 50 years of age, with a second peak in women more than 50 years of age.[1] Sarcoidosis is rare in the preadolescent period.[3] The lifetime risk for developing sarcoidosis has been estimated as 1.4% and 1.0% in women and men of Scandinavian countries, respectively, whereas one US study calculated a lifetime risk "in women and men of 2.7% and 2.1% in Blacks and 1.0% and 0.7% in Whites, respectively" in a midwestern city.[4] Based on autopsy studies, the prevalence of sarcoidosis is likely underestimated.[5] Whether the incidence of sarcoidosis is changing remains unknown given a lack of studies over the past decade.[6]

The frequency of different clinical manifestations of sarcoidosis also varies among geographic regions and ethnic groups, and is influenced by gender. Erythema nodosum is common in Scandinavian countries and Ireland, but found in less than 5% of Black or Japanese patients. In contrast, lupus pernio appears more frequently among Black populations. In Japan, over 50% of patients may have cardiac sarcoidosis.[7] Several studies suggest that race is an important determinant of disease severity with Black populations more likely to have persistent disease and greater mortality than White populations.[4,8] In the United States, 40% to 80% of mortality from sarcoidosis is from advanced pulmonary disease, with higher rates observed in Blacks and women.[9,10] In Sweden and Japan, cardiac involvement is the leading cause of death from sarcoidosis. Overall, mortality rates directly related to sarcoidosis approximate <1% to 5% depending on the study setting.[11,12]

ETIOLOGY

The cause of sarcoidosis remains uncertain. Since sarcoidosis was first described, investigators have postulated an infectious cause of the disease based on the clinical similarities to tuberculosis. Environmental exposures are linked to sarcoidosis due to seasonal clustering of the disease with a predilection for winter and early spring months in both northern and southern hemispheres.[13] Geographic variation and time–space clustering also support a role for environmental factors in sarcoidosis.[14] Occupational associations have been described for healthcare professionals, firefighters, military personnel, and workers involved in the lumber industry. Chronic beryllium disease causes a granulomatous pneumonitis histologically identical to pulmonary sarcoidosis in less than 5% of exposed workers following immunologic sensitization to beryllium.[15] However, there is no evidence that beryllium is a cause of systemic sarcoidosis.[16] An increased risk of a "sarcoidosis-like" pulmonary disease was documented in first-response rescue workers exposed to the heavy dust burden from the World Trade Center disaster; a minority of these workers had multisystem disease confirming a likely diagnosis of multisystem sarcoidosis.[17,18]

The US-based multicenter study of sarcoidosis etiology called ACCESS (A Case Control Etiologic Study of Sarcoidosis) compared 706 newly diagnosed, biopsy-proven sarcoidosis cases to age-, sex-, and race-matched controls.[19,20] Results from the study showed an absence of environmental or occupational associations positively linked to sarcoidosis risk that carried an odds ratio (OR) greater than 2.0 and an exposure prevalence of greater than 5% (prestudy goal). Weak positive associations (OR ~1.5) were found for insecticide use at work, mold/mildew exposures at work, and musty odors, suggesting possible links to microbial-rich environments. Sarcoidosis was not associated with exposure to heavy metals including beryllium, wood dusts, or rural residence as previously hypothesized. The ACCESS study found a robust negative association of smoking and sarcoidosis risk, confirming earlier studies. The lack of a single, dominant exposure associated with sarcoidosis risk is consistent with the concept that gene–environment interactions are important in causing disease.

Many studies have directly examined a role for infectious agents in sarcoidosis given the clinical similarities to mycobacterial disease. A meta-analysis of studies published between 1980 to 2006 identified a 10- to 20-fold greater likelihood of detecting mycobacterial nucleic acids (DNA, RNA) in sarcoidosis tissues than control tissues.[21] The authors and their colleagues used a limited proteomic approach to identify potential pathogenic antigens in sarcoidosis tissues based solely on the biochemical properties of the Kveim reaction, a delayed granulomatous skin reaction to sarcoidosis tissue extracts.[22] Using homogenized sarcoidosis tissue extracts, mass spectrometry, and protein immunoblotting, we identified the mycobacterial catalase-peroxidase protein (mKatG) as a candidate pathogenic antigen.[23] This unbiased approach was not predicated on any *a priori* hypothesis regarding specific pathogenic microbes or autoantigens, supporting a mycobacterial link to sarcoidosis etiology. Several groups have demonstrated that as many as 70% of sarcoidosis patients have lung and blood T-cell responses to mycobacterial antigens including mKatG, *Mycobacterium tuberculosis* ESAT-6, Ag85, superoxide dismutase.[24–26] Several studies report extensive overlap in peripheral blood gene expression between individuals with sarcoidosis and tuberculosis infection, further supporting a mycobacterial etiology of sarcoidosis.[27–29]

Japanese investigators find *Propionibacterium acnes* DNA in 80% to 98% of sarcoidosis tissues from Japan and Europe but also in 0% to 60% of control tissues.[30] An animal model of granulomatous lung inflammation induced by *P. acnes* has been reported.[31,32] However, a role for *Propionibacteria* in sarcoidosis remains unclear because of the frequent detection and recovery of these organisms from tissues and evidence of immune responses to these commensal organisms in nonsarcoidosis control individuals. Other microbial agents, such as *Borrelia burgdorferi, Chlamydia pneumonia,* or *Rickettsia helvetica* have been implicated in sarcoidosis from tissue or serologic studies, but these latter studies all lack wider confirmation. High titers of antibodies against lymphotropic DNA viruses (Epstein–Barr virus, cytomegalovirus, and human herpesvirus type 6) and HTLV1 have been described in patients with sarcoidosis but may reflect generalized B-cell activation in sarcoidosis, since a viral origin has not been substantiated by viral cultures or tissue analysis.

Despite the evidence for linking some microbes to sarcoidosis etiology, there is no histopathologic or microbiologic evidence that viable mycobacterial organisms or other pathogenic organisms are present in sarcoidosis tissues. Cell-wall deficient microbes have been suggested to cause sarcoidosis, but none are supported by independent, reproducible studies.[33] Although direct demonstration of an infectious etiology remains unproven, many investigators favor the hypothesis that certain classes of microbial organisms trigger sarcoidosis in those with genetic susceptibility.

Some investigators hypothesize an etiologic association with autoimmunity, perhaps triggered by an infectious agent through molecular mimicry. In support of this concept, sarcoidosis is associated with features of autoimmunity, such as antinuclear antibodies, rheumatoid factor, hypergammaglobulinemia, and immune complexes. Sarcoidosis patients often express low titer autoantibodies of unclear significance, although no disease-specific autoantibody profile has been identified. One recent study identified several potential autoantigens such as vimentin, ATP synthase, and lysyl-tRNA whose derived peptides stimulated Th1 lymphocytes in the blood or lung of sarcoidosis patients, suggesting these responses may help sustain chronic inflammation.[34]

GENETICS

Family and case control association studies provide strong evidence for a genetic influence on the risk of developing sarcoidosis and in determining clinical expression of the disease. Familial clustering of sarcoidosis occurs in 3% to 14% of patients, with a greater frequency among Black compared with White populations. The US ACCESS study found siblings of sarcoidosis cases have a higher relative risk (RR) (OR ~5.8) than parents (OR ~3.8).[35] The significantly higher adjusted familial RR estimates reported for Whites in both the US ACCESS study (RR ~18) and in a UK study with mostly Whites (RR ~36–73) and Blacks (RR ~2.8), suggest that genetic factors have a greater influence in susceptibility to sarcoidosis in Whites than Blacks.

Early studies examined the role of HLA class I alleles using serologic techniques. The HLA-B8 allele has most consistently been associated with disease susceptibility, increasing sarcoidosis risk in Whites from the United States and Europe but not in Blacks or Japanese.[36–38]

The role of HLA class II alleles has been intensively studied in sarcoidosis. HLA-DR3 has been associated with sarcoidosis susceptibility, while HLA-DR1 and -DR4 alleles have been associated with disease protection in Scandinavian and European populations. Using molecular genotyping, the ACCESS study found a significant association between HLA-DRB1*1101 in both Blacks and Whites, while HLA-DRB1*1501 was associated with sarcoidosis risk only in Whites.[39] Other studies find the class II HLA-DR17 (DR3) haplotype and specifically HLA DRB1*0301 or the closely linked DQB1*0201 alleles to be associated with favorable outcomes (Löfgren syndrome, acute arthritis, stage I chest radiograph, or remission within 2 years) in European and Japanese populations.[40,41] The DRB1*1501 or the closely linked DQB1*0602 alleles were associated with more severe or chronic disease in a Danish cohort. HLA-DPB1 and DQB1 alleles have been associated with disease susceptibility in some studies, although linkage disequilibrium makes it difficult to separate from effects of HLA-DR alleles.[42] One study identified four DR and nine DQ gene polymorphisms associated with increased risk of developing sarcoidosis.[43] Since the pockets within the HLA class II sequence determine specific antigenic peptide binding, these results are consistent with the existence of etiologically important antigens in sarcoidosis. Family linkage studies employing genome-wide microsatellite analysis confirm the importance of genes from the MHC locus in determining susceptibility to sarcoidosis.[44] These data support a consensus view that MHC class II alleles are the major contributor to disease susceptibility across different ethnic populations in sarcoidosis, likely through binding specific pathogenic antigens.

Non-HLA genes have been the subject of multiple case control studies but most candidate genes linked to sarcoidosis lack replication. A meta-analysis concluded that polymorphisms of the tumor necrosis factor (TNF) gene located within the MHC locus is associated with a 1.5-fold increase risk of developing sarcoidosis.[45] There appears to be no increased risk associated with polymorphisms in genes encoding angiotensin-converting enzyme (ACE) or vitamin D receptor.

Genome-wide association studies of both familial and sporadic sarcoidosis incident cases have identified multiple chromosomal regions that may contribute to sarcoidosis susceptibility, suggesting multiple small genetic effects may influence risk. German and US investigators reported that the butyrophilin-like 2 (*BTNL2*) gene is associated with sarcoidosis risk in White and to a lesser extent, Black populations.[46,47] In addition to increased risk for disease susceptibility, recent studies suggest that BTNL2 polymorphisms may associate with chronic active disease.[48,49] Since *BTNL2* is a member of the B7 receptor family that functions in T-cell costimulation, a plausible hypothesis links the *BTNL2* gene with T-cell immunity and sarcoidosis susceptibility.

German investigators reported novel genetic loci at chromosome 6p12.1, and 11q13.1 to be associated with sarcoidosis susceptibility.[50,51] This group also identified risk associations with annexin A11, which has been also associated with Crohn disease.[52] Other studies have

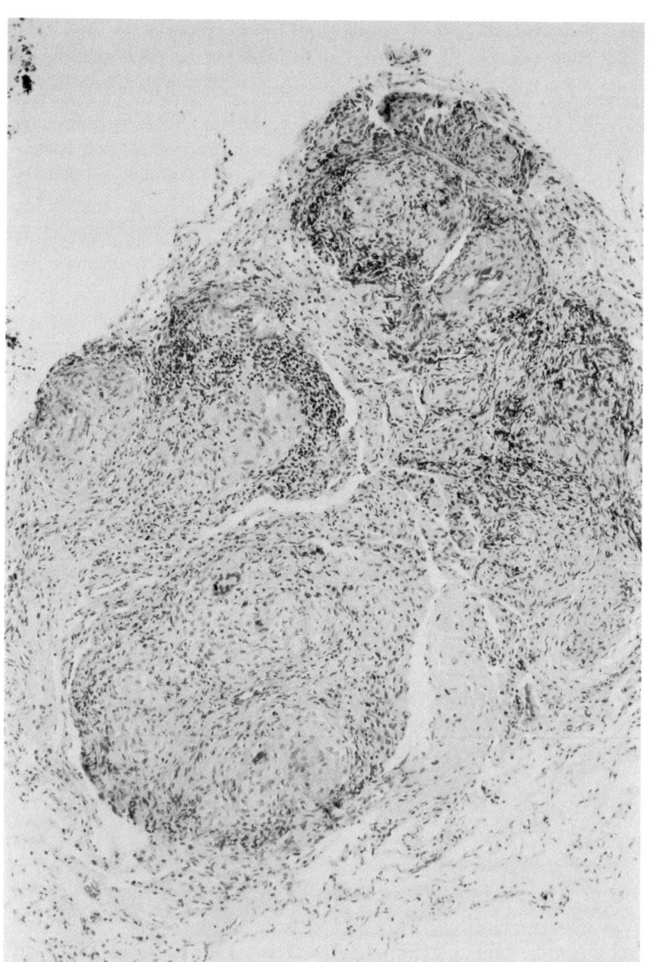

A

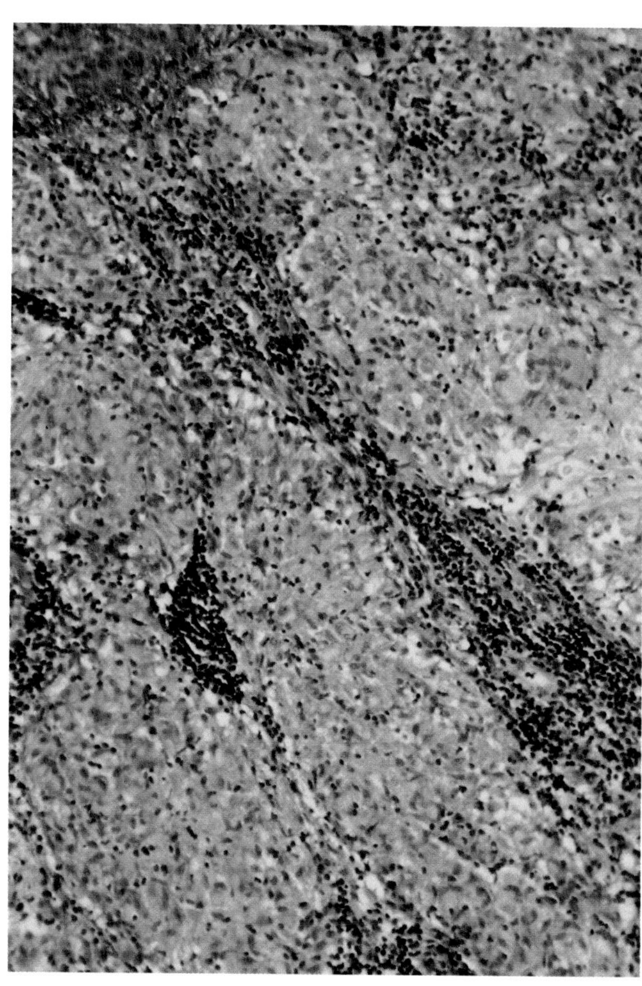

B

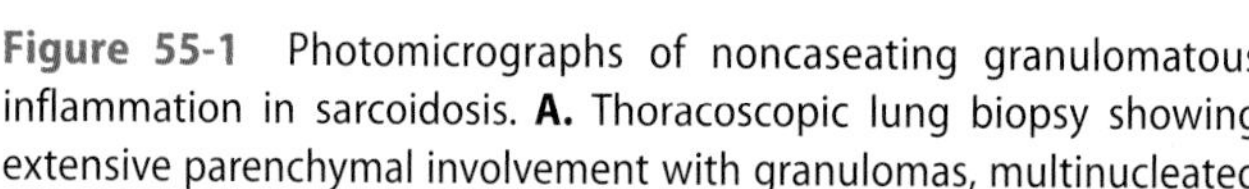

Figure 55-1 Photomicrographs of noncaseating granulomatous inflammation in sarcoidosis. **A.** Thoracoscopic lung biopsy showing extensive parenchymal involvement with granulomas, multinucleated giant cells, and mononuclear cell inflammation (×80). **B.** Mediastinal lymph node biopsy showing typical discrete epithelioid granulomas (×200).

identified additional loci including 10p12.2 to have associations with both sarcoidosis and inflammatory bowel disease.[53,54]

PATHOLOGY

The pathologic hallmark of sarcoidosis is the presence of discrete, noncaseating, epithelioid cell granulomas (Fig. 55-1). The dominant cell in the central core is the epithelioid cell, thought to be a differentiated form of a mononuclear phagocyte. CD4 lymphocytes and mature macrophages are typically interspersed throughout the epithelioid core, whereas both CD4+ and CD8+ T cells and B lymphocytes may be seen in the periphery of the granuloma. Occasionally, focal fibrinoid but not caseating necrosis may be seen. Giant cells, often containing cytoplasmic inclusions such as calcium and iron-laden Schaumann bodies and Hamazaki–Wesenberg bodies are scattered throughout the inflammatory locus. These features are not specific for sarcoidosis, as similar histopathologic findings can be seen in infections, berylliosis, Crohn disease, and local "sarcoid reactions" that occur near neoplastic, foreign body, or chronic inflammatory areas.

In the lung, granulomas tend to form along perivascular, peribronchial, and septal regions, areas rich in lymphatic vessels. In the lung, a mononuclear cell infiltration composed predominantly of lymphocytes is often present in the adjacent interstitium. Granulomas in sarcoidosis may resolve or undergo fibrosis, leaving a stellate scar or hyalinized ghost of a former granuloma.

PATHOPHYSIOLOGY

Important considerations in the pathophysiology of sarcoidosis are discussed below.

IMMUNOPATHOLOGY

Experimental models indicate that the first step in granuloma formation involves the tissue deposition of poorly soluble antigenic material. An initial innate immune response involves the recruitment and activation of antigen-presenting cells such as macrophages or dendritic cells expressing pattern recognition receptors and Toll-like receptors (TLRs). This results in the phagocytosis and degradation of antigenic proteins, generating peptide: MHC complexes that are displayed on the cell surface for analysis by CD4+ T cells. The resulting adaptive immune response is characterized by the expression of effector cytokines dominated by either a type 1 T helper cell (Th1; IFNγ), Th2 (IL4/IL13), or Th17 (IL17/IL21/IL22) response, depending on the nature of the antigen and host genetic/epigenetic factors.[55] Granuloma formation is orchestrated by the subsequent release of cytokines, chemokines, and other mediators by activated innate and adaptive immune cells. Granulomatous inflammation is downregulated with clearance of antigen along with release of anti-inflammatory mediators such as transforming growth factor-b (TGFβ) and IL10 by local immune cells.[56,57]

The immunopathology of sarcoidosis can be modeled in this experimental context (Table 55-1). Sites of granulomatous

TABLE 55-1 Hallmarks of the Pathobiology of Sarcoidosis

Pathology of noncaseating epithelioid granulomas
Genetic susceptibility determined primarily by HLA genes of MHC locus
Oligoclonal expansion of $\alpha\beta$+T cells consistent with antigen-driven inflammation
Polarized Th1 immunity with upregulated Th1 cytokines and chemokines at sites of disease
Potential contribution of Th17 immune responses
Reduced regulatory T-cell function
Microbial triggers with mycobacterial or propionibacterial organisms most commonly implicated
Serum amyloid A dysaggregation within granulomas provides a mechanism for chronic disease

inflammation such as the lung contain activated T cells and mononuclear phagocytes that express the same proinflammatory cytokines and chemokines that have been shown experimentally to be critical in granuloma formation.[58] Lung T cells are predominantly of the CD4 T helper, CD45R0 "memory" phenotype, express the activation markers, VLA-1 (very late activation antigen-1, CD49a) and HLA-DR molecules. Sarcoidosis alveolar macrophages (AMs) spontaneously produce TNF, interleukin-6 (IL6), IL1α, IL15, osteopontin, and the Th1 regulatory cytokines, IL12 and IL18 as well as increased amounts of lysozyme, ACE, and reactive oxygen species. Sarcoidosis AMs express increased density of the costimulatory molecules, CD80, CD86, and CD40, consistent with their enhanced antigen-presenting capability. Dendritic cells likely play a critical role in regulating local immune responses in sarcoidosis but have been the focus of few studies.[59-61] TNF is considered to be a major effector cytokine of granuloma formation in sarcoidosis (and therapeutic target) as enhanced release of TNF by BAL cells is associated with persistent disease.[62] Other proinflammatory cytokines such as IL1, macrophage migration inhibitory factor, IL6, and osteopontin are upregulated in sarcoidosis. Consistent with upregulated proinflammatory cytokine expression, there is increased activation of the transcription factor NF-κB in the lung of sarcoidosis patients,[63] and downregulation of the inflammation-suppressive transcription factor, peroxisome proliferator–activated receptor-γ.[64]

Studies of T-cell receptor (TCR) gene expression provide direct evidence that sarcoidosis is an antigen-driven disorder. Oligoclonal expansions of T cells expressing specific Vβ- or Vα-specific TCR gene segments have been found in the lung (BAL T cells), skin (Kveim biopsy sites), and blood.[65,66] The best studied example involves the remarkable expansion of Vα2.3 (AV2S3)+ BAL T cells from HLA-DRB1*0301-positive Scandinavian patients with sarcoidosis.[67] The specific antigens driving these clonally expanded T-cell populations remain uncertain but may include autoantigens such as vimentin and microbial antigens such as mKatG.[34] These studies provide evidence that oligoclonal T-cell expansions in sarcoidosis are driven by conventional antigens.

TH1 AND TH17 IMMUNITY

There are compelling data that sarcoidosis is characterized by dominant Th1 cytokine production compartmentalized to sites of inflammation.[68,69] Multiple studies confirm that pulmonary sarcoidosis is associated with enhanced expression of Th1 associated IFNγ, IL12, and IL18 in the lung but low or undetectable levels of IL4 or IL5. Characteristic of a Th1 response, the Th1-differentiation transcription factors, T-bet (T-box, expressed in T cells), and STAT-1 and its phosphorylated form are upregulated in sarcoidosis.[70,71] Consistent with Th1 polarization, most sarcoidosis BAL T cells express a functional, high-affinity IL12 receptor and the chemokine receptors CXCR3 and CCR5. This dominant Th1 polarization is characteristic of sarcoidosis at time of diagnosis and after years of known disease.

The role of Th17 responses in sarcoidosis is uncertain. Several studies show upregulated Th17 responses in sarcoidosis blood and tissues,[72,73] with release of IL17 and IL22,[74] but others show decreased or no upregulated Th17 responses in sarcoidosis compared to control subjects.[75-77] Despite an established role for Th17 effector T cells in granulomatosis with polyangiitis (GPA), (formerly known as Wegener granulomatosis) and tuberculosis,[78,79] whether Th17 responses play a critical role in disease outcome or can substitute for the polarized Th1 responses documented in sarcoidosis needs further study.

IMMUNOREGULATORY CELLS

Regulatory T cells (Tregs) maintain immune homeostasis by suppressing the function of antigen-presenting cells and effector T cells. Several groups have reported that FoxP3-positive natural Tregs (nTreg) accumulate at sites of granulomatous inflammation in sarcoidosis but may have reduced function in suppressing proinflammatory cytokine expression and granuloma formation.[80-82] Diminished numbers of immunoregulatory natural killer T (NKT) cells have also been reported and may contribute to chronic active sarcoidosis.[83] Whether the functional impairment of nTreg or NKT cells in sarcoidosis are primary defects or secondary to the hyperimmune Th1 responses in sarcoidosis remains uncertain.

One group studied the effects of nebulized vasoactive intestinal peptide (VIP) in sarcoidosis and found it significantly reduced TNF production by BAL cells.[84] This effect was associated with an increased frequency of lung CD4+CD127-CD25+ Tregs. Since VIP converted naïve CD4+CD25-T cells into CD4+CD25+FoxP3+ Tregs in vitro, the authors suggested inhaled VIP as a potential treatment of immune-mediated lung diseases including sarcoidosis.

MECHANISMS OF PULMONARY FIBROSIS

The mechanisms that promote pulmonary fibrosis in sarcoidosis remain uncertain. IFNγ has direct antifibrotic effects,[85] but this pleotropic cytokine may mediate fibrosis by enhancing lung injury.[86] There is evidence that sarcoidosis AMs transition to an alternative profibrotic M2-like phenotype in fibrotic pulmonary sarcoidosis with upregulated expression of chemokines such as CCL18.[87] The lack of evidence for IL4 upregulation in sarcoidosis suggests that IL10 or IL13 may foster this profibrotic macrophage phenotype.[88]

Increased expression of TGFβ, fibronectin, insulin-like growth factor-1 (IGF-1), laminin, and matrix metalloproteases by sarcoidosis AMs may promote a fibrosis-permissive environment in chronic active sarcoidosis through the recruitment and activation of fibroblasts.[69,89] While increased TGFβ is associated with the presence of structural lung disease among sarcoidosis patients,[90,91] the exact role of TGFβ in sarcoidosis remains unclear since it not only has profibrotic but immunoregulatory effects.

SERUM AMYLOID A DYSAGGREGATION HYPOTHESIS

The major challenge of sarcoidosis is to understand what drives chronic granulomatous inflammation given the lack of evidence for an active mycobacterial or other viable microbial infection in sarcoidosis tissues at any point in the disease. The lack of evidence of viable pathologic organisms in sarcoidosis tissues occurs in the context of often long-term treatment with corticosteroid, immunosuppressive or anti-TNF therapy in these patients. This observation, together with evidence of nonviable remnants of mycobacterial or other microbial DNA in sarcoidosis tissues, and relevant immune responses to these

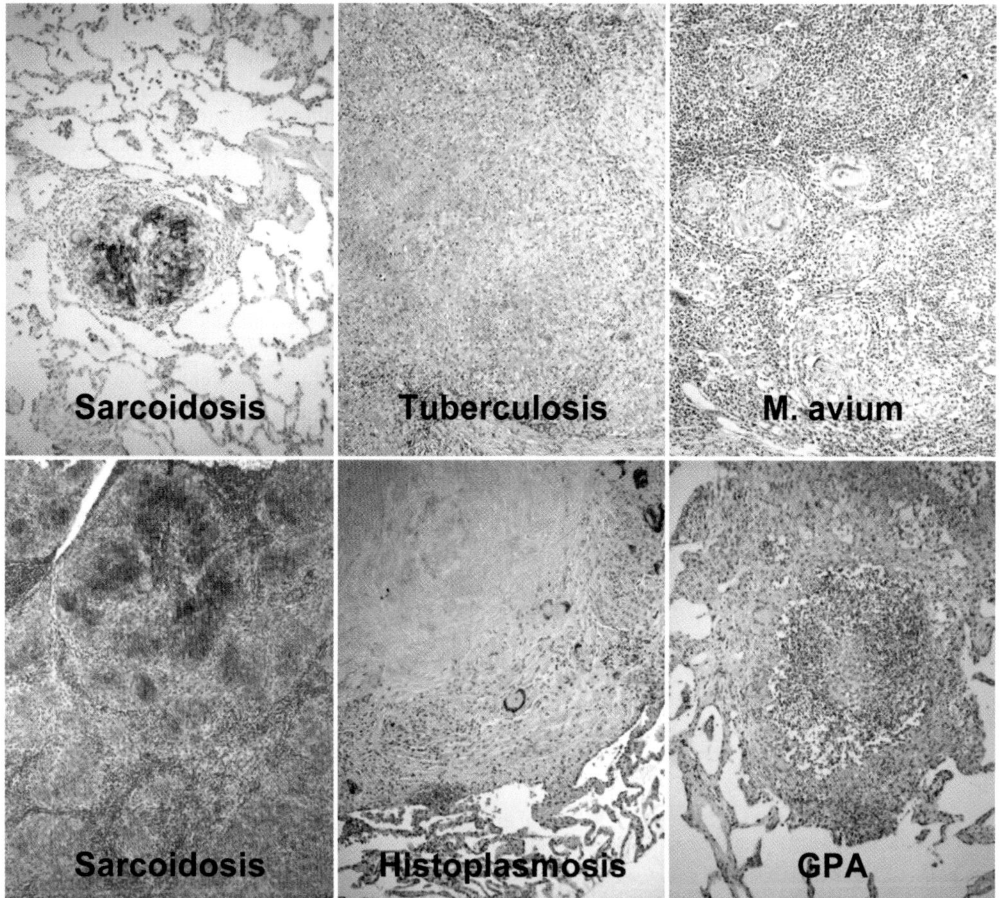

Figure 55-2 Immunohistochemistry showing focal deposition of serum amyloid A *(brownish stain)* in tissues from patients with sarcoidosis but little or no staining for SAA in tuberculosis, *Mycobacterium avium* infection, histoplasmosis, or granulomatosis with polyangiitis (GPA).

organisms, suggests that specific microbes may trigger sarcoidosis, but that a local hyperpolarized Th1 response results in permanent immune control of the triggering infectious agent.

The authors and their colleagues recently reported on a potential mechanism for chronic granulomatous inflammation in sarcoidosis involving the host protein serum amyloid A (SAA).[92,93] Our investigation of SAA was based on our recognition that the granuloma-inducing component in Kveim reagent had physicochemical properties that closely resemble amyloid or prion proteins.[94] SAA is an amyloid precursor protein and acute phase reactant[95] that was previously reported to be upregulated in the blood of sarcoidosis patients as an inflammatory biomarker.[96–98] We reported that SAA was highly concentrated within sarcoidosis granulomas unlike all other granulomatous disorders examined (Fig. 55-2). Our studies showed SAA could promote experimental granulomatous lung inflammation and stimulated the expression of TNF, Th1-related cytokines, and immunoregulatory IL10 by lung BAL cells from sarcoidosis patients, effects mediated in part through TLR-2. We hypothesized that the pathobiology of sarcoidosis is caused by the induction, misfolding, and progressive aggregation of insoluble SAA within granulomas in an amyloid-like process (Fig. 55-3). Tissue SAA and its released peptides then promote the subsequent feed-forward amplification of local Th1 responses to pathogenic antigens at sites of granulomatous inflammation to promote slowly progressive chronic inflammation centered around insoluble SAA as a nidus for granuloma formation.

CLINICAL FEATURES

The clinical features of sarcoidosis are discussed in detail below.

CLASSIFICATION

The clinical manifestations and course of sarcoidosis vary greatly (Table 55-2). Although any organ of the body can be affected, the lungs or intrathoracic lymph nodes are involved in more than 90% of patients with sarcoidosis. Patients may manifest with no symptoms or develop acute, subacute, or indolent manifestations. Systemic constitutional symptoms such as fever, fatigue, malaise, and weight loss are seen in over 50% of patients and may be disabling. One classification scheme with prognostic information categorizes patients based on their initial manifestations as follows: asymptomatic, acute sarcoidosis with or without erythema nodosum, sarcoidosis with symptoms or signs of pulmonary disease for less than 2 years, chronic pulmonary sarcoidosis of more than 2 years, and dominant extrapulmonary sarcoidosis. Two years represent an arbitrary but useful reference point for distinguishing patients who usually, but not always, have long-term disease.

Rare manifestations of sarcoidosis include unusual patterns of organ involvement, the result of granulomatous inflammation developing in unusual locations for sarcoidosis, or when sarcoidosis is associated with a second disorder (Table 55-2). In general, rarer manifestations reflect the known pathophysiology and clinical behavior of more common organ involvement.

ASYMPTOMATIC SARCOIDOSIS

Up to two-thirds of patients are asymptomatic but have sarcoidosis diagnosed after an incidental radiographic finding of bilateral hilar adenopathy. Occasionally, interstitial infiltrates are seen in association with intrathoracic adenopathy in asymptomatic patients, most commonly in Whites.

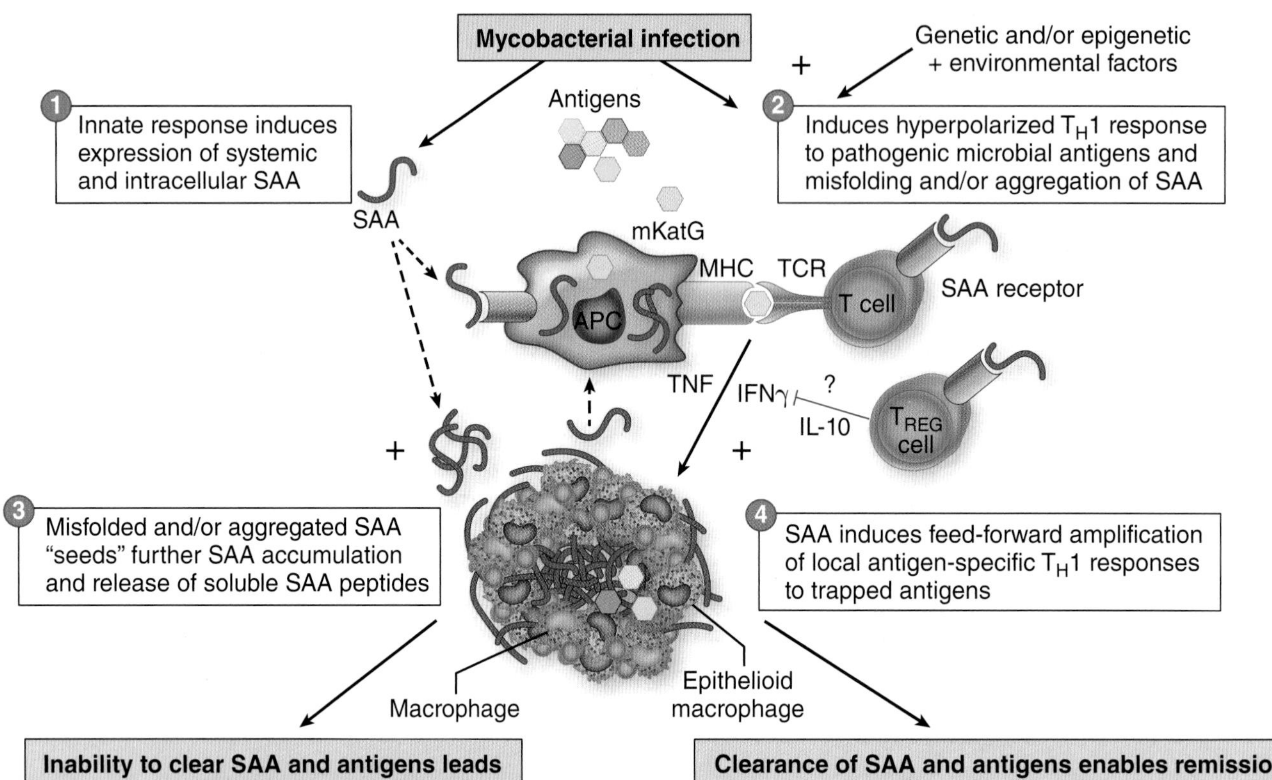

Figure 55-3 Serum Amyloid A dysaggregation as a disease-defining pathway for chronic sarcoidosis. In this scenario, misfolded amyloid-like SAA aggregates serve as "seed" that provides a poorly soluble nidus and a template for further SAA aggregation within sarcoidosis granulomas. SAA and SAA peptides released from the granulomas stoke a feed-forward stimulation of macrophages and T cells that amplifies polarized Th1 responses to local pathogenic antigens with production of TNF, Th1 promoting cytokines and IL10 (which partially dampens the inflammatory response). These effects are mediated in part through TLR2. Persistent tissue antigens may derive from degradation-resistant pathogenic microbial antigens such as mKatG, new antigens trapped by the granuloma matrix and cells or from induction of autoimmune responses. This pathobiologic course continues unabated unless there is clearance of SAA and local pathogenic antigens with downregulation of Th1 responses. Although the model depicts mycobacterial organisms as inciting agents, nonmycobacterial microbes or environmental agents could trigger a similar pathobiologic outcome. *(Reproduced with permission from Chen ES, Moller DR. Sarcoidosis–scientific progress and clinical challenges. Nat Rev Rheumatol. 2011;7(8):457–467.)*

■ ACUTE SARCOIDOSIS WITH OR WITHOUT ERYTHEMA NODOSUM

Sarcoidosis may manifest with the acute onset of erythema nodosum associated with bilateral hilar adenopathy, fevers, polyarthritis, and often uveitis, known as Löfgren syndrome. Erythema nodosum is characterized by tender reddish nodules several centimeters in diameter, usually located on the lower extremities; histologic examination shows panniculitis, not granulomas. The polyarthritis is often severe and incapacitating, typically involving the ankles, feet, knees, and occasionally, wrists, and elbows. Approximately 10% of patients with this syndrome have a normal chest radiograph. Löfgren syndrome is more common in European and White populations, but found in less than 5% of Blacks with sarcoidosis. Some patients manifest acute arthritis, bilateral hilar lymphadenopathy, and constitutional symptoms without erythema nodosum. In either case, the prognosis is excellent for remission in 70% to 80% of patients, typically within several months.

■ PULMONARY SARCOIDOSIS

Respiratory symptoms occur in 40% to 60% of patients.[99] The most common symptoms are cough and shortness of breath, usually of a progressive, insidious nature. The cough is usually nonproductive and may be severe. Dyspnea is typically worse with exertion. Sputum production and hemoptysis are frequent in patients with fibrocystic sarcoidosis that is often associated with bronchiectasis. Ill-defined chest pain is a frequent complaint, possibly caused by nerve irritation from inflammation, scarring, or lymph node enlargement in the chest. Chest tightness and wheezing are common with endobronchial disease or fibrocystic changes. These symptoms are usually poorly responsive to bronchodilators, except in those with reversible airway hyperreactivity. Physical findings are infrequent, with lung crackles heard in less than 20% of patients; clubbing is rare.

Chest Imaging

The chest radiograph is abnormal in more than 90% of known cases and carries prognostic information. Chest radiographs are categorized by international convention: stage 0 (<15%) denotes a normal chest X-ray; stage I (30% to 50%) shows symmetric bilateral hilar adenopathy often with right paratracheal adenopathy; stage II (40% to 60%) and stage III (10% to 20%) indicate the presence of pulmonary infiltrates with (stage II) or without (stage III) bilateral hilar adenopathy; stage IV (<15%) shows obvious scarring with fibrocystic changes with cephalad hilar retraction (Fig. 55-4). The hilar adenopathy often has a symmetric "potato node" appearance and calcifications are uncommon. Infiltrates most commonly appear as linear or reticulonodular markings in the middle and upper lung fields, but occasionally can present with patchy, focal alveolar consolidations mimicking infectious pneumonia, granulomatosis with polyangiitis (GPA), eosinophilic pneumonia, or malignancy. Less frequently, a miliary pattern is observed but would warrant exclusion

TABLE 55-2 Clinical Manifestations of Sarcoidosis

Organ System (Percent Clinical Disease)	Major/Uncommon Manifestations
Pulmonary (>90%)	Restrictive, obstructive impairment, reduced diffusing capacity, fibrocystic disease, bronchiectasis/ pulmonary vasculitis, mycetomas, cavitating nodules, lobar atelectasis, tracheal or bronchial stenosis, superior vena cavae syndrome, pleural disease, pneumothorax
Constitutional symptoms (>50%)	Fevers, night sweats, malaise, excessive fatigue, unintentional weight loss
Upper respiratory tract and oral cavity (5–10%)	Hoarseness, laryngeal or tracheal obstruction, nasal congestion, sinusitis/saddle nose deformity, respiratory failure from upper airway obstruction, sleep apnea
Ocular (20–30%)	Anterior and posterior uveitis, chorioretinitis, conjunctivitis, optic neuritis/granulomatous orbital inflammation
Skin (20–30%)	Erythema nodosum, chronic nodules and plaques, lupus pernio, alopecia/subcutaneous sarcoidosis, ichthyosis, alopecia, scar granulomas
Hepatic/Abdominal (10–20%)	Hepatosplenomegaly, jaundice, cirrhosis, abdominal/retroperitoneal lymphadenopathy/massive hepatomegaly, jaundice with pruritus, cirrhosis with portal hypertension, massive splenomegaly, pancreatic mass, gastric involvement, small or large intestine involvement, appendicitis
Cardiac (5–20%)	Arrhythmias, heart block, cardiomyopathy, sudden death/valvular disease, pericardial disease, ventricular or atrial mass
Neurologic (5–10%)	Facial and other cranial neuropathies (e.g., Bell palsy) aseptic meningitis brain mass, seizures, obstructing hydrocephalus, hypothalamic hypopituitarism, myelopathy, polyneuropathy, peripheral neuropathies, small fiber neuropathy/optic chiasmal involvement, cerebritis (white matter involvement), cerebral vascular occlusion, encephalitis, corpus callosum involvement, hydrocephalus, Horner syndrome, Argyll Robertson or Adie pupil, cerebellar involvement, pseudotumor cerebrei, brain stem involvement, transverse myelitis, intraspinal mass, cauda equina or spinal root involvement, mononeuritis multiplex
Exocrine gland (10–20%)	Salivary, lacrimal, and parotid gland enlargement, sicca syndrome/Heerfordt syndrome, hypopituitarism, diabetes insipidus, thyroid mass, thyroiditis, parotid mass, dacryoadenitis, sicca syndrome
Hematologic (20–30%)	Peripheral or retroperitoneal lymphadenopathy, splenomegaly, hypersplenism, anemia, lymphopenia/ hypogammaglobulinemia, lymphedema, idiopathic thrombocytopenic purpura (ITP)
Joints and musculoskeletal (10–20%)	Polyarthritis, Achilles tendinitis, heel pain, polydactylitis, bone cysts, myopathy/polymyositis, bone cysts—long bones, skull, vertebrae
Endocrine (10–30%)	Hypercalciuria, hypercalcemia, hypopituitarism, diabetes insipidus
Renal (<5–10%)	Renal calculi, nephrocalcinosis, renal failure
Genitourinary (<5%)	Ovarian or uterine mass, dysmenorrhea, testicular mass, epididymitis/uterine mass, ovarian involvement, menometrorrhagia, testicular mass, epididymitis, intermittent azoospermia
Psychosocial manifestations (30–60%)	Depression, pain, fatigue

of tuberculosis, hypersensitivity pneumonitis, chronic beryllium disease, or lymphangitic carcinomatosis. While stage IV sarcoidosis is associated with a poor prognosis, the recent ACCESS study affirms the weak correlation between stages I, II, or III chest radiographs and clinical status.[12,100] Unusual radiographic signs of sarcoidosis include pneumothorax, mycetoma, isolated nodule or mass, lobar atelectasis, or pleural effusions.

Chest computed tomography (CT) typically demonstrates that infiltrates tend to be central, following bronchovascular structures. Ground-glass infiltrates or honeycombing can also be seen. The adenopathy of sarcoidosis typically appears as multiple discrete enlarged lymph nodes rather than amorphous, mass-like growths more suggestive of malignancy. CT of the chest is often useful in the evaluation of patients with suspected sarcoidosis and to help plan bronchoscopic biopsy of enlarged lymph nodes, define unusual radiographic features, fibrocystic disease, or bronchiectasis.

Pulmonary Function Tests

Pulmonary function may be normal even when the chest radiograph demonstrates pulmonary infiltrates. However, restrictive impairment with reduction in lung volumes, forced vital capacity (FVC) and forced expiratory volume in 1 second (FEV_1), is common, particularly when pulmonary infiltrates are present on chest radiograph. Reduction in diffusing capacity can be seen in association with restrictive impairment or as an isolated deficit. Obstructive impairment is as common as restrictive impairment, particularly in advanced fibrocystic disease or endobronchial disease. A subgroup of patients have bronchial hyperresponsiveness and airway obstruction that may respond to bronchodilators. Resting hypoxemia and exercise O_2 desaturation are typical when there is severe obstructive or restrictive impairment. CO_2 retention is unusual except in advanced pulmonary disease.

Pulmonary Hypertension

Pulmonary hypertension represents an important complicating factor of pulmonary sarcoidosis because it is associated with increased mortality. In patients with end-stage pulmonary sarcoidosis awaiting lung transplantation, pulmonary hypertension is associated with a fivefold increased rate of mortality.[101,102] Overall, ~6% of patients with sarcoidosis have pulmonary hypertension, but is seen in over 70% of patients with advanced lung disease. In patients with dyspnea disproportionate to pulmonary function impairment, pulmonary hypertension may be seen in 50% of cases.[103] The causes of pulmonary hypertension include extensive interstitial lung disease with loss of pulmonary capillary bed, granulomatous pulmonary vasculitis, pulmonary arterial impingement by lymphadenopathy or traction lung scarring of bronchovascular bundles, left heart dysfunction, or rarely, pulmonary venous occlusion.[104] Patients typically present with progressive dyspnea. Echocardiography is a useful screening technique, but right heart catheterization is needed to confirm clinically significant pulmonary hypertension.

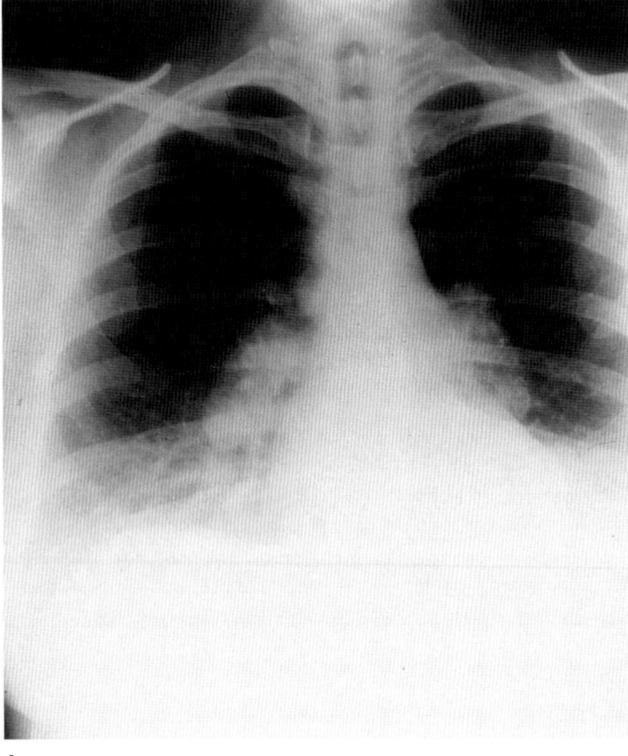

A

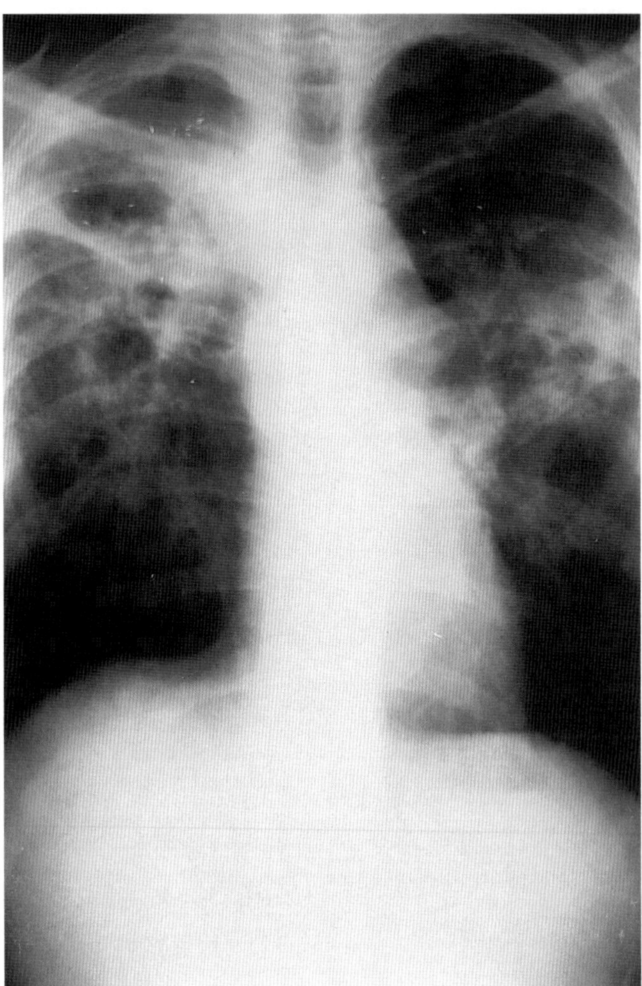

B

Figure 55-4 Chest radiographs of pulmonary sarcoidosis. **A.** Stage II sarcoidosis pattern with prominent, discrete "stand-away" hilar nodes, right paratracheal adenopathy, and fine reticulonodular infiltrates. **B.** Fibrocystic sarcoidosis with extensive scarring, bullous and cystic changes, hilar retraction, and parenchymal infiltrates.

Necrotizing Sarcoid Granulomatosis

This disorder is characterized by large, confluent, noncaseating granulomas involving both pulmonary arteries and veins but without systemic vasculitis, and is often considered a variant of pulmonary sarcoidosis.[105] Patients may be asymptomatic or have cough, dyspnea, fever, chest pain, or constitutional symptoms. Chest radiographs typically demonstrate multiple, usually noncavitating, nodules. Pleural disease with pleurisy or pleural effusions occurs in the majority of patients and may be a clue to the diagnosis. Most patients have spontaneous improvement or a rapid response to corticosteroid therapy.

EXTRAPULMONARY SARCOIDOSIS

Many patients have manifestations of granulomatous inflammation in one or more organ systems either in addition to pulmonary involvement or without evidence of pulmonary disease (Table 55-1). The presence of these characteristic extrapulmonary manifestations may help distinguish sarcoidosis from other systemic diseases. Defining clinically significant organ involvement remains a challenge despite improved imaging techniques.

Sarcoidosis of the Upper Respiratory Tract and Oral Cavity

Sarcoidosis of the upper respiratory tract (SURT) occurs in 5% to 10% of patients, usually involving the nasal sinuses or laryngeal structures. Symptoms of nasal congestion, sinusitis, and intermittent epistaxis are often chronic and unresponsive to decongestants or topical corticosteroids. Chronic disease or surgical intervention may result in destruction of the nasal septum and a "saddle nose" deformity. Laryngeal sarcoidosis may manifest with severe hoarseness, stridor, or acute respiratory failure secondary to upper airway obstruction. Frequently, laryngeal sarcoidosis is associated with chronic skin lesions, lupus pernio, or sinus disease. Oral and pharyngeal sarcoidosis is rare, but may manifest with macroglossia, tongue mass, or palatal mass with cartilaginous or bone destruction.

Ocular Sarcoidosis

Ocular involvement is detected in approximately 20% to 30% of patients, more frequently in Black populations.[1] Uveitis is the most common manifestation and is often associated with bilateral hilar adenopathy. The uveitis is more commonly anterior, and may be unilateral or bilateral, with either granulomatous or nongranulomatous features. Granulomatous conjunctivitis is less common. Optic neuritis, or severe chorioretinitis, may present dramatically with blindness. The International Workshop on Ocular Sarcoidosis (2006) has proposed seven clinical signs of ocular inflammation consistent with sarcoidosis including mutton-fat keratic precipitates, nodules in the iris, stroma, or trabecular meshwork, optic disk, and periphlebitis.[106]

Cardiac Sarcoidosis

Although myocardial sarcoidosis is clinically apparent in less than 10% of cases in the United States at initial diagnosis, autopsy studies

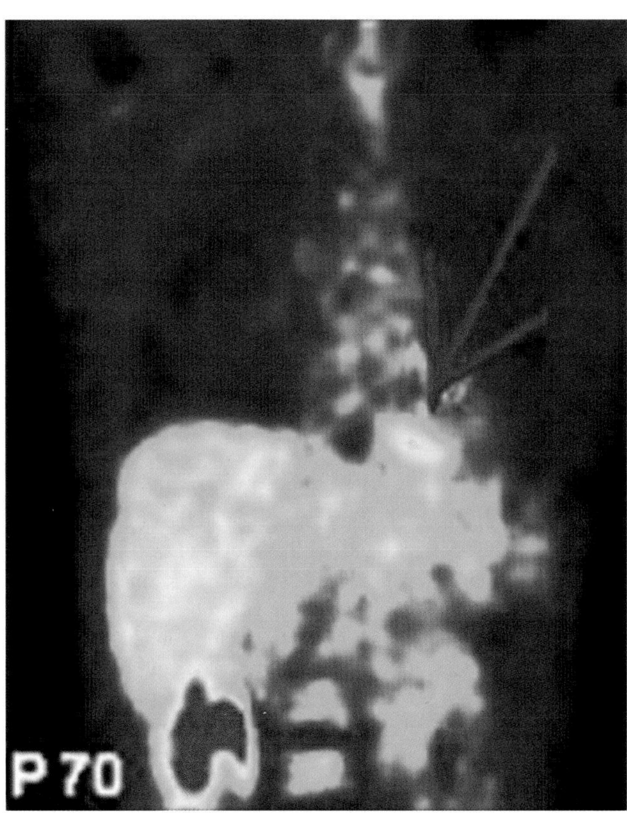

A

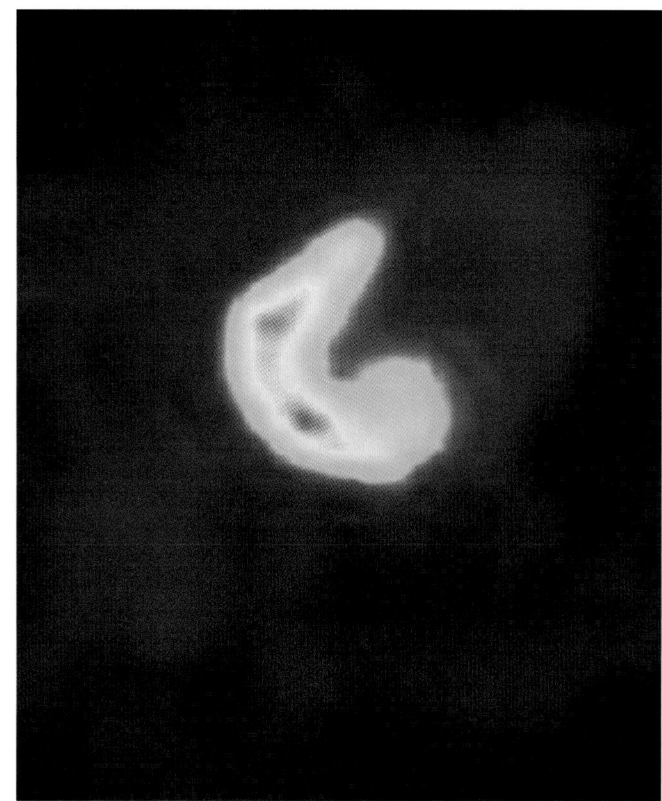

B

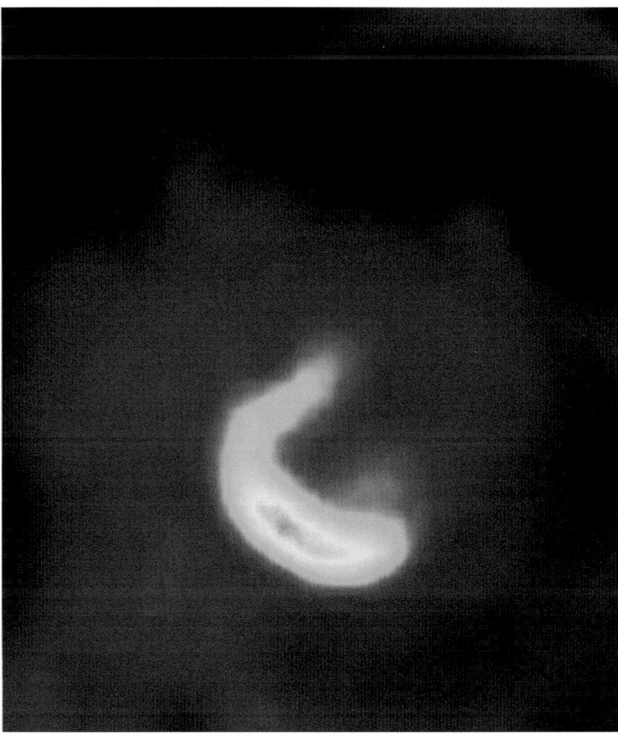

C

Figure 55-5 **A, B.** ^{18}F-Fluorodeoxyglucose (FDG)-PET scanning shows ^{18}F-FDG uptake in the inferior myocardium *(red arrow)*. **C.** ^{18}F-FDG uptake level is reduced by more than 50% after 1 month of corticosteroid therapy. *(Images used with permission of Jens Sorensen, MD of Uppsala University, Sweden.)*

suggest the prevalence may be greater than 20% in the United States and greater than 50% in Japan.[107,108] Arrhythmias, heart block, or sudden death may be the initial manifestation due to involvement of the conduction system. Myocardial inflammation can lead to dilated cardiomyopathy and congestive heart failure, local akinesia, or aneurysms. Myocardial mass, valvular dysfunction from papillary muscle dysfunction, pericarditis, and myocardial ischemia are rarer manifestations.[109] Radiographic scanning using thallium or technetium sestamibi myocardial scanning, cardiac MRI or cardiac PET reveal myocardial inflammation in a distribution not defined by normal coronary vascular anatomy (Fig. 55-5). The severity of pulmonary involvement does not appear to predict the presence or severity of cardiac sarcoidosis.

Neurosarcoidosis

Neurologic manifestations of sarcoidosis are varied and are estimated to occur in 10% to 20% of patients with sarcoidosis.[110] Cranial neuropathies, with unilateral or bilateral seventh nerve (Bell) palsy being the

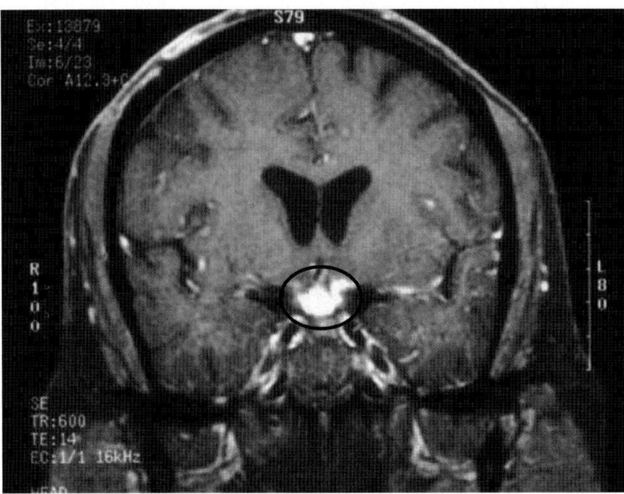

Figure 55-6 Sarcoidosis involving the optic chiasm *(circle)* resulting in blindness.

most common, often resolve spontaneously or with corticosteroids but may recur years later. Optic neuropathy may result in sudden blindness (Fig. 55-6). Impingement of the recurrent laryngeal nerve may cause vocal cord dysfunction. The more typical presentations of sarcoidosis in the brain include a basilar meningitis or aseptic encephalitis, sometimes associated with hypothalamic pituitary dysfunction leading to diabetes insipidus, hypogonadism, or hyperprolactinemia. Meningeal granulomatous masses may mimic meningioma. Spinal cord involvement is rare and can present as a transverse myelitis or mass-like lesion resulting in paraparesis, hemiparesis, back and leg pains mimicking radiculopathy. Peripheral neuropathies account for about 20% of cases of neurosarcoidosis, typically presenting as mononeuritis multiplex or a predominant sensory deficit. The presence of a small fiber neuropathy has been demonstrated in a subset of patients with sarcoidosis and can contribute to chronic pain, excessive fatigue, and autonomic dysfunction.[111]

Cutaneous Sarcoidosis

Chronic skin sarcoidosis is seen in approximately 25% of patients, usually manifesting as plaques or subcutaneous nodules and is more common and severe in Blacks. Typically, the plaques are located around the hairline, eyelids, ears, nose, and extensor surfaces of the arms and legs. Lupus pernio is a disfiguring form of cutaneous sarcoidosis of the face, with violaceous plaques and nodules covering the nose, nasal alae, malar areas, and areas around the eyes. Erythema nodosum is a nongranulomatous panniculitis seen in acute sarcoidosis.

Hepatic Sarcoidosis

Liver biopsies show granulomatous inflammation in over 50% of patients, but clinical manifestations are much less frequent. Active hepatic inflammation may be associated with fever, tender hepatomegaly, or pruritus that may mimic primary biliary cirrhosis except that autoimmune serologies are negative. Characteristically, the serum alkaline phosphatase and γ-glutamyltransferase are elevated proportionately higher than the transaminases or bilirubin, although the latter may be observed with advancing liver dysfunction. Progressive cirrhosis occurs in a subset of patients if not treated.

Gastrointestinal Sarcoidosis

Sarcoidosis involvement of the gastrointestinal tract is rare. Occasionally, direct esophageal involvement may cause dysphagia, but more commonly this symptom may be caused by extensive mediastinal lymphadenopathy that impinges esophageal motility. Gastric sarcoidosis may manifest as dyspepsia, abdominal pain, or gastric nodule. Although autopsy studies show scattered granulomas in the gut, clinically symptomatic intestinal sarcoidosis is rare.

Abdominal Sarcoidosis

A variant of sarcoidosis, often called abdominal sarcoidosis, manifests with liver, spleen, and often bone marrow involvement with hypercalcemia or abdominal lymphadenopathy. Constitutional symptoms are frequent with fevers and fatigue. This "triad" pattern may be seen with or without pulmonary involvement; in the latter instance, intra-abdominal malignancy must be excluded.

Hematologic Sarcoidosis

Persistent, bulky, painful, or disfiguring adenopathy is seen in <10% of patients, most commonly involving the cervical, supraclavicular, axillary, or epitrochlear lymph nodes. Splenomegaly occurs in <10% of patients, and may be massive and associated with hypersplenism. Because many of the clinical features of sarcoidosis and lymphoma are similar, clinicians should employ heightened awareness to exclude malignancy in patients with a known diagnosis of sarcoidosis who experience new onset of adenopathy and splenomegaly.[112]

Peripheral blood lymphopenia is common in sarcoidosis.[113] Granulomas in the bone marrow are found in about 20% of patients who come to autopsy but usually do not cause symptoms. A known feature of sarcoidosis is the impaired cutaneous response to common antigens that elicit delayed-type hypersensitivity reactions, seen in >30% of patients. The mechanism is unknown but may be related to alterations in regulatory T-cell function.

Joint and Musculoskeletal Sarcoidosis

Arthralgias are a frequent complaint in sarcoidosis. A short-lived polyarthritis is typical of acute sarcoidosis, usually associated with erythema nodosum. Chronic joint disease is found in less than 5% of patients. Joint cartilaginous erosion is rare, but "punched out" bony lesions with cystic changes and loss of bony trabeculae may be seen in subchondral locations. Cystic lesions of the long bones, pelvis, sternum, skull, and vertebrae are uncommon. Symptomatic myopathy with marked elevation of serum creatinine phosphokinase, aldolase, aspartate aminotransferase, weakness and tenderness is uncommon. Typically, the myositis from sarcoidosis is responsive to systemic immunosuppression, and recalcitrant cases prompt consideration of alternative diagnosis such as inclusion body myositis.[114]

Exocrine Gland Sarcoidosis

Granulomatous inflammation of salivary, parotid, and lacrimal glands results in enlarged, tender glands, and/or sicca syndrome with dry mouth and dry eyes in less than 5% of patients with sarcoidosis. The association of fever, parotid enlargement, facial palsy, and uveitis is known as uveoparotid fever, or Heerfordt syndrome, and is usually accompanied by bilateral hilar adenopathy.

Endocrine Sarcoidosis

Abnormal calcium metabolism is found in sarcoidosis; hypercalciuria is more frequent than hypercalcemia. These abnormalities are due primarily to increased conversion of 25(OH) vitamin D metabolites to active 1,25$(OH)_2$ vitamin D by tissue macrophages and epithelioid cells at sites of granulomatous inflammation.[115] Hypothalamic/pituitary insufficiency may be a manifestation of neurosarcoidosis.

Renal Sarcoidosis

Kidney stones are the most frequent manifestation of renal sarcoidosis, usually related to abnormal calcium metabolism. Renal failure due to nephrocalcinosis may result from chronic, often asymptomatic hypercalcemia or hypercalciuria. Granulomatous involvement of the kidneys occurs but is rarely the cause of significant renal dysfunction.

Genitourinary Sarcoidosis

Sarcoidosis of the reproductive system has been estimated to occur in less than 1% of clinically diagnosed cases and in 5% of autopsy cases. Genitourinary manifestations of sarcoidosis in men include testicular masses and acute epididymitis-orchiditis. In women, sarcoidosis may manifest with uterine or ovarian involvement that may cause dysmenorrhea or mimic malignancy or fibroids.

Psychosocial Manifestations

A Dutch study found the prevalence of depression was 4% in asymptomatic patients and 30% in symptomatic patients with sarcoidosis while the prevalence of depression was found to be 60% in a US study of both White and Black patients with sarcoidosis.[116,117] In this latter study, depression was associated with the female sex, lower socioeconomic status, poor access to care, and increased disease severity, but not race.

Fatigue is commonly reported and may be disabling for a subset of patients.[118] The prevalence of pain in sarcoidosis is unclear, but clinical experience suggests it is common with frequent reports of arthralgias, myalgias, headache, and chest pain. The cause of pain is often multifactorial with causes ranging from direct granulomatous inflammation of bones, joints, muscles, or peripheral nerves to small fiber neuropathy. A subset of patients meets diagnostic criteria for fibromyalgia. In addition to its association with pain, small fiber neuropathy may cause autonomic dysfunction with gastrointestinal dysmotility, incontinence or retention, sicca syndrome, flushing, sweats, orthostatic hypotension, and sexual dysfunction.[119]

■ ASSOCIATED CONDITIONS

Important selected conditions associated with sarcoidosis are discussed briefly below.

Sarcoidosis and Pregnancy

There is usually little long-term effect on the course of sarcoidosis from pregnancy. In contrast to diseases such as asthma and systemic lupus that may progress during pregnancy, spontaneous improvement in chronic sarcoidosis has been reported in some patients during pregnancy, although exacerbations often follow several months after delivery. The reasons for the temporary clinical improvement are not known but might be related to suppressed Th1 immunity during pregnancy associated with enhanced Treg function.

Altered Th1 Immunity

Sarcoidosis is associated with several clinically disparate situations associated with altered, enhanced Th1 immunity. The clearest example involves the administration of Th1-promoting therapeutics such as IFNα, IFNγ, IL2, and IFNβ that may be associated with initiation or recrudescence of sarcoidosis.

Common Variable Immunodeficiency Granulomatous inflammation has been identified in several immunodeficiency states, particularly in patients with hypogammaglobulinemia secondary to common variable immunodeficiency (CVID). Within subsets of patients with CVID, case series reports suggest that a diagnosis of concurrent sarcoidosis can be inferred by a compatible history of systemic illness and confirmed by biopsy.[120] In other CVID patients who present with dominant pulmonary manifestations, a recently described CVID-associated granulomatous-lymphocytic interstitial lung disease may be present and is often resistant to treatment.[121] Since CVID occurs at any age, a high index of suspicion must be maintained, particularly in sarcoidosis patients who have recurrent infections or in any child with sarcoidosis given the low frequency of sarcoidosis in this age group.

Human Immunodeficiency Virus Sarcoidosis may develop in HIV-infected patients with immune reconstitution following initiation of highly active antiretroviral therapy, perhaps from reconstituted Th1 immunity.[122] Granulomatous inflammation of the lungs or skin is most often reported.

Autoimmune Disorders Sarcoidosis is associated with a variety of disorders of the immune system, such as Crohn's disease, ulcerative colitis, primary biliary cirrhosis, scleroderma, Sjögren syndrome, autoimmune hemolytic anemia, and autoimmune endocrinopathies.[123] Given the rarity of some of these disorders, it is reasonable to postulate that these associations are the result of a common immune disturbance, with altered Th1 immunity that may predispose to both disorders.

Recently, a syndrome of immune-mediated disorders in patients with elevated serum IgG4 levels has been described, commonly presenting as adenopathy, constitutional symptoms, and mass-like tumors.[124] Granulomatous inflammation is observed in a subset of such patients and can mimic sarcoidosis.[125,126]

Cancer Noncaseating granulomas may be seen in or nearby 3% to 10% of tumors and in approximately 4% of regional draining lymph nodes. Less commonly, multi-system granulomas consistent with systemic sarcoidosis develop in patients with a recent or past diagnosis of cancer or following chemotherapy treatment. Often the diagnosis is established by biopsy of enlarged lymph nodes or lung where the presurgical diagnosis is recurrent malignancy. There is usually little functional lung impairment from pulmonary sarcoidosis in these instances, and treatment is often unnecessary with eventual remission. A possible link involves dysregulated Th1/Th2 immunity, a premise supported by several cases of sarcoidosis developing in patients with changes that result in deletion of several Th2 genes (IL4, IL13, CSF2).[127]

Pediatric Sarcoidosis

Sarcoidosis is rare in the preteen ages. In the teenage years, clinical manifestations and prognosis in children is similar to that of adults.[128] Early onset disease in children under 5 years of age typically involves skin, eye, and joint involvement that can mimic juvenile rheumatoid arthritis or Blau syndrome, an autosomal dominant granulomatous disease caused by a NOD2 mutation.[129] This form of sarcoidosis carries a much worse prognosis than disease presenting in older children.[130,131] Pediatric sarcoidosis may also be associated with CVID.

Sarcoidosis in the Elderly

There is a second peak incidence of sarcoidosis between 50 and 65 years. In the ACCESS study, one-third of patients were over the age of 50.[132] Recurrent sarcoidosis after many years, even decades of apparent remission, is also seen, often manifesting with new onset neurologic involvement, or recurrent manifestations of original organ involvement.

DIAGNOSTIC APPROACH

There is no reliable, noninvasive screening test to help confirm a diagnosis of sarcoidosis. A diagnosis of sarcoidosis is based on compatible clinical and radiologic manifestations together with a tissue biopsy demonstrating noncaseating granulomatous inflammation and exclusion of other granulomatous disorders. Exceptions to this approach include patients who manifest with Löfgren syndrome in areas with a low prevalence of histoplasmosis, which may mimic Löfgren syndrome, in which case most experts believe a biopsy is not necessary.[133] Many experts suggest that patients with asymptomatic bilateral hilar adenopathy with presumptive stage I sarcoidosis do not need biopsy unless atypical features are present, given a low pretest probability for alternative diagnoses and the risks for potential complications of a diagnostic biopsy.[134,135] Clinical involvement of more than one organ system helps exclude local granulomatous reactions to foreign bodies, infection, or malignancy.

In general, the easiest accessible biopsy site can be approached to confirm a diagnosis of sarcoidosis. Biopsy of a skin or conjunctival nodule, enlarged superficial lymph node, or lacrimal gland may help to establish a diagnosis. Noncaseating granulomas on a liver or bone marrow biopsy are nonspecific and support a diagnosis only when competing diagnoses such as infection, drug reaction, or malignancy are excluded.[136]

When a more easily accessible site is not available, biopsy by fiberoptic bronchoscopy remains the most common approach because of its high yield and relative safety. The diagnostic yield of transbronchial biopsy (TBB) is estimated to be >40% even in patients with a stage I chest radiograph and approaches 80% in the presence of lung infiltrates.[137] Transbronchial lung biopsy in advanced fibrocystic sarcoidosis has a low yield, owing to extensive fibrotic changes. Sampling by endobronchial mucosal biopsy (EMB) and transbronchial needle aspiration (TBNA) of thoracic lymph nodes provides additional sensitivity when combined with TBB.[137] The sensitivity of endoscopic bronchial ultrasound (EBUS)-guided TNBA has been found to be superior to standard TBNA in diagnosis of sarcoidosis, but in cases of suspected lymphoma, mediastinoscopy may be needed for histologic diagnosis.[138]

Bronchoalveolar lavage obtained as part of a diagnostic bronchoscopy remains an important method for excluding infectious causes of granulomatous inflammation. Some studies suggest a CD4:CD8 ratio >3.5 of BAL T cells supports a diagnosis of sarcoidosis, but may not differentiate some infectious or noninfectious inflammatory lung diseases.

A diagnosis of cardiac sarcoidosis is usually established by a noncardiac biopsy confirming systemic sarcoidosis along with consistent myocardial imaging studies or rhythm disturbances (Fig. 55-5). Endomyocardial biopsy is positive in <20% of cardiac sarcoidosis owing to sampling inefficiencies and the infrequency of right ventricular involvement; thus a negative biopsy never excludes cardiac sarcoidosis.[139]

A diagnosis of neurosarcoidosis is usually confirmed by biopsy of a non-CNS site. Rarely, brain biopsy is needed to exclude infectious or malignant disease.

For organs that are rarely involved in sarcoidosis, directed biopsy of the involved tissue is often recommended to exclude alternative causes, even when there is documentation of a prior biopsy that confirmed an original diagnosis of sarcoidosis. For organs that are difficult to biopsy, ^{18}F-fluorodeoxyglucose-positron emission tomography (FDG-PET) scanning, or contrast enhanced MRI scanning have replaced gallium^{67} scans in helping define sites of clinically occult inflammation that could provide an alternative biopsy approach.[140]

Laboratory tests are generally not helpful in confirming a diagnosis of sarcoidosis but may assist in establishing an alternative diagnosis, such as autoimmune disease. A diagnostic biomarker has not been identified for sarcoidosis. Serum ACE (SACE) levels are elevated in 30% to 80% of patients with clinically active disease from activated epithelioid cells and macrophages at sites of inflammation, but can be also seen in infectious granulomatous diseases, lymphoma, primary biliary cirrhosis, and thyroid disease and lack specificity for use as a diagnostic tool.[141]

CLINICAL ASSESSMENT

Once a diagnosis is established or suspected, an initial evaluation should consist of tests to evaluate the presence and extent of pulmonary involvement and assess the presence and severity of extrathoracic disease (Table 55-3).

Specialized testing is indicated when symptoms or signs suggest extrapulmonary sarcoidosis. Guidelines for when and how to screen for potential cardiac involvement remain uncertain.[142] Given the risk for sudden death, screening for cardiac sarcoidosis is recommended whenever symptoms such palpitations, near-syncope, or syncope are present.[143] A second-level screening may include a Holter monitor, signal-averaged ECG, and echocardiogram to detect conduction abnormalities, heart rate variability, or myocardial dysfunction. Advanced cardiac imaging with cardiac MRI with gadolinium enhancement or cardiac PET scanning is recommended for those patients with continued uncertainty of possible cardiac sarcoidosis.[144] Unexplained dyspnea or chest pain may also be suggestive for sarcoidosis but may also prompt investigations for other etiologies such as pulmonary hypertension. Thallium or technicium sestamibi myocardial scanning is useful to exclude coronary artery disease and may detect patchy fixed or reverse ischemia–perfusion defects consistent with myocardial inflammation or fibrosis.[145] Electrophysiologic testing may be indicated to exclude arrhythmias not detected by routine studies and assess indications for prophylactic cardiac pacemaker or implantable defibrillator to reduce the risk of sudden death. There is no consensus on risk stratification of patients with known cardiac sarcoidosis for placement of an implantable defibrillator, but is typically recommended for patients with moderate or severe cardiomyopathy or serious ventricular arrhythmias.[109,146]

Evaluation for possible CNS and spinal sarcoidosis should include MRI with gadolinium enhancement, now considered the optimal test to detect characteristic inflammatory lesions[147]. The distribution of inflammatory loci has a propensity for periventricular and leptomeningeal areas, although the images are nonspecific, and can be produced by infectious, malignant, or occasionally demyelinating disease. A normal scan does not exclude neurosarcoidosis, particularly for cranial neuropathies or in the presence of corticosteroid therapy. Examination of the cerebrospinal fluid is less often performed today, but may be useful by demonstrating characteristic lymphocytic pleocytosis and/or elevated protein levels. In suspected cases of peripheral neuropathy or myopathy, EMG or nerve conduction studies or rarely, tissue biopsy, may help to establish a link to sarcoidosis. Specialized evaluation including skin biopsy analysis of intraepidermal nerve fiber density may be considered to confirm cases of small fiber neuropathy.[148]

TABLE 55-3 Recommended Tests in the Clinical Evaluation of Systemic Sarcoidosis

All Patients	Organ-Specific Testing for Suspected Involvement
Chest radiograph or chest CT	Cardiac: Echocardiogram, Holter monitoring, thallium or sestamibi myocardial scan, cardiac MR, cardiac PET
Pulmonary function tests: Spirometry, diffusion capacity, lung volumes	Neurologic: Brain or spine MRI with gadolinium enhancement, cerebrospinal fluid examination, nerve conduction studies, small fiber nerve analysis
Ophthalmologic examination	Upper respiratory tract: Flow–volume loop, ENT evaluation
Complete metabolic panel	Endocrine: Pituitary function tests; thyroid function tests
Complete blood count with differential count	
Electrocardiogram	
Purified protein derivative (PPD) skin test	

CLINICAL COURSE AND PROGNOSIS

A clinical framework can be constructed to assist in decisions regarding monitoring and planning treatment strategies. First, organ involvement usually defines itself early in the disease. For example, only 23% of patients in the ACCESS study were found to have one or more new organ systems involved with sarcoidosis during a 2-year follow-up evaluation; the presence of extrapulmonary involvement at presentation was a risk factor for new organ development.[100] Second, patients who undergo remission usually do so within the first 2 to 3 years. Clinical experience suggests sarcoidosis rarely recurs after a prolonged period of remission, with exceptions most often involving neurologic or ocular manifestations. Third, patients with chronic sarcoidosis generally have progressive, unremitting organ impairment. High rates of relapse are observed in patients (>50%) requiring systemic immunosuppressive medications compared with those who experience spontaneous disease remission (<10%).[149–151] In these patients, the rate of progression varies from individual to individual, as does their response to treatment. A waxing–waning clinical course is uncommon except for a subset of patients with neurologic or ocular manifestations or occasionally recurrent erythema nodosum. Fourth, prognosis in sarcoidosis is strongly influenced by the initial manifestations of disease. Patients with Löfgren syndrome have remission rates of 70% to 80%. An initial stage I chest radiograph is associated with a 60% to 90% remission rate. Patients manifesting with type II chest radiographs have a poorer outcome, with spontaneous remission occurring 40% to 70% of the time. A stage III chest radiograph is associated with remission in only 10% to 20% of patients. Patients with extensive pulmonary fibrosis (stage IV) rarely undergo remission.

Currently, a consensus recommendation is that treatment decisions are best based on repeated clinical examinations and direct measurement of organ function and not on laboratory markers of disease "activity."[152] SACE levels tend to correlate with the extent of granulomatous inflammation throughout the body particularly when interpreted in the context of known polymorphisms of ACE alleles and usually decrease in response to corticosteroids or with disease remission, but the test is highly variable, correlates poorly with functional assessments of disease activity and has no prognostic value.[153] Similarly, BAL parameters such as the proportion of CD4 lymphocytosis or the CD4:CD8 ratio of BAL T cells have been inconsistent in predicting outcomes. Many inflammatory molecules have been proposed as helpful biomarkers for disease activity including sIL2R, TNF, and neopterin but are not reliable prognostic indicators. More recently, studies suggest transcriptomic signatures may be useful for prognosis, but there are no currently validated markers useful for clinical purposes.[154] Monitoring for at least 3 years following presumed "disease remission" is recommended; longer periods of observation are indicated for patients with serious pulmonary or extrapulmonary manifestations.

TREATMENT

A variety of approaches have been utilized in the treatment of sarcoidosis and are outlined in this section.

INDICATIONS

There have been attempts to provide evidence-based recommendations for treatment of sarcoidosis, but the lack of placebo-controlled clinical trials in this highly heterogeneous disease have made firm conclusions problematic. Most physicians agree that corticosteroid or other systemic therapy is indicated for the manifestations listed in Table 55-4.

Indications for treatment must take into account the overall excellent prognosis for most patients with sarcoidosis, particularly for patients with stage I disease, for whom systemic therapy is usually not required. Symptomatic or local therapy is recommended whenever possible. Löfgren syndrome is usually managed with bed rest and nonsteroidal anti-inflammatory drugs; corticosteroids are recommended when symptoms, particularly arthritis, are disabling and persistent. The following consensus recommendations from the British Thoracic Society and the Thoracic Societies of Australia, New Zealand, and Ireland are shown in Table 55-5.[155]

TABLE 55-4 Indications for Treatment of Sarcoidosis

Threatened organ failure—severe ocular, cardiac, or neurologic disease
Progressive or persistent pulmonary disease
Uveitis unresponsive to topical corticosteroids
Persistent hypercalcemia, renal or hepatic dysfunction
Palpable splenomegaly or hypersplenism
Severe myopathy
Disfiguring skin disease
Painful lymphadenopathy
Severe fatigue and weight loss

SYSTEMIC TREATMENT

There are no FDA-approved systemic therapies for sarcoidosis.

CORTICOSTEROID THERAPY

Corticosteroids remain the cornerstone of therapy for sarcoidosis. Although controversy exists regarding the overall effectiveness of corticosteroids in altering the long-term course of the disease, there is no disagreement that corticosteroids provide prompt symptomatic relief and reverse organ dysfunction in most patients with the degree of reversibility dependent on the extent of pre-existing fibrosis. Case series and several but not all clinical trials support the view that corticosteroids favorably affect disease outcome in chronic pulmonary sarcoidosis. One large study by the British Thoracic Society

TABLE 55-5 Consensus Approach to Treatment of Sarcoidosis

1. Treatment is not indicated for asymptomatic patient with only intrathoracic lymphadenopathy
2. Treatment is not indicated in asymptomatic patient with pulmonary infiltrates and mildly abnormal lung function and stable disease
3. Oral corticosteroids are the first line of therapy in patients with progressive disease determined by radiology or lung function, significant symptoms or extrapulmonary disease requiring treatment
4. Treatment with prednisone (or equivalent) 20–40 mg/d initially for 4 wk, then reduced to a maintenance dose that will control symptoms and disease progression for a period of 6–24 mo
5. Bisphosphonates are recommended to minimize steroid-induced osteoporosis
6. Inhaled corticosteroids are not of significant benefit as initial treatment or for maintenance therapy. Inhaled corticosteroids may be considered for symptom control (cough) or bronchial hyperreactivity in a subgroup of patients
7. Steroid-sparing immunosuppressive or anti-inflammatory treatments only have an undefined role in sarcoidosis, but should be considered in patients when corticosteroids are not controlling the disease or side effects are intolerable. At present, methotrexate is the treatment of choice if there are no relative contraindications for its use. Azathioprine is often used when methotrexate is contraindicated or not tolerated
8. Lung (and heart) transplantation should be considered in end-stage pulmonary and cardiac sarcoidosis

Source: Data from Bradley B, Branley HM, Egan JJ, et al. Interstitial lung disease guideline: the British Thoracic Society in collaboration with the Thoracic Society of Australia and New Zealand and the Irish Thoracic Society. Thorax. 2008;63(Suppl 5):v1–v58.

found long-term improved lung function in patients with stage II or III pulmonary disease treated with daily corticosteroid therapy compared with a group treated intermittently with corticosteroids based on symptoms.[149]

Optimal dosing of corticosteroid therapy has not been established by clinical trials. Most authorities suggest that initial treatment of pulmonary sarcoidosis usually does not require more than 20 to 40 mg per day of prednisone followed by a slow taper to a maintenance dose of 5 to 15 mg per day of prednisone. A qod regimen of prednisone in patients may be effective in some but not all patients. Treatment is usually continued for a minimum of 6 to 24 months, since premature attempts to taper off steroids are likely to result in relapse of disease. Inhaled steroids appear to have limited effectiveness in chronic pulmonary sarcoidosis and are not recommended as sole therapy. Overall, recurrent progressive pulmonary disease occurs in more than 20% of patients as oral corticosteroids are tapered or discontinued.

■ ALTERNATIVE AGENTS

Several classes of drugs have been reported to be beneficial in subgroups of patients with sarcoidosis but none of these drugs has been proved effective by rigorous clinical trials.

Nonimmunosuppressive Drugs

Case series suggest hydroxychloroquine is effective in many patients with mucocutaneous sarcoidosis, hypercalcemia and occasionally, as a steroid-sparing agent in systemic sarcoidosis. Ocular toxicity is rare, and its overall safety profile provides a rationale for an early trial of this drug. Chloroquine may be efficacious in treating lupus pernio, SURT, or sinus disease, which is often recalcitrant to other therapies, although ocular toxicity has limited its use.

The tetracyclines, minocycline, and doxycycline, may be effective in a subgroup of patients with mild cutaneous sarcoidosis but rarely as a steroid-sparing drug in systemic disease. These antibiotics have mild anti-inflammatory effects, which probably account for their mechanism of action given that other antibiotics with similar antimicrobial activity have not been found effective in sarcoidosis.

Pentoxifylline is a phosphodiesterase inhibitor with anti-inflammatory effects that was found to be effective in early pulmonary sarcoidosis in one study.[156] Other experiences have not been as favorable with responses in less than 10% of patients, generally those with mild pulmonary or systemic sarcoidosis.

Melatonin was found to be beneficial in a small case series of patients with generally mild disease but wider experience has not confirmed its efficacy.

Thalidomide was found in one study to be beneficial in over 80% of patients with severe skin sarcoidosis (lupus pernio unresponsive to other therapies), but was not effective in pulmonary sarcoidosis.[157] Given the drug's well-known teratogenicity and potential to cause peripheral neuropathy and sedation, the drug is recommended only in patients refractory to other treatments.

Immunosuppressive Drugs

Clinical experience in sarcoidosis suggests that all immunosuppressive therapies share the following characteristics: beneficial responses are seen in no more than 50% to 70% of patients; responses may take 3 to 6 months or longer; low-dose corticosteroid therapy is often needed for synergistic effect to obtain adequate suppression of granulomatous inflammation. Dosing and monitoring for these therapies should follow the recommendations of the American College of Rheumatology.[158]

Methotrexate is often the first immunosuppressive therapy used as an alternative therapy for refractory pulmonary or systemic sarcoidosis when corticosteroid and antimalarial therapies are ineffective or poorly tolerated. Hepatic, pulmonary, and renal toxicities limit the use of the drug. Azathioprine has shown benefit in small clinical trials and is used by some authorities as an initial potent steroid-sparing therapy. Clear advantages of methotrexate or azathioprine over low-dose corticosteroids in the routine management of sarcoidosis have not been established. Other immunosuppressive agents, such as mycophenylate mofetil, leflunomide, or cyclophosphamide, have been found beneficial in a small series of patients with manifestations of sarcoidosis refractory to corticosteroids.

Small studies have shown that cyclosporine and FK506, drugs known to inhibit T-cell activation, are not effective in pulmonary or ocular sarcoidosis or in suppressing recurrent sarcoidosis in transplants. Given their toxicities, consensus is to avoid these medications until new studies demonstrate potential benefits.

Anti-TNF Therapies

The scientific basis for the use of TNF inhibitors in sarcoidosis is firmly established based on the role of TNF in experimental models of granuloma formation. One multicenter study found infliximab to be effective in one of several primary end points (improved FVC after 24 weeks of therapy), although the effect was modest.[159] Etanercept was not shown to be effective in a smaller clinical trial of pulmonary sarcoidosis.[160] Anecdotal cases suggest adalimumab may be effective in some patients with sarcoidosis, although larger studies are lacking. Given the risk profiles of current immunosuppressive drugs, additional clinical trials of these agents are warranted but most authorities reserve these therapies after failure of one or more immunosuppressive drugs.

■ SPECIAL CIRCUMSTANCES

Several special considerations in the management of systemic sarcoidosis warrant particular mention.

Fibrocystic Sarcoidosis

Advanced pulmonary sarcoidosis may be complicated by mycetomas, usually from *Aspergillus fumigatus* that colonize pre-existing cystic spaces. The fungi rarely cause invasive disease. Spontaneous resolution may be seen. The benefit of antifungal agents has not been established but may be used for serious hemoptysis. Massive hemoptysis associated with mycetomas or bronchiectasis may be life-threatening, requiring therapeutic embolization of the appropriate bronchial or collateral artery for control. Surgery is usually not feasible because of the severe restrictive lung disease.

Pulmonary Hypertension

Moderate or severe pulmonary hypertension is an independent predictor of reduced survival in patients with advanced lung disease awaiting lung transplantation. Studies suggest drugs used to treat primary pulmonary hypertension may improve dyspnea and pulmonary hypertension but no study has yet demonstrated survival benefit.[161–163] Further studies are underway to determine the role of these therapies in sarcoidosis.

Cardiac Sarcoidosis

Several large case series find prognosis in cardiac sarcoidosis, and response to treatment is related to the degree of cardiac dysfunction. Treatment of cardiac sarcoidosis consists of antiarrhythmic therapy, diuretics, and afterload-reducing agents for specific cardiac abnormalities. Although randomized trials are lacking, studies from Asia, Europe, and the United States consistently report that corticosteroids in moderate doses are associated with improved cardiac function and outcomes.[164,165] Maintenance doses often range between prednisone 10 to 25 mg a day, although higher doses may be needed for intractable arrhythmias. Immunosuppressive drugs are frequently used as steroid-sparing agents since treatment often must be maintained for years. Automatic implantable cardioverter-defibrillators (ICDs) may prevent sudden death in patients with serious arrhythmias; guidelines for prophylactic placement of ICDs or pacemakers have not yet been established.

Neurosarcoidosis and Ocular Sarcoidosis

High doses of oral corticosteroids or high-dose pulse intravenous therapy are often indicated for serious ocular or CNS disease, such as optic neuritis or encephalitis followed by maintenance corticosteroid or immunosuppressive therapy. Anterior uveitis can usually be treated with topical ophthalmologic steroid drops. Systemic immunosuppression may be necessary in cases of severe or recurrent disease, but aggressive treatment of neurosarcoidosis is generally associated with favorable outcomes.[166] Small fiber neuropathy typically does not reliably respond to corticosteroid therapy, prompting trials of neuropathic drugs, TNF-inhibitors or other novel agents.[167,168]

Pregnancy

Corticosteroids are the only drugs recommended for use during pregnancy because of the potential of other steroid-sparing drugs to cause fetal toxicity or teratogenicity. Sometimes, spontaneous abatement of chronic sarcoidosis occurs in pregnant patients, allowing a temporary reduction in steroid dosage. After pregnancy, however, an exacerbation often occurs, requiring a return to the original maintenance dose.

Quality of Life

There is increasing recognition of the need to treat depression and pain to improve quality of life in patients with these manifestations. The utility of nonpharmacologic treatments, such as exercise training or rehabilitation, merits investigation because of the impact of these problems in sarcoidosis patients.

Lung and Heart Transplantation

Successful lung, heart–lung, and heart transplantations have been performed in patients with advanced pulmonary sarcoidosis or cardiomyopathy. Although noncaseating granulomas have been found in some transplanted lungs or hearts, these findings do not appear to significantly affect outcome. Outcomes for lung transplant in sarcoidosis are similar to other interstitial lung diseases.[169–171]

REFERENCES

1. Statement on sarcoidosis. Joint Statement of the American Thoracic Society (ATS), the European Respiratory Society (ERS) and the World Association of Sarcoidosis and Other Granulomatous Disorders (WASOG) adopted by the ATS Board of Directors and by the ERS Executive Committee, February 1999. *Am J Respir Crit Care Med.* 1999;160(2):736–755.
2. Rybicki BA, Iannuzzi MC. Epidemiology of sarcoidosis: recent advances and future prospects. *Semin Respir Crit Care Med.* 2007; 28(1):22–35.
3. Hoffmann AL, Milman N, Byg KE. Childhood sarcoidosis in Denmark 1979–1994: incidence, clinical features and laboratory results at presentation in 48 children. *Acta Paediatr.* 2004; 93(1):30–36.
4. Rybicki BA, Major M, Popovich J Jr, Maliarik MJ, Iannuzzi MC. Racial differences in sarcoidosis incidence: a 5-year study in a health maintenance organization. *Am J Epidemiol.* 1997; 145(3):234–241.
5. Reid JD. Sarcoidosis in coroner's autopsies: a critical evaluation of diagnosis and prevalence from Cuyahoga County, Ohio. *Sarcoidosis Vasc Diffuse Lung Dis.* 1998;15(1):44–51.
6. Erdal BS, Clymer BD, Yildiz VO, Julian MW, Crouser ED. Unexpectedly high prevalence of sarcoidosis in a representative U.S. Metropolitan population. *Respir Med.* 2012;106(6):893–899.
7. Morimoto T, Azuma A, Abe S, et al. Epidemiology of sarcoidosis in Japan. *Eur Respir J.* 2008;31(2):372–379.
8. Edmondstone WM, Wilson AG. Sarcoidosis in Caucasians, Blacks and Asians in London. *Br J Dis Chest.* 1985;79(1):27–36.
9. Rabin DL, Thompson B, Brown KM, et al. Sarcoidosis: social predictors of severity at presentation. *Eur Respir J.* 2004;24(4): 601–608.
10. Swigris JJ, Olson AL, Huie TJ, et al. Sarcoidosis-related mortality in the United States from 1988 to 2007. *Am J Respir Crit Care Med.* 2011;183(11):1524–1530.
11. Reich JM. Mortality of intrathoracic sarcoidosis in referral vs population-based settings: influence of stage, ethnicity, and corticosteroid therapy. *Chest.* 2002;121(1):32–39.
12. Nardi A, Brillet PY, Letoumelin P, et al. Stage IV sarcoidosis: comparison of survival with the general population and causes of death. *Eur Respir J.* 2011;38(6):1368–1373.
13. Wilsher ML. Seasonal clustering of sarcoidosis presenting with erythema nodosum. *Eur Respir J.* 1998;12(5):1197–1199.
14. Kern DG, Neill MA, Wrenn DS, Varone JC. Investigation of a unique time-space cluster of sarcoidosis in firefighters. *Am Rev Respir Dis.* 1993;148(4 Pt 1):974–980.
15. Maier LA, McGrath DS, Sato H, et al. Influence of MHC class II in susceptibility to beryllium sensitization and chronic beryllium disease. *J Immunol.* 2003;171(12):6910–6918.
16. Ribeiro M, Fritscher LG, Al-Musaed AM, et al. Search for chronic beryllium disease among sarcoidosis patients in Ontario, Canada. *Lung.* 2011;189(3):233–241.
17. Crowley LE, Herbert R, Moline JM, et al. "Sarcoid like" granulomatous pulmonary disease in World Trade Center disaster responders. *Am J Ind Med.* 2011;54(3):175–184.
18. Izbicki G, Chavko R, Banauch GI, et al. World Trade Center "sarcoid-like" granulomatous pulmonary disease in New York City Fire Department rescue workers. *Chest.* 2007;131(5): 1414–1423.
19. Newman LS, Rose CS, Bresnitz EA, et al. A case control etiologic study of sarcoidosis: environmental and occupational risk factors. *Am J Respir Crit Care Med.* 2004;170(12):1324–1330.
20. Barnard J, Rose C, Newman L, et al. Job and industry classifications associated with sarcoidosis in A Case-Control Etiologic Study of Sarcoidosis (ACCESS). *J Occup Environ Med.* 2005; 47(3):226–234.
21. Gupta D, Agarwal R, Aggarwal AN, Jindal SK. Molecular evidence for the role of mycobacteria in sarcoidosis: a meta-analysis. *Eur Respir J.* 2007;30(3):508–516.
22. Teirstein AS. Kveim antigen: what does it tell us about causation of sarcoidosis? *Semin Respir Infect.* 1998;13(3): 206–211.
23. Song Z, Marzilli L, Greenlee BM, et al. Mycobacterial catalase-peroxidase is a tissue antigen and target of the adaptive immune response in systemic sarcoidosis. *J Exp Med.* 2005; 201(5):755–767.
24. Chen ES, Wahlstrom J, Song Z, et al. T cell responses to mycobacterial catalase-peroxidase profile a pathogenic antigen in systemic sarcoidosis. *J Immunol.* 2008;181(12):8784–8796.
25. Drake WP, Dhason MS, Nadaf M, et al. Cellular recognition of *Mycobacterium tuberculosis* ESAT-6 and KatG peptides in systemic sarcoidosis. *Infect Immun.* 2007;75(1):527–530.
26. Dubaniewicz A, Trzonkowski P, Dubaniewicz-Wybieralska M, Singh M, Mysliwski A. Mycobacterial heat shock

protein-induced blood T lymphocytes subsets and cytokine pattern: comparison of sarcoidosis with tuberculosis and healthy controls. *Respirology.* 2007;12(3):346–354.

27. Koth LL, Solberg OD, Peng JC, Bhakta NR, Nguyen CP, Woodruff PG. Sarcoidosis blood transcriptome reflects lung inflammation and overlaps with tuberculosis. *Am J Respir Crit Care Med.* 2011;184(10):1153–1163.
28. Thillai M, Eberhardt C, Lewin AM, et al. Sarcoidosis and tuberculosis cytokine profiles: indistinguishable in bronchoalveolar lavage but different in blood. *PLoS One.* 2012;7(7):e38083.
29. Maertzdorf J, Weiner J 3rd, Mollenkopf HJ, et al. Common patterns and disease-related signatures in tuberculosis and sarcoidosis. *Proc Natl Acad Sci U S A.* 2012;109(20):7853–7858.
30. Eishi Y, Suga M, Ishige I, et al. Quantitative analysis of mycobacterial and propionibacterial DNA in lymph nodes of Japanese and European patients with sarcoidosis. *J Clin Microbiol.* 2002;40(1):198–204.
31. Nishiwaki T, Yoneyama H, Eishi Y, et al. Indigenous pulmonary Propionibacterium acnes primes the host in the development of sarcoid-like pulmonary granulomatosis in mice. *Am J Pathol.* 2004;165(2):631–639.
32. McCaskill JG, Chason KD, Hua X, et al. Pulmonary immune responses to Propionibacterium acnes in C57 BL/6 and BALB/c mice. *Am J Respir Cell Mol Biol.* 2006;35(3):347–356.
33. Brown ST, Brett I, Almenoff PL, Lesser M, Terrin M, Teirstein AS. Recovery of cell wall-deficient organisms from blood does not distinguish between patients with sarcoidosis and control subjects. *Chest.* 2003;123(2):413–417.
34. Wahlstrom J, Dengjel J, Winqvist O, et al. Autoimmune T cell responses to antigenic peptides presented by bronchoalveolar lavage cell HLA-DR molecules in sarcoidosis. *Clin Immunol.* 2009;133(3):353–363.
35. Rybicki BA, Iannuzzi MC, Frederick MM, et al. Familial aggregation of sarcoidosis. A case-control etiologic study of sarcoidosis (ACCESS). *Am J Respir Crit Care Med.* 2001;164(11):2085–2091.
36. Gardner J, Kennedy HG, Hamblin A, Jones E. HLA associations in sarcoidosis: a study of two ethnic groups. *Thorax.* 1984;39(1):19–22.
37. Hedfors E, Lindstrom F. HLA-B8/DR3 in sarcoidosis. Correlation to acute onset disease with arthritis. *Tissue Antigens.* 1983;22(3):200–203.
38. Grunewald J, Eklund A, Olerup O. Human leukocyte antigen class I alleles and the disease course in sarcoidosis patients. *Am J Respir Crit Care Med.* 2004;169(6):696–702.
39. Rossman MD, Thompson B, Frederick M, et al. HLA-DRB1*1101: a significant risk factor for sarcoidosis in blacks and whites. *Am J Hum Genet.* 2003;73(4):720–735.
40. Sato H, Grutters JC, Pantelidis P, et al. HLA-DQB1*0201: a marker for good prognosis in British and Dutch patients with sarcoidosis. *Am J Respir Cell Mol Biol.* 2002;27(4):406–412.
41. Berlin M, Fogdell-Hahn A, Olerup O, Eklund A, Grunewald J. HLA-DR predicts the prognosis in Scandinavian patients with pulmonary sarcoidosis. *Am J Respir Crit Care Med.* 1997;156(5):1601–1605.
42. Voorter CE, Drent M, van den Berg-Loonen EM. Severe pulmonary sarcoidosis is strongly associated with the haplotype HLA-DQB1*0602-DRB1*150101. *Hum Immunol.* 2005;66(7):826–835.
43. Voorter CE, Amicosante M, Berretta F, Groeneveld L, Drent M, van den Berg-Loonen EM. HLA class II amino acid epitopes as susceptibility markers of sarcoidosis. *Tissue Antigens.* 2007;70(1):18–27.
44. Muller-Quernheim J, Schurmann M, Hofmann S, et al. Genetics of sarcoidosis. *Clin Chest Med.* 2008;29(3):391–414, viii.
45. Medica I, Kastrin A, Maver A, Peterlin B. Role of genetic polymorphisms in ACE and TNF-alpha gene in sarcoidosis: a meta-analysis. *J Hum Genet.* 2007;52(10):836–847.
46. Valentonyte R, Hampe J, Huse K, et al. Sarcoidosis is associated with a truncating splice site mutation in BTNL2. *Nat Genet.* 2005;37(4):357–364.
47. Rybicki BA, Walewski JL, Maliarik MJ, Kian H, Iannuzzi MC. The BTNL2 gene and sarcoidosis susceptibility in African Americans and Whites. *Am J Hum Genet.* 2005;77(3):491–499.
48. Morais A, Lima B, Peixoto MJ, Alves H, Marques A, Delgado L. BTNL2 gene polymorphism associations with susceptibility and phenotype expression in sarcoidosis. *Respir Med.* 2012;106(12):1771–1777.
49. Wijnen PA, Voorter CE, Nelemans PJ, Verschakelen JA, Bekers O, Drent M. Butyrophilin-like 2 in pulmonary sarcoidosis: a factor for susceptibility and progression? *Hum Immunol.* 2011;72(4):342–347.
50. Hofmann S, Fischer A, Till A, et al. A genome-wide association study reveals evidence of association with sarcoidosis at 6p12.1. *Eur Respir J.* 2011;38(5):1127–1135.
51. Fischer A, Schmid B, Ellinghaus D, et al. A novel sarcoidosis risk locus for Europeans on chromosome 11q13.1. *Am J Respir Crit Care Med.* 2012;186(9):877–885.
52. Hofmann S, Franke A, Fischer A, et al. Genome-wide association study identifies ANXA11 as a new susceptibility locus for sarcoidosis. *Nat Genet.* 2008;40(9):1103–1106.
53. Franke A, Fischer A, Nothnagel M, et al. Genome-wide association analysis in sarcoidosis and Crohn's disease unravels a common susceptibility locus on 10p12.2. *Gastroenterology.* 2008;135(4):1207–1215.
54. Fischer A, Nothnagel M, Franke A, et al. Association of inflammatory bowel disease risk loci with sarcoidosis, and its acute and chronic subphenotypes. *Eur Respir J.* 2011;37(3):610–616.
55. Harrington LE, Hatton RD, Mangan PR, et al. Interleukin 17-producing CD4+ effector T cells develop via a lineage distinct from the T helper type 1 and 2 lineages. *Nat Immunol.* 2005;6(11):1123–1132.
56. Zissel G, Homolka J, Schlaak J, Schlaak M, Muller-Quernheim J. Anti-inflammatory cytokine release by alveolar macrophages in pulmonary sarcoidosis. *Am J Respir Crit Care Med.* 1996;154(3 Pt 1):713–719.
57. Bingisser R, Speich R, Zollinger A, Russi E, Frei K. Interleukin-10 secretion by alveolar macrophages and monocytes in sarcoidosis. *Respiration.* 2000;67(3):280–286.
58. Zissel G, Prasse A, Muller-Quernheim J. Immunologic response of sarcoidosis. *Semin Respir Crit Care Med.* 2010;31(4):390–403.
59. Mathew S, Bauer KL, Fischoeder A, Bhardwaj N, Oliver SJ. The anergic state in sarcoidosis is associated with diminished dendritic cell function. *J Immunol.* 2008;181(1):746–755.
60. Ten Berge B, Kleinjan A, Muskens F, et al. Evidence for local dendritic cell activation in pulmonary sarcoidosis. *Respir Res.* 2012;13:33.
61. Zaba LC, Smith GP, Sanchez M, Prystowsky SD. Dendritic cells in the pathogenesis of sarcoidosis. *Am J Respir Cell Mol Biol.* 2010;42(1):32–39.

62. Ziegenhagen MW, Benner UK, Zissel G, Zabel P, Schlaak M, Muller-Quernheim J. Sarcoidosis: TNF-alpha release from alveolar macrophages and serum level of sIL-2R are prognostic markers. *Am J Respir Crit Care Med.* 1997;156(5):1586–1592.
63. Drent M, van den Berg R, Haenen GR, van den Berg H, Wouters EF, Bast A. NF-kappaB activation in sarcoidosis. *Sarcoidosis Vasc Diffuse Lung Dis.* 2001;18(1):50–56.
64. Culver DA, Barna BP, Raychaudhuri B, et al. Peroxisome proliferator-activated receptor gamma activity is deficient in alveolar macrophages in pulmonary sarcoidosis. *Am J Respir Cell Mol Biol.* 2004;30(1):1–5.
65. Moller DR. T-cell receptor genes in sarcoidosis. *Sarcoidosis Vasc Diffuse Lung Dis.* 1998;15(2):158–164.
66. Klein JT, Horn TD, Forman JD, Silver RF, Teirstein AS, Moller DR. Selection of oligoclonal V beta-specific T cells in the intradermal response to Kveim-Siltzbach reagent in individuals with sarcoidosis. *J Immunol.* 1995;154(3):1450–1460.
67. Grunewald J, Wahlstrom J, Berlin M, Wigzell H, Eklund A, Olerup O. Lung restricted T cell receptor AV2 S3+ CD4+ T cell expansions in sarcoidosis patients with a shared HLA-DRbeta chain conformation. *Thorax.* 2002;57(4):348–352.
68. Moller DR, Forman JD, Liu MC, et al. Enhanced expression of IL-12 associated with Th1 cytokine profiles in active pulmonary sarcoidosis. *J Immunol.* 1996;156(12):4952–4960.
69. Zissel G, Prasse A, Muller-Quernheim J. Sarcoidosis–immunopathogenetic concepts. *Semin Respir Crit Care Med.* 2007;28(1):3–14.
70. Rosenbaum JT, Pasadhika S, Crouser ED, et al. Hypothesis: sarcoidosis is a STAT1-mediated disease. *Clin Immunol.* 2009;132(2):174–183.
71. Kriegova E, Fillerova R, Tomankova T, et al. T-helper cell type-1 transcription factor T-bet is upregulated in pulmonary sarcoidosis. *Eur Respir J.* 2011;38(5):1136–1144.
72. Dagur PK, Biancotto A, Wei L, et al. MCAM-expressing CD4(+) T cells in peripheral blood secrete IL-17 A and are significantly elevated in inflammatory autoimmune diseases. *J Autoimmun.* 2011;37(4):319–327.
73. Facco M, Cabrelle A, Teramo A, et al. Sarcoidosis is a Th1/Th17 multisystem disorder. *Thorax.* 2011;66(2):144–150.
74. Ten Berge B, Paats MS, Bergen IM, et al. Increased IL-17 A expression in granulomas and in circulating memory T cells in sarcoidosis. *Rheumatology (Oxford).* 2012;51(1):37–46.
75. Wiken M, Idali F, Al Hayja MA, Grunewald J, Eklund A, Wahlstrom J. No evidence of altered alveolar macrophage polarization, but reduced expression of TLR2, in bronchoalveolar lavage cells in sarcoidosis. *Respir Res.* 2010;11:121.
76. Judson MA, Marchell RM, Mascelli M, et al. Molecular profiling and gene expression analysis in cutaneous sarcoidosis: the role of interleukin-12, interleukin-23, and the T-helper 17 pathway. *J Am Acad Dermatol.* 2012;66(6):901–910, 910 e901–e902.
77. Furusawa H, Suzuki Y, Miyazaki Y, Inase N, Eishi Y. Th1 and Th17 immune responses to viable Propionibacterium acnes in patients with sarcoidosis. *Respir Investig.* 2012;50(3):104–109.
78. Abdulahad WH, Stegeman CA, Limburg PC, Kallenberg CG. Skewed distribution of Th17 lymphocytes in patients with Wegener's granulomatosis in remission. *Arthritis Rheum.* 2008;58(7):2196–2205.
79. Khader SA, Cooper AM. IL-23 and IL-17 in tuberculosis. *Cytokine.* 2008;41(2):79–83.
80. Miyara M, Amoura Z, Parizot C, et al. The immune paradox of sarcoidosis and regulatory T cells. *J Exp Med.* 2006;203(2):359–370.
81. Taflin C, Miyara M, Nochy D, et al. FoxP3+ regulatory T cells suppress early stages of granuloma formation but have little impact on sarcoidosis lesions. *Am J Pathol.* 2009;174(2):497–508.
82. Rappl G, Pabst S, Riemann D, et al. Regulatory T cells with reduced repressor capacities are extensively amplified in pulmonary sarcoid lesions and sustain granuloma formation. *Clin Immunol.* 2011;140(1):71–83.
83. Ho LP, Urban BC, Thickett DR, Davies RJ, McMichael AJ. Deficiency of a subset of T-cells with immunoregulatory properties in sarcoidosis. *Lancet.* 2005;365(9464):1062–1072.
84. Prasse A, Zissel G, Lutzen N, et al. Inhaled vasoactive intestinal peptide exerts immunoregulatory effects in sarcoidosis. *Am J Respir Crit Care Med.* 2010;182(4):540–548.
85. Elias JA, Freundlich B, Adams S, Rosenbloom J. Regulation of human lung fibroblast collagen production by recombinant interleukin-1, tumor necrosis factor, and interferon-gamma. *Ann N Y Acad Sci.* 1990;580:233–244.
86. Chen ES, Greenlee BM, Wills-Karp M, Moller DR. Attenuation of lung inflammation and fibrosis in interferon-gamma-deficient mice after intratracheal bleomycin. *Am J Respir Cell Mol Biol.* 2001;24(5):545–555.
87. Pechkovsky DV, Prasse A, Kollert F, et al. Alternatively activated alveolar macrophages in pulmonary fibrosis-mediator production and intracellular signal transduction. *Clin Immunol.* 2010;137(1):89–101.
88. Hauber HP, Gholami D, Meyer A, Pforte A. Increased interleukin-13 expression in patients with sarcoidosis. *Thorax.* 2003;58(6):519–524.
89. Henry MT, McMahon K, Mackarel AJ, et al. Matrix metalloproteinases and tissue inhibitor of metalloproteinase-1 in sarcoidosis and IPF. *Eur Respir J.* 2002;20(5):1220–1227.
90. Salez F, Gosset P, Copin MC, Lamblin Degros C, Tonnel AB, Wallaert B. Transforming growth factor-beta1 in sarcoidosis. *Eur Respir J.* 1998;12(4):913–919.
91. Szlubowski A, Soja J, Grzanka P, et al. TGF-beta1 in bronchoalveolar lavage fluid in diffuse parenchymal lung diseases and high-resolution computed tomography score. *Pol Arch Med Wewn.* 2010;120(7–8):270–275.
92. Chen ES, Song Z, Willett MH, et al. Serum amyloid A regulates granulomatous inflammation in sarcoidosis through Toll-like receptor-2. *Am J Respir Crit Care Med.* 2010;181(4):360–373.
93. Chen ES, Moller DR. Sarcoidosis–scientific progress and clinical challenges. *Nat Rev Rheumatol.* 2011;7(8):457–467.
94. Munro CS, Mitchell DN. The K veim response: still useful, still a puzzle. *Thorax.* 1987;42(5):321–331.
95. Uhlar CM, Whitehead AS. Serum amyloid A, the major vertebrate acute-phase reactant. *Eur J Biochem.* 1999;265(2):501–523.
96. Salazar A, Mana J, Fiol C, et al. Influence of serum amyloid A on the decrease of high density lipoprotein-cholesterol in active sarcoidosis. *Atherosclerosis.* 2000;152(2):497–502.
97. Rubinstein I, Knecht A, de Beer FC, Baum GL, Pras M. Serum amyloid-A protein concentrations in sarcoidosis. *Isr J Med Sci.* 1989;25(8):461–462.
98. Ehrenfeld M, Levartowsky D. Serum amyloid-A protein and sarcoidosis. *Isr J Med Sci.* 1989;25(8):418–420.

99. Lynch JP 3rd, Ma YL, Koss MN, White ES. Pulmonary sarcoidosis. *Semin Respir Crit Care Med.* 2007;28:53–74.

100. Judson MA, Baughman RP, Thompson BW, et al. Two year prognosis of sarcoidosis: the ACCESS experience. *Sarcoidosis Vasc Diffuse Lung Dis.* 2003;20(3):204–211.

101. Shorr AF, Helman DL, Davies DB, Nathan SD. Pulmonary hypertension in advanced sarcoidosis: epidemiology and clinical characteristics. *Eur Respir J.* 2005;25(5):783–788.

102. Arcasoy SM, Christie JD, Pochettino A, et al. Characteristics and outcomes of patients with sarcoidosis listed for lung transplantation. *Chest.* 2001;120(3):873–880.

103. Baughman RP, Engel PJ, Taylor L, Lower EE. Survival in sarcoidosis-associated pulmonary hypertension: the importance of hemodynamic evaluation. *Chest.* 2010;138(5):1078–1085.

104. Nunes H, Humbert M, Capron F, et al. Pulmonary hypertension associated with sarcoidosis: mechanisms, haemodynamics and prognosis. *Thorax.* 2006;61(1):68–74.

105. Popper HH, Klemen H, Colby TV, Churg A. Necrotizing sarcoid granulomatosis–is it different from nodular sarcoidosis? *Pneumologie.* 2003;57(5):268–271.

106. Herbort CP, Rao NA, Mochizuki M. International criteria for the diagnosis of ocular sarcoidosis: results of the first International Workshop On Ocular Sarcoidosis (IWOS). *Ocul Immunol Inflamm.* 2009;17(3):160–169.

107. Lagana SM, Parwani AV, Nichols LC. Cardiac sarcoidosis: a pathology-focused review. *Arch Pathol Lab Med.* 2010;134(7):1039–1046.

108. Uemura A, Morimoto S, Hiramitsu S, Kato Y, Ito T, Hishida H. Histologic diagnostic rate of cardiac sarcoidosis: evaluation of endomyocardial biopsies. *Am Heart J.* 1999;138(2 Pt 1):299–302.

109. Roberts WC, Vowels TJ, Ko JM, Capehart JE, Hall SA. Cardiac transplantation for cardiac sarcoidosis with initial diagnosis by examination of the left ventricular apical "core" excised for insertion of a left ventricular assist device for severe chronic heart failure. *Am J Cardiol.* 2009;103(1):110–114.

110. Stern BJ, Corbett J. Neuro-ophthalmologic Manifestations of Sarcoidosis. *Curr Treat Options Neurol.* 2007;9(1):63–71.

111. Voorter CE, Drent M, Hoitsma E, Faber KG, van den Berg-Loonen EM. Association of HLA DQB1 0602 in sarcoidosis patients with small fiber neuropathy. *Sarcoidosis Vasc Diffuse Lung Dis.* 2005;22(2):129–132.

112. Papanikolaou IC, Sharma OP. The relationship between sarcoidosis and lymphoma. *Eur Respir J.* 2010;36(5):1207–1209.

113. Sweiss NJ, Salloum R, Gandhi S, et al. Significant CD4, CD8, and CD19 lymphopenia in peripheral blood of sarcoidosis patients correlates with severe disease manifestations. *PLoS One.* 2010;5(2):e9088.

114. Larue S, Maisonobe T, Benveniste O, et al. Distal muscle involvement in granulomatous myositis can mimic inclusion body myositis. *J Neurol Neurosurg Psychiatry.* 2011;82(6):674–677.

115. Sharma OP. Vitamin D and sarcoidosis. *Curr Opin Pulm Med.* 2010;16(5):487–488.

116. Chang B, Steimel J, Moller DR, et al. Depression in sarcoidosis. *Am J Respir Crit Care Med.* 2001;163(2):329–334.

117. Goracci A, Fagiolini A, Martinucci M, et al. Quality of life, anxiety and depression in sarcoidosis. *Gen Hosp Psychiatry.* 2008;30(5):441–445.

118. Drent M, Lower EE, De Vries J. Sarcoidosis-associated fatigue. *Eur Respir J.* 2012;40(1):255–263.

119. Hoitsma E, Reulen JP, de Baets M, Drent M, Spaans F, Faber CG. Small fiber neuropathy: a common and important clinical disorder. *J Neurol Sci.* 2004;227(1):119–130.

120. Fasano MB, Sullivan KE, Sarpong SB, et al. Sarcoidosis and common variable immunodeficiency. Report of 8 cases and review of the literature. *Medicine (Baltimore).* 1996;75(5):251–261.

121. Bates CA, Ellison MC, Lynch DA, Cool CD, Brown KK, Routes JM. Granulomatous-lymphocytic lung disease shortens survival in common variable immunodeficiency. *J Allergy Clin Immunol.* 2004;114(2):415–421.

122. Mirmirani P, Maurer TA, Herndier B, McGrath M, Weinstein MD, Berger TG. Sarcoidosis in a patient with AIDS: a manifestation of immune restoration syndrome. *J Am Acad Dermatol.* 1999;41(2 Pt 2):285–286.

123. Sharma OP. Sarcoidosis and other autoimmune disorders. *Curr Opin Pulm Med.* 2002;8(5):452–456.

124. Stone JH, Zen Y, Deshpande V. IgG4-related disease. *N Engl J Med.* 2012;366(6):539–551.

125. Matsui S, Taki H, Shinoda K, et al. Respiratory involvement in IgG4-related Mikulicz's disease. *Mod Rheumatol.* 2012;22(1):31–39.

126. Michel L, Clairand R, Neel A, Masseau A, Frampas E, Hamidou M. Association of IgG4-related disease and sarcoidosis. *Thorax.* 2011;66(10):920–921.

127. Airaghi L, Montori D, Zorzi F, Miadonna A, Tedeschi A. Sarcoidosis in a patient with 5q-myelodysplasia. A possible pathogenetic link between the two diseases. *Monaldi Arch Chest Dis.* 2000;55(5):378–380.

128. Milman N, Hoffmann AL. Childhood sarcoidosis: long-term follow-up. *Eur Respir J.* 2008;31(3):592–598.

129. Blau EB. Familial granulomatous arthritis, iritis, and rash. *J Pediatr.* 1985;107(5):689–693.

130. Fink CW, Cimaz R. Early onset sarcoidosis: not a benign disease. *J Rheumatol.* 1997;24(1):174–177.

131. Sarigol SS, Hay MH, Wyllie R. Sarcoidosis in preschool children with hepatic involvement mimicking juvenile rheumatoid arthritis. *J Pediatr Gastroenterol Nutr.* 1999;28(5):510–512.

132. Baughman RP, Teirstein AS, Judson MA, et al. Clinical characteristics of patients in a case control study of sarcoidosis. *Am J Respir Crit Care Med.* 2001;164(10 Pt 1):1885–1889.

133. Mana J, Gomez-Vaquero C, Montero A, et al. Lofgren's syndrome revisited: a study of 186 patients. *Am J Med.* 1999;107(3):240–245.

134. Reich JM, Brouns MC, O'Connor EA, Edwards MJ. Mediastinoscopy in patients with presumptive stage I sarcoidosis: a risk/benefit, cost/benefit analysis. *Chest.* 1998;113(1):147–153.

135. Winterbauer RH, Belic N, Moores KD. Clinical interpretation of bilateral hilar adenopathy. *Ann Intern Med.* 1973;78(1):65–71.

136. Flamm SL. Granulomatous liver disease. *Clin Liver Dis.* 2012;16(2):387–396.

137. Bilaceroglu S, Perim K, Gunel O, Cagirici U, Buyuksirin M. Combining transbronchial aspiration with endobronchial and transbronchial biopsy in sarcoidosis. *Monaldi Arch Chest Dis.* 1999;54(3):217–223.

138. Tremblay A, Stather DR, Maceachern P, Khalil M, Field SK. A randomized controlled trial of standard vs endobronchial

ultrasonography-guided transbronchial needle aspiration in patients with suspected sarcoidosis. *Chest.* 2009;136(2):340–346.

139. Ardehali H, Howard DL, Hariri A, et al. A positive endomyocardial biopsy result for sarcoid is associated with poor prognosis in patients with initially unexplained cardiomyopathy. *Am Heart J.* 2005;150(3):459–463.

140. Braun JJ, Kessler R, Constantinesco A, Imperiale A. 18 F-FDG PET/CT in sarcoidosis management: review and report of 20 cases. *Eur J Nucl Med Mol Imaging.* 2008;35(8):1537–1543.

141. Hyldgaard C, Kaae S, Riddervold M, Hoffmann HJ, Hilberg O. Value of s-ACE, BAL lymphocytosis, and CD4+/CD8 +and CD103+CD4+/CD4 +T-cell ratios in diagnosis of sarcoidosis. *Eur Respir J.* 2012;39(4):1037–1039.

142. Hamzeh NY, Wamboldt FS, Weinberger HD. Management of cardiac sarcoidosis in the United States: a Delphi study. *Chest.* 2012;141(1):154–162.

143. Mehta D, Lubitz SA, Frankel Z, et al. Cardiac involvement in patients with sarcoidosis: diagnostic and prognostic value of outpatient testing. *Chest.* 2008;133(6):1426–1435.

144. Ohira H, Tsujino I, Ishimaru S, et al. Myocardial imaging with 18 F-fluoro-2-deoxyglucose positron emission tomography and magnetic resonance imaging in sarcoidosis. *Eur J Nucl Med Mol Imaging.* 2008;35(5):933–941.

145. Haywood LJ, Sharma OP, Siegel ME, et al. Detection of myocardial sarcoidosis by thallium 201 imaging. *J Natl Med Assoc.* 1982;74(10):959–964.

146. Donsky AS, Escobar J, Capehart J, Roberts WC. Heart transplantation for undiagnosed cardiac sarcoidosis. *Am J Cardiol.* 2002;89(12):1447–1450.

147. Stern BJ, Aksamit A, Clifford D, Scott TF. Neurologic presentations of sarcoidosis. *Neurol Clin.* 2010;28(1):185–198.

148. Bakkers M, Merkies IS, Lauria G, et al. Intraepidermal nerve fiber density and its application in sarcoidosis. *Neurology.* 2009; 73(14):1142–1148.

149. Gibson GJ, Prescott RJ, Muers MF, et al. British Thoracic Society Sarcoidosis study: effects of long term corticosteroid treatment. *Thorax.* 1996;51(3):238–247.

150. Gottlieb JE, Israel HL, Steiner RM, Triolo J, Patrick H. Outcome in sarcoidosis. The relationship of relapse to corticosteroid therapy. *Chest.* 1997;111(3):623–631.

151. Takada K, Ina Y, Noda M, Sato T, Yamamoto M, Morishita M. The clinical course and prognosis of patients with severe, moderate or mild sarcoidosis. *J Clin Epidemiol.* 1993;46(4):359–366.

152. Judson MA. A proposed solution to the clinical assessment of sarcoidosis: the sarcoidosis three-dimensional assessment instrument (STAI). *Med Hypotheses.* 2007;68(5):1080–1087.

153. Turner-Warwick M, McAllister W, Lawrence R, Britten A, Haslam PL. Corticosteroid treatment in pulmonary sarcoidosis: do serial lavage lymphocyte counts, serum angiotensin converting enzyme measurements, and gallium-67 scans help management? *Thorax.* 1986;41(12):903–913.

154. Zhou T, Zhang W, Sweiss NJ, et al. Peripheral blood gene expression as a novel genomic biomarker in complicated sarcoidosis. *PLoS One.* 2012;7(9):e44818.

155. Bradley B, Branley HM, Egan JJ, et al. Interstitial lung disease guideline: the British Thoracic Society in collaboration with the Thoracic Society of Australia and New Zealand and the Irish Thoracic Society. *Thorax.* 2008;63(Suppl 5):v1–v58.

156. Park MK, Fontana Jr, Babaali H, et al. Steroid-sparing effects of pentoxifylline in pulmonary sarcoidosis. *Sarcoidosis Vasc Diffuse Lung Dis.* 2009;26(2):121–131.

157. Baughman RP, Judson MA, Teirstein AS, Moller DR, Lower EE. Thalidomide for chronic sarcoidosis. *Chest.* 2002;122(1):227–232.

158. Singh JA, Furst DE, Bharat A, et al. 2012 update of the 2008 American College of Rheumatology recommendations for the use of disease-modifying antirheumatic drugs and biologic agents in the treatment of rheumatoid arthritis. *Arthritis Care Res (Hoboken).* 2012;64(5):625–639.

159. Baughman RP, Drent M, Kavuru M, et al. Infliximab therapy in patients with chronic sarcoidosis and pulmonary involvement. *Am J Respir Crit Care Med.* 2006;174(7):795–802.

160. Utz JP, Limper AH, Kalra S, et al. Etanercept for the treatment of stage II and III progressive pulmonary sarcoidosis. *Chest.* 2003;124(1):177–185.

161. Barnett CF, Bonura EJ, Nathan SD, et al. Treatment of sarcoidosis-associated pulmonary hypertension. A two-center experience. *Chest.* 2009;135(6):1455–1461.

162. Milman N, Svendsen CB, Iversen M, Videbaek R, Carlsen J. Sarcoidosis-associated pulmonary hypertension: acute vasoresponsiveness to inhaled nitric oxide and the relation to long-term effect of sildenafil. *Clin Respir J.* 2009;3(4):207–213.

163. Judson MA, Highland KB, Kwon S, et al. Ambrisentan for sarcoidosis associated pulmonary hypertension. *Sarcoidosis Vasc Diffuse Lung Dis.* 2011;28(2):139–145.

164. Yazaki Y, Isobe M, Hiroe M, et al. Prognostic determinants of long-term survival in Japanese patients with cardiac sarcoidosis treated with prednisone. *Am J Cardiol.* 2001;88(9): 1006–1010.

165. Chiu CZ, Nakatani S, Zhang G, et al. Prevention of left ventricular remodeling by long-term corticosteroid therapy in patients with cardiac sarcoidosis. *Am J Cardiol.* 2005;95(1): 143–146.

166. Scott TF, Yandora K, Valeri A, Chieffe C, Schramke C. Aggressive therapy for neurosarcoidosis: long-term follow-up of 48 treated patients. *Arch Neurol.* 2007;64(5):691–696.

167. Hoitsma E, Faber CG, van Santen-Hoeufft M, De Vries J, Reulen JP, Drent M. Improvement of small fiber neuropathy in a sarcoidosis patient after treatment with infliximab. *Sarcoidosis Vasc Diffuse Lung Dis.* 2006;23(1):73–77.

168. Heij L, Niesters M, Swartjes M, et al. Safety and efficacy of ARA 290 in sarcoidosis patients with symptoms of small fiber neuropathy: a randomized, double-blind pilot study. *Mol Med.* 2012;18:1430–1436.

169. Shorr AF, Helman DL, Davies DB, Nathan SD. Sarcoidosis, race, and short-term outcomes following lung transplantation. *Chest.* 2004;125(3):990–996.

170. Lingaraju R, Pochettino A, Blumenthal NP, et al. Lung transplant outcomes in white and African American recipients: special focus on acute and chronic rejection. *J Heart Lung Transplant.* 2009;28(1):8–13.

171. Shlobin OA, Nathan SD. Management of end-stage sarcoidosis: pulmonary hypertension and lung transplantation. *Eur Respir J.* 2012;39(6):1520–1533.

CHAPTER 56

Idiopathic Pulmonary Fibrosis

Robert M. Tighe
Eric B. Meltzer
Paul W. Noble

OVERVIEW

In simplest terms, pulmonary fibrosis equates with the growth of "scar" in the lung. Scarred lung can assume any one of a variety of patterns; these patterns define unique pathologic phenotypes. When scar assumes a patchy distribution and appears to emanate from the pleural surface, it is recognized as the "usual" type—otherwise known as usual interstitial pneumonia (UIP). The disease in which UIP manifests without cause or trigger is called idiopathic pulmonary fibrosis (IPF). IPF is, therefore, a type of pulmonary fibrosis (also known as interstitial lung disease [ILD]). IPF is recognized by a unique compilation of clinical, radiographic, and pathologic features. IPF causes breathlessness, disability due to respiratory insufficiency and, in most instances, eventually leads to death.

While there are many causes of ILD, IPF is the most common form of ILD and certainly the most serious. IPF is characterized by an inexorable progression of interstitial pulmonary fibrosis that results in restrictive lung disease and worsening gas exchange. Death from respiratory failure is reported to ensue within 5 years of diagnosis in the majority of patients.

By definition, IPF is UIP in the absence of cause or explanation. It is equally important to remember what IPF is not. IPF is not pulmonary fibrosis from chronic aspiration, drug toxicities, environmental exposures (such as chronic hypersensitivity pneumonitis), and collagen vascular diseases, even if the pattern of fibrosis resembles UIP. Therefore, the diagnosis of IPF can only be made by excluding other possibilities. One of the major challenges in diagnosing IPF is the reasonable exclusion of other potential causes of pulmonary fibrosis. This requires a careful clinical and diagnostic evaluation; and often verges on areas of clinical uncertainty.

IPF typically comes to medical attention later in life, beginning in the sixth decade. IPF is rarely the cause of ILD in patients under the age of 40. The predominant presenting symptoms of IPF are exertional breathlessness and a dry, harassing cough. These are nonspecific complaints shared by a variety of pulmonary and cardiac diseases. In particular, exertional breathlessness is often attributed to advancing age by patients in their sixties and seventies, leading to delays in seeking medical evaluation. In addition, many patients are poorly conditioned and overweight and attribute their symptoms of breathlessness to these circumstances. In addition to nonspecific clinical symptoms, initial nonspecific radiographic findings also fail to trigger prompt medical evaluation. Fine peripheral linear radiographic opacities on plain chest radiographs, predominantly in the lower lung zones, may be interpreted as chronic and nonspecific pulmonary fibrosis, which often does not elicit an alarming response. Delay in diagnosis is therefore the norm. However, in recent years important scientific advances have improved the understanding of IPF pathogenesis; new therapeutic trials are under way and this has increased the enthusiasm for an early diagnosis of IPF.

HISTORICAL PERSPECTIVE

A brief review of the evolution in our understanding of IPF illustrates the contributions made by earlier investigators and account for much of the confusion that many clinicians have regarding IPF. One of the challenges in defining IPF has been the variety of antiquated terms formerly used to describe pulmonary fibrosis. While there are many causes of ILD in general, and pulmonary fibrosis in particular, it is important to note that IPF is a unique disease, although it had not been formally codified until recently when a group of expert pulmonologists, radiologists, and pathologists collaborated on a classification of ILD. Reviewing the history of IPF will both clarify the present terminology and distinguish contemporary nomenclature from the outmoded terms encountered in earlier literature.

Fibrosis of the lung was long recognized in association with infection or dust inhalation. In the 19th century, pulmonary fibrosis was known as "cirrhosis" of the lung. Yet little attention was paid to this form of respiratory illness.[1] Interest in pulmonary fibrosis was ignited in 1944 when Drs. Louis Hamman and Arnold Rich published a seminal paper describing "acute diffuse interstitial fibrosis of the lungs."[2] Hamman and Rich reported a series of unusual cases that shared a unique clinical presentation featuring idiopathic subacute respiratory failure followed by death. Their report was complete with pathologic findings from autopsy. They described thickening of the alveolar interstitium and areas of dense fibrotic scar tissue within the lung. This was the first pathologic depiction of pulmonary fibrosis and, to this day, is considered an accurate portrayal. In retrospect, the cases of Hamman and Rich best fit a diagnosis of the fibrosing interstitial pneumonia now known as acute interstitial pneumonitis (AIP).[3] Yet in the 1940s, the "Hamman–Rich syndrome" became synonymous with IPF. So it remained for the next three decades.

Over the years, clinical reports of pulmonary fibrosis suggested a number of alternate presentations that were referred to as "variants" of the Hamman–Rich syndrome.[4] This included cases that exhibited a rather protracted duration of illness compared to the "classic" Hamman and Rich cases. It was also noted that pulmonary fibrosis occurred in patients who suffered from the "rheumatoid group of collagen diseases." An assortment of abnormal patterns was noted under the microscope. Eventually, the breadth of the Hamman–Rich syndrome encompassed a heterogeneous mixture of clinical manifestations and a variety of histologic forms of pulmonary fibrosis with no distinction made between systemic and limited illness nor any concession to the prognostic implications of an acute versus chronic presentation.

In the 1960s authors began to regularly substitute the term "IPF" for "acute diffuse interstitial fibrosis."[5,6] A debate began concerning the chronicity of this disease, with some authors suggesting a slow course punctuated by "terminal complications,"[5] while others reported an average illness of no more than 2 years.[6]

The term "fibrosing alveolitis" was introduced in England in 1964.[7] Cryptogenic fibrosing alveolitis (CFA) became the preferred term for pulmonary fibrosis in the European literature and it is essentially synonymous with IPF. This term was originally meant to improve upon its predecessor by capturing pathologic features in a manner that was more precise and descriptive. CFA refers to the interalveolar location of the inflammation in pulmonary fibrosing as compared with the intra-alveolar inflammation of infectious pneumonia. This interalveolar septal inflammation was dubbed "alveolitis." It was maintained that alveolitis was responsible for the subsequent development of fibrosis and it was first suggested that corticosteroids be used to treat alveolitis and therefore pulmonary fibrosis.

The most important advance came in 1964 with the publication of an improved and safe technique for performing open lung biopsy.[8] With this procedure, it became possible to carry out a widespread analysis of lung tissue from patients with suspected pulmonary fibrosis. Before long there were new insights into the pathology associated with fibrotic lung disease.

In 1969 Liebow and Carrington[9] heralded the modern era of ILD histopathology with the notion that idiopathic interstitial pneumonia (IIP) could be split into separate pathologic subtypes. They described distinct patterns of IIP that were identified by examination of lung biopsy specimens with light microscopy. Moreover, these subtypes were found to predict prognosis and response to treatment. Based on their research findings, Liebow and Carrington produced the first detailed histopathologic classification of IIP. They created five categories that were termed UIP, desquamative interstitial pneumonia (DIP), bronchiolitis obliterans interstitial pneumonia (BIP), lymphocytic interstitial pneumonitis (LIP), and giant cell interstitial pneumonia (GIP). More recent observations have led to a modification of this classification of IIP subtypes.[10,11] New categories have been added, such as respiratory bronchiolitis–associated interstitial lung disease (RB-ILD) and nonspecific interstitial pneumonia (NSIP).[10,11]

Simultaneously, a revolution in thinking about the pathogenesis of IPF affected the way in which experts talked about the disease. Researchers at the National Heart, Lung, and Blood Institute (NHLBI) were major proponents of an "inflammatory theory" of pathogenesis as originally proposed by European investigators. This theory was based on studies at the NHLBI throughout the 1970s during which excessive amounts of inflammatory cells were identified in bronchoalveolar lavage (BAL) fluid obtained from IPF patients.[12] The NHLBI agreed with European researchers who had coined the term "alveolitis" and the NHLBI also endorsed corticosteroid treatments. The inflammatory theory has since fallen from favor, mostly as a consequence of corticosteroid inefficacy, and the term "alveolitis" has also fallen out of vogue.

A new hypothesis has replaced the "inflammatory theory" of IPF. This new concept proposes that IPF is the result of alveolar epithelial injury, which is then followed by aberrant repair mechanisms. This theory emerged from landmark ultrastructural studies performed in the mid-1980s.[13,14] Using electron microscopy, it was discovered that the alveolar epithelial cells were injured in IPF. In addition, foci of subepithelial fibrosis were first described. This concept of injury and repair was modified and expand on by subsequent investigators.[15]

In 1997 a modified version of Liebow's pathologic classifications were proposed.[16] The new classification scheme reinforced acceptance of certain categories within the context of an updated understanding of ILD pathogenesis. For instance DIP and UIP categories were retained in the new classification scheme. Some original categories were discarded and two modern categories were added. RB-ILD was recognized in the spectrum of smoking-related lung diseases and a provisional category, NSIP, was also added.[16,17] This modern pathologic classification became the basis for a consensus statement that finally standardized the nomenclature of ILD and IPF for the very first time.

In 2002 a panel of experts convened sponsored jointly by the American Thoracic Society and the European Respiratory Society.[18] This panel released an official statement for the purpose of providing a new and comprehensive classification of IIP that considered all clinical, radiographic, and pathologic features. The diseases recognized by the 2002 ATS/ERS classification of IIP are IPF, NSIP, cryptogenic organizing pneumonia (COP), acute interstitial pneumonia, RB-ILD, DIP, LIP. Further classification of IPF has been undertaken by joint consensus statements of the American Thoracic Society, and European Respiratory Society, in 2000 and 2010.[19,20] These statements attempt to offer strict definitions for each subtype of IIP with practical guidelines for diagnostic purposes. The benefit of attempting to utilize precise definitions is to provide a uniformity of diagnostic decisions in both clinical practice and in research.

Despite the utility of rigorously defining IIP (and IPF), there are several potential pitfalls. For instance, the current classification system relies upon an assumption that each specific IIP is a discrete clinical entity. There has never been validation of this assumption by careful phenotyping and prospective trials. In addition, these definitions are heavily reliant on surgical pathology, suggesting that pathology be considered the "gold standard"; however, evidence shows even expert pathologists can have difficulty agreeing on pathologic classification.[21] This continues to create confusion and difficulty in the diagnosis of IIPs and IPF. Hopefully continued refinement of consensus guidelines, greater expertise of clinicians and greater identification and use of genetic signatures/biomarkers will lead to more confident separation of the IIPs and a clear definition of IPF.

EPIDEMIOLOGY

Below are considered the incidence and prevalence of IPF, along with risk factors and associated familial and genetic factors.

INCIDENCE, PREVALENCE, AND VITAL STATISTICS

The epidemiology of IPF is difficult to determine and the available data are of limited value. It has been principally assessed by large population studies using death certificates and/or medical coding as the principle component for determination of disease. The main criticism of these studies is that surgical lung biopsy (SLB) was rarely performed or incorporated into the criteria used for analysis, although SLB remains the gold standard of diagnosis. In addition, many of these studies have not incorporated the up-to-date definition of the disease and use disparate methodologies to develop their assessments of the epidemiology of IPF.[22,23] The most recent update of the diagnostic criteria for IPF may help to clarify these difficulties but will also make it difficult to compare data over time. Early studies from Great Britain and from the United States suggest that IPF is widely underreported.[24,25] Though this is probably still the case heightened clinical awareness of the disease and the greater availability of high-resolution computed tomography (HRCT) appear to be changing the landscape; and this may explain recent studies that suggest an increasing incidence of the disease.[22]

The precise incidence and prevalence of IPF remains difficult to determine. However, there are several studies worth considering. Coultas et al.[26] utilized a population-based registry in which cases were determined using a combination of medical records, pathology reports, and death certificates. With this data, the prevalence/annual incidence was estimated at 20.2/10.7 cases per 100,000 males and 13.2/7.4 per 100,000 females.

Recent studies by two different groups have attempted to update and further define these estimations.[27,28] Both studies employed sensitivity analyses to examine the impact of diagnostic reliability; they examined the epidemiology of IPF using both narrow- and broad case definitions. Fernandez et al.[27] reported a prevalence of 27.9 per 100,000 people, using a narrow case definition, and 63.0 per 100,000 people using a broad case definition; similarly, annual incidence was estimated at 8.8/100,000 and 17.43/100,000 using the narrow and broad definitions respectively. Raghu et al.[28] relied on yet another North American database and reported a prevalence of 14.0 per 100,000 persons with their narrow definition and 42.7 per 100,000 persons with their broad case definition; annual incidence was reported as 6.8 and 16.3 per 100,000 persons for narrow and broad definitions respectively. It is important to point out that Fernandez et al. and Raghu et al. used different definitions of IPF in their separate studies, which likely accounts for some of the difference in the incidence and prevalence between the two studies. In European epidemiologic studies, there is even wider variation in case definition and reported incidence and prevalence; though some authors have claimed that IPF is more common in the United States than in Europe.[23]

Mortality data is equally difficult to determine, as data is scant and varies by country and race. Retrospective longitudinal studies have suggested that median survival is 2 to 3 years from time of diagnosis.[29–33] However, new information is coming from the placebo arms of recent clinical trials. This data suggests that survival time may be greater than previously expected.[34–36] As a result of this emerging data, the actual mortality of IPF therefore remains without clear definition.

RISK FACTORS

IPF remains a disease without known pathogenesis, which makes the definition of risk factors problematic. Despite this shortcoming, a few case-control observational studies have identified potential risk factors that include age, gender, smoking status, environmental exposures, gastroesophageal reflux, and viral infections. The identification of these risk factors remains just associations as research identifying causality is either ongoing or inconclusive. Despite the lack of clear causality these risk factors can help to identify patients who have higher risk of developing IPF.

Age/Gender

The incidence of IPF undoubtedly increases with age and appears to have a higher predilection for men. Patients with IPF are usually between 40 and 70 years old. Two-thirds of IPF cases present in patients over the age of 60 years, with a mean age of 66 years at the time of diagnosis.[19] IPF occurs infrequently amongst those younger than 40 years and rarely affects children, if at all. Several studies stratified the incidence and prevalence of IPF by age.[26–28,37,38] Amongst adults aged 35 to 44 years the prevalence was 2.7 cases per 100,000 persons. In contrast, the prevalence for individuals older than 75 years was greater than 175 cases per 100,000.[26] Other studies in both USA and Europe have demonstrated similar findings.[23] In addition, there appears to be a higher incidence and prevalence of IPF in males than in females with the notable exception of a study in Norway, which identified a higher incidence and prevalence in females.[37]

Smoking

Another risk factor that emerges from case-control studies is a history of cigarette smoking. The prevalence of tobacco use in patients with IPF is high, ranging from 41% to 83%.[19,39] A meta-analysis of five case-control studies demonstrated that IPF patients were significantly more likely to report a history of smoking than controls with an odds ratio of 1.58 (95% CI 1.27–1.97).[40] There may even be a dose–response relationship. Baumgartner et al.[41] reported that IPF patients with a greater than 21-pack-year smoking history had an odds ratio of 2.26 (95% CI = 1.3–2.8) compared to individuals with less than a 20-pack-year history. This finding was corroborated in a subsequent study.[42] Despite the association, a mechanistic link between smoking and IPF remains undefined.[43]

Environmental Exposures

A number of papers have implicated environmental exposures to such particulate materials as metal and wood dusts.[20] In a related finding, an increased incidence of IPF was noted in industrial centers of the southeastern United States and central regions of the United Kingdom.[44] There is also an association between farming and risk of IPF.[40] A specific association exists between exposure to livestock and the risk of developing IPF though this seems to be strongest at exposures greater than 5 years.[45] At this point these types of risk factors are only associations as the causative link to environmental exposures remains undefined.

Viral Infections

Several articles have implicated a variety of viruses such as the Epstein–Barr virus, influenza virus, cytomegalovirus, and hepatitis C.[46–48] All are found with higher incidence amongst patients with IPF. The best studies are of herpes viruses (including EBV, CMV, human herpes virus 7 and 8). Tang et al.[49] identified DNA from herpes virus in 33 patients with IPF. Herpes virus antigens have also been detected by immunohistochemistry in type II alveolar epithelial cells from IPF patients but were not seen in cells from patients with normal lungs.[49–51] The significance of these findings remains unclear because there is still no evidence to support a pathogenic mechanism for IPF involving viruses. Interestingly, new animal models have shown a role for viral infection in the development of experimental fibrosis.[52,53] Despite the suggestive evidence of virus in human IPF cells and potential mechanistic links from animal modeling, direct causal links to human disease remain undefined.

FAMILIAL AND GENETIC FACTORS

Familial cases of IPF have been described in dozens of reports. The clinical features of familial IPF are indistinguishable from those of the nonfamilial form, except that the familial form may have an earlier age of onset.[54] Familial IPF or familial interstitial pneumonia (FIP) is defined by at least two members of a primary biologic family (parent, child, siblings) presenting with a characteristic appearance of IPF that is confirmed by biopsy. Familial IPF seems to account for 0.5% to 2% of all cases of IPF.[55]

In 2000, a report was published describing 25 families and comprising 67 cases of familial IPF.[55] In this report the mean age at time of diagnosis was 56 years. Only half of the patients were smokers. The male-to-female ratio was 2:1 in contrast to earlier reviews of FIP, which suggested an inverted male-to-female ratio. This was followed by a larger study of FIP published in 2005.[56] This impressive report described a much larger cohort of 111 families with 309 affected family members. Most of these subjects were identified as having probable or definite IPF by the American Thoracic Society/European Respiratory Society diagnostic criteria. Interestingly, correlation with biopsy specimens suggested that FIP could present with a variety of pathologic patterns (other than UIP), even within the same family. This study revealed a mean age at diagnosis of 68.3 years, with a slight male predominance (55%) and an increased association with cigarette smoking (even after controlling for age and gender differences). Analysis of pedigrees confirmed vertical transmission and provided strong evidence for an autosomal dominant inheritance pattern of disease with variable penetrance.

These accounts of FIP provide compelling evidence for genetic factors that predispose to the development of IPF. One such factor is a mutation in the gene that encodes surfactant protein C (SPC) gene.[57] Other studies have implicated mutations in the gene for surfactant protein A; and mutations in the genes that encode telomerase reverse transcriptase and the telomerase RNA template.[58,59] By leveraging genomic linkage, investigators have recently described a common polymorphism in the promoter of MUC5B, which is associated with both FIP and sporadic IPF.[60] This was followed by a large genome-wide association study of patients with IIPs, which identified additional genetic loci suggesting potential genetic markers of disease.[61] This data is opening up insights into potential genetic pathways of this disease and confirms a generally understood concept that there is a combination of genetic factors and environmental exposures, which account for the significant disease heterogeneity observed in individual patients. While these studies provide useful insights they do not define a direct causal link at present. Several candidate genes have been selected, because of their bearing on proposed mechanisms of the disease, and these genes are currently under investigation.

CLINICAL PRESENTATION

In this section, we discuss important aspects of the clinical presentation of IPF.

DIAGNOSIS

Differential

In the setting of exertional breathlessness, the hallmark of IPF is a predominance of radiographically visualized lower lung zone reticular opacities that spread out over time to involve an ever

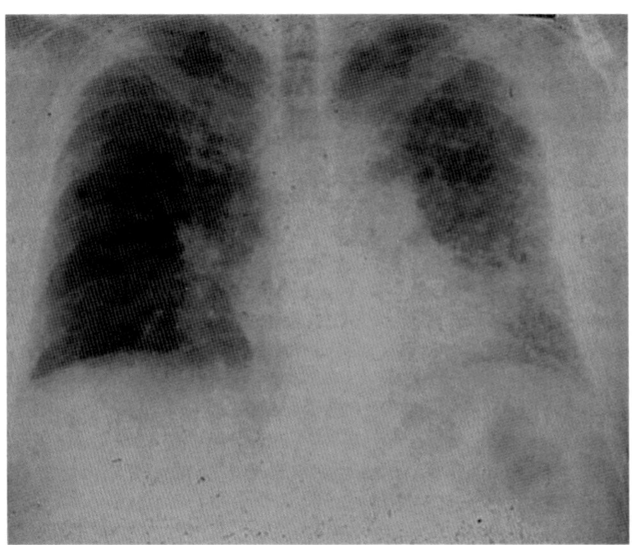

Figure 56-1 Posteroanterior chest radiograph of a 67-year-old man with progressive dyspnea revealing bilateral reticular infiltrates with lower lobe predominance.

enlarging area of lung parenchyma (Fig. 56-1). The differential diagnosis of IPF includes the other IIP, connective tissue diseases (principally scleroderma and rheumatoid arthritis), chronic hypersensitivity pneumonitis, environmental exposures, occupational exposures, chronic aspiration, and heritable conditions such as the Hermansky–Pudlak syndrome. The aforementioned disorders all present with exertional dyspnea coupled with radiographic abnormalities indicative of an interstitial pulmonary disorder.

HRCT has emerged as the single most important diagnostic modality in ILD. A number of diseases share a radiographic pattern that is similar to IPF, in other words, reticular abnormalities are demonstrated by HRCT with a tendency to involve the lower lobes. Examples include asbestosis, chronic aspiration, radiation pneumonitis, chronic hypersensitivity pneumonitis, end-stage sarcoidosis, and congenital disorders such as Gaucher disease, Niemann–Pick disease, and tuberous sclerosis–lymphangioleiomyomatosis. The presence of extensive ground-glass opacities on HRCT should prompt the consideration of an alternative diagnosis such as DIP, cellular NSIP, or acute hypersensitivity pneumonitis. Other IIP that are included in the differential diagnosis of IPF are fibrotic NSIP and COP.

History

Patients with IPF typically present with exertional dyspnea and a nonproductive cough. The dyspnea begins insidiously and is usually progressive. Dyspnea is the most prominent symptom in IPF. Associated systemic symptoms can occur but are not common. Systemic symptoms may include weight loss, low-grade fevers, fatigue, arthralgias, or myalgias.

Patients will often have symptoms for longer than 6 months before seeking medical attention. It is not unusual for symptoms to be present for up to 2 years before an initial consultation is arranged with a pulmonary specialist. Patients are frequently evaluated and treated for other ailments, such as asthma or heart failure, before IPF is identified as the final diagnosis. Because most patients present over the age of 60 where coronary artery disease is highly prevalent, many patients are referred for a cardiac evaluation before pursuing a pulmonary evaluation.

The patient's age is an essential clue to the recognition of IPF. While IPF mostly occurs in older patients (>50 years), the other ILDs are more common among the young or middle-aged (examples include sarcoidosis, lymphangioleiomyomatosis, and pulmonary Langerhans cell histiocytosis).

A history of cigarette smoking is a vital piece of information. While IPF, DIP, and PLCH are diseases found in former and current smokers, other diseases such as hypersensitivity pneumonitis are rare among the smoking population.

It is critical to obtain a detailed occupational history with particular attention to exposures such as asbestos, silica, or any other respiratory toxins. This history is necessary to exclude the presence of pneumoconiosis. It is equally important to inquire about exposure to molds and/or pets in the home environment as this information may suggest a diagnosis of hypersensitivity pneumonitis.

A general health history, including an accounting of all medications, can be revealing. A review of systems may uncover photosensitivity, Raynaud phenomenon, dry eyes, or dry mouth that implies a connective tissue disorder. Certain drugs have been associated with pulmonary fibrosis, most notably nitrofurantoin, bleomycin, and amiodarone.

Physical Examination

In most patients the physical examination reveals fine, bibasilar inspiratory crackles, known as "Velcro rales." As the disease progresses, rales can extend toward the upper lung zones. Clubbing is found in up to 50% of patients with IPF. Resting arterial oxygen saturation may be normal but desaturation is expected with exercise. Extrapulmonary involvement does not occur in IPF. Thus the physical examination is otherwise unremarkable in the early stages of the disease.

Later in the course of disease weight loss, cyanosis, and signs of pulmonary hypertension with cor pulmonale may become apparent. Findings at this stage include an accentuated pulmonic second heart sound, presence of a third heart sound, a right ventricular heave, and edema of the lower extremities.

Routine Laboratories

A routine laboratory evaluation is not helpful except for its role in ruling out other causes of diffuse parenchymal lung disease. Polycythemia is a rare finding despite the frequency of chronic hypoxemia. Elevation of systemic inflammatory markers (i.e., erythrocyte sedimentation rate or C-reactive protein level) or the presence of hypergammaglobulinemia is found in IPF yet such findings are nondiagnostic. The lactate dehydrogenase activity is often elevated but is also nonspecific. Up to 30% of patients with IPF may have positive tests for antinuclear antibodies or rheumatoid factor. These titers are not generally high. The presence of a high titer of autoantibodies suggests connective tissue disease while an elevated angiotensin-converting enzyme level or antineutrophil cytoplasmic antibodies indicates alternative diagnoses.

PULMONARY FUNCTION AND PHYSIOLOGY

Pulmonary function tests in IPF normally identify a restrictive ventilatory defect with reductions of total lung capacity (TLC), functional residual capacity (FRC), and the residual volume (RV). These changes are the result of diminished lung compliance. Pressure–volume studies will yield a curve that is shifted downward and to the right, indicative of lost lung compliance. As the disease progresses, compliance decreases further. Forced expiratory volume in 1 second (FEV_1) and forced vital capacity (FVC) will also be decreased.

Unless a complicating airways disease is present (e.g., chronic obstructive pulmonary disease [COPD]), isovolume flow rates are preserved. While functional alterations associated with small airways disease have been reported in IPF, this description is exclusive to smokers and likely represents a concurrent smoking-related airways disorder.[62]

Impaired gas exchange is demonstrated by the measurement of a lowered diffusing capacity. The decline of diffusion capacity may even precede the development of abnormal lung volumes. Resting arterial blood gases are usually normal in IPF or else they will reveal mild hypoxemia with a respiratory alkalosis. Patients with

IPF have tachypnea and often develop a pattern of rapid-shallow breathing. The work of breathing is increased in IPF. While no chemical changes can explain the observed hyperventilation, it is felt that rapid respiratory rates are secondary to altered mechanical reflexes resulting from an increase in elastic recoil and elastic load. The major cause of hypoxemia is ventilation and perfusion (V/Q) mismatching, not anatomic shunting or reduced oxygen diffusion as was previously suspected.[62]

During exercise, patients with IPF and may exhibit evidence of pulmonary hypertension, even in early cases that have preserved lung function at rest. Pulmonary hypertension can also be present at rest, and is an expected finding, once the vital capacity drops below 50% of predicted or the diffusing capacity falls below 45% of predicted. The presence of pulmonary hypertension may be a predictor of poor outcome yet may not correlate with lung function.[63]

RADIOLOGY

Conventional Chest Radiograph

The chest radiograph is abnormal in nearly all patients with IPF (Fig. 56-1). Yet, in up to 10% of patients with histologically proven IPF, the chest film might be normal. In most of these cases, the use of HRCT will uncover evidence of the disease.[20]

The most common abnormalities seen on a conventional chest film are reticular opacities. In other words there is an appearance of net-like linear and curvilinear densities. Reticular markings may be found bilaterally, in an asymmetrical distribution with a predilection for the lower lobes. A course reticular pattern on the plain radiograph, taking the form of translucent "honeycombing," will emerge late in the course of disease and portends a poor prognosis. The chest radiograph lacks specificity for the diagnosis of IPF. The correct diagnosis is made on the conventional radiograph in less than 50% of cases. In addition, the interpretation of conventional radiographs with an interstitial pattern shows poor interobserver agreement. Studies have examined this particular characteristic and report that concordance between radiologists is only 70%.[64,65]

High-Resolution Computed Tomography

Development of the high-resolution CT scanner has revolutionized the diagnostic evaluation of the ILDs. HRCT allows a detailed examination of the lung parenchyma by creating 1- to 2-mm thin slices of the chest. HRCT uses a computerized reconstruction algorithm to maximize spatial resolution. This generates much improved image clarity such that the specificity of interpretations is increased, interobserver variability is reduced, and the overall accuracy of diagnosis is enhanced. HRCT scanning allows for the earlier diagnosis of IPF and permits the identification of alternate patterns of disease. The primary role of HRCT in the diagnostic evaluation of ILD is the discrimination of typical IPF from the other ILDs. Given the utility and availability of scanners, HRCT has become the primary diagnostic tool for identifying IPF.

The HRCT appearance of IPF is characterized by patchy, predominantly peripheral, predominantly subpleural, and bibasilar reticular opacities (Fig. 56-2). Ground-glass opacities can be found, but should occupy no more than a limited amount of territory. Areas that are severely involved with reticular markings may also demonstrate traction bronchiectasis. The presence of subpleural honeycombing (small, round translucencies with a density equal to that of air), traction bronchiectasis, and thickened interlobular septae will increase the specificity of the CT scan for diagnosing IPF. Several studies have examined the diagnostic accuracy of HRCT scans in IPF.[64–68] Studies were conducted in which observers were asked to determine a radiographic diagnosis that was then compared with the histopathology of UIP as the "gold standard." In the hands of experienced observers, radiographic diagnosis of IPF has a reported specificity and positive predictive value for IPF histology that exceeds 90%.[66–68] However, the "confident" HRCT is not a sensitive tool for the diagnosis of IPF.[66] The full spectrum of a "confident" radiographic pattern will only be seen in two-thirds of biopsy-proven IPF. One-third of IPF cases will not show a definitive CT pattern and would be missed if the HRCT was relied upon exclusively (Fig. 56-3). In such cases, and in the right clinical context, an SLB should be considered to clarify the diagnosis. Nonetheless it has become apparent that, in the right clinical setting, an experienced radiologist can diagnose IPF by the HRCT with considerable accuracy, obviating the need for biopsy.

Given the evolving importance of HRCT in the diagnosis of IPF, CT scan criteria were defined during the most recent expert consensus statement on the diagnosis of IPF.[20] HRCT patterns were

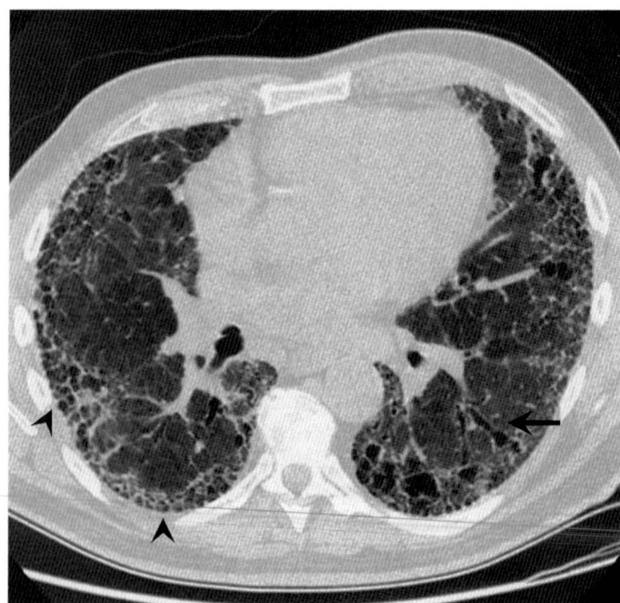

Figure 56-2 Computed tomography scan illustrates the "classic" features of idiopathic pulmonary fibrosis (IPF). Bilateral, peripheral, and subpleural reticular infiltrates are evident. The presence of advanced fibrosis is indicated by honeycomb changes *(arrowheads)* and traction bronchiectasis *(arrow)*. These features permit experienced clinicians to make a confident radiographic diagnosis of IPF.

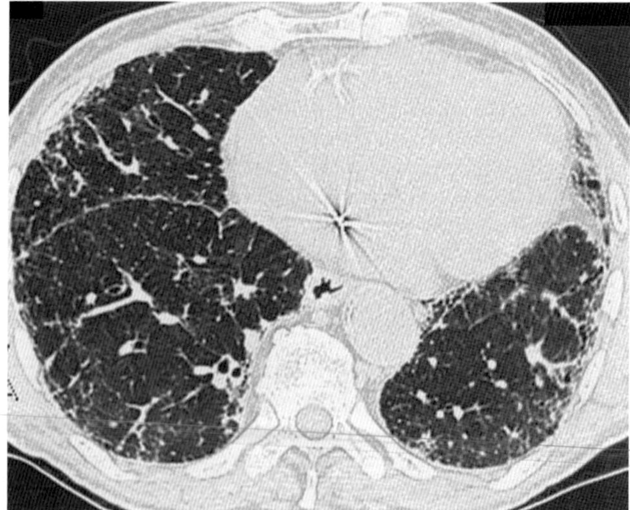

Figure 56-3 Computed tomography scan of an 81-year-old man with biopsy-proven idiopathic pulmonary fibrosis. A peripheral distribution of reticular opacities is demonstrated. Honeycombing and traction bronchiectasis are notably absent. In the absence of specific findings, a surgical lung biopsy was needed to make a diagnosis.

separated into three groups: A UIP pattern; a possible UIP pattern; and a pattern labeled "inconsistent with UIP." The UIP pattern has four features: (1) Subpleural, basal predominance of disease; (2) reticular abnormality; (3) honeycombing with or without traction bronchiectasis; and (4) absence of any inconsistent features. The inconsistent features include (1) upper or midlung predominance; (2) peribronchovascular predominance; (3) extensive ground-glass abnormalities that are greater than the amount of reticulation; (4) profuse micronodules; (5) multiple discrete cysts that are located away from areas of honeycombing; (6) diffuse mosaic attenuation/air trapping; and (7) consolidation in bronchopulmonary segments.[20] Features defined as consistent with a "possible UIP pattern" were those of the UIP pattern except without evidence of honeycombing.

BRONCHOALVEOLAR LAVAGE

An enormous amount of scientific information has been obtained by analyzing the content of BAL fluid from patients with IPF. Notable increases of immune cells (neutrophils, eosinophils, and activated alveolar macrophages) are present in BAL fluid from IPF. In addition, BAL has aided in the identification of cytokines, growth factors, and other cellular products that are now implicated in the pathogenesis of IPF. As a research tool, BAL has been immensely valuable. However, the role of BAL in the clinical diagnosis of IPF remains limited. Though much effort has been invested in evaluating the clinical utility of this modality, study results have been contradictory and generally disappointing.[69] Most samples of BAL from IPF patients demonstrate simultaneous increases of several effector cell types including neutrophils (70%–90% of patients); eosinophils (40%–60% of patients); and lymphocytes (10%–20% of patients).[20] Despite this finding, studies have failed to demonstrate a clear distinction amongst pulmonary diseases based upon the predominant type of cell in the BAL fluid.[62] As a consequence of this, in standard practice, BAL is no longer generally recommended for the routine evaluation of IPF.

PATHOLOGY

Previously, SLB was recommended to confirm all cases of suspected IPF. With the advent and availability of HRCT this is no longer the case, as the positive predictive value of HRCT is comparable and in some studies better than that of biopsy.[70] Despite this fact, SLB remains critical to the diagnosis of IPF in the context of HRCT scans that are equivocal (e.g., without the full complement of radiographic features that are expected in IPF). Biopsy may be achieved by either open thoracotomy or by video-assisted thoracoscopy (VATS). VATS is preferred as it has been associated with less morbidity and shorter hospital stays compared to open biopsy. An SLB provides the best sample from which to distinguish UIP from other forms of IIP. The recommendation is that the SLB be taken from at least two lobes, preferably the upper and lower lobes. The basis of this recommendation is from studies that identified that different pathologies could exist in different sections of the lung. Despite the coexisting patterns, if one of these had UIP pathology then the patient's clinical course followed that of the UIP pathology.[71] Transbronchial biopsies are less helpful in identifying IPF lesions because the small size of the sample prohibits the pathologist from identifying all the necessary features for a confident pathologic diagnosis of IPF.

The gross appearance of an IPF sample may be normal but often has a distinctive nodular pleural surface that has been likened to cirrhosis. The histopathologic lesion associated with IPF is UIP. This lesion is defined by a variegated structure. Normal lung alternates with patchy collagen fibrosis (Figs. 56-4 and 56-5). The fibrosis takes the form of alveolar septal thickening with a predominantly subpleural distribution. Whirls of fibroblasts embedded in a loose extracellular matrix embody the fibroblastic foci that are found in numerous quantities at the leading edge of dense scar (Figs. 56-4 and 56-5). Interstitial inflammation is present but remains scant and confined to areas of fibrosis. This limited inflammation consists of lymphocytes and plasma cells. Associated hyperplasia of the type 2 pneumocytes is found within areas of active inflammation. Areas that contain dense collagen may develop cystic structures, which may be filled with mucin or lined by bronchiolar epithelium. These cysts are referred to as microscopic honeycomb change. Hyaline membranes and organized alveolar exudates are absent. Occasionally alveolar macrophages are present.

The UIP pathologic pattern exhibits a wide range of severity with regards to the extent of honeycomb change and the extent of involved lung. A history of smoking may alter the histopathologic appearance of UIP. Emphysematous change can be superimposed upon UIP. Pigmented alveolar macrophages, the hallmark feature of RB-ILD and DIP pathologic patterns, may be present in small number in UIP lesions from former or current smokers.

The UIP pattern can be found in other diseases besides IPF. The presence of granulomas in a UIP lesion favors a diagnosis of fibronodular sarcoidosis or chronic hypersensitivity pneumonitis. Asbestos bodies found within a UIP pattern suggest the diagnosis of asbestosis.

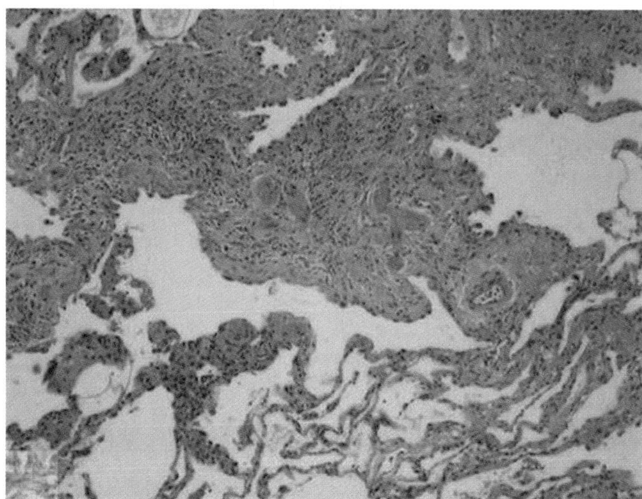

A

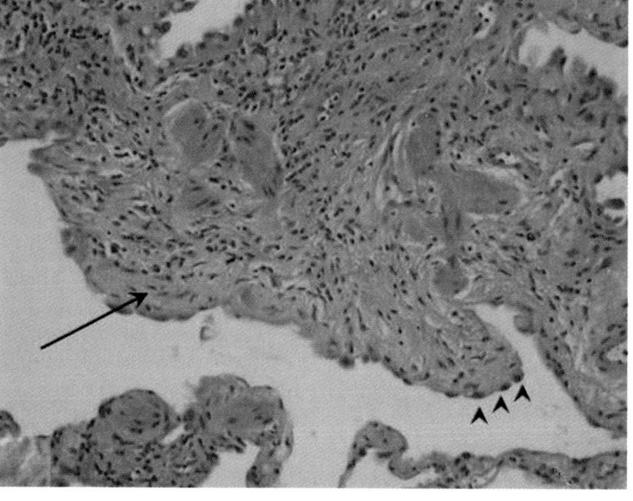

B

Figure 56-4 **A.** Low-magnification photomicrograph of usual interstitial pneumonia (UIP) showing the characteristic heterogeneous involvement of the parenchyma. Zones of interstitial fibrosis are seen alternating with areas of normal lung. **B.** Higher magnification demonstrates enlarged cystic air spaces lined with hyperplastic alveolar epithelium *(arrowheads)*. Beneath the mucosal layer is an advancing region of young fibrosis containing loose extracellular matrix *(pale pink staining)* and fibroblasts *(arrow)*.

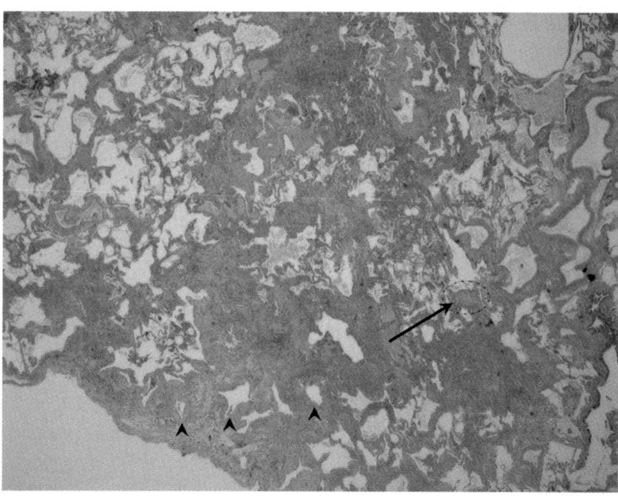

Figure 56-5 Scanning view of usual interstitial pneumonia (UIP) demonstrates the characteristic variegated appearance of UIP. Note the honeycomb change *(arrowheads)* present in the region of dense fibrosis adjacent to the pleural surface. A fibroblast focus *(arrow)* is seen at the leading edge of advancing fibrosis.

The histopathologic pattern of UIP can also be found in several conditions other than IPF. UIP can be found in association with connective tissue diseases, asbestosis, chronic hypersensitivity pneumonitis, the Hermansky–Pudlak syndrome, neurofibromatosis, or in the setting of a toxic drug reaction (typically after administration of either bleomycin, methotrexate, nitrofurantoin, or amiodarone; [this is a partial list]). The identification of these conditions is largely a matter of correlation with the clinical history. It is important to note that the presence of honeycombing on biopsy is a nonspecific finding with a broad differential. Honeycombing is a common endpoint for a myriad of pathologic processes. Although honeycombing carries the connotation of end-stage fibrosis it can also occur in a focal distribution after any lung injury. Seen alone, honeycombing is not indicative of IPF.

To standardize the pathologic definition of UIP, a set of consensus criteria were established to represent expert opinion.[20] The consensus definition allows for four pathologic categories: The UIP pattern; a probable UIP pattern; a possible UIP pattern; and a pattern referred to as "not UIP." The UIP pattern requires (1) evidence of marked fibrosis/architectural distortion generally with honeycombing in a predominant subpleural distribution; (2) patchy involvement of the fibrosis in the lung parenchyma; (3) presence of fibroblastic foci; and (4) absence of features such as hyaline membranes, organizing pneumonia, granulomas, predominant airway-centered pathology, inflammatory cell infiltrate away from honeycombing or pathologic features suggestive of another disorder. The "probable" UIP pattern requires (1) evidence of marked fibrosis/architectural distortion with or without honeycombing; (2) absence of either patchy involvement or fibroblastic foci but not both; plus (3) an absence of features such as hyaline membranes, organizing pneumonia, granulomas, etc. In the right clinical context, "probable" UIP can be considered when honeycomb changes alone are present in the SLB. The "possible" UIP pattern incorporates (1) patchy or diffuse fibrosis within the pulmonary parenchyma; (2) in the absence of other criteria for a UIP pattern; and (3) in the absence of the features such as hyaline membranes, etc.

DIAGNOSTIC ALGORITHM

The objective is to secure an accurate diagnosis of IPF. The task is critical, to provide patients with accurate prognostic information; and, also to define cohorts for clinical/therapeutic trials. As previously discussed, the central issue is that the diagnosis of IPF is a diagnosis of exclusion. However, complete exclusion of other diagnostic possibilities is a daunting challenge. For one, there are multiple studies demonstrating significant interobserver disagreement between pulmonologists, radiologists, and pathologists especially when their decisions are made in isolation from each other's expertise.[21,72,73] By corollary, a multidisciplinary approach to diagnosis has been shown to improve diagnostic accuracy. The multidisciplinary approach requires real-time collaboration between the diagnosing physicians: The pulmonologists, radiologists, and pathologists involved with the case. If these groups are not available, then referral of patients to a center where this expertise is available is recommended.[20]

Given the complexity of making an accurate diagnosis, and the lack of definitive molecular biomarkers to aid such a diagnosis, practical diagnostic algorithms have relied on the practices and opinions of a consensus of experts. It must be noted that such diagnostic criteria (adopted from expert opinion) have never been validated. The most recent expert diagnostic guideline was endorsed by the American Thoracic Society, European Respiratory Society, Japanese Respiratory Society, and the Latin American Thoracic Association (ATS/ERS/JRS/ALAT).[20] In the revised 2011 guidelines, SLB is no longer considered an absolute necessity for a definitive diagnosis. Rather, HRCT may qualify as a surrogate in appropriate circumstances. As per the ATS/ERS/JRS/ALAT statement, the diagnosis of IPF requires (1) exclusion of other known causes of ILD; and (2) either (a) UIP pattern from SLB, supported by a UIP pattern of fibrosis on HRCT; or (b) UIP pattern by HRCT alone (in patients not subjected to an SLB).[20] In clinical practice, the most critical (yet most challenging) factor is to exclude other known causes of ILD. This requires a careful history, physical examination, and evaluation with a focus on environmental/work place exposures; medication use; family history; clinical evidence connective tissue disease (oftentimes, the evidence is subtle); and other comorbidities.

A diagnostic algorithm follows: Patients with suspected IPF in whom there are no identifiable causes of ILD will undergo HRCT scans of the chest; if there is definitive evidence of a UIP pattern on the HRCT, then the diagnosis is complete. If the HRCT pattern is equivocal, SLB can be considered to clarify the diagnosis. Prior to SLB, the safety of such an invasive procedure must be weighed against the utility of a definitive diagnosis (in other words, a careful risk–benefit analysis is indicated). Expert consultation with a multidisciplinary group of ILD experts is recommended in this setting. A UIP or probable UIP pattern on biopsy was felt to confirm the diagnosis of IPF in the setting of a HRCT pattern, which is defined as a possible UIP pattern. An HRCT possible UIP pattern in the setting of a not UIP pathology pattern was defined as not IPF. In this algorithm, if the HRCT scan was inconsistent with UIP, and the pathology was a UIP pattern then this was determined to be possible IPF. Per the algorithm, these types of cases require a multidisciplinary discussion to resolve any potential inconsistencies and come to a consensus diagnosis.

Although this algorithm provides a clear path toward the diagnosis of IPF several caveats must be considered. This algorithm is based on experience and expert opinion; it has never been validated in prospective studies. It also requires a high level of expertise (to define the radiographic, clinical, and pathologic evidence) that may not be available in all clinical settings. Such diagnostic algorithms and diagnostic criteria are best suited to defining populations for clinical research. A much more elegant and streamlined approach is needed for standard clinical practice. As of yet, this state of art is lacking.

NATURAL HISTORY AND PROGNOSIS

The natural history of IPF has never been fully defined. IPF is felt to be a progressive disorder of subjective and objective decline in pulmonary function ultimately resulting in death. The exact length of time from diagnosis to mortality has been difficult to clearly define. Studies utilizing the modern definition of IPF first reported median survival between 2 and 5 years from the time of diagnosis.[29] Recent data from the placebo arms of clinical trials suggest longer survival.[34,36] There are few, if any, reports of long-term survival with biopsy-proven IPF/UIP.

Several factors have combined to create barriers preventing the further, more rigorous description of the natural history of IPF. First, the diagnosis of IPF can be challenging and, not infrequently, the presence of "early" disease gets overlooked. Patients develop IPF in the later decades of life and often attribute their symptoms to old age. When their disease eventually comes to medical attention, there may be further delay in diagnosis because the symptoms are nonspecific. Most patients with IPF are evaluated for other diseases before a diagnosis of pulmonary fibrosis is considered. Moreover, the interstitial markings found on a chest radiograph are subtle and tend to go unnoticed or else simply get disregarded as clinically unimportant. Experts in IPF agree that patients usually have symptoms for 2 or more years before receiving a definitive diagnosis. It is therefore apparent as to why many older cohorts are enriched with advanced, late-stage IPF. The epidemiology is shifting with the advent and more commonplace use of HRCT, which may detect interstitial markings and pick up the diagnosis of IPF at an earlier stage.

The other major issue is that there is clear heterogeneity in the clinical course of individual patients. This heterogeneity has led to the consideration that there are several possible natural histories of IPF.[20] This determination is the result of observations that have occurred over clinical trials especially in circumstances that placebo groups have had different clinical trajectories despite similar clinical definition of disease. The majority of patients appear to follow a slowly progressive clinical course, though others appear to have a more rapid course. Selman et al.[74] described different clinical groups based on the length of symptoms prior to diagnosis. The patients who had symptoms <6 months (rapid progression) prior to diagnosis had higher mortality than those who had symptoms for more than 24 months (slow progression). In the "rapid progression" patients there were associated alterations to their gene expression profile, as well as increased BAL active matrix metalloproteinase-9 and fibroblast migration. What influences these different clinical courses is not well known or understood.

■ ACUTE EXACERBATION OF IPF

Japanese investigators made the initial observation that patients with IPF can experience episodes of sudden decline, which they characterized as acute exacerbations.[75] Recent observations from the placebo arm of two randomized clinical trials have suggested that acute exacerbations may be more common that previously appreciated.[33,76,77] The acute exacerbation of IPF (AE-IPF) is characterized by a sudden worsening of symptoms and has been associated with hypoxemia and new radiographic infiltrates. It is important in making the diagnosis of AE-IPF to rule out infection, congestive heart failure, and pulmonary embolism. AE-IPF typically occurs in patients with established IPF however it has been recognized that AE-IPF can form the initial presentation of IPF as well, mimicking AIP. Patients with established IPF satisfy the criteria for an acute exacerbation if they have (1) previous or concurrent diagnosis of IPF; (2) unexplained development or worsening of dyspnea in the past 30 days; (3) HRCT with evidence of new ground-glass opacities superimposed on the background of a radiographic pattern of UIP; (4) no evidence of pulmonary infection; and (5) exclusion of alternative causes.[76] Histopathologic examination of AE-IPF commonly reveals a UIP pattern with superimposed diffuse alveolar damage (DAD) characterized by diffuse alveolar septal thickening within a pale matrix that includes hyaline membranes and fibrin. UIP with superimposed organizing pneumonia has also been reported in AE-IPF. The prognosis of AE-IPF is poor. Series of patients with AE-IPF reported in-hospital mortality rates between 78% and 96%.[77–80] Mortality is strongly associated with the need for mechanical ventilation. The etiology of AE-IPF is poorly understood and remains an area of active research.

■ PROGNOSIS

While accurate predictions of the prognosis of IPF are essential for clinical decision making, such predictions remain challenging for a variety of reasons. Still, rudimentary predictions can be based on pathologic, physiologic, and radiographic information. In addition, various composite scores have been developed for prognostic purposes.

■ PATHOLOGIC PREDICTORS

One of the most important features of the spectrum of illness encompassed by IIP is the fact that pathologic patterns predict survival. In the late 1990s it was recognized that the UIP pathologic pattern had a precise correlation with clinical parameters and with outcome.[17] Survival is significantly worse amongst patients whose biopsy contains a UIP pattern as compared to either NSIP or other patterns of fibrosis.[29] Within biopsy specimens, specific traits have also been correlated with survival.[33] The degree of cellularity does not seem to affect survival nor does the degree of fibrosis. However, the number of fibroblastic foci has been shown to predict survival. Fibroblastic foci have been linked to high mortality and large declines in physiologic measures such as the FVC and diffusion capacity.[81]

■ PHYSIOLOGIC PREDICTORS

Baseline pulmonary function as a determinant of prognosis has not been reproducible,[82–90] though more recent studies utilizing standardized definitions and involving patients with earlier disease suggest that it may have better prognostic value than initially appreciated.[91–93] Changes in pulmonary function over time have been more clearly correlated with measures of long-term survival. For instance, a 10% decline in FVC over 6 months, or a 15% decline in $D_{L_{CO}}$ over 6 months, predicts shortened survival.[91,94] For this reason, clinical trials in IPF have utilized changes in FVC as a clinical outcome measure to assess drug efficacy,[95] though some disagreement exists on this issue.[96] In clinical practice, at the present time, the use of decrements in pulmonary function remains an important objective means of assessing clinical disease progression.

An issue that affects the predictive value of physiologic variables in IPF is the confounding influence of coexistent emphysema. This problem is addressed by the composite physiologic index (CPI), which corrects for emphysema by combining several physiologic measures into a single-weighted score.[97] The formula for the CPI includes diffusion capacity, FVC, and FEV_1 in its calculations. The CPI was validated by comparison with HRCT. In addition, it was shown that the CPI is a more accurate prognostic determinant than any individual test of pulmonary function.

■ RADIOGRAPHIC PREDICTORS

The utility of HRCT in predicting the outcome of IPF is supported by a study, which compares HRCT patterns to biopsy.[98] Patients who had both an HRCT and a biopsy were analyzed and it was found that an HRCT pattern consistent with UIP correlated pathologically with the UIP pattern. However, an indeterminate HRCT pattern could be a manifestation of either UIP or NSIP. Patients with combined pathologic UIP and radiographic "confident UIP" had a worse outcome compared to patients with pathologic UIP and an indeterminate HRCT.

■ COMPOSITE SCORES

Some authors have proposed that a composite scoring system for IPF would have better predictive value than measuring individual disease-related factors. The first clinical, radiologic, and physiologic (CRP) scoring system was developed in 1986 and employed seven variables that accounted for parameters such as dyspnea, specific radiographic findings, and physiologic function.[99] This CRP score was validated through comparison to histopathology in a group of

26 patients. No single component of the CRP score had a better correlation than the composite score.

Over time further scoring systems have been developed. In 2001, a CRP score was derived to predict death rather than just histopathology.[82] A large cohort of patients was followed prospectively to devise the revised CRP score, utilizing multivariate statistical models to identify significant disease-related parameters. The revised CRP score incorporates age, smoking status, the presence of clubbing, TLC, arterial oxygen during maximal exercise, radiographic infiltrates, and radiographic findings consistent with pulmonary hypertension. The revised CRP score ranges from 0 to 100, with higher scores indicating more severe disease. Five-year survival can be predicted in individual patients by calculating a CRP score employing the published formulas and then referencing published survival curves. This system was felt to be cumbersome and therefore Collard et al. developed a simplified staging system from retrospective data of three large cohorts in California, Minnesota, and Italy (Ley B Annals of Internal Medicine 2012).[100] Utilizing gender; age; physiology, which included FVC and D_{LCO}(GAP) patients with IPF could be grouped into stages I, II, or III and that had defined 1-, 2-, and 3-year predicted mortality rates. This simple system using readily available clinical and physiologic data could provide important prognostic data for patients at the time of initial evaluation and assist with immediate management decisions.

PATHOGENESIS

IPF is a complex disorder and many pathogenic events have been observed. Despite significant research effort, no definitive, unifying hypothesis has yet emerged. Multiple pathways have been implicated in both experimental models of pulmonary fibrosis and patients with IPF. Despite this information, drug targets to modify these pathways have thus far been largely ineffectual. It remains distinctly possible that there is no single common pathway that results in the IPF phenotype; but rather, a combination of multiple factors that lead to aberrant wound healing, progressive fibrosis, and diffuse scar formation. Although more questions than answers currently exist, great strides are being made to elucidate new mechanisms in IPF pathogenesis.[101,102]

A primary change in our understanding of the pathogenesis of IPF has been a movement away from inflammation as the driver of the fibrotic response in the IPF lung. "Inflammation" dominated the field in the 1970s and 1980s and was based largely on the observation that BAL fluid from patients with IPF had increased numbers of inflammatory cells (mostly neutrophils and eosinophils) relative to normal individuals.[103–108] The concept that permeated the literature in that era was that IPF resulted from an unremitting inflammatory response to an exogenous insult, culminating in progressive fibrosis. By targeting the inflammatory response, the belief was that fibrosis could be limited or prevented. Unfortunately, it now appears that the data are more likely explained by structural abnormalities in lung architecture (traction bronchiectasis) that result in airway inflammation but do not appear to be causative of the fibrosis inflammation.[17,109] This is further supported by the pathologic observation that there is a lack of inflammation at the leading edge of the fibrosis and the fact that patients with IPF do not respond to systemic immunosuppression with corticosteroids. As a consequence of this understanding the overall research into mechanisms of IPF has made a clear transition from the belief of a primary "inflammatory-driven" process to one that focuses on dysfunctional repair of alveolar epithelial cells with generation of profibrotic mediators, activation of fibroblasts, and resultant scarring.[101]

BASEMENT MEMBRANE INJURY

A unique feature of the UIP pathologic pattern is a loss of integrity of the subepithelial basement membrane. This has been definitively demonstrated through the use of electron microscopy.[14] Basement membranes in IPF are denuded of the usual type I pneumocytes. It is theorized that loss of this protective epithelial barrier results in further oxidative injury that degrades basement membranes. At the same time it appears that hyperplastic type II pneumocytes are abundantly present. This likely represents an attempt at epithelial cell regeneration. While the exposed basement membrane may provide the signal for epithelial growth, new epithelial cells cannot attach to a damaged membrane. The result is a "frustrated" epithelial cell response with failure to signal a termination of epithelial cell proliferation. Further examination of tissue from patients with IPF has confirmed an irregular pattern of alveolar epithelial cell proliferation, concurrent with dysregulation of the proteins that control the cell cycle.[110,111]

An accumulation of growth factors in IPF may originate from the persistent proliferative response of epithelial cells. A downstream consequence of "frustrated" epithelial cell regeneration would be recruitment of fibroblasts and myofibroblasts through the release of such growth factors. In essence, the signal to recruit and maintain a pool of mesenchymal cells (fibroblasts) might originate from an inability to successfully re-epithelialize the alveolar lining surface.

ALVEOLAR EPITHELIUM

Multiple lines of investigation suggest that the alveolar epithelium is critically involved in the pathogenesis of IPF.[53,109,112] The prevailing hypothesis is that repetitive low-level injury to a vulnerable or susceptible alveolar epithelium drives the pathologic features of IPF.[102] Why IPF alveolar epithelium is more vulnerable appears to be from a combination of age-related and genetic factors that are not clearly defined but being actively investigated.

Epithelial Apoptosis/Injury

An emerging body of literature supports alveolar epithelial cell injury and apoptosis as important features of IPF and in the development of experimental pulmonary fibrosis. Electron microscopic studies of human IPF tissue demonstrate injury and apoptosis of alveolar epithelial cells.[14] BAL from patients with IPF has established the presence of proapoptotic proteins.[113] In the bleomycin model of lung injury and fibrosis in animals, fibrosis can be abrogated by various approaches to inhibit epithelial cell apoptosis.[114–116] These include a reduction in experimental fibrosis by inhibiting the Fas–Fas ligand pathway, angiotensin production, or caspase activation.

In addition direct inhibition of apoptotic pathways, factors that cause epithelial cell apoptosis are critical to the development of fibrosis. Evidence suggests that fibroblasts produce angiotensin peptides that lead to epithelial apoptosis. Other researchers have demonstrated that transforming growth factor-β (TGF-β) is involved with promoting epithelial cell apoptosis.[117] Oxidant injury may also promote epithelial cell death and several studies of IPF patients have confirmed excessive oxidant production as well as glutathione deficiency.[118–120] Tumor necrosis factor-α (TNF-α) has been shown to promote alveolar epithelial cell apoptosis in vitro.[121] In a mouse model, knockout of the TNF-α receptor confers resistance to bleomycin-induced lung fibrosis, while overexpression of TNF-α in the mouse has been associated with an increase in experimental fibrosis.[122] Patients with IPF are known to exhibit an exaggerated expression of TNF-α, which may contribute to epithelial injury.[123]

Evidence of direct injury to the alveolar epithelium suggests that this may be an important model of pulmonary fibrosis. Utilizing a transgenic mouse directing expression of human diphtheria toxin receptor in SPC-expressing cells, it was shown that targeted injury of type II epithelial cells resulted in the development of experimental lung fibrosis.[124] The development of fibrosis in this targeted epithelial cell injury is dependent on plasminogen activating factor 1 and the recruitment of monocytes and macrophages into the lung.[125,126]

Endoplasmic Reticulum Stress

Mutations of surfactant proteins A2 and C have been associated with familial types of pulmonary fibrosis and suggest a potential genetic mechanism for alveolar epithelial injury.[57,58,127–130] In alveolar epithelium, during both homeostatic and inflammatory conditions, surfactant proteins are regularly produced. This production requires appropriate and coordinated folding and packaging of the proteins in the endoplasmic reticulum (ER) prior to their release.[131] When this folding does not occur correctly, the cell experiences ER stress, which results in activation of the unfolded protein response (UPR) a cellular pathway designed to limit the deleterious consequences of misfolded proteins.[132] The fact that mutations in these proteins were associated with pulmonary fibrosis suggested that misfolding of these proteins could result in cellular stress and thereby enhance the vulnerability of the epithelium.[51] Using a mouse model that expressed a mutant form of SPC, Lawson et al.[133] demonstrated that misfolded SPC caused ER stress and thereby activating the UPR. Despite this activation the mice did not spontaneously develop pulmonary fibrosis but rather required a secondary challenge with bleomycin or viral infection.[133,134] With secondary challenge, the mice exhibiting enhanced ER stress were more susceptible to fibrosis. A growing body of literature suggests that the UPR response is defective with advancing age, which may provide a direct link to IPF as it is a disease of advanced age. ER stress and secondary insults provide an attractive model for IPF as this model system has the potential to link both genetic- and age-related disease factors to microinjuries and a vulnerable epithelium.

■ THE FIBROBLAST

The hallmark of pulmonary fibrosis is the development and expansion of scar tissue in the lung. In this context, patients develop progressive respiratory failure associated with unrelenting accumulation of extracellular matrix in the gas-exchanging regions. The generally accepted predominant sources of this matrix are fibroblasts. In IPF, fibroblasts accumulate in areas of advancing fibrosis and are associated with regions of alveolar epithelial hyperplasia, a.k.a. the fibroblast foci. Though not completely unique to IPF[101] (they can be found in small numbers in NSIP), fibroblastic foci are pathognomonic for IPF.[135] Supporting their importance two groups have observed that a large number of fibroblast foci within lung biopsies correlate with a worse prognosis in IPF.[33,81]

Myofibroblast

One of the hallmarks of IPF pathology is the development of a subset of cells called myofibroblasts.[136] Much attention has been focused recently on the role of the myofibroblast in the pathogenesis of IPF. The defining characteristics of myofibroblasts are positive staining for α-smooth muscle actin (α-SMA) and production of new collagen. Myofibroblasts have contractile properties critical to normal wound healing, though they only appear transiently in this circumstance.[137] In IPF lung biopsies, myofibroblasts have been described in abundance especially in the fibroblastic foci.[138] Myofibroblasts have also been shown to accumulate in bleomycin-induced lung fibrosis.[139] Immunohistochemical studies have suggested that they are important in the production of newly synthesized collagen.[139] The source of these myofibroblasts and the reasons for their persistence in IPF lung are just starting to be clarified.[140]

Origin of Fibroblasts and Myofibroblasts

The source of fibroblasts has been a subject of intense research and debate. Several possibilities include resident lung fibroblasts, bone marrow progenitors called fibrocytes, and epithelial cell transition in a process called epithelial to mesenchymal transition (EMT).

Evidence has accumulated over the past several years that suggests that bone marrow–derived cells may contribute to the pool of lung fibroblasts in IPF. In an animal model of experimental lung fibrosis it was shown that fluorescently tagged bone marrow–derived cells trafficked to the lung where they became a source of collagen expression.[141] Interestingly these bone marrow–derived cells did not express α-SMA, nor did they express α-SMA when stimulated in vitro with TGF-β, suggesting that they are not capable of acquiring the myofibroblast phenotype. Another group of researchers observed that a newly defined cell type migrated into the lungs of animals following bleomycin injury called fibrocytes.[142] Fibrocytes are a recently recognized cell type of hematopoietic origin that circulate in the peripheral blood and have been suggested to play a role in wound repair.[143] They also have been implicated in the pathogenesis of hypertrophic scars, scleroderma, and asthma-related airway fibrosis.[144] Fibrocytes are present in the blood of patients with IPF and appear to be a marker of disease progression.[145] Still, the exact role of these cells (and their relationship to the fibroblast) remains unclear due to the lack of specificity in lineage-tracing markers.

Another possibility is that the fibroblasts in IPF are derived from the alveolar epithelium. A transformation of cell type from epithelium to mesenchyme is a well-documented phenomenon that takes place during embryogenesis. In culture, it has been shown that isolated type II alveolar epithelial cells (AEC2) exhibit a loss of AEC2 markers and express fibroblast markers when stimulated with TGF-β, a critical fibrogenic factor. Whether this occurs in IPF remains a point of controversy with some studies demonstrating colocalization of AEC2 and fibroblast markers[146] and others that do not observe evidence of this phenomenon.[147] To address this question in vivo, lineage-tracing experiments were performed. Initial studies utilized a fragment of the human SPC promoter to drive the expression of a lineage label to track AEC2 cells.[148,149] Tracking AEC2 cells after TGF-β or bleomycin exposure suggested that these cells were a significant source of mesenchymal cells in experimental lung fibrosis. In contrast to these observations, alternative in vivo lineage tracing using a knock-in allele of the SPC gene directing inducible expression of a fluorescent lineage tag in mature AEC2 cells did not demonstrate evidence of EMT after bleomycin.[150] This work suggested a complex and heterogeneous proliferation of mesenchymal cells in experimental lung fibrosis. None of the cells that they explored appeared to be the origin of myofibroblasts.[150] Determining the origin of these cells remains an area of active investigation.

Fibroblast Phenotypes and Functions in IPF

Various growth factors that influence fibroblast function have been shown to be produced in the lung tissue of patients with IPF and also shown to mediate the pathogenesis of experimental fibrosis.[151,152] Examples include keratinocyte growth factor, TGF-β, insulin-like growth factor-1 (IGF-1), platelet-derived growth factors (PDGF-A and PDGF-B), fibroblast growth factor-2, and hepatocyte growth factor. Many of these growth factors activate tyrosine kinase signaling pathways that promote fibroblast proliferation and matrix production.

TGF-β is a critical mediator of lung fibrosis in animal models.[153] Several studies have shown that antagonizing TGF-β prevents the development of lung fibrosis.[154] Alternatively, targeted overexpression of TGF-β has been shown to produce progressive pulmonary fibrosis.[155] Evidence suggests that TGF-β has the capacity to promote epithelial cell transformation into a mesenchymal phenotype.[146] Studies have suggested that fibrosis is attenuated in the setting of targeted loss of TGF-β signaling in epithelial cells[156,157] and that epithelial expression of the integrin αvβ6 responsible for the activation of latent TGF-β is also critical to the development of fibrosis.[158] TGF-β also induces the differentiation of fibroblasts to myofibroblasts.[159,160] This effect appears to be dependent on NADPH oxidase 4.[161]

Secreted factors that influence fibroblast migration may also be important to fibrogenesis. The production of CXCL10 by innate immune cells may be critical to fibroblast migration and fibrogenesis.[162–164] Recent work highlighted lysophosphatidic acid (LPA) as an additional chemotactic factor for fibroblasts.[165] LPA interacting with its cognate receptor LPAR1 is critical for recruitment of fibroblasts. LPA was increased in the BALF from IPF patients and inhibition of LPAR1 markedly attenuated the migration of fibroblasts to IPF BALF.

It appears that IPF fibroblasts have an enhanced proliferative capacity as compared to non-IPF fibroblasts.[166,167] The mechanism of enhanced proliferation is not fully elucidated but data suggest that several pathways may be involved. These include defective fibroblast/extracellular matrix interactions, aberrant activation of PI3 K/Akt/S6K1 signaling pathways, and genome-wide derangements in translation control.[168–171] The derangements in transcriptional control have the potential to allow IPF fibroblasts to circumvent normal negative feedback signals that would inhibit fibroblast proliferation and therefore limit fibrogenesis.

It has also been suggested that IPF fibroblasts have the capacity to invade through tissue. Such an invasive capacity might lead to the destruction of the basement membrane and collapse of alveolar tissue, both hallmarks of IPF pathology. It was recently shown that IPF fibroblasts may spontaneously invade an artificial matrix in an in vitro model.[172] It was also shown that targeted overexpression of hyaluronan, an extracellular matrix component, in myofibroblasts resulted in enhanced invasive capacity.[173] The invasive capacity of human IPF fibroblasts could be abrogated by either blockade of CD44 (the receptor for hyaluronan) or inhibition of hyaluronan synthase 2 (the enzyme responsible for HA production).[173] The importance of fibroblast capacity to invade matrix was also demonstrated in mice where there was deletion in regulators of G-protein–coupled receptor functioning called β-arrestins. β-Arrestin null mice were protected from experimental fibrosis and both mouse and IPF fibroblasts had suppression of fibroblast invasion when β-arrestins were inhibited.[174]

TREATMENT

Treatment for IPF is discussed below. Both pharmacologic and nonpharmacologic approaches are considered.

■ PHARMACOTHERAPY

The management of patients presents several challenges, namely (1) whom to treat; (2) when to treat; and (3) how to select treatment. In IPF, selection of treatment has been a contentious issue due to lack of drugs conferring a survival benefit, physiologic improvement, or quality of life (QOL) benefit. Recently, this landscape has changed due to a combination of promising novel treatment pathways and two recent clinical trials demonstrating positive outcomes in the treatment of IPF.

Historically, treatment strategies have been directed at suppressing the inflammatory processes of IPF. This strategy was employed despite histologic evidence demonstrating that inflammation is but a meager component of this disease. Alternative therapeutic agents were then developed to inhibit cytokines, proteases, oxidants, and mesenchymal growth factors. Several clinical trials have been undertaken over recent years to study these pathways. More recently potential targets for treatment have shifted to targeted therapies directed at the specific pathways that appear to mediate fibrogenesis. The goal continues to remain to prevent the onset and progression of fibrosis as there remains little evidence to support the notion that mature fibrosis can ever be reversed.

Corticosteroids and Immunosuppressants

Corticosteroids have never been studied head-to-head against placebo to determine their benefit in treating IPF. Retrospective studies have failed to demonstrate benefit from steroid monotherapy.[175] The most recent consensus guidelines on IPF recommend against the use of steroid monotherapy for the treatment of IPF.[20] Combination immunosuppressant therapy (steroid plus azathioprine, for instance) is also lacking for evidence of efficacy. Current guidelines recommend against the use of combination immunosuppressant therapy as the limited evidence in support of its benefit does not outweigh concerns for associated morbidity and mortality with such treatment. This opinion relies heavily on new data from a trial that compared the use of prednisone and azathioprine to placebo (the PANTHER trial).[176] The study was halted early due to an excess of mortality in the arm of the trial receiving combination prednisone and azathioprine.

N-acetylcysteine

Previous studies have demonstrated both an increased oxidant burden in the epithelial-lining fluid from patients with IPF as well as diminished antioxidant capacity.[118,119] These studies formed the basis for a controlled study comparing prednisone and azathioprine to prednisone, azathioprine, and N-acetylcysteine (NAC).[177] The results of this study showed that NAC slowed the deterioration of FVC and diffusion capacity after 1 year to a statistically significant extent. There was a high dropout rate in both arms and there was no difference in mortality. In order to address these concerns, an arm of the PANTHER trial was designed to compare NAC to placebo. The results of this study failed to demonstrate a change in either the primary or secondary endpoints. These results suggest that NAC does not have a benefit in IPF patients who had evidence of mild-to-moderate impairment in pulmonary function (FVC >50% predicted and $D_{L_{CO}}$ >30% predicted). The effect on later stage disease and other interstitial lung diseases is not known.

Pirfenidone

Pirfenidone is an orally administered agent with anti-inflammatory, antioxidant, and antifibrotic properties. There is evidence to suggest that pirfenidone has efficacy in slowing the progression of IPF. The first study of pirfenidone evaluated 105 Japanese patients with IPF using a 2:1 randomization and a physiologic endpoint incorporating gas exchange with exertion.[178] The study was discontinued prematurely due to concern over excess morbidity in the placebo group though it failed to demonstrate efficacy as measured by the primary endpoint. However, there were differences in FVC at the end of the study that stimulated interest in further clinical trials. As a result of this observation, two large international efficacy trials were completed.[179] In one of these studies a statistically significant reduction in the decline of FVC was observed in the active arm (patients who took 2403 mg/d of pirfenidone daily). However, the other trial, with a nearly identical protocol, failed to demonstrate efficacy. Based on this data and the data from the Japanese trial, pirfenidone was approved for use in Japan and in the European Union. Similar approval did not occur in the United States. A new phase III trial was undertaken at the request of the United States Food and Drug Administration (FDA) to clarify the concern over the results of the CAPACITY trials. In the ASCEND trial, 555 patients with idiopathic pulmonary fibrosis were randomized to receive 2403 mg of oral pirfenidone or placebo and then followed for 52 weeks. The enrolled patients had: (1) mild to moderate functional impairment, defined by an FVC range from 50–90% perdicted; (2) $D_{L_{CO}}$ range from 30–90% predicted; (3) FEV_1/FVC >0.80; and (4) 6-minute walk distance >150 meters. In recently published data from the ASCEND trial, pirfenidone was associated with a significant reduction in the proportion of patients who had a decline of 10% or greater in their predicted FVC. Additionally, there was a significant increase in the numbers of patients who demonstrated no decline in FVC. In a combined analysis of the ASCEND and CAPACITY trials, pirfenidone was associated with a decrease in both all-cause and IPF-related mortality. On the basis of these results, pirfenidone is in the process of being re-evaluated by the FDA for approval as a therapy for IPF in the United States.

Thalidomide

Thalidomide is a drug with a variety of properties including anti-inflammatory, immunomodulatory, and antiangiogenic effects.[180–182] In animal models thalidomide has attenuated pulmonary fibrosis after bleomycin challenge.[183] When a small open label trial was performed, hoping to assess the safety and efficacy of this drug as a disease-modifying agent, a reduction of cough was serendipitously observed. This led to a follow-up randomized crossover design study in which thalidomide was shown to significantly reduce cough and improve QOL in patients with IPF.[184] Since cough is a particularly debilitating aspect of IPF this could represent a potential future therapy to impact QOL in this disease.

Tyrosine Kinase Inhibitor BIBF 1120 (Nintedanib)

BIBF 1120 is a triple tyrosine kinase inhibitor with efficacy on fibroblast growth factor (FGF), vascular endothelial growth factor (VEGF), and on platelet-derived growth factor (PDGF).[185] The activation of these pathways has been implicated in the pathogenesis of experimental fibrosis. In a 12-month phase II trial (the TOMORROW trial) patients who received 150 mg of BIBF 1120 twice daily had a trend toward reduction in the decline of FVC.[186] In addition, there was an improved QOL and a reduction in acute exacerbations of IPF. These results led to a phase III trial. This was designed as two identical phase III studies called INPULSIS-1 and INPULSIS-2. The INPULSIS trials tested the effect on IPF disease progression over 52 weeks using 150 mg of twice daily nintedanib (formerly BIBF 1200) versus placebo. The inclusion criteria included patients diagnosed with idiopathic pulmonary fibrosis based on established criteria.[20] In addition, the participants' HRCT scans and biopsies, if available, were reviewed by a central radiologist or pathologist to confirm the diagnosis. Enrolled subjects had a FVC which was >50% of the predicted value and a DL_{CO} from 30–79% of predicted values. Published data from the two trials indicated that patients who received nintedanib demonstrated a statistically significant reduction in the rate of decline in lung function compared with the placebo group. In the INPULSIS-2 trial, there was a significant reduction in the time to first acute exacerbation of IPF. This was not replicated in the INPULSIS-1 trial data. The most common side effect for the medication was diarrhea. On the basis of this study, nintedanib is pending evaluation for approval for use in the United States.

Gastroesophageal Reflux Therapy

It has been observed that IPF patients have a high prevalence of gastroesophageal reflux disease (GERD). A retrospective cohort study identified that GERD treatment in IPF patients was associated with an increased length of survival and reduced radiographic evidence of fibrosis.[187] The contribution of this observation to the pathogenesis of the disease is unknown as no rigorous prospective studies have been performed. Nevertheless, pursuing the diagnosis of GERD in IPF patients appears warranted and, when identified, treatment according to established practice guidelines is appropriate.

■ NONPHARMACOLOGIC THERAPY

The roles of lung transplantation and additional nonpharmacologic measures are presented briefly below.

Lung Transplantation

Lung transplant remains the only therapeutic intervention of proven benefit in IPF. Transplant has been reserved for patients at the advanced stages of IPF and the 5-year survival data approach 50%. However, complications of lung transplant remain common and severe. Among the most important complications and the major cause of long-term mortality following lung transplant is bronchiolitis obliterans syndrome (BOS). BOS is an enigmatic process characterized by progressive fibrosis of terminal and respiratory bronchioles leading to an inexorable decline in transplant function. New therapeutic approaches are sought to control BOS. Therapy for BOS is limited at this time.

Supplemental Oxygen

Patients with hypoxemia (Pa_{O_2} <55 mm Hg or Sp_{O_2} <88%) at rest or during exercise can be managed with supplemental oxygen. There is evidence in patients with COPD, which suggests that supplemental oxygen relieves exercise-induced hypoxemia and improves exercise performance. Studies examining QOL in patients with IPF emphasize the importance of maintaining a patient's independence and participation in physical activities. In one study that examined QOL in IPF patients, no difference was found between patients receiving supplemental oxygen compared to those who were not receiving oxygen. Thus, any concern can be put to rest that supplemental oxygen would have a deleterious effect on QOL domains such as "self-esteem," "dependence on therapy," and "body image."[188]

Pulmonary Rehabilitation

Patients with IPF should be encouraged to enroll in pulmonary rehabilitation programs. Although pulmonary rehabilitation has not yet been shown to be effective in the IPF population, recent evidence suggests the possibility of benefit from a tailored exercise program. Exercise capacity in the IPF population has been correlated with quadriceps strength, which implies that training of the lower extremities would increase exercise capacity in IPF much the same as it does in COPD.[189] Furthermore, it has been shown that overall QOL is impaired in IPF, with specific defects in areas of physical health and perceived social independence. Therefore it has been suggested that pulmonary rehabilitation programs for IPF be designed to include education and psychosocial support elements with the goal of improving coping skills affecting a better QOL.[188]

REFERENCES

1. Reynolds HY, Gail DB, Kiley JP. Interstitial lung diseases–where we started from and are now going. *Sarcoidosis Vasc Diffuse Lung Dis.* 2005;22(1):5–12.
2. Hamman L, Rich AR. Acute diffuse interstitial fibrosis of the lungs. *Bull Johns Hopkins Hosp.* 1944;74:177–212.
3. Noble PW, Homer RJ. Back to the future: historical perspective on the pathogenesis of idiopathic pulmonary fibrosis. *Am J Respir Cell Mol Biol.* 2005;33(2):113–120.
4. Rubin EH, Lubliner R. The Hamman-Rich syndrome: review of the literature and analysis of 15 cases. *Medicine.* 1957;36(4):397–463.
5. Gross P. The concept of the Hamman-Rich syndrome. A critique. *Am Rev Respir Dis.* 1962;85:828–832.
6. Sheridan LA, Harrison EG Jr, Divertie MB. The current status of idiopathic pulmonary fibrosis (Hamman-Rich Syndrome). *Med Clin North Am.* 1964;48:993–1010.
7. Scadding JG. Fibrosing alveolitis. *Br Med J.* 1964;2(5410):686.
8. Gaensler EA, Moister VB, Hamm J. Open-lung biopsy in diffuse pulmonary disease. *N Engl J Med.* 1964;270:1319–1331.
9. Liebow AA, Carrington CB. The interstitial pneumonias. In: Simon M, Potchen EJ, Lemay E, eds. *Frontiers in Pulmonary Radiology.* New York, NY: Grune and Stratton; 1969:102–141.
10. Myers JL, Veal CF Jr, Shin MS, Katzenstein AL. Respiratory bronchiolitis causing interstitial lung disease. A clinicopathologic study of six cases. *Am Rev Respir Dis.* 1987;135(4):880–884.
11. Katzenstein AL, Fiorelli RF. Nonspecific interstitial pneumonia/fibrosis. Histologic features and clinical significance. *Am J Surg Pathol.* 1994;18(2):136–147.
12. Crystal RG, Fulmer JD, Roberts WC, Moss ML, Line BR, Reynolds HY. Idiopathic pulmonary fibrosis. Clinical, histologic, radiographic, physiologic, scintigraphic, cytologic, and biochemical aspects. *Ann Intern Med.* 1976;85(6):769–788.
13. Myers JL, Katzenstein AL. Epithelial necrosis and alveolar collapse in the pathogenesis of usual interstitial pneumonia. *Chest.* 1988;94(6):1309–1311.
14. Katzenstein AL. Pathogenesis of "fibrosis" in interstitial pneumonia: an electron microscopic study. *Hum Pathol.* 1985;16(10): 1015–1024.

15. Kuhn C 3rd, Boldt J, King TE Jr, Crouch E, Vartio T, McDonald JA. An immunohistochemical study of architectural remodeling and connective tissue synthesis in pulmonary fibrosis. *Am Rev Respir Dis.* 1989;140(6):1693–1703.
16. Katzenstein A-LA, Askin FB. *Katzenstein and Askin's Surgical Pathology of Non-Neoplastic Lung Disease.* 3rd ed. Philadelphia, PA: WB Saunders; 1997.
17. Katzenstein AL, Myers JL. Idiopathic pulmonary fibrosis: clinical relevance of pathologic classification. *Am J Respir Crit Care Med.* 1998;157(4 Pt 1):1301–1315.
18. American Thoracic Society, European Respiratory Society. American Thoracic Society/European Respiratory Society International Multidisciplinary Consensus Classification of the Idiopathic Interstitial Pneumonias. This joint statement of the American Thoracic Society (ATS), and the European Respiratory Society (ERS) was adopted by the ATS board of directors, June 2001 and by the ERS Executive Committee, June 2001. *Am J Respir Crit Care Med.* 2002;165(2):277–304.
19. American Thoracic Society. Idiopathic pulmonary fibrosis: diagnosis and treatment. International consensus statement. American Thoracic Society (ATS), and the European Respiratory Society (ERS). *Am J Respir Crit Care Med.* 2000;161(2 Pt 1): 646–664.
20. Raghu G, Collard HR, Egan JJ, et al. An official ATS/ERS/JRS/ALAT statement: idiopathic pulmonary fibrosis: evidence-based guidelines for diagnosis and management. *Am J Respir Crit Care Med.* 2011;183(6):788–824.
21. Nicholson AG, Addis BJ, Bharucha H, et al. Inter-observer variation between pathologists in diffuse parenchymal lung disease. *Thorax.* 2004;59(6):500–505.
22. Olson AL, Swigris JJ. Idiopathic pulmonary fibrosis: diagnosis and epidemiology. *Clin Chest Med.* 2012;33(1):41–50.
23. Nalysnyk L, Cid-Ruzafa J, Rotella P, Esser D. Incidence and prevalence of idiopathic pulmonary fibrosis: review of the literature. *Eur Respir Rev.* 2012;21(126):355–361.
24. Johnston ID, Bleasdale C, Hind CR, Woodcock AA. Accuracy of diagnostic coding of hospital admissions for cryptogenic fibrosing alveolitis. *Thorax.* 1991;46(8):589–591.
25. Coultas DB, Hughes MP. Accuracy of mortality data for interstitial lung diseases in New Mexico, USA. *Thorax.* 1996;51(7): 717–720.
26. Coultas DB, Zumwalt RE, Black WC, Sobonya RE. The epidemiology of interstitial lung diseases. *Am J Respir Crit Care Med.* 1994;150(4):967–972.
27. Fernandez Perez ER, Daniels CE, Schroeder DR, et al. Incidence, prevalence, and clinical course of idiopathic pulmonary fibrosis: a population-based study. *Chest.* 2010;137(1):129–137.
28. Raghu G, Weycker D, Edelsberg J, Bradford WZ, Oster G. Incidence and prevalence of idiopathic pulmonary fibrosis. *Am J Respir Crit Care Med.* 2006;174(7):810–816.
29. Bjoraker JA, Ryu JH, Edwin MK, et al. Prognostic significance of histopathologic subsets in idiopathic pulmonary fibrosis. *Am J Respir Crit Care Med.* 1998;157(1):199–203.
30. Flaherty KR, Toews GB, Travis WD, et al. Clinical significance of histological classification of idiopathic interstitial pneumonia. *Eur Respir J.* 2002;19(2):275–283.
31. Nicholson AG, Colby TV, du Bois RM, Hansell DM, Wells AU. The prognostic significance of the histologic pattern of interstitial pneumonia in patients presenting with the clinical entity of cryptogenic fibrosing alveolitis. *Am J Respir Crit Care Med.* 2000;162(6):2213–2217.
32. Rudd RM, Prescott RJ, Chalmers JC, Johnston ID, Fibrosing Alveolitis Subcommittee of the Research Committee of the British Thoracic Society. British Thoracic Society Study on cryptogenic fibrosing alveolitis: Response to treatment and survival. *Thorax.* 2007;62(1):62–66.
33. King TE Jr, Schwarz MI, Brown K, et al. Idiopathic pulmonary fibrosis: relationship between histopathologic features and mortality. *Am J Respir Crit Care Med.* 2001;164(6): 1025–1032.
34. Raghu G, Brown KK, Bradford WZ, et al. A placebo-controlled trial of interferon gamma-1b in patients with idiopathic pulmonary fibrosis. *N Engl J Med.* 2004;350(2):125–133.
35. King TE Jr, Albera C, Bradford WZ, et al. Effect of interferon gamma-1b on survival in patients with idiopathic pulmonary fibrosis (INSPIRE): a multicentre, randomised, placebo-controlled trial. *Lancet.* 2009;374(9685):222–228.
36. King TE Jr, Behr J, Brown KK, et al. BUILD-1: a randomized placebo-controlled trial of bosentan in idiopathic pulmonary fibrosis. *Am J Respir Crit Care Med.* 2008;177(1):75–81.
37. von Plessen C, Grinde O, Gulsvik A. Incidence and prevalence of cryptogenic fibrosing alveolitis in a Norwegian community. *Respir Med.* 2003;97(4):428–435.
38. Navaratnam V, Fleming KM, West J, et al. The rising incidence of idiopathic pulmonary fibrosis in the U.K. *Thorax.* 2011;66 (6):462–467.
39. Ryu JH, Colby TV, Hartman TE, Vassallo R. Smoking-related interstitial lung diseases: a concise review. *Eur Respir J.* 2001;17(1): 122–132.
40. Taskar VS, Coultas DB. Is idiopathic pulmonary fibrosis an environmental disease? *Proc Am Thorac Soc.* 2006;3(4):293–298.
41. Baumgartner KB, Samet JM, Stidley CA, Colby TV, Waldron JA. Cigarette smoking: a risk factor for idiopathic pulmonary fibrosis. *Am J Respir Crit Care Med.* 1997;155(1):242–248.
42. Miyake Y, Sasaki S, Yokoyama T, et al. Occupational and environmental factors and idiopathic pulmonary fibrosis in Japan. *Ann Occup Hyg.* 2005;49(3):259–265.
43. Oh CK, Murray LA, Molfino NA. Smoking and idiopathic pulmonary fibrosis. *Pulm Med.* 2012;2012:808260.
44. Johnston I, Britton J, Kinnear W, Logan R. Rising mortality from cryptogenic fibrosing alveolitis. *BMJ.* 1990;301(6759):1017–1021.
45. Baumgartner KB, Samet JM, Coultas DB, et al. Occupational and environmental risk factors for idiopathic pulmonary fibrosis: a multicenter case-control study. Collaborating Centers. *Am J Epidemiol.* 2000;152(4):307–315.
46. Vergnon JM, Vincent M, de The G, Mornex JF, Weynants P, Brune J. Cryptogenic fibrosing alveolitis and Epstein-Barr virus: an association? *Lancet.* 1984;2(8406):768–771.
47. Jiwa M, Steenbergen RD, Zwaan FE, Kluin PM, Raap AK, van der Ploeg M. Three sensitive methods for the detection of cytomegalovirus in lung tissue of patients with interstitial pneumonitis. *Am J Clin Pathol.* 1990;93(4):491–494.
48. Irving WL, Day S, Johnston ID. Idiopathic pulmonary fibrosis and hepatitis C virus infection. *Am Rev Respir Dis.* 1993;148 (6 Pt 1):1683–1684.
49. Tang YW, Johnson JE, Browning PJ, et al. Herpesvirus DNA is consistently detected in lungs of patients with idiopathic pulmonary fibrosis. *J Clin Microbiol.* 2003;41(6):2633–2640.
50. Egan JJ, Stewart JP, Hasleton PS, Arrand JR, Carroll KB, Woodcock AA. Epstein-Barr virus replication within pulmonary epithelial cells in cryptogenic fibrosing alveolitis. *Thorax.* 1995;50(12):1234–1239.

51. Lawson WE, Crossno PF, Polosukhin VV, et al. Endoplasmic reticulum stress in alveolar epithelial cells is prominent in IPF: association with altered surfactant protein processing and herpesvirus infection. *Am J Physiol Lung Cell Mol Physiol.* 2008;294(6):L1119–L1126.
52. Mora AL, Torres-Gonzalez E, Rojas M, et al. Activation of alveolar macrophages via the alternative pathway in herpesvirus-induced lung fibrosis. *Am J Respir Cell Mol Biol.* 2006;35(4): 466–473.
53. Naik PK, Moore BB. Viral infection and aging as cofactors for the development of pulmonary fibrosis. *Expert Rev Respir Med.* 2010;4(6):759–771.
54. Garcia CK, Raghu G. Inherited interstitial lung disease. *Clin Chest Med.* 2004;25(3):421–433, v.
55. Marshall RP, Puddicombe A, Cookson WO, Laurent GJ. Adult familial cryptogenic fibrosing alveolitis in the United Kingdom. *Thorax.* 2000;55(2):143–146.
56. Steele MP, Speer MC, Loyd JE, et al. Clinical and pathologic features of familial interstitial pneumonia. *Am J Respir Crit Care Med.* 2005;172(9):1146–1152.
57. Thomas AQ, Lane K, Phillips J 3rd, et al. Heterozygosity for a surfactant protein C gene mutation associated with usual interstitial pneumonitis and cellular nonspecific interstitial pneumonitis in one kindred. *Am J Respir Crit Care Med.* 2002;165(9):1322–1328.
58. Wang Y, Kuan PJ, Xing C, et al. Genetic defects in surfactant protein A2 are associated with pulmonary fibrosis and lung cancer. *Am J Hum Genet.* 2009;84(1):52–59.
59. Armanios MY, Chen JJ, Cogan JD, et al. Telomerase mutations in families with idiopathic pulmonary fibrosis. *N Engl J Med.* 2007;356(13):1317–1326.
60. Seibold MA, Wise AL, Speer MC, et al. A common MUC5B promoter polymorphism and pulmonary fibrosis. *N Engl J Med.* 2011;364(16):1503–1512.
61. Fingerlin TE, Murphy E, Zhang W, et al. Genome-wide association study identifies multiple susceptibility loci for pulmonary fibrosis. *Nat Genet.* 2013;45(6):613–620.
62. Schwarz MI, King TE. *Interstitial Lung Disease.* 4th ed. Hamilton, Ontario; Lewiston, NY: B.C. Decker; 2003.
63. Lettieri CJ, Nathan SD, Barnett SD, Ahmad S, Shorr AF. Prevalence and outcomes of pulmonary arterial hypertension in advanced idiopathic pulmonary fibrosis. *Chest.* 2006;129 (3):746–752.
64. Grenier P, Valeyre D, Cluzel P, Brauner MW, Lenoir S, Chastang C. Chronic diffuse interstitial lung disease: diagnostic value of chest radiography and high-resolution CT. *Radiology.* 1991;179(1):123–132.
65. Mathieson JR, Mayo JR, Staples CA, Muller NL. Chronic diffuse infiltrative lung disease: comparison of diagnostic accuracy of CT and chest radiography. *Radiology.* 1989;171(1):111–116.
66. Hunninghake GW, Zimmerman MB, Schwartz DA, et al. Utility of a lung biopsy for the diagnosis of idiopathic pulmonary fibrosis. *Am J Respir Crit Care Med.* 2001;164(2): 193–196.
67. Hunninghake GW, Lynch DA, Galvin JR, et al. Radiologic findings are strongly associated with a pathologic diagnosis of usual interstitial pneumonia. *Chest.* 2003;124(4):1215–1223.
68. Raghu G, Mageto YN, Lockhart D, Schmidt RA, Wood DE, Godwin JD. The accuracy of the clinical diagnosis of new-onset idiopathic pulmonary fibrosis and other interstitial lung disease: a prospective study. *Chest.* 1999;116(5):1168–1174.
69. Veeraraghavan S, Latsi PI, Wells AU, et al. BAL findings in idiopathic nonspecific interstitial pneumonia and usual interstitial pneumonia. *Eur Respir J.* 2003;22(2):239–244.
70. Aalokken TM, Naalsund A, Mynarek G, et al. Diagnostic accuracy of computed tomography and histopathology in the diagnosis of usual interstitial pneumonia. *Acta Radiol.* 2012;53(3):296–302.
71. Flaherty KR, Travis WD, Colby TV, et al. Histopathologic variability in usual and nonspecific interstitial pneumonias. *Am J Respir Crit Care Med.* 2001;164(9):1722–1727.
72. Aziz ZA, Wells AU, Hansell DM, et al. HRCT diagnosis of diffuse parenchymal lung disease: inter-observer variation. *Thorax.* 2004;59(6):506–511.
73. Peckham RM, Shorr AF, Helman DL Jr. Potential limitations of clinical criteria for the diagnosis of idiopathic pulmonary fibrosis/cryptogenic fibrosing alveolitis. *Respiration.* 2004;71(2):165–169.
74. Selman M, Carrillo G, Estrada A, et al. Accelerated variant of idiopathic pulmonary fibrosis: clinical behavior and gene expression pattern. *PLoS One.* 2007;2(5):e482.
75. Kondoh Y, Taniguchi H, Kawabata Y, Yokoi T, Suzuki K, Takagi K. Acute exacerbation in idiopathic pulmonary fibrosis. Analysis of clinical and pathologic findings in three cases. *Chest.* 1993;103(6):1808–1812.
76. Collard HR, Moore BB, Flaherty KR, et al. Acute exacerbations of idiopathic pulmonary fibrosis. *Am J Respir Crit Care Med.* 2007;176(7):636–643.
77. Akira M, Hamada H, Sakatani M, Kobayashi C, Nishioka M, Yamamoto S. CT findings during phase of accelerated deterioration in patients with idiopathic pulmonary fibrosis. *AJR Am J Roentgenol.* 1997;168(1):79–83.
78. Ambrosini V, Cancellieri A, Chilosi M, et al. Acute exacerbation of idiopathic pulmonary fibrosis: report of a series. *Eur Respir J.* 2003;22(5):821–826.
79. Rice AJ, Wells AU, Bouros D, et al. Terminal diffuse alveolar damage in relation to interstitial pneumonias. An autopsy study. *Am J Clin Pathol.* 2003;119(5):709–714.
80. Douglas WW, Ryu JH, Schroeder DR. Idiopathic pulmonary fibrosis: Impact of oxygen and colchicine, prednisone, or no therapy on survival. *Am J Respir Crit Care Med.* 2000;161(4 Pt 1): 1172–1178.
81. Nicholson AG, Fulford LG, Colby TV, du Bois RM, Hansell DM, Wells AU. The relationship between individual histologic features and disease progression in idiopathic pulmonary fibrosis. *Am J Respir Crit Care Med.* 2002;166(2):173–177.
82. King TE Jr, Tooze JA, Schwarz MI, Brown KR, Cherniack RM. Predicting survival in idiopathic pulmonary fibrosis: scoring system and survival model. *Am J Respir Crit Care Med.* 2001;164(7):1171–1181.
83. Hubbard R, Venn A, Smith C, Cooper M, Johnston I, Britton J. Exposure to commonly prescribed drugs and the etiology of cryptogenic fibrosing alveolitis: a case-control study. *Am J Respir Crit Care Med.* 1998;157(3 Pt 1):743–747.
84. Enomoto N, Suda T, Kato M, et al. Quantitative analysis of fibroblastic foci in usual interstitial pneumonia. *Chest.* 2006;130(1):22–29.
85. Jegal Y, Kim DS, Shim TS, et al. Physiology is a stronger predictor of survival than pathology in fibrotic interstitial pneumonia. *Am J Respir Crit Care Med.* 2005;171(6):639–644.
86. Schwartz DA, Helmers RA, Galvin JR, et al. Determinants of survival in idiopathic pulmonary fibrosis. *Am J Respir Crit Care Med.* 1994;149(2 Pt 1):450–454.

87. Collard HR, King TE Jr, Bartelson BB, Vourlekis JS, Schwarz MI, Brown KK. Changes in clinical and physiologic variables predict survival in idiopathic pulmonary fibrosis. *Am J Respir Crit Care Med.* 2003;168(5):538–542.

88. Hallstrand TS, Boitano LJ, Johnson WC, Spada CA, Hayes JG, Raghu G. The timed walk test as a measure of severity and survival in idiopathic pulmonary fibrosis. *Eur Respir J.* 2005;25(1):96–103.

89. Hamada K, Nagai S, Tanaka S, et al. Significance of pulmonary arterial pressure and diffusion capacity of the lung as prognosticator in patients with idiopathic pulmonary fibrosis. *Chest.* 2007;131(3):650–656.

90. King TE Jr, Safrin S, Starko KM, et al. Analyses of efficacy end points in a controlled trial of interferon-gamma1b for idiopathic pulmonary fibrosis. *Chest.* 2005;127(1):171–177.

91. du Bois RM, Weycker D, Albera C, et al. Forced vital capacity in patients with idiopathic pulmonary fibrosis: test properties and minimal clinically important difference. *Am J Respir Crit Care Med.* 2011;184(12):1382–1389.

92. du Bois RM, Weycker D, Albera C, et al. Ascertainment of individual risk of mortality for patients with idiopathic pulmonary fibrosis. *Am J Respir Crit Care Med.* 2011;184(4):459–466.

93. Nathan SD, Shlobin OA, Weir N, et al. Long-term course and prognosis of idiopathic pulmonary fibrosis in the new millennium. *Chest.* 2011;140(1):221–229.

94. Zappala CJ, Latsi PI, Nicholson AG, et al. Marginal decline in forced vital capacity is associated with a poor outcome in idiopathic pulmonary fibrosis. *Eur Respir J.* 2010;35(4):830–836.

95. du Bois RM, Nathan SD, Richeldi L, Schwarz MI, Noble PW. Idiopathic pulmonary fibrosis: lung function is a clinically meaningful endpoint for phase III trials. *Am J Respir Crit Care Med.* 2012;186(8):712–715.

96. Raghu G, Collard HR, Anstrom KJ, et al. Idiopathic pulmonary fibrosis: clinically meaningful primary endpoints in phase 3 clinical trials. *Am J Respir Crit Care Med.* 2012;185(10): 1044–1048.

97. Wells AU, Desai SR, Rubens MB, et al. Idiopathic pulmonary fibrosis: a composite physiologic index derived from disease extent observed by computed tomography. *Am J Respir Crit Care Med.* 2003;167(7):962–969.

98. Flaherty KR, Thwaite EL, Kazerooni EA, et al. Radiological versus histological diagnosis in UIP and NSIP: survival implications. *Thorax.* 2003;58(2):143–148.

99. Watters LC, King TE, Schwarz MI, Waldron JA, Stanford RE, Cherniack RM. A clinical, radiographic, and physiologic scoring system for the longitudinal assessment of patients with idiopathic pulmonary fibrosis. *Am Rev Respir Dis.* 1986; 133(1):97–103.

100. Ley B, Ryerson CJ, Vittinghoff E, et al. A multidimensional index and staging system for idiopathic pulmonary fibrosis. *Ann Intern Med.* 2012;156(10):684–691.

101. Noble PW, Barkauskas CE, Jiang D. Pulmonary fibrosis: patterns and perpetrators. *J Clin Invest.* 2012;122(8):2756–2762.

102. Fernandez IE, Eickelberg O. New cellular and molecular mechanisms of lung injury and fibrosis in idiopathic pulmonary fibrosis. *Lancet.* 2012;380(9842):680–688.

103. Reynolds HY, Fulmer JD, Kazmierowski JA, Roberts WC, Frank MM, Crystal RG. Analysis of cellular and protein content of broncho-alveolar lavage fluid from patients with idiopathic pulmonary fibrosis and chronic hypersensitivity pneumonitis. *J Clin Invest.* 1977;59(1):165–175.

104. Weinberger SE, Kelman JA, Elson NA, et al. Bronchoalveolar lavage in interstitial lung disease. *Ann Intern Med.* 1978;89(4):459–466.

105. Watters LC, Schwarz MI, Cherniack RM, et al. Idiopathic pulmonary fibrosis. Pretreatment bronchoalveolar lavage cellular constituents and their relationships with lung histopathology and clinical response to therapy. *Am Rev Respir Dis.* 1987;135(3):696–704.

106. Haslam PL, Turton CW, Heard B, et al. Bronchoalveolar lavage in pulmonary fibrosis: comparison of cells obtained with lung biopsy and clinical features. *Thorax.* 1980;35(1):9–18.

107. Haslam PL, Turton CW, Lukoszek A, et al. Bronchoalveolar lavage fluid cell counts in cryptogenic fibrosing alveolitis and their relation to therapy. *Thorax.* 1980;35(5):328–339.

108. Bronchoalveolar lavage constituents in healthy individuals, idiopathic pulmonary fibrosis, and selected comparison groups. The BAL Cooperative Group Steering Committee. *Am Rev Respir Dis.* 1990;141(5 Pt 2):S169–S202.

109. Selman M, King TE, Pardo A, American Thoracic Society, European Respiratory Society, American College of Chest Physicians. Idiopathic pulmonary fibrosis: prevailing and evolving hypotheses about its pathogenesis and implications for therapy. *Ann Intern Med.* 2001;134(2):136–151.

110. Chilosi M, Poletti V, Murer B, et al. Abnormal re-epithelialization and lung remodeling in idiopathic pulmonary fibrosis: the role of deltaN-p63. *Lab Invest.* 2002;82(10):1335–1345.

111. Chilosi M, Poletti V, Zamo A, et al. Aberrant Wnt/beta-catenin pathway activation in idiopathic pulmonary fibrosis. *Am J Pathol.* 2003;162(5):1495–1502.

112. King TE Jr, Pardo A, Selman M. Idiopathic pulmonary fibrosis. *Lancet.* 2011;378(9807):1949–1961.

113. Kuwano K, Kawasaki M, Maeyama T, et al. Soluble form of fas and fas ligand in BAL fluid from patients with pulmonary fibrosis and bronchiolitis obliterans organizing pneumonia. *Chest.* 2000;118(2):451–458.

114. Kuwano K, Hagimoto N, Kawasaki M, et al. Essential roles of the Fas-Fas ligand pathway in the development of pulmonary fibrosis. *J Clin Invest.* 1999;104(1):13–19.

115. Kuwano K, Kunitake R, Maeyama T, et al. Attenuation of bleomycin-induced pneumopathy in mice by a caspase inhibitor. *Am J Physiol Lung Cell Mol Physiol.* 2001;280(2):L316–L325.

116. Wang R, Ibarra-Sunga O, Verlinski L, Pick R, Uhal BD. Abrogation of bleomycin-induced epithelial apoptosis and lung fibrosis by captopril or by a caspase inhibitor. *Am J Physiol Lung Cell Mol Physiol.* 2000;279(1):L143–L151.

117. Hagimoto N, Kuwano K, Inoshima I, et al. TGF-beta 1 as an enhancer of Fas-mediated apoptosis of lung epithelial cells. *J Immunol.* 2002;168(12):6470–6478.

118. Cantin AM, Hubbard RC, Crystal RG. Glutathione deficiency in the epithelial lining fluid of the lower respiratory tract in idiopathic pulmonary fibrosis. *Am Rev Respir Dis.* 1989;139(2):370–372.

119. Cantin AM, North SL, Fells GA, Hubbard RC, Crystal RG. Oxidant-mediated epithelial cell injury in idiopathic pulmonary fibrosis. *J Clin Invest.* 1987;79(6):1665–1673.

120. Saleh D, Barnes PJ, Giaid A. Increased production of the potent oxidant peroxynitrite in the lungs of patients with idiopathic pulmonary fibrosis. *Am J Respir Crit Care Med.* 1997; 155(5):1763–1769.

121. Wang R, Alam G, Zagariya A, et al. Apoptosis of lung epithelial cells in response to TNF-alpha requires angiotensin II generation de novo. *J Cell Physiol.* 2000;185(2):253–259.

122. Ortiz LA, Lasky J, Hamilton RF Jr, et al. Expression of TNF and the necessity of TNF receptors in bleomycin-induced lung injury in mice. *Exp Lung Res.* 1998;24(6):721–743.

123. Zhang Y, Lee TC, Guillemin B, Yu MC, Rom WN. Enhanced IL-1 beta and tumor necrosis factor-alpha release and messenger RNA expression in macrophages from idiopathic pulmonary fibrosis or after asbestos exposure. *J Immunol.* 1993; 150(9):4188–4196.

124. Sisson TH, Mendez M, Choi K, et al. Targeted injury of type II alveolar epithelial cells induces pulmonary fibrosis. *Am J Respir Crit Care Med.* 2010;181(3):254–263.

125. Osterholzer JJ, Christensen PJ, Lama V, et al. PAI-1 promotes the accumulation of exudate macrophages and worsens pulmonary fibrosis following type II alveolar epithelial cell injury. *J Pathol.* 2012;228(2):170–180.

126. Osterholzer JJ, Olszewski MA, Murdock BJ, et al. Implicating exudate macrophages and Ly-6 C(high) monocytes in CCR2-dependent lung fibrosis following gene-targeted alveolar injury. 2013;190(7):3447–3457.

127. Nogee LM, Dunbar AE 3rd, Wert SE, Askin F, Hamvas A, Whitsett JA. A mutation in the surfactant protein C gene associated with familial interstitial lung disease. *N Engl J Med.* 2001;344(8):573–579.

128. van Moorsel CH, van Oosterhout MF, Barlo NP, et al. Surfactant protein C mutations are the basis of a significant portion of adult familial pulmonary fibrosis in a dutch cohort. *Am J Respir Crit Care Med.* 2010;182(11):1419–1425.

129. Ono S, Tanaka T, Ishida M, et al. Surfactant protein C G100 S mutation causes familial pulmonary fibrosis in Japanese kindred*Eur Respir J.* 2011;38(4):861–869.

130. Kropski JA, Lawson WE, Young LR, Blackwell TS. Genetic studies provide clues on the pathogenesis of idiopathic pulmonary fibrosis. *Dis Model Mech.* 2013;6(1):9–17.

131. Beers MF, Lomax CA, Russo SJ. Synthetic processing of surfactant protein C by alveolar epithelial cells. The COOH terminus of proSP-C is required for post-translational targeting and proteolysis. *J Biol Chem.* 1998;273(24):15287–15293.

132. Mulugeta S, Nguyen V, Russo SJ, Muniswamy M, Beers MF. A surfactant protein C precursor protein BRICHOS domain mutation causes endoplasmic reticulum stress, proteasome dysfunction, and caspase 3 activation. *Am J Respir Cell Mol Biol.* 2005;32(6):521–530.

133. Lawson WE, Cheng DS, Degryse AL, et al. Endoplasmic reticulum stress enhances fibrotic remodeling in the lungs. *Proc Natl Acad Sci U S A.* 2011;108(26):10562–10567.

134. Torres-Gonzalez E, Bueno M, Tanaka A, et al. Role of endoplasmic reticulum stress in age-related susceptibility to lung fibrosis. *Am J Respir Cell Mol Biol.* 2012;46(6):748–756.

135. Larsen BT, Colby TV. Update for pathologists on idiopathic interstitial pneumonias. *Arch Pathol Lab Med.* 2012;136(10): 1234–1241.

136. Hinz B, Phan SH, Thannickal VJ, Galli A, Bochaton-Piallat ML, Gabbiani G. The myofibroblast: one function, multiple origins. *Am J Pathol.* 2007;170(6):1807–1816.

137. Tomasek JJ, Gabbiani G, Hinz B, Chaponnier C, Brown RA. Myofibroblasts and mechano-regulation of connective tissue remodelling. *Nat Rev Mol Cell Biol.* 2002;3(5):349–363.

138. Kuhn C, McDonald JA. The roles of the myofibroblast in idiopathic pulmonary fibrosis. Ultrastructural and immunohistochemical features of sites of active extracellular matrix synthesis. *Am J Pathol.* 1991;138(5):1257–1265.

139. Zhang K, Rekhter MD, Gordon D, Phan SH. Myofibroblasts and their role in lung collagen gene expression during pulmonary fibrosis. A combined immunohistochemical and in situ hybridization study. *Am J Pathol.* 1994;145(1):114–125.

140. Phan SH. Genesis of the myofibroblast in lung injury and fibrosis. *Proc Am Thorac Soc.* 2012;9(3):148–152.

141. Hashimoto N, Jin H, Liu T, Chensue SW, Phan SH. Bone marrow-derived progenitor cells in pulmonary fibrosis. *J Clin Invest.* 2004;113(2):243–252.

142. Phillips RJ, Burdick MD, Hong K, et al. Circulating fibrocytes traffic to the lungs in response to CXCL12 and mediate fibrosis. *J Clin Invest.* 2004;114(3):438–446.

143. Moore BB, Kolodsick JE, Thannickal VJ, et al. CCR2-mediated recruitment of fibrocytes to the alveolar space after fibrotic injury. *Am J Pathol.* 2005;166(3):675–684.

144. Quan TE, Cowper S, Wu SP, Bockenstedt LK, Bucala R. Circulating fibrocytes: collagen-secreting cells of the peripheral blood. *Int J Biochem Cell Biol.* 2004;36(4):598–606.

145. Moeller A, Gilpin SE, Ask K, et al. Circulating fibrocytes are an indicator of poor prognosis in idiopathic pulmonary fibrosis. *Am J Respir Crit Care Med.* 2009;179(7):588–594.

146. Willis BC, Liebler JM, Luby-Phelps K, et al. Induction of epithelial-mesenchymal transition in alveolar epithelial cells by transforming growth factor-beta1: potential role in idiopathic pulmonary fibrosis. *Am J Pathol.* 2005;166(5):1321–1332.

147. Yamada M, Kuwano K, Maeyama T, et al. Dual-immunohistochemistry provides little evidence for epithelial-mesenchymal transition in pulmonary fibrosis. *Histochem Cell Biol.* 2008;129(4):453–462.

148. Kim KK, Wei Y, Szekeres C, et al. Epithelial cell alpha3beta1 integrin links beta-catenin and Smad signaling to promote myofibroblast formation and pulmonary fibrosis. *J Clin Invest.* 2009;119(1):213–224.

149. Tanjore H, Xu XC, Polosukhin VV, et al. Contribution of epithelial-derived fibroblasts to bleomycin-induced lung fibrosis. *Am J Respir Crit Care Med.* 2009;180(7):657–665.

150. Rock JR, Barkauskas CE, Cronce MJ, et al. Multiple stromal populations contribute to pulmonary fibrosis without evidence for epithelial to mesenchymal transition. *Proc Natl Acad Sci U S A.* 2011;108(52):E1475–E1483.

151. Martinet Y, Rom WN, Grotendorst GR, Martin GR, Crystal RG. Exaggerated spontaneous release of platelet-derived growth factor by alveolar macrophages from patients with idiopathic pulmonary fibrosis. *N Engl J Med.* 1987;317(4):202–209.

152. Rom WN, Basset P, Fells GA, Nukiwa T, Trapnell BC, Crysal RG. Alveolar macrophages release an insulin-like growth factor I-type molecule. *J Clin Invest.* 1988;82(5):1685–1693.

153. Khalil N, Bereznay O, Sporn M, Greenberg AH. Macrophage production of transforming growth factor beta and fibroblast collagen synthesis in chronic pulmonary inflammation. *J Exp Med.* 1989;170(3):727–737.

154. Khalil N, Greenberg AH. The role of TGF-beta in pulmonary fibrosis. *Ciba Found Symp.* 1991;157:194–207; discussion 207–111.

155. Sime PJ, Xing Z, Graham FL, Csaky KG, Gauldie J. Adenovector-mediated gene transfer of active transforming growth factor-beta1 induces prolonged severe fibrosis in rat lung. *J Clin Invest.* 1997;100(4):768–776.

156. Li M, Krishnaveni MS, Li C, et al. Epithelium-specific deletion of TGF-beta receptor type II protects mice from bleomycin-induced pulmonary fibrosis. *J Clin Invest.* 2011;121(1):277–287.

157. Degryse AL, Tanjore H, Xu XC, et al. TGF-β signaling in lung epithelium regulates bleomycin-induced alveolar injury and fibroblast recruitment. *Am J Physiol Lung Cell Mol Physiol.* 2011;300(6):L887–L897.

158. Munger JS, Huang X, Kawakatsu H, et al. The integrin alpha v beta 6 binds and activates latent TGF beta 1: a mechanism for regulating pulmonary inflammation and fibrosis. *Cell.* 1999;96(3):319–328.

159. Desmouliere A, Geinoz A, Gabbiani F, Gabbiani G. Transforming growth factor-beta 1 induces alpha-smooth muscle actin expression in granulation tissue myofibroblasts and in quiescent and growing cultured fibroblasts. *J Cell Biol.* 1993;122(1):103–111.

160. Thannickal VJ, Lee DY, White ES, et al. Myofibroblast differentiation by transforming growth factor-beta1 is dependent on cell adhesion and integrin signaling via focal adhesion kinase. *J Biol Chem.* 2003;278(14):12384–12389.

161. Hecker L, Vittal R, Jones T, et al. NADPH oxidase-4 mediates myofibroblast activation and fibrogenic responses to lung injury. *Nat Med.* 2009;15(9):1077–1081.

162. Tager AM, Kradin RL, LaCamera P, et al. Inhibition of pulmonary fibrosis by the chemokine IP-10/CXCL10. *Am J Respir Cell Mol Biol.* 2004;31(4):395–404.

163. Jiang D, Liang J, Hodge J, et al. Regulation of pulmonary fibrosis by chemokine receptor CXCR3. *J Clin Invest.* 2004;114(2): 291–299.

164. Jiang D, Liang J, Campanella GS, et al. Inhibition of pulmonary fibrosis in mice by CXCL10 requires glycosaminoglycan binding and syndecan-4. *J Clin Invest.* 2010;120(6):2049–2057.

165. Tager AM, LaCamera P, Shea BS, et al. The lysophosphatidic acid receptor LPA1 links pulmonary fibrosis to lung injury by mediating fibroblast recruitment and vascular leak. *Nat Med.* 2008;14(1):45–54.

166. Mio T, Nagai S, Kitaichi M, Kawatani A, Izumi T. Proliferative characteristics of fibroblast lines derived from open lung biopsy specimens of patients with IPF (UIP). *Chest.* 1992;102(3):832–837.

167. Ramos C, Montano M, Garcia-Alvarez J, et al. Fibroblasts from idiopathic pulmonary fibrosis and normal lungs differ in growth rate, apoptosis, and tissue inhibitor of metalloproteinases expression. *Am J Respir Cell Mol Biol.* 2001;24(5): 591–598.

168. Xia H, Diebold D, Nho R, et al. Pathological integrin signaling enhances proliferation of primary lung fibroblasts from patients with idiopathic pulmonary fibrosis. *J Exp Med.* 2008; 205(7):1659–1672.

169. Schor SL. Cell proliferation and migration on collagen substrata in vitro. *J Cell Sci.* 1980;41:159–175.

170. Tian B, Lessan K, Kahm J, Kleidon J, Henke C. Beta 1 integrin regulates fibroblast viability during collagen matrix contraction through a phosphatidylinositol 3-kinase/Akt/protein kinase B signaling pathway. *J Biol Chem.* 2002;277(27):24667–24675.

171. Larsson O, Diebold D, Fan D, et al. Fibrotic myofibroblasts manifest genome-wide derangements of translational control. *PLoS One.* 2008;3(9):e3220.

172. White ES, Thannickal VJ, Carskadon SL, et al. Integrin alpha4beta1 regulates migration across basement membranes by lung fibroblasts: a role for phosphatase and tensin homologue deleted on chromosome 10. *Am J Respir Crit Care Med.* 2003; 168(4):436–442.

173. Li Y, Jiang D, Liang J, et al. Severe lung fibrosis requires an invasive fibroblast phenotype regulated by hyaluronan and CD44. *J Exp Med.* 2011;208(7):1459–1471.

174. Lovgren AK, Kovacs JJ, Xie T, et al. β-arrestin deficiency protects against pulmonary fibrosis in mice and prevents fibroblast invasion of extracellular matrix. *Sci Transl Med.* 2011;3(74): 74ra23.

175. Richeldi L, Davies HR, Ferrara G, Franco F. Corticosteroids for idiopathic pulmonary fibrosis. *Cochrane Database Syst Rev.* 2003;(3):CD002880.

176. Idiopathic Pulmonary Fibrosis Clinical Research Network, Raghu G, Anstrom KJ, King TE Jr, Lasky JA, Martinez FJ. Prednisone, azathioprine, and N-acetylcysteine for pulmonary fibrosis. *N Engl J Med.* 2012;366(21):1968–1977.

177. Demedts M, Behr J, Buhl R, et al. High-dose acetylcysteine in idiopathic pulmonary fibrosis. *N Engl J Med.* 2005;353(21): 2229–2242.

178. Azuma A, Nukiwa T, Tsuboi E, et al. Double-blind, placebo-controlled trial of pirfenidone in patients with idiopathic pulmonary fibrosis. *Am J Respir Crit Care Med.* 2005;171(9):1040–1047.

179. Noble PW, Albera C, Bradford WZ, et al. Pirfenidone in patients with idiopathic pulmonary fibrosis (CAPACITY): two randomised trials. *Lancet.* 2011;377(9779):1760–1769.

180. D'Amato RJ, Loughnan MS, Flynn E, Folkman J. Thalidomide is an inhibitor of angiogenesis. *Proc Natl Acad Sci U S A.* 1994;91(9):4082–4085.

181. Moreira AL, Sampaio EP, Zmuidzinas A, Frindt P, Smith KA, Kaplan G. Thalidomide exerts its inhibitory action on tumor necrosis factor alpha by enhancing mRNA degradation. *J Exp Med.* 1993;177(6):1675–1680.

182. Koch HP. Thalidomide and congeners as anti-inflammatory agents. *Prog Med Chem.* 1985;22:165–242.

183. Tabata C, Tabata R, Kadokawa Y, et al. Thalidomide prevents bleomycin-induced pulmonary fibrosis in mice. *J Immunol.* 2007;179(1):708–714.

184. Horton MR, Santopietro V, Mathew L, et al. Thalidomide for the treatment of cough in idiopathic pulmonary fibrosis: a randomized trial. *Ann Intern Med.* 2012;157(6):398–406.

185. Hilberg F, Roth GJ, Krssak M, et al. BIBF 1120: triple angiokinase inhibitor with sustained receptor blockade and good antitumor efficacy. *Cancer Res.* 2008;68(12):4774–4782.

186. Richeldi L, Costabel U, Selman M, et al. Efficacy of a tyrosine kinase inhibitor in idiopathic pulmonary fibrosis. *N Engl J Med.* 2011;365(12):1079–1087.

187. Lee JS, Ryu JH, Elicker BM, et al. Gastroesophageal reflux therapy is associated with longer survival in patients with idiopathic pulmonary fibrosis. *Am J Respir Crit Care Med.* 2011;184(12):1390–1394.

188. De Vries J, Kessels BL, Drent M. Quality of life of idiopathic pulmonary fibrosis patients. *Eur Respir J.* 2001;17(5): 954–961.

189. Nishiyama O, Taniguchi H, Kondoh Y, et al. Quadriceps weakness is related to exercise capacity in idiopathic pulmonary fibrosis. *Chest.* 2005;127(6):2028–2033.

CHAPTER 57

Idiopathic Interstitial Pneumonias Other Than Idiopathic Pulmonary Fibrosis

Erica L. Herzog
Ami N. Rubinowitz
Mridu Gulati

INTRODUCTION

The idiopathic interstitial pneumonias (IIPs) encompass a subcategory of interstitial lung diseases (ILDs) that pose significant diagnostic and management challenges. The general diagnostic approach to these disorders is discussed elsewhere in this textbook (Chapter 54), as is the diagnosis and management of idiopathic pulmonary fibrosis (IPF), (Chapter 56). This chapter details the classification, diagnosis, and management of non-IPF forms of IIPs including nonspecific interstitial pneumonia (NSIP), organizing pneumonia (OP), desquamative interstitial pneumonia (DIP), and respiratory bronchiolitis-associated interstitial lung disease (RB-ILD), acute interstitial pneumonia (AIP), and lymphocytic interstitial pneumonia (LIP). Historical perspectives, current definitions, and epidemiologic information will be provided along with clinical aspects, imaging, and pathologic findings. Each section ends with a discussion of current therapeutic options. This information is summarized in Table 57-1.

NONSPECIFIC INTERSTITIAL PNEUMONIA

The important entity of nonspecific interstitial pneumonia is discussed below.

DEFINITION AND HISTORICAL PERSPECTIVES

In 1994, the term "nonspecific interstitial pneumonia" (NSIP) was developed by Katzenstein and Fiorelli[1] to describe a histologic pattern that demonstrates a temporally uniform appearance of interstitial inflammation and fibrosis This definition was further refined in 1998, when Katzenstein went on to formally designate NSIP as a distinct category within the IIPs.[2] While most sources are in agreement about the presence of NSIP as a distinct *histologic* entity, the existence of NSIP as a distinct *clinical* entity remains controversial.[3–5] For example, the American Thoracic Society (ATS) reports that in one review of 193 cases of NSIP, only 67 cases (or approximately one-third) were truly idiopathic while the rest were associated with a discrete diagnosis. As a result, when a radiographic or pathologic diagnosis of NSIP is made, clinicians should search for one of the underlying conditions with which this pattern is known to be associated.

UNDERLYING DISEASE ASSOCIATIONS

Nonidiopathic NSIP is associated with a number of underlying causes.[5,6] NSIP is the most prevalent form of ILD to complicate connective tissue diseases (CTD) and as such is frequently the histologic pattern seen when ILD complicates polymyositis and dermatomyositis,[7] Sjögren syndrome,[8] and systemic sclerosis (SSc).[9] NSIP is seen in rheumatoid arthritis though far less commonly than is usual interstitial pneumonia (UIP).[10] NSIP is also encountered in the setting of hypersensitivity pneumonitis,[11] drug reactions,[12] and in some forms of familial ILD.[13] Some cases of apparently idiopathic NSIP may later develop CTD, indicating that NSIP is a forme fruste of CTD.[14]

CLINICAL PRESENTATION

NSIP most commonly affects nonsmoking middle-aged adults between 40 and 60 years of age and has a female predilection.[1,4,15] Like most other IIPs, NSIP tends to present with the subacute onset of dyspnea and cough. Lung examination frequently reveals bilateral crackles though in some settings lungs will be clear. Extrapulmonary examination may provide clues to an underlying CTD (Chapter 60). For example, the presence of a heliotrope rash, shawl-like rash, and digital edema/desquamation (the so-called "mechanic's hands") suggests underlying dermatomyositis. The presence of telangiectasis, calcinosis, and sclerodactyly suggests a diagnosis of scleroderma. The presence of joint effusions and radial deviation of the MCP joints suggests an underlying diagnosis of rheumatoid arthritis. Clubbing is seen only rarely.

Patients sometimes present without an established diagnosis. In this case, a complete history regarding occupational, environmental, and medication exposures must be obtained. In addition, because idiopathic NSIP is frequently associated with CTD, an exhaustive rheumatologic history should be obtained. This includes questions regarding the presence of arthralgias, swallowing difficulties, myopathic symptoms, rash and mechanic's hands commonly encountered in antisynthetase syndrome, ocular and/or salivary gland dryness associated with Sjögren syndrome, and Raynaud phenomenon and swallowing difficulties that are characteristic of SSc. While most sources recommend serologic testing in the diagnosis of NSIP, there exist no standardized practice guidelines in this area. At minimum, ANA and rheumatoid factor should be ordered, along with extractable nuclear antigens (which include Jo-1 and Scl-70) and anticyclic citrullinated peptide (anti-CCP). Serum creatine phosphokinase (CPK) and aldolase are useful in the diagnosis of myositis. Because hypersensitivity pneumonitis may also present with NSIP, antigen testing for mold or birds is sometimes performed though the clinical relevance of a positive (or negative) test is unclear and as such these tests are insufficient for diagnostic purposes.

PULMONARY FUNCTION TESTING

Pulmonary function testing demonstrates a restrictive ventilatory defect characterized by a preserved FEV_1/FVC ratio and a depressed FVC, TLC, and DL_{CO}. The presence of obstructive physiology should raise suspicion of an alternate or superimposed diagnosis.

CHEST IMAGING

The imaging appearance of NSIP may vary, depending on if it is cellular, fibrotic, or mixed. Chest radiograph may be normal in patients with early disease or show nonspecific interstitial markings and ground-glass opacities mostly in the lower lobes with more advanced disease. Distribution of disease at CT is typically peripheral and lower lobe predominant, but may also involve the upper lobes without an obvious apicobasal gradient and can be patchy or peribronchovascular in distribution as well.[16–19] The most common CT findings include ground-glass density and reticular markings with or without traction bronchiectasis (Figs. 57-1 and 57-2). Honeycombing is sometimes seen in fibrotic NSIP but is usually not the dominant feature.[18,19]

PATHOLOGY

When a tissue biopsy is required for diagnosis of NSIP, video-assisted thoracoscopic surgery (VATS) is the procedure of choice because this approach yields sufficient tissue to accurately diagnose the IIPs. The original description of NSIP categorizes its temporally uniform appearance of fibrosis and inflammation into three groups:

TABLE 57-1 Key Features of Idiopathic Interstitial Pneumonias

Features	IPF/UIP	NSIP	COP	AIP	DIP/RB-ILD	LIP
Mean age of onset	60s	50s	50s	50s	40s	50s
Duration of illness	Chronic	Subacute to chronic	Subacute	Acute	Subacute to chronic	Chronic
Frequency of diagnosis	47–64%	14–36%	4–12%	Rare	10–17%	Rare
Smoking	Up to 2/3	Uncommon	Up to 1/2	Unknown	Most	Unknown
HRCT	Peripheral, subpleural; basilar predominant; reticular opacities; traction bronchiectasis architectural distortion and honeycombing	Peripheral, subpleural; basal, symmetric; ground-glass opacities, reticular markings, traction bronchiectasis	Patchy, bilateral, subpleural and peribronchovascular consolidation	Diffuse consolidation and ground-glass opacities often with lobular sparing	DIP: peripheral or diffuse ground-glass opacities, reticular markings, +/− small cysts RB-ILD: bronchial wall thickening; centrilobular nodules; patchy ground-glass opacity	Diffuse; centrilobular nodules; ground-glass opacities; septal thickening; thin-walled cysts
Key pathologic features	Variegated temporal appearance; scant inflammation; patchy fibrosis; fibroblastic foci; honeycomb change	Uniform temporal appearance; prominent inflammation; variable, diffuse fibrosis; rare honeycomb	Uniform temporal appearance; moderate inflammation; intra-alveolar (Masson bodies) fibroblast proliferation; foamy macrophages	Structural cell death responses; acute inflammation; hyaline membranes may be present	Uniform temporal appearance DIP: diffuse variable moderate fibrosis with diffuse intra-alveolar macrophage accumulation RB-ILD: peribronchilar intra-alveolar macrophage accumulation with only focal, mild fibrosis	Diffuse interstitial infiltration, infiltrates comprises T and/or B cell lymphocytes, plasma cells, macrophages, lymphoid hyperplasia
Prognosis	50–70% mortality in 5 y	<10% mortality in 5 y	Rare deaths	50–60% mortality at 1 mo	5% mortality in 5 y	Not well defined
Response to steroids	Poor response	Responsive (particularly cellular)	Responsive	Unknown	Responsive	Not well defined

Source: Data from American Thoracic Society/European Respiratory Society International Multidisciplinary Consensus Classification of the Idiopathic Interstitial Pneumonias. This joint statement of the American Thoracic Society (ATS), and the European Respiratory Society (ERS) was adopted by the ATS board of directors, June 2001 and by the ERS Executive Committee. 2001. Am J Respir Crit Care Med. 2002;165(2):277–304.

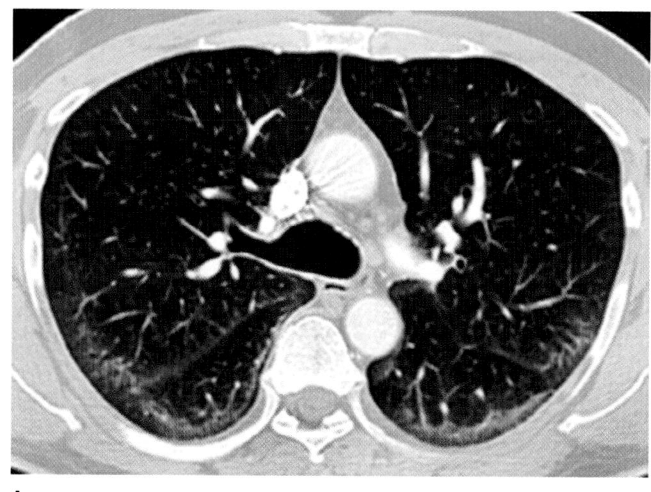

A

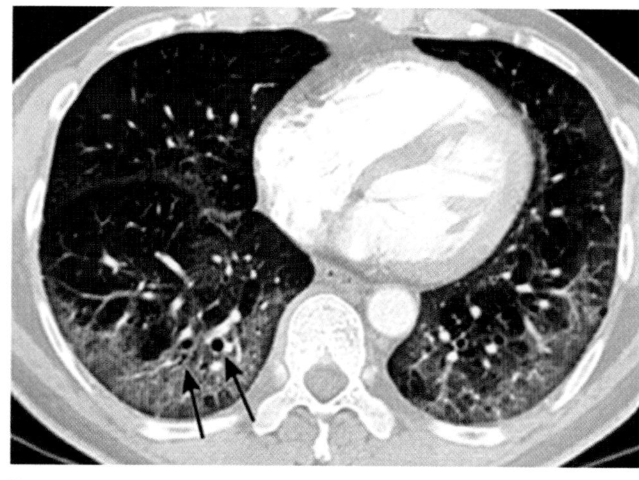

B

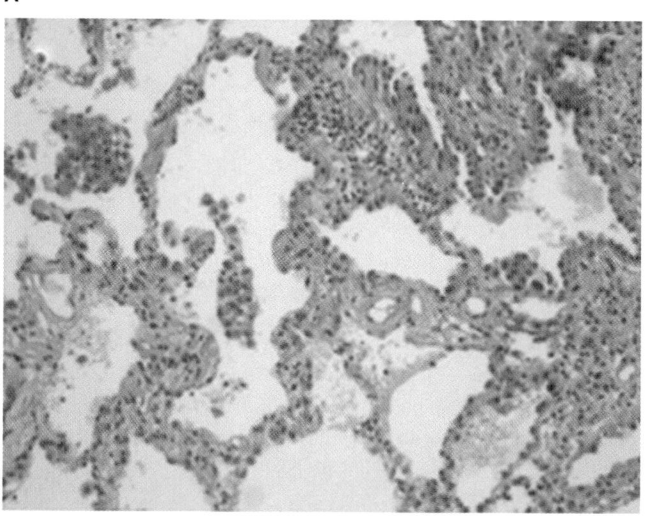

C

Figure 57-1 A 60-year-old male with antisynthetase syndrome and cellular nonspecific interstitial pneumonia (NSIP). High-resolution CT images through the upper (**A**) and lower (**B**) thorax demonstrate peripheral and lower lobe predominant ground-glass opacities with mild reticular markings and minimal traction bronchiectasis *(arrows)*. **C.** Open lung biopsy revealed temporally uniform septal thickening and inflammation consistent with a cellular NSIP. *(Pathology images used with permission of Robert J. Homer, MD, PhD, Yale School of Medicine.)*

those dominated by active inflammation (later called, "cellular" NSIP [Fig. 57-1]), those dominated by established fibrosis (later called, "fibrotic" NSIP [Fig. 57-2]), and those demonstrating a combination of inflammation and fibrosis (later called, "mixed" NSIP.[1])

CLINICAL COURSE, OUTCOME, AND TREATMENT

Patients with NSIP demonstrate a good to fair prognosis as shown by several studies. Those individuals with cellular NSIP can expect 74% survival at 5 years[20] and this specific pathologic pattern is associated with reduced event-free survival compared to the fibrotic forms.[21] Similarly, radiographic changes that would be expected to accompany fibrotic NSIP such as honeycombing have been associated with reduced survival, as have progressive dyspnea and desaturation during 6-minute walk test.[20]

PHARMACOLOGIC THERAPY

Immunosuppression is commonly employed in the management of NSIP but the lack of prospective, randomized controlled trials in this area means that evidence for a therapeutic effect of these agents is lacking. For cases of exposure-related NSIP related to drugs or inhalations, cessation of the offending agent is the initial treatment strategy. In very mild situations this intervention may be sufficient but oftentimes patients with significant disease burden radiographically or physiologically require treatment with systemically administered immunosuppressive agents. Patients with arterial hypoxemia at rest or during exercise require the administration of supplemental oxygen. Patients with exercise impairment may benefit from pulmonary rehabilitation. Finally, due to the rapid deterioration that is sometimes encountered in patients with NSIP, referral for orthotopic lung transplantation (OLT) should be considered for any eligible patient.

The use of immunosuppression is based on the rationale that the inflammation seen on pathology at least partially contributes to disease. Most of the immunosuppressive agents used to treat NSIP have not been formally evaluated in prospective, randomized clinical trials and all of them have significant toxicities. Thus, the decision to embark upon a course of immunosuppression should be considered in light of the risk–benefit ratio. Similarly, when treating a patient with NSIP in the setting of CTD, the management of these medications is best performed with the patient's rheumatologist because since the pulmonary and systemic involvement may demonstrate independent responses, systemic effects must be monitored as well. Patients should be seen frequently and should have lab monitored monthly in order that serious and potentially fatal side effects can be recognized in a timely fashion.

Corticosteroids

Despite a lack of clinical trials in this area, expert opinion recommends a trial of corticosteroid therapy in patients with NSIP. Patients are typically treated with 1 mg/kg per ideal body weight of oral prednisone for several months and then assessed for evidence of objective response on PFTs or HRCT.[16] The side effects of steroid therapy are well-known and include diabetes, bone complications, cataracts, hypertension, weight gain, and opportunistic infection so patients should be followed closely with serial monitoring blood chemistry and CBC. Due to these

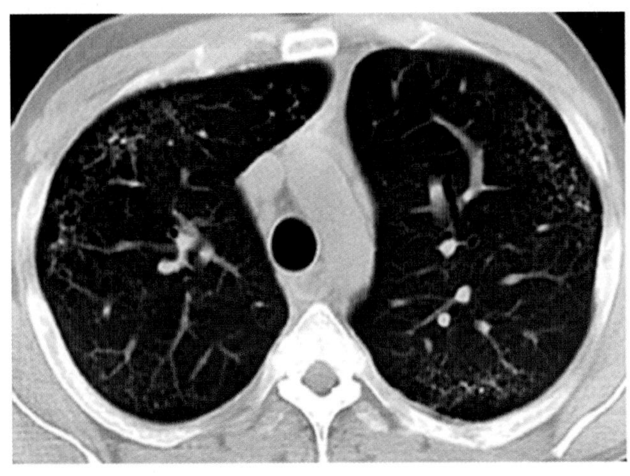
A

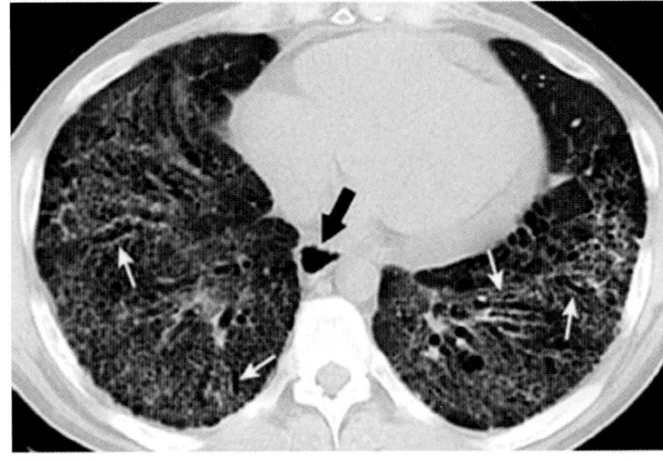
B

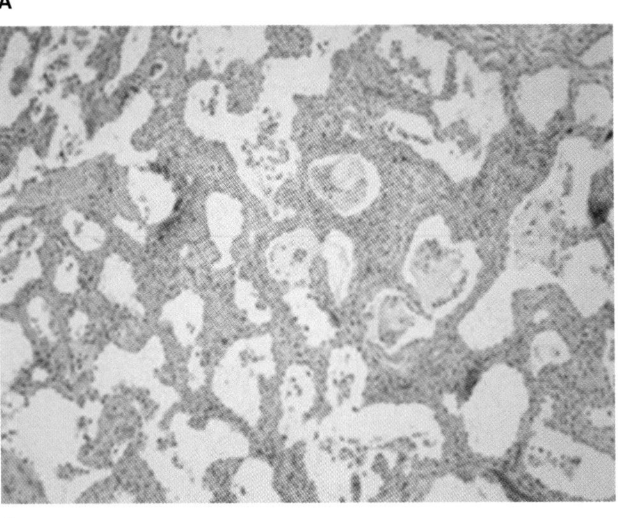
C

Figure 57-2 A 41-year-old male with fibrotic NSIP secondary to scleroderma. Axial CT images through the upper (**A**) and lower (**B**) thorax demonstrate extensive lower lobe predominant fibrotic changes with coarse reticular markings and traction bronchiectasis *(white arrows)*. Note also the presence of a dilated esophagus *(black arrow)*. The constellation of findings is compatible with a fibrotic NSIP pattern secondary to scleroderma. **C.** This patient eventually underwent lung transplantation and pathologic examination of the explanted lung revealed diffuse septal thickening and fibrosis with little inflammation, consistent with fibrotic NSIP. *(Pathology images used with permission of Robert J. Homer, MD, PhD, Yale School of Medicine.)*

toxicities, every attempt to transition the patient to a steroid-sparing agent is made once the patient has responded to therapy.

Azathioprine

Azathioprine is a commonly used alternate therapy used in patients with NSIP. The evidence for this approach derives from an early study of subjects with IIPs in which a small subset comprised in part of patients with NSIP were found to improve. There have since then been no large-scale clinical trials in this area though one small case series found that patients with fibrotic NSIP experienced improved outcomes when treated with combination therapy of prednisone and azathioprine.[20] Because azathioprine carries several risks including bone-marrow suppression and hepatotoxicity most centers perform genotyping for thiopurine methyltransferase prior to initiation of therapy and when a mutation is uncovered reduce dosage accordingly though evidence for this approach is currently lacking.

Cyclophosphamide

Cyclophosphamide (Cytoxan™) is used in patients with significant or rapidly progressive lung involvement. In a prospective study comparing patients with confirmed fibrotic NSIP versus those with UIP/IPF receiving pulse therapy with methylprednisolone followed by low-dose prednisone and cyclophosphamide, 33% of subjects with NSIP improved with steroids alone and 66% improved with combined therapy. In contrast, only 15% of the subjects with UIP/IPF demonstrated clinical improvement at either timepoint.[22] Further suggestion of efficacy was provided by a small retrospective study in which patients with known or suspected NSIP showed stabilization of lung function following 6 months of therapy. Perhaps the best evidence for a therapeutic benefit of Cytoxan™ was seen in patients with SSc-ILD (most of whom have NSIP) randomized to placebo or Cytoxan™. A small but significant improvement in lung function was noted in those subjects assigned to the treatment arm[23] though subsequent analysis found this effect to dissipate after 2 years.[24] Because cyclophosphamide is associated with many side effects including bone-marrow suppression, hemorrhagic cystitis, and the long-term risk of bladder cancer and hematologic malignancies, its use is reserved for severe and progressive cases of NSIP and it is recommended that it only be used by experienced practitioners with appropriate monitoring.

Other Immunosuppressive Agents

Several case series indicate that mycophenolate mofetil (MMF) may be efficacious in delaying lung function decline in patients with SSc-ILD.[25,26] Because most of these patients have NSIP, these studies are viewed as providing direct evidence of a potential role for MMF in the management of this form of ILD. A large-scale randomized controlled trial of MMF versus cyclophosphamide is currently underway in for the treatment of SSc-ILD. MMF is started at 500 mg b.i.d. and titrated up to a maximum dosage of 2000 mg b.i.d. This agent is pregnancy category D due to its teratogenic potential. A role for tacrolimus in the treatment of NSIP is supported by one retrospective series[27] of patients with polymyositis- and dermatomyositis-related ILD. However, because no large-scale studies have been performed, consideration of this agent for the treatment of NSIP should be considered on a case-by-case basis and patients should be managed with physicians who are experienced in the interpretation of serum levels. The most feared side effect is renal toxicity, which can in some cases be permanent and lead to kidney failure.

CRYPTOGENIC ORGANIZING PNEUMONIA

The entity of cryptogenic organizing pneumonia was described over 30 years ago. Important clinical aspects and associations are described below.

DEFINITION AND HISTORICAL PERSPECTIVES

First described by Davison[28] and Epler[29] in the early 1980s, cryptogenic organizing pneumonia (COP) was categorized as an IIP in a 2002 working group sponsored by the ATS and the European Respiratory Society (ERS).[16] The pathologic hallmark of COP consists of whorls of myofibroblasts and inflammatory cells in a connective tissue matrix within the distal airspaces. This nonspecific pathologic pattern is termed "organizing pneumonia" and is found in a variety of settings such as in the context of infection, drug toxicity, posttransplant, radiation exposure, or rheumatologic conditions. Therefore, it is only in the absence of an associated condition or inciting factor that clinicians may establish a diagnosis of COP. Thus, the diagnosis of COP rests on an integrated assessment of clinical symptoms, radiographic patterns, compatible histopathologic features, when available, and the exclusion of other associated causes and conditions.

The pathology was initially called "bronchiolitis obliterans organizing pneumonia" (BOOP) and this term initially dominated the North American literature and was included in the seminal paper by Katzenstein and Myers in 1998.[30] Given clinical confusion between the term BOOP and the distinct airway-centered disease of bronchiolitis obliterans syndrome ("BOS"), the terminology was changed in 2002. However, because many cases of COP are associated with an underlying etiology, the inclusion of COP as an "idiopathic" interstitial pneumonia has also been confusing for some. Perhaps most perplexing to clinicians is the fact that the disease in COP dominates the airspaces and not the interstitium. However, the working group justified the inclusion of COP within the IIPs because in clinical practice COP is part of the differential diagnosis of other IIPs, and because interstitial inflammation and fibrosis may be present in COP.

CLINICAL PRESENTATION

Similar to other IIPs, the epidemiology of COP is not well characterized though it seems to affect both genders equally with a mean age of onset of 58 years. Nonsmokers or former smokers may be affected more frequently than current smokers.[31] The classic presentation of COP includes an initial prodromal flu-like illness and symptoms of fever, cough, and dyspnea. Complaints such as hemoptysis, chest pain, arthralgias, or myalgias are uncommon. Chest auscultation may be clear or may reveal crackles. Patients are frequently treated with multiple courses of antibiotics before being diagnosed. The presence of systemic symptoms and/or findings consistent with CTD should lead to careful investigation for an associated underlying disease.[32]

UNDERLYING ASSOCIATIONS

A diagnosis of *COP* requires exclusion of associated causes. It has been suggested that gastroesophageal reflux with silent aspiration may play a role in the development of OP; however, this association has not been firmly established.[33] Many viral, bacterial, fungal, and parasitic infections have been implicated[31,34] as has influenza A H1N1 flu.[35] OP is a frequently encountered manifestation of drug-induced lung disease caused by antibiotics such as nitrofurantoin, medications such as phenytoin, amiodarone, sulfasalazine,[36] and illicit drugs such as cocaine.[37] Occupational exposures are also associated with an OP pattern of lung injury including but not limited to the aerosolized textile dye Acramin FWN, titanium nanoparticles in paint, and certain chemicals used in spice processing.[38–40] OP has been reported in patients with dermatomyositis-polymyositis[41–46] as well as other conditions such as rheumatoid arthritis,[47–49] scleroderma,[50–52] and systemic lupus erythematosus.[53–55] Rheumatologic serologies can be helpful in identifying the presence of disease because this form of lung injury may present as the initial manifestation of systemic disease. OP may be present in other inflammatory diseases such as in patients with Crohn's disease and ulcerative colitis.[56] Radiotherapy treatment is also associated with the development of OP particularly after treatment for breast cancer 3 to 6 months following therapy. Compared to radiation pneumonitis which is fairly well circumscribed and characterized by retracted lung and traction bronchiectasis, postradiotherapy OP occurs diffusely, is migratory, and is highly steroid responsive.[57] OP can also occur following transplantation of lung or bone marrow. While BOS is the most commonly reported lung injury pattern in patients experiencing lung transplant rejection, OP patterns have also been described.[58,59] Similarly, bone-marrow transplant recipients may develop OP as a manifestation of transplant rejection, graft-versus-host disease, or idiopathic pneumonia syndrome.[60–62] OP can also complicate malignant or hematologic conditions such as various forms of acute and chronic leukemias and lymphomas.[63]

PULMONARY FUNCTION TESTING

Similar to other IIPs, a restrictive ventilatory defect, characterized by a reduction in total lung capacity is generally present. In a subset of patients, an obstructive ventilatory defect can be found. Hypoxemia is typically mild although in a subgroup of patients with infiltrative opacities severe hypoxemia may be seen.[64,65]

CHEST IMAGING

OP displays a variable imaging appearance. The CXR usually shows nonspecific patchy areas of consolidation. Sometimes the imaging appearance mimics infectious pneumonia with lobar consolidation that is unresponsive to antibiotics. Peripheral, patchy, and peribronchovascular areas of ground-glass opacity and consolidation are the most classic CT appearance (Fig. 57-3).[16,17,66] Nodular areas of ground glass and consolidation as well as fleeting or migratory areas of consolidation can also be seen with OP.[16,17,66] Findings suggestive of fibrosis such as reticulation, architectural distortion, traction bronchiectasis, and honeycombing are not typically present with this entity. An area of ground-glass opacity surrounded by a rim of increased density, also known as the atoll (or reverse-halo) sign, when present, is strongly suggestive of OP[66] but can also be present with other entities such as vasculitis, certain infections, or pulmonary infarction.

PATHOLOGY

When the clinical presentation and chest imaging is insufficient for a confident diagnosis of COP, bronchoscopy with transbronchial biopsy or surgical lung biopsy can be employed. Bronchoalveolar lavage (BAL) typically reveals significant accumulation of lymphocytes, neutrophils, and eosinophils. Transbronchial biopsies may be performed to make a diagnosis; however, the quantity of lung tissue obtained during these procedures is quite small and may be insufficient to fully evaluate the spectrum of pathology that may exist within the lung parenchyma.[67–69] Thus, larger lung tissue specimens obtained by VATS are frequently used to provide the opportunity for more thorough analyses.

The pathology of OP is characterized by intraluminal plugs of inflammatory debris within the alveolar ducts and surrounding alveoli. The plugs consist of buds of granulation tissue, whorls of fibroblasts and myofibroblasts in a connective tissue matrix referred to as Masson bodies (Fig. 57-3). OP patterns can be seen concomitantly in patients with NSIP or UIP and may in certain patients represent an exacerbation of underlying ILD. In this setting, interpretation of the pathology in the context of the radiographic and clinical features can greatly aid in accurate diagnosis.

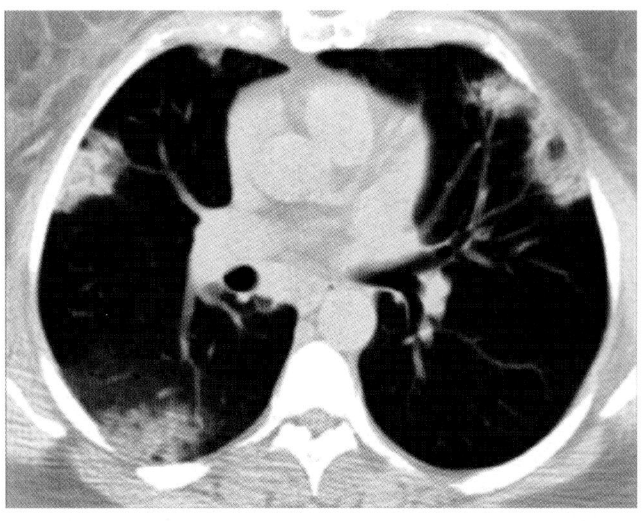
A

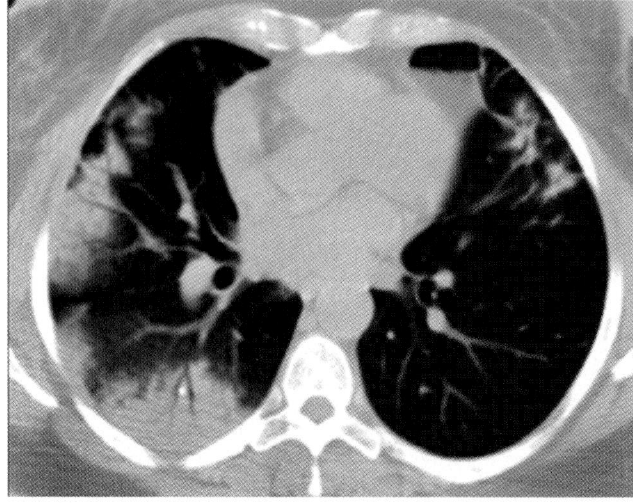
B

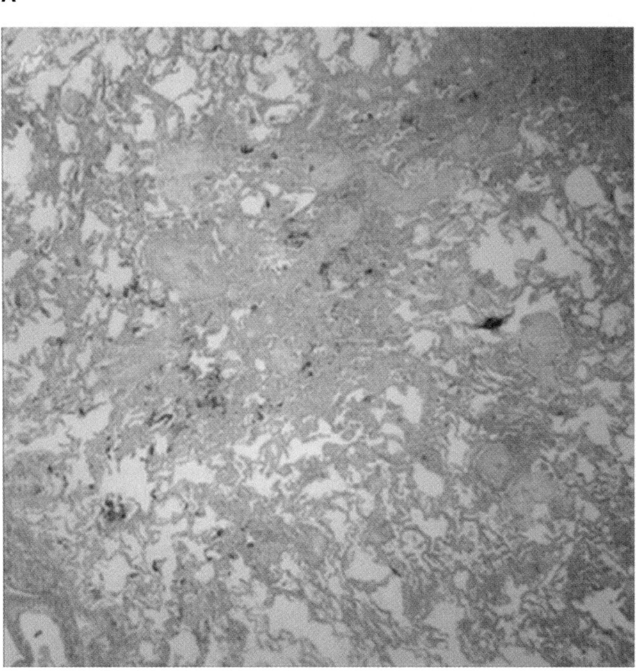
C

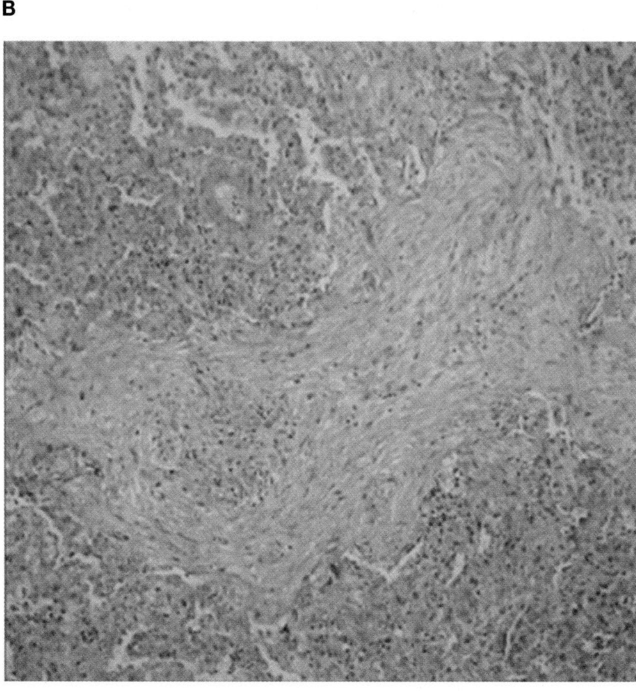
D

Figure 57-3 A 50-year-old female with cough and dyspnea secondary to organizing pneumonia (OP). Axial CT images through the mid (**A**) and mid to lower (**B**) thorax demonstrate multifocal, peripheral areas of consolidation with a distribution compatible with OP. Low (**C**) and high (**D**) power views of lung tissue from this patient reveal a patchy organizing pneumonia pattern of exudates, fibroblasts, and inflammatory cells. *(Pathology images used with permission of Robert J. Homer, MD, PhD, Yale School of Medicine.)*

■ CLINICAL COURSE, OUTCOME, AND TREATMENT

Patients with mild or asymptomatic disease may not require treatment.[70] When compared to other fibrotic lung diseases such as IPF, COP is impressively steroid responsive though a significant proportion of patients, ranging from 13% to 58%, experience relapse. Fortunately, relapses are not associated with poorer long-term outcomes and death is very infrequent.

■ PHARMACOLOGIC THERAPY

Historically, a 6-month course of treatment has been advised. More recently, shorter 3-month durations of corticosteroids have been recommended to avoid unnecessarily prolonged courses of steroids in patients who do not relapse.[32] Macrolide antibiotics[71] and steroid-sparing agents[72,73] have been used as alternative immunosuppressants for individuals with COP or secondary OP. However, the clinical utility of these approaches has not been completely validated. It is not known whether individuals with secondary causes of OP experience different long-term outcomes from individuals with COP.

While the majority of COP patients have favorable prognosis, a subset of patients present with a rapidly progressive and fatal form of OP. Some investigators have suggested that such cases represent an overlap group with acute interstitial pneumonia or acute respiratory distress syndrome (ARDS). In another series, AFOP, an acute fibrinous organizing pneumonia pattern was reported. In AFOP, organizing pneumonia and intra-alveolar fibrin balls are present.[74] Nonetheless, the literature does suggest that a small subgroup of COP patients suffer a progressive fibrotic course. Alternative forms of immunosuppression such as cyclophosphamide have been used in such rapidly deteriorating patients though experience with this approach is at best limited and the clinical utility is not entirely clear.[72]

RESPIRATORY BRONCHIOLITIS-ASSOCIATED INTERSTITIAL LUNG DISEASE AND DESQUAMATIVE INTERSTITIAL PNEUMONIA

The entities of respiratory bronchiolitis-associated interstitial lung disease and desquamative interstitial pneumonia are part of a spectrum of disorders affecting smokers. Important clinical and pathologic considerations in these two entities are described below.

DEFINITION AND HISTORICAL PERSPECTIVES

While regarded clinically as two discrete forms of IIPs, RB-ILD and DIP are generally thought of as representing ends of a continuous spectrum of disease primarily affecting tobacco smokers. The diagnostic distinction persists due to evidence indicating that RB-ILD and DIP have divergent natural histories and prognoses. The pathologic hallmark of both diseases features cytoplasmic accumulation of golden-brown pigment in macrophages. RB-ILD pathology appears to reflect inhalational exposure as findings center around the bronchioles with peribronchiolar inflammation and fibrosis. In contrast, DIP involves the airways but also extends into the alveolar space and may even include mild to moderate associated interstitial fibrosis. Because RB-ILD and DIP reactions are frequent and often incidental findings in the lung tissue of smokers, formal clinical diagnosis of RB-ILD or DIP hinges upon the presence of symptomatic, radiographic, and functional impairment. Taken together, DIP and RB-ILD account for up to 15% to 20% of patients with biopsied IIPs.[75–78]

CLINICAL PRESENTATION

Patients diagnosed with RB-ILD and DIP are typically males in the fourth or fifth decade of life with an average 30 pack-year smoking history. Affected patients report nonspecific complaints of progressive dyspnea and nonproductive cough. Physical examination may be normal but might reveal dry inspiratory crackles and clubbing as seen in other forms of ILDs. Extrapulmonary findings are usually absent.

UNDERLYING ASSOCIATIONS

Tobacco smoke exposure accounts for the most cases of RB-ILD and DIP, despite their categorization as "IIPs." In fact, it has been reported that up to 90% of RB-ILD and DIP cases are causatively linked to tobacco smoke.[75] However, in one review of 49 cases, it was noted that only 60% of DIP patients versus 93% of RB-ILD patients had a prior smoking history.[79] Although the lower prevalence of smoking in this study compared to prior studies may reflect referral bias, investigators should remain cognizant that such pathologies can occur independently of smoking. When viewed in this light, it is relevant that a number of exposures have been reported in association with DIP such as marijuana smoking, diesel fume, beryllium, copper, fire extinguisher powder, asbestos, and certain chemicals used to process textiles.[79–82] DIP has also been reported as a complication of autoimmune disorders including rheumatoid arthritis and scleroderma[50,52,80,83] and has occurred in association with infections such as hepatitis C, cytomegalovirus, and aspergillus.[84–86] Finally, idiopathic DIP has also been reported.[79] Genetic factors seem unlikely to play a dominant role; however, a few studies particularly among children and sibling studies have implicated genetic abnormalities of surfactant function, such as mutations in SP-B, SP-C, and ABCA-3 genes[87–89] though the applicability of these studies to the adult IIPs described herein remain uncertain. The difficulty in determining the contribution of other exposures may occur because when evaluating individuals with a smoking history, clinical providers dismiss the possible contribution of alternate etiologies. Furthermore, since many individuals with conditions such as rheumatologic disease do not proceed to lung biopsy, the specific underlying pathology of the associated IIP may remain unconfirmed and individuals may be assumed to have NSIP.

PULMONARY FUNCTION TESTING

Patients with RB-ILD often manifest a restrictive physiologic pattern with concomitant reduction in DL_{CO}. However, given the bronchiolocentric nature of the pathology, a mixed pattern with some elements of obstruction may also be seen. DIP patients generally demonstrate restrictive ventilatory defects along with reductions in diffusion capacity. Hypoxemia may be seen in more severely affected patients. On occasion spirometry and lung volume impairments seem less severe compared to the patient's clinical status. This phenomenon may be due to the mixed or obstructive patterns seen due to the airway-centered nature of RB-ILD or concomitant smoking-related lung pathologies such as chronic obstructive pulmonary disease (COPD).

CHEST IMAGING

The imaging findings of RB-ILD are usually subtle and not visualized on CXR. CT findings include subtle, mild diffuse or upper lobe predominant, centrilobular ground-glass nodules, and patchy ground-glass densities (Fig. 57-4).[16,17,90,91] Ancillary findings associated with cigarette smoking may also be present such as bronchial wall thickening from chronic bronchitis and tissue rarefaction and bullae reflecting emphysema. The main alternative diagnosis in a patient with centrilobular ground-glass nodules on CT is subacute hypersensitivity pneumonitis. However, the ground-glass nodules with hypersensitivity pneumonitis are usually not as subtle as those seen with RB-ILD. Similar to the CXR findings in RB-ILD, the CXR in DIP are usually quite faint and although sometimes hazy, nonspecific, ground-glass opacities may be present. Ground-glass opacities that are usually peripherally located (Fig. 57-5), but which can also be diffuse, are the most common finding seen on CT.[26,62,86,87] Other CT findings include reticular markings and small cysts, which may indicate a component of fibrosis[26,62,86,87] can be seen but more extensive fibrotic changes such as traction bronchiectasis and honeycombing are rare. In addition, bronchial wall thickening and emphysema may be seen here as well.[87] When peripheral ground-glass opacities exist in this disease, the differential diagnosis includes NSIP, OP, and chronic eosinophilic pneumonia.

PATHOLOGY

The diagnosis of RB-ILD and DIP hinges upon a comprehensive clinical assessment integrating history, physical examination, PFTs, and HRCT. Because the histopathology of DIP and RB-ILD may exist in the lung tissue of asymptomatic smokers, pathology alone does is not diagnostic. Bronchoscopy may have a role in ruling out other processes resembling RB-ILD or DIP. BAL reveals characteristic pigmented macrophages. A pronounced eosinophilia has also been reported in the BAL specimens of some DIP patients. Investigators have suggested that in the appropriate clinical setting and BAL profile, transbronchial biopsy showing RB may be sufficient to support the diagnosis of RB-ILD. Nonetheless, for both RB-ILD and DIP surgical lung biopsy may be necessary to formally establish the diagnosis as well as exclude alternative causes.

The pathologic hallmark of RB-ILD and DIP centers around the accumulation of pigmented macrophages, commonly referred to as smoker's macrophages. These macrophages contain iron and display glassy eosinophilic cytoplasm with a finely granular, yellowish-brown pigment that likely contains components of tobacco smoke. In heavy smokers, the pigmentation may become coarser making the distinction from hemosiderin deposition seen in chronic alveolar hemorrhage more challenging.[79,92] Clinicians must also differentiate the common pathologic finding of respiratory bronchiolitis (RB), first described by Niewoehner in 1974, from the specific disease entity referred to as RB-ILD.[93] In the 1980s, Myers described the phenomena of RB-ILD characterized by the intensified RB response.[94] Lung tissue from RB-ILD may demonstrate a chronic inflammatory

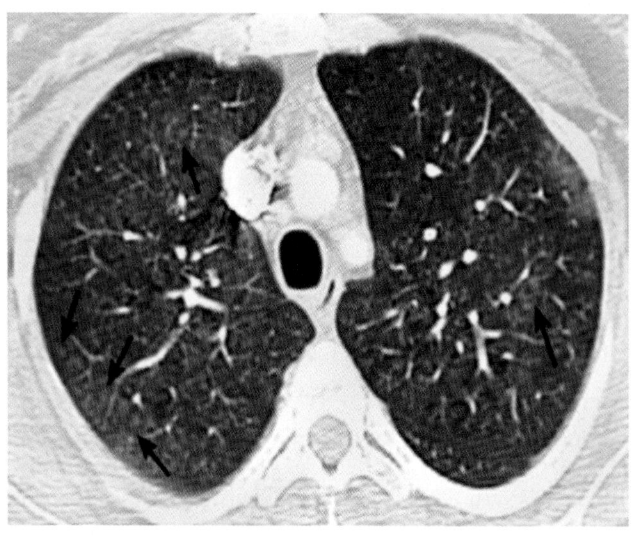
A

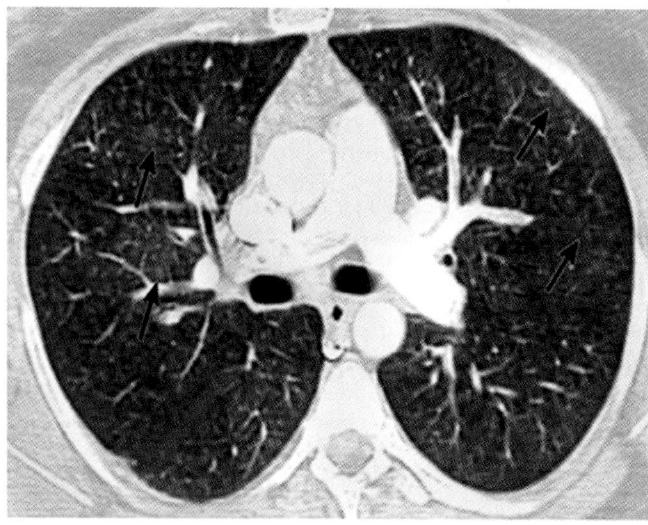
B

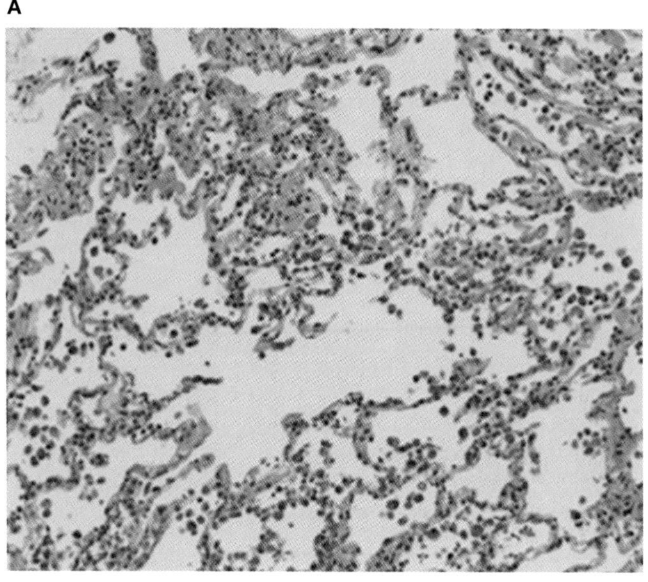
C

Figure 57-4 A 42-year-old male with smoking history and chronic cough secondary to respiratory bronchiolitis-interstitial lung disease (RB-ILD). High-resolution CT images through the upper (**A**) and mid (**B**) thorax show diffuse, centrilobular ground-glass nodules *(arrows)*. These findings are compatible with the pathologic pattern of RB-ILD, which features the peribronchial accumulation of pigmented macrophages. Note the relative sparing of the alveolar space (**C**). *(Pathology images used with permission of Robert J. Homer, MD, PhD, Yale School of Medicine.)*

cell infiltrate as well as a peribronchiolar fibrotic pattern more pronounced as compared to uncomplicated RB (Figs. 57-4 and 57-5). Churg has proposed that an RB-ILD diagnosis should be differentiated from RB in smokers when individuals demonstrate evidence of significant functional and physiologic impairment along radiographic abnormalities.[95]

First described by Liebow in 1965,[96] DIP was highlighted as a diagnostic entity in a 1978 study by Carrington.[97] Comparison of DIP and RB-ILD reveals that in DIP the macrophages extend more diffusely into the lobule in contrast to the more limited peribronchiolar involvement found in RB-ILD and that interstitial fibrosis, giant cells, and eosinophils are more commonly found in DIP (Fig. 57-5). Pathologists must exclude the presence of alternative ILDs on biopsy. A clinical diagnosis of RB-ILD or DIP necessitates overall assessment of the patient incorporating pathologic and radiographic findings, functional impairment and exclusion of other diagnostic considerations pathologically and radiographically.

CLINICAL COURSE, OUTCOMES, AND TREATMENT

Patients with RB-ILD or DIP are generally characterized by less fibrosis and experience a more favorable prognosis compared to IPF, perhaps in part due to the finding that smoking cessation and corticosteroids are often effective therapies in RB-ILD and DIP patients.[77,78,98] Progressive disease is uncommon in RB-ILD and is more often seen in patients with DIP as one study found that 33% of DIP patients versus 64% of RB-ILD patients experienced objective radiographic or physiologic improvement.[75] Similarly, another study found that 26% of patients with DIP died compared to no patients in the RB-ILD, a finding that confirmed prior work by Carrington and Yousem.[92,97,99]

Smoking Cessation

The cornerstone of treatment for these diseases includes tobacco smoking cessation. In patients with mild to moderate symptoms and impairment a period of observation after smoking cessation is reasonable. Many patients stabilize and improve; however, concomitant corticosteroid therapy often confounds interpretation of the efficacy of smoking cessation alone[77] and earlier studies by Carrington and Yousem failed to comprehensively characterize the effect of smoking cessation. Additional confounders that complicate assessment of improvement include the presence of other smoking-related lung pathologies such as emphysema whose contribution to impairment will not generally respond to any intervention.

Corticosteroids

When symptoms and impairment are severe, treatment with systemic corticosteroids may be of benefit. A 6- to 9-month course of therapy starting at a level of 40 to 60 mg/d for 6 weeks is reasonable.

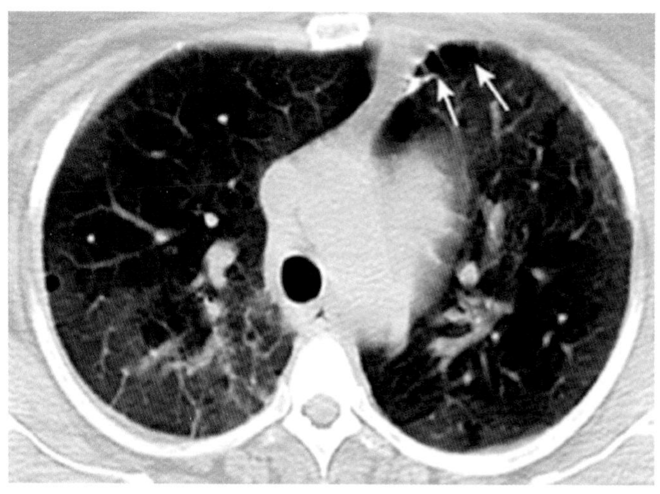

A

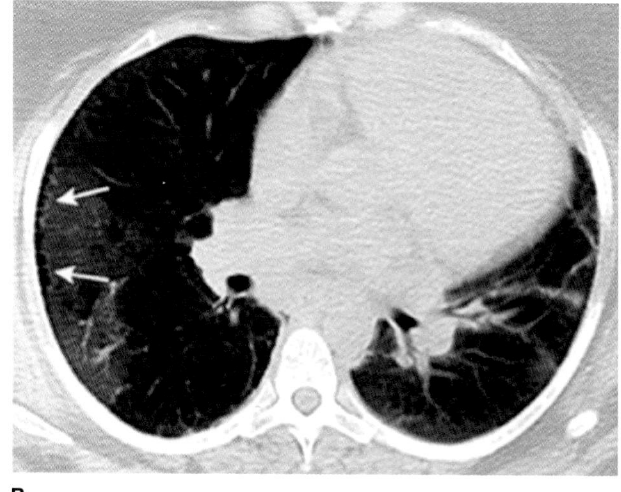

B

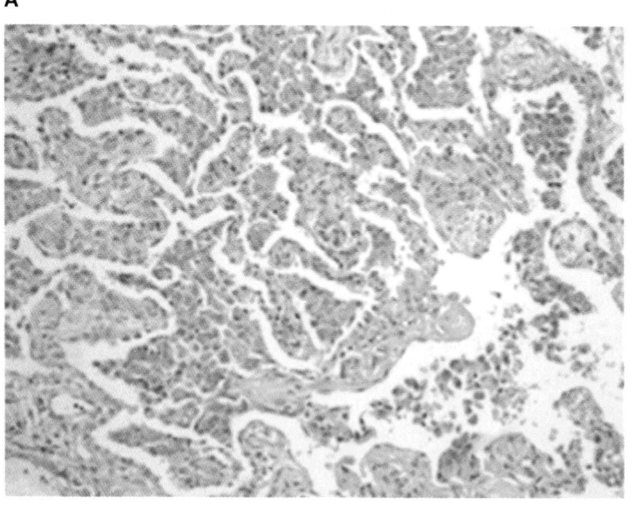

C

Figure 57-5 A 36-year-old female with significant cigarette smoking history, cough, and dyspnea. Axial CT images through the upper (**A**) and lower (**B**) thorax demonstrate bilateral, patchy, and peripheral ground-glass opacities. Small bullae along the pleural surfaces compatible with paraseptal emphysema are also present *(arrows)*. The ground-glass opacities did not resolve on follow-up imaging so the patient underwent video-assisted thoracoscopic surgery (VATS) and pathology revealed desquamative interstitial pneumonia (DIP) shown in (**C**), demonstrating the peribronchial and intra-alveolar accumulation of pigmented macrophages. *(Pathology image used with permission of Robert J. Homer, MD, PhD, Yale School of Medicine.)*

The role of alternative immunosuppressants that are used in other ILDs have been less well defined in RB-ILD and DIP although macrolide antibiotic therapy has been reported to be an effective steroid-sparing treatment in DIP.[100] Lung transplantation may be necessary for patients with severe progressive disease. Recurrence of disease after transplant has been reported.[99]

ACUTE INTERSTITIAL PNEUMONIA

The original description of acute interstitial pneumonia dates back over 75 years. Clinical hallmarks of this entity are described below.

■ DEFINITION AND HISTORICAL PERSPECTIVE

Acute interstitial pneumonia, also called "AIP" or "Hamman–Rich syndrome," was first described by Hamman and Rich in 1935 and is a rare and fulminant IIP.[101] Current ATS/ERS diagnostic criteria for AIP include the following[16]: (1) rapidly progressive clinical course (≤2 months) leading to respiratory failure; (2) exclusion of infectious, toxic, autoimmune, or any other known cause of ARDS; (3) diffuse alveolar damage (DAD) on biopsy specimens (see below); (4) radiologic findings consistent with ILD; and (5) absence of chronic lung disease.

■ CLINICAL PRESENTATION

AIP is quite rare and most frequently presents in previously healthy individuals with no prior lung disease. The disease has no gender predominance and most commonly affects patients over 40 years old with a mean age of 50 to 55 years.[102–104] Unlike most other IIPs,[102] AIP typically presents as the acute onset of fever (75%), cough (70%), and rapidly progressive dyspnea (90%)[105] with many patients reporting the sensation of an infectious prodrome. Most patients are hypoxemic upon presentation and rapidly progress to respiratory failure requiring mechanical ventilation. Physical examination frequently reveals tachypnea and bilateral crackles in all lung fields. Signs of chronic lung disease such as clubbing are uncommon and argue against a diagnosis of AIP while the presence of skin or joint abnormalities might suggest an underlying autoimmune process. While initial management focuses on stabilizing the patient's respiratory status, diagnostic evaluation should be undertaken. Once cardiogenic pulmonary edema has been ruled out by EKG, cardiac enzymes, and echocardiogram, causes of noncardiogenic pulmonary edema and ARDS should be evaluated. Given the broad array of diseases and exposures associated with the development of ARDS, this assessment should include careful exposure history including medications and occupational hazards, as well as a complete rheumatologic history. The serologic and muscle enzyme testing described earlier for NSIP may also be valuable in this setting.

■ UNDERLYING ASSOCIATIONS

The differential diagnosis of AIP is broad and includes left heart failure, diffuse alveolar hemorrhage, OP, hypersensitivity pneumonitis, UIP/IPF, and DIP. AIP can generally be distinguished from these entities based on careful history, examination of chest films, and ancillary tests described earlier. Once the AIP diagnosis has been established, it is imperative to further seek underlying causes

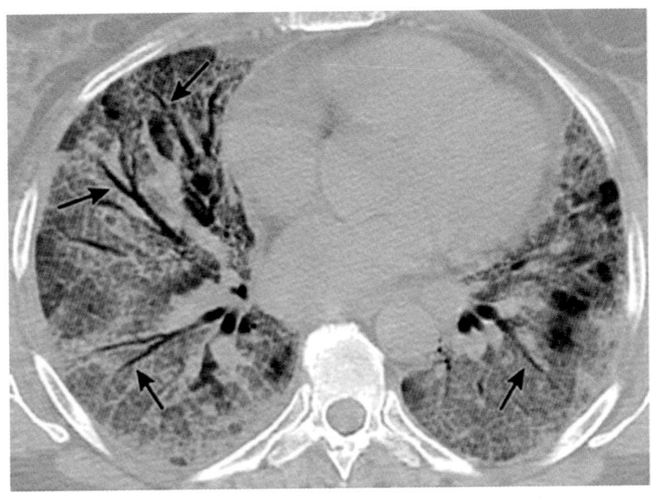

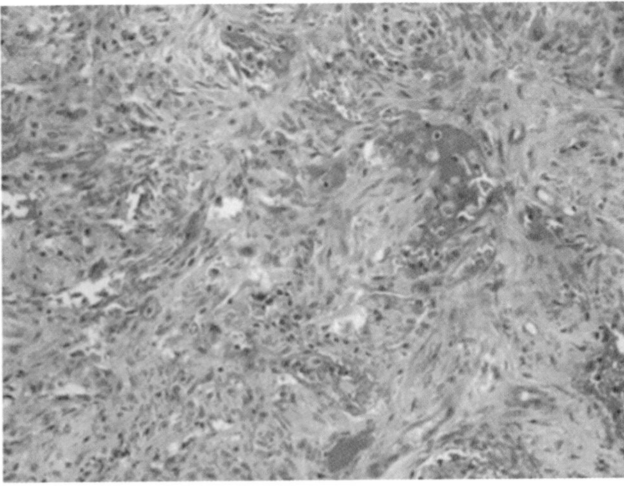

Figure 57-6 A 45-year-old female with acute shortness of breath. High-resolution CT image through the thorax (**A**) demonstrates diffuse ground-glass opacities involving every lobe. Within areas of ground-glass opacity are reticular markings and traction bronchiectasis *(arrows)* suggestive of organization and underlying fibrosis. Lung tissue obtained at autopsy revealed findings of diffuse alveolar damage which was including obliteration of the alveolar space with structural cell death responses, acute inflammation, and hyaline membrane formation (**B**). *(Pathology image used with permission of Robert J. Homer, MD, PhD, Yale School of Medicine.)*

such as collagen vascular disease such as antisynthetase syndrome[106] or lupus[107]; therapeutic exposures such as certain chemotherapies, biologic therapies, radiation, hyperoxia[108,109]; illicit drugs such as heroin or cocaine[110]; toxic exposures such as smoke inhalation and other gases[108]; massive transfusion,[111] fat embolism, aspiration,[112] and infections such as atypical pneumonias (mycoplasma[113] or legionella[114]) and viral infections (influenza).[115] AIP should also be differentiated from acute exacerbations of underlying IIPs or other pre-existing forms of underlying lung disease.

PULMONARY FUNCTION TESTING

Most patients are too ill to undergo pulmonary function testing but a restrictive ventilatory defect and impaired diffusion capacity would be expected.

CHEST IMAGING

AIP is radiographically and pathologically indistinguishable from ARDS. Imaging findings depend upon whether the early, exudative phase or chronic, fibrotic phase is present. Diffuse consolidation and ground-glass opacities are typically seen in the early, exudative phase, with the dependent areas of lung being more affected.[16,17,116] The early, exudative phase is difficult to distinguish radiographically from other entities such as cardiogenic or noncardiogenic edema, diffuse infection or diffuse hemorrhage. In patients who survive the acute phase (sometime after the first week), in addition to the lung consolidation, findings of underlying fibrosis such as architectural distortion, traction bronchiectasis, with or without honeycombing, become apparent at imaging and are usually more severe in the nondependent portions of the lung (Fig. 57-6).[16,17,116]

PATHOLOGY

If microbiologic testing yields negative sputum culture and viral studies, bronchoscopy with BAL is next performed to rule out undiagnosed infection or alternate diagnosis. There is generally no role for transbronchial biopsy in the diagnosis of AIP as when a tissue diagnosis is required, surgical lung biopsy is the preferred approach. A pathologic diagnosis of DAD demonstrates diffuse and extensive cell death accompanied hyaline membranes, which are histologically apparent layers of fibrin mixed with necrotic epithelium. This material lines the alveolus and reflects the severity and acuity of the injury (Fig. 57-6). As the injury progresses, it evolves into its organizing phase, which can either resolve into relatively normal lung or result in lung fibrosis.

CLINICAL COURSE, OUTCOMES, AND TREATMENT

The fulminant and often untreatable nature of AIP endows this disease with a particularly high mortality. More than 50% of patients die during hospitalization and most patients die within 6 months of diagnosis. Those who survive are at risk for disease recurrence or the development of other forms of ILD. However, a small fraction of survivors may experience complete recovery of lung function.[103,105] Treatment is detailed below and is aimed at supporting the patient and attempting to limit the acute injury and inflammation.

Nonpharmacologic Therapy

The mainstay of therapy for AIP is supportive care.[103,105] This includes supplemental oxygen or mechanical ventilation, adequate sedation, nutritional support, and prevention of ICU-related complications such as stress-induced ulcers, venous thromboembolism, catheter-related bloodstream infections, and ventilator-associated pneumonias.

Pharmacologic Therapy

High/pulse-dose glucocorticoid therapy is frequently administered to patients suffering from AIP though, due to the rarity and often grave nature of AIP, there have been no clinical trials assessing efficacy of this treatment.[105] Therefore, the evidence supporting this approach is anecdotal and is, in fact, based on case reports that showed a conflicting survival benefit.[102,105,117] For example, in the largest case series published in 1990, of 29 patients treated with glucocorticoids, survival was 45% in the treated group versus 33% in the untreated group.[102] Similarly, in smaller series of only eight patients treated with pulse-dose steroids, seven patients survived.[117] Conversely, a different study of nine patients treated with 8 mg/kg of methylprednisolone found a mortality of 100% with this regimen.[105] Despite this lack of clear benefit, expert opinion recommends continuation of high-dose steroids for several days followed by a maintenance dose of the equivalent of prednisone 60 mg/d that can be tapered over the ensuing weeks if the patient survives.[103,105]

The side effects of high-dose steroids cannot be understated. In addition to the long-term side effects described earlier, short-term risks in the ICU include hyperglycemia, immunosuppression, neuromuscular complications, and delirium. Thus, in some settings when steroids are contraindicated or a steroid-sparing agent is required, practitioners might employ a trial of nonsteroid-based therapy. Use of other agents such as azathioprine, cyclosporine,[118] Cytoxan™, and vincristine have been reported in AIP though these agents are not recommended for routine use.[112] OLT has been successful in several patients with respiratory failure attributed to AIP. However because these patients are frequently too unstable for transfer to a transplant center, the utility of OLT in AIP is at best limited.

LYMPHOID INTERSTITIAL PNEUMONIA

The final entity discussed within this group of idiopathic interstitial pneumonias is lymphoid interstitial pneumonia.

DEFINITION AND HISTORICAL PERSPECTIVES

In 1969, Liebow and Carrington developed the term "lymphoid interstitial pneumonia" (LIP) to describe a benign polyclonal infiltration of the alveolar space and interstitium with mature B or T cells. LIP exists within a spectrum of lymphoproliferative disorders affecting the lung and as such its classification as an IIP has been debated. Furthermore, the malignant potential of LIP is not well defined[119,120] but all sources agree that identification of monoclonal features effectively rules out LIP and points to a malignant etiology.[121,122] However, because the clinical and radiographic features overlap with the other IIPs in terms of differential diagnosis[123] and treatment approach, the most recent ATS and ERS statement on IIPs retained LIP within this classification.[16] LIP is also sometimes seen in children; however, because this chapter addresses the adult IIPs, pediatric LIP will not be discussed.

CLINICAL PRESENTATION

Given its rarity, the demographics of LIP are difficult to define but the available data indicate that this diagnosis is more commonly seen in women and that the mean age of onset is during the fifth decade of life.[16,124] LIP typically presents as slowly progressive cough and dyspnea over several years.[124] Systemic symptoms are rare though fever, weight loss, chest pain, and joint aches have been reported.[16,124] Chest auscultation may be normal or may reveal crackles as the disease progresses.[25,42] Extrapulmonary findings may include lymphadenopathy or joint findings consistent with an underlying diagnosis of Sjögren syndrome or rheumatoid arthritis. Findings consistent with severe lung disease such as clubbing, are rarely detected.[16] Laboratory examination may reveal mild anemia. Quantification of serum immunoglobulins reveals either a polyclonal gammaglobulinemia or a monoclonal increase in either IgG or IgM up to 75% of patients.[122,125] Immune complexes are sometimes seen but only infrequently.[126]

UNDERLYING DISEASE ASSOCIATIONS

Most cases of LIP are associated with an underlying cause such as Sjögren syndrome[127] or immunodeficiency such as severe combined immunodeficiency and HIV.[42,43] LIP has also been reported in association with rheumatoid arthritis,[128] Hashimoto disease,[129] pernicious anemia,[130] chronic active hepatitis,[131] systemic lupus erythematosus,[132] autoimmune hemolytic anemia,[125] primary biliary cirrhosis,[122] and hypogammaglobulinemia.[130,133] LIP is also seen in association with certain viral infections including Epstein–Barr[134,135] and human T cell lymphotropic virus type I (HTLV-I).[136,137] Truly idiopathic LIP accounts for less than 20% of cases.[124] Thus, as with NISP, a diagnosis of LIP should prompt a dedicated search for an underlying cause.

PULMONARY FUNCTION TESTING

When present, PFT abnormalities include a restrictive defect characterized by reduced FVC and TLC, an impaired DL_{CO}, and, potentially, hypoxemia.[138]

CHEST IMAGING

The imaging findings of LIP are variable and depend upon the underlying disease process. The CXR reveals nonspecific findings such as bilateral reticular markings and hazy, ground-glass opacities. As with the other IIPs, LIP is much better characterized by HRCT. Diffuse, patchy, or lower lobe predominant ground-glass opacities with reticular markings and small cysts is the pattern most commonly seen on CT in patients with AIDS, and can be difficult to distinguish from viral or opportunistic infections such as pneumocystis or CMV pneumonia.[17,139] Thickened bronchovascular bundles, septal thickening, and centrilobular nodules are less commonly present. LIP in patients with Sjögren syndrome typically manifests as bilateral, thin-walled cysts of varying sizes (but usually larger than the cysts seen in AIDS-associated LIP) scattered throughout the lungs with intervening normal lung parenchyma (Fig. 57-7).[16] Often times a vessel appears to be associated with (or adjacent to) the wall of a cyst, thus the term "perivascular cyst." Ground-glass opacities may exist as well.[16,123,140] The main differential diagnosis for this appearance would include other causes of cystic lung disease, such as lymphangioleiomyomatosis (in a female patient), Langerhans cell histiocytosis (in a cigarette smoker), and pneumocystis pneumonia (in immunocompromised patient) though the latter two entities usually manifest with upper lobe predominant cysts.

PATHOLOGIC FINDINGS

LIP pathology demonstrates a dense interstitial lymphoid infiltrate containing lymphocytes, plasma cells, and histiocytes, in combination with Type II cell hyperplasia (Fig. 57-7). The alveolar septa are extensively infiltrated. Lymphoid follicles with germinal centers are often seen.[16,122] Honeycombing and nonnecrotizing granulomas are sometimes detected[122] along with intra-alveolar organization and macrophage but when these latter aspects are the dominant pathologic feature, the diagnosis of LIP should be reconsidered.[16]

NATURAL HISTORY, CLINICAL COURSE, AND TREATMENT

Little is known about the clinical course and prognosis of LIP. The results of several case series suggest that approximately 50% of patients improve, 10% remain stable, and 40% will die of disease within 2 years even when treated with immunosuppression.[122,124,141] Those patients surviving are subject to a small but significant chance of progression to pulmonary lymphoma[122] as well as increased risk of serious and potentially fatal infections related either to the underlying cause of LIP (inherited or acquired immunodeficiency) or to the immunosuppressive therapies used to treat this disease.

Idiopathic LIP

Treatment for LIP in part depends upon the patient's symptoms and the underlying cause. Asymptomatic patients with mild, idiopathic disease are typically subject to careful longitudinal follow-up with serial PFTs and chest imaging because a small percentage of these patients will spontaneously improve.[16] Patients who deteriorate over time, or those who are highly symptomatic or significantly impaired upon initial diagnosis, are offered treatment with immunosuppression. While there exist no data regarding the safety or efficacy of glucocorticoids in patients with idiopathic LIP,[16] extrapolation of case series of patients with CTD-associated LIP (in which approximately 50% of patients show some evidence of response) suggests potential benefit.[141] Patients are typically started on the equivalent of 1 mg/kg (ideal body weight) oral prednisone for 8 to 12 weeks after

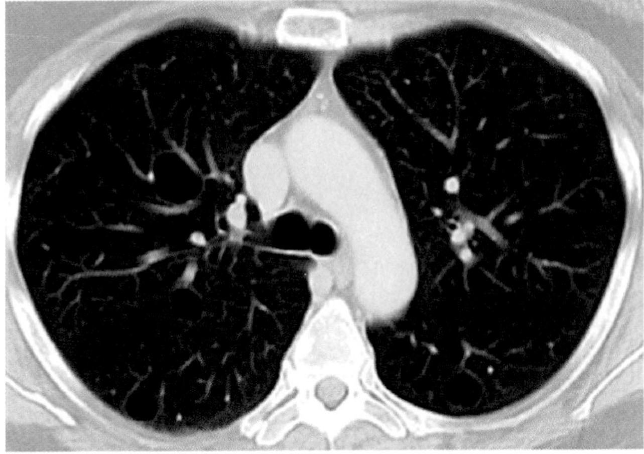

A

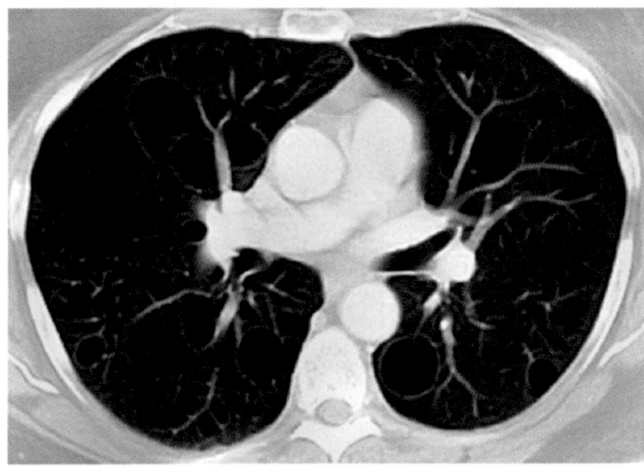

B

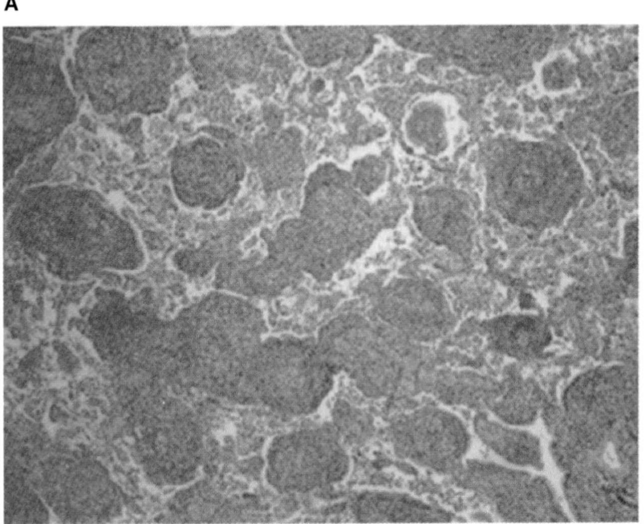

C

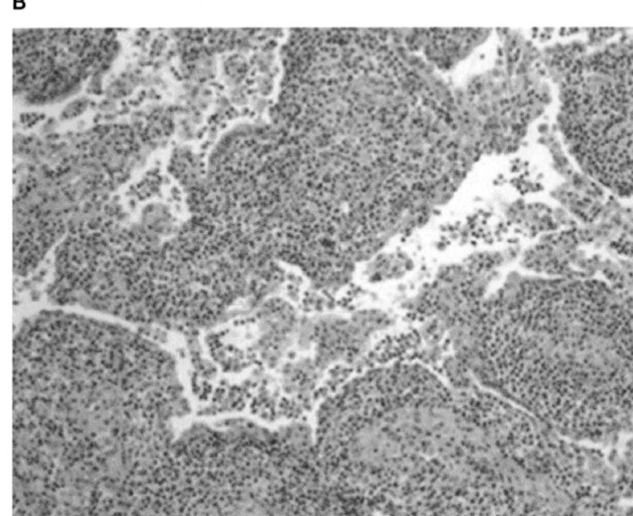

D

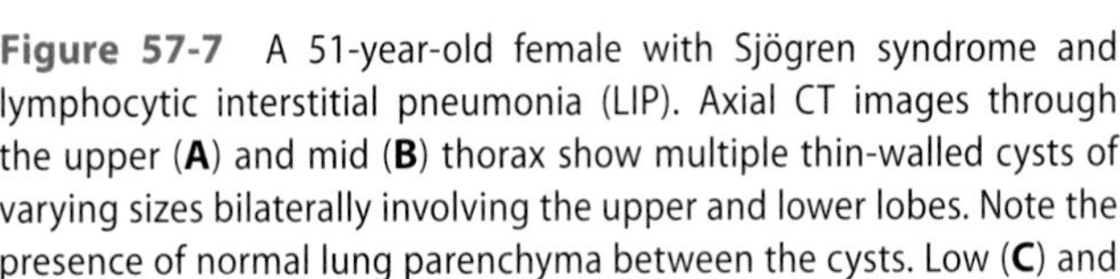

Figure 57-7 A 51-year-old female with Sjögren syndrome and lymphocytic interstitial pneumonia (LIP). Axial CT images through the upper (**A**) and mid (**B**) thorax show multiple thin-walled cysts of varying sizes bilaterally involving the upper and lower lobes. Note the presence of normal lung parenchyma between the cysts. Low (**C**) and high (**D**) power views of LIP lung tissue reveal a dense interstitial infiltrate containing lymphocytes, plasma cells, and histiocytes, combined with Type II cell hyperplasia and increased alveolar macrophages. *(Pathology images used with permission of Robert J. Homer, MD, PhD, Yale School of Medicine.)*

which chest imaging and PFTs are repeated. Those patients who demonstrate an objective response may continue their prednisone at a tapered dose for several months longer; those patients who do not respond generally have therapy discontinued or are offered an alternate disease modifying agent such as cyclosporine or azathioprine. Again, it should be noted that the evidence for this approach is scarce and the risk of side effects, and possible lack of efficacy, should be weighed against the potential benefit inherent in this class of drugs. In addition, patients on long-term steroid therapy should be offered prophylaxis against pneumocystis pneumonia and should be monitored for bone health.

Nonidiopathic LIP

Management of LIP in the setting of CTD is similar to that of idiopathic LIP and in fact the use of immunosuppression in this population is based on stronger evidence.[124,141] Treatment of LIP in the setting of HIV usually involves institution of HAART as in many patients this intervention will reduce symptoms and improve both radiographic disease burden and lung physiology.[142–144] For those patients whose disease persists despite use of HAART, glucocorticoids are commonly used though evidence for this regimen precedes the HAART era.[138,145] As with idiopathic and CTD-related LIP, pneumocystis prophylaxis should be strongly considered for patients with HIV-related LIP that are treated with immunosuppression.

CONCLUSION

The non-IPF IIPs are characterized by diverse presentations, underlying associations, natural history, and response to therapy. Given the complexity of diagnosis and management, these diseases are best managed by highly experienced practitioners using a multidisciplinary approach.

REFERENCES

1. Katzenstein AL, Fiorelli RF. Nonspecific interstitial pneumonia/fibrosis. Histologic features and clinical significance. *Am J Surg Pathol.* 1994;18(2):136–147.
2. Katzenstein AL, Myers JL. Nonspecific interstitial pneumonia and the other idiopathic interstitial pneumonias: classification and diagnostic criteria. *Am J Surg Pathol.* 2000;24(1):1–3.
3. Bradley B, Branley HM, Egan JJ, et al. Interstitial lung disease guideline: the British Thoracic Society in collaboration with the Thoracic Society of Australia and New Zealand and the Irish Thoracic Society. *Thorax.* 2008;63(Suppl 5):v1–v58.

4. Travis WD, Hunninghake G, King TE Jr, et al. Idiopathic nonspecific interstitial pneumonia: report of an American Thoracic Society project. *Am J Respir Crit Care Med.* 2008;177(12): 1338–1347.

5. Poletti V, Romagnoli M, Piciucchi S, Chilosi M. Current status of idiopathic nonspecific interstitial pneumonia. *Semin Respir Crit Care Med.* 2012;33(5):440–449.

6. Flaherty KR, Martinez FJ. Nonspecific interstitial pneumonia. *Semin Respir Crit Care Med.* 2006;27(6):652–658.

7. Arakawa H, Yamada H, Kurihara Y, et al. Nonspecific interstitial pneumonia associated with polymyositis and dermatomyositis: serial high-resolution CT findings and functional correlation. *Chest.* 2003;123(4):1096–1103.

8. Parambil JG, Myers JL, Lindell RM, Matteson EL, Ryu JH. Interstitial lung disease in primary Sjogren syndrome. *Chest.* 2006; 130(5):1489–1495.

9. Kim DS, Yoo B, Lee JS, et al. The major histopathologic pattern of pulmonary fibrosis in scleroderma is nonspecific interstitial pneumonia. *Sarcoidosis Vasc Diffuse Lung Dis.* 2002;19(2): 121–127.

10. Lee HK, Kim DS, Yoo B, et al. Histopathologic pattern and clinical features of rheumatoid arthritis-associated interstitial lung disease. *Chest.* 2005;127(6):2019–2027.

11. Ohtani Y, Saiki S, Kitaichi M, et al. Chronic bird fancier's lung: histopathological and clinical correlation. An application of the 2002 ATS/ERS consensus classification of the idiopathic interstitial pneumonias. *Thorax.* 2005;60(8):665–671.

12. Rossi SE, Erasmus JJ, McAdams HP, Sporn TA, Goodman PC. Pulmonary drug toxicity: radiologic and pathologic manifestations. *Radiographics.* 2000;20(5):1245–1259.

13. Kim HB, Lee SY, Kim JH, et al. Familial interstitial lung disease in two young Korean sisters. *J Korean Med Sci.* 2005;20(6): 1066–1069.

14. Sato T, Fujita J, Yamadori I, et al. Non-specific interstitial pneumonia; as the first clinical presentation of various collagen vascular disorders. *Rheumatol Int.* 2006;26(6):551–555.

15. Bjoraker JA, Ryu JH, Edwin MK, et al. Prognostic significance of histopathologic subsets in idiopathic pulmonary fibrosis. *Am J Respir Crit Care Med.* 1998;157(1):199–203.

16. American Thoracic Society, European Respiratory Society. American Thoracic Society/European Respiratory Society International Multidisciplinary Consensus Classification of the Idiopathic Interstitial Pneumonias. This joint statement of the American Thoracic Society (ATS), and the European Respiratory Society (ERS) was adopted by the ATS board of directors, June 2001 and by the ERS Executive Committee, June 2001. *Am J Respir Crit Care Med.* 2002;165(2):277–304.

17. Lynch DA. High-resolution CT of idiopathic interstitial pneumonias. *Radiol Clin North Am.* 2001;39(6):1153–1170.

18. MacDonald SL, Rubens MB, Hansell DM, et al. Nonspecific interstitial pneumonia and usual interstitial pneumonia: comparative appearances at and diagnostic accuracy of thin-section CT. *Radiology.* 2001;221(3):600–605.

19. Hartman TE, Swensen SJ, Hansell DM, et al. Nonspecific interstitial pneumonia: variable appearance at high-resolution chest CT. *Radiology.* 2000;217(3):701–705.

20. Park IN, Jegal Y, Kim DS, et al. Clinical course and lung function change of idiopathic nonspecific interstitial pneumonia. *Eur Respir J.* 2009;33(1):68–76.

21. Travis WD, Matsui K, Moss J, Ferrans VJ. Idiopathic nonspecific interstitial pneumonia: prognostic significance of cellular and fibrosing patterns: survival comparison with usual interstitial pneumonia and desquamative interstitial pneumonia. *Am J Surg Pathol.* 2000;24(1):19–33.

22. Kondoh Y, Taniguchi H, Yokoi T, et al. Cyclophosphamide and low-dose prednisolone in idiopathic pulmonary fibrosis and fibrosing nonspecific interstitial pneumonia. *Eur Respir J.* 2005; 25(3):528–533.

23. Tashkin DP, Elashoff R, Clements PJ, et al. Cyclophosphamide versus placebo in scleroderma lung disease. *N Engl J Med.* 2006; 354(25):2655–2666.

24. Tashkin DP, Elashoff R, Clements PJ, et al. Effects of 1-year treatment with cyclophosphamide on outcomes at 2 years in scleroderma lung disease. *Am J Respir Crit Care Med.* 2007;176(10): 1026–1034.

25. Swigris JJ, Olson AL, Fischer A, et al. Mycophenolate mofetil is safe, well tolerated, and preserves lung function in patients with connective tissue disease-related interstitial lung disease. *Chest.* 2006;130(1):30–36.

26. Simeon-Aznar CP, Fonollosa-Pla V, Tolosa-Vilella C, Selva-O'Callaghan A, Solans-Laque R, Vilardell-Tarres M. Effect of mycophenolate sodium in scleroderma-related interstitial lung disease. *Clin Rheumatol.* 2011;30(11):1393–1398.

27. Wilkes MR, Sereika SM, Fertig N, Lucas MR, Oddis CV. Treatment of antisynthetase-associated interstitial lung disease with tacrolimus. *Arthritis Rheum.* 2005;52(8):2439–2446.

28. Davison AG, Heard BE, McAllister WA, Turner-Warwick ME. Cryptogenic organizing pneumonitis. *Q J Med.* 1983;52(207): 382–394.

29. Epler GR. Bronchiolitis obliterans organizing pneumonia. *Semin Respir Infect.* 1995;10(2):65–77.

30. Katzenstein AL, Myers JL. Idiopathic pulmonary fibrosis: clinical relevance of pathologic classification. *Am J Respir Crit Care Med.* 1998;157(4 Pt 1):1301–1315.

31. Cordier JF. Bronchiolitis obliterans organizing pneumonia. *Semin Respir Crit Care Med.* 2000;21(2):135–146.

32. Cottin V, Cordier J-F. Cryptogenic organizing pneumonia. *Semin Respir Crit Care Med.* 2012;33(5):462–475.

33. Sadoun D, Valeyre D, Cargill J, Volter F, Amouroux J, Battesti JP. [Bronchiolitis obliterans with cryptogenetic-like organizing pneumonia. Demonstration of gastro-esophageal reflux in 5 cases]. *Presse Med.* 1988;17(45):2383–2385.

34. Llibre JM, Urban A, Garcia E, Carrasco MA, Murcia C. Bronchiolitis obliterans organizing pneumonia associated with acute Mycoplasma pneumoniae infection. *Clin Infect Dis.* 1997; 25(6):1340–1342.

35. Gomez-Gomez A, Martinez-Martinez R, Gotway MB. Organizing pneumonia associated with swine-origin influenza A H1N1 2009 viral infection. *AJR Am J Roentgenol.* 2011;196(1): W103–W104.

36. Epler GR. Drug-induced bronchiolitis obliterans organizing pneumonia. *Clin Chest Med.* 2004;25(1):89–94.

37. Patel RC, Dutta D, Schonfeld SA. Free-base cocaine use associated with bronchiolitis obliterans organizing pneumonia. *Ann Intern Med.* 1987;107(2):186–187.

38. Camus P, Nemery B. A novel cause for bronchiolitis obliterans organizing pneumonia: exposure to paint aerosols in textile workshops. *Eur Respir J.* 1998;11(2):259–262.

39. Alleman T, Darcey DJ. Case report: bronchiolitis obliterans organizing pneumonia in a spice process technician. *J Occup Environ Med.* 2002;44(3):215–216.

40. Cheng TH, Ko FC, Chang JL, Wu KA. Bronchiolitis obliterans organizing pneumonia due to titanium nanoparticles in paint. *Ann Thorac Surg.* 2012;93(2):666–669.

41. Akira M, Hara H, Sakatani M. Interstitial lung disease in association with polymyositis-dermatomyositis: long-term follow-up CT evaluation in seven patients. *Radiology.* 1999;210(2):333–338.

42. Douglas WW, Tazelaar HD, Hartman TE, et al. Polymyositis-dermatomyositis-associated interstitial lung disease. *Am J Respir Crit Care Med.* 2001;164(7):1182–1185.

43. Kalenian M, Zweiman B. Inflammatory myopathy, bronchiolitis obliterans/organizing pneumonia, and anti-Jo-1 antibodies–an interesting association. *Clin Diagn Lab Immunol.* 1997;4(2):236–240.

44. Knoell KA, Hook M, Grice DP, Hendrix JD Jr. Dermatomyositis associated with bronchiolitis obliterans organizing pneumonia (BOOP). *J Am Acad Dermatol.* 1999;40(2 Pt 2):328–330.

45. Oiwa H, Maeda A, Nishisaka T, Yamanishi Y, Yamana S, Takanashi A. A case of polymyositis complicated with organizing pneumonia: case report and literature review. *Mod Rheumatol.* 2004;14(5):388–393.

46. Xing M, Lansdale TF 3rd, McNamara CF, et al. Bronchiolitis obliterans with organizing pneumonia (BOOP) heralding anti-Jo-1-positive polymyositis. *J Clin Rheumatol.* 1999;5(4):219–223.

47. Komiya K, Teramoto S, Kurosaki Y, et al. Organizing pneumonia with a positive result for anti-CCP antibodies as the first clinical presentation of rheumatoid arthritis. *Inter Med.* 2010;49(15):1605–1607.

48. Konsta M, Bournia VK, Alexandrou P, Iliopoulos A. Cryptogenic organizing pneumonia mimicking malignancy in a patient with rheumatoid arthritis. *J Rheumatol.* 2011;38(9):2007–2008.

49. Nakamura Y, Suda T, Kaida Y, et al. Rheumatoid lung disease: prognostic analysis of 54 biopsy-proven cases. *Respir Med.* 2012; 106(8):1164–1169.

50. Bridges AJ, Hsu KC, Dias-Arias AA, Chechani V. Bronchiolitis obliterans organizing pneumonia and scleroderma. *J Rheumatol.* 1992;19(7):1136–1140.

51. Shimizu Y, Tsukagoshi H, Nemoto T, Honma M, Nojima Y, Mori M. Recurrent bronchiolitis obliterans organizing pneumonia in a patient with limited cutaneous systemic sclerosis. *Rheumatol Int.* 2002;22(5):216–218.

52. Taylor JG, Bolster MB. Bronchiolitis obliterans with organizing pneumonia associated with scleroderma and scleroderma spectrum diseases. *J Clin Rheumatol.* 2003;9(4):239–245.

53. Krishnappriya R, Gupta R, Christopher DJ, Balamugesh T, James P. Bronchiolitis obliterans organising pneumonia in systemic lupus erythematosus with anti-phospholipid antibody syndrome–an unusual presentation. *Clin Respir J.* 2010;4(2):125–126.

54. Min JK, Hong YS, Park SH, et al. Bronchiolitis obliterans organizing pneumonia as an initial manifestation in patients with systemic lupus erythematosus. *J Rheumatol.* 1997;24(11): 2254–2257.

55. Otsuka F, Amano T, Hashimoto N, et al. Bronchiolitis obliterans organizing pneumonia associated with systemic lupus erythematosus with antiphospholipid antibody. *Intern Med.* 1996; 35(4):341–344.

56. Camus P, Colby TV. The lung in inflammatory bowel disease. *Eur Respir J.* 2000;15(1):5–10.

57. Crestani B, Valeyre D, Roden S, Wallaert B, Dalphin JC, Cordier JF. Bronchiolitis obliterans organizing pneumonia syndrome primed by radiation therapy to the breast. The Groupe d'Etudes et de Recherche sur les Maladies Orphelines Pulmonaires (GERM"O"P). *Am J Respir Crit Care Med.* 1998;158(6): 1929–1935.

58. Milne DS, Gascoigne AD, Ashcroft T, Sviland L, Malcolm AJ, Corris PA. Organizing pneumonia following pulmonary transplantation and the development of obliterative bronchiolitis. *Transplantation.* 1994;57(12):1757–1762.

59. Siddiqui MT, Garrity ER, Husain AN. Bronchiolitis obliterans organizing pneumonia-like reactions: a nonspecific response or an atypical form of rejection or infection in lung allograft recipients? *Human Pathol.* 1996;27(7):714–719.

60. Pipavath SN, Chung JH, Chien JW, Godwin JD. Organizing pneumonia in recipients of hematopoietic stem cell transplantation: CT features in 16 patients. *J Comput Assist Tomogr.* 2012;36(4): 431–436.

61. Yanik G, Kitko C. Management of noninfectious lung injury following hematopoietic cell transplantation. *Curr Opin Oncol.* 2013;25(2):187–194.

62. Yoshihara S, Yanik G, Cooke KR, Mineishi S. Bronchiolitis obliterans syndrome (BOS), bronchiolitis obliterans organizing pneumonia (BOOP), and other late-onset noninfectious pulmonary complications following allogeneic hematopoietic stem cell transplantation. *Biol Blood Marrow Transplant.* 2007; 13(7):749–759.

63. Daniels CE, Myers JL, Utz JP, Markovic SN, Ryu JH. Organizing pneumonia in patients with hematologic malignancies: a steroid-responsive lesion. *Respir Med.* 2007;101(1):162–168.

64. Bellomo R, Finlay M, McLaughlin P, Tai E. Clinical spectrum of cryptogenic organising pneumonitis. *Thorax.* 1991;46(8):554–558.

65. Izumi T, Kitaichi M, Nishimura K, Nagai S. Bronchiolitis obliterans organizing pneumonia. Clinical features and differential diagnosis. *Chest.* 1992;102(3):715–719.

66. Lee KS, Kullnig P, Hartman TE, Muller NL. Cryptogenic organizing pneumonia: CT findings in 43 patients. *AJR Am J Roentgenol.* 1994;162(3):543–546.

67. Azzam ZS, Bentur L, Rubin AH, Ben-Izhak O, Alroy G. Bronchiolitis obliterans organizing pneumonia. Diagnosis by transbronchial biopsy. *Chest.* 1993;104(6):1899–1901.

68. Costabel U, Teschler H, Guzman J. Bronchiolitis obliterans organizing pneumonia (BOOP): the cytological and immunocytological profile of bronchoalveolar lavage. *Eur Respir J.* 1992; 5(7):791–797.

69. Jara-Palomares L, Gomez-Izquierdo L, Gonzalez-Vergara D, et al. Utility of high-resolution computed tomography and BAL in cryptogenic organizing pneumonia. *Respir Med.* 2010; 104(11):1706–1711.

70. Epler GR. Bronchiolitis obliterans organizing pneumonia. *Arch Intern Med.* 2001;161(2):158–164.

71. Stover DE, Mangino D. Macrolides: a treatment alternative for bronchiolitis obliterans organizing pneumonia? *Chest.* 2005; 128(5):3611–3617.

72. Purcell IF, Bourke SJ, Marshall SM. Cyclophosphamide in severe steroid-resistant bronchiolitis obliterans organizing pneumonia. *Respir Med.* 1997;91(3):175–177.

73. Laszlo A, Espolio Y, Auckenthaler A, Michel JP, Janssens JP. Azathioprine and low-dose corticosteroids for the treatment of cryptogenic organizing pneumonia in an older patient. *J Am Geriatr Soc.* 2003;51(3):433–434.

74. Beasley MB, Franks TJ, Galvin JR, Gochuico B, Travis WD. Acute fibrinous and organizing pneumonia: a histological pattern of lung injury and possible variant of diffuse alveolar damage. *Arch Pathol Lab Med.* 2002;126(9):1064–1070.

75. Ryu JH, Myers JL, Capizzi SA, Douglas WW, Vassallo R, Decker PA. Desquamative interstitial pneumonia and respiratory bronchiolitis-associated interstitial lung disease. *Chest.* 2005;127(1):178–184.

76. Davies G, Wells AU, du Bois RM. Respiratory bronchiolitis associated with interstitial lung disease and desquamative interstitial pneumonia. *Clin Chest Med.* 2004;25(4):717–726, vi.

77. Caminati A, Cavazza A, Sverzellati N, Harari S. An integrated approach in the diagnosis of smoking-related interstitial lung diseases. *Eur Respir Rev.* 2012;21(125):207–217.

78. Caminati A, Harari S. Smoking-related interstitial pneumonias and pulmonary Langerhans cell histiocytosis. *Proc Am Thorac Soc.* 2006;3(4):299–306.

79. Craig PJ, Wells AU, Doffman S, et al. Desquamative interstitial pneumonia, respiratory bronchiolitis and their relationship to smoking. *Histopathology.* 2004;45(3):275–282.

80. Aoki Y, Fukuoka M, Naitoh K, Kohsa K, Kawashima M, Hayashi S. [Desquamative interstitial pneumonitis accompanied by a variety of autoimmune abnormalities in an individual with a history of asbestos exposure]. *Nihon Kokyuki Gakkai Zasshi.* 1998;36(8):717–721.

81. Lougheed MD, Roos JO, Waddell WR, Munt PW. Desquamative interstitial pneumonitis and diffuse alveolar damage in textile workers. Potential role of mycotoxins. *Chest.* 1995;108(5):1196–1200.

82. Freed JA, Miller A, Gordon RE, Fischbein A, Kleinerman J, Langer AM. Desquamative interstitial pneumonia associated with chrysotile asbestos fibres. *Br J Ind Med.* 1991;48(5):332–337.

83. Ishii H, Iwata A, Sakamoto N, Mizunoe S, Mukae H, Kadota J. Desquamative interstitial pneumonia (DIP) in a patient with rheumatoid arthritis: is DIP associated with autoimmune disorders? *Intern Med.* 2009;48(10):827–830.

84. Schroten H, Manz S, Kohler H, Wolf U, Brockmann M, Riedel F. Fatal desquamative interstitial pneumonia associated with proven CMV infection in an 8-month-old boy. *Pediatr Pulmonol.* 1998;25(5):345–347.

85. Hasegawa H, Nakamura Y, Kaida Y, et al. [A case of desquamative interstitial pneumonia associated with hepatitis C virus infection]. *Nihon Kokyuki Gakkai zasshi.* 2009;47(8):698–703.

86. Iskandar SB, McKinney LA, Shah L, Roy TM, Byrd RP Jr. Desquamative interstitial pneumonia and hepatitis C virus infection: a rare association. *South Med J.* 2004;97(9):890–893.

87. Doan ML, Guillerman RP, Dishop MK, et al. Clinical, radiological and pathological features of ABCA3 mutations in children. *Thorax.* 2008;63(4):366–373.

88. Tsukahara M, Yoshii H, Imamura T, Kamei T, Koga M, Furukawa S. Desquamative interstitial pneumonia in sibs. *Am J Med Genet.* 1995;59(4):431–434.

89. Tal A, Maor E, Bar-Ziv J, Gorodischer R. Fatal desquamative interstitial pneumonia in three infants siblings. *J Pediatr.* 1984;104(6):873–876.

90. Heyneman LE, Ward S, Lynch DA, Remy-Jardin M, Johkoh T, Muller NL. Respiratory bronchiolitis, respiratory bronchiolitis-associated interstitial lung disease, and desquamative interstitial pneumonia: different entities or part of the spectrum of the same disease process? *AJR Am J Roentgenol.* 1999;173(6):1617–1622.

91. Attili AK, Kazerooni EA, Gross BH, Flaherty KR, Myers JL, Martinez FJ. Smoking-related interstitial lung disease: radiologic-clinical-pathologic correlation. *Radiographics.* 2008; 28(5):1383–1396; discussion 1396–1388.

92. Yousem SA, Colby TV, Gaensler EA. Respiratory bronchiolitis-associated interstitial lung disease and its relationship to desquamative interstitial pneumonia. *Mayo Clinic proceedings. Mayo Clinic.* 1989;64(11):1373–1380.

93. Niewoehner DE, Kleinerman J, Rice DB. Pathologic changes in the peripheral airways of young cigarette smokers. *N Engl J Med.* 1974;291(15):755–758.

94. Myers JL, Veal CF Jr, Shin MS, Katzenstein AL. Respiratory bronchiolitis causing interstitial lung disease. A clinicopathologic study of six cases. *Am Rev Respir Dis.* 1987;135(4):880–884.

95. Churg A, Muller NL, Wright JL. Respiratory bronchiolitis/interstitial lung disease: fibrosis, pulmonary function, and evolving concepts. *Arch Pathol Lab Med.* 2010;134(1):27–32.

96. Liebow AA, Steer A, Billingsley JG. Desquamative interstitial pneumonia. *Am J Med.* 1965;39:369–404.

97. Carrington CB, Gaensler EA, Coutu RE, FitzGerald MX, Gupta RG. Natural history and treated course of usual and desquamative interstitial pneumonia. *N Engl J Med.* 1978;298(15):801–809.

98. Vassallo R, Ryu JH. Tobacco smoke-related diffuse lung diseases. *Semin Respir Crit Care Med.* 2008;29(6):643–650.

99. Carrington CB, Gaensler EA, Coutu RE, Fitzgerald MX, Gupta RG. Usual and desquamative interstitial pneumonia. *Chest.* 1976;69(2 Suppl):261–263.

100. Knyazhitskiy A, Masson RG, Corkey R, Joiner J. Beneficial response to macrolide antibiotic in a patient with desquamative interstitial pneumonia refractory to corticosteroid therapy. *Chest.* 2008;134(1):185–187.

101. Hamman L, Rich AR. Fulminating diffuse interstitial fibrosis of the lungs. *Trans Am Clin Climatol Assoc.* 1935;51:154–163.

102. Olson J, Colby TV, Elliott CG. Hamman-Rich syndrome revisited. *Mayo Clin Proc.* 1990;65(12):1538–1548.

103. Vourlekis JS. Acute interstitial pneumonia. *Clin Chest Med.* 2004;25(4):739–747, vii.

104. Katzenstein AL, Myers JL, Mazur MT. Acute interstitial pneumonia. A clinicopathologic, ultrastructural, and cell kinetic study. *Am J Surg Pathol.* 1986;10(4):256–267.

105. Avnon LS, Pikovsky O, Sion-Vardy N, Almog Y. Acute interstitial pneumonia-Hamman-Rich syndrome: clinical characteristics and diagnostic and therapeutic considerations. *Anesth Analg.* 2009;108(1):232–237.

106. Guglielmi S, Merz TM, Gugger M, Suter C, Nicod LP. Acute respiratory distress syndrome secondary to antisynthetase syndrome is reversible with tacrolimus. *Eur Respir J.* 2008;31(1):213–217.

107. Singh A, Kaur R. Non-invasive ventilation in patients with acute lupus pneumonitis: a case report and review of literature. *Lung India.* 2012;29(3):270–272.

108. Katzenstein AL, Bloor CM, Leibow AA. Diffuse alveolar damage–the role of oxygen, shock, and related factors. A review. *Am J Pathol.* 1976;85(1):209–228.

109. Schwaiblmair M, Behr W, Haeckel T, Markl B, Foerg W, Berghaus T. Drug induced interstitial lung disease. *Open Respir Med J.* 2012;6:63–74.

110. Gotway MB, Marder SR, Hanks DK, et al. Thoracic complications of illicit drug use: an organ system approach. *Radiographics.* 2002;22 Spec No: S119–S135.

111. Gong MN, Thompson BT, Williams P, Pothier L, Boyce PD, Christiani DC. Clinical predictors of and mortality in acute respiratory distress syndrome: potential role of red cell transfusion. *Crit Care Med.* 2005;33(6):1191–1198.

112. Ware LB, Matthay MA. The acute respiratory distress syndrome. *N Engl J Med.* 2000;342(18):1334–1349.

113. Radisic M, Torn A, Gutierrez P, Defranchi HA, Pardo P. Severe acute lung injury caused by Mycoplasma pneumoniae: potential role for steroid pulses in treatment. *Clin Infect Dis.* 2000;31(6):1507–1511.

114. Demello D, Kierol-Andrews L, Scalise PJ. Severe sepsis and acute respiratory distress syndrome from community-acquired legionella pneumonia: case report. *Am J Crit Care.* 2007;16(3):320, 317.

115. Mauad T, Hajjar LA, Callegari GD, et al. Lung pathology in fatal novel human influenza A (H1N1) infection. *Am J Respir Crit Care Med.* 2010;181(1):72–79.

116. Tomiyama N, Muller NL, Johkoh T, et al. Acute respiratory distress syndrome and acute interstitial pneumonia: comparison of thin-section CT findings. *J Comput Assist Tomogr.* 2001;25(1):28–33.

117. Suh GY, Kang EH, Chung MP, et al. Early intervention can improve clinical outcome of acute interstitial pneumonia. *Chest.* 2006; 129(3):753–761.

118. Ogawa D, Hashimoto H, Wada J, et al. Successful use of cyclosporin A for the treatment of acute interstitial pneumonitis associated with rheumatoid arthritis. *Rheumatology (Oxford).* 2000;39(12): 1422–1424.

119. Banerjee D, Ahmad D. Malignant lymphoma complicating lymphocytic interstitial pneumonia: a monoclonal B-cell neoplasm arising in a polyclonal lymphoproliferative disorder. *Hum Pathol.* 1982;13(8):780–782.

120. Schuurman HJ, Gooszen HC, Tan IW, Kluin PM, Wagenaar SS, van Unnik JA. Low-grade lymphoma of immature T-cell phenotype in a case of lymphocytic interstitial pneumonia and Sjogren's syndrome. *Histopathology.* 1987;11(11):1193–1204.

121. Bragg DG, Chor PJ, Murray KA, Kjeldsberg CR. Lymphoproliferative disorders of the lung: histopathology, clinical manifestations, and imaging features. *AJR Am J Roentgenol.* 1994;163(2):273–281.

122. Koss MN, Hochholzer L, Langloss JM, Wehunt WD, Lazarus AA. Lymphoid interstitial pneumonia: clinicopathological and immunopathological findings in 18 cases. *Pathology.* 1987;19(2): 178–185.

123. Honda O, Johkoh T, Ichikado K, et al. Differential diagnosis of lymphocytic interstitial pneumonia and malignant lymphoma on high-resolution CT. *AJR Am J Roentgenol.* 1999;173(1):71–74.

124. Cha SI, Fessler MB, Cool CD, Schwarz MI, Brown KK. Lymphoid interstitial pneumonia: clinical features, associations and prognosis. *Eur Respir J.* 2006;28(2):364–369.

125. DeCoteau WE, Tourville D, Ambrus JL, Montes M, Adler R, Tomasi TB Jr. Lymphoid interstitial pneumonia and autoerythrocyte sensitization syndrome. A case with deposition of immunoglobulins on the alveolar basement membrane. *Arch Intern Med.* 1974;134(3):519–522.

126. Dreisin RB, Schwarz MI, Theofilopoulos AN, Stanford RE. Circulating immune complexes in the idiopathic interstitial pneumonias. *N Engl J Med.* 1978;298(7):353–357.

127. Strimlan CV, Rosenow EC 3rd, Divertie MB, Harrison EG Jr. Pulmonary manifestations of Sjogren's syndrome. *Chest.* 1976;70(03):354–361.

128. Yousem SA, Colby TV, Carrington CB. Follicular bronchitis/bronchiolitis. *Hum Pathol.* 1985;16(7):700–706.

129. Julsrud PR, Brown LR, Li CY, Rosenow EC 3rd, Crowe JK. Pulmonary processes of mature-appearing lymphocytes: pseudolymphoma, well-differentiated lymphocytic lymphoma, and lymphocytic interstitial pneumonitis. *Radiology.* 1978;127(2):289–296.

130. Levinson AI, Hopewell PC, Stites DP, Spitler LE, Fudenberg HH. Coexistent lymphoid interstitial pneumonia, pernicious anemia, and agammaglobulinemia. *Arch Intern Med.* 1976;136(2): 213–216.

131. Helman CA, Keeton GR, Benatar SR. Lymphoid interstitial pneumonia with associated chronic active hepatitis and renal tubular acidosis. *Am Rev Respir Dis.* 1977;115(1):161–164.

132. Yood RA, Steigman DM, Gill LR. Lymphocytic interstitial pneumonitis in a patient with systemic lupus erythematosus. *Lupus.* 1995;4(2):161–163.

133. Popa V. Lymphocytic interstitial pneumonia of common variable immunodeficiency. *Ann Allergy.* 1988;60(3):203–206.

134. Hanto DW. Classification of Epstein-Barr virus-associated posttransplant lymphoproliferative diseases: implications for understanding their pathogenesis and developing rational treatment strategies. *Annu Rev Med.* 1995;46:381–394.

135. Barbera JA, Hayashi S, Hegele RG, Hogg JC. Detection of Epstein-Barr virus in lymphocytic interstitial pneumonia by in situ hybridization. *Am Rev Respir Dis.* 1992;145(4 Pt 1): 940–946.

136. Setoguchi Y, Takahashi S, Nukiwa T, Kira S. Detection of human T-cell lymphotropic virus type I-related antibodies in patients with lymphocytic interstitial pneumonia. *Am Rev Respir Dis.* 1991;144(6):1361–1365.

137. Resnick L, Pitchenik AE, Fisher E, Croney R. Detection of HTLV-III/LAV-specific IgG and antigen in bronchoalveolar lavage fluid from two patients with lymphocytic interstitial pneumonitis associated with AIDS-related complex. *Am J Med.* 1987;82(3): 553–556.

138. Lin RY, Gruber PJ, Saunders R, Perla EN. Lymphocytic interstitial pneumonitis in adult HIV infection. *N Y State J Med.* 1988;88(5): 273–276.

139. Johkoh T, Muller NL, Pickford HA, et al. Lymphocytic interstitial pneumonia: thin-section CT findings in 22 patients. *Radiology.* 1999;212(2):567–572.

140. Ichikawa Y, Kinoshita M, Koga T, Oizumi K, Fujimoto K, Hayabuchi N. Lung cyst formation in lymphocytic interstitial pneumonia: CT features. *J Comput Assist Tomogr.* 1994;18(5): 745–748.

141. Strimlan CV, Rosenow EC 3rd, Weiland LH, Brown LR. Lymphocytic interstitial pneumonitis. Review of 13 cases. *Ann Intern Med.* 1978;88(5):616–621.

142. Innes AL, Huang L, Nishimura SL. Resolution of lymphocytic interstitial pneumonitis in an HIV infected adult after treatment with HAART. *Sex Transm Infect.* 2004;80(5):417–418.

143. Scarborough M, Lishman S, Shaw P, Fakoya A, Miller RF. Lymphocytic interstitial pneumonitis in an HIV-infected adult: response to antiretroviral therapy. *Int J STD AIDS.* 2000;11(2): 119–122.

144. Dufour V, Wislez M, Bergot E, Mayaud C, Cadranel J. Improvement of symptomatic human immunodeficiency virus-related lymphoid interstitial pneumonia in patients receiving highly active antiretroviral therapy. *Clin Infect Dis.* 2003;36(10):e127–e130.

145. Teirstein AS, Rosen MJ. Lymphocytic interstitial pneumonia. *Clin Chest Med.* 1988;9(3):467–471.

CHAPTER 58

Hypersensitivity Pneumonitis

Alex H. Gifford
Richard I. Enelow

EPIDEMIOLOGY AND ETIOLOGIES

Hypersensitivity pneumonitis (HP), or extrinsic allergic alveolitis, is a spectrum of interstitial, alveolar, and bronchiolar lung diseases resulting from immunologically induced inflammation in response to inhalation of a wide variety of different materials that are usually organic or low–molecular-weight chemical antigens (or haptens), which may lead to irreversible lung damage. Despite the terms *hypersensitivity* and *allergic,* HP is not an atopic disease and is not associated with increased IgE or eosinophils. The prevalence of HP is quite variable in different populations, presumably because of differing intensity, frequency, and duration of inhalation exposure, and also probably due to host factors that have yet to be identified. Once thought to be a relatively rare disease, it is becoming more frequently recognized as awareness is of the limitations of classical diagnostic criteria has increased. Among pigeon breeders, 8% to 30% of members of pigeon-breeding clubs who participated in surveys exhibited evidence of HP, so-called pigeon breeder's disease (Fig. 58-1). Among farmers, 0.5% to 5% have symptoms compatible with HP, so-called farmer's lung disease. The prevalence of symptoms is lower in farms that use hay-drying methods that decrease exposure to the responsible antigens and increased after a wet summer season.

The population at risk and the season of exposure vary with the type of HP. For example, most cases of farmer's lung disease occur in cold, damp climates in late winter and early spring, when farmers (usually male) use stored hay to feed their livestock. Pigeon breeder's disease occurs chiefly in men in Europe and the United States but predominantly in women in Mexico, owing to differing patterns of exposure, but without a seasonal preference in either population. Bird fancier's disease in Europe and the United States occurs in subjects who keep domestic birds and does not exhibit a predilection to either sex. Japanese summer-type HP occurs mostly in women without an occupation outside the home in June to September in warm, moist parts of the country. The disease has been reported in children as well, though rarely.

In contrast to other pulmonary diseases, there is a curious predominance (80%–95%) of nonsmokers in all examples of HP, which is substantially higher than the proportion of nonsmokers in similarly exposed individuals without HP.[1] The mechanisms of this phenomenon are unknown, but could include anti-inflammatory effects of nicotine. This clinical finding suggests that the presence of

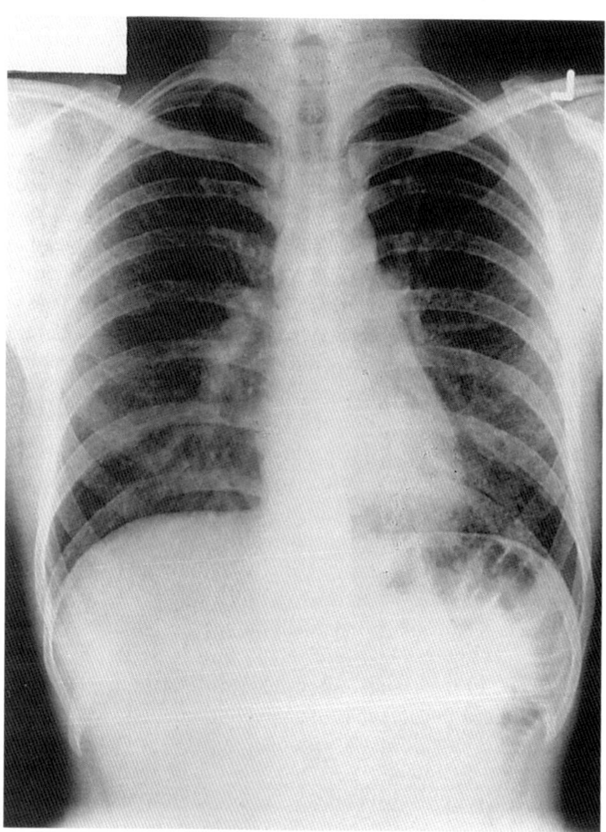

A

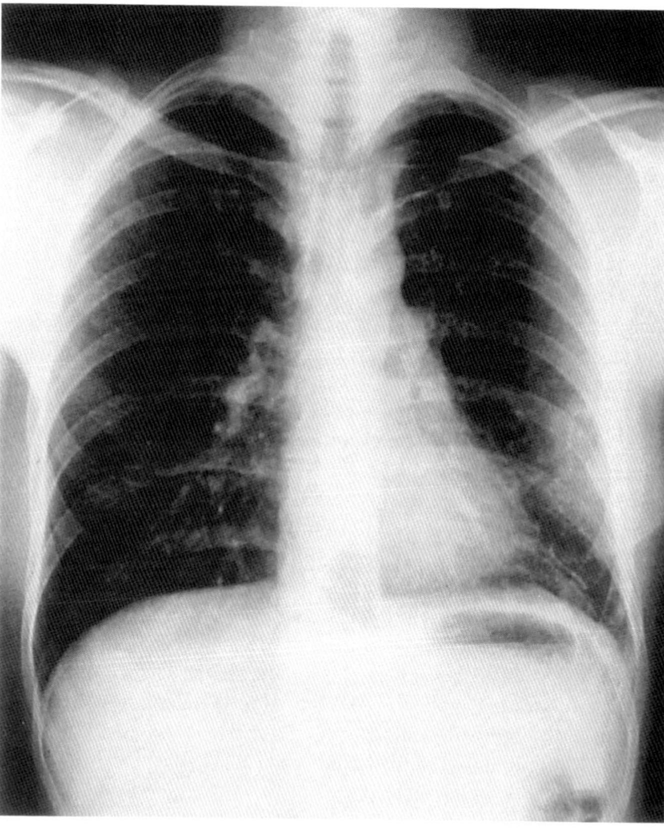

B

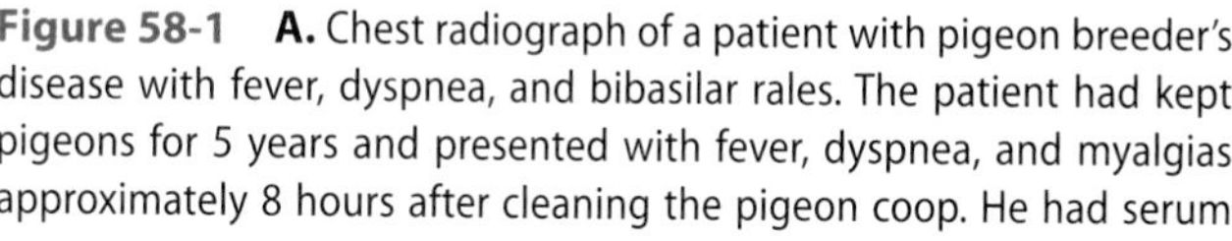

Figure 58-1 **A.** Chest radiograph of a patient with pigeon breeder's disease with fever, dyspnea, and bibasilar rales. The patient had kept pigeons for 5 years and presented with fever, dyspnea, and myalgias approximately 8 hours after cleaning the pigeon coop. He had serum antibody to pigeon dropping extract. Note bilateral lower lobe 2- to 3-mm nodules. **B.** Chest radiograph of the same patient 2 weeks later without specific treatment. Note clearing of the lower-lobe nodules and the staples in the left chest from the open lung biopsy.

active smoking may be evidence against the diagnosis of HP, although this has not been consistently observed.[2]

An important feature of HP is the great variability of susceptibility among exposed populations and the apparent resistance to illness of most exposed persons. Possible reasons include differences in exposure, or differences in the host response to exposure, which may be inborn and/or acquired. There are no differences in the prevalence of atopy or HLA-A, B, or C haplotypes in exposed subjects with and without HP,[1] although there may be an alteration in the prevalence of several HLA-DR and -DQ alleles.[3]

Several case-control studies have identified single nucleotide polymorphisms (SNPs) that are disproportionately represented in patients with HP and have accordingly garnered interest as potential pathogenetic determinants. Compared with healthy controls of the same ethnic heritage, a Mexican cohort with HP was found to have SNPs in MHC class II genes encoding a family of transporters associated with antigen processing (TAP).[4] Mexican HP patients also more frequently possess the KQ genotype of the PSMB8 gene, which codes for a constituent of the low–molecular-weight proteosome required for peptide processing and eventual presentation in the context of class I MHC.[5] SNPs in the interleukin-6 (IL-6) gene have been correlated with higher levels of epithelial neutrophil-activating protein (CXCL-5) in the BAL fluid of HP patients,[6] but the clinical implications of cytokine gene variation in this disease are undefined. An increased prevalence of a particular polymorphism in the tumor necrosis factor-α (TNF-α) promoter has been reported in patients with pigeon breeder's disease compared with exposed subjects without pigeon breeder's disease,[7] as well as protective variants in the tissue inhibitor of metalloproteinase-3 (TIMP3) promoter in exposed subjects without pigeon breeder's disease,[8] the possible significance of which is discussed below (see Immunopathogenesis).

A large number of agents are associated with HP, shown in Table 58-1. Some types of HP have apparently disappeared from their originally described clinical settings (e.g., bagassosis in Louisiana) but presumably exist in areas with similar agricultural or industrial settings. In addition, other forms of HP are being newly recognized (e.g., potato riddler's lung and machine operator's lung). Both the disappearance of previously described examples of HP and the appearance of new examples are due to changing agricultural or industrial practices that result in changes of exposure of subjects to antigenic material that can cause HP. At the present time farmer's lung disease, bird fancier's disease, ventilator lung, and Japanese summer-type HP are the most commonly recognized forms of HP.

Recognition of new examples of HP usually requires a cluster of new cases with a unifying exposure history, underscoring the importance of obtaining at least a basic occupational and avocational history whenever possible. Such diligence revealed that a group of musicians developed HP from instruments contaminated with *Mycobacteria* in the case of trombonists[9] and by molds in the case of a saxophonist.[10] Use of a new metalworking fluid (MWF) led to recognition of machine operator's lung in an auto parts–manufacturing facility due to clustering of cases and a common unusual exposure (*Pseudomonas* in cooling fluid). Highly sensitive genomic testing applied to MWF used in the automotive and nonautomotive industries suggests that HP risk may be associated with microbial colonization patterns,[11] particularly the presence of *Mycobacterium immunogenum*.

CLINICAL FEATURES

The manifestations of the disease may be acute, subacute, or chronic. The stereotypical acute clinical presentation includes transient fever, hypoxemia, myalgias, arthralgias, dyspnea, and cough that occur 2 to 9 hours after exposure and resolve in 12 to 72 hours without specific treatment (sometimes longer after a particularly intense exposure). Patients exhibit tachypnea, bibasilar rales, and occasionally cyanosis. There is usually peripheral blood leukocytosis with neutrophilia and lymphopenia (without eosinophilia), and BAL neutrophilia. Subacute or intermittent disease may result from repeated exposures, and manifest as productive cough, dyspnea, fatigue, and weight loss. There may be BAL lymphocytosis, frequently (though not always) with a predominance of $CD8^+$ T lymphocytes.

The chronic form is clinically more insidious, and patients may lack a history of acute episodes, but present with a gradual onset of cough, dyspnea, fatigue, and weight loss. Symptoms are usually present for months to years. There is typically no fever, but tachypnea and bibasilar dry rales are usually present. This form of the disease may be difficult to distinguish from idiopathic pulmonary fibrosis (IPF). Symptoms and signs of cor pulmonale are not uncommon at presentation.

The reasons for the different clinical presentations (i.e., acute, subacute, and chronic) of HP are not clear, but could include differences of intensity and duration of exposure (low-intensity long-duration exposure tending to cause chronic HP; high-intensity short-duration exposure tending to cause acute HP). This is most clearly demonstrated in HP due to bird exposure. Long-term exposure to low amounts of bird antigens is associated with chronic HP. Pigeon breeder's disease has different presentations in different geographic areas, manifesting as an acute HP in some and chronic HP in others. Intermittent exposure of pigeon breeders to large amounts of pigeon antigens in the United States and Europe is associated with acute disease and a good prognosis, whereas chronic exposure to a few household pigeons in Mexico is associated with chronic disease and a much poorer prognosis. In the United States and Europe, pigeon breeders keep their animals in an enclosure separate from their living areas, which they visit periodically so that exposure is intermittent. In Mexico, birds are often kept in living quarters so that exposure is constant. It is of interest that bird antigens can persist in a room for substantial lengths of time (>18 months) after removal of the birds,[12] so that Mexicans with pigeon breeder's disease might be exposed to pigeon antigens for prolonged periods even after removal of the pigeons. Therefore, pigeon breeder's disease in Mexico resembles bird fancier's disease in the United States and Europe in type of exposure, clinical presentation, and prognosis. It differs greatly from the acute HP that characterizes the pigeon breeder's disease in the United States and Europe. Since the relevant antigens are similar in these two examples of bird-associated HP, it is likely that the type of exposure, and not the antigen characteristics, determines clinical presentation and prognosis. The recognition of a new example of HP is usually associated with the acute form, which is likely related to the relative ease in making the association of acute disease and an acute exposure.

The previous discussion indicates that HP, and particularly chronic HP, may be more prevalent than is readily apparent and may often be confused with other diseases, such as chronic bronchitis or IPF. The latter may be particularly important because detailed histories are not always obtained from patients with IPF, the serum antibody levels to the agents responsible for HP tend to wane after cessation of exposure, and chest high-resolution computed tomography (CT) scans of chronic HP can resemble those of IPF.

RADIOGRAPHIC FEATURES

The chest radiographs of patients with acute and chronic HP differ significantly. In acute HP, chest radiographs demonstrate diffuse poorly defined nodular radiodensities, often with areas of ground-glass radiodensities or occasionally even consolidation. These radiodensities tend to occur in the lower lobes and spare the apices. Linear radiodensities (presumably representing

TABLE 58-1 Etiologies of Hypersensitivity Pneumonitis

Disease	Antigen Source	Probable Antigen
Farmer's lung disease	Moldy hay	*Thermophilic actinomycetes, M. faeni (S. rectivirgula), Thymus Vulgaris, Aspergillus* spp.
Bagassosis	Moldy pressed sugarcane (bagasse)	*Thermophilic actinomycetes, Thermoactinomyces Sacchari, T. vulgaris*
Mushroom worker's disease	Moldy compost and mushrooms	Thermophilic actinomycetes, *M. faeni, T. vulgaris, Aspergillus* spp., Mushroom spores
Suberosis	Moldy cork	*Penicillium* spp.
Malt worker's lung	Contaminated barley	*Aspergillus clavatus*
Maple bark disease	Contaminated maple logs	*Cryptostroma corticale*
Sequoisis	Contaminated	*Graphium* spp., redwood dust, *Pullularia* spp.
Soybean lung	Soybeans in animal feed	Soybean hull antigens
Wood pulp worker's disease	Contaminated wood pulp	*Alternaria* spp.
Wood dust HP	Contaminated wood dust	*Bacillus subtilis, Alternaria*
Compost lung	Compost	*Aspergillus* spp., *T. vulgaris*
Cheeseworker's disease	Cheese or cheese casings	*Penicillium* spp.
Wood trimmer's disease	Contaminated wood trimmings, at times in sawmills	*Rhizopus* spp., *Mucor* spp.
Thatched roof disease	Dried grasses and leaves	*Saccharomonospora viridis*
Greenhouse lung	Greenhouse soil	*Aspergillus* spp., *Penicillium* spp., *Cryptostroma corticale*
Coffee worker's lung	Green coffee dust	Unknown
Potato riddler's lung	Moldy hay around potatoes	*Thermophilic actinomycetes, M. faeni, T. vulgaris, Aspergillus* spp.
Tobacco worker's disease	Mold on tobacco	*Aspergillus* spp.
Wine grower's lung	Mold on grapes	*Botrytis cinerea*
Woodman's disease	Mold on bark and fuel chips	*Penicillium* spp.
Soy sauce brewer's lung	Fermentation starter for soy sauce	*Aspergillus oryzae*
Domestic allergic alveolitis	Decayed wood	*Serpula lacrymans, Leucogyrophana pinastr, Paecilomyces variotii, Aspergillus fumigatus*
Riding school lung	Hay in horse stall	*Thermophilic actinomycetes, M. faeni (S. rectivirgula), T. vulgaris*
Stipatosis	Esparto grass (Stipa tenacissima), used to make plaster	Esparto grass antigens
Pigeon breeder's disease	Avian droppings, feathers, serum	Altered serum/feather proteins
Turkey handler's disease	Turkey products	Turkey proteins
Chicken breeder's lung	Chicken feathers	Chicken feather proteins
Bird fancier's lung	Domestic and wild bird products	Bird proteins
Duvet lung	Duvet and pillow	Goose proteins
Laboratory worker's HP	Rat fur	Rat urine protein
Pituitary snuff taker's disease	Pituitary powder	Vasopressin
Shell lung	Oyster or mollusk shell	Shell proteins
Miller's lung	Grain weevils in wheat flour	*Sitophilus granarius* proteins
Sericulturist's lung	Silkworm larvae	Silkworm larvae proteins
TDI HP	Toluene di-isocyanate	Altered proteins (albumin + others)
MDI HP	Diphenylmethane diisocyanate	
HDI HP	Hexamethylene diisocyanate	
TMA HP	Trimetallic anhydride	Altered proteins
Ventilator lung	Contaminated humidifiers, dehumidifiers, air conditioners, heating systems	*Thermophilic actinomycetes, T. candidus, T. vulgaris, Penicillium* spp., *Cephalosporium* spp., *Amoebae, Klebsiella* spp., *Candida* spp.
Basement lung	Contaminated basement (sewage or mold)	*Cephalosporium spp., Penicillium* spp.
Sauna taker's disease	Sauna water	*Aureobasidium* spp.
Detergent worker's disease	Detergent enzymes	*Bacillus subtilis*
Japanese summer house HP	House dust, bird droppings	*Trichosporon cutaneum*
Hot-tub lung	Mold on ceiling	*Cladosporium* spp.
Tractor lung	Contaminated tractor, cab air conditioner	*Rhizopus* spp.
Machine operator's lung	Contaminated metal working fluid	*Pseudomonas* spp.
Fertilizer lung	Contaminated fertilizer	*Streptomyces albus*
Sax lung	Saxophone mouthpiece	*Candida albicans*

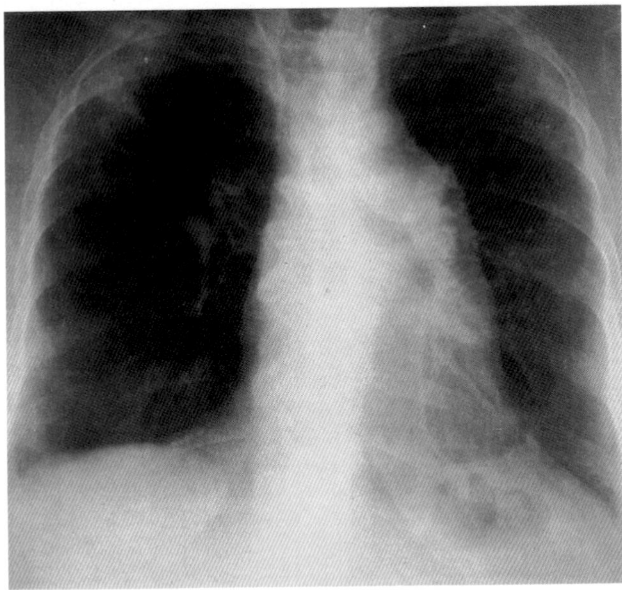

Figure 58-2 Chest radiograph of a patient with bird fancier's disease who presented with progressive dyspnea and weight loss. She had kept two to three parakeets in her home for 15 years and did not notice episodic fever or acute dyspnea. She had positive serum precipitins to parakeet serum, severe restrictive disease, and resting hypoxemia. Note the diffuse radiodensities, loss of volume of the upper lobes, and pulmonary hypertension.

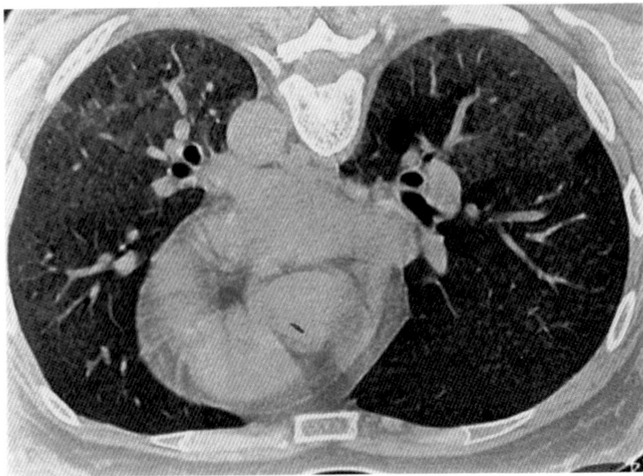

Figure 58-3 High-resolution CT scan of a nonsmoking patient with exposure to both birds and shells who presented with progressive dyspnea and weight loss and had hypoxemia and a restrictive ventilatory defect. Note the diffuse nodular radiodensities in the lower lobes, with areas of ground-glass densities posteriorly.

areas of fibrosis from previous episodes of acute HP) may also be present. The nodular and ground-glass densities tend to disappear after cessation of exposure, so the chest radiograph may be normal after resolution of an acute episode of HP (Fig. 58-2). High-resolution CT scans often demonstrate ground-glass densities better than chest radiographs and at times reveal diffusely increased pulmonary radiodensities. They may also become normal after resolution of an acute episode. Pleural effusions or thickening, calcification, cavitation, atelectasis, localized radiodensities (coin lesions or masses), and intrathoracic lymphadenopathy are rare.

In chronic HP, chest radiographs are notable for diffuse linear and nodular radiodensities, with sparing of the bases and upper-lobe predominance, and volume loss (Fig. 58-3). Pleural effusions and thickening are very unusual, although subcutaneous emphysema (presumably as a consequence of pleural rupture due to bronchiolitis and lobular overinflation) has been reported.

High-resolution CT scans of patients with chronic HP demonstrate several patterns. Most commonly there are multiple centrilobular nodules 2 to 4 mm in diameter throughout the lung fields, with some areas of ground-glass radiodensities, especially in the lower lobes (Fig. 58-4). Unlike sarcoidosis, the nodules are seldom attached to the pleura or bronchovascular bundles, and the border between the nodules and the surrounding lung is well demarcated. There are also well-delineated areas of increased radiolucency, which are presumably overinflated pulmonary lobules subserved by partly occluded bronchioles. The ground-glass densities and micronodules tend to resolve after cessation of exposure. Although these findings are suggestive of HP, they are found in only a subset (50%–75%) of patients with HP, and high-resolution CT scans of the lungs of patients with HP can resemble those of patients with IPF. In cases of chronic avian-related HP, honeycombing and airspace consolidation on high-resolution CT scans are independently associated with increased mortality risk, even after controlling for spirometric and demographic variables.[13] Emphysematous abnormalities are also commonly detected by high-resolution CT scans in nonsmoking patients with farmer's lung disease.

LABORATORY FINDINGS

Patients with acute HP often have a peripheral blood leukocytosis with neutrophilia and without eosinophilia. Prominent cellular abnormalities may also be seen in their BAL fluid, which may be useful in supporting the diagnosis of HP. At time points greater than 5 days after the last exposure, a two- to fourfold increase in BAL fluid leukocytes and lymphocytosis (typically 30%–70% of total cells) are frequently noted. In most instances of HP, the BAL fluid lymphocytes are virtually all $CD3^+$ (T lymphocytes), with a relative increase of $CD8^+$ cells, so that the CD4:CD8 ratio is usually less than 1 (normally 2–2.5, as in peripheral blood).[14] This profile varies considerably with the stage of disease. Indeed, only 33 of 98 HP patients (34%) in one case series displayed a lymphocytic $CD8^+$ alveolitis.[15] Findings of a higher $CD4^+$:$CD8^+$ ratio, fewer $\gamma\delta$ T cells,

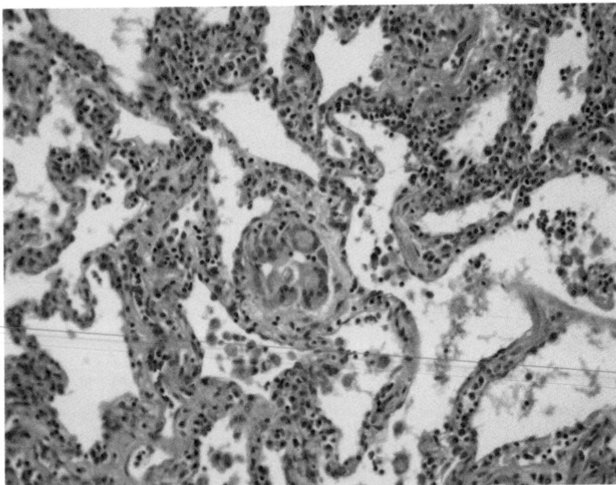

Figure 58-4 Low power view (20×) of H&E-stained section of surgical lung biopsy from a patient with bird fancier's disease. There are nonspecific interstitial mononuclear inflammation and loosely formed granulomatous lesions.

and more terminally differentiated memory CD4$^+$ and CD8$^+$T cell subsets in BAL fluid from patients with chronic HP compared to that from patients with subacute HP suggest that fibrosis may be related to a shift toward Th2 immunity in the lung.[16] Furthermore, BAL lymphocytosis may persist for years following clinical improvement and apparent removal from antigen exposure. Conversely, exposed asymptomatic individuals may exhibit BAL lymphocytosis, further limiting its utility in diagnostic evaluation. After recent (<48 h) exposure, as well as in advanced disease, the lavage is frequently characterized by BAL fluid neutrophilia.[17] The concentrations of IgG, IgM, IgG, and albumin are increased in BAL fluid, presumably a nonspecific manifestation of pulmonary inflammation.

Many patients with HP have easily demonstrable antibodies (typically IgG, IgM, and IgA) to the offending material in the serum, detectable by a variety of methods. Since antigen preparations are not standardized, it is difficult to be confident of the meaning of a negative result; therefore negative "HP panel" does not exclude the diagnosis of HP. Furthermore, since serum antibody is also present in many exposed, but not ill, subjects in virtually the same amounts as in patients with HP, the presence of antibody should be considered supporting data in the proper clinical context.

In asymptomatic pigeon breeders, the prevalence of antibody to pigeon antigens is 30% to 60%. In farmers, the prevalence of anti-*Micropolyspora faeni* serum antibody is 2% to 27%. The occurrence of serum antibody is not consistently related to apparent exposure (i.e., hours of exposure or intensity of exposure) in most instances of HP. This may be related to a threshold effect, so that most exposures are above the minimum required to induce antibody and increases above that threshold are not associated with increases of the prevalence of antibody. In addition, serum antibody tends to wane after cessation of exposure, so patients with chronic HP who have not been exposed for some time may not have demonstrable antibody. In farmer's lung disease, approximately 50% of patients with initially positive serum antibody to *M. faeni (Saccharopolyspora rectivirgula)* lose demonstrable antibody 6 years after cessation of exposure. Farmers who continue to farm also lose detectable antibody (35%–50% in 5 years),[18] and some asymptomatic farmers who were initially negative later develop antibody without farmer's lung disease. In pigeon breeder's disease and bird fancier's disease, approximately 50% of patients with initially positive serum antibody to avian antigens lose demonstrable antibody 2 to 3 years after cessation of exposure. Therefore, it is possible that patients with HP will have no detectable serum antibody owing to either use of an inappropriate antigen in the assay or the waning of antibody in time since the last exposure.

Nonspecific markers of inflammation, such as increased sedimentation rate and C-reactive protein, are often elevated during an acute episode of HP, though are quite nonspecific. In contrast to sarcoidosis, the serum angiotensin-converting enzyme levels are usually not elevated. Skin tests (either immediate or delayed type) to detect sensitization to the suspected antigens are not useful, since extracts of agents that cause HP produce nonspecific reactions that do not indicate sensitization and do not discriminate between sensitized and nonsensitized subjects.

Pulmonary function tests may be restrictive, obstructive, or mixed. There is an increased lung elastic recoil, and usually decreased diffusing capacity. Arterial hypoxemia with hypocapnia reflecting an increased alveolar-arterial oxygen gradient either at rest or after exercise is common. However, 39 of 177 patients (22%) with DL_{CO} data available to the HP Study Group displayed normal diffusion capacity, defined as a $DL_{CO} \geq 80\%$ predicted at the time of diagnosis.[19] Many patients with HP (20%–40%) exhibit increased nonspecific airway reactivity, and 5% to 10% also develop clinical asthma.[20] The increased airway reactivity and asthma tend to diminish after cessation of exposure.

DIAGNOSIS

The symptoms, signs, and laboratory findings of acute HP can resemble those of many other lung diseases, including pulmonary edema, organic dust toxic syndrome (ODTS), inhalation fever, chronic bronchitis, and some pneumoconioses. Acute HP is also often confused with infectious pneumonia (viral, mycoplasma, or chlamydia in subjects exposed to birds). Subacute HP is characterized by a more gradual onset of cough, fatigue, dyspnea, and weight loss, and such symptoms may also develop with intermittent acute attacks. There is considerable overlap in the presentations of acute and subacute HP, in contrast to chronic progressive HP (discussed below).

Chronic bronchitis in nonsmoking farmers and bird breeders is more common than HP, and may share overlapping immunopathogenic mechanisms with HP. The finding of serum precipitins is more frequent in farm workers with chronic bronchitis than those who are asymptomatic. ODTS has been seen in some of the same populations exposed to materials that cause HP, although its cause is likely mycotoxins from bioaerosols contaminated with toxin-producing fungi. ODTS can occur in a larger proportion of the exposed population than HP and is characterized by transient fever, dyspnea, nonproductive cough, peripheral blood leukocytosis, and BAL fluid neutrophilia. The manifestations commonly include diffuse opacities on chest radiograph, restrictive ventilatory defects, reduced DL_{CO}, and bronchiolitis obliterans without granulomas on lung biopsy. Diffuse alveolar damage may occur in severe cases. In contrast to HP, prior sensitization is not required (as indicated by the absence of serum antibodies). Patients presenting with ODTS tend to have more intense exposure of shorter duration than those who present with farmer's lung disease. Another disease caused by exposure to the some of the same agents associated with HP is inhalation fever. This is manifested as fevers, chills, malaise, headaches, and myalgias without prominent pulmonary findings, although mild dyspnea and cough may occur. The onset usually occurs 4 to 12 hours after exposure. Usually there are normal lung volumes and diffusing capacity. The clinical syndrome remits after 12 to 24 hours without specific therapy. Symptoms and signs are exaggerated following an exposure that occurs after a period of nonexposure (such as vacations or weekends), but then become blunted despite continued exposure ("Monday illness"). All signs and symptoms of inhalation fever remit after cessation of exposure, and there are no permanent physiologic or radiographic changes.

In contrast to acute and subacute HP, the classic or typical clinical findings are usually not present in chronic HP. The chronic form of HP often resembles IPF, and these entities may be extremely difficult to distinguish. The differential diagnoses also includes other causes of pulmonary fibrosis (e.g., drug reactions, rheumatologic disease, asbestosis, radiation). Further complicating matter is the frequent lack of clear history of acute episodes. In addition, removal from the presumptive offending agent may result in little or no clinical improvement at this stage.

A thorough and complete occupational and avocational history is essential to the diagnosis of all forms of HP. The history should seek to establish a link between a particular exposure (at work, at home, or elsewhere) and previous episodes of "pneumonia." Knowledge of other exposed persons with similar symptoms should be sought. Evidence of repetitive appropriate symptoms and laboratory and radiologic abnormalities associated with exposure to a particular environment is also highly suggestive of HP. In questionable instances, a "natural exposure" (i.e., documentation of appropriate symptoms and laboratory abnormalities after exposure to a suspect environment) can be used to diagnose HP. A "natural exposure" challenge should not be considered positive unless there is objective evidence of a change in temperature, total peripheral white blood cell count, chest radiograph (or high-resolution CT scan), or a decrease in diffusing capacity (or arterial P_{O_2}). If the history suggests a relationship between exposure and pulmonary symptoms, evidence of sensitization and the nature of the pulmonary inflammatory response should be determined. Sensitization is indicated by the presence of serum antibody to an agent known to cause HP. A large proportion of lymphocytes in BAL fluid (usually over 40%) is highly suggestive of, though not specific for, HP.

A variety of tools exist that have utility in the diagnosis of HP, all of which have advantages and disadvantages. One of the difficulties in assessing the value of diagnostic methods in HP is the vagueness of the "gold standard."[21] Though most would agree that the presence of poorly formed, airway-centered nonnecrotizing granuloma on lung biopsy in a patient with exposure to a known offending agent is supportive enough to be "diagnostic," these features are commonly absent, and a number of histologic variants have been described (see below).[22,23] Since the utility of lung biopsy, absent classic features, is largely supportive, several prediction rules have been devised to determine the probability of a diagnosis of HP based upon clinical features. One such model, developed by the Hypersentitivity Pneumonitis Study Group,[24] examined a cohort of 400 patients with suspected HP and found six significant predictors retrospectively (116 were ultimately diagnosed with HP). These were then validated prospectively in 261 patients (83 of whom were eventually given the diagnosis). It should be noted that the ultimate determination, or gold standard, was the consensus of experts, in many cases without tissue. Although not ideal, at the current level of understanding of the nature of HP, this may be the best method available.[21] The criteria used in this study were (1) exposure to a known offending antigen, (2) positive precipitating antibodies to the offending agent, (3) recurrent episodes of symptoms, (4) inspiratory crackles on physical examination, (5) symptoms occurring 4 to 8 hours after exposure, and (6) weight loss. The probability of having HP was determined based upon the presence or absence of these predictors. The probability of HP ranged from 0% in those patients with none of the predictors to 98% in patients with all six of these features. Exposure to a known offending antigen was the strongest clinical predictor with an odds ratio of 38.8. In cases lacking a compatible exposure history, the diagnosis of HP was made only after further investigation, including supportive findings on lung biopsy (discussed below). It should be emphasized that these clinical prediction rules are of little value in chronic HP, which is usually a more difficult diagnostic problem (often even when histopathology is available). Of course, in the evaluation of individual patients, the threshold for further investigation clearly depends upon the clinical setting and the consequences of the diagnosis.

HISTOPATHOLOGY

A lung biopsy specimen is generally required when there is significant doubt about the diagnosis. Transbronchial lung biopsies often do not provide sufficient material to fully establish the presence and interrelationships of granulomas, bronchiolitis, and interstitial inflammation, so either open or thoroscopically obtained lung biopsies may be necessary. These often reveal chronic interstitial and alveolar inflammation with infiltration of plasma cells, mast cells, macrophages, and lymphocytes, usually with poorly formed nonnecrotizing granulomas (Figs. 58-4 and 58-5). The inflammation usually extends from the terminal bronchioles into the parenchyma. Foamy macrophages are usually evident in the alveoli. There is often bronchiolitis as well as bronchiolitis obliterans. Organizing pneumonia is also present in up to 50% of patients with HP (Fig. 58-6). Conversely, patients with recognized bronchiolitis obliterans with organizing pneumonia (BOOP) may have underlying HP, whether or not other histologic manifestations are evident.

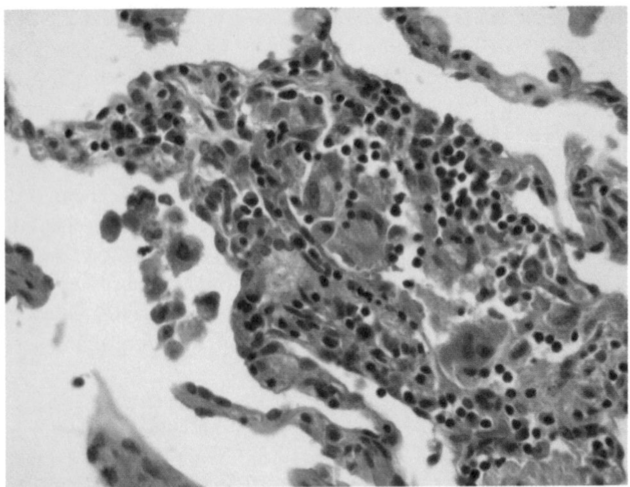

Figure 58-5 Higher power view (40×) of the section shown in Figure 58-4.

Varying degrees of interstitial fibrosis are also often present. The granulomatous interstitial inflammatory responses of HP and sarcoidosis can be difficult to differentiate, though in HP these are usually smaller, poorly differentiated, loosely arranged and contain more lymphocytes and fewer multinucleated giant cells. In contrast to sarcoidosis, the interstitial inflammatory cell infiltrate in HP occurs distal as well as proximal to the granulomas. The granulomas of HP also tend not to occur in groups and tend not to occur near bronchi or in subpleural locations. Instead, they are usually adjacent to bronchioles and are often single. In the absence of granulomas, the pattern may resemble that of nonspecific interstitial pneumonitis, though the bronchiolocentric nature of the lesions and the presence of giant cells or organizing pneumonia may be clues suggesting underlying HP.

The predominant pattern of inflammation and fibrosis in a patient's lung biopsy stands to inform his or her prognosis. In a study of 110 patients with pigeon breeder's lung, the survival rate was highest for those with biopsy specimens displaying a nonspecific interstitial pneumonia (NSIP) pattern and lowest for those with changes of UIP.[24] Interestingly, the survival prediction for patients with typical HP biopsy findings fell between the Kaplan–Meier curves for patients with NSIP and UIP in this investigation. Another

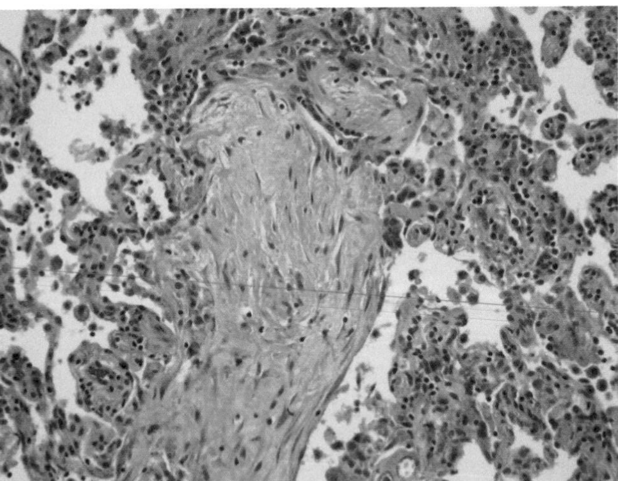

Figure 58-6 Organizing pneumonitis in a patient with bird fancier's disease.

study that considered more diverse causes of HP demonstrated that survival is considerably shorter for patients with UIP-like and fibrotic NSIP-like histology compared to those with isolated peribronchiolar fibrosis.[25] Therefore, lung biopsy results may play an important role in counseling patients about the anticipated natural history of their disease.

The specific histologic changes of HP, when present, are quite helpful in making the diagnosis. However, the granulomas and respiratory bronchiolitis may not be present years after cessation of exposure, so only interstitial inflammation and fibrosis remain in many subacute and most chronic cases.[26] Although these findings might be useful in supporting the clinical diagnosis of HP, they would be insufficient to confirm it.

IMMUNOPATHOGENESIS

Considerable evidence obtained over the past 25 years suggests a primary role for T cell–mediated events in the pathogenesis of HP. A contribution of humoral immunity, especially in acute HP, has not been excluded however. The presence of serum antibody in patients with HP and the timing of symptoms after exposure (2–9 hours) led to the hypothesis that HP represents an example of immune complex–mediated lung disease. Therefore, it is possible that immune complexes initiate the injury upon antigen exposure, which is then perpetuated and amplified by T cell activities. By the time the disease is clinically evident, lung tissue gene expression profiles indicate T cell–driven inflammation (in contrast to the profiles of IPF and NSIP).[27] The T cell responses evident in HP are notable for the predominance of $CD8^+$ cells and the expression of interferon-gamma (IFN-γ), the prototypic cytokine of type 1 inflammatory processes. Expression of IFN-γ–dependent chemokines, such as CXCL9 and CXCL10, is also observed in HP lungs, which undoubtedly serves to amplify the type 1 inflammation. Not unexpectedly, $CD8^+$ T cells in BAL of HP patients strongly express CXCR3, the receptor for both of these chemokine.[28]

Although the Th1 response has canonically defined HP, recent evidence suggests that dysfunctional regulatory T cells (Tregs) are involved with a loss of tolerance to inhaled antigens. Broadly speaking, these $CD4^+Foxp3^+$ lymphocytes suppress the activity of Th1 and Th2 effector cells, which is important for antigen self-recognition and the prevention of autoimmune diseases.[29] Compared to Tregs from BAL and blood of healthy controls, those obtained from HP patients cannot suppress T-lymphocyte activation in vitro, perhaps because of IL-17 production, given that significantly higher IL-17 levels are found in sera and BAL samples from the latter population.[30] The importance of Th17 polarized $CD4^+$ T cells in generating fibroinflammatory lung injury has been described in mice using *S. rectivirgula*.[31] This murine model has also been used to demonstrate that Tregs concurrently reduce IFN-γ production and pulmonary infiltration by $CD4^+$ and $CD8^+$ lymphocytes.[32] Whether Tregs and/or Th17 immunity explain the clinical heterogeneity of HP has yet to be determined.

In animal models of HP, macrophage-derived cytokines such as IL-1, IL-6, IL-12, and TNF-α (as well as a variety of chemokines) play a central role in models that entail intrapulmonary administration of various antigenic substances.[33] TNF-α, produced by activated macrophages as well as $CD8^+$ T cells, likely participates both in the amplification of the inflammation and the activation/degranulation of neutrophils recruited to the alveolar space.[34,35] Interestingly, polymorphisms in the TNF-α promoter have been reported in a group of patients with farmer's lung disease, which correlated with higher serum levels of TNF-α after challenge with hay dust, compared with a group of sensitized asymptomatic controls.[7] Two small genetic susceptibility studies in Mexican[8] and Dutch[36] patients with bird fancier's disease found protective polymorphisms in the tissue inhibitor of metalloproteinase-3 (TIMP-3) gene, which is involved in the inhibition of metalloproteinases associated with extracellular matrix turnover. TIMP-3 has also been identified recently as the primary inhibitor of TNF-α–converting enzyme (TACE/ADAM-17), and this enzyme is responsible for processing TNF-α to its soluble form, which is intensely proinflammatory.[37] The TIMP-3 polymorphism was not found in patients with IPF or NSIP.[8] It is therefore reasonable to speculate that the expression and/or proteolytic processing of TNF-α is important in the pathogenesis of HP, though clearly this leaves much to be explained concerning the varying clinical pictures of the disease.

PROGNOSIS AND TREATMENT

Prognosis varies considerably with the type of HP and even the geographic location. For example, farmer's lung disease has a good prognosis in Quebec, even in farmers who continue to farm. However, farmer's lung disease in Finland often results in significant physiologic impairment and even death. Pigeon breeder's disease has a good prognosis in the United States and Europe, whereas the same disease in Mexico has a 30% 5-year mortality.[38] The reasons for these differences are not clear but may include differences in the nature of the antigen and the exposure.

Identification of the offending antigen is critical to effective avoidance, which is the primary intervention in all forms of HP. This is not always practical when the exposure is occupational, such as in farmer's lung disease. In addition most farmers who continue to be exposed may fare no worse than those who leave their farms.[39] Nevertheless, removal from exposure to the offending antigen(s) is usually sufficient to resolve symptoms and physiologic abnormalities. Measures to reduce antigenic burden may include protective equipment and reducing microbial contamination of the home or work environment. Elimination of excess moisture, reduction in humidity, repair of water damaged materials, regular cleaning of humidifiers, ventilation, and air conditioning equipment all contribute to reduction in mold and other microbial colonization, which may predispose to sensitization. Removal of birds from the home of patients with bird fancier's disease is a critical aspect of treatment, but antigens may persist for extended periods despite thorough cleaning of the home environment.[12]

Systemic glucocorticosteroids are usually required to treat severely symptomatic patients, although there is no formal evidence that such treatment is associated with long-term abatement of symptoms or radiologic or pulmonary function test abnormalities.[30,40] The usual treatment is prednisone or prednisolone, 40 to 60 mg a day for 2 weeks, followed by a gradual decrease over 2 to 4 weeks. Patients with farmer's lung disease treated with prednisolone, compared with those not treated with prednisone, demonstrated slightly more rapid resolution of some radiologic (ground-glass opacities) and some physiologic abnormalities than untreated patients (slight improvement of diffusing capacity, no difference in lung volumes or arterial P_{O_2}). However, there were no differences between the groups 6 months after the diagnosis of HP. The evidence mentioned earlier suggests that systemic steroids may slightly increase the rate of resolution of acute pulmonary inflammation but have little or no effect on chronic residue of HP.

If patients are removed from exposure before there are permanent radiologic or physiologic abnormalities, the prognosis is excellent, with little evidence of long-term ill effects. If removal from exposure is impossible, the use of efficient masks during exposure can result in prevention of acute HP and an excellent prognosis. The prognosis varies considerably with different types of HP. In general, bird fancier's disease carries a worse prognosis than other forms of HP, though even this varies considerably depending on the specific nature of the exposure. It appears that long-term low-level exposure is associated with a poorer prognosis, whereas short-term intermittent exposure is associated with a more favorable one. Unfortunately, many patients with chronic HP present with pulmonary fibrosis and physiologic abnormalities that are only partly reversible after cessation of exposure. The specific nature of histopathologic findings on biopsy in these patients at the time of diagnosis may help predict subsequent clinical course of the disease.[41] Not surprisingly, patients with organizing pneumonia/BOOP or cellular NSIP have a better prognosis than those with fibrotic NSIP or other patterns of fibrosing pneumonitis.

SUMMARY

In conclusion, HP is an immunologically mediated lung disease likely mediated primarily by T cell responses to inhaled antigens. The diagnosis requires careful history, appropriate laboratory tests, and lung biopsy in selected cases. Avoidance of exposure is usually associated with a good prognosis, and corticosteroids are indicated in severely symptomatic patients. Because of constantly changing environmental exposures, new examples of HP are continually being described, and represent an ongoing challenge in patients presenting with undefined interstitial lung disease.

REFERENCES

1. Terho EO, Husman K, Vohlonen I. Prevalence and incidence of chronic bronchitis and farmer's lung with respect to age, sex, atopy, and smoking. *Eur J Respir Dis Suppl.* 1987;152:19–28.
2. Lacasse Y, Selman M, Costabel U, et al.; HP Study Group. Clinical diagnosis of hypersensitivity pneumonitis. *Am J Respir Crit Care Med.* 2003;168:952–958.
3. Camarena A, Juarez A, Mejia M, et al. Major histocompatibility complex and tumor necrosis factor-alpha polymorphisms in pigeon breeder's disease. *Am J Respir Crit Care Med.* 2001;163: 1528–1533.
4. Aquino-Galvez A, Camarena A, Montano M, et al. Transporter associated with antigen processing (TAP) 1 gene polymorphisms in patients with hypersensitivity pneumonitis. *Exp Mol Pathol.* 2008;84:173–177.
5. Camarena A, Aquino-Galvez A, Falfan-Valencia R, et al. PSMB8 (LMP7) but not PSMB9 (LMP2) gene polymorphisms are associated to pigeon breeder's hypersensitivity pneumonitis. *Respir Med.* 2010;104:889–894.
6. Vasakova M, Sterclova M, Kolesar L, et al. Cytokine gene polymorphisms and BALF cytokine levels in interstitial lung diseases. *Respir Med.* 2009;103:773–779.
7. Schaaf BM, Seitzer U, Pravica V, Aries SP, Zabel P. Tumor necrosis factor-alpha -308 promoter gene polymorphism and increased tumor necrosis factor serum bioactivity in farmer's lung patients. *Am J Respir Crit Care Med.* 2001;163: 379–382.
8. Hill MR, Briggs L, Montano MM, et al. Promoter variants in tissue inhibitor of metalloproteinase-3 (TIMP-3) protect against susceptibility in pigeon breeders' disease. *Thorax.* 2004;59: 586–590.
9. Metersky ML, Bean SB, Meyer JD, et al. Trombone player's lung: a probable new cause of hypersensitivity pneumonitis. *Chest.* 2010; 138:754–756.
10. Metzger F, Haccuria A, Reboux G, Nolard N, Dalphin JC, De Vuyst P. Hypersensitivity pneumonitis due to molds in a saxophone player. *Chest.* 2010;138:724–726.
11. Murat JB, Grenouillet F, Reboux G, et al. Factors influencing the microbial composition of metalworking fluids and potential implications for machine operator's lung. *Appl Environ Microbiol.* 2012;78:34–41.
12. Craig TJ, Hershey J, Engler RJ, Davis W, Carpenter GB, Salata K. Bird antigen persistence in the home environment after removal of the bird. *Ann Allergy.* 69:510–512.
13. Tateishi T, Ohtani Y, Takemura T, et al. Serial high-resolution computed tomography findings of acute and chronic hypersensitivity pneumonitis induced by avian antigen. *J Comput Assist Tomogr.* 2011;35:272–279.
14. Costabel U, Guzman J. Bronchoalveolar lavage in interstitial lung disease. *Curr Opin Pulm Med.* 2001;7:255–261.
15. Caillaud DM, Vergnon JM, Madroszyk A, Melloni BM, Murris M, Dalphin JC; French Group of Environmental Immunoallergic Bronchopulmonary Diseases. Bronchoalveolar lavage in hypersensitivity pneumonitis: a series of 139 patients. *Inflamm Allergy Drug Targets.* 2012;11:15–19.
16. Barrera L, Mendoza F, Zuniga J, et al. Functional diversity of T-cell subpopulations in subacute and chronic hypersensitivity pneumonitis. *Am J Respir Crit Care Med.* 2008;177:44–55.
17. Drent M, van Velzen-Blad H, Diamant M, Wagenaar SS, Hoogsteden HC, van den Bosch JM. Bronchoalveolar lavage in extrinsic allergic alveolitis: effect of time elapsed since antigen exposure. *Eur Respir J.* 1993;6:1276–1281.
18. Monkare S, Haahtela T. Farmer's lung–a 5-year follow-up of eighty-six patients. *Clin Allergy.* 1987;17:143–151.
19. Lacasse Y, Girard M, Cormier Y. Recent advances in hypersensitivity pneumonitis. *Chest.* 2012;142:208–217.
20. Kokkarinen JI, Tukiainen HO, Terho EO. Recovery of pulmonary function in farmer's lung. A five-year follow-up study. *Am Rev Respir Dis.*1993;147:793–796.
21. Morris DG. Gold, silver, and bronze: metals, medals, and standards in hypersensitivity pneumonitis. *Am J Respir Crit Care Med.* 2003;168:909–910.
22. Coleman A, Colby TV. Histologic diagnosis of extrinsic allergic alveolitis. *Am J Surg Pathol.* 1988;12:514–518.
23. Vourlekis JS, Schwarz MI, Cool CD, Tuder RM, King TE, Brown KK. Nonspecific interstitial pneumonitis as the sole histologic expression of hypersensitivity pneumonitis. *Am J Med.* 2002;112:490–493.
24. Gaxiola M, Buendia-Roldan I, Mejia M, et al. Morphologic diversity of chronic pigeon breeder's disease: clinical features and survival. *Res Med.* 2011;105:608–614.
25. Churg A, Sin DD, Everett D, Brown K, Cool C. Pathologic patterns and survival in chronic hypersensitivity pneumonitis. *Am J Surg Pathol.* 2009;33:1765–1770.
26. Churg A, Muller NL, Flint J, Wright JL. Chronic hypersensitivity pneumonitis. *Am J Surg Pathol.* 2006;30:201–208.
27. Selman M, Pardo A, Barrera L, et al. Gene expression profiles distinguish idiopathic pulmonary fibrosis from hypersensitivity pneumonitis. *Am J Respir Crit Care Med.* 2006;173: 188–198.
28. Agostini C, Calabrese F, Poletti V, et al. CXCR3/CXCL10 interactions in the development of hypersensitivity pneumonitis. *Respir Res.* 2005;6:20.
29. Ding Y, Xu J, Bromberg JS. Regulatory T cell migration during an immune response. *Trends Immunol.* 2012;33:174–180.
30. Girard M, Israel-Assayag E, Cormier Y. Impaired function of regulatory T-cells in hypersensitivity pneumonitis. *Eur Respir J.* 2011; 37:632–639.
31. Simonian PL, Roark CL, Wehrmann F, et al. Th17-polarized immune response in a murine model of hypersensitivity pneumonitis and lung fibrosis. *J Immunol.* 2009;182:657–665.

32. Park Y, Oh SJ, Chung DH. CD4(+)CD25(+) regulatory T cells attenuate hypersensitivity pneumonitis by suppressing IFN-gamma production by CD4(+) and CD8(+) T cells. *J Leukoc Biol.* 2009;86:1427–1437.

33. Schuyler M, Gott K, Cherne A. Mediators of hypersensitivity pneumonitis. *J Lab Clin Med.* 2000;136:29–38.

34. Chen B, Tong Z, Nakamura S, Costabel U, Guzman J. Production of IL-12, IL-18 and TNF-alpha by alveolar macrophages in hypersensitivity pneumonitis. *Sarcoidosis Vasc Diffuse Lung Dis.* 2004; 21:199–203.

35. Denis M, Bedard M, Laviolette M, Cormier Y. A study of monokine release and natural killer activity in the bronchoalveolar lavage of subjects with farmer's lung. *Am Rev Respir Dis.* 1993;147: 934–939.

36. Janssen R, Kruit A, Grutters JC, Ruven HJ, van Moorsel CM, van den Bosch JM. TIMP-3 promoter gene polymorphisms in BFL. *Thorax.* 2005;60:974.

37. Smookler DS, Mohammed FF, Kassiri Z, Duncan GS, Mak TW, Khokha R. . Tissue inhibitor of metalloproteinase 3 regulates TNF-dependent systemic inflammation. *J Immunol.* 2006;176: 721–725.

38. Perez-Padilla R, Salas J, Chapela R, et al. Mortality in Mexican patients with chronic pigeon breeder's lung compared with those with usual interstitial pneumonia. *Am Rev Respir Dis.* 1993;148:49–53.

39. Cormier Y, Belanger J. Long-term physiologic outcome after acute farmer's lung. *Chest.* 1985;87:796–800.

40. Kokkarinen JI, Tukiainen HO, Terho EO. Effect of corticosteroid treatment on the recovery of pulmonary function in farmer's lung. *Am Rev Respir Dis.* 1992;145:3–5.

41. Ohtani Y, Saiki S, Kitaichi M, et al. Chronic bird fancier's lung: histopathological and clinical correlation. An application of the 2002 ATS/ERS consensus classification of the idiopathic interstitial pneumonias. *Thorax.* 2005;60:665–671.

CHAPTER 59

Radiation Pneumonitis

Kenneth B. Roberts
Roy Decker
Sara Rockwell

INTRODUCTION

The discovery of X-rays by Roentgen in 1895 and of radium by the Curies in 1898 revolutionized medicine at the turn of the 20th century. Roentgen's first paper on X-rays illustrated the power of diagnostic imaging with a remarkably detailed radiographic image of Frau Roentgen's hand. As researchers around the world built vacuum tubes and acquired radioactive sources for their studies, it rapidly became apparent that these invisible radiations could produce dangerous, and even lethal, injuries.[1-3] Erythema, chronic dermatitis, ulceration, loss of hair, and eye injuries were soon reported in patients who received large doses of radiation during prolonged fluoroscopy procedures. Even greater injuries were reported among the physicians, technicians, and scientists who performed diagnostic procedures or laboratory studies using unshielded X-ray-generating equipment and highly radioactive sources. The development of these radiation injuries suggested that radiation might be useful in the treatment of cancer; indeed, patients with cancer were treated with radiation therapy as early as 1896.[1-3]

Radiation was found to inhibit the growth of tumors, but this benefit came with the cost of injury to normal tissues within the irradiated areas. Because of the very low energies of the early X-ray and gamma-ray sources, radiotherapy in its early days was limited to using poorly penetrating radiations, which delivered much higher doses of radiation to skin than to even very superficial tumors. As a result, severe early radiation reactions in the skin limited the doses of radiation that could be delivered to tumors. Studies of these skin reactions led to the development of the concept of normal tissue tolerance and an appreciation of the benefits of "fractionated" radiotherapy, using multiple treatments with small doses of radiation.[2] The relative sensitivity of the lung to injury from radiation became apparent early in the development of radiation oncology. The clinical syndromes of dyspnea, cough, fever, and radiographic infiltrates occurring weeks to months after irradiation of the thorax were dramatic enough to be described as early as 1922.[4]

The field of radiation oncology has matured immeasurably over the last century and has incorporated significant advances from fields as diverse as theoretical and applied physics, radiation biology, pathology, cell biology, and immunology.[1,2,5-7] The importance of advances in physics and engineering to the maturation of radiation oncology is especially notable.[2,7] These advances have led to the development of modern linear accelerators capable of delivering very high-energy, deeply penetrating radiations, which can be used to deliver high radiation doses with great precision to tumors deep within the body. Precise systems for radiation dose measurement, or *dosimetry,* rapid computers, and precise algorithms for the rapid computerized three-dimensional planning of individualized radiotherapy treatments based on computed tomography (CT) scans and magnetic resonance imaging (MRI) studies have been developed. These advances have changed the dose-limiting toxicities of radiation therapy from painful early reactions in the skin to life-threatening late reactions in the normal tissues invaded by and surrounding the tumors, including the lung.

For clinicians interested in pulmonary medicine, understanding radiation pneumonitis is important. An understanding of radiation injury to the lung can be useful in understanding other lung diseases. Because the chemical mediators of radiation effects, both beneficial and harmful, are free radicals, the pathway leading to radiation injury in the lung overlaps with those leading to many other lung injuries.[8,9] In addition, understanding radiation pneumonitis has practical value to physicians in many areas of medicine. Approximately one in three people in the United States will be diagnosed with cancer at some point in their lifetimes. Over half of these patients will be permanently cured of their malignancies. Approximately 65% of all patients with cancer receive radiotherapy at some point in the treatment of their malignancies, and radiotherapy seems destined to remain an important component of cancer treatment for the foreseeable future. Because of this, every physician can expect to care for many patients who are receiving radiotherapy or have received radiotherapy at some point in the past.

In addition to the association of radiation therapy with acute or subacute pulmonary disease, recent studies of plutonium workers have shown an excess incidence of pulmonary fibrosis.[10] These findings, which are supported by data from a large number of studies in experimental animals, show that lung injury may be produced by inhalation of insoluble particulate radionuclides that are deposited in lung tissue and produce long-term irradiation of the tissue.

Respiratory diseases are also known to be a cause of increased late morbidity and mortality in the survivors of the atomic bombs in Hiroshima and Nagasaki.[11] Therefore, radiation injury to lung is possible in cases in which people are exposed to high levels of inhaled radionuclides or external irradiation through their occupations, accidents, or acts of war or terrorism.[9] A working knowledge of the basics of radiobiology and radiation oncology is important to every physician and healthcare provider. An understanding of the potential toxicities of radiotherapy and other exposures to radiation, including radiation pneumonitis, can be critical to patient care.

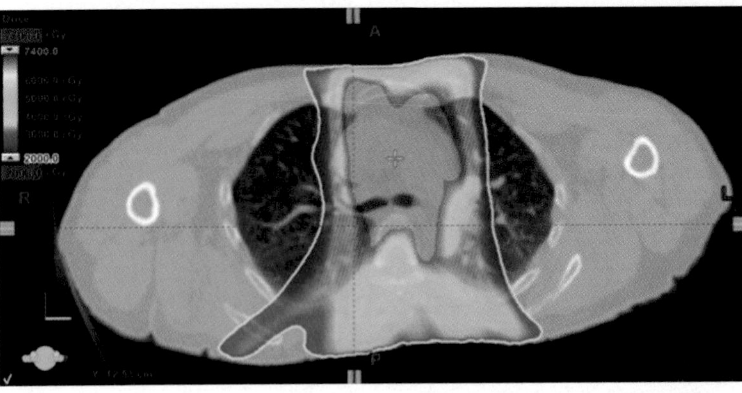

A

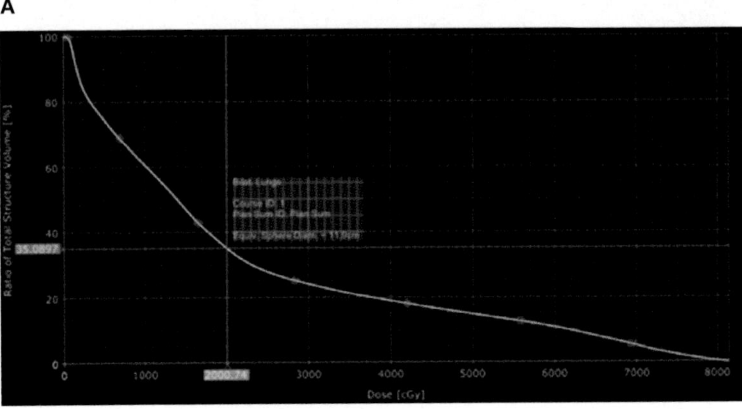

B

Figure 59-1 A 60-year-old man with stage IIIB non–small-cell lung cancer was treated with radiotherapy and concurrent cisplatin-based chemotherapy. The plans for his radiation treatments are summarized. **A.** The isodose distribution from a complex multifield radiation plan is overlaid on a treatment-planning CT scan. Using a color-wash format, radiation dose is demonstrated from 20 Gy *(green)* to 70 Gy *(red)*. **B.** Cumulative dose–volume histogram of the entire treatment course for bilateral lung tissue. The volume of normal lung receiving 20 Gy or more (V_{20}) is 35%.

Many neoplasms involving the thorax are treated with regimens that include the use of radiotherapy to produce either cure or palliation. Radiotherapy is principally a localized, anatomically based modality. The success of radiotherapy hinges on delivering radiation selectively to the sites of malignant disease, while sparing to the maximal extent possible the uninvolved normal tissues.[1,2,5] To plan radiotherapy treatments effectively, the radiation oncologist must have a sophisticated appreciation of the malignancy being treated and understand its biologic behavior, patterns of local and metastatic spread, radiosensitivity, and factors that influence the responses of individual patients to therapy. The radiation oncologist must also consider the effects of radiation on normal tissues within the treatment volumes.

Many factors, including radiation dose, fractionation pattern, volume of the tumor and involved margins, prior or planned use of other therapies such as surgery or systemic chemotherapy, and presence of other diseases influence both the probability of controlling the neoplasm and of producing toxic reactions. For cancers of the lung, esophagus, pleura, breast, and chest wall, as well as for lymphomas involving the thorax, optimal treatment frequently involves use of multiple overlapping X-ray beams and possibly electron beams, planned to encompass all of the cancer-containing tissues. Although treatments are carefully planned to include the smallest possible amount of healthy normal tissue, some normal tissue will necessarily be included in the radiation fields. The radiation sensitivity of the specific tissues in the irradiated fields and the acceptable level of risk for complications combine to limit the dose of radiation that can be administered. The planning of radiotherapy always involves a balance of benefit and risk, because the probabilities of controlling the malignancy increase with increasing radiation dose, but the probabilities and severities of the potential complications increase with dose as well.

To illustrate the mechanisms involved in planning radiotherapy treatments, a treatment plan is depicted in Figure 59-1A. The first panel shows the isodose distribution for treatment of a stage IIIB non–small-cell lung cancer, using a color-wash display in which the highest radiation dose is shown in red and lower doses in shades of yellow, green, and blue. This represents the sum of multiple radiation portals using intensity-modulated radiation therapy (IMRT), in which computer-based planning is used to deliver high dose to the tumor target with specific dose limits to normal tissue structures, such as the spinal cord, esophagus, heart, and lungs. The volume of normal lung receiving significant radiation can be readily appreciated.

The radiation dose delivered to the lung tissue is shown in a cumulative dose–volume histogram, in Figure 59-1B, which integrates the percentage of the volume of the organ at risk (on the vertical axis) receiving the specified cumulative radiation dose (on the horizontal axis). While this is a simplified representation of a complex dose/volume relationship, this formalism has become important in analyzing radiation dose delivery and correlating dosimetry with treatment outcome. In the illustration, the volume of lung receiving greater than or equal to 20 Gy is referred to as the V_{20}. In this case, the V_{20} is 35%, which predicts at least a 25% risk of grade 2 or greater pneumonitis (see discussion below, Clinical Syndromes). In Figure 59-2, the patient's pretreatment CT scan (panel A) is shown in comparison to a 3-month postradiation scan (panel B). The latter demonstrates radiation-induced inflammatory changes corresponding to the high-dose region of the radiotherapy. In this case, these changes were associated with increasing dyspnea, cough, and a decrease in diffusion capacity. Panel C shows slowly resolving changes, with persistent pulmonary fibrotic changes, on a CT scan obtained 1 year post treatment.

In the case presented, if the malignancy is cured, or the patient experiences the desired improvement in symptoms with minimal or manageable toxicity from the radiotherapy, the treatment is a success even if accompanied by radiographic changes or by other subclinical damage to the lung or other organs. Overt pulmonary toxicity is, however, a potential consequence of thoracic radiotherapy that sometimes overshadows the benefits of treatment.

BRIEF OVERVIEW OF RADIOLOGIC PHYSICS

External beam radiotherapy is generally delivered using X-rays or gamma rays. Both of these radiations are high-energy electromagnetic waves or photons that are able to cause ionizations when

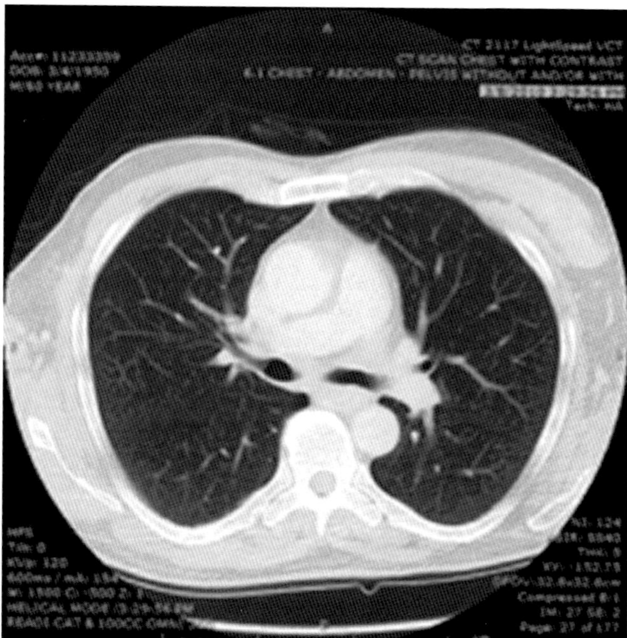

A

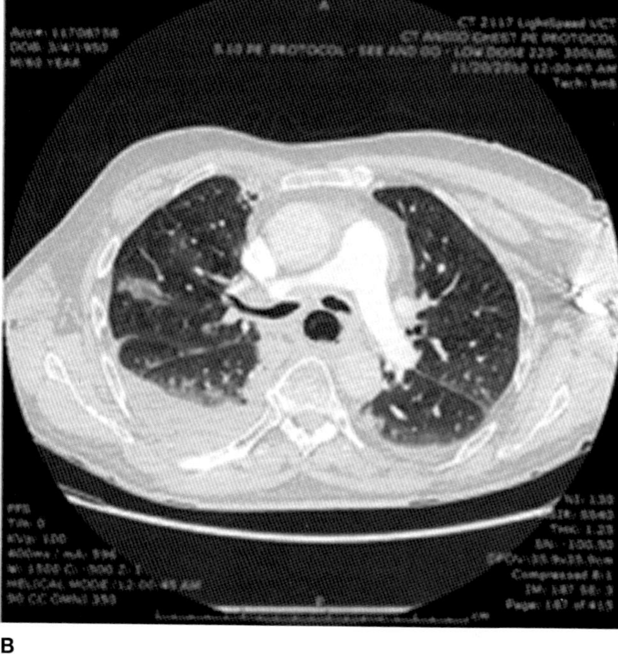

B

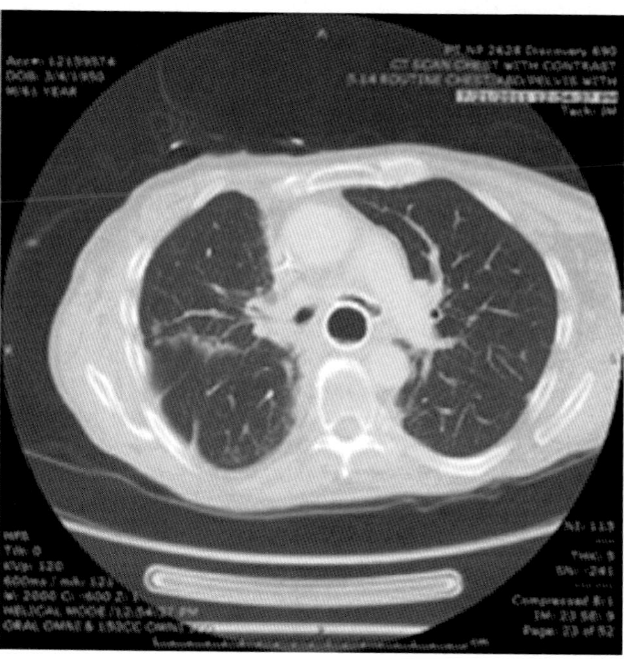

C

Figure 59-2 The same patient as in Figure 59-1, developed a progressive dyspnea and nonproductive cough. A comparison of chest CT imaging from before treatment (Panel A) and 3 months after treatment (**Panel B**) demonstrated interstitial infiltrates and ground-glass changes in a distribution consistent with the prior radiation, as well as the development of new pleural effusions. This is consistent with radiation pneumonitis, and the patient was treated with corticosteroids. He symptomatically improved over several months. A chest CT scan at 1 year (**Panel C**) shows residual fibrotic changes in the paramediastinal region. **Panels** (**B**) and (**C**) also show bronchial and esophageal stents placed for palliation of a tracheoesophageal fistula.

interacting with matter.[7] The only difference between them lies in the manner in which they are produced: Gamma-ray photons are emitted from atomic nuclei during the decay of radioactive atoms, and X-rays are produced when high-energy electrons strike a target material and interact with the electron shells of atoms in that target, causing them to emit X-ray photons (the *bremsstrahlung effect*). After its emission, an individual X-ray photon is indistinguishable from a gamma-ray photon. Thus, although the discussion below uses X-rays as examples, the principles are equally applicable to radiotherapy using high-energy gamma rays (e.g., from cobalt-60 teletherapy units or brachytherapy using implanted radioactive sources).

The X-rays used for diagnostic imaging are in a relatively low-energy range, in which the dominant interaction of photons with matter is through the "*photoelectric effect*." In this process, absorption of a photon causes an electron to be ejected from the inner shell of an atom. The probability of photoelectric interactions increases as a function of the cube of the atomic number, that is, as Z.[3] Consequently, large, heavy atoms absorb low-energy diagnostic X-rays much more efficiently than smaller, lighter atoms.

Diagnostic radiology capitalizes on the large differences between the absorption of low-energy X-rays in materials with different compositions, for example, air, soft tissue (which is 70% water and, therefore, composed primarily of the small atoms hydrogen and oxygen), bone (with its high calcium content), and administered contrast agents containing barium, iodine, or other heavy atoms. The differences in absorption are used to image anatomical structures. In contrast, high-energy X-rays used in radiotherapy interact with matter primarily by a phenomenon called the "*Compton effect*," in which X-rays cause ionization of atoms via interactions with their outer electron shells. The Compton effect is not dependent on the atomic number, but is, instead, a function of the electron density. Because the electron densities of most biologic tissues are relatively uniform, for the purposes of most radiotherapy dosimetry, it is reasonable to assume that a patient is of uniform density, equivalent to water.

An important caveat to radiation dosimetry involves the standard specification of doses in tissues that include a large proportion of air, such as the lung. As a single X-ray beam penetrates through water or tissue, the dose received by the tissue falls progressively, generally as an exponential function of distance. Because of its markedly lower density, air absorbs less radiation energy and, therefore, attenuates the X-rays less than does tissue or water. With the quantitative knowledge of lung density that can now be derived from CT scanning, algorithms have been devised to estimate the inhomogeneity in the absorbed dose resulting from differences in the density of lung and other soft tissues.[7,12] These heterogeneity corrections show that routine dosimetric calculations, which assume uniform density, underestimate the radiation doses to lung and tissues beyond the lung by 5% to 25%.

Although the effect of tissue heterogeneity is a very important consideration when quantifying the radiation dose delivered to the lungs, one must remember that doses delivered to the thorax and the lungs historically have been reported in the medical literature *without* heterogeneity corrections. Moreover, because the preponderance of clinical data concerning lung tolerance have been determined and reported using older dosimetric algorithms, which assume that lung has water-equivalent density, the impetus to change dose reporting is tempered by the desire to avoid confusion between the newer and older literature. The reader should assume, unless explicitly stated otherwise, that the historic radiation doses given in this chapter, or for that matter any publication, are not necessarily corrected for lung density. Most modern radiotherapy planning systems now include the ability to account for tissue heterogeneity. Without such corrections, actual dose delivery to the chest region is modestly higher than the nominal doses reported. However, the variability of the actual dose delivery is highly individual and only recently has been accounted on a routine basis with improvements in computerized treatment planning.

Radiation dose is currently reported using the unit of the Système International (SI), the gray (Gy). The Gy is a measure of the energy absorbed by 1 kg of tissue; 1 Gy = 1 J/kg. The former unit of absorbed dose, called the "rad" (an acronym for "radiation absorbed dose") was measured with the CGS system; by definition, 1 rad = 100 ergs per gram. To compare old and recent literature, one must remember that 1 Gy = 100 rad. Despite the fact that it is not an approved SI unit, some radiotherapy literature avoids this conversion by giving the dose in centigray (cGy), where 1 cGy = 0.01 and Gy = 1 rad. Other measures of radiation dose seen in the literature include the roentgen, the Sievert, and the rem.

The roentgen measures radiation *exposure,* rather than energy *absorption,* and refers specifically to the amount of ionization produced in air under standard conditions (1 R = 1 electrostatic unit/cc = 2.58×10^{-4} coulombs/kg of "standard air" at a density of 1.29×10^{-4} g/cm^3 at 0°C and 760 torr). This unit is frequently encountered in the radiation dosimetry literature, not only because it was historically used as a measure of dose, but also because many widely used radiation monitors (e.g., ionization chambers) directly measure radiation exposure at the surface of the body. The dose absorbed by tissue is then calculated from this exposure.

The radiation protection literature uses the unit of "equivalent dose," the Sievert (Sv), which is calculated as the absorbed dose (in Gy) multiplied by a "weighting factor" that considers the differing biologic effects of different radiations. Although the weighting factors for some radiations, such as neutrons and alpha particles, can be as high as 20, the weighting factors for X-rays, gamma rays, and electrons are all defined as 1. For most purposes in diagnostic and therapeutic radiology, therefore, 1 Sv = 1 Gy. The Sv replaces the older unit of equivalent dose, the rem (1 Sv = 100 rem). Unfortunately, the literature on radiation-induced lung injury includes papers using all of these different units, creating great confusion for readers. For simplicity, all doses in this chapter have been converted to Gy.

RADIOBIOLOGY OF RADIOTHERAPY

When X-rays pass through tissue, a complex series of physical and chemical reactions occurs.[1,13,14] As the X-rays interact with atoms along their path, energy is absorbed, and energetic fast electrons are ejected. These fast electrons travel through tissue, producing secondary ionizations, which lead within milliseconds to the generation of a variety of highly reactive free radical species. Because biologic materials are about 70% water, ions and free radicals derived from water (e.g., H, OH, H_2O^+, H_3O^+) are the main reactive species produced. These ions and radicals react with each other and with other nearby molecules, creating a wide variety of chemically reactive species and producing many kinds of damage in biologic macromolecules. Because DNA contains information that is critical to the cell, while most other molecules can be replaced readily, damage to DNA is the most important biologic effect of irradiation. Radiation produces a wide variety of lesions in DNA, including single- and double-strand breaks, damaged bases and loss of bases, as well as chromosomal breaks and rearrangements. If these lesions are not repaired, the result can be permanent mutations or changes in chromosomal structure that lead to the death of the cell or changes in its behavior.

The cytotoxic effects of radiation are the basis for both the antineoplastic effects and the toxicities of radiotherapy. A theoretical concern is that radiotherapy may produce a mutation in a previously normal cell that leads to the development of a new malignancy. Although radiation-induced malignancies do occur and are a primary concern in considerations of environmental and occupational exposures,[1,11,13] malignant transformation is, fortunately, a rare enough event at the doses used in radiotherapy that the risk of inducing a second cancer in an individual patient is very small relative to the great benefit of curing the existing malignancy.[5] The greater risk to the patient lies in the fact that radiation is not selectively toxic to the tumor cells, but instead, kills both normal and malignant cells within the treatment field.

Although the radiochemical reactions that lead to cytotoxic damage are complete within milliseconds after the end of irradiation, cells dying from radiation injury do not die immediately. In fact, soon after irradiation, radiation-sterilized cells are indistinguishable from cells that ultimately survive irradiation in their appearance, metabolic activities, and even rates and patterns of proliferation. Most radiation-sterilized cells ultimately die during mitosis, but they may first undergo one or even several divisions, producing an abortive clone of sterile cells, all of which ultimately die and disintegrate through apoptosis, necrosis, mitotic catastrophe, senescence, autophagy, or other pathways of cell death.[15,16] This delayed cytotoxicity underlies many of the effects seen in radiotherapy. Rapidly growing tumors, for example, generally begin shrinking sooner than slowly growing tumors, and many tumors continue to shrink progressively for months after radiotherapy.[13,17] Analogously, radiation reactions in normal tissues reflect the normal patterns of cell turnover in the tissue.

After irradiation, nonproliferating, terminally differentiated cells continue to perform their differentiated functions throughout their normal life spans. Other cells that are not proliferating at the time of irradiation likewise continue to function normally until they are recruited into proliferation, perhaps months or even years after irradiation; when they begin to proliferate, their progeny die. Rapidly proliferating cells, such as mucosal or intestinal epithelium or nucleated blood and bone marrow cells, die within a few days of irradiation, leading to the familiar early radiation reactions of epilation, desquamation, mucositis, and hematologic depression.[3,5] Some cell types, especially hematopoietic cells, may be induced by radiation-induced damage to enter a pathway of

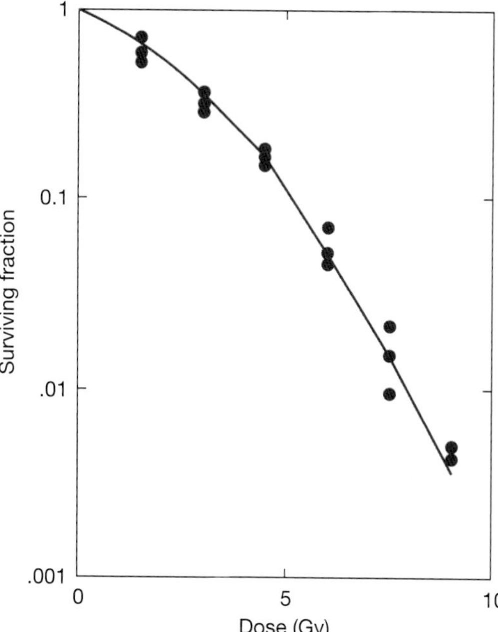

Figure 59-3 Survival of lung cells treated with different doses of radiation. Cells were explanted from mouse lungs, irradiated in vitro, and assayed for viability using a colony formation assay. *(Reproduced with permission from Guichard M, Deschavanne PJ, Malaise EP. Radiosensitivity of mouse lung cells measured using an in vitro colony method. Int J Radiat Oncol Biol Phys. 1980;6(4):441–447.)*

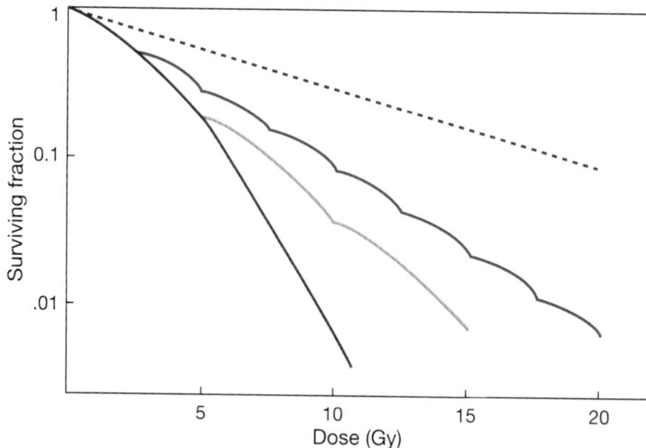

Figure 59-4 Effect of fractionated irradiation and low-dose rate irradiation on cell survival. The survival curve for lung cells treated with a single dose of radiation is redrawn from Fig. 59-3. The calculated effect of dividing the radiation dose into several daily treatments with 5 Gy/fraction or 2.5 Gy/fraction is illustrated. The *dashed line* illustrates the survival curve that would be expected for irradiation delivered continuously at a low-dose rate over several hours, allowing repair and proliferation to occur during treatment. Changes in the cytotoxicity of radiation with fractionation and at low-dose rates lead to decreased injury in lungs irradiated with analogous regimens.

programmed cell death that leads to apoptosis; the role of early and delayed apoptosis in determining the response of tumors and normal tissues to radiotherapy is the subject of intensive investigation.

A typical survival curve for mammalian cells, obtained using mouse lung cells, is shown in Figure 59-3. As a first approximation, cell survival falls exponentially as the radiation dose increases. Statistically, this implies that each incremental dose of radiation has the same cytotoxic effect; that is, each incremental dose kills the same proportion of the viable cells that were present in the population at the beginning of that irradiation. Very low doses of radiation have somewhat lesser effects; the shoulder on the cell survival curve reflects the ability of the cells to accumulate and tolerate or repair some of the damage produced by radiation.

The effect of the repair of radiation damage can be seen when the radiation dose is divided into two or more treatments separated by hours or days, rather than being delivered in a large single dose. Dividing, or "fractionating," the radiation dose allows cells to repair damage to their DNA and to proliferate between treatments.[1,5] As a result, there is less cytotoxicity from a fractionated treatment regimen than from the same total radiation dose delivered as a large single fraction (Fig. 59-4). Smaller fractions produce less cytotoxicity than larger fractions. Similarly, the cytotoxic effects of radiation are diminished when the radiation is delivered continuously at a low-dose rate, over hours or days, allowing repair and proliferation to occur during irradiation (Fig. 59-4).

Fractionating therapeutic irradiations or delivering the radiation at low-dose rates generally appears to increase the therapeutic ratio by protecting normal tissues against radiation injury, while producing a smaller increase in the relative radioresistance of the tumor; treatment outcomes are thereby improved. This increase in the therapeutic ratio is thought to reflect qualitative and quantitative differences between normal and malignant cell populations, including differences in the intrinsic radiosensitivity of the critical cells and in the patterns of cell proliferation and cell loss, as well as differences in the ability of the normal and malignant cells to repair radiation damage. Empiric observations of patients treated with radiotherapy, laboratory experiments with tumors and normal tissues in rodents, and studies with cells in culture have all been used to guide the development of the clinical fractionation schedules now in use. This optimization process is ongoing and will undoubtedly continue, incorporating new information about the repair of radiation damage in normal and malignant cells and about the physiologic factors that modulate development of late radiation injuries in specific normal tissues. In addition, efforts will continue in the development of new technologies for targeting and delivering radiation.

In this process, as in any change in cancer therapy, the critical parameter is the therapeutic ratio (Fig. 59-5). A new treatment regimen is superior *only* when it produces an increased effect on the tumor without an equivalent increase in toxicity to critical normal tissues, reflected in an increase in the therapeutic ratio and therapeutic gain. The art of radiotherapy lies in the design of treatment fields that minimize radiation doses to normal tissues and in the development of treatment regimens that use all available information on the biology of the tumor and of the critical normal tissues.

PATHOPHYSIOLOGY OF RADIATION PNEUMONITIS

Much of our current understanding of the pathophysiology of radiation injury to the lungs is derived from animal experimentation. Translation of animal data to human conditions is always problematic, because differences in the biology and physiology of different species may preclude direct and definitive extrapolation from animals to humans.[9,13,18] Instead, studies with experimental animals must be designed to identify physiologic factors and biologic mechanisms that can be used to interpret clinical data and suggest avenues for clinical investigations.

Data on radiation pneumopathy in humans is fragmentary and complicated by the variability in the patients treated with thoracic irradiation. Most studies of radiation pneumonitis include patients with a variety of malignancies who have been treated with different irradiation regimens, often in combination with chemotherapy and surgery. Moreover, patients vary widely in age and the presence of

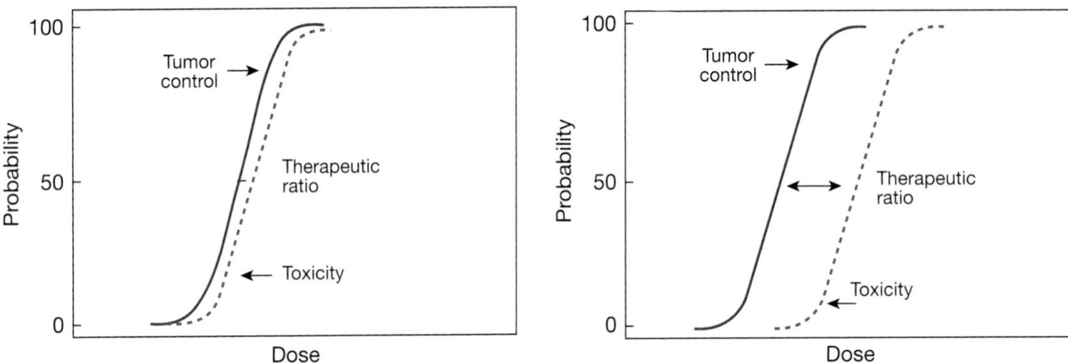

Figure 59-5 The therapeutic ratio is the critical factor determining the success of cancer therapy.

other diseases and risk factors. Therefore, our current understanding of radiation injury to the lung remains incomplete. What is known suggests a complex, multifactorial mechanism of injury and disease progression that reflects cytotoxic effects on both epithelial and endothelial tissues. Inflammatory responses involved in this injury cascade include transient increases in reactive oxygen and nitrogen species, macrophage infiltration and activation, oxidative stress, induction of interstitial fibrosis with regional tissue hypoxia, and disordered cytokine and cellular signaling—including profibrogenic transforming growth factor-beta (TGF-β), proangiogenic hypoxia-inducible factor-1 alpha (HIF-1α), and vascular endothelial growth factor (VEGF).[8,9,14,19–25] Similarities to lung injuries resulting from cancer chemotherapy, other drugs, inhaled chemicals, oxygen toxicity, immune reactions, and idiopathic pulmonary fibrosis are intriguing, especially when one considers that many of these diseases include pathologic responses to free radical chemical species and are likely to reflect similar underlying initial lesions.

Partial-lung resection and localized irradiation have certain similarities: Their effects are largely localized to the treated areas and, consequently, depend on the number of pulmonary lobules or alveolar–capillary units functionally destroyed. Thus, the volume of lung irradiated is an important determinant of toxicity. Consequently, the radiation oncologist plans treatment to minimize the volume of lung receiving high radiation doses, just as the thoracic surgeon plans lung resection with due consideration to anticipated residual lung function. Of course, this simple analogy has its limitations. For example, inactivation of enough lobules by radiation increases the ventilatory dead space and could lead to shunting and ventilation–perfusion mismatching. However, in clinical practice, extensive shunting generally is not observed.[26] In fact, postradiation radionuclide ventilation–perfusion scans tend to show both underperfusion and underventilation that is dose dependent in irradiated areas of partially irradiated lungs.[27] In most cases, radiation injury in lung conforms to the radiation treatment fields, but in some, effects outside the treated areas are observed, with localized radiation inducing a more generalized or diffuse hypersensitivity pneumonitis.[28]

The effects of radiotherapy on the lung reflect the proliferation patterns of the different cellular components of the terminal capillary–alveolar units.[29] Type I pneumocytes are the dominant epithelial cells of the lung, covering about 83% of the alveolar surface. Type I pneumocytes are normally nonproliferating and do not proliferate in response to injury. Consequently, they are thought to be relatively resistant to the cytotoxic effects of radiation.

Type II pneumocytes, which comprise about 16% of the cells in the human lung, are the principal source of surfactant that modifies alveolar surface tension to prevent atelectasis. Type II pneumocytes have turnover times of about 1 month. In response to certain injuries, these granular pneumocytes can be induced both to undergo rapid mitosis and differentiate into type I pneumocytes.

Endothelial cells comprise about 30% of the cells in human lungs and form a continuous layer between the blood and the lung tissue. Although endothelial cells are classified in most tissues as stromal cells, endothelial cells in lung are actually parenchyma, because they are critical to the function of this organ. Capillary endothelial cells are a constantly renewing population, with an estimated turnover time on the order of 2 months. Endothelial cells can be induced into rapid compensatory proliferation after injury; therefore, radiation may result in depletion of both type II pneumocytes and endothelial cells.

Several lines of evidence suggest that radiation injury is related primarily to cytotoxic damage, especially to the surfactant-producing type II pneumocytes and vascular endothelial cells. Although clinical signs of pneumonitis require weeks to develop, laboratory studies reveal evidence of lung injury within hours after large single doses of radiation.[6,22,30–32] Shortly after irradiation, electron microscopy may detect abnormalities in surfactant-containing lamellar bodies. There is an increase in surfactant in bronchoalveolar lavage specimens within hours of irradiation that persists for several weeks. Ultrastructural evidence of endothelial cell damage is also seen soon after lung irradiation, and a rapid increase in capillary permeability occurs, reflecting loss of integrity of cell junctions, intracellular vacuolization, cellular pleomorphism, and sloughing of the basement membrane. Capillary occlusion by cellular debris and microthrombi may occur at high doses.

The clinical course of lung injury occurs later and includes a pneumonitic phase, developing weeks to months after radiation, followed by a fibrotic phase, developing months to years later. To explain the two clinical phases, Rubin and Casarett's original model of radiation lung toxicity suggested that the pneumocytes and endothelium represented two separate and distinct cellular targets, and that damage to pneumocytes led to pneumonitis, while vascular damage led to fibrosis. This older model is now thought to be incorrect; current data[19,20,22,29,33–38] suggest that the pneumonitic and fibrotic processes both are manifestations of a common pathway of injury and response.

Histologically, one can recognize a typical sequence of events developing in the lung after large doses of radiation.[6,21,30] Within days to weeks, vascular congestion and intra-alveolar edema and exudation occur, followed by infiltration of inflammatory cells and epithelial desquamation. Weeks later, collagen fibrils are deposited within areas of injury and interstitial edema, leading to a thickening of alveolar septa similar to that in hyaline membrane disease. The probability and severity of these changes are quite variable and depend on such factors as the radiation dose and treatment volume. The severity of the damage and volume of tissue affected determine whether a pneumonitic picture becomes clinically evident. Resolution of inflammatory infiltrates and alveolar exudates, which can be improved by anti-inflammatory agents such as glucocorticoids, correlates with symptomatic improvement and resolution of radiographic opacities in the affected lung.

Inflammatory cells, particularly alveolar macrophages, migrate into areas of radiation injury. This induces an ensuing cytokine cascade and mediates the host response,[9,20,22,25] similar to that which occurs in other inflammatory conditions, which can lead to pulmonary fibrosis.

Rubin et al. have detected a biphasic increase in mRNA expression for the proinflammatory cytokines IL-1α, IL-1β, and TNF-α at 2 and 8 weeks after radiation.[22] Preliminary clinical trials also suggest that elevated serum levels of IL-6 before and during radiotherapy predict an elevated risk of radiation pneumonitis. Beginning 24 hours following radiation, TGF-β, a cytokine that mediates fibrotic responses, increases.[21] Elevated levels of VEGF may be detected 2 weeks later. Tissue hypoxia accompanies the inflammatory response. Clinical data implicating TGF-β as a predictive marker for pneumonitis, however, have been mixed. Collagen gene expression is also appreciably increased corresponding to the fibrotic changes seen histologically. These studies suggest that early and persistent elevations of cytokine production and alterations of intercellular signaling are critical to the development of radiation reactions in the lung. There is increasing evidence from studies with inbred mice that genetic differences, age, and past health and treatment history modulate the development and severity of fibrosis and hyaline membrane formation, thus determining the nature of the late toxic lesion and the time of development of radiation pneumotoxicity.[9,33,34]

The processes described earlier lead to pathologic changes that conform spatially to the areas to which localized radiation was administered. Interestingly, it has been discovered that radiation can also induce an allergic alveolitis. This is observed infrequently as a diffuse pneumonitis, or occasionally as a patchy, transient bronchiolitis obliterans organizing pneumonia (BOOP; see Chapter 57) occurring outside the treated fields. In its most severe form, the result is the acute respiratory distress syndrome (ARDS; see Chapter 141). Morgan and Breit[28] have suggested that this form of radiation-induced pneumonitis be termed "sporadic". The occurrence of the syndrome actually may be more common than appreciated. One series showed a 2.3% incidence of BOOP in women undergoing whole breast radiotherapy, occurring outside the radiotherapy fields four or more months after exposure.[39] Bronchoalveolar lavage in humans and in experimental animals frequently shows a significant increase in activated T-helper ($CD4^+$) lymphocytes, temporally related to irradiation and occurring equally in the irradiated lung and the contralateral, nonirradiated lung. Gallium scanning may also show bilateral uptake not corresponding to the treated regions. Frequent reports of autoantibodies, including antibodies to collagen, in the sera of patients with cancer even before treatment suggest the possibility that malignancy-associated autoimmune reactions may be involved in the syndrome.

CONFOUNDING EFFECTS OF CHEMOTHERAPY

Many cytotoxic drugs employed as antineoplastic agents can produce pulmonary toxicity (see Chapter 65).[40–42] Bleomycin, which has been extensively studied, kills cells by generating reactive free radical species similar to radiotherapy and may give rise to both pneumonitis and fibrosis.[42] Doxorubicin, mitomycin C, irinotecan, and gefitinib have been associated with lung toxicity, as have the antimetabolites (methotrexate, cytosine arabinoside, gemcitabine, fludarabine, and the nitrosamines) and the podophyllotoxins (etoposides, paclitaxel, and docetaxel). Interestingly, lung injury has also been reported after treatment with immune modulators, including interferons, IL-2, and TNF-α.

As high-dose alkylating agent chemotherapy is used more frequently in the setting of bone marrow or peripheral stem cell transplantation, agents such as cyclophosphamide, BCNU, and busulfan have been associated increasingly with clinically significant pneumonitis. The direct toxicity of many widely used anticancer drugs to the lungs sounds a note of caution for those considering development of treatment protocols combining systemic chemotherapy with lung irradiation. Moreover, the concurrent administration of antineoplastic agents and radiotherapy may make it difficult to discern to what degree pulmonary injury in an individual patient is related to radiotherapy alone.

Animal studies addressing changes in respiratory rates and/or death resulting from lung injury show that the severity of the lung injury can be increased when doxorubicin, bleomycin, cyclophosphamide, mitomycin C, dactinomycin, or vincristine are administered along with radiation.[43,44] No enhancement has been documented in studies with 5-fluorouracil, cisplatinum, carboplatinum, hydroxyurea, vinblastine, or methotrexate, despite reports of lung toxicity from methotrexate alone.

As a wide variety of cytokines and molecularly targeted agents are now available for pharmacologic administration, modulation of radiation injury by these biologic agents needs increased study. Interferons have been shown both to increase and decrease radiation lung toxicity, whereas interleukins 1 and 2 may have protective effects. Some radiation-drug interactions in the lung have been shown to be schedule dependent, with the effect of the combination varying with the sequence and the time between treatments with the two agents.[43,44] Additive, subadditive, and even supra-additive toxicities may be observed in rodents when single treatments with the same dose of radiation and drug are given over a 24-hour period, but in different sequences and different times between treatments. Such findings highlight the complexities of combined-modality therapy and the difficulty of using animal data to plan clinical treatment regimens.

Data from several specific clinical situations show that regimens combining radiation with particular chemotherapy agents can produce significant risks of pneumonitis. As summarized in reviews of chemotherapy and radiation-induced pneumonitis, docetaxel, mitomycin C, gemcitabine, and irinotecan given concurrently with radiotherapy seem to elevate the risk of pneumonitis or lung toxicity.[45,46] On the other hand, drugs that are commonly used in lung cancer concurrent with radiotherapy, such as cisplatin, carboplatin, paclitaxel, and etoposide, do not consistently elevate the risk of pneumonitis; alternatively, the clinical data regarding pneumonitis risk so commonly include these chemotherapy agents that the risk may already be incorporated into consideration.[47–51] Older clinical data from pediatric trials strongly suggest that administration of concurrent doxorubicin or actinomycin D with thoracic radiotherapy generally should be avoided or, alternatively, that the radiation doses should be reduced significantly where these drugs are used.

Sequential treatment with doxorubicin or actinomycin D and radiation is less likely to produce lung injury. However, a phenomenon termed "radiation recall" has been well described, in which either of these two drugs given even several months after radiotherapy will produce an inflammatory reaction in the region corresponding to the radiation treatment fields.[52] Although this reaction is best known in skin, it also has been well documented in the lungs in several case reports and has been produced in experimental animals. Radiation recall probably reflects the fact that the irradiated areas of the lung still retain residual, subclinical injury, which is exacerbated into clinical pneumonitis as a result of the additional injury from the drug. Therefore, the biologic basis of the recall phenomenon is analogous to that of the residual radiation injury, which decreases the ability of heavily irradiated lung tissue to tolerate a second course of radiotherapy delivered months or years later.[5,6,37]

CLINICAL SYNDROMES

Radiation oncologists conventionally divide clinical toxicities into acute and late effects,[5,6] with both radiation pneumonitis and fibrosis considered late toxicities. Several grading systems for pneumonitis

TABLE 59-1 Toxicity Criteria for Pneumonitis

Scoring System	Grade 1	2	3	4	5
CTCAE	Asymptomatic; radiographic findings only	Symptomatic; not interfering with ADL	Symptomatic; interfering with ADL; O_2 indicated	Life-threatening ventilatory support indicated	Death
RTOG/EORTIC (LENT-SOMA)	Asymptomatic or mild symptoms (dry cough), with radiographic findings	Moderately symptomatic (severe cough fever)	Severely symptomatic	Severe respiratory insufficiency; continuous oxygen/assisted ventilation	Death
SWOG (33)	Asymptomatic or symptoms not requiring steroids with radiographic findings	Initiation of or increase in steroids required	O_2 required	Assisted ventilation necessary	Death

CTCAE, common terminology criteria for adverse events; ADL, activities of daily living; RTOG, Radiation Therapy Oncology Group; EORTC, European Organization for the Research and Treatment of Cancer; LENT-SOMA, late effects on normal tissue-subjective, objective, management and analytic scales; SWOG, Southwest Oncology Group. Source: Reproduced with permission from Mehta V. Radiation pneumonitis and pulmonary fibrosis in non-small-cell lung cancer: pulmonary function, prediction, and prevention. Int J Radiat Oncol Biol Phys. 2005;63(1):5–24.

have been developed for scoring lung injury during clinical trials (Table 59-1).

ACUTE MANIFESTATIONS

It is relatively uncommon to observe acute pulmonary toxicity during the administration of fractionated radiotherapy. However, at relatively high therapeutic doses (50–60 Gy), acute radiation changes in the tracheobronchial tree can be expected. Bronchoscopic examination is likely to reveal erythematous mucosa, with thickened secretions that can accumulate in and obstruct the airways. Although a majority of patients remain asymptomatic, occasional patients experience an irritative, dry cough. Antitussive agents, such as codeine, adequate hydration, and reassurance are usually all that are required to manage this problem. Once radiotherapy has been completed, the bronchial epithelium regenerates and heals over several weeks, accompanied by resolution of symptoms.

LATE MANIFESTATIONS

The clinical course of late radiation injury to the lungs is biphasic, with both inflammatory and fibrotic components.[19,30,32]

Radiation Pneumonitis

A pneumonitic process frequently becomes evident 6 weeks to 6 months following radiotherapy. At this time, radiographs show alveolar opacities that generally conform to the treatment portals. The severity of radiation pneumonitis varies dramatically from patient to patient, even in those receiving identical therapeutic regimens. In most cases, the pneumonitis is asymptomatic, even though radiologic abnormalities are quite common, as noted in some prospective studies, in which as many as 50% of patients who have completed a course of thoracic radiotherapy were asymptomatic.

When symptomatic, this syndrome is often characterized by the abrupt onset of fever, cough, and dyspnea. The severity of symptoms depends on the extent of radiotherapy, increasing with the treated volume and with the radiation dose. Symptoms in patients irradiated to limited lung volumes or to relatively low doses may consist of low-grade fever, cough, congestion, and chest fullness or discomfort. Any hemoptysis tends to be minimal. In more severe situations, dyspnea, high fever, and cough occur. When large volumes of normal lung receive high radiation dose, acute radiation pneumonitis is more likely and can be extremely severe, producing respiratory distress. The radiation oncologist is probably most likely to see clinically significant radiation pneumonitis that can be life-threatening when it occurs as a rare and unanticipated consequence of standard treatment, despite appropriate treatment planning designed to minimize the volume of lung treated with high doses of radiation. Fortunately, with well-planned radiotherapy, severe radiation pneumonitis is a rare event. Milder pneumonitis is not uncommon, but is readily manageable.

It is important to distinguish radiation pneumonitis from infection, recurrent tumor (particularly with lymphangitic spread), drug reactions, congestive heart failure, and other respiratory disorders. These distinctions may not be easy; one series from Duke suggested that up to 28% of patients with radiation-associated lung toxicity have complex comorbidities that make it difficult to assign a definitive diagnosis.[53] Bacterial, fungal, viral, and pneumocystis pneumonias can be quite difficult to differentiate from pneumopathy induced by chemotherapy or radiation.

Aids in the differential diagnosis include the clinical course and temporal relationship between the irradiation and respiratory illness. Definition of the radiographic pattern of the infiltrate is also very useful, because radiation pneumonitis often conforms to the outline of the sharply demarcated radiation portal (Figs. 59-2 and 59-6). Bronchoscopy and lung biopsy can also be helpful diagnostic tools to direct therapeutic decisions. Ruling out infection is particularly important, because treatment of symptomatic radiation pneumonitis relies on supportive care in conjunction with corticosteroids.

Doses of glucocorticoids generally can be tailored to the severity of the symptoms. Asymptomatic pneumonitis may be managed with close observation. Severe cases generally warrant treatment with prednisone (or its equivalent) at a dose of 0.5 to 1 mg/kg per day in divided doses. Response rates between 20% and 100% have been reported, and dramatic clinical and radiographic responses are not infrequently seen. Steroids should be tapered slowly after the patient is stabilized, because it is common to see a recrudescence of symptomatology when steroids are discontinued too rapidly. Failure to respond to steroid therapy is an adverse prognostic factor that suggests the prospect of rapid disease progression.

Most studies show at least a transient decline in pulmonary function in patients who receive radiation to a significant lung volume (i.e., patients with lung cancer receiving a potentially curative course of fractionated radiotherapy). There may be a transient reduction in FEV_1 and FVC 3 to 6 months post radiation. Carbon monoxide diffusing capacity (DL_{CO}) may be reduced over a similar time course, but typically to a greater degree relative to baseline.[54] Absent the development of radiation fibrosis, these parameters tend to recover toward the patient's baseline, reaching maximal recovery at approximately 12 months.

Radiation Fibrosis

A more indolent fibrotic process may follow either subclinical or symptomatic radiation pneumonitis.[19,30,32] This begins several

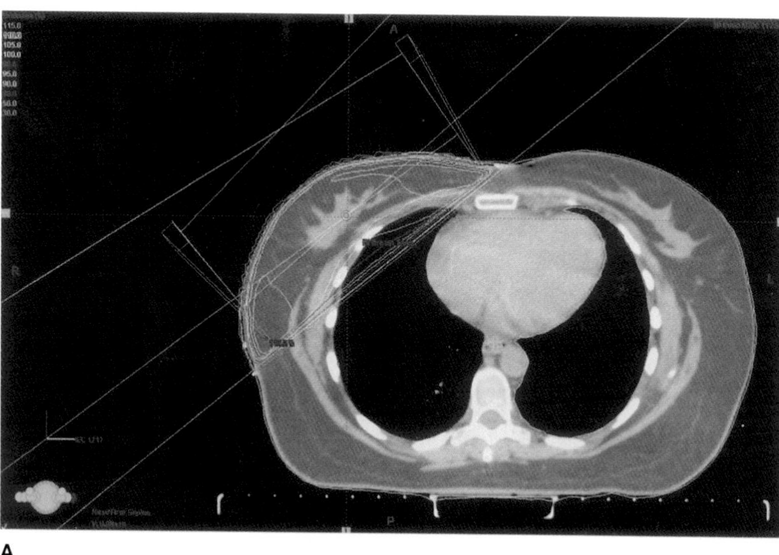

A

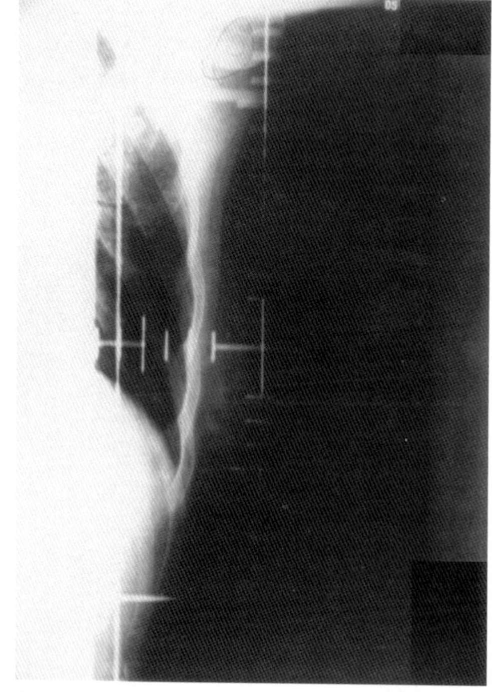

B

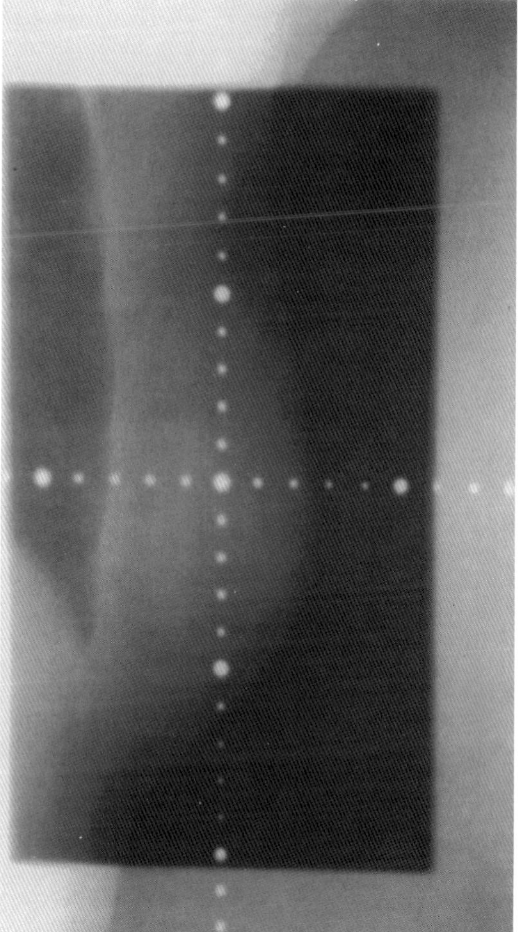

C

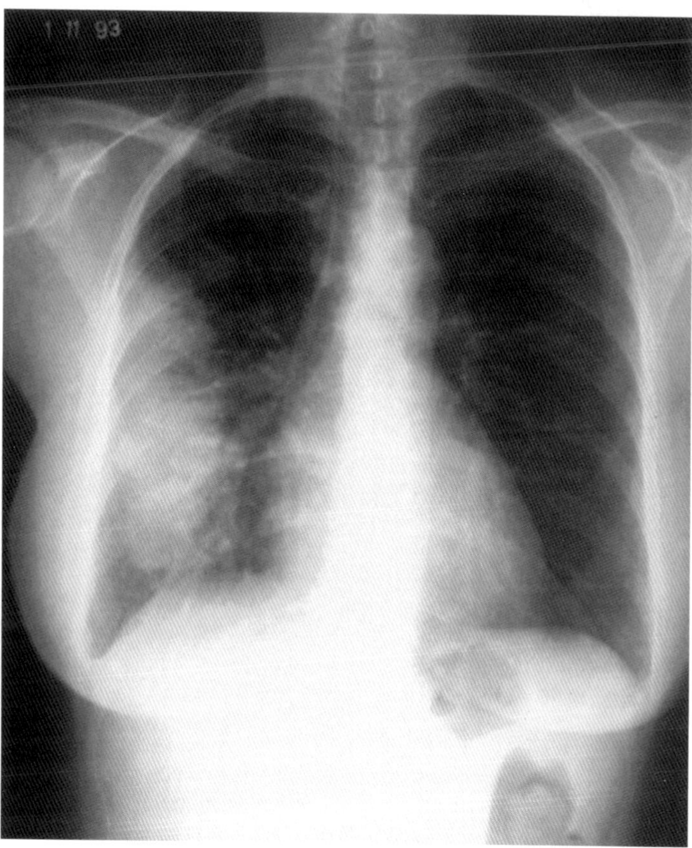

D

Figure 59-6 A 52-year-old woman found a nontender lump in her right breast and subsequently underwent a lumpectomy for a localized 1.4-cm diameter infiltrating ductal carcinoma. The axillary lymph nodes were negative. The patient was placed on Tamoxifen and underwent radiotherapy to the right breast, using tangential fields, to 50 Gy in 25 fractions over 36 days. **A.** A radiation dose distribution of the photon fields overlying the right breast and chest wall. This was followed by boost radiation treatments to the surgical bed for an additional 14 Gy in seven fractions. **B**, **C.** The simulation and port films, respectively, of the whole-breast treatments, highlighting the different interactions of low-energy and high-energy X-rays with tissues. Four months after radiotherapy, the patient developed radiation pneumonitis characterized by fever, cough, and dyspnea requiring hospitalization. **D.** A right-lung opacity that does not correspond to normal anatomic structures but does correspond to her treatment fields. *(continued)*

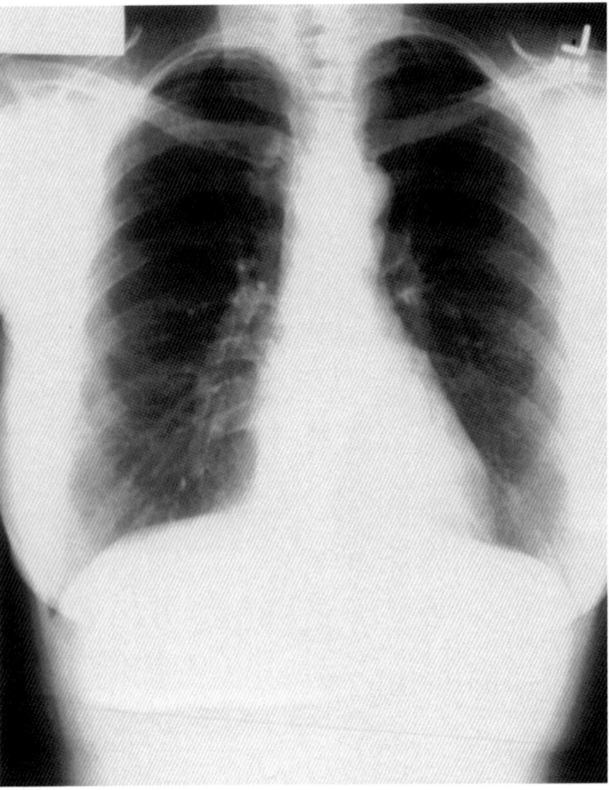

E

Figure 59-6 *(Continued)* **E.** The patient responded dramatically to steroids, with resolution of radiographic findings on follow-up chest radiographs.

months after radiotherapy and peaks in radiographic severity several years later. Fibrosis tends to occur in, or adjacent to, areas of prior pneumonitis,[33] but it can also occur in the absence of clinically overt radiation pneumonitis. Fibrotic changes and the retraction of the lung parenchyma from scarring occur in the irradiated regions (Fig 59-2). When the volume of lung irradiated is relatively small and the remaining lung parenchyma contains sufficient respiratory surface area, the changes tend to be asymptomatic.

With increasing relative volumes of pulmonary fibrosis, a spectrum of symptomatology is possible, ranging from mild dyspnea on exertion to severe fibrosis with respiratory compromise, chronic cor pulmonale, cyanosis, and finger clubbing. At the severe end of the spectrum, the syndrome can be life-threatening. In general, in the absence of other underlying lung disease, symptoms are mild when less than 25% to 30% of total lung parenchyma is involved.

Radiation-induced Pleural Reactions

Pleuritis may also be seen 2 to 6 months following radiation. It can be associated with pleuritic chest pain, a pleural friction rub, and an exudative pleural effusion. Large effusions are, however, distinctly unusual in the absence of other pathology. Like radiation pneumonitis, radiation-induced pleuritis may heal without significant residue, or it may proceed through a fibrotic phase that generates pleural thickening.

Radiation-induced Bronchial Stenosis

With improvements in the technical delivery of radiotherapy, recent clinical trials for lung cancer have emphasized escalation of the administered radiation dose. Stereotactic body radiotherapy (SBRT) utilizes —three to five large fractions (i.e., >10 Gy per fraction), delivering significantly higher biologically effective doses than are feasible with conventional fractionated radiotherapy.[55] As a result, there is an increasing appreciation that, particularly for perihilar tumors, radiation-induced fibrosis may result in bronchial stenosis or necrosis, causing postobstructive atelectasis, volume loss, and functional impairment.[56–58] Clinically, this complication needs to be differentiated from recurrent tumor; bronchoscopy or positron emission tomography (PET) imaging may be of help. One retrospective series in which radiation doses ranged from 60 Gy to as high as 86 Gy demonstrated that radiation-induced bronchial stenosis may occur in up to 25% of patients; the incidence directly correlates with radiation dose.[59] However, severe bronchial injury is rare with fractionated chest radiotherapy using conventional doses.

DEFINING THE RADIATION TOLERANCE OF THE LUNGS

While we customarily refer to radiation doses that can be delivered safely either to the whole body or to a particular organ, radiation *tolerance* is usually defined as the dose that yields a 5% risk of severe late radiation injury.[60] When discussing the tolerance of the lungs, one must consider several different therapeutic situations. The tolerance of the lung varies with the volume of lung tissue irradiated.[5,35,60,61] In addition, single-dose irradiations, fractionated irradiations, and irradiations given at low-dose rates each pose different risks of injury, and therefore, they must be considered separately.[5,38,62] Additional injury from surgery or chemotherapy or from a prior course of radiotherapy also must be considered, as must the confounding effects of injury to lung tissue from coexisting cardiopulmonary disease and from the underlying malignancy.

Infections and immunologic reactions are also important. The clinical endpoints used to define a case of radiation pneumonitis vary as well, because the severity of the lung injury spans a wide spectrum of diagnostic signs and clinical symptoms. Moreover, with improvements in imaging and three-dimensional dose-calculation algorithms, there is a concerted effort within the radiation oncology community to better define dose–volume determinants for a variety of organ radiation-related toxicities. Known as QUANTEC (quantitative analysis of normal tissue effects in the clinic), this broad compilation of data shows that there are strong correlations of pneumonitis risk with radiation dose, fractionation, and tissue volume.[63] Given the heterogeneity of clinical circumstances and biologic data in general, it is not surprising that the medical literature that defines the risks for radiation pneumonitis and fibrosis is extremely complex and often difficult to interpret.

■ WHOLE-LUNG IRRADIATION

A good starting point for considering lung tolerance is analysis of the effects of irradiating the entire lung. This construct has direct clinical relevance because there are several circumstances in which the entire lung is irradiated. These include total-body irradiation (TBI) for bone marrow or hematologic stem cell transplantation, hemibody irradiation for palliation of widespread metastatic disease, and whole-lung irradiation given electively or therapeutically for relatively radiosensitive tumors, such as Wilms tumor, Ewing sarcoma, or Hodgkin lymphoma. These are often circumstances in which chemotherapy is administered as well.

Published experience from the Princess Margaret Hospital in Toronto[12,64–67] provides some of the best data regarding whole-lung tolerance. Investigators from that institution have an extensive experience with delivering upper hemibody irradiation to different doses and varying fractionation patterns. They reported in 1978 on a cohort of 245 patients, most with metastatic solid tumors, who received single-fraction, upper hemibody irradiation at dose rates of 0.3 to 0.8 Gy/min to doses of up to 10 Gy.[64] The actuarial incidence of acute radiation pneumonitis, defined as the sudden onset of cough, dyspnea, and opacities visible on chest radiographs at about 16 weeks following treatment, was strikingly dose dependent

TABLE 59-2 Actuarial Incidence of Radiation Pneumonitis after Single-fraction Whole-lung Irradiation

Uncorrected Dose	Patients	Pneumonitis (%)
<6 Gy	49	2.7
6 Gy	24	17.5
8 Gy	149	35.6
10 Gy	23	83.9

Source: Data from Fryer Fitzpatrick PJ, Rider WD; CJH, et al. Int J Radiat Oncol Biol Phys. 1978;4:931–936.
Note: Doses are not corrected for heterogeneity in tissue density.

(Table 59-2). The doses shown in Table 59-2 were not corrected for heterogeneity in density.[12] When doses are corrected, resulting in an upward estimation of the doses actually received by the lungs, analysis yielded the sigmoid-shaped curve shown in Figure 59-7.

Using heterogeneity-corrected data, the incidence of pneumonitis is estimated to be negligible for single doses less than about 7.5 Gy. Other published data regarding upper hemibody single-fraction irradiation are in general agreement with these findings.

Careful analysis suggests that the single-fraction data might predict an unacceptable risk for pneumonitis when single-fraction TBI is utilized in the setting of bone marrow transplantation (BMT). The most important treatment factor making single-fraction TBI in the range of 8 to 10 Gy (uncorrected for heterogeneity) tolerable is that treatments generally are given at a low-dose rate (less than or equal to 0.1 Gy/min) over 1 to 2 hours.[38,68] In Seattle, where hundreds of patients with leukemia have undergone BMT after TBI, using single fractions of 10 Gy (uncorrected) delivered at dose rates on the order of 0.08 Gy/min, the incidence of pneumonitis is roughly 25%. Review of transplant-related single-fraction TBI with variable dose rates shows incidences of clinical lung injury varying from 25% to 70%.[65,69–71]

Studies in mice show that the toxicities of TBI can be improved further by fractionating the irradiation, as well as by delivering radiation at a low-dose rate. This concept is supported by a randomized clinical trial comparing low-dose rate, single-fraction TBI (10 Gy)

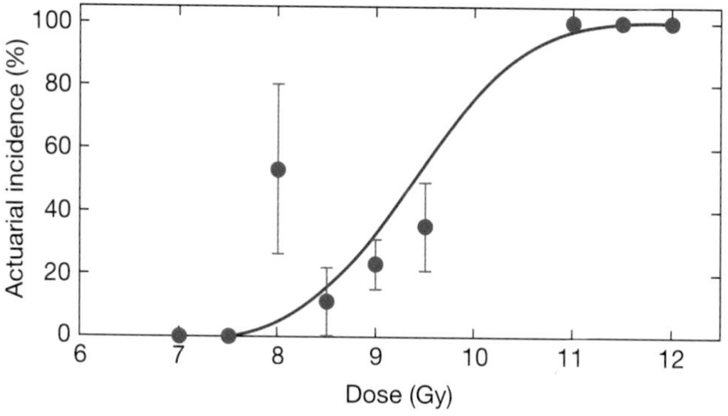

Figure 59-7 Incidence of radiation pneumonitis in patients receiving single-dose, whole-lung irradiation at dose rates of 0.3 to 0.8 Gy/min. Unlike most doses given in the text, doses on this figure *are* corrected for heterogeneity in density. The effect of this correction can be seen by comparing these data with those in Table 59-1, which were derived from an earlier analysis by the same group and are presented using uncorrected doses. *(Reproduced with permission from Van Dyk J, Keane TJ, Kan S, et al. Radiation pneumonitis following large single dose irradiation: a re-evaluation based on absolute dose to lung. Int J Radiat Oncol Biol Phys. 1981;7(4):461–467.)*

with low-dose rate, fractionated TBI (12 Gy in six fractions over three days) for patients with acute myelogenous leukemia in first remission. A significant improvement in event-free survival was noted with fractionation, mainly because of an improvement in early mortality.[68] Interstitial pneumonitis was decreased from 26% to 15% with fractionation. Other studies have corroborated a reduced incidence of pneumonitis to less than 20% without increasing the rate of tumor recurrence using fractionated TBI.[72–74] Within a range of 1.5 to 2 Gy per fraction given once or twice daily, there is no significant increase in pneumonitis risk using doses up to 15 Gy.[72,75,76] Nevertheless, total dose delivered to the lung is a key determinant of pneumonitis risk.[65,77] In addition, at many transplant centers it has become common practice to utilize lung transmission blocks to attenuate the lung dose and thereby reduce the risk of pneumonitis, in part by compensating for the heterogeneity in tissue density due to the air within the lungs.[71]

Another radiobiologic approach to reduce the incidence of interstitial pneumonitis has been to lower the dose rate at which the radiation is delivered—in essence, a kind of continuous fractionation. While efficacious,[78,79] treatment times of 2 to 3 hours are impractical and poorly tolerated by patients. Within the context of fractionated TBI schemes, instantaneous dose rates of 0.05 to 0.18 Gy/min generally have been employed due to practical considerations. Whether or not higher instantaneous dose rates are detrimental in the context of fractionated TBI remains unclear. One small study comparing dose rates of 0.075 versus 0.15 Gy/min for TBI prescribed to 12 Gy in six fractions reported pneumonitis risks of 13% and 43%, respectively, for these dose rates, although there were many confounding covariates.[80]

Pneumonitis in the BMT setting has a multifactorial etiology, reflecting not only the effects of radiation, but also the effects of chemotherapy, graft-versus-host disease (GVH), lung injury from tumor, opportunistic infections, and other risk factors.[69,71,81] Cyclophosphamide is almost universally given with TBI. The addition of other drugs is based on institutional treatment policies; many of these anticancer drugs are known to injure the lung.[41,42] BMT conditioning regimens that do not use TBI (which often use high-dose busulfan in place of radiation) in fact have rates of interstitial pneumonitis comparable to regimens that include TBI. The presence of GVH is also important, not only because GVH causes lung injury directly, but also because the drugs used to control GVH injure the lung. Perhaps, for this reason, T-cell-depleted transplants, which produce less GVH, tend to have lower risk for pneumonitis.[82]

Whole-lung irradiation has been used in the treatment of widespread lung metastases. In two published series, a combined total of 70 patients with osteosarcoma who received elective whole-lung irradiation to prevent pulmonary metastases (which is not currently a standard practice pattern) received 15 to 17.5 Gy in 10 fractions. None of these patients developed pneumonitis.[19] Similarly, in a series of 40 patients who received 20 to 25 Gy of thoracic irradiation in 1.5-Gy fractions to treat pulmonary metastasis, no cases of pneumonitis were reported.[19] This and other clinical experience with fractionated whole-lung irradiation in the nontransplant setting and in the absence of chemotherapy indicate that the following dose schemes should have a relatively low risk (<5%) for radiation pneumonitis: 25 Gy given in 20 fractions over 4 weeks or 20 Gy given in 10 fractions over 2 weeks. (All doses noted are without heterogeneity corrections.)

Historically, radiotherapy for Hodgkin disease has used whole-lung treatment in situations in which there is massive mediastinal adenopathy, hilar adenopathy, or overt pulmonary disease treated with chemotherapy. Risks of symptomatic pneumonitis ranging from 7% to 35% have been reported, with the risk highly dependent on the total radiation dose and the fractionation pattern.[19,83] When the whole lung is to be irradiated, available data suggest that the lungs should be treated through transmission blocks, rather than using open fields. This reduces both the total dose and the dose per fraction to the lungs, thereby reducing the risk of symptomatic pneumonitis to 4% to 7% over a broad range of total lung doses of 10 to 20 Gy.

There is a suggestion that the addition of mediastinal irradiation to fractionated whole-lung radiotherapy increases the risk of pneumonitis. To many oncologists, the risk of radiation pneumonitis from such a treatment seems too great. As a result, such patients are often treated primarily with chemotherapy (often with adjuvant low-dose radiotherapy), even though these regimens also produce significant risks for lung toxicity. In the setting of pulmonary metastases, the addition of low-dose radiotherapy to the whole lung after chemotherapy is controversial. There are few clinical data to quantify risks and benefits, but doses of 10 to 16 Gy, given in 0.7- to 1.5-Gy fractions, are associated with only modest risk.[19,83]

Lung radiotherapy using 12 to 14 Gy for pulmonary metastases in pediatric patients with Wilms tumor (who also receive sequential doxorubicin and actinomycin D) is associated with a 10% incidence of pneumonitis.[84] Long-term follow-up in such children also shows restrictive lung disease, with total lung and vital capacities approximately 70% of the predicted values. In children receiving thoracic irradiation, inhibition of normal growth and development of the lung parenchyma and bones as a result of radiotherapy also produces significant morbidity. The effects of radiation on growth and development and the radiosensitivity of growing tissues raise special concerns in the treatment of pediatric patients.[5]

PARTIAL-LUNG IRRADIATION

The role of partial-lung irradiation in the treatment of various malignancies and assessment of its risks are considered below.

Assessment of Risk

Estimating the risks of radiation pneumopathy for individual patients receiving fractionated external beam radiotherapy is a daunting task, because so many confounding factors must be considered. With lung cancer, the tumor size and location influence the volume of adjacent normal lung that must be irradiated. The volume irradiated should determine the number of capillary–alveolar units destroyed and, therefore, should influence the risk of symptomatic radiation pneumonitis and fibrosis.[29] This qualitative prediction is borne out by clinical experience, but quantifying the risks is not straightforward. The lung region irradiated is also important, because the upper lung regions contribute less to gas exchange than do the lower regions. Treatment-related factors such as total dose, dose per fraction, and overall treatment time are also important, as are the other confounding factors described in the preceding sections.[32]

Patients begin radiotherapy with a wide range of pulmonary function, reflecting age, smoking history, and the presence or absence of underlying cardiopulmonary disease. Because regional pulmonary fibrosis may be partially compensated by functional lung parenchyma, pretreatment lung status influences the severity of symptoms. The clinical endpoints used to measure lung injury are quite varied and include symptom and quality-of-life scores; radiographic changes, such as changes in CT-assessed lung density, pneumonitis, and fibrosis; and other objective measures.[32]

Pulmonary function tests are global measure of organ function that correlate imperfectly with symptomatology after partial-lung irradiation. A large tumor mass may cause localized obstructive or restrictive changes in lung function or phrenic nerve dysfunction, any of which may improve or worsen as the tumor shrinks with treatment. These factors add to the variability produced by patient-to-patient differences in the treatment volume, dose, fractionation, etc. Thus, radiotherapy-induced changes in global lung function with regard to gas exchange, physiologic dead space, shunting, ventilation–perfusion mismatch, and respiratory surface area, as measured by arterial blood gases, spirometry, and DL_{CO}, are complex and highly individualized.

Several clinical studies have attempted to predict radiotherapy-induced changes in FEV_1 by superimposing radiation treatment portals on quantitative ventilation and perfusion scans.[85–88] Unfortunately, the simple notion that the proportion of lung irradiated should match the drop in FEV_1, akin to the highly useful preoperative assessment of predicted postresection lung function, has not been verified. In fact, a report from the Massachusetts General Hospital[88] examining global and regional pulmonary function in patients with lung cancer showed improvement in pulmonary function in 52% of patients and a mild decline in 37%; the decline was predicted from changes in radionuclide scans in only 11%. Similar observations have been made in nonoperative lung cancer patients.[86] Whereas the mean pretreatment FEV_1 of 1.71 ± 0.67 L declined to an average of 1.15 ± 0.43 L after treatment, the change was not consistent: Posttreatment FEV_1 was improved in 19% of the patients, unchanged in 53%, mildly decreased in 22%, and decreased below predicted levels in 5%. The technique of superimposing radiation treatment portals over quantitative lung perfusion scans is, therefore, of limited utility in predicting pneumonitis in individual patients. In fact, it has been suggested that the diffusing capacity is a more sensitive indicator of tolerance to radiotherapy.[85]

Unfortunately, there are no firm tests or data to guide the development of tolerable regimens of radiotherapy for patients with borderline lung function, except that we know the treatment volumes should be minimized. If the initial FEV_1 is below 1.0 L or DL_{CO} is less than 50% of predicted, large-volume radiotherapy (e.g., elective nodal irradiation for lung cancer) may well be too hazardous. Despite its limitations, quantitative perfusion scanning in selected patients may give a worst-case scenario and help the radiation oncologist decide on dose and treatment volume.

The quantitative relationship between the volume of lung irradiated and toxicity has only recently been studied in any systematic fashion. An interesting set of mouse data published by investigators at MD Anderson showed a clear shift in dose–response curves for changes in respiratory rate and pulmonary death as a function of the volume of lung irradiated.[35] As expected, the region of the lung irradiated was important: Effects were more pronounced when the well-perfused base of the lung was irradiated, rather than the less well-perfused apex. The response to lung irradiation was quite heterogeneous, even within mice of the same age and sex, from a single highly inbred mouse strain, maintained in microbiologic isolation under rigorously controlled environmental conditions. The morbidity and symptomatology observed in the individual mice was not always reflected in the histology findings found after necropsy.

In patients, radiation dose–volume histogram analyses derived from detailed three-dimensional treatment evaluations and applied to an empirical normal tissue complication model show only a fair correlation between volume and risk of complications.[61,89] Nevertheless, it is common practice to evaluate dosimetric parameters, such as V_{dose} or mean lung dose (MLD), in an effort to predict the risk of pneumonitis prospectively. The V_{dose} (i.e., $V_{20\ Gy}$ or $V_{30\ Gy}$) parameter is defined as the percentage of total volume receiving greater than the threshold dose (i.e., 20 Gy or 30 Gy, respectively). The MLD is defined as the average dose delivered to the whole lungs. These simple metrics predict pulmonary risk based on a single-radiation dose point, used as a mean or threshold.

More complex dosimetric models have also been derived that fit observed normal tissue complication probabilities (NTCPs) to functions that include more comprehensive evaluations of low- and high-dose partial-volume organ exposures using standard radiobiologic models. These approaches may have broader applicability across various radiation treatment techniques, but they are infrequently used because of their complexity. Recently, a multidisciplinary effort, the QUANTEC (see above), was undertaken to summarize the published three-dimensional dose–volume/toxicity

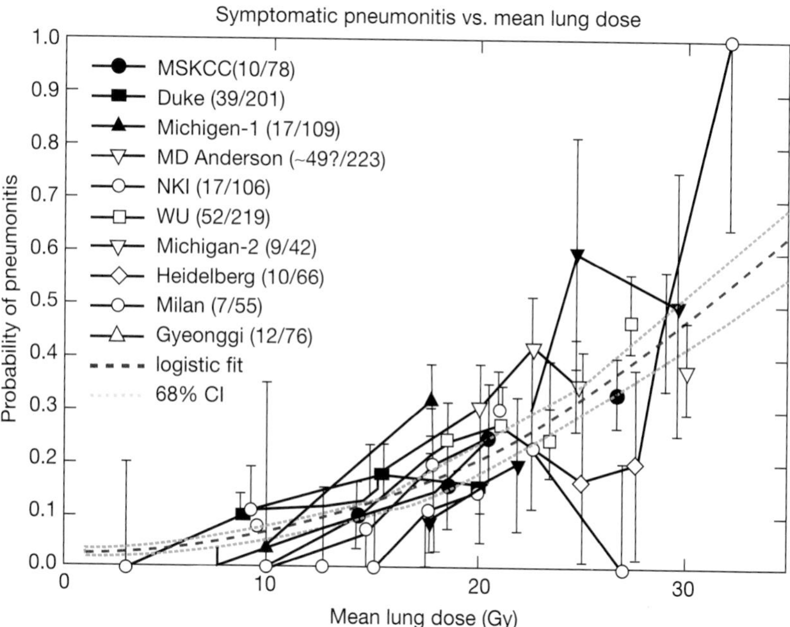

Figure 59-8 Probability of symptomatic pneumonitis versus mean lung dose; data from 10 clinical studies with *dashed line in red* fit by logistic Lyman–Kutcher–Burman dose–volume histogram model with one standard deviation shown in *light blue curves. (Reproduced with permission from Marks LB, Bentzen SM, Deasy JO, et al. Radiation dose-volume effects in the lung. Int J Radiat Oncol Biol Phys. 1;76(3 Suppl):S70–S76.)*

data in the literature, review NTCP modeling, and provide practical guidance for radiotherapy treatment planning.[63] From collected data in the QUANTEC effort, the risk of radiation pneumonitis is less than 20% when the MLD is less than approximately 20 Gy, when V_{20} <30 to 35 Gy, or when V_5 <60%. These predicted risks apply to patients receiving conventional fractionation of 1.8 to 2 Gy per day and are less relevant when the dose per day is greater than 2 Gy.

For hypofractionated treatments, such as SBRT, where doses in excess of 10 Gy per day are given in one to five fractions, the incidence of radiation pneumonitis is significantly lower.[90] This is primarily because the target volume for this type of treatment is quite small. While the risk of symptomatic pneumonitis does seem to follow a radiation dose-volume relationship similar to that seen in conventionally fractionated treatment, specific dose threshold guidelines have not yet been definitively elucidated. In one large series, the risk of grade 2 or greater pneumonitis was 17% when the MLD was >4 Gy, compared with 4% for lower values, and this risk was 16% when the V_{20} was >4% compared with 4% when V_{20} was <4%.[90] The American Association of Physicists in Medicine (AAPM) Task Group 101 report included a first approximation of tissue tolerance doses for SBRT.[91] For lung, they recommended 12.4 Gy to no more than 10 cc, and 11.6 Gy to no more than 15 cc of lung for three-fraction SBRT, and no more than 13.5 and 12.5 Gy to 10 and 15 cc for five-fraction SBRT.

In patients undergoing pneumonectomy for mesothelioma who will then require radiotherapy, dosimetric parameters to avoid pneumonitis of the remaining lung are even more stringent: V_{20} should be below 4% to 10% and MLD should be below 8 Gy.[92] QUANTEC has reviewed over 70 reports on dose–volume parameters and the risk of pneumonitis, selecting the largest series for use in performing a meta-analysis of complication probability models.[61] Such clinical data is challenging to interpret, owing to a host of confounding covariates. However, there are clear trends showing increasing pneumonitis risk with increasing radiation dose. Figure 59-8 shows the risk of symptomatic pulmonary complications as a function of MLD from 10 studies.

Investigators at Duke[93] and the Netherlands Cancer Institute[94,95] have attempted to refine the correlation of dose–volume histograms with toxicity by factoring out nonfunctioning lung using lung perfusion scans. In patients with lung cancer, particularly those with chronic obstructive pulmonary disease (COPD), areas of hypoperfusion separate from tumor are seen frequently; irradiation of such irreversibly hypoperfused lung may not contribute additional toxicity. Such a "functional" dose–volume histogram analysis has not been proven to be of clinical value, but it does provide an interesting analytical framework. The existing data show a direct correlation between regional changes in ventilation, perfusion, or CT density with increasing radiation dose to that region (Fig. 59-9).[96]

Perhaps the most accurate and clinically relevant approach to estimating risks for symptomatic radiation pneumopathy is to study a large group of patients who receive a relatively standard dose and fractionation scheme for a specific disease. As discussed earlier, the variability of the treatment volumes for individual patients with diseases such as lung cancer, as well as the frequent coexistence of other lung diseases, especially COPD from tobacco use, makes this a difficult task.

More complex prediction models that factor in baseline DL_{CO}, serum cytokine levels, or tumor locations in upper versus low lobes have yielded variable improvements in prognostication. Similar data regarding the incidence of radiation fibrosis are quite difficult to obtain, largely because of the wide spectrum of severity in symptomatology. Clinical experience suggests that radiographic fibrosis is rare below 20 Gy and common above 40 to 50 Gy, with symptoms of respiratory insufficiency dependent on the volume of injured lung and the presence of coexisting lung disease.

Lung Cancer: Local Tumor Boosting

In the treatment of lung (and, perhaps, esophageal) cancer, it is quite standard to boost the primary tumor and a small volume of the lung to total cumulative doses above 50 Gy, commonly to 60 to 70 Gy. Clinical data, notably the dose-escalation lung cancer trials of the

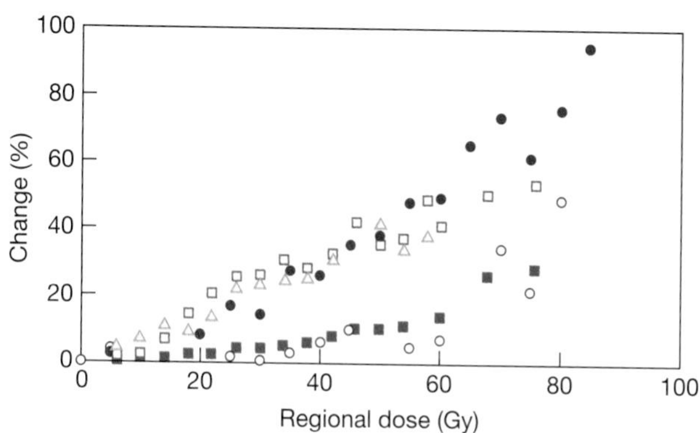

Figure 59-9 Regional changes in ventilation, perfusion, and computed tomography (CT) density from partial lung radiotherapy as a function of regional radiation dose: data from Duke University (Duke) and Netherlands Cancer Institute (NKI). Symbols in graph represent: (•) reduction in perfusion-Duke; (¡) increase in CT density-Duke; (■) change in air-filled fraction-NK; (□) reduction in perfusion-NKI; and (Δ) reduction in ventilation-NKI. *(Reproduced with permission from Marks LB, Yu X, Vujaskovic Z, et al. Radiation-induced lung injury. Semin Radiat Oncol. 2003;13(3):333–345.)*

Radiation Therapy Oncology Group, suggest that increasing doses to small volumes from approximately 50 to approximately 65 Gy is not associated with a significant increase in lung toxicity,[97] probably because the number of nonfunctional alveoli is not increased by this increase in dose. In most series of patients receiving radical thoracic radiotherapy, the risk of symptomatic radiation pneumonitis is usually about 10% to 20%, and some degree of radiographic fibrosis is almost universal.

Breast Cancer

Breast cancer radiotherapy, whether after lumpectomy or after mastectomy, typically uses opposed tangential beams, as depicted in Figure 59-6, which irradiate a volume of lung anterolateral to a plane demarcating the midchest to the lateral axillary line to doses of 45 to 50 Gy in 23 to 25 fractions. The volume of the ipsilateral lung irradiated can be estimated for individual patients from the simulator films and is typically about 20% of the lung volume. If the supraclavicular and axillary nodes are irradiated as well, the anterior treatment portals are matched to the tangential chest wall fields. As a result, the apex of the lung (roughly another 10%–15% of ipsilateral lung volume) is also irradiated. The incidence of symptomatic pneumonitis from tangential fields alone is roughly 0.5%, with some series documenting an increased risk with increasing lung volume.[98,99] It is desirable to keep the irradiated volume below approximately 25%, if possible. Nodal irradiation increases the risk for pneumonitis to 0.5% to 1.5%. Risk further increases to as high as 9% when chemotherapy is given concurrently. The risk of pneumonitis is much lower when chemotherapy and radiation are given sequentially.[98]

Early-stage Hodgkin Disease

Radiotherapy for early-stage Hodgkin lymphoma, using moderate doses (40–45 Gy in 1.5–2 Gy fractions) and large volumes to treat lymph node-bearing regions, has represented a remarkable success story in oncology.[5,100] Because it now has produced very high cure rates in a young patient population, allowing for extended follow-up over several decades, this experience also has produced considerable data regarding late radiation toxicities.

With the protocols employed, the chest is irradiated with treatment portals, generically called "mantle fields," as depicted in Figure 59-10. With modern radiation techniques that use sequential shrinking fields, the incidence of symptomatic radiation pneumonitis is 3% to 4%. The risk of pneumonitis increases to roughly 10% when full doses of both chemotherapy and radiation to a mantle field are given sequentially, even when bleomycin is not part of the regimen.

Studies on pulmonary function in patients with Hodgkin disease suggest that a transient reduction in FEV_1 and vital capacity, on the order of 5% to 20%, occurs 3 to 9 months after radiotherapy, corresponding to the period of pneumonitis. There tends to be some recovery by about 1 year. Late follow-up of pulmonary function in patients with Hodgkin disease[100] further suggests that mantle field radiotherapy is associated with small, and, for the most part, clinically insignificant, reductions in vital capacity and DL_{CO}. These decreases in pulmonary function tests were associated with minor, if any, symptomatology, even for treatment regimens that included sequential chemotherapy with doxorubicin or bleomycin.

Primary radiotherapy for Hodgkin disease is now rarely practiced. Decades of follow-up in patients cured of their lymphomas show a steady increase in secondary cancers as well as cardiac complications. As a consequence, clinical trials have shown improved disease-free survival over 5 to 10 years with primary chemotherapy. In this setting in which lower-dose (20–30 Gy) involved-field radiotherapy is often delivered after chemotherapy, the incidence of clinical pneumonitis is quite low, although small changes in spirometry and diffusion capacity may be detected in up to 50% of the patients. Longer-term follow-up of toxicities from combined-modality therapy in Hodgkin disease is in progress.

PROGNOSTIC ASSAYS AND FUTURE TRENDS

Our understandings of the molecular and cellular mechanisms of radiation injury in general, and radiation pneumonitis in particular, are still evolving and improving. We hope that increased understanding of these processes will lead to new approaches for avoiding radiation injury to the lung, for modulating the development of injury or ameliorating its symptomatology, and for identifying patients at unusually high risk of injury. Several different lines of investigation leading to these ends are being pursued.

Innovations in radiation therapy techniques are under active investigation. These include modifications in the dose rates, fractionation patterns, and radiation dose distributions used in radiation therapy regimens for specific diseases. Improvements in diagnostic imaging that allow better identification of tumor-involved regions, computerized treatment planning and dosimetry systems, improved patient immobilization systems, the use of multiple "noncoplanar, noncoaxial" radiation portals (three-dimensional conformal radiotherapy), and the use of multiple radiation fields that have variable rather than uniform spatial intensities (intensity-modulated radiotherapy) are now standard techniques in the radiotherapy clinic.

Proton radiotherapy takes advantage of the "Bragg peak," in which the radiation dose is deposited at a well-defined maximum depth that depends on the proton energy to produce very precise, highly localized dose distributions. This type of charged-particle radiation technique is being explored in the hope that the approach will enable the radiotherapist to increase the dose to the tumor while decreasing the volume of surrounding normal tissue irradiated to high doses.

Four-dimensional treatment planning to take into account respiratory motion, along with deep inspiration breath-hold methods, are also being examined in an effort to better limit the volume of normal tissue exposed to radiotherapy. In addition, refinements in combined-modality therapy may also lead to the development of regimens that increase the therapeutic ratio for the treatment of thoracic tumors and, therefore, decrease the risk and severity of radiation pneumonitis after effective antineoplastic therapy.

The risk of developing radiation pneumonitis varies dramatically in different patients. To a certain extent, increased risk can be predicted from identifiable risk factors, such as prior treatment with thoracic radiotherapy, treatment with pneumotoxic drugs, or the existence of lung disease from other causes. However, even when the known risk factors are considered, the risk of symptomatic injury after radiotherapy varies dramatically from patient to patient. Studies with mice indicate that genetic factors contribute to individual variability in the development of late radiation injury in the lung.[34] This raises the possibility that pretreatment measurements of genetic or proteomic polymorphisms or of enzyme or cytokine levels in the lung, analyses of changes in cytokine levels during treatment or of tissue response to cytokines, or some other relevant measure may be useful in predicting patients at high risk for the development for pneumotoxicity.[36]

Assays of surfactant levels shortly after irradiation predict radiation pneumonitis in some rodent studies but have not predicted radiation pneumonitis in individual patients in the clinical trials performed to date. TGF-β1, a cytokine that mediates fibrosis, is currently the subject of intense investigation. Serum levels of TGF-β1 have been reported to predict pulmonary toxicity after high-dose chemotherapy for breast cancer[101] and may also predict for breast fibrosis from radiotherapy,[102] but its application to predicting toxicities after radiotherapy for lung cancer has been tenuous and controversial due to the fact that TGF-β1 correlates with adverse dosimetric parameters, thus eliminating any independent prognostic importance as a biomarker.[32,103–106] Nevertheless, there is laboratory evidence that antagonists of TGF-β1 receptors may someday be useful in the clinic.[107]

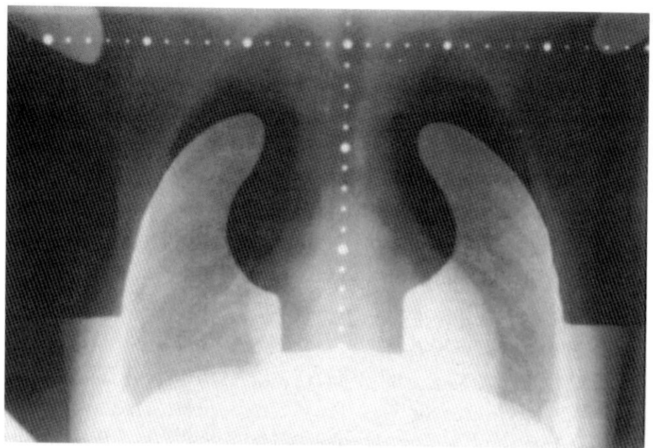

A

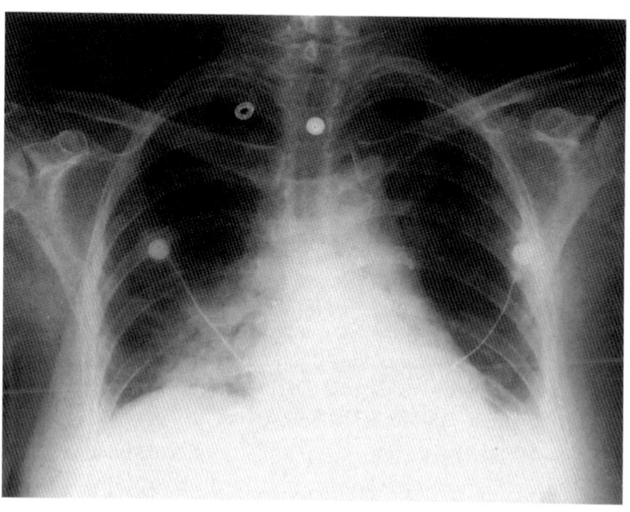

C

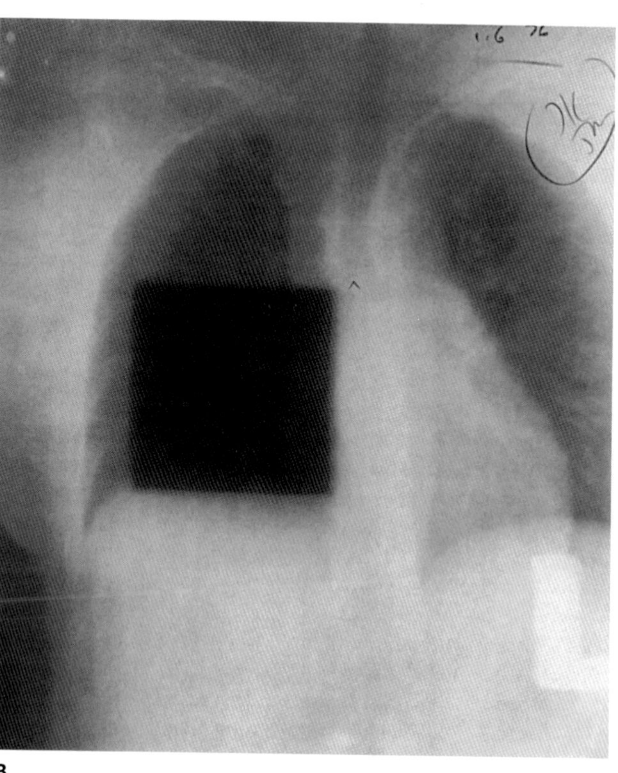

B

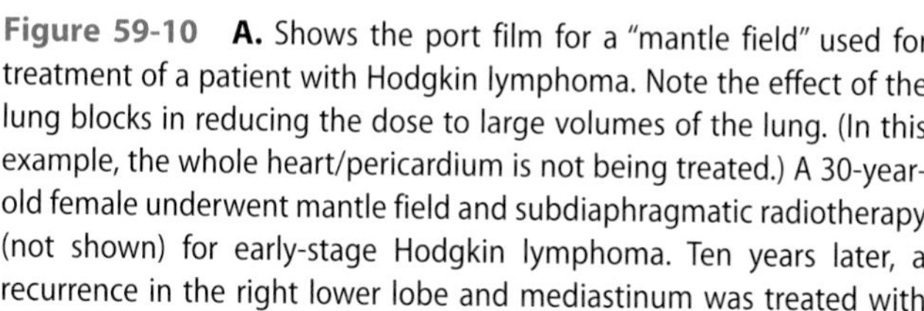

Figure 59-10 **A.** Shows the port film for a "mantle field" used for treatment of a patient with Hodgkin lymphoma. Note the effect of the lung blocks in reducing the dose to large volumes of the lung. (In this example, the whole heart/pericardium is not being treated.) A 30-year-old female underwent mantle field and subdiaphragmatic radiotherapy (not shown) for early-stage Hodgkin lymphoma. Ten years later, a recurrence in the right lower lobe and mediastinum was treated with MOPP-type chemotherapy and low-dose involved-field radiotherapy. The treatment field to the right lung, shown in (**B**), was irradiated to 15 Gy in 10 fractions, in addition to the 40 Gy given to the mantle field 10 years previous. Radiation pneumonitis occurred 6 months later, as seen in (**C**). This responded to prednisone. Twenty years later, the patient remains well and free of recurrence.

Assays of other cytokines such as interleukins, IL-6 and IL-1α are being explored clinically in studies that suggest high positive predictive values for pneumonitis.[108] Similarly, analyses of the intrinsic radiosensitivity in vitro of fibroblasts from patient biopsies have been suggested as a possible approach to measuring the general risks of individual patients for radiation injury. Such assays have proved useful in planning treatments for patients with the genetic disease ataxia telangiectasia (AT), which leads to unusual radiosensitivity. One intriguing study of AT polymorphisms in a cohort of lung cancer patients treated with chemoradiation does suggest increased susceptibility to radiation pneumonitis with certain genotypes.[109] Prognostic assays predicting high or low risks for radiation pneumopathy could be used to guide clinical decision making and plan optimal therapy for individual patients.

Insights into the physiology underlying the development of radiation pneumopathy may also lead to the development of regimens that prevent the development of this disease or ameliorate its symptomology.

The "radioprotector," amifostine (Ethyol, WR2721) has been examined extensively because of its widespread distribution into most normal tissues, limited distribution into tumors, and its activity as a free radical scavenger, which results in a decrease in radiation cytotoxicity. Amifostine has been of variable benefit in reducing mucositis or xerostomia in patients with head and neck cancer undergoing radiotherapy (without apparent effect on tumor control). This has led to analogous clinical investigations of amifostine to prevent pneumonitis.

Several small phase III trials in lung cancer suggested a benefit to amifostine during thoracic radiotherapy, with a decrease not only in pneumonitis, but also in radiation esophagitis as well.[110] A large multi-institutional trial sponsored by the Radiation Therapy Oncology Group involving 242 patients, however, failed to document a difference in pneumonitis rates with amifostine.[111] The trial has been criticized for its twice a day fractionation scheme, in which amifostine was administered with only one fraction each day, the unusually high patient dropout rate of 19% due to toxicity, and the fact that 52% of patients did not receive their intended dose of amifostine.

The development of radiation pneumopathy has not been appreciably altered by the use of prophylactic steroids, antibiotics, or anticoagulants. The use of gamma interferon in conjunction with radiation actually worsened pneumonitis in recent clinical trials.[112] Beta interferon is under clinical investigation. Nutritional factors and neutraceuticals merit further consideration, as subclinical vitamin

A deficiency has been shown to increase radiation injury in the rat lung[113] and genistein decreases effects in irradiated mouse lungs.[114]

Numerous other approaches are being investigated in laboratory studies, including the use of captopril, superoxide dismutase analogs, lovastatin, pentoxifylline, IL-11, and inhibitors of TGF-β.[9,115] Captopril, which is an angiotensin-converting enzyme (ACE) inhibitor used clinically for the treatment of hypertension and heart failure, is especially promising in laboratory studies. As a thiol compound, captopril can act as a free radical scavenger. It can also form copper complexes, which have superoxide dismutase-like activity. Moreover, in animal studies, captopril has vascular effects and can inhibit platelet aggregation, perhaps mediated by IL-2 release, which ameliorate radiation injury to pulmonary endothelium and decrease pulmonary fibrosis.[116,117]

One retrospective clinical review failed to demonstrate a benefit for ACE inhibitors in general, but it did not specifically evaluate captopril and may have been further confounded by including older radiation techniques.[118] Two clinical series of lung cancer patients treated with chemoradiation have shown a significant decrease in pneumonitis associated with the incidental use of ACE inhibitors.[119,120] Experiments in a mouse model suggest that captopril administration subsequent to radiation exposure may mitigate radiation lung injury.[121] In another mouse study, another experimental agent having superoxide dismutase activity, EUK-207, mitigated lung injury following thoracic irradiation.[122]

Lovastatin, a cholesterol-lowering drug that inhibits 3HMG coenzyme A reductase and also has potent anti-inflammatory effects, improved survival and reduced pulmonary infiltration by macrophages and lymphocytes in a murine model of whole-lung irradiation.[123] This approach has not yet been investigated in the clinic.

Pentoxifylline, with or without vitamin E, has been shown to reduce radiation-induced breast or soft tissue fibrosis[124–126] and has been proposed as a potential agent for mitigating pulmonary fibrosis. A number of promising compounds, some in clinical use for other indications, have been proposed for clinical testing as agents for mitigating radiation-induced lung injuries.

All attempts to modulate the development of radiation pneumonitis must be pursued cautiously, however, because these therapeutic strategies are based on biologic epiphenomena and rely on an incomplete understanding of the mechanisms by which radiation pneumopathies are produced. In testing such interventions, as with any alteration of cancer therapy, it will be critical to consider the effects of the intervention on the response of the malignancy, as well as its effects on normal tissue injury; the intervention will be of value only if it increases the therapeutic ratio.

REFERENCES

1. Hall EJ, Giacci AJ. *Radiobiology for the Radiologist*. 7th ed. Philadelphia, PA: Lippincott Williams and Wilkins; 2012.
2. Phillips TL. 50 years of radiation research: medicine. *Radiat Res*. 2002;158(4):389–417.
3. Rockwell S. Experimental radiotherapy: a brief history. *Radiat Res*. 1998;150(5 Suppl):S157–S169.
4. Groover TA, Christie AC, Merritt EA. Observations on the use of the copper filter in the roentgen treatment of deep-seated malignancies. *South Med J*. 1922;15(6):440–443.
5. Halperin EC, Perez CA, Brady LW, (eds). *Principles and Practice of Radiation Oncology*. 5th ed. Philadelphia, PA: Lippincott Williams and Wilkins; 2008.
6. Casarett GW. *Radiation Histopathology*. Boca Raton, FL: CRC Press; 1980.
7. Johns HE, Cunningham JR. *The Physics of Radiology*. 4th ed. Springfield, IL: Charles C Thomas; 1983.
8. McBride WH, Chiang CS, Olson JL, et al. A sense of danger from radiation. *Radiat Res*. 2004;162(1):1–19.
9. Williams JP, Jackson IL, Shah JR, Czarniecki CW, Maidment BW, DiCarlo AL. Animal models and medical countermeasures development for radiation-induced lung damage: report from an NIAID Workshop. *Radiat Res*. 2012;177(5):e0025–e0039.
10. Newman LS, Mroz MM, Ruttenber AJ. Lung fibrosis in plutonium workers. *Radiat Res*. 2005;164(2):123–131.
11. Ozasa K, Shimizu Y, Suyama A, et al. Studies of the mortality of atomic bomb survivors, Report 14, 1950–2003: an overview of cancer and noncancer diseases. *Radiat Res*. 2012;177(3):229–243.
12. Van Dyk J, Keane TJ, Kan S, Rider WD, Fryer CJ. Radiation pneumonitis following large single dose irradiation: a re-evaluation based on absolute dose to lung. *Int J Radiat Oncol Biol Phys*. 1981;7(4):461–467.
13. Rockwell S. Radiobiology. In: Dulbecco R, ed. *Encyclopedia of Human Biology*. 1st ed. Vol 6. San Diego, CA: Academic Press; 1991:441–453.
14. Mikkelsen RB, Wardman P. Biological chemistry of reactive oxygen and nitrogen and radiation-induced signal transduction mechanisms. *Oncogene*. 2003;22(37):5734–5754.
15. Thompson LH, Suit HD. Proliferation kinetics of x-irradiated mouse L cells studied WITH TIME-lapse photography. II. *Int J Radiat Biol*. 1969;15(4):347–362.
16. Chu K, Teele N, Dewey MW, Albright N, Dewey WC. Computerized video time lapse study of cell cycle delay and arrest, mitotic catastrophe, apoptosis and clonogenic survival in irradiated 14-3-3σ and CDKN1 A (p21) knockout cell lines. *Radiat Res*. 2004;162(3):270–286.
17. Steel GG. *Growth Kinetics of Tumours: Cell Population Kinetics in Relation to the Growth and Treatment of Cancer*. Oxford, England: Oxford University Press; 1977.
18. Williams JP, Brown SL, Georges GE, et al. Animal models for medical countermeasures to radiation exposure. *Radiat Res*. 2010;173(4):557–578.
19. Marks LB. The pulmonary effects of thoracic irradiation. *Oncology (Williston Park)*. 1994;8(6):89–106; discussion 100, 103–104.
20. Rubin P, Finkelstein J, Shapiro D. Molecular biology mechanisms in the radiation induction of pulmonary injury syndromes: interrelationship between the alveolar macrophage and the septal fibroblast. *Int J Radiat Oncol Biol Phys*. 1992;24(1):93–101.
21. Fleckenstein K, Zgonjanin L, Chen L, et al. Temporal onset of hypoxia and oxidative stress after pulmonary irradiation. *Int J Radiat Oncol Biol Phys*. 2007;68(1):196–204.
22. Rubin P, Johnston CJ, Williams JP, McDonald S, Finkelstein JN. A perpetual cascade of cytokines postirradiation leads to pulmonary fibrosis. *Int J Radiat Oncol Biol Phys*. 1995;33(1):99–109.
23. Vujaskovic Z, Anscher MS, Feng QF, et al. Radiation-induced hypoxia may perpetuate late normal tissue injury. *Int J Radiat Oncol Biol Phys*. 2001;50(4):851–855.
24. Ao X, Lubman DM, Davis MA, et al. Comparative proteomic analysis of radiation-induced changes in mouse lung: fibrosis-sensitive and -resistant strains. *Radiat Res*. 2008;169(4):417–425.
25. Johnston CJ, Hernady E, Reed C, Thurston SW, Finkelstein JN, Williams JP. Early alterations in cytokine expression in adult compared to developing lung in mice after radiation exposure. *Radiat Res*. 2010;173(4):522–535.
26. Prato FS, Kurdyak R, Saibil EA, Rider WD, Aspin N. Physiological and radiographic assessment during the development of pulmonary radiation fibrosis. *Radiology*. 1977;122(2):389–397.

27. Theuws JC, Kwa SL, Wagenaar AC, et al. Dose-effect relations for early local pulmonary injury after irradiation for malignant lymphoma and breast cancer. *Radiother Oncol.* 1998;48(1):33–43.

28. Morgan GW, Breit SN. Radiation and the lung: a reevaluation of the mechanisms mediating pulmonary injury. *Int J Radiat Oncol Biol Phys.* 1995;31(2):361–369.

29. Travis EL, Tucker SL. The relationship between functional assays of radiation response in the lung and target cell depletion. *Br J Cancer Suppl.* 1986;7:304–319.

30. Gross NJ. Pulmonary effects of radiation therapy. *Ann Intern Med.* 1977;86(1):81–92.

31. Gurley LR, London JE, Tietjen GL, van der Kogel AJ, Dethloff LA, Lehnert BE. Lung hyperpermeability and changes in biochemical constituents in bronchoalveolar lavage fluids following X irradiation of the thorax. *Radiat Res.* 1993;134(2):151–159.

32. McDonald S, Rubin P, Phillips TL, Marks LB. Injury to the lung from cancer therapy: clinical syndromes, measurable endpoints, and potential scoring systems. *Int J Radiat Oncol Biol Phys.* 1995;31(5):1187–1203.

33. Franko AJ, Sharplin J. Development of fibrosis after lung irradiation in relation to inflammation and lung function in a mouse strain prone to fibrosis. *Radiat Res.* 1994;140(3):347–355.

34. Franko AJ, Sharplin J, Ward WF, Hinz JM. The genetic basis of strain-dependent differences in the early phase of radiation injury in mouse lung. *Radiat Res.* 1991;126(3):349–356.

35. Liao ZX, Travis EL, Tucker SL. Damage and morbidity from pneumonitis after irradiation of partial volumes of mouse lung. *Int J Radiat Oncol Biol Phys.* 1995;32(5):1359–1370.

36. Rubin P, Finkelstein JN, Siemann DW, Shapiro DL, Van Houtte P, Penney DP. Predictive biochemical assays for late radiation effects. *Int J Radiat Oncol Biol Phys.* 1986;12(4):469–476.

37. Terry NH, Tucker SL, Travis EL. Residual radiation damage in murine lung assessed by pneumonitis. *Int J Radiat Oncol Biol Phys.* 1988;14(5):929–938.

38. Travis EL, Peters LJ, McNeill J, Thames HD Jr, Karolis C. Effect of dose-rate on total body irradiation: lethality and pathologic findings. *Radiother Oncol.* 1985;4(4):341–351.

39. Katayama N, Sato S, Katsui K, et al. Analysis of factors associated with radiation-induced bronchiolitis obliterans organizing pneumonia syndrome after breast-conserving therapy. *Int J Radiat Oncol Biol Phys.* 2009;73(4):1049–1054.

40. Collis CH. Lung damage from cytotoxic drugs. *Cancer Chemother Pharmacol.* 1980;4(1):17–27.

41. Limper AH. Chemotherapy-induced lung disease. *Clin Chest Med.* 2004;25(1):53–64.

42. Carver JR, Shapiro CL, Ng A, et al. American society of clinical oncology clinical evidence review on the ongoing care of adult cancer survivors: cardiac and pulmonary late effects. *J Clin Oncol.* 2007;25(25):3991–4008.

43. Kallman RF. The importance of schedule and drug dose intensity in combinations of modalities. *Int J Radiat Oncol Biol Phys.* 1994;28(3):761–771.

44. von der Maase H, Overgaard J, Vaeth M. Effect of cancer chemotherapeutic drugs on radiation-induced lung damage in mice. *Radiother Oncol.* 1986;5(3):245–257.

45. Abid SH, Malhotra V, Perry MC. Radiation-induced and chemotherapy-induced pulmonary injury. *Curr Opin Oncol.* 2001;13(4):242–248.

46. Meadors M, Floyd J, Perry MC. Pulmonary toxicity of chemotherapy. *Semin Oncol.* 2006;33(1):98–105.

47. Graham MV, Purdy JA, Emami B, et al. Clinical dose-volume histogram analysis for pneumonitis after 3D treatment for non-small cell lung cancer (NSCLC). *Int J Radiat Oncol Biol Phys.* 1999;45(2):323–329.

48. Robnett TJ, Machtay M, Vines EF, McKenna MG, Algazy KM, McKenna WG. Factors predicting severe radiation pneumonitis in patients receiving definitive chemoradiation for lung cancer. *Int J Radiat Oncol Biol Phys.* 2000;48(1):89–94.

49. Hernando ML, Marks LB, Bentel GC, et al. Radiation-induced pulmonary toxicity: a dose-volume histogram analysis in 201 patients with lung cancer. *Int J Radiat Oncol Biol Phys.* 2001;51(3):650–659.

50. Kong FM, Ten Haken R, Eisbruch A, Lawrence TS. Non-small cell lung cancer therapy-related pulmonary toxicity: an update on radiation pneumonitis and fibrosis. *Semin Oncol.* 2005;32(2 Suppl 3):S42–S54.

51. Hope AJ, Lindsay PE, El Naqa I, et al. Modeling radiation pneumonitis risk with clinical, dosimetric, and spatial parameters. *Int J Radiat Oncol Biol Phys.* 2006;65(1):112–124.

52. Ma LD, Taylor GA, Wharam MD, Wiley JM. "Recall" pneumonitis: adriamycin potentiation of radiation pneumonitis in two children. *Radiology.* 1993;187(2):465–467.

53. Kocak Z, Evans ES, Zhou SM, et al. Challenges in defining radiation pneumonitis in patients with lung cancer. *Int J Radiat Oncol Biol Phys.* 2005;62(3):635–638.

54. Myers JN, O'Neil KM, Walsh TE, Hoffmeister KJ, Venzon DJ, Johnson BE. The pulmonary status of patients with limited-stage small cell lung cancer 15 years after treatment with chemotherapy and chest irradiation. *Chest.* 2005;128(5):3261–3268.

55. Timmerman R, Papiez L, McGarry R, et al. Extracranial stereotactic radioablation: results of a phase I study in medically inoperable stage I non-small cell lung cancer. *Chest.* 2003;124(5):1946–1955.

56. Corradetti MN, Haas AR, Rengan R. Central-airway necrosis after stereotactic body-radiation therapy. *N Engl J Med.* 2012;366(24):2327–2329.

57. Rowe BP, Boffa DJ, Wilson LD, Kim AW, Detterbeck FC, Decker RH. Stereotactic body radiotherapy for central lung tumors. *J Thorac Oncol.* 2012;7(9):1394–1399.

58. Timmerman R, McGarry R, Yiannoutsos C, et al. Excessive toxicity when treating central tumors in a phase II study of stereotactic body radiation therapy for medically inoperable early-stage lung cancer. *J Clin Oncol.* 2006;24(30):4833–4839.

59. Miller KL, Shafman TD, Anscher MS, et al. Bronchial stenosis: an underreported complication of high-dose external beam radiotherapy for lung cancer? *Int J Radiat Oncol Biol Phys.* 2005;61(1):64–69.

60. Emami B, Lyman J, Brown A, et al. Tolerance of normal tissue to therapeutic irradiation. *Int J Radiat Oncol Biol Phys.* 1991;21(1):109–122.

61. Marks LB, Bentzen SM, Deasy JO, et al. Radiation dose-volume effects in the lung. *Int J Radiat Oncol Biol Phys.* 2010;76(3 Suppl):S70–S76.

62. Siemann DW, Rubin P, Penney DP. Pulmonary toxicity following multi-fraction radiotherapy. *Br J Cancer.* 1886;53(Suppl):365–367.

63. Marks LB, Fan M, Clough R, et al. Radiation-induced pulmonary injury: symptomatic versus subclinical endpoints. *Int J Radiat Biol.* 2000;76(4):469–475.

64. Fryer CJ, Fitzpatrick PJ, Rider WD, Poon P. Radiation pneumonitis: experience following a large single dose of radiation. *Int J Radiat Oncol Biol Phys.* 1978;4(11–12):931–936.

65. Keane TJ, Van Dyk J, Rider WD. Idiopathic interstitial pneumonia following bone marrow transplantation: the relationship with total body irradiation. *Int J Radiat Oncol Biol Phys.* 1981;7(10):1365–1370.

66. Mah K, Keane TJ, Van Dyk J, Braban LE, Poon PY, Hao Y. Quantitative effect of combined chemotherapy and fractionated radiotherapy on the incidence of radiation-induced lung damage: a prospective clinical study. *Int J Radiat Oncol Biol Phys.* 1994;28(3):563–574.

67. Mah K, Van Dyk J, Keane T, Poon PY. Acute radiation-induced pulmonary damage: a clinical study on the response to fractionated radiation therapy. *Int J Radiat Oncol Biol Phys.* 1987;13(2):179–188.

68. Deeg HJ, Sullivan KM, Buckner CD, et al. Marrow transplantation for acute nonlymphoblastic leukemia in first remission: toxicity and long-term follow-up of patients conditioned with single dose or fractionated total body irradiation. *Bone Marrow Transplant.* 1986;1(2):151–157.

69. Cardozo BL, Zoetelief H, van Bekkum DW, Zurcher C, Hagenbeek A. Lung damage following bone marrow transplantation: I. The contribution of irradiation. *Int J Radiat Oncol Biol Phys.* 1985;11(5):907–914.

70. Molls M, Budach V, Bamberg M. Total body irradiation: the lung as critical organ. *Strahlenther Onkol.* 1986;162(4):226–232.

71. Shank B. Radiotherapeutic principles of bone marrow transplantation. In: Forman S, Thomas ED, eds. *Bone Marrow Transplantation.* Boston, MA: Blackwell; 1994:96–113.

72. Phillips GL, Herzig RH, Lazarus HM, et al. Treatment of resistant malignant lymphoma with cyclophosphamide, total body irradiation, and transplantation of cryopreserved autologous marrow. *N Engl J Med.* 1984;310(24):1557–1561.

73. Shank B, Hopfan S, Kim JH, et al. Hyperfractionated total body irradiation for bone marrow transplantation: I. Early results in leukemia patients. *Int J Radiat Oncol Biol Phys.* 1981;7(8):1109–1115.

74. Thomas ED, Clift RA, Hersman J, et al. Marrow transplantation for acute nonlymphoblastic leukemic in first remission using fractionated or single-dose irradiation. *Int J Radiat Oncol Biol Phys.* 1982;8(5):817–821.

75. Clift RA, Buckner CD, Appelbaum FR, et al. Allogeneic marrow transplantation in patients with acute myeloid leukemia in first remission: a randomized trial of two irradiation regimens. *Blood.* 1990;76(9):1867–1871.

76. Clift RA, Buckner CD, Appelbaum FR, et al. Allogeneic marrow transplantation in patients with chronic myeloid leukemia in the chronic phase: a randomized trial of two irradiation regimens. *Blood.* 1991;77(8):1660–1665.

77. Weiner RS, Bortin MM, Gale RP, et al. Interstitial pneumonitis after bone marrow transplantation. Assessment of risk factors. *Ann Intern Med.* 1986;104(2):168–175.

78. Barrett A, Depledge MH, Powles RL. Interstitial pneumonitis following bone marrow transplantation after low dose rate total body irradiation. *Int J Radiat Oncol Biol Phys.* 1983;9(7):1029–1033.

79. Thomas E, Storb R, Clift RA, et al. Bone-marrow transplantation (first of two parts). *N Engl J Med.* 1975;292(16):832–843.

80. Carruthers SA, Wallington MM. Total body irradiation and pneumonitis risk: a review of outcomes. *Br J Cancer.* 2004;90(11):2080–2084.

81. Sampath S, Schultheiss TE, Wong J. Dose response and factors related to interstitial pneumonitis after bone marrow transplant. *Int J Radiat Oncol Biol Phys.* 2005;63(3):876–884.

82. Huisman C, van der Straaten HM, Canninga-van Dijk MR, Fijnheer R, Verdonck LF. Pulmonary complications after T-cell-depleted allogeneic stem cell transplantation: low incidence and strong association with acute graft-versus-host disease. *Bone Marrow Transplant.* 2006;38(8):561–566.

83. Tarbell NJ, Thompson L, Mauch P. Thoracic irradiation in Hodgkin's disease: disease control and long-term complications. *Int J Radiat Oncol Biol Phys.* 1990;18(2):275–281.

84. Green DM, Finklestein JZ, Tefft ME, Norkool P. Diffuse interstitial pneumonitis after pulmonary irradiation for metastatic Wilms' tumor. A report from the National Wilms' Tumor Study. *Cancer.* 1989;63(3):450–453.

85. Abratt RP, Willcox PA, Smith JA. Lung cancer in patients with borderline lung functions–zonal lung perfusion scans at presentation and lung function after high dose irradiation. *Radiother Oncol.* 1990;19(4):317–322.

86. Curran WJ Jr, Moldofsky PJ, Solin LJ. Observations on the predictive value of perfusion lung scans on post-irradiation pulmonary function among 210 patients with bronchogenic carcinoma. *Int J Radiat Oncol Biol Phys.* 1992;24(1):31–36.

87. Rubenstein JH, Richter MP, Moldofsky PJ, Solin LJ. Prospective prediction of post-radiation therapy lung function using quantitative lung scans and pulmonary function testing. *Int J Radiat Oncol Biol Phys.* 1988;15(1):83–87.

88. Choi NC, Kanarek DJ, Kazemi H. Physiologic changes in pulmonary function after thoracic radiotherapy for patients with lung cancer and role of regional pulmonary function studies in predicting postradiotherapy pulmonary function before radiotherapy. *Cancer Treat Symp.* 1985;2:119–130.

89. Martel MK, Ten Haken RK, Hazuka MB, Turrisi AT, Fraass BA, Lichter AS. Dose-volume histogram and 3-D treatment planning evaluation of patients with pneumonitis. *Int J Radiat Oncol Biol Phys.* 1994;28(3):575–581.

90. Barriger RB, Forquer JA, Brabham JG, et al. A dose-volume analysis of radiation pneumonitis in non-small cell lung cancer patients treated with stereotactic body radiation therapy. *Int J Radiat Oncol Biol Phys.* 2012;82(1):457–462.

91. Benedict SH, Yenice KM, Followill D, et al. Stereotactic body radiation therapy: the report of AAPM Task Group 101. *Med Phys.* 2010;37(8):4078–4101.

92. Miles EF, Larrier NA, Kelsey CR, et al. Intensity-modulated radiotherapy for resected mesothelioma: the Duke experience. *Int J Radiat Oncol Biol Phys.* 2008;71(4):1143–1150.

93. Marks LB, Spencer DP, Sherouse GW, et al. The role of three dimensional functional lung imaging in radiation treatment planning: the functional dose-volume histogram. *Int J Radiat Oncol Biol Phys.* 1995;33(1):65–75.

94. Borst GR, De Jaeger K, Belderbos JS, Burgers SA, Lebesque JV. Pulmonary function changes after radiotherapy in non-small-cell lung cancer patients with long-term disease-free survival. *Int J Radiat Oncol Biol Phys.* 2005;62(3):639–644.

95. De Jaeger K, Seppenwoolde Y, Boersma LJ, et al. Pulmonary function following high-dose radiotherapy of non-small-cell lung cancer. *Int J Radiat Oncol Biol Phys.* 2003;55(5):1331–1340.

96. Marks LB, Yu X, Vujaskovic Z, Small W Jr, Folz R, Anscher MS. Radiation-induced lung injury. *Semin Radiat Oncol.* 2003;13(3):333–345.

97. Cox JD, Azarnia N, Byhardt RW, Shin KH, Emami B, Pajak TF. A randomized phase I/II trial of hyperfractionated radiation therapy with total doses of 60.0 Gy to 79.2 Gy: possible survival

benefit with greater than or equal to 69.6 Gy in favorable patients with Radiation Therapy Oncology Group stage III non-small-cell lung carcinoma: report of Radiation Therapy Oncology Group 83-11. *J Clin Oncol.* 1990;8(9):1543–1555.

98. Lingos TI, Recht A, Vicini F, Abner A, Silver B, Harris JR. Radiation pneumonitis in breast cancer patients treated with conservative surgery and radiation therapy. *Int J Radiat Oncol Biol Phys.* 1991;21(2):355–360.
99. Rothwell RI, Kelly SA, Joslin CA. Radiation pneumonitis in patients treated for breast cancer. *Radiother Oncol.* 1985;4(1): 9–14.
100. Horning SJ, Adhikari A, Rizk N, Hoppe RT, Olshen RA. Effect of treatment for Hodgkin's disease on pulmonary function: results of a prospective study. *J Clin Oncol.* 1994;12(2): 297–305.
101. Anscher MS, Peters WP, Reisenbichler H, Petros WP, Jirtle RL. Transforming growth factor beta as a predictor of liver and lung fibrosis after autologous bone marrow transplantation for advanced breast cancer. *N Engl J Med.* 1993;328(22): 1592–1598.
102. Li C, Wilson PB, Levine E, Barber J, Stewart AL, Kumar S. TGF-beta1 levels in pre-treatment plasma identify breast cancer patients at risk of developing post-radiotherapy fibrosis. *Int J Cancer.* 1999;84(2):155–159.
103. Anscher MS, Marks LB, Shafman TD, et al. Risk of long-term complications after TFG-beta1-guided very-high-dose thoracic radiotherapy. *Int J Radiat Oncol Biol Phys.* 2003;56(4):988–995.
104. Anscher MS, Kong FM, Andrews K, et al. Plasma transforming growth factor beta1 as a predictor of radiation pneumonitis. *Int J Radiat Oncol Biol Phys.* 1998;41(5):1029–1035.
105. Evans ES, Kocak Z, Zhou SM, et al. Does transforming growth factor-beta1 predict for radiation-induced pneumonitis in patients treated for lung cancer? *Cytokine.* 2006;35(3–4): 186–192.
106. Zhao L, Wang L, Ji W, et al. Elevation of plasma TGF-beta1 during radiation therapy predicts radiation-induced lung toxicity in patients with non-small-cell lung cancer: a combined analysis from Beijing and Michigan. *Int J Radiat Oncol Biol Phys.* 2009;74(5):1385–1390.
107. Anscher MS, Thrasher B, Zgonjanin L, et al. Small molecular inhibitor of transforming growth factor-β protects against development of radiation-induced lung injury. *Int J Radiat Oncol Biol Phys.* 2008;71(3):829–837.
108. Chen Y, Hyrien O, Williams J, Okunieff P, Smudzin T, Rubin P. Interleukin (IL)-1A and IL-6: applications to the predictive diagnostic testing of radiation pneumonitis. *Int J Radiat Oncol Biol Phys.* 2005;62(1):260–266.
109. Xiong H, Liao Z, Liu Z, et al. ATM polymorphisms predict severe radiation pneumonitis in patients with non-small cell lung cancer treated with definitive radiation therapy. *Int J Radiat Oncol Biol Phys.* 2013;85(4):1066–1073.
110. Antonadou D, Petridis A, Synodinou M, et al. Amifostine reduces radiochemotherapy-induced toxicities in patients with locally advanced non-small cell lung cancer. *Semin Oncol.* 2003; 30(6 Suppl 18):2–9.
111. Movsas B, Scott C, Langer C, et al. Randomized trial of amifostine in locally advanced non-small-cell lung cancer patients receiving chemotherapy and hyperfractionated radiation: Radiation Therapy Oncology Group trial 98-01. *J Clin Oncol.* 2005;23(10):2145–2154.
112. Shaw EG, Deming RL, Creagan ET, et al. Pilot study of human recombinant interferon gamma and accelerated hyperfractionated thoracic radiation therapy in patients with unresectable stage IIIA/B nonsmall cell lung cancer. *Int J Radiat Oncol Biol Phys.* 1995;31(4):827–831.
113. Redlich CA, Rockwell S, Chung JS, Sikora AG, Kelley M, Mayne ST. Vitamin A inhibits radiation-induced pneumonitis in rats. *J Nutr.* 1998;128(10):1661–1664.
114. Calveley VL, Jelveh S, Langan A, et al. Genistein can mitigate the effect of radiation on rat lung tissue. *Radiat Res.* 2010;173(5):602–611.
115. Redlich CA, Gao X, Rockwell S, Kelley M, Elias JA. IL-11 enhances survival and decreases TNF production after radiation-induced thoracic injury. *J Immunol.* 1996;157(4): 1705–1710.
116. Molteni A, Moulder JE, Cohen EF, et al. Control of radiation-induced pneumopathy and lung fibrosis by angiotensin-converting enzyme inhibitors and an angiotensin II type 1 receptor blocker. *Int J Radiat Biol.* 2000;76(4):523–532.
117. Molteni A, Wolfe LF, Ward WF, et al. Effect of an angiotensin II receptor blocker and two angiotensin converting enzyme inhibitors on transforming growth factor-β (TGF-β) and α-Actomyosin (α SMA), important mediators of radiation-induced pneumopathy and lung fibrosis. *Curr Pharm Des.* 2007;13(13):1307–1316.
118. Wang LW, Fu XL, Clough R, et al. Can angiotensin-converting enzyme inhibitors protect against symptomatic radiation pneumonitis? *Radiat Res.* 2000;153(4):405–410.
119. Jenkins P, Watts J. An improved model for predicting radiation pneumonitis incorporating clinical and dosimetric variables. *Int J Radiat Oncol Biol Phys.* 2011;80(4):1023–1029.
120. Kharofa J, Cohen EP, Tomic R, Xiang Q, Gore E. Decreased risk of radiation pneumonitis with incidental concurrent use of angiotensin-converting enzyme inhibitors and thoracic radiation therapy. *Int J Radiat Oncol Biol Phys.* 2012;84(1):238–243.
121. Molthen RC, Wu Q, Fish BL, Moulder JE, Jacobs ER, Medhora MM. Mitigation of radiation induced pulmonary vascular injury by delayed treatment with captopril. *Respirology.* 2012;17(8):1261–1268.
122. Gao F, Fish BL, Szabo A, et al. Short-term treatment with a SOD/catalase mimetic, EUK-207, mitigates pneumonitis and fibrosis after single-dose total-body or whole-thoracic irradiation. *Radiat Res.* 2012;178(5):468–480.
123. Williams JP, Hernady E, Johnston CJ, et al. Effect of administration of lovastatin on the development of late pulmonary effects after whole-lung irradiation in a murine model. *Radiat Res.* 2004;161(5):560–567.
124. Okunieff P, Augustine E, Hicks JE, et al. Pentoxifylline in the treatment of radiation-induced fibrosis. *J Clin Oncol.* 2004;22(11):2207–2213.
125. Jacobson G, Bhatia S, Smith BJ, Button AM, Bodeker K, Buatti J. Randomized trial of pentoxifylline and vitamin E vs standard follow-up after breast irradiation to prevent breast fibrosis, evaluated by tissue compliance meter. *Int J Radiat Oncol Biol Phys.* 2013;85(3):604–608.
126. Magnusson M, Hoglund P, Johansson K, et al. Pentoxifylline and vitamin E treatment for prevention of radiation-induced side-effects in women with breast cancer: a phase two, double-blind, placebo-controlled randomised clinical trial (Ptx-5). *Eur J Cancer.* 2009;45(14):2488–2495.

CHAPTER 60

Pulmonary Manifestations of the Collagen Vascular Diseases

Gregory P. Cosgrove
Marvin I. Schwarz

Pleuropulmonary involvement associated with the collagen vascular diseases occurs frequently. All the structures within the respiratory tract may be affected, either separately or in combination. This includes the respiratory muscles, the pleura, the conducting airways, and the lung parenchyma—the small airways, the interstitium, or the pulmonary vessels. Moreover, these patients experience an increased incidence of community-acquired pneumonia as well as pneumonia associated with the immunosuppressive drugs employed for treatment. Anti–tumor necrosis factor-α (anti–TNF-α) agents increase the risk for infections, particularly mycobacterial pathogens, both tuberculous and nontuberculous. Cytotoxic drugs, particularly methotrexate and gold, can also induce various noninfectious interstitial reactions, which are often difficult to distinguish from a primary interstitial complication of a collagen vascular disease.[1]

Although most pulmonary complications appear in an established case of a collagen vascular disease, lung disease may precede the more typical systemic manifestations.[2] For example, in both rheumatoid arthritis and polymyositis–dermatomyositis, the interstitial lung disease may precede the joint and muscle disease for several months to several years. This is also the case, but to a lesser extent, for scleroderma. In one study, 19% of patients initially diagnosed with idiopathic pulmonary fibrosis developed a collagen vascular disease over a period of 1 to 11 years, primarily rheumatoid arthritis or polymyositis–dermatomyositis. These individuals were younger and more likely to be women. Pleuritis with or without effusion sometimes heralds the onset of rheumatoid arthritis or systemic lupus erythematosus (SLE). An acute immunologic pneumonitis or diffuse alveolar hemorrhage has been reported to be the signal event in SLE, polymyositis–dermatomyositis, and mixed connective-tissue disease.

The incidence of the pleuropulmonary complications (Table 60-1) is variable. Interstitial lung disease is reported to be as high as 60% in premortem and 100% in postmortem studies in scleroderma. In contrast, interstitial lung disease in ankylosing spondylitis is an uncommon event. In general, the incidence of interstitial lung disease is increasing for most of the collagen vascular diseases, primarily due to increased recognition and more sensitive screening techniques such as high-resolution computed tomography and bronchoalveolar lavage, which will detect abnormalities in both asymptomatic as well as symptomatic patients with normal chest radiographs. Prior studies assessing the incidence of disease relied on physiologic testing, which included spirometry, lung volumes, and diffusing capacity but did not measure rest and exercise gas exchange, which is the most sensitive physiologic marker of interstitial lung disease and pulmonary vascular disease.

PULMONARY PARENCHYMAL, VASCULAR, AND AIRWAY PATHOLOGY IN THE COLLAGEN VASCULAR DISEASES

The spectrum of pathologic changes in the lung parenchyma, pulmonary vasculature, and airways are considered below, prior to a discussion of clinical findings in individual collagen vascular diseases.

■ INTERSTITIAL LUNG DISEASE

Interstitial involvement is a common manifestation of the collagen vascular disorders, presenting with a number of different

TABLE 60-1 Pulmonary Complications of the Collagen Vascular Diseases

	Relative Frequency (0–4)						
Manifestation	SLE	RA	SS	PM-DM	MCTD	AS	Sjögren's
Respiratory muscle dysfunction	2	1	0	2	1	0	0
Aspiration pneumonia	0	0	3	3	2	0	2
Primary pulmonary hypertension	2	1	4	1	2	0	0
Vasculitis	2	2	0	1	1	0	0
Interstitial lung disease	2	3	4	3	2	1	3
Capillaritis + DAH	2	1	1	1	1	0	0
Bland DAH	2	0	0	0	1	0	0
Diffuse alveolar damage	2	0	0	2	1	0	0
Nonspecific interstitial pneumonitis	2	3	3	3	3	0	1
Lymphocytic interstitial pneumonitis	1	2	1	0	0	0	3
Usual interstitial pneumonitis	2	3	2	2	2	1	1
Honeycomb lung	1	2	4	3	2	1	1
Bronchiolitis obliterans organizing pneumonia	1	3	1	3	2	0	1
Bronchiolitis	1	2	1	0	1	0	1
Obliterative bronchiolitis	0	2	0	0	0	0	1
Pleural effusion	2	3	1	0	2	0	1
Parenchymal nodules	0	2	0	0	0	0	1

SLE, systemic lupus erythematosus; RA, rheumatoid arthritis; SS, systemic sclerosis (scleroderma); PM-DM, polymyositis-dermatomyositis; MCTD, mixed connective-tissue disease; AS, ankylosing spondylitis; Sjögren's, Sjögren syndrome; DAH, diffuse alveolar hemorrhage.

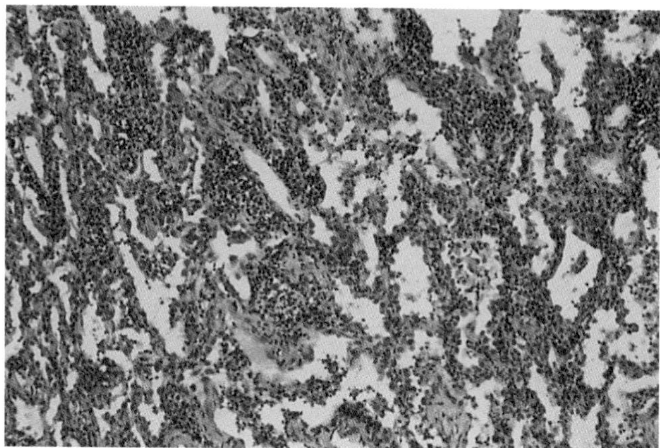

Figure 60-1 Nonspecific interstitial pneumonitis (NSIP) in rheumatoid arthritis. There is a lymphoplasmacytic infiltration of the interstitial compartment with minimal collagen deposition.

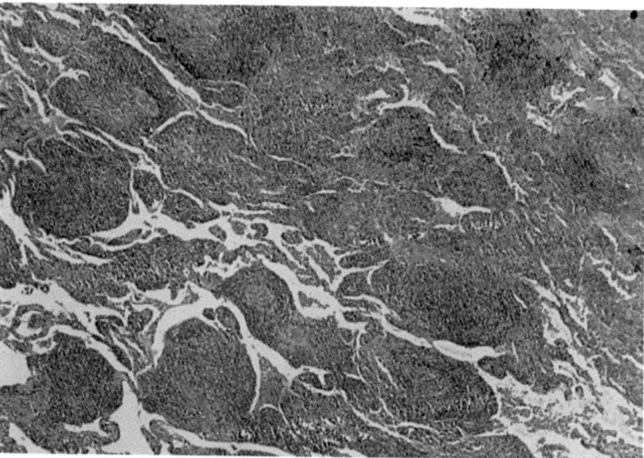

Figure 60-2 Lymphocytic interstitial pneumonitis in a patient with primary Sjögren syndrome. There is a dense lymphocytic infiltrate, broadening the interstitium and lymphoid follicles.

inflammatory responses within the lung. Each response may represent a different form of lung injury or response to injury. Defining which response is underlying a patient's interstitial lung disease has important prognostic and therapeutic significance.

Diffuse alveolar damage (DAD) is the underlying histologic lesion that is also seen in the acute respiratory distress syndrome, idiopathic acute interstitial pneumonitis (Hamman–Rich syndrome), severe viral pneumonias, and cytotoxicity from some drugs. This damage consists of a mixed interstitial inflammatory infiltrate, interstitial edema and fibrin deposition, and characteristic intra-alveolar hyaline membrane formation. Intra-alveolar red blood cells (diffuse alveolar hemorrhage) may be present in severe cases. With progression, there is intra-alveolar organization, intra-alveolar and interstitial fibrosis, alveolar collapse, and the development of an end-stage fibrotic or "honeycomb" lung. An acute immunologic pneumonia, seen in SLE (acute lupus pneumonitis) and in polymyositis–dermatomyositis, may also demonstrate this underlying histologic appearance.

Nonspecific interstitial pneumonitis (NSIP) refers to a spectrum of histologic features with varying degrees of lymphoplasmacytic infiltration of the interstitium and collagen deposition (Fig. 60-1). In the cellular form, lymphoplasmacytic interstitial inflammation exists with associated type II alveolar epithelial cell hyperplasia. In the fibrosing form, the inflammation is accompanied by a temporally and spatially homogeneous deposition of collagen (fibrosis). Architectural distortion or honeycombing may occur in advanced cases and the presence of fibrosis dramatically changes the clinical course and prognosis to one resembling that seen in usual interstitial pneumonitis (UIP) (see below). NSIP is most frequently seen in patients with rheumatoid arthritis, polymyositis–dermatomyositis, mixed connective-tissue disease, and scleroderma.

Lymphocytic interstitial pneumonitis refers to a monotonous infiltration of the interstitium by mature lymphocytes (Fig. 60-2). These lymphocytes tend to form germinal centers within the interstitium as well as displaying an angiocentric distribution. Other features of lymphocytic interstitial pneumonia include macrophagic giant cells, granuloma formation, and amyloid deposition. Lymphocytic interstitial pneumonitis can progress to UIP and end-stage honeycomb lung. Among the collagen vascular diseases, this pneumonitis most commonly accompanies the primary form of Sjögren syndrome and, to a lesser extent, the secondary form of Sjögren syndrome appearing with other collagen vascular diseases, particularly rheumatoid arthritis.

UIP is the underlying lesion of idiopathic pulmonary fibrosis and can also appear in all the collagen vascular diseases. It consists of varying degrees of mononuclear cell infiltration and fibroblastic proliferation leading to collagen deposition within the alveolar interstitium (Fig. 60-3). With progression, this fibrotic reaction results in marked distortion of the lung architecture and what remains are 2- to 3-mm cystic spaces lined by metaplastic epithelium, the so-called honeycomb lung (Fig. 60-4). Other features of UIP include type II epithelial cell hyperplasia producing a "hob-nailed" appearance on the alveolar surface, collections of intra-alveolar macrophages, and smooth-muscle proliferation within the interstitium. Additional abnormalities seen in collagen vascular disease-associated UIP but not in patients with idiopathic pulmonary fibrosis may include: focal chronic pleuritis, lymphoid follicles with germinal center formation, perivascular collagen deposition, and an increase in CD4+ T lymphocytes, especially in rheumatoid arthritis.

Organizing pneumonia, previously termed bronchiolitis obliterans organizing pneumonia, is a distinctive histologic lesion that follows a variety of insults to the alveolar structures including drugs, infection, radiation, and an idiopathic variety. Organizing pneumonia can also complicate the collagen vascular diseases, particularly rheumatoid arthritis and polymyositis–dermatomyositis. Three features comprise the histologic picture: (1) intra-alveolar space and intra-alveolar ductal fibroblastic proliferation with early collagen deposition (Masson bodies), (2) inflammatory polyps consisting of fibroblasts and mononuclear cells protruding into the lumens of respiratory and terminal

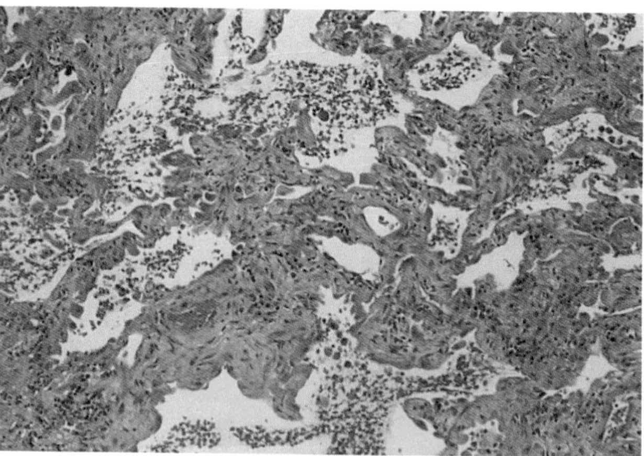

Figure 60-3 Usual interstitial pneumonia (UIP) in a patient with rheumatoid arthritis. There is broadening of the interstitium by varying degrees of mononuclear cell infiltration and collagen deposition.

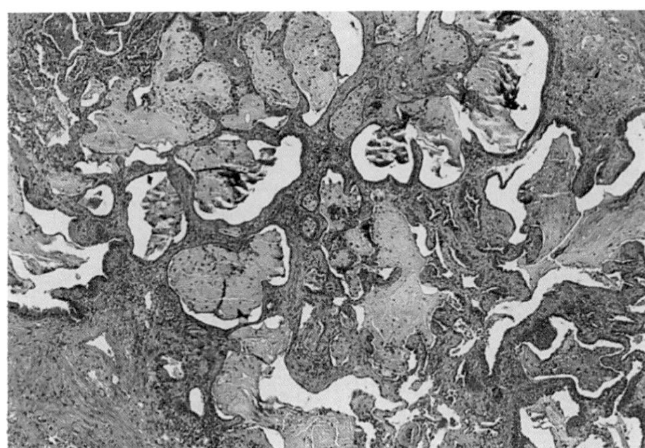

Figure 60-4 Advanced UIP in a patient with scleroderma (honeycomb lung). Normal alveolar tissue is replaced with broad bands of fibrous tissue lined by metaplastic epithelium and filled with inspissated mucus producing a cyst-like network. *(Used with permission of the Armed Forces Institute of Pathology [AFIP].)*

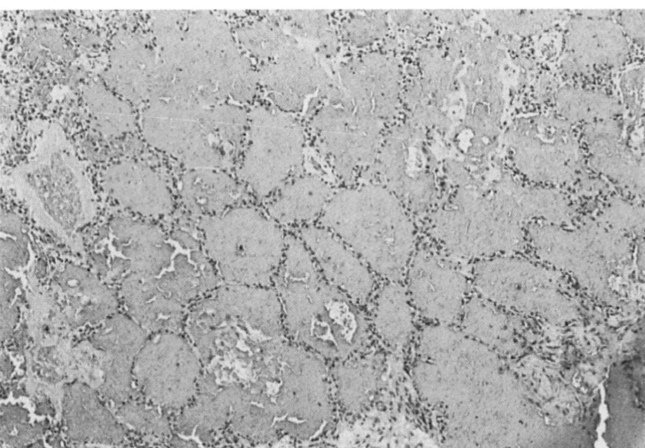

Figure 60-6 Bland diffuse alveolar hemorrhage in SLE. There is little if any interstitial reaction except for type II pneumocyte epithelial cell hyperplasia. The alveolar spaces are filled with red blood cells.

bronchioles, and (3) alveolar septal lymphoplasmacytic infiltrate with type II pneumocyte hyperplasia within affected areas (Fig. 60-5). Bronchiolitis obliterans organizing pneumonia has the potential for being a completely reversible lesion; however, with continuing injury it may progress to end-stage fibrosis and honeycomb lung.

PULMONARY VASCULAR DISEASE

A form of pulmonary artery hypertension, which most commonly appears in patients with scleroderma and is now being increasingly recognized in SLE, rheumatoid arthritis, and mixed connective-tissue disease, is histologically identical to the syndrome of idiopathic pulmonary artery hypertension (IPAH) seen in young women without collagen vascular disease, formerly known as primary pulmonary hypertension. This is a proliferative disorder (plexogenic arteriopathy) affecting the arterioles and small muscular pulmonary arteries. This form of pulmonary hypertension must be differentiated from secondary forms as a result of hypoxic vasoconstriction induced by interstitial lung disease or severe emphysema. In the plexogenic variety, there is endothelial cell intimal proliferation and smooth muscle cell proliferation causing medial thickening with a resultant "onion ring" configuration and luminal obliteration. In the secondary forms of pulmonary hypertension due to hypoxia, medial hypertrophy is the primary finding. In patients with SLE and the antiphospholipid syndrome, pulmonary artery hypertension may develop as a result of recurrent pulmonary emboli and mimic the clinical picture of IPAH.

Vasculitis refers to an acute inflammatory angiodestructive process resulting in fibrinoid necrosis of the vascular wall. In the collagen vascular diseases, this is most often a small-vessel vasculitis involving arterioles and small muscular pulmonary arteries. Although uncommon, this is seen with greatest regularity in SLE and less frequently in rheumatoid arthritis, polymyositis–dermatomyositis, and mixed connective-tissue disease. Often accompanying the arteriolitis is the lesion of pulmonary capillaritis (see below).

DIFFUSE ALVEOLAR HEMORRHAGE

Diffuse alveolar hemorrhage is recognized by the accumulation of red blood cells within the alveolar spaces, and with recurrent episodes, intra-alveolar and interstitial hemosiderin is deposited and fibrosis may result. There are two different histologic subtypes seen in diffuse alveolar hemorrhage. One is devoid of inflammation and is referred to as *bland hemorrhage* (Fig. 60-6). It is therefore similar in histologic appearance to idiopathic pulmonary hemosiderosis. The other, pulmonary capillaritis is a unique neutrophilic infiltration of the alveolar interstitium, which results in necrosis and loss of integrity

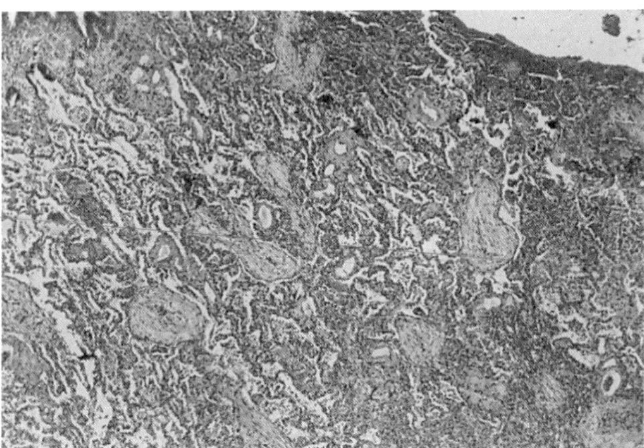

Figure 60-5 Bronchiolitis obliterans organizing pneumonia in a patient with rheumatoid arthritis. There is a mononuclear cellular infiltration of the interstitium without collagen deposition as well as alveolar duct and intra-alveolar fibroblastic proliferation and early collagen production.

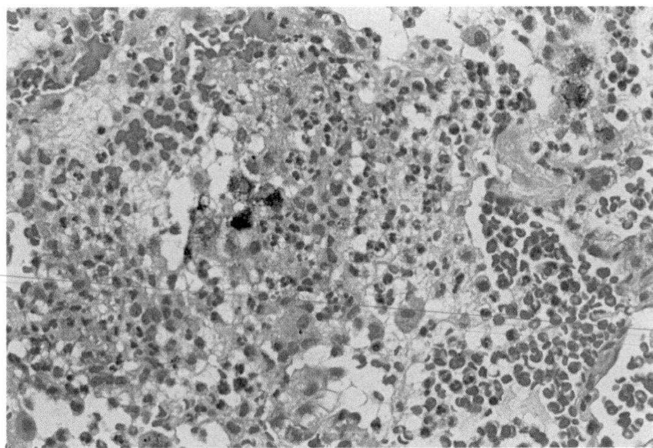

Figure 60-7 Low-power view of pulmonary capillaritis in a patient with SLE. There is marked thickening of the interstitial compartment and infiltration by acute and chronic inflammatory cells. The alveolar spaces are filled with red blood cells and neutrophils.

of the alveolar–capillary basement membrane, capillary destruction and thrombosis, and a leakage of red blood cells into the alveolar space (Fig. 60-7). A unique feature in pulmonary capillaritis is that many of the infiltrating neutrophils are undergoing fragmentation (leukocytoclasis), and others appear as densely staining apoptotic cells. Nuclear debris ("dust") subsequently accumulates within the necrotic, edematous interstitium, and intra-alveolar compartments while red blood cells freely leak into the interstitial matrix due to capillary destruction. Capillary and arteriolar thrombosis, organizing pneumonia, and type II epithelial cell hyperplasia may also be seen.

Capillaritis is most commonly seen in the systemic vasculitides, particularly granulomatosis with polyangiitis (GPA/Wegener granulomatosis) and microscopic polyangiitis (MPA), the small-vessel variant of polyarteritis nodosa. Of the collagen vascular diseases, both bland pulmonary hemorrhage and diffuse alveolar hemorrhage secondary to pulmonary capillaritis appear most commonly in SLE. Cases of pulmonary capillaritis have also been reported to occur in rheumatoid arthritis, Sjögren syndrome, polymyositis–dermatomyositis, and mixed connective-tissue disease.

BRONCHIOLITIS

Bronchiolitis refers to an inflammatory-fibrotic process involving the terminal and respiratory bronchioles and possibly the surrounding alveolar structures. Respiratory bronchiolitis is primarily seen in smokers with or without an associated collagen vascular disease. There is also a primary form of cellular bronchiolitis that complicates the collagen vascular diseases, most often appearing in rheumatoid arthritis and Sjögren syndrome. Histologically, there is a mononuclear cell infiltration of the wall of the bronchiole without impingement of the bronchiolar lumen. In contrast, in bronchiolitis obliterans, or obliterative bronchiolitis, there is a concentric fibrous obliteration of the bronchiolar lumen leading to a severe obstructive lung disease (Fig. 60-8). Bronchiolitis obliterans is most often reported as a complication of rheumatoid arthritis.

PARENCHYMAL NODULES

Noninfectious inflammatory parenchymal nodules occur in both rheumatoid arthritis and Sjögren syndrome. In rheumatoid arthritis the nodules are referred to as the *necrobiotic* or *rheumatoid nodules.* These lesions are found both in the pleura and lung parenchyma and are identical in appearance to a subcutaneous rheumatoid nodule. In the lung parenchyma, these nodules are located in the interlobular septa and in the subpleural parenchyma. The necrobiotic nodule is comprised of palisading histiocytes, giant cells, and other mononuclear cells surrounding an area of fibrinoid debris (Fig. 60-9). In Sjögren syndrome, a rounded lesion known as pseudolymphoma can occasionally be detected on the chest radiograph. Pseudolymphoma is considered to be a localized form of lymphocytic interstitial pneumonia and is made up of a dense infiltrate of lymphocytes and histiocytes with occasional granuloma formation. There is a potential risk for malignant transformation in pseudolymphoma as well as in the other forms of lymphocytic interstitial pneumonia.

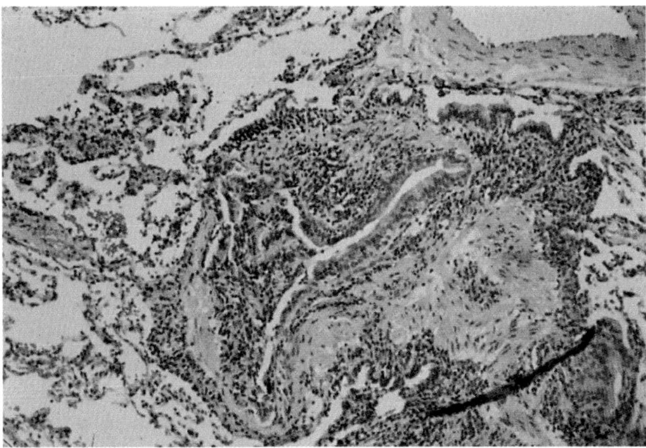

Figure 60-8 Obliterative bronchiolitis in rheumatoid arthritis. There is a marked reduction of the luminal diameter due to concentric fibrous obliteration and dense chronic inflammation. *(Reproduced with permission from Schwarz MI, Lynch DA, Tuder R. Bronchiolitis obliterans: The lone manifestation of rheumatoid arthritis. Eur Respir J. 1994;7(4):817–820.)*

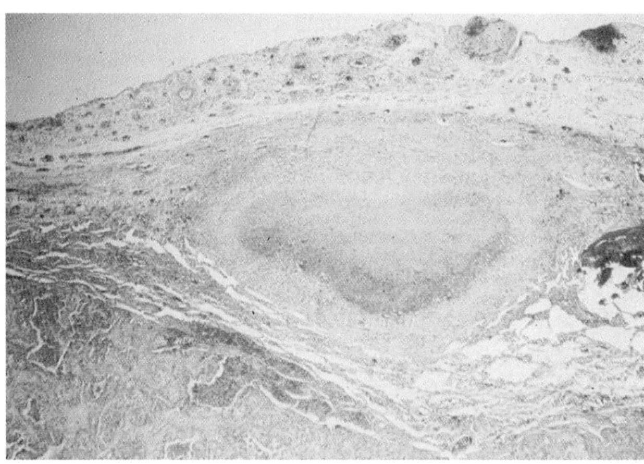

Figure 60-9 Typical subpleural location of a necrobiotic rheumatoid nodule. There is a central area of fibrinoid debris surrounded by palisading histiocytes.

SYSTEMIC LUPUS ERYTHEMATOSUS: CLINICAL FEATURES

SLE is characterized by the production of antibodies against various cellular antigens derived from the nucleus, cytoplasm, or cell membrane. Tissue injury appears to be associated with the development of immune complexes, the presence of low serum complement levels, and the production of antibodies to native DNA. Pleuropulmonary involvement in SLE occurs in the vast majority of patients (97.8%), with pleuritis (77%), bacterial infections (58%), and diffuse alveolar hemorrhage (26%) being the most common.[3,4] Lung injury is thought to be the result of an immune complex-mediated injury and appears to increase in incidence depending on the age of the patient, duration of illness, pleuritis, and the presence of specific autoantibodies. Pulmonary vascular and shrinking lung syndrome appear to be associated with the development of the anti-RNP autoantibody.[5] A number of syndromes (Table 60-2) are associated with acute respiratory-type illness in SLE. Patients with SLE who present with a febrile illness, cough with or without productive sputum, and new pulmonary infiltrates must be considered

TABLE 60-2 Acute Lung Syndromes in Systemic Lupus Erythematosus

Community-acquired or immunocompromised pneumonia
Pleurisy
Pulmonary embolization
Uremic pneumonitis
Cardiogenic pulmonary edema
Acute reversible hypoxemia syndrome
Acute lupus pneumonitis
Diffuse alveolar hemorrhage

to have an infectious pneumonia, although acute lupus pneumonitis and diffuse alveolar hemorrhage may have a similar presentation.[6] Infection can be community-acquired or a complication of immunosuppressive therapy. Infectious pneumonia represents the most common cause of pulmonary disease in SLE, and infections in general represent the most common reason for death (33%–77%).[7] Bronchoalveolar lavage is often helpful in excluding an infectious pneumonia in the immunocompromised SLE patient.

Another important consideration in an acutely dyspneic SLE patient is pulmonary embolism, a complication reportedly occurring in up to 25% of patients and a significant cause of mortality.[8] The occurrence of thromboembolic disease correlates with the presence in the serum of acquired antiphospholipid antibodies (lupus anticoagulant or anticardiolipin).[9] The most common epitope(s) to which antibodies exist in these patients is β_2-glycoprotein I. A more appropriate term may therefore be anti-β_2–glycoprotein syndrome. Up to a third of patients with SLE have the antiphospholipid syndrome. Thrombocytopenia, recurrent venous or arterial thrombosis, hemolytic anemia, leg ulcers, and recurrent fetal loss are also manifestations of antiphospholipid syndrome.

Other causes for acute respiratory failure in patients with SLE include a volume overload state, due either to renal failure or to congestive heart failure secondary to myocarditis. Uremic pneumonitis with underlying DAD is also a possible cause of an acutely dyspneic SLE patient with renal failure. A syndrome, *acute reversible hypoxemia*, occurring in acutely ill SLE patients who are experiencing systemic exacerbations has been described.[10] These patients have hypoxemia and a widened alveolar–arterial oxygen gradient, but both the chest radiograph and ventilation–perfusion lung scans are normal. It is postulated that there is complement-activated neutrophil aggregation in the pulmonary vasculature. The hypoxemia improves with immunosuppressive therapy. Given the high incidence of antiphospholipid syndrome in SLE, acute reversible hypoxemia should be considered only after excluding thromboembolic disease.

■ ACUTE LUPUS PNEUMONITIS

Acute lupus pneumonitis is a clinical syndrome with an underlying histology of DAD, bronchiolitis obliterans organizing pneumonia, NSIP, or a combination of these.[11] Acute lupus pneumonitis mimics an acute infectious pneumonia and may be the presenting manifestation of SLE in up to 50% of patients. In those with an established diagnosis, it also appears during a flare-up of the other systemic manifestations of SLE, particularly pleuritis, pericarditis, arthritis, and nephritis. Acute lupus pneumonitis is reportedly more common in the postpartum period. It frequently recurs and cases have been documented that have progressed to a more chronic interstitial lung disease (UIP). Fortunately, acute lupus pneumonitis is a relatively uncommon complication, occurring in less than 5% of patients.

Bilateral alveolar infiltrates, which can be patchy or densely consolidated and often accompanied by pleural effusions and cardiomegaly due to underlying pericardial effusion or myocarditis (Fig. 60-10A), are present on chest radiographs at presentation. White blood cell counts and sedimentation rates are elevated and serum complement is often low. Immunopathologic studies reveal the presence of complement as well as antibodies to IgG and DNA in some patients, supporting the concept of an immune complex pathogenesis (Fig. 60-10B). Because of the difficulty in distinguishing acute lupus pneumonitis from an infectious pneumonia, a bronchoalveolar lavage and sometimes an open (thoracoscopic) lung biopsy are indicated prior to instituting anti-inflammatory and immunosuppressive therapy. Acute respiratory failure in acute lupus pneumonitis often requires assisted mechanical ventilation. The mortality rate has been reported to be as high as 50%, with the causes of death in patients with acute lupus pneumonitis being due to respiratory failure, another complication of SLE (nephritis, cerebritis), or a superimposed infection.

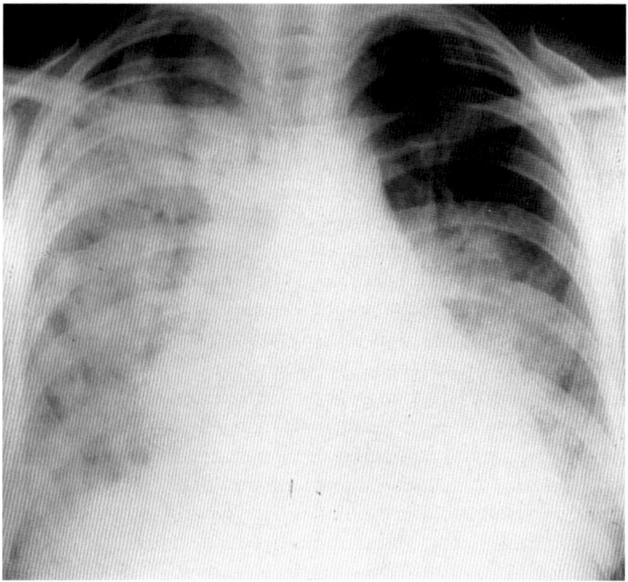

A

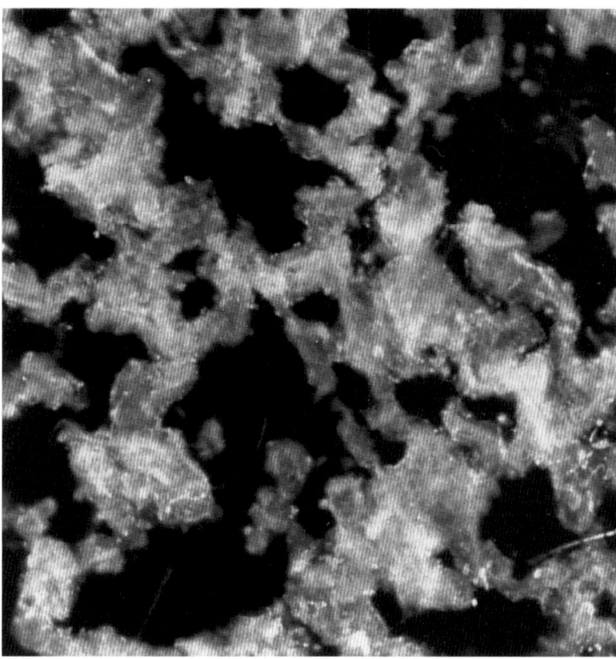

B

Figure 60-10 Acute lupus pneumonitis. **A.** The chest radiograph demonstrates diffuse alveolar filling with cardiomegaly (pericardial effusion vs. myocarditis). There is also a left pleural effusion. **B.** The immunofluorescent study demonstrates granular immune complex deposition in the alveolar interstitium.

■ DIFFUSE ALVEOLAR HEMORRHAGE

Diffuse alveolar hemorrhage, although rare, may be a presenting manifestation of SLE. In several cases, recurrent diffuse alveolar hemorrhage was present for years prior to the diagnosis of SLE.[12] The majority of cases, in contrast to acute lupus pneumonitis, first appear in a well-documented case of SLE. Diffuse alveolar hemorrhage accounts for 1% to 4% of SLE-related hospitalizations.

Diffuse alveolar hemorrhage can also present with symptoms reminiscent of an infectious pneumonia or acute lupus pneumonitis, and the additional symptom of hemoptysis raises the possibility of this diagnosis. Hemoptysis is present in 30% to 50% of patients during their initial presentation, but up to 90% will have hemoptysis

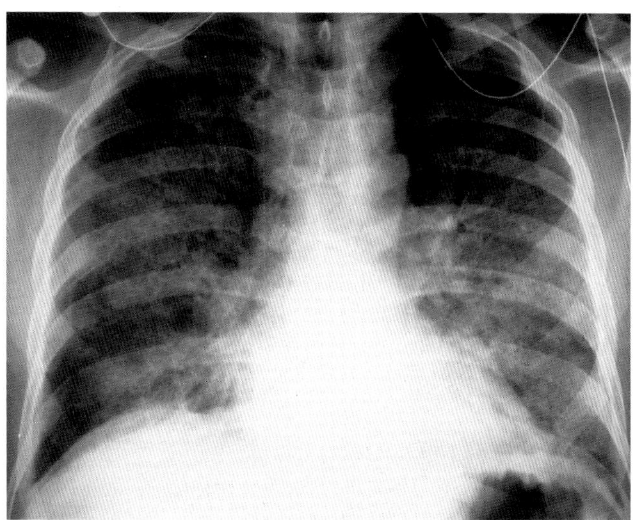

Figure 60-11 Diffuse alveolar hemorrhage in SLE. There are diffuse alveolar infiltrates without cardiomegaly or pleural effusions.

during their subsequent course. Routine laboratory work demonstrates a falling hematocrit, and in 60% to 90% of patients an active glomerulonephritis is invariably present. A progressive serosanguineous bronchoalveolar lavage may be the first clue to this diagnosis. Diffuse alveolar infiltrates are present on chest radiography (Fig. 60-11), but in contrast to acute lupus pneumonitis, pleuritis and pericarditis are not prominent features. Pathologic changes that are reminiscent of both acute lupus pneumonitis (DAD and NSIP) and diffuse alveolar hemorrhage with or without pulmonary capillaritis are not unusual in a single biopsy specimen.[13] The mortality rate is approximately 50% and is independent of the underlying histopathology (bland hemorrhage vs. pulmonary capillaritis). Recurrent DAH is common and should be expected in the absence of therapeutic intervention.

There are no controlled clinical trials for the treatment of either acute lupus pneumonitis or diffuse alveolar hemorrhage. Once infection has been excluded, corticosteroids are the mainstay of therapy. Intravenous methylprednisolone, 1 to 2 g daily in divided doses for 3 to 4 days before tapering, should be considered. Concomitant oral or parenteral cyclophosphamide or azathioprine is commonly administered, given the associated incidence of lupus nephritis. Plasmapheresis, immunoglobulin therapy, and rituximab have been used successfully, consistent with the proposed immune complex pathogenesis.[14-17]

LUPUS PLEURITIS

Pleurisy and pleural effusion are the most common primary pulmonary complications of SLE, occurring in 50% to 80% of patients. Pleurisy and/or a pleural effusion may also be the presenting and sole manifestation of the disease. They are usually recurrent and may accompany more severe complications such as acute lupus pneumonitis or nephritis. Patients complain of pleuritic pain, fever, and dyspnea. The chest radiograph may be normal (dry pleurisy) or demonstrate small to moderate pleural effusions (massive effusions are rare), which are bilateral in 50% of patients. When unilateral, there is no predilection for either side.

Effusions are serous or serosanguineous and exudative in nature. The white cell counts range from 5 to 10,000 cells/mm.^{3} Early on, neutrophils predominate, but with time mononuclear cells appear. These characteristics are nonspecific and are often seen with infectious parapneumonic effusions. In contrast to rheumatoid arthritis, the pleural fluid glucose concentration in lupus pleuritis is not reduced. Rheumatoid factor may be positive in lupus pleuritis. Pleural fluid complement levels are abnormally decreased in lupus, with both total complement activity and C3 and C4 reduced. A positive double-stranded pleural fluid DNA titer is nonspecific as opposed to the serum test, since it has been found in pleural effusions due to malignancy and tuberculosis. The most helpful measurement is the pleural fluid antinuclear antibody titer. Levels greater than 1:160 are very suggestive of lupus pleuritis. Examination of the pleural tissue reveals infiltration with plasma cells and lymphocytes, and, with repeated episodes, pleural fibrosis supervenes. Occasionally, a vasculitis of the pleural vessels is detected, and immune complex deposition has been reported. Corticosteroid treatment is effective for relief of pleural pain, but time to resolution of the pleural effusion is quite variable and probably unaffected by this treatment. In the unusual case, recurrent lupus pleuritis may result in massive pleural fibrosis and lung entrapment, necessitating a pleural stripping procedure.

While pleural effusions and pleurisy are common in patients with SLE, a broad differential diagnosis should be considered. The increased incidence of infectious complications, thromboembolic disease, and pulmonary hypertension in SLE predisposes patients to parapneumonic effusions and empyema, congestive heart failure, and effusions secondary to thromboembolic disease.

INTERSTITIAL LUNG DISEASE

Clinically significant interstitial lung disease is an uncommon pulmonary manifestation in SLE but UIP, lymphocytic interstitial pneumonitis, NSIP, and organizing pneumonia have all been reported. UIP is known to appear following acute lupus pneumonitis and in some cases has been documented to appear as an independent insidious disease. Using high-resolution computed tomography, 38% of patients with SLE patients with normal chest radiographs demonstrate pulmonary abnormalities consistent with some form of interstitial lung disease. In those who develop interstitial lung disease, a prior episode of acute lupus pneumonitis and an insidious onset of dyspnea are often noted. The prevalence of interstitial lung disease is increased in the subset of SLE patients with features suggestive of a mixed connective-tissue disease.

In patients who develop the insidious form of interstitial lung disease, the diagnosis of SLE is present for several years, and no other pattern of organ involvement predicts its appearance. These patients have progressive dyspnea and cough with interstitial infiltration on the chest radiograph. High-resolution computed tomography indicates combinations of ground-glass attenuation, inter- and intralobular septal thickening, and honeycomb change. Pulmonary function tests reveal a restrictive pattern with reduction in the diffusing capacity and hypoxemia accentuated by exercise. Response to therapy, either corticosteroids alone or in combination with cyclophosphamide or azathioprine, depends upon the underlying histology. Those cases with underlying NSIP or organizing pneumonia are more likely to respond to treatment than those who demonstrate excess collagen deposition and cystic honeycomb formation.

PULMONARY VASCULAR DISEASE

Idiopathic pulmonary hypertension due to plexogenic arteriopathy was previously thought to be an uncommon complication of SLE. It is now estimated to occur in 1% to 9% of patients.[18,19] This form of pulmonary hypertension is associated with Raynaud phenomenon, digital vasculitis, serositis, antibodies to ribonucleoprotein, rheumatoid factor, antiphospholipid antibodies, and most recently antiendothelial cell antibodies. Patients complain of dyspnea and fatigue but have normal chest radiographs. In advanced cases, pulmonary arterial enlargement appears. Spirometry and lung volumes are normal, but there is often an isolated reduction of the diffusing capacity for carbon monoxide as well as gas exchange abnormalities. Ventilation–perfusion lung scanning and, occasionally, pulmonary arteriography are indicated, particularly in those patients with the antiphospholipid syndrome who have a potential for recurrent small pulmonary emboli. Therapeutic options include vasodilator therapy, anticoagulation, immunosuppression with cyclophosphamide, and transplantation.

Vasculitis in SLE is more likely to be discovered in lung biopsy specimens, demonstrating either diffuse alveolar hemorrhage or acute lupus pneumonitis as opposed to being an isolated finding. Autopsy series indicate small-vessel vasculitis in 20% of cases.

BRONCHIOLITIS

Five percent of SLE patients are reported also to have obstructive physiology. Obliterative bronchiolitis has been documented in SLE, but is rare in contrast to rheumatoid arthritis. Organizing pneumonia, with inflammatory polyps protruding into bronchiolar lumens, is one of the interstitial patterns that occurs in acute lupus pneumonitis and in chronic interstitial lung disease in SLE, but this entity causes restriction rather than obstructive lung disease. Bronchiectasis may occur in up 20% of patients but is often asymptomatic. Large airway involvement including tracheal and subglottic stenosis, vocal fold paralysis, epiglottitis, and necrotizing tracheitis have all been reported, but are rare.

RESPIRATORY MUSCLE DYSFUNCTION

It is estimated that weakness of the diaphragm and other respiratory muscles is found in 25% of patients with SLE. This accounts for the previously unexplained findings of dyspnea without evidence of interstitial or pulmonary vascular disease. These patients have subsegmental atelectasis, an elevated diaphragm on chest radiograph (Fig. 60-12), and restrictive physiology. This has been referred to as *unexplained dyspnea and shrinking lungs syndrome.* Although there is a reduction in static lung volumes, the diffusing capacity, when corrected for alveolar volume, remains normal, thereby distinguishing respiratory muscle dysfunction from interstitial lung disease. The likely explanation for this is a reduction in the transdiaphragmatic pressure generated during maximal inspiration, which in turn reduces static lung compliance, producing the linear atelectasis seen on the chest radiograph. Moreover, in the patients with respiratory muscle weakness, no evidence for a generalized neuromuscular disease can be found. The pathogenesis of respiratory muscle dysfunction remains unexplained, although phrenic nerve conduction abnormalities have been excluded.[20] Abnormal diaphragmatic activation, due in part to voluntary inhibition due to pleuritic pain, may contribute to diaphragmatic dysfunction in this disorder. Clinical variables associated with the development of shrinking lung syndrome include: pleuritis, double-stranded DNA antibody and RNP antibody seropositivity, serositis, and a prolonged course of SLE.[5] Corticosteroids are not a frequently effective treatment modality. Rituximab has been used successfully in the treatment of shrinking lung syndrome, albeit anecdotally in nature.[21] Progression is uncommon and most patients stabilize. Positive-pressure ventilation, particularly at night, may improve these patients' daytime symptoms, although there is limited evidence available. Rituximab has been used successfully in patients with respiratory muscle dysfunction with significant physiologic improvement.[21]

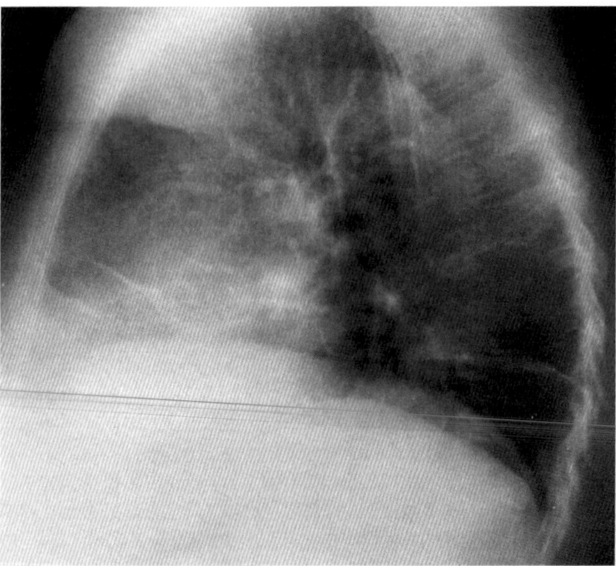

Figure 60-12 Diaphragmatic dysfunction in SLE. There is diaphragmatic elevation resulting in plate-like atelectasis.

RHEUMATOID ARTHRITIS: CLINICAL FEATURES

Rheumatoid arthritis classically affects the articular surfaces, but pleuropulmonary complications are responsible for significantly increased morbidity and mortality.[22] Most often cited is a 50% incidence for these complications, but it is likely that this underestimates their frequency.[23] Rheumatoid arthritis–associated interstitial lung disease abnormalities may be present in over 60% of patients with RA and are clinically asymptomatic during the initial assessment.[24] In those that manifest symptoms, the presence of RA-ILD, which approximates 10%, is associated with increased mortality.[25–27] Pleuropulmonary complications are more apt to occur in patients with more severe chronic articular disease, with high titers of rheumatoid factor, and in patients who have subcutaneous nodules, as well as other systemic complications such as cutaneous vasculitis, myocarditis, pericarditis, ocular inflammation, and Felty syndrome. An association between smoking and an increased risk for the development of pleuropulmonary disease, radiographic progression, and nodule formation in rheumatoid factor–seropositive patients has been reported. More recent observations series suggest that in those patients with anticitrullinated protein antibodies (anti-CCPs) there is an increase in parenchymal lung abnormalities, independent of current or prior tobacco exposure, supportive of the hypothesis that anti-CCPs are important in the pathogenesis of lung disease in RA.[28,29] Pleuropulmonary disease may occur in seronegative patients and both cytolytic and biologic therapies, commonly employed for treatment, can induce an interstitial lung disease, which is often difficult to distinguish from the primary forms complicating rheumatoid arthritis.[30] Moreover, interstitial lung disease, pleuritis, and occasionally obliterative bronchiolitis may be the first and only manifestation of the rheumatoid state in up to 20% of patients, preceding the articular manifestations by months to years.

PLEURISY AND PLEURAL EFFUSION

Pleural disease in a postmortem series was found in 40% of patients with rheumatoid arthritis. The incidence of clinically apparent pleural disease is closer to 5%, and the majority of patients experience mild symptoms. In approximately 20% of the patients who develop pleural complications, they do so prior to the onset of articular disease. In patients with rheumatoid arthritis, pleural complications are more common in men and occur most frequently during episodes of active articular disease and in patients with subcutaneous rheumatoid nodules.

Pleural disease is often first discovered on routine chest radiograph, and both pleural fibrosis and effusions have been reported to occur in asymptomatic patients. In more recent series using multidetector CT imaging, pleural thickening was noted in 49% of patients and did not correlate to the presence of symptoms.[31] Pleural effusions can be unilateral or bilateral and coexist with interstitial lung disease or necrobiotic nodules. Symptomatic patients present with pleuritic pain, dyspnea, and occasionally fever. The effusion is an exudate by protein and lactic dehydrogenase criteria, and, if chronic, cholesterol concentrations are increased. Other characteristics include a low pleural fluid pH (<7.2), thought to be due to impaired carbon dioxide exit from the pleural space. The leukocyte counts can be as high as 15,000 cells/mm^3 and consist of a mixture of neutrophils and mononuclear leukocytes. As in SLE, the total and individual complement components are low, and the rheumatoid factor level is increased. The presence of rheumatoid factor in pleural fluid has also been reported with tuberculosis, malignancy, and other infectious diseases. A low pleural fluid glucose concentration, thought to be due to a defect in glucose transport, is characteristic of rheumatoid effusions. Up to 40% of patients have pleural fluid glucose levels less than 10 mg/dL, and 75% have levels under 50 mg/dL. It has been stated that cytologic examination of the pleural fluid, which demonstrates a background of necrotic debris, spindle-shaped macrophages, and multinucleated histiocytes, is characteristic of a rheumatoid effusion. Necrobiotic nodules are thought to be involved in the pathogenesis of the pleural effusions, but transthoracic pleural biopsy only occasionally will demonstrate this finding.

Treatment is not indicated for asymptomatic cases; however corticosteroids, when used for active articular disease, are also effective in hastening the resolution of the pleural effusion. Rarely, is any other form of intervention such as intrapleural corticosteroids necessary for these patients. In the unusual case, pleural fibrosis with resultant lung entrapment occurs, requiring surgical intervention. Spontaneous pneumothorax due to rupture of a necrobiotic nodule, another uncommon complication, necessitates tube thoracostomy, and with persistence of the bronchopleural fistula, surgical intervention is indicated.

PULMONARY VASCULAR DISEASE

In general, pulmonary vascular disease is the least common pleuropulmonary complication in rheumatoid arthritis. The fibroproliferative plexogenic arteriopathy typical of scleroderma and SLE is an infrequent complication. When it does occur, Raynaud phenomenon is commonly present. The chest radiograph reveals normal lung fields and enlarged pulmonary arteries, and there is an isolated reduction of the diffusing capacity for carbon monoxide as well as hypoxemia.

Small-vessel vasculitis in rheumatoid arthritis occurs in the setting of diffuse alveolar hemorrhage due to pulmonary capillaritis and is a very rare event in rheumatoid arthritis. Several cases have been well documented and, in one, antineutrophilic cytoplasmic antibody to myeloperoxidase (p-ANCA) was present in the serum. Treatment with intravenous methylprednisolone, followed by oral corticosteroid preparations in addition to cyclophosphamide, is indicated for this complication.

NECROBIOTIC (RHEUMATOID) NODULE

Radiographically visible parenchymal rheumatoid nodules are infrequently seen in a rheumatoid population (1%). If present, necrobiotic nodules are more common in men, particularly those who smoke, with active articular disease and high rheumatoid factors, and in those who have subcutaneous nodules. The nodules are primarily a radiographic finding, subpleural in distribution, and asymptomatic in most. Cavitation and rupture may occur rarely and are associated with pneumothorax, pleural effusions, and hemoptysis. Radiographically, the nodules can be single or multiple with upper- and midzone predilection, and approximately 50% will undergo cavitation due to the large amounts of proteolytic enzymes in these lesions. The size is variable, and nodules up to 7 cm have been reported. Spontaneous resolution and recurrence are to be expected. Continuous growth, although possible, should prompt a more aggressive diagnostic approach. In most cases, no treatment is required. The major problem is differentiating the necrobiotic nodule from either malignant or infectious granulomatous disease, particularly given the increased risk of lung cancer in patients with RA.[32]

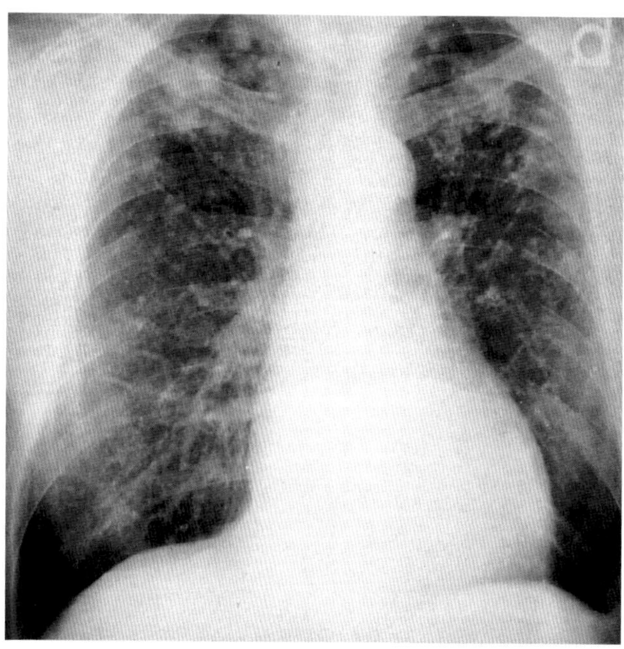

Figure 60-13 Caplan syndrome in a patient with rheumatoid arthritis and silicosis (hard-rock miner). There are multiple small nodules in the middle and upper lung representing the silicosis. In addition, multiple upper-zone rheumatoid nodules are present.

Caplan syndrome refers to a radiographic picture that developed in Welsh coal miners with rheumatoid arthritis and a pneumoconiosis.[33] It consists of the sudden appearance of discrete nodules primarily in the upper lobes that are histologically identical to the necrobiotic nodule (Fig. 60-13). The incidence of necrobiotic nodules is higher in rheumatoid patients with underlying pneumoconiosis, including coal workers' pneumoconiosis, silicosis, and asbestosis, than it is in a general rheumatoid population.

AIRWAY DISEASE

Upper airway involvement by the rheumatoid process most commonly involves the cricoarytenoid joint, causing difficulty with inspiration and occasionally resulting in stridor. A sore throat, hoarseness, and globus sensation are other common complaints. The prevalence of this complication, although asymptomatic in the majority of cases, approaches 50% when computed tomography screening is employed. Clinically significant disease can be detected by performing flow-volume loops, which indicate a variable extrathoracic obstruction of the inspiratory loop. Cricoarytenoid arthritis may further complicate endotracheal intubation and should be considered in all patients with rheumatoid arthritis requiring general anesthesia.

Bronchiolitis obliterans or obliterative bronchiolitis is a well-recognized cause of progressive and often severe obstructive lung disease in patients with rheumatoid arthritis.[34] The majority of patients develop bronchiolitis subsequent to the diagnosis of RA. Of note, bronchiolitis obliterans may be the initial manifestation of RA in a small group of patients.[35] This complication was first thought to be a consequence of either penicillamine or gold therapy, but many cases have appeared in the absence of either treatment. The onset of obliterative bronchiolitis is insidious, with patients complaining of progressive dyspnea and cough while having a normal or hyperinflated chest radiograph (Fig. 60-14A). It was thought that this complication was limited to women, but this is not the case. Physical examination reveals a generalized reduction of breath sounds and occasionally an inspiratory squeak. Physiologic testing reveals varying degrees of airflow limitation and hyperinflation, and the diffusing capacity may be normal or reduced. High-resolution computed tomography demonstrates adjacent areas of decreased and increased attenuation (geographic pattern), suggesting air trapping, which may be further identified by expiratory imaging (Fig. 60-14B). The response to therapy is poor. Some patients have responded to treatment with a combination of corticosteroids and cyclophosphamide, but the majority of cases progress to hypercapnic respiratory failure.

Another form of bronchiolitis seen in rheumatoid arthritis is a respiratory or follicular bronchiolitis, consisting of a dense infiltration of lymphocytes and plasma cells surrounding the terminal and respiratory bronchioles. Cough and dyspnea are common symptoms. Chest radiographs may be normal or demonstrate a fine nodular pattern more predominant in the middle and lower lung zones. High-resolution computed tomography reveals a pattern of follicular bronchiolitis in up to 33% of patients with RA, demonstrating centrilobular nodules and bronchiectasis (Fig. 60-15).[31] There is usually no physiologic evidence for airflow limitation or reduced lung volumes, but rather gas exchange abnormalities dominate the physiologic picture. Treatment with corticosteroids yields variable results.

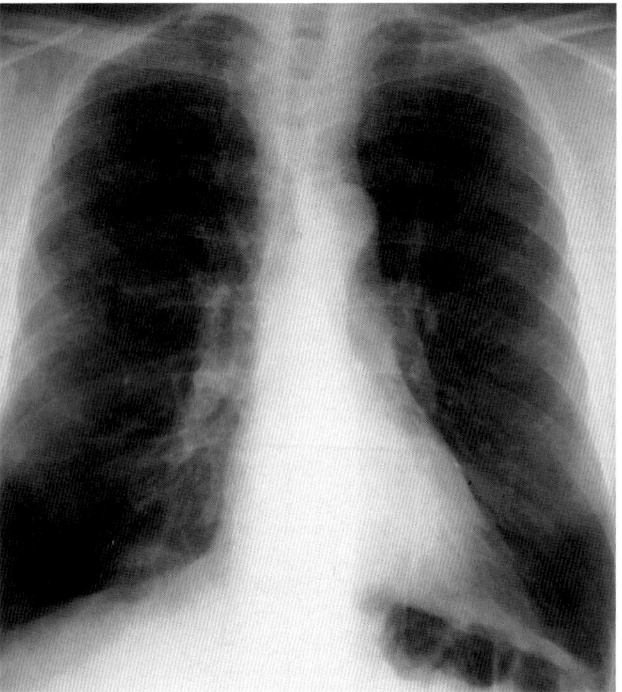

A

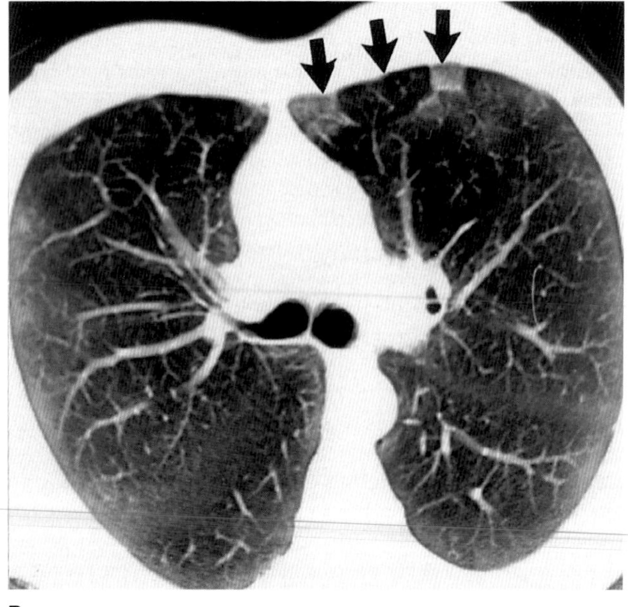

B

Figure 60-14 Obliterative bronchiolitis in a patient with rheumatoid arthritis. **A.** The chest radiograph is normal except for hyperinflation. **B.** A high-resolution computed tomography demonstrating areas of increased and decreased attenuation *(arrows)*.

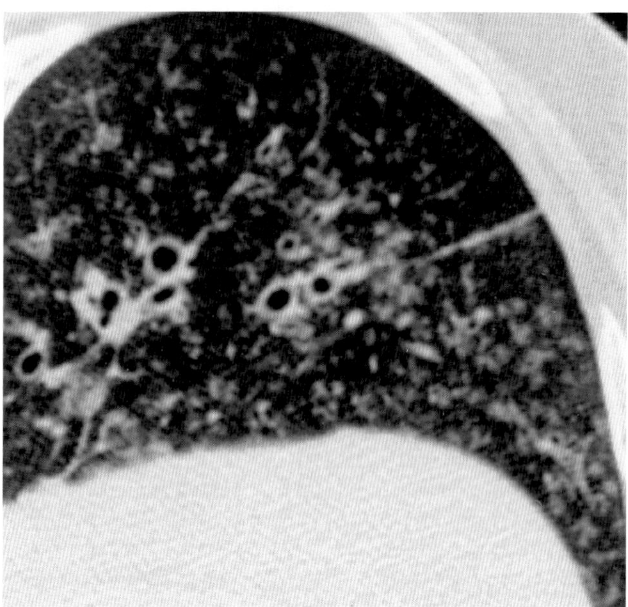

Figure 60-15 Follicular bronchiolitis in rheumatoid arthritis. High-resolution computed tomography demonstrating multiple centrilobular nodules.

Diffuse panbronchiolitis has been reported in Japanese patients with rheumatoid arthritis. In both diffuse panbronchiolitis and rheumatoid arthritis, an association with HLADR4 and B54 haplotypes has been reported, suggesting a common genetic predisposition.[36,37]

■ INTERSTITIAL LUNG DISEASE

Interstitial lung disease is a relatively common complication in patients with rheumatoid arthritis. In contrast to most connective-tissue diseases, interstitial lung disease is more common in males than females (3:1), individuals who have late-onset disease, high-titer rheumatoid factors, and in those who smoke. It is not unusual for interstitial lung disease to precede the articular manifestations for a period of months to years. The incidence of this complication in a rheumatoid population is difficult to determine, being reported in 5% to 40% of patients depending upon the methods of detection. The use of bronchoalveolar lavage indicating alveolar inflammation and high-resolution computed tomographic scans indicating various interstitial changes, often in the face of a negative chest radiograph, are difficult to interpret. This is because follow-up studies determining whether these patients developed clinically apparent interstitial lung disease are lacking. Furthermore, some parenchymal changes described on computed tomography such as bronchiectasis have very little, if any, clinical significance. It is likely that clinically important interstitial lung disease occurs in 5% to 10% of patients with rheumatoid arthritis, the most common forms being UIP and NSIP. These patients are dyspneic and complain of cough. Physical examination reveals bibasilar crackles, clubbing of the digits, and evidence of cor pulmonale when pulmonary hypertension appears secondary to hypoxic vasoconstriction. The chest

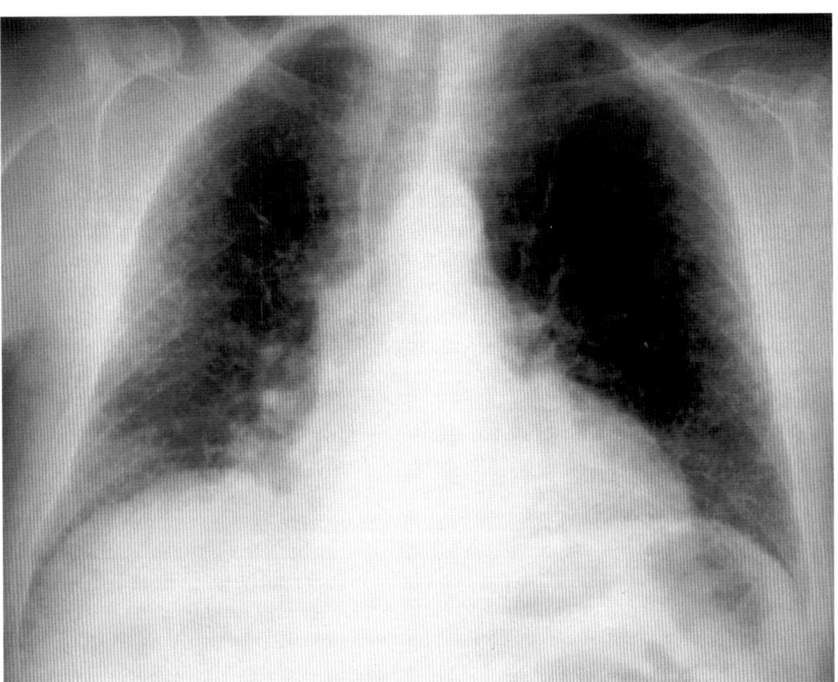

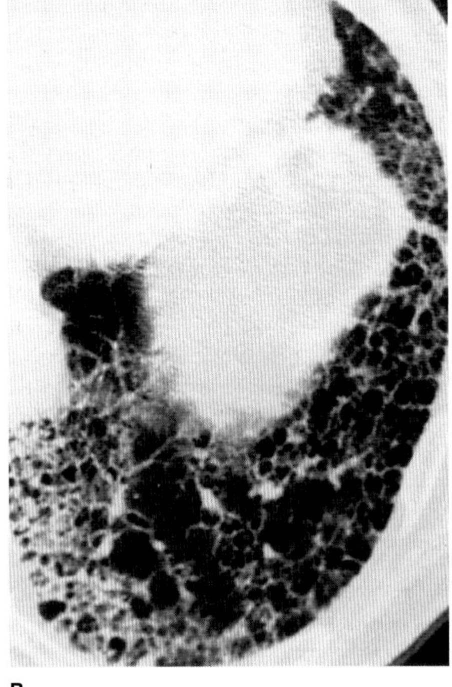

Figure 60-16 UIP in rheumatoid arthritis. **A.** Chest radiograph demonstrating lower zone and peripheral reticulonodular infiltrates. **B.** High-resolution computed tomography demonstrating a cystic network (honeycomb lung) at the lung base in a patient with advanced disease.

radiograph and computed tomographic scan demonstrate varying degrees of interstitial infiltrates with predilection for the lung bases and lung periphery (Fig. 60-16A). Other features include ground-glass attenuation on computed tomography with mixed alveolar–interstitial infiltrates on chest radiograph indicating a component of NSIP. Both imaging studies in advanced disease reveal the presence of honeycomb lung (Fig. 60-16B).

Several other interstitial reactions, which produce subacute or chronic symptoms, complicate rheumatoid arthritis. The first is organizing pneumonia, which can present with identical symptoms to UIP and preempt the onset of the articular disease as well. The chest radiograph (Fig. 60-17) and computed tomography scan differ from that seen in UIP because the infiltrates are primarily alveolar and localized, patchy, or diffuse. The second interstitial reaction is lymphocytic interstitial pneumonia, which occurs when rheumatoid arthritis is complicated by Sjögren syndrome. In addition to dyspnea and cough, these patients complain of dry mouth and eyes (xerophthalmia and xerostomia). The chest radiograph indicates patchy alveolar infiltrates primarily seen at the lung bases. In contrast to patients with primary Sjögren syndrome in which large cystic structure may develop within the lung, parenchymal cysts are uncommon in patients with RA-ILD. Eosinophilic pneumonia has been reported as a pleuroparenchymal complication of rheumatoid arthritis and may be the primary presentation of the disease. Acute interstitial pneumonitis is a rare, acute form of interstitial lung disease in rheumatoid arthritis. While it may occur as a result of an immunologic injury to the lung, medication-related pulmonary toxicity and opportunistic infections should be considered. Finally, fibrobullous disease, similar to that seen in ankylosing spondylitis, has been reported in rheumatoid arthritis and may precede the articular manifestations of the disease.

It is important to establish the underlying histology, since response to therapy and prognosis differs. Unless the imaging studies indicate end-stage honeycomb lung, which can also result from unresponsive or recurrent organizing pneumonia, lymphocytic interstitial pneumonia, or UIP, further evaluation is indicated. Bronchoalveolar lavage will not necessarily help differentiate between these three histologic pictures, but the finding of increased lymphocytic percentages as opposed to neutrophils and eosinophils indicates the potential for therapeutic responsiveness. Alveolar infiltrates and increased lymphocyte percentages are seen in lymphocytic interstitial pneumonitis. Organizing pneumonia is associated with increases in neutrophil, eosinophil, and lymphocyte percentages as well as radiographic alveolar infiltrates. The finding of increased

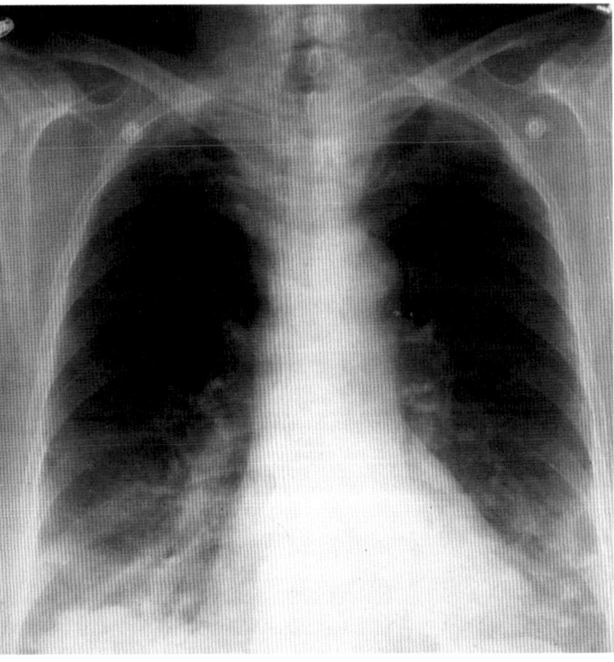

Figure 60-17 Bronchiolitis obliterans organizing pneumonia in rheumatoid arthritis. Chest radiograph demonstrating lower-zone mixed alveolar-interstitial infiltrates.

neutrophil and eosinophil percentages in suspected underlying UIP is an indicator of poor prognosis. Therefore, patients with lymphocytic interstitial pneumonitis and organizing pneumonia are more treatment-responsive when compared to those with UIP. If imaging studies and bronchoalveolar lavage cellular analysis are not definitive, thoracoscopic open lung biopsy should be considered. Treatment consists of a corticosteroid preparation and often the addition of cytotoxic drugs in the nonresponsive cases. As opposed to the idiopathic variety of organizing pneumonia, in which 66% of cases have favorable responses to corticosteroid medications, those associated with collagen vascular diseases are less responsive to treatment, often recur with tapering of the treatment regimen, and can progress to honeycomb lung. While the histopathology may be similar between rheumatoid arthritis and idiopathic pulmonary fibrosis, improved survival exists for those with rheumatoid arthritis–associated UIP but the long-term prognosis remains poor.[25,26,38]

Gold-induced pneumonitis must be differentiated from the primary forms of interstitial lung disease in patients with rheumatoid arthritis, particularly since the underlying histology can be similar, indicating varying degrees of NSIP and organizing pneumonia.[39] Dyspnea and cough usually begin 4 to 6 weeks following initiation of therapy, and peripheral eosinophilia occurs in a minority of cases. Occasionally, the chest radiograph will demonstrate upper- as opposed to lower-zone mixed alveolar interstitial infiltration. Bronchoalveolar lavage indicates a predominance of lymphocytes, and differentiation from rheumatoid interstitial lung disease can only be made after withdrawal of the drug results in remission. In severe cases with marked gas exchange abnormalities, corticosteroid therapy will occasion prompt reversal.

Methotrexate given in relatively low weekly doses (10–20 mg) is associated with the development of an interstitial disease in rheumatoid patients. No correlation with age, sex, duration of disease, or weekly or cumulative dose could be found. Conflicting data suggest that rheumatoid patients with underlying primary rheumatoid lung disease are predisposed to develop methotrexate pneumonitis. In rheumatoid patients treated with methotrexate, the incidence of methotrexate pneumonitis is 1% to 11%. The clinical onset is relatively acute with cough, fever, dyspnea, and new mixed alveolar and interstitial pulmonary infiltrates on chest radiograph. Increased white blood cell counts with mild eosinophilia, elevated sedimentation rates, and increased serum lactic dehydrogenase are nonspecific findings. Bronchoalveolar lavage indicates lymphocytosis and should be performed to rule out an infectious etiology. Lung tissue reveals an NSIP, organizing pneumonia, and granuloma formation reminiscent of a hypersensitivity pneumonitis. In patients who develop this clinical syndrome while on methotrexate, the drug should be discontinued since progression to end-stage fibrosis may occur. With life-threatening respiratory failure, corticosteroids given intravenously are an effective therapy.

The advent of TNF-α antagonists has revolutionized therapy for patients with rheumatoid arthritis. Their efficacy in the treatment of pleuroparenchymal complications remains unknown, with conflicting data having been reported. Of concern in those patients being treated with these agents should be the increased risk of infections, particularly both typical and atypical mycobacteria and fungi, as well as common bacterial pathogens. Several series suggest a temporal association between the use of biologic therapies and the development of ILD. It remains unclear if the association is temporal or causative.[30,40–43]

SCLERODERMA: CLINICAL FEATURES

Scleroderma or systemic sclerosis is an inflammatory-fibrotic disease that results in deposition of excessive extracellular matrix in the skin and several visceral organs including the lungs, heart, kidneys, and gastrointestinal tract. Two subtypes of systemic sclerosis exist: diffuse and limited. In diffuse systemic sclerosis, extensive skin involvement of the extremities, face, and torso exists with accompanying marked visceral involvement that is progressive in nature. The limited form, or CREST variant (*c*alcinosis, *R*aynaud phenomenon, *e*sophageal dysmotility, *s*clerodactyly, and *t*elangiectasias), has a more protracted course in most patients and usually affects an older subset of patients. Pulmonary disease contributes significantly to both the morbidity and mortality of patients. The pathogenesis, although not well understood, involves a complex interaction among immune cells, endothelial cells, and fibroblasts. In addition to the excessive extracellular matrix, which in the lung results in interstitial fibrosis, endothelial cell damage with intimal thickening of pulmonary and systemic arteries occurs, leading to luminal obliteration. This may result in a form of idiopathic pulmonary hypertension.

The lung is involved in the great majority of cases of scleroderma, with postmortem series indicating a 70% to 100% incidence.[44] Most patients with scleroderma develop dyspnea during the course of their illness due either to interstitial lung disease or pulmonary hypertension. Both bronchoalveolar lavage and high-resolution computed tomographic scans, in the face of normal chest radiographs, have indicated interstitial lung disease in both symptomatic and asymptomatic patients (Fig. 60-18). Although unusual, interstitial lung disease and pulmonary hypertension have preceded the dermatologic manifestations, defined as systemic sclerosis sine scleroderma.[45] Despite the lack of skin involvement, the course in systemic sclerosis sine scleroderma does not significantly differ from the more common forms, with exception of a greater tendency toward the development of pulmonary hypertension.

PLEURAL DISEASE

Although pleural fibrosis and adhesions are reported to be present in 40% of patients with scleroderma in postmortem studies, clinically apparent pleural thickening or pleural effusions on chest radiographs are considerably less frequent. The exception to this is pleural effusions secondary to congestive heart failure due to a scleroderma-associated cardiomyopathy.

INTERSTITIAL LUNG DISEASE

Interstitial lung disease, progressing to honeycomb lung, is the most common pulmonary complication of scleroderma, occurring in 30% to 100% of cases. A high-resolution computed tomographic study indicated a greater than 90% incidence of this abnormality with up to two-thirds of patients having normal chest radiographs. As many as 60% of patients who undergo bronchoalveolar lavage will demonstrate an abnormal inflammatory cell distribution. Chest radiographic and physiologic screenings indicate somewhat lower prevalence. The significance of the bronchoalveolar lavage and computed tomographic findings remain unclear, since no longitudinal follow-up is available. Following the histologic reclassification of idiopathic interstitial pneumonias, the most common underlying histology in systemic sclerosis is NSIP with honeycomb lung. UIP, unclassifiable fibrosing interstitial lung disease, and rarely, organizing pneumonia and granulomatous lung disease resembling sarcoidosis have also been reported.[46] It was previously thought that interstitial lung disease in scleroderma was primarily a fibrotic disorder. However, recent information derived from high-resolution computed tomography demonstrating ground-glass attenuation, which indicates more cellular disease, bronchoalveolar lavage revealing increased inflammatory cell populations, and biopsy material demonstrating cellular infiltration of the interstitium indicates the presence of a cellular inflammatory response.[47] This predates the development of fibrosis, consistent with the cellular subtype of NSIP. It is likely that the inflammatory phase in most cases is clinically silent.

Interstitial lung disease is more likely to occur in diffuse systemic sclerosis, although it may also complicate limited systemic sclerosis, formerly referred to as the CREST syndrome. Dyspnea on exertion

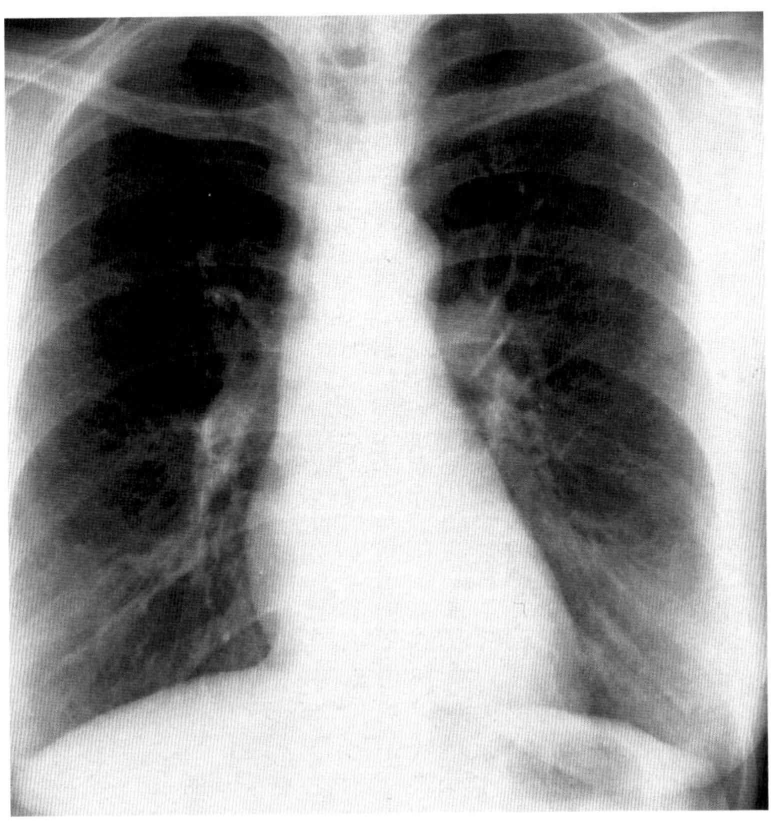

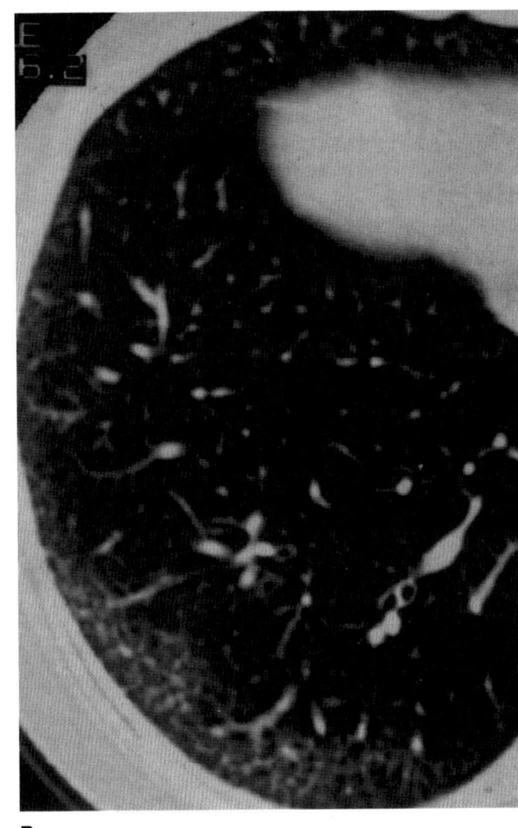

Figure 60-18 **A.** Normal chest radiograph in a dyspneic patient with scleroderma. **B.** High-resolution computed tomography of the same patient demonstrating reticular interstitial infiltrates.

progressing to dyspnea at rest and cough are the predominant symptoms. Bibasilar crackles are heard, but clubbing is unusual due to the capillary destruction in the nail beds. Physical findings of cor pulmonale eventually appear. Bibasilar interstitial infiltrates followed by more diffuse changes, loss of lung volume, honeycomb cysts, and pulmonary hypertension are the typical radiographic features. Scleroderma was the first interstitial lung disease in which scar carcinoma (adenocarcinoma or alveolar cell carcinoma) was reported. Several reports suggest an increased incidence of lung neoplasms in patients with scleroderma.[48,49] Physiologic testing eventually reveals restrictive lung disease, preserved flow rates, and a reduced diffusing capacity. Early on, the aforementioned measurements may be normal, and hypoxemia and a widened alveolar–arterial oxygen gradient at rest and heightened by exercise may be the only physiologic abnormality. A disproportionally greater reduction[50] of the diffusing capacity, when compared to lung volumes, most likely indicates the presence of idiopathic pulmonary hypertension due to plexogenic arteriopathy, particularly in the limited form of systemic sclerosis.

Other forms of interstitial lung disease seen in scleroderma include lymphocytic interstitial pneumonitis in those cases associated with Sjögren syndrome; rare cases of diffuse alveolar hemorrhage, and DAD in association with exacerbations of fibrotic lung disease in scleroderma have been reported.

Immunosuppression is the mainstay of treatment, with corticosteroids and cyclophosphamide being the agents of choice. The NHLBI-sponsored Scleroderma Lung Health Study confirmed prior retrospective studies suggesting improved lung function in those patients treated with cyclophosphamide. Although the improvement in lung function is of questionable clinical significance, a therapeutic effect is expected in those with ground-glass attenuation on HRCT imaging, a lymphocytic or eosinophilic predominant bronchoalveolar lavage, and a cellular interstitial pneumonia on lung biopsy.[51,52] Unfortunately, the durability of response to cyclophosphamide was limited as the majority of physiologic benefit waned after 12 months of discontinuation of treatment.[53] Mycophenolate mofetil and rituximab have been reported to benefits patients with progressive disease in scleroderma.[54–57] The efficacy of mycophenolate is currently the focus of an ongoing study sponsored by the National Institutes of Health.

■ PULMONARY VASCULAR DISEASE

Pulmonary hypertension, due to a plexogenic arteriopathy involving the pulmonary arteries, occurs in approximately 10% of cases of scleroderma and is primarily seen in the limited form (CREST syndrome). In this form of scleroderma, pulmonary hypertension may coexist with interstitial lung disease. Patients present with a gradual onset of dyspnea and increasing fatigue. Physical examination and chest radiograph may initially be normal, and, with disease progression, physical and radiographic signs of pulmonary hypertension appear. Lung volumes and airflow parameters are maintained, unless there is concomitant interstitial lung disease. Typically there is an isolated reduction in the diffusing capacity as well as progressive hypoxemia. Prior to the use of vasodilator therapy, the mean survival following a diagnosis of pulmonary hypertension was approximately 2 years. Treatment with continuous intravenous prostacyclin, phosphodiesterase type 5 inhibitors, and endothelin antagonists have improved the quality of life and exercise performance. Improved survival has been suggested with the use of these agents, specifically in those patients with isolated pulmonary arterial hypertension, in contrast to those with ILD-associated pulmonary hypertension.[58]

■ ASPIRATION PNEUMONIA

There is a high incidence of esophageal dilatation and decreased peristalsis (dysmotility) in patients with scleroderma, particularly in

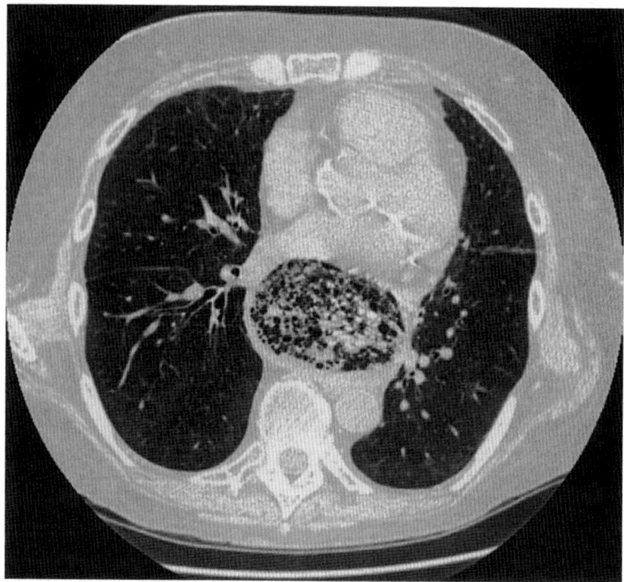

Figure 60-19 Mild peripheral, linear, ground-glass opacities in both lungs with marked thickening of the esophageal wall and severe dilatation of esophageal lumen with extensive debris filling the lumen in a patient with limited systemic sclerosis.

the limited variety (Fig. 60-19). This leads to dysphagia, heartburn, gastroesophageal reflux, and possibly aspiration with subsequent pneumonia.[59] It has long been held that reflux and aspiration contribute to the development of interstitial lung disease, albeit with a paucity of direct evidence.[60] In scleroderma, several different abnormalities contribute to the risk of reflux and aspiration: altered peristalsis, reduced lower esophageal pressure, presence of a hiatal hernia, gastroparesis, and autonomic nerve dysfunction.[61] Aggressive treatment to reduce the risk of reflux and aspiration is recommended despite inconclusive evidence to suggest an association. Behavioral modification and pharmacologic acid suppression are the initial interventions. In refractory situations, fundoplication may be considered in the appropriate patient, particularly in those with advanced lung fibrosis awaiting transplantation in an attempt to decrease the incidence posttransplantation bronchiolitis obliterans and chronic rejection.[62–64]

POLYMYOSITIS-DERMATOMYOSITIS: CLINICAL FEATURES

Polymyositis is a systemic autoimmune disorder characterized by an inflammatory myopathy. Dermatomyositis differs from polymyositis in that prominent skin involvement, characterized by a heliotropic rash and/or erythematosus scaling over the proximal interphalangeal joints, termed *Gottron papules* or *rash*, occurs with less severe myositis. In polymyositis–dermatomyositis, pulmonary complications are common and important causes of morbidity and mortality and as seen in other connective-tissue diseases, often predate or overshadow the muscle or skin manifestations. Pulmonary involvement has been reported in up to 40% of cases.[65] In contrast to the other collagen vascular diseases, in polymyositis–dermatomyositis primary involvement of the airways and pleura do not routinely occur. Pulmonary hypertension secondary to plexogenic arteriopathy has been reported on several occasions, most often in cases in which a crossover with scleroderma was suspected.

ASPIRATION PNEUMONIA

Aspiration pneumonia is a common pulmonary complication, occurring in 10% to 20% of patients with polymyositis–dermatomyositis; almost half of the patients complain of dysphagia as well. This complication results from an inflammatory myositis affecting the striated muscle of the hypopharynx and upper third of the esophagus. As a result, there is loss of normal swallowing function and failure to protect the airway. Aspiration is more likely in those patients with extensive skin or muscle involvement given the associated myositis.

RESPIRATORY MUSCLE DYSFUNCTION

Hypercapnic respiratory failure requiring assisted ventilation, due to extensive myositis involving the respiratory muscles and diaphragm, is an uncommon event (5% prevalence). In those patients presenting with unexplained hypercapnic respiratory failure, polymyositis–dermatomyositis as well as demyelinating neuromuscular disorders should be considered. With less extensive involvement of these muscles, however, there is a reduction in cough generation and the potential for the development of hypostatic pneumonia and atelectasis due to mucus plugging. Weakness can also cause a restricted physiologic defect with resulting tachypnea and dyspnea in the face of a normal diffusing capacity, normoxia, and hyperventilation. Respiratory muscle dysfunction as the cause of restrictive lung disease can best be demonstrated by measurement of the maximal pressure generated during both phases of the respiratory cycle. Sequential measurements are useful for monitoring the disease course and response to treatment.

INTERSTITIAL LUNG DISEASE

The prevalence of interstitial lung disease in polymyositis–dermatomyositis ranges from 5% to 30%.[66,67] The incidence is significantly higher in certain populations. In Japan, it approached 40% to 80% in one series. As in the other collagen vascular diseases, the use of bronchoalveolar lavage and high-resolution computed tomography for screening increases the documented incidence. In those screened with high-resolution CT imaging, the incidence approaches 78% within 3 years of diagnosis.[68]

Although UIP was previously reported to be the predominant histologic type of interstitial lung disease seen in polymyositis–dermatomyositis, NSIP now appears to be most common, based on the revised classification system for idiopathic interstitial pneumonias. DAD, organizing pneumonia, and diffuse alveolar hemorrhage secondary to pulmonary capillaritis may also occur.[69] All forms of interstitial lung disease may precede, appear simultaneously with, or follow the muscle or skin manifestations. There is no relationship between interstitial lung disease and the extent of muscle or skin disease, the level of creatinine phosphokinase elevation, or the presence of serum rheumatoid factor or antinuclear antibodies. There is, however, a relationship between interstitial lung disease and a serum antibody directed against the cellular enzymes tRNA-synthetases, the most common of which being known as anti–Jo-1.[70] This antibody appears in 25% of patients with polymyositis–dermatomyositis in total, but in 50% of patients with interstitial lung disease and in 13% of patients without lung disease. Depending on which tRNA-synthetase antibody is present, different clinical phenotypes may occur with varying degrees of myositis and lung involvement.[71,72]

All forms of interstitial lung disease in polymyositis–dermatomyositis are more common in women. Several clinical syndromes occur and are associated with the underlying interstitial lung disease. The most common presentation is chronic cough and progressive dyspnea due to NSIP with varying degrees of fibrosis.[73] Digital clubbing is rarely, if ever, seen. Chest radiographs demonstrate reticulonodular infiltrates, and with disease progression there is a reduction of the lung volume and the development of radiographic honeycomb lung and pulmonary hypertension. Physiologic testing indicates a restrictive pattern with a low diffusing capacity. Response to treatment depends upon the underlying histology, the more cellular disease being more responsive. In

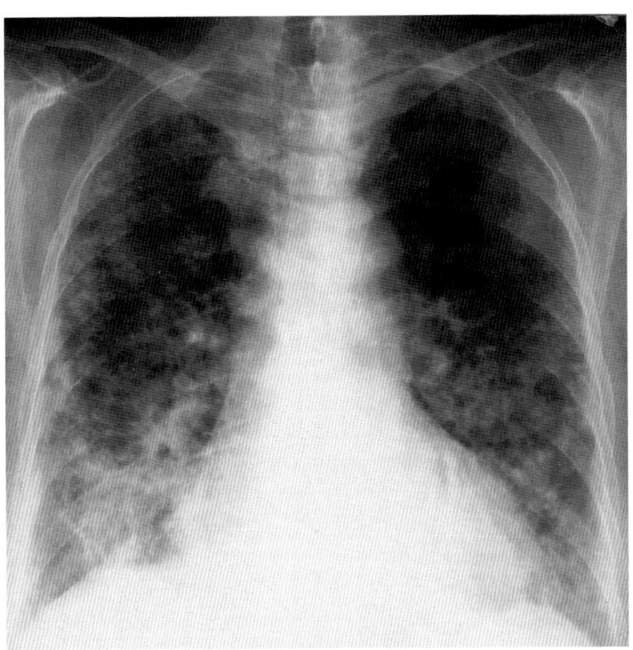

Figure 60-20 Bronchiolitis obliterans organizing pneumonia in a patient with polymyositis-dermatomyositis and acute symptoms. Chest radiograph demonstrating diffuse patchy alveolar infiltrates.

corticosteroid-resistant patients, cyclophosphamide, cyclosporine, tacrolimus, mycophenolate mofetil, intravenous immunoglobulins, and rituximab have been used with efficacy.[74]

In polymyositis–dermatomyositis, an acute pulmonary presentation with a clinical and radiographic picture reminiscent of a diffuse infectious pneumonia may occur and is associated with a poorer prognosis. The underlying lesion is DAD. Severe respiratory failure occurs, and recovery is unusual in spite of aggressive anti-inflammatory and immunosuppressive therapy. Organizing pneumonia may have either an acute or subacute presentation (Fig. 60-20). The differentiation from DAD becomes important because of the marked disparity in treatment outcome and survival. In organizing pneumonia, corticosteroid responsiveness with or without an additional agent is the rule rather than the exception. Diffuse alveolar hemorrhage due to pulmonary capillaritis may also occur.[75] This complication appears simultaneously with the onset of the muscle disease. Hemoptysis may or may not be present. As with other forms of pulmonary capillaritis, immunosuppression with corticosteroids and cyclophosphamide is utilized and been efficacious.

MIXED CONNECTIVE-TISSUE DISEASE: CLINICAL FEATURES

Patients with mixed connective-tissue disease have features of SLE, polymyositis–dermatomyositis, and scleroderma. Mixed connective-tissue disease is characterized by elevated titers of a specific antinuclear antibody directed against nuclear ribonucleoprotein (anti-RNP). Because of the similarity of mixed connective-tissue disease to the aforementioned collagen vascular diseases, pleuropulmonary complications are frequent, occurring in 20% to 80% of cases.[76,77]

PLEURAL DISEASE

Although pleurisy has been reported to occur in 40% of cases, pleural effusions are uncommon, appearing in approximately 5% of cases.[78] Effusions have been characterized as exudative in nature, but limited information is available in the literature.

PULMONARY VASCULAR DISEASE

Pulmonary hypertension may be caused by recurrent pulmonary emboli, hypoxic vasoconstriction secondary to interstitial lung disease, or plexogenic arteriopathy, as occurs in SLE and scleroderma. This is a significant problem for these patients; however, the incidence is unknown but may be less common than previously believed.[79] These patients, primarily women, present with dyspnea and fatigue. They have normal chest radiographs except for pulmonary arterial enlargement and an isolated reduction in the diffusing capacity for carbon monoxide. The prognosis in pulmonary hypertension secondary to mixed connective-tissue disease is similar to that noted in pulmonary hypertension seen in scleroderma and SLE. In contrast to patients without pulmonary arterial hypertension, 5-year survival is decreased from 96% to 73%.[80,81]

Medium-sized pulmonary artery vasculitis has been reported in mixed connective-tissue disease, with evidence suggesting immunologic-mediated injury with deposition (IgG, C_3) in the vascular walls. Circulating lupus anticoagulant (antiphospholipid syndrome) may also complicate the course of patients with mixed connective-tissue disease, predisposing them to thromboembolic disease.[82] It is in these patients that recurrent small pulmonary emboli may mimic the clinical picture of idiopathic pulmonary hypertension.

ASPIRATION PNEUMONIA

Patients with mixed connective-tissue disease, presenting with predominant features of scleroderma or polymyositis–dermatomyositis, are predisposed to esophageal dysmotility and dilatation, which can be a significant problem leading to reflux esophagitis and recurrent aspiration pneumonia. The presence of radiographic evidence of ILD closely associates with esophageal dilation and motor dysfunction, suggesting a common pathobiology.[83]

RESPIRATORY MUSCLE DYSFUNCTION

In those patients with features of polymyositis–dermatomyositis, an inflammatory myositis with respiratory muscle involvement may lead to hypercapnic respiratory failure or a restrictive lung disease with the development of hypostatic pneumonia.

INTERSTITIAL LUNG DISEASE

The incidence of interstitial lung disease in mixed connective-tissue disease is increased in comparison to other collagen vascular diseases, with greater than 50% of patients having abnormal high-resolution CT imaging abnormalities.[84] The histologic pattern of NSIP and/or UIP are noted, both of which may progress to honeycomb lung, particularly in those patients with the features of scleroderma. As with the other connective-tissue diseases, this interstitial lung disease manifests as progressive dyspnea, bibasilar reticulonodular infiltrates on chest radiograph, and physiologic parameters with low lung volumes and a reduction in the diffusing capacity for carbon monoxide.

Diffuse alveolar hemorrhage has been reported in a few cases of mixed connective-tissue disease and is similar in presentation to that in SLE. It is assumed that the histology is one of either bland pulmonary hemorrhage or pulmonary capillaritis but remains unknown.[85]

SJÖGREN SYNDROME

Sjögren syndrome refers to a triad of xerophthalmia, xerostomia, and polyarthritis. This autoimmune exocrinopathy is characterized by lymphocytic infiltration of the lacrimal and salivary glands.[86] A primary form, occurring in the absence of another collagen vascular disease, and a secondary form, associated with one of the other collagen vascular diseases, most frequently rheumatoid arthritis, exist.[87] A strong female predominance exists in Sjögren syndrome (90%). A positive rheumatoid factor (95%) and antinuclear antibodies in a speckled pattern (80%) are to be expected, as well as positive tests for antibodies to extractable nuclear antigens (anti-SSA, anti-SSB), which are specific for the primary form of the syndrome.

AIRWAY DISEASE

Lymphocytic infiltration and destruction of airway mucus glands result in desiccation of the tracheobronchial tree in Sjögren syndrome.[88] Patients may develop hoarseness, cough, inspissation of secretions resulting in luminal obstruction and atelectasis, recurrent pneumonias, and bronchiectasis. There is a high incidence of obstructive ventilatory dysfunction in these patients, secondary to follicular bronchiolitis. Obliterative bronchiolitis, constrictive bronchiolitis, and bronchiolectasis have also been reported.

INTERSTITIAL LUNG DISEASE

In primary Sjögren syndrome, patients present with a nonproductive cough, dyspnea on exertion, or asymptomatic radiographic abnormalities. As occurs in the lacrimal and salivary glands, interstitial lung disease in these patients is the result of lymphocytic infiltration of the lung parenchyma. This occurs in two forms, lymphocytic interstitial pneumonitis and, less commonly, pseudolymphoma. Both of these lesions have the potential for lymphomatous conversion. Lymphocytic interstitial pneumonitis is an interstitial lung disease in which cough, dyspnea, and restrictive physiology manifest. Because lymphocytes may also infiltrate the alveolar spaces as well as the interstitium, the radiologic studies indicate mixed alveolar and interstitial infiltrates. In a subset of patients, variably sized cystic lesions with associated ground glass may be the only radiographic abnormality (Fig. 60-21). The development of pleural effusions or the appearance of hilar or mediastinal adenopathy should be investigated further as it may suggest a malignant transformation to a lymphoma. Lymphocytic interstitial pneumonia is responsive to anti-inflammatory agents such as corticosteroids. Occasionally, cytolytic therapy, such as azathioprine or cyclophosphamide, is required but remains of unproven benefit. Cyclosporine has also been recommended as an additional agent in corticosteroid-resistant cases. Rituximab, an anti-CD20 monoclonal antibody, may be beneficial in selected patients but further controlled studies are required to better assess its efficacy in primary Sjögren syndrome. While the majority of patients will respond to immunosuppressive therapy, a subset of patients progress to fibrotic lung disease with honeycomb change.

Pseudolymphoma is a tumor-like proliferation appearing as single or multiple masses on the chest radiograph. It is often difficult to distinguish from a malignant lymphoma and it has been suggested that pseudolymphoma, which is considered to be a localized form of lymphocytic interstitial pneumonitis, is a premalignant lesion.[89] When associated with a monoclonal gammopathy, malignant transformation to lymphoma is suggested.[90]

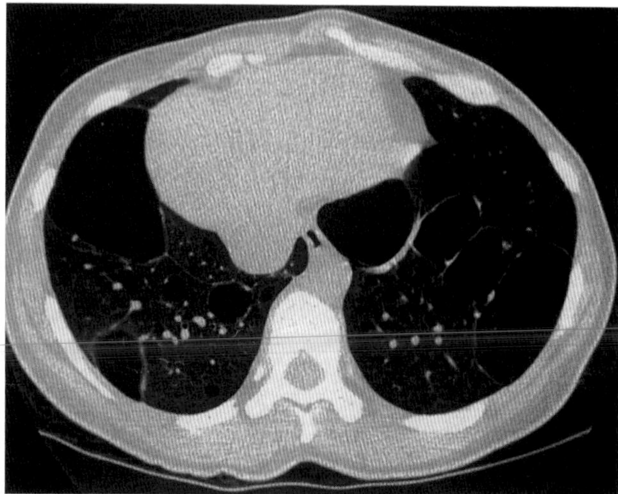

Figure 60-21 Multiple cysts of varying sizes scattered throughout both lungs in a patient with Sjögren syndrome and lymphocytic interstitial pneumonia.

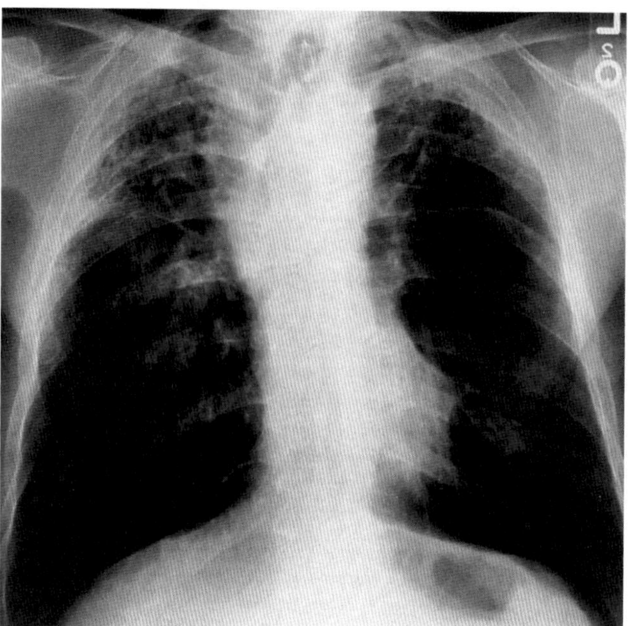

Figure 60-22 Ankylosing spondylitis. Chest radiograph demonstrating bilateral upper-zone fibronodular infiltrates.

Interstitial lung disease occurs more commonly in the secondary forms of Sjögren syndrome and most likely represents a complication of the associated collagen vascular disease.[2] The histologic pattern in secondary Sjögren syndrome mimics that seen in rheumatoid arthritis, with NSIP, UIP, and organizing pneumonia reported. UIP is uncommon in the primary form of Sjögren syndrome.

ANKYLOSING SPONDYLITIS

Ankylosing spondylitis is one of the seronegative spondyloarthropathies that may eventually result in fixation of the chest wall and a mild to moderate restrictive lung disease. Muscular involvement, in contrast to polymyositis–dermatomyositis, does not occur and diaphragmatic function is preserved, limiting ventilatory failure given the preserved respiratory muscle function.

The incidence of interstitial lung disease complication is reportedly less than 2%.[91] In contrast to the other collagen vascular diseases that primarily affect the basilar portion of the lung, ankylosing spondylitis has a predilection for the upper lung zones, only appears late in the course of the chronic spondylitis, and never precedes it.[92] Interstitial lung disease often appears as fibrocystic disease on the chest radiograph (Fig. 60-22) and is difficult to distinguish from apical lung infections such as tuberculosis. Histologically, it is a fibrosing process with cystic formation. Progressive dyspnea and cough are the predominant symptoms, and treatment with corticosteroids is ineffective and therefore not suggested. Etanercept may afford patient a short-term benefit with improvements in spinal mobility and pulmonary physiology.[93] The most serious complication of this apical fibrocystic disease is infection with invasive aspergilla species as well as atypical mycobacteria. Further, saprophytic colonization of the cysts by aspergilla species (aspergilloma) may induce life-threatening hemoptysis.

REFERENCES

1. Barrera P, Laan RF, van Riel PL, Dekhuijzen PN, Boerbooms AM, van de Putte LB. Methotrexate-related pulmonary complications in rheumatoid arthritis. *Ann Rheum Dis*. 1994;53:434–439.

2. Homma Y, Ohtsuka Y, Tanimura K, et al. Can interstitial pneumonia as the sole presentation of collagen vascular diseases be differentiated from idiopathic interstitial pneumonia? *Respiration*. 1995;62:248–251.

3. Gross M, Esterly JR, Earle RH. Pulmonary alterations in systemic lupus erythematosus. *Am Rev Respir Dis*. 1972;105:572–577.

4. Quadrelli SA, Alvarez C, Arce SC, et al. Pulmonary involvement of systemic lupus erythematosus: analysis of 90 necropsies. *Lupus*. 2009;18:1053–1060.

5. Allen D, Fischer A, Bshouty Z, et al. Evaluating systemic lupus erythematosus patients for lung involvement. *Lupus*. 2012;21:1316–1325.

6. Boulware DW, Hedgpeth MT. Lupus pneumonitis and anti-SSA(Ro) antibodies. *J Rheumatol*. 1989;16:479–481.

7. Rosner S, Ginzler EM, Diamond HS, et al. A multicenter study of outcome in systemic lupus erythematosus. II. Causes of death. *Arthritis Rheum*. 1982;25:612–617.

8. Brucato A, Baudo F, Barberis M, et al. Pulmonary hypertension secondary to thrombosis of the pulmonary vessels in a patient with the primary antiphospholipid syndrome. *J Rheumatol*. 1994;21:942–944.

9. Alarcón-Segovia D, Delezé M, Oria CV, et al. Antiphospholipid antibodies and the antiphospholipid syndrome in systemic lupus erythematosus. A prospective analysis of 500 consecutive patients. *Medicine (Baltimore)*. 1989;68:353–365.

10. Abramson SB, Dobro J, Eberle MA, et al. Acute reversible hypoxemia in systemic lupus erythematosus. *Ann Intern Med*. 1991;114:941–947.

11. Matthay RA, Schwarz MI, Petty TL, et al. Pulmonary manifestations of systemic lupus erythematosus: review of twelve cases of acute lupus pneumonitis. *Medicine (Baltimore)*. 1975;54:397–409.

12. Byrd RB, Trunk G. Systemic lupus erythematosus presenting as pulmonary hemosiderosis. *Chest*. 1973;64:128–129.

13. Myers JL, Katzenstein AA. Microangiitis in lupus-induced pulmonary hemorrhage. *Am J Clin Pathol*. 1986;85:552–556.

14. Claridge S, Das P, Dorling A, Robson MG. Plasmapheresis as rescue therapy for systemic lupus erthyematosus-associated diffuse alveolar haemorrhage. *BMJ Case Rep*. 2011;2011. pii:bcr0220113893.

15. Duxbury B, Combescure C, Chizzolini C. Rituximab in systemic lupus erythematosus: an updated systematic review and meta-analysis. *Lupus*. 2013;22:1489–1503.

16. Martinez-Martinez MU, Abud-Mendoza C. Recurrent diffuse alveolar haemorrhage in a patient with systemic lupus erythematosus: long-term benefit of rituximab. *Lupus*. 2012;21:1124–1127.

17. Witt M, Grunke M, Proft F, et al. Clinical outcomes and safety of rituximab treatment for patients with systemic lupus erythematosus (SLE) - results from a nationwide cohort in Germany (GRAID). *Lupus*. 2013;22:1142–1149.

18. Love PE, Santoro SA. Antiphospholipid antibodies: anticardiolipin and the lupus anticoagulant in systemic lupus erythematosus (SLE) and in non-SLE disorders. Prevalence and clinical significance. *Ann Intern Med*. 1990;112:682–698.

19. Asherson RA, Higenbottam TW, Dinh Xuan AT, Khamashta MA, Hughes GR. Pulmonary hypertension in a lupus clinic: experience with twenty-four patients. *J Rheumatol*. 1990;17:1292–1298.

20. Wilcox PG, Stein HB, Clarke SD, Pare PD, Pardy RL. Phrenic nerve function in patients with diaphragmatic weakness and systemic lupus erythematosus. *Chest*. 1988;93:352–358.

21. Benham H, Garske L, Vecchio P, Eckert BW. Successful treatment of shrinking lung syndrome with rituximab in a patient with systemic lupus erythematosus. *J Clin Rheumatol*. 2010;16:68–70.

22. Walker WC, Wright V. Pulmonary lesions and rheumatoid arthritis. *Medicine (Baltimore)*. 1968;47:501–520.

23. Shannon TM, Gale ME. Noncardiac manifestations of rheumatoid arthritis in the thorax. *J Thorac Imaging*. 1992;7:19–29.

24. Chen J, Shi Y, Wang X, Huang H, Ascherman D. Asymptomatic preclinical rheumatoid arthritis-associated interstitial lung disease. *Clin Dev Immunol*. 2013;2013:406927.

25. Olson AL, Swigris JJ, Sprunger DB, et al. Rheumatoid arthritis-interstitial lung disease-associated mortality. *Am J Respir Crit Care Med*. 2011;183:372–378.

26. Koduri G, Norton S, Young A, et al. Interstitial lung disease has a poor prognosis in rheumatoid arthritis: results from an inception cohort. *Rheumatology (Oxford)*. 2010;49:1483–1489.

27. Bongartz T, Nannini C, Medina-Velasquez YF, et al. Incidence and mortality of interstitial lung disease in rheumatoid arthritis: a population-based study. *Arthritis Rheum*. 2010;62:1583–1591.

28. Reynisdottir G, Karimi R, Joshua V, et al. Structural lung changes and local anti-citrulline immunity are early features of anti citrullinated-proteins antibodies positive rheumatoid arthritis. *Arthritis Rheum*.2013;66:31–39.

29. Giles JT, Danoff SK, Sokolove J, et al. Association of fine specificity and repertoire expansion of anticitrullinated peptide antibodies with rheumatoid arthritis associated interstitial lung disease. *Ann Rheum Dis*.2014;73(8):1487–1494.

30. Roubille C, Haraoui B. Interstitial lung diseases induced or exacerbated by DMARDS and biologic agents in rheumatoid arthritis: a systematic literature review. *Semin Arthritis Rheum*. 2014;43(5):613–626.

31. Yuksekkaya R, Celikyay F, Yilmaz A, et al. Pulmonary involvement in rheumatoid arthritis: multidetector computed tomography findings. *Acta Radiol*. 2013;54(10):1138–1149.

32. Khurana R, Wolf R, Berney S, Caldito G, Hayat S, Berney SM. Risk of development of lung cancer is increased in patients with rheumatoid arthritis: a large case control study in US veterans. *J Rheumatol*. 2008;35:1704–1708.

33. Caplan A. Certain unusual radiological appearances in the chest of coal-miners suffering from rheumatoid arthritis. *Thorax*. 1953;8:29–37.

34. Geddes DM, Corrin B, Brewerton DA, Davies RJ, Turner-Warwick M. Progressive airway obliteration in adults and its association with rheumatoid disease. *Q J Med*. 1977;46:427–444.

35. Devouassoux G, Cottin V, Lioté H, et al. Characterisation of severe obliterative bronchiolitis in rheumatoid arthritis. *Eur Respir J*. 2009;33:1053–1061.

36. Homma S, Kawabata M, Kishi K, et al. Diffuse panbronchiolitis in rheumatoid arthritis. *Eur Respir J*. 1998;12:444–452.

37. Sugiyama Y, Ohno S, Kano S, Maeda H, Kitamura S. Diffuse panbronchiolitis and rheumatoid arthritis: a possible correlation with HLA-B54. *Intern Med*. 1994;33:612–614.

38. Solomon JJ, Ryu JH, Tazelaar HD, et al. Fibrosing interstitial pneumonia predicts survival in patients with rheumatoid arthritis-associated interstitial lung disease (RA-ILD). *Respir Med*. 2013;107:1247–1252.

39. Levinson ML, Lynch JP 3rd, Bower JS. Reversal of progressive, life-threatening gold hypersensitivity pneumonitis by corticosteroids. *Am J Med*. 1981;71:908–912.

40. Picchianti Diamanti A, Germano V, Bizzi E, Lagana B, Migliore A. Interstitial lung disease in rheumatoid arthritis in the era of biologics. *Pulm Med.* 2011;2011:931342.

41. Dixon WG, Hyrich KL, Watson KD, Lunt M, Symmons DP. Influence of anti-TNF therapy on mortality in patients with rheumatoid arthritis-associated interstitial lung disease: results from the British Society for Rheumatology Biologics Register. *Ann Rheum Dis.* 2010;69:1086–1091.

42. Hagiwara K, Sato T, Takagi-Kobayashi S, Hasegawa S, Shigihara N, Akiyama O. Acute exacerbation of preexisting interstitial lung disease after administration of etanercept for rheumatoid arthritis. *J Rheumatol.* 2007;34:1151–1154.

43. Imaizumi K, Sugishita M, Usui M, Kawabe T, Hashimoto N, Hasegawa Y. Pulmonary infectious complications associated with anti-TNFalpha therapy (infliximab) for rheumatoid arthritis. *Intern Med.* 2006;45:685–688.

44. Schurawitzki H, Stiglbauer R, Graninger W, et al. Interstitial lung disease in progressive systemic sclerosis: high-resolution CT versus radiography. *Radiology.* 1990;176:755–759.

45. Fischer A, Meehan RT, Feghali-Bostwick CA, West SG, Brown KK. Unique characteristics of systemic sclerosis sine scleroderma-associated interstitial lung disease. *Chest.* 2006;130:976–981.

46. D'Angelo WA, Fries JF, Masi AT, Shulman LE. Pathologic observations in systemic sclerosis (scleroderma). A study of fifty-eight autopsy cases and fifty-eight matched controls. *Am J Med.* 1969;46:428–440.

47. Wells AU, Cullinan P, Hansell DM, et al. Fibrosing alveolitis associated with systemic sclerosis has a better prognosis than lone cryptogenic fibrosing alveolitis. *Am J Respir Crit Care Med.* 1994;149:1583–1590.

48. Colaci M, Giuggioli D, Sebastiani M, et al. Lung cancer in scleroderma: results from an Italian rheumatologic center and review of the literature. *Autoimmun Rev.* 2013;12:374–379.

49. Omair MA, Lee P. Development of adenocarcinoma of the lung in a transplanted lung of a scleroderma patient. *Clin Exp Rheumatol.* 2012;30:317–318.

50. Park IN, Kim DS, Shim TS, et al. Acute exacerbation of interstitial pneumonia other than idiopathic pulmonary fibrosis. *Chest.* 2007;132:214–220.

51. Tashkin DP, Elashoff R, Clements PJ, et al. Cyclophosphamide versus placebo in scleroderma lung disease. *N Engl J Med.* 2006;354:2655–2666.

52. Strange C, Bolster MB, Roth MD, et al. Bronchoalveolar lavage and response to cyclophosphamide in scleroderma interstitial lung disease. *Am J Respir Crit Care Med.* 2008;177:91–98.

53. Tashkin DP, Elashoff R, Clements PJ, et al. Effects of 1-year treatment with cyclophosphamide on outcomes at 2 years in scleroderma lung disease. *Am J Respir Crit Care Med.* 2007;176:1026–1034.

54. Zamora AC, Wolters PJ, Collard HR, et al. Use of mycophenolate mofetil to treat scleroderma-associated interstitial lung disease. *Respir Med.* 2008;102:150–155.

55. Gerbino AJ, Goss CH, Molitor JA. Effect of mycophenolate mofetil on pulmonary function in scleroderma-associated interstitial lung disease. *Chest.* 2008;133:455–460.

56. Yoo WH. Successful treatment of steroid and cyclophosphamide-resistant diffuse scleroderma-associated interstitial lung disease with rituximab. *Rheumatol Int.* 2012;32:795–798.

57. McGonagle D, Tan AL, Madden J, et al. Successful treatment of resistant scleroderma-associated interstitial lung disease with rituximab. *Rheumatology (Oxford).* 2008;47:552–553.

58. Mathai SC, Hummers LK, Champion HC, et al. Survival in pulmonary hypertension associated with the scleroderma spectrum of diseases: impact of interstitial lung disease. *Arthritis Rheum.* 2009;60:569–577.

59. Savarino E, Bazzica M, Zentilin P, et al. Gastroesophageal reflux and pulmonary fibrosis in scleroderma: a study using pH-impedance monitoring. *Am J Respir Crit Care Med.* 2009;179:408–413.

60. Lee JS, Ryu JH, Elicker BM, et al. Gastroesophageal reflux therapy is associated with longer survival in patients with idiopathic pulmonary fibrosis. *Am J Respir Crit Care Med.* 2011;184:1390–1394.

61. Ebert EC. Esophageal disease in scleroderma. *J Clin Gastroenterol.* 2006;40:769–775.

62. Kent MS, Luketich JD, Irshad K, et al. Comparison of surgical approaches to recalcitrant gastroesophageal reflux disease in the patient with scleroderma. *Ann Thorac Surg.* 2007;84:1710–1715; discussion 1715–1716.

63. Hartwig MG, Davis RD. Gastroesophageal reflux disease-induced aspiration injury following lung transplantation. *Curr Opin Organ Transplant.* 2012;17:474–478.

64. Mohammed A, Neujahr DC. Gastroesophageal reflux disease and graft failure after lung transplantation. *Transplant Rev.* 2010;24:99–103.

65. Dickey BF, Myers AR. Pulmonary disease in polymyositis/dermatomyositis. *Semin Arthritis Rheum.* 1984;14:60–76.

66. Schwarz MI. Pulmonary and cardiac manifestations of polymyositis-dermatomyositis. *J Thorac Imaging.* 1992;7:46–54.

67. Schwarz MI, Matthay RA, Sahn SA, Stanford RE, Marmorstein BL, Scheinhorn DJ. Interstitial lung disease in polymyositis and dermatomyositis: analysis of six cases and review of the literature. *Medicine (Baltimore).* 1976;55:89–104.

68. Fathi M, Vikgren J, Boijsen M, et al. Interstitial lung disease in polymyositis and dermatomyositis: longitudinal evaluation by pulmonary function and radiology. *Arthritis Rheum.* 2008;59:677–685.

69. Clawson K, Oddis CV. Adult respiratory distress syndrome in polymyositis patients with the anti-Jo-1 antibody. *Arthritis Rheum.* 1995;38:1519–1523.

70. Bernstein RM, Morgan SH, Chapman J, et al. Anti-Jo-1 antibody: a marker for myositis with interstitial lung disease. *Br Med J (Clin Res Ed).* 1984;289:151–152.

71. Hervier B, Wallaert B, Hachulla E, et al. Clinical manifestations of anti-synthetase syndrome positive for anti-alanyl-tRNA synthetase (anti-PL12) antibodies: a retrospective study of 17 cases. *Rheumatology (Oxford).* 2010;49:972–976.

72. Hamaguchi Y, Fujimoto M, Matsushita T, et al. Common and distinct clinical features in adult patients with anti-aminoacyl-tRNA synthetase antibodies: heterogeneity within the syndrome. *PLoS One.* 2013;8:e60442.

73. Tazelaar HD, Viggiano RW, Pickersgill J, Colby TV. Interstitial lung disease in polymyositis and dermatomyositis. Clinical features and prognosis as correlated with histologic findings. *Am Rev Respir Dis.* 1990;141:727–733.

74. Moolman JA, Bardin PG, Rossouw DJ, Joubert JR. Cyclosporin as a treatment for interstitial lung disease of unknown aetiology. *Thorax.* 1991;46:592–595.

75. Schwarz MI, Sutarik JM, Nick JA, Leff JA, Emlen JW, Tuder RM. Pulmonary capillaritis and diffuse alveolar hemorrhage. A primary manifestation of polymyositis. *Am J Respir Crit Care Med.* 1995;151:2037–2040.

76. Prakash UB. Lungs in mixed connective tissue disease. *J Thorac Imaging*. 1992;7:55–61.

77. Prakash UB, Luthra HS, Divertie MB. Intrathoracic manifestations in mixed connective tissue disease. *Mayo Clin Proc*. 1985; 60:813–821.

78. Sullivan WD, Hurst DJ, Harmon CE, et al. A prospective evaluation emphasizing pulmonary involvement in patients with mixed connective tissue disease. *Medicine (Baltimore)*. 1984;63: 92–107.

79. Gunnarsson R, Andreassen AK, Molberg Ø, et al. Prevalence of pulmonary hypertension in an unselected, mixed connective tissue disease cohort: results of a nationwide, Norwegian cross-sectional multicentre study and review of current literature. *Rheumatology (Oxford)*. 2013;52:1208–1213.

80. Ueda N, Mimura K, Maeda H, et al. Mixed connective tissue disease with fatal pulmonary hypertension and a review of literature. *Virchows Arch A Pathol Anat Histopathol*. 1984;404: 335–340.

81. Vegh J, Szodoray P, Kappelmayer J, et al. Clinical and immunoserological characteristics of mixed connective tissue disease associated with pulmonary arterial hypertension. *Scand J Immunol*. 2006;64:69–76.

82. Hainaut P, Lavenne E, Magy JM, Lebacq EG. Circulating lupus type anticoagulant and pulmonary hypertension associated with mixed connective tissue disease. *Clin Rheumatol*. 1986; 5:96–101.

83. Fagundes MN, Caleiro MT, Navarro-Rodriguez T, et al. Esophageal involvement and interstitial lung disease in mixed connective tissue disease. *Respir Med*. 2009;103:854–860.

84. Gunnarsson R, Aaløkken TM, Molberg Ø, et al. Prevalence and severity of interstitial lung disease in mixed connective tissue disease: a nationwide, cross-sectional study. *Ann Rheum Dis*. 2012;71:1966–1972.

85. Sanchez-Guerrero J, Cesarman G, Alarcon-Segovia D. Massive pulmonary hemorrhage in mixed connective tissue diseases. *J Rheumatol*. 1989;16:1132–1134.

86. Bloch KJ, Buchanan WW, Wohl MJ, Bunim JJ. Sjoegren's syndrome. A clinical, pathological, and serological study of sixty-two cases. *Medicine (Baltimore)*. 1965;44:187–231.

87. Tanoue LT. Pulmonary involvement in collagen vascular disease: a review of the pulmonary manifestations of the Marfan syndrome, ankylosing spondylitis, Sjogren's syndrome, and relapsing polychondritis. *J Thorac Imaging*. 1992;7:62–77.

88. Newball HH, Brahim SA. Chronic obstructive airway disease in patients with Sjogren's syndrome. *Am Rev Respir Dis*. 1977;115:295–304.

89. Schuurman HJ, Gooszen HC, Tan IW, Kluin PM, Wagenaar SS, van Unnik JA. Low-grade lymphoma of immature T-cell phenotype in a case of lymphocytic interstitial pneumonia and Sjogren's syndrome. *Histopathology*. 1987;11:1193–1204.

90. Walters MT, Stevenson FK, Herbert A, Cawley MI, Smith JL. Urinary monoclonal free light chains in primary Sjogren's syndrome: an aid to the diagnosis of malignant lymphoma. *Ann Rheum Dis*. 1986;45:210–219.

91. Fisher LR, Cawley MI, Holgate ST. Relation between chest expansion, pulmonary function, and exercise tolerance in patients with ankylosing spondylitis. *Ann Rheum Dis*. 1990;49: 921–925.

92. Rosenow E, Strimlan CV, Muhm JR, Ferguson RH. Pleuropulmonary manifestations of ankylosing spondylitis. *Mayo Clin Proc*. 1977;52:641–649.

93. Dougados M, Braun J, Szanto S, et al. Efficacy of etanercept on rheumatic signs and pulmonary function tests in advanced ankylosing spondylitis: results of a randomised double-blind placebo-controlled study (SPINE). *Ann Rheum Dis*. 2011;70:799–804.

CHAPTER 61

Pulmonary Langerhans' Cell Histiocytosis

Sergio Harari
Olga Torre
Talmadge E. King Jr.
Joel Moss

INTRODUCTION

Pulmonary Langerhans' cell histiocytosis is part of a large spectrum of disorders characterized by abnormal organ infiltration by Langerhans' cells, which are highly differentiated cells in the monocyte-macrophage line that are also found in the dermis of the skin, reticuloendothelial system, pleura, and lung. Clinically, these disorders vary greatly, ranging from mild, single-organ disease to acute, disseminated life-threatening presentations. Depending on the sites involved and severity, the entity now referred to as Langerhans' cell histiocytosis has been previously defined as eosinophilic granuloma, Hand–Schüller–Christian disease, and Letterer–Siwe disease. A more recent and simplified system of classification includes Langerhans' cell histiocytosis with single-organ involvement or with multisystem involvement.[1]

Pulmonary Langerhans' cell histiocytosis is an uncommon, smoking-related, interstitial lung disease that primarily affects young adults. Usually, lung involvement occurs in isolation; less frequently, involvement of other systems, for example, bone, skin, pituitary gland, is seen. Although there is some similarity to other diffuse interstitial lung diseases, pulmonary Langerhans' cell histiocytosis, as a specific disease entity, is distinct in its clinical, radiologic, and pathologic manifestations.

EPIDEMIOLOGY

The true incidence and prevalence of pulmonary Langerhans' cell histiocytosis are unknown. Studies in which diagnoses were confirmed by lung biopsy showed that pulmonary Langerhans' cell histiocytosis is an uncommon, if not rare, disease.[2,3] A Japanese study of discharge diagnoses in hospitals with 200 beds estimated the disease prevalence at 0.27 and 0.07 per 100,000 population in males and females, respectively.[4] These reports may underestimate the true incidence of the disease, as lung biopsy is not performed in all cases of pulmonary Langerhans' cell histiocytosis, and some patients exhibit no symptoms or experience spontaneous remission. Occupational or geographical predisposition has not been reported.

Of note, nearly all affected persons report a current or prior smoking history. Thus, tobacco smoke is thought to play a key role in the pathogenesis of pulmonary Langerhans' cell histiocytosis of adulthood. Other diffuse parenchymal lung diseases associated with cigarette smoking are respiratory bronchiolitis-associated interstitial lung disease and desquamative interstitial pneumonitis.[5]

Most patients with pulmonary Langerhans' cell histiocytosis present to medical attention in young adulthood (20–40 years of age). Pulmonary Langerhans' cell histiocytosis, however, may present in any age group. Older literature suggested a male preponderance; however, recent literature suggests an equal sex distribution, with increasing presentations in middle age. In general, women tend to present at an older age than men. These differences in prevalence may reflect the changing smoking habits of women in our society. For unknown reasons, whites are affected much more commonly than blacks or Asians, in whom this disease is very rare.

Pulmonary Langerhans' cell histiocytosis has reportedly been associated with a number of malignancies and may be a premalignant condition. Lymphoma, both Hodgkin's and non-Hodgkin's, and other hematologic and solid cancers have been reported in association with pulmonary Langerhans' cell histiocytosis.[6] However, the evidence regarding this association is inconclusive. Malignancies may precede, follow, or occur concomitantly with the diagnosis of the interstitial lung disease. The carcinogenic effects of cigarette smoke are probably responsible for some of these tumors; thus, other components of tobacco may be responsible for pulmonary Langerhans' cell histiocytosis. Given the complexity of factors involved in the pathogenesis of cancer and pulmonary Langerhans' cell histiocytosis, it has been difficult to define the effects of tobacco on the pathogenesis of malignancies in patients with pulmonary Langerhans' cell histiocytosis. Possibly, shared genetic predisposition factors may also have a role in the development of malignancies in patients with the disorder.[7]

NATURAL HISTORY AND CLINICAL PRESENTATION

Patients with pulmonary Langerhans' cell histiocytosis come to medical attention in a variety of ways: as an incidental diagnosis that is suggested by a screening chest radiograph, after pneumothorax, or with respiratory or constitutional symptoms. Symptomatic patients most often have a nonproductive cough (56%–70%), dyspnea (40%), chest pain (10%–21%), fatigue (~30%), weight loss (20%–30%), and fever (15%). Pleuritic pain and acute dyspnea with a spontaneous pneumothorax can be a recurrent problem in as many as 25% of patients. Pleural thickening or effusion is rarely seen in the absence of a history of pneumothorax. Hemoptysis (13%) is occasionally reported, and it should prompt consideration of superimposed infection (e.g., *Aspergillus*) or tumor.[8]

Cystic bone lesions are present in 4% to 20% of patients with pulmonary Langerhans' cell histiocytosis and may produce localized pain or a pathologic bone fracture. The precise number of patients with bone lesions is not known because complete bone surveys are not routinely performed. Skeletal involvement may be either the sole symptomatic manifestation of pulmonary Langerhans' cell histiocytosis or may precede the more typical pulmonary manifestations. The radiographic pattern is not diagnostic. In most instances, the lesions are solitary and affect the flat bones. Central nervous system involvement with diabetes insipidus (approximately 15% of patients) is also seen and is believed to portend a poor prognosis. Skin involvement may also be present in adults with pulmonary Langerhans' cell histiocytosis.

Skin lesions are usually erythematous, maculopapular, or nodular. In these patients, the scalp is often involved by characteristic seborrheic and crusted lesions.[9]

The physical examination is usually unremarkable. On chest examination, crackles are uncommon. Digital clubbing is also uncommon. Secondary pulmonary hypertension (PH) may occur and is probably underrecognized. Manifestations of cor pulmonale are seen in advanced stages. Routine laboratory studies are usually unrevealing; the peripheral eosinophil count is normal.[1]

PATHOGENESIS

The pathogenesis of adult pulmonary Langerhans' cell histiocytosis is still poorly understood. However, the nearly universal association with cigarette smoking strongly implies causation. Smoke may activate alveolar macrophages through bombesin-like peptides. Bombesin is a neuropeptide produced by neuroendocrine cells, which are increased in the lungs of smokers.[10] Bombesin-like peptides are chemotactic for monocytes, are mitogenic for epithelial cells and fibroblasts, and stimulate cytokine secretion. Several antigens in cigarette smoke, including tobacco glycoprotein, may stimulate macrophage and epithelial cell production of cytokines, such as granulocyte-macrophage colony-stimulating factor (GM-CSF), dendritic cell chemokines, for example, chemokine (C-C motif) ligand 20 (CCL20), osteopontin, and tumor necrosis factor-α (TNF-α) that promote recruitment and activation of Langerhans' cells.[11] In fact, GM-CSF and TNF-α have been found in the lesions of patients with Langerhans' cell histiocytosis and have been shown to facilitate the in vitro generation of Langerhans' cells from CD34+ hematopoietic stem cells.[12] TNF-α and other cytokines, for example, tumor necrosis factor-β (TNF-β), may also stimulate fibroblasts leading to fibrosis.[13] Moreover, tobacco glycoprotein may also cause an abnormal differentiation of T lymphocytes and a reduction in interleukin (IL)-2 release by lymphocytes, thereby enhancing survival or proliferation of Langerhans' cells (Fig. 61-1).[14]

Abnormalities in immune function, with a nonspecific increase in immunoglobulin G (IgG) in bronchoalveolar fluid, circulating and tissue-bound immune complexes, and abnormalities in T-cell function, have been observed in association with pulmonary Langerhans' cell histiocytosis and may be important in the pathophysiology of this disorder.[15] It is possible, however, that these findings represent nonspecific consequences of a generalized activation of immune effector cells.

Recent studies report high serum levels of IL-17A during active Langerhans' cell histiocytosis, IL-17A synthesis by dendritic cells of patients with multisystem Langerhans' cell histiocytosis, and an IL-17–dependent pathway for dendritic cells fusion, showing that IL-17 may play a role in pathogenesis, although its significance in pulmonary Langerhans' cell histiocytosis is not known.[16] Some studies suggest that the pathogenesis of pulmonary Langerhans' cell histiocytosis entails alterations of the expression of the adhesion molecules that regulate interactions between white blood cells and endothelial cells.[17,18] One important adhesion molecule for neutrophils that is expressed by endothelial cells is intercellular adhesion molecule-1 (ICAM-1). ICAM-1 expression by Langerhans' cells has been demonstrated in biopsy specimens of subjects with Langerhans' cell histiocytosis. Expression of other leukocyte adhesion molecules, such as the β_1 and β_2 integrins, has also been noted.[19] The significance of these findings and their relevance to pulmonary Langerhans' cell histiocytosis remain to be elucidated.

Alternatively, a viral infection has been suggested as the underlying cause of generalized Langerhans' cell histiocytosis. However, there are no convincing data to suggest a role for viral infection as a cause of pulmonary Langerhans' cell histiocytosis.[20] Although clonality of histiocytes has been shown in children and adults with multisystem Langerhans' cell histiocytosis or unifocal bone disease, pulmonary Langerhans' cell histiocytosis appears to be primarily a reactive process to cigarette smoke in which nonmalignant clonal evolution of LCH cells may occur in the setting of abnormal Langerhans' cell hyperplasia in the airways.[21,22]

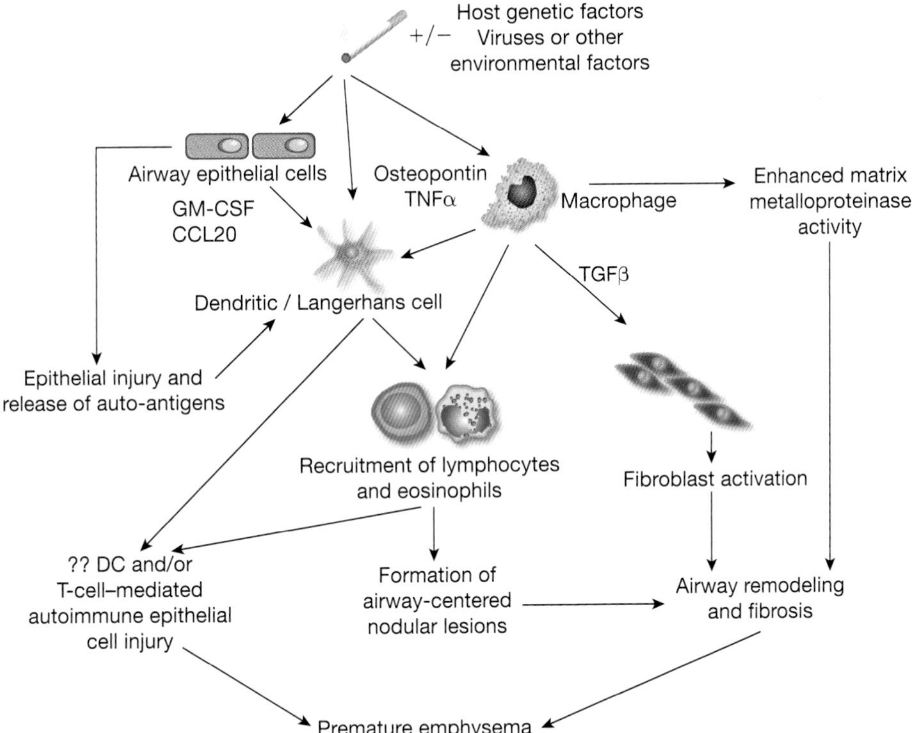

Figure 61-1 The primary event in the pathogenesis of pulmonary Langerhans' cell histiocytosis probably involves cigarette-smoke–induced recruitment to the lung and activation of Langerhans' cells, a process that may result from a variety of potential mechanisms. Antigens in cigarette smoke, including tobacco glycoprotein (TGP), may stimulate alveolar macrophages and epithelial cells to produce cytokines or other factors that enhance recruitment and activation of Langerhans' cells. Cigarette smoke may also directly activate Langerhans' cells to secrete cytokines (such as TNF or GM-CSF) that mediate local accumulation of inflammatory cells, with resultant formation of nodules. Uptake of cigarette-smoke antigens by alveolar macrophages or Langerhans' cells may also promote local expansion of T lymphocytes and further inflammation. Through the action of tobacco glycoprotein, reduced interleukin-2 secretion by lymphocytes may occur, thereby enhancing local survival and proliferation of Langerhans' cells. T lymphocytes may further stimulate B-lymphocyte activation, promoting secretion of antibodies and immune-complex formation. Fibroblast activation and fibrosis may result from the local synthesis of tumor growth factor-β (TGF-β) and by alveolar macrophages. *(Reproduced with permission from Suri HS, Yi ES, Nowakowski GS, Vassallo R. Pulmonary langerhans cell histiocytosis. Orphanet J Rare Dis. 2012;7:16.)*

HISTOPATHOLOGY

The pathologic cell type of pulmonary Langerhans' cell histiocytosis is the Langerhans' cell, a differentiated cell of the monocyte-macrophage line (Fig. 61-2). Langerhans' cells are distinguished by a pale-staining cytoplasm and large convoluted nucleus. Electron microscopy may demonstrate the classic pentalaminar cytoplasmic inclusion known as a Birbeck granule (Fig 61-3). Langerhans' cells are also characterized by the presence of the CD1a antigen on the cell surface, a feature not found in other cells of histiocytic origin. Langerhans' cells also react with anti-S-100 antibody, but this reactivity can also be observed in other cell types. More recently, langerin, a type II mannose lectin that is constitutively associated with Birbeck granules, has been identified as a specific marker of Langerhans' cells.[23] Although this cell can be found in association

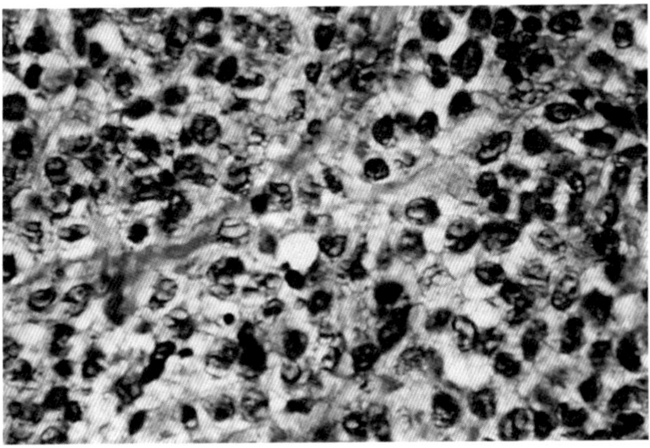

Figure 61-2 Lung tissue in pulmonary Langerhans' cell histiocytosis. The Langerhans' cells are typical. A characteristic longitudinal groove is seen along the center of some cells (×96.)

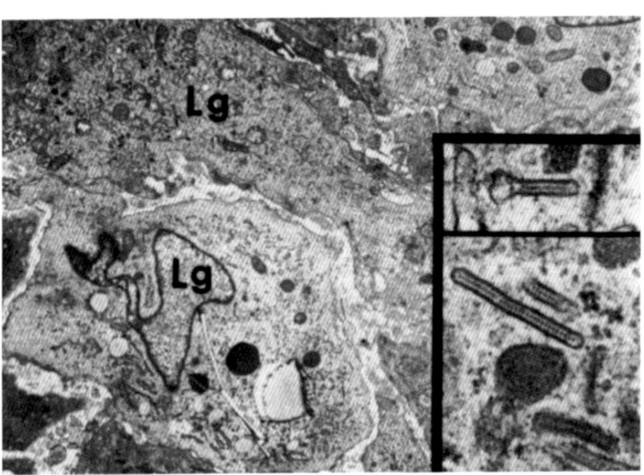

Figure 61-3 Electron micrograph of Langerhans' cell (Lg) of the lung. Typical X bodies (Birbeck granules) are seen in the two insets.

with cigarette smoking in otherwise healthy persons and with other pulmonary pathologies (e.g., idiopathic pulmonary fibrosis) or in normal lung, its presence is characteristic of pulmonary Langerhans' cell histiocytosis. In pulmonary Langerhans' cell histiocytosis, the Langerhans' cells are characteristically found in clusters and significantly outnumber those seen in other lung diseases. Absolute quantitative guidelines for diagnosis of pulmonary Langerhans' cell histiocytosis have not been established.

Early inflammatory lesions center around the smaller bronchioles and usually contain a mixture of Langerhans' cells, eosinophils, lymphocytes, and neutrophils. The cells appear to invade the bronchiole, destroying the bronchiolar wall in an eccentric fashion. The lesions often affect pulmonary arterioles and venules, so that the disorder can be described as having a bronchovascular distribution.

Pseudodesquamative interstitial pneumonia (characterized by the accumulation of alveolar macrophages in the alveolar parenchyma between pulmonary Langerhans' cell lesions) and respiratory (smoker's) bronchiolitis (with pigmented macrophages filling the lumen of bronchioles and the surrounding alveolar spaces) have also often been found on lung biopsy.[3,8] In addition, intraluminal fibrosis was often present (86% of specimens). The fibrosis was characterized by mural incorporation, alveolar obliteration, and intraluminal buds. It was mild in extent in 59% of specimens, moderate in 20%, and marked in 9%. These findings support the hypothesis that intraluminal fibrosis serves as a mechanism for alveolar collapse, with progression to interstitial fibrosis and lung remodeling.[8]

Interstitial fibrosis and small cyst formation with a middle- to upper-zone predominance occur in advancing disease. This middle- to upper-zone predominance differs from that of idiopathic pulmonary fibrosis, which generally has a lower-zone predominance. More advanced lesions extend widely into the lung parenchyma that surrounds the bronchovascular structures and produce the so-called stellate lesions that are characteristic of this disorder.[3] Kambouchner et al.[24] used three-dimensional reconstructions of serial histologic sections to demonstrate that pulmonary Langerhans' cell histiocytosis lesions are elongated, sheath-like structures of variable diameter that extend proximally and distally along bronchioles and do not necessarily have a spherical morphology (Fig. 61-4).

Older lesions are relatively acellular, lacking Langerhans' cells entirely and producing a diffuse interstitial pathology that can be difficult to distinguish from other forms of end-stage pulmonary fibrosis, with extensive areas of fibrosis and honeycombing accompanying the cystic lesions. The mechanism for cyst formation is unknown. It may be a consequence of central necrosis of older stellate lesions. Alternatively, the cysts may occur as a result of secondary inflammatory foci in relatively avascular areas distal to more advanced bronchovascular lesions. Finally, these cysts may form, in part, because of obstruction of the more proximal airway by the stellate lesions (traction emphysema).

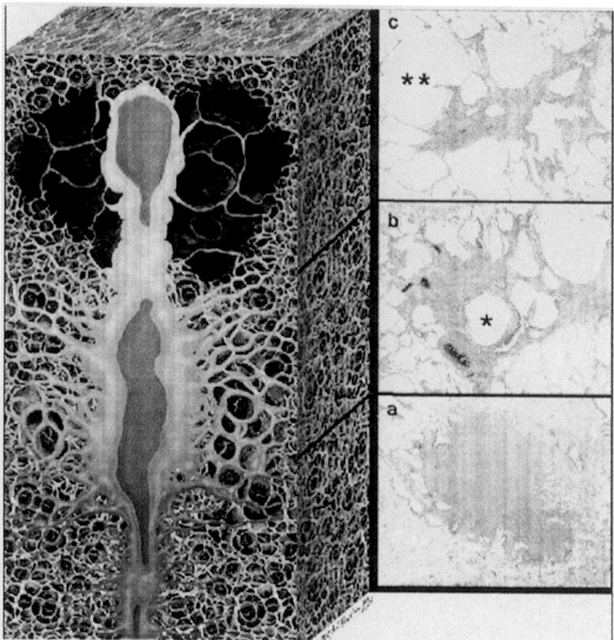

Figure 61-4 Three-dimensional appearance of a pulmonary Langerhans' cell histiocytosis (PLCH) lesion. Artist's rendering, based on the reconstructions by Kambouchner et al.,[24] illustrates the elongated morphology and variable cellular and fibrotic composition of PLCH with correlative histologic sections. As a PLCH lesion evolves, the nodule of densely packed cells (*bottom*, A) is centripetally replaced by fibrous tissue and ultimately becomes a stellate scar (*top*, C). This continuum of change may be evident within a single lesion. PLCH lesions are bronchiolocentric and propagate both proximally and distally along the small airways. The involved bronchiolar lumen may become either dilated or obliterated. The histologic sections correspond to the early, middle, and late phases of PLCH. In the early phase (*a*), there is a densely cellular nodule with delicate stellate extensions along the adjacent alveolar walls (original magnification, ×12; H&E stain). As the disease progresses (*b*), cellularity diminishes as fibroblasts replace the lesion (original magnification, ×19.2; H&E stain). Note that the stellate extensions have become more prominent, the central bronchiole (*) is dilated, and adjacent alveolar spaces have coalesced because of focal destruction of alveolar walls (paracicatricial airspace enlargement). In the final phase (*c*), the characteristic Langerhans' cell histiocytosis is absent and only a fibrous, stellate scar remains (original magnification, ×24; H&E stain). This phase is often accompanied by paracicatricial airspace enlargement (**). *(Used with permission of the Armed Forces Institute of Pathology (AFIP).)*

RADIOLOGY

The appearance of Langerhans' cell histiocytosis on routine chest x-ray, computed tomography (CT), magnetic resonance imaging (MRI), and positron emission tomography (PET) are described below.

■ CHEST RADIOGRAPH

The radiographic appearance of pulmonary Langerhans' cell histiocytosis may be very characteristic. The combination of ill-defined or stellate nodules (2–10 mm in size), reticular opacities, upper-zone cysts or honeycombing, preservation of lung volume, and costophrenic angle sparing are believed to be highly specific for this disorder.[25] Typically, in keeping with the pathology, the reticular or nodular opacities are seen in the middle to upper zone (Fig. 61-5). The total lung volume is most often normal, although both hyperinflation and reduced volume have been described. In addition to pulmonary Langerhans' cell histiocytosis, other interstitial diseases that may present with an increased lung volume are lymphangioleiomyomatosis, chronic hypersensitivity pneumonitis, stage III sarcoidosis, constrictive bronchiolitis, and any interstitial lung disease in an individual with emphysema.

Small cysts and nodules are the radiographic hallmark of pulmonary Langerhans' cell histiocytosis (Fig. 61-6A); occasionally miliary disease is seen. Hilar or mediastinal adenopathy in pulmonary Langerhans' cell histiocytosis is rare and should prompt consideration of malignancy as a secondary diagnosis. Pleural thickening is most often due to treated pneumothorax, since pleural involvement by the primary disease process is uncommon. Bone lesions can occur in any bone, including the ribs. On rare occasions, patients come to medical attention with a solitary pulmonary nodule that, on biopsy, proves to be pulmonary Langerhans' cell histiocytosis.[26]

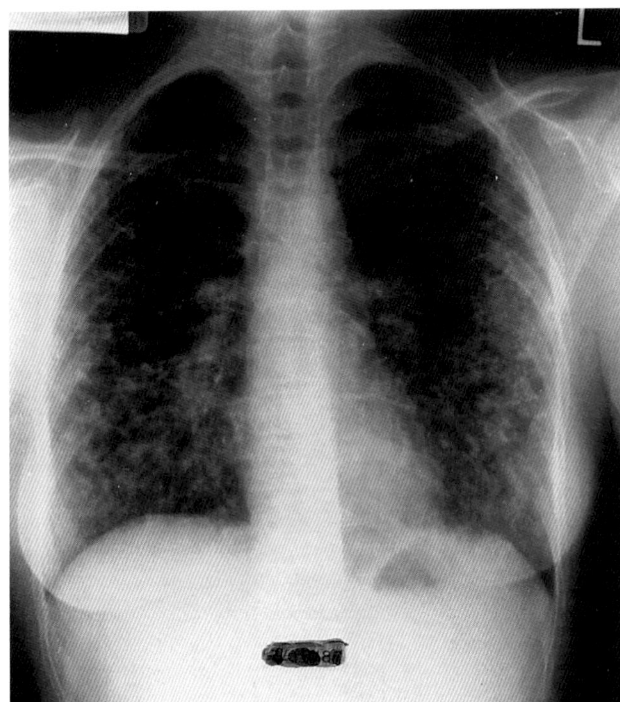

Figure 61-5 Pulmonary Langerhans' cell histiocytosis in a 22-year-old woman. Chest radiograph demonstrates the classic features of profuse ill-defined nodules, reticulonodular opacities, cysts, costophrenic angle sparing, and preservation of lung volumes.

COMPUTED TOMOGRAPHY

The combination of multiple cysts and nodules with a middle- to upper-zone predominance with interstitial thickening in a young smoker is so characteristic as to be diagnostic of pulmonary Langerhans' cell histiocytosis (Fig. 61-6B). The nodules can be well or poorly defined. Occasionally, they can be large and bizarrely shaped (Fig. 61-6C). Cysts may vary in shape, size, and wall thickness from a few to several millimeters. Honeycombing can be seen in advanced disease.[27,28] Serial chest CT scanning often suggests a sequence of progression from nodular to cavitating to cystic lesions over time.[29] Moreover, the CT pattern seems to reflect the histopathologic evolution of lung lesions, with cystic changes prominent in the advanced, fibrotic stages of the disease.[30]

The degree of cyst formation is often underappreciated with routine chest radiography. Thus, this progression may explain a number of "spontaneous remissions" in the literature reported before the routine use of thin-section CT scanning.[31] Although the extent of the cystic lesions present on HRCT at one point in time has been correlated with impaired lung function, the utility of serial CT scanning in managing these patients has yet to be determined.[32,33]

MAGNETIC RESONANCE IMAGING

The role of MRI in pulmonary Langerhans' cell histiocytosis is limited to evaluation of bone and central nervous system lesions.

POSITRON EMISSION TOMOGRAPHY

Fluorodeoxyglucose (FDG)-PET scan imaging has shown to be useful in quantifying disease activity, with positive scan results seen in patients with nodular, inflammatory lung disease. Moreover, FDG-PET scan may provide valuable information regarding extrapulmonary involvement in patients with a known diagnosis of pulmonary Langerhans cell histiocytosis. Nevertheless, the mean maximum standardized uptake value (SUV) of the PET scan-positive lesions may vary significantly, suggesting that PET scan imaging cannot reliably distinguish between the benign, inflammatory nodular lesions of Langerhans' cell histiocytosis and malignant lesions.[34]

PHYSIOLOGIC TESTING

Basic physiologic assessment in Langerhan's cell histiocytosis includes pulmonary function and exercise testing.

PULMONARY FUNCTION TESTING

Pulmonary function testing of subjects with pulmonary Langerhans' cell histiocytosis may demonstrate all possible patterns of function abnormality—normal, obstructive, restrictive, or mixed. In general, total lung capacity (TLC) is well preserved, with nearly normal airflow. Most often, the diffusing capacity (DL_{CO}) is disproportionately reduced.[7,22,24] This pattern of pulmonary function abnormality suggests pulmonary vascular involvement by the disease process.

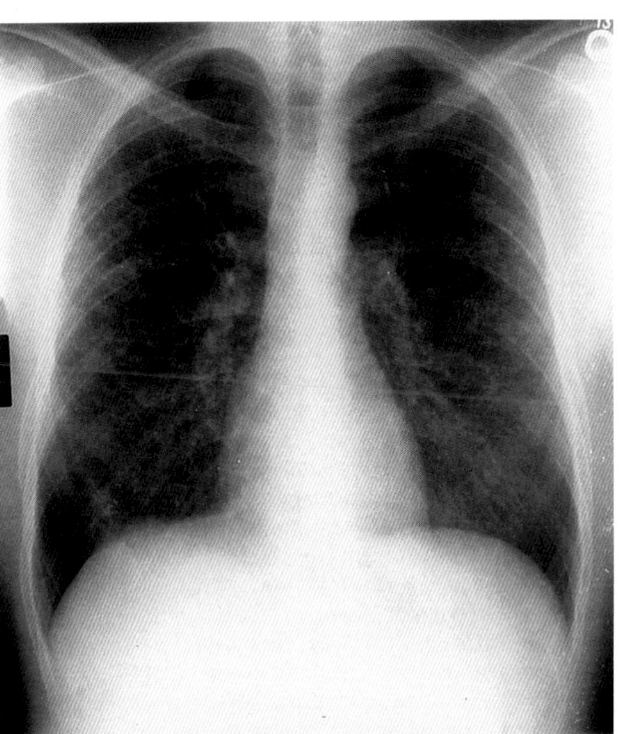

A

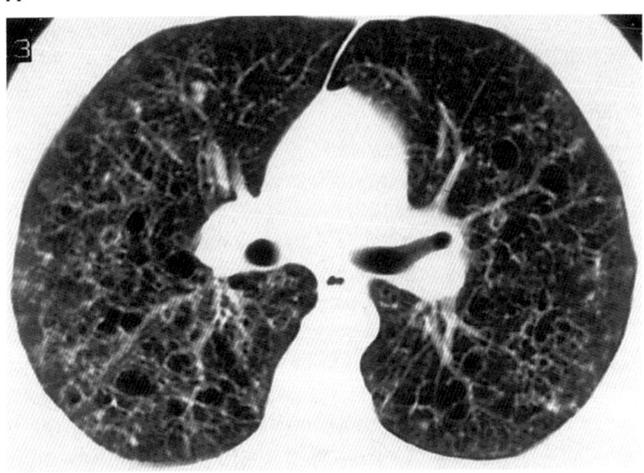

B

Figure 61-6 Pulmonary Langerhans' cell histiocytosis in a 33-year-old man. **A.** Chest radiograph reveals reticulonodular opacities in midlung zones, cysts, costophrenic angle sparing, and preservation of lung volumes. **B.** Conventional CT scan helps confirm the presence of bilateral reticulonodular opacities and cysts. *(continued)*

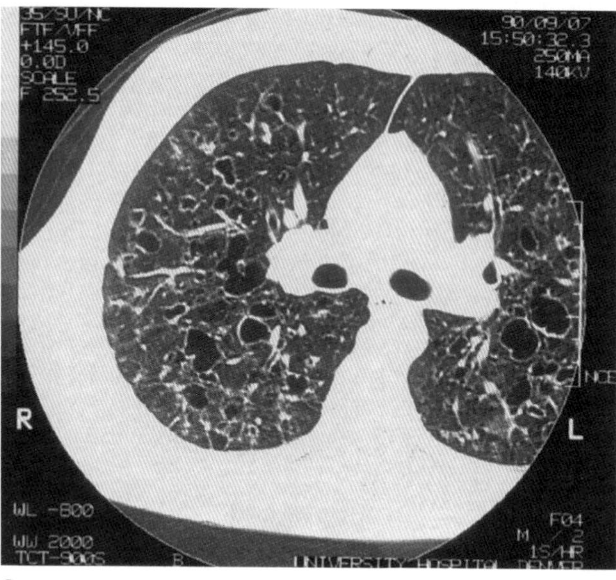

C

Figure 61-6 *(Continued)* **C.** High-resolution CT with thin section shows more clearly that the reticulonodular or emphysematous changes on chest radiography are actually cysts. In this instance, few nodules are present. The cysts vary markedly in size and may be larger than 10 mm. The cysts are bizarre in shape, and many are closely related to pulmonary arteries, often mimicking bronchiectasis.

In the experience at San Giuseppe Hospital in Milan, among 35 patients with pulmonary Langerhans' cell histiocytosis, an obstructive functional pattern was present in 43% of subjects. 10.5% of patients had a restrictive pattern and 3.5% a mixed pattern; 43% of patients showed normal airflow and volumes. A reduction in DL_{CO} was evident in 78% of patients.

Airflow limitation is sometimes associated with reactive airways; significant improvement may occur after administration of a bronchodilator. When present, reactive airways disease may reflect coexisting chronic obstructive pulmonary disease (COPD).

The mean alveolar–arterial difference in P_{O_2} (AaP_{O_2}) may be normal at rest, but the subset with more severe disease had a markedly elevated AaP_{O_2} and required supplemental oxygen. Resting pH and Pa_{CO_2} were most often normal. Thus, the resting arterial blood gas was a very insensitive indicator of disease.[35]

■ EXERCISE TESTING

Clinically, we have observed that patients with established pulmonary Langerhans' cell histiocytosis generally demonstrate a limitation in physical activity and intolerance for exercise that is out of proportion to their pulmonary function abnormalities.

In our cross-sectional study of 23 subjects with pulmonary Langerhans' cell histiocytosis, a marked decrease in exercise capacity, as measured by either work achieved (mean + SEM, 54 ± 4% of predicted) or oxygen utilization ($\dot{V}_{O_2}$, 44% ± 3) at maximal exercise, was found.[35] The oxygen pulse at maximal exercise was reduced to 56 ± 3%. The anaerobic threshold was decreased to 33% ± percent of expected $\dot{V}_{O_{2max}}$ (it was ≤40% in all subjects). The maximal ventilatory response ($\dot{V}_{E_{max}}$, 83 ± 5%) was excessive for the maximal level of work. The maximal ventilatory response was not limiting, and the $\dot{V}_{E_{max}}$ was well below predicted ventilatory ceilings. Gas exchange abnormalities were reflected in increasing AaP_{O_2} differences as the level of exercise increased. In addition, alveolar dead space to tidal volume ratio (V_D/V_T), a parameter believed to reflect pulmonary vascular function, was either abnormally elevated or failed to decrease in most patients (Fig. 61-7). This abnormality suggested either pathologic or functional involvement of the pulmonary vasculature.

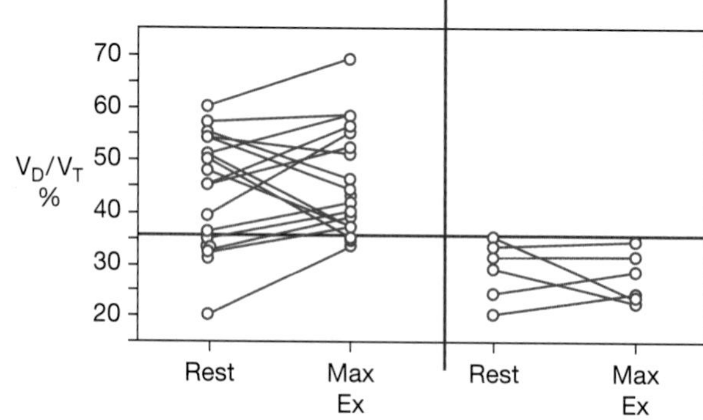

Figure 61-7 Dead space to tidal volume ratio (expressed as percentage, V_D/V_T%) at rest and maximal exercise (max ex) in patients with pulmonary Langerhans' cell histiocytosis (n = 23). Seventeen patients demonstrated either an abnormal V_D/V_T at rest or response to exercise *(left panel)*. Six patients had a normal V_D/V_T at rest and normal response to exercise *(right panel)*. *(Data from Crausman RS, Jennings CA, Tuder R, et al. Pulmonary histiocytosis X: Pulmonary function and exercise pathophysiology. Am J Respir Crit Care Med. 1996;153:426–435.)*

Two linear regression models derived from pulmonary function indices predicted 73% (r^2 = 0.73) and 75% (r^2 = 0.75) of the variability in the maximal achieved workload and predicted oxygen consumption at maximal exercise, respectively. The following equation was derived for the maximal achieved workload:

$$\text{Maximal achieved workload} = 0.884 - (0.0088 \times V_D/V_T \text{ baseline}) - (0.002 \times RV) + (0.0044 \times DL_{CO}) \quad (1)$$

Here the partial r^2 was V_D/V_T baseline (r^2 = 0.40, p = 0.0007), RV (0.19, 0.001), and DL_{CO} (0.15, 0.004). Figure 61-8 shows the regression model for the predicted oxygen consumption at maximal exercise.

Analysis of the composite results suggests that exercise intolerance in subjects with pulmonary Langerhans' cell histiocytosis is

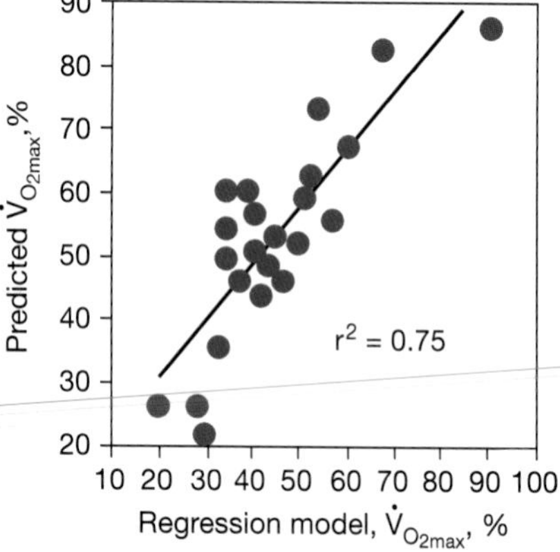

Figure 61-8 Correlation between predicted oxygen consumption at maximal exercise ($\dot{V}_{O_{2max}}$ and predicted $\dot{V}_{O_{2max}}$ from the linear regression model): $\dot{V}_{O_{2max}}$ = 0.062 − (0.0074 * baseline V_D/V_T) − (0.0014 * RV) + (0.0017 * baseline $P(Aa)_{O_2}$) + (0.0011 * D_{LCO}); r^2 = 0.75. *(Data from Crausman RS, Jennings CA, Tuder R, et al. Pulmonary histiocytosis X: Pulmonary function and exercise pathophysiology. Am J Respir Crit Care Med. 1996;153:426–435.)*

due to a combination of mechanical factors and pulmonary vascular involvement by pulmonary Langerhans' cell histiocytosis.[35]

Precapillary PH is a complication of advanced pulmonary Langerhans' cell histiocytosis and is associated with increased mortality.[36] Severe PH has been reported in a high percentage of patients referred for lung transplantation.[37,38]

In patients with respiratory insufficiency, chronic hypoxemia is a relevant factor, but the pathophysiology of PH in pulmonary Langerhans' cell histiocytosis is likely to be multifactorial, with other contributors including abnormal pulmonary mechanics and vascular remodeling. Histopathologic analysis of patients with end-stage disease shows proliferative vasculopathy involving muscular arteries and frequent venular involvement, with aspects of veno-occlusive disease.[37] The degree of PH appears not to be related to variables of pulmonary function; in a subgroup of patients, vasculopathy worsened, although parenchymal and bronchiolar lesions were unchanged, consistent with intrinsic pulmonary vascular disease.[37]

DIAGNOSTIC EVALUATION

The history and physical examination are the first steps in the diagnostic evaluation of a patient suspected of having pulmonary Langerhans' cell histiocytosis. Unfortunately, the signs and symptoms of pulmonary Langerhans' cell histiocytosis are generally nonspecific and often point to other, more common pulmonary diagnoses.[7,22] For example, wheezing, cough, and dyspnea in a 50-year-old patient with a prominent smoking history are much more commonly due to COPD than to pulmonary Langerhans' cell histiocytosis. However, when present, a history of recurrent pneumothorax, diabetes insipidus, or bone pain can be helpful. A smoking history is a consistent but not an essential component of the history, since pulmonary Langerhans' cell histiocytosis may occur without an antecedent smoking history especially in a young adult.

Most evaluations for pulmonary Langerhans' cell histiocytosis are prompted by an abnormal chest radiograph. As previously noted, the chest CT, if classic, may be diagnostic, and should, therefore, be obtained in all who are suspected of having this disease. We recommend high-resolution chest CT as a prebiopsy step in the evaluation of any patient with diffuse interstitial lung disease suspected of having pulmonary Langerhans' cell histiocytosis. A sufficiently characteristic chest CT, in association with the appropriate history, is believed by many to obviate the need for tissue confirmation. It should be noted that most often chest CT scans in pulmonary Langerhans' cell histiocytosis are not diagnostic and may be confused with chest CT scans of lymphangioleiomyomatosis, hypersensitivity pneumonitis, sarcoidosis, or idiopathic pulmonary fibrosis. In these instances, further diagnostic evaluation is warranted.

Bronchoalveolar lavage (BAL) fluid may be of diagnostic value in cases of suspected pulmonary Langerhans' cell histiocytosis.[39] The total number of cells recovered is usually increased (as expected in smokers), and a modest increase in the concentration of neutrophils and eosinophils is common. In active disease, the total number of lymphocytes recovered may also be increased, and the CD4:CD8 ratio may be decreased. Langerhans' cells in BAL fluid may be recognized by their characteristic reactivity with anti-S-100 protein antibodies or peanut agglutination antigen. These cells are also OKT-6 (CD1) positive, are identified by a specific monoclonal antibody (MT-1), and contain characteristic Birbeck or pentilaminar bodies on electron microscopic evaluation (Fig. 61-3).

Quantitative criteria for the definitive diagnosis of Langerhans' cell histiocytosis based on BAL fluid Langerhans' cell numbers have not been conclusively established. A BAL cell differential with more than 5% Langerhans' cells strongly suggests the diagnosis. Lower proportions of Langerhans' cells may be seen in current smokers, in patients with other interstitial lung disorders, in bronchoalveolar carcinoma, or even in normal subjects. Thus, the mere presence of Langerhans' cells is of little diagnostic value, and the effective sensitivity of this tool seems to be lower than previously believed.[40] BAL is also useful to exclude other inflammatory or infectious lung diseases.

When tissue confirmation is sought, transbronchial biopsy may be performed, but the patchy nature of the disease, with a focal distribution of the lesions, the potential for sampling error, and the inability to obtain sufficient tissue may account for the substantial number of false-negative or nondiagnostic biopsies.[41] Open, video-guided thoracoscopic lung biopsy, is generally definitive and may be done with a minimal operative risk. Tissue reactivity with the monoclonal antibody CD1 (OKT-6) distinguishes Langerhans' cells from other histiocytes and can be a useful diagnostic adjunct. It may be performed on routinely fixed tissue and is less expensive than electron microscopy.

In patients with progressive disease and extensive fibrosis, the number of Langerhans' cells in either tissue specimens or BAL fluid decreases dramatically. Diagnosis at this stage may be difficult, regardless of the laboratory methods used. In most cases, the combination of transbronchial lung biopsy and BAL, supplemented with the identification of CD1-positive cells in tissue and BAL fluid, is highly likely to result in the correct diagnosis.

TREATMENT AND PROGNOSIS

The natural history of pulmonary Langerhans' cell histiocytosis is extraordinarily variable, with some patients experiencing spontaneous remission of symptoms and others progressing to end-stage fibrotic lung disease and severe respiratory failure. A poor outcome in pulmonary Langerhans' cell histiocytosis has been associated with older age at the time of diagnosis, severe airway obstruction, reduced carbon monoxide diffusing capacity, and the need for corticosteroid therapy during follow-up.[42] Most subjects who continue to smoke demonstrate gradual progression; regression of disease is noted following smoking cessation.[43] Therefore, it is important to stress smoking cessation (Fig. 61-9). Patients with radiographic sparing of

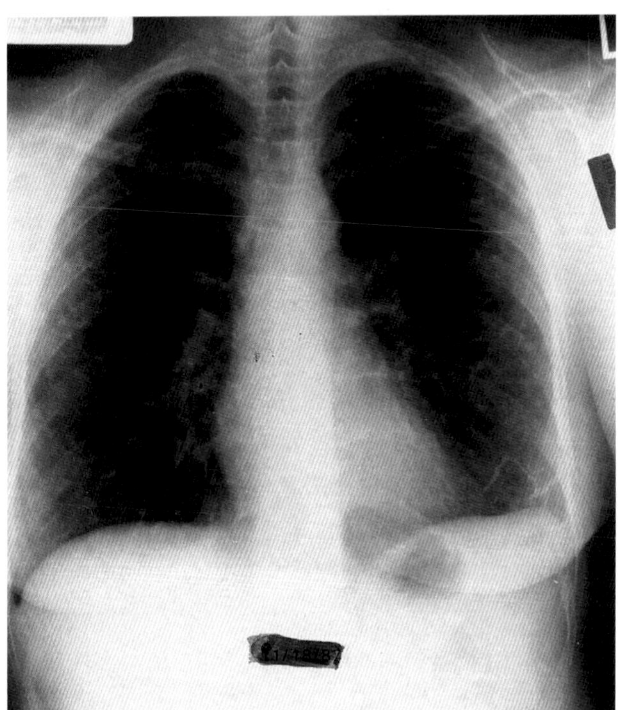

Figure 61-9 Follow-up chest radiograph in a 22-year-old woman obtained 4 months after the initial film shown in Figure 61-6. After an open lung biopsy performed on the left, she was told to stop smoking and treated with prednisone. The chest radiograph shows marked clearing of the ill-defined nodules and preservation of lung volumes.

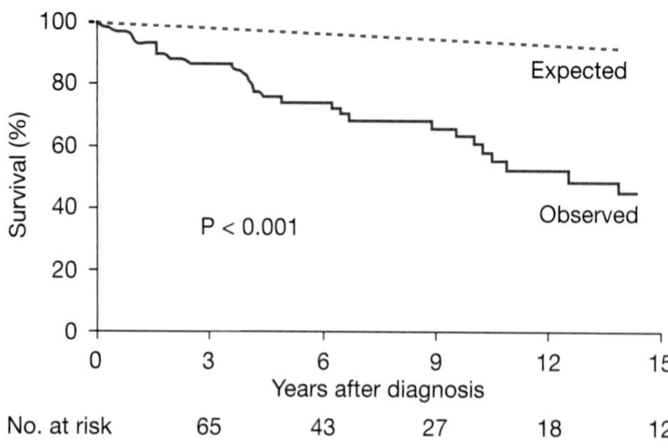

Figure 61-10 Kaplan–Meier analysis of expected and observed survival among 102 adults (40 men and 62 women) with pulmonary Langerhans' cell histiocytosis. The expected survival was defined as that for age- and sex-matched members of the general US population. The median follow-up period after the diagnosis of pulmonary Langerhans' cell histiocytosis was 4 years (range, 0–23). There were 33 deaths, 15 of which were attributable to respiratory failure. Survival was significantly shorter than that expected for healthy persons of the same sex and calendar year of birth ($p < 0.001$). *(Reproduced with permission from Vassallo R, Ryu JH, Schroeder DR, et al. Clinical outcomes of pulmonary Langerhans'-cell histiocytosis in adults. N Engl J Med. 2002;346(7):484–490.)*

the costophrenic angle are more likely to remain stable or to improve than are patients with involvement of the costophrenic angle.

Although corticosteroids have historically been employed in patients with progressive disease, their efficacy in the treatment of pulmonary Langerhans' cell histiocytosis has not been proved. Cytotoxic therapy, which may be of value in the treatment of disseminated disease, has not shown to be effective in pulmonary Langerhans' cell histiocytosis.

Recently, cladribine (2-chlorodeoxyadenosine), an agent cytotoxic for lymphocytes and monocytes, has been reported to have some efficacy in patients with progressive pulmonary Langerhans' cell histiocytosis.[44,45] Cladribine has been used successfully alone or in combination with an alkylating cytostatic agent and corticosteroids in a small number of adult patients with a multisystem or aggressive multifocal form of Langerhans' cell histiocytosis.[46] A randomized controlled trial is needed to assess the effectiveness and tolerance of cladribine in a larger population of patients. Successful use of therapy for PH has been reported in patients with Langerhans' cell histiocytosis.[47,48]

Radiotherapy for symptomatic bone lesions may be palliative. Radiation is not useful in the treatment of the pulmonary manifestations. Lung transplantation has been successfully accomplished in a number of centers. It is a viable option for selected patients with end-stage disease or severe PH. Recurrence of pulmonary Langerhans' cell histiocytosis after lung transplantation has been reported, especially in patients who resumed smoking after the transplant.[49]

The rate of recurrence of pneumothoraces is high in the absence of interventions to prevent additional episodes. Pleurodesis may be needed in patients with recurrences.[50]

Figure 61-10 shows a Kaplan–Meier analysis of expected and observed survival among adults with pulmonary Langerhans' cell histiocytosis.

ACKNOWLEDGMENT

This research was supported in part by the Intramural Research Program of the National Institutes of Health, National Heart, Lung, and Blood Institute.

REFERENCES

1. Vassallo R, Ryu JH, Colby TV, Hartman T, Limper AH. Pulmonary Langerhans'-cell histiocytosis. *N Engl J Med.* 2000; 342:1969–1978..
2. Gaensler EA, Carrington CB. Open biopsy for chronic diffuse infiltrative lung disease: clinical, roentgenographic, and physiological correlations in 502 patients. *Ann Thorac Surg.* 1980;30: 411–426.
3. Colby TV, Lombard C. Histiocytosis X in the lung. *Hum Pathol.* 1983;14:847–856.
4. Watanabe R, Tatsumi K, Hashimoto S, Tamakoshi A, Kuriyama T. Respiratory Failure Research Group of Japan. Clinico-epidemiological features of pulmonary histiocytosis X. *Intern Med.* 2001;40:998–1003.
5. Caminati A, Cavazza A, Sverzellati N, Harari S. An integrated approach in the diagnosis of smoking-related interstitial lung diseases. *Eur Respir Rev.* 2012;21(125):207–217.
6. Rodig SJ, Payne EG, Degar BA, et al. Aggressive Langerhans cell histiocytosis following T-ALL: clonally related neoplasms with persistent expression of constitutively active NOTCH1. *Am J Hematol.* 2008;83:116–121.
7. Vassallo R, Ryu JH, Schroeder DR, Decker PA, Limper AH. Clinical outcomes of pulmonary Langerhans'-cell histiocytosis in adults. *N Engl J Med.* 2002;346:484–490.
8. Travis WD, Borok Z, Roum JH, et al. Pulmonary Langerhans cell granulomatosis (histiocytosis X). A clinicopathologic study of 48 cases. *Am J Surg Pathol.* 1993;17:971–986.
9. Schönfeld N, Frank W, Wenig S, et al. Clinical and radiologic features, lung function and therapeutic results in pulmonary histiocytosis X. *Respiration.* 1993;60:38–44.
10. Aguayo SM, King TE Jr, Waldron JA, Sherritt KM, Kane MA, Miller YE. Increased pulmonary neuroendocrine cells with bombesin- like immunoreactivity in adult patients with eosinophilic granuloma. *J Clin Invest.* 1990;86:838–844.
11. Suri HS, Yi ES, Nowakowski GS, Vassallo R. Pulmonary Langerhans cell histiocytosis. *Orphanet J Rare Dis.* 2012;7:16.
12. Caux C, Dezutter-Dambuyant C, Schmitt D, Banchereau J. GM-CSF and TNF-alpha cooperate in the generation of dendritic Langerhans cells. *Nature.* 1992;360:258–261.
13. Letterio JJ, Roberts AB. Regulation of immune responses by TGF-beta. *Annu Rev Immunol.* 1998;16:137–161.
14. Youkeles LH, Grizzanti JN, Liao Z, Chang CJ, Rosenstreich DL. Decreased tobacco-glycoprotein induced lymphocyte proliferation in vitro in pulmonary eosinophilic granuloma. *Am J Respir Crit Care Med.* 1995;151:145–150.
15. Senecha B, Elain G, Jeziorski E, et al. Expansion of regulatory T cells in patients with Langerhans cell histiocytosis. *PLoS Medicine.* 2007;4:e253.
16. Coury F, Annels N, Rivollier A, et al. Langerhans cell histiocytosis reveals a new IL-17 A–dependent pathway of dendritic cell fusion. *Nat Med.* 2007;14:81–87.
17. Ruco LP, Stoppacciaro A, Vitolo D, Uccini S, Baroni CD. Expression of adhesion molecules in Langerhans' cell histiocytosis. *Histopathology.* 1993;23:29–37.
18. de Graaf JH, Tamminga RY, Kamps WA, Timens W. Langerhans' cell histiocytosis: expression of leukocyte cellular adhesion molecules suggests abnormal homing and differentiation. *Am J Pathol.* 1994;144:466–472.
19. McClain K, Weiss RA. Viruses and Langerhans cell histiocytosis: is there a link? *Br J Cancer Suppl.* 1994;23:S34–S36.

20. Mierau GW, Wills EJ, Steele PO. Ultrastructural studies in Langerhans cell histiocytosis: a search for evidence of viral etiology. *Pediatr Pathol.* 1994;14:895–904.

21. Willman CL, Busque L, Griffith BB, et al. Langerhans'-cell histiocytosis (histiocytosis X)—a clonal proliferative disease. *N Engl J Med.* 1994;331:154–160.

22. Yousem SA, Colby TV, Chen YY, Chen WG, Weiss LM. Pulmonary Langerhans' cell histiocytosis: molecular analysis of clonality. *Am J Surg Pathol.* 2001;25(5):630–636.

23. Smetana K Jr, Mericka O, Saeland S, Homolka J, Brabec J, Gabius HJ. Diagnostic relevance of Langerin detection in cells from bronchoalveolar lavage of patients with pulmonary Langerhans cell histiocytosis, sarcoidosis and idiopathic pulmonary fibrosis. *Virchows Arch.* 2004;444:171–174.

24. Kambouchner M, Basset F, Marchal J, Uhl JF, Hance AJ, Soler P. Three-dimensional characterization of pathologic lesions in pulmonary Langerhans cell histiocytosis. *Am J Respir Crit Care Med.* 2002;166(11):1483–1490.

25. Abbott GF, Rosado-de-Christenson ML, Franks TJ, Frazier AA, Galvin JR. From the archives of the AFIP: pulmonary Langerhans cell histiocytosis. *Radiographics.* 2004;24:821–841.

26. ten Velde GP, Thunnissen FB, van Engelshoven JM, Wouters EF. A solitary pulmonary nodule due to eosinophilic granuloma. *Eur Respir J.* 1994;7:1539–1540.

27. Bonelli FS, Hartman TE, Swenson SJ, Sherrick A. Accuracy of high resolution CT in diagnosing lung diseases. *AJR Am J Roentgenol.* 1998;170:1507–1512.

28. Brauner MW, Grenier P, Mouelhi MM, Mompoint D, Lenoir S. Pulmonary histiocytosis X: evaluation with high-resolution CT. *Radiology.* 1989;172:255–258.

29. Brauner MW, Grenier P, Tijani K, Battesti JP, Valeyre D. Pulmonary Langerhans cell histiocytosis: evolution of lesions on CT scans. *Radiology.* 1997;204:497–502.

30. Soler P, Bergeron A, Kambouchner M, et al. Is high-resolution computed tomography a reliable tool to predict the histopathological activity of pulmonary Langerhans cell histiocytosis? *Am J Resp Crit Care Med.* 2000;162:264–270.

31. Von Essen S, West W, Sitorius M, Rennard SI. Complete resolution of roentgenographic changes in a patient with pulmonary histiocytosis X. *Chest.* 1990;98:765–767.

32. Paciocco G, Uslenghi E, Bianchi A, et al. Diffuse cystic lung diseases: correlation between radiologic and functional status. *Chest.* 2004;125:135–142.

33. Canuet M, Kessler R, Jeung MY, Métivier AC, Chaouat A, Weitzenblum E. Correlation between high resolution computed tomography findings and lung function in pulmonary Langerhans cell histiocytosis. *Respiration.* 2007;74:640–646.

34. Krajicek BJ, Ryu JH, Hartman TE, Lowe VJ, Vassallo R. Abnormal fluorodeoxyglucose PET in pulmonary Langerhans cell histiocytosis. *Chest.* 2009;135:1542–1549.

35. Crausman RS, Jennings CA, Tuder R, Ackerson LM, Irvin CG, King TE Jr. Pulmonary histiocytosis X: pulmonary function and exercise pathophysiology. *Am J Respir Crit Care Med.* 1996;153:426–435.

36. Harari S, Brenot F, Barberis M, Simmoneau G. Advanced pulmonary histiocytosis X is associated with severe pulmonary hypertension. *Chest.* 1997;111:1142–1144.

37. Fartoukh M, Humbert M, Capron F, et al. Severe pulmonary hypertension in histiocytosis X. *Am J Respir Crit Care Med.* 2000;161:216–223.

38. Dauriat G, Mal H, Thabut G, et al. Lung transplantation for pulmonary Langerhans' cell histiocytosis: a multicenter analysis. *Transplantation.* 2006;81:746–750.

39. Danel C, Israel-Biet D, Costabel U, Rossi GA, Wallaert B. The clinical role of BAL in rare pulmonary diseases. *Eur Respir Rev.* 1991;2:83–88.

40. Harari S, Torre O, Cassandro R, et al. Bronchoscopic diagnosis of Langerhans cell histiocytosis and lymphangioleiomyomatosis. *Respir Med.* 2012;106:1286–1292.

41. Housini I, Tomashefski JF Jr, Cohen A, Taveira-DaSilva AM, Moss J. Transbronchial biopsy in patients with pulmonary eosinophilic granuloma. Comparison with findings on open lung biopsy. *Arch Pathol Lab Med.* 1994;118:523–530.

42. Mogulkoc N, Veral A, Bishop PW, Bayindir U, Pickering CA, Egan JJ. Pulmonary Langerhans' cell histiocytosis: radiologic resolution following smoking cessation. *Chest.* 1999;115:1452–1455.

43. Delobbe A, Durieu J, Duhamel A, Wallaert B. Determinants of survival in pulmonary Langerhans' cell granulomatosis (histiocytosis X). Groupe d'Etude en Pathologie Interstitielle de la Société de Pathologie Thoracique du Nord. *Eur Respir J.* 1996;9:2002–2006.

44. Lazor R, Etienne-Mastroianni B, Khouatra C, Tazi A, Cottin V, Cordier JF. Progressive diffuse pulmonary Langerhans cell histiocytosis improved by cladribine chemotherapy. *Thorax.* 2009;64:274–275.

45. Lorillon G, Bergeron A, Detourmignies L, et al. Cladribine is effective against cystic pulmonary Langerhans cell histiocytosis. *Am J Respir Crit Care Med.* 2012;186:930–932.

46. Adam Z, Szturz P, Vaníček J, et al. Cladribine (2-chlorodeoxyadenosine) in frontline chemotherapy for adult Langerhans cell histiocytosis: a single-center study of seven cases. *Acta Oncol.* 2013;52(5):994–1001.

47. Kiakouama L, Cottin V, Etienne-Mastroïanni B, Khouatra C, Humbert M, Cordier JF. Severe pulmonary hypertension in histiocytosis X: long-term improvement with bosentan. *Eur Respir J.* 2010;36:202–204.

48. Le Pavec J, Lorillon G, Jaïs X, et al. Pulmonary Langerhans cell histiocytosis associated pulmonary hypertension: clinical characteristics and impact of pulmonary arterial hypertension therapies. *Chest.* 2012;142(5):1150–1157.

49. Collins J, Hartman MJ, Warner TF, et al. Frequency and CT findings of recurrent disease after lung transplantation. *Radiology.* 2001;219:503–509.

50. Mendez JL, Nadrous HF, Vassallo R, Decker PA, Ryu JH. Pneumothorax in pulmonary Langerhans cell histiocytosis. *Chest.* 2004;125:1028–1032.

CHAPTER 62

Pulmonary Lymphangioleiomyomatosis

Angelo M. Taveira-DaSilva
Talmadge E. King Jr.
Joel Moss

Lymphangioleiomyomatosis (LAM) is a multisystem disorder, predominantly affecting women, which is characterized by cystic lung lesions, abdominal angiomyolipomas (AML) and lymphatic abnormalities, for example, lymphatic tumors, chylous effusions.[1–5] These pathologic features are caused by the proliferation of a neoplastic smooth muscle–like LAM cell that also has characteristics of melanocytes.[6] Inherited and sporadic forms of LAM have been described. Sporadic LAM is caused by somatic mutations in an unknown susceptible cell of the tuberous sclerosis complex (TSC) 2 (*TSC2*) gene.[7,8] LAM also occurs in TSC, an autosomal dominant disorder resulting from germline mutations in the *TSC1* or *TSC2* genes that is characterized by widespread hamartomas in several organs including the brain, heart, skin, kidney, eyes, lung, and liver, and occurs in 1 of 6000 live births.[9]

EPIDEMIOLOGY

Until the establishment of LAM registries,[1] LAM was considered to be a fatal disease of women of child-bearing age for which oophorectomy, antiestrogen therapy, and lung transplantation were the only therapeutic options.[10–13] LAM is now best defined as a chronic disease of post- and premenopausal women with a life expectancy spanning decades.[14] Sporadic LAM is an uncommon disease occurring in approximately 4.9/1,000,000 women.[15] Although the association of TSC and cystic lung disease has long been recognized,[11–13] little is known about the prevalence and the natural history of LAM in TSC (TSC-LAM). The prevalence of cystic lung disease in women with TSC was reported to range from 30% to 40%; in male patients, it has been estimated to be 13%.[16] Males with TSC tend to have milder, subclinical lung involvement.

CLINICAL PRESENTATION

Patients with LAM often present with a history of progressive dyspnea. Pneumothorax, another common presentation of LAM, is often recurrent, occurring in about 50% to 60% of patients.[1–4] The size of the lung cysts, as seen on high-resolution computed tomography (HRCT) scans (Fig. 62-1A), appears to parallel the incidence of pneumothorax; higher incidence of pneumothorax is seen in patients with larger cysts.[17] Other modes of presentation include chylothorax, abdominal lymphangioleiomyomas, chylous ascites, hemoptysis, chyluria, chyloptysis, and hemorrhage caused by renal AML (Table 62-1).[1,5,18] Lymphatic involvement in LAM occurs in the posterior mediastinum, retroperitoneal and pelvic areas and includes lymphadenopathy, chylous effusions, and lymphangioleiomyomas.[5,18] AML are benign tumors, usually localized in the kidneys and found in approximately 90% of patients with TSC-LAM and 30% of those with sporadic LAM (Table 62-1).[1,5,18] The physical examination of LAM patients may disclose wheezing, pleural effusions, ascites, or intra-abdominal masses. In patients with TSC, typical skin lesions or signs of brain involvement may be evident.[9]

PATHOLOGY

Gross examination of lung sections shows cysts ranging in size from 0.2 to 2 cm.[6,19] Microscopically, cysts characterize lung lesions and proliferation of LAM cells in the walls of cysts and along blood vessels, lymphatics, and bronchioles (Fig. 62-1B1,B2), causing airways narrowing, vascular wall thickening, lymphatic disruption, and venous occlusion are observed.[6,19] Focal hemosiderosis may be present. Often LAM cells grow in a haphazard, disorderly fashion.[6,19] Two types of LAM cells have been described. Small, spindle-shaped cells predominate in the center of the lung nodules; epithelioid cells with large cytoplasm predominate at the periphery.[6,19] Both cell types react with antibodies against smooth muscle–cell antigens (e.g., smooth muscle α-actin, vimentin, desmin). The epithelioid cells also react with human melanin black antibody (HMB-45), a monoclonal antibody that recognizes gp100, a premelanosomal protein encoded by the *Pmel17* gene (Fig. 62-1B2, inset).[6,19] Spindle-shaped LAM cells react with proliferating cell nuclear antigen, indicating that these cells are more proliferative.[6] Receptors for estrogen, progesterone, insulin-like growth factors, angiotensin II, hyaluronic acid (CD44), chemokines, and erythropoietin have been identified in LAM cells.[20–27]

AML are highly vascular tumors comprising smooth muscle–like cells, immature, poorly differentiated blood vessels, and fatty tissue (Fig. 62-1D).[6,19] Tumors vary in size from 1 mm to more than 15 cm in diameter.[18,19] Smooth muscle–like cells found in AML have the same immunocytochemical properties as lung LAM cells (Fig. 62-1D).[6,19] All the major cell types in AML (vascular, fat, smooth muscle) may have mutations in the TSC genes.[7,8] The blood supply of AML originates from the renal arteries or aberrant vessels and may completely disrupt normal kidney architecture.[18,19] Hilar, mediastinal, and retroperitoneal lymphadenopathy may be seen.[18,19] The thoracic duct may be thickened and dilated.[19] Lymphangioleiomyomas consist of encapsulated lymphatic masses of varying sizes comprising chyle-filled cysts, with infiltration of LAM cells, displaying the immunoreactivity profile of LAM lung cells, arranged in fascicular, trabecular or papillary patterns and associated with slit-like vascular channels (Fig. 62-1F).[6,19]

PATHOGENESIS

Sporadic LAM is caused by proliferation of neoplastic LAM cells that have mutations or deletions in the *TSC2* (16p13) gene.[7,8] Consistent with Knudson's "two-hit" hypothesis of tumor development,[28] loss of heterozygosity of *TSC2* has been reported in LAM cells isolated from lung, blood, chyle, urine, and AML from both sporadic LAM and TSC-LAM patients.[8,29–31] LAM cells having identical mutations were identified in AML and lungs of the same patient.[8,31] LAM cells from patients receiving lung transplantation have been detected in the donor lung, suggesting migration from other sites, such as the kidney or lymphatic system, to the lungs.[32,33] The metastatic properties of LAM cells were also demonstrated by the presence of LAM cells in blood, urine, expectorated chyle and pleural, or abdominal chylous fluid of LAM patients.[29,30] LAM cell clusters, consisting of LAM cell aggregates covered by lymphatic endothelial cells, which have been proposed to originate from lung LAM lesions, have also been identified in chylous fluid.[34] Potential sources of lung LAM cells include AML, the lymphatic system, and the uterus,[35] in which case they may originate from abnormal leiomyoma.

A role of estrogens in the pathogenesis of LAM has been suggested by its predominance in premenopausal women, worsening of lung disease during pregnancy or following the administration of estrogens[36,37] and the presence of estrogen and progesterone receptors in lung and angiomyolipoma LAM cells.[20–22] Estrogens promote the proliferation of TSC-null rat ELT3 leiomyoma–derived cells

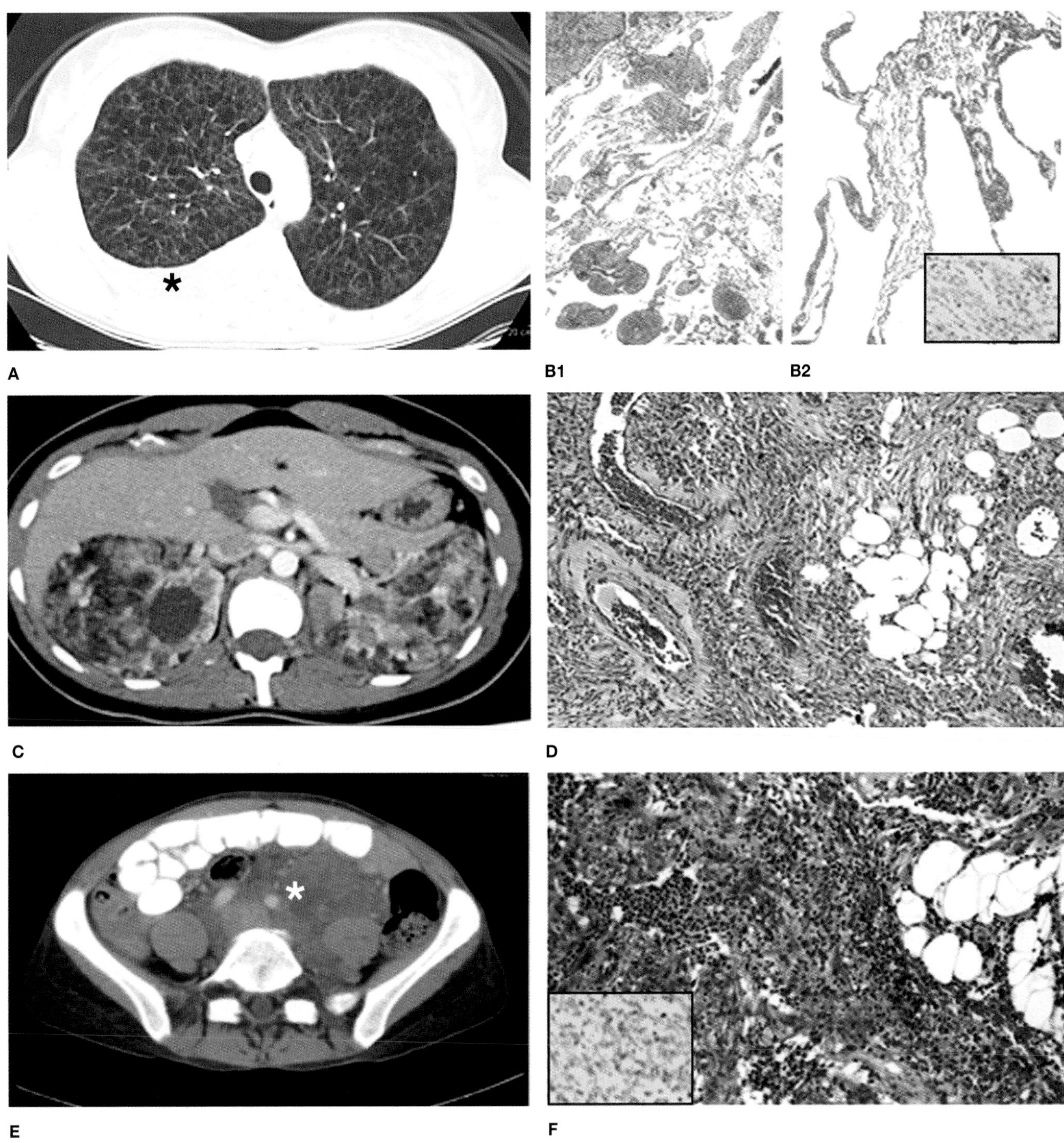

Figure 62-1 Computed tomography scans showing pulmonary and extrapulmonary images of patients with LAM, and the corresponding histopathologic findings. **A.** Multiple thin-walled cysts scattered throughout the lungs that have completely replaced the normal lung parenchyma. The *black asterisk* indicates the presence of a right pleural effusion. **B1 and B2.** Histopathology of the lung showing characteristic nodular smooth muscle cell–like infiltrates and cystic lesions. Inset image on **B2** shows immunocytochemistry of lung tissue showing reactivity with monoclonal antibody HMB45. **C.** Bilateral angiomyolipomas in a patient with TSC-LAM. The fatty, low-density component is clearly visualized. **D.** Histopathology of AML showing smooth muscle cell–like infiltrates, fatty tissue, and poorly differentiated vascular structures. **E.** Large, fluid-filled lymphangioleiomyoma (*white asterisk*) surrounding vascular structures. **F.** Histologic appearance of a lymphangioleiomyoma showing smooth muscle–like cells arranged in fascicular, trabecular or papillary patterns. Inset image on **F** shows immunocytochemistry of lymphangioleiomyoma tissue showing reactivity with monoclonal antibody HMB45.

in vitro, and the growth of subcutaneous tumors in a nude mouse xenograph system.[38] Estrogens stimulate the growth of human angiomyolipoma *TSC2*$^{-/-}$ cells, increase the survival and metastatic properties of *TSC2*$^{-/-}$ ELT3 cells in mice, and enhance matrix metalloproteinase (MMP)-2 activity of LAM lung-derived cells, thereby promoting cell invasiveness.[39–41]

The mechanism by which interstitial LAM cell proliferation causes lung cyst formation is unknown.[42] It has been proposed that compression of the airways by LAM cells leads to distention of the terminal airspaces and cyst formation.[6,19] It has also been proposed that degradation of lung elastic fibers is a major cause of the cystic lesions.[42] Matrix metalloproteinases, which play a role in

TABLE 62-1 Clinical and Physiologic Features of Patients with Sporadic LAM and TSC-LAM

Demographics	TSC-LAM	Sporadic LAM
Number of patients	34	196
Age of LAM diagnosis	39.0 ± 1.6	41.4 ± 0.7
Signs and symptoms		
Dyspnea	70.6%	73.5%
Pneumothorax	47.1%	56.9%
Wheezing	58.8%	44.4%
Cough	26.5%	31.6%
Hemoptysis	20.6%	32.1%
Pleural effusions	5.9%	23.5%
Lung function		
Airflow obstruction	37.5%	60.8%
Low diffusion capacity	38.2%	60.3%
Normal spirometry	53.1%	30.7%
Extra-pulmonary LAM		
Number of patients	67	256
Renal angiomyolipoma	32%	93%
Hepatic angiomyolipomas	2%	33%
Lymphangioleiomyomas	6%	29%
Ascites	6%	10%

TSC-LAM, Lymphangioleiomyomatosis associated with Tuberous Sclerosis Complex.
Source: Data from Ryu JH, Moss J, Beck GJ, et al. The NHLBI Lymphangioleiomyomatosis Registry, Characteristics of 230 Patients at Enrollment. Am J Respir Crit Care Med. 2006;173:105; Avila NA, Dwyer AJ, Rabel A, et al. Sporadic lymphangioleiomyomatosis and tuberous sclerosis complex with lymphangioleiomyomatosis, comparison of CT features. Radiology. 2007;242:277.

TABLE 62-2 Cardiopulmonary Exercise Abnormalities in LAM

Decreased $\dot{V}_{O_{2max}}$
Decreased work rate
Decreased oxygen pulse
Decreased breathing reserve
Decreased Pa_{O_2}
Increased $\dot{V}_E/\dot{V}_{CO_2}$ at AT
Increased $\dot{V}_D/\dot{V}_T$
Increased A-a/O_2 gradient

[a] $\dot{V}_{O_{2max}}$, peak oxygen uptake; Pa_{O_2}, arterial oxygen tension; $\dot{V}_E/\dot{V}_{CO_2}$, ventilatory equivalent for CO_2; AT, anaerobic threshold; $\dot{V}_D/\dot{V}_T$, dead space ventilation ratio; A-a/O_2, alveolar arterial oxygen tension difference.
Source: Data from Crausman RS, Jennings CA, Mortensen RL, et al. Lymphangioleiomyomatosis: the pathophysiology of diminished exercise capacity. Am J Respir Crit Care Med. 1996;153:1368; Taveira-DaSilva AM, Stylianou MP, Hedin CJ, et al. Maximal oxygen uptake and severity of disease in lymphangioleiomyomatosis. Am J Respir Crit Care Med. 2003;168:1427.

lung remodeling and lymphangiogenesis, are associated with LAM lesions.[43] LAM nodules contain MMP2, MMP9, MMP1, and MMP activators (MT1-MMP), and their inhibitors (TIMPs).[44,45] Levels of TIMP-3, which inhibits some MMP, were reportedly reduced in LAM lesions.[45,46] Compared with normal subjects, serum levels of MMP-9 were higher in patients with LAM,[47] suggesting that an imbalance between MMP and their inhibitors may contribute to lung destruction.[48] Growth of TSC2-null lesions was associated with an increase in MMP activity and vascular endothelium growth factor D (VEGF-D).[48] Elastic fibers were demonstrated in alveoli of mice with TSC2-null lesions[48] and human lung LAM nodules show disrupted elastic fibers. The presence of lymphatic spaces in the LAM nodules and strong immunoreactivity towards vascular endothelium growth factor C (VEGF-C), VEGF-D, vascular endothelium growth factor receptor (VEGFR) 3, and podoplanin, markers of lymphatic endothelial cells, led to the hypothesis that disorganized lymphangiogenesis enhances metalloproteinase expression and lung remodeling.[48] Some combination of these mechanisms may be the best explanation for the pathogenesis of cystic lung destruction.

PULMONARY PHYSIOLOGY

Airflow obstruction was seen in approximately 61% of patients with sporadic LAM[1,49]; normal spirometry was present in about 31%. The remaining patients had restrictive disease. By comparison, normal lung function was observed in 53% of patients with TSC-LAM (Table 62-1).[1] Increased gas trapping may be also present. The cause of airflow limitation in LAM has been attributed to alveolar destruction,[50] but a study of pulmonary mechanics showed that lung elastic recoil was not significantly reduced.[51] Instead, upstream airway resistance was increased, suggesting increased airways resistance as the major cause of airflow obstruction.[51,52] Reduced diffusing capacity (DL_{CO}) occurred in approximately 60% of sporadic LAM patients.[1] Most patients have both decreased FEV_1 and DL_{CO}, but some patients have only a reduced DL_{CO}.[49] Gas exchange, especially during exercise, is often abnormal (Table 62-2).[52,53] An abnormal ventilatory response with excessive minute ventilation and reduced breathing reserve are seen during exercise. Baseline and exercise dead space to tidal volume ratio and alveolar–arterial oxygen difference (A-a/O_2) are increased both at rest and during exercise.[52] The primary determinants of exercise limitation in LAM are airflow limitation, decreased breathing reserve, dynamic hyperinflation,[52–54] and limitation of oxygen transfer due to loss of alveolar capillary surface area. The latter exerts a significant effect upon exercise performance, because the increase in physiologic dead space produces excessive ventilation. The interdependence between airflow obstruction, which produces a decrease in the ventilatory reserve, and cystic lung destruction, which affects gas exchange during exercise, leads to severe impairment in exercise performance.[52,53] Pulmonary hypertension may also contribute to reduce oxygen transfer during exercise.[55]

RADIOLOGY

Chest radiographic findings in LAM range from being normal, to showing a reticular or nodular irregular shadowing or, in advanced stages, severe cystic changes. Computed tomography (CT) demonstrates diffuse, well-defined, round thin-walled cysts scattered throughout the lungs. Cysts vary in size from a few millimeters to up to 2 cm (Fig. 62-1A).[56,57] Additional findings are pleural effusions and lung opacities caused by chyle (Fig. 62-1A). Correlation between the extent of the cystic parenchymal replacement, as measured by high-resolution chest CT (HRCT), and the severity of the disease, as determined by spirometry, DL_{CO} or exercise performance, has been reported.[53,57–61] Computer analysis of HRCT can quantify the extent of cystic changes and detect abnormalities in areas adjacent to the cysts that may appear to be radiographically normal[60,61]; these emphysematous changes were also seen by histopathology.[61]

Abdominal CT and ultrasonography studies may show renal AML, abdominal lymphadenopathy, lymphangioleiomyoma, ascites, and dilatation of the thoracic duct.[18] AML occur predominantly in the kidney and liver and are recognized by their characteristic appearance consisting of areas of fatty density, intermixed with more dense areas and normal-appearing renal parenchyma (see Fig. 62-1C).[18] Atypical AML lacking adipose tissue have a predominance of epithelioid LAM cells and radiologically may mimic renal cell carcinoma. Lymphangioleiomyomas appear as well-circumscribed masses of variable dimensions, comprising a wall and a central fluid-rich region (Fig. 62-1E).[18] Diurnal variation in size of lymphangioleiomyomas has been demonstrated by CT and ultrasound, which may help differentiating them from malignant tumors and explain worsening of symptoms during day time.[62,63]

DIAGNOSIS

The characteristic CT scan appearance and its histologic features on open or thoracoscopic lung biopsy can diagnose LAM. Transbronchial lung biopsy may yield adequate sample size for pathologic diagnosis.[64,65] The diagnosis of LAM should be strongly suspected in any woman who presents with progressive dyspnea, recurrent pneumothorax, or a chylous pleural effusion.[1–5] The differential diagnosis includes pulmonary emphysema, asthma, chronic extrinsic allergic alveolitis, Langerhans cell histiocytosis, sarcoidosis, Birt–Hogg–Dubé syndrome, and follicular bronchiolitis. Definite LAM may be diagnosed in the presence of a characteristic HRCT and a lung biopsy showing the pathologic features of LAM or a characteristic lung HRCT and (1) angiomyolipoma, (2) chylous effusion, (3) lymphangioleiomyoma or lymphadenopathy, and (4) TSC.[66] A diagnosis of probable LAM may be established in the presence of a characteristic HRCT and a compatible clinical history or a characteristic HRCT and angiomyolipoma or chylous effusions. Possible LAM may be diagnosed in the presence of a characteristic or compatible HRCT.[66]

Serum VEGF-D, a lymphangiogenic factor, is increased in the serum of patients with LAM compared to normal individuals and is a measure of lymphatic involvement in LAM.[67–70] In the appropriate clinical and radiologic setting, a VEGF-D serum level equal or greater than 800 pg/mL is unlikely to be found in other cystic lung diseases and appears to be diagnostic of LAM.[69,70]

PROGNOSIS

The clinical course of LAM is highly variable. The estimated median transplant-free survival time for LAM patients in the United States is 29 years from symptom onset and 23 years from diagnosis.[71] The estimated 10-year transplant-free survival is 86%. Age appears also to affect survival, as rapid decline in lung function is more common in younger premenopausal patients.[49,72] Patients whose lung tissue shows predominance of cystic lesions tend to have worse lung function and prognosis than those with more LAM cell infiltrates.[73]

The severity of lung involvement in LAM may be assessed in patients who had a lung biopsy using the LAM Histology Score (LHS), which grades the extent of replacement of normal lung tissue by cystic lesions and LAM cell infiltrates.[74] The amount of tissue involvement is graded semiquantitatively based on percent of lung tissue involved: LHS-1, <25%; LHS-2, 25% to 50%; and LHS-3, >50% lung tissue. LHS-2 and LHS-3 scores and the presence of hemosiderin-laden macrophages are associated with decreased survival.[74] Patients with more cystic disease are likely to have lower FEV_1 and DL_{CO}, lower peak oxygen uptake ($\dot{V}_{O_{2max}}$), and more exercise-induced hypoxemia.[53,75]

The severity of lung disease in LAM can be also graded by HRCT. HRCT findings correlate with lung function tests, gas exchange, and exercise performance.[53,56–59] HRCT computer analysis can quantify the percentage of lung volume affected by cysts and evaluate the texture of areas not involved with cysts.[60,61] Using these methods, percentage of lung volume occupied by cysts was found to correlate with FEV_1, residual volume, and DL_{CO}.[60,61]

The simplest method of assessing the severity of lung disease in LAM is pulmonary function testing.[1,49] Most patients have airflow obstruction and impaired gas exchange. Early in the disease, a significant number of patients may have normal spirometry or only mild airflow obstruction, along with a marked decrease in diffusion capacity. In these patients, the severity of disease is best graded by tests of gas exchange such as DL_{CO}, arterial blood gases, A-a/O_2 gradient, cardiopulmonary exercise testing, and 6-minute walk test.[52,53,59] Exercise-induced hypoxemia may occur in the presence of near-normal DL_{CO} and FEV_1.[53] Correlation between $\dot{V}_{O_{2max}}$ and LHS scores, and between CT severity grade and A-a/O_2 gradient, dead space/tidal volume ratio, and $\dot{V}_{O_{2max}}$ have been demonstrated.[53,58–61] Rates of functional decline over time may help in defining the course of disease, that is, whether it is rapidly or slowly progressive. Sequential lung function testing every 3 to 6 months is warranted to assess the progression of disease.[49,72] A positive response to bronchodilators occurs in 25% to 30% of LAM patients.[75,76] Patients who respond to bronchodilators tend to have a predominantly cellular pattern of LAM lung lesions and greater rates of decline in FEV_1.[75] A low initial DL_{CO} was also reported to be a predictor of accelerated loss of FEV_1.[77]

OTHER PROGNOSTIC INDICATORS

There is some evidence that older age and/or menopause are associated with slower disease progression.[49,72] Patients who present with exertional dyspnea and hemoptysis tend to have more severe disease, greater rates of progression of disease, and lower survival than those with a history of pneumothorax.[78] This may be due to either a delay in diagnosis or an insidious course in those who present with dyspnea. Lymphatic involvement, for example, chylous effusions, lymphadenopathy, lymphangioleiomyomas, may be associated with a more severe form of disease.[68,79,80] Correlation between LHS and the expression of VEGF-C has been reported.[80] Serum levels of VEGF-D are especially elevated in patients with lymphatic abnormalities and show a correlation with DL_{CO} and HRCT scan grading of severity of lung disease.[68,79,80] Measurement of serum VEGF-D may be of value in establishing a diagnosis and grading the severity of disease and response to therapy.

TREATMENT

Treatment includes general principles of management and specific therapeutic interventions.

GENERAL PRINCIPLES OF MANAGEMENT

LAM patients should be told about the chronic nature of LAM and be advised to lead, as much as possible, a normal life. If there is an excess body mass, they should be encouraged to lose weight, engage in physical activities, and exercise regularly. The limits of exercise should be dictated only by the severity of their lung disease. Sports involving physical contact and martial arts should be avoided because of potentially causing bleeding from AML. Patients should be advised to continue with normal activities, and be allowed to travel by land or air except to high altitude locations, depending on disease severity. The risk of life-threatening pneumothorax associated with air travel is minor. However, if patients should experience sudden onset of breathlessness or chest pain, pneumothorax should be excluded prior to travelling. An arterial blood gas may help to determine whether a patient may travel by air without supplemental oxygen. A 6-minute walk test or a cardiopulmonary exercise test to uncover exercise-induced hypoxemia and determine the need for supplemental oxygen is recommended. Patients who desaturate during exercise should be given supplemental oxygen at flow rates adjusted to sustain oxygen saturation above 88% to 90%. Patients should be advised against using estrogen-containing contraceptives and avoid phytoestrogen-rich food.

SPECIFIC THERAPIES

Specific therapies include antiestrogen therapy, mTOR inhibitors, matrix metalloproteinase inhibitors, statins, and inhibitors of autophagy.

Antiestrogen Therapy

Oophorectomy, progesterone, and gonadotrophin-releasing hormone (GnRH) analogs have been employed in the treatment of LAM. Case reports and uncontrolled studies claimed a beneficial effect of antiestrogen therapies.[81] Taylor et al.[13] however, found no benefit from oophorectomy and improvement in dyspnea only in 2 of 19 patients treated with progesterone. A reduced rate of decline in FEV_1 and DL_{CO} was reported in premenopausal patients treated with progesterone.[72] However, when patients with short-term follow-up were excluded from the analysis, the effect of progesterone was not significant.[72] In a retrospective study, no difference was observed in disease progression between patients treated with or not treated with progesterone.[49] Data from studies that assessed the effect of GnRH analogs have also been inconclusive.[82,83] Experimental data however, appear to provide a rational for hormonal manipulations in the treatment of LAM.[38–41] Further studies aimed at suppressing estrogen secretion with aromatase inhibitors (i.e., letrozole) are undergoing a clinical trial (clinicaltrials.gov) in postmenopausal women in whom the main source of estrogens are the adrenal glands (Frank X. McCormack P.I. ClinicalTrials.gov Identifier:NCT01353209).

Mammalian Target of Rapamycin (mTOR) Inhibitors

Since the discovery that TSC genes *TSC1* and *TSC2* were involved in the pathogenesis of LAM, major advances were made in treatment of LAM. *TSC1* and *TSC2* are tumor suppressor genes that encode respectively, hamartin and tuberin (Fig. 62-2).[84–87] These proteins form a cytosolic complex that regulates the intracellular serine/threonine kinase mTOR, which integrates growth factor, energy, and stress signaling, thereby regulating cell growth, proliferation, and survival.[84,85] Two different complexes involving mTOR, mTORC1, and mTORC2, have been identified.[85–87] Tuberin, which exists in a complex with hamartin, is a GTPase-activating protein for the guanine nucleotide–binding protein Rheb (Ras homolog enriched in brain), promoting the formation of inactive Rheb-GDP from active Rheb-GTP.[85] Inhibition or absence of tuberin, as occurs with *TSC2* gene mutations, results in accumulation of active Rheb-GTP, leading to stimulation of mTORC1, which results in phosphorylation of S6 kinase and eukaryotic initiation factor 4E-binding protein, and increased translation and cell growth.[85]

Sirolimus is an immunosuppressant drug that forms a complex with FK506-binding protein-12 and inhibits mTORC1.[85,88] Sirolimus provides only partial inhibition of mTORC1 and has some inhibitory effect on mTORC2 signaling (Fig. 62-2B).[87,89,90] In experimental models, sirolimus was shown to decrease tumor size in animals with a germline mutation of *TSC2*.[91] Treatment with a sirolimus analog decreased the severity of renal cystadenomas and liver hemangiomas in *TSC2*$^{+/-}$ mice, and decreased tumor growth and improved survival of nude mice with *TSC2*$^{+/-}$ tumors.[92] In human subjects with TSC or LAM who had AML, treatment with sirolimus decreased tumor size by half after 1 year of therapy.[93] Following withdrawal of sirolimus, the angiolipomas partially regained their size. Subsequent studies have confirmed these findings.[94–96] The most recent study found that 42% of 79 patients with AML, treated with everolimus, responded with a 50% reduction in tumor size after 24 weeks of therapy.[96] Sirolimus also appears to be effective in reducing the size of giant-cell astrocytomas in patients with TSC.[97,98]

The effect of sirolimus on pulmonary function was examined in 89 patients with LAM (MILES trial). Forty-six patients were treated with sirolimus and 43 with placebo for 12 months and followed for an additional year after discontinuation of therapy.[99] Compared to the placebo group, the sirolimus group had improvements

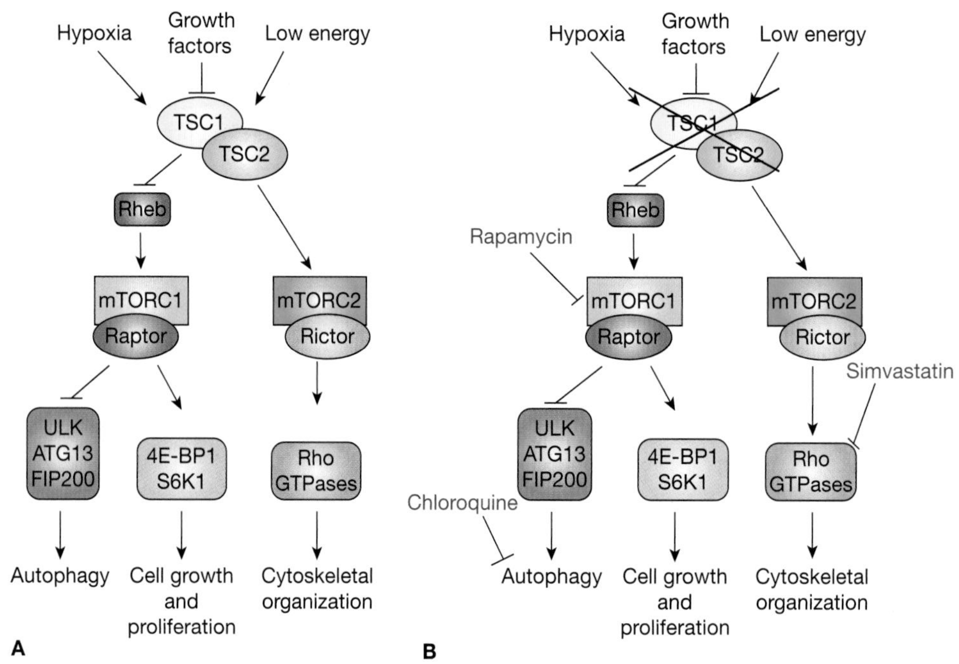

Figure 62-2 Simplified scheme of the mTOR signaling pathways. **A.** TSC1/2 integrates multiple signals, such as growth factors, energy state and hypoxia, to control cell growth and proliferation. Growth factors stimulate several signaling pathways leading to phosphorylation of TSC2 and its inactivation. TSC1/2 negatively regulates mTORC1 through its actions on Rheb, while it positively regulates mTORC2. Activation of mTORC1 leads to cell growth and proliferation and inhibition of autophagy. mTORC2 regulates the actin cytoskeleton through Rho GTPases, which affects cell migration and morphogenesis. **B.** mTORC1 is acutely inhibited by sirolimus (rapamycin) treatment. mTORC2 is sensitive to prolonged rapamycin treatment, which may affect mTORC2 assembly and function. Simvastatin inhibits Rho GTPases, whereas chloroquine inhibits autophagy by blocking fusion of autophagosomes with lysosomes. mTOR, mammalian target of rapamycin; Rheb GAP, Ras homolog enriched in brain GTPase-activating protein; S6K1, S6 kinase 1; 4E-BP1, factor 4E binding protein 1; raptor, regulatory associated protein of mTOR; rictor, rapamycin-insensitive companion of mTOR; ULK 1, UNC-51–like kinase 1; ATG13, autophagy-related protein 13; FIP200, focal adhesion kinase family interacting protein of 200 kDa.

from baseline of FVC, FEV_1, quality of life, and functional performance. After discontinuation of sirolimus, decline of lung function resumed and paralleled that of the placebo group.[99] In another study, 19 patients with either rapidly progressive lung disease or lymphangioleiomyomas and chylous effusions were treated with sirolimus for approximately 2.5 years. Instead of the expected decrease in lung function, an increase in FEV_1 and DL_{CO} was observed.[100] Nine patients experienced complete resolution of their chylous effusions and abdominal lymphangioleiomyomas.[100]

Based on the findings in the MILES trial we recommend that sirolimus be given to patients in whom lung function is declining rapidly. We also recommend sirolimus therapy for LAM patients with symptomatic lymphangioleiomyomas and chylous pleural effusions or ascites.[100,101] The role of sirolimus in patients with normal or stable lung function or very slow rates of decline is unclear. Currently the starting dose of sirolimus is 2 mg/d. Sirolimus serum levels must be monitored and dosage adjusted to attain serum trough levels between 5 and 15 ng/mm, a range thought to be therapeutic for patients with renal transplants.[99] Adverse events associated with sirolimus therapy include oral mucosa ulcers, hypertension, hyperlipidemia, proteinuria, increased serum creatinine, infections, acne, amenorrhea, and sirolimus-related interstitial pneumonitis. Close patient monitoring is recommended. Given the limited experience with sirolimus in the treatment of LAM, it is not known whether treatment must be continued for life or whether resistance to sirolimus may eventually develop.

Matrix Metalloproteinase Inhibitors

Doxycycline is a MMP inhibitor that affects MMP production in TSC-null ELT3 cells,[102] and inhibits MMP2 secretion by TSC-null mouse embryonic and human LAM cells.[103] A potential role of doxycycline in the treatment of LAM was suggested by a report of one patient with LAM in whom treatment with doxycycline decreased urinary MMP levels and improved lung function.[104] A decrease in serum and urine levels of MMP-9 and MMP-2 in 34 patients treated with doxycycline has been reported.[105] A controlled study showed that it is unlikely that doxycycline has a useful effect in LAM.[105A]

Statins

There is evidence that both mTORC1 and mTORC2 are necessary for tuberin-dependent cell proliferation and survival.[106] In the absence of tuberin, RhoA activity is increased, resulting in increased cell survival.[106] Since sirolimus primarily suppresses mTORC1 signaling, there is a rational for new therapies targeting mTORC2 signaling. Statins inhibit both sirolimus-sensitive and sirolimus-insensitive mechanisms of TSC-null cell growth by inhibiting RhoA GTPase activity.[107] In one study, atorvastatin was shown to inhibit the growth of *TSC2*$^{-/-}$ ELT-3 cells and mouse embryonic fibroblasts while decreasing Rheb-GTPase activity and function.[107] A synergistic effect of simvastatin and sirolimus in inhibiting proliferation of TSC2-null cells and TSC-null tumor growth has been described.[106] This effect appears to be specific for simvastatin; in a mouse model of TSC, atorvastatin failed to reduce the size of liver and renal tumors.[108] In a mouse model of LAM, simvastatin prevented alveolar space enlargement and, combined with sirolimus, blocked MMP upregulation, reducing TSC2-null lesions and alveolar destruction.[48] However, in a retrospective study, it was found that the rate of decline in lung diffusion for patients treated for hypercholesterolemia with statins was greater than that of their matched off-statin therapy controls.[109]

Inhibitors of Autophagy

Autophagy is a mechanism by which cells maintain energy homeostasis and recycle proteins and organelles.[110] Autophagosomes are formed that encapsulate damaged organelles or cellular debris and fuse with lysosomes to degrade their contents.[111] Autophagy is controlled by signaling from mTOR, and the human homolog of ATG1 (ULK1) kinase complex, comprising ULK1, Atg13, and Atg17; mTORC1 is a major regulator of autophagy.[111–113] Under conditions of cellular stress, mTORC1 is downregulated, triggering autophagy. mTOR inhibitors such as sirolimus stimulate autophagy by causing phosphorylation of Atg13, which interacts with ULK1 and inhibits the formation of autophagosomes which increases autophagy and, within limits, increases cell survival.[110–113] Since LAM cells have been shown to have low levels of autophagy, blockade of mTOR signaling with sirolimus may result in increased survival of LAM cells.[114,115] Hydroxychloroquine and its analogs inhibit the growth of cancer cells and induce cell death by blocking autophagy.[113–115] The combination of mTORC1 inhibition with sirolimus and inhibition of autophagy with hydroxychloroquine was found to be more effective than either treatment alone in inhibiting the survival of TSC2-null cells and the growth of TSC2-null xenograph tumors, as well as the spontaneous development of renal tumors in *TSC2*$^{+/-}$ mice.[115] Inhibition of autophagy with hydroxychloroquine could potentially complement the effect of sirolimus in the treatment of LAM. These observations provide a rational for testing the effect of chloroquine and sirolimus in LAM patients. A current study (SAIL trial) testing the effects of sirolimus and hydroxychloroquine is ongoing (Elizabeth Henske P.I.; ClinicalTrials.gov Identifier:NCT01687179).

TREATMENT OF COMPLICATIONS

Treatment of well recognized complications of LAM and special considerations are discussed below.

■ PNEUMOTHORAX

Small pneumothoraces may be treated conservatively by chest tube drainage. Because of the high rate of pneumothorax recurrence if air leak persists or the pneumothorax recurs, chemical or surgical pleurodesis by video-assisted thoracoscopy should be considered.[3,116] Chemical sclerosis, pleurectomy, mechanical abrasion, and talc poudrage are most effective.[116] Talc pleurodesis may result in fibrothorax that can complicate removal of the lung at the time of transplantation.[3,116] The risk of developing a pneumothorax during air travel appears to be small.[117]

■ CHYLOUS EFFUSIONS AND LYMPHANGIOLEIOMYOMAS

Chylous effusions and lymphangioleiomyomas may compromise respiratory function and cause abdominal pain, urinary frequency, obstipation, tenesmus, and peripheral edema. Abdominal symptoms may suggest malignancy.[63,118–120] Frequent drainage of chylous effusions may result in protein loss, lymphopenia, and weight loss.[100,121] Several treatments such as low fat diet, pleuro-peritoneal or peritoneal-venous shunts, have been employed but there is little experience with these therapeutic modalities in LAM.[122,123] The same is true of treatment with somatostatin and octreotide.[124,125] The finding that sirolimus is effective in decreasing the size of chylous effusions and lymphangioleiomyomas strongly suggests that instead of undertaking invasive procedures such as pleurodesis, symptomatic patients should be treated with sirolimus.[100,126]

■ ANGIOMYOLIPOMAS

AML occur primarily in the kidney, although other organs, for example, liver, may be involved.[127] Small AML, for example, less than 4 cm in diameter, are well tolerated and are associated with well-preserved renal function.[127] The principal complication of larger AML is bleeding. Embolization, rather than resection, is recommended to preserve kidney function.[128–130] Severe pain may be also an indication for selective embolization of the tumor. Prophylactic embolization may be undertaken in patients with large AML and no known episodes of bleeding but evidence favoring this approach is lacking. Indeed, embolization appears to be of little value in the long-term management of AML.[130] Since treatment with sirolimus reduces tumor size in about 44% to 50% of the patients, it may also prevent bleeding and

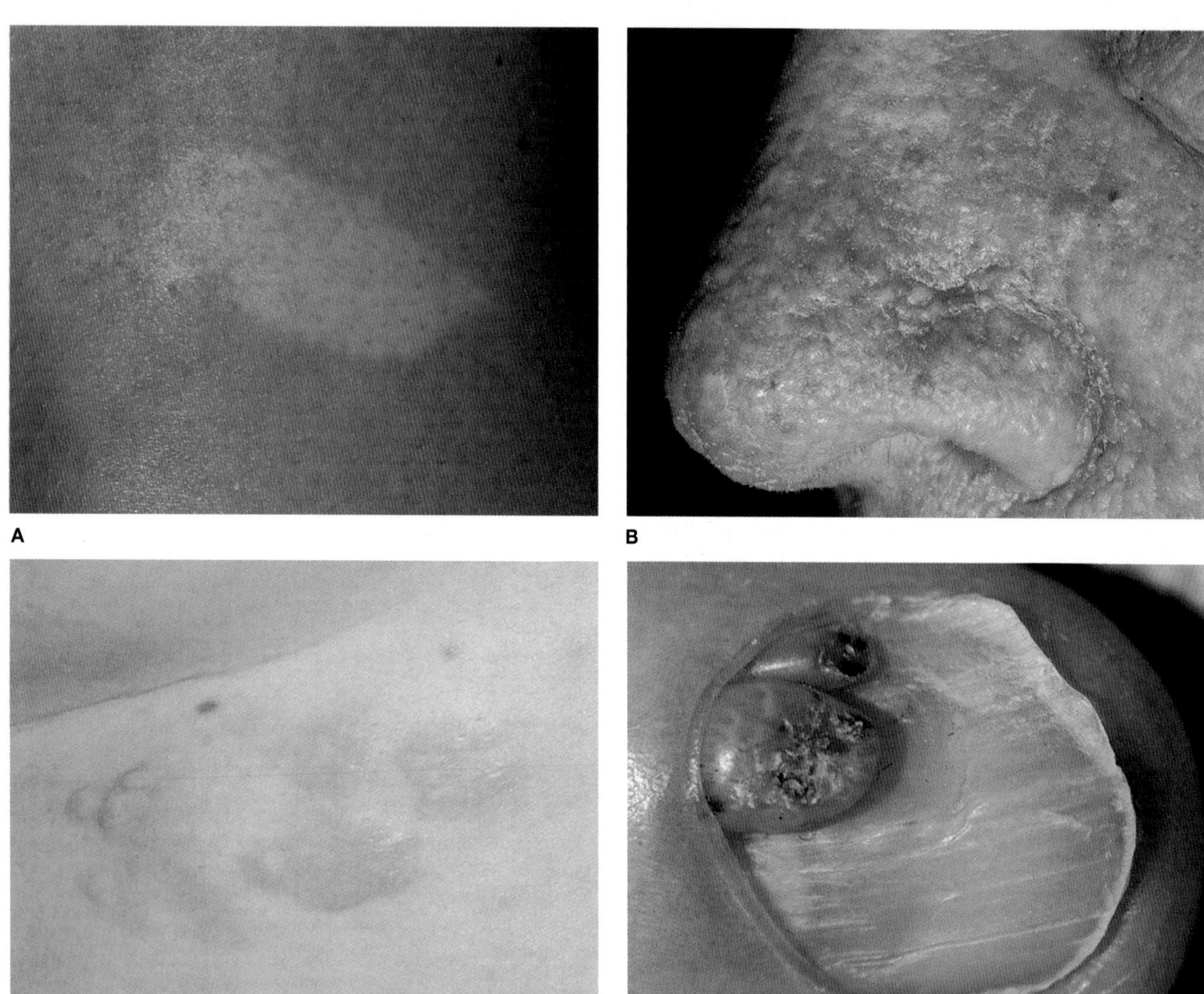

Figure 62-3 Skin manifestations of TSC in an adult women. **A.** Large hypomelanotic macule on the back. **B.** Multiple facial angiofibromas involving the nose and adjacent cheek. **C.** Shagreen patch on the lower back. **D.** Periungual fibroma near the fingernail.

the need for embolization or surgical intervention.[99-102] Accordingly, treatment with mTOR inhibitors is currently the initial approach for the treatment of large AML. Arterial embolization, which has a response rate similar to mTOR inhibitors, should be reserved for patients with acute bleeding or those who do not respond or do not tolerate sirolimus therapy.[93-95,130] Discontinuation of sirolimus therapy may result in return of the AML to its original a size.

■ PREGNANCY

Of 353 pregnancies recorded in the LAM registry, 66.9% resulted in live birth, 16.7% had spontaneous abortion and 15% had therapeutic abortion.[1] Twenty-two percent of those who had been pregnant experienced worsening of respiratory symptoms during pregnancy.[1] Patients who were diagnosed with LAM during pregnancy had more premature births, higher frequency of dyspnea, pneumothorax, and chylothorax than those diagnosed either before or after pregnancy.[131] These data, along with anecdotal reports of worsening symptoms during pregnancy,[132] raise the question whether LAM patients should be advised not to become pregnant. In patients with moderate to severe disease or those in whom lung function is declining rapidly, pregnancy should be discouraged. Instead, these patients should be treated with sirolimus. Patients with mild disease who wish to become pregnant should be told about the potential risks (e.g., pneumothorax, decline in lung function) and advised that with close medical and obstetrics monitoring they have a chance of having a normal pregnancy and delivering a normal child.

■ LUNG TRANSPLANTATION

Except in advance stages, dyspnea at rest is not a major feature of LAM. Exercise limitation and hypoxemia requiring supplemental oxygen are major factors affecting the ability of the patient to conduct activities of daily living. Consequently, patients with an FEV_1 less than 1 L and a DL_{CO} less than 30% predicted receiving supplemental oxygen might be comfortable at rest. In the series of Pechet et al.[133] preoperative FEV_1 and DL_{CO} were respectively, 20 ± 8 and 23 ± 9% predicted and there was resting hypoxemia prior to transplantation. The average 6-minute walk test distance was 250 m. The 5-year survival was 69%.[133-135] The European experience is similar to that of the USA.[136] Before transplantation is considered, lung function needs to be severely compromised because LAM patients with very low FEV_1 and DL_{CO} on supplemental oxygen may live for many years. We suggest that lung transplantation be considered when FEV_1

and DL_{CO} are less than 30% predicted, and the patient is on continuous supplemental oxygen and unable to carry out activities of daily living. Importantly, the patient should rate her quality of life as being poor and be certain that she wishes to undergo lung transplantation.

TUBEROUS SCLEROSIS COMPLEX

TSC is a multisystem autosomal-dominant disorder that affects men and women equally. Its frequency is 1 in 12,000 to 14,000 children under the age of 10, or 1 in 6000 births.[9] It is characterized by mental retardation, seizures, facial angiofibroma, periungual fibromas, Shagreen patches, cortical tubers, giant-cell astrocytomas, and cardiac rhabdomyomas (Fig. 62-3).[9] The association of TSC and cystic lung disease has long been reported in the literature,[137] but little is known about the natural history of LAM in the presence of TSC (TSC-LAM). Initially the prevalence of clinically significant LAM in TSC was thought to be relatively low, ranging from 0.6% to 2.3% of TSC patients.[137–140] However, subsequent studies showed that the prevalence of lung cysts in women with LAM ranges from 26% to 38%.[141–143] Lung cysts were demonstrated in only 13% of men with TSC.[16] If it is accepted that visualization of four or more cysts in the lungs of a TSC patient equates the presence of LAM, then the prevalence of LAM in males may be as high as 38% but the lung disease is mild.[144] The NHLBI LAM registry reported data from 34 TSC patients who were known to have LAM or were later confirmed to have LAM.[1] In a study comparing CT features of 67 patients with TSC-LAM and 256 patients with sporadic LAM,[145] severe disease was present in 25% of TSC-LAM patients versus 40% of sporadic LAM patients (Table 62-1). Renal AML occurred in 93% of TSC-LAM patients and in only 32% of sporadic LAM subjects. Lymphangioleiomyomas and chylous effusions were more common in sporadic LAM. Sclerotic bone lesions were very common in patients with TSC-LAM.[146]

Lung disease in TSC tends to be milder than in sporadic LAM, often comprising only a few cysts scattered throughout the lungs. These patients have subclinical disease and usually are diagnosed with LAM only because they have TSC. TSC patients who initially present with characteristic symptoms of pulmonary LAM may have more severe lung disease and a clinical course similar to patients with sporadic LAM.

REFERENCES

1. Ryu JH, Moss J, Beck GJ, et al; NHLBI LAM Registry Group. The NHLBI Lymphangioleiomyomatosis registry, characteristics of 230 patients at enrollment. *Am J Respir Crit Care Med.* 2006;173:105–111.
2. McCormack FX. Lymphangioleiomyomatosis: a clinical update. *Chest.* 2008;133:507–516.
3. Meraj R, Wikenheiser-Brokamp KA, Young LR, McCormack FX. Lymphangioleiomyomatosis: new concepts in pathogenesis, diagnosis, and treatment. *Semin Respir Crit Care Med.* 2012;33:486–497.
4. Urban T, Lazor R, Lacronique J, et al. Pulmonary lymphangioleiomyomatosis. A study of 69 patients. Groupe d'Etudes et de Recherche sur les Maladies "Orphelines" Pulmonaires (GERM "O"P). *Medicine (Baltimore).* 1999;78:321–337.
5. Matsui K, Tatsuguchi A, Valencia J, et al. Extrapulmonary lymphangioleiomyomatosis (LAM): clinicopathologic features in 22 cases. *Hum Pathol.* 2000;31:1242–1248.
6. Ferrans VJ, Yu ZX, Nelson WK, et al. Lymphangioleiomyomatosis (LAM). A review of clinical and morphological features. *J Nippon Med Sch.* 2000;67:311–329.
7. Smolarek TA, Wessner LL, McCormack FX, Mylet JC, Menon AG, Henske EP. Evidence that lymphangiomyomatosis is caused by TSC2 mutations, chromosome 16p13 loss of heterozygosity in angiomyolipomas and lymph nodes from women with lymphangiomyomatosis. *Am J Hum Genet.* 1998;62:810–815.
8. Carsillo T, Astrinidis A, Henske EP. Mutations in the tuberous sclerosis complex gene TSC2 are a cause of sporadic pulmonary lymphangioleiomyomatosis. *Proc Natl Acad Sci U S A.* 2000;97:6085–6090.
9. Curatolo P, Bombardieri R, Jozwiak S. Tuberous sclerosis. *Lancet.* 2008;372:657–668.
10. Silversteen EF, Ellis K, Wolff M, Jaretzki A 3rd. Pulmonary lymphangiomyomatosis. *Am J Roentgenol.* 1974;120:832–850.
11. Corrin B, Liebow AA, Friedman PJ. Pulmonary lymphangioleiomyomatosis: a review. *Am J Pathol.* 1975;79:348–382.
12. Carrington CB, Cugell DW, Gaensler EA, et al. Lymphangioleiomyomatosis. Physiologic-pathologic-radiologic correlations. *Am Rev Respir Dis.* 1977;116:977–995.
13. Taylor JR, Ryu J, Colby TV, Raffin TA. Lymphangioleiomyomatosis: clinical course in 32 patients. *N Engl J Med.* 1990;323:1254–1260.
14. Cohen MM, Pollock-BarZiv S, Johnson SR. Emerging clinical picture of lymphangioleiomyomatosis. *Thorax.* 2005;60:875–879.
15. Harknett EC, Chang WY, Byrnes S, et al. Use of variability in national and regional data to estimate the prevalence of lymphangioleiomyomatosis. *QJM.* 2011;104:971–979.
16. Adriaensen ME, Schaefer-Prokop CM, Duyndam DA, Zonnenberg BA, Prokop M. Radiological evidence of lymphangioleiomyomatosis in female and male patients with tuberous sclerosis complex. *Clin Radiol.* 2011;66:625–628.
17. Steagall WK, Glasgow CG, Hathaway OM, et al. Genetic and morphologic determinants of pneumothorax in lymphangioleiomyomatosis. *Am J Physiol Lung Cell Mol Physiol.* 2007;293:L800–L808.
18. Avila NA, Kelly JA, Chu SC, Dwyer AJ, Moss J. Lymphangioleiomyomatosis: abdominopelvic CT and US findings. *Radiology.* 2000;216:147–153.
19. Abbott GF, Rosado-de-Christenson ML, Frazier AA, Franks TJ, Pugatch RD, Galvin JR. From the archives of the AFIP: lymphangioleiomyomatosis: radiologic-pathologic correlation. *Radiographics.* 2005;25:803–828.
20. Berger U, Khaghani A, Pomerance A, Yacoub MH, Coombes RC. Pulmonary lymphangioleiomyomatosis and steroid receptors. *Am J Clin Pathol.* 1990;93:609–614.
21. Ohori NP, Yousem SA, Sonmez-Alpan E, Colby TV. Estrogen and progesterone receptors in lymphangioleiomyomatosis, epithelioid hemangioendothelioma, and sclerosing hemangioma of the lung. *Am J Clin Pathol.* 1991;96:529–535.
22. Logginidou H, Ao X, Russo I, Henske EP. Frequent estrogen and progesterone receptor immunoreactivity in renal angiomyolipomas from women with pulmonary lymphangioleiomyomatosis. *Chest.* 2000;117:25–30.
23. Valencia JC, Matsui K, Bondy C, et al. Distribution and mRNA expression of insulin-like growth factor system in pulmonary lymphangioleiomyomatosis. *J Investig Med.* 2001;49:421–433.
24. Valencia JC, Pacheco-Rodriguez G, Carmona AK, et al. Tissue-specific renin-angiotensin system in pulmonary lymphangioleiomyomatosis. *Am J Respir Cell Mol Biol.* 2006;35:40–47.
25. Pacheco-Rodriguez G, Steagall WK, Crooks DM, et al. TSC2 loss in lymphangioleiomyomatosis cells correlated with expression of CD44v6, a molecular determinant of metastasis. *Cancer Res.* 2007;67:10573–10581.
26. Pacheco-Rodriguez G, Kumaki F, Steagall WK, et al. Chemokine-enhanced chemotaxis of lymphangioleiomyomatosis cells with

mutations in the tumor suppressor TSC2 gene. *J Immunol.* 2009; 182:1270–1277.

27. Ikeda Y, Taveira-DaSilva AM, Pacheco-Rodriguez G, et al. Erythropoietin-driven proliferation of cells with mutations in the tumor suppressor gene TSC2. *Am J Physiol Lung Cell Mol Physiol.* 2011;300:L64–L72.
28. Knudson AG. Hereditary cancer: two hits revisited. *J Cancer Res Clin Oncol.* 1996;122:135–140.
29. Crooks DM, Pacheco-Rodriguez G, DeCastro RM, et al. Molecular and genetic analysis of disseminated neoplastic cells in lymphangioleiomyomatosis. *Proc Natl Acad Sci USA.* 2004;101:17462–17467.
30. Cai X, Pacheco-Rodriguez G, Fan QY, et al. Phenotypic characterization of disseminated cells with TSC2 loss of heterozygosity in patients with lymphangioleiomyomatosis. *Am J Respir Crit Care Med.* 2010;182:1410–1418.
31. Yu J, Astrinidis A, Henske EP. Chromosome 16 loss of heterozygosity in tuberous sclerosis and sporadic lymphangiomyomatosis. *Am J Respir Crit Care Med.* 2001;164:1537–1540.
32. Bittmann I, Rolf B, Amann G, Löhrs U. Recurrence of lymphangioleiomyomatosis after single lung transplantation, new insights into pathogenesis. *Hum Pathol.* 2003;34:95–98.
33. Karbowniczek M, Astrinidis A, Balsara BR, et al. Recurrent lymphangioleiomyomatosis after transplantation: genetic analyses reveal a metastatic mechanism. *Am J Respir Crit Care Med.* 2003;167:976–982.
34. Mitani K, Kumasaka T, Takemura H, et al. Cytologic, immunocytochemical and ultrastructural characterization of lymphangioleiomyomatosis cell clusters in chylous effusions of patients with lymphangioleiomyomatosis. *Acta Cytol.* 2009;53:402–409.
35. Hayashi T, Kumasaka T, Mitani K, et al. Prevalence of uterine and adnexal involvement in pulmonary lymphangioleiomyomatosis: a clinicopathologic study of 10 patients. *Am J Surg Pathol.* 2011;35:1776–1785.
36. Brunelli A, Catalini G, Fianchini A. Pregnancy exacerbating unsuspected mediastinal lymphangioleiomyomatosis and chylothorax. *Int J Gynaecol Obstet.* 1996;52:289–290.
37. Yano S. Exacerbation of pulmonary lymphangioleiomyomatosis by exogenous oestrogen used for infertility treatment. *Thorax.* 2002;57:1085–1086.
38. Howe SR, Gottardis MM, Everitt JI, Walker C. Estrogen stimulation and tamoxifen inhibition of leiomyoma cell growth in vitro and in vivo. *Endocrinology.* 1995;136:4996–5003.
39. Yu J, Astrinidis A, Howard S, Henske EP. Estradiol and tamoxifen stimulate LAM-associated angiomyolipoma cell growth and activate both genomic and nongenomic signaling pathways. *Am J Physiol Lung Cell Mol Physiol.* 2004;286:L694–L700.
40. Yu JJ, Robb VA, Morrison TA, Henske EP. Estrogen promotes the survival and pulmonary metastasis of tuberin-null cells. *Proc Natl Acad Sci U S A.* 2009;106:2635–2640.
41. Glassberg MK, Elliot SJ, Fritz J, et al. Activation of the estrogen receptor contributes to the progression of pulmonary lymphangioleiomyomatosis via matrix metalloproteinase-induced cell invasiveness. *J Clin Endocrinol Metab.* 2008;93: 1625–1633.
42. Henske EP, McCormack FX. Lymphangioleiomyomatosis - a wolf in sheep's clothing. *J Clin Invest.* 2012;122:3807–3816.
43. Matsui K, Takeda K, Yu Z-X, Travis WD, Moss J, Ferrans VJ. Role for activation of matrix metalloproteinases in the pathogenesis of pulmonary lymphangioleiomyomatosis. *Arch Pathol Lab Med.* 2000;124:267–275.
44. Krymskaya VP, Shipley JM. Lymphangioleiomyomatosis: a complex tale of serum response factor-mediated tissue inhibitor of metalloproteinase-3 regulation. *Am J Respir Cell Mol Biol.* 2003; 28:546–550.
45. Papakonstantinou E, Dionyssopoulos A, Aletras AJ, Pesintzaki C, Minas A, Karakiulakis G. Expression of matrix metalloproteinases and their endogenous tissue inhibitors in skin lesions from patients with tuberous sclerosis. *J Am Acad Dermatol.* 2004;51:526–533.
46. Zhe X, Yang Y, Jakkaraju S, Schuger L. Tissue inhibitor of metalloproteinase-3 downregulation in lymphangioleiomyomatosis: potential consequence of abnormal serum response factor expression. *Am J Respir Cell Mol Biol.* 2003;28:504–511.
47. Odajima N, Betsuyaku T, Nasuhara Y, Inoue H, Seyama K, Nishimura M. Matrix metalloproteinases in blood from patients with LAM. *Respir Med.* 2009;103:124–129.
48. Goncharova EA, Goncharov DA, Fehrenbach M, et al Prevention of alveolar destruction and airspace enlargement in a mouse model of pulmonary lymphangioleiomyomatosis (LAM). *Sci Transl Med.* 2012;4:154ra134.
49. Taveira-DaSilva AM, Stylianou MP, Hedin CJ, Hathaway O, Moss J Decline in lung function in patients with lymphangioleiomyomatosis treated with or without progesterone. *Chest.* 2004;126:1867–1874.
50. Sobonya RE, Quan SF, Fleishman JS. Pulmonary lymphangioleiomyomatosis: quantitative analysis of lesions producing airflow limitation. *Hum Pathol.* 1985;16:1122–1128.
51. Burger CD, Hyatt RE, Stats BA Pulmonary mechanics in lymphangioleiomyomatosis. *Am Rev Respir Dis.* 1991;143:1030–1033.
52. Crausman RS, Jennings CA, Mortensen RL, Ackerson LM, Irvin CG, King TE Jr. Lymphangioleiomyomatosis: the pathophysiology of diminished exercise capacity. *Am J Respir Crit Care Med.* 1996;153:1368–1376.
53. Taveira-DaSilva AM, Stylianou MP, Hedin CJ, et al. Maximal oxygen uptake and severity of disease in lymphangioleiomyomatosis. *Am J Respir Crit Care Med.* 2003;168:1427–1431.
54. Baldi BG, Albuquerque AL, Pimenta SP, Salge JM, Kairalla RA, Carvalho CR. Exercise performance and dynamic hyperinflation in lymphangioleiomyomatosis. *Am J Respir Crit Care Med.* 2012;186:341–348.
55. Taveira-DaSilva AM, Hathaway OM, Sachdev V, Shizukuda Y, Birdsall CW, Moss J. Pulmonary artery pressure in lymphangioleiomyomatosis: an echocardiographic study. *Chest.* 2007; 132:1573.
56. Avila NA, Chen CC, Chu SC, et al. Pulmonary lymphangioleiomyomatosis: correlation of ventilation-perfusion scintigraphy, chest radiography, and CT with pulmonary function tests. *Radiology.* 2000;214:441–446.
57. Avila NA, Kelly JA, Dwyer AJ, Johnson DL, Jones EC, Moss J. Lymphangioleiomyomatosis: correlation of qualitative and quantitative thin-section CT with pulmonary function tests and assessment of dependence on pleurodesis. *Radiology.* 2002; 223:189–197.
58. Crausman RS, Lynch DA, Mortensen RL, et al. Quantitative CT predicts the severity of physiologic dysfunction in patients with lymphangiomyomatosis. *Chest.* 1996;109:131–137.
59. Paciocco G, Uslenghi E, Bianchi A, et al. Diffuse cystic lung diseases. Correlation between radiologic and functional status. *Chest.* 2004;125:135–142.
60. Schmithorst VJ, Altes TA, Young LR, et al. Automated algorithm for quantifying the extent of cystic change on volumetric

chest CT: initial results in Lymphangioleiomyomatosis. *AJR Am J Roentgenol.* 2009;192:1037–1044.

61. Yao J, Taveira-DaSilva AM, Colby TV, Moss J. CT grading of lung disease in Lymphangioleiomyomatosis. *AJR Am J Roentgenol.* 2012;199:787.
62. Avila NA, Bechtle J, Dwyer AJ, Ferrans VJ, Moss J. Lymphangioleiomyomatosis: CT of diurnal variation of lymphangioleiomyomas. *Radiology.* 2001;221:415–421.
63. Avila NA, Dwyer AJ, Moss J. Imaging features of lymphangioleiomyomatosis: diagnostic pitfalls. *AJR Am J Roentgenol.* 2011;196:982–986.
64. Harari S, Torre O, Cassandro R, Taveira-DaSilva AM, Moss J. Bronchoscopic diagnosis of Langerhans cell histiocytosis and lymphangioleiomyomatosis. *Respir Med.* 2012;106:1286–1292.
65. Meraj R, Wikenheiser-Brokamp KA, Young LR, Byrnes S, McCormack FX. Utility of transbronchial lung biopsy in the diagnosis of lymphangioleiomyomatosis. *Front Med.* 2012;6:395–405.
66. Johnson SR, Cordier JF, Lazor R, et al; Review Panel of the ERS LAM Task Force. European Respiratory Society guidelines for the diagnosis and management of lymphangioleiomyomatosis. *Eur Respir J.* 2010;35:14–26.
67. Seyama K, Kumasaka T, Souma S, et al. Vascular endothelial growth factor-D is increased in serum of patients with lymphangioleiomyomatosis. *Lymphat Res Biol.* 2006;4:143–152.
68. Glasgow CG, Avila NA, Lin JP, Stylianou MP, Moss J. Serum vascular endothelial growth factor-D levels in patients with lymphangioleiomyomatosis reflect lymphatic involvement. *Chest.* 2009;135:1293–1300.
69. Young LR, Vandyke R, Gulleman PM, et al. Serum vascular endothelial growth factor-D prospectively distinguishes lymphangioleiomyomatosis from other diseases. *Chest.* 2010; 138:674–681.
70. Chang WY, Cane JL, Blakey JD, Kumaran M, Pointon KS, Johnson SR. Clinical utility of diagnostic guidelines and putative biomarkers in lymphangioleiomyomatosis. *Respir Res.* 2012; 13:34.
71. Oprescu N, McCormack FX, Byrnes S, Kinder BW. Clinical predictors of mortality and cause of death in lymphangioleiomyomatosis: a population-based registry. *Lung.* 2013;191:35–42.
72. Johnson SR, Tattersfield AE. Decline in lung function in lymphangioleiomyomatosis: relation to menopause and progesterone treatment. *Am J Respir Crit Care Med.* 1999;160: 628–633.
73. Kitaichi M, Nishimura K, Itoh H, Izumi T. Pulmonary lymphangiomyomatosis: a report of 46 patients including a clinicopathologic study of prognostic factors. *Am J Respir Crit Care Med.* 1995;151:527–533.
74. Matsui K, Beasley MB, Nelson WK, et al. Prognostic significance of pulmonary lymphangioleiomyomatosis histologic score. *Am J Surg Pathol.* 2001;25:479–484.
75. Taveira-DaSilva AM, Hedin CJ, Stylianou MP, et al. Reversible airflow obstruction, proliferation of abnormal smooth muscle cells and impairment of gas exchange as predictors of outcome in lymphangioleiomyomatosis. *Am J Respir Crit Care Med.* 2001;164:1072–1076.
76. Taveira-Dasilva AM, Steagall WK, Rabel A, et al. Reversible airflow obstruction in Lymphangioleiomyomatosis. *Chest.* 2009; 136:1596–1603.
77. Lazor R, Valeyre D, Lacronique J, Wallaert B, Urban T, Cordier JF; Groupe d'Etudes et de Recherche sur les Maladies "Orphelines" Pulmonaires. Low initial KCO predicts rapid FEV1 decline in pulmonary lymphangioleiomyomatosis. *Respir Med.* 2004;98:536–541.
78. Hayashida M, Seyama K, Inoue Y, Fujimoto K, Kubo K; Respiratory Failure Research Group of the Japanese Ministry of Health, Labor, and Welfare. The epidemiology of lymphangioleiomyomatosis in Japan: a nationwide cross-sectional study of presenting features and prognostic factors. *Respirology.* 2007;12:523–530.
79. Seyama K, Kumasaka T, Kurihara M, Mitani K, Sato T. Lymphangioleiomyomatosis: a disease involving the lymphatic system. *Lymphat Res Biol.* 2010;8:21–31.
80. Kumasaka T, Seyama K, Mitani K, et al. Lymphangiogenesis in lymphangioleiomyomatosis. Its implication in the progression of lymphangioleiomyomatosis. *Am J Surg Pathol.* 2004;28: 1007–1016.
81. Eliasson AH, Phillips YY, Tenholder MF. Treatment of lymphangioleiomyomatosis:a meta-analysis. *Chest.* 1989;96: 1352–1355.
82. Harari S, Cassandro R, Chiodini J, Taveira-DaSilva AM, Moss J. Effect of a gonadotrophin-releasing hormone analogue on lung function in lymphangioleiomyomatosis. *Chest.* 2007;133:448–454.
83. Baldi BG, Medeiros Junior P, Pimenta SP, Lopes RI, Kairalla RA, Carvalho CR. Evolution of pulmonary function after treatment with goserelin in patients with lymphangioleiomyomatosis. *J Bras Pneumol.* 2011;37:375–379.
84. Rosner M, Hanneder M, Siegel N, Valli A, Hengstschläger M. The tuberous sclerosis gene products hamartin and tuberin are multifunctional proteins with a wide spectrum of interacting partners. *Mutat Res.* 2008;658:234–246.
85. Sengupta S, Peterson TR, Sabatini DM. Regulation of the mTOR complex 1 pathway by nutrients, growth factors, and stress. *Mol Cell.* 2012;40:310–322.
86. Sarbassov DD, Ali SM, Kim DH, et al. Rictor, a novel binding partner of mTOR, defines a rapamycin-insensitive and raptor-independent pathway that regulates the cystoskeleton. *Curr Biol.* 2004;14:1296–1302.
87. Hung J, Manning BD. A complex interplay between Akt, TSC2 and the mTOR complexes. *Biochem Soc Trans.* 2009;37: 217–222.
88. Krymskaya VP, Goncharova EA. PI3 K/mTORC1 activation in hamartoma syndromes, therapeutic prospects. *Cell Cycle.* 2009;8:403–413.
89. Sarbassov DD, Ali SM, Sengupta S, et al. Prolonged rapamycin treatment inhibits mTORC2 assembly and Akt/PKB. *Mol Cell.* 2006;22:159–168.
90. Zeng Z, Sarbassov DD, Samudio IJ, et al. Rapamycin derivatives reduce mTORC2 signaling and inhibit Akt activation in AML. *Blood.* 2007;109:3509–3512.
91. Kenerson H, Dundon TA, Yeung RS. Effects of rapamycin in the Eker rat model of tuberous sclerosis complex. *Pediatr Res.* 2005;57:67–75.
92. Lee L, Sudentas P, Donohue B, et al. Efficacy of a rapamycin analog (CCI-779) and IFN-gamma in tuberous sclerosis mouse models. *Genes Chromosomes Cancer.* 2005;42:213–227.
93. Bissler JJ, McCormack FX, Young LR, et al. Sirolimus for angiomyolipoma in tuberous sclerosis complex or lymphangioleiomyomatosis. *N Engl J Med.* 2008;358:140–151.
94. Davies DM, de Vries PJ, Johnson SR, et al. Sirolimus therapy for angiomyolipoma in tuberous sclerosis and sporadic

lymphangioleiomyomatosis: a phase 2 trial. *Clin Cancer Res.* 2011;17:4071–4081.

95. Dabora SL, Franz DN, Ashwal S, et al. Multicenter phase 2 trial of sirolimus for tuberous sclerosis: kidney angiomyolipomas and other tumors regress and VEGF- D levels decrease. *PLoS One.* 2011;6(9):e23379.
96. Bissler JJ, Kingswood JC, Radzikowska E, et al. Everolimus for angiomyolipoma associated with tuberous sclerosis complex or sporadic lymphangioleiomyomatosis (EXIST-2): a multicentre, randomised, double-blind, placebo-controlled trial. *Lancet.* 2013;381(9869):817–824.
97. Krueger DA, Care MM, Holland K, et al. Everolimus for subependymal giant-cell astrocytomas in tuberous sclerosis. *N Engl J Med.* 2010;363:1801–1811.
98. Franz DN, Belousova E, Sparagana S, et al. Efficacy and safety of everolimus for subependymal giant cell astrocytomas associated with tuberous sclerosis complex (EXIST-1): a multicentre, randomised, placebo-controlled phase 3 trial. *Lancet.* 2013;381(9861):125–132.
99. McCormack FX, Inoue Y, Moss J, et al; National Institutes of Health Rare Lung Diseases Consortium; MILES Trial Group. Efficacy and safety of sirolimus in lymphangioleiomyomatosis. *N Engl J Med.* 2011;364:1595–1606.
100. Taveira-DaSilva AM, Hathaway O, Stylianou M, Moss J. Changes in lung function and chylous effusions in patients with lymphangioleiomyomatosis treated with sirolimus. *Ann Intern Med.* 2011;154:797–805.
101. Neurohr C, Hoffmann AL, Huppmann P, et al. Is sirolimus a therapeutic option for patients with progressive pulmonary lymphangioleiomyomatosis? *Respir Res.* 2011;12:66.
102. Chang WY, Clements D, Johnson SR. Effect of doxycycline on proliferation, MMP production, and adhesion in LAM-related cells. *Am J Physiol Lung Cell Mol Physiol.* 2010;299:L393–L400.
103. Moir LM, Ng HY, Poniris MH, et al. Doxycycline inhibits matrix metalloproteinase-2 secretion from tsc2-null mouse embryonic fibroblasts and lymphangioleiomyomatosis cells. *Br J Pharmacol.* 2011;164:83–92.
104. Moses MA, Harper J, Folkman J. Doxycycline treatment for lymphangioleiomyomatosis with urinary monitoring for MMPs. *N Engl J Med.* 2006;324:2621–2622.
105. Pimenta SP, Baldi BG, Acencio MM, Kairalla RA, Carvalho CR. Doxycycline use in patients with lymphangioleiomyomatosis, safety and efficacy in metalloproteinase blockade. *J Bras Pneumol.* 2011;37:424–430.

105A. Chang WY, Cane JL, Kumaran M, Lewis S, Tattersfield AE, Johnson SR. A 2-year randomised placebo-controlled trial of doxycycline for lymphangioleiomyomatosis. *Eur Respir J.* 2014; 43:1114–23.

106. Goncharova EA, Goncharov DA, Li H, et al. MTORC2 is required for proliferation and survival of TSC2-null cells. *Mol Cell Biol.* 2011;31:2484–2498.
107. Finlay GA, Malhowski AJ, Liu Y, Fanburg BL, Kwiatkowski DJ, Toksoz D. Selective inhibition of growth of tuberous sclerosis complex 2 null cells by atorvastatin is associated with impaired Rheb and Rho GTPase function and reduced mTOR/S6 kinase activity. *Cancer Res.* 2007;67:9878–9886.
108. Finlay GA, Malhowski AJ, Polizzi K, Malinowska-Kolodziej I, Kwiatkowski DJ. Renal and liver tumors in $Tsc2^{+/-}$ mice, a model of tuberous sclerosis complex, do not respond to treatment with atorvastatin, a 3-hydroxy-3-methylglutaryl coenzyme A reductase inhibitor. *Mol Cancer Ther.* 2009;8:1799–1807.
109. El-Chemaly S, Taveira-Dasilva AM, Stylianou MP, Moss J. Statins in lymphangioleiomyomatosis, A word of caution. *Eur Respir J.* 2009;34:513–514.
110. Yang ZJ, Chee CE, Huang S, Sinicrope FA. The role of autophagy in cancer. *Mol Cancer Ther.* 2011;10:1533–1541.
111. Pattingre S, Espert L, Biard-Piechaczyk M, Codogno P. Regulation of autophagy by mTOR and Beclin 1 complexes. *Biochimie.* 2008;90:313–323.
112. Mizushima N. The role of the Atg1/ULK1 complex in autophagy regulation. *Curr Opin Cell Biol.* 2010;22:132–139.
113. Takeuchi H, Kondo Y, Fujiwara K, et al. Synergistic augmentation of rapamycin-induced autophagy in malignant glioma cells by phosphatidylinositol 3-kinase/protein kinase B inhibitors. *Cancer Res.* 2005;65:3336–3346.
114. Yu J, Parkhitko AA, Henske EP. Mammalian target of rapamycin signaling and autophagy: roles in lymphangioleiomyomatosis therapy. *Proc Am Thorac Soc.* 2010;7:48–53.
115. Parkhitko A, Myachina F, Morrison TA, et al. Tumorigenesis in tuberous sclerosis complex is autophagy and p62/sequestosome 1 (SQSTM1)-dependent. *Proc Natl Acad Sci U S A.* 2011;108:12455–12460.
116. Almoosa KF, Ryu JH, Mendez J, et al. Management of pneumothorax in lymphangioleiomyomatosis: effects on recurrence and lung transplantation complications. *Chest.* 2006;29: 1274–1281.
117. Taveira-Dasilva AM, Burstein D, Hathaway OM, et al. Pneumothorax after air travel in Lymphangioleiomyomatosis, idiopathic pulmonary fibrosis, and sarcoidosis. *Chest.* 2009; 136:665–670.
118. Jaiswal VR, Baird J, Fleming J, Miller DS, Sharma S, Molberg K. Localized retroperitoneal lymphangioleiomyomatosis mimicking malignancy. A case report and review of the literature. *Arch Pathol Lab Med.* 2003;127:879–882.
119. Wong YY, Yeung TK, Chu WC. Atypical presentation of lymphangioleiomyomatosis as acute abdomen, CT diagnosis. *AJR Am J Roentgenol.* 2009;181:284–285.
120. Lu H-C, Wang J, Tsang Y-K, Lin MC, Li YW Lymphangioleiomyomatosis initially presenting with abdominal pain. A case report. *Clin Imaging.* 2003;27:166–170.
121. Ryu JH, Doerr CH, Fisher SD, Olson EJ, Sahn SA. Chylothorax in lymphangioleiomyomatosis. *Chest.* 2003;123:623–627.
122. Kimura M, Morikawa T, Takeuchi K, et al. Lymphangioleiomyomatosis with chylous ascites treatment successfully by peritoneovenous shunting. *Nihon Kyobu Shikkan Gakkai Zasshi.* 1996;34:557–562.
123. Makino Y, Shimanuki Y, Fujiwara N, et al. Peritoneovenous shunting for intractable chylous ascites complicated with lymphangioleiomyomatosis. *Intern Med.* 2008;47:281–285.
124. Mikroulis D, Didilis V, Bitzikas G, Bougioukas G. Octreotide in the treatment of chylothorax. *Chest.* 2002;121:2079–2080.
125. Makrilakis K, Pavlatos S, Giannikopoulos G, Toubanakis C, Katsilambros N. Successful octreotide treatment of chylous pleural effusion and lymphedema in the yellow nail syndrome. *Ann Intern Med.* 2004;141:246–247.
126. Piha-Paul SA, Hong DS, Kurzrock R. Response of lymphangioleiomyomatosis to a mammalian target of rapamycin inhibitor (temsirolimus)-based treatment. *J Clin Oncol.* 2011;29: e333–e335.
127. Bissler JJ, Kingswood JC. Renal angiomyolipomata. *Kidney Int.* 2004;66:924–934.

128. Williams JM, Racadio JM, Johnson ND, Donnelly LF, Bissler JJ. Embolization of renal angiomyolipomata in patients with tuberous sclerosis complex. *Am J Kidney Dis.* 2006;47:95–102.

129. Wong IY, Shortliffe LD. The management of renal angiomyolipomas in a patient with tuberous sclerosis. *Nat Clin Pract Urol.* 2009;6:168.

130. Sooriakumaran P, Gibbs P, Coughlin G, et al. Angiomyolipomata: challenges, solutions, and future prospects based on over 100 cases treated. *BJU Int.* 2009;105:101–106.

131. Cohen MM, Freyer AM, Johnson SR. Pregnancy experiences among women with lymphangioleiomyomatosis. *Respir Med.* 2009;103:766–772.

132. Fujimoto M, Ohara N, Sasaki H, et al. Pregnancy complicated with pulmonary lymphangioleiomyomatosis: case report. *Clin Exp Obstet Gynecol.* 2005;32:199–200.

133. Pechet TT, Meyers BF, Guthrie TJ, et al. Lung transplantation for lymphangioleiomyomatosis. *J Heart Lung Transplant.* 2004;23:301–308.

134. Kpodonu J, Massad MG, Chaer RA, et al. The US experience with lung transplantation for pulmonary lymphangioleiomyomatosis. *J Heart Lung Transplant.* 2005;24:1247–1253.

135. Maurer JR, Ryu J, Beck G, et al; National Heart, Lung, and Blood Institute LAM Registry Study Group. Lung transplantation in the management of patients with lymphangioleiomyomatosis: baseline data from the NHLBI LAM Registry. *J Heart Lung Transplant.* 2007;26:1293–1299.

136. Benden C, Rea F, Behr J, Corris PA, et al. Lung transplantation for lymphangioleiomyomatosis: the European experience. *J Heart Lung Transplant.* 2009;28:1–7.

137. Dwyer JM, Hickie JB, Garvan J. Pulmonary tuberous sclerosis. Report of three patients and a review of the literature. *Q J Med.* 1971;40:115–125.

138. Shepherd CW, Gomez MR, Lie JT, Crowson CS. Causes of death in patients with tuberous sclerosis. *Mayo Clin Proc.* 1991;66: 792–796.

139. Castro M, Shepherd CW, Gomez MR, Lie JT, Ryu JH. Pulmonary tuberous sclerosis. *Chest.* 1995;107:189–195.

140. Hancock E, Tomkins S, Sampson J, Osborne J. Lymphangioleiomyomatosis and tuberous sclerosis. *Respir Med.* 2002;96:7–13.

141. Costello LC, Hartman TE, Ryu JH. High frequency of pulmonary lymphangioleiomyomatosis in women with tuberous sclerosis complex. *Mayo Clin Proc.* 2000;75:591–594.

142. Moss J, Avila N, Barnes PM, et al. Prevalence and clinical characteristics of lymphangioleiomyomatosis (LAM) in patients with tuberous sclerosis complex. *Am J Respir Crit Care Med.* 2001;163:669–671.

143. Franz DN, Brody A, Meyer C, et al. Mutational and radiographic analysis of pulmonary disease consistent with lymphangioleiomyomatosis and micronodular pneumocyte hyperplasia in women with tuberous sclerosis. *Am J Respir Crit Care Med.* 2001;164:661–668.

144. Ryu JH, Sykes AM, Lee AS, Burger CD. Cystic lung disease is not uncommon in men with tuberous sclerosis complex. *Respir Med.* 2012;106:1586–1590.

145. Avila NA, Dwyer AJ, Rabel A, Moss J. Sporadic lymphangioleiomyomatosis and tuberous sclerosis complex with lymphangioleiomyomatosis, comparison of CT features. *Radiology.* 2007;242:277-285.

146. Avila NA, Dwyer AJ, Rabel A, Darling T, Hong CH, Moss J. CT of sclerotic bone lesions: imaging features differentiating tuberous sclerosis complex with lymphangioleiomyomatosis from sporadic lymphangioleiomymatosis. *Radiology.* 2010;254:851–857.

CHAPTER 63

Benign Metastasizing Leiomyoma

Gustavo Pacheco-Rodriguez
Angelo M. Taveira-DaSilva
Joel Moss

Benign metastasizing leiomyoma (BML) is a rare disease of women, which is characterized by noninvasive, well-circumscribed tumors composed of differentiated smooth muscle cells, localized to sites other than the uterus.[1–5] Lungs and lymph nodes[6] are the most common sites involved, but BMLs have also been identified in the mediastinum,[7,8] retroperitoneum,[9] vascular channels,[10] bone,[11] heart,[12] skeletal muscle,[13] and soft tissues.[14] Pulmonary BML has been associated primarily with uterine leiomyomas and has been mainly diagnosed in patients who have undergone uterine myomectomy or hysterectomy.[1,4]

The first report of BML, in 1939, described a 36-year-old woman who presented with dyspnea and wheezing. Chest X-rays showed multiple lung nodules. At autopsy, lymph nodes, uterus, and lungs showed nodules of smooth muscle cells with identical morphology[15] and the term "metastasizing fibroleiomyoma of the uterus" was adopted. This term was later abandoned and the name BML was proposed because of the metastatic behavior of this disease.

Pathologically, BML lung nodules resemble hamartomas (the most common benign lung tumor), low-grade leiomyosarcomas, and nodules of proliferating smooth muscle cells.[16] Pulmonary BML is usually asymptomatic and presents with either single or multiple lung nodules of varying sizes.[17] The tumors do not appear to invade adjacent tissues.[18] BML, however, represents a diagnostic and therapeutic challenge because of its pathogenesis and metastatic potential.

EPIDEMIOLOGY

The occurrence and prevalence of pulmonary BML is unknown. There are over 100 cases of BML reported in the literature but only a few studies reported more than one case. BML is a rare disease, found primarily in premenopausal women who have undergone surgical procedures for treatment of uterine leiomyomas.[1,4,18] However, cases of lung BML have also been reported in women with no history of these surgical procedures.[19] Leiomyomas, including BML of the lung, may be found in women and, to a lesser extent, in men and children.[20] There is no ethnic or racial preference for BML and this differs from uterine leiomyoma, which is more frequent in African-American women.[21] Cases of BML have been reported from countries all over the world[4,22] including, but not limited to, the United States,[19] Portugal,[23] Brazil,[24] China,[25] India,[14] South Korea,[13] Japan,[26] and Turkey.[6]

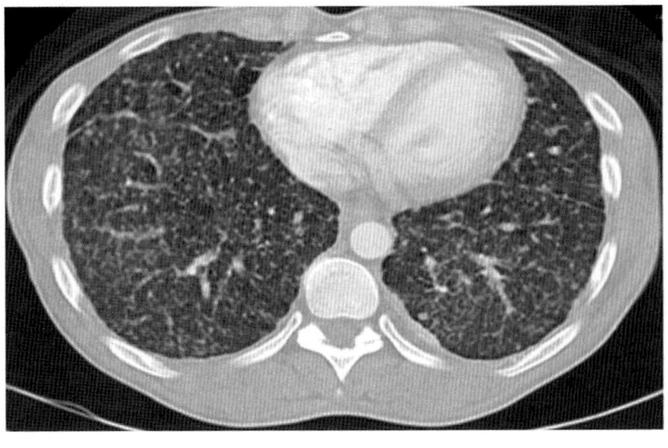

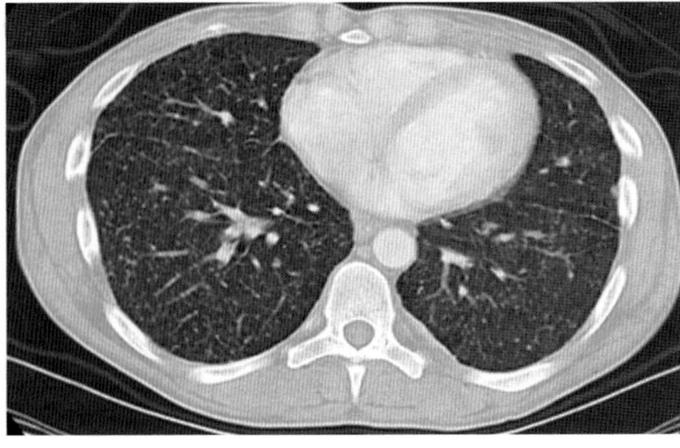

A B

Figure 63-1 Nodular structures in BML. High-resolution computed tomography (HRCT) shows multiple diffuse small bilateral nodules before (**A**) and after treatment (**B**). *(Reproduced with permission from Taveira-DaSilva AM, Alford CE, Levens ED, Kotz HL, Moss J. Favorable response to antigonadal therapy for a benign metastasizing leiomyoma. Obstet Gynecol. 2012;119(2 Pt 2):438–442.)*

CLINICAL PRESENTATION

Most cases of lung BML have been identified as an incidental finding on imaging procedures performed for other purposes (Fig. 63-1).[1] BML nodules may present in premenopausal women as unilateral or bilateral tumors with no specific lobar distribution.[17,27] A number of different types of uterine tumors (e.g., leiomyoma, smooth muscle tumors of uncertain malignant potential, leiomyosarcomas, other smooth muscle tumors, endometrial stromal tumors) are associated with the diagnosis of BML. BML may present with respiratory symptoms including cough, wheezing, dyspnea, and chest pain.[15,17,19,28,29] BML lung nodules have been detected in women in a few months to over 30 years after they have undergone uterine myomectomy or hysterectomy.[30]

PATHOLOGY

BML lung lesions consist of well-circumscribed nodules ranging in size from few millimeters to several centimeters in diameter.[1,4] The lung tumors are composed of well-differentiated proliferative smooth muscle cells that form intersecting fascicles and show positive immunoreactivity toward actin, desmin, and caldesmon (Fig. 63-2).[4,31] Most of these cells also react with antibodies against receptors for estrogen and progesterone.[1,3,22]

Benign lung nodular or mass lesions may be either of epithelial or mesenchymal origin.[32] BML lesions consist of well-differentiated smooth muscle cells, which form lung nodules with low cellularity, exhibiting low mitotic index and no nuclear atypism. The lung nodules do not invade the surrounding tissue and lack evidence of necrosis. Since most of the BML cases are discovered after hysterectomy or myomectomy, it would be important to identify the type of uterine cell causing the tumor. BML cells without a clearly distinct smooth muscle phenotype may exhibit unusual growth patterns.[33] In general, BMLs have been classified as benign tumors of mesenchymal origin.

BML lesions contain vascular structures as determined by anti-CD34 antibody reactivity within nodules adjacent to vessels. BML lesions express variable levels of p53, but the role of this tumor suppressor in BML cells has not been reported.[31] BML lung lesions also show reactivity with antibodies against proliferating cell nuclear

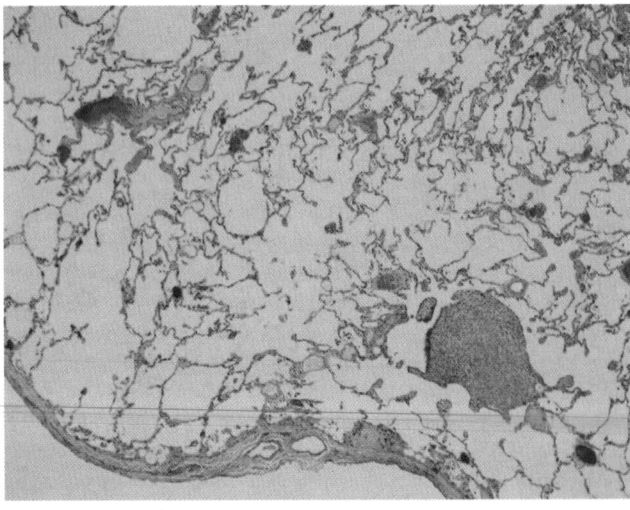

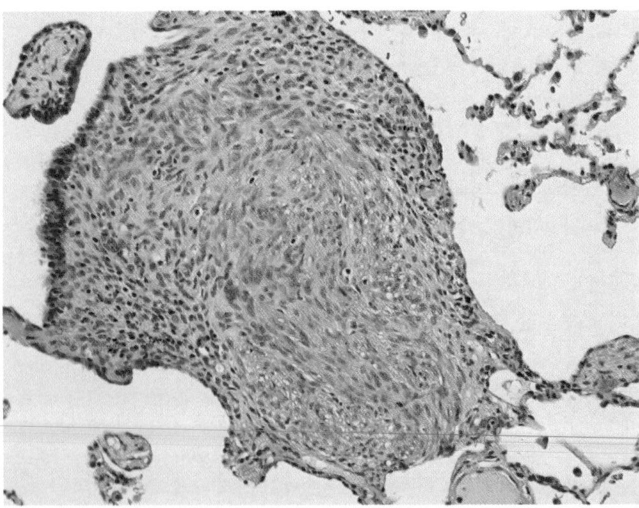

A B

Figure 63-2 Histologic section of proliferative areas of lung BML. Tissue section shows proliferative smooth muscle cells forming fascicles characteristic of leiomyomas and BML. **A, B.** Show low- and high- resolution pictures of lung proliferative nodules. *(Reproduced with permission from Taveira-DaSilva AM, Alford CE, Levens ED, Kotz HL, Moss J. Favorable response to antigonadal therapy for a benign metastasizing leiomyoma. Obstet Gynecol. 2012;119(2 Pt 2): 438–442.)*

antigen (PCNA). In contrast to what is seen in leiomyomatous hamartoma, most of the histopathologic sections of lung BML are not reactive with the monoclonal antibody Human Melanoma Black-45 (HMB-45), which recognizes Pmel17,[31] a melanosomal protein expressed in cells from lung hamartomas, PEComas (perivascular epithelioid cells), and lymphangioleiomyomatosis (LAM).[34] BML nodules are in most of the cases not reactive to antibodies against EMA, CD10, CD117, TTF-1, BCL-2 GPAP, calretinin, and cytokeratin chromogranin. S-100 is expressed at very low levels in BMLs. PEComas of the uterus with pulmonary metastases have a similar presentation to BML but the proliferating smooth muscle cells are mostly nonreactive to HMB-45.[19,35,36] Thus, BML lung nodules appear to have distinct pathologic characteristics.

It has been proposed that leiomyomas should be classified as benign or malignant based on the number of mitotic figures. If 10 mitotic figures per 10 high power field (HPF) are present, the tumor is classified as a neoplasm and if there are more than 5 mitotic figures per 10 HPF it should be considered a leiomyosarcoma. Benign lesions should have less than 5 mitotic figures per HPF.[37] The fact that BML lesions contain less than 5 mitotic figures per HPF, identifies them as a benign tumor.

It is possible to identify cancer cells based on their molecular phenotype,[38,39] however, the molecular characteristics of BML cells remain unknown. Expression of the micro-RNA 221 (miR-221), which has been correlated with different malignancies,[40] appears to differentiate leiomyosarcoma from BML.[41] Molecular assays of X-chromosome inactivation have shown that it is very likely that the lung and uterine cells have a similar origin.[42] BMLs proliferate without telomeric changes, suggesting that their proliferative behavior is independent of telomeric attrition as is the case in other malignant diseases.[43,44] Cytogenetic studies of BML lung tumors have shown that the cells have abnormalities in several chromosomes. BML tumors from five cases showed 19q and 22q terminal deletions.[45] Interestingly, a single case showed multiple chromosomal deletions from cells isolated from different metastatic sites.[46] Rearrangement of the 6p21 region was correlated with changes in the high mobility group A1 gene (*HMGA1*). Chromosomal translocation and mutations have been associated with HMGIC in leiomyomas but they have not been identified in the leiomyomas present in BML patients. It has been possible to correlate the proliferative behavior of BML cells with chromosomal translocations present in other noninvasive tumors.[45–47]

Some of the factors potentially involved in the development of uterine leiomyoma are basic fibroblast growth factor (bFGF), transforming growth factor-beta (TGF-β) and granulocyte macrophage colony–stimulating factor (GM-CSF),[48] although a role for these factors in the pathogenesis of BMLs has not been defined. Analysis of BML tumor cells from different sites suggests a clonal origin.[42] The balanced karyotype of BMLs is consistent with the findings seen with leiomyomas.[49] The clonality of these tumors should be interpreted with caution due to the fact that the founding mutation has not been identified in any case.

PATHOGENESIS

BMLs are considered mesenchymal tumors not mixed tumors of the uterus. Although there are different types of leiomyomas (e.g., mitotically active, cellular, hemorrhagic cellular, atypical, epitheliod, myxoid, vascular, lipoleiomyomas), the type of leiomyoma associated with BML has not been determined. Hamartomas, the most common tumor of the lung, are seen in both genders. PEComas of the uterus with pulmonary metastases may have a similar presentation to BML but these tumors express Pmel7, and are recognized by the monoclonal antibody HMB-45.

The source of the cells that form the lung nodules remains unknown, but due to the strong association with uterine leiomyomas, it is believed that the main source of the cells is the uterus. It has been proposed that those cells responsible for the formation of pulmonary BML are derived from (a) low-grade tumors; (b) cells dislodged from uterus at the time of myomectomy and hysterectomy; (c) metastasis from uterus or an unknown site; (d) proliferation of lung smooth muscle cells; and/or (e) simultaneous-independent development of multiple leiomyomas.

LOW-GRADE TUMORS

Although other tumors may occur in patients with BML including leiomyosarcoma, adenocarcinoma,[50] breast carcinoma, and skeletal muscle tumors, their association with BML is not clear. Leiomyomas of the esophagus, lung, and uterus are found in association with multiple endocrine neoplasia type I (MEN1) but loss of heterozygosity for MEN1 has not been investigated in BML, as is the case in many MEN cases.[51] Tumors characterized as low-grade leiomyosarcomas and high-grade leiomyosarcomas do not appear to metastasize to the lung; these tumors occur mainly in the abdominal cavity.[52] It has also been proposed that BML could be an intermediate tumor stage leading to a malignant leiomyosarcoma[7] but high-grade leiomyosarcomas involving the lung reappear in a short period of time following surgery.[52] Low-grade leiomyosarcomas do not express progesterone and estrogen receptors as is the case in BML. Thus, it is very unlikely that BMLs arise from low-grade malignancies.

CELLS DISLODGED FROM UTERUS AT THE TIME OF MYOMECTOMY AND HYSTERECTOMY

Since pulmonary BML has been associated with hysterectomy and myomectomies, it has been postulated that some of the uterine cells move into the blood circulation at the time of surgery and migrate to the lung where they remain and grow at a slow rate.[18] Lung BML has been associated with tumors in the retroperitoneal cavity,[9] pelvis, and the para-aortic lymph nodes arguing against the passive passage of cells from uterus to lung.[18] The presence of BML tumors in the pelvic region is not in agreement with the concept that uterine cells became dislodged and seeded the lung. Although most cases of BML report multiple pulmonary tumors after hysterectomy, few cases describe the occurrence of nodules before hysterectomy.[53] BML has been correlated with endometriosis as BMLs and endometriosis have a similar course and may develop after hysterectomy or myomectomy.[3,4] Estrogen and progesterone receptors are found in lung BML cells and uterine leiomyomas, which are the most likely source of the cells. However, it is not clear if lymphatics or blood vessels are involved in the metastatic process leading to pulmonary BML.

METASTASIS FROM UTERUS OR UNKNOWN SITE

Due to the fact that BMLs are present in multiple sites, it is possible that either uterine smooth muscle cells or cells from other non-uterine sites metastasize to the lung. Forty percent of leiomyomas or myomas possess specific chromosomal abnormalities.[49] Uterine leiomyomas comprise smooth muscle cells with the extracellular matrix containing a high collagen content. Lung BML nodules however, do not have a high content of extracellular matrix. Leiomyomas contain high concentrations of estrogen[54] and progesterone[55] receptors, which drive the proliferation of cells in response to their ligands. In addition, leiomyomas contain large amounts of aromatase,[56] an enzyme involved in estrogen synthesis.[57] The presence of leiomyomas in lung, lymph nodes, muscular tissue, heart, vascular structures, retroperitoneal cavity, and parietal pleura[58] suggest a metastatic process.[9,12] Leiomyomatosis of the uterus does not tend to metastasize to the lung[59] but BML can present with uterine vascular invasion,[25] supporting a metastatic model. Similar patterns of X-chromosome (human androgen receptor) inactivation suggest that there is a single BML cell source, which is the uterus.

PROLIFERATION OF LUNG SMOOTH MUSCLE CELLS

BML nodules could originate from proliferative lung smooth muscle cells as is the case in primary leiomyoma.[60] However, pathologic sections of a primary pulmonary leiomyoma lacked immunoreactivity for estrogen and progesterone receptors as is found in BML.[61]

SIMULTANEOUS INDEPENDENT DEVELOPMENT OF LEIOMYOMAS AT MULTIPLE SITES

Multiple BML tumors have been identified in some cases and it is possible that they occur independently or via a metastatic process.[13] Since initial mutations have not been identified, it is possible that the mutations occur independently in the different sites. Experimental models to study BML are not available. Interestingly, N-nitroso compounds promoted formation of tumors in lung, reproductive and mammary organs.[62] In fact, chronic treatment of mice with N6-(Methylnitroso) adenosine (m6(NO)Ado) caused tumors in lungs and reproductive tract.[62] These findings support the idea that BML could be promoted by carcinogenic processes.

Metastatic dissemination of BML cells appears to be the most accepted mechanism for localization of BML to the lungs. BML cells could metastasize via the lymphatics, hematologic spread, coelomic metaplasia, and intraperitoneal seeding.[3] Galactins have been identified in pathologic sections of BML lesions, suggesting that these proteins could play a role in cell transformation, regulation of apoptosis and cell growth, cell adhesion during metastasis, and regulation of tumor invasiveness.[63] Molecular studies support the notion that BML metastasis to the lung is promoted by the inherent properties of BML cells and is not a mere by-product of the surgical procedures.

PULMONARY PHYSIOLOGY

Few studies have evaluated lung function in patients with BML.[19,29,52,64] In one study, a patient was followed for more than 10 years and serial pulmonary function tests were obtained.[19] Initially, the patient presented with diminished vital capacity and total lung capacity (TLC) without any evidence of airflow obstruction or impairment in diffusion capacity (Fig. 63-3). As the disease progressed, the patient experienced a decline in diffusion capacity that could be accounted by the decline in lung volumes. In response to antiestrogen therapy, an increase in vital capacity and TLC were observed. In this case, the pathophysiologic profile was consistent with that of an interstitial lung disease.

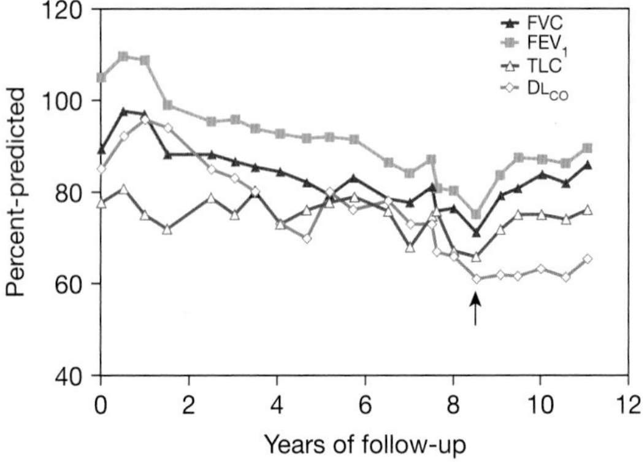

Figure 63-3 Changes in lung function before and after leuprolide acetate therapy. The patient was followed for 8.5 years before therapy and for over 2 years after therapy. Respiratory parameters, for example, forced vital capacity (FVC), force expiratory volume in the first second (FEV_1), total lung capacity (TLC), diffusion capacity for carbon monoxide (D_{LCO}), declined prior to therapy but improved following treatment with leuprolide. *(Reproduced with permission from Taveira-DaSilva AM, Alford CE, Levens ED, Kotz HL, Moss J. Favorable response to antigonadal therapy for a benign metastasizing leiomyoma. Obstet Gynecol. 2012;119(2 Pt 2):438–442.)*

RADIOLOGY

BML nodules may be identified by chest X-rays, computed tomography (CT), positron emission tomography (PET), and magnetic resonance imaging (MRI). The nodular structures observed in BML are well circumscribed. Bilateral pulmonary BML nodules are more common than unilateral nodules. Lung BML may occasionally present with cystic lung destruction.[19] Fluorodeoxyglucose-positron emission is negative in BML and may be used to differentiate BML from other tumors. BMLs and tumors such as adenomas, bronchoalveolar carcinomas, carcinoid tumors, and low-grade lymphomas also have low glycolytic activity.[65] ^{18}F-FDP-PET however, can distinguish a BML from leiomyosarcoma, which is a more glycolytically active tumor and may be found in association with BML.[6] CT and magnetic resonance has also been used to identify BML lesions in the retroperitoneal space and pelvic cavity.[66] Leiomyomas can be easily recognized on pelvic examination. The dimensions and locations of the fibroids may be identified by ultrasound.[67] Since, in most instances the lung nodules are detected by incidental X-rays, a chest X-ray may be warranted after a woman is diagnosed with uterine leiomyomas.

DIAGNOSIS

The differential diagnosis of BML nodular lesions include infectious or neoplastic metastatic lesions.[68] BMLs are usually asymptomatic but may result in lung-related symptoms.[69] Diagnosis requires a compatible medical history and pathologic analysis of biopsies and/or surgically removed tumor. CT-guided, transbronchial or open lung biopsy may be used to establish the diagnosis.[37] Although most cases of pulmonary BML are asymptomatic, some patients present with dyspnea, cough, wheezing, chest pain, chylothoraces, and pneumothoraces. The respiratory symptoms of BML are more prevalent in younger patients. The manifestations of BML in other sites such as uterus, heart, and lymph nodes, for the most part, may be nonspecific. The symptoms of uterine fibroids include abnormal uterine bleeding, pelvic pressure/pain, and reproductive dysfunction. Some of these symptoms have been reported in patients diagnosed with BML prior to myomectomy or hysterectomy.[3,19] BML patients do not present with dysregulated levels of tumor biomarkers, for example, carcinoembryonic antigen (CEA), carbohydrate antigen 19-9, also called cancer antigen 19-9 or sialylated Lewis (a) antigen (CA19-9), carcinoma antigen 15-3 (CA 15-3), cancer antigen-125 (CA-125), cytokeratin 19 fragment (CyFRA21-1), neuron-specific enolase (NSE), alpha-fetoprotein (AFP), hyperglycosylated hCG (HCG-β), beta-2-microglobulin *(β2-MG)*.

Differential diagnosis of BML includes primary pulmonary leiomyoma, primary pulmonary leiomyosarcoma, metastatic leiomyomatosis of an extrauterine source, pulmonary hamartomas, and lymphangioleiomyomatosis (LAM).[1] BML, depending on location, has been classified as intravenous leiomyomatosis and disseminated BML.[9] BML lung nodules have been associated primarily with leiomyomas. Lung hamartomas are associated with other cancers and express the melanogenic protein Pmel17.[70] High-grade leiomyosarcomas may involve the lung. In leiomyosarcomas, the mean time to recurrence is 19 months and metastasis to the lung is seen in 16% of patients for low-grade and 70% for high-grade leiomyosarcomas. Low-grade leiomyosarcomas do not express progesterone and estrogen receptors, which distinguish them from BML. Leiomyomatosis peritonealis disseminata could be one of the confounding diagnoses to consider when a BML patient presents with peritoneal lesions.[9] The slow growth of BMLs could be mistaken by other potential causes of lung nodules for example, infectious processes (fungal, parasitic and tuberculosis), metastatic cancers, benign neoplasms (e.g., chondrohamartomas, hamartomas, BML), amyloidosis, mucoid impaction syndromes, multiple arteriovenous malformation, paraffinoma, plasma cell granuloma, rheumatoid nodules, sarcoidosis, silicosis.[68]

PROGNOSIS

The prognosis of patients with BML is favorable. Although most cases of BML present with multiple pulmonary tumors after myomectomy and hysterectomy, few cases reported the presence of these nodules before hysterectomy.[53] There are only scattered reports where BML was described as a cause of death. Other cancers detected in association with BML could influence prognosis.

TREATMENT

There is no standard treatment for BML. Treatment involves tumor resection and manipulation of hormonal status. Lung tumors may regress at menopause and during/after pregnancy, supporting a role for estrogen in BML.[71] Treatments have been adapted from those used for uterine leiomyoma, and include hysterectomy, myomectomy, dilation of the cervix, uterine artery embolization and endometrial ablation, and scrapping of the uterus (curettage).

Oophorectomy has been reported to improve lung function and cause regression of the lung tumors.[29,64,72–76] Another line of treatment has involved antiestrogenic therapy. Gonadotropin-releasing hormone (GnRH) analogs (e.g., Lupron) have been used to reduce estrogen levels.[10,19,77] Other drugs include the selective estrogen receptor modulators (SERMs), e.g. raloxifene.[24,64,78] Aromatase inhibitors such as anastrozole[64] have been shown to be effective treatments. Progesterone therapy has also proven to be effective.[79–81] However, there have been some cases of BML refractory to progesterone and aromatase inhibitors.[82] Treatments of uterine leiomyoma have also included combination of GnRH analogs and aromatase inhibitors.[64,83] Patients with BML have been treated with a single drug or combination of drugs,[22,83] e.g. leuprolide acetate, letrazole, leuprolide acetate and aromatase inhibitors, and antiprogestin (CDB-2914)[22,83] e.g., In some cases total abdominal hysterectomy with bilateral salpingo-oophorectomy (TAH/BSO) has been combined with drugs. Although bilateral oophorectomy has been the most commonly used treatment, unilateral oophorectomy has been effective in treating some BML tumors.[74] It is important to consider loss of bone mineral density due to antiestrogenic therapies. The slow-growing behavior of BML suggests that these tumors can be left untreated unless the patient becomes symptomatic.

ACKNOWLEDGMENT

This research was supported by the Intramural Research Program of the NIH, National Heart, Lung, and Blood Institute.

REFERENCES

1. Pitts S, Oberstein EM, Glassberg MK. Benign metastasizing leiomyoma and lymphangioleiomyomatosis: sex-specific diseases? *Clin Chest Med.* 2004;25(2):343–360.
2. Patton KT, Cheng L, Papavero V, et al. Benign metastasizing leiomyoma: clonality, telomere length and clinicopathologic analysis. *Mod Pathol.* 2006;19(1):130–140.
3. Awonuga AO, Shavell VI, Imudia AN, Rotas M, Diamond MP, Puscheck EE. Pathogenesis of benign metastasizing leiomyoma: a review. *Obstet Gynecol Surv.* 2010;65(3):189–195.
4. Jautzke G, Muller-Ruchholtz E, Thalmann U. Immunohistological detection of estrogen and progesterone receptors in multiple and well differentiated leiomyomatous lung tumors in women with uterine leiomyomas (so-called benign metastasizing leiomyomas). A report on 5 cases. *Pathol Res Pract.* 1996;192(3):215–223.
5. Bakalianou K, Iavazzo C, Salakos N, Paltoglou G, Papadias K, Kondi-Pafiti A. Leiomyomatosis with multiple extrauterine pulmonary sites: an unusual case report. *Clin Exp Obstet Gynecol.* 2008;35(1):86–88.
6. Sapmaz F, Ergin M, Katrancioglu O, Gonlugur T, Gonlugur U, Elagoz S. Benign metastasizing leiomyoma. *Lung.* 2008;186(4): 271–273.
7. Ogawa M, Hara M, Ozawa Y, et al. Benign metastasizing leiomyoma of the lung with malignant transformation mimicking mediastinal tumor. *Clin Imaging.* 2011;35(5):401–404.
8. Cho KR, Woodruff JD, Epstein JI. Leiomyoma of the uterus with multiple extrauterine smooth muscle tumors: a case report suggesting multifocal origin. *Hum Pathol.* 1989;20(1):80–83.
9. Lim SY, Park JC, Bae JG, Kim JI, Rhee JH. Pulmonary and retroperitoneal benign metastasizing leiomyoma. *Clin Exp Reprod Med.* 2011;38(3):174–177.
10. Arif S, Ganesan R, Spooner D. Intravascular leiomyomatosis and benign metastasizing leiomyoma: an unusual case. *Int J Gynecol Cancer.* 2006;16(3):1448–1450.
11. Kang MW, Kang SK, Yu JH, et al. Benign metastasizing leiomyoma: metastasis to rib and vertebra. *Ann Thorac Surg.* 2011;91(3): 924–926.
12. Takemura G, Takatsu Y, Kaitani K, et al. Metastasizing uterine leiomyoma. A case with cardiac and pulmonary metastasis. *Pathol Res Pract.* 1996;192(6):622–629; discussion 630–633.
13. Jo JH, Lee JH, Kim DC, et al. A case of benign metastasizing leiomyoma with multiple metastasis to the soft tissue, skeletal muscle, lung and breast. *Korean J Intern Med.* 2006;21(3):199–201.
14. Ahmad SZ, Anupama R, Vijaykumar DK. Benign metastasizing leiomyoma – case report and review of literature. *Eur J Obstet Gynecol Reprod Biol.* 2011;159(1):240–241.
15. Steiner PE. Metastasizing fibroleiomyoma of the uterus: Report of a case and review of the literature. *Am J Pathol.* 1939;15(1): 89–110.7.
16. Gal AA, Brooks JS, Pietra GG. Leiomyomatous neoplasms of the lung: a clinical, histologic, and immunohistochemical study. *Mod Pathol.* 1989;2(3):209–216.
17. Wolff M, Silva F, Kaye G. Pulmonary metastases (with admixed epithelial elements) from smooth muscle neoplasms. Report of nine cases, including three males. *Am J Surg Pathol.* 1979;3(4):325–342.
18. Abell MR, Littler ER. Benign metastasizing uterine leiomyoma. Multiple lymph nodal metastases. *Cancer.* 1975;36(6): 2206–2213.
19. Taveira-DaSilva AM, Alford CE, Levens ED, Kotz HL, Moss J. Favorable response to antigonadal therapy for a benign metastasizing leiomyoma. *Obstet Gynecol.* 2012;119(2 Pt 2):438–442.
20. Martin E. Leiomyomatous lung lesions: a proposed classification. *AJR Am J Roentgenol.* 1983;141(2):269–272.
21. Kjerulff KH, Guzinski GM, Langenberg PW, Stolley PD, Moye NE, Kazandjian VA. Hysterectomy and race. *Obstet Gynecol.* 1993;82(5):757–764.
22. Lewis EI, Chason RJ, DeCherney AH, Armstrong A, Elkas J, Venkatesan AM. Novel hormone treatment of benign metastasizing leiomyoma: an analysis of five cases and literature review. *Fertil Steril.* 2013;99(7):2017–2024.
23. Silva I, Tome V, Oliveira J. Benign metastasising leiomyoma: a progressive disease despite chemical and surgical castration. *BMJ Case Rep.* 2012;2012.
24. Benetti-Pinto CL, Soares PM, Petta CA, De Angelo-Andrade LA. Pulmonary benign metastasizing leiomyoma: a report of 2 cases with different outcomes. *J Reprod Med.* 2006;51(9):715–718.

25. Fu Y, Li H, Tian B, Hu B. Pulmonary benign metastasizing leiomyoma: a case report and review of the literature. *World J Surg Oncol.* 2012;10(1):268.

26. Izumiyama N, Miki H, Saito Y, Suzuki H, Kikuchi Y. [A case of benign metastasizing leiomyoma medicating for 14 years]. *Nihon Kokyuki Gakkai Zasshi.* 2011;49(4):271–276.

27. Lefebvre R, Nawar T, Fortin R, Genest J. Leiomyoma of the uterus with bilateral pulmonary metastases. *Can Med Assoc J.* 1971;105(5):501–503.

28. Rao AV, Wilson J, Sylvester K. Pulmonary benign metastasizing leiomyoma following hysterectomy: a clinicopathologic correlation. *J Thorac Oncol.* 2008;3(6):674–676.

29. Banner AS, Carrington CB, Emory WB, et al. Efficacy of oophorectomy in lymphangioleiomyomatosis and benign metastasizing leiomyoma. *N Engl J Med.* 1981;305(4):204–209.

30. Kwon YI, Kim TH, Sohn JW, Yoon HJ, Shin DH, Park SS. Benign pulmonary metastasizing leiomvomatosis: case report and a review of the literature. *Korean J Intern Med.* 2006;21(3): 173–177.

31. Kayser K, Zink S, Schneider T, et al. Benign metastasizing leiomyoma of the uterus: documentation of clinical, immunohistochemical and lectin-histochemical data of ten cases. *Virchows Arch.* 2000;437(3):284–292.

32. Borczuk AC. Benign tumors and tumorlike conditions of the lung. *Arch Pathol Lab Med.* 2008;132(7):1133–1148.

33. Al-Nafussi A. Uterine smooth-muscle tumours: practical approach to diagnosis. *Curr Diagn Pathol.* 2004;10:140–156.

34. Folpe AL, Kwiatkowski DJ. Perivascular epithelioid cell neoplasms: pathology and pathogenesis. *Hum Pathol.* 2010;41(1): 1–15.

35. Huang PC, Chen JT, Chia-Man C, Kwan PC, Ho WL. Benign metastasizing leiomyoma of the lung: a case report. *J Formos Med Assoc.* 2000;99(12):948–951.

36. Yamazaki K. CD10- and CD34-positive periglandular stromal cells in pulmonary benign metastasizing leiomyoma with metaplastic adenomyomatous glands: an ultrastructural and immunohistochemical study. *Virchows Arch.* 2005;446(3):270–277.

37. Kishore R, Richards AP, Evans N. Benign metastasizing leiomyoma. *Clin Radiol Extra.* 2004;59:29–31.

38. Hanahan D, Weinberg RA. The hallmarks of cancer. *Cell.* 2000;100 (1):57–70.

39. Hanahan D, Weinberg RA. Hallmarks of cancer: the next generation. *Cell.* 2011;144(5):646–674.

40. Garofalo M, Quintavalle C, Romano G, Croce CM, Condorelli G. miR221/222 in cancer: their role in tumor progression and response to therapy. *Curr Mol Med.* 2012;12(1):27–33.

41. Nuovo GJ, Schmittgen TD. Benign metastasizing leiomyoma of the lung: clinicopathologic, immunohistochemical, and micro-RNA analyses. *Diagn Mol Pathol.* 2008;17(3):145–150.

42. Tietze L, Gunther K, Horbe A, et al. Benign metastasizing leiomyoma: a cytogenetically balanced but clonal disease. *Hum Pathol.* 2000;31(1):126–128.

43. Armanios M, Blackburn EH. The telomere syndromes. *Nat Rev Genet.* 2012;13(10):693–704.

44. Calado RT, Young NS. Telomere diseases. *N Engl J Med.* 2009;361 (24):2353–2365.

45. Nucci MR, Drapkin R, Dal Cin P, Fletcher CD, Fletcher JA. Distinctive cytogenetic profile in benign metastasizing leiomyoma: pathogenetic implications. *Am J Surg Pathol.* 2007;31(5): 737–743.

46. Bowen JM, Cates JM, Kash S, et al. Genomic imbalances in benign metastasizing leiomyoma: characterization by conventional karyotypic, fluorescence in situ hybridization, and whole genome SNP array analysis. *Cancer Genet.* 2012;205(5):249–254.

47. Hodge JC, Morton CC. Genetic heterogeneity among uterine leiomyomata: insights into malignant progression. *Hum Mol Genet.* 2007;16(Spec No 1):R7–R13.

48. Stewart EA. Uterine fibroids. *Lancet.* 2001;357(9252):293–298.

49. Sandberg AA. Updates on the cytogenetics and molecular genetics of bone and soft tissue tumors: leiomyoma. *Cancer Genet Cytogenet.* 2005;158(1):1–26.

50. Naito M, Kobayashi T, Yoshida M, et al. Solitary pulmonary nodule of benign metastasizing leiomyoma associated with primary lung cancer: a case report. *J Med Case Rep.* 2011;5:500.

51. Carnevale V, Romagnoli E, Remotti D, et al. Pulmonary lymphangioleiomyoma in a patient with multiple endocrine neoplasia type I. *J Endocrinol Invest.* 1997;20(5):282–285.

52. Posligua L, Silva EG, Deavers MT, Merino MJ, Malpica A. Low-grade smooth muscle tumors of the primary and the secondary mullerian system: a proposed concept of multicentricity. *Int J Gynecol Pathol.* 2012;31(6):547–555.

53. Rege AS, Snyder JA, Scott WJ. Benign metastasizing leiomyoma: a rare cause of multiple pulmonary nodules. *Ann Thorac Surg.* 2012;93(6):e149–e151.

54. Brandon DD, Erickson TE, Keenan EJ, et al. Estrogen receptor gene expression in human uterine leiomyomata. *J Clin Endocrinol Metab.* 1995;80(6):1876–1881.

55. Brandon DD, Bethea CL, Strawn EY, et al. Progesterone receptor messenger ribonucleic acid and protein are overexpressed in human uterine leiomyomas. *Am J Obstet Gynecol.* 1993;169(1):78–85.

56. Folkerd EJ, Newton CJ, Davidson K, Anderson MC, James VH. Aromatase activity in uterine leiomyomata. *J Steroid Biochem.* 1984;20(5):1195–1200.

57. Simpson ER, Clyne C, Rubin G, et al. Aromatase–a brief overview. *Annu Rev Physiol.* 2002;64:93–127.

58. Budde RB, Jr, Yankura JA. Leiomyomatosis with a solitary pleural metastasis. *Clin Imaging.* 1989;13(3):228–230.

59. Clement PB, Young RH, Scully RE. Intravenous leiomyomatosis of the uterus. A clinicopathological analysis of 16 cases with unusual histologic features. *Am J Surg Pathol.* 1988;12(12): 932–945.

60. Esteban JM, Allen WM, Schaerf RH. Benign metastasizing leiomyoma of the uterus: histologic and immunohistochemical characterization of primary and metastatic lesions. *Arch Pathol Lab Med.* 1999;123(10):960–962.

61. Cavazza A, Rossi G, Paci M, et al. [Primary leiomyoma of the lung, with clear-cell features and admixed alveolar spaces: description of a case presenting with pneumothorax]. *Pathologica.* 2003;95(2):108–114.

62. Anderson LM, Giner-Sorolla A, Greenbaum JH, Last-Barney K, Budinger JM. Induction of reproductive system tumors in mice by N6-(methylnitroso)-adenosine and a tumorigenic effect of its combined precursors. *Int J Cancer.* 1979;24(3):319–322.

63. Liu FT, Rabinovich GA. Galectins as modulators of tumour progression. *Nat Rev Cancer.* 2005;5(1):29–41.

64. Rivera JA, Christopoulos S, Small D, Trifiro M. Hormonal manipulation of benign metastasizing leiomyomas: report of two cases and review of the literature. *J Clin Endocrinol Metab.* 2004;89(7):3183–3188.

65. Lin X, Fan W, Lang P, Hu Y, Zhang X, Sun X. Benign metastasizing leiomyoma identified using 18 F-FDG PET/CT. *Int J Gynaecol Obstet*. 2010;110(2):154–156.

66. Park BK, Kim SH, Moon MH. Benign metastasizing leiomyoma involving multiple sites: CT and MR findings. *Eur J Radiol Extra*. 2003;48:19–22.

67. Van Voorhis B. A 41-year-old woman with menorrhagia, anemia, and fibroids: review of treatment of uterine fibroids. *JAMA*. 2009;301(1):82–93.

68. Allen MS. Multiple benign lung tumors. *Semin Thorac Cardiovasc Surg*. 2003;15(3):310–314.

69. Abramson S, Gilkeson RC, Goldstein JD, Woodard PK, Eisenberg R, Abramson N. Benign metastasizing leiomyoma: clinical, imaging, and pathologic correlation. *AJR Am J Roentgenol*. 2001; 176(6):1409–1413.

70. Abe Y, Shioya S, Ohshika Y, et al. [Clinicopathological study of pulmonary hamartoma with special reference to 6 patients who also had another tumor]. *Nihon Kyobu Shikkan Gakkai Zasshi*. 1996;34(12):1354–1358.

71. Arai T, Yasuda Y, Takaya T, Shibayama M. Natural decrease of benign metastasizing leiomyoma. *Chest*. 2000;117(3):921–922.

72. Abu-Rustum NR, Curtin JP, Burt M, Jones WB. Regression of uterine low-grade smooth-muscle tumors metastatic to the lung after oophorectomy. *Obstet Gynecol*. 1997;89(5 Pt 2): 850–852.

73. Ni Y, Shi G, Wan H, Shen J, Jiang X, Yuan F. Pulmonary benign metastasizing leiomyoma: case report and review of the literature. *Clin Exp Obstet Gynecol*. 2012;39(2):249–251.

74. Awonuga AO, Rotas M, Imudia AN, Choi C, Khulpateea N. Recurrent benign metastasizing leiomyoma after hysterectomy and bilateral salpingo-oophorectomy. *Arch Gynecol Obstet*. 2008;278(4):373–376.

75. Evans AJ, Wiltshaw E, Kochanowski SJ, Macfarlane A, Sears RT. Metastasizing leiomyoma of the uterus and hormonal manipulations. Case report. *Br J Obstet Gynaecol*. 1986;93(6):646–648.

76. Uchida T, Tokumaru T, Kojima H, Nakagawaji K, Imaizumi M, Abe T. A case of multiple leiomyomatous lesions of the lung: an analysis of flow cytometry and hormone receptors. *Surg Today*. 1992;22(3):265–268.

77. Hague WM, Abdulwahid NA, Jacobs HS, Craft I. Use of LHRH analogue to obtain reversible castration in a patient with benign metastasizing leiomyoma. *Br J Obstet Gynaecol*. 1986;93(5): 455–460.

78. Riggs BL, Hartmann LC. Selective estrogen-receptor modulators – mechanisms of action and application to clinical practice. *N Engl J Med*. 2003;348(7):618–629.

79. Motegi M, Takayanagi N, Sando Y, et al. [A case of so-called benign metastasizing leiomyoma responsive to progesterone]. *Nihon Kyobu Shikkan Gakkai Zasshi*. 1993;31(7):890–895.

80. Beck MM, Biswas B, D'Souza A, Kumar R. Benign metastasising leiomyoma after hysterectomy and bilateral salpingo-oophorectomy. *Hong Kong Med J*. 2012;18(2):153–155.

81. Londero AP, Perego P, Mangioni C, Lelle RJ, Londero F, Marchesoni D. Locally relapsed and metastatic uterine leiomyoma: a case report. *J Med Case Rep*. 2008;2:308.

82. Abramson S, Gilkeson RC. Multiple pulmonary nodules in an asymptomatic patient. *Chest*. 1999;116(1):245–247.

83. Martinez AM, Chason RJ, DeCherney AH, Venkatesan AM, Elkas J, Armstrong A. Medical treatment of benign metastasizing leiomyoma: a case series. *Fertil Steril*. 2010;94(4):S220.

CHAPTER 64

Depositional Diseases of the Lungs

Robert J. Homer

INTRODUCTION

Deposits of endogenous body constituents or exogenous materials in amounts sufficient to deform structure and impair function can occur virtually anywhere in the body. Deposits of endogenous materials in the lungs or airways cause a variety of diseases (Table 64-1). These may have different clinical manifestations, depending on localization (i.e., pulmonary parenchyma or conducting airways). This chapter deals with a few of these manifestations: amyloidosis; diffuse pulmonary calcification; alveolar microlithiasis; diffuse alveolar hemorrhage (DAH) syndromes; and idiopathic pulmonary hemosiderosis. Others are discussed elsewhere in this text.

AMYLOIDOSIS

Characteristics of amyloid and the various forms of pulmonary amyloid are considered below.

NATURE OF AMYLOID

Amyloidosis refers to the extracellular deposition of amyloid, a fibrillar, proteinaceous, insoluble material that has characteristic light, ultrastructural, and histochemical features (Fig. 64-1). Electron microscopic examination of amyloid reveals a dominant (95%) fibrillar component with distinctive periodicity, associated with a lesser (5%) pentagonal doughnut-shaped glycoprotein component, physically and chemically identical in all forms of amyloid, which is derived from a soluble plasma protein, soluble amyloid P protein (SAP). Amyloid also includes various glycosaminoglycans and certain apolipoproteins (E and J). Radiographic diffraction studies of amyloid show the fibrils to be arrayed in a β-pleated sheet configuration.

TABLE 64-1 Depositional Diseases of the Lungs

Biologic Material	Disease
Interstitial Deposition	
Amyloid	Amyloidosis
Water	Interstitial edema
Calcium	Metastatic calcification
Alveolar Deposition	
Surfactant	Alveolar proteinosis
Water	Alveolar edema
Calcium	Alveolar microlithiasis
Blood and hemosiderin	Alveolar hemorrhage syndromes

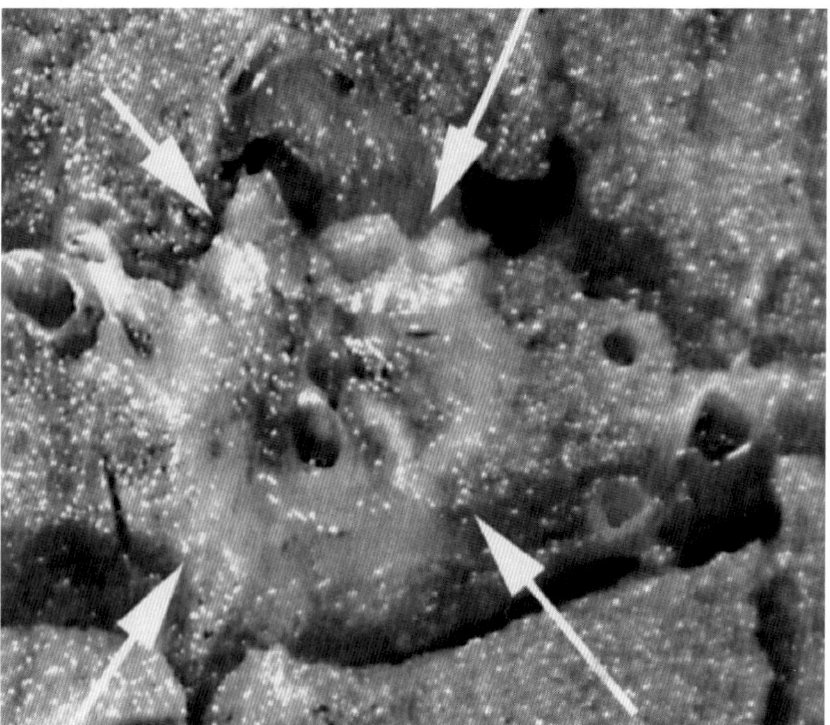

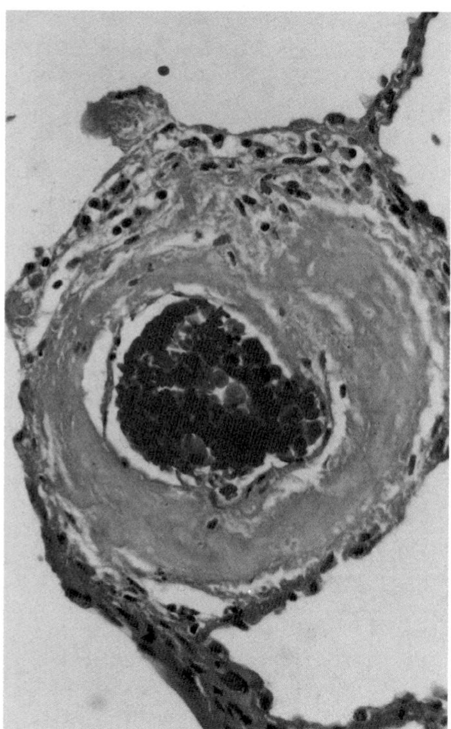

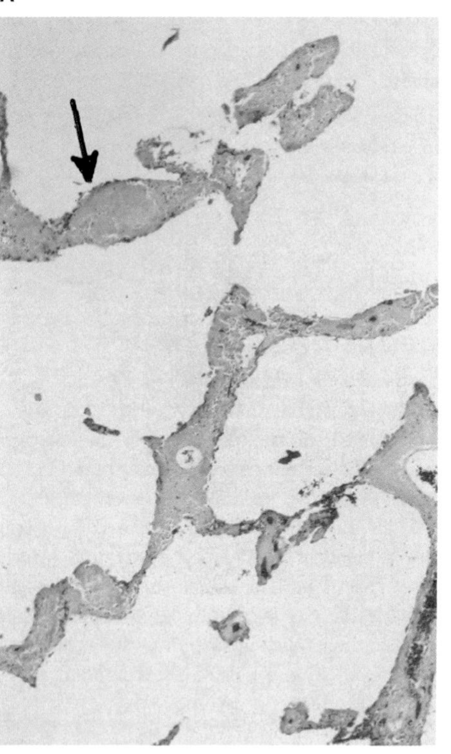

Figure 64-1 Amyloid deposition. **A.** Amyloidoma. Cut surface of lung with *white arrows* indicating a dense, wax-like lesion that is characteristic of nodular amyloid. Incidental finding at autopsy. *(Used with permission of Leslie A. Litzky, MD, Department of Pathology and Laboratory Medicine, Hospital of the University of Pennsylvania, Philadelphia.)* **B.** The typical amorphous appearance of amyloid is seen deposited within the wall of a pulmonary venule. *Green* birefringence on polarized light examination after staining with *Congo red* will confirm the amyloid nature of the deposit (H&E ×700). **C.** Amorphous amyloid in the alveolar interstitial space. *Arrow* indicates a thickened alveolar septum (H&E ×420).

This accounts for the ordered binding of the histochemical stain Congo red such that Congo red–stained amyloid appears apple-green under polarized light.[1,2] When amyloid is deposited in tissues it may produce atrophy of parenchymal cells (e.g., glomeruli), interference with mechanical function (e.g., heart and lungs), or impaired vasoconstriction of blood vessels, leading to hemorrhage (e.g., lungs and gastrointestinal tract). Other mechanisms of tissue injury are also hypothesized including direct tissue toxicity.[3]

While the main fibrillar component of amyloid can be derived from any one of 27 precursor proteins,[2] only a few are common in systemic disease, including immunoglobulin light-chain, serum amyloid-associated (SAA) protein (a family of acute phase reactants), transthyretin (TTR, a prealbumin molecule that binds and transports thyroxine and retinol), and β_2-microglobulin.[1,4–6] The established amyloid fibril nomenclature is based on the chemical nature of the fibril protein, where an A, for amyloid, is followed by a suffix that is an abbreviated form of the parent or precursor protein. These forms of amyloidosis are therefore known as AL, AA, ATTR, and $A\beta_2M$, respectively. An entity related to amyloidosis is light-chain deposition disease (LCDD) in which tissue deposits are also derived from immunoglobulin light chains and are similar to amyloid by light microscopy, but show granular deposition by electron microscopy and do not stain with Congo red.[7] It seems likely that the biochemical properties of the light chain determine the nature of the deposit produced.

AL amyloidosis usually occurs in association with a neoplastic clonal proliferation of B cells or plasma cells which produce a monoclonal immunoglobulin or immunoglobulin fragment (monoclonal gammopathy). The neoplastic clone may clinically manifest as multiple myeloma or lymphoma (generally lymphoplasmacytic lymphoma) or may be subclinical (formerly known as primary amyloidosis), causing bone-marrow plasmacytosis. Most often the protein source is a λ-light chain, either intact or the amino terminal fragment. Amyloid-associated (AA) amyloidosis (previously referred to as secondary amyloidosis) is associated with a chronic increase in serum acute-phase reactants. It was formerly seen predominantly in patients with chronic infections (e.g., tuberculosis, leprosy, and chronic osteomyelitis) but is now seen more commonly with noninfectious chronic inflammatory diseases (e.g., rheumatoid arthritis, familial Mediterranean fever, Crohn disease, and heroin abuse with "skin popping").[1,6] TTR is deposited in familial amyloid polyneuropathies and senile systemic amyloidosis (ATTR amyloidosis).[5] β_2-microglobulin deposition (Aβ_2M amyloidosis) is seen in patients with chronic renal failure on dialysis.

PULMONARY INVOLVEMENT IN AMYLOIDOSIS

It is important to distinguish secondary involvement of the respiratory tract in patients with systemic disease from localized pulmonary involvement with the latter being much less common than the former.[4,8,9] Tracheobronchial amyloid deposition and nodular parenchymal amyloid deposition (amyloidoma) (Fig. 64-1A) most often occur as isolated phenomena, whereas diffuse interstitial deposition is more often seen in systemic amyloidosis. In addition to pulmonary involvement per se, amyloidosis may also cause symptoms in any portion of the respiratory tract or there may be secondary effects from deposition in other organs. For example, deposits in the tongue may be extensive enough to cause obstructive sleep apnea. Persistent pleural effusions may be due to both pleural and cardiac disease.[10] Diaphragmatic deposition may lead to respiratory failure. Pulmonary hypertension is a rare complication.[11] The vast majority of cases of pulmonary amyloidosis can be categorized as tracheobronchial amyloidosis, nodular parenchymal amyloidosis, and diffuse septal amyloidosis.

Nodular Parenchymal Amyloidosis

Solitary amyloid nodules (amyloidomas) are commonly incidental radiographic findings in asymptomatic individuals (Fig. 64-1).[4,8] When multiple, such nodules may be associated with cough, dyspnea, or hemoptysis. These nodules have no distinctive features, although occasionally, they may show radiographic evidence of calcification or cavitation. Usually the diagnosis of an amyloid nodule is made after surgical resection. Occasionally, the diagnosis has been made by transbronchial biopsy or percutaneous fine-needle aspiration. However, surgical excision of one or more nodules may be prudent, since, on rare occasion, amyloid deposition occurs within a pulmonary neoplasm (e.g., a primary neoplasm such as atypical carcinoid or a metastatic neoplasm such as medullary carcinoma from the thyroid). It is possible that advances in biochemical analysis of the amyloid (see below) may influence this decision, but this is not yet commonly discussed in the literature.

Nodular parenchymal amyloidosis most often represents AL. Histologically, the amyloid deposit is often associated with an intense inflammatory reaction consisting of plasma cells, macrophages, and multinucleated giant cells. Interestingly, when the accompanying plasma cells have been analyzed for clonality, they are more often polyclonal than monoclonal. In such cases, the inflammatory cells may therefore be a local reaction to the presence of amyloid, rather than the source of the amyloid precursor light chains. In a few instances, nodular amyloidosis has been associated with a histologically apparent low-grade pulmonary lymphoma. Rare cases of AA amyloidosis have also been reported. Clinical follow-up of nodular parenchymal amyloidosis unassociated with systemic or, frankly, neoplastic disease is generally benign.[8]

Tracheobronchial Amyloidosis

Amyloid deposition in the tracheobronchial tree can produce either plaques or tumoral masses.[4,9] The more common presentation as plaques is diffuse and multifocal, and represents submucosal deposition of amyloid. Diffuse or proximal involvement of the airways is apt to be symptomatic, producing cough, stridor, or hemoptysis. Less commonly, deposition of amyloid in the tracheobronchial tree produces a solitary mass, which mimics an endobronchial neoplasm with signs of bronchial obstruction or hemorrhage. Tracheobronchial amyloid deposition, like parenchymal nodule amyloid, is most often of light-chain derivation and a localized phenomenon. Again, like nodular amyloidosis, this form is rarely associated with systemic disease. Both types of airways lesions can be readily identified by bronchoscopic examination. However, as is the case with amyloid deposition at all sites, with biopsy there is a risk of hemorrhage. Although localized tumoral masses may be treated by excision or observation, more diffuse involvement may be treated by laser ablation, stents, or radiation. Involvement of proximal airway leads to significant mortality while involvement of distal or mid airway has generally good prognosis.

Diffuse Interstitial Amyloidosis

Widespread, *diffuse interstitial amyloidosis* of the pulmonary parenchyma may produce either a reticulonodular or miliary pattern on the chest radiograph.[4,8,12] The deposition of amyloid may involve the alveolar septal interstitium, the walls of small blood vessels, or both (Fig. 64-1B,C). Such pulmonary involvement occurs most often in patients with systemic amyloidosis, derived from either immunoglobulin light-chain or AA protein. Pulmonary interstitial amyloid deposition in secondary involvement is rarely sufficiently severe to produce clinical manifestations but, uncommonly, it may produce progressive dyspnea, hemoptysis, or restrictive pulmonary function tests. It is thought that the morbidity and mortality of diffuse septal amyloidosis in patients with systemic disease is related to concurrent cardiac amyloidosis with which tissue burden closely correlates, possibly explaining why septal amyloidosis by itself in this setting is not of more significance.[4] On the other hand, primary diffuse interstitial pulmonary amyloidosis has been considered to have a relatively poor prognosis.[4,12]

DIAGNOSIS AND TREATMENT OF AMYLOIDOSIS

Diagnosis of amyloidosis requires tissue examination and Congo-red staining and/or electron microscopy. The biochemical nature of the amyloid fibril in patients with systemic amyloidosis cannot be predicted from clinical manifestations alone.[13–18] Even in patients with a known plasma cell dyscrasia, if amyloid is detected, it should not be assumed that this represents AL amyloid since a significant number of patients with familial or senile type amyloid also have plasma cell dyscrasias. Historically, a variety of immunohistochemical and immunofluorescence tests were used, combined with genetic testing; but these commonly required frozen tissue, which were technically challenging and did not always provide an answer. More recently, improved immunohistochemistry and biochemical techniques have become available and are applicable in formalin fixed paraffin embedded tissue.[13–17,19–21] Published data show these approaches are highly robust and generalizable to multiple clinical scenarios although they have not yet been reported in patients with isolated pulmonary disease.

While it is beyond the scope of this chapter to discuss therapy in depth, it is important to note that therapy for systemic disease is entirely dependent on the specific peptide responsible. In cases of systemic AL amyloidosis, there has been considerable progress in treatment with introduction of myeloma type therapy with high-dose prednisone and mephalan therapy combined with use of hematopoietic stem-cell transplantation. Newer agents also appear promising such as thalidomide and related compounds and especially bortezomib which targets plasma cells.[3] In contrast, treatment for AA amyloidosis focuses on the underlying inflammatory disease but may also include small molecule inhibitors.[6] Systemic senile amyloidosis due to deposition of transthyretin (ATTR) has also been approached with small molecule inhibitors.[5] In some cases of hereditary disease, either small molecule inhibitors or organ (liver, heart) transplantation has been explored.[5] The significance of these therapies for lung-limited disease is unclear since localized disease is typically treated with ablative therapy such as stents, radiation, laser treatment, resection, and other localized methods. The more recent systemic therapies have not yet been reported in patients with lung-limited disease.

DIFFUSE PULMONARY CALCIFICATION

Calcification of the pulmonary parenchyma can occur by a variety of mechanisms.[22] Dystrophic calcification refers to the deposition of calcium salts, most often crystalline hydroxyapatite, in dead tissue such as within the healing granulomas of tuberculosis or sarcoidosis. It can also be seen in various other conditions such as in pulmonary hypertension, other post infectious conditions or pneumoconiosis. This type of calcification is usually localized; its distinctive radiographic features are sometimes diagnostically helpful. It is rarely of any clinical significance beyond that of the underlying condition.

Metastatic calcification refers to the deposition of calcium salts, usually amorphous, in normal tissues (Fig. 64-2). This latter type of calcification occurs in association with some derangement of calcium metabolism, such as primary hyperparathyroidism, secondary hyperparathyroidism of chronic renal failure, hypervitaminosis D, the milk-alkali syndrome, sarcoidosis, or increased bone turnover due to multiple myeloma or metastatic carcinoma.

Although metastatic calcification can occur in almost any tissue of the body, it occurs most often in the lungs, kidneys, and the stomach (tissues with more alkaline pH), and the walls of blood vessels. Metastatic calcification in the lungs usually affects the interstitium of the alveolar septa and the walls of bronchioles and pulmonary vessels, sometimes localizing on elastic fibers.

Clinical manifestations of diffuse pulmonary calcification are unusual, occurring most often in patients who are in chronic renal failure, particularly in those on chronic hemodialysis. Radiographically, metastatic calcification usually takes the form of a diffuse interstitial infiltrate, sometimes with fine nodularity. Less often, confluent patchy consolidation mimicking pneumonia may be seen. Although the calcific nature of the infiltrate is often apparent on routine chest radiograph, computed tomography (CT) scan is more sensitive both in detecting the interstitial deposits and in revealing their calcific nature. Moreover, CT scan may also demonstrate calcification of chest wall blood vessels, circumstantially implicating calcification as the cause of pulmonary parenchymal abnormalities. Recognition of the calcific nature of the infiltrate is furthered by scanning with ^{99m}technetium.

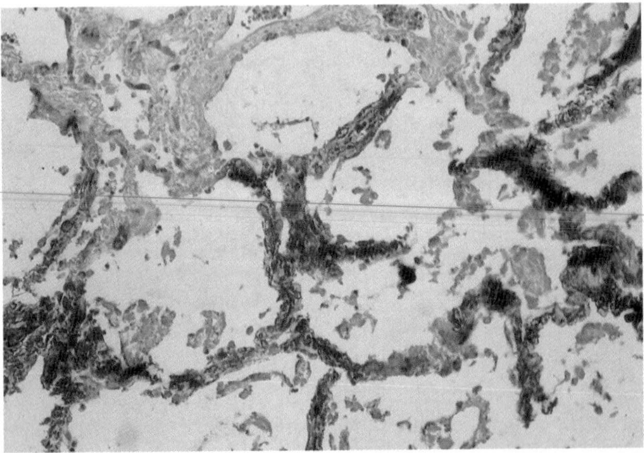

Figure 64-2 Metastatic calcification of alveolar septa in a renal dialysis patient. Photomicrograph shows calcium forming a *dark red* precipitate within the alveolar septa (Alizarin red ×280).

Only rarely do the patients manifest dyspnea or arterial hypoxemia, and pulmonary function tests tend to not show signs of restrictive pulmonary disease. Unexplained dyspnea in a patient with chronic renal failure or hypercalcemia in the presence of a normal chest radiograph should lead to consideration of high-resolution computed tomography (HRCT) or technetium scanning. Rarely, respiratory failure may develop although death from metastatic calcification is typically due to cardiac disease.

The mechanism responsible for diffuse pulmonary calcification is unknown. Although high levels of parathyroid hormone or a marked increase in the calcium-phosphate solubility product occur in some patients, diffuse calcification can occur in the absence of either. Ultrastructural observations of minimal, presumably early, lesions show selective deposition of calcium on elastic fibers, suggesting that they may serve as the initial nidus. In contrast to their apparent role in alveolar microlithiasis, extracellular matrix vesicles do not appear to be involved.

ALVEOLAR MICROLITHIASIS

Pulmonary alveolar microlithiasis (PAM) is a rare autosomal recessive disorder characterized by intra-alveolar accumulation of spherical calcified concretions (called calciferites, calcospherites, or microliths), in the absence of any known calcium metabolism disorder.[23] This disorder usually presents with an abnormal chest radiograph from an asymptomatic patient (Fig. 64-3). Presentation can occur at any age, although symptoms usually occur in third or fourth decade of life. The chest radiograph and/or HRCT are diagnostic, showing a sand-like micronodulation throughout the lung fields. This is caused by the presence of innumerable minute calcified spherules filling the alveolar spaces. Although not usually required, bronchoalveolar lavage or biopsy can confirm the diagnosis. Biopsy shows calcified spherules filling alveolar spaces (Fig. 64-3).

Although usually asymptomatic at the time of presentation, alveolar microlithiasis typically progresses to end-stage lung disease, but the rate of progression is highly variable. When it does, the findings are those of restrictive pulmonary disease or exercise-induced pulmonary hypertension. No therapy has proven effective but lung transplantation has been performed successfully in a few patients.

The disease is due to a mutation in a type IIb sodium-phosphate cotransporter (SLC34A2) gene. As surfactant phospholipids are metabolized, phosphate is liberated and the transporter is needed to eliminate the excess phosphate from the alveolar space. In the absence of this transporter, increased phosphate levels lead to microlith formation. While this is most dramatic in the lungs, other organs can also be affected. The accumulation of microliths ultimately leads to loss of vital capacity by mass effect as well as by inducing underlying parenchymal fibrosis.

ALVEOLAR HEMORRHAGE SYNDROMES

Pulmonary hemorrhage most commonly arises from endobronchial diseases (tumors, bronchiectasis, bronchitis).[24] However, there is a subset of patients in whom bleeding originates at the level of the alveoli and who are referred to as having DAH.[25] Symptoms range from cough, fever, and dyspnea alone to respiratory failure. While hemoptysis is common, it is not universal, even when DAH is severe. In these

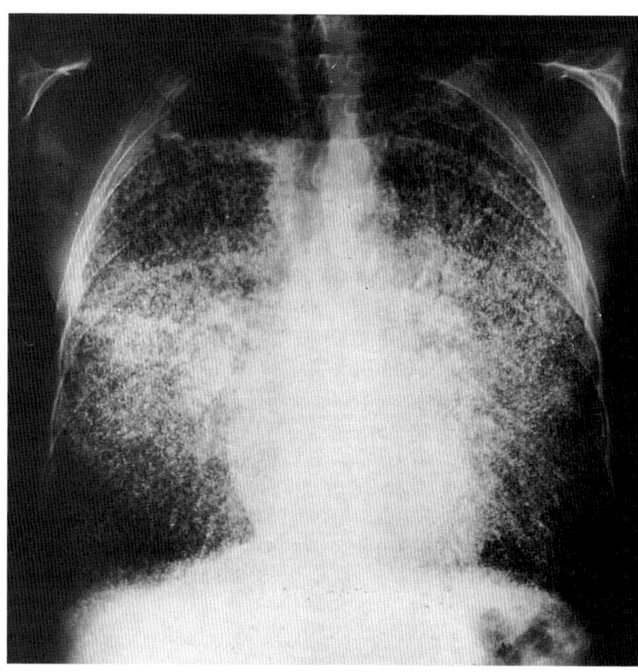

A

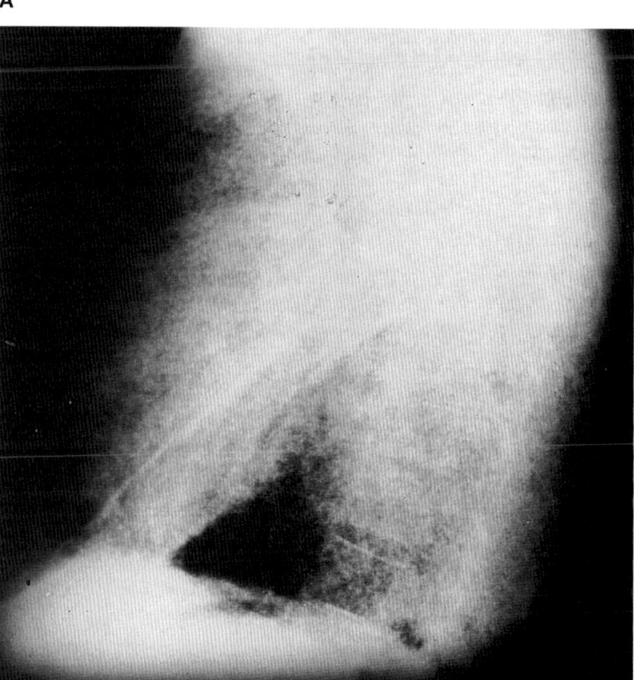

B

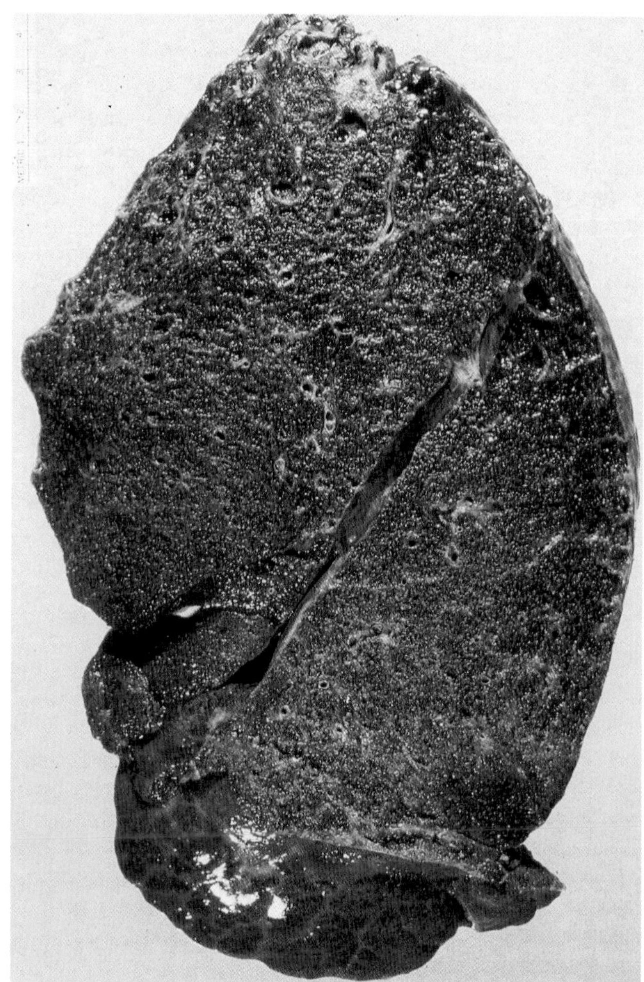

C

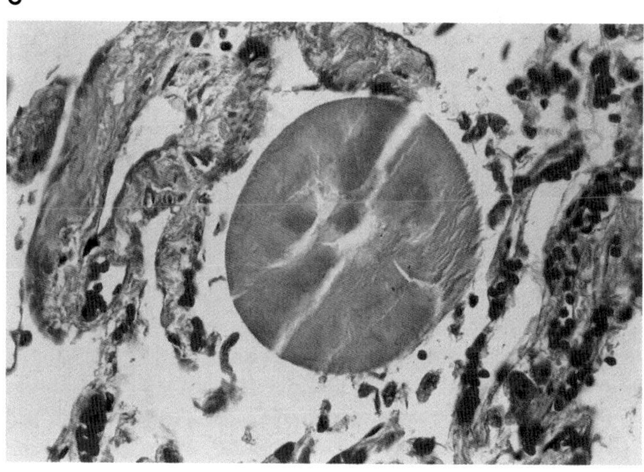

D

Figure 64-3 Alveolar microlithiasis in a 46-year-old man admitted for nonpulmonary problems. History included slight dyspnea on exertion and previous episodes of "pneumonia" in 1947, 1950, and 1952. Clinical examination revealed severe restrictive lung disease, pulmonary hypertension, and cor pulmonale. Diagnosis confirmed by lung biopsy. **A and B.** Posterior–anterior and lateral chest radiographs demonstrate innumerable, tiny calcified nodules throughout both lung fields. Thin, lucent lines on each side represent normal pleura visualized between the calcified pulmonary parenchyma and the chest wall. Emphysematous blebs in the apices displace the calcifications. **C.** Cut surface of explanted lung from a patient undergoing lung transplantation for primary alveolar microlithiasis. Note the fine nodularity which correlated with the chest radiographs. *(Used with permission of Leslie A. Litzky, MD, Department of Pathology and Laboratory Medicine, Hospital of the University of Pennsylvania, Philadelphia.)* **D.** Photomicrograph demonstrating a typical calcospherite in an alveolar space (H&E ×1120).

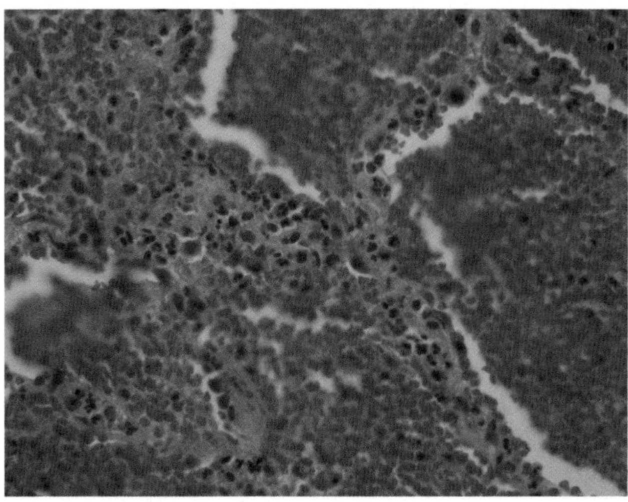

Figure 64-4 Capillaritis as a cause of pulmonary hemorrhage. Note the neutrophils in the alveolar septum (in *center* of image) and the blood and fibrin in the alveolar spaces (H&E ×100).

cases, the diagnosis can be suspected due to a falling hemoglobin level. Evaluation of serial bronchoalveolar lavage aliquots in such patients may show a progressive increase in bloody return, as opposed to endobronchial disease, in which bleeding tends to clear. Bronchoalveolar lavage is also useful to exclude infection in patients with DAH.

The damage to alveolar septa may either be due to immunologic mechanisms (immune complex, antineutrophil cytoplasmic antibody [ANCA], antiglomerular basement antibodies, antiphospholipid antibodies) or to nonimmunologic causes. This distinction is largely, although not perfectly, captured in the presence or absence of the pathologic finding of capillaritis (Fig. 64-4 and Table 64-2).[26]

TABLE 64-2 Causes of Diffuse Alveolar Hemorrhage

Diffuse Alveolar Hemorrhage without Pulmonary Capillaritis
Inhalational toxins (trimetallic anhydride, crack cocaine)
Mitral stenosis
Severe coagulopathy (iatrogenic, renal failure, thrombocytopenia)
Nonspecific inflammation (diffuse alveolar damage, pulmonary gangrene, endocarditis)
Neoplasm/hamartomatous (angiosarcoma, lymphangioleiomyomatosis, tuberous sclerosis)
Pulmonary vascular disease (pulmonary veno-occlusive disease, capillary hemangiomatosis)
Idiopathic pulmonary hemosiderosis
Diffuse Alveolar Hemorrhage with Pulmonary Capillaritis
ANCA-associated vasculitis (granulomatosis with polyangiitis [formerly known as Wegener granulomatosis], microscopic polyangiitis, Churg–Strauss syndrome)
Immune complex—associated with vascular disease (Behçet disease, Henoch–Schönlein purpura, systemic lupus erythematosus, rheumatoid arthritis, mixed connective-tissue disease, polymyositis)
Isolated pauci-immune pulmonary capillaritis
Diffuse Alveolar Hemorrhage with or without Capillaritis
Goodpasture syndrome
Systemic lupus erythematosus
Primary or secondary antiphospholipid syndrome
Drug-induced pulmonary hemorrhage

Capillaritis is characterized by infiltration of alveolar walls by inflammatory cells, usually neutrophils, but sometimes eosinophils or monocytes, with fibrinoid necrosis of the alveolar and vessel wall. However, due to the absence of supporting structures, alveolar necrosis leads to wall breakdown so rapidly that this latter feature may be hard to appreciate. In order to distinguish this process from simple margination of neutrophils, there should be evidence for neutrophils undergoing apoptosis (pyknosis and nuclear fragments). Distinction from infection requires determination that there is minimal accumulation of inflammatory cells within alveoli. The pathologic diagnosis of pulmonary hemorrhage itself requires that there is either hemosiderin-laden macrophages or evidence of hemophagocytosis, since the blood that is commonly seen in lung biopsies may be due to surgery alone. If this evidence is absent, clinical criteria for DAH should be used.

Nonimmunologic mechanisms are quite diverse and include diffuse alveolar damage, inhalation of toxins, coagulopathy, and mitral valve disease, among others listed (Table 64-2).[25] While the presence or absence of capillaritis is a useful way to think about these diseases, the decision about whether to actually perform a biopsy in these cases is challenging as interpretation of these biopsies is difficult, there is potential sampling error, and there is a significant risk of surgery to these patients. These problems limit this procedure's utility while alternative diagnostic schemes usually allow diagnosis in absence of biopsy.

GOODPASTURE SYNDROME

This entity was originally described as an association of alveolar hemorrhage with glomerulonephritis.[27,28] It was later determined that pulmonary and renal damage in many such patients was mediated by antibodies that are specifically directed against a component of glomerular and other capillary basement membranes, most often the α_3-chain of type IV (basement membrane) collagen. The anti-basement membrane antibodies cause pulmonary hemorrhage only in genetically predisposed individuals, after some injury such as cigarette smoke, viral respiratory infection, or hydrocarbon vapor inhalation exposes alveolar capillary basement membranes to the immune system.[29] Although there are other causes of concomitant alveolar hemorrhage and glomerulonephritis, Goodpasture syndrome is generally reserved for disease mediated by antiglomerular basement membrane antibodies (anti-GBM antibodies).

Goodpasture syndrome can present with a broad spectrum of clinical findings. The "classic" patient presents with massive hemoptysis, dyspnea, diffuse alveolar infiltrates on chest radiograph (Fig. 64-5) and overt glomerulonephritis, often with acute renal failure.[30] However, some patients present with only hemoptysis and subsequently develop overt renal disease months or even years later. On occasion, patients present with acute glomerulonephritis due to anti-GBM antibodies and either develop pulmonary hemorrhage subsequently or never develop pulmonary hemorrhage. Without pulmonary hemorrhage, the entity should not be called "Goodpasture syndrome."

The histologic findings on lung biopsy in Goodpasture syndrome are not diagnostic. Routine light microscopy reveals intra-alveolar hemorrhage, usually associated with intra-alveolar hemosiderin-laden macrophages (Fig. 64-5).[24,31] There may be no evidence of vasculitis, capillaritis, interstitial or intra-alveolar inflammation, or necrosis. In some cases, subtle capillaritis may be present. In either case, nonspecific reparative proliferation of the alveolar-lining cells may be present.

While the diagnosis of Goodpasture syndrome can be made by detecting anti-GBM antibodies in the patient's serum, the sensitivity and specificity of various methods to detect these antibodies vary considerably. The gold standard remains the detection of the linear pattern of immunofluorescence on a lung or kidney biopsy. However, only occasionally will immunofluorescence microscopy

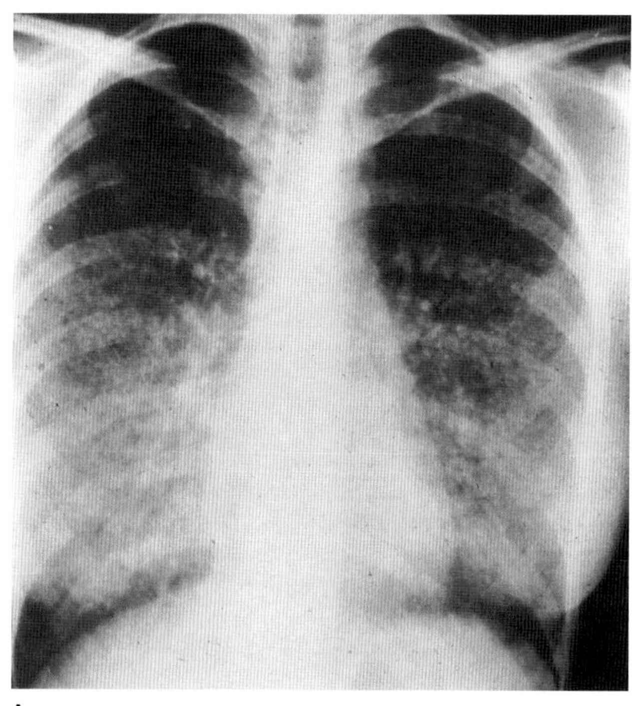

A

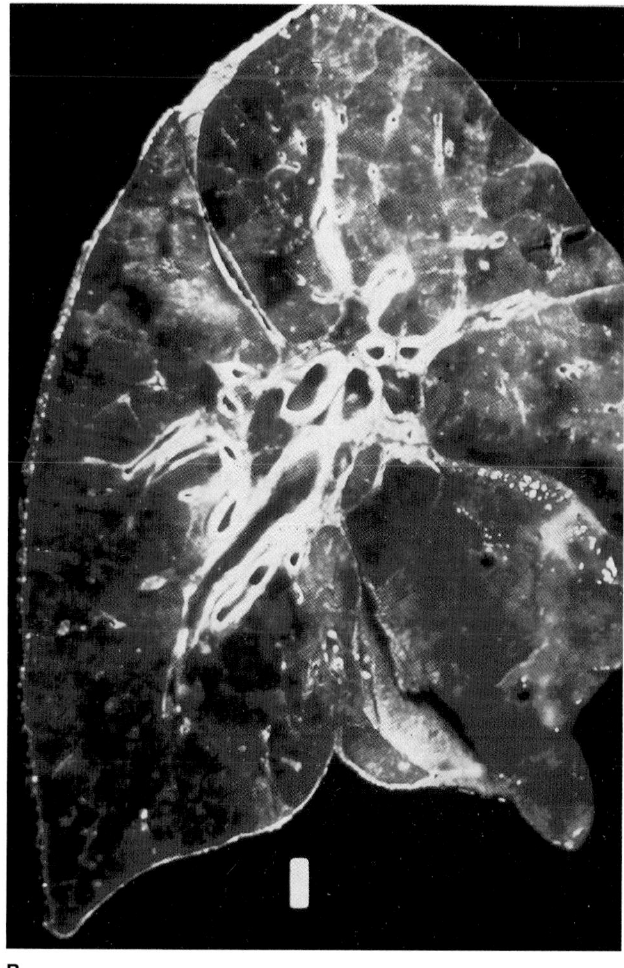

B

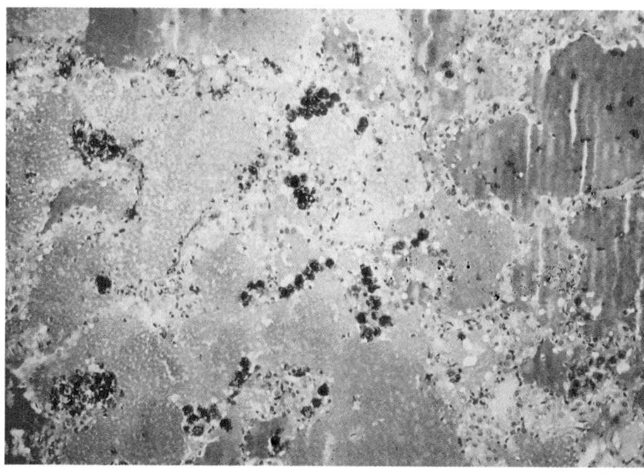

C

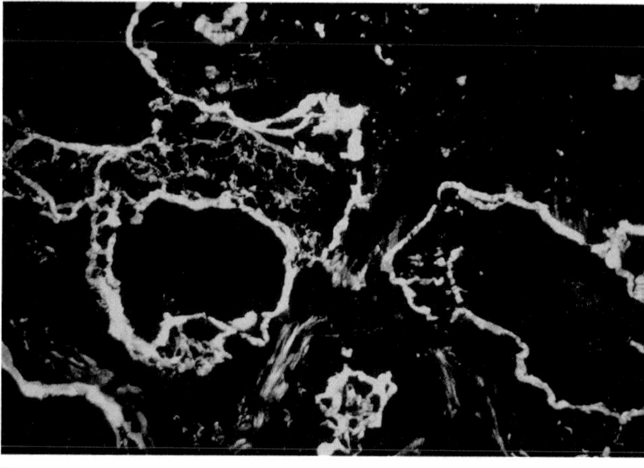

D

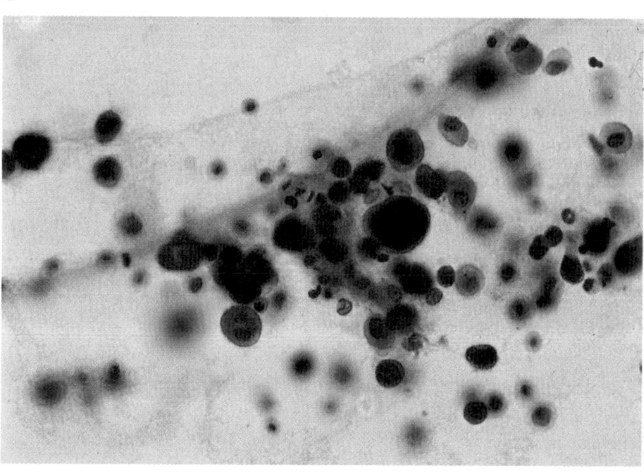

E

Figure 64-5 Goodpasture syndrome. **A.** Chest radiograph showing bilateral alveolar infiltrates, predominantly in the middle and lower lung fields. **B.** Autopsy specimen showing cut surface of lung with massive alveolar hemorrhage. *(Used with permission of Dr. Richard Garnett, Reid Memorial Hospital, Richmond, IN.)* **C.** Photomicrograph of intact alveoli, containing both red blood cells and hemosiderin-laden macrophages (H&E ×45). **D.** Immunofluorescent demonstration of immunoglobulin-lining alveolar surfaces in a uniform distribution (fluoresceinated anti-IgG ×113). **E.** Smear of bronchoalveolar lavage demonstrating hemosiderin-laden macrophages (*Prussian blue stain*; original magnification ×132). *(Used with permission of Dr. David Lyon, lankenau Lankenau Hospital, Wynnewood, PA.)*

show diagnostic linear deposits of immunoglobulin and/or complement along alveolar capillary walls (Fig. 64-5D). In contrast, kidney biopsy in Goodpasture syndrome is usually diagnostic. Conventional light microscopy shows nonspecific focal or diffuse glomerulonephritis which may be crescentic and necrotizing.

When pulmonary hemorrhage due to Goodpasture syndrome is life-threatening, plasmapheresis for rapid lowering of circulating levels of anti-GBM antibody and administration of intravenous corticosteroids and cyclophosphamide to suppress antibody synthesis can be life-saving.[25,28,30] If the patient is not in advanced renal failure at the time of diagnosis, chronic immunosuppression with a combination of corticosteroids and cyclophosphamide can prevent progressive renal damage. If irreversible renal failure has already occurred, the patient can eventually be successfully transplanted once anti-GBM antibodies have disappeared from the serum. Elimination of the antibodies usually can be achieved by immunosuppression alone; in some instances, pretransplant nephrectomy may be required.

ANCA-ASSOCIATED PULMONARY VASCULITIS

The ANCA-associated vasculitides, granulomatosis with polyangiitis (GPA, formerly known as Wegener granulomatosis) and microscopic polyangiitis (MPA), represent the most common cause of immunologically mediated DAH.[25,26,30,32] These have been associated with the development of autoantibodies directed against cytoplasmic components of neutrophils (and monocytes), the ANCAs. Detection of ANCAs entails the use of indirect immunofluorescence and heterologous antibodies against human immunoglobulin to detect autoantibodies bound to neutrophils of affected patients. Ethanol fixation of the neutrophils prior to antibody staining produces one of two patterns when autoantibodies are present: (1) a finely granular centrally accentuated cytoplasmic localization (c-ANCA); or (2) a perinuclear localization (p-ANCA). The usual targets of these antibodies have been identified as proteinase 3 for c-ANCA and myeloperoxidase for p-ANCA. Both antigens are found in the primary azurophilic granules of neutrophils. When ethanol is used as the fixative, the cellular granules are disrupted; the positively charged myeloperoxidase molecules then migrate toward the negatively charged nucleus to produce the perinuclear pattern, and the neutral proteinase 3 molecules remain dispersed in the cytoplasm to produce the cytoplasmic pattern. To maximize diagnostic accuracy, dual testing by fluorescence and an antigen-specific solid phase assay is required. Otherwise, a high degree of clinicopathologic correlation is required for correct interpretation of these tests. Some patients with ANCA-associated alveolar hemorrhage also have antibasement membrane antibodies in the serum. These antibodies are directed against basement antigens other than those seen in Goodpasture syndrome and are thought to be a secondary phenomenon, rather than of pathogenic significance.

Overt DAH occurs in approximately 15% of patients with GPA or MPA. Depending on the specific syndrome present, alveolar hemorrhage may be isolated, associated with glomerulonephritis, or associated with widespread systemic vasculitis. In patients with ANCA-associated vasculitis, the occurrence of DAH is a poor prognostic indicator, although among survivors, complete recovery of lung function is common. Therapy does not depend on diagnosis of MPA versus GPA, and is based on immunosuppression with steroids and cyclophosphamide possibly augmented with plasmapheresis. Nevertheless, patients with GPA/c-ANCA/proteinase 3 have worse outcomes with higher mortality and recurrence rate. While Churg–Strauss syndrome (CSS) is classified among the ANCA-associated vasculitides, DAH due to CSS is extraordinarily rare.

Rarely, patients present with isolated pulmonary capillaritis with no serologic or clinical evidence for a systemic disorder.[33] These patients respond to immunosuppression but relapses occur.

ANTIPHOSPHOLIPID ANTIBODY–ASSOCIATED ALVEOLAR HEMORRHAGE

Patients with serum antibodies directed against membrane phospholipid (antiphospholipid syndrome or APS) display hypercoagulability.[25,34] Clinically, this manifests as peripheral arterial and venous thrombosis, fetal wastage in pregnant women, and thrombocytopenia. Pulmonary involvement can include pulmonary thromboembolism, pulmonary hypertension, diffuse alveolar damage, or rarely DAH. The latter produces fever, dyspnea, and diffuse pulmonary infiltrates on chest radiograph. Alveolar hemorrhage in APS has been associated with alveolar capillaritis with or without immune complex deposition and with microvascular thrombosis in the lungs. The combination of both thrombosis and hemorrhage greatly complicates therapy.

Antiphospholipid antibodies were first detected in patients with systemic lupus erythematosus (SLE) and were formerly known as the lupus anticoagulant because they prolong some laboratory tests of clotting. APS can occur in the absence of SLE. How often these antibodies play a role in pulmonary hemorrhage due to SLE is unknown, as there are other possible mechanisms in that syndrome (see below). In patients with isolated APS and alveolar hemorrhage, corticosteroid treatment, sometimes supplemented by cyclophosphamide, can result in a favorable outcome.

COLLAGEN VASCULAR DISEASE AND IMMUNE COMPLEX–ASSOCIATED PULMONARY HEMORRHAGE

DAH also occurs as a rare complication of certain connective-tissue disease syndromes, most often SLE but also rheumatoid arthritis, progressive systemic sclerosis, and mixed connective-tissue disease.[35] Particularly in SLE, other causes of alveolar hemorrhage must be considered, including infection, uremia, and coagulopathy. When such causes have been eliminated, alveolar hemorrhage is sometimes found to be associated with capillaritis, with interstitial pneumonitis, or with immunofluorescent or ultrastructural evidence of immune complex deposition in alveolar septa. However, none of these disorders are consistently associated with pulmonary hemorrhage in SLE. Early diagnosis and treatment with corticosteroids and cytotoxic drugs are associated with favorable outcomes, although relapse is not uncommon.

DRUG-INDUCED PULMONARY HEMORRHAGE

There is a long list of drugs, both therapeutic and drugs of abuse, associated with vasculitis. The clinical spectrum ranges from isolated mild skin disease to severe multiorgan systemic disease, usually due to a small vessel vasculitis. Some of these drugs can induce an ANCA-associated vasculitis. DAH due to ANCA-associated pulmonary capillaritis is well documented for propylthiouracil, D-penicillamine, allopurinol, diphenylhydantoin, and minocycline. Drug-induced ANCA-associated vasculitis should be treated with cessation of all potential causative agents as well as immunosuppression. Once the offending drug has been eliminated, the possibility of relapse seems low.

NONIMMUNOLOGIC CAUSES OF DIFFUSE ALVEOLAR HEMORRHAGE

There is a wide range of conditions that are associated with DAH with no capillaritis seen on biopsy and which are due to a wide variety of specific conditions, including toxins, neoplasms, nonspecific inflammation, infection, coagulopathy, and pulmonary vascular disease.[25] While all the previously mentioned diseases and syndromes have been excluded as likely possibilities, there still remains a small group of patients who develop recurrent DAH in the absence of extrapulmonary disease and with no evidence of an immune etiology. These patients are considered to have idiopathic pulmonary

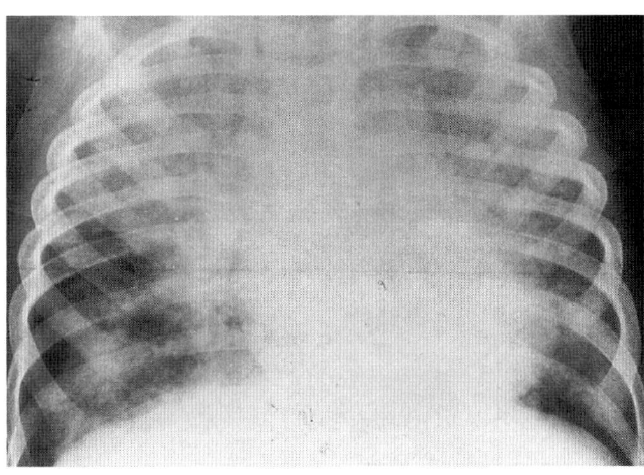

A

B

Figure 64-6 Idiopathic pulmonary hemosiderosis in a 21-month-old child with anemia soon after birth. Iron stain of the sputum showed hemosiderin-laden macrophages. **A.** Chest radiograph showing extensive, bilateral, almost punctate densities throughout both lung fields, most prominent in the perihilar regions where an alveolar filling pattern appears. **B.** Photomicrograph of lung at autopsy, showing intact alveoli containing degenerating red blood cells and hemosiderin-laden macrophages. Immunofluorescence studies for immunoglobulin and complement deposition were negative (H&E ×31). *(Used with permission of Department of Pathology, St. Christopher's Hospital for Children, Philadelphia.)*

hemosiderosis, a diagnosis of exclusion (Fig. 64-6).[30,36] Clinically, the patients form a heterogeneous group with respect to the onset and course of disease, which range from fulminant and fatal to chronic relapse with eventual chronic pulmonary insufficiency due to interstitial fibrosis, to spontaneous remission with little or no residual deficit. The disease usually affects children and young adults. Pathologic examination reveals nonspecific alveolar hemorrhage without evidence of inflammation, vasculitis, or immune complex deposition. Only a few observations on ultrastructure are available. These include focal disruption, smudging, or lamination of alveolar capillary basement membranes.

The pathogenesis of this condition remains unknown, and there are no associated antibodies or other serum markers in the idiopathic cases. However, the clinical and morphologic similarities to some cases of alveolar hemorrhage of known immune pathogenesis, the occasional responsiveness to immunosuppressive therapy, the occasional association with celiac sprue – a presumably immunologic disease of the small intestine – and frequent association with a nonspecific elevation of serum IgA, all point to an as yet unelucidated immune pathogenesis. Rarely, children with hypersensitivity to cow's milk (Heiner syndrome) can present with DAH.

If the diagnosis proves to be idiopathic pulmonary hemosiderosis, high-dose corticosteroid therapy with or without cyclophosphamide and plasmapheresis is useful in controlling acute bleeding, but the long-term effectiveness of these measures in preventing recurrence or progression of this disease is unknown.

REFERENCES

1. Pettersson T, Konttinen YT. Amyloidosis-recent developments. *Semin Arthritis Rheum.* 2010;39:356–368.
2. Sipe JD, Benson MD, Buxbaum JN, et al. Amyloid fibril protein nomenclature: 2010 recommendations from the nomenclature committee of the International Society of Amyloidosis. *Amyloid.* 2010;17:101–104.
3. Merlini G, Seldin DC, Gertz MA. Amyloidosis: pathogenesis and new therapeutic options. *J Clin Oncol.* 2011;29:1924–1933.
4. Berk JL, O'Regan A, Skinner M. Pulmonary and tracheobronchial amyloidosis. *Semin Respir Crit Care Med.* 2002;23:155–165.
5. Ruberg FL, Berk JL. Transthyretin (TTR) cardiac amyloidosis. *Circulation.* 2012;126:1286–1300.
6. Obici L, Merlini G. AA amyloidosis: basic knowledge, unmet needs and future treatments. *Swiss Med Wkly.* 2012;142:w13580.
7. Khoor A, Myers JL, Tazelaar HD, Kurtin PJ. Amyloid-like pulmonary nodules, including localized light-chain deposition: clinicopathologic analysis of three cases. *Am J Clin Pathol.* 2004;121:200–204.
8. Utz JP, Swensen SJ, Gertz MA. Pulmonary amyloidosis. The Mayo Clinic experience from 1980 to 1993. *Ann Intern Med.* 1996;124:407–413.
9. O'Regan A, Fenlon HM, Beamis JF Jr., Steele MP, Skinner M, Berk JL. Tracheobronchial amyloidosis. The Boston University experience from 1984 to 1999. *Medicine (Baltimore).* 2000;79:69–79.
10. Berk JL, Keane J, Seldin DC, et al. Persistent pleural effusions in primary systemic amyloidosis: etiology and prognosis. *Chest.* 2003;124:969–977.
11. Dingli D, Utz JP, Gertz MA. Pulmonary hypertension in patients with amyloidosis. *Chest.* 2001;120:1735–1738.
12. BoydKing A, Sharma O, Stevenson K. Localized interstitial pulmonary amyloid: a case report and review of the literature. *Curr Opin Pulm Med.* 2009;15:517–520.
13. Chee CE, Lacy MQ, Dogan A, Zeldenrust SR, Gertz MA. Pitfalls in the diagnosis of primary amyloidosis. *Clin Lymphoma Myeloma Leuk.* 2010;10:177–180.
14. Lachmann HJ, Booth DR, Booth SE, et al. Misdiagnosis of hereditary amyloidosis as AL (primary) amyloidosis. *N Engl J Med.* 2002;346:1786–1791.
15. Leung N, Nasr SH, Sethi S. How I treat amyloidosis: the importance of accurate diagnosis and amyloid typing. *Blood.* 2012;120:3206–3213.
16. Seldin DC, Sanchorawala V. Amyloidomics comes of age. *Blood.* 2012;119:1795–1796.
17. Brambilla F, Lavatelli F, Di Silvestre D, et al. Reliable typing of systemic amyloidoses through proteomic analysis of subcutaneous adipose tissue. *Blood.* 2012;119:1844–1847.
18. Picken MM. New insights into systemic amyloidosis: the importance of diagnosis of specific type. *Curr Opin Nephrol Hypertens.* 2007;16:196–203.

19. Linke RP. On typing amyloidosis using immunohistochemistry. Detailed illustrations, review and a note on mass spectrometry. *Prog Histochem Cytochem*. 2012;47:61–132.

20. Schonland SO, Hegenbart U, Bochtler T, et al. Immunohistochemistry in the classification of systemic forms of amyloidosis: a systematic investigation of 117 patients. *Blood*. 2012;119:488–493.

21. Lavatelli F, Vrana JA. Proteomic typing of amyloid deposits in systemic amyloidoses. *Amyloid*. 2011;18:177–182.

22. Chan ED, Morales DV, Welsh CH, McDermott MT, Schwarz MI. Calcium deposition with or without bone formation in the lung. *Am J Respir Crit Care Med*. 2002;165:1654–1659.

23. Ferreira Francisco FA, Pereira e Silva JL, Hochhegger B, Zanetti G, Marchiori E. Pulmonary alveolar microlithiasis. State-of-the-art review. *Respir Med*. 2013;107:1–9.

24. Colby TV, Fukuoka J, Ewaskow SP, Helmers R, Leslie KO. Pathologic approach to pulmonary hemorrhage. *Ann Diagn Pathol*. 2001;5:309–319.

25. Krause ML, Cartin-Ceba R, Specks U, Peikert T. Update on diffuse alveolar hemorrhage and pulmonary vasculitis. *Immunol Allergy Clin North Am*. 2012;32:587–600.

26. Lee AS, Specks U. Pulmonary capillaritis. *Semin Respir Crit Care Med*. 2004;25:547–555.

27. Nachman PH, Henderson AG. Pathogenesis of lung vasculitis. *Semin Respir Crit Care Med*. 2011;32:245–253.

28. Cui Z, Zhao MH. Advances in human antiglomerular basement membrane disease. *Nat Rev Nephrol*. 2011;7:697–705.

29. Gibelin A, Maldini C, Mahr A. Epidemiology and etiology of Wegener granulomatosis, microscopic polyangiitis, churg-strauss syndrome and goodpasture syndrome: vasculitides with frequent lung involvement. *Semin Respir Crit Care Med*. 2011;32: 264–273.

30. Ioachimescu OC, Stoller JK. Diffuse alveolar hemorrhage: diagnosing it and finding the cause. *Cleve Clin J Med*. 2008;75:258, 260, 264–265.

31. Lombard CM, Colby TV, Elliott CG. Surgical pathology of the lung in anti-basement membrane antibody-associated Goodpasture's syndrome. *Hum Pathol*. 1989;20:445–451.

32. Manganelli P, Fietta P, Carotti M, et al. Respiratory system involvement in systemic vasculitides. *Clin Exp Rheumatol*. 2006; 24:S48–S59.

33. Jennings CA, King TE Jr., Tuder R, Cherniack RM, Schwarz MI. Diffuse alveolar hemorrhage with underlying isolated, pauciimmune pulmonary capillaritis. *Am J Respir Crit Care Med*. 1997;155:1101–1109.

34. Espinosa G, Cervera R, Font J, Asherson RA. The lung in the antiphospholipid syndrome. *Ann Rheum Dis*. 2002;61: 195–198.

35. Zamora MR, Warner ML, Tuder R, Schwarz MI. Diffuse alveolar hemorrhage and systemic lupus erythematosus. Clinical presentation, histology, survival, and outcome. *Medicine (Baltimore)*. 1997;76:192–202.

36. Ioachimescu OC, Sieber S, Kotch A. Idiopathic pulmonary haemosiderosis revisited. *Eur Respir J*. 2004;24:162–170.

PART 6

Drug-Induced Lung Diseases

CHAPTER 65

Pulmonary Toxicity Related to Chemotherapeutic Agents

Lynn T. Tanoue
John McArdle
Jennifer Possick

INTRODUCTION

Toxicities related to medications comprise a major category of iatrogenic illness. Many agents used for cancer treatment have the potential to cause pulmonary toxicity. As the horizon for treatment options has broadened with our ever-expanding understanding of biological mechanisms fundamental to neoplasia, so has the spectrum of pulmonary complications related to new therapies. Further, with availability of new therapeutic modalities, patients with cancer are living longer, and may, in their long-term survivorship, display delayed toxicities related to treatment. Consequently, for the pulmonologist, drug-induced lung disease is an area of growing complexity.

Chemotherapeutic agents, therapeutic radiation, and biological response modifiers are used in a wide range of regimens, and their use is further complicated by the use of hematopoietic support and bone marrow or stem cell transplantation. Many are, directly or indirectly, associated with pulmonary toxicity. An estimated 5% to 10% of patients undergoing chemotherapy ultimately develop therapy-related pulmonary complications.[1-3] This chapter reviews the evaluation of patients with suspected chemotherapy-induced pulmonary toxicity, as well as the potential toxicities associated with specific classes of drugs.

APPROACH TO THE PATIENT WITH SUSPECTED CHEMOTHERAPY-INDUCED PULMONARY TOXICITY

The differential diagnosis of patients with cancer receiving treatment who develop pulmonary complications is often very challenging, particularly as the diagnosis of drug-induced pulmonary toxicity is typically one of exclusion. Patients most often present with nonspecific constitutional or respiratory complaints. In many cases, symptoms and physical signs may be minimal or even absent. In these situations, the only evidence of an ongoing pulmonary process may be an abnormal chest radiograph (Table 65-1).

The diagnosis of lung disease caused by chemotherapeutic agents poses a particular challenge to the clinician, as there are several complicating features inherent to the oncology patient population.

First, treatment may be given in multidrug regimens or in combination with other modalities such as radiation therapy, bone marrow transplantation, or stem cell transplantation. Assigning pulmonary toxicity to a single drug or modality within such a regimen is often impossible. Moreover, the combined toxicity of two or more drugs or a single drug with radiation therapy may exceed the individual toxicities of those drugs.

Second, patients undergoing chemotherapy are often immune suppressed, either from the malignancy itself or from myelosuppressive or immunosuppressive effects of their treatment. These patients are therefore susceptible to opportunistic infection, which may be indistinguishable radiographically from drug toxicity. This is particularly challenging, as the lung is the most common site of serious infection in patients with cancer. It has been estimated that a relative minority (5%–30%) of pulmonary complications in immunocompromised patients are actually due to drug toxicity; hence it is important to remember that infection is still the most likely culprit when pulmonary decompensation occurs. Since changing a treatment regimen may affect the chance for cure or prolongation of survival, reasonable certainty of drug-related complications necessarily involves exclusion of infection.

Third, cancers themselves may mimic lung disease. This is particularly true in cases of lymphangitic tumor spread or metastases to the lung parenchyma or pleura.

Fourth, toxicity from some drugs appears to be related to cumulative dosage levels. However, adverse reactions may occur even with a low cumulative dose, when clinical suspicion for toxicity is low.

Finally, pulmonary toxicity due to a single chemotherapeutic agent may present with several different syndromes that vary clinically, radiographically, and temporally. While a severe pulmonary reaction acutely following drug administration usually raises suspicion of drug toxicity, as patients survive for longer periods of time it is becoming increasingly clear that toxicity due to some chemotherapeutic agents may be delayed by months to even years after treatment. In such situations, clinical suspicion of drug toxicity may be low.

Monitoring for potential pulmonary toxicity in the patient undergoing chemotherapy requires ongoing clinical vigilance. Symptoms such as cough, dyspnea, or chest discomfort may be mild or even absent. Radiographic findings may be equally subtle. Even if clinical symptoms and radiographic abnormalities are present and severe, they are usually nonspecific. The possibility of adverse drug effects must be considered within the complex medical context inherent to the patient with cancer undergoing physically challenging or immunosuppressive treatment.

PULMONARY PHYSIOLOGICAL TESTING

Pulmonary physiological testing has been utilized in surveillance of patients receiving drugs with potential for pulmonary toxicity. A multitude of investigations studying the utility of pulmonary function testing (PFT) in monitoring pulmonary effects related to administration of chemotherapy have been reported, but the

TABLE 65-1 Differential Diagnosis of Radiographic Abnormalities in Cancer Patients

Pulmonary toxicity related to chemotherapy or other medication
Infection
Primary malignancy
Lymphangitic tumor, metastatic disease, leukemic infiltration
Radiation lung injury
Acute respiratory distress syndrome
Interstitial lung disease, unrelated to drug toxicity
Pulmonary edema (cardiogenic)
Pulmonary thromboembolism
Pulmonary hemorrhage
Transfusion-related acute lung injury

application of these findings to clinical management has been a subject of debate.

Various physiological abnormalities have been described, the most common of which are decreases in lung volumes and diffusing capacity for carbon monoxide (DL_{CO}). Patients receiving chemotherapy who are monitored serially by PFT frequently demonstrate physiological abnormalities in the absence of clinical signs of toxicity.[4–6] Abnormalities in DL_{CO} in particular have been thought by some to be indicative of early-onset, drug-related pulmonary injury. Most such studies have been performed in patients receiving bleomycin, busulfan, or carmustine. Discontinuation of drug, with or without initiation of treatment, including corticosteroids, typically results in improvement. Whether early intervention based on DL_{CO} abnormalities in the absence of clinical symptoms decreases the likelihood of long-term pulmonary impairment related to toxicity is unclear. Conversely, in situations of clinically evident drug toxicity accompanied by PFT abnormalities, withdrawal of culprit therapy may not be paralleled by improvement in physiological measurements. For example, in a study examining pulmonary function in 116 long-term (5–13 years after treatment) survivors of Hodgkin disease in Norway, nearly 30% of patients had exertional dyspnea with associated pulmonary function abnormalities.[7] Multivariate analysis of these patients identified chemotherapy with a combination of bleomycin and anthracyclines as the sole significant predictor of lung function impairment. In all patients in whom drug toxicity is of concern, consideration must be given to the possibility that discontinuation of a specific treatment might result in substitution of less effective therapy.

A number of factors further complicate the practice and interpretation of PFT in the oncology population. Many physiological parameters are effort dependent. The ability of a patient to consistently perform test maneuvers may be affected by weakness, pain, or the use of analgesic or sedating medications. Reproducibility of results therefore may be a significant concern in patients whose functional status and strength are impaired by their malignancy or its treatment. Many patients have anemia induced by malignancy, medication, or chronic illness. Since DL_{CO} is affected by hemoglobin concentration, it is critical that appropriate corrections for anemia be made. Patients with cancers may also be subject to processes other than drug toxicity that will affect PFT results. Primary pulmonary malignancy, metastatic lung disease, infection, thoracic or abdominal surgical procedures, and a host of other clinical situations may all independently cause variation in physiological measurements. Therefore, identifying pulmonary physiological abnormalities specific to drug effect may prove very difficult.

Ultimately, even though the predictive value of baseline or serial PFT remains unclear, most clinicians will continue to rely on such testing as screening and monitoring tools. Though there are no definitive data that toxicity can be averted by physiological monitoring, we are limited by the absence of other means of identifying toxicity early enough to prevent severe pulmonary disease. Though the presence of subclinical abnormalities does not imply that patients will develop irreversible lung disease, these abnormalities may dictate closer monitoring, or even the withdrawal of drug. Conversely, normal physiology cannot predict abrupt toxicity that may produce profound pulmonary injury. As always, medical decisions based on pulmonary physiological findings must be made in the context of the patient's clinical situation as a whole.

DIAGNOSTIC EVALUATION

Given the potential impact of pulmonary drug toxicity on a patient's present and future cancer treatment, it is important to establish this diagnosis as firmly as possible. Thoughtful and judicious use of invasive procedures plays an important role in that evaluation.

The approach to the cancer patient in whom drug toxicity is suspected should parallel the approach to any immunocompromised patient with diffuse or localized lung disease (see Chapter 123). Because clinical features are usually not specific, sampling of respiratory tract secretions and/or lung tissue may be critical to this evaluation. Direct sputum examination or culture may suggest specific pathogens or may be diagnostic of infections such as invasive fungal disease, *Pneumocystis jiroveci* pneumonia, or tuberculosis. In the absence of diagnostic sputum findings, invasive procedures may be necessary. Fine-needle aspiration of the lung may be useful with focal lesions. However, the utility of this procedure in diffuse lung disease is relatively low. This is particularly problematic for patients with drug-induced pulmonary toxicity, which often presents with a diffuse interstitial pattern on chest radiograph. Fiberoptic bronchoscopy with bronchoalveolar lavage (BAL) and transbronchial biopsy has become central to the evaluation of both diffuse and localized lung disease in the immunocompromised host. The procedure is associated with a low rate of major complications. Diagnostic yield varies widely, reflecting the broad range of disease processes that can involve the lung in the immunocompromised patient. Highest diagnostic yields are obtained in patients with infections; lower yields are seen in interstitial inflammatory processes, which may include toxicity from drugs. However, even in situations in which a specific etiology is not identified, exclusion of infection by bronchoscopy often provides clinically useful information.

Open or thoracoscopic lung biopsy is associated with the highest diagnostic yield and can be performed with low complication rates even in critically ill patients. If drug-induced pulmonary injury is suspected, surgical biopsy may be necessary to definitively exclude other causes of lung disease.

The evaluation of a patient in whom chemotherapy-related pulmonary toxicity is a consideration clearly presents significant challenges. Clinicians must be vigilant in the evaluation and management of patients receiving chemotherapeutic regimens. An awareness of potential iatrogenic complications related to drug therapy is, therefore, essential.

CYTOTOXIC ANTIBIOTICS

A variety of cytotoxic antibiotics have been associated with pulmonary toxicity (Table 65-2). Important examples are discussed below.

BLEOMYCIN

Bleomycin, a cytotoxic antibiotic produced by *Streptomyces verticillus*, is used in the treatment of various malignancies, including lymphomas, germ cell tumors, and squamous cell cancers of the head and neck.[8] Unfortunately, it has significant potential for pulmonary toxicity due to relative lack of the inactivating enzyme bleomycin hydrolase in the lungs.[9] The most severe complication is interstitial pneumonitis progressing to fibrosis and respiratory failure, though there are also less severe syndromes, including organizing pneumonia and hypersensitivity pneumonitis.[10]

The pulmonary toxicities of bleomycin have been studied extensively, primarily in animal models. Endothelial injury via oxidative stress is the sentinel event, followed by the influx of inflammatory cells (predominantly macrophages, neutrophils, and lymphocytes), development of perivascular edema, elaboration of inflammatory cytokines, and, ultimately, fibroblast activation and fibrosis (Fig. 65-1).[11] A variety of mediators have been implicated in bleomycin-induced lung injury, including tumor necrosis factor α (TNFα), transforming growth factor-β (TGF-β), interleukin-6 (IL-6), and interleukin-1 (IL-1).[10] Human studies have demonstrated activation of in vitro alveolar macrophages in response to bleomycin,[12] and patients treated with bleomycin for testicular cancer demonstrate a rise in serum TNFα 3 to 24 hours after drug administration.[13] The continued expression of TNFα and IL-1 may predispose to the production of TGF-β and promotion of dysregulated collagen production and fibrosis. Animal studies have shown that bleomycin-induced pulmonary toxicity can

TABLE 65-2 Cytotoxic Antibiotics

Drug	Pulmonary Syndrome	Treatment	Comments
Bleomycin	Chronic pneumonitis; pulmonary fibrosis; rare fulminant variant with acute respiratory failure	Discontinue drug; corticosteroids	Risk factors: Cumulative dose >400 units; supplemental oxygen; therapeutic radiation; renal insufficiency; age >70 y; additional cytotoxic drugs
	Hypersensitivity-type lung disease	Discontinue drug; corticosteroids	Dyspnea, cough, skin rash, and peripheral eosinophilia
	Chest pain syndrome	Discontinue drug	Associated with drug infusion
Mitomycin C	Chronic pneumonitis; pulmonary fibrosis; rare fulminant variant after single dose	Discontinue drug; corticosteroids	Risk factors: Oxygen therapy; therapeutic radiation; additional cytotoxic drugs May relapse after withdrawal of corticosteroids
	Acute dyspnea and/or bronchospasm	Discontinue drug; bronchodilators; supportive care; consider corticosteroids	Risk factors: Vinca alkaloid use; may develop noncardiogenic pulmonary edema and/or chronic interstitial disease Can recur with rechallenge of vinca alkaloids
	Hemolytic uremic syndrome	Discontinue drug; supportive care; poor response to plasmapheresis or corticosteroids	Microangiopathic hemolytic anemia thrombocytopenia, renal insufficiency, noncardiogenic pulmonary edema; rare hemorrhage
Actinomycin D	"Radiation recall" pneumonitis	Discontinue drug	Effect may be longstanding

be ameliorated or prevented by antibodies to TNFα and TGF-β, or receptor antagonists to IL-1; knockout of the TNFα receptor has also demonstrated protective effects.[14–16] Bleomycin also induces direct free-radical damage after oxidation of the bleomycin-Fe (II) complex; this effect has been mitigated by iron depletion with chelators both in vitro and in vivo.[10]

The incidence of bleomycin-induced pneumonitis varies from 6% to 18%, though this figure may be higher depending on the criteria used for diagnosis and the presence of other chemotherapeutic agents in a multidrug regimen; overall mortality is estimated at 3% or less, depending on risk factor subgroup.[10,17]

Several risk factors for severe bleomycin-induced pneumonitis have been identified: (1) Toxicity appears to correlate with higher cumulative dosages. While fatal injury has been observed after administration of <100 units, there is a significant escalation in toxicity with total doses over 400 units, and severe toxicity develops in 20% of patients receiving >500 units.[18] (2) Exposure to high concentrations of supplemental oxygen, particularly in the setting of general anesthesia, may create a synergistic toxic effect. This is primarily based on animal data, including a study which demonstrated a 75% increase in mortality in hamsters treated with bleomycin and 70% oxygen for 72 hours versus bleomycin alone.[19] As a result, high fractions of supplemental oxygen are generally avoided whenever possible in clinical practice, and the evidence substantiating human risk has been largely anecdotal. There have also been case reports of recrudescence in patients exposed to even modest levels of supplemental oxygen several months after bleomycin exposure, so caution in limiting oxygen exposure for at least 6 months after treatment appears warranted.[20] (3) Thoracic irradiation prior to, concomitant with, or subsequent to, bleomycin administration may be associated with an increase in toxicity. This "radiation recall" may extend outside the original port of irradiation, and may last for years after bleomycin therapy. More recent data suggests that the augmented risk from consolidative radiation therapy may be attenuated if there is an interval of at least 28 days between chemotherapy and radiation.[21] While there is still certainly an increase in pulmonary symptoms during treatment for patients receiving combined therapy, and patients must be closely monitored, long-term sequelae may be less pronounced than originally feared.[22] (4) Since bleomycin is excreted by the kidneys, and is often coadministered with potentially nephrotoxic agents, decreased creatinine clearance below 35 mL/min is associated with increased risk of toxicity.[23] (5) The risk for pulmonary toxicity rises proportionately for every decade after 30 years, and patients over 70 years of age are at particular risk.[24] (6) Concurrent use of

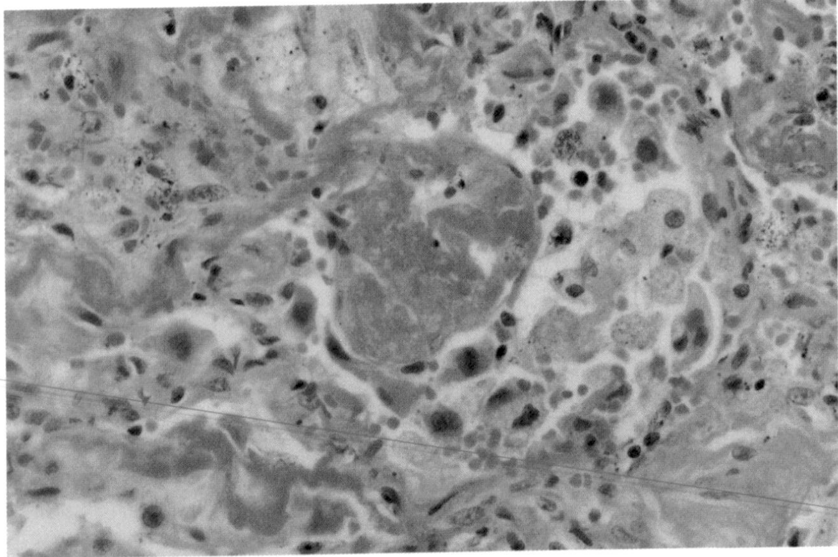

Figure 65-1 Lung biopsy specimen from a patient with clinical and radiographic evidence of bleomycin-induced pulmonary toxicity shows drug effect with acute and chronic changes. The alveolus contains an exudate of fibrin, which is undergoing organization and is surrounded by alveolar macrophages. The large and atypical cells are markedly reactive alveolar type II pneumocytes. The alveolar wall itself is scarred with collagen deposition by the spindle-shaped fibroblasts. *(Used with permission of Dr. Darryl Carter, Professor of Pathology, Yale University School of Medicine.)*

other chemotherapeutic regimens, including gemcitabine, cisplatin, and drugs in the ABVD regimen, may result in synergistic toxicity.[21,22] Though these effects have not been clearly reproducible in all cases, convention has been to reduce bleomycin dosage in drug regimens in which this synergy is a concern. (7) Smoking appeared to confer an increased risk of bleomycin toxicity in one study,[25] however this has not been confirmed in other studies, and may be confounded by the presence of other risk factors. (8) Similarly, though there have been case reports of increased incidence of bleomycin toxicity in patients receiving granulocyte colony–stimulating factor (G-CSF), likely due to increased cytokine induction, larger series have not clearly demonstrated a relationship.[26]

The clinical presentation of bleomycin-induced pneumonitis is usually subacute and insidious, occurring within a few weeks to 6 months after treatment.[10] A more fulminant presentation with acute respiratory failure has been reported but is far less common. Patients generally present with dyspnea, nonproductive cough, and low-grade fever, though some patients may be asymptomatic. Substernal or pleuritic chest pain occurs, but is infrequent. Common physical findings include hypoxemia and fine bibasilar crackles; rhonchi and a pleural rub may also develop.[27] Chest radiograph usually shows bilateral reticular or fine nodular infiltrates with a basilar predominance, often beginning at the costophrenic angles (Fig. 65-2A,B). Loss of lung volume with diaphragmatic elevation is also commonly seen. However, various radiographic patterns including alveolar infiltrates, lobar consolidation, organizing pneumonia, asymmetric lung involvement, pneumothorax, pneumomediastinum, and even lung nodules have been described. Computed tomographic (CT) scanning, particularly high-resolution computed tomography (HRCT) scanning, is more sensitive in the evaluation of radiographic abnormalities and may be useful in patients who have spirometric or clinical evidence of toxicity but negative chest radiographs (Fig. 65-3); CT scanning provides more accurate assessment of anatomic distribution of disease that correlates well with lung function impairment.[28] Most patients receiving bleomycin demonstrate a decrease in $D_{L_{CO}}$ over the course of therapy, though only a small percentage of these patients will go on to manifest clinical signs of pulmonary toxicity, which is typically also associated with restrictive ventilatory defect.[29]

Bleomycin may also cause an acute hypersensitivity syndrome of dyspnea, cough, and rash immediately following administration of drug. Lung biopsy in these cases shows eosinophilic infiltration, and changes consistent with hypersensitivity pneumonitis; peripheral eosinophilia may also be observed. These cases show a particularly favorable response to steroid therapy.[30] An acute chest pain syndrome has also been reported in 1% of patients; it occurs during infusion, resolves with termination of drug, and does not appear to predict other pulmonary toxicity from bleomycin.[31]

Discontinuation of drug is recommended for patients with clinically significant bleomycin-induced toxicity, and may be sufficient treatment for individuals with mild presentations. For more significant disease, corticosteroids are usually given in the range of 60 to 100 mg of prednisone per day for 4 to 8 weeks, with slow taper over the following 4 to 6 months guided by clinical stability of the patient. It should be noted that the steroid responsiveness of bleomycin-induced pulmonary toxicity is highly variable, with more responsive cases likely representing hypersensitivity pneumonitis or organizing pneumonia.[10] Improvement often occurs within weeks of drug cessation, but complete resolution may take up to 2 years; patients may be left with residual radiographic and/or physiological abnormalities, particularly if fibrosis has developed. Though a number of promising agents have been explored in animal models, none have yet been shown to be effective in humans.

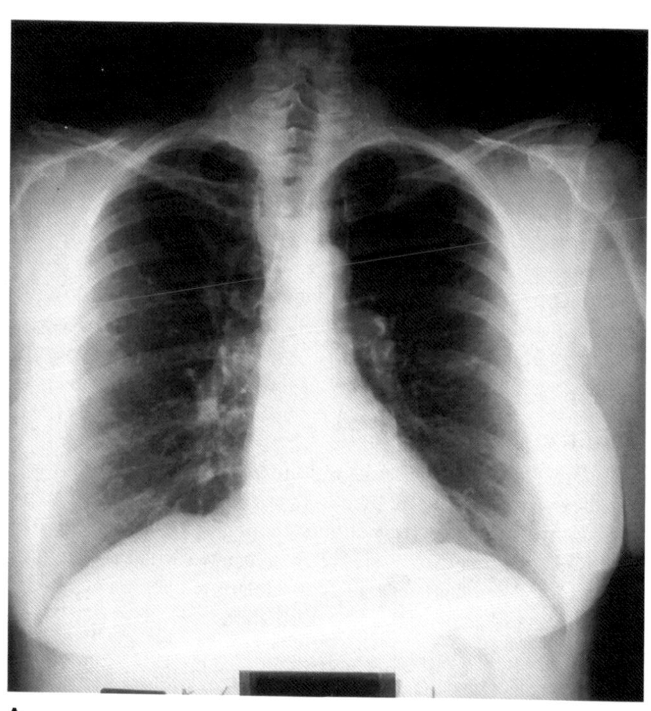

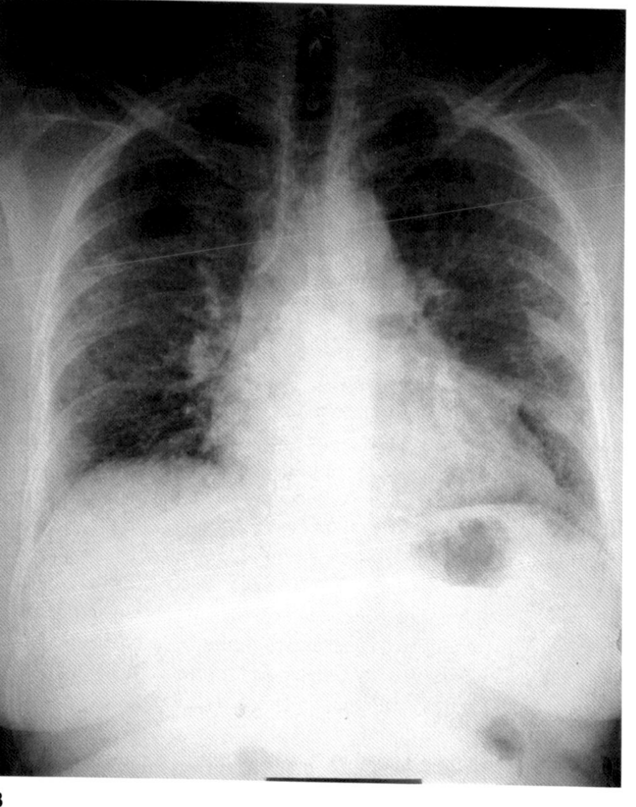

Figure 65-2 Posteroanterior chest radiographs of a 56-year-old woman with cervical carcinoma (**A**) before and (**B**) after chemotherapy with a bleomycin-containing regimen. Note the decrease in lung volume and diffusely increased interstitial lung markings in the post-chemotherapy radiograph.

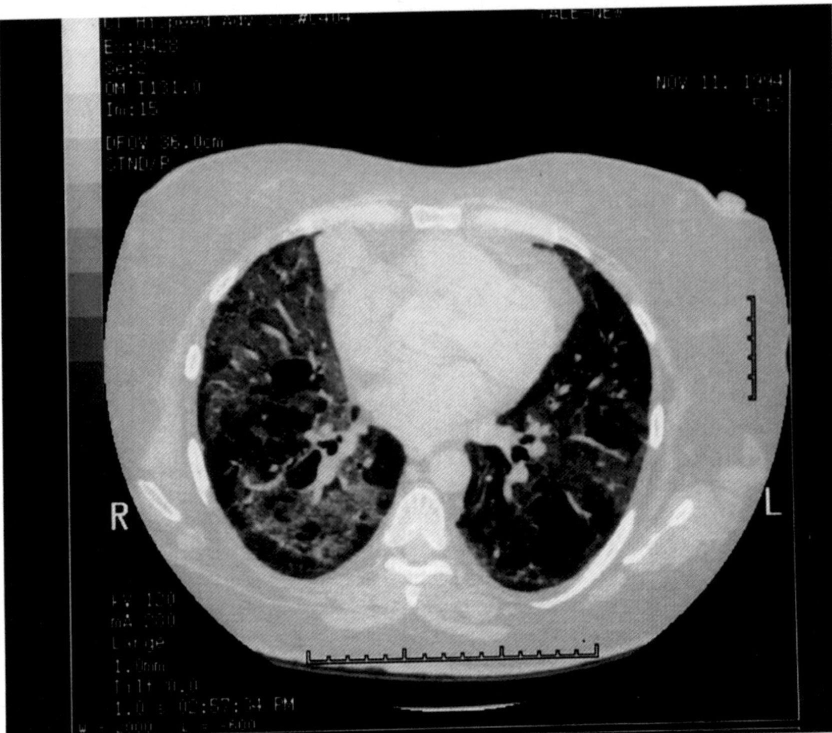

Figure 65-3 Chest computed tomography (CT) scan of same patient as in Figure 65-2, taken at the time of radiograph in Figure 65-2. Note the patchy distribution of bilateral infiltrates, whose extent is clearly delineated by CT.

Histologically, biopsy specimens show mononuclear cell infiltration, alveolar-lining cell hypertrophy, collagen deposition, and alveolar septal thickening; type II pneumocyte enlargement and lymphocytic or eosinophilic infiltration have also been described. This syndrome may respond to discontinuation of drug and institution of corticosteroids at an initial dose of 60 mg/d tapered over a 4- to 6-week period; patients may demonstrate relapse once steroids are discontinued.[37]

The second syndrome of mitomycin-induced pulmonary toxicity is primarily seen in patients who have also received vinca alkaloids. While drugs of this latter category (vinblastine, vinorelbine, and vindesine) confer little in the way of risk of pulmonary toxicity when used alone, they may precipitate a syndrome of acute pulmonary toxicity when given concurrently with or subsequent to administration of mitomycin C.[38] Patients present with rapid onset of dyspnea or bronchospasm hours to weeks after exposure; symptoms generally abate in 12 to 24 hours with cessation of drug, supportive care, and bronchodilators. In some cases, however, bilateral interstitial infiltrates or noncardiogenic pulmonary edema may also develop, and patients may go on to develop chronic interstitial lung disease with permanent physiological impairment.[39] Rechallenge with vinca alkaloids alone, independent of mitomycin C, can also result in recrudescence of symptoms.[38]

The third syndrome of mitomycin C toxicity is a microangiopathy, with a presentation similar to thrombotic thrombocytopenic purpura and hemolytic uremic syndrome (TTP–HUS); in the case of mitomycin C microangiopathy, it is also associated with acute lung injury and respiratory failure in 50% of cases.[40] Pulmonary alveolar hemorrhage in this setting has also been described.[41] The mechanism of toxicity appears related to endothelial injury in the pulmonary vasculature. Unfortunately, prognosis is poor, and patients with chemotherapy-induced TTP–HUS respond poorly to the plasma exchange and corticosteroids that are the mainstay of therapy; there are case reports of successful treatment with rituximab, though it should be noted that these patients did not have respiratory failure.[42,43]

In addition, mitomycin C has been implicated in two cases of fatal pulmonary hypertension caused by pulmonary venoocclusive disease in patients with non–small-cell lung cancer (NSCLC) treated prior to surgical resection.[44] There have also been reports of pleural toxicity, with exudative effusions and pleural fibrosis.[6]

■ MITOMYCIN C

Mitomycin C is an alkylating agent derived from *Streptomyces caespitosus*. It is used in multidrug regimens for multiple solid organ malignancies including non–small-cell lung, breast, gastric, pancreatic, cervical, prostate, and bladder cancers.[32] The incidence of pulmonary toxicity due to mitomycin is variably reported between 2% and 38% (with clinically relevant toxicity likely <10%), and appears to be potentiated by concurrent administration of other agents, particularly vinca alkaloids.[32] Though typically associated with intravenous therapy, cases of significant pulmonary toxicity have been reported in patients receiving both intravesicular and intraperitoneal mitomycin C.[33,34] Mitomycin C lung injury presents with multiple distinct pulmonary syndromes, including interstitial pneumonitis and fibrosis, bronchospasm, acute lung injury, thrombotic microangiopathy, venoocclusive disease with pulmonary hypertension, and pleural disease.

The most common form of mitomycin-induced lung toxicity is a chronic pneumonitis with pulmonary fibrosis similar to that seen with bleomycin; it similarly appears potentiated by exposure to supplemental oxygen and radiation.[35] Some studies have suggested a dose–response effect, with increased risk of toxicity after cumulative doses ranging from 20 to 39 mg/m^2, though this finding has not been consistently reproducible.[28,29] The exact mechanism of injury is unknown, though several have been proposed, including lipid peroxidant injury, hypersensitivity reactions, or immune complex–mediated disease.[36] Pulmonary toxicity usually occurs after 2 to 12 months of therapy, though a more fulminant form of acute lung injury has been reported after a single dose.[36]

Clinically, patients present with a subacute syndrome of cough and progressive dyspnea, often with fatigue and sometimes with pleuritic chest pain.[37] Fever is less common. Chest radiographs usually show bilateral interstitial infiltrates, occasionally with alveolar or fine nodular patterns. PFTs demonstrate a restrictive pattern with impairment in $D_{L_{CO}}$, though degree of impairment correlates poorly with prognosis.[6]

■ ACTINOMYCIN D

Actinomycin D is an older antitumor antibiotic derived from *Streptomyces*, which is still used in the treatment of Ewing sarcoma, rhabdomyosarcoma, Wilms tumor, and gestational choriocarcinomas. While this drug is not often associated with primary lung toxicity, it may potentiate "radiation recall" pneumonitis in patients who have received prior thoracic irradiation.[45]

ALKYLATING AGENTS

Alkylating agents (Table 65-3) have been implicated in chemotherapeutic agent–related lung disease. Important examples are described below.

The chemotherapeutic properties of the alkylating agents result from the formation of covalent linkages (alkylation) of DNA

TABLE 65-3 Alkylating Agents

Drug	Pulmonary Syndrome	Treatment	Comments
Cyclophosphamide	Chronic pneumonitis; pulmonary fibrosis	Discontinue drug; corticosteroids	Risk factors: High cumulative dose; additional cytotoxic drugs; supplemental oxygen; therapeutic radiation Toxicity may occur years after treatment is completed Pleural fibrosis may occur in late-stage disease
Busulfan	Chronic pneumonitis; pulmonary fibrosis	Discontinue drug; consider corticosteroids	Risk factors: Cumulative dose >500 mg Often occurs after cessation of drug; prognosis poor
Oxaliplatin	Eosinophilic pneumonitis; organizing pneumonia; diffuse alveolar damage	Discontinue drug; corticosteroids	Risk factors: Pre-existing interstitial lung disease
Chlorambucil Melphalan Ifosfamide	Chronic pneumonitis; pulmonary fibrosis	Discontinue drug; consider corticosteroids for patients with hypersensitivity features	Clinical pulmonary toxicity is rare with exception of high-dose melphalan (>200 mg/m^2)

components.[46] Nitrogen mustards are the prototypic alkylating agents and were the first drugs to be used as modern cancer chemotherapy, but many other drugs also exert antineoplastic effects by alkylation. Alkylating agents that have been associated with pulmonary toxicity include derivatives of nitrogen mustards (cyclophosphamide, melphalan, chlorambucil, ifosfamide), alkyl sulfonates (busulfan), platinum-based therapies (oxaliplatin), and the nitrosoureas (carmustine/BCNU, lomustine/CCNU). The nitrosoureas are considered in a separate section below.

■ CYCLOPHOSPHAMIDE

Cyclophosphamide is widely used in the treatment of many malignancies, including lymphomas, breast and ovarian cancers, and a variety of other solid tumors. It may be used as part of myeloablative conditioning regimens prior to bone marrow or peripheral blood stem cell transplantation. It is also used alone or in combination with corticosteroids in the treatment of autoimmune diseases and systemic vasculitides.[3] The overall incidence of cyclophosphamide-induced lung injury is less than 1%, though as with other agents, increased pulmonary toxicity may occur in the setting of radiation therapy, oxygen supplementation, or combination treatment with other cytotoxic agents.[47]

Cyclophosphamide is administered as an inactive prodrug that is metabolized by the liver, and to lesser extent, in the lung, to 4-hydroxycyclophosphamide, phosphoramide mustard (responsible for alkylation and DNA cross-linking), and acrolein (responsible for the hemorrhagic cystitis which can complicate therapy).[48] Though the exact mechanism of cyclophosphamide-induced injury to the lung is unknown, in vitro models suggest contributions from oxidative stress, and upregulation of TGF-β, increase in collagen synthesis and, ultimately, fibrosis.[49] Cyclophosphamide toxicity lacks a clear dose–response relationship in humans, possibly due to genetic variations in drug metabolism.[50] In addition, the pharmacokinetics of both the inactive parent compound and the active alkylating derivative can be affected by variations in the cytochrome P450 superfamily of enzymes, as well as by interactions with other drugs. Therefore, functionally higher exposure to active drug may occur in the setting of substances that induce hepatic enzyme activity, such as rifampin, phenytoin, and alcohol, or with decreased renal clearance.

As with a number of other chemotherapeutic agents, cyclophosphamide-induced pulmonary toxicity may present either early in the course of treatment or in a delayed, progressive fashion that may begin years after treatment is completed. In cases where pulmonary symptoms occur long after exposure, an association with the drug may be difficult to identify. Clinical features are nonspecific, including nonproductive cough, dyspnea, fatigue, and fever. Occasionally, patients are asymptomatic but are discovered to have radiographic abnormalities compatible with drug toxicity. Chest radiographs and CT scans usually show evidence of bilateral interstitial lung disease (either bilateral reticular or nodular markings with ground-glass opacities or, later, fibrosis) but may also show pleural fibrosis in late-stage disease.[51] This latter radiographic finding may be helpful in distinguishing cyclophosphamide-associated interstitial lung disease from the idiopathic interstitial pneumonias.

Histological findings in the lung are not specific. Lung biopsy in these patients is primarily useful for exclusion of other identifiable causes of interstitial lung disease in immunocompromised patients, including infection and malignancy. When used to treat nonneoplastic lung disease, the distinction between underlying lung disease from a systemic syndrome and lung disease exacerbated by drug toxicity is often very difficult to delineate. When cyclophosphamide is used as a chemotherapeutic agent, its identification as the specific etiology of lung injury may also be difficult, as it is rarely used alone, pinpointing specific toxicity to a single agent may be impossible. Like other agents, cyclophosphamide may have synergistic toxicity with therapeutic thoracic radiation, high levels of supplemental oxygen, and other chemotherapeutic drugs with potential for lung injury.[52]

Cyclophosphamide-induced lung injury may cause significant morbidity, and a high clinical suspicion for pulmonary toxicity should result in prompt discontinuation of the drug. Early-onset pneumonitis can occasionally be fatal, but when recognized quickly, prognosis is generally favorable and recovery, though slow, is expected for most individuals. Discontinuation of the drug alone may be sufficient, though most patients also receive glucocorticoid therapy. The optimal regimen and magnitude of benefit in these cases remain unclear.[53] Unfortunately, late-onset toxicity follows an irreversible and progressive course, which appears steroid unresponsive; mortality due to progressive respiratory failure exceeds 60%.[51]

■ BUSULFAN

Busulfan, previously used as a treatment for chronic myelogenous leukemia (CML) prior to the advent of oral tyrosine kinase inhibitors, is now mainly used as a component of conditioning regimens for bone marrow and stem cell transplantation. Toxicity may develop within weeks of exposure, but is more typically insidious, with the average onset of symptoms more than 3 years after treatment.[3] Estimates of frequency vary widely, with an average of approximately 6%.[54] Because of the indolent nature of CML, patients were often treated for months to years with busulfan. Though it was generally well tolerated in this setting, patients receiving a cumulative dose above 500 mg appeared to be at higher risk for pulmonary complications.[55]

Currently, busulfan is used in combination with other chemotherapeutic agents in conditioning regimens prior to bone marrow and stem cell transplantation. Pulmonary complications in this situation are not uncommon though it is difficult to clearly attribute toxicity to busulfan rather than other causes including infection (notably cytomegalovirus), radiation therapy, and other drugs (particularly etoposide).[56,57] In long-term comparisons of patients receiving busulfan and cyclophosphamide versus total body irradiation prior to allogeneic transplantation, bronchiolitis obliterans was far more frequent in the former group (26% vs. 5%), while rates of pneumonitis were similar; this raises the concern that the main source of pulmonary toxicity in busulfan-based conditioning regimens may be an increase in chronic pulmonary graft versus host disease.[58]

Symptoms of busulfan lung injury usually present insidiously, weeks to years after exposure, with cough, progressive dyspnea, fever, fatigue, and weight loss. Chest radiographs typically show bilateral interstitial infiltrates with a basilar predominance. Pathological findings are consistent with other cytotoxic drug–induced pulmonary injuries, with type II pneumocyte hyperplasia, dysplasia, and desquamation into alveolar spaces. Fibroblast proliferation, collagen deposition, and fibrosis are usually evident. Desquamation and accumulation of alveolar debris can be severe in some cases, yielding a pattern similar to pulmonary alveolar proteinosis; unfortunately, total lung lavage is usually ineffective in such cases.[3,59]

There is no specific treatment for busulfan-induced pulmonary injury, except withdrawal of the drug. However, due to the delayed nature of presentation, patients are often no longer on therapy by the time toxicity is detected; thus, treatment is largely supportive. Though some spontaneous improvement may occur, when there is clinically evident busulfan-induced pulmonary toxicity the prognosis for recovery is generally poor. Corticosteroids have anecdotally been reported to be of benefit but, as with most chemotherapeutic agents, no prospective studies are available.[3] Given the possibility of late-onset pulmonary toxicity, it seems prudent that long-term follow-up of recipients of bone marrow or peripheral blood stem cell transplants with busulfan-based conditioning regimens should include pulmonary evaluation. However, guidelines for identification or treatment of pulmonary toxicity in this situation are lacking.

■ OTHER ALKYLATING AGENTS

Chlorambucil and melphalan are both slow-acting nitrogen mustards. Chlorambucil has an important role in the treatment of lymphoreticular malignancies including chronic lymphocytic leukemia (CLL) and has also been used in the treatment of nonneoplastic diseases, such as rheumatoid arthritis and sarcoidosis. Though pulmonary toxicity is less common than with other alkylating agents, occurring in less than 1% of patients, mortality from irreversible fibrosis when it occurs exceeds 50%.[60] As with busulfan, chlorambucil may be administered over a prolonged time in the treatment of CLL, but there does not appear to be a clear relationship between toxicity and either cumulative dose or duration of therapy. The number of cases of reported chlorambucil pulmonary toxicity is relatively small, thus no distinct clinical pattern has emerged. In cases of chlorambucil-related interstitial pneumonitis, BAL has demonstrated a CD8+ T cell alveolitis suggestive of hypersensitivity reaction.[61] Given the possibility of hypersensitivity pneumonitis, clinical suspicion should prompt immediate discontinuation of the drug, and administration of corticosteroids can be considered in patients with progressive pulmonary disease.

Melphalan has traditionally been used in the treatment of multiple myeloma, but, like other alkylating agents, it is now used to treat a variety of malignancies. High-dose melphalan (200 mg/m^2 or more) is used in conditioning regimens prior to stem cell transplantation and has been associated with fatal pneumonitis and fibrosis.[62] Since large series of such patients are not available, the incidence of pulmonary toxicity associated with high-dose melphalan given in these situations is not known. As these types of treatments become more widely available, new data should define whether pulmonary toxicity related to melphalan or other alkylating agents is indeed more prevalent than has been historically appreciated.

Ifosfamide is an alkylating agent that is structurally related to cyclophosphamide. It is used in the treatment of lymphoma and acute and chronic leukemias, as well as in solid tumors including sarcomas, ovarian cancer, and breast cancer. Dose limitation is usually related to bladder toxicity. Clinically evident ifosfamide-induced pulmonary toxicity appears to be rare and typically presents as interstitial pneumonitis.[63] It has also been described as a cause of acquired methemoglobinemia; this should be considered in the differential for patients on ifosfamide presenting with dyspnea, cyanosis, or altered mental status.[64]

Oxaliplatin is a platinum-derivative cytotoxic agent primarily used as part of multidrug regimens with 5-fluorouracil and leucovorin (FOLFOX) for treatment of colorectal cancer, as well as for treatment of pancreatic, breast, ovarian, and NSCL cancers. Though pulmonary complications are relatively rare, variable patterns of lung toxicity have been reported with FOLFOX regimens, including eosinophilic pneumonia, organizing pneumonia, and diffuse alveolar damage.[65–68] The timing, severity, progression, and prognosis of individual cases have been heterogeneous, probably owing to the diversity in pathological mechanisms. Some cases have demonstrated complete resolution with withdrawal of drug, with or without administration of corticosteroids, but others have nonetheless progressed rapidly to respiratory failure and death.[66,68] In some cases, patients were successfully rechallenged with 5-fluorouracil and leucovorin, indicating oxaliplatin as the likely culprit in the original drug reaction.[65,67] Mechanism of toxicity is still poorly understood, and likely multifactorial; glutathione depletion has been suggested based on the mechanistic role in oxaliplatin-induced hepatic injury, and an anecdotal case report of an individual who improved when treated with a combination of corticosteroids and N-acetylcysteine.[69,70] Patients with pre-existing interstitial lung disease, even when subclinical, may be at increased risk for oxaliplatin toxicity, progression of underlying interstitial disease, or both.[70] Individuals with baseline physiological and radiographic abnormalities, even in absence of symptoms, should be monitored carefully, and the threshold for withdrawal of drug and trial of corticosteroids should be low. It is unclear whether prophylactic N-acetylcysteine might be of benefit in these cases.

ANTIMETABOLITES

Antimetabolites are associated with lung injury (Table 65-4). Representative examples are discussed below.

■ METHOTREXATE

Methotrexate is an antimetabolite used to treat malignancies, as well as connective tissue diseases and other inflammatory conditions, including sarcoidosis and psoriasis. When used in high doses for the treatment of cancers, the incidence of pulmonary toxicity is estimated at 1% to 8%. The exact nature of methotrexate causing pulmonary toxicity in the context of cancer treatment is less well defined than in treatment of inflammatory diseases. Methotrexate, as a chemotherapeutic agent, would rarely be used alone, making interpretation of its role in any pulmonary syndrome challenging. In patients with rheumatoid arthritis, polymyositis, and other collagen vascular diseases, the potential for a variety of pulmonary manifestations related to the underlying disease can make the diagnosis of methotrexate-induced pneumonitis challenging.

The diagnostic criteria of Searles and McKendry (Table 65-5) are frequently employed in an effort to determine whether pulmonary involvement is related to methotrexate.[71] Though the criteria have

TABLE 65-4 Antimetabolites

Drug	Pulmonary Syndrome	Treatment	Comments
Methotrexate	Chronic pneumonitis; pulmonary fibrosis	Corticosteroids; discontinue drug	Most common syndrome of methotrexate-induced lung toxicity; risk factors: older age, pre-existing lung disease, diabetes, previous use of disease-modifying drugs, hypoalbuminemia
	Hypersensitivity-type lung disease	Corticosteroids; discontinue drug	May resolve even if drug is continued, but can progress to fibrosis
	Acute chest pain syndrome	Discontinue drug	Often accompanied by pleural effusions
	Noncardiogenic pulmonary edema	Supportive care; discontinue drug	Associated with intrathecal administration
Cytosine arabinoside	Noncardiogenic pulmonary edema	Supportive care; discontinue drug	Onset of symptoms usually occurs within days of initiation of treatment; risk factor: cumulative dose
	Cryptogenic organizing pneumonia	Discontinue drug; corticosteroids	Risk factors: combined therapy with anthracyclines or interferon-α
Fludarabine	Hypersensitivity-type lung disease; interstitial pneumonitis	Discontinue drug	Toxicity is uncommon; treatment associated with increased incidence of delayed opportunistic infections
Gemcitabine	Dyspnea	Occurs within hours of dose	Usually self-limited
	Interstitial lung disease; noncardiogenic pulmonary edema	Discontinue drug; corticosteroids; diuretics	Risk factors: combination treatment with taxanes or bleomycin

not been validated in a prospective cohort, they may be useful in situations where methotrexate pulmonary toxicity is a consideration.

In a multicenter case-control study of methotrexate-induced lung toxicity in patients with rheumatoid arthritis, Alarcon et al.[72] identified risk factors associated with the development of pneumonitis, including age greater than 60 years (associated with a sixfold increase in risk of pneumonitis compared with those <50 years of age), prior history of rheumatoid pleuropulmonary disease, diabetes, previous use of disease-modifying antirheumatic drugs, and hypoalbuminemia. Toxicity does not appear to have dose dependency, but daily versus weekly administration and higher weekly doses of methotrexate have been suggested as associated with increased risk, as well as pre-existing lung disease, prior PFT abnormalities, and the presence of renal insufficiency.[1,73–75] Synergistic toxicity has been reported with combination therapy using cyclophosphamide. Tapering of corticosteroid therapy or adrenalectomy may also increase the risk of methotrexate-induced toxicity.[1,76]

Methotrexate is a folate analog; its therapeutic effect is related to its ability to inhibit cellular proliferation by inducing deficiencies of folate coenzymes, and ultimately to decreased synthesis of DNA and RNA.[77] The mechanism(s) of methotrexate-induced lung injury is unknown. Clinically, toxicity presents with several syndromes. The most common of these is development of a symptom complex characterized by fever, dyspnea, cough, malaise, and myalgias, usually within weeks after initiation of therapy. Chest radiography usually shows diffuse interstitial infiltrates. Chest radiography may demonstrate unilateral or bilateral effusion, a nodular appearance, or hilar and/or mediastinal adenopathy, or may be normal. Rash is present in up to 17% of patients and peripheral blood eosinophilia in up to 40% of patients. BAL in this setting may show a lymphocytic alveolitis, suggestive of a hypersensitivity reaction. However, illness may resolve even with continuation of the drug, and rechallenge does not necessarily result in relapse, suggesting that hypersensitivity may not be the true mechanism of injury. This presentation of methotrexate-induced pulmonary toxicity parallels the hypersensitivity-type syndrome that is sometimes observed with bleomycin. As some patients may go on to develop chronic pneumonitis and pulmonary fibrosis, the drug is generally withdrawn when toxicity occurs.

Pulmonary toxicity from methotrexate may also present as a more insidious subacute syndrome of interstitial lung disease. Symptoms including cough, fever, dyspnea, headache, and malaise typically occur within 4 months after the initiation of treatment. Radiographically and clinically this syndrome more closely resembles the type of chronic pneumonitis seen with other cytotoxic drugs and has been reported with all routes of methotrexate administration (oral, intravenous, intrathecal). In contrast to the lung injury associated with many other chemotherapeutic agents, the pneumonitis caused by methotrexate appears, in general, to be responsive to corticosteroids. Pathological findings in the lung parallel those seen with lung injury due to other cytotoxic drugs, with interstitial and alveolar inflammation and fibrosis.[3] In addition, eosinophilic

TABLE 65-5 Diagnosis of Methotrexate Pneumonitis

Diagnostic criteria:

- Acute onset of shortness of breath
- Fever (>38.0°C)
- Tachypnea (≥28 breaths/min) with nonproductive cough
- Radiographic evidence of interstitial or alveolar infiltrates
- WBC ≤15,000
- Negative blood or sputum cultures for pathogenic organisms (required)
- Pulmonary function tests demonstrating restrictive disease with low diffusion capacity
- Pa_{O_2} <55 mm Hg on room air (at presentation)
- Biopsy histopathology consistent with bronchiolitis or interstitial pneumonitis with giant cells and without evidence of pathogenic microorganisms

Presence of methotrexate pneumonitis:

- Definite: at least 6 of 9 criteria
- Probable: 5 of 9 criteria
- Possible: 4 of 9 criteria

Source: Data from Searles G, McKendry RJ. Methotrexate pneumonitis in rheumatoid arthritis: potential risk factors. Four case reports and a review of the literature. J Rheumatol. 1987;14(6):1164–1171.

infiltration of the interstitium, as well as granulomatous inflammation, may be observed. These latter findings are again suggestive of a potential hypersensitivity-type mechanism of inflammation.

Methotrexate-induced lung injury may also appear as an acute syndrome with pleuritis and pleural effusion. Respiratory distress progressing to noncardiogenic pulmonary edema has been described after intrathecal administration of the drug and may be neurogenic in origin.

The prognosis with methotrexate-associated lung toxicity is generally thought to be favorable. As noted, symptoms and radiographic abnormalities may resolve even with continuation of treatment. The use of corticosteroids is generally recommended, though prospective trials of this intervention are not available.

CYTOSINE ARABINOSIDE

Cytosine arabinoside (Ara-C) is a pyrimidine nucleoside analog that rapidly inhibits DNA synthesis. It is important in the treatment of acute leukemias and non-Hodgkin lymphoma. Pulmonary toxicity parallels intensity of treatment; high-dose regimens are associated with a 5% to 44% incidence of acute or subacute respiratory insufficiency.[1,78,79] Symptoms include fever, cough, dyspnea, and tachypnea; their onset may coincide with chemotherapeutic treatment or may be delayed for up to several weeks after treatment is initiated. Hypoxemia may be present. The chest radiograph generally shows a diffuse interstitial or alveolar pattern.

The pathogenesis of pulmonary toxicity due to Ara-C is unknown, but it appears to result in a syndrome of noncardiogenic pulmonary edema. In an autopsy series of 181 patients who died of acute leukemia, Haupt et al.[80] described a group of 42 patients who had received Ara-C within 30 days of death and who had moderate to severe pulmonary edema. Lung pathology showed protein-rich infiltrates in both alveoli and interstitium. Twenty-eight of these 42 patients had no other identifiable cause of their pulmonary edema. In these cases, Ara-C was thought to be the most likely precipitant. Treatment for Ara-C lung toxicity is standard supportive care for noncardiogenic pulmonary edema. Administration of corticosteroids has been recommended by some authors but is of unclear benefit.

Ara-C has also been associated with cryptogenic organizing pneumonia when administered with anthracyclines or interferon-α.[81,82] The pulmonary manifestations typically occur within a few weeks to 2 months after drug exposure and are characterized by fever, shortness of breath, and radiographic infiltrates that may be either lobar or nodular. All patients reported to date have achieved resolution of their pulmonary disease, either spontaneously or with the use of corticosteroids. Overall mortality associated with Ara-C–induced pulmonary toxicity ranges from 6% to 13%.[1,3,78,80–82]

FLUDARABINE

Fludarabine monophosphate is a purine nucleotide analog used in the treatment of CLL, low-grade non-Hodgkin lymphoma, and a variety of other lymphoproliferative disorders. A major clinical issue related to pulmonary complications with fludarabine therapy is the profound immunosuppression that may persist for months after treatment. The persistent nature of this immunosuppression is unusual when compared to other chemotherapeutic agents. The risk of opportunistic infections, including *P. jiroveci* pneumonia is increased by the use of corticosteroids in this setting. Therefore, symptomatic pulmonary disease in patients treated with fludarabine within this time frame is most likely to be related to infection.

Pulmonary toxicity from fludarabine, including interstitial pneumonitis and acute eosinophilic pneumonitis, is uncommon but has been described.[83–85] Helman et al.[83] reported the largest series to date, which included nine patients with fludarabine-related pulmonary toxicity out of a total of 105 patients (8.6%) treated with fludarabine over an 11-year period at a single institution. Toxicity did not correlate with age, prior treatment regimens, or history of prior lung disease, but occurred more frequently in patients with CLL compared to those with other lymphoproliferative disorders. The onset of symptoms ranged from 3 to 6 days after therapy, with radiographs notable for new interstitial or mixed interstitial and alveolar infiltrates. BAL fluid revealed increased cellularity without a consistently predominant cell type. Multifocal nodular pulmonary infiltrates have also been described.[85]

Biopsy specimens most commonly reveal diffuse, chronic interstitial inflammation and fibrosis, although in some cases granulomas have been observed, suggesting the possibility of a hypersensitivity reaction. In the report by Helman et al., patients with fludarabine-associated pulmonary toxicity generally demonstrated subjective and objective improvement with corticosteroid therapy. Most patients responded within days, although more delayed responses were possible. Recrudescence of noninfectious pulmonary infiltrates has been described with fludarabine retreatment; thus, fludarabine should be avoided in future regimens in patients who have developed drug-related pulmonary toxicity.

GEMCITABINE

Gemcitabine is a pyrimidine analog used in the treatment of cancers of the lung, pancreas, ovary, and uroepithelium. It is structurally similar to cytosine arabinoside. Gemcitabine is generally well tolerated when used as a single agent, which may make it appealing for use in older patients. Myelosuppression is its major toxicity. The most common respiratory complaint is dyspnea, which occurs in less than 1% of patients.[86] Dyspnea may occur within hours to days of treatment and is generally self-limited. More serious pulmonary side effects, including interstitial lung disease, pulmonary fibrosis, and acute respiratory distress syndrome, are reported much more frequently when gemcitabine is used in combination with other chemotherapeutic agents. Gemcitabine appears to have a reasonable safety profile when given with carboplatin, a treatment regimen often used for NSCLC.[5] However, severe pulmonary toxicity appears to be much more common when gemcitabine is given in combination with taxanes or bleomycin.[87–90] Acute respiratory distress has been reported with these regimens, with development of noncardiogenic pulmonary edema characterized radiographically by mixed interstitial and alveolar infiltrates. Though responses to diuretics and corticosteroids have been noted, severe pulmonary complications in this setting can be fatal. Histological evaluation most commonly reveals type II pneumocyte hyperplasia, interstitial inflammation, and hyaline membrane formation, consistent with acute lung injury. Some patients with ultimately fatal outcome have demonstrated early symptomatology, including dyspnea, hypoxemia, and radiographic infiltrates to a milder degree with prior doses of gemcitabine. Such findings should raise consideration for discontinuation of gemcitabine.

NITROSOUREAS

The nitrosoureas (Table 65-6) include carmustine or BCNU (1,3-bis-(2-chloroethyl)-1-nitrosourea), lomustine or CCNU (1-(2-chloroethyl)-3-cyclohexyl-1-nitrosourea), semustine or methyl-CCNU, and chlorozotocin. These cytotoxic drugs are active against a variety of neoplasms. BCNU and CCNU are highly lipophilic and can cross the blood–brain barrier, which makes them particularly useful in the treatment of central nervous system malignancies. BCNU is also used in high-dose conditioning regimens prior to bone marrow or stem cell transplantation for a variety of malignancies, including breast cancer, Hodgkin and non-Hodgkin lymphomas, multiple myeloma, and gliomas.

CARMUSTINE (BCNU)

Of the nitrosoureas, BCNU has been most extensively studied. Like bleomycin, this drug has been used in animal models of lung injury.

TABLE 65-6 Nitrosoureas

Drug	Pulmonary Syndrome	Treatment	Comments
Carmustine (BCNU)	Early-onset interstitial lung disease	Discontinue drug; corticosteroids	Risk factors: total dose, female sex, underlying lung disease, cigarette smoking, combination treatment with other cytotoxic drugs
	Late-onset pulmonary fibrosis	May appear years after treatment	
Lomustine Semustine Chlorozotocin	Interstitial lung disease	Discontinue drug	By extrapolation, toxicities and risk factors probably parallel BCNU

Intraperitoneal injection of BCNU in rats results in granulomatous inflammation and interstitial fibrosis, which progresses even after withdrawal of drug. Oxidant lung injury may play a role in the pathogenesis of toxicity as BCNU is known to inhibit glutathione reductase in pulmonary macrophages and reduces lung glutathione stores; however, the exact mechanisms by which pulmonary fibrosis occur are not well defined.

Like bleomycin, the toxicity of BCNU appears to be dose related. In a study of 94 patients with Hodgkin lymphoma who received chemotherapeutic regimens including BCNU, doses less than 475 mg/m^2 were associated with a 15% incidence of pulmonary toxicity; doses ranging between 475 and 525 mg/m^2 with a 32% incidence; and doses in excess of 525 mg/m^2 with a 47% incidence of pulmonary toxicity.[91] Treatment of intracranial gliomas may result in substantially higher cumulative BCNU doses. Very high doses (>1200–1500 mg/m^2) result in pulmonary toxicity in as many as 20% to 50% of patients.[91–93] Of note, BCNU may be used in single high doses pre–bone marrow or stem cell transplantation or may be given sequentially over longer periods of time. Whether the pattern of administration of a given total dosage has an impact on the potential for lung injury is unknown. Reported risk factors contributing to the development of pulmonary toxicity with BCNU include underlying lung disease, a history of smoking, previous or simultaneous treatment with other chemotherapy agents (including cyclophosphamide or bleomycin), chest radiotherapy, and female sex; of these, higher dose of drug and female sex are most consistently reported as related to development of pulmonary fibrosis.[92,94–98]

Pulmonary fibrosis related to BCNU falls into two patterns: An early-onset group that typically occurs within days to weeks of treatment or up to 3 years, and a late-onset group that may present years later. Early-onset pulmonary injury appears to be an underappreciated event. In a study of 152 patients treated for breast cancer with a regimen of BCNU (600 mg/m^2), cyclophosphamide, and cisplatin followed by stem cell transplantation, 59% developed a significant decrease in DL_{CO} at a median time after treatment of 45 days.[92] The vast majority of patients had subclinical disease and appeared to have improvement in their pulmonary status with initiation of corticosteroid therapy. Early-onset toxicity can also present as fulminant lung injury with progression in some cases to fatal pulmonary fibrosis.[97–99]

Late-onset pulmonary toxicity, typically presenting as pulmonary fibrosis, may occur years after BCNU treatment. In 1990, O'Driscoll et al.[95] first reported their observations on this phenomenon in survivors of childhood brain tumors. Of 31 original patients, 14 died of their tumors. In their last report in 2004 of a 25-year follow-up of the 17 survivors, 9 (53%) had died of complications related to pulmonary fibrosis.[100,101] Two patients died within the first 3 years after chemotherapy, four died between 6 and 13 years after chemotherapy, and three died between 13 and 25 years after chemotherapy. Furthermore, of the remaining eight patients still surviving, seven had radiographic and physiological evidence of pulmonary fibrosis. Thus, in this population of children treated with high-dose BCNU, late toxicity in the lung was extremely common and of severe clinical consequence.

The clinical presentation of BCNU-induced lung toxicity is variable. As noted, it may present as fulminant acute respiratory failure but more commonly presents insidiously with asymptomatic physiological abnormalities or radiographic evidence of pulmonary fibrosis. Symptoms of this latter subacute course include cough, fatigue, and progressive dyspnea. Chest radiograph is rarely normal in symptomatic patients, usually showing bilateral interstitial infiltrates with a basilar predominance. However, in O'Driscoll's series of patients with childhood brain tumors treated with high-dose BCNU and who developed late-onset pulmonary fibrosis, patients demonstrated an upper lobe predominance to the distribution of fibrotic changes.[95,100,101] Patients with an acute presentation may present with confluent alveolar infiltrates. Pneumothorax has been described in a number of cases and may be bilateral (Fig. 65-4). Pulmonary physiology generally shows a restrictive ventilatory defect, with diffusion abnormalities and eventually hypoxia. As with bleomycin-related lung injury, DL_{CO} may decrease without radiographic or clinical evidence of disease. While it has been suggested that a decrease in DL_{CO} may be the earliest sign of pulmonary toxicity, prospective evaluation of screening pulmonary function studies in the diagnosis of BCNU-induced lung toxicity has not been adequately studied. However, in light of the frequency and severity with which BCNU-associated pulmonary injury appears to occur, PFT may be helpful in identifying patients at risk and in whom administration of corticosteroids might be considered. Since BCNU toxicity is, unfortunately, common, and the likelihood of progression of BCNU-related lung injury to significant pulmonary fibrosis is seemingly high, it could be argued that surveillance with PFT should be considered, particularly if high doses of drug are to be given.

Pathological changes in the lung from BCNU parallel those seen with other cytotoxic agents. Type II pneumocyte hyperplasia and dysplasia, fibroblast proliferation, and deposition of proteinaceous material in alveoli have been described. However, inflammation tends not to be a prominent histological feature, and the cardinal feature of BCNU-induced lung toxicity appears to be interstitial fibrosis. In some cases, angiocentric necrotizing granulomatous inflammation or, more rarely, pulmonary venoocclusive disease may be seen.

The prognosis for patients with BCNU-induced lung injury is poor. For patients with early-onset lung toxicity, treatment with corticosteroids may be effective. One study of patients with breast cancer for whom BCNU was administered as part of treatment with high-dose chemotherapy followed by stem cell transplantation suggested that inhaled corticosteroids might be helpful in preventing pulmonary toxicity.[102] Late-onset pulmonary fibrosis related to BCNU does not appear to respond to corticosteroid therapy. The primary approach to BCNU toxicity should be to administer the lowest possible effective dose and monitor closely for signs of toxicity. Long-term treatment remains supportive. With the known long potential delay in the onset of signs of toxicity, long-term pulmonary follow-up is also warranted.

OTHER NITROSOUREAS

The other nitrosoureas used as chemotherapeutic agents, lomustine (CCNU), semustine (methyl CCNU), and chlorozotocin, have also been described to cause pulmonary toxicity. In general, these drugs have been used less widely than BCNU and in smaller cumulative doses. Their described lower incidence of pulmonary toxicity is likely due to these factors. As with BCNU, toxicity tends to present

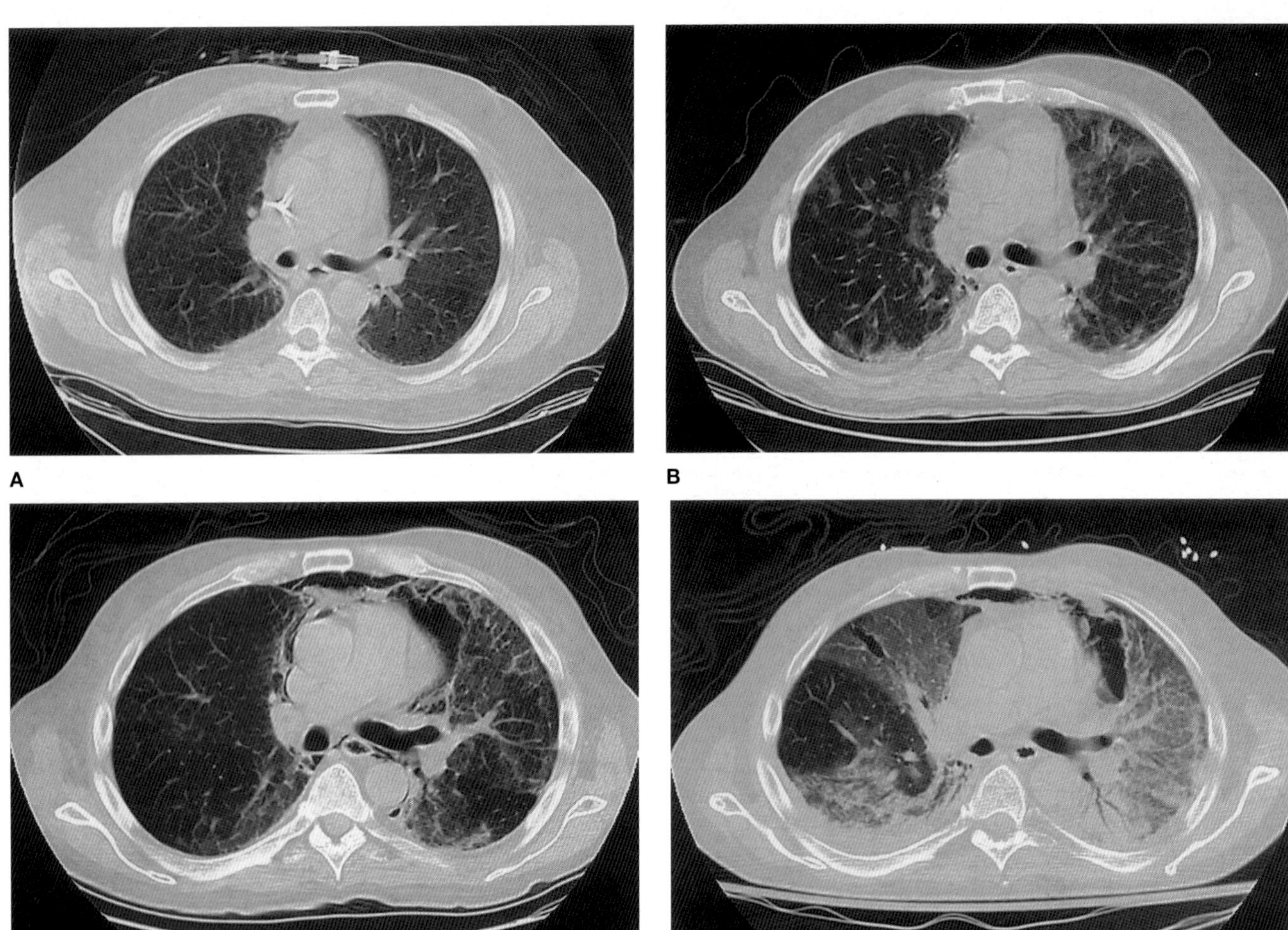

Figure 65-4 Serial chest computed tomography scans of a 54-year-old man with a history of Hodgkin lymphoma, treated with a BCNU-containing regimen. The dates of the examinations span 6 months from (**A**) to (**D**). Note the progression of diffuse interstitial patchy infiltrates, starting with the baseline normal study in (**A**). Pneumomediastinum and left pneumothorax are seen in (**C**) and (**D**). Bronchoscopy was performed between examinations (**B**) and (**C**), and demonstrated no evidence of infection. The patient had progressive dyspnea and respiratory insufficiency and eventually died of respiratory failure.

insidiously with interstitial pneumonitis and pulmonary fibrosis. However, given their close chemical relation, the potential for severe lung toxicity as seen with BCNU must be taken into consideration when using other drugs of this class.

MOLECULARLY TARGETED AGENTS

Examples of molecularly targeted agents (Table 65-7) include epidermal growth factor receptor (EGFR) tyrosine kinase inhibitors (gefitinib and erlotinib), BCR-Abl tyrosine kinase inhibitors (imatinib and dasatinib), and anaplastic lymphoma kinase (ALK) inhibitors (crizotinib).

EGFR TYROSINE KINASE INHIBITORS: GEFITINIB AND ERLOTINIB

Small molecule inhibitors of the EGFR tyrosine kinase were the first successful molecularly targeted agents effective for patients with NSCLC and virtually revolutionized the approach to treatment of this group of patients (Fig. 65-5).

Gefitinib was the first EGFR tyrosine kinase inhibitor available for clinical use. In a prospective study involving over 3000 patients treated with gefitinib for NSCLC in Japan, 4% of patients developed interstitial lung disease by 12 weeks of treatment with gefitinib, compared with 2.1% in patients treated with cytotoxic chemotherapy.[103] Studies done around the world have noted that pulmonary toxicity appears to vary geographically, being seen more commonly in Asian, as opposed to Caucasian or African populations.[104–106] Toxicity typically occurs fairly early in the course of treatment, with median exposure from 24 to 42 days. Withdrawal of drug appears in most cases to be helpful, but inexorable progression to end-stage respiratory failure and death occurs in approximately 31% of patients with gefitinib-induced pulmonary toxicity. Histological evaluation in patients who have succumbed to this illness has revealed diffuse alveolar damage. Risk factors associated with a higher likelihood of developing toxicity include older age, cigarette smoking, pre-existing interstitial lung disease, and poor performance status.[103,106]

The mechanism of gefitinib-induced lung injury remains a subject of investigation. EGFR is known to be upregulated in response to lung injury, and may be important in promoting type II pneumocyte hyperplasia in response to injury. In murine models, gefitinib has been demonstrated to result in more severe lung fibrosis in animals exposed to bleomycin. The increased frequency of this toxicity in patients with pre-existing pulmonary fibrosis lends credence to the hypothesis that gefitinib impairs the regeneration of alveolar epithelial cells in response to injury.

Erlotinib is the EGFR tyrosine kinase inhibitor used most commonly in the United States, as gefitinib is not available for clinical

TABLE 65-7 Molecularly Targeted Agents

Drug	Pulmonary Syndrome	Treatment	Comments
Gefitinib	Interstitial lung disease; pulmonary fibrosis	Discontinue drug	Usually occurs within first 3 mo of treatment; risk factors: older age, cigarette smoking, pre-existing lung disease, Asian ethnicity
Erlotinib	Interstitial lung disease	Discontinue drug	Risk factors: pre-existing lung disease
Imatinib	Pleural effusions	Diuretics	
	Interstitial lung disease	Discontinue drug; corticosteroids	Risk factors: pre-existing interstitial lung disease
Dasatinib	Pleural effusions	Diuretics	
	Pulmonary arterial hypertension	Discontinue drug	
Bevacizumab	Pulmonary hemorrhage	Supportive care; discontinue drug	Risk factors: cavitary tumor, squamous cell histology
Cetuximab	Bronchospasm, stridor	Discontinue drug; supportive care; corticosteroids	May occur during infusion; risk factors: asthma, atopy, history of allergic reactions
Rituximab	Interstitial pneumonitis; cryptogenic organizing pneumonia	Discontinue drug; corticosteroids	
	Bronchospasm, stridor, angioedema	Discontinue drug; supportive care; corticosteroids	May occur during infusion
Trastuzumab	Bronchospasm, hemodynamic instability	Discontinue drug	May occur during infusion
	Interstitial lung disease	Discontinue drug; corticosteroids	

treatment purposes.[93,107,108] While pulmonary toxicity manifesting as interstitial lung disease is also described with erlotinib, the incidence of this complication appears to be lower compared to gefitinib. This may reflect geography, as erlotinib has predominantly been used outside of Asia, but the exact incidence of erlotinib-associated interstitial disease is not clearly defined. In a study comparing treatment of patients with advanced NSCLC with erlotinib combined with carboplatin and paclitaxel followed by maintenance erlotinib versus placebo in combination with the two cytotoxic agents, there were no differences in overall survival.[109] However, five severe cases of interstitial disease occurred in the erlotinib group, compared to one in the placebo group; three cases were fatal, were all in the erlotinib group and were thought to be related to drug toxicity.[110] The time course of lung injury appears to be similar to gefitinib, with appearance of pulmonary injury typically occurring within weeks of initiation of treatment. The presence of underlying interstitial lung disease appears to be a risk factor for the development of drug toxicity.[111]

■ BCR-Abl TYROSINE KINASE INHIBITORS: IMATINIB AND DASATINIB

Imatinib was the first clinically available and prototypic molecularly targeted therapy. Developed in the 1990s, it is a small molecule tyrosine kinase inhibitor that suppresses proliferation of cells expressing the BCR-Abl fusion protein. The fusion gene created by translocation of the Abl-1 ("Abelson") gene on chromosome 9 to a part of the "breakpoint cluster region" (BCR) gene on chromosome 22 is the "Philadelphia chromosome," a hallmark for CML. Imatinib is used for treatment of patients with CML as well as gastrointestinal stromal tumors.

The most common pulmonary complication related to administration of imatinib is the development of pleural effusions. This reflects the propensity of patients receiving imatinib to retain fluid in various anatomic compartments.[112] Less commonly, imatinib has been associated with the development of interstitial lung disease; underlying fibrotic lung disease may be a predisposing factor.[113,114] In small series, corticosteroids have been reported as potentially beneficial; rechallenge is generally not recommended, but has been reported without recurrent lung disease.[113]

Almost inevitably, tumor resistance to the small molecule tyrosine kinase inhibitors occurs, due to development of new point mutations in the tumor kinase, resulting in resistant clones of cells and relapse of disease. Second generation BCR-Abl tyrosine kinase inhibitors include dasatinib and nilotinib. Like imatinib, these drugs may cause fluid retention and pleural effusions and have generated reports of associated interstitial lung disease.[115,116] Perhaps more concerning, a number of case reports have been published identifying pulmonary hypertension in patients treated with dasatinib.[117,118] Withdrawal of drug does not necessarily result in reversal of the elevation of pulmonary pressures, so rechallenge should not be attempted. Pulmonary hypertension has not been reported as a complication of imatinib.

■ ALK INHIBITORS: CRIZOTINIB

Crizotinib inhibits the ALK and has been useful in patients with NSCLC demonstrating the EML4-ALK fusion oncogene. Interstitial lung disease has been reported with crizotinib treatment.[119] As this drug is used only in a relatively small population of lung cancer patients with the specific targetable mutation, clinical information relating to potential lung injury is limited.

MONOCLONAL ANTIBODIES

Monoclonal antibodies have been increasingly employed to treat a variety of malignancies. Pulmonary toxicity has been reported with their use.

■ BEVACIZUMAB

Bevacizumab is a monoclonal antibody directed against vascular endothelial growth factor (VEGF) with activity against breast, colon, renal, and NSCL cancers. Improved response rates for locally advanced and metastatic NSCLC are observed when bevacizumab is added to traditional chemotherapy.[120] In a series including 99 patients

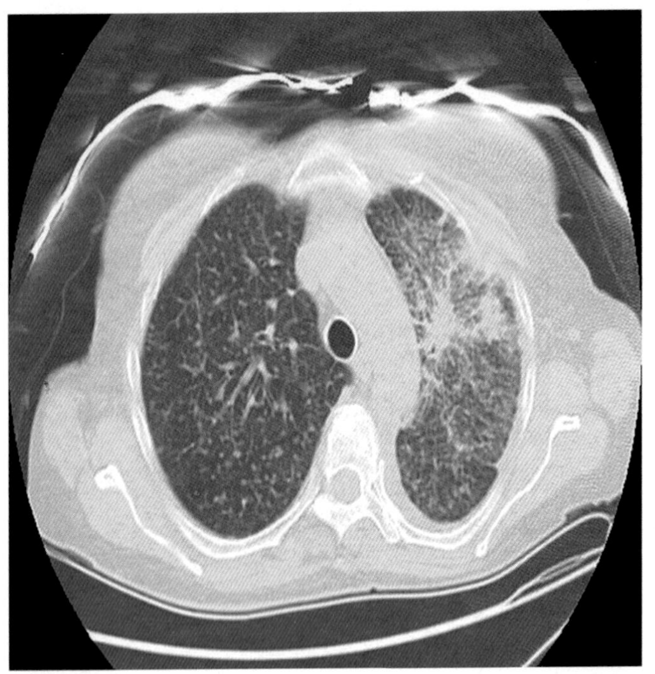

A

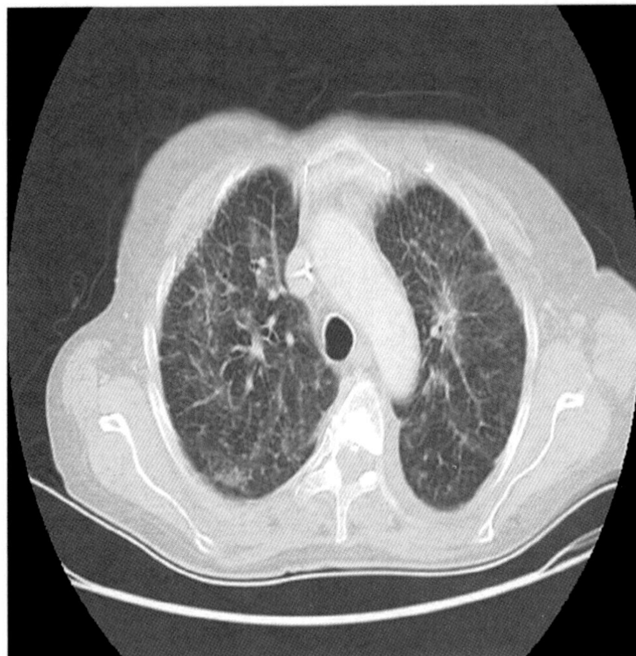

B

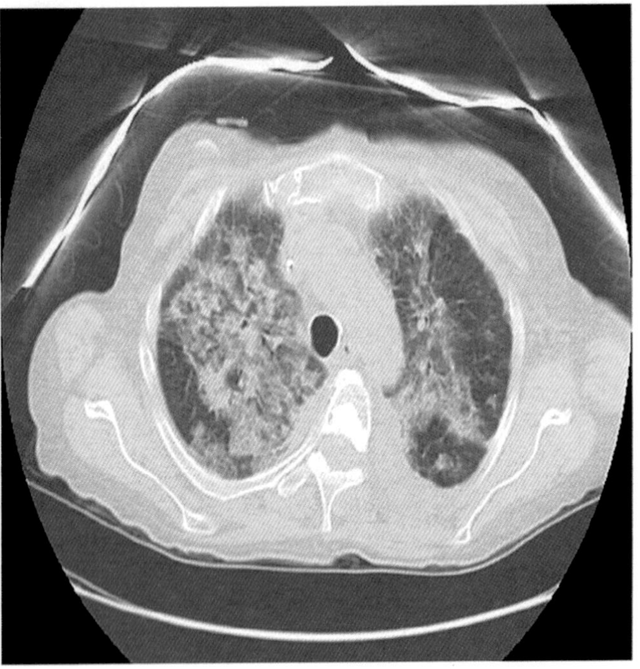

C

Figure 65-5 Serial chest computed tomography scans of a 79-year-old Caucasian woman with Stage IV adenocarcinoma of the lung, with primary site in the left upper lobe. The tumor was positive for an EGFR exon 19 deletion mutation, and the patient was treated with erlotinib. **A.** Chest CT scan performed at the time of diagnosis, demonstrating tumor in the left upper lobe. **B.** Chest CT scan after 2 months of erlotinib therapy, demonstrating improvement in the primary tumor site in the left upper lobe. **C.** Chest CT scan after 4 months of erlotinib therapy, demonstrating diffuse interstitial infiltrates in the right upper lobe and left upper lobe. The patient had no evidence of tumor relapse or infection at that time. The clinical picture was thought to be consistent with erlotinib-induced interstitial lung disease. Erlotinib was withdrawn, but the patient had relentless progression of respiratory insufficiency and eventually died of respiratory failure.

with newly diagnosed stage IIIB or IV or recurrent NSCLC, six patients developed serious bleeding complications including hemoptysis or hematemesis.[121] Four of the six patients died as a result of the hemorrhage. All six cases of hemorrhage appeared to be tumor related, with four of the six patients having squamous cell histology. Radiographically visible cavitation or necrosis was seen in five of the six cases of hemorrhage. As a result, current clinical investigations of regimens including bevacizumab generally exclude patients with cavitary pulmonary disease or squamous cell histology.

CETUXIMAB

Cetuximab is a chimeric monoclonal antibody directed against EGFR. Infusion of cetuximab may be associated with symptoms suggestive of anaphylaxis, including bronchospasm or stridor. In severe cases, respiratory compromise may be life-threatening. Risk factors for the development of these complications include a history of asthma, atopy, or allergic reactions.[122,123]

RITUXIMAB

Rituximab is a chimeric monoclonal antibody directed against the CD-20 antigen on B lymphocytes; it has demonstrated activity against non-Hodgkin lymphoma. It is increasingly used in inflammatory processes, including connective tissue diseases, autoimmune disorders, and solid organ transplantation. Like cetuximab, rituximab can be associated with infusion reactions, which, in severe form, may include bronchospasm and angioedema. Pulmonary parenchymal toxicity, while rare, is well described.[124–126] In one series of 107 patients with NHL receiving a regimen including rituximab, 9 of 107 patients developed interstitial pneumonitis associated with fever, dyspnea, and cough.[126] Treatment with glucocorticoids resulted in improvement. Retreatment was attempted in four patients, two of whom developed recurrence of interstitial disease; therefore, rechallenge is usually not recommended.

The clinical syndrome of rituximab-induced pulmonary toxicity typically begins insidiously with cough and dyspnea, which may progress with subsequent reexposure to rituximab. Development of hypoxemia in association with parenchymal ground-glass opacification on CT scan has been noted. Histological examinations have revealed reactions typical of cryptogenic organizing pneumonia/bronchiolitis obliterans organizing pneumonia, as well as interstitial inflammation with T lymphocytes and extensive arterial thrombosis. While fatal outcomes have been reported, generally this entity has responded well to withdrawal of rituximab and administration of corticosteroids.

TRASTUZUMAB

Trastuzumab is a humanized monoclonal antibody directed against the HER2 protein expressed by some breast and gastroesophageal tumors. Infusion reactions with trastuzumab are common; in severe cases, symptoms may include bronchospasm and hemodynamic instability. Rarely, patients with breast cancer receiving trastuzumab may develop acute pulmonary toxicity, with interstitial pneumonitis, organizing pneumonia, or acute respiratory distress syndrome; in some cases, glucocorticoids have been used successfully.[127,128]

MISCELLANEOUS AGENTS

A number of other agents used in treating malignant disease have been reported to be associated with pulmonary toxicity (Table 65-8). Representative examples are discussed below.

ALL-TRANS RETINOIC ACID

All-*trans* retinoic acid (ATRA) is a vitamin A derivative that has proved beneficial in the treatment of acute promyelocytic leukemia (APL). Activity of ATRA occurs through the induction of maturation of malignant cells into mature neutrophils. A constellation of symptoms and signs called the "differentiation (retinoic acid) syndrome," characterized by fever, weight gain related to volume overload and edema, respiratory distress with interstitial or alveolar infiltrates, pleural or pericardial effusions, hemodynamic instability, and renal insufficiency may occur from 2 to 21 days after drug initiation.[129,130] Pulmonary alveolar hemorrhage has been described as a rare complication.[131] The syndrome is frequently, although not universally, seen coincident with the development of a pronounced leukocytosis.[132]

Differentiation syndrome is not described with treatment on non-APL malignancies with ATRA. Radiographic features of the syndrome include pleural effusions, cardiomegaly, increased pulmonary blood volume, and widened vascular pedicle. Less frequently seen are prominent septal lines, nodules, ground-glass opacities, or parenchymal consolidation with air bronchograms. In the setting of diffuse alveolar hemorrhage, HRCT reveals poorly defined centrilobular nodules and diffuse ground-glass opacification.

Histological examination most commonly reveals infiltration of the lung parenchyma with maturing myeloid cells, with or without pulmonary hemorrhage. Fibrinoid necrosis and pulmonary capillaritis have also been described. The syndrome is thought to result from endothelial damage resulting in edema, hemorrhage, fibrinous exudates, and infiltration of neutrophils. The mechanism of ATRA-mediated pulmonary toxicity is poorly understood, but is thought to reflect systemic release of inflammatory cytokines.[133] Increased expression of cell adhesion molecules on leukemic cells has been demonstrated after ATRA administration, as has increased endothelial expression of intracellular adhesion molecule-1 (ICAM-1) and vascular cell adhesion molecule-1 (VCAM-1). In addition, elevated levels of interleukin-1β (IL-1β), IL-6, and TNFα have been observed and may promote leukocyte activation, contributing to tissue injury.

The incidence of the differentiation syndrome varies between 5% and 27% in the published literature.[129,132,134] Mortality rates vary from 5% to 29%. Prompt initiation of corticosteroids may be associated with improved outcome. Continuation of ATRA does not appear to be absolutely contraindicated, as long as corticosteroids are administered in a timely fashion. In cases with severe manifestations, discontinuation of ATRA seems reasonable, although reintroduction of drug on resolution of the syndrome is only infrequently met with recurrence.

INTERLEUKIN-2

Interleukin-2 (IL-2) is a glycoprotein secreted by activated lymphocytes. IL-2 therapy alone, or in conjunction with lymphokine-activated

TABLE 65-8 Miscellaneous Agents

Drug	Pulmonary Syndrome	Treatment	Comments
All-*trans* retinoic acid	"Differentiation syndrome"	Discontinue drug; corticosteroids	Treatment regimens for acute promyelocytic leukemia using all-*trans* retinoic acid should include corticosteroids
Interleukin-2	Cardiogenic edema, pleural effusions	Diuretics; supportive care	Vascular leak syndrome; risk factors: cumulative dose; administration of LAK cells
Procarbazine	Hypersensitivity-type pneumonitis	Discontinue drug	
	Interstitial lung disease	Discontinue drug	
Paclitaxel	Dyspnea, bronchospasm	Decrease infusion rate; corticosteroids and/or histamine antagonists	Pretreatment with histamine antagonists and/or corticosteroids reduces incidence
	Interstitial pneumonitis	Discontinue drug	Tends to occur within days to weeks after administration of drug
Docetaxel	Pleural effusions; noncardiogenic pulmonary edema	Discontinue drug; diuretics; supportive care	Pretreatment with corticosteroids may decrease incidence
	Interstitial pneumonitis	Discontinue drug	
Vinca alkaloids	Noncardiogenic pulmonary edema, interstitial pneumonitis, bronchospasm	Discontinue drug; corticosteroids	Risk factor: concurrent treatment with mitomycin C

killer (LAK) cells, has proved beneficial in patients with metastatic renal cell carcinoma or melanoma. Pulmonary complications related to IL-2 largely relate to cardiovascular instability with a vascular leak syndrome. This can result in cardiogenic, as well as noncardiogenic, pulmonary edema and may be associated with hypotension, renal insufficiency, and pleural effusions.

Several mechanisms have been identified that may explain the increase in capillary permeability. IL-2–activated lymphocytes produce a variety of cytokines, including tumor necrosis factor and IL-1. These may alter endothelial permeability and are thought, for example, to contribute to the septic shock syndrome. IL-2 also may promote the adhesion of natural killer cells to the capillary endothelium, thus altering vascular integrity. Furthermore, IL-2 is also associated with toxicity in multiple other organs, including the heart. Therefore, IL-2–induced cardiac dysfunction may contribute to the development of pulmonary interstitial edema.

IL-2 appears to have a cumulative dose-dependent lung toxicity that seems to be compounded by LAK cell administration.[135,136] Lung toxicity does appear to be reversible. In most cases, clinical and radiographic abnormalities resolve within several days after cessation of therapy. IL-2 has also been administered via inhalation to treat pulmonary metastases in patients with renal cell carcinoma and melanoma. The inhalational route of IL-2 appears to abrogate the risk of pulmonary toxicity, while demonstrating efficacy against intrapulmonary metastatic disease.[137]

PROCARBAZINE

Procarbazine is a cytotoxic drug used primarily in the treatment of lymphoma; it is associated with hypersensitivity pneumonitis in a small number of patients. This syndrome typically is seen after the second or third cycle of chemotherapy, although earlier as well as later occurrences have been described. Cough, dyspnea, and fever are typical symptoms, with the development of radiographic interstitial and/or alveolar infiltrates. A variable response to corticosteroids is reported, and rechallenge with procarbazine is associated with recurrence of the syndrome in the majority of patients.

TAXANES

Paclitaxel is a member of the taxane family, which functions through inhibition of microtubule disassembly and disruption of the G2 and M phases of the cell cycle. Paclitaxel has activity against a variety of carcinomas, including breast, ovarian, and NSCL cancers. There is a high incidence (up to 30%) of acute hypersensitivity reactions associated with paclitaxel infusion, with symptoms including dyspnea, bronchospasm, urticaria, and hypotension. Decreasing the infusion rate and/or administration of corticosteroids and histamine antagonists greatly reduces the frequency of this reaction to 1% to 2%. Paclitaxel has also been associated with the development of interstitial pneumonitis occurring days to weeks after paclitaxel administration, and should be suspected in those who develop interstitial infiltrates following paclitaxel therapy.[138–140]

Docetaxel has a much lower incidence of acute hypersensitivity reactions than paclitaxel.[90,141–143] Docetaxel is, however, associated with a syndrome of fluid retention related to capillary leak.[142] This syndrome is characterized by the development of peripheral edema, pleural effusions, or ascites, and is mitigated by pretreatment with corticosteroids. Interstitial pneumonitis has been associated with docetaxel administration, and may progress to respiratory failure and death.[90,141,143] This syndrome may occur as early as 1 to 2 weeks after administration of the drug. Biopsies have been reported to reveal histological changes consistent with drug-induced hypersensitivity pneumonitis or diffuse alveolar damage. As opposed to many cases of drug-induced hypersensitivity, this reaction may have a protracted course prior to recovery.

VINCA ALKALOIDS

The vinca alkaloids given as sole agents are rarely associated with pulmonary toxicity. However, the combination of vinblastine, vindesine, or vinorelbine with mitomycin C has been reported to be associated with noncardiogenic pulmonary edema, interstitial pneumonitis, and bronchospasm, often in conjunction with more diffuse endothelial dysfunction (see earlier section on mitomycin C).[36] Vinorelbine as a sole agent has been associated with dyspnea in less than 5% of cases; it occurs within hours of dosing, and generally responds to bronchodilators and corticosteroids.[144] Respiratory distress with pulmonary edema and interstitial pneumonitis has also been rarely described.

REFERENCES

1. Cooper JA Jr, White DA, Matthay RA. Drug-induced pulmonary disease. Part 1: cytotoxic drugs. *Am Rev Respir Dis.* 1986;133(2):321–340.
2. Flieder D, Travix W. Pathologic characteristics of drug-induced lung disease. In: Camus P, Rosenow EC 3rd, eds. *Clinics in Chest Medicine.* Vol 25. Philadelphia, PA: WB Saunders; 2004:37–45.
3. Limper AH. Chemotherapy-induced lung disease. *Clin Chest Med.* 2004;25(1):53–64.
4. Rivera MP, Detterbeck FC, Socinski MA, et al. Impact of preoperative chemotherapy on pulmonary function tests in resectable early-stage non-small cell lung cancer. *Chest.* 2009;135(6):1588–1595.
5. Dimopoulou I, Efstathiou E, Samakovli A, et al. A prospective study on lung toxicity in patients treated with gemcitabine and carboplatin: clinical, radiological and functional assessment. *Ann Oncol.* 2004;15(8):1250–1255.
6. Castro M, Veeder MH, Mailliard JA, Tazelaar HD, Jett JR. A prospective study of pulmonary function in patients receiving mitomycin. *Chest.* 1996;109(4):939–944.
7. Lund MB, Kongerud J, Nome O, et al. Lung function impairment in long-term survivors of Hodgkin's disease. *Ann Oncol.* 1995;6(5):495–501.
8. Umezawa H, Maeda K, Takeuchi T, Okami Y. New antibiotics, bleomycin A and B. *J Antibiot (Tokyo).* 1966;19(5):200–209.
9. Lazo JS, Merrill WW, Pham ET, Lynch TJ, McCallister JD, Ingbar DH. Bleomycin hydrolase activity in pulmonary cells. *J Pharmacol Exp Ther.* 1984;231(3):583–588.
10. Sleijfer S. Bleomycin-induced pneumonitis. *Chest.* 2001;120(2):617–624.
11. Hay J, Shahzeidi S, Laurent G. Mechanisms of bleomycin-induced lung damage. *Arch Toxicol.* 1991;65(2):81–94.
12. Scheule RK, Perkins RC, Hamilton R, Holian A. Bleomycin stimulation of cytokine secretion by the human alveolar macrophage. *Am J Physiol.* 1992;262(4 Pt 1):L386–L391.
13. Sleijfer S, Vujaskovic Z, Limburg PC, Schraffordt Koops H, Mulder NH. Induction of tumor necrosis factor-alpha as a cause of bleomycin-related toxicity. *Cancer.* 1998;82(5):970–974.
14. Piguet PF, Collart MA, Grau GE, Kapanci Y, Vassalli P. Tumor necrosis factor/cachectin plays a key role in bleomycin-induced pneumopathy and fibrosis. *J Exp Med.* 1989;170(3):655–663.
15. Piguet PF, Vesin C, Grau GE, Thompson RC. Interleukin 1 receptor antagonist (IL-1ra) prevents or cures pulmonary

fibrosis elicited in mice by bleomycin or silica. *Cytokine*. 1993;5(1):57–61.

16. Giri SN, Hyde DM, Hollinger MA. Effect of antibody to transforming growth factor beta on bleomycin induced accumulation of lung collagen in mice. *Thorax*. 1993;48(10):959–966.
17. Jules-Elysee K, White DA. Bleomycin-induced pulmonary toxicity. *Clin Chest Med*. 1990;11(1):1–20.
18. Collis CH. Lung damage from cytotoxic drugs. *Cancer Chemother Pharmacol*. 1980;4(1):17–27.
19. Tryka AF, Skornik WA, Godleski JJ, Brain JD. Potentiation of bleomycin-induced lung injury by exposure to 70% oxygen. Morphologic assessment. *Am Rev Respir Dis*. 1982;126(6):1074–1079.
20. Gilson AJ, Sahn SA. Reactivation of bleomycin lung toxicity following oxygen administration. A second response to corticosteroids. *Chest*. 1985;88(2):304–306.
21. Macann A, Bredenfeld H, Muller RP, Diehl V, Engert A, Eich HT. Radiotherapy does not influence the severe pulmonary toxicity observed with the administration of gemcitabine and bleomycin in patients with advanced-stage Hodgkin's lymphoma treated with the BAGCOPP regimen: a report by the German Hodgkin's Lymphoma Study Group. *Int J Radiat Oncol Biol Phys*. 2008;70(1):161–165.
22. Hirsch A, Vander Els N, Straus DJ, et al. Effect of ABVD chemotherapy with and without mantle or mediastinal irradiation on pulmonary function and symptoms in early-stage Hodgkin's disease. *J Clin Oncol*. 1996;14(4):1297–1305.
23. Crooke ST, Comis RL, Einhorn LH, Strong JE, Broughton A, Prestayko AW. Effects of variations in renal function on the clinical pharmacology of bleomycin administered as an iv bolus. *Cancer Treat Rep*. 1977;61(9):1631–1636.
24. Simpson AB, Paul J, Graham J, Kaye SB. Fatal bleomycin pulmonary toxicity in the west of Scotland 1991–95: a review of patients with germ cell tumours. *Br J Cancer*. 1998;78(8):1061–1066.
25. Lower EE, Strohofer S, Baughman RP. Bleomycin causes alveolar macrophages from cigarette smokers to release hydrogen peroxide. *Am J Med Sci*. 1988;295(3):193–197.
26. Saxman SB, Nichols CR, Einhorn LH. Pulmonary toxicity in patients with advanced-stage germ cell tumors receiving bleomycin with and without granulocyte colony stimulating factor. *Chest*. 1997;111(3):657–660.
27. De Lena M, Guzzon A, Monfardini S, Bonadonna G. Clinical, radiologic, and histopathologic studies on pulmonary toxicity induced by treatment with bleomycin (NSC-125066). *Cancer Chemother Rep*. 1972;56(3):343–356.
28. Bellamy EA, Husband JE, Blaquiere RM, Law MR. Bleomycin-related lung damage: CT evidence. *Radiology*. 1985;156(1):155–158.
29. Comis RL, Kuppinger MS, Ginsberg SJ, et al. Role of single-breath carbon monoxide-diffusing capacity in monitoring the pulmonary effects of bleomycin in germ cell tumor patients. *Cancer Res*. 1979;39(12):5076–5080.
30. Holoye PY, Luna MA, MacKay B, Bedrossian CW. Bleomycin hypersensitivity pneumonitis. *Ann Intern Med*. 1978;88(1):47–49.
31. White DA, Schwartzberg LS, Kris MG, Bosl GJ. Acute chest pain syndrome during bleomycin infusions. *Cancer*. 1987;59(9):1582–1585.
32. Verweij J, Pinedo HM. Mitomycin C: mechanism of action, usefulness and limitations. *Anticancer Drugs*. 1990;1(1):5–13.
33. Wada H, Nakano Y, Yamada H, Saiga T, Yamanaka A, Sakai N. Intravesical mitomycin-C-induced interstitial pneumonia. *Respiration*. 2010;80(3):256–259.
34. Gonzalez-Moreno S, Lambert LA, Mansfield PF. Interstitial pneumonitis: an exceptional toxicity of hyperthermic intraperitoneal mitomycin C. *Eur J Surg Oncol*. 2008;34(4):482–484.
35. Okuno SH, Frytak S. Mitomycin lung toxicity. Acute and chronic phases. *Am J Clin Oncol*. 1997;20(3):282–284.
36. Rivera MP, Kris MG, Gralla RJ, White DA. Syndrome of acute dyspnea related to combined mitomycin plus vinca alkaloid chemotherapy. *Am J Clin Oncol*. 1995;18(3):245–250.
37. Chang AY, Kuebler JP, Pandya KJ, Israel RH, Marshall BC, Tormey DC. Pulmonary toxicity induced by mitomycin C is highly responsive to glucocorticoids. *Cancer*. 1986;57(12):2285–2290.
38. Luedke D, McLaughlin TT, Daughaday C, et al. Mitomycin C and vindesine associated pulmonary toxicity with variable clinical expression. *Cancer*. 1985;55(3):542–545.
39. Rouzaud P, Estivals M, Pujazon MC, Carles P, Lauque D. [Respiratory complications of the vinorelbine-mitomycin combination]. *Rev Mal Respir*. 1999;16(1):81–84.
40. Jolivet J, Giroux L, Laurin S, Gruber J, Bettez P, Band PR. Microangiopathic hemolytic anemia, renal failure, and non-cardiogenic pulmonary edema: a chemotherapy-induced syndrome. *Cancer Treat Rep*. 1983;67(5):429–434.
41. Torra R, Poch E, Torras A, Bombi JA, Revert L. Pulmonary hemorrhage as a clinical manifestation of hemolytic-uremic syndrome associated with mitomycin C therapy. *Chemotherapy*. 1993;39(6):453–456.
42. Hong MJ, Lee HG, Hur M, Kim SY, Cho YH, Yoon SY. Slow, but complete, resolution of mitomycin-induced refractory thrombotic thrombocytopenic purpura after rituximab treatment. *Korean J Hematol*. 2011;46(1):45–48.
43. Gourley BL, Mesa H, Gupta P. Rapid and complete resolution of chemotherapy-induced thrombotic thrombocytopenic purpura/hemolytic uremic syndrome (TTP/HUS) with rituximab. *Cancer Chemother Pharmacol*. 2010;65(5):1001–1004.
44. Gagnadoux F, Capron F, Lebeau B. Pulmonary veno-occlusive disease after neoadjuvant mitomycin chemotherapy and surgery for lung carcinoma. *Lung Cancer*. 2002;36(2):213–215.
45. Ma LD, Taylor GA, Wharam MD, Wiley JM. "Recall" pneumonitis: adriamycin potentiation of radiation pneumonitis in two children. *Radiology*. 1993;187(2):465–467.
46. Hall AG, Tilby MJ. Mechanisms of action of, and modes of resistance to, alkylating agents used in the treatment of haematological malignancies. *Blood Rev*. 1992;6(3):163–173.
47. Twohig KJ, Matthay RA. Pulmonary effects of cytotoxic agents other than bleomycin. *Clin Chest Med*. 1990;11(1):31–54.
48. Kachel DL, Martin WJ 2nd. Cyclophosphamide-induced lung toxicity: mechanism of endothelial cell injury. *J Pharmacol Exp Ther*. 1994;268(1):42–46.
49. Hoyt DG, Lazo JS. Early increases in pulmonary mRNA encoding procollagens and transforming growth factor-beta in mice sensitive to cyclophosphamide-induced pulmonary fibrosis. *J Pharmacol Exp Ther*. 1989;249(1):38–43.
50. Hoyt DG, Lazo JS. Acute pneumocyte injury, poly(ADP-ribose) polymerase activity, and pyridine nucleotide levels after in vitro exposure of murine lung slices to cyclophosphamide. *Biochem Pharmacol*. 1994;48(9):1757–1765.

51. Malik SW, Myers JL, DeRemee RA, Specks U. Lung toxicity associated with cyclophosphamide use. Two distinct patterns. *Am J Respir Crit Care Med.* 1996;154(6 Pt 1): 1851–1856.
52. Spector JI, Zimbler H, Ross JS. Early-onset cyclophosphamide-induced interstitial pneumonitis. *JAMA.* 1979;242(26): 2852–2854.
53. Mark GJ, Lehimgar-Zadeh A, Ragsdale BD. Cyclophosphamide pneumonitis. *Thorax.* 1978;33(1):89–93.
54. Fernandez HF, Tran HT, Albrecht F, Lennon S, Caldera H, Goodman MS. Evaluation of safety and pharmacokinetics of administering intravenous busulfan in a twice-daily or daily schedule to patients with advanced hematologic malignant disease undergoing stem cell transplantation. *Biol Blood Marrow Transplant.* 2002;8(9):486–492.
55. Ginsberg SJ, Comis RL. The pulmonary toxicity of antineoplastic agents. *Semin Oncol.* 1982;9(1):34–51.
56. Brockstein BE, Smiley C, Al-Sadir J, Williams SF. Cardiac and pulmonary toxicity in patients undergoing high-dose chemotherapy for lymphoma and breast cancer: prognostic factors. *Bone Marrow Transplant.* 2000;25(8):885–894.
57. Crilley P, Topolsky D, Styler MJ, et al. Extramedullary toxicity of a conditioning regimen containing busulphan, cyclophosphamide and etoposide in 84 patients undergoing autologous and allogenic bone marrow transplantation. *Bone Marrow Transplant.* 1995;15(3):361–365.
58. Ringden O, Remberger M, Ruutu T, et al. Increased risk of chronic graft-versus-host disease, obstructive bronchiolitis, and alopecia with busulfan versus total body irradiation: long-term results of a randomized trial in allogeneic marrow recipients with leukemia. Nordic Bone Marrow Transplantation Group. *Blood.* 1999;93(7):2196–2201.
59. Aymard JP, Gyger M, Lavallee R, Legresley LP, Desy M. A case of pulmonary alveolar proteinosis complicating chronic myelogenous leukemia. A peculiar pathologic aspect of busulfan lung? *Cancer.* 1984;53(4):954–956.
60. Khong HT, McCarthy J. Chlorambucil-induced pulmonary disease: a case report and review of the literature. *Ann Hematol.* 1998;77(1–2):85–87.
61. Crestani B, Jaccard A, Israel-Biet D, Couderc LJ, Frija J, Clauvel JP. Chlorambucil-associated pneumonitis. *Chest.* 1994;105(2): 634–636.
62. Akasheh MS, Freytes CO, Vesole DH. Melphalan-associated pulmonary toxicity following high-dose therapy with autologous hematopoietic stem cell transplantation. *Bone Marrow Transplant.* 2000;26(10):1107–1109.
63. Baker WJ, Fistel SJ, Jones RV, Weiss RB. Interstitial pneumonitis associated with ifosfamide therapy. *Cancer.* 1990;65(10): 2217–2221.
64. Hadjiliadis D, Govert JA. Methemoglobinemia after infusion of ifosfamide chemotherapy: first report of a potentially serious adverse reaction related to ifosfamide. *Chest.* 2000;118(4): 1208–1210.
65. Garrido M, O'Brien A, Gonzalez S, Clavero JM, Orellana E. Cryptogenic organizing pneumonitis during oxaliplatin chemotherapy for colorectal cancer: case report. *Chest.* 2007; 132(6):1997–1999.
66. Hannan LM, Yoong J, Chong G, McDonald CF. Interstitial lung disease in a patient treated with oxaliplatin, 5-fluorouracil and leucovorin (FOLFOX) for metastatic colorectal cancer. *Radiol Oncol.* 2012;46(4):360–362.
67. Gagnadoux F, Roiron C, Carrie E, Monnier-Cholley L, Lebeau B. Eosinophilic lung disease under chemotherapy with oxaliplatin for colorectal cancer. *Am J Clin Oncol.* 2002;25(4): 388–390.
68. Watkins J, Slade JH, Phan A, Eng C, Weissferdt A, Overman MJ. Fatal diffuse alveolar damage associated with oxaliplatin administration. *Clin Colorectal Cancer.* 2011;10(3):198–202.
69. Rubbia-Brandt L, Audard V, Sartoretti P, et al. Severe hepatic sinusoidal obstruction associated with oxaliplatin-based chemotherapy in patients with metastatic colorectal cancer. *Ann Oncol.* 2004;15(3):460–466.
70. Wilcox BE, Ryu JH, Kalra S. Exacerbation of pre-existing interstitial lung disease after oxaliplatin therapy: a report of three cases. *Respir Med.* 2008;102(2):273–279.
71. Searles G, McKendry RJ. Methotrexate pneumonitis in rheumatoid arthritis: potential risk factors. Four case reports and a review of the literature. *J Rheumatol.* 1987;14(6):1164–1171.
72. Alarcon GS, Kremer JM, Macaluso M, et al. Risk factors for methotrexate-induced lung injury in patients with rheumatoid arthritis. A multicenter, case-control study. Methotrexate-Lung Study Group. *Ann Intern Med.* 1997;127(5): 356–364.
73. Golden MR, Katz RS, Balk RA, Golden HE. The relationship of preexisting lung disease to the development of methotrexate pneumonitis in patients with rheumatoid arthritis. *J Rheumatol.* 1995;22(6):1043–1047.
74. Sany J, Anaya JM. Predictive value of pulmonary function tests in methotrexate induced pneumonitis in rheumatoid arthritis. *Arthritis Rheum.* 1992;35:S147.
75. The effect of age and renal function on the efficacy and toxicity of methotrexate in rheumatoid arthritis. Rheumatoid Arthritis Clinical Trial Archive Group. *J Rheumatol.* 1995;22(2): 218–223.
76. Sostman HD, Matthay RA, Putman CE, Smith GJ. Methotrexate-induced pneumonitis. *Medicine (Baltimore).* 1976;55(5): 371–388.
77. Cronstein BN, Merrill JT. Mechanisms of the effects of methotrexate. *Bull Rheum Dis.* 1996;45(5):6–8.
78. Andersson BS, Luna MA, Yee C, Hui KK, Keating MJ, McCredie KB. Fatal pulmonary failure complicating high-dose cytosine arabinoside therapy in acute leukemia. *Cancer.* 1990;65(5):1079–1084.
79. Rubio C, Hill ME, Milan S, O'Brien ME, Cunningham D. Idiopathic pneumonia syndrome after high-dose chemotherapy for relapsed Hodgkin's disease. *Br J Cancer.* 1997;75(7): 1044–1048.
80. Haupt HM, Hutchins GM, Moore GW. Ara-C lung: noncardiogenic pulmonary edema complicating cytosine arabinoside therapy of leukemia. *Am J Med.* 1981;70(2):256–261.
81. Patel M, Ezzat W, Pauw KL, Lowsky R. Bronchiolitis obliterans organizing pneumonia in a patient with chronic myelogenous leukemia developing after initiation of interferon and cytosine arabinoside. *Eur J Haematol.* 2001;67(5–6): 318–321.
82. Battistini E, Dini G, Savioli C, et al. Bronchiolitis obliterans organizing pneumonia in three children with acute leukaemias treated with cytosine arabinoside and anthracyclines. *Eur Respir J.* 1997;10(5):1187–1190.
83. Helman DL Jr, Byrd JC, Ales NC, Shorr AF. Fludarabine-related pulmonary toxicity: a distinct clinical entity in chronic lymphoproliferative syndromes. *Chest.* 2002;122(3):785–790.

84. Kane GC, McMichael AJ, Patrick H, Erslev AJ. Pulmonary toxicity and acute respiratory failure associated with fludarabine monophosphate. *Respir Med.* 1992;86(3):261–263.

85. Levin M, Aziz M, Opitz L. Steroid-responsive interstitial pneumonitis after fludarabine therapy. *Chest.* 1997;111(5): 1472–1473.

86. Roychowdhury DF, Cassidy CA, Peterson P, Arning M. A report on serious pulmonary toxicity associated with gemcitabine-based therapy. *Invest New Drugs.* 2002;20(3):311–315.

87. Barlesi F, Villani P, Doddoli C, Gimenez C, Kleisbauer JP. Gemcitabine-induced severe pulmonary toxicity. *Fundam Clin Pharmacol.* 2004;18(1):85–91.

88. Belknap SM, Kuzel TM, Yarnold PR, et al. Clinical features and correlates of gemcitabine-associated lung injury: findings from the RADAR project. *Cancer.* 2006;106(9):2051–2057.

89. Li J, Juliar B, Yiannoutsos C, et al. Weekly paclitaxel and gemcitabine in advanced transitional-cell carcinoma of the urothelium: a phase II Hoosier Oncology Group study. *J Clin Oncol.* 2005;23(6):1185–1191.

90. Binder D, Hubner RH, Temmesfeld-Wollbruck B, Schlattmann P. Pulmonary toxicity among cancer patients treated with a combination of docetaxel and gemcitabine: a meta-analysis of clinical trials. *Cancer Chemother Pharmacol.* 2011;68(6): 1575–1583.

91. Schmitz N, Diehl V. Carmustine and the lungs. *Lancet.* 1997;349(9067):1712–1713.

92. Cao TM, Negrin RS, Stockerl-Goldstein KE, et al. Pulmonary toxicity syndrome in breast cancer patients undergoing BCNU-containing high-dose chemotherapy and autologous hematopoietic cell transplantation. *Biol Blood Marrow Transplant.* 2000; 6(4):387–394.

93. Spigel DR, Lin M, O'Neill V, Hainsworth JD. Final survival and safety results from a multicenter, open-label, phase 3b trial of erlotinib in patients with advanced nonsmall cell lung cancer. *Cancer.* 2008;112(12):2749–2755.

94. Durant JR, Norgard MJ, Murad TM, Bartolucci AA, Langford KH. Pulmonary toxicity associated with bischloroethylnitrosourea (BCNU). *Ann Intern Med.* 1979;90(2):191–194.

95. O'Driscoll BR, Hasleton PS, Taylor PM, Poulter LW, Gattameneni HR, Woodcock AA. Active lung fibrosis up to 17 years after chemotherapy with carmustine (BCNU) in childhood. *N Engl J Med.* 1990;323(6):378–382.

96. Parish JM, Muhm JR, Leslie KO. Upper lobe pulmonary fibrosis associated with high-dose chemotherapy containing BCNU for bone marrow transplantation. *Mayo Clin Proc.* 2003;78(5): 630–634.

97. Selker RG, Jacobs SA, Moore PB, et al. 1,3-Bis(2-chloroethyl)-1-nitrosourea (BCNU)-induced pulmonary fibrosis. *Neurosurgery.* 1980;7(6):560–565.

98. Wong R, Rondon G, Saliba RM, et al. Idiopathic pneumonia syndrome after high-dose chemotherapy and autologous hematopoietic stem cell transplantation for high-risk breast cancer. *Bone Marrow Transplant.* 2003;31(12):1157–1163.

99. Clark JG, Hansen JA, Hertz MI, Parkman R, Jensen L, Peavy HH. NHLBI workshop summary. Idiopathic pneumonia syndrome after bone marrow transplantation. *Am Rev Respir Dis.* 1993;147(6 Pt 1):1601–1606.

100. O'Driscoll BR, Kalra S, Gattameneni HR, Woodcock AA. Late carmustine lung fibrosis. Age at treatment may influence severity and survival. *Chest.* 1995;107(5):1355–1357.

101. Lohani S, O'Driscoll BR, Woodcock AA. 25-year study of lung fibrosis following carmustine therapy for brain tumor in childhood. *Chest.* 2004;126(3):1007.

102. McGaughey DS, Nikcevich DA, Long GD, et al. Inhaled steroids as prophylaxis for delayed pulmonary toxicity syndrome in breast cancer patients undergoing high-dose chemotherapy and autologous stem cell transplantation. *Biol Blood Marrow Transplant.* 2001;7(5):274–278.

103. Kudoh S, Kato H, Nishiwaki Y, et al. Interstitial lung disease in Japanese patients with lung cancer: a cohort and nested case-control study. *Am J Respir Crit Care Med.* 2008;177(12): 1348–1357.

104. Cohen MH, Williams GA, Sridhara R, Chen G, Pazdur R. FDA drug approval summary: gefitinib (ZD1839) (Iressa) tablets. *Oncologist.* 2003;8(4):303–306.

105. Endo M, Johkoh T, Kimura K, Yamamoto N. Imaging of gefitinib-related interstitial lung disease: multi-institutional analysis by the West Japan Thoracic Oncology Group. *Lung Cancer.* 2006;52(2):135–140.

106. Takano T, Ohe Y, Kusumoto M, et al. Risk factors for interstitial lung disease and predictive factors for tumor response in patients with advanced non-small cell lung cancer treated with gefitinib. *Lung Cancer.* 2004;45(1):93–104.

107. Mok TS, Wu YL, Yu CJ, et al. Randomized, placebo-controlled, phase II study of sequential erlotinib and chemotherapy as first-line treatment for advanced non-small-cell lung cancer. *J Clin Oncol.* 2009;27(30):5080–5087.

108. Reck M, van Zandwijk N, Gridelli C, et al. Erlotinib in advanced non-small cell lung cancer: efficacy and safety findings of the global phase IV Tarceva Lung Cancer Survival Treatment study. *J Thorac Oncol.* 2010;5(10):1616–1622.

109. Herbst RS, Prager D, Hermann R, et al. TRIBUTE: a phase III trial of erlotinib hydrochloride (OSI-774) combined with carboplatin and paclitaxel chemotherapy in advanced non-small-cell lung cancer. *J Clin Oncol.* 2005;23(25):5892–5899.

110. Yoneda KY, Shelton DK, Beckett LA, Gandara DR. Independent review of interstitial lung disease associated with death in TRIBUTE (paclitaxel and carboplatin with or without concurrent erlotinib) in advanced non-small cell lung cancer. *J Thorac Oncol.* 2007;2(6):537–543.

111. Liu V, White DA, Zakowski MF, et al. Pulmonary toxicity associated with erlotinib. *Chest.* 2007;132(3):1042–1044.

112. Ishii Y, Shoji N, Kimura Y, Ohyashiki K. Prominent pleural effusion possibly due to imatinib mesylate in adult Philadelphia chromosome-positive acute lymphoblastic leukemia. *Intern Med.* 2006;45(5):339–340.

113. Ohnishi K, Sakai F, Kudoh S, Ohno R. Twenty-seven cases of drug-induced interstitial lung disease associated with imatinib mesylate. *Leukemia.* 2006;20(6):1162–1164.

114. Ma CX, Hobday TJ, Jett JR. Imatinib mesylate-induced interstitial pneumonitis. *Mayo Clin Proc.* 2003;78(12):1578–1579.

115. Latagliata R, Breccia M, Fava C, et al. Incidence, risk factors and management of pleural effusions during dasatinib treatment in unselected elderly patients with chronic myelogenous leukaemia. *Hematol Oncol.* 2013;31(2):363–369.

116. Bergeron A, Rea D, Levy V, et al. Lung abnormalities after dasatinib treatment for chronic myeloid leukemia: a case series. *Am J Respir Crit Care Med.* 2007;176(8):814–818.

117. Montani D, Bergot E, Gunther S, et al. Pulmonary arterial hypertension in patients treated by dasatinib. *Circulation.* 2012; 125(17):2128–2137.

118. Dumitrescu D, Seck C, ten Freyhaus H, Gerhardt F, Erdmann E, Rosenkranz S. Fully reversible pulmonary arterial hypertension associated with dasatinib treatment for chronic myeloid leukaemia. *Eur Respir J.* 2011;38(1):218–220.

119. Tamiya A, Okamoto I, Miyazaki M, Shimizu S, Kitaichi M, Nakagawa K. Severe acute interstitial lung disease after crizotinib therapy in a patient with EML4-ALK-positive non-small-cell lung cancer. *J Clin Oncol.* 2013;31(1):e15–e17.

120. Sandler A, Gray R, Perry MC, et al. Paclitaxel-carboplatin alone or with bevacizumab for non-small-cell lung cancer. *N Engl J Med.* 2006;355(24):2542–2550.

121. Johnson DH, Fehrenbacher L, Novotny WF, et al. Randomized phase II trial comparing bevacizumab plus carboplatin and paclitaxel with carboplatin and paclitaxel alone in previously untreated locally advanced or metastatic non-small-cell lung cancer. *J Clin Oncol.* 2004;22(11):2184–2191.

122. O'Neil BH, Allen R, Spigel DR, et al. High incidence of cetuximab-related infusion reactions in Tennessee and North Carolina and the association with atopic history. *J Clin Oncol.* 2007;25(24):3644–3648.

123. Pointreau Y, Commins SP, Calais G, Watier H, Platts-Mills TA. Fatal infusion reactions to cetuximab: role of immunoglobulin e-mediated anaphylaxis. *J Clin Oncol.* 2012;30(3):334; author reply 335.

124. Bitzan M, Anselmo M, Carpineta L. Rituximab (B-cell depleting antibody) associated lung injury (RALI): a pediatric case and systematic review of the literature. *Pediatr Pulmonol.* 2009;44(9):922–934.

125. Burton C, Kaczmarski R, Jan-Mohamed R. Interstitial pneumonitis related to rituximab therapy. *N Engl J Med.* 2003; 348(26):2690–2691; discussion 2690–2691.

126. Liu X, Hong XN, Gu YJ, Wang BY, Luo ZG, Cao J. Interstitial pneumonitis during rituximab-containing chemotherapy for non-Hodgkin lymphoma. *Leuk Lymphoma.* 2008;49(9): 1778–1783.

127. Radzikowska E, Szczepulska E, Chabowski M, Bestry I. Organising pneumonia caused by transtuzumab (Herceptin) therapy for breast cancer. *Eur Respir J.* 2003;21(3):552–555.

128. Pepels MJ, Boomars KA, van Kimmenade R, Hupperets PS. Life-threatening interstitial lung disease associated with trastuzumab: case report. *Breast Cancer Res Treat.* 2009;113(3): 609–612.

129. De Botton S, Dombret H, Sanz M, et al. Incidence, clinical features, and outcome of all trans-retinoic acid syndrome in 413 cases of newly diagnosed acute promyelocytic leukemia. The European APL Group. *Blood.* 1998;92(8):2712–2718.

130. Sanz MA, Grimwade D, Tallman MS, et al. Management of acute promyelocytic leukemia: recommendations from an expert panel on behalf of the European LeukemiaNet. *Blood.* 2009;113(9):1875–1891.

131. Nicolls MR, Terada LS, Tuder RM, Prindiville SA, Schwarz MI. Diffuse alveolar hemorrhage with underlying pulmonary capillaritis in the retinoic acid syndrome. *Am J Respir Crit Care Med.* 1998;158(4):1302–1305.

132. Tallman MS, Andersen JW, Schiffer CA, et al. Clinical description of 44 patients with acute promyelocytic leukemia who developed the retinoic acid syndrome. *Blood.* 2000;95(1): 90–95.

133. Luesink M, Jansen JH. Advances in understanding the pulmonary infiltration in acute promyelocytic leukaemia. *Br J Haematol.* 2010;151(3):209–220.

134. Wiley JS, Firkin FC. Reduction of pulmonary toxicity by prednisolone prophylaxis during all-trans retinoic acid treatment of acute promyelocytic leukemia. Australian Leukaemia Study Group. *Leukemia.* 1995;9(5):774–778.

135. Sznol M, Dutcher JP, Atkins MB, et al. Review of interleukin-2 alone and interleukin-2/LAK clinical trials in metastatic malignant melanoma. *Cancer Treat Rev.* 1989;16(Suppl A):29–38.

136. Margolin KA, Rayner AA, Hawkins MJ, et al. Interleukin-2 and lymphokine-activated killer cell therapy of solid tumors: analysis of toxicity and management guidelines. *J Clin Oncol.* 1989;7(4):486–498.

137. Huland E, Heinzer H, Huland H, Yung R. Overview of interleukin-2 inhalation therapy. *Cancer J Sci Am.* 2000;6(Suppl 1): S104–S112.

138. Graziano SL, Herndon JE 2nd, Socinski MA, et al. Phase II trial of weekly dose-dense paclitaxel in extensive-stage small cell lung cancer: cancer and leukemia group B study 39901. *J Thorac Oncol.* 2008;3(2):158–162.

139. Yasuda K, Igishi T, Kawasaki Y, et al. Phase II trial of weekly paclitaxel in previously untreated advanced non-small-cell lung cancer. *Oncology.* 2003;65(3):224–228.

140. Wong P, Leung AN, Berry GJ, et al. Paclitaxel-induced hypersensitivity pneumonitis: radiographic and CT findings. *AJR Am J Roentgenol.* 2001;176(3):718–720.

141. Read WL, Mortimer JE, Picus J. Severe interstitial pneumonitis associated with docetaxel administration. *Cancer.* 2002;94(3):847–853.

142. Semb KA, Aamdal S, Oian P. Capillary protein leak syndrome appears to explain fluid retention in cancer patients who receive docetaxel treatment. *J Clin Oncol.* 1998;16(10):3426–3432.

143. Wang GS, Yang KY, Perng RP. Life-threatening hypersensitivity pneumonitis induced by docetaxel (taxotere). *Br J Cancer.* 2001;85(9):1247–1250.

144. Furuse K, Kubota K, Kawahara M, et al. A phase II study of vinorelbine, a new derivative of vinca alkaloid, for previously untreated advanced non-small cell lung cancer. Japan Vinorelbine Lung Cancer Study Group. *Lung Cancer.* 1994;11(5–6):385–391.

CHAPTER 66

Drug-Induced Pulmonary Disease Due to Nonchemotherapeutic Agents

Hilary C. Cain

INTRODUCTION

Drugs have long been recognized as having the potential to cause pulmonary injury. The precise incidence of drug-induced lung disease is difficult to ascertain, because the signs and symptoms of disease are shared by many other pulmonary conditions and diseases. An analysis of a database of approximately 9 million patients from the United Kingdom describes an incidence density of 0.7 per 100,0000 patient years for interstitial disease related to drugs over a 12-year period (1997–2008).[1] These data reflect only a portion of the impact of drug-induced respiratory disease, because the alveoli, upper and lower airways, pleura, pulmonary vasculature, muscles of respiration, and the central nervous system governing respiratory control are all susceptible to injury from ingested, inhaled, and parenterally administered agents. As the categories and varieties of therapeutic drugs continue to increase, clinicians will encounter disease from new culprit drugs in addition to well-established drug reactions. Web-based data repositories, such as www.pneumotox.com, can serve as useful tools for the clinician, as they provide frequent updates based on the emerging literature on drug toxicities.

As the clinician-scientist explores the literature on drug-induced lung injury, it is critical to recognize that not all associations between drug use and respiratory dysfunction imply a definitive causal link between a specific drug and the injury pattern described. The literature needs to be cautiously interpreted before concluding that the reported associations are actually due to the implicated drug rather than a confluence of clinical conditions. This chapter addresses a broad array of drug classes implicated in pulmonary toxicity. Chemotherapeutic agents are discussed separately.

GENERAL PRINCIPLES OF DRUG-INDUCED LUNG DISEASE

The lung has an enormous surface area on which blood-borne substances (therapeutic medications, nutritional supplements, illicit drugs, or toxins) actively interact with lung tissue. Drug-related pulmonary toxicity, however, is a rare event. Reactions typically occur in a small minority of individuals exposed to a given agent. In most cases, lung injury appears to be an idiosyncratic event and cannot be predicted by dose, latency from drug initiation, duration of exposure, or pharmacologic characteristics of the drug. Often, there is no characteristic clinical presentation or pathognomonic histologic pattern of injury associated with a given drug, although certain histologic patterns of lung injury may occur more frequently than others. Thus, establishment of a diagnosis of lung toxicity is frequently a diagnosis of exclusion (see Table 66-1).

It may be inferred from the idiosyncratic nature of toxicity that there are host-specific risk factors that influence development of pulmonary toxicity. The factors influencing individual susceptibility may be: (1) genetically determined, (2) due to concurrent exposures to medications or environmental factors, (3) related to the individual's comorbid disease, or (4) a function of a combination of these factors.

Genetic predisposition to drug-induced injury is not fully characterized. While drug metabolism occurs primarily in the liver, through the action of the cytochrome P450 family of enzymes, the lung also is an active site of drug biotransformation, with cytochrome P450 enzyme levels estimated as 10% to 15% of those in the liver. In addition, the existence of lung-specific cytochrome P450 isoenzymes implies lung-specific metabolism of drugs.[2] Host-specific enzyme polymorphisms affecting drug metabolism may confer increased risk of toxicity on certain individuals.[3,4]

MECHANISMS OF PULMONARY INJURY

Mechanisms of lung injury include: (1) oxidant injury, (2) immunological and inflammatory cell–mediated injury (including immune complex–mediated injury), (3) interference with matrix formation, (4) abnormal protease/antiprotease balance, and (5) interference with lipid metabolism.

Mechanisms of lung toxicity are less well characterized than are other organ toxicities. The role of drug-induced oxidant injury is well established for nitrofurantoin, and it may be the mechanism of injury of other drugs, as well. Biotransformation of these drugs results in generation of reactive oxygen species, including hydrogen peroxide (H_2O_2), the hydroxyl radical (•HO), and superoxide anion (O_2^-•), which promote lipid peroxidation, glutathione depletion, and, consequently, cellular dysfunction or cell death.[2]

Immunologically mediated injury is undoubtedly important as well. The observation that drug metabolite–protein adducts can act as immunogens, resulting in hypersensitivity reactions or other immunologically mediated tissue injury likely applies to the lung, as well as to other organs.[5,6] Lymphocytic or neutrophilic alveolitis and inflammatory cell interstitial infiltrates are present in many cases of drug-induced lung injury, and the elaboration of chemokines and proteases by these cells may lead to cellular injury. Complement-mediated injury has been implicated for drugs causing noncardiogenic pulmonary edema (ARDS), particularly opiates and β-agonists.

Amphiphilic compounds, such as amiodarone, quinidine, and some β-blockers are passively sequestered in the lung within macrophages and type II alveolar cells. The role of disruption of phospholipid metabolism as a consequence of this sequestration has been well established for amiodarone-mediated lung injury, as discussed below.

TABLE 66-1 General Principles of Drug-Induced Lung Injury

Clinical presentation is nonspecific
Injury occurs with variable latency from drug initiation
Lung injury is often dose-independent
Pulmonary toxicity may be unrelated to the drug's pharmacologic properties
Acute, subacute, and chronic reactions may be caused by a drug
A variety of histopathologic patterns may be induced by a drug
Diagnosis of drug-induced injury is often made by exclusion
Resolution of injury may occur with drug discontinuation alone
Rechallenge with the suspected culprit drug is *not* recommended

IMPACT OF CONCURRENT EXPOSURES OR CONDITIONS

The harmful effect of concurrent oxygen administration in association with the chemotherapeutic agent, bleomycin, has been well established. It has been suggested that the apparent increased risk of amiodarone toxicity in patients who have had thoracic surgery (see below) may be a result of the impact of intraoperative high oxygen tensions.[7] However, high oxygen tension does not substantially increase the risk of toxicity for most nonchemotherapeutic agents. It is plausible that the additive effect of oxidant injury may be more relevant for some individuals than others. There are evolving data that other exogenous factors, such as cigarette smoke, may influence lung injury through induction of cytochrome P450 enzymes.

DIAGNOSTIC APPROACH TO THE PATIENT WITH SUSPECTED DRUG-INDUCED LUNG DISEASE

Confirmation of suspected drug-induced pulmonary toxicity is often a diagnostic challenge. No definitive criteria exist by which to establish the diagnosis of drug-induced disease, but the diagnosis may be inferred if: (1) there is a history of drug exposure; (2) clinical, radiologic, and histopathology are consistent with previously reported toxicity; (3) alternate diagnoses are excluded (e.g., infection, systemic or idiopathic diseases); and (4) findings regress with drug discontinuation and/or treatment. Recrudescence of the lung injury following rechallenge with the culprit drug is further confirmation of drug-induced disease, but rechallenge is *not* recommended due to the substantial risk of morbidity and/or mortality.

Recognition of a patient's risk of drug-induced injury is the first step in the diagnostic process. Drug-induced lung disease occurs with prescribed drugs, over-the-counter drugs, herbal or alternative medicine preparations (many of which contain a variety of substances that could be implicated as culprit agents), and illicit drugs. Patients may be reluctant to offer accurate information about their use of alternative medicines or supplements, and the clinician must skillfully elicit the history.

The challenge of diagnosis is further compounded by the fact that the latency from the onset of drug use to development of a toxic reaction can be highly variable, such that the temporal relationship between the pulmonary findings and the culprit drug is not readily apparent. Furthermore, many drugs (e.g., amiodarone and nitrofurantoin) can cause acute, subacute, or chronic pulmonary toxicity. Moreover, new drugs will continue to come on the market, some of which will inevitably cause lung disorders. Often the potential for drugs to cause toxic reactions will only be recognized once the drug has been in use for a sufficient length of time to allow a low frequency event, such as drug-induced toxicity, to be recognized.

In many cases, drug reactions are idiopathic, rather than dose-dependent reactions, and are unpredictable in that they are unrelated to the drug's intended pharmacologic properties. Exceptions to these observations include (1) amiodarone, for which there is an increased risk of toxicity with higher daily maintenance dosages, and for which the associated histopathology is related to amiodarone's pharmacologic properties; and (2) heroin, methadone, aspirin, propoxyphene, ethchlorvynol, and colchicine that cause pulmonary toxicity only in the setting of overdose.

A diagnosis of drug-induced lung toxicity is often difficult to establish, because patients with this condition typically come to medical attention with nonspecific symptoms, radiologic findings, and laboratory data. The clinical presentation of drug-induced lung disease may be similar to that of other disorders, including infection, hypersensitivity pneumonitis due to environmental antigens, eosinophilic lung disease, systemic rheumatologic or collagen vascular disease, and idiopathic interstitial pneumonias. High-resolution computed tomography (HRCT) has utility in characterizing the lung injury, but it does not confidently predict the histologic pattern of drug-induced injury.[8,9] Even in cases in which lung tissue is obtained by biopsy, the histopathologic features may not fully distinguish drug-induced disease from the disorders or conditions mentioned earlier.

An additional consideration is that the underlying disease for which a drug is given may produce pulmonary findings similar to drug-induced lung disease. For example, rheumatoid arthritis may cause pulmonary infiltrates with similar radiographic appearance and histology to toxic reactions induced by the methotrexate, gold, or penicillamine used to treat the rheumatoid arthritis.

Once the clinician has established that a patient has (1) a recognized, identifiable risk of drug-induced lung toxicity, and (2) history, physical examination, laboratory data, and radiographic findings compatible with known patterns of lung injury, then further cytopathologic or histologic evidence may be warranted to further establish the diagnosis. The technique of bronchoalveolar lavage (BAL) is used in the diagnostic evaluation of patients with interstitial lung diseases (ILDs). Analysis of BAL fluid is most useful when it is used in conjunction with a comprehensive clinical history and HRCT.[10] BAL cytologic analysis and culture can be particularly useful to exclude typical or atypical bacterial, fungal, viral, or parasitic infections in patients with suspected drug-induced lung injury. BAL may be helpful in diagnosing diffuse lung malignancies, such as lymphangitic spread of tumor or diffuse pulmonary lymphoma.[11] BAL can also provide evidence of alveolar hemorrhage, whether bland or vasculitic in origin. The grossly cloudy BAL fluid that settles with gravity is consistent with pulmonary alveolar proteinosis, which is a reported pattern of injury associated with disease-modifying, antirheumatoid arthritis drugs.[12]

The cellular differential of the BAL fluid may help narrow the diagnosis in suspected drug-induced pulmonary disease. The most common BAL cellular profile in drug-induced disease is lymphocytosis; a cell differential of ≥25% lymphocytes should earn drug-induced ILD a place on the differential diagnosis of any presentation of ILD. Recent guidelines for the use of BAL do not recommend routine measurement of lymphocyte subsets on all patients with ILD. However, if a lymphocyte alveolitis is suspected or confirmed, the subset measurement may be justified.[10] The T suppressor (CD8+) lymphocyte subset is commonly reported in drug-induced lung disease, as seen in hypersensitivity pneumonitis. BAL T helper (CD4+) predominance has been associated with immunomodulatory drug injury, including methotrexate, sirolimus, and temsirolimus.[13,14] Other cellular profiles occur in drug-induced disease: Eosinophils and neutrophils are variably present.[15–17] A percentage of eosinophils ≥25% is consistent with acute or chronic eosinophilic pneumonia, which may be seen as a result of drug injury.

Lung tissue obtained bronchoscopically or surgically may help characterize the injury pattern and may support the diagnosis of drug-induced injury. However, lung biopsy is not essential to establish the diagnosis. The histologic patterns seen in drug-induced injury, whether usual or nonspecific interstitial pneumonia (NSIP), organizing pneumonia with or without bronchiolitis obliterans, eosinophilic pneumonia, or granulomatous inflammation are histologically indistinguishable from other etiologies of these lung injury patterns.

Adjunctive testing for serum markers has been studied in the context of drug-induced lung injury. Serum markers, including surfactant proteins (SP-A, SP-D), KL-6, and ADAM8 have been associated with drug-induced injury but have not entered into the diagnostic armamentarium for most routine clinical evaluations.[18–21] Similarly, drug-specific lymphocyte stimulation testing and lymphocyte migration inhibition testing have been shown to be useful in the diagnosis of drug-induced lung disease by some investigators, but have not been found to be sufficiently and clinically helpful to enter mainstream clinical practice.[22–25]

CLINICAL AND HISTOPATHOLOGIC PATTERNS OF INJURY

The entire respiratory system – upper and lower airway, pleura, lung parenchyma, pulmonary vasculature, muscles of respiration, and the central nervous system governing respiratory control – is susceptible to the adverse effects of drugs. Of these areas, injury to the parenchyma is the most important cause of morbidity and mortality.

Respiratory disease may occur as the sole consequence of drug toxicity, or it may be one manifestation of a systemic drug-induced syndrome. For example, systemic hypersensitivity syndromes, such as drug rash with eosinophilia and systemic symptoms (DRESS), may be induced by drugs, particularly the aromatic anticonvulsants.[26] Drug-induced systemic lupus erythematosus (SLE) may occur, with or without pulmonary involvement, from exposure to β-blockers, amiodarone, angiotensin-converting enzyme inhibitors (ACEIs), hydralazine, procainamide, isoniazid, methyldopa, minocycline, and tetracycline, among others. In addition, drugs (e.g., phenytoin, hydralazine, propylthiouracil, D-penicillamine, and cocaine, among others) can cause the clinical picture of a pulmonary–renal syndrome, with evidence for pulmonary and renal vasculitis with renal failure.

Parenchymal injury may manifest itself in the interstitial, alveolar, and/or vascular compartments. Of the processes affecting the lung parenchyma, interstitial involvement is the most common. The major histopathologic forms of ILD – cellular and fibrotic NSIP and usual interstitial pneumonia (UIP) – have been reported to occur as an adverse effect of drugs. Unfortunately for diagnostic clarity, among the many case reports citing the presence of ILD, many have no tissue confirmation of the precise lung histology, and older case reports were published before the current guidelines for classification of ILDs were established. However, it seems likely that much of the previously reported drug-induced ILD would now be classified as either cellular or fibrotic NSIP. Virtually all histopathologic types of ILD have been reported to occur in association with drugs, including organizing pneumonia (with and without obliterative bronchiolitis), usual interstitial pneumonitis, eosinophilic pneumonia, desquamative interstitial pneumonitis, and hypersensitivity pneumonitis. It is important to recognize that few drugs have been reported to cause a single histopathologic pattern of parenchymal injury, and in the cases of many drugs, several patterns of injury may occur (Table 66-2).

■ NONSPECIFIC AND USUAL INTERSTITIAL PNEUMONIAS

The radiographic and histologic definitions of NSIP and UIP have been defined in the American Thoracic Society/European Respiratory Society (ATS/ERS) international, multidisciplinary consensus statements of 2002 and 2013.[27,28] Whether drug-induced, idiopathic, or due to systemic disease, the radiographic and histologic features are largely indistinguishable, and it is the clinical scenario that is critical to the differential diagnosis. Older literature on drug-induced lung disease does not necessarily conform to recent consensus definitions of NSIP, UIP, or otherwise unclassified interstitial pneumonias, making older case series somewhat difficult to interpret. Culprit drugs leading to these interstitial pneumonias include antimicrobials, antirheumatics, tumor necrosis factor (TNF) antagonsists, β-adrenergic antagonists, antiarrhythmics, anti-inflammatory drugs, antipyretics, and immunosupressants (see Table 66-2).

■ BRONCHIOLITIS OBLITERANS AND ORGANIZING PNEUMONIA

Organizing pneumonia (OP) with or without histopathologic evidence of obliterative bronchiolitis is a frequently reported pulmonary reaction to medications. The histologic pattern seen in drug-induced parenchymal injury is indistinguishable from cryptogenic organizing pneumonia (COP) or other causes of bronchiolitis obliterans organizing pneumonia (BOOP). The histology consists of plugs of loose connective tissue, or granulation tissue that fills respiratory bronchioles, alveolar ducts, and alveolar spaces. This may be accompanied by mild interstitial inflammation with preserved architecture. Radiographic findings of BOOP are typically bilateral, patchy areas of consolidation that are often subpleural, with a tendency to lower lobe predominance or distribution along the bronchovascular bundle.

Many of the drugs that have been reported to cause BOOP are commonly used medications. Among the implicated antimicrobials are cephalosporins, minocycline, nitrofurantoin, amphotericin B, and interferons. One of the most utilized antiarrhythmic agents, amiodarone, is known to cause BOOP, as are the anticonvulsants, carbamazepine and phenytoin, and the anti-inflammatory agents, gold, penicillamine, and sulfasalazine. In patients treated for rheumatoid arthritis (RA) with gold or penicillamine, it is important to distinguish between drug-induced OP and infiltrates reflecting a pulmonary manifestation of the underlying RA itself. A variety of other agents reported to cause obliterative bronchiolitis are listed in Table 66-2.

The clinical presentation of drug-associated OP or BOOP is similar to that of the idiopathic disease, which is now referred to as COP. Symptoms include shortness of breath, nonproductive cough, and, in some cases, low-grade fever and/or pleuritic chest pain. The chest radiograph typically shows bilateral patchy infiltrates that may be migratory over serial radiographs, with interval normal chest radiographs despite continuous drug exposure. As with other interstitial lung disease, the utility of BAL is primarily to exclude an infectious etiology of the infiltrates. There is no specific BAL cellular profile characteristic of OP or BOOP. Lung biopsy reveals characteristic histopathology, identical to that of COP. Patients with drug-induced OP or BOOP may have spontaneous resolution of disease when the offending drug is discontinued, but oral corticosteroids may be used to accelerate disease resolution if the patient is symptomatic.

■ EOSINOPHILIC LUNG DISEASE

Drug-induced eosinophilic lung disease may mimic other eosinophilic pulmonary syndromes, including simple eosinophilic pneumonitis (Loeffler's syndrome), chronic eosinophilic pneumonia, acute eosinophilic pneumonia, pulmonary infiltrates with peripheral eosinophilia (PIE), and Churg–Strauss syndrome (see Chapter 71). The differential diagnosis of eosinophilic lung disease includes drug-induced injury and a search for the culprit drug is an integral part of the diagnostic evaluation. Although the clinical presentation of drug-induced eosinophilic pneumonia may be identical to idiopathic conditions, several distinctions can be made. In idiopathic eosinophilic pneumonia, symptoms affect the lung exclusively, while in drug-induced eosinophilic pneumonia, respiratory symptoms may be accompanied by systemic symptoms, such as rash and fever. Marked peripheral blood eosinophilia (>1000 cells/mL) suggests drug-induced pneumonitis, rather than acute idiopathic eosinophilic pneumonia, in which the eosinophilia tends to be more modestly elevated or normal.

The diagnosis of drug-induced eosinophilic pneumonia is supported by peripheral blood and/or pulmonary eosinophilia in a setting of exposure to a suspect drug. The diagnosis may be established when other eosinophilic lung diseases are excluded. When evaluating a patient with pulmonary eosinophilia, it is particularly important to exclude infectious causes of eosinophilia so as to avoid promoting progressive infection and/or death by use of corticosteroid treatment for presumptive drug-induced eosinophilic pneumonia. Tropical pulmonary eosinophilia caused by filarial infection should be suspected if the patient has a consistent travel history. Schistosoma and Paragonimus westermani are other potential pathogens to be excluded. Strongyloides, Ascaris, and Toxocara are indigenous to the United States and are known to cause pulmonary

TABLE 66-2 Histopathologic Diagnosis or Clinical Syndrome and Strength of Association with Drug

Histopathologic Diagnosis or Syndrome	Drug	Strength of Association
Interstitial Infiltrate/ Fibrosis (acute, subacute, or chronic)	Amiodarone	++++
	ACE Inhibitor	+
	Azathioprine	++
	β-Adrenergic blockers	+
	Carbamazepine	+
	Cocaine	++
	Erlotinib	++
	Flecainide	++
	Fluoxitine	++
	Gold salts	++
	Hydrochlorothiazide	++
	Interferon-α/β	+
	mTOR inhibitors	+++
	Mesalamine	+
	Methotrexate	+++++
	Nitrofurantoin	++++
	Penicillins	+
	Phenytoin	++
	Rifampicin	+
	Rituximab	++
	Statins	++
	Sulfasalizine	+
	TNF-α antagonists	++
	Venlafexine	+
OP/BOOP	Amiodarone	++
	Amphotericin B	+
	β-Adrenergic blockers	++
	Carbamazepine	+
	Cephalosporins	+
	Cocaine	++
	Gold	+
	Interferon-α/β	+
	mTOR inhibitors	++
	Methotrexate	+
	Minocycline	+
	Nitrofurantoin	++
	D-Penicillamine	+
	Phenytoin	+
	Rituximab	++
	Sulfasalazine	+
	Talc	+
Eosinophilic lung disease	Antibiotics	++
	Carbamazepine	+
	Cocaine	++
	Ethambutol	+
	Fluoxitine	+
	Heroin	+
	Infliximab	+
	Minocycline	++
	NSAIDs	++
	Penicillins	++
	Sulfonamides	++
	Tacrolimus	+
	Tetracycline	++
	L-tryptophan (OTC preparation)[a]	++
	Venlafexine	+
Pulmonary and/or systemic hypersensitivity	Aspirin	+++
	Carbamazepine	+
	HAART	+
	Hydralazine	++
	Infliximab	+
	Minocycline	+
	NSAIDs	+
	Phenytoin	++
	Sulfasalazine	+
	Sulfonamides	+
	Valproate	++
	Vancomycin	+
	Venlafexine	+
Lupus-like Syndrome	ACE inhibitor	++
	Amiodarone	++
	β-Adrenergic blockers	++
	Carbamazepine	+++
	Hydralazine	++
	Infliximab	++
	Interferon-α/β	+
	Isoniazid	++
	Methyldopa	+++
	Minocycline	++
	Procainamide	++
	Statins	+
	Sulfasalazine	++
	TNF-α antagonists	+++
	Zafirlukast	+
Bronchospasm/Cough	Acetylcysteine	++
	Amiodarone (cough)	++
	Aspirin	++++
	ACE inhibitor	+++++
	Adenosine	++
	β-Adrenergic blockers	++++
	ARB (cough)	+
	Carbamazepine	+
	Cephalosporins	++
	Clarithromycin	+
	Cocaine	+++
	Etanercept	+
	Heroin	+++
	Interferon-α/β	++
	NSAIDs	++++
	Penicillins	+
	Proton pump inhibitors	++
	Radiocontrast	+
	Statins (cough)	++
	Venlafexine	+

TABLE 66-2 Histopathologic Diagnosis or Clinical Syndrome and Strength of Association with Drug *(Continued)*

Histopathologic Diagnosis or Syndrome	Drug	Strength of Association
Noncardiogenic pulmonary edema/ ARDS	Amiodarone	+++
	Amitriptyline	++
	Amphotericin	++
	Aspirin/NSAID overdose	++
	Carbamazepine	+
	Cocaine	++
	Cyclosporin	+
	HCTZ	++
	Heparins	+
	Interferon-α/β	+
	Methotrexate	++
	Neuroleptics	++
	Nitrofurantoin	+
	Opiate overdose	+++
	Propofol	+
	Propylthiouracil	+
	Radiographic contrast	++
	Rituximab	++
	Tocolytic agents (e.g., terbutaline, ritodrine)	+
	Tricyclic antidepressants	+++
DAH: Bland or vasculitis	Amiodarone	++
	Aspirin	+
	Azathioprine	+
	Clopidigrel	+
	Cocaine	+
	Epoprostenol	++
	Etanercept	+
	Heparin	++
DAH: Bland or vasculitis	Heroin	+
	Hydralazine	+ (vasculitis)
	Immunoglobulins	+
	LTRAs	++ (vasculitis)
	mTOR inhibitors	++
	Methotrexate	++
	Minocycline	+ (vasculitis)
	Nitrofurantoin	+ (vasculitis)
	Penicillamine	++ (bland/ vasculitis)
	Phenytoin	+ (vasculitis)
	Propylthiouracil	++ (vasculitis)
	Radiocontrast	+
	Sildenafil	+
	Sulfonamides	+++ (vasculitis)
	TNF-α antagonists	+
	Thrombolytics	++
	Warfarin	++
	Valproate	+
	Pulmonary hypertension	++++
	Aminorex	+++
	Buprenorphine	++
	Flenfluramine	+++
	Metamphetamine	++
	Methadone	+
	SSRI	++
	Talc	++
	L-tryptophan (OTC preparation)[a]	++

ACE, angiotensin converting enzyme; ARB, angiotensin II receptor blocker; ARDS, acute respiratory distress syndrome; BOOP, bronchiolitis obliterans organizing pneumonia; LTRA, leukotriene receptor antagonist; mTOR, mammalian target of rapamycin; NSAIDs, nonsteroidal anti-inflammatory drugs; OTC, over the counter; TNF, tumor necrosis factor.
[a]Withdrawn from the market.

infiltrates and peripheral blood eosinophilia. Missing the diagnosis of a fungal infection can be lethal. Aspergillus is a ubiquitous fungus that can be difficult to diagnose as a pulmonary pathogen. BAL eosinophilia may be present without definitive evidence of invasive fungal infection, which may require a tissue biopsy for diagnosis. Coccidioides immitis is endemic in the southwestern United States, and infection can result in peripheral blood eosinophilia and pulmonary infiltrates. Serologic testing for antibodies to Coccidioides and sputum or BAL cultures are useful studies to exclude coccidioidomycosis.

Specific testing for drug reactions, such as drug-specific lymphocyte transformation tests, has been used to implicate a culprit drug. However, the clinical utility of such tests is uncertain, especially because a negative assay does not exclude the diagnosis.

Successful management of drug-induced eosinophilic lung disease is achieved by identification and discontinuation of the inciting drug. Typically, resolution of symptoms in drug-induced eosinophilic lung disease occurs with discontinuation of the culprit drug, frequently without the need for corticosteroids. In contrast, idiopathic chronic eosinophilic pneumonia may require months of treatment with corticosteroids, and relapse may occur as steroids are tapered. Relapse of the disease as steroids are tapered is rare in drug-induced eosinophilic disease; recrudescence of the lung infiltrates suggests an alternate diagnosis.

HYPERSENSITIVITY SYNDROMES

Systemic hypersensitivity syndromes with granulomatous inflammation of the lung may be caused by a number of drugs, most commonly the aromatic anticonvulsants, phenytoin, and carbamazepine, as well as nonsteroidal anti-inflammatory drugs (NSAIDs), minocycline, and sulfonamides, among others. DRESS has been reported primarily with the anticonvulsants and, in some cases, is accompanied by pulmonary histopathology consistent with BOOP, ILD, or granulomatous inflammation.

Not all cases of pulmonary hypersensitivity are accompanied by rash or other systemic symptoms. The clinical presentation of drug-related pulmonary hypersensitivity typically consists of acute onset of dyspnea, cough, and fever. The radiographic pattern is one of diffuse reticular or peripheral alveolar infiltrates, sometimes accompanied by pleural effusion. In most cases, drug discontinuation results in disease resolution. A minority of individuals (10%) have persistent radiographic abnormalities after several months, and rarely, progressive disease may occur despite drug withdrawal. In these cases, a trial of corticosteroids is reasonable if the diagnosis has been well established.

■ ALVEOLAR INJURY: NONCARDIOGENIC PULMONARY EDEMA AND ACUTE RESPIRATORY DISTRESS SYNDROME

Alveolar disease occurs in the form of noncardiogenic pulmonary edema, diffuse alveolar damage (DAD) or acute respiratory distress syndrome (ARDS), and both bland and vasculitic diffuse alveolar hemorrhage (DAH). (Vasculitis due to drugs is discussed in the separate section below.)

Noncardiogenic pulmonary edema may be precipitated by numerous drugs, including aspirin, opiates, calcium channel blockers, some diuretics (e.g., hydrochlorothiazide and acetazolamide), intravenous and inhaled pulmonary vasodilators (e.g., epoprostenol and nitric oxide), methotrexate, TNF-alpha radiographic contrast media, tocolytics, and oxytocin, among others.[29] The onset of drug-induced pulmonary edema typically occurs in close temporal proximity to ingestion of the culprit drug and does not have a variable latency of onset.

A variety of mechanisms are implicated in the development of pulmonary edema. Increased pulmonary capillary permeability is the likely cause of aspirin-induced, interleukin-2–induced, and ethchlorvynol-induced edema. Volume expansion and sodium retention likely cause the pulmonary edema associated with the use of β2-sympathomimetic tocolytic agents. Opioid-induced edema is mediated by neurogenic reflex and deposition of immunoglobulin and complement in the lung.[30] Although the mechanisms of pulmonary edema may vary, frequently the resolution of symptoms is prompt within days of drug discontinuation.

Pulmonary edema is common in salicylate intoxication, and the risk is correlated with the degree of intoxication. A prevalence of alveolar edema as high as 20% to 30% has been reported for aspirin-intoxicated adults. An increased risk of edema is associated with chronic aspirin ingestion, older age, positive smoking history, neurologic disease, and proteinuria.[31,32]

In many cases reported as drug-induced ARDS, this condition is considered as a clinical syndrome of lung injury, rather than a specific histopathologic pattern of disease. If we examine the more specific histopathology of DAD, many cases of drug-induced injury have been reported to have these histologic characteristics and diffuse ground-glass attenuation on CT imaging of the lung. The more commonly implicated drugs associated with DAD are amiodarone, methotrexate, rituximab, and many chemotherapeutic agents.

■ DIFFUSE ALVEOLAR HEMORRHAGE, VASCULITIS, AND PULMONARY–RENAL SYNDROMES

Drug-induced DAH is infrequently reported in the literature on drug-induced pulmonary disease. DAH should be suspected in patients with unexplained ground-glass infiltrates or consolidation, accompanied by anemia. Hemoptysis is not required for the diagnosis, and may be absent in as many as one-third of patients with DAH.

The classification of DAH is based on histopathologic findings and includes (1) capillaritis, (2) bland hemorrhage due to drug-induced coagulopathies, and (3) DAD, the histopathologic finding in ARDS.

Pulmonary capillaritis has been described as an adverse effect of many drugs, but strong associations with its development are reported for relatively few drugs. One of the best-characterized toxicities presenting as DAH is that from propylthiouracil.[33] The DAH is a manifestation of a systemic vasculitic syndrome characterized by leukocytoclastic vasculitis, glomerulonephritis, and pulmonary capillaritis. Use of propylthiouracil induces antineutrophil cytoplasmic antibodies (ANCAs) in as many as 46% of patients, although only a minority of these develop pulmonary toxicity; pathogenesis may be mediated by antimyeloperoxidase antibodies.[34,35] Cases of pulmonary or systemic vasculitis also have been reported for diphenylhydantoin, hydralazine, nitrofurantoin, and leukotriene receptor antagonists. In the case of the last group of drugs noted, there has been considerable discussion as to whether the vasculitis is a toxic effect of the leukotriene antagonists or whether withdrawal of oral corticosteroids leads to identification of pre-existing Churg–Strauss granulomatous vasculitis. At least some reported cases of Churg–Strauss syndrome are unrelated to steroid withdrawal and appear to represent a rare complication of leukotriene antagonists.

Bland hemorrhage without capillaritis can occur (1) in the setting of therapeutic and supratherapeutic anticoagulation, (2) with the use of inhibitors of platelet aggregation (e.g., clopidigrel), and platelet glycoprotein IIa/IIIb inhibitor therapy, and (3) as a complication of thrombolysis. Drug combinations may increase the risk of pulmonary hemorrhage. For example, when therapeutic anticoagulation is combined with epoprostenol for management of pulmonary hypertension, the risk of hemorrhage is compounded.[36] Bland DAH related to D-penicillamine, amiodarone, and cocaine is discussed in the sections on individual drugs in later sections.

Drug-induced DAD may lead to bland DAH and has been reported for amiodarone, nitrofurantoin, minocycline, methotrexate, gold, cocaine, and chemotherapeutic agents.

■ COUGH AND ANGIOEDEMA

Cough induced by ACEIs is well characterized in several case series.[36–40] The overall reported incidence of cough ranges from 5% to 25%. Women are more at risk of developing cough than are men.[37,39,41] The latency from initiation of use to the onset of cough is variable, ranging from 1 week to 15 months. A prior diagnosis of asthma has not been found to be a significant risk factor for the development of ACEI-associated cough. While some series have reported increased nonspecific bronchial hyperresponsiveness among subjects with cough, others have not. Symptoms typically resolve promptly after a week to 1 month after discontinuation of the drug, but occasionally resolution may take as long as 3 months.[41] Angiotensin receptor blockers induce cough in approximately one-third of patients in whom ACEI-induced cough has been diagnosed.[42] Less frequent side effects of ACEIs include PIE, SLE, and subacute ILD, but these do not typically appear in conjunction with ACEI-induced cough.

Angioedema to ACEIs is a potentially life-threatening complication of these medications. Edema more commonly affects the face (57%) and less commonly affects the floor or roof of mouth and tongue (26%). In 17%, the oropharynx and glottis are involved.[43] Presenting symptoms may range from simple edema of the lips and/or face to respiratory failure requiring ventilatory support. The latency for onset is even wider than that for cough, ranging from 4 weeks to 4 years after onset of ACEI use. In one series, 70% presented within the first month of treatment.[44]

Numerous case series have reported a higher incidence of angioedema among African Americans, and a higher risk of intubation among those affected in this racial group.[43,44] Angioedema formation is likely due to elevation of circulating bradykinin as a result of ACEI-induced inhibition of its degradation, leading to vasodilatation and capillary leak. The effect of impaired bradykinin degradation may be compounded in individuals with genetically based deficiency of other bradykinin metabolizing enzymes. Most experts recommend treatment for angioedema with corticosteroids, H1- and H2-blockers, and, in some case, epinephrine.

■ BRONCHOSPASM AND ANAPHYLAXIS

Drug-induced bronchospasm is a relatively common side effect of many categories of medications (see Table 66-2).[45] Bronchospasm is mediated by a variety of mechanistic pathways including (1) IgE-mediated anaphylaxis, (2) non–IgE-mediated anaphylactoid reactions, (3) alteration in the cyclooxygenase (COX) and lipoxygenase pathways, and (4) other pharmacologic mechanisms, such as β-blockade.[46,47]

Brochospasm triggered by drugs is more common in subjects with underlying asthma, atopy, or bronchial hyperreactivity. These reactions are more common in women than in men, and there appears to be familial predisposition to reactions to some drugs.[48] Symptoms range from mild chest tightness and dyspnea on exertion to respiratory failure in susceptible individuals.

In the United States, medications are the primary cause of anaphylaxis in adults and antimicrobials have been implicated as the cause of 0.7% to 10% of cases of severe bronchospasm. Penicillin remains the most important cause of anaphylaxis, accounting for up to 75% of cases annually.[49,50] Aspirin and NSAIDs are commonly implicated in bronchospasm, in one series accounting for as many as 24% of bronchoconstrictive reactions, ranging from mild to severe reactions.[49,51] (Aspirin and NSAIDs are discussed in the sections below.) Other agents more commonly implicated in bronchospasm and anaphylaxis include sulfonamides, omalizumab, halothane, heparins, protamine, insulin, and neuromuscular blocking agents.

■ BRONCHIOLITIS

Agents that have been reported to cause small airway inflammation (bronchiolitis) include medications used in the treatment of RA, such as D-penicillamine, gold, and tiopronin. The bronchiolitis in these cases may be fatal.[52–55] Interpretation of earlier literature on D-penicillamine and gold-induced bronchiolitis is complicated by the fact that RA itself can cause bronchiolitis.[56] Use of these agents has been largely supplanted by disease modifying antirheumatic drugs, immunosuppressants, and biologics, but the implicated agents may still be used in certain cases. Drug-induced bronchiolitis typically causes shortness of breath, with or without wheezing, and cough. Spirometry may not detect small airway disease until obstruction is severe, but high-resolution CT imaging protocols may show centrilobular nodules and/or tree-in-bud opacities, as well as mosaic attenuation of the lung parenchyma, reflective of airtrapping.[57]

■ PULMONARY HYPERTENSION

Pulmonary hypertension (see Chapter 72) is a relatively infrequent complication of drug therapy, but because of the subtlety of the onset of disease, paucity of symptoms until significant vascular compromise has occurred, and potential for eventual vascular collapse and death, it is critical to recognize drug-induced pulmonary hypertension early in its course. Among the drugs known to cause pulmonary hypertension are cocaine, other illicit stimulants, anorexigens, and toxic contaminants of food and nutritional supplements (e.g., tryptophan).[58]

The association of appetite suppressants with pulmonary hypertension dates to the late 1970s when reports of unexplained "primary" pulmonary hypertension were first published. The "epidemic" of pulmonary hypertension was linked to the use of aminorex fumarate, an amphetamine-derived appetite suppressant that came into use because its potential for addiction and abuse was lower than that of amphetamine. The use of aminorex was associated with a significant rise in the incidence of pulmonary hypertension, primarily among women in Germany, Austria, and Switzerland. Development of disease occurred as early as weeks to months from the onset of use of the drug, with a dose-dependent risk as high as 2 in 100. The mechanism of action on the pulmonary vasculature is through the release of catecholamines, including dopamine. The epidemic subsided as the drug's use declined.

The aminorex epidemic was followed by the introduction of fenfluramine, a phenylethylamine, like amphetamine and aminorex. Fenfluramine had been shown to be equally effective for weight reduction as an amphetamine, without the potential for abuse.

Satiety is normally accompanied by the release of serotonin, which acts on central serotonin 2_C receptors. Fenfluramine and racemic dexfenfluramine mimic normal satiety through competitive inhibition of the serotonin transporter, leading to release of serotonin from intracellular stores. These agents were used primarily in Europe throughout the 1980s. Case reports of users with pulmonary hypertension were published in Britain as early as 1981, but use of these agents persisted through the 1980s.

Two landmark reports supported a causal relationship between pulmonary hypertension and the use of fenfluramine and dexfenfluramine. The first was published in 1993, describing a cohort of young-to-middle–aged users of the anorexigens who developed pulmonary hypertension indistinguishable from idiopathic primary arterial pulmonary hypertension.[59] This was followed in 1996 by the findings of the International Primary Pulmonary Hypertension Study Group, which published a case-control series of 95 patients with pulmonary arterial hypertension.[60] An odds ratio (OR) of 23.1 for development of disease was found among those who had used an anorexigen for more than 3 months, with an estimated incidence of one to two cases per million users per year. Further support for a causal link is contained in the surveillance study of pulmonary hypertension among anorexigen users in the United States. Fenfluramine was withdrawn from the market in 1995 due to its association with increased risk for pulmonary hypertension, as well as its role in the development of valvular heart disease in users of the fenfluramine–phentermine combination anorexigen, known as "fen-phen."[61]

Epidemics of pulmonary hypertension also have been reported due to contaminants in a specific manufacturer's rapeseed oil in Spain, and from use of an over-the-counter L-tryptophan preparation that resulted in the eosinophilic myalgia syndrome, characterized by a systemic syndrome, which included acute lung injury and pulmonary hypertension.

The reason(s) that some individuals develop drug-related pulmonary hypertension while others do not has not been clearly defined. One putative risk may be polymorphisms of a cytochrome P450 enzyme, CYP 2D6, which is the primary enzyme for metabolism of fenfluramine.[62] Other risk factors have yet to be characterized.

TOXICITY ASSOCIATED WITH SELECTED DRUGS

The following drugs have been selected for discussion because (1) they are very commonly used, or (2) have important forms of toxicity associated with their use, or (3) have more recently entered into our pharmacologic armamentarium and, therefore, are likely associated a lower level of awareness of their potential toxicity to the respiratory system.

■ CARDIOVASCULAR DRUGS

Important examples of cardiovascular agents associated with pulmonary toxicity are highlighted in the sections that follow.

Amiodarone

Amiodarone is an iodinated, benzofuran-derivative antiarrhythmic used for management of life-threatening supraventricular and ventricular arrhythmias. Both amiodarone and its major metabolite, desethylamiodarone, are cationic, amphiphilic compounds with high lipid solubility, causing the drug to accumulate in a variety of tissues. The elimination half-life of amiodarone is 30 to 60 days. However, the concentration of amiodarone in lung tissue can be 100- to 500-fold higher than serum levels and the drug has been found in lung tissue as long as 1 year after discontinuation of therapy. These pharmacokinetic characteristics contribute to the drug's potential toxicity and impact treatment strategies.

One of amiodarone's biochemical effects is to impair normal phospholipid catabolism by phospholipases, thereby leading to cellular phospholipidosis. The accumulation of phospholipids in the cell may cause direct cellular injury and secondary tissue inflammation. Evidence supports cellular injury through production of the unstable aryl radical as amiodarone is deiodinated, leading to reactive oxygen species formation and cell death.[63] The impairment of phospholipid metabolism results in the lamellar inclusions and lipid-laden foamy macrophages that characterize the histology seen on lung biopsy and BAL. These findings are characteristic of amiodarone exposure and are not indicative of toxicity unless accompanied by the lung injury patterns discussed below.

Adverse reactions to amiodarone have been reported in a variety of tissues, including the lung, liver (liver function abnormalities and increased tissue attenuation on radiographic imaging), thyroid (thyrotoxicosis), skin (discoloration), and cornea. The first reports of amiodarone pulmonary toxicity were published in 1980 and were followed by larger series of patients as amiodarone was tested in the United States in early-to-middle 1980s. Based on two trials published in 1987, the clinical picture of amiodarone pulmonary toxicity emerged as a syndrome of pulmonary infiltrates and respiratory symptoms, most often cough and dyspnea of subacute or chronic onset, accompanied by fever, malaise, and chest discomfort in 50% of those affected. In one series, 11 of 171 patients (6.4%) treated with 400 to 1200 mg of amiodarone developed pulmonary disease. In the other series, 15 of 154 subjects (9.7%) developed disease.[64–66] The time from initiation of therapy to development of symptoms was 61 to 465 days in one series and 30 to 720 days in the other. Subsequent reports have further refined these initial observations.[67]

Disease Prevalence and Risk Factors for Amiodarone Toxicity Based on the analysis of administrative databases in Quebec, approximately 4% of amiodarone users with atrial fibrillation carry a diagnosis of pulmonary fibrosis, alveolar or interstitial lung disease or ARDS.[68] Earlier studies reported the incidence of pulmonary toxicity to range from 0.1% to 10%. Predisposing risk factors for the identification of amiodarone pulmonary toxicity include older age, higher daily dosages, male gender, renal disease, and pre-existing lung disease.[68] The risk of pulmonary toxicity is dependent on daily dose: In one series, 0.1% to 0.5% of patients on 200 mg per day developed amiodarone pulmonary toxicity, while as many as 50% of those using the highest dosages (e.g., 1200 mg per day) were affected.[69] Most reports of amiodarone toxicity have been of subjects receiving doses greater than 400 mg daily. The lower doses of amiodarone that are more commonly used are considered to be safer than higher doses; however, toxicity has been reported at doses as low as 200 mg per day.[68,70]

Pre-existing lung disease may enhance the risk of toxicity, but not all studies have shown this to be the case. It is not clear whether there is actually higher incidence of toxicity in those with pre-existing lung disease, or if prior disease results in earlier perception of symptoms and attention to pulmonary causes of dyspnea. The AFFIRM (Atrial Fibrillation Follow-up of Rhythm Management) trial reported a higher risk of diagnosis of amiodarone lung toxicity if the patient had pre-existing pulmonary disease; however, there was no higher risk of either pulmonary death or all-cause mortality.[71] Patients with atrial fibrillation and amiodarone used in the setting of chronic obstructive pulmonary disease (COPD) had a hazard ratio of 2.53 (2.2–2.89) compared to those without COPD.[68] It is acceptable to use amiodarone in the setting of pre-existing lung disease if vigilance is maintained for the development of symptoms suggestive of amiodarone toxicity. Prospective studies have suggested that a decrement in diffusing capacity from baseline is a poor predictor of amiodarone toxicity. Therefore, there are no formal recommendations for screening pulmonary function tests during amiodarone use. However, it is reasonable to obtain a baseline pulmonary function test, including diffusing capacity measurement, and to follow the patient with symptom-driven testing, thereafter.

Exposure to high concentrations of supplemental oxygen may increase the risk of amiodarone pulmonary toxicity. Several authors have suggested that amiodarone pulmonary toxicity may be triggered by administration of high concentrations of supplement oxygen, or that oxygen may act in synergy with amiodarone to enhance cellular injury.[72–74] A high index of suspicion for amiodarone toxicity, therefore, should be maintained especially if high concentrations of oxygen were used perioperatively, and if high loading doses of amiodarone were initiated for the management of perioperative cardiac arrhythmias. Similarly, serious consideration to amiodarone lung toxicity is warranted if high concentrations of oxygen are used for management of respiratory failure. A less substantiated risk factor may include use of intravenous iodinated contrast media. Rapidly progressive, fatal ARDS attributed to amiodarone toxicity has been reported following pulmonary angiography.[75] A protective effect against amiodarone pulmonary toxicity by ACEIs is supported in several publications.[76–78]

Clinical Presentation of Amiodarone Toxicity The typical clinical presentation of amiodarone pulmonary toxicity is nonproductive cough and dyspnea, sometimes accompanied by pleuritic chest pain, fever, malaise, and/or weight loss. Symptom onset is most often 6 to 24 months into treatment (100–150 g cumulative dose), but ranges from a few days to 10 years into therapy. Most subjects have an insidious onset of symptoms over several months, but fatal amiodarone-induced pulmonary toxicity occurring 2 weeks into therapy has been reported.[79]

The earliest abnormality identifiable on pulmonary function testing of affected individuals is impairment in diffusing capacity for carbon monoxide (DL_{CO}) There may be an accelerated decline in the DL_{CO} as the disease progresses, accompanied by mild restrictive physiology. Since a low DL_{CO} is not specific for amiodarone toxicity, a decline should not necessarily prompt discontinuation of the drug, but should trigger evaluation for possible cause(s) of the impairment.

Radiographic and Histologic Findings of Amiodarone Toxicity The radiographic and histologic findings associated with amiodarone pulmonary toxicity are not stereotypic (Fig. 66-1). While the most common pattern observed is subacute ILD, there are also many reports of organizing pneumonia and pulmonary fibrosis, and fewer reports of nodules (which can be fluorodeoxyglucose [FDG]-avid on PET imaging), ARDS, and SLE. Reports of PIE and DAH are rare.[67,80]

Typical radiographic findings in patients with subacute or chronic onset of disease are diffuse or patchy, interstitial or mixed alveolar–interstitial infiltrates, which are either bilateral or unilateral. Mild cases of toxicity may be characterized by a diffuse ground-glass pattern on HRCT, often in a peripheral, subpleural distribution.[81] Focal and patchy areas of higher attenuation may be superimposed on the ground-glass opacification. Alveolar opacities may correspond to areas of organizing pneumonia that are indistinguishable from idiopathic BOOP. Amiodarone toxicity should be considered in cases of migratory infiltrates that are consistent with BOOP but that are poorly responsive to steroids. Amiodarone-induced fibrosis occurs in 5% to 7% of patients diagnosed with amiodarone pneumonitis and may be present at disease presentation. A coarse interstitial pattern in the periphery of the lung, accompanied by traction bronchiectasis, is characteristic. Honeycombing is rare.

Laboratory Analysis in Amiodarone Toxicity Laboratory analyses have little utility in the differential diagnosis of amiodarone-associated lung toxicity. Common laboratory abnormalities include mild leukocytosis and elevation in serum lactate dehydrogenase (LDH). Earlier trials of amiodarone identified elevated sedimentation rates (ESRs) (i.e., a range of 39–150 mm/h) in 9 of 11 patients with pulmonary toxicity,[64] but nonspecificity of the ESR makes this test less useful in the clinical setting. Identification of a value for brain natriuretic peptide (BNP) that is normal, or at a patient's baseline, may be useful in distinguishing pulmonary causes of dyspnea from congestive heart

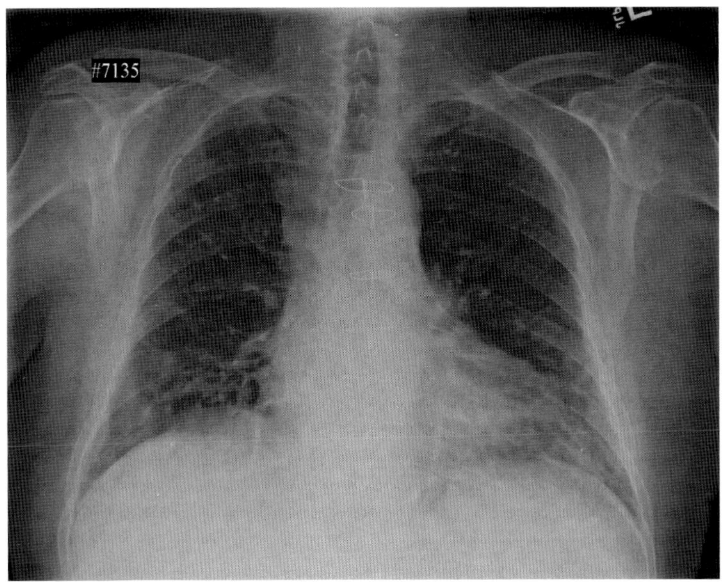

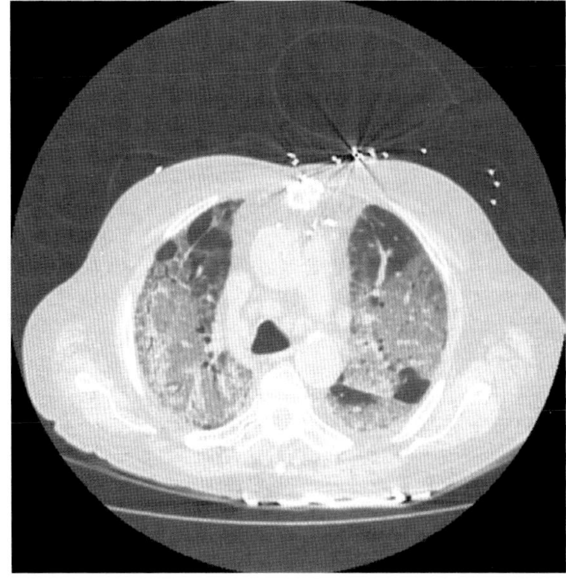

A B

Figure 66-1 **A.** Baseline chest radiograph before initiation of amiodarone. **B.** Amiodarone lung toxicity. ARDS superimposed on mild underlying fibrosis at 3 months after initiation of amiodarone in an 80-year-old man with progressive dyspnea. Dyspnea began insidiously approximately 1 month after amiodarone load.

failure. Laboratory findings that are investigational include elevated serum levels of KL-6, a mucin glycoprotein secreted by proliferating type II pneumocytes, and surfactant protein SP-D.[21,82] Elevations of the latter may be an early marker of amiodarone pulmonary toxicity, but the sensitivity and specificity of these tests is uncertain, and neither has a place in routine clinical evaluation of amiodarone toxicity.

Diagnostic Evaluation and Management of Amiodarone Toxicity The challenge to the practitioner considering the diagnosis of amiodarone pulmonary toxicity is that the differential diagnosis is extensive for dyspnea with pulmonary infiltrates in patients with known cardiac disease. Cardiogenic and noncardiogenic etiologies must be excluded. Consideration must be given to cardiac conditions, including ischemic and nonischemic cardiomyopathies, diastolic dysfunction, mitral valve disease, aortic stenosis, and atrial fibrillation. Noncardiogenic causes may include infections; the broad range of idiopathic interstitial pneumonias; malignant causes of infiltrates (e.g., lymphangitic spread of tumor or lymphoma); systemic diseases, such as sarcoidosis, amyloidosis, or autoimmune disease; exposures to inhaled agents (e.g., occupational inorganic dust exposures, or organic inhalations, with subsequent development of hypersensitivity pneumonitis); and exposures to drugs other than amiodarone.

The risk of invasive workup must be weighed against those of empiric therapy, which includes drug discontinuation and, possibly, corticosteroids. BAL may reveal a lymphocytosis, often with a predominance of CD8+ lymphocytes, reflective of a lymphocytic alveolitis. This finding, however, is not consistently reported, and some affected individuals may have elevated BAL neutrophils as well. Significant BAL eosinophilia is rare. Abundant alveolar macrophages with a "foamy" cytoplasm, indicative of undigested phospholipids, are found in all subjects chronically exposed to amiodarone and are not indicative of pulmonary toxicity per se. Hemosiderin laden macrophages are infrequently found, since alveolar hemorrhage is rare. As the BAL findings are neither sensitive nor specific for amiodarone pulmonary toxicity, the role of BAL in the diagnosis is controversial.

Lung biopsy findings, however, may support the diagnosis of amiodarone toxicity. Earlier reports of amiodarone pulmonary toxicity describe DAD of variable severity in all affected subjects. Those more severely affected had evidence of acute DAD, with abundant hyaline membranes and reactive type II pneumonocytes lining the alveoli, while others showed organizing DAD with interstitial and intra-alveolar proliferation of fibroblasts and prominent type II pneumocytes. All cases had abundant "foamy" macrophages in the alveolar spaces. The foamy appearance of the cytoplasm is due to the presence of lamellar bodies (~1 μm in diameter) containing lipid particles, reflecting the disrupted lipid metabolism caused by amiodarone. The foamy macrophages or histiocytes are not indicative of toxicity; in fact, similar vacuolated histiocytes and parenchymal cells may be found in the thyroid, liver, and skin of treated individuals without clinical evidence of cellular dysfunction.

The diagnosis of amiodarone pulmonary toxicity is supported by the presence of lamellar bodies in macrophages, pneumocytes, bronchiolar epithelium, and/or endothelial cells, but the diagnosis cannot be made unless there is also evidence of interstitial lymphocytic infiltrates or fibrosis with alveolar distortion. Histologic findings may also fit the description of fibrotic NSIP or bronchiolitis with organizing pneumonia, and combinations of histologic findings may occur. Despite the early reports, few patients with amiodarone pulmonary toxicity have DAD pathologically unless they fit the clinical picture of ARDS. Alveolar hemorrhage may be present, but it is not a common feature of amiodarone toxicity.[83]

In contrast to other types of drug-induced pulmonary toxicity, resolution of amiodarone-induced toxicity does not often occur with discontinuation of the drug alone. Amiodarone becomes sequestered in tissues and the clearance of drug is typically prolonged. Depending on the severity of respiratory symptoms, practitioners often may need to treat affected patients with corticosteroids. Specific dosages of prednisone have not been studied for efficacy, but 0.5 to 1 mg/kg is a reasonable starting point in most cases. Due to the pharmacokinetic characteristics of amiodarone, the required duration of therapy may be as long as several months, and recrudescent disease after tapering of corticosteroids is not uncommon.

β-Adrenergic Receptor Blockers

The most common adverse effect of β-adrenergic blockers on the respiratory system is precipitation of bronchospasm in asthmatics and patients with reactive airway disease. The high frequency of clinically significant bronchospasm in hypertensive asthmatics treated with nonselective β-adrenergic blockers, such as propranolol, requires that these agents be avoided in asthmatics. β1-Receptor–selective agents and the mixed α- and β-receptor blockers, labetalol, are better tolerated but should be used with considerable caution in asthmatics. The use of β-adrenergic blockers is not contraindicated in patients with COPD. Many individuals with COPD tolerate β-adrenergic blockers without significant decrement in their lung function. Patients with COPD who have clinical or spirometric evidence of variable airflow obstruction responsive to bronchodilators should be observed carefully for bronchospasm upon initiation of these agents; the cardiac benefit of β-blockade in these subjects may outweigh any risk.

Pulmonary parenchymal injury associated with the use of β-adrenergic blockers is not common, but it warrants mention because of the ubiquitous use of these agents. Subacute interstitial infiltrates, PIE, and pulmonary edema have been reported in conjunction with the use of acebutolol, propranolol, labetalol, nadolol, and pindolol. Thus, the clinician should be vigilant for these reactions from using β-adrenergic blockers as a class. SLE has reported with the use of acebutolol, propranolol, labetalol, and pindolol.

Hydralazine

Hydralazine-induced pulmonary disease is not common, but it can be associated with systemic autoimmune disease that is potentially fatal even when recognized.[84] Half of the patients on daily doses of greater than 200 mg have a positive ANA, however only 10% of these patients develop clinical symptoms. The most important reported complication of long-term use of hydralazine is drug-inducedLE, which occurs more frequently if daily dosing is greater than 200 mg or the cumulative dose exceeds 100 g. In addition, there have been cases of pulmonary–renal syndrome associated with the use of hydralazine.[85] Pleuropulmonary manifestations occur in 30% of affected subjects, and isolated pulmonary parenchymal disease is rare. Subacute ILD/NSIP, organizing pneumonia, and DAH also have been documented.

Hydrochlorothiazide

The most commonly reported pulmonary side effect of the diuretic hydrochlorothiazide (HCTZ) is noncardiogenic pulmonary edema or ARDS.[86] Pulmonary edema was first reported in 1968 as a potentially life-threatening complication of HCTZ use. The onset of symptoms is typically acute and less often occurs later in the course of HCTZ use. Typical symptoms and signs include acute dyspnea and hypoxemia; fever, tachycardia, hypotension, and shock may accompany the dyspnea. Immunologically mediated capillary leak has been suggested as a possible mechanism of action. IgG deposition in the alveolar membrane and elevated serum IgM have been reported. Management is supportive, and symptom resolution typically occurs in a few days. Rechallenge with HCTZ can cause recrudescent pulmonary edema and is not recommended. Since HCTZ is a widely used diuretic, frequently used in patients with cardiovascular disease who are prone to pulmonary edema, the true incidence of drug-induced noncardiogenic pulmonary edema may be underreported.

Procainamide

Procainamide, used in the treatment of supraventricular and ventricular arrhythmias, is frequently cited as a cause of drug-induced lupus (DIL). Among patients using procainamide for over 2 months, as many as 50% to 90% develop serum antinuclear antibodies (ANAs), and of these, 10% to 30% may develop symptomatic DIL. Slow acetylators develop DIL at lower doses of procainamide and earlier in their course of treatment.[87] Symptoms associated with drug-induced disease are indistinguishable from those of idiopathic SLE, and may include fever, rash, arthralgias, Raynaud disease, myositis, vasculitis, and serositis. Among affected subjects, 40% to 80% exhibit pleuropulmonary manifestations characteristic of SLE, such as pleuritis, with pleural effusion and/or diffuse parenchymal infiltrates. Of these findings, pleural disease is more common, while parenchymal infiltrates are present in fewer than half of affected individuals.[88] The pleuritis of DIL may produce pleural fluid with characteristics indistinguishable from those of spontaneous SLE: high pleural fluid ANA (≥1:160), high pleural fluid to serum ratio of ANA (≥1), and LE cells. More severe myositis also may affect respiratory muscle function and result in ventilatory insufficiency, perhaps potentiated by competitive blockade of the acetylcholine receptor by procainamide. The absence of renal or central nervous system involvement is suggestive of DIL, but it is otherwise difficult to differentiate drug-induced disease from other SLEs on clinical grounds. The absence of anti–double-stranded DNA, normal complement levels, and identification of antibodies to histone complex H2A-H2B support the diagnosis of DIL.

Unlike idiopathic SLE, DIL may resolve over several weeks simply with discontinuation of the drug and without the use of corticosteroids or immunosuppressants. More severely affected patients may benefit from oral corticosteroids, which appear to accelerate symptom resolution. A positive ANA without signs or symptoms of local or systemic disease need not warrant discontinuation of procainamide. Relapse after symptom resolution does not occur unless the drug is reintroduced.

STATINS

Statins are widely used 3-hydroxy-3-methylglutaryl coenzyme A (HMG-CoA) reductase inhibitors. Injury has been reported for various statin compounds and appears to be a class effect. Clinicians are more familiar with the well-reported myositis and hepatotoxicity associated with statins than they are pulmonary side effects.[89] Based on Food and Drug Administration reports of adverse events and the medical literature, lung injury occurs in 0.01% to 0.04% of patients with side effects attributed to statin use.[90] Although the incidence of adverse pulmonary events among all statin users is low, the widespread use of this class of drugs makes lung injury a potentially important side effect.

As with other drugs, the latency, radiographic and histopathologic pleuropulmonary manifestations associated with statins are variable. The latency between initial use and onset of injury ranges from 1 week to 120 months (mean, 34 months; SD, ±35 months).[91] The most common presenting complaints are nonspecific: dyspnea, cough, and fever. The predominant radiographic findings are ground-glass and alveolar opacities that are diffuse in distribution, sometimes with patchy consolidation. Fewer subjects exhibit interstitial infiltrates or fibrosis, and pleural effusion is reported, but is rare.[91,92] Analysis of BAL fluid shows no characteristic predominant cellular profile. Foamy macrophages suggesting pulmonary phospholipidosis have been observed in some, but not all cases. When obtained, biopsies demonstrate histopathology consistent with NSIP or hypersensitivity pneumonitis.[90,92–94] The mechanism of lung injury from statins is not fully characterized, but a role of NLRP3 inflammasome activation has been proposed.[95]

Resolution of statin-induced lung disease has been achieved with drug discontinuation, with or without corticosteroid therapy.

ANTICONVULSANTS

Various types of pulmonary injury may result from exposure to phenytoin. Among the reported patterns of injury are pulmonary hypersensitivity reactions, which may be a component of systemic hypersensitivity (see the prior discussion of DRESS). Two fatal cases of apparent polyarteritis nodosum and necrotizing vasculitis have been reported. The histologic findings in subacute phenytoin lung toxicity are most consistent with NSIP, but lymphocytic interstitial pneumonitis and BOOP have been described, as well. In some cases, parenchymal findings are accompanied by peripheral blood eosinophilia, suggesting PIE syndrome. The presence of cold hemagglutinins has been reported. Carbamazepine has also been reported to cause systemic and pulmonary hypersensitivity syndromes.

ANTIRHEUMATIC AND ANTI-INFLAMMATORY DRUGS

Pulmonary toxicity has been reported with aspirin non-steroidal anti-inflammatory drugs (NSAIDs), and a number of drugs used in the management of rheumatologic disorders.

Aspirin

The most common pulmonary reaction associated with aspirin use is bronchospasm, which may occur with therapeutic dosing in aspirin-sensitive individuals. Aspirin and NSAIDs induce bronchoconstriction by diverting arachidonic acid metabolites toward the lipoxygenase metabolic pathway, thereby leading to enhanced leukotriene-mediated airway inflammation and bronchoconstriction. Less commonly reported pulmonary complications of aspirin use include PIE syndrome, DAH, pulmonary hypersensitivity, vasculitis, and ARDS.

Acute salicylate poisoning produces symptoms of central nervous system toxicity (tinnitus, vertigo, nausea, vomiting, and hyperventilation) in mild to moderate overdose, and may result in coma, severe metabolic acidosis, and noncardiogenic pulmonary edema with critical overdoses. Pulmonary edema occurs in as many as 30% of patients with severe salicylate poisoning and may result in respiratory failure, often exacerbated by severe metabolic acidosis. Risk factors for salicylate toxicity include increased age and chronic aspirin ingestion. Management of severe toxicity includes supportive intensive care and sodium bicarbonate infusion to promote drug excretion.

Non-Steroidal Anti-Inflammatory Drugs

NSAIDs are widely used and generally well tolerated. However, NSAIDs may cross react with aspirin, producing a variety of allergic and pseudoallergic reactions affecting upper and lower airways.[96] NSAIDs cause bronchospasm in susceptible individuals with symptoms range from mild to severe. NSAIDs also cause anaphylactic reactions through the same mechanisms as that for aspirin.

The bleeding tendency induced by NSAIDs is well known, and reports exist of pulmonary hemorrhage associate with their use. DAH has been reported for ketorolac tromethamine in subjects without an underlying bleeding diathesis, but the histopathology leading to DAH has not been characterized.[97]

Methotrexate

Methotrexate is a dihydrofolate reductase inhibitor used as an anti-inflammatory and immunosuppressant, as well as a chemotherapeutic agent when used in higher doses. Despite the availability of newer antirheumatic drugs, methotrexate has retained its position as a first-line disease-modifying agent for the management of RA. Methotrexate affects cell replication through inhibition of dihydrofolate reductase, the enzyme that converts folic acid to its active coenzyme, tetrahydrofolate, allowing it to serve as one-carbon carriers in the synthesis and repair of DNA. The major nonpulmonary side effects of methotrexate correlate with the degree of folate deficiency. In contrast, pulmonary toxicity does not correlate with folate deficiency and may be seen at doses as low as 7.5 mg/wk, a conventional starting dose for treatment of RA. Conditions that have been identified as risk factors for toxicity include diabetes (OR, 35.6), hypoalbuminemia (OR, 19.5), rheumatoid pleuropulmonary disease (OR, 7.1), previous use of other disease-modifying agents (e.g., gold, sulfasalazine, or penicillamine), and older age (OR, 5.1).[98]

Methotrexate-induced pulmonary toxicity typically occurs within the first 2 years of treatment, but it can occur as early as 1 month into therapy. Pulmonary symptoms are most often subacute in onset, presenting over days to weeks, and include dyspnea, cough, fever, and less frequently, chest pain (<10%).[99] Symptoms may also develop acutely.[100] Radiographic changes are interstitial and bilateral in 50% of cases, but may also include a mixed alveolar–interstitial pattern that may appear as ground-glass opacities on high-resolution CT imaging.[99] Fibrotic changes are less common.

Diagnosis is challenging in cases of suspected methotrexate-induced pulmonary toxicity and RA, because similar clinical presentations may occur as a manifestation of RA itself. The most important diagnosis to exclude is infectious pneumonia, including that from opportunistic organisms. A diagnosis of methotrexate-induced lung disease is suggested by a predominance of lymphocytes, rather than neutrophils, on BAL.[14,22] The lymphocytic BAL fluid of methotrexate-induced hypersensitivity pneumonitis often has a CD8-predominant profile (low CD4:CD8 ratio), but not exclusively so. It appears that the type inflammatory cells may predict disease severity. In one study of 56 cases of methotrexate pulmonary toxicity, a lymphocyte-predominant BAL fluid was associated with late onset of symptoms (>6 months from drug initiation) and lower mortality than in those with neutrophil-predominant BAL.[101] Histopathology is varied and may demonstrate ill-formed granulomas suggestive of hypersensitivity pneumonitis, changes of chronic interstitial pneumonitis, BOOP, and/or DAD. PIE syndrome has also been reported.[99]

As with other pulmonary toxicities, prompt drug withdrawal is critical; resolution follows in the majority of patients. Corticosteroids may accelerate recovery in those with severe disease or symptoms refractory to drug withdrawal alone. Fatalities have been reported in subjects rechallenged with methotrexate, but rechallenge has been tolerated in others, arguing against hypersensitivity as the mechanism of injury in some subjects.

D-Penicillamine

D-Penicillamine is used as an anti-inflammatory agent in the management of rheumatoid arthritis. Although currently used less frequently than disease-modifying antirheumatic drugs (DMARDs), its pulmonary manifestations are important to recognize, as mortality from penicillamine pulmonary toxicity can be as high as 5%.

Penicillamine is a heavy metal chelating agent that has inhibitory effects on T-lymphocytes, impairs fibroblast proliferation, and decreases levels of rheumatoid factor and immune complexes. DAH and subacute interstitial infiltrates are the two most frequently reported histologic patterns of penicillamine-induced lung toxicity. Other patterns of pulmonary injury associated with its use include chronic alveolitis, PIE, and hypersensitivity pneumonitis.

Penicillamine is one of the few drugs that cause a pulmonary–renal syndrome, including a clinical presentation similar to Goodpasture syndrome.[102,103] The syndrome occurs infrequently among patients on penicillamine therapy for rheumatic disease, and also has been reported in patients given penicillamine as a chelating agent in Wilson disease—findings which support the hypothesis that the pulmonary findings are not simply a manifestation of the underlying collagen vascular disease.[104] Diagnosis is supported by high serum titers of ANA; antiglomerular basement membrane (anti-GBM) antibodies are typically absent from the serum. Pulmonary vasculitis is absent. Renal histopathology is that of crescentic glomerulonephritis, similar to that of Goodpasture syndrome; immunoglobulin deposition is absent. No specific risk factors have been identified for penicillamine-induced pulmonary–renal syndrome.

Symptoms at presentation include cough, dyspnea, hemoptysis, and hematuria. Symptom onset has been reported from 10 months to 20 years after drug initiation. No definitive dose–response relationship has been defined but there are reports of toxicity at doses as low as 300 mg per day and as high as 3.5 g per day. Coalescing, bilateral alveolar infiltrates characterize the radiographic findings, resulting in severe hypoxemia. BAL reveals an increase in the concentration of red blood cells on serial lavage and the presence of hemosiderin-laden macrophages, both of which characterize DAH. The syndrome may progress to include respiratory and/or renal failure. Mortality from penicillamine-induced pulmonary–renal disease has been reported to be as high as 50%. Survivors in one series were all left with residual radiographic abnormalities. Many patients become hemodialysis dependent despite treatment. Therefore, prompt identification and treatment are warranted.

Drug withdrawal, accompanied by high-dose corticosteroids, is the cornerstone of therapy. Adjunctive treatment with cyclophosphamide or azathioprine is often offered, although studies definitively supporting their use do not exist. In the absence of anti-GBM antibodies, plasmapheresis is not warranted.

Penicillamine may also induce interstitial lung disease, including hypersensitivity pneumonitis and/or bronchiolitis obliterans. In some cases, the findings are accompanied by alveolitis. A sister drug, bucillamine, has also been reported to cause centrilobular, ground-glass opacities and thickening of interlobular septae.

Gold Salts

The immunomodulatory properties of gold have been recognized since the 1920s, when the first cases of RA treated with chrysotherapy were reported. The first reports of gold-induced pulmonary toxicity followed in 1948.

Gold remains a therapeutic option for the treatment of RA that is refractory to other agents. It also has a role in the management of juvenile RA, ankylosing spondylitis, and pemphigus. As with methotrexate and penicillamine, the toxic reaction of gold must be distinguished from pulmonary disease related directly to the underlying RA.

One of the largest reviews of 140 patients with gold-related pulmonary toxicity identified distinguishing features.[25] The pattern that emerged from this review is one of cough and dyspnea as the most common presenting symptoms, with half of the patients exhibiting fever, as well. More than one-third of patients have an erythematous skin rash. Peripheral blood eosinophilia is a common finding. The onset of symptoms is typically early in the course of treatment, often within the first 4 months. Gold-induced pulmonary toxicity affects women more often than men (4:1). The mean age of onset of disease is in the sixth decade of life. A restrictive ventilatory defect is characteristic. The diffusing capacity is reduced in over 90% of affected individuals. The radiographic injury patterns seen include ILD, hypersensitivity pneumonitis, and BOOP.[105,106]

Diagnostic evaluation may include BAL, which typically shows a lymphocytic-predominant fluid, including CD8+ lymphocyte predominance.[106,107] This finding, in conjunction with a positive in vitro gold lymphocyte proliferation assay, strongly supports the diagnosis of gold-induced pulmonary toxicity. The diagnostic features suggest that the gold-induced toxicity can be a hypersensitivity reaction.

Treatment of gold-induced lung toxicity necessitates discontinuation of the drug. Longitudinal data reveal that gold-induced impairments in diffusing capacity may take months to resolve. Rarely, disease progression may occur after discontinuation of the gold. Refractory or progressive symptoms may be treated with prednisone at 30 to 60 mg per day.

Sulfasalazine and Mesalazine

Sulfasalazine is used as a DMARD and also is commonly employed in the treatment of inflammatory bowel disease, as is mesalazine. Both agents have been associated with pulmonary toxicity, most commonly interstitial pneumonias, including NSIP.[108,109] Sulfasalazine has been reported to cause BOOP.[110,111] BOOP has been associated with mesalazine, as well.[112] Mesalazine has been associated with eosinophilic pneumonia when taken orally and when it is used as a suppository.[113]

Biologic Agents

Rituximab is a CD20-directed, B-cell–depleting monoclonal antibody used in the treatment of RA. granulomatosis with polyangiitis (formerly known as Wegener granulomatosis), and microscopic polyangiitis. Many case reports regarding its pulmonary toxicity have been reported in the literature, with clinical presentations ranging from dyspnea and mild hypoxemia to fatal respiratory failure.[114] Clinical disease occurs in three different time courses, most commonly as a subacute onset of dyspnea 2 weeks following rituximab infusion, often several cycles into therapy.[115–117] Radiographic imaging shows bilateral diffuse interstitial infiltrates or ground-glass opacities. Less common presentations include acute onset of ARDS within hours of first infusion of the drug and chronic, insidious onset of disease.[115] Histopathology may include obliterative bronchiolitis.[118]

TNF antagonists are used in the management of rheumatic diseases. The most important pulmonary side effects of these agents are pneumonias due to bacteria, mycobacteria, Pneumocystis jiroveci, and fungi, occurring in 1.4% of patients treated with etanercept and 2.4% of those treated with infliximab. Among noninfectious pulmonary disorders associated with the use of anti-TNF therapies, interstitial pneumonitis is the most common manifestation of drug-induced disease. Interstitial pneumonitis was reported in 0.5% of 5000 Japanese subjects treated with infliximab and in 0.6% of over 7000 subjects who received etanercept.[119,120]

The reliability of case reports for demonstrating a definite causal link between monoclonal antibody use and pulmonary toxicity is complicated by the fact that interstitial pneumonitis is part of the spectrum of disease in patients with rheumatologic disorders. In addition, biologics are often administered to those with more severe manifestations of disease in whom lung disease is often present. In a large case series of autoimmune disease induced by TNF antagonists, 24 cases of interstitial pneumonitis were noted among 233 subjects studied.[121] In a review summarizing case series and reports published between 1990 and 2010, the mean time of onset of respiratory symptoms for subjects receiving biologic was 26 weeks, with 50% of cases occurring within the first 2 months.[122] Sarcoid-like granulomatosis has been frequently reported with the use of etanercept.[122,123] Among cases of sarcoid-like disease associated with monoclonal antibody therapies, 50% were compatible with stage 2 sarcoidosis, and two-thirds of all cases resolved with discontinuation of biologic therapy.[122]

Etanercept and infliximab have also been associated with development of drug-induced lupus, presenting with pleural effusion and/or pericarditis, along with positive ANA and antihistone or anti–double-stranded DNA antibodies.[124,125] The lupus-like conditions subside with drug discontinuation.

Adalimumab, a new TNF-α antagonist used in management of RA , also has been reported to cause pulmonary toxicity. Reports indicate lung injury occurring months to years into therapy. Patients usually present with dyspnea, cough, and a radiographic pattern are consistent with interstitial pneumonitis. Acute onset of lung injury has reported within 1 hour of dosing of this agent.[126] Symptoms may begin subtly as mild cough following a treatment cycle and progress with each subsequent injection.[127] Imaging shows patchy ground-glass opacities, with or without consolidation and patchy fibrosis.[127,128] In one case, patchy fibrotic interstitial disease was seen initially, followed by resolution after drug withdrawal, and then recurrent injury characterized by areas of ground-glass opacification after rechallenge.[129] Patients usually require corticosteroids to achieve clinical resolution.

■ IMMUNOSUPPRESSANTS

Sirolimus and everolimus are immunosuppressive agents used in the management of patients with solid organ transplants. They function as inhibitors of mammalian target of rapamycin (mTOR) and suppress organ rejection through inhibition of growth factor–induced smooth muscle cell proliferation and migration; they also inhibit T- and B-cell activation.

Sirolimus was introduced into clinical use in the late 1990s. Sirolimus-induced pneumonitis in solid organ transplant recipients is an important consideration in the differential diagnosis of dyspnea with interstitial infiltrates after exclusion of infection. Case reports of sirolimus-induced pulmonary toxicity began to appear in the literature in 2000, when the drug was first implicated as the cause of biopsy-proven BOOP in a renal transplant recipient. A dose–response relationship is suggested, because dose reduction appears to ameliorate the pneumonitis. However, toxicity may occur despite therapeutic serum sirolimus levels and can occur as early as 2 weeks into therapy. However, it occurs more often after at least 6 weeks of therapy.

A case series of 24 patients further characterized the drug reaction. Most patients in the series exhibited a radiographic pattern of patchy peripheral consolidations consistent with BOOP, while four patients had reticular and ground-glass opacities.[130]

The BAL of subjects with sirolimus lung toxicity is typically lymphocytic (19 of 24 subjects); ≥5% eosinophilia was present in four cases.[130] Lymphocyte subsets have not been consistently reported, but some authors have described CD4+ predominance in the BAL.

The histology is consistent with BOOP and/or granulomatous interstitial pneumonitis, characterized by noncaseating granulomas in the bronchial wall and surrounding granulomatous inflammation.[131,132]

Cases of DAH have also been reported associated with sirolimus, and in some cases have been fatal.[133,134]

Discontinuation of sirolimus is necessary for syndrome resolution. Complete recovery is typically achieved in all patients by 6 months.

Everolimus has been shown to cause mild, reversible pulmonary toxicity.[135] It has also been implicated in fatal respiratory failure presenting initially with cough and dyspnea and accompanied by patchy alveolar infiltrates. Despite drug withdrawal and treatment with corticosteroids, the patient described in the case report progressed to respiratory failure and DAH.[136]

ANTIMICROBIAL DRUGS

The most commonly reported clinical syndrome for all classes of antimicrobials is pulmonary infiltrates with PIE. Among the reports of antibiotic-associated PIE syndrome are many cases of minocycline- and erythromycin-induced PIE, and fewer cases associated with penicillins, tetracyclines, sulfonamides, and cephalosporins. Cases of PIE have also been reported with the use of antituberculous drugs, including isoniazid, rifampin, and ethambutol.

Nitrofurantoin

Nitrofurantoin is one of the most commonly implicated antimicrobial agents that causes pulmonary toxicity. Although its peak usage worldwide was probably in the 1980s, it remains a widely used antibiotic for management of chronic urinary tract infections. Pulmonary toxicity may have significant clinical impact if the affected patient has underlying cardiopulmonary disease. Since the drug is used primary in the elderly population, in whom cardiopulmonary disease is common, recognition of its potential contribution to a patient's respiratory decline is important.

The clinical spectrum of respiratory disease caused by nitrofurantoin is broad. The onset of symptoms is highly unpredictable and of variable latency. The severity of disease varies; and the histopathology is diverse. Ninety percent of the earliest reported cases of nitrofurantoin pulmonary toxicity were acute in onset, occurring within days to weeks of treatment initiation. These patients presented with fever (80%), cough, dyspnea, rash (20%), arthralgias, and peripheral eosinophilia. As reports of toxicity have continued to populate the literature, it has become clear that subacute and chronic presentations also are common (Fig. 66-2).

It is inevitable that many cases may be missed due to the long latency between the initial dose and the onset of clinical symptoms. The median time to diagnosis in one series was 4 months; however, some diagnoses were made as long as 5 years after drug initiation. Among those with chronic symptoms, the most common histopathologic pattern is that of chronic interstitial pneumonitis, with fewer reported cases of BOOP and granulomatous interstitial disease.[137] High-resolution CT findings in 18 patients with chronic nitrofurantoin lung injury showed bilateral ground-glass opacities in all subjects (diffuse in 30%, and with a middle to upper lung zone predominance in 40%). Irregular linear opacities were present in 30%, consolidation in 30%, and traction bronchiectasis in 10% (one subject).[138]

Many other histopathologic patterns and clinical syndromes have been reported, including pulmonary edema, ARDS, vasculitis, DAH, SLE, PIE, and nodules. Bronchospasm and anaphylaxis related to antimicrobials is discussed in the section on those conditions.

INTERFERON-α AND PEGYLATED INTERFERON-α_2b

The rising prevalence of chronic hepatitis C worldwide, and its treatment with interferon-α and pegylated interferon-α_2b, has brought with it reports of pulmonary toxicity, most commonly interstitial infiltrates and BOOP. Systemic side effects are common among patients using interferon, and typically include flu-like symptoms of fatigue, headache, anorexia and myalgias. Pulmonary symptoms occur infrequently. Ribavirin, a synthetic nucleoside analog is often used in conjunction with either interferon-α or pegylated interferon-α_2b to enhance the antiviral activity of the interferons. Ribavirin is associated with dyspnea and cough, but it has not been reported to cause pulmonary toxicity when used alone. The reported rate of significant pulmonary interstitial disease and/or BOOP is as high as 6% among patients receiving high-dose daily interferon for hepatitis C, and <1% among patients on conventional three-times-weekly dosing schedules of interferon-α and ribavirin.[139]

The occurrence of interstitial disease among users of interferon-α is not exclusive to those with hepatitis, and it has been reported in patients on interferon therapy for chronic myelogenous leukemia and myelofibrosis as well. Most cases of pulmonary toxicity occur within several weeks of initiation of therapy and resolve with discontinuation of the medications.

Several case reports or small series of cases characterize the association of de novo sarcoidosis or recrudescent sarcoidosis with interferon-α and interferon-α_2a used in chronic hepatitis C.[140] The incidence of sarcoidosis among patients receiving interferon is not well established, but has been reported to be as high as 5% among patients receiving treatment with interferon-α_2a for hepatitis C.[141] Although most of the reports of sarcoidosis have been in patients undergoing treatment for hepatitis C, it also can occur in the setting of treatment of hematological malignancy. Interferon-associated pulmonary sarcoidosis occurs along with manifestations of disease involvement of other sites, including cutaneous, parotid, liver, ocular, and cardiac diseases. Prompt withdrawal of the drug is advised, and corticosteroids may be necessary for disease resolution.

OPIATES AND ILLICIT DRUGS

Complications of illicit drug use are numerous and encompass toxic injury to the lung related to use of the drug itself, and the associated infectious sequelae of venous cannulation, including endocarditis, septic embolization, and HIV-associated opportunistic infection. The prevalence of tuberculosis among drug users puts these individuals at high risk of active tuberculosis as well. Opiates or other sedatives may cause altered mental status and impairment of the gag reflex, substantially increasing the risk of aspiration pneumonia. Pulmonary parenchymal disease may also be caused by talc or other inert substances used to "cut" the drugs. Recognition of these

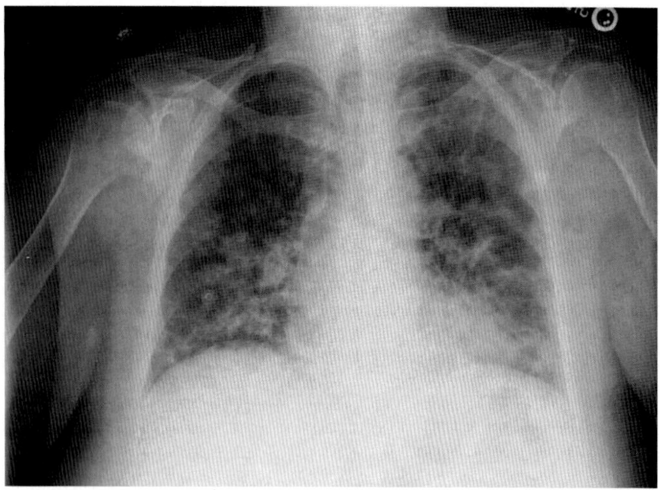

A

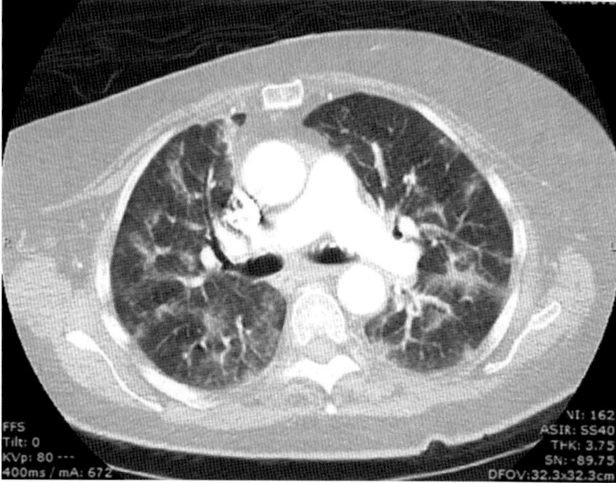

B

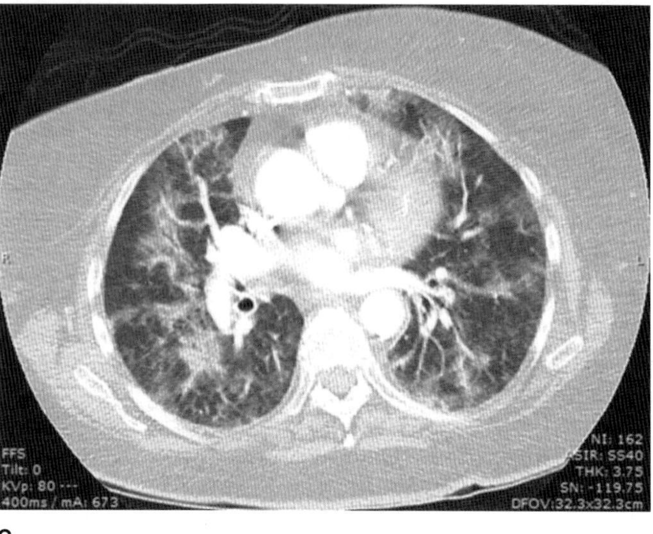

C

Figure 66-2 **A.** Chest radiograph of an 80-year-old woman 1 year after initiation of nitrofurantoin for recurrent urinary tract infection. **B, C.** CT scan: Patchy ground-glass opacities and consolidation consistent with nitrofurantoin-induced bronchiolitis obliterans—organizing pneumonia. *(Used with permission of Ami Rubinowitz, MD.)*

conditions unrelated to direct toxicity of the drug broadens the differential diagnosis of respiratory symptoms in users of illicit drugs.[142]

Heroin

Overdoses of heroin and other narcotics have long been known to cause pulmonary edema. One of the earliest reports of drug-induced lung disease was by Osler in 1880, in which he described pulmonary edema in an opiate addict and ascribed the edema to the opiate use. For unknown reasons, the frequency with which heroin-induced pulmonary edema (HIPE) occurs appears to have decreased in recent decades. In one series of patients compiled between 1968 and 1970, 48% of 149 patients with heroin overdose had pulmonary edema on presentation.[143] The presence of pulmonary edema was associated with increased mortality (18.3% vs. 8.7% if pulmonary edema was absent). A more recent case series describes a much lower incidence of pulmonary edema: 2.1% cases of heroin overdose.[144] It is unclear whether the change in epidemiology of HIPE relates to a change in the additives to illicit heroin or other factors. In the latter series, one-third of the patients required intubation and mechanical ventilation, but the hypoxemia of HIPE resolved within 48 hours of presentation.

The literature does not conclusively indicate the mechanism of HIPE. Some studies have reported higher protein levels in pulmonary edema fluid of HIPE than in cardiogenic pulmonary edema, supporting increased capillary permeability as the mechanism.[145] There are reports of significant acute inflammation in the lung tissue of narcotic abusers who were examined postmortem.[146] Other reactions associated with heroin use include acute bronchospasm.

Pulmonary disease associated with illicit injection drug use may be unrelated to the drug itself. Talc used to cut heroin or inert substances used in pills that are crushed and injected produce foreign-body granulomatous reactions in the pulmonary vasculature and interstitium. A longitudinal study of six patients with pulmonary talcosis described characteristic radiographic findings, consisting of a diffuse, micronodular pulmonary infiltrate that evolved into coalescent conglomerates, often in the upper lobes, similar in appearance to those of progressive massive fibrosis. These alterations may be accompanied by emphysematous changes in the lower lobes, which may result in pneumothoraces. Other pulmonary complications of injection drug use include septic emboli, abscess formation, bronchiectasis, and bullae independent of apical fibrotic reactions.

Cocaine

Cocaine may be injected intravenously, inhaled nasally, or smoked. It is the last noted route that is most frequently associated with respiratory symptoms and pulmonary injury. Cocaine is typically smoked as "crack" cocaine, an alkaloid derivative of cocaine hydrochloride that is mixed with ether or alcohol. Respiratory symptoms typically develop acutely, within hours of use, and include cough, hemoptysis, chest pain, and shortness of breath. Bronchospasm, which may be severe enough to precipitate respiratory failure, has been reported with and without a prior history of asthma. The radiographic appearance may be consistent with ARDS, and the histopathology that of DAD, with or without alveolar hemorrhage.[147] Capillaritis, accompanied by glomerulonephritis, has been reported, but is not typically present.

PRINCIPLES OF TREATMENT AND DISEASE RESOLUTION

Prompt recognition of drug-induced lung disease affords patients the greatest chance of clinical and radiographic recovery, before irreversible lung injury occurs. In most cases of drug-induced pulmonary injury, discontinuation of the culprit drug is sufficient for regression of clinical symptoms and most or all of the radiographic findings. The decision to treat with corticosteroids must be individualized, based on the severity of the clinical picture and the expected rapidity of symptom resolution. For example, amiodarone pulmonary toxicity frequently requires oral corticosteroid administration unless the symptoms are very mild, because of the long serum half-life of the drug. Recrudescence of lung injury is rare among other implicated drugs in the absence of reexposure to the culprit drug. Overall, corticosteroids are used with apparent success, but controlled studies to determine therapeutic efficacy are lacking, and the infrequent occurrence of most drug toxicities will not allow this treatment to be convincingly studied in clinical trials.

REFERENCES

1. Amar RK, Jick SS, Rosenberg D, Maher TM, Meier CR. Drug-/radiation-induced interstitial lung disease in the United Kingdom general population: incidence, all-cause mortality and characteristics at diagnosis. *Respirology*. 2012;17(5):861–868.
2. Delaunois LM. Mechanisms in pulmonary toxicology. *Clin Chest Med*. 2004;25(1):1–14.
3. Baillie TA, Rettie AE. Role of biotransformation in drug-induced toxicity: influence of intra- and inter-species differences in drug metabolism. *Drug Metab Pharmacokinet*. 2011;26(1):15–29.
4. Wijnen PA, Bekers O, Drent M. Relationship between drug-induced interstitial lung diseases and cytochrome P450 polymorphisms. *Curr Opin Pulm Med*. 2010;16(5):496–502.
5. Park BK, Kitteringham NR. Drug-protein conjugation and its immunological consequences. *Drug Metab Rev*. 1990;22(1):87–144.
6. Pohl LR, Satoh H, Christ DD, Kenna JG. The immunologic and metabolic basis of drug hypersensitivities. *Annu Rev Pharmacol Toxicol*. 1988;28:367–387.
7. Lardinois D, Handschin A, Weder W. Acute amiodarone-induced pulmonary toxicity after lung operation. *Ann Thorac Surg*. 2002;73(6):2033–2034; author reply 2034.
8. Akira M, Ishikawa H, Yamamoto S. Drug-induced pneumonitis: thin-section CT findings in 60 patients. *Radiology*. 2002;224(3):852–860.
9. Cleverley JR, Screaton NJ, Hiorns MP, Flint JD, Muller NL. Drug-induced lung disease: high-resolution CT and histological findings. *Clin Radiol*. 2002;57(4):292–299.
10. Meyer KC, Raghu G, Baughman RP, et al. An official American Thoracic Society clinical practice guideline: the clinical utility of bronchoalveolar lavage cellular analysis in interstitial lung disease. *Am J Respir Crit Care Med*. 2012;185(9):1004–1014.
11. Semenzato G, Poletti V. Bronchoalveolar lavage in lung cancer. *Respiration*. 1992;59(Suppl 1):44–46.
12. Wardwell NR Jr, Miller R, Ware LB. Pulmonary alveolar proteinosis associated with a disease-modifying antirheumatoid arthritis drug. *Respirology*. 2006;11(5):663–665.
13. Duran I, Siu LL, Oza AM, et al. Characterisation of the lung toxicity of the cell cycle inhibitor temsirolimus. *Eur J Cancer*. 2006;42(12):1875–1880.
14. White DA, Rankin JA, Stover DE, Gellene RA, Gupta S. Methotrexate pneumonitis. Bronchoalveolar lavage findings suggest an immunologic disorder. *Am Rev Respir Dis*. 1989;139(1):18–21.
15. Akoun GM, Cadranel JL, Milleron BJ, D'Ortho MP, Mayaud CM. Bronchoalveolar lavage cell data in 19 patients with drug-associated pneumonitis (except amiodarone). *Chest*. 1991;99(1):98–104.
16. Akoun GM, Cadranel JL, Rosenow EC 3rd, Milleron BJ. Bronchoalveolar lavage cell data in drug-induced pneumonitis. *Allerg Immunol (Paris)*. 1991;23(6):245–252.
17. Costabel U, Uzaslan E, Guzman J. Bronchoalveolar lavage in drug-induced lung disease. *Clin Chest Med*. 2004;25(1):25–35.
18. Inomata S, Takahashi H, Nagata M, et al. Acute lung injury as an adverse event of gefitinib. *Anti-cancer drugs*. 2004;15(5):461–467.
19. Matsuno O, Ono E, Ueno T, et al. Increased serum ADAM8 concentration in patients with drug-induced eosinophilic pneumonia-ADAM8 expression depends on a the allergen route of entry. *Respir Med*. 2010;104(1):34–39.
20. Ohnishi H, Yokoyama A, Yasuhara Y, et al. Circulating KL-6 levels in patients with drug induced pneumonitis. *Thorax*. 2003;58(10):872–875.
21. Umetani K, Abe M, Kawabata K, et al. SP-D as a marker of amiodarone-induced pulmonary toxicity. *Intern Med*. 2002;41(9):709–712.
22. Akoun GM, Gauthier-Rahman S, Mayaud CM, Touboul JL, Denis MF. Leukocyte migration inhibition in methotrexate-induced pneumonitis. Evidence for an immunologic cell-mediated mechanism. *Chest*. 1987;91(1):96–99.
23. Gauthier-Rahman S, Akoun GM, Milleron BJ, Mayaud CM. Leukocyte migration inhibition in propranolol-induced pneumonitis. Evidence for an immunologic cell-mediated mechanism. *Chest*. 1990;97(1):238–241.
24. Hirata S, Hattori N, Kumagai K, Haruta Y, Yokoyama A, Kohno N. Lymphocyte transformation test is not helpful for the diagnosis of methotrexate-induced pneumonitis in patients with rheumatoid arthritis. *Clin Chim Acta*. 2009;407(1–2):25–29.
25. Tomioka R, King TE Jr. Gold-induced pulmonary disease: clinical features, outcome, and differentiation from rheumatoid lung disease. *Am J Respir Crit Care Med*. 1997;155(3):1011–1020.
26. Cacoub P, Musette P, Descamps V, et al. The DRESS syndrome: a literature review. *Am J Med*. 2011;124(7):588–597.
27. American Thoracic Society, European Respiratory Society. International Multidisciplinary Consensus Classification of the Idiopathic Interstitial Pneumonias. This joint statement of the American Thoracic Society (ATS), and the European Respiratory Society (ERS) was adopted by the ATS board of directors, June 2001 and by the ERS Executive Committee, June 2001. *Am J Respir Crit Care Med*. 2002;165(2):277–304.
28. Travis WD, Costabel U, Hansell DM, et al. An official American Thoracic Society/European Respiratory Society statement: Update of the international multidisciplinary classification of the idiopathic interstitial pneumonias. *Am J Respir Crit Care Med*. 2013;188(6):733–748.
29. Lee-Chiong T Jr, Matthay RA. Drug-induced pulmonary edema and acute respiratory distress syndrome. *Clin Chest Med*. 2004;25(1):95–104.
30. Bruera E, Miller MJ. Non-cardiogenic pulmonary edema after narcotic treatment for cancer pain. *Pain*. 1989;39(3):297–300.
31. Heffner JE, Sahn SA. Salicylate-induced pulmonary edema. Clinical features and prognosis. *Ann Intern Med*. 1981;95(4):405–409.

32. Walters JS, Woodring JH, Stelling CB, Rosenbaum HD. Salicylate-induced pulmonary edema. *Radiology*. 1983;146(2): 289–293.

33. Bonaci-Nikolic B, Nikolic MM, Andrejevic S, Zoric S, Bukilica M. Antineutrophil cytoplasmic antibody (ANCA)-associated autoimmune diseases induced by antithyroid drugs: comparison with idiopathic ANCA vasculitides. *Arthritis Res Ther*. 2005;7(5):R1072–R1081.

34. Slot MC, Links TP, Stegeman CA, Tervaert JW. Occurrence of antineutrophil cytoplasmic antibodies and associated vasculitis in patients with hyperthyroidism treated with antithyroid drugs: a long-term followup study. *Arthritis Rheum*. 2005;53(1):108–113.

35. Ye H, Gao Y, Guo XH, Zhao MH. Titre and affinity of propylthiouracil-induced anti-myeloperoxidase antibodies are closely associated with the development of clinical vasculitis. *Clin Exp Immunol*. 2005;142(1):116–119.

36. Ogawa A, Matsubara H, Fujio H, et al. Risk of alveolar hemorrhage in patients with primary pulmonary hypertension–anticoagulation and epoprostenol therapy. *Circ J*. 2005;69(2):216–220.

37. Coulter DM, Edwards IR. Cough associated with captopril and enalapril. *Br Med J (Clin Res Ed)*. 1987;294(6586):1521–1523.

38. Dicpinigaitis PV. Angiotensin-converting enzyme inhibitor-induced cough: ACCP evidence-based clinical practice guidelines. *Chest*. 2006;129(Suppl 1):169S–173S.

39. Israili ZH, Hall WD. Cough and angioneurotic edema associated with angiotensin-converting enzyme inhibitor therapy. A review of the literature and pathophysiology. *Ann Intern Med*. 1992;117(3):234–242.

40. Sebastian JL, McKinney WP, Kaufman J, Young MJ. Angiotensin-converting enzyme inhibitors and cough. Prevalence in an outpatient medical clinic population. *Chest*. 1991;99(1):36–39.

41. Gibson GR. Enalapril-induced cough. *Arch Intern Med*. 1989; 149(12):2701–2703.

42. Lacourciere Y, Brunner H, Irwin R, et al. Effects of modulators of the renin-angiotensin-aldosterone system on cough. Losartan Cough Study Group. *J Hypertens*. 1994;12(12):1387–1393.

43. Chiu AG, Newkirk KA, Davidson BJ, Burningham AR, Krowiak EJ, Deeb ZE. Angiotensin-converting enzyme inhibitor-induced angioedema: a multicenter review and an algorithm for airway management. *Ann Otol Rhinol Laryngol*. 2001;110(9):834–840.

44. Gibbs CR, Lip GY, Beevers DG. Angioedema due to ACE inhibitors: increased risk in patients of African origin. *Br J Clin Pharmacol*. 1999;48(6):861–865.

45. Babu KS, Marshall BG. Drug-induced airway diseases. *Clin Chest Med*. 2004;25(1):113–122.

46. Brown SG. Anaphylaxis: clinical concepts and research priorities. *Emerg Med Australas*. 2006;18(2):155–169.

47. Gruchalla R. Understanding drug allergies. *J Allergy Clin Immunol*. 2000;105(6 Pt 2):S637–S644.

48. Vervloet D, Durham S. Adverse reactions to drugs. *BMJ*. 1998; 316(7143):1511–1514.

49. Lieberman P, Nicklas RA, Oppenheimer J, Kemp SF, Lang DM. The diagnosis and management of anaphylaxis practice parameter: 2010 Update. Joint Task Force on Practice Parameters: American Academy of Allergy, Asthma and Immunology; American College of Allergy, Asthma and Immunology; and the Joint Council of Allergy, Asthma and Immunology. *J Allergy Clin Immunol*. 2010;126:477–480.

50. Neugut AI, Ghatak AT, Miller RL. Anaphylaxis in the United States: an investigation into its epidemiology. *Arch Intern Med*. 2001;161(1):15–21.

51. Leuppi JD, Schnyder P, Hartmann K, Reinhart WH, Kuhn M. Drug-induced bronchospasm: analysis of 187 spontaneously reported cases. *Respiration*. 2001;68(4):345–351.

52. Brewerton D. D-Penicillamine. *Br Med J*. 1976;2(6050):1507.

53. Demaziere A, Maugars Y, Chollet S, Prost A. Non-fatal bronchiolitis obliterans possibly associated with tiopronin. A case report with long-term follow-up. *Br J Rheumatol*. 1993;32(2):172–174.

54. Epler GR, Snider GL, Gaensler EA, Cathcart ES, FitzGerald MX, Carrington CB. Bronchiolitis and bronchitis in connective tissue disease. A possible relationship to the use of penicillamine. *JAMA*. 1979;242(6):528–532.

55. Pegg SJ, Lang BA, Mikhail EL, Hughes DM. Fatal bronchiolitis obliterans in a patient with juvenile rheumatoid arthritis receiving chrysotherapy. *J Rheumatol*. 1994;21(3):549–551.

56. Devouassoux G, Cottin V, Liote H, et al. Characterisation of severe obliterative bronchiolitis in rheumatoid arthritis. *Eur Respir J*. 2009;33(5):1053–1061.

57. Devakonda A, Raoof S, Sung A, Travis WD, Naidich D. Bronchiolar disorders: a clinical-radiological diagnostic algorithm. *Chest*. 2010;137(4):938–951.

58. Higenbottam T, Laude L, Emery C, Essener M. Pulmonary hypertension as a result of drug therapy. *Clin Chest Med*. 2004; 25(1):123–131.

59. Brenot F, Herve P, Petitpretz P, Parent F, Duroux P, Simonneau G. Primary pulmonary hypertension and fenfluramine use. *Br Heart J*. 1993;70(6):537–541.

60. Abenhaim L, Moride Y, Brenot F, et al. Appetite-suppressant drugs and the risk of primary pulmonary hypertension. International Primary Pulmonary Hypertension Study Group. *N Engl J Med*. 1996;335(9):609–616.

61. Connolly HM, Crary JL, McGoon MD, et al. Valvular heart disease associated with fenfluramine-phentermine. *N Engl J Med*. 1997;337(9):581–588.

62. Gross AS, Phillips AC, Rieutord A, Shenfield GM. The influence of the sparteine/debrisoquine genetic polymorphism on the disposition of dexfenfluramine. *Br J Clin Pharmacol*. 1996;41(4): 311–317.

63. Yano T, Itoh Y, Yamada M, Egashira N, Oishi R. Combined treatment with L-carnitine and a pan-caspase inhibitor effectively reverses amiodarone-induced injury in cultured human lung epithelial cells. *Apoptosis*. 2008;13(4):543–552.

64. Dean PJ, Groshart KD, Porterfield JG, Iansmith DH, Golden EB Jr. Amiodarone-associated pulmonary toxicity. A clinical and pathologic study of eleven cases. *Am J Clin Pathol*. 1987;87(1):7–13.

65. Kennedy JI, Myers JL, Plumb VJ, Fulmer JD. Amiodarone pulmonary toxicity. Clinical, radiologic, and pathologic correlations. *Arch Intern Med*. 1987;147(1):50–55.

66. Myers JL, Kennedy JI, Plumb VJ. Amiodarone lung: pathologic findings in clinically toxic patients. *Hum Pathol*. 1987;18(4): 349–354.

67. Camus P, Martin WJ 2nd, Rosenow EC 3rd. Amiodarone pulmonary toxicity. *Clin Chest Med*. 2004;25(1):65–75.

68. Jackevicius CA, Tom A, Essebag V, et al. Population-level incidence and risk factors for pulmonary toxicity associated with amiodarone. *Am J Cardiol*. 2011;108(5):705–710.

69. Ott MC, Khoor A, Leventhal JP, Paterick TE, Burger CD. Pulmonary toxicity in patients receiving low-dose amiodarone. *Chest*. 2003;123(2):646–651.

70. Fung RC, Chan WK, Chu CM, Yue CS. Low dose amiodarone-induced lung injury. *Int J Cardiol*. 2006;113(1):144–145.

71. Olshansky B, Sami M, Rubin A, et al. Use of amiodarone for atrial fibrillation in patients with preexisting pulmonary disease in the AFFIRM study. *Am J Cardiol.* 2005;95(3):404–405.

72. Handschin AE, Lardinois D, Schneiter D, Bloch K, Weder W. Acute amiodarone-induced pulmonary toxicity following lung resection. *Respiration.* 2003;70(3):310–312.

73. Kay GN, Epstein AE, Kirklin JK, Diethelm AG, Graybar G, Plumb VJ. Fatal postoperative amiodarone pulmonary toxicity. *Am J Cardiol.* 1988;62(7):490–492.

74. Saussine M, Colson P, Alauzen M, Mary H. Postoperative acute respiratory distress syndrome. A complication of amiodarone associated with 100 percent oxygen ventilation. *Chest.* 1992;102(3):980–981.

75. Wood DL, Osborn MJ, Rooke J, Holmes DR Jr. Amiodarone pulmonary toxicity: report of two cases associated with rapidly progressive fatal adult respiratory distress syndrome after pulmonary angiography. *Mayo Clin Proc.* 1985;60(9):601–603.

76. Kosseifi SG, Halawa A, Bailey B, Micklewright M, Roy TM, Byrd RP Jr. Reduction of amiodarone pulmonary toxicity in patients treated with angiotensin-converting enzyme inhibitors and angiotensin receptor blockers. *Ther Adv Respir Dis.* 2009;3(6):289–294.

77. Nikaido A, Tada T, Nakamura K, et al. Clinical features of and effects of angiotensin system antagonists on amiodarone-induced pulmonary toxicity. *Int J Cardiol.* 2010;140(3): 328–335.

78. Uhal BD, Wang R, Laukka J, Zhuang J, Soledad-Conrad V, Filippatos G. Inhibition of amiodarone-induced lung fibrosis but not alveolitis by angiotensin system antagonists. *Pharmacol Toxicol.* 2003;92(2):81–87.

79. Kharabsheh S, Abendroth CS, Kozak M. Fatal pulmonary toxicity occurring within two weeks of initiation of amiodarone. *Am J Cardiol.* 2002;89(7):896–898.

80. Azzam I, Tov N, Elias N, Naschitz JE. Amiodarone toxicity presenting as pulmonary mass and peripheral neuropathy: the continuing diagnostic challenge. *Postgrad Med J.* 2006;82(963): 73–75.

81. Vernhet H, Bousquet C, Durand G, Giron J, Senac JP. Reversible amiodarone-induced lung disease: HRCT findings. *Eur Radiol.* 2001;11(9):1697–1703.

82. Endoh Y, Hanai R, Uto K, et al. Diagnostic accuracy of KL-6 as a marker of amiodarone-induced pulmonary toxicity. *Pacing Clin Electrophysiol.* 2000;23(11 Pt 2):2010–2013.

83. Vizioli LD, Cho S. Amiodarone-associated hemoptysis. *Chest.* 1994;105(1):305–306.

84. Yokogawa N, Vivino FB. Hydralazine-induced autoimmune disease: comparison to idiopathic lupus and ANCA-positive vasculitis. *Mod Rheumatol.* 2009;19(3):338–347.

85. Marina VP, Malhotra D, Kaw D. Hydralazine-induced ANCA vasculitis with pulmonary renal syndrome: a rare clinical presentation. *Int Urol Nephrol.* 2012;44(6):1907–1909.

86. Goetschalckx K, Ceuppens J, Van Mieghem W. Hydrochlorothiazide-associated noncardiogenic pulmonary oedema and shock: a case report and review of the literature. *Acta Cardiol.* 2007;62(2):215–220.

87. Henningsen NC, Cederberg A, Hanson A, Johansson BW. Effects of long-term treatment with procaine amide. A prospective study with special regard to ANF and SLE in fast and slow acetylators. *Acta Med Scand.* 1975;198(6):475–482.

88. Cush JJ, Goldings EA. Drug-induced lupus: clinical spectrum and pathogenesis. *Am J Med Sci.* 1985;290(1):36–45.

89. Bellosta S, Paoletti R, Corsini A. Safety of statins: focus on clinical pharmacokinetics and drug interactions. *Circulation.* 2004;109(23 Suppl 1):III50–III57.

90. Fernandez AB, Karas RH, Alsheikh-Ali AA, Thompson PD. Statins and interstitial lung disease: a systematic review of the literature and of food and drug administration adverse event reports. *Chest.* 2008;134(4):824–830.

91. Huang LK, Tsai MJ, Tsai HC, Chao HS, Lin FC, Chang SC. Statin-induced lung injury: diagnostic clue and outcome. *Postgrad Med J.* 2013;89(1047):14–19.

92. De Groot RE, Willems LN, Dijkman JH. Interstitial lung disease with pleural effusion caused by simvastin. *J Intern Med.* 1996;239(4):361–363.

93. Lantuejoul S, Brambilla E, Brambilla C, Devouassoux G. Statin-induced fibrotic nonspecific interstitial pneumonia. *Eur Respir J.* 2002;19(3):577–580.

94. Liscoet-Loheac N, Andre N, Couturaud F, Chenu E, Quiot JJ, Leroyer C. [Hypersensitivity pneumonitis in a patient taking pravastatin]. *Rev Mal Respir.* 2001;18(4 Pt 1):426–428.

95. Xu JF, Washko GR, Nakahira K, et al. Statins and pulmonary fibrosis: the potential role of NLRP3 inflammasome activation. *Am J Respir Crit Care Med.* 2012;185(5):547–556.

96. Kowalski ML, Makowska JS, Blanca M, et. al. Hypersensitivity to nonsteroidal anti-inflammatory drugs (NSAIDs)-classification, diagnosis and management: review of the EAACI/ENDA and GA2LEN/HANNA. *Allergy.* 2011;66:818–829.

97. Marak CP, Alappan N, Shim C, Guddati AK. Diffuse alveolar hemorrhage due to ketorolac tromethamine. *Pharmacology.* 2013;92(1–2):11–13.

98. Alarcon GS, Kremer JM, Macaluso M, et al. Risk factors for methotrexate-induced lung injury in patients with rheumatoid arthritis. A multicenter, case-control study. Methotrexate-Lung Study Group. *Ann Intern Med.* 1997;127(5):356–364.

99. Imokawa S, Colby TV, Leslie KO, Helmers RA. Methotrexate pneumonitis: review of the literature and histopathological findings in nine patients. *Eur Respir J.* 2000;15(2): 373–381.

100. Hargreaves MR, Mowat AG, Benson MK. Acute pneumonitis associated with low dose methotrexate treatment for rheumatoid arthritis: report of five cases and review of published reports. *Thorax.* 1992;47(8):628–633.

101. Chikura B, Sathi N, Lane S, Dawson JK. Variation of immunological response in methotrexate-induced pneumonitis. *Rheumatology.* 2008;47(11):1647–1650.

102. Gavaghan TE, McNaught PJ, Ralston M, Hayes JM. Penicillamine-induced "Goodpasture's syndrome": successful treatment of a fulminant case. *Aust N Z J Med.* 1981;11(3): 261–265.

103. Gibson T, Burry HC, Ogg C. Letter: Goodpasture syndrome and D-penicillamine. *Ann Intern Med.* 1976;84(1):100.

104. Sternlieb I, Bennett B, Scheinberg IH. D-penicillamine induced Goodpasture's syndrome in Wilson's disease. *Ann Intern Med.* 1975;82(5):673–676.

105. Sinha A, Silverstone EJ, O'Sullivan MM. Gold-induced pneumonitis: computed tomography findings in a patient with rheumatoid arthritis. *Rheumatology (Oxford).* 2001;40(6):712–714.

106. Agarwal R, Sharma SK, Malaviya AN. Gold-induced hypersensitivity pneumonitis in a patient with rheumatoid arthritis. *Clin Exp Rheumatol.* 1989;7(1):89–90.

107. Breton JL, Garnier G, Toulouse J, Depierre A. Bronchoalveolar lavage and gold salt-induced pneumonitis. *Chest.* 1985;87(3):410.

108. Foster RA, Zander DS, Mergo PJ, Valentine JF. Mesalamine-related lung disease: clinical, radiographic, and pathologic manifestations. *Inflamm Bowel Dis.* 2003;9(5):308–315.

109. Parry SD, Barbatzas C, Peel ET, Barton JR. Sulphasalazine and lung toxicity. *Eur Respir J.* 2002;19(4):756–764.

110. Camus P, Colby TV. The lung in inflammatory bowel disease. *Eur Respir J.* 2000;15(1):5–10.

111. Ulubas B, Sahin G, Ozer C, Aydin O, Ozgur E, Apaydin D. Bronchiolitis obliterans organizing pneumonia associated with sulfasalazine in a patient with rheumatoid arthritis. *Clin Rheumatol.* 2004;23(3):249–251.

112. Haralambou G, Teirstein AS, Gil J, Present DH. Bronchiolitis obliterans in a patient with ulcerative colitis receiving mesalamine. *Mt Sinai J Med.* 2001;68(6):384–388.

113. Kim JH, Lee JH, Koh ES, et al. Acute eosinophilic pneumonia related to a mesalazine suppository. *Asia Pac Allergy.* 2013;3(2):136–139.

114. Hadjinicolaou AV, Nisar MK, Parfrey H, Chilvers ER, Ostor AJ. Non-infectious pulmonary toxicity of rituximab: a systematic review. *Rheumatology.* 2012;51(4):653–662.

115. Liote H, Liote F, Seroussi B, Mayaud C, Cadranel J. Rituximab-induced lung disease: A systematic literature review. *Eur Respir J.* 2010;35(3):681–687.

116. O'Connor MB, Abdullah MF, O'Donovan N, Phelan MJ. Rituximab-induced pulmonary disease. *Rheumatol Int.* 2012;32(9):2955–2956.

117. Subramanian M, Manjunath R, Kilara N, Mohan Rao KN. Rituximab-induced subacute interstitial pneumonitis: a case report and review of literature. *J Cancer Res Ther.* 2010;6(3):344–346.

118. Shen T, Braude S. Obliterative bronchiolitis after rituximab administration: a new manifestation of rituximab-associated pulmonary toxicity. *Intern Med J.* 2012;42(5):597–599.

119. Koike T, Harigai M, Inokuma S, et al. Postmarketing surveillance of the safety and effectiveness of etanercept in Japan. *J Rheumatol.* 2009;36(5):898–906.

120. Takeuchi T, Tatsuki Y, Nogami Y, et al. Postmarketing surveillance of the safety profile of infliximab in 5000 Japanese patients with rheumatoid arthritis. *Ann Rheum Dis.* 2008;67(2):189–194.

121. Ramos-Casals M, Brito-Zeron P, Munoz S, et al. Autoimmune diseases induced by TNF-targeted therapies: analysis of 233 cases. *Medicine (Baltimore).* 2007;86(4):242–251.

122. Ramos-Casals M, Perez-Alvarez R, Perez-de-Lis M, Xaubet A, Bosch X, Group BS. Pulmonary disorders induced by monoclonal antibodies in patients with rheumatologic autoimmune diseases. *Am J Med.* 2011;124(5):386–394.

123. Daien CI, Monnier A, Claudepierre P, et al. Sarcoid-like granulomatosis in patients treated with tumor necrosis factor blockers: 10 cases. *Rheumatology (Oxford).* 2009;48(8):883–886.

124. Abunasser J, Forouhar FA, Metersky ML. Etanercept-induced lupus erythematosus presenting as a unilateral pleural effusion. *Chest.* 2008;134(4):850–853.

125. Benucci M, Li Gobbi F, Fossi F, Manfredi M, Del Rosso A. Drug-induced lupus after treatment with infliximab in rheumatoid arthritis. *J Clin Rheumatol.* 2005;11(1):47–49.

126. Kohli R, Namek K. Adalimumab (Humira) induced acute lung injury. *Am J Case Rep.* 2013;14:173–175.

127. Yamazaki H, Isogai S, Sakurai T, Nagasaka K. A case of adalimumab-associated interstitial pneumonia with rheumatoid arthritis. *Mod Rheumatol.* 2010;20(5):518–521.

128. Huggett MT, Armstrong R. Adalimumab-associated pulmonary fibrosis. *Rheumatology (Oxford).* 2006;45(10):1312–1313.

129. Dascalu C, Mrejen-Shakin K, Bandagi S. Adalimumab-induced acute pneumonitis in a patient with rheumatoid arthritis. *J Clin Rheumatol.* 2010;16(4):172–174.

130. Champion L, Stern M, Israel-Biet D, et al. Brief communication: sirolimus-associated pneumonitis: 24 cases in renal transplant recipients. *Ann Intern Med.* 2006;144(7):505–509.

131. Avitzur Y, Jimenez-Rivera C, Fecteau A, Jones N, Ngan BY, Ng VL. Interstitial granulomatous pneumonitis associated with sirolimus in a child after liver transplantation. *J Pediatr Gastroenterol Nutr.* 2003;37(1):91–94.

132. Howard L, Gopalan D, Griffiths M, Mahadeva R. Sirolimus-induced pulmonary hypersensitivity associated with a CD4 T-cell infiltrate. *Chest.* 2006;129(6):1718–1721.

133. Patel AV, Hahn T, Bogner PN, et al. Fatal diffuse alveolar hemorrhage associated with sirolimus after allogeneic hematopoietic cell transplantation. *Bone Marrow Transplant.* 2010;45(8):1363–1364.

134. Khalife WI, Kogoj P, Kar B. Sirolimus-induced alveolar hemorrhage. *J Heart Lung Transplant.* 2007;26(6):652–657.

135. White DA, Camus P, Endo M, et al. Noninfectious pneumonitis after everolimus therapy for advanced renal cell carcinoma. *Am J Respir Crit Care Med.* 2010;182(3):396–403.

136. Depuydt P, Nollet J, Benoit D, Praet M, Caes F. Fatal acute pulmonary injury associated with everolimus. *Ann Pharmacother.* 2012;46(3):e7.

137. Sakata KK, Larsen BT, Boland JM, et al. Nitrofurantoin-induced granulomatous interstitial pneumonia. *Int J Surg Pathol.* 2013;22(4):352–357.

138. Mendez JL, Nadrous HF, Hartman TE, Ryu JH. Chronic nitrofurantoin-induced lung disease. *Mayo Clin Proc.* 2005;80(10):1298–1302.

139. Kumar KS, Russo MW, Borczuk AC, et al. Significant pulmonary toxicity associated with interferon and ribavirin therapy for hepatitis C. *Am J Gastroenterol.* 2002;97(9):2432–2440.

140. Celik G, Sen E, Ulger AF, et al. Sarcoidosis caused by interferon therapy. *Respirology.* 2005;10(4):535–540.

141. Marzouk K, Saleh S, Kannass M, Sharma OP. Interferon-induced granulomatous lung disease. *Curr Opin Pulm Med.* 2004;10(5):435–440.

142. Wolff AJ, O'Donnell AE. Pulmonary effects of illicit drug use. *Clin Chest Med.* 2004;25(1):203–216.

143. Duberstein JL, Kaufman DM. A clinical study of an epidemic of heroin intoxication and heroin-induced pulmonary edema. *Am J Med.* 1971;51(6):704–714.

144. Sporer KA, Dorn E. Heroin-related noncardiogenic pulmonary edema : a case series. *Chest.* 2001;120(5):1628–1632.

145. Katz S, Aberman A, Frand UI, Stein IM, Fulop M. Heroin pulmonary edema. Evidence for increased pulmonary capillary permeability. *Am Rev Respir Dis.* 1972;106(3):472–474.

146. Byers JM 3rd, Soin JS, Fisher RS, Hutchins GM. Acute pulmonary alveolitis in narcotics abuse. *Arch Pathol.* 1975;99(5):273–277.

147. Murray RJ, Albin RJ, Mergner W, Criner GJ. Diffuse alveolar hemorrhage temporally related to cocaine smoking. *Chest.* 1988;93(2):427–429.

PART 7

Other Infiltrative and Airspace Disorders

CHAPTER 67

The Lungs in Patients with Inborn Errors of Metabolism

Timothy Craig Allen

INTRODUCTION

Inborn errors of metabolism, also termed "inherited metabolic disorders," are a group of inherited systemic conditions involving various types of chemical imbalances that cause disease and affect essentially all organs to a greater or lesser degree.[1-9] Each of the diseases is characterized by a specific genetic defect that causes an abnormality of an enzyme necessary for the degradation of some chemical substance.[2] The disruption of degradation leads to disease due to the deficiency of a substance or to the pathologic accumulation of a substance.[2,5] The first inborn errors of metabolism were identified about a century ago. Sir Archibald Garrod coined the phrase in 1902.[10] Today, there are over 500 inborn errors of metabolism identified.[11]

The diseases that comprise the inborn errors of metabolism are individually rare; however, taken together, they affect about 1 in 1000 people.[2] The majority of the diseases making up the inborn errors of metabolism exhibit autosomal recessive inheritance; however, X-linked recessive inheritance occurs with some diseases, and, less commonly, autosomal dominant inheritance is seen.[5] The majority of these diseases are pediatric; however, with the identification of attenuated variants, and with improved survival, they are today's conditions that must be considered in patients of all ages.[2] Tissue biopsy may be necessary for specific diagnosis; however, given that these disorders typically present with unexpected findings, high clinical suspicion and careful radiologic evaluation are usually the key to faster and more accurate diagnoses. Particularly as newer and more effective therapies being designed require earlier diagnoses, radiology plays a central role in diagnosis, and clinical–radiologic correlations are increasingly important.[2] Although metabolic specialists with expertise in the various inborn errors of metabolism are present in large academic centers and tertiary care centers, pediatricians and primary care physicians are typically the first physicians to whom patients with these diseases present themselves.[5]

Some of the diseases that make up the inborn errors of metabolism can be placed into a few broad groups; these include disorders of amino acid metabolism, organic acidurias, urea cycle defects, disorders of ketogenesis and ketolysis, disorders of fatty acid oxidation, lysosomal storage disorders, and mitochondrial disease.[2] While the lung is not typically a primary site of clinical disease in patients with inborn errors of metabolism, the lungs are involved with many inborn errors of metabolism, and in some diseases, clinically significant lung disease may occur.[1,12] Of course, the lungs may be involved with infections as a secondary feature in many types of chronic diseases, including inborn errors of metabolism; however, this chapter focuses on several specific inborn errors of metabolism for which lung disease may be a clinically significant feature.

ACID SPHINGOMYELINASE DEFICIENCY (NIEMANN–PICK DISEASE TYPES A AND B)

Acid sphingomyelinase (ASM) deficiency, an autosomal recessive condition, has a phenotype that occurs in a continuum, with severe, neuropathic disease with early symptoms and resulting in death in infancy or early childhood designated as Niemann–Pick disease type A (NPA), and nonneuropathic disease with generally later onset and milder symptoms designated as Niemann–Pick disease type B (NPB).[13-17] Patients with NPA typically show hepatosplenomegaly by about 3 months of age. The hepatosplenomegaly may ultimately become massive, and children are often dead within 3 years. Psychomotor development in patients with NPA typically is limited to not more than the 12-month level, after which deterioration occurs. NPB patients generally show milder hepatosplenomegaly and may survive to adulthood; however, progressive and clinically significant pulmonary changes are frequent in these patients.[14,18,19] Diagnosis is made by showing less than 10% normal residual ASM activity in peripheral blood lymphocytes or cultured skin fibroblasts.

Patients with NPA often exhibit radiographic changes of interstitial lung disease due to sphingomyelin storage within pulmonary macrophages, and they may exhibit low arterial blood oxygen levels. Respiratory infections are common, and not infrequently culminate in respiratory failure and death.[13,20,21] Patients with NPB, who have generally milder disease, may develop pulmonary complications at any age.[21,22] Most patients with NPB exhibit radiographic changes of interstitial lung disease, even while their individual symptoms may vary dramatically; their radiographic changes often do not correlate with the severity of pulmonary function abnormalities.[14,18] Cystic lung disease has also been reported in association with NPB.[23] Whole lung lavage has been attempted for symptomatic treatment of patients with NPB.[24]

Radiographically, patients show nodular infiltrates and linear strands, with a predominantly basilar honeycomb pattern.[19,25] Histologically, the lungs demonstrate predominantly normal architecture, with airspaces filled with Niemann–Pick cells—enlarged histiocytes with finely vacuolated cytoplasm (Figs. 67-1 and 67-2).[26] If necessary, CD68 immunostain may be used to establish their presence. These collections of cells have been termed "sea blue histiocytosis," due to the vivid blue staining with May–Grunwald Giemsa stain. Pulmonary fibrosis may occur over time (Fig. 67-3).

NIEMANN–PICK DISEASE TYPE C

Niemann–Pick disease type C (NPC) is a rare, autosomal recessive inborn error of metabolism characterized by impaired intracellular lipid trafficking and accumulation of cholesterol and glycosphingolipids in the brain and other tissues.[27-34] It is diagnosed by

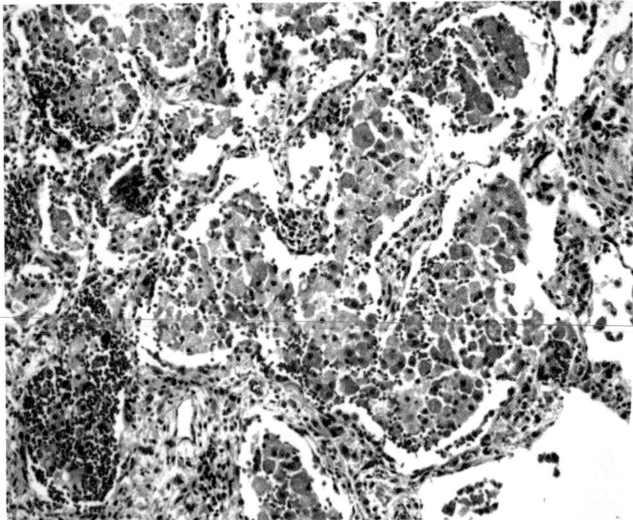

Figure 67-1 Low power image of lung in Niemann–Pick disease showing collections of foam cells within alveoli.

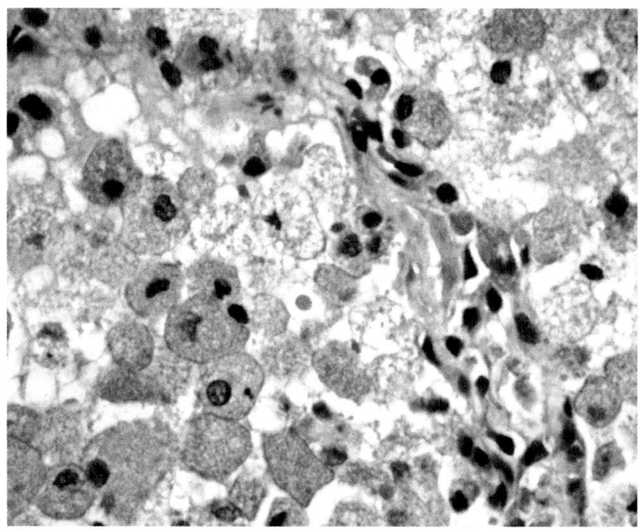

Figure 67-2 High power image of lung in Niemann–Pick disease showing enlarged histiocytes with finely vacuolated cytoplasm within the alveolar spaces.

biochemical tests that show impaired cholesterol esterification and positive filipin staining in cultured fibroblasts. Patients typically have saccadic eye movement abnormalities or vertical supranuclear gaze palsy; cerebellar signs, such as ataxia, dystonia/dysmetria, dysarthria, and dysphagia; gelastic cataplexy; and epileptic seizures[27,33] are given symptomatic treatment for cataplexy, dystonia, and seizures, as well as physical therapy to maintain as much independent mobility as possible. Approximately 95% of NPC cases are due to mutations of the NPC1 gene, with the remainder due to mutations of the NPC2 gene.[27]

NPC may produce symptoms in patients of any age; and initial presentation may occur from neonatal to adult periods. Infants often have nonspecific symptoms that make exact diagnosis difficult. Along with liver disease, infants may present with often-fatal pulmonary failure due to impaired gas exchange due to lung infiltration with foam cells. Patients presenting in childhood or adolescence, or as adults, typically do not have pronounced pulmonary involvement.[30–32,35] Pulmonary alveolar proteinosis may occur in patients with NPC2 disease; possibly due to loss of normal NPC2 protein expression in alveolar macrophages

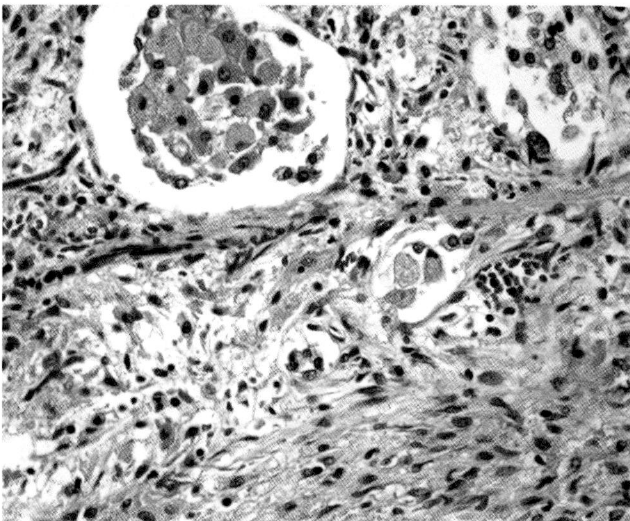

Figure 67-3 High power image of lung in long-standing Niemann–Pick disease showing developing pulmonary fibrosis.

and accumulation of functionally inactive cholesterol-rich surfactant.[33,34,36] Bronchoalveolar lavage has been reported to improve pulmonary symptoms in children with foam cell infiltrates.[37] Histologic features are similar to those seen in patients with NPA and NPB.

GAUCHER DISEASE

Gaucher disease (GD), an autosomal recessive disease, is due to inadequate lysosomal enzyme glucosylceramidase activity, with the resulting accumulation of glucosylceramide, the enzyme's undegraded substrate, as well as other glycolipids.[12,15,38–40] The substrate arises primarily from the breakdown of red blood cells and other tissue cells. The undegraded substrate is then taken up by monocytes and macrophages. Central nervous system involvement with GD may be caused by membrane ganglioside turnover; however, neuron death may also play a role.[41]

GD encompasses three main clinical subtypes, as well as two additional subtypes, each with characteristic features. Type 1, 2, and 3 GD frequently show lung involvement. Type 1 GD is characterized clinically by bone disease, including osteonecrosis, lytic and sclerotic lesions, and osteopenia; anemia; thrombocytopenia; and hepatosplenomegaly; however, affected patients do not typically show central nervous system involvement. Type 2 and type 3 GD are both characterized by central nervous system involvement with disease; however, type 2 GD patients typically present with disease before age 2, exhibit poor psychomotor development, and rapidly deteriorate, with death occurring usually between ages 2 and 4. Patients with Type 3 GD, in contrast, typically present before age 2, but progress slowly, with some patients surviving to adulthood. There are also two additional subtypes, for which lung involvement is not characteristic. Cardiovascular GD shows mitral value and aortic valve calcification, corneal opacities, and supranuclear opthalmoplegia. Perinatal lethal GD shows nonimmune hydrops fetalis or skin abnormalities.

GD may be caused by mutations in Saposin C and acid-β-glucosidase.[42] Diagnosis of GD requires the demonstration of inadequate glucosylceramidase activity in peripheral blood leukocytes or other cells. Treatments include enzyme replacement therapy or substrate reduction therapy.[43–46]

Pulmonary involvement in patients with GD includes pulmonary hypertension, lobar consolidation, and interstitial lung disease.[1,12,15,38,47,48] Pulmonary hypertension is a typical finding in GD patients with hepatic disease, perhaps because of the patients' inability to detoxify gut-derived factors that affect pulmonary endothelium, with resultant pulmonary hypertension. Pulmonary hypertension may also occur in patients with GD without liver disease.[47] Some patients with type 1 GD without pulmonary disease may, nonetheless, exhibit rapid fatigability, possibly due to GD-caused circulatory impairment.[12,48,49]

Histologically, GD cells infiltrate liver, spleen, and bone marrow. Lung involvement is common in pediatric patients and less common in adults.[50] Lung involvement may be clinically significant in as many as one-third of patients.[51] GD cells most often involve septal capillaries; this is thought to be the cause of GD-associated pulmonary hypertension.[51] Infants and children may also demonstrate intra-alveolar involvement. GD cells have also been found to cause substantial septal thickening and patchy involvement in a lymphatic distribution.[51] The characteristic Gaucher cell has a "wrinkled paper" appearance (Fig. 67-4), highlighted with Periodic acid-Schiff (PAS) staining. Gaucher cells are CD68 negative, in contrast to alveolar macrophages, which show CD68 positivity.[52]

FABRY DISEASE

Fabry disease (FD) is an X-linked lysosomal storage disease caused by a deficiency of α-galactosidase A enzyme activity, resulting in globotriaosylceramide accumulation in a variety of tissues, including cardiomyocytes, smooth muscle cells, and endothelial cells.[53–55]

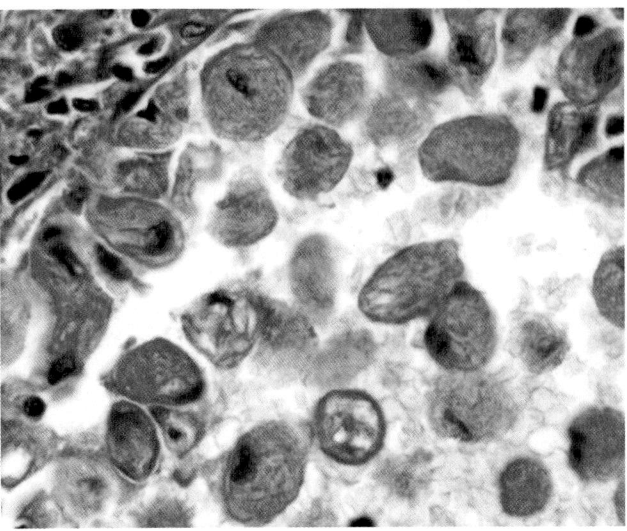

Figure 67-4 High power image of Gaucher cells within an alveolar space showing its characteristic "wrinkled paper" appearance.

Males with less than 1% enzyme activity develop the classic form of FD, which typically present in childhood or adolescence and is characterized by proteinuria, corneal and lenticular opacities, angiokeratomas, hypohidrosis, and periodic episodes of markedly painful extremities. By the third to fifth decades, gradually worsening renal function usually leads to end-stage renal disease. If an adult with FD survive their renal disease, they typically succumb to cerebrovascular or cardiovascular disorders. If men exhibit greater than 1% enzyme activity, however, they typically exhibit a renal variant, with resultant end-stage renal disease, but without extremity pain or skin lesions. Alternatively, they may exhibit a cardiac variant, which typically presents in men in their 50s to 70s. Findings include proteinuria, mitral value insufficiency, cardiomyopathy, and left ventricular hypertrophy; end-stage renal disease is absent.

Female patients with FD, who are heterozygous for the disease, often exhibit later onset of findings and milder symptoms than males; however, their presentations may range from essentially asymptomatic throughout life to symptoms mimicking their male counterparts with classic FD.

Diagnosis in males is made by showing α-galactosidase A enzyme deficiency in leukocytes, cultured cells, or plasma. Enzyme measurement is not a reliable test for females; some carriers have decreased enzyme activity, but others show normal activity. Enzyme testing for a mutation in *GLA*, the gene associated with FD, is necessary for diagnosis in female carriers. Males essentially always show a *GLA* mutation. Enzyme replacement therapy is typically used in male patients and symptomatic female carriers.[49,53,54]

Pulmonary involvement may occur in both males and females with FD.[12,56–58] Patients typically exhibit dyspnea, wheezing, and findings of chronic bronchitis; pulmonary function tests may show obstruction.[59] Radiologic changes may be minimal and do not correlate with the severity of pulmonary dysfunction. Histologic diagnosis of FD typically involves identification of laminated inclusions in type II pneumocytes and capillary endothelium.[58] Lamellar inclusions have been reportedly identified cytologically in alveolar macrophages, ciliated epithelial cells, and goblet cells by examination of induced sputum, bronchial brushings, and bronchoalveolar lavage specimens.[58,60,61]

HERMANSKY–PUDLAK SYNDROME

Hermansky–Pudlak syndrome (HPS), also termed oculocutaneous albinism syndrome, is a rare autosomal recessive multisystem disease involving disorders of intercellular trafficking. HPS is characterized by tyrosinase-positive oculocutaneous albinism, a platelet storage pool deficiency that causes bleeding diatheses, and, in some cases, pulmonary fibrosis.[62–71] Patients with HPS exhibit congenital nystagmus, decreased visual acuity, iris transillumination, and variable skin and hair hypopigmentation.[72] Approximately 15% of patients may also develop granulomatous colitis.[63–65,73] HPS is diagnosed based on clinical characteristics and ultrastructural absence of platelet-dense bodies.[74] Patients often exhibit easy bruising and prolonged bleeding.

HPS, including its subtypes, has been shown to be caused by mutations in several genes. These include *HPS1*, causing HPS-1; *AP3B1*, causing HPS-2, *HPS3*, causing HPS-3; *HPS4*, causing HPS-4; *HPS5*, causing HPS-5; *HPS6*, causing HPS-6; *DTNBP1*, causing HPS-7; *BLOC1 S3*, causing HPS-8; and *BLOC1 S*, causing HPS-9.[65,66,75]

Pulmonary involvement in patients with HPS generally presents clinically and radiologically as pulmonary fibrosis. Patients generally become symptomatic by the fourth decade; lung disease is progressive and restrictive in nature. Death may ensue within a few years following onset of pulmonary symptoms.[76] Pulmonary fibrosis is typically found in HPS1, HPS2, and HPS4; it is particularly prevalent in patients with HPS1 from Puerto Rico.[64,72,77–83] Pulmonary fibrosis is not characteristic of HPS3, HPS5, or HPS6. Lung transplantation may be appropriate for some patients with HPS.[84]

The basis for the pulmonary fibrosis is unknown; however, a postinflammatory response has been hypothesized as the causative factor.[85] Pirfenidone treatment has been attempted in patients with HPS with pulmonary function greater than 50% of normal, with some benefit.[77] Histologically, the pulmonary fibrosis may show a pattern of usual interstitial pneumonia or nonspecific interstitial pneumonia.[72,86] Ceroid–filled macrophages fill airspaces and the lung interstitium (Figs. 67-5–67-7) and may be identified with bronchoalveolar lavage.[86]

CHOLESTERYL ESTER STORAGE DISEASE

Cholesteryl ester storage disease (CESD), a rare autosomal recessive disease, is characterized by lysosomal acid lipase/cholesteryl ester hydrolase deficiency.[87] Most patients with CESD have some enzyme activity; individuals with complete enzyme deficiency are diagnosed as having Wolman disease.[88] In patients with CESD, there is deposition of cholesteryl ester generally in the liver, bone marrow, bowel, and spleen. Gastrointestinal bleeding, often occult, and hepatomegaly are frequently identified.[89] Patients usually survive well into adulthood, ultimately dying from chronic hepatic failure or premature atherosclerosis.[87]

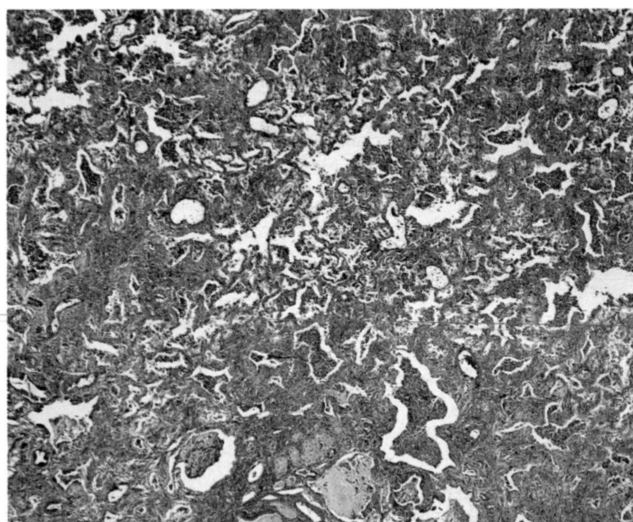

Figure 67-5 Lower power image of lung in Hermansky–Pudlak syndrome showing a nonspecific interstitial pneumonia-like pattern.

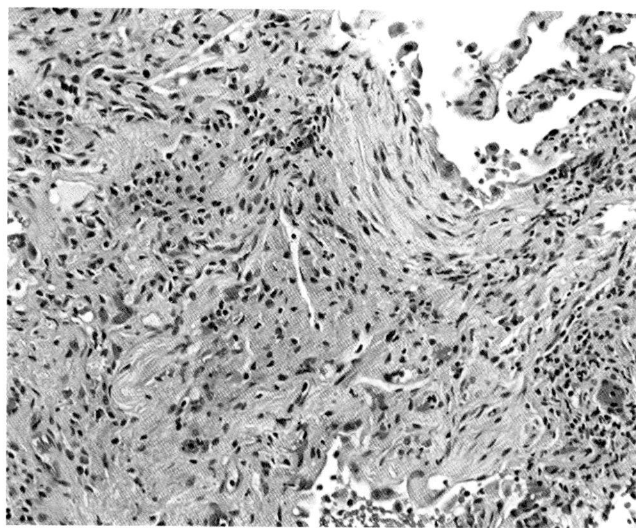

Figure 67-6 Medium power image of lung in Hermansky–Pudlak syndrome showing a usual interstitial pneumonia-like pattern.

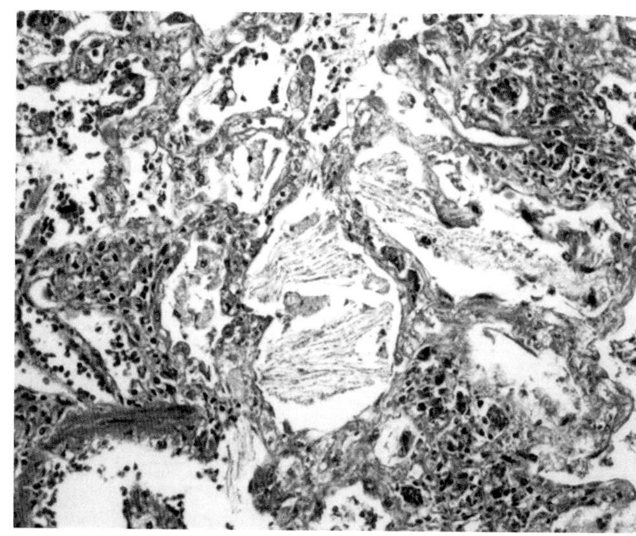

Figure 67-8 Medium power image of lung in cholesteryl ester storage disease showing cholesteryl ester accumulation within alveolar macrophages, and interstitial fibroblasts.

Pulmonary involvement in CESD is uncommon; however, it may occur due to accumulation of cholesteryl esters within alveolar macrophages and interstitial fibroblasts (Figs. 67-8 and 67-9). Pulmonary arteries may also develop from cell deposits within the intima, which may be complicated by associated reactive fibrosis.[90,91] Treatment of pulmonary involvement in patients with CESD is supportive; however, for most patients, pulmonary involvement is not life-threatening.[90]

MUCOPOLYSACCHARIDOSIS TYPE I

Mucopolysaccharidosis Type I (MPS1), an autosomal recessive disease, is a progressive multisystem disease due to a lysosomal storage disorder caused by deficiency of the enzyme α-L-iduronidase.[92,93] Patients with MPS1 show varying levels of severity. The diagnoses of Hurler syndrome, Hurler–Scheie syndrome, and Scheie syndrome have shown generally overlapping clinical features and no biochemical differences; therefore, currently, patients are clinically diagnosed as having either Severe MPS1 (formerly Hurler syndrome) or Attenuated MPS1 (formerly Hurler–Scheie syndrome and Scheie syndrome). The diagnosis of MPS1 is based on demonstration of insufficient α-L-iduronidase activity in plasma, in cultured fibroblasts, or peripheral blood leukocytes. Treatment may include enzyme replacement therapy and bone marrow transplantation.[92–95] Attenuated MPS1 patients may show pulmonary disease, including changes in forced vital capacity, and respiratory complications are often the cause of death.[96]

MUCOPOLYSACCHARIDOSIS TYPE II

Muopolysaccharidosis type II (MPSII), also termed Hunter syndrome, is inherited as an X-linked recessive disease. MPSII is a multisystem disease characterized by the pathologic lysosomal storage of glycosaminoglycans.[97–99] Most patients are males, with carrier females showing clinical features only rarely. Patients with MPSII typically show central nervous system involvement, predominantly a progressive deterioration of cognitive functions. Patients generally have macrocephaly, with or without communicating hydrocephalus, hoarseness, hearing loss, macroglossia, splenomegaly, hepatomegaly, short stature, dysostosis multiplex, and joint contractures.[98,99] Patients may also exhibit cardiac findings and progressive airway disease in severe cases. Patients frequently do not survive their second decade.

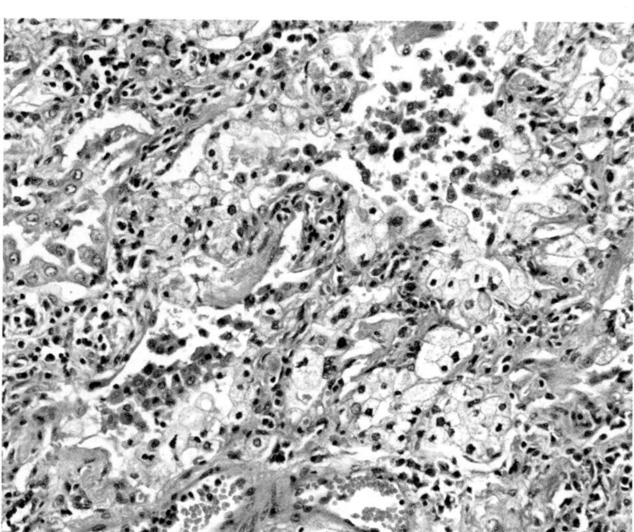

Figure 67-7 High power image of lung in Hermansky–Pudlak syndrome showing ceroid-filled histiocytes within alveolar spaces.

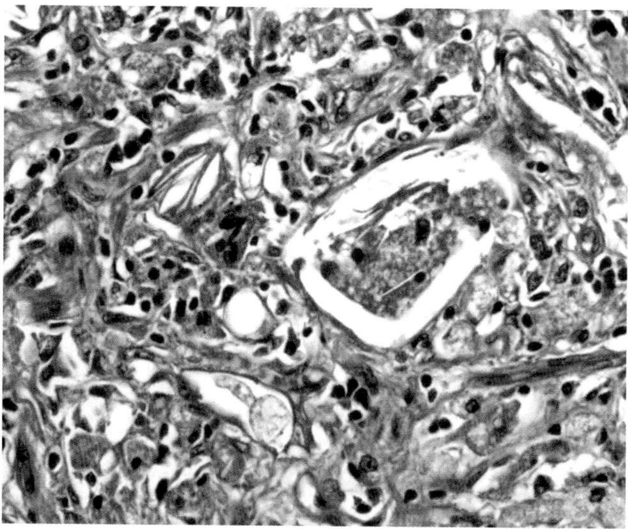

Figure 67-9 High power image of lung in cholesteryl ester storage disease showing alveolar macrophages containing cholesteryl esters.

Clinical manifestations and progression may vary significantly; severity should be considered to be on a continuum. Some patients with milder forms of disease show normal intelligence into early adulthood and survive into the sixth decade.[97,98]

To confirm clinical suspicion, testing for deficient iduronate sulfatase enzyme activity in plasma, fibroblasts, or white blood cells may be performed. Diagnosis may be confirmed by molecular testing of *IDS*, the gene associated with MPSII. Until recently, treatment has been supportive only.[97] Bone marrow transplantation has been attempted, but has not been successful.[100] Treatment with enzyme replacement therapy is currently being studied in patients with MPSII.[98,101–104]

Patients with MPSII often show frequent upper respiratory infections as an early feature of disease. Progressive airway narrowing due to accumulation of glycosaminoglycans in the tongue, upper airway, and trachea usually cause symptomatic airway obstruction.[97,99] Ultimately, progressive airway obstruction with associated sleep apnea requires tracheostomy. Along with airway obstruction, hepatomegaly and splenomegaly, thick pulmonary secretions, and chest wall stiffness.[98]

REFERENCES

1. Pletcher BA, Turcios NL. Pulmonary complications of genetic disorders. *Paediatr Respir Rev.* 2012;13(1):2–9.
2. Hendriksz CJ. Inborn errors of metabolism for the diagnostic radiologist. *Pediatr Radiol.* 2009;39(3):211–220.
3. Raghuveer TS, Garg U, Graf WD. Inborn errors of metabolism in infancy and early childhood: an update. *Am Fam Physician.* 2006;73(11):1981–1990.
4. Chung MJ, Lee KS, Franquet T, Muller NL, Han J, Kwon OJ. Metabolic lung disease: imaging and histopathologic findings. *Eur J Radiol.* 2005;54(2):233–245.
5. Kamboj M. Clinical approach to the diagnoses of inborn errors of metabolism. *Pediatr Clin North Am.* 2008;55(5):1113–1127, viii.
6. Cakir B, Teksam M, Kosehan D, Akin K, Koktener A. Inborn errors of metabolism presenting in childhood. *J Neuroimaging.* 2011;21(2):e117–e133.
7. Prust MJ, Gropman AL, Hauser N. New frontiers in neuroimaging applications to inborn errors of metabolism. *Mol Genet Metab.* 2011;104(3):195–205.
8. Ellaway CJ, Wilcken B, Christodoulou J. Clinical approach to inborn errors of metabolism presenting in the newborn period. *J Paediatr Child Health.* 2002;38(5):511–517.
9. Lanpher B, Brunetti-Pierri N, Lee B. Inborn errors of metabolism: the flux from Mendelian to complex diseases. *Nat Rev Genet.* 2006;7(6):449–460.
10. Garrod AE. The incidence of alkaptonuria: a study in chemical individuality. 1902 [classical article]. *Yale J Biol Med.* 2002; 75(4):221–231.
11. Saudubray JM, Chappentier C. Clinical phenotypes: diagnosis/algorithms. In: Scriver CR, Beaudet AL, Sly WS, et al., eds. *Metabolic and Molecular Bases of Inherited Disease.* 8th ed. New York, NY: McGraw Hill; 2001:1327–1403.
12. Dinwiddie R, Sonnappa S. Systemic diseases and the lung. *Paediatr Respir Rev.* 2005;6(3):181–189.
13. Guillemot N, Troadec C, de Villemeur TB, Clement A, Fauroux B. Lung disease in Niemann-Pick disease. *Pediatr Pulmonol.* 2007;42(12):1207–1214.
14. Iaselli F, Rea G, Cappabianca S, et al. Adult-onset pulmonary involvement in Niemann-Pick disease type B. *Monaldi Arch Chest Dis.* 2011;75(4):235–240.
15. Gulhan B, Ozcelik U, Gurakan F, et al. Different features of lung involvement in Niemann-Pick disease and Gaucher disease. *Respir Med.* 2012;106(9):1278–1285.
16. Schuchman EH. The pathogenesis and treatment of acid sphingomyelinase-deficient Niemann-Pick disease. *Int J Clin Pharmacol Ther.* 2009;47(Suppl 1):S48–S57.
17. Schuchman EH. Acid sphingomyelinase, cell membranes and human disease: lessons from Niemann-Pick disease. *FEBS Lett.* 2010;584(9):1895–1900.
18. Castanon Martinez R, Fernandez-Velilla Pena M, Gonzalez Montano MV, Gomez Carrera L, Torres Sanchez MI. Lung affectation in an adult patient with Niemann-Pick disease, type B. *Arch Bronconeumol.* 2012;48(6):213–215.
19. Ferretti GR, Lantuejoul S, Brambilla E, Coulomb M. Case report. Pulmonary involvement in Niemann-Pick disease subtype B: CT findings. *J Comput Assist Tomogr.* 1996;20(6): 990–992.
20. Mendelson DS, Wasserstein MP, Desnick RJ, et al. Type B Niemann-Pick disease: findings at chest radiography, thin-section CT, and pulmonary function testing. *Radiology.* 2006;238(1):339–345.
21. Uyan ZS, Karadag B, Ersu R, et al. Early pulmonary involvement in Niemann-Pick type B disease: lung lavage is not useful. *Pediatr Pulmonol.* 2005;40(2):169–172.
22. Alymlahi E, Dafiri R. Pulmonary involvement in Niemann-Pick type B disease. *J Postgrad Med.* 2004;50(4):289–290.
23. Baldi BG, Santana AN, Takagaki TY, Fujita C, Kairalla RA, Carvalho CR. Lung cyst: an unusual manifestation of Niemann-Pick disease. *Respirology.* 2009;14(1):134–136.
24. Nicholson AG, Wells AU, Hooper J, Hansell DM, Kelleher A, Morgan C. Successful treatment of endogenous lipoid pneumonia due to Niemann-Pick Type B disease with whole-lung lavage. *Am J Respir Crit Care Med.* 2002;165(1):128–131.
25. Gonzalez-Reimers E, Sanchez-Perez MJ, Bonilla-Arjona A, et al. Case report. Pulmonary involvement in an adult male affected by type B Niemann-Pick disease. *Br J Radiol.* 2003;76(911):838–840.
26. Minai OA, Sullivan EJ, Stoller JK. Pulmonary involvement in Niemann-Pick disease: case report and literature review. *Respir Med.* 2000;94(12):1241–1251.
27. Patterson MC, Hendriksz CJ, Walterfang M, et al. Recommendations for the diagnosis and management of Niemann-Pick disease type C: an update. *Mol Genet Metab.* 2012;106(3):330–344.
28. Roszell BR, Tao JQ, Yu KJ, Huang S, Bates SR. Characterization of the Niemann-Pick C pathway in alveolar type II cells and lamellar bodies of the lung. *Am J Physiol Lung Cell Mol Physiol.* 2012;302(9):L919–L932.
29. Erickson RP. Current controversies in Niemann-Pick C1 disease: steroids or gangliosides; neurons or neurons and glia. *J Appl Genet.* 2013;54(2):215–224.]
30. Vanier MT. [Niemann-Pick C disease: history, current research topics, biological and molecular diagnosis]. *Arch Pediatr.* 2010;17 (Suppl 2):S41–S44.
31. Vanier MT. Niemann-Pick disease type C. *Orphanet J Rare Dis.* 2010;5:16.
32. Bi X, Liao G. Cholesterol in Niemann-Pick Type C disease. *Subcell Biochem.* 2010;51:319–335.
33. Tang Y, Li H, Liu JP. Niemann-Pick Disease Type C: from molecule to clinic. *Clin Exp Pharmacol Physiol.* 2010;37(1):132–140.

34. Karten B, Peake KB, Vance JE. Mechanisms and consequences of impaired lipid trafficking in Niemann-Pick type C1-deficient mammalian cells. *Biochim Biophys Acta.* 2009;1791(7):659–670.
35. Peake KB, Vance JE. Defective cholesterol trafficking in Niemann-Pick C-deficient cells. *FEBS Lett.* 2010;584(13):2731–2739.
36. Griese M, Brasch F, Aldana VR, et al. Respiratory disease in Niemann-Pick type C2 is caused by pulmonary alveolar proteinosis. *Clin Genet.* 2010;77(2):119–130.
37. Palmeri S, Tarugi P, Sicurelli F, et al. Lung involvement in Niemann-Pick disease type C1: improvement with bronchoalveolar lavage. *Neurol Sci.* 2005;26(3):171–173.
38. Rosenbloom BE, Weinreb NJ. Gaucher disease: a comprehensive review. *Crit Rev Oncog.* 2013;18(3):163–175.
39. Thomas AS, Mehta AB, Hughes DA. Diagnosing Gaucher disease: an on-going need for increased awareness amongst haematologists. *Blood Cells Mol Dis.* 2013;50(3):212–217.
40. Pastores GM. Neuropathic Gaucher disease. *Wien Med Wochenschr.* 2010;160(23–24):605–608.
41. de Fost M, Aerts JM, Hollak CE. Gaucher disease: from fundamental research to effective therapeutic interventions. *Neth J Med.* 2003;61(1):3–8.
42. Lieberman RL. A Guided Tour of the Structural Biology of Gaucher Disease: Acid-β-Glucosidase and Saposin C. *Enzyme Res.* 2011;2011:973231.
43. Zimran A, Elstein D. No justification for very high-dose enzyme therapy for patients with type III Gaucher disease. *J Inherit Metab Dis.* 2007;30(6):843–844.
44. Lukina E, Watman N, Arreguin EA, et al. Improvement in hematological, visceral, and skeletal manifestations of Gaucher disease type 1 with oral eliglustat tartrate (Genz-112638) treatment: 2-year results of a phase 2 study. *Blood.* 2010;116(20):4095–4098.
45. Lukina E, Watman N, Arreguin EA, et al. A phase 2 study of eliglustat tartrate (Genz-112638), an oral substrate reduction therapy for Gaucher disease type 1. *Blood.* 2010;116(6):893–899.
46. Hollak CE, Aerts JM, Belmatoug N, et al. Guidelines for the restart of imiglucerase in patients with Gaucher disease: recommendations from the European Working Group on Gaucher disease. *Blood Cells Mol Dis.* 2010;44(2):86–87.
47. Mistry PK, Sirrs S, Chan A, et al. Pulmonary hypertension in type 1 Gaucher's disease: genetic and epigenetic determinants of phenotype and response to therapy. *Mol Genet Metab.* 2002;77(1–2):91–98.
48. Miller A, Brown LK, Pastores GM, Desnick RJ. Pulmonary involvement in type 1 Gaucher disease: functional and exercise findings in patients with and without clinical interstitial lung disease. *Clin Genet.* 2003;63(5):368–376.
49. Ohashi T. Enzyme replacement therapy for lysosomal storage diseases. *Pediatr Endocrinol Rev.* 2012;10 Suppl 1:26–34.
50. Zimran A, Kay A, Gelbart T, et al. Gaucher disease. Clinical, laboratory, radiologic, and genetic features of 53 patients. *Medicine (Baltimore).* 1992;71(6):337–353.
51. Amir G, Ron N. Pulmonary pathology in Gaucher's disease. *Hum Pathol.* 1999;30(6):666–670.
52. Shamburek RD, Brewer HB Jr, Gochuico BR. Erdheim-Chester disease: a rare multisystem histiocytic disorder associated with interstitial lung disease. *Am J Med Sci.* 2001;321(1):66–75.
53. Mehta A, Beck M, Eyskens F, et al. Fabry disease: a review of current management strategies. *QJM.* 2010;103(9):641–659.
54. Koskenvuo JW, Kantola IM. Evaluating enzyme replacement therapy in fabry disease. *Arch Intern Med.* 2010;170(6):573–574; author reply 574.
55. Koskenvuo JW, Kantola IM, Nuutila P, et al. Cardiopulmonary involvement in Fabry's disease. *Acta Cardiol.* 2010;65(2):185–192.
56. Zarate YA, Hopkin RJ. Fabry's disease. *Lancet.* 2008;372(9647):1427–1435.
57. Kariman K, Singletary WV Jr, Sieker HO. Pulmonary involvement in Fabry's disease. *Am J Med.* 1978;64(5):911–912.
58. Brown LK, Miller A, Bhuptani A, et al. Pulmonary involvement in Fabry disease. *Am J Respir Crit Care Med.* 1997;155(3):1004–1010.
59. Magage S, Lubanda JC, Susa Z, et al. Natural history of the respiratory involvement in Anderson-Fabry disease. *J Inherit Metab Dis.* 2007;30(5):790–799.
60. Kelly MM, Leigh R, McKenzie R, Kamada D, Ramsdale EH, Hargreave FE. Induced sputum examination: diagnosis of pulmonary involvement in Fabry's disease. *Thorax.* 2000;55(8):720–721.
61. Rosenberg DM, Ferrans VJ, Fulmer JD, et al. Chronic airflow obstruction in Fabry's disease. *Am J Med.* 1980;68(6):898–905.
62. Mahavadi P, Guenther A, Gochuico BR. Hermansky-Pudlak syndrome interstitial pneumonia: it's the epithelium, stupid! *Am J Respir Crit Care Med.* 2012;186(10):939–940.
63. Ciledag A, Cirit Kocer B, Kokturk N, Kaya A, Celik G, Numanoglu N. A rare cause of interstitial lung disease: Hermansky-Pudlak syndrome. *Tuberk Toraks.* 2011;59(1):85–88.
64. Gochuico BR, Huizing M, Golas GA, et al. Interstitial lung disease and pulmonary fibrosis in Hermansky-Pudlak syndrome type 2, an adaptor protein-3 complex disease. *Mol Med.* 2012; 18:56–64.
65. Young LR, Gulleman PM, Bridges JP, et al. The alveolar epithelium determines susceptibility to lung fibrosis in Hermansky-Pudlak syndrome. *Am J Respir Crit Care Med.* 2012;186(10):1014–1024.
66. Wei AH, Li W. Hermansky-Pudlak syndrome: pigmentary and non-pigmentary defects and their pathogenesis. *Pigment Cell Melanoma Res.* 2013;26(2):176–192.
67. Hurford MT, Sebastiano C. Hermansky-pudlak syndrome: report of a case and review of the literature. *Int J Clin Exp Pathol.* 2008;1(6):550–554.
68. Nurden AT, Freson K, Seligsohn U. Inherited platelet disorders. *Haemophilia.* 2012;18(Suppl 4):154–160.
69. Carter BW. Hermansky-Pudlak syndrome complicated by pulmonary fibrosis. *Proc (Bayl Univ Med Cent).* 2012;25(1):76–77.
70. Walker M, Payne J, Wagner B, Vora A. Hermansky-Pudlak syndrome. *Br J Haematol.* 2007;138(6):671.
71. Huizing M, Anikster Y, Gahl WA. Hermansky-Pudlak syndrome and Chediak-Higashi syndrome: disorders of vesicle formation and trafficking. *Thromb Haemost.* 2001;86(1):233–245.
72. Brantly M, Avila NA, Shotelersuk V, Lucero C, Huizing M, Gahl WA. Pulmonary function and high-resolution CT findings in patients with an inherited form of pulmonary fibrosis, Hermansky-Pudlak syndrome, due to mutations in HPS-1. *Chest.* 2000;117(1):129–136.
73. O'Brien K, Troendle J, Gochuico BR, et al. Pirfenidone for the treatment of Hermansky-Pudlak syndrome pulmonary fibrosis. *Mol Genet Metab.* 2011;103(2):128–134.

74. Witkop CJ, Krumwiede M, Sedano H, White JG. Reliability of absent platelet dense bodies as a diagnostic criterion for Hermansky-Pudlak syndrome. *Am J Hematol.* 1987;26(4):305–311.

75. Thielen N, Huizing M, Krabbe JG, et al. Hermansky-Pudlak syndrome: the importance of molecular subtyping. *J Thromb Haemost.* 2010;8(7):1643–1645.

76. Harmon KR, Witkop CJ, White JG, et al. Pathogenesis of pulmonary fibrosis: platelet-derived growth factor precedes structural alterations in the Hermansky-Pudlak syndrome. *J Lab Clin Med.* 1994;123(4):617–627.

77. Gahl WA, Brantly M, Troendle J, et al. Effect of pirfenidone on the pulmonary fibrosis of Hermansky-Pudlak syndrome. *Mol Genet Metab.* 2002;76(3):234–242.

78. Hermos CR, Huizing M, Kaiser-Kupfer MI, Gahl WA. Hermansky-Pudlak syndrome type 1: gene organization, novel mutations, and clinical-molecular review of non-Puerto Rican cases. *Hum Mutat.* 2002;20(6):482.

79. Avila NA, Brantly M, Premkumar A, Huizing M, Dwyer A, Gahl WA. Hermansky-Pudlak syndrome: radiography and CT of the chest compared with pulmonary function tests and genetic studies. *AJR Am J Roentgenol.* 2002;179(4):887–892.

80. Anderson PD, Huizing M, Claassen DA, White J, Gahl WA. Hermansky-Pudlak syndrome type 4 (HPS-4): clinical and molecular characteristics. *Hum Genet.* 2003;113(1):10–17.

81. Bachli EB, Brack T, Eppler E, et al. Hermansky-Pudlak syndrome type 4 in a patient from Sri Lanka with pulmonary fibrosis. *Am J Med Genet A.* 2004;127 A(2):201–207.

82. Carmona-Rivera C, Golas G, Hess RA, et al. Clinical, molecular, and cellular features of non-Puerto Rican Hermansky-Pudlak syndrome patients of Hispanic descent. *J Invest Dermatol.* 2011;131(12):2394–2400.

83. Carmona-Rivera C, Hess RA, O'Brien K, et al. Novel mutations in the HPS1 gene among Puerto Rican patients. *Clin Genet.* 2011;79(6):561–567.

84. Lederer DJ, Kawut SM, Sonett JR, et al. Successful bilateral lung transplantation for pulmonary fibrosis associated with the Hermansky-Pudlak syndrome. *J Heart Lung Transplant.* 2005;24(10):1697–1699.

85. Nakatani Y, Nakamura N, Sano J, et al. Interstitial pneumonia in Hermansky-Pudlak syndrome: significance of florid foamy swelling/degeneration (giant lamellar body degeneration) of type-2 pneumocytes. *Virchows Arch.* 2000;437(3):304–313.

86. Reynolds SP, Davies BH, Gibbs AR. Diffuse pulmonary fibrosis and the Hermansky-Pudlak syndrome: clinical course and postmortem findings. *Thorax.* 1994;49(6):617–618.

87. Elleder M, Chlumska A, Ledvinova J, Poupetova H. Testis—a novel storage site in human cholesteryl ester storage disease. Autopsy report of an adult case with a long-standing subclinical course complicated by accelerated atherosclerosis and liver carcinoma. *Virchows Arch.* 2000;436(1):82–87.

88. Wolman M, Sterk VV, Gatt S, Frenkel M. Primary familial xanthomatosis with involvement and calcification of the adrenals. Report of two more cases in siblings of a previously described infant. *Pediatrics.* 1961;28:742–757.

89. Elleder M, Chlumska A, Hyanek J, et al. Subclinical course of cholesteryl ester storage disease in an adult with hypercholesterolemia, accelerated atherosclerosis, and liver cancer. *J Hepatol.* 2000;32(3):528–534.

90. Cagle PT, Ferry GD, Beaudet AL, Hawkins EP. Pulmonary hypertension in an 18-year-old girl with cholesteryl ester storage disease (CESD). *Am J Med Genet.* 1986;24(4):711–722.

91. Michels VV, Driscoll DJ, Ferry GD, Duff DF, Beaudet AL. Pulmonary vascular obstruction associated with cholesteryl ester storage disease. *J Pediatr.* 1979;94(4):621–623.

92. Miebach E. Enzyme replacement therapy in mucopolysaccharidosis type I. *Acta Paediatr Suppl.* 2005;94(447):58–60; discussion 57.

93. Wraith JE, Clarke LA, Beck M, et al. Enzyme replacement therapy for mucopolysaccharidosis I: a randomized, double-blinded, placebo-controlled, multinational study of recombinant human alpha-L-iduronidase (laronidase). *J Pediatr.* 2004;144(5):581–588.

94. Valayannopoulos V, de Blic J, Mahlaoui N, et al. Laronidase for cardiopulmonary disease in Hurler syndrome 12 years after bone marrow transplantation. *Pediatrics.* 2010;126(5):e1242–e1247.

95. Tolar J, Grewal SS, Bjoraker KJ, et al. Combination of enzyme replacement and hematopoietic stem cell transplantation as therapy for Hurler syndrome. *Bone Marrow Transplant.* 2008;41(6):531–535.

96. Murray JF. Pulmonary disability in the Hurler syndrome (lipochondrodystrophy): a study of two cases. *N Engl J Med.* 1959;261:378–382.

97. Wraith JE, Scarpa M, Beck M, et al. Mucopolysaccharidosis type II (Hunter syndrome): a clinical review and recommendations for treatment in the era of enzyme replacement therapy. *Eur J Pediatr.* 2008;167(3):267–277.

98. Beck M. Mucopolysaccharidosis Type II (Hunter Syndrome): clinical picture and treatment. *Curr Pharm Biotechnol.* 2011;12(6):861–866.

99. Sohn YB, Choi EW, Kim SJ, et al. Retrospective analysis of the clinical manifestations and survival of Korean patients with mucopolysaccharidosis type II: emphasis on the cardiovascular complication and mortality cases. *Am J Med Genet A.* 2012;158 A(1):90–96.

100. Vellodi A, Young E, Cooper A, Lidchi V, Winchester B, Wraith JE. Long-term follow-up following bone marrow transplantation for Hunter disease. *J Inherit Metab Dis.* 1999;22(5):638–648.

101. Burrow TA, Leslie ND. Review of the use of idursulfase in the treatment of mucopolysaccharidosis II. *Biologics.* 2008;2(2):311–320.

102. Glamuzina E, Fettes E, Bainbridge K, et al. Treatment of mucopolysaccharidosis type II (Hunter syndrome) with idursulfase: the relevance of clinical trial end points. *J Inherit Metab Dis.* 2011;34(3):749–754.

103. Hoffmann B, Schulze-Frenking G, Al-Sawaf S, Beck M, Mayatepek E. Hunter disease before and during enzyme replacement therapy. *Pediatr Neurol.* Sep 2011;45(3):181–184.

104. da Silva EM, Strufaldi MW, Andriolo RB, Silva LA. Enzyme replacement therapy with idursulfase for mucopolysaccharidosis type II (Hunter syndrome). *Cochrane Database Syst Rev.* 2011;(11):CD008185.

CHAPTER 68

Alveolar Hemorrhage Syndromes

Joseph P. Lynch
Michael C. Fishbein
Tisha Wang

Diffuse alveolar hemorrhage (DAH) is a potentially catastrophic complication of myriad immune and nonimmune disorders.[1–3] Clinical features are broad, but hemoptysis, infiltrates on chest radiographs, hypoxemia, and progressive respiratory insufficiency are common to diverse etiologies.[2] Nonimmune causes of alveolar hemorrhage include endobronchial tumors, arteriovenous malformations or aneurysms, ulcerative tracheobronchitis, hemorrhagic pneumonia, bronchiectasis, congestive heart failure, uremia, thrombocytopenia or coagulopathy, pulmonary venoocclusive disease, infections, and massive pulmonary embolism.[4,5] These nonimmune causes need to be excluded in patients with severe alveolar hemorrhage. Depending upon the clinical scenario, coagulation profiles and ancillary tests (e.g., echocardiogram, chest computed tomographic [CT] pulmonary angiography, fiberoptic bronchoscopy) may be required to establish a specific diagnosis. In addition, other causes of diffuse parenchymal infiltrates (but without severe alveolar hemorrhage) share features in common with DAH syndromes (e.g., cryptogenic organizing pneumonia, hypersensitivity pneumonia, pulmonary alveolar proteinosis, and diverse interstitial or alveolar lung disorders). A discussion of these disorders is beyond the scope of this chapter, which focuses primarily on immune-mediated causes of DAH.

AUTOIMMUNE CAUSES OF ALVEOLAR HEMORRHAGE: DIFFERENTIAL DIAGNOSIS

Autoimmune DAH results from diffuse injury to the pulmonary microvasculature (termed *capillaritis* or *endotheliitis*) (Table 68-1).[6,7] Systemic necrotizing vasculitides[8,9] (principally microscopic polyangiitis [MPA][10,11] and Wegener's granulomatosis [12] account for most cases of autoimmune DAH.* Other causes of autoimmune DAH include antiglomerular basement membrane (anti-GBM) antibody disease,[13–15] connective tissue disease (CTD) (principally systemic lupus erythematosus [SLE]),[16] exogenous agents or drugs.[17] In many of these disorders, rapidly progressive glomerulonephritis (RPGN) is present concomitantly.[18,19] In most patients with autoimmune DAH and glomerulonephritis (GN), anti-GBM antibody and immune complexes are lacking.[19] The term *pauci-immune glomerulonephritis* has been used to refer to this group of patients, who encompass a heterogeneous group of disorders.[20,21] (discussed in detail below).

Idiopathic pulmonary hemosiderosis (IPH), a rare cause of recurrent DAH with no renal or extrapulmonary component, occurs primarily in children[22–24] and remains a diagnosis of exclusion.

Differentiation of these diverse syndromes can usually be accomplished by serological studies and by kidney biopsy. In such cases, lung biopsy is not required. GN can be demonstrated in the great majority of patients with DAH complicating granulomatosis with polyangiitis (GPA)[12] or MPA.[7,10,11] By contrast, the kidneys may be spared in DAH associated with CTD,[16] bone marrow transplant recipients,[25,26] or immunocompromised patients.[27,28] Urinalysis (to look for microscopic hematuria, red cell casts, and proteinuria) and measurement of renal function should always be done in the diagnostic evaluation of DAH. Findings consistent with GN warrant a prompt and aggressive evaluation that should include percutaneous needle biopsy of the kidney.

CLINICAL FEATURES OF AUTOIMMUNE ALVEOLAR HEMORRHAGE

Irrespective of etiology, the clinical, radiographic, and histopathological features of DAH may be similar.[1,2,6] Classical findings are hemoptysis, diffuse alveolar infiltrates, hypoxemia, renal failure, and iron-deficiency anemia.[2,7] However, the clinical spectrum is wide, and many of these features may be subtle or absent. In this context, the diagnosis of DAH may be difficult, as signs and symptoms overlap with diverse etiologies of diffuse alveolar infiltrates. Prompt diagnosis and institution of therapy is vital to avert early mortality from DAH and late sequelae from end-stage renal failure. Chest radiographs typically reveal bilateral alveolar infiltrates, often with a batwing appearance. However, focal, and even unilateral, patterns indistinguishable from pneumonia may occur. Following cessation of bleeding, infiltrates markedly improve or normalize within 24 to 72 hours (Fig. 68-1). A presumptive diagnosis of DAH can often be made by a combination of clinical and serological findings and bronchoalveolar lavage (BAL) fluid. Grossly bloody BAL fluid (with progressively more blood with serial aliquots),[1,2,7] large numbers of hemosiderin-laden macrophages,[8,27] and the absence of purulent secretions or ancillary evidence for infection strongly support DAH as a cause of pulmonary infiltrates. Ancillary studies including serologies, renal function tests, and urinalysis may support the diagnosis.

TABLE 68-1 Etiology of Autoimmune Diffuse Alveolar Hemorrhage

Antiglomerular basement membrane antibody disease (Goodpasture's syndrome)
Antineutrophil cytoplasmic antibody (ANCA)-mediated vasculitis (e.g., granulomatosis with polyangiitis, microscopic polyangiitis, Churg–Strauss syndrome, pauci-immune glomerulonephritis)
Idiopathic rapidly progressive glomerulonephritis
Collagen vascular disease (e.g., systemic lupus erythematosus)
Immunocompromised status (e.g., bone marrow transplant, AIDS)
Exogenous agents or drugs (e.g., trimellitic anhydride, isocyanates, D-penicillamine, cocaine)
Idiopathic pulmonary hemosiderosis (pathogenesis unknown)

*The Boards of Directors of the American College of Rheumatology (ACR), American Society of Nephrology (ASN), and the European League Against Rheumatism (EULAR) have recommended a gradual shift from honorific eponyms to disease-descriptive or aetiology-based nomenclature. The leadership of these three organizations tasked an international group of senior academicians expert in the care of patients with vasculitis and engaged in research in the field to provide the medical community with proper descriptive terms instead of the names for Wegener's granulomatosis, Churg–Strauss syndrome, and Behçet syndrome. The move toward a vasculitis terminology based on pathology, rather than historical reference, was triggered by evidence that Dr Friedrich Wegener was a member of the Nazi party before and during World War II. Falk RJ, Gross WL, Guillevin L, Hoffman GS, Jayne DR, Jennette JC, Kallenberg CG, Luqmani R, Mahr AD, Matteson EL, Merkel PA, Specks U, Watts RA; American College of Rheumatology; American Society of Nephrology; European League Against Rheumatism. Granulomatosis with polyangiitis (Wegener's): an alternative name for Wegener's granulomatosis. *Arthritis Rheum.* 2011:863–4.

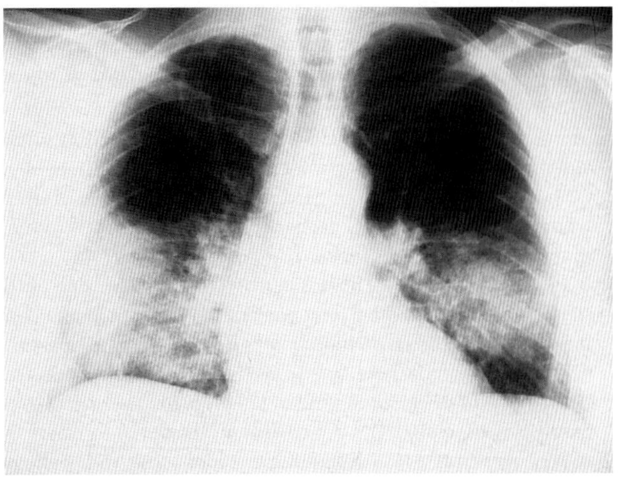

A

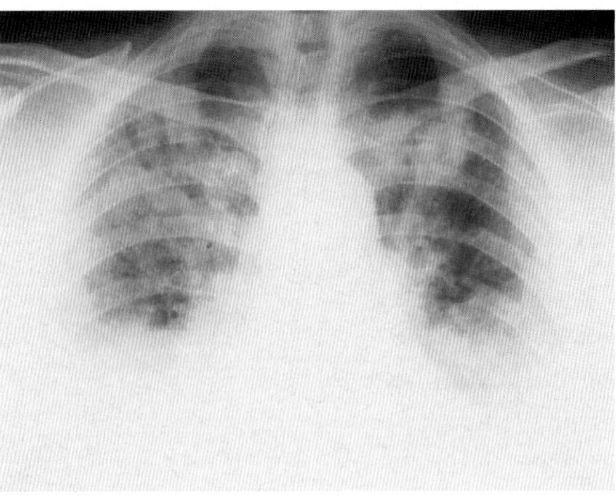

B

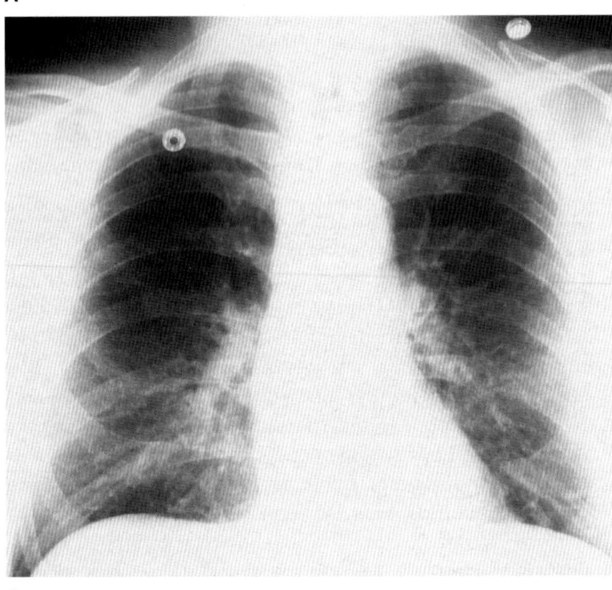

C

Figure 68-1 **A.** Idiopathic rapidly progressive glomerulonephritis. Posterior–anterior (PA) chest radiograph from a 52-year-old man with rapidly progressive glomerulonephritis, hemoptysis, and bilateral alveolar infiltrates, consistent with alveolar hemorrhage. Bronchoalveolar lavage demonstrated blood-tinged fluid and numerous hemosiderin-laden macrophages. **B.** Idiopathic rapidly progressive glomerulonephritis. PA chest radiograph from the same patient 18 months later with diffuse bilateral alveolar infiltrates representing recurrent massive alveolar hemorrhage. He was treated with pulse methylprednisolone (1 g daily for 3 days), followed by a gradual corticosteroid taper. **C.** PA chest radiograph from the same patient 3 weeks later demonstrating complete resolution of the alveolar infiltrates.

DIAGNOSIS

THE ROLE OF LUNG BIOPSY

The role of lung biopsy in the diagnosis of DAH and the determination of its etiology is controversial. We believe the risks of open or thoracoscopic lung biopsy are excessive in patients with severe DAH and respiratory failure. Postoperative complications such as infection and air leaks may be exacerbated by the corticosteroid or immunosuppressive agents used to treat many of these immune-mediated DAH syndromes. Furthermore, histological features are usually nonspecific. Predominant findings are extensive intra-alveolar hemorrhage and necrotizing pulmonary capillaritis (endotheliitis) (Fig. 68-2).[6–8] Capillaritis is characterized by neutrophilic infiltration of capillaries, fragmented neutrophils (leukocytoclasis), and necrosis of the capillary walls (Fig. 68-3).[8] Loss of the integrity of the alveolar–capillary basement membrane results in leakage of red blood cells and neutrophils into the alveolar space.[2] Hemosiderin-laden macrophages (siderophages) accumulate within the alveolar spaces and interstitium; their presence is a clue to prior episodes of alveolar hemorrhage (Figs. 68-2B,C and 68-4).[8]

Capillaritis was initially described as a marker of systemic vasculitis, but may also be observed in myriad disorders associated with DAH (e.g., SLE,[16] CTD,[2] anti-GBM disease,[14] bone marrow[25,26] or lung[29] transplant recipients, and drug-induced DAH).[1,6,7] An associated venulitis and arteriolitis may sometimes be present, but larger vessels are spared.[8] Capillaritis is subtle and often overshadowed by DAH filling the alveolar spaces.

Pulmonary capillaritis can be diagnosed by transbronchial biopsy, but this diagnosis is made with greater confidence when larger biopsy specimens are obtained by video-assisted thoracoscopy or limited thoracotomy.[6] Additional pathological features may be seen in patients with underlying granulomatous vasculitis (e.g., granulomas, necrosis, or eosinophils).[6,8] Nongranulomatous inflammation in airways and lung interstitium, interstitial fibrosis, diffuse alveolar damage (DAD), fibrinous pleuritis, and organizing pneumonia have also been described in DAH associated with antineutrophil cytoplasmic antibody (ANCA) vasculitic syndromes.[8] It should be emphasized that histological findings of alveolar hemorrhage and capillaritis, although distinctive, are nonspecific.[7] Immunofluorescent (IF) stains (of lung or kidney) or serological markers (e.g., anti-GBM antibody or ANCA) are required to differentiate the various causes of autoimmune DAH (Table 68-2).[6–8] Linear deposits of immunoglobulin G (IgG) along alveolar septa is pathognomonic for anti-GBM disease.[13,14] A granular, or "lumpy-bumpy" pattern of immune complex deposits may be seen in SLE, systemic necrotizing vasculitis, or immune complex–mediated idiopathic RPGN.[6] In ANCA-associated capillaritis, immune complexes are usually lacking (hence the term *pauci-immune*).[10,11,30] When immune DAH is suspected, a portion of the lung biopsy can

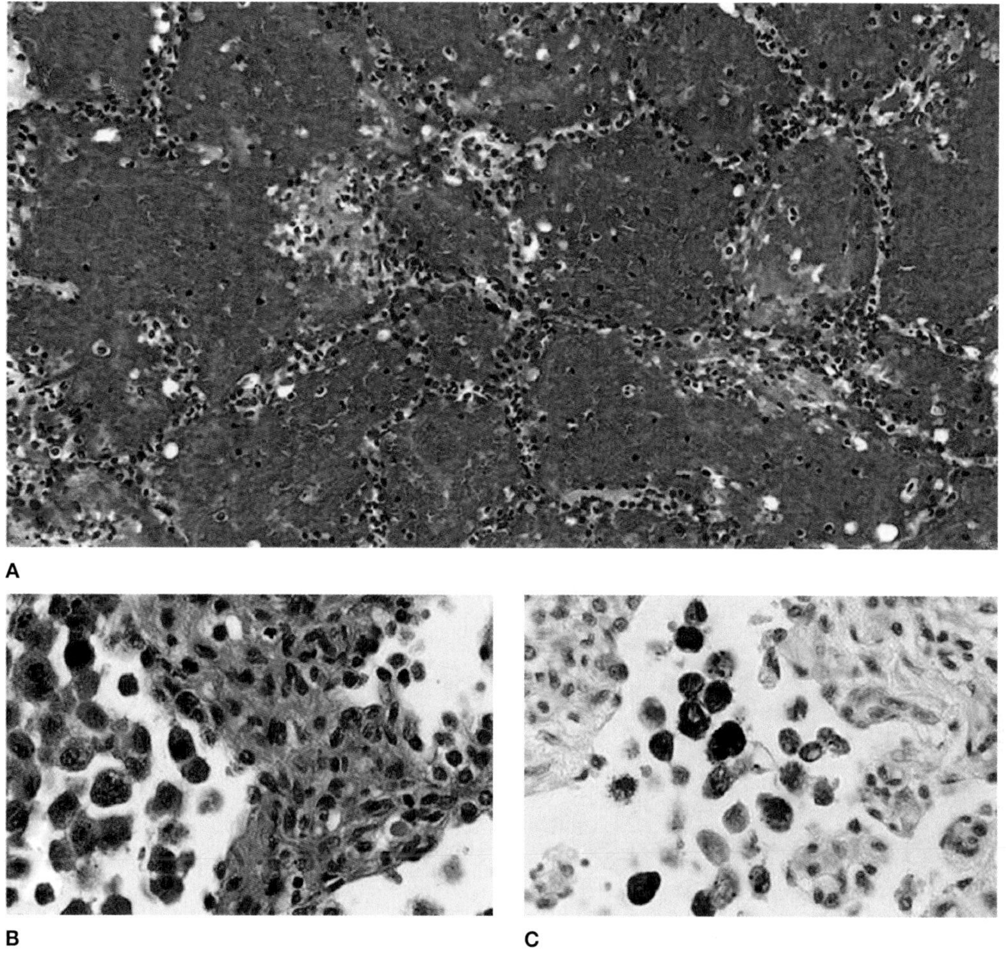

Figure 68-2 Alveolar hemorrhage. **A.** Acute hemorrhage with blood-filling alveolar spaces (H&E stain, ×40). **B.** Pigment-laden alveolar macrophages (H&E, ×200) shown in (**C**) to be full of iron (blue cytoplasm) indicative of prior hemorrhage (Prussian blue stain, ×200).

be frozen for IF stains, but IF stains of lung tissue are logistically difficult, and nonspecific background staining may lead to misinterpretation. When GN is present concomitantly, kidney IF stains are more sensitive and reliable.

Despite the greater accuracy of surgical lung biopsy in evaluating DAH, fiberoptic bronchoscopy with BAL is usually adequate to exclude infectious etiologies and support the diagnosis of DAH.[1] Bloody or serosanguinous BAL fluid (consistent with active or recent bleeding)[1,2,7] or hemosiderin-laden macrophages[8,27] (a clue to prior episodes of alveolar hemorrhage) may be sufficient to justify initiation of therapy provided clinical and serological features are consistent. Thoracoscopic lung biopsy may be useful in *noncritically ill* patients with suspected DAH when ancillary studies, kidney biopsy, and BAL are nondiagnostic.

■ THE ROLE OF PERCUTANEOUS KIDNEY BIOPSY

Necrotizing GN is a cardinal (albeit nonspecific) feature of most immune-mediated DAH syndromes.[19,31] The histological spectrum is varied, ranging from mild mesangial thickening to severe crescentic GN. Vasculitis of renal arterioles is rarely found, even in granulomatous vasculitides. Because of the strong association of autoimmune DAH and GN, percutaneous kidney biopsy should be performed in any patient with suspected DAH who has abnormalities on urinalysis or renal function tests. Conventional hematoxylin and eosin (H&E) stains are nonspecific, but the demonstration of glomerular inflammation with necrosis and crescents supports the diagnosis of an immune-mediated etiology (Fig. 68-5).[19,31,32] IF stains may clarify the nature of the underlying disorder. Bright linear IF staining along glomerular basement membranes (GBMs) is pathognomonic for anti-GBM disease (Fig. 68-6).[13,33] A lumpy-bumpy IF pattern, consistent with deposits of immune complexes, is found in some cases of CTD[16] and in idiopathic immune complex–mediated GN.[34] Negative IF stains are characteristic of the pauci-immune GN of necrotizing vasculitis.[19,30,35,36] Serologies are critically important in defining the underlying disorder responsible for DAH (particularly ANCA, anti-GBM antibody, and antinuclear antibodies). Recognizing the different pathogenetic mechanisms of these DAH syndromes is important, as the prognosis and treatment strategies differ.

■ THERAPY OF IMMUNE-MEDIATED ALVEOLAR HEMORRHAGE

Irrespective of etiology, the most immediate concern in patients with severe immune DAH is to control intrapulmonary bleeding, which may be fatal. Besides general supportive measures, corticosteroids are considered part of standard therapy for all immune-mediated DAH syndromes. For severe cases (e.g., severe hypoxemia, respiratory failure), high-dose "pulse" methylprednisolone (1000 mg daily for 3 days) should be given (irrespective of underlying etiology), even while pursuing a diagnostic workup.[1,7] Delaying pulse therapy in a critically ill patient for even a few hours may be catastrophic. Rapid resolution of bleeding can occur, often within 24 to 72 hours of initiation of therapy (Fig. 68-7). Following the 3-day pulse, corticosteroids (dose of methylprednisolone 60 to 120 mg per day or equivalent) should be continued for a few days, until control of the

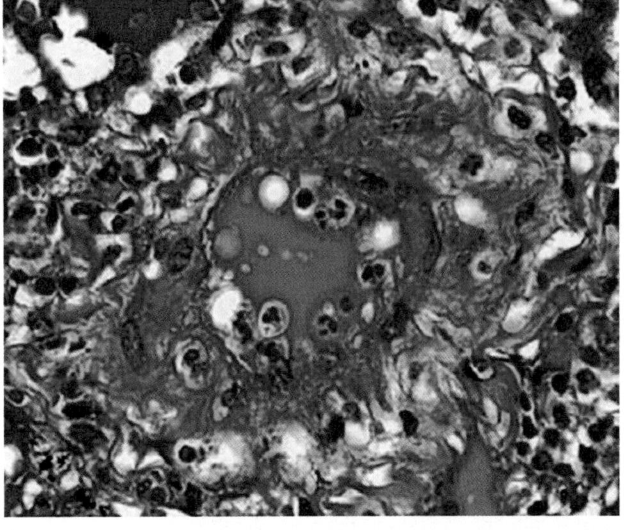

A

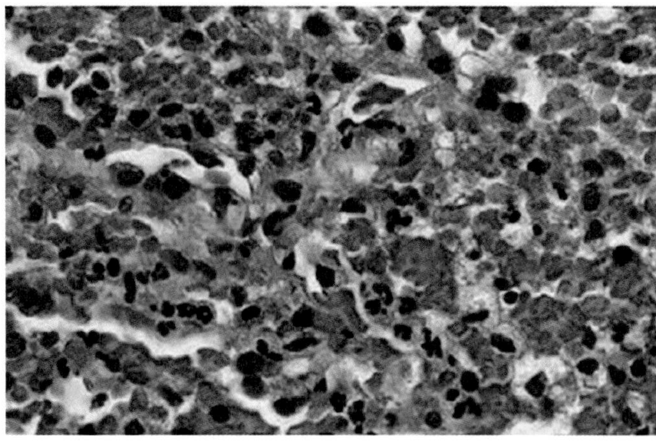

B

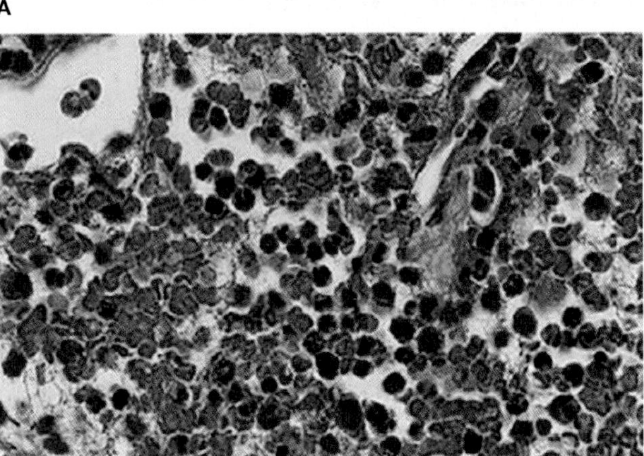

C

Figure 68-3 Pulmonary capillaritis. **A.** Necrotizing arteritis in microscopic polyangiitis (H&E, ×400); (**B**) capillaritis with intact alveolar septae in Wegener's granulomatosis (granulomatosis with polyangiits) (H&E, ×400); and (**C**) capillaritis with destruction of alveolar septae (H&A, ×400).

bleeding and extrapulmonary manifestations has been achieved. The subsequent dose and rate of corticosteroid taper need to be individualized, based upon clinical, radiographic, and serological response. The presence of renal involvement, vasculitis, or progression of DAH on corticosteroids is an indication for adding cyclophosphamide (CYC) (or occasionally other immunosuppressive agents).[1,18,37] Rituximab may be as effective, and possibly more effective than CYC for ANCA-associated vasculitis,[38,39] but data are limited for DAH.

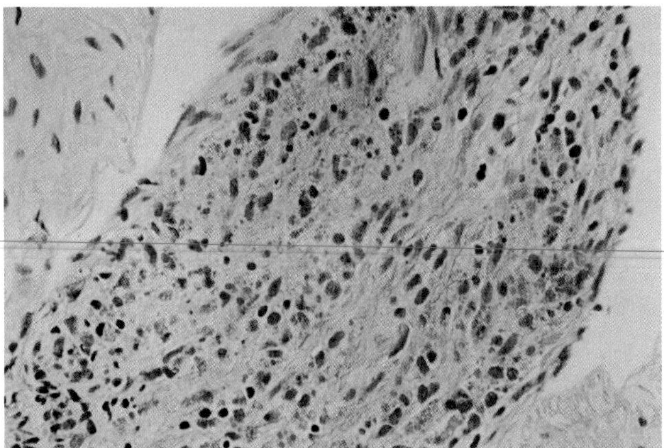

Figure 68-4 Hemosiderin-laden macrophages (siderophages) are prominent in the alveolar interstitium in a patient with recurrent alveolar hemorrhage (H&E). *(Used with permission of Joseph Fantone, MD.)*

Plasmapheresis is a central component of therapy for anti-GBM disease[13,14] but has no *routine* role for other disorders.[11,12,40,41] However, plasmapheresis may have an adjunctive role in patients with autoimmune DAH and severe renal insufficiency (i.e., serum creatinine >4 mg%)[41,42] and in patients with severe or progressive DAH refractory to corticosteroids or immunosuppressive agents.[43] Measures to ensure adequate oxygenation are also essential. Mechanical ventilatory support, often with positive end-expiratory pressure, may be necessary in fulminant cases of DAH, to prevent death due to refractory hypoxemia. Transfusion of red blood cells may be required to maintain an acceptable hematocrit (more than 25%) and adequate blood pressure. In the sections that follow, we discuss each of the autoimmune DAH syndromes individually.

SPECIFIC SYNDROMES

GOODPASTURE'S SYNDROME

Clinical Features

Anti-GBM disease (Goodpasture's syndrome), the prototype of pulmonary renal syndromes, accounts for 18% to 32% of immune-mediated DAH.[3,13,15,31,44] Classically, anti-GBM disease manifests as DAH and RPGN.[13,14,33,45] In 30% to 50% of patients with anti-GBM disease, GN occurs *without* DAH; DAH alone is rare (<5%).[14,15] Anti-GBM disease typically affects individuals between 20 and 45 years of age with a distinct male predominance.[14,45] The incidence has been estimated as 1 to 3 cases per million population per year.[46,47] The etiology is not known, but exposure to inhaled hydrocarbons,[46] cigarette smoke,[45] cocaine,[15] and antecedent viral

TABLE 68-2 Autoimmune Diffuse Alveolar Hemorrhage: Pathology and Serology

	Lung Pathology		Renal Pathology		
	Histopathology	Immunofluorescence	Histopathology	Immunofluorescence	Serology
ABMA disease (Goodpasture's syndrome)	±Capillaritis	Linear	Variable	Linear	ABMA (±p-ANCA)
Granulomatosis with polyangiitis	Capillaritis (±granulomatous)	Negative	Segmental necrosis, crescents	Pauci-immune	ANCA (c-ANCA ⋙ p-ANCA)
Microscopic polyangiitis	Capillaritis	Negative	Segmental necrosis, crescents	Pauci-immune	ANCA (p-ANCA or c-ANCA)
Systemic lupus erythematosus	Capillaritis	Granular	Variable	Granular	ANA
Idiopathic pulmonary hemosiderosis	±Capillaritis	Negative	Normal	—	Negative

ABMA, antibasement membrane antibody; ANA, antinuclear antibody; ANCA, antineutrophil cytoplasmic antibody; p-ANCA, perinuclear antineutrophilcytoplasmic antibody; c-ANCA, cytoplasmic antineutrophil cytoplasmic antibody.

illnesses, particularly influenza, have been cited as risk factors.[14] The demonstration of anti-GBM antibodies in tissue (typically kidney)[33] or in serum[13,14] is the cornerstone of the diagnosis.

The clinical expression of anti-GBM disease is highly variable. Most patients present with progressive dyspnea, diffuse alveolar infiltrates, and hypoxemia; hemoptysis occurs in 45% to 94%.[13–15,48] GN is a cardinal feature.[33,47,49,50] Microscopic hematuria, red cell casts, or proteinuria are almost always present. Gross hematuria occurs in up to 41% of patients.[14] Azotemia is noted in 55% to 71% of patients at presentation.[13,48] Fatigue and weakness are common.[14] In the absence of therapy, progressive renal insufficiency ensues, often resulting in end-stage renal failure within days to weeks of the onset of symptoms.[13] Oliguria, severe renal failure, or greater than 50% crescents on renal biopsy are associated with a poor prognosis and low rate of recovery of renal function.[13,14,33,51] The course may be fulminant, with severe renal failure and explosive, life-threatening DAH.[13,14] Chest radiographs typically reveal dense bilateral alveolar infiltrates, often with air-bronchograms. With cessation of bleeding, infiltrates may resolve within 24 to 36 hours. Pleural effusions are rare and suggest an alternative diagnosis. Pulmonary function tests are rarely helpful in the acute setting of DAH.[14,15] Bloody or serosanguineous BAL fluid (that worsens with serial aliquots) suggests DAH but is nonspecific.[8] Anemia is present in more than 90% of cases and may be profound. Serum iron and ferritin levels are usually decreased, reflecting diminished iron stores. Factors associated with a higher incidence of DAH include cigarette smoking,[15] exposure to high concentrations of oxygen, upper respiratory tract infections, and increased hydrostatic (pulmonary capillary) pressures.[13,14]

Serological assays for anti-GBM antibody are invaluable in confirming the diagnosis and monitoring the adequacy of therapy.[14,47] Radioimmunoassays or enzyme-linked immunosorbent assays (ELISA) for anti-GBM antibody are highly sensitive (>95%) and specific (>97%)[13,14] but are performed in only a few laboratories. Results are usually not available for several days. Since delay in institution of therapy may preclude a favorable outcome, percutaneous renal biopsy is usually performed while awaiting the results of serum assays. Although disparate results have been reported, the height of serum anti-GBM antibody titer correlated with the prognosis of renal disease in some studies.[48,52] Further, changes in anti-GBM titer over time may be a guide to efficacy of therapy.[14] Treatment can be tapered and discontinued after the antibody has disappeared from the circulation (usually within 3–6 months).[15] Up to one-third of patients with circulating anti-GBM antibodies have concomitant ANCA (usually MPO).[13,32,53] Other serological studies are negative or nondiagnostic.

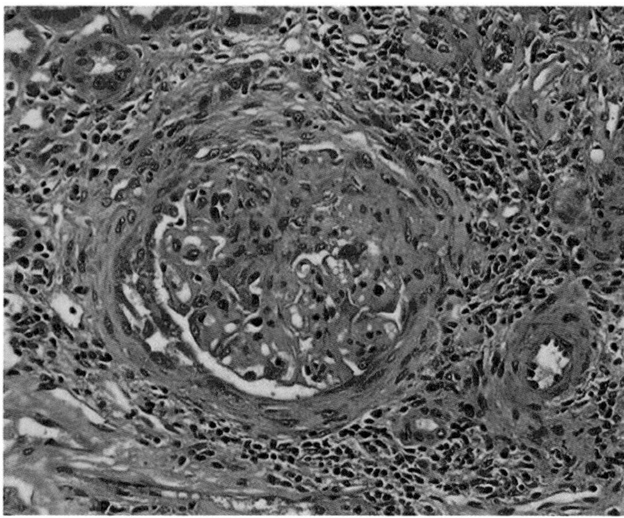

Figure 68-5 Segmental necrotizing and crescentic glomerulonephritis due to vasculitis (H&E).

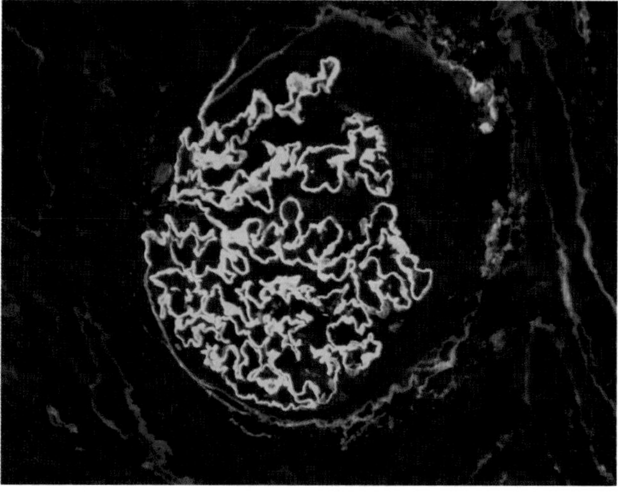

Figure 68-6 Linear immunofluorescent staining along glomeruli due to deposition of anti-glomerular basement membrane (anti-GBM) antibody.

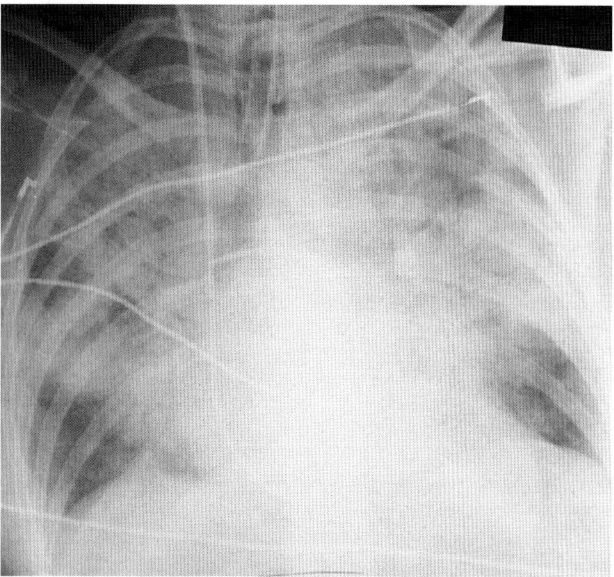

A

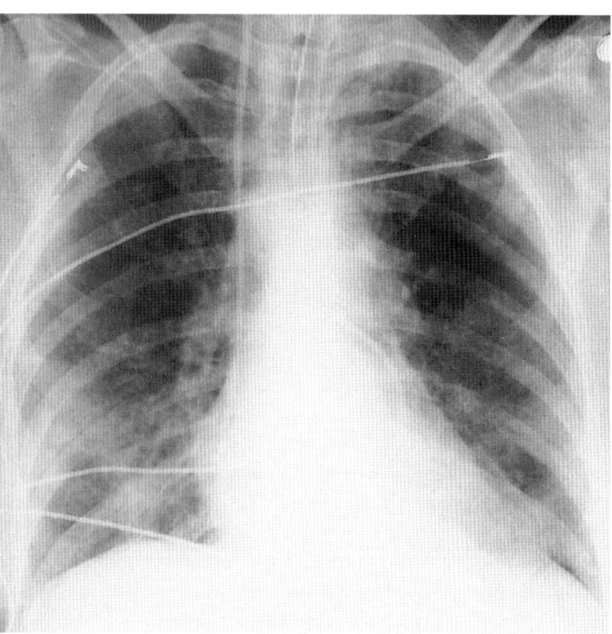

B

Figure 68-7 **A.** Alveolar hemorrhage due to microscopic polyarteritis (MPA). Posterior–anterior (PA) chest radiograph demonstrating massive alveolar infiltrates involving all lobes. Because of the severity of respiratory failure (requiring 16 cmH_2O of positive end-expiratory pressure to achieve acceptable oxygenation), no lung biopsy was performed. Urinalysis demonstrated numerous red cells and occasional red cell casts. Serum creatinine was 1.4 mg%. Pulse methylprednisolone (1 g daily × 3 days) was initiated, and renal biopsy was scheduled for the following morning. **B.** Alveolar hemorrhage due to MPA. PA chest radiograph from the same patient 12 hours following initiation of pulse methylprednisolone. Marked improvement in alveolar infiltrates is evident. Renal biopsy demonstrated glomerulonephritis and a necrotizing vasculitis involving renal arterioles; no granulomas were present. Cyclophosphamide (2 mg/kg per day) was instituted, and corticosteroids were continued. Within 5 days, the infiltrates had cleared completely and serum creatinine was 0.6 mg%.

■ HISTOPATHOLOGY

Percutaneous kidney biopsy is the preferred invasive procedure to substantiate the diagnosis of anti-GBM disease.[15] Light microscopy demonstrates a proliferative or necrotizing GN, often with cellular crescents.[14,33] Over time, the crescents may fibrose, and frank glomerulosclerosis, interstitial fibrosis, and tubular atrophy may be observed.[33] Although these microscopic features are nonspecific, IF stains are the cornerstone of the diagnosis. Bright linear deposits of IgG and complement (C3) along GBM are pathognomonic of anti-GBM disease (Fig. 68-6).[14,33] All four subclasses of IgG are represented, but IgG_1[54,55] and IgG_3[55] predominate in anti-GBM disease. Rare cases of linear deposits of IgM or IgA have been described.[15] Lung biopsies are rarely necessary,[14] as the histological features on renal biopsy are usually adequate to establish the diagnosis. When lung biopsy has been done, extensive hemorrhage predominates[6,8] with accumulation of hemosiderin-laden macrophages within the alveolar spaces.[14] Foci of DAD and capillaritis may also be found.[6] Interstitial or intra-alveolar inflammation is minimal or absent. Extensive necrosis or large-vessel vasculitis is not found. Similar histopathological features may be seen with a wide gamut of immune-mediated DAH syndromes.[6,8] IF stains of lung tissue may be diagnostic, provided a clear linear pattern of immunofluorescence is present. However, IF stains are technically difficult in lung tissue and autofluorescence may obscure the linear IgG deposits.

■ PATHOGENESIS

Antibodies are directed against the α3 chain of type IV collagen, an antigen highly expressed in both alveolar and GBMs.[13,15,54] Anti-GBM antibodies bind the GBM and activate complement, initiating an inflammatory pathway that elicits injury.[13] In addition to circulating antibodies, autoreactive T lymphocytes directed against the α3 antigen are key mediators for development of RPGN.[15,56] Immunoglobulin synthesis and deposits of IgG along the alveolar and glomerular capillary basement membranes then ensue. Anti-GBM disease is monophasic, and during the course of the disease, self-tolerance is restored.[13] Late relapses are rare.[13] This tolerance may be achieved by regulatory CD4+ and CD25+ T cells[15,57] or anti-idiotypic (blocking) antibodies,[54] but this remains speculative.

The pathogenesis of anti-GBM disease is unknown, but both genetic[15,58] and environmental factors[54] may play roles. Patients with anti-GBM disease preferentially express certain immunoglobulin Gm allotypes and links between anti-GBM disease and the HLA-DR2 histocompatibility antigen have been noted.[13,15] Exposure to cigarette smoke, hydrocarbon-containing solvents, hard-metal dust, influenza A2 virus, chlorine gas, and D-penicillamine have been associated with anti-GBM disease.[13–15] These exogenous factors may injure the basement membrane, resulting in increased capillary permeability, exposing the Goodpasture's antigen (α3 chain), which is then recognized as foreign, eliciting a T-helper cell response.[15,54]

■ TREATMENT

Before the availability of the current therapy and renal dialysis, mortality exceeded 90%.[13] Plasmapheresis was introduced as a therapeutic option for anti-GBM disease in the 1970s,[49] and was quickly adopted worldwide and incorporated in all clinical trials. Currently, with the combination of plasmapheresis, corticosteroids (CSs), and CYC, mortality has been reduced to less than 20%.[13–15] Because of the rarity of anti-GBM syndrome, only one small randomized trial compared immunosuppressive therapy with the *combination* of immunosuppressive therapy *plus* plasma exchange.[49] In that study, plasmapheresis plus immunosuppressive therapy was associated with more rapid disappearance of anti-GBM antibody and improved renal function than treatment with immunosuppressive agents *alone*.[49] The optimal extent and duration of plasma exchanges have not been defined. Most investigators advocate plasma exchange daily or every other day for 2 to 3 weeks, until the clinical course has improved and serum anti-GBM antibodies are nondetectable.[13,41] Immunosuppressive therapy is required to inhibit antibody production and rebound hypersynthesis, which may occur following discontinuation of plasma exchange.[13] Treatment of acute, life-threatening DAH in Goodpasture's syndrome is similar to other autoimmune disorders. Pulse methylprednisolone (1 g daily for 3 days) is given, followed by a gradual corticosteroid taper.[14] Either CYC (oral or IV pulse) or azathioprine should be initiated once the diagnosis of anti-GBM disease is substantiated. Most investigators favor CYC over azathioprine,[13–15] but studies comparing these agents have not been done. CYC is maintained for the duration of therapy, unless complications such as leukopenia necessitate dose reduction. The corticosteroid dose is gradually tapered over several months. Immunosuppressive or cytotoxic therapy may be discontinued within 3 to 6 months provided a sustained remission has been achieved and anti-GBM antibodies have disappeared.[13,15] Circulating anti-GBM antibodies usually clear within 8 weeks, irrespective of the initial titer. Early relapse (within the first 2 months) may occur when circulating antibodies are still present. This typically manifests as DAH. Risk factors for relapse include infection, volume overload, and cigarette smoking.[15] Late recurrence, associated with renewed antibody synthesis following a remission, is rare.[14] In summary, aggressive therapy with plasmapheresis, corticosteroids, and immunosuppressive agents has dramatically improved prognosis.[14,15,51] With this approach, 5-year survival exceeds 80%, and fewer than 30% of patients require chronic dialysis.[14,15] Early recognition and treatment of this syndrome are critical, as the prognosis for recovery of renal function depends upon the initial extent of injury.[32,50] Recovery of renal function can be expected in patients with minor functional impairment. By contrast, patients manifesting initial serum creatinine greater than 4 mg/dL, oliguria, or greater than 50% crescents on renal biopsy rarely recover and usually progress to end-stage renal failure requiring chronic dialysis.[32,50] In one study of 71 patients with anti-GBM disease (all were treated with steroids, immunosuppressive agents, and plasmapheresis), renal survival was linked to extent of renal failure at presentation.[51] Renal survival rates at 1 year were as follows: 8% among 39 patients requiring dialysis at presentation; 82% among 13 patients with creatinine >5.7 but not requiring dialysis; 95% among 19 patients with initial serum creatinine <5.7 mg%. Renal transplantation has been successful in patients with irreversible renal failure, provided serum anti-GBM antibodies are undetectable.[59,60]

Systemic Vasculitis

DAH is a common complication of MPA[10,11] and granulomatosis with polyangiitis (GPA) (formerly called Wegener's syndrome)[12,61] and rarely complicates Churg–Strauss syndrome (CSS),[62,63] Behçet disease,[64] mixed cryoglobulinemia,[65] Henoch–Schöenlein purpura,[66] and other systemic necrotizing vasculitides.[1,37] Classic polyarteritis nodosa (PAN) rarely involves the lung.[8,67] Necrotizing small-vessel vasculitis accounts for the majority of autoimmune DAH syndromes.[1,8] RPGN is usually present in each of these DAH syndromes, but the disease is sometimes limited to the kidneys or lungs. Circulating antibodies directed against cytoplasmic components of neutrophils and monocytes (ANCA) have been detected in most patients with these "pulmonary–renal syndromes,"[7,34,37,68] suggesting a common pathogenesis and mechanism of lung injury in these diverse vasculitic disorders.

ANCA-Associated Vasculitides

Goodpasture's syndrome (anti-GBM disease) was the first of the pulmonary–renal syndromes to be immunologically characterized.[14,15] Subsequent studies documented immune complexes in serum or renal tissue in subsets of patients with pulmonary–renal syndromes, particularly SLE[16] and immune complex–mediated GN.[69] However, more than two-thirds of patients with pulmonary–renal syndromes are mediated by ANCA antibodies without anti-GBM or immune complexes (i.e., pauci-immune).[1,34,37] Depending upon clinicopathological features, some patients with pauci-immune GN and DAH may meet criteria for GPA or CSS, while others exhibit a multisystemic small-vessel vasculitis but lack granulomatous inflammation of the respiratory tract. In this context, the term *microscopic polyangiitis* is used.[10,11,70] The availability of serum assays for ANCAs has profoundly influenced the classification of immune DAH and GN. ANCA-positive patients with pauci-immune DAH and GN (*formerly* given a diagnosis of idiopathic RPGN and DAH) are now considered to have MPA.[11] The spectrum of ANCA-associated diseases is not limited to patients with pulmonary–renal syndromes but includes individuals with MPA limited to the lung (i.e., manifesting as DAH) or kidney (i.e., necrotizing GN).[11] To avoid further confusion, brief definitions of the major ANCA-associated vasculitides are outlined below.

GRANULOMATAOSIS WITH POLYANGIITIS, GPA (FORMERLY CALLED WEGENER'S GRANULOMATOSIS)

GPA, the most common of the pulmonary vasculitides, typically involves the upper respiratory tract (e.g., sinuses, ears, nasopharynx, oropharynx, trachea), lower respiratory tract (bronchi and lung), and kidney, with varying degrees of disseminated vasculitis (see Chapter 83).[12] The annual incidence of GPA has been estimated at 4 to 12 cases per million.[12,46,71,72] Alveolar hemorrhage is a rare complication of GPA, reflecting diffuse injury to the lung microvasculature (i.e., capillaritis) (Fig. 68-8).[1,6] In this context, RPGN is present in more than 90% of patients.[6,12] The salient histopathological features of GPA include small-vessel vasculitis (involving capillaries, arterioles, venules), geographic necrosis, hemorrhagic infarcts, a mixed inflammatory cellular infiltrate, and a granulomatous component.[6,8,12] Circulating c-ANCAs (PR3 epitope) have been detected in more than 90% of patients with active generalized GPA and in 40% to 70% with active regional GPA.[12,68,73–75] Oral CYC (2 mg/kg per day) plus prednisone has been the initial treatment of choice for GPA for more than 3 decades.[12,76,77] With this regimen, remissions are achieved in 70% to 93% of patients, with early mortality rates of less than 15%.[76–81]

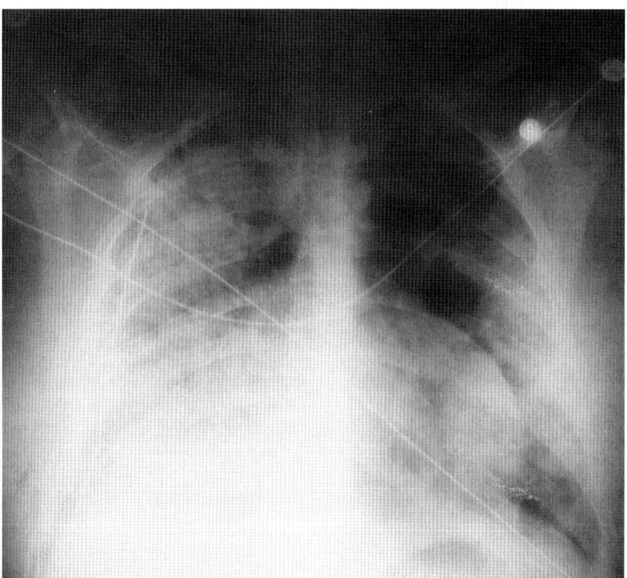

Figure 68-8 Granulomatosis with polyangiitis (GPA) (formerly called Wegener's granulomatosis. Posterior–anterior (PA) chest radiograph demonstrated bilateral alveolar infiltrates in a 13-year-old girl with hemoptysis and respiratory failure. A right chest tube is in place from an open lung biopsy performed 2 days earlier. Open lung biopsy demonstrated capillaritis and massive alveolar hemorrhage. Pulse methylprednisolone, followed by oral cyclophosphamide and prednisone, was associated with a complete remission.

By 3 to 6 months, assuming complete remissions are achieved, azathioprine[78,79] or methotrexate[79] can be substituted for CYC. Treatment should be continued for a minimum of 12 to 18 months (total duration).[12,77] Relapses can be treated with CYC and prednisone. Methotrexate may be used in patients with limited disease or those experiencing significant toxicity from CYC.[82,83] Rituximab may be as effective, and possibly more effective than CYC for GPA and AAV.[38,39,84–86] However, whether rituximab should be used with corticosteroids alone or corticosteroids combined with CYC has not been clarified. Further, the role for long-term maintenance therapy with rituximab has not been studied.[84–86] Additional studies are required to assess indications for rituximab, appropriate dosing and frequency of administration, role for concomitant therapy, and long-term side effects. Trimethoprim/sulfamethoxazole may have an adjunctive role (together with CYC and prednisone) to reduce relapse rates,[87] but should not be considered as primary therapy.

■ CHURG–STRAUSS SYNDROME (ALLERGIC ANGIITIS AND GRANULOMATOSIS)

CSS, also termed *allergic angiitis* and *granulomatosis,* is a rare, small-vessel vasculitis associated with a prominent allergic component, asthma, and eosinophils in blood or involved tissues (see Chapter 83).[63,88] CSS involves capillaries, venules, and arterioles.[63] Granulomas, eosinophils, and palisading histiocytes in extravascular tissues are hallmarks of the disorder[88,89] and distinguish CSS from other vasculitides.[8,63] The annual incidence of CSS has been estimated at 0.6 to 6.8 cases per million.[46,71,88,90] In the classic form of CSS, vasculitis develops after a several-year history of atopy or asthma.[89] Pulmonary involvement is nearly invariably present.[63,88,89] Asthma is present in 96% to 100%; focal infiltrates on chest radiographs, in 30% to 70% of cases.[63,88,89] DAH is a rare complication of CSS. In a French series of 112 patients with CSS, moderate DAH was observed in 3/43 ANCA-(+) patients and in 5/69 ANCA-negative patients.[91] DAH was cited in only 1/32 patients in a Spanish series,[92] and 1/19 in an Italian series.[93] Severe DAH has only rarely been reported in CSS.[94,95] Constitutional symptoms may herald the onset of vasculitis.[88] Extrapulmonary manifestations include mononeuritis multiplex (63%–93%); skin (50%–78%); cardiac (16%–56%); kidney (16%–49%); skin (50%–78%); gastrointestinal (GI) tract (17%–58%).[63,88] Factors associated with a worse prognosis include cardiac or GI tract involvement, renal insufficiency; age >65 years.[96]

The erythrocyte sedimentation rate (ESR), C-reactive protein (CRP), and blood eosinophil count are elevated in more than 80% of patients during the acute phase of vasculitis or exacerbations.[62,70,88,89] Circulating ANCAs (primarily p-ANCA) have been detected in 40% of patients with CSS.[88,91,97] Interestingly, the presence of ANCA was associated with a higher incidence of renal involvement and pulmonary hemorrhage, but a lower frequency of cardiac involvement.[97]

A variety of treatment regimens have been employed for CSS including corticosteroids, immunosuppressive or cytotoxic agents, and plasmapheresis (alone or in combination).[62,88,96] Corticosteroids achieve remissions in more than 80% of patients with CSS and are first-line therapy for mild to moderate cases of CSS.[88,98,99] Oral or pulse CYC (or other immunosuppressive agents such as azathioprine or mycophenolate mofetil) should be added for severe or multisystemic disease or corticosteroid-recalcitrant cases or when unfavorable prognostic factors are present.[40,62,88,96,98] Plasmapheresis should be considered as adjunctive therapy for ANCA-positive CSS patients with severe pulmonary–renal syndrome.[42]

■ MICROSCOPIC POLYANGIITIS

MPA (formerly termed *microscopic polyarteritis* or *polyangiitis overlap syndrome*) typically presents with GN and pulmonary capillaritis manifesting as DAH.[10,11] Clinical and serological features of MPA overlap with GPA and CSS.[11,70] MPA is rare, with an annual incidence of 2.1 to 17.5 cases per million.[46,71,90] As its name implies, MPA involves small vessels (arterioles, venules, or capillaries); extension to larger vessels occurs in a minority of cases.[100] Small vessels are always spared in classic PAN.[67,100] In contrast to GPA or CSS, neither granulomas nor eosinophils are prominent in MPA.[11,100] Circulating ANCAs are present in 50% to 90% of patients with MPA,[11,70,100] suggesting a relationship with other ANCA-associated vasculitides. By contrast, circulating ANCAs are present in fewer than 20% of patients with classic (macroscopic) PAN.[100] A necrotizing, crescentic pauci-immune GN is nearly invariably present in MPA[11,100] but is rare in classic PAN.[67] Alveolar hemorrhage, which is rarely observed in classic PAN, occurs in 30% to 50% of patients with MPA and is often the dominant and most life-threatening manifestation.[10,11,70]

Corticosteroids, CYC, and plasmapheresis, alone or in combination, have been used to treat MPA.[11,70,78] Response rates and long-term survival have generally been similar with the various regimens. Most investigators use oral CYC (2 mg/kg per day) plus prednisone (1 mg/kg per day, with gradual taper), similar to the regimen used for GPA. With this approach, favorable responses are achieved in more than 80% of patients; 10-year survival exceeds 70%.[11,70,78] By 3 to 6 months, once complete remissions have been achieved, azathioprine, methotrexate, or mycophenolate mofetil may be substituted for CYC.[11,78] As was discussed in the section on GPA, rituximab may be as efficacious as CYC-containing regimens for AAV,[38,39,84–86] but data are limited.

ANCA-ASSOCIATED PULMONARY RENAL SYNDROMES: CLINICAL FEATURES

The clinical and radiologic manifestations of ANCA-associated DAH are similar to other immune causes. Acute necrotizing GN is nearly always present, but the renal lesion is nonspecific.[34,35,101] Distinguishing the specific underlying disorder may be difficult. The pathological lesions in ANCA-associated diseases share characteristic features, regardless of the organ affected. The three key histopathological findings are a segmental (focal) distribution of vascular injury, infiltration with neutrophils, and fibrinoid necrosis.[11,70,100] The latter results from lysis of the vascular wall, allowing plasma coagulation factors to enter the interstitium and come into contact with thrombogenic substances, generating fibrin. Neutrophils that infiltrate vessel walls undergo disruption and karyorrhexis, leading to the typical leukocytoclastic pattern of injury in capillaries and venules.[100] ANCA-associated vascular injury is accompanied by few, if any, immune deposits (pauci-immune).[19] However, the presence of immune deposits may be associated with more severe renal injury.[34] The salient lesion of renal vasculitis is a segmental necrotizing GN, usually accompanied by extracapillary proliferation of Bowman capsule (crescents) (Fig. 68-5).[11] Depending on the duration and extent of renal injury, varying degrees of glomerular fibrosis and sclerosis may be seen.[19] Vasculitis affecting the kidney often involves only the glomerular capillaries; macroscopic arteritis is seldom apparent.[100] When the lung is involved, the histopathology is nonspecific, demonstrating only capillaritis and intra-alveolar hemorrhage.[7] Immune deposits are absent.

Clinical features of ANCA-associated DAH syndromes overlap. Striking elevations in the ESR and CRP may be observed in all the syndromes, particularly when disseminated vasculitis is present.[11,88] Anemia and leukocytosis are common. Marked eosinophilia is characteristic of CSS[89] but is not a feature of MPA[11] or GPA.[12] Extrapulmonary and extrarenal manifestations suggesting small-vessel vasculitis (e.g., palpable purpura, leukocytoclastic vasculitis, mononeuritis multiplex, arthralgias or arthritis, ocular disease, sinusitis) may direct biopsies at these sites. Histological features of granulomatous vasculitis are consistent with GPA or CSS whereas granulomas are lacking in MPA.[11,100] Radiographic features may discriminate granulomatous vasculitides from MPA. In GPA (and less commonly in CSS), focal nodular or cavitary mass lesions may be seen.[12] These are not found in MPA.[11] The diagnosis of CSS can usually be readily established by a pronounced eosinophilic component in the blood or in extravascular sites.[67,89] However, discriminating GPA from MPA may be difficult or impossible as small-vessel vasculitis is common to both disorders. By definition, GPA is associated with concomitant granulomatous inflammation, typically, but not invariably involving the upper and lower respiratory tracts.[12] The latter may lead to the highly distinctive features attributed to GPA including sinusitis, otitis media, nasal or laryngotracheal ulcerations, subglottic stenosis, and cavitary pulmonary nodules.[12]

Characteristics of ANCA

The identification of circulating antibodies directed against cytoplasmic components of neutrophils and monocytes (i.e., ANCA) represented a major advance in the classification and understanding of vasculitis.[68,75] Using ethanol-fixed granulocytes incubated with patient serum, two distinct patterns of ANCA are identified by IF techniques: cytoplasmic (c-ANCA) and perinuclear (p-ANCA) (Fig. 68-9). The p-ANCA pattern is an artifact of fixation causing movement of the target antigens to a perinuclear location. These differing IF patterns reflect distinct antigenic specificities.

In both radioimmunoassays and ELISA, the antibody responsible for c-ANCA is directed against proteinase 3 (PR3).[68,75] The p-ANCA pattern is usually due to an antibody to myeloperoxidase (MPO).[68,75] MPO-ANCA is usually associated with small-vessel vasculitis, but multiple p-ANCA antibodies directed against a variety of antigens (e.g., cathepsin G, lactoferrin, and elastin) may be seen in nonvasculitic inflammatory disorders including CTD and inflammatory bowel or liver disease.[68,75] Therefore, while c-ANCA is more than 90% specific for small-vessel vasculitis, p-ANCA is nonspecific. In untreated GPA, circulating c-ANCA (PR3-ANCA) is detected in more than 70% of patients; the incidence is lower (40% to 65%) in patients with limited disease (e.g., involvement confined to the upper respiratory tract).[12] By contrast, p-ANCA (MPO-ANCA) is rarely found in GPA. Circulating ANCAs are present in more than 70% of patients with MPA[7,11,70] and 30% to 70% of patients with CSS.[62,67,88] In MPA either c-ANCA or MPO-ANCA may be present, but MPO is more common.[70] Circulating ANCAs have been found in fewer than 20% of patients with classic PAN.[67] When present, antibodies have shown MPO antigenic specificity. Individual patients almost never have both c-ANCA and p-ANCA. Most ANCAs are of the IgG class. However, IgM ANCAs associated with severe DAH have been described, either concomitant with IgG-ANCA or in the absence of IgG-ANCA.[102] It is unknown how often patients with ANCA-negative vasculitis would be ANCA-positive if reagents that detected IgM antibodies were used.

The antigenic specificities of ANCA (i.e., PR3 or MPO) may provide clues to the nature of the underlying disorder and may assist in categorizing the type of disease, but overlap exists.[68,75] Biopsies are important to differentiate the nature of the underlying vasculitic disorder. For example, patients with c-ANCA and small-vessel vasculitis may be misclassified as MPA if clinically inapparent areas of granulomatous inflammation are overlooked. For clinical purposes, distinguishing GPA from MPA is not critical, because therapy and management are similar.[78] Circulating p-ANCA (MPO) or c-ANCA (PR3) are present in more than 70% of patients with pauci-immune necrotizing GN (renal vasculitis).[30,68,75,103] ANCA-negative patients usually have disease limited to the kidney. Nearly all patients with concomitant DAH have circulating ANCA. Indeed, a negative ANCA provides strong evidence against vasculitis as the cause of DAH and GN. When applied to patients with RPGN, a positive ANCA almost invariably predicts pauci-immune necrotizing GN. In the setting of clinical, laboratory, and radiologic features that are highly suggestive of DAH and RPGN, a positive c-ANCA or MPO-ANCA, together with a negative anti-GBM and ANA assay, is virtually diagnostic of systemic vasculitis (e.g., GPA or MPA). Similarly, a positive ANCA (usually MPO-ANCA) is sufficient to diagnose lung-limited MPA, provided the clinical presentation is typical of DAH and nonimmune causes of DAH have been excluded. Most patients previously diagnosed as having idiopathic IPH likely had lung-limited MPA or ANCA-associated pulmonary capillaritis.

Problems with using serum ANCA to diagnose vasculitis arise when the clinical presentation is ambiguous. The low incidence of vasculitis in the general population dictates that the positive predictive value of ANCA will be low when applied indiscriminately. Routine assay of serum ANCA in patients with nonspecific respiratory complaints yields a high rate of false-positive results. Given the risks of immunosuppressive therapy, misinterpretation of ANCA may lead to devastating consequences. Accordingly, results of serum ANCA assays must be interpreted in light of the entire clinical picture.

Anti-GBM disease and vasculitis have traditionally been viewed as distinct clinicopathological entities. However, up to 30% of patients with anti-GBM disease (as evidenced by anti-GBM antibody in serum and linear deposits of IgG in kidney biopsy) also have serum MPO-ANCA.[7,32,15] The coexistence of ANCA and anti-GBM antibodies is almost certainly not a chance occurrence, given the rarity of both antibodies in the general population.[15] It is possible that ANCA initiates vascular injury, and anti-GBM antibody then forms in response to the damaged basement membrane.

The role of ANCA in the pathogenesis of vasculitis is uncertain, but these antibodies probably mediate vascular damage.[68,74,75,104] Sera from patients with either c-ANCA or MPO-ANCA induce neutrophils to undergo

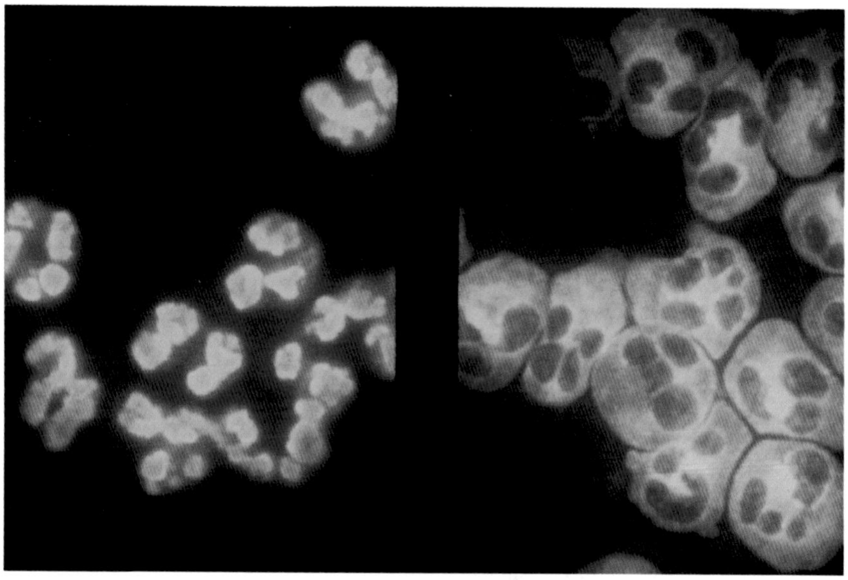

Figure 68-9 Indirect immunofluorescent stains demonstrating two distinct types of anti-neutrophil antibodies. On the left panel, note the perinuclear pattern of immunofluorescence characteristic of p-ANCA (myeloperoxidase epitope). On the right panel, a coarse granular pattern of immunofluorescence within the cytoplasm is evident, characteristic of c-ANCA (proteinase-3 epitope).

a respiratory burst with release of reactive oxygen species and proteolytic enzymes.[104] Cytokine-primed neutrophils are stimulated by ANCA to damage human endothelial cells in vitro.[104] These observations, together with correlations of ANCA titer with clinical disease in humans (although imperfect), suggest that ANCAs are not innocent markers of vasculitis but play a crucial role in mediating vessel injury.[68,75,104]

Therapy

Therapy of DAH due to ANCA-associated syndromes depends on the underlying disorder and the extent and severity of symptoms. Irrespective of etiology, the most immediate concern in patients with severe immune DAH is to control intrapulmonary bleeding, which may be fatal. Besides general supportive measures, high-dose "pulse" methylprednisolone (followed by a tapering regimen of corticosteroids) should be given. The presence of renal involvement *or* progression of DAH on corticosteroids is an indication for adding CYC (with or without empiric plasma exchange).[18] Plasma exchange has been used, with anecdotal successes, as therapy for ANCA-associated systemic vasculitis with severe renal insufficiency[43,105–109] or DAH.[43] Because ANCA may play a pivotal role in mediating tissue injury, plasmapheresis may be beneficial in selected patients (particularly those with DAH[43] or severe renal failure, i.e., serum creatinine >4 mg%[41,42] or dialysis-dependent).[105,107,109,110] When plasma exchange is used to treat ANCA-associated DAH, it may be preferable to use an apparatus that efficiently removes both IgM and IgG, because of the reported association of IgM-ANCA and DAH.[110] Protein A immunoadsorption has also been used to treat patients with DAH and GN,[111] in the hope of removing pathogenic antibodies without producing the side effects of plasma exchange. Additional strategies for patients resistant to conventional therapies include high-dose, intermittent intravenous immunoglobulin G (IVIG).[112] The mechanism of action is uncertain but may involve binding of ANCA idiotype by anti-idiotype antibodies in the intravenous IgG preparation.[112]

The role of serial ANCA determinations in following patients with vasculitis is controversial. We do not base therapeutic decisions on the ANCA titer alone. However, a rising titer should alert the clinician to the possibility of disease exacerbation and clinical follow-up should be intensified. Serial ANCA titers may help differentiate disease relapse from nonimmune causes of pulmonary infiltrates. However, ANCA titers do not obviate the need to aggressively evaluate patients with vasculitis presenting with a new pulmonary process while receiving immunosuppressive therapy.

CONNECTIVE TISSUE DISORDERS

■ SYSTEMIC LUPUS ERYTHEMATOSUS

Alveolar hemorrhage is a rare, but potentially catastrophic, complication of SLE, with mortality rates as high as 50%.[16,113–115] In one large tertiary care center, 19 episodes of DAH were observed among 15 patients with SLE, accounting for 3.7% of hospitalizations for complications of SLE.[16] Alveolar hemorrhage complicating SLE is almost invariably accompanied by other manifestations of active SLE.[16,113,114,116] Alveolar hemorrhage is rarely the sole or presenting feature of SLE.[16,116] Clinical and radiographic features of DAH complicating SLE are similar to other DAH syndromes. However, in SLE-associated DAH, GN is usually, but not uniformly, present.[16,113,114] Diffuse, bilateral alveolar infiltrates, dyspnea, and hypoxemia are characteristic (Fig. 68-10). Hemoptysis is noted in a minority of patients at presentation, obscuring the diagnosis.[16,114,116] The diffuse pulmonary infiltrates must be differentiated from other pulmonary complications of SLE[117] including lupus pneumonitis, opportunistic infections, congestive heart failure, uremia, or pulmonary embolism.

Lung biopsy may be needed to exclude alternative diagnoses and corroborate the diagnosis of DAH. However, the risk of lung biopsy

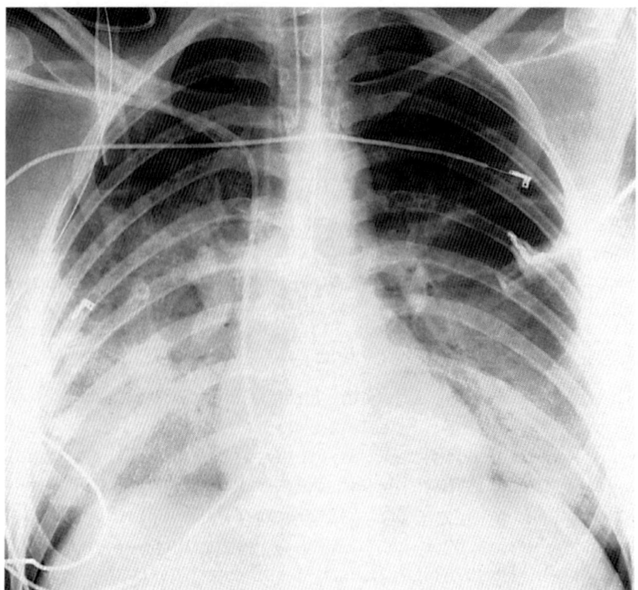

Figure 68-10 Systemic lupus erythematosus (SLE). Posterior–anterior (PA) chest radiograph reveals extensive bilateral alveolar infiltrates in a 22-year-old woman with SLE, hemoptysis, and anemia.

may be substantial in critically ill patients with fulminant DAH and respiratory failure. In addition, as with other immune DAH syndromes, histopathological features of DAH complicating SLE are nonspecific. The dominant feature is intra-alveolar hemorrhage and capillaritis, without macroscopic necrosis.[16] The small-vessel necrotizing vasculitis rarely extends to arterioles and small muscular arteries in addition to capillaries. Granular deposits of IgG or C3 (consistent with immune complexes) have been found in up to 50% of cases of DAH complicating SLE.[16,118] Because of its potential morbidity, we rarely advise surgical lung biopsy to diagnose DAH. Provided clinical features are consistent, the diagnosis of DAH can often be established by fiberoptic bronchoscopy with BAL and transbronchial lung biopsies. Transbronchial biopsies may demonstrate foci of capillaritis with intra-alveolar hemorrhage, but due to sampling error, these features may be missed. However, the presence of gross blood in the airways or serosanguineous BAL fluid, large numbers of hemosiderin-laden macrophages, absence of purulent sputum, and lack of infectious organisms by appropriate stains strongly supports the diagnosis of autoimmune DAH and justifies institution of therapy. Transbronchial lung biopsies may be deferred in acutely ill patients with severe DAH and respiratory failure. In this context, BAL alone is adequate, primarily to exclude local or infectious causes of bleeding.

Due to the rarity of this syndrome, prospective, controlled trials evaluating therapy have not been performed. As with other causes of immune DAH, high-dose IV pulse methylprednisolone (1 g daily for 3 days), followed by gradual steroid taper is the mainstay of therapy.[16,115,116] Immunosuppressive or cytotoxic agents may be considered for DAH refractory to corticosteroids.[114–116,119] The role of plasmapheresis has not been elucidated, but anecdotal successes have been cited for severe DAH complicating SLE.[16,110,115,120] We reserve plasmapheresis for patients with severe DAH refractory to corticosteroids and/or cytotoxic agents. Rituximab was efficacious in anecdotal cases of SLE-associated DAH refractory to immunosuppressive agents.[119]

■ OTHER CONNECTIVE TISSUE DISORDERS

Anecdotal reports of DAH, with or without capillaritis, have been described in association with rheumatoid arthritis,[121] scleroderma,[122] mixed connective tissue disease,[121] polymyositis,[123] antiphospholipid antibody syndrome,[124] Henoch–Schönlein syndrome,[125] and Behçet disease.[64] The clinical spectrum ranges from minimal hemoptysis to life-threatening respiratory failure. In addition to capillaritis and DAH, additional histopathological features on lung biopsies include vasculitis of small and medium muscular pulmonary arteries, DAD, and organizing pneumonia. In view of the rarity of DAH complicating these diverse CTDs, data regarding therapy are limited. High-dose (pulse) intravenous methylprednisolone is advised as initial treatment. In patients with fulminant or corticosteroid-recalcitrant disease, CYC, alone or combined with plasmapheresis,[110,122] should be added.

ALVEOLAR HEMORRHAGE IN IMMUNOCOMPROMISED HOSTS

Alveolar hemorrhage may occur in immunocompromised patients.[27,126] Alveolar hemorrhage may reflect injury to pulmonary endothelial or epithelial cells (secondary to chemotherapy or radiation toxicity), thrombocytopenia (secondary to bone marrow toxicity), pulmonary edema, pulmonary malignancies, and diverse infectious and nonspecific interstitial pneumonias.[126] The incidence of DAH in severely immunocompromised hosts with hematologic malignancies or bone marrow transplants has varied from 11% to 64%.[25,126] The variable frequency in large part is due to differing diagnostic criteria for the diagnosis of DAH. Subclinical alveolar hemorrhage (as evidenced by increased numbers of hemosiderin-laden macrophages in BAL) occurs in up to one-third of immunocompromised hosts with pulmonary infiltrates and may reflect pulmonary endothelial or epithelial injury from diverse causes.[27] Nonimmune causes of DAH in this patient population include coagulopathy, thrombocytopenia or platelet dysfunction, renal failure, congestive heart failure, bronchopulmonary Kaposi sarcoma, and diverse infections.[27,28]

ALVEOLAR HEMORRHAGE COMPLICATING BONE MARROW TRANSPLANTATION

DAH occurs in approximately 5% (range 2%–31%) of hematopoietic stem cell transplantation (HSCT) or bone marrow transplant (BMT) recipients receiving pre-BMT conditioning with high-dose chemotherapy or radiation therapy.[25,26,127–130] Opportunistic infections or thrombocytopenia account for some cases of DAH,[26,128,129] but a distinct syndrome of DAH in this population unrelated to infection is well accepted.[126,127] The incidence of DAH is similar among autologous and allogeneic HSCT recipients.[25,127,130] Risk factors for DAH include age >40 years,[128,130] myeloablative conditioning,[25,128,130] thoracic[131] or total body irradiation,[25,132] acute severe graft versus host disease (GVHD),[128,132] severe oral mucositis,[133] renal failure,[25,133] airway inflammation or increased proportions of bronchial neutrophils and eosinophils,[134] and leukocyte recovery.[25,134] Thrombocytopenia or coagulopathy do not predict DAH.[25,131,133] DAH usually develops within 10 to 40 days after BMT, but may develop earlier or later.[127,131,132] Case reports of DAH developing immediately following autologous bone marrow transfusion suggest that components within the transfusion (e.g., dimethylsulfoxide [DMSO] for cryopreservation of blood stem cells) may mediate acute lung injury in some cases.[135]

Progressive dyspnea, hypoxemia, and respiratory failure are typical.[25,128,130] Even with extensive DAH, hemoptysis is uncommon (<20%).[127,130,134] Chest radiographs *initially* demonstrate predominantly interstitial opacities, which evolve to diffuse alveolar opacities, with a confluent alveolar pattern involving all lobes. Serosanguineous or frankly bloody BAL fluid,[127,128,130] with negative stains for infectious organisms, support the diagnosis of DAH. Lung biopsies or necropsies typically reveal histological features of both DAD and DAH.[129,133,134,136] However, the risk of lung biopsy is excessive in critically ill patients, many of whom are thrombocytopenic.[130] Hence the diagnosis is made by clinical, radiographic, and BAL findings.[127,130]

The clinical course of DAH is variable, but severe respiratory failure requiring mechanical ventilation is common.[127,133] Mortality rates in patients with DAH are high (60-day mortality ranging from 48% to 84%).[26,127,128,133] In one study, hospital mortality was lower among autologous (28%) compared to allogeneic (70%) SCT recipients and early onset DAH (within 30 days of transplant) (32% mortality) compared to 70% for late-onset DAH.[127] Secondary infections are serious and potentially lethal.[26,126,128,129]

Multiple mechanisms may mediate alveolar hemorrhage in this patient population. Diffuse injury to the pulmonary microvasculature, secondary to chemotherapy or radiation therapy, coupled with a heightened inflammatory response in the airways, appear to be operative.[25] Bleeding may be amplified by a precipitating factor such as coagulopathy, pulmonary edema, GVHD, or infections. DAD, a pathological hallmark seen in toxic lung injury from chemotherapy, radiation therapy, or viral infections, is frequently observed in lung biopsies or necropsies in bone marrow recipients with DAH.[127] An association between microangiopathy and DAH in patients receiving BMT for hematologic malignancies was cited.[137] Neutrophils and other inflammatory cells likely play important roles in the pathogenesis of DAH. The onset of DAH frequently coincides with marrow recovery and reappearance of neutrophils within the circulation or BAL fluid. Influx of neutrophils may promote the lung injury by release of oxygen radicals, proteases, and other phlogistic mediators.[25,134] Hematopoietic growth factors (e.g., granulocyte colony–stimulating factor) may exacerbate alveolar damage and capillary leakage by increasing neutrophil influx into the lungs.[25]

High-dose pulse IV corticosteroids are considered standard of care for DAH,[25,26,127,129] but randomized, controlled studies are lacking and a survival benefit has not been established. Unfortunately, DAH or bloody BAL fluid may be seen in infectious causes of pneumonia (particularly due to cytomegalovirus [CMV] or *Aspergillus* spp.),[130] and high-dose corticosteroids could be disastrous under these circumstances. Infectious etiologies must be rigorously excluded. Among patients who respond favorably to corticosteroids, the dose can be gradually tapered over 2 to 6 weeks.[25,127] A more prolonged course is appropriate for patients with GVHD or other complications requiring long-term corticosteroid therapy. Anecdotal response to recombinant factor VIIa was cited in one allogeneic SCT recipient with DAH.[138]

ALVEOLAR HEMORRHAGE COMPLICATING HIV INFECTION

DAH can complicate human immunodeficiency virus (HIV) infection. The incidence and clinical significance of DAH is not clear, as additional pulmonary processes (e.g., opportunistic infections;[139] Kaposi sarcoma[140]) are usually present.[28] Subclinical episodes of alveolar hemorrhage are common, as studies in HIV-infected patients with pulmonary infiltrates detected more than 20% hemosiderin-laden macrophages in BAL fluid in 15% to 44% of patients.[27,28] In one study of 203 HIV-infected patients with pulmonary symptoms who underwent BAL, alveolar hemorrhage (AH) was detected in 73; however, AH was severe in only eight patients and AH did not affect survival.[28] Thrombocytopenia, coagulopathy, renal failure, hydrostatic pulmonary edema, CMV pneumonia, and Kaposi sarcoma were more frequent in patients with AH compared to HIV-infected controls without AH.[28] Pulmonary capillaritis has been cited in occasional patients, most of whom had concomitant opportunistic infections. CMV pneumonia has been implicated as a cause of DAH in HIV-infected patients.[139] CMV exhibits tropism for endothelial cells, and CMV may induce vascular injury or thrombotic microangiopathy. Antiviral therapy (e.g., ganciclovir) may be curative for CMV-associated DAH. Opportunistic pathogens[139] or endobronchial Kaposi sarcoma[140] account for most cases of DAH in HIV-infected individuals. The incidence and appropriate therapy of DAH of unknown etiology in the setting of acquired immunodeficiency syndrome (AIDS) has not been defined.

ALVEOLAR HEMORRHAGE DUE TO EXOGENOUS AGENTS

Certain exogenous agents or drugs[7,17] (e.g., trimellitic anhydride,[141] isocyanates,[142] D-penicillamine,[143] cocaine,[144] diphenylhydantoin,[145] propylthiouracil,[146] hydralazine,[147] sulfasalazine,[147] allopurinol,[1,147] all-*trans*-retinoic acid (ATRA),[148] minocycline[149] are rare causes of DAH. An exhaustive list of drugs capable of causing DAH is available on www.pneumotox.com. Circulating ANCAs, GN, and DAH have been linked with some agents (particularly d-penicillamine,[143] hydralazine,[150] propylthiouracil,[146] methimazole, and carbimazole[151]). Lung biopsies have rarely been performed in these cases of DAH. However, pulmonary capillaritis (without immune deposits) is the most common finding.[7,17]

ATRA, a therapeutic agent for acute promyelocytic leukemia, may be associated with "retinoic acid syndrome," characterized by fever, thrombosis, pulmonary infiltrates, and DAH.[148,152] The onset is 2 to 21 days after initiation of treatment. In this circumstance, ATRA is continued but high-dose IV corticosteroids should be administered.

Propylthiouracil can cause a systemic small-vessel vasculitis with necrotizing GN, leukocytoclastic vasculitis, ANCAs, and DAH secondary to pulmonary capillaritis.[146,147] Withdrawal of the drug may be associated with resolution of the disease, but corticosteroids or immunosuppressive agents are indicated in patients with severe DAH or renal failure.

A variety of chemotherapeutic agents (e.g., bischloroethyl nitrosourea [BCNU], carmustine, CYC, methotrexate, mitomycin C, bleomycin, or busulfan) may cause lung injury and fibrosis.[17,153] In some cases, DAH may result from epithelial injury and injury to the alveolar capillary basement membranes.[17] In this context, fatality rates are high (more than 50%).[17,153] High-dose corticosteroids are recommended, but efficacy is uncertain.

Trimellitic anhydride (TMA), a chemical used in manufacturing plastics and epoxy resins, may elicit pulmonary hemorrhage and anemia.[141,142] Most patients with DAH secondary to TMA exposure recover within a few days following removal from the offending environment. An immune mechanism is likely, as circulating IgG antibodies against trimellitic protein were found in some patients with DAH, suggesting TMA acts as a hapten.[142] TMA may cause asthma, rhinitis, and hemolytic anemia mediated by IgE antibodies directed against trimellitic protein. Animal models of TMA-induced lung disease have also been developed.[141] Induction of serum antibodies against epitopes of TMA produced acute lung injury in animals, mediated by at least two types of humoral antibodies. It is also possible that TMA may exert a direct toxic effect on alveolar endothelium. This syndrome is exceptionally rare, as only sporadic cases have been described. Exposure to isocyanates in spray paint has been linked to occupational asthma and (in a few cases) DAH.[154] The mechanism is likely mediated by high levels of IgE and IgG antibodies against diisocyanates.[142] Thus, exposure to TMA or isocyanates, and possibly other chemicals, can elicit hemorrhagic pneumonitis, likely mediated by circulating antibodies (IgG or IgE) and immune complexes.

Smoking, snorting, or intravenous "crack" cocaine has been associated with hemoptysis and varying degrees of DAH,[144,155] including rare fatalities. Histopathological features of cocaine-induced DAH are nonspecific, but include DAD, acute or chronic DAH, interstitial pneumonitis/fibrosis, and intra-alveolar edema.[156] The mechanism of DAH is not clear but may relate to direct toxic injury from cocaine or its contaminants, vasospasm, or a combination of both mechanisms. This syndrome typically reverses with cessation of exposure. The frequency of clinically significant DAH associated with inhaled or intravenous use of cocaine has not been established.

When drug- or hapten-induced DAH is suspected, immediate avoidance of the implicated agent or drug is essential. For acute or severe cases, a brief course of high-dose corticosteroids is warranted. Plasmapheresis or cytotoxic agents may be considered for fulminant cases refractory to corticosteroids, but data supporting their use are lacking.

Finally, coagulopathies, severe thrombocytopenia, or the use of anticoagulants, thrombolytic agents, or platelet inhibitors may rarely cause DAH.[157–159] In this context, the histology is "bland" without evidence for capillaritis or acute inflammation.

ALVEOLAR HEMORRHAGE DUE TO MOLDS

Acute, life-threatening DAH in infants identified fungal contamination as the etiology.[160,161] Exposure to *Stachybotrys chartarum* and other toxigenic fungi elicits the syndrome.[160] *Stachybotrys chartarum* produces several classes of toxins including hemolysins, proteinases, macrocyclic trichothecenes, phenylspirodrimanes, and others.[160] Acute respiratory distress, progressing to respiratory failure requiring mechanical ventilatory support, may occur.[160] High-dose IV corticosteroids are warranted for acute DAH. Long-term management mandates removal of infants from the residential environment to avoid relapse.[160,161] This syndrome has rarely been reported in adults, but must be considered in water-damaged homes or environs where mold/fungal contamination exists.[161]

IDIOPATHIC PULMONARY HEMOSIDEROSIS

IPH is an exceptionally rare cause of DAH that occurs primarily in infants and children.[23,162–164] The estimated incidence is 0.2 to 1.2 cases per million.[22,165] Many children with IPH have a history of milk or gluten sensitivity.[166] A subset of adults with celiac sprue manifest IPH,[167] which may respond to elimination of gluten from the diet.[168] Clinical features of IPH are similar to immune causes of DAH, but extrapulmonary or renal involvement is lacking.[23] Serum or tissue antibodies (including ANCA, immune complexes, anti-GBM antibody) are also absent. A diagnosis of IPH can be made *only* when other specific causes of DAH have been *reliably* excluded. Most early series of IPH, published in the 1960s and 1970s, antedated the availability of serologies and immunohistochemical assays (e.g., ANCA, anti-GBM antibody, etc.).[169,170] It is likely that most cases formerly diagnosed as IPH in adults had ANCA-associated vasculitis, MPA, or underlying CTD.

The onset of the disease is typically in infants and young children (<5 years old).[23,162] The clinical course of IPH is variable, but recurrent episodes of DAH over several years are characteristic.[23,164,171] Spontaneous remissions without long-term sequelae have been cited in up to 25% of cases.[164] Sequelae of recurrent episodes of DAH include pulmonary fibrosis, progressive respiratory failure, and cor pulmonale.[23,164,171] Early studies cited median survival rates of 3 to 6 years,[162,165] but more recent studies suggest a more favorable prognosis, with many patients surviving >10 to 15 years.[164,171] During acute episodes, chest radiographs demonstrate bilateral alveolar infiltrates. Following cessation of bleeding, chest radiographs may normalize within 1 to 2 weeks. Reticulonodular infiltrates may be observed as the process is resolving or with recurrent episodes (Fig. 68-11). CT reveals areas of ground-glass opacification, representing foci of alveolar hemorrhage. Thickening of interlobular septae and honeycombing may be observed in a subset of patients who progress to pulmonary fibrosis.[172] Hemoptysis may be absent, particularly in young children who may be unable to expectorate blood. Iron-deficiency anemia is characteristic and can be profound.[23,164,171,173] Iron deficiency may persist despite normal total body iron stores, because hemosiderin within alveolar macrophages is not available to developing erythrocytes. Siderophages may be found in sputum, BAL fluid, or tracheal or gastric aspirates in patients with recent episodes of DAH.[22,164,171] Lung biopsies may reveal fresh areas of alveolar hemorrhage or patchy interstitial fibrosis and aggregates of hemosiderin-laden macrophages from prior episodes of alveolar hemorrhage (Fig. 68-12).[23,164]

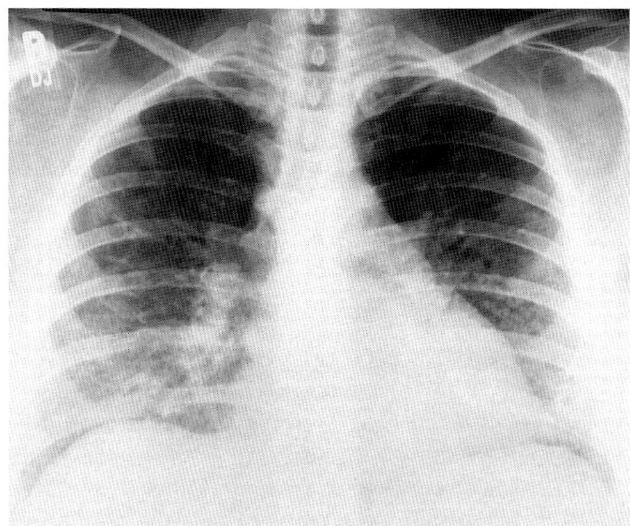

Figure 68-11 Idiopathic pulmonary hemosiderosis (IPH). Posterior–anterior (PA) chest radiograph demonstrates bilateral reticulonodular infiltrates in a 28-year-old woman with IPH confirmed 10 years earlier by open lung biopsy.

The pathogenesis of IPH is not known. In children, associations between IPH and cow's milk hypersensitivity, celiac disease,[173] IgA monoclonal gammopathy, autoimmune hemolytic anemia, and autoimmune thyrotoxicosis have been suggested,[164] but a pathogenetic link has not been substantiated. Resolution of pulmonary symptoms following elimination of milk products or gluten from diet[167,173] supports a role for exogenous factors in the pathogenesis in at least some cases. No genetic basis has been found, but clusters within families have been described.[170,174]

In view of the rarity of IPH, optimal therapy is not clear. Corticosteroids are considered the mainstay of therapy,[22–24,163] but controlled studies evaluating therapeutic regimens have not been done. Because IPH is life-threatening, most physicians treat acute episodes with daily corticosteroids and taper to the lowest dose that appears to control the disease. Long-term (and possibly indefinite) therapy may be required to prevent recurrences. Favorable responses have been cited with azathioprine,[175] CYC,[176] or other immunosuppressive agents[171] in patients failing corticosteroids. Chronic immunosuppressive agents may improve prognosis for patients with corticosteroid-recalcitrant disease or patients experiencing repetitive relapses of DAH.[171] In this context, we prefer azathioprine over CYC given the heightened risk of neoplasia and gonadal toxicities associated with the long-term use of CYC.[177]

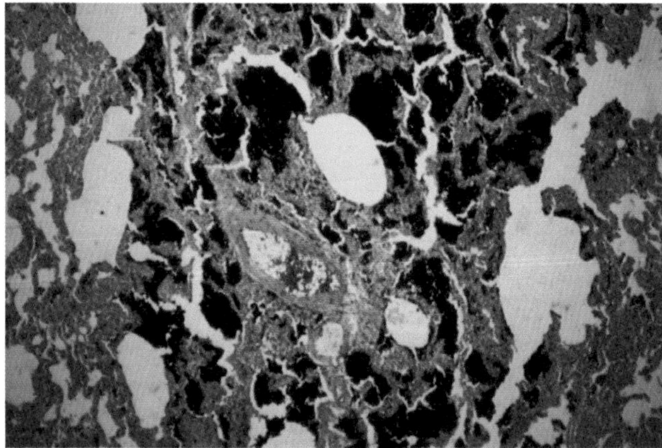

Figure 68-12 Idiopathic pulmonary hemosiderosis (IPH). Photomicrograph demonstrating extensive deposits of hemosiderin within alveolar interstitium (Prussian blue stain).

REFERENCES

1. Cordier JF, Cottin V. Alveolar hemorrhage in vasculitis: primary and secondary. *Semin Respir Crit Care Med.* 2011;32:310–321.
2. Lara AR, Schwarz MI. Diffuse alveolar hemorrhage. *Chest.* 2010;137:1164–1171.
3. Leatherman JW, Davies SF, Hoidal JR. Alveolar hemorrhage syndromes: diffuse microvascular lung hemorrhage in immune and idiopathic disorders. *Medicine (Baltimore).* 1984;63:343–361.
4. Rhee H, Song SH, Lee YJ, et al. Pandemic H1N1 influenza A viral infection complicated by atypical hemolytic uremic syndrome and diffuse alveolar hemorrhage. *Clin Exp Nephrol.* 2011;15:948–952.
5. de Prost N, Parrot A, Cuquemelle E, et al. Diffuse alveolar hemorrhage in immunocompetent patients: etiologies and prognosis revisited. *Respir Med.* 2012;106:1021–1032.
6. Travis WD, Colby TV, Lombard C, Carpenter HA. A clinicopathologic study of 34 cases of diffuse pulmonary hemorrhage with lung biopsy confirmation. *Am J Surg Pathol.* 1990;14:1112–1125.
7. Lee AS, Specks U. Pulmonary capillaritis. *Semin Respir Crit Care Med.* 2004;25:547–555.
8. Fishbein GA, Fishbein MC. Lung vasculitis and alveolar hemorrhage: pathology. *Semin Respir Crit Care Med.* 2011;32:254–263.
9. Frankel SK, Jayne D. The pulmonary vasculitides. *Clin Chest Med.* 2010;31:519–536.
10. Lauque D, Cadranel J, Lazor R, et al. Microscopic polyangiitis with alveolar hemorrhage. A study of 29 cases and review of the literature. Groupe d'Etudes et de Recherche sur les Maladies "Orphelines" Pulmonaires (GERM"O"P). *Medicine (Baltimore).* 2000;79:222–233.
11. Smyth L, Gaskin G, Pusey CD. Microscopic polyangiitis. *Semin Respir Crit Care Med.* 2004;25:523–533.
12. Lynch JP 3rd, Tazelaar H. Wegener granulomatosis (granulomatosis with polyangiitis): evolving concepts in treatment. *Semin Respir Crit Care Med.* 2011;32:274–297.
13. Sanders JS, Rutgers A, Stegeman CA, Kallenberg CG. Pulmonary: renal syndrome with a focus on anti-GBM disease. *Semin Respir Crit Care Med.* 2011;32:328–334.
14. Lazor R, Bigay-Game L, Cottin V, et al. Alveolar hemorrhage in anti-basement membrane antibody disease: a series of 28 cases. *Medicine (Baltimore).* 2007;86:181–193.
15. Chan AL, Louie S, Leslie KO, Juarez MM, Albertson TE. Cutting edge issues in Goodpasture's disease. *Clin Rev Allergy Immunol.* 2011;41:151–162.
16. Zamora MR, Warner ML, Tuder R, Schwarz MI. Diffuse alveolar hemorrhage and systemic lupus erythematosus. Clinical presentation, histology, survival, and outcome. *Medicine (Baltimore).* 1997;76:192–202.
17. Schwarz MI, Fontenot AP. Drug-induced diffuse alveolar hemorrhage syndromes and vasculitis. *Clin Chest Med.* 2004;25:133–140.
18. Kokolina E, Alexopoulos E, Dimitriadis C, et al. Immunosuppressive therapy and clinical evolution in forty-nine patients with antineutrophil cytoplasmic antibody-associated glomerulonephritis. *Ann N Y Acad Sci.* 2005;1051:597–605.
19. Hauer HA, Bajema IM, van Houwelingen HC, et al. Renal histology in ANCA-associated vasculitis: differences between diagnostic and serologic subgroups. *Kidney Int.* 2002;61:80–89.

20. Beirne GJ, Wagnild JP, Zimmerman SW, Macken PD, Burkholder PM. Idiopathic crescentic glomerulonephritis. *Medicine (Baltimore)*. 1977;56:349–381.
21. Cole E, Cattran D, Magil A, et al. A prospective randomized trial of plasma exchange as additive therapy in idiopathic crescentic glomerulonephritis. The Canadian Apheresis Study Group. *Am J Kidney Dis*. 1992;20:261–269.
22. Ioachimescu OC, Sieber S, Kotch A. Idiopathic pulmonary haemosiderosis revisited. *Eur Respir J*. 2004;24:162–170.
23. Milman N, Pedersen FM. Idiopathic pulmonary haemosiderosis. Epidemiology, pathogenic aspects and diagnosis. *Respir Med*. 1998;92:902–907.
24. Kjellman B, Elinder G, Garwicz S, Svan H. Idiopathic pulmonary haemosiderosis in Swedish children. *Acta Paediatr Scand*. 1984;73:584–588.
25. Afessa B, Tefferi A, Litzow MR, Krowka MJ, Wylam ME, Peters SG. Diffuse alveolar hemorrhage in hematopoietic stem cell transplant recipients. *Am J Respir Crit Care Med*. 2002;166: 641–645.
26. Gupta S, Jain A, Warneke CL, et al. Outcome of alveolar hemorrhage in hematopoietic stem cell transplant recipients. *Bone Marrow Transplant*. 2007;40:71–78.
27. De Lassence A, Fleury-Feith J, Escudier E, Beaune J, Bernaudin JF, Cordonnier C. Alveolar hemorrhage. Diagnostic criteria and results in 194 immunocompromised hosts. *Am J Respir Crit Care Med*. 1995;151:157–163.
28. Vincent B, Flahault A, Antoine M, et al. AIDS-related alveolar hemorrhage: a prospective study of 273 BAL procedures. *Chest*. 2001;120:1078–1084.
29. Badesch DB, Zamora M, Fullerton D, et al. Pulmonary capillaritis: a possible histologic form of acute pulmonary allograft rejection. *J Heart Lung Transplant*. 1998;17:415–422.
30. Chen M, Kallenberg CG, Zhao MH. ANCA-negative pauci-immune crescentic glomerulonephritis. *Nat Rev Nephrol*. 2009;5: 313–318.
31. Gallagher H, Kwan JT, Jayne DR. Pulmonary renal syndrome: a 4-year, single-center experience. *Am J Kidney Dis*. 2002;39: 42–47.
32. Levy JB, Hammad T, Coulthart A, Dougan T, Pusey CD. Clinical features and outcome of patients with both ANCA and anti-GBM antibodies. *Kidney Int*. 2004;66:1535–1540.
33. Fischer EG, Lager DJ. Anti-glomerular basement membrane glomerulonephritis: a morphologic study of 80 cases. *Am J Clin Pathol*. 2006;125:445–450.
34. Haas M, Eustace JA. Immune complex deposits in ANCA-associated crescentic glomerulonephritis: a study of 126 cases. *Kidney Int*. 2004;65:2145–2152.
35. Chen M, Xing GQ, Yu F, Liu G, Zhao MH. Complement deposition in renal histopathology of patients with ANCA-associated pauci-immune glomerulonephritis. *Nephrol Dial Transplant*. 2009;24:1247–1252.
36. Zauner I, Bach D, Braun N, et al. Predictive value of initial histology and effect of plasmapheresis on long-term prognosis of rapidly progressive glomerulonephritis. *Am J Kidney Dis*. 2002;39:28–35.
37. Casian A, Jayne D. Management of alveolar hemorrhage in lung vasculitides. *Semin Respir Crit Care Med*. 2011;32: 335–345.
38. Stone JH, Merkel PA, Spiera R, et al. Rituximab versus cyclophosphamide for ANCA-associated vasculitis. *N Engl J Med*. 2010;363:221–232.
39. Jones RB, Cohen Tervaert JW, Hauser T, et al. Rituximab versus cyclophosphamide in ANCA-associated renal vasculitis. *N Engl J Med*. 2010;363:211–220.
40. Guillevin L, Lhote F, Gayraud M, et al. Prognostic factors in polyarteritis nodosa and Churg-Strauss syndrome. A prospective study in 342 patients. *Medicine (Baltimore)*. 1996;75:17–28.
41. Casian A, Jayne D. Plasma exchange in the treatment of Wegener's granulomatosis, microscopic polyangiitis, Churg-Strauss syndrome and renal limited vasculitis. *Curr Opin Rheumatol*. 2011;23:12–17.
42. Jayne DR, Gaskin G, Rasmussen N, et al. Randomized trial of plasma exchange or high-dosage methylprednisolone as adjunctive therapy for severe renal vasculitis. *J Am Soc Nephrol*. 2007;18:2180–2188.
43. Klemmer PJ, Chalermskulrat W, Reif MS, Hogan SL, Henke DC, Falk RJ. Plasmapheresis therapy for diffuse alveolar hemorrhage in patients with small-vessel vasculitis. *Am J Kidney Dis*. 2003;42:1149–1153.
44. Saxena R, Bygren P, Arvastson B, Wieslander J. Circulating autoantibodies as serological markers in the differential diagnosis of pulmonary renal syndrome. *J Intern Med*. 1995;238:143–152.
45. Shah MK, Hugghins SY. Characteristics and outcomes of patients with Goodpasture's syndrome. *South Med J*. 2002;95: 1411–1418.
46. Gibelin A, Maldini C, Mahr A. Epidemiology and etiology of wegener granulomatosis,microscopic polyangiitis, Churg-Strauss syndrome and goodpasture syndrome: vasculitides with frequent lung involvement. *Semin Respir Crit Care Med*. 2011;32:264–273.
47. Salama AD, Levy JB, Lightstone L, Pusey CD. Goodpasture's disease. *Lancet*. 2001;358:917–920.
48. Yang R, Hellmark T, Zhao J, et al. Levels of epitope-specific autoantibodies correlate with renal damage in anti-GBM disease. *Nephrol Dial Transplant*. 2009;24:1838–1844.
49. Johnson JP, Moore J Jr, Austin HA 3rd, Balow JE, Antonovych TT, Wilson CB. Therapy of anti-glomerular basement membrane antibody disease: analysis of prognostic significance of clinical, pathologic and treatment factors. *Medicine (Baltimore)*. 1985;64:219–227.
50. Hirayama K, Yamagata K, Kobayashi M, Koyama A. Anti-glomerular basement membrane antibody disease in Japan: part of the nationwide rapidly progressive glomerulonephritis survey in Japan. *Clin Exp Nephrol*. 2008;12:339–347.
51. Levy JB, Turner AN, Rees AJ, Pusey CD. Long-term outcome of anti-glomerular basement membrane antibody disease treated with plasma exchange and immunosuppression. *Ann Intern Med*. 2001;134:1033–1042.
52. Segelmark M, Hellmark T, Wieslander J. The prognostic significance in Goodpasture's disease of specificity, titre and affinity of anti-glomerular-basement-membrane antibodies. *Nephron Clin Pract*. 2003;94:c59–c68.
53. Rutgers A, Slot M, van Paassen P, van Breda Vriesman P, Heeringa P, Tervaert JW. Coexistence of anti-glomerular basement membrane antibodies and myeloperoxidase-ANCAs in crescentic glomerulonephritis. *Am J Kidney Dis*. 2005;46: 253–262.
54. Pedchenko V, Vanacore R, Hudson B. Goodpasture's disease: molecular architecture of the autoantigen provides clues to etiology and pathogenesis. *Curr Opin Nephrol Hypertens*. 2011;20:290–296.

55. Zhao J, Yan Y, Cui Z, Yang R, Zhao MH. The immunoglobulin G subclass distribution of anti-GBM autoantibodies against rHalpha3(IV)NC1 is associated with disease severity. *Hum Immunol.* 2009;70:425–429.

56. Wu J, Hicks J, Borillo J, Glass WF 2nd, Lou YH. CD4(+) T cells specific to a glomerular basement membrane antigen mediate glomerulonephritis. *J Clin Invest.* 2002;109:517–524.

57. Wolf D, Hochegger K, Wolf AM, et al. CD4+CD25+ regulatory T cells inhibit experimental anti-glomerular basement membrane glomerulonephritis in mice. *J Am Soc Nephrol.* 2005;16:1360–1370.

58. Zhou XJ, Lv JC, Zhao MH, Zhang H. Advances in the genetics of anti-glomerular basement membrane disease. *Am J Nephrol.* 2010;32:482–490.

59. Deegens JK, Artz MA, Hoitsma AJ, Wetzels JF. Outcome of renal transplantation in patients with pauci-immune small vessel vasculitis or anti-GBM disease. *Clin Nephrol.* 2003;59:1–9.

60. Khandelwal M, McCormick BB, Lajoie G, Sweet J, Cole E, Cattran DC. Recurrence of anti-GBM disease 8 years after renal transplantation. *Nephrol Dial Transplant.* 2004;19:491–494.

61. Travis WD, Carpenter HA, Lie JT. Diffuse pulmonary hemorrhage. An uncommon manifestation of Wegener's granulomatosis. *Am J Surg Pathol.* 1987;11:702–708.

62. Guillevin L, Cohen P, Gayraud M, Lhote F, Jarrousse B, Casassus P. Churg-Strauss syndrome. Clinical study and long-term follow-up of 96 patients. *Medicine (Baltimore).* 1999;78:26–37.

63. Conron M, Beynon HL. Churg-Strauss syndrome. *Thorax.* 2000;55:870–877.

64. Uzun O, Akpolat T, Erkan L. Pulmonary vasculitis in Behcet disease: a cumulative analysis. *Chest.* 2005;127:2243–2253.

65. Amital H, Rubinow A, Naparstek Y. Alveolar hemorrhage in cryoglobulinemia–an indicator of poor prognosis. *Clin Exp Rheumatol.* 2005;23:616–620.

66. Matsubayashi R, Matsubayashi T, Fujita N, Yokota T, Ohro Y, Enoki H. Pulmonary hemorrhage associated with Henoch-Schonlein purpura in a child. *Clin Rheumatol.* 2008;27:803–805.

67. Mouthon L, Le Toumelin P, Andre MH, Gayraud M, Casassus P, Guillevin L. Polyarteritis nodosa and Churg-Strauss angiitis: characteristics and outcome in 38 patients over 65 years. *Medicine (Baltimore).* 2002;81:27–40.

68. Kallenberg CG. Antineutrophil cytoplasmic autoantibody-associated small-vessel vasculitis. *Curr Opin Rheumatol.* 2007; 19:17–24.

69. Couser WG. Rapidly progressive glomerulonephritis: classification, pathogenetic mechanisms, and therapy. *Am J Kidney Dis.* 1988;11:449–464.

70. Guillevin L, Durand-Gasselin B, Cevallos R, et al. Microscopic polyangiitis: clinical and laboratory findings in eighty-five patients. *Arthritis Rheum.* 1999;42:421–430.

71. Mahr A, Guillevin L, Poissonnet M, Ayme S. Prevalences of polyarteritis nodosa, microscopic polyangiitis, Wegener's granulomatosis, and Churg-Strauss syndrome in a French urban multiethnic population in 2000: a capture-recapture estimate. *Arthritis Rheum.* 2004;51:92–99.

72. Watts RA, Al-Taiar A, Scott DG, Macgregor AJ. Prevalence and incidence of Wegener's granulomatosis in the UK general practice research database. *Arthritis Rheum.* 2009;61:1412–1416.

73. Boomsma MM, Stegeman CA, van der Leij MJ, et al. Prediction of relapses in Wegener's granulomatosis by measurement of antineutrophil cytoplasmic antibody levels: a prospective study. *Arthritis Rheum.* 2000;43:2025–2033.

74. Gomez-Puerta JA, Bosch X. Anti-neutrophil cytoplasmic antibody pathogenesis in small-vessel vasculitis: an update. *Am J Pathol.* 2009;175:1790–1798.

75. Kallenberg CG. Pathogenesis of PR3-ANCA associated vasculitis. *J Autoimmun.* 2008;30:29–36.

76. Fauci AS, Haynes BF, Katz P, Wolff SM. Wegener's granulomatosis: prospective clinical and therapeutic experience with 85 patients for 21 years. *Ann Intern Med.* 1983;98:76–85.

77. Hoffman GS, Leavitt RY, Kerr GS, Fauci AS. The treatment of Wegener's granulomatosis with glucocorticoids and methotrexate. *Arthritis Rheum.* 1992;35:1322–1329.

78. Jayne D, Rasmussen N, Andrassy K, et al. A randomized trial of maintenance therapy for vasculitis associated with antineutrophil cytoplasmic autoantibodies. *N Engl J Med.* 2003;349:36–44.

79. Pagnoux C, Mahr A, Hamidou MA, et al. Azathioprine or methotrexate maintenance for ANCA-associated vasculitis. *N Engl J Med.* 2008;359:2790–2803.

80. de Groot K, Harper L, Jayne DR, et al. Pulse versus daily oral cyclophosphamide for induction of remission in antineutrophil cytoplasmic antibody-associated vasculitis: a randomized trial. *Ann Intern Med.* 2009;150:670–680.

81. Seror R, Pagnoux C, Ruivard M, et al. Treatment strategies and outcome of induction-refractory Wegener's granulomatosis or microscopic polyangiitis: analysis of 32 patients with first-line induction-refractory disease in the WEGENT trial. *Ann Rheum Dis.* 2010;69(12):2125–2130.

82. De Groot K, Rasmussen N, Bacon PA, et al. Randomized trial of cyclophosphamide versus methotrexate for induction of remission in early systemic antineutrophil cytoplasmic antibody-associated vasculitis. *Arthritis Rheum.* 2005;52:2461–2469.

83. Villa-Forte A, Clark TM, Gomes M, et al. Substitution of methotrexate for cyclophosphamide in Wegener granulomatosis: a 12-year single-practice experience. *Medicine (Baltimore).* 2007;86:269–277.

84. Cartin-Ceba R, Fervenza FC, Specks U. Treatment of anti-neutrophil cytoplasmic antibody-associated vasculitis with rituximab. *Curr Opin Rheumatol.* 2012;24:15–23.

85. Rees F, Yazdani R, Lanyon P. Long-term follow-up of different refractory systemic vasculitides treated with rituximab. *Clin Rheumatol.* 2011;30:1241–1245.

86. Roubaud-Baudron C, Pagnoux C, Meaux-Ruault N, et al. Rituximab maintenance therapy for granulomatosis with polyangiitis and microscopic polyangiitis. *J Rheumatol.* 2012;39: 125–130.

87. Stegeman CA, Cohen Tervaert JW, de Jong PE, Kallenberg CG. Trimethoprim-sulfamethoxazole (co-trimoxazole) for the prevention of relapses of Wegener's granulomatosis. Dutch Co-Trimoxazole Wegener Study Group. *N Engl J Med.* 1996;335: 16–20.

88. Dunogue B, Pagnoux C, Guillevin L. Churg-strauss syndrome: clinical symptoms, complementary investigations, prognosis and outcome, and treatment. *Semin Respir Crit Care Med.* 2011;32: 298–309.

89. Lanham JG, Elkon KB, Pusey CD, Hughes GR. Systemic vasculitis with asthma and eosinophilia: a clinical approach to the Churg-Strauss syndrome. *Medicine (Baltimore).* 1984;63: 65–81.

90. Watts RA, Carruthers DM, Scott DG. Epidemiology of systemic vasculitis: changing incidence or definition? *Semin Arthritis Rheum.* 1995;25:28–34.

PART 7

Other Infiltrative and Airspace Disorders

91. Sable-Fourtassou R, Cohen P, Mahr A, et al. Antineutrophil cytoplasmic antibodies and the Churg-Strauss syndrome. *Ann Intern Med.* 2005;143:632–638.

92. Solans R, Bosch JA, Perez-Bocanegra C, et al. Churg-Strauss syndrome: outcome and long-term follow-up of 32 patients. *Rheumatology (Oxford).* 2001;40:763–771.

93. Della Rossa A, Baldini C, Tavoni A, et al. Churg-Strauss syndrome: clinical and serological features of 19 patients from a single Italian centre. *Rheumatology (Oxford).* 2002;41:1286–1294.

94. Clutterbuck EJ, Pusey CD. Severe alveolar haemorrhage in Churg-Strauss syndrome. *Eur J Respir Dis.* 1987;71:158–163.

95. Ciledag A, Deniz H, Eledag S, et al. An aggressive and lethal course of Churg-Strauss syndrome with alveolar hemorrhage, intestinal perforation, cardiac failure and peripheral neuropathy. *Rheumatol Int.* 2012;32:451–455.

96. Guillevin L, Pagnoux C, Seror R, Mahr A, Mouthon L, Le Toumelin P. The Five-Factor Score revisited: assessment of prognoses of systemic necrotizing vasculitides based on the French Vasculitis Study Group (FVSG) cohort. *Medicine (Baltimore).* 2011;90:19–27.

97. Sinico RA, Di Toma L, Maggiore U, et al. Prevalence and clinical significance of antineutrophil cytoplasmic antibodies in Churg-Strauss syndrome. *Arthritis Rheum.* 2005;52:2926–2935.

98. Bourgarit A, Le Toumelin P, Pagnoux C, et al. Deaths occurring during the first year after treatment onset for polyarteritis nodosa, microscopic polyangiitis, and Churg-Strauss syndrome: a retrospective analysis of causes and factors predictive of mortality based on 595 patients. *Medicine (Baltimore).* 2005;84:323–330.

99. Ribi C, Cohen P, Pagnoux C, et al. Treatment of Churg-Strauss syndrome without poor-prognosis factors: a multicenter, prospective, randomized, open-label study of seventy-two patients. *Arthritis Rheum.* 2008;58:586–594.

100. Jennette JC, Falk RJ. Small-vessel vasculitis. *N Engl J Med.* 1997;337:1512–1523.

101. Weidner S, Geuss S, Hafezi-Rachti S, Wonka A, Rupprecht HD. ANCA-associated vasculitis with renal involvement: an outcome analysis. *Nephrol Dial Transplant.* 2004;19:1403–1411.

102. Esnault VL, Soleimani B, Keogan MT, Brownlee AA, Jayne DR, Lockwood CM. Association of IgM with IgG ANCA in patients presenting with pulmonary hemorrhage. *Kidney Int.* 1992;41:1304–1310.

103. Chen M, Yu F, Wang SX, Zou WZ, Zhao MH, Wang HY. Antineutrophil cytoplasmic autoantibody-negative Pauci-immune crescentic glomerulonephritis. *J Am Soc Nephrol.* 2007;18:599–605.

104. Nachman PH, Henderson AG. Pathogenesis of lung vasculitis. *Semin Respir Crit Care Med.* 2011;32:245–253.

105. Pusey CD, Rees AJ, Evans DJ, Peters DK, Lockwood CM. Plasma exchange in focal necrotizing glomerulonephritis without anti-GBM antibodies. *Kidney Int.* 1991;40:757–763.

106. Frasca GM, Soverini ML, Falaschini A, Tampieri E, Vangelista A, Stefoni S. Plasma exchange treatment improves prognosis of antineutrophil cytoplasmic antibody-associated crescentic glomerulonephritis: a case-control study in 26 patients from a single center. *Ther Apher Dial.* 2003;7:540–546.

107. Yamagata K, Hirayama K, Mase K, et al. Apheresis for MPO-ANCA-associated RPGN-indications and efficacy: lessons learned from Japan nationwide survey of RPGN. *J Clin Apher.* 2005;20:244–251.

108. de Lind van Wijngaarden RA, Hauer HA, Wolterbeek R, et al. Chances of renal recovery for dialysis-dependent ANCA-associated glomerulonephritis. *J Am Soc Nephrol.* 2007;18:2189–2197.

109. de Lind van Wijngaarden RA, Hauer HA, Wolterbeek R, et al. Clinical and histologic determinants of renal outcome in ANCA-associated vasculitis: a prospective analysis of 100 patients with severe renal involvement. *J Am Soc Nephrol.* 2006;17:2264–2274.

110. Sanchez AP, Ward DM. Therapeutic apheresis for renal disorders. *Semin Dial.* 2012;25:119–131.

111. Laczika K, Knapp S, Derfler K, Soleiman A, Horl WH, Druml W. Immunoadsorption in Goodpasture's syndrome. *Am J Kidney Dis.* 2000;36:392–395.

112. Bayry J, Negi VS, Kaveri SV. Intravenous immunoglobulin therapy in rheumatic diseases. *Nat Rev Rheumatol.* 2011;7:349–359.

113. Kwok SK, Moon SJ, Ju JH, et al. Diffuse alveolar hemorrhage in systemic lupus erythematosus: risk factors and clinical outcome: results from affiliated hospitals of Catholic University of Korea. *Lupus.* 2011;20:102–107.

114. Martinez-Martinez MU, Abud-Mendoza C. Predictors of mortality in diffuse alveolar haemorrhage associated with systemic lupus erythematosus. *Lupus.* 2011;20:568–574.

115. Araujo DB, Borba EF, Silva CA, et al. Alveolar hemorrhage: distinct features of juvenile and adult onset systemic lupus erythematosus. *Lupus.* 2012;21:872–877.

116. Canas C, Tobon GJ, Granados M, Fernandez L. Diffuse alveolar hemorrhage in Colombian patients with systemic lupus erythematosus. *Clin Rheumatol.* 2007;26:1947–1949.

117. Keane MP, Lynch JP 3rd. Pleuropulmonary manifestations of systemic lupus erythematosus. *Thorax.* 2000;55:159–166.

118. Hughson MD, He Z, Henegar J, McMurray R. Alveolar hemorrhage and renal microangiopathy in systemic lupus erythematosus. *Arch Pathol Lab Med.* 2001;125:475–483.

119. Martinez-Martinez MU, Abud-Mendoza C. Recurrent diffuse alveolar haemorrhage in a patient with systemic lupus erythematosus. long term benefit of Rituximab. *Lupus.* 2012;21(10):1124–1127.

120. Pagnoux C. Plasma exchange for systemic lupus erythematosus. *Transfus Apher Sci.* 2007;36:187–193.

121. Schwarz MI, Zamora MR, Hodges TN, Chan ED, Bowler RP, Tuder RM. Isolated pulmonary capillaritis and diffuse alveolar hemorrhage in rheumatoid arthritis and mixed connective tissue disease. *Chest.* 1998;113:1609–1615.

122. Arad U, Balbir-Gurman A, Doenyas-Barak K, Amit-Vazina M, Caspi D, Elkayam O. Anti-neutrophil antibody associated vasculitis in systemic sclerosis. *Semin Arthritis Rheum.* 2011;41:223–229.

123. Schwarz MI, Sutarik JM, Nick JA, Leff JA, Emlen JW, Tuder RM. Pulmonary capillaritis and diffuse alveolar hemorrhage. A primary manifestation of polymyositis. *Am J Respir Crit Care Med.* 1995;151:2037–2040.

124. Gertner E, Lie JT. Pulmonary capillaritis, alveolar hemorrhage, and recurrent microvascular thrombosis in primary antiphospholipid syndrome. *J Rheumatol.* 1993;20:1224–1228.

125. Nadrous HF, Yu AC, Specks U, Ryu JH. Pulmonary involvement in Henoch-Schonlein purpura. *Mayo Clin Proc.* 2004;79:1151–1157.

126. Afessa B, Abdulai RM, Kremers WK, Hogan WJ, Litzow MR, Peters SG. Risk factors and outcome of pulmonary

complications after autologous hematopoietic stem cell transplant. *Chest.* 2012;141:442–450.

127. Afessa B, Tefferi A, Litzow MR, Peters SG. Outcome of diffuse alveolar hemorrhage in hematopoietic stem cell transplant recipients. *Am J Respir Crit Care Med.* 2002;166:1364–1368.
128. Majhail NS, Parks K, Defor TE, Weisdorf DJ. Diffuse alveolar hemorrhage and infection-associated alveolar hemorrhage following hematopoietic stem cell transplantation: related and high-risk clinical syndromes. *Biol Blood Marrow Transplant.* 2006;12:1038–1046.
129. Roychowdhury M, Pambuccian SE, Aslan DL, et al. Pulmonary complications after bone marrow transplantation: an autopsy study from a large transplantation center. *Arch Pathol Lab Med.* 2005;129:366–371.
130. Peters SG, Afessa B. Acute lung injury after hematopoietic stem cell transplantation. *Clin Chest Med.* 2005;26:561–569, vi.
131. Jules-Elysee K, Stover DE, Yahalom J, White DA, Gulati SC. Pulmonary complications in lymphoma patients treated with high-dose therapy autologous bone marrow transplantation. *Am Rev Respir Dis.* 1992;146:485–491.
132. Wojno KJ, Vogelsang GB, Beschorner WE, Santos GW. Pulmonary hemorrhage as a cause of death in allogeneic bone marrow recipients with severe acute graft-versus-host disease. *Transplantation.* 1994;57:88–92.
133. Robbins RA, Linder J, Stahl MG, et al. Diffuse alveolar hemorrhage in autologous bone marrow transplant recipients. *Am J Med.* 1989;87:511–518.
134. Metcalf JP, Rennard SI, Reed EC, et al. Corticosteroids as adjunctive therapy for diffuse alveolar hemorrhage associated with bone marrow transplantation. University of Nebraska Medical Center Bone Marrow Transplant Group. *Am J Med.* 1994;96:327–334.
135. Corso S, Vukelja SJ, Wiener D, Baker WJ. Diffuse alveolar hemorrhage following autologous bone marrow infusion. *Bone Marrow Transplant.* 1993;12:301–303.
136. Sisson JH, Thompson AB, Anderson JR, et al. Airway inflammation predicts diffuse alveolar hemorrhage during bone marrow transplantation in patients with Hodgkin disease. *Am Rev Respir Dis.* 1992;146:439–443.
137. Srivastava A, Gottlieb D, Bradstock KF. Diffuse alveolar haemorrhage associated with microangiopathy after allogeneic bone marrow transplantation. *Bone Marrow Transplant.* 1995;15:863–867.
138. Hicks K, Peng D, Gajewski JL. Treatment of diffuse alveolar hemorrhage after allogeneic bone marrow transplant with recombinant factor VIIa. *Bone Marrow Transplant.* 2002;30:975–978.
139. Herry I, Cadranel J, Antoine M, et al. Cytomegalovirus-induced alveolar hemorrhage in patients with AIDS: a new clinical entity? *Clin Infect Dis.* 1996;22:616–620.
140. Hughes-Davies L, Kocjan G, Spittle MF, Miller RF. Occult alveolar haemorrhage in bronchopulmonary Kaposi's sarcoma. *J Clin Pathol.* 1992;45:536–537.
141. Zeiss CR, Leach CL, Smith LJ, et al. A serial immunologic and histopathologic study of lung injury induced by trimellitic anhydride. *Am Rev Respir Dis.* 1988;137:191–196.
142. Patterson R, Nugent KM, Harris KE, Eberle ME. Immunologic hemorrhagic pneumonia caused by isocyanates. *Am Rev Respir Dis.* 1990;141:226–230.
143. Derk CT, Jimenez SA. Goodpasture-like syndrome induced by D-penicillamine in a patient with systemic sclerosis: report and review of the literature. *J Rheumatol.* 2003;30:1616–1620.
144. Baldwin GC, Choi R, Roth MD, et al. Evidence of chronic damage to the pulmonary microcirculation in habitual users of alkaloidal ("crack") cocaine. *Chest.* 2002;121:1231–1238.
145. Yermakov VM, Hitti IF, Sutton AL. Necrotizing vasculitis associated with diphenylhydantoin: two fatal cases. *Hum Pathol.* 1983;14:182–184.
146. Dhillon SS, Singh D, Doe N, Qadri AM, Ricciardi S, Schwarz MI. Diffuse alveolar hemorrhage and pulmonary capillaritis due to propylthiouracil. *Chest.* 1999;116:1485–1488.
147. Choi HK, Merkel PA, Walker AM, Niles JL. Drug-associated antineutrophil cytoplasmic antibody-positive vasculitis: prevalence among patients with high titers of antimyeloperoxidase antibodies. *Arthritis Rheum.* 2000;43:405–413.
148. Nicolls MR, Terada LS, Tuder RM, Prindiville SA, Schwarz MI. Diffuse alveolar hemorrhage with underlying pulmonary capillaritis in the retinoic acid syndrome. *Am J Respir Crit Care Med.* 1998;158:1302–1305.
149. Elkayam O, Yaron M, Caspi D. Minocycline-induced autoimmune syndromes: an overview. *Semin Arthritis Rheum.* 1999;28:392–397.
150. Short AK, Lockwood CM. Antigen specificity in hydralazine associated ANCA positive systemic vasculitis. *QJM.* 1995;88:775–783.
151. Calanas-Continente A, Espinosa M, Manzano-Garcia G, Santamaria R, Lopez-Rubio F, Aljama P. Necrotizing glomerulonephritis and pulmonary hemorrhage associated with carbimazole therapy. *Thyroid.* 2005;15:286–268.
152. Frankel SR, Eardley A, Lauwers G, Weiss M, Warrell RP Jr. The "retinoic acid syndrome" in acute promyelocytic leukemia. *Ann Intern Med.* 1992;117:292–296.
153. Agusti C, Ramirez J, Picado C, et al. Diffuse alveolar hemorrhage in allogeneic bone marrow transplantation. A postmortem study. *Am J Respir Crit Care Med.* 1995;151:1006–1010.
154. Wisnewski AV, Jones M. Pro/Con debate: is occupational asthma induced by isocyanates an immunoglobulin E-mediated disease? *Clin Exp Allergy.* 2010;40:1155–1162.
155. Garcia-Rostan y Perez GM, Garcia Bragado F, Puras Gil AM. Pulmonary hemorrhage and antiglomerular basement membrane antibody-mediated glomerulonephritis after exposure to smoked cocaine (crack): a case report and review of the literature. *Pathol Int.* 1997;47:692–697.
156. Bailey ME, Fraire AE, Greenberg SD, Barnard J, Cagle PT. Pulmonary histopathology in cocaine abusers. *Hum Pathol.* 1994;25:203–207.
157. Barnett VT, Bergmann F, Humphrey H, Chediak J. Diffuse alveolar hemorrhage secondary to superwarfarin ingestion. *Chest.* 1992;102:1301–1302.
158. Kilaru PK, Schweiger MJ, Kozman HA, Weil TR. Diffuse alveolar hemorrhage after clopidogrel use. *J Invasive Cardiol.* 2001;13:535–537.
159. Ikeda M, Tanaka H, Sadamatsu K. Diffuse alveolar hemorrhage as a complication of dual antiplatelet therapy for acute coronary syndrome. *Cardiovasc Revasc Med.* 2011;12:407–411.
160. Dearborn DG, Smith PG, Dahms BB, et al. Clinical profile of 30 infants with acute pulmonary hemorrhage in Cleveland. *Pediatrics.* 2002;110:627–637.
161. Elidemir O, Colasurdo GN, Rossmann SN, Fan LL. Isolation of Stachybotrys from the lung of a child with pulmonary hemosiderosis. *Pediatrics.* 1999;104:964–966.

162. Chryssanthopoulos C, Cassimos C, Panagiotidou C. Prognostic criteria in idiopathic pulmonary hemosiderosis in children. *Eur J Pediatr*. 1983;140:123–125.

163. Poggi V, Lo Vecchio A, Menna F, Menna G. Idiopathic pulmonary hemosiderosis: a rare cause of iron-deficiency anemia in childhood. *J Pediatr Hematol Oncol*. 2011;33:e160–e162.

164. Le Clainche L, Le Bourgeois M, Fauroux B, et al. Long-term outcome of idiopathic pulmonary hemosiderosis in children. *Medicine (Baltimore)*. 2000;79:318–326.

165. Ohga S, Takahashi K, Miyazaki S, Kato H, Ueda K. Idiopathic pulmonary haemosiderosis in Japan: 39 possible cases from a survey questionnaire. *Eur J Pediatr*. 1995;154:994–995.

166. Torres MJ, Giron MD, Corzo JL, et al. Release of inflammatory mediators after cow's milk intake in a newborn with idiopathic pulmonary hemosiderosis. *J Allergy Clin Immunol*. 1996;98:1120–1123.

167. Mayes DH, Guerrero ML. A few good men: a Marine with hemoptysis and diarrhea. Idiopathic pulmonary hemosiderosis and celiac sprue. *Chest*. 2008;134:644–647.

168. Pacheco A, Casanova C, Fogue L, Sueiro A. Long-term clinical follow-up of adult idiopathic pulmonary hemosiderosis and celiac disease. *Chest*. 1991;99:1525–1526.

169. Soergel K, Sommers SC. Idiopathic pulmonary hemosiderosis and related syndromes. *Am J Med*. 1962;32:499–511.

170. Breckenridge RL Jr, Ross JS. Idiopathic pulmonary hemosiderosis: a report of familial occurrence. *Chest*. 1979;75:636–639.

171. Nuesslein TG, Teig N, Rieger CH. Pulmonary haemosiderosis in infants and children. *Paediatr Respir Rev*. 2006;7:45–48.

172. Buschman DL, Ballard R. Progressive massive fibrosis associated with idiopathic pulmonary hemosiderosis. *Chest*. 1993;104:293–295.

173. Malhotra P, Aggarwal R, Aggarwal AN, Jindal SK, Awasthi A, Radotra BD. Coeliac disease as a cause of unusually severe anaemia in a young man with idiopathic pulmonary haemosiderosis. *Respir Med*. 2005;99:451–453.

174. Thaell JF, Greipp PR, Stubbs SE, Siegal GP. Idiopathic pulmonary hemosiderosis: two cases in a family. *Mayo Clin Proc*. 1978;53:113–118.

175. Rossi GA, Balzano E, Battistini E, et al. Long-term prednisone and azathioprine treatment of a patient with idiopathic pulmonary hemosiderosis. *Pediatr Pulmonol*. 1992;13:176–180.

176. Colombo JL, Stolz SM. Treatment of life-threatening primary pulmonary hemosiderosis with cyclophosphamide. *Chest*. 1992;102:959–960.

177. Wang T, Weigt SS, Belperio JA, Lynch JP 3rd. Immunosuppressive and cytotoxic therapy: pharmacology, toxicities, and monitoring. *Semin Respir Crit Care Med*. 2011;32:346–370.

CHAPTER 69

Aspiration-Related Pulmonary Disorders

Paul E. Marik

Pneumonia—"Captain of the Men of Death"

—William Osler[1]

Aspiration is defined as the misdirection of oropharyngeal or gastric contents into the larynx and lower respiratory tract.[2] An assortment of pulmonary syndromes may occur following aspiration depending on the quantity and nature of the aspirated material, the chronicity of aspiration, as well as the nature of the host's defense mechanisms and the host's response to the aspirated material. The most important syndromes include "*aspiration pneumonitis*" or Mendelson's syndrome, which is a chemical pneumonitis caused by the aspiration of gastric contents, and *"aspiration pneumonia,"* an infectious process caused by the aspiration of oropharyngeal secretions colonized by pathogenic bacteria.[2] While there is some overlap between these two syndromes they are distinct clinical entities. In addition, a variety of pulmonary conditions have been described from chronic recurrent occult aspiration, most notably "*diffuse aspiration bronchiolitis*."[3] Other aspiration syndromes include airway obstruction, lung abscess, exogenous lipoid pneumonia, chronic interstitial fibrosis, and *Mycobacterium fortuitum* pneumonia. This chapter will focus on the pathophysiology, clinical features and management of aspiration pneumonitis, aspiration pneumonia, and diffuse aspiration bronchiolitis.

ASPIRATION PNEUMONITIS

Aspiration pneumonitis is best defined as acute lung injury following the aspiration of regurgitated gastric contents.[2] This syndrome occurs in patients with a marked disturbance of consciousness such as drug overdose, seizures, coma due to acute neurologic insults, massive cerebrovascular accident, following head trauma and during anesthesia. It is important to emphasize that aspiration pneumonitis only occurs in patients who have a depressed level of consciousness with impairment of airway protective reflexes. In clinical practice, drug overdose is the most common cause of aspiration pneumonitis, occurring in approximately 10% of patients hospitalized following a drug overdosage. Adnet and Baud[4] demonstrated that the risk of aspiration increases with the degree of impairment in consciousness (as measured by the Glasgow Coma Scale). Historically, the syndrome most commonly associated with aspiration pneumonitis is Mendelson's syndrome, reported in 1946 in obstetric patients who aspirated while receiving general anesthesia.[5] Mendelson's original report consisted of 44,016 nonfasted obstetric patients whom he studied between 1932 and 1945, of whom more than half received an "operative intervention" with ether by mask without endotracheal intubation. He described aspiration in 66 patients (1:667). Although several of the patients were critically ill from their aspiration, recovery was usually complete within 24 to 36 hours and only two patients died (1:22,008).

Although aspiration is a widely feared complication of general anesthesia, clinically apparent aspiration in modern anesthesia practice is exceptionally rare, and in healthy patients the overall morbidity and mortality are low (see section below). The risk of aspiration is greatly increased in patients intubated emergently in the field, emergency room or in the ICU. In these patients every effort should be made to reduce the risk of aspiration; this includes removing dentures and clearing the airway and in certain circumstances placing a nasogastric tube to empty the stomach prior to intubation. If there is an immediate risk of airway compromise endotracheal intubation should be performed prior to placement of a nasogastric tube. However, if the patient is likely to have a full stomach (upper GI bleed, small bowel obstruction, ileus, etc.) it may be prudent to place a nasogastric tube prior to endotracheal intubation. When intubating emergently, suction equipment must be immediately available and rapid-sequence induction using cricoid pressure should be performed.

■ PATHOPHYSIOLOGY

Mendelson emphasized the importance of acid when he showed that unneutralized gastric contents introduced into the lungs of rabbits caused severe pneumonitis indistinguishable from that caused by an equal amount of 0.1 N hydrochloric acid.[5–7] However, if the pH of the vomitus was neutralized before aspiration, the pulmonary injury was minimal. Experimental studies have demonstrated that the severity of lung injury increases significantly with the volume of the aspirate and inversely with its pH, with a pH of less than 2.5 being required to cause aspiration pneumonitis. However, the stomach contains a variety of other substance in addition to acid. Several experimental studies have revealed that aspiration of small, particulate food matter from the stomach may cause severe pulmonary damage, even if the pH of the aspirate is above 2.5.[8,9] These studies suggest that cell recruitment and expression of inflammatory mediators are most pronounced after injury with combined acid and small food particles. These data are supported by findings in patients where the most severe lung injury was observed in patients following aspiration with particulate food matter.[10,11]

Aspiration of gastric contents results in a chemical burn of the tracheobronchial tree and pulmonary parenchyma with an intense parenchymal inflammatory reaction. The proinflammatory cytokines including tumor necrosis factor-α and CXC chemokines are crucial to the development of aspiration pneumonitis by mediating neutrophil recruitment. Once localized to the lung, neutrophils play a key role in the development of lung injury through the release of oxygen radicals and proteases. Gastric acid prevents the growth of bacteria and therefore the contents of the stomach are normally sterile. Bacterial infection, therefore, does not play a significant role in the early stages of acute lung injury following aspiration of gastric contents. However, acid aspiration pneumonitis reduces host defenses against infection increasing the risk of superinfection.[12] The incidence of this complication has, however, not been well studied. Furthermore, experimental models suggest that acid aspiration pneumonitis "primes the lung" making secondary infection more severe.[12,13] Colonization of the gastric contents by potentially pathogenic organisms may occur when the gastric pH is increased by the use of antacids, histamine-2 (H2) receptor blockers, or proton pump inhibitors. In addition, gastric colonization by gram-negative bacteria occurs in patients receiving enteral feedings, as well as in patients with gastroparesis and small bowel obstruction. In these circumstances the pulmonary inflammatory response is likely to result from both bacterial infection and the inflammatory response of the gastric particulate matter.

■ ANESTHESIA AND ASPIRATION PNEUMONIA

Aspiration pneumonitis has traditionally been regarded as the major cause of serious anesthetic complications. However, with the recognition of the importance of this complication, and the fact that it is largely preventable, the risk of aspiration pneumonitis in modern anesthesia is very low. Nevertheless, aspiration pneumonitis is an important perioperative complication and remains the commonest cause of anesthesia-related death. The risk of aspiration with modern anesthesia is reported to be between 2.9 and 4.7 per 10,000 general anesthetics (about 1 in 3000 anesthetics) with a mortality of approximately 1:125,000, accounting for between 10% and 30% of all anesthetic deaths.[14,15] Warner et al.[7] published data from a study of 215,488 anesthetics and observed 67 episodes of aspiration in adults (3.1 per 10,000 patients) undergoing general anesthesia. In a recent study involving 99,441 patients undergoing nonobstetrical anesthesia, perioperative pulmonary aspiration occurred in 14 patients (1 in 7103 procedures).[16] All 14 patients has one or more risk factors for aspiration. The Thai Anesthesia Incident Monitoring Study prospectively recorded reports on aspiration from 51 hospitals across Thailand during a 6-month period in 2007.[17] Twenty-eight reports met the definition of pulmonary aspiration (denominator not reported). Most of the incidents occurred in American Society of Anesthesiology (ASA) class 1 to 2 patients (85.7%), during day time hours (64.3%), and when the anesthesiologists were in charge (67.9%). Eleven incidents (39.3%) occurred during induction, seven (25%) during maintenance, and seven (25%) during the emergence phase. All the incidents except one (96.4%) were considered human error and 25 (89.2%) were preventable. Thirteen patients (46.4%) had major physiologic changes and 10 (35.7%) of them required unplanned ICU admission. Ten patients (35.7%) needed prolonged ventilator support and two (7.14%) of them died.

The most definitive and extensive review on the risk of airway problems associated with intubation was reported by Cook et al.[18,19] who summarized the findings of the 4th National Audit Project of the Royal College of Anaesthetists. In this 1-year prospective audit, the authors examined the occurrence of serious airway complications in anesthesia, ICUs, and emergency departments of all the National Health Service hospitals in the United Kingdom. The authors found 184 cases that met the inclusion criteria: 133 from anesthesia, 36 from ICUs, and 15 from emergency departments. A concurrent national census of anesthesia activity over a 2-week period was performed to provide denominator data for anesthesia, which indicated 2.9 million anesthetic procedures annually, resulting in a nominal incidence (using the 133 anesthesia events) of one serious airway complication per 22,000 anesthetics. In total, 38 deaths were attributable to airway complications, and the death rate was 16 of 133 (12%) in anesthesia, 18 of 36 (50%) in the ICUs, and 4 of 16 (25%) in the emergency departments. Pulmonary aspiration of gastric contents was the commonest cause of death and brain damage. A supraglottic airway was the planned technique in more than 50% of death or brain damage cases. A statistical analysis of the reports suggested that as few as 25% of relevant incidents may have been reported. The authors therefore suggest that this audit provides an indication of the lower limit for the incidence of such complications.

Emergency surgery (particularly, trauma and abdominal surgery with delayed gastric emptying) procedures performed at night, inadequate anesthesia, obesity, elderly immobilized patients, and obstructive sleep apnea have been associated with a higher risk of aspiration.[15,20] Obtunded adults and children with known gastroesophageal reflux are more likely to aspirate even without narcotic or sedative impairment of airway reflexes. The factors increasing the risk for aspiration are listed in Table 69-1. Patients who are at risk before surgery are also at increased risk during the postoperative period when immobility, residual effects of anesthetic agents, and narcotics combine to decrease protective airway reflexes.[21–23]

The incidence of aspiration appears higher in obstetric patients as highlighted by the pioneering study of Mendelsohn.[5] A study from 1973 reported an incidence of 1 in 6000 obstetric patients receiving general anesthesia for vaginal deliveries and 1 in 430 for cesarean section patients.[24] In more recent studies, an aspiration incidence of 1 in 1547 and 1 in 1431, respectively, were described for cesarean section under general anesthesia,[21,23] and a recent audit showed an incidence of 1 in 900 women undergoing cesarean section.[22] The risk of pulmonary aspiration is, therefore, at least double or three times as high as in general surgical patients. Pregnant women are at increased risk of aspiration because of gastroesophageal reflux and delay in gastric emptying.[25,26]

TABLE 69-1 Factors Increasing the Risk of Perioperative Aspiration

Recent eating
Delayed gastric emptying
Diabetic neuropathy
Opioids
Paralytic ileus
Small bowel obstruction
Pregnancy
Emergency surgery
Obesity
Obstructive sleep apnea
Reflux esophagitis
Achalasia
Esophageal stricture
Previous gastric bypass surgery
Traumatic brain injury
Cerebral infarction/bleed

Gastroesophageal reflux is common in pregnancy and can be demonstrated even in the absence of symptoms. There is no difference in basal and evoked gastric acid secretion in pregnancy but there is a reduction in lower esophageal barrier pressure, which is likely to be a progesterone effect present from early pregnancy. The surgical procedure may itself increase aspiration risk through the adoption of lithotomy or Trendelenburg positions or the creation of a pneumoperitoneum.

The laryngeal mask airway (LMA) does not reliably protect the lungs from regurgitated stomach contents and should be avoided in patients at an increased risk for aspiration.[27,28] In a meta-analysis of 12,901 low-risk cases, where the standard contraindications to the use of the LMA were followed (e.g., absence of gastrointestinal pathology, obesity, history of reflux, or emergency surgery), only 3 cases of aspiration were identified, an incidence of 2.3 per 10,000.[29]

Inadequate reversal of neuromuscular blockage at the end of surgery is an important risk factor for aspiration. After the administration of nondepolarizing neuromuscular blocking agents, it is essential to ensure adequate return of normal neuromuscular function. Residual paralysis decreases upper esophageal tone, coordination of the esophageal musculature during swallowing, and the hypoxic ventilatory drive.[30] These factors significantly increase the risk for aspiration. Adequate recovery of postoperative neuromuscular function cannot be guaranteed without objective neuromuscular monitoring. Good evidence-based practice dictates that clinicians should always quantitate the extent of neuromuscular blockade by objective monitoring (train-of-four monitoring).[30] To exclude clinically significant residual neuromuscular blockade, the train-of-four ratio, when measured mechanically or by electromyography, must exceed 0.9. If sufficient recovery (i.e., train-of-four $\geq$0.9) has not been documented objectively at the end of the surgical procedure, the neuromuscular block should be antagonized.

Prevention of Aspiration During Anesthesia

In recent years more liberal preoperative fasting guidelines have been promoted. In healthy adults without an increased risk of regurgitation or aspiration solids should be avoided after midnight; however, a light meal such as dry toast may be considered up to 6 hours before anesthesia and clear liquids such as water, coffee without milk, or fruit juice can be given up to 2 hours before induction.[31,32] Meta-analyses of randomized controlled trials comparing fasting times of 2 to 4 hours *versus* more than 4 hours report smaller gastric volumes and higher gastric pH values in adult patients given clear liquids 2 to 4 hours before a procedure and this approach is currently endorsed by the ASA.[33]

Preoperative antacids, H2 receptor blockers, proton pump inhibitors, and prokinetic agents have been used to reduce the volume and/or acidity of the gastric contents. There is, however, a lack of data indicating that any of these drugs reduce the risk of aspiration pneumonitis.[34] The routine use of these drugs is not recommended by the ASA guidelines.[33] However, it is not unreasonable to use these drugs in patients at an increased risk of aspiration. It is however important to realize that it takes time for the clinical effects of the acid suppressive drugs to manifest and these drugs should therefore be dosed at least 2 hours prior to induction.[35]

Standard teaching suggests that rapid-sequence induction with cricoid pressure should be performed when intubating patients at an increased risk of aspiration. Cricoid pressure, known as the Sellick maneuver, is designed to occlude the cervical esophagus by compressing it between the cricoid cartilage and the vertebral bodies.[36] Passively regurgitated gastric contents are therefore prevented from entering the pharynx. Neither rapid-sequence induction nor cricoid pressure has been prospectively studied and proven to decrease the incidence of aspiration. Rapid-sequence induction shortens the time between the onset of unconsciousness and securing the airway, which may be of benefit if the aspiration risk is high. However, the use of cricoid pressure is controversial.[37] The esophagus cannot be reliably occluded between the cricoid cartilage and the vertebral bodies. Studies in volunteers (men and nonpregnant women) clearly show that the esophagus often does not lie in the midline or that cricoid pressure displaces the esophagus laterally without occluding it.[38] More recent data suggest that the hypopharynx posterior to the cricoid cartilage is in continuity with the esophageal inlet and this hypopharyngeal area is occluded with the Sellick maneuver.[39] Cricoid pressure is often applied incorrectly or without the appropriate amount of force and may reduce visualization of the vocal cords and impede intubation. Although not proven to reduce the risk of aspiration during emergent intubations, cricoid pressure is currently considered the standard of care in this situation.

CLINICAL PRESENTATION

Aspiration of gastric contents can present dramatically with a full-blown picture that includes gastric contents in the oropharynx, wheezing, coughing, shortness of breath, cyanosis, pulmonary edema, hypotension, and hypoxemia; this may progress rapidly to severe ARDS and death (see Fig. 69-1). However, many patients may not develop signs or symptoms associated with aspiration, while others may develop a cough or wheeze. In some patients aspiration may be clinically silent manifesting only as arterial desaturation with radiologic evidence of aspiration. Warner et al.[7] studied 67 patients who aspirated while undergoing anesthesia. Forty-two (64%) of these patients were totally asymptomatic, 13 required mechanical ventilatory support for more than 6 hours and 4 died.

MANAGEMENT OF ASPIRATION PNEUMONITIS

The upper airway should be suctioned following a witnessed aspiration. Endotracheal intubation should be considered in patients who are unable to protect their airway. While common practice, the prophylactic use of antibiotics in patients with suspected or witnessed aspiration is not recommended. Similarly, the use of antibiotics shortly after an aspiration episode in a patient who develops a fever, leukocytosis, and a pulmonary infiltrate is discouraged as it may select for more resistant organisms in a patient with an

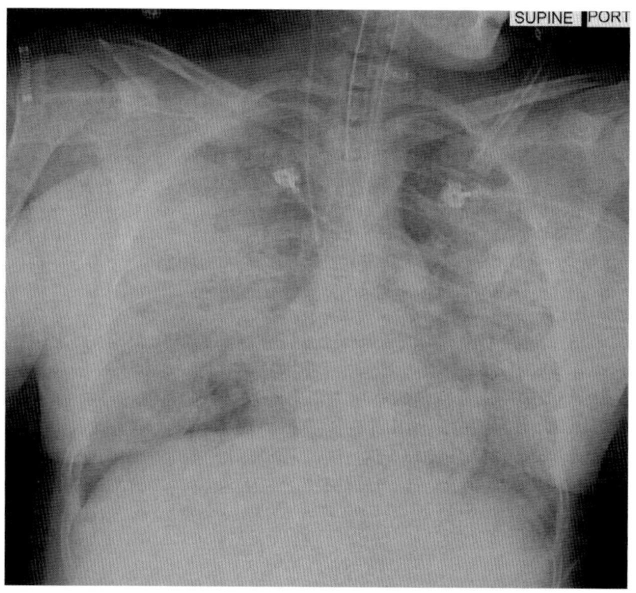

Figure 69-1 Anteroposterior chest radiograph demonstrating bilateral alveolar infiltrates following aspiration of gastric contents (aspiration pneumonitis).

uncomplicated chemical pneumonitis. However, empiric antimicrobial therapy is appropriate in patients who aspirate gastric contents in the setting of small bowel obstruction or in other circumstances associated with colonization of gastric contents (acid-suppressive therapy, tube feeds). Antimicrobial therapy should be considered in patients with an aspiration pneumonitis that fails to resolve within 48 hours. Empiric therapy with broad-spectrum agents is recommended. Antimicrobials with anaerobic activity are not routinely required. Recently serum procalcitonin has emerged as a biomarker that has been postulated to be able to discriminate bacterial infections from nonbacterial inflammatory disorders.[40] El-Solh et al.[41] investigated the predictive accuracy of serum procalcitonin in distinguishing aspiration with bacterial pneumonia from "sterile" aspiration pneumonitis. In this study serum procalcitonin levels had poor diagnostic value in separating bacterial pneumonia from aspiration pneumonitis based on quantitative bronchoalveolar lavage culture.

■ IMMUNOMODULATING AGENTS

Corticosteroids have been used in the management of aspiration pneumonitis since 1955.[42] However, limited data exist on which to evaluate the role of these agents, with only a single prospective, placebo-controlled study having been performed. In this study, Sukumaran et al.[43] randomized 60 patients with "aspiration pneumonitis" to methylprednisolone (15 mg/kg/day for 3 days) or placebo. The patients were subdivided into two groups; a younger group with drug overdose as the predominant diagnosis and an older group with neurologic disorders. Radiographic abnormalities improved more rapidly in the steroid group, as did oxygenation. The number of ventilator and ICU days was significantly shorter in the overdose patients who received corticosteroids; however, these variables were longer in the neurologic group receiving this therapy. There was no significant difference in the incidence of complications or mortality. The results of this study are somewhat difficult to interpret as it is likely that the patients in the overdose group had true "aspiration pneumonitis" while many patients in the neurologic group probably developed "aspiration pneumonia." Wolfe et al.[44] performed a case-controlled study of 43 patients with aspiration pneumonitis, of whom 25 received high-dose corticosteroids (approximately 600 mg prednisolone/day for 4 days). While there was no difference in mortality, secondary gram-negative pneumonia was reported to be more frequent in the steroid group (7/20 vs. 0/13); however, ventilator days tended to be less in this group (4.3 vs. 9.8 days). Based on this limited data it is not possible to make evidence-based recommendations on the use of corticosteroids in patients with aspiration pneumonitis.

In animal models, a number of pharmacologic interventions including inhaled B_2 agonists, pentoxifylline, antiplatelet drugs, and omega-3 fatty acids have been shown to attenuate the acute lung injury following acid aspiration.[45–50] The role of these interventions in patients remains to be tested; however, due to their inherent safety, these agents should be considered in patients with severe acid aspiration pneumonitis.

ASPIRATION PNEUMONIA

Aspiration pneumonia refers to the development of a radiographic infiltrate and clinical features consistent with pneumonia in a patient with risk factors for increased oropharyngeal aspiration (see Fig. 69-2). Approximately half of all healthy adults aspirate small amounts of oropharyngeal secretions during sleep. Presumably, the low virulent bacterial burden of normal pharyngeal secretions together with forceful coughing, active ciliary transport, and normal humoral and cellular immune mechanisms result in clearance of the inoculum, without sequelae. However, if the mechanical, humoral, or cellular mechanisms are impaired or if the aspirated inoculum is large enough, pneumonia may follow. Any condition that increases the volume and/or bacterial burden of oropharyngeal secretions in the setting of impaired host defense mechanism may lead to aspiration pneumonia. Indeed, in stroke patients undergoing swallow evaluation there is a strong correlation between the volume of the aspirate and the development of pneumonia.[51] Factors that increase oropharyngeal colonization with potentially pathogenic organisms and that increase the bacterial load may augment the

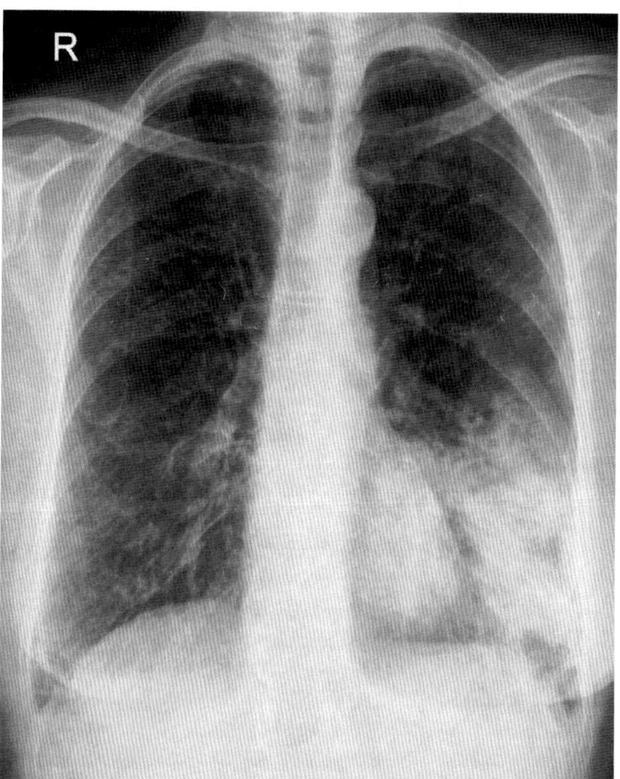

Figure 69-2 Anteroposterior chest radiograph demonstrating a left lower lobe aspiration pneumonia.

risk of aspiration pneumonia. The clinical setting in which pneumonia develops largely distinguishes aspiration pneumonia from other forms of pneumonia. However, there is much overlap. This is illustrated by the fact that otherwise healthy elderly patients with "community-acquired pneumonia" (CAP) have been demonstrated to have a significantly higher incidence of silent aspiration when compared with age-matched controls.[52]

■ EPIDEMIOLOGY

The lack of specific and sensitive markers of aspiration makes the epidemiologic study of aspiration syndromes difficult. Furthermore, most studies do not make the distinction between aspiration pneumonitis and aspiration pneumonia. Nevertheless, several studies list "aspiration pneumonia" as the cause of CAP in 5% to 15% of cases.[53,54] CAP is a major cause of morbidity and mortality in the elderly and it is likely that aspiration is the major cause of pneumonia in these patients. Epidemiologic studies have demonstrated that the incidence of pneumonia increases with aging, with the risk being almost six times higher in those over the age of 75, compared to those less than 60 years of age.[55,56] The attack rate for pneumonia is highest among those in nursing homes.[57]

■ DYSPHAGIA IN PATIENTS WITH ASPIRATION PNEUMONIA

Swallowing is a complex function, with both voluntary and reflexive components. Five cranial nerves and more than 50 muscles in the head and neck are involved in oropharyngeal swallowing. Both brainstem and cortical areas are involved in the neural processing of swallowing. The coordination of swallowing requires bilateral input from the sensorimotor cortex with descending input to the brainstem medullary swallowing center.[58] Functional and anatomic imaging studies have identified several sites that play an important role in swallowing, including the primary sensorimotor cortex, insula, anterior cingulate, internal capsule, basal ganglia, and thalamus. The swallowing process can be divided into oropharyngeal phase and esophageal phase.[59] The oropharyngeal phase includes biting and chewing in the oral cavity, and the transport of food into the pharynx. In simplified terms, this process is accompanied by elevation and anterior movement of the larynx to meet with the epiglottis for protection of the airway. It is followed by passage of the bolus through the upper esophageal sphincter into the esophagus (esophageal phase). During the esophageal phase, the lower esophageal sphincter relaxes and food is pushed into the stomach by peristalsis and gravity.

Dysphagia refers to the difficulty in swallowing. The severity of dysphagia varies from moderate difficulty to complete inability to swallow. Dysphagia is the major risk factor leading to aspiration pneumonia. In addition, dysphagia contributes significantly to protein-energy malnutrition and dehydration. Impairment in any component of the swallow mechanism including anatomical abnormities of the upper airway or esophagus can lead to dysphagia. Dysphagia has traditionally been associated with brainstem and bilateral cerebral infarction, though it has more recently been shown to occur in isolated cerebral infarctions as well. Furthermore, dysphagia is commonly associated with silent cerebral infarction.

Dysphagia is remarkably common in Westernized nations and is a major cause of morbidity and mortality. Indeed, aspiration pneumonia is probably the final common pathway by which most chronically ill patients die. It has been estimated that over 16 million senior citizens in the United States suffer from dysphagia.[60] Furthermore, an additional 300,000 to 600,000 patients develop dysphagia each year in the United States from neurologic disorders.[61] Dysphagia affects more than 30% of patients who have had a cerebrovascular accident; 52% to 82% of patients with Parkinson disease; 84% of patients with Alzheimer disease, up to 40% adults aged 65 years and older, and more than 60% of elderly institutionalized patients.[62] The efficiency of the swallow mechanism decreases with aging, increasing the risk of aspiration and pneumonia in the elderly. Kikuchi et al. evaluated the occurrence of silent aspiration in otherwise "healthy elderly patients" with CAP and age-matched control subjects using indium[111] chloride scanning.[52] Silent aspiration was demonstrated in 71% of patients with CAP compared to 10% in control subjects. The impaired swallow mechanism in the elderly can be attributed to diminished sensation, silent cerebral infarction, cerebral atrophy, a delay in the synapse conduction in the afferent inputs to the central nervous system, and lingual weakness (sarcopenia) caused by aging.[63,64]

■ RISK FACTOR FOR DYSPHAGIA

The major risk factors for dysphagia are listed in Table 69-2. In patients with an acute stroke the incidence of dysphagia ranges from 40% to 70%.[65] Dysphagic patients who aspirate are at an increased risk of developing pneumonia.[66,67] Although dysphagia improves in most patients following a stroke, in many the swallowing difficulties follow a fluctuating course with 10% to 30% continuing to have dysphagia with aspiration.[68,69]

The Cough Reflex in Patients with Aspiration Pneumonia

An intact cough reflex is an important respiratory defense mechanism. Sekizawa et al.[70] demonstrated a marked depression of the cough reflex in elderly patients with pneumonia. Furthermore, the greater the derangement of the cough reflex, the greater the risk of pneumonia.[71] Nakazawa et al.[72] demonstrated impairment of the swallow and the cough reflex in elderly patients with aspiration pneumonia but not in patients with dementia who had no prior history of aspiration pneumonia. Angiotensin-converting enzyme (ACE) modulates the cough reflex. Along with its effects that cleave angiotensin I to angiotensin II, ACE also metabolizes the protussive peptides, substance *P* and bradykinin. Substance P, which is released from vagal sensory nerves in the pharynx and upper airways, mediates the cough reflex. One study found that substance *P* levels in sputum were reduced substantially in elderly patients with pneumonia.[73] Bradykinin, an inflammatory peptide that mediates cough due

TABLE 69-2 Risk Factors for Dysphagia and Aspiration Pneumonia

Cerebrovascular disease
Ischemic stroke
Hemorrhagic stroke
Subarachnoid hemorrhage
Degenerative neurologic disease
Alzheimer dementia
Multi-infarct dementia
Parkinson disease
Amyotrophic lateral sclerosis (motor neuron disease)
Multiple sclerosis
Head and neck cancer
Oropharyngeal malignancy
Oral cavity malignancy
Esophageal malignancy
Other
Scleroderma
Diabetic gastroparesis
Reflux esophagitis
Presbyesophagus
Achalasia

to ACE inhibitors, sensitizes airway sensory nerves and enhances the cough reflex. A number of reports indicate that the insertion/deletion (*I/D*) polymorphism of the ACE gene (ACE DD allele) is associated with an increased risk of pneumonia.[74,75] Furthermore, the use of ACE inhibitors is associated with a reduced risk of aspiration pneumonia (see the section that follows).

FACTORS THAT INCREASE THE RISK OF PNEUMONIA IN PATIENTS WHO ASPIRATE

While the presence of dysphagia and the volume of the aspirate are key factors that predispose patients to aspiration pneumonia, a number of other factors play an important role.[51] Colonization of the oropharynx is an important step in the pathogenesis of aspiration pneumonia. The elderly have increased oropharyngeal colonization with pathogens such as *Staphylococcus aureus* and aerobic gram-negative bacilli (e.g., *Klebsiella pneumoniae* and *Escherichia coli*). Although this increased colonization may be transient, it underlies the increased risk in the elderly of pneumonia with these pathogens. Furthermore, colonization of dental plaque may be an important risk factor for aspiration pneumonia.[76] The defects in host defenses that predispose to enhanced colonization with these organisms are uncertain; however, dysphagia with a decrease in salivary clearance and poor oral hygiene may be major risk factors.[77] Residents of long-term care facilities are prone to poor oral health due to lack of oral hygiene care as well as conditions of peridental and/or dental disease. Langmore et al.[78] reported that in elderly patients the number of decayed teeth and never or only occasionally brushing teeth were independent predictors of aspiration pneumonia. Similarly, Azarpazhooh and Leake [79] performed a systematic review that demonstrated that the presence of cariogenic and periodontal pathogens in dental plaque and saliva and decayed teeth were independent predictors of aspiration pneumonia. Awano et al.[80] demonstrated that persons with 10 or more periodontal pockets had an increased risk of death from pneumonia. Proton pump inhibitors increase gastric and oropharyngeal colonization with potentially pathogenic organisms. Gulmez et al.[81] reported that the concurrent use of proton pump inhibitors in patients over the age of 60 increased the risk for community-acquired (aspiration) pneumonia.

DIAGNOSIS AND MANAGEMENT OF ASPIRATION PNEUMONIA

There is no "gold standard" test to diagnose aspiration pneumonia. Furthermore, in patients with aspiration pneumonia, unlike the case of aspiration pneumonitis, the episode of aspiration is generally not witnessed. The diagnosis is therefore inferred when a patient with known risk factors for aspiration develops clinical features compatible with pneumonia (fever, shortness of breath, purulent sputum) with an infiltrate in a characteristic bronchopulmonary segment (see Fig. 69-2). In patients who aspirate in the recumbent position the commonest sites of involvement are the posterior segments of the upper lobes and the apical segments of the lower lobes. In patients who aspirate in the upright or semirecumbent position the basal segments of the lower lobes are favored. The usual picture is that of an acute pneumonic process, which runs a course similar to that of a typical CAP. Untreated, however, these patients appear to have a higher incidence of cavitation and lung abscess formation.[82]

Antimicrobial therapy is indicated in patients with aspiration pneumonia. The choice of antibiotics should depend on the setting in which the aspiration occurs as well as the patient's premorbid condition. This includes such factors as whether the aspiration occurred in the community or in a healthcare facility (healthcare-associated pneumonia [HCAP]) and patient characteristics such as alcoholism, oral hygiene, intravenous drug abuse, and the recent use of antibiotics or acid suppressive therapy.[83] In otherwise "healthy" outpatients a narrow-spectrum antibiotic which targets organisms such as *Streptococcus pneumoniae, S. aureus,* and *Haemophilus influenzae* is recommended. However, most patients with aspiration pneumonia have risk factors for colonization and infection with aerobic gram-negative organisms and require treatment with antimicrobials such as third generation cephalosporins, fluoroquinolones, piperacillin, or carbapenems.[83–86] In addition, vancomycin or linezolid should be considered in patients at risk of infection with methicillin-resistant *S. aureus* (MRSA). Although commonly prescribed (and often considered the standard of care) antimicrobials with specific anaerobic activity are not routinely warranted. The anaerobic bacteria that colonize the oropharynx are intrinsically of low virulence. In an experiment dating back to 1930, Smith introduced bacteria isolated from patients with Vincent angina into the lungs of rabbits.[87] Cultures of a single organism failed to produce pneumonia; only when multiple different organisms were instilled into the lungs did the animals develop pneumonia (synergistic anaerobic infection). In the most rigorous study to date, El-Sohl et al.[86] performed protected quantitative bronchial sampling in 95 patients with severe aspiration pneumonia. Out of the 67 pathogens identified, gram-negative enteric bacteria were the predominant organisms isolated (49%), followed by anaerobic bacteria (16%) and *S. aureus* (12%). A single anaerobic bacterium was isolated from 11 patients usually in association with a gram-negative pathogen. Although seven cases with anaerobic isolates received initially inadequate antimicrobial therapy, six had effective clinician response. Antimicrobials with specific anaerobic activity may only be indicated in patients with periodontal disease, patients expectorating putrid sputum and patients with a necrotizing pneumonia or lung abscess on chest radiograph.[2,83–85]

ASSESSMENT AND MANAGEMENT OF DYSPHAGIA

All elderly patients with CAP, as well as patients with a recent cerebrovascular accident and those with degenerative neurologic diseases should be referred to a speech and language pathologist (SLP) for a formal swallow evaluation (Video 69-1).[67,88] Those patients with dysphagia require the formulation and implementation of an individualized management strategy. A clinician's bedside assessment of the cough and gag reflex is unreliable in screening for patients at risk of aspiration. Because objective swallowing evaluation can be performed with a nasogastric tube or feeding tube in place, it is not necessary to remove the tube (and interrupt enteral feedings) to evaluate dysphagia. Similarly, there is no contraindication to leaving a nasogastric tube in place to supplement oral alimentation.[89]

The management of patients with dysphagia requires the coordinated expertise of a number of healthcare professionals, including the patient's primary care physician, pulmonologist, SLP, clinical dietician, occupational therapist, physiotherapist, nurse, oral

Video 69-1 An 82 year-old male admitted with PNA, required multiple intubations and eventual tracheostomy. Fiberoptic endoscopic evaluation of swallowing (FEES) completed with #5XLT proximal/cuffless tracheostomy (patient capped on room air) and Dobhoff feeding tube in place. FEES revealed a severe pharyngeal dysphagia. There is pooling of secretions throughout pharynx/larynx (valleculae and pyriform sinuses) with aspiration of secretions. With pureed texture there is residue throughout the pharynx suggestive of generalized reduced pharyngeal contraction. The residue in the valleculae is a result of reduced base of tongue retraction, epiglottis dysfunction, and poor hyoid elevation. The residue in the pyriform sinuses is a result of cricopharyngeus dysfunction/inadequate upper esophageal sphincter opening. There is a delayed pharyngeal swallow response with nectar consistency with bolus spilling to the pyriform sinuses resulting in + aspiration before/during/after the swallow response due to reduced arytenoid tilt and vocal fold adduction. *(Used with permission of Randy Dubin.) Access at www.fishmansonline.com*

hygienist, dentist, as well as the patient's primary caregivers. The goal is to optimize the safety, efficiency, and effectiveness of the oropharyngeal swallow to maintain adequate nutrition and hydration and to improve oral hygiene. Enhanced quality of life, wherever possible, should direct management and oral intake (when possible) is preferred over tube feeding. A fundamental principle of rehabilitation is that the best therapy for any activity is the activity itself; as swallowing may be considered the best therapy for swallowing disorders, rehabilitation should be aimed at identifying ways of ensuring safe and effective swallowing in individual patients. Current treatment for dysphagia includes prevention of aspiration in the form of diet and fluid modifications, compensatory maneuvers, position changes, and rehabilitation exercises.[90] Diet modification is a common treatment for dysphagia. Modifications in food consistency are individually determined by means of the clinical swallow and/or videofluoroscopic swallow evaluation. Reduction in bolus volume and enhancement of bolus viscosity significantly improve the safety of swallowing and reduce the risk of aspiration.[63] The SI physical unit of dynamic viscosity is the pascal-second (Pa·s). The prevalence of aspiration is maximal with water and thin fluids (20 Pa·s) and decreases with nectar (270 Pa·s) and pudding (3900 Pa·s) viscosity boluses.[63] By increasing the viscosity or thickness of the food or liquid bolus in patients with oral sensory or motor deficits, the material is less likely to escape from the oral cavity, fall into the laryngeal inlet, or penetrate the incompletely sealed larynx during the delay before pharyngeal swallowing starts. Videofluoroscopic studies have demonstrated that increasing viscosity of liquids to pudding viscosity significantly reduces the risk of aspiration.[91,92] In addition to changes in diet, maintenance of oral feeding often requires compensatory techniques to reduce aspiration or to improve pharyngeal clearance. A variety of behavioral techniques are used, including modifications in posture, head position and respiration, as well as specific swallowing maneuvers. The chin-down posture has been suggested to reduce the risk of aspiration.[92–94] Welch et al.[95] noted that the posterior shift of anterior pharyngeal structures with the chin-down posture improved airway protection. The preferred intervention in patients with dysphagia and the impact of these interventions on the risk of aspiration pneumonia is however unclear.[96]

Neuromuscular electrical stimulation (NMES) is a relatively new treatment for oropharyngeal dysphagia.[97–99] NMES for dysphagia entails applying electrodes to the muscles of the head and neck, and stimulating those muscles that are weakened or hemiparetic by means of electric pulses. This is generally combined with the subject swallowing food or fluids that are predetermined to represent the most appropriate consistency that the person can tolerate without aspiration. Further research on the effects of NMES is warranted before surface electrical stimulation can be recommended as treatment of dysphagia

Tube Feeding

Tube feeding is not essential in all patients who aspirate. Short-term tube feeding, however, may be indicated in elderly patients with severe dysphagia and aspiration in whom improvement of swallowing is likely to occur. Nakajoh et al.[71] demonstrated that the incidence of pneumonia was significantly higher in stroke patients with dysphagia who were fed orally compared to those who received tube feeding (54.3 vs. 13.2%, $p < 0.001$), despite the fact that the orally fed patients had a higher functional status (higher Barthel index). The *FOOD* trials consisted of two large randomized studies that enrolled dysphagic stroke patients.[100] In the first trial, patients enrolled within 7 days of admission were randomly allocated to early tube feeding or no tube feeding. Early tube feeding was associated with an absolute reduction in risk of death of 5.8%. The second trial allocated patients to early nasogastric feeding or early feeding via a percutaneous endoscopic gastrostomy (PEG) tube. PEG feeding was associated with an absolute increase in the risk of death of 1% and an increased risk of death or poor outcome of 7.8%. Patients with a PEG were less likely to be transitioned to oral feeding than the nasogastric group and were more likely to be living in an institution. This may in part explain the higher mortality of the PEG-fed patients. Furthermore, it was interesting to note that PEG-fed patients were more likely to develop pressure sores, suggesting that these patients may have been nursed differently. The results of the FOOD trials suggest that dysphagic stroke patients should be fed early via a nasogastric or feeding tube and transitioned to oral feeding as their dysphagia resolves. Those patients whose dysphagia does not resolve may be candidates for placement of a PEG tube.

Oral Hygiene

Dental plaque as well as "tongue coating" serves as a reservoir of potentially pathogenic organisms.[76] Occupants of residential homes have been shown to have poor oral hygiene and rarely receive treatment from dentists and oral hygienists.[101] An aggressive protocol of oral care will reduce colonization with potentially pathogenic organisms and decrease the bacterial load, measures that have been demonstrated to reduce the risk of aspiration pneumonia.[102–105] Oral care should not be overlooked in edentulous patients as "tongue cleaning" is associated with a decreased oropharyngeal bacterial load.[106,107]

Pharmacologic Management

The neurotransmitter, Substance P, is believed to play a major role in both the cough and swallow sensory pathways. ACE inhibitors prevent the breakdown of Substance P and may theoretically be useful in the management of patients with aspiration pneumonia. A number of studies have demonstrated a lower risk of aspiration pneumonia in stroke patients treated with an ACE inhibitor compared to other antihypertensive agents.[108,109] This observation was initially noted in Japanese patients and it has been suggested that this benefit was restricted to Asian populations.[110] Furthermore, it has been postulated that lipophilic ACE inhibitors may be more beneficial than hydrophilic ACE inhibitors.[111] However, a population-based case-control study from the United Kingdom demonstrated that the current prescription for an ACE inhibitor was associated with a reduction of the risk of pneumonia in the general population (OR 0.75, 95% CI 0.65–0.86).[112] Nicergoline (Sermion, Pfizer), an ergot alkaloid derivative, has been demonstrated to upregulate Substance P and improve dysphagia with an efficacy similar to that of ACE inhibitors.[113] Additional studies are required with this drug to determine its role in preventing aspiration pneumonia.

Sedative medication has been demonstrated to increase the risk of pneumonia in residents of long-term-care facilities and should, therefore, be avoided.[114] The prescription of phenothiazines and haloperidol should be very carefully considered, as they reduce oropharyngeal swallow coordination, causing dysphagia.[115,116] Medications that dry up secretions, including antihistamines and drugs with anticholinergic activity, make it more difficult for patients to swallow and should therefore also be avoided.[115,117]

DIFFUSE ASPIRATION BRONCHIOLITIS

Occult aspiration can result in lung damage with a variety of radiographic, clinical, and histologic manifestations. Occult aspiration in the elderly is usually associated with esophageal dysmotility, gastroesophageal reflux disease (GERD) as well as neurologic impairment (dysphagia) and frequently presents with acute onset of symptoms while sleeping.[118] Diffuse aspiration bronchiolitis is a distinct clinical entity that was first defined by Matsuse et al.[3] in 1996 as a syndrome characterized by chronic bronchiolar inflammation from recurrent aspiration of foreign matter (food). Their case series was based on autopsy findings and represented an elderly, chronically debilitated

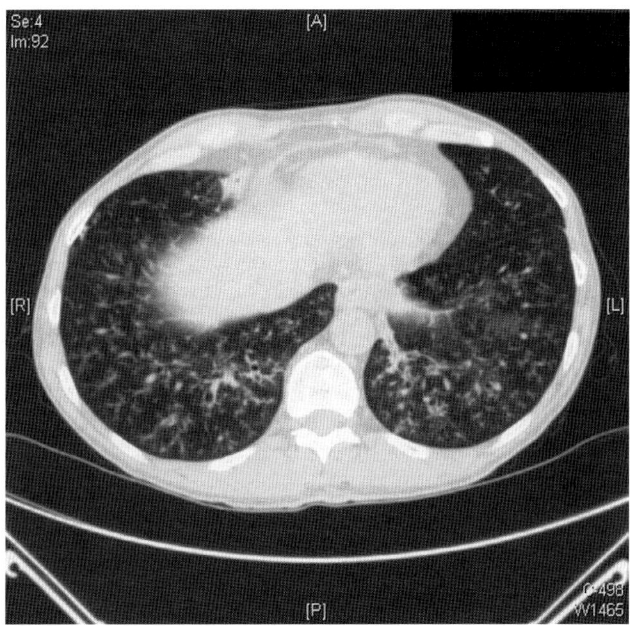

Figure 69-3 CT scan of patient with diffuse aspiration bronchiolitis.

population. Dysphagia was recorded in over half of the patients with two-thirds being bedridden. Diffuse aspiration bronchiolitis should be suspected in elderly patients with recurrent episodes of bronchorrhea, bronchospasm, and dyspnea. However, this syndrome has been reported in middle-aged patients (mean age 50 years) with "asymptomatic" GERD.[119] Typical findings on the chest radiograph include the presence of regional or disseminated small nodular shadows and hyperlucency. Airspace consolidation is relatively rare. Chest CT scans demonstrate diffuse centrilobular nodules with a tree-in-bud pattern (Fig. 69-3).[120] It is likely that this disease is underrecognized and therefore often inappropriately managed.

CONCLUSIONS

Aspiration pneumonitis and pneumonia are common clinical syndromes. Aspiration pneumonitis follows the aspiration of gastric contents, usually in patients with a marked decreased level of consciousness. Treatment of aspiration pneumonitis is essentially supportive, however, corticosteroids and other immunomodulating agents may have a role in these patients. Aspiration pneumonia occurs in patients with dysphagia and usually presents as a "CAP" with a focal infiltrate in a dependent bronchopulmonary segment. Patients with aspiration pneumonia require treatment with broad-spectrum antibiotics and management of the underlying dysphagia. Diffuse aspiration bronchiolitis presents with radiographic evidence of widespread centrilobular and tree-in-bud opacities; clinicians must be aware of the possibility of occult aspiration in order to make the correct diagnosis.

REFERENCES

1. Osler W. *Pneumonias and Pneumococcic Infections. The Principles and Practice of Medicine*. 8th ed. New York, NY: D. Appleton & Co.; 1918; 74–108.
2. Marik PE. Aspiration pneumonitis and pneumonia: a clinical review. *N Engl J Med*. 2001;344:665–671.
3. Matsuse T, Oka T, Kida K, Fukuchi Y. Importance of diffuse aspiration bronchiolitis caused by chronic occult aspiration in the elderly. *Chest*. 1996;110:1289–1293.
4. Adnet F, Baud F. Relation between Glasgow Coma Scale and aspiration pneumonia [letter]. *Lancet*. 1996;348:123–214.
5. Mendelson CL. The aspiration of stomach contents into the lungs during obstetric anesthesia. *Am J Obstet Gynecol*. 1946;52:191–205.
6. Teabeaut JR. Aspiration of gastric contents. An experimental study. *Am J Pathol*. 1952;28:51–67.
7. Warner MA, Warner ME, Weber JG. Clinical significance of pulmonary aspiration during the perioperative period. *Anesthesiol*. 1993;78:56–62.
8. Knight PR, Rutter T, Tait AR, Coleman E, Johnson K. Pathogenesis of gastric particulate lung injury: a comparison and interaction with acidic pneumonitis. *Anesth Analg*. 1993;77:754–760.
9. Knight PR, Davidson BA, Nader ND, et al. Progressive, severe lung injury secondary to the interaction of insults in gastric aspiration. *Exp Lung Res*. 2004;30:535–557.
10. Pepe PE, Potkin RT, Reus DH, Hudson LD, Carrico CJ. Clinical predictors of the adult respiratory distress syndrome. *Am J Surg*. 1982;144:124–130.
11. Fowler AA, Hamman RF, Good JT, et al. Adult respiratory distress syndrome: risk with common predispositions. *Ann Intern Med*. 1983;98:593–597.
12. Rotta AT, Shiley KT, Davidson BA, Helinski JD, Russo TA, Knight PR. Gastric acid and particulate aspiration injury inhibits pulmonary bacterial clearance. *Crit Care Med*. 2004;32:747–754.
13. van Westerloo DJ, Knapp S, van't Veer C, et al. Aspiration pneumonitis primes the host for an exaggerated inflammatory response during pneumonia. *Crit Care Med*. 2005;33:1770–1778.
14. Olsson GL, Hallen B, Hambraeus-Jonzon K. Aspiration during anaesthesia: a computer-aided study of 185,358 anaesthetics. *Acta Anaesthesiol Scand*. 1986;30:84–92.
15. Beck-Schimmer B, Bonvini JM. Bronchoaspiration: incidence, consequences and management. *Eur J Anaesthesiol*. 2011;28:78–84.
16. Sakai T, Planinsic RM, Quinlan JJ, Handley LJ, Kim TY, Hilmi IA. The incidence and outcome of perioperative pulmonary aspiration in a university hospital: a 4-year retrospective analysis. *Anesth Analg*. 2006;103:941–947.
17. Klanarong S, Suksompong S, Hintong T, Chau-In W, Jantorn P, Werawatganon T. Perioperative pulmonary aspiration: an analysis of 28 reports from the Thai Anesthesia Incident Monitoring Study (Thai AIMS). *J Med Assoc Thai*. 2011;94:457–464.
18. Cook TM, Woodall N, Frerk C. Major complications of airway management in the UK: results of the Fourth National Audit Project of the Royal College of Anaesthetists and the Difficult Airway Society. Part 1: anaesthesia. *Br J Anaesth*. 2011;106:617–631.
19. Cook TM, Woodall N, Harper J, Benger J. Major complications of airway management in the UK: results of the Fourth National Audit Project of the Royal College of Anaesthetists and the Difficult Airway Society. Part 2: intensive care and emergency departments. *Br J Anaesth*. 2011;106:632–642.
20. Memtsoudis S, Liu SS, Ma Y, et al. Perioperative pulmonary outcomes in patients with sleep apnea after noncardiac surgery. *Anesth Analg*. 2011;112:113–121.
21. Dindelli M, La RM, Rossi R, et al. Incidence and complications of the aspiration of gastric contents syndrome during cesarean section in general anesthesia [Italian]. *Ann Ostet Ginecol Med Perinat*. 1991;112:376–384.
22. Soreide E, Bjornestad E, Steen PA. An audit of perioperative aspiration pneumonitis in gynaecological and obstetric patients. *Acta Anaesthesiol Scand*. 1996;40:14–19.

23. La Rosa M, Piva L, Ravanelli A, Dindelli M, Pagnoni B. Aspiration syndrome in cesarean section. Our experience from 1980 to 1990 [Italian]. *Minerva Anestesiol.* 1992;58:1213–1220.

24. Krantz ML, Edwards WL. The incidence of nonfatal aspiration in obstetric patients. *Anesthesiol.* 1973;39:359.

25. Levy DM, Williams OA, Magides AD, Reilly CS. Gastric emptying is delayed at 8–12 weeks' gestation. *Br J Anaesth.* 1994;73: 237–238.

26. Vanner RG. Gastro-oesophageal reflux and regurgitation during general anaesthesia for termination of pregnancy. *Int J Obstet Anesth.* 1992;1:123–128.

27. Keller C, Brimacombe J, Bittersohl J, Lirk P, von Goedecke A. Aspiration and the laryngeal mask airway: three cases and a review of the literature. *Br J Anaesth.* 2004;93:579–582.

28. Hirani A, Cavallazzi R, Shnister A, Marik PE. Airway pressure release ventilation (APRV) for treatment of severe life-threatening ARDS in a morbidly obese patient. *Crit Care Shock.* 2008;11:132.

29. Brimacombe JR, Berry A. The incidence of aspiration associated with the laryngeal mask airway: a meta-analysis of published literature. *J Clin Anesth.* 1995;7:297–305.

30. Viby-Mogensen J. Neuromuscular monitoring. In: Miller RD, Eriksson LI, Fleisher LA, et al., eds. *Miller's Anesthesia.* 7th ed. Orlando, FL: Churchill Livingstone; 2009:1515–1531.

31. Miller M, Wishart HY, Nimmo WS. Gastric contents at induction of anaesthesia. Is a 4-hour fast necessary? *Br J Anaesth.* 1983;55:1185–1188.

32. Brady M, Kinn S, Stuart P. Preoperative fasting for adults to prevent perioperative complications. *Cochrane Database Syst Rev.* 2003;(4):CD004423.

33. American Society of Anesthesiologists Committee. Practice guidelines for preoperative fasting and the use of pharmacologic agents to reduce the risk of pulmonary aspiration: application to healthy patients undergoing elective procedures. An updated report by the American Society of Anesthesiologists Committee on Standards and Practice Parameters. *Anesthesiology.* 2011;114:495–511.

34. Engelhardt T, Webster NR. Pulmonary aspiration of gastric contents in anaesthesia. *Br J Anaesth.* 1999;83:453–460.

35. Ryan JR, Vargas R, McMahon FG, Chremos AN. Comparison of effects of oral and intravenous famotidine on inhibition of nocturnal gastric acid secretion. *Am J Med.* 1986;81:60–64.

36. Sellick BA. Cricoid pressure to control regurgitation of stomach contents during induction of anaesthesia. *Lancet.* 1961;2: 404–406.

37. Neilipovitz DT, Crosby ET. No evidence for decreased incidence of aspiration after rapid sequence induction. *Can J Anaes.* 2007;54:748–764.

38. Smith KJ, Dobranowski J, Yip G, Dauphin A, Choi PT. Cricoid pressure displaces the esophagus: an observational study using magnetic resonance imaging. *Anesthesiology.* 2003;99:60–64.

39. Rice MJ, Mancuso AA, Gibbs C, Morey TE, Gravenstein N. Cricoid pressure results in compression of the postcricoid hypopharynx: the esophageal position is irrelevant. *Anesth Analg.* 2009;109:1546–1552.

40. Agarwal R, Schwartz DN. Procalcitonin to guide duration of antimicrobial therapy in intensive care units: a systematic review. *Clin Infect Dis.* 2011;53:379–387.

41. el-Solh AA, Vora H, Knight PR III, Porhomayon J. Diagnostic use of serum procalcitonin levels in pulmonary aspiration syndromes. *Crit Care Med.* 2011;39:1251–1256.

42. Haussmann W, Lunt RL. Problem of treatment of peptic aspiration pneumonia following obstetric anesthesia (Mendelson's syndrome). *J Obstet Gynaecol Br Emp.* 1955;62:509–512.

43. Sukumaran M, Granada MJ, Berger HW, Lee M, Reilly TA. Evaluation of corticosteroid treatment in aspiration of gastric contents: a controlled clinical trial. *Mt Sinai J Med.* 1980;47: 335–340.

44. Wolfe JE, Bone RC, Ruth WE. Effects of corticosteroids in the treatment of patients with gastric aspiration. *Am J Med.* 1977;63: 719–722.

45. Kudoh I, Miyazaki H, Ohara M, Fukushima J, Tazawa T, Yamada H. Activation of alveolar macrophages in acid-injured lung in rats: different effects of pentoxifylline on tumor necrosis factor-alpha and nitric oxide production. *Crit Care Med.* 2001;29:1621–1625.

46. Zarbock A, Singbartl K, Ley K. Complete reversal of acid-induced acute lung injury by blocking of platelet-neutrophil aggregation. *J Clin Invest.* 2006;116:3211–3219.

47. Kinniry P, Amrani Y, Vachani A, et al. Dietary flaxseed supplementation ameliorates inflammation and oxidative tissue damage in experimental models of acute lung injury in mice. *J Nutr.* 2006;136:1545–1551.

48. Terao Y, Nakamura T, Morooka H, Sumikawa K. Effect of cyclooxygenase-2 inhibitor pretreatment on gas exchange after hydrochloric acid aspiration in rats. *J Anesth.* 2005;19: 257–259.

49. Pawlik MT, Schreyer AG, Ittner KP, et al. Early treatment with pentoxifylline reduces lung injury induced by acid aspiration in rats. *Chest.* 2005;127:613–321.

50. Pawlik MT, Schubert T, Hopf S, et al. The effects of fenoterol inhalation after acid aspiration-induced lung injury. *Anesth Analg.* 2009;109:143–150.

51. Croghan JE, Burke EM, Caplan S, Denman S. Pilot study of 12-month outcomes of nursing home patients with aspiration on videofluoroscopy. *Dysphagia.* 1994;9:141–146.

52. Kikuchi R, Watabe N, Konno T, Mishina N, Sekizawa K, Sasaki H. High incidence of silent aspiration in elderly patients with community-acquired pneumonia. *Am J Respir Crit Care Med.* 1994;150:251–253.

53. Torres A, Serra-Batlles J, Ferrer A, et al. Severe community-acquired pneumonia epidemiology and prognostic factors. *Am Rev Respir Dis.* 1991;144:312–318.

54. Moine P, Vercken JP, Chevret S, Chastang C, Gajdos P. Severe community-acquired pneumonia: etiology, epidemiology, and prognosis factors. *Chest.* 1994;105:1487–1495.

55. Jokinen C, Heiskanen L, Juvonen H, et al. Incidence of community-acquired pneumonia in the population of four municipalities in eastern Finland. *Am J Epidemiol.* 1993;137: 977–988.

56. Koivula I, Stenn M, Makela PH. Risk factors for pneumonia in the elderly. *Am J Med.* 1994;96:313–320.

57. Loeb M, McGreer A, McArthur M, Walter S, Simor AS. Risk factors for pneumonia and other lower respiratory tract infections in elderly residents of long-term care facilities. *Arch Intern Med.* 1999;159:2058–2064.

58. Daniels SK, Foundas AL. Lesion localization in acute stroke patients with risk of aspiration. *J Neuroimaging.* 1999;9: 91–98.

59. Australian and New Zealand Society for Geriatric Medicine. Position statement - dysphagia and aspiration in older people*. *Australas J Ageing.* 2011;30:98–103.

60. Robbins J, Langmore S, Hind JA, Erlichman M. Dysphagia research in the 21st century and beyond: proceedings from Dysphagia Experts Meeting, August 21, 2001. *J Rehabil Res Dev*. 2002;39:543–548.

61. Agency for Health Care Policy and Research. *Diagnosis and Treatment of Swallowing Disorders (Dysphagia) in Acute Care Stroke. Patients Summary*. Agency for Health Care Policy and Research;1999. http:www.ahcpr.gov/clinic/dysphsum.htm.

62. Ekberg O, Hamdy S, Woisard V, Wuttge-Hannig A, Ortega P. Social and psychological burden of dysphagia: its impact on diagnosis and treatment. *Dysphagia*. 2002;17:139–146.

63. Rofes L, Arreola V, Almirall J, et al. Diagnosis and management of oropharyngeal dysphagia and its nutritional and respiratory complications in the elderly. *Gastroenterol Res Pract*. 2011; 2011.

64. Robbins J, Levine R, Wood J, Roecker EB, Luschei E. Age effects on lingual pressure generation as a risk factor for dysphagia. *J Gerontol A Biol Sci Med Sci*. 1995;50:M257–M262.

65. Holas MA, DePippo KL, Reding MJ. Aspiration and relative risk of medical complications following stroke. *Arch Neurol*. 1994;51:1051–1053.

66. Smithard DG, O'Neill PA, Parks C, Morris J. Complications and outcome after acute stroke. Does dysphagia matter? *Stroke*. 1996;27:1200–1204.

67. Agency for Health Care Policy and Research Guidelines. *Post-Stroke Rehabilitation Clinical Guidelines*; 1996. http://www.ncbi.nlm.nih.gov/bookshelf/br.fcgi?book=hsarchive&part=A27305. Accessed September 1, 2009.

68. Smithard DG, O'Neill PA, England RE, et al. The natural history of dysphagia following a stroke. *Dysphagia*. 1997;12: 188–193.

69. Mann G, Hankey GJ, Cameron D. Swallowing function after stroke: prognosis and prognostic factors at 6 months. *Stroke*. 1999;30:744–748.

70. Sekizawa K, Ujiie Y, Itabashi S, Sasaki H, Takishima T. Lack of cough reflex in aspiration pneumonia. *Lancet*. 1990;335:1228–1229.

71. Nakajoh K, Nakagawa T, Sekizawa K, Matsui T, Arai H, Sasaki H. Relation between incidence of pneumonia and protective reflexes in post-stroke patients with oral or tube feeding. *J Intern Med*. 2000;247:39–42.

72. Nakazawa H, Sekizawa K, Ujiie Y, Sasaki H, Takishima T. Risk of aspiration pneumonia in the elderly. *Chest*. 1993;103:1636–1637.

73. Nakagawa T, Ohrui T, Sekizawa K, Sasaki H. Sputum substance P in aspiration pneumonia. *Lancet*. 1995;345:1447.

74. Morimoto S, Okaishi K, Onishi M, et al. Deletion allele of the angiotensin-converting enzyme gene as a risk factor for pneumonia in elderly patients. *Am J Med*. 2002;112:89–94.

75. Takahashi T, Morimoto S, Okaishi K, et al. Reduction of pneumonia risk by an angiotensin I-converting enzyme inhibitor in elderly Japanese inpatients according to insertion/deletion polymorphism of the angiotensin I-converting enzyme gene. *Am J Hypertens*. 2005;18:1353–1359.

76. el-Solh AA, Pietrantoni C, Bhat A, et al. Colonization of dental plaques: a reservoir of respiratory pathogens for hospital-acquired pneumonia in institutionalized elders. *Chest*. 2004;126: 1575–1582.

77. Palmer LB, Albulak K, Fields S, Filkin AM, Simon S, Smaldone GC. Oral clearance and pathogenic oropharyngeal colonization in the elderly. *Am J Respir Crit Care Med*. 2001;164:464–468.

78. Langmore SE, Terpenning MS, Schork A, et al. Predictors of aspiration pneumonia: how important is dysphagia? *Dysphagia*. 1998;13:69–81.

79. Azarpazhooh A, Leake JL. Systematic review of the association between respiratory diseases and oral health. *J Periodontol*. 2006; 77:1465–1482.

80. Awano S, Ansai T, Takata Y, et al. Oral health and mortality risk from pneumonia in the elderly. *J Dent Res*. 2008;87: 334–339.

81. Gulmez SE, Holm A, Frederiksen H, Jensne TG, Pedersen C, Hallas J. Use of proton pump inhibitors and the risk of community-acquired pneumonia. *Arch Intern Med*. 2007;167:950–955.

82. Bartlett JG, Gorbach SL, Feinegold SM. The bacteriology of aspiration pneumonia. *Am J Med*. 1974;56:202–207.

83. American Thoracic Society; Infectious Diseases Society of America. Guidelines for the management of adults with hospital-acquired, ventilator-associated, and healthcare-associated pneumonia. *Am J Respir Crit Care Med*. 2005;171:388–416.

84. Mier L, Dreyfuss D, Darchy B, et al. Is penicillin G an adequate initial treatment for aspiration pneumonia? A prospective evaluation using a protected specimen brush and quantitative cultures. *Intensive Care Med*. 1993;19:279–284.

85. Marik PE, Careau P. The role of anaerobes in patients with ventilator-associated pneumonia and aspiration pneumonia. A prospective study. *Chest*. 1999;115:178–183.

86. El-Sohl AA, Pietrantoni C, Bhat A, et al. Microbiology of severe aspiration pneumonia in institutionalized elderly. *Am J Respir Crit Care Med*. 2003;167:1650–1654.

87. Smith DT. Fusospirochetal disease of the lungs produced with cultures from Vincent's angina. *J Infect Dis*. 1930;46:303.

88. Murray J. *Manual of Dysphagia Assessment in Adults*. San Diego, CA: Singular Publishing Group; 1999.

89. Leder SB, Suiter DM. Effect of nasogastric tubes on incidence of aspiration. *Arch Phys Med Rehabil*. 2008;89:648–651.

90. Cecconi E, Di Piero V. Dysphagia–pathophysiology, diagnosis and treatment. *Front Neurol Neurosci*. 2012;30:86–89.

91. Clave P, de Kraa M, Arreola V, et al. The effect of bolus viscosity on swallowing function in neurogenic dysphagia. *Aliment Pharmacol Ther*. 2006;24:1385–1394.

92. Longemann JA, Gensler G, Robbins JA, et al. A randomized study of three interventions for aspiration of thin liquids in patients with dementia or Parkinson's disease. *J Speech Lang Hear Res*. 2008;51:173–183.

93. Shanahan TK, Logemann JA, Rademaker AW, Pauloski BR, Kahrilas PJ. Chin-down posture effect on aspiration in dysphagic patients. *Arch Phys Med Rehabil*. 1993;74:736–739.

94. Rasley A, Logemann JA, Kahrilas PJ, Rademaker AW, Pauloski BR, Dodds WJ. Prevention of barium aspiration during videofluoroscopic swallowing studies: value of change in posture. *AJR Am J Roentgenol*. 1993;160:1005–1009.

95. Welch MV, Logemann JA, Rademaker AW, Kahrilas PJ. Changes in pharyngeal dimensions effected by chin tuck. *Arch Phys Med Rehabil*. 1993;74:178–181.

96. Robbins J, Gensler G, Hind J, et al. Comparison of 2 interventions for liquid aspiration on pneumonia incidence: a randomized trial. *Ann Intern Med*. 2008;148:509–518.

97. Langdon C, Blacker D. Dysphagia in stroke: a new solution. *Stroke Res Treat*. 2010;2010:pii: 570403. doi:10.4061/2010/570403

98. Heijnen BJ, Speyer R, Baijens LW, Bogaardt HC. Neuromuscular electrical stimulation versus traditional therapy in patients

with Parkinson's disease and oropharyngeal dysphagia: effects on quality of life. *Dysphagia*. 2012;27:336–345.

99. Bogaardt H, van DD, Wever NM, Bruggeman CE, Koops J, Fokkens WJ. Use of neuromuscular electrostimulation in the treatment of dysphagia in patients with multiple sclerosis. *Ann Otol Rhinol Laryngol*. 2009;118:241–246.
100. Dennis MS, Lewis SC, Warlow C. Effect of timing and method of enteral tube feeding for dysphagic stroke patients (FOOD): a multicentre randomised controlled trial. *Lancet*. 2005;365: 764–772.
101. Simons D, Kidd EA, Beighton D. Oral health of elderly occupants in residential homes. *Lancet*. 1999;353:1761.
102. Yoneyama T, Yoshida M, Matsui T, Sasaki H. Oral care and pneumonia [letter]. *Lancet*. 1999;354:515.
103. Bassim CW, Gibson G, Ward T, Paphides BM, Denucci DJ. Modification of the risk of mortality from pneumonia with oral hygiene care. *J Am Geriatr Soc*. 2008;56:1601–1607.
104. Ishikawa A, Yoneyama T, Hirota K, Miyake Y, Miyatake K. Professional oral health care reduces the number of oropharyngeal bacteria. *J Dent Res*. 2008;87:594–598.
105. Adachi M, Ishihara K, Abe S, Okuda K, Ishikawa T. Effect of professional oral health care on the elderly living in nursing homes. *Oral Surg Med Oral Path Oral Radiol Endod*. 2002;94:191–195.
106. Yonezawa H, Takasaki K, Teraoka K, Asaka T, Sato C, Tsuchiya K. Effects of tongue and oral mucosa cleaning on oral Candida species and production of volatile sulfur compounds in the elderly in a nursing home. *J Med Dent Sci*. 2003;50:1–8.
107. Abe S, Ishihara K, Adachi M, Okuda K. Tongue-coating as risk indicator for aspiration pneumonia in edentate elderly. *Arch Gerontol Geriatr*. 2008;47:267–275.
108. Arai T, Yasuda Y, Toshima S, Yoshimi N, Kashiki Y. ACE inhibitors and pneumonia in elderly people. *Lancet*. 1998;352: 1937–1938.
109. Arai T, Yasuda Y, Takaya T, et al. Angiotensin-converting enzyme inhibitors, angiotensin-II receptor antagonists, and pneumonia in elderly hypertensive patients with stroke. *Chest*. 2001;119: 660–661.
110. Ohkubo T, Chapman N, Neal B, Woodward M, Omae T, Chalmers J. Effects of an angiotensin-converting enzyme inhibitor-based regimen on pneumonia risk. *Am J Respir Crit Care Med*. 2004;169:1041–1045.
111. Mortensen EM, Restrepo MI, Copeland LA, Pugh JA, Anzueto A. Association of hydrophilic versus lipophilic angiotensin-converting enzyme inhibitor use on pneumonia-related mortality. *Am J Med Sci*. 2008;336:462–466.
112. Myles PR, Hubbard RB, McKeever TM, Pogson Z, Smith CJ, Gibson JE. Risk of community-acquired pneumonia and the use of statins, ace inhibitors and gastric acid suppressants: a population-based case-control study. *Pharmac Drug Saf*. 18:269–275.
113. Nakashima T, Hattori N, Okimoto M, Yanagida J, Kohno N. Nicergoline improves dysphagia by upregulating substance P in the elderly. *Medicine*. 2011;90:279–283.
114. Vergis EN, Brennen C, Wagener M, Muder RR. Pneumonia in long-term care: a prospective case-control study of risk factors and impact on survival. *Arch Intern Med*. 2001;161:2378–2381.
115. Stoschus B, Allescher HB. Drug-induced dysphagia. *Dysphagia*. 1993;8:154–159.
116. Sokoloff LG, Pavlakovic R. Neuroleptic-induced dysphagia. *Dysphagia*. 1997;12:177–179.
117. Liedenberg B, Owall B. Masticatory ability in experimentally induced xerostomia. *Dysphagia*. 1991;6:211–213.
118. Friedlander AL, Fessler MB. A 70-year-old man with migratory pulmonary infiltrates. *Chest*. 2006;130:1269–1274.
119. Barnes TW, Vassallo R, Tazelaar HD, Hartman TE, Ryu JH. Diffuse bronchiolar disease due to chronic occult aspiration. *Mayo Clinic Proc*. 2006;81:172–176.
120. Okada F, Ando Y, Yoshitake S, et al. Clinical/pathologic correlations in 553 patients with primary centrilobular findings on high-resolution CT scan of the thorax. *Chest*. 2007;132: 1939–1948.

CHAPTER 70

Pulmonary Alveolar Proteinosis Syndrome

Bruce C. Trapnell

Takuji Suzuki

Pulmonary alveolar proteinosis (PAP) syndrome is characterized by the accumulation of surfactant in alveoli and terminal airways resulting in hypoxemic respiratory failure.[1] This fascinating syndrome continues to serve as a paradigm for disease discovery and development due to a globalized collaborative network, employment of diverse clinical, basic, and translational research approaches, and active patient involvement. While PAP occurs in many clinical settings including recently identified genetic etiologies, its molecular basis is now known in more than 90% of cases, and the molecular basis of the role of granulocyte macrophage colony-stimulating factor (GM-CSF) in surfactant homeostasis has been defined. Diseases associated with PAP can be grouped into primary PAP, secondary PAP, and congenital PAP based primarily on pathogenesis involved. Primary PAP is caused by impairment of GM-CSF–dependent surfactant clearance by alveolar macrophages and accounts for approximately 90% of all cases.[2] Secondary PAP occurs as a consequence of a comorbid condition that impair surfactant clearance by alveolar macrophages and accounts for about 5% of cases.[3] Congenital PAP is a clinically distinct and pathogenically heterogeneous group of genetic disorders associated with the production of abnormal surfactant and accounts for about 5% of cases.[4] Because of its increased frequency and greater research attention, primary PAP will be the focus of this chapter and data for secondary and congenital PAP will be provided where available.

PATHOGENESIS

In their initial description of PAP in 1958, Rosen et al.[5] established that the material accumulating within alveoli in PAP was composed of lipids, proteins, and a small amount of carbohydrate. Research over the past two decades has shown that in more than 90% of patients pathogenesis is driven by disruption of GM-CSF signaling, which blocks terminal differentiation of alveolar macrophages thereby impairing their ability to clear surfactant.[2] GM-CSF is a 23-kDa cytokine produced by respiratory epithelium and other cells[6,7] initially identified by its ability to stimulate the formation of macrophage and granulocyte colonies from hematological progenitors and subsequently shown to stimulate functions in mature myeloid and other cells. GM-CSF is expressed similarly in humans and mice and its effects are mediated by binding to cell surface receptors composed of a GM-CSF–binding α-chain (CD116) and an affinity-enhancing β-chain (CD131). Ligand binding activates intracellular signaling via multiple pathways including signal transducer and activator of transcription 5 (STAT5) regulating diverse functions of myeloid cells including survival, differentiation, proliferation, and priming of specific host defense functions.[8,9] GM-CSF also has poorly understood effects of alveolar epithelium. In primary PAP, pathogenesis is caused by disruption of GM-CSF signaling by neutralizing GM-CSF autoantibodies in autoimmune PAP or by recessive mutations in *CSF2RA* or *CSF2RB* (encoding GM-CSF receptor α-chain [CD116] or β-chain [CD131], respectively) in hereditary PAP.[1,2,10–13]

SURFACTANT HOMEOSTASIS

Surfactant is vital to lung function and acts at the air–liquid–tissue interface to prevent alveolar wall collapse. It is composed of 90% lipids (largely phospholipids), 10% proteins (surfactant protein [SP]-A, -B, -C and -D), and less than 1% carbohydrate.[14] SP-B and SP-C are hydrophobic phosphoproteins that contribute significantly to the surface active properties of surfactant.[15] SP-A and SP-D are hydrophilic collectin family members that contribute to lung host defense.[16] Surfactant lipids and proteins are synthesized, stored, and secreted into the alveoli by type II alveolar epithelial cells. In the extracellular space, surfactant "large aggregates" contribute to formation of a film that lowers surface tension and stabilizes the alveolus.[17] Surfactant is expelled from the film as "small aggregates" that are internalized by type II cells and alveolar macrophages in roughly equal amounts (Fig. 70-1). Type II cells recycle and catabolize internalized surfactant equally via mechanisms that are poorly understood but do not appear to involve regulation by GM-CSF.[17–19] In contrast, alveolar macrophages exclusively catabolize internalized surfactant under the positive regulatory control of GM-CSF.[20,21]

ANIMAL MODELS OF PAP

The discovery that GM-CSF knockout (GM-CSF^{KO}) mice develop a pulmonary disease indistinguishable from primary PAP provided the first real pathogenic clue (Fig. 70-2).[22,23] In these mice, neither production of surfactant by type II cells, nor its uptake by alveolar macrophages was impaired.[22,24] Rather, surfactant clearance by alveolar macrophages was impaired.[25] Replacement of GM-CSF in the lungs by direct instillation or expression of its cDNA in airway epithelium corrected the lung disease.[26–28] Disruption of the GM-CSF receptor β gene (i.e., *Csf2rb*^{KO} mice) caused a similar lung phenotype[29] that could be corrected by bone marrow transplantation, which indicated the critical cell type driving pathogenesis was myeloid (i.e., alveolar macrophages) not epithelial (i.e., type II cells) in origin.[30] Surfactant clearance in GM-CSF^{KO} alveolar macrophages could be corrected by retroviral expression of PU.1, a transcription factor normally expressed in murine alveolar macrophages in vivo under tight regulatory control of pulmonary GM-CSF.[31] These studies established that GM-CSF, via PU.1, was required for surfactant clearance in alveolar macrophages (Fig. 70-3).[20] Recently, passive immunization with human PAP patient–derived neutralizing GM-CSF autoantibodies resulted in recapitulation of the cardinal pathological features

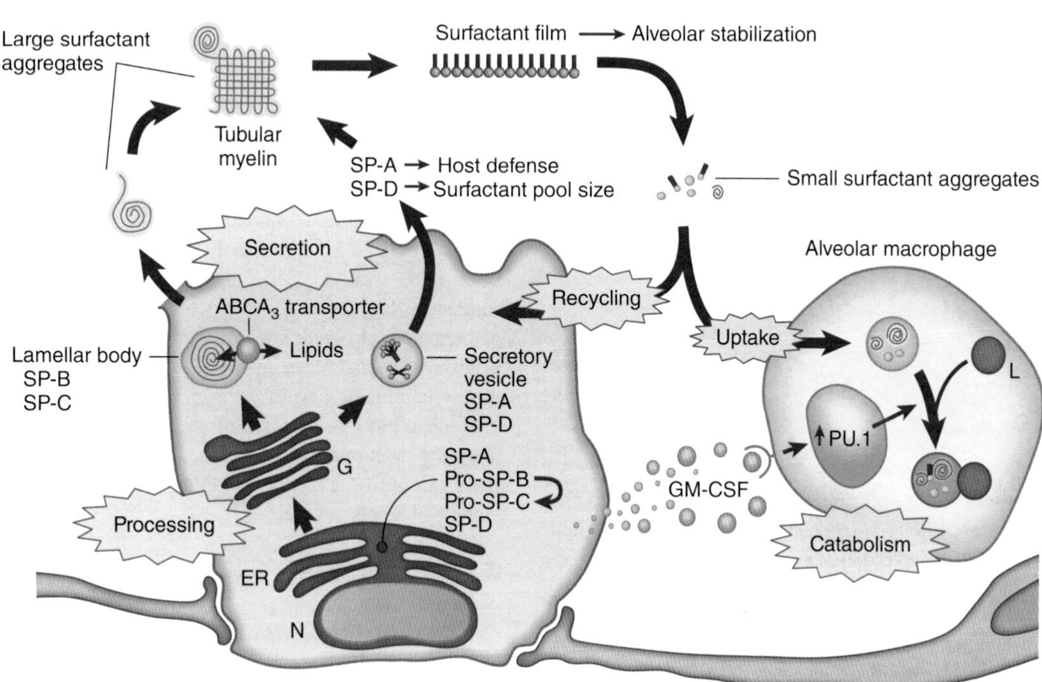

Figure 70-1 Schematic illustration depicting mechanisms of surfactant production, recycling, and catabolism. Surfactant phospholipids and proteins are synthesized in type II alveolar epithelial cells that line pulmonary alveoli. Surfactant B and C precursor proteins are processed, transported to lamellar bodies, and then secreted into the alveolar space where they interact with surfactant protein A to form tubular myelin. Surfactant monolayers and multilayers are formed from tubular myelin and function to reduce surface tension at the air–liquid–tissue interface, thus stabilizing the alveoli. Surfactant remnants are taken up and either catabolized or reutilized by type II alveolar epithelial cells. Alveolar macrophages play a critical role in surfactant homeostasis by taking up and catabolizing surfactant remnants. GM-CSF is required to maintain surfactant homeostasis and acts by stimulating catabolism of surfactant lipids and proteins in alveolar macrophages. *(Reproduced with permission from Whitsett JA, Wert SE, Trapnell BC. Genetic disorders influencing lung formation and function at birth. Hum Mol Genet. 2004;13[Spec No 2]:R207–R215.)*

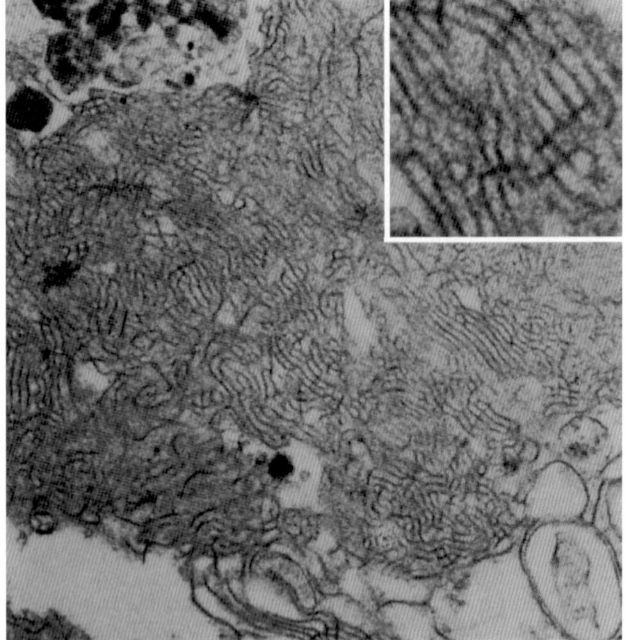

A

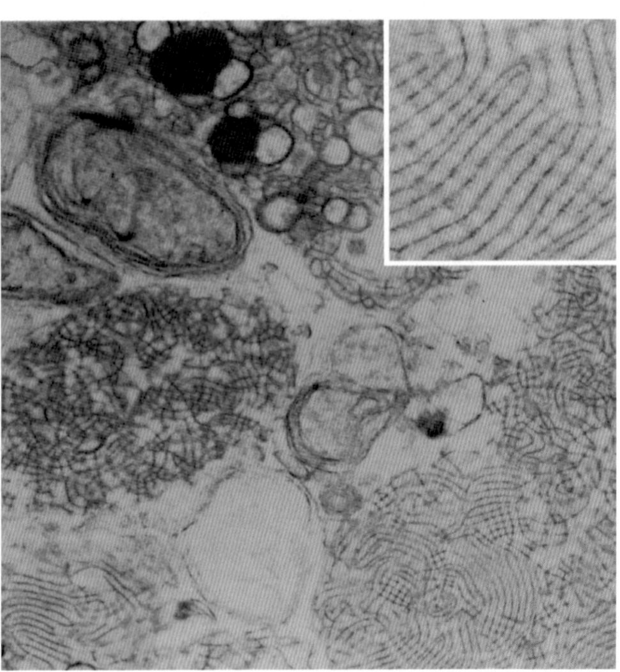

B

Figure 70-2 Ultrastructural appearance of the sediment from the lungs of a human patient with primary PAP (**A**) and a GM-CSF–deficient mouse (**B**). Note the presence of lamellated, fused membrane structures and amorphous debris (uranyl acetate, ×30,000).

of autoimmune PAP in nonhuman primates.[32,33] The abnormalities induced in alveolar macrophage included impaired GM-CSF signaling, GM-CSF–dependent gene expression (including PU.1), and surfactant clearance and increased neutral lipid accumulation resulting in foamy appearing alveolar macrophages. These animal models provide strong support for disruption of GM-CSF signaling as the critical driver of PAP pathogenesis. As a model of secondary PAP, depletion of alveolar macrophages has been shown to increase lung surfactant pool size in rats.[34] Congenital PAP models have been created in mice by disruption of the genes required for normal surfactant production *(Sftpb, Sftpc, Abca3)*.[35–37]

PRIMARY PAP

Autoimmune and hereditary forms of primary PAP are considered below.

Autoimmune PAP

In 1999, the Nakata group discovered that idiopathic PAP (also reported as acquired PAP) was specifically associated with high levels of neutralizing anti–GM-CSF autoantibodies (Fig. 70-4).[10] Subsequently, these autoantibodies were shown to be (1) polyclonal, primarily comprised of immunoglobulin G subclass 1 (IgG_1) and IgG_2 with smaller amounts of IgG_3 and IgG_4, (2) have a very high affinity for GM-CSF in the 3 to 20 pM range, and (3) capable of neutralizing GM-CSF, and (4) eliminating GM-CSF bioactivity in vivo.[38,39] Notwithstanding, several findings were difficult to reconcile. GM-CSF autoantibodies were also present in healthy individuals, albeit at lower levels,[39] and the antibody levels in PAP patients did not correlate with disease severity.[40] The recapitulation of PAP in healthy nonhuman primates by passive immunization with PAP patient–derived GM-CSF autoantibodies firmly established their critical role in pathogenesis.[32,33] The low autoantibody levels in healthy individuals and lack of correlation with disease severity in PAP patients was explained by a model in which constitutive in vivo stimulation of GM-CSF–dependent myeloid cell functions (including surfactant clearance) declined with increasing GM-CSF autoantibody level until a critical threshold was reached where function became zero.[39,41] The threshold level was identified and similar in humans and nonhuman primates.[33,39] These studies provide strong evidence that GM-CSF autoantibodies were pathogenic and led to a recommendation to change the name from "idiopathic PAP" to "autoimmune PAP."[41]

Hereditary PAP

While humans with GM-CSF deficiency have not been identified to date, in 2008, a GM-CSF autoantibody-negative child was found to have compound heterozygous mutations in *CSF2RA* (encoding GM-CSF receptor α) as the cause of familial PAP.[11] Additional patients were identified by exploiting use of a biomarker, increased serum GM-CSF, to screen sera from a repository including patients with PAP of unknown etiology, which identified a cohort of patients with PAP-causing *CSF2RA* mutations (Fig. 70-4).[42] Subsequently, *CSF2RB* mutations were identified as a cause of hereditary PAP.[12,43] Detailed characterization were done including molecular cloning and expression studies to recapitulate the receptor dysfunction established that the pathogenesis of hereditary PAP is caused by recessive or compound heterozygous mutations in the *CSF2RA* or *CSF2RB* genes.[11,12,42,43] A variety of mutation types were identified as the cause of hereditary PAP including missense mutations, nonsense mutations, small insertions and deletions, exon deletion, and gene deletion.[2] Together, these studies defined the clinical presentation, pathogenesis, diagnosis, and therapy of hereditary PAP.

SECONDARY PAP

Results from a national registry recently confirmed that secondary PAP occurs in association with a heterogeneous group of underlying diseases including hematological disorders, primarily myelodysplasia (76%–88% of cases), infectious diseases (2%–3%), other autoimmune diseases (7%), immunosuppression after organ transplantation (7%), and in nonhematological malignancies (5%).[44] Secondary PAP also occurs in association with (and presumably due to) heavy inhalation exposure to inorganic dusts (e.g., silica, titanium, aluminum) and other gasses and fumes, or as a consequence of systemic infections, for example, during human immunodeficiency virus (HIV) infection.[45] Secondary PAP appears to be caused by a reduction in the numbers or clearance capacity of alveolar macrophages, consistent with macrophage depletion studies in rats.[34]

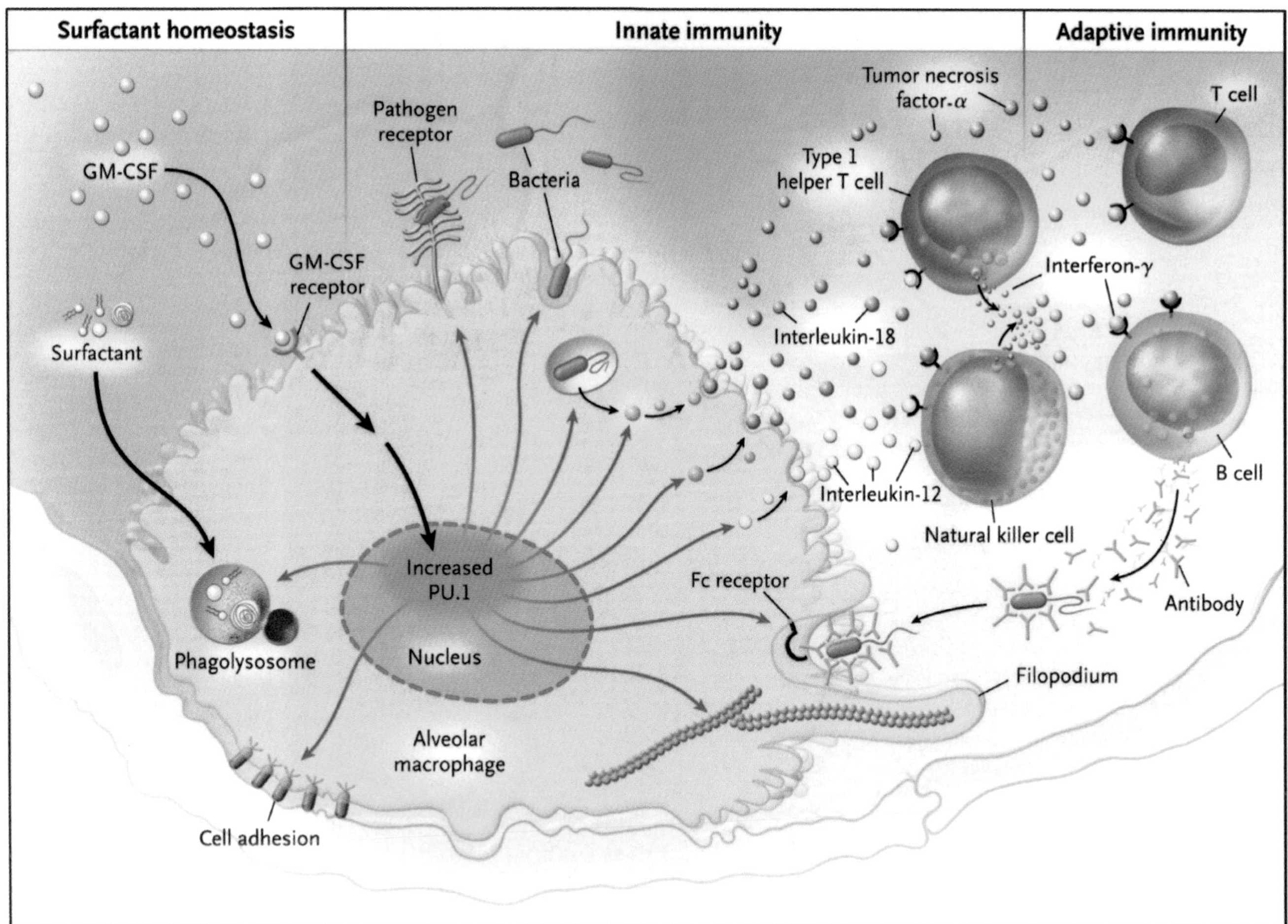

Figure 70-3 Role of GM-CSF in modulating the function of alveolar macrophages in mice. Pulmonary GM-CSF stimulates increased levels of the transcription factor PU.1 in alveolar macrophages in the lungs in vivo. Alveolar macrophages from mice deficient in GM-CSF have a number of functional defects including defects in cellular adhesion, catabolism of surfactant proteins and surfactant lipids, expression of pathogen-associated molecular pattern receptors (e.g., toll-like receptors and the mannose receptor), toll-like–receptor signaling, phagocytosis of pathogens, intracellular killing of bacteria (independent of uptake), pathogen-stimulated secretion of cytokines (tumor necrosis factor-α, interleukin [IL]-12, and IL-18), and Fc-receptor–mediated phagocytosis. Cytoskeletal organization is abnormal and may in part account for defects in phagocytosis. The ability of alveolar macrophages to release IL-12 and IL-18 severely impairs the interferon-γ response to pulmonary infection, thus impairing an important molecular connection between innate and adaptive immunity in the lung. Retroviral-mediated expression of PU.1 in alveolar macrophages from GM-CSF knockout mice corrects all these defects, suggesting that GM-CSF stimulates terminal differentiation of the macrophages primarily through the master transcription factor PU.1. The *blue arrows* represent the functions regulated by PU.1 that are affected by the absence of GM-CSF. *(Reproduced with permission from Trapnell BC, Whitsett JA, Nakata K. Pulmonary alveolar proteinosis. N Engl J Med. 2003;349(26):2527–2539.)*

■ CONGENITAL PAP

PAP occurs in neonates, infants, and children in association with various defects in the genes encoding SP-B, SP-C, ABCA3 – a lipid transporter expressed in type II alveolar epithelial cells, or TTF-1 – a transcription factor essential for lung development and surfactant expression.[4,46–49] In contrast to primary and secondary PAP that are caused by reduced surfactant clearance, these disorders result from production of abnormal surfactant. While surfactant accumulation does occur to varying degrees in surfactant production disorders, these disorders are clinically, histopathologically, and pathogenically distinct from primary and secondary PAP (see below).

■ THE EMERGING ROLE OF GM-CSF IN INNATE IMMUNITY

GM-CSF^{KO} mice have increased susceptibility to a broad range of microbial pathogens, increased mortality from spontaneous infections,[50,51] and numerous host defense defects in macrophages and neutrophils.[31,52] In macrophages, all these diverse defects could be corrected by forced expression of PU.1 (Fig. 70-3).[31] Similar defects are present in alveolar macrophages and neutrophils from humans and nonhuman primates with disruption of GM-CSF signaling.[2] GM-CSF^{KO} mice also have systemic immune and inflammatory abnormalities[51] including reduced severity in arthritis models,[53] an observation that has led to conduct the human trials of GM-CSF signaling disruption as therapy of rheumatoid arthritis.[54,55] These and other studies lead to an emerging understanding of the important roles that GM-CSF plays in the regulation of alveolar macrophage terminal differentiation, the basal functional capacity of circulating neutrophils, and in autoimmune and inflammatory diseases.[56]

EPIDEMIOLOGY

The epidemiology of PAP remains poorly defined. Results from a national registry study estimated the incidence and prevalence of autoimmune PAP in Japan to be approximately 0.49 and 6.2 per million in the general population, respectively.[57] In a subsequent report from the registry,[44] 40 cases of secondary PAP were identified premortem resulting in a prevalence estimate of approximately 0.3 per million. The incidence and prevalence of congenial PAP are unknown. In recent reports from specialized clinical centers, the

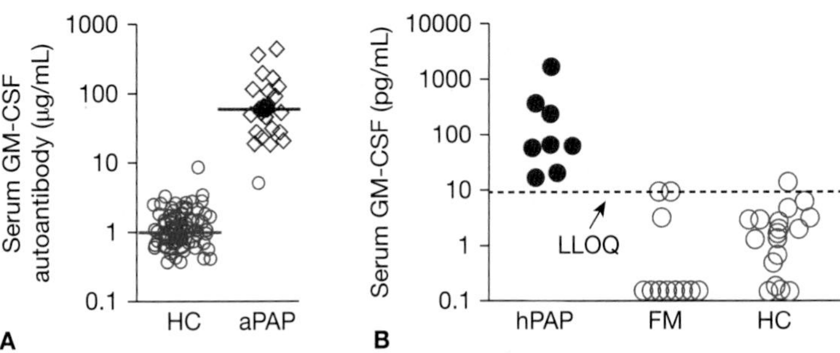

Figure 70-4 Biomarkers of use in identifying individuals with primary PAP. **A.** Serum GM-CSF autoantibody concentration. Shown are data for healthy controls (HCs) and patients with aPAP (autoimmune PAP). *(Reproduced with permission from Uchida K, Nakata K, Suzuki T, et al. GM-CSF autoantibodies and myeloid cell immune functions in healthy individuals. Blood. 2009;113(11):2547–2556.)* **B.** Serum GM-CSF concentration. Shown are data for children with hereditary PAP (hPAP) caused by recessive *CSF2RA* or *CSF2RB* mutations, members of their immediate family who were health (FM), or unrelated HCs. The lower limit of quantification (LLOQ) of the assay was 7.8 pg/mL *(dashed line)*. The serum levels of GM-CSF (median, interquartile range) in children with hPAP (52 pg/mL [28–101 pg/mL]) were increased compared with healthy family members (0.0 pg/mL [0.0–3 pg/mL]) and unrelated health controls (0.0 pg/mL [0.0–1.9 pg/mL]) (n = 8, 11, 30, respectively; $P < 0.001$; Kruskal–Wallis analysis of variance on ranks with comparisons using Dunn's method). *(Reproduced with permission from Suzuki T, Sakagami T, Young LR, et al. Hereditary pulmonary alveolar proteinosis: pathogenesis, presentation, diagnosis, and therapy. Am J Crit Care Med. 2010;182(10):1292–1304.)*

age at the time of diagnosis of autoimmune PAP in years (median/mean, number of patients, country) were 52 (248, Japan),[57] 42 (241, China),[58] 43 (70, Germany),[59] 40 (81, Italy),[60] although the diagnosis has been made in children as young as 3 years (unpublished). In these reports, the male/female ratio varied from 1.3 to 2.2 overall but was close to one in nonsmokers. Autoimmune PAP occurs in various ethnic backgrounds including Hispanic, Asian, Black, and white and in wide geographic distribution.

CLINICAL FEATURES

PRESENTATION

Autoimmune PAP typically presents as progressive dyspnea of insidious onset in previously healthy adults between the ages of 20 and 50 years, but has presented in children as young as 3 years old and in the elderly. In several series, dyspnea occurred in 67% to 94% of patients, followed by cough (23%–66%) and fatigue (49%) whereas fever (4%–11%) and sputum production (1%–4%) were less common.[57–60] In the Japanese registry study, one-third of patients were asymptomatic and identified only by mandatory health screening programs.[57] A history of diffuse pneumonia that is poorly responsive or unresponsive to antibiotic therapy is sometimes present and should raise the suspicion of PAP. The physical examination is often normal but commonly includes crackles especially in dependent areas and cyanosis is occasionally present in severe cases. Digital clubbing is typically absent. Hereditary PAP presents in remarkably similar fashion but at a mean age of 4.8 ± 1.6 years.[42] Secondary PAP has been reported to present at a median age of 49 years, most frequently accompanied by exertional dyspnea (40% of cases) followed by fever (38% of cases).[44] In patients with lung disease associated with abnormal surfactant production, dyspnea, crackles, and digital clubbing may be present.

RADIOGRAPHIC APPEARANCE

The chest radiograph in primary PAP usually reveals bilateral symmetrical alveolar opacities located centrally in mid- and lower-lung zones, often with a perihilar predominance resembling the "bat wing" appearance of pulmonary edema but without other signs of left-sided heart failure (Fig. 70-5A,C). The peripheral lung is commonly spared, resulting in lucency along the diaphragmatic, mediastinal, and peripheral borders. High-resolution computed tomography (HRCT) scanning reveals a characteristic geographical pattern of ground-glass opacification with superimposed interlobular septal and intralobular thickening, commonly referred to as "crazy paving" (Fig. 70-5B,D) that is characteristic of PAP but not diagnostic.

LABORATORY FINDINGS

In primary PAP, routine blood counts and chemistries are usually normal in primary PAP with the exception of serum lactate dehydrogenase (LDH), which is increased two- to threefold and correlates well with the degree of functional impairment as determined by physiological testing and arterial blood gas analysis. A number of biomarkers have been identified in autoimmune PAP including increased serum levels of GM-CSF autoantibody, SP-A, SP-B, SP-D, KL-6, CEA, Cyfra-21-1, cytokeratin 19, and others.[1,57,59–61] Many of these biomarkers are also increased in hereditary PAP.[11–13,42,43] Importantly, serum GM-CSF is specifically elevated in hereditary PAP but not in autoimmune PAP, which was important in identifying an initial cohort of patients for study (Fig. 70-4).[42] Biomarkers of secondary and congenital PAP have been less well studied.

LUNG FUNCTION

In primary PAP, spirometry and lung volume testing is usually normal or near normal but may show a restrictive pattern of impairment with modest reduction in the vital capacity and total lung capacity (TLC) and a disproportionate reduction of the carbon monoxide diffusing capacity (DL_{CO}). Arterial blood gas analysis in symptomatic patients reveals hypoxia caused by ventilation–perfusion inequality and intrapulmonary shunting, resulting in a widened alveolar–arterial diffusion gradient ($A\text{-}a_{DO_2}$).

BRONCHOSCOPIC FINDINGS

The bronchoscopic appearance of the airways in primary PAP is normal but white, frothy proteinosis material is occasionally seen.[42,59,60,62] The bronchoalveolar lavage (BAL) fluid is opaque and has a milky or waxy appearance and develops a thick layer of sediment upon standing overnight (Fig. 70-6). The sediment consists of large, acellular, eosinophilic bodies in a diffuse background of granular material that stains with periodic acid-Schiff (Fig. 70-7A). The cellular fraction contains large, foamy macrophages (Fig. 70-7B), smaller monocyte-like macrophages, and lymphocytes with relatively few neutrophils unless infection is also present. SP is increased and electron microscopy reveals the presence of lamellar bodies and tubular myelin that are characteristic of surfactant (Fig. 70-2).

LUNG PATHOLOGY

Macroscopically, the cut surface of the lung in autoimmune PAP reveals a patchwork of 2- to 3-cm grayish-yellow regions of firm consolidation that exudes fatty material. Microscopically, alveoli and terminal airspaces are filled with a fine eosinophilic material (Fig. 70-7C) that stains strongly for SPs (Fig. 70-7D).[1] In primary PAP, the alveolar wall and interstitial architecture are usually well preserved but occasionally, lymphocytosis and fibrosis can be seen. The vasculature appears normal. Electron microscopy reveals characteristic, concentrically laminated surfactant structures within the granular material and in alveolar macrophages. The gross and microscopic appearance of the lung in hereditary PAP

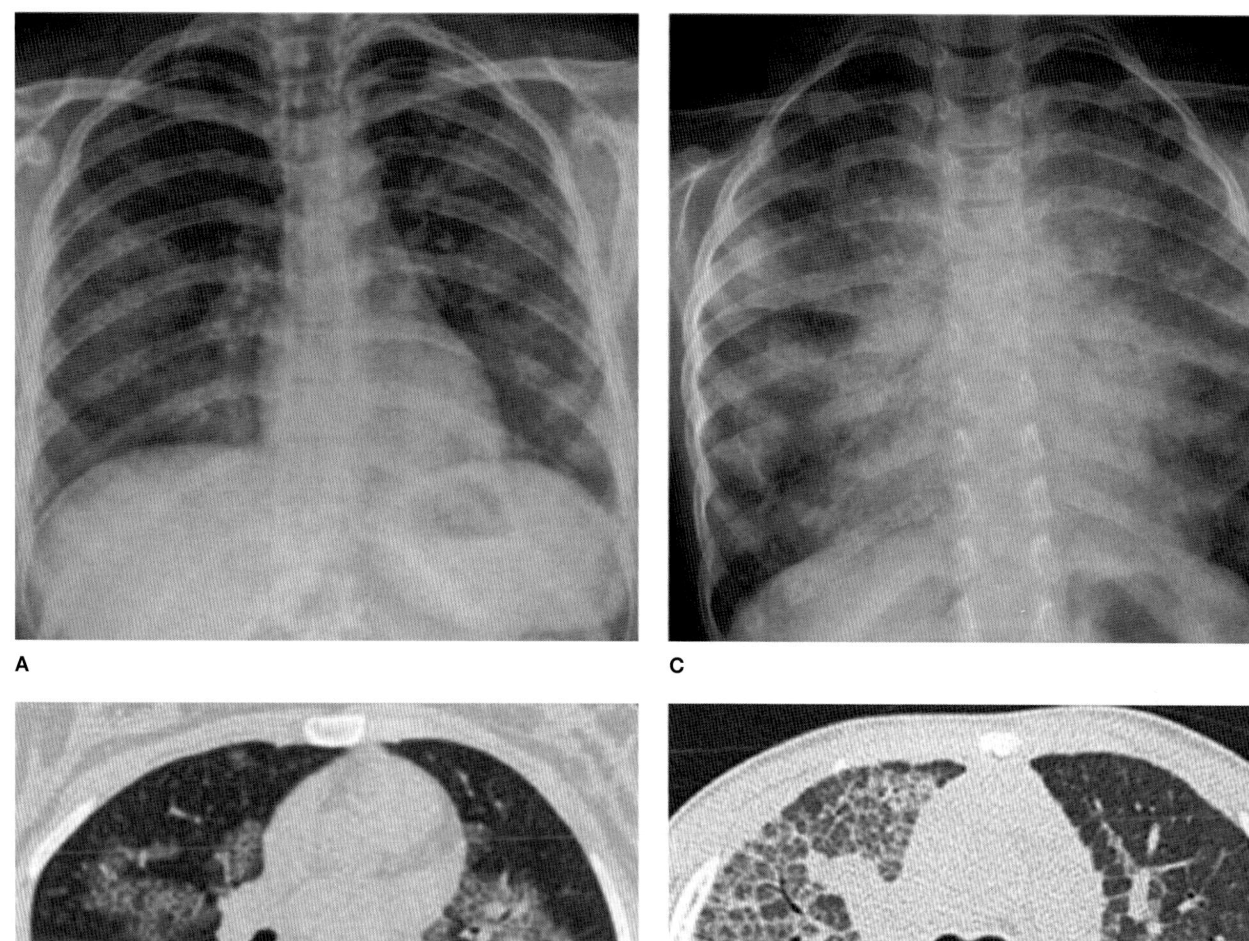

Figure 70-5 Radiographic appearance of primary PAP. **A.** Chest radiograph of a 25-year-old woman autoimmune PAP. **B.** Corresponding chest high-resolution computed tomographic (HRCT) scan. **C.** Chest radiograph of a 6-year-old girl with compound heterozygous *CSF2RA* mutations. **D.** HRCT of a 3-year-old girl with recessive null *CSF2RA* mutations.

is similar.[11–13,42,43] The lung pathology in secondary and congenital PAP varies significantly depending on the disease.

SECONDARY INFECTIONS

Individuals with autoimmune PAP have an increased risk of infections, which contribute significantly to increased morbidity and mortality.[1,61] Although pathogens commonly seen in community- and hospital-acquired lung infections are sometimes identified, opportunistic organisms are often responsible and can include Nocardia, Mycobacterium, Aspergillus, Cryptococcus, and others. Infections can occur at both pulmonary and extrapulmonary sites supporting the concept that a systemic defect in host defense is present secondary to defects in the antimicrobial functions of macrophages and neutrophils.[31,51,52,63]

DIAGNOSIS

While PAP syndrome can be suspected based on historical, physical, radiographic lung function findings, further studies are needed to exclude other conditions in the differential diagnosis such as hypersensitivity pneumonitis, pulmonary edema, pneumonia, and interstitial lung diseases. Traditionally, transbronchial or surgical lung biopsy have been considered necessary and are commonly used to identify the syndrome. However, none of these approaches *including lung biopsy* are capable of identifying the specific disease causing PAP. In contrast, the development and testing of several disease-specific and semi-specific biomarkers is particularly useful. The serum-based GM-CSF autoantibody ELISA initially established by Nakata[10] has been refined[38,39,52,62] and recently evaluated in a multinational validation study that demonstrated a sensitivity and specificity for a diagnosis of autoimmune PAP of 100%.[64] Similarly, an increase in serum GM-CSF appears to be both sensitive and specific for a diagnosis of hereditary PAP.[65] In both these diseases, the STAT5-phosphorylation index test can be helpful in establishing disruption of GM-CSF signaling.[66] Secondary PAP can usually be distinguished from primary PAP on the basis of the clinical context and histological or immunohistochemical evaluation of lung biopsy

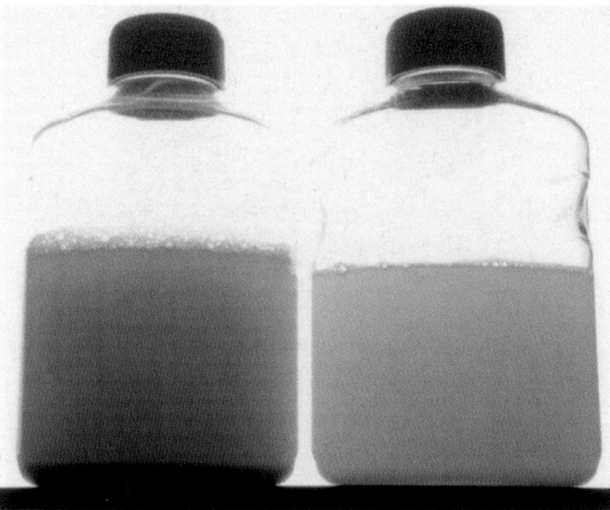

Figure 70-6 Lavage fluid obtained during the whole lung lavage procedure of a patient with autoimmune PAP has a characteristic turbid appearance and a sediment that forms upon standing. The marked opacity and sediment of the fluid observed at the beginning (left bottle) shows progressive clearing by the end of the procedure (right bottle).

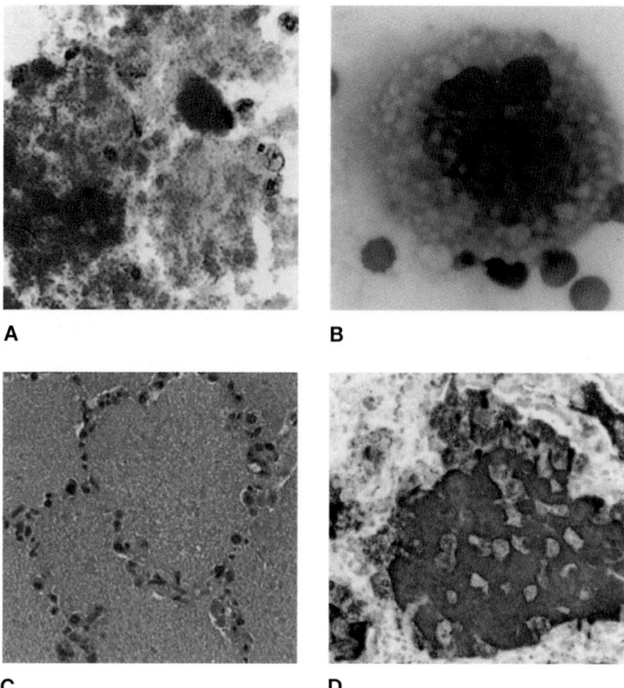

Figure 70-7 Cytological, pathological, and immunohistochemical appearance of the lipoproteinaceous material from patients with autoimmune alveolar proteinosis. **A.** Positive periodic acid-Schiff staining of the sediment from bronchoalveolar lavage (×100). **B.** Cytological appearance of a typical "foamy" alveolar macrophage. **C.** Histopathological appearance of the lung biopsy specimen from a 10-year-old child with primary PAP. Note the homogeneous staining pattern, normal alveolar wall architecture, and the absence of inflammatory cells (H&E, ×200). **D.** Immunohistochemical staining reveals the presence of abundant accumulation of surfactant protein A in a lung biopsy specimen (human anti–surfactant protein A immunostain, ×200).

specimens. Further, disease mimics like *Pneumocystis pneumonia* can be distinguished by specific histological staining. That radiographic abnormalities are often increased out of proportion to the severity suspected on clinical grounds is of diagnostic utility but its practical application requires a high degree of clinical suspicion.

NATURAL HISTORY

Prospective, longitudinal studies of the natural history of PAP have not been done. However, experience from several large retrospective and cross-sectional PAP cohorts (number of patients) at tertiary referral centers in Japan (248), China (241), Germany (70), and Italy (81) have recently been reported.[57–60] The "time-to-diagnosis" ranged from 9 to 11 months similar to a prior report by Seymour.[57–61] Most patients had stable disease with mild, persistent symptoms while some had spontaneous remission or progressive disease. Spontaneous remissions occurred in 5% to 7% of 399 patients[57,59,60] confirming a previous estimate of 6% in 410 patients by Seymour.[61] In Seymour's study, the 5-year survival was 85% without therapy and 95% with whole lung lavage therapy.[61] Of the deaths attributable to PAP among 303 patients, 47 were due to respiratory failure from PAP, 12 were from infections, and 1 was from cardiac arrest during whole lung lavage (WLL) therapy (see below).[61] The prognosis of secondary PAP is worse than primary PAP due to linkage with the underlying disease with an estimated 5-year survival of between 20% to 40%.[44] The prognosis of congenital PAP varies, ranging widely from death at birth for SP-B deficiency and some ABCA3 mutations to respiratory insufficiency or failure from interstitial lung disease in adolescence or adulthood for SP-C mutations and some ABCA3 mutations.[4,48]

THERAPY

Therapy of PAP varies by disease. In autoimmune PAP, therapy is required by most but not all patients and is usually initiated when symptoms become limiting. In secondary PAP, treatment is aimed at the underlying clinical condition although WLL can be effective. In congenital PAP, therapy is generally limited to supportive care although SP-B deficiency has been treated successfully by lung transplantation.[67]

■ WHOLE LUNG LAVAGE

WLL remains the most widely used therapy of primary PAP[57–61] and is still the recommended standard approach. It can be helpful in secondary PAP but has little to no utility in congenital PAP, likely due to the extensive parenchymal derangement present in these latter patients. In independent cohorts, WLL was used in 54% to 90% of a combined total of 899 patients.[51,57–60] While indications vary among centers, some of the recommendations include a histopathological diagnosis of PAP; Pa_{O_2} <60 mm Hg; A-a_{DO_2} gradient >40 mm Hg; shunt fraction >10% to 12%; or severe dyspnea at rest or with exercise. The WLL procedure itself also varies among centers. It requires general anesthesia, endotracheal intubation, and simultaneous mechanical ventilation of one lung while repeatedly filling and draining the other lung with warm saline with or without chest percussion to emulsify and physically remove the alveolar surfactant. Infusion volumes of up to 50 L per lung have been used in adults but may reach diminishing return above 20 L. Other variations include use of extracorporeal or hyperbaric oxygen. While specific therapeutic response criteria have not been defined, most patients experience clinical, physiological, and radiographic improvement following WLL.[68] Physiological parameters demonstrated to improve with lavage include increases in forced vital capacity (FVC), TLC, DL_{CO}, Pa_{O_2} at rest and with exercise, and a decrease in A-a_{DO_2} and shunt fraction. WLL improves the 5-year survival from 85±5% to 94±2%.[61] Two studies have reported a duration of response to WLL of 15 months.[60,61] Sequential lobar lavage has been used although its clinical utility is unclear.

■ EXPERIMENTAL APPROACHES

Our improved understanding of PAP as a disease driven by reduced GM-CSF–dependent surfactant clearance in alveolar macrophages has stimulated the development of specific pharmacological therapy. One such strategy is based on augmentation with recombinant human GM-CSF and several clinical studies have demonstrated therapeutic efficacy with this approach.[62,69–75] Both subcutaneous and inhaled administration have been used but the latter appears more efficacious. In 39 patients with unremitting/progressive autoimmune PAP, 62% of the patients receiving inhaled GM-CSF therapy had improvement in the A-a_{DO_2} gradient.[69] Radiographic improvement was also seen,[69] which in a separate study, was documented by quantitative densitometry of the chest HRCT.[75] Notwithstanding, GM-CSF therapy of autoimmune PAP is still in development and many questions remain unanswered including the optimal dosage, frequency of administration, duration of therapy. While no drug-emergent toxicities have been identified, formal safety studies of inhaled GM-CSF therapy have not been done but have been requested by the FDA and are currently underway with support from the National Institutes of Health Therapeutics for Rare and Neglected Diseases (TRND) program. Another approach aimed at GM-CSF autoantibodies is anti–B lymphocyte immunotherapy, which is used to deplete anti–GM-CSF autoantibody-producing cells.[76–78] While results are encouraging, the number of patients is small and results should be interpreted cautiously.

REFERENCES

1. Trapnell BC, Whitsett JA, Nakata K. Pulmonary alveolar proteinosis. *N Eng J Med.* 2003;349(26):2527–2539.
2. Carey B, Trapnell BC. The molecular basis of pulmonary alveolar proteinosis. *Clin Immunol.* 2010;135(2):223–235.
3. Ishii H, Trapnell BC, Tazawa R, et al.; Japanese Center of the Rare Lung Disease Consortium. Comparative study of high-resolution CT findings between autoimmune and secondary pulmonary alveolar proteinosis. *Chest.* 2009;136(5):1348–1355.
4. Nogee LM. Genetic basis of children's interstitial lung disease. *Pediatr Allergy Immunol Pulmonol.* 2010;23(1):15–24.
5. Rosen SH, Castleman B, Liebow AA. Pulmonary alveolar proteinosis. *N Eng J Med.* 1958;258:1123–1142.
6. Lieschke GJ, Burgess AW. Granulocyte colony-stimulating factor and granulocyte-macrophage colony-stimulating factor (2). *N Eng J Med.* 1992;327(2):99–106.
7. Lieschke GJ, Burgess AW. Granulocyte colony-stimulating factor and granulocyte-macrophage colony-stimulating factor (1). *N Eng J Med.* 1992;327(1):28–35.
8. Hansen G, Hercus TR, McClure BJ, et al. The structure of the GM-CSF receptor complex reveals a distinct mode of cytokine receptor activation. *Cell.* 2008;134(3):496–507.
9. Hercus TR, Thomas D, Guthridge MA, et al. The granulocyte-macrophage colony-stimulating factor receptor: linking its structure to cell signaling and its role in disease. *Blood.* 2009;114(7):1289–1298.
10. Kitamura T, Tanaka N, Watanabe J, et al. Idiopathic pulmonary alveolar proteinosis as an autoimmune disease with neutralizing antibody against granulocyte/macrophage colony-stimulating factor. *J Exp Med.* 1999;190(6):875–880.
11. Suzuki T, Sakagami T, Rubin BK, et al. Familial pulmonary alveolar proteinosis caused by mutations in CSF2RA. *J Exp Med.* 2008;205(12):2703–2710.
12. Suzuki T, Maranda B, Sakagami T, et al. Hereditary pulmonary alveolar proteinosis caused by CSF2RB mutations. *Eur Respir J.* 2011;37(1):201–204.
13. Martinez-Moczygemba M, Doan ML, Elidemir O, et al. Pulmonary alveolar proteinosis caused by deletion of the GM-CSFRalpha gene in the X chromosome pseudoautosomal region 1. *J Exp Med.* 2008;205(12):2711–2716.
14. Jobe AH, Ikegami M. Surfactant metabolism. *Clin Perinatol.* 1993;20(4):683–696.
15. Whitsett JA, Weaver TE. Hydrophobic surfactant proteins in lung function and disease. *N Eng J Med.* 2002;347(26):2141–2148.
16. Wright JR. Host defense functions of pulmonary surfactant. *Biol Neonate.* 2004;85(4):326–332.
17. Perez-Gil J, Weaver TE. Pulmonary surfactant pathophysiology: current models and open questions. *Physiology.* 2010;25(3): 132–141.
18. Gurel O, Ikegami M, Chroneos ZC, Jobe AH. Macrophage and type II cell catabolism of SP-A and saturated phosphatidylcholine in mouse lungs. *Am J Physiol Lung Cell Mol Physiol.* 2001;280(6):L1266–L1272.
19. Wright JR. Clearance and recycling of pulmonary surfactant. *Am J Physiol.* 1990;259(2 Pt 1):L1–L12.
20. Trapnell BC, Whitsett JA. GM-CSF regulates pulmonary surfactant homeostasis and alveolar macrophage-mediated innate host defense. *Annu Rev Physiol.* 2002;64:775–802.
21. Wright JR, Youmans DC. Degradation of surfactant lipids and surfactant protein A by alveolar macrophages in vitro. *Am J Physiol.* 1995;268(5 Pt 1):L772–L780.
22. Dranoff G, Crawford AD, Sadelain M, et al. Involvement of granulocyte-macrophage colony-stimulating factor in pulmonary homeostasis. *Science.* 1994;264(5159):713–716.
23. Stanley E, Lieschke GJ, Grail D, et al. Granulocyte/macrophage colony-stimulating factor-deficient mice show no major perturbation of hematopoiesis but develop a characteristic pulmonary pathology. *Proc Natl Acad Sci U S A.* 1994;91(12):5592–5596.
24. Yoshida M, Ikegami M, Reed JA, Chroneos ZC, Whitsett JA. GM-CSF regulates protein and lipid catabolism by alveolar macrohpages. *Am J Physiol Lung Cell Mol Physiol.* 2001;280(3): L379–L386.
25. Ikegami M, Ueda T, Hull W, et al. Surfactant metabolism in transgenic mice after granulocyte macrophage-colony stimulating factor ablation. *Am J Physiol.* 1996;270(4 Pt 1):L650–L658.
26. Ikegami M, Jobe AH, Huffman Reed JA, Whitsett JA. Surfactant metabolic consequences of overexpression of GM-CSF in the epithelium of GM-CSF-deficient mice. *Am J Physiol.* 1997;273(4 Pt 1):L709–L714.
27. Reed JA, Ikegami M, Cianciolo ER, et al. Aerosolized GM-CSF ameliorates pulmonary alveolar proteinosis in GM-CSF-deficient mice. *Am J Physiol.* 1999;276(4 Pt 1):L556–L563.
28. Zsengeller ZK, Reed JA, Bachurski CJ, et al. Adenovirus-mediated granulocyte-macrophage colony-stimulating factor improves lung pathology of pulmonary alveolar proteinosis in granulocyte-macrophage colony-stimulating factor-deficient mice. *Hum Gene Ther.* 1998;9(14):2101–2109.
29. Robb L, Drinkwater CC, Metcalf D, et al. Hematopoietic and lung abnormalities in mice with a null mutation of the common beta subunit of the receptors for granulocyte-macrophage colony-stimulating factor and interleukins 3 and 5. *Proc Natl Acad Sci U S A.* 1995;92(21):9565–9569.
30. Nishinakamura R, Nakayama N, Hirabayashi Y, et al. Mice deficient for the IL-3/GM-CSF/IL-5 beta c receptor exhibit lung pathology and impaired immune response, while beta IL3 receptor- deficient mice are normal. *Immunity.* 1995;2(3): 211–222.

31. Shibata Y, Berclaz PY, Chroneos ZC, Yoshida M, Whitsett JA, Trapnell BC. GM-CSF regulates alveolar macrophage differentiation and innate immunity in the lung through PU.1. *Immunity*. 2001;15(4):557–567.

32. Sakagami T, Uchida K, Suzuki T, et al. Human GM-CSF autoantibodies and reproduction of pulmonary alveolar proteinosis. *N Eng J Med*. 2009;361(27):2679–2681.

33. Sakagami T, Beck D, Uchida K, et al. Patient-derived granulocyte/macrophage colony-stimulating factor autoantibodies reproduce pulmonary alveolar proteinosis in non-human primates. *Am J Respir Crit Care Med*. 2010;182(1):49–61.

34. Forbes A, Pickell M, Foroughian M, Yao LJ, Lewis J, Veldhuizen R. Alveolar macrophage depletion is associated with increased surfactant pool sizes in adult rats. *J Appl Physiol*. 2007;103(2):637–645.

35. Clark JC, Wert SE, Bachurski CJ, et al. Targeted disruption of the surfactant protein B gene disrupts surfactant homeostasis, causing respiratory failure in newborn mice. *Proc Natl Acad Sci U S A*. 1995;92(17):7794–7798.

36. Glasser SW, Detmer EA, Ikegami M, Na CL, Stahlman MT, Whitsett JA. Pneumonitis and emphysema in sp-C gene targeted mice. *J Biol Chem*. 2003;278(16):14291–14298.

37. Cheong N, Zhang H, Madesh M, et al. ABCA3 is critical for lamellar body biogenesis in vivo. *J Biol Chem*. 2007;282(33): 23811–23817.

38. Uchida K, Nakata K, Trapnell BC, et al. High-affinity autoantibodies specifically eliminate granulocyte-macrophage colony-stimulating factor activity in the lungs of patients with idiopathic pulmonary alveolar proteinosis. *Blood*. 2004;103(3): 1089–1098.

39. Uchida K, Nakata K, Suzuki T, et al. Granulocyte/macrophage-colony-stimulating factor autoantibodies and myeloid cell immune functions in healthy subjects. *Blood*. 2009;113(11): 2547–2556.

40. Seymour JF, Doyle IR, Nakata K, et al. Relationship of anti-GM-CSF antibody concentration, surfactant protein A and B levels, and serum LDH to pulmonary parameters and response to GM-CSF therapy in patients with idiopathic alveolar proteinosis. *Thorax*. 2003;58(3):252–257.

41. Bendtzen K, Svenson M, Hansen MB. GM-CSF autoantibodies in pulmonary alveolar proteinosis. *N Eng J Med*. 2007;356: 2001–2002.

42. Suzuki T, Sakagami T, Young LR, et al. Hereditary pulmonary alveolar proteinosis: pathogenesis, presentation, diagnosis, and therapy. *Am J Respir Crit Care Med*. 2010;182(10): 1292–1304.

43. Tanaka T, Motoi N, Tsuchihashi Y, et al. Adult-onset hereditary pulmonary alveolar proteinosis caused by a single-base deletion in CSF2RB. *J Med Genet*. 2011;48(3):205–209.

44. Ishii H, Tazawa R, Kaneko C, et al. Clinical features of secondary pulmonary alveolar proteinosis: pre-mortem cases in Japan. *Eur Respir J*. 2011;37(2):465–468.

45. Ruben FL, Talamo TS. Secondary pulmonary alveolar proteinosis occurring in two patients with acquired immune deficiency syndrome. *Am J Med*. 1986;80(6):1187–1190.

46. Galambos C, Levy H, Cannon CL, et al. Pulmonary pathology in thyroid transcription factor-1 deficiency syndrome. *Am J Respir Crit Care Med*. 2010;182(4):549–554.

47. Whitsett JA, Wert SE, Trapnell BC. Genetic disorders influencing lung formation and function at birth. *Hum Mol Genet*. 2004;13 Spec No 2:R207–R215.

48. Hamvas A. Inherited surfactant protein-B deficiency and surfactant protein-C associated disease: clinical features and evaluation. *Sem Perinatol*. 2006;30(6):316–326.

49. Garmany TH, Moxley MA, White FV, et al. Surfactant composition and function in patients with ABCA3 mutations. *Pediatr Res*. 2006;59(6):801–805.

50. LeVine AM, Reed JA, Kurak KE, Cianciolo E, Whitsett JA. GM-CSF-deficient mice are susceptible to pulmonary group B streptococcal infection. *J Clin Invest*. 1999;103(4):563–569.

51. Seymour JF. Extra-pulmonary aspects of acquired pulmonary alveolar proteinosis as predicted by granulocyte-macrophage colony-stimulating factor-deficient mice. *Respirology*. 2006;11 Suppl:S16–S22.

52. Uchida K, Beck DC, Yamamoto T, et al. GM-CSF autoantibodies and neutrophil dysfunction in pulmonary alveolar proteinosis. *N Engl J Med*. 2007;356(6):567–579.

53. Campbell IK, Bendele A, Smith DA, Hamilton JA. Granulocyte-macrophage colony stimulating factor exacerbates collagen induced arthritis in mice. *Ann Rheum Dis*. 1997;56(6):364–368.

54. Burmester GR, Feist E, Sleeman MA, Wang B, White B, Magrini F. Mavrilimumab, a human monoclonal antibody targeting GM-CSF receptor-α, in subjects with rheumatoid arthritis: a randomised, double-blind, placebo-controlled, phase I, first-in-human study. *Ann Rheum Dis*. 2011;70(9):1542–1549.

55. Burmester GR, Weinblatt ME, McInnes IB, et al. Efficacy and safety of mavrilimumab in subjects with rheumatoid arthritis. *Ann Rheum Dis*. 2012;72(9):1445–1452.

56. Hamilton JA. Colony-stimulating factors in inflammation and autoimmunity. *Nat Rev Immunol*. 2008;8(7):533–544.

57. Inoue Y, Trapnell BC, Tazawa R, et al. Characteristics of a large cohort of patients with autoimmune pulmonary alveolar proteinosis in Japan. *Am J Respir Crit Care Med*. 2008;177(7): 752–762.

58. Xu Z, Jing J, Wang H, Xu F, Wang J. Pulmonary alveolar proteinosis in China: a systematic review of 241 cases. *Respirology*. 2009;14(5):761–766.

59. Bonella F, Bauer PC, Griese M, Ohshimo S, Guzman J, Costabel U. Pulmonary alveolar proteinosis: new insights from a single-center cohort of 70 patients. *Respir Med*. 2011;105(12):1908–1916.

60. Campo I, Mariani F, Rodi G, et al. Assessment and management of pulmonary alveolar proteinosis in a reference center. *Orphanet J Rare Dis*. 2013;8:40.

61. Seymour JF, Presneill JJ. Pulmonary alveolar proteinosis: progress in the first 44 years. *Am J Respir Crit Care Med*. 2002; 166(2):215–235.

62. Schoch OD, Schanz U, Koller M, et al. BAL findings in a patient with pulmonary alveolar proteinosis successfully treated with GM-CSF. *Thorax*. 2002;57(3):277–280.

63. Berclaz PY, Shibata Y, Whitsett JA, Trapnell BC. GM-CSF, via PU.1, regulates alveolar macrophage Fcgamma R-mediated phagocytosis and the IL-18/IFN-gamma-mediated molecular connection between innate and adaptive immunity in the lung. *Blood*. 2002;100(12):4193–4200.

64. Carey B, Uchida K, Nakata K, et al. A multicenter, international evaluation of blood testing for the diagnosis of autoimmune pulmonary alveolar proteinosis. *Am J Respir Crit Care Med*. 2012;183:A1624.

65. Carey B, Heald C, Chalk C, Suzuki T, Uchida K, Trapnell BC. Use of serum GM-CSF for diagnosis of patients with hereditary pulmonary alveolar proteinosis. *Am J Respir Crit Care Med*. 2013;187:A850.

66. Sakagami T, Suzuki T, Carey B, Chalk C, Trapnell BC. A novel assay to measure GM-CSF signling in clinical blood specimens. *Am J Respir Crit Care Med.* 2010;181:A2984.

67. Hamvas A, Nogee LM, Mallory GB Jr, et al. Lung transplantation for treatment of infants with surfactant protein B deficiency. *J Pediatr.* 1997;130(2):231–239.

68. Beccaria M, Luisetti M, Rodi G, et al. Long-term durable benefit after whole lung lavage in pulmonary alveolar proteinosis. *Eur Respir J.* 2004;23(4):526–531.

69. Tazawa R, Trapnell BC, Inoue Y, et al. Inhaled granulocyte/macrophage-colony stimulating factor as therapy of pulmonary alveolar proteinosis. *Am J Respir Crit Care Med.* 2010;181(12):1345–1354.

70. Tazawa R, Nakata K, Inoue Y, Nukiwa T. Granulocyte-macrophage colony-stimulating factor inhalation therapy for patients with idiopathic pulmonary alveolar proteinosis: a pilot study; and long-term treatment with aerosolized granulocyte-macrophage colony-stimulating factor: a case report. *Respirology.* 2006;11 Suppl:S61–S64.

71. Tazawa R, Hamano E, Arai T, et al. Granulocyte-macrophage colony-stimulating factor and lung immunity in pulmonary alveolar proteinosis. *Am J Respir Crit Care Med.* 2005;171(10):1142–1149.

72. Venkateshiah SB, Yan TD, Bonfield TL, et al. An open-label trial of granulocyte macrophage colony stimulating factor therapy for moderate symptomatic pulmonary alveolar proteinosis. *Chest.* 2006;130(1):227–237.

73. Seymour JF, Presneill JJ, Schoch OD, et al. Therapeutic efficacy of granulocyte-macrophage colony-stimulating factor in patients with idiopathic acquired alveolar proteinosis. *Am J Respir Crit Care Med.* 2001;163(2):524–531.

74. Seymour JF, Dunn AR, Vincent JM, Presneill JJ, Pain MC. Efficacy of granulocyte-macrophage colony-stimulating factor in acquired alveolar proteinosis. *N Eng J Med.* 1996;335(25):1924–1925.

75. Robinson TE, Trapnell BC, Goris ML, Quittell LM, Cornfield DN. Quantitative analysis of longitudinal response to aerosolized granulocyte-macrophage colony-stimulating factor in two adolescents with autoimmune pulmonary alveolar proteinosis. *Chest.* 2009;135(3):842–848.

76. Amital A, Dux S, Shitrit D, Shpilberg O, Kramer MR. Therapeutic effectiveness of rituximab in a patient with unresponsive autoimmune pulmonary alveolar proteinosis. *Thorax.* 2010;65(11):1025–1026.

77. Borie R, Debray MP, Laine C, Aubier M, Crestani B. Rituximab therapy in autoimmune pulmonary alveolar proteinosis. *Eur Respir J.* 2009;33(6):1503–1506.

78. Malur A, Kavuru MS, Marshall I, et al. Rituximab therapy in pulmonary alveolar proteinosis improves alveolar macrophage lipid homeostasis. *Respir Res.* 2012;13:46.

CHAPTER 71 The Eosinophilic Pneumonias

Carolyn L. Rochester

INTRODUCTION

The association between pulmonary infiltrates and eosinophilia was first identified by Loeffler in 1932. It is now recognized that the eosinophilic pneumonias are a heterogeneous group of disorders characterized by varying degrees of pulmonary parenchymal and/or blood eosinophilia.[1] The precise role that eosinophils play in the pathogenesis of the different eosinophilic pneumonias is not clear. Normally, less than 2% of the leukocyte cell differential in bronchoalveolar lavage (BAL) are eosinophils. The presence of increased BAL and/or tissue eosinophils, and our knowledge of the biology of eosinophils (see Chapter 22) does, however, suggest that they play a variety of roles, including initiation, perpetuation, and amplification of tissue inflammation and injury. These effector functions are no doubt the result of the ability of the eosinophils to release numerous soluble mediators, including granule-derived proteins, arachidonic acid metabolites, proinflammatory cytokines, superoxide anions, metalloproteases, and hydroxyl radicals. The different roles of eosinophils in these disorders can be appreciated when comparisons are made of parasitic infections and disorders such as asthma or allergic bronchopulmonary aspergillosis (ABPA). In the former, eosinophils play a crucial role in eradicating the infectious pathogen; in the latter, the eosinophils accumulate in the lung as a result of immune hypersensitivity and are prominent mediators of tissue injury.

The spectrum of diseases that can be primarily or secondarily associated with blood or pulmonary eosinophilia is shown in Table 71-1. It is beyond the scope of this chapter to discuss each of these disease entities in detail. Instead, discussion will focus on diseases of known or unknown causes in which eosinophilic infiltration of lung tissue is a characteristic feature, including acute eosinophilic pneumonias, tropical pulmonary eosinophilia (TPE), chronic eosinophilic pneumonia (CEP), ABPA, Churg–Strauss syndrome (now termed as eosinophilic granulomatosis with polyangiitis [EGPA]), and idiopathic hypereosinophilic syndrome (HES). Since eosinophilic granuloma of the lung is frequently seen in the absence of blood or tissue eosinophilia, it is considered separately (Chapter 74).

EOSINOPHILIC PNEUMONIAS WITH ACUTE PRESENTATIONS

Acute presentations of eosinophilic pneumonia center on several primary considerations, including Loeffler Syndrome, parasitic infections, drug- and toxin-related disorders, and idiopathic varieties. Each is discussed in the following sections.

LOEFFLER SYNDROME (SIMPLE PULMONARY EOSINOPHILIA)

In 1932, Loeffler first described a clinical syndrome characterized by mild respiratory symptoms, peripheral blood eosinophilia, and transient, migratory pulmonary infiltrates. The term *Loeffler syndrome,* or *simple pulmonary eosinophilia,* has been used to define the numerous similar cases reported subsequently. Immune hypersensitivity to *Ascaris lumbricoides* has been recognized as the likely cause of most of the earliest reported cases, although several other parasitic infections, including hookworms (*Ancylostoma duodenale, Necator Americanus, Necator Brasilensis*), *Strongyloides, Trichinella Spiralis, and Toxocara Canis*[2–4] and exposures to numerous drugs and other agents have also been recognized to induce a Loeffler-like syndrome (see below and Tables 71-2 and 71-3). An identifiable etiologic agent may be lacking in up to one-third of patients.

TABLE 71-1 Diseases Associated with Pulmonary Infiltrates and Eosinophilia

Pulmonary Eosinophilic Syndromes of Known Cause
Parasitic-induced eosinophilic pneumonias (including Loeffler syndrome)
Drug- or toxin-induced eosinophilic pneumonias
Tropical pulmonary eosinophilia
Allergic bronchopulmonary mycosis
Pulmonary Eosinophilic Syndromes of Unknown Cause
Idiopathic acute eosinophilic pneumonia
Chronic eosinophilic pneumonia
EGPA (allergic granulomatosis and angiitis)
Idiopathic hypereosinophilic syndrome
Other Lung Diseases Variably Associated with Eosinophilia
Asthma/allergy
Bronchocentric granulomatosis
Bronchiolitis obliterans–organizing pneumonia
Infections
Fungal (esp. coccidioidomycosis, *Aspergillus, Pneumocystis jirovecii*)
Tuberculosis
Viral
Interstitial lung disease
Idiopathic pulmonary fibrosis
Collagen vascular disease associated
Sarcoidosis
Hypersensitivity pneumonitis
Eosinophilic granuloma (pulmonary histiocytosis X)
Malignancy
Non–small-cell cancer of lung
Non-Hodgkin lymphoma
Myeloblastic leukemia
Metastatic disease
Miscellaneous (e.g., lung transplantation, lung allograft rejection, ulcerative colitis)

Loeffler syndrome affects people of all ages. It is characterized clinically by the presence of low-grade fever, nonproductive cough, dyspnea (mild to severe), chest discomfort with coughing or deep breathing, and, occasionally, hemoptysis.[3,5] The respiratory manifestations of Loeffler syndrome are usually self-limited, typically resolving in 1 to 2 weeks. Laboratory examination of peripheral

TABLE 71-2 Parasitic Infections Associated with Eosinophilic Pneumonia

Ancylostoma spp.	*Opisthorchis* spp.
Ascaris spp.	*Paragonimus westermani*
Brugia malayi	*Schistosoma* spp.
Clonorchis sinensis	*Strongyloides stercoralis*
Dirofilaria immitis	*Toxocara gondii*
Echinococcus spp.	*Trichinella spiralis*
Entamoeba histolytica	*Trichosporon terrestre*
Necator americanus	*Wuchereria bancrofti*

TABLE 71-3 Drugs and Other Exposures Causing Eosinophilic Pneumonia

Acetaminophen
Acetylsalicylic acid[a]
Aluminum
Amiodarone[a]
Amitriptyline[a]
Ampicillin
Angiotensin-converting enzyme inhibitors[a]
Azathioprine
Beclomethasone dipropionate
Beryllium
β-Blockers
Bleomycin[a]
Captopril[a]
Carbamazepine[a]
Chloroquine
Chlorpromazine
Chlorpropamide
Clarithromycin
Clofibrate
Cocaine (inhalation)
Contrast agents
Cromolyn (inhalation)
Dantrolene
Dapsone
Daptomycin[a]
Desipramine
Diclofenac
D-penicillamine
Dust (inhalation), e.g., World Trade Center
Ethambutol
Fenbarbamate
Fenbufen
Fludarabine
Glafenine
Gold salts[a]
Granulocyte macrophage colony–stimulating factor
Heroin (inhalation)
Hydrochlorothiazide
Ibuprofen
Imipramine
Indomethacin
Infliximab
Interferon-alpha
Interleukins
Iodinated contrast agents[a]
Isoniazid
Levofloxacin
L-Tryptophan[a]
Maloprim
Mecamylamine
Mephenesin carbamate
Mesalazine
Methotrexate[a]
Methylphenidate
Minocycline[a]
Montelukast
Naproxen
Nickel dust (inhalation)
Nilutamide[a]
Nitrofurantoin[a]
Nomifensine
Oxaliplatin
Para-aminosalicylic acid
Penicillamine[a]
Penicillin
Pentamidine (inhaled)
Phenytoin[a]
Piroxicam
Procarbazine
Progesterone
Prontosil
Propylthiouracil[a]
Pyramethamine
Radiation exposure
Ranitidine
Rapeseed oil
Red spider antigens
Salicylazosulfapyridine
Scorpion stings
Sertraline
Smoke exposure
Streptomycin
Sulfa-containing antibiotics[a]
Sulfasalazine[a]
Sulindac
Tamoxifen
Tetracycline
Thiazides
Tolazamide
Tolfenamic acid
Trazodone
Trichloroethane
Venlafaxine

[a]*Drugs commonly or occasionally reported to cause pulmonary eosinophilia.*

blood from patients reveals moderate-to-extreme eosinophilia, which may be at peak levels as respiratory symptoms resolve and which resolves over several weeks.[4] Expectorated sputum, if present, frequently contains eosinophils and/or Charcot–Leyden crystals.[4,5] Transient, migratory, nonsegmental, bilateral, interstitial, and alveolar infiltrates (often peripheral or pleural based) are evident on the chest radiograph.[3] Infiltrates typically clear after several weeks. Pulmonary function evaluation typically reveals a mild-to-moderate restrictive ventilatory defect with a reduced diffusing capacity for carbon monoxide (DL_{CO}).

When Loeffler syndrome is due to *A. Lumbricoides*, hookworms or other parasites, the pulmonary manifestations are believed to result from a hypersensitivity reaction to the parasite larvae. Following ingestion of *Ascaris* ova, larvae hatch within the small intestine, then cross the intestinal wall to enter the splanchnic, and ultimately the pulmonary circulation. Subsequently, the larvae migrate across pulmonary capillaries into alveoli, mature into adult worms, ascend the large airways, and are swallowed into the gastrointestinal (GI) tract, where they complete their life cycle. The pulmonary manifestations of Loeffler syndrome begin approximately 9 to 14 days following ingestion and occur during the migration of larvae through the lung. *Ascaris suum*, a large roundworm endemic to pigs, can cause a nearly identical syndrome. Cutaneous penetration of larvae is the principal relevant mode of tissue entry for hookworms.

During the pneumonic stage of the illness, *Ascaris* or hookworm larvae may be identified in sputum or gastric aspirates.[4] In keeping with the life cycle of *Ascaris* or hookworms, stool examination for ova and parasites is typically negative until 8 weeks after the onset of the respiratory syndrome.[6] Histologic evaluation of lung tissue is not required for confirmation of the diagnosis. When tissue has been obtained, a characteristic and striking eosinophilic infiltration of interstitium and alveolar–capillary units has been noted. Increased numbers of macrophages have also been appreciated. Tissue necrosis and vasculitis are not features of the disorder. *Ascaris* or hookworm larvae may be identified in the tissue specimen.[4]

Since Loeffler syndrome may be induced by a variety of exposures, a search for an etiologic agent (e.g., parasitic infection or drug reaction) should be undertaken. Bronchodilators and rarely corticosteroids may be used for alleviation of pulmonary symptoms, although these are usually self-limited. In cases due to *Ascaris*, treatment with oral mebendazole (100 mg twice a day for 3 days or a single dose of 500 mg) should be given to prevent late GI manifestations of *Ascaris* infestation, which may include malnutrition, diarrhea, abdominal pain, and/or intestinal obstruction typically 8 weeks or more after onset of respiratory symptoms. Pyrantel pamoate, albendazole, or ivermectin are alternate treatment options.[4] Since stool specimens are negative for ova and parasites early in the illness, clinical follow-up over a 2- to 3-month period is indicated.

■ PARASITIC INFECTIONS

Infections with parasites other than *Ascaris* species are also commonly associated with pulmonary infiltrates and blood or pulmonary eosinophilia.[3–5] The parasites associated with the development of pulmonary eosinophilic syndromes are listed in Table 71-2. The prevalence of infection with each of these organisms varies with geographical location, socioeconomic status, and host immunity. Parasites may infect the lung via direct pulmonary invasion or via hematogenous seeding. In addition to *Ascaris* species, *Strongyloides stercoralis* (an intestinal nematode), *Ancylostoma brasiliensis* (cutaneous helminthiasis, "creeping eruption"), *Ancylostoma duodenale,* and *T. canis* (dog roundworm, "visceral larva migrans") are the parasitic agents most commonly associated with pulmonary eosinophilia in the United States.

Strongyloides is widely distributed in the tropical and subtropical regions.[3] Following initial transcutaneous infection, a Loeffler-like syndrome may occur as larvae migrate through the lungs. Chronic strongyloidiasis occurs as a result of autoinfection, whereby the noninfectious rhabditiform larvae transform within the GI tract into infectious filariform larvae, penetrate the colonic wall or perianal skin, and reinfect the host.[4,5] Chronic strongyloidiasis may be associated with recurrent asthma-like symptoms that may worsen with the administration of corticosteroids. The hyperinfection syndrome results from accelerated autoinfection, and usually occurs in persons with defects in cell-mediated immunity[3] (such as lymphoma, human immunodeficiency virus [HIV] or human-T lymphotropic virus type 1 [HTLV-1] infection, and with chronic corticosteroid use), as well as in persons with underlying GI disease, chronic lung disease, malnutrition, and use of H2 blockers or antacids.[7] It may also occur in healthy persons. Respiratory manifestations include cough, dyspnea, chronic bronchitis, wheezing, hemoptysis, and patchy pulmonary infiltrates, in association with blood eosinophilia. Rarely, acute respiratory distress syndrome (ARDS) has been reported in patients with hyperinfection. GI manifestations are also common, including abdominal pain, paralytic ileus, nausea and vomiting, bowel perforation, and secondary sepsis from gram-negative bacteria. Central nervous system (CNS) manifestations such as meningitis have also been noted.

The diagnosis of *Strongyloides* infection may be established by identification of larvae in sputum, BAL fluid, bronchial brushings, or transbronchial biopsy specimens, pleural fluid or stool. Several stool samples are often required to identify the pathogen.[5] Serologic testing, such as ELISA to detect IgG antibody to *Strongyloides stercoralis* can also be used to establish a diagnosis.[4] Patients at risk for *Strongyloides* hyperinfection syndrome should be screened for the parasite prior to initiation of immunosuppressive therapy.[3]

Thiabendazole (25 mg/kg twice a day for 2 days) or ivermectin (200 μg/kg given orally for 1–2 days) may be used for the treatment of uncomplicated or disseminated strongyloidias.[4] Ivermectin is generally better tolerated in terms of side effects.[5] Albendazole is an alternative agent. Higher dose and longer duration of thiabendizole treatment are needed to treat disseminated strongyloidiasis in immunocompromised persons.[5] The hyperinfection syndrome associated with *Strongyloides* can be difficult to cure. Therapy should be continued until the clinical syndrome resolves and larvae are no longer detectable in the GI tract.

Ancylostomiasis is a nematodal infection endemic to the southeastern coastal regions of the United States, Mexico, and Central and South America.[4,5] The organism is present in soil contaminated by stool from infected domestic animals. It penetrates human skin most commonly through the feet. This results in the development of the "creeping eruption" lesion – a raised, erythematous, serpiginous, tunnel-like, and often itchy lesion on areas of exposed skin.[8] A Loeffler-like syndrome occurs in up to 50% of cases of "creeping eruption." Specific treatment for pulmonary involvement is typically not required as illness is usually self-limited.

Infection with *T. canis* may occur throughout the world and leads to the clinical syndrome of "visceral larva migrans."[4] This syndrome is characterized by hepatomegaly, leukocytosis, fever, hypergammaglobulinemia, and persistent blood eosinophilia.[9] Because the disease most commonly affects young children, a high degree of clinical suspicion is necessary to establish the diagnosis in adults. Respiratory symptoms, including cough and severe wheezing, may occur after ingestion of substantial numbers of larvae. Laboratory evaluation reveals peripheral blood and BAL eosinophilia, elevated serum levels of immunoglobulin E (IgE), and poorly defined, diffuse nodular alveolar infiltrates on chest radiograph.[4] ELISA testing for larval antigens is diagnostic. Although the disease may be self-limited, treatment with thiabendazole, albendazole, mebendazole, diethylcarbamazine, or corticosteroids may hasten recovery in patients who are severely ill.[3–5]

DRUG AND TOXIN-INDUCED PULMONARY EOSINOPHILIC SYNDROMES

A vast number of drugs and toxic exposures have been associated with the development of pulmonary infiltrates and blood or pulmonary eosinophilia.[1,10–13] A partial list of these medications and exposures is given in Table 71-3, and information regarding pulmonary drug toxicities may also be found on the Internet on the regularly updated web site, www.pneumotox.com. Of the medications implicated, many are commonly used antibiotics, nonsteroidal anti-inflammatory agents, anticonvulsants, cardiovascular medications, and antidepressants.

In addition to medications, a number of toxic exposures may also be associated with eosinophilic pneumonia.[10] For example, eosinophilic pneumonia has been described following radiation therapy for breast cancer, dust or smoke exposure,[14–17] exposure to iodinated contrast agents or 1,1,1-trichloroethane (Scotchguard),[18] and after inhalation of cocaine or heroin.[19–21]

Whereas most cases of drug- or toxin-induced pulmonary eosinophilia are sporadic, outbreaks of pulmonary eosinophilia have occurred following ingestion of rapeseed oil (contaminated with aniline derivatives)[22] or L-tryptophan.[23] The precise incidence of drug- or toxin-induced pulmonary eosinophilia is difficult to assess, since most of the literature pertaining to these syndromes is published in the form of case reports, rather than large series or controlled trials. For the same reason, the precise pathogenesis and the definition of the clinical syndromes associated with individual exposures are difficult to characterize.

In general, drug-induced pulmonary eosinophilic syndromes have an acute or subacute onset and are not always related to either the cumulative dose of drug used or the duration of treatment. Respiratory symptoms vary widely in severity, from a mild Loeffler-like illness with dyspnea, cough, and fever to severe fulminant respiratory failure. The DRESS syndrome consists of acute eosinophilic pneumonia with drug rash and systemic manifestations.[24] Wheezing may be present, but obstructive physiology is not common on pulmonary function testing. Although radiographic findings are not specific, interstitial or alveolar infiltrates are typically evident on chest radiograph (Fig. 71-1), and common high-resolution chest computed tomographic (CT) findings include bilateral consolidation and ground-glass opacities, both of which are frequently peripherally located.

A diagnosis of drug- or toxin-induced eosinophilic pneumonia is based upon a careful review of drug and other exposures (including nonprescription drugs, herbal preparations, street drugs, and environmental exposures). Other causes of eosinophilic lung disease must be excluded. A concurrent skin rash and pleural effusion can support the diagnosis of drug-induced eosinophilic pneumonia. In some cases, testing with lymphocyte proliferation assays may reveal T-cell sensitization to specific drugs. However, the utility of such assays is limited as negative tests do not rule out a drug-induced disorder, and these assays are not widely available for routine clinical use. The prognosis is favorable in most cases. Elimination of exposure to the drug or other toxin usually leads to resolution of symptoms, eosinophilia, pulmonary infiltrates, and normalization of lung function within a month. Supplemental therapy with corticosteroids is not universally required, but it may hasten recovery in patients who are severely ill.

IDIOPATHIC ACUTE EOSINOPHILIC PNEUMONIA

In contrast to the typically benign Loeffler syndrome, a more severe idiopathic form of eosinophilic pneumonia termed *acute eosinophilic pneumonia* (AEP) has been recognized as a distinct clinical entity.[25–28] Although seen in patients of both genders and any age group, AEP tends to occur in patients between the age of 20 and 40[26,29,30] and is more common in men.[25] AEP is usually idiopathic, occurs commonly in previously healthy persons, and may represent an acute hypersensitivity reaction to an inhaled agent.[28] Similar cases have been reported in persons with a history of chronic myelogenous leukemia, hematopoietic stem cell transplantation[31,32] or HIV infection.[33] Many cases have been reported in patients who have recently commenced smoking,[27,34–36] used flavored tobacco products,[37] or had other changes in smoking habits. The disease may recur when former smokers resume smoking.[35,38] Overall up to 70% of patients with AEP have a history of smoking.[26,39] In addition, cases have been reported in persons treated with venlafexine,[40] minocycline,[26] daptomycin,[11,41] and several other drugs.[26] It has also been reported among persons who have been involved in activities with unusual exposures (including exposure to dust from the World Trade Center collapse in New York City,[14] after military deployment in Iraq,[17] cave exploration, gasoline tank cleaning, plant repotting, woodpile moving, and indoor renovations).[26,42] AEP has also been seen following inhalation of cocaine or heroin[21,43] and in association with H1N1 influenza infection.[1,44] Although none of the patients in the original reported series had atopy or asthma, cases have since been described in persons with a history of atopy. No definite seasonal variation has been identified.

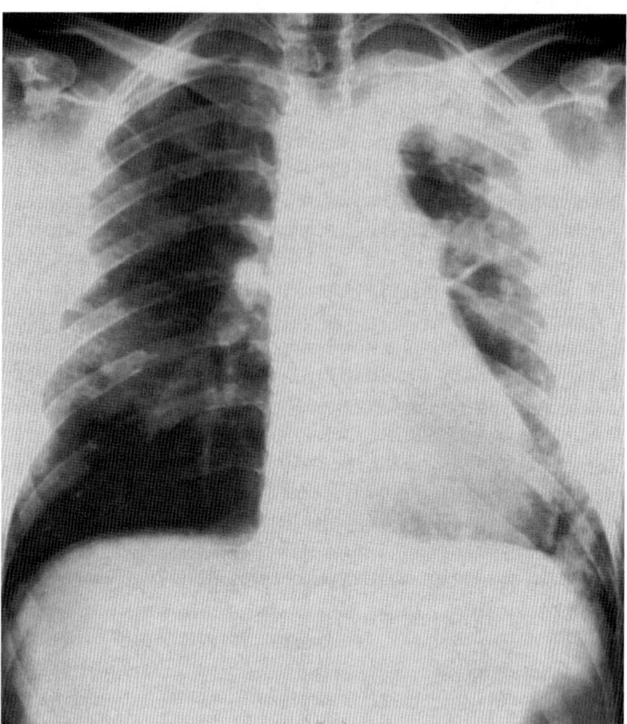

Figure 71-1 Chest radiograph of a 23-year-old woman with acute sulfasalazine-induced eosinophilic pneumonia. Bilateral interstitial and alveolar infiltrates are present.

Idiopathic AEP presents as an acute illness with dyspnea, fever, nonproductive cough, tachypnea, pleuritic chest pain, and hypoxemia (arterial Pa_{O_2} under 60 mm Hg) at times with myalgias.[25,26,39] Symptom duration is typically less than 7 days,[1] although longer courses of up to 30 days have been described. Patients usually have diffuse inspiratory crackles on chest auscultation, wheezing may be present, and rapid progression from mild dyspnea to overt respiratory failure requiring mechanical ventilation is common.[17,26,27] A moderate leukocytosis with left shift is typical,[27] but blood eosinophilia is usually absent at the onset of disease.[17,25,26] Early clinical features may be mistaken for community-acquired pneumonia. Blood eosinophilia may develop later in the course of the disease and may

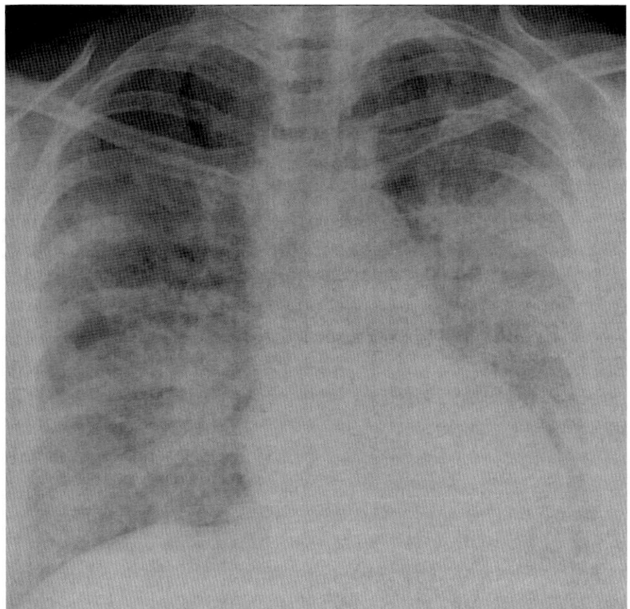

A

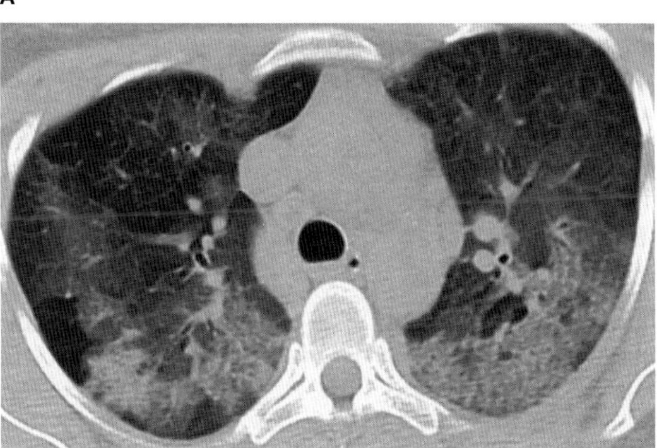

B

Figure 71-2 Radiographic apœpearance of idiopathic acute eosinophilic pneumonia (AEP). **A.** Diffuse bilateral alveolar and interstitial infiltrates apparent on chest radiograph. **B.** Diffuse parenchymal ground-glass opacity and consolidation evident on computed tomography scan.

provide a clue to the diagnosis.[27,45] Serum IgE levels may be moderately elevated.[26,46] The erythrocyte sedimentation rate (ESR) may be elevated as well. Serum levels of thymus and activation-regulated chemokine (TARC)/CCL17 (a ligand for CCR4 on Th2 lymphocytes) may be elevated and may help to distinguish AEP from other cause of acute lung injury(ALI).[47] Striking eosinophilia (25%–55%) is present in BAL fluid.[17,26,27,45,48] Increased numbers of lymphocytes (up to 20%) and neutrophils (up to 15%) are commonly also present in BAL fluid in AEP.[48] Pulmonary function tests reveal a restrictive ventilatory defect with a reduced $D_{L_{CO}}$ that typically normalize following treatment.[48]

Early in the course of illness, the chest radiograph reveals subtle, patchy infiltrates with Kerley B lines.[26,49] Diffuse, symmetric alveolar and interstitial infiltrates resembling ARDS with a ground-glass or micronodular or reticular appearance (Fig. 71-2A) develop within 48 hours.[50,51] Infiltrates are typically bilateral, although AEP with unilateral infiltrates has been described. Small-to-moderate bilateral pleural effusions are common (affecting up to 50%–70% of patients).[27] Fluid analysis typically reveals a high pH and marked eosinophilia.[51] CT scanning confirms the presence of diffuse parenchymal ground-glass attenuation, inerlobular septal thickening and/or consolidation (Fig. 71-2B), with prominence along bronchovascular bundles, with or without pleural effusion.[49,52] Lymphadenopathy may also be seen.

Light microscopic examination of lung tissue reveals prominent eosinophil infiltration in interstitium and/or alveolar spaces, and bronchial walls.[53] The pathologic pattern of diffuse alveolar damage with hyaline membranes and eosinophilic infiltrates should suggest the possibility of AEP. Lymphocytic infiltration of interstitium, type 2 pneumocyte hyperplasia, and intra-alveolar fibrinous exudate are also common. Granulomas, alveolar hemmorhage, and nonnecrotic perivascular inflammation have been reported.[53] Basal lamina damage is unusual.[49] Extrapulmonary involvement is rare.

The pathogenesis of idiopathic AEP is poorly understood.[26,39] The occurrence of cases following unusual environmental exposures (as noted earlier) suggests these exposures as possible disease-inciting events, perhaps as triggers for a hypersensitivity reaction to an unidentified antigen in susceptible persons. Of note, elevated levels of the fungal cell wall component β-D-glucan have been described in the BAL fluid of some patients with AEP, suggesting a possible association between exposure to fungus and development of disease.

However, the roles of lymphocytes and eosinophils in this disorder have not been fully elucidated. Elevated levels of interleukin (IL)-5, a Th2 lymphocyte–derived cytokine involved in activation and recruitment of eosinophils, have been described in the BAL of patients with AEP.[54] Levels of vascular endothelial growth factor (VEGF), a cytokine induced by IL-5, have also been shown to be elevated in BAL and to correlate with number of eosinophils and levels of IL-5.[55] Elevated BAL levels of IL-18, a cytokine capable of inducing several cytokines known to induce or enhance eosinophilia, have also been identified among patients with acute (and other) forms of eosinophilic pneumonia.[26] Collectively, these findings suggest a role for Th2 lymphocytes and eosinophils in disease pathogenesis. It remains unknown, however, whether the eosinophils initiate the disease process or are a secondary manifestation of the disorder. Alveolar macrophage–derived cytokines may also play a role in the development of AEP.[56]

Idiopathic AEP is a diagnosis of exclusion[51] and should be considered in a patient who presents with an acute febrile illness less than 1 week in duration, apparent ALI or ARDS without a typical antecedent illness. A careful search must be undertaken for other causes of pulmonary infiltrates, especially fungal or other infection, and drug or other exposures. Specimens of blood, sputum, stool, BAL, and often transbronchial biopsy specimens should be obtained for stain and culture as well as serologic testing to rule out viral, bacterial, mycobacterial, fungal, and parasitic infection.[26,39] BAL cell differential should be performed. Elevated blood levels of TARC/CCL17 may distinguish AEP from other causes of ALI, even in the early phase of disease before blood esoinophilia is present.[47] In contrast, levels of KL-6, a marker for alveolar cell damage, tend to be lower in AEP than in other forms of ALI.[47] An elevated fraction of exhaled nitric oxide (FeNO; e.g., levels >23.5 ppb) may also help to distinguish AEP from non-AEP disorders[57] and FeNO levels decreased following corticosteroid treatment. Lower serum IgG levels have also been reported in AEP as compared with other causes of pulmonary eosinophilia.[58]

Idiopathic AEP generally carries an excellent prognosis. Although fatalities have been reported, most patients demonstrate rapid dramatic responses to corticosteroid therapy,[25,26,59] with abatement of fever and respiratory symptoms within 12 to 48 hours and complete resolution of infiltrates, pleural effusion, and pulmonary function impairment usually within 1 month.[27,48] The optimal steroid regimen for the treatment of AEP has not been determined. However, initial doses of methylprednisolone typically used range from 60 to 125 mg administered every 6 hours. After resolution of respiratory failure, oral prednisone (in doses of 40–60 mg per day) may be continued for 2 to 4 weeks with a subsequent slow taper over the next several weeks.[26,51] Despite the apparent clinical success of steroid treatment, there is no definitive proof that steroids alter the natural history of the disease. Spontaneous disease regression has been reported,[27] and in contrast to idiopathic CEP, absence of clinical relapse is characteristic. Follow-up pulmonary function testing is generally normal, although a small number of patients may demonstrate mild reductions in DL_{CO} or lung volumes.

TROPICAL PULMONARY EOSINOPHILIA

TPE was first described in the early 1940s[60] as a syndrome characterized by fevers, malaise, anorexia, weight loss, paroxysmal dry cough with dyspnea or wheezing, marked peripheral blood eosinophilia, and spontaneous resolution over several weeks' time. In the 1950s and 1960s, filarial infections were recognized as the cause of this disorder.[61] TPE is most prominent in India, Africa, and Southeast Asia, but it may be seen worldwide in filarial-endemic regions.[3,4,62] Disease may also present in nonendemic regions among immigrants or travelers.[62,63] A rare manifestation of parasitic infection, TPE occurs in less than 1% of patients infected with lymphatic filariae (usually introduced by mosquito bite) and results from a hypersensitivity reaction to microfilariae from *Wuchereria bancrofti* and *Brugia malayi*.[5,62,64] Illnesses resembling TPE have also been reported following infection with other parasites. Approximately four times more common in men, most patients with TPE manifest the disease between the age of 25 and 40 years,[4,62] although children and older adults may also be affected. There is no known seasonal or genetic propensity to this disease, and it remains unclear why only such a small percentage of patients with filarial infection develop TPE.

Clinical manifestations of TPE develop months to years after the infection.[4] The most common distinguishing symptom of TPE is spasmodic cough that usually occurs at night.[62] Other typical early symptoms include low-grade fevers, weight loss, fatigue, and malaise. Dyspnea and wheezing, which can be severe, are common, and the clinical presentation may resemble status asthmaticus. Chest pain, muscle tenderness, and cardiac, pericardial, and CNS involvement have also been reported. Rarely, patients remain asymptomatic. Physical examination of patients with TPE is notable for coarse rales or rhonchi and wheezing,[62] although no abnormalities are found in approximately 20% of patients. Generalized lymphadenopathy and hepatosplenomegaly, pericarditis, musculoskeletal or CNS manifestations may be present,[4,62] but they are less common in adults than in children.

Laboratory findings in TPE include extreme peripheral blood eosinophilia[4,5,62] (usually more than 3000 eosinophils per cubic millimeter and up to 90% of the leukocyte differential) that persists for several weeks, although the degree of eosinophilia generally does not correlate well with clinical disease severity or radiographic findings. Blood eosinophils appear degranulated and contain cytoplasmic vacuoles.[62] Total serum IgE is usually elevated (more than 1000 U/mL), and the presence of high titers of filarial-specific IgE and IgG, measured by complement fixation or hemagglutination techniques, confirms the diagnosis.[3,5] Hypergammaglobulinemia results from polyclonal activation of B cells.[4] The ESR, circulating immune complexes, serum IgG, IgM and IgA, and complement (CH50) may be moderately elevated,[4,5] and patients may also have an abnormal electrocardiogram (ECG). Eosinophils may be identified in the sputum,[4,62] and, in those with active disease, BAL typically reveals intense eosinophilia (upto 50% of the differential), elevated levels of total IgE, and filarial-specific IgE, IgM, IgG and fibronectin.[4,5,62] BAL may also contain IgE antibodies to *B. Malayi* BM 23–25 antigen[4,62,65] as well as eosinophil-derived neurotoxin.[5] Pleural fluid, when present, is eosinophilic and also contains elevated IgE.[4] Serum α1-antitrypsin levels are reduced and return to normal with treatment.[4,66] Microfilariae are not found in blood or sputum,[4] and examination of stool or urine for ova and parasites is negative (although patients from endemic countries may be simultaneously infected with other parasites). In contrast, microfilariae have been identified in lung and lymph node tissue, especially when lymphadenopathy is present.

Pulmonary function test findings vary with the duration of disease: They reveal an obstructive ventilatory defect in up to 30% of patients, particularly when symptoms have been present less than 1 month. A restrictive ventilatory defect and reduced DL_{CO}, with or without a concomitant obstructive defect, are typical of long-standing disease.[3–5] Mild arterial hypoxemia may be present.[62] Ill-defined, diffuse reticulonodular infiltrates with a mottled appearance primarily affecting the mid to lower lung fields are characteristic radiographic findings in TPE.[3,4,62] Bronchovascular markings may be prominent and hilar adenopathy and pleural effusions have occasionally been reported.[4,62] The chest radiograph may be normal at the time of presentation in as many as 20% of patients.[62] In rare cases where *Dirofilaria* is the causative agent, the chest radiograph may reveal solitary or multiple nodules thought to represent infarcts caused by parasitic emboli. CT scanning may show mediastinal adenopathy, bronchiectasis, and areas of calcification.[67]

The histopathologic findings in TPE depend on the tissue examined, as well as the stage and duration of the disease.[62] Studies of lung pathology have shown that the early stage of the disease (within the first 2 weeks) is characterized by histiocytic inflammation in the alveolar, interstitial, peribronchial, and perivascular spaces, with preservation of lung architecture.[4] Tiny nodules may be palpable within the lung tissue. One to three months after symptom onset, eosinophilic infiltration with eosinophilic bronchopneumonia and microabscesses is present in lungs of untreated patients. Degenerating microfilariae may be present within the center of the microabscesses, and some destruction of alveolar walls may be evident. Local bronchial walls are also edematous and inflamed, with evidence of epithelial disruption. Long-standing untreated disease is associated with the presence of chronic mixed-cell inflammation (histiocytes, eosinophils, and lymphocytes) in a nodular pattern and the development of pulmonary fibrosis.[4,62] Foreign body–type granulomatous lesions are often present. Lymph node biopsies may reveal degenerating microfilariae or adult worms, surrounded by aggregates of eosinophils, their granule products, and giant cells.

The clinical features of TPE are believed to result from an intense hypersensitivity reaction to microfilarial antigens of *W. bancrofti* and *Brugia malayi*. Although a broad spectrum of clinical disease may be caused by filaria, patients with TPE rarely have other systemic features of filariasis. Canine filarial forms (e.g., *Dirofilaria immitis*) are rarely transmitted to humans but also may be recovered from lung and lymph node specimens. Disease occurs when larvae introduced into the body via insect bites develop into mature filariae.[4] The adult worms, dwelling within the lymphatics, produce microfilariae, which are then trapped in the pulmonary vasculature. The release of antigens from degenerating microfilariae leads to an intense local and systemic inflammatory response. A striking antibody and eosinophilic response, similar to that seen in peripheral blood, is also present within the lung.[4,5,62] Although little is known about the precise mechanisms by which filariae are cleared in patients with TPE, both antibody-dependent mechanisms and eosinophils probably play a role.[4,62] In vitro, both granulocytes and macrophages can bind microfilariae in the presence of IgG, IgE, or complement leading to the death of the organism. The finding of an intense lymphocytic- and plasma-cell infiltrate around microfilariae in tissues suggests that lymphocytes may be important for clearance of the organism. In vitro lymphocyte transformation in response to stimulation with microfilarial antigens can be demonstrated in some cases. The transcription factor NFkB[68]

TABLE 71-4 Diagnostic Criteria for Tropical Pulmonary Eosinophilia

Relevant exposure in endemic area
Paroxysmal nocturnal cough, dyspnea
Infiltrate on chest radiograph
Leukocytosis with eosinophilia
Elevated serum IgE
Elevated serum antifilarial IgE, IgG (*W. bancrofti, B. malayi*)
Clinical improvement with diethylcarbamazine treatment

and oxidants[69] are also reported to play an important role in the inflammatory response to TPE. The precise mechanisms by which eosinophils accumulate in the lung and contribute to tissue inflammation in patients with TPE are incompletely understood. Lung (as well as blood) eosinophils appear degranulated by microscopy.[62,70] Elevated levels of eosinophil-derived neurotoxin, an RNase capable of damaging the lung epithelium, have been observed in the BAL fluid of patients with TPE. IgE and eosinophil-, lymphocyte-, mast cell-, or basophil-derived products may contribute to the wheezing and airway hyperresponsiveness that can occur in this disorder.

The diagnosis of TPE is usually established on the basis of the clinical and laboratory findings described earlier including pertinent exposure history. Lung or other tissue biopsies are not typically required. The diagnostic criteria for TPE are summarized in Table 71-4.[62] Biopsy of enlarged lymph nodes (e.g., scalene) may assist in establishing the diagnosis in some cases. A rapid treatment response may provide confirmatory evidence that the correct diagnosis has been made. The differential diagnosis includes Loeffler syndrome, CEP, ABPA, drug reactions, other parasitic infections, HES, and lymphangitic spread of carcinoma. In nonendemic areas, the disease may also masquerade as asthma, atypical pneumonia, sarcoidosis, EGPA, granulomatosis with polyangiitis (formerly known as Wegener's granulomatosis, WG), or tuberculosis (TB). Diagnosis in nonendemic regions is often delayed, and a careful review of travel history and a high index of suspicion are necessary to prompt the diagnosis.

Diethylcarbamazine, a piperazine derivative used widely in the treatment of filarial infections, is the therapy of choice for TPE, typically at a dose of 6 mg/kg/d for 14 to 21 days.[4,5,62] Diethylcarbamazine acts by both direct and indirect mechanisms. It is directly filaricidal to both adult worms and microfilariae. It can also enhance the binding of granulocytes, macrophages, antibodies, and complement to the surface of microfilariae. A marked clinical improvement and decrease in eosinophil count usually occurs in the first 7 to 14 days of therapy. Clinical improvement following diethylcarbamazine treatment has been correlated temporally with the resolution of eosinophilic alveolitis. In addition, improvement in pulmonary function, reduction in BAL eosinophilia, a decrease in total and filarial-specific IgE and IgG, increase in serum α1-antitrypsin levels, and radiographic clearing generally occur within 1 to 4 weeks of treatment.[4,62]

The course and prognosis of the acute disease in patients treated with diethylcarbamazine are generally benign, and 3 weeks of diethylcarbamazine therapy is curative in most patients. However, acute relapses related to reinfection or release of microfilaria from existing adult worms do occur in up to 20% of patients.[4] Persons whose α1-antitrypsin levels remain low after initial treatment may be at greater risk of relapse .[4,66] Patients who experience acute relapses often respond to additional treatment with diethylcarbamazine at higher doses of 2 to 4 mg/kg three times a day for 21 to 30 days. Alternatively, mild, chronic inflammation may persist, causing chronic interstitial lung disease, with persistent respiratory symptoms, radiographic findings, and hematologic and serologic abnormalities.[62] Persistent clinical symptoms have been reported over 2- to 5-year follow-up periods in up to 13% of patients with TPE treated with a standard course of therapy. BAL in these patients reveals a mild, persistent eosinophilia. Persons with symptoms of longer duration are less likely to have a favorable treatment response. Alternative antifilarial drugs (e.g., ivermectin) or a trial of corticosteroids may be useful therapies for the chronic variant of the disease,[4,62] although controlled studies of these agents are lacking. A subset of patients with apparent TPE may fail to respond to diethylcarbamazine; whether these patients have diethylcarbamazine-resistant TPE or disease due to other parasites is unclear, as current serologic testing does not distinguish between human lymphatic filarial antigens and antigens on certain other parasites.

Untreated disease usually persists for weeks to months. Untreated TPE may remit spontaneously, but it commonly recurs within months to years. It is important to treat TPE early in the course of the disease, since although seldom fatal, untreated TPE often leads to the development of irreversible pulmonary fibrosis.[63,71]

CHRONIC EOSINOPHILIC PNEUMONIA

CEP was first described as a clinical entity by Carrington et al.[72] in 1969. Although CEP may develop in people of any age, the peak incidence occurs in persons 30 to 45 years of age.[1,73,74] Women are affected approximately twice as often as men, and CEP has been reported during pregnancy and following radiation therapy for breast cancer.[75] The female predominance is less obvious among patients whose disease begins after the age of 60. Most cases occur in Caucasians. Up to two-thirds have adult-onset asthma preceding (by several weeks to years) or arising concurrently with the occurrence of CEP.[1,74,76,77] The asthma is often severe and may lead to fixed airflow obstruction (approximately 10% of patients) despite medical therapy.[76] Most patients with CEP are nonsmokers. In addition, approximately one-third to one-half of patients have antecedent atopy, allergic rhinitis, nasal polyps, or urticaria.[1]

In contrast to idiopathic AEP, CEP typically has a subacute presentation, with symptoms present for weeks to several months before diagnosis.[1,74] Common presenting complaints include dyspnea, low-grade fevers, malaise, drenching night sweats, and moderate (10 to 50 lb) weight loss.[74,77] Cough, often dry initially and later productive of small amounts of mucoid sputum, is a virtually universal finding.[74] Rhinitis or sinusitis may be present. Two of the nine patients described in Carrington's original series had minor hemoptysis. Patients ultimately develop progressive dyspnea, which may be associated with wheezing in those with adult-onset asthma. Very rarely, patients with CEP may also have severe acute respiratory failure or ARDS, with severe hypoxemia requiring mechanical ventilation. There are no major extrapulmonary manifestations of CEP. Rarely, arthralgias, skin rash, diarrhea or colitis, mononeuritis, hepatitis, pericarditis or unexplained heart failure have been described, raising suspicion that there may be a continuum between CEP and EGPA.[74] Indeed, cases have been reported wherein patients initially diagnosed with CEP later developed EGPA.[78,79]

Patients with CEP frequently manifest a moderate leukocytosis. The majority (66%–95%) have peripheral blood eosinophilia (usually >1000/mm^3),[74] with eosinophils constituting more than 6%, and typically up to 20% to 30% of their leukocyte differential.[73,80] Leukocyte differentials with up to 90% eosinophils have been noted in this disorder. However, a lack of peripheral blood eosinophilia does not rule out the diagnosis, since eosinophilia may be absent in 10% to 30% of cases.[73,77] Normochromic, normocytic anemia and thrombocytosis may be present. The C-reactive protein levels and the

ESR are typically elevated (greater than 20 mm per hour),[74] and IgE levels are elevated in up to one-half of cases. Analysis of BAL fluid reveals increased eosinophils, typically accounting for 40% or more of the white blood cell (WBC) differential, with a range from 12% to 95% reported.[1,74,77,81] Urinary eosinophil-derived neurotoxin levels are also elevated.[82] Blood and sputum cultures routinely fail to identify an infectious etiology in these patients.

The severity of pulmonary function abnormalities depends on the stage and severity of the disease. In the initial stage prior to treatment with corticosteroids, testing may reveal restrictive, obstructive, or normal physiology.[74] Obstructive ventilatory defects, while more common in patients with a history of asthma, are also encountered in patients without pre-existing asthma. Restrictive physiology may result from changes in lung compliance due to acute eosinophilic infiltration of lung parenchyma. Diffusing capacity may be reduced and the alveolar–arterial oxygen gradient may be mildly elevated.[74,77]

In the original series, Carrington et al. described three radiographic features that are characteristic for CEP: (1) peripherally based, progressive dense infiltrates; (2) rapid resolution of infiltrates following corticosteroid treatment, with recurrences in identical locations; and (3) the appearance of infiltrates as the "photographic negative of pulmonary edema."[72,83,84] The pulmonary infiltrates associated with CEP are typically dense and patchy areas of airspace consolidation with ill-defined margins usually affecting the outer two-thirds of the lung fields (Fig. 71-3). Infiltrates are most commonly bilateral, tend to be located in the mid to upper lung zones, and may mimic loculated pleural fluid. They are frequently nonsegmental, subsegmental, or lobar in distribution. The characteristic "photographic negative of pulmonary edema" appearance (which occurs in <50% of cases) results if extensive infiltrates surround major portions of or the entire lung. Pleural effusions and cavitation are rare.[73,85,86] The infiltrates may be migratory in up to 25% of cases. Occasionally, the chest radiograph can be normal.

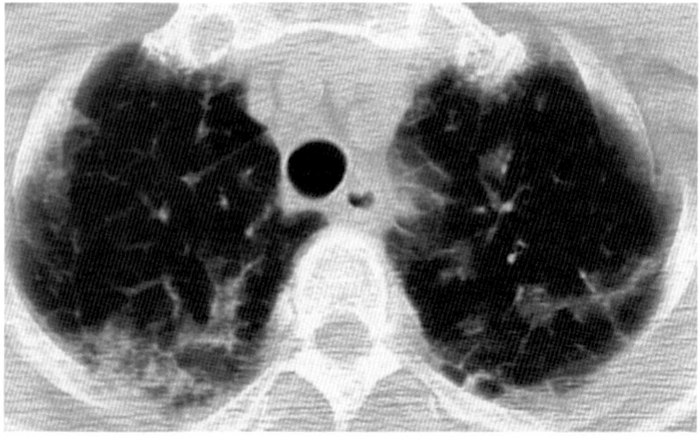

A

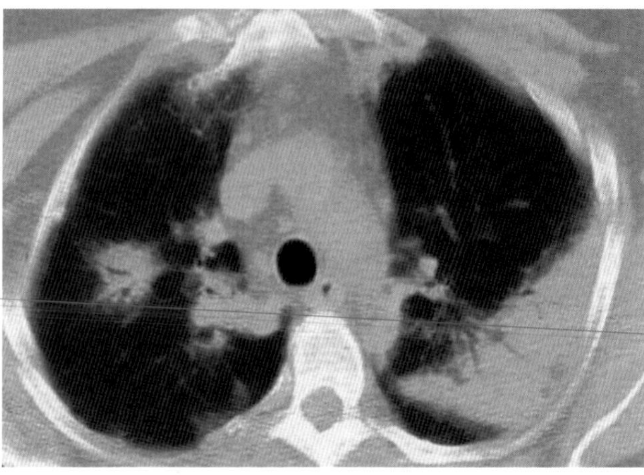

B

Figure 71-3 Radiographic appearance of chronic eosinophilic pneumonia (CEP). Variable computed tomography appearance of infiltrates in two patients with chronic eosinophilic pneumonia. Peripheral upper lobe–predominant infiltrates may have a ground-glass appearance (**A**) or may appear as regions of dense consolidation or nodular opacity (**B**).

Common CT scan findings include ground-glass opacities and areas of consolidation involving the middle and/or upper lung zones in peripheral regions of the lung.[73,87–90] In addition, apparent unilateral or isolated lower lung zone involvement noted on chest radiography may prove to be bilateral and diffuse on CT scanning. Mediastinal adenopathy, which may be evident on conventional chest radiograph, may also be identified on CT scan.[90] Less typical radiographic findings include nodular infiltrates, linear oblique or vertical densities, bronchial wall thickening, pleural effusion, and areas of fibrosis unassociated with anatomic divisions. Findings on CT scan may vary depending on the timing of the CT relative to the onset of symptoms. Typical areas of dense, peripherally located airspace consolidation are found in most cases within the first several weeks of disease onset. Streaky bandlike opacities may appear when symptoms have been present for more than 2 months.

The pulmonary lesions of CEP are characterized histopathologically by varying degrees of leukocytic infiltration of the alveolar airspaces and alveolar septae. These infiltrates are predominantly eosinophilic,[49,72,77] with some associated macrophages, a small-to-moderate number of lymphocytes, occasional plasma cells, multinucleated giant cells, and an associated fibrinous exudate. Unlike AEP, the basal lamina may be disrupted[49] but frank alveolar necrosis is absent. Eosinophilic microabscesses can be found. Focal edema of the capillary endothelium, focal type II epithelial cell hyperplasia, proteinaceous and fibrinous alveolar exudates can also be appreciated. Histologic evidence of proliferative bronchiolitis obliterans or bronchiolitis obliterans–organizing pneumonia may occur in up to one-third of cases, and a mild, nonnecrotizing microangiitis affecting predominantly the small venules may be seen. Biopsy specimens of lymph nodes from patients with intrathoracic lymphadenopathy reveal lymphoid hyperplasia and eosinophil infiltration.

The cause of CEP is unknown. No specific genetic predisposition for the disease has been identified, although CEP has been reported in identical twins, raising the question of a familial tendency toward the disease. An association has been reported between rheumatoid arthritis and CEP[91] but no clear causal relationship has been identified.[92] Although the precise immunopathogenesis of CEP is unknown, evidence suggests that Th2 helper T cells likely have a role in disease pathogenesis. Levels of the cytokines TARC-CCL17 and macrophage-derived cytokine 22 (MDC-22) and macrophage inflammatory protein 1-beta (MIP-1β/CCL14), which help recruit Th2 T cells are increased in CEP.[74,84] Increased levels of the T-cell–derived eosinophil chemoattractant cytokines IL-5, eotaxin, and RANTES (CCL-5) are also elevated in BAL fluid of patients with CEP.[74] Thus Th2 cells likely recruit and attract eosinophils to the lung.[84] The number of regulatory (CD4+CD25+) T-cells is also increased in peripheral blood and BAL in CEP.[93] The potential role of blood and lung tissue lymphocytes in the pathogenesis of CEP requires further study.

Several lines of evidence suggest that eosinophils also play a primary pathogenetic role in the pulmonary tissue damage seen in this disorder. Increased numbers of eosinophils appear in the peripheral blood and bone marrow before the onset of clinical disease, and eosinophilia is the predominant abnormality in BAL fluid. These eosinophils appear to be activated, since they show evidence of degranulation on electron microscopy,[94] eosinophil-derived granule proteins (EDGPs) have been identified microscopically within the pulmonary parenchyma and microvasculature, increased concentrations of EDGP are identified in BAL fluid from patients with CEP compared to controls, and BAL-derived eosinophils express activation markers including class II major histocompatibility (MHC) antigens.[95] Also, eosinophil-derived neurotoxin[82] and leukotriene E4[96] are identified in the urine of patients with CEP, and inducible nitric oxide synthase (iNOS) is expressed on lung eosinophils.[97] The processes that regulate eosinophil activation and degranulation in CEP are not clear. Evidence showing that class II MHC and other activation markers are expressed by BAL- but not blood-derived eosinophils suggests the presence of an immune inflammatory response compartmentalized within the lung. Data also suggest that eosinophils from the BAL fluid are more resistant to apoptosis than peripheral blood eosinophils in subjects with CEP.[98]

Of interest are the findings that immunoglobulins can augment eosinophil chemotaxis and degranulation in vitro, and that circulating immune complexes and elevated titers of IgE are noted in the context of clinical flares of the disease. To date, however, no clear causal relationship has been established between immunoglobulins and eosinophil activation in CEP. An association between CEP and diffuse pulmonary neuroendocrine cell hyperplasia has also been reported.[99]

The diagnosis of CEP is based on the presence of compatible clinical, radiographic, and BAL findings, and on the inability to document pulmonary or systemic infection or other known causes of eosinophilic lung disease. The clinical signs and symptoms of CEP are nonspecific, however, and blood eosinophilia and typical radiographic features may be absent in some cases. In most reported series, open lung biopsy has been required only rarely to establish the diagnosis. Transbronchial biopsy, usually performed to rule out other diagnostic entities, may reveal eosinophil and mononuclear cell infiltrates. Because of the rapid and dramatic responsiveness of CEP to steroid treatment, a therapeutic trial of steroids is often useful in establishing the diagnosis. Failure to document rapid clinical improvement should alert the clinician to consider other diagnoses. The differential diagnosis of CEP includes drug-induced eosinophilic pneumonia, infection (especially TB, fungal diseases such as cryptococcosis and parasitic disease), sarcoidosis, Loeffler syndrome, desquamative interstitial pneumonitis, cryptogenic organizing pneumonia, ABPA, chronic hypersensitivity pneumonitis, acute idiopathic eosinophilic pneumonia, EGPA, and eosinophilic granuloma.

CEP rarely resolves without therapy and if left untreated may result in pulmonary fibrosis.[100] Corticosteroids are the mainstay of therapy for CEP. Dramatic clinical, radiographic, and physiologic improvements have been documented following steroid treatment in all series reported.[1,74,87] Even patients presenting with severe respiratory failure may respond well to steroid treatment. In most cases, treatment with steroids leads to defervescence within 6 hours, reduced dyspnea, cough, and blood eosinophilia within 24 to 48 hours, resolution of hypoxia in 2 to 3 days, radiographic improvement within 1 to 2 weeks, complete resolution of symptoms within 2 to 3 weeks, and normalization of the chest radiograph within 2 months.[1,73,77] No comparative studies exist to determine optimum treatment doses or duration of steroids, but one recommended regimen is prednisone 0.5 mg/kg/d (40–60 mg a day) continued until 2 weeks after resolution of symptoms and radiographic abnormalities, generally for 4 to 6 weeks. The dose of prednisone can then be tapered slowly by 0.25 mg/kg/d and then continued for the subsequent 8 weeks. Treatment is usually maintained for at least 3 months and optimally for 6 to 9 months; during this phase prednisone dosing can be decreased by 5 mg every 4 weeks. Shorter courses of prednisone may also be effective.[74]

The prognosis of CEP is generally favorable.[101] In steroid-treated patients, morbidity and mortality directly related to CEP are low. Patients may require 1 to 3 years of initial steroid treatment to control the disease,[1] and up to 50% may require long-term maintenance treatment (2.5–10 mg prednisone a day) to remain disease-free.[74] The lowest possible dose of steroid that suppresses disease activity should be used. Some patients may respond to high doses (e.g., 1000–1500 μg/24 h) of inhaled corticosteroids, allowing discontinuation of oral steroids, although inhaled steroids alone as initial therapy are inadequate.

Clinical, hematologic, or radiographic evidence of relapses are common, occurring in 50% to 80% of cases when steroids are tapered or discontinued.[1,73,74,77] Relapses may involve radiographic infiltrates in the same or different anatomic distribution compared to the original disease. Relapsing CEP must be distinguished from the development of new or worsening asthma. No obvious factors exist to identify persons who are likely to relapse or require long-term steroids, although relapses are more common in persons treated initially with a short course (<6 months) of steroids. Regular long-term treatment of patients with CEP and asthma with inhaled corticosteroids may reduce the risk of CEP relapses.[76] Multiple recurrences may occur in anyone. Relapses should be managed by increasing the prednisone dose to ≥40 mg per day until 2 weeks after symptom control has been achieved, with gradual taper thereafter. The reinstitution of steroids generally leads to improvement, and relapses do not appear to indicate a worse prognosis, increased likelihood of treatment failure, or increased morbidity. The anti–IL-5 monoclonal antibody omalizumab has also been used successfully as a steroid-sparing agent in the treatment of CEP.[102]

ALLERGIC BRONCHOPULMONARY ASPERGILLOSIS (MYCOSIS)

ABPA is a disorder caused by a complex hypersensitivity response to inhaled fungal antigens.[103–110] Since the disease is most commonly induced by *Aspergillus* species, it is usually known as ABPA. When induced by non-*Aspergillus* species, the syndrome is called allergic bronchopulmonary mycosis. A comprehensive discussion of ABPA is provided in Chapter 48. Highlights of the disorder are discussed here.

ABPA occurs most commonly in immunocompetent patients and complicates 1% to 2% of cases of persistent asthma and 7% to 14% of cases of chronic steroid-dependent asthma,[111] most often among patients in their third to fourth decade. It also complicates up to 15% of patients with cystic fibrosis (CF), most often during the teen years.[105,112] Rare cases lacking a history of asthma but meeting the other major diagnostic criteria (summarized in Table 71-5) have

TABLE 71-5 Diagnostic Criteria for Allergic Bronchopulmonary Aspergillosis

Major[a]
Asthma (ABPA is also common in persons with cystic fibrosis)
Positive immediate hypersensitivity skin-prick test to *Aspergillus*
Precipitating antibodies against *Aspergillus*
Elevated total IgE
Elevated serum *Aspergillus*–specific IgE, IgG
History of pulmonary infiltrates
Peripheral blood eosinophilia
± Central bronchiectasis
Minor
Expectoration of thick brown mucus plugs
Aspergillus in sputum
Dual cutaneous reaction to *Aspergillus*

[a]*The presence of 6 of eight major criteria strongly suggests the diagnosis.*

been reported.[113] The diagnosis of ABPA is based on appropriate clinical features in combination with supporting serologic and radiologic findings.[104]

Patterson and Greenberger[114] proposed five minimal essential criteria needed to establish the diagnosis, including (1) asthma, (2) positive immediate hypersensitivity skin test to *Aspergillus,* (3) total IgE greater than 1000 ng/mL (or >417 IU/mL), (4) elevated serum anti-AF IgE and IgG (more than twofold greater than for asthmatic controls), and (5) serum precipitins to *Aspergillus fumigatus* (AF) or other relevant fungus. These features, as well as a history of current or previous pulmonary infiltrates and/or central bronchiectasis evident on high-resolution CT scan (HRCT) and peripheral blood eosinophils (~10,000 cells/mL), comprise the major diagnostic criteria of ABPA.[103,106,115–118] Expectoration of brown mucus plugs, identification of *Aspergillus* (or other relevant fungus) in the sputum, and dual (immediate and delayed) cutaneous reactions to challenge with *Aspergillus* are also common clinical features of ABPA.

Five clinical stages of ABPA have been recognized: acute illness (stage 1); remission (stage II); exacerbation (stage III); steroid-dependent asthma (stage IV); and fibrotic lung disease (stage V).[104,105,114] The clinical features of these stages are shown in Table 71-6. Two variants of ABPA have been recognized: seropositive ABPA (ABPA-S), wherein the preceding essential criteria are met and there is no evidence of central bronchiectasis; and ABPA with central bronchiectasis (ABPA-CB), wherein the above criteria are met and CB is present.[105,119] It is unclear whether ABPA-S is an earlier stage of disease that precedes ABPA-CB or whether it is perhaps a milder form of the disease.

Typical radiographic manifestations of ABPA include transient, irregular pulmonary infiltrates with a predilection for the upper lobes (Fig. 71-4).[88,120] Other common radiographic features include "finger-in-glove opacities," "tramline shadows," "parallel lines," "toothpaste shadows," "ring shadows," and lobar consolidation (Fig. 71-4). These findings result from bronchial and bronchiolar wall inflammation, edema, and remodeling, and from mucoid impaction of the bronchi with or without parenchymal involvement. As noted, central (proximal) bronchiectasis, another characteristic radiographic manifestation of ABPA, occurs in many, although not all, patients. The presence of high attenuation mucus on HRCT may be a marker for disease severity.[121] ABPA is not typically diagnosed by tissue sampling. Nevertheless, histopathologic findings of ABPA include intense bronchocentric inflammation with eosinophils, lymphocytes, plasma cells, and monocytes, bronchocentric granulomatosis, as well as mucoid impaction of bronchi.[112,116] Fungal hyphae are typically present in mucus plugs without bronchial tissue invasion. The histologic findings may vary in differing parts of the lung and in different stages of the disease.

The features of ABPA are believed to result from a complex immunologic reaction to chronic airway colonization by *Aspergillus* (or other relevant fungal species) that includes features of type I, type III, and type IV immune responses.[104] T-helper lymphocytes, neutrophils, eosinophils, genetic susceptibility factors, and the fungus itself all also likely contribute to the pathogenesis of the disease.[103,122]

Typical symptoms include wheeze, cough, dyspnea, and sputum production, at times with expectoration of brownish/black mucus plugs. Other symptoms may include malaise, myalgias, low-grade fever, chest pain, weight loss, or hemoptysis. Respiratory symptoms may at times be absent despite serologic and radiologic evidence of active disease. The diagnosis of ABPA should be considered in any patient with asthma or CF who experiences frequent and/or recurrent exacerbations of respiratory symptoms, and/or the combination of asthma and eosinophilia. Worsening of lung function and/or steroid dependence or failure to improve clinically following antibiotic therapy for a suspected bacterial infection may also suggest the diagnosis in patients with CF.[112,123] The differential diagnosis of ABPA is broad, and in addition to other pulmonary eosinophilic disorders, includes asthma with fungal sensitization without ABPA, refractory asthma without fungal sensitization, aspergillus bronchitis, and other nonfungal infectious bronchitis or pneumonia. ABPA often goes unrecognized, due to overlap of clinical features with these disorders. ABPA may also be challenging to recognize due to the varying clinical presentations at different stages of disease.

Goals of treatment are to control symptoms, preserve normal lung function, and prevent exacerbations and disease progression. Early recognition and aggressive treatment are essential to prevent development of permanent airway remodeling, bronchiectasis, and pulmonary fibrosis.[105] Systemic corticosteroids, with careful patient monitoring of clinical symptoms, IgE levels, and chest radiograph, are the mainstay of therapy.[124–126] Corticosteroid doses that reduce IgE levels by at least half of acute stage levels within 6 to 8 weeks and induce clearing of radiographic infiltrates must be used to control the disease. These doses are typically higher than those needed to control symptoms alone.

The recommended initial prednisone dose is 0.5 mg/kg/d for 2 weeks followed by every other day dosing for 6 to 12 weeks, followed by a gradual taper of 5 to 10 mg every 2 weeks over 3 to 6 months.[105] Children with CF may require higher doses and/or longer duration of treatment. Total serum IgE levels should be measured at the time of diagnosis, at 4 and 8 weeks, and every 2 months thereafter for 1 year.

TABLE 71-6 Clinical Stages of Allergic Bronchopulmonary Aspergillosis

Stage I: Acute
Acute asthma symptoms ± constitutional symptoms
Elevated serum IgE (typically >1000 ng/mL)
Elevated *Aspergillus*-specific IgE and IgG
Infiltrate on chest radiograph
Peripheral blood eosinophilia
Immediate skin reactivity to *Aspergillus*
Positive precipitating antibodies to *Aspergillus fumigatus*
Stage II: Remission
Resolution of symptoms (concurrent decrease in total IgE needed to confirm remission)
Radiographic clearing
Reduction or stabilization of IgE levels (normalization rare)
Stage III: Exacerbation
Recurrence of elevated IgE levels (greater than twofold over baseline)
± Development of a new pulmonary infiltrate on chest radiograph
± Escalation of asthma symptoms
Stage IV: Steroid-dependent Asthma
Difficult to control, steroid-dependent asthma
Persistently elevated total IgE, *Aspergillus* precipitins and *Aspergillus*-specific IgE and IgG despite corticosteroid therapy
± Transient infiltrates and/or bronchiectasis on chest radiograph or CT
Stage V: Fibrotic lung disease
Persistent steroid-dependent asthma
Fibrotic lung disease with gas exchange disturbances
Chronic sputum production and frequent infections common

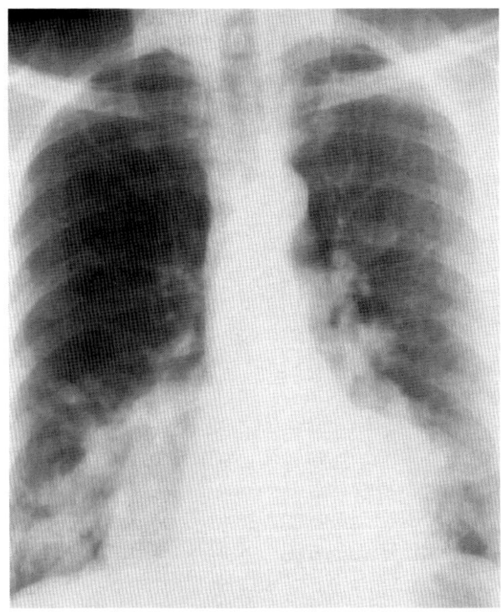

A

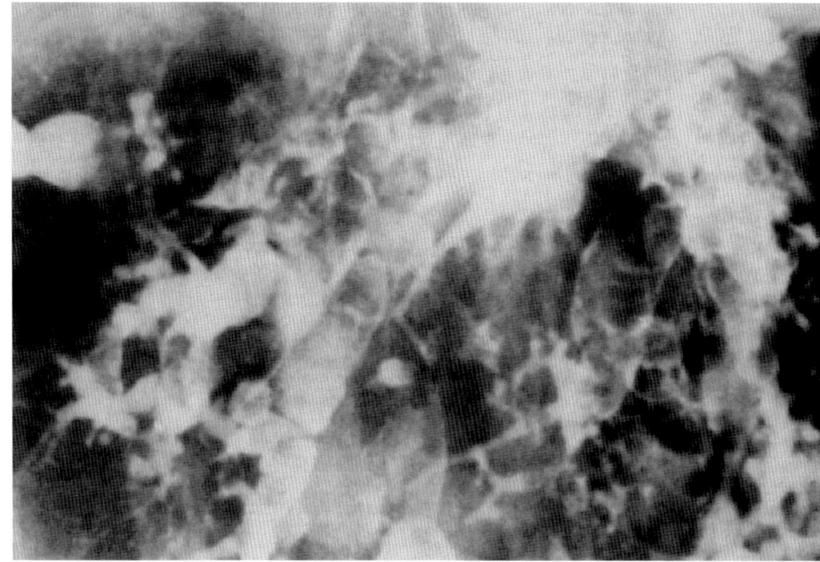

B

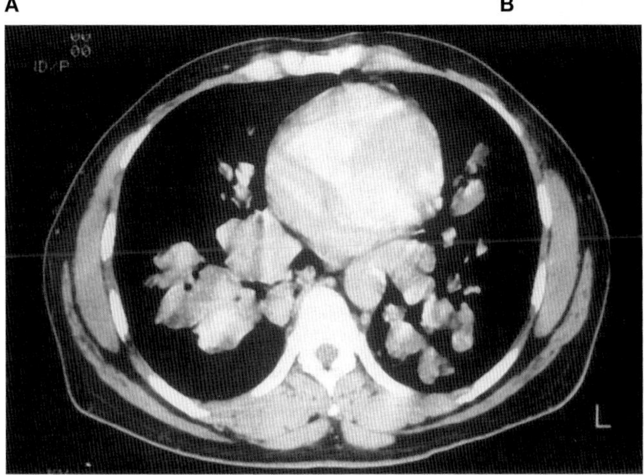

C

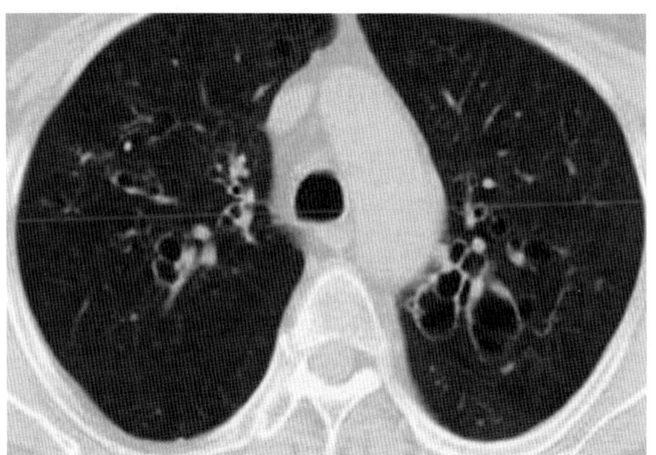

D

Figure 71-4 Radiographic appearance of allergic bronchopulmonary aspergillosis (ABPA). Extensive infiltrates with tubular configuration and "gloved finger" appearance are present, in this case predominantly in the lower lobes (**A**), the bronchogram (**B**), and computed tomography (CT) of the chest (**C**) reveal extensive proximal bronchiectasis. Extensive mucoid impaction of the bronchi is evident on CT scan (**C**). Central bronchiectasis and tram-track shadows in a patient with ABPA may also be present without mucoid impaction (**D**).

Treatment with the antifungal agent itraconazole can also help control the symptoms and immunologic features and exacerbations of the disease[127–129] and may enable reduction of the systemic corticosteroid dose.[130,131] Voriconazole may be a suitable alernate antifungal agent.[132,133] In case series, the anti-IgE antibody omalizumab has helped to control the disease in steroid-dependent patients with ABPA who have failed itraconazole treatment.[134–137] Bronchodilators and antibiotics help control bronchospasm and secondary respiratory infections. Inhaled corticosteroids alone are inadequate to prevent or treat acute episodes of ABPA. Yearly spirometry should be performed and patients should be monitored for concurrent gastroesophageal reflux, rhinosinusitis, or environmental mold exposures.[105]

CHURG–STRAUSS SYNDROME (EOSINOPHILIC GRANULOMATOSIS WITH POLYANGIITIS)

In 1939, Rackemann and Greene reported a subgroup of patients with polyarteritis nodosa and concomitant allergic disease. Similar findings were reported in the early 1940s by Harkavy. The histopathology and clinical features associated with this disease entity were first described in 1951 by Churg and Strauss, who reported a form of necrotizing vasculitis in several organs, associated with eosinophilic tissue inflammation and extravascular granulomas, occurring in asthmatics, with associated fever and peripheral hypereosinophilia (Churg–Strauss syndrome).[138] This disease entity, now termed eosinophilic granulomatosis with polyangiitis (EGPA), is an uncommon systemic disease.[139–141] An overall prevalence of 10.7 to 13 cases per million inhabitants is estimated among the general population,[142] and up to 64 cases per million persons per year is estimated among patients with a history of asthma. The mean annual incidence has been estimated at 0.5 to 6.8 per million population across various countries.[142]

Approximately 10% of all patients with vasculitis prove ultimately to have EGPA (see also Chapter 74). Nevertheless, the precise incidence of EGPA is unknown due to uncertainties regarding diagnosis and variable clinical presentation. The true incidence of EGPA may be higher than is generally recognized, since the syndrome has many clinical, radiographic, and histologic features in common with other vasculitic, eosinophilic, and granulomatous disease states. The diagnosis of EGPA may be missed if not carefully entertained.

EGPA may occur in patients of any age, but it develops most commonly in patients between the ages of 38 and 50.[1,143,144] It is rare in persons older than age 65, as well as children and adolescents. However, among affected children, it tends to follow a more aggressive clinical course.[145] There is no clear gender predominance.[142,144] Among women, disease onset has been reported during pregnancy. The MHC complex DRB4 allele may confer genetic risk for the disease.[146,147]

EGPA tends to follow a subacute course, with symptoms ranging over months to years. Historically, three distinct clinical phases of the disease have been recognized: the prodromal phase, the eosinophilic phase, and the vasculitic phase.[148,149] The *prodromal phase* has been characterized by "late-onset" (in the second or third decade) allergic rhinitis and atopy in persons often lacking a family history of atopy. Severe allergic rhinitis, sinusitis, and drug sensitivity are usually present for 8 to 10 years, and up to 30 years before EGPA disease recognition. Asthma is a feature of EGPA in all cases. It typically precedes the onset of vasculitis by 3 to 6 years.[148] The *eosinophilic phase* is typified by the development of marked peripheral blood eosinophilia and eosinophilic tissue infiltration, most commonly of the lung, GI tract, and skin. The *vasculitic phase* is characterized by vasculitis of the small and medium vessels with vascular and extravascular granulomas. The onset of the vasculitic phase is often heralded by development of constitutional symptoms, including fever, malaise, weight loss, arthralgias, myalgias, and increased allergic or asthmatic symptoms. Although the vasculitis tends to occur several years after the onset of allergic manifestations of the disease, in some cases it develops within months of, or concomitant with, the onset of asthma. A short duration between the onset of asthma and vasculitis has been associated with increased severity of vasculitis. During the vasculitic stage, the asthma symptoms may persist and worsen, or they may diminish. When asthma dissipates, it often flares later in the course of illness and may require prolonged steroid treatment. Importantly, not all patients progress sequentially through these phases, and overlap of clinical features between phases is often present. Although EGPA typically affects multiple organ systems, limited forms of disease have also been described.[142,150] Manifestations in the lungs, heart, skin, and nervous system are most common.

Lung involvement occurs in nearly all patients with EGPA.[142] Most of the respiratory manifestations of EGPA occur in the prodromal and eosinophilic phases of the disease. As noted earlier, all patients have asthma at some point in the illness. Upper airway allergic disease, including sinusitis, rhinitis, and polyposis, is seen in 75% to 85% of patients and may be the presenting symptom.[1,142] Unlike granulomatosis with polyangiitis, necrotizing granulomas involving the upper airway are unusual in EGPA. The asthma and upper airway disease usually are long-standing, severe, and often require steroid therapy (systemic or inhaled) to maintain control of symptoms.[142] Spirometry may reveal an obstructive ventilatory defect.[151] A Loeffler-like syndrome with eosinophilic infiltration of the lung parenchyma is seen in 50% to 70% of patients. These patients may develop dyspnea, cough, and wheezing. Their chest radiographs have transient, migratory, patchy, nonlobar, nonsegmental, often peripheral pulmonary infiltrates, with no regional predilection.[152–154] Nodular lesions, reticular opacities, bronchial wall thickening, bronchiectasis, and hilar adenopathy are less common findings. In contrast to granulomatosis with polyangiitis, the allergic granulomas cavitate more rarely. Up to 50% of patients develop unilateral or bilateral pleural effusions,[154] which may be associated with pleuritic chest pain. The chest radiograph may occasionally be normal. HRCT scanning has demonstrated bronchial wall thickening, pulmonary artery enlargement (in comparison to the corresponding bronchi), irregular stellate configuration of some vessels, adenopathy, areas of interlobular septal thickening, and scattered patchy parenchymal opacities with ground-glass, nodular, consolidated, or tree-in bud appearance.[1] Nodules may be present within areas of ground glass.[90,154,155] These findings have been reported to correlate with pathologic findings evident on open lung biopsy such as eosinophilic pneumonia, alveolar hemorrhage, eosinophilic infiltration of the bronchial wall, and septum.[153] Further studies are necessary to determine whether high-resolution CT is useful to stage the disease or establish the diagnosis without tissue biopsy.

Cardiac manifestations generally are not evident on initial presentation of EGPA. However, they typically occur during the vasculitic phase of the disease and are a major source of morbidity and the principal cause of death (in up to 50% of cases) from the disorder.[142,143,156] Patients may be asymptomatic. Progressive congestive heart failure (CHF) occurs in up to 47% of cases because of endomyocardial infiltration by eosinophils[1,157] or ischemic cardiomyopathy resulting from necrotizing vasculitis of the coronary arteries.[158] This coronary vasculitis is fatal up to 60% of the time. Acute pericarditis is present in approximately one-third of cases, and cardiac tamponade has been reported. Constrictive pericarditis may develop over time. Cardiac involvement is more common in persons with EGPA who lack serum ANCA (see below).[159,160]

A wide array of neurologic manifestations may develop in EGPA. Mono- or polyneuropathy (most notably mononeuritis multiplex) is present in 69% to 75% of cases. The common peroneal, ulnar, and internal popliteal nerves are most frequently affected.[142] CNS manifestations occur more rarely and include cranial nerve impairment (especially optic neuritis), seizure, subarachnoid hemorrhage, and cerebral infarction. Skin, GI, renal, and other systemic alterations have been well described in EGPA. Skin findings are present in 40% to 70% of cases and may develop in localized crops. They can manifest as nonthrombocytopenic purpura (particularly on the lower extremities), urticaria, a maculopapular rash, petechiae, ecchymoses, or livedo reticularis. Skin biopsies typically demonstrate eosinophilic infiltration and leukocytoclastic vasculitis.[161] Tender cutaneous or subcutaneous nodules (which may ulcerate) containing extravascular granulomas may preferentially involve the fingers, scalp, and extensor surface of the elbow.[142] GI manifestations of EGPA are present in up to 60% of cases. They can include eosinophilic gastroenteritis or vasculitis that can lead to diarrhea, abdominal pain, intestinal obstruction, cholecystitis, pancreatitis, bleeding, liver function test abnormalities, and bowel perforation.[142] GI disease also carries a poor prognosis[142] and is the second leading cause of death in patients with EGPA. A degree of renal insufficiency occurs in 25% to 50% of patients with EGPA. Eosinophilic interstitial nephritis with necrotizing features is the most common histopathologic finding, but focal segmental glomerulosclerosis, hematuria, and proteinuria also occur.[143,162,163] Severe, difficult-to-control hypertension is also a major sequela of EGPA (in 25%–75% of cases) and may be due to recurrent renal infarction. In contrast to granulomatosis with polyangiitis, overt renal failure is not commonly seen in EGPA.[143] Mild lymphadenopathy (in 30%–40%), rheumatologic manifestations (migratory polyarthralgias, myalgias, temporal arteritis), urologic disease (ureteral, urethral, prostatic), and ocular manifestations (scleritis, uveitis, optic neuropathy, conjunctival nodules)[142] have also been described.

The diagnosis of EGPA is based on clinical features with corroborating laboratory and/or histologic findings. There is no single laboratory test specific for a diagnosis of EGPA. A majority of patients with EGPA have a striking but fluctuating degree of peripheral blood eosinophilia (mean values between 5 and 20,000/mm^3; 20% to 90% of the WBC differential) at diagnosis,[1,142] generally greater than that seen with asthma alone. The degree of eosinophilia tends to parallel the vasculitis activity[1] and may be suppressed by corticosteroid treatment of asthma. Serum C-reactive protein levels and total IgE levels are elevated (range, 500–1000 U/mL) in 75% of patients. Elevated exhaled breath condensate and BAL fluid concentrations of the eicosanoid 12-HETE can help distinguish EGPA from asthma without EGPA.[164] Elevated blood levels of the Th2 T lymphocyte cytokines IL-4, IL-5, and IL-13[165] as well as serum IgG4,[166] TARC/CCL17,[167] urinary eosinophil-derived neurotoxin,[168] and serum eotaxin-3 levels[169,170] also correlate with disease activity. BAL fluid of patients with active EGPA also contains increased levels of the Th2 cytokines IL-4, IL-5, and IL-10 as compared with inactive EGPA.[171,172] Most patients have a normochromic, normocytic anemia, and moderate elevation of their ESR. Rheumatoid factor titers may be positive, but antinuclear antibodies are usually negative.[142] Hypergammaglobulinemia and circulating immune complexes may also be seen.

Approximately 40% to 60% of patients have positive antinuclear cytoplasmic antibody with a perinuclear staining pattern (pANCA).[159,160,173] The majority of these are directed against myeloperoxidase (MPO-ANCA) and a minority against proteinase 3 (PR3-ANCA). The absence of ANCA does not exclude the diagnosis. Indeed, recent case series suggest that persons positive for ANCA have different clinical features than those without.[174] Persons with positive ANCA (the "vasculitic phenotype") tend to manifest evidence of biopsy-proven vasculitis, purpura, ENT manifestations, peripheral neuropathy, and renal disease but have less cardiac involvement.[159,160,175] In contrast, those without ANCA (the "eosinophilic tissue infiltration phenotype") manifest predominantly with fever, eosinophilic pneumonia, and eosinophilic myocarditis.[159,160,176]

Laboratory examination of pleural fluid, if present, reveals an eosinophil-predominant exudate with low glucose levels.[142] Pleural biopsy shows chronic pleuritis with eosinophilic infiltration. BAL reveals an increased percentage of eosinophils,[177] the magnitude of which is generally less than that seen with CEP or idiopathic HES. However, patients have been described whose BAL fluid leukocyte differential contained 81% eosinophils. Electrocardiogram, echocardiography, N-terminal pro-brain natriuretic peptide and tropinin-1 levels, and/or cardiac MRI are recommended to evaluate patients with suspected EGPA for the presence of cardiac involvement.[142,178,179] ^{18}FDG/^{13}N ammonia positron emission tomography (PET) imaging may also be useful to identify cardiac involvement in EGPA. Magnetic resonance imaging may show T2-weighted signals in subcortical matter suggestive of CNS vasculitis.[142]

Although lung biopsy is rarely required for diagnosis, the histopathologic hallmarks of EGPA vary depending on the stage of illness but include tissue (interstitial, blood vessel, and alveolar) infiltration by eosinophils, eosinophilic necrotizing giant cell vasculitis of small arteries, arterioles, and, to a lesser extent, small veins, venules, and capillaries and perivascular and interstitial eosinophilic granulomas (typically microscopic).[180–182] Both pulmonary and systemic vessels may be affected. The precise histopathology of vascular impairment depends on the stage of the lesion. Early lesions demonstrate eosinophilic infiltration of the vessels and perivascular region (Fig. 71-5). Later lesions are characterized by necrotizing arteritis or vessel obliteration and scarring. The extent of vascular impairment varies from mild, eosinophilic perivascular cuffing to severe transmural inflammation with necrotization. Lesions may be sparse or widespread. In the lung the allergic granulomas may have central necrosis with eosinophilic infammation, may involve interlobular septae and extend along the pleura. Diffuse capillaritis and alveolar hemmorhage has been reported. Eosinophilic lymphadenopathy may also be present. Biopsies of skin, nerve, or muscle may also confirm the diagnosis.[156]

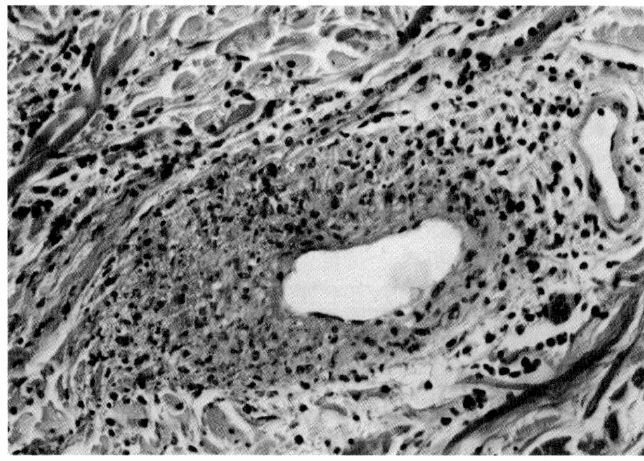

Figure 71-5 Pathologic appearance of small arteriole in Churg–Strauss vasculitis. Intense perivascular inflammation with eosinophilia is present.

The pathogenesis of EGPA remains poorly understood. A possible pathogenic role of antineutrophil cytoplasmic antibody (ANCA) is suggested by the finding of ANCA in 40% to 60% of patients with EGPA.[144] ANCA may contribute to tissue inflammation and injury by activation of inflammatory cells, release of proteolytic enzymes, and generation of oxidative stress[142] but its presence may be a consequence rather than a cause of the tissue injury. As noted previously, the clinical features of EGPA differ between persons with versus without ANCA.[159,160] The strong association with allergy, atopy, eosinophilia, and elevated blood levels of Th2 T lymphocyte-derived cytokines and IgE (especially during the vasculitic phase of the disease) has raised the likelihood of augmented Th2 immunity.[142,172,183–185]

Reductions in T regulatory cells[183,186] and augmented Th1 immunity[187] have also been demonstrated. Eosinophils likely also contribute significantly to the tissue injury[188] since blood, BAL, and urine specimens contain eosinophil-derived cytotoxic granule proteins.[142] Based on these collective findings, it has been proposed that repeated antigenic stimulation in patients with a heightened T-cell and eosinophil response may be important in the development of the disorder. Heightened humoral immunity with immune complex disease may also play a role. Genetic factors including polymorphisms in the IL-10 gene[189] and HLA-DRB107 and HLA-DRB4[146] may be important in predilection to develop EGPA.

The relationship between the pathophysiology of asthma in EGPA to that of asthma without EGPA also remains uncertain. CEP with asthma may precede EGPA in up to 50% of cases. A decrease in the number of blood regulatory T cells (Treg) occurs in persons who develop EGPA following CEP, but not in those with CEP who do not later develop EGPA or in persons with asthma without EGPA.[186,190] This suggests that maintenance of normal numbers of Treg cells may protect against the development of EGPA. Also, a strong association has been noted between the use of leukotriene receptor antagonists (LTRA) and 5-lipoxygenase inhibitors,[172,191–194] as well as other asthma therapies including inhaled glucocorticoids[195,196] and omalizumab[197] and the development of EGPA. These findings raise question as to whether these agents may serve as triggers for the disease. The appearance of EGPA following reduction in systemic corticosteroid dosing in many of these reports raises the likelihood that pre-existing, underlying EGPA that was being treated with corticosteroids is unmasked by the administration of these agents and the reduction in corticosteroid dose. Thus, it remains uncertain whether any of these agents may be causally related to the onset of EGPA. Patients with steroid-dependent asthma, in whom the diagnosis of EGPA has not been demonstrated or entertained, should be monitored closely for evidence of EGPA when steroid doses are tapered, or when symptoms escalate despite systemic corticosteroid treatment and require intensification of medical therapy. EGPA has also been reported following inhalational use of cocaine,[198] following exposure to other medications, birds, vaccinations, and various infectious pathogens.[13,142]

The diagnosis of EGPA is generally based on clinical features. Various diagnostic criteria have been reported.[148,182] In 1990, the American College of Rheumatology published diagnostic criteria for EGPA,[182] based on assessments of the sensitivity and specificity of the diagnostic criteria used previously. The presence of at least four out of six of the following criteria yielded 85% sensitivity and 99.7% specificity in establishing the diagnosis: (1) asthma, (2) peripheral eosinophilia greater than 10%, (3) mono- or polyarthropathy, (4) migratory or transient pulmonary infiltrates, (5) paranasal sinus abnormality, and (6) extravascular eosinophils in a blood vessel on a biopsy specimen. The presence of asthma or allergy as well as more than 10% eosinophilia was 95% sensitive and 99% specific in distinguishing EGPA among a subgroup of patients with well-documented systemic vasculitis. Subsequently, the Chapel Hill Consensus Conference recommended that diagnostic criteria for EGPA include[1] appropriate clinical setting and histopathology and[2] eosinophil-rich and granulomatous inflammation involving the respiratory tract and necrotizing vasculitis affecting small and medium vessels with associated asthma and eosinophilia.[199] However, these criteria require tissue biopsy and are less sensitive for EGPA than others that have been proposed; hence, they may be less useful to assist diagnosis in the routine clinical setting. Open lung biopsy is the gold standard for tissue biopsy but is rarely necessary. Transbronchial biopsy may reveal the diagnosis if there is alveolar involvement, but is often nondiagnostic. Biopsy of other sites (e.g., skin, pericardium, muscle, nerve, gut), with or without immunostaining, may assist in establishing the diagnosis in selected cases, although demonstration of characteristic histopathologic changes are not essential for establishing the diagnosis. The diagnosis may be elusive since EGPA may be suppressed by corticosteroid treatment for asthma.

The differential diagnosis of EGPA includes polyarteritis nodosa, microscopic angiitis, granulomatosis with polyangiitis, CEP, ABPA, idiopathic HES, Loeffler syndrome, asthma, fungal or parasitic infection, drug-induced vasculitis, sarcoidosis, and Hodgkin lymphoma. EGPA can be distinguished from granulomatosis with polyangiitis since compared with the latter, patients with EGPA have nasal polyps and allergic rhinitis but lack significant necrotizing upper airway lesions and cavitation of lung nodules, and are more likely to have pANCA (in contrast to the c-ANCA seen in granulomatosis with polyangiitis). Also, patients with EGPA are less likely to develop renal failure, and vasculitic neuropathy and asthma/eosinophilia are not typical features of granulomatosis with polyangiitis. EGPA can be distinguished from MPO-ANCA–positive microscopic angiitis since patients with the latter syndrome have leukocytoclastic vasculitis without granulomas and do not have upper airway involvement, asthma, and eosinophilia. Further, unlike EGPA, cardiac involvement is rare in MPO-ANCA–positive vasculitis. EGPA may be difficult to distinguish from idiopathic HES among persons who lack ANCA and/or neuropathy without overt vasculitis.[200] EGPA is more likely among those with lower eosinophil counts who later develop vasculitis.

Patients in whom EGPA goes untreated have a poor prognosis; up to 50% die within 3 months after the onset of vasculitis. As such, efforts at early recognition and treatment are important.

Two randomized controlled trials of therapy for EGPA have been conducted recently.[201,202] The choice of treatment depends in part on the clinical features at the time of diagnosis, since the presence of some features portends a worse prognosis and requires a more aggressive treatment approach.[201–203] Poor prognostic features include age >65 years, cardiac, GI, CNS, and renal involvement (with serum creatinine >150 μmol/L) and absence of ENT involvement.[175,203] In persons *without* poor prognostic features, corticosteroids are the mainstay of treatment and generally lead to dramatic clinical improvement, with disease stabilization or cure. Prednisone, 1 to 1.5 mg/kg/d (or 60 mg per day in adults) is given for 3 to 12 weeks, aiming to eliminate constitutional symptoms and cardiac, renal, neurologic, or other vasculitic manifestations. Higher doses (e.g., 15 mg/kg/d methylprednisolone) are occasionally required for control of life-threatening symptoms. Severe hypertension and mononeuritis multiplex often require prolonged steroid treatment and may be difficult to eliminate. Once the vasculitic phase is controlled, steroids may be tapered, with doses titrated to maintain disease control. Low-dose prednisone (e.g., 5–10 mg) is often given every day or every other day for up to 1 year. Although relapses are uncommon, patients should be followed closely for evidence of clinical deterioration, and should have periodic screening of total WBC and differential, ESR, and IgE levels. Most reports suggest the pANCA is not useful to monitor disease activity or direct therapeutic intervention, but one recent case series demonstrated that ANCA-positive persons had more frequent relapses and lower 5-year relapse-free survival rates than ANCA-negative persons.[175] Treatment with cytotoxic immunosuppressive agents, such as cyclophosphamide or azathioprine, should be administered in patients whose condition fails to improve or have relapses despite steroid treatment.

Persons who have poor prognostic features at the time of disease presentation,[142,204] or who have severe systemic involvement should receive high-dose intravenous methylprednisolone or oral prednisone for 3 days plus induction therapy with cyclophosphamide (2 mg/kg/d orally or 0.6–0.7 g/m^2 intravenously day 1, 15, and 30 and then every 3 to 4 weeks theareafter).[205] Patients treated with cyclophosphamide should be monitored closely for hemorrhagic cystitis, renal insufficiency, bone marrow suppression, bladder fibrosis, and urologic malignancies. Patients with severe disease treated with corticosteroids and cyclophosphamide have better survival than those treated with corticosteroids alone. Azathioprine maintenance therapy (2 mg/kg/d) for 18 to 24 months may be beneficial once remission of disease has been achieved.[142,143,202]

Intravenous immunoglobulin (IvIg) may be beneficial for use in pregnant women and for reducing symptoms and organ involvement and improving long-term disease control among persons with severe organ involvement. The number of blood Treg cells was increased among persons with EGPA treated with IV Ig and conventional therapy.[206] The anti-IL5 antibody mepolizumab has also demonstrated efficacy as a steroid-sparing agent in small uncontrolled case series.[207,208] The immunoregulatory cytokine interferon-α (IFN-α) has led to improved pulmonary function tests, reduction in corticosteroid dose, and decreased WBC count and may be considered as another alternative treatment in persons with refractory disease[209] but may be of limited efficacy and can cause cardiac toxicity. Plasma exchange may also be a successful adjunct treatment in some patients,[142,210] particularly those with ANCA positivity and glomerulonephritis. Finally, rituximab may be effective as an alternate therapeutic agent but further studies are needed to clarify benefits of treatment in EGPA as compared with other forms of ANCA-positive vasculitis.[211] β-Blockers should be avoided in the management of EGPA-related hypertension, owing to the risk of bronchospasm and CHF. Persons undergoing immunosuppressive treatment for EGPA should receive prophylactic treatment to prevent infection with pneumocystis jirovecii.

Prolonged treatment may be necessary to maintain disease control. Long-term overall remission can be achieved in approximately 81% to 92% of patients[142,156]; relapses occur in 25% of cases and are most common within 1 year.[142] In a series of 30 patients collected over the period 1950 to 1974, a median survival of more than 9 years was reported in patients treated with steroids; 1-year survival was 90%, 3-year survival was 76%, and 62% survival was noted at 5 years. More recent studies suggest 85% to 100% survival at 5 years.[1,175,205]

IDIOPATHIC HYPEREOSINOPHILIC SYNDROME

Idiopathic HES is a rare disorder first described in 1968 by Hardy and Anderson. Over the ensuing years, many case reports of severe peripheral eosinophilia and diffuse organ infiltration with eosinophils were described. Several names – including *eosinophilic leukemia, Loeffler fibroplastic endocarditis,* and *disseminated eosinophilic cardiovascular disease* – were used to describe this disease entity. In 1975, Chusid et al. [212] revised the definition of HES to include only cases in which no other underlying cause of hypereosinophilia could be found. HES is now recognized as a clinically heterogeneous syndrome with a wide range of disease severity. Whereas some patients experience a mild, limited form of the disease with minimal involvement of noncritical organs (e.g., skin), others have life-threatening multiorgan dysfunction. Emerging evidence suggests that HES may indeed represent several diseases of distinct etiology that share several features in common.[213–215]

Current consensus defines hypereosinophilia as blood eosinophils $>1.5 \times 10^9$/L on two examinations separated by ≥1 month and/or tissue eosinophilia (defined as >20% of cells in a bone marrow specimen, tissue infiltration defined by a pathologist, and/or marked deposition of EDGP in tissue).[216] The term HES is defined as the presence of hypereosinophilia together with eosinophilic tissue infiltration and organ damage (in the absence of other identifiable cause). HES is a rare disorder. Although persons of any age may be affected, disease onset is most common between 20 and 50 years of age.[217,218] When it occurs in children it often heralds a clonal hematologic disturbance.[218] There is no known racial or ethnic predisposition. Familial cases with autosomal dominant transmission have been reported.

Clinical features and symptoms vary according to the organ system(s) affected. Presenting complaints are often nonspecific and include weakness, fatigue, low-grade fevers, myalgias, cough, angioedema, rash, retinal lesions, and dyspnea. Involvement of virtually every organ system has been described.

Several distinct clinical variants of HES have been recognized.[216,219] Three of the most common are:

1. The myeloproliferative variant (primary/neoplastic HES): In this variant there is clonal expansion of eosinophils related to stem cell, myeloid, or eosinophil neoplasms. Clinical features inlcude anemia, thrombocytopenia, hepatosplenomegaly, elevated leukocyte alkaline phosphatase, circulating immature leukocytes, and elevated B_{12} levels.[220] The most common chromosomal abnormality noted is deletion on 4q12, leading to fusion of genes for and constitutive activation of the tyrosine kinase fusion protein FIP1L1-PDGFRA.[221] Other chromosomal abnormalities have also been reported.
2. The lymphocytic variant (secondary, reactive HES, ~30% of cases): This variant is related to clonal expansion of Th2 T cells with an abnormal surface antigen phenotype (CD3–/CD4+) and increased production of IL-5.[222,223] Increased amounts of IL-4, IL-13, GMCSF, and hypergammaglobulinemia may be present.[224] Skin and soft tissue involvement are the predominant clinical features of this variant.
3. The idiopathic variant (~50% of cases): The disturbances present in the previously noted variants are lacking, but end-organ damage is present.[215]

The respiratory system is affected in an estimated 63% of patients with HES.[225] The most common symptoms include a predominantly nocturnal cough, which is either nonproductive or productive of small quantities of nonpurulent sputum, wheezing, and dyspnea (without evidence of airflow obstruction on spirometric examination). In general, respiratory manifestations are mild.[225] Pulmonary hypertension, ARDS, and pleural effusions (which may be due to CHF) have been reported but are rare. In patients with pulmonary manifestations, the chest radiograph or CT may reveal transient focal consolidation, ground glass opacities or diffuse pulmonary infiltrates (with no predilection for any particular distribution), small nodules, pleural effusion(s), adenopathy, or pulmonary emboli.[212,225] Histopathologic examination of affected lung specimens most commonly reveals intense interstitial infiltration with eosinophils. Less commonly, necrotic areas of parenchyma are found. These are believed to be due to pulmonary microemboli. In contrast to EGPA, significant vasculitis is not present.

Cardiac disease is the major cause of morbidity and mortality in patients with HES.[217,226] The most common cardiac manifestations are relentlessly progressive CHF due to eosinophilic myocarditis and endocarditis, intracardiac thrombi, and endocardial fibrosis.[217] Cardiac involvement in HES, which may be clinically silent, is believed to progress from an initial acute necrosis stage, followed by endocardial thrombus formation and eventually development of fibrosis, which may lead to restrictive cardiomyopathy or valvular dysfunction such as mitral regurgitation.[217] Intracardiac thrombus formation can lead to ischemic embolic events. Bacterial endocarditis has also been noted. The cardiac damage is believed to be mediated at least in part by EDGP . Elevation in serum troponin level can provide a clue to the presence of cardiac involvement in HES.[227] Disturbingly, cardiac involvement correlates poorly with the peripheral blood eosinophilia, hence echocardiographic follow-up at 6-month intervals is recommended. Cardiac MRI also detects eosinophil-mediated cardiac injury[228] or intracardiac thrombus.

Involvement of the central or peripheral nervous system, which occurs in up to 60% of patients, is also a major cause of morbidity.[229] Neurologic manifestations of HES include encephalopathy with neuropsychiatric dysfunction, memory loss, gait disturbances with or without signs of upper motor neuron injury, visual changes, and sequelae of thromboembolic events, including hemiparesis. Peripheral neuropathy with sensory and/or motor axonal loss (no vasculitic or eosinophilic infiltration) is extremely common in HES.

The bone marrow is universally affected with a striking eosinophilia (up to 25%–75% of the differential). Other hematologic manifestations are venous and arterial thromboembolism,[230] anemia, thrombocytopenia, elevated vitamin B_{12} levels, hepatosplenomegaly, and lymphadenopathy (in 12%–20%).

Cutaneous manifestations may include eczema, uritcaria, angioedema, nodular or papular lesions, skin thickening, erythroderma or dermatographia.[217,231] Mucosal ulcerations may develop. As noted, cutaneous manifestations are more likely seen among persons with the lymphocyte HES variant.[223] Urticaria or angioedema generally portend a benign prognosis. Persons with papules are likely to have the FIP1L1-PDGFRA variant.[232] GI (20–30% of patients), renal (10–20%), musculoskeletal, ocular, and endocrine manifestations are all also well described.

Laboratory findings associated with HES include peripheral blood eosinophilia >1.5 × 10^9/L,[212] an elevated total serum IgE (25%–38%), hypergammaglobulinemia, circulating immune complexes (32%–50%), and an ESR above 15 mm/h (68%). Anemia is likely in patients with the myeloproliferative variant.[233] Elevated serum B_{12} and leukocyte alkaline phosphatase levels are also noted. Fungal and parasitic serologies, as well as aspirates of body fluids for ova and parasites, are negative. Of interest is that whereas blood and BAL eosinophilia are both prominent in persons with pulmonary involvement, blood eosinophilia is present and BAL eosinophilia is absent in persons lacking pulmonary manifestations of the disease. This finding has raised the question whether BAL eosinophilia may serve as a marker for the development of pulmonary disease associated with HES.

The organ damage in HES is believed to be due to both eosinophilic infiltration of tissues[234,235] and tissue injury caused by thromboembolic events. Eosinophils probably contribute to tissue damage via antibody-mediated cytotoxicity and the release of toxic granule products such as major basic protein and eosinophil cationic protein. Elevated serum levels of eosinophil cationic protein and major basic protein have been reported, but they do not correlate universally with clinical disease severity. The precise events inciting the extreme eosinophilia in HES are unknown, but several mechanisms have been proposed, including overproduction or abnormal activity of cytokines leading to eosinophilia, and defects in cytokine signaling or signal transduction.

The diagnosis of HES is established by demonstrating multiorgan dysfunction, severe peripheral blood eosinophilia (>1.5 × 10^9/L) on two separate occasions in the absence of any other known causes of peripheral blood eosinophilia. Occasionally, the disease presents with the incidental finding of blood eosinophilia before development of other complications. The total peripheral leukocyte count is typically elevated to above 10,000 (typical range, 10,000 to 30,000), with a preponderance of eosinophils (up to 70%). The leukocytosis may be progressive. Eosinophilic blast transformation was reported to occur at some time during the course of the disease in 28% of 51 patients in one series. Tests recommended to assess for end-organ damage also include serum chemistries, liver function tests, CPK, troponin, EKG, echocardiogram, chest x-ray and/or CT, pulmonary function tests, abdominal CT scan, and tissue biopsy as indicated. Serum tryptase, vitamin B_{12} and Ig levels may also support the diagnosis.[236] In addition, patients with suspected HES should undergo bone marrow aspirate and biopsy, FIP1L1/PDGFRA mutation analysis, and T lymphocyte phenotyping by flow cytometry or karyotype analysis to evaluate for the HES subtypes noted earlier. Proper diagnosis of the HES subtypes has implications for choosing therapy for the disease.

The differential diagnosis of HES includes parasitic infection, acute eosinophilic leukemia, drug-induced hypersensitivity, EGPA, episodic angioedema with eosinophilia, tuberculous or fungal infection, allergic or autoimmune disease, other acute or CEPs, TPE, other lymphoproliferative disorders, and paraneoplastic syndromes. Patients with eosinophilic leukemia have immature eosinophils or blasts in the bone marrow and/or blood, whereas patients with HES typically do not. Patients with HES do not have asthma or vasculitis characteristically associated with EGPA, and patients with episodic angioedema typically lack the multiorgan involvement associated with HES.

Before the discovery of an effective therapy, the prognosis of HES was poor. In one early series, 81% of 48 patients died within 1 year of diagnosis. Overall, without therapy, average survival was 9 months, and 3- to 4-year survival was estimated at 10% to 12%.[212] The greatest mortality occurs within the first year after diagnosis. Death may occur from refractory CHF, azotemia, hepatic failure, venous thromboembolism, a perforated abdominal viscus, or infection. Persons with the myeloproliferative variant of HES (especially those with FIP1L1/PDGFRA positive disease) tend to have an aggressive course with high mortality without treatment. The advent of effective therapy for HES has led to a marked improvement in median survival to more than 10 years.

Patients with the incidental finding of peripheral eosinophilia but without evidence of end-organ dysfunction can be followed closely at 3- to 6-month intervals without specific treatment, as they tend to follow a benign course. Patients should be monitored routinely at 6-month intervals with chemistries, EKG, echocardiogram, and pulmonary function tests as well as monitored for clinical signs of thrombotic complications. Additional monitoring and testing should be done as indicated depending on symptoms and other known organ involvement.

The tyrosine kinase inhibitor imatinib mesylate (initial dose 400 mg per day) is the first line therapy for all patients with the PDGFRA-positive variant of HES.[214,221,237,238] Persons with cardiac involvement should receive concomitant systemic corticosteroid therapy, to avoid further cardiac damage potentially induced by imatinib.[239] Case reports have suggested other tyrosine kinase inhibitors, nilotinib and sorafenib, can be effective alternate therapies in cases of resistance to imatinib therapy.[240,241]

A mainstay of therapy for persons with HES and organ involvement who lack FIP1L1/PDGFRA fusion or other imatinib responsive mutation includes corticosteroids such as prednisone at 1 mg/kg/d for several weeks, with taper of dose attempted to an every-other-day regimen once eosinophil levels are reduced. The mechanisms by which steroids are effective in this disorder are not fully clear. If the disease stabilizes or resolves (e.g., if blood eosinophilia and symptoms are controlled), corticosteroids can be tapered gradually to alternate-day dosing, and should be continued for approximately 1 year at the minimal dose that effectively controls disease activity.[214]

IFN-α, a mediator that suppresses eosinophil function in vitro, has been beneficial in management of HES, perhaps by inhibiting eosinophil proliferation and differentiation. IFN-α should be tried as a second-line agent among patients with HES who fail to respond to corticosteroid treatment or as a steroid-sparing agent for persons requiring high-dose corticosteroids.[214] IFN-α monotherapy should be avoided among persons with lymphocyte-variant disease.[242] Pegylated interferon may be an effective alternate therapy in selected cases.[243] Existing data suggest that another anti-eosinophil strategy, the anti–IL-5 antibody mepolizumab, may reduce symptoms and eosinophilic organ involvement associated with HES, and may be particularly helpful as a steroid-sparing agent in patients with high IL-5 levels (e.g., persons with lymphocyte variant HES lacking the FIP1L1/PDGFRA fusion gene).[244,245] Case reports have also demonstrated efficacy of the anti–CD-52 antibody alemtuzumab that targets eosinophils and T cells in the lymphocyte variant of HES.[246–248]

Hydroxyurea (0.5–1.5 g per day) may be added to the regimen if there is evidence of further disease progression or steroid toxicity,[214] with the aim of reducing the peripheral leukocyte count to the range of 5000 to 10,000. Vincristine may be used as a chemotherapeutic inducing agent in patients with extremely high peripheral WBC counts. Etoposide, chlorambucil, and other chemotherapeutic agents may be effective alternative agents for cases that prove refractory to standard treatment with corticosteroids. Cyclosporine may also be of benefit in controlling the disease, especially when used in combination with corticosteroids.

Allogeneic bone marrow transplantation has also been reported anecdotally to be successful in selected severe cases of HES in which end-organ damage is potentially reversible.[249]

Leukapheresis affords no clear benefit unless there is elevated blood viscosity with associated coagulation. Antiparasitic agents and radiation therapy are ineffective. Anticoaguation with warfarin and/or antiplatelet agents may be needed for management of thromboembolic events.

Favorable prognostic features include a rapid clinical response to treatment with reduction in blood eosinophilia, the presence of angioedema, an elevated IgE, and absence of findings associated with myeloproliferative disorder.[217,236,250,251] Factors associated with a poor prognosis include presence of total blood WBC greater than 100,000/mm^3, myeloblasts in the peripheral blood, refractory CHF, basophilia above 3%, identifiable chromosomal abnormalities in bone marrow cells, and elevated serum B_{12} levels. The mechanisms by which these features are associated with a given prognosis are largely unknown.

APPROACH TO THE EVALUATION OF EOSINOPHILIC PNEUMONIAS

In approaching the patient with pulmonary infiltrates and eosinophilia, one must first establish whether the patient has one of the eosinophilic disorders described in this chapter or a disease process that is secondarily associated with eosinophilia (Table 71-1). A useful algorithmic approach to the evaluation of patients with pulmonary infiltrates and eosinophilia (blood or lung) is shown in Figure 71-6. A careful search for the cause of the disease should be undertaken. A comprehensive medical history should be elicited, with particular attention paid to any antecedent illness (e.g., atopy, rhinitis, asthma, steroid use, immunosuppression), disease exposures, travel, and the duration and nature of the patient's symptoms. One should take special notice of the sequence and timing of events during the course of the illness. In addition to a careful chest examination, a search should be undertaken for physical findings suggestive of extrapulmonary disease (e.g., skin lesions, CHF, hypertension, neurologic abnormalities, musculoskeletal disorders, or GI illness). The nature, distribution, and duration of infiltrates on chest radiograph should be noted. CT scanning of the chest can also provide additional information that may not be apparent on the chest radiograph.

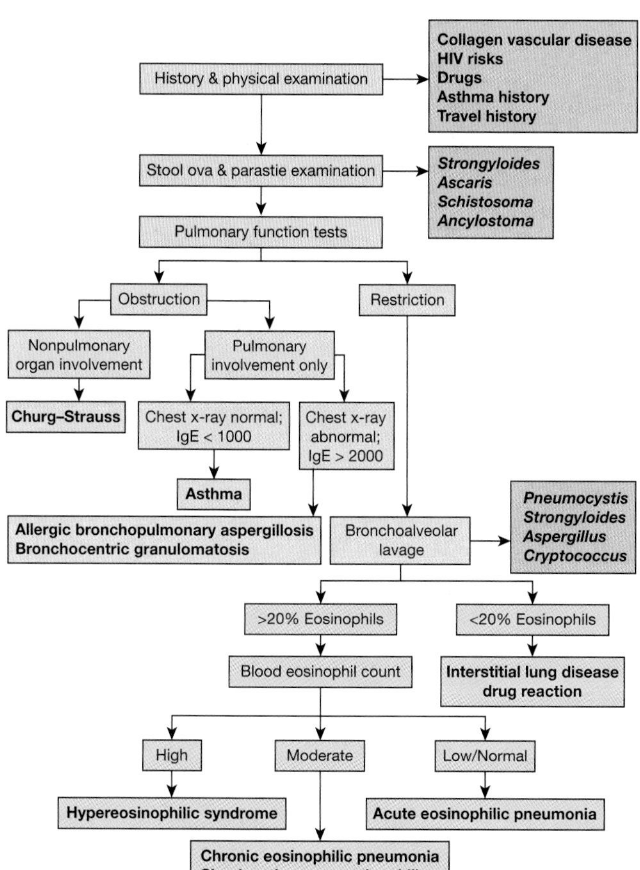

Figure 71-6 Algorithmic approach to evaluation of patients with pulmonary infiltrate and eosinophilia. *(Data from Allen JN, Davis WB. Eosinophilic lung diseases. Am J Respir Crit Care Med. 1994;150: 1423–1438.)*

The workup should include the following additional laboratory data: complete blood count (CBC) with differential, ESR, IgE level, ECG, blood urea nitrogen (BUN), creatinine, liver function tests, urinalysis, sputum cultures, and, when appropriate, sputum cytology. Serologies (e.g., *Aspergillus* precipitins, ANCA, antiparasitic antibodies) are indicated in selected cases. Bronchoscopy with BAL or transbronchial biopsy is important in the evaluation of pulmonary eosinophilic syndromes. The advent of BAL has allowed diagnosis of most cases of eosinophilic pneumonia without open lung biopsy. Normally, BAL fluid contains less than 2% eosinophils. In contrast to diseases associated secondarily with eosinophilia, all the primary pulmonary eosinophilic syndromes are characterized by prominent BAL eosinophilia (more than 20% of the BAL leukocyte differential). The finding of more than 20% BAL eosinophils, viewed in combination with appropriate clinical and radiographic features, is strongly suggestive of the diagnosis of one of these syndromes. BAL and transbronchial biopsy are also useful in ruling out infections (bacterial, fungal, tuberculous, and parasitic), malignancies, and other causes of eosinophil-associated disease. It must be kept in mind that in the context of the overall list of pulmonary diseases associated with more than 5% BAL eosinophilia, the true pulmonary eosinophilic syndromes are rare.

The pulmonary eosinophilic syndromes are at times difficult to distinguish from one another, owing to the substantial amount of overlap among their clinical, radiographic, and histologic features, as well as variable features at different stages of disease. The comparative features of the eosinophilic pneumonias described in this chapter, with regard to several key features, are shown in Table 71-7. The clinical presentation may be acute, subacute, or chronic. Disease may range from mild and self-limited to severe and life-threatening illness. To varying degrees in all the pulmonary eosinophilic syndromes, dyspnea, malaise, low-grade fever, cough, and wheezing are common presenting complaints. Of the diseases considered in detail in this chapter, only EGPA and HES are consistently associated with significant extrapulmonary manifestations. Radiographic infiltrates may be transient in Loeffler syndrome, TPE, EGPA, ABPA, and HES. Blood eosinophilia is present in all the diseases discussed except idiopathic AEP and in a minority of cases of CEP. Variable degrees of elevation of serum IgE are also present. Pulmonary function abnormalities are not specific for these disorders. Except for the diseases caused by parasites, corticosteroids are the mainstay of therapy.

Although the eosinophilic pneumonias can, at times, pose diagnostic difficulties, it is crucial to establish an accurate diagnosis whenever possible. An accurate diagnosis is important because the dose and duration of steroid treatment, prognosis, and follow-up measures for each of these diseases vary widely, and initiation of other specific therapeutic interventions improves outcomes in selected situations. Furthermore, chronic fibrotic lung disease may result from failure to accurately diagnose and treat some of these disorders in a timely fashion, and misdiagnosis with resultant inappropriate therapy (e.g., high-dose steroid treatment of invasive fungal infection masquerading as CEP) may be catastrophic.

TABLE 71-7 Comparative Features of the Pulmonary Eosinophilic Syndromes

	Loeffler's	AEP	TPE	CEP	ABPA	EGPA	HES
Clinical course	Acute	Acute	Acute, subacute, chronic	Subacute	Acute, subacute, chronic	Acute, subacute, chronic	Subacute, chronic
Respiratory Symptoms	Self-limited, mild	Severe	Severe	Mod.–severe	Mod.—severe	Mod.–severe	Mild
H/o allergic disease/asthma	—	±	—	+(30–60%)	Nearly 100%	100%	—
Blood eosinophilia	Mod. to extreme, transient	Absent (delayed)	Extreme	Moderate in most	Typical	Extreme, fluctuating	Extreme, persistent
Sputum/BAL eosinophilia	Prominent	Striking	Prominent	Striking	In some	Prominent	Striking
Elevated serum IgE	±	Moderate elev. in some	High elev.	Mod.–elev. in 50%	Marked elev., fluctuates w/disease	Mod.–elev.	Mod.–elev. in some
Etiologic agent	*Ascaris* spp. *Ancylostoma*, *Strongyloides*, drugs	Unknown	Filarial infection	Unknown	*Aspergillus* (or other fungus)	Unknown	Unknown
Radiographic findings (CXR, CT)	Patchy, often peripheral unilateral or bilateral consolidation and GGO; usually transient, migratory, nonsegmental	Diffuse, alveolar and interstitial GGO and airspace opacities, interlobular septal thickening, pleural effusion	Diffuse, reticulonodular	Predominately, peripheral consolidation and GGO; "photographic negative of pulmonary edema"	Upper lobe–predominant proximal bronchiectasis	Transient, migratory peripheral, rarely diffuse; patchy peribronchial and septal thickening, patchy parenchymal GGO or consolidation, pleural effusion	Transient, focal or diffuse GGO or consolidation
PFTs	± Mild RVD	RVD	OVD early, RVD late, or mixed pattern	Normal, OVD, or RVD	OVD ± RVD	OVD ± RVD	Mild RVD in some
Characteristic diagnostic findings	*Ascaris* larvae in sputum, BAL, gastric aspirate	None	Filaria-specific IgE, IgG, microfilaria in LN/lung	None	See Table 71-5	Histopathology plus appropriate clinical setting	Extreme persistent eosinophilia and multiorgan dysfunction (no other evident cause)
Vasculitis	None	None	None	Occasionally mild, nonnecrotic	None	Characteristic (see text)	None
Extrapulmonary manifestations	GI late, if untreated	None	Cardiac, CNS rare	Very rarely reported	None	Typical of vasculitic phase	Cardiac, neurologic, GI, hematologic, other
Therapy	Mebendazole, if *Ascaris* or hookworm; removal of drug or toxin exposure ± steroids	Corticosteroids	Diethylcarbamazine, Ivermectin	Corticosteroids	Corticosteroids, bronchodilators, antibiotics, antifungals	Corticosteroids, other immunosuppressives (see text)	Depends on disease variant (see text)
Chronic/recurrent disease	None	None	May occur	Common	Typical	May occur (∼25%)	Chronicity typical

+, yes or present; –, no or not present; BAL, bronchoalveolar lavage; CT, computed tomography; elev., elevated; GGO, ground-glass opacity; GI, gastrointestinal; h/o, history of; LN, lymph node; mod., moderately; OVD, obstructive ventilatory defect; CXR, chest x-ray (radiograph); PFTs, pulmonary function tests; RVD, restrictive ventilatory defect.

REFERENCES

1. Cottin V, Cordier JF. Eosinophilic lung diseases. *Immunol Allergy Clin North Am.* 2002;32:557–586.
2. Wilson ME, Weller PF. Eosinophilia. In: Guerrant RL, Walker DH, Weller PF, eds. *Tropical Infectious Diseases: Principles, Pathogens and Practice.* 2nd ed. Philadelphia, PA: Elsevier; 2006:1478.
3. Kuzucu A. Parasitic diseases of the respiratory tract. *Curr Opin Pulm Med.* 2006;12:212–221.
4. Chitkara RK, Krishna G. Parasitic pulmonary eosinophilia. *Semin Respir Crit Care Med.* 2006;27:171–184.
5. Vijayan VK. How to diagnose and manage common parasitic pneumonias. *Curr Opin Pulm Med.* 2007;13:218–224.
6. Butts C, Henderson SO. Ascariasis. *Top Emerg Med.* 2003; 25:38–43.
7. Tsai HC, Lee SS, Liu YC, et al. Clinical manifestations of strongyloidiasis in southern Taiwan. *J Microbiol Immunol Infect.* 2002;35:29–36.
8. Inoue K, Inoue Y, Arai T, et al. Chronic eosinophilic pneumonia due to visceral larva migrans. *Intern Med.* 2002;41:478–482.
9. Figueiredo SD, Taddei JA, Menezes JJ, et al. Clinical-epidemiological study of toxocariasis in a pediatric population. *J Pediatr (Rio J).* 2005;81:126–132.
10. Solomon J, Schwarz M. Drug-, toxin-, and radiation therapy-induced eosinophilic pneumonia. *Semin Respir Crit Care Med.* 2006;27:192–197.
11. Kim PW, Sorbiello AF, Wassei RT, Pham TM, Tonning JM, Nambiar S. Eosinophilic pneumonia in patients treated with daptomycin: review of the literature and US FDA adverse event reporting system reports. *Drug Saf.* 2012;35:447–457.
12. Foucher P, Camus P. Pneumotox online: the drug-induced lung diseases. Available at http://www.pneumotox.com. Accessed August 10, 2013.
13. Cottin V, Bonniaud P. Drug-induced infiltrative lung disease. *Eur Respir Mon.* 2009;46:28.
14. Rom WN, Weiden M, Garcia R, et al. Acute eosinophilic pneumonia in a New York City firefighter exposed to World Trade Center dust. *Am J Respir Crit Care Med.* 2002;166:797–800.
15. Hirai K, Yamazaki Y, Okada K, Furuta S, Kubo K. Acute eosinophilic pneumonia associated with smoke from fireworks. *Intern Med.* 2000;39:401–403.
16. Shintani H, Fujimura M, Yasui M, et al. Acute eosinophilic pneumonia caused by cigarette smoking. *Intern Med.* 2000;39: 66–68.
17. Shorr AF, Scoville SL, Cersovsky SB, et al. Acute eosinophilic pneumonia among US Military personnel deployed in or near Iraq. *JAMA.* 2004;292:2997–3005.
18. Kelly KJ, Ruffing R. Acute eosinophilic pneumonia following intentional inhalation of Scotchguard. *Ann Allergy.* 1993;71:358–361.
19. Nadeem S, Nasir N, Israel RH. Loeffler's syndrome secondary to crack cocaine. *Chest.* 1994;105:1599–1600.
20. Sauvaget E, Dellamonica J, Arlaud K, et al. Idiopathic acute eosinophilic pneumonia requiring ECMO in a teenager smoking tobacco and cannabis. *Pediatr Pulmonol.* 2010;45:1246–1249.
21. Brander PE, Tukiainen P. Acute eosinophilic pneumonia in a heroin smoker. *Eur Respir J.* 1993;6:750–752.
22. Alonso-Ruiz A, Calabozo M, Perez-Ruiz F, et al. Toxic oil syndrome. A long-term follow-up of a cohort of 332 patients. *Medicine (Baltimore).* 1993;72:285–295.
23. Swygert LA, Maes EF, Sewell LE, Miller L, Falk H, Kilbourne EM. Eosinophilia-myalgia syndrome. Results of national surveillance. *JAMA.* 1990;264:1698–1703.
24. Favrolt N, Bonniaud P, Collet E, et al. Severe drug rash with eosinophilia and systemic symptoms after treatment with minocycline (in French). *Rev Mal Respir.* 2007;24:892–895.
25. Allen JN, Pacht ER, Gadek JE, Davis WB. Acute eosinophilic pneumonia as a reversible cause of noninfectious respiratory failure. *N Engl J Med.* 1989;321:569–574.
26. Allen J. Acute eosinophilic pneumonia. *Semin Respir Crit Care Med.* 2006;27:142–147.
27. Philit F, Etienne-Mastroianni B, Parrot A, Guérin C, Robert D, Cordier JF. Idiopathic acute eosinophilic pneumonia: a study of 22 patients. *Am J Respir Crit Care Med.* 2002;166:1235–1239.
28. Badesch DB, King TE Jr, Schwarz MI. Acute eosinophilic pneumonia: a hypersensitivity phenomenon? *Am Rev Respir Dis.* 1989;139:249–252.
29. Ricker DH, Taylor SR, Gartner JC Jr, Kurland G. Fatal pulmonary aspergillosis presenting as acute eosinophilic pneumonia in a previously healthy child. *Chest.* 1991;100:875–877.
30. Buchheit J, Eid N, Rodgers G Jr, Feger T, Yakoub O. Acute eosinophilic pneumonia with respiratory failure: a new syndrome? *Am Rev Respir Dis.* 1992;145:716–718.
31. Wagner T, Dhedin N, Phillipe B, Rivaud E, Vernant JP, Couderc LJ. Acute eosinophilic pneumonia after allogeneic hematopoietic stem cell transplantation. *Ann Hematol.* 2006;85: 202–203.
32. Yoshimi M, Nannya Y, Watanabe T, et al. Acute eosinophilic pneumonia is a non-infectious lung complication after allogeneic hematopoietic stem cell transplantation. *Int J Hematol.* 2009;89:244–248.
33. Glazer CS, Cohen LB, Schwarz MI. Acute eosinophilic pneumonia in AIDS. *Chest.* 2001;120:1732–1735.
34. Miki K, Miki M, Nakamura Y, et al. Early-phase neutrophilia in cigarette smoke-induced acute eosinophilic pneumonia. *Intern Med.* 2003;42:839–845.
35. Uchiyama H, Suad T, Nakamura Y, et al. Alterations in smoking habits are associated with acute eosinophilic pneumonia. *Chest.* 2008;133:1174–1180.
36. Vahid B, Marik PE. An 18 year-old woman with fever, diffuse pulmonary opacities and rapid onset of respiratory failure: idiopathic acute eosinophilic pneumonia. *Chest.* 2006;130: 1938–1941.
37. Al-Saieg N, Moammar O, Kartan R. Flavored cigar smoking induces acute eosinophilic pneumonia. *Chest.* 2007;131:1234–1237.
38. Watanabe K, Fujimura M, Kasahara K, et al. Acute eosinophilic pneumonia following cigarette smoking: a case report including cigarette-smoking challenge test. *Intern Med.* 2002;41:1016–1020.
39. Janz DR, O'Neal HR Jr, Ely EW. Acute eosinophilic pneumonia: a case report and review of the literature. *Crit Care Med.* 2009;37(4):1470–1474.
40. Paparrigopoulos T, Tzavellas E, Karaiskos D, Ilias I, Liappas I. Acute eosinophilic pneumonia after venlafexine overdose. *J Clin Psychopharmacol.* 2011;31(2):258–259.
41. Miller BA, Gray A, LeBlanc TW, Sexton DJ, Martin AR, Slama TG. Acute eosinophilic pneumonia secondary to daptomycin: a report of three cases. *Clin Infect Dis.* 2010;50(11):e63–e68.
42. Imokawa S, Sato A, Hayakawa H, Toyoshima M, Taniguchi M, Chida K. Possible involvement of an environmental agent in

the development of acute eosinophilic pneumonia. *Ann Allergy Asthma Immunol.* 1996;76:419–422.

43. McCormick M, Nelson T. Cocaine-induced fatal acute eosinophilic pneumonia: a case report. *WMJ.* 2007;106:92–95.
44. Jeon EJ, Kim KH, Min KH. Acute eosinophilic pneumonia associated with 2009 influenza A (H1N1). *Thorax.* 2010;65:268–270.
45. Hayakawa H, Sato A, Toyoshima M, Imokawa S, Taniguchi M. A clinical study of idiopathic eosinophilic pneumonia. *Chest.* 1994;105:1462–1466.
46. Umeki S, Soejima R. Acute and chronic eosinophilic pneumonia: clinical evaluation and the criteria. *Intern Med.* 1992;31:847–856.
47. Miyazaki E, Nureki S, Ono E, et al. Circulating thymus-and activation-regulated chemokine/CCL 17 is a useful biomarker for discriminating acute eosinophilic pneumonia from other causes of acute lung injury. *Chest.* 2007;131:1726–1734.
48. Pope-Harman AL, Davis WB, Allen ED, Christoforidis AJ, Allen JN. Acute eosinophilic pneumonia. A summary of 15 cases and review of the literature. *Medicine (Baltimore).* 1996;75:334–342.
49. Mochimaru J, Kawamoto M, Fukuda Y, Kudoh S. Clinicopathological differences between acute and chronic eosinophilic pneumonia. *Respirology.* 2005;10:76–85.
50. Cheon JE, Lee KS, Jung GS, Chung MH, Cho YD. Acute eosinophilic pneumonia: radiographic and CT findings in six patients. *AJR Am J Roentgenol.* 1996;167:1195–1199.
51. Allen JN, Davis WB. Eosinophilic lung diseases. *Am J Respir Crit Care Med.* 1994;150(5 Pt 1):1423–1438.
52. Daimon T, Johkoh T, Sumikawa H, et al. Acute eosinophilc pneumonia: thin-section CT findings in 29 patients. *Eur J Radiol.* 2008;65:462–467.
53. Tazelaar HD, Linz LJ, Colby TV, Myers JL, Limper AH. Acute eosinophilic pneumonia: histopathologic findings in nine patients. *Am J Respir Crit Care Med.* 1997;155:296–302.
54. Allen JN, Liao Z, Wewers MD, Altenberger EA, Moore SA, Allen ED. Detection of IL-5 and IL-1 receptor antagonist in bronchoalveolar lavage fluid in acute eosinophilic pneumonia. *J Allergy Clin Immunol.* 1996;97:1366–1374.
55. Nishigaki Y, Fujiuchi S, Yamazaki Y, et al. Increased vascular endothelial growth factor in acute eosinophilic pneumonia. *Eur Respir J.* 2003;21:774–778.
56. Nureki S, Miyazaki E, Ando M, Kumamoto T, Tsuda T. CC Chemokine receptor 4 ligand production by bronchoalveolar lavage fluid cells in cigarette-smoke-associated acute eosinophilic pneumonia. *Clin Immunol.* 2005;116:83–93.
57. Lee JE, Rhee CK, Lim JH, et al. Fraction of exhaled nitric oxide in patients with acute eosinophilic pneumonia. *Chest.* 2012;141(5):1267–1272.
58. Matsuno O, Takenaka R, Hiroshige S, et al. Reduced IgG levels found during acute eosinophilic pneumonia, which normalize during recovery from disease. *Respir Med.* 2008;102:899–903.
59. Jantz MA, Sahn SA. Corticosteroids in acute respiratory failure. *Am J Respir Crit Care Med.* 1999;160:1079–1100.
60. Weingarten RJ. Tropical eosinophilia. *Lancet.* 1943;1:103.
61. Donohugh DL. Tropical eosinophilia. An etiologic inquiry. *N Engl J Med.* 1969;269:1357–1364.
62. Vijayan VK. Tropical pulmonary eosinophilia: pathogenesis, diagnosis and management. *Curr Opin Pulm Med.* 2007;13:428–433.
63. Boggild AK, Keystone JS, Kain KC. Tropical pulmonary eosinophilia: a case series in a setting of nonendemicity. *Clin Infect Dis.* 2004;39:1123–1128.
64. Ottesen EA, Nutman TB. Tropical pulmonary eosinophilia. *Annu Rev Med.* 1992;43:417.
65. Lobos E, Nutman TB, Hothersall JS, Moncada S. Elevated immunoglobulin E against recombinant Brugia malayi γ-glutaryl transpeptidase in patients with bancroftian filariasis: association with tropical pulmonary eosinophilia or putative immunity. *Infect Immun.* 2003;71:747–753.
66. Ray D, Sri Krishna K. Alpha 1 antitrypsin in tropical pulmonary eosinophilia. *Chest.* 1993;104:487–492.
67. Sandhu M, Mukhopadhyay S, Sharma SK. Tropical pulmonary eosinophilia: a comparative evaluation of plain chest radiography and computed tomography. *Australas Radiol.* 1996;40:32–37.
68. Narayanan K, Balakrishnan A, Miyamoto S. NF-kappaB is essential for induction of proinflammatory cytokine genes by filarial parasite sheath proteins. *Mol Immunol.* 2000;37:115–123.
69. Rom WN. Role of oxidants in interstitial lung diseases: pneumoconioses, constrictive bronchiolitis, and chronic tropical pulmonary eosinophilia, Hindawi Publishing Corp. *Mediators Inflamm.* 2011;2011:407657; doi:10.1155/2011/407657
70. O'Bryan L, Pinkston P, Kumaraswami V, et al. Localized eosinophil degranulation mediates disease in tropical pulmonary eosinophilia. *Infect Immun.* 2003;71:1337–1342.
71. Ong RK, Doyle RL. Tropical pulmonary eosinophilia. *Chest.* 1998;113:1673–1679.
72. Carrington CB, Addington WW, Goff AM, et al. Chronic eosinophilic pneumonia. *N Engl J Med.* 1969;280:787–798.
73. Marchand E, Reynaud-Gaubert M, Lauque D, Durieu J, Tonnel AB, Cordier JF. Idiopathic chronic eosinophilic pneumonia. A clinical and follow-up study of 62 cases. The Groupe d'Etudes et de Recherche sur les Maladies "Orphelines" Pulmonaires (GERM"O"P). *Medicine (Baltimore).* 1998;77:299–312.
74. Marchand E, Cordier JF. Idiopathic chronic eosinophilic pneumonia. *Semin Respir Crit Care Med.* 2006;27:134–141.
75. Cottin V, Frognier R, Monnot H, et al. Chronic eosinophilic pneumonia after radiation therapy for breast cancer. *Eur Respir J.* 2004;23:9–13.
76. Marchand E, Etienne-Mastroianni B, Chanez P, et al. Idiopathic chronic eosinophilic pneumonia and asthma: how do they influence each other? The Groupe d'Etudes et de Recherche sur les Maladies "Orphelines" Pulmonaires (GERM"O"P). *Eur Respir J.* 2003;22:8.
77. Jederlinic PJ, Sicilian L, Gaensler EA. Chronic eosinophilic pneumonia: a report of 19 cases and a review of the literature. *Medicine (Baltimore).* 1988;67:154–162.
78. Hueto-Perez-de Heredia JJ, Dominguez-del-Valle FJ, Garcia E, Gomez ML, Gallego J. Chronic eosinophilic pneumonia as a presenting feature of Churg-Strauss syndrome. *Eur Respir J.* 1994;7:1006–1008.
79. Golstein MA, Steinfeld S. Chronic eosinophilic pneumonia followed by Churg-Strauss syndrome. *Rev Rheum Engl Ed.* 1996;63:624–628.
80. Matsuse H, Shimoda T, Fukushima C, et al. Diagnostic problems in chronic eosinophilic pneumonia. *J Int Med Res.* 1997;25:196–201.

81. Danel C, Israel-Biet D, Costabel U, et al. The clinical role of BAL in rare pulmonary diseases. *Eur Respir Rev.* 1991;2:83.

82. Cottin V, Deviller P, Tardy F, Cordier JF. Urinary eosinophil-derived neurotoxin/protein X: a simple method for assessing eosinopil degranulation in vivo. *J Allergy Clin Immunol.* 1998;101:116–123.

83. Gaensler EA, Carrington CB. Peripheral opacities in chronic eosinophilic pneumonia: the photographic negative of pulmonary edema. *AJR Am J Roentgenol.* 1977;128:1–13.

84. Alam M, Burki NK. Chronic eosinophilic pneumonia: a review. *So Med J.* 2007;100(1)49–53.

85. Samman YS, Wali SO, Abdelaal MA, Gangi MT, Krayem AB. Chronic eosinophilic pneumonia presenting with recurrent massive bilateral pleural effusion: case report. *Chest.* 2001; 119:968–970.

86. Laufs U, Schneider C, Wasserman K, Erdmann E. Chronic eosinophilic pneumonia with atypical radiographic presentation. *Respiration.* 1998;65:323–326.

87. Ebara H, Ikezoe J, Johkoh T, et al. Chronic eosinophilic pneumonia: evolution of chest radiograms and CT features. *J Comput Assist Tomogr.* 1994;18:737.

88. Johkoh T, Muller NL, Akira M, et al. Eosinophilic lung diseases: diagnostic accuracy of thin-section CT in 111 patients. *Radiology.* 2000;216:773–780.

89. Mayo JR, Muller NL, Road J, Sisler J, Lillington G. Chronic eosinophilic pneumonia: CT findings in six cases. *AJR Am J Roentgenol.* 1989;153:727.

90. Furuiye M, Yoshimura N, Kobayashi A, et al. Churg-Strauss syndrome versus chronic eosinophilic pneumonia on high-resolution computed tomographic findings. *J Comut Assist Tommogr.* 2010;34(1)19–22.

91. Payne CR, Connellan SJ. Chronic eosinophilic pneumonia complicating long-standing rheumatoid arthritis. *Postgrad Med J.* 1980;56:519–520.

92. Jaimes-Hernández J, Mendoza-Fuentes A, Meléndez-Mercado CI, Aranda-Pereira P. Chronic eosinophilic pneumonia: autoimmune phenomenon or immunoallergic disease? Case report and literature review. *Reumatol Clin.* 2012;8(3):145–148.

93. Albera C, Ghio P, Solidoro P, Mabritto I, Marchetti L, Pozzi E. Activated and memory alveolar T-lymphocytes in idiopathic eosinophilic pneumonia. *Eur Respir J.* 1995;8:1281–1285.

94. Janin A, Torpier G, Courtin P, et al. Segregation of eosinophil proteins in alveolar macrophage compartments in chronic eosinophilic pneumonia. *Thorax.* 1993;48:57–62.

95. Cottin V, Cordier JF. Idiopathic eosinophilic pneumonias. *Eur Respir Mon.* 2012;134:118.

96. Ono E, Taniguchi M, Mita H, et al. Increased urinary leukotriene E4 concentration in patients with eosinophilic pneumonia. *Eur Respir J.* 2008;32:437–442.

97. Nakaji H, Matsumoto H, Niimi A, et al. Eosinophils and macrophages are involved in nitrosative stress in chronic eosinophilic pneumonia. *Nitric Oxide.* 2011;24:173–175.

98. Saita N, Yamanaka T, Kohrogi H, Ando M, Hirashima M. Difference in apoptotic function between eosinophils from peripheral blood and bronchoalveolar lavage in chronic eosinophilic pneumonia. *Int Arch Allergy Immunol.* 1999;120 (Suppl 1):91–94.

99. Sanaee MS, O'Byrne PM, Nair P. Diffuse idiopathic neuroendocrine hyperplasia, chronic eosinophilic pneumonia, and asthma. *Eur Respir J.* 1489;34(6):1489–1492.

100. Yoshida K, Shijubo N, Koba H, et al. Chronic eosinophilic pneumonia progressing to lung fibrosis. *Eur Respir J.* 1994;7:1541–1544.

101. Naughton M, Fahy J, FitzGerald MX. Chronic eosinophilic pneumonia. A long-term follow-up of 12 patients. *Chest.* 1993;103:162–165.

102. Kaya H, Gumus S, Ucar E, et al. Omalizumab as a steroid-sparing agent in chronic eosinophilic pneumonia. *Chest.* 2012;142(2)513.

103. Teba C, Rochester CL. Allergic bronchopulmonary aspergillosis. In: Grippi MA, Heffner J, Kotloff R. *Clinical Decision Support: Pulmonary Medicine and Sleep Disorders.* Wilmington, DE: Decision Support in Medicine, LLC; 2013. (On-line Publication)

104. Bains SN, Judson MA. Allergic bronchopulmonary aspergillosis. *Clin Chest Med.* 2012;33:265–281.

105. Greenberger PA. Allergic bronchopulmonary aspergillosis. *Allergy Asthma Proc.* 2012;33:S61–S6.

106. Agarwal R. Allergic bronchopulmonary aspergillosis. *Chest.* 2009;135:805–826.

107. Vining C, Bush RK. Allergic bronchopulmonary aspergillosis: a US perspective. *Curr Opin Pulm Med.* 2007;13:67–71.

108. Patterson K, Strek ME. Allergic bronchopulmonary aspergillosis. *Proc Am Thorac Soc.* 2010;7:237–244.

109. Knutsen AP, Slavin RG. Allergic bronchopulmonary aspergillosis in asthma and cystic fibrosis. *Clin Devel Immunol.* 2011;2011:843763.

110. Gibson PG. Allergic bronchopulmonary aspergillosis. *Semin Respir Crit Care Med.* 2006;27(2):185–191.

111. Agarwal R, Aggarwal AN, Gupta D, Jindal SK. Aspergillus hypersensitivity and allergic bronchopulmonary aspergillosis in patients with bronchial asthma: systematic review and meta-analysis. *Int J Tuberc Lung Dis.* 2009;13: 936–944.

112. Stevens DA, Moss RB, Kurup VP, et al. Allergic bronchopulmonary aspergillosis in cystic fibrosis—state of the art. Cystic Fibrosis Foundation Consensus Conference. *Clin Infect Dis.* 2003;37(Suppl 3):S225–S264.

113. Glancy JJ, Elder JL, McAleer R. Allergic bronchopulmonary fungal disease without clinical asthma. *Thorax.* 1981;36: 345–349.

114. Patterson R, Greenberger PA, Radin RC, Roberts M. Allergic bronchopulmonary aspergillosis. Natural history and classification of early disease by serologic and roentgenographic studies. *Ann Intern Med.* 1982;96(3)286–291.

115. Greenberger PA. Allergic bronchopulmonary aspergillosis. *J Allergy Clin Immunol.* 2002;110:685–692.

116. Riscilli BP, Wood KL. Noninvasive pulmonary Aspergillus infections. *Clin Chest Med.* 2009;30:315–335.

117. Greenberger PA, Patterson R. Diagnosis and management of allergic bronchopulmonary aspergillosis. *Ann Allergy.* 1986; 56:444–448.

118. Vlahakis NE, Aksamit TR. Diagnosis and treatment of allergic bronchopulmonary aspergillosis. *Mayo Clin Proc.* 2001;76: 930–938.

119. Greenberger PA, Miller TP, Roberts M, Smith LL. Allergic bronchopulmonary aspergillosis in patients with and without bronchiectasis. *Ann Allergy.* 1993;70(4):333–338.

120. Buckingham SJ, Hansell DM. Aspergillus in the lung: diverse and coincident forms. *Eur Radiol.* 2003;13:1786–1800.

121. Agarwal R, Gupta D, Aggarwal AN, Saxena AK, Chakrabarti A, Jindal SK. Clinical significance of hyperattenuating mucoid impaction in allergic bronchopulmonary aspergillosis: an analysis of 155 patients. *Chest.* 2007;132:1183–1190.

122. Wark PAB, Gibson P. Pathogenesis of ABPA. In: Pasqualotto AC, ed. *Aspergillosis: From Diagnosis to Prevention.* Springer Science and Business Media; Heidelberg, London, New York 2010:695–706.

123. Moss RB. Allergic bronchopulmonary aspergillosis and aspergillus infection in cystic fibrosis. *Curr Opin Pulm Med.* 2010;16:598–603.

124. Ricketti AJ, Greenberger PA, Patterson R. Serum IgE as an important aid in management of allergic bronchopulmonary aspergillosis. *J Allergy Clin Immunol.* 1984;74:68–71.

125. Gilley SK, Goldblatt MR, Judson MA. The treatment of ABPA. In: Pasqualotto AC, ed. *Aspergillosis: From Diagnosis to Prevention*, Springer Science and Business Media; Heidelberg, London, New York 2010:747–759.

126. Agarwal R, Gupta D, Aggarwal AN, et al. Clinical significance of decline in serum IgE levels in allergic bronchopulmonary aspergillosis. *Respir Med.* 2010;104:204–210.

127. Stevens DA, Schwartz HJ, Lee JY, et al. A randomized trial of itraconazole in allergic broncopulmonary aspergillosis. *N Engl J Med.* 2000;342(11):756–762.

128. Pasqualotto AC, Powell G, Niven R, Denning DW. The effects of antifungal therapy on severe asthma with fungal sensitization and allergic bronchopulmonary aspergillosis. *Respirology.* 2009;14:1121–1127.

129. Wark PA, Gibson PG, Wilson AJ. Azoles for allergic bronchopulmonary aspergillosis associated with asthma. *Cochrane Database Syst Rev.* 2004;(3):CD001108.

130. Walsh TJ, Anaissie EJ, Denning DW, et al. Treatment of aspergillosis: clinical practice guidelines of the Infectious Diseases Society of America. *Clin Infect Dis.* 2008;46:327–360.

131. Knutsen AP, Bush RK, Demain JG, et al. Fungi and allergic lower respiratory tract diseases. *J Allergy Clin Immunol.* 2012;129:280–891.

132. Erwin GE, Fitzgerald JE. Case report: allergic bronchopulmonary aspergillosis and allergic fungal sinusitis successfully treated with voriconazole. *J Asthma.* 2007;44:891–895.

133. Glackin L, Leen G, Elnazir B, et al. Voriconazole in the treatment of allergic bronchopulmonary aspergillosis in cystic fibrosis. *Ir Med J.* 2009;102:29.

134. Tillie-Leblond I, Germaud P, Leroyer C, et al. Allergic bronchopulmonary aspergillosis and omalizumab. *Allergy.* 2011;66(9):1254–1256. doi: 10.1111/j.1398-9995.2011.02599.x

135. Zirbes JM, Milla CE. Steroid-sparing effect of omalizumab for allergic bronchopulmonary aspergillosis and cystic fibrosis. *Pediatr Pulmonol.* 2008;43:607–610.

136. Kanu A, Patel K. Treatment of allergic bronchopulmonary aspergillosis (ABPA) in CF with anti-IgE antibody (omalizumab). *Pediatr Pulmonol.* 2008;43:1249–1251.

137. Lebecque P, Leonard A, Pilette C. Omalizumab for treatment of ABPA exacerbations in CF patients. *Pediatr Pulmonol.* 2009;44:516.

138. Blanchard C, Rothenberg ME. Biology of the eosinophil. *Adv Immunol.* 2009;101:81–121.

139. Sinico RA, Bottero P. Churg-Strauss angiitis. *Best Pract Res Clin Rheumatol.* 2009;23:355–366.

140. Pagnoux C, Guilpain P, Guillevin L. Churg-Strauss syndrome. *Curr Opin Rheumatol.* 2007;19:25–32.

141. Keogh KA, Specks U. Churg-Strauss syndrome. *Semin Respir Crit Care Med.* 2006;27:148–157.

142. Dunogue B, Pagnoux C, Guillevin L. Churg-Strauss syndrome: clinical symptoms, complementary investigations, prognosis, outcome, and treatment. *Semin Respir Crit Care Med.* 2011;32:298–309.

143. Baldini C, Talarico R, Della Rossa A, Bombardieri S. Clinical manifestations and treatment of Churg-Strauss syndrome. *Rheum Dis Cln N Am.* 2010;36:527–543.

144. Conron M, Beynon HL. Churg-Stauss syndrome. *Thorax.* 2000;55:870–877.

145. Zwerina J, Eger G, Englbrecht M, Manger B, Schett G. Churg-Strauss syndrome in childhood: a systematic literature review and clinical comparison with adult patients. *Semin Arth Rheum.* 2009;39:108–115.

146. Vaglio A, Martorana D, Maggiore U, et al. HLA-DRB4 as a genetic risk factor for Churg-Strauss syndrome. *Arthritis Rheum.* 2007;56:3159–3166.

147. Wieczorek S, Holle JU, Epplen JT. Recent progress in the genetics of Wegener's granulomatosis and Churg-Strauss syndrome. *Curr Opin Rheumatology.* 2010;22:8–14.

148. Lanham JG, Elkon KB, Pusey CD, Hughes GR. Systemic vasculitis with asthma and eosinophilia: a clinical approach to the Churg-Strauss syndrome. *Medicine (Baltimore).* 1984;63:65–81.

149. Abril A. Churg-strauss syndrome: an update. *Curr Rheumatol Rep.* 2011;13:489–495.

150. Lie JT. Limited forms of Churg-Strauss sydrome. *Pathol Annu.* 1993;28:199–120.

151. Cottin V, Khoutra C, Dubost R, Glérant JC, Cordier JF. Persistent airflow obstruction in asthma of patients with Churg-Strauss syndrome and long-term follow-up. *Allergy.* 2009;64:589–595.

152. Choi YH, Im JG, Han BK, Kim JH, Lee KY, Myoung NH. Thoracic manifestation of Churg-Strauss syndrome: radiologic and clinical findings. *Chest.* 2000;117:117–124.

153. Kim YK, Lee KS, Chung MP, et al. Pulmonary involvement in Churg-Strauss syndrome: an analysis of CT, clinical and pathologic findings. *Eur Radiol.* 17:2007;3157–3165.

154. Chung MP, Yi CA, Lee HY, Han J, Lee KS. Imaging of pulmonary vasculitis. *Radiology.* 2010;255:322–341.

155. Szczeklik W, Sokolowska B, Mastalerz L, et al. Pulmonary findings in Churg-Strauss syndrome in chest X-rays and high resolution computed tomography at the time of initial diagnosis. *Clin Rheumatol.* 2010;29:1127–1134.

156. Guillevin L, Cohen P, Gayraud M, Lhote F, Jarrousse B, Casassus P. Churg-Strauss syndrome. Clinical study and long-term follow-up of 96 patients. *Medicine (Baltimore).* 1999;78:26–37.

157. Neumann T, Manger B, Schmid M, et al. Cardiac involvement in Churg-Strauss syndrome: impact of endomyocarditis. *Medicine (Baltimore).* 2009;88:236–243.

158. Ginsberg F, Parillo JE. Eosinophilic myocarditis. *Heart Fail Clin.* 2005;1:419–429.

159. Sable-Fourtassou R, Cohen P, Mahr A, et al. French Vasculitis Study Group. Antineutrophil cytoplasmic antibodies and the Chrug-Strauss syndrome. *Ann Intern Med.* 2005;143(9):632–638.

160. Sinico RA, Di Toma L, Maggiore U, et al. Prevalence and clinical significance of antineutrophil cytoplasmic antibodies in

Churg-Strauss syndrome. *Arthritis Rheum.* 2005;52(9):2926–2935.

161. Kawakami T, Soma Y, Kawasaki K, Kawase A, Mizoguchi M. Initial cutaneous manifestations consistent with mononeuritis multiplex in Churg-Strauss syndrome. *Arch Dermatol.* 2005;141: 873–878.
162. Sinico RA, DiToma L, Maggiore U, et al. Renal involvement in Churg-Strauss syndrome. *Am J Kidney Dis.* 2006;47:770–779.
163. Clutterbuck EJ, Evans DJ, Pusey CD. Renal involvement in Churg-Strauss Syndrome. *Nephrol Dial Transplant.* 1990;5: 161–167.
164. Szczeklik W, Sanak L, Mastalerz B, et al. 12-hydroxy-eicosatetraenoic acid (12-HETE): a biomarker of Churg-Strauss syndrome. *Clin Exp Allergy.* 2011;42:513–522.
165. Nachmann PH, Henderson AG. Pathogenesis of lung vasculitis. *Semin Resp Crit Care Med.* 2011;32:245–253.
166. Vaglio A, Strehl JD, Manger B, et al. IgG4 immune response in Churg-Strauss syndrome. *Ann Rheum Dis.* 2012;71:390–393.
167. Dallos T, Heiland GR, Strehl J, et al. CCL17/thymus and activation-related chemokine in Churg-Strauss syndrome. *Arthritis Rheum.* 2010;62:3496–3503.
168. Cottin V, Tardy F, Gindry D, Vernet G, Deviller P, Cordier JF. Urinary eosinophil-derived neurotoxin in Churg-Strauss syndrome. *J Allergy Clin Immnol.* 1995;96:261–264.
169. Zwerina J, Bach C, Martorana D, et al. Eotaxin-3 in Churg-Strauss syndrome: a clinical and immunogenetic study. *Rheumatology.* 2011;50:1823–1827.
170. Polzer K, Karonitsch T, Neumann T, et al. Eotaxin-3 is involved in Churg-Strauss syndrome—a serum marker closely correlating with disease activity. *Rheumatology (Oxford).* 2008;47(6): 804–808.
171. Jakiela B, Szczeklik W, Plutecka H, et al. Increased production of IL-5 and dominant Th2-type response in airways of Churg-Strauss syndrome patients. *Rheumatology.* 2012;51:1887–1893.
172. Zwerina J, Axmann R, Jatzwauk M, Sahinbegovic E, Polzer K, Schett G. Pathogenesis of Churg-Strauss syndrome: recent insights. *Autoimmunity.* 42(4):2009;376–379.
173. Kallenberg CG. Churg-Strauss syndrome: just one disease entity? *Arthritis Rheum.* 2005;52:2589–2593.
174. Pagnoux C, Guillevin L. Churg-Strauss syndrome: evidence for disease subtypes? *Curr Opin Rheumatol.* 2010;22:21–28.
175. Comarmond C, Pagnoux C, Khellaf M, et al. Eosinophilic granulomatosis with polyangiitis (Churg-Strauss), clinical characteristics and long-term followup of the 383 patients enrolled in the French Vasculitis Study Group Cohort. *Arthritis Rheum.* 2013;65(1):270–281.
176. Sinico RA, Bottero P, Guillevin L. Antineutrophil cytoplasmic autoantibodies and clinical phenotype in patients with Churg-Strauss syndrome (letter). *J Allergy Clin Immunol.* 2012;130(6):1440.
177. Wallaert B, Gosset P, Prin L, Bart F, Marquette CH, Tonnel AB. Bronchoalveolar lavage in allergic granulomatosis and angiitis. *Eur Respir J.* 1993;6:413–417.
178. Bhagirath KM, Paulson K, Ahmadie R, Bhalla RS, Robinson D, Jassal DS. Clinical utility of cardiac magnetic resonance imaging in Churg-Strauss syndrome: case report and review of the literature. *Rheumatol Int.* 2009;29(4):445–449.
179. Baccouche H, Yilmaz A, Alscher D, Klingel K, Val-Bernal JF, Mahrholdt H. Magnetic resonance assessment and therapy monitoring of cardiac involvement in Churg-Strauss syndrome. *Circulation.* 2008;117:1745–1749.
180. Churg A. Recent advances in the diagnosis of Churg-Strauss Syndrome. *Mod Pathol.* 2001;14:1284–1293.
181. Katzenstein AL. Diagnostic features and differential diagnosis of Churg-Strauss syndrome in the lung. A review. *Am J Clin Pathol.* 2000;114:767–772.
182. Lie JT. Illustrated histopathologic classification criteria for selected vasculitis syndromes. American College of Rheumatology Subcommittee on Classification of Vasculitis. *Arthritis Rheum.* 1990;33:1074–1087.
183. Saito H, Tsurikisawa N, Tsuburai T, Oshikata C, Akiyama K. The proportion of regulatory T cells in the peripheral blood reflects the relapse or remission status of patients with Churg-Strauss syndrome. *Int Arch Allergy Immunol.* 2011;155(1): 46–52.
184. Schmitt WH, Csernok E, Kobayashi S, Klinkenborg A, Reinhold-Keller E, Gross WL. Churg-Strauss syndrome: serum markers of lymphocyte activation and endothelial damage. *Arth Rheum.* 1998;41:445–452.
185. Vaglio A, Moosig F, Zwerina J. Churg-Strauss syndrome: update on pathophysiology and treatment. *Curr Opin Rheumatol.* 2012;24:24–30.
186. Tsurikisawa N, Saito H, Tsuburai T, et al. Differences in regulatory T cells between Churg-Strauss syndrome and chronic eosinophilic pneumonia with asthma. *J Allergy Clin Immunol.* 2008;122:610–616.
187. Hellmich B, Csernok E, Gross WL. Proinflammatory cytokines and autoimmunity in Churg-Strauss syndrome. *Ann NY Acad Sci.* 2005;1051:121–131.
188. Hellmich B, Ehlers S, Csernok E, Gross WL. Update on the pathogenesis of Churg-Strauss syndrome. *Clin Exp Rheumatol.* 2003;21:S69–S77.
189. Wieczorek S, Hellmich B, Arning L, et al. Functionally relevant variations of the interleukin-10 gene associated with antineutrophil cytoplasmic antibody-negative Churg-Strauss syndrome, but not with Wegener's granulomatosis. *Arth Rheum.* 2008;58:1839–1848.
190. Saito H, Tsurikisawa N, Tsuburai T, Akiyama K. Involvement of regulatory T cells in the pathogenesis of Churg-Strauss syndrome. *Int Arch Allergy Immunol.* 2008;146(1):73–76.
191. Green RL, Vayonis AG. Churg-Strauss syndrome after zafirlukast in two patients not receiving systemic steroid treatment. *Lancet.* 1999;353:725–726.
192. Wechsler ME, Finn D, Gunawardena D, et al. Churg-Strauss syndrome in patients receiving montelukast as treatment for asthma. *Chest.* 2000;117:708–713.
193. Nathani N, Little MA, Kunst H, Wilson D, Thickett DR. Churg-Strauss syndrome and leukotriene antagonist use: a respiratory perspective. *Thorax.* 2008;63:883–888.
194. Keogh KA, Specks U. Churg-Strauss syndrome: clinical presentation, antineutrophil cytoplasmic antibodies, and leukotriene receptor antagonists. *Am J Med.* 2003;115: 284–290.
195. Le Gall C, Pham S, Vignes S, et al. Inhaled corticosteroids and Churg-Strauss syndrome: a report of five cases. *Eur Respir J.* 2000;15:978–981.
196. Cooper SM, Libman BS, Lazarovich M. Churg-Strauss syndrome in a group of patients receiving fluticasone for asthma. *J Rheumatol.* 2002;29:2651–2652.

197. Wechsler ME, Wong DA, Miller MK, Lawrence-Miyasaki L. Churg-Strauss syndrome in patients treated with omalizumab. *Chest.* 2009;136:507–518.

198. Orriols R, Munoz X, Ferrer J, Huget P, Morell F. Cocaine-induced Churg-Strauss vasculitis. *Eur Respir J.* 1996;9:175–177.

199. Jennette JC, Falk RJ, Andrassy K, et al. Nomenclature of systemic vasculitides. Proposal of an international consensus conference. *Arthritis Rheum.* 1994;37:187–192.

200. Khoury P, Zagallo P, Talar-Williams C, et al. Serum biomarkers re similar in Churg-Strauss syndrome and hypereosinophilic syndrome. *Allergy.* 2012;67:1149–1156.

201. Ribi C, Cohen P, Pagnoux C, et al; French Vasculitis Study Group. Treatment of Churg-Strauss syndrome without poor prognosis factors: a multicenter, prospective, randomized, open-label study of seventy-two patients. *Arth Rheum.* 2008;58(2):586–594.

202. Guillevin L, Cohen P, Mahr A, et al. Treatment of polyarteritis nodosa and microscopic polyangiitis with poor prognosis factors: a prospective trial comparing glucocorticoids and six or twelve cyclophosphamide pulses in sixty-five patients. *Arthritis Rheum.* 2003;49(1):93.

203. Guillevin L, Pagnous C, Seror R, et al. The five-factor score revisited: assessment of prognoses of systemic necrotizing vasculitides based on the French Vasculitis Study Group (FVSG) cohort. *Medicine (Baltimore).* 2011;90(1):19.

204. Rich EN, Brown KK. Treatment of antineutrophil cytoplasmic antibody-associated vasculitis. *Curr Opin Pulm Med* 2012;18: 447.

205. Bourgarit A, Le Toumelin P, Pagnoux C, et al. French Vasculitis Study Group. Deaths occuring during the first year after treatment onset for polyarteritis nodosa, microscopic polyangiitis, and Churg-Strauss syndrome: a retrospective analysis of causes and factors predictive of mortality based on 595 patients. *Medicine (Baltimore).* 2005;84(5): 323–330.

206. Tsurikisawa N, Saito H, Oshikata C, Tsuburai T, Akiyama K. High-dose intravenous immunoglobulin treatment increases regulatory T cells in patients with eosinophilic granulomatosis with polyangiitis. *J Rheumatol.* 2012;39:1019–1025.

207. Moosig F, Gross WL, Hellmich B, Bremer JP, Hellmich B. Targeting interleukin-5 in refractory and relapsing Churg-Strauss syndrome. *Ann Intern Med.* 2011;155(5):341–343.

208. Kim S, Marigowda G, Oren E, Israel E, Wechsler ME. Mepolizumab as a steroid-sparing treatment option in patients with Churg-Strauss syndrome. *J Allergy Clin Immunol.* 2010;125:1336–1343.

209. Metzler C, Schnabel A, Gross WL, Hellmich B. A phase II study of interferon-alpha for the treatment of refractory Churg-Strauss syndrome. *Clin Exp Rheumatol.* 2008;26(3 Suppl 49):S35–S40.

210. Cottin V, Cordier JF. Eosinophilic pneumonias. *Allergy.* 2005;60:841–857.

211. Niles J. Rituximab in induction therapy for anti-neutrophil cytoplasmic antibody (ANCA) vasculitis. *Clin Exp Immunol.* 2011;164(Suppl 1):27–30.

212. Chusid MJ, Dale DC, West BC, Wolff SM. The hypereosinophilic syndrome: analysis of fourteen cases with review of the literature. *Medicine (Baltimore).* 1975;54:1–27.

213. Klion A. Hypereosinophilic syndrome: current approach to the diagnosis and treatment. *Annu Rev Med.* 2009;60:293–306.

214. Ogbogu PU, Bochner BS, Butterfield JH, et al. Hypereosinophilic syndrome: a multicenter retrospective analysis of clinical characteristics and response to therapy. *J Allergy Clin Immunol.* 2009;124:1319–1325.

215. Klion AD, Bochner BS, Gleich GJ, et al. Approaches to the treatment of hypereosinophilic syndromes: a workshop summary report. *J Allergy Clin Immunol.* 2006;117: 1292–1302.

216. Valent P, Klion AD, Horny HP, et al. Contemporary consensus proposal on criteria and classification of eosinophilic disorders and related syndromes. *J Allergy Clin Immunol.* 2012;130: 607–612.

217. Weller PF, Bubley GJ. The idiopathic hypereosinophilic syndrome. *Blood.* 1994;83:2759–2779.

218. Rapanotti MC, Caruso R, Ammatuna E, et al. Molecular characterization of paediatric idiopathic hypereosinophilia. *Br J Haematol.* 2010;151:440–446.

219. Simon HU, Rothenberg ME, Bochner BS, et al. Refining the definition of hypereosinophilic syndrome. *J Allergy Clin Immunol.* 2010;126:45–49.

220. Bain BJ, Fletcher SH. Chronic eosinophilic leukemias and the myeloproliferative variant of the hypereosinophilic syndrome. *Immunol Allergy Clin North Am.* 2007;27:377–388.

221. Cools J, DeAngelo DJ, Gotlib J, et al. A tyrosine kinase created by fusion of the PDGFRA and FIP1L1 genes as a therapeutic target of imatinib in idiopathic hypereosinophilic syndrome. *New Engl J Med.* 2003;348:1201–1214.

222. Roufosse F, Cogan E, Goldman M. Lymphocytic variant hypereosinophilic syndromes. *Immunol Allergy Clin North Am.* 2007;27:389–413.

223. Simon HU, Plotz SG, Dummer R, Blaser K. Abnormal clones of T cells producing interleukin-5 in idiopathic eosinophilia. *N Engl J Med.* 1999;341:1112–1120.

224. Roufosse F, Schandene L, Sibille C, et al. Clonal Th2 lymphocytes in patients with the idiopathic hypereosinophilic syndrome. *Br J Haematol.* 2000;109:540–548.

225. Dulohery MM, Patel RR, Schneider F, Ryu JH. Lung involvement in hypereosinophilic syndromes. *Respir Med.* 2011;105:114–121.

226. Ogbogu PU, Rosing DR, Horne MK 3rd. Cardiovascular manifestations of hypereosinophilic syndromes. *Immunol Allergy Clin North Am.* 2007;27:457–475.

227. Gertz MA. Troponin in hematologic oncology. *Leuk Lymphoma.* 2008;49:194–203.

228. Syed IS, Martinez MW, Feng DL, Glockner JF. Cardiac magnetic resonance imaging of eosinophilic endomyocardial disease. *Int J Cardiol.* 2008;126:e50–e52.

229. Moore PM, Harley JB, Fauci AS. Neurologic dysfunction in the idiopathic hypereosinophilic syndrome. *Ann Intern Med.* 1985;102:109–114.

230. Kawata E, Kuroda J, Wada K, et al. Hypereosinophilic syndrome accompanied by Buerger's disease-like femoral artery occlusions. *Intern Med.* 2007;46:1919–1922.

231. Leiferman KM, Gleich GJ, Peters MS. Dermatologic manifestations of the hypereosinophilic syndromes. *Immunol Allergy Clin North Am.* 2007;27:415–441.

232. McPherson T, Cowen EW, McBurney E, Klion AD. Platelet-derived growth factor receptor-alpha-associated hypereosinophilic syndrome and lymphomatoid papulosis. *Br J Dermatol.* 2006;155:824–826.

233. Flaum MA, Schooley RT, Fauci AS, Grainick HR. A clinicopathologic correlation of the idiopathic hypereosinophilic syndrome. I. Hematologic manifestations. *Blood.* 1981;58:1012–1020.

234. Spry CJF. Idiopathic hypereosinophilic syndrome. In: Makino S, Fukuda T, eds. *Eosiophils: Biological and Clinical Aspects.* Boca Raton, FL: CRC; 1992:403.

235. Ackerman SJ, Bochner BS. Mechanisms of eosinophilia in the pathogenesis of hypereosinophilic disorders. *Immunol Allergy Clin North Am.* 2007;27:537–575.

236. Klion AD, Noel P, Akin C, et al. Elevated serum tryptase levels identify a subset of patients with a myeloproliferative variant of idiopathic hypereosinophilic syndrome associated with tissue fibrosis, poor prognosis, and imatinib responsiveness. *Blood.* 2003;101:4660–4666.

237. Griffin JH, Leung J, Bruner RJ, Caligiuri MA, Briesewitz R. Discovery of a fusion kinase in EOL-1 cells and idiopathic hypereosinophilic syndrome. *Proc Natl Acad Sci USA.* 2003;100:7830–7835.

238. Baccarani M, Cilloni D, Rondoni M, et al. The efficacy of imatinib mesylate in patients with FIP1L1-PDGFRalpha-positive hypereosinophilic syndrome. Results of a multicenter prospective study. *Haematologica.* 2007;92:1173–1179.

239. Pitini V, Arrigo C, Azzarello D, et al. Serum concentration of cardiac Troponin T in patients with hypereosinophilic syndrome treated with imatinib is predictive of adverse outcomes. *Blood.* 2003;102:3456–3457.

240. Ikezoe T, Togitani K, Tasaka T, Nishioka C, Yokoyama A. Successful treatment of imatinib-resistant hypereosinophilic syndrome with nilotinib. *Leuk Res.* 2010;34:e200–e201.

241. Lierman E, Michaux L, Beullens E, et al. FIP1L1-PDGFRalpha D842 V, a novel panresistant mutant emerging after treatment of FIP1L1-PDGFRalpha T674I eosinophilic leukemia with single agent sorafenib. *Leukemia.* 2009;23:845–851.

242. Roufosse F, Cogan E, Goldman M. Recent advances in the pathogenesis and management of hypereosinophilic syndromes. *Allergy.* 2004;59:673–689.

243. Butterfield JH, Weiler CR. Treatment of hypereosinophilic syndromes—the first 100 years. *Semin Hematol.* 2012;49:182–191.

244. Rothenberg ME, Klion AD, Roufosse FE, et al; Mepolizumab HES Study Group. Treatment of patients with the hypereosinophilic syndrome with mepolizumab. *New Eng J Med.* 2008;358:1215–1228.

245. Roufosse FE, Kahn JE, Gleich GJ, et al. Long-term safety of mepolizumab for the treatment of hypereosinophilic syndromes. *J Allergy Clin Immunol.* 2012;131(2):461–467. e1–e5.

246. Verstovsek S, Tefferi A, Kantarjian H, et al. Alemtuzumab therapy for hypereosinophilic syndrome and chronic eosinophilic leukemia. *Clin Cancer Res.* 2009;15:368–373.

247. Kalac M, Quintas Cardama A, Vrhovac R, Kantarjian H, Verstovsek S. A critical appraisal of conventional and investigational drug therapy in patients with hypereosinophilic syndrome and clonal eosinophilia. *Cancer.* 2007;110:955–964.

248. Pitini V, Teti D, Arrigo C, Righi M. Alemtuzumab therapy for refractory idiopathic hypereosinophilic syndrome with abnormal T cells: a case report. *Br J Haematol.* 2004;127:477.

249. Halaburda K, Prejzner W, Szatkowski D, Limon J, Hellmann A. Allogeneic bone marrow transplantation for hypereosinophilic syndrome: long-term follow-up with eradication of FIP1L1-PDGFRA fusion transcript. *Bone Marrow Transplant.* 2006;38:319–320.

250. Parillo JE, Lawley TJ, Frank MM, Kaplan AP, Fauci AS. Immunologic reactivity in the hypereosinophilic syndrome. *J Allergy Clin Immunol.* 1979;64:113–121.

251. Parillo JE, Fauci AS, Wolff SM. Therapy of the hypereosinophilic syndrome. *Ann Intern Med.* 1978;89:167–172.

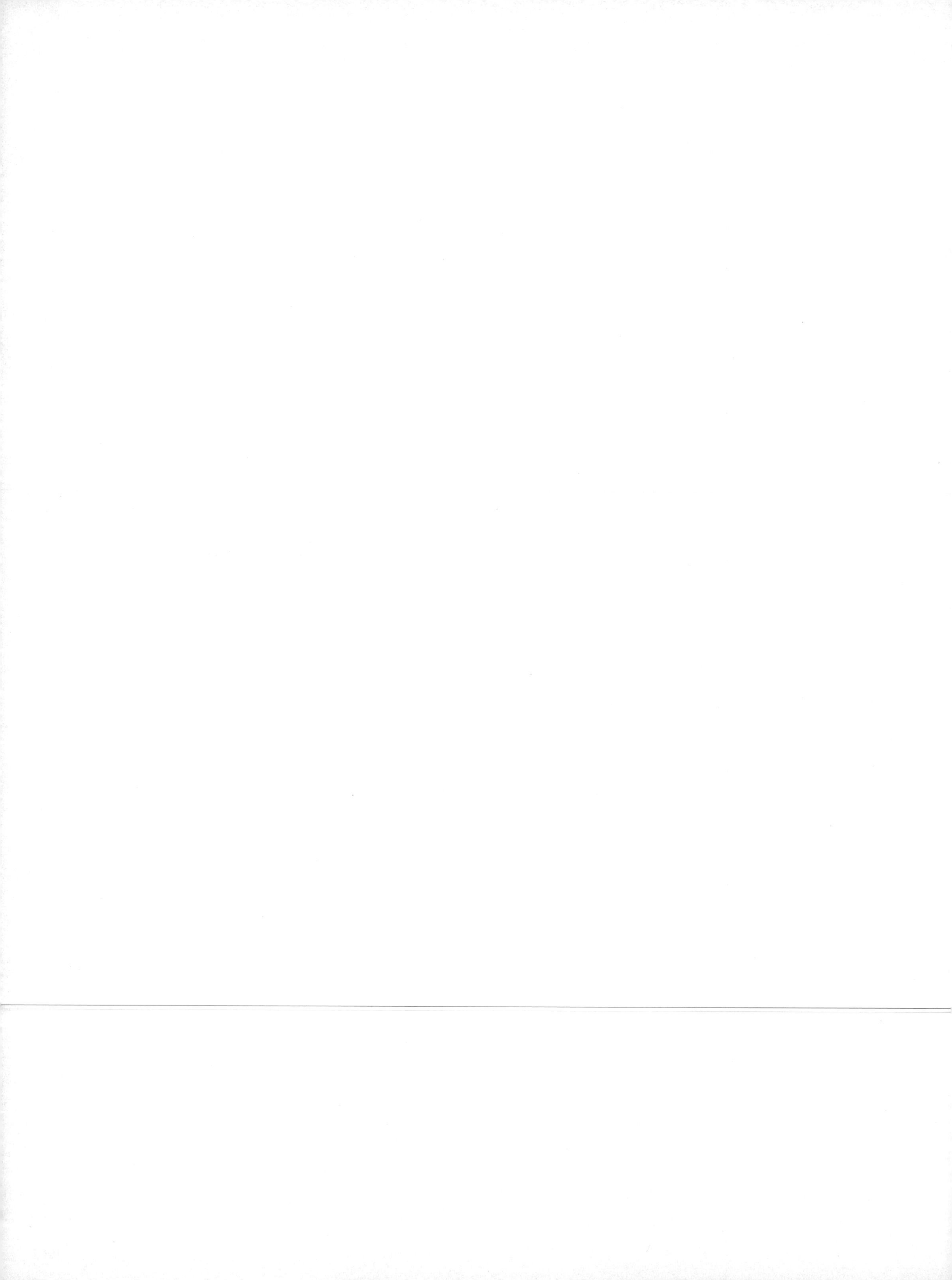

PART 8

Disorders of the Pulmonary Circulation

CHAPTER 72

Pulmonary Arterial Hypertension

Darren B. Taichman
Jess Mandel
Kimberly A. Smith
Jason X.-J. Yuan

Pulmonary arterial hypertension (PAH) is a progressive disease of the pulmonary vasculature in which an ever increasing resistance to circulatory flow imposes a mounting afterload for the right heart to overcome. Without therapy, and frequently despite it, patients with PAH suffer progressive and inexorable right heart failure, functional decline, and ultimately die. Although rapid progress has resulted in the availability of therapy that can improve the outlook for many patients, long delays in disease recognition are common, exposing patients to prolonged suffering and potentially irreversible harm.

PAH is one of several possible causes of pulmonary hypertension. Pulmonary hypertension is defined as a mean pulmonary artery pressure greater than or equal to 25 mm Hg at rest. It can be due to diseases primarily isolated to the pulmonary vasculature itself, as in PAH, or can be a complication of other diseases, including hypoxemic lung disorders (e.g., chronic obstructive pulmonary disease [COPD]), left heart disease (e.g., systolic, diastolic, or valvular dysfunctions), or thromboembolism.[1,2] Identification of its cause is essential, as appropriate therapy for pulmonary hypertension is aimed at its underlying cause—be that repair of a stenotic mitral valve, bronchodilators for obstructive lung disease or, in the case of PAH, the use of advanced therapies targeted at the pulmonary vasculature.

CLASSIFICATION OF THE PULMONARY HYPERTENSIVE DISEASES

A "sclerosis of the pulmonary arteries" ("Uber Sklerose der Lungen Arterie") without identifiable cause was first described by Ernst von Romberg in 1891.[3] Exclusively descriptive reports of pathologic findings continued until the 1950s when the development of catheterization techniques allowed for hemodynamic evaluation. Using such methods, Dresdale and colleagues described a hypertensive vasculopathy of the pulmonary circulation involving vasoconstriction, elevation of pulmonary arterial pressures (PAPs), and a measurable response to the injection of the nonselective alpha adrenergic antagonist tolazoline.[4] No cause could be identified for the pulmonary arteriopathy and the term primary pulmonary hypertension (PPH) was introduced.[5]

Subsequent classification schemes for diseases-causing pulmonary hypertension have been adopted by international consensus panels. These have evolved from systems based primarily on histopathologic findings to a current model that emphasizes the grouping of entities according to similarities in hemodynamic and clinical characteristics (Table 72-1).[6] Importantly, accurate classification of pulmonary hypertension is essential to guide the rational and appropriate use of medications.

It is important to note the specific nomenclature purposefully adopted in the current classification scheme. The group of patients with PAH is identified as distinct from those patients with other causes of pulmonary hypertension (e.g., due to chronic left heart or respiratory disease). This grouping recognizes similarities in the histologic and many clinical features of patients with identifiable genetic causes of PAH (i.e., those with heritable PAH), collagen vascular or other diseases known to be associated with PAH (Associated PAH), and patients in whom no known associated entity or genetic cause has

TABLE 72-1 Updated Classification of Pulmonary Hypertension[a]

1.	Pulmonary arterial hypertension
1.1	Idiopathic PAH
1.2	Heritable PAH
1.2.1	BMPR2
1.2.2	ALK-1, ENG, SMADS, CAV1, KCNK3
1.2.3	Unknown
1.3	Drug and toxin induced
1.4	Associated with:
1.4.1	Connective tissue disease
1.4.2	HIV infection
1.4.3	Portal hypertension
1.4.4	Congenital heart diseases
1.4.5	Schistosomiasis
1′	Pulmonary veno-occlusive disease and/or pulmonary capillary hemangiomatosis
1″.	Persistent pulmonary hypertension of the newborn (PPHN)
2.	Pulmonary hypertension due to left heart disease
2.1	Left ventricular systolic dysfunction
2.2	Left ventricular diastolic dysfunction
2.3	Valvular disease
2.4	Congenital/acquired left heart inflow/outflow tract obstruction and congenital cardiomyopathies
3.	Pulmonary hypertension due to lung diseases and/or hypoxia
3.1	Chronic obstructive pulmonary disease
3.2	Interstitial lung disease
3.3	Other pulmonary diseases with mixed restrictive and obstructive pattern
3.4	Sleep-disordered breathing
3.5	Alveolar hypoventilation disorders
3.6	Chronic exposure to high altitude
3.7	Developmental lung diseases
4.	Chronic thromboembolic pulmonary hypertension (CTEPH)
5.	Pulmonary hypertension with unclear multifactorial mechanisms
5.1	Hematologic disorders: chronic hemolytic anemia, myeloproliferative disorders, splenectomy
5.2	Systemic disorders: sarcoidosis, pulmonary histiocytosis, lymphangioleiomyomatosis
5.3	Metabolic disorders: glycogen storage disease, Gaucher disease, thyroid disorders
5.4	Others: tumoral obstruction, fibrosing mediastinitis, chronic renal failure, segmental PH

[a]5th WSPH Nice 2013. Main modifications to the previous Dana Point classification are in bold.
BMPR2, bone morphogenetic protein receptor type II; CAV1, caveolin 1; ENG, endogin; HIV, human immunodeficiency virus; PAH, pulmonary arterial hypertension.
Source: Adapted with permission from Simonneau G, Robbins IM, Beghetti M, et al. Updated clinical classification of pulmonary hypertension. J Am Coll Cardiol. 2009;54(1 Suppl):S43–S54.

been found. This last group is referred to as having idiopathic PAH (IPAH). IPAH replaces the previously (and often loosely) used term "PPH." Abandonment of the term "primary" also is important as a means of discouraging the use of the confusing and clinically inappropriate term "secondary" pulmonary hypertension. Use of such "primary" and "secondary" groupings may inappropriately suggest clinical similarities among the many very different diseases previously referred to as "secondary" pulmonary hypertension (e.g., patients with COPD and those with congenital heart disease). It may also promote a failure to recognize important similarities in clinical features (including appropriate treatment) between what was previously called "primary" pulmonary hypertension and entities inappropriately labeled "secondary" (e.g., patients with Eisenmenger syndrome or HIV infection).

DETERMINANTS OF PULMONARY ARTERY PRESSURE AND PULMONARY VASCULAR RESISTANCE

The pulmonary circulation normally is a high-flow, low-resistance, low-pressure system that carries blood into the pulmonary microcirculation where the blood takes up oxygen and unloads excess carbon dioxide. From early childhood to the fifth decade of life, the mean PAP is approximately 20 mm Hg.[7] PAP is the product of cardiac output (CO) and pulmonary vascular resistance (PVR) as shown in equation 1 (Eq. 1), where PVR is the vascular resistance of the entire lung, including the pulmonary arteries, capillaries, and veins.

$$PAP = CO \times [PVR_{arteries} + PVR_{capillaries} + PVR_{veins}] \quad \text{(Eq. 1)}$$

From this equation, it is clear that PAP can be raised by an increase in CO or an increase in arterial, capillary, or venous resistance. It would be expected then, that during periods of increased CO, such as during strenuous exercise, there would be a significant increase in PAP. However, in a normal healthy individual, the PAP is only slightly increased during periods of increased CO due to the compensatory increase in the cross-sectional area of the pulmonary vascular bed (due to recruitment of previously unperfused vessels and distension of vessels) resulting in a decreased PVR. Arterial distension and optimal recruitment are dependent upon the compliance of the blood vessel walls. Loss of this compliance due to vascular remodeling leads to pulmonary hypertension. As demonstrated in Eq. 1, an increase in PVR of any of the three components of the pulmonary vasculature can lead to an increase in PAP.[8]

Eq. 1 demonstrates the physical laws that govern blood flow in the lungs. To further understand and use this equation, we must know its physical and anatomical foundations. When a liquid (e.g., blood) flows through a cylindrical tubular structure (e.g., a blood vessel), the resistance (e.g., PVR) is inversely proportional to the fourth power of the radius of the lumen of the tube. This is demonstrated by the Poiseuille equation (Eq. 2), where L is the length of the tube (or vessel), r is the inner radius of the tube, and η is the coefficient of viscosity of the liquid (blood). Therefore, even small changes in the radius of a vessel can significantly change the PVR.[8]

$$PVR = (8L\eta)/\pi \times 1/r^4 \quad \text{(Eq. 2)}$$

PULMONARY VASCULAR STRUCTURAL AND FUNCTIONAL CHANGES IN PULMONARY HYPERTENSION

Regardless of the initial genetic or pathogenic trigger, the increased PVR seen in pulmonary hypertension can be attributed to the collective effects of sustained vasoconstriction, vascular remodeling, in situ thrombosis, and increased arterial wall stiffness (Fig. 72-1).[8–13] A rise in cytosolic free Ca^{2+} concentration ($[Ca^{2+}]_{cyt}$)

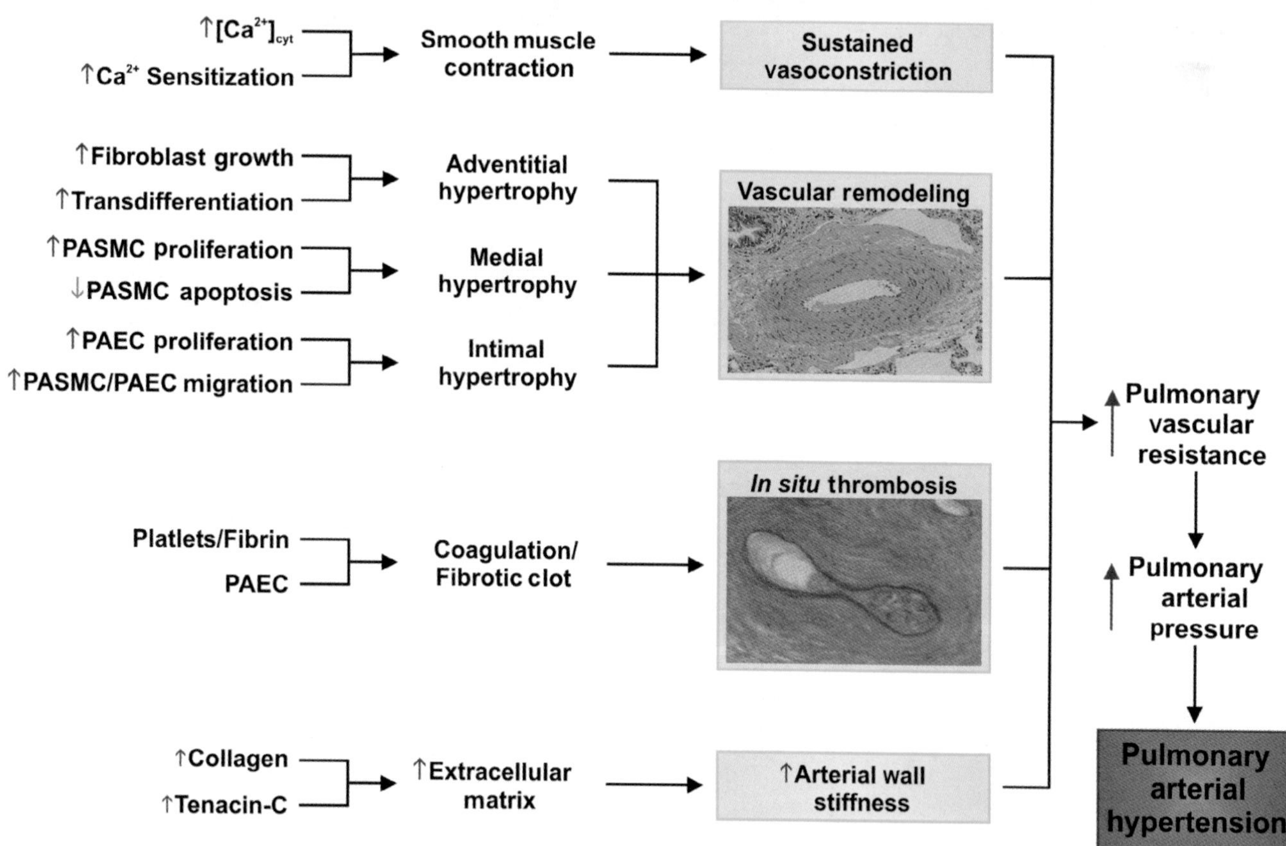

Figure 72-1 Schematic illustration of pathophysiologic components contributing to the development of increased pulmonary vascular resistance, pulmonary arterial pressure, and pulmonary arterial hypertension. *(In situ thrombosis figure reproduced with permission from Zwicke D. PAH and pregnancy: Physiological changes, challenges, and outcomes. Advances in Pulmonary Hypertension. Fall; 2011;10(3).)*

in pulmonary arterial smooth muscle cells is a major trigger for vasoconstriction and a key stimulus for pulmonary arterial smooth muscle cell proliferation and migration, which contributes to vascular remodeling.

■ SUSTAINED VASOCONSTRICTION

Pulmonary vasoconstriction can be a major contributor to increased PVR and hence PAP. Vasoconstrictive lesions include medial hypertrophy involving an increase in the number and size of pulmonary arterial smooth muscle cells. The elevated PAP and sustained vasoconstriction in PAH can, in turn, enhance pulmonary arterial smooth muscle cell hypertrophy and hyperplasia.[14] Marked smooth muscle hypertrophy can eventually cause medial atrophy, fibrosis, and the subsequent thinning of the media and dilation of the vessel lumen. Extension of pulmonary arterial smooth muscle cells into vessels normally only partially muscularized or nonmuscularized is a common and often prominent feature of precapillary vessels (Fig. 72-2).[15]

Hypoxic pulmonary vasoconstriction is an adaptive mechanism important for redirecting blood flow away from poorly ventilated areas of the lung and into the better ventilated areas to maximize the ventilation–perfusion matching and optimize oxygenation of blood.[16–19] Hypoxia induces vasoconstriction in isolated pulmonary arteries without the endothelium and also induces contraction in a single isolated pulmonary arterial smooth muscle cell model, indicating that hypoxic pulmonary vasoconstriction is an intrinsic property of pulmonary arterial smooth muscle cells. In chronic hypoxia, two factors contribute to increased PAP: vascular remodeling due to pulmonary arterial smooth muscle cell proliferation and sustained vasoconstriction and structural changes that develop within a matter of weeks.[20,21] This remodeling is characterized by thickening of the media of the small pulmonary arteries and arterioles, and by peripheral extension of muscle into minute pulmonary vessels that are normally devoid of muscle (Fig. 72-2).[22] Although the precise mechanism by which hypoxia induces pulmonary vasoconstriction is still somewhat unclear, the signaling pathways initiated in response to acute and chronic hypoxia seem to relate, at least in part, to disrupted Ca^{2+} homeostasis.[8,23]

■ VASCULAR REMODELING

The thickness and tissue mass of the pulmonary arterial walls are maintained at an appropriate level by a fine balance between proliferation and apoptosis of fibroblasts, pulmonary arterial smooth muscle cells, and pulmonary arterial endothelial cells. Thickening of the wall and luminal narrowing and eventual obliteration can occur if the balance is tipped in favor of cell proliferation. These structural changes that lead to hypertrophy and/or luminal occlusion are referred to as pulmonary vascular remodeling.[24–26] The precise cellular and molecular mechanisms contributing to vascular remodeling are extremely complex. However, vasoconstriction and cellular proliferation share a common pathway. Increased proliferation and hypertrophy of pulmonary arterial smooth muscle cells have been implicated in the development of PAH and these processes, like vasoconstriction, relate in part to disturbed Ca^{2+} homeostasis.[7] Resting $[Ca^{2+}]_{cyt}$ is increased in proliferating pulmonary artery smooth muscle cells compared to growth-arrested cells, demonstrating a role for enhanced Ca^{2+} in both proliferation and vasoconstriction.[27,28] In addition to increased proliferation, decreased apoptosis has been implicated in the development and maintenance of severe pulmonary hypertension,[29] and induction of apoptosis has been shown to promote the regression of hypertrophied pulmonary vascular walls in animal experiments.[30] Hypoxia can induce proliferation of pulmonary arterial adventitial fibroblasts, and in pulmonary hypertension patients, hypoxia induces the appearance of α-smooth muscle actin in the proliferative and matrix-producing fibroblasts, suggesting these cells have transdifferentiated into myofibroblasts.[31] Therefore, fibroblasts may play an important role in vascular remodeling due to hypoxia.

Complex lesions such as plexiform lesions also contribute to vascular remodeling. Plexiform lesions are aneurysmatic dilations of a muscular artery that can occur in very small arteries and arterioles.[8,32] These lesions are often found in patients with IPAH, but they

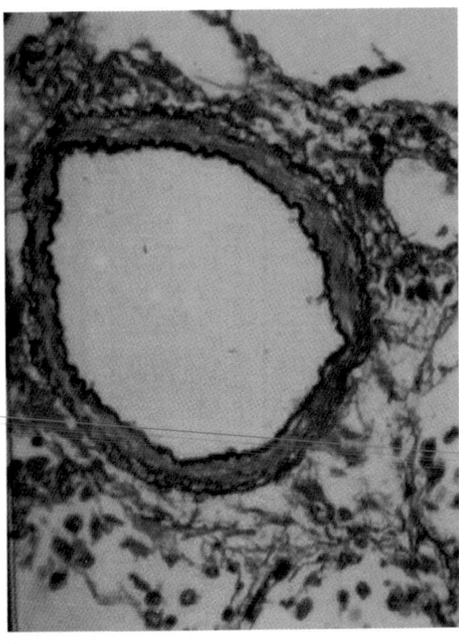

A

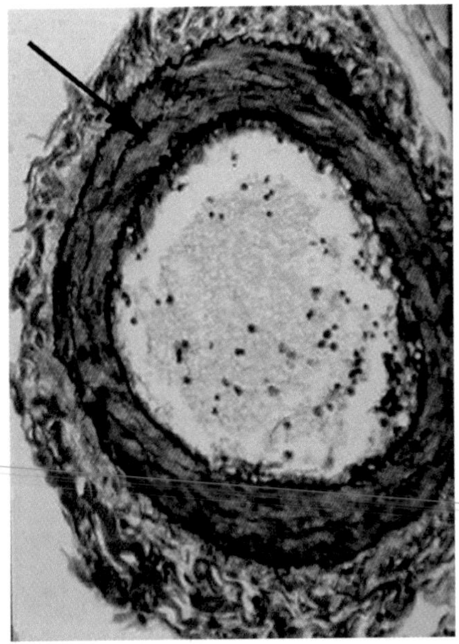

B

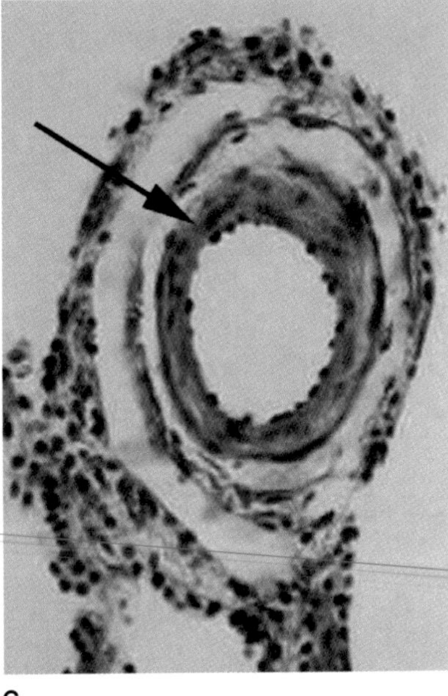

C

Figure 72-2 Vascular remodeling. As compared with a normal vessel (**A**), hypertrophy of smooth muscle cells *(arrow)* is seen in the pulmonary artery of a patient with pulmonary arterial hypertension (**B**). Extension of muscle *(arrow)* into normally nonmuscularized small intra-acinar pulmonary vessels is another prominent feature of pulmonary arterial hypertension (**C**). *(Reproduced with permission from Taichman DB, Snow JL, Pietra GG. Histopathology of pulmonary arterial hypertension. In: Pulmonary Vascular Disease, Mandel J, Taichman DB. Philadelphia: WB. Saunders; 2006.)*

also occur in the lungs of patients with severe PAH associated with left-to-right cardiac shunts, HIV infection, liver cirrhosis, and scleroderma. Although not pathognomonic, the plexiform lesion has been the focus of many studies of the cellular and molecular pathogenesis of PAH.[33–36] They contain collections of proliferating endothelial and smooth muscle cells, together with myofibroblasts and matrix proteins that can partially or completely occlude the vessel lumen. Narrowing or complete obliteration of the parent vessel by intimal thickening is a frequent associated finding, as is destruction of its media. Plexiform lesions often coexist with other obliterative vascular changes such as concentric laminar intimal thickening.[37]

The origin of plexiform lesions is complex and somewhat controversial. Originally, plexiform lesions were considered a congenital malformation.[38] Currently, there are investigators who believe that plexiform lesions develop due to the proliferation of pulmonary arterial smooth muscle cells that transform into myofibroblasts.[39–41] Other investigators propose that, in IPAH patients, plexiform lesions develop due to an endothelial-initiated response to cytokines, growth factors, or vascular injury.[39,41,42] Endothelial cells isolated from the plexiform lesions of IPAH patients proliferate in a monoclonal fashion. However, plexiform lesions from patients with forms of pulmonary hypertension other than IPAH develop from a polyclonal cell population, suggesting different mechanisms contribute to plexiform lesion development in different forms of PAH.[8,43]

■ IN SITU THROMBOSIS

Monoclonal proliferation of pulmonary arterial endothelial cells, pulmonary arterial smooth muscle cell migration, and accumulation of circulating inflammatory cells, platelets, and progenitor cells can result in occlusion of smaller vessels.[11,42] Thrombosis is frequently seen within the small vessels of patients with PAH. This occurs without evidence of a remote (embolic) source of the thrombus,[44–47] suggesting a local imbalance of pro- and anticoagulant forces. Activation and altered function of the endothelium leading to a shift from anti- to procoagulant activities might be due to the effects of shear stress associated with elevated pressure and/or flow. In addition to altered endothelial cell activity, platelets also promote thrombus formation by releasing vasoactive and mitogenic factors such as thromboxane metabolites and serotonin.[48] These, as well as other platelet-derived products (e.g., platelet-derived growth factor [PGDF], transforming growth factor-beta (TGFβ), and vascular endothelial growth factor [VEGF]) likely also contribute to the remodeling of vessel walls seen in PAH.

■ INCREASED ARTERIAL WALL STIFFNESS

Increased arterial wall stiffness can also contribute to increased PVR.[49,50] The normal turnover of extracellular matrix proteins is accelerated with remodeling of the vasculature in PAH patients.[51,52] The expression of tenascin-C, for example, is increased in experimental pulmonary hypertension induced by either monocrotaline in rats or increased blood flow in swine.[53–55] Indeed, inhibition of tenascin-C expression by antisense RNA ameliorates monocrotaline-induced pulmonary vascular lesions.[56] Elevated levels of this extracellular matrix protein are also seen on pulmonary arteries of patients with PAH.[57,58] Decreased vascular compliance resulting in the inability to recruit previously unperfused vessels due to increased parenchymal stiffness can also contribute to the development of PAH.[11,42] As a result, there is little capacity for distention and modest increases in pulmonary blood flow can elicit disproportionate elevations in PAPs. This situation is in marked contrast to that of the normal pulmonary circulation, in which an amputation of considerable lung parenchyma rarely suffices, per se, to raise PAPs to pulmonary hypertensive levels, as the remaining vessels retain their normal high capacitance. In some interstitial lung diseases, such as progressive systemic sclerosis, the parenchymal disease and the pulmonary vascular disease can evolve independently. In other connective tissue disorders, such as systemic lupus erythematosis, combinations of interstitial disease and intrinsic vascular abnormalities can contribute to pulmonary hypertension. While there are many structural changes in the pulmonary vasculature that lead to the development of PAH, vasoconstriction and vascular remodeling characterized by intimal, medial, and adventitial hypertrophy are the major structural changes that contribute to the increased PVR/PAP seen in PAH patients.

No single histologic feature distinguishes between the clinical PAH diagnoses. Each of the changes described can be seen in varying proportions in all clinical forms of PAH. For example, the vascular remodeling seen in chronic hypoxia-induced pulmonary hypertension is virtually indistinguishable from that seen in IPAH.[8] The predominant causes of the increased PVR in patients with PAH are sustained vasoconstriction, vascular remodeling, in situ thrombosis, and increased arterial wall stiffness. Persistent pulmonary hypertension, regardless of the cause, can ultimately lead to the development of cor pulmonale with hypertrophy of the right ventricle, its eventual dilation, and ultimately its failure (Fig. 72-3).

PATHOGENIC MECHANISMS OF PULMONARY HYPERTENSION

The pathogenic mechanisms leading to pulmonary hypertension have been conceptualized in six categories (Table 72-2): (1) *passive,* due to obstruction to pulmonary venous outflow (e.g., fibrosing mediastinitis, mitral stenosis, or left heart failure); (2) *hyperkinetic,* due to abnormally high pulmonary blood flow (e.g., left-to-right shunts); (3) *obstructive,* due to pulmonary thromboembolic disease; (4) *obliterative,* due to destruction of the pulmonary vascular bed by parenchymal proliferative disease; (5) *vasoconstrictive,* due to hypoxic vasoconstriction; and (6) *idiopathic* (i.e., without discernible cause).[59] Each mechanism leads to pulmonary vascular remodeling discussed previously, though the progression and reversibility may vary between entities. Other anatomic alterations can be seen in several categories and, over time, distinctions between categories tend to become blurred (e.g., thrombosis may complicate obliterative vascular disease). Also, by the time pulmonary hypertension becomes manifest clinically, the pulmonary arterial tree has undergone considerable remodeling that limits its area and distensibility.

These mechanisms share commonality with the clinical classification of pulmonary hypertension, though overlap of mechanisms occur. The most clearly linked is chronic thromboembolic pulmonary hypertension (CTEPH) with the obstructive mechanism. The most common form of pulmonary hypertension, that related to left heart failure, can also closely be tied to its passive mechanism along with fibrosing mediastinitis, which is classified in group 5 with unclear multifactorial mechanisms. Pulmonary hypertension owing to lung diseases and/or hypoxia, group 3, can be understood as having two primary pathogenic mechanisms, vasoconstrictive in the chronic hypoxic subset and obliterative in the parenchymal disease/fibrosis subset, though these two often overlap. Group 5, pulmonary hypertension with unclear multifactorial mechanisms by definition contains multiple pathogenic mechanisms. Group 1 remains the most diverse and difficult to equate to a particular mechanism as hyperkinetic, vasoconstrictive, obliterative, and other idiopathic mechanisms all contribute to disease pathophysiology.

GENETIC, CELLULAR, AND MOLECULAR MECHANISMS OF PULMONARY ARTERIAL HYPERTENSION

The development of PAH involves increased PVR due to sustained vasoconstriction, vascular remodeling, in situ thrombosis, and increased atrial wall stiffness (Fig. 72-1). Abnormalities in the expression of numerous vasoactive mediators, vasoconstriction mediators, growth factors, and cytokines cause, or result from

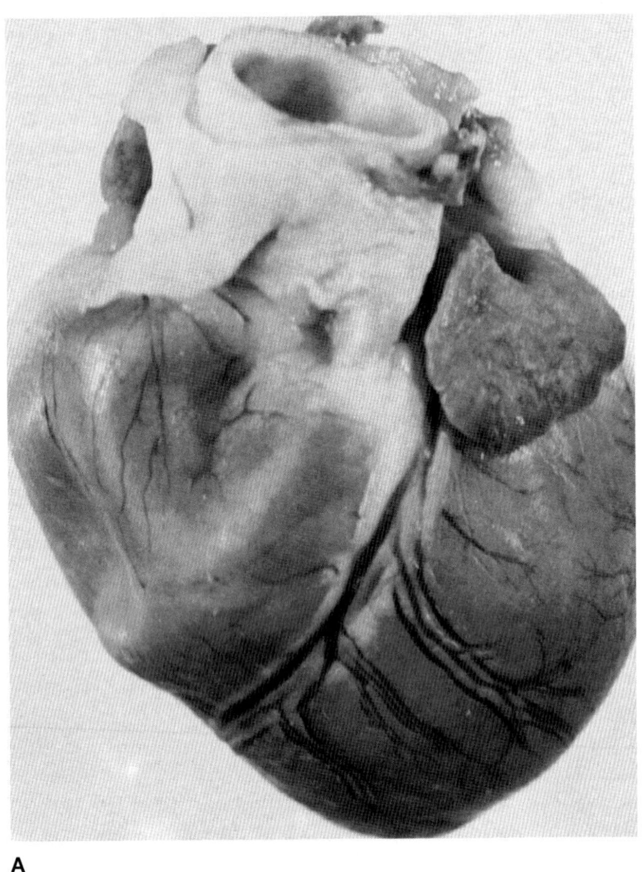
A

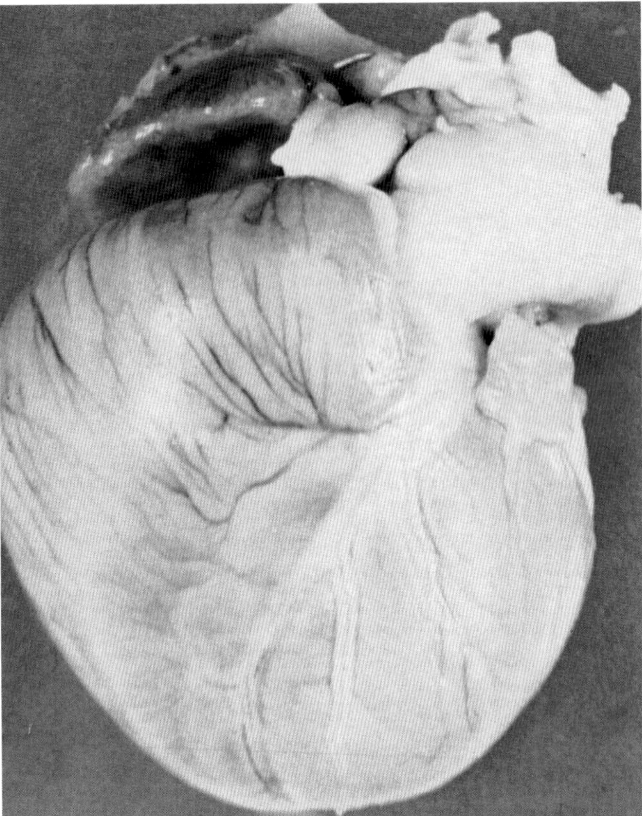
B

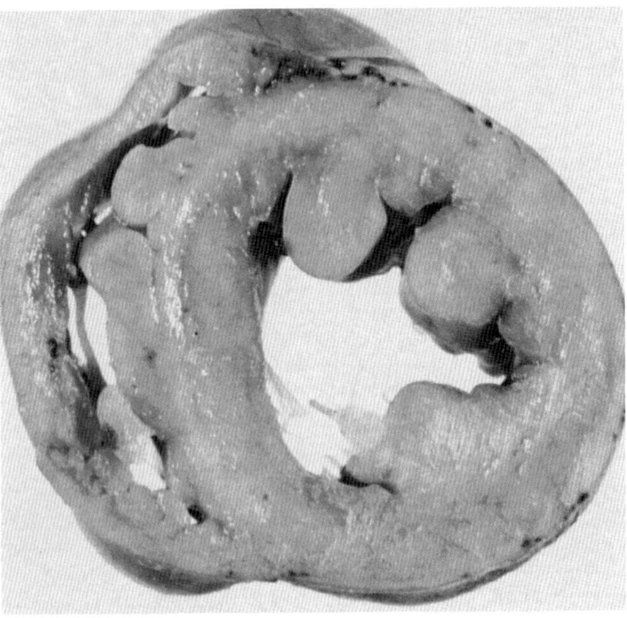
C

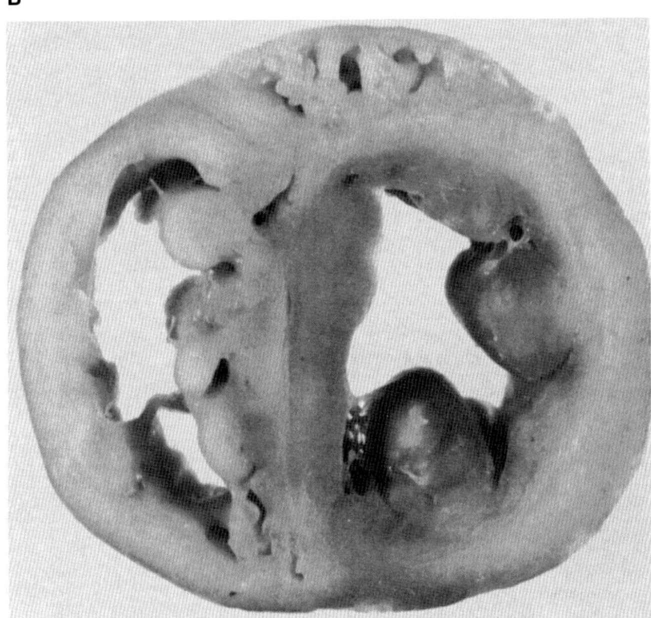
D

Figure 72-3 Cor pulmonale in experimental pulmonary arterial hypertension in the dog. **A.** Normal heart. **B.** Chronic cor pulmonale secondary to severe pulmonary arterial hypertension. **C.** Cross section of normal heart to show thin wall of the right ventricular cavity. **D.** Cross section of heart with chronic cor pulmonale to show hypertrophy of the right ventricular myocardium and enlargement of the right ventricular cavity. *(Used with permission of Dr. B. Atkinson.)*

changes in pulmonary arterial endothelial cells, pulmonary arterial smooth muscle cells, and platelet function and together result in a thickened vessel wall and markedly narrowed or even completely obliterated lumen. Some of the mechanisms for this combination of uncontrolled vasoconstriction, cell proliferation, and thrombosis are highlighted here.

■ IMBALANCE OF VASOACTIVE MEDIATORS

Relative deficiencies of factors with vasodilatory properties and a simultaneous excess in those promoting vasoconstriction have been noted in both animal models and patients with PAH. In addition to vasoconstriction/dilation, these same factors influence cell proliferation and thrombosis. Deficiencies in the production

TABLE 72-2 Pathogenetic Mechanisms of Pulmonary Hypertension

	Mechanism	Examples
Passive	Pulmonary venous hypertension	Mitral stenosis, left atrial myxoma, fibrosing mediastinitis, pulmonary venoocclusive disease
Hyperkinetic	Increased pulmonary blood flow[a]	Left-to-right intracardiac shunts
Obstructive	Thromboembolic pulmonary vascular disease	High grade obstruction of large pulmonary arteries by organized thromboemboli, multiple pulmonary emboli
Obliterative	Inflammatory and/or proliferative pulmonary vascular disease	Interstitial lung disease, pulmonary arterial hypertension, schistosomiasis
Venoconstrictive	Hypoxia	High altitude, chronic bronchitis and emphysema (COPD)
Idiopathic	Unknown	Drug-associated pulmonary hypertension, portopulmonary hypertension, HIV infection

[a]Most categories overlap to some extent. For example, increased pulmonary blood flow is usually coupled with anatomic changes in the resistance vessels to produce pulmonary hypertension.

of the potent vasodilators nitric oxide (NO) and prostacyclin have each been observed, and indeed both substances have been used as a basis for effective therapies for PAH. Normally produced by vascular endothelial cells, each promotes the formation of cyclic nucleotides (cGMP and cAMP) by pulmonary arterial smooth muscle cells resulting in their relaxation and vasodilation. In addition, both prostacyclin and NO inhibit pulmonary arterial smooth muscle cell proliferation and platelet aggregation. In patients with PAH, the chronic administration of prostacyclin analogs improves hemodynamics, exercise capacity, and survival. The overexpression of NO synthase (NOS) by transgenic animals protects against the development of hypoxia-induced pulmonary hypertension, whereas mice lacking the gene for this enzyme develop severe pulmonary hypertension upon exposure to mild hypoxia.[60–62] In rats, monocrotaline-induced pulmonary hypertension can be prevented, or even reversed, with the administration of endothelial progenitor cells overexpressing human endothelial NOS (eNOS).[63] Inhaled NO has been proposed for the treatment of PAH and persistent pulmonary hypertension of the newborn,[64] however, inhaled NO has limitations regarding dose and duration of the exposure.[65] The inorganic anion nitrite (NO_2^-) is an oxidative product of NO metabolism and can function as an intravascular reservoir of NO bioactivity that can be converted to NO under physiologic and pathologic conditions.[65] Studies have shown that inhaled nebulized nitrite can prevent and reverse established pulmonary hypertension in the monocrotaline-induced rat pulmonary hypertension model.[66,67]

Vasoactive intestinal protein (VIP) also promotes vasodilation and inhibits smooth muscle proliferation and platelet aggregation. VIP levels are reduced in patients with PAH. In a preliminary study of 8 patients with IPAH, treatment with inhaled VIP improved hemodynamics and exercise capacity.[68] The acute effect of inhaled VIP was confirmed in a subsequent study that included patients with multiple etiologies of pulmonary hypertension including IPAH, congenital heart disease, CTEPH, and pulmonary hypertension related to parenchymal lung disease, although the modest effect on hemodynamics had questionable clinical relevance.[69]

INCREASE IN VASOCONSTRICTION MEDIATORS

In addition to deficiencies in vasodilators, excesses of other mediators capable of promoting vasoconstriction, smooth muscle proliferation, or platelet aggregation have been noted in patients with PAH. Thromboxane, an arachidonic acid metabolite produced by endothelial cells and platelets, causes vasoconstriction, platelet aggregation, and is a smooth muscle mitogen. Increased thromboxane metabolites have been documented in the urine of patients with PAH.[48] Attention was focused on the effects of serotonin (5-HT) on the pulmonary circulation by the epidemic of PAH in patients who ingested the appetite suppressants aminorex and fenfluramine.[70] These agents increase plasma 5-HT levels by inducing the release of 5-HT from platelets and interfering with its reuptake.[71] The 5-HT hypothesis was supported by the occurrence of pulmonary hypertension in fawn-hooded rats with an inherited defect in the platelet storage of 5-HT, and by an increase in circulating 5-HT in a patient with platelet storage disease and PAH.[72] 5-HT causes vasoconstriction and is a smooth muscle mitogen (Fig. 72-4). A key regulator of 5-HT action is the 5-HT transporter (5-HTT) whose expression is increased above normal in platelets and the pulmonary arteries of patients with IPAH. The overexpression of the 5-HTT gene in recombinant mice results in worsened hypoxia-induced pulmonary hypertension[73] whereas loss of the gene's function is protective against hypoxia or monocrotaline-induced disease.[74,75] A polymorphism in the 5-HTT gene that increases its activity may confer an increased susceptibility to the development of pulmonary hypertension in patients with COPD.[76] While some studies have suggested a similar role in IPAH,[77] larger data sets have not found such an association.[78] Blockade of the 5-HT receptor has successfully prevented the development and progression of experimental pulmonary hypertension in rats, yet a human trial was not able to show significant decreases in PVR.[79,80]

Endothelin-1 (ET-1) is one of the most potent endogenous vasoconstrictors known. Its expression is increased in the blood and tissues of patients with idiopathic and other forms of PAH and correlates with disease severity.[81–83] In addition to its vasoconstricting properties, ET-1 is mitogenic for both pulmonary arterial smooth muscle cells and fibroblasts (Fig. 72-4).[84,85] ET-1 administration or overexpression in animal models has been shown to result in fibrosis, inflammation, and platelet aggregation.[86,87] ET-1 binds endothelin A (ET_A) and B (ET_B) receptors on the surface of pulmonary arterial smooth muscle cells, resulting in potent vasoconstriction. ET_B receptors on pulmonary arterial endothelial cells increase the production of nitric oxide, resulting in vasodilatation. ET_B receptors are also active in the clearance of endothelin. The net effect of endothelin's vasoconstricting or dilating actions may be both site and context dependent, as both the distribution and relative expression of the ET_A and ET_B receptors differ according to vessel location in normal lung tissue, and are altered in patients with IPAH.[88,89] Indeed, both selective ET_A and dual ET_A/ET_B inhibition improve the hemodynamic derangements and clinical outcome of patients with PAH.[90–92]

INCREASED EXPRESSION OF GROWTH FACTORS

Growth factors that promote the maturation and stabilization of the developing vasculature have also been implicated in the

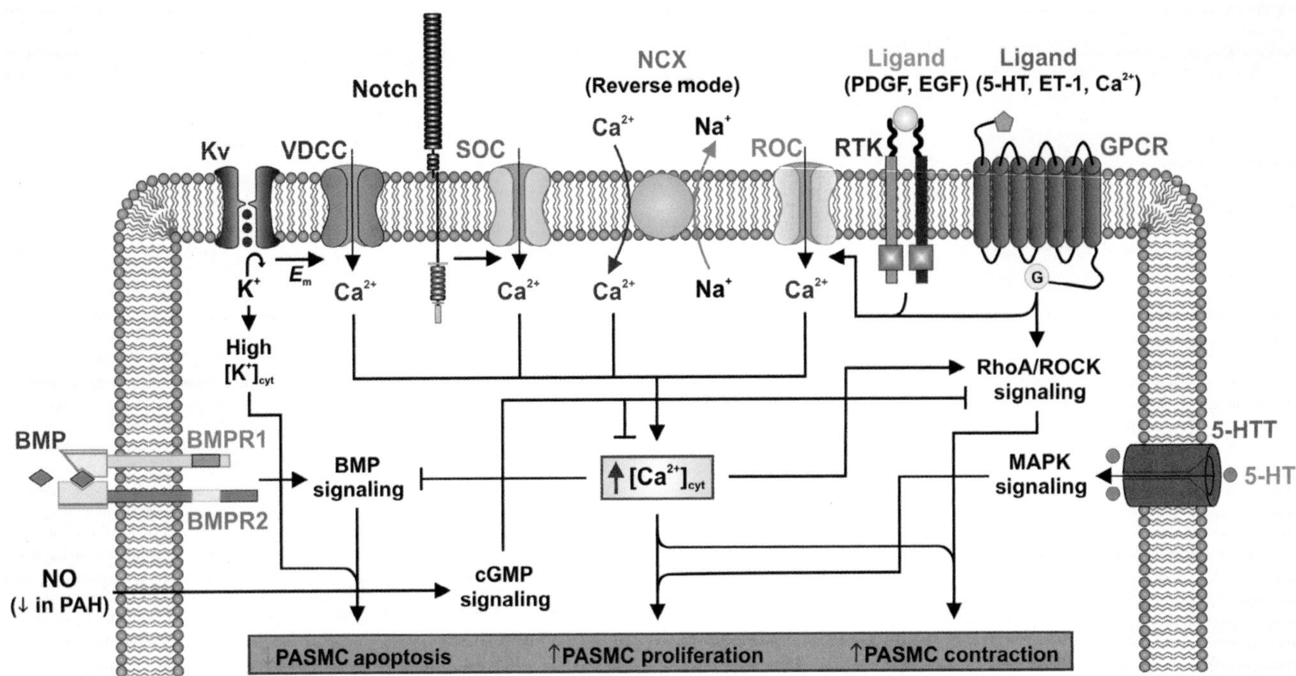

Figure 72-4 Potential mechanisms involved in the development of pulmonary arterial hypertension. Schematic diagram depicting potential mechanisms involved in the development of pulmonary arterial hypertension. BMP, bone morphogenic protein; BMPR, bone morphogenic protein receptor; cGMP, cyclic guanosine monophosphate; E_m, membrane potential; ET-1, endothelin 1; EGF, epidermal growth factor; GPCR, G-protein–coupled receptor; 5-HT, hydroxytryptamine (serotonin); 5-HTT, hydroxytryptamine (serotonin) transporter; Kv, voltage-gated K^+ channel; MAPK, mitogen-activated protein kinase; NO, nitric oxide; NCX, Na^+/Ca^{2+} exchanger; PAH, pulmonary arterial hypertension; PASMC, pulmonary arterial smooth muscle cell; PDGF, platelet-derived growth factor; ROC, receptor-operated Ca^{2+} channel; RTK, receptor tyrosine kinase; SOC, store-operated Ca^{2+} channel; VDCC, voltage-dependent Ca^{2+} channel.

pathogenesis of PAH. Elevations in angiopoietin 1 and its ligand TIE2 correlate with disease severity in patients with multiple forms of PAH.[93] Angiopoietin 1 is overexpressed in most forms of nonfamilial PAH,[93,94] however, how angiopoietin becomes elevated in these patients is not clear. Several lines of evidence suggest that angiopoietin 1 regulates pulmonary arterial smooth muscle cell hyperplasia in PAH.[9] Interestingly, in an animal model of PAH induced by monocrotaline, the overexpression of angiopoietin is actually protective.[95] Whether this discrepancy represents differences in human versus animal tissues or the differing insults to the vasculature involved is not clear. Another modulator of development, VEGF and its target, tyrosine kinase receptor, are increased in the pulmonary vasculature of patients with PAH. Increased VEGF expression has been reported specifically within plexiform lesions[34,96] where its proangiogenic properties are hypothesized to mediate disordered endothelial cell proliferation.[97] Whether such changes are primary, secondary, or indeed detrimental is not entirely clear. Like elevations in angiopoietin, increases in the expression of VEGF thought to be deleterious in some situations might be beneficial in others that promote the development of pulmonary hypertension. In animal models of hypoxia, the inhibition of VEGF signaling results in proliferative vascular abnormalities[98] and promotion of VEGF signaling is protective against the development of monocrotaline-induced PH.[99]

PDGF along with its receptor, tyrosine kinase, are also found to be increased in the pulmonary vasculature of patients with PAH (Fig. 72-4).[100] PDGF has been implicated in smooth muscle cell proliferation and migration, which is thought to contribute to PAH pathogenesis. The tyrosine kinase inhibitor imatinib has a particular affinity for the PDGF receptor and several small studies have identified a potential benefit in PAH patients.[101] Early human trials have also shown improvements in hemodynamic measurements after treatment.[102]

Cellular microparticles recently have been implicated as vasoactive mediators in PAH. Microparticles represent vesicle fragments of the cell membrane containing various proteins and antigens that are involved in cellular communication.[103] These small particles are released during cell activation or apoptosis and can be derived from multiple cell lines including endothelial cells, platelets, leukocytes, red blood cells, and fibroblasts. Circulating levels of endothelial microparticles are increased in PAH, which may represent endothelial dysfunction and has also been correlated with disease survival.[104] Microparticles, when isolated from rats with hypoxia-induced pulmonary hypertension, have been shown to impair endothelium-dependent vasorelaxation in pulmonary arteries and decrease NO production.[105] Circulating microparticles have also been linked to inflammatory signaling in the lung.[106]

■ INCREASED CYTOKINES AND INFLAMMATION

The close association of systemic inflammatory disorders to IPAH has implicated inflammation as an important factor in vascular remodeling. Numerous cytokines have been implicated in the pathogenesis of PAH including tumor necrosis factor alpha, and interleukins 1b, 2, 4, 6, 8, 10, and 12p70. Early data showed increased levels of IL-1β and IL-6 in IPAH patients[107] and higher IL-6 levels were later found to be associated with mortality.[108] The chemokine fractalkine (CX3CL1) is elevated in CD4 and CD8 T-cells of PAH patients and further studies have shown that CX3CL1 may promote proliferation in pulmonary arterial smooth muscle cells.[109,110] Monocyte chemotactant protein (MCP)-1 is also elevated in serum and lung samples from IPAH patients and may influence monocyte and T-cell recruitment to the diseased lung.[111] Increased expression of Regulated upon Activation, Normal T cell Expressed and Secreted (RANTES) has been found in lung samples from PAH patients.[112] As a chemoattractant for monocytes and T-cells, RANTES is thought to promote inflammation, but may also play a role in the synthesis of endothelin-1, a potent vasoconstrictor.

FUNCTIONAL CHANGES IN MEMBRANE RECEPTORS AND ION CHANNELS

Important functional changes in membrane receptors and ion channels in IPAH are discussed below.

Ca^{2+} CHANNELS IN IPAH

Sustained vasoconstriction and vascular remodeling are both directly mediated by pulmonary arterial smooth muscle cell contraction and proliferation. A rise in $[Ca^{2+}]_{cyt}$ due to Ca^{2+} influx through various Ca^{2+}-permeable channels in the plasma membrane is a major trigger for pulmonary arterial smooth muscle cell contraction and a key stimulus for pulmonary arterial smooth muscle cell proliferation.[113] Therefore, understanding how the regulation of Ca^{2+} homeostasis is disrupted in IPAH is important to understanding how IPAH develops. Pulmonary arterial smooth muscle cells isolated from IPAH patients have an elevated $[Ca^{2+}]_{cyt}$.[114–117] Ca^{2+} influx through the plasma membrane in pulmonary arterial smooth muscle cells involves multiple Ca^{2+}-permeable channels including (a) voltage-dependent Ca^{2+} channels (VDCC) regulated by changes in membrane potential,[118] (b) receptor-operated Ca^{2+} channels (ROC) activated by interaction of agonist with membrane receptors, and (c) store-operated Ca^{2+} channels (SOC) activated by depletion of Ca^{2+} from the intracellular stores (Fig. 72-4).[8] Decreased expression and/or function of K^+ channels leads to sustained membrane depolarization, activation of VDCC, and increased $[Ca^{2+}]_{cyt}$. Ca^{2+} influx through ROC, termed receptor-operated Ca^{2+} entry (ROCE), and through SOC, referred to as store-operated Ca^{2+} entry (SOCE) is enhanced in IPAH-associated pulmonary arterial smooth muscle cells compared to those from normal controls.[114–117] Several experimental studies have demonstrated increased expression of several proteins involved in ROCE/SOCE such as, TRPC3, TRPC6, STIM2, and Orai2, in pulmonary arterial smooth muscle cells from IPAH patients.[114–117,119,120] In addition, a single-nucleotide polymorphism (SNP) has been identified in IPAH patients that results in enhanced expression and function of TRPC6.[115]

K^+CHANNELS IN IPAH

Vascular tone might also be altered in IPAH by changes in the expression of voltage-gated K^+ (Kv) channels as well as other types of K^+ channels (Fig. 72-4). Their activation normally allows an efflux of K^+ and resultant changes in intracellular Ca^{2+} that promote vasodilation.[121] Gene expression of Kv channel family members is downregulated by hypoxia-induced pulmonary hypertension in rats,[122,123] whereas induction of their expression can reverse the hemodynamic effects of hypoxia.[122,124] The expression of specific Kv channels is also decreased in the lungs of patients with IPAH[125–127] possibly contributing to heightened vasoconstriction resulting from a more depolarized membrane leading to increased $[Ca^{2+}]_{cyt}$ due to activation of VDCC. Kv channels may also mediate the effects of certain drugs. The anorexigens dexfenfluramine and aminorex inhibit smooth muscle Kv channel activity, thus causing pulmonary vasoconstriction.[128] In contrast, enhanced activity of Kv channels may be one mechanism by which sildenafil promotes vasodilation in addition to its activity as an inhibitor of phosphodiesterase-5.[122] One final way in which decreased activity of Kv channels might promote the development of PAH is by inhibiting apoptosis, thus enabling unchecked pulmonary arterial smooth muscle cell proliferation. Apoptosis requires a loss in cell volume as well as the function of specific caspases, both of which require appropriate K^+ movement via Kv channels.[129,130]

G-PROTEIN–COUPLED RECEPTORS IN IPAH

The Ca^{2+}-sensing receptor is a G-protein–coupled receptor in the plasma membrane that can be activated by extracellular Ca^{2+} (and Mg^{2+}), polyamines (e.g., spermine), amino acids and neomycin.[131–134] Activation of the Ca^{2+}-sensing receptor results in activation of intracellular Ca^{2+} signaling pathways that lead to pulmonary arterial smooth muscle cell contraction, proliferation, and migration (Fig. 72-4).[135,136] Like some G-protein–coupled receptors coupled to Gq (e.g., endothelin receptors), Ca^{2+}-sensing receptor activation increases the synthesis of inositol 1,4,5 triphosphate (IP_3) and diacylglycerol via phospholipase C. IP_3 binds to the IP_3 receptor on the sarcoplasmic reticulum (SR) membrane and releases Ca^{2+} from the SR to the cytosol. Depletion of Ca^{2+} from the SR induces Ca^{2+} entry via SOCE, and diacylglycerol directly activates ROCE. In addition to increasing $[Ca^{2+}]_{cyt}$ via ROCE and SOCE, the extracellular Ca^{2+}-induced activation of CaSR also activates other signal transduction pathways (e.g., Akt/mTOR and MAPK/ERK) to induce cellular proliferation.[137–139] A recent study[135] indicates that the extracellular Ca^{2+}-induced increase in $[Ca^{2+}]_{cyt}$ by activation of the Ca^{2+}-sensing receptor is enhanced and the Ca^{2+}-sensing receptor protein expression is upregulated in IPAH-pulmonary arterial smooth muscle cells compared to normal pulmonary arterial smooth muscle cells. These observations suggest that upregulated expression and enhanced function of Ca^{2+}-sensing receptor in pulmonary arterial smooth muscle cells are involved in the development of sustained pulmonary vasoconstriction and pulmonary vascular remodeling in patients with IPAH and animals with experimental pulmonary hypertension. In addition to Ca^{2+}-sensing receptor, many other G-protein–coupled receptors are reported to be involved in PAH such as endothelin receptor, prostacyclin receptor, and serotonin receptor.[48,140,141]

Na^+/Ca^{2+} EXCHANGER IN IPAH

The Na^+/Ca^{2+} exchanger (NCX) is a ubiquitously expressed protein that transports Ca^{2+} across the plasma membrane along the electrochemical gradient of Na^+ and Ca^{2+}.[142] The NCX can operate in either forward mode, transporting 3 Na^+ ions into the cell and 1 Ca^{2+} ion out of the cell, or the reverse mode, transporting 1 Ca^{2+} ion into the cell and 3 Na^+ ions out of the cell, based on the Na^+ and Ca^{2+} concentration gradients and membrane potential. Due to the reverse mode of the NCX, a small increase in the cytosolic Na^+ concentration ($[Na^+]_{cyt}$) can greatly increase $[Ca^{2+}]_{cyt}$. The canonical transient receptor potential (TRPC) channels, such as TRPC6, which is overexpressed in IPAH patients, are permeable to both Na^+ and Ca^{2+}, and for many TRPC channels, the permeability to Na^+ is greater than the permeability to Ca^{2+}. The reverse mode of the NCX has been shown to couple to TRPC6 and localized increases in $[Na^+]_{cyt}$ result in transport of Ca^{2+} into the cell resulting in increased $[Ca^{2+}]_{cyt}$ in pulmonary arterial smooth muscle cells.[143] The NCX is overexpressed in PASMC isolated from patients with IPAH, and is found localized in caveolae along with other G-protein–coupled receptors, ROC, and SOC resulting in a functional coupling of these receptors and contributing to increased $[Ca^{2+}]_{cyt}$, resulting in increased proliferation and contraction of PASCM in patients with IPAH.[116,144]

ALTERED SIGNALING PATHWAYS IN IPAH

Alterations in signaling pathways have been observed in IPAH and are discussed below.

CYCLIC GUANOSINE MONOPHOSPHATE IN IPAH

IPAH is associated with abnormally low levels of the potent pulmonary arterial smooth muscle cell relaxant NO. In pulmonary arterial endothelial cells, NO produced by eNOS freely diffuses across the cell membrane to pulmonary arterial smooth muscle cells and activates intracellular soluble guanylate cyclase (sGC), which catalyzes the conversion of guanosine 5′-triphosphate (GTP) to cyclic guanosine monophosphate (cGMP). cGMP then activates cGMP-dependent kinases, which can reduce $[Ca^{2+}]_{cyt}$, inhibit Rho signaling, and inhibit phosphorylation of myosin-binding protein, all of which lead to smooth muscle relaxation.[145,146] In the lung, metabolism of cGMP is controlled by phosphodiesterase 5 (PDE-5). PDE-5 inhibitors block the breakdown of cGMP, leading to vasodilation due to an accumulation of cGMP in the tissue.[147] In 2005, following several clinical studies, sildenafil was approved for the treatment of PAH.[148] Tadalafil was approved for the treatment of PAH in 2009.[149] Both sildenafil and tadalafil share structural similarities with cGMP and inhibit PDE-5 by competitively binding to the catalytic site.[147]

■ PDGF AND Akt/mTOR SIGNALING IN IPAH

PDGF and its receptor PDGFR have been implicated in the pathogenesis of IPAH. Previous studies have indicated that PDGF increases SOCE in rat and human pulmonary arterial smooth muscle cells, thereby promoting cell proliferation (Fig. 72-4).[119,150] Binding of PDGF to PDGFR leads to activation of phosphatidylinositol 3-kinase (PI3K),[151] which activates Akt. Akt promotes cell growth through the downstream mediator mammalian target of rapamycin (mTOR) or by directly phosphorylating proteins involved in cell cycle regulation and apoptosis.[152] The Akt/mTOR pathway has been shown to be important for pulmonary arterial smooth muscle cell proliferation[150,153] and the development of PAH.[154] Inhibition of mTOR and Akt by rapamycin and Akt inhibitor VIII, respectively, abrogated the PDGF-induced increased SOCE and Ca^{2+} channel expression in normal and PAH-pulmonary arterial smooth muscle cells,[150,155] suggesting that the PDGF-mediated increase in SOCE occurs via the Akt/mTOR pathway. Clinical trials have shown some benefit to the use of imatinib, an orally active PDGFR inhibitor, in patients with severe PAH.[102]

■ RhoA/ROCK SIGNALING IN IPAH

The RhoA/ROCK signaling pathway is a major mediator of Ca^{2+}-sensitization/desensitization and a key regulator of vascular tone (Fig. 72-4).[156,157] RhoA is a GTP-binding protein that is activated following activation of G-protein–coupled receptors by vasodilators. In addition, RhoA can be activated by serotonin, which enters the cell through its transporter 5-HTT, and by an increase in $[Ca^{2+}]_{cyt}$.[158] Activation of RhoA leads to activation of Rho kinase (ROCK), which increases the Ca^{2+} sensitivity of contraction in pulmonary arterial smooth muscle cells by inhibiting myosin light chain phosphatase and increasing the phosphorylation of myosin light chain kinase, leading to increased contraction of pulmonary arterial smooth muscle cells.[20,21] Recent studies have indicated that the RhoA/ROCK signaling pathway is enhanced in patients with IPAH.[159,160] Small clinical studies have demonstrated that inhibition of the RhoA/ROCK signaling pathway with fasudil, a selective ROCK inhibitor, results in acutely improved pulmonary hemodynamic variables in patients with IPAH.[161,162]

■ NOTCH SIGNALING IN IPAH

Notch signaling is involved in vascular development and has been implicated in the development of IPAH (Fig. 72-4).[163,164] Both Notch receptors (Notch1-Notch4) and their ligands, Jagged (Jag1 and Jag2) and Delta-like (Dll1, Dll3, and Dll4), are single-transmembrane–spanning proteins that restrict Notch signaling to adjacent cells. After ligand binding, Notch undergoes a series of proteolytic cleavages resulting in the release of the Notch intracellular domain, which translocates to the nucleus where it interacts with recombination signal binding protein for immunoglobulin kappa j region (RBPjκ) to function as a transcription factor resulting in activation of transcription of Notch target genes.[163,165–167] The most commonly induced Notch target genes are the basic helix–loop–helix transcriptional repressors of the *Hes* (*Hairy/Enhancers of Split*) and *Hrt* (*Hes-related transcription factor*) gene families. In addition, Notch signaling has been shown to upregulate expression of PDGFR-β,[168] which is known to be upregulated in IPAH.[155,169] Notch3 signaling has recently been implicated in PAH. Lung tissue from IPAH patients displays increased Notch3 and Notch3 intracellular domain (N3ICD) expression when compared to normotensive patients.[164] In addition, Notch3 and N3ICD expression is increased in two animal models of pulmonary hypertension, hypoxic-induced pulmonary hypertension in mice and monocrotaline-induced pulmonary hypertension in rats.[164] This suggests that the Notch signaling pathway may be an important pathway to target for the development of new drugs for the treatment of IPAH.

GENETIC ALTERATIONS RELATED TO IDIOPATHIC AND FAMILIAL PAH

Identification of bone morphogenetic protein receptor II (BMPR2) gene mutations has led to increasing interest in genetic susceptibility to pulmonary hypertension. As a receptor for the TGFβ super family, BMPR2 is involved in diverse cell growth and differentiation processes in multiple systems. Engagement of a BMP receptor with its ligand normally results in the activation of intracellular mediators (Smads) and their translocation to the cell nucleus and regulation of the transcription of target genes. The resulting activation of some genes and the inhibition of others varies according to the BMP pathway and tissue involved. BMP signaling is essential to both normal vascular development and the maintenance of the normal adult pulmonary vasculature, likely by regulating the growth and apoptosis of endothelial and smooth muscle cells (Fig. 72-4). Loss of such regulation gives rise to pulmonary hypertension.[170] Normally found primarily on endothelium and to a lesser extent smooth muscle cells, the expression of BMPR2 is reduced and its function abnormal in patients with various types of PAH, most notably those with mutations of the *BMPR2* gene.[171] The ability of BMP to inhibit smooth muscle proliferation and induce apoptosis is suppressed in cells isolated specifically from smaller pulmonary vessels in patients with IPAH (e.g., 1 to 2 mm, where occlusive vascular pathologic changes predominate).[29,172,173] Germline mutations in *BMPR2* have been identified in up to 70% of patients with familial PAH, and in 20% of patients with IPAH,[174–180] as well as disease associated with anorexigens,[181] congenital heart disease,[182] and pulmonary venoocclusive disease (PVOD).[183] Nearly 300 different mutations of BMPR2 have been identified.[177]

Further work has identified other genetic alterations in the TGFβ pathway including activin receptor kinase-like 1 (*ALK1*), endoglin (*Eng*), and Smad 8.[184] ALK1 is a receptor for TGFβ and endoglin is its coreceptor; while Smad 8 is a downstream second messenger of BMPR2. Mutations in *ALK1* and *Eng* have been shown to confer susceptibility to the development of PAH in patients with hereditary hemorrhagic telangiectasia.[185,186] In addition, concomitant Thrombospondin-1 gene mutation (*THBS1*) has been detected in a small subset of familial PAH patients with BMPR2 mutations; this mutation has been proposed to further promote pulmonary hypertension development and increase genetic penetrance.[187]

CLINICAL EVALUATION OF PULMONARY HYPERTENSION

The symptoms and signs of PAH are nonspecific, overlapping with many more common entities. As a result, patients experience problematic delays between the time of symptom onset and appropriate diagnosis.[188,189] The problem is usually first suggested by findings suggestive of pulmonary hypertension on an echocardiogram. The evaluation of PAH is predominantly,

TABLE 72-3 Presenting Symptom(s) Attributable to PAH

Symptom	Percentage of Patients at Presentation
Abdominal distention	4%
Chest pain/discomfort	2%
Cough	14%
Dizziness/lightheadedness	15%
Dyspnea at rest	11%
Dyspnea on exertion	86%
Edema	21%
Fatigue	27%
Presyncope/syncope	17%
Palpitations	13%

Source: Data from Brown LM, Chen H, Halpern S, et al. Delay in recognition of pulmonary arterial hypertension: factors identified from the REVEAL registry. Chest. 2011;140(1):19–26 and represent percentage of patients with each indicated symptom at the time of initial presentation, from among 2493 patient enrolled in a multicenter United States national registry of patients with pulmonary hypertension (Registry to Evaluate Early and Long-term PAH Disease Management).

TABLE 72-4 World Health Organization Functional Classification of Patients with Pulmonary Hypertension

Class I: Patients with PH but without resulting limitation of physical activity. Ordinary physical activity does not cause undue dyspnea or fatigue, chest pain, or near syncope.

Class II: Patients with PH resulting in slight limitation of physical activity. They are comfortable at rest. Ordinary physical activity causes undue dyspnea or fatigue, chest pain, or near syncope.

Class III: Patients with PH resulting in marked limitation of physical activity. They are comfortable at rest. Less than ordinary activity causes undue dyspnea or fatigue, chest pain, or near syncope.

Class IV: Patients with PH with inability to carry out any physical activity without symptoms. These patients manifest signs of right heart failure. Dyspnea and/or fatigue may even be present at rest. Discomfort is increased by any physical activity.

Source: Adapted with permission from Rich S. Primary Pulmonary hypertension: executive summary. Evian, France. World Health Organization, 1998.

therefore, the evaluation of pulmonary hypertension more generically: a step-wise process to establishing whether pulmonary hypertension is likely present, and if so confirmation and careful evaluation of the specific cause and classification so as to guide rational therapy.

PATIENT HISTORY IN PULMONARY HYPERTENSION

Except for mild breathlessness – often attributed to being "out of shape" – PAH is generally asymptomatic until severe. Because of the nonspecific nature of the symptoms (Table 72-3), underrecognition of the disease by healthcare providers, and its confusion with other conditions, a significant delay between the onset of symptoms and the diagnosis of PAH is common. The mean time from symptom onset until PAH diagnosis was over 2 years in a National Institutes of Health (NIH) registry assembled in the 1980s.[190] Twenty years later, registries in China, France, Germany, and the United States each found that similarly disappointing delays of over 2 years persist.[189,191–193] As a result, diagnosis is delayed until most patients have severe functional impairment, with more than one-half reporting World Health Organization (WHO) functional class III or IV symptoms (Table 72-4).

Symptoms due to pulmonary hypertension are generally difficult to dissociate from symptoms of underlying pulmonary or cardiac disease. In IPAH, the first symptoms generally occur during exertion, usually as dyspnea and, less often, chest pain, dizziness, or syncope.[194] Dyspnea on exertion is by far the most common presenting complaint. Often, because of the lack of other signs or symptoms, it is attributed to physical deconditioning or anxiety. Other initial complaints, particularly easy fatigability and chest discomfort, are often similarly dismissed. Angina-like or nonspecific chest pain is common in patients with severe pulmonary hypertension and generally attributed to right ventricular overload and myocardial ischemia. Chest pain might also occur due to the extrinsic compression of the left main coronary artery by an enlarged pulmonary artery.[195]

In time, in the absence of amelioration of the pulmonary hypertension, right-sided heart failure evolves. Syncope, or light-headedness on exertion, are less common but more ominous complications of pulmonary hypertension. They occur in patients with severe pulmonary hypertension and a fixed low CO. The cause is inadequate cerebral blood flow due to a combination of failure to increase the CO, along with diversion of systemic blood flow toward the exercising muscles. Syncope may also occur at rest in association with the onset of bradycardia, presumably vagal in origin. Hoarseness, due to paralysis of the left recurrent laryngeal nerve, may result from trapping of the nerve between the aorta and the dilated left pulmonary artery (a form of Ortner syndrome). If the right ventricle should fail, lower extremity swelling is common, as are abdominal signs and symptoms including a sensation of "bloating," early satiety, tender hepatomegaly, ascites, and abdominal pain. Symptoms of right ventricular failure and the presence of syncopal events are associated with a worse prognosis. Hemoptysis in the setting of pulmonary hypertension is most often due to pulmonary venous congestion but when mitral stenosis is present, it is generally attributed to bleeding from bronchial veins. Occasionally, hemoptysis occurs in other forms of pulmonary hypertension and may originate in alveolar capillaries, precapillaries, or elsewhere in the pulmonary arterial tree.

Not infrequently, the suspicion of pulmonary hypertension is raised by the presence of a known risk for pulmonary hypertension (e.g., systemic sclerosis) or by serendipitous discovery of right ventricular enlargement by an electrocardiogram or chest radiograph taken for other reasons (Figs. 72-5 and 72-6). Initial recognition of the presence of pulmonary hypertension also frequently occurs in the absence of reported symptoms when an echocardiogram is performed for the evaluation of a murmur. Alternatively, echocardiographic evidence of pulmonary hypertension may be found unsuspectedly when the study is obtained as "routine" evaluation of a patient complaining of any of a number of chest symptoms, including dyspnea. Patients with severe pulmonary hypertension are prone to sudden death and its occurrence may be the first (and last) indication of disease. Death has occurred unexpectedly during normal activities, cardiac catheterization, and surgical procedures, and after the administration of sedatives or anesthetic agents. In a few instances, bradycardia leading to cardiac arrest has preceded sudden death.

An important hint to the presence of pulmonary hypertension is a history of long-standing dyspnea that has not responded to treatment for other more common disorders. Patients have often seen several clinicians before an appropriate diagnosis is made.

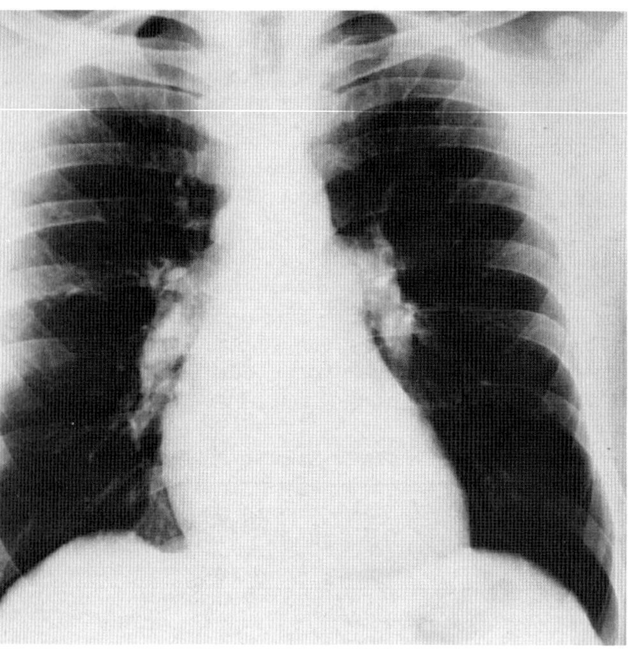

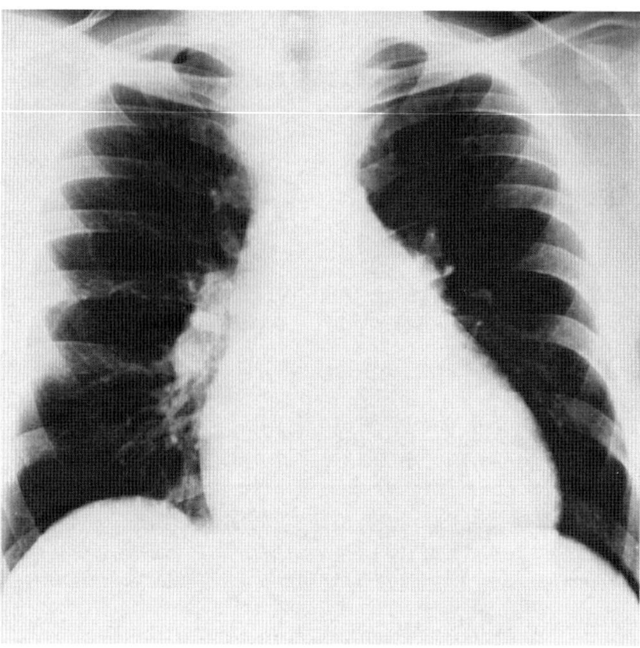

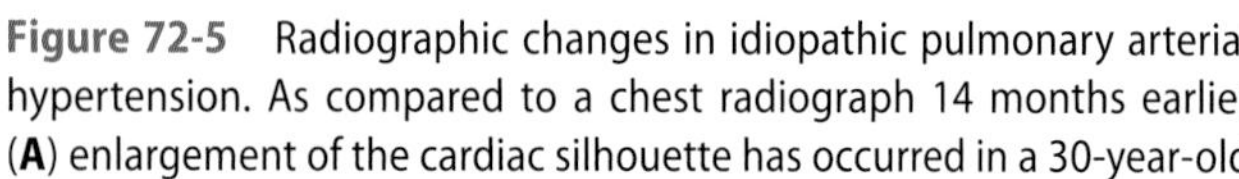

Figure 72-5 Radiographic changes in idiopathic pulmonary arterial hypertension. As compared to a chest radiograph 14 months earlier (**A**) enlargement of the cardiac silhouette has occurred in a 30-year-old man in association with increasing dyspnea (**B**). Decrease in the cardiac silhouette occurred in response to chronic pulmonary vasodilator therapy.

Younger patients have frequently been told their symptoms are due to asthma, yet failed to improve significantly with aggressive anti-inflammatory and bronchodilator therapies. In older patients, dyspnea or exercise limitation may have been blamed on COPD, often despite a trivial history of tobacco use. Unfortunately, a further clue in such patients is learning that these "diagnostic" labels were never investigated with pulmonary function testing. Patients should be asked about important symptoms or risk factors that might suggest the presence and cause of pulmonary hypertension. These include symptoms of collagen vascular disease (e.g., dysphagia, skin or joint changes, Raynaud's phenomenon), sleep apnea (e.g., witnessed apneic events, daytime hypersomnolence), history of risks for thromboembolism, HIV infection, liver disease, or anorectic agent use. A history of tobacco use and chronic sputum production, or a known history of asthma with poor control might be important clues to the presence of obstructive airway disease and hypoxia as the cause of pulmonary hypertension. A prior history of interstitial lung disease or any cause of chronic hypoxia must be noted. A careful family history should be taken including inquiring about relatives who suffer(ed) poorly understood cardiopulmonary conditions.

PHYSICAL EXAMINATION

A careful physical examination is necessary to recognize the presence of pulmonary hypertension and begin elucidating its cause (Table 72-5). In mild-to-moderate pulmonary hypertension, the physical examination is apt to be unrevealing unless suspicion has been aroused that pulmonary hypertension may be present. Right ventricular enlargement is an important clue but notoriously difficult to detect in its early stages on physical examination. Evidence of pulmonary hypertension, such as prominent closure of the pulmonary valve, is apt to be overlooked or discounted, especially in younger people; recognition of tricuspid insufficiency or a right ventricular gallop is often delayed until pulmonary hypertension becomes severe and has led to heart failure.

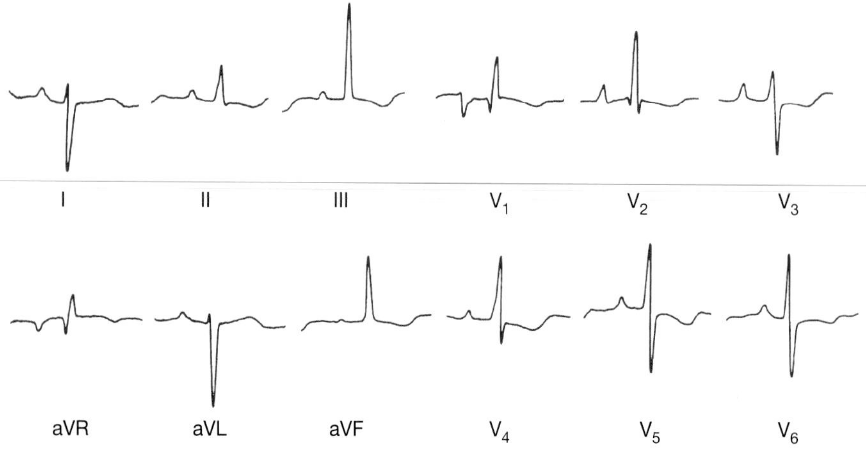

Figure 72-6 Twenty-six-year-old woman in whom the first evidence of primary pulmonary hypertension was by electrocardiography. The record shows marked right axis deviation and dominant R waves over the right precordium consistent with right ventricular hypertrophy.

TABLE 72-5 Physical Examination Findings in Pulmonary Hypertension

Sign	Implication
Physical Signs that Reflect Severity of PH	
Accentuated pulmonary component of S2 (audible at apex in over 90%)	High pulmonary pressure increases force of pulmonic valve closure
Early systolic click	Sudden interruption of opening of pulmonary valve into high-pressure artery
Midsystolic ejection murmur	Turbulent transvalvular pulmonary outflow
Left parasternal lift	High right ventricular pressure and hypertrophy present
Right ventricular S4 (in 38%)	High right ventricular pressure and hypertrophy present
Increased jugular "a" wave	Poor right ventricular compliance
Physical Signs that Suggest Moderate-to-Severe PH	
Sign	**Implication**
Moderate-to-severe PH	Tricuspid regurgitation
Holosystolic murmur that increases with inspiration tricuspid regurgitation	
Increased jugular v waves	
Pulsatile liver	
Diastolic murmur	Pulmonary regurgitation
Hepatojugular reflux	High central venous pressure
Advanced PH with right ventricular failure	
Right ventricular S3 (in 23%)	Right ventricular dysfunction
Distention of jugular veins	Right ventricular dysfunction or tricuspid regurgitation or both
Hepatomegaly	
Peripheral edema (in 32%)	
Ascites	
Low blood pressure, diminished pulse pressure, cool extremities	Reduced cardiac output, peripheral vasoconstriction
Physical Signs that Suggest Possible Underlying Cause or Associations of PH	
Sign	**Implication**
Central cyanosis	Abnormal V/Q, intrapulmonary shunt, hypoxemia, pulmonary-to-systemic shunt
Clubbing	Congenital heart disease, pulmonary venoocclusive disease
Cardiac systolic murmurs, diastolic murmurs, opening snap, and gallop	Congenital or acquired heart or valvular disease
Crackles, dullness, or decreased breath sounds	Pulmonary congestion or effusion or both
Crackles, accessory muscle use, wheezing, protracted expiration, productive cough	Pulmonary parenchymal disease
Obesity, kyphoscoliosis, enlarged tonsils, narrowed pharyngeal opening, macroglossia	Disordered ventilation, sleep apnea
Sclerodactyly, arthritis, telangiectasia, Raynaud phenomenon, rash	Connective tissue disorder
Peripheral venous insufficiency or obstruction	Possible venous thrombosis
Venous stasis ulcers	Possible sickle cell disease
Pulmonary vascular bruits	Chronic thromboembolic PH
Splenomegaly, spider angiomata, palmary erythema, icterus, caput medusa, ascites	Portal hypertension

PH, Pulmonary hypertension.
Source: Adapted with permission from McLaughlin VV, Archer SL, Badesch DB, et al. ACCF/AHA 2009 expert consensus document on pulmonary hypertension a report of the American College of Cardiology Foundation task force on expert consensus documents and the American Heart Association developed in collaboration with the American College of Chest Physicians; American Thoracic Society, Inc.; and the Pulmonary Hypertension Association. J Am Coll Cardiol. 2009;53(17):1573–1619.

Once pulmonary hypertension is suspected, the physical examination can offer important signs. When symptoms first become manifest, a large *a* wave generally can be detected in the jugular venous pulse. Auscultation usually discloses splitting of the second heart sound with accentuation of the pulmonic component. A sharp systolic ejection click over the region of the pulmonary artery is usually heard. As pulmonary hypertension persists, enlargement of the right ventricle becomes evident as a palpable cardiac impulse near the left sternal border and in the hypogastrium. An important sign of cor pulmonale is a right-sided (ventricular) diastolic (S_3) gallop; it is accentuated by inspiration. Less helpful is the right atrial gallop (S_4), which occurs immediately before the first heart sound and suggests an increase in the filling pressure of the right side of the heart.

In time, tricuspid insufficiency develops. It is manifested by a holosystolic murmur, best heard in the fourth interspace to the left of the sternum; the murmur characteristically increases in intensity during inspiration (as do the third and fourth heart sounds). A prominent *v* wave appears in the jugular pulse, and distended neck veins pulsate with each heartbeat. The onset of right ventricular failure is often marked by discomfort in the right upper quadrant due to hepatic engorgement as well as edema in the lower extremities. The liver often also shows expansive pulsations that are synchronous with the heartbeat. Hydrothorax and ascites are uncommon, even after right ventricular failure has progressed to the stage of hepatomegaly and pedal edema. Systemic arterial hypoxemia is often present. Assessment of oxyhemoglobin desaturation with activity is an important component of the patient evaluation; if desaturation is noted, formal exercise testing to titrate oxygen therapy should be pursued promptly. Late in the disease, many patients develop peripheral cyanosis secondary to a reduced CO and peripheral vasoconstriction; central cyanosis also occurs preterminally in some patients because of right-to-left shunting through a patent foramen ovale.

The physical examination should be focused on the presence of additional signs to indicate a possible cause of pulmonary hypertension. Systemic hypertension, a risk factor for coronary artery disease or diastolic dysfunction, may suggest left-sided heart disease. Abnormal lung sounds might include wheezing suggesting airway obstruction, or crackles suggesting either pulmonary edema or interstitial disease. Additional findings suggestive of lung disease include hyperresonance to percussion or hyperinflation of the thorax (barrel chest) suggestive of COPD or kyphoscoliosis causing a restrictive pattern. Skin changes such as rash or telangiectasias are clues to the presence of collagen vascular disease, as are digital ulcers in patients with the CREST variant of systemic sclerosis. The presence of digital clubbing should also be noted as it may indicate congenital heart disease, certain forms of chronic hypoxic lung disease (e.g., cystic fibrosis or certain interstitial lung diseases) or PVOD.[196] Narrowing of the posterior oropharynx, macroglossia, and a large neck size may suggest obstructive sleep apnea.

DIAGNOSTIC STUDIES

Diagnostic testing is used to confirm the presence of pulmonary hypertension, identify the etiology, assess severity and prognosis, and to help guide appropriate therapy. Table 72-6 lists tests that are essential in the evaluation of pulmonary hypertension.[197] Table 72-7 lists the criteria required for a diagnosis of PAH.

Following a detailed history and physical examination, an electrocardiogram, chest radiograph, and echocardiogram are indicated if there is suspicion of pulmonary hypertension, and often as logical tests to evaluate symptoms such as dyspnea even if concern for pulmonary hypertension has not been raised.

Chest Radiograph and Electrocardiogram

Early in the evolution of pulmonary hypertension, the chest radiograph appears normal. In time, the central pulmonary arteries become increasingly prominent as the peripheral vessels become attenuated, and the cardiac silhouette enlarges (Fig. 72-7). The chest radiograph (together with pulmonary function tests) may also suggest the presence of underlying lung disease. An electrocardiogram should be obtained and may indicate signs of ischemic heart disease or conduction abnormalities. Findings suggestive of the presence of pulmonary hypertension include right axis deviation, right atrial enlargement, and right

TABLE 72-6 Evaluation of Patients with Pulmonary Hypertension

Detection of pulmonary hypertension	Detailed history and physical examination	Suspicion of pulmonary hypertension and possible causes/associations
	Electrocardiogram	Exclude other causes of cardiopulmonary symptoms
	Chest radiograph	
	Echocardiogram (at rest, to consider repeat with exertion)	Evaluate for presence of pulmonary hypertension, assess chamber sizes and function, valvular abnormalities, contrast (bubble) study to evaluate possible shunt
Essential testing	Pulmonary function testing	Exclude intrinsic lung disease
	Overnight oximetry	Screen for sleep-disordered breathing
	Lung (V/Q) scan	Exclude thromboembolism
	Blood serologies (e.g., CBC, liver function, renal function, HIV, ANA, antiphospholipid antibodies)	Exclude collagen vascular disease, liver disease, infection, and other possible causes of pulmonary hypertension
	Oxygen desaturation study	Assess need for supplemental oxygen (rest and exertion)
	6-Minute walk test	Establish baseline
	Right cardiac catheterization	Confirm diagnosis, assess other cardiac causes (shunt); consider left heart catheterization
Contingent testing	Transesophageal echocardiogram	Assess patent foramen ovale (PFO)
		Characterize valvular function
	Computed tomogram of chest	Assess interstitial lung disease, adenopathy
	Polysomnogram	Diagnosis and treatment of sleep-disordered breathing
	Pulmonary angiogram	Assess presence and location of organized thromboemboli and suitability for pulmonary thromboendarterectomy
	Blood studies (BNP, clotting studies, genetic testing)	
	Lung biopsy	Exclude subtle interstitial lung disease vasculitis and other uncommon diseases (PVOD, PCH) to assist planning

Source: Data from Barst RJ, McGoon M, Torbicki A, et al. Diagnosis and differential assessment of pulmonary arterial hypertension. J Am Coll Cardiol. 2004;43 (12 Suppl S):40S–47S.

TABLE 72-7 Requirements for the Diagnosis of Pulmonary Arterial Hypertension

Required Testing	Rationale
Cardiac catheterization: • A mean pulmonary artery pressure ≥25 mm Hg • Pulmonary artery wedge or left ventricular end diastolic pressure ≤15 mm Hg • Pulmonary vascular resistance >3 Wood units[a]	Confirm presence of pulmonary hypertension Exclude left heart disease as the cause of pulmonary hypertension (pulmonary venous hypertension) (Group 2 PH)
PFTs, chest imaging without evidence of more than mild lung disease	Exclude chronic hypoxemic lung disease as cause of PH (Group 3 PH)
Ventilation–perfusion scan without evidence of unmatched perfusion defects	Exclude chronic thromboembolic pulmonary hypertension (Group 4 PH)

[a]*An elevated pulmonary vascular resistance is not included in all published criteria for the diagnosis of PAH.*

ventricular hypertrophy (Fig. 72-6). Arrhythmias are uncommon until late in the course of the disease, when they may contribute to syncopal episodes.

Echocardiogram

When there is suspicion, the echocardiogram is the appropriate first test to assess if pulmonary hypertension is present.[194,198] Indeed, as noted earlier, the unsuspected finding of pulmonary hypertension on an echocardiogram often first brings the issue to attention. A carefully performed Doppler examination is able to quantify the tricuspid regurgitant jet in the majority of cases.[199] A modified Bernoulli equation is used to estimate right ventricular systolic (RVSP = $4v^2$ + right atrial pressure; v = tricuspid jet velocity in meters per second) and is assumed equal to the pulmonary artery systolic pressure when the pulmonic valve is normal. Normal RVSP has been reported as 28 ± 5 mm Hg. Echocardiographic evaluation with exercise is an additional consideration when estimates of RVSP at rest are normal and there is a high suspicion of pulmonary hypertension (e.g., dyspnea in a patient with systemic sclerosis and no other obvious cause). Echocardiographic measurements taken at peak exercise may reveal undue elevations, perhaps signaling the presence of earlier disease. However, normative echocardiographic values of RVSP with exercise have not been well established and whether patients with "exercise-induced" pulmonary hypertension require or benefit from therapies useful for patients with resting pulmonary hypertension is debated.

The echocardiogram also reveals important anatomical and functional information that may assist in identifying the cause of pulmonary hypertension (Table 72-8). Evaluation for a patent foramen ovale and intracardiac or intrapulmonary shunting of blood should be performed (e.g., using "bubble" contrast). Echocardiography can help to rule out related anatomic abnormalities, such as acquired or congenital mitral valve disease or left atrial myxoma. Left ventricular hypertrophy, signs of diastolic noncompliance, decreased systolic function or focal hypokinesis as well as mitral or aortic valvular

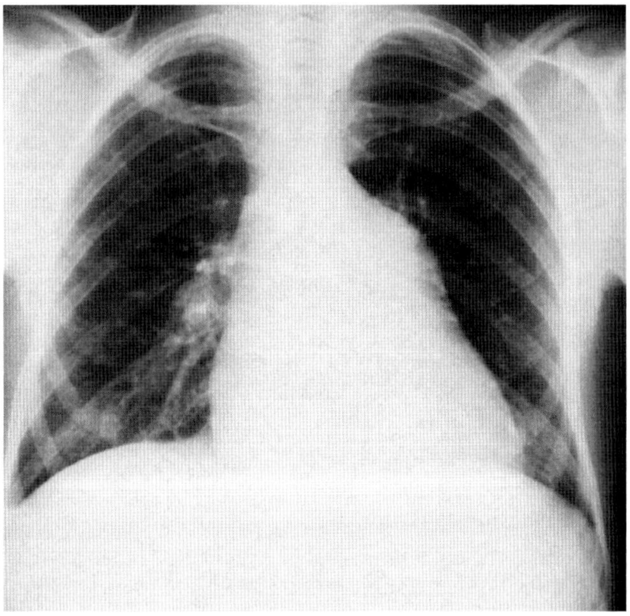

Figure 72-7 Chronic thromboembolic pulmonary hypertension. Prominent central pulmonary arteries in conjunction with the marked pruning of the peripheral tree reflect marked pulmonary hypertension in a patient with a history of multiple pulmonary thromboemboli.

TABLE 72-8 Potential Causes of Pulmonary Hypertension that may be Identified by Echocardiography

Conditions that Predispose to Pulmonary Hypertension
Congenital or acquired valvular disease (MR, MS, AS, prosthetic valve dysfunction)
Left ventricular systolic dysfunction
Impaired left ventricular diastolic function (hypertensive heart disease, HCM, Fabry disease, infiltrative cardiomyopathies)
Other obstructive lesions (aortic coarctation, supravalvular AS, subaortic membrane, cor triatriatum)
Congenital disease with shunt (ASD, VSD, coronary fistula, patent ductus arteriosus, anomalous pulmonary venous return)
Pulmonary embolus (thrombus in IVC, right-sided cardiac chamber, or PA; tricuspid or pulmonic valve vegetation)
Pulmonary vein thrombosis/stenosis
Findings that Suggest Specific Disease Entity
Left-sided valve changes (SLE, anorexigen use)
Intrapulmonary shunts (hereditary hemorrhagic telangiectasia)
Pericardial effusion (IPAH, SLE, systemic sclerosis)

Source: Reproduced with permission from McLaughlin VV, Archer SL, Badesch DB, et al. ACCF/AHA 2009 expert consensus document on pulmonary hypertension: a report of the American College of Cardiology Foundation task force on expert consensus documents and the American Heart Association developed in collaboration with the American College of Chest Physicians; American Thoracic Society, Inc. and the Pulmonary Hypertension Association. J Am Coll Cardiol. 2009;53(17):1573–1619.

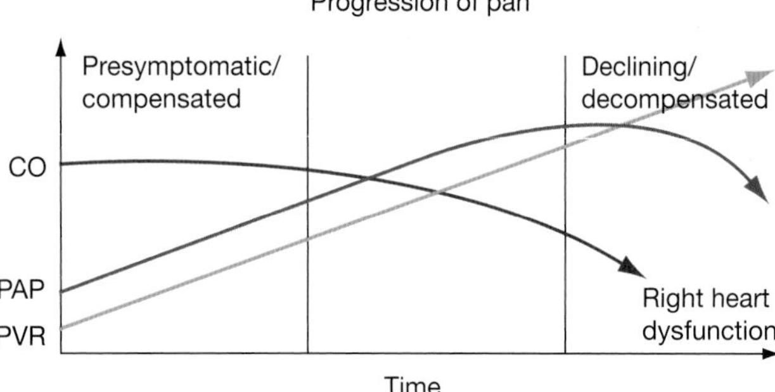

Figure 72-8 Hemodynamic changes during the progression of pulmonary arterial hypertension. With progressive increase in the pulmonary vascular resistance (PVR), the pulmonary artery pressure (PAP) initially increase until a failing right heart can no longer generate the required pressures to maintain cardiac output (CO). At this late stage both the cardiac output and pulmonary pressures may fall. *(Reproduced with permission from Friedman EB, Palevsky HI, Taichman DB. Classification and prognosis of pulmonary arterial hypertension. In: Pulmonary Vascular Disease, Taichman DB. Philadelphia: WB. Saunders; 2006.)*

defects all are vital observations when evaluating the likely cause of pulmonary hypertension. Assessment of right ventricular size and function is essential, as the symptoms caused by pulmonary hypertension and the prognosis of patients with PAH are determined in large measure by the status of the right heart (Fig. 72-8). Indeed, unexplained echocardiographic findings of RV dilation and/or decreased function warrant further investigation regardless of whether pulmonary hypertension appears to be present by echocardiographic estimate. The degree of RV function is often evaluated subjectively, but more quantitative approaches to assessment are becoming more commonly reported, have variably been shown to predict right ventricular output and patient prognosis, and may provide better means of assessing change with disease progression or in response to therapy. Such approaches include evaluation of the tricuspid annular plane systolic excursion, tissue Doppler imaging, and myocardial performance index (Tei-Doppler index).[200] The presence and greater size of a pericardial effusion are also poor prognostic signs.[201–204] Flattening of the intraventricular septum is seen with advanced right heart dilation and failure, and the leftward movement of the septum may impair left ventricular filling (Videos 72-1 and 72-2).

Video 72-1 Short-axis view of an echocardiogram of a patient with pulmonary hypertension demonstrating flattening of the interventricular septum with bowing toward the left ventricle during diastole. The right ventricle is hypocontractile. A small pericardial effusion is demonstrated as well. *(Used with permission of Drs. Lissa Sugeng and Wassim Fares, Yale School of Medicine.)* Video 1, still shot 1: An echocardiogram performed during diastole in the short-axis view demonstrates an enlarged right ventricle (RV), a flattened interventricular septum (IVS) with bowing toward the left ventricle (LV), and a small pericardial effusion (PE). *(Used with permission of Drs. Lissa Sugeng and Wassim Fares, Yale School of Medicine.)* Video 1, still shot 2: An echocardiogram performed during systole in the short-axis view demonstrates an enlarged right ventricle (RV), a flattened interventricular septum (IVS), and a small pericardial effusion (PE). Impaired filling of the left ventricle (LV) during diastole compromises stroke volume. *(Used with permission of Drs. Lissa Sugeng and Wassim Fares, Yale School of Medicine.) Access at www.fishmansonline.com*

Video 72-2 A four-chamber view of an echocardiogram in a patient with pulmonary hypertension. The right ventricle (RV) is enlarged, dilated, and hypocontractile. The right atrium (RA) is enlarged. The interventricular septum (IS) moves paradoxically toward the left ventricle (LV) during diastole, impairing LV filling. A small pericardial effusion (PE) is demonstrated. *(Used with permission of Drs. Lissa Sugeng and Wassim Fares, Yale School of Medicine.)* Video 2, still shot 1: An echocardiogram in the four-chamber view demonstrating an enlarged, dilated RV and RA, as well as a relatively underfilled left ventricle LV and a small PE. The moderator band (MB) of the right ventricle is well visualized. *(Used with permission of Drs. Lissa Sugeng and Wassim Fares, Yale School of Medicine.) Access at www.fishmansonline.com*

While the correlation between echocardiographic estimates of pulmonary arterial systolic pressure and measurements taken at right heart catheterization is generally good, there is significant variability and confirmation by catheterization is absolutely required when the presence of pulmonary hypertension will influence the approach to treatment. For example, in the setting of some patients with severe COPD in whom an echocardiogram reveals evidence of pulmonary hypertension, confirmation by right heart catheterization might not impact medical therapy. If, on the other hand, there is consideration of surgical interventions for the COPD (e.g., transplantation or volume reduction), confirmation of the presence of pulmonary hypertension with catheterization may be important. When the diagnosis might be PAH, diagnostic catheterization is absolutely required to confirm the diagnosis and to guide appropriate therapy. Cardiac catheterization in the evaluation of pulmonary hypertension is described in the following section.

Pulmonary Function Testing, Ventilation–Perfusion Scanning, Sleep Studies

Once echocardiographic evidence of pulmonary hypertension has been established, testing for possible causes is in order. Pulmonary function tests, a radionuclide ventilation–perfusion scan, and overnight oximetry are essential to screen for possible underlying obstructive/restrictive lung disease, occult thromboembolism, and sleep-disordered breathing, respectively. Although computed tomographic angiography may reveal the presence of organized thrombus and is frequently useful for evaluation of other possible causes of the patient's symptoms, it is not established to be sufficiently sensitive to exclude CTEPH. Since a diagnosis of CTEPH as a cause of pulmonary hypertension will markedly alter therapeutic approach, its exclusion with a ventilation–perfusion scan remains an essential test (Fig. 72-9). A history or examination findings suggestive of sleep-disordered breathing should prompt performance of overnight oximetry and/or polysomnography. Treatment of significant sleep apnea may be all that is required to treat mild pulmonary hypertension in some patients with preserved right ventricular function who are followed closely for compliance and resolution of pulmonary hypertension.

LABORATORY TESTING

Blood tests including HIV antibody, rheumatologic serologies (e.g., ANA), liver function tests, and a complete blood count are essential. Dyspnea due to PAH may the presenting symptom leading to the initial diagnosis of systemic sclerosis or HIV infection, and the presence of either would alter required therapeutic plans. Abnormal liver function should prompt further evaluation for possible portal hypertension as an explanation for PAH.

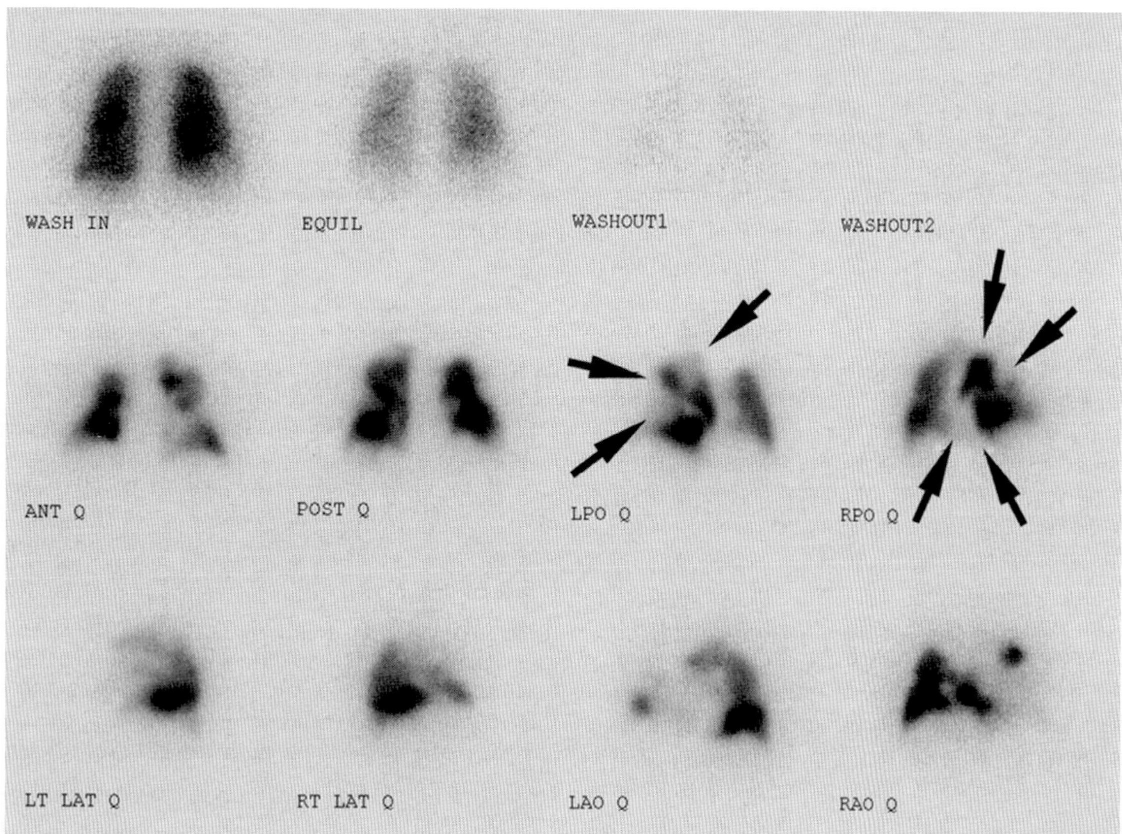

Figure 72-9 Ventilation–perfusion scan in chronic thromboembolic pulmonary hypertension. The top row of images shows normal ventilation; images in the following two rows reveal multiple unmatched perfusion defects, indicated by arrows in the posterior oblique views. *(Image used with permission of Kim Kerr, MD.)*

EXERCISE TESTING AND ASSESSMENT OF OXYHEMOGLOBIN SATURATION

Baseline testing should also include assessments of exercise tolerance and a determination of whether supplemental oxygen is required. A 6-minute walk test is a useful means of assessing exercise capacity and prognosis. It may be useful when choosing initial therapy and serial testing can be helpful in evaluating the response to therapy. Measurements of arterial oxyhemoglobin saturation both at rest and with exertion are important to ensure adequate levels are maintained, and to titrate supplemental oxygen appropriately.

CARDIAC CATHETERIZATION

Right heart cardiac catheterization is required to confirm the diagnosis of pulmonary hypertension, test for important cardiac causes, and in appropriate patients perform vasodilator trials to determine an initial approach to therapy. Both to ensure appropriate interpretation and avoid the need to subject the patient to repeated invasive testing when initial testing is inadequately performed, cardiac catheterization should be performed under the direction of expert operators sufficiently familiar with the evaluation of pulmonary hypertension. Except in those considered to be at very low risk of coronary artery disease, many expert centers also perform a left heart catheterization in all patients. In addition to coronary angiography, measurement of the left ventricular end diastolic pressure (LVEDP) is important to exclude left atrial hypertension (e.g., as seen in diastolic dysfunction) as an important cause of pulmonary hypertension (pulmonary venous hypertension). Although pulmonary artery wedge pressure (PAWP) is routinely obtained during right heart catheterization, it does not always provide an accurate estimate of LVEDP. To maximize the chance of an accurate measurement, PAWP should be made at end expiration and not on the basis of digitally computed "mean" PAWP.[205,206] The PAWP should be measured with equipment leveled at the midchest position (halfway between the table surface and skin surface at the sternum). Discrepant readings between the PAWP and the LVEDP may occur frequently, and so the need for left heart catheterization to directly measure left-sided pressures should be carefully considered given the therapeutic implications of the findings.[207]

During right heart catheterization, serial measurements of blood oxygen saturation should be performed for evidence of a "step up" in oxyhemoglobin saturation suggesting the presence of left to right shunting of blood as an etiology of PAH. Attention should also be paid to the right atrial pressure as significant elevation has been associated with a poorer prognosis. When suspicion of pulmonary hypertension is high and resting pressures are normal, some centers assess values with exercise (e.g., with serial leg lifts, arm raising with weights, or with a stationary bicycle). As noted previously, however, normative values for pressures with exercise have not been well established and whether exercise-induced PAH represents an early stage of disease or alone warrants treatment remains debated.

A diagnosis of PAH requires a mean pulmonary artery pressure greater than or equal to 25 mm Hg, an adequately measured PAWP or a directly recorded LVEDP of less than or equal to 15 mm Hg; an elevated PVR >3 Wood units is also seen and required in some published diagnostic criteria for PAH. The CO is obtained by either thermodilution or use of measured arterial and venous hemoglobin saturations and the Fick principle; the latter is likely more accurate when either significant tricuspid or pulmonary regurgitation is present or the CO is very low. The PVR is calculated as (mean

PA pressure – PCWP)/CO. A normal PVR may be seen if pulmonary hypertension is due to pulmonary venous hypertension, or abnormally high CO (as may occur, for example, in patients with hyperthyroidism, thiamine deficiency, Paget disease of the bone, or arteriovenous fistulae in hereditary hemorrhagic telangiectasia). PH with an elevated CO and normal PVR may also be found in some patients with liver disease (which is to be distinguished from those with PAH associated with liver disease, termed portopulmonary hypertension (POPH) and characterized by an elevated PVR, PH, and a variable CO). It must also be noted that although the hemodynamic profile of patients with PAH (an elevated mean PA with a normal PAWP) may be seen in patients with pulmonary hypertension and pulmonary parenchymal disease (Group 3) but pulmonary function testing and chest imaging distinguish these patients from those with PAH.

In patients with PAH, vasodilator testing is often performed at the time of right heart catheterization to identify those few patients in whom a trial of treatment with oral calcium channel antagonists is appropriate (discussed below). Agents commonly used for acute vasodilator testing include inhaled nitric oxide, intravenous adenosine, or epoprostenol administered by either route.[208–214] Although the definition has varied, a decrease in the mPAP of at least 10 mm Hg to a value less than 40 mm Hg, together with a CO that is unchanged or increased (but not decreased) is generally considered a "positive" acute vasodilator response.[194,215]

Acute vasodilator testing carries significant risk and deaths have been reported.[216] It should not be performed when PVOD is suspected, as the inability of the venous system to accommodate an acute increase in flow may precipitate pulmonary edema.[217] Acute vasodilator testing should be performed only at experienced centers and when the results will influence therapy. Patients who do not demonstrate acute vasoreactivity at the time of right heart catheterization should not receive calcium channel antagonist therapy.

EPIDEMIOLOGY OF PAH

Estimates of the incidence of PAH in studies from France, Scotland, Spain, and the United States range between 2.4 and 7.6 cases per million people. Prevalence estimates range between 15 and 26 cases per million people.[189,191,218–221] Overall, PAH appears to occur more frequently among women (around 2:1) and at a mean age of approximately 50. IPAH and PAH associated with connective tissue diseases appear to be the most commonly recognized in published studies, although limited studies suggest that the burden of schistosomiasis-related disease is likely large.

In the largest such study to date, the mean (±SD) age of patients enrolled in a multicenter US-based national registry of 2525 patients with PAH was 50.1 ± 14.4 years and 79.5% were female. Nearly half of the patients were diagnosed with idiopathic disease (Fig. 72-10). It is important to note that 86% of these were prevalent patients, with a mean of almost 3 years from the time of initial PAH diagnosis until enrollment in the study, thus limiting the ability to extrapolate these data to incident disease.[191]

The prognosis of patients with PAH is worse when hemodynamic variables indicate right heart dysfunction (e.g., elevated right atrial pressure or a depressed CO), and varies according to the specific diagnosis, with PAH associated with scleroderma and portal hypertension portending a worse prognosis than other forms of PAH. Although the outlook appears to have improved with advances in disease management and the availability of multiple drug classes for therapy, many patients continue to require consideration of lung transplantation, and many continue to die. Several risk prediction tools have been recently developed, derived using data from both incident and prevalent patients managed with currently available therapies.[222] One such tool derived and validated with patients in a large US-based cohort is shown in Figure 72-11. This, as well as other risk prediction models, have been validated in populations from other countries.[222–225]

SPECIFIC PAH DISEASE SUBTYPES

In the sections to follow, the various PAH disease subtypes will be discussed in detail.

IDIOPATHIC PULMONARY ARTERIAL HYPERTENSION

IPAH is a rare disease with an estimated incidence of 1 to 2 cases per million in industrialized countries.[226–228] The paucity of numbers of patients with IPAH and the likelihood that diverse causes and pathogenetic mechanisms can produce the same clinical syndrome have complicated descriptions of its natural history. In the past, certain stereotypes were regarded as the norm: young women with Raynaud's syndrome, with acute onset of dyspnea and fatigue, and death within 3 years. Now it is appreciated that even though there

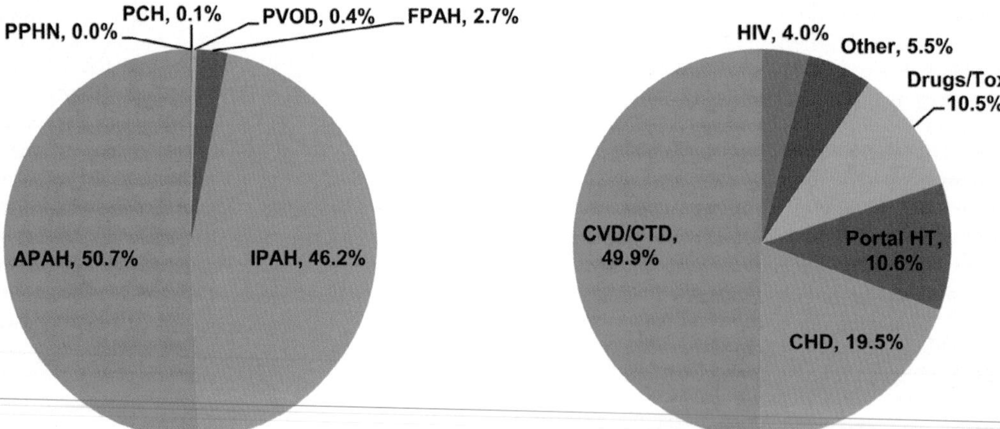

Figure 72-10 Distribution of pulmonary arterial hypertension diagnoses among 2525 prevalent patients in a United States national registry. World Health Organization (WHO) Group I pulmonary arterial hypertension classification of REVEAL patients at enrollment. **A.** WHO Group I PAH classification. **B.** Breakdown of associated PAH subgroup. APAH, associated PAH; CHD, congenital heart disease; CVT/CTD, collagen vascular disease/connective tissue disease; FPAH, familial PAH; PAH, pulmonary arterial hypertension; PCH, pulmonary capillary hemangiomatosis; PPHN, persistent pulmonary hypertension of the newborn; PVOD, pulmonary venoocclusive disease; REVEAL, Registry to Evaluate Early And Long-term PAH Disease Management.

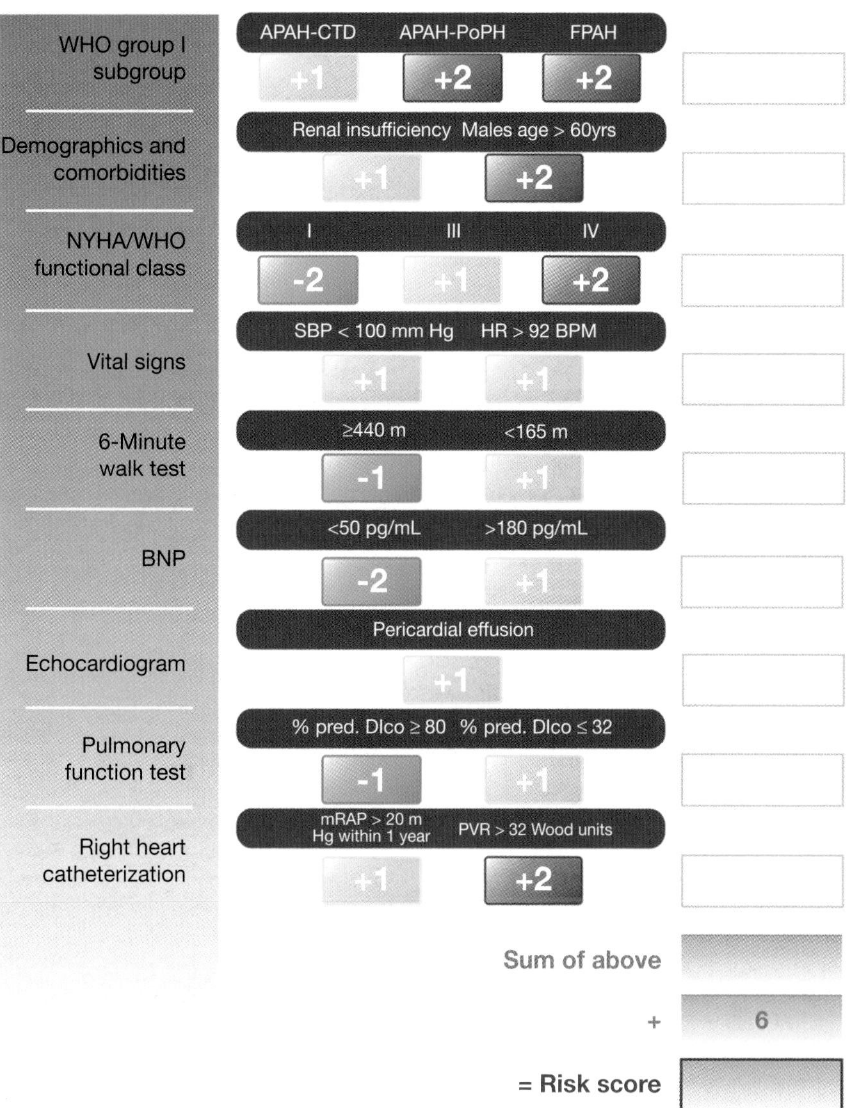

Figure 72-11 REVEAL Registry PAH Risk Score Calculator. Calculated risk scores can range from 0 (lowest risk) to 22 (highest risk). In the REVEAL cohort, the average predicted 1-year survival was 95% to 100% in the low-risk group (score <7), 90% to <95% in the average-risk group (score 8), 85% to <90% in the moderately high-risk group (score 9), 70% to <85% in the high-risk group (score 10–11), and <70% in the very high-risk group (score >12). If N-terminal proBNP is available and BNP is not, listed cut points are replaced with <300 pg/mL and >1500 pg/mL. APAH, associated pulmonary arterial hypertension; BNP, brain natriuretic peptide; BPM, beats per minute; CTD, connective tissue disease; $D_{L_{CO}}$, diffusing capacity of lung for carbon monoxide; FPAH, familial pulmonary arterial hypertension; HR, heart rate; mRAP, mean right atrial pressure; NYHA, New York Heart Association; PAH, pulmonary arterial hypertension; PoPH, portopulmonary hypertension; PVR, pulmonary vascular resistance; REVEAL Registry, Registry to Evaluate Early and Long-term Pulmonary Arterial Hypertension Disease Management; SBP 5 systolic BP; WHO, World Health Organization. *(Reproduced with permission from Benza RL, Gomberg-Maitland M, Miller DP, et al. The REVEAL Registry risk score calculator in patients newly diagnosed with pulmonary arterial hypertension. Chest. 2012;141(2):354–362.)*

is such a subset, prolonged survival in response to medical therapy is not unusual and the disease may affect all ages, both sexes, and different ethnic groups.[229,230]

To overcome the limitations of sporadic reports, the NIH established a nationwide registry in 1981 to collect and analyze data on IPAH (then called PPH). Criteria for entry of a patient into the national registry included normal pulmonary function tests (except for a moderate reduction in diffusing capacity); a right heart catheterization to exclude congenital or left heart disease; perfusion scans and, if inconclusive, pulmonary angiography to exclude CTEPH; and serologic testing to rule out collagen vascular disease. Included in the registry were certain associated diseases, such as hepatic cirrhosis, because the reason for the association was unclear and because of the suspicion that the association might provide a clue to etiology.

By the close of the registry in 1987, data were available on 187 patients.[231] The mean age was 36.4 years and similar for women and men, although the female-to-male ratio was 1.7:1. Few patients were older than 60 years, although race and ethnicity of the cohort was similar to that of the general population. Similar demographic trends have been reported in series from France, Israel, Japan, and Mexico.[228,232,233] Dyspnea was the most common initial symptom and the mean time to diagnosis among patients in the NIH registry was 2 years.

Prognosis of IPAH

Without effective therapy the prognosis of IPAH is very poor. The median survival of patients in the NIH registry was 2.8 years; estimated survival at 1, 3, and 5 years was 68%, 48%, and 34%, respectively.[231] Similar or even poorer figures have been reported absent effective treatment in other series from various countries.[46,234] Most patients die of right heart failure.

The outlook is worse with more advanced symptoms. NIH registry patients with WHO functional classes III and IV symptoms had a median survival of only 31.5 months, as compared with 58.6 months in patients with milder impairment (Class I or II; Table 72-4). Although the figures have improved, functional status remains a significant indicator of prognosis even with effective advanced therapy.[228,235-238] Functional assessment with a 6-minute walk test, for example, is a useful means of following response to therapy and independently predicts prognosis.[237,239-241] Maximal oxygen consumption has also been used to assess response to therapy and can correlate with survival.[241]

On echocardiogram, an enlargement of the right atrium, the presence of a pericardial effusion and its severity are each associated with an increased risk of death.[201-204] A relative increase in the isovolumetric contraction and relaxation times of the RV as compared to RV ejection time is indicative of RV dysfunction and a significantly poorer prognosis.[242]

Levels of endothelin, catecholamines, and atrial natriuretic peptide have been correlated with disease severity, whereas elevations of uric acid, von Willebrand factor, D-dimer, troponin-T, and brain natriuretic peptide have each been associated with a poorer survival in patients with IPAH.[243-249] More recently, a low serum albumin has been associated with an increased risk of death, independent other measures that would reflect passive hepatic congestion or right heart dysfunction.[204] None of these putative prognostic markers is currently incorporated into clinical decision making.

Hemodynamic variables reflecting the development of right heart failure (an increased right atrial pressure and decreased cardiac index) are associated with a poorer prognosis.[228,233,250,251] Worsened survival has been seen in association with both increasing and decreasing mean pulmonary artery pressures (mPAPs). These observations are not necessarily contradictory. Rather, they reflect the natural history of right heart failure in PAH: mPAP rises initially as the vascular derangements worsen only to fall later as the right heart fails and is no longer able to generate an increased pressure (Figs. 72-8 and 72-12.)

A regression equation based on hemodynamic data from the NIH registry has been used to predict survival.[233,252] Because of the dismal prognosis expected, long-term "control" groups without treatment in clinical trials are unethical and assessments of survival with new therapies have been compared with outcome as predicted by the NIH equation. Such comparisons have suggested improved survival with epoprostenol and endothelin receptor antagonists. These improvements are addressed in the discussion of individual therapies in the following sections. As a growing number of effective drugs are now routinely employed, the relevance of survival estimates based on data from an era lacking effective treatment is questionable. The NIH registry equation may no longer be sufficient for predicting survival given current standards of care and background therapies. Indeed, when applied to a more recent cohort of patients treated with current agents, the NIH equation underestimated survival.[204]

It is not surprising that the prognosis of patients with IPAH who have suffered cardiac arrest is dismal even when resuscitative efforts are initiated promptly. In a retrospective review of the records of over 3000 patients, 132 episodes of attempted cardiopulmonary resuscitation (CPR) following cardiac arrest were identified. Survival at 90 days following CPR was only 6%.[253]

■ HERITABLE PULMONARY ARTERIAL HYPERTENSION

A family of patients with what was then termed "PPH" was first described by Dresdale in 1951.[4] Thereafter additional families were reported, and Loyd and Newman identified an autosomal dominant pattern of inheritance, a greater tendency for female carriers to manifest clinical disease, and an earlier onset in successive generations (genetic anticipation).[254,255] Linkage analysis led to a marker at chromosome 2q31–32, and mutations in the gene for a member of the TGFβ family of receptors, bone morphogenetic protein receptor II (BMPRII), were identified as the cause of heritable PAH.[175,176,256,257] Mutations in another member of the TGFβ family, ALK1 predispose patients with hereditary hemorrhagic telangiectasia to develop PAH.[185,186,258,259]

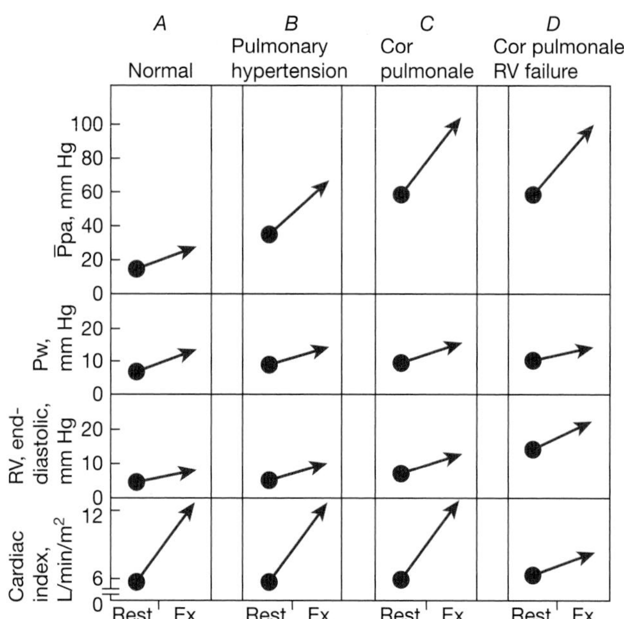

Figure 72-12 Schematic representation of evolution of chronic cor pulmonale. Hemodynamic studies at rest and during exercise in a normal subject (**A**). The stage of pulmonary arterial hypertension (**B**) is succeeded by cor pulmonale (**C**), in which the right ventricle performs normally despite pulmonary arterial hypertension but is known to be enlarged because of radiographic and electrocardiographic findings. Once right ventricular failure supervenes (**D**), cardiac output fails to increase normally during exercise, despite an increase of right ventricular filling pressure (end-diastolic) to abnormally high levels.

TGFβ receptors control an array of cell growth and differentiation systems. BMP signaling is involved in the control of normal vascular development as well as the homeostasis of the adult pulmonary vasculature, likely by regulating the growth and apoptosis of endothelial and smooth muscle cells.[170] In an assessment of mutations from the coding sequence of *BMPRII* in 210 patients, over 140 distinct mutations were identified, the majority predicting premature truncation of the gene transcript. Disease is believed to result from haploinsufficiency, where inadequate quantities of BMPR2 protein are produced for normal function.[177] In addition, the low penetrance observed in heritable PAH suggests that additional environmental factors likely contribute to disease development in genetically susceptible individuals.[260] Up to 70% of patients with heritable PAH have germline mutations in a *BMPRII* allele as do some patients with idiopathic and other associated forms of PAH.[175,176,178-183] Clinically asymptomatic carriers may have evidence of mild pulmonary hypertension on echocardiogram.[261] Common ancestries have been identified that link previously assumed "sporadic" cases of IPAH. Failure to recognize heritable cases of PAH may arise due to incomplete family history taking or reporting, and low disease penetrance, particularly in smaller families.[179,262]

There are no established differences in the approach to treating patients with heritable PAH as compared with IPAH. At present, the clinical evaluation of patients remains the same. Genetic testing of family members should be considered to assess the risk of developing PAH. As a rough guide, there is a one in five chance of PAH developing in a first-order relative who carries a disease-causing *BMPRII* mutation. If genetic testing has not been performed, the risk of disease developing in the first-order relative of a patient with known heritable PAH is approximately one in ten. In the absence of a disease-causing *BMPRII* mutation, the risk of disease is the same as in the general population (estimated at one in a million).[260] Because of the potential interpersonal, psychological, and economic implications of identifying an at-risk genotype, genetic testing should only be performed in conjunction with professional genetic counseling.

■ PULMONARY ARTERIAL HYPERTENSION ASSOCIATED WITH SPECIFIC CONDITIONS

Pulmonary arterial hypertension has been reported in a wide variety of disorders, as discussed below.

Collagen Vascular Diseases

The lungs and the pleura are commonly affected in patients with collagen vascular diseases. Although the incidence in each of the collagen vascular diseases varies, interstitial lung disease is more common than isolated involvement of the pulmonary vasculature. When present, however, PAH is frequently a more rapidly lethal development than interstitial lung disease. It is important in this population to differentiate between pulmonary hypertension associated with interstitial lung disease and the true development of PAH that occurs in the absence of significant interstitial changes. Pulmonary hypertension may also develop due to left heart ischemia or diastolic dysfunction, or to thromboembolic complications of collagen vascular disease.[263] Unfortunately, both interstitial lung disease and true PAH coexist in many patients. Most clinical studies of PAH therapy have excluded patients with collagen vascular diseases and evidence of "significant" restriction (usually defined as an FVC of <70% of predicted values) or interstitial changes on radiographs. Drugs that are efficacious in PAH have not proven effective in the treatment of pulmonary hypertension that accompanies interstitial lung disease. Among patients with systemic sclerosis, PAH occurs most commonly in those with limited disease or the CREST syndrome. Prevalence estimates have ranged significantly, but when investigated with right heart catheterization, PAH has been found in between 7% and 12% of patients.[264,265] The prognosis of patients with scleroderma is worse when their disease is complicated by PAH than by pulmonary fibrosis, even when the latter is severe. Nearly one-half of patients with PAH in the context of scleroderma die within 1 year, compared with a 3-year 50% mortality when the lung is affected by fibrosis alone.[266,267] Even with the use of equivalent therapies, the outcome of patients with PAH associated with systemic sclerosis is less favorable than for IPAH (Fig. 72-13).[90,236,266,268,269]

When estimated by echocardiography, pulmonary hypertension has been identified in approximately 4% to 10% of patients with systemic lupus erythematosis, but as many as 43% when patients are followed prospectively.[270–275] Estimates of prevalence are variable and most were obtained without confirmation by catheterization in patients with mixed connective tissue disease. Regardless of frequency, however, when it is present, PAH appears to be a significant cause of death in these patients. PAH occurs in numerous other rheumatologic disorders, including Sjögren's syndrome and rheumatoid arthritis although firm data on incidence or impact on survival are lacking.

Human Immunodeficiency Virus

Patients infected with the human immunodeficiency virus (HIV) are at increased risk of developing PAH. The mechanism by which

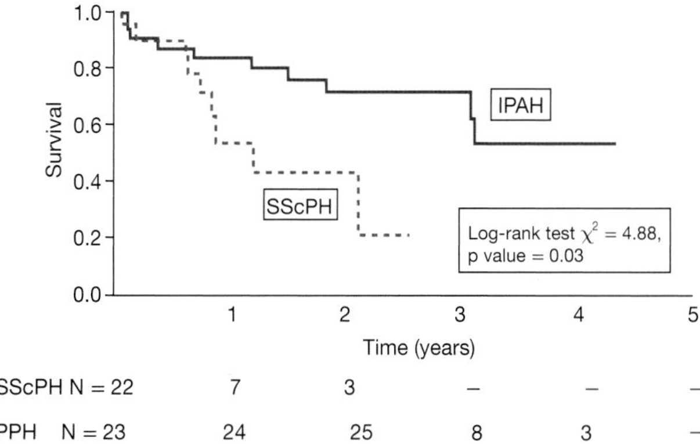

Figure 72-13 Survival of patients with systemic sclerosis–associated pulmonary arterial hypertension is worse than that of patients with idiopathic pulmonary arterial hypertension despite equivalent therapies. *(Reproduced with permission from Kawut SM, Taichman DB, Archer-Chicko CL, et al. Hemodynamics and survival in patients with pulmonary arterial hypertension related to systemic sclerosis. Chest. 2003;123(2):344–350.)*

HIV predisposes to the development of PAH is not known, but it does not appear to be due to direct viral infection of pulmonary vascular endothelial cells.[276] Infection may cause elevations in local concentrations of growth factors or other mediators such as endothelin to indirectly result in the development of PAH.[277–279]

The estimated annual incidence of PAH among HIV-infected patients is approximately 0.5%, significantly higher than the estimated annual incidence of 1.7 per million in the general population.[226,280] The annual incidence of pulmonary hypertension in a large Swiss cohort of HIV-positive patients appears to be declining, having peaked at 0.24% in 1993 as compared with 0.02% in 2001; this decline was hypothesized to relate to the introduction of highly effective antiretroviral therapies.[281] However, no such change was seen in a French study population, comparing rates of HIV-associated PAH between the early 1990s and 2008.[282] It is unclear, therefore, if better control of HIV infection alters the risk of developing PAH.

Symptoms, hemodynamic findings, and survival of PAH associated with HIV appear to be similar to IPAH.[283] Like IPAH, the prognosis is worse with more advanced symptoms (e.g., WHO functional class III or IV as compared with either I or II). A CD4 lymphocyte count below 212 cells/mm^3 has also been associated with a poorer prognosis.[284] Mortality is more often directly attributable to PAH and right heart failure than to infectious complications.[283,284]

Portal Hypertension

The lung may be affected by chronic liver disease in several ways, including the hepatopulmonary syndrome with the development of vascular dilatations and resultant hypoxemia, the development of pleural effusions (hepatic hydrothorax), and pulmonary hypertension. Liver disease is frequently characterized by a low systemic vascular resistance and high CO; the accompanying increased flow and blood volume result in pulmonary hypertension although the PVR is normal or even decreased. Vascular changes resulting in an elevated PVR, on the other hand, are seen with the development of PAH associated with portal hypertension, also termed POPH. Evaluation of pulmonary hypertension in these patients may be difficult as the high CO state of liver disease may precede or accompany the developmental POPH. Thus, as compared with patients with IPAH, patients with similar degrees of clinical impairment and POPH may display numerically smaller elevations in PVR or decrements in CO.[285]

The pathologic changes seen in POPH are similar to those described in other forms of PAH: vasoconstrictive, proliferative, and obliterative changes including both plexiform and thrombotic lesions.[286,287] The pathogenesis is not well understood and may involve abnormal proliferative (or other) vascular responses, but inducing triggers are not well defined. Portal hypertension might alter the vasoactive mediators to which the pulmonary circulation is exposed because of blood bypassing the liver via portosystemic shunts and returning to the systemic circulation.[288] As in other forms of PAH, altered levels of vasodilators and vasoconstrictors have been observed in patients with POPH.[289,290] Women with portal hypertension appear to be at greater risk for the development of POPH than men, as do patients with autoimmune hepatitis. The severity of portal hypertension does not appear to influence the risk of POPH.[291,292] Predisposing, likely genetic, factors are also believed to determine why only some patients with liver disease develop POPH.[293] The degree to which mutations in *BMPRII* are involved in the development of POPH remains unclear.

The prevalence of PAH in patients with liver disease has not been established. Estimates of up to 16% have been reported in studies screening patients with advanced liver disease.[289,294] In one series of patients evaluated for liver transplantation, the prevalence of POPH was 8.5%.[286] Incidence has not been evaluated. Without effective treatment the prognosis of POPH is poor, with a mean survival of only 15 months reported in one retrospective series of 78 patients.[295] Survival with current therapies is worse for patients with POPH than IPAH. In the REVEAL cohort, despite less severe hemodynamic derangements at the time of enrollment, 5-year survival of 174 patients with POPH was significantly worse than of 1478 patients with IPAH/HPAH (40% vs. 64%, respectively), although the initiation of therapy appeared to have been delayed in POPH as compared to IPAH.[285]

The symptoms and findings on physical examination of POPH reflect the presence of both PAH and of chronic liver disease. While shortness of breath may be overshadowed by abdominal complaints and fatigue, dyspnea becomes prominent as POPH progresses. Differentiating between the contributions of PAH-related cor pulmonale and cirrhosis as the cause of fatigue, edema, and abdominal complaints such as satiety, bloating, and ascites can be difficult.

Compared with IPAH, relatively little is known regarding effective treatments for POPH, due to the small number of patients with POPH and their exclusion from clinical trials. Mild disease usually does not require specific treatment; whether early therapy will prevent progression is unknown. Treatment for more severe disease differs from that of other patients with PAH in that some experts have advised against the use of calcium channel antagonists even if acute vasoreactivity is documented during cardiac catheterization. This concern is based upon the potential worsening of intrahepatic venous gradients by calcium channel antagonists.[296–299] Diuretics are particularly important in POPH due to the frequent presence of both cor pulmonale and cirrhosis causing fluid retention, edema, and ascites. Anticoagulation is less frequently employed due to pre-existing coagulopathy related to underlying hepatic synthetic deficiencies or the presence of splenomegaly and significant thrombocytopenia.

The experience with inhaled or parenteral prostenoids or oral endothelin antagonists or phosphodiesterase-5 inhibitors in the treatment of POPH has been reported in small case series.[300–309] Given the significant incidence of liver function abnormalities associated with endothelin antagonist treatment, there has been concern for their use in patients with POPH. However, bosentan was successfully used in a nonrandomized study of 11 patients with POPH and Child Class A resulting in improvements in hemodynamic values, exercise capacity, and no significant liver toxicity.[310] The potentially more favorable liver toxicity profile of ambrisentan may permit therapy in additional patients with POPH, and the safe use of the drug in this setting has been reported.[311,312]

Many patients with advanced hepatic dysfunction require liver transplantation. The perioperative mortality is significantly increased by the presence of severe PAH, however, and therefore a mean PA pressure above 50 mm Hg is considered a contraindication to transplantation at most centers.[313,314] Effective treatment to lower PAPs has been used in some patients who subsequently underwent orthotopic liver transplantation successfully.[300–303,307,315] It is therefore essential that POPH be recognized in patients being considered for liver transplantation prior to surgery. All potential liver transplant patients should be assessed by echocardiography, and cardiac catheterization should be undertaken when the estimated right ventricular systolic pressure approaches 50 mm Hg. Serial monitoring for the development of pulmonary hypertension should be performed in patients listed for liver transplantation.[316] Unlike the hepatopulmonary syndrome in which liver transplantation results in resolution of the pulmonary vascular abnormality, liver transplantation is not reliably curative of POPH. While some cases of reversal have been reported, POPH has progressed in other patients following transplantation.[296]

Drugs and Toxins

The term "dietary pulmonary hypertension" refers to the fact that substances taken by mouth can damage the pulmonary circulation. In animals, ingestion of *Crotalaria spectabilis*, an annual shrub, causes multiorgan injury, including damage to the lungs. In humans, certain appetite suppressant drugs exert similar effects.

Anorectic Agents—Aminorex and Fenfluramine Derivative

Between 1966 and 1968, an epidemic of PAH erupted in Switzerland, Austria, and Germany where the incidence increased 20-fold.[317] The epidemic followed the introduction in these countries of an appetite-depressant agent, aminorex (2-amino-5-phenyl-2-oxazoline), in November 1965. Although only 2% of those exposed to the drug developed PAH, the relative risk compared to unexposed individuals was 52:1.[318] Aminorex resembles epinephrine and amphetamine in chemical structure; both of these agents release endogenous stores of catecholamines. Aminorex was banned in 1968, and the epidemic subsided. After stopping the drug, the level of pulmonary hypertension decreased or stabilized at a tolerable level in some patients and completely reversed in others. However, in many patients, the disease continued inexorably from pulmonary hypertension to cor pulmonale and death despite discontinuation of the drug. The pathology produced by aminorex in humans was identical with that of IPAH, including plexiform lesions and intimal fibrosis. Unfortunately, attempts to produce pulmonary hypertension by administering aminorex to experimental animals were consistently unsuccessful.

This outbreak had several important epidemiologic implications: (1) A medication taken by mouth could damage pulmonary arteries and arterioles; (2) because only few of the many individuals who used the agent developed pulmonary hypertension, the possibility was raised of genetic susceptibility to injury by aminorex; (3) other anorectic medications that resemble the catecholamines and amphetamines in structure might have similar effects in predisposed individuals (this possibility was reinforced by experience with phenformin, an antidiabetic agent that resembles the amphetamines in structure); and (4) pulmonary hypertension can be reversible, particularly when detected early in its course and before pressures reach systemic levels.

After the aminorex epidemic, a variety of appetite-suppressant medications were used with little heed to the possibility that these agents might cause PAH. Then, in the early 1990s, Brenot et al.[319] called attention to possible association in Europe of PAH and the use of fenfluramine derivatives for weight reduction, prompting the establishment of an international registry in Europe to assess the incidence and risks of IPAH. Among the 95 patients enrolled in the registry, anorectic agent use was clearly associated with an increased risk of PAH, especially when taken longer than 3 months (odds ratio 23.8). In 1996, Abenheim sounded the alarm that an epidemic might be in the making: the Food and Drug Administration in the United States had approved the use of dexfenfluramine, a fenfluramine derivative, for the long-term treatment of obesity even though experience with long-term use was extremely sparse.[226]

Approval of dexfenfluramine by the FDA was followed by a tremendous increase in sales of this and other anorectic agents. A registry of idiopathic and anorectic agent associated PAH in the United States revealed that use of fenfluramine was strongly associated with the development of PAH (odds ratio 7.5 with greater than 6 months use). A high prevalence of anorectic agent use in patients with other forms of PAH was also seen, suggesting these agents might also precipitate disease in the presence of other risks such as a collagen vascular disease.[320]

Several points were illustrated: (1) Although aminorex and the fenfluramines differ in their pharmacologic characteristics, the pulmonary vascular lesions in the patients who die of pulmonary hypertension after taking either drug are identical; (2) the longer the anorectic agent is used, the more likely pulmonary hypertension is to develop; and (3) the occurrence of pulmonary hypertension in users of anorectic agents likely is related to other determinants of susceptibility, perhaps genetic.

Aminorex and fenfluramine derivatives may cause PAH by altering blood levels of serotonin (5-HT). These agents cause the release of serotonin from storage in platelets and inhibit its reuptake,[71] and serotonin is a potent vasoconstrictor and induces the aggregation of platelets. An additional mechanism by which aminorex and fenfluramine derivatives might contribute to pulmonary vasoconstriction is via the inhibition of potassium channels that mediate vasodilation.[128] An inductive role of anorexigens in promoting the development of PAH in genetically susceptible individuals has also been hypothesized. Genotyping for the presence of mutations in *BMPRII* (with familial PAH) has not revealed a significant number of abnormalities among patients with anorexigen-associated PAH.[181,321]

In one series of 62 patients with fenfluramine-associated PAH evaluated over a 10-year period at a single center in France, the interval from drug exposure to the development of dyspnea was approximately 4 years. Hemodynamic values at the time of diagnosis were similar to a control group of patients with IPAH, although the anorectic agent–exposed patients were less likely to demonstrate acute vasoreactivity and thus be treated with calcium channel antagonists.[322] The approach to therapy for PAH associated with anorectic agent use, however, is similar as for IPAH.

Relatively little is known regarding the prognosis of anorectic agent–associated disease. Data conflict regarding prognosis as compared with IPAH. In one retrospective study of 104 patients with aminorex-associated PAH and 69 with IPAH, survival was better in both groups for patients treated with warfarin, and better overall for the anorectic-agent associated disease patients.[323] With the use of advanced therapies, survival in fenfluramine-exposed patients with PAH appears similar to that of IPAH patients.[322] When matched according to treatments and disease severity, however, a separate study of IPAH and fenfluramine-exposed patients found poorer survival in the anorectic agent group.[324]

Toxic Oil Syndrome

Another episode of dietary pulmonary hypertension unfolded with the occurrence of the "toxic oil syndrome." In May and June 1981, rapeseed oil adulterated with aniline was sold door to door as olive oil in Spain and caused an outbreak of noncardiogenic pulmonary edema.[325] Twenty thousand persons were affected, and approximately 375 died. About 2000 individuals experienced sequelae. As a consequence of close surveillance, the features of three stages of the disease were categorized as early (first 6 months), intermediate (6 months to 2 years), and chronic (persisting years). From the outset, it was clear that the damage was widespread (affecting lungs, liver, skin, nervous system, immune system, muscle, and fat) and that pervasive endothelial injury featured prominently in the pathogenesis of the clinical syndromes.

The early stage was characterized by noncardiogenic pulmonary edema, eosinophilia, and pulmonary hypertension in a subset of patients; these findings resolved within 6 months. The intermediate stage was marked by thromboembolic events, weight loss, and neuromuscular dystrophies; PAH developed in some but often resolved. The chronic stage (particularly 4 and 5 years after the oil was ingested) involved progressive PAH and cor pulmonale. Increasingly evident were vascular lesions of intimal fibrosis and proliferation in association with organized pulmonary thromboemboli. Plexiform lesions were also seen.

Unfortunately, the exact chemical ingredients in the toxic oil responsible for the syndrome remain enigmatic and are unlikely to be identified, since the bootleggers could provide no recipe for the adulterated cooking oil. Nonetheless, the outbreak did show that material taken by mouth – often in small quantities – could cause widespread endothelial injury in the lungs. It also underscored the spontaneous reversibility of the pulmonary hypertension (as well as the ineffectiveness of vasodilators tried at different stages in the disease).

Hemoglobinopathies

Patients with sickle cell anemia and other hemoglobinopathies are at increased risk for the development of pulmonary hypertension. Pulmonary hypertension in this setting has been variably categorized as WHO Group 1 (PAH) or as WHO Group 5 disease. Multiple factors likely contribute to the pathogenesis of pulmonary hypertension in patients with hemolytic states, including recurrent thromboembolism, recurrent infectious or hemolytic crises causing lung damage and hypoxia, asplenia, and the microvascular effects of intravascular hemolysis itself. Hemolysis contributes to the development of pulmonary hypertension by reducing the bioavailability of NO. Hemoglobin is released into the plasma from destroyed red blood cells where it can bind and sequester NO. There is also destruction of the substrate for NO production, L-arginine, by increased levels the enzyme arginase, also released into plasma by hemolysis. Further effects of hemolysis include an increase in the expression of vascular adhesion molecules, platelet activation, the production of free radicals, and elevated levels of endothelin, all of which might contribute to the vasculopathy.[326–328]

The reported prevalence of pulmonary hypertension in patients with sickle cell anemia has ranged from 0% to 40%. Factors influencing this wide range include the age of patients examined, whether the study involved asymptomatic or symptomatic patients, and whether testing involved echocardiography or cardiac catheterization. In one prospective study of 195 adult patients with sickle cell anemia, 32% of patients had echocardiographic evidence of pulmonary hypertension, of which over 90% had the SS phenotype.[329] Pulmonary hypertension is associated with a poorer prognosis in patients with sickle cell anemia.[326,329] Pulmonary hypertension has also been noted in patients with other chronic hemolytic disorders, including thalassemias, hereditary spherocytosis, and paroxysmal nocturnal hemoglobinuria.[330–335]

The hemodynamic findings of pulmonary hypertension associated with sickle cell anemia differ from those seen in patients with idiopathic or other forms of associated PAH. Specifically, the mean PAP tends to be lower and CO higher in patients with sickle cell anemia diagnosed with pulmonary hypertension than in patients with IPAH. In addition, many patients with hemoglobinopathy and pulmonary hypertension demonstrate a combination of intrinsic pulmonary vascular disease suggested by an elevated vascular resistance together with left heart diastolic dysfunction with an elevated PAWP.[336] As an example, in 20 patients with pulmonary hypertension associated with sickle cell anemia the mean PAP was 36 mm Hg, CO 8.6 L/min, and PCWP 16 mm Hg; one-half of the patients had PAWP values above 15 mm Hg.[337]

The optimal treatment of patients with pulmonary hypertension associated with a hemoglobinopathy has not been established. As markers of ongoing hemolysis correlate with the severity of pulmonary hypertension as well as survival in patients with sickle cell disease, maximizing treatment of the hemolytic anemia is likely an important therapeutic consideration.[326,329] Treatment includes the use of hydroxyurea or transfusions to minimize anemia and ongoing hemolysis. Intravenous prostacyclin can acutely decrease the mean PAP and PVR in patients with PAH associated with sickle cell anemia, but its long-term benefits have not been established.[337] Oral sildenafil has been shown to acutely improve the mPAP, PVR and cardiac index; however, conflicting effects on 6-minute walk distance have been reported.[338,339] Safety concerns such as headache, priapism, and increased hospitalization rates for pain remain incompletely resolved. Improvement with sildenafil has also been reported in a small, uncontrolled series of patients with other hemoglobinopathies but large trials are lacking.[340] Supplemental oxygen to prevent hypoxia should be used as in other forms of pulmonary hypertension. While not studied in patients with hemoglobinopathy for treatment of pulmonary hypertension itself, anticoagulation to prevent thromboembolic complications of sickle cell anemia is also a consideration.

PULMONARY VENOOCCLUSIVE DISEASE

PVOD is a rare form of PAH in which there is even less understanding of mechanisms and less experience with therapy.[217,341] Some combination of pathologic changes on both the arterial and venous sides of the pulmonary circulation is found in all forms of PAH, but arterial changes tend to predominate in most cases. There is patchy occlusion of pulmonary veins by fibrous tissue, intimal thickening, and large numbers of hemosiderin-laden macrophages. Lymphatic dilation in the lung and pleura are additional features, likely related to pulmonary capillary hypertension and consequent chronically increased hydrostatic movement of fluid from the capillaries into the interstitium.

The incidence and prevalence of PVOD are unknown owing at least in part to frequent misdiagnosis as IPAH. Thirteen percent of cases in the NIH registry had histologic changes of PVOD.[37] In a pooling of IPAH patient series in which cases meeting criteria for a diagnosis of PVOD were reported, an incidence of 0.1 to 0.2 cases per million persons in the general population has been estimated.[217] Prospective studies have not been performed, however, and this figure likely underestimates the true incidence of PVOD, as some cases are likely misclassified as either interstitial lung disease or heart failure because of similarities in radiographic appearance.[341] There is no apparent predilection for women (as is seen in IPAH) and patients have been diagnosed from infancy to the seventh decade of life.[342]

The risk factors for PVOD are not well known. As familial cases of this apparently rare disease have been reported, a genetic predisposition has been postulated. Indeed, mutations in *BMPRII* have been identified in several patients with PVOD.[183,342] Case reports of PVOD complicating treatment of cancer with various chemotherapeutic agents (notably mitomycin, bleomycin, carmustine, and gemcitabine) or following bone marrow transplantation suggest that toxic exposures might elicit pathologic vascular responses.[343–356] Other case reports have noted the development of PVOD in association with various thrombophilic states, autoimmune disorders, or following bacterial or viral infection, including HIV.[357–364] More recently, abnormal circulating cytotoxic lymphocyte subpopulations and epigenetic dysregulation within the GNLY gene have been reported in individuals with PVOD, although the significance of such observations remains unclear.[365]

Patients with PVOD usually present with dyspnea and fatigue; symptoms less typical of other forms of PAH such as cough, orthopnea, and hemoptysis have also been observed.[196,366–370] The presence of basilar inspiratory crackles on physical examination favors a diagnosis of PVOD over other forms of PAH although these are clearly nonspecific. Decreased basilar breath sounds might suggest the presence of pleural effusions, which tend to occur more commonly in PVOD.[371,372]

The diagnosis of PVOD is suggested by the triad of pulmonary hypertension, radiographic evidence of pulmonary edema, and a normal PCWP. Unfortunately, all three are not universally present in cases of PVOD and the diagnosis frequently is delayed because of confusing findings during evaluation. As an example, "high probability" findings on ventilation–perfusion scanning, a frequent finding in PVOD, may lead to an erroneous diagnosis of CTEPH.[373] Findings on plain radiographs and CT scans in PVOD include enlargement of the central pulmonary arteries, peribronchial cuffing, Kerley B lines, interstitial infiltrates, and pleural effusions that in other circumstances might suggest left heart failure.[196,374]

In the appropriately placed pulmonary artery catheter with its balloon inflated, there is a static column of blood from the catheter tip to the left atrium and the pressure transduced is reflective of left heart chamber filling pressures (which should be normal in patients with PVOD).[375,376] Obtaining an adequate tracing, however, can be difficult and may require positioning the catheter in multiple areas. Of note, there may be a marked rise in measured pressure and a subsequent slow decline back to normal when saline is flushed through the wedged catheter; this is presumed due to impaired run-off of fluid through the restricted pulmonary venous vessels.

The antemortem diagnosis of PVOD often requires surgical biopsy but this frequently is avoided due to increased operative and anesthetic risk in the setting of severe pulmonary hypertension, particularly given the questionable impact on therapy that establishing the diagnosis produces. However, establishing a diagnosis does provide prognostic information to the patient, may influence the urgency of evaluation for lung transplantation, and may be helpful in avoiding needless and possibly harmful therapies.

The features atypical of other forms of PAH (e.g., radiographic abnormalities "normally" consistent with left heart failure) should prompt caution when considering acute vasodilator testing.[196,374] Acute pulmonary edema, at times life-threatening, has been precipitated by the administration of vasodilators to patients with PVOD.

There are no established therapies for PVOD. Controlled studies have not been performed and only anecdotal reports are available. These describe both positive and negative responses to various agents. Some patients have experienced benefit while others have died with the use of calcium channel antagonists, intravenous epoprostenol, or other advanced therapies.[196,377–382] Glucocorticoids and other immunosuppressive agents have been attempted but experience has been anecdotal, with mixed results, and their use is not generally recommended except in rare cases where a concomitant inflammatory condition exists.[341,383,384] As in other forms of PAH, diuretics and supplemental oxygen should be employed as indicated. Lung transplantation is the only therapeutic option for many patients. The prognosis of patients with PVOD is poor, with most dying within 2 years of diagnosis.

PULMONARY CAPILLARY HEMANGIOMATOSIS

Pulmonary capillary hemangiomatosis is another rare form of PAH with predominant involvement of the pulmonary veins. Pathologically, the findings are those of "pulmonary microvasculopathy" marked by angioproliferative capillary lesions that appear to invade the pulmonary vessels, interstitium, and in some cases the airways.[385,386] The etiology is unknown. Descriptive studies have reported the presence of vascular growth factors as well as markers of altered endothelial cell proliferation; altered expression of nitric oxide synthase has also been noted.[387–389] A heritable form has been reported to have occurred in three siblings but specific genetic linkage has not been established.[390]

Epidemiologic features of the disease are unknown, as only scattered case reports are available for evaluation. Pulmonary capillary hemangiomatosis may present with dyspnea and episodes of hemoptysis, and cases both with and without associated pulmonary hypertension have been reported. The radiographic findings are described as diffuse bilateral reticulonodular infiltrates, often associated with enlargement of the central pulmonary arteries.[391,392] The prognosis is poor, with most cases reported as fatal, often rapidly. Attempts at treatment with intravenous epoprostenol have resulted in pulmonary edema.[393–395] Successful treatment of several patients has been described with α-interferon; another patient with superimposed endotheliomatosis was stabilized with doxycycline.[396,397] Urgent evaluation for lung transplantation is recommended.

■ SCHISTOSOMIASIS

Schistosomiasis, also referred to as bilharzia or snail fever, is caused by infection with any of several species of the trematode flatworm fluke *Schistosoma*. Typically, humans contract schistosomiasis by contact with shallow water that contains snails that are intermediate hosts of the *Schistosoma* pathogen. Cercariae, the life-cycle stage released from infected snails, may penetrate human skin and after a conformational change to become schistosomulae, reach the lungs.[398] Lung involvement tends to develop after extensive chronic liver involvement and there is debate about the relative contributions of POPH, periovular granulomas in the lungs, and host immunologic changes in producing PAH-like pathologic changes in up to 9% of patients.[399] It is estimated that up to 300 million individuals worldwide have schistosomiasis and as such it is likely to be one of the most numerically important causes of PAH. Patients generally present clinically with dyspnea on exertion and other features similar to PAH due to other causes. Diagnosis requires documentation of PAH via hemodynamic assessments along with clinical and serologic evidence of *Schistosoma* infection.

Much remains unknown regarding the prognosis and optimal approach to therapy. One series of 54 patients in Brazil suggested a more benign course than IPAH patients at the same institution.[400] Treatment with prostenoids, endothelin antagonists, and phosphodiesterase-5 inhibitors appears efficacious in improving hemodynamics and 6-minute walk distance although large randomized trials are lacking.[401] The antischistosomal agent, praziquantel, can reverse pulmonary hypertension and vascular remodeling in murine schistosomiasis although its efficacy in human disease is not documented.[402]

THERAPY FOR PULMONARY ARTERIAL HYPERTENSION

The many facets and challenges in treating pulmonary arterial hypertension are presented below.

■ A CAUTIONARY NOTE: NON-PAH FORMS OF PULMONARY HYPERTENSION

Therapy must be driven by an appropriately established diagnosis.[403] As is noted previously, PAH is but one form of pulmonary hypertension and overall less common than pulmonary hypertension due to parenchymal lung or left heart disorders. Appropriate therapy for pulmonary hypertension due to left heart disease or parenchymal lung disease centers on optimal management of the underlying left heart disorder or lung disease, respectively. Far too often focus on the presence of pulmonary hypertension distracts clinicians' attention from the underlying cause. This not only leads to inappropriate use of drugs that are of established benefit only among patients with PAH, but may be accompanied by a failure to pursue appropriate therapies more likely to relieve a patient's symptoms (such as appropriate fluid management for left heart failure, interventions for coronary artery disease, correction of a mitral or aortic valvular dysfunction, bronchodilators and other inhaled medications for obstructive lung disease, or control of systemic hypertension). Other times, when underlying lung or left heart disorders have been maximally treated and symptoms remain, frustrated clinicians and patients may be driven to "blame" persistent problems on the presence of pulmonary hypertension. They may try drugs approved for treatment of PAH reasoning, "there is nothing else to do," or that, "it couldn't hurt." Unfortunately, such an approach is currently ill-informed and potentially harmful. The use of drugs approved for treatment of PAH in patients with other forms of pulmonary hypertension has not been found to be beneficial and is associated with known harms including exposure to well-established side effects. For example, randomized trials of patients with decreased left ventricular systolic function have raised concerns for worsened heart failure with the use of endothelin receptor antagonists, and have resulted in an increased risk for death with epoprostenol infusion.[404,405] Another randomized trial of patients with COPD and echocardiographic evidence of pulmonary hypertension found use of bosentan worsened hypoxemia and quality of life, and failed to improve exercise capacity.[406] Despite suggestion of improved exercise capacity among patients with left heart dysfunction and pulmonary hypertension treated with sildenafil in a preliminary study, a larger randomized trial found no improvement, and there were more adverse events among the participants who received sildenafil.[407,408] Finally, the high expense of these drugs often must be borne by the patient as well as the healthcare system.

■ GENERAL MANAGEMENT

A variety of pharmacologic and nonpharmacologic interventions are used in treatment of pulmonary arterial hypertension. PAH-specific pharmacotherapy is discussed in a separate section, below.

Exercise and the Avoidance of Deconditioning

Regardless of the cause, patients with pulmonary hypertension and cor pulmonale should be encouraged to maintain as active a lifestyle as possible. Recommendations that the patient minimize exertion for fear of further raising pulmonary pressures generally result only in deconditioning of the muscles and an increase in fatigue and breathlessness when an activity is attempted. Regular, steady aerobic exercise should be encouraged, and is often best initiated under guidance of a pulmonary or cardiac rehabilitation program. Indeed, randomized trials of exercise rehabilitation in patients with PAH or CTEPH have demonstrated not only the safety of exercise in these patients, but improvements in exercise capacity (e.g., 6-minute walk distance) greater than that observed in randomized clinical trails of currently available pharmacologic treatments for PAH. Clinically significant improvements in exercise capacity as well as health-related quality of life occurred in both an intensive exercise regimen beginning with inpatient therapy, as well as a 10-week outpatient program of treadmill walking similar in intensity to that commonly used in pulmonary and cardiac rehabilitation programs.[409,410] In addition to improving strength and endurance, the benefits of a supervised rehabilitation program may include a decrease in the fear many patients with dyspnea experience when initiating exercise programs. Many rehabilitation programs teach techniques to cope with dyspnea when it occurs, allowing exercise to continue. Importantly, activities that cause patients to experience lightheadedness or syncope should be avoided, including hot showers or baths and bending over to lift heavy objects.

Oxygen Therapy

Although controlled studies analogous to those performed in the treatment of COPD have not been conducted,[411] it is recommended that patients with pulmonary hypertension avoid acute hypoxia, as hypoxic pulmonary vasoconstriction will add to the burden on the right ventricle. Oxygen relieves hypoxic pulmonary vasoconstriction, thus decreasing vascular resistance and improving CO.

It also lessens renal vasoconstriction, improving urinary sodium excretion, and alleviates tissue hypoxia by improving oxygen delivery. Measurements of arterial oxyhemoglobin saturation should be performed at rest, with exertion, and with sleep. Levels of arterial oxygen saturation below 90% should prompt supplemental oxygen. Maintenance of adequate oxygen saturation may be difficult in patients with severe pulmonary hypertension in whom a patient foramen ovale allows right-to-left shunting.

Air travel is a particular concern because of the threat of hypoxic pulmonary vasoconstriction. Measurements made during commercial airline flights lasting a mean of 3.6 hours in a series of patients with PAH or CTEPH found that oxyhemoglobin desaturation below 85% occurred in 26% of participants, at a mean cabin pressure of 1971 ± 73 m (6467 ± 240 ft) with the lowest occurring at 1829 m (6000 ft).[412] Over one-third of patients developed symptoms during flight. Although more definitive studies have not been performed, it seems prudent to evaluate pulmonary hypertension patients who plan air travel that will last more than a few hours for in-flight oxygen use, particularly among patients with prior need of supplemental oxygen (including with sleep only). Many pulmonary function laboratories can simulate conditions of high altitude with an inspired oxygen concentration of 15% to determine whether the patient requires supplemental oxygen to maintain adequate oxyhemoglobin saturation. Patients should contact airlines in advance of travel as requirements differ, as do costs (which regrettably may not be covered by insurance). An attractive alternative to stored oxygen systems are portable concentrators, which most airlines will permit patients to carry on board without special arrangements.

Immunizations

Immunizations against influenza and pneumococcal pneumonia are important preventive measures in all patients with pulmonary hypertension and cor pulmonale. Influenza vaccination should occur annually, and administration of the 23-valent polysaccharide pneumococcal vaccine should occur once at the time PH is diagnosed and again when the patient turns 65.

Fluid Management and Diuretics

Careful attention to avoid fluid overload is central to the management of cor pulmonale of any cause. Patients must be educated regarding appropriate dietary habits and to restrict sodium intake to minimize fluid retention and the development of right heart failure. Patients should weigh themselves daily so that any trend toward fluid retention can be reversed before progressive right ventricular overload results in failure that may then be more difficult to reverse and require inpatient treatment.

Management of right heart failure relies heavily on diuretic therapy. Spironolactone is often used to manage mild fluid retention. It may also have beneficial effects in heart failure by modulating neurohormones. Loop diuretics are often required to prevent more significant fluid retention and right heart failure. Indeed, high doses and combinations of diuretics are often required to maintain appropriate fluid balance, but must be used cautiously to avoid electrolyte imbalances and volume depletion.

Digitalis

It is unsettled whether cardiac glycosides should play a role in treating right heart failure. In one series of 17 patients with PAH and right ventricular failure, the intravenous administration of 1 mg of digoxin resulted in a modest increase in CO after 2 hours[413] but longer-term data are lacking. Approximately 25% of patients in the REVEAL registry were using digoxin, [191] but many physicians avoid use of this agent even when right-sided heart failure is evident on account of a lack of sufficient evidence regarding its use in PAH and the potential for toxicity.

Anticoagulation

In the absence of contraindications, anticoagulation with warfarin is recommended for patients with significant IPAH.[191,197] This is reasoned to be of benefit on the basis of autopsy studies revealing in situ thrombosis in both venous and arterial vessels without evidence of an embolic source in a significant proportion of patients with PAH.[44–46] Anticoagulation is also justified on the basis of the increased risk of venous thromboembolic disease in patients with severe heart failure and immobility, and their expected poor tolerance of embolic events. The efficacy of anticoagulant therapy in patients with PAH has never been studied in randomized controlled trials. Uncontrolled observational reports, however, have demonstrated an association between warfarin use and increased survival. In a study of 64 IPAH patients randomized to treatment with calcium channel antagonists or placebo, survival after 5 years was greater among those patients in either group who at their provider's discretion had received warfarin.[414] In a retrospective evaluation of 173 patients with either idiopathic or anorexigen-associated PAH, anticoagulation was associated with a statistically greater survival among the anorexigen agent patients and a trend toward improvement after 5 years of therapy in patients with idiopathic disease.[323] Extrapolating from such studies, warfarin is often prescribed to patients with other forms of PAH but disease-specific data supporting this practice is nonexistent.

The generally recommended target international normalized ratio (INR) for warfarin therapy in patients with PAH is 1.5 to 2.5.[415] The severity of disease (e.g., threshold mean PAP or PVR) at which anticoagulation should be initiated has not been determined. A role for newer, non-warfarin oral anticoagulants (e.g., rivaroxaban, dabigatran, apixaban) has not been defined in patients with PAH.

Contraception and Pregnancy

Pregnancy in women with IPAH is associated with a high mortality, on the order of 30% to 50%.[416–418] Expert consensus is that pregnancy should be avoided, and early termination recommended on account of the high maternal mortality.[191,197] Effective contraception should be ensured; if hormonal contraception is chosen, anticoagulation may be advisable to reduce the risk of venous thromboembolism. Although the successful management of pregnancy has been reported,[419] single and multicenter series continue to report high rates of maternal death despite the use of aggressive treatments including intravenous prostenoids.[420–422]

Other Considerations

Patients should be queried about the concomitant use of medications and herbs. Warfarin is particularly apt to be associated with drug–drug interactions. The use of vasoconstrictor or serotonergic medications for unrelated illnesses, such as migraine, should also be undertaken cautiously. Patients taking bosentan are at risk of interaction with such medications as cyclosporine and azole-type antimicrobial agents, and care must be taken to avoid glyburide-containing diabetic therapies. Surgical procedures may entail considerable operative and postoperative risk in patients with hemodynamic compromise from PAH.

Vulnerability of patients with severe PAH to vasovagal events has to be kept in mind. An attack can be precipitated by pain, nausea, vomiting, or straining (Fig. 72-14). The induction of anesthesia and intubation may be a particularly troublesome time. The combination of bradycardia and systemic vasodilation can lead to a precipitous drop in systemic blood pressure. Atropine or a similar agent should be kept at hand during invasive procedures.

■ PAH-SPECIFIC PHARMACOTHERAPY

Treatment of PAH aims to decrease PVR, thereby improving CO. Acute improvements occur in some patients with certain vasodilators. Used chronically, some agents also appear to have cellular

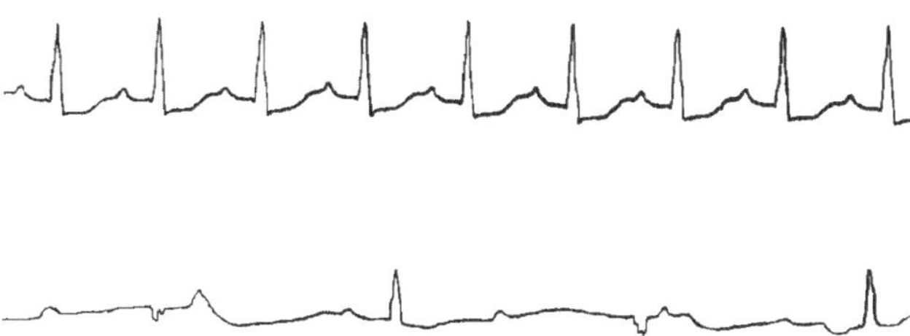

Figure 72-14 Idiopathic pulmonary arterial hypertension. Bradycardia and prolongation of atrioventricular conduction progressed to atrioventricular dissociation while patient was on bedpan. Associated with syncope.

effects that may ameliorate some of the vascular derangements seen in untreated disease. Remarkable progress in the treatment of IPAH has resulted in the availability of multiple therapies and a significantly improved outlook, with many long-term survivors. No currently available medical treatment, however, is curative and despite clinical improvement in many patients that is durable in some, histopathologic changes of vasculopathy remain.[423] Lung transplantation remains an option for some failing medical therapy.

The majority of subjects studied in controlled clinical trials of treatment with calcium channel antagonists, prostenoids, endothelin receptor antagonists, or phosphodiesterase inhibitors have been patients with either IPAH or PAH associated with scleroderma. Since most of these studies compared a single agent to placebo, our knowledge regarding the relative efficacy of available agents is limited by the lack of head-to-head comparisons. In addition, patients treated in earlier studies with epoprostenol were generally sicker than those treated in more recent studies of oral therapies. Finally, only small numbers of patients with heritable or various other forms of PAH have been studied, limiting our ability to draw firm conclusions about efficacy in these less common disorders.

Care must be taken in comparing and applying the results of clinical trials of different pharmacologic agents. Most clinical trials have enrolled patients and assessed response at least in part on the basis of a WHO modification of the New York Heart Association functional assessment of patients with heart failure (Table 72-4), and there appears to be substantial variability in even expert clinicians' judgments of functional class.[424] The 6-minute walk distance has been the most commonly used primary end point in trials of PAH drugs currently available, and with several exceptions improvements in this parameter have been the basis for their approval by the US Food and Drug Administration. The minimal clinically meaningful change in 6-minute walk distance in patients with PAH has been estimated to be between 33 and 42 meters.[425,426] These estimates, however, have been made using data from trials of predominantly treatment naïve patients, and may not be applicable when additional therapies are added.[427,428] Further, trials have mostly been of short duration (12–16 weeks). Additional endpoints such as threshold levels of exercise capacity, indications of clinical deterioration and long-term morbidity or even mortality may emerge as more important metrics to assess individual and combinations of drugs. Assessments of clinical deterioration have been reported as endpoints in several trials of PAH-specific therapy, including, for example, the time until PAH-related hospitalization, death, need for transplantation, or escalation of therapy, but the definitions used have varied.

In addition, the results of long-term follow-up studies (discussed below) must be interpreted with caution. In addition to being open-label (nonblinded) therapy, the selection of patients for therapy was determined at the physician's discretion (nonrandomized) and nonprotocol changes in other therapies occurred. Thus, confident assessments of the benefit or adverse effects of a given agent, comparison to others, and generalization of the findings are not possible. These results are, however, the best descriptions currently available regarding long-term use of these agents.

In general, the choice of initial therapy depends upon an assessment of disease severity and the patient's prognosis and risk for further, rapid deterioration. This judgment involves an assessment of a combination of variables, including hemodynamic and echocardiographic findings, exercise capacity, functional classification, and recent clinical stability of deterioration (Table 72-9). Although more or less "aggressive" approaches have not been compared directly in randomized studies, in general, patients thought to be at lower risk are first treated with an oral agent, whereas

TABLE 72-9 Assessment of Risk in PAH[a]

Determinants of Risk	Lower Risk (Good Prognosis)	Higher Risk (Poor Prognosis)
Clinical evidence of RV failure	No	Yes
Progression of symptoms	Gradual	Rapid
WHO class[b]	II, III	IV
6MW distance[c]	Longer (>400 m)	Shorter (<300 m)
CPET	Peak $\dot{V}_{O_2}$ greater than 10.4 mL/kg/min	Peak $\dot{V}_{O_2}$ less than 10.4 mL/kg/min
Echocardiography	Minimal RV dysfunction	Pericardial effusion, significant RV enlargement/dysfunction, right atrial enlargement
Hemodynamics	RAP less than 10 mm Hg, CI greater than 2.5 L/min/m^2	RAP greater than 20 mm Hg, CI less than 2.0 L/min/m^2
BNP[d]	Minimally elevated	Significantly elevated

[a]Most data available pertains to IPAH. Little data is available for other forms of PAH. One should not rely on any single factor to make risk predictions.
[b]WHO class is the functional classification for PAH and is a modification of the New York Heart Association functional class.
[c]6MW distance is also influenced by age, gender and height.
[d]As there is currently limited data regarding the influence of BNP on prognosis, and many factors including renal function, weight, age, and gender may influence BNP, absolute numbers are not given for this variable.
natriuretic peptide. CI, cardiac index; CPET, cardiopulmonary exercise testing; peak $\dot{V}_{O_2}$, average peak oxygen uptake during exercise; RAP, right atrial pressure; RV, right ventricle; WHO, World Health Organization.
Source: Reproduced with permission from McLaughlin VV, Archer SL, Badesch DB, et al. ACCF/AHA 2009 expert consensus document on pulmonary hypertension a report of the American College of Cardiology Foundation task force on expert consensus documents and the American Heart Association developed in collaboration with the American College of Chest Physicians; American Thoracic Society, Inc. and the Pulmonary Hypertension Association. J Am Coll Cardiol. 2009;53(17):1573–1619.

higher-risk patients are started on parenteral therapy. No single variable determines the choice of therapy. For example, a WHO functional class III patient without rapid recent clinical change and a cardiac index above 2.5 L/min/m^2 might be appropriately treated initially with oral therapy. A WHO class III patient who is either rapidly declining clinically or who has a more severely depressed cardiac index (e.g., below 2 L/min/m^2), however, might be more appropriately managed initially with intravenous prostenoid therapy. Personal preferences often influence a patient's willingness to undertake intravenous therapy. In addition, psychosocial issues, cognitive abilities, and other determinants of patient compliance may make certain therapies unsafe even if otherwise medically indicated.[429]

How best to follow patients treated for PAH, and to adjust medications, also are not well established. In addition to the clinical evaluation, most expert referral centers monitor patients with varying combinations of 6-minute walk distance measurements, echocardiograms, and serum NT-BNP. Some practitioners will repeat the right heart catheterization at regular intervals, while others do so only when a change in clinical status requires repeat diagnostic evaluation to guide further treatment. Which tests and frequencies are best at improving outcomes have not been studied in an organized manner, nor has the relative cost effectiveness of different approaches.

Note that additional therapies approved for the treatment of PAH by the FDA since the completion of this volume include an endothelin receptor antagonist (macitentan), an oral prostenoid (treprostinil) and a soluble guanylate cyclase inhibitor (riociguat). In addition, an up-dated guideline to pharmacotherapy for PAH has been released.[430]

Calcium Channel Antagonists

The calcium channel antagonists diminish vascular tone by preventing an increase in cytosolic calcium concentration through inhibition of both the influx of extracellular calcium and the release of calcium from intracellular stores. The long-term prognosis is good for some IPAH patients who respond acutely to the administration of short-acting pulmonary vasodilators and are treated subsequently with calcium channel antagonists. In one study, the survival rate of acutely vasoresponsive patients treated chronically with oral calcium antagonists was maintained at 94% when measured at 1, 3, and 5 years.[414] Unfortunately, relatively few patients demonstrate acute vasoreactivity (~10% by recent estimates) and of these only about one-half experience a sustained clinical response.[431] Oral calcium antagonists should not be used as vasodilator therapy in the absence of documented acute vasoreactivity. Those failing to demonstrate acute vasoreactivity not only fail to benefit from calcium channel antagonist therapy, but are also prone to adverse side effects including systemic hypotension, decreased CO because of a negative inotropic effects, arrhythmias, salt and water retention, syncope, and death. Acute vasodilator testing as described earlier is therefore required to determine whether a clinical trial of calcium channel antagonist therapy is appropriate.

Patients who do manifest a significant acute pulmonary vasodilator response to short-acting agents should undergo monitored trials of oral calcium channel antagonists while the pulmonary artery catheter is still in place. Increasing doses of nifedipine or diltiazem are usually administered until pulmonary hemodynamics are improved (i.e., there is a significant decrease in PVR and PAP and, ideally, an increase in CO). Agents such as verapamil, which exert negative inotropic effects, should be avoided. Testing is stopped if systemic hypotension or a trend of worsening hemodynamic values is seen. Relatively high doses of calcium channel antagonists are required to promote sufficient pulmonary vasodilation. In some instances, the required daily doses of nifedipine and diltiazem have exceeded 200 mg and 700 mg, respectively.[432] The total daily dose should be divided and administered in two or three doses of long-acting formulations to minimize peak and trough drug effects throughout the day. Patients treated with oral calcium antagonists must be monitored for the development of side effects including systemic hypotension or peripheral edema, as well as for evidence of continued benefit.

Endothelin Receptor Antagonists

Endothelin-1 (ET-1) is a member of the endothelin family of peptides secreted by endothelial cells that promote vasoconstriction and modulate the proliferation of vascular smooth muscle and endothelial cells. ET-1 is overexpressed in the vasculature of patients with various forms of PAH and antagonists of its interaction with its receptors (ET_A and ET_B) have been developed for oral use. A dual ET_A/ET_B and a relatively ET_A-selective antagonist are available.

Bosentan is a dual ET_A/ET_B antagonist that improves hemodynamics, exercise capacity, WHO functional class, and the time to clinical worsening (defined as death, PAH-related hospitalization, need for altered therapy or lung transplantation).[90,433] In a double-blind, randomized, placebo-controlled trial of patients with IPAH and PAH associated with collagen vascular disease (predominantly systemic sclerosis), bosentan improved the 6-minute walk distance by 44 m as compared with placebo at 16 weeks. Exercise capacity improved in IPAH patients, while stabilization or a slowing in the rate of deterioration was observed in patients with systemic sclerosis.[90] The beneficial effects of bosentan on exercise capacity and functional class persist at 1 year with open-label use.[434] In a double-blind, randomized placebo-controlled trial of PAH patients with less severe symptoms (WHO functional class II), bosentan treatment for 6 months improved hemodynamics and 6-minute walk distance as compared to placebo.[435] Survival of IPAH patients treated with bosentan in these trials and their open-label extensions was 96% at 1 year and 89% at 2 years as compared with "expected" survival of 69% and 57%, respectively, as predicted by the NIH registry equation.[92]

Improved hemodynamics and exercise capacity have also been demonstrated with bosentan use in a 16-week randomized controlled trial of patients with Eisenmenger syndrome, with persistent effects seen during a 24-week open-label extension.[436,437] Nonrandomized reports have suggested a benefit of bosentan in other specific PAH populations. A prospective open-label study of 16 patients with PAH associated with HIV infection reported improved hemodynamics, exercise capacity, and quality of life after 16 weeks.[438] Retrospective observational studies have reported the successful use of bosentan in pediatric patients with PAH.[439–442]

Ambrisentan is a relatively ET_A-selective antagonist. In concurrent double-blind, placebo-controlled studies of patients with PAH, 5 and 10 mg daily of ambrisentan for 12 weeks resulted in placebo-corrected improvements in 6-minute walk distance of 31 and 51 m, respectively, in one trial, and 32 and 59 m with 2.5 and 5 mg treatments, respectively, in the other trial. A delay in the time to clinical worsening was seen in one of the trials, and health-related quality of life improved in both.[443] In open-label extension studies, ambrisentan therapy was accompanied by improved hemodynamic values at a median duration of over 1 year and persistent improvements in exercise capacity at 2 years.[444,445]

Bosentan therapy is initiated at 62.5 mg orally twice daily and, if liver function remains normal, increased after 1 month to 125 mg twice daily. Liver function must be monitored monthly as significant elevations may occur; severe elevations (transaminase levels greater than eight times normal) require discontinuation of therapy. Lower rates of elevated transaminases are observed with ambrisentan than bosentan and the FDA-label requirement for monthly liver function monitoring has been removed for ambrisentan, although experts continue to recommend intermittent evaluations. Notable side effects include peripheral edema (usually readily responsive to diuretics), anemia, and nasal congestion. Bosentan is contraindicated with either cyclosporine or glyburide. Both ambrisentan and bosentan are teratogenic and contraception and pregnancy testing are required for use in women with childbearing potential.

Phosphodiesterase Inhibitors

The relative deficiency of NO-mediated vasodilation and modulation of cell growth in patients with PAH has led to attempts to augment its effects therapeutically. NO acts through the second messenger cGMP, which is metabolized in the lung predominantly by phosphodiesterase 5. Specific inhibitors of phosphodiesterase type 5 (e.g., sildenafil, vardenafil, and tadalafil) can promote acute pulmonary vasodilation.[446]

In a double-blind, randomized placebo-controlled trial of 267 patients predominantly with IPAH but also some with congenital heart or collagen vascular disease, sildenafil administered orally at 20, 40, or 80 mg three times daily improved hemodynamics, exercise capacity, and functional class.[148] Although the time to clinical worsening was not affected in this single trial, the improvement in exercise capacity (51 m as compared with baseline) was maintained over 1 year among the subset of patients continuing open-label use of sildenafil at 80 mg three times daily. No statistically significant dose response was seen in the primary end point, exercise capacity, of this trial and the FDA-approved dosage for treatment of PAH is 20 mg by mouth three times daily. In open-label follow-up of a subset of patients up to 3 years following 12 weeks of randomized therapy with sildenafil, 46% demonstrated continued improvement over baseline exercise capacity, although additional therapies had been added to sildenafil during this period. In a posthoc analysis of patients in this randomized trial who had PAH associated with connective tissue disease (predominantly scleroderma and lupus erythematosis), improvements in exercise capacity, functional class, and hemodynamics were seen. An initial 12-week, double-blind, placebo-controlled trial of sildenafil for treatment of PAH in children aged 1 to 18 years demonstrated efficacy in improving exercise capacity and hemodynamics at some doses, although the optimal regimen requires further study.[447]

A 12-week, double-blind, placebo-controlled trial of four different doses of tadalafil found an overall placebo-corrected increase in 6-minute walk distance of 33 m (although statistically significant only for the highest dose group, 40 mg daily). The time to clinical worsening and quality of life also improved.[149] The trial included both treatment naïve patients with PAH, as well as those already receiving bosentan treatment. The mean improvement in 6-minute walk distance was greater among the treatment naïve participants (44 m) than those already receiving bosentan (23 m). During open-label extension for up to 1 year, improvements in 6-minute walk distance in patients receiving either 20 or 40 mg daily of tadalafil appeared to be maintained.[448] In a 12-week, double-blind, placebo-controlled trial of an additional phosphodiesterase type 5 inhibitor, vardenafil, improved 6-minute walk distance and hemodynamic values.[449]

Common side effects of phosphodiesterase type 5 inhibitors when used to treat PAH are headache, flushing, diarrhea, epistaxis, and myalgias. Systemic hypotension has also occurred, particularly with concomitant nitrate use, and this combination should be avoided.

Prostenoid Therapies

Prostacyclin analogs have played a key role in the management of idiopathic and other forms of PAH. Prostacyclin is a powerful vasodilator (both pulmonary and systemic) as well as an inhibitor of smooth muscle proliferation and platelet aggregation. It is a product of arachidonic acid metabolism and acts, at least in part, by stimulating the intracellular production of cAMP. Its major source is the vascular endothelial cell and deficiencies are noted in patients with PAH. Several synthetic prostacyclin analogs are currently available in the United States for the long-term treatment of PAH, including formulations administered by continuous intravenous infusion (epoprostenol and treprostinil), subcutaneous infusion (treprostinil), and via inhalation (treprostinil and iloprost).

Prostenoid infusion therapy requires a relatively highly functional and compliant patient for safe administration, preferably in conjunction with a strong social support system at home. Intensive patient and family education is required for safe initiation of therapy and, particularly for intravenous infusions, is often performed with the patient hospitalized until appropriate understanding and proficiency in self-care is demonstrated. While appropriate expertise in the management of PAH is required for nonparenteral treatments, parenteral prostenoid therapy in particular requires the support of a dedicated team of nurses and physicians at a program with sufficient expertise, typically with the additional assistance of nurses from specialty pharmacies.[450]

Intravenous Prostenoid Therapy (Epoprostenol, Iloprost, and Treprostinil) The first prostenoid therapy shown in randomized clinical trials to be beneficial in the treatment of PAH was epoprostenol. Because of its short half-life (on the order of only minutes) it requires continuous intravenous infusion. In an initial study, 81 patients with IPAH were randomized to receive epoprostenol infusion or treatment considered "standard" at the time (oral vasodilators, diuretics, cardiac glycosides, and anticoagulants).[451] After 12 weeks of treatment, hemodynamic values were improved in the epoprostenol group (e.g., a 21% decrease in PVR as compared with an increase in control patients) as was the 6-minute walk distance (increased by 31 m compared with a decrease of 29 m). None of the patients treated with epoprostenol died during the study, as compared to a 20% mortality by 12 weeks with conventional therapy. Intravenous epoprostenol therapy for IPAH was approved by the FDA in 1995.

Additional reports have confirmed and extended these observations. Indeed, originally conceived as a "bridge" to lung transplantation in patients with severe PAH, the long-term use of epoprostenol and other treatments was followed by a decrease in the demand for lung transplantation for this indication.[452] In a cohort of 162 IPAH patients treated with intravenous epoprostenol at a center in the United States, the observed 1- and 3-year survival rates were 88% and 62%, compared to rates of 59% and 35% predicted by the NIH registry equation.[238] Remarkably similar results were observed in a cohort in France of 178 epoprostenol-treated patients with IPAH at 1 and 3 years, and somewhat lower survival rates in a cohort of 91 patients at a second United States center. In each case survival was improved over that predicted by the NIH registry equation.[236,237] Unfortunately, however, one-third of patients with IPAH died within 3 years and nearly half by 5 years (Fig. 72-15).[234]

Epoprostenol infusion therapy has also been used in other forms of PAH. A randomized multicenter trial in patients with systemic sclerosis associated PAH (without significant interstitial lung disease) showed improvements in both hemodynamics and exercise capacity.[453] Favorable results of epoprostenol treatment have also been reported in uncontrolled series of patients with systemic lupus erythematosis,[454] congenital left-to-right shunts,[455] anorectic agent use,[322] patients with HIV, POPH,[300] and inoperable CTEPH.[456] Epoprostenol has been used successfully in isolated reports of patients with PVOD. The use of epoprostenol in patient with PVOD must be approached with extreme caution, however, as its use in patients with impeded venous blood flow might precipitate pulmonary edema.[217] Isolated attempts at treating patients with pulmonary capillary hemangiomatosis (also characterized by predominant involvement of the pulmonary veins) have resulted in death.[397] In a single randomized trial of patients with left ventricular dysfunction, the use of epoprostenol was associated with a trend toward increased mortality.

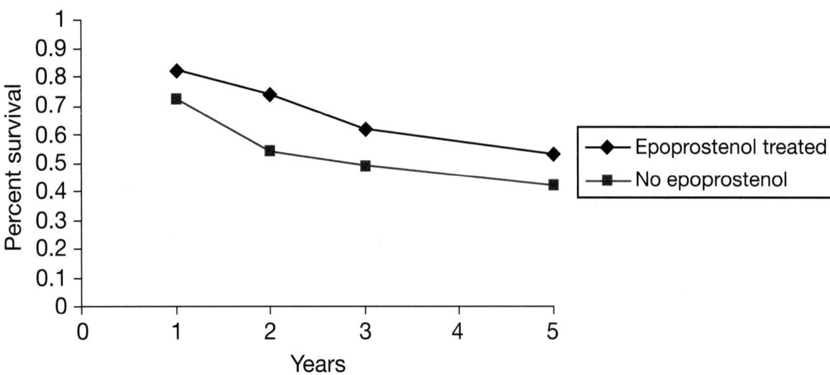

Figure 72-15 The effect of chronically infused epoprostenol therapy on survival in patients ($n = 431$) from multiple series with idiopathic pulmonary arterial hypertension. Survival in the absence of epoprostenol was estimated using a prediction equation derived from observation in the NIH registry of primary pulmonary hypertension at which time effective therapy was not available. *(Reproduced with permission from McLaughlin VV, Presberg KW, Doyle RL, et al. Prognosis of pulmonary arterial hypertension: ACCP evidence-based clinical practice guidelines, Chest. 2004;126(1 Suppl):78S–92S.)*

A longer half-life (3 hours) and stability at room temperature prompted the development of treprostinil as an alternative prostenoid analog for intravenous therapy. Treprostinil appears to have acute hemodynamic effects similar to those of epoprostenol.[457] In an uncontrolled 12-week, open-label study of 16 PAH (8 with IPAH and 6 and 2 associated with connective tissue and congenital heart disease, respectively) intravenous treprostinil infusion resulted in an 82-m improvement in 6-minute walk distance as well as improvements in hemodynamic values.[458] In a subsequent 12-week placebo-controlled randomized trial of 44 PAH patients continuously infused treprostinil resulted in an 83-m placebo-corrected increase in 6-minute walk distance and improvements in functional class.[459] Importantly, this randomized study involved the placement of central venous catheters for placebo infusions (that indeed were associated with harm, including a death). This has raised ethical concerns and questions that must be addressed as investigators of therapy in this rare disease face difficulties with recruitment and aim to extend their reach.[460,461]

Intravenously administered iloprost, another prostanoid, is available in some European countries, but not in the United States. In uncontrolled trials it has been used in patients with IPAH, collagen vascular disease associated PAH, and CTEPH.[462–464] The acute hemodynamic effects are similar to those of epoprostenol, but no controlled trials of its efficacy are available. In a retrospective analysis of 50 patients with PAH treated at multiple centers in Germany with intravenous iloprost following insufficient or deteriorating clinical status after the use of oral therapy with endothelin receptor or phosphodiesterase type 5 inhibitors, only approximately 25% had an improved functional class at 3 months, and more than 50% of patients died or required lung transplantation within 1 year.[465]

Epoprostenol therapy is initiated at 1 to 4 ng/kg/min and progressively increased in 0.5 to 1 ng/kg/min increments at intervals dictated by patient response and side effects. Treprostinil is initiated at 0.625 or 1.25 ng/kg/min and similarly increased as dictated by clinical response, typically in increments of 1.25 ng/kg/min. Induced metabolism mandates a need for continuous increases in dosage to maintain improvements in symptoms. Increases are usually required at more frequent intervals initially to relieve symptoms due to PAH (e.g., dyspnea and lightheadedness) although many patients will reach a more stable dosing with less frequently required increases after several weeks to months. Such titration must be closely monitored for prostenoid side effects (nausea, tachycardia, diarrhea, masticatory jaw pain).[450] Even patients lacking an acute vasodilator response (e.g., to infused epoprostenol) have shown improved hemodynamics and exercise capacity after sustained treatment, suggesting that the beneficial effects are not mediated merely through acute vasodilation, but also by altering cell growth.

Intravenous treatment with epoprostenol or treprostinil requires a tunneled venous catheter and thus is associated with a significant risk of bacterial infection. In an evaluation of 1146 patients who received intravenous prostenoid therapy during over 3 years of the multicenter observational US-based REVEAL cohort, an approximate threefold increase in blood stream infections of any type and over sixfold increase in those due to gram-negative organisms was observed among patients receiving intravenous treprostinil as compared with intravenous epoprostenol.[466] A retrospective study by the US Center for Disease Control of data from seven PAH treatment centers also concluded that rates of bloodstream infection were higher with continuous intravenous infusions of treprostinil than epoprostenol. The higher rate of infection did not appear to be due to intrinsic drug contamination,[467] but may have been related to the neutral pH of the treprostinil diluent, as substitution with the basic pH epoprostenol diluent appeared to eliminate the increase in infection rates with treprostinil at one institution.[468]

Prostenoid infusion requires the use of a battery-powered portable infusion pump that must be carried at all times. A back-up medication cassette and pump must also be immediately available as an interruption of only minutes can result in hemodynamic compromise. In theory, the risk with interrupted treprostinil infusion is somewhat lower on account of its longer half-life. The originally available formulation of epoprostenol is unstable at room temperature and must be mixed daily and kept cool with ice packs. Like treprostinil, a more recently approved formulation of epoprostenol has greater stability at room temperature and does not require continuous cooling with ice packs.[469] Treprostinil may be administered with the same infusion pump used for epoprostenol therapy but smaller equipment is available that may potentially allow for more convenient therapy. Preliminary experience suggests that a higher dosage of treprostinil is required than epoprostenol to maintain an improvement in symptoms. Further observation is required to establish whether survival is similarly improved with treprostinil as with epoprostenol. Experience and established duration of benefit is greatest with epoprostenol infusion and it remains an important treatment for severe PAH, and a benchmark against which other therapies are often compared.

Subcutaneous Prostenoid Therapy (Treprostinil) Treprostinil is also available for subcutaneous administration. In a large randomized double-blind placebo-controlled trial of 470 patients with IPAH or PAH associated with congenital heart or collagen vascular disease, subcutaneous treprostinil resulted in improvements in hemodynamic parameters and a modest improvement in 6-minute walk distance of 16 m at 12 weeks.[470] In an open-label extension study of participants previously enrolled in the randomized trial, together with de novo patients, survival up to 4 years was evaluated in 332 IPAH patient for whom baseline hemodynamic measurements were available. Observed survival was 91% and 72% at 1 and 4 years, respectively, compared with survival rates of 69% and 38% at 1 and 4 years predicted by the NIH registry equation.[471]

The major advantage of subcutaneous treprostinil is avoidance of an intravenous catheter and the associated risk of life-threatening bacteremia. While infections can occur at the subcutaneous infusion site, these are usually mild and manageable with oral antibiotics. Other side effects are similar to those seen with intravenous prostenoid therapy (nausea, diarrhea, flushing, and jaw discomfort). In addition, however, the major drawback of treprotinil has been a significant incidence of troublesome infusion site pain. This occurred in 85% of patients in the pivotal clinical trial and led to discontinuation in 8%.[470] Out of 860 total patients in the previously noted open-label study, 196 (23%) discontinued subcutaneous therapy due to infusion site pain or reactions.[471] Management strategies to reduce the occurrence and severity of pain have been reported, including initial "dry" catheter insertions with delayed infusion of medication, less frequent site rotations, and the application of topical analgesics and anti-inflammatory agents.[472] For those with severe pain refractory to these measures, narcotic analgesics may be required. Another relative disadvantage is a slower rate of dosage titration as compared to intravenous therapy, making it less attractive for severely ill patients in need of a rapid response. In select patients, however, subcutaneous treprostinil has proven to be effective therapy with minimal side effects and has allowed for avoidance of the risks and inconveniences of intravenous therapy.

Inhalational Prostenoid Therapy (Iloprost and Treprostinil) Inhaled prostenoid therapies have been developed in the hopes of avoiding the need for an invasive delivery system. Iloprost is an inhaled prostacyclin analog. Conflicting results of efficacy were seen in uncontrolled studies,[473–475] but a 12-week randomized, placebo-controlled trial of 203 patients demonstrated a placebo-corrected improvement of 36 m in 6-minute walk distance.[476] Most of the patients studied had IPAH; the remainder had PAH associated with anorectic agent or collagen vascular disease, or had CTEPH. Functional class and quality-of-life measures also improved in association with treatment. Hemodynamic variables were improved at 12 weeks when measured following a dose of iloprost, although preinhalation values were unchanged. As in other trials of PAH therapies, hemodynamic variables were worse compared to baseline following 12 weeks of placebo. Following another 3-month placebo-controlled study, 52 patients received open-label iloprost therapy. At 2 years, 36 (69%) remained on iloprost while treatment was discontinued in 16 patients due to death, lack of efficacy, and adverse events in 2, 6, and 6 patients, respectively. The study included patients with PAH and non-PAH forms of disease. The 2-year event-free survival was 74% in the IPAH patients, as compared to a predicted survival of 63% according to the NIH formula.[477]

Treprostinil is also available for inhalational therapy. A 12-week double-blind, placebo-controlled randomized trial of 235 patients with PAH already receiving either endothelin receptor or phosphodiesterase type 5 inhibition therapies demonstrated an overall 20-m improvement in postinhalation 6-minute walk distance as compared to baseline (14 m in preinhalational distance), as well as improved measures of quality of life. There was no difference in the time until clinical worsening.[478] An open-label extension of 206 patients from this trial found a median 18-m improvement over baseline 6-minute walk distance after 24 months.[479]

In addition to the lack of need for invasive administration equipment, inhaled prostenoid therapy is easier to initiate. Frequent dosing, however, is required (four times daily for treprostinil and between 6 and 9 while awake for iloprost) and compliance may be a challenge. In addition, as the hemodynamic effects wane prior to each administration, whether patients receive the same benefit as with continuously infused prostenoid therapy is unclear.[480]

Iloprost inhalational therapy is initiated at a dosage of 2.5 and increased to 5 μg with the subsequent dose if tolerated. Treprostinil is started at 18 μg (3 breaths) four times a day, with dose escalation suggested every 1 to 2 weeks to a maximum and target dose of 54 μg (nine breaths) four times daily. Inhaled prostenoids are each administered with drug-specific portable delivery devices. Prostenoid side effects are seen with inhalational therapy, including headache, nausea, diarrhea, flushing, and jaw discomfort. Systemic hypotension and syncope may also occur although have not been associated with further clinical deterioration in clinical trials.[476]

Oral Prostenoid Therapy An orally active prostacyclin analog, beroprost, has been studied in two randomized placebo-controlled trials of patients with various forms of PAH and appears to result in a nonsustained improvement in exercise capacity. An initial trial of 130 patients demonstrated an improvement in 6-minute walk distance after 12 weeks of therapy but in a subsequent study of 116 patients the effect was not sustained beyond 6 months.[481,482] Neither trial demonstrated significant hemodynamic improvement as compared with placebo, and beroprost is currently only approved for use in Japan. An oral formulation of treprostinil was ineffective at improving exercise capacity in patients already receiving oral endothelin receptor antagonists or phosphodiesterase type 5 inhibitors.[483]

Combination Pharmacotherapy

Despite the improvements in exercise capacity and functional status that many patients achieve with individual agents, PAH a life-threatening disease and many patients fail to improve with or maintain a positive response to initial treatment, or suffer progressive decline. With further clinical deterioration it is tempting to replace one agent for another. Alternatively, additional agents are added and used in combination. Indeed, 41% of 2438 patients enrolled in the multicenter US-based REVEAL cohort were receiving two PAH-specific therapies (excluding calcium channel antagonists) and 7.5% were receiving three.[191] Unfortunately, despite such widespread adoption of combination therapy, data regarding the most efficacious and safest approach to using multiple drugs in patients with PAH are limited.

In the only randomized controlled study of upfront combination therapy for PAH, 33 patients with IPAH were randomized to receive either bosentan or placebo 2 days after the initiation of epoprostenol. Both groups demonstrated improved exercise capacity and hemodynamics, but no statistically significant difference was seen as a result of the combination therapy. The small sample size may have precluded identification of differences in efficacy or safety.[484] Other randomized trials of combination therapy have involved sequential ("add-on") therapy in which a second PAH-specific agent has been added to the regimen of a patient already on at least one other drug. In a 12-week trial of 67 patients with PAH, the addition of inhaled iloprost to background bosentan therapy resulted in a 26-m increase in 6-minute walk distance as compared with placebo over 12 weeks. Iloprost also delayed the time to clinical worsening in this study.[485] In a 16-week study of 267 PAH patients, the addition of sildenafil (up to 80 mg three times daily) to continuous intravenous epoprostenol infusion increased 6-minute walk distance by 29 m and improved hemodynamic variables and measures of health-related quality of life.[486] Patients on background bosentan therapy experienced a 23-m placebo-corrected increase in 6-minute walk distance when tadalafil was added in a 16-week trial.[149] In contrast, the addition of oral treprostinil to background endothelin and/or phosphodiesterase type 5 inhibitors for 16 weeks did not improve 6-minute walk distance.[483]

■ SURGICAL INTERVENTIONS FOR PULMONARY ARTERIAL HYPERTENSION

Lung transplantation is addressed in detail in Chapter 107. Here, it will suffice to note that lung transplantation remains an important consideration for some patients with PAH whose disease fails to respond adequately to medical therapy. Although changes in the method of allocating donor lungs within the United States have improved wait times, mortality on the wait list for patients with PAH remains excessive compared to patients with other indications for lung transplantation.[487] To address this issue, PAH patients who are deteriorating despite optimal medical therapy and who have a cardiac index <1.8 L/min/m^2 or a right atrial pressure >15 mm are now granted special priority.

Atrial septostomy has been performed as a palliative measure, as well a "bridge" to lung transplantation in some patients with severe PAH and symptoms refractory to other therapies. The creation of a right-to-left shunt is aimed at decreasing the pressure overload of the right ventricle, and simultaneously increasing preload of the left ventricle thereby improving systemic perfusion. Controlled studies have not been performed, and evidence-based selection criteria have not been established. Significant palliation of patients has been reported, but deaths have been reported as well.[488] The procedure should only be performed at experienced institutions.[489]

ACUTE COR PULMONALE OR RESPIRATORY FAILURE IN PULMONARY ARTERIAL HYPERTENSION

Patients with PAH may become acutely unstable due to a number of factors, including infection, volume overload with dietary indiscretion, or complications of medicines (Table 72-10). Often a clear acute precipitating source of decompensation is not identified. Regardless of the inciting event,[490] in many patients an acute stress will convert stable cor pulmonale into rapidly progressive hemodynamic failure. Acutely worsened hypoxemia, if not the precipitating cause of the hemodynamic instability will usually develop quickly as well.[491] Although the precipitating events may differ, each tends to lead to a vicious cycle that will result in worsening right ventricular function and hypotension (Fig. 72-16). Increased work of the right heart, be it from acute hypoxia and pulmonary vasoconstriction, or due to fever and infection, will increase ventricular wall stress further impeding ventricular performance. A decreased CO will impede myocardial perfusion, as will the increase in intraventricular pressure. Increases in right ventricular volume and pressure will, through displacement of the interventricular septum and increases in pericardial pressure, impede left ventricular filling and function. The resultant hypoxemia and ventricular ischemia, as well as acidemia from either respiratory insufficiency or poor systemic perfusion, can worsen the situation.

The goals of management are the same as for any patient who is hemodynamically unstable or in respiratory distress: to decrease the demand for oxygen while improving its delivery. Supportive care therefore aims to reverse the hypotension and hypoxemia through judicious fluid management, the reduction of RV afterload, support of cardiac function, and provision of supplemental oxygen and, if necessary, ventilator support (Fig. 72-17). Few data are available to guide the management of acute hemodynamic instability in patients with PAH. Available studies of various agents have frequently been performed in patients with acute right heart dysfunction following cardiac surgery, who generally do not suffer from severe underlying pulmonary vasculature disease. It is similarly important to recognize the limitations in extrapolating data from acute vasodilator trials performed on an elective basis in patients with PAH to the care of a hemodynamically unstable PAH patient.

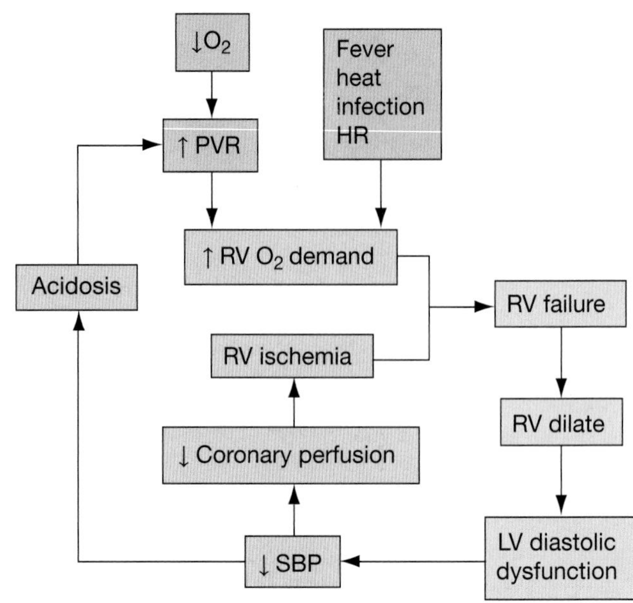

Figure 72-16 Interacting mechanisms in the acute development of worsened right heart function in patients with pulmonary arterial hypertension. A vicious cycle frequently results in both respiratory failure and hemodynamic instability. *(Reproduced with permission from Jeffery ME, Taichman DB. Management of the acutely ill patient with pulmonary arterial hypertension. In: Pulmonary Vascular Disease, Mandel J, Taichman DB. Philadelphia: Elsevier Science; 2006.)*

TABLE 72-10 Clinical Presentations of Patients with Pulmonary Arterial Hypertension with Acute Hemodynamic Instability

Acute recognition/late presentation • Syncope, shock, renal failure, ascities, hypoxemia
Acute medication failure • Medical noncompliance, interrupted infusions • Intolerance (calcium channel antagonist)
Dietary indiscretion/fluid retention
Infection (sepsis with infused therapy)
Fever (environmental causes, infection)
Venous thromboembolism
Medical/surgical procedures/anesthesia
Pregnancy
Tachydysrhythmia (atrial fibrillation, atrial flutter)
Increased activity of underlying disease (flare of systemic lupus erythematosis with worsened PAH that may be responsive to increase immunosuppression)

Source: Adapted with permission from Jeffery ME, Taichman DB. Management of the acutely ill patient with pulmonary arterial hypertension. In: Mandel J, Taichman DB, eds. Pulmonary Vascular Disease. Philadelphia, PA: Saunders/Elsevier; 2006.

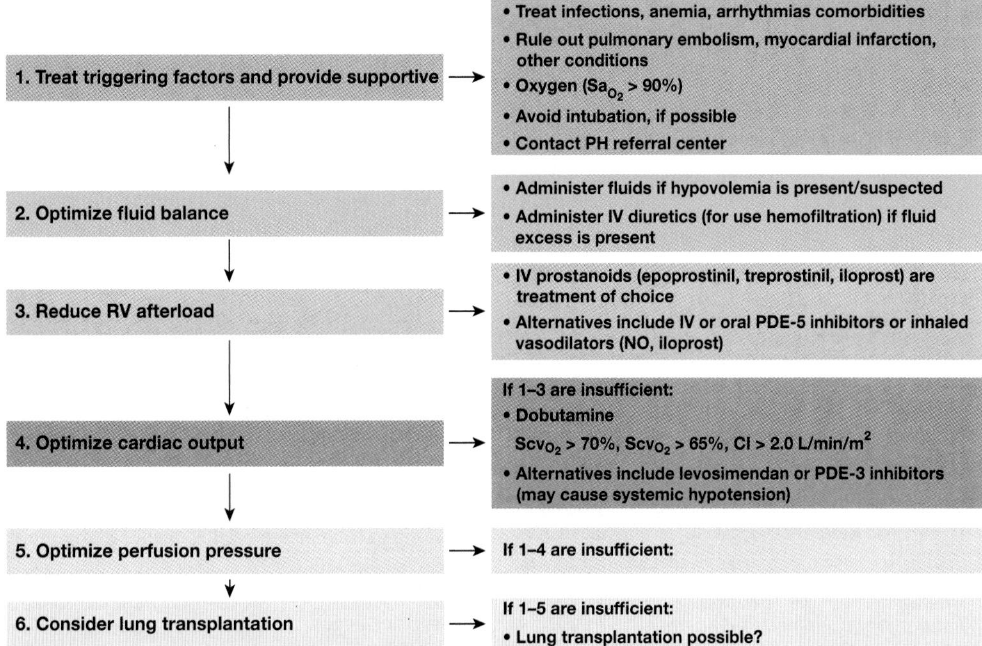

Figure 72-17 Hemodynamic management of critically ill patients with right ventricular failure due to pulmonary arterial hypertension. Which measures are necessary will depend on the individual patient. On many occasions, these treatment strategies need to be administered simultaneously rather than sequentially. CI, cardiac index; IV, intravenous; PDE-5, phosphodiesterase-5; PH, pulmonary hypertension; RV, right ventricular; Scv_{O_2}, central venous oxygen saturation; Sv_{O_2}, mixed venous oxygen saturation. *(Reproduced with permission from Hoeper MM, Granton J. Intensive care unit management of patients with severe pulmonary hypertension and right heart failure. Am J Respir Crit Care Med. 2011;184(10):1114–1124.)*

Although administration of intravenous fluids is the usual first, and frequently most important, intervention for hypotension causing critical illness, fluid challenges for hypotension in the patient with PAH and right ventricular failure must be pursued cautiously with the clinician paying close attention to the potential for making the situation worse. A fluid challenge is often an appropriate initial measure for hypotension, especially when infection or other factors that might predispose to hypovolemia exist. In many patients with PAH and chronic cor pulmonale, however, acute hypotension is caused or complicated by worsened right heart dilation further impairing both right and left ventricular functions. In such cases, fluid removal is required to recover right ventricular function. Vasopressors may be needed for hemodynamic support while fluid removal is accomplished with diuretics.

There are few data to firmly guide the choice of vasopressors.[492] Norepinephrine or dobutamine are often employed for their inotropic properties, while agents that may constrict pulmonary vessels such as phenylephrine are usually avoided if possible.[493–495] Tachycardia and a resultant further impairment of ventricular filling and output may limit the use of any of these agents. If tolerated, the use of intravenous pulmonary vasodilators (e.g., epoprostenol) may result in significant improvement both acutely and longer term. Attempts to promote pulmonary vasodilatation with intravenous or oral agents are, however, frequently complicated by hypotension from the systemic effects of the drugs. In the setting of acute hemodynamic instability, the use of inhaled agents (iloprost, nitric oxide, aerosolized epoprostenol, or milrinone) is often preferable.[496–498] The phosphodiesterase type 5 inhibitor sildenafil has been administered intravenously in a small series of hemodynamically stable patients with PAH; whether it might prove useful for therapy of critically ill patients has not been studied.[499]

Oxygen is a potent pulmonary vasodilator and should be administered at concentrations adequate to prevent hypoxemia. Mechanical ventilation is avoided if possible due to the hemodynamic effects of positive pressure ventilation as well as required sedatives. Unfortunately, invasive ventilator support may be unavoidable. When mechanical ventilation is required, the same principles apply as in other patients with respiratory failure, although certain points are worth noting in the management specifically of patients with PAH. While intra-alveolar vessels are stretched and their resistance increased with overdistention of alveoli, compression of extra-alveolar vessels with atelectasis at low lung volumes might increase their vascular resistance. Thus, at either extreme PVR might increase. The application of positive end-expiratory pressure must also be done with attention to possible overdistention of alveolar vessels and a resultant increase in their resistance. As hypercarbia tends to promote pulmonary vasoconstriction, lung-protective strategies that permit hypoventilation (and hypercapnea) must be carefully monitored to be certain of overall benefit.[500] Hyperventilation to induce mild alkalemia and pulmonary vasodilation has been used empirically, but with attention to avoid dynamic hyperinflation. Finally, care must be taken to avoid agitation with noxious procedures (such as endotracheal suctioning) that might promote further surges in vascular resistance; sedation and analgesia should be employed judiciously with such procedures.[501]

Some acutely ill patients may be candidates for lung transplantation. Although experience is limited, extracorporeal membrane oxygenation (ECMO) has been used in the successful support of individual acutely ill patients with PAH and right ventricular failure awaiting transplantation.[502,503] Newer dual channel cannulas inserted into the internal jugular vein permit patients to remain ambulatory while on ECMO. A pumpless oxygenation system implanted between the pulmonary artery and left atrium has been used to provide support to acutely ill patients while awaiting lung transplantation.[504]

REFERENCES

1. Mandel J, Taichman DB, eds. *Pulmonary Vascular Disease.* 1st ed. Philadelphia, PA: Elsevier Inc; 2006.
2. Yuan JX, Garcia JG, Hales CA, et al., eds. *Textbook of Pulmonary Vascular Disease.* New York, NY: Springer; 2011.
3. Romberg E. [Uber Sklerose der Lungen Arterie]. *Dtsch Arch Klin Med.* 1891;48:197–206.
4. Dresdale DT, Schultz M, Michtom RJ. Primary pulmonary hypertension. I. Clinical and hemodynamic study. *Am J Med.* 1951;11(6):686–705.
5. Runo JR, Loyd JE. Primary pulmonary hypertension. *Lancet.* 2003;361(9368):1533–1544.
6. Simonneau G, Gatzoulis MA, Adatia I, et al. Updated clinical classification of pulmonary hypertension. *J Am Coll Cardiol.* 2013;62(25 Suppl):D34–D41.
7. Yuan JX, Rubin LJ. Pathophysiology of pulmonary hypertension. In: Scharf SM, ed. *Respiratory-Circulation Interactions in Health and Disease.* New York, NY: Marcel Dekker, Inc; 2001: 447–477.
8. Mandegar M, Fung YC, Huang W, Remillard CV, Rubin LJ, Yuan JX. Cellular and molecular mechanisms of pulmonary vascular remodeling: role in the development of pulmonary hypertension. *Microvasc Res.* 2004;68(2):75–103.
9. Morrell NW, Adnot S, Archer SL, et al. Cellular and molecular basis of pulmonary arterial hypertension. *J Am Coll Cardiol.* 2009;54(1 Suppl):S20–S31.
10. Pietra GG. Histopathology of primary pulmonary hypertension. *Chest.* 1994;105(2 Suppl):2S–6S.
11. Rubin LJ. Primary pulmonary hypertension. *N Engl J Med.* 1997;336(2):111–117.
12. Wagenvoort CA, Wagenvoort N. Pulmonary vascular bed: normal anatomy and responses to disease. In: Moser KM, ed. *Pulmonary Vascular Diseases: Lung Biology in Health and Disease.* New York, NY: Marcel Dekker, Inc; 1979:1–109.
13. Wagenvoort CA, Wagenvoort H. Primary pulmonary hypertension: a pathologic study of the lung vessels in 156 classically diagnosed cases. *Circulation.* 1970;42:1163–1184.
14. Hishikawa K, Nakaki T, Marumo T, et al. Pressure promotes DNA synthesis in rat cultured vascular smooth muscle cells. *J Clin Invest.* 1994;93(5):1975–1980.
15. Heath D, Smith P, Gosney J, et al. The pathology of the early and late stages of primary pulmonary hypertension. *Br Heart J.* 1987;58(3):204–213.
16. Ward JP, McMurtry IF. Mechanisms of hypoxic pulmonary vasoconstriction and their roles in pulmonary hypertension: new findings for an old problem. *Curr Opin Pharmacol.* 2009;9 (3):287–296.
17. Fishman AP. Hypoxia on the pulmonary circulation. How and where it acts. *Circ Res.* 1976;38(4):221–231.
18. Sylvester JT, Shimoda LA, Aaronson PI, et al. Hypoxic pulmonary vasoconstriction. *Physiol Rev.* 2012;92(1):367–520.
19. Yuan JX. *Hypoxic Pulmonary Vasoconstriction: Cellular and Molecular Mechanisms.* Boston: Kluwer Academic Publishers; 2004.
20. Fagan KA, Oka M, Bauer NR, et al. Attenuation of acute hypoxic pulmonary vasoconstriction and hypoxic pulmonary hypertension in mice by inhibition of Rho-kinase. *Am J Physiol Lung Cell Mol Physiol.* 2004;287(4):L656–L664.
21. Nagaoka T, Morio Y, Casanova N, et al. Rho/Rho kinase signaling mediates increased basal pulmonary vascular tone in chronically hypoxic rats. *Am J Physiol Lung Cell Mol Physiol.* 2004;287(4):L665–L672.
22. de Meer K, Heymans HS, Zijlstra WG. Physical adaptation of children to life at high altitude. *Eur J Pediatr.* 1995;154(4): 263–272.
23. Shimoda LA, Wang J, Sylvester JT. Ca2+ channels and chronic hypoxia. *Microcirculation.* 2006;13(8):657–670.
24. Masri FA, Xu W, Comhair SA, et al. Hyperproliferative apoptosis-resistant endothelial cells in idiopathic pulmonary arterial hypertension. *Am J Physiol Lung Cell Mol Physiol.* 2007;293(3):L548–L554.
25. Stenmark KR, Davie N, Frid M, Gerasimovskaya E, Das M. Role of the adventitia in pulmonary vascular remodeling. *Physiology (Bethesda).* 2006;21:134–145.
26. Stenmark KR, Fagan KA, Frid MG. Hypoxia-induced pulmonary vascular remodeling: cellular and molecular mechanisms. *Circ Res.* 2006;99(7):675–691.
27. Golovina VA, Platoshyn O, Bailey CL, et al. Upregulated TRP and enhanced capacitative Ca^{2+} entry in human pulmonary artery myocytes during proliferation. *Am J Physiol Heart Circ Physiol.* 2001;280(2):H746–H755.
28. Platoshyn O, Golovina VA, Bailey CL, et al. Sustained membrane depolarization and pulmonary artery smooth muscle cell proliferation. *Am J Physiol Cell Physiol.* 2000;279(5): C1540–C1549.
29. Zhang S, Fantozzi I, Tigno DD, et al. Bone morphogenetic proteins induce apoptosis in human pulmonary vascular smooth muscle cells. *Am J Physiol Lung Cell Mol Physiol.* 2003; 285(3):L740–L754.
30. Rabinovitch M. Elastase and the pathobiology of unexplained pulmonary hypertension. *Chest.* 1998;114(3 Suppl): 213S–224S.
31. Stenmark KR, Durmowicz AG, Dempsey EC. Modulation of vascular wall cell phenotype in pulmonary hypertension. In: Bishop JE, Reeves JJ, Laurent GJ, eds. *Pulmonary Vascular Remodeling.* London, UK: Portland Press; 1995.
32. Pietra GG. The pathology of primary pulmonary hypertension. In: Rubin LJ, Rich S, ed. *Primary Pulmonary Hypertension.* New York, NY: Marcel Dekker, Inc; 1997:19–61.
33. Voelkel NF, Tuder RM, Weir EK. Pathophysiology of primary pulmonary hypertension: from physiology to molecular mechanisms. In: Rubin LJ, Rich S, eds. *Primary Pulmonary Hypertension.* New York, NY: Marcel Dekker, Inc; 1997: 83–129.
34. Cool CD, Stewart JS, Werahera P, et al. Three-dimensional reconstruction of pulmonary arteries in plexiform pulmonary hypertension using cell-specific markers. Evidence for a dynamic and heterogeneous process of pulmonary endothelial cell growth. *Am J Pathol.* 1999;155(2):411–419.
35. Yeager ME, Halley GR, Golpon HA, Voelkel NF, Tuder RM. Microsatellite instability of endothelial cell growth and apoptosis genes within plexiform lesions in primary pulmonary hypertension. *Circ Res.* 2001;88(1):E2–E11.
36. Jamison BM, Michel RP. Different distribution of plexiform lesions in primary and secondary pulmonary hypertension. *Hum Pathol.* 1995;26(9):987–993.
37. Pietra GG. The histopathology of primary pulmonary hypertension. In: Fishman AP, ed. *The Pulmonary Circulation:*

Normal and Abnormal. Mechanisms, Management, and the National Registry. Philadelphia, PA: University of Pennsylvania Press; 1990:459–472.

38. Moschowitz E, Rubin E, Strauss L. Hypertension of the pulmonary circulation due to congenital glomoid obstruction of the pulmonary arteries. *Am J Pathol.* 1961;39:75–93.
39. Cool CD, Kennedy D, Voelkel NF, Tuder RM. Pathogenesis and evolution of plexiform lesions in pulmonary hypertension associated with scleroderma and human immunodeficiency virus infection. *Hum Pathol.* 1997;28(4):434–442.
40. Smith P, Heath D, Yacoub M, Madden B, Caslin A, Gosney J. The ultrastructure of plexogenic pulmonary arteriopathy. *J Pathol.* 1990;160(2):111–121.
41. Yi ES, Kim H, Ahn H, et al. Distribution of obstructive intimal lesions and their cellular phenotypes in chronic pulmonary hypertension. A morphometric and immunohistochemical study. *Am J Respir Crit Care Med.* 2000;162(4 Pt 1):1577–1586.
42. Tuder RM, Groves B, Badesch DB, Voelkel NF. Exuberant endothelial cell growth and elements of inflammation are present in plexiform lesions of pulmonary hypertension. *Am J Pathol.* 1994;144(2):275–285.
43. Lee SD, Shroyer KR, Markham NE, Cool CD, Voelkel NF, Tuder RM. Monoclonal endothelial cell proliferation is present in primary but not secondary pulmonary hypertension. *J Clin Invest.* 1998;101(5):927–934.
44. Bjornsson J, Edwards WD. Primary pulmonary hypertension: a histopathologic study of 80 cases. *Mayo Clin Proc.* 1985; 60(1):16–25.
45. Cohen M, Fuster V, Edwards WD. Anticoagulation in the treatment of pulmonary hypertension. In: Fishman AP, ed. *The Pulmonary Circulation: Normal and Abnormal. Mechanisms, Management, and the National Registry*. Philadelphia, PA: University of Pennsylvania Press; 1990:501–510.
46. Fuster V, Steele PM, Edwards WD, Gersh BJ, McGoon MD, Frye RL. Primary pulmonary hypertension: natural history and the importance of thrombosis. *Circulation.* 1984;70(4):580–587.
47. Herve P, Humbert M, Sitbon O, et al. Pathobiology of pulmonary hypertension. The role of platelets and thrombosis. *Clin Chest Med.* 2001;22(3):451–458.
48. Christman BW, McPherson CD, Newman JH, et al. An imbalance between the excretion of thromboxane and prostacyclin metabolites in pulmonary hypertension. *N Engl J Med.* 1992;327(2):70–75.
49. Wang Z, Chesler NC. Pulmonary vascular wall stiffness: an important contributor to the increased right ventricular afterload with pulmonary hypertension. *Pulm Circ.* 2011;1(2): 212–223.
50. Davies H, Williams J, Wood P. Lung stiffness in states of abnormal pulmonary blood flow and pressure. *Br Heart J.* 1962;24: 129–138.
51. Humbert M, Morrell NW, Archer SL, et al. Cellular and molecular pathobiology of pulmonary arterial hypertension. *J Am Coll Cardiol.* 2004;43(12 Suppl S):13S–24S.
52. Jeffery TK, Morrell NW. Molecular and cellular basis of pulmonary vascular remodeling in pulmonary hypertension. *Prog Cardiovasc Dis.* 2002;45(3):173–202.
53. Jones PL, Rabinovitch M. Tenascin-C is induced with progressive pulmonary vascular disease in rats and is functionally related to increased smooth muscle cell proliferation. *Circ Res.* 1996;79(6):1131–1142.
54. Ivy DD, McMurtry IF, Colvin K, et al. Development of occlusive neointimal lesions in distal pulmonary arteries of endothelin B receptor-deficient rats: a new model of severe pulmonary arterial hypertension. *Circulation.* 2005;111(22): 2988–2996.
55. Jones PL, Chapados R, Baldwin HS, et al. Altered hemodynamics controls matrix metalloproteinase activity and tenascin-C expression in neonatal pig lung. *Am J Physiol Lung Cell Mol Physiol.* 2002;282(1):L26–L35.
56. Cowan KN, Jones PL, Rabinovitch M. Elastase and matrix metalloproteinase inhibitors induce regression, and tenascin-C antisense prevents progression, of vascular disease. *J Clin Invest.* 2000;105(1):21–34.
57. Jones PL, Cowan KN, Rabinovitch M. Tenascin-C, proliferation and subendothelial fibronectin in progressive pulmonary vascular disease. *Am J Pathol.* 1997;150(4):1349–1360.
58. Ihida-Stansbury K, McKean DM, Gebb SA, et al. Paired-related homeobox gene Prx1 is required for pulmonary vascular development. *Circ Res.* 2004;94(11):1507–1514.
59. Wood P. Pulmonary hypertension with special reference to the vasoconstrictive factor. *Br Heart J.* 1958;20(4):557–570.
60. Steudel W, Ichinose F, Huang PL, et al. Pulmonary vasoconstriction and hypertension in mice with targeted disruption of the endothelial nitric oxide synthase (NOS3) gene. *Circ Res.* 1997;81(1):34–41.
61. Ozaki M, Kawashima S, Yamashita T, et al. Reduced hypoxic pulmonary vascular remodeling by nitric oxide from the endothelium. *Hypertension.* 2001;37(2):322–327.
62. Fagan KA, Fouty BW, Tyler RC, et al. The pulmonary circulation of homozygous or heterozygous eNOS-null mice is hyperresponsive to mild hypoxia. *J Clin Invest.* 1999;103(2):291–299.
63. Zhao YD, Courtman DW, Deng Y, Kugathasan L, Zhang Q, Stewart DJ. Rescue of monocrotaline-induced pulmonary arterial hypertension using bone marrow-derived endothelial-like progenitor cells: efficacy of combined cell and eNOS gene therapy in established disease. *Circ Res.* 2005;96(4): 442–450.
64. Clark RH, Kueser TJ, Walker MW, et al. Low-dose nitric oxide therapy for persistent pulmonary hypertension of the newborn. Clinical inhaled nitric oxide research group. *N Engl J Med.* 2000;342(7):469–474.
65. Bueno M, Wang J, Mora AL, Gladwin MT. Nitrite signaling in pulmonary hypertension: mechanisms of bioactivation, signaling, and therapeutics. *Antioxid Redox Signal.* 2013; 18(14): 1797–1809.
66. Zuckerbraun BS, George P, Gladwin MT. Nitrite in pulmonary arterial hypertension: therapeutic avenues in the setting of dysregulated arginine/nitric oxide synthase signalling. *Cardiovasc Res.* 2011;89(3):542–552.
67. Zuckerbraun BS, Shiva S, Ifedigbo E, et al. Nitrite potently inhibits hypoxic and inflammatory pulmonary arterial hypertension and smooth muscle proliferation via xanthine oxidoreductase-dependent nitric oxide generation. *Circulation.* 2010;121 (1):98–109.
68. Petkov V, Mosgoeller W, Ziesche R, et al. Vasoactive intestinal peptide as a new drug for treatment of primary pulmonary hypertension. *J Clin Invest.* 2003;111(9):1339–1346.
69. Leuchte HH, Baezner C, Baumgartner RA, et al. Inhalation of vasoactive intestinal peptide in pulmonary hypertension. *Eur Respir J.* 2008;32(5):1289–1294.

70. Fishman AP. *The Pulmonary Circulation: Normal and Abnormal.* Philadelphia, PA: University of Pennsylvania Press; 1990.

71. Rothman RB, Ayestas MA, Dersch CM, Baumann MH. Aminorex, fenfluramine, and chlorphentermine are serotonin transporter substrates. Implications for primary pulmonary hypertension. *Circulation.* 1999;100(8):869–875.

72. Herve P, Launay JM, Scrobohaci ML, et al. Increased plasma serotonin in primary pulmonary hypertension. *Am J Med.* 1995;99(3):249–254.

73. MacLean MR, Deuchar GA, Hicks MN, et al. Overexpression of the 5-hydroxytryptamine transporter gene: effect on pulmonary hemodynamics and hypoxia-induced pulmonary hypertension. *Circulation.* 2004;109(17):2150–2155.

74. Eddahibi S, Hanoun N, Lanfumey L, et al. Attenuated hypoxic pulmonary hypertension in mice lacking the 5-hydroxytryptamine transporter gene. *J Clin Invest.* 2000;105(11):1555–1562.

75. Guignabert C, Raffestin B, Benferhat R, et al. Serotonin transporter inhibition prevents and reverses monocrotaline-induced pulmonary hypertension in rats. *Circulation.* 2005;111(21):2812–2819.

76. Eddahibi S, Chaouat A, Morrell N, et al. Polymorphism of the serotonin transporter gene and pulmonary hypertension in chronic obstructive pulmonary disease. *Circulation.* 2003;108(15):1839–1844.

77. Eddahibi S, Humbert M, Fadel E, et al. Serotonin transporter overexpression is responsible for pulmonary artery smooth muscle hyperplasia in primary pulmonary hypertension. *J Clin Invest.* 2001;108(8):1141–1150.

78. Machado RD, Koehler R, Glissmeyer E, et al. Genetic association of the serotonin transporter in pulmonary arterial hypertension. *Am J Respir Crit Care Med.* 2006;173(7):793–797.

79. Dumitrascu R, Kulcke C, Konigshoff M, et al. Terguride ameliorates monocrotaline-induced pulmonary hypertension in rats. *Eur Respir J.* 2011;37(5):1104–1118.

80. Ghofrani HA, Al-Hiti H, Vonk-Noordegraaf A, et al. Proof-of-concept study to investigate the efficacy, hemodynamics and tolerability of terguride vs. placebo in subjects with pulmonary arterial hypertension: results of a double blind, randomised, prospective phase IIa study. *Am J Respir Crit Care Med* 2012; 185:1. MeetingAbstracts.

81. Giaid A, Yanagisawa M, Langleben D, et al. Expression of endothelin-1 in the lungs of patients with pulmonary hypertension. *N Engl J Med.* 1993;328(24):1732–1739.

82. Rubens C, Ewert R, Halank M, et al. Big endothelin-1 and endothelin-1 plasma levels are correlated with the severity of primary pulmonary hypertension. *Chest.* 2001;120(5):1562–1569.

83. Yamakami T, Taguchi O, Gabazza EC, et al. Arterial endothelin-1 level in pulmonary emphysema and interstitial lung disease. Relation with pulmonary hypertension during exercise. *Eur Respir J.* 1997;10(9):2055–2060.

84. Cambrey AD, Harrison NK, Dawes KE, et al. Increased levels of endothelin-1 in bronchoalveolar lavage fluid from patients with systemic sclerosis contribute to fibroblast mitogenic activity in vitro. *Am J Respir Cell Mol Biol.* 1994;11(4): 439–445.

85. Yang Z, Krasnici N, Lüscher TF. Endothelin-1 potentiates human smooth muscle cell growth to PDGF: effects of ETA and ETB receptor blockade. *Circulation.* 1999;100(1):5–8.

86. Helset E, Lindal S, Olsen R, Myklebust R, Jørgensen L. Endothelin-1 causes sequential trapping of platelets and neutrophils in pulmonary microcirculation in rats. *Am J Physiol.* 1996;271(4 Pt 1):L538–L546.

87. Hocher B, Schwarz A, Fagan KA, et al. Pulmonary fibrosis and chronic lung inflammation in ET-1 transgenic mice. *Am J Respir Cell Mol Biol.* 2000;23(1):19–26.

88. Davie N, Haleen SJ, Upton PD, et al. ETA and ETB receptors modulate the proliferation of human pulmonary artery smooth muscle cells. *Am J Respir Crit Care Med.* 2002;165(3): 398–405.

89. Kuc RE, Davenport AP. Endothelin-A-receptors in human aorta and pulmonary arteries are downregulated in patients with cardiovascular disease: an adaptive response to increased levels of endothelin-1? *J Cardiovasc Pharmacol.* 2000;36 (5 Suppl 1):S377–S379.

90. Rubin LJ, Badesch DB, Barst RJ, et al. Bosentan therapy for pulmonary arterial hypertension. *N Engl J Med.* 2002;346(12): 896–903.

91. Barst RJ, Rich S, Widlitz A, Horn EM, McLaughlin V, McFarlin J. Clinical efficacy of sitaxsentan, an endothelin-A receptor antagonist, in patients with pulmonary arterial hypertension: open-label pilot study. *Chest.* 2002;121(6):1860–1868.

92. McLaughlin V, Sitbon O, Rubin LJ. The effect of first-line bosentan on survival of patients with primary pulmonary hypertension. *Am J Respir Crit Care Med.* 2003;167(7).

93. Du L, Sullivan CC, Chu D, et al. Signaling molecules in nonfamilial pulmonary hypertension. *N Engl J Med.* 2003; 348(6): 500–509.

94. Thistlethwaite PA, Lee SH, Du LL, et al. Human angiopoietin gene expression is a marker for severity of pulmonary hypertension in patients undergoing pulmonary thromboendarterectomy. *J Thorac Cardiovasc Surg.* 2001;122(1):65–73.

95. Zhao YD, Campbell AI, Robb M, Ng D, Stewart DJ. Protective role of angiopoietin-1 in experimental pulmonary hypertension. *Circ Res.* 2003;92(9):984–991.

96. Hirose S, Hosoda Y, Furuya S, Otsuki T, Ikeda E. Expression of vascular endothelial growth factor and its receptors correlates closely with formation of the plexiform lesion in human pulmonary hypertension. *Pathol Int.* 2000;50(6):472–479.

97. Tuder RM, Chacon M, Alger L, et al. Expression of angiogenesis-related molecules in plexiform lesions in severe pulmonary hypertension: evidence for a process of disordered angiogenesis. *J Pathol.* 2001;195(3):367–374.

98. Christou H, Yoshida A, Arthur V, Morita T, Kourembanas S. Increased vascular endothelial growth factor production in the lungs of rats with hypoxia-induced pulmonary hypertension. *Am J Respir Cell Mol Biol.* 1998;18(6):768–776.

99. Campbell AI, Zhao Y, Sandhu R, Stewart DJ. Cell-based gene transfer of vascular endothelial growth factor attenuates monocrotaline-induced pulmonary hypertension. *Circulation.* 2001;104(18):2242–2248.

100. Perros F, Montani D, Dorfmuller P, et al. Platelet-derived growth factor expression and function in idiopathic pulmonary arterial hypertension. *Am J Respir Crit Care Med.* 2008; 178(1):81–88.

101. Ghofrani HA, Seeger W, Grimminger F. Imatinib for the treatment of pulmonary arterial hypertension. *N Engl J Med.* 2005;353(13):1412–1413.

102. Ghofrani HA, Morrell NW, Hoeper MM, et al. Imatinib in pulmonary arterial hypertension patients with inadequate response to established therapy. *Am J Respir Crit Care Med.* 2010;182(9):1171–1177.

103. Diamant M, Tushuizen ME, Sturk A, Nieuwland R. Cellular microparticles: new players in the field of vascular disease? *Eur J Clin Invest*. 2004;34(6):392–401.

104. Amabile N, Heiss C, Real WM, et al. Circulating endothelial microparticle levels predict hemodynamic severity of pulmonary hypertension. *Am J Respir Crit Care Med*. 2008;177 (11):1268–1275.

105. Tual-Chalot S, Guibert C, Muller B, et al. Circulating microparticles from pulmonary hypertensive rats induce endothelial dysfunction. *Am J Respir Crit Care Med*. 2010; 182(2): 261–268.

106. Densmore JC, Signorino PR, Ou J, et al. Endothelium-derived microparticles induce endothelial dysfunction and acute lung injury. *Shock*. 2006;26(5):464–471.

107. Humbert M, Monti G, Brenot F, et al. Increased interleukin-1 and interleukin-6 serum concentrations in severe primary pulmonary hypertension. *Am J Respir Crit Care Med*. 1995; 151(5):1628–1631.

108. Soon E, Holmes AM, Treacy CM, et al. Elevated levels of inflammatory cytokines predict survival in idiopathic and familial pulmonary arterial hypertension. *Circulation*. 2010;122(9):920–927.

109. Balabanian K, Foussat A, Dorfmuller P, et al. CX3 C chemokine fractalkine in pulmonary arterial hypertension. *Am J Respir Crit Care Med*. 2002;165(10):1419–1425.

110. Perros F, Dorfmuller P, Souza R, et al. Dendritic cell recruitment in lesions of human and experimental pulmonary hypertension. *Eur Respir J*. 2007;29(3):462–468.

111. Sanchez O, Marcos E, Perros F, et al. Role of endothelium-derived CC chemokine ligand 2 in idiopathic pulmonary arterial hypertension. *Am J Respir Crit Care Med*. 2007;176(10): 1041–1047.

112. Dorfmuller P, Zarka V, Durand-Gasselin I, et al. Chemokine RANTES in severe pulmonary arterial hypertension. *Am J Respir Crit Care Med*. 2002;165(4):534–539.

113. Kuhr FK, Smith KA, Song MY, Levitan I, Yuan JX. New mechanisms of pulmonary arterial hypertension: role of Ca^{2+} signaling. *Am J Physiol Heart Circ Physiol*. 2012;302(8):H1546–H1562.

114. Yu Y, Fantozzi I, Remillard CV, et al. Enhanced expression of transient receptor potential channels in idiopathic pulmonary arterial hypertension. *Proc Natl Acad Sci U S A*. 2004; 101(38):13861–13866.

115. Yu Y, Keller SH, Remillard CV, et al. A functional single-nucleotide polymorphism in the TRPC6 gene promoter associated with idiopathic pulmonary arterial hypertension. *Circulation*. 2009;119(17):2313–2322.

116. Zhang S, Dong H, Rubin LJ, Yuan JX. Upregulation of $Na+/Ca^{2+}$ exchanger contributes to the enhanced Ca^{2+} entry in pulmonary artery smooth muscle cells from patients with idiopathic pulmonary arterial hypertension. *Am J Physiol Cell Physiol*. 2007;292(6):C2297–C2305.

117. Zhang S, Patel HH, Murray F, et al. Pulmonary artery smooth muscle cells from normal subjects and IPAH patients show divergent cAMP-mediated effects on TRPC expression and capacitative Ca^{2+} entry. *Am J Physiol Lung Cell Mol Physiol*. 2007; 292(5):L1202–L1210.

118. Firth AL, Remillard CV, Platoshyn O, Fantozzi I, Ko EA, Yuan JX. Functional ion channels in human pulmonary artery smooth muscle cells: voltage-dependent cation channels. *Pulm Circ*. 2011;1(1):48–71.

119. Yu Y, Sweeney M, Zhang S, et al. PDGF stimulates pulmonary vascular smooth muscle cell proliferation by upregulating TRPC6 expression. *Am J Physiol Cell Physiol*. 2003;284(2): C316–C330.

120. Song MY, Makino A, Yuan JX. STIM2 contributes to enhanced store-operated Ca^{2+} entry in pulmonary artery smooth muscle cells from patients with idiopathic pulmonary arterial hypertension. *Pulm Circ*. 2011;1(1):84–94.

121. Makino A, Firth AL, Yuan JX. Endothelial and smooth muscle cell ion channels in pulmonary vasoconstriction and vascular remodeling. *Compr Physiol*. 2011;1(3):1555–1602.

122. Michelakis ED, McMurtry MS, Wu XC, et al. Dichloroacetate, a metabolic modulator, prevents and reverses chronic hypoxic pulmonary hypertension in rats: role of increased expression and activity of voltage-gated potassium channels. *Circulation*. 2002;105(2):244–250.

123. Platoshyn O, Yu Y, Golovina VA, et al. Chronic hypoxia decreases Kv channel expression and function in pulmonary artery myocytes. *Am J Physiol Lung Cell Mol Physiol*. 2001; 280(4):L801–L812.

124. Pozeg ZI, Michelakis ED, McMurtry MS, et al. In vivo gene transfer of the O2-sensitive potassium channel Kv1.5 reduces pulmonary hypertension and restores hypoxic pulmonary vasoconstriction in chronically hypoxic rats. *Circulation*. 2003;107(15):2037–2044.

125. Geraci MW, Moore M, Gesell T, et al. Gene expression patterns in the lungs of patients with primary pulmonary hypertension: a gene microarray analysis. *Circ Res*. 2001;88(6): 555–562.

126. Yuan JX, Aldinger AM, Juhaszova M, et al. Dysfunctional voltage-gated K+ channels in pulmonary artery smooth muscle cells of patients with primary pulmonary hypertension. *Circulation*. 1998;98(14):1400–1406.

127. Yuan XJ, Wang J, Juhaszova M, Gaine SP, Rubin LJ. Attenuated K+ channel gene transcription in primary pulmonary hypertension. *Lancet*. 1998;351(9104):726–727.

128. Weir EK, Reeve HL, Huang JM, et al. Anorexic agents aminorex, fenfluramine, and dexfenfluramine inhibit potassium current in rat pulmonary vascular smooth muscle and cause pulmonary vasoconstriction. *Circulation*. 1996;94(9): 2216–2220.

129. Remillard CV, Yuan JX. Activation of K^+ channels: an essential pathway in programmed cell death. *Am J Physiol Lung Cell Mol Physiol*. 2004;286(1):L49–L67.

130. Krick S, Platoshyn O, Sweeney M, Kim H, Yuan JX. Activation of K^+ channels induces apoptosis in vascular smooth muscle cells. *Am J Physiol Cell Physiol*. 2001;280(4):C970–C979.

131. Brown EM, Butters R, Katz C, Kifor O. Neomycin mimics the effects of high extracellular calcium concentrations on parathyroid function in dispersed bovine parathyroid cells. *Endocrinology*. 1991;128(6):3047–3054.

132. Conigrave AD, Quinn SJ, Brown EM. L-amino acid sensing by the extracellular Ca^{2+}-sensing receptor. *Proc Natl Acad Sci U S A*. 2000;97(9):4814–4819.

133. Gowen M, Stroup GB, Dodds RA, et al. Antagonizing the parathyroid calcium receptor stimulates parathyroid hormone secretion and bone formation in osteopenic rats. *J Clin Invest*. 2000;105(11):1595–1604.

134. Hu J, McLarnon SJ, Mora S, et al. A region in the seven-transmembrane domain of the human Ca^{2+} receptor critical for response to Ca^{2+}. *J Biol Chem*. 2005;280(6):5113–5120.

135. Yamamura A, Guo Q, Yamamura H, et al. Enhanced Ca^{2+}-sensing receptor function in idiopathic pulmonary arterial hypertension. *Circ Res.* 2012;111(4):469–481.

136. Zhang J, Zhou J, Cai L, et al. Extracellular calcium-sensing receptor is critical in hypoxic pulmonary vasoconstriction. *Antioxid Redox Signal.* 2012;17(3):471–484.

137. Brown EM, MacLeod RJ. Extracellular calcium sensing and extracellular calcium signaling. *Physiol Rev.* 2001;81(1):239–297.

138. Hofer AM, Brown EM. Extracellular calcium sensing and signalling. *Nat Rev Mol Cell Biol.* 2003;4(7):530–538.

139. Magno AL, Ward BK, Ratajczak T. The calcium-sensing receptor: a molecular perspective. *Endocr Rev.* 2011;32(1):3–30.

140. Yu J, Taylor L, Wilson J, Comhair S, Erzurum S, Polgar P. Altered expression and signal transduction of endothelin-1 receptors in heritable and idiopathic pulmonary arterial hypertension. *J Cell Physiol.* 2013;228(2):322–329.

141. Launay JM, Herve P, Peoc'h K, et al. Function of the serotonin 5-hydroxytryptamine 2B receptor in pulmonary hypertension. *Nat Med.* 2002;8(10):1129–1135.

142. Blaustein MP, Lederer WJ. Sodium/calcium exchange: its physiological implications. *Physiol Rev.* 1999;79(3):763–854.

143. Lemos VS, Poburko D, Liao CH, Cole WC, van Breemen C. Na+ entry via TRPC6 causes Ca^{2+} entry via NCX reversal in ATP stimulated smooth muscle cells. *Biochem Biophys Res Commun.* 2007;352(1):130–134.

144. Schach C, Firth AL, Xu M, et al. Regulation of pulmonary vasoconstriction by agonists and caveolae. *Exp Lung Res.* 2008;34(4): 195–208.

145. Sauzeau V, Le Jeune H, Cario-Toumaniantz C, et al. Cyclic GMP-dependent protein kinase signaling pathway inhibits RhoA-induced Ca^{2+} sensitization of contraction in vascular smooth muscle. *J Biol Chem.* 2000;275(28):21722–21729.

146. Sawada N, Itoh H, Yamashita J, et al. cGMP-dependent protein kinase phosphorylates and inactivates RhoA. *Biochem Biophys Res Commun.* 2001;280(3):798–805.

147. Chen CN, Watson G, Zhao L. Cyclic guanosine monophosphate signalling pathway in pulmonary arterial hypertension. *Vascul Pharmacol.* 2012;58(3):211–218.

148. Galie N, Ghofrani HA, Torbicki A, et al. Sildenafil citrate therapy for pulmonary arterial hypertension. *N Engl J Med.* 2005;353(20):2148–2157.

149. Galie N, Brundage BH, Ghofrani HA, et al. Tadalafil therapy for pulmonary arterial hypertension. *Circulation.* 2009;119(22): 2894–2903.

150. Ogawa A, Firth AL, Smith KA, Maliakal MV, Yuan JX. PDGF enhances store-operated Ca^{2+} entry by upregulating STIM1/Orai1 via activation of Akt/mTOR in human pulmonary arterial smooth muscle cells. *Am J Physiol Cell Physiol.* 2012; 302(2):C405–C411.

151. Ross R. Platelet-derived growth factor. *Annu Rev Med.* 1987; 38: 71–79.

152. Brunet A, Bonni A, Zigmond MJ, et al. Akt promotes cell survival by phosphorylating and inhibiting a Forkhead transcription factor. *Cell.* 1999;96(6):857–868.

153. Krymskaya VP, Snow J, Cesarone G, et al. mTOR is required for pulmonary arterial vascular smooth muscle cell proliferation under chronic hypoxia. *Faseb J.* 2011;25(6):1922–1933.

154. Wessler JD, Steingart RM, Schwartz GK, Harvey BG, Schaffer W. Dramatic improvement in pulmonary hypertension with rapamycin. *Chest.* 2010;138(4):991–993.

155. Ogawa A, Firth AL, Yao W, et al. Inhibition of mTOR attenuates store-operated Ca^{2+} entry in cells from endarterectomized tissues of patients with chronic thromboembolic pulmonary hypertension. *Am J Physiol Lung Cell Mol Physiol.* 2009;297(4):L666–L676.

156. Somlyo AP, Somlyo AV. Ca^{2+} sensitivity of smooth muscle and nonmuscle myosin II: modulated by G proteins, kinases, and myosin phosphatase. *Physiol Rev.* 2003;83(4):1325–1358.

157. Uehata M, Ishizaki T, Satoh H, et al. Calcium sensitization of smooth muscle mediated by a Rho-associated protein kinase in hypertension. *Nature.* 1997;389(6654):990–994.

158. Sakurada S, Takuwa N, Sugimoto N, et al. Ca^{2+}-dependent activation of Rho and Rho kinase in membrane depolarization-induced and receptor stimulation-induced vascular smooth muscle contraction. *Circ Res.* 2003;93(6):548–556.

159. Do e Z, Fukumoto Y, Takaki A, et al. Evidence for Rho-kinase activation in patients with pulmonary arterial hypertension. *Circ J.* 2009;73(9):1731–1739.

160. Guilluy C, Eddahibi S, Agard C, et al. RhoA and Rho kinase activation in human pulmonary hypertension: role of 5-HT signaling. *Am J Respir Crit Care Med.* 2009;179(12):1151–1158.

161. Fukumoto Y, Matoba T, Ito A, et al. Acute vasodilator effects of a Rho-kinase inhibitor, fasudil, in patients with severe pulmonary hypertension. *Heart.* 2005;91(3):391–392.

162. Ishikura K, Yamada N, Ito M, et al. Beneficial acute effects of Rho-kinase inhibitor in patients with pulmonary arterial hypertension. *Circ J.* 2006;70(2):174–178.

163. Gridley T. Notch signaling in the vasculature. *Curr Top Dev Biol.* 2010;92:277–309.

164. Li X, Zhang X, Leathers R, et al. Notch3 signaling promotes the development of pulmonary arterial hypertension. *Nat Med.* 2009;15(11):1289–1297.

165. Bray SJ. Notch signalling: a simple pathway becomes complex. *Nat Rev Mol Cell Biol.* 2006;7(9):678–689.

166. Kopan R, Ilagan MX. The canonical Notch signaling pathway: unfolding the activation mechanism. *Cell.* 2009;137(2): 216–233.

167. Thistlethwaite PA, Li X, Zhang X. Notch signaling in pulmonary hypertension. *Adv Exp Med Biol.* 2010;661:279–298.

168. Jin S, Hansson EM, Tikka S, et al. Notch signaling regulates platelet-derived growth factor receptor-β expression in vascular smooth muscle cells. *Circ Res.* 2008;102(12):1483–1491.

169. Overbeek MJ, Boonstra A, Voskuyl AE, et al. Platelet-derived growth factor receptor-b and epidermal growth factor receptor in pulmonary vasculature of systemic sclerosis-associated pulmonary arterial hypertension versus idiopathic pulmonary arterial hypertension and pulmonary veno-occlusive disease: a case-control study. *Arthritis Res Ther.* 2011;13(2): R61.

170. Stewart DJ. Bone morphogenetic protein receptor-2 and pulmonary arterial hypertension: unraveling a riddle inside an enigma? *Circ Res.* 2005;96(10):1033–1035.

171. Atkinson C, Stewart S, Upton PD, et al. Primary pulmonary hypertension is associated with reduced pulmonary vascular expression of type II bone morphogenetic protein receptor. *Circulation.* 2002;105(14):1672–1678.

172. Morrell NW, Yang X, Upton PD, et al. Altered growth responses of pulmonary artery smooth muscle cells from patients with primary pulmonary hypertension to transforming growth factor-b1 and bone morphogenetic proteins. *Circulation.* 2001;104(7):790–795.

173. Yang X, Long L, Southwood M, et al. Dysfunctional Smad signaling contributes to abnormal smooth muscle cell proliferation in familial pulmonary arterial hypertension. *Circ Res*. 2005;96(10):1053–1063.

174. Cogan JD, Pauciulo MW, Batchman AP, et al. High frequency of BMPR2 exonic deletions/duplications in familial pulmonary arterial hypertension. *Am J Respir Crit Care Med* 2006;174(5):590–598.

175. Deng Z, Morse JH, Slager SL, et al. Familial primary pulmonary hypertension (gene PPH1) is caused by mutations in the bone morphogenetic protein receptor-II gene. *Am J Hum Genet*. 2000;67(3):737–744.

176. Lane KB, Machado RD, Pauciulo MW, et al. Heterozygous germline mutations in BMPR2, encoding a TGF-b receptor, cause familial primary pulmonary hypertension. *Nat Genet*. 2000;26(1):81–84.

177. Machado RD, Aldred MA, James V, et al. Mutations of the TGF-b type II receptor BMPR2 in pulmonary arterial hypertension. *Hum Mutat*. 2006;27(2):121–132.

178. Newman JH, Trembath RC, Morse JA, et al. Genetic basis of pulmonary arterial hypertension: current understanding and future directions. *J Am Coll Cardiol*. 2004;43(12 Suppl S):33S–39S.

179. Newman JH, Wheeler L, Lane KB, et al. Mutation in the gene for bone morphogenetic protein receptor II as a cause of primary pulmonary hypertension in a large kindred. *N Engl J Med*. 2001;345(5):319–324.

180. Thomson JR, Machado RD, Pauciulo MW, et al. Sporadic primary pulmonary hypertension is associated with germline mutations of the gene encoding BMPR-II, a receptor member of the TGF-b family. *J Med Genet*. 2000;37(10):741–745.

181. Humbert M, Deng Z, Simonneau G, et al. BMPR2 germline mutations in pulmonary hypertension associated with fenfluramine derivatives. *Eur Respir J*. 2002;20(3):518–523.

182. Roberts KE, McElroy JJ, Wong WP, et al. BMPR2 mutations in pulmonary arterial hypertension with congenital heart disease. *Eur Respir J*. 2004;24(3):371–374.

183. Runo JR, Vnencak-Jones CL, Prince M, et al. Pulmonary veno-occlusive disease caused by an inherited mutation in bone morphogenetic protein receptor II. *Am J Respir Crit Care Med*. 2003;167(6):889–894.

184. Shintani M, Yagi H, Nakayama T, Saji T, Matsuoka R. A new nonsense mutation of SMAD8 associated with pulmonary arterial hypertension. *J Med Genet*. 2009;46(5):331–337.

185. Trembath RC, Thomson JR, Machado RD, et al. Clinical and molecular genetic features of pulmonary hypertension in patients with hereditary hemorrhagic telangiectasia. *N Engl J Med*. 2001;345(5):325–334.

186. Chaouat A, Coulet F, Favre C, et al. Endoglin germline mutation in a patient with hereditary haemorrhagic telangiectasia and dexfenfluramine associated pulmonary arterial hypertension. *Thorax*. 2004;59(5):446–448.

187. Maloney JP, Stearman RS, Bull TM, et al. Loss-of-function thrombospondin-1 mutations in familial pulmonary hypertension. *Am J Physiol Lung Cell Mol Physiol*. 2012;302(6): L541–L554.

188. Brown LM, Chen H, Halpern SD, et al. Delay in recognition of pulmonary arterial hypertension: factors identified from the REVEAL registry. *Chest*. 2011;140(1):19–26.

189. Humbert M, Sitbon O, Chaouat A, et al. Pulmonary arterial hypertension in France: results from a national registry. *Am J Respir Crit Care Med*. 2006;173(9):1023–1030.

190. Lee K, Mize R, Lowenstein SR. Glyburide-induced hypoglycemia and ranitidine. *Ann Intern Med*. 1987;107(2):261–262.

191. Badesch DB, Raskob GE, Elliott CG, et al. Pulmonary arterial hypertension: baseline characteristics from the REVEAL Registry. *Chest*. 2010;137(2):376–387.

192. Jing ZC, Xu XQ, Han ZY, et al. Registry and survival study in Chinese patients with idiopathic and familial pulmonary arterial hypertension. *Chest*. 2007;132(2):373–379.

193. Wilkens H, Grimminger F, Hoeper M, et al. Burden of pulmonary arterial hypertension in Germany. *Respir Med*. 2010;104(6):902–910.

194. McGoon M, Gutterman D, Steen V, et al. Screening, early detection, and diagnosis of pulmonary arterial hypertension: ACCP evidence-based clinical practice guidelines. *Chest*. 2004;126(1 Suppl):14S–34S.

195. Kawut SM, Silvestry FE, Ferrari VA, et al. Extrinsic compression of the left main coronary artery by the pulmonary artery in patients with long-standing pulmonary hypertension. *Am J Cardiol*. 1999;83(6):984–986.

196. Holcomb BW Jr, Loyd JE, Ely EW, Johnson J, Robbins IM. Pulmonary veno-occlusive disease: a case series and new observations. *Chest*. 2000;118(6):1671–1679.

197. McLaughlin VV, Archer SL, Badesch DB, et al. ACCF/AHA 2009 expert consensus document on pulmonary hypertension a report of the American College of Cardiology Foundation task force on expert consensus documents and the American Heart Association developed in collaboration with the American College of Chest Physicians; American Thoracic Society, Inc.; and the Pulmonary Hypertension Association. *J Am Coll Cardiol*. 2009;53(17):1573–1619.

198. Barst RJ, McGoon M, Torbicki A, et al. Diagnosis and differential assessment of pulmonary arterial hypertension. *J Am Coll Cardiol*. 2004;43(12 Suppl S):40S–47S.

199. Borgeson DD, Seward JB, Miller FA Jr, Oh JK, Tajik AJ. Frequency of doppler measurable pulmonary artery pressures. *J Am Soc Echocardiogr*. 1996;9(6):832–837.

200. Forfia PR, Vachiery JL. Echocardiography in pulmonary arterial hypertension. *Am J Cardiol*. 2012;110(6 Suppl):16S–24S.

201. Eysmann SB, Palevsky HI, Reichek N, Hackney K, Douglas PS. Two-dimensional and Doppler-echocardiographic and cardiac catheterization correlates of survival in primary pulmonary hypertension. *Circulation*. 1989;80(2):353–360.

202. Hinderliter AL, Willis PW 4th, Long W, et al. Frequency and prognostic significance of pericardial effusion in primary pulmonary hypertension. PPH Study Group. Primary pulmonary hypertension. *Am J Cardiol*. 1999;84(4):481–484.

203. Raymond RJ, Hinderliter AL, Willis PW, et al. Echocardiographic predictors of adverse outcomes in primary pulmonary hypertension. *J Am Coll Cardiol*. 2002;39(7):1214–1219.

204. Kawut SM, Horn EM, Berekashvili KK, et al. New predictors of outcome in idiopathic pulmonary arterial hypertension. *Am J Cardiol*. 2005;95(2):199–203.

205. Ryan JJ, Rich JD, Thiruvoipati T, et al. Current practice for determining pulmonary capillary wedge pressure predisposes to serious errors in the classification of patients with pulmonary hypertension. *Am Heart J*. 2012;163(4):589–594.

206. Tonelli AR, Mubarak KK, Li N, Carrie R, Alnuaimat H. Effect of balloon inflation volume on pulmonary artery occlusion pressure in patients with and without pulmonary hypertension. *Chest*. 2011;139(1):115–121.

207. Halpern SD, Taichman DB. Misclassification of pulmonary hypertension due to reliance on pulmonary capillary wedge pressure rather than left ventricular end-diastolic pressure. *Chest.* 2009;136(1):37–43.

208. Morgan JM, Griffiths M, du Bois RM, Evans TW. Hypoxic pulmonary vasoconstriction in systemic sclerosis and primary pulmonary hypertension. *Chest.* 1991;99(3):551–556.

209. Krasuski RA, Warner JJ, Wang A, Harrison JK, Tapson VF, Bashore TM. Inhaled nitric oxide selectively dilates pulmonary vasculature in adult patients with pulmonary hypertension, irrespective of etiology. *J Am Coll Cardiol.* 2000;36(7):2204–2211.

210. Rubin LJ, Groves BM, Reeves JT, Frosolono M, Handel F, Cato AE. Prostacyclin-induced acute pulmonary vasodilation in primary pulmonary hypertension. *Circulation.* 1982;66(2):334–338.

211. Sitbon O, Brenot F, Denjean A, et al. Inhaled nitric oxide as a screening vasodilator agent in primary pulmonary hypertension. A dose-response study and comparison with prostacyclin. *Am J Respir Crit Care Med.* 1995;151(2 Pt 1):384–389.

212. Galie N, Ussia G, Passarelli P, Parlangeli R, Branzi A, Magnani B. Role of pharmacologic tests in the treatment of primary pulmonary hypertension. *Am J Cardiol.* 1995;75:55A–62A.

213. Nootens M, Schrader B, Kaufmann E, Vestal R, Long W, Rich S. Comparative acute effects of adenosine and prostacyclin in primary pulmonary hypertension. *Chest.* 1995;107(1):54–57.

214. Palevsky HI, Long W, Crow J, Fishman AP. Prostacyclin and acetylcholine as screening agents for acute pulmonary vasodilator responsiveness in primary pulmonary hypertension. *Circulation.* 1990;82(6):2018–2026.

215. Barst RJ, Maislin G, Fishman AP. Vasodilator therapy for primary pulmonary hypertension in children. *Circulation.* 1999;99(9):1197–1208.

216. Partanen J, Nieminen MS, Luomanmaki K. Death in a patient with primary pulmonary hypertension after 20 mg of nifedipine. *N Engl J Med.* 1993;329(11):812–813.

217. Mandel J, Mark EJ, Hales CA. Pulmonary veno-occlusive disease. *Am J Respir Crit Care Med.* 2000;162(5):1964–1973.

218. Escribano Subias P, Barbera Mir JA, Suberviola V. Current diagnostic and prognostic assessment of pulmonary Hypertension. *Rev Esp Cardiol.* 2010;63(5):583–596.

219. Fraser K, Wright B, Girard L, et al. Simulation training improves diagnostic performance on a real patient with similar clinical findings. *Chest.* 2011;139(2):376–381.

220. Peacock AJ, Murphy NF, McMurray JJ, Caballero L, Stewart S. An epidemiological study of pulmonary arterial hypertension. *Eur Respir J.* 2007;30(1):104–109.

221. Soria JM. The genetic component of disorders of coagulation and thrombosis. *Revista Española de Cardiología.* 2009;09(Suppl B):58–65.

222. Benza RL, Gomberg-Maitland M, Miller DP, et al. The REVEAL Registry risk score calculator in patients newly diagnosed with pulmonary arterial hypertension. *Chest.* 2012;141(2):354–362.

223. Humbert M, Sitbon O, Yaici A, et al. Survival in incident and prevalent cohorts of patients with pulmonary arterial hypertension. *Eur Respir J.* 2010;36(3):549–555.

224. Ling Y, Johnson MK, Kiely DG, et al. Changing demographics, epidemiology, and survival of incident pulmonary arterial hypertension: results from the pulmonary hypertension registry of the United Kingdom and Ireland. *Am J Respir Crit Care Med.* 2012;186(8):790–796.

225. Thenappan T, Shah SJ, Rich S, et al. Survival in pulmonary arterial hypertension: a reappraisal of the NIH risk stratification equation. *Eur Respir J.* 2010;35(5):1079–1087.

226. Abenhaim L, Moride Y, Brenot F, et al. Appetite-suppressant drugs and the risk of primary pulmonary hypertension. International primary pulmonary hypertension study group. *N Engl J Med.* 1996;335(9):609–616.

227. Group IPPHS. The international primary pulmonary hypertension study. *Chest.* 1994;105(2 Suppl):37S–41S.

228. Appelbaum L, Yigla M, Bendayan D, et al. Primary pulmonary hypertension in Israel: a national survey. *Chest.* 2001;119(6):1801–1806.

229. Braman SS, Eby E, Kuhn C, Rounds S. Primary pulmonary hypertension in the elderly. *Arch Intern Med.* 1991;151(12):2433–2438.

230. Yigla M, Kramer MR, Bendayan D, Reisner SA, Solomonov A. Unexplained severe pulmonary hypertension in the elderly: report on 14 patients. *Isr Med Assoc J.* 2004;6(2):78–81.

231. Rich S, Dantzker DR, Ayres SM, et al. Primary pulmonary hypertension. A national prospective study. *Ann Intern Med.* 1987;107(2):216–223.

232. Brenot F. Primary pulmonary hypertension: case series from France. *Chest.* 1994;105(2 Suppl):33S–36S.

233. Sandoval J, Bauerle O, Palomar A, et al. Survival in primary pulmonary hypertension. Validation of a prognostic equation. *Circulation.* 1994;89(4):733–744.

234. McLaughlin VV, Presberg KW, Doyle RL, et al. Prognosis of pulmonary arterial hypertension: ACCP evidence-based clinical practice guidelines. *Chest.* 2004;126(1 Suppl):78S–92S.

235. Bossone E, Paciocco G, Iarussi D, et al. The prognostic role of the ECG in primary pulmonary hypertension. *Chest.* 2002;121(2):513–518.

236. Kuhn KP, Byrne DW, Arbogast PG, Doyle TP, Loyd JE, Robbins IM. Outcome in 91 consecutive patients with pulmonary arterial hypertension receiving epoprostenol. *Am J Respir Crit Care Med.* 2003;167(4):580–586.

237. Sitbon O, Humbert M, Nunes H, et al. Long-term intravenous epoprostenol infusion in primary pulmonary hypertension: prognostic factors and survival. *J Am Coll Cardiol.* 2002;40(4):780–788.

238. McLaughlin VV, Shillington A, Rich S. Survival in primary pulmonary hypertension: the impact of epoprostenol therapy. *Circulation.* 2002;106(12):1477–1482.

239. Barst RJ, Rubin LJ, Long WA, et al. A comparison of continuous intravenous epoprostenol (prostacyclin) with conventional therapy for primary pulmonary hypertension. The primary pulmonary hypertension study group. *N Engl J Med.* 1996;334(5):296–301.

240. Miyamoto S, Nagaya N, Satoh T, et al. Clinical correlates and prognostic significance of six-minute walk test in patients with primary pulmonary hypertension. Comparison with cardiopulmonary exercise testing. *Am J Respir Crit Care Med.* 2000;161(2 Pt 1):487–492.

241. Wensel R, Opitz CF, Anker SD, et al. Assessment of survival in patients with primary pulmonary hypertension: importance of cardiopulmonary exercise testing. *Circulation.* 2002;106(3):319–324.

242. Yeo TC, Dujardin KS, Tei C, Mahoney DW, McGoon MD, Seward JB. Value of a Doppler-derived index combining systolic and diastolic time intervals in predicting outcome in primary pulmonary hypertension. *Am J Cardiol.* 1998;81(9):1157–1161.

243. Lopes AA, Maeda NY, Goncalves RC, Bydlowski SP. Endothelial cell dysfunction correlates differentially with survival in primary and secondary pulmonary hypertension. *Am Heart J.* 2000;139(4):618–623.

244. Nagaya N, Nishikimi T, Uematsu M, et al. Plasma brain natriuretic peptide as a prognostic indicator in patients with primary pulmonary hypertension. *Circulation.* 2000;102(8): 865–870.

245. Nagaya N, Uematsu M, Satoh T, et al. Serum uric acid levels correlate with the severity and the mortality of primary pulmonary hypertension. *Am J Respir Crit Care Med.* 1999; 160(2):487–492.

246. Nootens M, Kaufmann E, Rector T, et al. Neurohormonal activation in patients with right ventricular failure from pulmonary hypertension: relation to hemodynamic variables and endothelin levels. *J Am Coll Cardiol.* 1995;26(7):1581–1585.

247. Shitrit D, Bendayan D, Bar-Gil-Shitrit A, et al. Significance of a plasma D-dimer test in patients with primary pulmonary hypertension. *Chest.* 2002;122(5):1674–1678.

248. Torbicki A, Kurzyna M, Kuca P, et al. Detectable serum cardiac troponin T as a marker of poor prognosis among patients with chronic precapillary pulmonary hypertension. *Circulation.* 2003;108(7):844–848.

249. Voelkel MA, Wynne KM, Badesch DB, Groves BM, Voelkel NF. Hyperuricemia in severe pulmonary hypertension. *Chest.* 2000;117(1):19–24.

250. Okada O, Tanabe N, Yasuda J, et al. Prediction of life expectancy in patients with primary pulmonary hypertension. A retrospective nationwide survey from 1980–1990. *Intern Med.* 1999;38(1):12–16.

251. Rajasekhar D, Balakrishnan KG, Venkitachalam CG, et al. Primary pulmonary hypertension: natural history and prognostic factors. *Indian Heart J.* 1994;46(3):165–170.

252. D'Alonzo GE, Barst RJ, Ayres SM, et al. Survival in patients with primary pulmonary hypertension. Results from a national prospective registry. *Ann Intern Med.* 1991;115(5):343–349.

253. Hoeper MM, Galie N, Murali S, et al. Outcome after cardiopulmonary resuscitation in patients with pulmonary arterial hypertension. *Am J Respir Crit Care Med.* 2002;165(3): 341–344.

254. Loyd JE, Primm RK, Newman JH. Familial primary pulmonary hypertension: clinical patterns. *Am Rev Respir Dis.* 1984;129(1):194–197.

255. Loyd JE, Butler MG, Foroud TM, Conneally PM, Phillips JA 3rd, Newman JH. Genetic anticipation and abnormal gender ratio at birth in familial primary pulmonary hypertension. *Am J Respir Crit Care Med.* 1995;152(1):93–97.

256. Nichols WC, Koller DL, Slovis B, et al. Localization of the gene for familial primary pulmonary hypertension to chromosome 2q31-32. *Nat Genet.* 1997;15(3):277–280.

257. Morse JH, Jones AC, Barst RJ, Hodge SE, Wilhelmsen KC, Nygaard TG. Mapping of familial primary pulmonary hypertension locus (PPH1) to chromosome 2q31-q32. *Circulation.* 1997;95(12):2603–2606.

258. Abdalla SA, Gallione CJ, Barst RJ, et al. Primary pulmonary hypertension in families with hereditary haemorrhagic telangiectasia. *Eur Respir J.* 2004;23(3):373–377.

259. Harrison RE, Flanagan JA, Sankelo M, et al. Molecular and functional analysis identifies ALK-1 as the predominant cause of pulmonary hypertension related to hereditary haemorrhagic telangiectasia. *J Med Genet.* 2003;40(12):865–871.

260. Elliott CG. Genetics of pulmonary arterial hypertension. In: Mandel J, Taichman D, eds. *Pulmonary Vascular Disease.* Philadelphia, PA: WB Saunders; 2006:50–65.

261. Grunig E, Janssen B, Mereles D, et al. Abnormal pulmonary artery pressure response in asymptomatic carriers of primary pulmonary hypertension gene. *Circulation.* 2000;102(10): 1145–1150.

262. Elliott G, Alexander G, Leppert M, et al. Coancestry in apparently sporadic primary pulmonary hypertension. *Chest.* 1995;108(4):973–977.

263. Fox BD, Shimony A, Langleben D, et al. High prevalence of occult left heart disease in scleroderma-pulmonary hypertension. *Eur Respir J.* 2013;42(4):1083–1091.

264. Hachulla E, Gressin V, Guillevin L, et al. Early detection of pulmonary arterial hypertension in systemic sclerosis: a French nationwide prospective multicenter study. *Arthritis Rheum.* 2005;52(12):3792–3800.

265. Mukerjee D, St George D, Coleiro B, et al. Prevalence and outcome in systemic sclerosis associated pulmonary arterial hypertension: application of a registry approach. *Ann Rheum Dis.* 2003;62(11):1088–1093.

266. Kawut SM, Taichman DB, Archer-Chicko CL, Palevsky HI, Kimmel SE. Hemodynamics and survival in patients with pulmonary arterial hypertension related to systemic sclerosis. *Chest.* 2003;123(2):344–350.

267. Steen VD, Medsger TA Jr. Severe organ involvement in systemic sclerosis with diffuse scleroderma. *Arthritis Rheum.* 2000;43(11):2437–2444.

268. Benza RL, Miller DP, Barst RJ, Badesch DB, Frost AE, McGoon MD. An evaluation of long-term survival from time of diagnosis in pulmonary arterial hypertension from the REVEAL Registry. *Chest.* 2012;142(2):448–456.

269. Launay D, Sitbon O, Hachulla E, et al. Survival in systemic sclerosis-associated pulmonary arterial hypertension in the modern management era. *Ann Rheum Dis.* 2013;72(12):1940–1946.

270. Badui E, Garcia-Rubi D, Robles E, et al. Cardiovascular manifestations in systemic lupus erythematosus. Prospective study of 100 patients. *Angiology.* 1985;36(7):431–441.

271. Li EK, Tam LS. Pulmonary hypertension in systemic lupus erythematosus: clinical association and survival in 18 patients. *J Rheumatol.* 1999;26(9):1923–1929.

272. Simonson JS, Schiller NB, Petri M, Hellmann DB. Pulmonary hypertension in systemic lupus erythematosus. *J Rheumatol.* 1989;16(7):918–925.

273. Winslow TM, Ossipov MA, Fazio GP, Simonson JS, Redberg RF, Schiller NB. Five-year follow-up study of the prevalence and progression of pulmonary hypertension in systemic lupus erythematosus. *Am Heart J.* 1995;129(3):510–515.

274. Prabu A, Patel K, Yee CS, et al. Prevalence and risk factors for pulmonary arterial hypertension in patients with lupus. *Rheumatology (Oxford).* 2009;48(12):1506–1511.

275. Shen JY, Chen SL, Wu YX, et al. Pulmonary hypertension in systemic lupus erythematosus. *Rheumatol Int.* 1999;18(4):147–151.

276. Mette SA, Palevsky HI, Pietra GG, et al. Primary pulmonary hypertension in association with human immunodeficiency virus infection. A possible viral etiology for some forms of hypertensive pulmonary arteriopathy. *Am Rev Respir Dis.* 1992;145(5):1196–1200.

277. Ehrenreich H, Rieckmann P, Sinowatz F, et al. Potent stimulation of monocytic endothelin-1 production by HIV-1 glycoprotein 120. *J Immunol.* 1993;150(10):4601–4609.

278. Humbert M, Monti G, Fartoukh M, et al. Platelet-derived growth factor expression in primary pulmonary hypertension: comparison of HIV seropositive and HIV seronegative patients. *Eur Respir J.* 1998;11(3):554–559.

279. Voelkel NF, Tuder RM. Cellular and molecular mechanisms in the pathogenesis of severe pulmonary hypertension. *Eur Respir J.* 1995;8(12):2129–2138.

280. Speich R, Jenni R, Opravil M, Pfab M, Russi EW. Primary pulmonary hypertension in HIV infection. *Chest.* 1991;100(5): 1268–1271.

281. Zuber JP, Calmy A, Evison JM, et al. Pulmonary arterial hypertension related to HIV infection: improved hemodynamics and survival associated with antiretroviral therapy. *Clin Infect Dis.* 2004;38(8):1178–1185.

282. Sitbon O, Lascoux-Combe C, Delfraissy JF, et al. Prevalence of HIV-related pulmonary arterial hypertension in the current antiretroviral therapy era. *Am J Respir Crit Care Med.* 2008;177(1):108–113.

283. Petitpretz P, Brenot F, Azarian R, et al. Pulmonary hypertension in patients with human immunodeficiency virus infection. Comparison with primary pulmonary hypertension. *Circulation.* 1994;89(6):2722–2727.

284. Nunes H, Humbert M, Sitbon O, et al. Prognostic factors for survival in human immunodeficiency virus-associated pulmonary arterial hypertension. *Am J Respir Crit Care Med.* 2003; 167(10):1433–1439.

285. Krowka MJ, Miller DP, Barst RJ, et al. Portopulmonary hypertension: a report from the US-based REVEAL Registry. *Chest.* 2012;141(4):906–915.

286. Ramsay MA, Simpson BR, Nguyen AT, Ramsay KJ, East C, Klintmalm GB. Severe pulmonary hypertension in liver transplant candidates. *Liver Transpl Surg.* 1997;3(5): 494–500.

287. Edwards BS, Weir KE, Edwards WD, Ludwig J, Dykoski RK, Edwards JE. Coexistent pulmonary and portal hypertension: morphologic and clinical features. *J Am Coll Cardiol.* 1987; 10:1233–1238.

288. Hoeper MM, Krowka MJ, Strassburg CP. Portopulmonary hypertension and hepatopulmonary syndrome. *Lancet.* 2004; 363:1461–1468.

289. Benjaminov FS, Prentice M, Sniderman KW, Siu S, Liu P, Wong F. Portopulmonary hypertension in decompensated cirrhosis with refractory ascites. *Gut.* 2003;52(9):1355–1362.

290. Tuder RM, Cool CD, Geraci MW, et al. Prostacyclin synthase expression is decreased in lungs from patients with severe pulmonary hypertension. *Am J Respir Crit Care Med.* 1999;159(6):1925–1932.

291. Hadengue A, Benhayoun MK, Lebrec D, et al. Pulmonary hypertension complicating portal hypertension: prevalence and relation to splanchnic hemodynamics. *Gastroenterology.* 1991;100(2):520–528.

292. Kawut SM, Krowka MJ, Trotter JF, et al. Clinical risk factors for portopulmonary hypertension. *Hepatology.* 2008;48(1): 196–203.

293. Roberts KE, Fallon MB, Krowka MJ, et al. Genetic risk factors for portopulmonary hypertension in patients with advanced liver disease. *Am J Resp Crit Care Med.* 2009;179(9): 835–842.

294. McDonnell PJ, Toye PA, Hutchins GM. Primary pulmonary hypertension and cirrhosis: are they related? *Am Rev Respir Dis.* 1983;127(4):437–441.

295. Robalino BD, Moodie DS. Association between primary pulmonary hypertension and portal hypertension: analysis of its pathophysiology and clinical, laboratory and hemodynamic manifestations. *J Am Coll Cardiol.* 1991;17(2):492–498.

296. Rodriguez-Roisin R, Krowka MJ, Herve P, Fallon MB, ERS Task Force Pulmonary-Hepatic Vascular Disorders (PHD) Scientific Committee. Pulmonary-hepatic vascular disorders scientific committee ERS task force. *Eur Respir J.* 2004;24:861–880.

297. Ota K, Shijo H, Kokawa H, et al. Effects of nifedipine on hepatic venous pressure gradient and portal vein blood flow in patients with cirrhosis. *J Gastroenterol Hepatol.* 1995;10(2):198–204.

298. Navasa M, Bosch J, Reichen J, et al. Effects of verapamil on hepatic and systemic hemodynamics and liver function in patients with cirrhosis and portal hypertension. *Hepatology.* 1988;8(4):850–854.

299. Swanson K, Krowka M. Portopulmonary hypertension. In: Mandel J, Taichman DB, eds. *Pulmonary Vascular Disease.* Philadelphia, PA: Elsevier Science; 2006.

300. Kuo PC, Johnson LB, Plotkin JS, Howell CD, Bartlett ST, Rubin LJ. Continuous intravenous infusion of epoprostenol for the treatment of portopulmonary hypertension. *Transplantation.* 1997;63:604–606.

301. Findlay JY, Plevak DJ, Krowka MJ, Sack EM, Porayko MK. Progressive splenomegaly after epoprostenol therapy in portopulmonary hypertension. *Liver Transpl Surg.* 1999;5(5):362–365.

302. Krowka MJ, Frantz RP, McGoon MD, Severson C, Plevak DJ, Wiesner RH. Improvement in pulmonary hemodynamics during intravenous epoprostenol (prostacyclin): a study of 15 patients with moderate to severe portopulmonary hypertension. *Hepatology.* 1999;30(3):641–648.

303. Kahler CM, Graziadei I, Wiedermann CJ, Kneussl MP, Vogel W. Successful use of continuous intravenous prostacyclin in a patient with severe portopulmonary hypertension. *Wien Klin Wochenschr.* 2000;112(14):637–640.

304. Chua R, Keogh A, Miyashita M. Novel use of sildenafil in the treatment of portopulmonary hypertension. *J Heart Lung Transplant.* 2005;24(4):498–500.

305. Halank M, Kolditz M, Miehlke S, Schiemanck S, Schmeisser A, Hoeffken G. Combination therapy for portopulmonary hypertension with intravenous iloprost and oral bosentan. *Wien Med Wochenschr.* 2005;155(15–16):376–380.

306. Kett DH, Acosta RC, Campos MA, Rodriguez MJ, Quartin AA, Schein RM. Recurrent portopulmonary hypertension after liver transplantation: management with epoprostenol and resolution after retransplantation. *Liver Transpl.* 2001;7(7):645–648.

307. Makisalo H, Koivusalo A, Vakkuri A, Hockerstedt K. Sildenafil for portopulmonary hypertension in a patient undergoing liver transplantation. *Liver Transpl.* 2004;10(7):945–950.

308. Rafanan AL, Maurer J, Mehta AC, Schilz R. Progressive portopulmonary hypertension after liver transplantation treated with epoprostenol. *Chest.* 2000;118(5):1497–1500.

309. Schroeder RA, Rafii AA, Plotkin JS, Johnson LB, Rustgi VK, Kuo PC. Use of aerosolized inhaled epoprostenol in the treatment of portopulmonary hypertension. *Transplantation.* 2000;70(3):548–550.

310. Hoeper MM, Halank M, Marx C, et al. Bosentan therapy for portopulmonary hypertension. *Eur Respir J.* 2005;25(3): 502–508.

311. Cartin-Ceba R, Swanson K, Iyer V, Wiesner RH, Krowka MJ. Safety and efficacy of ambrisentan for the treatment of portopulmonary hypertension. *Chest.* 2011;139(1):109–114.

312. McGoon MD, Frost AE, Oudiz RJ, et al. Ambrisentan therapy in patients with pulmonary arterial hypertension who discontinued bosentan or sitaxsentan due to liver function test abnormalities. *Chest.* 2009;135(1):122–129.

313. Krowka MJ, Mandell MS, Ramsay MA, et al. Hepatopulmonary syndrome and portopulmonary hypertension: a report of the multicenter liver transplant database. *Liver Transpl.* 2004;10(2):174–182.

314. Krowka MJ, Plevak DJ, Findlay JY, Rosen CB, Wiesner RH, Krom RA. Pulmonary hemodynamics and perioperative cardiopulmonary-related mortality in patients with portopulmonary hypertension undergoing liver transplantation. *Liver Transpl.* 2000;6(4):443–450.

315. Minder S, Fischler M, Muellhaupt B, et al. Intravenous iloprost bridging to orthotopic liver transplantation in portopulmonary hypertension. *Eur Respir J.* 2004;24(4):703–707.

316. Kim WR, Krowka MJ, Plevak DJ, et al. Accuracy of doppler echocardiography in the assessment of pulmonary hypertension in liver transplant candidates. *Liver Transpl.* 2000;6: 453–458.

317. Gurtner HP. Aminorex pulmonary hypertension. In: Fishman AP, ed. *The Pulmonary Circulation: Normal and Abnormal.* Philadelphia, PA: University of Pennsylvania Press; 1990:397–411.

318. Brenot F. Risk factors for primary pulmonary hypertension. In: Rubin LJ, Rich S, eds. *Primary Pulmonary Hypertension.* New York, NY: Marcel Dekker; 1996:131–149.

319. Brenot F, Herve P, Petitpretz P, Parent F, Duroux P, Simonneau G. Primary pulmonary hypertension and fenfluramine use. *Br Heart J.* 1993;70(6):537–541.

320. Rich S, Rubin L, Walker AM, Schneeweiss S, Abenhaim L. Anorexigens and pulmonary hypertension in the United States: results from the surveillance of North American pulmonary hypertension. *Chest.* 2000;117(3):870–874.

321. Scholand MB, Singh NA, Leppert M, et al. BMPR2 mutations are uncommon in North American patients with appetite suppressant associated pulmonary arterial hypertension. *Am J Resp Crit Care Med.* 2003;167.

322. Simonneau G, Fartoukh M, Sitbon O, Humbert M, Jagot JL, Hervé P. Primary pulmonary hypertension associated with the use of fenfluramine derivatives. *Chest.* 1998;114(3 Suppl):195S–199S.

323. Frank H, Mlczoch J, Huber K, Schuster E, Gurtner HP, Kneussl M. The effect of anticoagulant therapy in primary and anorectic drug-induced pulmonary hypertension. *Chest.* 1997;112(3):714–721.

324. Rich S, Shillington A, McLaughlin V. Comparison of survival in patients with pulmonary hypertension associated with fenfluramine to patients with primary pulmonary hypertension. *Am J Cardiol.* 2003;92(11):1366–1368.

325. Lopez-Sendon J, Gomez-Sanchez MA, Mestre de Juan MJ, et al. Pulmonary hypertension in the toxic oil syndrome. In: Fishman AP, ed. *The Pulmonary Circulation: Normal and Abnormal. Mechanisms, Management, and the National Registry.* Philadelphia, PA: University of Pennsylvania Press; 1990:385–395.

326. Morris CR, Kato GJ, Poljakovic M, et al. Dysregulated arginine metabolism, hemolysis-associated pulmonary hypertension, and mortality in sickle cell disease. *JAMA.* 2005;294(1):81–90.

327. Castro O. Pulmonary hypertension in sickle cell disease and thalassemia. In: Peackock AJ, Rubin L, eds. *Pulmonary Circulation – Diseases and their Treatment.* London: Arnold Publishers; 2004:237–243.

328. Machado RF, Gladwin MT. Hemolytic anemia associated pulmonary hypertension. In: Mandel J, Taichman DB, eds. *Pulmonary Vascular Disease.* Philadelphia, PA: Elsevier; 2006.

329. Gladwin MT, Sachdev V, Jison ML, et al. Pulmonary hypertension as a risk factor for death in patients with sickle cell disease. *N Engl J Med.* 2004;350(9):886–895.

330. Jootar P, Fucharoen S. Cardiac involvement in b-thalassemia/hemoglobin E disease: clinical and hemodynamic findings. *Southeast Asian J Trop Med Public Health.* 1990;21(2): 269–273.

331. Du Z, Roguin N, Milgram E, et al. Pulmonary hypertension in patients with thalassemia major. *Am Heart J.* 1997;134(3): 532–537.

332. Aessopos A, Farmakis D, Deftereos S, et al. Thalassemia heart disease: a comparative evaluation of thalassemia major and thalassemia intermedia. *Chest.* 2005;127(5):1523–1530.

333. Aessopos A, Farmakis D. Pulmonary hypertension in b-thalassemia. *Ann N Y Acad Sci.* 2005;1054:342–349.

334. Heller PG, Grinberg AR, Lencioni M, Molina MM, Roncoroni AJ. Pulmonary hypertension in paroxysmal nocturnal hemoglobinuria. *Chest.* 1992;102(2):642–643.

335. Verresen D, De Backer W, Van Meerbeeck J, Neetens I, Van Marck E, Vermeire P. Spherocytosis and pulmonary hypertension coincidental occurrence or causal relationship? *Eur Respir J.* 1991;4(5):629–631.

336. Fitzgerald M, Fagan K, Herbert DE, Al-Ali M, Mugal M, Haynes J Jr. Misclassification of pulmonary hypertension in adults with sickle hemoglobinopathies using Doppler echocardiography. *South Med J.* 2012;105(6):300–305.

337. Castro O, Hoque M, Brown BD. Pulmonary hypertension in sickle cell disease: cardiac catheterization results and survival. *Blood.* 2003;101(4):1257–1261.

338. Machado RF, Martyr S, Kato GJ, et al. Sildenafil therapy in patients with sickle cell disease and pulmonary hypertension. *Br J Haematol.* 2005;130(3):445–453.

339. Machado RF, Barst RJ, Yovetich NA, et al. Hospitalization for pain in patients with sickle cell disease treated with sildenafil for elevated TRV and low exercise capacity. *Blood.* 2011;118(4): 855–864.

340. Derchi G, Forni GL, Formisano F, et al. Efficacy and safety of sildenafil in the treatment of severe pulmonary hypertension in patients with hemoglobinopathies. *Haematologica.* 2005;90(4):452–458.

341. Mandel J. Pulmonary veno-occlusive disease. In: Mandel J, Taichman DB, eds. *Pulmonary Vascular Disease.* Philadelphia, PA: WB Saunders; 2006:157–169.

342. Montani D, Achouh L, Dorfmuller P, et al. Pulmonary veno-occlusive disease: clinical, functional, radiologic, and hemodynamic characteristics and outcome of 24 cases confirmed by histology. *Medicine (Baltimore).* 2008;87(4):220–233.

343. Doll DC, Yarbro JW. Vascular toxicity associated with chemotherapy and hormonotherapy. *Curr Opin Oncol.* 1994;6(4): 345–350.

344. Joselson R, Warnock M. Pulmonary veno-occlusive disease after chemotherapy. *Hum Pathol.* 1983;14(1):88–91.

345. Knight BK, Rose AG. Pulmonary veno-occlusive disease after chemotherapy. *Thorax.* 1985;40(11):874–875.

346. Swift GL, Gibbs A, Campbell IA, Wagenvoort CA, Tuthill D. Pulmonary veno-occlusive disease and Hodgkin's lymphoma. *Eur Respir J.* 1993;6(4):596–598.

347. Waldhorn RE, Tsou E, Smith FP, Kerwin DM. Pulmonary veno-occlusive disease associated with microangiopathic hemolytic anemia and chemotherapy of gastric adenocarcinoma. *Med Pediatr Oncol.* 1984;12(6):394–396.

348. Gagnadoux F, Capron F, Lebeau B. Pulmonary veno-occlusive disease after neoadjuvant mitomycin chemotherapy and surgery for lung carcinoma. *Lung Cancer.* 2002;36(2):213–215.

349. Vansteenkiste JF, Bomans P, Verbeken EK, Nackaerts KL, Demedts MG. Fatal pulmonary veno-occlusive disease possibly related to gemcitabine. *Lung Cancer.* 2001;31(1):83–85.

350. Hackman RC, Madtes DK, Petersen FB, Clark JG. Pulmonary veno-occlusive disease following bone marrow transplantation. *Transplantation.* 1989;47(6):989–992.

351. Kuga T, Kohda K, Hirayama Y, et al. Pulmonary veno-occlusive disease accompanied by microangiopathic hemolytic anemia 1 year after a second bone marrow transplantation for acute lymphoblastic leukemia. *Int J Hematol.* 1996;64(2):143–150.

352. Mukai M, Kondo M, Bohgaki T, Notoya A, Kohno M. Pulmonary veno-occlusive disease following allogeneic peripheral blood stem cell transplantation for chronic myeloid leukaemia. *Br J Haematol.* 2003;123(1):1.

353. Salzman D, Adkins DR, Craig F, Freytes C, LeMaistre CF. Malignancy-associated pulmonary veno-occlusive disease: report of a case following autologous bone marrow transplantation and review. *Bone Marrow Transpl.* 1996;18(4): 755–760.

354. Seguchi M, Hirabayashi N, Fujii Y, et al. Pulmonary hypertension associated with pulmonary occlusive vasculopathy after allogeneic bone marrow transplantation. *Transplantation.* 2000;69(1):177–179.

355. Trobaugh-Lotrario AD, Greffe B, Deterding R, Deutsch G, Quinones R. Pulmonary veno-occlusive disease after autologous bone marrow transplant in a child with stage IV neuroblastoma: case report and literature review. *J Pediatr Hematol Oncol.* 2003;25(5):405–409.

356. Williams LM, Fussell S, Veith RW, Nelson S, Mason CM. Pulmonary veno-occlusive disease in an adult following bone marrow transplantation. Case report and review of the literature. *Chest.* 1996;109(5):1388–1391.

357. Ruchelli ED, Nojadera G, Rutstein RM, Rudy B. Pulmonary veno-occlusive disease. Another vascular disorder associated with human immunodeficiency virus infection? *Arch Pathol Lab Med.* 1994;118(6):664–666.

358. Escamilla R, Hermant C, Berjaud J, Mazerolles C, Daussy X. Pulmonary veno-occlusive disease in a HIV-infected intravenous drug abuser. *Eur Respir J.* 1995;8(11):1982–1984.

359. Hourseau M, Capron F, Nunes H, et al. Pulmonary veno-occlusive disease in a patient with HIV infection. A case report with autopsy findings. *Ann Pathol.* 2002;22(6):472–475.

360. Kishida Y, Kanai Y, Kuramochi S, Hosoda Y. Pulmonary venoocclusive disease in a patient with systemic lupus erythematosus. *J Rheumatol.* 1993;20(12):2161–2162.

361. Saito A, Takizawa H, Ito K, et al. A case of pulmonary veno-occlusive disease associated with systemic sclerosis. *Respirology.* 2003;8(3):383–385.

362. Scully R, Mark E, McNeely B. Case records of the Massachusetts General Hospital: weekly clinicpatholigic exercises. Case 14–1983: a 67-year-old woman with pulmonary hypertension. *N Engl J Med.* 1983;308:823–834.

363. Townend JN, Roberts DH, Jones EL, Davies MK. Fatal pulmonary venoocclusive disease after use of oral contraceptives. *Am Heart J.* 1992;124(6):1643–1644.

364. Tsou E, Waldhorn RE, Kerwin DM, Katz S, Patterson JA. Pulmonary venoocclusive disease in pregnancy. *Obstet Gynecol.* 1984;64(2):281–284.

365. Perros F, Cohen-Kaminsky S, Gambaryan N, et al. Cytotoxic cells and granulysin in pulmonary arterial hypertension and pulmonary veno-occlusive disease. *Am J Respir Crit Care Med.* 2013;187(2):189–196.

366. Thadani U, Burrow C, Whitaker W, Heath D. Pulmonary veno-occlusive disease. *Q J Med.* 1975;44(173):133–159.

367. Heath D, Segel N, Bishop J. Pulmonary veno-occlusive disease. *Circulation.* 1966;34(2):242–248.

368. Calderon M, Burdine JA. Pulmonary veno-occlusive disease. *J Nucl Med.* 1974;15(6):455–457.

369. Glassroth J, Woodford DW, Carrington CB, Gaensler EA. Pulmonary veno-occlusive disease in the middle-aged. *Respiration.* 1985;47(4):309–321.

370. Chawla SK, Kittle CF, Faber LP, Jensik RJ. Pulmonary venoocclusive disease. *Ann Thorac Surg.* 1976;22(3):249–253.

371. Swensen SJ, Tashjian JH, Myers JL, et al. Pulmonary venoocclusive disease: CT findings in eight patients. *AJR Am J Roentgenol.* 1996;167(4):937–940.

372. Wiener-Kronish JP, Goldstein R, Matthay RA, et al. Lack of association of pleural effusion with chronic pulmonary arterial and right atrial hypertension. *Chest.* 1987;92(6):967–970.

373. Bailey CL, Channick RN, Auger WR, et al. "High probability" perfusion lung scans in pulmonary veno-occlusive disease. *Am J Respir Crit Care Med.* 2000;162(5):1974–1978.

374. Dufour B, Maitre S, Humbert M, Capron F, Simonneau G, Musset D. High-resolution CT of the chest in four patients with pulmonary capillary hemangiomatosis or pulmonary venoocclusive disease. *AJR Am J Roentgenol.* 1998;171(5): 1321–1324.

375. Weed HG. Pulmonary "capillary" wedge pressure not the pressure in the pulmonary capillaries. *Chest.* 1991;100(4): 1138–1140.

376. Rambihar VS, Fallen EL, Cairns JA. Pulmonary veno-occlusive disease: antemortem diagnosis from roentgenographic and hemodynamic findings. *Can Med Assoc J.* 1979;120(12): 1519–1522.

377. Salzman GA, Rosa UW. Prolonged survival in pulmonary veno-occlusive disease treated with nifedipine. *Chest.* 1989;95(5):1154–1156.

378. Palevsky HI, Pietra GG, Fishman AP. Pulmonary veno-occlusive disease and its response to vasodilator agents. *Am Rev Respir Dis.* 1990;142(2):426–429.

379. Okumura H, Nagaya N, Kyotani S, et al. Effects of continuous IV prostacyclin in a patient with pulmonary veno-occlusive disease. *Chest.* 2002;122(3):1096–1098.

380. Davis LL, deBoisblanc BP, Glynn CE, Ramirez C, Summer WR. Effect of prostacyclin on microvascular pressures in a patient with pulmonary veno-occlusive disease. *Chest.* 1995;108(6):1754–1756.

381. Hoeper MM, Eschenbruch C, Zink-Wohlfart C, et al. Effects of inhaled nitric oxide and aerosolized iloprost in pulmonary veno-occlusive disease. *Respir Med.* 1999;93(1):62–64.

382. Palmer SM, Robinson LJ, Wang A, Gossage JR, Bashore T, Tapson VF. Massive pulmonary edema and death after prostacyclin infusion in a patient with pulmonary veno-occlusive disease. *Chest.* 1998;113(1):237–240.

383. Gilroy RJ Jr, Teague MW, Loyd JE. Pulmonary veno-occlusive disease. Fatal progression of pulmonary hypertension despite

steroid-induced remission of interstitial pneumonitis. *Am Rev Respir Dis.* 1991;143(5 Pt 1):1130–1133.

384. Sanderson JE, Spiro SG, Hendry AT, Turner-Warwick M. A case of pulmonary veno-occlusive disease respondong to treatment with azathioprine. *Thorax.* 1977;32(2):140–148.

385. Wagenvoort CA, Beetstra A, Spijker J. Capillary haemangiomatosis of the lungs. *Histopathology.* 1978;2(6):401–406.

386. Eltorky MA, Headley AS, Winer-Muram H, Garrett HE Jr, Griffin JP. Pulmonary capillary hemangiomatosis: a clinicopathologic review. *Ann Thorac Surg.* 1994;57(3):772–776.

387. Kawut SM, Assaad AM, Arcasoy SM, Rosenzweig EB, Sonett JR, Borczuk AC. Pulmonary capillary hemangiomatosis: results of gene expression analysis. *Chest.* 2005;128(6 Suppl): 575S–576S.

388. Sullivan A, Chmura K, Cool CD, Voelkel N, Chan ED. Pulmonary capillary hemangiomatosis: an immunohistochemical analysis of vascular remodeling in a fatal case. *Chest.* 2005;128(6 Suppl):576S.

389. Kradin R, Matsubara O, Mark EJ. Endothelial nitric oxide synthase expression in pulmonary capillary hemangiomatosis. *Exp Mol Pathol.* 2005;79(3):194–197.

390. Langleben D, Heneghan JM, Batten AP, et al. Familial pulmonary capillary hemangiomatosis resulting in primary pulmonary hypertension. *Ann Intern Med.* 1988;109(2):106–109.

391. Lippert JL, White CS, Cameron EW, Sun CC, Liang X, Rubin LJ. Pulmonary capillary hemangiomatosis: radiographic appearance. *J Thorac Imaging.* 1998;13(1):49–51.

392. Lawler LP, Askin FB. Pulmonary capillary hemangiomatosis: multidetector row CT findings and clinico-pathologic correlation. *J Thorac Imaging.* 2005;20(1):61–63.

393. Humbert M, Maitre S, Capron F, Rain B, Musset D, Simonneau G. Pulmonary edema complicating continuous intravenous prostacyclin in pulmonary capillary hemangiomatosis. *Am J Respir Crit Care Med.* 1998;157(5 Pt 1):1681–1685.

394. Ito K, Ichiki T, Ohi K, et al. Pulmonary capillary hemangiomatosis with severe pulmonary hypertension. *Circ J.* 2003;67(9):793–795.

395. Gugnani MK, Pierson C, Vanderheide R, Girgis RE. Pulmonary edema complicating prostacyclin therapy in pulmonary hypertension associated with scleroderma: a case of pulmonary capillary hemangiomatosis. *Arthritis Rheum.* 2000;43(3):699–703.

396. White CW, Sondheimer HM, Crouch EC, Wilson H, Fan LL. Treatment of pulmonary hemangiomatosis with recombinant interferon a-2 a. *N Engl J Med.* 1989;320(18):1197–1200.

397. Almagro P, Julia J, Sanjaume M, et al. Pulmonary capillary hemangiomatosis associated with primary pulmonary hypertension: report of 2 new cases and review of 35 cases from the literature. *Medicine (Baltimore).* 2002;81(6):417–424.

398. Gray DJ, Ross AG, Li YS, McManus DP. Diagnosis and management of schistosomiasis. *BMJ.* 2011;342:d2651.

399. Andrade ZA, Andrade SG. Pathogenesis of schistosomal pulmonary arteritis. *Am J Trop Med Hyg.* 1970;19(2):305–310.

400. dos Santos Fernandes CJ, Jardim CV, Hovnanian A, et al. Survival in schistosomiasis-associated pulmonary arterial hypertension. *J Am Coll Cardiol.* 2010;56(9):715–720.

401. Fernandes CJ, Dias BA, Jardim CV, et al. The role of target therapies in schistosomiasis-associated pulmonary arterial hypertension. *Chest.* 2012;141(4):923–928.

402. Crosby A, Jones FM, Kolosionek E, et al. Praziquantel reverses pulmonary hypertension and vascular remodeling in murine schistosomiasis. *Am J Respir Crit Care Med.* 2011;184(4): 467–473.

403. Galiè N, Hoeper MM, Humbert M, et al. Guidelines for the diagnosis and treatment of pulmonary hypertension: The Task Force for the Diagnosis and Treatment of Pulmonary Hypertension of the European Society of Cardiology (ESC) and the European Respiratory Society (ERS), endorsed by the International Society of Heart and Lung Transplantation (ISHLT). *Eur Heart J.* 2009;30(20):2493–2537.

404. Califf RM, Adams KF, McKenna WJ, et al. A randomized controlled trial of epoprostenol therapy for severe congestive heart failure: The Flolan International Randomized Survival Trial (FIRST). *Am Heart J.* 1997;134(1):44–54.

405. Guazzi M, Borlaug BA. Pulmonary hypertension due to left heart disease. *Circulation.* 2012;126(8):975–990.

406. Stolz D, Rasch H, Linka A, et al. A randomised, controlled trial of bosentan in severe COPD. *Eur Respir J.* 2008;32(3):619–628.

407. Lewis GD, Shah R, Shahzad K, et al. Sildenafil improves exercise capacity and quality of life in patients with systolic heart failure and secondary pulmonary hypertension. *Circulation.* 2007;116(14):1555–1562.

408. Redfield MM, Chen HH, Borlaug BA, et al. Effect of phosphodiesterase-5 inhibition on exercise capacity and clinical status in heart failure with preserved ejection fraction: a randomized clinical trial. *JAMA.* 2013;309(12):1268–1277.

409. Chan L, Chin LM, Kennedy M, et al. Benefits of intensive treadmill exercise training on cardiorespiratory function and quality of life in patients with pulmonary hypertension. *Chest.* 2012;143(2):333–343.

410. Mereles D, Ehlken N, Kreuscher S, et al. Exercise and respiratory training improve exercise capacity and quality of life in patients with severe chronic pulmonary hypertension. *Circulation.* 2006;114(14):1482–1489.

411. NOTTG. Continuous or nocturnal oxygen therapy in hypoxemic chronic obstructive lung disease: a clinical trial. Nocturnal Oxygen Therapy Trial Group. *Ann Intern Med.* 1980;93(3):391–398.

412. Roubinian N, Elliott CG, Barnett CF, et al. Effects of commercial air travel on patients with pulmonary hypertension. *Chest.* 2012;142(4):885–892.

413. Rich S, Seidlitz M, Dodin E, et al. The short-term effects of digoxin in patients with right ventricular dysfunction from pulmonary hypertension. *Chest.* 1998;114(3):787–792.

414. Rich S, Kaufmann E, Levy PS. The effect of high doses of calcium-channel blockers on survival in primary pulmonary hypertension. *N Engl J Med.* 1992;327(2):76–81.

415. Badesch DB, Abman SH, Simonneau G, Rubin LJ, McLaughlin VV. Medical therapy for pulmonary arterial hypertension: updated ACCP evidence-based clinical practice guidelines. *Chest.* 2007;131(6):1917–1928.

416. McCaffrey RM, Dunn LJ. Primary pulmonary hypertension in pregnancy. *Obstet Gynecol Surv.* 1964;19:567–591.

417. Weiss JR, Pietra GG, Scharf SM. Primary pulmonary hypertension and the human immunodeficiency virus. Report of two cases and a review of the literature. *Arch Intern Med.* 1995;155(21):2350–2354.

418. Weiss BM, Zemp L, Seifert B, Hess OM. Outcome of pulmonary vascular disease in pregnancy: a systematic overview from 1978 through 1996. *J Am Coll Cardiol.* 1998;31(7):1650–1657.

419. Kiely DG, Condliffe R, Webster V, et al. Improved survival in pregnancy and pulmonary hypertension using a multiprofessional approach. *BJOG.* 2010;117(5):565–574.

420. Bedard E, Dimopoulos K, Gatzoulis MA. Has there been any progress made on pregnancy outcomes among women with pulmonary arterial hypertension? *Eur Heart J*. 2009;30(3):256–265.

421. Jais X, Olsson KM, Barbera JA, et al. Pregnancy outcomes in pulmonary arterial hypertension in the modern management era. *Eur Respir J*. 2012;40(4):881–885.

422. Rosengarten D, Blieden LC, Kramer MR. Pregnancy outcomes in pulmonary arterial hypertension in the modern management era. *Eur Respir J*. 2012;40(5):1304–1305.

423. Rich S, Pogoriler J, Husain AN, Toth PT, Gomberg-Maitland M, Archer SL. Long-term effects of epoprostenol on the pulmonary vasculature in idiopathic pulmonary arterial hypertension. *Chest*. 2010;138(5):1234–1239.

424. Taichman DB, McGoon MD, Harhay MO, et al. Wide variation in clinicians' assessment of New York Heart Association/World Health Organization functional class in patients with pulmonary arterial hypertension. *Mayo Clin Proc*. 2009;84(7):586–592.

425. Gabler NB, French B, Strom BL, et al. Validation of 6-minute walk distance as a surrogate end point in pulmonary arterial hypertension trials. *Circulation*. 2012;126(3):349–356.

426. Mathai SC, Puhan MA, Lam D, Wise RA. The minimal important difference in the 6-minute walk test for patients with pulmonary arterial hypertension. *Am J Respir Crit Care Med*. 2012;186(5):428–433.

427. McLaughlin VV. Has the 6-min walk distance run its course? *Chest*. 2012;142(6):1363–1364.

428. Rubin LJ. The 6-minute walk test in pulmonary arterial hypertension: how far is enough? *Am J Respir Crit Care Med*. 2012; 186(5):396–397.

429. Taichman DB, Christie J, Biester R, et al. Validation of a brief telephone battery for neurocognitive assessment of patients with pulmonary arterial hypertension. *Respir Res*. 2005;6(1):39.

430. Taichman DB, Ornelas J, Chung L, et al. Pharmacologic therapy for pulmonary arterial hypertension in adults: CHEST guideline and expert panel report. *Chest*. 2014;146(2):449–475.

431. Sitbon O, Humbert M, Jais X, et al. Long-term response to calcium channel blockers in idiopathic pulmonary arterial hypertension. *Circulation*. 2005;111(23):3105–3111.

432. Rich S, Kaufmann E. High dose titration of calcium channel blocking agents for primary pulmonary hypertension: guidelines for short-term drug testing. *J Am Coll Cardiol*. 1991;18(5):1323–1327.

433. Channick RN, Simonneau G, Sitbon O, et al. Effects of the dual endothelin-receptor antagonist bosentan in patients with pulmonary hypertension: a randomised placebo-controlled study. *Lancet*. 2001;358(9288):1119–1123.

434. Sitbon O, Badesch DB, Channick RN, et al. Effects of the dual endothelin receptor antagonist bosentan in patients with pulmonary arterial hypertension: a 1-year follow-up study. *Chest*. 2003;124(1):247–254.

435. Galie N, Rubin L, Hoeper M, et al. Treatment of patients with mildly symptomatic pulmonary arterial hypertension with bosentan (EARLY study): a double-blind, randomised controlled trial. *Lancet*. 2008;371(9630):2093–2100.

436. Galie N, Beghetti M, Gatzoulis MA, et al. Bosentan therapy in patients with Eisenmenger syndrome: a multicenter, double-blind, randomized, placebo-controlled study. *Circulation*. 2006;114(1):48–54.

437. Gatzoulis MA, Beghetti M, Galie N, et al. Longer-term bosentan therapy improves functional capacity in Eisenmenger syndrome: results of the BREATHE-5 open-label extension study. *Int J Cardiol*. 2008;127(1):27–32.

438. Sitbon O, Gressin V, Speich R, et al. Bosentan for the treatment of human immunodeficiency virus-associated pulmonary arterial hypertension. *Am J Respir Crit Care Med*. 2004;170(11):1212–1217.

439. Maiya S, Hislop AA, Flynn Y, Haworth SG. Response to bosentan in children with pulmonary hypertension. *Heart*. 2006;92(5):664–670.

440. Rosenzweig EB, Ivy DD, Widlitz A, et al. Effects of long-term bosentan in children with pulmonary arterial hypertension. *J Am Coll Cardiol*. 2005;46(4):697–704.

441. Gilbert N, Luther YC, Miera O, et al. Initial experience with bosentan (Tracleer) as treatment for pulmonary arterial hypertension (PAH) due to congenital heart disease in infants and young children. *Z Kardiol*. 2005;94(9):570–574.

442. Ivy DD, Rosenzweig EB, Lemarie JC, Brand M, Rosenberg D, Barst RJ. Long-term outcomes in children with pulmonary arterial hypertension treated with bosentan in real-world clinical settings. *Am J Cardiol*. 2010;106(9):1332–1338.

443. Galie N, Olschewski H, Oudiz RJ, et al. Ambrisentan for the treatment of pulmonary arterial hypertension: results of the ambrisentan in pulmonary arterial hypertension, randomized, double-blind, placebo-controlled, multicenter, efficacy (ARIES) study 1 and 2. *Circulation*. 2008;117(23):3010–3019.

444. Klinger JR, Oudiz RJ, Spence R, Despain D, Dufton C. Long-term pulmonary hemodynamic effects of ambrisentan in pulmonary arterial hypertension. *Am J Cardiol*. 2011;108(2):302–307.

445. Oudiz RJ, Galie N, Olschewski H, et al. Long-term ambrisentan therapy for the treatment of pulmonary arterial hypertension. *J Am Coll Cardiol*. 2009;54(21):1971–1981.

446. Ghofrani HA, Voswinckel R, Reichenberger F, et al. Differences in hemodynamic and oxygenation responses to three different phosphodiesterase-5 inhibitors in patients with pulmonary arterial hypertension: a randomized prospective study. *J Am Coll Cardiol*. 2004;44(7):1488–1496.

447. Barst RJ, Ivy DD, Gaitan G, et al. A randomized, double-blind, placebo-controlled, dose-ranging study of oral sildenafil citrate in treatment-naive children with pulmonary arterial hypertension. *Circulation*. 2012;125(2):324–334.

448. Oudiz RJ, Brundage BH, Galie N, et al. Tadalafil for the treatment of pulmonary arterial hypertension: a double-blind 52-week uncontrolled extension study. *J Am Coll Cardiol*. 2012;60(8):768–774.

449. Jing ZC, Yu ZX, Shen JY, et al. Vardenafil in pulmonary arterial hypertension: a randomized, double-blind, placebo-controlled study. *Am J Respir Crit Care Med*. 2011;183(12):1723–1729.

450. Archer-Chicko C, Housten-Harris T, Palevsky HI. Practical nursing issues in the outpatient management of pulmonary vascular disease. In: Mandel J, Taichman DB, eds. *Pulmonary Vascular Disease*. Philadelphia, PA: Elsevier Science; 2006 p.

451. Barst RJ, Rubin LJ, McGoon MD, Caldwell EJ, Long WA, Levy PS. Survival in primary pulmonary hypertension with long-term continuous intravenous prostacyclin. *Ann Intern Med*. 1994;121(6):409–415.

452. Lang G, Klepetko W. Lung transplantation for end-stage primary pulmonary hypertension. *Ann Transplant*. 2004;9(3):25–32.

453. Badesch DB, Tapson VF, McGoon MD, et al. Continuous intravenous epoprostenol for pulmonary hypertension due to the scleroderma spectrum of disease. A randomized, controlled trial. *Ann Intern Med*. 2000;132(6):425–434.

454. Robbins IM, Gaine SP, Schilz R, Tapson VF, Rubin LJ, Loyd JE. Epoprostenol for treatment of pulmonary hypertension

in patients with systemic lupus erythematosus. *Chest.* 2000;117(1):14–18.

455. Rosenzweig EB, Kerstein D, Barst RJ. Long-term prostacyclin for pulmonary hypertension with associated congenital heart defects. *Circulation.* 1999;99(14):1858–1865.

456. McLaughlin VV, Genthner DE, Panella MM, Hess DM, Rich S. Compassionate use of continuous prostacyclin in the management of secondary pulmonary hypertension: a case series. *Ann Intern Med.* 1999;130(9):740–743.

457. McLaughlin VV, Gaine SP, Barst RJ, et al. Efficacy and safety of treprostinil: an epoprostenol analog for primary pulmonary hypertension. *J Cardiovasc Pharmacol.* 2003;41(2):293–299.

458. Tapson VF, Gomberg-Maitland M, McLaughlin VV, et al. Safety and efficacy of IV treprostinil for pulmonary arterial hypertension: a prospective, multicenter, open-label, 12-week trial. *Chest.* 2006;129(3):683–688.

459. Hiremath J, Thanikachalam S, Parikh K, et al. Exercise improvement and plasma biomarker changes with intravenous treprostinil therapy for pulmonary arterial hypertension: a placebo-controlled trial. *J Heart Lung Transplant.* 2010;29(2): 137–149.

460. Farber HW, Walkey AJ, O'Donnell MR. Ethical issues associated with globalization of placebo-controlled in pulmonary arterial hypertension. *J Heart Lung Transplant.* 2010;29(7):825–826.

461. Park MH, Rubin LJ. The globalization of clinical trials in pulmonary arterial hypertension. *J Heart Lung Transplant.* 2010;29(2):157–158.

462. de la Mata J, Gomez-Sanchez MA, Aranzana M, Gomez-Reino JJ. Long-term iloprost infusion therapy for severe pulmonary hypertension in patients with connective tissue diseases. *Arthritis Rheum.* 1994;37(10):1528–1533.

463. Higenbottam T, Butt AY, McMahon A, Westerbeck R, Sharples L. Long-term intravenous prostaglandin (epoprostenol or iloprost) for treatment of severe pulmonary hypertension. *Heart.* 1998;80(2):151–155.

464. Scott JP, Higenbottam T, Wallwork J. The acute effect of the synthetic prostacyclin analogue iloprost in primary pulmonary hypertension. *Br J Clin Pract.* 1990;44(6):231–234.

465. Knudsen L, Schurawlew A, Nickel N, et al. Long-term effects of intravenous iloprost in patients with idiopathic pulmonary arterial hypertension deteriorating on non-parenteral therapy. *BMC Pulm Med.* 2011;11:56.

466. Kitterman N, Poms A, Miller DP, Lombardi S, Farber HW, Barst RJ. Bloodstream infections in patients with pulmonary arterial hypertension treated with intravenous prostanoids: insights from the REVEAL REGISTRY(R). *Mayo Clin Proc.* 2012;87(9):825–834.

467. Centers for Disease Control and Prevention (CDC). Bloodstream infections among patients treated with intravenous epoprostenol or intravenous treprostinil for pulmonary arterial hypertension–seven sites, United States, 2003–2006. *MMWR Morb Mortal Wkly Rep.* 2007;56(8):170–172.

468. Rich JD, Glassner C, Wade M, et al. The effect of diluent pH on bloodstream infection rates in patients receiving IV treprostinil for pulmonary arterial hypertension. *Chest.* 2012;141(1):36–42.

469. Fuentes A, Coralic A, Dawson KL. A new epoprostenol formulation for the treatment of pulmonary arterial hypertension. *Am J Health Syst Pharm.* 2012;69(16):1389–1393.

470. Simonneau G, Barst RJ, Galie N, et al. Continuous subcutaneous infusion of treprostinil, a prostacyclin analogue, in patients with pulmonary arterial hypertension: a double-blind, randomized, placebo-controlled trial. *Am J Respir Crit Care Med.* 2002;165(6):800–804.

471. Barst RJ, Galie N, Naeije R, et al. Long-term outcome in pulmonary arterial hypertension patients treated with subcutaneous treprostinil. *Eur Respir J.* 2006;28(6):1195–1203.

472. Mathier MA, McDevitt S, Saggar R. Subcutaneous treprostinil in pulmonary arterial hypertension: practical considerations. *J Heart Lung Transplant.* 2010;29(11):1210–1217.

473. Olschewski H, Walmrath D, Schermuly R, Ghofrani A, Grimminger F, Seeger W. Aerosolized prostacyclin and iloprost in severe pulmonary hypertension. *Ann Intern Med.* 1996;124(9):820–824.

474. Olschewski H, Ghofrani HA, Schmehl T, et al. Inhaled iloprost to treat severe pulmonary hypertension. An uncontrolled trial. German PPH Study Group. *Ann Intern Med.* 2000;132(6): 435–443.

475. Machherndl S, Kneussl M, Baumgartner H, et al. Long-term treatment of pulmonary hypertension with aerosolized iloprost. *Eur Respir J.* 2001;17(1):8–13.

476. Olschewski H, Simonneau G, Galie N, et al. Inhaled iloprost for severe pulmonary hypertension. *N Engl J Med.* 2002;347(5):322–329.

477. Olschewski H, Hoeper MM, Behr J, et al. Long-term therapy with inhaled iloprost in patients with pulmonary hypertension. *Respir Med.* 2010;104(5):731–740.

478. McLaughlin VV, Benza RL, Rubin LJ, et al. Addition of inhaled treprostinil to oral therapy for pulmonary arterial hypertension: a randomized controlled clinical trial. *J Am Coll Cardiol.* 2010;55(18):1915–1922.

479. Benza RL, Seeger W, McLaughlin VV, et al. Long-term effects of inhaled treprostinil in patients with pulmonary arterial hypertension: the Treprostinil Sodium Inhalation Used in the Management of Pulmonary Arterial Hypertension (TRIUMPH) study open-label extension. *J Heart Lung Transplant.* 2011;30(12):1327–1333.

480. Fruhwald FM, Kjellstrom B, Perthold W, et al. Continuous hemodynamic monitoring in pulmonary hypertensive patients treated with inhaled iloprost. *Chest.* 2003;124(1):351–359.

481. Barst RJ, McGoon M, McLaughlin V, et al. Beraprost therapy for pulmonary arterial hypertension. *J Am Coll Cardiol.* 2003;41(12):2119–2125.

482. Galie N, Humbert M, Vachiery JL, et al. Effects of beraprost sodium, an oral prostacyclin analogue, in patients with pulmonary arterial hypertension: a randomized, double-blind, placebo-controlled trial. *J Am Coll Cardiol.* 2002;39(9): 1496–1502.

483. Tapson VF, Torres F, Kermeen F, et al. Oral treprostinil for the treatment of pulmonary arterial hypertension in patients on background endothelin receptor antagonist and/or phosphodiesterase type 5 inhibitor therapy (The FREEDOM-C Study): a randomized controlled trial. *Chest.* 2012;142(6):1383–1390.

484. Humbert M, Barst RJ, Robbins IM, et al. Combination of bosentan with epoprostenol in pulmonary arterial hypertension: BREATHE-2. *Eur Respir J.* 2004;24(3):353–359.

485. McLaughlin VV, Oudiz RJ, Frost A, et al. Randomized study of adding inhaled iloprost to existing bosentan in pulmonary arterial hypertension. *Am J Respir Crit Care Med.* 2006;174(11): 1257–1263.

486. Simonneau G, Rubin LJ, Galie N, et al. Addition of sildenafil to long-term intravenous epoprostenol therapy in patients

with pulmonary arterial hypertension: a randomized trial. *Ann Intern Med.* 2008;149(8):521–530.

487. Chen H, Shiboski SC, Golden JA, et al. Impact of the lung allocation score on lung transplantation for pulmonary arterial hypertension. *Am J Respir Crit Care Med.* 2009;180(5): 468–474.

488. Sandoval J, Gaspar J, Pena H, et al. Effect of atrial septostomy on the survival of patients with severe pulmonary arterial hypertension. *Eur Respir J.* 2011;38(6):1343–1348.

489. Sandoval J, Rothman A, Pulido T. Atrial septostomy for pulmonary hypertension. *Clin Chest Med.* 2001;22(3):547–560.

490. Sztrymf B, Souza R, Bertoletti L, et al. Prognostic factors of acute heart failure in patients with pulmonary arterial hypertension. *Eur Respir J.* 2010;35(6):1286–1293.

491. Jeffery ME, Taichman DB. Management of the acutely ill patient with pulmonary arterial hypertension. In: Mandel J, Taichman DB, eds. *Pulmonary Vascular Disease.* Philadelphia, PA: Elsevier Science; 2006.

492. Price LC, Wort SJ, Finney SJ, Marino PS, Brett SJ. Pulmonary vascular and right ventricular dysfunction in adult critical care: current and emerging options for management: a systematic literature review. *Crit Care.* 2010;14(5):R169.

493. Kwak YL, Lee CS, Park YH, Hong YW. The effect of phenylephrine and norepinephrine in patients with chronic pulmonary hypertension*. *Anaesthesia.* 2002;57(1):9–14.

494. Holloway EL, Polumbo RA, Harrison DC. Acute circulatory effects of dopamine in patients with pulmonary hypertension. *Br Heart J.* 1975;37(5):482–485.

495. Kerbaul F, Rondelet B, Motte S, et al. Effects of norepinephrine and dobutamine on pressure load-induced right ventricular failure. *Crit Care Med.* 2004;32(4):1035–1040.

496. Hoeper MM, Olschewski H, Ghofrani HA, et al. A comparison of the acute hemodynamic effects of inhaled nitric oxide and aerosolized iloprost in primary pulmonary hypertension. German PPH study group. *J Am Coll Cardiol.* 2000;35(1): 176–182.

497. Olschewski H, Ghofrani HA, Walmrath D, et al. Inhaled prostacyclin and iloprost in severe pulmonary hypertension secondary to lung fibrosis. *Am J Respir Crit Care Med.* 1999;160(2):600–607.

498. Buckley MS, Feldman JP. Nebulized milrinone use in a pulmonary hypertensive crisis. *Pharmacotherapy.* 2007;27(12): 1763–1766.

499. Vachiery JL, Huez S, Gillies H, et al. Safety, tolerability and pharmacokinetics of an intravenous bolus of sildenafil in patients with pulmonary arterial hypertension. *Br J Clin Pharmacol.* 2011;71(2):289–292.

500. Amato MB, Barbas CS, Medeiros DM, et al. Beneficial effects of the "open lung approach" with low distending pressures in acute respiratory distress syndrome. A prospective randomized study on mechanical ventilation. *Am J Respir Crit Care Med.* 1995;152(6 Pt 1):1835–1846.

501. Hickey PR, Hansen DD, Wessel DL, Lang P, Jonas RA. Pulmonary and systemic hemodynamic responses to fentanyl in infants. *Anesth Analg.* 1985;64(5):483–486.

502. Gregoric ID, Chandra D, Myers TJ, Scheinin SA, Loyalka P, Kar B. Extracorporeal membrane oxygenation as a bridge to emergency heart-lung transplantation in a patient with idiopathic pulmonary arterial hypertension. *J Heart Lung Transplant.* 2008;27(4):466–468.

503. Olsson KM, Simon A, Strueber M, et al. Extracorporeal membrane oxygenation in nonintubated patients as bridge to lung transplantation. *Am J Transplant.* 2010;10(9):2173–2178.

504. Fischer S, Simon AR, Welte T, et al. Bridge to lung transplantation with the novel pumpless interventional lung assist device NovaLung. *J Thorac Cardiovasc Surg.* 2006;131(3):719–723.

CHAPTER 73

Pulmonary Thromboembolic Disease

Peter F. Fedullo
Gordon L. Yung

INTRODUCTION

Pulmonary thromboembolic disease refers to the condition in which blood clot(s) (thrombus or multiple thrombi) migrate from the systemic circulation to the pulmonary vasculature. Most of these thrombi arise from the deep veins of the lower and upper extremities (deep venous thrombosis [DVT]). From the clinical standpoint, DVT and pulmonary embolism (PE) can be considered a continuum of the same disease, and the two terms are often collectively referred to as venous thromboembolism.

The annual incidence of PE in the United States remains uncertain. In a retrospective analysis of data involving 2218 Olmsted County residents over a 10-year period, community residents who were not hospitalized within a 90 days period had an incidence of PE of 3.6 per 10,000 person-years.[1] A slightly lower incidence of 2.3 per 10,000 person-years was reported in an earlier study in Massachusetts.[2] This translates to an annual incidence of approximately 100,000 cases in the United States. However, the true incidence of PE is likely to be much higher since many cases remain undiagnosed. A recent systematic review revealed that silent PE was present in 32% of patients with DVT.[3] An earlier report estimated that as many as 630,000 patients develop PE every year in the United States with 200,000 related deaths, the majority in patients in whom the diagnosis was never made (Fig. 73-1).[4] Although considerable effort is directed toward the development of new diagnostic techniques and therapeutic agents, a considerable impact on mortality related to the disease would arise from the routine use of prophylactic strategies, an understanding of the often subtle clinical presentation of the disease, and the appropriate application of existing diagnostic techniques.

SOURCES OF EMBOLI

Most cases (80%–95%) of PE occur as a result of thrombus originating in the lower extremity. Thrombus often begins at a site where blood flow is turbulent, such as at a venous bifurcation, or behind a venous valve (Fig. 73-2). When thrombus propagation exceeds the rate of thrombus organization and adherence to the endothelium, part or all of thrombus may break away and migrate via the venous system to the lungs. Most thrombi originate in the deep veins of the

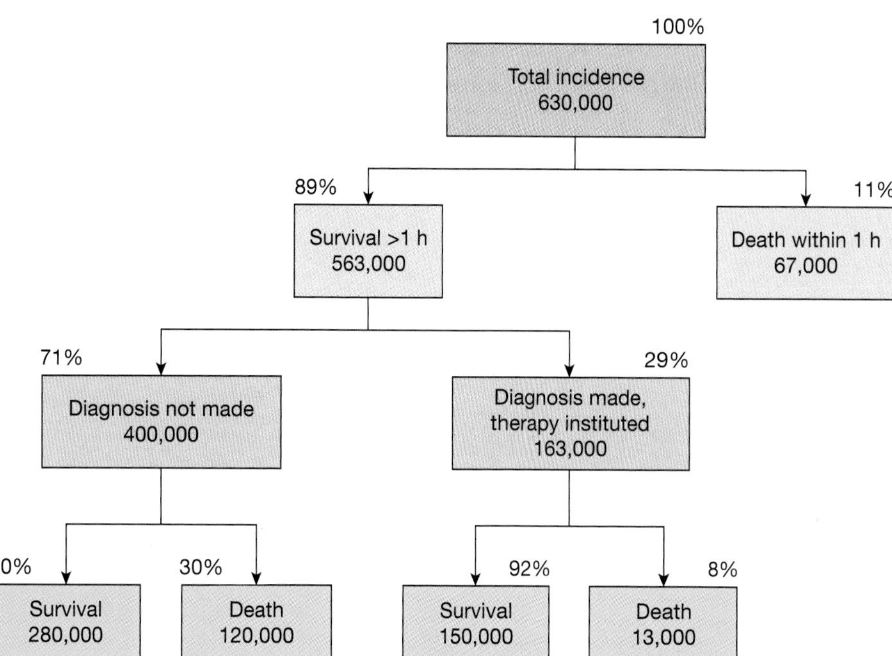

Figure 73-1 Estimated incidence and survival statistics for pulmonary embolism in the United States. *(Reproduced with permission from Dalen JE, Alpert JS. Natural history of pulmonary embolism. Prog Cardiovasc Dis. 1975;17(4):259–270.)*

calf and propagate proximally to the popliteal and femoral veins. Calf-limited thrombi pose a minimal embolic risk while those that extend into and above the popliteal vein represent the most common source of acute symptomatic PE. This is not meant to imply that calf-limited thrombosis represents a benign condition. Proximal propagation may occur in as many as 15% of untreated patients along with a higher risk of thrombotic recurrence and postphlebitic syndrome.[5]

Emboli may originate from other sources, most often from the pelvic veins, in which case a predisposing factor such as pregnancy, pelvic thrombophlebitis or pelvic infection, prostate disease, or recent pelvic surgery can often be identified. Emboli may also originate from upper extremity thrombosis associated with central venous catheters or intravascular cardiac devices, or may be associated with thoracic outlet obstruction or effort thrombosis (Paget–von Schroetter syndrome).[6] A small number of patients with PE may have evidence of right ventricular thrombus at presentation and this has been associated with more hemodynamic instability and an increase in mortality.[7]

Although the majority of cases of PE are the result of thrombus migration (hence, *thromboembolism*), other materials may occasionally obstruct the pulmonary vascular bed. These include blood-borne parasites (such as schistosomiasis), sickle cell disease, and various "contaminants" of illicit injected drugs (talc, cloth fibers, etc.). Air embolism is usually iatrogenic and typically enters the blood stream accidentally through a central venous catheter. Less commonly, a patient's own tissues or cells may enter the blood stream and lodge in the pulmonary vasculature. Examples include amniotic fluid embolism, which can occur during or immediately after labor or late-term abortion; fat embolism, which is usually associated with long bone fractures; and tumor embolism. PE due to sickle cell disease is caused by "clumping" of abnormal red blood cells in the setting of hypoxia and stress, and can cause both acute respiratory distress as well as a more progressive disease with secondary pulmonary hypertension.

PREDISPOSING FACTORS

Rudolf Virchow first described the phenomena of "embolism" and "thrombosis" in the mid-nineteenth century, and identified three main factors contributing to the formation of venous thrombosis (Virchow's triad): venous stasis, hypercoagulability, and injury to the venous wall (endothelium). One hundred and fifty years later, this basic classification remains useful in helping clinicians stratify individual patient's risk of developing venous thromboembolism (Table 73-1). It is important to recognize that there is an interplay between acquired and genetic risk factors, that multiple mechanisms lead to the development of DVT and/or PE, and that multiple factors can often be found in individual patients.

■ ACQUIRED RISK FACTORS

The risk imposed by a major surgical procedure is well recognized. Without prophylaxis, venous thrombosis occurs after approximately 20% of all major surgical procedures with associated embolism after 1% to 2%.[8] The incidence of thromboembolism without prophylaxis is even higher in orthopedic patients with over 50% of major orthopedic procedures complicated by venous thrombosis.[9] In the absence of prophylaxis, the frequency of fatal postoperative PE ranges from 0.1% to 0.4% in patients undergoing elective general surgery and from 1% to 5% in patients undergoing elective hip or knee surgery, emergency hip surgery, major trauma, or spinal cord injury.

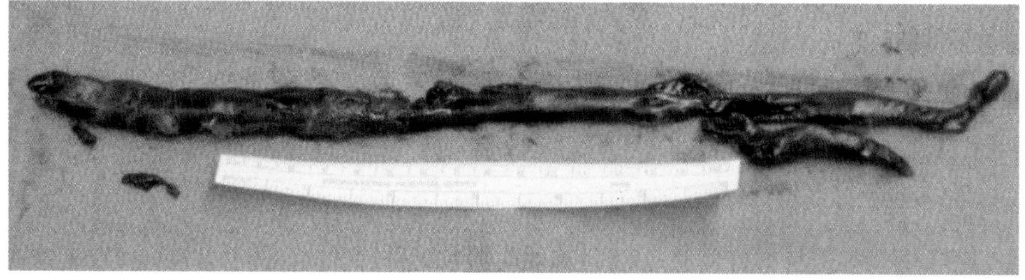

Figure 73-2 Large, well-organized embolus representing "cast" of a lower extremity vein removed from pulmonary artery at pulmonary embolectomy.

TABLE 73-1 Virchow's Triad: Clinical States Predisposing to Venous Thrombosis

Stasis	Immobility
	Bed rest
	Anesthesia
	Congestive heart failure/cor pulmonale
	Prior venous thrombosis
Hypercoagulability	Malignancy
	Anticardiolipin antibody
	Nephrotic syndrome
	Essential thrombocytosis
	Estrogen therapy
	Heparin-induced thrombocytopenia
	Inflammatory bowel disease
	Paroxysmal nocturnal hemoglobinuria
	Disseminated intravascular coagulation
	Protein C and S deficiencies
	Antithrombin III deficiency
Vessel wall injury	Trauma
	Surgery

Major traumatic injuries, most notably those of the head, spine, and pelvis, are also associated with high risk. The basis for this risk is multifactorial, involving all three components of Virchow's triad.

Although initially recognized and studied in surgical patients, it is now appreciated that hospitalized medical patients may be equally prone to develop DVT.[10] In about 80% of the cases, one or more risk factors may be present when extensive investigative testing is performed. Major risk factors include New York Heart Association class III and IV congestive heart failure, chronic obstructive pulmonary disease, sepsis and other inflammatory disorders, advanced age, stroke, critical illness, and prolonged bed rest.

Any prolonged period of immobilization may increase thromboembolic risk and explains the occurrence of thrombosis under such circumstances as paralysis, bed rest, and prolonged air travel. Long distance traveling (economy class syndrome) is associated with a 1.5- to 3-fold increase in thromboembolic risk, depending on the travel duration.[11] Despite the relative increase in risk, the actual incidence of PE associated with air travel is quite low.[12]

Pregnancy is the most common cause of venous thromboembolism in women younger than 40 years old, and if untreated may account for 20% to 50% of all pregnancy-related deaths. Compared with nonpregnant women, the risk of venous thrombotic events is increased fivefold during pregnancy and 60-fold in the first 3 months after delivery.[13,14] The increase may be a result of decreased mobility, pregnancy-related hypercoagulable state (increases in factors II, VII, VIII, X, acquired activated protein C resistance, and decreased free protein S level), and venous obstruction from uterine compression. The incidence is estimated at 0.76 to 1.72 cases per 1000 pregnancies and occurs in roughly equal distribution over all trimesters. Most cases of postpartum DVT occur within the first 6 weeks after delivery. Cesarean section, premature birth, multiple births, preeclampsia, advance maternal age, and maternal history of cardiac disease have all been identified as contributing factors. Interestingly, 90% of all DVT cases are noted in the left leg, presumably because of the anatomic relationship between the uterus and inferior vena cava (IVC).

The use of oral contraceptive agents and hormonal replacement therapy has also been associated with an increased risk of venous thromboembolism.[14,15] Although the risk of venous thromboembolism is higher among users of oral estrogen-containing contraceptives, the absolute risk is low. In terms of oral contraceptive agents, the relative risk of developing venous thrombosis is a four- to sixfold increased risk. There appears to be a synergistic effect of oral contraceptives with obesity.[16]

Hormone replacement therapy appears to be associated with a two- to fourfold increased risk of venous thromboembolism.[17] Studies have suggested that venous thromboembolic risk is lower with transdermal hormone preparations. However, none of these studies are randomized trials. Given that the baseline risk of thrombosis increases with age, the use of hormonal replacement therapy in a postmenopausal population has a considerably higher impact on absolute rates of thrombosis.

Obesity has been associated with venous thromboembolism, particularly in women. The Nurses' Health Study found that a body mass index greater than or equal to 29 kg/m^2 was an independent risk factor.[18] The metabolic syndrome, defined by abdominal obesity, elevation of blood pressure, elevated fasting blood sugar and triglycerides, and low levels of high-density lipoprotein cholesterol, appears to be associated not only with an increased risk of atherosclerotic disease but also of venous thromboembolism.[19]

The risk of venous thromboembolism increases with age. A recent study, using hospital discharge surveys over a 21-year period, found that patients 70 years or older have an approximately 25-fold increased risk, compared with those 20 to 29 years of age.[20] Presumably the difference may be due to decrease in mobility and increase in comorbidities in this population. Elderly patients also appear to have a higher mortality due to PE, and PE is suspected less commonly prior to death in the elderly patient.

Cancer patients, particularly those with primary malignancies from lung, pancreas, breast (mucin-secreting adenocarcinoma), prostate, stomach/colorectal, and genitourinary tracts are at a high risk for venous thromboembolism. Cancer is estimated to increase the risk of venous thromboembolism by four- to sixfold. Patients with cancer also have a higher risk of thromboembolic recurrence and those with venous thromboembolism have a higher overall mortality rate than cancer patients without thrombosis. Multiple factors are probably involved and include the development of abnormalities in the hemostatic system related to the malignancy itself, hemostatic alterations induced by chemotherapeutic agents, immobility, infectious complications, and the presence of chronic indwelling central venous catheters. Although most instances of cancer-associated venous thromboembolism occur after the diagnosis of the malignancy, approximately 5% to 10% of patients with "idiopathic" venous thrombosis have a malignancy diagnosed within the next 2 to 3 years. There is no evidence at this time to recommend an aggressive search for cancer in patients with idiopathic or unprovoked thrombosis. Recent data suggest that a limited approach (routine laboratory testing, chest radiograph, tumor markers, abdominal ultrasound) may have the capacity to identify approximately one-half of malignancies in patients who were negative on routine examination.[21] More extensive screening utilizing chest and abdominal computed tomography (CT) appears to result in excessive false-positive results without an effect on outcome.[22]

Various hematologic conditions such as polycythemia vera, essential thrombocytosis, and acute leukemia may result in significant overproduction of different cell lines, which in turn may increase the risk of venous thromboembolism by increasing blood viscosity (hyperviscosity syndromes) and through the release of procoagulants.[23] This type of thrombosis seems to occur more frequently in the hepatic or portal veins and may be the presenting symptoms of the underlying disorder.

Paroxysmal nocturnal hemoglobinuria is a rare condition associated with an incidence of venous thromboembolism of approximately 40%.[24] Many cases involve nonlower extremity sites, particularly in the intra-abdominal vessels. The reason for thrombosis is not clear but may be related to a decrease in blood complement levels in these patients.

The presence of antiphospholipid antibodies, most notably the lupus anticoagulant, appears to be an independent risk factor for venous thromboembolism.[25] Among patients with venous thrombosis, a lupus anticoagulant has been reported in 5% to 15% and this abnormality has been estimated to lead to a ninefold increased risk of thrombosis.

The frequency of venous thromboembolism in patients with nephrotic syndrome may be as high as 40%.[26] There is a higher tendency for the thrombosis to present in unusual locations such as the cerebral sinus or as arterial thrombosis. Rarely, thrombosis may also be the presenting symptom of the nephrotic syndrome. The mechanism for venous thromboembolism in these patients is not clear but various factors such as functional or quantitative changes in coagulation factors, diminished fibrinolytic activity, platelet hyperreactivity, and increased blood viscosity have been proposed.

Patients with inflammatory bowel disease are at substantially increased risk of both venous and arterial thromboses.[27,28] The exact pathogenetic mechanism remains unclear. The majority of thrombotic complications occur during an active phase of the disease and inflammatory mechanisms have been proposed.

■ INHERITED RISK FACTORS

Many patients who develop venous thromboembolism are found to have an inherited risk factor due to either abnormal levels of or functional abnormalities in coagulation factors (inherited thrombophilia). The relative risk of thrombosis varies widely depending on the hemostatic defect. In general, this group of patients tends to be younger (less than 50 years) and has a tendency to develop recurrent venous thromboembolism.

The first known inherited thrombophilic trait was antithrombin III deficiency, originally described in 1965. Subsequently, a number of other genetic mutations associated with venous thromboembolism have been reported. The most common of these inherited predispositions was first described in 1993 by Dahlback and designated as a factor V Leiden mutation.[29] It is the consequence of a single point mutation on the factor V gene (adenine for guanine) resulting in factor Va with diminished sensitivity to the natural anticoagulant effect of activated protein C. Approximately 5% of Caucasians in Europe and North America are heterozygous for this genetic defect; lower rates of carrier frequency have been reported among Native American, African, and Asian populations. The heterozygous state carries a 5- to 10-fold increase in lifetime risk for venous thromboembolism, whereas the risk among patients homozygous for this mutation may be increased 80-fold. Factor V Leiden mutation appears to be an important risk factor for venous thromboembolism during pregnancy, in the postpartum period, and during oral contraceptive use.[30] Compared with women who do not use oral contraceptives and are not carriers of the factor V mutation, the risk of thrombosis among those with both risk factors is increased approximately 30-fold.[31]

Another common mutation has been identified in the 3' untranslated region of the prothrombin gene (substitution of A for G at position 20210) and is present in 2% to 4% of the general population.[32] This mutation results in an overproduction of prothrombin, which is otherwise normal. It is associated with a three- to fourfold increased risk of lower extremity venous thrombosis and appears to act in a synergistic manner with other forms of thrombophilia in increasing both the initial and recurrent thrombosis risk.

In clinical practice, factor V Leiden mutation and prothrombin gene mutation are the most common inherited conditions and account for more than half of the cases of inherited thrombophilia-related venous thromboembolism; three other conditions (deficiencies in antithrombin III, protein C, or protein S) account for most of the remainder. Occasionally one may also encounter venous thromboembolism patients who may have other conditions, particularly related to dysfibrinogenemias. It is important to recognize that, when multiple inherited risk factors coexist (such as factor V Leiden and prothrombin gene mutation), the risk of recurrent venous thromboembolism may increase substantially, and lifelong anticoagulation may be necessary in these patients.

PATHOPHYSIOLOGY

Once detached from their point of origin, emboli travel via the systemic venous system, through the right chambers of the heart, and eventually reach the pulmonary arterial system. The physiologic effects and clinical consequences of pulmonary thromboembolism vary widely, ranging from asymptomatic disease to hemodynamic collapse and death. Major factors that determine the outcome include (1) size and location of emboli; (2) coexisting cardiopulmonary diseases; (3) secondary humoral mediator release and vascular hypoxic responses; and (4) the rate of resolution of emboli.

■ HEMODYNAMIC CONSEQUENCES

Obstruction of the pulmonary vascular bed by embolism acutely increases right ventricular afterload. The normal pulmonary arterial system is a low-pressure system capable of accommodating substantial increases in blood flow with only modest increases in pressure. The thin-walled right ventricle is poorly equipped to generate the pressure necessary to overcome any significant increase in pulmonary vascular resistance. Compensatory mechanisms exist that allow up to 70% obstruction of the pulmonary vascular bed before right ventricular failure develops.[33–36]

In the absence of pre-existing cardiopulmonary disease, obstruction of less than 20% of the pulmonary vascular bed results in minimal hemodynamic consequences as a result of recruitment and distention of pulmonary vessels. When the degree of pulmonary vascular obstruction exceeds 30% to 40%, modest increases in right ventricular pressure occur, but cardiac output is maintained through an increase in heart rate and myocardial contractility. Compensatory mechanisms begin to fail when the degree of pulmonary artery obstruction exceeds 50% to 60%. Cardiac output begins to fall and right atrial pressure increases dramatically. Mixed venous oxygen saturation falls and a lactic acidosis may develop. With further acute obstruction, the right heart dilates, right ventricular wall tension increases, right ventricular ischemia may develop, the cardiac output falls, and systemic hypotension develops. In patients without prior cardiopulmonary disease, the maximal mean pulmonary artery pressure capable of being generated by the right ventricle appears to be 40 mm Hg (pulmonary artery systolic pressure of approximately 70 mm Hg).[34]

Other factors may affect the hemodynamic consequences of PE. Patients with pre-existing cardiopulmonary disease often have diminished pulmonary vascular reserve and even a relatively minor embolus may result in significant hemodynamic instability (Fig. 73-3). Alternatively, if the right ventricle has had time (months to years) to hypertrophy in response to a gradual increase in demand (left ventricular disease, idiopathic pulmonary arterial hypertension, chromic thromboembolism, etc.) a significantly higher pulmonary artery pressure may be seen.

Several observations suggest that other mechanisms are involved in hemodynamic consequences of acute PE. For example, patients

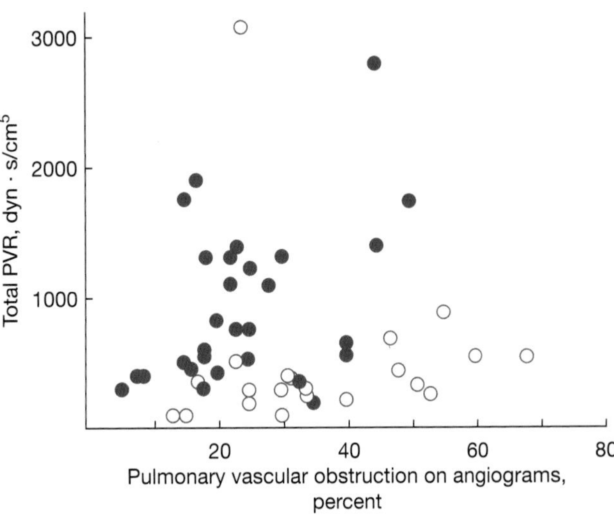

Figure 73-3 Hemodynamic consequences of pulmonary embolism and the underlying state of the pulmonary vasculature. Patients in whom the pulmonary vasculature was previously normal (*open circles*) develop little increase in pulmonary vascular resistance (PVR) until the clot burden exceeds 50%. In those with antecedent cardiopulmonary disease (*solid circles*), the PVR increases appreciably with only modest clot burden. *(Reproduced with permission from Sharma GV, McIntyre KM, Sharma S, Sasahara AA. Clinical and hemodynamic correlates in pulmonary embolism. Clin Chest Med. 1984;5(3):421–437.)*

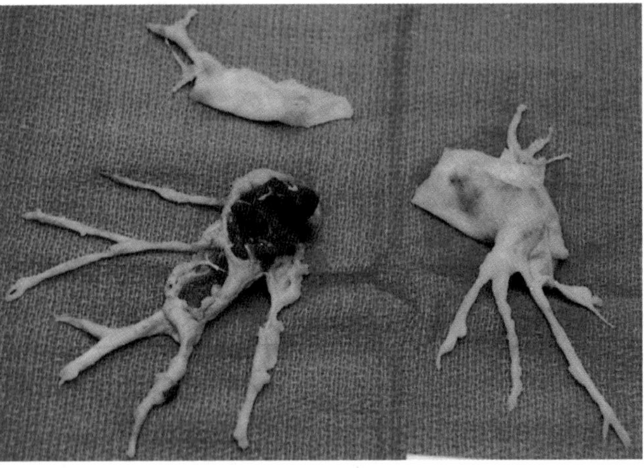

Figure 73-4 Chronic thromboembolic material dissected from pulmonary arteries at pulmonary thromboendarterectomy. Resolution of emboli is occasionally complete but certain patients may be left with significant emboli residua.

develop only minimal hemodynamic instability during elective lobectomy, pneumonectomy, or even single lung transplantation despite complete and acute interruption of blood supply during cross-clamping. In the experimental setting, cyproheptadine (a nonselective serotonin antagonist) and ketanserin (a selective serotonin antagonist) have been shown to diminish some of the hemodynamic and airway responses that occur after pulmonary embolization. Certain patients develop disproportionately large and fluctuating pulmonary hemodynamic changes in response to relatively small emboli, suggesting that other mechanisms such as reflex vasoconstriction and release of vasoactive compounds may also be involved.[37,38]

As expected, large or multiple emboli tend to cause more severe symptoms and changes in oxygenation and hemodynamics. Given the large surface area of the peripheral pulmonary vascular bed compared to the central, symptomatic improvement may occur when a large central embolus is fragmented by forces generated by cardiac contractions or even with chest compressions during cardiopulmonary resuscitation. Eventually, the emboli may either resolve by fibrinolysis, or organize and become scar-like tissue that adheres to the vascular endothelium (Fig. 73-4). Recent data suggest that complete resolution is uncommon and that as many as 50% of patients have some residual obstruction 6 months after the embolic event.[39,40]

■ GAS-EXCHANGE ABNORMALITIES

Hypoxemia is the most common immediate physiologic consequence of PE. Obstruction of the pulmonary vasculature prevents systemic venous blood from reaching the pulmonary capillaries of the involved vessels and redirects the blood flow to other parts of the pulmonary vascular bed. This results in an increase in ventilation–perfusion (V/Q) inequality, intrapulmonary shunting, and decreases in the mixed venous O_2 level, thereby magnifying the effect of the normal venous admixture.[41,42] Further shunting and increase in alveolar dead space can also occur as a result of alveolar hemorrhage or to atelectasis related to loss of surfactant. Despite an increase in alveolar dead space, patients with PE often develop hypocapnia. This is thought to be due to hypoxia-induced intrapulmonary reflex vagal stimulation, with resulting hyperventilation. Finally, embolic events large enough to increase right atrial pressure may result in intracardiac right-to-left shunting through a patent foramen ovale.

One uncommon consequence of PE is pulmonary infarction. Infarction is uncommon because the pulmonary parenchyma has three potential sources of oxygen: the pulmonary arteries, bronchial arteries, and airways. Two of these three sources apparently must be compromised before infarction develops (Fig. 73-5). Therefore, in a patient with no coexisting cardiopulmonary disease, infarction is rare.[43] Infarction occurs in approximately 20% of patients with significant cardiac or pulmonary disease that compromise either bronchial arterial flow or airway patency. In patients with left ventricular failure, increased pulmonary venous pressure may decrease bronchial flow and infarction may occur.

DIAGNOSIS OF PULMONARY EMBOLISM

The diagnostic approach to PE has undergone a fundamental transition over the past decade. V/Q scanning, the mainstay of diagnosis for almost three decades, has been relegated to a secondary role. The prospective investigation of pulmonary embolism diagnosis (PIOPED) trial demonstrated the shortcomings of this technique while providing valuable insight into the diagnostic utility of clinical assessment.[44] CT, highly sensitive D-dimer assays, stratification according to clinical assessment, and the application of Bayesian analysis to the diagnostic pathway have become the cornerstones of the current diagnostic approach. What has not changed is the understanding that clinical evidence per se, although capable of raising suspicion of the disease, is incapable of reliably confirming or excluding the diagnosis in the absence of objective testing. Recognition of the clinical signs and symptoms associated with embolism is valuable because clinical findings and clinical suspicion represent an essential first step in the diagnostic pathway.

■ CLINICAL PRESENTATION

The mainstay for the diagnosis of PE is a high index of suspicion tempered by the reality that most patients with embolism have one or more factors predisposing them to the condition. These predisposing factors need not be major or readily apparent. Advancing age, a period of bed rest, a prolonged air flight, or a minor traumatic injury can result in the development of venous thromboembolism. The absence of a known clinical or thrombophilic predisposition, however, should not dissuade an objective evaluation if the clinical presentation is consistent with embolism.

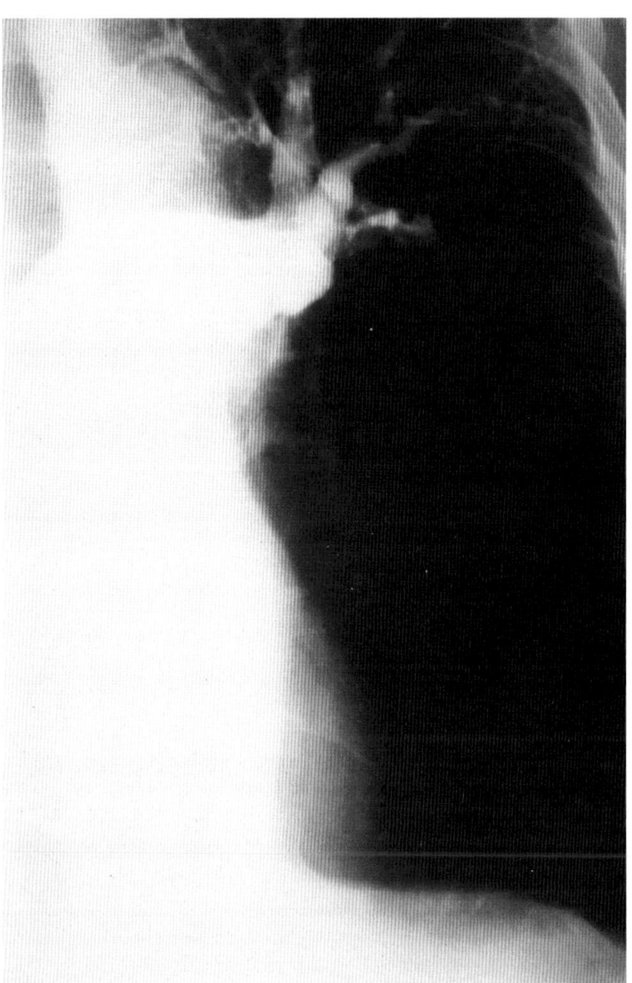

Figure 73-5 Pulmonary angiogram demonstrating thromboembolic obstruction of left pulmonary artery with absent blood flow to lingula and lower lobe. Despite extension obstruction, infarction did not occur as a result of lung's dual blood supply.

Although a somewhat arbitrary classification (as presenting symptoms and signs of embolism frequently overlap), the presentation of acute PE can be categorized into one of the three clinical syndromes: (1) isolated dyspnea; (2) pleuritic pain or hemoptysis; and (3) circulatory collapse.[45,46] Among patients without prior cardiopulmonary disease in the PIOPED study, the syndrome of pleuritic pain or hemoptysis was found to be the most common mode of presentation, occurring in approximately 60% of patients. Isolated dyspnea occurred in approximately 25%, whereas circulatory collapse occurred in 10%.

Two additional modes of presentation are also possible: subclinical clot and chronic, nonresolving or propagating clot. With the increasing use of computed tomographic studies, incidental emboli are occasionally found.[47] Typically, these emboli are found in the peripheral segments of the pulmonary arterial vasculature and do not correlate with any clinical symptoms. At this time, the short- and long-term significance of these incidental findings is not clear. In patients who are known to be at high risk of recurrent disease, such as those with inherited thrombophilia and hormonal use or those with poor cardiopulmonary reserve, it is reasonable to consider treatment with anticoagulation or at least the use of more aggressive prophylactic therapies during at-risk situations, such as prolonged hospitalization or air travel.

Complete anatomic resolution of PE appears to be uncommon. When there is sufficient residual pulmonary vascular obstruction, some patients may develop chronic thromboembolic pulmonary hypertension (CTEPH).[48] Although exact values for frequencies vary, it is estimated that approximately 0.5% to 1% of patients may develop this condition following an initial, symptomatic episode of PE.[49] The diagnosis should be considered even in the absence of a history of acute embolism. Approximately 30% of patients who present with CTEPH do not have a history of precedent acute embolism and are diagnosed during the evaluative process for unexplained dyspnea or pulmonary hypertension.

The most common presenting symptom of acute PE is the sudden onset of dyspnea.[45,46] Dyspnea usually occurs over minutes to hours but in approximately 15% occurs over days. Although usually present at rest, dyspnea may only be noted with exertion. It is important to recognize that dyspnea does not occur in approximately 25% of patients ultimately proven to have embolism. Other symptoms include pleuritic chest pain, cough, leg swelling or pain, and hemoptysis. The most common physical finding is unexplained tachypnea (respiratory rate greater than 20/min) present in approximately 70% of patients with embolism. Less frequent physical findings include rales, tachycardia, and an increased pulmonic component of the second heart sound. Fever may develop some hours after the event and often reaches, but rarely exceeds, 38.3°C.[50]

Obviously, these symptoms and signs are nonspecific (Table 73-2). In the PIOPED study, none of the presenting symptoms or

TABLE 73-2 Incidence of Signs and Symptoms of Pulmonary Embolism

	Massive PE[a] (%)	Submassive PE[a] (%)	Without Pre-existing Cardiopulmonary Disease (%)[b]
Dyspnea	85	82	73
Pleuritic chest pain	64	85	66
Cough	53	52	37
Hemoptysis	23	40	13
Tachypnea	95 (>16 breaths/min)	87 (>16 breaths/min)	70 (>20 breaths/min)
Tachycardia (>100 beats/min)	48	38	30
Increased pulmonic component of second heart sound	58	45	23
Rales	57	60	51
Phlebitis	36	26	11

[a]*Data from NIH-sponsored urokinase and streptokinase clinical trials (Am J Med. 1977;62:355–360).*
[b]*Data from NIH-sponsored PIOPED study (Chest. 1991;100:598–603).*

TABLE 73-3 The Wells' Clinical Prediction Score

Variable	Points
DVT symptoms/signs	3.0
PE likely or more likely than alternative diagnosis	3.0
Heart rate >100	1.5
Immobilization/surgery previous 4 wk	1.5
Previous DVT or PE	1.5
Hemoptysis	1.0
Malignancy	1.0
Total Score	**Pretest Probability**
<2.0	Low
2.0–6.0	Moderate
>6.0	High
Dichotomized Score	
≤4	PE unlikely
>4	PE likely

Source: Data from Wells PS, Anderson DR, Rodger M, et al. Derivation of a simple clinical model to categorize patients probability of pulmonary embolism: increasing the models utility with the SimpliRED D-dimer. Thromb Haemost. 2000;83(3):416–420.

signs with the exception of the presence of rales, a fourth heart sound, and an increased pulmonic component of the second heart sound could differentiate between those with positive and negative angiograms.[45]

■ CLINICAL ASSESSMENT

A major advance in the diagnostic approach to PE has been a transition from a purely technique-oriented approach to one that uses Bayesian analysis. In doing so, the pretest probability of the disease, calculated independently of a particular test result using either empiric means or a standardized prediction rule, is calculated. This pretest probability aids in the selection and interpretation of further diagnostic tests to create a posttest probability of the disease. This posttest probability can then be used as a basis for clinical decision making. For PE, a number of such scores have been developed and validated (Tables 73-3–73-5). Wells et al.[51] have prospectively tested a rapid seven-item bedside assessment to estimate the clinical pretest probability for PE. An alternative scoring system, the Geneva score, involved seven variables and required gas exchange and radiographic information.[52] A revised Geneva score requiring eight clinical variables without gas exchange or radiographic information was validated and published.[53] Other clinical decision rules include the PISA rule, the PERC (pulmonary embolism rule-out criteria) rule, and the Charlotte rule.[54–56] Although such scoring systems have not proved to be more accurate than clinical assessment, they do provide a method of standardization that compensates for variability in physician experience and judgment.

■ LABORATORY FINDINGS

Routine laboratory testing is not useful in confirming or excluding the diagnosis of PE but may be helpful in suggesting other diagnoses. A modest leukocytosis may accompany embolism but rarely exceeds 20,000/mm^3.[57]

As noted, hypoxemia is common in acute PE although the diagnosis cannot be excluded based upon a normal P_{O_2}.[58,59] The more massive the obstruction, the more severe the hypoxemia is likely to be. However, many other conditions also cause hypoxemia and,

TABLE 73-4 The Original Geneva Clinical Prediction Score

Variable	Point Score
Age	
60–79 y	1
>80 y	2
Previous DVT or PE	2
Recent surgery	3
Pulse rate >100	1
Pa_{CO_2}, kPa (mm Hg)	
<4.8 (36)	2
4.8–5.19 (36–38)	1
Pa_{CO_2}, kPa (mm Hg)	
<6.5 (<48)	4
6.5–7.99 (48–60)	3
8.0–9.49 (61–71)	2
9.5–10.99 (72–82)	1
Chest radiograph appearance	
Plate-like atelectasis	1
Elevated hemidiaphragm	1
Total Score	**Pretest Probability**
0–4	Low
5–8	Moderate
9–16	High

Source: Data from Ageno W, Becattini C, Brighton T, et al. Cardiovascular Risk Factors and Venous Thromboembolism: a Meta-Analysis. Circulation. 2008;117(1):93–102.

TABLE 73-5 The Revised Geneva Clinical Prediction Score

Variable	Points
Age >65 y	1
Previous DVT or PE	3
Surgery (under general anesthesia) or lower limb fracture within 1 mo	2
Active malignancy (currently active or considered cured <1 y)	2
Symptoms	
Unilateral lower limb pain	3
Hemoptysis	2
Clinical signs	
Heart rate: 75–94 beats/min	3
≥95 beats/min	5
Pain on lower limb deep venous palpation or unilateral edema	4
Total Score	**Pretest Probability**
0–3	Low
4–10	Moderate
≥11	High

Source: Data from Stein PD, Hull RD, Kayali F, et al. Venous thromboembolism according to age: the impact of an aging population. Arch Intern Med. 2004;164(20):2260–2265.

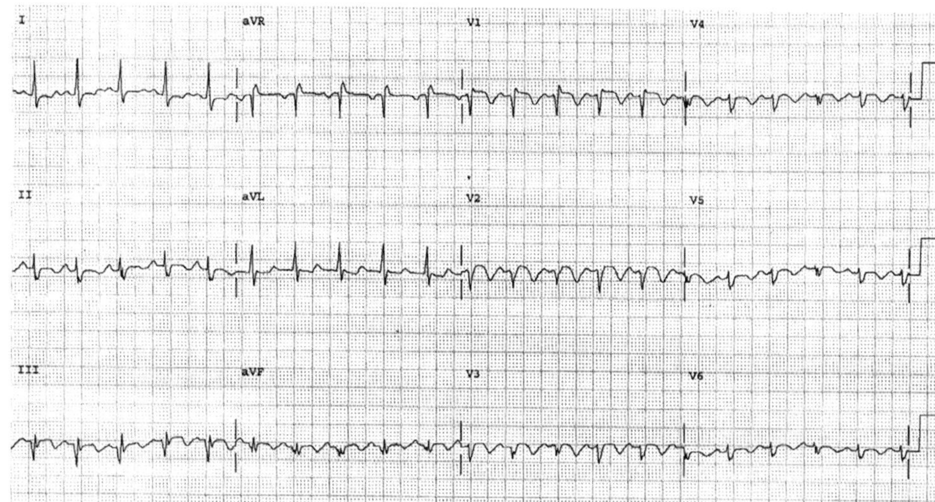

Figure 73-6 Electrocardiogram demonstrating findings consistent with embolism including sinus tachycardia, incomplete right bundle branch block, S1Q3T3 pattern, and inverted precordial T waves.

conversely, acute PE does not necessarily cause hypoxemia or even a widening of the $(A\text{-}a)_{O_2}$ gradient.[58] In the PIOPED trial, no combinations of blood–gas abnormalities were identified that reliably excluded PE. Although most patients with embolism have a low Pa_{O_2}, low Pa_{CO_2}, or high $P(A\text{-}a)_{O_2}$ gradient, the absence of such abnormal values, alone or in combination, did not exclude PE. Hypercapnia resulting from increased dead space ventilation is rare and appears with PE only in patients with marked antecedent ventilatory limitation or when such limitation has been imposed because the patient is on controlled mechanical ventilation when the embolism occurs.

■ ELECTROCARDIOGRAM

The electrocardiogram is nonspecific in the diagnosis of PE, and its major value may be in identifying other clinical disorders (e.g., acute myocardial infarction and pericarditis) that may be confused with PE. Findings in acute PE are generally nonspecific and include T-wave changes, ST-segment abnormalities, and left- or right-axis deviation (Fig. 73-6).[46] Atrial arrhythmias may occur but appear to be more common in patients with underlying cardiopulmonary disease. The S1Q3T3 pattern, commonly considered to be specific for PE, is seen in only a minority of patients. Electrocardiographic findings can offer insight into the extent and hemodynamic consequence of the embolism. The electrocardiogram is rarely normal in the setting of PE associated with right ventricular dysfunction. The presence of an S1Q3T3 pattern, right bundle branch block, or T-wave inversion in leads V1 toV3 in a patient with PE should suggest the presence of right ventricular dysfunction.[60,61]

■ CHEST RADIOGRAPHY

Most patients with PE have abnormal but nonspecific chest radiographic findings.[46,62] Common radiographic findings include atelectasis, pleural effusion, pulmonary infiltrates, and mild elevation of a hemidiaphragm. Classic findings of pulmonary infarction – such as Hampton's hump or decreased vascularity (Westermark sign) – are suggestive but infrequent. There is some confusion about the diagnostic configuration of infiltrates due to embolism. These infiltrates, although usually abutting a pleural surface, can be of any shape, not necessarily wedge shaped. Although pleural effusions occur in almost half of the patients, the majority of effusions are small and involve only blunting of the costophrenic angle. The main use of the chest radiograph in suspected PE is to exclude alternative diagnostic possibilities such as pneumothorax, which may simulate the disease. A normal chest radiograph in a patient with otherwise unexplained acute tachypnea, dyspnea, or hypoxemia should raise the possibility of PE.

■ D-DIMER

The development of a rapid and accurate blood test capable of diagnosing venous thromboembolism has been the subject of considerable investigative interest. A number of different hemostasiologic markers have been investigated. Of these, D-dimer, alone and in combination with other noninvasive studies has been subjected to the most rigorous clinical evaluation.[63,64] D-dimer testing has proven to be highly sensitive but not specific. Increased levels are present in nearly all patients with venous thromboembolism, but also occur in a wide range of other circumstances, including advancing age, pregnancy, trauma, infections, the postoperative period, inflammatory states, and malignancy. Therefore, the role of D-dimer testing is limited to one of venous thromboembolism exclusion. The study is of limited utility in inpatients given the high frequency of positive results in this population.[65]

Multiple assays for D-dimer have been developed with a range of sensitivities and specificities.[66] Highly sensitive assays such as the enzyme-linked immunosorbent assay (ELISA) are capable of excluding venous thromboembolism but are associated with such a high frequency of false-positive results, especially when applied to an inpatient population, as to limit their clinical utility. Less sensitive assays (e.g., latex agglutination, red cell agglutination) lack the ability to exclude venous thromboembolism in isolation but have been used successfully in combination with either a clinical probability estimate or noninvasive diagnostic study. D-dimer testing has been used successfully as part of a number of different diagnostic strategies. Negative results of standardized, highly sensitive assays (ELISA) have proved capable of safely excluding PE in outpatients presenting with a low or intermediate clinical likelihood of the disease. Certain non-ELISA assays are capable of excluding embolism as a stand-alone study in outpatients with a low probability of disease but are more appropriately used in a multibranch diagnostic pathway.

■ VENTILATION–PERFUSION SCANNING

V/Q scanning had been the pivotal diagnostic test for suspected PE for many years but has been replaced by CT imaging. Despite limitations, V/Q lung scanning can provide valuable information if used and interpreted appropriately. The PIOPED trial provided valuable insight into the strengths and limitations of V/Q scanning.[44] A negative study is capable of ruling out the diagnosis of PE with the same degree of certainty as a negative pulmonary angiogram and with a higher degree of certainty than can be achieved by a negative CT scan (Fig. 73-7). The positive predictive value of a "high probability" study (one characterized by multiple, segmental-sized, mismatched

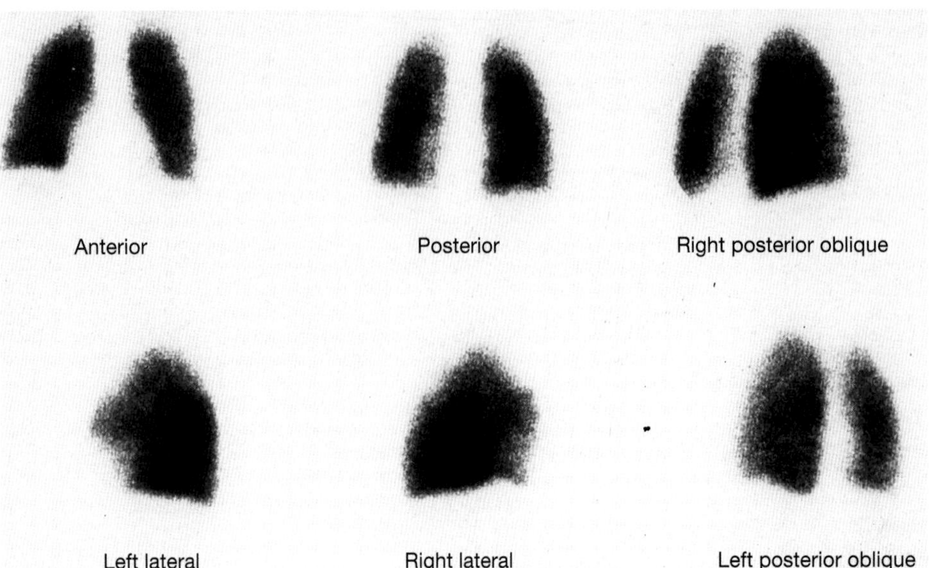

Figure 73-7 Normal six-view perfusion scan. Such a scan finding has a negative predictive value equivalent to a negative pulmonary angiogram and higher than that of a negative computed tomographic study.

defects) approximates 88%; when coupled with a high clinical probability of embolism, the positive predictive value increased to 96% (Fig. 73-8). However, only 28% of patients in PIOPED had scans characterized as high probability or normal, the only categories that can be considered definitive. The majority of patients with PE do not have a high probability scan, whereas the majority of those without embolism do not have a normal scan.

The PIOPED study also undertook to correlate the clinical impression of the likelihood of PE with the interpretation of the lung scan (Table 73-6). When interpretation of the lung scan and clinical assessment were concordant (both high and low probability), diagnostic accuracy was greater than that of the lung scan alone. In contrast, when interpretation of the lung scan and clinical assessment were discordant, the predictive value of the lung scan was decreased. In as many as two-thirds of patients suspected of PE, the combination of the lung scan and clinical assessment were either discordant or indeterminate and failed to diagnose or exclude PE.

There are certain situations in which V/Q scanning may be preferred over CT-pulmonary angiography (CT-PA). IV contrast is not required for V/Q scanning making it a more desirable option in patients with renal dysfunction or a severe iodinated contrast allergy. In addition, with a portable gamma scintillation camera the perfusion portion of the study can be performed at the bedside, which may be a major advantage in a critically ill patient for whom transportation to the CT scanner may be deemed too high risk. The role of V/Q scanning versus CT-PA in pregnancy remains unsettled but V/Q scanning appears to offer similar diagnostic performance in this setting with significantly lower levels of maternal radiation.[67]

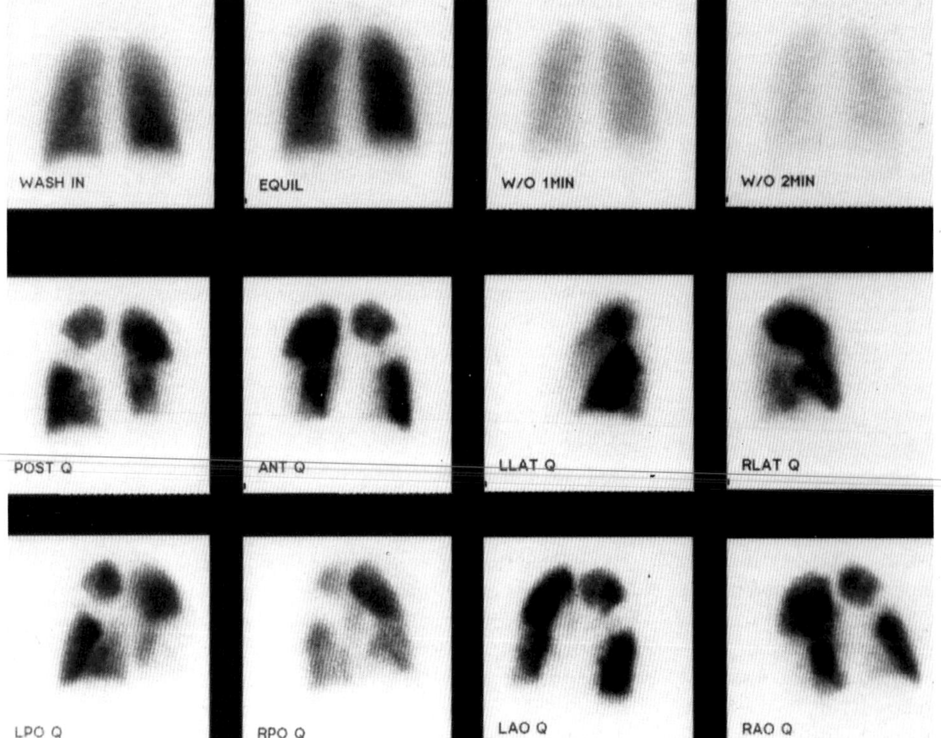

Figure 73-8 "High probability" ventilation/perfusion scan demonstrating normal ventilation and multiple mismatched segmental and larger defects.

TABLE 73-6 Prevalence of Pulmonary Embolism in PIOPED: Value of Correlating Lung Scan Interpretation with Clinical Assessment

		Clinical Assessment		
		High No./Total (%)	Intermediate No./Total (%)	Low No./Total (%)
Lung Scan Interpretation	**High Probability**	28/29 (96%)	70/80 (88%)	5/9 (56%)
	Intermediate Probability	27/41 (66%)	66/236 (28%)	11/68 (16%)
	Low Probability	6/15 (40%)	30/191 (16%)	4/90 (4%)

Source: Data from Pomp ER, Lenselink AM, Rosendaal FR, et al. Pregnancy, the postpartum period and prothrombotic defects: risk of venous thrombosis in the MEGA study. J Thromb Haemost. 2008;6(4):632–637.

■ ECHOCARDIOGRAM

The overall sensitivity of transthoracic echocardiography in PE approximates 50%.[68] Under appropriate clinical circumstances, the detection of unexplained right ventricular volume or pressure overload should suggest the possibility of PE and lead to confirmatory testing. Transthoracic echocardiography has emerged as a potentially important tool for risk assessment and treatment guidance in patients with acute PE. The presence of right ventricular dysfunction on a baseline echocardiogram in normotensive patients appears to represent an independent predictor of an adverse outcome or early death.[69,70] Properly performed transesophageal echocardiography has demonstrated sensitivity and specificity exceeding 90% in the detection of proximal emboli involving the pulmonary trunk and the right and left main pulmonary arteries.[71] Echocardiography also may prove valuable in the evaluation of competing diagnostic possibilities such as right ventricular infarction, endocarditis, pericardial tamponade, and aortic dissection in patients with unexplained shock and evidence of elevated central venous pressure.

■ LOWER EXTREMITY EVALUATION

Duplex ultrasonography, which refers to the combination of Doppler venous flow detection and real-time B-mode imaging, has assumed a central role in the noninvasive diagnosis of symptomatic lower extremity DVT.[72] A number of criteria are used to diagnose DVT, the most reliable of which is noncompressibility of a venous segment. Secondary, less reliable criteria include the presence of echogenic material within the venous lumen, loss of phasicity with respiration, attenuated increase in venous diameter in response to Valsalva, and lack of augmentation of flow in response to calf compression. The absence of an echogenic luminal mass cannot be considered useful in excluding the diagnosis of venous thrombosis because acute thrombus may not demonstrate echogenicity. Multiple studies over the past decade have demonstrated sensitivities and specificities exceeding 95% in *symptomatic* patients with proximal DVT.

While duplex ultrasonography is highly sensitive and specific in the diagnosis of DVT in symptomatic patients, its accuracy in the diagnosis of asymptomatic DVT is less clear. A meta-analysis of studies comparing ultrasound to contrast venography in asymptomatic patients found that ultrasound was accurate for the detection of asymptomatic proximal DVT, but the data was limited almost entirely limited to postoperative orthopedics patients.[73] Approximately 30% to 40% of patients with PE will also have signs and/or symptoms of DVT and 60% to 80% will have evidence of proximal DVT when subject to duplex ultrasonography. However, given that the overwhelming majority of patients with suspected PE will not prove to have that diagnosis, duplex ultrasonography as the initial diagnostic study should be reserved for those patients with clinical evidence of DVT and for special populations in which avoidance of radiation or contrast material is preferred.[74–77]

The role of CT venography as a stand-alone test for DVT is limited. CT venography appears to be comparable to ultrasonography with respect to sensitivity and specificity, but it requires contrast injection with its associated risks and radiation exposure. A potential advantage of CT venography is the ability to visualize the pelvic veins and vena cava. The concept of combined CT-PA and venography is attractive. Such an approach would provide visualization of the embolus and its source in a single study as well as potentially increase diagnostic yield in comparison with the use of CT-PA alone.[78] However, the absolute increase in diagnostic yield appears to be modest and comes at the cost of increased expense, substantial pelvic radiation exposure, and the risk of hemorrhagic complications from providing anticoagulation to patients with false-positive studies.

■ MAGNETIC RESONANCE IMAGING

Magnetic resonance imaging (MRI) techniques for detecting DVT and PE have been investigated. The PIOPED III trial was the largest, multicenter study designed to assess magnetic resonance angiography (MRA) for the diagnosis of PE.[79] Three hundred and seventy-one patients were enrolled in whom PE was confirmed or excluded by CT-PA or V/Q. Approximately 25% of studies were technically inadequate and could not be interpreted. However, this seemed to vary by site (11%–52%) suggesting that some sites may have had more experience and were able to limit their number of inadequate scans. The sensitivity and specificity of MRA among patients with technically adequate scans was 78% and 99%, respectively. These figures fell considerably when the technically inadequate scans were included in the calculations. Sensitivity for PE involving the main or lobar pulmonary arteries was only 79%.

There are patients in whom CT-PA may not be possible due to IV contrast allergy or in whom avoidance of radiation is preferred (e.g., pregnancy). In these patients it seems that MRA may be a reasonable alternative. The risk of gadolinium-related nephrogenic systemic fibrosis has dampened the initial enthusiasm for MRI scanning in patients with renal insufficiency.[80]

■ COMPUTED TOMOGRAPHY

CT-PA has become the first-line imaging test for PE (Fig. 73-9). CT technology has evolved from single detector scanners to 64-multidetector-row CT (MDCT) scanners. Using the latest generation scanners, visualization of the entire chest with submillimeter resolution extending to the sixth generation arteries can now be performed within a single breath hold. The PIOPED II trial, which used predominantly 4-MDCT technology and a composite reference standard, demonstrated sensitivity for the diagnosis of PE of 83%, specificity of 96%, positive predictive value of 86%, and negative predictive value of 97% (Table 73-7).[46] The predictive value of CT-PA varied substantially when clinical assessment was taken into account, with the major variance occurring when there was discordance between the clinical assessment and CT-PA finding. Both the positive predictive value in patients with a low clinical probability and the negative predictive value in those with a high clinical probability were in the range of 60%.

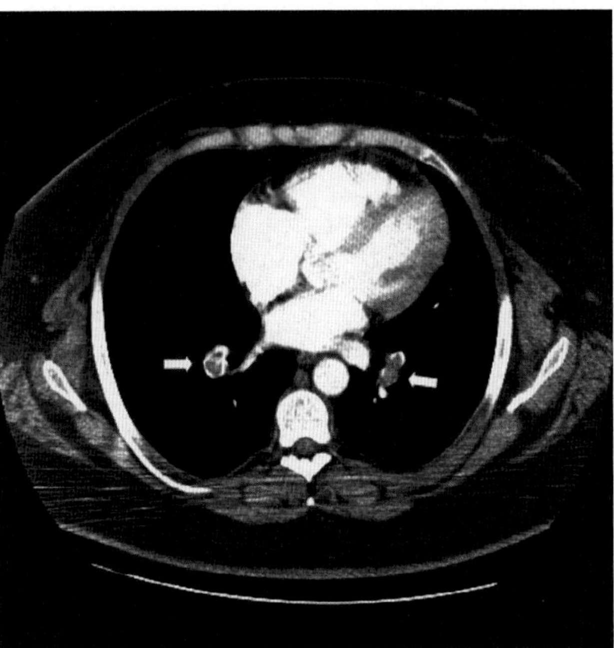

Figure 73-9 Computed tomographic angiogram demonstrating nearly occlusive thrombus in both lower lobe pulmonary arteries (*arrows*).

At the present time, CT can be considered confirmatory in excluding embolism in patients with a low or intermediate likelihood of disease and confirming embolism in patients with intermediate or high probability of disease. When discordance exists between the clinical assessment and CT findings, additional studies should be considered.

Concerns have been raised that the widespread utilization of CT-PA is resulting in the overdiagnosis of PE, defined as diagnosing clinically insignificant disease. The highest level of evidence thus far is a randomized controlled trial by Anderson et al.[81] of pulmonary CT-PA versus V/Q scan for suspected PE that showed comparable mortality and false-negative rates for the two imaging modalities with a 51% higher rate of PE diagnosis for CT. It has been suggested, based on the known natural history of subsegmental embolism, that patients with isolated subsegmental PE do not necessarily need to be treated with anticoagulants provided they meet the following criteria: (1) good cardiopulmonary reserve; (2) no evidence of DVT with serial lower extremity studies; (3) a transient (reversible) major risk factor for PE that is no longer present; (4) no history of central venous catheterization and no history of atrial fibrillation; and (5) a compliant and trustworthy patient who would return for serial noninvasive lower extremity studies.[82] Concerns have also been raised that CT-PA, as a result of its easy availability, is being overutilized in outpatients without adequate patient screening through validated methods such as the Wells criteria/D-dimer model or the PERC.[55,83]

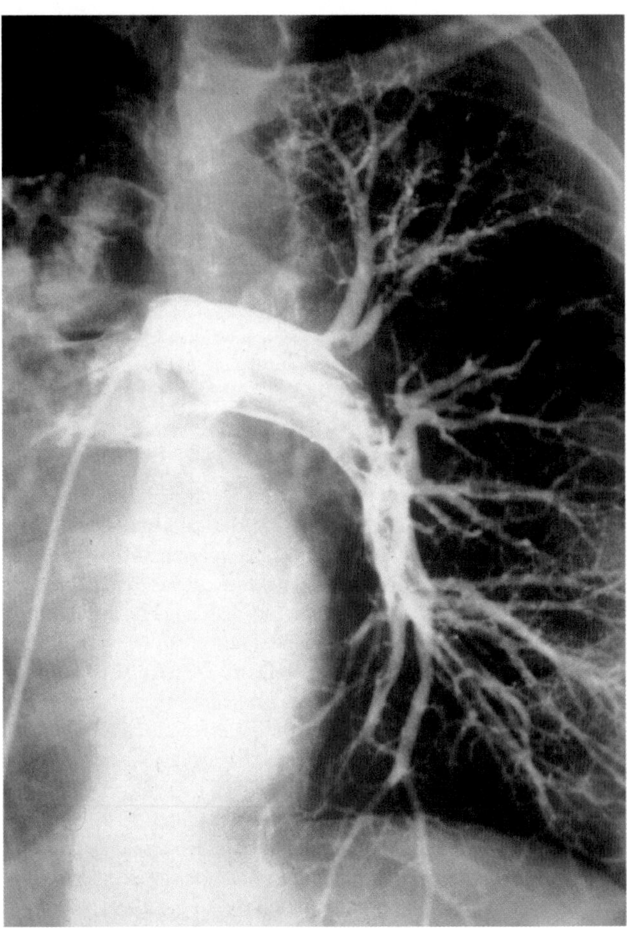

Figure 73-10 Conventional contrast pulmonary angiogram demonstrating extensive embolus within the left main pulmonary artery and extending into lobar branches.

CONVENTIONAL PULMONARY ANGIOGRAPHY

Prior to widespread acceptance of CT-PA, pulmonary angiography was considered the accepted "gold standard" for PE diagnosis although it had a number of limitations (Fig. 73-10). It requires expertise in study performance and interpretation. It is invasive and

TABLE 73-7 Prevalence of Pulmonary Embolism in PIOPED II: Value of Correlating CT Interpretation with Clinical Assessment

		Clinical Assessment		
		High No./Total (%)	Intermediate No./Total (%)	Low No./Total (%)
CT Scan Interpretation	**PPV of CTA**	22/23 (96%)	93/101 (92%)	22/38 (58%)
	PPV of CTA-CTV	27/28 (96%)	100/111 (90%)	24/42 (57%)
	NPV of CTA	9/15 (60%)	121/136 (89%)	158/164 (96%)
	NPV of CTA-CTV	9/11 (82%)	114/124 (92%)	146/151 (97%)

PPV of CTA, positive predictive value of computed tomographic angiography; PPV of CTA-CTV, positive predictive value of combined computed tomography angiography + venography; NPV of CTA, negative predictive value of computed tomographic angiography; NPV of CTA-CTV, negative predictive value of computed tomographic angiography + venography.

Source: Data from Galli M, Luciani D, Bertolin G, et al. Lupus anticoagulants are stronger risk factors for thrombosis than anticardiolipin antibodies in the antiphospholipid syndrome: a systematic review of the literature. Blood. 2003;101(5):1827–1832.

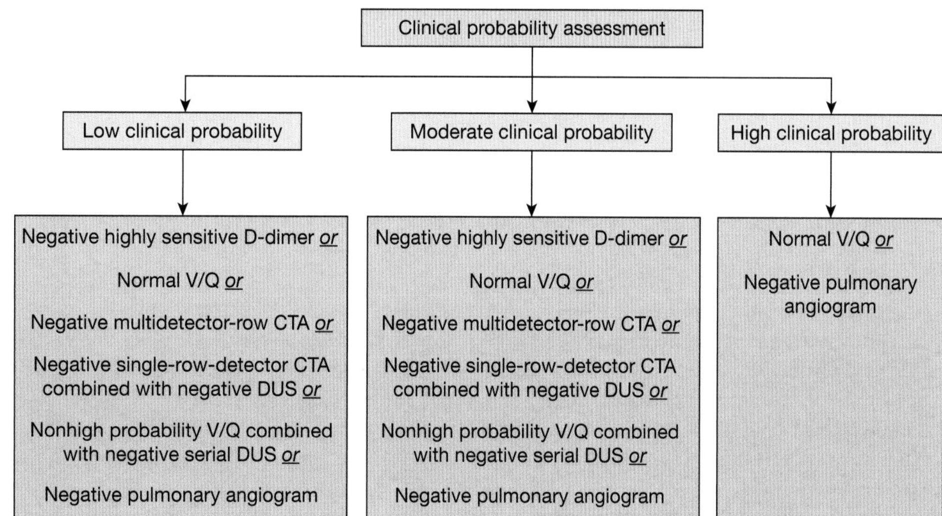

Figure 73-11 Current diagnostic strategies capable of excluding diagnosis of pulmonary embolism.

has associated risks, although published studies suggest that the use of modern techniques and contrast materials has reduced the risk well below its lingering perception. Pulmonary angiography can be performed quite safely if certain safeguards are observed and experienced personnel are involved. In the 1111 angiograms performed in the original PIOPED trial, pulmonary angiography was nondiagnostic in 3% of patients and associated with a major complication rate of 1% and death rate of 0.5%.[84] Major complications occurred more frequently among patients sent for angiography from the medical intensive care unit than in patients from elsewhere (4% vs. 1%). The procedure has other limitations. One is accessibility and the need for transportation. The other limitation is interpretation. Interpretation of pulmonary angiograms is heavily influenced by three factors: the location of the thromboembolic obstruction, the quality of the images, and the experience of the interpreters. Only two angiographic findings are diagnostic of acute embolism: a filling defect and abrupt cutoff of a vessel. Technical adequacy of the angiogram is critical to accurate identification of both. Flow artifacts can falsely suggest a filling defect. It is essential that good vessel opacification be obtained and that the filling defects be identified as real on a sequence of films.

Angiography is reserved for the small subset of patients in whom the diagnosis of PE cannot be established or excluded by less invasive means and for the evaluation of suspected chronic thromboembolic disease.

DIAGNOSTIC APPROACH

The diagnostic approach to PE should be targeted toward the patient population being studied (Figs. 73-11 and 73-12). For outpatients, the use of a clinical prediction rule coupled with D-dimer testing or the use of the PERC criteria can substantially reduce the number of imaging studies performed. In the outpatient setting, D-dimer results would not alter the need for an objective imaging study in patients with a high probability of PE. In patients with a low or intermediate clinical likelihood of PE, a negative D-dimer study is sufficient to exclude the diagnosis, assuming a highly sensitive assay is used. An imaging study should be performed in all patients with a high probability of disease as well as those with a low or intermediate probability whose D-dimer tests are positive.

Patients with signs or symptoms of lower extremity DVT should initially undergo lower extremity duplex ultrasonography. A positive lower extremity study, although not proving PE has occurred, has the same therapeutic implications. Although such an approach will yield a confirmatory study in only about 20% of patients suspected of having PE, it avoids the cost and radiation exposure associated with CT-PA. A negative study is insufficient to exclude the possibility of PE.[77]

In patients without lower extremity symptoms or signs who have a high or intermediate clinical probability of PE, a positive CT-PA confirms the diagnosis. In patients with a low or intermediate clinical probability, a negative CT-PA excludes the diagnosis. The only patients who may require additional testing (duplex ultrasonography and/or conventional angiography) are those in whom the clinical assessment and CT findings are discordant (low clinical probability and positive CT scan or high clinical probability and negative CT scan) unless the CT scan is of adequate quality and demonstrates evidence of PE in the main or lobar arteries in a patient with a low clinical probability assessment.

An approach utilizing V/Q scanning as the primary imaging tool can be used in settings such as pregnancy, contrast allergy,

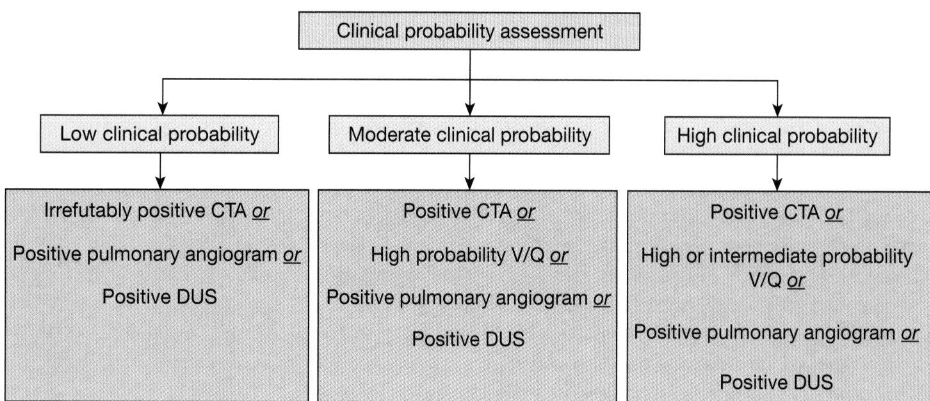

Figure 73-12 Current diagnostic strategies capable of confirming diagnosis of pulmonary embolism.

or renal insufficiency. This approach should be reserved for those with normal chest radiographs and no history of chronic pulmonary disease. Lower extremity evaluation should be considered before chest imaging given the likelihood that the V/Q scan will not be diagnostic. A negative V/Q scan is capable of excluding the diagnosis regardless of the clinical assessment as does a low probability scan in conjunction with a low clinical suspicion. A high probability scan is capable of confirming the diagnosis in patients with a high clinical suspicion. All other circumstances (high clinical probability with low or intermediate V/Q result, intermediate clinical probability regardless of V/Q result, and low clinical probability with a high or intermediate V/Q scan result) require additional testing.[44]

Whatever approach is undertaken, the treating physician should be aware of the type of D-dimer assay, discriminant value of that particular assay, and generation of CT scanner used. "Negative" findings on a low-sensitivity D-dimer assay or a single-row CT scanner have very different implications than similar findings using a highly sensitive D-dimer assay or 64-MDCT scanner.

The role of D-dimer testing and clinical assessment in hospitalized patients is limited. A substantial proportion of hospitalized patients have a positive highly sensitive D-dimer result related to an active inflammatory process, malignancy, recent surgery, liver disease, and even advancing age.[85] In a recent study that evaluated the use of the Wells prediction rule in conjunction with a latex agglutination or rapid ELISA D-dimer assay in hospitalized patients, only 10% of over 600 patients tested fell into the low probability category.[85] Furthermore, comorbid conditions affect the clinical likelihood assessment. Therefore, a far higher proportion of hospitalized patients require an imaging study to confirm or exclude the diagnosis of venous thromboembolism. In patients with limited cardiopulmonary reserve, high clinical probability assessment, and negative CT scan, pulmonary angiography should be considered given the potentially fatal consequences of a recurrent embolic event. In patients with adequate cardiopulmonary reserve under the same circumstances, a strategy incorporating sequential lower extremity evaluation can be undertaken.

TREATMENT

Management of acute PE consists of a systematic approach that involves early intervention, patient risk stratification, selection of therapy, and determination of treatment duration. The goals of therapy in PE are severalfold—to assure adequate oxygenation, provide hemodynamic support, and prevent thrombus propagation and embolic recurrence.

When a diagnosis of venous thromboembolism is suspected, empiric treatment should be considered until the diagnosis is either objectively excluded or confirmed. Given the ready availability of rapid D-dimer assays and CT, diagnostic confirmation or exclusion should require a relatively short period of time. Early empiric treatment should be initiated if diagnostic tests are not readily available. An exception can be made in those patients with a low clinical likelihood of disease, adequate cardiopulmonary reserve, and a high risk of bleeding complications.

The availability of low-molecular-weight heparin (LMWH) potentially allows carefully selected patients to be managed in the outpatient setting as demonstrated in the recently published study.[86] Although there are good data to support treating uncomplicated cases of DVT entirely in the outpatient setting, most physicians still advocate a short period of hospitalization in patients with newly diagnosed acute PE. Hospitalization should be mandatory for older patients who may have less cardiopulmonary reserve, or significant coexisting illnesses, or those who may not be able to follow instructions or have adequate follow-up. Other indications for hospitalization include hypoxemia, hypotension, hemodynamic instability, or sufficient renal disease to contraindicate the use of LMWH or a factor Xa inhibitor.

HEPARIN

Anticoagulation with heparin remains the standard initial therapy. The major anticoagulant effect of heparin is to reduce thrombus propagation and prevent embolic recurrence. Choices include either intravenous unfractionated heparin (UFH) or subcutaneous LMWH preparations. Given that failure to achieve rapid therapeutic levels of anticoagulation appears to be associated with an increased recurrence rate, it is reasonable to attempt to ensure adequate anticoagulation as soon as possible.[87]

Physician practices in the administration of intravenous unfractionated heparin have often resulted in substantial delays before adequate prolongation of the activated partial thromboplastin time (aPTT) is achieved. To overcome these problems, standardized protocols for unfractionated heparin administration and monitoring have been recommended. One commonly employed dosing regimen using an initial intravenous bolus of 80 units of heparin per kilogram followed by a continuous infusion initiated at 18 U/kg/h has been demonstrated to reach therapeutic thresholds more quickly than regimens using fixed dosing.[88] The heparin drip is adjusted based on monitoring of the aPTT, drawn 6 hours after the initial bolus dose, then 6 hours after each dose adjustment, with a target aPTT ratio of 1.5 to 2.5. Because attempts to straddle the lower therapeutic range may result in periods of inadequate anticoagulation, it is prudent to maintain the ratio in the upper range of the recommended target.

More recently, an approach using a fixed dose of subcutaneous unfractionated heparin without aPTT monitoring, administered as an initial dose of 333 U/kg followed by a dose of 250 U/kg every 12 hours, has been demonstrated to be as safe and effective as LMWH in patients presenting with DVT and PE.[89]

With the exception of special circumstances, LMWH preparations have displaced unfractionated heparin as the anticoagulant of choice in uncomplicated venous thromboembolism including PE.[90] Situations in which the use of UFH is appropriate include renal insufficiency, extremes of body weight, and circumstances in which a rapid adjustment or reversal of anticoagulation is needed, such as women in the late stage of pregnancy who may need Cesarean sections, patients with recent surgery or recent history of bleeding, and hemodynamically unstable patients with venous thromboembolism who may need surgical procedures such as emergency embolectomy.

Available evidence suggests that LMWH is at least as effective as unfractionated heparin in treating acute PE.[91] Advantages of LMWH compared with UFH include (1) longer half-life and ease of use; (2) ability to consistently achieve early therapeutic anticoagulation; (3) no need to monitor anticoagulant effects; and (4) reduced incidence of major bleeding complications. There are few data comparing different LMWH preparations. Even though there are differences in their Food and Drug Administration (FDA)-approved indications in the United States, it is not clear if their actions differ significantly.

In general, therapeutic monitoring is not needed with LMWH, but there are situations where the therapeutic effects may be less predictable and monitoring with anti-Xa levels is indicated. Typical examples include (1) patients with antiphospholipid antibodies or other circulating anticoagulants who have elevated baseline aPTT; (2) extremes of body weight (less than 40 kg and greater than 150 kg); (3) significant renal disease (creatinine clearance less than 30 mL/min); (4) pregnancy; and (5) unexplained bleeding or recurrent thrombosis during therapy. A therapeutic target range for peak anti-Xa levels ranges from 0.6 to 1.0 IU/mL, 4 hours after administration. The target range for peak anti-Xa levels with once daily enoxaparin is likely to be greater than1.0 IU/mL whereas it is greater than 0.85 IU/mL with tinzaparin and 1.3 IU/mL and 1.05 IU/mL with nadroparin and dalteparin, respectively.[92]

FACTOR XA INHIBITORS

Fondaparinux, a synthetic pentasaccharide, represented the first in a new class of antithrombotic agents. Unlike unfractionated heparin and LMWH, the antithrombotic properties of fondaparinux are selective for factor Xa. By binding rapidly and strongly to antithrombin, fondaparinux catalyzes specifically the inhibition of factor Xa, which results in inhibition of thrombin generation. It does not bind to other plasma components or platelets, has a half-life of approximately 17 hours, and is excreted almost completely by the kidneys. Fondaparinux was shown to be as effective and safe as intravenous unfractionated heparin in a large, open-label study.[93] It has been approved for prophylaxis in patients undergoing hip, knee, and abdominal surgery as well as for treatment of DVT and PE in conjunction with warfarin.

Rivaroxaban represents the first in a new generation of oral factor Xa inhibitors. In a large, open-label randomized study, rivaroxaban proved noninferior to conventional therapy (LMWH followed by a vitamin K antagonist) in patients with symptomatic DVT.[94] Patients with acute PE were excluded from the acute phase of the study. Although not specifically designed to determine efficacy in acute PE, the incidence of subsequent PE was equivalent between the two study groups. In a subsequent study involving 4832 patients, a fixed-dose regimen of rivaroxaban alone was noninferior to standard therapy for the initial and long-term treatment of PE with or without DVT.[95] Ongoing trials are underway evaluating the efficacy and safety of other oral factor Xa inhibitors, including apixaban and edoxaban in venous thromboembolism.[96]

Intravenously administered direct thrombin inhibitors (lepirudin, argatroban) represent another class of anticoagulant agents that have been approved for the management of patients with venous thromboembolism in the setting of heparin-induced thrombocytopenia (HIT).[97] Their mechanism of action differs from that of heparin and the synthetic pentasaccharides in that they directly inhibit the active site of thrombin and do not require interaction with antithrombin to produce an anticoagulant effect. Argatroban is a synthetic agent derived from arginine. It has a half-life of approximately 45 minutes and is cleared by the liver. Lepirudin is a recombinant polypeptide similar to hirudin. It has a half-life of 40 to 60 minutes and is cleared by the kidneys. Both agents are administered by continuous intravenous infusion and dose adjustments made with monitoring of the aPTT. Both agents affect the international normalized ratio (INR), thereby complicating the transition to oral warfarin therapy. Although demonstrating promise, data supporting the use of fondaparinux in the management of HIT is far less robust than that of the intravenous direct thrombin inhibitors.[98] Based on its size, the drug is less immunogenic than unfractionated heparin or LMWH. Fondaparinux has not been approved by the FDA for this indication.

THROMBOLYTIC THERAPY

Unlike anticoagulants, thrombolytic drugs cause direct lysis of thrombi by increasing plasmin production through plasminogen activation. The potential benefits, however, are often offset by the relatively high incidence of hemorrhagic complications.

Multiple thrombolytic agents are available. Those most studied for the management of acute PE include streptokinase, alteplase (rt-PA), and urokinase, all of which are FDA approved for use in the United States. The PEITHO (pulmonary embolism thrombolysis) trial, a large multicenter study designed to enroll 1000 patients, is currently underway and will evaluate the efficacy and safety of tenecteplase in normotensive patients with evidence of right ventricular (RV) dysfunction.[99]

The exact role of thrombolytic agents in acute PE remains controversial. While thrombolytic therapy does appear to accelerate the rate of thrombolysis, there is no convincing evidence to suggest that it decreases mortality, increases the ultimate extent of embolic resolution when measured at 7 days, reduces thromboembolic recurrence rates, improves symptomatic outcome, or decreases the incidence of thromboembolic pulmonary hypertension.[100] The one issue about which there can be little controversy is that the use of thrombolytic agents is associated with a substantially increased risk of bleeding, including intracranial hemorrhage. Intracranial hemorrhage has occurred in 0.5% to 3.0% of patients treated with thrombolytic agents in trials evaluating the use of these agents in both PE and myocardial infarction.[101]

Based on these data, and assuming there is no contraindication to its use, the use of thrombolytic therapy in PE appears to be appropriate when an accelerated rate of thrombolysis may be considered lifesaving. Specifically, this applies to patients with PE who present with hemodynamic compromise (in whom the mortality rate approaches 30%), patients who develop hemodynamic compromise during conventional therapy with heparin, and patients with PE associated with intracavitary right heart thrombi.[36]

The role of thrombolytic therapy in patients with anatomically massive embolism or echocardiographic evidence of right ventricular dysfunction in the absence of systemic hypotension is less well defined. Risk stratification strategies using echocardiography, troponin levels, or brain natriuretic peptide (BNP) levels are currently under investigation and may help resolve this area of controversy.[102] At the present time, the finding of right ventricular dysfunction on echocardiography in the absence of hemodynamic instability would not appear to serve as a justification for the routine use of thrombolytic therapy. Approximately 40% to 50% of patients with symptomatic PE have echocardiographic evidence of right ventricular dysfunction.[103] Clinical scoring systems have also been constructed capable of estimating 30-day mortality rates in patients with acute PE (Table 73-8).[104,105] However, these scoring systems appear best suited in identifying patients with a low mortality risk who may be suitable for home management rather than those with a sufficiently high mortality risk to justify the use of thrombolytic therapy.

Normotensive patients with evidence of right ventricular dysfunction, as determined by echocardiography or an elevated BNP or troponin level, appear to be at risk for an adverse outcome when

TABLE 73-8 Original and Simplified Pulmonary Embolism Severity Index

Variable	Original PESI	Simplified PESI
Age >80 y	Age in years	1
Male sex	+10	
History of cancer	+30	1
History of heart failure	+10	1[a]
History of chronic lung disease	+10	
Pulse ≥110 beats/min	+20	1
Systolic blood pressure <100	+30	1
Respiratory rate ≥30 breaths/min	+20	
Temperature <36°C	+20	
Altered mental status	+60	
Arterial oxyhemoglobin saturation <90%	+20	1

Original PESI: Class I, 65 or less; Class II, 66–85; Class III, 86–105; Class IV, 106–125; Class V, >125.
Modified PESI: 0, low risk; 1 or more, high risk.
[a]Variables combined into a single category of chronic cardiopulmonary disease.
Source: Modified with permission from Aujesky D, Obrosky DS, Stone RA, et al. Derivation and validation of a prognostic model for pulmonary embolism. Am J Respir Crit Care Med. 2005;172(8):1041–1046.

compared with patients without right ventricular dysfunction. However, until criteria have been established that more clearly define that subset of patients who will benefit from thrombolytic therapy, there is little basis for exposing all such patients to the considerable risk of hemorrhagic complications associated with this intervention. It is hoped that the ongoing PEITHO trial will help resolve this uncertainty.[99]

Because of the side effects and the prolonged period of infusion required, many physicians are reluctant to use thrombolytics in cases of DVT, whether delivered systemically or by local catheter-directed infusion. In selected patients with symptomatic iliofemoral thrombosis, catheter-directed thrombolysis either alone or combined with angioplasty or stent placement may result in increased venous patency and may improve quality of life.[106]

■ INTERVENTIONAL RADIOLOGIC TECHNIQUES

Interventional thrombus fragmentation represents a potential alternative to systemic thrombolysis or surgical embolectomy for treatment of PE.[107] If the bleeding risk is not exceedingly high, catheter fragmentation may be combined with local or systemic thrombolysis. A wide variety of devices designed to either fragment and/or remove fresh embolic material have been tested in patients with PE.[108] In general, the devices use either pressured saline or a rotating impeller to fragment central thrombi. The fragments are either aspirated through a separate port on the catheter or allowed to migrate distally. Most of the devices appear to be effective, safe, and potentially lifesaving in the presence of central, acute clots. However, none of the devices has been investigated in a large controlled trial, and all commercially available devices have important limitation. These limitations include a risk of paradoxical embolism from the clot fragments. Therefore, the intervention is contraindicated in patients who have an intracardiac communication, such as a patent foramen ovale.

■ PULMONARY EMBOLECTOMY

Embolectomy has been used for the emergency removal of PE. Small observational studies comparing surgical embolectomy and thrombolytics did not show significant advantage using embolectomy, although there was a trend toward better survival and lower bleeding rates in the surgical group. In a recent review of 3770 patients undergoing surgical embolectomy for acute PE between 1999 and 2008, all-cause inhospital case fatality rate was 28%; mortality was 24% in patients considered stable and 40% in those unstable.[109] Based on current data, it is reasonable to consider surgical embolectomy in patients with persistent hypotension, shock, or cardiac arrest who either failed thrombolysis or have a contraindication to thrombolytic management.

LONG-TERM MANAGEMENT

Long-term management includes use of traditional anticoagulants, including warfarin and heparin, as well as a variety of new pharmacologic agents. In addition, insertion of devices in the inferior vena cava to prevent additional embolic events has been employed.

■ WARFARIN

Recurrence is common following an acute thromboembolic event. Therefore, treatment should be continued until the benefits of ongoing therapy no longer outweigh the potential risks.

Oral anticoagulation using warfarin, a vitamin K antagonist, is generally used for long-term treatment of venous thromboembolism because of its proven efficacy. Warfarin inhibits gamma carboxylation activation of coagulation factors II, VII, IX, and X as well as proteins C and S. With proper monitoring, less than 3% of patients using warfarin develop significant bleeding. The drug is usually started soon after the initiation of heparin therapy. Use of warfarin without heparin is strongly discouraged as it generally takes 3 to 5 days of warfarin to achieve full therapeutic efficacy. In patients with protein C deficiency, skin necrosis or paradoxical thrombosis may occur in the absence of concurrent heparin therapy.

Warfarin has a narrow therapeutic index and patients are generally monitored closely by measuring the prothrombin time corrected to the reagent being used (the INR). To maximize efficacy while minimizing side effects, an INR range between 2 and 3 is recommended for most patients. Even in the setting of an antiphospholipid antibody, high-intensity warfarin therapy does not appear superior to standard treatment but is associated with an increased incidence of minor bleeding complications.[110,111] Besides bleeding complications, warfarin has been associated with fetal abnormalities particularly when given during the 6th to 12th weeks of gestation. Another rare complication of warfarin use is cholesterol microembolism ("purple toes" syndrome), which is thought to be due to cholesterol crystal release from ulcerated intravascular plaques.[112]

Individuals metabolize warfarin differently and age, genetic variations in CYP2C9 alleles, nutritional factors, and concomitant medications can affect anticoagulant levels significantly. Multiple mechanisms of drug interaction are possible including alterations of absorption (cholestyramine), induction of hepatic CYP450 (barbiturates, carbamazepine), inhibition of CYP3A4 (amiodarone), inhibition of CYP2C9 (metronidazole, clotrimazole), and displacement of protein-bound warfarin (phenytoin).[113]

Suggested dosing regimens involve an initial daily dose of 5 or 10 mg with use of a standardized nomogram to dose adjust based on INR values obtained on days 3 and 5.[114] Beginning with a 10-mg dose appears to hasten the achievement of a therapeutic INR without an increase in bleeding complications.[115,116] Elderly, malnourished, and debilitated patients tend to require less warfarin and the initial dose should be lowered accordingly. Some medical conditions, such as concomitant liver or kidney failure, alcoholism, malignancy, and recent history of gastrointestinal bleeding or trauma, are additional factors that may predict dose titration difficulties and higher risk of bleeding.

To minimize potential subtherapeutic anticoagulation, it is generally recommended that patients should receive at least 5 days of combined heparin and warfarin therapy, including at least 2 days in which the INR is in a therapeutic range before stopping heparin. The safety and effectiveness of both short- and long-term anticoagulation can be optimized by a systematic, evidence-based approach to therapy, often in the context of dedicated anticoagulation management services.[117] In carefully selected patients, self-management of warfarin therapy using INR measurement with "point of care" devices may also be done.[118]

■ HEPARIN

There are occasional instances in which heparin should be considered for long-term anticoagulation despite the cost and inconvenience associated with subcutaneous administration. Because of the teratogenic potential of warfarin, unfractionated heparin or LMWH should be used in pregnant women who developed venous thromboembolism in the first and possibly early second trimesters. Since the risk of venous thromboembolism may be highest in the postpartum period, anticoagulation should be continued for at least 3 to 6 months, including a minimum of 4 to 6 weeks after delivery. Patients with cancer complicated by thromboembolism appear to have fewer recurrent thromboembolic events and bleeding complications when treated with LMWH compared with warfarin.[119] Whether this is a specific effect of LMWH or simply a reflection of fluctuating INR levels in patients with cancer treated with warfarin is uncertain. LMWH therapy is now recommended over warfarin as a first-line treatment to reduce the risk of recurrent venous thromboembolism in patients with active cancer.[120]

NOVEL AGENTS

Novel agents have been used successfully for long-term management of patients with venous thromboembolism. As noted previously, rivaroxaban alone was noninferior to standard therapy for the initial and long-term treatment of PE with or without DVT.[95] Dabigatran, an oral direct inhibitor of thrombin, has also proven effective for long-term management. In the RE-COVER trial involving 2539 patients with acute venous thromboembolism, 786 of whom had PE, dabigatran administered at a dose of 150 mg twice daily after initial treatment with heparin was as effective as warfarin therapy in preventing thromboembolic recurrence while significantly reducing nonmajor bleeding.[121] In the AMPLIFY-EXT (apixaban after the initial management of PE and deep vein thrombosis with first-line therapy-extended treatment) trial, apixaban reduced the risk of recurrent venous thromboembolism without increasing the rate of major bleeding in patients with venous thromboembolism who had completed 6 to 12 months of anticoagulation therapy and for whom there was clinical equipoise regarding the continuation or cessation of anticoagulation therapy.[122]

The role of aspirin in the long-term management of patients with venous thromboembolism remains incompletely defined. In the WARFASA (the warfarin and aspirin study) trial, the use of aspirin reduced the risk of thromboembolic recurrence by 40% when given to patients with unprovoked venous thromboembolism following discontinuation of anticoagulant therapy.[123] In the ASPIRE (aspirin to prevent recurrent venous thromboembolism) trial, however, aspirin, as compared with placebo, did not significantly reduce the rate of recurrence of venous thromboembolism but resulted in a significant reduction in the rate of major vascular events, with improved net clinical benefit.[124]

DURATION OF THERAPY

Over the past decade, data have emerged that have significantly changed our recommendation regarding duration of anticoagulation after venous thromboembolism. Central to this change has been awareness that venous thromboembolism often represents a recurrent disease and that the risk for recurrence is based on the initiating factors, persistence or resolution of those factors, and anatomic consequences of the initial event.

Patients with venous thromboembolism associated with a transient risk factor appear to be at a low risk of recurrence. Patients who experience postoperative venous thromboembolism appear to be at lowest risk. However, the annualized risk of recurrent disease is still in the region of 3%.[125] A 3-month course of anticoagulation appears to be adequate in this group (assuming the risk factor has resolved). Patients with idiopathic (unprovoked) thromboembolism have a substantially higher rate of recurrence, corresponding to an annualized event rate of 7.9% per patient-year.[125] In these patients, anticoagulation may simply delay subsequent recurrent thromboembolic events and ongoing risk factors may be present that have yet to be identified. Therefore, it is recommended that strong consideration be given to extended therapy in those with a low risk of bleeding complications.[126] Determining which patients remain at increased risk of thromboembolic recurrence is the target of ongoing investigative efforts. A number of clinical and serologic factors have been identified that predict a higher likelihood of recurrent venous thromboembolism following an initial course of therapy. These include PE as the initial presenting manifestation, age greater than 65, male gender, evidence of residual lower extremity DVT by ultrasonography, and elevated D-dimer levels measured at the end of warfarin therapy and then 1 month after its discontinuation.[127] How these factors should influence decisions about duration of anticoagulation in an individual patient remains to be determined.

In patients with venous thromboembolism associated with an irreversible risk factor, the absolute recurrence risk depends on the underlying disease or condition.[128,129] Patients heterozygous for the factor V Leiden mutation or the prothrombin G20210A mutation, although at higher recurrence risk than those without the mutation, do not appear to warrant prolonged anticoagulation while those homozygous for either of these mutations, or with a combined thrombophilia (i.e., heterozygous factor V Leiden combined with heterozygous prothrombin mutation), do. Patients with antiphospholipid antibody syndrome, those with active cancer, and those with deficiencies of protein S, protein C and antithrombin III are at considerable risk for thromboembolic recurrence and consideration should be given to lifelong therapy. In patients with two or more episodes of recurrent venous thromboembolism, the current recommendation is to consider lifelong anticoagulation with interval reassessment of the risk–benefit ratio. In summary, long-term anticoagulation should be individualized based on the risk for recurrent thromboembolism and bleeding. This is especially true in patients with cancer in whom the recurrent thrombosis risk and bleeding risk are substantially increased.[130] The appropriateness of ongoing therapy should be continuously re-evaluated, and the prophylaxis stopped if the benefit no longer appears to exceed the risk.

VENA CAVA INTERRUPTION AND VENA CAVA FILTER

The concept of vena cava interruption came from the historical practice of surgical ligation (by complete vascular ligation or partial interruption using surgical suture) of the IVC in an attempt to prevent thrombus migration. A variety of vena cava filters are now available, both permanent and temporary, and surgical ligation is rarely performed in the modern era.

The central indication for IVC filter placement is to prevent PE in patients who have a contraindication to anticoagulation. Recent data suggests that the utilization of IVC filters has dramatically expanded over the past decade and that IVC filters are being placed for alternative reasons, including prophylaxis.[131] Much of this expansion in utilization can be attributed to the development of retrievable IVC filters, which in many instances are not removed.[132] Guidelines for filter placement, albeit based on limited data, have been established by the American College of Chest Physicians and the Society of Interventional Radiologists.[133,134] These recommendations are somewhat disparate with the recommendations of the latter society being considerably more liberal than those of the former.

Despite the obvious theoretical benefit, carefully controlled trials that demonstrate the ability of IVC filters to decrease recurrence rates or mortality from PE have not been performed.[135] In one of the largest trials to date examining the effectiveness of IVC filters, 400 patients with proximal DVT were randomly assigned to either standard anticoagulation alone or anticoagulation plus insertion of a Vena Tech, Greenfield, Bird's Nest, or Cardial IVC filter.[136] During the first 12 days after randomization, significantly fewer patients in the IVC filter group suffered PE (1% vs. 5%). However, after a 2-year follow-up period, there were no significant differences in survival or symptomatic PE between the two groups, and a significantly higher rate of recurrent DVT was observed among patients who had received an IVC filter (21% vs. 12%).[137]

Given that IVC filters may decrease the incidence of early, recurrent PE, an argument can be made for their use in patients with residual lower extremity DVT who have suffered hemodynamically massive PE or who have poor cardiopulmonary reserve. Data on the effectiveness of IVC filters purely for prophylactic reasons are limited and randomized controlled trials are warranted to provide better practice-based evidence for or against this indication. Placement of an IVC filter is not a benign procedure and carries several possible risks including potential DVT formation, filter migration, filter tilt, filter thrombosis, and the possibility of a higher incidence of lower extremity thrombotic events and postthrombotic syndrome.[138,139]

CHRONIC THROMBOEMBOLISM

Anatomic resolution of PE is rarely complete.[39,140] However, resolution in most patients is adequate to permit normalization of pulmonary hemodynamics and exercise tolerance. In some cases, however, the residual thromboembolic burden is sufficiently extensive to cause CTEPH. Estimates of the incidence of CTEPH range from 0.5% to 3.8% following an initial episode of PE to 13.4% following recurrent episodes of venous thromboembolism.[141–143] Approximately 30% of patients who develop CTEPH have no documented history of acute DVT or PE, and this feature greatly impedes the diagnosis. Anticardiolipin antibodies or lupus anticoagulants have been detected in approximately 10% to 20% of patients and elevated factor VIII levels detected in 40%.[144,145] No other defined thrombophilic or fibrinolytic abnormality has been encountered in this population. Age greater than 70, systolic pulmonary artery pressure greater than 50 mm Hg at the time of diagnosis of acute PE or at the time of hospital discharge following acute PE, previous PE, prior splenectomy, ventriculoatrial shunts, the presence of antiphospholipid antibodies, and a larger degree of pulmonary vascular obstruction at the time of acute PE have been identified as risk factors for CTEPH.[146]

The mortality of untreated CTEPH is high, with a 5-year survival of only about 10% in those who have a mean pulmonary artery pressure exceeding 50 mm Hg.[147,148] The treatment of choice for CTEPH is pulmonary thromboendarterectomy, which involves the dissection of endothelialized thrombi under cardiopulmonary bypass and deep hypothermia.[149] For the majority of patients, successful pulmonary thromboendarterectomy is considered curative. However, the hemodynamic outcome is incomplete in approximately 20% of patients. These patients have been successfully treated with medical therapies that are used in patients with idiopathic pulmonary arterial hypertension.[150] Indications for medical therapy in CTEPH include: (1) surgically accessible CTEPH in patients who elect not to undergo surgery for personal choice or where comorbidities are so substantial as to exclude the patient from consideration of thromboendarterectomy; (2) distal chronic thromboembolic disease or limited central disease that is so disproportionate to the severity of the pulmonary hypertension that the surgical mortality risk is prohibitive; (3) use as a preoperative therapeutic "bridge" to surgery in patients with severe right ventricular dysfunction; and (4) management of persistent pulmonary hypertension following pulmonary thromboendarterectomy. Patients with inoperable CTEPH or persistent pulmonary hypertension despite thromboendarterectomy may be considered for lung transplantation.

PROPHYLAXIS

The use of prophylactic strategies in hospitalized patients represents a major opportunity to prevent the morbidity and mortality associated with venous thromboembolism. Current data suggests, however that thrombosis prophylaxis is underutilized in patients at risk, especially medical patients whose risk approximates that of their moderate-risk surgical counterparts.[10,151,152]

Patients should be stratified according to DVT risk, and certain prophylactic measures are more appropriate for some patients than for others. The intensity of a prophylactic regimen should take into account the relative risk for thrombosis. Initial assessment should focus on the following questions: (1) What is the risk of venous thromboembolism in this patient? (2) What type(s) and intensity of prophylaxis should be used? (3) When is the best time to use prophylaxis? A patient's thrombotic risk may change over time and periodic assessment of the best prophylactic strategy should also be done. Most hospitalized patients are at risk of venous thromboembolism and should receive some form of prophylaxis unless its use is contraindicated. Prophylaxis may not be necessary in rare instances, as in the case of a young (less than 40 years) ambulatory patient who is admitted for a short (less than 48–72 hours) hospital stay without a history of prior venous thromboembolism history or recent surgery.

Four categories of drugs have been used successfully: unfractionated heparin, LMWH (enoxaparin, dalteparin), factor Xa inhibitors (fondaparinux, rivaroxaban), and the vitamin K antagonist warfarin. With the exception of warfarin, prophylactic dosing is subtherapeutic but sufficient to decrease the likelihood of thrombus formation. Recommended, evidence-based prophylactic strategies for a wide range of clinical circumstances in medical, surgical, and orthopedic patients have been published by the American College of Chest Physicians.[153–155]

When administered correctly in appropriate patients, prophylactic anticoagulation is safe and effective with an absolute reduction in the incidence of venous thromboembolism in the range of 40% to 60%. Major bleeding complications occur in less than 1% of patients.

Prevention of venous thromboembolism may also be achieved by the use of mechanical devices. These devices fall into two categories, graduated compression stockings and intermittent pneumatic compression stockings. Although studied less rigorously than pharmacologic methods of prophylaxis, the use of pneumatic compression has been shown in selected patients to be as effective as subcutaneous unfractionated heparin in preventing thrombosis. Mechanical methods of prophylaxis are especially useful in patients at bleeding risk and as an adjunct to pharmacologic methods in patients at high risk of thrombosis.[156]

Whatever form of prophylaxis is used, its intensity should be based on a patient's thrombotic risk determined by both individual and clinical circumstances. Prophylaxis adequate for a 41-year-old patient undergoing an elective appendectomy would be inadequate for a 70-year-old patient with cancer undergoing hip replacement surgery. Risk scores have been developed in an attempt to objectively and quantitatively describe the relative risk of venous thromboembolism in hospitalized patients and to help define the intensity of the prophylactic regimen.[157] The introduction of electronic medical records provides the opportunity to identify patients at risk, to alert the physician, and to develop decision-support, evidence-based recommendations for prophylaxis.

Thromboembolic risk does not necessarily end at the time of hospital discharge. The trend toward early hospital discharge has only served to transfer risk to the outpatient setting. Whether on an inpatient or outpatient basis, prophylaxis should continue until the thrombotic risk has resolved.[158]

The potential for bleeding complications associated with prophylaxis is a common dilemma in surgical or trauma patients, for whom bleeding may occur from the surgical site, especially in the immediate postoperative period. On the other hand, effective prophylaxis depends on timely administration of therapy before a thrombus develops. Recommendations can be drawn from multiple studies with regard to the appropriate timing for anticoagulation in different surgical settings. In cases in which anticoagulation may be delayed, it is customary to use either graduated compression stockings or pneumatic compression devices before surgery begins or as soon as surgery has been completed. Although evidence-based data are lacking, it may be reasonable to consider placement of a retrievable IVC filter in high-risk patients in whom pharmacologic prophylaxis is absolutely contraindicated.

OTHER VARIETIES OF EMBOLIC DISEASE

Because the lung receives all of the blood flow returned from the venous system, the pulmonary vascular bed serves as a "sieve" for all particulate substances entering the venous blood and is the first vascular bed to be exposed to any toxic substance injected intravenously. As a result of its strategic position, the pulmonary vascular bed is, therefore, exposed to a wide variety of potentially obstructing and injurious agents.

■ VENOUS AIR EMBOLISM

An increasingly common form of nonthrombotic embolism in the United States is venous air embolism. The increasing frequency of the problem reflects the wide variety of invasive surgical and medical procedures now available, the broad use of indwelling central venous catheters, the use of positive pressure ventilation with high levels of positive end-expiratory pressure, and the frequency of thoracic and other forms of trauma. The simple inadvertent transection or loss of closure of a large-bore intravenous catheter, particularly in the jugular or subclavian vein, can result in ingress of substantial quantities of air. Air bubbles enter the pulmonary vascular bed and, from there, can enter the arterial system and are diffusely distributed throughout the body by way of either an intracardiac shunt (atrial septal defect, patent foramen ovale) or, more likely, through microvascular pulmonary shunts.

Physiologic consequences are related to the volume of air entrainment and rate of accumulation. An abrupt rise in pulmonary artery pressure and noncardiogenic pulmonary edema may develop, lung compliance falls, and hypoxemia ensues. The symptoms of venous air embolism are variable and nonspecific, and may include alterations in sensorium, chest pain, dyspnea, or a sense of impending doom.[159] These and other consequences appear to be due to two phenomena: actual lodgment of the bubbles in capillary beds that interfere with nutrient supply to the affected organs, and the formation of platelet–fibrin aggregates, creating diffuse microthrombi. Thrombocytopenia may be seen as a consequence of this latter event. The most serious consequences result from cerebral or coronary artery air embolism, the severity of the consequences depending upon the rate and volume of air gaining access to the circulation.

The best approaches to air embolism are prevention and early detection. Treatment consists of measures designed to restore flow and promote reabsorption of the intravascular air.[160] Measures designed to restore flow include patient positioning (Trendelenburg position with the left side down), removal of air through central venous catheters or direct needle aspiration, and closed chest cardiac massage. Measures designed to increase absorption include the use of 100% oxygen and hyperbaric oxygen therapy. Using such aggressive measures, mortality from venous air embolism has been dramatically reduced.

■ FAT EMBOLISM

Fat embolism represents another form of nonthrombotic embolism.[161,162] In its full-blown form, a rather characteristic syndrome follows entry of neutral fat into the vascular system, consisting of dyspnea, hypoxemia, petechiae, and mental confusion. Seizures and focal neurologic deficits have been described. There is a variable lag time of 24 to 72 hours in the onset of the syndrome following the inciting event; rarely, cases occur within 12 hours or as late as 2 weeks after the event.

By far, the most common inciting event is traumatic fracture of long bones, with incidence rising with the number of fractures. However, orthopedic procedures and trauma to other fat-laden tissues (e.g., fatty liver) occasionally can lead to the same syndrome. Although considerably less common, fat embolism syndrome has been reported following both liposuction and lipoinjection procedures.

The basis for the variability in the incidence and severity of the syndrome after apparently comparable injuries has not been well defined, nor has the delay in clinical presentation. The pathophysiologic consequences appear to derive from two events: (1) actual vascular obstruction by neutral particles of fat; and (2) the injurious effects of free fatty acids released by the action of lipases on the neutral fat. The latter effect is probably the more important, causing diffuse vasculitis with leakage from cerebral, pulmonary, and other vascular beds. The time necessary to produce toxic intermediaries may explain the delay from the inciting event to clinical presentation.

The diagnosis of fat embolism syndrome is a clinical one suggested by the constellation of dyspnea, neurologic abnormalities, petechiae, and fever in the proper clinical context. Petechiae, typically distributed over the head, neck, anterior chest, and axillae, are present in only 20% to 50% of cases. Therefore, their absence should not preclude consideration of the disease. No laboratory test is diagnostic of the syndrome. Fat can be demonstrated in the serum of a majority of fracture patients with evidence of fat embolism syndrome. The finding of lipid-laden cells in bronchoalveolar lavage fluid appears to occur commonly in patients with traumatic injuries irrespective of the presence of fat embolism syndrome.

Although a variety of treatments have been suggested (e.g., intravenous ethanol, albumin, dextran, heparin), none has proved effective. The role of corticosteroid therapy to prevent the onset of fat embolism syndrome after an inciting event remains controversial.[163] Supportive treatment, including mechanical ventilatory support when necessary, is the primary approach, and survival is now the rule with meticulous support.

■ AMNIOTIC FLUID EMBOLISM

Another special form of embolism is amniotic fluid embolism, a rare, unpredictable and potentially catastrophic complication of pregnancy. Amniotic fluid embolism is reported to occur in approximately 2.0 per 100,000 deliveries and represents a leading cause of maternal mortality.[164] This disorder occurs during or after delivery when amniotic fluid gains access to uterine venous channels and, therefore, to the pulmonary and general circulations. The delivery may be either spontaneous or by Cesarean section and usually has been uneventful. Most cases occur during labor, but delayed onset of symptoms up to 48 hours after delivery can occur. Advanced maternal age, multiparity, premature placental separation, fetal death, and meconium staining of amniotic fluid have been associated with increased risk of amniotic fluid embolism.

Amniotic fluid embolism syndrome should be suspected with the sudden onset of severe respiratory distress, cyanosis, hypotension, cardiovascular collapse and, often, disseminated intravascular coagulation.[165] Occasionally, seizure activity occurs. It has been postulated that there is a biphasic pattern of hemodynamic disturbance: an initial period of pulmonary hypertension, commonly seen in animal models, followed by left ventricular dysfunction and cardiogenic shock. Patients who survive the first several hours develop noncardiogenic pulmonary edema coincident with improvement in left ventricular dysfunction.[166]

Amniotic fluid contains particulate materials that can cause pulmonary vascular obstruction, but the major pathogenetic mechanism of the syndrome remains uncertain. Amniotic fluid has thromboplastic activity that leads to extensive fibrin deposition in the pulmonary vasculature and, occasionally, other organs. As a consequence of fibrin deposition, severe consumptive coagulopathy develops, including marked hypofibrinogenemia and thrombocytopenia. Following the acute event, an enhanced fibrinolytic state often occurs.

The diagnosis of amniotic fluid embolism is based on a compatible clinical picture, often enhanced by finding amniotic fluid components in the pulmonary circulation. The presence of squamous cells in pulmonary arterial blood, once considered pathognomonic, has proved to be a nonspecific finding. Serologic assays and immunohistochemical staining techniques have been described as having high sensitivity for amniotic fluid embolism.

Although various forms of therapy have been suggested (e.g., antifibrinolytic agents such as aminocaproic acid, cryoprecipitate), the best approach is supportive. Pulmonary artery catheterization is useful to monitor left ventricular function and volume status and to guide the appropriate use of inotropic and vasoactive agents. Even in the setting of aggressive supportive measures, however, maternal mortality has approached 80%.

SEPTIC EMBOLISM

Septic embolism is another special disorder that, unfortunately, is increasing in frequency owing to widespread intravenous drug abuse and the expanding use of indwelling intravenous devices. Previously, septic embolism was almost exclusively a complication of septic pelvic thrombophlebitis due to either septic abortion or postpuerperal uterine infection.[167] However, almost any venous structure can be involved, either as a focus of primary infection or from intravascular or contiguous spread: septic cavernous sinus thrombosis resulting from meningitis, sinusitis, or facial cellulitis; septic portal venous thrombosis resulting from diverticulitis or liver abscess; septic tonsillar or internal jugular venous thrombosis (Lemmiere syndrome) resulting from oropharyngeal infection. Increasingly common causes are those related to intravenous drug use and those that are iatrogenic; namely, infections secondary to indwelling catheters inserted for a variety of diagnostic or therapeutic purposes.[168–170]

Microscopically, septic phlebitis consists of purulent material admixed with fibrin thrombus. Embolization from such material does occur and can result in obstruction of small pulmonary vessels, but the major consequence is pulmonary infection. Characteristically, the chest roentgenogram displays scattered pulmonary infiltrates that undergo cavitation. An increasing number of such infiltrates develop over periods of hours to a few days. Symptoms and signs include fever, dyspnea, cough, pleuritic chest pain, and hemoptysis. Initial treatment consists of appropriate antibiotics. If an indwelling catheter is the source of the infection, it should be removed. If there is not a prompt response to this regimen, surgical isolation of the septic vein, if present, should be considered. The role of systemic anticoagulation remains uncertain. Endocarditis may complicate septic phlebitis, or mimic it, particularly in drug addicts.

TUMOR EMBOLISM

Involvement of the pulmonary vascular bed by tumor cells is not unusual given the frequency with which circulating tumor cells can be identified in patients with a wide range of malignancies and the frequency with which tumor emboli are discovered as an incidental finding at autopsy.[171] Tumor embolism becomes clinically apparent, however, in only a minority of patients with malignancy.

Microvascular tumor embolism is associated with a wide range of malignancies, the most common of which are breast, lung, prostate, stomach, and liver cancer. Tumor embolism of large fragments occurs rarely and may mimic acute thromboembolic disease. In this setting, survival following tumor embolectomy has been reported.

The clinical presentation of microvascular tumor embolism is typically subacute and involves progressive dyspnea, tachycardia, and tachypnea. Jugular venous distention, a prominent P2, tricuspid regurgitation or a right-sided S3 may be present on physical examination if the extent of pulmonary vascular obstruction is sufficient to cause pulmonary hypertension.

The development of pulmonary hypertension is a common accompaniment of symptomatic, microvascular tumor embolism and remains a major cause of mortality. Pulmonary hypertension appears to result from an obliteration of the pulmonary vascular bed by an admixture of tumor cells and thrombus as well as the development of medial hypertrophy, intimal fibrosis, and fibrinoid necrosis encountered in other etiologies of pulmonary hypertension.

Hypoxemia and a compensated respiratory alkalosis are commonly present. The chest radiograph is most often normal but focal or diffuse infiltrates, which may be fleeting, have been described. V/Q scanning most commonly demonstrates a mottled appearance or peripheral, subsegmental defects; segmental or larger defects, indistinguishable from those associated with thromboembolic embolism, may occur in those rare instances of large-vessel involvement. CT may demonstrate peripheral, wedge-shaped defects consistent with infarcts; a pattern of multifocal dilatation and beading of the peripheral pulmonary arteries has been described.[172]

Pulmonary angiographic findings may include delayed vascular filling, pruning, and tortuosity, similar to that seen in other forms of small-vessel pulmonary hypertension. The angiographic findings in large fragment tumor embolism may be indistinguishable from those seen in acute thromboembolic disease.

Pulmonary microvascular cytology on specimens aspirated through a wedged pulmonary artery catheter may demonstrate malignant cells. Positive cytologies, however, can also be obtained in the setting of lymphangitic carcinomatosis. The misidentification of megakaryocytes as tumor cells obtained in this manner has been reported to lead to false-positive results.

Although diagnosis by transbronchial biopsy has been reported, diagnostic confirmation may require surgical lung biopsy. Before proceeding to that step, however, it must be stressed that the impact of early diagnosis on outcome is uncertain. This intervention should only be considered in the setting of a primary malignancy for which effective chemotherapeutic options are available.

The differential diagnosis of tumor embolism includes thrombotic embolism, parenchymal metastasis, lymphangitic carcinomatosis, malignant pericardial effusion, and chemotherapy-related lung toxicity. The premortem diagnosis is often one of exclusion. Parenchymal metastasis, lymphangitic carcinomatosis and chemotherapy-related lung toxicity can be differentiated from tumor embolism by findings on high-resolution CT. Differentiation of tumor embolism from thrombotic embolism may be somewhat more problematic, especially if there is large-vessel involvement.

SICKLE CELL DISEASE

Sickle cell disease affects the lungs by causing local thrombosis and occasionally by embolization of bone marrow elements. Small pulmonary arteries, arterioles, and capillaries are generally affected.[173,174] Thrombosis in the pulmonary circulation is part of the general proclivity of red blood cells containing S hemoglobin to sickle under appropriate circumstances, particularly hypoxia; stagnation and clotting follow sickling. In some instances, the thrombus organizes, the vascular lumen is obliterated, and perivascular fibrosis ensues in the adjacent lung; in others, the thrombus recanalizes. Occasionally, infarction occurs.

Of the factors that predispose to thrombosis in the lungs in sickle cell disease, the most important is the low oxygen saturation of mixed venous blood. Not only is the mixed venous oxygen inordinately low but also the O_2 dissociation curve is shifted to the right, thereby handicapping O_2 uptake in the lungs. Patients with sickle cell disease are prone to develop pneumonia, which, in turn, can lead to local areas of hypoxia favoring sickling and thrombosis in the lung. Patients with severe sickle cell anemia and large fractions of hemoglobin S in their red blood cells are particularly susceptible to intense sickling and thrombosis anywhere, including the lungs. However, vulnerability is not restricted to states of hemoglobin S. In some heterozygous sickle states – for example, hemoglobin SC, S-thalassemia, and hemoglobin SA – enough hemoglobin S is present to cause extensive thrombosis and infarction during an episode of severe hypoxemia, acidosis, or septicemia associated with fever and leukocytosis.

The clinical picture of pulmonary infarction in patients with sickle cell disease can mimic or coexist with bronchopneumonia. An episode often begins with chest pain, fever, and sputum that is blood streaked but fails to disclose any specific bacterial cause. A fleeting episode of breathlessness is usually overlooked. The subsequent course is characterized by an unconvincing response to antibiotics and slow clearing; often a linear scar in the lungs remains as a residue of the infarction.

Distinguishing between in situ thrombosis and thromboembolism can be difficult clinically and even with invasive procedures such as angiography, although in situ thrombosis tends to be in small, distal vessels. Moreover, because radiographic contrast materials may promote sickling, they have to be used cautiously. To complicate matters, some patients with sickle cell disease are also at increased risk of thromboembolism because of predisposing factors, such as bed rest, congestive heart failure, and dehydration.

Sometimes, occlusive disease is sufficiently extensive to cause pulmonary hypertension and cor pulmonale. For this sequence to evolve, many severe episodes of sickling are required. The cor pulmonale that results is unusual because of its association with a high cardiac output (due to anemia) and with the intrinsic myocardial damage that generally complicates sickle cell disease.[175]

Management of the patient with pulmonary thrombosis and infarction in sickle cell disease is largely supportive and includes supplemental oxygen, intravenous hydration, and pain control.

Simple or exchange transfusions are recommended for patients with significant hypoxemia and pulmonary infiltrates (i.e., acute chest syndrome). Anticoagulants are generally not used in sickle cell crisis. Their utility in larger-vessel pulmonary artery thrombosis is uncertain since there are no data to substantiate their effectiveness. Because it implicates large vessels' occlusion, pulmonary artery thrombosis during acute chest syndrome should be amenable to the same therapeutic approach as currently used for venous thromboembolic disease.[174]

■ OTHER EMBOLI

Because of its sieve function, the lung may also be the target of embolization by a wide variety of other materials.[176–179] Trophoblastic tissue can escape the uterus and lodge in the pulmonary circulation during pregnancy. After head trauma, brain tissue has been found in the lungs; the same is true of liver cells following abdominal trauma and bone marrow after cardiopulmonary resuscitation.

Finally, noninfectious vasculitic–thrombotic complications are seen in association with the intravenous use of drugs intended for oral use. Medications associated with pulmonary complications include methylphenidate hydrochloride, oral opiates (pentazocine, meperidine), and antihistamines. Particulate and irritant drug carriers (e.g., talc, cellulose) and occasionally the drugs themselves may cause vascular inflammation and secondary thrombosis. The clinical presentation may be diverse and includes lower lobe emphysema, diffuse interstitial fibrosis, and progressive massive fibrosis. Repetitive insults may lead to severe and irreversible pulmonary hypertension. In many intravenous drug users, perfusion scans demonstrate segmental or smaller defects. Distinguishing these defects from those due to venous thromboembolism may be difficult.

The diagnosis is often suggested by the clinical history. Radiographic findings include small, diffuse, well-defined nodular densities. These nodules can progress and massive fibrosis may ensue. Lower lobe emphysematous changes may also be present. Diagnostic confirmation often requires transbronchial or surgical lung biopsy. Occasionally, fine crystalline deposits may be seen in the retinal microvasculature on funduscopic examination, confirming the diagnosis noninvasively. The prognosis is generally poor with most patients experiencing progressive pulmonary disease.

REFERENCES

1. Silverstein MD, Heit JA, Mohr DN, Petterson TM, O'Fallon WM, Melton LJ IIIrd. Trends in the incidence of deep vein thrombosis and pulmonary embolism: a 25-year population-based study. *Arch Intern Med.* 1998;23:585–593.
2. Anderson FA Jr, Wheeler HB, Goldberg RJ, et al. A population-based perspective of the hospital incidence and case-fatality rates of deep vein thrombosis and pulmonary embolism: the Worcester DVT Study. *Arch Intern Med.* 1991;151:933–938.
3. Stein PD, Matta F, Muzammil MH, Diaczok B. Silent pulmonary embolism in patients with deep venous thrombosis: a systematic review. *Am J Med.* 2010;123:426–431.
4. Dalen JE, Alpert JS. Natural history of pulmonary embolism. *Prog Cardiovasc Dis.* 1975;17:259–270.
5. Masuda EM, Kistner RL, Musikasinthorn C, Liquido F, Geling O, He Q. The controversy of managing calf vein thrombosis. *J Vasc Surg.* 2012;55:550–561.
6. Mai C, Hunt D. Upper-extremity deep venous thrombosis: a review. *Am J Med.* 2011;124:402–407.
7. Torbicki A, GaliéN MD, Covezzoli A, et al. Right heart thrombi in pulmonary embolism. Results from the international cooperative pulmonary embolism registry. *J Am Coll Cardiol.* 2003;41:2245–2251.
8. Prevention of fatal postoperative pulmonary embolism by low doses of heparin. An international multicentre trial. *Lancet.* 1975;2:45–51.
9. Freedman KB, Brookenthal KR, Fitzgerald RH Jr., Williams S, Lonner JH. A meta-analysis of thromboembolic prophylaxis following elective total hip arthroplasty. *J Bone Joint Surg Am.* 2000;82-A:929–938.
10. Samama MM, Cohen AT, Darmon JY, et al. A comparison of enoxaparin with placebo for the prevention of venous thromboembolism in acutely ill medical patients. Prophylaxis in Medical Patients with Enoxaparin Study Group. *N Engl J Med.* 1999;341:793–800.
11. Chandra D, Parisini E, Mozaffarian D. Meta-analysis: travel and risk for venous thromboembolism. *Ann Intern Med.* 2009;151:180–190.
12. Kuipers S, Schreijer AJM, Cannegieter SC, Büller HR, Rosendaal FR, Middeldorp S. Travel and venous thrombosis: a systematic review. *J Intern Med.* 2007;262:615–634.
13. Marik PE. Venous thromboembolism in pregnancy. *Clin Chest Med.* 2010;31:731–740.
14. Pomp ER, Lenselink AM, Rosendaal FR, Doggen CJ. Pregnancy, the postpartum period and prothrombotic defects: risk of venous thrombosis in the MEGA study. *J Thromb Haemost.* 2008;6:632–637.
15. Vandenbroucke JP, Rosing J, BloemenkampK W, et al. Oral contraceptives and the risk of venous thrombosis. *N Engl J Med.* 2001;344:1527–1535.
16. Pomp ER, le Cessie S, Rosendaal FR, et al. Risk of venous thrombosis: obesity and its joint effect with oral contraceptive use and prothrombotic mutations. *Br J Haematol.* 2007;139:289–296.
17. Canonico M, Plu-Bureau G, Lowe GD, Scarabin PY. Hormone replacement therapy and risk of venous thromboembolism in postmenopausal women: systematic review and meta-analysis. *BMJ.* 2008;336:1227–1231.
18. Goldhaber SZ, Grodstein F, Stampfer MJ, et al. A prospective study of risk factors for pulmonary embolism in women. *JAMA.* 1997;277:642–645.

19. Ageno W, Becattini C, Brighton T, Selby R, Kamphuisen PW. Cardiovascular risk factors and venous thromboembolism: a meta-analysis. *Circulation*. 2008;117:93–102.

20. Stein PD, Hull RD, Kayali F, Ghali WA, Alshab AK, Olson RE. Venous thromboembolism according to age: the impact of an aging population. *Arch Intern Med*. 2004;164:2260–2265.

21. Monreal M, Lensing AW, Prins MH, et al. Screening for occult cancer in patients with acute deep vein thrombosis or pulmonary embolism. *J Thromb Haemost*. 2004;2:876–881.

22. Kleinjan A, van Doormaal FF, Prins MH, Büller HR, Otten JM. Limitations of screening for occult cancer in patients with idiopathic venous thromboembolism. *Neth J Med*. 2012;70(7): 311–317.

23. Leone G, Sica S, Chiusolo P, Teofili L, De Stefano V. Blood cell diseases and thrombosis. *Haematologica*. 2001;86: 1236–1244.

24. Hillmen P, Lewis SM, Bessler M, Luzzatto L, Dacie JV. Natural history of paroxysmal nocturnal hemoglobinuria. *N Engl J Med*. 1995;333:1253–1258.

25. Galli M, Luciani D, Bertolin G, Barbui T. Lupus anticoagulants are stronger risk factors for thrombosis than anticardiolipin antibodies in the antiphospholipid syndrome: a systematic review of the literature. *Blood*. 2003;101:1827–1832.

26. Fadi Kayali F, Najjar R, Aswad F, Matta F, Stein PD. Venous thromboembolism in patients hospitalized with nephrotic syndrome. *Am J Med*. 2008;121:226–230.

27. Saleh T, Matta F, Yaekoub AY, Danescu S, Stein PD. Risk of venous thromboembolism with inflammatory bowel disease. *Clin Appl Thromb Hemost*. 2011;17:254–258.

28. Ha C, Magowan S, Accorrt N, Chen J, Stone CD. Risk of arterial thrombotic events in inflammatory bowel disease. *Am J Gastroenterol*. 2009;104:1445–1451.

29. Dahlback B, Carlsson M, Svensson PJ. Familial thrombophilia due to a previously unrecognized mechanism characterized by poor anticoagulant response to activated protein C: prediction of a cofactor to activated protein C. *Proc Natl Acad Sci*. 1993;90:1004–1008.

30. Jacobsen AF, Dahm A, Bergrem A, Jacobsen EM, Sandset PM. Risk of venous thrombosis in pregnancy among carriers of the factor V Leiden and the prothrombin gene G20210 A polymorphisms. *J Thromb Haemost*. 2010;8:2443–2449.

31. Vandenbroucke JP, Koster T, Rosendall FR, Reitsma PH, Bertina RM, Rosendaal FR. Increased risk of venous thrombosis in oral-contraceptive users who are carriers of factor V Leiden mutation. *Lancet*. 1994;344:1453–1457.

32. Poort SR, Rosendaal FR, Reitsma PH, Bertina RM. A common genetic variation in the 3′-untranslated region of the prothrombin gene is associated with elevated plasma prothrombin and an increase in venous thrombosis. *Blood*. 1996;88: 3698–3703.

33. McIntrye KM, Sasahara AA. Hemodynamic and ventricular response to pulmonary embolism. *Prog Cardiovasc Dis*. 1974;17: 175–180.

34. McIntrye KM, Sasahara AA. The hemodynamic response to pulmonary embolism in patients without prior cardiopulmonary disease. *Am J Cardiol*. 1971;17:288–294.

35. Elliott CG. Pulmonary physiology during pulmonary embolism. *Chest*. 1992;101:163S–171S.

36. Wood KE. Major pulmonary embolism: review of a pathophysiologic approach to the golden hour of hemodynamically significant pulmonary embolism. *Chest*. 2002;121:877–905.

37. Smulders YM. Pathophysiology and treatment of haemodynamic instability in acute pulmonary embolism: the pivotal role of pulmonary vasoconstriction. *Cardiovasc Res*. 2000;48:23–33.

38. Tsang JY, Lamm WJ. Estimation of endothelin-mediated vasoconstriction in acute pulmonary thromboembolism. *Pulm Circ*. 2012;2:67–74.

39. Nijkeuter M, Hovens MM, Davidson BL, Huisman MV. Resolution of thromboemboli in patients with acute pulmonary embolism. A systematic review. *Chest*. 2006;129: 192–197.

40. Wartski M, Collignon MA. Incomplete recovery of lung perfusion after 3 months in patients with acute pulmonary embolism treated with antithrombotic agents. *J Nucl Med*. 2000;41: 1043–1048.

41. Santolicandro A, Prediletto R, Fornai E, et al. Mechanisms of hypoxemia and hypocapnia in pulmonary embolism. *Am J Respir Crit Care Med*. 1995;152:336–347.

42. Manier G, Castaing Y, Guenard H. Determinants of hypoxemia during the acute phase of pulmonary embolism in humans. *Am J Respir Crit Care Med*. 1985;132:332–338.

43. Katsumura Y, Ohtsubo KI. Correlation between clinical and pathological features of pulmonary thromboemboli and the development of infarcts. *Respirology*. 1998;3:203–206.

44. The PIOPED Investigators. Value of the ventilation/perfusion scan in acute pulmonary embolism. Results of the prospective investigation of pulmonary embolism diagnosis (PIOPED). *JAMA*. 1990;263:2753–2759.

45. Stein PD, Terrin ML, Hales CA, et al. Clinical, laboratory, roentgenographic, and electrocardiographic findings in patients with acute pulmonary embolism and no pre-existing cardiac or pulmonary disease. *Chest*. 1991;100:598–603.

46. Stein PD, Beemath A, Matta F, et al. Clinical characteristics of patients with acute pulmonary embolism: data from PIOPED II. *Am J Med*. 2007;120:871–879.

47. Wiener RS, Schwartz LM, Woloshin S. Time trends in pulmonary embolism in the United States. *Arch Intern Med*. 2011;171: 831–837.

48. Fedullo PF, Auger WR, Kerr KM, Rubin LJ. Chronic thromboembolic pulmonary hypertension. *N Engl J Med*. 2001;345: 1465–1472.

49. Daniela Poli D, Grifoni E, Antonucci E, et al. Incidence of recurrent venous thromboembolism and of chronic thromboembolic pulmonary hypertension in patients after a first episode of pulmonary embolism. *J Thromb Thrombolysis*. 2010;30: 294–299.

50. Stein PD, Afzal A, Henry JW, Villareal CG. Fever in acute pulmonary embolism. *Chest*. 2000;117;39–42.

51. Wells PS, Anderson DR, Rodger M, et al. Derivation of a simple clinical model to categorize patients probability of pulmonary embolism: increasing the models utility with the SimpliRED D-dimer. *Thromb Haemost*. 2000;83:416–420.

52. Wicki J, Perneger TV, Junod AF, Bounameaux H, Perrier A. Assessing clinical probability of pulmonary embolism in the emergency ward: a simple score. *Arch Intern Med*. 2001;161: 92–97.

53. Le Gal G, Righini M, Roy PM, et al. Prediction of pulmonary embolism in the emergency department: the revised Geneva score. *Ann Intern Med*. 2006;144:165–171.

54. Miniati M, Monti S, Bottai M. A structured clinical model for predicting the probability of pulmonary embolism. *Am J Med*. 2003;114:173–179.

55. Kline JA, Courney DM, Kabrhel C, et al. Prospective multicenter evaluation of the pulmonary embolism rule-out criteria. *J Thromb Haemost.* 2008;6:772–780.

56. Kline JA, Nelson RD, Jackson RE, Courtney DM. Criteria for the safe use of D-dimer testing in emergency department patients with suspected pulmonary embolism. A multicenter US study. *Ann Emerg Med.* 2002;39:144–152.

57. Afzal A, Noor HA, Gill SA, Brawner C, Stein PD. Leukocytosis in acute pulmonary embolism. *Chest.* 1999;115:1329–1332.

58. Rodger MA, Carrier M, Jones GN, et al. Diagnostic value of arterial blood gas measurement in suspected pulmonary embolism. *Am J Respir Crit Care Med.* 2000;162:2105–2108.

59. Stein PD, Goldhaber SZ, Henry JW, Miller AC. Arterial blood gas analysis in the assessment of suspected acute pulmonary embolism. *Chest.* 1996;109:78–81.

60. Daniel KR, Courtney DM, Kline JA. Assessment of cardiac stress from massive pulmonary embolism with 12-lead ECG. *Chest.* 2001;120:474–481.

61. Ferrari E, Imbert A, Chevalier T, Mihoubi A, Morand P, Baudouy M. The ECG in pulmonary embolism. Predictive value of negative T waves in precordial leads–80 case reports. *Chest.* 1997;111:537–543.

62. Worsley DF, Alavi A, Aronchick JM, Chen JT, Greenspan RH, Ravin CE. Chest radiographic findings in patients with acute pulmonary embolism: observations from the PIOPED Study. *Radiology.* 1993;189:133–136.

63. Roy PM, Colombet I, Durieux P, Chatellier G, Sors H, Meyer G. Systematic review and meta-analysis of strategies for the diagnosis of suspected pulmonary embolism. *BMJ.* 2005;331: 259.

64. Lucassen W, Geersing GJ, Erkens PM, et al. Clinical decision rules for excluding pulmonary embolism: a meta-analysis. *Ann Intern Med.* 2011;155:448–460.

65. Rathbun SW, Whitsett TL, Vesely SK, Raskob GE. Clinical utility of D-dimer in patients with suspected pulmonary embolism and nondiagnostic lung scans or negative CT findings. *Chest.* 2004;125:851–855.

66. Heim SW, Schectman JM, Siadaty MS, Philbrick JT. D-dimer testing for deep venous thrombosis: a metaanalysis. *Clin Chem.* 2004;50:1136–1147.

67. Revel MP, Cohen S, Sanchez O, et al. Pulmonary embolism during pregnancy: diagnosis with lung scintigraphy or CT angiography. *Radiology.* 2011;258:590–598.

68. Miniati M, Monti S, Pratali L, et al. Value of transthoracic echocardiography in the diagnosis of pulmonary embolism: results of a prospective study in unselected patients. *Am J Med.* 2001;110:528–535.

69. Konstantinides S, Geibel A, Heusel G, et al. Heparin plus alteplase compared with heparin alone in patients with submassive pulmonary embolism. *N Engl J Med.* 2002;347:1143–1150.

70. Grifoni S, Olivotto I, Cecchini P, et al. Short-term clinical outcome of patients with acute pulmonary embolism, normal blood pressure, and echocardiographic right ventricular dysfunction. *Circulation.* 2000;101:2817–2822.

71. Pruszczyk P, Torbicki A, Kuch-Wocial A, Szulc M, Pacho R. Diagnostic value of transoesophageal echocardiography in suspected haemodynamically significant pulmonary embolism. *Heart.* 2001;85:628–634.

72. Kearon C, Ginsberg JS, Hirsh J. The role of venous ultrasonography in the diagnosis of suspected deep venous thrombosis and pulmonary embolism. *Ann Intern Med.* 1998;129:1044–1049.

73. Kassai B, Boissel JP, Cucherat M, Sonie S, Shah NR, Leizorovicz A. A systematic review of the accuracy of ultrasound in the diagnosis of deep venous thrombosis in asymptomatic patients. *Thromb Haemost.* 2004;91:655–666.

74. Girard P, Sanchez O, Leroyer C, et al. Deep venous thrombosis in patients with acute pulmonary embolism. Prevalence, risk factors, and clinical significance. *Chest.* 2005;128:1593–1600.

75. Pomero F, Brignone C, Serraino C, et al. Venous lower-limb evaluation in patients with acute pulmonary embolism. *South Med J.* 2011;104:405–411.

76. Barrellier MT, Lezin B, Landy S, Le Hello C. Prevalence of duplex ultrasonography detectable venous thrombosis in patients with suspected or acute pulmonary embolism. *J Mal Vasc.* 2001;26:23–30.

77. Turkstra F, Kuijer PM, van Beek EJ, Brandjes DP, ten Cate JW, Büller HR. Diagnostic utility of ultrasonography of leg veins in patients suspected of having pulmonary embolism. *Ann Intern Med.* 1997;126:775–781.

78. Goodman LR, Stein PD, Matta F, et al. CT venography and compression sonography are diagnostically equivalent: data from PIOPED II. *AJR Am J Roentgenol.* 2007;189:1071–1076.

79. Stein PD, Chenevert TL, Fowler SE, et al. Gadolinium-enhanced magnetic resonance angiography for pulmonary embolism: a multicenter prospective study (PIOPED III). *Ann Intern Med.* 2010;152:434–443.

80. Kaewlai R, Abujudeh H. Neprhogenic systemic fibrosis. *AJR Am J Roentgenol.* 2012;199:W17–W23.

81. Anderson DR, Kahn SR, Rodger MA, et al. Computed tomographic pulmonary angiography vs ventilation-perfusion lung scanning in patients with suspected pulmonary embolism: a randomized controlled trial. *JAMA.* 2007;298:2743–2753.

82. Stein PD, Goodman LR, Hull RD, Dalen JE, Matta F. Diagnosis and management of isolated subsegmental pulmonary embolism: review and assessment of the options. *Clin Appl Thromb Hemost.* 2012;18:20–26.

83. Crichlow A, Cuker A, Mill AM. Overuse of computed tomography pulmonary angiography in the evaluation of patients with suspected pulmonary embolism in the emergency department. *Acad Emerg Med.* 2012;19:1220–1226.

84. Stein PD, Athanasoulis C, Alavi A, et al. Complications and validity of pulmonary angiography in acute pulmonary embolism. *Circulation.* 1992;85:462–468.

85. Bruinstroop E, van de Ree MA, Huisman MV. The use of D-dimer in specific clinical conditions: a narrative review. *Eur J of Intern Med.* 2009;20:441–446.

86. Zondag W, Mos IC, Creemers-Schild D, et al. Outpatient treatment in patients with acute pulmonary embolism: the Hestia Study. *J Thromb Haemost.* 2011;9:1500–1507.

87. Hull RD, Raskob GE, Brant, RF, Pineo GF, Valentine KA. Relation between the time to achieve the lower limit of the APTT therapeutic range and recurrent venous thromboembolism during heparin treatment for deep vein thrombosis. *Arch Intern Med.* 1997;157:2562–2568.

88. Raschke RA, Reilly BM, Guidry JR, Fontana JR, Srinivas S. The weight-based heparin dosing nomogram compared with a "standard care" nomogram. A randomized controlled trial. *Ann Intern Med.* 1993;119(9):874–881.

89. Kearon C, Ginsberg JS, Julian JA, et al. Comparison of fixed-dose weight-adjusted unfractionated heparin and low-molecular-weight heparin for acute treatment of venous thromboembolism. *JAMA.* 2006;296(8):935–942.

90. Quinlan DJ, McQuillan A, Eikelboom JW. Low-molecular-weight heparin compared with intravenous unfractionated heparin for treatment of pulmonary embolism. A meta-analysis of randomized, controlled trials. *Ann Intern Med.* 2004;140:175–183.

91. Erkens PM, Prins MH. Fixed dose subcutaneous low molecular weight heparins versus adjusted dose unfractionated heparin for venous thromboembolism. *Cochrane Database Syst Rev.* 2010;9:CD001100.

92. Hirsh J, Bauer KA, Donati MB, Samama MM, Weitz JI; American College of Chest Physicians. Parenteral anticoagulants. American College of Chest Physicians Evidence-Based Clinical Practice Guidelines (8th edition). *Chest.* 2008;133: 141S–159S.

93. The Matisse Investigators. Subcutaneous fondaparinux versus intravenous unfractionated heparin in the initial treatment of pulmonary embolism. *N Engl J Med.* 2003;349:1695–702.

94. Bauersachs R, Berkowitz SD, Brenner B, et al. Oral rivaroxaban for symptomatic venous thromboembolism. *N Engl J Med.* 2010;363: 2499–2510.

95. EINSTEIN-PE investigators. Oral rivaroxaban for the treatment of symptomatic pulmonary embolism. *N Engl J Med.* 2012;366: 1287–1297.

96. Becattini C, Vedovati MC, Agnelli G. Old and new oral anticoagulants for venous thromboembolism and atrial fibrillation: a review of the literature. *Thromb Res.* 2012;129:392–400.

97. Linkins L-A, Dans AL, Moores LK, et al. Treatment and prevention of heparin-induced thrombocytopenia: Antithrombotic Therapy and Prevention of Thrombosis, 9th ed: American College of Chest Physicians Evidence-Based Clinical Practice Guidelines. *Chest.* 2012;141:e495S–e530S.

98. Nagler M, Haslauer M, Wuillemin WA. Fondaparinux – data on efficacy and safety in special situations. *Thromb Res.* 2012;129: 407–417.

99. The Steering Committee. Single-bolus tenecteplase plus heparin compared with heparin alone for normotensive patients with acute pulmonary embolism who have evidence of right ventricular dysfunction and myocardial injury: Rationale and design of the Pulmonary Embolism Thrombolysis (PEITHO) trial. *Am Heart J.* 2012;163:33–38.

100. Wan S, Agnelli G, Quinlan DJ, Eikelboom JW. Thrombolysis compared with heparin for the initial treatment of pulmonary embolism: a meta-analysis of the randomized controlled trials. *Circulation.* 2004;110:744–749.

101. Goldhaber SZ, Visani L, De Rosa M. Acute pulmonary embolism: clinical outcomes in the international cooperative pulmonary embolism registry (ICOPER). *Lancet.* 1999;353: 1386–1389.

102. Jimenez D, Aujesky D, Yusen RD. Risk stratification of normotensive patients with acute symptomatic pulmonary embolism. *Br J Haematol.* 2010;151:415–424.

103. Sanchez O, Trinquart L, Colombet I, et al. Prognostic value of right ventricular dysfunction in patients with haemodynamically stable pulmonary embolism: a systematic review. *Eur Heart J.* 2008;29:1569–1577.

104. Aujesky D, Obrosky DS, Stone RA, et al. Derivation and validation of a prognostic model for pulmonary embolism. *Am J Respir Crit Care Med.* 2005;172:1041–1046.

105. Jimenez D, Aujesky S, Moores L, et al. Simplification of the pulmonary embolism severity index for prognostication in patients with acute symptomatic pulmonary embolism. *Arch Intern Med.* 2010;170:1383–1389.

106. Lin PH, Ochoa LN, Duffy P. Catheter-directed thrombectomy and thrombolysis for symptomatic lower-extremity deep vein thrombosis: review of current interventional treatment strategies. *Perspect Vasc Surg Endovasc Ther.* 2010;22:152–163.

107. Kuo WT, Gould MK, Louie JD, Rosenberg JK, Sze DY, Hofmann LV. Catheter-directed therapy for the treatment of massive pulmonary embolism: systematic review and meta-analysis of modern techniques. *Vasc Interv Radiol.* 2009;20:1431–1440.

108. Uflacker R. Interventional therapy for pulmonary embolism. *J Vasc Interv Radiol.* 2001;12:147–164.

109. Stein PD, Matta F. Case fatality rate with pulmonary embolectomy for acute pulmonary embolism. *Am J Med.* 2012;125:471–477.

110. Finazzi G, Marchioli R, Brancaccio V, et al. A randomized clinical trial of high-intensity warfarin vs. conventional antithrombotic therapy for the prevention of recurrent thrombosis in patients with the antiphospholipid syndrome (WAPS). *J Thromb Haemost.* 2005;3:848–853.

111. Crowther MA, Ginsberg JS, Julian J, et al. A comparison of two intensities of warfarin for the prevention of recurrent thrombosis in patients with the antiphospholipid antibody syndrome. *N Engl J Med.* 2003;349:1113–1138.

112. Sallah S, Thomas D, Roberts HR. Warfarin and heparin induced skin necrosis and the purple toe syndrome: infrequent complications of anticoagulant treatment. *Thromb Haemost.* 1997;78:785–790.

113. Holbrook AM, Pereira JA, Labiris R, et al. Systematic overview of warfarin and its drug and food interactions. *Arch Intern Med.* 2005;165:1095–1106.

114. Crowther MA, Ginsberg JB, Kearon C, et al. A randomized trial comparing 5-mg and 10-mg warfarin loading doses. *Arch Intern Med.* 1999;159:46–48.

115. Kovacs MJ, Rodger M, Anderson DR, et al. Comparison of 10-mg and 5-mg warfarin initiation nomograms together with low-molecular weight heparin for outpatient treatment of acute venous thromboembolism. A randomized, double-blind, controlled trial. *Ann Intern Med.* 2003;138:714–719.

116. Monkman K, Lazo-Langner A, Kovacs MJ. A 10 mg warfarin initiation nomogram is safe and effective in outpatients starting oral anticoagulant therapy for venous thromboembolism. *Thromb Res.* 2009;124:275–280.

117. Garcia DA, Witt DM, Hylek E, et al. Delivery of optimized anticoagulant therapy: consensus statement from the anticoagulation forum. *Ann Pharmacother.* 2008;42:979–988.

118. Heneghan C, Alonso-Coello P, Garcia-Alamino JM, et al. Self-monitoring of oral anticoagulation: a systematic review and meta-analysis. *Lancet.* 2006;367:404–411.

119. Prandoni P, Lensing AW, Piccioli A, et al. Recurrent venous thromboembolism and bleeding complications during anticoagulant treatment in patients with cancer and venous thrombosis. *Blood.* 2002;100:3484–3488.

120. Kearon C, Kahn SR, Agnelli G, Goldhaber S, Raskob GE, Comerota AJ. Antithrombotic therapy for venous thromboembolic disease: American College of Chest Physicians Evidence-Based Clinical Practice Guidelines (8th edition). *Chest.* 2008;133(Suppl 6):454S–545S.

121. Schulman S, Kearon C, Kakkar AK, et al. Dabigatran versus warfarin in the treatment of acute venous thromboembolism. *N Engl J Med.* 2009;361:2342–2352.

122. Agnelli G, Buller HR, Cohen A, et al. Apixaban for extended treatment of venous thromboembolism. *N Engl J Med.* 2013;368: 699–708.

123. Becattini C, Agnelli GA, Schenone A, et al. Aspirin for preventing the recurrence of venous thromboembolism. *N Engl J Med.* 2012;366:1959–1967.

124. Brighton TA, Eikelboom JW, Mann K, et al. Low-dose aspirin for preventing recurrent venous thromboembolism. *N Engl J Med.* 2012;367:1979–1987.

125. Lorio A, Kearon C, Filippucci E, et al. Risk of recurrence after a first episode of symptomatic venous thromboembolism provoked by a transient risk factor. *Arch Intern Med.* 2010;170:1710–1716.

126. Kearon C. Extended anticoagulation for unprovoked venous thromboembolism: a majority of patients should be treated. *J Thromb Thrombolysis.* 2011;31:295–300.

127. Bauer KA. Long-term management of venous thromboembolism: a 61-year-old woman with unprovoked venous thromboembolism. *JAMA.* 2011;305:1336–1345.

128. Ho WK, Hankey GJ, Quinlan DJ, Eikelboom JW. Risk of recurrent venous thromboembolism in patients with common thrombophilia: a systematic review. *Arch Intern Med.* 2006; 166:729–736.

129. Kyrle PA, Rosendaal FR, Eichinger S. Risk assessment for recurrent venous thrombosis. *Lancet.* 2010;376:2032–2039.

130. Pabinger I, Schneider B. Thrombotic risk in hereditary antithrombin III, protein C, or protein S deficiency. A cooperative, retrospective study. Gesellschaft fur Thrombose- und Hamostaseforschung (GTH) Study Group on Natural Inhibitors. *Arterioscler Thromb Vasc Biol.* 1996;16:742–748.

131. Stein PD, Matta F, Hull RD. Increasing use of vena cava filters for prevention of pulmonary embolism. *Am J Med.* 2011;124: 655–661.

132. Mission JF, Kerlan RK, Tan JH, Fang MC. Rates and predictors of plans for inferior vena cava filter retrieval in hospitalized patients. *J Gen Intern Med.* 2010;25:321–325.

133. Hirsch J, Guyatt G, Albers GW, Harrington R, Schunemann HJ; American College of Chest Physicians. Executive summary: American College of Chest Physicians Evidence-Based Clinical Practice Guidelines (8th edition). *Chest.* 2008;133 (6 Suppl):71S–109S.

134. Kaufman JA, Kinney TB, Streiff MB, et al. Guidelines for the use of retrievable and convertible vena cava filters: report from the Society of Interventional Radiology multidisciplinary consensus conference. *J Vasc Interv Radiol.* 2006;17: 449–459.

135. Girard P, Stern JB, Parent F. Medical literature and vena cava filters: so far so weak. *Chest.* 2002;122:963–967.

136. Decousus H, Leizorovicz A, Parent F, et al. A clinical trial of vena caval filters in the prevention of pulmonary embolism in patients with proximal deep-vein thrombosis. *N Engl J Med.* 1998;338:409–415.

137. PREPIC Study Group. Eight-year follow-up of patients with permanent vena cava filters in the prevention of pulmonary embolism: the PREPIC (Prevention du Risque d'Embolie Pulmonaire par Interruption Cave) randomized study. *Circulation.* 2005;112:416–422.

138. Gorman PH, Qadri SFA, Rao-Patel A. Prophylactic inferior vena cava (IVC) filter placement may increase the relative risk of deep venous thrombosis after acute spinal cord injury. *J Trauma.* 2009;66:707–712.

139. Fox MA, Kahn SR. Postthrombotic syndrome in relation to vena cava filter placement: a systematic review. *J Vasc Interv Radiol.* 2008;19:981–985.

140. Miniati M, Monti S, Bottai M, et al. Survival and restoration of pulmonary perfusion in a long-term follow-up of patients after pulmonary embolism. *Medicine (Baltimore).* 2006;85:253–262.

141. Pengo V, Lensing AWA, Prins MH, et al. Incidence of chronic thromboembolic pulmonary hypertension after pulmonary embolism. *N Engl J Med.* 2004;350;2257–2264.

142. Becattini C, Agnelli G, Pesavento R, et al. Incidence of chronic thromboembolic pulmonary hypertension after a first episode of pulmonary embolism. *Chest.* 2006;130:172–175.

143. Klok F, van KK, van DA, Heyning FH, Vliegen HW, Huisman MV. Prospective cardiopulmonary screening program to detect chronic thromboembolic pulmonary hypertension in patients after acute pulmonary embolism. *Haematologica.* 2010;95:970–975.

144. Lang I, Kerr KM. Risk factors for chronic thromboembolic pulmonary hypertension. *Proc Am Thorac Soc.* 2006;3:568–570.

145. Wolf M, Boyer-Neumann C, Parent F, et al. Thrombotic risk factors in pulmonary hypertension. *Eur Resp J.* 2000;15:395–399.

146. Fedullo PF, Kerr KM, Kim NH, Auger WR. Chronic thromboembolic pulmonary hypertension. *Am J Resp Crit Care Med.* 2011;183:1605–1613.

147. Riedel M, Stanek V, Widimsky J, Prerovsky I. Long-term follow-up of patients with pulmonary thromboembolism: late prognosis and evolution of hemodynamic and respiratory data. *Chest.* 1982;81:151–158.

148. Lewczuk J, Piszko P, Jagas J, et al. Prognostic factors in medically treated patients with chronic pulmonary embolism. *Chest.* 2001;119:818–823.

149. Madani MM, Auger WR, Pretorius P, et al. Pulmonary endarterectomy: recent changes in a single institution's experience of more than 2,700 patients. *Ann Thorac Surg.* 2012;94:97–103.

150. Freed DH, Thomson BM, Berman M, et al. Survival after pulmonary thromboendarterectomy: effect of residual pulmonary hypertension. *J Thorac Cardiovasc Surg.* 2011;141:383–387.

151. Tapson VF, Decousus H, Pini M, et al. Venous thromboembolism prophylaxis in acutely ill hospitalized medical patients. Findings from the International Medical Prevention Registry on Venous Thromboembolism. *Chest.* 2007;132:936–945.

152. Bergmann JF, Cohen AT, Tapson VF, et al. Venous thromboembolism risk and prophylaxis. *Thromb Haemost.* 2010;103(4): 736–748.

153. Gould MK, Garcia DA, Wren SM, et al. Prevention of venous thromboembolism in nonorthopedic surgical patients. Antithrombotic Therapy and Prevention of Thrombosis, 9th ed: American College of Chest Physicians Evidence-Based Clinical Practice Guidelines. *Chest.* 2012;141(2 Suppl):e227S–e277S.

154. Falck-Ytter Y, Francis CW, Johanson NA, et al. Prevention of venous thromboembolism in orthopedic surgery patients. Antithrombotic Therapy and Prevention of Thrombosis, 9th ed: American College of Chest Physicians Evidence-Based Clinical Practice Guidelines. *Chest.* 2012;141(2 Suppl):e278S–e325S.

155. Kahn SR, Lim W, Dunn AS, et al. Prevention of venous thromboembolism in nonsurgical Patients. Antithrombotic Therapy and Prevention of Thrombosis, 9th ed: American College of Chest Physicians Evidence-Based Clinical Practice Guidelines. *Chest.* 2012;141(2 Suppl):e195S–e226S.

156. Lippi G, Favaloro EJ, Cervellin G. Prevention of venous thromboembolism: focus on mechanical prophylaxis. *Semin Thromb Hemost.* 2011;37(3):237–251.

157. Caprini JA. Risk assessment as a guide for the prevention of the many faces of venous thromboembolism. *Am J Surg*. 2010;199: S3–S10.

158. Huo MH, Muntz J. Extended thromboprophylaxis with low-molecular-weight heparins after hospital discharge in high-risk surgical and medical patients: a review. *Clin Ther*. 2009;31: 1129–1141.

159. van Hulst RA, Klein J, Lachmann B. Gas embolism: pathophysiology and treatment. *Clin Physiol Funct Imaging*. 2003;23: 237–246.

160. Mirski MA, Lele AV, Fitzsimmons L, Toung T. Diagnosis and treatment of vascular air embolism. *Anesthesiology*. 2007;106: 164–177.

161. Gossling HR, Pellegrin VD. Fat embolism syndrome. A review of the pathophysiology and physiological basis of treatment. *Clin Orthop*. 1982;165:68–82.

162. Parisi DM, Koval K, Egol K. Fat embolism syndrome. *Am J Orthop*. 2002;31:507–512.

163. Bederman SS, Bhandari M, McKee MD, Schemitsch EH. Do corticosteroids reduce the risk of fat embolism syndrome in patients with long bone fractures? A meta-analysis. *Can J Surg*. 2009;52:386–393.

164. Knight M, Tuffnell D, Brocklehurst P, Spark P, Kurinczuk JJ; UK Obstetric Surveillance System. Incidence and risk factors for amniotic-fluid embolism. *Obstet Gynecol*. 2010;115:910–917.

165. Conde-Agudelo A, Romero R. Amniotic fluid embolism: an evidence-based review. *Am J Obstet Gynecol*. 2009;201:445.e1–13.

166. Clark SL, Montz FJ, Phelan JP. Hemodynamic alterations associated with amniotic fluid embolism: a reappraisal. *Am J Obstet Gynecol*. 1985;151:617–621.

167. Julander I. Staphylococcal septicaemia and endocarditis in 80 drug users. *Scand J Infect Dis*. 1983;41:49–54.

168. Raad I, Hanna H, Maki D. Intravascular catheter-related infections: advances in diagnosis, prevention and management. *Lancet Infec Dis*. 2007;7:645–657.

169. Oim GM, Jeffrey RB Jr, Ralls PW, Marn CS. Septic thrombophlebitis of the portal vein: CT and clinical observations. *J Comput Assist Tomogr*. 1989;13:656–658.

170. Ebright JR, Pace MT, Niazi AF. Septic thrombosis of the cavernous sinuses. *Arch Intern Med*. 2001;161:2671–2676.

171. Roberts KE, Hamele-Bena D, Saqu A, Stein CA, Cole RP. Pulmonary tumor embolism: a review of the literature. *Am J Med*. 2003;115:228–232.

172. Shepard JA, Moore EH, Templeton PA, McLoud TC. Pulmonary intravascular tumor emboli: dilated and beaded peripheral pulmonary arteries at CT. *Radiology*. 1993;187:797–801.

173. Adedeji MO, Cespedes J, Allen K, Subramony C, Hughson MD. Pulmonary thrombotic arteriopathy in patients with sickle cell disease. *Arch Pathol Lab Med*. 2001;125: 1436–1441.

174. Dessap AM, Deux JF, Abidi N, et al. Pulmonary artery thrombosis during acute chest syndrome in sickle cell disease. *Am J Respir Crit Care Med*. 2011;184:1022–1029.

175. Parent F, Bachir D, Inamo J, et al. A hemodynamic study of pulmonary hypertension in sickle cell disease. *N Engl J Med*. 2011;365:44–53.

176. Montagnana M, Cervellin G, Franchini M. Pathophysiology, clinics and diagnostics of non-thrombotic pulmonary embolism. *J Thromb Thrombolysis*. 2011;31:436–444.

177. Marchiori E, Lourenco S, Gasparetto TD, Zanetti G, Mano CM, Nobre LF. Pulmonary talcosis: imaging findings. *Lung*. 2010; 188:165–171.

178. Wai CT, Lin M, Tan KC. Hepatobiliary and pancreatic: pulmonary embolism after injection therapy for gastric varices. *J Gastroenterol Hepatol*. 2008;23:1306.

179. Bonardel G, Pouit B, Gontier E, et al. Pulmonary cement embolism after percutaneous vertebroplasty: a rare and nonthrombotic cause of pulmonary embolism. *Clin Nucl Med*. 2007;32: 603–606.

CHAPTER 74 Pulmonary Vasculitis

Ulrich Specks

NOMENCLATURE AND DEFINITIONS

Pulmonary vasculitis is usually a manifestation of a systemic disorder leading to inflammation of vessels of different sizes by a variety of immunological mechanisms. Vasculitis can be categorized into primary vasculitis and secondary vasculitis. The primary systemic vasculitides are a heterogeneous group of syndromes of unknown etiology, which share a clinical response to immunosuppressive therapy (Table 74-1). Their wide spectrum of frequently overlapping clinical manifestations is defined by the size and location of the affected vessels as well as the nature of the inflammatory infiltrate. Secondary vasculitis may represent significant management problems in the context of a well-defined underlying disorder, such as diffuse alveolar hemorrhage caused by systemic lupus erythematosus (SLE). Alternatively, secondary vasculitis may be an incidental histopathological finding, for instance, in the context of an infection or necrotizing sarcoid granulomatosis.

Classification schemes and definitions of the various forms of vasculitis have evolved over the past decades. Historically, the classification of the vasculitis has been based on the size of the most prominently affected vessels. The primary purpose of classification and nomenclature is to standardize communication between clinicians and investigators and to facilitate more uniform treatment approaches. Ideally, they reflect the current understanding of pathogenesis. The first international consensus conference on the nomenclature of systemic vasculitides held in 1992 in Chapel Hill aimed to reconcile definitions and classification schemes used by European and American investigators. The resulting nomenclature and definitions were based mainly on histopathological criteria, particularly the size of the vessels involved, but allowed for radiographic and clinical surrogates to fulfill the definitions. These definitions, nomenclature, and classification found wide acceptance. The terminology was recently revised and updated at the second 2012 Chapel Hill International Consensus Conference so that it reflects novel insights into the pathogenesis of various vasculitides while avoiding the use of eponyms as much as possible.[1] In this chapter, the specific definition of each form of vasculitis is discussed in detail as part of the description of the clinical manifestations and differential diagnosis of each entity.

TABLE 74-1 Chapel Hill Consensus Nomenclature of the Primary Systemic Vasculitides

Name	Respiratory Manifestations	Presence of ANCA
Large vessel vasculitis		
Giant cell arteritis	Rare	No
Takayasu arteritis	Frequent	No
Medium-sized vessel vasculitis		
Polyarteritis nodosa	Rare	No
Kawasaki disease	No	No
Small vessel vasculitis *ANCA-associated vasculitis*		
Granulomatosis with polyangiitis (formerly Wegener's)	Frequent	>80%
Microscopic polyangiitis	Frequent	>80%
Eosinophilic granulomatosis with polyangiitis (formerly Churg–Strauss syndrome)	Frequent	>50%
Immune complex small vessel vasculitis		
Anti-GBM disease	Frequent	No
IgA vasculitis	Rare	IgA-ANCA reported
Cryoglobulinemic vasculitis	No	No
Hypocomplementemic urticarial vasculitis	Frequent	No
Variable vessel vasculitis		
Behçet disease	Rare	No

The 2012 Chapel Hill nomenclature is clinically very useful to pulmonologists as it reflects the clinical and histopathological pulmonary features and facilitates the therapeutic approach to individual patients. The three small vessel vasculitides that present most often with respiratory symptoms are granulomatosis with polyangiitis (GPA [formerly Wegener granulomatosis]), microscopic polyangiitis (MPA), and eosinophilic granulomatosis with polyangiitis (EGPA [formerly Churg–Strauss syndrome]). Most patients with these syndromes have antineutrophil cytoplasmic autoantibodies (ANCA) detectable in the serum at the time of initial presentation.[2] Consequently, this group of small vessel vasculitides is referred to *in cumulo* as "ANCA-associated vasculitis." In patients with vasculitis, two types of ANCA are of clinical significance. In more than 80% of patients with GPA (Fig. 74-1), ANCA occur and are associated with a cytoplasmic immunofluorescence pattern (C-ANCA) on ethanol-fixed neutrophils that react with the neutrophil granule enzyme, proteinase 3 (PR3-ANCA). In contrast, ANCA that cause a perinuclear immunofluorescence pattern (P-ANCA) on ethanol-fixed neutrophils and react with myeloperoxidase (MPO-ANCA) occur in fewer than 10% of patients with GPA but in the majority of patients with MPA (Fig. 74-2). MPO-ANCA are also the predominant type of ANCA encountered in patients with EGPA, in which PR3-ANCA are the exception. Despite these circulating autoantibodies, hardly any immunoglobulin deposits can be detected in the tissue lesions of ANCA-associated vasculitis, and they are consequently called "pauci-immune" lesions.

EPIDEMIOLOGY

The primary systemic vasculitides are rare and few epidemiological studies have been conducted, mostly in ethnically homogeneous populations.[3] Giant cell arteritis is the most frequent form of systemic vasculitis with an annual incidence of 13 per million adults (40 per million over the age of 60). It appears to be increasing in frequency and becoming cyclical over time. The latter observation has been interpreted as possibly suggesting a relationship with

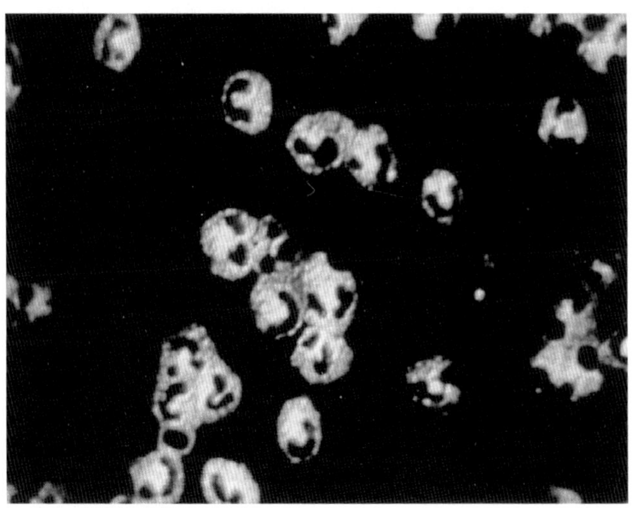

Figure 74-1 Cytoplasmic indirect immunofluorescence (C-ANCA) pattern in ethanol-fixed neutrophils caused by ANCA reacting with PR3.

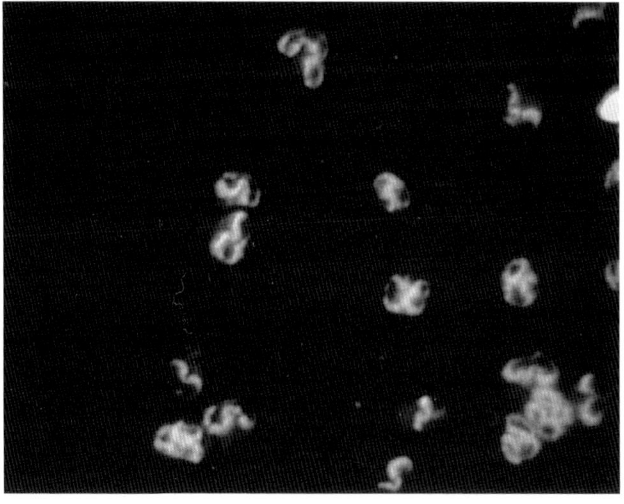

Figure 74-2 Perinuclear indirect immunofluorescence (P-ANCA) pattern in ethanol-fixed neutrophils caused by ANCA reacting with MPO.

TABLE 74-2 Organ Systems Affected by ANCA-Associated Vasculitis

Feature	Granulomatosis with Polyangiitis (formerly Wegener's)	Microscopic Polyangiitis	Eosinophilic Granulomatosis with Polyangiitis (formerly Churg–Strauss)
Upper airway disease	90–95%	No	50–60%
Pulmonary parenchymal disease	54–85%	20%	30%
Alveolar hemorrhage	5–15%	10–50%	<3%
Glomerulonephritis	51–80%	60–90%	10%–25%
Gastrointestinal tract	<5%	30%	30–50%
Eyes	35–52%	<5%	<5%
Nervous system	20–50%	60–70%	70%–80%
Heart	8–16%	10–15%	10–15%
Skin	33–46%	62%	50–60%
Eosinophilia	Rare	Rare	Yes
Asthma	No[a]	No[a]	Yes
Granulomatous inflammation	Yes	No	Yes

[a]*Not more than general population.*

infections. Respiratory manifestations rarely represent significant management problems in these patients. Various studies from different regions of the world report a fairly uniform annual incidence of one to two cases per million for Takayasu arteritis. Pulmonary vascular complications occur in about half of the afflicted patients. The estimated annual incidence of GPA has been rising over the decades from 0.5 to 0.7 per million during the 1970s and early 1980s to current estimates of about 10 to 12 per million. Similar increases in annual incidence have been observed for MPA and EGPA. The average frequency of MPA is similar to that of GPA; for EGPA it is estimated to be of the order of one to three per million. The ANCA-associated vasculitides have different ethnic predilections: GPA affects predominantly whites, and northern Europeans appear more prone to develop GPA. In contrast, individuals of southern European and Mediterranean descent appear to be relatively more apt to develop MPA. GPA and MPA can affect individuals of any age. However, the incidence of GPA plateaus after age 50, whereas the likelihood of developing MPA continues to increase with age.

The annual incidence of the secondary vasculitides varies widely. The reported frequencies for rheumatoid vasculitis and vasculitis in SLE are 12.5 per million and 3.6 per million, respectively. Behçet disease has a peculiar geographic distribution along the old Silk Road, with the highest prevalence being reported from Turkey, Central and far eastern Asia, where the frequencies range from 100 to 380 per 100,000, compared with only 1 per 100,000 in western Europe.

The available population-based studies need to be interpreted with some caution because they do not distinguish between whether the observed increased incidence of systemic vasculitis is true, or the result of more frequent recognition of the disease. Moreover, whether individual diagnoses are accurate and consistent is challenged by the changing definitions of the syndromes over time.

ANCA-ASSOCIATED VASCULITIS

The ANCA-associated vasculitides include granulomatosis with polyangiitis, microscopic polyangiitis, and eosinophilic granulomatosis with polyangiitis. The clinical presentation, diagnosis, pathophysiology, and treatment of these entities are discussed below.

■ GRANULOMATOSIS WITH POLYANGIITIS: CLINICAL PRESENTATION AND DIAGNOSIS

GPA is the most common form of vasculitis to involve the lung. The Chapel Hill Consensus Conference defined GPA as "necrotizing granulomatous inflammation usually involving the respiratory tract, and necrotizing vasculitis affecting predominantly small- to medium-sized vessels."[1] However, it is important to recognize that GPA is a systemic disease that can affect almost any organ (Table 74-2). The most frequently involved sites are the upper airways, lungs, and kidneys.[4] Symptoms and clinical disease manifestations are the result of necrotizing granulomatous inflammation and small vessel vasculitis that occur in variable degrees of combination.

In the 1960s the term "limited Wegener granulomatosis" was introduced to indicate patients with GPA who lacked renal disease. The use of this term and its implications have evolved over the last two decades. Even in the absence of renal involvement, patients may have life-threatening pulmonary or neurological disease requiring aggressive immunosuppressive treatment. For instance, a patient who "only" has alveolar hemorrhage in the absence of glomerulonephritis should never be classified as having "limited" GPA. Consequently, today, the use of the term "limited GPA" implies that (a) the pathology is predominantly a necrotizing granulomatous inflammation, and the vasculitis seen on biopsy is of lesser clinical significance; and (b) there is no immediate threat either to the patient's life or that the affected organ is at risk for irreversible damage. In this sense, the terms "limited" or "nonsevere" GPA are now used interchangeably as distinction from "severe" GPA, which by definition either threatens the patient's life (alveolar hemorrhage) or a vital organ with the risk of irreversible damage (rapidly progressive glomerulonephritis, scleritis, or mononeuritis multiplex). These definitions and distinctions form the basis for stratification of current standard therapy.

Over 90% of patients with GPA first seek medical attention for symptoms arising from either the upper and/or lower airway. Nasal and sinus disease is characterized by congestion and epistaxis due to mucosal friability, ulceration, and thickening. Patients may also have features of chronic sinusitis and recurrent or chronic serous otitis. Perforation of the nasal septum and/or saddle nose deformity may result from ischemia of the nasal cartilage (Fig. 74-3). Oral manifestations include gingival hyperplasia (Fig. 74-4) and oropharyngeal ulcerations. Subglottic stenosis occurs in approximately 20% of patients and can cause life-threatening compromise of the airway. Subglottic stenosis may occur in the absence of other features of active GPA, and its symptoms may be nonspecific, for example, dyspnea, hoarseness, cough or stridor; the latter is occasionally mistaken for wheezing.

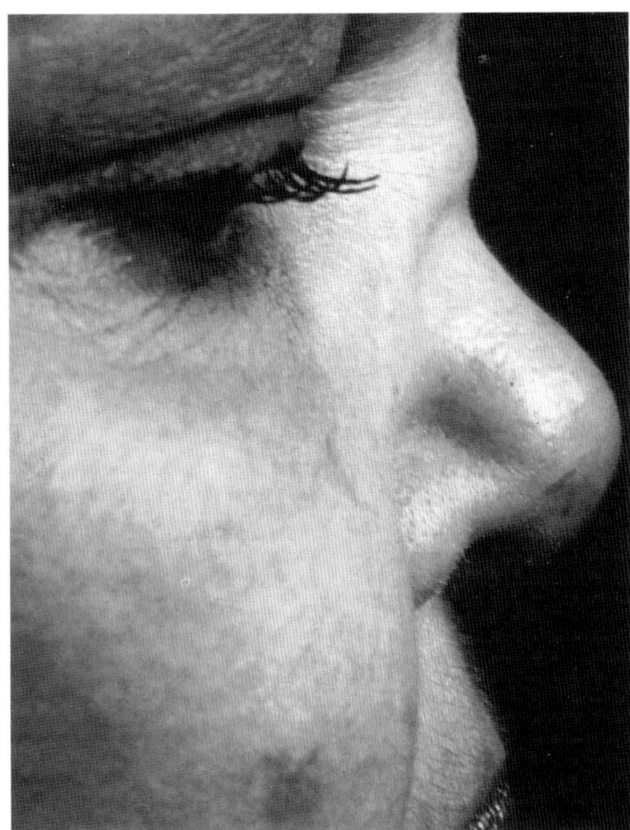

Figure 74-3 Saddle nose deformity of granulomatosis with polyangiitis.

GPA involving the lower airways can affect the pulmonary parenchyma, the bronchi, and rarely the pleura. Presenting features of parenchymal involvement may include cough, dyspnea, chest pain, or hemoptysis. However, some patients may be completely asymptomatic. Patients with diffuse alveolar hemorrhage usually present with progressive dyspnea and anemia (Fig. 74-5). Hemoptysis is absent in about one-third of patients. Patients with diffuse alveolar hemorrhage may deteriorate rapidly and experience respiratory failure, which has a mortality rate up to 50%.

The clinical presentation of alveolar hemorrhage is caused by pulmonary capillaritis (Fig. 74-6). The predominant inflammatory cells are neutrophils. However, eosinophils or monocytes may also be present. Capillaritis usually causes fibrinoid necrosis of alveolar and vessel walls and may culminate in the destruction of the underlying architecture of the lung. An important hallmark of capillaritis is the presence of pyknotic cells and nuclear fragments from

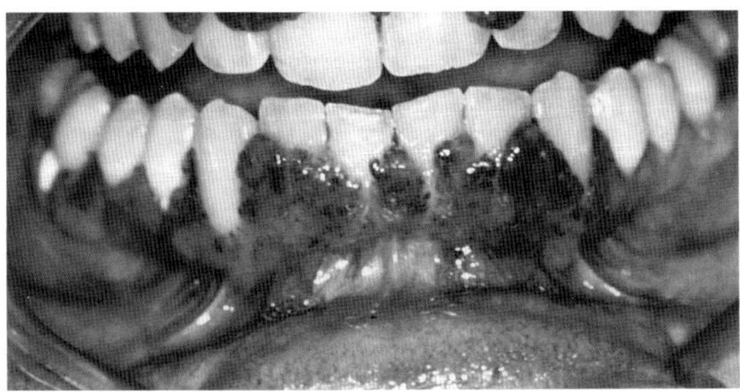

Figure 74-4 Strawberry or mulberry gums in a patient with granulomatosis with polyangiitis.

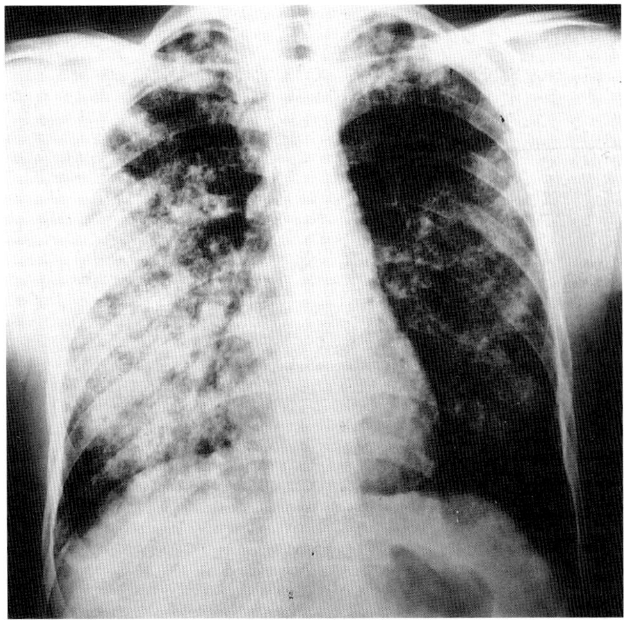

Figure 74-5 Chest radiograph of a patient with granulomatosis with polyangiitis displaying an alveolar filling pattern indicative of diffuse alveolar hemorrhage.

neutrophils undergoing apoptosis, a feature called leukocytoclasis. This hallmark enables distinction between true capillaritis and margination of neutrophils related to surgical trauma. Depending on the acuteness and duration of alveolar hemorrhage, hemosiderin-laden macrophages and interstitial hemosiderin deposits may be present.

The most common form of pulmonary involvement in GPA is caused by necrotizing granulomatous inflammation and presents radiographically as nodules or mass lesions, which may cavitate (Figs. 74-7–74-9). These lesions may be incidental findings on thoracic imaging studies as they cause little symptoms and do not result in significant abnormalities of pulmonary function. Prominent air–fluid levels can be seen when the necrotic center of the inflammatory lesion gets superinfected (Fig. 74-8). These necrotizing granulomatous lesions are a disease-defining feature of GPA. Their presence easily separates GPA from MPA. In the absence of other features of small vessel vasculitis in other organs, the differential diagnosis of these lesions consists primarily of infections, particularly caused by fungal or mycobacterial organisms, and less likely of malignancies or necrotizing sarcoid granulomatosis.

The lung nodules of GPA have very characteristic histopathological features. Small necrotizing microabscesses appear to be the earliest lesion. They enlarge and coalesce until the typical geographic and basophilic appearance of the necrosis has developed (Fig. 74-10). The necrotic center is surrounded by palisading histiocytes and scattered giant cells. Occasionally the necrosis may be bronchocentric. When this type of necrotizing granulomatous inflammation extends into the walls of small vessels it is referred to as granulomatous vasculitis (Fig. 74-11). In contrast to capillaritis, this type of vasculitis seems to be a secondary phenomenon of the necrotizing granulomatous inflammation affecting the lung parenchyma. The inflammatory background of the granulomatous necrosis and vasculitis consists of a mixed cellular infiltrate containing lymphocytes, plasma cells, scattered giant cells, and eosinophils. It may cause extensive parenchymal consolidation mimicking organizing pneumonia. Well-defined sarcoid-like nonnecrotizing granulomas are not found in GPA.

Inflammation and stenosis of the tracheobronchial tree occur in at least 15% of patients with lung involvement.[5,6] Endobronchial disease may be an incidental finding on bronchoscopy or present

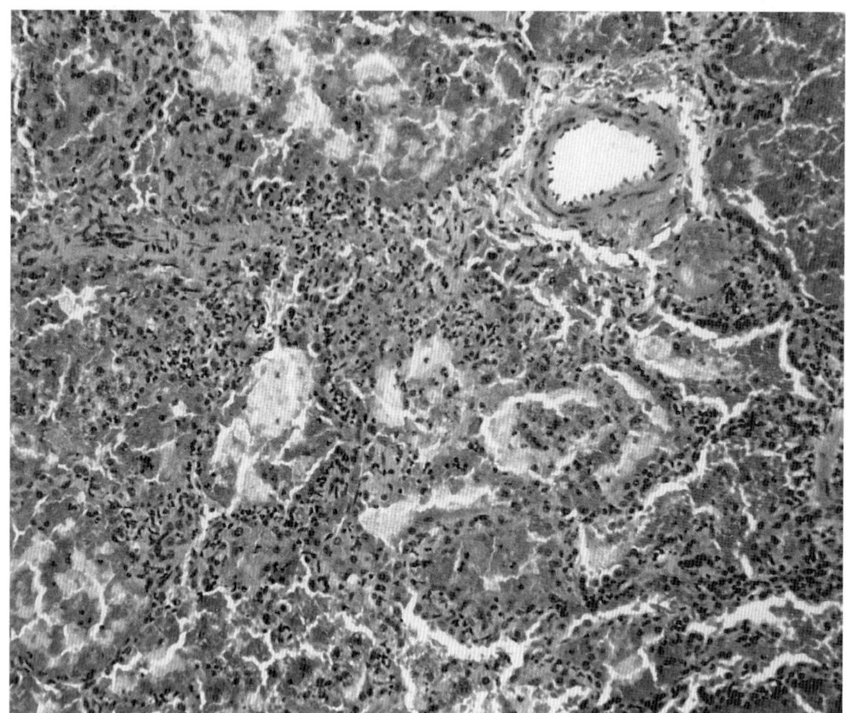

Figure 74-6 Alveolar capillaritis causing pulmonary hemorrhage in granulomatosis with polyangiitis.

with cough, hemoptysis, wheezing, dyspnea, or symptoms related to parenchymal collapse or postobstructive infection. Spirometry including inspiratory and expiratory flow–volume loops may show characteristic abnormalities indicative of degree and location of airway narrowing. Subglottic stenosis represents a fixed airway obstruction resulting in flattening of both the inspiratory and expiratory loops. If the intrathoracic trachea, or more commonly, one or both mainstem bronchi are affected, flattening of the expiratory curve can be found. Pleural effusions may occur, but are usually small, asymptomatic, and incidental findings (Fig. 74-9). Other thoracic manifestations of GPA include inflammatory pleural pseudotumors or hilar adenopathy. The latter should raise the suspicion of infection, sarcoidosis, or lymphoma.

Glomerulonephritis is among the most concerning disease manifestations of GPA as it can progress to complete renal failure in the absence of symptoms. It is usually detected by the presence of abnormal laboratory results such as active urine sediment with microscopic hematuria and red cell casts, proteinuria, and declining renal function. Continued vigilance for glomerulonephritis is essential as it is present at diagnosis in less than half of all patients. However, over the course of their disease, the kidneys are affected in 80% of patients.

A renal biopsy is useful to establish a diagnosis of ANCA-associated vasculitis and to determine the renal prognosis. The glomeruli are not affected uniformly (focal) by segmental, necrotizing inflammation (Fig. 74-12), and cellular crescents (Fig. 74-13) are frequently found. The number of glomeruli affected, degree of crescent formation, and destruction of individual glomeruli as well as the amount of sclerosis found determine the chance of recovery of renal function. In addition, tubular fibrosis and atrophy affect renal outcomes. Direct immunofluorescence reveals no or only scant immune deposits (pauci-immune glomerulonephritis). Granulomatous inflammation affecting the renal parenchyma and tubulointerstitial nephritis can also be found rarely.

A wide spectrum of ocular manifestations has been observed in GPA, which may threaten vision by affecting the eye directly or involving its contiguous structures. Manifestations may include conjunctivitis, episcleritis, scleritis, keratitis, corneal ulceration, uveitis, and retinal vasculitis. Involvement of the lacrimal system

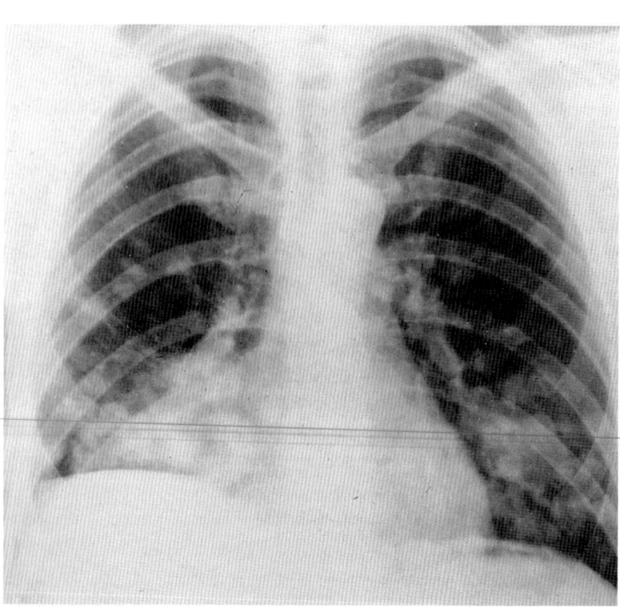

Figure 74-7 Chest radiograph of a patient with granulomatosis with polyangiitis displaying multiple nodules with and without cavitation.

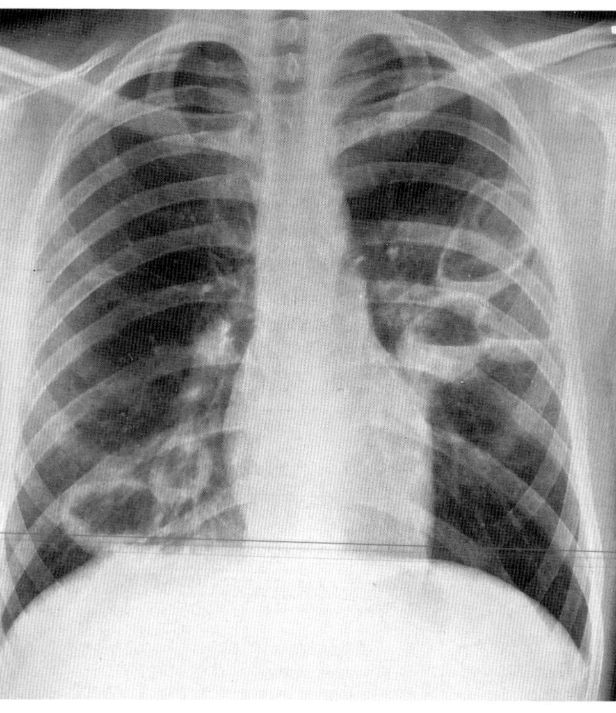

Figure 74-8 Chest radiograph of a patient with granulomatosis with polyangiitis showing multiple large cavities, some with air–fluid levels.

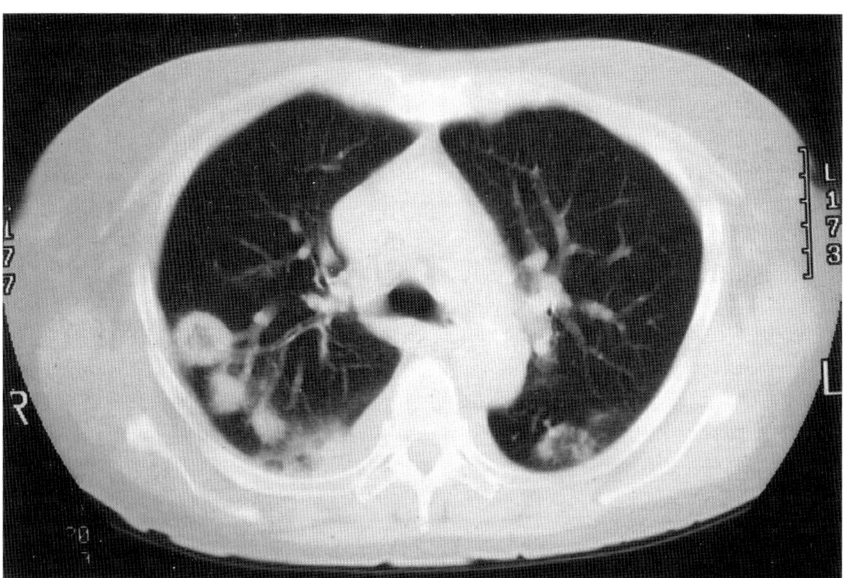

Figure 74-9 Computed tomography scan of a patient with granulomatosis with polyangiitis showing multiple nodules, some with cavitation. There are also small bilateral pleural effusions.

may result in epiphora, dacryocystitis, and fistula. Retro-orbital inflammatory pseudotumors may affect one or both the eyes, threaten the vision, and represent the most difficult challenge in the management of GPA (Figs. 74-14 and 74-15). Any patient with GPA who presents with eye pain or redness, proptosis, change in visual acuity, diplopia, or loss of visual field should be referred for emergent ophthalmological consultation.

Nervous system involvement may occur in up to one-third of patients. Mononeuritis multiplex of the peripheral nervous system caused by inflammation of the vasa nervorum as well as central nervous system vasculitis and pachymeningitis represent severe disease manifestations with substantial risk of irreversible damage, persisting even after the acute inflammation is adequately controlled.

Cardiac involvement may be occult. Regional wall motion abnormalities with a noncoronary distribution pattern are frequent echocardiographic findings.[7] It is unclear whether this type of cardiomyopathy is the result of small vessel disease or inflammatory infiltration of the cardiac muscle. Pericarditis, valvulitis, and inflammatory pseudotumor have also been described.

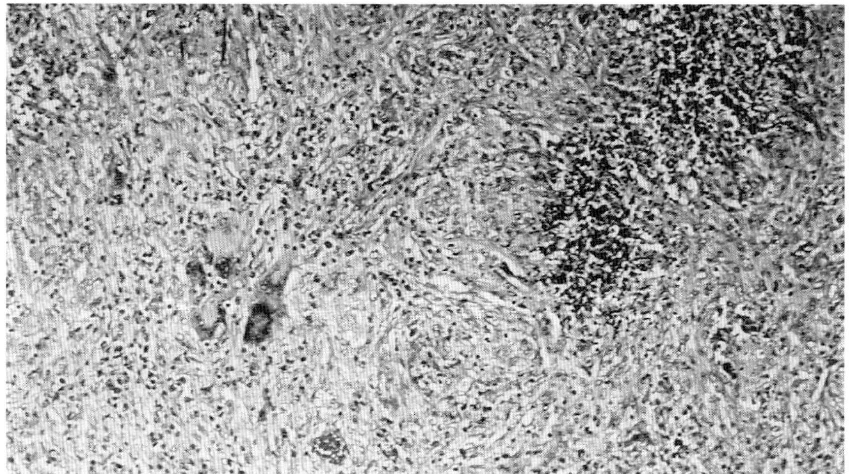

Figure 74-10 Geographic basophilic necrosis with palisading histiocytes and giant cells from a lung nodule in a patient with granulomatosis with polyangiitis.

A wide spectrum of cutaneous manifestations may be observed in GPA. Leukocytoclastic vasculitis presenting as palpable purpura is most common, followed by pyoderma gangrenosum–like lesions (Fig. 74-16) and so-called Churg–Strauss granulomas.

MICROSCOPIC POLYANGIITIS: CLINICAL PRESENTATION AND DIAGNOSIS

Histopathologically, the necrotizing small vessel vasculitis of MPA causing necrotizing crescentic glomerulonephritis and pulmonary capillaritis is indistinguishable from that encountered in GPA.[8] Consequently, there is substantial overlap in organ manifestations and symptoms between the two syndromes (Table 74-2). A timely diagnosis of MPA may be delayed by a gradual onset or the nonspecific nature of symptoms such as fever, malaise, and weight loss. All organ systems may be involved. The kidneys are most commonly affected in up to 80% of patients. Other commonly encountered disease manifestations include diffuse alveolar hemorrhage due to pulmonary capillaritis affecting 10% to 30% of patients. MPA is the most frequent cause of pulmonary renal syndrome. Several cases of MPA in association with severe obstructive airway disease or bronchiectasis have also been described. More recently, several case series have highlighted an association between usual interstitial pneumonia and MPO-ANCA–positive MPA. In these cases, the fibrotic changes either precede the development of MPA or are already present at the time of diagnosis of MPA.

Palpable purpura caused by leukocytoclastic vasculitis of the skin, and musculoskeletal complaints, such as arthralgias and myalgias, are also common. Gastrointestinal involvement occurs in about one-third of patients. This is in contrast to GPA, in which gastrointestinal involvement is very rare. Visceral angiography is generally not helpful for the evaluation of abdominal symptoms as the vessels involved are too small to be visualized. CT with or without contrast injection may be more helpful if gastrointestinal involvement is suspected. However, the use of contrast is relatively contraindicated in patients with active renal involvement. Sinusitis and asthma are rarely found in MPA, and should lead to the consideration of an alternative diagnosis.

Most patients with MPA have ANCA, and in 40% to 80% they are of the P-ANCA variety, reacting with MPO. C-ANCA reacting with PR3 is seen less frequently. Occasionally patients with MPA later develop granulomatous inflammation and are reclassified as having GPA; this is more likely to occur in patients with C-ANCA.

As in GPA, a histopathological diagnosis may be necessary to confirm the diagnosis before the patient is committed to prolonged immunosuppressive therapy. The biopsy specimen should be sought from the most accessible site. Renal biopsy shows pauci-immune focal segmental–necrotizing glomerulonephritis, with extracapillary proliferation forming crescents. In contrast to GPA, granulomatous inflammation is not a feature of MPA. All other histopathological features are indistinguishable from those of

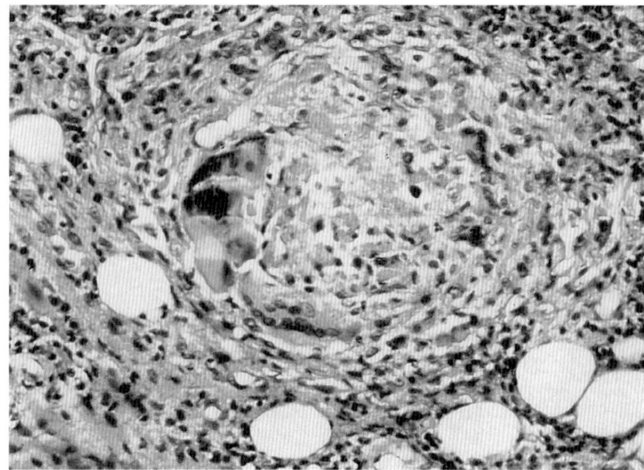

Figure 74-11 Granulomatous vasculitis with giant cells in a lung biopsy of a patient with granulomatosis with polyangiitis.

GPA. Treatment of MPA should follow the principles applied to the management of GPA. Consequently, most cases of MPA require immunosuppressive therapy used for patients with severe GPA.

EOSINOPHILIC GRANULOMATOSIS WITH POLYANGIITIS: CLINICAL PRESENTATION AND DIAGNOSIS

EGPA is the third type of vasculitis that commonly affects the lung. The 2012 Chapel Hill Consensus definition for the disease is "eosinophil-rich and necrotizing granulomatous inflammation often involving the respiratory, and necrotizing vasculitis predominantly affecting small- to medium-sized vessels, and associated with asthma and eosinophilia."[1] EGPA is included among the ANCA-associated vasculitides even though only 40% to 70% of patients with active EGPA are ANCA positive.[9–11] EGPA is primarily distinguished from GPA and MPA by a high prevalence of asthma and peripheral blood and tissue eosinophilia. Three distinct phases of the disease have been described. The first is a prodromal allergic phase with asthma. This phase may last for a number of years. The second is an eosinophilic phase with prominent peripheral and tissue eosinophilia. This phase may also last a number of years and the manifestations may remit and recur over this time period. The differential diagnosis for patients in this phase of the disease includes parasitic infection and chronic eosinophilic pneumonia. The third vasculitic phase consists of systemic vasculitis and may be life threatening. The three phases are not seen in all patients and do not necessarily occur in this order; they may even concur. However, asthma usually predates vasculitic symptoms by a mean of 7 years (range 0–61). Formes frustes of EGPA have also been described with eosinophilic vasculitis and/or eosinophilic granulomas in isolated organs without evidence of systemic disease.

Pulmonary parenchymal involvement occurs in 38% of patients. Transient alveolar-type infiltrates are most common (Fig. 74-17). These have a predominantly peripheral distribution and are indistinguishable from infiltrates seen in chronic eosinophilic pneumonia. Occasionally, nodular lesions may be seen in EGPA. In contrast

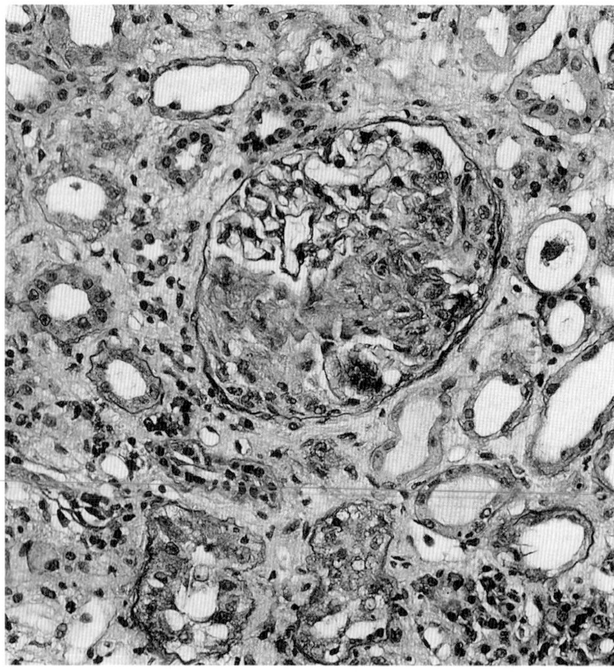

Figure 74-12 Focal necrotizing glomerulitis of granulomatosis with polyangiitis.

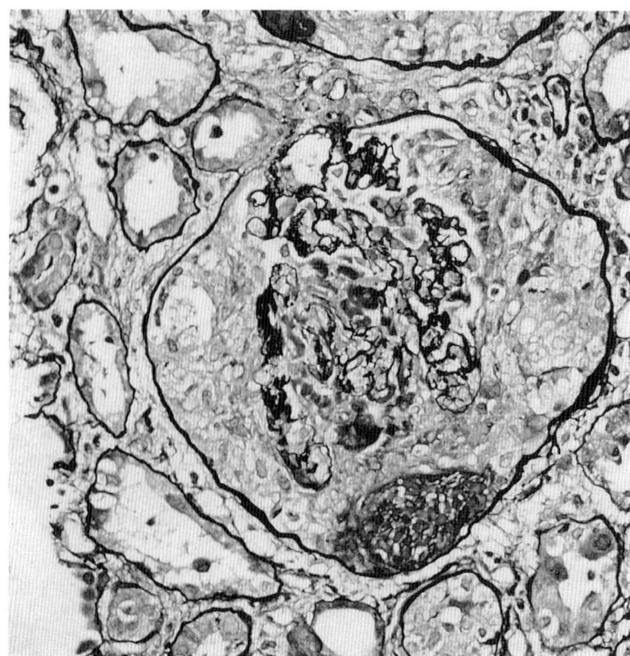

Figure 74-13 Rapidly progressive crescentic glomerulonephritis in granulomatosis with polyangiitis.

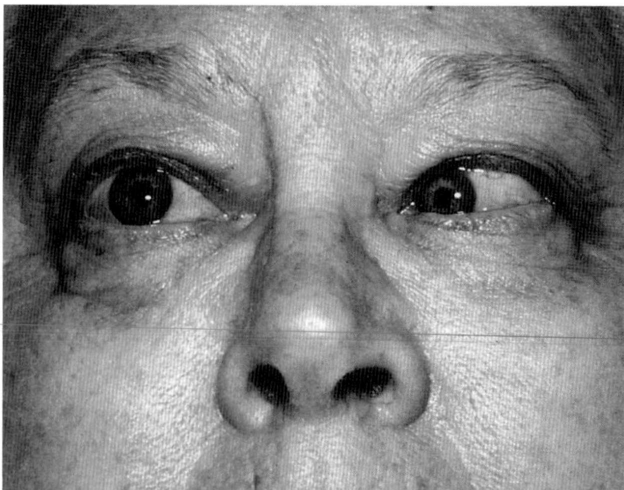

Figure 74-14 External ophthalmoplegia of the left eye due to orbital involvement with granulomatosis with polyangiitis.

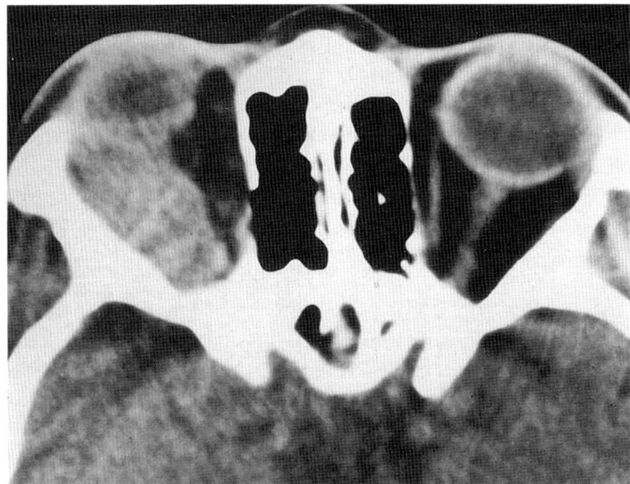

Figure 74-15 Computed tomography scan of the orbits in a patient with granulomatosis with polyangiitis showing a mass in the right orbit causing external ophthalmoplegia.

to GPA and MPA, alveolar hemorrhage is exceedingly rare. Renal involvement in EGPA is less prominent than in GPA and MPA and does not generally lead to renal failure. In contrast, peripheral nerve involvement, typically in the form of mononeuritis multiplex, is more frequent. The peripheral nerve involvement can result from both capillaritis and direct toxicity from eosinophil granule proteins. Skin, heart, central nervous system, and abdominal viscera may also be involved.

The classic histopathological picture consists of necrotizing vasculitis, eosinophilic tissue infiltration, and extravascular granulomas. However, not all features are found in every case, and they are not pathognomonic of the condition. Particularly the finding of a "Churg–Strauss granuloma" on skin biopsy should not be confused with the diagnosis of EGPA. While this type of necrotizing extravascular granuloma may be seen in EGPA, it may occur in other systemic autoimmune diseases, including GPA and rheumatoid arthritis.

If ANCA are present, they are usually P-ANCA reacting with MPO. The ANCA status appears to correlate with disease activity. Recent studies suggest a more vasculitic disease phenotype in the presence of ANCA, with ANCA being particularly frequent among patients with glomerulonephritis. Patients with heart involvement are less likely to be ANCA positive. However, not all studies have found this consistently, and there remains substantial overlap of organ manifestations between patients with EGPA who are ANCA positive and those who are ANCA negative.

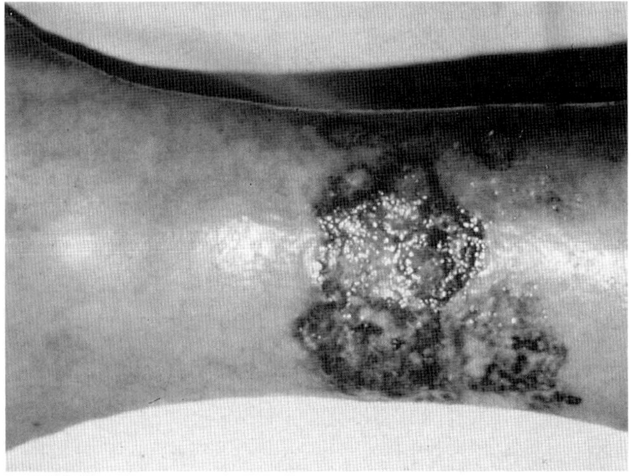

Figure 74-16 Pyoderma gangrenosum of the leg in a patient with granulomatosis with polyangiitis.

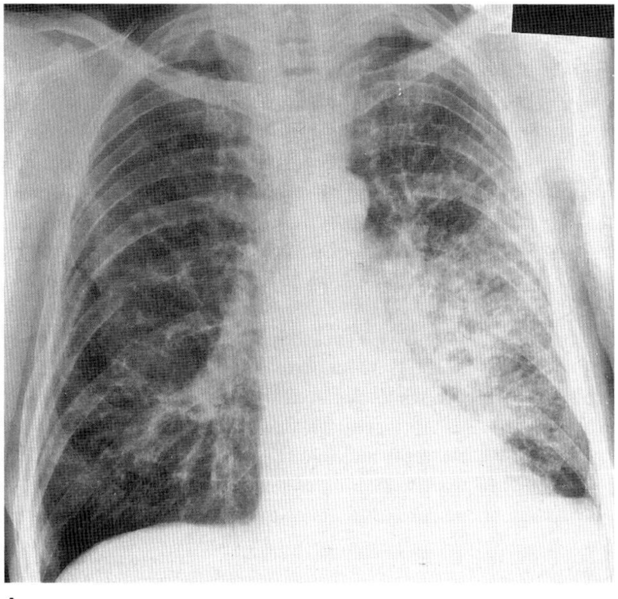

A

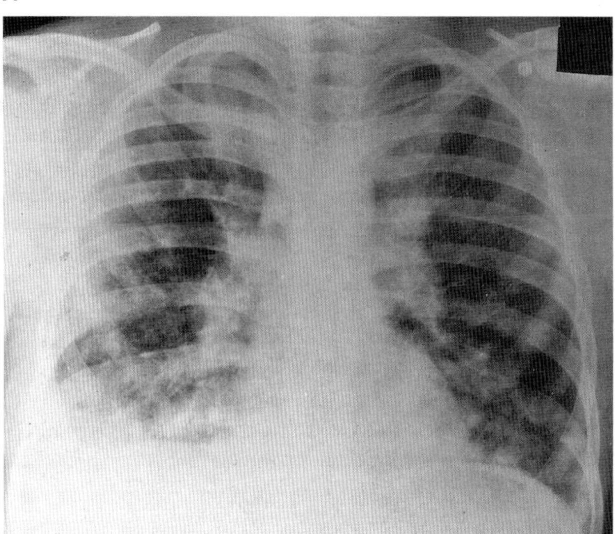

B

Figure 74-17 Chest radiographs of patients with eosinophilic granulomatosis with polyangiitis (Churg–Strauss): (**A**) Nonspecific gnomonic infiltrates; (**B**) Multiple vague, patchy infiltrates. *(Reproduced with permission from Chumbley LC, Harrison EG, DeRemee RA. Allergic Granulomatosis and angiitis (Churg-Strauss syndrome): report and analysis of 30 cases. Mayo Clin Proc. 1977;52(8):477–484.)*

In recent years significant attention has been devoted to EGPA detected in patients using leukotriene receptor antagonists. Available case studies and limited population-based incidence estimates suggest that these agents may lead to unmasking of vasculitic symptoms in asthmatics, by allowing dose reductions or discontinuation of oral glucocorticoid therapy. There is no evidence suggesting that these agents cause EGPA.

The prognosis of EGPA is better than that of GPA and MPA, as the overall mortality is lower and not significantly different from the normal population. Most deaths are secondary to cardiac involvement.

PATHOPHYSIOLOGY OF ANCA-ASSOCIATED VASCULITIS

The etiology of ANCA-associated vasculitis remains unknown. Several different pathways and mechanisms have been proposed for the pathogenesis.[12] A genetic predisposition for autoimmunity, epigenetic factors and environmental triggers seem to play a role in the development of ANCA-associated vasculitis. Currently available clinical and experimental evidence support that infections or other environmental exposures can lead to the loss of tolerance and an inflammatory environment that is conducive for the production of autoantibodies (ANCA) in predisposed patients. In the context of an inflammatory milieu, ANCA can cause specific tissue inflammation and injury by a variety of different mechanisms which involve direct interactions with PR3 or MPO.

Multiple studies have reported skewing in polymorphisms of a variety of immune response genes and genes encoding for ANCA-target antigens and α1-proteinase inhibitor with potential effects on disease outcome. A recent genome-wide association study found major histocompatibility complex (MHC) and non-MHC associations with GPA and MPA and that these syndromes are genetically distinct.[13] Moreover, the associations with the specific ANCA types (PR3-ANCA vs. MPO-ANCA) and the differences between them were stronger than those between patients diagnosed with GPA versus MPA. For PR3-ANCA–positive patients strong associations were found with *HLA-DP*, the serpin A1 gene (*SERPINA1*), which codes for the α1-antitrypsin, the major inhibitor of PR3, and with the *PRTN3* gene which encodes PR3. In patients with MPO-ANCA only an association with *HLA-DQ* was found.

The expression of ANCA-target antigens on the neutrophil surface, particularly PR3, is increased in patients with GPA and genetically determined. Moreover, epigenetic modifications that interfere with the normal silencing of genes coding for the ANCA autoantigens in mature neutrophils may also contribute to the observed inappropriately increased expression of PR3 or MPO by these cells in patients with GPA or MPA.

Many clinical observations suggest that the presence or absence of ANCA as well as the specific type of ANCA (PR3-ANCA vs. MPO-ANCA) defines the disease phenotype. Patients with limited GPA who remain ANCA negative rarely develop systemic vasculitic disease manifestations. Patients with glomerulonephritis and PR3-ANCA lose their renal function much more rapidly than patients with MPO-ANCA. Patients with PR3-ANCA also have a higher relapse rate than patients with MPO-ANCA. Experimental data and animal models support a pathogenic role of ANCA in the development of vasculitis. A couple of recent studies have also suggested a different clinical phenotype of ANCA-positive patients with Churg–Strauss syndrome compared with ANCA-negative patients.

In GPA, the presence of PR3-ANCA appears most closely related to the development of vasculitic complications. Furthermore, systemic vasculitic relapses without recurrence of ANCA are extremely rare. Yet, remission may be maintained for extended periods of time in up to one-half of the patients despite the presence of ANCA. These clinical observations suggest that ANCA alone are not sufficient to cause disease activity, but ANCA seem to be required for the development of vasculitic complications of GPA and systemic relapses.

Many in vitro studies have demonstrated proinflammatory effects of PR3-ANCA and MPO-ANCA on neutrophils, monocytes, and endothelial cells, which enhance and perpetuate endothelial cell and tissue damage. ANCA may increase the adhesion of neutrophils to endothelial cells by enhancing the expression of cell adhesion molecules on endothelial cells. ANCA can activate primed neutrophils, resulting in the release of oxygen radicals and proteolytic enzymes. The latter may in turn induce endothelial cell apoptosis. ANCA-mediated neutrophil activation involves both Fc-γ–receptor engagement and recognition of expressed target antigen on the surface of primed neutrophils. ANCA may also cause endothelial cell damage by direct cytotoxicity or localized immune complex formation with target antigens bound to the endothelial cell surface. The latter may initiate localized complement activation. Finally, ANCA are thought to contribute to the recruitment of more inflammatory cells to the area of tissue injury by stimulating the release of chemotactic chemokines and agents from neutrophils, monocytes, and endothelial cells. For a detailed description of pathways and mechanisms by which ANCA may directly and indirectly contribute to damage of the vascular endothelium, the reader is referred to other recent reviews.

Many patients with ANCA-associated vasculitis relate the onset or recurrence of their disease to preceding infectious episodes. The following link to infection has been hypothesized. Most ANCA-mediated effects on neutrophils and monocytes require priming of the cells. This cytokine-dependent process is not unique to vasculitis. Cytokine stimulation of neutrophils and monocytes, typically by tumor necrosis factor (TNF), with resulting increased surface expression of ANCA-target antigens, occurs normally in the context of infections. Patients with active vasculitis have indeed been shown to have both increased expression of ANCA-target antigens on the surface of their neutrophils and elevated levels of TNF. In combination, these observations allow the hypothesis that neutrophil priming, which occurs in response to cytokine stimulation during infection, enables ANCA to interact with their target antigen on the neutrophil surface. This in turn sets the documented proinflammatory effects of ANCA in motion, which aggravate and perpetuate the inflammatory reaction at the endothelial cell interphase.

Rodent models of MPO-ANCA–associated vasculitis support this hypothesis of a pathogenic role of ANCA. They clearly indicate that ANCA contribute directly to the development of vasculitis and glomerulonephritis, and that the interaction of ANCA with its target antigen is required for the development of lesions. Furthermore, the localization of lesions is determined by the site of this interaction. At the same time, animal models support the significance of genetic determinants for the development of autoimmunity, vasculitis, and a specific phenotype with characteristic organ involvement and histopathological features. Finally, animal model studies indicate that infections may be significant disease modifiers. Even though proinflammatory effects of murine PR3-ANCA could also be documented in vivo, the animals did not develop organ pathology typical for GPA or MPA, and good animal model for PR3-ANCA–associated vasculitis remains elusive. This may be due to substantial differences between human and murine PR3, as the latter behaves more like human elastase than human PR3.

To date, the causes of the production and persistence of ANCA remain poorly understood. Yet infections may be instrumental for the development of this specific type of autoimmunity. ANCA directed against a broad variety of target antigens have been documented in association with viral, fungal, bacterial, and protozoal infections. In the rare instances of C-ANCA/PR3-ANCA observed in infections, the ANCA disappeared with appropriate antimicrobial therapy. These observations may suggest that ANCA can occur transiently in the setting of infection, and that the persistent ANCA response in patients with vasculitis may be the result of molecular mimicry in susceptible hosts. Subsequent diversification of T- and B-cell responses ("epitope spreading") may lead to responses against different epitopes on the same target molecule (intramolecular spreading) or extend to other molecules (intermolecular spreading. Bacterial superantigens have also been implicated in the pathogenesis of ANCA-associated vasculitis. GPA patients colonized with superantigen-producing *Staphylococcus aureus* are at high risk for relapse. GPA patients had expansion of T-cell clones expressing Vβ genes specific for *S. aureus* superantigens more frequently than controls. This supports the theory that *S. aureus* contributes to the pathogenesis of vasculitis. By inducing potent T- and B-cell activity, superantigens produced during an *S. aureus* infection could initiate and maintain both ANCA production and cytokine release, thought to be required for the cascade that results in necrotizing granulomatous inflammation and vasculitis.

■ TREATMENT OF ANCA-ASSOCIATED VASCULITIS

Treatment of granulomatosis with polyangiitis and microscopic polyangiitis, including management of patients who are refractory to standard therapy, is described below. In addition, treatment of eosinophilic granulomatosis with polyangiitis is considered.

Treatment of Granulomatosis with Polyangiitis and Microscopic Polyangiitis

The first goal of therapy for patients with ANCA-associated vasculitis is to induce a remission as quickly as possible, so that irreversible organ damage is minimized. To this end, early diagnosis and prompt application of an appropriate immunosuppressive regimen are crucial. At the same time the treatment plan needs to include the prevention of treatment-related toxicity. Once remission has been induced, the second goal of therapy is to maintain remission with as few side effects as possible. Finally, once the patient has enjoyed a stable remission, surgical interventions aiming to repair damage may proceed as necessary. These overarching principles apply to the therapy of both GPA and MPA.

Remission Induction Therapy

Remission induction therapy is best tailored to the patient's degree of disease severity, extent, and acuity. Patients who present with indolent GPA localized to the upper and/or lower airways and who are ANCA negative can be treated with trimethoprim/sulfamethoxazole (T/S) at a dose of 160/800 mg twice daily. The mechanism of action of T/S is unclear, but possibly related to antimicrobial effects on *S. aureus,* the organism most frequently cultured from the nostrils of patients with GPA. It is also possible that this agent has immune-modulatory effects not shared with other antibiotics. T/S monotherapy should not be used in ANCA-positive patients, in the setting of glomerulonephritis or any other severe disease manifestation, and patients treated with T/S need continued long-term observation, as some will later develop more severe disease manifestations requiring immunosuppressive therapy.

Standard remission induction therapy for most patients categorized as having "limited" or "nonsevere" or "early-systemic" GPA or MPA consists of oral prednisone at doses of 0.5 to 1 mg/kg per day (generally not to exceed 80 mg/d) in combination with methotrexate with a target dose of 20 to 25 mg once a week.[14,15] This dose can be applied orally or subcutaneously. To minimize toxicity and the risk of *Pneumocystis* pneumonia (PCP), this immunosuppressive regimen should be supplemented by folic acid, 1 mg/d and standard PCP prophylaxis.

For the last four decades standard remission induction therapy for patients with severe disease (also called "generalized" or "organ-threatening" disease) has consisted of oral prednisone in combination with oral cyclophosphamide at a dose of 2 mg/kg daily for 3 to 6 months.[16] One randomized controlled trial has shown that intravenous pulse therapy with cyclophosphamide consisting of three pulses of 15 mg/kg given 2 weeks apart followed by 15 mg/kg pulses given every 3 weeks for 6 months, is equally effective to induce remission in severe GPA or MPA.[17] Based on results from a large multicenter randomized double-dummy–controlled trial that compared four once-weekly doses (375 mg/m^2 of body surface) of rituximab to standard oral cyclophosphamide for remission induction in severe ANCA-associated vasculitis, rituximab has now been approved for this indication by most regulatory agencies across the globe.[18] The long-term follow-up of this study has shown that the efficacy of a single course of four once-weekly doses of rituximab (375 mg/m^2 of body surface) remains equivalent to continued standard daily oral immunosuppressive therapy with cyclophosphamide followed by azathioprine for 18 months.[19] These three remission induction regimens have been shown to be equivalent for newly diagnosed patients with severe GPA or MPA. Remission can be achieved in up to 90% of patients with either of these regimens. For patients presenting with a severe disease relapse, rituximab was found to be superior to cyclophosphamide.[18,19] Rituximab is also the preferred agent for young patients in whom fertility needs to be preserved. If oral cyclophosphamide is used, patients need to be monitored carefully to minimize the risk of bone marrow toxicity. The dose of cyclophosphamide should be adjusted in patients with impaired renal function, and the patient's complete blood counts need to be monitored at least biweekly for the duration of therapy. Optimal dosing with oral cyclophosphamide is achieved when the lymphocyte count is reduced, but the total white blood count is maintained above 3500. To avoid bladder toxicity of cyclophosphamide, the entire dose is applied in the morning and patients are instructed to drink at least 3 L of fluid per day.

In patients with rapidly progressive fulminant disease, such as those presenting with alveolar hemorrhage or rapidly deteriorating renal function, intravenous methylprednisolone, 1000 mg per day for 3 to 5 days may be necessary for effective control of inflammation. If this therapy does not generate the desired effects, plasma exchange should be implemented.[20,21]

Remission Maintenance Therapy

Once remission has been induced the prednisone dose is tapered gradually over the course of 5 to 6 months with the goal of complete discontinuation. Patients with limited or "nonsevere" disease should be maintained on methotrexate for remission maintenance.[15] Patients treated with cyclophosphamide for remission induction should be switched to either methotrexate or azathioprine for remission maintenance.[22] Azathioprine is preferred in patients with any degree of renal insufficiency. Mycophenolate mofetil is an alternative for patients who cannot tolerate either methotrexate or azathioprine for remission maintenance. However, mycophenolate mofetil appears less effective than azathioprine for remission maintenance. Remission maintenance therapy is continued for at least 12 months beyond achievement of remission, and longer in patients who have suffered relapses. Early discontinuation of immunosuppressive therapy is associated with an unduly high relapse rate. The need for remission maintenance therapy following remission induction with rituximab in newly diagnosed patients remains unclear. Over 18 months a single remission induction course of rituximab is as effective as oral cyclophosphamide followed by azathioprine, but PR3-ANCA–positive patients with GPA are at risk for relapse once peripheral blood B lymphocytes are reconstituted (after 6–12 months) and may benefit from long-term remission maintenance therapy.[23]

Long-term remission maintenance therapy with T/S beyond immunosuppression may also be beneficial. In one study, patients who received T/S at a dose of 160/800 mg twice daily had a lower rate of disease relapse than those who received placebo.[24]

Treatment of Patients Refractory to Standard Therapy

About 10% of patients do not respond adequately to therapy with cyclophosphamide and fail to achieve remission. These patients are particularly challenging. Anti–TNF-α agents have not been shown to be effective in such patients. One large multicenter, double-blind, placebo-controlled, randomized trial conducted in GPA, has shown no efficacy of etanercept when added to standard therapy.[25] Moreover, a higher frequency of malignancies was observed in the treatment arm compared with the control arm of that trial. All patients with malignancies had also received cyclophosphamide. For this reason, the use of etanercept in patients who have received cyclophosphamide is now strongly discouraged. Smaller, uncontrolled open-label studies with infliximab conducted in Europe have suggested some efficacy of that agent, but many complicated infections were observed in these patients. Over the last decade many cohort studies have found rituximab to be very effective in such patients, and rituximab has now become the *de facto* standard of care for refractory GPA.[26]

Supportive Therapy

PCP still carries a mortality of up to 35%. Therefore, PCP with T/S is recommended for all non–sulfa allergic patients with ANCA-associated vasculitis receiving immunosuppressive therapy including rituximab. Patients who have a sulfa allergy manifesting itself with a skin rash can be desensitized against the drug. Those who fail this approach or have other contraindications for the use of this drug should be given other agents for PCP prophylaxis. Patients receiving methotrexate for remission induction or maintenance should also receive PCP. This can be safely accomplished with T/S at recommended doses for this purpose, provided that folic acid, 1 mg daily, is also given. Patients undergoing intense immunosuppression during the remission induction phase may also benefit from prophylactic antifungal therapy. Finally, every patient treated with glucocorticoids for ANCA-associated vasculitis should receive osteoporosis prophylaxis with calcium and vitamin D supplements and possibly bisphosphonates.

TREATMENT OF EOSINOPHILIC GRANULOMATOSIS WITH POLYANGIITIS

Even though mortality of EGPA is lower than that of GPA or MPA, the management of EGPA remains a challenge. Systemic glucocorticoids are the cornerstone of therapy. There are no clinical trials that provide clear guidance. The reports from the French Vasculitis Study Group are difficult to interpret with respect to this disease, because patients with EGPA were not separated from those with polyarteritis nodosa and MPA, two diseases with distinct clinical manifestations, pathophysiology, and prognosis.[27,28] Yet, these studies suggest that it is appropriate to treat EGPA according to the principles applied to the management of GPA and MPA. Accordingly, cyclophosphamide should be added to glucocorticoids for remission induction in all patients with disease manifestations that threaten the patient's life or the function of a vital organ, that is, particularly those with central or peripheral nerve involvement, glomerulonephritis, heart involvement, or alveolar hemorrhage. Methotrexate, azathioprine, and mycophenolate mofetil have been used as glucocorticoid-sparing agents in less severe disease and for remission maintenance. Refractory disease and disease dominated by difficult-to-control eosinophilic inflammation may respond to interferon-α therapy.[29] However, continued long-term interferon-α therapy may be necessary, and this treatment carries the risk of substantial toxicity. More recently, small case series and a formal pilot trial have shown beneficial effects of rituximab, particularly in ANCA-positive patients with renal involvement.[30,31] Two pilot trials have documented substantial glucocorticoid-sparing effects of anti–interleukin-5 therapy with mepolizumab.[32,33]

OTHER DISORDERS PRESENTING WITH PULMONARY VASCULITIS

A broad spectrum of other disorders which may include pulmonary vasculitis is described below.

GIANT CELL ARTERITIS

Giant cell arteritis is a generalized inflammatory disorder involving large- and medium-sized arteries.[34] It is the most common form of vasculitis in the white population, and appears to affect predominantly elderly patients. Respiratory symptoms have been reported in up to 25% of patients. However, pulmonologists rarely see patients with giant cell arteritis for the management of its respiratory complications. Cough, hoarseness, and throat pain usually resolve promptly with prednisone therapy.[35] Chest roentgenograms and pulmonary function tests rarely show abnormalities attributable to the disease. Occasionally respiratory symptoms are the initial manifestations of giant cell arteritis. Therefore, this possibility should be considered in any elderly patient with new onset of cough, hoarseness, or throat pain without other identifiable cause, and it is reasonable to measure the erythrocyte sedimentation rate in such patients. Isolated cases with pleural effusion or multinodular pulmonary lesions have also been reported in giant cell arteritis. Such cases are difficult to interpret. Particularly in the latter situation, Wegener granulomatosis should be considered in the differential diagnosis, because it may also present with temporal arteritis.

TAKAYASU ARTERITIS

Takayasu arteritis is a large vessel vasculitis affecting predominantly the aorta and its major branches in young patients.[34] Pulmonary complications are the result of a unique arteriopathy predominantly of the large- and medium-sized pulmonary vessels. Progressive defects in the outer media of the arteries and ingrowth of granulation tissue–like capillaries associated with thickened intima and subendothelial smooth muscle proliferation lead to pulmonary artery stenoses and occlusion as well as pulmonary hypertension in up to one-half of all patients. The involvement of pulmonary arteries is common but often asymptomatic. It is detectable by conventional angiography, perfusion scan, or magnetic resonance angiography. CT may show areas of low attenuation as a result of regional hypoperfusion, subpleural reticulolinear changes, and pleural thickening. Fistula formation between pulmonary artery branches and bronchial arteries, as well as nonspecific inflammatory interstitial lung disease, has also been reported.

Therapy for Takayasu arteritis consists primarily of immunosuppression with glucocorticoids. Other immunosuppressive agents, including methotrexate are used as in conjunction with glucocorticoids for remission induction and as glucocorticoid-sparing agents for remission maintenance. Unfortunately, many patients relapse when the glucocorticoid dose is reduced below 15 mg daily. Most recently, the use of anti–TNF-α agents has been reported as beneficial in patients who are refractory to standard therapy. Vascular bypass or stenting procedures may be beneficial in severe disease, but their long-term benefits remain unclear.

CLASSIC POLYARTERITIS NODOSA

Since its formal separation from microscopic polyangiitis, this form of vasculitis affecting predominantly medium-sized vessels is diagnosed rarely. Because it does not affect capillaries, it does not cause either glomerulonephritis or alveolar hemorrhage. However, classic polyarteritis nodosa can affect the bronchial or bronchiolar arteries on rare occasions. Most cases of classic polyarteritis nodosa diagnosed today are associated with viral infections, specifically hepatitis B and C. Consequently, antiviral therapy plays a prominent role in the management of such cases in addition to immunosuppression. Classic polyarteritis nodosa is far less likely to relapse than microscopic polyangiitis, and therefore can generally be treated with a shorter course of immunosuppression.

BEHÇET DISEASE

Behçet disease is a rare chronically relapsing systemic inflammatory disorder characterized by aphthous oral ulcers and at least two or more of the following: aphthous genital ulcers, uveitis, cutaneous nodules or pustules, or meningoencephalitis. Respiratory manifestations are common in Behçet disease and include cough, hemoptysis, chest pain, and dyspnea.[36] Hemoptysis is often massive and fatal. The vasculitis of Behçet disease is immune complex mediated, and may affect vessels of all sizes. If the veins are affected secondary thrombosis with major venous occlusion can occur. This type of thrombosis may not be preventable by anticoagulation, but the use of aspirin 80 mg/d has been advocated. Massive hemoptysis is the result of destruction of the elastic lamina of pulmonary arteries leading to the characteristic aneurysm formation, secondary erosion of bronchi, and arterial–bronchial fistulae. Pulmonary artery aneurysms are detectable by CT or MR angiography, and pulmonary angiography is no longer necessary. Recurrent pneumonia as well as bronchial obstruction as a consequence of mucosal inflammation has also been described.

Therapy of the underlying disease consists of immunosuppression. Prednisone alone may not be sufficient to control the vasculitis. The addition of other drugs, such as colchicine, chlorambucil, methotrexate, cyclosporin, or azathioprine is recommended. The addition of azathioprine or cyclophosphamide to glucocorticoids has resulted in resolution of pulmonary aneurysms. Once pulmonary arteritis has been identified in these patients, anticoagulation should be avoided. The prognosis of pulmonary involvement is poor. About one-third of patients die within 2 years of developing pulmonary involvement, most from fatal pulmonary hemorrhage. Embolization therapy may be used as treatment and prevention of hemorrhage from pulmonary artery aneurysms.

IDIOPATHIC PAUCI-IMMUNE PULMONARY CAPILLARITIS

Diffuse alveolar hemorrhage as a result of capillaritis in the absence of symptoms or serological evidence of any detectable underlying systemic disorder may occur rarely.[37] Direct immunofluorescence studies of the lung tissue did not reveal any immune deposits. This isolated pauci-immune pulmonary capillaritis is histopathologically indistinguishable from that of ANCA-associated vasculitis. It is a diagnosis of exclusion, and such patients are best treated with an immunosuppressive regimen according to the guidelines for severe Wegener granulomatosis or microscopic polyangiitis.

SYSTEMIC LUPUS ERYTHEMATOSUS AND OTHER COLLAGEN VASCULAR DISORDERS

The disease manifestations of SLE are highly variable. Pulmonary capillaritis leading to diffuse alveolar hemorrhage is rare in patients with SLE. However, it represents one of the most serious complications of the disease. In contrast to the pauci-immune pathology of ANCA-associated vasculitis, prominent immune complex deposits can be detected by direct immunofluorescence in the affected tissue of patients with SLE (Fig. 74-18). Hence, the development of pulmonary capillaritis in SLE is thought to be immune complex mediated. The onset of diffuse alveolar hemorrhage in patients with SLE is usually abrupt, and it is seldom the first sign of SLE. In the overwhelming majority of patients the rapid development of pulmonary infiltrates is associated with fever. Hemoptysis may be absent in up to one-half of the patients. Consequently, the differentiation of diffuse alveolar hemorrhage from infection may be difficult in patients with SLE, and may require a diagnostic bronchoalveolar lavage. Mechanical ventilation, infection, and cyclophosphamide therapy were identified as negative prognostic factors in one cohort.[38] However, no multivariate analysis was performed, and these factors may simply identify patients with more severe disease. The reported mortality from diffuse alveolar hemorrhage in SLE varies widely, between 0% and 90%. Treatment consists of glucocorticoids and cyclophosphamide.[39] The use of plasma exchange has been suggested, but its benefit remains unproved.

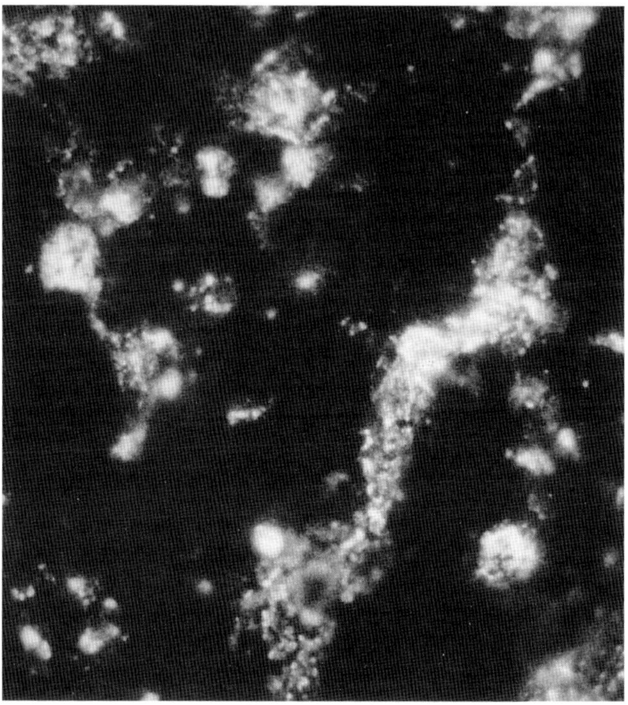

Figure 74-18 Lung biopsy of a patient with lupus erythematosus and alveolar hemorrhage showing so-called lumpy, bumpy deposition of immune complexes as demonstrated by direct immunofluorescence.

Respiratory complications are very common in all other types of collagen vascular or connective tissue disorders. However, pulmonary capillaritis presenting as diffuse alveolar hemorrhage is rare. Isolated cases have been reported with polymyositis, rheumatoid arthritis, and mixed connective tissue disease. Consequently, serological testing performed as part of an evaluation of diffuse alveolar hemorrhage should include studies aimed at the identification of these potential underlying disease entities.

ANTIPHOSPHOLIPID SYNDROME

Antiphospholipid syndrome is defined by arterial and venous thromboses, or recurrent miscarriages occurring in patients with antiphospholipid antibodies (anticardiolipin antibodies, lupus anticoagulant, or both). If antiphospholipid syndrome in the context of another autoimmune disease, malignancy, or drug exposure, it is labeled secondary antiphospholipid syndrome. In the absence of other coexisting disorders, it is considered primary. Hypercoagulability can cause pulmonary embolism and infarction, pulmonary microthrombosis, and pulmonary arterial thrombosis with secondary pulmonary hypertension as consequence. However, primary pulmonary hypertension has also been reported in antiphospholipid syndrome. Acute respiratory distress syndrome (ARDS) is another possible complication of antiphospholipid syndrome. Antiphospholipid syndrome can also be complicated by diffuse alveolar hemorrhage, presenting with cough, dyspnea, fever, and bilateral pulmonary infiltrates. Because of this nonspecific clinical presentation, the possible occurrence of diffuse alveolar hemorrhage in the context of ARDS, and the lack of hemoptysis in over one-half of the reported antiphospholipid syndrome patients with alveolar hemorrhage, and early bronchoalveolar lavage may help in the differential diagnosis. Tissue necrosis from microthrombosis as well as pulmonary capillaritis has been implicated as the cause of alveolar hemorrhage in antiphospholipid syndrome. As in SLE, the capillaritis of antiphospholipid syndrome appears to be immune complex mediated. Most patients respond to glucocorticoids.[40,41] Yet, the coexistence of thrombosis and capillaritis with alveolar hemorrhage represents a therapeutic dilemma, as anticoagulation may need to be interrupted to control the hemorrhage. Early plasma exchange in addition to immunosuppressive therapy should be considered in patients with antiphospholipid syndrome and alveolar hemorrhage.[42]

ANTI–GLOMERULAR BASEMENT MEMBRANE DISEASE

Historically, the syndrome of alveolar hemorrhage and glomerulonephritis has been called Goodpasture syndrome. Today's terminology restricts the use of the term Goodpasture disease to alveolar hemorrhage or necrotizing glomerulonephritis caused by autoantibodies directed against the NC1-domain of the $\alpha3$ chain of basement membrane collagen type IV. This epitope is only accessible for autoantibodies in the basement membranes of kidneys and lungs. Diffuse alveolar hemorrhage is common in anti–glomerular basement membrane (anti-GBM) disease but is thought

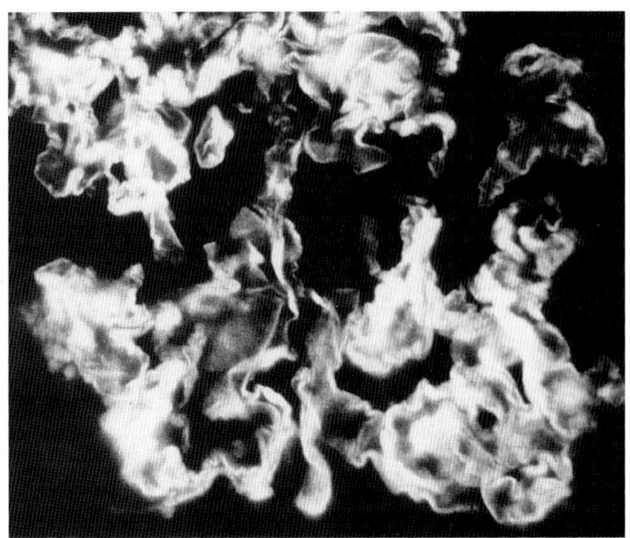

Figure 74-19 Kidney biopsy of a patient with anti–glomerular basement membrane (anti-GBM) disease showing linear immunofluorescence of the GBM due to fixation of IgG anti-GBM antibodies.

to require an additional inhalational injury, particularly smoking for the development of the pulmonary manifestation of this disease. Isolated alveolar hemorrhage in the absence of renal disease is rare in anti-GBM disease. The finding of circulating anti-GBM autoantibodies in the serum may facilitate the early implementation of appropriate therapy. However, methods used for their detection are of highly variable sensitivity and specificity, and a definitive diagnosis depends on the documentation of linear anti-GBM deposits in the kidney or lung (Fig. 74-19). In most patients, tissue from the kidney is more easily accessible for histopathological evaluation than lung tissue. Anti-GBM is arguably not a vasculitis. Bland pulmonary hemorrhage is the most frequently described histopathological pattern in diffuse alveolar hemorrhage associated with anti-GBM disease. However, capillaritis as a secondary histopathological feature has been encountered in some patients. Early implementation of immunosuppressive therapy in conjunction with plasma exchange is the key to a favorable outcome in patients with anti-GBM disease.[43]

IgA VASCULITIS (HENOCH–SCHÖNLEIN)

Henoch–Schönlein purpura has been renamed into IgA vasculitis (Henoch–Schönlein) as at the 2012 Chapel Hill Consensus Conference to reflect the evolving understanding of its pathogenesis. Pulmonary manifestations of IgA vasculitis are rare. Only 26 cases have been reported to date, and capillaritis has been documented histopathologically only in a minority of them.[44] IgA deposits along the pulmonary capillary walls, analogous to those found in vessels of the skin and glomeruli of affected kidneys are pathognomonic features of IgA vasculitis, detectable by direct immunofluorescence.

DRUG-INDUCED VASCULITIS

The list of drugs described in association with vasculitis includes a long list of therapeutic agents as well as drugs of abuse.[45] The clinical spectrum of drug-induced vasculitis ranges from isolated and mild vasculitis of the skin to severe multiorgan system disease. Small- to medium-sized vessels are usually affected. Based on clinical manifestations, drug-induced vasculitis cannot be distinguished from the primary vasculitis syndromes.

The following drug-induced syndromes merit special attention. First, a variety of drugs including propyl-thiouracil, D-penicillamine, hydralazine, sulfasalazine, minocycline, allopurinol, and others can induce an ANCA-associated vasculitis. Pulmonary capillaritis as a manifestation of an ANCA-associated vasculitis induced by these agents is well documented. Drug-induced ANCA-associated vasculitis should be treated with immunosuppression according to the principles for primary ANCA-associated vasculitis. However, once the offending drug has been eliminated, the likelihood of a relapse seems low.

The use of all-*trans*-retinoic acid in acute promyelocytic leukemia can cause a syndrome of fever, leukocytosis, fluid retention, hemorrhage, thrombosis, and organ failure. Pulmonary complications of this syndrome are frequent, and pulmonary capillaritis has been reported in this context.

Some chronic nasal cocaine abusers develop severe midline destructive lesions. In its early stage, such a lesion is clinically and histopathologically difficult to differentiate from limited Wegener granulomatosis, particularly in patients who do not volunteer the history of abuse.[46] The presence of ANCA reacting with human neutrophil elastase (HNE) appears to be an immunological marker separating patients with cocaine-induced midline destructive lesions from those with Wegener granulomatosis.[47]

More recently levamisole has become a common adulterant of cocaine.[48] Levamisole is a polyclonal B-cell–stimulating agent that can induce a variety of autoantibodies including antigranulocyte antibodies, antiphospholipid antibodies, and ANCA. The ANCA reactivity is directed against multiple target antigens including MPO, PR3, and HNE.[49] The clinical picture of patients exposed to levamisole can mimic systemic vasculitis.

PULMONARY CAPILLARITIS AFTER LUNG TRANSPLANTATION

Five cases of acute rejection after lung transplantation with prominent pulmonary capillaritis, histopathologically distinct from typical rejection, have been reported. In these cases, the capillaritis was

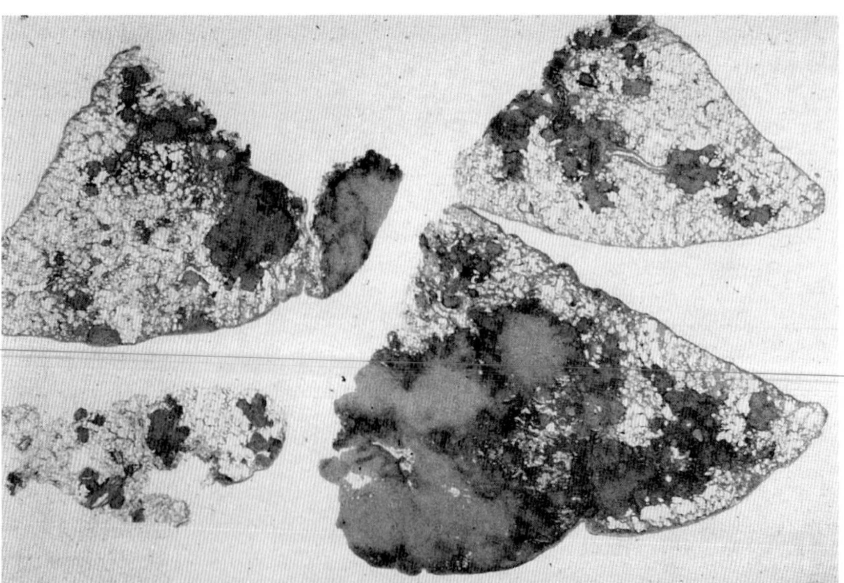

Figure 74-20 Low-power photomicrograph of lung revealing coalescing necrotizing granulomas in a patient with necrotizing sarcoid granulomatosis.

thought to represent a form of severe, acute vascular rejection. Early histological diagnosis and aggressive immunosuppression, possibly in conjunction with plasma exchange, was suggested to control the inflammatory activity and prevent relapses.

NECROTIZING SARCOID GRANULOMATOSIS

Vasculitis is a prominent histopathological feature of necrotizing sarcoid granulomatosis. The disease is usually limited to the lungs. The characteristic pulmonary nodules are bilateral, and may be an incidental finding in asymptomatic patients. Alternatively, patients may complain of cough, dyspnea, or phlegm production. Generalized constitutional symptoms occur rarely. The differential diagnosis of necrotizing sarcoid granulomatosis includes primarily infectious processes. Special sputum and tissue stains and cultures should always be obtained to exclude mycobacterial or fungal disease. Clinically, these patients are difficult to differentiate from limited Wegener granulomatosis. Histopathologically, there are characteristic necrotizing epithelioid granulomas that may form aggregates (Fig. 74-20). In contrast to Wegener granulomatosis, these granulomas are well circumscribed. Vasculitis is a central histopathological feature of necrotizing sarcoid granulomatosis. Liebow originally described three types of vasculitis: an epithelioid-granulomatous form, a form reminiscent of giant cell arteritis with prominent histiocytes and multinucleated giant cells in the inflammatory infiltrate of the vessel wall, and a lymphocytic form lacking granuloma formation and giant cells. The separation from sarcoidosis remains controversial. Yet, the extensive vasculitis and necrosis seen in necrotizing sarcoid granulomatosis are unusual for sarcoidosis. The chest roentgenographic appearance of pulmonary nodules, or masses and pleural involvement are also atypical for sarcoidosis. Finally, extrapulmonary involvement has only rarely been documented in necrotizing sarcoid granulomatosis.

It is debatable whether necrotizing sarcoid granulomatosis should be included with the systemic vasculitides. Most authors would argue against this inclusion because of its limitation to the lungs and good prognosis (spontaneous remission may occur). Therapeutically, necrotizing sarcoid granulomatosis can be approached as cases with chronic pulmonary sarcoidosis. Decisions about the use of oral glucocorticoid therapy should be individualized based on symptoms, pulmonary function data, and their evolution over time.

REFERENCES

1. Jennette JC, Falk RJ, Bacon PA, et al. 2012 revised International Chapel Hill Consensus Conference Nomenclature of Vasculitides. *Arthritis Rheum.* 2013;65(1):1–11.
2. Hoffman GS, Specks U. Anti-neutrophil cytoplasmic antibodies. *Arthritis Rheum.* 1998;41:1521–1537.
3. Watts RA, Scott DG. Epidemiology of the vasculitides. *Semin Respir Crit Care Med.* 2004;25(5):455–464.
4. Hoffman GS, Kerr GS, Leavitt RY, et al. Wegener granulomatosis: an analysis of 158 patients. *Ann Intern Med.* 1992;116:488–498.
5. Daum DE, Specks U, Colby TV, et al. Tracheobronchial involvement in Wegener's granulomatosis. *Am J Respir Crit Care Med.* 1995;151:522–526.
6. Polychronopoulos VS, Prakash UB, Golbin JM, Edell ES, Specks U. Airway involvement in Wegener's granulomatosis. *Rheum Dis Clin North Am.* 2007;33(4):755–775.
7. Oliveira GH, Seward JB, Tsang TS, Specks U. Echocardiographic findings in patients with Wegener granulomatosis. *Mayo Clin Proc.* 2005;80(11):1435–1440.
8. Guillevin L, Durand-Gasselin B, Cevallos R, et al. Microscopic polyangiitis: clinical and laboratory findings in eighty-five patients. *Arthritis Rheum.* 1999;42(3):421–430.
9. Keogh KA, Specks U. Churg-Strauss syndrome: clinical presentation, antineutrophil cytoplasmic antibodies, and leukotriene receptor antagonists. *Am J Med.* 2003;115(4):284–290.
10. Sinico RA, Di Toma L, Maggiore U, et al. Prevalence and clinical significance of antineutrophil cytoplasmic antibodies in Churg-Strauss syndrome. *Arthritis Rheum.* 2005;52(9):2926–2935.
11. Comarmond C, Pagnoux C, Khellaf M, et al. Eosinophilic granulomatosis with polyangiitis (Churg-Strauss): clinical characteristics and long-term followup of the 383 patients enrolled in the French Vasculitis Study Group cohort. *Arthritis Rheum.* 2013;65(1):270–281.
12. Cartin-Ceba R, Peikert T, Specks U. Pathogenesis of ANCA-associated vasculitis. *Curr Rheumatol Rep.* 2012;14(6):481–493.
13. Lyons PA, Rayner TF, Trivedi S, et al. Genetically distinct subsets within ANCA-associated vasculitis. *N Engl J Med.* 2012;367(3):214–223.
14. De Groot K, Rasmussen N, Bacon PA, et al. Randomized trial of cyclophosphamide versus methotrexate for induction of remission in early systemic antineutrophil cytoplasmic antibody-associated vasculitis. *Arthritis Rheum.* 2005;52(8):2461–2469.
15. Specks U. Methotrexate for Wegener's granulomatosis: what is the evidence? *Arthritis Rheum.* 2005;52(8):2237–2242.
16. Jayne D, Rasmussen N, Andrassy K, et al. A randomized trial of maintenance therapy for vasculitis associated with antineutrophil cytoplasmic autoantibodies. *N Engl J Med.* 2003;349(1):36–44.
17. de Groot K, Harper L, Jayne DR, et al. Pulse versus daily oral cyclophosphamide for induction of remission in antineutrophil cytoplasmic antibody–associated vasculitis: a randomized trial. *Ann Intern Med.* 2009;150(10):670–680.
18. Stone JH, Merkel PA, Spiera R, et al. Rituximab versus cyclophosphamide for ANCA-associated vasculitis. *N Engl J Med.* 2010;363(3):221–232.
19. Specks U, Merkel PA, Seo P, et al. Efficacy of remission induction regimens for ANCA-associated vasculitis. *N Engl J Med.* 2013;369(5):417–427.
20. Klemmer PJ, Chalermskulrat W, Reif MS, Hogan SL, Henke DC, Falk RJ. Plasmapheresis therapy for diffuse alveolar hemorrhage in patients with small-vessel vasculitis. *Am J Kidney Dis.* 2003;42(6):1149–1153.
21. Jayne DR, Gaskin G, Rasmussen N, et al. Randomized trial of plasma exchange or high-dosage methylprednisolone as adjunctive therapy for severe renal vasculitis. *J Am Soc Nephrol.* 2007;18(7):2180–2188.
22. Pagnoux C, Mahr A, Hamidou MA, et al. Azathioprine or methotrexate maintenance for ANCA-associated vasculitis. *N Engl J Med.* 2008;359(26):2790–2803.
23. Cartin-Ceba R, Golbin JM, Keogh KA, et al. Rituximab for remission induction and maintenance in refractory granulomatosis with polyangiitis (Wegener's): a single-center ten-year experience. *Arthritis Rheum.* 2012;64(11):3770–3778.
24. Stegeman CA, Cohen Tervaert JW, de Jong PE, Kallenberg CG. Trimethoprim-sulfamethoxazole (co-trimoxazole) for the prevention of relapses of Wegener's granulomatosis. *N Engl J Med.* 1996;335(1):16–20.
25. Wegener's Granulomatosis Etanercept Trial (WGET) Research Group. Etanercept plus standard therapy for Wegener's granulomatosis. *N Engl J Med.* 2005;352(4):351–361.
26. Cartin-Ceba R, Fervenza FC, Specks U. Treatment of antineutrophil cytoplasmic antibody-associated vasculitis with rituximab. *Curr Opin Rheumatol.* 2012;24(1):15–23.

27. Gayraud M, Guillevin L, le Toumelin P, et al. Long-term followup of polyarteritis nodosa, microscopic polyangiitis, and Churg-Strauss syndrome: analysis of four prospective trials including 278 patients. *Arthritis Rheum.* 2001;44(3):666–675.

28. Ribi C, Cohen P, Pagnoux C, et al. Treatment of Churg-Strauss syndrome without poor-prognosis factors: a multicenter, prospective, randomized, open-label study of seventy-two patients. *Arthritis Rheum.* 2008;58(2):586–594.

29. Tatsis E, Schnabel A, Gross WL. Interferon-a treatment of four patients with the Churg-Strauss syndrome. *Ann Intern Med.* 1998;129:370–374.

30. Pepper RJ, Fabre MA, Pavesio C, et al. Rituximab is effective in the treatment of refractory Churg-Strauss syndrome and is associated with diminished T-cell interleukin-5 production. *Rheumatology (Oxford).* 2008;47(7):1104–1105.

31. Cartin-Ceba R, Keogh KA, Specks U, Sethi S, Fervenza FC. Rituximab for the treatment of Churg-Strauss syndrome with renal involvement. *Nephrol Dial Transplant.* 2011;26(9):2865–2871.

32. Kim S, Marigowda G, Oren E, Israel E, Wechsler ME. Mepolizumab as a steroid-sparing treatment option in patients with Churg-Strauss syndrome. *J Allergy Clin Immunol.* 2010; 125(6):1336–1343.

33. Moosig F, Gross WL, Herrmann K, Bremer JP, Hellmich B. Targeting interleukin-5 in refractory and relapsing Churg-Strauss syndrome. *Ann Intern Med.* 2011;155(5):341–343.

34. Seo P, Stone JH. Large-vessel vasculitis. *Arthritis Rheum.* 2004; 51(1):128–139.

35. Larson TS, Hall S, Hepper NGG, Hunder GG. Respiratory tract symptoms as a clue to giant cell arteritis. *Ann Intern Med.* 1984;101:594–597.

36. Uzun O, Akpolat T, Erkan L. Pulmonary vasculitis in behcet disease: a cumulative analysis. *Chest.* 2005;127(6):2243–2253.

37. Jennings CA, King TE Jr, Tuder R, Cherniack RM, Schwarz MI. Diffuse alveolar hemorrhage with underlying isolated, pauciimmune pulmonary capillaritis. *Am J Respir Crit Care Med.* 1997;155(3):1101–1109.

38. Zamora MR, Warner ML, Tuder R, Schwarz MI. Diffuse alveolar hemorrhage and systemic lupus erythematosus. Clinical presentation, histology, survival, and outcome. *Medicine (Baltimore).* 1997;76(3):192–202.

39. Santos-Ocampo AS, Mandell BF, Fessler BJ. Alveolar hemorrhage in systemic lupus erythematosus: presentation and management. *Chest.* 2000;118(4):1083–1090.

40. Gertner E, Lie JT. Pulmonary capillaritis, alveolar hemorrhage, and recurrent microvascular thrombosis in primary antiphospholipid syndrome. *J Rheumatol.* 1993;20(7): 1224–1228.

41. Crausman RS, Achenbach GA, Pluss WT, O'Brien RF, Jennings CA. Pulmonary capillaritis and alveolar hemorrhage associated with the antiphospholipid antibody syndrome. *J Rheumatol.* 1995;22(3):554–556.

42. Waterer GW, Latham B, Waring JA, Gabbay E. Pulmonary capillaritis associated with the antiphospholipid antibody syndrome and rapid response to plasmapheresis. *Respirology.* 1999;4(4):405–408.

43. Levy JB, Turner AN, Rees AJ, Pusey CD. Long-term outcome of anti-glomerular basement membrane antibody disease treated with plasma exchange and immunosuppression. *Ann Intern Med.* 2001;134(11):1033–1042.

44. Nadrous HF, Yu AC, Specks U, Ryu JH. Pulmonary involvement in Henoch-Schonlein purpura. *Mayo Clin Proc.* 2004;79(9): 1151–1157.

45. Merkel PA. Drug-induced vasculitis. *Rheum Dis Clin North Am.* 2001;27(4):849–862.

46. Trimarchi M, Gregorini G, Facchetti F, et al. Cocaine-induced midline destructive lesions: clinical, radiographic, histopathologic, and serologic features and their differentiation from Wegener granulomatosis. *Medicine (Baltimore).* 2001;80(6): 391–404.

47. Wiesner O, Russell KA, Lee AS, et al. Antineutrophil cytoplasmic antibodies reacting with human neutrophil elastase as a diagnostic marker for cocaine-induced midline destructive lesions but not autoimmune vasculitis. *Arthritis Rheum.* 2004;50(9):2954–2965.

48. Specks U. The growing complexity of the pathology associated with cocaine use. *J Clin Rheumatol.* 2011;17(4):167–168.

49. McGrath MM, Isakova T, Rennke HG, Mottola AM, Laliberte KA, Niles JL. Contaminated cocaine and antineutrophil cytoplasmic antibody-associated disease. *Clin J Am Soc Nephrol.* 2011; 6(12):2799–2805.

CHAPTER 75

Pulmonary Arteriovenous Malformations

Daniel M. Goodenberger
Murali Chakinala

HISTORY

Pulmonary arteriovenous malformations (PAVMs) were first described in the late 19th century; Churton[1] reported the autopsy findings in a young boy with cyanosis in 1897. Based on the correlation of physical with postmortem findings, the triad of cyanosis, clubbing, and polycythemia was identified with PAVM in 1932.[2] Hereditary hemorrhagic telangiectasia (HHT) was first connected to PAVM in 1938.[3] As described below (Causes and Disease Associations), HHT is often intimately related to PAVMs—a fact that prompts the following discussion of the history of HHT.

Hereditary epistaxis was first described in 1864,[4] though neither that nor Babbington's description a year later report an association with telangiectasia.[5] These reports were not generally recognized; nor were subsequent descriptions of telangiectasia, hereditary transmission, and epistaxis by Legg[6] in 1876, or a similar kindred reported by Chiari in 1887.[7] The first widely recognized connection of epistaxis to telangiectasia was made by Rendu in 1896.[8] Osler[9] added three cases, and recognized familial occurrence in 1901. Weber[10] elucidated the familial nature and lack of coagulation abnormality, and thus earned his eponymic association. By precedence of description, this eponym should be Rendu–Osler–Weber, even though Osler–Weber–Rendu is the most common usage.

Hanes[11] was responsible for naming the syndrome HHT, the designation now most often preferred, in 1909.

GENETICS

The genetic basis, if any, of isolated PAVMs remains unknown. HHT is an autosomal dominant disease. Its frequency was believed until relatively recently to be less than 3 per 100,000 people.[12] Newer studies suggest a much higher prevalence. The highest frequency reported, 1:1331, occurs in the Afro-Caribbean population of the Netherlands Antilles, presumably due to a founder effect.[13] Other estimates vary geographically; 1:6410 in Denmark,[14] 1:8000 in Japan,[15] and 1:16,500 in Vermont.[16] Phenotypic variation is extreme, ranging from asymptomatic to severely symptomatic, and from cases with no or few mucocutaneous lesions to those with diffuse cutaneous telangiectasias. For many patients, the disease remains undiagnosed by their primary care physicians, suggesting that disease frequency may be greater than reported, and that some patients with "isolated" PAVMs may actually have HHT.

A gene for HHT was first localized to chromosome 9, region q^{33-34} ($9q^{33-34}$).[17–19] Investigation revealed the protein product to be endoglin, which associates with the transforming growth factor-beta (TGF-β) bone morphogenetic protein (BMP) receptor complex and binds TGF-β-1 and -3.[20] The same work showed the disease to be genetically heterogeneous, with multiple mutations in the responsible gene. It rapidly became clear that there were other chromosomal mutations resulting in the same syndrome, and the endoglin mutation disease was designated HHT-I; it was noted to be associated more often with PAVMs than were those with non-$9q^3$ mutations.[21,22] A haploinsufficient mouse model also demonstrated phenotypic heterogeneity which was very dependent on the genetic background.[23]

The activin receptor–like kinase 1 gene (ALK-1 or ACVRL1) on chromosome 12 is the second locus for HHT.[24,25] It produces a TGF-β superfamily type I receptor. Mice heterozygous for a loss-of-function mutation in ALK-1 develop age-dependent vascular lesions in the skin, extremities, oral cavity and in the lung, liver, intestine, spleen, and brain, similar to those seen in HHT patients.[26] Disease resulting from mutations in this gene has been designated HHT-2.

A small number of patients with juvenile polyposis also have HHT. This is due to mutations in MADH4 (encoding SMAD4); SMAD proteins influence the cellular response to TGF-β through interactions with other SMADs as transcription factors.[27,28]

A fourth gene abnormality producing clinical HHT in one family has been described on chromosome 5. The gene product is as yet unidentified.[29]

A fifth genetic abnormality in a family with HHT has been described on the short arm of chromosome 7.[30] The gene product of this mutation is also unknown at present.

Most HHT appears to be caused by mutations in endoglin and ALK-1. Mutations can be identified in up to 88% of affected individuals[31,32]; in one series, 61% were in endoglin, 37% in ALK-1, and 2% in MADH4.[33] ALK-1 mutations appear to be more common in France and Italy, with endoglin mutations more frequent in northern Europe and North America.[31,32,34] PAVMs are more frequent and on the average of larger size in HHT-1.[35]

Genetic testing for mutations in endoglin, ALK-1, and MADH-4 is currently available from six laboratories in North America, and a number of other laboratories in Europe. An up-to-date list with contact information is maintained at http://hht.org. The primary role for testing is to identify a mutation in an index case who meets criteria for a diagnosis of HHT. If this is possible, the index case's children and other first-degree relatives may be screened. Those with negative tests may be reassured, and those with positive tests may be evaluated for complications of HHT. On occasion, a diagnosis may be confirmed in an index case when clinical criteria are insufficient for clinical diagnosis. As with all genetic diseases, testing should be accompanied by genetic counseling.

PATHOPHYSIOLOGY

Important pathophysiologic considerations of PAVM are discussed below.

STRUCTURE

The three essential structural elements of PAVMs are the arterial supply ("feeder vessel"), a draining vein, and the intervening aneurysmal sac. Because of this simple relationship, the label of "AVM" is a bit of a misnomer as these malformations are more characteristic of a fistulous connection between arterial and venous branches without a customary intervening capillary network that is vital for gas exchange. PAVMs appear to develop between precapillary arterioles and venules, with intervening epithelial dysplasia.[36,37]

Approximately 80% of PAVMs have a single feeding and a single draining vessel; the remaining 20% are complex, with two or more of each.[38] By far the most common form of PAVM has a pulmonary arterial supply and pulmonary venous drainage.[39] In one series, 60 of 63 PAVMs had a pulmonary arterial blood supply[40] but arteries from the systemic circulation can also be involved, including arterial branches from the internal mammary artery, intercostal arteries, and subdiaphragmatic arteries. While systemic "feeders" are prone to develop as sequelae of chronic suppuration in the lung (e.g., sequestration), postpulmonary infarction after pulmonary embolism, or postembolization of pulmonary artery-to-vein malformations,[41] this chapter will focus on the classic form PAVMs involving the pulmonary arteries.

PATHOGENESIS

Our evolving understanding of PAVM development was summarized in a recent and thorough review of HHT.[42] Briefly, pathogenesis of PAVMs is presumed to initiate from periods of increased angiogenic activity, possibly triggered at sites of vascular injury,[43] and likely spurred on by an imbalance between proangiogenic signaling and reduced antiangiogenic activity. Angiogenesis is dysregulated due to altered expression of TGF-β–mediated pathways in endothelial cells of the pulmonary circulation, which plays a critical role in endothelial cell homeostasis. Mutations in one of the HHT-causative genes (described earlier) leads to either altered ligand-receptor interaction at the endothelial cell surface (ENG or ACVR1) or intracellular signaling (SMAD4) within endothelial cells. Downregulation of TGF-β expression is postulated to permit excessive endothelial cell proliferation and increase blood vessel formation[44] (under the influence of proangiogenic signals from molecules such as vascular endothelial growth factor [VEGF]), form persistent direct arteriovenous connections,[45] and destabilize vessels due to interactions between endothelial and mural cells (e.g., pericytes, smooth muscle cells).[46] The lack of a capillary network within a PAVM and the direct communication between arterioles and venules exposes thin-walled conduits to arterial blood flow and increased shear forces. Again, genetic defects and dysregulated angiogenesis lead to a muted compensatory response within these "arterialized" veins that must dilate. Furthering this concept, work in an animal model of HHT suggests a two-step dysregulatory sequence culminating in AVM formation, whereby the initial endothelial cell proliferation is mediated by HHT-causing mutations[44] and the subsequent dilation and persistence of downstream arteriovenous communications is independent of the mutations and, indeed, may be a homeostatic response to altered upstream blood flow pattern.[47] Over time, these initial microscopic communications grow into macroscopic communications[48] notable for relatively increased flow and passage of material normally sequestered or cleared in the pulmonary microcirculation (e.g., air bubbles, thrombi, bacteria). Further work in this area should clarify the molecular steps from altered gene expression to dysregulated

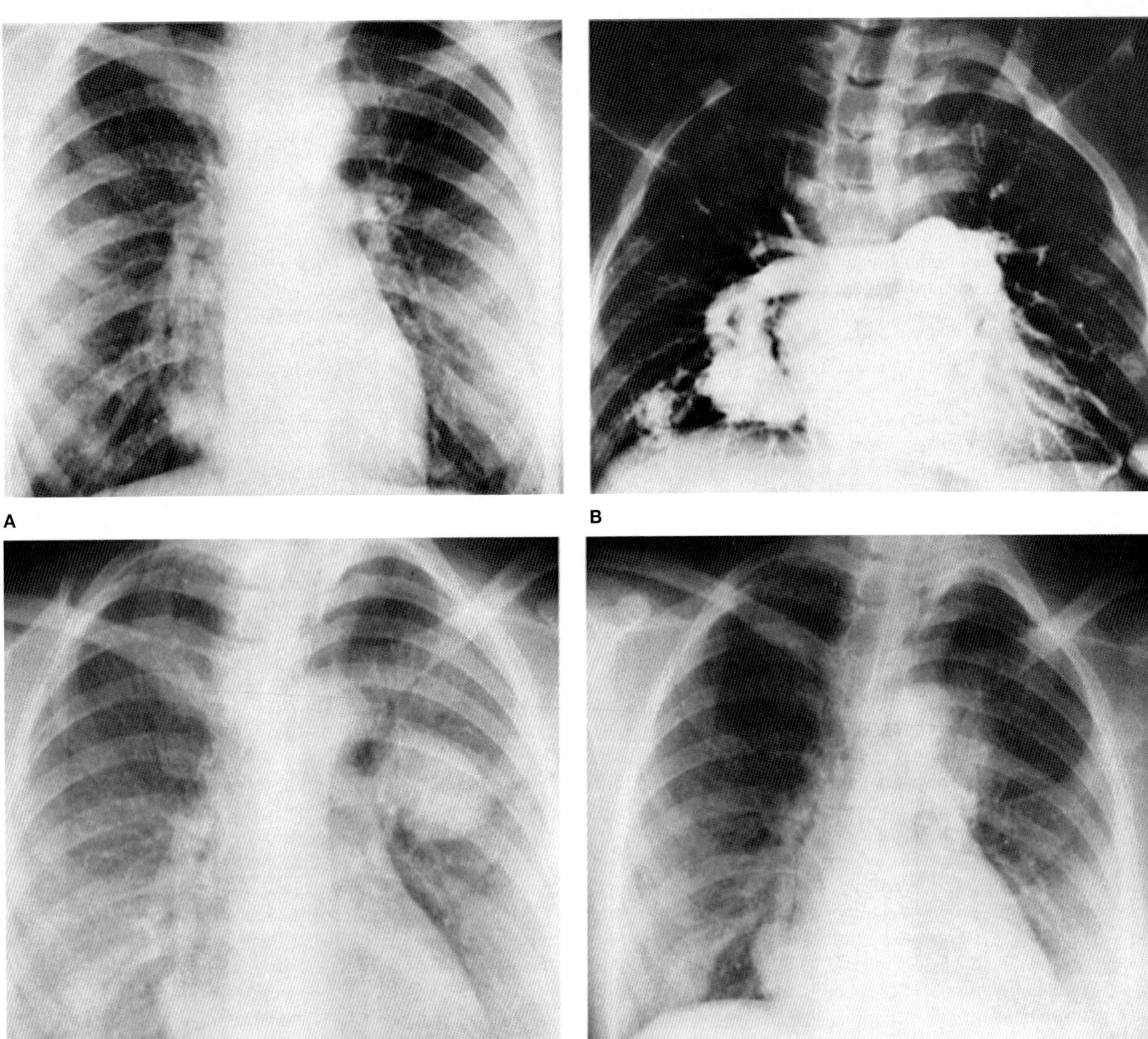

Figure 75-1 Pulmonary arteriovenous fistulas in a pregnant 24-year-old woman with hereditary hemorrhagic telangiectasia. **A.** Before pregnancy. Small nodular densities are seen at both bases and in the left hilus. The shunt was estimated to be 49% of the cardiac output. **B.** Arteriogram before pregnancy demonstrates arteriovenous fistulas of both lower lobes. **C.** Seven months pregnant, the patient was admitted to the hospital with hemoptysis and left hemothorax. The enlargement of the arteriovenous fistulas is striking. The pregnancy was terminated. **D.** Two weeks after termination of pregnancy, the nodular densities have decreased in size. *(Used with permission of Dr. M. Rossman.)*

multistep angiogenesis, discover precipitants of the dysregulated angiogenesis, and identify comediators, associated pathways, and environmental factors that influence angiogenesis.

Growth rates of AVMs remain unknown but is likely subject to intersubject variability and overall blood flow. One observed phenomenon of PAVM growth is accelerated growth during pregnancy leading to potential peripartum hemorrhagic complications,[49] which in part is theorized to occur due to increased blood flow and higher cardiac output of pregnancy but customary hormonal alterations of pregnancy could also be influential (Fig. 75-1).[50]

NUMBER

In one series, more than 60% of individuals present with more than one PAVM.[51] In general, multiple PAVMs correlate with HHT. A small percentage have diffuse, multilobar PAVMs that are typically bilateral and associated with marked hypoxemia.[52,53]

SIZE

PAVMs may vary from malformations too small to be seen by radiography or angiography[54,55] to those greater than 5 cm in diameter.[56]

LOCATION

Up to 65% of PAVMs are located in the lower lobes[55]—a phenomenon that may be due to the increased pulmonary blood flow and pressure, and subsequent “stretch” due to hydrodynamic forces. A recent small series noted less selectivity for the lower lobes in cases of “idiopathic” PAVMs.[57] The lower lobe location is the likely cause of the orthodeoxia (desaturation in an upright position) and platypnea (dyspnea in an upright position) which are sometimes seen. These symptoms may also occur with cirrhosis, which has pulmonary vascular abnormalities see below "Other Associations". Location may also account for an increase in right-to-left shunt which occurs at total lung capacity.[58]

CAUSES AND DISEASE ASSOCIATIONS

Early observers thought that all PAVMs were due to HHT.[38] The estimates of frequency with which PAVMs are due to HHT have varied substantially, from 36% to 95%.[38,40,50,59,60] Most recent series report HHT in well over 90%.

Estimates of the percentage of patients with HHT who have associated PAVMs have varied widely. Different series have reported frequencies of 15%,[50] 20%,[61] 24%,[36] 33%,[62] 49%,[63] and 57%.[64] Frequency of PAVMs appears to be significantly greater in cases with ENG mutations, as opposed to ACVRL1 mutations.[65] Furthermore, overall PAVM detection rates are being influenced by improving imaging techniques that provide clearer resolution of the vasculature in the peripheral areas of the lung.

OTHER ASSOCIATIONS

Cirrhosis may result in diffuse small arteriovenous connections.[66] Nearly all such patients have cutaneous spider angiomas. The right-to-left shunt is probably due not to true PAVMs but, rather, to vasodilation of pleural vessels, which resemble cutaneous spiders, and increased numbers of peripheral small arteriolar branches with precapillary arteriole-to-venous connections in the peripheral respiratory lobule. As many as 44% to 60% may have positive contrast echocardiography indicative of intrapulmonary shunt;[67,68] many of these patients have shunt eliminated by liver transplantation. A PAVM of significant size, known as a Rasmussen aneurysm, may also develop as a result of tuberculosis.[69] Metastatic thyroid carcinoma, a highly vascular tumor, may mimic pulmonary arteriovenous fistula.[70] Cavopulmonary anastomosis, used in the palliation of functionally univentricular heart disease, results in pulmonary arteriovenous connections similar to those in cirrhosis, in approximately 10% of patients. The reasons are unclear.[71] Rarely, penetrating chest trauma may result in subsequent PAVM.[72]

PRESENTATION AND COMPLICATIONS

PRESENTATION

The occurrence and frequency of symptoms related to PAVMs depend on how the patients are found—that is, whether they present with manifestations of disease or whether they are discovered as a result of screening. When detection occurs as a result of screening in patients with HHT, between 25% and 59% are asymptomatic.[50,73–75]

The age at onset is usually in the third or fourth decade.[38] The mean age at detection in various series is remarkably constant at 38 to 40 years.[50,51,73,74] In one series, the patients ranged in age from 5 to 76 years, with a mean of 36; 26% presented at an age less than 21 years.[55] PAVMs are, however, uncommon in childhood; only 4% of affected persons are under 10.[78,79]

Pulmonary symptoms include dyspnea on exertion, with a frequency ranging from 27% to 71%.[21,40,55,80] Platypnea and orthodeoxia also may occur. Hemoptysis ranges in frequency from 4% to 18%.[21,51,55] Extrapulmonary symptoms include chest pain in 6%[81] and epistaxis (largely seen in HHT), ranging from 32% to 85%.[37,80,82] The mean age at onset of epistaxis in HHT is 12 years, with 54% of patients presenting by age 10. Severity of epistaxis ranges from mild to severe, with up to 45 episodes per month.[76] Headache is also remarkably common in HHT patients, occurring in 43%.[55] Transient ischemic attack (TIA) occurs in up to 57% of patients with PAVM, and symptomatic cerebrovascular accident in 18%.[55,76]

Physical signs due to the PAVM itself are relatively uncommon. As many as 25% of patients may exhibit no findings at all.[40] Hypoxemia, when present, is secondary to the right-to-left shunt, and may result in cyanosis and secondary polycythemia. This tends to occur in advanced disease, and has been reported in 9% to 73% (mean 30%).[40,59,76] The frequency of clubbing has been reported in an average of 32%[76]; it is much less common in our experience.[49,56] Clubbing is nearly always associated with cyanosis. Clubbing may resolve after the PAVM is removed[83] or occluded. A pulmonary bruit, which is often described, is also variable; its frequency, probably influenced by selection bias, ranges from less than 10% to 58%.[40,49,76,80]

Telangiectasia have been reported in up to 66% of patients with PAVM, depending on the frequency of HHT.[84] These small red vascular blemishes occur most frequently on the face, followed in descending order by the lips, nares, tongue, ears, hands, chest, and feet. They often increase in size and number with age, and cutaneous telangiectasias are seldom identifiable until the second or third decade.[37] We have been struck by the frequency with which classic tongue and lip telangiectasias have been passed off as nonspecific blemishes by primary care physicians.

Laboratory results are nonspecific. A complete blood count may show polycythemia, although in patients with HHT, this tendency may be overshadowed by iron deficiency anemia. Anemia was present in 94 of 292 (34%) in our series. This was more often due to GI bleeding when severe. GI blood loss of variable severity was present in 65 of 292 (22%).[56]

The severely affected person may have arterial hypoxemia at rest; those less severely affected may have orthodeoxia documented by supine and upright arterial blood gases.[85] Arterial blood gases, determined on blood samples drawn while the patient is breathing room air, followed by 100% oxygen, may reveal a significant right-to-left shunt.[86]

COMPLICATIONS

Pulmonary and neurologic complications of PAVMs are important considerations.

Pulmonary Complications

Significant hemoptysis occurs in fewer than 10% of patients; in our most recent series, it occurred in 5 of 142 (<4%). Two of five occurred during pregnancy.[56] It may be massive and life-threatening. Bronchial telangiectasias may be the cause,[62] but all cases in untreated patients in our experience have been due to PAVMs. An increasingly frequent problem in recent years is hemoptysis following extensive embolotherapy after a delay of months to years. This has generally been due to postembolization bronchial collateral formation.

Hemothorax has been reported in up to 9% of patients,[87] but is usually less than 2%.[76] Pregnancy has been associated with hemothorax on several occasions, perhaps related to PAVM enlargement.[88–90] Hemothorax may also occur without any other predisposing factors, presumably caused by rupture of large subpleural PAVMs into the pleural space.

Typically, PAVMs are associated with a normal or low pulmonary vascular resistance (PVR) as the direct arteriovenous communications are low-resistance circuits. However, pulmonary hypertension is encountered, albeit uncommonly, in the setting of PAVMs and HHT.[91] Pulmonary hypertension most often develops from increased pulmonary blood flow, which occurs in HHT because of massive hepatic arteriovenous malformations that rapidly return blood to the right side of the heart and lead to a high cardiac output state. The high output can be aggravated by concomitant chronic anemia from blood loss. In this situation, the PVR will be low as the entire pulmonary circuit, not just the PAVM, dilates to accommodate increased pulmonary blood flow; but the capacitance of the circuit has limits and additional blood flow will lead to mild pulmonary hypertension. In distinction, another more devastating but rarer form of pulmonary hypertension can be seen in the setting of PAVMs, whereby the PVR is quite high due to a proliferative vasculopathy of small pulmonary arterioles.[92] In these rare cases, mutations occur primarily in ACVRL1 gene and represent a form of heritable pulmonary arterial hypertension (HPAH),[93] which is a form of Group I pulmonary hypertension in the Dana Point classification of pulmonary hypertension.[94] When PAH patients are discovered to have ACVRL1 or endoglin mutations during the genetic workup, PAVMs should be excluded as other clues for HHT can be subtle or absent in this rare population and PAH can be detected prior to a diagnosis of HHT being made.[95,96] When PAVMs coexist with significant PAH, caution must be exercised with PAVM embolization (see Treatment section) as sudden obliteration of the low-resistance circuit could significantly increase the PVR and unsettle an already fragile right ventricle or lead to other hemorrhagic complications[97,98]; these rare cases should be managed in a multidisciplinary fashion by individuals familiar with the management of PAVMs and PAH.

Central Nervous System Complications

The pulmonary capillary vascular bed appears to be an important filter for otherwise asymptomatic small emboli, and may also have a significant role in cleansing the bloodstream during transient bacteremia. Most neurologic complications, which occur in 8% to 12% of patients with HHT, are complications of PAVMs. In one series, 60% were due to PAVM, including brain abscess, paradoxical embolus, and hypoxemia.[37,99]

TIAs occur in approximately 37% of patients with PAVMs.[55] PAVMs can cause symptomatic cerebrovascular accidents (Fig. 75-2); the frequency of this complication ranges from 6% to 27%.[40,55,76] In our clinic, 28 of 132 patients screened by magnetic resonance imaging (MRI) had evidence of prior paradoxical embolic stroke.[56] Unfortunately, paradoxical embolization to the brain may be the first manifestation of an occult pulmonary venous malformation. This has been a particularly regrettable repetitive problem in young women who smoke and take oral contraceptives. Care should be taken to avoid air embolism; IV should be free of air and a micropore inline filter used.

Brain abscess occurs in 3% to 10% of patients with PAVMs.[37,76] In a series in our clinic, 5/132 (4%) had prior brain abscess.[56] Up to 1% of HHT patients may have brain abscesses (1000 times the incidence in the general population). In one series, 5 of 31 patients had recurrent abscess[100]; in another, 6 of 128.[101] Up to 8% of brain abscesses in the general population may be due to PAVMs.[102] Unfortunately, brain abscess may also be the first symptom of an occult PAVM (Fig. 75-3), and many years may elapse before diagnosis of PAVM (Fig. 75-4). Most occur following dental work. For that reason, antibiotic prophylaxis following the standard American Heart Association protocol for prevention of endocarditis is recommended.[103]

Migraine is more common in HHT than in the general population, and appears to be more common in those with PAVM. In one series, migraine occurred in 88 patients with HHT, a prevalence of 16.4%. The prevalence of migraine in patients with PAVM was 21.2%, which

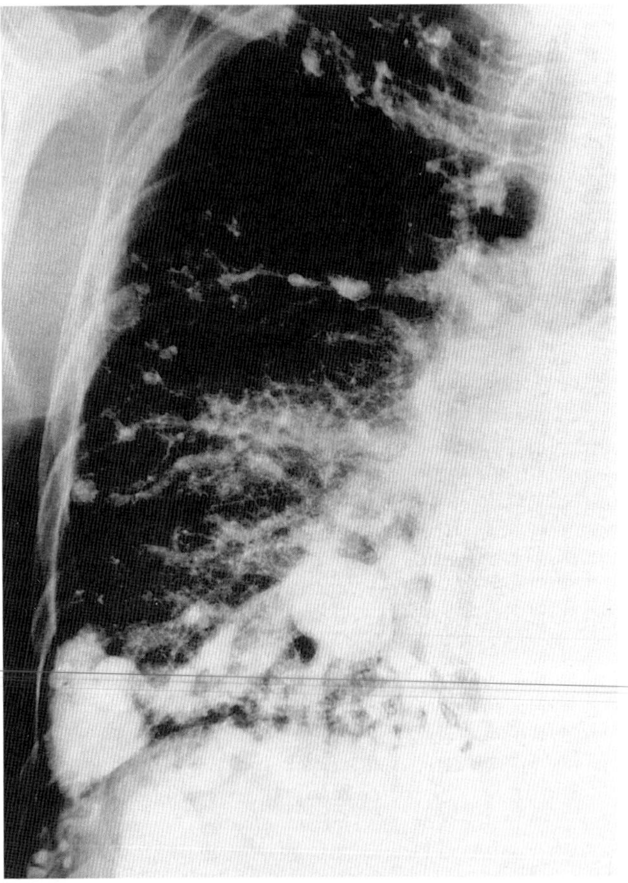

Figure 75-2 Right-sided pulmonary angiogram showing multiple PAVMs in a middle-aged man with clubbing, polycythemia, and CT evidence of several prior strokes.

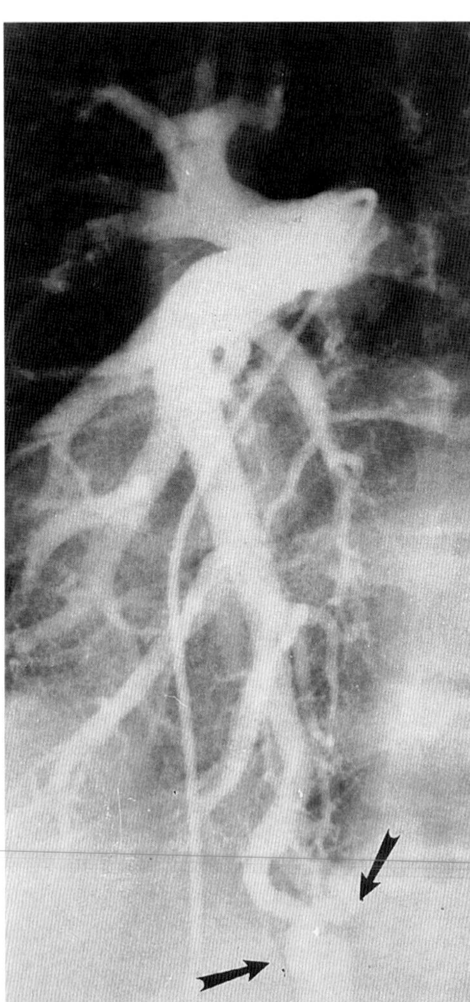

Figure 75-3 PAVM detected in patient with HHT after initial presentation with brain abscess. The PA and lateral chest radiographs were normal on several occasions. Right pulmonary angiogram with inferomedial PAVM *(arrows)*.

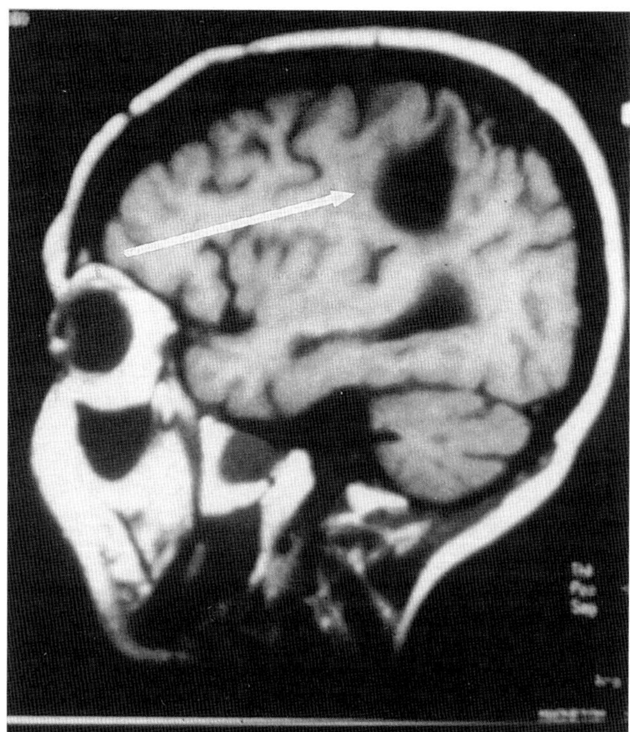

Figure 75-4 MRI showing brain abscess residua in patient whose brain abscess preceded diagnosis of pulmonary arteriovenous fistula by 17 years.

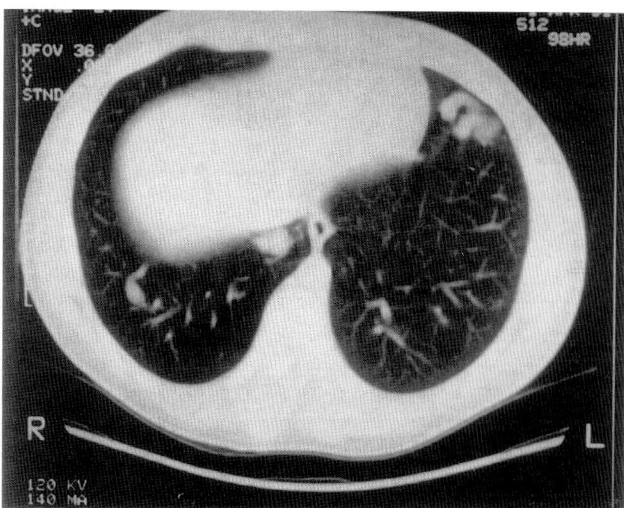

Figure 75-5 Characteristic CT image appearance of PAVM in left hemithorax. Portions of two PAVMs are seen in right hemithorax.

was significantly higher than in patients without PAVM (13.3%).[104] In our experience, migraines occurred in 74/292 (25%) with HHT.[56]

Cerebral arteriovenous malformations (CAVMs) occur in 4% to 8% of patients with HHT[55,105] and tend to run in families.[106] Although CAVMs are not complications of PAVMs, they occur more frequently in patients with endoglin mutations, as do PAVMs. In our series of 149 patients screened by MRI, 11 had CAVM (7%). An additional 16 (11%) had telangiectasia or venous angioma (11%).[56] It is recommended that individuals with HHT, including children, be screened for CAVM.[103] The hemorrhage rate in individuals with cerebral AV malformations appears to be 0.5% annually, less than that in the non-HHT population with cerebral AVMs.[107] Cerebral MRI is currently the most sensitive noninvasive test, although it will fail to detect a significant proportion of AVMs.[105] MRI may be performed in patients with pulmonary AVMs embolized with both stainless steel coils and platinum Nester coils in machine with fields up to 3.0 T[108]; we have performed many such cerebral MRI examinations without complications, although the MRI is not done for a minimum of 6 weeks after embolotherapy.

DIAGNOSIS

Diagnostic evaluation of suspected PAVMs includes assessment of chest radiographs and CT scans, supplemented by additional studies, as warranted.

■ EVALUATION OF A RADIOGRAPHIC ABNORMALITY

Discovery of a nodule on chest x-ray is typically followed by CT scan of the chest. This may show the typical lesion with feeding and draining veins (Fig. 75-5),[3] but vascular tumors may cause false-positive results. Evidence of intrapulmonary right-to-left shunt confirms the diagnosis. A perfusion lung scan may detect a right-to-left shunt. Ordinarily, 95% of the technetium-labeled macroaggregated albumin, with an average diameter of approximately 35 μ, is trapped in the pulmonary capillaries. When there is an intracardiac or intrapulmonary shunt, unusually large amounts may pass through the lung and travel to the brain and kidneys, resulting in excess radioactivity in those areas. However, this method cannot differentiate intracardiac from intrapulmonary shunt.

Echocardiography, using indocyanine green as a contrast material, was found to be effective in the diagnosis of intrapulmonary shunt, with delayed appearance of the contrast material in the left side of the heart.[109] This was simplified and improved by the use of agitated saline as contrast (Fig. 75-6) (Video 75-1).[110] The intrapulmonary nature of the shunt can be determined by the delay, averaging four to five cardiac cycles, of left heart contrast appearance. If contrast echocardiography is negative, a PAVM is very unlikely, and an alternative cause of the pulmonary nodule should be sought. On rare occasions, if the PAVM is fed by a systemic artery, the contrast echocardiogram will be negative, and bronchial and/or internal mammary angiography should be undertaken if suspicion is high.

■ SCREENING OF PROBANDS OR RELATIVES WITH HHT

Because the majority of PAVMs occur in HHT, it is important to evaluate individuals with PAVMs for HHT, and to screen individuals with HHT for PAVMs. Criteria for diagnosis of HHT include (1) spontaneous and recurrent epistaxis; (2) multiple characteristic telangiectasia (typically found on lips, tongue, malar eminence, pinnae, and digits); (3) visceral lesions (gastrointestinal telangiectasia with or without GI bleeding, PAVMs, hepatic arteriovenous malformations, CAVMs, and spinal AVMs); (4) family history with a first-degree relative with HHT.[111] In addition, relatives of patients with HHT should be evaluated for that diagnosis. Those found to have HHT should be screened for PAVMs. Consensus of an international panel was that screening should occur at the time of diagnosis, including children.[103]

The reported sensitivity of chest radiographs varies widely, depending on whether they are used for screening or in patients with symptomatic disease. Rates of abnormality on the chest radiograph range from 41%[75] to 100%.[40] In our experience, chest

Video 75-1 Saline contrast echocardiogram demonstrating characteristic delay of left-sided contrast in patient with intrapulmonary shunt. *(Used with permission of Dr. Daniel Goodenberger) Access at www.fishmansonline.com*

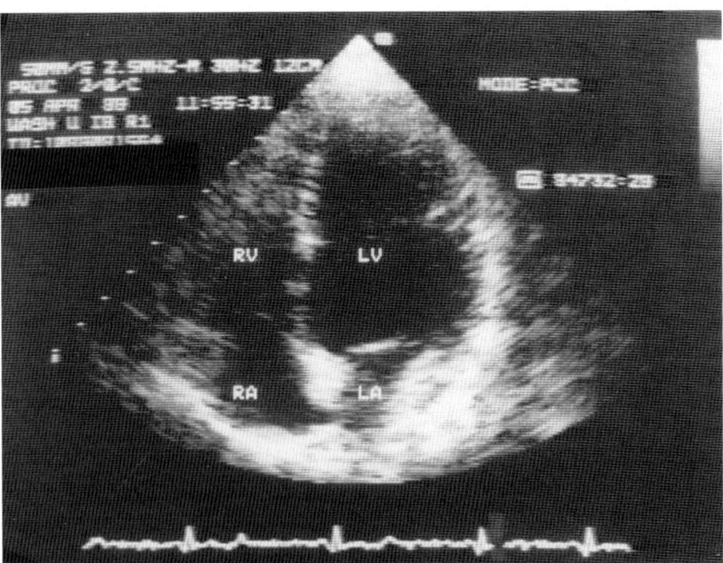

A

B

C

Figure 75-6 Echocardiographic images using saline contrast. **A.** Before contrast. **B.** Right-sided chamber opacification. **C.** Delayed high-degree left-sided chamber opacification indicative of large intrapulmonary shunt.

radiography does not reliably detect PAVMs less than 20 mm in size (Fig. 75-7), and it may miss larger PAVMs when they are located in radiographically inopportune places, such as the costophrenic sulci, the retrocardiac region, or the proximal hila (Fig. 75-8).[86]

Arterial blood gases, determined on samples drawn while the patient is supine and upright, have been advocated for screening.[85] However, this technique has not proved useful. Various combinations of shunt measurement utilizing albumin microspheres labeled with technetium-99m, Pa_{O_2} on room air, shunt measurement in subjects breathing 100% oxygen, and erect oxygen saturation measurement have been utilized, but all have insufficient sensitivity, specificity, or both.[14,78,112–114]

Contrast echocardiography is more sensitive than symptoms, plain radiography, measurements of Sa_{O_2}, Pa_{O_2} on room air, and Pa_{O_2} breathing 100% oxygen.[14,63] It is positive in 55% to 73% of those with HHT,[56,112] and may be the only positive screening study in 31% of patients.[113] Eighty percent or more will have persistently positive contrast echo findings after undergoing embolotherapy.[115] In patients with diffuse small PAVMs or telangiectasia, transesophageal contrast echocardiography may provide the definitive evidence.[116] On the basis of the preceding information, a screening algorithm based on contrast echocardiography and anteroposterior chest radiograph, followed by chest CT if either test is positive, is used in many centers.[63] This algorithm is based on studies in which CT without contrast was used as the "gold standard," with confirmatory pulmonary angiogram only if positive, and has been recommended by the international HHT working group.[103]

The sensitivity and specificity of chest CT are unknown, although this modality is significantly more sensitive than are chest radiographs.[85] One early study suggested that CT enabled identification more than 98% of PAVMs and was superior to pulmonary angiography.[117] CT has also been advocated for pretherapy planning.[118]

Our center for many years followed a scheme in which patients with HHT are screened with saline contrast echocardiography. Those with positive findings underwent pulmonary angiography. This approach identified PAVMs in 57% of patients screened. In combination with our observations regarding false-negative chest CT, we believed the frequency of PAVMs identified, greater than in any other series, justified this approach. In ~15% of patients with angiographically detectable PAVMs using this approach, no therapeutic embolization results. These PAVMs represent an opportunity to more fully understand the natural history and complication rates of PAVMs.[64]

Technology has an impact on this approach. Contrast-enhanced 64-row multidetector array chest CT with reconstruction is now used in our center as an alternative to diagnostic angiography (Video 75-2). Results to

Video 75-2 CT angiogram of right lower lobe pulmonary arteriovenous malformation in patient with hereditary hemorrhagic telangiectasia. *(Used with permission of Dr. Daniel Goodenberger) Access at www.fishmansonline.com*

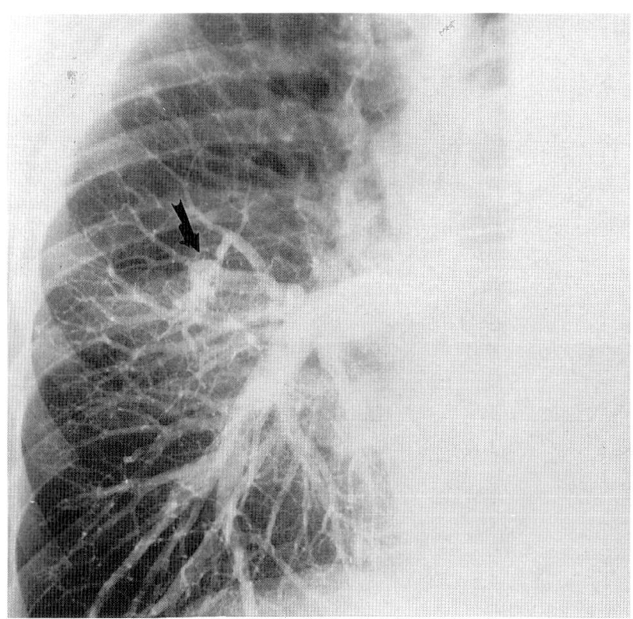

Figure 75-7 Example of PAVM not seen on standard chest radiography. Right pulmonary angiogram showing small PAVM *(arrow)*.

date suggest that this technique is at least equivalent to pulmonary angiography (Fig. 75-9).

TREATMENT

The earliest treatment of PAVMs was thoracotomy and resection. Pneumonectomy was the first successful surgical approach, reported in 1942.[119] As thoracic surgery improved, the extent of resections diminished; by 1959, local excision was the procedure of choice.[62] Surgical removal of a PAVM inevitably results in loss of viable lung tissue, a problem for patients with multiple PAVMs; the record is probably held by a patient who underwent staged bilateral thoracotomies with removal of 23 PAVMs, with substantial symptomatic improvement.[120] Thoracoscopic resection has more recently been described.[121] Although surgical mortality can be as low as 0%,[62] the general anesthesia, morbidity of thoracotomy, and loss of viable lung tissue made a new approach desirable.

Embolization of PAVMs has proved to be an excellent alternative. This procedure was first performed using homemade coils. The procedure was refined and perfected at Johns Hopkins by Terry et al.[122] The original procedure utilized silicone balloons unless the feeding vessel was larger than 9 mm in diameter, in which case embolization

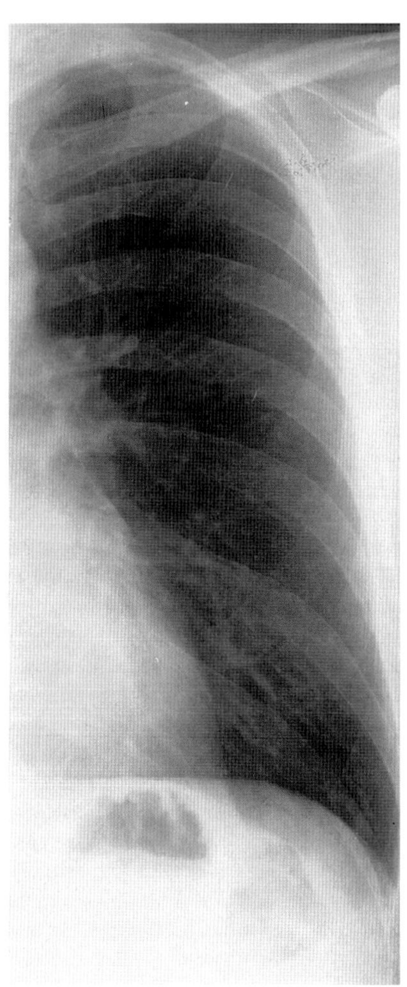

A

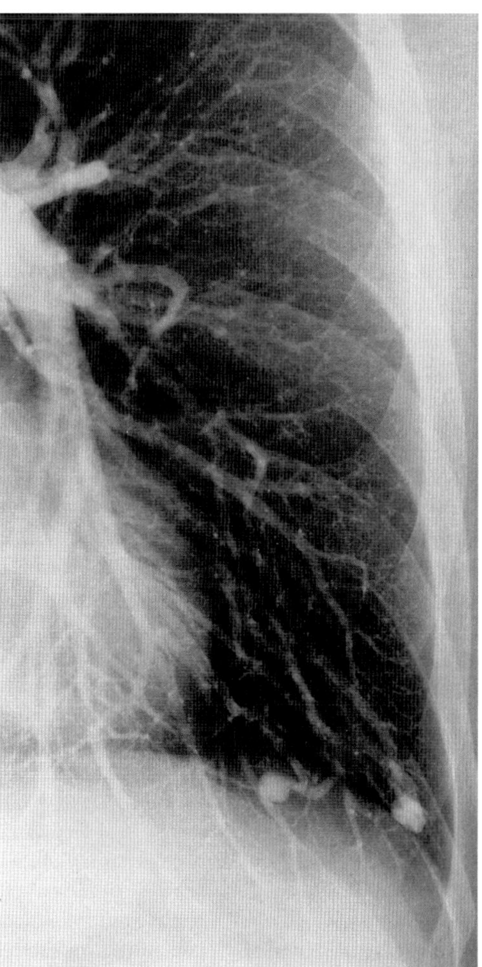

B

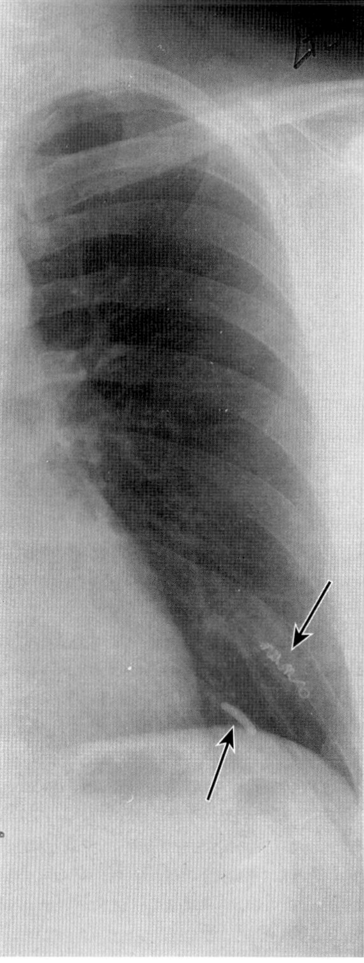

C

Figure 75-8 Example of patient with PAVMs that were not seen on standard radiography but were detected by echocardiographic screening. **A.** Before embolization. **B.** Angiogram. **C.** After embolization, showing both coil and balloon emboli.

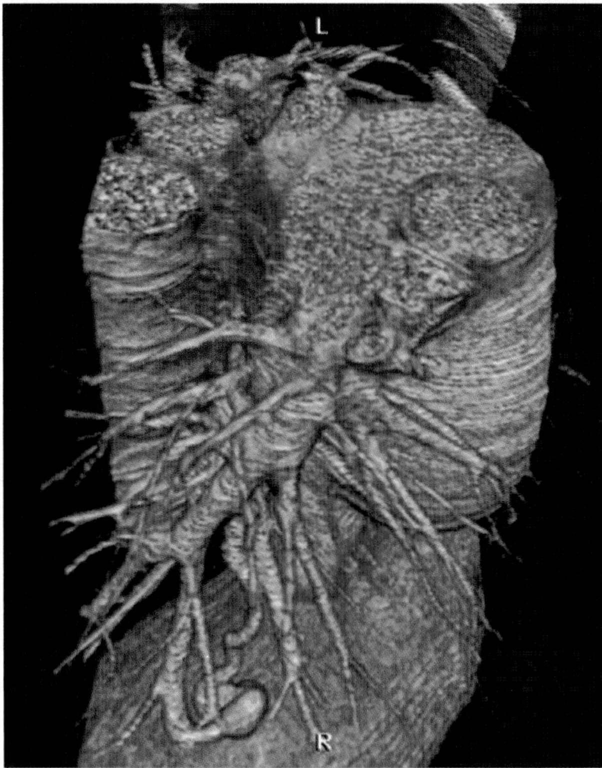

A

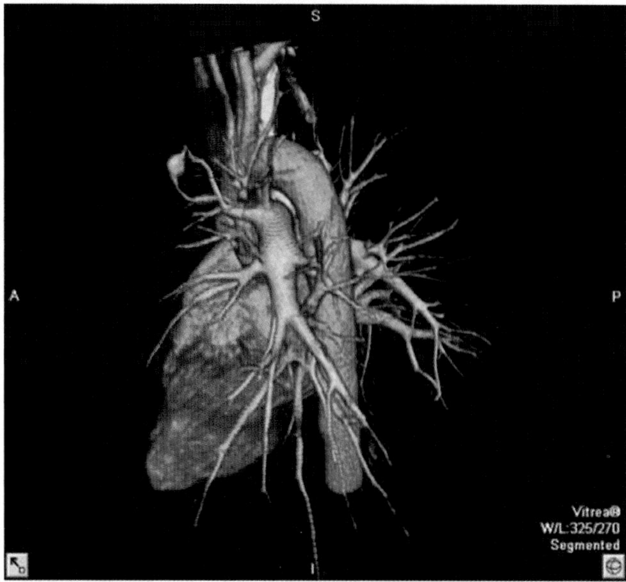

B

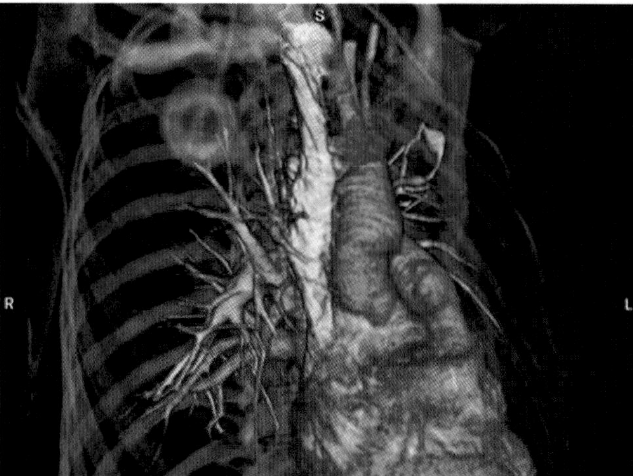

C

Figure 75-9 **A–C.** Three-dimensional reconstruction of PAVMs on 64-row multidetector array CT.

coils with thrombogenic Dacron tails were used (Fig. 75-10A–C).[55] Generally, all PAVMs with feeding vessel diameter of 3 mm or larger are embolized. Results have been very good, with success rates greater than 93%,[123] and embolization therapy is now the procedure of choice, with an apparent mortality of 0%, few serious complications, minimal loss of pulmonary parenchyma, and no exposure to anesthesia or thoracotomy. Silicone balloons are no longer available and are of historic interest only. Recently, many interventional radiologists have preferred using vascular plugs for larger feeding vessels, reserving coils for small or more tortuous vessels. Advantages include occlusion with a single device, allowing decreased operative time, and possible reduction in reperfusion (Fig. 75-11A–C).[124]

Pregnant women requiring urgent embolotherapy because of hemoptysis or hemothorax may safely undergo embolization, with radiation exposure to the fetus acceptable after 16 weeks of gestational age, with successful pregnancy outcome.[77] Absent those complications, embolotherapy may be deferred until the patient is postpartum.

Embolotherapy may also be performed safely and effectively in children.[125]

There are some limitations. The feeding vessel must be 2 to 3 mm in diameter or larger. It is technically feasible to embolize most PAVMs, but occasionally this is not possible. All but three patients in our 24-year experience have been able to be treated with embolotherapy (2/132 in the most recent series).[56] A majority will have persistent intrapulmonary shunt and should receive predental antibiotic prophylaxis.[115]

Reperfusion of the embolized vessel may occur in up to 15%.[80,126,127] This may require repeated embolotherapy. The current standard is follow-up by CT at 6 months, and if negative, every 3 years thereafter.[103]

While observations documenting serial growth of small PAVMs are somewhat limited, there is published evidence to support their growth with time.[12,40,60,80,128,129] Progression of PAVMs appears more likely in those with multiple PAVMs.[75] It has been suggested that patients with treated PAVM need follow-up every 5 years to detect growth of small PAVMs that could become large enough to cause paradoxical embolization and stroke.[103]

In general, successful embolization of most or all visible PAVMs results in abatement of hypoxemia and its complications,[128,130] but a

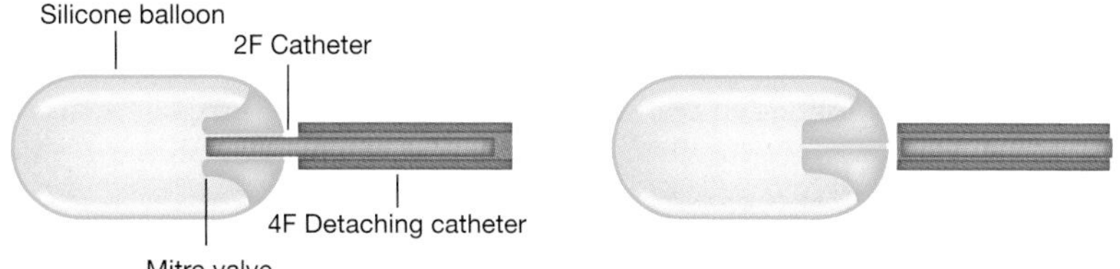

A

B

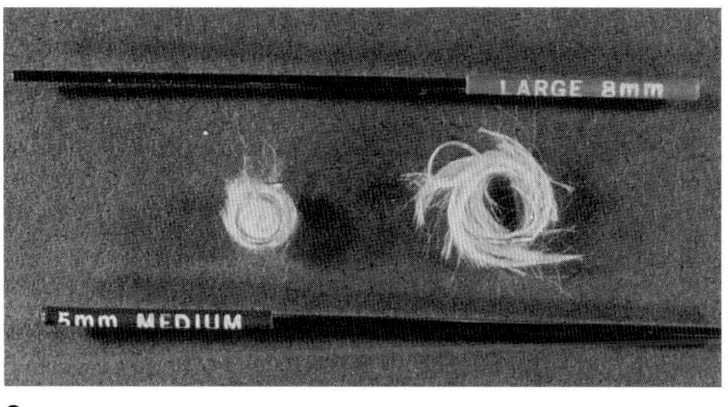

C

Figure 75-10 Embolotherapy devices. **A.** Detachable balloon mechanism from catheter. **B.** Fluoroscopic image of balloon in vivo. **C.** Embolization coils of two sizes.

small number of patients have diffuse small PAVMs not amenable to embolization.

Occlusion of all PAVMs with feeding vessels 3 mm or larger greatly reduces the risk of embolic stroke. Complex PAVMs must have all feeding vessels embolized for success. Embolotherapy may reduce the risk of brain abscess, but abscess may recur even after successful therapy.[129] Although no data regarding efficacy exist, standard American Heart Association endocarditis guidelines for antibiotic prophylaxis before embolotherapy is recommended.[103] Because of the frequent observation of small persistent left-to-right shunt demonstrated by echocardiography even after successful embolotherapy, antibiotic prophylaxis is recommended for dental and other surgical procedures.[103]

In general, those PAVMs which may feasibly be embolized should be occluded at or around the time of discovery, as immediate embolotherapy on detection results in improved life expectancy and quality-adjusted survival.[131]

Serious complications of embolotherapy are rare. Because of the potential for systemic air and particulate embolism, all intravenous tubing is equipped with micropore filters and embolization precautions are taken. Air embolism during the procedure is rare, occurring in less than 5% in one series. It is generally manifested by perioral paresthesias or angina without permanent effect.[55] The most common postembolization symptom is pleurisy, and has been reported at rates ranging from 10% to 31%.[55,80,132] The onset may be delayed for up to 17 days in our experience, and severity may range from mild pain to a level of discomfort requiring hospitalization. These episodes are sometimes accompanied by large pleural effusions. The effusions and resulting hypoxemia always resolve within several weeks. Other complications have included migration of an embolic device, PAVM perforation, TIA, early cerebral infarction after embolization, and paradoxical embolization of a device during deployment (4%).[128,129,132–134]

Diffuse PAVMs resulting in hypoxemia are difficult to treat with embolization therapy. Multiple embolizations tend to result in modest improvement at best, and posttherapy complications may be severe.[53,135] Those which are not amenable to embolotherapy represent a particularly difficult problem. A few such cases have been successfully treated with lung transplantation.[136,137]

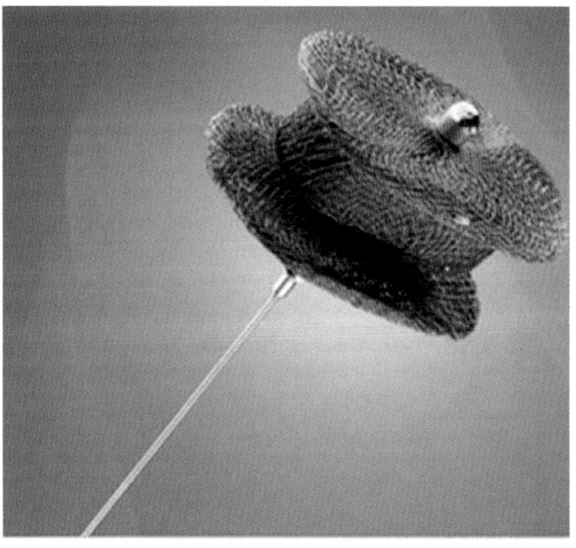

A

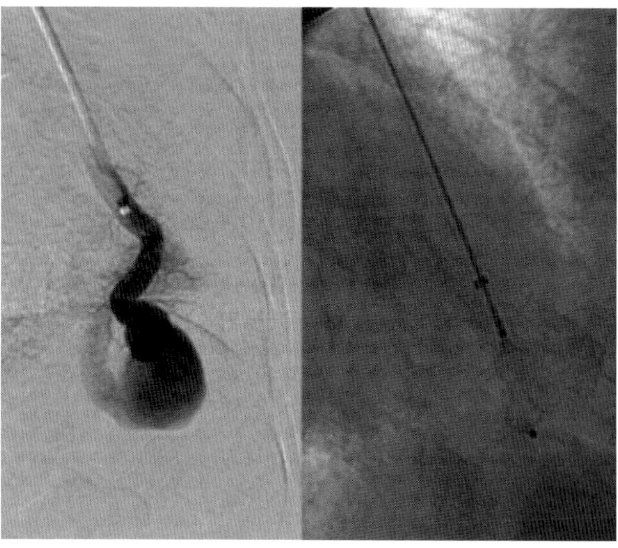

B

Figure 75-11 Vascular occlusion plugs. **A.** Amplatzer vascular occlusion plug. **B.** Pulmonary AVM before and after deployment. *(continued)*

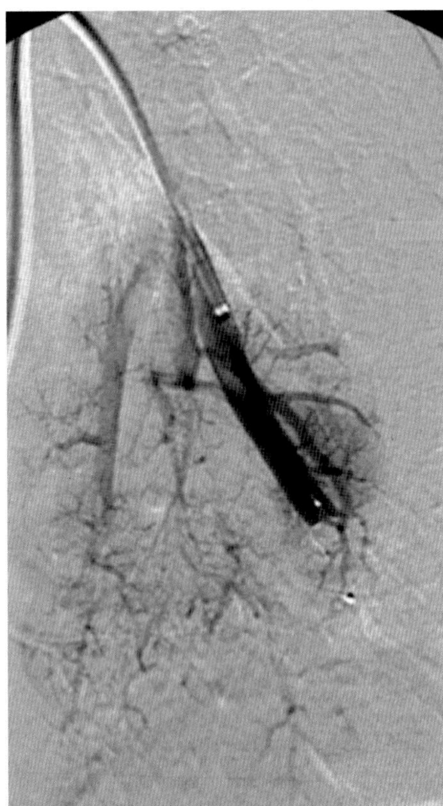

Figure 75-11 *(Continued)* **C.** Pulmonary angiogram after deployment.

FOLLOW-UP AND PROGNOSIS

Patients with HHT and screening negative for PAVM should have repeat screening (a) after puberty; (b) after pregnancy; (c) within 5 years of planned pregnancy; and (d) every 5 to 10 years routinely.[103]

Early reports suggested a high mortality for patients who did not undergo treatment of PAVMs. Examination of family trees in older reports impresses one with the frequency of death from meningitis, brain abscess, and stroke. Some of this apparently high mortality may have been due to selection bias. More recent studies suggest that the prognosis may be more benign, and complications may be nonexistent when PAVMs are discovered by screening.[75] In one series, mortality was approximately 10%. Two-thirds of deaths were due to cerebrovascular accident, and all of these patients were cyanotic and polycythemic.[40]

In summary, patients with PAVM can be successfully treated, with resolution of essentially all symptoms and substantial reduction in risk of complications. Embolotherapy is the treatment of choice for most patients. The relatives of patients with PAVMs or HHT should be screened with contrast echocardiography to prevent central nervous system complications as the first manifestation of disease. Patients with PAVMs should be fully educated about their diagnosis, potential clinical complications, and the often hereditary nature of the problem. Educational materials for patients with HHT, and the location of specialized centers for managing HHT and PAVM are available from the HHT Foundation International at http://hht.org. Caregivers are also urged to consult the website for updated recommendations.

REFERENCES

1. Churton T. Multiple aneurysm of pulmonary artery. *Br Med J.* 1897;1:1223.
2. Reading B. Case of congenital telangiectasia of lung, complicated by brain abscess. *Tex St J Med.* 1932;28:462.
3. Rodes CB. Cavernous hemangiomas of the lung with secondary polycythemia. *JAMA.* 1938;110:1914.
4. Sutton HG. Epistaxis as an indication of impaired nutrition and of degeneration of the vascular system. *Med Mirror.* 1864;1:769.
5. Babbington BG. Hereditary epistaxis. *Lancet.* 1865;2:362–363.
6. Legg W. A case of haemophilia complicated with multiple naevi. *Lancet.* 1876;2:856–857.
7. Chiari O. *Enfahrungen auf dem Gebiete der Hals und Nasenkrankheiten.* Wien, 1887.
8. Rendu M. Épistaxis répétées chez un sujet porteur de petits angiomes cutanés et muqueux. *Bull Et Mém Soc Méd Hôp Paris.* 1896;13:731–733.
9. Osler W. On a family form of recurring epistaxis, associated with multiple telangiectases of the skin and mucous membranes. *Bull Johns Hopkins Hosp.* 1901;12:333–337.
10. Weber FP. Multiple hereditary developmental angiomata (telangiectases) of the skin and mucous membranes associated with recurring hemorrhages. *Lancet.* 1907;2:160–162.
11. Hanes FM. Multiple hereditary telangiectases causing hemorrhage (hereditary hemorrhagic telangiectasia). *Bull Johns Hopkins Hosp.* 1909;20:63–73.
12. Vase P, Holm M, Arendrup H. Pulmonary arteriovenous fistulas in hereditary hemorrhagic telangiectasia. *Acta Med Scand.* 1985;218:105–109.
13. Westermann CJ, Rosina AF, De Vries V, de Coteau PA. The prevalence and manifestations of hereditary hemorrhagic telangiectasia in the Afro-Caribbean population of the Netherlands Antilles: a family screening. *Am J Med Genet A.* 2003;116:324–328.
14. Kjeldsen AD, Vase P, Green A. Hereditary haemorrhagic telangiectasia: a population-based study of prevalence and mortality in Danish patients. *J Intern Med.* 1999;245:31–39.
15. Dakeishi M, Shioya T, Wada Y, et al. Genetic epidemiology of hereditary hemorrhagic telangiectasia in a local community in the northern part of Japan. *Hum Mutat.* 2002;19:140–148.
16. Guttmacher AE, Marchuk DA, White RI Jr. Hereditary hemorrhagic telangiectasia. *N Engl J Med.* 1995;333:918–924.
17. Heutink P, Haitjema T, Breedveld GJ, et al. Linkage of hereditary haemorrhagic telangiectasia to chromosome 9q34 and evidence for locus heterogeneity. *J Med Genet.* 1994;31:933–936.
18. McDonald MT, Papenberg KA, Ghosh S, et al. A disease locus for hereditary haemorrhagic telangiectasia maps to chromosome 9q33–34. *Nat Genet.* 1994;6:197–204.
19. Shovlin CL, Hughes JM, Tuddenham EG, et al. A gene for hereditary haemorrhagic telangiectasia maps to chromosome 9q3. *Nat Genet.* 1994;6:205–209.
20. McAllister KA, Grogg KM, Johnson DW, et al. Endoglin, a TGF-beta binding protein of endothelial cells, is the gene for hereditary haemorrhagic telangiectasia type 1. *Nat Genet.* 1994;8:345–351.
21. McAllister KA, Lennon F, Bowles-Biesecker B, et al. Genetic heterogeneity in hereditary haemorrhagic telangiectasia: possible correlation with clinical phenotype. *J Med Genet.* 1994;31:927–932.
22. Porteous ME, Curtis A, Williams O, Marchuk D, Bhattacharya SS, Burn J. Genetic heterogeneity in hereditary hemorrhagic telangiectasia. *J Med Genet.* 1994;31:925–926.

23. Bourdeau A, Faughnan ME, Letarte M. Endoglin-deficient mice, a unique model to study hereditary hemorrhagic telangiectasia. *Trends Cardiovasc Med.* 2000;10:279–285.

24. Berg JN, Gallione CJ, Stenzel TT, et al. The activin receptor-like kinase 1 gene: genomic structure and mutations in hereditary hemorrhagic telangiectasia type 2. *Am J Hum Genet.* 1997;61: 60–67.

25. Johnson DW, Berg JN, Baldwin MA, et al. Mutations in the activin receptor-like kinase 1 gene in hereditary haemorrhagic telangiectasia type 2. *Nat Genet.* 1996;13:189–195.

26. Srinivasan S, Hanes MA, Dickens T, et al. A mouse model for hereditary hemorrhagic telangiectasia (HHT) type 2. *Hum Mol Genet.* 2003;12:473–482.

27. Gallione CJ, Repetto GM, Legius E, et al. A combined syndrome of juvenile polyposis and hereditary haemorrhagic telangiectasia associated with mutations in MADH4 (SMAD4). *Lancet.* 2004;363:852–859.

28. Gallione CJ, Richards JA, Letteboer TGW, et al. SMAD4 mutations found in unselected HHT patients. *J Med Genet.* 2006; 43:793–797.

29. Cole SG, Begbie ME, Wallace GM, Shovlin CL. A new locus for hereditary haemorrhagic telangiectasia (HHT3) maps to chromosome 5. *J Med Genet.* 2005;42:577–582.

30. Bayrak-Toydemir P, McDonald J, Akarsu N, et al. A fourth locus for hereditary hemorrhagic telangiectasia maps to chromosome 7. *Am J Med Genet A.* 2006;140:2155–2162.

31. Lesca G, Burnichon N, Raux G, et al. Distribution of ENG and ACVRL1 (ALK1) mutations in French HHT patients. *Hum Mutat.* 2006;27:598.

32. Fernandez A, Sanz-Rodriguez F, Zarrabeitia R, et al. Mutation study of Spanish patients with hereditary hemorrhagic telangiectasia and expression analysis of Endoglin and ALK1. *Hum Mutat.* 2006;27:295.

33. Prigoda NL, Savas S, Abdalla SA, et al. Hereditary haemorrhagic telangiectasia: mutation detection, test sensitivity and novel mutations. *J Med Genet.* 2006;43:722–728.

34. Letteboer TGW, Zewald RA, Kamping EJ, et al. Hereditary hemorrhagic telangiectasia: ENG and ALK-1 mutations in Dutch patients. *Hum Genet.* 2005;116:8–16.

35. Bayrak-Toydemir P, McDonald J, Markewitz B, et al. Genotype-phenotype correlation in hereditary hemorrhagic telangiectasia: mutations and manifestations. *Am J Med Genet A.* 2006;140:463–470.

36. McCue CM, Hartenberg M, Nance WE. Pulmonary arteriovenous malformations related to Rendu-Osler-Weber syndrome. *Am J Med Genet.* 1984;19:19–27.

37. Peery WH. Clinical spectrum of hereditary hemorrhagic telangiectasia (Osler-Weber-Rendu disease). *Am J Med.* 1987;82: 989–997.

38. White RI Jr, Mitchell SE, Barth KH, et al. Angioarchitecture of pulmonary arteriovenous malformations: an important consideration before embolotherapy. *AJR Am J Roentgenol.* 1983;140:681–686.

39. Anabtawi IN, Ellison RG, Ellison LT. Pulmonary arteriovenous aneurysms and fistulas: anatomical variations, embryology, and classification. *Ann Thorac Surg.* 1965;1:277–285.

40. Dines DE, Arms RA, Bernatz PE, Gomes MR. Pulmonary arteriovenous fistulas. *Mayo Clin Proc.* 1974;49:460–465.

41. Brillet PY, Dumont P, Bouaziz N, et al. Pulmonary arteriovenous malformation treated with embolotherapy: systemic collateral supply at multidetector CT angiography after 2–20 year follow-up. *Radiology.* 2007;242:267–276.

42. Shovlin CL. Hereditary hemorrhagic telangiectasia: pathophysiology, diagnosis, and treatment. *Blood Rev.* 2010;24:203–219.

43. Park SO, Wankhede M, Lee YJ, et al. Real-time imaging of de novo arteriovenous malformation in a mouse model of hereditary hemorrhagic telangiectasia. *J Clin Invest.* 2009;119: 3487–3496.

44. Roman BL, Pham VN, Lawson ND, et al. Disruption of ACVRL1 increases endothelial cell number in zebra fish cranial vessels. *Development.* 2002;129:3009–3019.

45. Kim JH, Peacock R, George SC, Hughes CC. BMP9 induces EphrinB2 expression in endothelial cells through an Alk1-BMPRII/ActRII-ID1/ID3-dependent pathway: implications for hereditary hemorrhagic telangiectasia type II. *Angiogenesis.* 2012;15:497–509.

46. Chen W, Guo Y, Walker EJ, et al. Reduced mural cell coverage and impaired vessel integrity after angiogenic stimulation in the ALK-1 deficient brain. *Arterioscler Thromb Vasc Biol.* 2013;33:305–310.

47. Corti P, Young S, Chen CY, et al. Interaction between ALK1 and blood flow in the development of arteriovenous malformations. *Development.* 2011;138:1573–1582.

48. Braverman IM, Keh H, Jacobson BJ. Ultrastructure and three-dimensional organization of the telangiectases of hereditary hemorrhagic telangiectasia. *J Invest Dermatol.* 1990;95:422–427.

49. Shovlin CL, Sodhi V, McCarthy A, Lasjaunias P, Jackson JE, Sheppard MN. Estimates of risk of pregnancy for women with hereditary hemorrhagic telangiectasia. *BJOG.* 2008;115: 1108–1115.

50. Burke CM, Safai C, Nelson DP, Raffin TA. Pulmonary arteriovenous malformations: a critical update. *Am Rev Respir Dis.* 1986;134:334–339.

51. Swanson KL, Prakash UB, Stanson AW. Pulmonary arteriovenous fistulas: Mayo Clinic experience 1982–1997. *Mayo Clin Proc.* 1999;74:671–680.

52. Faughnan ME, Lui YW, Wirth JA, et al. Diffuse pulmonary arteriovenous malformations: characteristics and prognosis. *Chest.* 2000;117:31–38.

53. Pierucci P, Murphy J, Henderson KJ, Chyun DA, White RI Jr. New definition and natural history of patients with diffuse pulmonary arteriovenous malformations: twenty-seven year experience. *Chest.* 2008;133:653–661.

54. Hales MR. Multiple small arteriovenous fistulae of the lungs. *Am J Pathol.* 1956;32:927–943.

55. White RI Jr, Lynch-Nyhana A, Terry P, et al. Pulmonary arteriovenous malformations: techniques and long-term outcome of embolotherapy. *Radiology.* 1988;169:663–669.

56. Goodenberger DM. Unpublished data. 11/99-08/06. 354 patients with HHT Age range 10 months to 83 years.

57. Wong HH, Chan RP, Klatt R, Faughnan ME. Idiopathic pulmonary arteriovenous malformations: clinical and imaging characteristics. *Eur Respir J.* 2011;38:368–375.

58. Huseby JS, Culver BH, Butler J. Pulmonary arteriovenous fistulas: increase in shunt at high lung volume. *Am Rev Respir Dis.* 1977;115:229–232.

59. Barzilai B, Waggoner A, Spessert C, Picus D, Goodenberger D. Two-dimensional contrast echocardiography in the detection and follow-up of congenital pulmonary arteriovenous malformations. *Am J Cardiol.* 1991;68:1507–1510.

60. Pollak JS, Saluja S, Thabet A, Henderson KJ, Denbow N, White RI Jr. Clinical and anatomic outcomes after embolotherapy of pulmonary arteriovenous malformations. *J Vasc Interv Radiol.* 2006;17:35–44.

61. Reilly PJ, Nostrant TT. Clinical manifestations of hereditary hemorrhagic telangiectasia. *Am J Gastroenterol.* 1984;79:363–367.

62. Haitjema T, Disch F, Overtoom TT, Westermann CJ, Lammers JW. Screening family members of patients with hereditary hemorrhagic telangiectasia. *Am J Med.* 1995;99:519–524.

63. Cottin V, Plauchu H, Bayle JY, Barthelet M, Revel D, Cordier JF. Pulmonary arteriovenous malformations in patients with hereditary hemorrhagic telangiectasia. *Am J Respir Crit Care Med.* 2004;169:994–1000.

64. Goodenberger D, Picus D. Pulmonary Arteriovenous Malformation Frequency in Hereditary Hemorrhagic Telangiectasia – Impact of Screening Procedure. *Sixth International HHT Scientific Conference*. Lyon, France: 2005.

65. van Gent MW, Post MC, Snijder RJ, Westermann CJ, Plokker HW, Mager JJ. Real prevalence of pulmonary right-to-left shunt according to genotype in patients with hereditary hemorrhagic telangiectasia: a transthoracic contrast echocardiography study. *Chest.* 2010;138:833–839.

66. Bertholet P, Walker JG, Sherlock S, Reid L. Arterial changes in the lung in cirrhosis of the liver – lung spider nevi. *N Engl J Med.* 1966;274:291–298.

67. Aller R, Moya JL, Moreira V, et al. Diagnosis of hepatopulmonary syndrome with contrast transesophageal echocardiography: advantages over contrast transthoracic echocardiography. *Digest Dis Sci.* 1999;44:1243–1248.

68. Langiulli M, Aronow WS, Das M, et al. Prevalence and prognosis of intrapulmonary shunts in patients with hepatic cirrhosis. *Cardiol Rev.* 2006;14:53–54.

69. Lundell M, Finck E. Arteriovenous fistulas originating from Rasmussen aneurysms. *Am J Roentgenol.* 1983;140:687–688.

70. Pierce JA, Reagan WP, Kimball RW. Unusual cases of pulmonary arteriovenous fistulas, with a note on thyroid carcinoma as a cause. *N Engl J Med.* 1959;260:901–907.

71. Marianeschi SM, McIlhinney DB, Reddy VM. Pulmonary arteriovenous malformations in and out of the setting of congenital heart disease. *Ann Thorac Surg.* 1998;66:688–691.

72. Manganas C, Iliopoulos J, Pang L, Grant PW. Traumatic pulmonary arteriovenous malformation presenting with massive hemoptysis 30 years after penetrating chest injury. *Ann Thorac Surg.* 2003;76:942–944.

73. Dines DE, Seward JB, Bernatz PE. Pulmonary arteriovenous fistulas. *Mayo Clin Proc.* 1983;58:176–181.

74. Gomes MR, Bernatz PE, Dines DE. Pulmonary arteriovenous fistulas. *Ann Thorac Surg.* 1969;7:582–593.

75. Sluiter-Eringa H, Orie NGM, Sluiter HJ. Pulmonary arteriovenous fistula: diagnosis and prognosis in noncomplainant patients. *Am Rev Respir Dis.* 1969;100:177–188.

76. Shovlin CL, Letarte M. Hereditary haemorrhagic telangiectasia and pulmonary arteriovenous malformations: issues in clinical management and review of pathogenic mechanisms. *Thorax.* 1999;54:714–729.

77. Gershon AS, Faughnan ME, Chon KS, et al. Transcatheter embolotherapy of maternal pulmonary arteriovenous malformations during pregnancy. *Chest.* 2001;119:470–477.

78. Goodenberger D, Barzilai B, Waggoner A, et al. Frequency of intrapulmonary shunt in relatives of patients with Osler-Weber-Rendu and pulmonary arteriovenous malformation (abstract). *Chest.* 1990;98:59S.

79. Shumacker HB, Waldhausen JA. Pulmonary arteriovenous fistulas in children. *Ann Surg.* 1963;158:713–720.

80. Mager JJ, Overtoom TT, Blauw H, Lammers JW, Westermann CJ. Embolotherapy of pulmonary arteriovenous malformations: long-term results in 112 patients. *J Vasc Intervent Radiol.* 2004;15:451–456.

81. Dinsmore BJ, Gefter WB, Hatabu H, Kressel HY. Pulmonary arteriovenous malformations: diagnosis by gradient refocused MR imaging. *J Comput Assist Tomogr.* 1990;14:918–923.

82. Assar OS, Friedman CM, White RI. The natural history of epistaxis in hereditary hemorrhagic telangiectasia. *Laryngoscope.* 1991;101:977–980.

83. Maher CO, Piepgras DG, Brown RD Jr, Friedman JA, Pollock BE. Cerebrovascular manifestations in 321 cases of hereditary hemorrhagic telangiectasia. *Stroke.* 2001;32:877–882.

84. Przybojewski JZ, Maritz F. Pulmonary arteriovenous fistulas: a case presentation and review of the literature. *S Afr Med J.* 1980;57:366–373.

85. White RI Jr. Pulmonary arteriovenous malformations: how do we diagnose them and why is it important to do so? *Radiology.* 1992;182:633–635.

86. Goodenberger D, Spessert C, Waggoner A, et al. Size and location of occult pulmonary arteriovenous malformations (PAVM's) in individuals with Osler-Weber-Rendu (OWR) (abstract). *Am Rev Respir Dis.* 1991;143:A663.

87. Dalton ML, Goodwin FC, Bronwell AW, Rutledge R. Intrapleural rupture of pulmonary arteriovenous aneurysm: report of a case. *Dis Chest.* 1967;52:97–100.

88. Ference BA, Shannon TM, White RI Jr, Zawin M, Burdge CM. Life-threatening pulmonary hemorrhage with pulmonary arteriovenous malformations and hereditary hemorrhagic telangiectasia. *Chest.* 1994;106:1387–1390.

89. Gammon RB, Miksa AK, Keller FS. Osler-Weber-Rendu disease and pulmonary arteriovenous fistulas: deterioration and embolotherapy during pregnancy. *Chest.* 1990;98:1522–1524.

90. LaRoche CM, Wells F, Shneerson J. Massive hemothorax due to enlarging arteriovenous fistula in pregnancy. *Chest.* 1992;101:1452–1454.

91. Faughnan ME, Granton JT, Young LH. The pulmonary vascular complications of hereditary haemorrhagic telangiectasia. *Eur Respir J.* 2009;33:1186–1194.

92. Trell E, Johansson BW, Linell F, Ripa J. Familial pulmonary hypertension and multiple abnormalities of large systemic arteries in Osler's disease. *Am J Med.* 1972;53:50–63.

93. Trembath RC, Thomson JR, Machado RD, et al. Clinical and molecular genetic features of pulmonary hypertension in patients with hereditary hemorrhagic telangiectasia. *N Engl J Med.* 2001;345:325–334.

94. Simonneau G, Robbins IM, Beghetti M, et al. Updated clinical classification of pulmonary hypertension. *J Am Coll Cardiol.* 2009;54(1 Suppl):S43–S54.

95. Girerd B, Montani D, Coulet F, et al. Clinical outcomes of pulmonary arterial hypertension in patients carrying ACVRL1 (ALK1) mutation. *Am J Respir Crit Care Med.* 2010;181:851–861.

96. Smoot LB, Obler D, McElhinney DB, et al. Clinical features of pulmonary arterial hypertension in young people with an

ALK1 mutation and hereditary haemorrhagic telangiectasia. *Arch Dis Child*. 2009;94:506–511.

97. Shovlin CL, Gibbs JS, Jackson JE. Management of pulmonary arteriovenous malformations in pulmonary hypertensive patients: a pressure to embolize? *Eur Respir Rev*. 2009;18:4–6.
98. Montani D, Price LC, Girerd B, et al. Fatal rupture of pulmonary arteriovenous malformation in hereditary hemorrhagic telangiectasis and severe PAH. *Eur Respir Rev*. 2009;18:42–46.
99. Roman G, Fisher M, Perl DP, Poser CM. Neurological manifestations of hereditary hemorrhagic telangiectasia (Rendu-Osler-Weber disease): report of two cases and review of the literature. *Ann Neurol*. 1978;4:130–144.
100. Press OW, Ramsey PG. Central nervous system infections associated with hereditary hemorrhagic telangiectasia. *Am J Med*. 1984;77:86–92.
101. Gallitelli M, Guastamacchia E, Resta F, Guanti G, Sabbà C. Pulmonary arteriovenous malformations, hereditary hemorrhagic telangiectasia, and brain abscess. *Respiration*. 2006;73:553–557.
102. Gelfand MS, Stephens DS, Howell EI, Alford RH, Kaiser AB. Brain abscess: association with pulmonary arteriovenous fistula and hereditary hemorrhagic telangiectasia: report of three cases. *Am J Med*. 1988;85:718–720.
103. Faughnan ME, Palda VA, Garcia-Tsao, et al. International guidelines for the diagnosis and management of hereditary haemorrhagic telangiectasia. *J Med Genet*. 2011;48:73–87.
104. Post MC, Letteboer TG, Mager JJ, Plokker TH, Kelder JC, Westermann CJ. A pulmonary right-to-left shunt in patients with hereditary hemorrhagic telangiectasia is associated with an increased prevalence of migraine. *Chest*. 2005;128:2485–2489.
105. Fulbright RK, Chaloupka JC, Putman CM, et al. MR of hereditary hemorrhagic telangiectasia: prevalence and spectrum of cerebrovascular malformations. *AJNR Am J Neuroradiol*. 1998;19:477–484.
106. Jessurun GA, Kamphuis DJ, van der Zande FH, Nossent JC. Cerebral arteriovenous malformations in the Netherlands Antilles: high prevalence of hereditary hemorrhagic telangiectasia-related single and multiple cerebral arteriovenous malformations. *Clin Neurol Neurosurg*. 1993;95:193–198.
107. Easey AJ, Wallace GMF, Hughes JMB, Jackson JE, Taylor WJ, Shovlin CL. Should asymptomatic patients with hereditary haemorrhagic telangiectasia (HHT) be screened for cerebral vascular malformations? Data from 22,061 years of HHT patient life. *J Neurol Neurosurg Psychiatry*. 2003;74:743–748.
108. Cook Medical MRI Information. http://www.cookmedical.com/product/-/catalog/nester-embolization-coils-platinum?ds=di_mwcen_webds#tab=mri. Accessed October 19, 2014.
109. Shub C, Tajik AJ, Seward JB, Dines DE. Detecting intrapulmonary right-to-left shunt with contrast echocardiography: observations in a patient with diffuse pulmonary arteriovenous fistulas. *Mayo Clin Proc*. 1976;51:81–84.
110. Hernandez A, Strauss AW, McKnight R, Hartmann AF Jr. Diagnosis of pulmonary arteriovenous fistula by contrast echocardiography. *J Pediatr*. 1978;93:258–261.
111. Shovlin CL, Guttmacher AE, Buscarini E, et al. Diagnostic criteria for hereditary hemorrhagic telangiectasia (Rendu-Osler-Weber Syndrome). *Am J Med Genet*. 2000;91:66–67.
112. Oxhoj H, Kjeldsen AD, Nielsen G. Screening for pulmonary arteriovenous malformations: contrast echocardiography versus pulse oximetry. *Scand Cardiovasc J*. 2000;34:281–285.
113. Nanthakumar K, Graham AT, Robinson TI, et al. Contrast echocardiography for detection of pulmonary arteriovenous malformations. *Am Heart J*. 2001;141:243–246.
114. Thompson RD, Jackson J, Peters AM, Doré CJ, Hughes JM. Sensitivity and specificity of radioisotope right-left shunt measurements and pulse oximetry for the early detection of pulmonary arteriovenous malformations. *Chest*. 1999;115:109–113.
115. Lee WL, Graham AF, Pugash RA, et al. Contrast echocardiography remains positive after treatment of pulmonary arteriovenous malformations. *Chest*. 2003;123:351–358.
116. Oliveira GH, Seward JB, Cortese DA, Dines DE. Contrast transesophageal echocardiography in the diagnosis and localization of diffuse pulmonary telangiectasias. *Chest*. 2000;118:557–559.
117. Remy J, Remy-Jardin M, Wattinne L, Deffontaines C. Pulmonary arteriovenous malformations: evaluation with CT of the chest before and after treatment. *Radiology*. 1992;182:809–816.
118. Remy J, Remy-Jardin M, Giraud F, Wattinne L. Angioarchitecture of pulmonary arteriovenous malformations: clinical utility of three-dimensional helical CT. *Radiology*. 1994;191:657–664.
119. Hepburn J, Dauphinee JA. Successful removal of hemangioma of the lung followed by the disappearance of polycythemia. *Am J Med Sci*. 1942;204:681.
120. Brown SE, Wright PW, Renner JW, Riker JB. Staged bilateral thoracotomies for multiple pulmonary arteriovenous malformations complicating hereditary hemorrhagic telangiectasia. *J Thorac Cardiovasc Surg*. 1982;83:285–289.
121. Watanabe N, Munakata Y, Ogiwara M, Miyatake M, Nakagawa F, Hirayama J. A case of pulmonary arteriovenous malformation in a patient with brain abscess successfully treated with video-assisted thoracoscopic resection. *Chest*. 1995;108(6):1724–1727.
122. Terry PB, White RI, Barth KH, Kaufman SL, Mitchell SE. Pulmonary arteriovenous malformations: physiologic observations and results of therapeutic balloon embolization. *N Engl J Med*. 1983;308:1197.
123. Prasad V, Chan RP, Faughnan ME. Embolotherapy of pulmonary arteriovenous malformations: efficacy of platinum versus stainless steel coils. *J Vasc Interv Radiol*. 2004;15:153–160.
124. Hart JL, Aldin Z, Braude P, Shovlin CL, Jackson J. Embolization of pulmonary arteriovenous malformations using the Amplatzer vascular plug: successful treatment of 69 consecutive patients. *Eur Radiol*. 2010;20:2663–2670.
125. Faughnan ME, Thabet A, Mei-Zahav M, et al. Pulmonary arteriovenous malformations in children: outcomes of transcatheter embolotherapy. *J Pediatr*. 2004;145:826–831.
126. Milic A, Chan RP, Cohen JH, Faughnan ME. Reperfusion of pulmonary arteriovenous malformations after embolotherapy. *J Vasc Interv Radiol*. 2005;16:1675–1683.
127. Remy-Jardin M, Dumont P, Brillet PY, Dupuis P, Duhamel A, Remy J. Pulmonary arteriovenous malformations treated with embolotherapy: helical CT evaluation of long-term effectiveness after 2–21-year follow-up. *Radiology*. 2006;239:576–585.
128. Remy-Jardin M, Wattinne L, Remy J. Transcatheter occlusion of pulmonary arterial circulation and collateral supply: failures, incidents, and complications. *Radiology*. 1991;180:699–705.
129. White RI Jr, Pollak JS, Wirth JA. Pulmonary arteriovenous malformations: diagnosis and transcatheter embolotherapy. *J Vasc Interv Radiol*. 1996;7:787–804.

130. Chilvers ER, Whyte MK, Jackson JE, Allison DJ, Hughes JM. Effect of percutaneous transcatheter embolization on pulmonary function, right-to-left shunt, and arterial oxygenation in patients with pulmonary arteriovenous malformations. *Am Rev Respir Dis*. 1990;142:420–425.

131. Gupta S, Faughnan ME, Bayoumi AM. Embolization for pulmonary arteriovenous malformations in hereditary hemorrhagic telangiectasia: a decision analysis. *Chest*. 2009;36:849–858.

132. Hartnell GG, Jackson JE, Allison DJ. Coil embolization of pulmonary arteriovenous malformations. *Cardiovasc Intervent Radiol*. 1990;13:347–350.

133. Lee DW, White RI Jr, Egglin TK, et al. Embolotherapy of large pulmonary arteriovenous malformations: long-term results. *Ann Thorac Surg*. 1997;64:930–940.

134. Gossage JR, Kanj G. Pulmonary arteriovenous malformations. A state of the art review. *Am J Respir Crit Care Med*. 1998;158: 643–661.

135. Lacombe P, Lagrange C, Beauchet A, El Hajjam M, Chinet T, Pelage JP. Diffuse pulmonary arteriovenous malformations in hereditary hemorrhagic telangiectasia: long term results of embolization according to extent of lung involvement. *Chest*. 2009;135:1031–1037.

136. Reynaud-Gaubert M, Thomas P, Gaubert JY, et al. Pulmonary arteriovenous malformations: lung transplantation as a therapeutic option. *Eur Respir J*. 1999;14:1425–1428.

137. Svetliza G, De la Canal A, Beveraggi E, et al. Lung transplantation in a patient with arteriovenous malformations. *J Heart Lung Transplant*. 2002;21:506–508.

APPENDIXES

APPENDIX A

Terms and Symbols in Respiratory Physiology

GENERAL SYMBOLS

P	Partial pressure in blood or gas P_{O_2} = partial pressure of O_2
$\bar{X}$	A bar over the symbol indicates a mean value. $\bar{P}$ = mean pressure, as distinct from instantaneous pressure
$\dot{X}$	A time derivative (rate) is indicated by a dot above the symbol $\dot{V}_{O_2}$ = oxygen consumption per minute, mL $\dot{V}_{CO_2}$ = CO_2 production per minute, mL
% X	Percent sign preceding a symbol indicates percentage of the predicted normal value
X/Y%	Percent sign following a symbol indicates a ratio function with the ratio expressed as a percentage. Both components of the ratio must be designated FEV_1/FVC, % = 100 × FEV_1/FVC
XA, Xa	A small capital letter or a lower-case letter on the same line following a primary symbol is a qualifier to further define the primary symbol. Alternatively, subscript letters may be used XA = X_A, Xa = X_a Additional qualifiers of the primary symbol may be identified as shown PE_{O_2} = Pressure of CO_2 in the expired air, mm Hg

GAS PHASE SYMBOLS

PRIMARY SYMBOLS

V	Volume of gas
$\dot{V}$	Flow of gas
F	Fractional concentration of a gas

QUALIFYING SYMBOLS

I	Inspired VI = inspired volume
E	Expired VE = expired volume $\dot{V}$E = expired volume per minute
A	Alveolar VA = alveolar volume $\dot{V}$ = alveolar ventilation per minute
T	Tidal VT = tidal volume
D	Dead space VD = volume of dead space $\dot{V}$D = dead-space ventilation per minute
B	Barometric PB = barometric pressure
STPD	Standard conditions: temperature 0°C, pressure 760 mm Hg, and dry (0 mm Hg water vapor)
BTPS	Body conditions: body temperature and ambient pressure, saturated with water vapor at these conditions
ATPD	Ambient temperature and pressure, dry
ATPS	Ambient temperature and pressure, saturated with water vapor at these conditions
an	Anatomic
p	Physiological
f	Respiratory frequency, per minute
max	Maximum
t	Time

BLOOD PHASE SYMBOLS

PRIMARY SYMBOLS

Q	Volume of blood
$\dot{Q}$	Blood flow $\dot{Q}$ = cardiac output, L/min
C	Concentration in the blood phase C_{O_2} = concentration of oxygen in blood, mL of O_2 per 100 mL of blood
S	Saturation in the blood phase S_{O_2} = Saturation of hemoglobin with O_2, percent

QUALIFYING SYMBOLS

a	Arterial Ca_{O_2} = concentration of O_2 in arterial blood, mL of O_2 per 100 mL of blood
c	Capillary Cc_{O_2} = concentration of O_2 in capillary blood, mL of O_2 per 100 mL of blood
C′	Pulmonary end-capillary Pc'_{O_2} = partial pressure of O_2 in end-capillary blood, mm Hg
v	Venous Cv_{O_2} = concentration of O_2 in venous blood, mL of O_2 per 100 mL of blood
$\bar{v}$	Mixed venous $C\bar{v}_{O_2}$ = concentration of O_2 in mixed venous blood, mL of O_2 per 100 mL of blood

VENTILATION AND LUNG MECHANICS TESTS AND SYMBOLS

STATIC LUNG VOLUMES*

RV — Residual volume. Volume of air remaining in the lungs after maximum expiration.

CV — Closing volume. Volume of air expired from the onset of airways closure to residual volume. May be expressed as a fraction of VC: CV/VC,%.

ERV — Expiratory reserve volume. Maximum volume of air expired from the resting end-expiratory level.

VT — Tidal volume. Volume of air inspired or expired with each breath during quiet breathing. When tidal volume is used in gas-exchange formulations, this symbol is used.

IRV — Inspiratory reserve volume. Maximum volume of air inspired from the end-tidal inspiratory level.

LUNG CAPACITIES**

IC — Inspiratory capacity. The sum of IRV and TV.

IVC — Inspiratory vital capacity. Maximum volume of air inspired from the point of maximum expiration, i.e., from RV.

VC — Vital capacity. Maximum volume of air expired from the point of maximum inspiration, i.e., from TLC.

FRC — Functional residual capacity. Sum of RV and ERV. FRC is the volume of air remaining in the lungs at the resting end-expiratory position.

TLC — Total lung capacity. Volume of air in the lungs after maximum inspiration. Also, the sum of all volume compartments of the lungs.

RV/TLC,% — Residual volume to total lung capacity ratio, expressed as a percentage.

CC — Closing capacity. Closing volume plus residual volume, may be expressed as a percentage of TLC: CC/TLC, %.

FORCED RESPIRATORY MANEUVERS DURING SPIROMETRY†

FVC — Forced vital capacity. The maximum volume of air forcibly expired from total lung capacity

FIVC — Forced inspiratory vital capacity. Maximum volume of air forcibly inspired starting from residual volume.

FEV*t* — Timed forced expiratory volume. Volume of air expired in a specified time in the course of the forced vital capacity maneuver. FEV_1 = volume of air expired during the first second of the FVC.

FEV*t*/FVC,% — Ratio of timed forced expiratory volume to forced vital capacity, expressed in percentage.

FEF*x* — Forced expiratory flow, related to some portion of the FVC curve. Modifiers refer to the amount of the FVC that has been expired at the time of measurement.

$FEF_{200-1200}$ — Forced expiratory flow between 200 and 1200 mL of the FVC (formerly called the maximum expiratory flow rate).

FEF_{25-75} — Forced expiratory flow during middle half of the FVC (formerly called the maximum midexpiratory flow rate or MMEF)

PEF — Peak expiratory flow. Highest value for expiratory flow.

$\dot{V}_{max_x}$ — Maximum flow when *x* percent of the FVC has been expired.

$\dot{V}_{max\,75}$ = flow (instantaneous) when 75% of the FVC has been expired.

FIF*x* — Forced inspiratory flow. As in the case of the FEF, appropriate modifiers designate the volume at which flow is being measured.

Unless otherwise specified, the volume qualifiers indicate the volume inspired from RV at the point of measurement.

FIF_{25-75} = forced inspiratory flow during the middle half of the FIVC.

MVV — Maximum voluntary ventilation. Volume of air exhaled during maximum breathing efforts within a specified time period. Formerly called the maximum breathing capacity (MBC)

MVV_{60} = MVV at a breathing frequency of 60 per minute.

PImax — Maximum inspiratory pressure. The maximum pressure generated during a maximal inspiratory effort made at RV.

PEmax — Maximum expiratory pressure. The maximum pressure generated during a maximal expiratory effort made at TLC.

MEASUREMENTS RELATED TO VENTILATION

$\dot{V}_E$ — Expired volume per minute (BTPS)

$\dot{V}_I$ — Inspired volume per minute (BTPS)

$\dot{V}_{CO_2}$ — Carbon dioxide production per minute (STPD)

$\dot{V}_{O_2}$ — Oxygen consumption per minute (STPD)

R — Respiratory exchange ratio, the ratio of CO_2 output to O_2 intake in the lungs

$\dot{V}_A$ — Alveolar ventilation per minute (BTPS)

$\dot{V}_D$ — Ventilation per minute of the physiological dead space (BTPS) defined by the equation

$$\dot{V} = \dot{V}_E \frac{Pa_{CO_2} - P_{A_{CO_2}}}{Pa_{CO_2} - P_{I_{CO_2}}}$$

V_D — Volume of the physiological dead space, calculated as $\dot{V}_D$/f.

V_D/V_T — Ratio of dead space to tidal volume. The fraction, usually expressed as a percentage, of each breath that does not contribute to CO_2 elimination.

MECHANICS OF BREATHING*

Pressure Terms

Paw — Pressure at any point along the airways

Pao — Pressure at the airway opening

Ppl — Pleural pressure

P_A — Alveolar pressure

*Expressed as BTPS.

**Combinations of volumes for practical purposes.

†All values at BTPS.

*All pressures expressed relative to ambient pressure unless otherwise specified.

Pbs	Pressure at the body surface
Pes	Esophageal pressure: used to estimate Ppl
PA–Pbs	Transthoracic pressure
PA–Ppl	Transpulmonary pressure
Ppl–Pbs	Pressure difference across the chest wall
Paw–Ppl	Transbronchial pressure, estimated as difference between airway and pleural pressures.

Flow–Pressure Relationships[†]

R	General symbol for frictional resistance, defined as the ratio of pressure difference to flow.
Raw	Airway resistance, calculated from pressure difference between airway opening (Pa_o) and alveoli (Pa) divided by the airflow, cm H_2O/L/s.
Rl	Total pulmonary resistance, measured by relating flow-dependent transpulmonary pressure to airflow at the mouth.
Rti	Tissue resistance (viscous resistance of lung tissue), calculated as difference between Rl and Raw.
Rus	Resistance of the airways on the upstream (alveolar) side of the point in the airways where intraluminal pressure equals Ppl, i.e., equal pressure point. Measured during a forced expiration.
Rds	Resistance of the airways on the downstream (mouth) side of the point in the airways where intraluminal pressure equals Ppl, i.e., equal pressure point. Measured during a forced expiration.
Gaw	Airway conductance, reciprocal of Raw.
Gaw/Vl	Specific conductance, airway conductance, expressed per liter of lung volume at which Gaw is measured.

Volume–Pressure Relationships

C	General symbol for compliance of the lungs, chest wall, or total respiratory system. Volume change per unit change in applied pressure. For the lungs, the applied pressure is the pressure difference across the lungs, or transpulmonary pressure, Pao–Ppl; for the chest wall, the applied pressure is the transthoracic pressure, Ppl–Pbs; for the entire respiratory system, the applied pressure is Pao–Pbs.
Cl	Lung compliance. Value for the volume change divided by the transpulmonary pressure.
Cw	Chest wall compliance. Value for the volume change divided by the transthoracic pressure.
Cdyn	Dynamic compliance. Value for compliance determined at time of zero gas flow at the mouth during uninterrupted breathing. The respiratory frequency appears as a qualifier. $Cdyn_{40}$ = dynamic compliance at a respiratory frequency of 40 per minute.
Cst	Static compliance, value for compliance determined on the basis of measurements made during a period of zero airflow.
C/Vl	Specific compliance. Compliance divided by the lung volume at which it is determined, usually FRC.

[†]Unless otherwise specified, resistance measurements are assumed to be made at FRC.

Pst	Static pulmonary pressure at a specified lung volume. $P{\rm ST}_{TLC}$ = static recoil pressure of the lung measured at TLC (maximum recoil pressure)

DIFFUSING CAPACITY TESTS AND SYMBOLS

DL*x*	Diffusing capacity of the lung expressed as volume (STPD) of gas (*x*) uptake per minute per unit alveolar-capillary pressure difference for the gas used. A modifier can be used to designate the technique: DL_{CO}/SB = Single-breath CO diffusing capacity; DL_{CO}/SS = Steady-state CO diffusing capacity
DM	Diffusing capacity of the alveolar-capillary membrane (STPD).
θ	Reaction rate coefficient for red blood cells. Determined as the volume of gas (STPD) that will combine per minute with 1 unit volume of blood per unit of gas tension. If the specific gas is not stated, θ is assumed to refer to CO and is a function of existing O_2 tension.
Vc	Pulmonary capillary blood volume. This should be Qc for consistency with other symbols, but Vc is entrenched in the literature. In the equation that follows for 1/DL, Vc represents the effective pulmonary capillary blood volume, i.e., capillary blood volume in intimate association with alveolar gas.
1/DL	Total resistance to diffusion, including resistance to diffusion of test gas across the alveolar-capillary membrane, through plasma in the capillary, and across the red blood cell membrane (1/Dm), with the resistance to diffusion within the red blood cell arising from the chemical reaction of the test gas and hemoglobin (1/θVc), according to the formulation

$$\frac{1}{D_L} = \frac{1}{D_M} + \frac{1}{\theta V_C}$$

DL/VA	Diffusing capacity per unit of alveolar volume. DL is expressed STPD, and VA is expressed in liters, BTPS.

BLOOD GAS SYMBOLS

Symbols for these values are readily composed by combining general symbols. Some examples include the following:

Pa_{CO_2}	Arterial CO_2 tension, mm Hg
Sa_{O_2}	Arterial O_2 saturation, percent
$Cc{O_2}$	Oxygen content of pulmonary end-capillary blood, mL of O_2 per 100 mL of blood
$(A\text{-}a)Po_2$	Alveolar–arterial difference in the partial pressure of O_2, mm Hg
$Ca_{O_2} - C\bar{v}_{O_2}$	O_2 content difference between arterial and mixed venous blood (arteriovenous O_2 difference), mL of O_2 per 100 mL of blood

PULMONARY SHUNT SYMBOLS

$\dot{Q}s$	Flow of blood via shunts. This is usually determined as percent of cardiac output ($\dot{Q}$) while breathing 100% O_2, according to the equation

$$\frac{\dot{Q}s}{\dot{Q}} = \frac{Cc{O_2} - Ca_{O_2}}{Ca_{O_2} - C\bar{v}_{O_2}} \times 100$$

Where

$Cc{O_2}$ = O_2 content of end-capillary blood

$Ca{O_2}$ = O_2 content of arterial blood

$C\bar{v}_{O_2}$ = O_2 content of mixed venous blood

APPENDIX B

Normal Values for a Healthy 20-Year Old Seated Man

Ventilation (BTPS)

Tidal volume (V_T), L	0.6
Frequency (f), breaths/min	12
Minute ventilation (V_E), L/min	7.2
Respiratory dead space (V_D), mL	150
Alveolar ventilation, V_A, L/min	5.4

Lung Volumes and Capacities (BTPS)

Inspiratory capacity (IC), L	3.0
Expiratory reserve volume (ERV), L	1.9
Vital capacity (VC), L	4.9
Residual volume (RV), L	1.4
Functional residual capacity (FRC), L	3.2
Total lung capacity (TLC), L	6.3
Residual volume/total lung capacity × 100 (RV/TLC), %	22

Mechanics of Breathing

Forced vital capacity (FVC), L	4.9
Forced expiratory volume, first second (FEV_1), L	4.0
Maximum voluntary ventilation (MVV), L/min	170
Forced expiratory volume in 1 s/forced vital capacity × 100 (FEV_1/FVC), %	83
Forced expiratory volume in 3 s/forced vital capacity × 100 (FEV_3/FVC), %	97
Forced expiratory flow during middle half of FVC (FEF_{25-75}), L/s	4.7
Forced inspiratory flow at the middle of forced inspiratory capacity (FIF_{50}), L/s	5.0
Static compliance of the lungs (Cst, l), L/cm H_2O	0.2
Compliance of lungs and thoracic cage (CRS, respiratory system compliance) L/cm H_2O	0.1
Airway resistance at FRC (Raw), cm H_2O/L/s	1.5
Pulmonary resistance at FRC, cm H_2O/L/s	2.0
Airway conductance at FRC (G_{aw}), L/s/cm H_2O	0.66
Specific conductance (G_{aw}/V_1)	0.22
Maximum inspiratory pressure, mm Hg	– 75
Maximum expiratory pressure, mm Hg	120

Distribution of Inspired Gas

Single-breath N_2 test (ΔN_2 from 750 to 1250 mL in expired gas), % N_2	<1.5
Alveolar N_2 after 7 min of breathing O_2, % N_2	<2.5
Closing volume (CV), mL	400
CV/VC × 100, %	8
Closing capacity (CC), mL	1900
CC/TLC × 100,%	30
Slope of phase III in single-breath N_2 test, % N_2/L	<2

Gas Exchange

O_2 consumption at rest (STPD), mL/min	240
CO_2 output at rest (STPD), mL/min	192
Respiratory exchange ratio (R), CO_2 output/O_2 uptake	0.8
ALVEOLAR GAS	
$P_{A_{O_2}}$, mm Hg	105
$P_{A_{CO_2}}$, mm Hg	40
ARTERIAL BLOOD	
Pa_{O_2}, mm Hg	95
Sa_{O_2}, %	98
pH	7.40
Pa_{CO_2}, mm Hg	40
Pa_{O_2}, while breathing 100% O_2, mm Hg	640

Alveolar Ventilation and Gas Exchange

Alveolar ventilation, L/min	4.2
Physiological dead space/tidal volume × 100 (V_D/V_T), %	<30
Alveolar–arterial oxygen-gradient, (A-a) P_{O_2}, mm Hg	10

Diffusing Capacity

Diffusing capacity at rest for CO, single-breath (DL_{COsb}), mL CO/min/mm Hg	29
Diffusing capacity per unit alveolar volume (D_L/V_A)	4.8

Control of Ventilation

Ventilatory response to hypercapnia, L/min/per ΔPa_{CO_2} mm Hg	>1.5

Pulmonary Hemodynamics

Pulmonary blood flow (cardiac output), L/min	5.4
Pulmonary artery systolic/diastolic pressure, mm Hg	25/8
Pulmonary capillary blood volume, mL	100
Pulmonary "capillary" (wedge) blood pressure, mm Hg	<10

INDEX

Note: Page numbers followed by *f* and *t* indicate figures and tables, respectively.

INDEX

INDEX

INDEX

INDEX

INDEX

INDEX

INDEX

INDEX

INDEX

INDEX

INDEX

INDEX

INDEX

INDEX

INDEX

INDEX

INDEX

E

INDEX

INDEX

INDEX

INDEX

INDEX

INDEX

INDEX

INDEX

INDEX

INDEX

J

K

L

INDEX

INDEX

INDEX

INDEX

INDEX

INDEX

M

INDEX

INDEX

INDEX

INDEX

INDEX

INDEX

INDEX

INDEX

INDEX

INDEX

INDEX

INDEX

INDEX

Q

R

INDEX

INDEX

INDEX

INDEX

INDEX

INDEX

INDEX

INDEX

U

INDEX